FOURTH EDITION

Understanding

Medical Surgical Nursing

FOURTH EDITION

Understanding Medical Surgical Nursing

LINDA S. WILLIAMS, MSN, RN
Professor of Nursing
Jackson Community College
Jackson, Michigan

PAULA D. HOPPER, MSN, RN
Professor of Nursing
Jackson Community College
Jackson, Michigan

F.A. Davis Company • Philadelphia

UNDERSTANDING Medical Surgical Nursing,

Fourth Edition

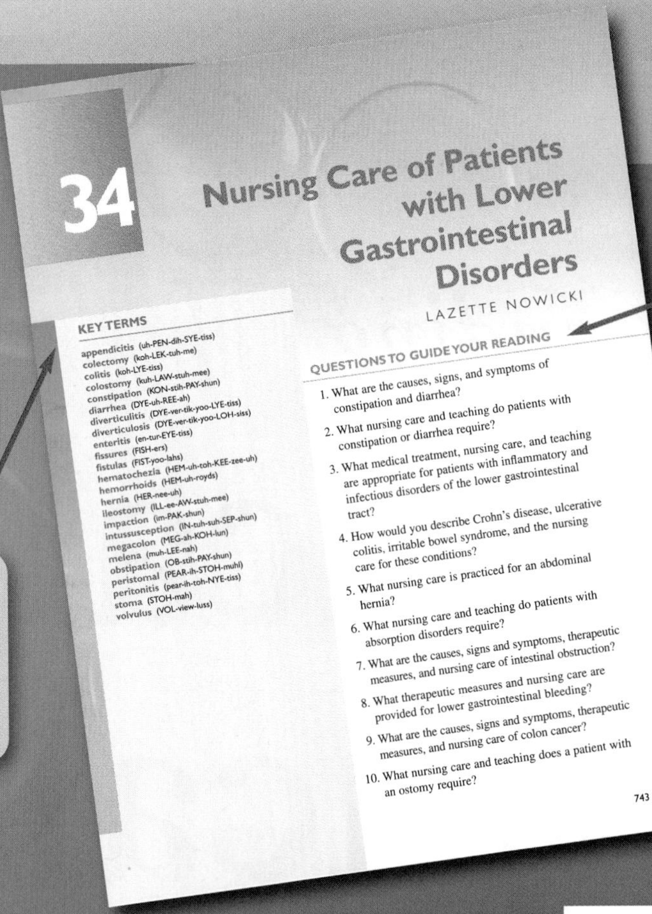

34 Nursing Care of Patients with Lower Gastrointestinal Disorders

LAZETTE NOWICKI

KEY TERMS

appendicitis (uh-PEN-dih-SYE-tiss)
colectomy (koh-LEK-tuh-me)
colitis (koh-LYE-tiss)
colostomy (kuh-LAW-stuh-mee)
constipation (KON-stih-PAY-shun)
diarrhea (DYE-uh-REE-ah)
diverticulitis (DYE-ver-tik-yoo-LYE-tiss)
diverticulosis (DYE-ver-tik-yoo-LOH-siss)
enteritis (en-tur-EYE-tiss)
fissures (FISH-ers)
fistulas (FIST-yoo-lahs)
hematochezia (HEM-uh-toh-KEE-zee-uh)
hemorrhoids (HEM-uh-royds)
hernia (HER-nee-uh)
ileostomy (ILL-ee-AW-stuh-mee)
impaction (im-PAK-shun)
intussusception (IN-tuh-suh-SEP-shun)
megacolon (MEG-ah-KOH-lun)
melena (muh-LEE-nah)
obstipation (OB-stih-PAY-shun)
peristomal (PEAR-ih-STOH-muhl)
peritonitis (pear-ih-toh-NYE-tiss)
stoma (STOH-mah)
volvulus (VOL-view-luss)

QUESTIONS TO GUIDE YOUR READING

1. What are the causes, signs, and symptoms of constipation and diarrhea?
2. What nursing care and teaching do patients with constipation or diarrhea require?
3. What medical treatment, nursing care, and teaching are appropriate for patients with inflammatory and infectious disorders of the lower gastrointestinal tract?
4. How would you describe Crohn's disease, ulcerative colitis, irritable bowel syndrome, and the nursing care for these conditions?
5. What nursing care is practiced for an abdominal hernia?
6. What nursing care and teaching do patients with absorption disorders require?
7. What are the causes, signs and symptoms, therapeutic measures, and nursing care of intestinal obstruction?
8. What therapeutic measures and nursing care are provided for lower gastrointestinal bleeding?
9. What are the causes, signs and symptoms, therapeutic measures, and nursing care of colon cancer?
10. What nursing care and teaching does a patient with an ostomy require?

743

Each chapter begins with questions that will increase comprehension and begin the critical thinking process. Excellent tool for review after the chapter has been read.

A list of key terms, with pronunciations, are provided at the beginning of each chapter.

Concept Maps provide a visual interpretation of a care plan or concept.

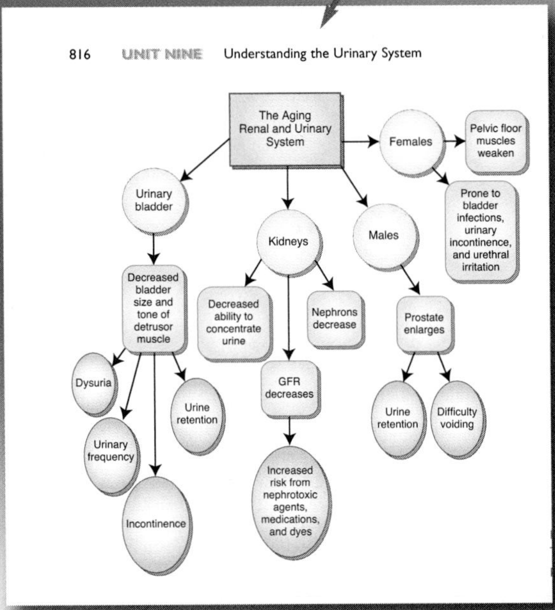

816 UNIT NINE Understanding the Urinary System
The Aging Renal and Urinary System
Females
Pelvic floor muscles weaken
Prone to bladder infections, urinary incontinence, and urethral irritation
Urinary bladder
Kidneys
Males
Decreased bladder size and tone of detrusor muscle
Decreased ability to concentrate urine
Nephrons decrease
Prostate enlarges
Dysuria
GFR decreases
Urine retention
Urinary frequency
Incontinence
Increased risk from nephrotoxic agents, medications, and dyes
Urine retention
Difficulty voiding

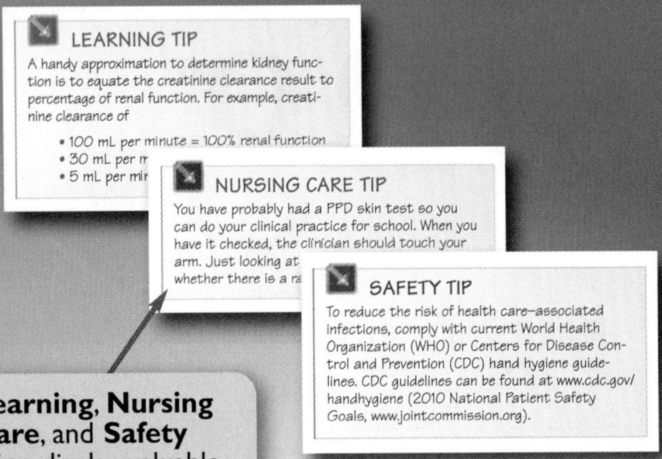

LEARNING TIP

A handy approximation to determine kidney function is to equate the creatinine clearance result to percentage of renal function. For example, creatinine clearance of

- 100 mL per minute = 100% renal function
- 30 mL per m
- 5 mL per mi

NURSING CARE TIP

You have probably had a PPD skin test so you can do your clinical practice for school. When you have it checked, the clinician should touch your arm. Just looking at whether there is a ra

SAFETY TIP

To reduce the risk of health care–associated infections, comply with current World Health Organization (WHO) or Centers for Disease Control and Prevention (CDC) hand hygiene guidelines. CDC guidelines can be found at www.cdc.gov/handhygiene (2010 National Patient Safety Goals, www.jointcommission.org).

Learning, Nursing Care, and **Safety Tips** display valuable advice on patient care.

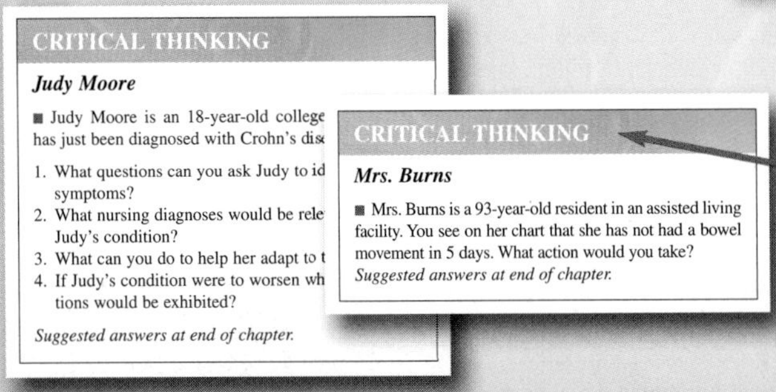

CRITICAL THINKING

Judy Moore

■ Judy Moore is an 18-year-old college has just been diagnosed with Crohn's dis

1. What questions can you ask Judy to id symptoms?
2. What nursing diagnoses would be rele Judy's condition?
3. What can you do to help her adapt to t
4. If Judy's condition were to worsen wh tions would be exhibited?

Suggested answers at end of chapter.

CRITICAL THINKING

Mrs. Burns

■ Mrs. Burns is a 93-year-old resident in an assisted living facility. You see on her chart that she has not had a bowel movement in 5 days. What action would you take?
Suggested answers at end of chapter.

Case Studies with critical-thinking questions are featured throughout, allowing you to apply what you've just learned. Suggested answers are provided at the end of each chapter.

ALL OF THE TOOLS YOU NEED TO THINK CRITICALLY AND LEARN REAL-WORLD NURSING CARE!

Patient Perspectives, stories written by patients, highlight their experiences with illness.

Nursing Care Plans are easy to read and clearly present the rationale for each action.

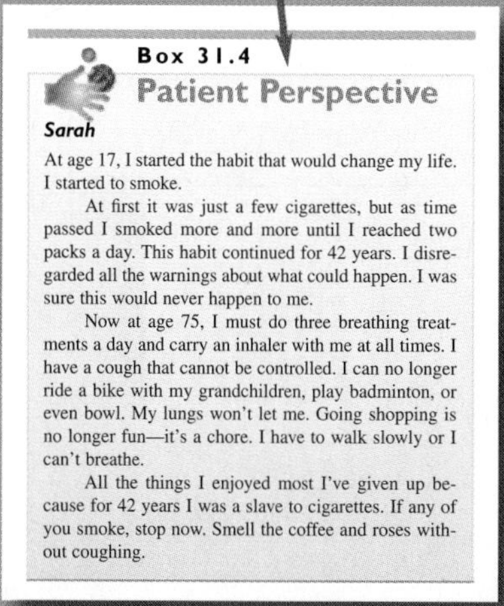

Box 31.4

Patient Perspective

Sarah

At age 17, I started the habit that would change my life. I started to smoke.

At first it was just a few cigarettes, but as time passed I smoked more and more until I reached two packs a day. This habit continued for 42 years. I disregarded all the warnings about what could happen. I was sure this would never happen to me.

Now at age 75, I must do three breathing treatments a day and carry an inhaler with me at all times. I have a cough that cannot be controlled. I can no longer ride a bike with my grandchildren, play badminton, or even bowl. My lungs won't let me. Going shopping is no longer fun—it's a chore. I have to walk slowly or I can't breathe.

All the things I enjoyed most I've given up because for 42 years I was a slave to cigarettes. If any of you smoke, stop now. Smell the coffee and roses without coughing.

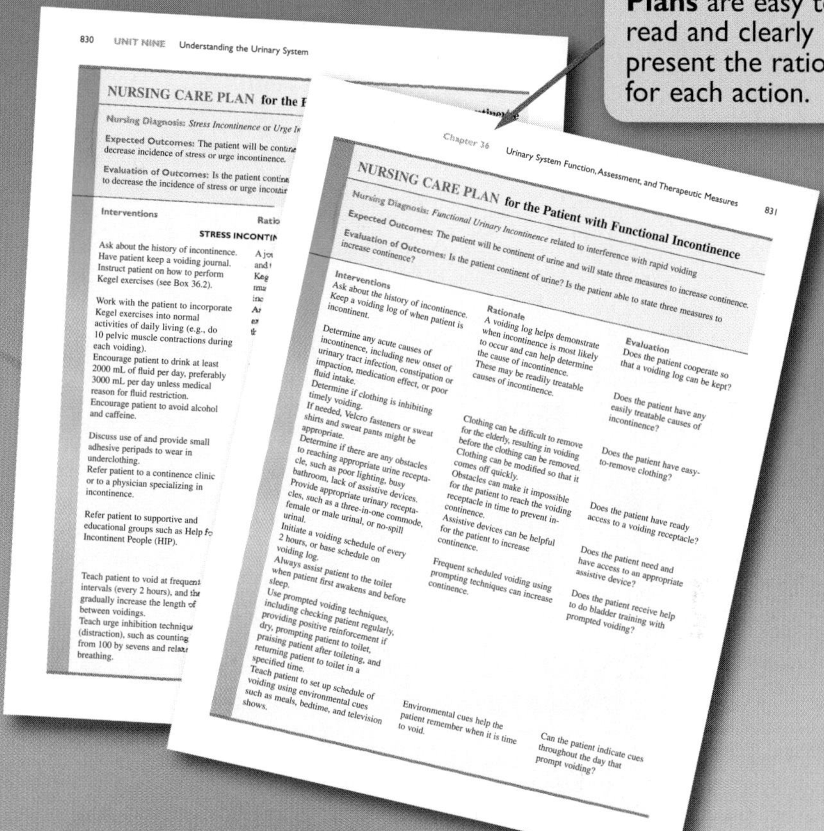

830 UNIT NINE Understanding the Urinary System

Chapter 36 Urinary System Function, Assessment, and Therapeutic Measures 831

NURSING CARE PLAN for the Patient with Functional Incontinence

Nursing Diagnosis: *Functional Urinary Incontinence related to interference with rapid voiding*

Expected Outcomes: The patient will be continent of urine and will state three measures to increase continence.

Evaluation of Outcomes: Is the patient continent of urine? Is the patient able to state three measures to increase continence?

Interventions	Rationale	Evaluation
Ask about the history of incontinence. Keep a voiding log of when patient is incontinent.	A voiding log helps demonstrate when incontinence is most likely to occur and can help determine the cause of incontinence.	Does the patient cooperate so that a voiding log can be kept?
Determine any acute causes of incontinence, including new onset of urinary tract infection, constipation or impaction, medication effect, or poor fluid intake.	These may be readily treatable causes of incontinence.	Does the patient have any easily treatable causes of incontinence?
Determine if clothing is inhibiting timely voiding. If needed, Velcro fasteners or sweat shirts and sweat pants might be appropriate.	Clothing can be difficult to remove for the elderly, resulting in voiding before the clothing can be removed. Clothing can be modified so that it comes off quickly.	Does the patient have easy-to-remove clothing?
Determine if there are any obstacles to reaching appropriate urine receptacle, such as poor lighting, busy bathroom, lack of assistive devices. Provide appropriate urinary receptacles, such as a three-in-one commode, female or male urinal, or no-spill urinal.	Obstacles can make it impossible for the patient to reach the voiding receptacle in time to prevent incontinence. Assistive devices can be helpful for the patient to increase continence.	Does the patient have ready access to a voiding receptacle? Does the patient need and have access to an appropriate assistive device?
Initiate a voiding schedule of every 2 hours, or base schedule on voiding log. Always assist patient to the toilet when patient first awakens and before sleep. Use prompted voiding techniques, including checking patient regularly, providing positive reinforcement if dry, prompting patient to toilet, praising patient after toileting, and returning patient to toilet in a specified time.	Frequent scheduled voiding using prompting techniques can increase continence.	Does the patient receive help to do bladder training with prompted voiding?
Teach patient to set up schedule of voiding using environmental cues such as meals, bedtime, and television shows.	Environmental cues help the patient remember when it is time to void.	Can the patient indicate cues throughout the day that prompt voiding?

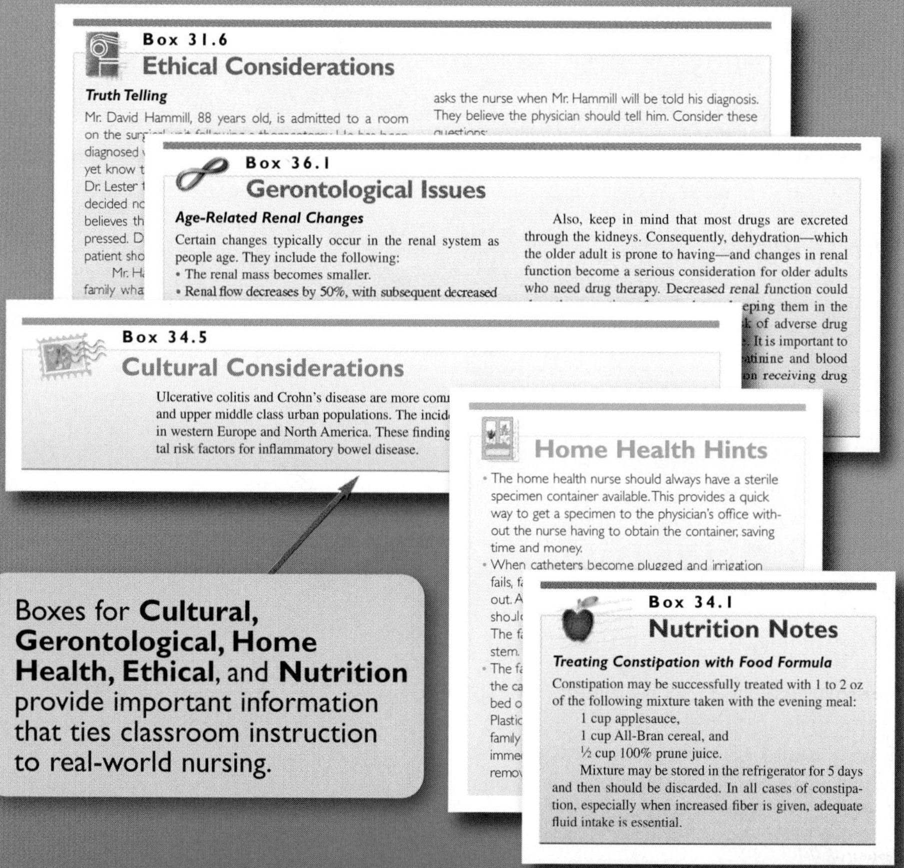

Box 31.6

Ethical Considerations

Truth Telling

Mr. David Hammill, 88 years old, is admitted to a room on the sur... asks the nurse when Mr. Hammill will be told his diagnosis. They believe the physician should tell him. Consider these questions:

Box 36.1

Gerontological Issues

Age-Related Renal Changes

Certain changes typically occur in the renal system as people age. They include the following:

- The renal mass becomes smaller.
- Renal flow decreases by 50%, with subsequent decreased

Also, keep in mind that most drugs are excreted through the kidneys. Consequently, dehydration—which the older adult is prone to having—and changes in renal function become a serious consideration for older adults who need drug therapy. Decreased renal function could ...

Box 34.5

Cultural Considerations

Ulcerative colitis and Crohn's disease are more com... and upper middle class urban populations. The incid... in western Europe and North America. These finding... tal risk factors for inflammatory bowel disease.

Home Health Hints

- The home health nurse should always have a sterile specimen container available. This provides a quick way to get a specimen to the physician's office without the nurse having to obtain the container, saving time and money.
- When catheters become plugged and irrigation fails, ...

Box 34.1

Nutrition Notes

Treating Constipation with Food Formula

Constipation may be successfully treated with 1 to 2 oz of the following mixture taken with the evening meal:

1 cup applesauce,
1 cup All-Bran cereal, and
½ cup 100% prune juice.

Mixture may be stored in the refrigerator for 5 days and then should be discarded. In all cases of constipation, especially when increased fiber is given, adequate fluid intake is essential.

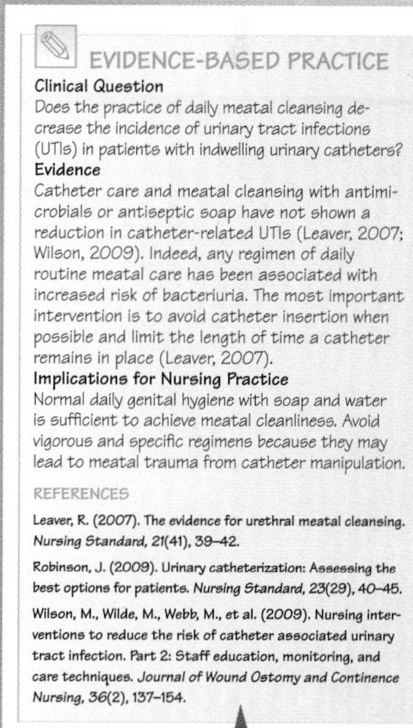

EVIDENCE-BASED PRACTICE

Clinical Question

Does the practice of daily meatal cleansing decrease the incidence of urinary tract infections (UTIs) in patients with indwelling urinary catheters?

Evidence

Catheter care and meatal cleansing with antimicrobials or antiseptic soap have not shown a reduction in catheter-related UTIs (Leaver, 2007; Wilson, 2009). Indeed, any regimen of daily routine meatal care has been associated with increased risk of bacteriuria. The most important intervention is to avoid catheter insertion when possible and limit the length of time a catheter remains in place (Leaver, 2007).

Implications for Nursing Practice

Normal daily genital hygiene with soap and water is sufficient to achieve meatal cleanliness. Avoid vigorous and specific regimens because they may lead to meatal trauma from catheter manipulation.

REFERENCES

Leaver, R. (2007). The evidence for urethral meatal cleansing. *Nursing Standard, 21*(41), 39–42.

Robinson, J. (2009). Urinary catheterization: Assessing the best options for patients. *Nursing Standard, 23*(29), 40–45.

Wilson, M., Wilde, M., Webb, M., et al. (2009). Nursing interventions to reduce the risk of catheter associated urinary tract infection. Part 2: Staff education, monitoring, and care techniques. *Journal of Wound Ostomy and Continence Nursing, 36*(2), 137–154.

Boxes for **Cultural, Gerontological, Home Health, Ethical,** and **Nutrition** provide important information that ties classroom instruction to real-world nursing.

Evidence-Based Practice boxes provide an in-depth look at research that supports best practices.

EXPERIENCE A WEALTH OF MULTI-MEDIA LEARNING TOOLS!

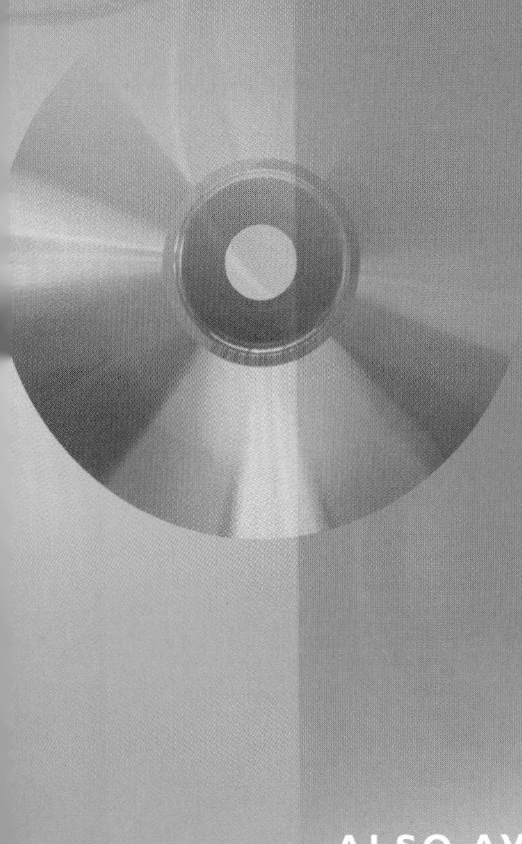

For Students...

Student CD-ROM

(MAC & PC compatible)

- **IQ Question Bank**
  - 500 NCLEX-style questions (with descriptors and rationales) covering a variety of topics found in the book and on the NCLEX-PN exam.
- **Media Bank**
  - Listen and learn with audio clips of heart, lung, and bowel sounds.
- **Interactive Exercises**
  - Fill-in-the-Blank, Picture Match, Flash Cards, and Case Studies.
- **NCLEX Prep Guide**
  - A certification prep "how-to" guide that provides test taking tips and strategies for the NCLEX-PN exam.

DavisPlus
Instructor and Student Online Resource Center

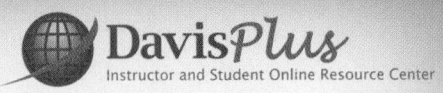

Davis*Plus* Online Resources

(No fee. No password. No registration.)

- **Chapter Summary Podcasts**
- **Concept Map Generator**
- **Review Question Rationales**
- **Animations**
- **Calculation Practice Problems**
- **Calculation Practice Answers**
- **Medication Math Using Unit Analysis**
- **Clinical Simulation Resource**

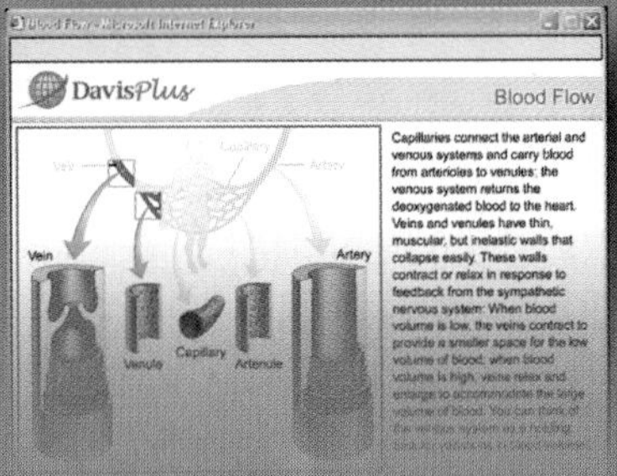
DavisPlus
Blood Flow
Vein
Artery
Venule
Capillary
Arteriole

For Instructors Upon Adoption...

Online at Davis*Plus* and on CD-ROM

- **Instructor's Guide**
- **Electronic Test Bank**
- **PowerPoint Presentations**
- **Guide to Better PowerPoint Presentations**
- **Guide to Better NCLEX Questions**
- **Image Bank**
- **Clinical Simulation (Davis*Plus* Only)**
- **Resource Kits for Learning Management Systems (Davis*Plus* Only)**

ALSO AVAILABLE...

Study Guide for UNDERSTANDING MEDICAL SURGICAL NURSING*

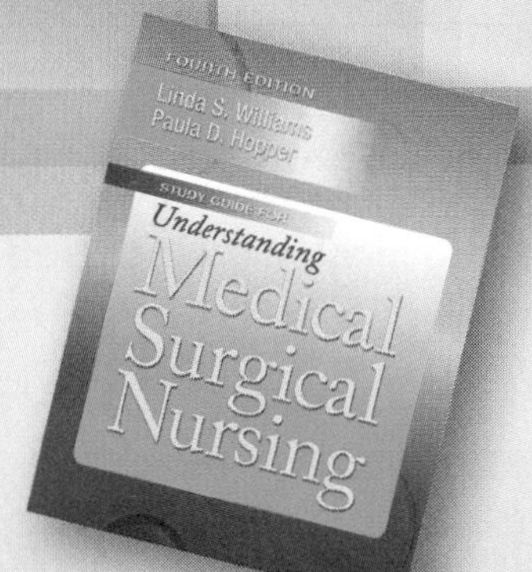
FOURTH EDITION
Linda S. Williams
Paula D. Hopper
STUDY GUIDE FOR
Understanding
Medical
Surgical
Nursing

Practice, practice, and more practice! Each chapter corresponds to the textbook and features critical-thinking exercises, basic matching and true/false tests, word scrambles, crossword puzzles, vocabulary review exercises, and NCLEX-PN-style questions.

**Sold separately or as part of a package.*

Contents In Brief

F. A. Davis Company
1915 Arch Street
Philadelphia, PA 19103
www.fadavis.com

Printed in the United States of America

Last digit indicates print number: 10 9 8 7 6 5 4 3 2 1

Acquisitions Editor: Jonathan Joyce
Director of Content Development: Darlene D. Pedersen
Senior Project Editor: Padraic J. Maroney
Art and Design Manager: Carolyn O'Brien

As new scientific information becomes available through basic and clinical research, recommended treatments and drug therapies undergo changes. The author(s) and publisher have done everything possible to make this book accurate, up to date, and in accord with accepted standards at the time of publication. The author(s), editors, and publisher are not responsible for errors or omissions or for consequences from application of the book, and make no warranty, expressed or implied, in regard to the contents of the book. Any practice described in this book should be applied by the reader in accordance with professional standards of care used in regard to the unique circumstances that may apply in each situation. The reader is advised always to check product information (package inserts) for changes and new information regarding dose and contraindications before administering any drug. Caution is especially urged when using new or infrequently ordered drugs.

ISBN 13: 978-0-8036-2219-7
ISBN 10: 0-8036-2219-8

Library of Congress Cataloging-in-Publication Data
Understanding medical surgical nursing / [edited by] Linda S. Williams, Paula D. Hopper. — 4th ed.
p. ; cm.
Includes bibliographical references and index.
ISBN-13: 978-0-8036-2219-7
ISBN-10: 0-8036-2219-8
1. Nursing. 2. Surgical nursing. I. Williams, Linda S. (Linda Sue), 1954- II. Hopper, Paula D.
[DNLM: 1. Nursing Care. 2. Nursing. WY 100.1]
RT41.W576 2011
610.73—dc22 2010033147

For practical and vocational nursing students everywhere.

You are valuable members of the health care team.

We hope this text helps you achieve your dreams.

Linda and Paula

Preface

Welcome to the fourth edition of *Understanding Medical Surgical Nursing!* We have fully updated all the material, and have added exciting new information on evidence-based practice, safety, and more. An all-new Chapter 2 introduces the concepts of evidence-based practice, and boxed materials throughout the text present actual evidence-based care guidelines.

We continue to work hard to provide a text written at an understandable level, with features that help students understand, apply, and practice the challenging content required to function as practical/vocational nurses. We are thankful to the many students who tell us they find the book very readable, and actually enjoyable. We are overjoyed to hear from several nursing programs that their NCLEX scores soared after adopting this textbook. We welcome and value your comments on this edition.

We continue to emphasize understanding, critical thinking, and application throughout the book. We believe that a student who learns to think critically will be better able to apply information to new situations. We hope both students and instructors find this fourth edition a practical tool for learning and understanding the principles of medical-surgical nursing.

Features of the Book

We have kept our most popular features from the first three editions and have added new ones based on reader input. Based on feedback, we have kept the following:

- Questions to Guide Your Reading at the beginning of each chapter. In our experience, the standard objectives found in many textbooks have little meaning and provide little assistance to students. Literature suggests that comprehension increases when students read guiding questions before reading the text. So we have provided a series of questions that students should keep in mind as they read. These questions can be translated easily back into objectives by instructors who prefer this format.
- Web links in the text to help students do further research on topics of interest. Every effort was made to use only major, established Web sites that are unlikely to change in the near future.
- One of our most popular features, Critical Thinking Exercises. These have been expanded to help students practice and think about what they are learning.
- Review questions at the end of each chapter. Questions have been updated and include alternate format items to reflect the NCLEX-PN.
- Suggested Answers for the Critical Thinking Exercises and Review Questions. Research supports the importance of immediate feedback to reinforce learning, so we feel strongly that students should have access to correct answers while they are studying, without having to wait for their next instructor contact. Since there may be many answers to some of the critical thinking questions, we have provided sample answers to help stimulate students' thinking.
- Easy to read tips. Patient Care Tips, Safety Tips, and Learning Tips help make learning easy. The Joint Commission's National Patient Safety Goals are reflected in many of the safety tips.
- Pronunciation keys for new words at the beginning of each chapter.
- A review of anatomy and physiology at the beginning of each unit.
- Word-building footnotes throughout the chapters.
- Nursing care plans with geriatric considerations. These have been updated to reflect current practice.
- Boxed presentations of Cultural Considerations, Gerontological Issues, Home Health Hints, Ethical Considerations, and Nutrition Notes. Additional boxes have been added where needed.
- A comprehensive, updated glossary of new words is included in the appendix.
- New to this edition are Evidence-Based Practice boxes throughout the text.

To Students: How to use this Book

As you begin each chapter, carefully read the section labeled *Questions to Guide your Reading.* Then, when you are finished reading each chapter, go back and make sure you can answer each question.

You will find a list of new words and their pronunciations at the beginning of each chapter. These words appear in bold at their first use in a chapter, and they also appear in the glossary at the end of the book. By learning the meanings of these words as you encounter them, you will increase your understanding of the material. Many of these words are also broken down at the bottom of the page, so you can see how the parts of each word make up the whole.

You also will find learning tips to increase your understanding and retention of the material. You may want to develop your own memory techniques in addition to those provided. (If you think of a good one, send it to us and you may find it in the next edition!) Many of the learning tips have been developed and used in our own classrooms. We find them helpful in fostering understanding of complex concepts or as memory aids. However, we want to stress that memorization is not the primary focus of the text but rather a foundation for understanding and thinking about more complex information. Understanding and application will serve you far better than memorization when dealing with new situations.

Each chapter includes critical thinking case studies designed to help you apply material that has been presented. A series of questions related to the case study will help you integrate the material with what you already know. These questions emphasize critical thinking, which is based on a foundation of recall and understanding of material. To enhance your learning, try to answer the questions before reading the answers.

Review questions appear at the end of each chapter to help you prepare for chapter tests, and also for the NCLEX-PN. Again, to assess your learning, try to answer the questions before looking up the answers at the back of the book.

Chapter reference lists provide sources for additional reading material at the back of the book. Web sites have been included in many chapters. We believe it is important for you to interact with current technology to expand your information resources.

The following appendices are included for easy reference:

- NANDA nursing diagnoses
- Normal adult reference laboratory values
- Answers to chapter review questions
- Common medical abbreviations (Although it is still important to know medical abbreviations, many can increase risk of errors. Check http://www.jointcommision.org for a list of abbreviations to avoid.)
- Common prefixes and suffixes to help learn word-building techniques
- Glossary of new words

Supplemental Materials

- An *Electronic Student Guide* is included with the book. This provides practice in the form of objective (fill-in, labeling, and flashcard) exercises and case studies. There are also review questions and a practice NCLEX-style test. These questions have been reviewed and revised by an item writing expert. We have also included a brief math tutorial using Unit Analysis, and practice calculation problems. Answers are provided to all exercises for immediate feedback.
- A paperback *Student Workbook* is available to provide additional contact and practice with the material. Each chapter includes vocabulary practice, objective exercises, a case study or other critical thinking practice and review questions written in NCLEX-PN format. These questions have been reviewed and revised by an item writing expert. Updated review questions have been organized according to Content Review and Test Preparation categories. Answers provide immediate feedback. Rationales are provided for applicable review question answers.
- New with this edition is a brief podcast for each chapter. These are presented in a fun and interesting format to help students review key concepts while they carry on their busy lives.
- An *Instructor's Resource Disk* includes an *Electronic Instructor's Guide* that provides materials for use in the classroom. Each chapter has a chapter outline with suggested classroom activities. New to the IRD are a PowerPoint tutorial and NCLEX-style item writing tutorial. Also included are student activities for printing and using for individual practice or for collaborative learning activities. These activities help the student to interact with the material, understand it, and apply it. Many of the activities are based on real patient cases and have been used with our own nursing students. Feedback from students has helped to refine the exercises. We believe the use of collaborative learning has greatly enhanced our students' success in achieving their educational and licensure goals. Another benefit is the sense of community the students develop as a result of working in groups. A brief introduction and guidelines for using collaborative learning techniques is included.
- Also included is an expanded *Electronic Test Bank,* available to instructors who adopt the textbook, which provides test questions that assist students to prepare for NCLEX-PN. These questions have been reviewed and revised by an item writing expert. The questions are in multiple choice and alternate formats, and they test understanding, application, and analysis of material. The program allows instructors to choose and modify the questions that best suit their classroom needs.
- Finally, for the instructor's convenience, there is a comprehensive *PowerPoint* program for classroom presentations. Images from the text are included in the presentations. Each presentation can be modified, reduced, or expanded by individual instructors to suit their needs.

Acknowledgments

Many people helped us make this book a reality. First and foremost are the students, who provide us with the inspiration to undertake this project. We hope that students everywhere continue to find this text worth reading.

The F.A. Davis Company has been an exceptional publishing partner. We feel fortunate to have had their continued enthusiasm and confidence in our book. The staff at F.A. Davis has guided us through this project for four editions to help us create a student-friendly book that truly promotes understanding of medical-surgical nursing.

Jonathan Joyce, Catherine Harold, Kim DePaul, Padraic Maroney, and many others have been extremely patient and kind as we worked hard to provide a quality text and meet deadlines.

Contributors from across the United States, including many well-known experts in their fields, brought expertise and diversity to the content. Their hard work is much appreciated. Reviewers from throughout the United States provided insights that enhanced the quality of the text. Elizabeth Hopper provided invaluable organizational assistance.

Many of our co-workers have contributed to this book and given us ongoing encouragement and validation of the worthiness of this project. Elizabeth Ackley, Marina Martinez-Kratz, Carroll Lutz, Erin Mazur, Sharon Nowak, Debra Perry-Philo, Susanne Fox, and Linda Nabozny were especially helpful in providing material, advice, and encouragement.

We would also like to thank several educators who have graciously provided input when we have needed it: Peggy Flener, Penny Snyder, and Terri Waisanen. Marcella Williams was a godsend as our item writing expert. Finally, we are thankful to Gay Alcenius, PharmD, for her expertise in updating all medications materials.

We wish to thank everyone who played a role, however large or small, in helping us to provide a tool to help students realize their dreams of becoming LPN/LVNs. We hope this book will help educate nurses who can provide safe and expert care because we have helped them to learn to think critically.

Contributors

Betty Ackley, BSN, MSN, EdS, RN
Professor Emeritus
Jackson Community College
Jackson, Michigan

Nancy Ahern, PhD, RN
Associate Professor
California State University, Fullerton
Fullerton, California

Debra Aucoin-Ratcliff, BSN, MN, DNP, RN
Professor
American River College
Sacramento, California

Cynthia Barrere, PhD, RN
Associate Professor
Quinnipiac University
Hamden, Connecticut

Kathy Berchem, MSN, RN, FNP-BC
Assistant Professor
Lake Superior State University
Sault Ste. Marie, Michigan

Michelle Block, MS, RN
Associate Professor
Purdue University Calumet
Hammond, Indiana

Janice L. Bradford, MS
Associate Professor
Jackson Community College
Jackson, Michigan

Lucy L. Colo, MSN, RN
Faculty
Huron School of Nursing
East Cleveland, Ohio

Colleen Delaney, PhD, RN, AHN-BC
Associate Professor
University of Connecticut
Storrs, Connecticut

Mary Dillinger, MSN, RN, ACRN
Clinical Nurse Specialist (Retired)
Munson Medical Center
Traverse City, Michigan

Susan Garbutt, DNP, RN, CIC
RN Program Director
Galen Health Institute
St. Petersburg, Florida

Karen P. Hall, RN-C, MSHSA, NE-BC
Pain Management and Palliative Care Program Manager
Doctors Medical Center
Modesto, California

Wendy Hockley, BS, MA, LPN
Manager
W.A. Foote Memorial Hospital
Jackson, Michigan

Paula D. Hopper, MSN, RN
Professor of Nursing
Jackson Community College
Jackson, Michigan

Elaine Kennedy, EdD, RN
Professor
Wor-Wic Community College
Salisbury, Maryland

Marty Kohn, BSN, MS, RN, FNP, CWOCN
Nurse Practitioner
Wound Care Center, Allegiance Health
Jackson, Michigan

Bobbi M. Martin, MSN, RN, CNE
Assistant Dean
Galen School of Nursing
St. Petersburg, Florida

Marina Martinez-Kratz, BSN, MS, RN
Professor
Jackson Community College
Jackson, Michigan

Diane Mayo, MSN, RN
Nurse Educator
Healthcare Ventures Alliance
Erie, Pennsylvania

Erin Mazur, MSN, RN, FNP-BC
Assistant Professor
Jackson Community College
Jackson, Michigan

Laura L. McCully, MS, RN, CNM
Certified Nurse Midwife
Women First Health Services
Jackson, Michigan

Maureen McDonald, MS, RN, CCRN
Assistant Clinical Professor
University of California, San Francisco
San Francisco, California

Kelly McManigle, BSN, MSN, RN
Nursing Faculty
Manatee Technical Institute
Bradenton, Florida

Kelly Ann Morris, DNP, RN
Associate Professor
Owensboro Community and Technical College
Owensboro, Kentucky

Betsy Murphy, FNP, CHPN, RN
Business Relations
Capital Hospice
Fairfax, Virginia

Sharon M. Nowak, MSN, EdD (ABD), RN
Associate Professor
Jackson Community College
Jackson, Michigan

Lazette V. Nowicki, BA, MSN, RN
Assistant Professor
American River College
Sacramento, California

Debra Perry-Philo, BSN, MSN, RN
Nursing Faculty
Jackson Community College
Holt, Michigan

Lynn D. Phillips, MSN, CRNI, RN
Nursing Instructor
Butte College
Oroville, California

Maryanne Pietraniec-Shannon, PhD, APRN-BC
Professor
Lake Superior State University
Sault Ste. Marie, Michigan

Patrick M. Shannon, JD, EdD, MPH
Attorney
Bay Mills Community College
Brimley, Michigan

John Sturtevant, MSN, RN
Clinical Quality Specialist
Allegiance Health
Jackson, Michigan

Rita Bolek Trofino, MNEd, RN
Associate Academic Dean
Chairperson, AD Nursing Program
Mount Aloysius College
Cresson, Pennsylvania

Deborah L. Weaver, PhD, RN
Associate Professor
Valdosta State University
Valdosta, Georgia

Linda S. Williams, MSN, RN
Professor of Nursing
Jackson Community College
Jackson, Michigan

Bruce K. Wilson, CRNA
Nurse Anesthesiologist
Lapeer, Michigan

CONTRIBUTORS TO PREVIOUS EDITIONS

We would like to acknowledge and thank the following individuals for their contributions to prior editions. All contributions have helped to make *Understanding Medical Surgical Nursing* what it has evolved into today.

Jeanette Acker

Brenda Anderson

Cynthia Francis Bechtel

Virginia Birnie

Joseph Catalano

Elizabeth Chapman

Kathleen R. Culliton

Constance Monlezun Darbonne

Sharon Gordon Dawson

Vera Dutro

Rowena Elliott

Mary Friel Fanning

Donna D. Ignatavicius

Cheryl L. Ivey

Lenetra Jefferson

Jean Jeffries

Josephine Whitney Johns

Rodney B. Kebicz

Gail Ladwig

Diane Lewis

Gary S. Lott

Sharon D. Martin

Deborah J. Mauffray

Cindy Meredith

Marsha A. Miles

Debbie Millar

Kathy Neeb

Debra Perry-Philo

Winifred J. Ellenchild Pinch

Larry Purnell

Ruth Remington

Deborah L. Roush

Valerie C. Scanlon

Kate Schmitz

Sally Schnell

Jill Secord

George B. Smith

Susan Smith

Martha Spray

Rose Utley

Kathleen Kelley Walsh

JoAnn Widner

Reviewers

Susan F. Bond, MSN, RN
Nursing Instructor
Pima Community College
Tucson, Arizona

Barbara Brown-McKenzie, BScN, MSN, RN
Associate Professor
UBC Okanagan
Kelowna, British Columbia
Canada

Betty L. Brunner, BSN, MSN
Adjunct Faculty
Northeastern Junior College
Sterling, Colorado

Gina L. Doyle, MEd, MS, RN
Practical Nursing Coordinator/ Instructor
Mid-America Technology Center
Wayne, Oklahoma

Evelyn F. Grigsby, MSN, RN
Program Coordinator
Bluegrass Community and Technical College – Danville Campus
Danville, Kentucky

Karen S. Lotz, MSN, Ed, RN
Nursing Instructor
Pasco-Hernando Community College
Brooksville, Florida

Maria Metcalf, MSN, RN
Assistant Professor
Allen College
Waterloo, Iowa

Sallie Noto, MS, MSN, RN
Director, School of Practical Nursing
Career Technology Center
Scranton, Pennsylvania

LeiLani Tacia, MSN, RN
Clinical Nurse Specialist
Allegiance Health
Jackson, Michigan

Rose M. Veith, MSN, FNP-BC, CNE
Coordinator, Practical Nursing Program
Assabet Valley Regional Technical School
Marlborough, Massachusetts

Rita Waller, MSN, RRT, RPSGT
Program Director, Respiratory Care Technology
Augusta Technical College
Augusta, Georgia

Catherine B. Wardlow, MS, MEd, RN
Nursing Instructor
Francis Tuttle Technology Center
Oklahoma City, Oklahoma

Christina R. Wilson, BA, PHN, RN
Faculty
Anoka Technical College
Anoka, Minnesota

Contents

unit ONE

UNDERSTANDING HEALTH CARE ISSUES

1

Critical Thinking and the Nursing Process

PAULA D. HOPPER AND
LINDA S. WILLIAMS

KEY TERMS

assessment (ah-SESS-ment)
collaborative (koh-LAB-rah-tiv)
critical thinking (KRIT-i-cull THING-king)
data (DAY-tuh)
evaluation (e-VAL-yoo-AY-shun)
evidence-based practice (EH-va-dense baste PRACK-tis)
intervention (in-ter-VEN-shun)
nursing diagnosis (NER-sing DYE-ag-NOH-sis)
nursing process (NER-sing PRAH-sess)
objective data (ob-JEK-tiv DAY-tuh)
subjective data (sub-JEK-tiv DAY-tuh)
vigilance (VIH-jih-lents)

QUESTIONS TO GUIDE YOUR READING

1. Why is critical thinking important in nursing?
2. What attitudes and skills promote good critical thinking?
3. What occurs in each step of the nursing process?
4. What is the role of a licensed practical nurse/licensed vocational nurse in using the nursing process?
5. What are objective and subjective data?
6. What is the best way to document objective and subjective data?
7. How would you prioritize patient care based on Maslow's hierarchy of human needs?

Excellence in the delivery of nursing care requires good thinking. Each day nurses make many decisions that affect the care of their patients. For those decisions to be effective, the thinking behind them must be sound.

CRITICAL THINKING

Nursing students must learn to think critically; in other words, to think like a nurse. This means they must use their knowledge and skills to make the best decisions possible in patient care situations. Halpern (1996) says that "**critical thinking** is the use of those cognitive [knowledge] skills or strategies that increase the probability of a desirable outcome" (p. 5). Critical thinking is sometimes called *directed thinking* because it focuses on a goal. Other terms used when talking about critical thinking include *reasoning, reflection, common sense, problem solving, analysis,* and *inquiry.* Good thinking requires critical thinking attitudes and skills, which are described below. It also requires a good knowledge base, so your thinking is based on correct factual material. This text will provide you with medical-surgical knowledge on which to base good decisions.

Critical Thinking Attitudes

It is important for nurses to possess an attitude that promotes good thinking. Researchers have identified attitudes associated with good critical thinking. Green (2000) identifies seven attitudes, as summarized next.

Intellectual Humility

Have you ever known people who think they know it all? They do not have intellectual humility. People with intellectual humility have the ability to say, "I'm not sure about that.... I need more information." Certainly, we want our patients to think we are smart and know what we are doing, but patients also respect nurses who can say, "I don't know, but I'll find out." It is unsafe to care for patients when you are unsure of what you need to do.

Intellectual Courage

Intellectual courage allows you to look at other points of view even when you do not agree with them at first. Maybe you really believe that 8-hour shifts are best for nurses, and you have a lot of good reasons for your belief. But if you have intellectual courage, you will be willing to really listen to the arguments for changing to 12-hour shifts. Maybe you will even be convinced. Sometimes you have to have the courage to say, "Okay, I see you were right after all."

Intellectual Empathy

Consider the patient who snaps as you enter her room, "I've been waiting all morning for my bath. If you don't help me with it right now I'm going to call your supervisor." The first response that comes into your head is, "I have five other patients; you're lucky I am here!" If you have intellectual empathy, however, you will be able to think, "If I were this patient, who is in chronic pain and is tired of being in the hospital, how would I feel?" Such thinking might change how you respond.

Intellectual Integrity

One of your patients asks a hundred questions when you bring her a medication that has been newly prescribed for her high blood pressure. But later you notice she is taking an herbal remedy from her purse. It is good that she asks a lot of questions about her drug, which has been tested extensively by the Food and Drug Administration (FDA). Herbal remedies, however, are not held to the same standards as medications in the United States. Someone with intellectual integrity would want the same level of proof applied to both medications and herbal remedies to determine if they are safe and effective before using them.

Intellectual Perseverance

Perseverance means you do not give up. Consider this scenario: You have concerns about some side effects you noticed after giving a new drug to a patient. You mention it to the physician, who says not to worry about it, but you are still concerned. If you have intellectual perseverance, you might do some research on the Internet, then go to your supervisor or the pharmacist to further discuss your concerns.

Faith in Reason

If you have faith in reason, you believe in your heart that good thinking, and reason, will result in the best outcomes for your patients. And if you really believe, you will be more likely to attend a seminar or read an article on developing your critical thinking skills.

Intellectual Sense of Justice

One of your coworkers wants to change the medication administration schedule on your unit. She says it will be better for the patients, but you think it might be because it fits her coffee break schedule better. If you have an intellectual sense of justice, you will be sure that your thinking is not biased by something that you just want for yourself, as seems to be happening with your coworker. You should examine your own motives as well as those of others when you are making decisions.

So, what does this all mean to you as a nursing student? The term *metacognition* means to "think about thinking." It is important for you to try to develop the attitudes of a critical thinker and to learn to think clearly and critically about your patient care. To do that, you need to constantly reflect on how you are thinking. Are you practicing intellectual humility? Are you trying to be courageous and empathetic? These attitudes create an excellent base on which to build nursing knowledge and develop further thinking skills.

Nursing Knowledge Base

Nurses must have a good knowledge base to safely care for patients. You would not drive a car without first learning the basics of how a car works and the rules of the road. In the same way, you must understand the human body in health and illness before you can understand how to take care of an ill patient. This is the reason you are going to school and studying this book.

Information is found in many places; some information is good, and some is not as good. For example, health information found on a website may have been put there by a major university medical school or other reputable source, or it may have been put there by a patient who has a particular disorder. You may learn about a patient's experience by reading his or her website, but you certainly would not base your patient care on someone's personal story.

The best knowledge on which to base your practice comes from research. Nurse researchers try new methods of caring for patients and compare them with traditional methods to determine what works best. For example, for many years nurses were taught to massage patients' reddened bony prominences to prevent pressure ulcers. Through research, we now know that this practice should be avoided because it can further harm the damaged tissue.

When nursing care is based on good, well-designed research studies, it is called **evidence-based practice**. As nurses, we need to use as many research-based **interventions** (actions) as we can. Other interventions, until they are confirmed by research, have to be based on traditional nursing practice. It is nice to be able to tell a patient or family member that their loved one is being cared for based on the latest research recommendations!

Critical Thinking Skills

Problem Solving

Problem solving is one type of critical thinking skill. Nurses solve problems every day. However, a problem can be handled in a way that may or may not help the patient. For instance, consider Mr. Frank, who is in pain and asks for pain medication. You check the medication record and find that his analgesic is not due for another 40 minutes. You can choose to manage this problem in several ways. One obvious approach is to tell Mr. Frank that it is not time for the pain medication and that he will have to wait. This may solve your problem (you can move on to the next patient), but it does not solve the problem in an acceptable way for Mr. Frank. He is still in pain! Another approach is to use a standard problem-solving method:

1. Gather **data**, or factual information, to help you think critically about Mr. Frank's request for pain medication. As a good critical thinker, you can use intellectual empathy as well as your knowledge base about pain to decide what data you need. You decide to use a pain-rating scale on which the patient rates pain on a scale of 0 (no pain) to 10 (the greatest pain possible). Mr. Frank says that his pain is in his back and rates it as an 8 on the 10-point scale. You check his history and find that he has compression fractures of his spine. Your empathetic attitude tells you that waiting for 40 minutes to relieve his pain is not acceptable. You next go to the medication record and find that he has no alternative pain medications ordered.
2. Identify the problem. Here you use your knowledge base to draw the conclusion that Mr. Frank is in acute pain, and the current medication orders are not sufficient to provide pain relief.
3. Decide what outcome (sometimes called a goal) is desirable. The outcome should be determined by you (the nurse) and the patient working together. The patient is intimately involved in this situation and deserves to be consulted. In this case you talk to Mr. Frank and determine that he needs pain relief now; he cannot wait until the next scheduled dose of medication. He states that he can tolerate a pain rating of 3 or less on a 10-point scale.
4. Plan what to do. Formulate and consider some alternate solutions. For example, you can decide to tell Mr. Frank that he has to wait 40 minutes; however, this will not help him reach his desired outcome of pain control. You could give the medication early, but this would not be following the physician's orders and may have harmful effects for Mr. Frank. You could decide to try some nondrug pain-control methods, such as relaxation, distraction, or imagery. These might be helpful, but you recall from pharmacology class that complementary methods should be used in conjunction with, not in place of, medications. Another option is to report to the registered nurse (RN) or physician that Mr. Frank's pain is not controlled with the current pain-control regimen. Once you have several alternative courses of action, decide which will best help the patient. Then you can discuss those options with the RN and together decide the best thing to do; in this case, you might decide to have the RN contact the physician while you work with the patient on relaxation exercises. You might decide to ask Mr. Frank if he would like to listen to some of the music his wife brought for him. You should also tell Mr. Frank that the physician is being contacted. This would assure him that his pain-relief needs are being taken seriously.
5. Implement the plan of care. The RN enters the room and informs you and the patient that the physician has changed the analgesic orders. You obtain and administer the first dose of the new analgesic, being sure to explain its effects and side effects to Mr. Frank. The RN also informs Mr. Frank that the physician has ordered a consultation with the pain clinic.
6. Evaluate the plan of care. Did the plan work? As you reassess Mr. Frank 30 minutes later, he rates his pain level at 2 on the 0-to-10 scale. You think back to the desired outcome, compare it with the current data collected, and determine that your interventions were successful.

Can you see how using good thinking attitudes, a good knowledge base, and the problem-solving process led to a better outcome than simply choosing the first obvious option? You were able to achieve a desirable outcome: assisting Mr. Frank in relieving his pain. And you have undoubtedly earned Mr. Frank's trust in the process. Problem solving is how nurses make decisions on a daily basis. You may already know this method as the nursing process.

Other Critical Thinking Skills

Problem solving is just one critical thinking skill. Another way you can use critical thinking in patient care is by anticipating what might go wrong, watching carefully for signs that a problem might be occurring, and then preventing it or notifying the RN or physician in time to intervene. Nurses save many lives each year by anticipating and preventing problems. Sometimes this is called **vigilance**. An example would be knowing the signs and symptoms of low blood glucose (because of an excellent knowledge base) and watching for them carefully (being vigilant) in a patient taking medication for diabetes. If early symptoms occur, you can intervene before the problem becomes severe. In addition, you could teach the patient and family about low blood glucose and how to prevent it, further reducing the risk to the patient.

There are many other thinking skills that are beyond the scope of this book. A few questions follow that you can ask yourself as you continue to develop your critical thinking. There are many more questions you might ask. These are not in any order, nor would they all be asked for in a given situation. They are just some ideas to get you started.

- Have I thought this through?
- What information do I need?
- How do I know?
- Is someone influencing my thinking in ways I am not aware of?
- What conclusions can I draw from the information I have?
- Am I basing this decision on assumptions that may or may not be true?
- Am I thinking creatively about this, or am I in a rut?
- What do I need to watch for in order to prevent complications?
- Is there an expert I can consult who can help me think this through?
- Is there any supporting research or evidence that this is true?
- Am I too stressed or tired to think carefully about this right now?

NURSING PROCESS

You have just used the nursing process to solve a real problem. The **nursing process** is an organizing framework that links the process of thinking with actions in nursing practice. The nursing process can be used to assess patient needs, formulate nursing diagnoses, and plan, implement, and evaluate care. As a nursing student, you consciously apply the nursing process to each patient problem. With experience, you will internalize the nursing process and use it without as much conscious effort.

Role of the Licensed Practical Nurse and Licensed Vocational Nurse

The licensed practical nurse (LPN) or licensed vocational nurse (LVN) carries out a specific role in the nursing process, as described in Table 1.1. The role of the LPN/LVN is to provide direct patient care. The LPN/LVN often spends more time at the bedside than the RN, which allows the LPN/LVN to develop a therapeutic relationship and understand the patient's needs. The LPN/LVN and the RN work as a team to analyze data and develop, implement, and evaluate the plan of care (Fig. 1.1).

Data Collection

The first step in the nursing process is data collection. This **assessment** is a way to evaluate a patient's condition. The LPN/LVN assists the RN in collecting data from a variety of

TABLE 1.1 ROLE OF THE LPN/LVN IN THE NURSING PROCESS

Steps of the Process	Role of the LPN/LVN
Assessment	Assists RN in collecting data.
Nursing Diagnosis	Assists RN in choosing appropriate nursing diagnoses.
Planning Care	Assists RN in planning care and developing outcomes to meet patient needs.
Implementation	Carries out portions of the plan of care that are within the LPN/LVN's scope of practice.
Evaluation	Assists RN in evaluation and revision of the plan of care.

Note: There may be slight variations by state.

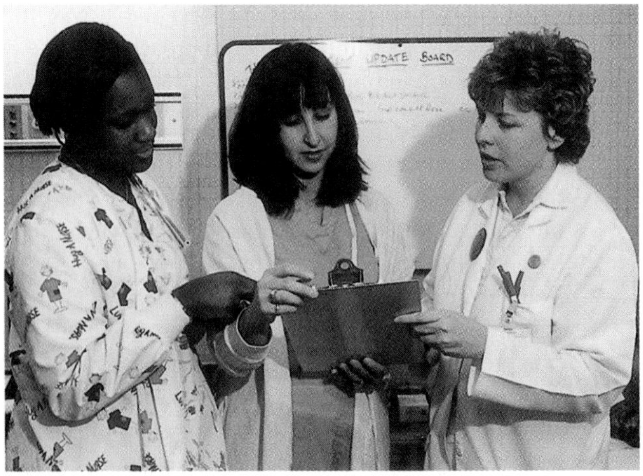

FIGURE 1.1 The nursing care team collaborating on a nursing care plan.

sources. Data are divided into two types: subjective data and objective data.

Subjective Data

Information provided verbally by the patient is called **subjective data**. Symptoms are subjective data. Often, subjective data are placed in quotes, such as "I have a headache" or "I feel out of breath." You must listen carefully to the patient and understand that only the patient truly knows how he or she feels.

When collecting subjective data, start with the patient's main concern. Focus on the reason the patient is seeking health care. The question "What happened that made you decide to come to the hospital (clinic, office)?" can be helpful.

Once the patient has identified the main concern, further questioning can reveal more pertinent information. Use the phrase "WHAT'S UP?" as a handy way to remember questions to ask the patient (Box 1.1). Asking the right questions can help you obtain better data with which to make the best decisions.

Next, obtain a patient history. This is done by asking the patient and family questions about the patient's past and present health problems, including specific questions about each body system, family health problems, and risk factors for health problems. The patient's medical record may also be consulted for background history information.

LEARNING TIP

Practice assessing a symptom on a classmate. Ask the WHAT'S UP? questions.

In addition to assessment of physiological function, ask the patient about personal habits that relate to health, such as exercise, diet, and the presence of stressors, according to institutional assessment guidelines. Finally, assess the patient's family role, support systems, and cultural and spiritual beliefs.

Objective Data

Objective data are pieces of factual information obtained through physical assessment and diagnostic tests that are observable or knowable through the five senses. For example, a rash can be observed with the eyes and palpated with the fingers. Objective data are sometimes called *signs*. Examples of objective data include the following:

- 3-cm red lesion
- Respiratory rate 36 per minute
- Blood glucose 326 mg/dL
- Patient is moaning.

These are all observable or measurable by a nurse and do not need explanation by the patient.

Objective data are gathered through physical assessment. Inspection, palpation, percussion, and auscultation techniques are used to collect objective data (Fig. 1.2). You can find more on these techniques, as well as how to obtain a complete history, in a nursing assessment text. Give special attention to areas that the patient has identified as potential problems.

Box 1.1

WHAT'S UP? Guide to Symptom Assessment

W—Where is it?
H—How does it feel? Describe the quality.
A—Aggravating and alleviating factors. What makes it worse? What makes it better?
T—Timing. When did it start? How long does it last?
S—Severity. How bad is it? This can often be rated on a scale of 0 to 10.
U—Useful other data. What other symptoms are present that might be related?
P—Patient's perception of the problem. The patient often has an idea about what the problem is, or the cause, but may not believe that his or her thoughts are important to share unless specifically asked.

Documentation of Data

Collected data are documented in the patient's medical record. If you identify any significant problem, change in the patient's status, or variation from normal, report it immediately to an RN or physician and then document it. Recorded data should be accurate and concise. When documenting objective data, include exactly what you observed. Avoid interpreting the data and using words that have vague meanings. For example, "nailbed color is pink" gives clearer information than "nailbed color is normal." "Normal" is an

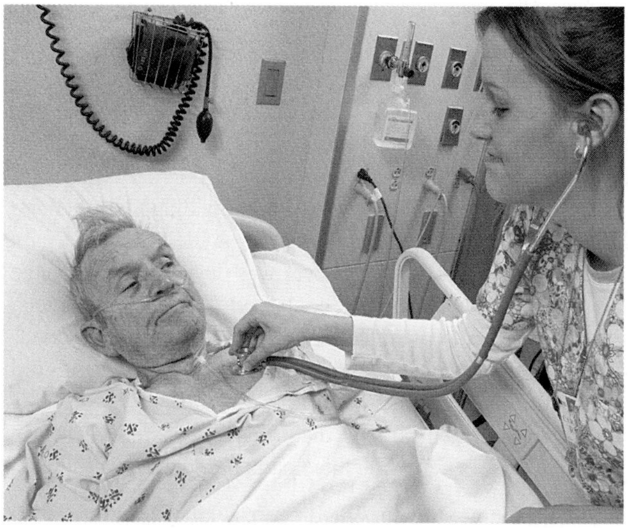

FIGURE 1.2 Nurse auscultating a patient's chest.

interpretation of data, rather than true data. "Capillary refill is 2 seconds" is more precise than "capillary refill is good." The statement "the wound looks better" is not meaningful unless the wound has been previously observed by the reader. Stating that "the wound is 1 by 2 inches, red, with no drainage or odor" provides data with which to compare the future status of the wound and determine whether it is responding to treatment.

When documenting subjective data, use what was stated by the patient or significant other. Use direct quotations whenever possible, such as "I feel sad." Quotes accurately represent the patient's view and are least open to interpretation. Meaningful documentation promotes continuity of patient care.

> **LEARNING TIP**
>
> Beginners may be tempted to search for elaborate phrases or words to document, when simple, direct words are best. Simply stating exactly what you saw or heard provides the most clear and accurate information.

Nursing Diagnosis

Once data have been collected, the LPN/LVN assists the RN to compare the findings with what is considered "normal." Data are then grouped, or clustered, into sets of related information that identify problems. Problems are then labeled as nursing diagnoses.

According to the North American Nursing Diagnosis Association (NANDA-I), a **nursing diagnosis** is a clinical judgment about individual, family, or community responses to actual or potential health problems or life processes (NANDA-I, 2009). Nursing diagnoses are standardized labels that make an identified problem understandable to all nurses. Nursing diagnoses guide the selection of interventions that will help achieve a desired outcome. A list of NANDA-I–approved nursing diagnoses can be found in Appendix A of this book.

A diagnosis is considered "medical" when the physician directs most of the care. A diagnosis is considered "nursing" if the interventions needed to treat the problem are mainly independent nursing functions.

One example of a NANDA-I nursing diagnosis is *Acute Pain*. In Mr. Frank's example, the nurse identified that pain was a problem, and a plan of care was developed to manage the pain. The physician was contacted for analgesic orders, and independent nursing actions were used, including relaxation and distraction. These independent nursing actions did not require a physician's order.

A well-written nursing diagnosis helps guide development of a plan of care. The three parts of a diagnosis follow:

- Problem—the nursing diagnosis label from the NANDA-I list
- Etiology—the cause or related factor (usually preceded by the words "related to")
- Signs and symptoms—the subjective or objective data that provide evidence that this is a valid diagnosis (often preceded by the words "as evidenced by").

The statement of problem, etiology, and signs and symptoms is called the PES format. Look again at the case study of Mr. Frank. A diagnosis using this format might read: "*Acute Pain* related to muscle spasms and nerve compression as evidenced by patient's pain rating of 8 on a 0-to-10 scale." Note how the complete diagnosis gives you more helpful information than simply the label "pain." This additional information helps determine an appropriate outcome and guides the selection of interventions.

Many patient problems are **collaborative—**that is, the nurse, physician, and other members of the health team all work together to reach the desired outcome. For example, a patient with pneumonia (a medical diagnosis) has many needs that depend on physician orders, such as respiratory treatments and antibiotics. The role of the LPN/LVN is to collect important data on the patient's respiratory status and to provide nursing measures such as encouraging fluid intake, coughing, and deep breathing.

> **CRITICAL THINKING**
>
> ***Nursing Diagnosis***
>
> ■ Which of the following are NANDA-I nursing diagnoses? Which are medical diagnoses? (Hint: Check Appendix A for help figuring these out!)
>
> 1. Impaired Physical Mobility
> 2. Ineffective Coping
> 3. Herniated Disk
> 4. Fractured Femur
> 5. Diabetes
> 6. Impaired Gas Exchange
> 7. Appendicitis
> 8. Activity Intolerance
>
> *Suggested answers at end of chapter.*

Plan of Care

Once nursing diagnoses have been identified, an individualized plan of care is designed to help meet the patient's care needs. Planning involves setting priorities, establishing outcomes, and identifying interventions that will help the patient meet the outcomes. It is important to include the patient in the development of the plan of care. The plan will be most successful if the patient agrees with and understands the interventions.

Prioritizing Care

Once you know what problems need to be addressed, you must decide which problem or intervention should be taken care of first. You and the patient decide together which problems take priority. Maslow's hierarchy of human needs is one commonly used system that can be used as a basis for determining priorities (Fig. 1.3). According to Maslow, humans must meet their most basic needs (those at the bottom of the triangle) first. They can then move up the hierarchy to meet higher level needs.

Physiological needs are the most basic. For example, a person who is short of breath cannot attend to higher level needs because the physiological need for oxygen is not being met. Once physiological needs are met, the patient can concentrate on meeting safety and security needs. Love, belonging, and self-esteem needs are next; self-actualization needs are generally the last priority when planning care.

Throughout life, people move up and down Maslow's hierarchy in response to life events. If a need occurs on a level below the patient's current level, the patient will move down to the level of that need. Once the need is fulfilled, the person can move upward on the hierarchy again.

In a nursing plan of care, the patient's most urgent problem is listed first. According to Maslow's hierarchy of human needs, this usually involves a physiological need such as oxygen or water because these are life-sustaining needs. If several physiological needs are present, life-threatening needs are ranked first, health-threatening needs are second, and health-promoting needs, although important, are last.

LEARNING TIP

If you are stuck wondering which physiological need should take priority, ask yourself, "Which problem is most threatening to my patient's life?"

Once physiological needs have been met, needs related to the next level of the hierarchy, safety and security, can be addressed. Remaining diagnoses are listed in order of urgency as they relate to the hierarchy. Needs can occur simultaneously on different levels and must be addressed in a holistic manner, with prioritization guiding the care provided.

LEARNING TIP

If you are developing a plan of care for a patient with complex needs and are not sure where to start, go back to the assessment phase. Often, additional information can help you better understand the patient's needs and develop a plan of care individualized to the patient's specific problem areas.

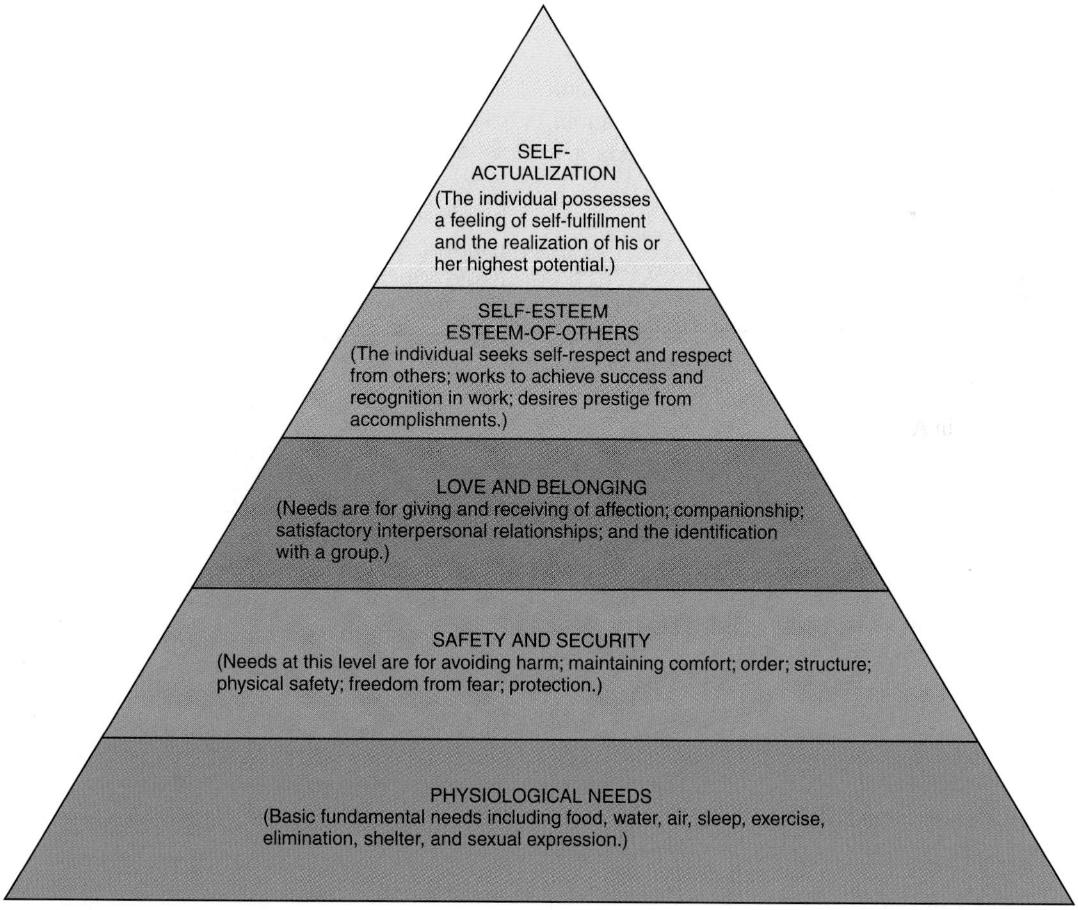
SELF-ACTUALIZATION
(The individual possesses a feeling of self-fulfillment and the realization of his or her highest potential.)
SELF-ESTEEM ESTEEM-OF-OTHERS
(The individual seeks self-respect and respect from others; works to achieve success and recognition in work; desires prestige from accomplishments.)
LOVE AND BELONGING
(Needs are for giving and receiving of affection; companionship; satisfactory interpersonal relationships; and the identification with a group.)
SAFETY AND SECURITY
(Needs at this level are for avoiding harm; maintaining comfort; order; structure; physical safety; freedom from fear; protection.)
PHYSIOLOGICAL NEEDS
(Basic fundamental needs including food, water, air, sleep, exercise, elimination, shelter, and sexual expression.)

FIGURE 1.3 Maslow's hierarchy of human needs.

Establishing Outcomes

An outcome is a statement that describes the patient's desired goal for a problem area. It should be measurable, be realistic for the patient, and have an appropriate time frame for achievement. *Measurable* means that the outcome is objective, or can be observed. It should not be vague or open to interpretation, with the use of subjective words such as *normal, large, small,* or *moderate.* Consider, for example, two outcomes:

- The patient's shortness of breath will improve.
- The patient will be less short of breath within 15 minutes as evidenced by the patient rating the shortness of breath at less than 3 on a scale of 0 to 10, respiratory rate between 16 and 20 per minute, and relaxed appearance.

Although the first outcome seems appropriate, in reality it is difficult to know when it has been met. There is nothing to objectively indicate when the problem has been resolved. The second outcome is objective. You can see that when the patient rates his or her shortness of breath at less than 3, is breathing at a rate of 16 to 20 per minute, and appears relaxed, the desired outcome will have been met. The outcome is realistic, and the 15-minute time frame ensures that the patient's distress is minimized. If the plan of care does not achieve the desired outcome in the given time frame, it should be evaluated and revised as needed.

When determining criteria for a measurable outcome, look at the signs and symptoms portion of the nursing diagnosis. The resolution of signs and symptoms identified in the NANDA-I nursing diagnoses is evidence that nursing interventions were effective. If the desired outcome is not achieved, the problem and interventions need reevaluation. Look at another outcome example to see how criteria are used for measurement:

Nursing diagnosis—*Ineffective Airway Clearance* related to excess secretions as evidenced by coarse crackles and nonproductive cough

Outcome—Patient will have effective airway clearance within 8 hours, as evidenced by clear lung sounds and productive cough.

> **CRITICAL THINKING**
>
> ***Prioritizing Care***
>
> ■ Based on Maslow's hierarchy of needs, list the following nursing diagnoses in order from highest (1) to lowest (5) priority. Give rationales for your decisions.
>
> ____ *Deficient Knowledge*
>
> ____ *Constipation*
>
> ____ *Disabled Family Coping*
>
> ____ *Readiness for Enhanced Self-Concept*
>
> ____ *Ineffective Airway Clearance*
>
> *Suggested answers at end of chapter.*

Identifying Interventions

Interventions are the actions you take to help a patient meet a desired outcome. Therefore, interventions are considered goal directed. Any intervention that does not contribute to meeting the outcome should not be part of the plan of care.

One way to create a care plan is to include interventions that can be categorized as "take, treat, and teach." In the first intervention category, "take," or identify, data related to the problem that should be routinely collected. Next, "treat" the problem by identifying deliberate actions to help reach the outcome. Last, identify what to "teach" the patient and family for the patient to learn to care for himself or herself.

Look again at the nursing diagnosis of *Ineffective Airway Clearance.* A plan of care for this problem using the take, treat, and teach method might look like this:

Take: Auscultate lung sounds every 4 hours and as needed.
Assess respiratory rate every 4 hours and as needed.

Treat: Provide 2 L of fluids every 24 hours.
Offer expectorant as ordered.
Provide cool mist vaporizer in room.

Teach: Teach the patient the importance of fluid intake.
Teach the patient to cough and deep breathe every 1 to 2 hours.

In addition to identifying interventions, it is important to understand how and why they will work. The "why" is called a *rationale.* For example, you should assess lung sounds and respiratory rate every 4 hours *because increased crackles and respiratory rate indicate retained secretions.* Fluids are provided *to help liquefy secretions and ease their removal.* Sound rationales that are evidence based (research based) should guide the selection of each nursing intervention. You will find rationales with interventions throughout this book, to help you understand why interventions will be effective.

Like nursing diagnoses, nursing interventions can be either independent or collaborative. Independent nursing actions can be initiated by the nurse. Examples of independent nursing actions include teaching the patient deep-breathing exercises, turning a patient every 2 hours, teaching about medications, and giving a back rub for comfort. Collaborative actions require a physician's order to perform, and may include both nursing and medical diagnoses. Examples of collaborative interventions include giving prescribed medications, applying elastic stockings, requesting a referral to physical therapy, and inserting a urinary catheter.

Implementation

Once the plan of care has been identified, it must be communicated to the patient, family, and health team members and then implemented. One way a plan of care is communicated is by writing it as a nursing care plan. The nursing care plan is documented on the patient's medical record, to communicate to all nurses the patient's priority problems, the desired outcomes, and the plan for meeting the outcomes. Many institutions have standardized care plans that are individualized for each patient by the nurse.

Implementation of the plan of care involves performing the interventions. The patient's response to each intervention is noted and documented. This documentation provides the basis for evaluation and revision of the plan of care.

Evaluation

The last step of the nursing process is **evaluation**. The nurse continuously evaluates the patient's progress toward the desired outcomes and the effectiveness of each intervention. If the outcomes are not reached within the given time frame, or if the interventions are ineffective, the plan of care is revised. Any part of the plan of care can be revised, from the diagnosis or desired outcome to the interventions. Acute care institutions require routine review and updating of the plan of care.

SUGGESTED ANSWERS TO CRITICAL THINKING

■ *Nursing Diagnosis*

1. Impaired Physical Mobility = nursing
2. Ineffective Coping = nursing
3. Herniated Disk = medical
4. Fractured Femur = medical
5. Diabetes = medical
6. Impaired Gas Exchange = nursing
7. Appendicitis = medical
8. Activity Intolerance = nursing

■ *Prioritizing Care*

1. *Ineffective Airway Clearance*—physiological need that can be life threatening
2. *Constipation*—physiological need that can be health threatening
3. *Deficient Knowledge*—safety and security need
4. *Disabled Family Coping*—love and belonging need
5. *Readiness for Enhanced Self-Concept*—self-esteem need

REVIEW QUESTIONS

1. In which of the following ways is critical thinking useful to the nursing process?
   a. It highlights the obvious solution to a problem.
   b. It can lead to a better outcome for the patient.
   c. It simplifies the process.
   d. It helps the nurse arrive at a solution more quickly.

2. Which nurse is exhibiting intellectual humility?
   a. The nurse who is an expert at wound care.
   b. The nurse who reports an error to the supervisor.
   c. The nurse who tries to empathize with the patient.
   d. The nurse who asks a coworker about a new procedure.

3. Which of the following pieces of information is considered objective data?
   a. The patient's respiratory rate is 28.
   b. The patient states, "I feel short of breath."
   c. The patient is short of breath.
   d. The patient is feeling panicky.

4. An LPN/LVN is collecting data on a newly admitted patient who has an ulcerated area on his left hip. It is 2 inches in diameter and 1 inch deep, with yellow exudate. Which of the following statements best documents the findings in the patient's database?
   a. Wound on left hip, 2 inches diameter, 1 inch deep, infected
   b. Left hip wound is large, deep, and has yellow drainage
   c. Pressure ulcer on left hip, yellow drainage
   d. Wound on left hip, 2 inches in diameter, 1 inch deep, yellow exudate

5. A 34-year-old mother of three children is admitted to a respiratory unit with pneumonia. Based on Maslow's hierarchy of needs, which of the following patient problems should the nurse address first?
   a. Frontal headache from stress of hospital admission
   b. Anxiety related to concern about leaving children
   c. Shortness of breath from newly diagnosed pneumonia
   d Deficient knowledge about treatment plan

Continued

REVIEW QUESTIONS—cont'd

6. Place the steps of the nursing process in correct chronological order of use. Use all options.
   a. Nursing diagnosis
   b. Evaluation
   c. Assessment
   d. Planning care
   e. Implementation

7. Which of the following parts of the nursing process can be carried out by an LPN/LVN?
   a. Implementation of interventions
   b. Nursing diagnosis
   c. Analysis of data
   d. Evaluation of outcomes

8. Which of the following is a nursing diagnosis?
   a. Stroke
   b. Renal Failure
   c. Fracture
   d. Acute Pain

9. A nurse teaches a patient the importance of stopping smoking. Which of the following patient responses indicates to the nurse that the teaching was effective?
   a. "I have a brother who died of lung cancer. I know smoking is bad."
   b. "I tried to quit 5 years ago, and I really would like to, but it is very hard."
   c. "Thank you for the information. I will call the Smoke Stoppers organization today."
   d. "I know you are right; I should stop smoking."

References

Green, C. J. (2000). *Critical thinking in nursing.* Upper Saddle River, NJ: Prentice Hall Health.

Halpern, D. (1996). *Thought and knowledge: An introduction to critical thinking* (3rd ed., p. 5). Mahwah, NJ: Lawrence Erlbaum Associates.

North American Nursing Diagnosis Association (NANDA-I). (2009). *Nursing diagnosis: Definitions and classification, 2009–2011.* Hoboken, NJ: Wiley.

DavisPlus | For additional resources and information visit http://davisplus.fadavis.com

2 Evidence-Based Practice

BETTY ACKLEY

KEY TERMS

evidence-based practice (EH-va-dense baste PRACK-tis)
randomized controlled trial (RAN-dumb-eyesd cun-TROLLD TRY-ull)
research (re-SURCH)
systematic review (SISS-tem-AT-ick re-VIEW)

QUESTIONS TO GUIDE YOUR READING

1. What is evidence-based practice (EBP)?
2. Why should EBP be used?
3. How do you identify nursing evidence that should be put into practice?
4. What is the EBP process?
5. What are the six steps of EBP?
6. What is the best method for oral care?

Amanda, LPN, is charge nurse of the fourth wing with 23 residents in an extended care agency. One of the residents, Mr. Samuel, had a right-sided stroke and currently has a gastrostomy tube going into his stomach, through which feeding formula is administered 12 hours per day. He has halitosis, and his teeth look fuzzy. He currently receives oral care twice daily with sponge foam Toothettes. What does the evidence say should be done for oral care for Mr. Samuel? (See discussion and answers throughout the chapter.)

Evidence-based practice (EBP) is a systematic process that employs current evidence to make decisions about patient care. It includes evaluation of the quality and applicability of existing research, patient preferences, costs, clinical expertise, and clinical settings. Evidence gives assurance that nursing practice will be effective. Using evidence-based nursing practice will increase your power to give the best nursing care possible.

EBP involves much more than just evaluating **research** (scientific study, investigation, or experimentation) to determine which results apply to nursing care. Clinical reality can be very different than a research setting. It could be unsafe to apply a research study that was done in a controlled environment to the very different environment found in an actual clinical situation. Or it could be unsafe to apply research results obtained on people of one age or medical diagnosis to those of another age or with multiple diagnoses. The context in which the evidence will be used must be considered. This includes the health care environment, the patient involved, the nurse's expertise, and the cost. Using EBP is a complex process, but it is an important way to ensure quality care and optimal patient outcomes.

REASONS FOR USING EBP

The use of EBP allows nurses to give patients the best care possible, which is the goal of all caring nurses. The reasons given for nursing care used to be "This is how it was taught in nursing school" or "This is what they told us in orientation" or "That's the way it is done here." Now the rationale behind the best nursing care is "Nursing care is based on evidence and how it applies to an individual patient in a specific setting." EBP is considered the gold standard of health care.

Evidence-based outcome measurement is built into the EBP process as a way to measure and confirm the value of a change in nursing practice. For example, nurses are measuring the number of new pressure ulcers, new cases of pneumonia, and new urinary tract infections in health care settings. Measuring outcomes as a part of EBP reenergizes nursing by helping nurses see the results of their nursing care. Measured outcomes show nurses that they are giving the best care possible, based on the evidence available at the time.

Evidence comes from multiple sources. Medical research and research from many other professions such as psychology, gerontology, and social work are utilized in addition to nursing research to develop EBP nursing care guidelines.

IDENTIFYING NURSING EVIDENCE

How do you identify nursing evidence that should be put into practice? It depends in part on the strength of the evidence. Evidence ranges from strong to weak, and levels can be assigned to rate its strength and quality. The rating scale used to label the quality of evidence ranges from level I to level IV (Table 2.1). Level I is the best evidence. It includes **systematic reviews** and analysis of many high-quality **randomized controlled trials** (studies designed to assess the effects of a variable by randomly assigning subjects to experimental, placebo, or control groups). Level IV evidence is the weakest and includes the non–research-based opinions of experts or published but non–research-based clinical articles. Two of the best known sources for level I evidence are the Cochrane Reviews (www.cochrane.org/reviews) for medical evidence and the Joanna Briggs Best Practice reviews (www.joannabriggs.edu.au/pubs/best_practice.php) for nursing practice.

TABLE 2.1 LEVELS OF EVIDENCE

Level	Type of Evidence
Level I	**Systematic reviews, such as Cochrane Reviews and Joanna Briggs Best Evidence Guidelines** Evidence from a systematic review of all relevant randomized clinical trials or evidence-based clinical practice guidelines that are based on systematic reviews of randomized controlled trials. Three or more randomized controlled trials of good quality that have similar results also have been considered level I evidence.
Level II	**Randomized controlled trials** Evidence obtained from at least one well-designed randomized controlled trial. These are true experimental studies where as many factors that could falsely change the results are controlled as possible.
Level III	**Quasi-experimental studies** Evidence obtained from quasi-experimental research studies. These studies do not control factors that could falsely change the results and, as a result, are less predictive of effectiveness of nursing care.
Level IV	**Expert opinion** Evidence from the opinion of authorities and/or reports of expert committees. Also nursing journal articles that are opinion based, not research based.

THE EBP PROCESS

Evidence that guides nursing care can be used in two ways, generally based on whether the evidence is an independent or a dependent nursing intervention. Dependent nursing interventions are those that are delegated by a physician. Here any change in practice must go through a committee, such as the policy and procedure committee, to determine if it is appropriate for adoption. If the intervention is independent, however, the nurse can implement an evidence-based change based on personal knowledge of the value of the intervention, as long as the change is safe and cannot harm the patient. An example is the intervention of reality orientation. Excellent research shows that the use of reality orientation can improve thinking ability in patients with dementia and delirium. The nurse can implement this intervention independently, because it does not require an order. Other intervention examples include the use of hand massage, music therapy, and other anxiety-relieving interventions.

A simplified version of the EBP process is discussed next and shown in Figure 2.1. The acronym "ASKMME!" is designed to help you remember the six essential steps: Ask, Search, thinK, Measure, Make it happen, and Evaluate.

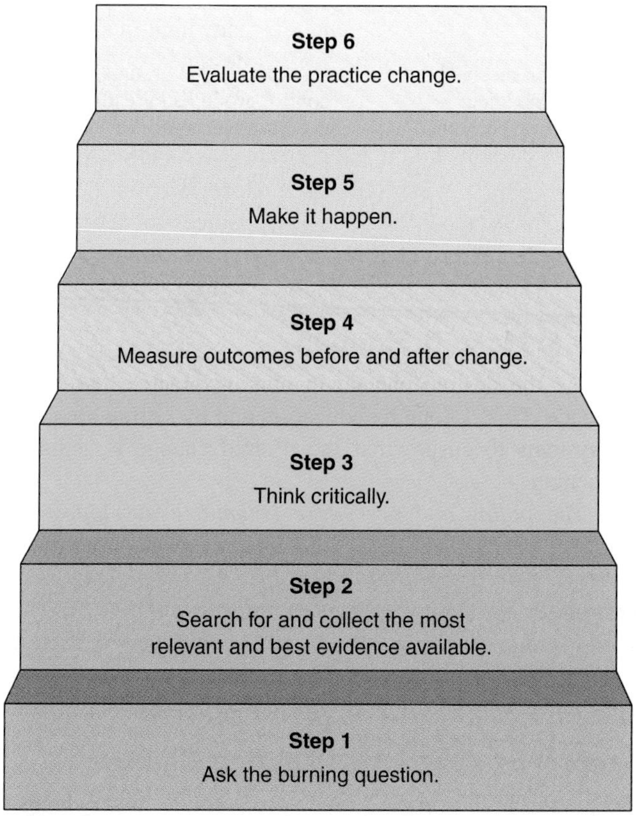
Step 6
Evaluate the practice change.
Step 5
Make it happen.
Step 4
Measure outcomes before and after change.
Step 3
Think critically.
Step 2
Search for and collect the most relevant and best evidence available.
Step 1
Ask the burning question.

FIGURE 2.1 The six steps of the EBP process. (*Source:* Ackley, B. J., Ladwig, G. B., Swan, B. A., & Tucker, S. J. (2008). *Evidence-based nursing care guidelines: Medical-surgical interventions.* Philadelphia: Mosby, with permission.)

Step 1: Ask the Burning Question

EBP begins with questioning the status quo, trying to solve a problem, or learning about new evidence that should be used in nursing practice. The initial question nurses often ask is "Why do we do it that way?" or "How could we do this better?" Questioning the existing way of doing things is part of critical thinking. It helps ensure that the patient receives the best care possible. As a student nurse you can do this as well.

For Mr. Samuel, in the case study at the start of the chapter, Amanda was motivated to find the best way to give oral care, because her instincts told her the current care was not sufficient. Amanda took her clinical question to the policy and procedure committee and, working with members, they began the evidence-based process to find the best way to give oral care to all tube-fed patients at their agency.

Step 2: Search For and Collect the Most Relevant and Best Evidence Available

A thorough search of the literature in the subject area needs to be conducted. As a student nurse, you will find medical librarians most helpful. It is important that you learn basic computer skills so that you also have the ability to search the nursing and medical literature. Several databases can help you find journal articles and reviews.

For nursing literature, the best known database is CINAHL, which stands for Cumulative Index to Nursing and Allied Health Literature (www.ebscohost.com/cinahl). CINAHL is available through school libraries and hospital libraries. For best practice nursing reviews, visit the Joanna Briggs Best Practices website at www.joannabriggs.edu.au/pubs/best_practice.php.

For medical literature, the comprehensive Medline/Pubmed database can be accessed at www.ncbi.nlm.nih.gov/sites/entrez?db=pubmed. Cochrane Reviews are available at www.cochrane.org/reviews. An easy way to find Cochrane Reviews is to type in "Cochrane" when searching for a topic.

Amanda worked with a medical librarian and other members of her agency's policy and procedure committee to conduct a search. They then summarized the research articles they found in this area (Table 2.2).

Step 3: Think Critically

Always appraise the evidence you find for validity, relevance to the situation, and applicability. First, evaluate the quality of the evidence you find. It is helpful to determine the level of the evidence to make sure you have the best information available (see Table 2.1). Then, using critical thinking, evaluate the evidence as it applies to the individual patient or patient population, the clinical expertise of the nurse(s) involved, the values in the situation, and agency policies that affect making a change in practice.

Amanda found many research articles on the value of oral care, and the results were exciting. When the research was analyzed, it became obvious that all tube-fed patients

TABLE 2.2 ORAL CARE FOR PATIENTS WHO ARE BEING TUBE FED

Study	Population	Interventions	Key Findings
Pearson, L. S., & Hutton, J. L. (2002). A controlled trial to compare the ability of foam swabs and toothbrushes to remove dental plaque. *Journal of Advanced Nursing, 39*(5), 480–489.	34 volunteers	Group 1 received oral care in the a.m. using a toothbrush. Group 2 received oral care in the a.m. using foam swabs (Toothettes).	Use of toothbrushes for oral care was much more effective than foam swabs in removing plaque from the teeth.
Yoneyama, T., Yoshida, M., Ohrui, T., et al. (2002). Oral care reduces pneumonia in older patients in nursing homes. *Journal of the American Geriatrics Society, 50*(3), 584–585.	417 subjects (older patients in long-term care facilities in Japan)	Experimental group received toothbrushing after each meal plus professional care from a dental hygienist or a dentist once a week. Control group received regular care.	The experimental group had decreased febrile days, decreased incidence of pneumonia, decreased deaths from pneumonia, increased activities of daily living, and increased cognitive function.
Leibovitz, A., Plotnikov, G., Habot, B., et al. (2003). Pathogenic colonization of oral flora in frail elderly patients fed by nasogastric tube or percutaneous enterogastric tube. *Journal of Gerontology Series A: Biological Sciences and Medical Sciences, 58*(1), 52–55.	215 subjects (patients in long-term care facilities)	Group 1: Patients fed via nasogastric (NG) tube had 81% pathogenic bacteria in mouth. Group 2: Patients fed by percutaneous enterogastric (PEG) tube had 51% pathogenic bacteria in mouth. Group 3: Patients fed orally had 17.5% pathogenic bacteria in mouth.	Patients fed by NG tube had more pathogenic bacteria in their mouths than those fed by PEG tube or those fed orally. If oral secretions are aspirated, the risk of pneumonia increases.
Adachi, M., Ishihara, K., Abe, S., et al. (2007). Professional oral health care by dental hygienists reduced respiratory infections in elderly persons requiring nursing care. *International Journal of Dental Hygiene, 5*(2), 69–74.	190 subjects	Experimental group received professional oral health care by dental hygienists. Control group received regular oral care.	Oral care reduced pathogenic organisms in mouth, reduced fever above 103.5°F (37.9°C), reduced onset of influenza, and reduced fatal pneumonia.
Panchabhai, T. S., Dangayach, N. S., Krishnan, A., et al. (2009). Oropharyngeal cleansing with 0.2% chlorhexidine for prevention of nosocomial pneumonia in critically ill patients. *Chest, 135*(5), 1150–1156.	512 subjects	Experimental group received oral care with chlorhexidine. Control group received oral care with 0.2% potassium permanganate.	Both experimental group and control group had greatly decreased incidence of pneumonia as compared with "usual" oral care.

needed better oral care and that oral care for Mr. Samuel should be given with a toothbrush and toothpaste. Since he had trouble swallowing, it was also important that suction be readily available as oral care was given. Plus, the studies found that inadequate oral care resulted in more than just halitosis and fuzzy teeth; it could result in pneumonia. Amanda felt a renewed sense of purpose.

Step 4: Measure Outcomes Before and After Change

Next, determine the outcomes that are likely to occur as a result of a change in nursing care. Usually, a small pilot study is done within the agency before any widespread change in practice is made. That way, it can be determined if the change will be effective, as intended, when the change is implemented across the agency.

The committee decided to measure the number of new pneumonia cases in their agency, which is a very important outcome.

Step 5: Make It Happen

Institute the desired change in nursing practice based on evidence. This is done by education and by setting up quality systems to ensure that the desired change is actually happening.

The policy and procedure committee developed an evidence-based procedure guideline for oral care of all patients, with a separate policy for tube-fed patients. The new policy and procedure was introduced and then became a care requirement for all patients at the agency. Then a quality audit was done at intervals on selected patients to ensure the appropriate oral care was being given.

Step 6: Evaluate the Practice Change

Evaluation is the process used to determine if the change made a significant difference. What were the results of the initial small study? Was the change in practice effective in improving patient outcomes? If it did make a difference, was the difference worth the extra cost or time it required?

Wow! Because of Amanda's concern about oral care, a change had been made that improved the care for every patient with teeth. Also, after making the change in oral care and evaluating the outcome, it was clear that Amanda's agency had a decrease in new-onset pneumonia. This was very exciting and reinforcing to the committee, and especially to Amanda.

EBP, QUALITY, AND SAFETY: THEY BELONG TOGETHER!

At this time, multiple quality initiatives are having a positive impact on health care. Insurance companies, businesses, patients, and the government are demanding quality care. All quality initiatives require collection of data, which is greatly facilitated by the health care agency having an EBP framework. Some quality initiatives are required, such as those of the Joint Commission that accredits health care agencies. Others are voluntary but desirable for the agency's well-being. All quality initiatives should begin with a literature search to determine the most effective interventions.

Quality and Safety Education for Nurses Project

In 2005, the Quality and Safety Education for Nurses (QSEN) project was funded by the Robert Wood Johnson Foundation. This project focuses on nursing education that promotes the continual improvement of quality and safety in patient care. The goal is for students to develop understanding, attitudes, skills, and the desire to continually improve the quality and safety of patient care. Information on the QSEN project can be found at www.qsen.org.

The development of teaching strategies for nursing students involves six areas of focus:

- *Evidence-based practice:* EBP is introduced in this chapter. Look for Evidence-Based Practice boxes throughout the book that provide information on research studies that tell us how best to care for our patients.
- *Safety:* We all want our patients to be safe! Many interventions are available that can help us reach this goal. Look for Safety Tips throughout the chapters and the section on safety in Chapter 3.
- *Teamwork and collaboration:* These are important aspects of providing safe and quality care. You are introduced to members of the health care team in Chapter 3 with whom you may work and collaborate. For example, you may talk with the pharmacist if you have a question about a patient's medication to ensure it is given safely, or alert the registered nurse to a change in a patient's vital signs so the physician can be informed for treatment orders. This illustrates teamwork to ensure the patient receives safe, high-quality care.
- *Patient-centered care:* When collaborating on the development of nursing care plans, it is important to individualize interventions to provide patient-centered care. As nursing interventions are performed, they should meet the patient's needs and preferred schedules rather than the institution's or caregiver's. You will find Nursing Care Plans throughout the chapters, but always remember that no plan fits all patients. You will always evaluate each suggested intervention to see if it fits your patient and then individualize it to the patient's needs.
- *Quality improvement:* Quality improvement (QI) is an ongoing process to improve patient care (see Fig. 3.3). You might participate in a QI project by collecting data, which is one aspect of a QI project.
- *Informatics:* Informatics is a growing area in health care because of the increasing use of technology to provide safer care. Examples you may use include computerized medical records, medication dispensing systems, medication barcoding systems, or computerized resources.

Concern for Patient Safety

Safety is on everyone's mind. Many people know of someone who has been affected by a medical error or who has been unhappy with his or her care. Health care providers are being held accountable for safe care by society. As a result, guidelines to reduce errors in health care and improve patient outcomes have been developed and based on evidence when available. The Joint Commission's 2010 National Patient Safety Goals can be found at www.jointcommission.org/patientsafety/nationalpatientsafetygoals. As you will see at the website, these goals address care in various types of health care settings.

SAFETY TIP

One important safety goal is to use at least two patient identifiers—but not the patient's room number or location—when providing care, treatment, or services. This is because wrong-patient errors occur in virtually all stages of diagnosis and treatment. The intent for this goal is twofold: first, to reliably identify the patient as the person for whom the service or treatment is intended; second, to match the service or treatment to that patient (2010 National Patient Safety Goals, www.jointcommission.org).

You will find other national patient safety goals in the Safety Tips features throughout the text of this book. These goals are included to increase your awareness and understanding of patient safety. They address important areas of concern, such as administering medications safely, identifying patients correctly, identifying operative sites correctly, improving communication, reducing fall injuries, and reducing the risk of infection in institutionalized elderly persons, to name a few. You will want to become familiar with them, and look for updates at the Joint Commission website. Of course, it takes critical thinking to use them at the right times and in the right circumstances. Using them appropriately helps you provide safer care with fewer errors, which your patients appreciate.

EBP is critical thinking at its finest, working to determine the best care for the patient based on the evidence. The evidence provides core information to direct safe, quality-driven, excellent patient care.

REVIEW QUESTIONS

1. Which of the following describes evidence-based practice? **Select all that apply.**
   a. Is a systematic process
   b. Uses current evidence
   c. Applies only to medical treatment
   d. Limits patient preferences
   e. Does not consider costs
   f. Evaluates quality of research

2. Which of the following is the best way to give excellence in nursing care?
   a. Base nursing care on what was taught in a nursing program.
   b. Base nursing care on what was taught in the orientation to the health care agency.
   c. Base nursing care on what is in textbooks and the nurse's assessment of each patient.
   d. Base nursing care on evidence that is reviewed and evaluated for practice at the health care agency and for each patient.

3. Which of the following sources of evidence would be generally safe for a hospital or extended care agency to implement?
   a. A Joanna Briggs Best Practices Guideline
   b. One randomized controlled trial
   c. Four quasi-experimental studies that show similar results
   d. The opinion of a national nursing expert on the subject

4. An LVN reads about a research study that affects nursing care and could lead to decreased wound infections. Which of the following actions should the LVN take regarding the information in the study?
   a. Put the information into practice while performing wound care.
   b. Discuss the research with a trusted coworker and, if the coworker agrees, put the information into practice at work.
   c. Present the proposed practice change to the policy and procedure committee at work for evaluation and possible adoption.
   d. Do a journal search to look for similar studies, and if three similar studies are found, incorporate the information into practice.

5. A policy and procedure committee is revising the nursing intervention of insertion of a retention catheter. Where should the committee begin looking for evidence to write an effective policy and procedure on this intervention?
   a. In current nursing skills textbooks.
   b. In nursing articles written by national nursing experts based on opinion.
   c. In research articles, preferably systematic reviews of randomized controlled trials.
   d. In the policies and procedures of other nursing facilities.

6. An LPN is caring for a patient with a tube feeding in the morning and is preparing to give oral care. Which of the following would be the best way to give oral care based on the case study in this chapter?
   a. Use Toothettes with a good mouthwash and then swab the teeth and the mouth.
   b. Use a soft toothbrush and fluoride toothpaste to brush the teeth.
   c. Use a tongue scraper to remove debris from the tongue twice daily.
   d. Skip oral care, recognizing that a tube-fed patient needs much more important care than that, such as checking for placement of the nasogastric tube.

Reference

Joint Commission. (2010). *2010 national patient safety goals.* Retrieved January 13, 2010, from http://www.jointcommission.org/patientsafety/nationalpatientsafetygoals

3 Issues in Nursing Practice

DIANE MAYO, MICHELLE BLOCK, AND PATRICK M. SHANNON

KEY TERMS

administrative laws (ad-MIN-i-STRAY-tive LAWZ)
autocratic leadership (AW-tuh-KRAT-ik LEE-der-ship)
autonomy (aw-TAWN-uh-MEE)
beneficence (buh-NEF-i-sens)
civil law (SIH-vil LAW)
code of ethics (KOHD OF ETH-icks)
confidentiality (KON-fi-den-she-AL-i-tee)
criminal law (KRIM-i-nuhl LAW)
delegation (DELL-a-GAY-shun)
democratic leadership (DEM-ah-KRAT-ik LEE-der-ship)
deontology (DEE-on-TOL-o-gee)
diagnosis-related groups (DYE-ag-NOH-sis ree-LAY-ted GROOPS)
distributive justice (dis-TRIB-yoo-tiv JUSS-tiss)
empathy (EM-puh-thee)
ethics (ETH-icks)
justice (JUSS-tiss)
laissez-faire leadership (LAYS-ay-FAIR LEE-der-ship)
leadership (LEE-der-ship)
liability (LYE-uh-BIL-i-tee)
limitation of liability (LIM-i-TAY-shun OF LYE-uh-BIL-i-tee)
maleficence (ma-LEF-i-cence)
malpractice (mal-PRAK-tiss)
morality (moh-RAL-i-tee)
negligence (NEG-li-jens)
nonmaleficence (NON-muh-LEF-i-sens)
paternalism (puh-TER-nuhl-izm)
principles (PRIN-sih-pulz)
respondeat superior (res-POND-ee-et sue-PEER-ee-or)
standard of best interest (STAN-derd OF BEST IN-ter-est)
summons (SUH-muns)
torts (TORTS)
utilitarian (yoo-TILL-ih-TAR-ee-en)
values (VAL-yooz)
welfare rights (WELL-fare RITES)

QUESTIONS TO GUIDE YOUR READING

1. What factors are influencing changes in the health care delivery system?
2. What is the significance of "never events" and hospital-acquired conditions?
3. What is the LPN/LVNs role in the health care delivery system?
4. What are four leadership styles?
5. What is the LPN/LVNs role in leadership?
6. Why are ethics important in health care?
7. What is an example of a character trait and how does it relate to nursing?
8. What are the definitions of two major principles in ethics and how do they relate to ethical dilemmas?
9. What are the steps of the ethical decision-making model?
10. What is moral distress and how does it affect nursing?
11. Where is the regulation of nursing practice defined?
12. How can you provide quality care and limit your liability?
13. How would you define the Health Insurance Portability and Accountability Act of 1996?

HEALTH CARE DELIVERY

Health–Illness Continuum

The term *health–illness continuum* describes the continually shifting levels of health experienced by each person. One end of the continuum represents high-level health. The other end represents poor health and impending death. We all move about the continuum throughout our lives.

Health Care Delivery Systems

A focus on prevention and providing services from birth to death under one integrated system is used for some health care systems. Hospital consolidations have resulted in development of health care systems that may cover large geographic areas. The hospital then provides the integrated care delivery network for the system (Fig. 3.1).

Factors Influencing Health Care Change

Today's health care delivery system is being influenced by the use of evidence to guide practice (see Chapter 2), health information technology, the expanding use of robotics in surgery and other areas of health care, and resistant infectious organisms that continue to emerge. Nursing informatics is a newer specialty area that deals with how to use information technology within nursing practice. These changes make learning a constant in today's health care environment.

The changing characteristics of the American population are also influencing the health care delivery system: the increasing size of the national population, the increasing number of elderly people, the increasing number of people who are uninsured or underinsured, and increased cultural diversity. The size of the American population is projected to increase to more than 363 million people by the year 2030, with those over age 62 increasing by 50% from 2000 (U.S. Census Bureau, 2005). The health care needs of the elderly can be complex, with chronic diseases most common, which places increased demands on the health care system. The increase in the number of uninsured patients places additional strains on the system, and the increase in cultural diversity impacts how health care is delivered.

Safe Practice

There has been a growing movement to promote and enhance safe health care practices to prevent harmful adverse events. A culture of safety should exist within the health care system and nursing. The Joint Commission's National Patient Safety Goals (www.jointcommission.org/patientsafety/nationalpatientsafetygoals) are updated annually, and sentinel events identify safety concerns and interventions for them.

The National Quality Forum (NQF) has identified serious reportable adverse events (also called *never events*). These 28 events are so devastating to patients that they should never occur in a health care setting. The Joint Commission considers never events to be sentinel events. An example of a never event is surgery on the wrong body part or death/disability associated with a fall within a facility. Visit www.qualityforum.org/Topics/Safety.aspx for more information.

The Centers for Medicare & Medicaid Services has implemented a new policy related to hospital-acquired conditions (taken from NQF's never event list) that is discussed below. The new trend is that, for ethical and patient safety reasons, hospitals should not receive payment for medical errors that should never have happened. For more information and examples of these events, visit www.cms.hhs.gov/apps/media/press/factsheet.asp?counter=3043.

Medication errors are of primary concern, and interventions to prevent them are being researched and implemented.

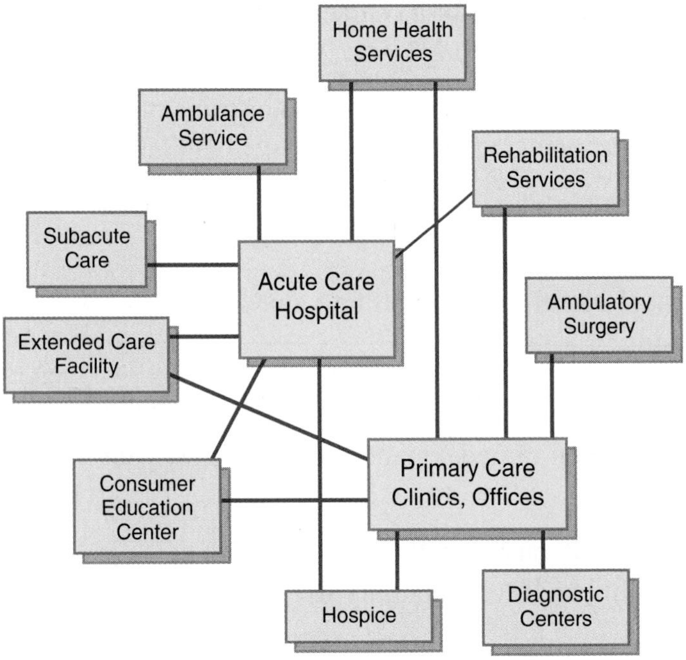
Home Health Services
Ambulance Service
Rehabilitation Services
Subacute Care
Acute Care Hospital
Ambulatory Surgery
Extended Care Facility
Consumer Education Center
Primary Care Clinics, Offices
Hospice
Diagnostic Centers

FIGURE 3.1 An integrated health care system.

Distractions during medication administration may increase errors, so you should stay focused and avoid interruptions during this time. Reducing errors requires everyone to be engaged and vigilant at all times during patient care. Continue to look for new initiatives for safe care.

LEARNING TIP

To learn more about safe health care practices, visit the Institute for Healthcare Improvement website at www.ihi.org/IHI/Programs/IHIOpenSchool.

ECONOMIC ISSUES

The health care system is funded primarily by the government and private insurers. Costs have risen dramatically in recent years. Access to care is not available to everyone and is often linked to availability of resources. Preventive care is not an option for many people. Treatment is often sought in costly emergency room settings after a medical problem has become complex.

Medicare and Diagnosis-Related Groups

Medicare was created in 1965 to provide health insurance as part of the Social Security Act. It is run by the U.S. government and currently covers all people ages 65 and over and people younger than age 65 who have disabilities and are eligible for Social Security. It is funded by a deduction from every person's paycheck that is matched by the government. Several Medicare plan options are offered, including Original Medicare, Medicare Health Plans, Medigap policies, and prescription drug coverage for everyone with Medicare. There are two parts of coverage in the Original Medicare plan. Part A covers inpatient hospital care, skilled nursing facilities, hospice services, and some home care. There is no premium or deductible for Part A. Part B is medical insurance that covers physician costs, outpatient services, some home care, supplies, and other things not covered by Part A. Some preventive services may also be covered. A monthly premium and yearly deductible are paid for Part B coverage. For more information, visit www.medicare.gov.

Congress created the **diagnosis-related group** (DRG) payment system in 1983 for 470 diagnostic categories to help control costs in the Medicare program, which previously had no reimbursement limits. All hospitals were paid the same fee for patients in the same diagnostic category regardless of length of stay and supply costs. The original DRG system has undergone modifications through the years and today several DRG systems are in use that take into consideration all populations, complications, and comorbidities. Hospitals lose money if the patient's costs exceed the DRG payment, but make money if the costs are less than the payment.

Hospital-Acquired Conditions and Present-on-Admission Reporting

On October 1, 2008, the Centers for Medicare & Medicaid Services implemented a change for Medicare Severity DRG payments to acute inpatient prospective payment system hospitals. This policy is called the Hospital-Acquired Conditions (HAC) and Present on Admission (POA) Indicator Reporting. Box 3.1 shows the 10 categories of HACs (also see www.cms.hhs.gov/HospitalAcqCond). At discharge, if certain conditions were not POA, hospitals do not receive additional reimbursement for those conditions. For example, if a patient was admitted with a stroke (primary diagnosis), and then developed a pressure ulcer that was not present on admission (secondary diagnosis) and could have been prevented, the hospital would receive reimbursement only for the primary diagnosis of stroke. The hospital would have to absorb the cost of care for the pressure ulcer.

With this new requirement, nurses must carefully assess and document patient conditions that are POA to show that they did not occur during the hospitalization. Providing safe, quality care and educating patients to prevent complications, such as the need to do leg exercises, turn every 2 hours, or ambulate, are essential to prevent these conditions. Documenting interventions, education provided, and the patient's refusal to participate (when applicable) are essential to help ensure reimbursement for secondary diagnoses.

Medicaid

The Medicaid payment system was also created in 1965 to provide health insurance as part of the Social Security Act for low-income or disabled persons younger than age 65 and their dependent children. Some low-income people older than age 65 may also qualify. Medicaid funding comes from federal, state, and local taxes. Medicaid benefits vary from state to state.

Managed Health Care

Some organizations consist of groups of health care providers who provide health care for a group of people in an effort to contain costs. Health maintenance organizations (HMOs) deliver health care services to individuals who enroll in this type of prepaid group practice health program. The purpose of an HMO is to reduce overlapping services and provide quality and cost-effective care. Healthy patients require fewer services so preventive care is promoted. Preferred provider organizations (PPOs) are networks of providers who offer care to plan members at set discounted rates. PPOs are designed to reduce costs to businesses that insure employees. Hospitals and physicians develop a contract with employers to provide services at a negotiated fee.

LEARNING TIP

To understand what the term *managed care* means, reverse the words: *care management*.

Box 3.1

Categories of Hospital-Acquired Conditions

The Centers for Medicare & Medicaid Services identified the following 10 categories of hospital-acquired conditions as those that increase health care costs or that could have been prevented by using evidence-based guidelines.

Foreign Object Retained After Surgery
Air Embolism
Blood Incompatibility
Stage III and IV Pressure Ulcers
Falls and Trauma
- Fractures
- Dislocations
- Intracranial Injuries
- Crushing Injuries
- Burns
- Electric Shock

Manifestations of Poor Glycemic Control
- Diabetic Ketoacidosis
- Nonketotic Hyperosmolar Coma
- Hypoglycemic Coma
- Secondary Diabetes with Ketoacidosis
- Secondary Diabetes with Hyperosmolarity

Catheter-Associated Urinary Tract Infection (UTI)
Vascular Catheter-Associated Infection
Surgical Site Infection Following:
- Coronary Artery Bypass Graft (CABG)—Mediastinitis
- Bariatric Surgery
  - Laparoscopic Gastric Bypass
  - Gastroenterostomy
  - Laparoscopic Gastric Restrictive Surgery
- Orthopedic Procedures
  - Spine
  - Neck
  - Shoulder
  - Elbow

Deep Vein Thrombosis (DVT)/Pulmonary Embolism (PE)
- Total Knee Replacement
- Hip Replacement

Source: Centers for Medicare & Medicaid. (n.d.). *Hospital-acquired conditions.* Retrieved August 1, 2009, from http://www.cms.hhs.gov/HospitalAcqCond/06_Hospital-Acquired_Conditions.asp.

Managed care has changed the delivery of health care. Hospitalizations have decreased. Lengths of stay are shorter for more acutely ill patients. After discharge, patients need more home care for more complex needs. Case management is being used to oversee and coordinate patient care to ensure that the best patient outcome is achieved while controlling costs.

NURSING AND THE HEALTH CARE TEAM

Nursing is an integral part of the health care network. Nurses work as *licensed practical nurses* (LPNs) or *licensed vocational nurses* (LVNs), *registered nurses* (RNs), or registered nurses with advanced practice skills that include *certified registered nurse practitioners* (CRNPs), *clinical nurse specialists* (CNSs), *certified nurse midwives* (CNMs), and *certified registered nurse anesthetists* (CRNAs). The LPN/LVN provides patient care under the direct supervision of an RN, physician, or dentist. Certified nursing assistants (CNAs) are trained to assist nurses in providing health care.

Nurses work in collaboration with other members of the health care team, such as those listed below, to meet patient health care needs:

Licensed *physicians* provide medical care to patients after graduating from a college of medicine (MD) or osteopathic medicine (DO).

Physician assistants (PA-C [certified]), after graduating from a physician's assistant program, work under the supervision of a physician and perform certain physician duties, such as history taking, physical examinations, and suturing of wounds.

Licensed *pharmacists* complete 5 or 6 years of college and dispense medications from prescriptions, consult with physicians, and provide medication information to patients.

Social workers usually have a master's degree in social work and treat psychosocial problems in patients and their families.

Dietitians provide nutrition information, analyze nutritional needs, and calculate special dietary needs.

Licensed *physical therapists* complete a college physical therapy program and assist patients in reducing physical disability, bodily malfunction, movement dysfunction, and pain through evaluation, education, and treatment.

Physical therapy assistants, whose educational requirements vary, may complete 2 years of education and be licensed and then work under the supervision of a physical therapist.

Occupational therapists complete a bachelor's or master's program, may be registered (OTR), and assist patients in restoring self-care, work, and leisure skills that have been diminished as a result of developmental deficits or injury.

Speech and language pathologists typically complete a master's program. They provide direct clinical services to those with communication or swallowing problems.

Respiratory therapists have a 2-year college degree, may be registered (RRT), and work with patients who have respiratory problems.

Respiratory therapy technicians have 1 year of education, may be certified (CRTT), and work under the supervision of a respiratory therapist to provide respiratory care.

Health unit secretaries manage the clerical work.

Student nurses are enrolled in a nursing program and work under the supervision of nursing faculty in the clinical setting.

LEADERSHIP IN NURSING PRACTICE

A leader seeks to influence, motivate, and enable others to achieve goals. **Leadership** skills are necessary for the LPN/LVN to effectively guide patient care and achieve patient care goals.

Effective leaders in a health care setting must be knowledgeable about management and supervisory processes. They must use critical thinking and be able to make decisions. They should be role models and an inspiration to others. A positive attitude and the use of humor are valuable assets of good leaders. Ultimately, leaders must earn the respect of their coworkers to be successful. To prepare for a leadership role, you should learn and apply the following principles of leadership, supervision, and management.

Leadership Styles

There are three traditional leadership styles: autocratic, democratic, and laissez-faire. A fourth style called coaching has emerged recently in health care settings.

Autocratic Leadership

An autocratic leader has a high degree of control. Almost no control is given to others. In **autocratic leadership**, the leader determines the goals and plans for achieving the goals. Others are instructed on what to do and are not asked to provide input. The group usually achieves high-quality outcomes under this style of leadership. This is an efficient leadership style for emergency situations when decisions must be made quickly, such as when evacuating a building or responding to a code for cardiac arrest.

Democratic Leadership

A democratic leader has a moderate degree of control. Others are given some control and freedom. In **democratic leadership**, participation is encouraged in determining goals and plans for achieving the goals (Fig. 3.2). Decisions are made within the group. The leader assists the group by steering and teaching rather than dominating. The leader shares responsibility with the group. The group usually achieves high-quality outcomes and is more creative under this style of leadership. This is an efficient leadership style for most situations. With this type of leadership, group members are more satisfied and motivated to achieve goals because they are active participants.

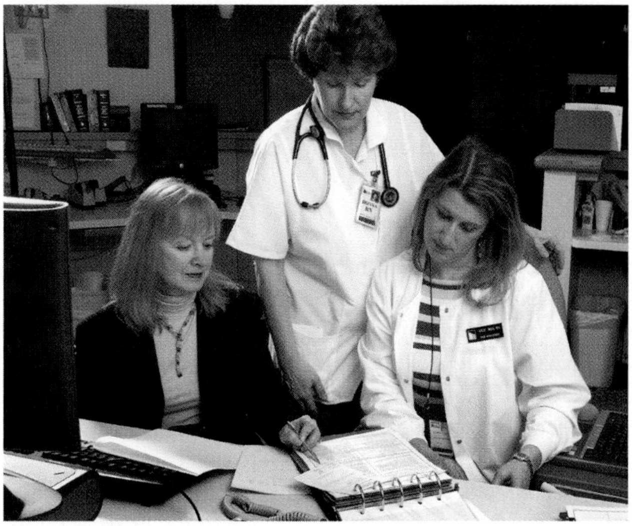

FIGURE 3.2 Group participation in decision making.

Laissez-Faire Leadership

A laissez-faire leader exerts no control over the group. Others are given complete freedom under this leadership style. With **laissez-faire leadership**, no one is responsible for determining goals and plans for achieving the goals. This produces a feeling of chaos. Very little is accomplished under this leadership and the quality of outcomes is often poor.

Coaching Leadership

By emphasizing active listening, clear communication, support, and accountability, coaching leaders work with others to develop problem-solving skills that facilitate critical thinking, prioritization, and effective communication. This leadership style helps direct-care employees feel more empowered, valued, and respected.

Management Functions

The five major components in the management process are planning, organizing, directing, coordinating, and controlling.

Planning

In the first step of the management process, a plan must be developed to ensure that desired patient care outcomes are achieved. To formulate the plan, desired outcomes or problems are identified and data are collected about them. Alternatives or solutions are considered using the collected data and input from others. A decision is then made about the best option or course of action. The leader should ensure that the choice is realistic and can be implemented. Involving others in the planning and decision-making process from beginning to end can increase acceptance at the time of implementation.

Organizing

The purpose of organizing, the second step in the management process, is to provide an orderly environment that promotes cooperation and goal achievement. Providing a framework for goals and the activities that accomplish them is the initial step in organization. Policies and procedures provide this framework as well as guidance for those carrying out tasks designed to accomplish the organization's goals.

Directing

Making assignments is the primary function of directing. One person, usually the nurse in charge or the team leader, makes the assignments for patient care. The nurse practice act in each state defines who can make assignments and delegate care. Communication is important in directing. Assignments must be clearly and specifically stated. The person making assignments must be sure that each assignment is correctly understood and should seek out the receiving person for clarification. Effective directing can be accomplished by providing verbal and written assignment information, making requests rather than giving orders, and giving instructions as needed.

Coordinating

Coordination is the process of looking at a situation to ensure that it is being handled in the most effective way for the organization or coordinating services for a patient. The nurse may assess a particular activity or issues related to patient care assignments. In a long-term care facility, for example, the nurse may want to review skin assessment and care throughout the facility to see if it is being done consistently and uniformly. If a concern is found, problem-solving techniques are used.

Controlling

The final phase of the management process is controlling to evaluate the accomplishment of the organization's goals. Continuous quality improvement is linked with controlling. If the organization's efficiency or ability to reach its goals is impaired, the use of the continuous quality improvement model can facilitate correction of the concern (Fig. 3.3).

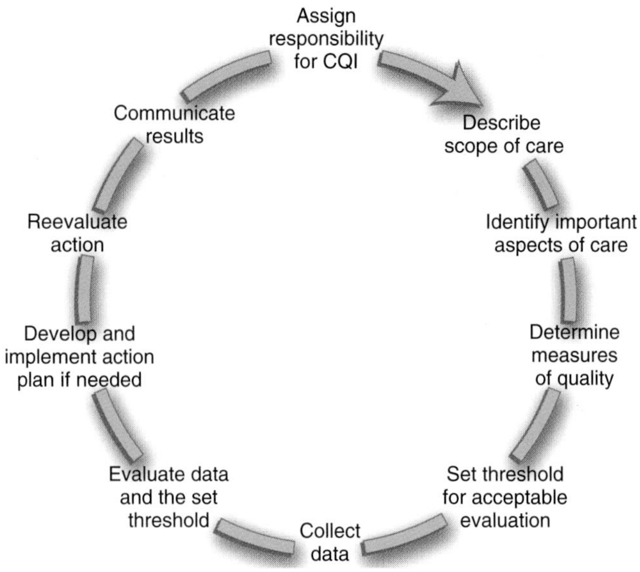
Assign responsibility for CQI
Describe scope of care
Identify important aspects of care
Determine measures of quality
Set threshold for acceptable evaluation
Collect data
Evaluate data and the set threshold
Develop and implement action plan if needed
Reevaluate action
Communicate results

FIGURE 3.3 A continuous quality improvement model.

Leadership and Delegation for the LPN/LVN

LPN/LVNs are leaders and managers of care for the patients to whom they are assigned, under the supervision of an RN, a physician, or a dentist. Beyond this application of a leader and manager role for the LPN/LVN, state nurse practice acts specify if the LPN/LVN can assume other leader or manager roles. Within this dependent role, some aspect of delegation may be allowed.

> **LEARNING TIP**
>
> Review your state's nurse practice act. Does your state allow LPN/LVNs to delegate? If so, to whom and what can be delegated?

Delegation is the act of empowering another person to act. Delegation occurs in a downward manner, meaning RNs delegate to LPN/LVNs and unlicensed assistive personnel (UAP), and LPN/LVNs, in certain circumstances, delegate to LPN/LVNs and UAPs (see below). When delegation occurs, responsibility for care is transferred to the delegatee, but accountability for the care remains with the delegator.

The LPN/LVN might function as a team leader or charge nurse mainly in the long-term care setting, requiring some use of delegation to UAPs. When the LPN/LVN acts as a team leader or charge nurse, an RN delegates the authority to provide supervision and delegation of tasks. Team leaders are responsible for the coordination and delivery of care to each of the patients assigned to the team. They assess the patients assigned to the team to plan appropriate care and contribute to the nursing care plan. Team leaders receive information from team members and communicate patients' needs to appropriate individuals. Since team leaders guide patient care provided by the team, they must be knowledgeable about safety policies, patients' rights, and the accountability of being a team leader.

All patients are entitled to quality care and treatment with dignity and respect. The team leader is accountable for all care provided by the team. Supervision involves initial direction for the task and then monitoring of the task and outcome at intervals. At the end of the team's work shift, team leaders are responsible for transferring patient care to the oncoming team in a way that prevents communication breakdowns that result in patient harm. This handoff communication is accomplished by reporting the patient's condition, status, and needs to the oncoming team leader (Fig. 3.4). Institutional policy specifies whether the RN or LPN/LVN communicates the report.

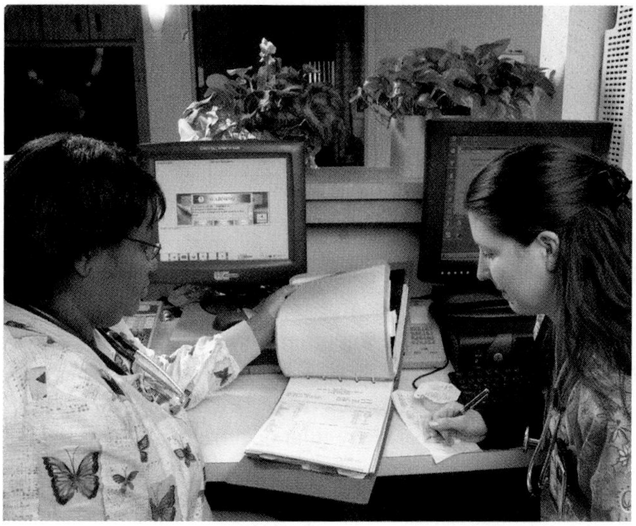

FIGURE 3.4 Communication of the patient's status when transferring the patient's care to another team leader.

Within the leadership role, the LPN/LVN must decide when delegation would most benefit the situation and the patient. All nurses must follow the state practice act and the scope of practice when making any decisions regarding delegation. Consult the charge nurse, team leader, and nurse practice act for your state when deciding if delegation is appropriate. Ultimately, you must ask several important questions to determine when delegation would best benefit the situation. These questions include:

- Does the state practice act allow for delegation in this situation?
- Does the person to whom I am delegating have the knowledge and education to perform this skill, and is it documented for me to make the decisions regarding delegation?
- Would it benefit the patient if I delegated this skill to the support person?

Delegation Process

Delegation is a complex process. In each case, take the following steps, which encompass the decision to delegate, what to delegate, and to whom delegation can be made:

1. Know your state practice act rules for delegation. The LPN/LVN scope of practice usually does not provide legal authority for an LPN/LVN to delegate. However, some state board rules allow LPN/LVNs to delegate tasks that are within the LPN/LVNs scope of practice as long as the RN has given the LPN/LVN authority to delegate the tasks.
2. Identify the skills of the person to whom you may delegate to determine if he or she has the knowledge and ability to carry out the task. When selecting a team member to delegate tasks to, consider if there is potential for harm to the patient during the task, whether it is a complex task that will require problem solving, how predictable the outcome is, and how much interaction with the patient is needed. Match the skills and talents of the team member to the task being delegated. Remember, nursing judgment can never be delegated.
3. Use the National Council of State Boards of Nursing's (1995) five rights of delegation. Following these guidelines provides a framework for your decision-making process and comfort in knowing you used them to make good choices:
   - Right task—is it appropriate to delegate?
   - Right circumstances—is this situation safe and appropriate for delegating?
   - Right person—is this delegatee the appropriate person for the task and this patient's needs?
   - Right communication—is there clear understanding between you and the delegatee for terms used, communication, and reporting needs?
   - Right supervision—is it defined how and when direct supervision will occur?

Delegation requires trust. You should be comfortable with which tasks can be delegated and the team member to whom you are delegating the tasks. Also, it is important to know and understand each other's methods of communicating so that miscommunications do not occur.

When you first begin your career, the process of delegating may seem difficult. As with any skill, it takes practice to feel confident in carrying out the process.

CAREER OPPORTUNITIES FOR LPN/LVNS

Because of the health care needs of the increasing elderly population and an increased need overall for health care services, the need for LPN/LVNs is expected to grow 14% between 2006 and 2016, which is faster than the average for other occupations (Bureau of Labor Statistics, n.d.). LPN/LVNs work in long-term care, physician offices, clinics, schools, child day care centers, hospitals, home care, and public administration. Employment of LPN/LVNs is declining in hospitals, but it is growing in settings outside of hospitals.

Travel nursing is one of the fastest growing areas in the health care delivery system. It is an exciting way to see the world while working. Private companies and the federal government offer travel nursing opportunities.

LPN/LVNs may seek additional education. Many schools provide for an accelerated educational tract for LPN/LVNs seeking to become RNs with either an associate degree or a bachelor's degree. Advanced educational opportunities include a master's degree in nursing or a doctoral degree. Check with colleges/universities to see which program would best meet your needs for continuing your education.

The LPN/LVN of today must be equipped with knowledge and skills to function successfully in a health care delivery system. An understanding of leadership, delegation, and career opportunities will provide a basis to begin your journey in practicing as a LPN/LVN. We wish you well on your journey!

ETHICS AND VALUES

Ethics is a code of values which guide our choices and actions and determine the purpose and course of our lives.

AYN RAND, RUSSIAN-AMERICAN NOVELIST AND PHILOSOPHER (1905–1982)

The study and practice of ethics is grounded in philosophy and dates back to the time of Hippocrates. **Ethics** is the practice of applying moral philosophy in order to conclude what should be done in a given situation. This practice is influenced by factors that are both philosophical and social (Burkhardt & Nathaniel, 2008). Bioethics is a branch of ethics that studies moral values in the biomedical sciences and has come to be most closely associated with health care.

Although ethics is concerned with "good" and "bad," this is only a small part of any ethical equation. Many considerations must be examined when confronted with an ethical dilemma. Morals or **morality** are also related to ethics. Some use the terms *ethics* and *morals* interchangeably; however, *morals* refers more specifically to our personal values, the standards set by our own conscience, and our personal choices of what we consider good and bad, right and wrong.

Values are unwritten standards, ideals, or concepts that give meaning to a person's life. Values are commonly derived from societal norms, religion, and family traditions. They serve as a guide for making decisions and setting priorities in daily life. Value systems can change when people experience life-changing events. Value conflicts often occur in everyday life, and people make decisions based on their values. For example, a nurse who values both her career and her family may be forced to decide between going to work or staying home with a sick child.

Values exist on many levels. Individuals have personal values that govern their lives and actions. Many groups and organizations have values that represent the group as a whole, but may or may not be identical to personal values. When a person becomes a member of a group or organization, he or she agrees to accept the values of the group. Examples of groups include clubs, churches and other religious organizations, political parties, and professions. Society as a whole has values. As a member of a society or country, an individual accepts the values of that culture. Finally, societal values may change with the adoption of new laws. The values of a profession are usually outlined in a **code of ethics**. This code is a comprehensive set of guidelines that outlines the behavioral expectations for the profession.

Ethical issues surround us throughout our entire lifetime. Bioethical issues are particularly prevalent in our professional lives for several reasons. To begin with, advances in technology and treatment regimes offer more complicated options for treating diseases and conditions. Often, these options promise to prolong life. Thus, questions arise related to medical futility: Should a patient receive a treatment because it is available or because it will be effective? How many health care resources should be used for the treatment of terminal illnesses? Does quantity or length of life matter more than quality of life? In addition, many of these advances come at a substantial cost. In turn, financial resources are limited. Therefore, it becomes both difficult and important to decide how and when these resources will be allocated.

Not all bioethical issues make headline news. In fact, many ethical dilemmas are regular occurrences in the clinical setting. Nurses are involved in decision making every day based on the traditional ethical principles of autonomy, beneficence, maleficence, and justice. Consider these examples: You might promise to return to a patient and assess whether or not his pain medication was effective. Patients might share information that they want to remain confidential. A family agrees to a "do not resuscitate" (DNR) order for their loved one when they believe there is no hope for recovery. A young man in the prime of life is given cardiopulmonary resuscitation (CPR) when he suddenly goes into respiratory failure on the day of his proposed discharge. Each of these examples has the potential to present an ethical dilemma if the circumstances were different. For example, a family may not agree to a DNR order if some family members believe there is hope for recovery. Then the questions must be asked, What should be done? Whose wishes should be honored? Does the patient have the capacity to make an informed decision?

An ethical dilemma is created when:

- The required moral action is not clear.
- Persons in the situation do not agree on the proposed solution.
- Neither of the available choices seems to offer a "best" option.

Decision making in the acute care setting is a complex process involving many members of the health care team. As a result of carrying out orders, nurses must handle consequences that arise from clinical problems. In addition, there is no one-size-fits-all solution for ethical problems. Even if dilemmas share a common thread, each has individual influences that make it unique.

Potential solutions may appear to be equally good or, worse, equally risky: A promise cannot be kept; information cannot remain confidential; DNR orders may not be acceptable for some people. Not all patients should receive CPR, even those who are very young. When patients are conscious, their choices are usually respected, but on occasion even that premise can be difficult to apply. Often, groups of individuals must work together to resolve a conflict if there is disagreement between physicians and families, nurses and physicians, or among family members. Nurses may experience moral distress as a result of being an integral part of this team (see *Evidence-Based Practice*). Moral distress can be defined as distress experienced by those who carry out actions they believe are wrong or those who are unable to carry out actions they believe are right (McCarthy & Deady, 2008). In response to increasing ethical and moral conflicts in the clinical setting, many hospitals and facilities have created an ethics committee that helps address especially difficult cases. The multidisciplinary committee may include physicians, nurses, therapists, social workers, and an ethicist.

EVIDENCE-BASED PRACTICE

Clinical Question

How does moral distress affect nurses and patient care?

Evidence

In a study of 1,215 nurses and social workers, moral distress contributed to feelings of powerlessness (32.5%), overwhelm (34.7%), frustration (52.8%), and fatigue (40%) (Ulrich et al., 2007). However, a positive ethical climate with adequate resources for support decreased the chance of this sample leaving their job.

In a study of 100 registered nurses, morally distressing events reported according to distress and frequency included unsafe staffing levels, implementing patient care based on family wishes when they were in conflict with personal feelings, continuing life support despite poor patient prognosis, and carrying out orders for unnecessary tests and treatments (Zuzelo, 2007). Nurses in this study requested more formal ethics training as well as ethics rounds.

A grounded theory study supports the need for inclusion of ethics in nursing education (Nathaniel, 2006). In addition, Nathaniel developed the theory of moral reckoning, which provides a more in-depth explanation of moral distress in nursing practice.

Implications for Nursing Practice

Moral distress is present in clinical practice and has a direct impact on job satisfaction. Supportive resources for ethical issues can help prevent nurses from resigning. If more nurses leave clinical practice, an increase in fiscal resources will be needed to replace and train those who have left.

REFERENCES

Nathaniel, A. K. (2006). Moral reckoning in nursing. *Western Journal of Nursing Research, 28*, 419–428.

Ulrich, C., O'Donnell, P., Taylor, C., et al. (2007). Ethical climate, ethical stress, and job satisfaction of nurses and social workers in the United States. *Social Science & Medicine, 65*, 1708–1719.

Zuzelo, P. R. (2007). Exploring the moral distress of registered nurses. *Nursing Ethics, 14*(3), 344–359.

A basic mastery of several elements enhances your ability to perform competently when bioethical issues arise and decision making is the focus. Understanding the ethical component of your nursing role is a first step. Discovering how your personal value set influences your nursing practice is another. Acquiring knowledge about relevant ethical material is also essential. An ethical decision-making process is a useful tool for examining ethical dilemmas. Together these elements provide a foundation from which you can begin to explore the meaning of bioethics in nursing practice today. For more information about bioethics, visit The Center for Bioethics and Human Dignity at www.cbhd.org.

Ethical Obligations and Nursing

As a nurse, you are an invaluable member of the health care team, contributing to patient care according to your educational preparation and assigned responsibilities. The nurse is guided by the law and the standards set forth by the profession. A professional code of ethics provides a framework. In addition to practicing within the law, nurses have ethical obligations related to the law. First, if the law is considered unethical or has serious limitations, a basic moral obligation of the nurse is to make an effort to change that law. This may be done as an individual, but it is more commonly achieved through political activism guided by professional organizations. Becoming involved in a professional organization is one way to change the laws that govern health care and nursing.

Nursing Code of Ethics

Some of the major ethical obligations of nursing practice are addressed in the nursing code of ethics. As a professional guide for ethical practice, the National Association for Practical Nurse Education and Service (NAPNES) developed a code of ethics for the LPN/LVN. Like all codes of ethics, this code is an important document because it is a public statement of the basic ethical principles and standards for LPN/LVNs. An organization's code of ethics should be supported by the majority of its members. The code should provide guidance for appropriate decision making based on current laws and professional standards. A code of ethics not only provides a base for professional self-evaluation and reflection, but also acts as a tool by which the public can hold the profession accountable.

A code does not dictate a particular action, nor is it a legal document, although the code should not be in conflict with the law. The code is not enforced by any organization, and no punishment exists if a nurse fails to adhere to it. A code must be interpreted because it usually contains broad statements, but it does serve as a general guideline for professional ethical issues. Ethical codes are updated to reflect current practice, responsibilities, and obligations set forth by the profession.

Virtues

Ethics based on virtues relies on the innate and acquired character traits of each individual. Virtues are character traits most often associated with one's values and morality or conscience and are different from the skills that we acquire as nurses. Skills are used to implement various actions, something we do, whereas virtues define who we are. Beauchamp and Childress (2008) outline four focal virtues that underpin a virtuous person: compassion, discernment, trustworthiness, and integrity. Although we may strive to act as virtuous people, we are human and may not always succeed. A code of ethics acts as a constant reminder of that high standard we should always strive to maintain.

FIDELITY (ALSO A PRINCIPLE). Fidelity is the obligation to be faithful to commitments made to self and others. In health care, fidelity includes faithfulness or loyalty to agreements and responsibilities accepted as part of the practice of nursing. It also means not promising a patient something that one cannot deliver or cannot control (for example, a patient asks not to be resuscitated if she has a cardiac arrest, but the physician has not been consulted). Fidelity is the main support for the concept of accountability, although conflicts in fidelity might arise because of obligations owed to different individuals or groups. For example, nurses have an obligation of fidelity to the patients they care for to provide the highest quality care possible, as well as an obligation of fidelity to their employing institution to follow its rules and policies. Nurses can have an ethical dilemma when a hospital's policy on staffing creates a situation that does not allow nurses to provide the quality of care they feel is needed.

Maintaining a patient's privacy and **confidentiality** is related to fidelity (Fig. 3.5). Privacy and confidentiality may or may not be explicit promises. Nurses are obligated to only discuss the patient under circumstances in which it is necessary to deliver high-quality holistic health care, such as:

- When given specific instructions to do so by the patient
- When there is the grave possibility of harm to either the patient or others
- When legally mandated to do so.

Maintaining confidentiality also applies to the necessary communication of information through the posting of unit censuses and various schedules for tests, procedures, or special examinations (operating room, physical therapy, radiology), storage and access of patient information in computers, and the transmission of patient information via fax machines. Many people other than direct caregivers have legitimate access to a patient's chart: faculty members in the course of making student assignments, accrediting agencies, risk managers, quality assurance personnel, insurance companies, and researchers. Each is obligated to maintain patient confidentiality to the extent that concealing information:

- Does not compromise mandated reports (communicable diseases or gunshot wounds).
- Considers various releases already granted by the patient (such as when insurance coverage was obtained).
- Ensures gathering data in the aggregate without identifying specific patients (research or institutional statistics).

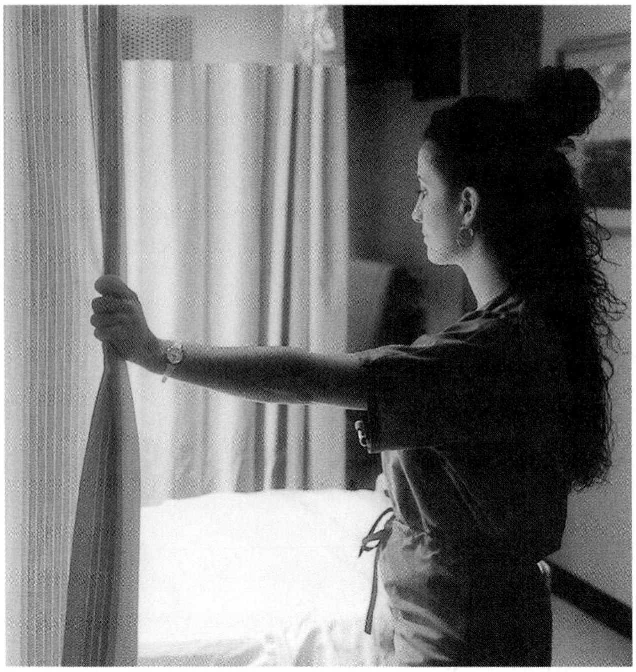

FIGURE 3.5 Maintaining privacy is a patient right and conveys caring to the patient.

Other forms of necessary communication include regular shift changes and case conferences. Care must be taken to hold these information-sharing events in settings where the discussion remains private.

VERACITY. Veracity is the virtue of truthfulness. Within health care, it requires health care providers, whenever possible, to tell the truth and not intentionally deceive or mislead patients. As with other rights and obligations, there are limitations to this virtue. The primary limitation occurs when telling patients the truth would seriously harm their ability to recover, or when the truth may produce greater illness (this can be considered under the principle of **nonmaleficence** or doing no harm, which finds its origins in the Hippocratic oath).

Another difficult situation may be created in relation to diagnostic information. Although giving diagnostic information is the responsibility of the physician or RN, LPN/LVNs sometimes find themselves caught in situations in which they must deal with patients' questions. If LPN/LVNs feel uncomfortable about reinforcing physician or RN explanations, they may avoid answering patients' questions directly. However, patients do have a right to know this information. The LPN should inform the physician or RN of the patient's request for information, and agency policy on patient information sharing should be followed.

INTEGRITY. Integrity is a holistic, unwavering moral sense of self. Each person has a cluster of values, beliefs, and

• WORD • BUILDING •

nonmaleficence: non—not + maleficentia—evil doing

traditions that forms the basis for moral decision making; in a sense, it is the conscience. This sense of self can be compromised when the nurse is requested to act in a manner that requires setting aside or acting against personal values, beliefs, or traditions. The nurse who believes in the sanctity of life and that human life begins at conception may not be able to maintain integrity if required to participate in abortion procedures. However, this nurse also has the responsibility not to accept a professional position where abortion is an issue, because a nurse cannot abandon a patient in need of nursing services. The nurse with integrity is faithful to professional responsibilities and obligations.

COMPASSION. Compassion or caring is a central virtue in nursing. Some label this **empathy** and connect it to the ability of a nurse to identify with a patient's suffering, pain, or disability. The difference between the two virtues, however, is that in compassion, the nurse wishes to alleviate discomfort. Patients are comforted by the compassionate nurse, and such nurturing can assist in the healing process. A nurse without any emotion robs patients of the full potential for healing that is only possible when all parties are actively engaged in all aspects of the relationship. Compassion should not be so dominant that it clouds judgment and prevents effective and efficient provision of nursing services. Compassion, in order to be effective, needs to be tempered with rationality.

DISCERNMENT. Discernment has been described as practical wisdom or common sense. This is the ability to understand, to have insight into the hidden as well as the obvious elements of a situation. A nurse who has a discerning approach is one who is sensitive to the patient's actions and responses and does not necessarily accept what is seen at face value. Verbal, nonverbal, and subconscious communication, as well as concrete signs and symptoms, all contribute to the overall evaluation of the patient by the discerning nurse. This is sometimes translated as practical wisdom because this type of nurse has a depth of understanding of patients that leads to the selection of the appropriate action, which in turn is implemented in a caring manner. It can be argued that possessing a discerning nature is a product of experience and knowledge, because in nursing it is not enough to act on gut instinct; a nurse must base opinion and action on accepted approaches.

TRUSTWORTHINESS. It is vital that as health care workers we inspire confidence in the patients we care for. We need to be considered trustworthy in order to have a true partnership with our patients. Sometimes, certain nurses may be preferred by patients because they convey a sense of confidence when providing care, and when one considers that in many situations, patients' lives are truly in the nurse's hands, this preference is well grounded.

When a patient feels that a nurse is worthy of trust, an ease develops within the relationship that decreases the stress and anxiety that diagnoses and treatment plans often create. As a result, the patient develops more effective coping mechanisms. Indeed, studies have shown that the erosion of trust is cited as a major factor in the escalating lawsuits that have been initiated against health professionals.

RESPECTFULNESS. A nurse who practices respectfulness displays an attitude toward the patient that conveys value for the patient and the patient's feelings. All patients should be treated with dignity and their autonomy acknowledged. Nurses are obligated to make an effort to identify their own biases and prejudices and work to avoid stereotyping and "isms" in patient relationships (e.g., classism, sexism, racism, ageism, and ethnocentrism). They should also eliminate discrimination based on religion, sexual orientation, or disability. Attentiveness to bias and discrimination is not limited to private interactions; nurses are also responsible for drawing attention to unacceptable statements or negative actions that reflect disrespect for race, religion, gender, class, age, culture, sexual orientation, or disability in any health care situation.

Rights

Rights represent ways to think about what we are owed or what we deserve. Harris (2001) puts forward the position that if all people are considered valuable and equal, then it follows that there are rights possessed by people by virtue of their humanity. These basic rights could be translated into goods and services (such as the right to clean water, the right to food). They are viewed positively and because something needs to be provided, there is a responsibility for someone to furnish these items. Second, other rights can be determined to protect us (e.g., right to privacy, right to self-determination). These are negative rights in that they are aimed at preventing some action that would intrude on our lives or prevent us from acting as we choose.

Laws guarantee some rights, whereas other rights are moral rights, which means they are based on values and ethical principles but are not enforceable by law. "Basic human rights" is a common phrase that we hear when discussing the condition of various people around the world, especially when those rights are compromised. A United Nations document titled *The Universal Declaration of Human Rights* serves to represent what all people should be provided with or protected from (see www.un.org/en/documents/udhr).

In health care, the topic of patient rights is ever present. The American Hospital Association's (AHA's) bill of rights recognizes what patients are entitled to but may not always receive. This bill of rights, *The Patient Care Partnership: Understanding Expectations, Rights and Responsibilities,* includes statements on confidentiality, informed consent, and the right to refuse treatment (AHA, 2009). The 2009 version is available as an easy-to-understand brochure in eight languages at www.aha.org/aha/issues/Communicating-With-Patients/pt-care-partnership.html. Many health care organizations use the AHA's patient bill of rights along with a more specific bill of rights, such as those developed by nursing homes and veterans' hospitals.

In bioethics many issues can be framed within a rights context. Whether people have a right to health care is a frequently debated topic. Such a right is discussed at every level of society, from local governments, which determine services they will provide in city clinics and public schools, to the federal government, which enacted a health care reform bill in 2010. Another prominent dispute is the right to die with dignity, which is arousing more interest as the largest population cohort (the baby boomers) edges toward the later decades of life. The loss of autonomy coupled with the growing number of treatment options further confounds this "right." By contrast, the right to life is another central concept in our society as groups organize politically to prevent abortions and overturn the *Roe v. Wade* decision of the Supreme Court (available at http://tourolaw.edu/patch/roe/#rop). This right also extends to discussions of reproductive rights and the health care of pregnant women. These are but a few examples of rights issues and potential conflicts. Others can be identified as various areas in medical-surgical nursing are explored.

Building Blocks of Ethics

The discipline of ethics, especially health care ethics, provides us with useful tools and knowledge that can assist us when we encounter difficult situations. An understanding of basic concepts, presented here in the form of ethical principles and ethical theories, helps specifically target the ethical components of the problem. Principles and theories offer frameworks for ethical problem solving. However, knowledge about ethics cannot in itself provide all of the answers to a problem or dilemma. What such knowledge does do is assist us in focusing on the ethical aspects of each case. When we apply appropriate ethical rationales to our problem solving, we become grounded in this analytical framework. Such frameworks have the ability to make us look at many facets of an ethical problem, and presenting a particular position relative to a situation or describing values, beliefs, and traditions using these common ethical terms helps clarify discussions and possibly prevents escalating arguments. When one becomes familiar with health care ethics, problems with communication, management of the unit, and legislation or the law can more easily be separated from the ethical dimension and resolved in their own problem-solving session.

Ethical Principles

Ethical **principles** derive from moral theory and have two purposes. The first is to provide some framework for society's moral conduct. The second is to help us take consistent positions and approaches to moral dilemmas. Ethical principles can be found in many professional codes of conduct and are key components of ethical decision making. The ethical principles widely used when examining bioethical and health care dilemmas include autonomy, beneficence, nonmaleficence, and justice. Given these ethical principles' prominence in the bioethical literature, a basic understanding of them is necessary.

AUTONOMY. According to ethicists (and behaviorists, social scientists, and psychologists), what makes human beings different from nonhumans is that people have dignity based on their ability to choose freely what they will do with their lives. **Autonomy** is the right of self-determination, independence, and freedom founded on the notion that humans have value, worth, and moral dignity. Autonomy in health care applies to all people capable of and competent in making health care decisions for themselves. Health care providers do not need to agree with another person's decisions, but we must respect the autonomy of the person making the choice. Preventing patients from making autonomous decisions or deciding for patients without regard for their preferences is **paternalism**. Autonomy also encompasses the professional's self-determination and freedom.

Autonomy, as with most rights, is not an absolute right, and under certain conditions, limitations can be imposed. Typically, these limitations arise when a person's autonomy interferes with the rights, health, or well-being of others. For example, patients generally have an autonomous right to make decisions regarding their care and level of independence. This autonomous right is guaranteed by federal legislation known as the Patient Self-Determination Act, which can be found at https://www.abanet.org/publiced/practical/patient_self_determination_act.html. However, if a person is no longer capable of self-care upon discharge, a request to live independently will not be granted. A person unable to care for himself cannot live alone at the expense of his health and well-being. The principle of beneficence (see next section), in this case, outweighs the principle of autonomy (Fry & Veatch, 2006).

BENEFICENCE. The beneficence principle proposes that one must take a positive action that does good for another and act in a way that will prevent harm to others. Within health care, **beneficence** is the principle of considering and offering treatments and care options that are likely to provide benefit to the patient (Fry & Veatch, 2006). The provision of good care not only means the provision of technologically competent care, but also care that respects the patient's beliefs, feelings, and wishes, as well as those of their family and significant others. A common problem encountered when applying the principle of beneficence is deciding what is good for another and who is the best person to make this decision.

NONMALEFICENCE. Nonmaleficence, one of the oldest obligations in health care, dating back to the Hippocratic oath (400 B.C.), is related to beneficence and in a sense it is the opposite side of the coin because it is difficult to speak of one concept without mentioning the other. According to Burkhardt and Nathaniel (2008), nonmaleficence

> *. . . requires us to act in such a manner as to avoid causing harm to patients. Included in this principle are deliberate harm, risk of harm, and harm that occurs during the performance of beneficial acts.*

• WORD • BUILDING •
autonomy: auto—self + nimos—rule
beneficence: bene—good + facere—to do

Health care providers are required to do no harm to their patients either *intentionally* or *unintentionally.* In current health care practice, the principle of nonmaleficence may be intentionally violated in order to produce a greater good in the patient's long-term treatment. For example, a patient may undergo a painful and debilitating or disfiguring surgery to remove a cancerous growth, thereby avoiding death and prolonging life.

By extension, the principle of nonmaleficence also requires a nurse to protect from harm those who are considered vulnerable. Vulnerable groups include children, the elderly, and those who are mentally incompetent, unconscious, or too weak or debilitated to protect themselves.

JUSTICE. **Justice** is based on the principles of fairness and equality. Concerns for justice may focus on how we treat individuals and groups in society (psychologically, socially, legally, politically). How we distribute material resources such as health care (**distributive justice**) and burdens (taxes) equitably, and the appropriate compensation to those who have been harmed. When a patient makes an appointment for 9 a.m. at an outpatient clinic, the patient expects to be seen by the primary care provider at the designated time unless an emergency occurs. Unequal treatment would result if a walk-in who has no pressing problem is seen by the provider in place of the 9 a.m. appointment, forcing subsequent appointments to be delayed. Distribution of material resources can be complex because it involves not only benefits (what we receive), but also burdens (what we may be taxed for but then do not receive). Burdens are not just monetary, but also include such factors as the unequal participation of individuals in medical research and the sacrifices family members make when caring for individuals with disabilities in the home.

USE OF PRINCIPLES. One of the most serious limitations of these principles is the lack of any built-in priority when applying them to an ethical dilemma. Autonomy is not automatically prioritized over justice or beneficence over nonmaleficence. However, these principles are helpful in categorizing various preferences and positions when examining a dilemma to clarify positions within it. Working with principles moves the discussion to a focus on ethics rather than a particular personal viewpoint or feeling. Such a strategy can also avoid a power struggle between those who simply want to win the argument.

Here is an example of an ethical dilemma. A nurse attempts to support a patient's refusal of surgery, while the physician claims that the patient must have surgery or she will lose her leg. When you shift your thinking to realizing that the nurse is arguing the case from the perspective of the patient's autonomy (self-determination) and the physician's actions are motivated by beneficence (to act in a way that benefits the patient), the discussion becomes one based on conflicting principles rather than conflict between individuals. Consequently, the discussion can focus on autonomy and beneficence and their respective rationales. This strategy does not resolve the dilemma but makes it less personal and forces participants to develop sound, ethical rationales for their solutions.

Ethical Theories

Ethical theories are concepts that are more complete than principles for analyzing ethical dilemmas. Theories are used to explain variables, guide inquiry, and provide a foundation with which to conduct decision making. We provide only a brief description of ethical theories here; a more in-depth understanding can be obtained from other resources, such as Web links, journals, and many books on ethics.

Two of the major theories used in bioethics—utilitarianism and deontology—are defined and explained next. Other theoretical approaches to ethical decision making exist, and theories are often combined to address ethical dilemmas. This section also explores the relationship of theology or religion to bioethics.

UTILITARIANISM. **Utilitarian** theory is grounded in the premise that actions are judged right or wrong based purely on their consequences and, therefore, outcomes are the most important elements to consider when making decisions. Right actions are morally preferred if they produce more happiness or greater benefits than unhappiness or burdens, and in utilitarianism, each person's happiness is equally important. This approach may be used by institutions and organizations under the guise of cost-benefit ratios. A hospital responsible for the care for hundreds of patients is not as concerned with the individual patient who unfortunately is caught in the bureaucracy of its functioning. This is not to say that all institutions operate on this theory at all times, but in general, rules, policies, and procedures are developed with the majority in mind.

There are several major criticisms of the utilitarian theory. One is that an individual is often sacrificed for the good of the majority (often seen in wartime). The second is that it can be difficult to predict outcomes, especially when human nature is involved.

DEONTOLOGY. **Deontology** is a philosophical theory requiring human actions and attitudes to be based on duty, and the moral worth of an action (the result) should not be judged only in terms of its consequences. For example, health professionals might operate by a rule that indicates that a moral person never lies. No matter how much the truth might hurt, the truth is revealed. Another rule might be to never use people as a means to an end. Translated this means that regardless of the benefits, individuals cannot be forced to participate in medical research studies to benefit others. An individual's right to voluntarily participate in research must be respected. Research does not have to benefit the individual participant as long as this is understood by the individual. However, the individual cannot be used simply to meet the investigator's needs. Acting morally only because one has a duty to do so, without any consideration of the outcome, is a serious limitation of this theory.

THEOLOGICAL PERSPECTIVES. Theological perspectives include the many religious traditions represented in our culture. Religious teachings are key concepts for ethical decision making for some people. In fact, many consider these teachings a divine source of values and morals. Jehovah's Witnesses' rejection of blood transfusions is a common example of how religious beliefs affect health care decision making. This religious group has collected a large amount of information about blood substitutes and alternative therapies. Leaders of Jehovah's Witnesses are prepared to provide education for health professionals about their beliefs and acceptable interventions.

In another area, a number of religious traditions oppose abortion, which affects both health professionals and patients. Euthanasia is another issue addressed by numerous organized religious groups, which in turn can affect how patients make decisions regarding end-of-life issues. One of the difficulties with religious traditions is that it is not simply the official church teaching that is involved, but the individual member's interpretation of that teaching. Assessment of the importance of this dimension of the patient's life is important in the ethical analysis.

Ethical Decision Making

A variety of models and frameworks are available for ethical decision making. The steps listed in this section are a combination of several ideas that have been suggested. In its simplest form, ethical decision making is an informed logical problem-solving process. Similar to the nursing process, as discussed in the first chapter, the steps described in this section take the user through a set of strategies that assist in approaching a problem in an organized and systematic manner. Nurses applying the steps of the nursing process use critical thinking skills in order to be as logical and objective as possible. Ethical decision making is a similar process. The goal is to have a balanced perspective that respects emotions but does not let them overshadow the process or the outcome.

Addressing ethical dilemmas is not a simple or easy process. However, the final decision may be more acceptable if the nurse feels the situation was thoroughly examined and all viable options weighed before the decision was made. To illustrate the process, a sample case will be examined using each step.

The case: Consider a dilemma that involves informing someone regarding health information following an automobile accident. Suppose the Smith family was in an automobile accident out of state. The family was on their way home from vacation. Mrs. Smith is in critical condition, Mr. Smith was pronounced dead in the emergency department, and their 12-year-old daughter, Melissa, is in critical condition. Mrs. Smith is still able to speak and asks you, the nurse, how her husband and daughter are doing. What should you do?

Step 1: Identify the Ethical Dilemma

The initial step is to identify the ethical dilemma. What makes it a true dilemma? Separating the ethical and non-ethical aspects facilitates the decision-making process. A conflict can arise because of gaps in communication rather than a conflict of ethical principles. Ethical dilemmas are different from clinical problems that have clear interventions and rationale.

Our sample case is an ethical dilemma because there is no obvious right answer. Do you tell the mother that her spouse is dead and her child is critically injured?

Step 2: Identify the Stakeholders and Their Values

The values, beliefs, and traditions of all participants are important because they will all influence the decision-making process. The patient is at the center of the process. Therefore, the patient's autonomy is important to the steps of the process. An advance directive or a living will can often help guide the decision-making process when the patient no longer has autonomy (the ability to express his or her own wishes). Even if there is a pre-existing advance directive, it may not match the wishes of the family for clinical decision making.

In our sample case, who are the stakeholders? Obviously, family members are all stakeholders, as well as the health care team of nurses, physicians, surgeons, therapists, and others. To answer the initial question, the mother is the patient and at the center of the process. We will keep in mind that the daughter is also a patient, but her role in this situation is not the ethical dilemma. So, what is the autonomy of our patient? At the present time, the patient is not fully autonomous because she suffered head trauma.

Step 3: Gather and Verify the Information

All facets of the dilemma need to be examined. Besides knowing who is involved, the context of the problem must be fully explored. How did the situation arise? Is there objective data to support various parts of the decision-making process? For example, determining competency can be an involved and frustrating process, especially when there are competing parties involved (such as a family disagreement about the competency of a parent). However, objective data such as a mental evaluation can support this fact and ease family disagreements. Both the medical record and health care professionals caring for the patient can provide clinically relevant data. In addition, health care records from previous hospitalizations and from other institutions may also be needed. The law, facility policies and procedures, and available resources also impact the overall context of the problem. Therefore, it is necessary to be comprehensive in examining all of these areas.

In our sample case, what do we know? The objective data tells us the following: (1) The spouse is dead; (2) the daughter, who is 12 years old, is in critical condition; (3) the family is from out of state; and (4) on assessment, we find that the mother experienced head trauma and although she is asking about her spouse and daughter, her vital signs are unstable and her condition is also critical. So, in considering the objective information, we must also gather more information. What comes to mind? Does Mrs. Smith or her daughter have any significant health history or take medications that the health care team should know about? What are the policies regarding contacting family in such an emergency? What resources or departments need to be called to assist in this case?

Step 4: Examine Possible Actions and the Consequences of Each Action

Bringing perspective to an ethical dilemma requires the development of a comprehensive set of all possible actions. In turn, each of the proposed actions should have identified consequences, both positive and negative. This makes the process more transparent and allows anyone to analyze each action by weighing the risks and benefits of implementing that action.

In our sample case, what are all of the possible actions or alternatives to resolve the dilemma? If you consider the extremes, the choices appear clear: You either tell Mrs. Smith about her husband and child or you do not. If you tell Mrs. Smith that her husband is dead and her child is in critical condition, what are the positive and negative consequences of this action? Conversely, if you do not tell Mrs. Smith about her spouse and child, what are the consequences, both positive and negative? These are considered the extremes in the case, but there are other options. For example, we could calm Mrs. Smith by saying that her husband and daughter are both still being evaluated or we could call a chaplain to assist the staff in telling her the truth. Even if partial truths seem unacceptable at first glance, they ought to be added to the list of possible actions. There are times when being completely truthful would violate the principle of beneficence (Fry & Veatch, 2006). So, as you can see, each proposed action should have corresponding consequences that allow those involved to ultimately choose the best action to be implemented. Can you think of any more actions appropriate for this scenario? What are the consequences for these actions?

Step 5: Determine the Ethical Foundation for Each Action

Each action should be based on ethical values, principles, or theories. In addition, the code of ethics can lend support as an ethical rationale. One strategy that is proposed for an incompetent or unconscious patient is the **standard of best interest**. This standard involves determination of the best outcome for the patient, given the information known about the patient and the context of the situation. Typically, family members together with health care providers make this determination. Ideally, the decision is made in an objective manner, setting aside any special interests of the family or health professionals.

In our sample case, if we revisit the actions proposed in the previous section, we can see that telling the truth supports veracity, but may also violate the principle of beneficence, while also supporting maleficence. In contrast, by not telling the truth, we violate the principle of veracity, but uphold beneficence. Lastly, if we entertain the idea of only telling part of the truth, once again we are violating veracity, but the difference is that we are striving to meet the principle of beneficence. We realize that by telling the whole truth, Mrs. Smith's condition may worsen from the stress of the situation.

Step 6: Determine the Best Action with the Strongest Ethical Support

Each action is judged based on its risks, benefits, and supporting rationale. The actions are then ranked in priority order. Strong ethical support for the first priority is required, as well as a reasonable potential for the action to be implemented.

In our sample case, what do you think is the best outcome? Everyone needs to examine the actions and their respective consequences, supporting ethical principles before making a final decision.

Utilitarians and deontologists may disagree about the important principles in decision making. However, it should not be assumed that different theoretical positions cannot reach a mutually agreeable decision. Although their rationale for the decision may differ, the final solution each proposes may be identical.

Step 7: Implement the Action

Needless to say, the selected action needs to be implemented in a logical way. Responsibilities for carrying out the plan can be assigned, especially if there are multiple steps in the process. In addition, a well-implemented plan can ensure that the plan is fully operationalized and also increases the potential for success.

In our sample case, each person must implement a plan based on the stakeholders, the chosen action, and the underlying ethical principles. How would you implement your action? What resources would you need? Which members of the health care team would you work with?

Step 8: Evaluate the Outcome

The evaluative process is most effective when the details of the care are still fresh. The resolution of an ethical dilemma, whether it has been successful or not, provides us with knowledge and experience to address the next ethical dilemma. Although each dilemma is unique in many ways, similarities between cases may provide insight into the best way to approach the decision-making process when a comparable case arises.

In our sample case, the outcome can be evaluated only after an action is implemented.

CRITICAL THINKING

Ethical Decisions

1. Identify a health care–related ethical dilemma you have encountered as a student. How did you solve the dilemma? What expert resources did you use?
2. Apply the ethical decision-making model to your ethical dilemma. How are your decision-making process and proposed actions different when using the model?

LEGAL CONCEPTS

To promote harmony, safety, and productivity as members of a society, we create rules. The rules of society can be informal or formal. An informal social rule, for example, is opening a door for someone. A criminal statute (law) is an example of a formal rule of society. Social rules or codes promote our social well-being. It would be unsafe to live in a community that existed without rules. All societies must require minimum standards of conduct for their members. Laws are the governmental mandates of a society that define individuals' duties to themselves, their neighbors, and the government. The failure to adhere to laws can result in punishment that may include imprisonment or monetary fines.

Regulation of Nursing Practice

Nursing is a licensed health care profession. Nurses must be licensed by their state to practice nursing. The rationale for state licensure is to improve the quality of health care services and to protect the public. As such, state governments have created licensing boards to establish entry-level requirements for nurses. These licensing boards also establish regulations that define the scope of appropriate nursing practice for licensed nurses. These licensing regulations are found in state nurse practice laws and within regulations that are made by the licensing agency.

State nurse practice laws and the attendant nursing regulations establish the parameters within which nurses must practice to obtain and maintain state license. These regulations are referred to as **administrative laws**. These considerations and mandates can be the basis for disciplinary actions by the licensing body. Failure to adhere to the regulatory mandates of the nursing licensing body can result in loss of the privilege to practice nursing. Unprofessional conduct and conviction of a crime are examples of possible violations of nursing regulations that could result in a loss of license.

Health Insurance Portability and Accountability Act of 1996

Since 1996, the federal government has regulated the distribution of personal health information. Licensed nurses along with other health workers are required to follow the requirements established by the Health Insurance Portability and Accountability Act of 1996 (HIPAA). This act creates civil and criminal liability for health care workers who wrongfully disclose a person's health information. HIPAA has created a national standard for the protection of individual health information. The U.S. Department of Health and Human Services has developed a privacy rule that has, for the first time, established a basis for the federal protection of private health information.

Licensed nurses must be sensitive to these legal limitations for the distribution of personal health information. Depending on the seriousness of the violation of HIPAA standards, a person may be sentenced to up to 10 years in prison. HIPAA establishes very stringent guidelines. Licensed nurses should review their employer's HIPAA compliance policies and adhere to them. For more information on HIPAA and how it impacts health care information and workers, see the U.S. Department of Health and Human Services website at www.hhs.gov/ocr/hipaa.

Nursing Liability and the Law

Liability refers to the level of responsibility that society places on individuals for their actions. In recent years, this responsibility has been interpreted to mean the financial responsibility owed to those who are injured by wrongful actions. Laws establish liability or responsibility for these wrongful actions. Following the law is a major part of the practice of nursing.

Administrative laws establish the licensing authority of the state to create, license, and regulate the practice of nursing. Criminal law regulates behaviors for citizens within this country. Civil law provides the rules by which individuals seek to protect their personal and property rights.

Criminal and Civil Law

Everyone, regardless of occupation, is required to obey the criminal laws of the government. **Criminal laws** establish the rules of social behavior and define the punishment for breaking those rules, which can result in imprisonment or monetary fines.

Criminal law is different from civil law in the nature of remedies that are used for punishment. A crime is viewed as an action taken by a person against society that the government will prosecute and punish. The breaking of a criminal law may result in criminal punishment and civil liability. For instance, an intoxicated driver may go to jail for a crime and also be held liable in a civil court for any personal injury that resulted. Examples of criminal acts are assault, battery, rape, murder, and larceny.

Civil laws dictate how disputes are settled among individuals and how liability is assigned for wrongful actions. For health care workers, civil liability is a constant concern. The potential for civil liability is demonstrated by an increased use of health care procedures such as diagnostic testing, which results in higher health care costs. Civil liability is a method by which a patient can seek financial recovery for injuries and losses caused by the wrongful action or lack of action by a health care worker.

A civil liability suit begins with the filing of a complaint with a court. A copy of the complaint must be given or served by the plaintiff to the defendant. The person claiming a civil cause of action and injury is the plaintiff, and the person alleged to have caused the injury is the defendant. A **summons**, which is a notice to defendants that they are being sued, is attached to the complaint. The complaint describes the claim being made by the plaintiff, and the summons instructs the defendant that the complaint must be answered within a specified period, usually 20 to 30 days.

Nurses served with a work-related summons should notify their employers and take these documents seriously.

The nurse must ensure that the summons is answered. If the employer does not answer the summons, the nurse must seek legal counsel to answer the summons within the specified time. If the nurse fails to answer the summons and complaint, it may result in a default judgment, which is acknowledgment of liability.

Civil wrongs caused by the act or omission of a health care worker can be physical, emotional, and financial in nature. Lawsuits involving civil wrongs are called **torts**. The institution that employs the worker may also become liable for the acts or omissions of its employees. This theory of law is called ***respondeat superior***. It is important for employees to understand that their work may result in civil liability for their employers.

Civil or tort liability for health care workers can be based on intentional actions, unintentional actions, and even the omission of action. **Malpractice** may be defined as a breach of the duty that arises out of the relationship between patient and health care worker. This term includes liability that may arise from intentional torts and unintentional torts. Intentional torts are lawsuits wherein the defendant is accused of intentionally causing injury to the plaintiff. Examples of intentional torts are assault, battery, defamation, false imprisonment, outrage, invasion of privacy, and wrongful disclosure of confidential information (Table 3.1).

Negligence

An unintentional tort is known as **negligence**. Negligence occurs when injury results from the failure of the wrongdoer to exercise care. This failure to follow due care in the protection of the injured person is referred to as a breach of duty. Professionals owe a higher duty of care to their patients. The failure of a health care professional to follow a prescribed duty of care is malpractice. Professional negligence, therefore, is referred to as malpractice (Box 3.2). All professionals, including LPN/LVNs, are responsible for their own actions whether they are intentional or negligent in nature. Although the employing agency is also responsible for the actions of its employees, employees always remain responsible for their own actions as well.

TABLE 3.1 INTENTIONAL TORTS

Assault	Unlawful conduct that places another in immediate fear of an unlawful touching or battery; real threat of bodily harm
Battery	Unlawful touching of another
Defamation	Wrongful injury to another's reputation or standing in a community; may be written (libel) or spoken (slander)
False imprisonment	Unlawful restriction of a person's freedom
Outrage	Extreme and outrageous conduct by a defendant in the care of the patient or the body of a deceased individual
Invasion of privacy and wrongful disclosure of confidential information	Liability when a patient's privacy is invaded physically or when records are released without authority

Box 3.2

Components Needed for a Finding of Negligence

- A duty of care owed to patients
- A breach of duty to exercise care
- Injury and damages occurring from this breach of duty

Limitation of Liability

All professions are concerned with the **limitation of liability**. Ways to limit liability include ensuring patient rights, accurately documenting procedures, following institutional policies, acquiring individual malpractice or liability insurance, pursuing continuing education, and practicing in accordance with the current standards of the nursing profession. Some states have enacted tort reform legislation. Much of this legislation is directed at limiting liability for health care professionals and institutions. Examples of this reform legislation are limitations on the dollar amount allowable for a patient's damages, shortening the time in which a patient can file a lawsuit, and requiring stringent expert medical evaluation of a claim before a lawsuit can be filed.

All patients are entitled to quality care and to be treated with dignity and respect. To provide quality care and limit liability, understand and provide the rights your patient is entitled to and question directions that are controversial, given verbally, concern situations of high liability, or involve a discrepancy between the direction and standard policy. Rights are defined as something due an individual according to just claims, legal guarantees, or moral and ethical principles. **Welfare rights**, also called legal rights, are rights that are based on a legal entitlement to some good or benefit. These rights are guaranteed by laws such as the Bill of Rights and, if violated, can come under the powers of the legal system. For example, citizens of the United States have a right to equal access to employment regardless of race, sex, or religion. The type of treatment and care a patient has the right to expect is outlined in the patient bill of rights. Stay informed about the status of patient rights' legislation because you will be expected to follow it. Knocking before entering a patient's room and introducing oneself to the patient are examples of a patient's rights.

Documentation is a legal record of your actions. Document nursing actions based on orders given, as well as the name and title of the person who gave the direction if it was verbal. Documentation must be clear, honest, and accurate. Always practice at a level that is generally accepted by the nursing profession. Failure to maintain acceptable practice standards is cause for concern and can create potential liability for both you and the health care institution.

It is important to understand that some employers do not provide malpractice insurance for their nursing employees. Always ask an employer exactly who is covered under the employer's liability insurance. If nursing employees are covered, the employer's insurance provides coverage from liability only as long as the employee follows the employer's work policies. For this reason, employer-provided liability insurance is not personal liability insurance. As a result, LPN/LVNs often carry personal liability insurance.

REVIEW QUESTIONS

1. Factors influencing health care changes include which of the following?
   a. Decreasing use of evidence
   b. Increasing elderly population
   c. Decreasing cultural diversity
   d. Decreasing population size in America

2. Which of the following should the nurse do during admission and throughout a patient's hospitalization to help ensure reimbursement for a secondary diagnosis occurrence? **Select all that apply.**
   a. Do not document conditions present on admission.
   b. Photograph wounds that are present on admission.
   c. Educate patients about methods used to prevent complications.
   d. Document interventions, such as turning and ambulating patients.
   e. Explain to patient that participation in preventive interventions is optional.
   f. Document patient education related to complication prevention.

3. Which of these actions would the nurse correctly interpret as falling within the scope of practice of the LPN/LVN?
   a. Performing a physical assessment on admission for a critical care patient
   b. Administering IV push morphine
   c. Ambulating a 1-day postoperative patient
   d. Developing the plan of care for a newly admitted surgical patient

4. Which of the following describes how an autocratic leader makes decisions?
   a. Seeks information from all staff members.
   b. Uses own knowledge to decide.
   c. Forms focus groups to gather information.
   d. Forms a staff committee to provide input.

5. Which of these situations would be an appropriate example of a leadership role for the LPN/LVN?
   a. Consulting with an RN to modify care for assigned patient
   b. Performing an annual employee evaluation for a nursing assistant
   c. Supervising the RN and LPN/LVN staff on a surgical unit
   d. Interviewing a new graduate RN for a staff position

6. As a nurse provides care to patients, it is important to have an understanding of ethics for which of the following reasons?
   a. Resources are unlimited and available to everyone.
   b. Technological interventions are always desirable.
   c. Health care systems are being simplified.
   d. A health crisis can occur at any stage of human development.

7. The nurse is planning quality care for a patient without regard to race, ethnicity, or gender. Which of the following ethical obligations does this exhibit?
   a. Fidelity
   b. Integrity
   c. Respectfulness
   d. Compassion

8. A patient's family requests that a feeding tube be inserted. The patient has an advance directive indicating that a feeding tube is not to be inserted. As the nurse and physician consider what is best for the patient in this ethical dilemma, which of the following principles is represented?
   a. Autonomy
   b. Beneficence
   c. Justice
   d. Nonmaleficence

9. The nurse reviews the advance directive for a patient who is comatose. Which of the steps in the ethical decision-making process is the nurse performing?
   a. Implementing the outcome
   b. Clarifying the values of all participants
   c. Determining the best action with the strongest ethical support
   d. Examining possible actions and the consequences of each

10. Which of the following situations could create moral distress for a nurse?
    a. Agreeing with a family's end-of-life care choices
    b. Believing that inserting a feeding tube for a DNR patient is wrong
    c. Supporting a patient's advance directive
    d. Supporting a family's decision to stop life support

REVIEW QUESTIONS—cont'd

11. A nurse has a question about how a nursing license is regulated. In which of the following documents will the nurse find this information?
    a. An institutional policy
    b. Nursing ethics code
    c. State nurse practice law
    d. National nursing standards

12. In providing professional nursing care, the nurse understands that the law of negligence requires which of the following to create liability? **Select all that apply.**
    a. A duty of care owed
    b. Assault
    c. Ethical violations
    d. A breach of duty
    e. Injury and damages
    f. A crime

13. The Health Insurance Portability and Accountability Act of 1996 (HIPAA) requires licensed professional nurses to do which of the following?
    a. Maintain continuing nursing education credit hours.
    b. Protect the privacy of an individual's personal health information.
    c. Limit nursing work hours to no more than 35 per week.
    d. Forgo membership in any union or collective bargaining agreement unit.

References

American Hospital Association. (2009). *The patient care partnership: Understanding expectations, rights and responsibilities.* Retrieved August 10, 2009, from http://www.aha.org/aha/issues/Communicating-With-Patients/pt-care-partnership.html

Beauchamp, T. L., Childress, J. F. (2008). *Principles of biomedical ethics* (6th ed.). New York: Oxford University Press.

Bureau of Labor Statistics, U.S. Department of Labor. (n.d.). *Occupational outlook handbook, 2008–09 edition, licensed practical and licensed vocational nurses.* Retrieved May 31, 2009, from http://www.bls.gov/oco/ocos102.htm

Burkhardt, M. A., & Nathaniel, A. K. (2008). *Ethics & issues in contemporary nursing* (3rd ed.). New York: Delmar.

Fry, S. T., & Veatch, R. M. (2006). *Case studies in nursing ethics* (3rd ed.). Boston: Jones and Bartlett Publishers.

Harris, J. (2001). *The value of life: An introduction to medical ethics.* London: Routledge.

McCarthy, J., & Deady, R. (2008). Moral distress reconsidered. *Nursing Ethics, 15*(2), 254–262.

National Council of State Boards of Nursing. (1995). Delegation: Concepts and decision-making process. *Issues, 16*(4), 1.

U.S. Census Bureau, Population Division, Interim State Population Projections. (2005, April 21). *Interim projections of the population by selected age groups for the United States and states: April 1, 2000 to July 1, 2030.* Retrieved April 21, 2009, from http://www.census.gov/population/projections/SummaryTabB1.pdf

Resources

American Hospital Association, One North Franklin, Chicago, IL 60606-4321 (www.aha.org/aha/issues/Communicating-With-Patients/pt-care-partnership.html)

National Association for Practical Nurse Education and Service, Inc., P.O. Box 25647, Alexandria, VA 22313 (www.napnes.org)

National Federation of Licensed Practical Nurses, Inc., 605 Poole Dr., Garner, NC 27529 (www.nflpn.org)

Nursing Ethics Network provides a host of links to information on ethical decision making for health care professionals (http://jmrileyrn.tripod.com/nen/nen.html)

DavisPlus | For additional resources and information visit http://davisplus.fadavis.com

4 Cultural Influences on Nursing Care

NANCY AHERN AND
BOBBI M. MARTIN

KEY TERMS

acculturation (uh-KUL-chur-AY-shun)
beliefs (bee-LEEFS)
cultural (KUL-chur-uhl)
cultural assimilation (KUL-chur-uhl uh-SIM-ih-LAY-shun)
cultural awareness (KUL-chur-uhl a-WEAR-ness)
cultural competence (KUL-chur-uhl KOM-pe-tents)
cultural conflict (KUL-chur-uhl KON-flikt)
cultural diversity (KUL-chur-uhl dih-VER-sih-tee)
cultural sensitivity (KUL-chur-uhl SEN-sih-TIV-ih-tee)
cultural shock (KUL-chur-uhl SHOK)
culture (KUL-chur)
customs (KUS-tums)
ethnic (ETH-nick)
ethnocentrism (ETH-noh-SEN-trizm)
generalizations (JEN-er-al-ih-ZAY-shuns)
stereotype (STARE-ee-oh-TIGHP)
traditions (tra-DISH-uns)
values (VAL-yooz)
worldview (WERLD-vyoo)

QUESTIONS TO GUIDE YOUR READING

1. What are the meanings of the concepts common to culture and ethnicity?
2. What are examples of cultural characteristics, values, beliefs, and practices?
3. What are attributes of culturally diverse patients and their families, and how do they affect nursing care?
4. What data should you collect from culturally diverse patients and their families?
5. How can you provide a holistic approach to patient care that respects cultural characteristics and attributes?

Your clinical instructor has assigned you to provide care to Mary Williams, a 72-year-old African American woman. Ms. Williams has diabetes and hypertension (high blood pressure). She was admitted to the hospital for gangrene of her left foot. When you enter her room, you find Ms. Williams anxious and crying. She tells you that she is scheduled for surgery later in the day. When asked about her foot, she tells you that she has been applying a poultice to draw out the germs but it has not worked yet. She adds that she has been praying for the cure that she knows will come. As you are collecting history information about her diabetes, Ms. Williams admits that her doctor told her to attend diabetes classes years ago but she stopped going because she didn't like what she heard. She quickly changes the subject, wanting to talk about nothing but her grandchildren. Your attempts to complete preoperative teaching are unsuccessful.

Cultural diversity in the United States is increasing. According to the U.S. Census Bureau, minorities, now roughly one-third of the U.S. population, are expected to become the majority during the next 30 years (Bernstein & Edwards, 2008). Immigration from Spanish-speaking and Asian countries has resulted in dramatic shifts in census numbers. Figure 4.1 illustrates the changes and projections in racial and ethnic makeup in the United States by the year 2050. As a result, **cultural** and **ethnic** differences between nurses and their patients are becoming more evident and must be recognized. Thus, there is a need for you to become knowledgeable about cultures other than your own. This chapter provides you with the basics of culture and its impact on health promotion and wellness.

CONCEPTS RELATED TO CULTURE

Culture refers to the socially transmitted behavior patterns, beliefs, values, customs, arts, and all other characteristics of people that guide their view of the world (**worldview**). Cultural beliefs, values, **customs**, and **traditions** are primarily learned within the family on an unconscious level. They can also be learned from the community in which one lives, from religious organizations, and in schools. As you try to understand more about culture, keep in mind that it contains a number of characteristics (Box 4.1). All individuals and groups have the right to maintain cultural practices that they feel are appropriate. Culture has strong influences on a patient's understanding of health and responses to nursing care. You must understand the impact diversity can have on health behaviors in order to better meet the needs of your patients (Fig. 4.2). As you learn more about ethnic and cultural groups, you will be challenged to look at the differences and similarities across cultures.

Consider our patient, Ms. Williams. Did she behave as you would have in a similar situation? How do you think the characteristics of her culture affected her behavior?

While the terms *cultural sensitivity*, *cultural awareness*, and *cultural competence* are similar, they have different meanings. **Cultural sensitivity** is knowing politically correct language and not making statements that may offend another person's cultural beliefs. **Cultural awareness** focuses on history and ancestry and emphasizes an appreciation for and attention to arts, music, crafts, celebrations, foods, and traditional clothing. **Cultural competence** includes the skills and

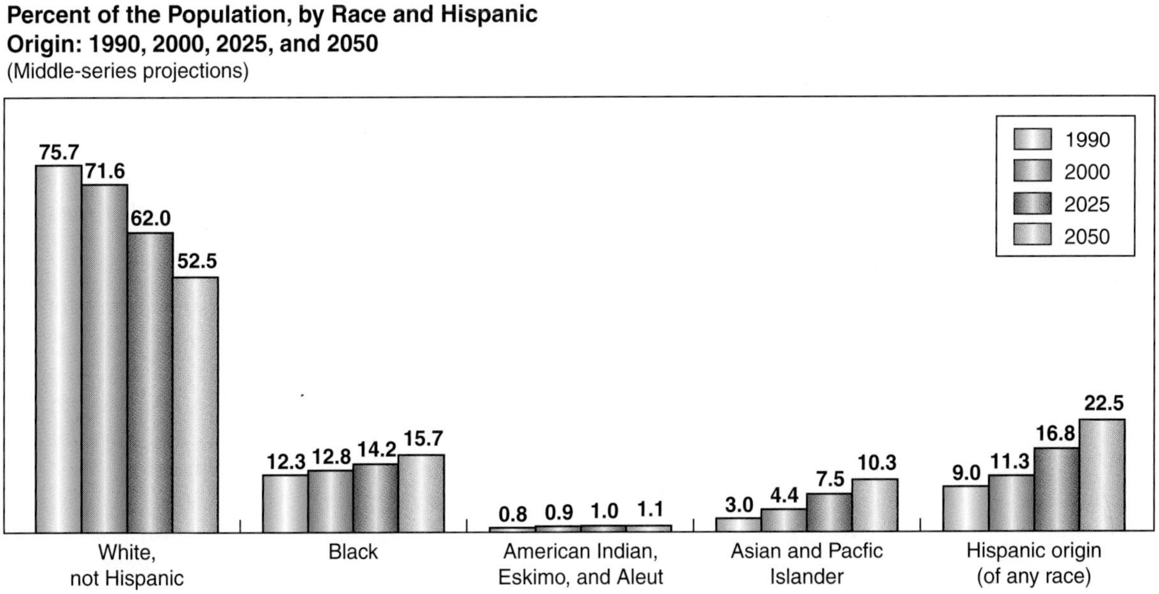
Percent of the Population, by Race and Hispanic Origin: 1990, 2000, 2025, and 2050
(Middle-series projections)
1990
2000
2025
2050
75.7
71.6
62.0
52.5
12.3
12.8
14.2
15.7
0.8
0.9
1.0
1.1
3.0
4.4
7.5
10.3
9.0
11.3
16.8
22.5
White, not Hispanic
Black
American Indian, Eskimo, and Aleut
Asian and Pacfic Islander
Hispanic origin (of any race)

Figure 4.1 Percent of the population of the United States, by race and Hispanic origin. (*Source:* U.S. Census Bureau, Population Division. Retrieved August 15, 2009, from http://www.census.gov/population/www/pop-profile/natproj.html.)

Box 4.1

Characteristics of Culture

- *Culture is learned.* Learning occurs through life experiences shared with other members of the culture.
- *Culture is taught.* Cultural values, beliefs, and traditions are passed down from generation to generation either formally (e.g., in schools) or informally (e.g., in families)
- *Culture is shared by its members.* Cultural norms are shared through teachings and social interactions.
- *Culture is dynamic and adaptive.* Cultural customs, beliefs, and practices are not static, but change over time and at different rates. Cultural change occurs with adaptation in response to the environment.
- *Culture is complex.* Cultural assumptions and habits are unconscious, which may make them difficult for members of the culture to explain to others.
- *Culture is diverse.* Culture demonstrates the variety that exists between groups and among members of a particular group.
- *Culture exists at many levels.* Culture exists at material (e.g., art, dress, or artifacts) and nonmaterial (as language, traditions, customs, beliefs, and practices) levels.
- *Culture has common beliefs and practices.* Members of a culture share the same beliefs, traditions, customs, and practices as long as they continue to be adaptive and satisfy their needs. Some members do not always follow all of these, but many do.
- *Culture is all encompassing.* Culture can affect everything its members think and do.
- *Culture provides identity.* Cultural beliefs provide identity for members as long as there is no conflict with the dominant culture or lack of gratification by its members.

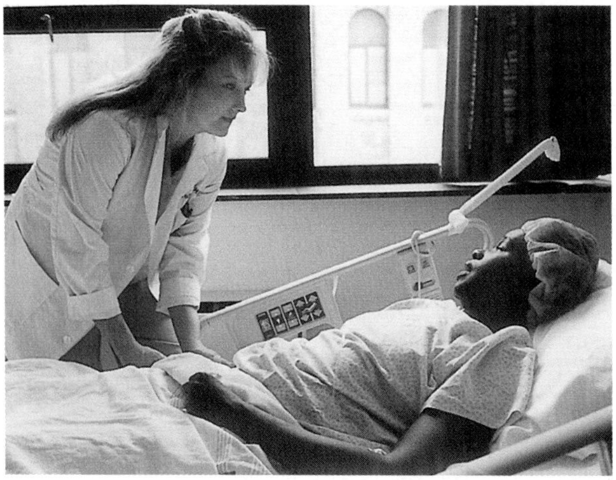

Figure 4.2 The nurse must assess patients' unique needs related to their cultural backgrounds.

knowledge required to provide effective nursing care. In order for you to be culturally competent, you need to:

- Have an awareness of your own culture and not let it have an undue influence on your patient care.
- Have specific knowledge about your patient's culture.
- Accept and respect cultural differences.
- Adapt your nursing care (when appropriate) to your patient's culture.

We will discuss more about cultural competence later in the chapter.

Even though you may have knowledge about another culture, barriers such as ethnocentrism and stereotyping can cause you not to appreciate cultural differences. **Ethnocentrism** is the tendency for humans to think that their ways of thinking, acting, and believing are the only right, proper, and natural ways. Ethnocentrism perpetrates an attitude that beliefs that differ greatly from your own are strange or bizarre and therefore wrong. Additionally, you must be careful not to stereotype your patient. A **stereotype** is an opinion or belief about a group of people that is ascribed to an individual. For example, the statement "All Chinese people prefer traditional Chinese medicine" is a stereotype. This stereotype is not true. Although many Chinese people may prefer traditional Chinese medicine for some health conditions, not all Chinese people prefer traditional Chinese medicine. Some Chinese people prefer the Western medicine that is practiced in the United States.

However, you can still make **generalizations** about an ethnic person without stereotyping. Although a generalization or assumption may be true for the group, it does not necessarily fit every individual. Therefore, you must seek additional information to determine whether the generalization fits the individual. The challenge is for you to understand the patient's cultural perspective. If you have specific cultural knowledge, you can improve therapeutic interventions by becoming a coparticipant with patients and their families. To do this, it is very important that you develop a personal, open style of communication and be receptive to learning from patients from cultures other than your own (Fig. 4.3).

A few additional terms important for your understanding of culture relate to the socialization process of those who are learning to become a member of a society or group. When people immigrate to a new country, they gradually accept the new culture through a learning process. They learn to accept their own beliefs and those of their new country. This is known as **acculturation**. This occurs because the new member must learn enough of the new culture to survive. A step further is when **cultural assimilation** occurs. This happens when the new member takes on the dominant culture's values, beliefs, and practices. This process could potentially be viewed as negative because the person may lose some of his rich heritage to become more like the dominant culture.

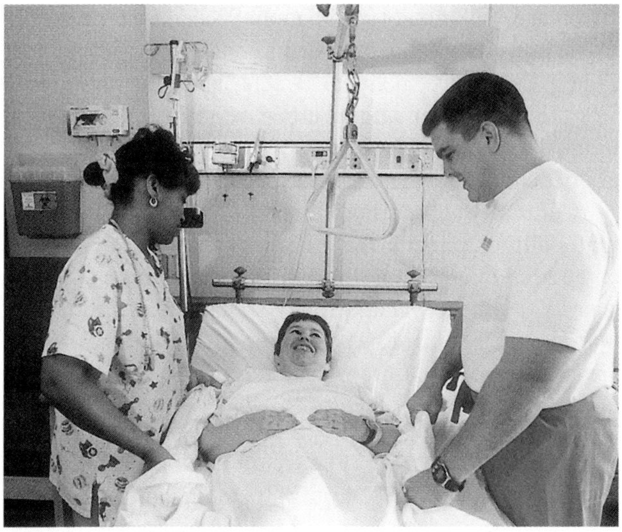

Figure 4.3 Health care workers and patients may come from a variety of cultural backgrounds.

Imagine for a moment that you have moved to China. At first you eat the food and try to understand the language of your new country. Over time, you may learn to cook the food, speak the language, and perhaps blend some of the Chinese beliefs, traditions, and practices with your own. As this practice continues to occur, acculturation is evident. This process may not always be smooth. When one's culture conflicts with the new culture, **cultural conflict** occurs. Worse than that, **cultural shock** happens when values, beliefs, and practices sanctioned by the new culture are very different from the ones of the native culture. Let's look at another example. Ling Chi is a 4-year-old boy who is a recent immigrant enrolled in a new school. He is alone and afraid even though he is surrounded by other boys and girls his age. It is lunchtime and while his teacher is trying to help him with his food, he starts crying. The fork and spoon are foreign to him. At home he is used to eating his lunch with chopsticks. In addition, he does not understand the words spoken to him. Little Chi is experiencing cultural shock.

HEALTH CARE VALUES, BELIEFS, AND PRACTICES

Cultural values, beliefs, and practices are important in health care. Values can help shape one's beliefs and practices. Do you know what your values are regarding health and illness? A **value** can be defined as a principle or standard that has meaning or worth to an individual (Purnell & Paulanka, 2008). "Cleanliness" is an example of a value. A **belief** is something that a person accepts as true (e.g., "I believe that germs cause illness and disease"). A *practice* is a set of behaviors that one follows—for example, washing hands before eating. It is important for you to understand the differences between these terms because we will be discussing them as they relate to cultural groups.

For you to be able to provide culturally competent care, you need to know how the people you encounter define health and illness. In general, people follow one of three major health belief systems: scientific (Western medicine or biomedical), spiritual, or holistic. You are already familiar with the scientific health system, which dominates health care in Western societies. Belief in supernatural forces dominates the spiritual system, which is considered by many to be an alternative health care system. (Some experts call this magicoreligious, but this is an offensive term to some religious persons.) The holistic belief system focuses on the need for balance and harmony of the body and spirit with nature.

Health care typically focuses on health promotion, the prevention of illness, and acute care practices while considering traditional, religious, and biomedical (scientific) beliefs. Additionally, individual responsibility for health, self-medicating practices, views toward mental illness, and the patient's response to pain and the sick role are shaped by one's culture. Most societies combine biomedical health care with traditional, folk, and religious practices, such as praying for good health or wearing charms or amulets to ward off diseases and illnesses. There are many examples of individual and family folklore practices for curing or treating specific illnesses. Think for a minute about such practices that you may perform. What do you do for a fever or a sore throat? Does chicken noodle soup come to mind? Many times folk therapies are handed down from family members and may have their roots in religious beliefs. Examples of folk medicines include covering a boil with axle grease, wearing copper bracelets for arthritic pain, and drinking herbal teas. As an addition to biomedical treatments, many people use complementary therapies, such as acupressure, reflexology, and other traditional therapies specific to the cultural group.

Often folk practices are not harmful and can be added to the patient's plan of care. However, some may conflict with prescription medications, intensify the treatment effect, or cause an overdose. It is essential to inquire about the full range of therapies being used by your patients, such as food items, teas, herbal remedies, nonfood substances, over-the-counter (OTC) medications, medications prescribed by others, and medications borrowed from others.

If patients feel that you do not accept their beliefs and practices, they may be less open to sharing information and less compliant with prescribed treatment. You should try to encourage your patients' practices that could be helpful and discourage those that may be harmful. Before encouraging or discouraging such practices, you will need to discuss them with the appropriate health care team member. *Think about Ms. Williams. Does she use any folk practices? How would you address this specific situation?*

Before moving on, we need to discuss the subjects of mental illness and cultural responses to pain and the sick role. Mental illness may be seen by many as being unimportant compared with physical illness. Mental illness is culture bound. What may be perceived as a mental illness in one society may not be considered a mental illness in another society. Among some cultures, having a mental illness or an emotional difficulty is considered a disgrace and is taboo. As a result, a family is likely to keep a person who is mentally ill at home as long as they possibly can.

Cultural responses to pain and the sick role can vary among cultures. For example, some people are expected to openly express their pain. Others are expected to suffer their pain in silence. For some, the sick role is readily accepted, and any excuse is accepted for not fulfilling daily obligations. Others minimize their illness and make extended efforts to fulfill their obligations.

Nursing Assessment and Strategies

To begin your assessment of your patient's health beliefs, ask the following questions:

- What do you usually do to maintain your health?
- What do you usually do when you are sick?
- What kind of home treatments do you use when you are sick?
- Who is the first person you see when you are sick?
- What do you do when you have pain?
- Do you wear charms or bracelets to ward off illness?
- Do you take herbs or drink special teas when you are sick? If so, what are they?
- Do you practice special rituals or prayers to maintain your health?

Cultural Self-Enrichment Exercise

HOW YOUR CULTURAL BELIEFS AFFECT YOUR HEALTH BEHAVIORS

- How do you define health for yourself?
- How do you define illness for yourself?
- Identify preventive health care practices that you use.
- When you see a health care provider for a minor illness, what do you expect the health care provider to do for you?
- Identify your self-medicating behaviors.
- What home remedies do you use when you are ill?
- What meaning does pain have to you? What measures do you use when you are in pain?
- What are your personal views toward autopsy, organ donation, organ transplantation, and receiving blood or blood products?

CHARACTERISTICS OF CULTURAL DIVERSITY

Primary and secondary characteristics of diversity affect how people view their culture. The primary characteristics of **cultural diversity** include nationality, race, skin color, gender, age, and religious affiliation. Secondary characteristics include socioeconomic status, education, occupation, military experience, political beliefs, length of time away from the country of origin, urban versus rural residence, marital status, parental status, physical characteristics, sexual orientation, and gender issues.

Culturally appropriate care needs to take into account eight cultural phenomena that may vary with use but can be seen in all cultural groups: (1) communication, (2) space, (3) time orientation, (4) social organization, (5) environmental control/health beliefs, (6) choice of health care practitioner, (7) biological variations, and (8) death and dying issues.

Communication Styles

Communication styles include verbal and nonverbal variations. Verbal communication includes spoken language, dialects, and voice volume. Dialects are variations in grammar, word meanings, and pronunciation of spoken language. Nonverbal communication includes the use and degree of eye contact, the perception of time, and physical closeness when talking with peers and perceived superiors. In some societies, people are expected to maintain eye contact without staring, which denotes that they are listening and can be trusted. However, in other societies, as a sign of respect, people should not maintain eye contact with superiors such as teachers and those in positions of higher status.

Nursing Assessment and Strategies

Ask the following questions:

- By what name do you prefer to be called?
- What language do you speak at home?

Cultural Self-Enrichment Exercise

WHAT IS YOUR CULTURAL BACKGROUND?

- How do you identify yourself in terms of racial, cultural, or ethnic background? From what country did your ancestors originate? Were your parents from the same or similar ethnic backgrounds?
- What stories do you remember that your parents, grandparents, or other relatives told about relocating in the United States? Do you know why they originally came to America?
- How do these stories compare with those of others from similar backgrounds?
- How do these stories compare with those of others from different backgrounds?
- Remember, one person's values and beliefs are not better than another person's—they are just different.

Cultural Self-Enrichment Exercise

COMMUNICATION

- How many languages do you speak? Do you speak a dialect of your dominant language? Does it interfere with communication with your patients?
- Do you speak in a soft, medium, or loud tone of voice? Does this tone change in different situations? How close do you stand when you speak with close friends? Does this distance change when you converse with your teacher, your religious leader, or a politician?
- Identify characteristics from your worldview in terms of being present, past, and future oriented.
- By what name do you prefer to be called? Why? Does this change in different situations?

Be sure to do the following:

- Take cues from the patient for voice volume.
- Be an active listener, and become comfortable with silence.
- Avoid appearing rushed.
- Be formal with greetings until told to do otherwise.
- Take greeting cues from the patient.
- Speak slowly and clearly. Do not speak loudly or with exaggerated mouthing.
- Explain why you are asking specific questions.
- Give reasons for treatments.
- Repeat questions if needed.
- Provide written instructions in the patient's preferred language.
- Obtain an interpreter if needed.

Health care providers should refrain from relying on untrained individuals to interpret, especially family members (see *Evidence-Based Practice*). Although it may seem logical that a patient's best advocate is his or her family, it is risky to rely on family members to interpret medical or health information for the following reasons:

- Family members may not be proficient in medical terminology.
- They may not possess the skills needed to interpret.
- They may unintentionally or intentionally omit or alter important information.
- Using family members to interpret may raise privacy issues protected by the Health Insurance Portability and Accountability Act of 1996 (HIPAA).
- If children are used, they may not be emotionally mature enough to handle the information being conveyed.

EVIDENCE-BASED PRACTICE

Clinical Question

Do patients with limited English proficiency who have professional interpreters experience improved clinical care over those who use ad hoc or family member interpreters?

Evidence

Multiple studies demonstrate that the use of professional interpreters is associated with improved care and that ad hoc interpreters were much more likely to make errors that led to serious medical problems than professionally trained interpreters (Karliner et al., 2007).

Implications for Nursing Practice

Organizations are required by law to provide language access services to individuals with limited English proficiency (Joint Commission, 2008). Addressing communication barriers is an important task for nurses as caregivers and patient advocates. Nurses can be aware of the population they serve and have interpreters available to facilitate communication. This is done through face-to-face interpretation, via phone, or via video. Nurses can also ensure there are written materials in the patients' native language, especially for discharge instructions.

REFERENCES

Joint Commission. (2008). Promoting effective communication: Language access services in health care. *Joint Commission Perspectives, 28*(2), 811. Retrieved March 24, 2009, from http://www.jointcommission.org/NR/rdonlyres/ACAFA57F-5F50-427A-BB98-73431D68A5E4/0/Perspectives_Article_Feb_2008.pdf.

Karliner, L. S., Jacobs, E. A., Chen, A. H., & Mutha, S. (2007). Do professional interpreters improve clinical care for patients with limited English proficiency? A systematic review of the literature. *Health Services Research, 42*(4), 727–754.

Space

Space refers to one's "personal space." Are you aware of your comfort zone? In other words, how close can someone get to you before you feel less safe and secure? Like you, most people have such a comfort zone. Personal space tends to be different when speaking with close friends versus strangers. For example, people from the Middle East tend to stand close together when talking, while others from European countries such as Germany require a much larger space. The need for space is important for the patient's privacy, autonomy, security, and self-identity. Understanding what space means for your patients can be important when you are trying to assess, treat, and teach them.

> **Cultural Self-Enrichment Exercise**
>
> **SPACE**
>
> - Are you aware of your comfort zone? Is it different for close friends/family and strangers?
> - How does it make you feel when someone violates your comfort zone?
> - Do you respect other individuals' space when you communicate with them?
> - How do you determine that you are protecting another's personal space?
> - How do you feel when someone touches you?
> - Do you have a firm handshake?

Nursing Assessment and Strategies

Ask the following questions:

- Are you comfortable?
- Do you have any concerns you would like to discuss?

Be sure to do the following:

- Make sure your patients are comfortable before you interview them.
- Maintain appropriate physical distance (observe for cues).
- Be aware of cultural differences.
- Be aware of physical objects that may be a barrier to comfort.
- Make sure that the patient's physical environment is arranged to ensure safety, security, and familiarity.

Time Orientation

Time orientation can vary among people from different cultures. The perception of time has two dimensions. The first dimension is related to clock time versus social time. For example, some cultures have a flexible orientation to time and events, and appointments take place when the person arrives. An event scheduled for 2 p.m. may not begin until 2:30 or when a majority of the people arrive. For others, time is less flexible, and appointments and social events are expected to start at the agreed-on time. For many, social events may be flexible, whereas medical appointments and business engagements start on time.

The second dimension of time relates to whether the culture is predominantly concerned with the past, present, or future. Past-oriented individuals maintain traditions that were meaningful in the past, and may worship ancestors. Present-oriented people accept the day as it comes, with little regard for the past; the future is unpredictable. Future-oriented people anticipate a bigger and better future and place a high value on change. Some people balance all three views—they respect the past, enjoy living in the present, and plan for the future.

Hospitals, clinics, and physicians' offices maintain a tight time schedule. It is therefore important that you understand patients' time orientation so you can prepare them for the timing of appointments, tests, and treatments. In addition, it is important that you assess their usual routines so that you can incorporate these as much as possible into their daily care.

> **Cultural Self-Enrichment Exercise**
>
> **TIME ORIENTATION**
>
> - Are you aware of your time orientation (past, present, future)?
> - Are you usually on time for appointments?
> - Are your biological capacities (e.g., sleep and rest, eating) affected by your body rhythms?
> - Do you have routines that you need to follow at certain times of the day?

Nursing Assessment and Strategies

Ask the following questions to understand your patients' time orientation:

- Are you normally on time for appointments?
- Are there any routines that you need to follow?
- What time do you usually eat your meals? Take your bath?

Be sure to do the following:

- Have a clock in the patient's room.
- Assess for orientation, and reorient to time as needed.
- Prepare patients prior to a procedure or test.
- Give time options when appropriate. ("Would you like to take a walk now or in an hour?")

Social Organization

Family organization includes the perceived head of the household, gender roles, and roles of the elderly and extended family members. The head of the household may be patriarchal (male dominated), matriarchal (female dominated), or egalitarian (shared equally between men and women). An awareness of the family dominance pattern is important for determining which family member to speak to when health care decisions have to be made. Confidentiality issues can complicate this issue. Be sure to follow your institution's policies when communicating with family members. You may need to obtain the patient's permission before planning care with family members.

In some cultures, specific roles are outlined for men and women. Men are expected to protect and provide for the family, manage finances, and deal with the outside world. Women are expected to maintain the home environment, including child care and household tasks. You must accept that not all societies share or even desire an egalitarian family structure.

Roles for the elderly and extended family vary among culturally diverse groups. In some cultures, the elderly are seen as being wise, are deferred to for decision making, and are held in high esteem. Their children are expected to provide for them when they are no longer able to care for themselves. In other cultures, although the elderly may be loved by family members, they may not be given such high regard and may be cared for outside the home when self-care becomes a concern.

The extended family is very important in some groups, and a single household may include several generations living together out of desire rather than out of necessity. The extended family may include both blood-related and non–blood-related persons who are given family status. In other families, each generation lives in a separate home or living space.

You can assist your patients with their treatment plans when you have a better understanding of their family dynamics. It is important to know who to include for planning of care, discharge planning, and patient teaching. This will also help the appropriate hospital personnel to assist the patient and family to plan for home care.

Nursing Assessment and Strategies

Ask the following questions:

- Who makes the decisions in your household?
- Who takes care of money matters, does the cooking, or is responsible for child care?
- Who decides when it is time to see a health care provider?
- Who lives in your household? Are they all blood related?

Be sure to do the following:

- Observe the use of touch between family members.
- Let family members decide where they want to stand or sit for comfort.

Cultural Self-Enrichment Exercise

SOCIAL ORGANIZATION

- Who is considered the head of the household in your family?
- Are there specified gender roles for family members?
- What are the roles of the elderly in your family?
- Do you identify with an extended family? Are they all blood relatives? What roles do they play?
- What kind of decisions do men make and what kind of decisions do women make?

Environmental Control

Environmental control refers to a person's perception of his or her ability to plan for activities that control nature or direct environmental factors. This concept is broader than where a person lives. It implies the systems and processes that affect individuals. While systems can include such things as cultural health beliefs and practices, processes can consist of interactions among individuals, families, and groups. Consideration is given to cultural values and beliefs, especially as they are different from those of the dominant health care view (scientific, biomedical).

Distinctions are made between health and illness and what people do to promote or maintain health and to prevent and treat illnesses. Not all of your patients will turn to a scientific health care system or provider. In fact, many people try some form of alternative therapy before seeking treatment. If you use herbs or over-the-counter medications, for example, you are doing just that. People also use alternative therapies and religious systems such as prayer in combination with the scientific medical system. Religious beliefs and practices may be very important to patients (Fig. 4.4).

Nursing Assessment and Strategies

Ask the following questions:

- How do you define health? Illness?
- Do you have any special beliefs about health and illness?
- What do you do to keep well?
- When you feel ill, what is the first thing you do to get better?
- How do you deal with pain?
- How do you and your family express grief?
- Are there any cultural beliefs or practices that I need to know about in order to plan your care?

Be sure to do the following:

- Be aware of possible cultural beliefs and practices.
- Never stereotype what you know about different cultures; always ask for specifics.
- Perform a cultural assessment on all of your patients.
- Determine how your patients view health and illness.
- Ask if they have received treatments of any kind for their illness.
- Ask about religions beliefs and practices.
- Encourage helpful practices and discourage those that are harmful.

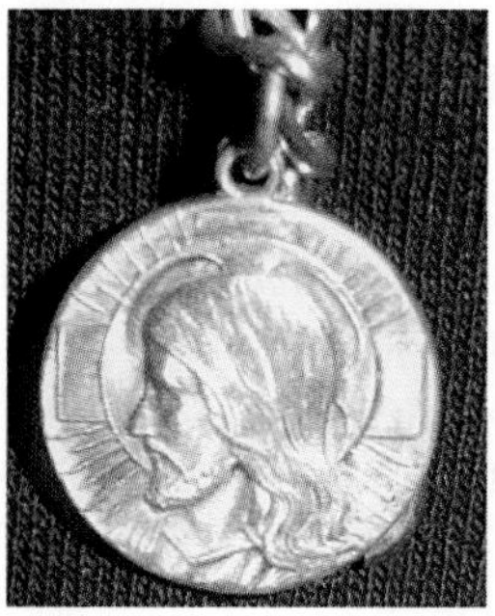

Figure 4.4 Religious artifacts are central to many people's health and illness practices.

Cultural Self-Enrichment Exercise
ENVIRONMENTAL CONTROL

- How do you define health and illness?
- What are your health and illness values, beliefs, and practices?
- What do you do when you are sick?
- Do you use alternative or religious practices for healing?
- How do you tolerate pain? What do you do for pain?
- How do you handle grief?
- How are your health and illness values, beliefs, and practices different from others in your dominant culture?

Health Care Practitioners

Health care practitioner choices are made based on the patient's perceived status and previous use of traditional, religious, and biomedical health care providers. In Western societies, educated health care providers are treated with great respect. However, some people prefer traditional healers because they are known to the patient, family, and community.

It is important to respect differences in gender relationships when providing care. Some people may be especially modest because of their religion, seeking out same-gender nurses and physicians for intimate care. Respect these patients' modesty by providing privacy and assigning a same-gender care provider when possible.

Nursing Assessment and Strategies

Ask the following questions of your patients:

- What health care providers besides physicians and nurses do you see when you are ill?
- Do you object to male or female health care providers giving physical care to you?

Be sure to do the following:

- Watch for alternative care providers who may visit the patient in the health care facility.

Cultural Self-Enrichment Exercise
HEALTH CARE PRACTITIONERS

- What complementary health care practitioners have you used? Were they successful?
- Identify complementary health care practitioners used by your friends. Were they successful?
- When you are ill and need to see a health care provider, do you prefer a same-gender provider? Why or why not?

Biological Variations

Biological variations refers to ways in which people are different from one another physiologically and genetically. These differences can make them more susceptible to certain illnesses and diseases and may also influence the effectiveness of different medications. Biological variations can include differences in (1) body build and structure, (2) skin color, (3) vital signs, (4) laboratory values, (5) susceptibility to disease, and (6) nutrition. Darker skin color can challenge you to be more observant when you are assessing the skin color of your patient. Laboratory test results can also be different in a number of cultures. For example, American Indians and Hispanic Americans may have higher blood glucose levels than whites.

The term *biological variations* also refers to differences in nutritional practices. Nutritional practices are currently being scrutinized in our society. These practices include the personal meaning of food, food choices and rituals, food taboos, and how food and food substances are used for health promotion and wellness. Cultural beliefs influence what people eat or avoid. In addition to being important for survival, food offers security and acceptance, plays a significant role in socialization, and can serve as an expression of love.

Culturally congruent dietary counseling, such as changing amounts and preparation practices and including ethnic food choices, can reduce health risks. Whenever possible, you should determine a patient's current dietary practices. Culturally diverse patients may refuse to eat on a schedule of American mealtimes or eat American foods. Counseling about food group requirements or dietary restrictions must respect an individual's cultural background. Most cultures have their own nutritional practices for health promotion and disease prevention. For many, a balance of different types of foods is important for maintaining health and preventing illness. Common folk practices recommend specific foods during illness and for prevention of illness or disease. A thorough history and assessment of dietary practices can be an important diagnostic tool to guide health promotion.

Nursing Assessment and Strategies

Ask the following questions of your patients:

- Are you at risk for any diseases or genetic disorders related to your cultural background?
- Are you satisfied with your weight?
- Are you active? What is your normal exercise pattern?
- Do you protect your eyes and skin from the sun? From possible injuries?
- Do you have any drug or food allergies?
- Has anyone in your family had any major illnesses?
- What do you eat to stay healthy?
- What do you eat when you are ill?
- Are there certain foods that you do not eat? Why?
- Do certain foods cause you to become ill? What are they?
- Who purchases the food in your household?
- Who prepares the food in your household?

Be sure to do the following:

- Teach about biological variations that may pertain to your patient.
- Determine and respect usual eating patterns whenever possible.
- Teach good nutrition habits, taking into account patient preferences. Refer to a dietitian if appropriate

Cultural Self-Enrichment Exercise

BIOLOGICAL VARIATIONS

- Do you know of any diseases or illnesses you are prone to because of your cultural background?
- Are you at ideal body weight for your height?
- What are your activity habits? Do they need to be improved?
- What is the meaning of food in your culture?
- Do you have any dietary deficiencies or food limitations?
- What cultural or ethnic foods do you prepare at home?
- When you eat out for lunch or dinner, what are your favorite ethnic foods? Which ethnic foods do you not like? Why?
- What dietary practices do you engage in when you are ill?
- What kinds of foods do you eat to stay healthy?
- In your culture or personal belief system, are there any foods that are restricted or taboo?

Death and Dying and End-of-Life Issues

Death rituals of cultural groups are the least likely to change over time. To avoid cultural taboos, you must become knowledgeable about rituals surrounding death and bereavement. For some, the body should be buried whole. Therefore, an amputated limb may be buried in the amputee's future grave site, and organ donation would probably not be acceptable. Cremation may be preferred for some, whereas for others it is taboo and burial is the preferred practice. Views on autopsy vary accordingly. Some cultural groups have elaborate ceremonies that last for days in commemoration of the dead. To some these rituals appear to be a celebration, and in a sense they are a celebration of the person's life rather than a mourning of the person's death. If you are uncertain, find out from the family if there is anything that the health care team can do to facilitate cultural practices.

The expression of grief in response to death varies within and among cultural and ethnic groups. For example, in some cultures, loved ones are expected to suffer the grief of death in silence, with little display of emotion. In other cultures, loved ones are expected to display elaborate emotions to show that they cared for the deceased. These variations in the grieving process may cause confusion if you perceive some people as overreacting and others as not caring. You must accept that culturally diverse behaviors are associated with the grieving process. Bereavement support strategies include being physically present, encouraging reality orientation, openly acknowledging the family's right to grieve as they need to, helping the family express their feelings, encouraging interpersonal relationships, promoting interest in a new life, and making referrals to other staff and spiritual leaders as appropriate.

At times you may be somewhat involved with other end-of-life decisions. Some of these may include advance directives, resuscitation status, and organ transplantation.

Nursing Assessment and Strategies

Ask the following questions of your patients:

- What are the usual burial practices in your family?
- What are your feelings about autopsy?

Be sure to do the following:

- Observe expressions of grief. Support the family in their expression of grief.
- Observe for differences in the expression of grief among family members.
- Offer to obtain a religious counselor/spiritual leader if the family wishes.

Cultural Self-Enrichment Exercise

DEATH AND DYING

- What are the usual burial practices in your family?
- What is expected of family members and friends after a loved one dies?
- How is grief expressed in your family? Are there different expectations for men and women?
- Are any specific rituals associated with death?
- Do you believe in organ transplantation?
- Do you have advance directive?

ETHNIC AND CULTURAL GROUPS IN THE UNITED STATES

This section describes selected attributes of some of the cultural groups in the United States. These groups include European Americans (white), Spanish/Hispanics/Latinos, African Americans (black), American Indians/Alaskan Native, Arab Americans, and Asian Americans/Pacific Islanders. The groups described here by no means represent all the cultural groups in North America; they do, however, represent the largest population percentages in the United States. As of the 2000 census, the federal government initiated new terminology for classifying people of diverse racial and ethnic backgrounds. This terminology is used in this section.

Attributes presented for each group include communication styles, space, time orientation, social organization, environmental control, biological variation, health care beliefs, traditional health care practitioners, and death and dying issues. Traditional health care practitioners are those practitioners from the patient's native culture, such as shamans, herbalists, and other traditional healers. Racial and ethnic biological variations, susceptibility to disease, and genetic diseases are covered to a greater extent elsewhere in this textbook. (See Box 4.2, *Ethical Considerations,* and Box 4.3, *Gerontological Issues.*)

Cultural Self-Assessment Exercise

CULTURAL CHARACTERISTICS

- Identify your primary and secondary cultural characteristics. How do they affect your worldview?
- Share these views with others in your class.

European Americans

European Americans is the term used to describe people living in the United States whose heritage is from England, Scotland, Wales, Ireland, Norway, Switzerland, France, Germany, Sweden, the Netherlands, Belgium, or other northern European countries. European American groups include the white ethnic groups. Many of the descendants of these original European immigrants practice the unique attributes of the subcultures from which they originate. There is much diversity in the primary and secondary characteristics of diversity within this cultural group.

Many European Americans maintain the value of individualism over group norms and are activity oriented. Most European Americans practice Western medicine that uses advanced technology and emphasizes scientific discovery. (See Table 4.1, *Cultural Considerations.*)

Spanish/Hispanics/Latinos

The term *Spanish/Hispanics/Latinos* is used to describe people whose cultural heritage has a strong Spanish influence. However, many people in this group prefer to identify themselves as Chicano or with terms that provide a country of origin, such as Mexican, Peruvian, Puerto Rican, and Cuban (Purnell & Paulanka, 2008). The population breakdown of Spanish/Hispanic/Latino populations in the United States is Mexican Americans (64.3%), Puerto Ricans (10.6%), Central and South Americans (13.4%), Cubans (4.7%), and other groups, including Caribbean (7%) (del Pinal, 2008). Hispanics immigrate from any number of Central and South American countries, the Caribbean, and other Spanish-speaking countries. Thus, there is much diversity in this population in the United States.

Some Spanish/Hispanics/Latinos speak only Spanish, only English, or both Spanish and English, while others speak neither Spanish nor English but rather an Indian dialect. The spoken language depends on individual circumstances and

Box 4.2

Ethical Considerations

Cultural Stereotyping

Sharon, an experienced licensed practical nurse, was on duty on the labor and delivery unit when Ruth and her husband Aaron arrived. Ruth was flushed and distressed and obviously in labor. Aaron was bending over his wife, attempting to coach her breathing, and trying to keep calm. Aaron was wearing a yarmulke, so Sharon assumed they were Jewish.

Despite the expectation of delivering a healthy baby, their infant son was stillborn due to prematurity (30 weeks' gestation) and a "true knot" in the cord that had denied oxygen to the baby during the later stages of the labor and delivery. After the delivery, Ruth was transferred to the medical-surgical unit for postpartum care, a practice commonly followed when stillbirths occur.

Sharon decided to assist the grieving couple by starting the funeral planning. She had done this many times before with positive results, so she expected that the parents would appreciate her efforts.

Sharon told Ruth she had made some preliminary phone calls to start the process of funeral planning. Ruth looked distressed, and Sharon misinterpreted this expression as her unfamiliarity with the funeral home that would be handling the arrangements. Sharon tried to reassure Ruth, stating that she had been present at many funerals of children who had died either before, during, or after birth and the funeral home she had called was reputable and respectful. Sharon recounted her personal experience with these events and stated that sometimes the ritual of the wake, the burial, and the gathering afterward were therapeutic, bringing some closure. Aaron, who was visiting at the time, called Sharon out of the room and indicated his very strong displeasure that Sharon had begun arrangements. He explained rather tersely that he had contacted his rabbi, who as *mara d'atra* [halakhic authority] held the position of authority in Aaron and Ruth's community. The rabbi had made a *p'sak* [ruling/decision]. This *p'sak* meant that although the child was both premature and dead at birth, it was to be treated as a fetus. For this reason, it would be the family that would conduct the funeral, and there would be no ceremony attached. Aaron turned his back on Sharon and went back into the room.

Sharon completed her shift without additional communication with the couple, and Ruth was discharged before Sharon returned the next day. Sharon was plagued with a feeling that she had made a major error in judgment and had failed to meet Ruth's emotional and religious needs.

It is evident from this case that several major ethical principles were either ignored or transgressed. What do you think they were and why?

Discussion and suggested answers at end of chapter.

Box 4.3
Gerontological Issues

Aging, Ethnicity, Health, and Illness

Compared with white or European American older adults, ethnic minorities are more likely to:

- Live in poverty
- Experience debilitating disease processes or functional disability at a higher rate and at an earlier age
- Have greater difficulty accessing health care services
- Be underserved for physical and mental health problems.

By 2030, the number of elderly adults will double. The largest growth will be among minorities. Remember that in order to provide culturally competent care older adults need to be assessed within their personal cultural context. Avoid generalizing cultural practices to individuals or families without first assessing whether this practice or belief is true for the individual. For example, it would be wrong to assume that an older Mexican American woman who lives with her extended family will receive the family's support for assistance with bathing and other activities of daily living. If an older Chinese woman uses herbs and folk treatments for common complaints, it does not mean that she will not use the services, treatments, or medications of Western medicine. Always assess individual and family preferences.

the length of time spent in the United States. Spanish is the second most commonly spoken language in the United States.

Spanish/Hispanics/Latinos compose approximately 15% of the U.S. population (Bernstein, 2008); they recently became the majority minority population. They live in all 50 states with more than 90% living in and around cities. Four of every five Spanish/Hispanics/Latinos are born and raised in the United States. Many of these individuals have come from poverty, and for them money has little value. They sacrifice for their basic needs (Figs. 4.5 and 4.6).

Most Spanish/Hispanics/Latinos practice adaptations of the Roman Catholic religion. Their close relationship with God makes it acceptable for people to have visions and dreams in which God or the saints speak directly to them. Thus, health care providers must be careful not to attribute these culture-bound visions to hallucinations that indicate a need for psychiatric services. (See Table 4.1, *Cultural Considerations.*)

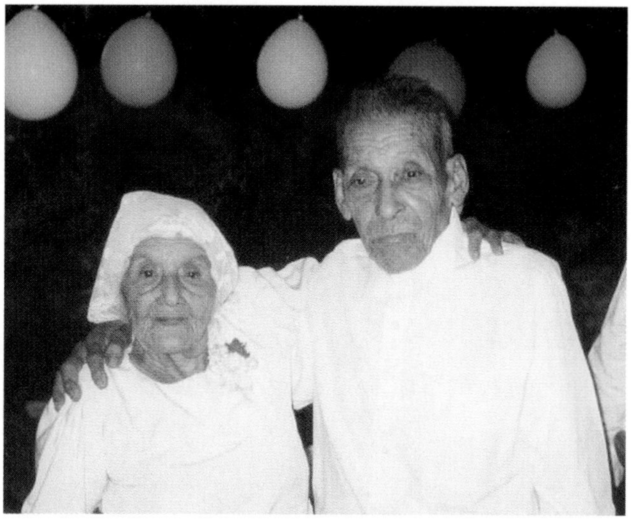

Figure 4.5 Honduran couples wait to get married until they can afford a celebration—at 100 years young in this case.

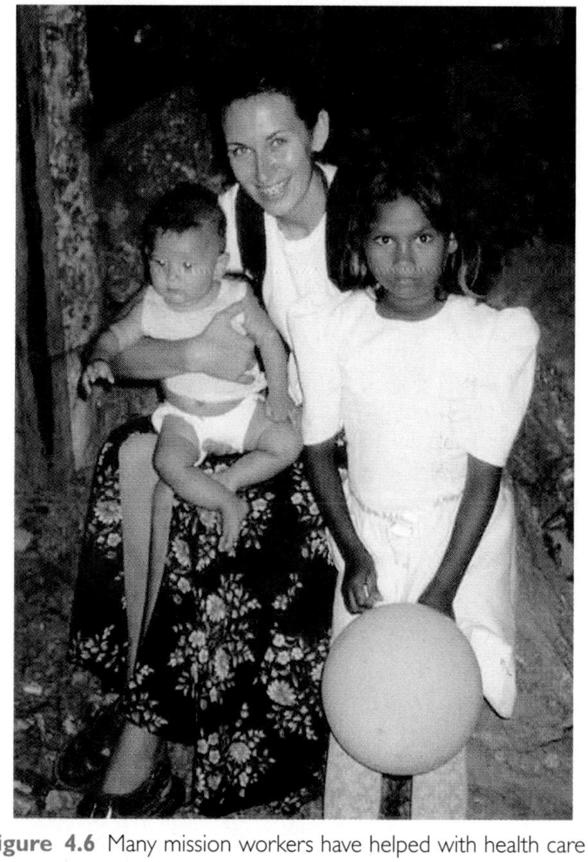

Figure 4.6 Many mission workers have helped with health care needs in Central and South American countries.

African Americans/Blacks

African Americans/blacks are the third largest ethnic group in the United States and represent more than 100 racial strains. They make up 12.3% of the population (Bernstein & Edwards, 2008). Although African Americans/blacks live in all 50 states, more than half live in the South. It is important to understand that not all people with black skin identify themselves as African American. Many black-skinned people from the Caribbean use terms more specific to their identity, such as *Haitian, Jamaican,* or *West Indian.*

African Americans/blacks have been called by many names. Their ancient African name is Nehesu or Nubian.

TABLE 4.1 CULTURAL CONSIDERATIONS*

	European Americans (White)	Spanish/Hispanics/ Latinos	African Americans (Black)	American Indian/ Alaskan Natives	Arab Americans	Asian Americans/ Pacific Islanders
Communication	Primary language is usually English; often speak own national language. Eye contact should be maintained, without staring. Loud voice volume is the norm. Readily shares personal information.	Primary language either English, Spanish, or Portuguese (many dialects). Dramatic body language. Some believe direct eye contact can cause illness ("evil eye").	Primary language is usually English. May speak "black English" occasionally depending on the situation. Usually loud voice volume. Nonverbal communication important; direct eye contact may be interpreted as aggression.	English, tribal languages. Talking loudly may be considered rude. Use body language. Avoid eye contact. Comfortable with long periods of silence. Information should be given over time, allowing adequate time to process information.	Primary language is Arabic. Most speak some English. May use spirited, loud voice. May be reluctant to disclose personal information. Maintain intense eye contact.	English (may prefer national language and specific to each country); many dialects. Loud talking is considered rude. Silence is acceptable. Avoid eye contact. Avoid use of "no."
Space	Depends on area; tend to avoid physical closeness. Handshake proper.	Value physical closeness and touching.	Close personal space. Touch frequently with friends, less so with strangers. Touching another's hair considered improper.	Space very important; has no boundaries. Touch is not acceptable from strangers. Pointing and direct eye contact may be considered rude.	Stand very close when talking. Touch only between same gender.	Avoid physical closeness and touching.
Time Orientation	Future over present.	Present.	Present over future.	Usually present.	Present or future.	Present.
Social Organization	Nuclear family basic, extended family important. Man dominant figure. Judeo-Christian religions. Community social organizations important. Many concerned with status.	Nuclear family basic, extended family highly valued. Man is decision maker; woman is homemaker. Catholicism.	Many female single-parent families, often matriarchal. Large, extended families important. Strong social and church affiliations. Protestant (often Baptist).	Extended family basic unit. Very family oriented. Elders honored. Strong community affiliations. Sacred myths and legends.	Patriarchal household, with well-defined gender roles. Elders respected and cared for by family. Extended family important; may live in close proximity to each other. May be Christian, Jewish, or Muslim.	High value on immediate and extended family. Hierarchical family structure. Family honor and loyalty honored. Tradition important. Male has power; woman is obedient. High value placed on children and education. Christianity, Buddhism, Taoism, and Islamic religions.
Environmental Control/Health Beliefs	Rely mainly on modern health care system. Value individual responsibility for health.	Traditional health and illness beliefs. Folk medicine traditions. Health beliefs are strongly affected by religion, believing in God's will.	Traditional health and illness beliefs. General distrust of health care professionals, practitioners, and the health care system.	Traditional health and illness beliefs. Folk medicine traditions. Promote harmony with nature. Inanimate objects ward off evil spirits.	Focus on acute care over prevention. Illness may be considered punishment for sins. May pray five times a day for health.	Traditional health and illness beliefs. Traditional medicine traditions. Good health is a gift from ancestors.

	Believe humans can control nature. Have strong belief and value in technology. Most use alternative remedies or OTCs before seeing a health care provider. Use prayers and religious symbols for good health. Have controlled expression of pain but need little encouragement to accept pain relief. Sick role not well accepted except with a major illness.	May have shrines or statues in the home to pray for good health. Theory of hot and cold foods used for health maintenance and treatment of disease. Expressive with pain. Easily enter the sick role.	Folk medicine tradition. May believe that serious illness sent from God. Use prayers for prevention and health recovery. Pain is seen as a sign of illness. Sick role not seen as a burden. Folk healers. A respected elderly female community member commonly sought for initial health care.	Elderly may request same-gender direct-care provider. Pain is something to be endured. Sick role not usually supported.	Acceptable to purchase organs for transplantation. Sick role supported. Food is eaten with the right hand, which is considered "clean." May fast while hospitalized. Eating and drinking at the same time is considered unhealthy.	Imbalances in the yin and yang cause illness. Believe blood is the source of life and is not replenished. Amulets worn to ward off disease.
Health Care Practitioners	Traditional healers: Western-educated health care providers; recent trend to use complementary therapists.	Traditional healers: curandero, espiritista, patera, senora.	Traditional healers: spiritualists, voodoo priest or priestess, root doctor.	Traditional healers: shamans, medicine man, diviners, crystal gazers.	Traditional healers: Western-educated health care providers; may prefer same sex caregivers.	Traditional healers: doctors, herbalists, acupuncturists who use such therapies as acupuncture, acumassage, coining, and cupping.
Biological Variations	Nutritional preferences include meats (especially red) and carbohydrates. Diets tend to be high in fat and sodium. Eating and drinking may be social rituals. Culture stresses thinness as attractive. Susceptibility: heart disease, breast cancer, diabetes mellitus, thalassemia, Tay-Sachs disease (Eastern European Jewish).	Nutritional preferences include spicy and fried foods, beans, and rice. Important for food to be served warm. May subscribe to hot and cold theory of illness (e.g., caused when body is exposed to imbalance of hot/cold substances). Food choices vary by specific country. Being overweight may be considered healthy. Susceptibility: lactose intolerance, diabetes mellitus, parasites, coccidioidomycosis, gout.	Nutritional preferences include fried foods, barbecued foods, greens, legumes. Diet commonly high in fat and sodium. Food selections may vary according to socioeconomic status and rural versus urban residence. Being overweight is seen as positive. Food is seen as a symbol of health and wealth.	Nutritional preferences vary greatly depending on location and tribe. Nontraditional diets tend to be high in fat and commonly lack fruits and vegetables. Herbs used to cleanse the body of evil spirits and poison. Susceptibility: heart disease, alcoholism, liver disease, diabetes mellitus, tuberculosis, arthritis, glaucoma.	Nutritional preferences include fresh meats and vegetables; may avoid pork and alcohol (Islam). Less likely than general population to smoke, drink alcohol, or use illicit drugs. High risk for diabetes, hypertension, hypercholesterolemia.	Nutritional preferences include raw fish and rice. Foods are balanced between yin and yang. Diet is high in salt. Food is fundamental form of socialization. Susceptibility: lactose intolerance, thalassemia, liver and stomach cancer, hypertension, coccidioidomycosis.

Continued

TABLE 4.1 CULTURAL CONSIDERATIONS*—cont'd

	European Americans (White)	Spanish/Hispanics/ Latinos	African Americans (Black)	American Indian/ Alaskan Natives	Arab Americans	Asian Americans/ Pacific Islanders
			Susceptibility: keloid formation, lactose intolerance, sickle cell anemia, glucose-6-phosphate dehydrogenase deficiency, thalassemia, sarcoidosis, hypertension, coccidioidomycosis, esophageal and stomach cancers.			
Death and Dying Issues	Autopsy and burial or cremation usually connected with religious practices or individual preferences. Have varied expressions of grief. Men are expected to be in more control during grief than women.	Burial is the usual practice, rarely cremation; many resist autopsy, the body should be buried whole. May have elaborate ceremonial burial. Women very expressive with grief; men are expected to maintain control.	Death does not end connection between people; body is kept intact after death; prefer no autopsy. Relatives may communicate with the dead person. Offer eulogy at burial with religious songs. Usually prefer burial. Express grief openly.	Believe body should go into the afterlife whole. Some engage in a cleansing ceremony after touching a dead body. Tribal laws may dictate cremation versus burial. Openly express grief.	Believe death is God's will. At time of death, bed should face the holy city of Mecca (for Muslims). May perform ritual washing of the body after death. Cremation or autopsy not acceptable. May weep with grief, but limited.	Autopsy not understood by many. Cremation acceptable, but burial also common. Extended grieving time (7 to 30 days) for the more traditional. Expression of grief is highly varied between men and women and among specific countries.
Nursing Considerations	Respect personal space. Encourage health screening and preventive health care strategies. Encourage low-fat, low-cholesterol, high-fiber diet.	Ask who makes decisions for the family. Reinforce need to be on time for appointments. Collaborate on decision of what is an acceptable weight.	Negotiate acceptable weight. When possible, encourage participation of similar ethnic minorities in planning care and to promote healthy interactions.	Incorporate time for processing information. Use silence therapeutically. Monitor body language.	Respect nutritional requests, and try to obtain specific dietary requests. Attempt to provide same-sex caregiver. Screen for domestic violence.	Monitor for cues of expression and body language. Inquire in a nonjudgmental manner regarding use of traditional medicine. Provide same-sex care provider when possible.

*Although many other cultural groups are represented in the United States, the most common are presented here.
Sources: Bernstein, 2008; Purnell & Paulanka, 2008.

During slavery days in America, they were called *Negro,* a Spanish-Portuguese word meaning "black." After emancipation in 1863, they were called *colored,* a term adopted by the First Colored Men's Convention in the United States in 1831. The U.S. Bureau of the Census adopted the word *Negro* in 1880. During the civil rights movements in the 1960s, the term *black* was used to signify a philosophy of life instead of color. In the 1970s, these ethnic peoples referred to themselves as African Americans because they were proud of both their African and American heritages. In 1988, the term *African American* was widely adopted in the United States by those whose ancestry originated from Africa. These terms continue to cause confusion when people try to use the "politically correct" term for this group in the United States. Additionally, titles such as the National Black Nurses Association and the National Association for the Advancement of Colored People (NAACP) still exist.

African Americans/blacks are underrepresented in colleges and universities, managerial and administrative positions, and the health care professions. They are overrepresented in high-risk, hazardous occupations such as the steel and tire industries, construction industries, and high-pollution factories. (See Table 4.1, *Cultural Considerations.*) The election of an African American president of the United States in 2008, whose education initiatives include outreach programs for low-income families and increased availability of advance placement classes nationwide, will likely have an impact on such issues in the future.

CRITICAL THINKING

Ms. Williams

■ Now that you have learned more about culture, let's look at Ms. Williams again. Review Table 4.1, *Cultural Considerations,* and answer the following questions:

1. What does your interaction with Ms. Williams tell you about her time orientation?
2. What is evident about her social organization?
3. What biological variations may Ms. Williams demonstrate that are likely part of her culture?

Suggested answers at end of chapter.

American Indians/Alaskan Natives

There are more than 400 American Indian/Alaskan Native tribes in the United States, totaling 1.6% of the population (Bernstein & Edwards, 2008). Although there are similarities among Native Americans, each tribe has its own unique perspective on health and illness. Many traditional American Indians/Alaskan Natives live on reservations; others live in urban areas and practice few of their traditions. Many American Indians/Alaskan Natives have a strong belief that illness is caused by an imbalance with nature and the universe. Tribal identity is maintained through powwows, ceremonial events, and arts and crafts that are taught to children at a young age. Communicating with nature is important for maintaining life forces. American Indians/Alaskan Natives are the original inhabitants of North America.

American Indians/Alaskan Natives are underrepresented in all of the health professions. They are consistently identified as the most underrepresented minority group in institutions of higher learning (Bernstein, 2008). (See Table 4.1, *Cultural Considerations.*)

Arab Americans

Arab Americans are a large and diverse population, with more than 3,000,000 in the United States. Some common bonds include the Arabic language and the Islamic religion. Arab Americans include people from Morocco, Algeria, Tunisia, Libya, Sudan, Egypt and the western Asian countries of Lebanon, occupied Palestine, Syria, Jordan, Iraq, Iran, Kuwait, Bahrain, Qatar, United Arab Emirates, Saudi Arabia, Oman, and Yemen. Many early Arab immigrants were Christians from Lebanon and Syria.

Although many Arab Americans favor professional occupations, many are underemployed, have their own businesses, and work in a variety of other occupations. Arab Americans, whether born in the United States or in Arab countries, are more educated than the average American. They are more likely to be in managerial and professional specialty occupations than any other ethnic group in America. However, a significant number of primarily foreign-born Arab Americans are unemployed and live in poverty.

Asian Americans/Pacific Islanders

This large group is far from homogeneous. The term *Asian,* as used in most references, includes 32 different groups. These groups include Asians, Pacific Islanders, Indochinese, and other Asian groups. Asians include people from Korea, Japan, and 54 ethnic groups from China. Pacific Islanders include Hawaiians, Polynesians, Filipinos, Malaysians, and Guamanians. Indochinese populations include Cambodian, Vietnamese, Hmong, and Laotian. Other Asian groups include Asian Indian, Pakistani, and Thai. Although it is difficult to determine exact numbers of Asians from specific countries because of the method of keeping population statistics, they are a significant and fast-growing population in the United States.

It is important for many Asian patients to "save face." Individual shame is shared with the family and community. Most Asians see the nurse as an authority figure. Although known by different names, most Asian cultures practice the *yin* and *yang* balance of forces for illness prevention and maintaining health. Yin is considered female and represents cold and weakness. Yang is considered male and represents strength and warmth. Foods and all forces are classified as yin or yang and must be balanced or illness occurs. Yin and yang forces are major components of traditional Chinese medicine, which includes acupressure, acupuncture, and cupping. (See Table 4.1, *Cultural Considerations.*)

CULTURALLY COMPETENT CARE

The American Nurses Association supports the need for nurses to understand cultural diversity and to become culturally competent. However, there is no real agreement as to how your knowledge, skills, and attitudes will best help these diverse populations. You certainly cannot achieve cultural competence overnight; it is a developmental process. Each time you care for a patient from a different culture, you learn more, become more aware and sensitive to individual needs, and move toward becoming culturally competent.

There are a number of models and theories that describe cultural competence. In addition, you will find that a number of good resource books and websites are available to assist you on this journey.

The following strategies for providing culturally competent care may be helpful:

- Consider each of your patients as unique, influenced but not defined by his or her culture.
- Know your own cultural values, beliefs, and practices, and appreciate how they may be different from those of others.
- Never let your own biases about people and groups stand in the way of culturally competent care.
- Learn as much as you can about cultural groups in your community.
- Make an effort to include beliefs and practices from other cultures into your care when appropriate.
- Try to encourage helpful cultural practices and discourage harmful ones.
- Be aware of how you communicate with others; be aware of verbal and nonverbal patterns.
- Respect your patients regardless of their cultural backgrounds.
- Learn from your mistakes.

This list does not include everything you can do. Can you think of other strategies?

CRITICAL THINKING

The Lopez Family

■ Jose, age 23, and his wife, Louisa, age 19, immigrated to the United States 3 years ago from Mexico. They have two children, Maria, 3 years old, and Jesus, 6 months old. The young couple has brought the children to the emergency room for the treatment of ear infections. Jose informs you that Maria has a sore throat and ear pain and Jesus is "fussy" and not eating. He states that he has been to his *curandero,* but neither child has improved. You also notice that the children are dressed in heavy clothing, although it is quite warm outside. When you question the parents, Louisa responds that they are "cold."

Jesus is admitted to the hospital for dehydration. As you are admitting the infant to your unit, you are aware that Jose is answering all of your questions and making decisions for Jesus's care. He states that they will all need to spend the night with Jesus. Jose further adds that Jesus needs more clothes on and that the temperature in the room needs to be increased. The parents refuse the warmed bottle of formula for Jesus but ask for it to be chilled. Louisa sits in the corner of the room chanting, crying, and rubbing some beads.

1. What nonverbal communication characteristics do these parents display that are common among people of Spanish descent?
2. Why do you think the children are dressed inappropriately for the weather?
3. Do Jose's demands mean that he is uncooperative and trying to control the care of his son?
4. Why do you think Jose refused his son's warm bottle?
5. What is the significance of Louisa's behavior?
6. What might you do to improve Jesus's care?
7. How will you handle the father's request for the entire family to stay in your patient's room?
8. How can you become more culturally competent in this situation?

Suggested answers at end of chapter.

LEARNING TIP

Take a trip to BALI:

Be aware of your own cultural heritage.

Appreciate that your patient is unique; influenced but not defined by his or her culture.

Learn about your patients' cultural groups.

Incorporate your patients' cultural values, beliefs, and practices into their plan of care.

REFLECTIONS ON MS. WILLIAMS

After learning more about culture, how do you think the characteristics of Ms. Williams' culture affected her behavior? At her age, it is evident that she has learned many of her beliefs and practices about health and illness from others. While many of her behaviors can be explained by fear and denial, it is probable that other things are going on in this situation. Ms. Williams may feel more comfortable with people of her own culture, at least when it comes to asking for health information. She may not trust biomedical or Western medicine treatments. She may be more comfortable with the practices and healers that she knows better. Can you think of other explanations?

Rarely do practicing nurses have the luxury to assess each patient comprehensively on a first encounter. The essentials for culturally competent care are obtained as needed. As you meet patients from other cultures, continue to learn about theses new cultures. Astute observations, openness to diversity, and willingness to learn from patients are what you need for effective cross-cultural competence in clinical practice. Through these avenues, you can provide culturally competent nursing care. Cultural competence is not a luxury; it is a necessity.

Remember that it is important that you acknowledge that there are similarities within a group. This does not mean that *all* of the people in the group have all of those characteristics. You must see each of your patients as being unique.

Home Health Hints

- The effects of a patient's cultural beliefs and practices related to health care are more evident when care is provided in the home. The nurse must adapt care to the patient's environment rather than the patient adapting to the nurse's hospital environment. The nurse is a guest in the patient's home.
- When scheduling a home visit, it is important to find out the primary language spoken in the home. It is also helpful to carry a translation book when the language is known. If necessary, arrange to have an interpreter available to ensure understanding of what is discussed.
- If you have a personal digital assistant (PDA), you can also download a language translator to have available to assist with communication. Many translation programs are available; a simple Web search can help you to determine what best meets your needs.
- Be aware of the cultural significance of family hierarchy. Avoid having children translate for parents.

ETHICAL CONSIDERATIONS DISCUSSION

It is evident from this story that the traditional American or Christian conception of the rituals associated with the death of a child may not be held by other cultures, including this Jewish patient and her husband. Upon reflection, Sharon realized that she had not respected this couple's *autonomy*, or provided an environment that would foster the *creation of autonomy*. She had failed to *minimize harm*, failed to produce the most *beneficial outcome* for Aaron and Ruth, and had not familiarized herself with the wishes of the couple.

Sharon did not serve her clients' needs first. She should have determined what Ruth and Aaron needed at that sensitive time. Instead, she assumed she knew what was required and subsequently made choices that were offensive to her clients. Were her clients harmed? If Sharon had known that there were significant religious protocols to be observed in this situation, would she have initiated the funeral planning? Sharon could have been more helpful by asking the parents if they needed assistance in the initial stages of funeral planning. Aaron and Ruth may indeed have asked Sharon to be involved in the preparations and funeral.

Instead of acting on assumptions and applying our own vision of what a client may need, nurses need to assess a family's values, gather appropriate information about their culture, and find what the role expectations are in each situation, creating an atmosphere of mutual respect and open communication. Patients' values and preferences cannot be assumed, even when nurses can correctly identify the culture of the family. Cultural stereotyping is a mistake that is easy to make. However, if we approach our clients with an open and nonjudgmental attitude, we will be able to gather the data that is essential to providing culturally competent nursing care.

SUGGESTED ANSWERS TO CRITICAL THINKING

■ *Ms. Williams*

1. African Americans may be present oriented. Her seeming lack of concern about her diabetes may reflect hesitance to worry about a future that is not here yet.
2. Family is very important. She prays for healing.
3. We do not know Ms. Williams weight, but overweight may be seen as positive and excess weight is a risk factor for diabetes and hypertension.

■ *The Lopez Family*

1. Jose's behavior indicates that he is the primary decision maker and in charge of this situation. Louisa's crying is normal. She is most likely praying.

SUGGESTED ANSWERS TO—cont'd

■ *The Lopez Family*

2. This may relate to the couple's beliefs in the hot and cold theory.
3. His role as father may dictate that he should maintain control. He probably does not mean to be uncooperative.
4. Again, this may be related to hot and cold beliefs about treatment of diseases.
5. Louisa's culture-bound role does not dictate that she assume control of the situation. She is upset and praying.
6. Attempt to incorporate the family's cultural beliefs and practices when possible.
7. Explain that it would not be good for Maria to remain in the hospital, because she will be at greater risk for exposure to infection. Ask if there are other relatives who can care for Maria. Find out if the parents can divide their time with their son.
8. Be aware of your own cultural beliefs, appreciate your patient's culture, learn more about the Lopez family's culture (ask questions), and include their beliefs and practices when possible. Explain when other practices cannot be followed. Ask for alternatives.

REVIEW QUESTIONS

1. A nurse who assumes all patients have the same beliefs as his or her own culture is exhibiting which one of the following?
   a. Cultural stereotyping
   b. Ethnocentrism
   c. Cultural sensitivity
   d. Cultural dominance

2. A 12-year-old Mexican child needs an appendectomy. His parents bring in the priest from their church to pray over the child. The prayers are continuing when it is time to take the child to surgery. How should the nurse respond?
   a. Gently tell the parents that they must stop praying so the child can be taken to surgery.
   b. Give the parents and priest as much time as they need for prayers before surgery.
   c. Tell the parents that the child could die from a ruptured appendix if surgery is delayed.
   d. Permit the parents and priest to stay and pray as the child goes into surgery.

3. An Osage American Indian woman is slow at giving responses and does not maintain eye contact with the nurse when her admission interview is being conducted. Which of the following interpretations of her behavior is most likely accurate?
   a. Direct eye contact may be interpreted as rude in her culture.
   b. She does not want to answer personal questions.
   c. She does not understand the nurse.
   d. She does not want to talk with a nurse and prefers a physician.

4. An Arab American man is refusing his dinner tray, which consists of potatoes with cheese, a slice of ham, and green beans. What knowledge should guide the nurse's data collection related to this incident?
   a. Arabs do not like foods from different sources on the same plate.
   b. Some Arabs do not eat dairy products.
   c. Islamic Arabs may not eat pork.
   d. Arabs typically do not eat vegetables.

5. A Puerto Rican man has been admitted for reconstructive orthopedic surgery on his knee. His wife brings jars of special blends of spices that he wants to put on his food because the hospital food is too bland. He is on a general diet. What action should the nurse take?
   a. Let him use them.
   b. Carefully explain that family cannot bring food items to the hospital.
   c. Have the dietitian speak with the family.
   d. Report the situation to the physician.

References

Bernstein, R. (2008). *Hispanic population surpasses 45 million. Now 15 percent of total.* Washington, DC: U.S. Census Bureau and U.S. Department of Commerce. Retrieved March 22, 2009, from http://www.census.gov/Press-Release/www/releases/archives/population/011910.html

Bernstein, R., & Edwards, T. (2008). *An older and more diverse nation by midcentury.* Washington, DC: U.S. Census Bureau, U.S. Department of Commerce. Retrieved March 16, 2009, from http://www.census.gov/Press-Release/www/releases/archives/population/012496.html

del Pinal, J. (2008). *The Hispanic population.* Washington, DC: U.S. Census Bureau, Population Division and Housing and Household Economic Statistics Division. Retrieved May 8, 2009, from http://www.census.gov/population/www/pop-profile/hisppop.html

Purnell, L., & Paulanka, B. (Eds.). (2008). *Transcultural health care: A culturally competent approach.* Philadelphia: F.A. Davis Company.

5

Complementary and Alternative Modalities

CYNTHIA BARRERE AND
COLLEEN DELANEY

KEY TERMS

acupuncture (ak-yoo-PUNGK-chur)
allopathic (AL-oh-PATH-ik)
Ayurvedic (AY-YUR-VAY-dik)
chiropractic (ky-roh-PRAK-tik)
homeopathy (HO-mee-AH-pa-thee)
naturopathy (NAY-chur-AH-pa-thee)
osteopathic (AHS-tee-ah-PATH-ik)

QUESTIONS TO GUIDE YOUR READING

1. What is the difference between a complementary and an alternative modality?
2. What are some systems of health care that have contributed to the development of new modalities?
3. How are the different types of modalities classified?
4. What are some safety issues in complementary and alternative modalities?
5. What is the role of the licensed practical nurse/licensed vocational nurse (LPN/LVN) in assisting a patient with complementary and alternative modalities?

Health care in the 21st century requires that nurses recognize the shift toward the inclusion of complementary and alternative approaches to care. Nurses at all levels and in every area of practice are answering the call to use new methods to care for those who are ill and enhance the health of those who are well.

Holistic nursing was a precursor to many of the now popular complementary and alternative modalities. It was introduced in the 1970s and has been growing ever since. Holistic nursing is simply defined as caring for the whole person—body, mind, and spirit—in a constantly changing environment.

Box 5.1

Gerontological Issues

About 88% of older adults use some form of alternative therapy, but most are unlikely to report the use of these therapies to their physician. Alternative therapies are commonly used to treat arthritis, back pain, heart disease, allergies, and diabetes. Personal beliefs and lifestyle are motivating factors for those who chose to use alternative therapies (Cuellar, Rogers, & Hisghman, 2007).

COMPLEMENTARY OR ALTERNATIVE: WHAT'S THE DIFFERENCE?

The words *complementary* and *alternative* are sometimes used interchangeably, but they are not the same. *Complementary therapy* refers to a therapy used in addition to a conventional therapy. For example, a nurse might suggest guided imagery, music, and relaxation techniques for pain control in addition to prescribed drug therapy. *Alternative therapy*, sometimes called "unconventional" therapy, refers to a therapy used instead of conventional or mainstream therapy. An example is using acupuncture instead of analgesics.

A good resource for current information about complementary and alternative modalities is the National Center for Complementary and Alternative Medicine at www.nccam.nih.gov. To learn about holistic nursing and complementary modalities, visit the American Holistic Nurses Association at www.ahna.org.

INTRODUCTION OF NEW SYSTEMS INTO TRADITIONAL AMERICAN HEALTH CARE

There are many new and different philosophies within the scope of expanded medical and nursing practice. These systems reflect cultures and attitudes in healing that range from East to West and from ancient to modern. In a landmark study, Eisenberg et al. (1993) reported that unconventional therapy use in the United States far exceeded previous estimates. Of the 1,539 adults interviewed, one in three (34%) reported using at least one unconventional modality during the previous year. More recent findings confirm that this trend is increasing, indicating a need for health care providers to ask patients about their use of complementary and alternative modalities (Eisenberg et al., 1998; Tindle et al., 2005) (Box 5.1, *Gerontological Issues*).

In the United States, the primary system of medicine is just called *medicine,* although some people refer to it as **allopathic** medicine. A number of other schools of thought and philosophies are also being increasingly used. The most frequently seen new systems include Ayurvedic, Chinese, chiropractic, naturopathic, American Indian, and osteopathic medicine. Each philosophical system can stand alone or, as in most instances in the United States, be used in combination with other systems. Most of these recently introduced systems use complementary and alternative modalities.

Allopathic/Western Medicine

The most common name for allopathic medicine is *Western medicine.* Other commonly used terms for Western medicine are *conventional medicine* and *mainstream medicine.* Many people have not heard the term *allopathic* because most doctors and nurses do not refer to themselves or their practice by this name. Practitioners of other systems of medicine more often use the term when referring to what most people consider mainstream medicine. Allopathy is a method of treating disease with remedies that produce effects different from those caused by the disease itself. For example, when a patient has a bacterial infection, a Western medical practitioner prescribes an antibiotic to eliminate the invading pathogen.

Practitioners of Western medicine are medical doctors, nurses, and allied health personnel. This system of medicine uses scientific data to determine the validity of a diagnosis and the effectiveness of treatment—this is called evidence-based medicine. Peer-reviewed medical literature is very important. In scientific investigations, results can be verified and reproduced through various types of studies and statistical analyses. Practitioners use a variety of therapies, including drugs, surgery, and radiation therapy. Western medicine practitioners have made most of the significant advances and developments in modern medicine.

For further information see the American Medical Association site at www.ama-assn.org.

Ayurvedic Medicine

Ayurveda is the ancient Hindu system of medicine, which originated in India. **Ayurvedic** medicine's main goals are to maintain the health of healthy people and cure the illnesses

• WORD • BUILDING •

allopathic: allos—other + pathic—disease or suffering

Ayurvedic: ayu—life + veda—knowledge or science

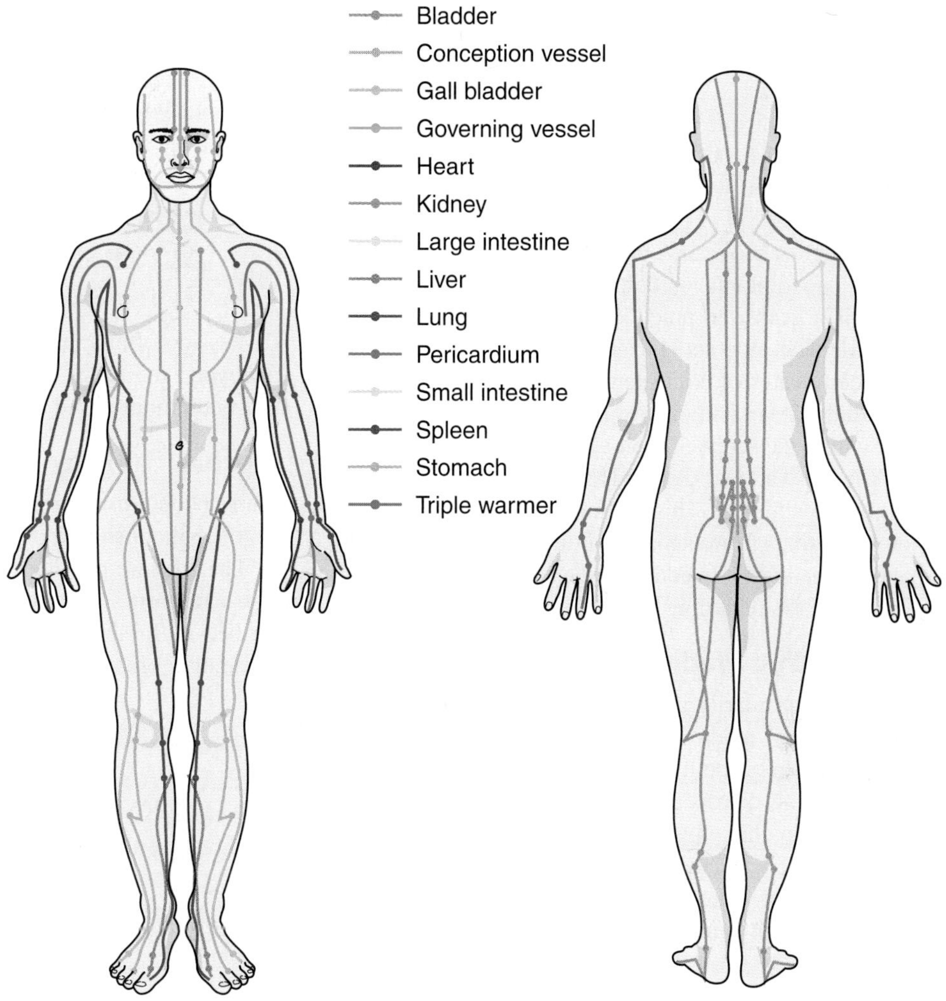
Bladder
Conception vessel
Gall bladder
Governing vessel
Heart
Kidney
Large intestine
Liver
Lung
Pericardium
Small intestine
Spleen
Stomach
Triple warmer

FIGURE 5.1 Qi meridians are used in the Chinese medicine techniques of acupressure and acupuncture.

of sick people. Ayurveda maintains that illness is the result of falling out of balance with nature. Diagnosis is based on three metabolic body types called *doshas.* An Ayurvedic doctor determines which dosha type is most appropriate for the patient: *vata*, *pitta*, or *kapha*. Treatment usually involves prescribing a diet, herbal remedies, breath work, physical exercise, yoga, meditation, massage, and a rejuvenation or detoxification program.

Ayurveda is rapidly becoming more popular in America. The books and videos of Deepak Chopra are examples of this increasingly popular system of therapy. An introduction to Ayurveda can be found at www.ayurveda.org.

Traditional Chinese Medicine

Traditional Chinese medicine is thousands of years old and involves such techniques and practices as acupuncture, acupressure, herbs, massage, and qi gong. The diagnosis and treatment of disturbances of qi (pronounced "chee")—or vital energy—are distinctive characteristics of Chinese medicine.

Acupuncturists, one type of traditional Chinese medicine practitioners, claim to be able to tell much about a patient's state of health by checking pulses, looking at the color of the tongue, checking facial color, assessing voice and smell, and asking a variety of questions. To treat patients with **acupuncture**, acupuncturists insert one or more needles along the meridians (pathways) where qi flows (Fig. 5.1). Many acupuncturists prescribe herbal remedies as well. Find information on how acupuncture is being integrated into Western medicine at www.medical-acupuncture.org.

Chiropractic Medicine

Daniel David Palmer founded chiropractic therapy in 1895. **Chiropractic** medicine is based on the belief that illness is a result of nerve dysfunction. The main treatment modality of chiropractors is manual adjustment and manipulation of the vertebral column and the limbs. They use direct hand contact and mechanical and electrical treatment methods to manipulate joints. The goal is to remove interference with nerve function so the body can heal itself. Chiropractors do not perform surgery, nor do they prescribe drugs. Review the American Chiropractic Association site at www.amerchiro.org for additional information.

• WORD • BUILDING •

acupuncture: acus—needle + punctura—puncture
chiropractic: cheir—hand + pracktos—to do

Homeopathic Medicine

Homeopathy was developed by Samuel Hahnemann in Germany in the early 19th century. Homeopathy is based on Hahnemann's principle that "like cures like," meaning that tiny doses of a substance that create the symptoms of disease in a healthy person will relieve those symptoms in a sick person.

Although schools and courses do exist for training homeopaths, no diploma or certificate from any school or program is a license to practice homeopathy in the United States. Medical doctors and doctors of osteopathy are granted certificates of competency to practice homeopathy. Other health care practitioners may be allowed to use homeopathy within the scope of their state licenses.

Visit the National Center for Homeopathy website at www.homeopathic.org. This site has a research section with annotated listings from the medical literature discussing the value of homeopathy. In addition, the site has a good review of licensing laws regarding homeopathy.

Naturopathic Medicine

Naturopathy primarily uses natural therapies such as nutrition, botanical medicine (herbs), hydrotherapy (water-based therapy), counseling, physical medicine, and homeopathy to treat disease, promote healing, and prevent illness. Naturopathic physicians have a doctor of naturopathy (ND) degree and can be licensed in 11 states. There are three schools of naturopathic medicine in the United States. For more information about naturopathy, visit www.naturopathic.org.

American Indian Medicine

American Indian medical practices vary from tribe to tribe. In general, American Indian medicine is a community-based system with rituals and practices such as the sweat lodge, herbal remedies, the medicine wheel, the sacred hoop, the "sing," and shamanistic healing. For example, an ill person may be placed in a small, enclosed sweat lodge while singing or chanting is done outside the lodge. It is believed that toxic substances are drawn out in the sweat of the person inside the lodge. After the ceremony, the ill person may be placed on a cot outside and be prayed over. Learn more about American Indian medicine at the Association of American Indian Physicians' website at www.aaip.org.

Osteopathic Medicine

Osteopathic medicine was founded in the United States in 1874 by Andrew Taylor Still, a frontier physician who was dissatisfied with the state of medicine at that time. This practice of medicine emphasizes the interrelationship of the body's nerves, muscles, bones, and organs. The osteopathic philosophy involves treating the whole person, recognizes the body's ability to heal itself, and stresses the importance of diet, exercise, and fitness with a focus on prevention. For more information about osteopathy, visit the American Osteopathic Association website at www.aoa-net.org.

• WORD • BUILDING •

homeopathy: homeo—like + pathos—disease
naturopathy: naturo—nature + pathy—disease
osteopathic: osteo—bone + pathy—disease

COMPLEMENTARY AND ALTERNATIVE MODALITIES

Discussion of all complementary and alternative modalities is beyond the scope of this text. Table 5.1 summarizes the most commonly used modalities.

Herbal Therapy

Many people use herbs for healing. However, when doing so, the patient should only take herbs under the supervision of a health care provider. Herbs can aid in healing, but they also can harm. Some of the more common herbs are described in Table 5.2. Figure 5.2 shows echinacea, an herb commonly prepared for use as an immune system booster.

TABLE 5.1 CATEGORIES AND TYPES OF COMPLEMENTARY AND ALTERNATIVE MODALITIES

Category of Therapy	Types of Individual Therapies
Biologically based modalities	Herbal medicine Nutrition and special diet therapies Nutritional supplements
Mind-body modalities	Art therapy Dance therapy Guided imagery Hypnosis and hypnotherapy Meditation and relaxation Music/sound therapies Prayer Tai chi and qi gong Yoga
Manipulative and body-based modalities	Acupressure Chiropractic Massage and related massage therapies Osteopathic manipulation
Energetic modalities	Biofeedback Healing touch Magnet therapy Polarity therapy Reiki Spiritual healing Therapeutic touch
Miscellaneous therapies	Aquatherapy/hydrotherapy Aromatherapy Chanting Chelation therapy Colon therapy Kinesiology Light therapy Pet therapy

TABLE 5.2 COMMON HERBS AND THEIR INTENDED PROPERTIES AND USES

Herb	Purported Properties/Uses
Aloe vera	Soothing agent, used for skin lesions Toxin absorber
Bee pollen	Increases energy, stamina, and strength
Capsaicin	For tenderness and pain of osteoarthritis, fibromyalgia, diabetic neuropathy, and shingles
Chamomile	For anxiety, stomach distress, and infant colic
Echinacea	Antiviral Used for colds, flu, and other infections
Feverfew	Anti-inflammatory Used for migraine headaches and as an appetite stimulant Promotes menstruation, eliminates worms, suppresses fever
Garlic	Reduces low-density lipoprotein and raises high-density lipoprotein cholesterol Reduces blood pressure Suppresses platelet aggregation, increases arterial elasticity, and decreases atherosclerotic plaque formation
Ginger	Reduces nausea and vomiting, hypertension, and high cholesterol
Ginkgo	May improve memory and help cognitive function in Alzheimer's disease
Ginseng	Reduces stress and increases alertness Numerous other claims, such as lowers cholesterol, balances blood glucose levels, slows the aging process, treats memory loss
Kava	For anxiety, insomnia, low energy, muscle tension
St. John's wort	For mild to moderate depression; viral infections, including human immunodeficiency virus (HIV); and herpes

Warning: Herbs may have many side effects and may interact with many prescribed and over-the-counter medications. Urge patients to consult health care providers before self-prescribing.

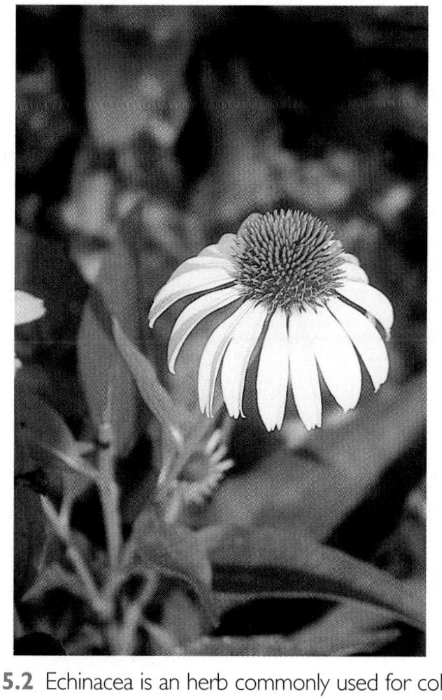

FIGURE 5.2 Echinacea is an herb commonly used for colds and flu.

It is important to note that herbal remedies are not foods. They have potent medicinal effects and can interact with prescribed medications and even complicate surgery. This can be problematic, both because herbs are readily available in health food stores and drugstores and because many patients do not tell their doctors or nurses about their herb use. For example, three common herbs, garlic, ginkgo, and ginseng, can each increase the risk of bleeding when taken with anticoagulant or antiplatelet medications. Another popular herb is St. John's wort, widely used for depression. It can interact adversely with many drugs, including other antidepressant agents and digoxin (Lanoxin). Be sure to assess patients' use of herbs and supplements, and educate them about the need to inform health care providers when using herbs.

A great website for you and your patients is www.mayoclinic.com. Just click on the *Drugs and Supplements* link and type in the herb you want to know about. They even have an *Evidence* section that grades the evidence of the herb's effectiveness for each disorder it is supposed to treat. Grades range from A, which indicates strong evidence for the herb's use, to F, which indicates strong evidence against its use.

Relaxation Therapies

Progressive Muscle Relaxation

Progressive muscle relaxation is a simple technique to learn. It is the process of alternately tensing and relaxing muscle groups. Often this process is performed in a systematic manner, such as from toes to head. The purpose of the technique is to help the participant identify subtle levels of mental and physical tension that accompany mental and emotional stress. When our conscious awareness of the tensions increases, we can learn to relax and thus reduce the effects of stress and tension.

LEARNING TIP

Try using progressive muscle relaxation the next time you are anxious during a nursing examination.

Guided Imagery

Guided imagery is another example of a complementary therapy that many nurses use. Guided imagery involves using mental images to promote physical healing or changes in attitudes or behavior. Practitioners may lead patients through visualization exercises or offer instruction in using imagery as a self-help tool. Guided imagery is often used to alleviate stress and to treat stress-related conditions such as insomnia and high blood pressure. People with cancer, acquired immunodeficiency syndrome (AIDS), chronic fatigue syndrome, and other disorders can use specific images to boost the immune system. Guided imagery is often an added layer of therapy for someone who has learned the progressive relaxation skill discussed previously.

A common guided imagery technique begins with a general relaxation process. For those new to the process, it is good to begin with the progressive muscle relaxation as explained above. Guided imagery works best when all of the senses are used. The exercise in Box 5.2 is very basic but gives an idea of how the technique works. When used for healing, many more steps are involved. It is important to note that appropriate training and skills are needed before using complementary and alternative modalities with patients. Find more on guided imagery at www.nccam.nih.gov; type "guided imagery" into the search window.

Box 5.2

Guided Imagery

Assist your patient to progress through the following steps:

- Assume a comfortable position in a quiet environment.
- Close your eyes and keep them closed until the exercise is completed.
- Breathe in and out deeply to the count of four, repeating this step four times.
- When relaxed, think of a favorite peaceful place and prepare to take an imaginary journey there.
- Picture what this place looks like and how comfortable you feel being there.
- Listen to all the sounds; feel the gentle, clean air; and smell the pleasant aromas.
- Continue to breathe deeply, and appreciate the feeling of being in this special place.
- Feel the sense of deep relaxation and peace of this place.
- As you continue to breathe deeply, slowly and gently bring your consciousness back to the setting in this room.
- Slowly and gently open your eyes, stretch, and think about how relaxed you feel.

LEARNING TIP

When you are stumped on a test question, close your eyes and imagine yourself asking the question of your favorite instructor. Imagine what his or her answer would be.

Biofeedback

Biofeedback could be considered the third tier of learning progressive relaxation. This technique is used especially for stress-related conditions such as asthma, migraines, insomnia, and high blood pressure. Biofeedback is a way of monitoring and controlling tiny metabolic changes in one's body with the aid of sensitive machines that provide feedback (Box 5.3, *Patient Perspective*).

Massage Therapy

Massage is the use of touch to achieve therapeutic results, and can include pressure, friction, and kneading of the body. Massage can be used to relax muscles, reduce anxiety, increase circulation, and reduce pain.

Massage also provides a caring form of touch. In the past, a back massage was a nightly routine for hospitalized patients, helping them relax for sleep. Sadly, today, patients are often not touched except during technical procedures.

You can learn basic massage techniques in nursing school. You may also choose to obtain formal massage therapy education in order to practice more advanced techniques.

SAFETY TIP

Do not use firm massage on a patient taking an anticoagulant or a patient with a low platelet level. Tissue injury could cause bleeding.

Aquatherapy

Sitting in a warm tub can feel good as aching, tired muscles relax and mental stress is decreased. People who suffer from arthritis or other chronic pain understand how warm water can ease their discomfort. Relaxing in water feels good for three reasons: warmth, water movement causing massage, and buoyancy.

Long before analgesics were developed, the human body relied on its own naturally occurring, internally generated, pain-killing chemicals called endorphins. Endorphins are released in response to both acute and chronic pain. Through research we now know that warm water also stimulates the release of endorphins.

The most recognized methods to release endogenous (naturally occurring) endorphins are physical exercise, acupuncture, and electrical nerve stimulation. Any type of skin

Box 5.3

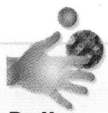

Patient Perspective

Polly

I'm scared to death of flying. The minute I get on an airplane, I feel jittery, my heart races, and I can't calm down until we're safely back on the ground. Several years ago, I decided to try biofeedback therapy to overcome this fear.

My therapist was wonderful. She immediately put me at ease and assured me I wasn't a crazy person to be afraid to fly. She then put a temperature sensor on my finger (my hands were usually pretty cold). In her calm, soft voice, she guided me through a relaxation exercise using imagery and progressive muscle relaxation. By the time we were finished, my hands would be several degrees warmer than when we started! This showed my vessels were dilating, a sign that my sympathetic nervous system was slowing down its activity. So, I felt calmer. The sensor gave me feedback that told me when my relaxation was working well. We did this every week for a couple of months, until I got really good at warming my hands and relaxing.

Now when I fly, I close my eyes, imagine a peaceful scene and use my relaxation techniques. I still don't like flying much, but at least I feel a bit calmer!

stimulation (even the mechanical impact of water) can cause the release of endorphins. However, pain reduction is only part of the healing process. Ultimately, blood flow is what brings nutrients to damaged cells and facilitates healing. When the body is immersed in warm water, the blood vessels nearest the skin relax, allowing more blood to flow. The results are faster tissue repair and relief of pain and fatigue.

Heat and Cold Application

Local application of heat or cold provides additional ways to stimulate the skin. A warm compress can soothe sore muscles and dilate vessels in a defined area, bringing healing circulation as well as endorphin release. Ice or a cold gel pack can help numb an area. They can also cause overdilated vessels to constrict, yielding relief from pain and throbbing of overstimulated nerve endings. Ice can be helpful on an acute injury and for some types of headaches. Check institution policy before applying heat or cold—a physician's order may be required.

SAFETY AND EFFECTIVENESS OF ALTERNATIVE MODALITIES

Safety generally means that the benefits outweigh the risks of a treatment or therapy. If a patient is interested in using complementary and alternative modalities, the nurse first needs to counsel the patient to talk with the primary care provider. The patient also should ask the practitioner of the therapy about its safety and effectiveness. Patients should tell their primary care providers and alternative practitioners about all therapies they are receiving because this information may be used to consider the safety of their entire treatment plan.

The patient should be as informed as possible and continue gathering information even after a practitioner has been selected (see Box 5.4).

ROLE OF THE LPN/LVN

Patients may ask you about the use of a complementary or alternative modality. Because the safety and effectiveness of many therapies is still unknown, advising patients presents a challenge. The following steps are suggestions for helping to advise patients regarding the use of these kinds of therapies:

1. Take a close look at the background, qualifications, and competence of the proposed practitioner. Check credentials with a state or local regulatory agency with authority over the area of practice in which the patient is interested. Is the practitioner licensed or certified? By whom?
2. Visit the practitioner's office, clinic, or hospital. Evaluate the conditions of the setting.
3. Talk with others who have used this practitioner.
4. Consider the costs. Are the treatments covered by insurance, or is it direct pay?
5. Discuss use of the modality with his or her primary care provider.

Box 5.4

Questions Patients Should Ask Before Starting a Complementary or Alternative Modality

1. What will this modality do for me?
2. What are its advantages?
3. What are its disadvantages?
4. What are its side effects?
5. What are its risks?
6. How much will it cost? Will my insurance cover the cost?
7. How long will it take? How many treatments will I need?
8. How will it interact with my other therapies and medications?
9. What research has been done on this modality?

NURSING APPLICATIONS

There are ways to gain confidence with complementary and alternative modalities:

1. Begin by trying one or two of these modalities yourself. Start by choosing a basic therapy such as massage, music, or guided imagery. Follow the guidelines listed in Box 5.4 to make sure it is a safe strategy. Not only will you encounter the benefits firsthand, but you will also come away with a better understanding of what patients experience.
2. Ask your patients if they use any complementary or alternative modalities and what their responses to them have been. Try to eliminate any preconceived notions you might have. Your patients will feel more comfortable mentioning them to you if they feel you understand the treatment and why they decided to use it.
3. If you decide to become involved, get adequate instruction in the therapies before you administer them. Many universities and agencies offer continuing education courses on these therapies, and some nursing schools incorporate complementary and alternative modalities in their skills courses.

Home Health Hints

- When taking a health history, ask the patient or caregiver about the use of complementary and alternative modalities because these may influence the effects or side effects of some prescription medications.
- Be mindful of the importance of complementary and alternative modalities to the patient's health care belief system.
- Consider the alternative practitioner as part of the patient's health care team.
- Discuss concerns regarding potential interactions with the registered nurse or physician.

Before incorporating complementary and alternative modalities into practice, be sure to check your state's nurse practice act for any regulations. Discuss these therapies with the patient and his or her primary care provider before using them. If you work for a hospital or other health care institution, also check institutional policy. See *Evidence-Based Practice* for ways nurses are implementing various modalities in practice.

EVIDENCE-BASED PRACTICE

Clinical Question

How are complementary and alternative modalities used by nurses to improve health outcomes?

Evidence

The following are examples of how complementary and alternative modalities have been used by nurses to enhance health outcomes in various patient populations.

In a recent study by Delaney and Barrere (2008), the effectiveness of a music/imagery CD titled *Blessings* improved psychospiritual outcomes in a cardiovascular population.

Imagery and, even more so, progressive muscle relaxation were found to be more effective in pain management than standard methods in patients with cancer-related pain (Kwekkeboom, Wanta, & Bumpus, 2008).

In a randomized controlled trial of patients recovering from coronary bypass surgery, those who received healing touch showed significantly decreased anxiety scores and decreased outpatient lengths of stay when compared to patients who did not receive healing touch (MacIntyre et al., 2008).

A study by Billhult and others (2007) revealed the positive effect of massage on relieving nausea in women who had breast cancer and were undergoing chemotherapy.

Implications for Nursing Practice

Complementary and alternative modalities such as music, muscle relaxation, imagery, and healing touch can improve health outcomes in diverse patient populations. After learning these healing modalities, nurses can easily implement them in a variety of patient settings.

REFERENCES

Billhult, A., Bergbom, I., & Stener-Victorin, E. (2007). Massage relieves nausea in women with breast cancer who are undergoing chemotherapy. *Journal of Alternative and Complementary Medicine, 13*(1), 53–57.

Delaney, C., & Barrere, C. (2008). Blessings: The influence of a spirituality-based intervention on psychospiritual outcomes in a cardiac population. *Holistic Nursing Practice, 22*, 210–219.

Kwekkeboom, K., Wanta, B., & Bumpus, M. (2008). Individual difference variable and the effects of progressive muscle relaxation and analgesic imagery interventions on cancer pain. *Journal of Pain and Symptom Management, 36*(6), 604–615.

MacIntyre, B., Hamilton, J., Fricke, T., et al. (2008). The efficacy of healing touch in coronary bypass surgery recovery: A randomized clinical control trial. *Alternative Therapies in Health and Medicine, 14*(4), 24–32.

As the public learns more about complementary and alternative modalities, there is likely to be an even greater demand for them. Nurses have been in the forefront of developing the holistic philosophy that has now become an accepted standard of care.

CRITICAL THINKING

Mr. Jones

■ Mr. Jones asks you whether he should stop his chemotherapy and try magnet therapy for his prostate cancer. How do you respond?

Suggested answer at end of chapter.

SUGGESTED ANSWERS TO

CRITICAL THINKING

■ *Mr. Jones*

As with all medical treatments, it is important to support the established therapy the health care provider has prescribed. Therefore a good response might be the following: "Mr. Jones, chemotherapy is an established medical treatment for your condition. There is a lot of evidence for its effectiveness in the medical literature. If you want to supplement your therapy, there may be some other treatments you can add. I suggest that you discuss your feelings about seeking some additional treatments with your health care provider."

REVIEW QUESTIONS

1. Which of the following statements best defines a complementary modality?
   a. An alternative treatment that is used in place of a conventional treatment
   b. A treatment that is often dangerous and should be avoided
   c. A treatment that can be used in addition to a conventional treatment
   d. A treatment that is used after conventional treatments have failed

2. Which of the following therapies is most likely to use research-based interventions?
   a. Naturopathy
   b. Osteopathy
   c. Allopathy
   d. Homeopathy

3. A patient who has high blood pressure tells his nurse he has been taking a ginger supplement in addition to his prescribed medications at home. What is the best response by the nurse?
   a. "Nonprescription supplements can interact with prescription medications. You should not take it any longer."
   b. "Ginger can be effective for hypertension. Be sure to monitor your blood pressure while you are taking it."
   c. "Ginger is a safe supplement because it is a food. It should not interact with your medications."
   d. "You should check with your physician to make sure the ginger doesn't interact with your other medications before you continue to take it."

4. Which of the following complementary modalities are considered relaxation therapies? **Select all that apply.**
   a. Progressive muscle relaxation
   b. Tai chi
   c. Biofeedback
   d. Homeopathic therapies
   e. Guided imagery

5. Which of the following statements best describes the most important role of the LPN in complementary and alternative modalities?
   a. The LPN should become familiar enough to recommend at least one complementary or alternative modality.
   b. The LPN should become adept at collecting and reporting data related to patients' use of complementary or alternative modalities.
   c. The LPN should discourage use of complementary or alternative modalities because they can interact negatively with conventional therapies.
   d. The LPN does not need to become involved in complementary and alternative modalities.

References

Cuellar, N. G., Rogers, A. E., & Hisghman, V. (2007). Evidenced based research of complementary and alternative medicine (CAM) for sleep in the community dwelling older adult. *Geriatric Nursing, 28*(1), 46–52.

Eisenberg, D. M., Kessler, R. C., Foster, C., et al. (1993). Unconventional medicine in the United States—Prevalence, costs, patterns of use. *New England Journal of Medicine, 328*(4), 246–252.

Eisenberg, D. M., Davis, R. B., Ettner, S. L., et al. (1998). Trends in alternative medicine use in the United States, 1990–1997. *Journal of the American Medical Association, 280*(18), 1569–1575.

Tindle, H. A., Davis, R. B., Phillips, R. S., & Eisenberg, D. M. (2005). Trends in use of complementary and alternative medicine by U.S. adults: 1997–2002. *Alternative Therapies in Health and Medicine, 11*(1), 42–49.

unit TWO

UNDERSTANDING HEALTH AND ILLNESS

6 Nursing Care of Patients with Fluid, Electrolyte, and Acid-Base Imbalances

BRUCE K. WILSON

KEY WORDS

acidosis (as-ih-DOH-sis)
alkalosis (al-kah-LOH-sis)
anion (AN-eye-on)
antidiuretic (AN-tee-DYE-yuh-RET-ik)
cation (KAT-eye-on)
dehydration (DEE-hye-DRAY-shun)
diffusion (dih-FEW-zhun)
dysrhythmia (dis-RITH-mee-yah)
edema (eh-DEE-mah)
electrolytes (ee-LEK-troh-lites)
extracellular (EX-trah-SELL-yoo-lar)
filtration (fill-TRAY-shun)
hydrostatic (HYE-droh-STAT-ik)
hypercalcemia (HYE-per-kal-SEE-mee-ah)
hyperkalemia (HYE-per-kuh-LEE-mee-ah)
hypermagnesemia (HYE-per-MAG-nuh-SEE-mee-ah)
hypernatremia (HYE-per-nuh-TREE-mee-ah)
hypertonic (HYE-per-TAWN-ik)
hyperventilation (HYE-per-VEN-tih-LAY-shun)
hypervolemia (HYE-per-voh-LEE-mee-ah)
hypocalcemia (HYE-poh-kal-SEE-mee-ah)
hypokalemia (HYE-poh-kuh-LEE-mee-ah)
hypomagnesemia (HYE-poh-MAG-nuh-SEE-mee-ah)
hyponatremia (HYE-poh-nuh-TREE-mee-ah)
hypotonic (HYE-poh-TAWN-ik)
hypovolemia (HYE-poh-voh-LEE-mee-ah)
interstitial (IN-tur-STISH-uhl)
intracellular (IN-trah-SELL-yoo-ler)
intracranial (IN-trah-KRAY-nee-uhl)
intravascular (IN-trah-VAS-kyoo-ler)
isotonic (EYE-so-TAWN-ik)
osmosis (ahs-MOH-sis)
osteoporosis (AHS-tee-oh-por-OH-sis)
semipermeable (SEM-ee-PER-mee-uh-bull)
transcellular (trans-SELL-yoo-lar)

QUESTIONS TO GUIDE YOUR READING

1. What are the purposes of fluids and electrolytes in the body?
2. What are the signs and symptoms of common fluid imbalances?
3. Which patients are at the highest risk for dehydration and fluid excess?
4. What data should you collect in patients with fluid and electrolyte imbalances?
5. What therapeutic measures are used for patients with fluid and electrolyte disturbances?
6. What are the education needs of patients with fluid imbalances?
7. What are common causes, signs and symptoms, and treatments for sodium, potassium, calcium, and magnesium imbalances?
8. Which foods have high sodium, potassium, and calcium contents?
9. What are common causes of acidosis and alkalosis?
10. How do arterial blood gases change for each type of acid-base imbalance?

The body undergoes continuous dynamic change. The proper amount of fluid is needed to support these changes and to transport building and waste materials. Approximately 60% of a young adult's body weight is water. Elderly people are less than 50% water, and infants are between 70% and 80% water. Women have less body water because they typically have more fat than men. Fat cells do not contain water.

In addition to water, body fluids also contain solid substances that dissolve, called solutes. Some solutes are **electrolytes** and some are nonelectrolytes. Electrolytes are chemicals that can conduct electricity when dissolved in water. Examples of electrolytes are sodium, potassium, calcium, magnesium, acids, and bases; these are discussed later in this chapter. Nonelectrolytes do not conduct electricity; for example, glucose and urea.

FLUID BALANCE

Fluids are located in various compartments within the body. Fluid inside the cells is referred to as **intracellular** fluid (ICF), and fluid outside the cells is called **extracellular** fluid (ECF). ECF can be further divided into three types: interstitial fluid, intravascular fluid, and transcellular fluid (Fig. 6.1).

Interstitial fluid is the water that surrounds the body's cells and includes lymph. **Intravascular** fluid, or blood plasma, is the fluid within arteries, veins, and capillaries. Fluids and electrolytes move between the interstitial fluid and the intravascular fluid. **Transcellular** fluids are those in specific compartments of the body, such as cerebrospinal fluid, digestive juices, and synovial fluid in joints.

Control of Fluid Balance

The primary control of water in the body is through pressure sensors in the vascular system, which stimulate or inhibit the release of **antidiuretic** hormone (ADH) from the pituitary gland. A diuretic is a substance that causes the kidneys to excrete more fluid. ADH works in just the opposite way. ADH causes the kidneys to retain fluid. If fluid pressures within the vascular system decrease, more ADH is released and water is retained. If fluid pressures increase, less ADH is released and the kidneys eliminate more water.

Movement of Fluids and Electrolytes in the Body

Fluids and electrolytes move in the body by active and passive transport systems. Active transport depends on the presence of adequate cellular adenosine triphosphate (ATP) for energy. The most common examples of active transport are the sodium-potassium pumps. These pumps, located in the cell membranes, cause sodium to move out of the cells and potassium to move into the cells when needed.

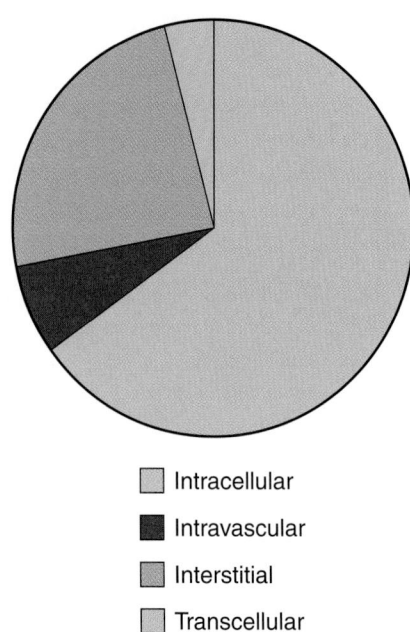

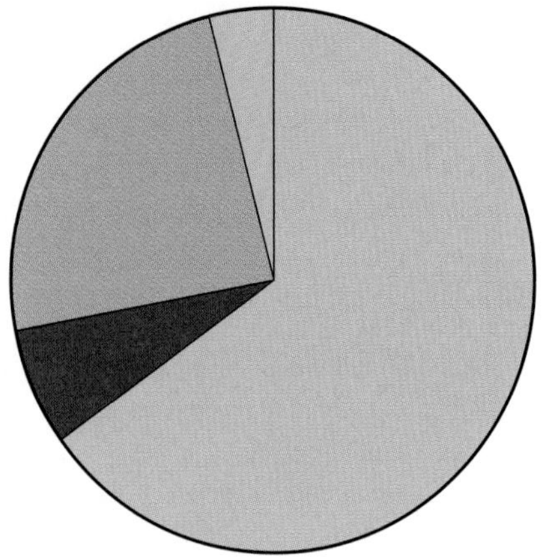
Intracellular
Intravascular
Interstitial
Transcellular

FIGURE 6.1 Normal distribution of total body water.

In passive transport, no energy is expended specifically to move the substances. General body movements aid passive transport. The three passive transport systems are diffusion, filtration, and osmosis.

Diffusion is a process in which the substance moves from an area of higher concentration to an area of lower concentration. If you pour cream into a cup of coffee, the movement of the molecules will eventually cause the cream to be dispersed throughout the beverage. If you stir the coffee, this process occurs at a faster rate. Body movement assists passive transport, like stirring the coffee. It causes diffusion to occur at a faster rate.

Filtration is the movement of both water and smaller molecules through a semipermeable membrane. A **semipermeable** membrane works like a screen that keeps larger substances on one side and permits only smaller molecules to filter to the other side of the membrane. Filtration is promoted by hydrostatic pressure differences between areas.

Hydrostatic pressure, sometimes called water-pushing pressure, is the force that water exerts. In the body, filtration

• WORD • BUILDING •

electrolyte: electro—electricity + lyte—dissolve
intracellular: intra—within + cellular—cell
extracellular: extra—outside of + cellular—cell
interstitial: inter—between + stitial—tissue
intravascular: intra—within + vascular—blood vessel
transcellular: trans—across + cellular—cell
antidiuretic: anti—against + diuretic—urination
diffusion: diffuse—spread, scattered
filtration: filter—strain through
semipermeable: semi—half or part of + permeable—passing through
hydrostatic: hydro—water + static—standing

is important for the movement of water, nutrients, and waste products in the capillaries. The capillaries serve as semipermeable membranes allowing water and smaller substances to move from the vascular system to the interstitial fluid, but larger molecules and red blood cells remain inside the capillary walls.

Osmosis is the movement of water from an area of lower substance concentration to an area of higher concentration. The substances exert an osmotic pressure sometimes called water-pulling pressure. The term *osmolarity* refers to the concentration of the substances in body fluids. The normal osmolarity of the blood is between 270 and 300 milliosmoles per liter (mOsm/L).

Another term for osmolarity is *tonicity*. Fluids or solutions can be classified as isotonic, hypotonic, or hypertonic. A fluid that has the same osmolarity as the blood is called **isotonic**. For example, a 0.9% (normal) saline solution is isotonic to the blood and is often used as a solution for intravenous (IV) therapy. A solution that has a lower osmolarity than blood is called **hypotonic**. When a hypotonic solution is given to a patient, the water in the solution leaves the blood and other ECF areas and enters the cells. **Hypertonic** solutions exert greater osmotic pressure than blood. When a hypertonic solution is given to a patient, water leaves the cells and enters the bloodstream and other ECF spaces.

Fluid Gains and Fluid Losses

Water is very important to the body for cellular metabolism, blood volume, body temperature regulation, and solute transport. Although people can survive without food for several weeks, they can survive only a few days without water.

Water is gained and lost from the body every day. In addition to liquid intake, some fluid is obtained from solid foods. When too much fluid is lost, the brain's thirst mechanism tells the individual that more fluid intake is needed. Older adults are more prone to fluid deficits because they have a diminished thirst reflex and their kidneys do not function as effectively. An adult loses as much as 2500 mL of sensible and insensible fluid each day. Sensible losses are those of which the person is aware, such as urination. Insensible losses may occur without the person recognizing the loss. Perspiration and water lost through respiration and elimination of feces are examples of insensible losses.

FLUID IMBALANCES

Fluid imbalances are common in all clinical settings. Elderly people are at the highest risk for life-threatening complications that can result from either fluid deficit, more commonly called **dehydration**, or fluid excess. Infants are at risk for fluid deficit because they take in and excrete a large proportion of their total body water each day.

Dehydration

Although there are several types of dehydration, only the most common type is discussed in this chapter. Dehydration occurs when there is not enough fluid in the body, especially in the blood (intravascular area).

Pathophysiology and Etiology

The most common form of dehydration results from loss of fluid from the body, resulting in decreased blood volume. This decrease is referred to as **hypovolemia**. Hypovolemia occurs when the patient is hemorrhaging or when fluids from other parts of the body are lost. For example, severe vomiting and diarrhea, severely draining wounds, and profuse diaphoresis (sweating) can cause dehydration. See Box 6.1.

Hypovolemia can also occur when fluid from the intravascular space moves into the interstitial fluid space. This process is called third spacing. Examples of conditions in which third spacing is common include burns, liver cirrhosis, and extensive trauma.

As described previously in this chapter, the body initially attempts to compensate for fluid loss by a number of mechanisms. If the cause of dehydration is not resolved or the patient is not able to replace the fluid, a state of dehydration occurs.

Box 6.1

Common Causes of Dehydration

Cecostomy
Diabetes insipidus
Diarrhea
Diuretic therapy
Draining abscesses
Draining fistulas
Fever
Frequent enemas
Gastrointestinal suction
Hemorrhage
Ileostomy
Long-term nothing by mouth (NPO) status
Profuse diaphoresis (sweating)
Severely draining wounds
Systemic infection
Vomiting

• WORD • BUILDING •

osmosis: osmo—impulse + osis—condition
isotonic: iso—equal + tonic—strength
hypotonic: hypo—less than + tonic—strength
hypertonic: hyper—more than + tonic—strength
dehydration: de—down + hydration—water
hypovolemia: hypo—less than + vol—volume + emia—blood

Prevention

You can help prevent dehydration by identifying patients who have the highest risk for developing this condition and intervening quickly to correct the cause. High-risk patients include the elderly, infants, children, and any patient with one of the conditions listed in Box 6.1. Also see Box 6.2, *Gerontological Issues.*

Adequate hydration is another important intervention to help prevent dehydration. You should encourage patients to drink adequate fluids. Adults need 30 mL/kg/day of fluids. If a patient is unable to take enough fluid by mouth, alternate routes may be necessary.

Signs and Symptoms

Thirst is the initial symptom experienced by otherwise healthy adults in response to hypovolemia. As the percentage of water in the blood goes down, the percentage of other substances goes up, resulting in the thirst response. As the blood volume decreases, the heart pumps the remaining blood faster but not as powerfully, resulting in a rapid, weak pulse and a low blood pressure. The body pulls water into the vascular system from other areas, resulting in decreased tear formation, dry skin, and dry mucous membranes.

A dehydrated person will have poor skin turgor. Turgor is considered to be poor if the skin is pinched and a small "tent" remains (called *tenting*). A dehydrated person's temperature increases because the body is less able to cool itself through perspiration. Temperature may not appear elevated in an elderly person because an elder's normal body temperature is often lower than a younger person's. Urine output decreases and the urine becomes more concentrated as water is conserved. Dehydration should be considered in any adult with a urine output of less than 30 mL per hour. The urine may appear darker because it is less diluted. The patient becomes constipated as the intestines absorb more water from the feces. A major method of evaluating dehydration is weight loss. A pint of water weighs approximately 1 pound. Symptoms of dehydration in the elderly may be atypical (see Box 6.2, *Gerontological Issues*).

> **LEARNING TIP**
>
> Do you remember your grandmother saying, "a pint's a pound the world around"? It's a great way to remember how much fluid loss is represented by each lost pound.

Complications

If dehydration is not treated, lack of sufficient blood volume causes organ function to decrease and eventually fail. The brain, kidneys, and heart must be adequately supplied with blood (perfused) to function properly. The body protects these organs by decreasing blood flow to other areas. When these organs no longer receive their minimum requirements, death results.

> **Box 6.2**
> **Gerontological Issues**
>
> As a person ages, total body water decreases from 60% to 50% of total body weight. The age-related decrease in total body water is secondary to an increase in body fat and a decrease in thirst sensation. These factors increase the risk of developing dehydration.
>
> Manifestations of dehydration in an older adult are different from typical manifestations in a younger person, and may include altered mental status, lightheadedness, and syncope. These occur because a patient with hypovolemia has an inadequate circulatory volume and, therefore, oxygen supply to the brain.

> **LEARNING TIP**
>
> The magic fluid number is 30: Healthy adults should drink approximately 30 mL of fluid per kilogram of body weight per day, and they should urinate at least 30 mL per hour. Of course, this is just a basic rule of thumb and will vary based on individual circumstances.

Diagnostic Tests

A patient with dehydration usually has an elevated blood urea nitrogen (BUN) level and elevated hematocrit. Both values are increased because there is less water in proportion to the solid substances being measured. The specific gravity of the urine also increases as the kidneys attempt to conserve water, resulting in a more concentrated urine.

Therapeutic Measures

The goals of therapeutic measures are to replace fluids and resolve the cause of dehydration. In a patient with moderate or severe dehydration, IV therapy is used. Isotonic fluids that have the same osmolarity as blood, such as normal saline, are typically administered.

> **SAFETY TIP**
>
> Use at least two patient identifiers when providing care, treatment, and services. The patient's room number or physical location is not used as an identifier. (2010 National Patient Safety Goals, www.jointcommission.org.)

Nursing Process for the Patient Experiencing Dehydration

Nurses can play a major role in identifying and caring for patients who are dehydrated.

DATA COLLECTION. Assess the patient for signs and symptoms of dehydration. All the classic signs and symptoms may not be present.

When assessing an elderly patient for skin turgor (tenting), assess the skin over the forehead or sternum. The skin over these areas usually retains elasticity and is therefore a more reliable indicator of skin turgor. Also check mucous membranes, which should be moist.

Weight is the most reliable indicator of fluid loss or gain. A loss of 1 to 2 pounds or more per day suggests water loss rather than fat loss. The patient in the hospital setting should be weighed every day. The patient in the nursing home or home setting should be weighed at least three times a week if the patient is at risk for fluid imbalance. Weigh the patient before breakfast using the same scale each time. Intake and output are also typically measured (Box 6.3, *Cultural Considerations*).

NURSING DIAGNOSES, PLANNING, AND IMPLEMENTATION. The primary nursing diagnosis and interventions for the patient with dehydration may include:

Risk for Deficient Fluid Volume or Deficient Fluid Volume Related to Fluid loss or Inadequate Fluid Intake

EXPECTED OUTCOME: The patient will be adequately hydrated as evidenced by stable weight, moist mucous membranes, and elastic skin turgor.

- Monitor daily weights and intake and output (I&O) so problems can be detected and corrected early.
- Plan with the patient and other members of the health care team the type and timing of fluid intake. Planning with the patient increases the likelihood that the plan will be followed.
- Offer fluids often to the confused patient since he or she may not drink independently.
- Correct the underlying cause of the fluid deficit, so it does not recur.
- Be careful not to overhydrate the patient, so fluid excess does not occur.

See Box 6.4 for best practices for maintaining oral hydration in older people.

EVALUATION. The patient who is adequately hydrated will have elastic skin turgor, moist mucous membranes, and stable weight.

Patient Education

The patient, family, and significant others need to be taught the importance of reporting early signs and symptoms of dehydration to a physician or other health care provider. At home or in the nursing home, infections often cause fever and sepsis, a serious condition in which the infection invades the bloodstream. The body attempts to decrease the temperature through perspiration. The patient becomes dehydrated as a result and can become increasingly ill.

Box 6.4

Best Practice Recommendations for Maintaining Oral Hydration in Older People

- A fluid intake sheet is the best method of monitoring daily fluid intake.
- Urine specific gravity may be the simplest, most accurate method to determine patient hydration status.
- Evidence of a dry furrowed tongue and mucous membranes, sunken eyes, confusion, and upper body muscle weakness may indicate dehydration.
- Regular presentation of fluids to bedridden older people can maintain adequate hydration status.
- Owing to the observation that medication time can be an important source of fluids, fluids should be encouraged at this time.

Source: Adapted from *Joanna Briggs Best Practice Recommendations: Maintaining Oral Hydration in Older People*, 5:6, 2001. Retrieved May 17, 2009, from http://www.joannabriggs.edu.au.

Box 6.3

Cultural Considerations

Muslims who celebrate Ramadan fast for 1 month from sunup to sundown. Although the ill are not required to fast, ill Muslims may still wish to do so. Fasting may include not taking fluids and medications during daylight hours. Therefore, the nurse may need to alter times for medication administration, including intramuscular medication. Special precautions may need to be taken to prevent dehydration in Muslim patients.

CRITICAL THINKING

Mrs. Levitt

■ Mrs. Levitt is a 92-year-old widow who has been in a nursing home for 4 years. Today she mentions that her urine smells bad and that her heart feels like it is beating faster than usual. You suspect that she is becoming dehydrated. You check her urine and find that it is a dark amber color and has a strong odor. Her heart rate is 98 beats per minute, blood pressure 126/74 mm Hg, respiratory rate 20 per minute, and temperature 99.2°F (37.3°C).

1. What other data should you collect, and what results do you expect?
2. Which interventions should you provide at this time?
3. How should you document your findings?

Suggested answers at end of chapter.

Fluid Excess

Fluid excess, sometimes called overhydration, is a condition in which a patient has too much fluid in the body. Most of the problems related to fluid excess result from too much fluid in the bloodstream or from dilution of electrolytes and red blood cells.

Pathophysiology and Etiology

The most common result of fluid excess is **hypervolemia** in which there is excess fluid in the intravascular space. Healthy adult kidneys can compensate for mild to moderate hypervolemia. The kidneys increase urinary output to rid the body of the extra fluid. Sometimes, however, the kidneys cannot keep up with the excess fluid.

Conditions that can cause excessive fluid intake are poorly controlled IV therapy, excessive irrigation of wounds or body cavities, and excessive ingestion of water. Conditions that can result in inadequate excretion of fluid include renal (kidney) failure, heart failure, and the syndrome of inappropriate antidiuretic hormone. These conditions are discussed elsewhere in this book.

Prevention

One of the best ways to prevent fluid excess is to avoid excessive fluid intake. For example, you should monitor the patient receiving IV therapy for signs and symptoms of fluid excess. In at-risk patients, an electronic infusion pump or a quantity-limiting device, such as a burette, should be used to control the rate of infusion.

Also monitor the amount of fluid used for irrigations. For example, when a patient's stomach is being irrigated (gastric lavage), be sure an excessive amount of fluid is not absorbed.

Signs and Symptoms

The vital sign changes seen in the patient with fluid excess are the opposite of those found in patients with dehydration. The blood pressure is elevated, pulse is bounding, and respirations are increased and shallow. The neck veins may become distended, and pitting **edema** in the feet and legs may be present. The skin is pale and cool. The kidneys increase urine output, and the urine appears diluted, almost like water. The patient rapidly gains weight. In severe fluid excess, the patient develops moist crackles in the lungs, dyspnea, and ascites (excess peritoneal fluid).

Complications

Acute fluid excess typically results in congestive heart failure. As the fluid builds up in the heart, the heart is not able to properly function as a pump. The fluid then backs up into the lungs, causing a condition known as pulmonary edema. Other major organs of the body cannot receive adequate oxygen, and organ failure can lead to death.

Diagnostic Tests

In the patient experiencing fluid excess, the BUN and hematocrit levels tend to decrease from hemodilution. The plasma content of the blood is proportionately increased when compared with the solid substances. The specific gravity of the urine also diminishes as the urinary output increases.

Therapeutic Measures

Once the patient's breathing has been supported, the goal of treatment is to rid the body of excessive fluid and resolve the underlying cause of the excess. Drug therapy and diet therapy are commonly used to decrease fluid retention.

POSITIONING. To facilitate ease in breathing, the head of the patient's bed should be in semi-Fowler's or high Fowler's position (Fig. 6.2). These positions allow greater lung expansion and thus aid respiratory effort. Once the patient has been properly positioned, oxygen therapy may be necessary.

OXYGEN THERAPY. Oxygen therapy is typically used to ensure adequate perfusion of major organs and to minimize dyspnea. If the patient has a history of chronic obstructive pulmonary disease, such as emphysema or chronic bronchitis, be cautious if you need to administer more than 2 L per minute of oxygen. At higher oxygen doses, the patient may lose the stimulus to breathe and may suffer respiratory arrest. Monitor pulse oximetry and respiratory rate carefully.

DRUG THERAPY. Diuretics are commonly administered to rapidly rid the body of excess water. A diuretic is a drug that increases elimination by the kidneys. The drug of choice for fluid excess when the patient has adequately functioning kidneys is usually a loop diuretic such as furosemide (Lasix). Loop diuretics cause the kidneys to excrete sodium and water. Sodium (Na^+) and water tend to move together in the body. Potassium (K^+), another electrolyte, is also lost, which can lead to a potassium deficit, which is discussed later in this chapter.

• WORD • BUILDING •

hypervolemia: hyper—more than + vol—volume + emia—blood
edema: swelling

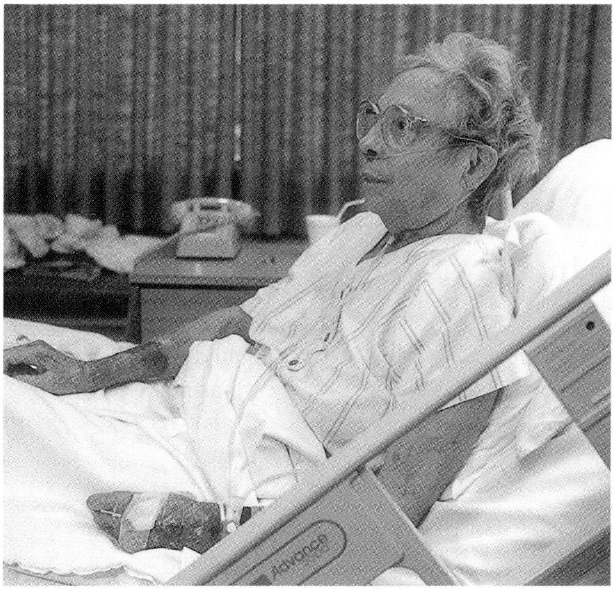

FIGURE 6.2 Patient in high Fowler's position with oxygen.

Furosemide may be given by the oral, intramuscular, or IV route. The oral route is used most commonly for mild fluid excess. IV furosemide is administered by a registered nurse (RN) or physician for severe excess. The patient should begin diuresis within 30 minutes after receiving IV furosemide. If not, another dose is given. Strict intake and output should be monitored, as well as daily weight, when a patient is receiving IV furosemide.

DIET THERAPY. Mild to moderate fluid restriction may be necessary, as well as a sodium-restricted diet. In collaboration with the dietitian, a physician prescribes the specific restriction necessary, usually a 1- to 2-g sodium restriction for severe excess. Different diuretics result in differing electrolyte elimination. Specific diet therapy depends on the medications the patient is receiving and the patient's underlying medical problems.

Nursing Process for the Patient Experiencing Fluid Excess

The nurse plays a pivotal role in the care of a patient with fluid excess. Prompt action is needed to prevent life-threatening complications.

DATA COLLECTION. Observe a patient who is at high risk for fluid excess and monitor fluid I&O carefully. If the patient is drinking adequate amounts of fluid (1500 mL per day or more) but is voiding in small amounts, the fluid is being retained by the body.

Assess for edema, which is fluid that accumulates in the interstitial tissues. If the edema is pitting, a finger pressed against the skin over a bony area such as the tibia leaves a temporary indentation. For patients in bed, check the sacrum for edema. For patients in the sitting position, check the feet and legs. Also assess lung sounds since excess fluid accumulation in the lungs can cause crackles (see Chapter 29).

As mentioned earlier, weight is the most reliable indicator of fluid gain. Weigh at-risk patients daily. A gain of 1 to 2 pounds or more per day indicates fluid retention even though other signs and symptoms may not be present.

NURSING DIAGNOSES, PLANNING, AND IMPLEMENTATION

Excess Fluid Volume Related to Excessive Fluid Intake or Inadequate Excretion of Body Fluid

EXPECTED OUTCOME: Patient will return to a normal hydration status as evidenced by return to weight that is normal for patient, absence of edema, and clear lung sounds.

- Report any increase in weight to the physician. Increased weight indicates fluid retention.
- Implement fluid restriction as ordered to reduce excess intake. Work with the patient and RN to determine how it should be implemented. For example, if a patient is on a 1000 mL per day fluid restriction, you might plan for 150 mL with each meal, 450 mL to be given to the patient to use as he or she likes during the day, and 100 mL to be used during the night. Be sure to include the patient in your planning, and remember to reserve enough fluid for swallowing medications. Post a sign in the patient's room so other caregivers know how much fluid the patient can have.
- Administer diuretics as ordered, and monitor patient response. Be sure to monitor potassium in patients receiving potassium-losing loop or thiazide diuretics. Diuretics promote diuresis.
- Report urinary output below 30 mL per hour to the physician or RN because it may signify increasing renal complications.

EVALUATION. If interventions have been effective, the patient will return to his or her normal weight with clear lung sounds and no edema. Many patients must remain on drug and diet therapy after hospital discharge to prevent the problem from recurring.

Patient Education

In collaboration with the dietitian, instruct the patient, family, or other caregiver about any fluid or sodium restrictions to prevent further problems (Box 6.5, *Nutrition Notes*). High-sodium foods to avoid are listed in Table 6.1.

Teaching about diuretic therapy is essential to prevent electrolyte imbalances. If a potassium-losing diuretic is prescribed, teach the patient to eat foods that are high in potassium (Table 6.2). The patient's serum potassium level must be periodically monitored by a physician or home care nurse. If it becomes too low, an oral potassium supplement is needed.

The patient or caregiver also needs to be taught common signs and symptoms of fluid excess that should be reported to a physician or other health care provider. Of special importance is weight gain. A patient at high risk for fluid

Box 6.5

Nutrition Notes

Reducing Sodium Intake

Many foods, such as dairy products, grain products, and some vegetables, are naturally high in sodium, but the major sources of dietary sodium are salted and processed foods, including baked goods and condiments. For example, American cheese has more sodium than cheddar, and cured ham has more than fresh pork.

Drinking water may contain significant amounts of sodium, particularly if it is softened or mineral water. Because of the numerous "hidden" sources of sodium, patients on low-sodium diets benefit from education by a dietician.

The adequate intake (AI) of sodium is

- 1.5 g daily for adults through age 49
- 1.3 g daily for those ages 50 to 70
- 1.2 g daily for those ages 71 and older.

The upper tolerable intake level (UL) for sodium is 2.3 g daily, which is contained in slightly more than a teaspoon of salt. None of these amounts applies to those losing large amounts of sweat daily or to unacclimatized persons exercising in a hot environment.

Specific definitions for reduced-sodium food products have been adopted. Note that serving size is an important variable.

- Salt or sodium free: <5 mg sodium per serving
- Very low sodium: <35 mg sodium per serving (per 100 g if main dish)
- Low sodium: <140 mg sodium per serving (per 100 g if main dish)

excess should be weighed at least three times a week in the home or nursing home, at the same time each day, and on the same scale. Weight gain should be reported.

CRITICAL THINKING

Mr. Peters

■ Mr. Peters is a 32-year-old man with a congenital heart problem. He has been recovering from congestive heart failure and fluid excess. Today, his blood pressure is higher than usual and his pulse is bounding. He is having trouble breathing and presses the call light for your assistance.

1. What should you do first when you assess Mr. Peters' condition?
2. What questions should you ask him?
3. What objective data should you collect?
4. What should you do with your findings?

Suggested answers at end of chapter.

TABLE 6.1 COMMON FOOD SOURCES OF SODIUM*

Food Group	Serving Size	Range (mg)
Breads, all types	1 oz	95–210
Frozen pizza, plain, cheese	4 oz	450–1200
Frozen vegetables, all types	½ cup	2–160
Salad dressing, regular fat, all types	2 tbsp	110–505
Salsa	2 tbsp	150–240
Soup (tomato), reconstituted	8 oz	700–1260
Tomato juice	8 oz (∼1 cup)	340–1040
Potato chips[†]	1 oz (28.4 g)	120–180
Tortilla chips[†]	1 oz (28.4 g)	105–160
Pretzels[†]	1 oz (28.4 g)	290–560

*Ranges of sodium content are for selected foods available in the retail market. This table is provided to exemplify the importance of reading the food label to determine the sodium content of food, which can vary by several hundreds of milligrams in similar foods.

[†]All snack foods are regular flavor, salted.

Note: None of the examples provided was labeled "low sodium."

Source: Agricultural Research Service Nutrient Database for Standard Reference, Release 17, and recent manufacturers' label data from retail market surveys. Serving sizes were standardized to be comparable among brands within a food. Pizza and bread slices vary in size and weight across brands.

TABLE 6.2 FOOD SOURCES OF POTASSIUM*

Food, Standard Amount	Potassium (mg)	Calories
Sweet potato, baked, 1 potato (146 g)	694	131
Beet greens, cooked, ½ cup	655	19
Potato, baked, flesh, 1 potato (156 g)	610	145
Yogurt, plain, nonfat, 8-oz container	579	127
Prune juice, 3/4 cup	530	136
Soybeans, green, cooked, ½ cup	485	127
Bananas, 1 medium	422	105
Spinach, cooked, ½ cup	419	21
Tomato juice, ¾ cup	417	31
Tomato sauce, ½ cup	405	39
Milk, nonfat, 1 cup	382	83
Pork chop, center loin, cooked, 3 oz	382	197
Apricots, dried, uncooked, ¼ cup	378	78
Cantaloupe, ¼ medium	368	47
1% or 2% milk, 1 cup	366	102–122
Kidney beans, cooked, ½ cup	358	112
Orange juice, ¾ cup	355	85
Split peas, cooked, ½ cup	355	116

*Food sources of potassium ranked by milligrams of potassium per standard amount, also showing calories in the standard amount. (The adequate intake for adults is 4700 mg/day of potassium.)

Source: Nutrient values from Agricultural Research Service (ARS) Nutrient Database for Standard Reference, Release 17. Foods are from ARS single nutrient reports, sorted in descending order by nutrient content in terms of common household measures. Food items and weights in the single nutrient reports are adapted from those in the 2002 revision of USDA Home and Garden Bulletin No. 72, *Nutritive Value of Foods*. Mixed dishes and multiple preparations of the same food item have been omitted from this table.

ELECTROLYTE BALANCE

Natural minerals in food become electrolytes or ions in the body through digestion and metabolism. Electrolytes are usually measured in milliequivalents per liter (mEq/L) or in milligrams per deciliter (mg/dL).

Electrolytes are one of two types: **cations**, which carry a positive electrical charge, and **anions**, which carry a negative electrical charge. Although there are many electrolytes in the body, this chapter discusses the most important ones, including sodium (Na^+), potassium (K^+), calcium (Ca^{2+}), and magnesium (Mg^{2+}). These electrolytes are maintained in different concentrations inside the cell and outside the cell because of pumps in the cell wall (Fig. 6.3).

ELECTROLYTE IMBALANCES

At times, a patient may experience problems because of too much or too little of an electrolyte. In general, if a patient experiences a deficit of an electrolyte, the electrolyte is replaced either orally or intravenously. If the patient experiences an excess of an electrolyte, treatment focuses on getting rid of the excess, often via the kidneys. The underlying cause of the imbalance must also be treated.

The most important aspects of nursing care are preventing and assessing electrolyte imbalances. You must be vigilant in watching for signs of imbalance in high-risk patients. Serum electrolytes are measured on a regular basis. As a general rule, patients should be checked for electrolyte imbalance when there is a change in their mental state (either increased irritability or decreased responsiveness) or when muscle function changes. Patient education is another important nursing role.

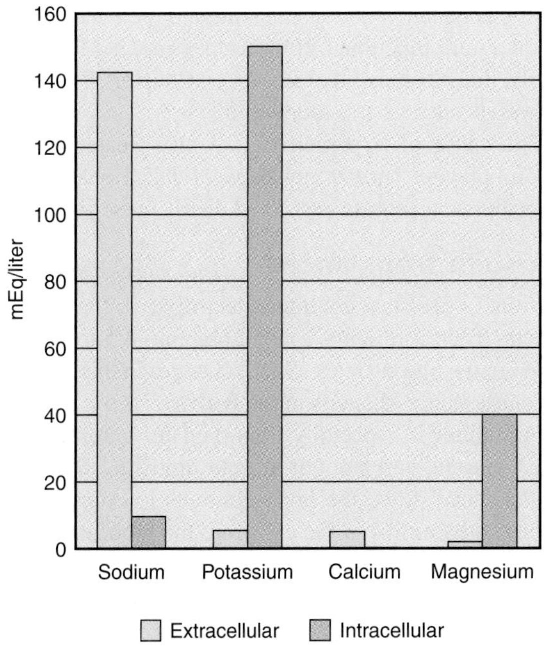
160
140
120
100
80
60
40
20
0
mEq/liter
Sodium
Potassium
Calcium
Magnesium
Extracellular
Intracellular

FIGURE 6.3 Extracellular and intracellular electrolytes.

Sodium Imbalances

The normal level of serum sodium is 135 to 145 mEq/L. Because sodium is the major cation in the blood, it helps maintain serum osmolarity. Therefore, sodium imbalances are often associated with fluid imbalances, described earlier in this chapter. Sodium is also important for cell function, especially in the central nervous system. The two sodium imbalances are **hyponatremia** (sodium deficit) and **hypernatremia** (sodium excess).

Hyponatremia

Hyponatremia occurs when the serum sodium level is less than 135 mEq/L.

PATHOPHYSIOLOGY AND ETIOLOGY. Many conditions can lead to either an actual or a relative decrease in sodium. In an actual decrease, the patient has inadequate intake of sodium or excessive sodium loss from the body. As the percentage of sodium in the ECF decreases, water is pulled by osmotic pressure into the cells. In a relative decrease, the sodium is not lost from the body but may leave the intravascular space and move into the interstitial tissues (third spacing). Another cause of a relative decrease occurs when the plasma volume increases (fluid excess), causing a dilutional effect. The percentage of sodium compared with the fluid is diminished.

PREVENTION. Additional sodium is commonly administered to patients at high risk for hyponatremia (see Box 6.6), usually by the IV route. Individuals who have high fevers or who engage in strenuous exercise or physical labor, especially in the heat, need to replace both sodium and water. Hyponatremia is especially dangerous for the elderly patient.

SIGNS AND SYMPTOMS. Unfortunately, the signs and symptoms of hyponatremia are vague and depend somewhat on whether a fluid imbalance accompanies the hyponatremia. The patient with sodium and fluid deficits has signs and symptoms of dehydration (discussed previously). The patient with a sodium deficit and relative fluid excess has signs and symptoms associated with fluid excess.

With more severe sodium deficit, the patient experiences mental status changes, including disorientation, confusion, and personality changes. This occurs because the low sodium and decrease in osmolarity cause more "water-pushing pressure," which causes water to collect in and around the brain and increase pressure (cerebral edema). Weakness, nausea, vomiting, and diarrhea may also occur.

• WORD • BUILDING •

cation: cat—descending + ion—carrying
anion: an—without + ion—carrying
hyponatremia: hypo—less than + natr—sodium + emia—blood
hypernatremia: hyper—more than + natr—sodium + emia—blood

Box 6.6

Conditions that Place Patients at High Risk for Hyponatremia

Nothing by mouth (NPO)
Excessive diaphoresis (sweating)
Diuretics
Gastrointestinal suction
Syndrome of inappropriate antidiuretic hormone
Excessive ingestion of hypotonic fluids
Freshwater near-drowning
Decreased aldosterone

COMPLICATIONS. In severe hyponatremia, respiratory arrest or coma can lead to death. The patient who also has fluid excess may develop pulmonary edema, another life-threatening complication.

DIAGNOSTIC TESTS. The primary diagnostic test is a serum sodium level, which is lower than the normal value when hyponatremia is present. The serum osmolarity also decreases in patients with hyponatremia. Other laboratory results may be affected if the patient experiences an accompanying fluid imbalance. Serum chloride (Cl^-), an anion, is often depleted when sodium decreases because these two electrolytes commonly combine as NaCl (salt in solution, or saline).

THERAPEUTIC MEASURES. Therapeutic measures focus on resolving the underlying cause of hyponatremia and replacing the lost sodium. The physician orders IV saline for patients who have hyponatremia without fluid excess.

For patients who have a fluid excess, a fluid restriction is often ordered. Diuretics that rid the body of fluid but do not cause sodium loss may also be used. For patients with cerebral edema, steroids may be prescribed to reduce **intracranial** swelling. I&O are strictly monitored, and the patient is weighed daily. Also implement interventions to keep the patient safe if mental status is affected.

Hypernatremia

Hypernatremia occurs when the serum sodium level is above 145 mEq/L.

PATHOPHYSIOLOGY AND ETIOLOGY. A serum sodium increase may be an actual increase or a relative increase. In an actual increase, the patient receives too much sodium or is unable to excrete sodium, as seen in renal failure. In a relative increase, the amount of sodium does not change but the amount of fluid in the intravascular space decreases. Therefore, the percentage of sodium (solid) is increased in relationship to the amount of plasma (water).

In mild hypernatremia, most excitable tissues, such as muscle and neurons of the brain, become more stimulated. The patient becomes irritable and has tremors. In severe cases, these tissues fail to respond.

PREVENTION. Prevention of hypernatremia is not as simple as prevention of hyponatremia. Most patients have a sodium excess as a result of an acute or chronic illness. Patients with a potential for electrolyte imbalance must always have their IV fluids carefully regulated.

SIGNS AND SYMPTOMS. Thirst is usually one of the first symptoms to appear. If you eat salty foods, such as potato chips, the amount of sodium in the body increases and you become thirsty. Other signs and symptoms of hypernatremia are vague and nonspecific until severe excess is present. Like the patient with a sodium deficit, the patient experiencing sodium excess has mental status changes, such as agitation, confusion, and personality changes—but this time, the cause is too little fluid in the brain tissues. Seizures may also occur.

At first, muscle twitches and unusual contractions may be present. Later, skeletal muscle weakness occurs that can lead to respiratory failure if it affects the diaphragm. If fluid deficit or fluid excess accompanies the hypernatremic state, the patient also has signs and symptoms associated with these imbalances.

COMPLICATIONS. A patient with severe hypernatremia may become comatose or have respiratory arrest as skeletal muscles weaken.

DIAGNOSTIC TESTS. The most reliable diagnostic test is the serum sodium level, which indicates an increase above the normal level. Serum osmolarity may also increase. If the patient has a fluid imbalance, other laboratory values, such as BUN, hematocrit, and urine specific gravity, are also affected (see earlier discussion).

THERAPEUTIC MEASURES. If a fluid imbalance accompanies hypernatremia, it is treated first. For example, fluid replacement without sodium in a patient with dehydration should correct a relative sodium excess. If the kidneys are not excreting adequate amounts of sodium, diuretics may help if the kidneys are functional. If the kidneys are not functioning properly, dialysis may be ordered (see Chapter 37). I&O and daily weights are strictly monitored.

The cause of hypernatremia is also treated in an attempt to prevent further episodes of this imbalance. For some patients, a sodium-restricted diet is prescribed.

Potassium Imbalances

Potassium is the most common electrolyte in the ICF compartment. Therefore, only a small amount, 3.5 to 5 mEq/L, is found in the bloodstream. Small changes in this laboratory value cause major changes in the body.

Potassium is especially important for cardiac muscle, skeletal muscle, and smooth muscle function. If the serum potassium level falls, the body attempts to compensate by moving potassium from the cells into the bloodstream.

• WORD • BUILDING •

intracranial: intra—within + cranial—cranium (skull)

The two potassium imbalances are **hypokalemia** (potassium deficit) and **hyperkalemia** (potassium excess). Hypokalemia is the most commonly occurring imbalance.

Hypokalemia

Hypokalemia occurs when the serum potassium level falls below 3.5 mEq/L.

PATHOPHYSIOLOGY AND ETIOLOGY. Most cases of hypokalemia result from inadequate intake of potassium or excessive loss of potassium through the kidneys. Hypokalemia most often occurs as a result of medications. Potassium-losing diuretics (e.g., furosemide [Lasix]), digitalis preparations (e.g., digoxin [Lanoxin]), and corticosteroids (e.g., prednisone [Deltasone]) are examples of drugs that cause increased excretion of potassium from the body. Potassium may also be lost through the gastrointestinal (GI) tract, which is rich in potassium and other electrolytes. Severe vomiting, diarrhea, and prolonged GI suction cause hypokalemia (Box 6.7, *Patient Perspective*). Major surgery and hemorrhage can also lead to potassium deficit.

PREVENTION. Most patients having major surgery receive potassium supplements in their IV fluids to prevent hypokalemia. For patients receiving drugs known to cause hypokalemia, foods high in potassium may prevent a deficit (see Table 6.2). Patients receiving digitalis must be closely monitored because digitalis can cause hypokalemia, which in turn can enhance the action of digitalis and cause digitalis toxicity.

SIGNS AND SYMPTOMS. Many body systems are affected by a potassium imbalance. Muscle cramping or muscle fatigue can occur with either a deficit or an excess of potassium. Vital signs change because the respiratory and cardiovascular systems need potassium to function properly. Diminished skeletal muscle activity results in shallow, ineffective respirations. The pulse is typically weak, irregular, and thready because the heart muscle is depleted of potassium. A major danger is an irregular heartbeat (**dysrhythmia**), which can lead to cardiac arrest. Orthostatic (postural) hypotension may also be present.

The nervous system is usually affected as well. The patient experiences changes in mental status followed by lethargy. The motility of the GI system is slowed, causing nausea, vomiting, abdominal distention, and constipation. Vomiting may further increase potassium loss.

COMPLICATIONS. If not corrected, hypokalemia can result in death from dysrhythmia, respiratory failure and arrest, or coma. The patient must be treated promptly before these complications occur.

DIAGNOSTIC TESTS. The primary laboratory test is to obtain a serum potassium level. The patient's electrocardiogram (ECG) may show cardiac dysrhythmias associated with potassium deficit. In addition to a decrease in the serum potassium level, the patient may have an acid-base imbalance known as metabolic **alkalosis**, which commonly accompanies hypokalemia. In metabolic alkalosis, the serum pH of the blood increases (above 7.45) so that the blood is more alkaline than usual. Acid-base imbalances are discussed later in this chapter.

THERAPEUTIC MEASURES. The goal of treatment is to replace potassium in the body and resolve the underlying cause of the imbalance. For mild to moderate hypokalemia, oral potassium supplements are given.

For severe hypokalemia, IV potassium supplements are given. Because the kidneys eliminate excess potassium, potassium should be added to IV fluids only after the patient has voided. Potassium is a potentially dangerous drug, especially when administered intravenously. In too high a concentration, it causes cardiac arrest. Only IV solutions that are premixed and carefully labeled should be used, and they are administered very slowly. Potassium is never given by IV push. The patient's laboratory values must be monitored carefully to prevent giving too much potassium. Administration of IV potassium is done by a registered nurse.

• WORD • BUILDING •

hypokalemia: hypo—less than + kal—potassium + emia—blood
hyperkalemia: hyper—more than + kal—potassium + emia—blood
dysrhythmia: dys—bad or disordered + rhythmia—measured motion
alkalosis: alkal—alkaline + osis—condition

Box 6.7

Patient Perspective

Patricia

I take hydrochlorothiazide for my high blood pressure. Since it can make me lose potassium, I also take a potassium supplement. So I thought I was all set. But recently I ate something that did not agree with me, and I had diarrhea for a couple of days. One morning as I was driving to work, I felt so weak it made me frightened. I drove back home and asked my husband to drive me to work. I arrived safely, but as I walked down the hallway, I again felt so weak I had to sit down. I felt like I could not put one foot in front of the other. I kept thinking, "This is all in my head." I decided maybe I was dehydrated from the diarrhea, so I drank a bottle of Gatorade and a glass of orange juice. Slowly I began to feel a bit better, and I made it through the day. After work I had to take my daughter to the doctor, so I asked about my symptoms. I was sent to the lab where I had my potassium level checked, and it was 3.1! Normal is 3.5 to 5 mEq/L. Mine must have been even lower before I drank the juice and Gatorade. I learned that I probably lost a lot of potassium because of the diarrhea. I also learned that low potassium made my muscles weak and could have affected my heart function. Next time I have diarrhea, I plan to call my doctor.

Teach the patient about the side effects of oral potassium and precautions associated with potassium administration. Box 6.8 summarizes the precautions the patient should be aware of when taking oral potassium supplements.

Hyperkalemia

Hyperkalemia is a condition in which the serum potassium level exceeds 5 mEq/L. It is rare in a person with healthy kidneys.

PATHOPHYSIOLOGY AND ETIOLOGY. Hyperkalemia may result from an actual increase in the amount of total body potassium or from the movement of intracellular potassium into the blood. Overuse of potassium-based salt substitutes or excessive intake of oral or IV potassium supplements can cause hyperkalemia. Use of potassium-sparing diuretics (e.g., spironolactone [Aldactone]) may also contribute to hyperkalemia. Patients with renal failure are at risk for hyperkalemia because the kidneys cannot excrete potassium.

Movement of potassium from the cells into the blood and other ECF is common in massive tissue trauma and metabolic acidosis. Metabolic **acidosis** is an acid-base imbalance commonly seen in patients with uncontrolled diabetes mellitus. Acid-base imbalances are discussed later in this chapter.

PREVENTION. For patients receiving potassium supplements, hyperkalemia can be prevented by monitoring serum electrolyte values and the patient's signs and symptoms and adjusting the dose accordingly.

Box 6.8

Tips for Patients Taking Oral Potassium Supplements

- Do not substitute one potassium supplement for another.
- Dilute powders and liquids in juice or other desired liquid to improve taste and to prevent gastrointestinal irritation. Follow manufacturer's recommendations for the amount of fluid to use for dilution, most commonly 4 oz per 20 mEq of potassium.
- Do not drink diluted solutions until mixed thoroughly.
- Do not crush potassium tablets, such as Slow-K or K-tab tablets. Read manufacturer's directions regarding which tablets can be crushed.
- Take slow-release tablets with 8 oz of water to help them dissolve.
- Do not take potassium supplements if taking potassium-sparing diuretics such as spironolactone or triamterene.
- Do not use salt substitutes containing potassium unless prescribed by the physician.
- Take potassium supplements with meals.
- Report adverse effects, such as nausea, vomiting, diarrhea, and abdominal cramping, to the physician.
- Have frequent laboratory testing for potassium levels as recommended by the physician.

Source: Adapted from Lee, C. A., Barrett, C. A., & Ignatavicius, D. D. (1996). *Fluids and electrolytes: A practical approach* (4th ed.). Philadelphia: F. A. Davis.

SIGNS AND SYMPTOMS. Most cases of hyperkalemia occur in patients who are hospitalized or those undergoing therapeutic measures for a chronic condition. The classic manifestations are muscle twitches and cramps, later followed by profound muscular weakness; increased GI motility (diarrhea); slow, irregular heart rate; and decreased blood pressure.

COMPLICATIONS. Cardiac dysrhythmias and respiratory failure can occur in severe hyperkalemia, causing death.

DIAGNOSTIC TESTS. In addition to an elevated serum potassium level, an irregular ECG is associated with hyperkalemia. If the patient also has metabolic acidosis, the serum pH falls below 7.35.

THERAPEUTIC MEASURES. For mild, chronic hyperkalemia, dietary limitation of potassium-rich foods may be helpful. Potassium supplements are discontinued, and potassium-losing diuretics are given to patients with healthy kidneys. For patients with renal problems, a cation exchange resin, such as sodium polystyrene sulfonate (Kayexalate), is administered either orally or rectally. This drug releases sodium and absorbs potassium for excretion through the feces and out of the body.

In cases in which cellular potassium has moved into the bloodstream, administration of glucose and insulin can facilitate the movement of potassium back into the cells. During treatment of moderate to severe hyperkalemia, the patient should be in the hospital on a cardiac monitor.

Calcium Imbalances

Calcium is a mineral that is primarily stored in bones and teeth. A small amount is found in ECF. The normal value for serum calcium is 9 to 11 mg/dL, or 4.5 to 5.5 mEq/L. Minimal changes in serum calcium levels can have major negative effects in the body.

Calcium is needed for the proper function of excitable tissues, especially cardiac muscle. The two calcium imbalances are **hypocalcemia** and **hypercalcemia.**

Hypocalcemia

Hypocalcemia occurs when the serum calcium level falls below 9 mg/dL, or 4.5 mEq/L.

PATHOPHYSIOLOGY AND ETIOLOGY. Although calcium deficit can be acute or chronic, most patients develop hypocalcemia slowly as a result of chronic disease or poor intake. The woman who is postmenopausal is most at risk for hypocalcemia. As a woman ages, calcium intake typically declines. The parathyroid glands recognize this decrease and stimulate bone to release some of its stored calcium into the

• WORD • BUILDING •

acidosis: acid—acidic + osis—condition
hypocalcemia: hypo—less than + calc—calcium + emia—blood
hypercalcemia: hyper—more than + calc—calcium + emia—blood
osteoporosis: osteo—bone + porosis—porous

blood for replacement. The result is a condition known as **osteoporosis**, in which bones become porous and brittle and fracture easily. The woman who is postmenopausal has a decreased level of estrogens, hormones that help prevent bone loss in the younger woman. Immobility or decreased mobility also contributes to bone loss in many patients. The patients at highest risk for osteoporosis are thin, petite, Caucasian women.

Hypocalcemia can also result from inadequate absorption of calcium from the intestines, as seen in patients with Crohn's disease, a chronic inflammatory bowel disease. Insufficient intake of vitamin D prevents calcium absorption as well. Conditions that interfere with the production of parathyroid hormone, such as partial or complete surgical removal of the thyroid or parathyroids, can also cause hypocalcemia.

Finally, patients with hyperphosphatemia (usually those with renal failure) often experience hypocalcemia. Calcium and phosphate have an inverse relationship. When one of these electrolytes increases, the other tends to decrease and vice versa.

PREVENTION. In the United States, the typical daily calcium intake is less than 550 mg. The adequate intake (AI) of calcium for adults ages 19 to 50 is 1000 mg; the AI for adults over age 50 is 1200 mg.

Hypocalcemia can be prevented by consuming calcium-rich foods and by taking calcium supplements. These supplements can be purchased over the counter in any pharmacy or large food store. An inexpensive source of calcium for patients who do not require vitamin D supplementation is calcium carbonate (Tums), which provides 240 mg of elemental calcium in each tablet.

Vitamin D supplementation may be required in addition to calcium for patients whose sun exposure is limited (see *Evidence-Based Practice*). The sun's ultraviolet light causes the skin to manufacture vitamin D.

EVIDENCE-BASED PRACTICE

Clinical Question

Should long-term care residents be supplemented with vitamin D?

Evidence

Research conducted in both Canada and the United States provides sufficient evidence to indicate that older people living in long-term care facilities are at high risk for vitamin D deficiency and should receive a minimum daily supplement of 800 IU (Lister, 2008).

Implications for Nursing Practice

To prevent complications related to calcium and vitamin D deficiencies, request orders for vitamin D supplements for nursing home residents.

REFERENCE

Lister, M. (2008). Should long-term care residents be supplemented with vitamin D? *Canadian Journal of Dietetic Practice and Research, 69*(1), 29–31.

SIGNS AND SYMPTOMS. Chronic hypocalcemia is usually not diagnosed until the patient breaks a bone, usually a hip. Acute hypocalcemia, which can occur after surgery or in patients with acute pancreatitis, has several signs and symptoms. These include increased and irregular heart rate, mental status changes, hyperactive deep tendon reflexes, and increased GI motility, including diarrhea and abdominal cramping. Two classic signs that can be used to assess for hypocalcemia are Trousseau's sign and Chvostek's sign.

To test for Trousseau's sign, inflate a blood pressure cuff around the patient's upper arm for 1 to 4 minutes. In a patient with hypocalcemia, the hand and fingers become spastic and go into palmar flexion (Fig. 6.4). A positive Chvostek's sign test also indicates calcium deficit. To test for this sign, tap the face just below and in front of the ear. Facial twitching on that side of the face indicates a positive test (Fig. 6.5).

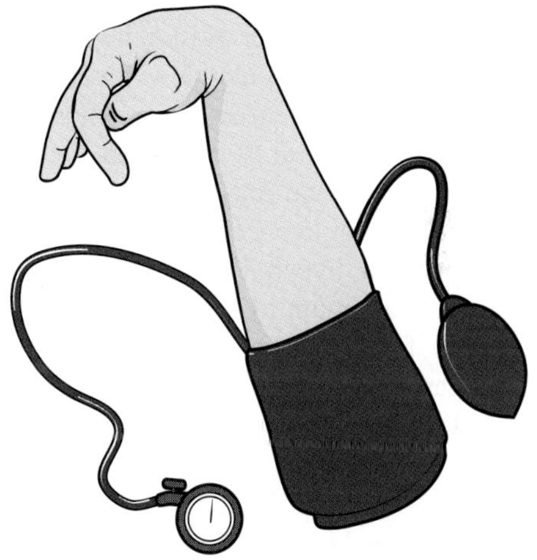

FIGURE 6.4 Trousseau's sign.

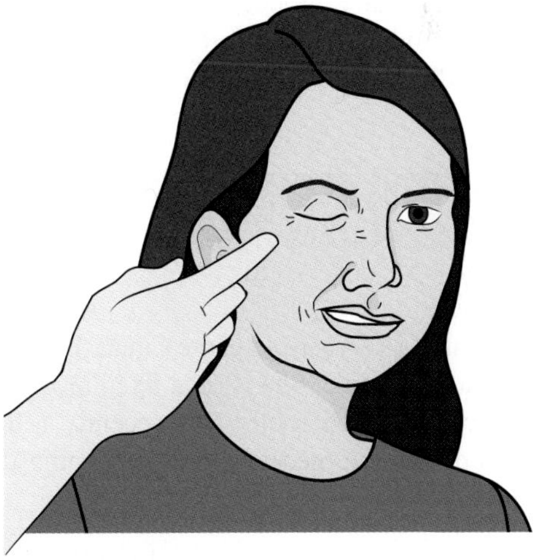

FIGURE 6.5 Chvostek's sign.

LEARNING TIP

You can remember which sign is **CH**vostek's sign because it causes spasm near the **CH**eek.

COMPLICATIONS. In severe hypocalcemia, neuromuscular irritability can lead to tetany, or continuous muscle contraction. The patient may have a sudden laryngospasm that will stop air from entering the lungs. Seizures, respiratory failure, or cardiac failure can occur and lead to death if not aggressively treated.

DIAGNOSTIC TESTS. The patient with hypocalcemia has a lowered serum calcium level and an abnormal ECG. The parathyroid hormone level may be increased as it attempts to stimulate bone to release more calcium into the blood.

THERAPEUTIC MEASURES. In addition to treating the cause of hypocalcemia, calcium is replaced. For mild or chronic hypocalcemia, oral calcium supplements with or without vitamin D are given. Calcium supplements should be administered 1 to 2 hours after meals to increase intestinal absorption. Be sure to check compatibility when administering calcium with other medications.

For patients with acute or severe hypocalcemia, IV calcium gluconate or calcium chloride is given. When a patient has had thyroid or parathyroid surgery, there is a danger that parathyroid hormone will be decreased, causing serum calcium to drop. IV calcium must be readily available for emergency use if signs of hypocalcemia occur

For patients with hyperphosphatemia, usually those with renal failure, aluminum hydroxide is used to bind the excess phosphate for elimination via the GI tract. As the phosphate decreases, the serum calcium level begins to approach normal levels.

Diet therapy is an important part of treatment. Teach the patient, family, or other caregiver which foods are high in calcium (Table 6.3). Many foods today are fortified with calcium. Vitamin D foods are also encouraged, especially milk and other dairy products. For patients experiencing difficulty digesting dairy products and those who choose not to use dairy products, special attention must be paid to including other dietary calcium sources in the diet.

CRITICAL THINKING

Mrs. Wright

■ Mrs. Wright is a 77-year-old petite Caucasian woman who lives alone at home. She is on a fixed income and rarely eats calcium-rich foods. She recently fell and broke her hip. After surgery she returned home under the care of a home health agency.

1. What made the patient at high risk for a fracture?
2. What would you expect her serum calcium level to have been before the fall?
3. What patient teaching related to diet and calcium supplements should the home health nurse include during his or her home visits?

Suggested answers at end of chapter.

Hypercalcemia

Hypercalcemia occurs when the serum calcium is above 11 mg/dL, or 5.5 mEq/L.

PATHOPHYSIOLOGY AND ETOLOGY. Chronic hypercalcemia can result from excessive intake of calcium or vitamin D, renal failure, hyperparathyroidism, cancers, and overuse or prolonged use of thiazide diuretics, such as hydrochlorothiazide (HydroDIURIL). Acute hypercalcemia can occur as an emergency in patients with invasive or metastatic cancers, especially cancers of the blood or bone.

PREVENTION. Although many causes of increased calcium cannot be prevented, a person receiving calcium supplements should be monitored carefully. Some patients believe that if two or three tablets a day are helpful, consuming twice that much will help even more. The result can be serum calcium excess. Educating the public about the proper amount of calcium needed each day and the danger of too much calcium is very important.

SIGNS AND SYMPTOMS. Patients who have mild hypercalcemia or a slowly progressing calcium increase may have no obvious signs and symptoms. However, acute hypercalcemia is associated with increased heart rate and blood pressure, skeletal muscle weakness, and decreased GI motility.

COMPLICATIONS. In some cases, the patient may experience renal or urinary calculi (stones) resulting from the buildup of calcium. In more severe cases of acute hypercalcemia, the patient may experience respiratory failure caused by profound muscle weakness or heart failure caused by dysrhythmias.

THERAPEUTIC MEASURES. Patients with severe hypercalcemia should be hospitalized and placed on a cardiac monitor. Unless contraindicated by other conditions, the primary treatment is to give large amounts of fluids and promote diuresis. Saline infusions are the most useful solutions to promote renal excretion of calcium.

The physician also discontinues thiazide diuretics if the patient was receiving them and prescribes diuretics that promote calcium excretion, such as furosemide (Lasix). Drugs that slow calcium movement from bones to the blood may also be used, such as pamidronate (Aredia), zoledronic acid (Zometa), or calcitonin.

If hypercalcemia is so severe that cardiac problems are present, hemodialysis, peritoneal dialysis, or ultrafiltration may be necessary to cleanse the blood of excess calcium. (See Chapter 37 for discussion of these procedures.)

Magnesium Imbalances

Magnesium and calcium work together for the proper functioning of excitable cells, such as cardiac muscle and nerve

• WORD • BUILDING •

hypomagnesemia: hypo—less than + magnes—magnesium + emia—blood

hypermagnesemia: hyper—more than + magnes—magnesium + emia—blood

TABLE 6.3 Food Sources of Calcium*

Food, Standard Amount	Calcium (mg)	Calories
Fortified ready-to-eat cereals (various), 1 oz	236–1043	88–106
Soy beverage, calcium fortified, 1 cup	368	98
Tofu, firm, prepared with nigari†, ½ cup	253	88
Pink salmon, canned, with bone, 3 oz	181	118
Collards, cooked from frozen, ½ cup	178	31
Spinach, cooked from frozen, ½ cup	146	30
Turnip greens, cooked from frozen, ½ cup	124	24
Ocean perch, Atlantic, cooked, 3 oz	116	103
Oatmeal, plain and flavored, instant, fortified, 1 packet prepared	99–110	97–157
Okra, cooked from frozen, ½ cup	88	26
Pak-choi, Chinese cabbage, cooked from fresh, ½ cup	79	10
Dandelion greens, cooked from fresh, ½ cup	74	17
Rainbow trout, farmed, cooked, 3 oz	73	144
Dairy Sources	**Calcium (mg)**	**Calories**
Plain yogurt, low-fat (12 g protein/8 oz), 8-oz container	415	143
Fruit yogurt, low-fat (10 g protein/8 oz), 8-oz container	345	232
Swiss cheese, 1.5 oz	336	162
Mozzarella cheese, part-skim, 1.5 oz	311	129
Cheddar cheese, 1.5 oz	307	171
Fat-free (skim) milk, 1 cup	306	83
2% reduced fat milk, 1 cup	285	122
Whole milk, 1 cup	276	146

*Both calcium content and bioavailability should be considered when selecting dietary sources of calcium. Some plant foods have calcium that is well absorbed, but the large quantity of plant foods that would be needed to provide as much calcium as in a glass of milk may be unachievable for many. Many other calcium-fortified foods are available, but the percentage of calcium that can be absorbed is unavailable for many of them.

†Calcium sulfate and magnesium chloride.

Source: Nutrient values from Agricultural Research Service (ARS) Nutrient Database for Standard Reference, Release 17. Foods are from ARS single nutrient reports, sorted in descending order by nutrient content in terms of common household measures. Food items and weights in the single nutrient reports are adapted from those in the 2002 revision of USDA Home and Garden Bulletin No. 72, *Nutritive Value of Foods*. Mixed dishes and multiple preparations of the same food item have been omitted from this table.

cells. Therefore, an imbalance of magnesium is usually accompanied by an imbalance of calcium.

The normal value for serum magnesium is 1.5 to 2.5 mEq/L. The magnesium imbalances are called **hypomagnesemia** and **hypermagnesemia**.

Hypomagnesemia

Hypomagnesemia occurs when the serum magnesium level falls below 1.5 mEq/L. It results from either a decreased intake or an excessive loss of magnesium. Causes of inadequate intake include malnutrition and starvation diets. Patients with severe diarrhea and Crohn's disease are unable to absorb magnesium in the intestines.

One of the major causes of hypomagnesemia is alcoholism, which causes both a decreased intake and an increased renal excretion of magnesium. Certain drugs, such as loop and osmotic diuretics, aminoglycosides (e.g., gentamicin), and some anticancer agents (e.g., cisplatin), can increase renal excretion of magnesium.

The signs and symptoms of hypomagnesemia are similar to those for hypocalcemia, including positive Trousseau's and Chvostek's signs, described earlier in this chapter.

The goal of management is to treat the underlying cause and replace magnesium in the body. Magnesium sulfate is administered intravenously. If the serum calcium is also low, calcium replacement is prescribed. The patient is placed on a cardiac monitor because of magnesium's effect on the heart. Life-threatening dysrhythmias can lead to cardiac failure and arrest.

Hypermagnesemia

Hypermagnesemia results when the serum magnesium level increases above 2.5 mEq/L. The most common cause of hypermagnesemia is increased intake coupled with decreased renal excretion caused by renal failure.

Signs and symptoms are usually not apparent until the serum level is greater than 4 mEq/L. Then the signs and symptoms include bradycardia and other dysrhythmias, hypotension, lethargy or drowsiness, and skeletal muscle weakness. If not treated, the patient experiences coma, respiratory failure, or cardiac failure.

When kidneys are functioning properly, loop diuretics such as furosemide (Lasix) and IV fluids can help increase magnesium excretion. For patients with renal failure, dialysis may be the only option.

ACID-BASE BALANCE

The cells of the body function best when the body fluids and electrolytes are within a very narrow range. Hydrogen (H^+) is another ion that must stay within its normal limits. The amount of hydrogen determines whether a fluid is an acid or base.

An acid is a substance that releases a hydrogen ion. The stronger the acid, the more hydrogen ions are released. A common acid in the body is hydrochloric acid (HCl), which is found in the stomach. A base is a substance that binds hydrogen. A common base in the body is bicarbonate (HCO_3^-). Alkali is another word for base.

Sources of Acids and Bases

Acids and bases are formed in the body as part of normal metabolic processes. Acids are formed as end products of glucose, fat, and protein metabolism. These are called fixed acids because they do not change once they are formed. A weak acid, carbonic acid, can be formed when the carbon dioxide resulting from cellular metabolism combines with water. This acid can change to bicarbonate (a base) and hydrogen and therefore is not a fixed acid.

The ECF maintains a delicate balance between acids and bases. The strength of the acids and bases can be measured by pH. The pH of a solution can vary from 0 to 14, with 7 being neutral, 0 to 6.99 being acid, and 7.01 to 14 being base, also called alkaline. The normal serum pH level is 7.35 to 7.45, which is slightly alkaline. It must remain in an extremely narrow range to sustain life. A pH lower than 6.9 or higher than 7.8 is usually fatal.

Control of Acid-Base Balance

As discussed in the sections on fluid and electrolyte balance, the body has several ways in which it tries to compensate for changes in the serum pH. Three major mechanisms are used: cellular buffers, the lungs, and the kidneys.

Cellular buffers are the first to attempt a return of the pH to its normal range. Examples of cellular buffers are proteins, hemoglobin, bicarbonate, and phosphates. These buffers act as a type of sponge to "soak up" extra hydrogen ions if there are too many (too acidic) or release hydrogen ions if there are not enough (too alkaline).

The lungs are the second line of defense to restore normal pH. When the blood is too acidic (pH is decreased), the lungs "blow off" additional carbon dioxide through rapid, deep breathing. This reduces the amount of carbon dioxide available to make carbonic acid in the body. If the blood is too alkaline (pH is increased), the lungs try to conserve carbon dioxide through shallow respirations.

The kidneys are the slowest to respond to changes in serum pH, taking as long as 24 to 48 hours to assist with compensation. The kidneys help in a number of ways, including regulating the amount of bicarbonate (base) that is kept in the body. If the serum pH lowers and becomes too acidic, the kidneys reabsorb additional bicarbonate rather than excreting it so that it can help neutralize the acid. If the serum pH increases and becomes too alkaline, the kidneys excrete additional bicarbonate to get rid of the extra base. The kidneys also buffer pH by forming acids and ammonium (a base).

Acidosis or alkalosis that is corrected for by the body is referred to as *compensated*. The pH is returned to normal or near normal, but the gases that monitor acid-base balance (Pco_2 and HCO_3^-) are abnormal.

ACID-BASE IMBALANCES

Acid-base imbalances are caused by a number of acute and chronic illnesses or conditions. The primary treatment for each of the imbalances is to manage the underlying cause, which corrects the imbalance. The role of the nurse is to identify patients at risk and monitor laboratory test values for significant changes.

The laboratory tests that are used to evaluate acid-base balance are called arterial blood gases (ABGs). As the name implies, the blood sample that is analyzed must be from an artery rather than a vein. The femoral, brachial, and radial arteries are most often used to obtain the sample. Table 6.4 lists ABG values and what they indicate.

The two broad types of acid-base imbalance are acidosis and alkalosis. Each of these imbalances can occur suddenly, which is called an acute imbalance, or develop over a long period, referred to as a chronic imbalance.

TABLE 6.4 ARTERIAL BLOOD GAS VALUES AND CHANGES IN ACID-BASE IMBALANCES

	pH	Pco_2	HCO_3^-
Normal values	7.35–7.45	32–45 mm Hg	20–26 mEq/L
Respiratory acidosis	↓	↑	Normal
Respiratory acidosis with compensation	Nearly normal	↑	↑
Respiratory alkalosis	↑	↓	Normal
Respiratory alkalosis with compensation	Nearly normal	↓	↓
Metabolic acidosis	↓	Normal	↓
Metabolic acidosis with compensation	Nearly normal	↓	↓
Metabolic alkalosis	↑	Normal	↑
Metabolic alkalosis with compensation	Nearly normal	↑	↑

When the serum pH level falls below 7.35, the patient has acidosis because the blood becomes more acidic than normal. Too much acid or too little base in the body causes acidosis. Acidosis can be divided into two types: respiratory and metabolic. Respiratory acidosis is caused by problems occurring in the respiratory system. Metabolic acidosis is the result of problems in the rest of the body.

When the serum pH level increases above 7.45, the patient has alkalosis because the blood becomes more alkaline or basic. Alkalosis is caused by too little acid in the body or too much base. It can also be divided into two types: respiratory alkalosis and metabolic alkalosis.

Respiratory Acidosis

As the name indicates, the primary cause of this type of acidosis is respiratory problems. Carbon dioxide is not adequately "blown off" during expiration, causing a buildup of carbon dioxide in the blood. As mentioned earlier, carbon dioxide mixes with water to create a weak acid in the body, thus increasing the acidity of the blood.

Acute respiratory acidosis is caused by hypoventilation, usually as a result of an acute flare-up of chronic respiratory disease, drugs, or neurologic problems that depress breathing. Patients with chronic respiratory disease such as emphysema or chronic bronchitis may have chronic respiratory acidosis.

The signs and symptoms of respiratory acidosis involve the central nervous system and the musculoskeletal system. As carbon dioxide increases, mental status is altered, progressing from confusion and lethargy to stupor and coma if not treated. The lungs are not able to get rid of excess carbon dioxide. Instead respirations become more depressed and shallow as muscle weakness worsens.

Treatment of respiratory acidosis is aggressive management of the underlying respiratory problem, discussed in the respiratory unit (Unit 7) of this text.

Metabolic Acidosis

Metabolic acidosis can result from too much acid in the body (usually fixed acids) or too little bicarbonate in the body. Uncontrolled diabetes mellitus and end-stage renal failure are the two most common causes of metabolic acidosis resulting from increased fixed acids.

The GI tract is rich in bicarbonate. Patients experiencing severe diarrhea or prolonged intestinal suction are at high risk for metabolic acidosis as a result of bicarbonate (base) loss. The serum pH decreases as the bicarbonate level decreases (see Table 6.4). As mentioned earlier in the discussion on hyperkalemia, serum potassium tends to increase in the presence of metabolic acidosis. Excess hydrogen in the ECF moves into the cells in exchange for potassium, which leaves the cells and enters the blood. In a sense, this is a way of compensating for the acidotic state.

The signs and symptoms are similar to those associated with respiratory acidosis, with the exception of the respiratory pattern. To help compensate for the acidotic state, the lungs get rid of extra carbon dioxide through Kussmaul's respirations. Kussmaul's respirations are deep and rapid and can occur only in patients with healthy lungs.

The treatment for the patient with metabolic acidosis is management of the underlying disease or condition. Information about disease management, such as diabetes, is found elsewhere in this book.

Respiratory Alkalosis

Respiratory alkalosis occurs when there is excessive loss of carbon dioxide through **hyperventilation**. Patients may hyperventilate when they are severely anxious or fearful. Patients who hyperventilate have rapid shallow respirations, are light-headed, and may become confused. The heart rate increases and the pulse becomes weak and thready. The serum pH is increased and the $Paco_2$ is very low. Mechanical ventilation can also cause respiratory alkalosis, and it can occur as a result of being at high altitudes. You may have experienced this while deep breathing during a pulmonary examination.

Respiratory alkalosis is treated by having patients hold their breath or rebreathe their own carbon dioxide with the use of either a rebreathing mask or a plain paper bag. The underlying cause must also be treated.

Metabolic Alkalosis

Metabolic alkalosis results from excessive ingestion of bicarbonate or other bases into the body or loss of acids from the body. Overuse or abuse of antacids or baking soda (sodium bicarbonate) can lead to metabolic alkalosis. Because the stomach contains hydrochloric acid, prolonged vomiting or gastric suction can cause loss of acid and also lead to metabolic alkalosis.

The serum pH is increased, as is bicarbonate. As discussed under potassium imbalances, the serum potassium decreases. Hydrogen from the ICF moves into the blood in exchange for potassium, which moves from the blood into the cells. This is one way that the body works to keep an acid-base balance. Hypocalcemia may also accompany hypokalemia.

The signs and symptoms of metabolic alkalosis are related to hypokalemia and hypocalcemia rather than the alkalotic state itself. Treatment involves identifying the underlying cause and managing it as quickly as possible.

Compensation

If the respiratory system is compensating for metabolic acidosis, the Pco_2 will be decreased to return the pH level to normal or near normal. In a similar fashion, if there is metabolic alkalosis, the breathing pattern will change to conserve CO_2 and restore the pH level. In chronic respiratory conditions, the kidneys conserve HCO_3^- to buffer in the case of respiratory acidosis and excrete HCO_3^- in cases of chronic respiratory alkalosis.

• WORD • BUILDING •

hyperventilation: hyper—more than + ventilation—air

SUGGESTED ANSWERS TO CRITICAL THINKING

■ *Mrs. Levitt*

1. Check her weight and compare it with her previous weights. Dehydration is associated with weight loss. Monitor mental status for disorientation. Check skin turgor for tenting. Continue to monitor vital signs.
2. Encourage increased fluid intake; notify the RN or physician if Mrs. Levitt is unable to take in additional fluids or if the fluids do not normalize assessment findings.
3. S: "My urine smells bad, and my heart is beating fast."
   O: Pt's urine is dark amber and strong smelling. (Also document weight and skin turgor findings.) VS: P 98 beats per minute, BP 126/74 mm Hg, RR 20 per minute, T 99.2. Fluids encouraged. RN notified.

■ *Mr. Peters*

1. Raise the head of the bed to assist breathing.
2. Using the WHAT'S UP? format as a guide, ask the following questions: How are you feeling? Did anything aggravate your symptoms? When did your symptoms begin? On a scale of 0 to 10, how difficult is your breathing? Are you having any problems besides shortness of breath? What do you think might be happening? (If the patient is too dyspneic to answer, do not ask many questions.)
3. Check breath sounds for crackles, observe for dependent edema and ascites, observe for distended neck veins, assess skin for color and temperature, check weight and compare with previous weight, and monitor I&O. Continue to monitor vital signs.
4. Notify RN or physician of your findings.

■ *Mrs. Wright*

1. The patient is at high risk for osteoporosis, and thus fracture, because she is an elderly, petite, Caucasian woman. In addition, she does not get much calcium in her diet.
2. Her serum calcium levels would be low or low normal, since the body will mobilize calcium in the bones in an attempt to maintain serum calcium levels.
3. Teach her about consuming foods high in calcium, the need to be compliant with taking her calcium supplements, and to take the supplements 1 to 2 hours after meals for best absorption by the body.

REVIEW QUESTIONS

1. Which of the following are functions of sodium in the body? **Select all that apply.**
   a. Maintenance of serum osmolarity
   b. Formation of bones and teeth
   c. Control of bronchodilation
   d. Control of serum glucose
   e. Maintenance of cellular function

2. A 93-year-old patient with diarrhea and dehydration is admitted to the hospital from an extended care facility. For which of the following symptoms of dehydration should the nurse assess?
   a. Pale-colored urine, bradycardia
   b. Disorientation, poor skin turgor
   c. Decreased hematocrit, hypothermia
   d. Lung congestion, abdominal discomfort

3. Which patient is most at risk for fluid excess?
   a. An infant with pneumonia
   b. A teen with multiple injuries following an automobile accident
   c. A middle-aged man who has just had surgery
   d. An elderly patient receiving IV therapy

4. Which of the following is the most reliable way to monitor a patient's fluid status?
   a. I&O
   b Skin turgor
   c. Daily weights
   d. Lung sounds

5. When caring for a patient with fluid excess, which of the following interventions will best help relieve respiratory distress?
   a. Elevate the head of the bed.
   b. Encourage the patient to cough and deep breathe.
   c. Increase fluids to promote urine output.
   d. Perform percussion and postural drainage.

6. A patient is being discharged following hospitalization for fluid imbalance. Which instruction by the nurse should take priority?
   a. "Weigh yourself at the same time every day and report changes."
   b. "Call your doctor immediately if you feel weak or fatigued."
   c. "Drink eight glasses of water a day."
   d. "Measure everything you drink, and measure how much you urinate each day."

REVIEW QUESTIONS—cont'd

7. A patient is being treated for hypokalemia. When evaluating his response to potassium replacement therapy, which of the following changes in his assessment should the nurse observe for?
   a. Improving visual acuity
   b. Worsening constipation
   c. Decreasing serum glucose
   d. Increasing muscle strength

8. A patient is being placed on a potassium-losing diuretic. Which foods are high in potassium and should be recommended to the patient by the nurse? **Select all that apply.**
   a. Bread
   b. Potato
   c. Tomato juice
   d. Banana
   e. Gelatin

9. Which patient is at risk for respiratory acidosis?
   a. The patient with uncontrolled diabetes mellitus
   b. The patient with chronic pulmonary disease
   c. The patient who is very anxious
   d. The patient who overuses antacids

10. Which pH value represents acidosis?
    a. 7.26
    b. 7.35
    c. 7.4
    d. 7.49

Reference

Joint Commission. (2010). *2010 national patient safety goals*. Retrieved January 13, 2010, from http://www.jointcommission.org/patientsafety/nationalpatientsafetygoals

7

Nursing Care of Patients Receiving Intravenous Therapy

LYNN D. PHILLIPS

KEY TERMS

cannula (KAN-yoo-lah)
extravasation (eks-TRAH-vah-ZAY-shun)
hematoma (HEE-muh-TOH-mah)
infiltration (in-fil-TRAY-shun)
intravenous (IN-trah-VEE-nuss)
macrodrop (MACK-roh-DROP)
microdrop (MIKE-roh-DROP)
parenteral (pah-REN-ter-ul)
phlebitis (fla-BYE-tis)

QUESTIONS TO GUIDE YOUR READING

1. How is the practice of intravenous therapy regulated?
2. What are the indications for intravenous therapy?
3. What factors influence the condition, size, and long-term use of veins?
4. What steps are used for insertion of an intravenous cannula?
5. What techniques can be used for visualization of difficult veins?
6. How will you know if your nursing interventions to prevent complications of intravenous therapy have been effective?
7. How do you calculate a drip rate for a patient receiving a primary solution?
8. What is the difference between isotonic, hypertonic, and hypotonic solutions?
9. How would you explain the basic differences between central venous access devices: non-tunneled catheter, peripherally inserted central catheter, tunneled catheter, and implanted port?

Mrs. Brown, 85 years old, is admitted to the hospital with weight loss of 6% of her total body weight due to gastroenteritis and diarrhea. Her blood pressure is 102/80, pulse is 96 beats per minute, and respirations are 14 per minute. Her physical assessment shows decreased skin turgor over the sternum; dry, cracked lips; and a weak, thready pulse. The physician has ordered an IV to be started of 5% dextrose and 0.45% sodium chloride at 100 mL per hour. As you read this chapter, reflect on the challenges of fluid volume deficit in the elderly and initiation of infusion therapy.

Intravenous (IV) therapy is the administration of fluids or medication via a needle or catheter (also called a **cannula**) directly into the bloodstream. The practice of IV therapy is governed by state nurse practice acts as statutory laws. Some states now include IV therapy within the licensed practical nurse (LPN) and licensed vocational nurse (LVN) roles. The practice acts define the parameters within which individuals are qualified and licensed to practice nursing in a particular state and serve to codify the nursing obligation to act in the best interest of society.

Various specialty organizations, such as the Infusion Nurses Society (INS, www.ins1.org), set forth guidelines for standards of practice for infusion therapy. The Centers for Disease Control and Prevention (CDC, www.cdc.gov) provides the newest guidelines for isolation precautions. The Institute for Healthcare Improvement (IHI, www.ihi.org) provides information related to central line care. The National Institute for Occupational Safety and Health (NIOSH, www.cdc.gov/NIOSH) oversees workplace safety, including safety issues related to IV therapy, and the American Society for Parenteral and Enteral Nutrition (ASPEN, www.nutritioncare.org) provides resources related to IV nutrition.

INDICATIONS FOR INTRAVENOUS THERAPY

Patients receive a variety of substances via IV therapy, including fluids, electrolytes, nutrients, blood products, and medications. Patients can receive life-sustaining fluids, electrolytes, and nutrition via an IV when they are unable to eat or drink adequate amounts. The IV route also allows rapid delivery of medication in an emergency. Many medications are faster acting and more effective when given via the IV route. Other medications can be administered continuously via IV to maintain a therapeutic blood level. Patients with anemia or blood loss can receive lifesaving IV blood transfusions. Patients who are unable to eat for an extended period can have their nutritional needs met with peripheral parenteral nutrition (PPN) or total parenteral nutrition (TPN). The term **parenteral** refers to any medication route other than the digestive tract.

When a patient needs intermittent rather than continuous IV therapy, access to the bloodstream can be provided by an intermittent device, sometimes called a *saline lock,* in which an IV cannula is inserted and covered with a cap or valve that seals after each use. (See the *Intermittent Infusion* section later in this chapter.) This provides access to the bloodstream for intermittent or emergency medications, without the need for continuous fluid infusion.

TYPES OF INFUSIONS

Continuous Infusion

A continuous infusion is a large-volume infusion of parenteral solution (typically 250 to 1000 mL) administered over 2 to 24 hours. For a continuous infusion, the authorized prescriber orders the infusion in milliliters (mL) to be delivered over a specific amount of time, such as 100 mL per hour; or a total amount over a specified time, such as 1000 mL over 8 hours. The infusion is kept running constantly until ordered to be discontinued.

Continuous infusions are used when a medication must be highly diluted, a constant plasma concentration of a drug must be maintained, or a large volume of fluids and electrolytes must be administered. Rate control is important in the delivery of continuous infusions and can be achieved by electronic infusion device (EID), mechanical controller, or roller clamp.

Intermittent Infusion

Piggyback/Secondary Infusion

Some IV medications, such as antibiotics, need to be infused over a short period of time. For example, an antibiotic may be mixed with 50 mL of dextrose or 0.9% sodium chloride solution and infused over 30 minutes. This may be done as an intermittent infusion. If the patient already has a primary continuous IV infusing, the antibiotic (secondary) infusion can be "piggybacked" into the primary IV line. In order for the piggyback medication to infuse, it must hang higher than the primary infusion (Fig. 7.1). Piggyback medications can be infused using either a mechanical controller or an electronic infusion device. The medication in the piggyback must be compatible with any other solution that is in the primary IV tubing. (Check with your pharmacy for compatibilities.)

Injection/Access Caps

Peripheral cannulas that are covered with an injection cap are sometimes called saline locks. Intermittent IV lines can be "capped off" with an injection or access cap; this makes them available for intermittent or emergency access. This add-on device has a resealable diaphragm that can be accessed by a needle or a needleless system device. Intermittent infusions are small volumes of fluid or medication administered over 15 minutes to 2 hours by IV push or infusion through the resealable diaphragm.

• WORD • BUILDING •

intravenous: intra—within + venous—vein

cannula: tube or sheath

parenteral: para—beside + enteral—intestines

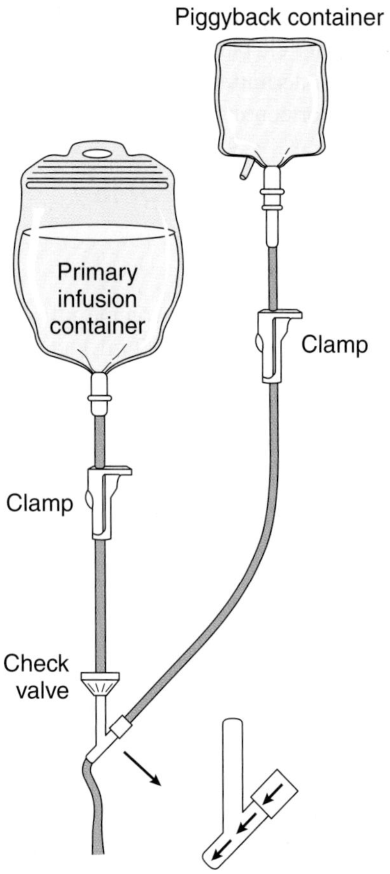
Piggyback container
Primary infusion container
Clamp
Clamp
Check valve

FIGURE 7.1 Gravity drip setup with piggyback infusion.

The patency of an intermittent cannula must be maintained by flushing at periodic intervals. Always check for patency of an intermittent device before administering a medication by inserting a syringe and drawing back to check for backflow of blood. To maintain patency of a cannula, normal saline solution (0.9% sodium chloride USP) is used to "flush" the cannula after each use, or every 12 hours if not in use or according to institution policy. In addition to ensuring patency, flushing with saline also prevents the mixing of incompatible medications and solutions. In *Infusion Nursing Standards of Practice* (2006), the Infusion Nurses Society (INS) recommends the use of sodium chloride for maintaining peripheral intermittent devices, whereas heparin, an anticoagulant, is recommended for flushing central venous access devices. Remember that heparin is a medication and may be incompatible with other medications. Check your institution's policy for specific guidelines.

Positive pressure must be maintained in the lumen of the cannula during the administration of the flush solution to prevent a backflow of blood into the cannula lumen, which could lead to occlusion of the lumen with a blood clot. This is accomplished by continuing to slowly inject the sodium chloride even as the syringe is withdrawn from the cap or valve. Intermittent cannulas should be flushed after administration of IV medication, taking a blood sample, and conversion from continuous to intermittent IV therapy.

If resistance is met while a cannula is being flushed, a clot may be occluding the cannula. Do not exert pressure on the syringe plunger in an attempt to restore patency because doing so may dislodge the clot into the vascular system or rupture the cannula.

NURSING CARE TIP

Always check for cannula patency before injecting any substance into the circulatory system.

Note: Some states require that registered nurses (RNs) administer medications given by the IV route; be sure to check your state's scope of practice policy regarding LVN/LPNs administering IV therapy.

Direct Injection/IV Push

An IV push (or IVP) medication is injected slowly via a syringe into an IV site or tubing port. It provides a rapid effect because it is delivered directly into the patient's bloodstream. IV push drugs can be dangerous if they are given incorrectly, and a drug reference should always be checked to determine the safe amount of time over which the drug can be injected. IV push drugs are usually administered by RNs and are not within the scope of practice of the LPN/LVN in some states. However, you should be aware of the drugs being given so you can assist in observing the patient for desired or adverse effects. (IVP administration is sometimes referred to as a *bolus*, which means "all at once.")

METHODS OF INFUSION

Gravity Drip

Gravity can be used to administer a solution into a vein (see Fig. 7.1). The solution is positioned about 3 feet above the infusion site. If it is positioned too high above the patient, the infusion may run too fast. Positioned too low, it may run too slowly. Flow is controlled with a roller, screw, or slide clamp. A mechanical flow device can be added to achieve accurate delivery of fluid with minimal deviation.

Calculating Drip Rates

When using a gravity set, you must calculate the drops (gtt, L. *guttae*) required per minute to deliver fluid at the ordered rate. Commercial parenteral administration sets vary in the number of drops delivering 1 mL. Sets typically deliver 10, 15, 20, or 60 drops per milliliter of fluid. For example, to deliver 100 mL per hour using a set with 10-drop factor tubing, a flow rate of 17 drops per minute is needed. To administer the same amount using a set with 15-drop factor tubing, a flow rate of 25 drops per minute is needed. Check the label on the administration set to determine how many drops per milliliter (drop factor) are delivered by the set. Sets delivering 10, 15, or 20 drops per milliliter are called

macrodrop sets, and are used for fluids that need to be infused more quickly. Sets delivering 60 drops per milliliter are called **microdrop** or minidrop sets and are used for solutions that need to be infused more slowly.

To determine drops per minute of an IV solution, the nurse needs to know the amount of fluid to be given in a specified time interval and the drop factor of the administration set to be used. The formula for determining drops per minute is as follows:

$$\frac{\text{mL}}{\text{hr or hrs}} \times \frac{1\text{ hr}}{60\text{ min}} \times \frac{\text{gtt}}{1\text{ mL}} = \text{gtt per minute}$$

If a controller or pump is being used, the calculation is even easier:

$$\frac{\text{mL}}{\text{Total number of hrs}} = \text{mL per hour}$$

SAMPLE PROBLEMS

Order: 125 mL of 5% dextrose and 0.45% sodium chloride per hour.

Drop factor: 15 gtt/mL.

$$\frac{125\text{ mL}}{1\text{ hr}} \times \frac{1\text{ hr}}{60\text{ min}} \times \frac{15\text{ gtt}}{1\text{ mL}} = 31\text{ gtt per minute}$$

Order: Normal saline 1000 mL over 8 hours.

$$\frac{1000\text{ mL}}{8\text{ hours}} = 125\text{ mL per hour}$$

LEARNING TIP

If you are having trouble with IV and drug calculations, check out the Calculating Drug Doses tutorial on your Student CD!

Factors Affecting Flow Rates of Gravity Infusions

CHANGE IN CANNULA POSITION. A change in the cannula's position may push the bevel either against the wall of the vein, which will decrease the flow rate, or away from the wall of the vein, which may increase the flow rate. Careful cannula securement and avoidance of joint flexion (usually bending the wrist or elbow) above the site minimize this problem. Patients may need to be reminded to keep flexion to a minimum when an IV is placed near a joint.

HEIGHT OF THE SOLUTION. Because infusions flow by gravity, a change in the height of the infusion bag or bottle or a change in the level of the bed can increase or decrease the flow rate. The flow rate increases as the distance between the solution and the patient increases. A patient may alter the flow rate greatly simply by standing up. The ideal height for a solution is 3 feet above the level of the patient's heart.

PATENCY OF THE CANNULA. A small clot or fibrin sheath may occlude the cannula lumen and decrease the flow rate or stop the flow. Clot formation can result from irritation, increased venous pressure, or backup of blood into the line. Avoid use of a blood pressure cuff on the affected limb because of the resulting transient increase in venous pressure. A regular flush schedule helps maintain patency. NEVER exert pressure with a saline or heparin flush in an attempt to restore patency; doing so may dislodge a clot into the vascular system or rupture the cannula.

Mechanical and Electronic Infusion Devices

Electronic infusion devices (EIDs) and mechanical controllers regulate the rate of infusion (Fig. 7.2). Mechanical controllers measure the amount of solution delivered and depend on gravity to deliver the infusion. Electronic infusion devices, sometimes called pumps, use positive pressure to deliver the solution.

Pumps and controllers are used for infusing precise volumes of solution. Institution policy often dictates use of controllers for infusion of potent medications, such as heparin, concentrated morphine, and chemotherapy solutions, and for very fast or slow rates. Some electronic infusion devices are portable and are designed to be worn on the body. These are called ambulatory infusion devices. It is important to know the type of pump being used and to follow its manufacturer's guidelines.

Filters

Filters can either be add-on devices to administration sets or built into the set during manufacturing. Various types of filters are available. The INS standards (2006) favor inline filters to remove bacteria, fungi, particulate matter, air, and some endotoxins from IV fluids.

A 0.22-micron (µm) filter removes bacteria and fungi from IV fluids. Blood infusion requires a 170-micron filter,

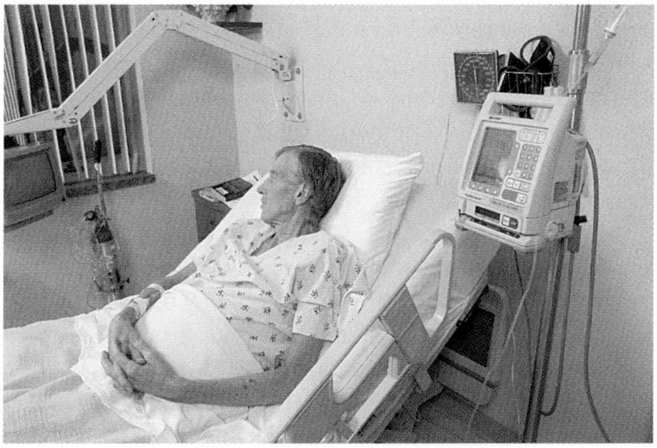

FIGURE 7.2 Infusion pump.

• WORD • BUILDING •

macrodrop: macro—large + drop

microdrop: micro—small + drop

which is built into the Y-administration set. Leukocyte-depleting filters are available for blood administration sets when concern for febrile reactions to leukocytes is anticipated (Roback et al., 2008). Other types of filters are used for nutritional products such as parenteral nutrition and fat emulsions. Check institution policy and manufacturers' guidelines for use of filters.

TYPES OF FLUIDS

Fluids and electrolytes administered intravenously pass directly into the plasma space of the extracellular fluid compartment. They are then absorbed based on the characteristics of the fluid and the hydration status of the patient. The most commonly infused fluids are dextrose and sodium solutions. These are called crystalloid solutions.

Dextrose Solutions

Dextrose in water is available in many concentrations and provides carbohydrates in a readily usable form. Solutions of 2.5%, 5%, and 10% dextrose in water are used for continuous peripheral infusions. Dextrose solutions provide calories for energy, reducing breakdown of glycogen and catabolism of protein to help prevent negative nitrogen balance. Dextrose is a nonelectrolyte and is well metabolized by all tissues.

The main disadvantage of dextrose solutions is vein irritation, which is caused by the slightly acidic pH of the solution. Vein irritation, damage, and thrombosis may result when hypertonic dextrose solutions are administered in a peripheral vein. Therefore, concentrations of 20% and above must be infused via a central line into a large vein. These high concentrations can be used for treating hypoglycemia or in combination with TPN because they supply a large number of calories.

Sodium Chloride Solutions

Sodium chloride solutions are available in concentrations of 0.25%, 0.33%, 0.45%, 0.9% (normal saline), 3%, and 5%. Sodium chloride 0.9% and 0.45% solutions are used most commonly. Sodium chloride solutions have many clinical uses, including replacement of fluid; treatment of shock, hyponatremia, and metabolic acidosis; and use as a primer for blood transfusions and during resuscitation after trauma. According to the American Association of Blood Banks, blood component administration sets can be primed only with 0.9% sodium chloride solution (Roback et al., 2008).

Combination dextrose and sodium chloride solutions, such as 5% dextrose with 0.45% sodium chloride (often referred to as "D_5 and a half"), are commonly used for hydration and to check for kidney function prior to administration of potassium replacement therapy.

Disadvantages of sodium chloride solutions include circulatory overload, if the prescribed rate is not monitored, and hypernatremia.

Balanced Electrolyte Solutions

Electrolyte solutions are used to replace lost fluids and electrolytes. A variety of balanced electrolyte solutions are available commercially. Maintenance electrolyte solutions, such as lactated Ringer's solution, approximate normal body electrolyte needs. Balanced solutions often contain lactate or acetate (yielding bicarbonate), which helps combat acidosis and provide a truly "balanced" solution. Potassium is an electrolyte that is commonly added to balanced solutions to replace potassium deficits. The patient must be monitored for signs and symptoms related to potassium imbalance (see Chapter 6). Guidelines for potassium administration must be reviewed prior to administration of any potassium-containing solution.

Osmolarity of IV Solutions

The osmolarity of IV solutions refers to the osmotic activity of a solution. Intravenous fluids may be classified as isotonic, hypotonic, or hypertonic. (See Chapter 6 to review these concepts.) Isotonic fluids have the same concentration of solutes to water as body fluids. Hypertonic solutions have more solutes (are more concentrated) than body fluids. Hypotonic solutions have fewer solutes (are less concentrated) than body fluids. Water moves from areas of lesser concentration to areas of greater concentration. Therefore, hypotonic solutions send water into areas of greater concentration (cells), and hypertonic solutions pull water from the more highly concentrated cells.

Isotonic Solutions

Normal saline (0.9% sodium chloride) solution is an isotonic solution that has the same tonicity as body fluid. When administered to patients requiring water, it neither enters cells nor pulls water from cells; it therefore expands the extracellular fluid volume. A solution of 5% dextrose in water (D_5W) is also isotonic when infused, but the dextrose is quickly metabolized, making the solution hypotonic.

Hypotonic Solutions

Hypotonic fluids are used when fluid is needed to enter the cells, as in the patient with cellular dehydration. They are also used as fluid maintenance therapy. An example of a hypotonic solution is 0.45% sodium chloride solution.

Hypertonic Solutions

Examples of hypertonic solutions include 5% dextrose in 0.9% sodium chloride and 5% dextrose in lactated Ringer's solution. Hypertonic solutions are used to expand the plasma volume, for example, in a hypovolemic patient. They are also used to replace electrolytes.

INTRAVENOUS ACCESS

Intravenous therapy can be administered into the systemic circulation via the peripheral or central veins. Peripheral veins lie beneath the epidermis, dermis, and subcutaneous tissue of the skin. They usually provide easy access to the venous system. Central veins are located close to the heart. Special catheters that end in a large vessel near the heart are called central lines. This chapter primarily discusses short peripheral catheters. The definitions of the various central venous access devices are discussed briefly at the end of the chapter.

ADMINISTERING PERIPHERAL INTRAVENOUS THERAPY

Starting a Peripheral (Short-Cannula) Infusion

The Phillips 15-step approach to starting a peripheral short-cannula infusion, described in Table 7.1, is organized and thorough (Phillips, 2010). Remember to always check your institution's policy before performing any procedure.

Precannulation (Steps 1–5)

STEP 1: CHECK AUTHORIZED PRESCRIBER'S ORDER. A physician or authorized prescriber's order is needed to start IV therapy. The nurse must verify that the order is clear, legible, and complete before starting therapy. According to the INS (2006), a prescriber's verbal order written by a nurse in the medical record in a hospital setting should be signed by the prescriber within an appropriate time (according to institution policy). The order should include solution, volume, rate, and route. If medication is ordered, the order should also include the medication, dosage, and frequency.

TABLE 7.1 THE PHILLIPS 15-STEP METHOD FOR STARTING A PERIPHERAL IV CANNULA

Phase	Step
Precannulation (preparation)	1. Check the authorized prescriber's order. 2. Perform hand hygiene with soap and water or alcohol-based hand gel for 15 to 20 seconds. 3. Inspect and prepare the equipment. 4. Identify, assess, and prepare the patient. 5. Select the site and dilate the vein.
Cannulation (venipuncture)	6. Select the needle (cannula). 7. Put on gloves. 8. Prepare the site using chlorhexidine for 30 seconds; let dry. 9. Enter the vein using the direct or indirect method. 10. Stabilize the cannula with a manufactured stabilization device or sterile tape, and apply a dressing.
Post-cannulation (cleanup)	11. Label the site, tubing, and bag. 12. Properly dispose of used equipment. 13. Educate the patient. 14. Calculate the drip rate, if applicable. 15. Document the procedure.

Source: Phillips, L. D. (2005). *Manual of IV therapeutics* (4th ed.). Philadelphia: F. A. Davis.

STEP 2: PERFORM HAND HYGIENE. Hand hygiene has been shown to significantly decrease the risk of contamination and cross-contamination. Before beginning the procedure, wash your hands for 15 to 20 seconds. Wear gloves when inserting the cannula and any time you have a risk of exposure to body fluid. The CDC (Siegel et al., 2007) recommends the following:

- Decontaminate hands after removing gloves.
- Antimicrobial-impregnated wipes may be considered an alternative to washing hands with non-antimicrobial soap and water.
- When using an alcohol-based hand gel, apply product to palm of one hand and rub hands together, covering all surfaces of hands and fingers until hand are dry.
- Do not wear artificial fingernails or extenders when having direct contact with patients at risk (those in intensive care units or operating rooms). Keep natural tips less than ¼ inch long.
- Limit jewelry when delivering health care to patients. Several studies have shown that skin underneath rings is more heavily colonized than comparable areas of skin on fingers without rings. (Trick et al., 2003).

STEP 3: INSPECT AND PREPARE EQUIPMENT. Obtain the following equipment and inspect it for integrity:

- Clean gloves
- Prepping solution (70% isopropyl alcohol, or chlorhexidine gluconate)
- Sterile 2" × 2" gauze pads
- Securement device
- Dressing material (gauze or transparent semipermeable membrane [TSM] dressing)
- Disposable nonlatex tourniquet
- Cannulas (over-the-needle sizes 18, 20, 22, and 24 are the most common)
- Appropriate administration set
- IV solution (Inspect and gently squeeze soft plastic bags for puncture holes or breaks; check expiration date; inspect solution for visible contamination or particles; ensure that outer wrap is dry.)
- Intermittent device (access cap) if the cannula is to be maintained as a saline lock
- IV pole if needed.

Some institutions have IV start kits that contain a tourniquet, gloves, alcohol, chlorhexidine gluconate, semipermeable membrane dressing, and 2" × 2" gauze pads.

Once the solution is verified and inspected for integrity, the administration set is spiked into the solution bag or bottle, taking care to keep the spike and the bag opening sterile. The prescribed IV fluid is then run through the tubing to eliminate all air; this is called priming.

STEP 4: IDENTIFY, ASSESS, AND PREPARE THE PATIENT.

Patient Identification. The 2010 National Patient Safety Goals established by the Joint Commission (www.jointcommission.org) specify that two patient identifiers should be used when administering medications, blood, or blood components. The patient's room number or physical location should not be used as an identifier.

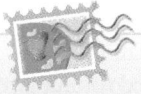

Patient Assessment. Several factors must be considered before venipuncture: the type of solution, condition of vein, duration of therapy, cannula size needed, patient age, patient activity, presence of disease or previous surgery, presence of a dialysis shunt or graft, medications being taken by the patient (such as anticoagulants), and allergies. In addition, be sure to assess specific needs related to the patient's culture (Box 7.1, *Cultural Considerations*).

Psychological Preparation. Provide privacy, explain the procedure, and evaluate the patient's knowledge of the procedure before assessing the patient's arms for suitable venipuncture sites. Ask if the patient has had experience with infusions before and if any difficulties were encountered with venipuncture or the infusion.

STEP 5: SELECT SITE AND DILATE VEIN.

Site Selection. Proper vein selection is important to accommodate the prescribed therapy and to minimize potential complications (Box 7.2). Avoid use of an arm on the side where the patient has had a mastectomy, has a dialysis access site, or is scheduled for a surgical procedure. The patient's condition and diagnosis; age; vein condition, size, and location; and type and duration of therapy should be considered before starting intravenous therapy (Box 7.3). The vein should be able to accommodate the gauge and length of cannula used.

The first cannula should be started in the most distal site that supports therapy. This allows each successive venipuncture to be made proximal to the site of the previous one, which eliminates the passage of irritating fluids through a previously injured vein and minimizes leakage through old puncture sites. Hand veins can be used successfully for most hydrating solutions, but they are best avoided when irritating solutions of potassium or antibiotics are anticipated.

Vein size must also be considered. Small veins do not tolerate large volumes of fluid, high infusion rates, or irritating solutions. Large veins should be used for these purposes. Figure 7.3 shows peripheral veins that may be used for IV therapy.

Vein Dilation. If veins are constricted, venipuncture is more difficult. Fever, anxiety, and cold temperatures can cause veins to constrict. Smoking before the insertion of an IV line also causes veins to constrict.

A tourniquet helps to dilate and stabilize the vein, easing venipuncture and threading of the cannula. Place the tourniquet

Box 7.2

Considerations for Vein Selection

- Age of patient
- Availability of sites
- Size of cannula to be used
- Purpose of infusion therapy
- Osmolarity of solution to be infused
- Volume, rate, and length of infusion
- Degree of mobility desired

Box 7.3

General Considerations for Initiating Intravenous Therapy

1. Use veins in the upper extremities.
2. When multiple sticks are anticipated, make the first venipuncture distally and work proximal with subsequent punctures. Make no more than two attempts at venipuncture before getting help.
3. Use only one cannula per cannulation attempt.
4. If therapy will be prescribed for longer than 6 days, a peripherally inserted central catheter (PICC) should be considered.
5. Avoid using venipunctures in affected arms of patients with radical mastectomy or a dialysis access site.
6. If possible, avoid taking a blood pressure on the arm receiving an infusion because the cuff interferes with blood flow and forces blood back into the cannula. This may cause a clot or cause the vein or cannula to rupture.
7. Select the smallest cannula in gauge and length that supports prescribed therapy. All cannulas should be radiopaque.
8. All peripheral cannulas should be stabilized with a stabilization device to preserve the integrity of the access device and prevent migration.

Box 7.1

Cultural Considerations

Among the Vietnamese, the head is considered sacred. Thus, the practice of starting IV lines in the scalp may cause a Vietnamese patient significant anxiety. Consider other sites first. If the patient must have an IV line in the scalp, carefully explain why it is needed.

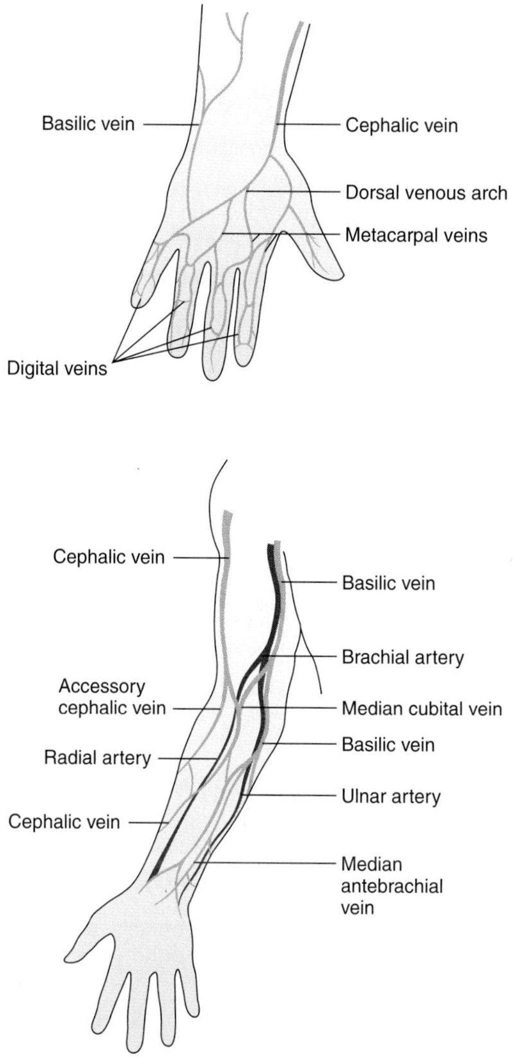
Basilic vein
Cephalic vein
Dorsal venous arch
Metacarpal veins
Digital veins
Cephalic vein
Basilic vein
Brachial artery
Accessory cephalic vein
Median cubital vein
Basilic vein
Radial artery
Ulnar artery
Cephalic vein
Median antebrachial vein

FIGURE 7.3 Peripheral veins used for IV therapy. (Modified from Phillips, L. D. [2005]. *Manual of IV therapeutics* [4th ed.]. Philadelphia: F.A. Davis.)

6 to 8 inches above the insertion site. If the tourniquet is too close to the insertion site, it can create too much pressure and cause a **hematoma**, which is a localized collection of blood in the subcutaneous tissue. The tourniquet should be tight enough to impede venous flow while maintaining arterial flow. A tourniquet should be at least 1 inch wide and should not be left on for more than 3 minutes to prevent impaired blood flow to the extremity. In general, use of nonlatex tourniquets is advised.

NURSING CARE TIP

Many patients know from experience whether their veins are difficult to access. Asking a patient to indicate which is his or her "best vein" may decrease the number of attempts before successful IV cannulation. In addition, when selecting a hand vein, consider avoiding the patient's dominant hand to avoid possible accidental patient removal of the IV.

Occasionally, additional techniques are needed to distend a vein. Placing the arm in a dependent position or placing a warm towel over the site for several minutes before applying the tourniquet helps to dilate a vein. The whole extremity must be warmed to improve blood flow to the area. Opening and closing the fist pumps blood to the extremity and increases blood flow to help dilate the vein. A blood pressure cuff inflated to 30 mm Hg is an appropriate method for vein dilation, especially with fragile veins in the elderly. Box 7.4 lists additional tips for difficult-to-find veins.

NURSING CARE TIP

Use a tourniquet only once to avoid cross-contamination between patients. Tourniquets may also be sources of latex exposure; use a nonlatex tourniquet or blood pressure cuff technique for patients whenever appropriate.

Box 7.4

Techniques for Patients with Difficult Venous Access

Impaired Skin Integrity related to lesions, burns, or disease process

- Use light directed toward the side of the patient's extremity (tangential lighting) to illuminate blue veins. (This technique can also be used on dark-skinned people.)
- Do not flatten veins or cause damage to skin.

Hard sclerosed vessels related to disease process, personal misuse, frequent drug therapy

- Assess for collateral circulation.
- Use multiple tourniquet technique to increase oncotic pressure inside the tissue, forcing small vessels of periphery to be visualized:
  - Place one tourniquet high on arm for 2 minutes and leave in place; stroke downward toward hand.
  - After 2 minutes, place a second tourniquet at midarm just below the antecubital fossa; leave along with first tourniquet for 2 minutes.
  - This should bring peripheral veins into view; if needed, place a third tourniquet at wrist.
  - Do not leave on for more than 6 minutes total.

Obesity or edema

- Use a 2-inch cannula.
- Use multiple tourniquet technique.
- Displace edema to side to visualize veins.

Source: Phillips, L. D. (2005). *Manual of IV therapeutics* (4th ed.). Philadelphia: F. A. Davis.

• **WORD** • **BUILDING** •
hematoma: hemat—blood + oma—tumor

Cannulation (Steps 6–10)

STEP 6: SELECT CANNULA. Needles have been largely replaced with flexible plastic catheters (cannulas) that are inserted over a needle (Fig. 7.4B). The needle (or stylet) is removed after the cannula is in place. These are available in a variety of sizes (gauges) and lengths. For patient comfort, choose the smallest gauge cannula that will work for the intended purpose. Use smaller gauge cannulas (22 to 24 gauge) for fluids and slow infusion rates. Use larger cannulas (18 to 20 gauge) for rapid fluid administration and viscous solutions such as blood. Also consider vein size when choosing a cannula gauge. Refer to institution policy and equipment stock for specific recommendations. The INS (2006) recommends that short peripheral cannulas be removed and replaced every 72 hours and immediately upon suspected contamination.

STEP 7: PUT ON GLOVES. The CDC recommends following standard precautions whenever exposure to blood or body fluids is likely. Wearing latex or vinyl gloves provides basic protection from blood and body fluids (Seigel et al., 2007). Remove gloves after contact with a patient, using proper technique to prevent hand contamination; wash hands after glove removal.

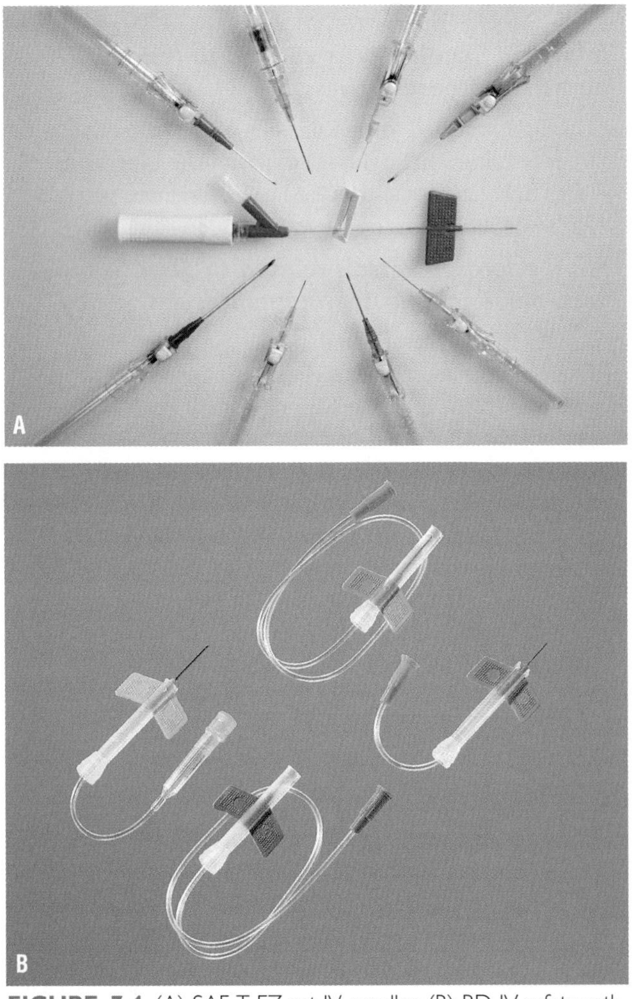
A
B

FIGURE 7.4 (A) SAF-T EZ set IV needles. (B) BD IV safety catheters. (Courtesy of Becton Dickinson, Franklin Lakes, NJ.)

STEP 8: PREPARE THE SITE. Some agency policies allow the use of a local anesthetic agent prior to insertion of a peripheral IV cannula. Be sure to check your agency's policy. Local anesthetic agents include lidocaine, iontophoresis low-frequency ultrasonification, pressure-accelerated lidocaine, and topical transdermal agents.

Clean the peripheral insertion site with an antimicrobial solution before cannula placement. If the patient's skin is dirty, wash it with soap and water before applying the antimicrobial solution. If the patient has excess hair, it can be clipped with scissors. Be sure to follow institution policy when choosing a solution. Most institutions use 70% alcohol or chlorhexidine gluconate. Chlorhexidine gluconate does not stain the skin or cause skin irritation, and is now recommended as the prep solution of choice (O'Grady et al., 2002). (See *Evidence-Based Practice.*) Avoid using alcohol after an antimicrobial preparation because alcohol negates the antimicrobial action of the skin prep agent.

EVIDENCE-BASED PRACTICE

Clinical Question

What technique can the nurse use to help decrease catheter-related bloodstream infections (CRBSI)?

Evidence

A meta-analysis of 4143 catheters evaluating a chlorhexidine-containing cutaneous antiseptic regimen in comparison with povidone-iodine or alcohol for care of catheter insertion sites resulted in reduced catheter related infection by 49% (Chaiyakunapruk et al., 2002).

To prevent bloodstream infections, the Institute for Healthcare Improvement (IHI) recommends as part of the central line bundle the use of 2% chlorhexidine gluconate as the solution to use to prepare for venipuncture. Results from Regions' Hospital implementation of the 100,000 Lives Campaign found that use of bundled care (which includes chlorhexidine gluconate as prep solutions) was associated with reductions in infections from 8.2% per 1000 device days in 2002 to 0 per 1000 device days in 2005 (IHI, n.d.).

Recent studies (Pronovost et al., 2006) have confirmed dramatic reductions in CRBSI with the use of chlorhexidine skin antisepsis, along with central line bundles.

Implications for Nursing Practice

Chlorhexidine gluconate 2% is useful for prevention of serious bloodstream infection complications related to peripheral and central infusion therapy. This solution for preparation of venipuncture site is recommended by the Centers for Disease Control and Prevention for skin preparation prior to venipuncture based on above studies.

EVIDENCE-BASED PRACTICE cont'd

REFERENCES

Chaiyakunapruk, N., Veenstra, D. L., Lipsky, B. A., & Saint, S. (2002). Chlorhexidine compared with povidone-iodine solution for vascular catheter site care: A meta-analysis. *Annals of Internal Medicine, 126*(11), 792–801.

Pronovost, P., Needham, D., Berenholtz, S., et al. (2006). An intervention to decrease catheter-related blood stream infections in the ICU. *New England Journal of Medicine, 355*(26), 2725–2732.

Institute for Healthcare Improvement. (n.d.). *Pursuing perfection. Report from HealthPartners' Regions Hospital on reducing hospital-acquired infection: Ventilator-associated pneumonia and catheter-related bloodstream infection.* Retrieved March 2, 2009, from http://www.ihi.org.

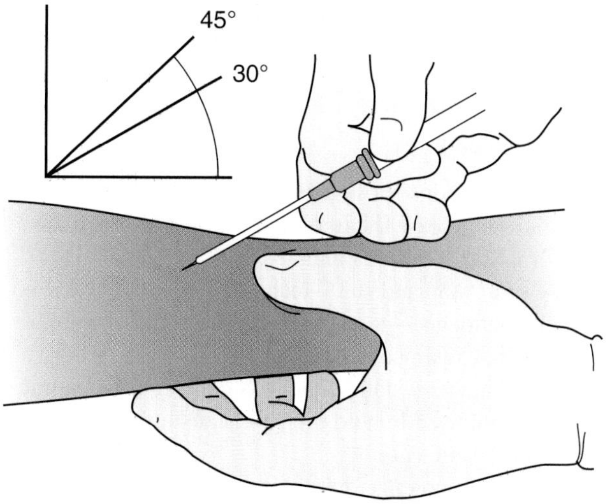
45°
30°

FIGURE 7.5 Insert the needle of choice bevel up at a 30- to 45-degree angle, depending on the vein location and catheter.

Apply the solution in a circular motion, starting at the intended site and working outward to clean an area 2 to 3 inches in diameter. Whether using alcohol or chlorhexidine, it should be applied with friction for at least 30 seconds. Blotting of excess solution at the insertion site is not recommended. Let solution air dry completely.

STEP 9: INSERT THE CANNULA. Venipuncture can be performed using a direct (one-step) or indirect (two-step) method. The direct method is appropriate for small-gauge cannulas, fragile hand veins, or rolling veins. The indirect method can be used for all venipunctures.

Hold the cannula with the bevel (slanted opening) of the needle facing up. With the tourniquet in place, enter the vein using either the direct or indirect approach. When using the direct entry approach, hold the needle at a 30- to 45-degree angle directly above the vein and then penetrate the skin and vein in one motion (Fig. 7.5). With some newer cannulas, the angle of insertion may be even less than 30 degrees.

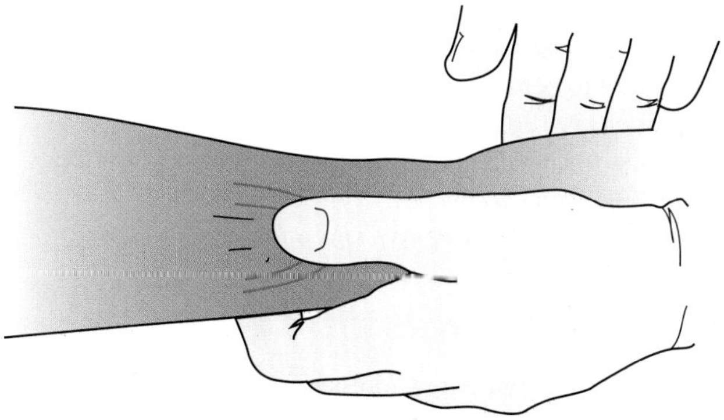

FIGURE 7.6 Pull skin below the intended puncture site using a downward motion to stabilize the skin and prevent the vein from rolling.

NURSING CARE TIP

Use traction (a downward pulling motion that makes the skin taut below the puncture site) to stabilize the skin before venipuncture and prevent the vein from rolling during venipuncture (Fig. 7.6).

The indirect approach may help decrease vein collapse. To use it, hold the needle at a 30- to 45-degree angle over the skin next to (not over) the vein. Once the skin is punctured, lower the needle angle and locate and puncture the vein. Depending on the type of device used, a small flash of blood may be seen in the tubing or at the hub of the cannula when the needle is in the vein. Lower the angle of the needle so that it is parallel with the skin as you thread it into the lumen of the vein. If a cannula-over-needle device is used, advance the needle ¼ inch and then advance the cannula for its remaining length as you withdraw the metal needle (stylet).

Once the cannula is in place, release the tourniquet and connect the IV solution or injection cap to the hub of the cannula. Blood may ooze from the hub at this time, so be sure to follow precautions against exposure. If an injection cap is being used, the cannula is flushed with 0.9% sodium chloride solution to check for patency. A smooth, easy flush and no signs of infiltration indicate that the cannula is patent and that the prescribed solution can be administered. Box 7.5 lists troubleshooting tips for peripheral cannula insertions.

STEP 10: STABILIZE THE CANNULA AND DRESS THE SITE. A common problem in IV therapy is dislodgement of the cannula. The purpose of cannula stabilization is to preserve the integrity of the access device and to prevent cannula movement, or migration. Stabilization should not interfere with visualization and evaluation of the insertion site. Several methods can be used to stabilize the cannula

Box 7.5

Troubleshooting Tips for Peripheral IV Therapy

Common reasons for failure of venipuncture include:

- Failure to release the tourniquet promptly when the vein is sufficiently cannulated
- Use of a "stop and start" technique by beginners who lack confidence—a tentative approach that can injure the vein, causing a hematoma
- Inadequate vein stabilization, as can occur when traction is not used to hold the vein, causing the stylet to push the vein aside
- Failure to recognize that the cannula has gone through the opposite vein wall
- Stopping too soon after insertion of only the stylet so that the cannula does not enter the lumen of the vein (causing blood return to disappear when the stylet is removed because the cannula is not in the lumen of the vein)
- Inserting the cannula too deep, below the vein
- Failure to penetrate the vein wall because of improper insertion angle (too steep or not steep enough), causing the cannula to ride on top of or below the vein.

Source: Phillips, L. D. (2005). *Manual of IV therapeutics* (4th ed.). Philadelphia: F. A. Davis.

hub, including transparent dressings, gauze and tape, and specialized securement devices.

A transparent, semipermeable membrane dressing allows stabilization of the cannula, allows the venipuncture site to be monitored for redness or swelling, and provides an occlusive dressing for the site. Another acceptable method of dressing management is the use of sterile gauze over the venipuncture site and a piece of 1-inch tape over the gauze. Band-Aids are not acceptable dressings over cannulas.

Arm boards are not used routinely. However, if a confused patient places the IV site in danger, the extremity can be immobilized as a last resort; this requires a physician's order.

NURSING CARE TIP

Gauze and tape should be changed every 2 days and transparent semipermeable membrane dressings should be changed at the time of cannula site rotation and immediately if the integrity of the dressing is compromised (INS, 2006).

Post-Cannulation (Steps 11–15)

STEP 11: LABEL THE SITE. The IV setup should be labeled in three areas: the insertion site, the tubing, and the solution container. Once the venipuncture procedure is completed, label the insertion site dressing with the date, time, cannula type and size, and your initials; label tubing and solution (if applicable) with date, time, and initials.

STEP 12: DISPOSE OF EQUIPMENT. Equipment disposal should follow CDC guidelines for biohazards. All needles, cannulas, and blood-contaminated equipment should be disposed of according to institution policy in a tamper-proof, nonpermeable, biohazard waste container.

STEP 13: EDUCATE THE PATIENT. Patients have the right to receive information on all aspects of their care in a manner they can understand. They also have the right to accept or refuse treatment. The following information should be included in education and documentation:

- Inform the patient of any limitations on movement or mobility that results from the IV placement.
- Explain all alarms if an electronic infusion device is used.
- Instruct the patient to call for assistance if the venipuncture site becomes tender or sore or if redness or swelling develops.

STEP 14: CALCULATE DRIP RATE. All IV infusions should be monitored frequently for accurate flow rates and complications associated with infusion therapy. See the section on calculating drip rates earlier in this chapter.

STEP 15: DOCUMENT. After implementation of infusion therapy the procedure must be documented in the medical record. Document your actions and the patient's response according to institution policy. All IV solutions are also documented on the medication administration record. Include the following:

- Date and time of insertion
- Manufacturer's brand name and style of device
- Gauge and length of the device
- Location of the accessed vein
- Solution infusing and rate of flow
- Method of infusion (gravity or pump)
- Number of attempts needed for a successful IV start
- Patient's response and specific comments related to the procedure
- Signature.

CRITICAL THINKING

Mrs. Green

■ Mrs. Green is admitted with a diagnosis of symptomatic anemia and has an atrioventricular (AV) dialysis shunt in her left arm. An IV line is ordered for administration of 2 units of packed red blood cells. What must be taken into consideration when assessing Mrs. Green for an appropriate venipuncture site?

Suggested answers at end of chapter.

NURSING PROCESS FOR THE PATIENT RECEIVING IV THERAPY

Data Collection

IV therapy is a medical intervention, and the nurse is responsible for appropriate assessment, monitoring, documentation, and reporting related to the therapeutic goals. Some institutions require assessment as often as every hour. Assessment should be systematic and thorough, and include physiological and psychosocial data, critical laboratory values, allergies and environmental issues, and presence of adverse reactions or complications related to infusion therapy. Older adults are at increased risk for complications, making careful assessment essential (Box 7.6, *Gerontological Issues*).

Physical assessments such as daily weights and measurement of intake and output help determine whether the patient is retaining too much fluid. Skin turgor, mucous membrane moisture, vital signs, and level of consciousness also indicate hydration status. New onset of fine crackles in the lungs can indicate fluid retention. Table 7.2 lists other symptoms of complications, along with prevention and treatment strategies.

Inspect the insertion site for redness or swelling, evaluate the integrity of the dressing, and document your findings. Inspect the tubing to ensure tight connections and the absence of kinks or defects. Inspect the solution container and compare it with the physician's order for type, amount, and rate. Report concerns to the RN or physician.

Nursing Diagnoses, Planning, and Implementation

Priority nursing diagnoses for IV-related issues may include:

Fear Related to Insertion of IV Cannula

EXPECTED OUTCOME: The patient will be able to cooperate with the procedure; patient will verbalize minimal fear.

- Explain the IV therapy (rationale for therapy, insertion procedure, care of the IV, and importance of reporting pain, swelling, or pump alarm) to the patient. *Lack of knowledge is associated with fear.*
- Use techniques to minimize discomfort. *Pain may increase fear.*

Impaired Physical Mobility Related to Placement and Maintenance of IV Cannula

EXPECTED OUTCOME: The patient will experience minimal inability to move; the patient will not experience complications related to immobility.

- Use insertion site away from joints if at all possible. *Joint areas are mobile, making it difficult to maintain an intact site.*
- If you must use a mobile site, such as the antecubital fossa or wrist area, immobilize with arm board or gauze wrapping *to reduce cannula movement.*
- If site must be wrapped, be sure to leave insertion site visible or remove dressing to view site according to agency policy. *The site must still be visualized for complications even if it is covered.*
- Assist patient with activities of daily living (ADLs). *The patient may have difficulty with ADLs if movement is limited.*

Risk for Infection Related to Broken Skin or Traumatized Tissue

EXPECTED OUTCOME: The patient will be free from infection as evidenced by no redness, swelling, or purulence at IV insertion site, no fever, and normal white cell count.

- Watch for signs of infection *so the IV can be changed and infection treated quickly if it occurs.*
- Use good hand washing and strict aseptic techniques during cannula insertion *to prevent introduction of pathogens.*
- Change cannula, tubing, and solutions regularly according to agency policy *to prevent growth of microorganisms.*

Box 7.6

Gerontological Issues

Care of the Older Adult Receiving Intravenous Therapy

When an older patient is receiving IV fluids, the nurse must regularly assess the patient for potential fluid volume excess. Symptoms of fluid volume excess include:

- Elevated blood pressure
- Increasing weight
- Full bounding pulse
- Shallow, rapid respirations
- Jugular venous distention
- Increased urine output
- Development of moist crackles in the lungs.

If these signs are present:

- Immediately notify the RN or turn down the IV to a minimum drip rate (1 mL per minute); do not discontinue the IV because the physician may want to order IV diuretics.
- Position the patient to maximize lung expansion.
- Check peripheral oxygen saturation with an oximeter.
- Apply oxygen by mask or nasal cannula if indicated and per institution guidelines.
- Closely monitor patient's vital signs, level of consciousness, and oxygen saturation along with fluid output.
- Assist the physician or RN with IV push administration of diuretic medication such as furosemide if ordered.

TABLE 7.2 COMPLICATIONS OF PERIPHERAL IV THERAPY

Complication	Signs and Symptoms	Prevention	Treatment
Local Complications of IV Therapy			
Hematoma	• Ecchymoses • Swelling • Inability to advance cannula • Resistance during flushing	Use indirect method of venipuncture. Choose smallest cannula appropriate. Apply tourniquet just before venipuncture.	Remove cannula. Apply pressure with 2" × 2" gauze. Elevate extremity.
Thrombosis	• Slowed or stopped infusion • Fever/malaise • Inability to flush cannula	Use an electronic infusion device (EID). Choose microdrop sets with gravity flow if rate is less than 50 mL/hr. Avoid use of flexion areas for insertion site.	Discontinue cannula. Apply cold compress to site. Assess for circulatory impairment.
Phlebitis	• Redness/warmth at site • Local swelling • Pain • Palpable cord • Sluggish infusion rate	Use larger veins for hypertonic solutions. Choose smallest cannula appropriate. Use good hand hygiene. Add buffer to irritating solutions. Change solutions and containers every 24 hr. Rotate infusion sites every 72–96 hr.	Discontinue cannula. Apply cold compress initially; then warm. Consult physician if severe.
Infiltration (Extravasation)	• Coolness of skin at site • Taut skin • Dependent edema • Absent backflow of blood • Sluggish infusion rate	Stabilize cannula. Place cannula in appropriate site. Avoid antecubital fossa. Stabilize cannula carefully.	Discontinue cannula. Apply cool compress. Elevate extremity slightly. Follow agency extravasation guidelines. Have antidote available (if medication extravasates).
Local Infection	• Redness and swelling at site • Possible exudate • Elevated WBC count • Elevated T lymphocytes	Inspect all solutions. Use sterile technique during venipuncture and site maintenance.	Discontinue cannula. Culture site and cannula. Apply sterile dressing over site. Administer antibiotics if ordered.
Venous Spasm	• Sharp pain at site • Sluggish infusion	Take thorough history. Verify allergies. Use proper patient identification. Warm solutions with appropriate warming device if appropriate.	Apply warm compress to site. Restart infusion in new site if spasm continues.
Systemic Complications of Peripheral IV Therapy			
Septicemia	• Fluctuating temperature • Profuse sweating • Nausea/vomiting • Diarrhea • Abdominal pain • Tachycardia • Hypotension • Altered mental status	Use good hand hygiene. Carefully inspect fluids. Use Luer-Lok devices. Cover infusion sites with appropriate dressings. Follow standards of practice related to rotation of sites and hang time of infusions. Use appropriate preparation solutions.	Restart new IV system. Obtain cultures. Notify physician. Initiate antimicrobial therapy as ordered. Monitor patient closely.
Circulatory Overload	• Weight gain • Puffy eyelids • Edema • Hypertension • Changes in input and output (I&O) • Rise in central venous pressure (CVP) • Shortness of breath • Crackles in lungs • Distended neck veins	Monitor infusion. Maintain flow at prescribed rate. Monitor I&O. Know patient's cardiovascular history. Do not "catch up" infusion if behind schedule.	Decrease IV flow rate. Place patient in high Fowler's position. Keep patient warm. Monitor vital signs. Administer oxygen. Use a microdrop set or an EID.
Venous Air Embolism	• Light-headedness • Dyspnea, cyanosis, tachypnea, expiratory wheezes, cough • Mill wheel murmur, chest pain, hypotension • Changes in mental status	Remove all air from administration sets. Use Luer-Loks. Attach piggyback to appropriate port.	Call for help! Place patient in Trendelenburg position. Administer oxygen. Monitor vital signs. Notify physician.

TABLE 7.2 COMPLICATIONS OF PERIPHERAL IV THERAPY—cont'd

Complication	Signs and Symptoms	Prevention	Treatment
Speed Shock	• Dizziness • Facial flushing • Headache • Tightness in chest • Hypotension • Irregular pulse • Progression of shock	Reduce the size of drops by using micro-drop set. Use an EID. Monitor infusion sites. Dilute IV push mediations if possible; give slowly.	Call for help! Give antidote or resuscitation medications.

Source: Adapted from Phillips, L. D. (2005). *Manual of IV therapeutics* (Table 9-9, pp. 396–398). Philadelphia: F. A. Davis.

Evaluation

The RN is responsible for evaluation and thus monitors the patient for evidence that the goals of therapy are being met and that complications are avoided. The LPN/LVN collects data that contribute to the evaluation. For example, if antibiotic therapy is administered, monitor the patient's temperature and other signs that the infection is resolving. If IV therapy is ordered to correct dehydration, monitor daily weights, skin turgor, vital signs, and other appropriate signs of improved fluid balance. Document all findings and report them to the RN.

COMPLICATIONS OF IV THERAPY

Complications of infusion therapy fall into two categories: local complications and systemic complications. Any complication or unusual incident should be reported to the RN or physician, and an incident report should be prepared according to institution policy. This applies to hospital, long-term care, and home care settings.

The most common peripheral local complications are hematoma, **phlebitis**, and **infiltration**. Systemic complications can be very serious and include circulatory overload, septicemia, venous air embolism, and speed shock. The nurse delivering infusion therapy must be knowledgeable in preventing, recognizing, and treating all complications of IV therapy (see Table 7.2).

CRITICAL THINKING

Mr. Rick

■ Mr. Rick's IV has blood backed up in the tubing. When you open the clamp to increase the flow, nothing happens. What should you do?

Suggested answer at end of chapter.

CRITICAL THINKING

Mrs. Gonzalez

■ Mrs. Gonzalez is receiving 5% dextrose in water at 83 mL per hour. One hour after the infusion starts, she reports pain at the site. The site is cool to the touch and swollen, and the infusion rate is sluggish.

1. What might be happening?
2. What additional data should you collect?
3. What action do you take?
4. How should you document your findings?

Suggested answers at end of chapter.

CENTRAL VENOUS ACCESS DEVICES

The role of the LPN/LVN in central venous access care in most states is limited to assisting the RN with assessments. Therefore, it is important for you to be familiar with the different central venous access devices so you can recognize and report problems.

Central venous catheters terminate in the superior vena cava near the heart (Fig. 7.7). They are used when peripheral sites are inadequate or when large amounts of fluid or irritating medication must be given. Central catheter devices include tunneled and non-tunneled catheters, peripherally inserted central catheters (PICCs), and implanted ports. These devices can have one, two, or three lumens in the catheter or one or more port chambers. Each lumen exits the site in a separate line, called a tail. Multilumen catheters allow for the administration of incompatible solutions at the same time.

• WORD • BUILDING •

phlebitis: phleb—vein + itis—inflammation

infiltration: in—inside + filtrate—to strain through + tion—condition

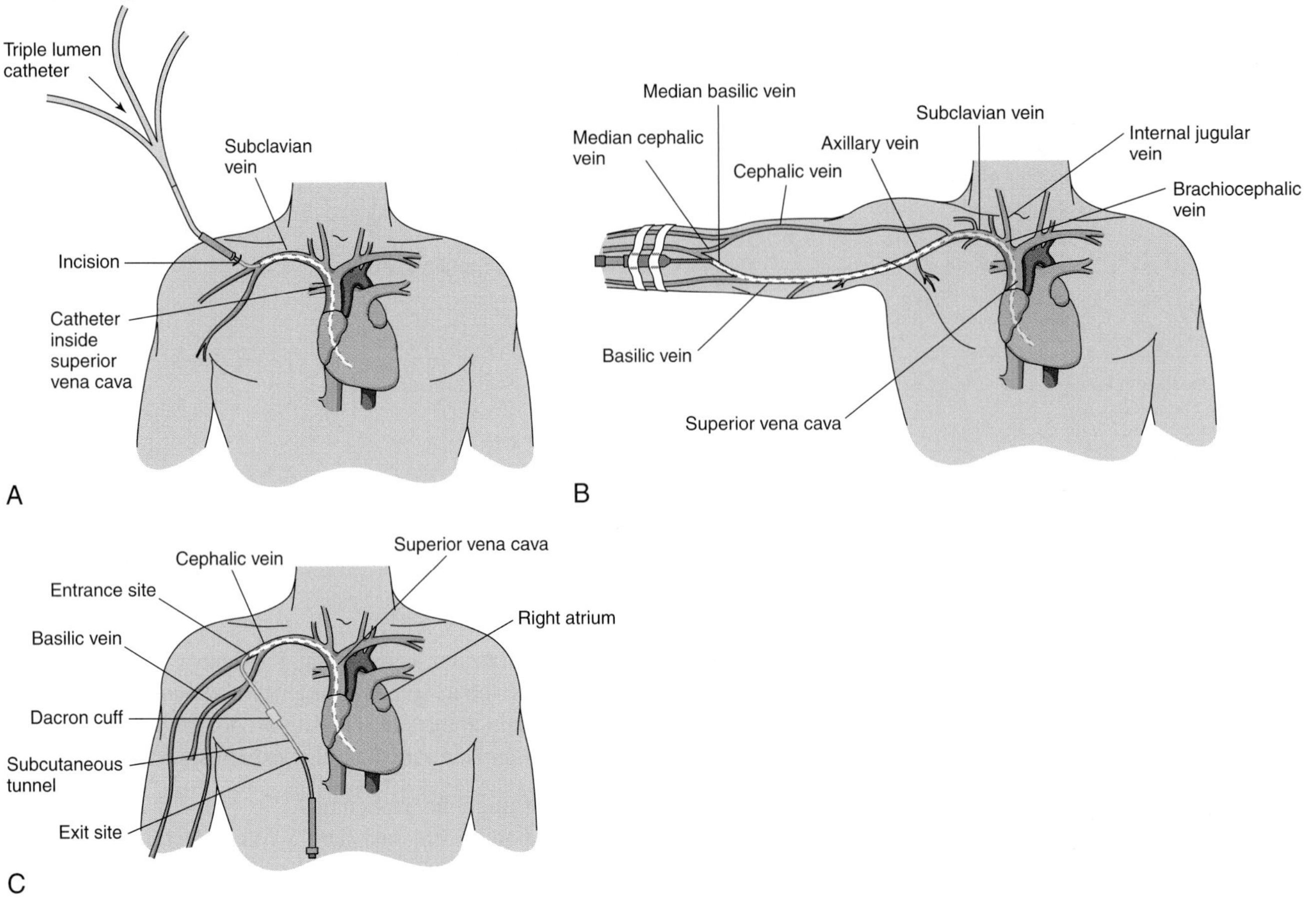
Triple lumen catheter
Subclavian vein
Incision
Catheter inside superior vena cava
A
Median basilic vein
Subclavian vein
Median cephalic vein
Axillary vein
Cephalic vein
Internal jugular vein
Brachiocephalic vein
Basilic vein
Superior vena cava
B
Superior vena cava
Cephalic vein
Entrance site
Right atrium
Basilic vein
Dacron cuff
Subcutaneous tunnel
Exit site
C

FIGURE 7.7 Central lines. (A) Triple-lumen subclavian catheter. (B) PICC line. (C) Tunneled catheter. (B and C modified from Phillips, L. D. [2005]. *Manual of IV therapeutics* [4th ed.]. Philadelphia: F. A. Davis.)

Be careful not to confuse a central catheter with a dialysis catheter. Dialysis catheters should be used only for dialysis and not for IV therapy, and should be accessed only by physicians or specially trained dialysis nurses.

Non-Tunneled Central Catheter

A non-tunneled central catheter is inserted by a physician into the jugular or subclavian vein. After insertion, correct placement is determined by x-ray before the catheter is used. These short-term central venous catheters may remain in place up to several weeks, but usual placement time is 7 days. These catheters are inserted at the bedside and are cost effective for short-term central venous access in the acute care setting.

Tunneled Catheters

Central venous tunneled catheters (CVTCs) are intended for use for months to years to provide long-term venous access. CVTCs are composed of polymeric silicone with a Dacron polyester cuff that anchors the catheter in place subcutaneously. The catheter tip is placed in the superior vena cava (see Fig. 7.7C).

Advantages of a CVTC are that a break or tear in a catheter is easy to repair, and they can be used for many purposes. Disadvantages include weekly site care, cost of maintenance supplies, and the effect on the patient's body image.

Peripherally Inserted Central Catheter

A peripherally inserted central catheter (called a PICC line) is a long catheter that is inserted in the arm and terminates in the central circulation (see Fig. 7.7B). This device is used when therapy will last more than 2 weeks or the medication is too caustic for peripheral administration. Specially trained RNs insert PICC lines. They can be left in place for long periods, minimizing the trauma of frequent IV insertions. Consult with a physician for a PICC order if long-term therapy is anticipated.

It is important to follow the manufacturer's recommended guidelines for flushing the catheter, and to be aware of your institution's policy. An RN removes the PICC catheter when therapy is terminated. An LPN/LVN may assist the RN with this procedure if the state nursing practice act permits.

Ports

A port is a reservoir that is surgically implanted into a pocket created under the skin, usually in the upper chest. An attached catheter is tunneled under the skin into a central vein. An advantage of a port is that, when not in use, it can be flushed and left unused for long periods. Because the port is under the skin, the patient can swim and shower without risk of contaminating the site.

Ports come in a variety of sizes and styles and are now being used in many areas of the body. Ports can be used to administer chemotherapeutic agents and antibiotics that are toxic to tissues and are suitable for long-term therapy. Ports should be accessed only by specially trained RNs. Most ports require the use of special noncoring needles that are specifically designed for this purpose.

SAFETY TIP

Implement best practices or evidence-based guidelines to prevent central line–related bloodstream infections (2010 National Patient Safety Goals, www.jointcommission.org). Vascular catheter–related infections are considered "never events" because they can be prevented. Hospitals will not be paid by Medicare for such infections acquired during hospitalization.

OTHER THERAPIES

Nutritional Support

Total parenteral nutrition (TPN) is complete IV nutrition that is administered to patients who cannot take adequate nutrients via the enteral route (by mouth or tube feeding). TPN may be used to promote wound healing or to help a patient achieve optimal weight before surgery, or it may be used to avoid malnutrition from chronic disease or after surgery. Patients with ulcerative colitis, trauma, or cancer cachexia are candidates for TPN. Every effort should be made to return a patient on TPN to oral or tube feedings as soon as possible

TPN provides and maintains the essential nutrients required by the body. Solutions contain carbohydrates, amino acids, lipid emulsions, electrolytes, trace elements, and vitamins in varied amounts according to the patient's needs. Parenteral nutrition requires filtration and an electronic infusion device for administration. In the home setting an ambulatory infusion device is used to allow the patient more mobility.

Initial assessment includes the patient's height, daily weight, nutritional status, and current laboratory values. Because of the high glucose concentration of TPN, the patient is at risk for infection and blood glucose disturbances. Insulin therapy may be necessary during TPN administration. Ongoing assessments include blood glucose levels according to institution policy and monitoring for signs and symptoms of infection, hyperglycemia, and hypoglycemia. When TPN therapy is begun, the rate is increased gradually to the prescribed rate to help prevent hyperglycemia. When it ends, the rate is gradually decreased to prevent hypoglycemia.

When nutritional solutions contain final concentrations exceeding 10% dextrose or 5% protein, they must be administered via a central catheter. When final concentrations are less than 10% dextrose or 5% protein, they may be administered through a peripheral vein. Peripheral parenteral nutrition (PPN) therapy is a short-term intervention because it does not provide adequate nutrition over an extended period. Some states allow LVN/LPNs to initiate PPN.

The entire health care team must be involved in TPN or PPN therapy. The pharmacist, dietitian, physician, and nurse communicate in a team conference to discuss the assessment, plan, and outcome criteria. Many institutions have nutrition teams that assess the appropriateness of TPN for individual patients.

Home Intravenous Therapy

As health care costs continue to rise, patients are using more alternatives to hospitalization. Subacute care, skilled nursing care in long-term care facilities, and home health care are growing. Home IV therapy allows many patients the benefit of early discharge and the ability to accomplish health care in the privacy and comfort of their own homes. Some home health agencies employ nurses to instruct patients and their families in the administration of home IV therapy (see *Home Health Hints*).

Home Health Hints

Prior to discharge:

- If IV therapy is to be continued after hospital discharge, assist the RN in teaching the patient and caregiver the skills to oversee the IV therapy.
- Obtain a referral for a home care nurse to continue monitoring and teaching after discharge.
- Teach the patient and caregiver the effects and side effects of any medication, along with signs and symptoms to report to the home care nurse or physician.

At home:

- Instruct the patient to refrain from smoking for at least 30 minutes before IV insertion to prevent vasoconstriction and ensure successful venipuncture.
- Instruct the patient to keep the IV site dry. If showering is permitted, instruct the patient to cover the IV with plastic (such as a grocery bag) and seal with tape on both ends to prevent water from entering the site.
- Assist the patient and caregiver to identify a safe place to store supplies. Make sure they understand correct storage—some solutions or medications require refrigeration.
- Provide a biohazard container. The nurse is responsible for returning filled boxes to the home health agency for disposal.

Home IV antibiotic therapy is becoming the method of choice in the long-term treatment of a number of infections, including bacterial endocarditis, osteomyelitis, and septic arthritis. Other patients with chronic diseases may choose to receive TPN at home. The health team can assess patients and their families for their ability to manage home IV therapy.

REFLECTIONS ON MRS. BROWN

Think again about Mrs. Brown from the beginning of the chapter. She will need monitoring of intake and output, daily weights, and close monitoring of her IV infusion. You should anticipate that serum electrolytes, BUN, and creatinine laboratory studies will be ordered. When initiating the infusion, use care in application of a tourniquet because elderly skin is thin and bruising can occur. Choose a number 20- or 22-gauge cannula to start the infusion. Once it is started, continue to monitor weights and lung sounds because elderly patients can quickly go from fluid depletion to fluid overload. (See Box 7.6, *Gerontological Issues.*)

SUGGESTED ANSWERS TO CRITICAL THINKING

■ *Mrs. Green*

Consider the following when assessing the patient for an appropriate venipuncture site:

1. An 18-gauge cannula should be used for blood administration whenever possible.
2. The cannula should not be inserted in the arm that has the dialysis access site.
3. The cannula should be placed in the forearm. Hand veins are too small to accommodate the delivery of blood.

■ *Mr. Rick*

Your patient's IV line is likely clotted. If it has been so for a long time, it will not be salvageable. Do not flush it because doing so can dislodge the clot into the circulation. Discontinue the IV and insert a new cannula.

■ *Mrs. Gonzalez*

1. The IV fluid may be leaking at the insertion site and flowing into the subcutaneous tissue, a problem known as infiltration or **extravasation**.
2. Consider whether the pain could be caused by the buildup of fluid under the skin. Compare the insertion site with the opposite limb.
3. If the IV solution has infiltrated, stop the infusion, discontinue the cannula, and restart the cannula in a new site.
4. "Patient reports pain at IV site in right arm; area is cool to touch and edematous in 4.5-cm area around site. Flow rate sluggish. Infusion discontinued; IV restarted in left arm with 22-gauge cannula. Infusing well with no signs of infiltration."

REVIEW QUESTIONS

1. Which resource is best for the nurse who has a question about implementation of IV therapy at a specific institution?
   a. An experienced nurse
   b. Institution policy
   c. The physician
   d. INS standards
2. Which patients have a need for IV therapy? **Select all that apply.**
   a. An 88-year-old man admitted to the hospital with dehydration
   b. A 21-year-old woman with an eating disorder and severe weight loss
   c. A 58-year-old woman with pneumonia who has been unresponsive to oral antibiotics
   d. A 37-year-old man recovering from a fall and broken arm
   e. A 4-year-old brought to the emergency room because of prolonged vomiting
   f. A patient with fluid overload who requires fast-acting diuretic therapy

• WORD • BUILDING •

extravasation: extra—outside + vas—vessel + tion—condition

REVIEW QUESTIONS—cont'd

3. A patient requests that an IV not be initiated in his hand. Which site is the next best choice?
   a. Forearm
   b. Antecubital fossa
   c. Upper arm
   d. Lower extremity

4. Place the steps for insertion of a peripheral IV cannula in chronological order. Use all of the options.
   a. Put on gloves
   b. Check physician's order.
   c. Prepare insertion site.
   d. Label the dressing.
   e. Wash hands.
   f. Dilate the vein.
   g. Document the procedure.
   h. Insert the cannula.
   i. Stabilize the site with tape.

5. The nurse must initiate an infusion on a 21-year-old man who has a history of sclerosed veins due to personal misuse, and multiple tattoos over both his arms. What would be the best approach to be able to visualize and initiate a peripheral IV?
   a. Place the arm in a dependent position.
   b. Use a blood pressure cuff.
   c. Use the multiple tourniquet technique.
   d. Have another nurse hold the patient's arm.

6. A patient receiving IV therapy via a central line develops hypotension, cyanosis, and dyspnea. The nurse notes a crack in the IV tubing. Which of the following actions should the nurse take first?
   a. Have the RN call the physician.
   b. Clamp the tubing and administer oxygen.
   c. Raise the head of the bed.
   d. Slow the infusion and lay the patient flat.

7. Which of the following solutions can be administered with a blood component?
   a. Lactated Ringer's solution
   b. D_5/0.2% NS
   c. D_5/0.45% NS
   d. 0.9% NS

8. While assessing a patient, the nurse notes a silicone catheter taped to his chest and can feel the catheter under the skin. This type of catheter would be a:
   a. Peripherally inserted central catheter
   b. Implanted port
   c. Central venous tunneled catheter
   d. Non-tunneled catheter

9. The physician orders 5% dextrose in water at 100 mL per hour. What is the drip rate using tubing with a drop factor of 20?
   Answer: ___ gtt per minute

10. A patient is to receive 1000 mL normal saline over 12 hours. How many milliliters per hour should be set on the EID?
   Answer: ___ mL per hour

References

Infusion Nurses Society. (2006). *Infusion nursing standards of practice.* Norwood, MA: Author.

Joint Commission. (2010). *2010 national patient safety goals.* Retrieved January 13, 2010, from http://www.jointcommission.org/patientsafety/nationalpatientsafetygoals

O'Grady, N. P., Alexander, M., Dellinger, E. P., et al. (2002). *Guidelines for the prevention of intravascular catheter-related infections.* Centers for Disease Control and Prevention. *MMWR, 51*(RR-10), 1. Retrieved August 1, 2009, from http://www.cdc.gov/mmwr/preview/mmwrhtml/rr5110a1.htm

Phillips, L. D. (2010). *Manual of IV therapeutics* (5th ed.). Philadelphia: F. A. Davis Company.

Roback, J. D., Combs, M. R., Grossman, B., & Hillyer, C. D. (2008). *Technical manual* (16th ed.). Bethesda, MD: American Association of Blood Banks.

Siegel, J. D., Rhinehart, E., Jackson, M., & Chiarello, L. (2007). *Guideline for isolation precautions: Preventing transmission of infectious agents in healthcare settings 2007.* Retrieved February 27, 2009, from http://www.cdc.gov/ncidod/dhqp/hai.html

Trick, W. E., Vernon, M. O., Hayes, R. A., et al. (2003). Impact of ring wearing on hand contamination and comparison of hand hygiene agents in a hospital. *Clinical Infectious Diseases, 36*(11), 1383–1390.

8 Nursing Care of Patients with Infections

SUSAN GARBUTT

KEY TERMS

aerobic (air-OH-bick)
anaerobic (ann-er-OH-bick)
antibodies (AN-ti-baw-dees)
antigen (AN-tih-jen)
asepsis (ah-SEP-sis)
bacteria (back-TEER-ee-ah)
Clostridium difficile (klo-STRIH-dee-um dih-fih-SEEL)
colonization (coll-in-ih-ZAY-shun)
dormant (DOOR-mant)
flora (FLOOR-ah)
fungi (FUNG-guy)
hand hygiene (HAND HY-jeen)
host (HOE-st)
morbidity (more-BIH-dih-tee)
mortality (more-TAH-lih-tee)
nosocomial infection (no-zoh-KOH-mee-uhl in-FECK-shun)
pathogen (PATH-o-jen)
personal protective equipment (PUR-sun-al pro-TEK-tiv i-KWIP-ment)
phagocytosis (fay-go-sy-TOH-sis)
probiotic (pro-buy-AH-tick)
protozoa (pro-tow-ZOH-ah)
reservoir (REZ-er-vwar)
rickettsiae (rah-KET-see-ah)
sepsis (SEP-sis)
standard precautions (STAN-derd pre-KAW-shuns)
Staphylococcus (staff-il-oh-KOCK-us)
trichinosis (TRICK-in-OH-sis)
vector (VECK-tur)
virulence (VEER-you-lence)
virus (VIGH-rus)

QUESTIONS TO GUIDE YOUR READING

1. What are the links in the chain of infection?
2. How can you interrupt the routes of transmission of infectious disease?
3. How can you assist the body's defense mechanisms to fight infectious disease?
4. What are the signs and symptoms of a localized versus a generalized infection?
5. What are the principles of anti-infective medication administration?
6. What nursing care will you provide for a patient with an infectious disease?
7. How will you know if your nursing care has been effective?

THE INFECTIOUS PROCESS

To prevent an infection, links in the chain of events leading to an infection must be broken (Fig. 8.1). If an infection occurs, treatment focuses on breaking the chain of infection to prevent the spread of infection to others (Box 8.1, *Cultural Considerations*).

A **pathogen** causes disease. **Colonization** occurs when pathogenic microbes are present in the body without causing symptomatic infection (fever, elevated white blood cell count [WBC]). An infection that does not produce symptoms is known as a *subclinical infection*. Identification of a subclinical infection is made when the **host** (the infected organism, in this case a person) has an increased antibody level for the microbe. An infection causes signs, symptoms, and injury to the host.

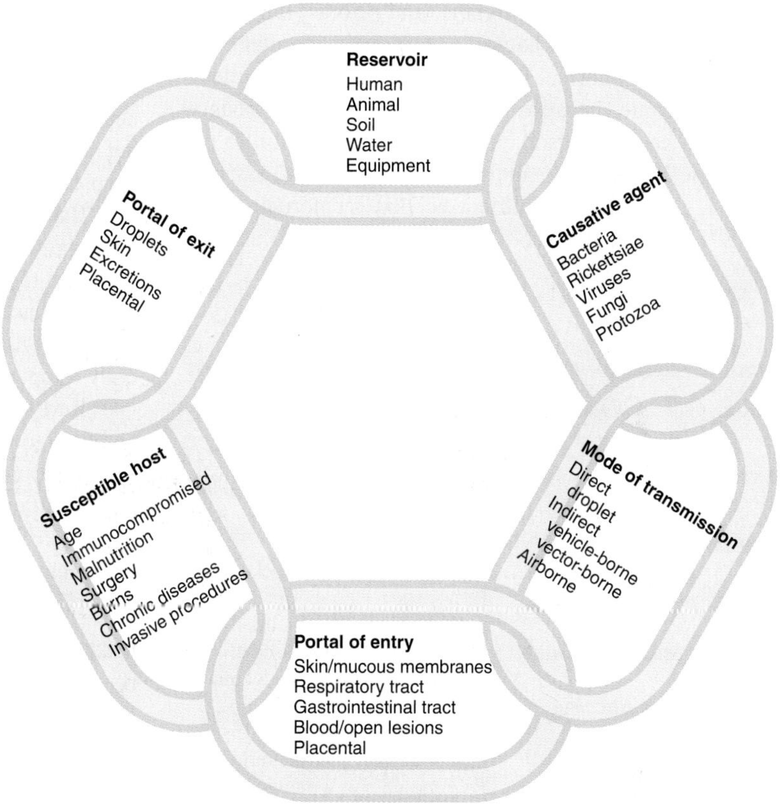
Reservoir
Human
Animal
Soil
Water
Equipment
Causative agent
Bacteria
Rickettsiae
Viruses
Fungi
Protozoa
Mode of transmission
Direct
droplet
Indirect
vehicle-borne
vector-borne
Airborne
Portal of entry
Skin/mucous membranes
Respiratory tract
Gastrointestinal tract
Blood/open lesions
Placental
Susceptible host
Age
Immunocompromised
Malnutrition
Surgery
Burns
Chronic diseases
Invasive procedures
Portal of exit
Droplets
Skin
Excretions
Placental

FIGURE 8.1 Chain of events in the infectious process.

Box 8.1

Cultural Considerations

One concern when caring for refugees, migrant workers, and immigrants is treating infectious conditions that jeopardize both the patient and the resident population. Some immigrants may suffer from a number of infectious such as malaria, gastrointestinal parasites, or tuberculosis. Standard precautions are a must when working with any patient.

Among Native Americans, infectious health problems include the plague and tick fever. Many of these illnesses stem from a reservation's rodent population, which can include prairie dogs and deer mice.

Some Appalachians live in rural areas that lack electricity, plumbing, and running water, putting them at increased risk of infection. Teach all patients to thoroughly wash their hands after toileting and coming in contact with raw food or contaminated water.

The drug isoniazid (INH), used in the treatment of tuberculosis, may be metabolized differently by some ethnic and racial groups. Half of European Americans and a smaller percentage of Asians are slow eliminators of INH. These individuals may have high blood concentrations of this medicine, leading to harmful reactions. Carefully monitor these patients for reactions to INH.

Reservoir

A **reservoir** is the place in the environment where infectious agents live, multiply, and reproduce so they can be transmitted to a susceptible host. A reservoir can be animate, such as people, insects, animals, and plants, or inanimate, such as water, soil, or medical devices.

Causative Agents

Microorganisms that cause infection include bacteria, viruses, fungi, protozoa, helminths, and prions (Table 8.1). The organisms that occur naturally in or on a particular body part are known as normal **flora**. They are usually harmless, or nonpathogenic, because they do not normally produce disease in a healthy person. Normal flora are helpful to the human host. For example, intestinal flora (bacteria) assist in vitamin K production, a nutrient needed for normal blood clotting. However, if these same bacteria get into another area of the body, such as the blood, they may produce disease and are then referred to as pathogens.

TABLE 8.1 COMMON INFECTIONS

Microorganism	Type or Site of Infection
Gram-Positive Bacteria	
Staphylococcus aureus	Pneumonia, cellulitis, peritonitis, toxic shock
Staphylococcus epidermidis	Postoperative bone/joints, IV line–related phlebitis
Staphylococcus pneumoniae	Pneumonia, meningitis, otitis media, sinusitis, septicemia
Gram-Negative Bacteria	
Escherichia coli	Urinary tract, pyelonephritis, septicemia, gastroenteritis
Klebsiella pneumoniae	Pneumonia and wounds
Legionella pneumophila	Pneumonia
Neisseria gonorrhoeae	Gonorrhea
Pseudomonas aeruginosa	Wounds, urinary tract, pneumonia, IV lines
Salmonella enteritidis	Gastroenteritis, food poisoning
Viruses	
Herpes virus group	Cold sores/fever blisters, genital herpes
Epstein-Barr	Infectious mononucleosis
Varicella zoster	Skin (chickenpox and shingles)
Hepatitis (A, B, C, D, E)	Liver
Human immunodeficiency virus	Acquired immunodeficiency syndrome
Influenza (A, B, C)	Bronchiolitis, pneumonia
Rubella	German measles
Rubeola	Measles
Fungi	
Candida albicans	Nailbed, thrush, vaginitis
Histoplasma capsulatum	Pneumonia
Protozoa	
Giardia lamblia	Gastroenteritis
Trichomonas vaginalis	Trichomoniasis
Dientamoeba fragilis	Diarrhea, fever
Entamoeba histolytica	Amebic dysentery
Toxoplasma gondii	Toxoplasmosis
Plasmodium falciparum	Malaria

Bacteria

Bacteria are single-celled organisms. They may depend on a host or live and reproduce outside a host. Most bacteria produce cell walls that are susceptible to antibiotics. However, bacteria can mutate in order to survive.

Bacteria are named according to their shape (spherical [coccus], rod [bacillus], and spiral [spirillum]) and classified according to their staining properties (Gram's method, acid-fast staining). Bacteria respond to stains in one of three ways: gram-positive bacteria stain purple; gram-negative bacteria lose purple stain when exposed to alcohol but stain pink with a second dye; and acid-fast bacteria keep purple stain when an acid is applied.

Bacterial growth depends on oxygen, nutrition, light, temperature, and humidity. **Aerobic** bacteria, such as those found on the skin, need oxygen to live. **Anaerobic** bacteria, such as bacteria in the gastrointestinal tract, live without oxygen. Most bacteria that inhabit humans grow best at body temperature, 98.6°F (37°C).

Rod-shaped bacteria form spores that are thick walled and hard to kill. Spores remain in a resting state until favorable conditions exist that allow the organism to resume normal function. Prolonged exposure to high temperature destroys spores on surgical equipment. Bleach is used in patient rooms to kill spores from ***Clostridium difficile*** (*C. difficile*).

RICKETTSIAE. Rickettsiae are a type of bacteria that must be inside living cells to reproduce. Rickettsiae **vectors** (living organisms that transmit disease) are infected fleas, ticks, mites, and lice that bite humans. Several diseases are caused by rickettsiae. Rocky Mountain spotted fever, caused by *Rickettsia rickettsii,* whose reservoirs (the places in nature where the organism usually lives and multiplies without causing disease) are rodents and dogs, is transmitted to humans by a tick bite.

Viruses

Viruses are organisms smaller than bacteria that depend on host cells to live and reproduce (see Table 8.1). Invaded host cells make more of the virus material. The new viral particles are then released either by destroying the host cell or by forming small buds that break away to infect other cells.

When a virus enters a cell, it may immediately trigger disease or remain **dormant** (inactive) for years without causing illness. An example of this is *human herpesvirus 3* (varicella zoster virus), which can cause disease quickly (chickenpox) or remain dormant for years, eventually erupting in the disease called shingles. Antibiotics are not effective against viruses. Antiviral drugs are used to decrease symptoms caused by viruses and to decrease the viral load (the number of viral cells in the patient's blood).

Fungi

Fungi are a group of organisms that includes yeasts, molds, and mushrooms and can produce highly resistant spores (see Table 8.1). Because fungi do not contain chlorophyll, they must obtain food from living organisms or dead organic matter. Normal flora of the mouth, skin, vagina, and intestinal tract include many fungi. Most fungi are not pathogenic, and serious fungal infections are rare. Antifungal medications treat fungal infections.

Protozoa

Protozoa are single-celled parasitic organisms with flexible membranes that live in the soil and obtain nourishment from dead or decaying organic material (see Table 8.1). Protozoa infect humans through fecal-oral contamination or through ingestion of food or water contaminated with cysts or spores, through host-to-host contact, or by the bite of a mosquito or other insect that has previously bitten an infected person.

Helminths

Helminths are wormlike parasitic animals: roundworms, flatworms, tapeworms, pinworms, hookworms, and flukes. Disease transmission occurs through skin penetration of larvae or ingestion of helminth eggs. **Trichinosis** (caused by the roundworm *Trichinella spiralis*) is a disease caused by eating raw or undercooked meat of pigs or wild animals that contain *Trichinella* larvae.

Prions

Prions are more recently identified organisms or agents thought to be unique proteins with long incubation periods. How they reproduce is unknown. Research will shed light on these unusual organisms or protein particles, which are thought to cause mad cow disease and the human dementia known as *Creutzfeldt-Jakob disease.*

Mode of Transmission

Once the causative agent exits the reservoir, a means of transfer to a susceptible host is needed. Transmission of microorganisms occurs through direct contact, indirect contact, or through the air.

Direct Contact

Direct transmission occurs through touching, kissing, sexual contact, biting, or droplet spray into the eyes or on mucous membranes through sneezing, coughing, spitting, singing, or talking. Droplet spread is usually limited to 3 feet or less. Illnesses spread by direct transmission may include influenza, impetigo, scabies, conjunctivitis, pediculosis, herpes, *C. difficile,* and all sexually transmitted diseases, including human immunodeficiency virus (HIV). Protect yourself and your patients from direct transmission with hand washing, aseptic technique, and use of **personal protective equipment** (PPE) such as gloves, surgical masks, goggles, gowns, and booties. PPE is selected and used based on the task to be performed. and the applicable isolation precautions (standard precautions and/or transmission-based precautions; see the *Infection Prevention Guidelines* discussion later in the chapter).

• WORD • BUILDING •

protozoa: proto—first + zoon—animal

Indirect Contact

Indirect transmission is either vehicleborne or vectorborne. Vehicleborne transmission is the spread of an infectious organism by contact with a contaminated object, such as a toy, soiled bedding, dressings from a wound, surgical instruments, water, food, and biological products such as blood, serum, plasma, tissues, and organs. Vehicleborne illnesses include conjunctivitis, trichinosis, HIV, and hepatitis A, B, C, D, and E. Vehicle transmission can be avoided through proper hand washing, thorough cleaning of the patient environment, and provision of clean water and food supplies.

Vectorborne transmission is the spread of infectious organisms through a living source other than humans, such as an insect, flea, mouse, or rat. Diseases spread through vectors include malaria, plague, and Lyme disease. Vector transmission can be reduced with insect repellants, avoidance of infested areas, and rodent control.

Airborne

Airborne transmission is different from droplet transmission (see direct contact discussed earlier) because the particles floating in the air are much smaller, remain suspended in the air for a long time, and may travel large distances. Airborne organisms can be inhaled or deposited on the mucous membrane of a susceptible host. Measles, chickenpox, and tuberculosis are transmitted by airborne transmission. Airborne transmission is prevented with the use of high-efficiency particulate air (HEPA) respirators (also known as a tuberculosis [TB] mask). HEPA respirators filter the tiniest particles from the air, unlike surgical masks, which can allow such particles to pass into the respiratory system of a host. Institutions provide individual-fit testing and training for HEPA respirator use for each health care worker.

> **SAFETY TIP**
>
> If you provide care for patients with suspected or confirmed diseases that are spread through airborne transmission, such as TB, be sure you have your own fit-tested HEPA mask to wear. Do not use other masks because they do not provide adequate protection. If you cannot obtain your own fit-tested mask, you should not enter the patient's room.

Multiple Modes of Transmission

Many diseases have multiple modes of transmission requiring a variety of protective techniques. For example, chickenpox is transmitted by direct contact, indirect contact, and airborne transmission. It is no wonder 80% to 90% of susceptible persons exposed to it develop the disease. Understanding the modes of transmission of a particular disease allows you to use the appropriate means of protection without using unnecessary supplies that increase costs.

Portal of Entry

To produce disease, organisms must gain entry into a susceptible host. Routes of entry into a susceptible host include the respiratory tract, skin (usually nonintact), mucous membranes, gastrointestinal tract, genitourinary tract, and placenta. Once the organism enters the host, it may lead to disease, depending on the condition of the host and many other factors, such as the **virulence** (ability to produce infection) of the organism.

Susceptible Host

The body has many defense mechanisms to prevent infection, such as intact skin and mucous membranes and a functioning immune system. A breakdown in these defenses increases the possibility of infection. Factors that increase susceptibility to infection are very young age, old age, malnourishment, immunocompromise, chronic disease, stress, burns and invasive procedures (Box 8.2, *Gerontological Issues*).

Portal of Exit

The portal of exit is the route by which the infectious agent leaves the host, who has become a reservoir for infection: respiratory tract, skin, mucous membranes, gastrointestinal tract, genitourinary tract, blood, open lesions, or placenta.

THE HUMAN BODY'S DEFENSE MECHANISMS

Skin and Mucous Membranes

Intact skin and mucous membranes are the body's first line of defense against infection. Preventing skin dryness and cracking with lotion keeps the skin intact so organisms do not have an entry point. Oral mucous membranes have many layers, making it difficult for organisms to enter the body. The skin has acidic (pH < 7) properties that render some organisms unable to produce disease. For example, many bacteria prefer an alkaline (pH >7) environment for reproduction. The body also has an abundance of normal flora that impairs the growth of pathogens both on the skin and in the gastrointestinal (GI) tract.

Cilia

Cilia are hairlike structures lining the upper respiratory tract mucous membranes that protect the lungs. Cilia trap mucus, pus, dust, and foreign particles to prevent them from entering the lungs. Then the cilia push the trapped particles up to the pharynx with wavelike movements for expectoration.

Gastric Juices

Gastric juices inside the stomach are very acidic (pH 1 to 5). This acidic environment destroys most organisms that enter the stomach.

Immunoglobulins

Immunoglobulins are proteins found in serum and body fluids that may act as antibodies to destroy invading organisms and prevent the development of infectious disease. **Antibodies** are proteins that are produced by B lymphocytes when foreign antigens of invading cells are detected. **Antigens** are markers on the surface of cells that identify cells as being the body's own cells (autoantigens) or as being foreign cells (foreign antigens). Antibodies combine with specific foreign antigens on the surface of the invading organisms, such as bacteria or viruses, to control or destroy them. Antigens are neutralized or destroyed by antibodies in several ways. Antibodies can initiate destruction of the antigen, neutralize toxins released by bacteria, promote antigen clumping with the antibody, or prevent the antigen from adhering to host cells.

Leukocytes and Macrophages

Leukocytes (white blood cells) are the primary cells that protect against infection and tissue damage. There are five types of leukocytes:

- Neutrophils are phagocytic cells that focus on bacteria and small particles.
- Monocytes become macrophages and are mainly phagocytic on tissue debris and large particles.
- Lymphocytes' functions include antigen recognition and antibody production.
- Basophils respond to inflammation from injury.
- Eosinophils destroy parasites and respond in allergic reactions.

After recognizing a foreign antigen, neutrophils and macrophages engulf and digest it, a process known as

---

Box 8.2

Gerontological Issues

Infection and Older Adults

Older patients may not have typical symptoms of infection. For example, a serious bacterial infection may cause no elevation in temperature. In fact, a fever is not a common sign of an infection for an older adult.

This difference among older adults may cause significant delay in providing appropriate treatment and care. Be alert for the following in older patients, which may indicate an infection:

- Behavioral change, such as pacing or irritability.
- Masking of the symptoms of infection by a chronic disease. For example, the inflammation and pain of degenerative joint disease may make it difficult for a patient to recognize an infection in an affected joint.

phagocytosis. The macrophages move the antigen fragments to their surface to be recognized by T lymphocytes to further stimulate action of the immune system. Phagocytes ingest and destroy bacteria, damaged or dead cells, cellular debris, and foreign substances.

Lysozymes

Lysozymes are bactericidal enzymes present in white blood cells and most body fluids, such as tears, saliva, and sweat. These enzymes dissolve the walls of bacteria, destroying them.

Interferon

If an invading organism is a virus, white blood cells and fibroblasts release interferon (a group of antiviral proteins). Interferon helps destroy infected cells and inhibits production of the virus within infected cells. Tumor cell growth may also be inhibited by interferon.

Inflammatory Response

The inflammatory response occurs with any injury to the body. This response can be caused by pathogens, trauma, or other events causing injury to tissues. Infection may or may not be present.

Vascular Response

The first step of the inflammatory process is local vasodilation, which increases blood flow to the injured area. Pathogenic organisms can trigger the first step of the inflammatory process. Increased blood flow creates redness and heat at the injury. The increase in blood flow brings more plasma to the area to nourish tissue and carry waste and debris away.

Inflammatory Exudate

The second step of the inflammatory process is increased permeability of the blood vessels, which allows plasma to move out of the capillaries and into the tissues. Swelling occurs, resulting in pain from pressure on nearby nerve endings.

Phagocytosis and Purulent Exudate

The final step of the inflammatory process is the destruction of pathogenic organisms and their toxins by leukocytes. During this process, a purulent exudate (pus) may form that contains protein, cellular debris, and dead leukocytes.

Immune System

The immune system is the body's final line of defense against infection (see Chapter 18). Immune cells and lymphoid tissue work with the body's other defense mechanisms. The immune system is a finely tuned network that functions together to protect the body from invasion by pathogenic organisms. When this network breaks down, infectious disease can result.

• WORD • BUILDING •

phagocytosis: phagein—to eat + cytos—cell + osis—condition

INFECTIOUS DISEASE

General Clinical Manifestations of Infection

Localized Infection

Localized infection is caused by an increase of microbes in one area that triggers the inflammatory response. Manifestations of a local infection include pain, redness, swelling, and warmth at the site. Pain is most severe when the infection occurs in closed cavities. Redness and swelling are seen when surface structures are involved. Warmth may be felt at the site. Body temperature may rise, producing an antimicrobial effect.

Generalized Infection

Generalized infections occur when there is systemic or whole body involvement. Symptoms of generalized infection may include headache, malaise, muscle aches, fever, and anorexia. As the infection progresses, there can be an increase in fever, elevated white blood cell count, decreased blood pressure, mental confusion, tachycardia, and shock. **Sepsis** is the term used for an infection that has spread to the bloodstream.

Laboratory Assessment

Several methods are used to identify pathogens. One method is to perform a microscopic examination, such as Gram's method of staining using gentian violet, to identify bacterial species. Gram-positive bacteria turn purple and Gram-negative bacteria are pink. Another method is culture and sensitivity (C&S). Organisms found in the culture specimen are grown on a laboratory plate and identified within 24 to 48 hours. A sensitivity examination is then done, which exposes any organism to many antibiotics to determine which antibiotic will be most effective for treatment.

A serum antibody test measures the reaction to a certain antigen. A positive result on this test does not always mean an active infection is present. It can simply mean there has been an exposure to the antigen, so it is not as accurate as a culture.

A complete blood cell count with differential (CBC with diff) is usually obtained when an infectious disease is suspected. The five different types of leukocytes and their levels are identified. Elevations in specific leukocytes occur based on the type and severity of the pathogen.

Erythrocyte sedimentation rate (ESR, sed rate) is an early screening test for inflammation but not a definitive test for infection. During the inflammatory process, red blood cells become heavier. The ESR measures in millimeters per hour the speed at which the red blood cells settle in a tube. The faster the settling, the greater the inflammation.

Other tests such as x-rays, computed tomography (CT), and magnetic resonance imaging (MRI) are helpful in identifying abscesses (walled-off infections). Skin tests diagnose infections. For example, the purified protein derivative (PPD) skin test screens for tuberculosis (see Chapter 31).

Immunity

Immunity is the ability of the body to protect itself from disease (see Chapter 18). There are several types of immunity:

- Natural immunity occurs in species and prevents one species from contracting illnesses found in another species.
- Innate immunity is genetic; hereditary immunity is that which a person is born with.
- Acquired immunity is obtained either actively or passively through exposure to an organism, from a vaccine, or from an injection of immunoglobulins (antibodies) or is passed from mother to baby.

Types of Diseases

The various types of infectious diseases are discussed in the chapters related to the body system they affect. For HIV, see Chapter 20; for respiratory diseases such as tuberculosis, see Chapter 31; for hepatitis, see Chapter 35. Mononucleosis is discussed below.

Mononucleosis

Infectious mononucleosis (referred to as mono or the kissing disease) is an infection that is usually caused by the Epstein-Barr virus (a herpes virus). Mononucleosis is a contagious disease that anyone can develop. However, it is mainly diagnosed in young adults. Most adults have been exposed to the virus and have antibodies to it but never develop the disease. The virus remains in the body for a lifetime but rarely causes another infection.

Mononucleosis is spread primarily through person-to-person contact, mainly through saliva. Sharing utensils, food, or beverages can also transmit the disease. Coughing or sneezing of small droplets of infected saliva or mucus into the air allows the virus to be inhaled by others.

The incubation period for mononucleosis is 4 to 8 weeks after exposure. Symptoms during the first 3 days include extreme fatigue, loss of appetite, and chills. Then a severe sore throat, headache, high fever, reddened throat and tonsils with a white coating, generalized lymphadenopathy (enlarged lymph nodes in two different sites other than inguinal nodes), or diarrhea occur. The spleen enlarges 50% of the time. Occasionally, a rash develops that is similar to the rash seen with measles.

Signs and symptoms, as well as diagnostic tests, confirm mononucleosis. Lymphocyte levels are elevated. The monospot and heterophile antibody tests confirm mononucleosis.

Usually no specific treatment is needed. The illness runs its course as other viral illnesses do. Antiviral drugs are not effective. Symptoms are treated as needed with supportive care. Fatigue may last for months. Rest is important. If the spleen is enlarged, lifting, straining and contact sports are avoided to prevent trauma and rupture. Mild inflammation of the liver or hepatitis may occur, but no treatment is usually required. Other complications are rare.

INFECTION CONTROL IN THE COMMUNITY

Many levels of organizations work closely together to control communicable diseases. The World Health Organization (WHO) and the Centers for Disease Control and Prevention (CDC) teach standards to prevent and control diseases and monitor disease outbreaks. Local health departments teach how to prevent and control the spread of disease. Community immunization programs have helped reduce infectious diseases.

Although requirements vary from state to state, most elementary schools require some proof of childhood immunization. Many colleges also require or recommend immunization to help control the outbreak of diseases such as measles and meningitis. In addition, educating the public about the importance of **hand hygiene**, the CDC's respiratory hygiene/cough etiquette measures (including the CDC's *Cover Your Cough* campaign), immunization, clean water, safe food handling techniques, and safer sex precautions in preventing the spread of disease is essential.

NURSING CARE TIP

For infection control, teach respiratory hygiene/cough etiquette to patients and family members who have a cough, congestion, rhinorrhea, or increased respiratory secretions. Provide these *Cover Your Cough* instructions:

- Cover your mouth and nose with a tissue when you cough or sneeze.
- Put your used tissue in the waste basket.
- If you don't have a tissue, cough or sneeze into your upper sleeve, not your hands.
- Clean your hands after coughing or sneezing. Wash with soap and water or clean with alcohol-based hand cleaner.
- If asked, put on a surgical mask to protect others.

Source: Centers for Disease Control and Prevention. (2009). *Cover your cough.* Retrieved January 21, 2010, from http://www.cdc.gov/flu/protect/covercough.htm.

Both the hospital and home health care nurse have a responsibility to provide infection control teaching for the patient with an infection and his or her family. Such techniques may include use of disposable dishes, utensils, and gloves, and proper disposal of contaminated items. Techniques used should be specific to the interruption of the transmission of the particular disease.

INFECTION CONTROL IN HEALTH CARE AGENCIES

If on admission to a hospital or health care agency a patient already has an infection, it is referred to as a community-acquired infection. An infection that develops as a result of a patient's stay in the hospital or health care agency is called a **nosocomial infection**. The host's condition plays a major role in whether or not an infection is acquired. Patients in the hospital are commonly debilitated, malnourished, or immunocompromised. Multiple antibiotic therapy also increases susceptibility to other types of infection and promotes the resistance of pathogens to antibiotics. Therefore, the risk of developing a nosocomial infection is very high. Some areas within an institution tend to have an increased number of nosocomial infections, such as intensive care, neonatal, dialysis, oncology, and burn units. Patients in these areas tend to undergo more invasive procedures and are debilitated, increasing susceptibility to infection.

Several pathogens are commonly responsible for causing nosocomial infections:

- *Escherichia coli* (*E. coli*) is the most common pathogen causing nosocomial urinary tract infections. *E. coli* normally lives in the healthy intestinal tract of humans. *E. coli* can be spread by the patient, by the unwashed hands of a health care worker, or through contaminated food and water.
- ***Staphylococcus** aureus* (commonly known as staph) is the most common pathogen causing nosocomial surgical wound infections and nosocomial septicemia. Staph usually lives in the nose and on the skin of healthy people.
- *Pseudomonas aeruginosa* is the most common pathogen in nosocomial pneumonia. It is found in soil, around water, and in the health care setting around sinks, water, irrigating solutions, and nebulizers on respiratory equipment.

Hand Hygiene

The single most effective way to prevent and control the spread of infection is with effective hand hygiene, which easily removes the transient organisms that cause most hospital infections that result from cross-transmission. Most of these organisms are transmitted via the hands of health care workers. Hands must be cleansed before and after every patient contact to help prevent the direct transmission of organisms (Fig. 8.2). The use of gloves decreases the transmission of organisms, but CDC guidelines also require hand washing before and after glove use because hands may still become contaminated. Patients may also transmit organisms with inadequate hand hygiene. Teach patients the importance of hand hygiene after handling their own secretions.

> **SAFETY TIP**
>
> The Joint Commission's 2010 National Patient Safety Goals emphasize the importance of preventing health care–associated infections with hand hygiene guideline compliance and the use of evidence-based practices to prevent infections (see www.jointcommission.org). You are responsible for using appropriate hand hygiene in the health care setting. Hand hygiene can include either the use of hand washing or an alcohol-based hand rub. For visibly soiled hands, wash with soap and water. Using alcohol-based hand rubs is preferred to kill bacteria in many cases and may increase compliance by saving time and reducing dry skin.
>
> **Hand Washing**
>
> Proper hand washing requires wetting the hands with warm—not hot—water, soaping, and lathering, with at least 15 seconds of rubbing your hands together, covering all surfaces. Interlace your fingers to cleanse between them, rub your nails against your palms to clean under the nails, and then rinse your hands with fingertips pointed downward under running water. Dry your hands with clean disposable paper towels. Use the paper towel to turn off the faucet. Use only facility-supplied lotions because others may reduce the effectiveness of soap or break down latex gloves (water-based lotion only). Apply lotion to your hands to prevent drying and cracking in which infection could develop (CDC, 2002).
>
> **Alcohol-Based Hand Rubs**
>
> Apply specified amount of the hand rub to the palm of one hand. Rub both hands together, covering all surfaces until the hands are completely dry to ensure the alcohol has evaporated. Do not wash off hand rub. For an informative presentation, visit www.cdc.gov/handhygiene/download/hand_hygiene_supplement_minus_notes.pdf

Asepsis

The concept of **asepsis** (freedom from organisms) is important for all health care workers who have direct or indirect patient contact. For hospitalized patients, the most common

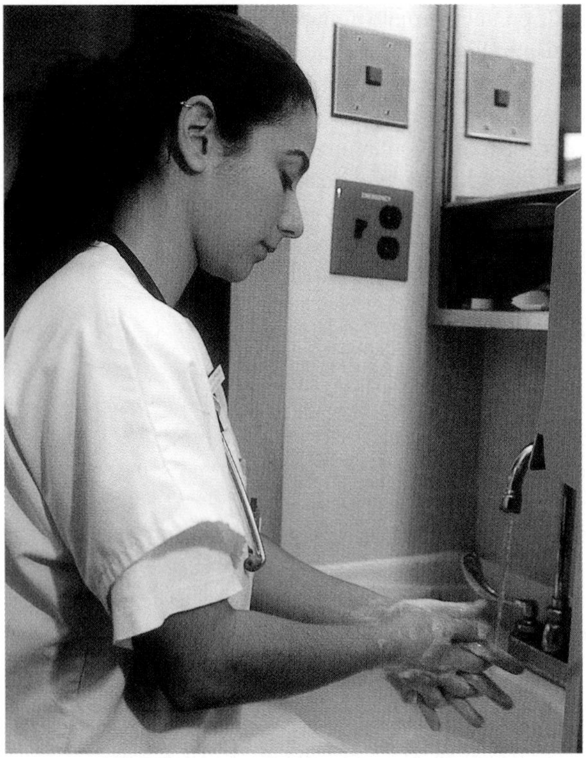

FIGURE 8.2 Frequent hand washing by health care workers helps reduce the spread of microorganisms.

sites for infectious diseases are the genitourinary tract, respiratory tract, bloodstream, and surgical wounds. Be aware of patients at risk of developing these infections and protect them with aseptic techniques.

CRITICAL THINKING

Mrs. Sampson

■ Mrs. Sampson has neutropenia from chemotherapy treatments.

1. Why is hand hygiene the most important intervention you can do to help prevent infection for Mrs. Sampson?
2. What would be a priority nursing diagnosis for Mrs. Sampson?
3. What type of isolation could be beneficial to Mrs. Sampson?

Suggested answers at end of chapter.

Medical Asepsis

Medical asepsis is commonly referred to as clean technique. The goal is to reduce the number of pathogens or prevent the transmission of pathogens from one person to another. Frequent, proper hand hygiene is one of the best ways to achieve this goal. The use of gowns, gloves, masks, and protective eyewear or rooms with special ventilation may also be helpful (Fig. 8.3). Disinfectants and precautions as defined by the CDC are also crucial tools. Techniques used should be appropriate to interrupt the spread of the known pathogen. As part of medical asepsis, you should keep your own body and clothing clean to prevent spread of infection to patients, yourself, and your family (Box 8.3).

Surgical Asepsis

Surgical asepsis (sterile technique) refers to an item or area that is free of all microorganisms and spores. Surgical asepsis is used in surgery and to sterilize equipment. Articles can be subjected to intense heat or chemical disinfectants to destroy all organisms. The use of pressurized steam sterilizers, called autoclaves, kills even the most powerful organisms. Some equipment cannot be exposed to moist heat, so gas sterilizers are used instead. Once these articles are sterilized, they are dated, packaged, and sealed. Once a package is opened or outdated, it is no longer considered sterile. Sterile technique is rarely required in the home care setting.

Infection Prevention Guidelines

CDC guidelines for infection control and isolation precautions are used in hospital and health care agency policies. CDC and agency guidelines are continuously updated and should be followed for your patients' and your own

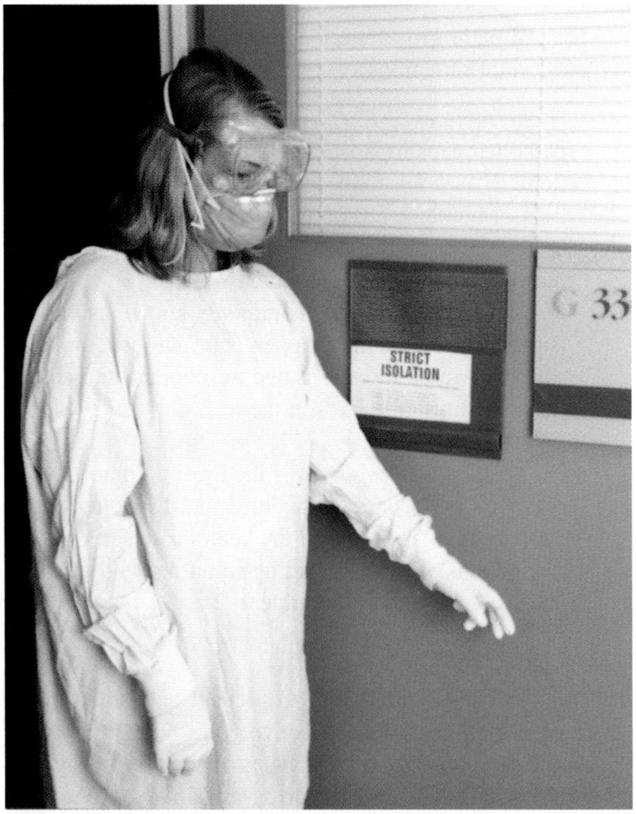
G 33
STRICT ISOLATION

FIGURE 8.3 Gloves, gown, mask, goggles, and face shield help prevent the spread of infection to health care workers and patients.

Box 8.3

Guidelines to Prevent the Spread of Infection to Patients, Self, and Family

- Bathe daily and wear a clean uniform/clothing every day.
- Keep your natural fingernail tips less than ¼ inch long, and do not wear artificial nails. Both long nails and artificial nails have been associated with spread of infection to patients because they can be colonized with harmful bacteria. Multiple studies have shown that long fingernails and artificial nails harbor bacteria and have caused infections in patients that sometimes have resulted in death.
- Avoid wearing rings and bracelets because they harbor organisms.
- Cleanse your stethoscope at least daily and in between patient use with alcohol. Vancomycin-resistant *Enterococcus* bacteria have been cultured from stethoscopes in a hospital setting.
- Use hand hygiene between each patient contact. The use of an alcohol-based hand gel or hand washing is recognized as the single most important action to take to prevent spread of infection.
- Follow prescribed isolation precautions for your protection, as well as that of the patient.
- Perform hand hygiene before going home to prevent transfer of bacteria to your home.
- Remove your uniform in a contained area of your home to launder it, and bathe/shower when you come home from work. This will decrease the spread of antibiotic-resistant bacteria to your home and your family. Keep your nursing shoes clean and stored away from the rest of the family.

protection. Current CDC guidelines for isolation precautions in hospitals include two tiers of precautions: standard precautions and transmission-based precautions (Table 8.2). Visit www.cdc.gov/ncidod/dhqp/pdf/guidelines/Isolation2007 for more details.

Standard Precautions

Standard precautions are used in the care of all patients. These precautions require you to assume that all patients are infectious regardless of their diagnosis. Standard precautions apply to blood, secretions, excretions, open skin, mucous membranes, and all body fluids, excluding sweat. All patients with draining wounds or secretions of body fluids are considered infectious until an infection is confirmed or ruled out. Using gloves, gowns, masks, goggles, face shields, and, most important, hand hygiene helps prevent the spread of infection to health care workers and other patients.

CRITICAL THINKING

Who Is at Greatest Risk of Infection?

■ Which of the following patients is at greatest risk for infection and why?

1. Mr. Ashland, age 55, is hospitalized for a hernia repair. He is overweight and has adult-onset diabetes.
2. Mrs. Burrows, age 72, is hospitalized for a broken hip. She is thin, frail, has dementia, and has undergone placement of a urinary catheter.
3. Jackson Dunn, age 22, is hospitalized for major surgery. Jackson is thin and small.

Suggested answers at end of chapter.

TABLE 8.2 STANDARD PRECAUTIONS AND TRANSMISSION-BASED PRECAUTIONS

Standard Precautions	
Use standard precautions for all patient care. Combine standard precautions with transmission-based precautions as needed based on the patient's illness.	
Hand hygiene	Use alcohol-based hand rub or wash hands with nonmicrobial soap unless specifically contraindicated before and after using gloves, between patients, and between procedures on the same patient.
Gloves	Wear gloves before contact with any body fluids or substances. Change gloves after each use.
Mask, eye protection, face shield	Use personal protective equipment for patient care if splashes or sprays of blood or body fluids are likely.
Gown	Wear gown to protect skin/prevent soiling of clothing for patient care if splashes or sprays of blood or body fluids are likely.
Occupational health and bloodborne pathogens	Dispose of sharps properly. Do not recap needles.
Patient care equipment	Clean reusable equipment before reuse. Discard single-use items properly.

Continued

TABLE 8.2 STANDARD PRECAUTIONS AND TRANSMISSION-BASED PRECAUTIONS—cont'd

Standard Precautions	
Linen	Handle linen to avoid clothing contamination.
Patient placement	Use private room for infectious patients.
Transmission-Based Precautions	
Airborne Precautions	
Examples: measles, tuberculosis, varicella (chickenpox, shingles)	
Patient placement	Provide private room with regulated airflow. Keep door closed.
Respiratory protection	Do not enter room if susceptible to measles or chickenpox unless no caregivers who are immune are available. If susceptible, wear a fit-tested (N95) disposable respirator. Do not enter room of patient with tuberculosis (TB) unless wearing a fit-tested (N95) disposable respirator. Have patient with TB also wear surgical mask during times that care is performed. Offer visitors an N95 respirator per agency policy. Teach patient respiratory hygiene/cough etiquette.
Patient transport	Limit patient transport to essential purposes. Place surgical mask on patient (may not contain all TB organisms)
Droplet Precautions	
Examples: adenovirus, diphtheria (pharyngeal), *Haemophilus influenzae* (epiglottitis, meningitis, pneumonia, sepsis), influenza, mumps, mycoplasma pneumonia, *Neisseria meningitidis* (meningitis, pneumonia, sepsis), pertussis, pneumonic plague, rubella, group A streptococcus.	
Patient placement	Provide private room, or separation greater than 3 feet between the infected patient and other patients and close privacy curtain.
Respiratory protection	Wear mask upon entering patient area. Teach patient respiratory hygiene/cough etiquette.
Patient transport	Limit patient transport to essential purposes. Place surgical mask on patient.
Contact Precautions	
Examples: cellulitis, *Clostridium difficile,* skin infections (diphtheria, herpes simplex virus, impetigo, pediculosis, scabies, conjunctivitis, viral hemorrhagic infections (Ebola, Lassa, or Marburg), herpes zoster	
Patient placement	Provide private room or place with patient with same infection and no other infection.
Hand washing, gloves, gown	Protect self and others from contaminated items.
Patient transport	Limit patient transport.
Patient care equipment	Dedicate the use of noncritical patient care equipment to a single patient.

Source: Data from Siegel, J. D., Rhinehart, E., Jackson, M., Chiarello, L., and the Healthcare Infection Control Practices Advisory Committee. (2007). *2007 guideline for isolation precautions: Preventing transmission of infectious agents in healthcare settings.* Atlanta, GA: Centers for Disease Control and Prevention. Retrieved September 22, 2009, from http://www.cdc.gov/ncidod/dhqp/pdf/guidelines/Isolation2007.pdf.

Transmission-Based Precautions

Transmission-based precautions are used for patients with specific communicable diseases that can be transmitted to others. Transmission-based precautions add an additional layer of protection to the standard precautions.

Prevention of Respiratory Tract Infections

Nosocomial pneumonia has been linked with the highest infection mortality rate in hospitalized patients. Patients who are at highest risk for pneumonia are those with endotracheal, nasotracheal, or tracheostomy tubes because these invasive tubes bypass the normal defenses of the upper respiratory tract. Strategies to prevent infections such as ventilator-associated pneumonia (VAP) are "bundled" together so nurses remember to use these strategies. For more information on VAP bundles visit www.qualitymeasures.ahrq.gov/summary/summary.aspx?view_id51&doc_id512124.

Prevention of Genitourinary Tract Infections

The most common hospital-acquired infection is a urinary tract infection. Patients with urinary catheters are at greatest risk. The urinary tract is sterile, but insertion of a catheter into the bladder may allow organisms to enter. Institutional policies on appropriate use of urinary catheters differ, so follow your agency's policy. Appropriate reasons for use of a urinary catheter may include urinary obstruction, a neurogenic bladder condition, shock, and palliative care.

Indwelling urinary catheters should be removed as soon as possible. For patients who need long-term catheter use, intermittent catheterization is preferred because it significantly reduces the risk of infection. Using strict aseptic technique while inserting and caring for the catheter in the health care agency is imperative. The catheter tubing must be securely anchored to the patient's leg, according to agency protocol, so it does not move in and out of the urethra. Movement can encourage organisms to enter the urinary tract.

The closed urinary drainage system seal should never be opened. (If intermittent irrigation is ordered, sterile technique must be used to protect both ends of the system from contamination.) The drainage bag should be positioned so that it is never higher than the level of the bladder to prevent backflow of urine into the bladder, which could contaminate the sterile urinary tract. If an indwelling urinary catheter and a drainage system are used long term, the catheter and the entire system should be changed regularly using sterile technique. All long-term indwelling urinary catheters are considered colonized. Standards in home care differ from institutional care because patients are generally at lower risk of infection within their own environment.

Remember that the most crucial point at which bacteria may enter the patient is during insertion of the catheter, so excellent sterile technique is required. Another point to remember is that the urinary tract is highly vascular (many blood vessels close to the surface), so that an infection in this tract can easily result in bacteremia (bacteria in the blood), which can then progress to septicemia (infection in the blood), a potentially life-threatening condition. For more information on prevention of urinary tract infections in adults, visit http://kidney.niddk.nih.gov/kudiseases/pubs/utiadult/index.htm.

SAFETY TIP

Catheters should be used only when necessary because of the **morbidity** (sickness) and **mortality** (death) associated with infections that can develop from them. The continued need for an indwelling catheter should be monitored daily, and the catheter should be discontinued as soon as it is no longer needed.

CRITICAL THINKING

Mr. Carson

■ While working in an extended care facility, you see Mrs. Brandt, nursing assistant, wheeling Mr. Carson to activities. He has a long-term urinary catheter. The urine bag is hung on the arm of the wheelchair. What is your responsibility in this situation?

Suggested answers at end of chapter.

Prevention of Surgical Wound Infections

The initial dressing for surgical wounds is applied in the operating room using sterile aseptic technique. Postoperative orders indicate when to change the dressing using sterile technique. Monitor the wound with every dressing change for signs of infection.

Protection from Sepsis

Sepsis (also known as septicemia or blood poisoning) is a blood infection with a variety of causes, including infection in another body site and contamination of invasive catheters and solutions (central lines, arterial lines, pulmonary artery catheters, urinary catheters). Insertion and care of these catheters require sterile technique and careful observation for infection signs. All solutions should be examined for expiration date, signs of contamination, cloudiness, particles, or discoloration before use. Indications of sepsis, fever, tachypnea, tachycardia, hypotension, and elevated white blood cell count should be reported promptly to the physician for immediate treatment. Blood cultures may be ordered before giving antibiotics to treat sepsis. In severe sepsis when death is likely, the intravenous drug drotrecogin alfa (activated) is given for 96 hours. It may reduce mortality in patients due to its anti-inflammatory effects. For more information, visit www.xigris.com.

ANTIBIOTIC-RESISTANT INFECTIONS

Antibiotic-resistant infections are on the rise. These types of infections result in increased health care costs, morbidity (death), and mortality (illness). Methods to prevent these infections include not using antibiotics in animal feed, teaching patients to take all prescribed medications exactly as ordered, and avoiding the use of antibiotics for viral infections (common cold or flu). American College of Physicians/American Society of Internal Medicine guidelines suggest that most upper respiratory infections do not require antibiotic treatment. For healthy adults with the symptoms of bronchitis, sinusitis, pharyngitis, and other upper respiratory infections, over-the-counter cold symptom remedies and saltwater gargles should be used for symptom relief.

Two infections that continue to rise include methicillin-resistant *Staphylococcus aureus* (MRSA) and vancomycin-resistant enterococci (VRE). For more information on antibiotic resistance, visit www.cdc.gov/drugresistance/index.htm.

Methicillin-Resistant *Staphylococcus Aureus*

A serious antibiotic-resistant infection, MRSA is difficult to treat and has a high mortality rate. It affects mainly the elderly and the chronically ill. Vancomycin hydrochloride, a potent and expensive antibiotic, can be used intravenously to treat MRSA. However, experts fear that the bacteria will further mutate and become resistant to all currently available antibiotics. A few isolated cases of this mutation have been documented worldwide. The risk that these resistant organisms will spread is real, which will return us to the preantibiotic days when *S. aureus* was a killer.

NURSING CARE TIP

Antibiotics are not effective against viral infections such as colds or the flu. When health care providers give antibiotics to treat viral infections, this misuse of antibiotics increases the risk of developing antibiotic-resistant "superbugs." Use of antibacterial products such as antibacterial soaps may also contribute to the superbug problem. People need to be educated that antibiotics do not work on viral infections. Nurses play a vital role in educating people about this growing problem.

Vancomycin-Resistant Enterococci

Vancomycin-resistant enterococci (VRE) infections are common. Although enterococci are normal flora in the GI and female genital tracts, VRE are a new pathogenic strain. VRE are transmitted via direct or indirect contact. Patients at risk for VRE infections include those with indwelling urinary or central venous catheters, the immunocompromised or critically ill, those receiving multiple antibiotics or vancomycin therapy, surgical patients, and those with extended hospital stays. Preventive VRE measures focus on proper hand hygiene, education of health care workers, aggressive infection control methods, and restricting use of vancomycin. Patients with VRE should be isolated, and current CDC and institutional isolation policies should be strictly followed (Fig. 8.4). Treatment is difficult, involving combination antibiotic therapy, although VRE may also be resistant to other antibiotics.

Quinupristin/dalfopristin (Synercid) is an intravenous drug for VRE treatment. After Synercid is given, the IV is flushed with 5% dextrose in water rather than normal saline solution or heparin due to compatibility issues. Linezolid (Zyvox) can treat both VRE and MRSA and should ideally be used only for these serious infections to decrease the risk that resistance will develop. Antibiotic-resistant bacteria remain a very serious threat to the health of the world population.

Antibiotic-Resistant Organism Precautions

Visitors: Report to the Nurses' Station before entering the room.

1. **Private** room required.
2. **Gloves** must be worn by all hospital personnel entering room.
3. **Wash Hands** on entering and leaving room.
4. **Gowns:** required **IF** contamination of clothing is likely.
5. **Decontaminate All Equipment** used in the room before removal from the room.

FIGURE 8.4 Antibiotic-resistant organism precautions for vancomycin-resistant enterococci (VRE).

THERAPEUTIC MEASURES FOR INFECTIOUS DISEASES

Once an infectious organism and the affected body system have been identified, the appropriate medication can be selected and treatment begun (Table 8.3). The drug of choice must be able to destroy (or control) the pathogen:

- Antibiotics treat bacterial infections, not viruses, fungi, helminths, or prions.
- Antiviral medications treat viral infections, but their use is aimed at symptom control rather than cure.
- Antifungal drugs are available for fungal infections, but cure may require extended use.

Cost effectiveness is another concern when selecting a medication. Newer anti-infectives can be very expensive.

Antibiotics can be classified as either bactericidal or bacteriostatic. Bactericidal agents kill bacteria, whereas bacteriostatic agents inhibit or retard bacterial growth, leaving the final destruction of the bacteria up to the infected host's immune system. Bacteriostatic agents may be less helpful for the patient who is immunocompromised.

SAFETY TIP

Whenever preparing to give an antibiotic, especially for the first time, ask what allergies a patient may have. Patients may have allergies to one antibiotic group that prevents the use of chemically similar drugs. Therefore, all allergies should be reported to the health care provider.

Many antibiotics are metabolized by the liver and excreted by the kidneys. Disorders of these organs may require lower doses. Antibiotic levels fluctuate greatly depending on organ function, age, sex, health, and other factors. Antibiotic peak and trough levels (highest and lowest blood levels) may need to be monitored according to agency protocol to ensure therapeutic levels and to prevent toxicity and damage to major organs.

Antibiotic-Associated Diarrhea

Antibiotic therapy may cause antibiotic-associated diarrhea (AAD) because antibiotics upset the delicate balance of natural bacteria normally found in the intestine. Any antibiotic can cause AAD, but ampicillin, cephalosporins, and clindamycin are the most common. Patients who are hospitalized or in nursing homes and on antibiotic therapy commonly develop AAD.

TABLE 8.3 MEDICATIONS USED TO TREAT INFECTIOUS DISEASE

Medication Class, Action	Examples	Route	Side Effects	Nursing Implications
Bactericidal Antibiotics				
Penicillins				
Most effective against gram-positive organisms.	amoxicillin (Amoxil), ticarcillin (Ticar), penicillin G, ampicillin (Omnipen)	PO, IM, IV	Allergic reaction, superinfection	Review signs of allergic reactions with patient. Monitor patient for allergic reaction (rash, hives, itching) or anaphylactic shock (fever, chills, trouble breathing, lower blood pressure, tight throat). Keep epinephrine available Teach patient and family to stop drug and call primary care provider if allergy signs occur If signs of allergic reaction occur, stop parenteral drug and notify primary care provider immediately. Teach patient to notify primary care provider if white patches appear in mouth or if vagina becomes irritated.
Carbapenems				
• Broad-spectrum antibacterial agents used to treat moderate to severe infection.	ertapenem (Invanz), imipenem and cilastatin (Primaxin), meropenem (Merrem)	IM (ertapenem), IV (others)	GI upset, rash, fever, seizures	Ertapenem: Check for lidocaine (diluent) allergy. Monitor patient for seizures and, if applicable, serum valproic acid level.
Cephalosporins				
• First-generation drugs are most effective against gram-positive organisms. • Second- and third-generation drugs are more effective against gram-negative organisms	cephalothin (Keflin), cefazolin (Ancef), cefaclor (Ceclor), ceftriaxone (Rocephin)	PO, IM, IV	GI disturbance, phlebitis, pain at injection site, rash, hives Less common but serious: kidney and liver damage, superinfection	Patients with penicillin allergy may have 10% risk of cross allergy to cephalosporins. Teach patient to take drug on an empty stomach, 1 hr before or 2 hr after meals, to increase absorption. Teach patient to take drug at specified intervals over 24-hr period. Monitor blood urea nitrogen, creatinine, lactic dehydrogenase, aspartate aminotransferase, and alanine aminotransferase to detect kidney or liver damage.
Aminoglycosides				
• Used to treat gram-negative organisms.	amikacin (Amikin), gentamicin (Garamycin), tobramycin (Nebcin)	Parenteral, topical	Nephrotoxicity, ototoxicity (ringing in ears, deafness)	Monitor peak and trough levels to keep drug in therapeutic range. Teach patient to report signs of allergy, tinnitus, vertigo, or hearing loss.
Fluoroquinolones				
• Used to treat a variety of infections, such as bronchitis, bone and joint infection, pneumonia, tuberculosis, sexually transmitted disease, and urinary tract infection.	moxifloxacin (Avelox), ciprofloxacin (Cipro), levofloxacin (Levaquin), norfloxacin (Noroxin), ofloxacin (Floxin)	PO, IV	GI upset, dizziness, headache, CNS disturbances, flatulence, rash, photosensitivity Rare but serious: tendon rupture	Give drug on an empty stomach. Teach patient to take with a full glass of water. Do not give with antacids that contain aluminum, calcium, or magnesium. Monitor liver function, and report signs of dysfunction (fatal hepatitis may occur). Encourage fluids. Explain side effects, and advise sun protection. Teach patient to report joint or muscle pain immediately.
Nitroimidazoles				
• Used to treat anaerobic bacterial and parasitic infections.	metronidazole (Flagyl)	PO, IV, topical	Nausea, diarrhea, metallic taste, thrombophlebitis	May be taken with or without food. Tell patient to avoid alcohol use.

Continued

TABLE 8.3 MEDICATIONS USED TO TREAT INFECTIOUS DISEASE—cont'd

Medication Class, Action	Examples	Route	Side Effects	Nursing Implications
Glycopeptides				
• Used to treat serious gram-positive infections.	vancomycin	IV, PO for pseudomembranous colitis	IV site pain, red man syndrome (flushing, rash on upper body, neck, head), thrombocytopenia	Administer over 1 hr to prevent red man syndrome. Monitor trough levels. Monitor IV site for thrombophlebitis.
Bacteriostatic Antibiotics				
Tetracyclines				
• Used to treat most gram-positive and gram-negative organisms.	tetracycline HCl, doxycycline (Vibramycin), minocycline HCl (Minocin)	PO (tetracycline HCl), IV (others)	GI upset, photosensitivity	Give 1 hr before or 2 hr after meals. Do not give with milk, milk products, or antacids because they impair absorption. Suggest eating crackers and juice (but not a full meal) to reduce GI upset. Teach patient to avoid prolonged sun exposure during therapy.
Macrolides				
• Broad-spectrum antibiotics used effectively against many gram-negative and gram-positive organisms.	azithromycin (Zithromax)	PO	GI upset, photosensitivity, chest pain	Give with a full glass of water. Capsules must be taken on an empty stomach. Do not give with aluminum or magnesium antacids within 2 hr before or after. Teach patient to avoid sun exposure.
	clarithromycin	PO	GI upset, chest pain, severe taste disturbance, hearing problems	Give with a full glass of water. May be taken with or without food except for time-release capsules.
	Erythromycin (E-mycin, EES)	PO, IV	GI upset	When giving drug IV, administer slowly to decrease vein irritation. Give orally on an empty stomach, 1 hr before or 2 hr after meals. Give with a full glass of water (not with acidic fruit juices, such as orange juice or grapefruit juice). Urge patient to take drug around the clock and to complete entire course of treatment. Explain that gastric distress is common but not a reason to stop the drug. Suggest that patient contact primary care provider if side effects are intolerable.
Lincomycins				
• Used to treat serious anaerobic bacterial infections, acne, methicillin-resistant *Staphylococcus aureus,* and some protozoal infections.	clindamycin (Cleocin)	PO, topical, IV, IM (deep)	GI upset, diarrhea, fever	Monitor patient for foul odor diarrhea, fever, and abdominal pain indicating possible *Clostridium difficile* infection, which is associated with clindamycin.
Streptogramins				
• Used to treat vancomycin-resistant *Enterococcus faecium* bacteremia and severe skin infections. • Combination drugs are bactericidal.	quinupristin/dalfopristin (Synercid)	IV infusion	Vein irritation, rash, nausea, arthralgia and myalgia, pruritus	After infusion, flush with 5% dextrose in water solution to minimize vein irritation (incompatible with saline or heparin).

TABLE 8.3 MEDICATIONS USED TO TREAT INFECTIOUS DISEASE—cont'd

Medication Class, Action	Examples	Route	Side Effects	Nursing Implications
Sulfonamides				
• Effective against most gram-positive and many gram-negative organisms. • Commonly used for urinary tract infections, *Pneumocystis jiroveci* (formerly *carinii*) pneumonia, and otitis media.	trimethoprim sulfamethoxazole (Bactrim, Septra)	PO, IV	Common: rash, pruritus, nausea, vomiting, phlebitis, bleeding, hypoglycemia, photosensitivity Increased bleeding time (use caution with anticoagulants), increased phenytoin (Dilantin) toxicity	IV drug should be given over 1 hr. Instruct patient to take oral drug on an empty stomach 1 hr before or 2 hr after meals with a full glass of water. Monitor intake and output. Fluid intake should be at least 1,500 mL daily. Advise against prolonged exposure to the sun. Teach patient to stop drug and call primary care provider if signs of allergic reaction or bleeding occur.
Oxazolidinones				
• Used to treat complicated infections caused by gram-negative microorganisms.	linezolid (Zyvox)	PO, IV	Diarrhea, headache, taste alteration	Before IV use, check compatibilities. Oral form may be taken with or without food. Teach patient to avoid tyramine found, for example, in aged cheeses, smoked foods, tap beer, red wine, soy sauce, sauerkraut.
Antifungals				
Amphotericin B				
• Interferes with the cell wall structure of the fungus, causing it to die.		IV, for life-threatening fungal infections	Nausea, vomiting, diarrhea, nephrotoxicity	Explain the purpose of treatment and need for long-term IV therapy. Instruct patient and family on side effects and possible discomfort at IV site. Monitor patient during first hour of infusion for febrile reaction. Monitor injection site often because drug is very irritating to tissues. Monitor intake and output, blood urea nitrogen (BUN), and creatinine levels for signs of kidney damage. Obtain daily weight because fluid retention follows kidney damage. Encourage 2,000–3,000 mL of fluid daily to help flush drug through kidneys.
Triazoles				
• Used to treat yeast or fungus infections.	fluconazole (Diflucan), itraconazole (Sporanox), voriconazole (Vfend)	PO, IV	Hepatotoxicity, nausea, vomiting, diarrhea, abdominal discomfort	Obtain cultures before giving drug. Monitor BUN and creatinine levels and liver function. Teach patient and family to notify physician at the first sign of yellow skin, dark urine, or pale stools (signs of liver damage). Explain that Vfend causes blurry vision about 20 minutes after dose and that patient should not drive.
Echinocandins				
• Disrupt fungal cell wall integrity. • Used to treat candidal infection.	caspofungin (Cancidas), micafungin (Mycamine), anidulafungin (Eraxis)	IV infusion	Diarrhea, nausea, rash	Monitor patient's liver function.

Antibiotics destroy helpful bacteria along with harmful bacteria. With fewer good bacteria to keep potentially harmful bacteria in check, harmful bacteria that are resistant to the antibiotic used increase in number. These bacteria can produce toxins that harm the intestinal wall and cause inflammation. Watery bowel movements result. When AAD occurs, the antibiotic therapy may be stopped, and the diarrhea usually resolves. For severe diarrhea, colitis (colon inflammation), or pseudomembranous colitis, metronidazole (Flagyl) or vancomycin (Vancocin) is given. A **probiotic** (a substance with health-promoting effects, such as yogurt in this case) may help prevent AAD (see *Evidence-Based Practice*).

EVIDENCE-BASED PRACTICE

Clinical Question

Are probiotics effective in preventing antibiotic-associated diarrhea (AAD)?

Evidence

Patients with AAD who consumed probiotics found in fermented milk products and yogurt starter cultures showed a significant reduction in AAD (Hickson et al., 2007). In a recent research review of 25 randomized controlled trials, probiotics were found effective in both preventing and treating AAD (McFarland, 2006).

Implications for Nursing Practice

Probiotics may be useful in treating or preventing AAD for non-immunocompromised patients. Nurses can encourage patients on antibiotic therapy to consult a health care provider, pharmacist, or dietitian about the use and appropriate dosage of probiotics (Yantis & Velander, 2009).

REFERENCES

Hickson, M., D'Souza, A. L., Muthu, N., et al. (2007). Use of probiotic *Lactobacillus* preparation to prevent diarrhoea associated with antibiotics: Randomised double blind placebo controlled trial. *British Medical Journal, 335*(7610), 80.

McFarland, L. V. (2006). Meta-analysis of probiotics for the prevention of antibiotic associated diarrhea and the treatment of *Clostridium difficile* disease. *American Journal of Gastroenterology, 101*(4), 812–822.

Yantis, M. A., & Velander, R. (2009). Antibiotics can thwart antibiotic-associated diarrhea. *Nursing, 38*(3), 58–59.

Clostridium difficile

Clostridium difficile is a gram-positive bacteria that can be one of the most serious causes of AAD. *C. difficile,* normally found in the intestine, overgrows and releases toxins that cause diarrhea, fever, bloating, and abdominal pain. Healthy people usually do not get *C. difficile* overgrowth. It occurs after antibiotic therapy, usually in those who are hospitalized or in nursing homes, with older adults being at greatest risk. *C. difficile* overgrowth can lead to pseudomembranous colitis, a serious and sometimes life-threatening condition with fever, diarrhea, and abdominal pain. The bacteria are transmitted by touching feces-contaminated surfaces and so can be transmitted from health care workers or from patient to patient. Hand washing is essential to reduce its spread. To treat diarrhea caused by *C. difficile,* antibiotic treatment is stopped and metronidazole (Flagyl) or vancomycin (Vancocin) is given.

• WORD • BUILDING •

probiotic: pro—for + biotic—life

Nursing Responsibilities

Nurses are responsible for administering medications correctly and for teaching patients the importance of taking these medications properly (Box 8.4). Follow these general guidelines and consult drug references for further information before giving anti-infectives:

- Note all patient allergies, and inform the primary care provider.
- Obtain ordered samples for culturing before starting ordered anti-infectives, so culture accuracy is not affected.
- Monitor and report any side effects or signs of allergic response, especially anaphylactic reactions.
- Observe and report any signs of superinfection (one that occurs as a result of antibiotic use). For example, thrush may develop because antibiotics disrupt the normal flora of the GI tract.

SAFETY TIP

Always review and know the normal dose of a medication before giving it. You are responsible for any medication you give, even if the dose was ordered incorrectly and you were following the order. If the dose is outside the normal range, do not give the drug. Consult with the RN, pharmacist, or supervisor, who should contact the ordering physician for clarification. Always review medication doses before giving them to keep your patient and your nursing license safe.

NURSING PROCESS FOR THE PATIENT WITH AN INFECTION

General Infections

Data Collection

It is important to recognize the earliest signs and symptoms of infection. Early detection can help provide early treatment

Box 8.4

Patient Teaching

Anti-Infective Medications

- Stress to the patient and family the need to take all of the medication exactly as prescribed.
- Explain that stopping treatment before the prescription is finished, even if the patient feels better, increases the risk of relapse and the growth of antibiotic-resistant organisms.
- Explain the signs and symptoms of side effects (allergic and nonallergic) to watch for and what to do about them.
- Explain when to call the primary care provider to report signs and symptoms.

to prevent major complications and reduce costs. Providing emotional support to the patient is also important (Box 8.5, *Patient Perspective*). Patients who are prone to infection because of immunosuppression should take special precautions to prevent infection (Box 8.6).

Box 8.5

Patient Perspective

Edie: Emotions of Chronic Infection

It was back! I wasn't sure I could deal with it one more time. I've been hospitalized four times with this same infection (cellulitis) in my leg. It feels like I've lost my life. I can't count on being able to do anything or go anywhere because the infection just keeps coming back.

My left leg is now all swollen, red, discolored, and very painful. I can tell when I'm infected by more than the pain in the leg. I feel weak, kind of spacey, and once I passed out. I'm so sick of going to the emergency room—waiting forever to get admitted, all the IV starts and blood draws. With these infections, I've had a PICC (peripherally inserted central catheter) line twice. I've been sent home on IV antibiotics, sometimes for weeks at a time. I've learned how to hang my own IV antibiotics; in fact, I've learned much more than I ever wanted to know.

My cellulitis is associated with chronic lymphedema, causing swelling in my legs. I'm working hard to keep the swelling down so the infection doesn't recur. Wish me luck and keep giving me psychosocial support during your nursing care. I'm not sure how I will be able to deal with this much longer.

Box 8.6

Patient Education

Prevention of Infection in Older, Debilitated, or Immunocompromised Patients

- Wash your hands often, using proper technique.
- Avoid crowds or anyone with an infection.
- Stay well nourished because food helps keep the immune system healthy.
- Have a flu shot yearly and a pneumonia shot as recommended by your primary care provider.
- Wash raw fruits and vegetables thoroughly, cook food thoroughly, and store food safely to prevent food poisoning. (*Note:* If you are severely immunocompromised, raw foods, soft cheeses, and yogurt may be contraindicated because of the risk of bacterial infection.)
- If your immune system is depressed, notify your primary care provider if you have an elevated temperature, even if you have no other symptoms. People with depressed immune function cannot mount the usual immune response to infection, and a low-grade fever may be the only sign of infection.

CRITICAL THINKING

Mr. Cheevers

■ Mr. Cheevers is admitted to the hospital for IV antibiotic therapy. He states that he has no allergies. One hour after the infusion begins, you happen to meet the nursing assistant coming down the hall with a blanket. He casually says, "Mr. Cheevers is very cold. I'm taking him a blanket. He is also restless and a bit short of breath." What is your responsibility in this situation?

Suggested answers at end of chapter.

Nursing Diagnoses, Planning, and Implementation

Risk for Infection Related to External Factors

EXPECTED OUTCOME: The patient will remain free from symptoms of infection.

- Follow current hand hygiene guidelines *to reduce spread of infection.*
- Use standard precautions and transmission-based precautions *to prevent the transmission of organisms.*
- Observe and report signs of infection such as redness, warmth, and fever, especially for neutropenic patients *because they do not have normal inflammatory response and low-grade fever is often the only sign.*

- Monitor laboratory values of white blood cell counts and cultures *because they correlate to patient's immune function for planning care.*

Evaluation
If interventions have been successful, the patient remains free from symptoms of infection.

Imbalanced Nutrition: Less Than Body Requirements Related to Problems Eating or Digesting Food
EXPECTED OUTCOME: The patient will maintain ideal body weight for height and weight and eat a balanced diet.

- Identify and provide foods patient enjoys with pleasant presentation *because patient will be more likely to try eating enjoyable foods in a clean, odor-free environment.*
- Explain and ensure that a balanced diet with protein, fatty acids, and vitamins is available and should be eaten. *These nutrients are needed for healthy immune system function.*
- Monitor and document patient intake *to provide accurate nutritional assessment.*
- Provide antiemetics, as ordered, *to control nausea and vomiting and improve nutritional intake.*

Evaluation
If interventions have been effective, patient's body weight will be maintained within ideal body weight range and patient will eat a balanced diet.

Deficient Knowledge Related to Disease Process and Treatment
EXPECTED OUTCOME: The patient will describe therapy and carry out treatment.

- Explain infection and prevention of infectious diseases. *Patients' understanding of how infections occur helps them in controlling their risk of infection.*
- Recommend responsible use of antibiotics *to prevent resistant organisms.*
- Explain medications, side effects, and symptoms to report *to promote compliance with treatment and safe medication use.*
- Teach patients how to participate in their own care and have them assist in the development of their plan of care *to promote compliance with treatment.*

Evaluation
If interventions have been effective, the patient will state understanding of therapy and plan and carry out treatment plan.

Respiratory Tract Infection
Data Collection
Patients with respiratory tract infections may have a cough, a congested or runny nose, a sore throat, chest congestion, or chest pain. The throat may be reddened, or there may be white patches in the back of the throat. Lung sounds can include crackles, rhonchi, or wheezing. Ask patients if they have a productive cough and the amount, frequency, and color of the sputum. A sputum culture is obtained to identify the presence of pathogenic organisms for appropriate treatment.

Nursing Diagnoses, Planning, and Implementation
Risk for Infection Related to External Factors
EXPECTED OUTCOME: The patient will remain free from symptoms of infection.

- Encourage coughing and deep breathing *to keep airways clear and prevent atelectasis.*
- Provide oral care with toothbrush or suction-type toothbrush regularly *to remove plaque, which has been found to contribute to pneumonia development.* (Toothettes do not remove plaque.)
- Encourage fluids if not contraindicated. *Dehydration is associated with dry, sticky secretions that are difficult to cough up.*
- Provide pain relief *so patient will take deep breaths.*
- Elevate head of bed 30 degrees or more when a tube feeding is infusing *to prevent aspiration pneumonia.*
- Use sterile water rather than tap water from faucet for oral care for immunocompromised patients *to prevent nosocomial pneumonia infection.*

Evaluation
If interventions have been effective, oxygen saturation will be above 90%, with report of decreased dyspnea. Respirations will be even and unlabored and patient will be free of signs and symptoms of infection.

Gastrointestinal Tract Infection
Data Collection
The symptoms of GI tract infections may include nausea, vomiting, diarrhea, cramping, and anorexia. Patients may have frequent episodes of emesis and diarrhea and need to be monitored for signs of dehydration resulting from the loss of fluid. Stool cultures may be ordered.

Nursing Diagnoses, Planning, and Implementation
Risk for Infection Related to External Factors
EXPECTED OUTCOME: The patient will remain free from symptoms of infection.

- Encourage fluid intake *to replace fluid lost during fever, vomiting, and diarrhea.*
- Follow standard precautions, especially for older and immunocompromised patients, *to prevent the spread of C. difficile. C. difficile* usually does not cause infection in healthy adults.
- Teach hand washing with antimicrobial soap and water if contact with *C. difficile* spores is likely *because alcohols, chlorhexidine, iodophors, and other antiseptic agents have poor activity against C. difficile spores, which transmit infection.*

Evaluation
Patient will be free of infection and nausea, vomiting, diarrhea, cramping, anorexia, and dehydration if interventions have been successful.

Genitourinary Tract Infection
Data Collection
Symptoms of a urinary tract infection (UTI) can include voiding urgency, frequency, burning, flank pain, change in urine color, foul urine odor, and confusion or change in mental status in an older adult. Monitor frequency, amount, color, and odor of the urine. Urinalysis and urine cultures may be ordered.

Nursing Diagnoses, Planning, and Implementation
Risk for Infection Related to External Factors

EXPECTED OUTCOME: The patient will remain free from symptoms of infection.

- Do not request and avoid use of urinary catheters unless no other options are available *because patients are more likely to develop bacteremia.*
- Use sterile technique for inserting urinary catheters *to prevent nosocomial infections.*
- Avoid contamination when emptying urinary catheter bags *to prevent nosocomial infections.*
- Use evidence-based facility policy for identifying and managing symptoms related to the urinary tract. *Evidence-based practice improves quality of care and reduces variability in management.*
- Standard diagnostic criteria should be used to identify, document, and communicate to physicians detailed symptoms such as fever or hematuria and not urine odor, urine color, clarity, or culture results alone *because they cannot distinguish symptomatic from asymptomatic infections and the need for medication.*
- Patients, residents, families, and staff should be taught to identify and manage UTIs using evidence-based practice *to promote appropriate practices.*

Evaluation
If interventions have been effective, the patient will have normal urine output without such symptoms of infection as urgency, frequency, burning, flank pain, change in urine color, foul urine odor, or confusion or change in mental status.

SUGGESTED ANSWERS TO CRITICAL THINKING

■ *Mrs. Sampson*
1. Hand hygiene reduces the microorganisms on the nurse's hands to help reduce their transmission from patient to patient. This helps prevent exposure to pathogens and infection.
2. *Risk for Infection.*
3. Reverse isolation, the goal of which is to protect the patient from exposure to organisms rather than to protect others from exposure to the patient.

■ *Who Is at Greatest Risk of Infection?*
1. Mr. Ashland has two risk factors: chronic disease and probably stress.
2. Mrs. Burrows has many risk factors, including older age, debilitated condition, probable malnourishment, probable stress, and an invasive procedure. This patient is at greatest risk.
3. Jackson has three risk factors: probable stress, possible malnourishment, and an invasive procedure.

■ *Mr. Carson*
1. Ask the nursing assistant about the urinary bag placed above the patient's bladder. Explain that the bag should always stay below the level of the bladder both for proper drainage and for infection control.
2. Assist the nursing assistant in repositioning the bag properly.
3. Let Mr. Carson's primary nurse know about the potential backflow of urine so that he can be assessed in the next few days for signs of a bladder infection.

■ *Mr. Cheevers*
Mr. Cheevers may be experiencing signs of allergic reaction to the medication. The fact that he has no history of allergy is no guarantee that he is not experiencing one now. If allergy is suspected, the IV should be stopped. He needs to be evaluated immediately and the primary care provider notified. Epinephrine should be on hand to treat the patient for anaphylaxis. The primary nurse needs to be alerted to the situation in the event that it worsens. Later, the nursing assistant can be instructed about the signs of allergic response.

REVIEW QUESTIONS

1. Place the links in the chain of infection in their proper order of occurrence in causing an infection.
   a. Portal of entry
   b. Causative agents
   c. Mode of transmission
   d. Portal of exit
   e. Reservoir
   f. Susceptible host

2. Which of the following is the most important technique for the nurse to use during patient care to prevent infection transmission?
   a. Wear gloves.
   b. Wear a gown.
   c. Wash hands.
   d. Wear a mask.

3. Which of the following nursing actions should the nurse include in the plan of care to help maintain the body's first line of defense against infection?
   a. Help the patient cough and deep-breathe.
   b. Apply lotion to clean skin.
   c. Give an antibiotic as ordered
   d. Help the patient void.

4. Which of the following patient temperature readings would be the priority for the LPN/LVN to report to the registered nurse?
   a. Temperature 97°F (36.1°C) for an older patient with hypertension
   b. Temperature 98.9°F (37°C) for a first-day postoperative patient
   c. Temperature 99.6°F (37.5°C) for a patient with neutropenia
   d. Temperature 100°F (37.7°C) for a patient with appendicitis

5. The nurse is to give a newly ordered antibiotic to a patient with a wound infection. Which of the following is essential to do before giving the medication?
   a. Check all patient allergies.
   b. Check the patient's temperature.
   c. Change dressing and note wound appearance.
   d. Give antibiotic before mealtime.

6. Which of the following is the most important action for the nurse to use to prevent a hospital-acquired urinary tract infection in a patient with an indwelling urinary catheter?
   a. Ensure an adequate intake of IV and oral fluids.
   b. Use clean technique for catheter insertion.
   c. Position the drainage bag higher than bladder level.
   d. Maintain a closed urinary drainage system.

7. Which of the following statements indicates to the nurse that the patient understands the general principles of appropriate antibiotic use?
   a. "I'll take this until I start feeling better."
   b. "I have pills left over from the last time I had this infection."
   c. "I'll take all of this as it says to on the medication label."
   d. "I take only half of a pill to reduce the cost of the pills."

References

Centers for Disease Control and Prevention. (2002). Guideline for Hand Hygiene in Health-Care Settings. *MMWR 51*(RR16):1-44. Retrieved April 19, 2009, from http://www.cdc.gov/mmwr/preview/mmwrhtml/rr5116a1.htm

Joint Commission. (2010). *2010 national patient safety goals.* Retrieved January 13, 2010, from http://www.jointcommission.org/patientsafety/nationalpatientsafetygoals

9 Nursing Care of Patients in Shock

BOBBI M. MARTIN

KEY TERMS

acidosis (AS-ih-DOH-sis)
acute pulmonary hypertension (ah-KEWT PULL-muh-NAIR-ee HY-per-TEN-shun)
anaerobic (AN-air-ROH-bick)
anaphylaxis (AN-uh-fih-LAK-sis)
bronchospasm (BRONG-koh-spazm)
cardiac output (KAR-dee-ack OWT-put)
cardiogenic (KAR-dee-oh-JEN-ick)
cyanosis (SY-uh-NOH-sis)
distributive (diss-TRIB-yoo-tiv)
dysrhythmia (diss-RITH-mee-yah)
epinephrine (EP-ih-NEFF-rin)
extracardiac (EX-trah-KAR-dee-ack)
hypoperfusion (HY-poh-per-FEW-shun)
hypotension (HY-poh-TEN-shun)
hypovolemic (HY-poh-voh-LEE-mick)
ischemia (iss-KEY-mee-ah)
lactic acid (LAK-tik AS-id)
laryngeal edema (lah-RIN-jee-uhl eh-DEE-muh)
myocarditis (MY-oh-kar-DYE-tiss)
myocardium (MY-oh-KAR-dee-um)
neurogenic (NEW-roh-JEN-ick)
norepinephrine (NOR-ep-ih-NEFF-rin)
oliguria (AWH-lih-GYOO-ree-ah)
perfusion (per-FEW-zhun)
pericardial tamponade (PER-ih-KAR-dee-uhl TAM-pon-AID)
sepsis (SEP-sis)
tachycardia (TAK-ih-KAR-dee-yah)
tachypnea (TAK-ip-NEE-ah)
tension pneumothorax (TEN-shun NEW-moh-THOR-raks)
thrombi (THROM-bye)
toxemia (tock-SEE-me-ah)
trauma (TRAW-mah)
urticaria (UR-ti-CARE-ee-ah)

QUESTIONS TO GUIDE YOUR READING

1. How would you explain the pathophysiology of shock and compensatory mechanisms?
2. What are the etiologies, signs, and symptoms of the four categories of shock?
3. What data should you collect when caring for patients with shock?
4. What current therapeutic measures are used for shock?
5. What nursing care should you provide for patients with shock?
6. How would you prioritize care for a client in shock?
7. What findings would demonstrate a positive response to therapeutic measures for shock?

Shock is a life-threatening condition. A patient in shock is in a state of circulatory collapse that results in organ damage and death without immediate treatment. Massive bleeding, overwhelming infection, severe allergic reactions, and cardiac failure are examples of conditions that may lead to shock. No matter what its source, shock is a medical emergency that requires rapid, comprehensive intervention in collaboration with the health care team.

Shock is defined as "inadequate tissue **perfusion**," in which there is insufficient delivery of oxygen and nutrients to the body's tissues and inadequate removal of waste products from these tissues or, more simply, an imbalance between oxygen supply and demand. The decrease in tissue perfusion leads to impaired cellular metabolism, which in turn leads to tissue hypoxia. Tissue hypoxia results in **hypoperfusion** of vital organs and cell death. All body systems are affected by reduced oxygen supplies. The resulting injury to the body can be treated in the early stages of shock, but if shock is prolonged, it leads to irreversible cell damage and death. By the time blood pressure drops, cellular and tissue damage have already occurred. Therefore, it is important to identify patients at risk for shock and carefully assess them to detect early symptoms.

PATHOPHYSIOLOGY OF SHOCK

Tissue perfusion and blood pressure are maintained in the body by three mechanisms: (1) adequate blood volume, (2) an effective cardiac pump, and (3) effective blood vessels. The body is able to compensate for failure of one of these mechanisms by making a change in one or both of the other two. Shock occurs when compensatory mechanisms fail, resulting in inadequate tissue perfusion. Common causes of shock include inadequate **cardiac output** caused by heart failure, a sudden loss of blood volume resulting from hemorrhage, or a sudden decrease in peripheral vascular resistance caused by **anaphylaxis** (a life-threatening allergic reaction), **sepsis** (an infection that has spread to the bloodstream), and neurologic alterations.

Metabolic and Hemodynamic Changes in Shock

When blood pressure falls, the body responds by activating the sympathetic nervous system. **Epinephrine** and **norepinephrine** are released from the adrenal medulla and increase cardiac output by causing the heart to beat faster and stronger. Blood is shunted away from the skin, kidneys, and intestines to preserve blood flow to the brain, liver, and heart. Epinephrine, cortisol, and glucagon raise blood glucose levels to supply cells with fuel. Stimulation of the renin-angiotensin-aldosterone system from decreased cardiac output causes vasoconstriction and retention of sodium and water to decrease further fluid loss. Respiratory rate increases to deliver more oxygen to the tissues. Together these compensatory responses produce the classic signs and symptoms of the initial stage of shock: **tachycardia, tachypnea**, restlessness, anxiety, and cool, clammy skin with pallor. If oxygen delivery remains inadequate, signs and symptoms of progressive and irreversible shock are seen (Table 9.1).

TABLE 9.1 CHARACTERISTICS OF SHOCK STAGES

Characteristics	Stages		
	• *Mild/compensated* • *Able to maintain blood pressure and tissue perfusion*	• *Moderate/progressive* • *Compensatory mechanisms start to fail*	• *Severe irreversible/ decompensated* • *No response to treatment* • *Death is imminent*
Heart rate	Tachycardia	Tachycardia Greater than 150 bpm	Slowing
Pulses	Bounding	Weak, thready	Absent
Systolic blood pressure	Normal	Below 90 mm Hg In hypertensive patient, 25% below baseline	Below 60 mm Hg
Diastolic blood pressure	Normal	Decreased	Decreasing to 0
Respirations	Increased rate, deep	Tachypnea, crackles, shallow	Slowing, irregular, shallow
Temperature	Varies	Decreased, may rise in septic shock	Decreasing
Level of consciousness	Anxious, restless, irritable, alert, oriented, sense of impending doom	Confused, lethargic	Unconscious, comatose
Skin and mucous membranes	Cool, clammy, pale	Moist, cold, clammy, pale	Cyanosis, mottled, cold, clammy
Urine output	Normal	Decreasing to less than 20 mL/hr	15 mL/hr, decreasing to anuria
Bowel sounds	Normal	Decreasing	Absent

CRITICAL THINKING

Classic Signs of Shock

■ What is the cause and compensatory purpose of each of the classic signs of shock: tachycardia, tachypnea, **oliguria**, pallor, and cool, clammy skin?

Suggested answer at end of chapter.

LEARNING TIP

Tachycardia is a compensatory mechanism that is usually the first sign of shock. When a patient develops sustained tachycardia, it is a signal that the patient's condition is changing. Be aware that elderly patients cannot tolerate tachycardia very long because their ability to adapt to stress is reduced.

Consider the cause of the tachycardia. For example, a surgical patient who develops tachycardia may be hemorrhaging and should be assessed for bleeding. Be aware that with internal hemorrhaging there may not be any visible signs of bleeding. Changes in vital signs may be the only evidence.

Provide prompt intervention, such as applying direct pressure to an area of hemorrhage, and implement the physician's orders immediately.

Inadequate tissue blood flow causes an important change in cellular metabolism. When cells are deprived of oxygen, they shift from aerobic metabolism to anaerobic metabolism to continue to receive nutrition and energy. **Anaerobic** metabolism is an inefficient form of metabolism that can supply the energy needs of the cell for only a few minutes. After that, the body's metabolic rate and temperature begin to fall as a result of reduced energy production.

Anaerobic metabolism results in the production of **lactic acid** as an unwanted by-product. Unless the lactic acid can be circulated to the liver and thus removed from the bloodstream, the blood becomes increasingly acidic. **Acidosis**, which is a decrease in blood pH below 7.35, is one of the classic signs of shock.

• WORD • BUILDING •

hypoperfusion: hypo—low + perfuser—to pour over or through
anaphylaxis: an—without + phylaxis—protection
tachycardia: tachy—fast + cardia—heart
tachypnea: tachy—fast + pnea—breathing
oliguria: olig—few + uria—urine
anaerobic: an—without + aerobic—presence of oxygen
acidosis: acid—sour + osis—condition

Effect on Organs and Organ Systems

Prolonged shock causes extensive damage to the organs and organ systems (Table 9.2). Inadequate blood flow results in tissue **ischemia** and injury. Because blood is shunted away from the kidneys early in shock to save fluid and provide oxygen to vital organs, the kidneys commonly are injured first. The kidneys can tolerate reduced blood flow for about 1 hour before cells in the kidneys die from a lack of oxygen and nutrients. If there is widespread damage to the kidneys, complete renal failure is likely. Renal failure resulting from inadequate blood flow to the kidneys can be prevented and treated by replacing lost fluids.

CRITICAL THINKING

Anaerobic Metabolism

■ Why is anaerobic metabolism necessary and helpful if it produces the complication of metabolic acidosis?

Suggested answer at end of chapter.

Several organs of the gastrointestinal system may be injured early in shock. Inadequate circulation to the intestines may result in injury of the mucosa and may even cause paralytic ileus (paralysis of the intestine). **Toxemia** may result when the body absorbs normally occurring bacteria and endotoxins from inside the bowel into the circulation. The liver may be injured both by ischemia and by toxins created by the

TABLE 9.2 EFFECT OF SHOCK ON ORGANS AND ORGAN SYSTEMS

Organ or Organ System	Effect
Lungs	Acute respiratory failure Acute respiratory distress syndrome
Renal system	Renal failure
Heart	Dysrhythmias Myocardial ischemia Myocardial depression
Liver	Abnormal clotting Decreased production of plasma proteins Elevated serum levels of ammonia, bilirubin, and liver enzymes
Immune system	Depletion of defense components
Gastrointestinal system	Mucosal injury Paralytic ileus Pancreatitis Absorption of endotoxins and bacteria
Central nervous system	Ischemic damage, necrosis, brain death

shock state as blood is circulated through it for cleansing. Signs and symptoms of liver injury include decreased production of plasma proteins, abnormal clotting (because clotting factor production by the liver is impaired), and elevated serum levels of ammonia, bilirubin, and liver enzymes.

The immune system is also affected by shock leaving the body vulnerable to infection. Also, if the liver has been damaged, it is unable to assist the immune system in providing defense.

The body attempts to preserve blood supply to the heart and brain because these are vital organs that require a continuous supply of oxygen. Shock places extra demands on the heart itself, creating a situation in which the heart is in extra need of oxygen at a time when oxygen supplies are already low. When the **myocardium** (the middle layer of the heart wall) receives inadequate oxygenation, cardiac output decreases and shock worsens. The pumping ability of the heart can be further depressed by acidosis, toxins released into the blood from ischemic tissues, or ischemia-induced **dysrhythmia** (abnormal heart rhythm). If the brain is deprived of circulation for more than 4 minutes, brain cells die from a lack of oxygen and glucose. Prolonged shock may result in brain death.

COMPLICATIONS FROM SHOCK

Acute respiratory distress syndrome (ARDS), disseminated intravascular coagulation (DIC), and multiple organ dysfunction syndrome (MODS) are three especially grave conditions that may follow a prolonged episode of shock. Patients with ARDS usually develop respiratory failure despite high levels of supplemental oxygen and mechanical ventilation. DIC results from ischemic damage to the endothelial lining of blood vessels. The formation of multiple tiny **thrombi** (blood clots), microscopic debris, and depletion of tissue-clotting factors cause abnormal bleeding and additional tissue damage. DIC itself may cause shock and death. MODS is a major cause of death following shock. When an organ has inadequate perfusion it fails, which may increase the rate of failure of other organs. It usually begins with respiratory failure, followed by failure of the kidneys, heart, liver, and finally cerebral and gastrointestinal function.

LEARNING TIP

To understand what *disseminated intravascular coagulation* (DIC) means, define each of the words and then put the definitions together.

Disseminated: scattered or widespread

Intravascular: intra = inside + vascular = vessels

Coagulation: clotting.

These definitions put together tell you that DIC is scattered, widespread, clotting inside the vessels.

At first, hemorrhage does not seem likely in light of a clotting problem, but if you think about what is occurring, it does make sense. When many clots form throughout the body in response to stressors, few clotting factors remain available to form the clots needed to prevent hemorrhage. As a result, hemorrhage is a risk in DIC.

CLASSIFICATION OF SHOCK

The four types of shock are classified by their cardiovascular characteristics (Table 9.3):

- **Hypovolemic** shock is caused by a decrease in the circulating blood volume.
- **Cardiogenic** shock is caused by cardiac failure.
- **Extracardiac** obstructive shock is caused by a blockage of blood flow in the cardiovascular circuit outside the heart.
- **Distributive** shock is caused by excessive dilation of the venules and arterioles.

TABLE 9.3 CATEGORIES OF SHOCK

Category	Causes	Signs and Symptoms
Hypovolemic Shock	Any severe loss of body fluid, including dehydration; internal or external hemorrhage; fluid loss from burns, vomiting, or diarrhea; or loss of intravascular fluid into the interstitium	Tachycardia; tachypnea; hypotension; cyanosis; oliguria; flat, nondistended peripheral veins; decreased jugular veins; altered mental status
Cardiogenic Shock	Myocardial infarction, myocarditis, end-stage cardiomyopathy, severe dysrhythmias, valvular disease, severe electrolyte imbalance, drug overdose	Dysrhythmias, labored respirations, hypotension, cyanosis, oliguria, altered mental status, possibly distended jugular and peripheral veins, symptoms of congestive heart failure
Extracardiac Obstructive Shock	Any block to the cardiovascular flow, such as pericardial tamponade, tension pneumothorax, intrathoracic tumor, massive pulmonary embolus, large systemic embolus	Tachycardia, tachypnea, hypotension, cyanosis, oliguria, altered mental status, possibly distended jugular veins

TABLE 9.3 CATEGORIES OF SHOCK—cont'd

Category	Causes	Signs and Symptoms
Distributive Shock	Any condition causing massive vasodilation of peripheral circulation, including the subcategories anaphylactic, septic, and neurogenic shock	*See subcategories below.*
• Anaphylactic shock	Reaction to an allergen, such as an insect sting, antibiotic, anesthetic, contrast dye, or blood product	• Tachycardia, tachypnea, wheezing, hypotension, cyanosis, oliguria, altered mental status. • May have urticaria, pruritus, angioedema, laryngeal edema, and severe bronchospasm. • If conscious, may be extremely apprehensive and report a metallic taste.
• Septic shock	Loss of vascular autoregulatory control and loss of fluid into the interstitium caused by massive release of chemical mediators and endotoxins from bacteria, especially gram-negative strains, protozoans, viruses	• *Early or warm phase:* Blood pressure, urine output, and neck veins may be normal. Skin warm and flushed with full veins. Fever usually present, although temperature may be subnormal. • *Late phase:* Tachycardia, tachypnea, hypotension, oliguria, flat jugular and peripheral veins, and cool clammy skin. Normal or subnormal temperature.
• Neurogenic shock	Dysfunction or injury to the nervous system from, for example, spinal cord injury, general anesthesia, fever, metabolic disturbance, brain injury	• *Early phase:* Hypotension and altered mental status, bradycardia, and skin that is warm and dry • *Late phase:* Tachycardia, tachypnea, and cool, clammy skin

Most cases of clinical shock show only some components of each of these categories. However, this classification system is helpful in understanding shock. The hallmark characteristic, seen in all forms of shock, is a decrease in blood pressure usually below the level needed to provide enough blood to the tissues.

Hypovolemic Shock

Any severe loss of body fluid may lead to hypovolemic shock. Hypovolemic shock can be caused by dehydration; internal or external hemorrhage; fluid loss from burns, vomiting, or diarrhea; or loss of intravascular fluid into the interstitial space as a result of sepsis or **trauma** (physical injury caused by an external force). Heat exhaustion or heatstroke can also cause hypovolemic shock by excessive water loss through sweating. Clinical signs and symptoms include restlessness; pale, cool, clammy skin; tachycardia; tachypnea; flat, nondistended peripheral veins; decreased jugular vein circumference; decreased urine output; and altered mental status. The body is usually able to compensate for blood loss of less than 15%, or 750 mL. The initial symptom may only be tachycardia, although there may be an initial rise in systolic blood pressure, then a fall to below 80 mm Hg. At 20% to 25% blood loss, tachycardia and mild to moderate **hypotension** are present. With a loss of 40% or greater (2000 mL), all clinical signs and symptoms of shock are present. Volume loss may not be the only contributing factor to hypovolemic shock. The patient's age, health status, and the time frame for fluid loss can also be factors.

Cardiogenic Shock

Cardiogenic shock results when the heart fails as a pump. It occurs in 5% to 10% of patients with acute myocardial infarction (AMI). In most cases, about 40% of the myocardium must be lost to produce cardiogenic shock. Patients with cardiogenic shock have signs and symptoms similar to hypovolemic shock, except that they may display distended jugular and peripheral veins, as well as other symptoms of heart failure, such as pulmonary edema. The presence of pulmonary edema is what differentiates cardiogenic shock from other forms of shock. Other causes of cardiogenic shock include rupture of heart valves, acute **myocarditis** (inflammation of the heart muscle), end-stage heart disease, severe dysrhythmias, or traumatic injury to the heart.

Extracardiac Obstructive Shock

Extracardiac obstructive shock occurs when there is a blockage of blood flow in the cardiovascular circuit outside the heart. Several conditions may cause obstructive shock. **Pericardial tamponade**, which is the filling of the pericardial sac with blood, compresses the heart and limits its filling capacity. **Tension pneumothorax** is compression of the heart from an abnormal collection of air in the pleural space, which interferes with normal cardiac function. **Acute pulmonary hypertension**, a sudden abnormally elevated pressure in the pulmonary artery, increases resistance for blood flowing out the right side of the heart. All of these conditions decrease cardiac output, which can lead to shock. Tumors or a pulmonary embolism may also cause shock. Signs and symptoms of obstructive shock are similar to those of hypovolemic shock, except that jugular veins are usually distended.

Distributive Shock

Distributive shock occurs when peripheral vascular resistance is lost because of massive vasodilation of the peripheral circulation. Unlike hypovolemic shock whereby there is an actual loss of blood volume, distributive shock occurs when the body's fluid distribution is abnormally altered within the body. Distributive shock includes anaphylactic, septic, and neurogenic shock.

Anaphylactic Shock

Anaphylactic shock, the most severe type of distributive shock, occurs when the body has an extreme hypersensitivity reaction to an antigen (Box 9.1, *Patient Education*). Death from anaphylactic shock can occur in minutes. It occurs most commonly from insect stings, antibiotics (especially penicillins), shellfish, peanuts, anesthetics, contrast dye, and blood products. The signs and symptoms are similar to those seen in hypovolemic shock. Additionally, patients may have symptoms specific to allergic reactions, including **urticaria** (hives), pruritus, wheezing, **laryngeal edema** (swelling of the larynx), angioedema (edema of skin, mucous membranes, or internal organs), and severe **bronchospasm** (narrowing of bronchi in the lungs). If conscious, patients may be extremely apprehensive and short of breath, and they may report a metallic taste.

Septic Shock

Septic shock, the most common type of distributive shock, is caused by systemic infection and inflammation. Extensive release of chemical mediators and endotoxins causes dilation of blood vessels and loss of fluid into the interstitial space. Most cases of sepsis are caused by gram-negative bacteria, although other bacteria and viruses may be the cause. In recent years, the number of cases of gram-negative shock has been decreasing, whereas there has been an alarming increase in the number of cases of septic shock from multidrug-resistant bacteria and fungi. Septic shock is the leading cause of death among critical care patients, and the incidence of sepsis is increasing year by year (Qureshi & Rajah, 2008). Predisposing conditions include trauma, diabetes mellitus, corticosteroid therapy, being immunocompromised (e.g., as seen in patients with human immunodeficiency virus [HIV] and in those undergoing chemotherapy treatment for cancer), burns, malnutrition, and invasive catheters (Box 9.2, *Gerontological Issues*).

Early recognition and rapid response are essential in the successful treatment of shock (see *Evidence-Based Practice*). The progression of sepsis to septic shock is subtle and rapid, requiring frequent monitoring of patients susceptible to septic shock. During the early, or warm, phase of septic shock (which may be referred to as "pink" shock), blood pressure, urine output, and neck vein size may be normal, but the skin is warm and flushed owing to vasodilation. Fever is present in the majority of patients, although some may have a subnormal temperature. A heart rate greater than 90 beats per minute, a respiratory rate greater than 20, and an elevated white blood cell count in addition to a fever may indicate a systemic inflammatory response syndrome that often leads to septic shock (Nelson et al., 2009). Left untreated, septic shock progresses to a second phase with signs and symptoms similar to hypovolemic shock: hypotension, oliguria, tachycardia, tachypnea, flat jugular and peripheral veins, and cold, clammy skin. Body temperature may be normal or subnormal.

Box 9.1

Patient Education

Teach patients who have allergies and are at risk for anaphylaxis to request a prescription for an allergy kit containing an epinephrine syringe and an oral antihistamine. The kit should be carried at all times for use if needed, because life-threatening reactions can occur rapidly.

EVIDENCE-BASED PRACTICE

Clinical Question

What are the best ways to manage sepsis and severe septic shock?

Evidence

The 2008 international guidelines for management of severe sepsis and septic shock provide evidence-based interventions (Dellinger et al., 2008). Interventions impacting nursing care include the following: Obtain blood cultures prior to antibiotic therapy; give broad-spectrum antibiotics within 1 hour of septic shock diagnosis or severe sepsis without septic shock; administer ordered crystalloid or colloid fluids, or fluid challenge; elevate head of bed for mechanically ventilated patients unless contraindicated; maintain ordered glycemic control; administer ordered deep venous thrombosis prophylaxis and stress ulcer prophylaxis.

Implications for Nursing Practice

Nurses should recognize that prompt performance of any ordered intervention included in the 2008 guidelines is important in the care of patients with septic shock or sepsis.

REFERENCES

Dellinger, R. P., Levy, M. M., Carlet, J. M., et al. (2008). Surviving sepsis campaign: International guidelines for management of severe sepsis and septic shock. *Critical Care Medicine, 36*(1), 296–327.

Box 9.2

Gerontological Issues

The older adult population is the most vulnerable to sepsis. People in this age group also have many of the predisposing conditions placing them at risk for sepsis. As more people live longer, the incidence of sepsis is likely to rise in this age group. Early recognition of signs of shock is essential for successful treatment in this high-risk population.

Neurogenic Shock

Neurogenic shock occurs when dysfunction or injury to the nervous system causes extensive dilation of peripheral blood vessels. It is a rarer form of shock, and results most commonly from an injury to the spinal cord (referred to as spinal shock). It occurs due to factors that either stimulate the parasympathetic nervous system or block the sympathetic nervous system. Other causes include general anesthesia, fever, metabolic disturbances, and brain contusions and concussions. Signs and symptoms include hypotension and altered mental status and, during the early phases, bradycardia and warm, dry skin. As shock progresses, however, tachycardia and cool, clammy skin develop.

THERAPEUTIC MEASURES FOR SHOCK

Because of the emergency nature of shock, the exact nature of the shock must be determined while interventions such as ventilatory and circulatory support are being implemented (Table 9.4). Life-threatening symptoms must be treated immediately (Table 9.5). Medications that are used in shock are listed in Table 9.6. The order of interventions and testing is guided by the stability of the patient. Intervention priorities are as follows:

1. Airway
2. Breathing and respiratory support
3. Cardiovascular support
4. Maintenance of circulatory volume
5. Control of bleeding if present
6. Assessment of neurologic status
7. Treatment of life-threatening injuries
8. Determination and treatment of the cause of shock.

NURSING CARE TIP

Trendelenburg Position

Traditionally, the Trendelenburg position, in which the body is laid flat on the back with the feet higher than the head, was used to try to increase cardiac output to increase blood pressure. The Trendelenburg position used to be first-line treatment for shock. However, research has shown that the Trendelenburg position is not helpful in improving cardiac output for patients in shock. In fact, this position may have negative effects, including compromising respirations.

Although you may still see this position used, it is important to use valid research results in practice for the best patient outcomes. In cardiogenic shock, any position that increases blood flow to the compromised heart increases the heart's workload. This could overwhelm or flood the heart, making it unable to keep up with the blood volume returning to it. The result could be death.

NURSING PROCESS FOR THE PATIENT IN SHOCK

Data Collection

Recognizing patients at risk for shock and being vigilant in monitoring their condition is vital. Early detection and prevention of shock in patients at risk for shock are the desired goals. Rapid response teams may be helpful in providing quick assessment and management of patients at risk of developing shock.

For the patient in shock, assessment must be carried out quickly and should always start with ABCD: airway, breathing, circulation, and disability.

Airway is assessed for patency and opened as necessary. A compromised airway must be treated immediately with the head-tilt/chin-lift method, an oral or nasal airway, or endotracheal intubation.

TABLE 9.4 ASSESSMENT OF THE PATIENT IN SHOCK

Signs and symptoms	Tachycardia, tachypnea, hypotension, oliguria, cyanosis, altered mental status
Laboratory tests	Complete blood count, serum osmolarity, blood chemistries, prothrombin time, partial thromboplastin time, blood typing and crossmatch, serum lactate, arterial blood gases, cardiac isoenzymes, urinalysis
Imaging	Chest x-ray, spinal films, computed tomography, echocardiogram
Monitoring	Electrocardiogram, arterial pressure monitor, central venous pressure, pulmonary artery catheter, gastric pH

TABLE 9.5 THERAPEUTIC MEASURES FOR SHOCK

Respiratory support	Oxygen (nasal cannula, face mask, partial nonrebreather mask, assisted ventilations with bag-valve-mask, ventilator) Spo_2 greater than 95% Venous lactic acid less than 2.2 mmol/L
Cardiovascular support	Vasopressor medication (dopamine) if fluid resuscitation not effective Revascularization of heart in cardiogenic shock via angioplasty, with or without stent or fibrinolytic therapy (alteplase) Antidysrhythmics Positive inotropes
Adequate circulatory volume	1–3 L IV fluids Crystalloid fluids: normal saline (0.9% sodium chloride) or lactated Ringer's solution; 3 mL crystalloid solution for every 1 mL fluid lost Blood or blood products Urine output greater than 30 mL/hr Hemoglobin greater than 10 g/dL
Control of bleeding	Pressure dressings Surgical intervention
Treatment of life-threatening injuries	Surgical intervention Medications
Determination and treatment of causes of shock	*Septic shock:* broad spectrum antibiotic within 1 hr of diagnosis *Cardiogenic shock:* morphine, diuretics, nitrates *Anaphylactic shock:* epinephrine, diphenhydramine (Benadryl), methylprednisolone (Solu-Medrol), aminophylline

TABLE 9.6 MEDICATIONS USED FOR SHOCK

Medication Class/Action	Examples	Route	Side Effects	Nursing Implications
Autonomic Nervous System Agents				
Alpha- and Beta-Adrenergic Agents				
Strengthens myocardial contraction, increases systolic blood pressure, and increases cardiac output.	epinephrine, dopamine, norepinephrine	IV	Nervousness, palpitations, tachycardia, tremors	Correct hypovolemia before giving medications in shock. Monitor VS often. Vasopressor use should include arterial blood pressure monitoring. Monitor intake and output.
Used to bronchodilate.	epinephrine	Subcutaneously, IM		First drug given in anaphylactic shock. Give with TB syringe.
Beta-Adrenergic Agent				
Increases cardiac output in cardiogenic shock.	dobutamine	IV	Increased heart rate, anginal pain	Monitor VS often. Monitor intake and output.
Antihistamine				
Inhibits histamine release.	diphenhydramine (Benadryl)	IV, PO	Drowsiness, tachycardia, dry mouth	Monitor VS. Caution about drowsiness.
Anti-Inflammatory				
Control of severe allergic reactions.	methylprednisolone (Solu-Medrol), hydrocortisone (Solu-Cortef), dexamethasone (Decadron)	IV	Side effects usually occur with long-term use.	Monitor patient for signs and symptoms of infection.
Protein C Derivative				
Inhibits coagulation, decreases inflammatory response, and promotes fibrinolysis in sepsis.	drotrecogin alfa (Xigris), recombinant human activated protein C (rhAPC)	IV infusion for 96 hr	Bleeding	Contraindicated in patients with active bleeding or high risk of bleeding.

TB = tuberculin; VS = vital signs.

Breathing is assessed for rate, depth, and symmetry of chest movement. The patient is observed for use of accessory muscles. Lung sounds are auscultated. Wheezing may be present in the patient with anaphylactic shock. Crackles may be found in the patient with cardiogenic shock or in the patient who has received too much intravenous (IV) fluid.

Circulation is assessed with blood pressure. A narrowing pulse pressure may be present before a drop in systolic pressure and indicates a decrease in cardiac stroke volume and peripheral vasoconstriction. Peripheral pulses are palpated. Tachycardia is the first sign of shock. However, patients on medications that block the sympathetic nervous system response will not exhibit tachycardia. The pulse is assessed for quality; commonly it is weak and thready in a patient with shock. As shock progresses, the peripheral pulses become bradycardic or absent. A capillary refill greater than 3 seconds indicates inadequate circulation, although it has been found to be an unreliable indicator of shock in adults, especially older adults. Other observations regarding circulation include distended neck veins; skin that may be cool, pale, and diaphoretic; presence of **cyanosis** (bluish color of the skin and mucous membranes due to decreased oxygen in the blood); mucous membranes that may be pale and dry; and thirst. Rapidly scan the entire body for evidence of bleeding or other injuries. Palpation of the abdomen can reveal signs of internal bleeding, such as a tender, distended, boardlike abdomen.

NURSING CARE TIP

There is usually a loss of peripheral pulses in the patient whose systolic blood pressure has dropped below 80. If you are able to palpate radial pulses on your patient, the systolic blood pressure is usually at least 80.

CRITICAL THINKING

Beta Blockers

■ A patient who takes a beta-blocker medication is being monitored for septic shock. What sign of shock do you understand will not be present in a patient taking a beta blocker?

Suggested answer at end of chapter.

Disability is assessed by determining the patient's level of consciousness (LOC). A decrease in LOC indicates disability. This disability can range from lethargy to coma.

All four limbs are assessed for circulation, sensation, and mobility (CSM). Bilateral responses are compared for equality. Circulation is assessed by palpating pulses for presence and quality. Sensation is determined by touching the patient's hands and feet and asking what the patient feels and if there is any numbness or tingling. Mobility (motor ability) is assessed by having the patient move all four limbs and wiggle the fingers and toes. Have the patient push with his or her feet against your hands and squeeze two of your fingers to assess strength.

NURSING CARE TIP

To assess level of consciousness, determine if the patient is alert by asking his or her name, the date, and the location. If the patient can answer all three questions correctly, he or she is "alert and oriented × 3 (person, place, time)."

A "head-to-toe" approach can follow the primary ABCD assessment. The presence, severity, and location of pain or nausea and vomiting are assessed. Body temperature is noted. Bowel sounds are auscultated to determine whether they are normal, absent, hyperactive, or hypoactive. When an indwelling urinary catheter has been placed, the color of the urine and the rate of urine output are noted.

Nursing Diagnoses, Planning, Implementation, and Evaluation

See Table 9.7 for a summary of shock. Also see the *Nursing Care Plan for the Patient Experiencing Shock.*

TABLE 9.7 SHOCK SUMMARY

Signs and Symptoms	Tachycardia Tachypnea Hypotension Oliguria Cyanosis Altered mental state
Diagnostic Tests	Decreased hemoglobin Increased lactic acid Decreased hematocrit in hemorrhage Increased WBC in sepsis Decreased pH in metabolic acidosis
Therapeutic Measures	Oxygen IV fluids Vasopressor medications Treat underlying cause
Complications	Acute respiratory distress syndrome (ARDS) Disseminated intravascular coagulation (DIC) Multiple organ dysfunction syndrome (MODS)
Priority Nursing Diagnoses	*Ineffective Tissue Perfusion (renal, cerebral, cardiopulmonary, gastrointestinal, peripheral)* *Decreased Cardiac Output* *Fear*

NURSING CARE PLAN for the Patient Experiencing Shock

Nursing Diagnosis: *Ineffective Tissue Perfusion (renal, cerebral, cardiopulmonary, gastrointestinal, peripheral)* related to hypovolemia or inadequate cardiac output or changes in circulatory volume or inadequate vascular tone possibly evidenced by altered level of consciousness, changes in skin color/temperature, tachycardia, reduced blood pressure, and decreased urine output.

Expected Outcomes: Patient will demonstrate adequate tissue perfusion as evidenced by warm dry skin, peripheral pulses strong, vital signs within normal parameters of baseline, breath sounds without adventitious sounds, and balanced intake and output, and patient will be alert and oriented to person, place, time within specified time frame.

Evaluation of Outcomes: Is patient's skin warm/dry and peripheral pulses present/strong? Are vital signs within patient's normal range? Are lung sounds normal, intake/output balanced, edema absent, pain/discomfort absent? Is patient alert and oriented?

Interventions	Rationale	Evaluation
Maintain airway and provide oxygenation.	Ensures adequate oxygenation and tissue perfusion.	Is Spo_2 greater than 95%? Are skin and mucous membranes pink? Are respirations between 12 and 20 per minute? Are lung sounds clear?
Monitor vital signs.	Changes in vital signs, which indicate change in condition, can be detected early and treated promptly.	Is heart rate between 60 and 100 beats per minute? Is heart rhythm regular? Are peripheral pulses strong? Is systolic blood pressure greater than 100 mm Hg? Is patient alert and oriented × 3?
Monitor intake and output.	Provides adequate cardiac output to perfuse tissues. Assesses renal function. Urine output is an indicator of renal function.	Is urinary output greater than 30 mL/hr?
Provide adequate fluid intake.	Maintains volume.	Are mucous membranes moist? Is skin turgor less than 3 seconds?
Position patient appropriately (head elevated for patients with shortness of breath, increased intracranial pressure).	Proper positioning promotes circulation and helps prevent skin breakdown.	Is edema noted? Is skin breakdown noted?
Provide quiet, restful environment.	Conserves energy and lowers tissue oxygen demands.	Is patient resting comfortably without anxiety?
Maintain body temperature with warmed IV fluids, room temperature, blankets.	Recovery is aided by normal body temperature.	Is body temperature within normal limits?
Assess for pain, and provide pain relief measures.	Pain increases tissue demands for blood and oxygen.	Is patient pain free?
	GERIATRIC	
Change positions slowly.	Age-related losses of cardiovascular reflexes can result in hypotension.	Is systolic blood pressure greater than 100 mm Hg?

NURSING CARE PLAN for the Patient Experiencing Shock—cont'd

Nursing Diagnosis: *Decreased Cardiac Output* related to reduced circulating blood volume, structural damage, or decreased myocardial contractility as evidenced by abnormal vital signs and irregular cardiac rhythm strip.

Expected Outcomes: Patient will have adequate cardiac output as evidenced by vital signs and cardiac rhythm within normal limits (WNL) within specified time frame.

Evaluation of Outcomes: Are blood pressure, heart rate, and cardiac rhythm within normal limits? Are nailbeds and/or skin pink? Is skin warm and dry?

Interventions	Rationale	Evaluation
Monitor heart rate and cardiac rhythm with electrocardiogram, and report abnormalities.	Changes in heart rate and cardiac rhythm can be detected immediately and treated appropriately.	Is heart rate and rhythm normal?
Assess skin/nailbed color, capillary refill, and peripheral pulses and report abnormalities.	Inadequate perfusion is first evident in skin/nailbeds and peripheral pulses.	What color and temperature is the skin/nailbeds? Is capillary refill less than 3 seconds? Are peripheral pulses present?
Give cardiovascular medications and oxygen as ordered.	Cardiac function can be supported with medications. Supplemental oxygen increases oxygenation of heart and tissues.	Is heart rate and rhythm normal?
Reduce myocardial oxygen demand by utilizing comfort measures to alleviate pain and anxiety, and by keeping the body at an appropriate temperature.	Pain, anxiety, and cold all increase tissue demands for blood and oxygen, which increases the workload on the heart to supply it.	Is body temperature within normal limits? Is the patient free of pain and anxiety?

Nursing Diagnosis: *Fear* related to severity of condition and unknown outcome as evidenced by verbalization of fear (e.g., "Am I going to die?")

Expected Outcomes: Patient will state fear is reduced after nurse provides information related to patient's condition.

Evaluation of Outcomes: Does patient state fear is decreased?

Interventions	Rationale	Evaluation
Explore patient's level of fear and knowledge of condition. Provide explanations for procedures, the condition and its treatment.	Knowledge allows a feeling of control and reduces fear.	Does patient state fear is reduced?

Nursing Diagnosis: *Deficient Knowledge* related to unfamiliar condition of shock as evidenced by verbalization of deficient knowledge (e.g., "I don't understand what's happening to me.")

Expected Outcomes: Patient will explain shock and its treatment.

Evaluation of Outcomes: Can patient explain shock and how it is treated?

Continued

NURSING CARE PLAN for the Patient Experiencing Shock—cont'd

Interventions	Rationale	Evaluation
Assess patient's ability to learn and identify barriers to learning.	For learning, the patient must be ready to learn. Barriers such as lifestyle changes or the shock of the diagnosis may decrease learning.	Is patient alert and stable? Does patient indicate willingness to learn? Does patient express concerns about condition?
Provide information that is most relevant to patient first.	Giving necessary information first meets patient's immediate needs.	Does patient state understanding of important information?
Allow time for questions and clarification.	Clarification ensures accurate information is learned.	Does the patient state accurate information?
	GERIATRIC	
Speak slowly and clearly in a low tone/pitch.	Older adults have difficulty hearing high-pitched tones.	Does the patient acknowledge when being spoken to?
Provide materials in large print.	Visual changes that accompany aging may require a patient to use larger print materials.	Can the patient restate and/or read aloud information that has been given?
Attempt to involve family members in teaching.	Family members can reinforce education provided.	Do family members verbalize understanding of material presented?

LEARNING TIP

Here is a saying to help you remember blood pressure effects in shock: If they're 90 over 60, they're getting kind of sickly. Say it again! If they're 90 over 60, they're getting kind of sickly.

CRITICAL THINKING

Mr. Hall

■ Mr. Hall, who is 58 years old, has had an acute myocardial infarction. He is reporting chest pain (rated 10/10 on the pain rating scale) and difficulty breathing. His Spo_2 is 89%. Crackles are heard on auscultation of breath sounds. The electrocardiogram shows an irregular and rapid heartbeat. He is restless and apprehensive.

1. Name three nursing priorities for Mr. Hall's care.
2. What type of IV fluid and rate are appropriate for Mr. Hall?
3. What signs and symptoms indicate Mr. Hall is in cardiogenic shock?

Suggested answers at end of chapter.

CRITICAL THINKING

Mrs. Neal

■ Mrs. Neal, who is 45 years old, came to the emergency room in severe hypovolemic shock after sustaining several bleeding wounds in an automobile accident. Her shock is resolving after receiving several transfusions and surgical repair of her injuries. She has just been admitted to the surgical unit for postoperative care.

1. What postoperative nursing assessments should be performed first?
2. Mrs. Neal's family is very alarmed by her condition. What interventions can be provided to decrease their anxiety?
3. What postoperative complications may develop in Mrs. Neal?
4. What documentation is appropriate for Mrs. Neal?

Suggested answers at end of chapter.

SUGGESTED ANSWERS TO CRITICAL THINKING

■ *Classic Signs of Shock*
Tachycardia is caused by decreased cardiac output and reduced tissue oxygenation. Its purpose is to increase cardiac output and oxygen delivery by causing more heartbeats to pump out blood from the heart.

Tachypnea is caused by decreased tissue oxygenation. Its purpose is to increase respirations so more oxygen is for delivery to tissues.

Oliguria is caused by a reduced blood flow to the kidneys. Its purpose as a compensatory mechanism is to conserve as much fluid as possible to help maintain a normal blood pressure.

Pallor is caused by reduced blood volume or flow. When pallor results from compensation, it is due to peripheral vasoconstriction that occurs to shunt blood volume to the vital organs.

Cool, clammy skin is the result of decreased blood flow to the skin and the release of moisture (sweat) from the skin. The sympathetic nervous system causes these compensatory mechanisms; peripheral vasoconstriction shunts blood to the vital organs, and sweating cools the body in anticipation of the fight-or-flight response, which generates body heat when it occurs.

■ *Anaerobic Metabolism*
Anaerobic metabolism is the source of nutrition and energy for the cell that prevents cellular death when oxygen is not available. It is a short-term compensatory mechanism to save the cell until oxygen becomes available again.

■ *Beta Blockers*
Tachycardia will not be present. Beta blockers block the response of the sympathetic nervous system, which is activated in shock.

■ *Mr. Hall*
1. Nursing priorities for Mr. Hall include adequate tissue perfusion, relief of chest pain and anxiety, and stabilization of cardiac rhythm and vital signs.
2. Because Mr. Hall's lung sounds reveal crackles, indicating fluid in the lungs, he should not be given IV fluids. He already has too much fluid for his heart to handle, and giving him IV fluids could be life threatening. He should have an IV access for IV medications as needed.
3. Signs of cardiogenic shock include decreased blood pressure; increased heart and respiratory rates; cyanosis; decreased urine output; cool, pale skin; and decreased mental status.

■ *Mrs. Neal*
1. Assessment of respiratory status and cardiovascular status, inspection of surgical wounds for bleeding, and assessment of mental status and the need for pain relief should be performed first.
2. Explain the cause of shock and all interventions, rationales, and desired outcomes. Keep the environment calm, provide for privacy, and answer all questions in a matter-of-fact and reassuring manner. Allow Mrs. Neal's family to visit.
3. Unrelieved pain, bleeding, infection, and respiratory complications are possible.
4. *Airway:* rate, depth, regularity of respirations; breath sounds, Spo_2. *Vital signs:* cardiac rhythm, quality of pulses, skin color, blood pressure, body temperature. *Urine output:* oral and IV intake, fluid balance. *Pain:* measures to relieve pain and evaluation of those measures. *Dressings:* any bleeding. *Bowel sounds.*

REVIEW QUESTIONS

1. Which of the following mechanisms does the body use to compensate for shock?
   a. Peripheral nervous system depression
   b. Central nervous system depression
   c. Sympathetic nervous system stimulation
   d. Parasympathetic nervous system stimulation

2. Which of the following findings would the nurse recognize as specifically occurring in anaphylactic shock? **Select all that apply.**
   a. Wheezing
   b. Hypotension
   c. Tachycardia
   d. Oliguria
   e. Urticaria
   f. Bronchospasm

Continued

REVIEW QUESTIONS—cont'd

3. Which of the following conditions causes the decreased level of consciousness commonly found in patients with shock?
   a. Severe pain
   b. Endotoxins
   c. Cerebral edema
   d. Cerebral hypoxia

4. Which of the following nursing diagnoses is most appropriate to include in the plan of care for a patient with shock?
   a. *Fatigue*
   b. *Ineffective Tissue Perfusion*
   c. *Ineffective Health Maintenance*
   d. *Hopelessness*

5. A patient who is found lying in a pool of blood from a leg incision that has opened is restless and confused. The nurse calls for help and takes vital signs. Which of the following treatments for shock would the nurse anticipate being ordered first?
   a. IV fluids
   b. Oxygen
   c. Vasopressor medications
   d. Antibiotics

6. Which patient would be a priority for the nurse to see?
   a. A patient who was in a motor vehicle accident with blood pressure 140/80 mm Hg, pulse 98 beats per minute, respirations 20 per minute.
   b. A patient who has a migraine with blood pressure 108/68 mm Hg, pulse 84 beats per minute, respirations 16 per minute.
   c. A patient who slipped and fell with blood pressure 112/74 mm Hg, pulse 68 beats per minute, respirations 14 per minute.
   d. A patient who is one day post-op with blood pressure 88/58 mm Hg, pulse beats 152 per minute, respirations 24 per minute.

7. Which of the following findings would indicate that therapeutic measures are effective in shock?
   a. Heart rate 110 beats per minute
   b. Spo_2 89%
   c. Systolic blood pressure 118 mm Hg
   d. Respiratory rate 22 per minute

8. Place in correct order of occurrence systolic blood pressure progression through the three stages of shock beginning with mild, moderate, and severe. Use all options.
   a. Below 60 mm Hg
   b. Normal
   c. Below 90 mm Hg

References

Nelson, D. P., LeMaster, T. H., Plost, G. N., et al. (2009). Recognizing sepsis in the adult patient. *American Journal of Nursing, 109*(3), 40–45.

Qureshi, K., & Rajah, A. (2008). Septic shock: A review article. *British Journal of Medical Practitioners, 1*(2), 7–12.

10

Nursing Care of Patients in Pain

KAREN P. HALL

KEY TERMS

addiction (uh-DIK-shun)
adjuvant (ad-JOO-vant)
agonist (AG-un-ist)
analgesic (AN-uhl-JEE-zik)
antagonist (an-TAG-on-ist)
breakthrough (BRAYK-THROO)
ceiling effect (SEE-ling ee-FEKT)
endorphins (en-DOOR-fins)
enkephalins (en-KEFF-e-lins)
equianalgesic (EH-kwee-AN-uhl-JEE-zik)
malingerer (muh-LING-gur-er)
neuropathic (NEW-roh-PATH-ik)
nociception (NOH-sih-SEP-shun)
opioid (OH-pee-OYD)
pain (PAYN)
patient-controlled analgesia (PAY-shunt kon-TROHLD AN-uhl-JEE-zee-ah)
physical dependence (FIZZ-ik-uhl dee-PEN-dense)
prostaglandins (PRAHS-tah-GLAND-ins)
pseudoaddiction (soo-doh-ah-DIK-shun)
psychological dependence (SY-ko-LAW-jik-al dee-PEN-dense)
suffering (SUH-fur-ing)
tolerance (TAWL-ur-ens)
transdermal (trans-DER-mal)

QUESTIONS TO GUIDE YOUR READING

1. How is pain defined?
2. What are common myths and barriers to the effective management of pain?
3. What are the differences between addiction, physical dependence, and tolerance?
4. What is the current knowledge about the basic physiology of the pain response?
5. What characteristics help to define acute, chronic nonmalignant, and cancer pain?
6. What should be included in a basic pain assessment?
7. How is the World Health Organization analgesic ladder used for the treatment of pain?
8. What are the three classes of analgesics and their uses?
9. What are commonly used pain medication treatment modalities and their appropriate use?
10. How and when are nondrug pain management techniques utilized?
11. How does ethical decision making play a role in the care of the patient in pain?

THE PAIN PUZZLE

Pain is an unpleasant sensory and emotional experience and is the most common reason patients seek medical advice. However, despite the widespread nature of the problem, pain is often untreated or undertreated. The care of patients with pain is challenging and requires a systematic approach to assessment and treatment.

Decisions about pain management require careful assessment of the patient's condition and attention to the ethical principles that influence patient care. Providing information and offering choices helps patients to maintain autonomy. Just as risks, benefits, and alternatives to surgery and anesthesia are discussed with the patient, so should pain management options be discussed in the process of obtaining informed consent.

Nurses often worry about overmedicating patients, thinking that they are "doing good" (beneficence) or "doing no harm" (nonmaleficence) by withholding medication from a patient they do not believe is in pain (Box 10.1, *Ethical Considerations*). It is important to learn as much as you can about pain and pain management so you can effectively advocate for your patients, assist with patient education, and provide appropriate resources.

The Joint Commission (formerly the Joint Commission for Accreditation of Healthcare Organizations) published pain management standards in 2000 and began assessing the management of pain in hospitals and other health care organizations based on these standards in January 2001. The standards support the importance of appropriate and effective management of pain. They address assessment and the safe pharmacological management of pain, as well as patient and family teaching, postoperative pain, management of opioid-induced side effects, discharge planning, and process improvement. These guidelines are available through the Joint Commission website at www.jointcommission.org.

For more information on pain management, visit the following websites. For some sites, you may need to type "pain" in the search window.

www.ahrq.gov
www.ampainsoc.org
www.cancer.org
www.iasp-pain.org
www.aspmn.org

Cultural differences must be considered when planning care for the patient in pain. People from various cultures have different ways of expressing pain (Box 10.2, *Cultural Considerations*). Some may be dramatic and emotional; others tend to be stoic and quiet. Knowledge of widely accepted information about different ethnic and cultural groups can be useful in understanding a patient's experience and what care might be considered acceptable. It is important, however, to assess a patient's pain care needs individually and not make assumptions based on culture or ethnicity alone.

Box 10.1 Ethical Considerations

Controlling Pain

A patient was admitted from home to a medical unit 2 days after his 83rd birthday with a diagnosis of metastatic cancer of the pancreas. He had several full-course treatments of chemotherapy and radiation during the previous year with only temporary remissions of the disease. His condition deteriorated rapidly during the previous month, and his family was no longer able to care for him. The patient's physician expected him to die within a few weeks and admitted him to the hospital, primarily for pain control. On admission, the physician ordered morphine sulfate 5 mg IV to be given every 2 hours around the clock.

Although this seemed like a relatively large dose of a strong opioid medication to be given this often, the patient tolerated the treatment for the first 36 hours and reported a significant reduction in his pain. On the third morning after his admission, he was difficult to arouse for his morning vital signs and breakfast. When his nurse, Kathy, finally did manage to awaken him, he was disoriented, his blood pressure was 82/50, and his respirations were shallow and 10/min. He still reported generalized pain and asked for more medication.

Kathy did not give the patient his scheduled 0800 dose of morphine sulfate. She phoned the physician and reported her assessment of the patient, expressing her belief that continuing the medication at the previously prescribed dose and frequency would be fatal to the patient. The physician, who had been up most of the night with an emergency patient, told her that the patient was dying and that she should administer the medication immediately. In this situation:

- What are Kathy's ethical obligations in this case (to self, patient, and community)?
- How should she weigh the risks and benefits of providing adequate pain medication given the possible side effect of hastening the patient's death?
- If Kathy has a moral objection to carrying out a physician's order, what are her options?
- How can Kathy find a way to start meaningful dialogue about such issues with the physician?

Discussion and suggested answers at end of chapter.

Because of the importance of controlling health care costs, the entire health team must provide care in the most cost-effective manner possible while continuing to provide the best quality of care. Effective pain management can help reach those goals by enhancing comfort, by minimizing the side effects of opioids and complications related to inadequate pain control, and by reducing the length of hospital stay or period of recovery.

Box 10.2

Cultural Considerations

The pain experience may differ between and among individuals of differing cultural, ethnic, or religious groups. Remember that people within groups vary, and not all fit the general descriptions provided below. (See Chapter 4.)

Culture	Expression and Meaning of Pain	Patient Preferences	Assessment	Interventions
Arab American	See pain as something to be controlled. May express pain openly to family with elaborate verbal expressions, less so with caregivers. May use terms such as *fire*, *hot*, and *cold*.	Intramuscular or intravenous usually preferred over oral medications.	Compare verbal and nonverbal characteristics of pain to determine degree of pain.	Engage family to help with distraction and relaxation techniques. Administer medication promptly.
Asian American	Chinese and Koreans tend to be stoical, and describe pain in terms of diverse body symptoms instead of locally. Filipinos may view pain as a part of living an honorable life. Some view this as an opportunity to reach a fuller life and to atone for past transgressions. Frequently stoic and tolerate pain to a high degree. Some moan as an expression of pain. For Asians, bearing pain is a virtue and a matter of family honor. Some, especially older individuals, may fear addiction.	Prefer oral or intravenous pain medications. May like warm compresses. For Koreans, intramuscular injections may be seen as an invasion of privacy. Vietnamese maintain self-control as a means of pain relief.	Observe for nonverbal signs of pain. Vietnamese may not understand numerical scale of rating pain. Observing facial expression may provide an indicator of pain.	Incorporate traditional healing methods as much as possible. Offer and encourage pain medicines to promote healing.
African American	May openly and publicly display pain, but this is highly variable. Many, especially the elderly, fear that medication may be addictive. Many believe that suffering and pain are inevitable and should be endured.	May focus on spirituality and religious beliefs to endure pain. Prayers and the laying on of hands are thought to relieve pain if the client has enough faith.	Observe for verbal and nonverbal expressions of pain. Use of pain scales is helpful.	Offer pain medication as needed. Allow meditation and prayer along with pain medication. Support patient's spiritual practices.

Continued

Box 10.3
Cultural Considerations—cont'd

Culture	Expression and Meaning of Pain	Patient Preferences	Assessment	Interventions
European American	Strong sense of stoicism, especially in men. Fear of being dependent may decrease use of pain medicine. Many have fear of addiction. May continue to work and carry out daily activities and minimize pain.	May prefer relaxation and distractions as means of pain control.	Observe for nonverbal signs of pain. Use visual analog or numerical pain scales to assess severity of pain.	Encourage use of pain medicine as needed. Incorporate distraction and relaxation techniques.
Hispanic American	Puerto Ricans tend to be expressive of pain and discomfort. Moaning, groaning, and crying are culturally accepted ways of dealing with and reducing pain. Mexicans may bear pain stoically because it is "God's will." Many feel that pain and suffering are a consequence of immoral behavior. For men, expressing pain shows weakness. The Spanish word for pain is *dolar.*	Prefer oral or intravenous medication for pain. Heat, herbal teas, and prayer are used to manage pain.	Visual analog and numerical scales may be helpful. Observe and compare verbal and nonverbal behaviors indicating pain.	Incorporate traditional practices as permitted. For individuals who are stoic about pain, encourage pain medicine frequently. Explain that pain control can hasten healing.
Native American	Frequently do not request pain medicine and are undertreated. May not realize that they can ask for pain medicine. Many believe pain is something that must be endured. May describe pain in general terms such as "not feeling good." The word for *pain* varies according to the tribal language.	Many prefer traditional herbal medicines. May mention pain to family member or visitor, who relays message to caregiver.	Frequently ask patient and family members or visitors if patient has pain. Observe for nonverbal clues of pain.	Explain that the control of pain can promote healing. Offer pain medicine as needed. Allow adequate time for response; silence is valued. Maintain a calm, relaxing environment. Incorporate traditional practices for pain relief if not harmful.

A patient's pain cannot be recorded on a machine or measured like a blood or urine sample. It is difficult to objectively gauge the effect of a nursing intervention on pain, whether the intervention is medication or nondrug therapy. Pain and its treatment can be likened to a difficult puzzle that requires many pieces to solve.

In this chapter, the many challenges of pain assessment and treatment are discussed. Some of the tools needed to effectively deal with these challenges are presented. Common myths and barriers that continue to affect nursing practice are clarified.

DEFINITIONS OF PAIN

According to Margo McCaffery, a well-known consultant in the care of patients with pain, "Pain is whatever the experiencing person says it is, existing whenever the experiencing person says it does" (McCaffery & Pasero, 1999, p. 17). This is a reminder to nurses to accept the patient's report of pain.

The International Association for the Study of Pain (IASP) describes pain as "an unpleasant sensory and emotional experience associated with actual or potential tissue damage or described in terms of such damage" (2009).This definition indicates that pain is complex, and is not only physical but has emotional and other components as well.

Why does pain exist? It is a protective mechanism or a warning. In the presence of injury, pain may help to prevent further injury. Consider the patient who has a fracture and holds it still to prevent further damage, or a child who touches a hot stove and pulls his or her hand away before a serious burn occurs.

Why is untreated or undertreated pain a bad thing? Complications can occur when pain is experienced. The body produces a stress response to pain during which harmful substances are released from injured tissue. Reactions include breakdown of tissue, increased metabolic rate, impaired immune function, and negative emotions. In addition, pain prevents the patient from participating in self-care activities such as walking, deep breathing, and coughing. Consider the patient who has had chest surgery and then has to cough and deep breathe. It hurts! Pain may make the patient want to avoid coughing, turning, or even moving. Retained pulmonary secretions and pneumonia can develop. If the patient is less active, return of bowel function is delayed and an ileus (disruption in the normal propulsive gastrointestinal activity) can result. When pain is well controlled, complications can be avoided and patients are able to do what they need to do to get well and go home from the hospital or continue with recovery activities.

Suffering often accompanies pain. In a study of suffering, Ferrel and Coyle (2008) conclude that "suffering is not synonymous with pain but is closely associated with it. Physical pain is closely related to psychological, social, and spiritual distress. Pain that persists without meaning becomes suffering" (p. 246). Pain can be a constant reminder for patients with cancer that they have a life-threatening illness. Suffering can often be relieved if patients believe that their pain can be relieved.

MYTHS AND BARRIERS TO EFFECTIVE PAIN MANAGEMENT

Treatment of patients in pain is influenced by a number of factors, including the nurse's personal experience with pain. Why are some patients not believed when they report pain? Why do some nurses and other health care team members insist that patients behave a certain way before they can be believed? Common myths about pain may impair the nurse's ability to be objective about pain and may create barriers to effective treatment. Because there is no objective measure for pain, nurses may rely on what is comfortable rather than what has been proven effective.

Myth: A person who is laughing and talking is not in pain.

Fact: A person in pain is likely to use laughing and talking as a form of distraction. This can be very effective in managing pain, especially when used with appropriate drug therapies. Patients may be more easily distracted when they have visitors and may ask for pain medication as soon as their family or significant other goes home.

Myth: If morphine is given too early to the patient with cancer pain, it will not work when the patient really needs it, toward the end, when the pain is worse.

Fact: Morphine is an opioid, a class of drugs that has properties similar to opium. Opioid doses can be escalated (titrated upward) indefinitely as needed as the patient's pain increases. There is no ceiling effect or maximum effective dose. Side effects such as sedation or clinically significant respiratory depression may temporarily limit the dose or the rate to which the dose can be increased.

Myth: Respiratory depression is common in patients receiving opioid pain medications.

Fact: Respiratory depression is uncommon in patients receiving opioid pain medications. If patients are monitored carefully when they are at risk, such as with the first dose of an opioid or when a dose is increased, respiratory depression is preventable. A patient's respiratory status and level of sedation (LOS) should be routinely monitored using an LOS scale.

Myth: Pain medication is more effective when given by injection.

Fact: Oral administration is the first choice if possible, or whenever the intravenous (IV) route is not an option. The IV route has the most rapid onset of action and is the preferred route for postoperative administration. Intramuscular (IM) injections are not recommended because they are painful, have unreliable absorption from the muscle, and have a lag time to peak effect and rapid falloff compared with oral administration.

Myth: Teenagers are more likely to become addicted than older patients.

Fact: Addiction to opioids is very uncommon in all age groups when taken for pain by patients without a prior drug abuse history.

MORE PAIN-RELATED DEFINITIONS

Nurses often express concern about patients who need large amounts of pain medication or know exactly when their next dose of pain medication is due. Nurses may worry that such patients are addicted or that they are "clock watchers," but do we really know what that means? Patients are expected to be informed about their medications and involved in their care, but when they know when their medications are due, we may become suspicious. In truth, if a patient is watching the clock, the most likely reason is because he or she is in pain. The most common reason that patients ask for more pain medicine is because they have increased pain. Similarly, patients are expected to know the effects of other medications they take such as blood pressure medications and insulin. Yet when they ask for a specific analgesic, concern regarding "drug seeking" is sometimes raised.

CRITICAL THINKING

Mrs. Smithers and Mr. Brown

■ Mrs. Smithers had an abdominal hysterectomy and is sitting up in bed the morning after surgery, putting on her makeup. On morning rounds she is smiling but reports that her pain is at 6 on a scale of 0 to 10. Mr. Brown has just been transferred from the surgical intensive care unit the day after surgery for multiple injuries. He is moaning and reports his pain at 6 on a scale of 0 to 10. Which of these patients is really having as much pain as they say they are? How can you make that judgment?

Suggested answers at end of chapter.

It is important to understand the differences between **addiction**, **tolerance**, and **physical dependence**. When talking with patients and teaching them about their medications, it is important to help them understand these differences as well. Addiction is something many patients fear.

Tolerance is a normal biological adaptation. Exposure to a drug induces changes that result in a decrease of one or more of the drug's effects over time. Simply put, this means it takes a larger dose to provide the same level of pain relief. *Physical dependence* is a normal physiological phenomenon that most people experience after a few weeks of continuous opioid use. If an opioid is discontinued abruptly after a few weeks of use, or if an opioid antagonist such as naloxone (Narcan) is administered, the patient experiences a withdrawal syndrome that includes such symptoms as sweating, tearing, runny nose, restlessness, irritability, tremors, dilated pupils, sleeplessness, nausea, vomiting, and diarrhea. These symptoms can be prevented by weaning a patient slowly from an opioid rather than stopping it suddenly.

According to the American Pain Society (n.d.), addiction or **psychological dependence** is characterized by "behaviors that include one or more of the following: impaired control over drug use, compulsive use, continued use despite harm, and craving." However, pain must be treated, even in patients with a history of addiction. Careful assessment and monitoring of treatment is essential in these patients. If such patients require opioids for pain control, remember that they will be tolerant to therapeutic and side effects and may need higher doses to control pain.

Pseudoaddiction has been described in patients who are receiving opioid doses that are too low or spaced too far apart to relieve their pain, and certain behavioral characteristics resembling psychological dependence, such as drug-seeking behaviors, have developed. In contrast to the addicted patient, a patient with pseudoaddiction stops drug-seeking behaviors when the pain is relieved.

MECHANISMS OF PAIN TRANSMISSION

Many theories of how pain is transmitted and perceived (called *nociception*) are described in the literature. The *specificity theory*, developed by Descartes in 1644, proposed that body trauma sends a message directly to the brain, causing a sort of "bell" to ring, prompting a response from the brain. In 1965, Melzack and Wall proposed the *gate control theory*, which describes the dorsal horn of the spinal cord as a gate, allowing impulses to go through when there is a pain stimulus and closing the gate when those impulses are inhibited. The gate control theory stimulated massive research on the physiology of pain and is still considered in current research. However, much more is known about the transmission of pain today.

Pain is transmitted through four distinct processes:

1. *Transduction* represents the initiation of the stimulus and conversion of that stimulus into an electrical impulse at the time of the injury. Chemical

• WORD • BUILDING •

pseudoaddiction: pseudo—false + addiction—psychological dependence substances called *neurotransmitters* are released from damaged tissue. These substances include **prostaglandins**, bradykinin, serotonin, and substance P.

2. *Transmission* is the process of moving a painful message from the peripheral nerve endings through the dorsal root ganglion and the ascending tract of the spinal cord to the brain.
3. The third process is *perception,* or actually feeling the pain. During perception, the hypothalamus activates and controls emotional input and also generates purposeful goal-directed behavior while the cerebral cortex receives the pain message.
4. Last in the process of nociception is *modulation*, or the body's attempt to interrupt pain impulses by releasing endogenous (naturally occurring) opioids. **Endorphins** are endogenous chemicals that act like opioids, inhibiting pain impulses in the spinal cord and brain. Endorphins are the chemicals that stimulate the long-distance runner's "high." Unfortunately, they degrade too quickly to be considered effective analgesics. **Enkephalins** are one type of endorphin.

Mechanisms of pain transmission are nociceptive and neuropathic. **Nociception** refers to the body's normal reaction to noxious stimuli, such as tissue damage, with the release of pain-producing substances. Nociceptive pain in the visceral organs may be felt in other parts of the body, a process called *referred pain* (Fig. 10.1). **Neuropathic** pain is pain associated with injury to either the peripheral or central nervous system. Unlike nociceptive pain, it is not usually localized, and it may spread to involve other areas along the nerve pathway.

TYPES OF PAIN

Pain is often categorized according to whether it is acute, cancer related, or chronic nonmalignant. *Acute pain* is described as pain that follows injury to the body, prompting an inflammatory response, and subsides as healing takes place. It may be associated with short-term, objective, physical signs, such as increased heart rate and elevated blood pressure. Examples of acute pain include pain related to fractures, burns, or other trauma.

Cancer-related pain may be acute, chronic, or intermittent and often has a definable cause such as tumor invasion or neuropathy caused by the cancer treatment.

Chronic nonmalignant pain persists beyond the time when healing usually takes place, such as low back pain, the pain accompanying arthritis, and phantom limb pain. Chronic nonmalignant pain may have nociceptive as well as neuropathic components and may require a variety of medications and nondrug treatments. Because of the body's ability to adapt, patients with chronic nonmalignant pain or chronic cancer pain may not appear to be in pain. The physiological responses that accompany acute pain, such as elevated heart rate and blood pressure, cannot be sustained without harm to the body, so the body adapts and vital signs return to normal. The nurse must guard against labeling such a patient a **malingerer** (pretending to be in pain) or drug seeker.

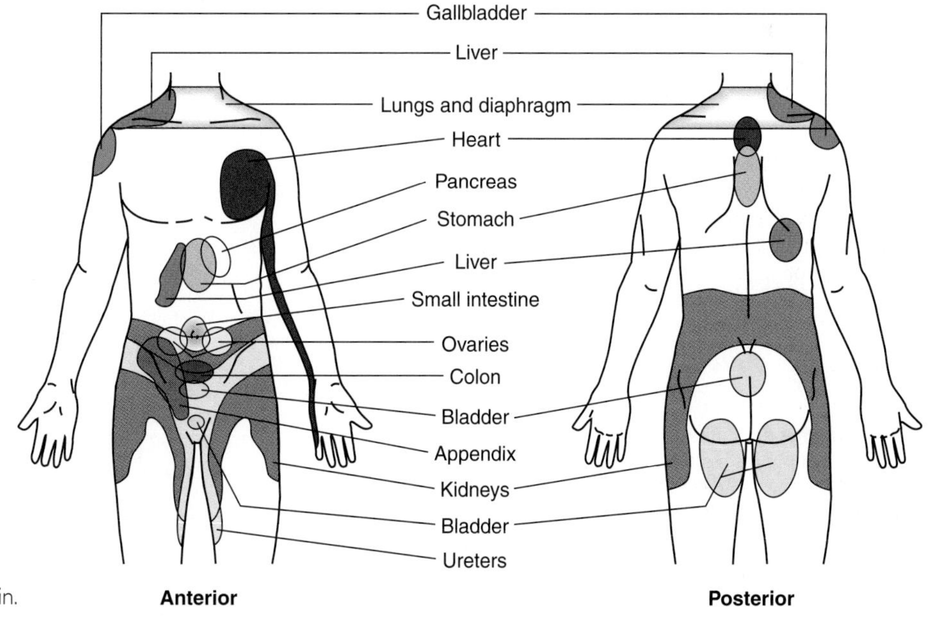
Gallbladder
Liver
Lungs and diaphragm
Heart
Pancreas
Stomach
Liver
Small intestine
Ovaries
Colon
Bladder
Appendix
Kidneys
Bladder
Ureters
Anterior
Posterior

FIGURE 10.1 Sites of referred pain.

• WORD • BUILDING •
nociception: noci—pain + ception—reception

• WORD • BUILDING •
neuropathic: neuro—nerves + pathy—disease, suffering

OPTIONS FOR TREATMENT OF PAIN

Analgesics

Medications that relieve pain are called analgesics. An **analgesic** is something—usually a drug—that relieves pain. Analgesics make up the largest pieces of the pain management puzzle. There are three main classes of analgesics: opioids, nonopioids, and adjuvants.

Opioids are classified by their ability to bind to opioid receptors in the brain, spinal cord, and other areas of the body, inhibiting the perception of pain. Nonopioids include nonsteroidal anti-inflammatory drugs (NSAIDs) and acetaminophen (Tylenol). Adjuvants include categories of drugs that were originally developed for a different purpose but have been found to have pain-relieving properties in certain painful conditions.

Nonopioid Analgesics

Nonopioids are typically the first class of drugs used to treat mild pain (Table 10.1). They can be useful for acute and chronic pain from a variety of causes, such as surgery, trauma, arthritis, and cancer. These drugs are limited in their use because they have a ceiling effect to analgesia. A **ceiling effect** means that there is a dose beyond which there is no improvement in the analgesic effect, but there may be an increase in adverse effects. When used with opioids, care must be taken to ensure that the nonopioid dose does not exceed the maximum safe dose for a 24-hour period. For example, if a patient receiving two Vicodin (acetaminophen and hydrocodone) tablets every 4 hours continues to experience pain, the dose cannot be increased because of the potentially toxic effects of acetaminophen at that dosage. (See Table 10.1 for side effects and nursing implications.) Nonopioids do not produce tolerance or physical dependence. Most do have antipyretic (fever-reducing) effects.

Nonopioids work mainly peripherally, at the site of injury, rather than in the central nervous system, as opioids do. The exception in this class is acetaminophen, which is believed to act on the central nervous system. NSAIDs block the synthesis of prostaglandins, one of many chemicals needed for pain transmission.

TABLE 10.1 ANALGESIC AGENTS

Medication Class/Action	Examples	Route	Side Effects	Nursing Implications
Salicylates				
Peripherally acting analgesics; reduce pain, fever, inflammation	aspirin	PO, PR	Tinnitus, GI upset and bleeding, renal impairment	Give with food. Decrease platelet aggregation, so watch for bleeding.
NSAIDs				
Peripherally acting analgesics; reduce pain, fever, inflammation	ibuprofen (Motrin) ketorolac (Toradol) naproxen (Naprosyn, Aleve)	PO PO, IM, IV PO	GI upset and bleeding, renal impairment	Give with food. Decrease platelet aggregation, so watch for bleeding. Do not give ketorolac longer than 5 days.
Second-Generation NSAIDs				
COX-2 inhibitor; reduces pain and inflammation, no effect on platelet aggregation	celecoxib (Celebrex)	PO	Abdominal pain, renal impairment GI upset and bleeding, but less risk for bleeding than first-generation NSAIDs Possible increased risk of stroke and heart attack	Give with food.
Acetaminophen				
Relieves pain and fever; no anti-inflammatory or antiplatelet effect	acetaminophen (Tylenol)	PO, PR	Few common side effects Liver toxicity and failure	Maximum safe dose is 4 g per day; less for those who use alcohol. Be aware of other drugs that contain acetaminophen, such as cold remedies, to prevent accidental overdose.

TABLE 10.1 ANALGESIC AGENTS—cont'd

Medication Class/Action	Examples	Route	Side Effects	Nursing Implications
Opioids				
Bind to opioid receptors in the central nervous system (CNS) to alter perception of pain	codeine	PO, IM	Sedation, nausea, vomiting, hypotension, constipation, respiratory depression, pupil constriction Cerebral irritation from toxic metabolite of meperidine (normeperidine)	May be combined with nonopioid (e.g., acetaminophen). Monitor vital signs, level of sedation, and respiratory status. Avoid fentanyl patch in patient with fever; heat increases absorption. Encourage fluids and fiber to prevent constipation. Meperidine should be avoided in older adults and those with renal dysfunction.
	fentanyl (Sublimaze, Duragesic)	PO, lozenge, IV, IM, patch, epidural		
	hydromorphone (Dilaudid)	PO, PR, IV, IM		
	meperidine (Demerol)	PO, IV, IM, subcutaneously		
	methadone (Dolophine)	PO, IM, subcutaneously		
	morphine	PO, IM, subcutaneously, IV		
	oxycodone (OxyIR, OxyContin)	PO		
	hydrocodone and acetaminophen (Vicodin)	PO		

In general, it is helpful to include a nonopioid agent in any analgesic regimen, even if the pain is severe enough to require the addition of an opioid. (See later section titled *Balanced Approach to Analgesia.*)

Opioid Analgesics

Opioids are drugs that have actions similar to those of morphine. Although opioids are extremely important in pain management, they are also on a short list of "high alert" drugs that can harm or even kill patients if they are not administered carefully (Federico, 2007). Institutions must have policies and procedures in place related to opioids to prevent medication errors and reduce the risk of serious side effects. It is especially important to be vigilant for side effects in patients unaccustomed to opioids. Such patients are sometimes called "opioid naïve."

Opioids are added to nonopioids for pain that cannot be managed effectively by nonopioids alone. Opioids are classified as full **agonists** (stimulators), partial agonists, or mixed agonists and **antagonists** (blockers). Full agonists have a complete response at the opioid receptor site; a partial agonist has a lesser response. A mixed agonist and antagonist activates one type of opioid receptor while blocking another.

• WORD • BUILDING •

analgesic: an—not + gesia—pain

antagonist: ant—against + agonist—stimulates receptor site

equianalgesic: equi—equal + analgesic—relieving pain

Opioids alone have no ceiling effect to analgesia. Doses can safely be increased to treat increasing pain if the patient's respiratory status and level of sedation are stable. See Table 10.1 for additional information and adverse effects of opioids. Controlled-release opioids such as oxycodone (OxyContin) and morphine (MS Contin) are effective for prolonged, continuous pain.

SAFETY TIP

Never crush a controlled- or time-release tablet. Because the tablet is designed to deliver a dose of medication over time, crushing it could deliver the entire dose at once, resulting in overdose.

Whenever a controlled-release form is used, it is important to have an immediate-release medication available for **breakthrough** pain (transient pain that arises during generally effective pain control), such as oral morphine solution or oxycodone immediate-release (OxyIR).

Morphine is commonly the drug of choice for treating moderate to severe pain. It is the standard to which all other analgesics are compared. (See Table 10.2 for **equianalgesic** doses of medications.) Morphine is long acting (4 to 5 hours) and available in many forms, making it convenient and affordable for patients. It has a slower onset than many other opioid agonists.

CRITICAL THINKING

Mrs. Zales

■ Mrs. Zales, a 32-year-old woman, was admitted for a hysterectomy after being treated for painful endometriosis for 12 months. After her surgery she had a patient-controlled analgesia (PCA) pump with hydromorphone, which was effective in relieving her pain. Forty-eight hours after surgery, the surgeon discontinued the PCA pump and ordered oral hydrocodone with acetaminophen. It was ineffective, so an order was added for hydromorphone 2 mg orally every 3 to 4 hours, as needed. The nurses gave only one dose of the hydromorphone. Then, thinking that her pain should be lessening, switched Mrs. Zales back to the hydrocodone with acetaminophen. By the next morning the patient was in severe pain, and the on-call physician ordered IM meperidine and promethazine (Phenergan). Mrs. Zales' discharge was delayed until her pain could be controlled.

What do you think happened? How could the delayed discharge have been avoided?

Suggested answers at end of chapter.

TABLE 10.2 EQUIANALGESIC CHART

Drug	Parenteral Dose*	Oral Dose
Morphine	5 mg	15 mg
Codeine	60 mg	100 mg
Hydromorphone (Dilaudid)	1.5 mg	4 mg
Methadone (Dolophine)	5 mg	10 mg
Meperidine (Demerol)	50 mg	150 mg
Oxycodone	Not applicable	10 mg

* Intramuscular, intravenous, subcutaneous.

Note: Approximate doses of medications in milligrams to equal same amount of pain relief between drugs or same drug–different route. Consult pharmacist and physician before changing drugs or routes.

Hydromorphone (Dilaudid) is another drug commonly used for moderate to severe pain. It is shorter acting than morphine and has a somewhat faster onset. It is a good option for pain management in most patients.

Meperidine (Demerol) was at one time a commonly used opioid, but is no longer recommended in most cases. Meperidine is an opioid agonist, and when broken down in the body, it produces a toxic metabolite called normeperidine. Normeperidine is a cerebral irritant that can cause adverse effects ranging from dysphoria and irritable mood to seizures. Normeperidine has a long half-life even in healthy patients, so those with impaired renal function are at increased risk. Meperidine use should be avoided in patients over age 65, patients with impaired renal function, and patients taking a monoamine oxidase inhibitor (MAOI) antidepressant. In general, the use of meperidine should be limited to young, healthy patients who need an opioid for a short period and to those who have unusual reactions or allergic responses to other opioids. The effective dose of oral meperidine is three to four times the parenteral dose and is never recommended.

SAFETY TIP

It is important to monitor the patient's level of sedation and respiratory status when administering opioids. Increased sedation, decreased respiratory effort, and constricted pupils can be signs of opioid overdose. Careful monitoring and dosage adjustments of opioids can prevent opioid-induced respiratory depression.

Fentanyl (Sublimaze, Duragesic) can be given parenterally, intraspinally, or by **transdermal** (across the skin) patch (Duragesic). Fentanyl is commonly used intravenously with anesthesia for surgery. It also is used to relieve postoperative pain via the intravenous route, patient-controlled analgesia (PCA) pump, or epidural route (discussed later in this chapter). IV fentanyl has a short duration of action and must be given more often than other opioids to maintain an effective level of analgesia. The fentanyl patch is useful for a patient with stable cancer pain; the patient needs a new patch every 3 days.

CRITICAL THINKING

Mrs. Shepard

■ Mrs. Shepard is 92 years old and has undergone an open cholecystectomy. Her continuous epidural infusion of analgesic is discontinued at 1400 on her second postoperative day. The physician orders oral acetaminophen with hydrocodone every 3 to 4 hours as needed for pain. At 1700 Mrs. Shepard refuses to get out of bed because her pain is 7 on a scale of 0 to 10. The nurse checks the medication administration record and notes that she has not yet received a dose of acetaminophen and hydrocodone.

1. Why is Mrs. Shepard in so much pain?
2. What complications can occur as a result of her pain?
3. Each analgesic tablet contains 500 mg of acetaminophen and 5 mg of hydrocodone. The maximum daily dose of acetaminophen is 4 g. If she takes one tablet every 3 hours, is her dose safe?
4. What can be done to relieve her pain and better prevent it in the future?

Suggested answers at end of chapter.

• WORD • BUILDING •

transdermal: trans—across + dermal—skin

Methadone (Dolophine) is a potent analgesic that has a longer duration of action than morphine. It has a very long half-life and accumulates in the body with continued dosing. Dosing intervals may be extended after pain relief has been achieved. Methadone is well absorbed from the gastrointestinal tract and is very effective when given orally at doses similar to the parenteral dose.

Methadone is also used in drug treatment programs during detoxification from heroin and other opioids. Patients on methadone maintenance can present a unique challenge when admitted to the hospital. It is important to continue the maintenance dose even if additional pain medications are required after surgery or trauma. See Table 10.1 for examples of opioids.

Opioid Antagonists

Naloxone (Narcan) is a pure opioid antagonist that counteracts, or antagonizes, the effect of opioids. Often, it is used in emergency departments for treating the effects of opioid overdose, such as sedation and respiratory depression. Caution must be used when giving naloxone to a patient who is receiving opioids for pain control. If too much naloxone is given too fast, it can reverse not only the unwanted effects—such as respiratory depression and sedation—but the desired effect of analgesia as well.

Some antagonists are shorter acting than the opioid that is being used. If the antagonist is given because of respiratory depression, the dose may need to be repeated because its effect may wear off before the opioid wears off. Some analgesics are classified as combined agonists and antagonists or partial agonists. These drugs bind with some opioid receptors and block others. The most commonly used drugs in this class are butorphanol (Stadol) and nalbuphine (Nubain).

How does this information translate into nursing practice? Consider, for example, a patient who receives sustained-release morphine every 12 hours to control metastatic bone pain, but the patient develops breakthrough pain between doses. You observe that butorphanol has been ordered for pain by another doctor and administer it. The butorphanol will antagonize, or counteract, some of the effects of the morphine, and the patient may experience acute pain. It is important to be informed about the actions of all drugs that are administered and to be aware of possible drug interactions that may interfere with patient care.

Analgesic Adjuvants

Adjuvants are classes of medications that may potentiate the effects of opioids or nonopioids, have analgesic activity themselves, or counteract the unwanted effects of other analgesics. Adjuvants are especially important when treating pain that does not respond well to traditional analgesics alone. Examples of adjuvants are corticosteroids, benzodiazepines, antidepressants, and anticonvulsants.

Corticosteroids can be used to treat a variety of painful conditions, including acute and chronic cancer-related pain. They may be used as part of actual cancer treatment because of their toxicity to some cancer cells, or they may reduce pain by decreasing inflammation and the resulting compression of healthy tissues.

Benzodiazepines such as midazolam (Versed) or diazepam (Valium) are effective for treating anxiety or muscle spasms associated with pain. These drugs do not provide pain relief alone but are effective in treating pain caused by muscle spasms. Benzodiazepines may cause sedation, which limits the amount of opioid that can be safely given at the same time.

Tricyclic antidepressants such as amitriptyline, imipramine, desipramine, and doxepin can relieve the pain of neuropathy and other painful nerve-related conditions. These drugs must be taken for days to weeks before they are fully effective, and patients must be told to continue the medication even if it seems ineffective at first. Additional benefits of this class of medications may include mood elevation and improved ability to sleep, but significant side effects often limit their use.

Anticonvulsants such as carbamazepine (Tegretol) and gabapentin (Neurontin) are often used to relieve the sharp or cutting pain caused by peripheral nerve syndromes. Again, these medications must be taken regularly to realize their full benefit.

Stimulants such as methylphenidate hydrochloride (Ritalin) or caffeine-containing medications may be used to counteract the sedating effects of opioids in some patients.

Balanced Approach to Analgesia

A *balanced analgesia* approach should be used, combining analgesics and adjuvants from different classes to minimize the adverse effects of opioids, such as nausea and vomiting or sedation, while maximizing pain relief. For example, an opioid and a nonopioid given together can provide pain relief with an overall lower dose of each medication than if each was given alone. Because these drugs have different mechanisms of action and different adverse effects, it is possible to give lower doses of each. If doses can be reduced in this manner, additional sedating medications such as antiemetics and antihistamines (to treat side effects) may not be needed.

Scheduling Options

Analgesics of any kind can be administered either as needed (prn) or on a scheduled basis. Intermittent, unpredictable pain may be best treated with prn doses. Pain that is predictable can be more effectively treated, or prevented, with scheduled doses of medication. Around-the-clock (ATC) dosing is an effective way to schedule doses evenly over a 24-hour period to prevent pain from spiraling out of control. It is important to use ATC dosing after surgery or trauma, with chronic pain, or in any other circumstance in which preventing pain will allow the patient to participate in daily or other recovery activities.

Patient-controlled analgesia (PCA) involves an opioid on an IV controller. The patient has a button on a cord that can be pushed to activate a dose of IV medication. The RN programs the pump to the dose and dosing interval ordered by the physician. A "lock-out" mechanism prevents the patient from receiving the medication more often than ordered. PCA is an excellent option after surgery because it gives the patient some control over pain management. Teach the patient and family that only the patient should push the button, never the nurse or a family member. If the patient is too sedated to push the button, a dose of opioid could be dangerous and likely is not needed.

World Health Organization Analgesic Ladder

In 1990, the World Health Organization (WHO) developed the WHO analgesic ladder, which involves choosing among three levels of treatments based on intensity of pain (Fig. 10.2). The ladder, which helps direct the interventions required when using medications to treat pain, was developed for the treatment of cancer pain but can be used when treating other types of pain as well.

When experiencing mild pain (level 1 on the WHO ladder), the patient can usually sleep, perform activities of daily living, and even work. The first level of the ladder addresses the use of nonopioid analgesics. When pain is unrelieved by maximum ATC dosing, the treatment moves up the ladder to level 2 (mild to moderate pain) and adds an opioid analgesic. A patient with mild to moderate pain may not be able to sleep and may have trouble working and staying focused. If pain increases beyond that which is controlled by the level 2 analgesics, it is time to move on to level 3. At this level, the pain is moderate to severe and is affecting the quality of the patient's life. The patient may not be able to perform activities of daily living. At any level, an adjuvant analgesic may be appropriate.

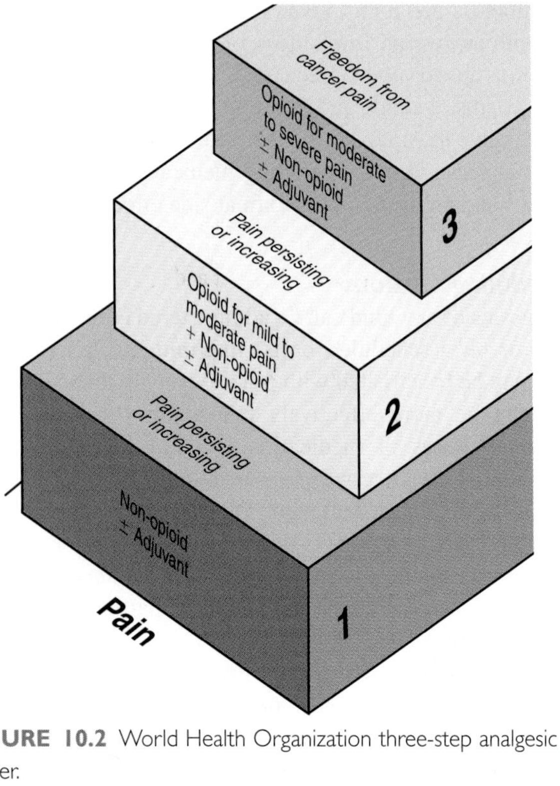
Freedom from cancer pain
Opioid for moderate to severe pain
± Non-opioid
± Adjuvant
3
Pain persisting or increasing
Opioid for mild to moderate pain
+ Non-opioid
± Adjuvant
2
Pain persisting or increasing
Non-opioid
± Adjuvant
1
Pain

FIGURE 10.2 World Health Organization three-step analgesic ladder.

Analgesics should be given on an ATC basis to prevent breakthrough pain, especially for cancer and chronic nonmalignant pain. For patients with surgical or traumatic pain, analgesics should be given ATC until the pain decreases to a level that allows medications to be given less often (e.g., prn, such as before physical therapy). When using the WHO ladder, it is important to keep in mind that it is not necessary to start at level 1 if the patient is having severe pain. Analgesics from level 3 on the WHO ladder may be the starting point for some patients.

> **CRITICAL THINKING**
>
> ***Ms. Jackson***
>
> ■ Ms. Jackson had abdominal surgery 2 days ago. She has been receiving morphine via IV PCA at an average of 2.5 mg per hour for the last 6 hours. She rates her pain at 3 on a scale of 0 to 10. She is to be discharged today. Her physician has ordered codeine 30 mg with acetaminophen (Tylenol with codeine No. 3), one or two tablets every 4 hours as needed for pain at home.
>
> Will Ms. Jackson be comfortable at home? Why or why not?
>
> *Suggested answers at end of chapter.*

Other Interventions

Other pain treatments include radiation therapy or antineoplastic chemotherapy to help shrink tumors that are causing pain for a patient with cancer. Chemotherapy is also used for treating pain associated with connective tissue disorders such as rheumatoid arthritis or systemic lupus erythematosus. Laxatives, enemas, or antigas medication to decrease abdominal fullness may also be considered pain treatments. In patients with osteoporosis, drugs that promote calcium uptake by the bones can aid in pain relief. These may include hormonal agents and medications that decrease calcium resorption from bone.

Lidocaine/prilocaine cream (EMLA) is a topical local anesthetic that decreases the pain of procedures such as venipuncture and lumbar puncture. It is most effective if covered with a semipermeable membrane dressing, such as Tegaderm, and left in place for 1 hour before the needlestick. EMLA and tetracaine gel are effective topical local anesthetics and safe for use in children. A lidocaine patch may be effective for patients with post-herpetic or other nerve pain.

Placebos

Use of placebos involves the administration of an inactive substitute such as normal saline in place of an active medication. In the past, placebos were sometimes given in an attempt to determine whether a patient's pain was "real." This is unethical and inappropriate unless the patient has given written consent. The use of placebos is a denial of the patient's report of pain. If a placebo is ordered for a patient, discuss concerns with the physician and nurse supervisor. Placebos are only to be used in drug studies (clinical trials) to compare a new drug with an inactive substance. In this situation patients are informed that they may be receiving a placebo.

Routes for Medication Administration

Analgesics can be administered by almost any route. The oral route is desired in most instances because it is easy and painless for the patient and can be used at home. See Table 10.3 for a comparison of the various routes.

TABLE 10.3 ROUTES FOR ANALGESIC ADMINISTRATION

Uses	Advantages	Disadvantages	Nursing Considerations
Oral			
Preferred route in most cases	Convenient Less expensive than other forms Immediate- and controlled-release forms available	Slower onset than IV form	Can provide consistent blood levels when given around the clock. Controlled-release form recommended for long-term use in chronic pain.
Rectal			
May be used to provide local or systemic pain relief	Can be used when patient cannot take oral medication	May be difficult for patient or family to self-administer	Some oral preparations can be given rectally. (Place in empty gel cap for ease of use.)
Transdermal Patch			
Chronic pain	Easy to apply Delivers pain relief for 3 days without patch change	May take up to 3 days before maximum effective drug level reached, and delay in excreting once removed. Patient must be closely monitored and alternative routes may be needed when starting and stopping therapy.	May be less effective in smokers and very thin people. Absorption may be erratic. Absorption may be increased with fever. Avoid heat application over patch. Do not touch medication when applying patch. Keep used patches away from pets and children.
Intramuscular			
Acute pain	Rapid pain relief, although slower than IV	Painful Inconsistent absorption	Use only if other routes cannot be used.
Intravenous			
Preferred route for postoperative and chronic cancer pain in patients who cannot tolerate oral route	Provides rapid relief Continuous infusion to achieve steady drug level	Difficult to use in home care setting Requires training and special equipment	Follow drug manufacturer's instructions for administration.
Patient-Controlled Intravenous			
Allows patient some control over administration schedule	Patient pushes a button to administer a dose of opioid.	Requires special training Pump must be programmed correctly.	An hourly limit and lock-out interval are programmed into the pump to keep the patient from receiving too much drug. Caution patient and family that only the patient should push the button.
Subcutaneous			
May be used if IV route is problematic	Can deliver effective pain relief Some opioids may be given as continuous infusion.	Injection may be painful.	May be effective for treatment of chronic cancer pain
Intraspinal (Epidural or Subarachnoid)			
Catheter into epidural or subarachnoid space used for traumatic injuries or chronic pain unrelieved by other methods May also be used for orthopedic, chest, and abdominal surgical procedures	May be able to control pain with lower doses of opioid because relief is delivered closer to site of pain Fewer systemic side effects	Requires single or continuous injection in back May be associated with intense itching Motor function must be assessed especially when local anesthetic is used	Steroids may be given with opioid to reduce pain by treating inflammation. Local anesthetic may be paired with opioid to enhance pain relief. Avoid use of anticoagulant and antiplatelet agents (including aspirin) because of risk of epidural hematoma.

Nondrug Therapies

Nondrug treatments are usually classified as cognitive-behavioral interventions or physical agents. The goals of these two groups of treatments differ. Cognitive-behavioral interventions can help patients understand and cope with pain and take an active part in its assessment and control. The goals of physical agents may include providing comfort, correcting physical dysfunction, altering physiological responses, and reducing fear that might be associated with immobility. Nondrug therapies should be used in conjunction with drug therapies and are not expected to relieve pain on their own.

Cognitive-Behavioral Interventions

Included in this group are interventions such as educational information, relaxation exercises, guided imagery, distraction (e.g., music, television), and biofeedback. These treatments require extra time for detailed instruction and demonstration. The use of these modalities must be acceptable to the patient to be useful. Educating patients about what to expect and how they can participate in their own care has been shown to decrease patients' reports of postoperative pain and analgesic use.

Relaxation can be accomplished through a variety of methods. The patient may prefer a relaxation exercise with a script that can be practiced and used the same way each time or simply the use of a favorite piece of music that allows a state of muscle relaxation and freedom from anxiety (See *Evidence-Based Practice*). Guided imagery uses the patient's imagination to take the patient away from the pain to a favorite place, such as a beach in Tahiti. The success of guided imagery does not mean that the pain is in any way imaginary. See Chapter 5 for more information on relaxation and imagery.

EVIDENCE-BASED PRACTICE

Clinical Question

Can music help relieve pain and reduce the need for opioid analgesics?

Evidence

Fifty-one studies were reviewed to determine the effectiveness of music on pain and analgesic use. Results were variable.

Implications for Nursing Practice

"Listening to music reduces pain intensity levels and opioid requirements, but the magnitude of these benefits is small and, therefore, its clinical importance unclear" (Cepeda et al., 2006). Listening to music is inexpensive, easy to try, and may work for some patients.

REFERENCE

Cepeda, M. S., Carr, D. B., Lau, J., et al. (2006). Music for pain relief. *Cochrane Database of Systematic Reviews, Issue 1* (Art. No. CD004843; DOI 10.1002/14651858.CD004843.pub2).

Distraction is commonly used by patients to focus their attention on something other than the pain. They may watch a favorite television program or laugh with visitors when they are in pain. When the program is over or the visitors leave, the patient may focus on the pain again and ask for a dose of pain medication.

Biofeedback is sometimes used in chronic-pain programs to teach patients how to train their bodies to respond to different signals. Biofeedback has been very useful in patients with migraine headaches. When an aura (a warning sign) occurs before a migraine headache, patients are prompted to begin the exercise that relaxes them and may allow them to prevent the headache.

Physical Agents

Physical agents can contribute directly to the patient's comfort. Examples of physical agents include applications of heat or cold, massage, exercise, immobilization, and transcutaneous electrical nerve stimulation (TENS).

The application of heat to sore muscles and joints is effective for pain relief. Heat works to increase circulation, induce muscle relaxation, and decrease inflammation when applied to a painful area. Heat can be applied using dry or moist packs or wraps, or in a bath or whirlpool. Heat is contraindicated in conditions that would be worsened by its use, such as in an area of trauma, because of the possibility of increased swelling caused by vasodilation. To prevent burns, heat should not be applied over areas of decreased sensation.

Cold can reduce swelling, bleeding, and pain when used to treat a new injury. Cold can be applied by a variety of methods, such as cold wraps and cold packs, as well as localized ice massage. Patients often choose heat over cold if they have the choice, because cold can be uncomfortable. Cold may be better tolerated over a small area. Alternating heat and cold therapies is most effective if not contraindicated.

Massage and exercise are used to stretch and regain muscle and tendon length and to relax muscles. Massage pressure can be superficial or deep. It is important that massage is acceptable and not offensive to the patient. Immobilization is used following a variety of orthopedic procedures, as well as fractures and other injuries worsened by movement.

Physical agents are readily available, inexpensive, and require little preparation or instruction. But always remember, it is important to use nondrug treatments to enhance appropriate drug treatments, not as a substitute.

NURSING PROCESS FOR THE PATIENT EXPERIENCING PAIN

Data Collection

Accurate assessment of pain is essential to effective treatment. Without appropriate assessment, it is not possible to intervene in a way that meets the patient's needs. In 1999, the Joint Commission and the Veterans Health Administration recommended that nurses consider pain the "fifth vital sign," and include a pain rating with each assessment of vital signs. Others are now finding that this has not made a significant difference in pain control, because more complete assessment is needed to manage pain effectively (Mularski et al., 2006). The WHAT'S UP? format introduced in Chapter 1 can help you perform a complete and effective assessment (Table 10.4). The following sections provide some additional key points for assessing pain and putting together more pieces of the pain puzzle.

Accept the Patient's Report of Pain

Pain is what the patient says it is, not what the nurse or physician thinks it should be. When a member of the health care team distrusts the patient's report of pain, the patient can usually sense that he or she is not believed. The patient may compensate by either underreporting pain or, less commonly, anxiously overreporting. Patients may try to hide their pain for fear of being thought of as complainers or drug seekers.

Obtain a Pain History

Obtain information from the patient about the pain he or she is experiencing. Letting the patient describe the pain in his or her own words helps establish a trust relationship between you and the patient. This is also the time to discover the effects the pain is having on the patient's quality of life. Does the pain prevent the patient from eating, sleeping, or participating in work or family activities? Are there adverse effects such as nausea and vomiting or constipation that need to be addressed? Also assess emotional and spiritual distress and coping abilities. Ask the patient about how he or she has coped with pain previously and what treatments have been effective and ineffective in the past. A thorough history is essential so you can individualize pain interventions to fit the patient's needs.

Various tools are available to assist with accurate and complete pain assessment. You should become familiar with the tool used in your setting and use it consistently. It is of utmost importance that all health care personnel caring for a particular patient use the same pain rating scale, whether it is a numerical scale (e.g., 0 to 5 or 0 to 10), a visual analog scale (Fig. 10.3), or the Wong-Baker faces scale (Fig. 10.4).

Whatever scale is used, it must be one that has been validated with research. The faces scale was developed for use in children, but it may also be helpful for others having difficulty with communicating their needs. Some scales are cute and interesting but may not be valid or even useful. The best tools are simple and easy to use. Longer questionnaires, although valid, require more time and may cause distress for a patient in acute pain, but they may be helpful when doing a complete pain history (Fig. 10.5). A scale should also be used to monitor the patient's level of sedation after opioid administration (Fig. 10.6). Any unexpected increase in the patient's level of sedation should be reported promptly to the RN or physician.

It is important to use the patient's own descriptions and words when documenting the pain history, such as *aching*, *knifelike*, or *throbbing*. This is also true when the patient is experiencing neuropathic (nonphysiological) pain, which can be difficult to describe. Some terms commonly used to describe neuropathic pain include *burning*, *shocklike*, and *tingling*. Finally, a pain diary may help the patient to document pain ratings, interventions, and responses, which can in turn help the nurse with planning.

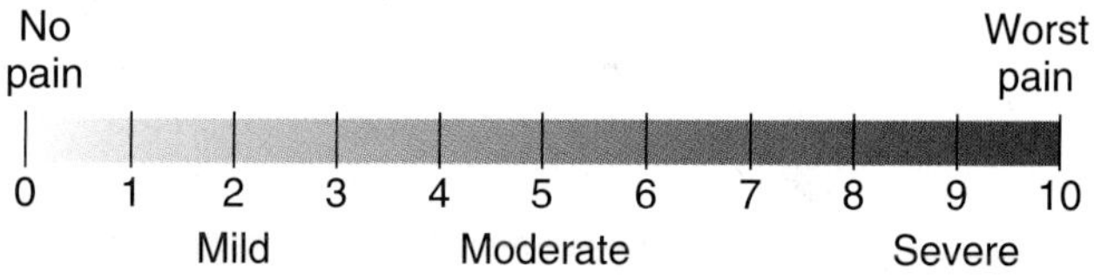
No pain
Worst pain
0 1 2 3 4 5 6 7 8 9 10
Mild
Moderate
Severe

FIGURE 10.3 Pain scale.

TABLE 10.4 WHAT'S UP? GUIDE FOR PAIN ASSESSMENT

Acronym	Key	Pain Assessment
W	Where is the pain?	Be specific. Use a drawing of the body if needed.
H	How does the pain feel?	Is the pain shooting, burning, dull, sharp?
A	Aggravating and alleviating factors	What makes the pain better? What makes it worse?
T	Timing	When did the pain start? Is it intermittent? Continuous?
S	Severity	How bad is the pain on a scale of 0 to 10? Use a different tool, such as the Wong-Baker faces scale, if needed.
U	Useful other data	Are any other symptoms associated with the pain or pain treatment? Itching, nausea, sedation, constipation? How does the pain affect lifestyle (inability to eat, sleep, work, enjoy sex, etc.)?
P	Perception	What is the patient's perception of what caused the pain?

0
1
2
3
4
5

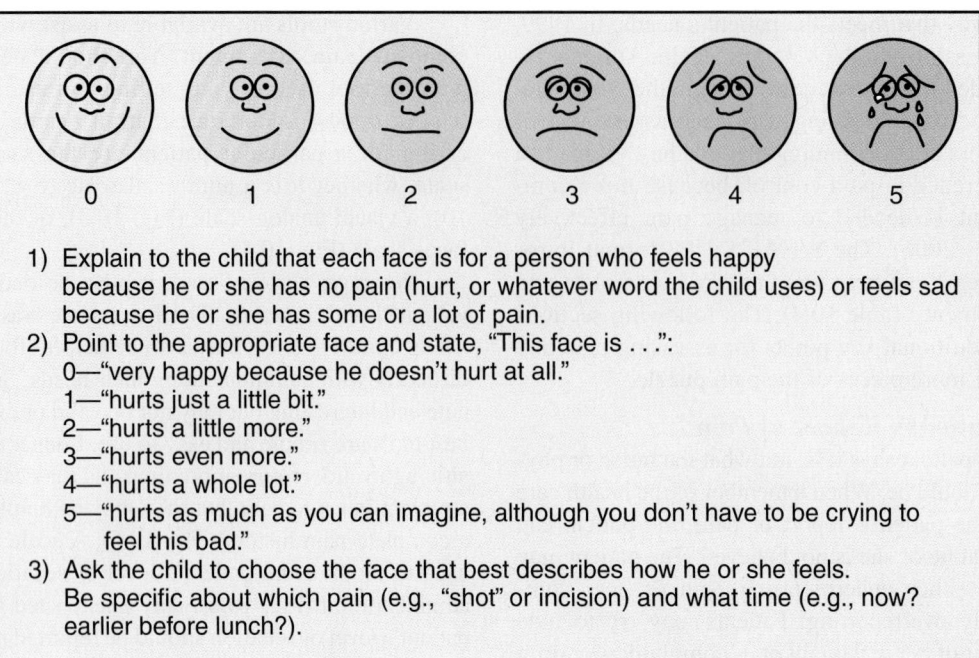

1) Explain to the child that each face is for a person who feels happy because he or she has no pain (hurt, or whatever word the child uses) or feels sad because he or she has some or a lot of pain.
2) Point to the appropriate face and state, "This face is . . .":
   0—"very happy because he doesn't hurt at all."
   1—"hurts just a little bit."
   2—"hurts a little more."
   3—"hurts even more."
   4—"hurts a whole lot."
   5—"hurts as much as you can imagine, although you don't have to be crying to feel this bad."
3) Ask the child to choose the face that best describes how he or she feels. Be specific about which pain (e.g., "shot" or incision) and what time (e.g., now? earlier before lunch?).

FIGURE 10.4 Wong-Baker faces scale. (From Wong, D. L. [1997]. *Whaley & Wong's essentials of pediatric nursing* [5th ed.]. St. Louis: Mosby.)

Pain Assessment Chart (For Admission and/or Follow-up)

1. Patient ____________________ 2. DX ____________

Assessment on Admission

Date ___/___/___ Pain ☐ No Pain ☐ Date of Pain Onset ___/___/___

1. Location of Pain (indicate on drawing)
2. Description of Predominant Pain (in patient's words) ____________________
3. Intensity [Scale 0 (no pain) — 10 (most intense)] ____________________
4. Duration and when occurs ____________________
5. Precipitating Factors ____________________
6. Alleviating Factors ____________________

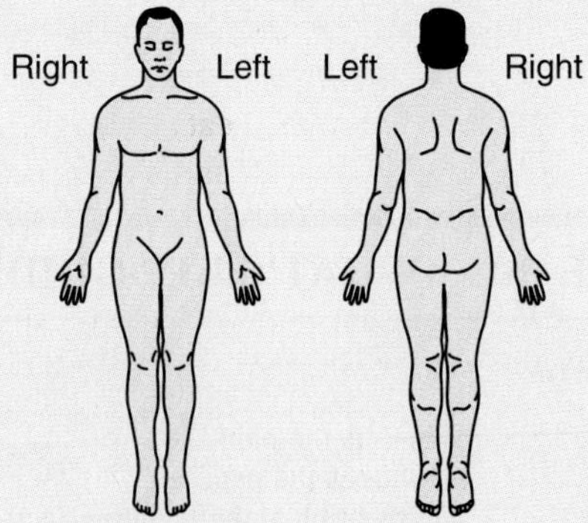
Right
Left
Left
Right

FIGURE 10.5 Pain assessment chart. (Modified from The Purdue Frederik Company, Norwalk, CT.)

7. Accompanying Symptoms

GI: Nausea ☐ Emesis ☐ Constipation ☐ Anorexia ☐

CNS: Drowsiness ☐ Confusion ☐ Hallucinations ☐

Psychosocial: Mood ____________ Anger ____________

Anxiety ____________ Depression ____________

Relationships ____________

____

8. Other Symptoms

Sleep ____________ Fatigue ____________

Activity ____________ Other ____________

9. Present Medications ____________

____

____

Doses and times medicated last 48 hours ____________

____

10. Breakthrough Pain ____________

____

Signature: ____________

FIGURE 10.5 cont'd

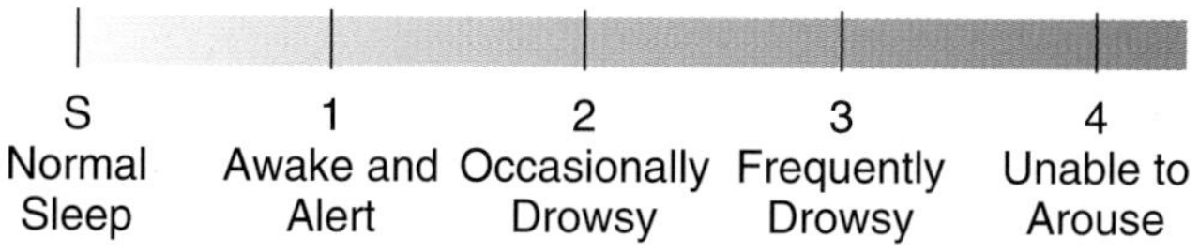
S
Normal Sleep
1
Awake and Alert
2
Occasionally Drowsy
3
Frequently Drowsy
4
Unable to Arouse

FIGURE 10.6 Level of sedation scale.

Do a Complete Physical Assessment

A good physical assessment is needed to determine the effect of the pain and pain treatments on the body. It helps identify all of the pain sites and helps prioritize the seemingly overwhelming task of helping the patient achieve acceptable pain relief and good quality of life. As discussed previously, the patient with acute pain may exhibit signs such as grimacing and moaning or elevated pulse and blood pressure, but these signs cannot be relied on to "prove" that the patient is in pain. The only reliable source of pain assessment is the patient's self-report (Box 10.3, *Gerontological Issues*). It is also important to monitor for side effects of analgesic and adjuvant agents.

Nursing Diagnoses, Planning, and Implementation

See the *Nursing Care Plan for the Patient in Pain.* Some additional principles to consider during planning and implementation follow.

Box 10.3

Gerontological Issues

Older patients may have different manifestations of pain than younger patients. Older patients who are confused may be unable to tell you that they are feeling pain. Consider incidents of restlessness and confusion as possible signs of pain. Pulling at dressings, tugging at IV sites, and trying to climb over the side rails to get out of bed can also be symptoms of discomfort. Any change in the patient's behavior may be indicative of discomfort. Remember to take more time when assessing pain in older patients because they may need more time to process what you are asking. Also take into consideration the patients' cultural backgrounds.

You can anticipate pain and provide relief measures to prevent severe pain. A trial dose of pain medication may help to determine if the patient's behavior is because of pain. Pain medications and basic comfort care can be administered routinely if pain is likely. Nagging achiness in hands and feet is often noted as a reason for decreased activity, inability to sleep, and altered functional ability. A hand or foot massage using lotion and gentle massage strokes is often a very relaxing comfort measure.

Opioid analgesic doses may need to be decreased by 25% to 50% initially because they tend to work longer and stronger in the older patient.

NURSING CARE PLAN for the Patient in Pain

Nursing Diagnosis: *Pain (acute or chronic)*

Expected Outcomes: Pain will be at a level that is acceptable to the patient. Patient will be able to participate in activities that are important to him or her.

Evaluation of Outcomes: Is pain at a level that is acceptable to the patient? Is the patient able to participate in activities that he or she has identified as important?

Intervention	Rationale	Evaluation
Assess pain based on patient report. Use the WHAT'S UP format.	Patient's pain is defined as what the patient says it is, when the patient says it is occurring.	Does the patient verbalize his or her pain? Does the patient use verbal or nonverbal messages that imply trust in nurse's belief of pain report?
Teach the patient to use a pain rating scale. Use the same scale consistently.	A rating scale is the most reliable method for assessing pain severity.	Does the patient understand the use of the scale and use it to report pain?
Have the patient keep a pain diary, documenting time of pain, interventions, and pre- and post-pain ratings.	A diary can show patterns of pain and pain relief, and help in planning care.	Does the diary reveal patterns that help with planning?
Determine with patient what is an acceptable pain level.	Only the patient can decide what pain level is acceptable.	Is the patient's pain at an acceptable level?
Assess whether pain is acute, chronic, or both.	Acute and chronic pain may present differently and may require different interventions.	Has acute versus chronic pain been identified? Are treatments appropriate?
Assess need for and offer emotional and spiritual support for the experience of pain and suffering.	Pain, as well as disease processes, can be accompanied by feelings of powerlessness and distress.	Does the patient appear emotional, angry, or withdrawn? Does the patient have difficulty making decisions? Is the patient–nurse relationship therapeutic?
Give analgesics before pain becomes severe. For moderate to severe pain, give analgesics around the clock.	Severe pain may be more difficult to relieve than to prevent.	Is analgesic schedule effective?
Combine opioid and nonopioid analgesics as ordered.	Balanced analgesia provides optimum pain relief with fewer side effects.	Is the analgesic combination effective?
Assess for pain relief approximately 1 hr after administration of oral analgesics, or 30 min after IV analgesics.	If pain is not relieved, additional measures will be needed.	Does patient report acceptable level of relief?
Observe for anticipated adverse effects of pain medication.	Many pain medications cause nausea and constipation. The nausea usually subsides after several days but constipation persists.	Are adverse effects occurring? Can they be managed? Does medication regimen need to be adjusted?
If opioids are being used, assess for respiratory depression and level of sedation at regular intervals.	If patient is opioid naïve or dose is increased, monitor patient carefully for sedation. Sedation always precedes respiratory depression.	Is the patient's respiratory rate greater than 8 per minute or above the parameter ordered by the physician? Is the patient alert and oriented?

NURSING CARE PLAN for the Patient in Pain—cont'd

Intervention	Rationale	Evaluation
Institute measures to prevent constipation: 8 to 10 glasses of fluid daily (unless contraindicated), fiber in meals, fiber or bulk laxatives, and exercise as tolerated.	Constipation is a common side effect of opioids.	Are the patient's bowels moving according to his or her usual pattern?
Teach patient alternative (nondrug) pain relief interventions, such as relaxation and distraction, to be used with medication.	Alternative interventions can help the patient feel in control and may help reduce the perception of pain.	Does the patient use alternative interventions effectively?
Assess whether patient is taking pain medications appropriately, and if not, assess reasons. Instruct in how to manage pain interventions.	Pain medications must be taken appropriately to be effective.	Is the patient able to manage the pain control regimen? Are adjustments necessary?

Set Goals with the Patient

Establish a pain control goal during the planning phase. The patient should be asked to determine an acceptable level of pain if complete freedom from pain is not possible. Education is important when helping the patient set a realistic pain control goal. Although a goal of zero pain is desirable, it may not be possible or safe. On the other hand, a patient may choose a pain goal of 6 but be unable to get out of bed and do other recovery activities.

Patients should also identify activity goals. After surgery, goals may include the ability to ambulate and sleep without pain. For patients with chronic pain, the goals may be different. For example, if a patient with terminal cancer wants to be able to attend her granddaughter's wedding, you can assist the patient in reaching that goal. She can be taught to reserve energy that day for the activity that is most important to her. Instructing her in optimal timing of her pain medication will also assist her in reaching a good comfort level for the activity.

Allow the Patient as Much Control as Possible

Pain can prompt feelings of helplessness and hopelessness. Giving patients pain management options allows them to maintain some control. It is also the nurse's responsibility to teach patients about the goals of pain management and why it is an important part of care. When patients understand that the health care provider's goals and theirs are the same, they are able to cooperate with and contribute to the pain management plan.

Understand that Pain Affects the Whole Family

It is important to include the whole family in the pain management plan. Understanding family dynamics helps the nurse in implementing an effective plan. Cultural influences are also important to consider (see Chapter 4). It is difficult for family members to see loved ones in pain. Including them in the planning helps them feel that they can help make the patient more comfortable.

Pain Is Exhausting

Pain may keep the patient from sleeping. This cycle of sleeplessness and pain must be interrupted to help the patient. Sleep difficulties are often an ongoing problem for the patient with chronic nonmalignant pain or chronic cancer pain, and they complicate the treatment process. The patient must get at least 4 to 6 hours of uninterrupted sleep to be relaxed enough to break the cycle. Controlled-release opioids may help maintain pain relief, allowing the patient to sleep. If controlled-release medications are not used, it may be necessary to wake a patient to administer pain medication so that the pain does not get out of control. The addition of a sedative may be needed to allow the patient to sleep.

A Team Approach to Pain Management

A plan must be developed using an interdisciplinary approach, including the patient and family, the nurse, and the physician. Other team members, such as occupational and physical therapists, chaplain, social worker, and pharmacist, should be included as appropriate. Communication is the important link allowing the team to be effective in creating a plan that works for the patient. As the nurse, you play an important role in ensuring effective communication among team members.

Patient Education

Patients must be informed about the medications they are taking for pain management so they can take an active role in their care. Patients informed about the goals of pain management are more likely to report unrelieved pain so that they can receive prompt and effective treatment. Goals include a satisfactory comfort level with minimal side effects and complications of pain and its treatment, as well as a reduced period of recovery.

The patient should be provided with information about a drug's effects, common adverse effects, frequency of the dose and duration of action, and potential drug–drug and drug–food interactions if indicated. There are many special considerations for medications, such as controlled-release oral agents and transdermal patches; care must be taken to include these considerations in the education plan for the patient taking these drugs at home. Drug-specific instructions are found in drug handbooks. Education must be presented at a level that the patient can understand. Informed patients use their medications more effectively and safely.

CRITICAL THINKING

Mr. Sebastian

■ Mr. Sebastian is a 75-year-old man who has been diagnosed with lung cancer and is anxious about leaving the hospital to return home following a thoracotomy. The nursing assessment reveals the need for home health care for dressing changes and teaching about the medications he will need at home. While in the hospital, Mr. Sebastian has required 5 mg of IV morphine every 4 hours around the clock.

1. The morphine is available in syringes prefilled with morphine grains 1/6 per mL. How many milliliters should the nurse administer while Mr. Sebastian is in the hospital?
2. What discharge instructions must be given to Mr. Sebastian and his wife before sending him home?
3. How might his pain be managed at home to prevent unnecessary readmissions to the hospital?

Suggested answers at end of chapter.

NURSING CARE TIP

Many medication interventions are available for the treatment of pain. Whenever possible, administer analgesics by the mouth, by the WHO ladder, and by the clock.

Evaluation

The final phase of the nursing process is evaluation. Once the plan of care has been implemented, evaluate whether the patient's goals have been met. What is the patient's pain rating? Has the patient's identified goal for an acceptable level of pain been met? How were the pain treatments tolerated? Was the patient able to participate in activities that he or she identified as important? The plan should be continuously updated based on the evaluation.

Home Health Hints

- Emotional or spiritual distress and fear related to dependence on family caregivers may alter the patient's perception or report of pain. Some patients may feel pain more intensely because of the influence of fear, and others may underreport if they are trying to protect family members.
- Several alternative measures are easily taught to patients and caregivers in the home. For example, ice can be made in paper cups and used for a cold massage of a painful area.
- Massage is commonly used for the treatment of chronic pain, especially musculoskeletal pain. Remember a physician's order might be necessary for this type of treatment. Discuss this option with the registered nurse, patient, and caregiver to help determine if this intervention is appropriate for your patient.

ETHICAL CONSIDERATIONS DISCUSSION

This is a complex case. In addition to looking at professional ethical obligations as dictated by her regulatory body, we also have to consider Kathy's personal values. There may be a conflict. Kathy may believe that life is valuable and worth preserving at any cost, and that the administration of a medication that will shorten life or even precipitate a death cannot be an activity that she can become involved in. Her beliefs about beneficence and nonmaleficence may prohibit her from taking many jobs where end-of-life issues are part of the daily routine (such as abortion clinics, palliative care units, long-term care units, and emergency rooms).

ETHICAL CONSIDERATIONS DISCUSSION—cont'd

If Kathy has moral objections to administering what she considers to be a lethal dose of medication, she should seek out her supervisor and explain her difficulty with the order. She may be able to withdraw from assisting with or performing procedures that are against her personal moral values. The supervisor may choose to administer the medication herself or to pursue alternate outcomes, such as contacting the palliative care team or an alternate physician if possible. Kathy might also consider talking with the physician or forming a group on the unit to discuss the issues and develop some unit guidelines for such cases. The case could be referred to the hospital ethics committee for guidance. It is important to remember the intent of the order. Was the intent in this case to relieve pain or to shorten life?

SUGGESTED ANSWERS TO CRITICAL THINKING

■ *Mrs. Smithers and Mr. Brown*

It is important to accept both patients' pain reports. Assessment should be based on what the patient says rather than what is observed. Each patient copes with his or her pain in a unique way, and the nurse cannot judge whether one is in more pain than the other.

■ *Mrs. Zales*

Mrs. Zales may have been tolerant to opioids because of her need for medication for chronic pain during the past year. For this reason, she needed more medication than a nontolerant patient who does not usually use opioids. Also, the belief that promethazine and other phenothiazines potentiate opioids is a myth. They do cause increased levels of sedation and may limit the amount of opioid that can be given safely. IM injections are not recommended because they are painful, absorption is not predictable, and there is a delay between injection and relief. A more rational approach to Mrs. Zales' pain management would have been regular pain assessment with ATC treatment until the pain began to subside. If her pain level had been better controlled, she might have been discharged on oral analgesics without the delay.

■ *Mrs. Shepard*

1. Pain medication is most effective when given on a routine schedule around the clock to avoid breakthrough pain. Mrs. Shepard's epidural infusion should continue to relieve her pain for a time, up to several hours after it is discontinued, depending on the medication used. The oral medication is most effective when given at the time the epidural is stopped so that it is taking effect as the epidural effects wear off. See Box 10.3 (*Gerontological Issues*) for special considerations for the older patient.
2. Pain prevents patients from moving freely. Postoperative complications such as retained pulmonary secretions and ileus can occur when patients are immobile. Effective pain management can help prevent these complications.
3. If she takes a dose every 3 hours, then she will receive eight doses in 24 hours: 500 mg × 8 = 4000 mg or 4 g, which is the maximum safe dose. Recall that elderly patients metabolize and excrete medications more slowly than younger patients. If she will need the hydrocodone/acetaminophen for more than a few days, it would be wise to consult with the physician about giving the opioid and acetaminophen separately.
4. Mrs. Shepard should be instructed about what her role will be when her pain management regimen is altered. Does she have to ask for the pain medication or will it just be brought to her? Patient and family education are vital to success in management of a patient's pain.

■ *Ms. Jackson*

Using an equianalgesic conversion, we can determine whether Ms. Jackson is likely to have good pain relief based on her requirement with the PCA. Her current pain level of 3 shows that the morphine has been effective. Remember that the pump keeps a history of what the patient uses, which is the best indicator of what the patient needs. Ms. Jackson has used 15 mg of morphine during the past 6 hours. An equianalgesic dose of Tylenol with codeine No. 3 would be almost 200 mg of codeine, but only 30 to 60 mg has been ordered. In addition, if Ms. Jackson takes enough Tylenol with codeine No. 3 to get 200 mg of codeine, she will receive a dangerous dose of both the codeine and the acetaminophen. The physician needs to be contacted for different analgesic orders.

■ *Mr. Sebastian*

1. $\dfrac{5\text{ mg}}{} \Big| \dfrac{1\text{ grain}}{60\text{ mg}} \Big| \dfrac{1\text{ mL}}{\text{grains } 1/6} = 0.5\text{ mL}$
2. Home instruction regarding around-the-clock administration of pain medication is indicated, as well as effects and side effects to report. He will also need to implement measures to prevent constipation.
3. MS Contin, a long-acting form of morphine, may be an option for Mr. Sebastian, along with an immediate-release preparation for breakthrough pain. Also, information about what to do and whom to contact if pain becomes unmanageable is necessary to help prevent readmissions to the hospital.

REVIEW QUESTIONS

1. A patient is walking up and down the hall and visiting with other patients. He is laughing and joking. He approaches the nurse's station, asks for his pain shot, and reports that his pain is 6 on a scale of 0 to 10. Based on McCaffery's definition of pain, which of the following assumptions by the nurse is most likely correct?
   a. The patient is not really in pain but just wants his medication.
   b. The patient is having pain at a level of 6 on a scale of 0 to 10.
   c. The patient is in minimal pain and should receive a pill instead of a shot.
   d. The patient is in pain but does not need his pain medication yet.

2. A patient with terminal cancer has been requiring 5 mg of IV morphine every 1 to 2 hours to control pain, yet is engrossed in a movie on television and appears to be in no pain. Which of the following explanations of this behavior is most likely correct?
   a. Denial of pain is common in patients with cancer.
   b. The cancer treatment is working and the pain is improving.
   c. The patient is hiding the pain in order to finish watching the movie undisturbed.
   d. Distraction can be an effective treatment for pain when used with appropriate drug treatments.

3. Which patient is showing tolerance to opioid analgesics?
   a. The patient who requests opioid analgesics frequently because of severe acute pain
   b. The patient who refuses opioid analgesics because of fear of addiction
   c. The patient who needs increasing doses of opioids to achieve the same level of pain relief
   d. The patient who requests opioid analgesics even when not in pain in order to feel euphoric

4. A patient has incisional pain following total hip replacement surgery. Which of the following types of pain is the patient experiencing?
   a. Nociceptive
   b. Neuropathic
   c. Chronic nonmalignant
   d. Suffering

5. With which type of pain is the patient least likely to present with outward signs such as moaning or changes in vital signs?
   a. Acute pain
   b. Chronic nonmalignant pain
   c. Cancer pain

6. Which of the following methods is the most reliable way to assess the severity of a patient's pain?
   a. Ask the patient to describe the pain.
   b. Observe the patient for physical signs of pain such as moaning or grimacing.
   c. Ask the patient to rate his or her pain using a valid assessment scale.
   d. Ask a family member to rate the patient's pain.

7. According to the World Health Organization's analgesic ladder, at what point in a patient's pain experience is it appropriate to use adjuvant treatments? **Select all that apply.**
   a. In addition to analgesics for early, mild pain
   b. As an alternative to analgesics for mild to moderate pain
   c. As an alternative to analgesics for severe pain
   d. In addition to analgesics for pain that is persistent despite treatment
   e. In addition to analgesics for pain that is growing increasingly more severe

8. A patient is hospitalized following a motor vehicle accident. He has multiple orthopedic injuries and is in acute pain. He has an order for morphine 6 mg IV every 4 hours as needed. He can also have a nonopioid oral analgesic every 4 hours as needed. To reduce the risk of adverse effects and maintain an acceptable level of sedation and pain control, which of the following analgesic schedules will be most effective?
   a. Offer the opioid every 4 hours.
   b. Tell him to put on his light when he feels pain, and give the drugs immediately when he requests them.
   c. Give both the IV opioid and the PO nonopioid every 4 hours around the clock.
   d. Alternate the IV analgesic with the nonopioid oral analgesic.

9. Mr. Lawrence is an 88-year-old man admitted with a broken hip after a fall. He has an order for meperidine 50 to 75 mg IM every 4 hr prn for pain. As his nurse, which of the following actions should you take?
   a. Give the meperidine every 4 hours around the clock.
   b. Offer the meperidine every 6 hours because you know that his liver and kidney function may be diminished.
   c. Administer an NSAID with the meperidine for added pain relief.
   d. Talk to the RN or physician about getting an order for a different analgesic.

REVIEW QUESTIONS—cont'd

10. A patient is started on gabapentin (Neurontin) 300 mg by mouth three times daily for chronic nerve pain related to diabetic neuropathy. Which instruction should the nurse provide?
    a. "Take the medication at the first sign of any pain, up to three times daily."
    b. "Take one capsule every eight hours continuously to keep the pain under control."
    c. "Take the medication only when you need it, to prevent becoming addicted."
    d. "Take one capsule three times a day, then stop it when the pain is under control."

11. A nurse receives an order to administer 1 mL of sterile normal saline solution IM to a patient suspected of opioid abuse. Which response by the nurse is appropriate first?
    a. Administer the saline and carefully document the patient's response in the medical record.
    b. Administer the saline but inform the patient exactly what it is and why it was ordered.
    c. Refuse to administer the medication and inform the physician that the order is inappropriate.
    d. Share concerns about the order with the supervisor and explain why the nurse cannot in good conscience administer the saline.

12. A nurse needs to administer morphine 10 mg IM. It is supplied as grains ¼ per mL. How many milliliters should the nurse prepare for injection?
    Answer: _________ mL

References

American Pain Society. (n.d.). *Definitions related to the use of opioids for the treatment of pain.* Retrieved May 30, 2009, from http://www.ampainsoc.org/advocacy/opioids2.htm

Federico, F. (2007). Preventing harm from high-alert medications. *Joint Commission Journal on Quality and Patient Safety, 33*(9), 537–542.

Ferrell, B. R., & Coyle, N. (2008). The nature of suffering and the goals of nursing. *Oncology Nursing Forum, 35*(2), 241–247.

Flaherty, E. (2008). Using pain-rating scales with older adults. *American Journal of Nursing, 108*(6), 40–48.

International Association for the Study of Pain. (n.d.). Retrieved May 30, 2009, from http://www.iasp-pain.org

Kurtzman, E. T. (2008). Pain diaries. *American Journal of Nursing, 108*(6), 36–39.

McCaffery, M., & Pasero, C. (1999). *Pain: Clinical manual* (2nd ed.). St. Louis: Mosby.

Mularski, R. A., White-Chu, F., Overbay, D., et al. (2006). Measuring pain as the 5th vital sign does not improve quality of pain management. *Journal of General Internal Medicine, 21*(6), 607–612.

11

Nursing Care of Patients with Cancer

LUCY L. COLO AND
JANICE L. BRADFORD

KEY TERMS

alopecia (AL-oh-PEE-she-ah)
anemia (uh-NEE-mee-yah)
anorexia (AN-oh-REK-see-ah)
benign (bee-NINE)
biopsy (BY-opp-see)
cancer (KAN-sir)
carcinogen (kar-SIN-oh-jen)
chemotherapy (KEE-moh-THAIR-uh-pee)
contact inhibition (kon-takt in-huh-BIH-shun)
cytotoxic (SY-toh-TOCK-sik)
desquamation (dee-skwa-MAY-shun)
in situ (in-SY-too)
leukopenia (LOO-koh-PEE-nee-ah)
malignant (muh-LIG-nunt)
metastasis (muh-TASS-tuh-sis)
mucositis (MYOO-koh-SY-tis)
nadir (NAY-dur)
neoplasm (NEE-oh-PLAZ-uhm)
neutropenia (noo-troh-PEE-nee-ah)
oncology (on-CAW-luh-gee)
oncovirus (ON-koh-VY-russ)
palliation (pal-ee-AY-shun)
radiation therapy (RAY-dee-AY-shun THAIR-uh-pee)
stomatitis (STOH-mah-TY-tis)
thrombocytopenia (THROM-boh-SY-toh-PEE-nee-ah)
tumor (TOO-merr)
vesicant (VESS-ih-kent)
xerostomia (ZEE-roh-STOH-mee-ah)

QUESTIONS TO GUIDE YOUR READING

1. What are the normal structures and functions of the cell?
2. What changes occur in the cell when it becomes malignant?
3. Which medications are commonly used as chemotherapeutic agents?
4. What are the special nursing needs of the patient receiving chemotherapy or radiation therapy?
5. Which data should you collect when caring for a patient with cancer?
6. What nursing interventions are used for common oncological emergencies?
7. How will you know if your nursing interventions have been effective?
8. What is the role of hospice in providing care for patients with advanced cancer?

REVIEW OF NORMAL ANATOMY AND PHYSIOLOGY OF CELLS

Cells are the smallest living structural and functional subunits of the body. Although human cells vary in size, shape, and certain metabolic activities, they have many characteristics in common.

Cell Structure

Human cells have a cell membrane, cytosol, cell organelles, and, with the exception of mature red blood cells, a nucleus. Mature red blood cells don't have nuclei. Each cell structure has a specific and vital function. The cell membrane forms the outer boundary of the cell and is made of phospholipids, proteins, and cholesterol. Proteins serve four different purposes: (1) some are channels or transporters that permit movement of materials, (2) some are enzymes that catalyze reactions, (3) some are receptor sites for hormones that trigger a cell's activity, and (4) some are antigens that identify the cell as belonging in the body.

A cell membrane is selectively permeable, meaning that not all substances pass through equally. The lipids in the membrane permit the diffusion of lipid-soluble materials into or out of the cell. Materials may enter or leave a cell in a variety of ways, such as diffusion, osmosis, active transport, pinocytosis, and phagocytosis.

Cytosol and Cell Organelles

Cytosol is a watery solution of minerals, gases, and organic molecules found between the cell membrane and the nucleus. Chemical reactions (such as the synthesis of adenosine triphosphate [ATP] in glycolysis) take place in the cytosol. Cell organelles, shown in Figure 11.1, are subcellular structures with specific functions. Many cell organelles are found in the cytosol.

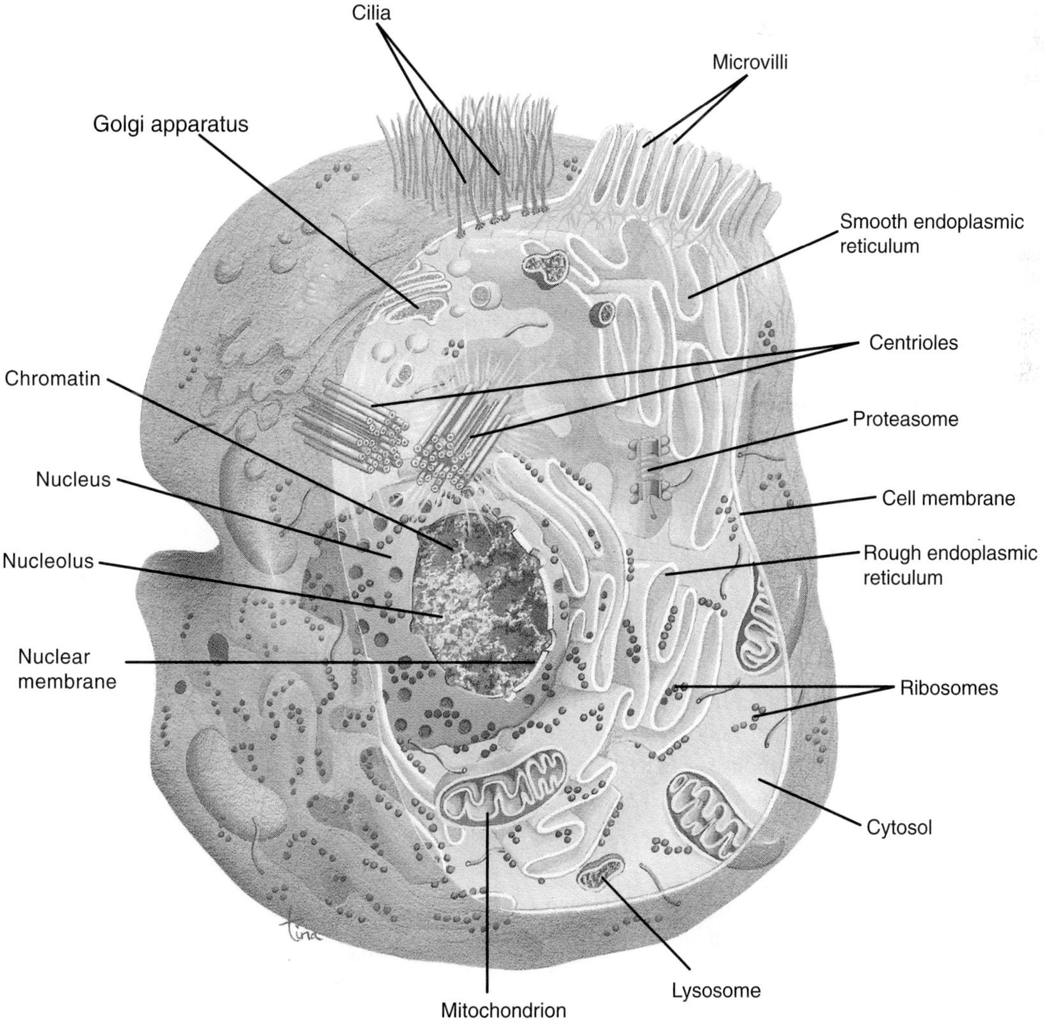
Cilia
Microvilli
Golgi apparatus
Smooth endoplasmic reticulum
Centrioles
Chromatin
Proteasome
Nucleus
Cell membrane
Nucleolus
Rough endoplasmic reticulum
Nuclear membrane
Ribosomes
Cytosol
Lysosome
Mitochondrion

FIGURE 11.1 Schematic diagram of a typical human cell. (From Scanlon, V. C., & Sanders, T. [2007]. *Essentials of anatomy and physiology* [5th ed.]. Philadelphia: F. A. Davis.)

Nucleus

The nucleus of a cell is surrounded by a double-layered nuclear membrane with many pores. Inside the nucleus are one or more nucleoli and the deoxyribonucleic acid (DNA) of the cell.

A nucleolus is a small sphere made of DNA, ribonucleic acid (RNA), and protein. The nucleoli form a type of RNA called ribosomal RNA, which is part of the cell organelle called the ribosome and is involved in protein synthesis.

Because it contains the DNA, the nucleus is the control center of the cell. DNA and protein make the 46 chromosomes of a human cell. DNA carries the genetic code for the characteristics and activities of the cell as specific regions called genes; a gene is the code for one protein. Not all of the genes in a particular cell are active—only those needed for the proteins required to carry out their specific functions. These proteins may be structural, such as the collagen of connective tissue, or functional, such as the hemoglobin of red blood cells. Important functional proteins are the enzymes that catalyze the specific reactions characteristic of each type of cell.

Genetic Code and Protein Synthesis

The genetic code of DNA is the code for the amino acid sequences needed to synthesize a cell's proteins. A complementary copy of the DNA's gene is made by a molecule called messenger RNA (mRNA). The mRNA then moves to the cytoplasm of the cell and attaches to the ribosomes. Transfer RNA (tRNA) molecules bring the necessary amino acids to the proper places on the mRNA molecule, and enzymes of the ribosomes catalyze the formation of peptide bonds to link the amino acids into the primary structure of a protein.

As with any complex process, mistakes are possible. Should there be a mistake in the DNA code, the process of protein synthesis may go on anyway, but the resulting protein will not function normally; this is the basis for genetic diseases. DNA mistakes acquired during life are called *mutations*. A mutation is any change in the DNA code. Ultraviolet rays or exposure to certain chemicals may cause structural changes in the DNA code. These changes may kill the affected cells or may irreversibly alter their function. Such altered cells may become malignant, being unable to function normally. These cells actively replicate the mutated DNA during division, creating a mass of faulty cells. This is the basis of some forms of cancer, which is a general term for many different types of malignant growths.

Mitosis

Mitosis is the process by which a cell reproduces itself. One cell, after its 46 chromosomes have replicated, divides into two cells, each with a membrane, cytosol, and organelles from the original cell and a complete set of chromosomes. Mitosis is necessary for the growth of the body and the replacement of dead or damaged cells. Some cells are capable of mitosis and others are not. Cells of the epidermis of the skin undergo mitosis continuously to replace the superficial cells that are constantly worn off the skin surface. The same is true of cells that line the stomach and intestines. Cells in the red bone marrow also divide frequently; red blood cells have a fixed life span (about 120 days) and must be replaced. Some cells seem to be capable of only a limited number of divisions, and when that limit has been reached, the cells die and are not replaced.

Other cells do not undergo mitosis to any great extent after birth. Nerve cells (neurons) are unable to divide (except for in the hippocampus), and muscle cells have very limited mitotic capability. When such cells are lost through injury or disease, the loss of their functions in the individual is usually permanent.

Cell Cycle

The cell cycle involves a series of changes through which a cell progresses, starting from the time it develops until it reproduces itself. The duration of the cell's life, the time it takes for mitosis to occur, the growth ratio (percentage of cycling cells), the frequency of cell loss, and the doubling time (the time for a **tumor**—an abnormal mass—to double its size) are important concepts related to tumor growth and treatment strategies.

Cells can occupy three places in the cell cycle: cells that are actively dividing, cells that leave the cycle after a certain point and die, and cells that temporarily leave the cycle and remain inactive until reentry into the cycle. Inactive cells continue to synthesize RNA and protein (Fig. 11.2).

Cells and Tissues

A tissue is a group of like cells with the same structure and function. The four groups of human tissues are epithelial, connective, muscle, and nervous tissue.

Epithelial tissues form coverings and linings throughout the body. Often the cells are capable of mitosis, and damage to the tissue may be repaired. The healing of a cut to the skin is a typical example. Epithelial tissue also forms glands.

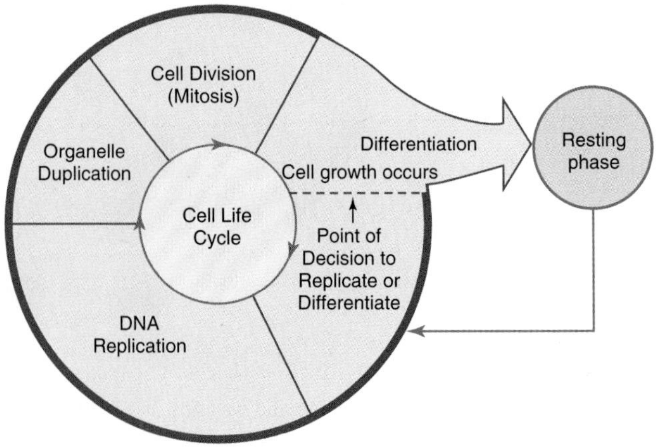
Cell Division
(Mitosis)
Organelle
Duplication
Differentiation
Cell growth occurs
Resting
phase
Cell Life
Cycle
Point of
Decision to
Replicate or
Differentiate
DNA
Replication

FIGURE 11.2 Cell cycle.

The many types of connective tissues have varied functions. For example, blood is a connective tissue involved in the transportation of materials throughout the body. Fibrous connective tissue, made mostly of the protein collagen, forms strong membranes such as those around muscles, attaching structures such as ligaments and tendons and the dermis of the skin. Bone and cartilage support connective tissues. Adipose connective tissue stores fat as potential energy. Some kinds of connective tissue cells are capable of mitosis.

The three kinds of muscle tissue are skeletal muscle, smooth muscle, and cardiac muscle. Skeletal muscle tissue makes up the voluntary muscles attached to the skeleton. Smooth muscle is found in visceral walls such as in the stomach and intestines, arteries and veins, the bronchial tubes, and the uterus. Cardiac muscle forms the walls of the heart. As mentioned, the cells of muscle tissue have little ability to reproduce themselves.

Nervous tissue is made of neurons and supporting neuroglial cells. Although mature neurons are not capable of mitosis, many neuroglia are capable. It is the neuroglia, not neurons, that usually form the tumors that develop in the central nervous system.

INTRODUCTION TO CANCER CONCEPTS

Oncology is the branch of medicine dealing with tumors. Oncology nursing is also called cancer nursing; it is an important component of medical-surgical nursing care. Cancer is second only to heart disease in mortality rates in the United States. The American Cancer Society (ACS) reports that an estimated 10 million Americans alive today have a history of cancer. Box 11.1 lists some helpful cancer resources.

Box 11.1

Cancer Resources

American Cancer Society
800-227-2345
www.cancer.org
CancerCare
800-813-4673
www.cancercare.org
www.lungcancer.org
National Cancer Institute
301-496-8531
www.nci.nih.gov
http://cis.nci.nih.gov
Oncology Nursing Society
412-921-7373
www.ons.org

Early accounts of cancer date back to the 17th century B.C. Documentation of the benefits of early cancer detection and treatment exist from the beginning of the 19th century. Today, microscopic technology and genetic engineering provide physicians with a better understanding of tumor growth and cell activity and a means for early cancer detection and intervention.

Benign Tumors

Cells that reproduce abnormally result in **neoplasms**, or tumors. *Neoplasm* is a term that combines the Greek word *neo,* meaning "new," and *plasia,* meaning "form," to suggest new tissue growth. The new growth results in enlargement of tissue and the formation of an abnormal mass. Not all neoplasms contain cancer cells; however, a neoplastic cell is responsible for producing a tumor and is a lively growing cell. A neoplastic growth is very difficult to detect until it contains about 500 cells and is about 1 cm in diameter.

A **benign** tumor is defined as a cluster of cells that is not normal to the body but is noncancerous. Benign tumors grow more slowly than malignant ones and have cells that are the same as the original tissue. An organ containing a benign tumor usually continues to function normally.

Cancer

Cancer is a group of cells that grows out of control, taking over the function of the affected organ. Cancer cells are described as poorly constructed, loosely formed, and without organization. A simplistic definition is "confused cell." An organ with a cancerous tumor eventually ceases to function. **Malignant**, a term often used to describe cancer, means that the tumor resists treatment and tends to worsen and threaten life. A comparison of benign and malignant tumors is found in Table 11.1.

NURSING CARE TIP

Teach patients and families that cancer is not contagious.

Pathophysiology

Cancer is not one disease, but many diseases with different causes, manifestations, treatments, and prognoses. There are more than 100 different types of cancer caused by mutation of cellular genes. Cancer takes on the characteristics of the cell it mutates and then takes on the characteristics of the mutation. Growth-regulating signals in the cells' surrounding environment are ignored as the abnormal cell growth

• WORD • BUILDING •

oncology: onco—mass + logy—word, reason
neoplasm: neo—new + plasm—form

TABLE 11.1 COMPARING BENIGN AND MALIGNANT TUMORS

	Benign	Malignant
Growth rate	Typically slow expansion	Often rapid growth; malignant cells infiltrate surrounding tissue
Cell features	Typical of the tissue of origin	Atypical in varying degrees compared to the tissue of origin; altered cell membrane; contains tumor-specific antigens
Tissue damage	Minor	Often causes necrosis and ulceration of tissue
Metastasis	Not seen; remains localized at site of origin	Often spreads to form tumors in other parts of the body
Recurrence after treatment	Seldom recurs after surgical removal	Recurrence can be seen after surgical removal and following radiation and chemotherapy
Related terminology	Hyperplasia, polyp, benign neoplasia	Cancer, malignancy, malignant neoplasia
Prognosis	Not injurious unless location causes pressure or obstruction to vital organs	Death if uncontrolled

increases. Normal cells are limited to about 50 to 60 divisions before they die. Cancer cells do not have a division limit and are considered to be immortal.

The progression from a normal cell to a malignant cell follows a pattern of mutation, defective division and abnormal growth cycles, and defective cell communication. Cell mutation occurs when a sudden change affects the chromosomes, causing the new cell to differ from its parent. The malignant cell's enzymes destroy the gluelike substance found between normal cells, which disrupts the transfer of information used for normal cell structure.

Cancer cells also lack **contact inhibition**. This is a property of normal cells in which contact by the cell with another cell or tissue signals them to stop dividing. Because cancer cells do not possess contact inhibition, they continue to divide and invade surrounding tissues.

Etiology

Cancer cell growth and reproduction involve a two-step process. The first step in cancer growth is called *initiation.* Initiation causes an alteration in the genetic structure of the cell (DNA). Cell alteration is associated with exposure to a **carcinogen**, which is a substance or agent that increases the risk of cancer. The cellular change primes the cell to become cancerous.

Promotion is the second step of cancer cell growth. It occurs after repeated exposure to carcinogens causes the initiated cells to mutate. During the promotion step, a tumor forms from mutated cell reproduction.

A healthy immune system can often destroy cancer cells before they replicate and become a tumor. It is important to remember that any substance that weakens or alters the immune system puts the individual at risk for cell mutation. Medical researchers support the theory that cancer is a symptom of a weakened immune system.

Risk Factors

Increased risk of cancer is linked to many environmental factors. An evaluation of cancer begins with assessment of well-known risk factors such as specific viruses; exposure to radiation, chemicals, and irritants; genetics; diet; hormones; and general immunity. Certain racial and ethnic groups also are at higher risk for some types of cancer (Box 11.2, *Cultural Considerations*).

VIRUSES. Certain viruses, such as the **oncoviruses** (RNA-type viruses), are linked to cancer in humans. A retrovirus is an enzyme produced by RNA tumor viruses and is found in human leukemia cells.

The Epstein-Barr virus (EBV), which causes infectious mononucleosis, is associated with Burkitt's lymphoma. Herpes simplex virus 2 has been associated with cervical and penile cancers. Human papillomavirus (HPV) is associated with genital warts and causes of cervical cancer in women. Vaccination against HPV (Gardasil) is recommended for girls age 11 to 12. Chronic hepatitis B is linked with liver cancer.

RADIATION. There is an increased incidence of cancer in persons exposed to prolonged or large amounts of radiation. Ionizing radiation involving ultraviolet rays such as sunlight, x-rays, and alpha, beta, and gamma rays plays a major role in promoting leukemia and skin cancers, primarily melanomas.

Persons exposed to radioactive materials in large doses, such as a radiation leak or an atomic bomb, are at risk for leukemia and breast, bone, lung, and thyroid cancer. Controlled **radiation therapy** is used to treat cancer patients by destroying rapidly dividing cancer cells. Radiation can also damage normal cells. The decision to use radiation is made after careful evaluation of the tumor's location and vulnerability to other treatments.

CHEMICALS. Chemicals are present in air, water, soil, food, drugs, and tobacco smoke. Chemical carcinogens are

• WORD • BUILDING •

carcinogen: karkinos—cancer, crab + genesis—birth
oncovirus: onco—mass + virus

Box 11.2

Cultural Considerations

Many racial and ethnic groups in the United States have high rates of cancer. Although risk factors for the development of specific cancers are similar, barriers to prevention and nursing strategies to reduce risk factors vary among ethnicities.

Europeans

Foreign-born and first-generation white men from Norway, Sweden, and Germany have an increased risk of stomach cancer. This suggests an interrelation among ethnic, geographical, and dietary risk factors. Assessing for these data among these populations may assist in the diagnostic process.

Recent Eastern European immigrants may be at risk for thyroid cancer and leukemia because of the current industrial pollution and radiation exposure from the Chernobyl nuclear disaster in the former USSR in 1986. Some contamination occurred in Estonia, Latvia, Lithuania, and Poland. This may constitute a health hazard and may affect both recent immigrants and visitors to these countries. It is essential for health care providers to carefully screen individuals for these cancers.

African Americans

Common cancer sites among African Americans include the prostate, breast, lung, colon, rectum, cervix, pancreas, and esophagus. Because African Americans are overrepresented in the working class, they experience increased exposure to hazardous occupations. For example, African American men are at a higher risk for developing cancer related to their work in the steel and tire industries and in factories manufacturing chemicals and pesticides. They have the highest overall cancer rate, the highest overall mortality rate, and their 5-year survival rate is 30% lower than that of European Americans. In general, African Americans report later for treatment than European Americans. Colon tumors may be deeper in African Americans, making detection on digital examination more difficult. Poverty, a diet high in fat and low in fiber, and lower levels of thiamine, riboflavin, vitamins A and C, and iron may increase cancer risk among African Americans. Additionally, cigarette smoking, inner city living with pollution, obesity, and alcohol consumption increase their risk for developing cancer.

Lack of access to medical care acts as a barrier to prevention among African Americans. Survival, not prevention, is the priority for some. Additional barriers include a lack of cancer risk teaching and detection in some African American communities, lack of health insurance, and little stigma attached to alcohol consumption and smoking. Strong family ties encourage seeking health care advice from family members before professionals.

Primary strategies for preventing cancer and increasing survival among African Americans include using African American professionals as speakers in community activities, using church-based information dissemination, providing forums in African American communities, and addressing smoking advertisements in African American communities. Additional strategies include involving granny healers and ministers, changing food preparation practices and amounts rather than changing cultural food habits, involving extended family members in educational campaigns, and using high-profile African Americans leaders in media campaigns.

Hispanics

Hispanic populations in the United States have an increased incidence for some types of cancer. Cervical cancer is increased among Central and South American women. Pancreatic, liver, and gallbladder cancer is increased among Mexican Americans. Many Mexican Americans are less aware of the early warning signs of cancer; many are more fearful of getting cancer than the general public; and many work in mining, factories using chemicals, and farming using pesticides.

Barriers to preventive health care among many Hispanics include high poverty rates, low educational rates, a preference for health care providers who understand Spanish, a preference for health care information presented in Spanish, a delay in seeking treatments for symptoms, and using lay healers as a first choice in health care. Additionally, many have a fear of surgical intervention because the body will be exposed to air, and many have decreased access to health care. For some, an undocumented immigration status creates a fear of reprisal.

Continued

Box 11.2

Cultural Considerations—cont'd

Nursing approaches effective among Hispanics include educating lay healers regarding cancer prevention and early warning signs of cancer, using bilingual health care providers, using Hispanic health care providers whenever available, using respected Hispanic community leaders in educational programs, presenting videos in Spanish using Hispanic actors, educating the entire family because of close family networks, and connecting with Hispanic community churches, restaurants, and stores. Additionally, the nurse can use the 1-800-4-CANCER telephone number for Spanish translation and counseling, become involved with Hispanic community movements, and provide information in community and regional Hispanic newspapers and community publications.

Asians and Pacific Islanders

Cervical, liver, lung, stomach, multiple myeloma, esophageal, pancreatic, and nasopharyngeal cancers are higher among Chinese Americans. Chinese American women have a 20% higher rate of pancreatic cancer. High rates of stomach and liver cancer in Korea predispose recent immigrants to these conditions. Thus, the nurse needs to assess and teach newer immigrants regarding these types of cancer.

High rates of stomach, breast, colon, and rectal cancer common among Japanese people may be related to the high sodium content of the Japanese diet, a genetic predisposition, consumption of salted fish and contaminated grain, hepatitis B, smoking, vitamin A deficiency, low vitamin C intake, chronic esophagitis, and pulmonary sequelae of cigarette smoking. Various barriers to prevention exist: Prevention models are not native to their culture; they may lack trust in Western medicine; they have decreased access to health care; some are unable to speak the English language; and for some, an undocumented immigration status creates a fear of reprisal.

Nursing approaches to improve cancer risk prevention among Asians and Pacific Islanders include education about prevention versus acute care practice, educating native healers, involvement in the community with respected native leaders, videos and literature in the native language, and incorporating native healing practices such as traditional Chinese medicine.

Arab Americans

Arab Americans are mainly at risk for lung cancer and other cancers related to smoking. Although many Arab Americans are Islamic and Islamic beliefs discourage tobacco use as well as alcohol or drug use, cigarette smoking continues to be a risk behavior among this population. Arab American women are considered very modest and rates of breast cancer screening and cervical Pap smears are low. Arab Americans tend to lead a sedentary lifestyle with high fat intake, which places them at higher risk for cardiovascular disease as well as certain cancers.

Nursing approaches with this population include promoting awareness and primary prevention strategies. Nurses should encourage cancer screenings and smoking cessation. Because of their modesty, nurses should attempt to ensure women are given same-sex caregivers to promote breast and cervical cancer screenings.

Native Americans

Native American populations have an increased risk for skin, pancreatic, gallbladder, liver, and prostate cancer. Risk factors for the development of cancer include obesity, a diet high in fat, high rates of alcohol consumption, and high rates of smoking. Barriers to prevention include a lack of Native American health care providers, health care providers' unfamiliarity with Native American cultures, lack of financial resources, and a lack of integration of Native American healing practices into prevention practices.

Nursing approaches to decrease cancer risk prevention among Native American populations include the following: incorporate prevention into Native American healing practices; educate Native American lay healers regarding cancer prevention practices; work with tribal community leaders; respect modesty, gender roles, and tribal customs; work with the Indian Health Service and Bureau of Indian Affairs; encourage traditional customs of physical fitness and exercise; and encourage dietary portion control and healthy food preparation practices instead of changing cultural food habits.

implicated as triggering mechanisms in malignant tumor development. Length of exposure time and degree of exposure intensity to chemical carcinogens are associated with risk for cancer development.

Smoking accounts for 87% of lung cancer worldwide (American Cancer Society, 2008a). Chemical agents, such as those in tobacco, are more toxic when used with alcohol. Alcohol and tobacco are the most frequent causes of cancers of the mouth and throat. Chemicals used in manufacturing, such as vinyl chloride, are associated with liver cancer.

IRRITANTS. Chronic irritation or inflammation caused by irritants such as snuff or pipe smoke often cause cancer in local areas. Nevi (moles) that are chronically irritated by clothing, especially clothing contaminated by chemical residue, may become malignant. Asbestos found in temperature and sound insulation has been proven to cause a particularly destructive type of lung cancer.

GENETICS. Genetics plays a large part in cancer formation. Certain breast cancers are linked to a specific gene mutation. Skin, colon, ovarian, and prostate cancers have a genetic tendency. People with Down syndrome (a chromosomal abnormality) have a higher risk of developing acute leukemia.

DIET. Diet is a large factor in both cause and prevention of malignancies. People who eat high-fat, low-fiber diets are more prone to develop colon cancers. Diets high in fiber reduce the risk of colon cancer. High-fat diets are linked to breast cancer in women and prostate cancer in men. Consumption of large amounts of pickled, smoked, and charbroiled foods has been linked with esophageal and stomach cancers. A diet low in vitamins A, C, and E is associated with cancers of the lungs, esophagus, mouth, larynx, cervix, and breast.

HORMONES. Hormonal agents that disturb the balance of the body may also promote cancer. Long-term use of the female hormone estrogen is associated with cancer of the breast, uterus, ovaries, cervix, and vagina. It has been found that children born of mothers who took diethylstilbestrol (DES) during pregnancy have an increased incidence of reproductive cancers. DES is a synthetic hormone with estrogen-like properties used in the past to prevent miscarriage.

Tumors of the breast and uterus are tested for estrogen or progesterone influence. If a breast tumor is malignant, the tumor is tested and treatment varies depending on whether it is positive for estrogen or progesterone dependence.

IMMUNE FACTORS. A healthy immune system destroys mutant cells quickly on formation. An individual with altered immunity is more susceptible to cancer formation when exposed to small amounts of carcinogens compared to someone with a healthy immune system. Immune system suppression allows malignant cells to develop in large numbers.

Altered immunity is noted in persons with chronic illness and stress. An increased risk of cancer follows a traumatic, stressful period in life, such as the loss of a mate or a job. Failure to decrease stress productively contributes to a higher incidence of chronic illnesses. Thus, a cycle of stress, illness, and increased cancer risk develops. People with acquired immunodeficiency syndrome (AIDS) have a compromised immune system and an increased risk for certain cancers. A decline in the immune system is also noted as the body ages. A weaker immune system contributes to chronic illnesses and cancers associated with the elderly population.

Cancer Classification

Cancers are identified by the tissue affected, speed of cell growth, cell appearance, and location. Neoplasms occurring in the epithelial cells are called carcinomas. *Carcinoma* is the most common type of cancer and includes cells of the skin, gastrointestinal system, and lungs (Figs. 11.3 and 11.4). Cancer cells affecting connective tissue, including fat, the sheath that contains nerves, cartilage, muscle, and bone, are called *sarcomas*. *Leukemia* is the term used to describe the abnormal growth of white blood cells. Cancers involving cells of the lymphatic system, lymph nodes, and spleen are called *lymphomas*. See Table 11.2 for cancer types based on origin.

> **LEARNING TIP**
>
> A person's cancer risk is viewed as the balance between exposure and susceptibility to carcinogens.

Spread of Cancer

Neoplastic cells that remain in one area are considered localized, or **in situ**, cancers. These tumors may be difficult to visualize on clinical examination and are detected through microscopic cell examination. In situ tumors are often removed surgically and may require no further treatment. **Metastasis** is the term used to describe the spread of the tumor from the primary site into separate and distant areas.

Metastasis is the stage at which cancer cells acquire invasive behavior characteristics and cause the surrounding tissue to change (Fig. 11.5). Metastasis occurs mainly because cancer cells break away more easily than normal cells and can survive for a time independently from other cells. There are three steps in the formation of a metastasis. Cancer cells are able to (1) invade blood or lymph vessels, (2) move by mechanical means, and (3) lodge and grow in a new location.

• WORD • BUILDING •

in situ: in—in + situ—position

metastasis: meta—beyond + stasis—stand

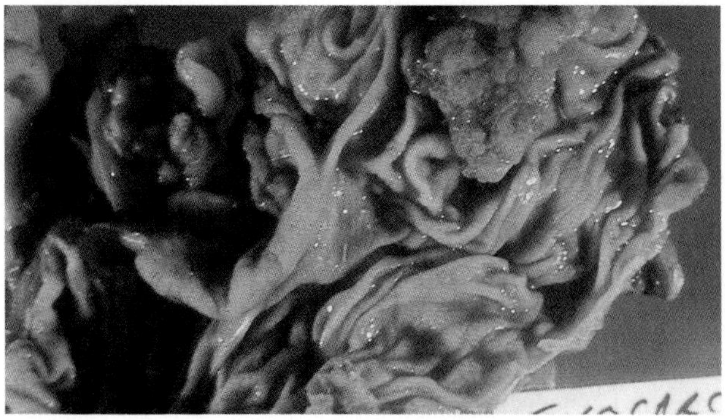

FIGURE 11.3 Adenocarcinoma of the cecum. (Photo courtesy of Dinesh Patel, MD, Medical Oncology, Internal Medicine, Zanesville, OH.)

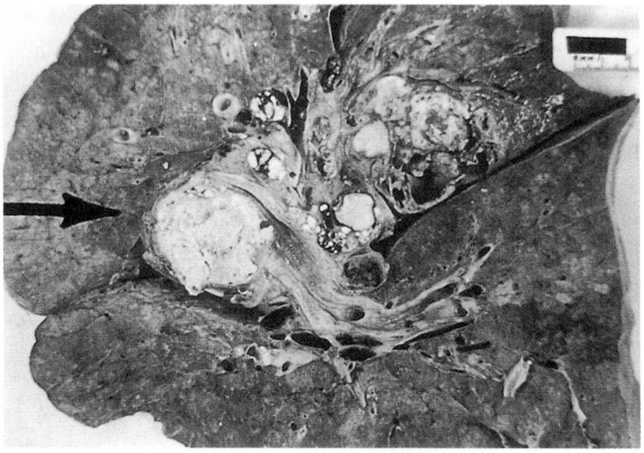

FIGURE 11.4 Lung cancer. (Photo courtesy of Dinesh Patel, MD, Medical Oncology, Internal Medicine, Zanesville, OH.)

Metastatic tumors carry with them the cell characteristics of the original or primary tumor site. As a result, surgeons are able to determine the original tumor site based on metastatic cell characteristics. For example, lung tissue found in the brain suggests a primary lung tumor with metastasis to brain tissue. Common sites of metastasis are the lungs, liver, bones, and brain.

TABLE 11.2 TUMOR DESCRIPTIONS

Tumor Type	Character	Origin
Fibroma	Benign	Connective tissue
Lipoma	Benign	Fat tissue
Carcinoma	Cancerous	Tissue of the skin, glands, and digestive, urinary, and respiratory tract linings
Leukemia	Cancerous	Blood, plasma cells, and bone marrow
Lymphoma	Cancerous	Lymph tissue
Melanoma	Cancerous	Skin cells
Sarcoma	Cancerous	Connective tissue, including bone and muscle

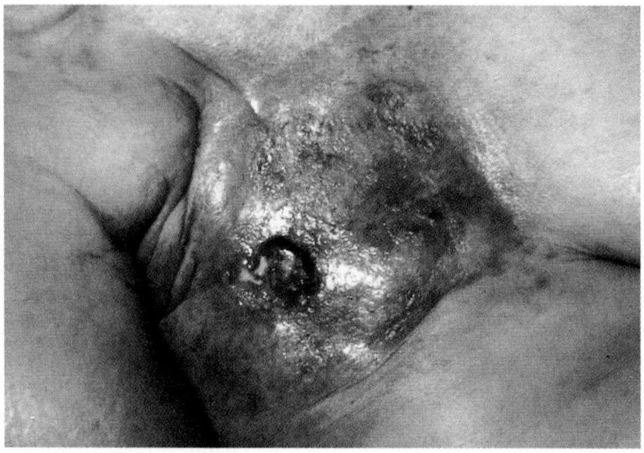

FIGURE 11.5 Invasive metastasis to skin area following mastectomy for breast cancer. (Photo courtesy of Dinesh Patel, MD, Medical Oncology, Internal Medicine, Zanesville, OH.)

Incidence of Cancer

Cancer affects all age groups, although the incidence is higher in people ages 60 to 69. The second highest age group is ages 70 to 79. Men have a higher incidence of cancer than women. Cancer in people over age 60 is thought to occur from a combination of exposure to carcinogens and weakening of the body's immune system.

Some cancers, such as Wilms' tumor of the kidney and acute lymphocytic leukemia, are more common in young people. The cause of tumors in young people is not well understood, but genetic predisposition tends to be a major factor.

The most common type of cancer in adults is skin cancer; it is also considered to be the most preventable. Exposure to ultraviolet radiation (sunlight) increases the risk of skin cancer. Wearing protective clothing and sunscreen can greatly reduce the risk of skin cancer.

Lung cancer has the highest of the cancer mortality rates in both men and women and also is commonly preventable. Cigarette smoking is the main cause, along with air pollution and exposure to radon and other chemicals.

Men have a high incidence of prostate cancer between ages 60 and 79. Cancer of the colon and rectum has been linked to consumption of high-fat, low-fiber diets and ranks as the third highest cancer in men.

The highest incidence of cancer in women is in the breast. Women with a family history of breast cancer have a greater risk than those with no family history. Commercial testing for the oncogene linked with breast cancer is available and marketed for high-risk women, especially those in the Ashkenazi Jewish population. Genetic testing is done through genetic counseling programs, and the cost ranges from $700 to $2400, depending on the geographical region. See Figure 11.6 for estimated new cancer cases and deaths for 2009.

Mortality Rates

Cancer survival rates have improved during the past 30 years and, since the 1990s, the number of cancer deaths has decreased for both men and women. A 5-year period is

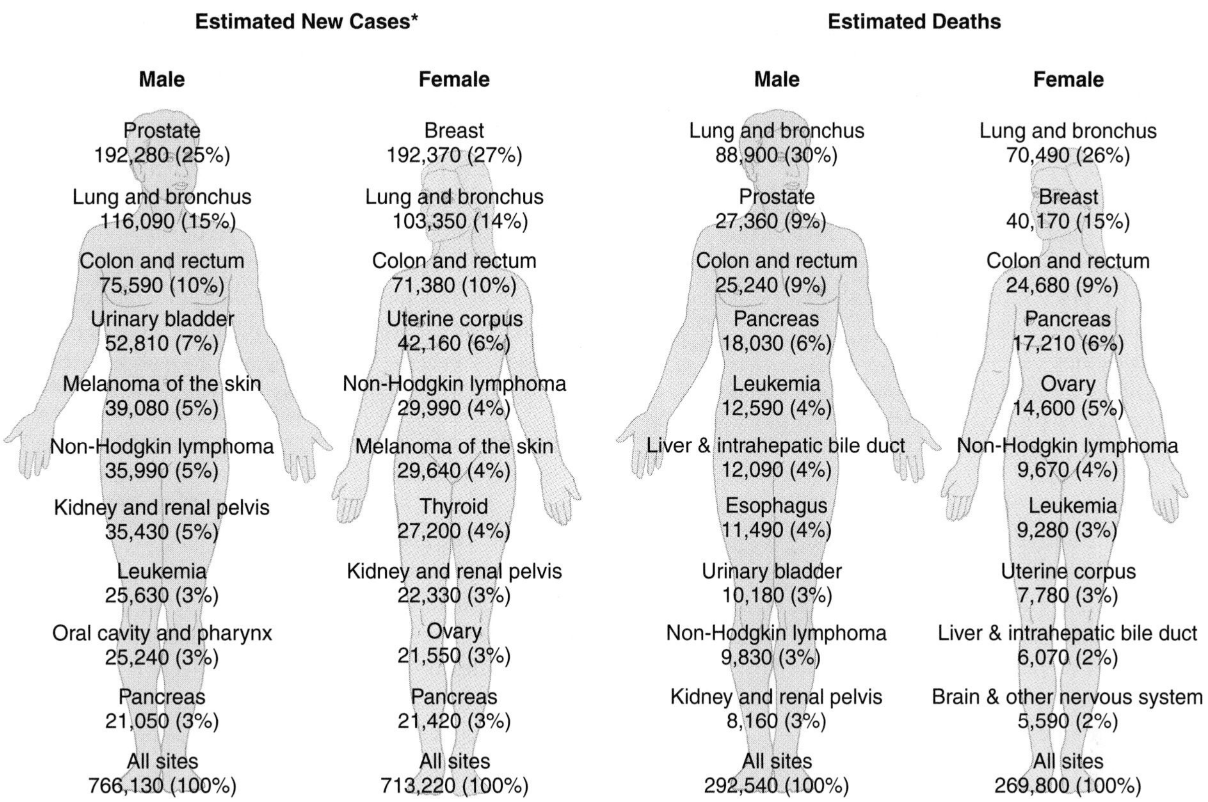

Estimated New Cases*
Male
Prostate
192,280 (25%)
Lung and bronchus
116,090 (15%)
Colon and rectum
75,590 (10%)
Urinary bladder
52,810 (7%)
Melanoma of the skin
39,080 (5%)
Non-Hodgkin lymphoma
35,990 (5%)
Kidney and renal pelvis
35,430 (5%)
Leukemia
25,630 (3%)
Oral cavity and pharynx
25,240 (3%)
Pancreas
21,050 (3%)
All sites
766,130 (100%)
Female
Breast
192,370 (27%)
Lung and bronchus
103,350 (14%)
Colon and rectum
71,380 (10%)
Uterine corpus
42,160 (6%)
Non-Hodgkin lymphoma
29,990 (4%)
Melanoma of the skin
29,640 (4%)
Thyroid
27,200 (4%)
Kidney and renal pelvis
22,330 (3%)
Ovary
21,550 (3%)
Pancreas
21,420 (3%)
All sites
713,220 (100%)
Estimated Deaths
Male
Lung and bronchus
88,900 (30%)
Prostate
27,360 (9%)
Colon and rectum
25,240 (9%)
Pancreas
18,030 (6%)
Leukemia
12,590 (4%)
Liver & intrahepatic bile duct
12,090 (4%)
Esophagus
11,490 (4%)
Urinary bladder
10,180 (3%)
Non-Hodgkin lymphoma
9,830 (3%)
Kidney and renal pelvis
8,160 (3%)
All sites
292,540 (100%)
Female
Lung and bronchus
70,490 (26%)
Breast
40,170 (15%)
Colon and rectum
24,680 (9%)
Pancreas
17,210 (6%)
Ovary
14,600 (5%)
Non-Hodgkin lymphoma
9,670 (4%)
Leukemia
9,280 (3%)
Uterine corpus
7,780 (3%)
Liver & intrahepatic bile duct
6,070 (2%)
Brain & other nervous system
5,590 (2%)
All sites
269,800 (100%)

*Excludes basal and squamous cell skin cancers and in situ carcinoma except urinary bladder.
Note: Percentages do not total 100% because not all cancers are included.

FIGURE 11.6 Estimated new cancer cases and deaths by sex, United States, 2009. (From American Cancer Society [2009]. *Cancer facts and figures, 2009*. Retrieved January 29, 2010, from http://www.cancer.org/downloads/STT/500809web.pdf.)

used to monitor cancer patients' progress following diagnosis and treatment. Survival statistics are based on those who live 5 years in remission. Remission is considered to have occurred when all signs and symptoms of cancer have disappeared, even though there may still be cancer in the body.

For more information about cancer incidence and mortality data, visit the National Cancer Institute website at www.nci.nih.gov or the American Cancer Society at www.cancer.org.

Early Detection and Prevention

Nurses play an important role in preventing and detecting cancer. You can help educate patients about risk factors, self-examination, and cancer screening programs. Early diagnosis and treatment provide time to stop the progression of cancer.

EARLY DETECTION. Regular physical examinations help medical personnel detect early warning signs of cancer. Mammography (a special x-ray of breast tissue used to detect a mass too small for palpation) is recommended every 1 to 2 years in women after age 40 (some sources say after age 50). A clinical breast exam (CBE) is recommended every 3 years for women in their 20s and 30s and annually after age 40 (ACS, 2008b). However, if a woman has a high risk for breast cancer because of family history, the type and frequency of screening should be discussed with her doctor.

Initial Papanicolaou testing (Pap smear) for cervical cancer is currently recommended to begin no later than age 21, and every 1 to 2 years thereafter. After age 30, most women who have had three normal results in a row can be screened every 2 to 3 years, unless risk factors are present. After age 70, a woman who has had three normal Pap tests in a row within the past 10 years can choose to stop screening.

Some women choose not to be screened, even when they have access to health care. Barriers to screening include fear of health care personnel and testing procedures and lack of knowledge. Women who fear cancer but trust their health providers and seek information are more likely to be screened. As a nurse, you can help by developing a trusting relationship and providing information to your female patients.

The ACS considers monthly breast self-examinations to be optional for women and testicular self-exams to be optional for men. ACS guidelines encourage everyone to be familiar with their bodies and to report changes to their care providers. Offer men and women instruction in breast and testicular self-exams if they are interested in doing self-examinations.

The ACS (2008b) recommends one of the following five options to screen for colorectal cancer, beginning at age 50:

- Fecal occult blood test every year using a take-home, multiple sample test, not a digital rectal exam (DRE) in the doctor's office. Screening should begin earlier and take place more often in high-risk people.
- Flexible sigmoidoscopy every 5 years
- Colonoscopy every 10 years
- Double-contrast barium enema every 5 years
- Colonography (virtual colonoscopy using computed tomography) every 5 years.

Before 2009, the ACS recommended annual DRE and prostate-specific antigen (PSA) blood testing for men older than age 50 with a life expectancy of at least 10 years and for younger men at higher risk. More recently, ACS withdrew this recommendation because routine screening has not been shown to prolong lives (ACS, 2008b). It seems reasonable, however, to still offer these tests as options to men in these populations.

GENETIC TESTING. Currently, much attention is directed toward genetic testing and identification of persons at risk for cancer. Genetic testing technology poses both legal and ethical questions concerning confidentiality and insurance cost issues. The cooperation of family members is important because genetic testing is done after a family member has been diagnosed with cancer. Family members may experience a variety of emotions surrounding the increased risk for themselves and their guilt over the role they may have played in increasing the risk for their children.

HEALTHY LIFESTYLE. Promotion of healthy lifestyles, including proper diet and exercise, helps strengthen the immune system and reduce cancer risk. Smoking is the most preventable cause of death from lung cancer, and smoking cessation is the subject of ongoing campaigns by the American Cancer Society. Second-hand smoke contributes to a significant increased risk of lung cancer in nonsmokers as well.

PROTECTANT FOODS. Much research is being done related to diet and cancer risk. A diet poor in folate, a B vitamin, can lead to development of cancers of the colon, rectum, and breast. Folate is best obtained by eating fruits, vegetables, and enriched grain products.

People who ingest a diet high in saturated fat are at a greater risk of obesity, which can be a risk factor for colon, prostate, and breast cancers.

A diet rich in vegetables and fruits can reduce the risk of lung, oral, esophageal, stomach, and colon cancer. The American Cancer Society recommends eating a variety of fresh fruits and vegetables daily. Because it is not known which compounds in vegetables and fruits are actually beneficial, there are no supplements that can take the place of eating whole foods. Frozen and canned foods can be healthy alternatives, but be careful to read labels for ingredients. See www.cancer.org and Box 11.3, *Nutrition Notes,* for additional dietary recommendations.

VACCINES. Preventive vaccines are being developed for cancers associated with specific viruses. Gardasil (human papillomavirus vaccine) can be given to young girls and women to protect against HPV and cervical cancer. However, most cancer vaccines are therapeutic rather than prophylactic and are used to stimulate the patient's immune system to destroy cancer cells. Vaccine therapy for malignant melanoma and lymphoma is being tested.

Diagnosis of Cancer

A cancer diagnosis is a very frightening experience (Box 11.4, *Patient Perspective*). Often, people try to mask symptoms because they are so frightened of the disease. A careful and thorough assessment of the patient's current status, medical and surgical histories, and pertinent family history should be completed. A complete physical examination provides both objective and subjective data. The most conclusive information about the health of tissue is acquired by examining cell activity through biopsy.

BIOPSY. Accurate identification of a cancer can be made only by **biopsy**. Microscopic examination of a sample of suspected tissue or aspirated body fluid can confirm the presence of mutant cells. A biopsy is commonly done in a physician's office or outpatient surgery department.

Box 11.3

Nutrition Notes

Reducing Cancer Risk

Encourage patients to consume these foods:
- Whole grains
- Vegetables and fruits, especially those rich in vitamin C (oranges, cantaloupe, strawberries)
- Cruciferous vegetables (cabbage, broccoli, Brussels sprouts, cauliflower)
- Grilled meats that have been:
  - Precooked in a microwave oven
  - Marinated but basted only with fresh marinade, not that used to steep raw meat

Encourage patients to avoid these foods:
- Excessive meat, especially when:
  - Processed (smoked, salted)
  - Charbroiled or cooked at high temperatures
- Excessive fat, especially saturated fat
- Excessive calories, leading to obesity

Encourage patients to limit:
- Alcohol intake to one (women) or two (men) standard drinks per day

Box 11.4

Patient Perspective

Robyn

I am a 43-year-old woman with three children and in the prime of my life—at least I thought. That was before I was diagnosed with cancer in my left breast. I was breastfeeding at the time I felt the lump and, although I went for a biopsy, I felt sure the lump resulted from a blocked milk duct or fibroid cyst. But, unbelievably, the biopsy came back positive for cancer. My whole life flipped upside down. I was devastated.

I was scheduled for surgery within a week, and my emotions were in complete turmoil. I felt nauseated all the time, vomited almost every morning, and had diarrhea daily. My stomach felt like it had a pot of bees inside. I never cried so much in my life. Thinking about all the tests, the surgery, and the untold ways my life could be affected made me a nervous wreck. Finally, I got down on my knees and turned this whole crisis over to God. I couldn't handle it anymore, so I asked God to give me peace, and I placed all my trust and faith in Him. It worked, and I was finally able to get control and face this thing head-on.

As I went for further testing, the nurses and technicians I met were all very helpful and informative. Some actually broke down with me because they had endured this same disease. We would hold each other and then exchange phone numbers just to "talk" if I needed it. It was very encouraging to know these women had made it through, and I could too.

The surgery went smoothly, and I was released the next day. There wasn't much discomfort, and I felt good physically. The nerve was removed and a scar runs from the center of my chest down under my armpit. I was able to return to work in 3 weeks. The doctor gave me a prescription for a prosthesis as soon as the drains were removed and I began healing. We went to a specialty place to be fitted, and, although the prosthesis was nothing like the real thing, I looked normal and it helped to build my confidence.

The impact on my family was one of complete bewilderment because I had no family history of this type of cancer. Everyone tried to help with positive sentiments like we caught it early, breast cancer has a high cure rate, periodic follow-up can keep you cancer free, and so on. My husband and children supported and comforted me. I tried to focus on them because I want to be there for them when they graduate, get married, etc. My mother and sister helped get me to all my appointments and filled my prescriptions.

Chemo was advised as a follow-up treatment, and I was scheduled for four rounds, one every 3 weeks. This was undoubtedly the worst thing I have ever endured. Not even giving birth can compare to the way chemo makes you feel. I had a very bad experience the first round and was extremely sick and unable to eat for 5 days. I wondered why I didn't just die from the cancer because I felt that this was killing me. Before the second round, I told the doctor how violently ill I'd been and she adjusted the dosages of some of the drugs. I was very groggy; although I didn't vomit, I still wasn't feeling myself. For the third round, they changed a medication and I withstood the side effects a lot better—although I was still nauseated, light-headed, fatigued, and unable to focus, eat, or taste anything. At times, it was hard just to put one foot in front of the other. They prepared me for the loss of my hair, but you really don't know how hard that is until it starts coming out in globs. Not just the loss, but then you have such a long time to wait for it to grow back. When the chemo is over, it's hard to look back and feel the way you did then, but when you look in the mirror and your hair is still gone, it's a hard reminder.

All through being diagnosed and dealing with breast cancer I have felt a tremendous outpouring of love and caring, not only from my immediate family but also from my church family. I was never so well taken care of. All the hugs, cards, calls, food, and flowers brought to the house encouraged me tremendously. It makes it a little easier to cope when you know you have so many people who care and are concerned enough to take time out of their daily lives to give you support.

I'm lucky because my sister is an RN and prepared me for many of the side effects and difficulties. She also was there to help ask questions and get information from other survivors that kept me in a positive frame of mind. I know that without her help and God's grace and peace my recovery would not have been so easy. Looking back I can't really feel all those terrible emotions and symptoms, but I still am afraid of the unknown. It is not easy when it is you and not someone else this happens to.

Now that I'm through the worst part of this, I take positive steps every day to enjoy the little things in life. I feel that the more you keep involved in everyday activities and become educated about the disease and its treatments, the easier it is to deal with. I am taking a drug called tamoxifen now and will be for 5 years. Two of the side effects are hot flashes and sweats. If this is all I have to deal with, however, praise God. My prognosis is very good, and I am expecting a complete cure because I am a survivor.

Incisional biopsy is an invasive procedure that involves surgical removal of a small amount of tissue for inspection. Tissue also can be removed during endoscopic procedures (insertion of a tube to observe the inside of a hollow organ or cavity), such as a lung biopsy done during bronchoscopy. Excisional biopsy is used to remove an entire tissue mass.

Needle aspiration biopsy involves insertion of a needle into tissue for fluid or tissue aspiration (Fig. 11.7). This procedure is less invasive than incisional or excisional biopsy. Transcutaneous aspiration involves insertion of a fine needle into tissue such as breast, prostate, or salivary gland and is used for diagnosing metastatic cancers. Frozen section biopsy provides immediate evaluation of a tissue sample during a surgical procedure. By freezing the tissue sample for microscopic examination, a quick analysis is possible, which helps direct the remainder of the surgical procedure. Frozen section biopsy is especially useful in the diagnosis of and surgical intervention for breast cancer.

Stereotactic biopsy is a safe and efficient procedure for evaluating lesions in the brain and breast. The procedure is done by a specially trained radiologist. The biopsy site must be firmly immobilized. The lesion is scanned for location, and a small incision is made for easy insertion of a small fiber-optic instrument (Fig. 11.8). Stereotactic biopsy of the brain involves a local anesthetic because a small hole in the skull is made. Breast stereotactic biopsy uses pressure exerted by a mammogram machine to secure the breast; anesthesia may not be necessary.

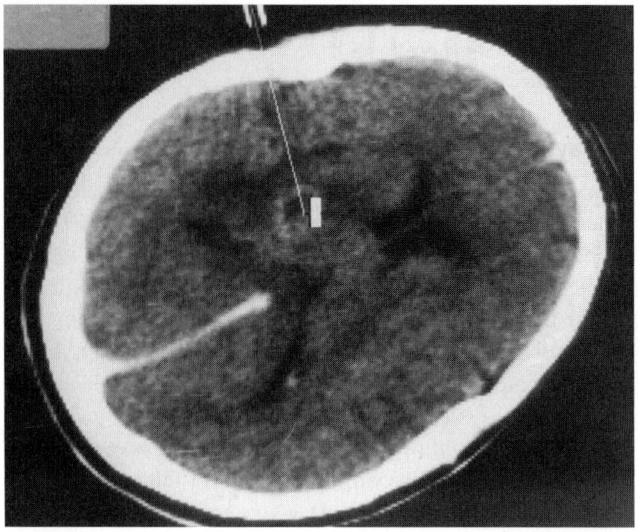

FIGURE 11.8 Stereotactic biopsy of a brain lesion. (Photo courtesy of Dinesh Patel, MD, Medical Oncology, Internal Medicine, Zanesville, OH.)

LABORATORY TESTS. Blood, serum, and urine tests are important in establishing baseline values and general health status. Laboratory values are used with other assessment findings. An elevated white blood cell (WBC) count is expected if the patient has evidence of infection; however, an increase in WBCs without infection raises suspicion of leukemia. Fifty percent of patients with liver cancer have increased levels of bilirubin, alkaline phosphatase, and glutamic-oxaloacetic transaminase.

Bone marrow aspiration is done to learn the number, size, and shape of red and white blood cells and platelets. Bone marrow aspiration is a major tool for diagnosis of leukemia. (See Chapter 27 for a description of this test and related nursing care.)

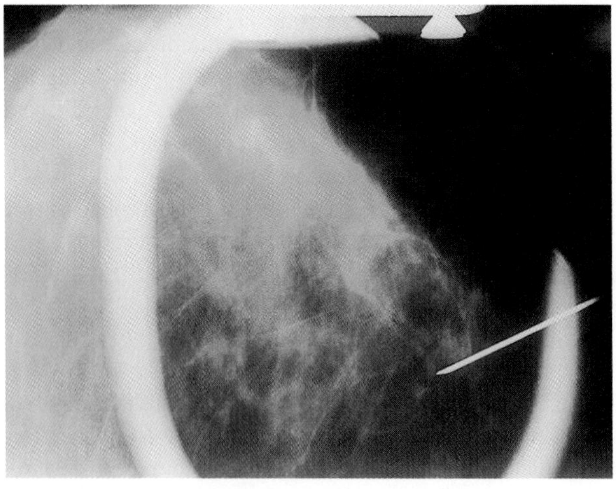

FIGURE 11.7 Fine-needle breast biopsy. (Photo courtesy of Dinesh Patel, MD, Medical Oncology, Internal Medicine, Zanesville, OH.)

Tumor markers, also called biochemical markers, are proteins, antigens, genes, hormones, and enzymes produced and secreted by tumor cells. Tumor markers help confirm a diagnosis of cancer, detect cancer origin, monitor the effect of cancer therapy, and determine cancer remission. Some examples of tumor markers are shown in Table 11.3.

CYTOLOGICAL STUDY. Cytology is the study of the formation, structure, and function of cells. Cytological diagnosis of cancer is obtained mainly through Pap smears of cells shed from a mucous membrane (e.g., cervical, anal, or oral). Test results are based on the degree of cell

TABLE 11.3 TUMOR MARKERS AND ASSOCIATED CANCERS

Tumor Marker	Associated Cancer
Alpha-fetoprotein (AFP)	Hepatocellular cancer
Cancer antigen (CA) 15-3	Breast cancer (useful in monitoring patient response to therapy for metastatic breast cancer)
CA 125	Ovarian, cervical, liver, and pancreatic cancers
CA 19-9	Colorectal, pancreatic, and hepatobiliary cancers (used to aid diagnosis and evaluation)
Carcinoembryonic antigen (CEA)	Colon and rectal cancers
Prostatic acid phosphatase (PAP)	Prostate cancer
Prostate-specific antigen (PSA)	Prostate cancer

abnormality. Normal results reflect no cellular changes. Slight cellular changes are considered normal, with a possible link to abnormal cells seen in infection. Significant cellular changes reflect a higher probability of precancerous or cancerous activity. Infection causes cellular changes and contributes to an increase in abnormal cells detected.

RADIOLOGICAL PROCEDURES. X-ray examination is a valuable diagnostic tool in detecting cancer of the bones and hollow organs. Routine chest x-ray examination is one diagnostic test used in detecting lung cancer. Mammography is a reliable and noninvasive low-radiation x-ray procedure for detecting breast masses (Fig. 11.9). During a mammogram, breast tissue is compressed to allow better visualization of the soft tissue. (See Chapter 41 for more information on mammography.)

Contrast media x-ray studies are used to detect abnormalities of bone and the gastrointestinal and urinary systems. Contrast media can be given by various methods. Barium is given orally for visualization of the esophagus and stomach or rectally as a barium enema for visualization of the colon. Intravenous injection of contrast media is used for lung and brain scans.

Computed tomography (CT) provides a three-dimensional, cross-sectional, computerized picture of the body. CT scans are important in the diagnosis and staging of malignancies and can detect minor variations in tissue thickness. The use of a contrast medium enhances the accuracy of an abdominal CT scan. CT scans are also used to improve the accuracy of inserting a fine needle for biopsy.

NUCLEAR IMAGING PROCEDURES. Nuclear medicine imaging involves camera imaging of organs or tissues containing radioactive media. Radioactive compounds are given intravenously or by mouth. These studies are highly sensitive and can detect sites of abnormal cell growth months before changes are seen on an x-ray.

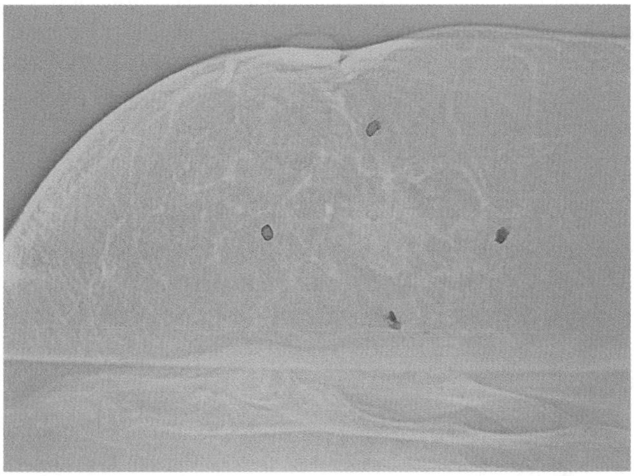

FIGURE 11.9 Mammogram. (Photo courtesy of Dinesh Patel, MD, Medical Oncology, Internal Medicine, Zanesville, OH.)

Positron emission tomography (PET) scanning provides information about cellular function. Patients are given biochemical compounds, and images are made of the tissue through gamma-camera tomography. PET scans have been useful in brain imaging as well as the detection of the spread of cancers of the lung, ovaries, colon, rectum, and breast.

ULTRASOUND PROCEDURES. Ultrasonography uses high-frequency sound waves to produce images of deep soft-tissue structures. The procedure is noninvasive and uses no x-rays. Echoes from high-frequency sound waves outline tissue density and masses. This technology helps detect tumors of the pelvis and breast. Ultrasound also may be used to distinguish between benign and malignant breast tumors.

MAGNETIC RESONANCE IMAGING. Magnetic resonance imaging (MRI) creates sectional images of the body. MRI can be done with or without contrast dye and does not use radiation. The patient is placed in a cylinder-shaped magnetic field. The magnetic field aligns the nuclei of body cells in one direction. The magnetized cells are then excited by radio-frequency pulses. Images are made as cell nuclei change their alignment. MRI is valuable in the detection, localization, and staging of malignant tumors in the central nervous system, spine, head, and musculoskeletal system. MRI cannot be used in patients with pacemakers, implanted pumps, surgical clips, metal knees or hips, or some types of tattoos and permanent makeup because metals are attracted by the powerful MRI magnets and injury can result.

ENDOSCOPIC PROCEDURES. An endoscopic examination allows the direct visualization of a body cavity or opening. The procedure involves the insertion of a flexible endoscope containing fiber-optic glass bundles that transmit light and can produce an image. Endoscopy enables the surgeon to biopsy tissue and is used to detect lesions of the throat, esophagus, stomach, colon, and lungs.

Oral endoscopic procedures require patient preparation to reduce the risk of aspirating stomach secretions. The patient is given nothing to eat or drink before and immediately after the examination. A local anesthetic is used during the examination to anesthetize the throat. Following the procedure, oral food and fluids are withheld until the gag reflex returns to prevent aspiration. The gag reflex is assessed by touching a cotton-tipped swab to the back of the throat to stimulate the reflex after the procedure.

Staging and Grading

Tumor staging is used to determine the stage of solid-tumor masses, providing valuable information to guide treatment plans. The most common system used for staging tumors is the tumor-node-metastasis (TNM) system, an international system that allows comparison of statistics among cancer centers. This staging system classifies solid tumors by size and degree of spread (Table 11.4). For example, a breast cancer staged as T3 N2 MX is a large breast cancer that has spread to regional lymph nodes, but metastasis cannot be evaluated at this time.

TABLE 11.4 TNM SYSTEM FOR CANCER STAGING

Primary Tumor (T)	
TX	Primary tumor cannot be evaluated
T0	No evidence of primary tumor
Tis	Carcinoma in situ (early cancer that has not spread to neighboring tissue)
T1, T2, T3, T4	Size and/or extent of the primary tumor
Regional Lymph Nodes (N)	
NX	Regional lymph nodes cannot be evaluated
N0	No regional lymph node involvement (no cancer found in the lymph nodes)
N1, N2, N3	Involvement of regional lymph nodes (number and/or extent of spread)
Distant Metastasis (M)	
MX	Distant metastasis cannot be evaluated
M0	No distant metastasis (cancer has not spread to other parts of the body)
M1	Distant metastasis (cancer has spread to distant parts of the body)

Source: U.S. National Institutes of Health. [2004]. *Staging: Questions and answers.* Retrieved January 29, 2010, from http://www.cancer.gov.

The TNM ratings correspond with one of five stages, but stages may differ based on the type of cancer. In general, the lower the number of the stage, the less the cancer has spread. A higher number means a more serious situation exists. Stages range from stage 0 (tumor in situ, no invasion of other tissues) to stage IV (distant metastasis to other sites).

A rating system has also been established to define the cell types of tumors. Tumors are classified according to the percentage of cells that are differentiated (mature). If the tissue of a neoplastic tumor closely resembles normal tissue, it is called *well differentiated.* A *poorly differentiated* tumor is a malignant neoplasm that contains some normal cells, but most of the cells are abnormal. The better defined or differentiated the tumor, the easier it is to treat.

Treatment for Cancer

There are three main types of treatment for cancer: surgery, radiation therapy, and chemotherapy. To find out more about cancer treatment options, visit the American Cancer Society website at www.cancer.org.

SURGERY. Surgery can be curative when it is possible to remove the entire tumor. Skin cancers and well-defined tumors without metastasis can be removed without any additional intervention. For some tumors, as much of the tumor is removed as possible (this is called debulking), and follow-up chemotherapy or radiation is used to treat the remaining tumor cells.

Prophylactic surgery is used to remove moles or lesions that have the potential to become malignant. Colon polyps are often removed to prevent malignancies from developing, especially if the polyps are considered premalignant. An extreme example of prophylactic surgery is a woman who elects to have a mastectomy (surgical removal of the breast) because of a high incidence of breast cancer in her family.

Surgery also may be done for **palliation** (symptom control). Surgical removal of tissue to reduce the size of the tumor mass is helpful, especially if the tumor is compressing nerves or blocking the passage of body fluids. The goals of palliative surgery are to increase comfort and quality of life.

Reconstructive surgery can be done for cosmetic enhancement or for return of function of a body part. Facial reconstruction is important for a patient's self-image after removal of head or neck tumors. Women can elect to have breast reconstruction after mastectomy.

Nurses should encourage patients to express and discuss their fears. Patients with a limited understanding of cancer may fear that tissues will not heal postoperatively. Provide information about wound care, including dressing changes and drainage tubes, to increase the patient's knowledge base and sense of control. Visual aids concerning tumor site and surgical procedures are valuable teaching tools.

Patients who are undernourished are poor surgical candidates and require intervention such as enteral or parenteral nutrition before and after surgery. Patients with cancer also are at increased risk for postoperative deep venous thrombosis (DVT). Preoperative teaching includes the importance of leg movement, early ambulation, wearing antiembolism stockings, and recognizing symptoms of DVT, such as calf redness, warmth, or pain.

RADIATION. Radiation is used commonly in cancer control and palliation, and it can be curative if the disease is localized. The decision to use radiation is commonly based on cancer site and size. Radiation destroys cancer cells by affecting cell structure and the cell environment. It is used in fractionated (divided) doses to prevent destructive side effects; however, side effects can occur in the area being treated because of damage to normal cells.

Radiation can be used before surgery to decrease the size of a large tumor, making surgical intervention more effective and less dangerous, or it can be used after surgery as adjuvant treatment. Palliative radiation is used to reduce the size of a large cancerous lesion and consequently reduce pressure and pain. Radioisotopes can be inserted into cancerous tissue during surgery to help destroy cancerous cells without removing the organ.

Nursing Care of the Patient Receiving Radiation Treatment. Symptoms of tissue reaction to radiation can be expected about 10 to 14 days after treatment starts and continue for up to 2 weeks after treatment ends. Typical reactions and appropriate nursing interventions include the following:

- *Fatigue:* Encourage the patient to nap often and prioritize activities. Reassure the patient that the feeling will go away when the treatments are completed.

- *Nausea, vomiting, and* ***anorexia:*** Encourage the patient to take prescribed medication for nausea and vomiting. Anorexia can be eased by giving small amounts of high-carbohydrate, high-protein foods and avoiding foods high in fiber.
- ***Mucositis*** *(inflammation of mucous membranes, especially of the mouth and throat):* Urge the patient to avoid irritants such as smoking, alcohol, acidic food or drinks, extremely hot or cold foods and drinks, and commercial mouthwash. Advise the patient to perform mouth care before meals and every 3 to 4 hours. A neutral mouthwash can be made by using 1 ounce of diphenhydramine hydrochloride (Benadryl) elixir diluted in 1 quart of water or normal saline solution. Agents that coat the mouth, such as Maalox, are sometimes used. Lidocaine hydrochloride 2% viscous has an anesthetic effect on the mouth and throat.
- ***Xerostomia*** *(dry mouth):* Encourage frequent mouth care. Saliva substitute is available over the counter and is helpful, especially at night when patients describe a choking sensation from extreme dryness.
- *Skin reactions:* These can vary from mild redness to moist **desquamation** (peeling skin) similar to a second-degree burn. Skin surfaces that are warm and moist, such as the groin, perineum, and axillae, are especially vulnerable. Prophylactic skin care includes keeping skin dry; keeping it free from irritants, such as powder, lotions, deodorants, and restrictive clothing; and protecting it against exposure to direct sunlight. Irradiated skin can be fragile during treatment. It is important to wash these areas gently with mild soap and water, rinse well, and pat dry. The skin may have markings or tattoos to delineate the treatment field. Take care not to wash off the markings.
- *Bone marrow depression:* Low blood cell counts occur with both radiation and chemotherapy because they can attack all rapidly dividing cells, not just cancer cells. Weekly blood cell counts are done to detect low levels of white blood cells, red blood cells, and platelets. Transfusions of whole blood, platelets, or other blood components may be needed.

Safety Considerations. Radiation may be administered externally or internally. External radiation is given by a trained medical specialist in a designated area in the hospital or clinic. Internal radiation is administered to patients admitted to a health care facility.

Safety guidelines must be followed when caring for a patient with internal radioactive materials that have been implanted into tissue or body cavities or administered orally or intravenously, because the patient will be radioactive. Nursing responsibilities include knowledge about the following:

- Radiation source being used
- Method of administration
- Start of treatment
- Length of treatment
- Prescribed nursing precautions.

Personnel involved with radiation therapy must recognize three primary factors to protect themselves: time, distance, and shielding. These three factors depend on the type of radiation used. *Time* involves the time spent administering care, *distance* involves the amount of space between the radioisotope and the nurse, and *shielding* involves the use of a barrier such as a lead apron.

You must work efficiently when caring for patients who are receiving radioisotopes that are releasing gamma rays. Your exposure to radiation is proportionate to the time spent and the distance from the radiation source. For example, you will receive less exposure standing at the foot of the bed of a patient with radioisotopes inserted into the head than if you stand at the head of the bed (Fig. 11.10). Principles of time and distance are used to protect the nurse, visitors, and other personnel.

It is important to teach the patient and family members the reason nursing care focuses on providing only essential care. Speedy nursing encounters and visitor restrictions are better accepted and less likely to promote feelings of isolation when patients understand the reasons behind them.

Drainage from the site of a radioactive colloid injection is considered radioactive, and the physician must be informed immediately if it occurs. Dressings contaminated with radioactive seepage must be removed with long-handled forceps. Radioactive materials must never be touched with unprotected hands; shielding is required to prevent exposure to radiation. Contamination from radioisotope applicators or interstitial implants cannot occur when the capsule is intact; contamination occurs when the capsule is broken.

SAFETY TIP

Remember to use the principles of time, distance, and shielding to protect yourself from radiation exposure.

CHEMOTHERAPY. Chemotherapy is chemical therapy that uses **cytotoxic** (destructive to cells) drugs to treat cancer. Cytotoxic drugs can be used for cure, control, or palliation of cancerous tumors. They are classified according to how they affect cell activity. For example:

- Alkylating agents bind with DNA to stop production of RNA.

• WORD • BUILDING •

anorexia: an—not + orexis—appetite
mucositis: muco—mucous (membrane) + itis—inflammation
xerostomia: xero—dry + stoma—mouth
desquamation: de—down, from + squamation—epidermis
chemotherapy: chemo—chemistry + therapy—treatment
cytotoxic: cyto—cell + toxic—poison

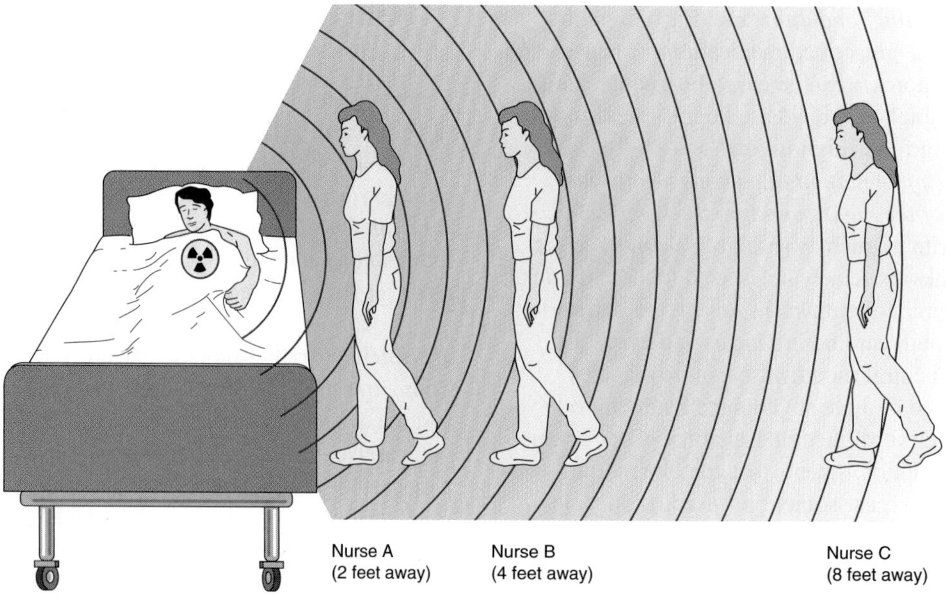

Nurse A
(2 feet away)
Nurse B
(4 feet away)
Nurse C
(8 feet away)

FIGURE 11.10 Radiation distancing. Nurse B receives less radiation than Nurse A, and Nurse C receives less radiation than Nurse B.

- Antimetabolites substitute for nutrients or enzymes in the cell life cycle
- Mitotic inhibitors interfere with cell division.
- Antibiotics inhibit DNA and RNA synthesis.
- Hormonal agents alter the hormonal structure of the body.

Examples of specific drugs and their adverse effects are listed in Table 11.5.

The effects of chemotherapy are systemic unless used topically for skin lesions. Chemotherapy is used preoperatively to shrink tumors and postoperatively to treat residual tumors. Factors influencing the effectiveness of chemotherapy are tumor type, available chemotherapeutic drugs, and genetics. Age is also a consideration, but treatment should be based on physiological age rather than chronological age. That is, just because a patient might be 70 years old doesn't mean his body is the same as that of other 70-year-olds.

TABLE 11.5 CANCER CHEMOTHERAPY MEDICATIONS

Medication Class/ Action	Examples	Route	Side Effects	Nursing Implications
Antitumor Antibiotics				
Damage cells' DNA and the ability to make DNA and RNA.	doxorubicin (Adriamycin, Doxil)	IV	Red urine, nausea and vomiting, alopecia, cardiac damage, radiation recall skin changes, decreased white blood cell and platelet counts	This drug is a vesicant and should be given through a running IV or a central line if it is a continuous infusion. Doxil is less irritating than Adriamycin. Monitor cardiac status. Lifetime dose is 550 mg/m^2.
Antimetabolites				
Resemble normal metabolites needed for cell function. Once they gain entry into the cell, cell division becomes impaired.	capecitabine (Xeloda)	PO	Bone marrow depression, nausea, vomiting, stomatitis, hand and foot syndrome	Monitor WBC and platelet count throughout therapy. Teach the patient signs of infection and bleeding. Teach the patient about mouth care. Drug should be taken after a meal with plenty of water. Teach the patient about hand and foot syndrome and to notify primary care provider if it occurs.

TABLE 11.5 CANCER CHEMOTHERAPY MEDICATIONS—cont'd

Medication Class/ Action	Examples	Route	Side Effects	Nursing Implications
	cytarabine (Cytosar, Ara-C)	IV	Fever, chills, unusual bleeding or bruising, sore throat, tiredness, nausea and vomiting	Check CBC before each dose. Review the signs of infection or bleeding. Instruct patient to call primary care provider for any temperature increases greater than 100.0°F (37.8°C).
	fluorouracil (5-FU)	IV	Diarrhea, loss of appetite, alopecia, nausea and vomiting, skin sensitivity, stomatitis	Check CBC before the dose. Nadir occurs in 10–14 days. Instruct about mouth care.
	gemcitabine (Gemzar)	IV	Dyspnea, edema, nausea, vomiting, diarrhea, stomatitis, hematuria, alopecia, bone marrow suppression	Check CBC before each dose. Premedicate with antiemetics. Instruct patient to report flu-like symptoms to primary care provider.
Alkylating Agents Cause the DNA strands to bind together and prevent the cell from dividing.	cisplatin (Platinol)	IV	Ototoxicity, fever and chills, tinnitus, nausea and vomiting	Monitor neurologic status, renal function studies. Premedicate with antiemetics. Monitor for signs of anaphylaxis. Nadir occurs in 2–3 weeks; check CBC before each dose. Ensure adequate hydration to prevent renal failure.
	cyclophosphamide (Cytoxan)	IV, PO	Nausea and vomiting, hematuria, alopecia, bone marrow depression	Check CBC before each dose. Monitor BUN and creatinine levels. Ensure adequate hydration to prevent renal failure. Oral form should be taken early in the morning to keep drug from building up in the bladder at night.
	ifosfamide (Ifex)	IV	CNS toxicity, nausea, vomiting, hemorrhagic cystitis, alopecia	Monitor urine for blood. Given with Mesna (Mesnex) to prevent hemorrhagic cystitis. Ensure adequate hydration before and after each dose. Premedicate with antiemetics. Monitor CBC.
Antimitotic Agents Come from plant sources. Prevent mitosis from occurring in the cell and then cells cannot divide.	docetaxel (Taxotere)	IV	Fatigue, edema, nausea and vomiting, stomatitis, anemia, thrombocytopenia, myalgia, alopecia, hypersensitivity, anaphylaxis, bone marrow depression, neuropathy	Patient must take dexamethasone starting 1 day before scheduled chemotherapy to prevent hypersensitivity. Monitor CBC. Nadir occurs on day 7. Monitor weight. Assess skin for changes. Watch for changes in neurologic status from baseline.
	paclitaxel, nanoparticle albumin bound (Abraxane)	IV	Nausea, vomiting, myalgia, cardiac toxicities, hypersensitivity/anaphylaxis, neuropathy, alopecia, stomatitis, anemia, neutropenia, thrombocytopenia, peripheral neuropathy	Watch for signs of hypersensitivity. Monitor CBC and platelet counts. Watch for changes in neurologic status from baseline. Teach mouth care. Monitor vital signs for changes.

Continued

TABLE 11.5 CANCER CHEMOTHERAPY MEDICATIONS—cont'd

Medication Class/ Action	Examples	Route	Side Effects	Nursing Implications
	vincristine (Oncovin)	IV	Constipation, difficulty walking, tingling in fingers and toes, death if given intrathecally	Drug is a vesicant and should be given through a running IV. Assess for neuropathies and changes in neurologic status from baseline. Monitor CBC and platelets.
	vinorelbine (Navelbine)	IV	Fatigue, constipation, nausea, alopecia, bone marrow suppression, neuropathy, nausea, vomiting, stomatitis	Drug is a vesicant. When giving through a running IV, use the port closest to the IV bag rather than the patient. Check CBC before each dose. Nadir occurs in 7–10 days. Teach signs of infection and bleeding. Monitor neurologic status and changes from baseline. Teach mouth care.
Topoisomerase Inhibitors				
Inhibit enzyme topoisomerase to interfere with DNA synthesis.	irinotecan (Camptosar)	IV	Dizziness, headache, insomnia, dyspnea, edema, nausea, vomiting, diarrhea, stomatitis, alopecia, bone marrow suppression, weight loss	Teach measures to control diarrhea, and patient to contact primary care provider if it occurs. Dose of loperamide may be higher than normal—verify with provider. Check CBC before each dose.
	topotecan (Hycamtin)	IV	Headache, dyspnea, nausea, vomiting, diarrhea, hair loss, bone marrow suppression	Monitor CBC. Premedicate for nausea.
Hormones				
Antagonize effects of androgen.	exemestane (Casodex)	PO	Weakness, hot flashes, constipation, diarrhea, generalized pain	Monitor PSA and liver function tests.
Synthetic analog of luteinizing hormone-releasing hormone, causes decrease in testosterone levels.	leuprolide (Lupron)	Subcutaneously, IM, implant	Hot flashes	Monitor PSA results.
Competes with estrogen for binding sites in breast and other tissues.	tamoxifen (Nolvadex)	PO	Hot flashes, weight gain, nausea, bone pain	Anticoagulants increase PT. Instruct the patient not to take antacids within 2 hours of tamoxifen. May cause bony pain but the discomfort is temporary.
Angiogenesis Inhibitors				
Blocks formation of new blood vessels to slow growth and spread of cancer.	bevacizumab (Avastin)	IV	Poor wound healing, increased risk for infection, reproductive problems, damage to fetus if pregnant	Assess for pregnancy. Avoid administration after surgery.
Monoclonal Antibodies				
Bind to receptor sites on cancer cells to inhibit proliferation.	alemtuzumab (Campath), trastuzumab (Herceptin), gemtuzumab (Mylotarg)	IV	Usually mild; risk for allergic reaction; fever, chills, nausea, vomiting, diarrhea	Watch for signs of allergic reaction.

TABLE 11.5 CANCER CHEMOTHERAPY MEDICATIONS—cont'd

Medication Class/ Action	Examples	Route	Side Effects	Nursing Implications
Miscellaneous Agents				
Work by interfering with enzyme systems or metabolic pathways in the cells.	hydroxyurea (Hydrea)	PO	Fever and chills, sore throat, drowsiness, diarrhea, nausea and vomiting	Monitor WBC count. Monitor metabolic panel for signs of tumor lysis syndrome. Monitor neurologic status and changes from baseline.
	thalidomide (Thalomid)	PO	Birth defects, peripheral neuropathy, drowsiness, rash, constipation, neutropenia	Pregnancy test is done before therapy starts. **Drug is contraindicated in pregnancy.** Monitor neurologic status and changes from baseline. Teach patient to report any rash. Teach measures to prevent constipation. Monitor CBC throughout therapy.

BUN = blood urea nitrogen; CBC = complete blood count; CNS = central nervous system; DNA = deoxyribonucleic acid; IM = intramuscular; IV = intravenous; PO = by mouth; PSA = prostate-specific antigen; PT = prothrombin time; WBC = white blood cell.

Combination Chemotherapy. In this kind of therapy, two or more antineoplastics are used together to treat the patient's cancer. This can expose a larger number of cells at different points in the cell cycle to more than one kind of chemotherapy. Combining drugs also decreases the side effects of therapy and decreases the possibility of the tumor becoming resistant to the therapy.

For drugs to be combined this way, several criteria must be met. Each drug must be effective when used alone to treat the cancer, and each must have a different toxicity that would limit its use. For example, if three drugs that are all cardiotoxic are given, the patient is more likely to develop cardiotoxicity. Patients are still monitored for toxic effects from the treatment as well as improvement in their status.

Routes of Administration. Chemotherapy may be given by the oral, intramuscular, intravenous, or topical route. The dosage is determined by the size of the patient and the toxicities of the drug. Intravenous administration requires specialized training and knowledge of antineoplastic drugs.

Vesicant drugs are given only by the intravenous route into a large vein. These drugs cause blistering of tissue that eventually leads to necrosis if they infiltrate, or leak, out of the blood vessel and into soft tissue (Fig. 11.11). Skin grafts may be needed if tissue damage is extensive.

Central Lines. Central lines are intravenous catheters that terminate in the superior vena cava near the right atrium of the heart. This is a large vessel that allows for dilution of vesicant drugs and reduces the risk of infiltration. Central lines may be external, with the distal end of the catheter exiting the skin, or internal, with the distal catheter ending in an implanted port. (See Chapter 7 for additional information on central lines.)

Side Effects. Toxicities in patients receiving chemotherapy vary with the medications given; however, some general side effects are common to chemotherapeutic drugs. Chemotherapy affects all rapidly growing cells. Fast-growing epithelial cells, such as those of the hair, blood, skin, and gastrointestinal tract, are usually the most affected by both chemotherapy and radiation.

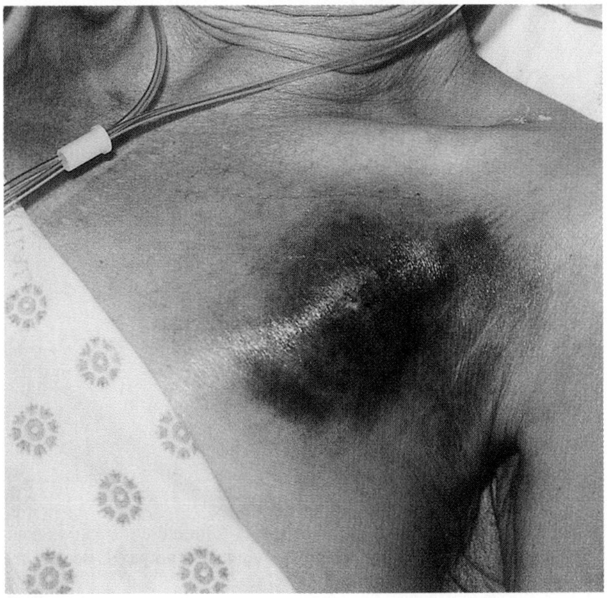

FIGURE 11.11 Necrosis of skin tissue resulting from administration of a vesicant chemotherapy drug. (Photo courtesy of Dinesh Patel, MD, Medical Oncology, Internal Medicine, Zanesville, OH.)

• **WORD • BUILDING** •
vesicant: vesicate—to blister

Hematologic System. Chemotherapy is toxic to bone marrow, which is where blood cells are produced. The number of blood cells (especially white cells) drops after about 7 to 14 days of chemotherapy, depending on the drug. This period when the cell counts are lowest is called the **nadir**, and it is when patients are most at risk for complications. Patients may develop low white blood cell counts (**leukopenia**), increasing their susceptibility to infection and sepsis. Sometimes this is called **neutropenia** because neutrophils are the most plentiful white cells. A reduction in platelets (**thrombocytopenia**) increases the risk of bruising and bleeding and can require platelet transfusions. Increased risk of **anemia** occurs with the reduction of red blood cells and may require blood transfusions. See Table 11.6 for medications that can be used to stimulate production of these cells.

LEARNING TIP

When assessing patients with possible side effects of chemotherapy and radiation, use the mnemonic BITES:
B—Bleeding suggests low platelet count.
I—Infection suggests low WBC count and a risk for infection.
T—Tiredness suggests anemia.
E—Emesis places the patient at risk for altered nutrition and fluid and electrolyte imbalance.
S—Skin changes may be evidence of radiation reaction or skin breakdown.

TABLE 11.6 COLONY-STIMULATING FACTORS

Medication Class/Action	Examples	Route	Side Effects	Nursing Implications
Granulocyte Colony-Stimulating Factor (G-CSF)				
Stimulates proliferation of stem cells into granulocytes (neutrophils).	filgrastim (Neupogen) pegfilgrastim (Neulasta)	IV, subcutaneously	Bone pain	Monitor CBC. Teach Sub-Q administration if drug will be given at home.
Granulocyte-Macrophage Colony-Stimulating Factor (GM-CSF)				
Stimulates proliferation of stem cells into neutrophils, monocytes, macrophages, and eosinophils.	sargramostim (Leukine)	IV, subcutaneously	Headache, itching, rash, bone or joint pain, muscle ache, dyspnea	Monitor vital signs and respiratory status during IV infusion. Monitor CBC. Teach Sub-Q administration if drug will be given at home.
Erythropoietin				
Stimulates proliferation of stem cells into red blood cells.	epoetin alfa (Epogen, Procrit) darbepoetin alpha (Aranesp)	IV, subcutaneously	Hypertension, seizure	Monitor blood pressure and hematocrit. Teach Sub-Q administration if drug will be given at home. Aranesp is long acting.
Interleukin-11				
Stimulates production of platelets.	oprelvekin (Neumega)	Subcutaneously	Dizziness, weakness, conjunctival hemorrhage, dyspnea, cough, pleural effusion, dysrhythmia, edema, syncope, anorexia, constipation, diarrhea, vomiting, alopecia, rash, bone and muscle pain, chills, fever, infection, pain	Watch for fluid retention. Monitor CBC, platelet count. Teach Sub-Q administration if drug will be given at home.

CBC = complete blood count; IV = intravenous.

Note: Because these drugs are proteins, they all require refrigeration and you cannot shake them. Many thousands of dollars have been lost because a drug was not returned to the refrigerator when it was not used. Be sure to check package instructions.

• WORD • BUILDING •

leukopenia: leuko—white cells + penia—lack
neutropenia: neutron—neutrophils + penia—lack

• WORD • BUILDING •

thrombocytopenia: thrombo—clot + cyte—cell + penia—lack
anemia: an—not + emia—blood

Gastrointestinal System. Because the lining of the gastrointestinal tract is made up of rapidly dividing cells, it is susceptible to the toxicity of chemotherapy drugs. Patients often become nauseated and vomit or experience diarrhea. **Stomatitis** (inflammation of the mouth) is a common complaint and is discussed under side effects of radiation. These side effects can be controlled with medication.

Hair. **Alopecia**, or hair loss, is common with many (but not all) chemotherapeutic drugs. This is a temporary condition, and growth of the new hair usually starts when the chemotherapeutic medication is stopped. Alopecia involves the entire body and includes eyebrows, eyelashes, and axillary and pubic hair. Hair that regrows may be a different color or texture than the original hair. It is not uncommon for individuals who originally had straight hair to regrow curly hair.

Reproductive System. The effects of chemotherapy or radiation can cause temporary or permanent changes in the reproductive system. Chemotherapy can damage sperm and ova. Issues concerning fertility should be discussed with the patient before treatment. Measures such as freezing ova and using a sperm bank can provide options for the patient and his or her partner. Patients should also talk to their physicians before engaging in intercourse during chemotherapy, and use protection against pregnancy.

Neurologic System. Drugs may affect the neurologic system. An adverse reaction to vincristine (Oncovin) is neurotoxicity, which may result in tingling or numbness in the extremities and in severe cases can cause footdrop from muscle weakness.

Less common complications include renal toxicities, such as pain and burning on urination, and hematuria. Doxorubicin (Adriamycin) has been associated with permanent heart damage, and bleomycin can cause pulmonary fibrosis.

Severe toxic side effects can be controlled by carefully limiting the amount of medication given and constantly monitoring the patient for complications.

CYTOPROTECTIVE AGENTS. Cytoprotective agents protect healthy cells from some side effects of certain chemotherapeutic drugs. For example, dexrazoxane helps prevent cardiac damage associated with doxorubicin. Amifostine (Ethyol) helps protect the kidneys from platinum-based chemotherapy. It also protects normal cells in parts of the body against damage from radiation treatments. Mesna (Mesnex) protects the bladder against chemotherapy drugs such as cyclophosphamide (Cytoxan).

New Treatments Being Researched

New therapies for cancer are constantly being researched. For example, hyperthermia has been used with radiation and chemotherapy. It has been beneficial in some types of cancer but is usually used only in investigational studies.

• WORD • BUILDING •

stomatitis: stoma—mouth + itis—inflammation

Biological response modifiers (such as interferons) are drugs used to stimulate the immune system. These drugs are used commonly for specific types of cancer and have produced some beneficial results. They are also being used in many investigational studies. Go to www.cancer.gov for information on current clinical trials.

NURSING PROCESS FOR THE PATIENT WITH CANCER

Data Collection

Patients with cancer are assessed for many different problems associated with the disease and its treatment. Thorough assessment will help the health team build a plan of care relevant to the patient's needs.

Monitor laboratory studies. The normal platelet level is 150,000 to 300,000/mm^3. Potential for bleeding exists when the platelet count is 50,000/mm^3 or less; risk for spontaneous bleeding occurs when the count is less than 20,000/mm^3. Monitor the white blood cell count for risk of infection and the red cell count for anemia.

Monitor the patient's weight, and note reports of nausea, changes in taste, vomiting, and diarrhea related to either the disease or treatment. Monitor the oral mucosa for lesions or inflammation. Also watch for signs of dehydration. Box 11.5 (*Nutrition Notes*) presents criteria for determining whether a patient needs nutritional support.

Psychosocial issues related to cancer are as varied as the persons afflicted with the disease. Help the patient explore perceptions about quality of life. Culture and age

Box 11.5

Nutrition Notes

Assessing the Need for Nutritional Support

Intensive nutritional support may not benefit all cancer patients because the tumor interferes with the patient's utilization of nutrients. Clinical judgment is required to analyze the patient's needs and expected response. In general, if any of the following findings are present, you should talk with the dietitian or physician about the need for nutritional support.

- Weight 5 kg (11 lb) below a healthy body weight
- Intolerance of oral/enteral feedings for more than 7 days
- Serum albumin level of less than 3 g/dL
- Location of cancer in head and neck or gastrointestinal system
- Severe gastrointestinal injury in patients with cured/controlled cancer.

affect cancer perceptions (e.g., in a culture in which life expectancy is short, possible death from cancer in the later years is a less significant threat). Assess the patient's ability to cope and coping strategies that have been effective in the past. Determine what information the patient has received and understands about his or her disease and prognosis.

Assess the roles of the patient and caregiver in the family. Be aware of whether the caregiver can be at home or whether he or she must work outside the home and also care for the patient. Isolation can be either self-imposed or imposed by friends and family, as terminal illness issues are confronted. It can be very distressing to see a loved one decline with cancer; often people say they are "afraid of saying or doing the wrong thing" so they "just stay away." Listen for cues from patients expressing self-blame, anger, or depression. It is important to recognize signs of depression and suicidal tendencies.

Assess for fatigue and anxiety in a patient being treated for cancer. A decline in sexual desire is not uncommon during cancer treatment. Assess for anxiety about sexual intercourse, including fears concerning contracting cancer from the patient and fears that sexual intercourse will make the cancer worse.

Assess the patient's feelings about any actual or perceived change in appearance due to surgery, radiation, or chemotherapy.

Nursing Diagnoses, Planning, and Implementation

See the *Nursing Care Plan for the Patient with Cancer,* for top nursing care priorities. Additional nursing diagnoses are presented below.

EVIDENCE-BASED PRACTICE

Clinical Question

Is oral morphine effective for cancer pain?

Evidence

A review of 54 studies found that various formulations of oral morphine were effective at relieving cancer pain, but had unwanted side effects, primarily constipation, nausea, and vomiting (Wiffen & McQuay, 2007).

Implications for Nursing Practice

Administer oral morphine as ordered for pain. Be sure to institute preventive measures against constipation before it becomes a problem. Talk with the physician about medications for nausea if it occurs.

REFERENCE

Wiffen, P. J., & McQuay, H. J. (2007). Oral morphine for cancer pain. ***Cochrane Database of Systematic Reviews 2007, Issue 4*** **(Art. No. CD003868; DOI 10.1002/14651858.CD003868.pub2).**

Ineffective Protection Related to Thrombocytopenia Associated with Chemotherapy and Radiation

EXPECTED OUTCOME: The patient will be free of bleeding as evidenced by stable blood counts and the absence of bruising or frank bleeding.

- Monitor platelet counts. *A platelet count of less than 50,000 indicates potential for bleeding.*
- Teach self-administration of oprelvekin (Neumega) as ordered. *Oprelvekin stimulates production of platelets.*
- Test all urine and stool for occult blood *to detect the presence of blood.*
- Avoid giving intramuscular, subcutaneous, or rectal medications. *Medications given via invasive routes can cause bleeding.*
- Apply pressure for at least 5 minutes to venipuncture or injection sites. *Pressure for a longer time is needed at sites of invasive procedures to stop bleeding.*
- Teach the patient about gentle mouth care including no flossing, a soft toothbrush, and wearing properly fitting dentures *to help prevent trauma and bleeding.*
- Avoid trauma to rectal tissue by avoiding rectal temperatures and enemas. Teach importance of avoiding anal intercourse. *Trauma to rectal tissue can cause bleeding.*
- Instruct the patient not to take any salicylates or nonsteroidal anti-inflammatory drugs *because they can interfere with platelet function and cause bleeding in the GI tract.*
- Observe for bruising, petechiae, bleeding gums, tarry stools, and black emesis. *These are signs of bleeding.*
- Advise the patient to use an electric razor *to decrease risk for trauma and bleeding.*
- Teach the patient to avoid forcefully blowing his or her nose or inserting objects into the nose *to reduce trauma to nasal mucosa to prevent spontaneous bleeding.*
- Teach the patient to avoid intercourse for the duration of the thrombocytopenia *to decrease the probability of bleeding after intercourse.*

Imbalanced Nutrition: Less Than Body Requirements Related to Anorexia, Nausea, or Vomiting Associated with Disease, Pain, and Treatment

EXPECTED OUTCOME: The patient will have caloric intake that is adequate to meet body requirements and balanced intake and output, as evidenced by stable weight and albumin level of 3 g/dL or greater.

- Monitor food and fluid intake and output every 8 hours. *This will provide objective data for the amount of nutrients and fluids taken in.*
- Weigh the patient daily. *Weight is an objective measurement to determine if intake is adequate enough to maintain weight.*

NURSING CARE PLAN for the Patient with Cancer—cont'd

Interventions	Rationale	Evaluation
Use good hand washing technique before interaction with the patient.	Appropriate hand hygiene can reduce the transmission of antimicrobial organisms.	Are you careful with your hand washing? Have you also instructed the patient, family, and nursing assistants about careful hand washing?
Limit visitors to only healthy adults.	Viral infection in an immunosuppressed patient has a high mortality rate.	Are the patient and family aware of visiting restrictions and rationale? Is there a sign on the door reminding visitors?
Keep fresh flowers and potted plants out of the patient's room.	*Aspergillus* is a fungus found in soil and water and can cause pneumonia.	Is the room free from potential sources of infection?

ATC = around the clock; G-CSF = granulocyte colony-stimulating factor; GM-CSF = granulocyte macrophage colony-stimulating factor; GU = genitourinary; PCA = patient-controlled analgesia.

- Consult a dietitian for dietary supplements. *Dietitians can calculate the calories needed for adequate nutrition and make recommendations for supplements.*
- Consult with the primary care provider for medications to control nausea, vomiting, and diarrhea. *If these symptoms are controlled, then the patient is better able to eat.*
- Keep the environment free of strong odors, such as disinfectants, perfumes, deodorizers, and body wastes. *Strong odors can induce nausea.*
- Provide room-temperature or cold foods and clear liquids. *These foods have fewer odors and may be more comfortable for the patient to eat.*
- Offer sour foods such as hard candy and lemon. *These may help control nausea.*
- Encourage listening to music or doing relaxation exercises. *These may provide distraction from pain and nausea.*
- Add nutmeg to foods. *Nutmeg may help slow the motility of the gastrointestinal tract and decrease the risk of nausea and vomiting.*
- Provide mouth care before meals. *Oral care allows for a better taste in the mouth, and saliva is needed for digestion of food.*
- Provide small, high-calorie meals. *Eating smaller, more frequent meals prevents the patient from feeling full and nauseated.*
- Administer pain medication before meals *to help reduce the impact of pain on the appetite.*
- Instruct the patient to avoid fluids with meals *to prevent premature feelings of fullness.*
- Teach the patient to avoid exercise before meals. *If the patient is fatigued, he or she will not have the energy to eat and digest food.*

See Box 11.6 (*Nutrition Notes*) for additional nutrition interventions.

Self-Care Deficit Related to Weakness and Fatigue

EXPECTED OUTCOME: Care needs will be met at all times as evidenced by statement that needs are being met by self or caregiver.

- Assess what self-care activities the patient can do independently (bathing, grooming, feeding, toileting, ambulating). *By assessing what the patient can do independently, you can develop goals and interventions appropriate for this patient.*
- Teach self-administration of epoetin alfa (Epogen, Procrit) as ordered. *Epoetin alfa stimulates production of red cells and can help reduce fatigue related to anemia.*
- Identify and include the patient's strengths in self-care activities *to help increase the patient's independence.*
- Provide the tools needed for the patient to assist with his or her own bathing, grooming, feeding, toileting, and ambulation. Physical and occupational therapy departments may be able to help identify assistive devices. *Adaptive and assistive devices can promote independence.*

Box 11.6

Nutrition Notes

Treating Problems Related to Nutrition

Early Satiety and Anorexia

- Select nutrient-dense foods. For example, fortify puddings and milkshakes with dry skim milk powder.
- Encourage appropriate exercise.
- Present food attractively.
- Remove covers from food containers away from the bedside if strong odors annoy the patient.
- Offer small, frequent meals.
- Encourage family to provide home-cooked food.
- If meals are not tolerated, offer 1 oz of a complete nutritional supplement every hour.

Bitter or Metallic Taste

- Cook in glass containers in a microwave oven.
- Use nonmetallic utensils when eating meals.
- Serve food cold or at room temperature.
- See if the patient prefers eggs, fish, poultry, and dairy products to beef and pork.
- Experiment with sauces and seasonings. Sweet sauces and marinades may improve the palatability of meats.

Local Oral Effects

- *Ulcerations:* Offer soft, mild foods; cream sauces, gravies, and dressings for lubrication; cold foods for numbing; and straws for liquids. Avoid hot items, salty or spicy foods, and acidic juices. If an anesthetic mouthwash is prescribed, the mouth may be numb; caution the patient to chew carefully to avoid biting the lips, tongue, or cheeks.
- *Dry mouth:* Offer frequent sips of water or artificial saliva. Lubricate with gravies, butter, margarine, milk, cream, or bouillon. Sugarless hard candy, chewing gum, or popsicles may stimulate saliva production.
- *Dysphagia:* Teach the patient to make swallowing a conscious act (inhale, swallow, exhale) and to experiment with head position. Offer foods with a smooth, even consistency. Thick liquids are easier to swallow than thin. Encourage dunking breads in a beverage to soften.

Nausea and Vomiting

- Administer antiemetics on a regular prophylactic schedule.
- Suggest dry crackers.
- Offer liquids between instead of with meals to reduce stomach volume, and low-fat meals to facilitate stomach emptying.
- Instruct the patient to chew thoroughly, eat slowly, and rest afterward.
- Arrange meal schedule to take advantage of times when patient feels better.
- Avoid serving favorite foods when the patient is nauseous to avoid an association between those foods and vomiting.

Diarrhea

- Suggest a low-residue diet. Citrotein and Enlive are supplements for clear liquid diets.
- Try a lactose-free diet for temporary lactose intolerance.
- Propose pectin-containing foods (apples, strawberries, citrus fruits) to absorb water in the bowel.
- Recommend active cultures of yogurt to repopulate intestine (see below).

Altered Immune Response

- Restrict fresh fruits and vegetables that cannot be peeled or adequately disinfected.
- Avoid raw and undercooked entrees and smoked or pickled fish.
- Consider avoiding yogurt to prevent translocation of the bacteria to the bloodstream.

- Teach the patient about options available for when he or she is no longer able to care for his or her own needs. *Support from other sources will help the patient conserve energy. Planning ahead can help reduce anxiety.*
- Instruct family members in how to assist in daily care. *Allowing family members to assist in the daily care will promote their role as caregivers.*
- Consult home health care or hospice nurses to assist with care needs upon discharge from the acute setting. *Support from these sources will assist the patient to maintain dignity when independence is no longer possible.*

Grieving Related to Potential Disease Outcome

EXPECTED OUTCOME: The patient will be able to grieve as evidenced by ability to express feelings of guilt, anger, or sorrow and to share anticipated needs related to end-of-life care.

- Use therapeutic communication techniques to ask open-ended questions such as "What are your thoughts and fears?" *This can assist the patient to identify concerns, and also help the nurse to individualize nursing care.*
- Actively listen to the patient's grief. *Being present for the patient and just listening helps the patient communicate needs and fears.*
- Encourage family members to spend time with the patient to make end-of-life decisions. *More people would rather rely on family and friends than physicians to make end-of-life decisions.*

- Ask the patient about end-of-life decisions. Provide information as needed. *Knowing what a dying patient wants will help the nurse to develop the end-of-life care plan.*
- Contact the patient's minister or clergy if the patient agrees. *Religious beliefs can influence the patient's and/or family's grieving process.*
- If the patient wishes, involve family members in building memories, such as by helping write letters, planning the funeral, or writing an obituary. *These are ways to nurture the patient's relationship with family and to leave a memento behind.*

Risk For Ineffective Role Performance Related to Needs of Patient and Anticipated Outcome

EXPECTED OUTCOME: The caregiver will be prepared to provide care effectively as evidenced by (1) identification of resources available to assist in providing care for the patient and (2) maintenance of physical and psychological health.

- Observe the caregiver's ability to provide care for the patient. *The nurse needs to know if the caregiver will be able to handle the care needs.*
- Observe the quality of the relationship between the patient and caregiver. *The quality of the relationship impacts the care delivered.*
- Teach appropriate caregiving skills as needed. *The caregiver may not be aware of how to bathe a patient or how to provide basic or advanced care.*
- Assist the caregiver to identify available supports. *Assistance can provide a break and decrease the risk of exhaustion and depression in the caregiver.*
- Instruct the caregiver in the resources available in the community. *Support groups can help the caregiver by providing an outlet for sharing concerns and finding support.*
- Consult the multidisciplinary team to provide the services needed at time of discharge. *Preparing the caregiver for discharge needs/care with the proper resources will help the caregiver feel empowered to deliver the care.*
- Watch for signs of depression in the caregiver, and intervene to help coping. *The caregiver can develop a weakened immune system secondary to stress and depression.*
- Arrange for respite for the caregiver or encourage the caregiver to utilize this service. *Respite care can provide a break for the caregiver.*
- Encourage the caregiver to grieve over the patient. *Caregivers will grieve for the loved one's loss of function or role in the family, even before death.*
- Assist the caregiver with ways to decrease stress. *Encouraging caregivers to take time to care for themselves will leave them with the energy they need to continue providing care.*
- Actively listen to the caregiver's concerns. *Doing so can assist the nurse in assessing the caregiver's ability to cope, and can help in planning care.*

Social Isolation Related to Changing Relationships

EXPECTED OUTCOME: The patient will manage social isolation as evidenced by (1) ability to identify feelings of isolation and (2) ability to participate in chosen activities.

- Observe the patient for signs of barriers to social interaction, such as incontinence, lack of transportation, and inadequate money or support system. *Why a patient feels isolated can vary from one person to another, but knowing the reason can help the nurse plan appropriate interventions.*
- Discuss causes of perceived or actual isolation. *How the patient is dealing with the illness will have an impact on how he or she manages the illness.*
- Listen to the patient describe reasons for isolation. *Listening and being present are ways to show caring.*
- Promote opportunities for the patient to interact socially, such as at mealtimes or during therapy sessions. *The patient will feel less isolated if given an opportunity to participate in diversional activities.*
- Provide positive reinforcement when the patient starts conversation with others. *Positive feedback from the nurse can impact the patient's sense of confidence.*
- Provide information about support groups, and encourage the patient to contact them. *Support groups can help the patient cope better with stressful events in life.*

Ineffective Sexuality Pattern Related to Change In Body Functions

EXPECTED OUTCOME: The patient will have knowledge about limitations or changes in sexual activity during cancer treatment as evidenced by statement of understanding.

- Provide a private environment to discuss issues of sexuality. *Privacy promotes a comfort level that allows the patient to express concerns.*
- Assess what the patient understands about sexuality during cancer treatment. *This discussion can clear up any misinformation the patient and partner may have.*
- Encourage the patient to discuss concerns about sexuality with his or her partner. *Communication is a key component of emotional intimacy.*
- Stress to the patient that cancer cannot be passed from person to person through sexual intimacy. *Cancer is not contagious.*
- Instruct the patient that sexual activity is usually safe during and after cancer treatment. *Sexual activity does not necessarily hurt the patient.*

- Advise the patient to abstain from sexual intercourse while the blood count is low to prevent secondary infections and bleeding. *A low white blood cell count can raise the risk of infection, and a low platelet count can raise the risk of bleeding.*
- Advise men to ask their primary care provider about using condoms for intercourse during chemotherapy *because some chemotherapy agents can be found in semen.*
- Advise the patient to consult the primary care provider about birth control during treatment *because of chemotherapy effects on sperm and ova.*
- Discuss with the patient and partner that closeness and touching may still be desired even if sexual intercourse is not. *Closeness and touching are ways to be intimate without intercourse.*
- Instruct the patient and partner that pain during intercourse can be related to surgery or treatment, and advise taking pain medication before intercourse *to help make the patient more comfortable.*

Disturbed Body Image Related to Cancer and Its Treatment (e.g., Surgical Procedures Such As Mastectomy, Ostomy, or Loss of Hair From Chemotherapy)

EXPECTED OUTCOME: The patient will be able to accept the changes in body image as evidenced by willingness to participate in care and adjust to change in lifestyle.

- Allow the patient to discuss feelings of anger or depression, and confirm that these feelings are normal when adjusting to body changes. *A patient may be better able to cope with body changes if he or she can talk about feelings and understand that they are normal.*
- Encourage the patient to select a wig before hair loss *so the patient can find one resembling his or her own hair color and style.*
- Provide education, and urge the patient to care for the ostomy site or surgical wound when ready *to promote independence.*
- Provide information about resources such as Reach to Recovery (www.cancer.org; type in Reach to Recovery) and Look Good . . . Feel Better support groups (www.lookgoodfeelbetter.org). *Support groups provide a forum for patients to share their experiences with others undergoing similar changes.*
- Provide information about community assistance and financial aid for programs or services. *Social workers can help with community resources that can provide equipment or supplies for the patient.*

Evaluation

If the interventions have been effective, the patient will have no unusual bleeding or bruising. The patient and family will be knowledgeable about risk factors for bleeding and about signs of bleeding to report promptly.

The patient will be nourished and maintain weight within normal limits. The patient will maximize the potential for self-care activities. The patient and caregiver will know about available resources to assist with self-care activities in the home setting. Caregivers will know how to provide care for the patient. The patient will be able to openly discuss feelings and be able to spend time with family and loved ones to resolve any issues.

Effective interventions will allow the caregiver to make use of resources in the community to assist with patient care and to maintain her or his own physical and psychological health while caring for the patient. The patient will be able to discuss feelings of isolation and seek out activities to participate in. The patient will maintain a healthy sexuality and be able to discuss feelings openly and honestly with her or his partner.

The patient will be able to openly discuss concerns regarding body changes and be able to maintain control of his or her body. The patient will know about community resources and support groups to assist with needs related to body image.

CRITICAL THINKING

Mrs. Jones

■ Mrs. Jones is admitted to your unit after a simple mastectomy for breast cancer. The tumor was staged as a T2, N0, M0. A bone scan was negative for metastasis. She is scheduled for four chemotherapy treatments, 3 weeks apart. The medications prescribed are high doses of doxorubicin (Adriamycin) and cyclophosphamide (Cytoxan). A central line is inserted for chemotherapy.

1. What does the staging of Mrs. Jones' tumor mean?
2. What major side effects of her medications should you look for?
3. Why was a central line inserted?
4. What nursing diagnoses are appropriate for Mrs. Jones?

Suggested answers at end of chapter.

HOSPICE CARE OF THE PATIENT WITH CANCER

Patients who are considered terminal and have a life expectancy of 6 months or less are eligible for hospice care, which provides humanistic care for dying people and their families. The dying person is provided care in a home or homelike setting that promotes comfort and quality of life until death. Hospice care is offered as an inpatient or outpatient service. (See *Home Health Hints.*)

Home Health Hints

- The home health or hospice nurse helps manage cancer pain in the home. Oral, transdermal, or intravenous analgesics are preferred. For moderate to severe pain, doses should be given around the clock with as-needed doses for breakthrough pain. Intramuscular delivery of pain medication should be avoided because of the pain of the injections and the burden it places on the caregiver.
- The nurse should anticipate constipation from opioid administration and treat prophylactically.
- Some patients are fearful of taking prescribed pain medications. Explain the importance of taking the medications as ordered, and note that it is easier to maintain pain relief than to reverse severe pain.
- Home health nurses are in key positions for making timely referrals for hospice care. Eligible patients are those who have a life expectancy of 6 months or less, have a desire for supportive palliative care rather than continued treatments, and have a friend or relative who is willing to coordinate the care.

Inpatient services are used for symptom control and respite care for the family. Family and pets may be allowed to stay with the patient. Hospice care assists the family in crisis and continues for up to 1 year after the patient dies, with follow-up counseling, listening, nurturing, and referrals.

Outpatient care is given in the home with family members providing the primary care. Support care is given by the hospice staff. Medications and supplies are furnished by the hospice service. At home, the patient can enjoy loved ones, pets, plants, music, and personal surroundings for as long as possible. See Chapter 17, *Nursing Care of Patients at the End of Life*, for more information.

ONCOLOGICAL EMERGENCIES

Superior Vena Cava Syndrome

Superior vena cava syndrome (SVCS) occurs in patients with lung cancer or cancers of the mediastinum when the tumor or enlarged lymph nodes block circulation in the vena cava. This results in edema of the head, neck, and arms. Symptoms include shortness of breath, cough, chest pain, facial redness, and swollen neck veins. Radiation therapy can be used to shrink the tumor and allow circulation to resume naturally. Nursing interventions for the patient with SVCS include removing rings and restrictive clothing, avoiding taking blood pressure and venipunctures in the arms, and elevating the head of the bed to decrease feeling of dyspnea.

Spinal Cord Compression

Spinal cord compression occurs when a malignant growth presses on the spinal cord. This is a very painful problem and requires pain management while radiation is given to relieve the symptoms. Patients may develop some motor loss when this occurs. Commonly, a myelogram or bone scan is used for diagnosis. Nursing care includes providing a safe environment, assisting with activity, and watching for changes in neurologic status as well as changes in the location or intensity of pain. Patients at risk include those with cancers that spread to the bone and spinal cord, such as lung, breast, and prostate cancer.

Hypercalcemia

In hypercalcemia, the serum calcium level exceeds 11 mg/dL. Hypercalcemia may result from the release of calcium into the blood from bone deterioration, or from ectopic secretion of parathyroid hormone by a tumor. It is common in patients with bone metastasis, especially metastasis from breast cancer. It can be treated with intravenous medication and hydration to lower the calcium level. Nursing care includes maintaining safety and monitoring intake and output, pain control, and changes in pulse rate and rhythm.

Pericardial Effusion and Cardiac Tamponade

In pericardial effusion, usually caused by direct invasion of the cancer, the pericardial sac fills with fluid and may lead to life-threatening compression of the heart (called tamponade). Treatment involves draining the fluid from the heart sac by pericardiocentesis and using sclerosing agents to keep the pericardial sac from refilling with fluid. Nursing care for the patient with cardiac tamponade includes monitoring respiratory status, keeping the head of the bed elevated for maximum lung expansion, monitoring vital signs, monitoring intake and output, and assessing for edema.

Disseminated Intravascular Coagulation

Disseminated intravascular coagulation (DIC) involves an abnormal activation of the clot formation and fibrin mechanisms in the blood, resulting in the consumption of coagulation factors and platelets. Patients with DIC are at high risk for thrombus formation, infarctions, and bleeding. Treatment includes fresh frozen plasma and cryoprecipitates with heparin. Nursing interventions for a patient with DIC include assessing for bleeding, monitoring vital signs, assessing skin for signs of bleeding, keeping accurate intake and output data, and watching for changes in mental status.

SUGGESTED ANSWERS TO

CRITICAL THINKING

■ *Mr. Jones*

1. Mrs. Jones's tumor is beginning to invade surrounding tissue. There is no lymph node involvement and no metastasis.
2. Doxorubicin is commonly associated with red urine and also poses a risk for cardiac toxicity. Cyclophosphamide can cause blood in the urine and a risk for hemorrhagic cystitis. Therefore the patient should take in plenty of fluids and void often (every 2 hours). Both medications can cause nausea, vomiting, and alopecia. Both are vesicants.
3. Because the drugs are vesicants, it is important to inject them into a large vein.
4. Many diagnoses are appropriate, including *Acute Pain* related to surgical incision, *Disturbed Body Image* related to alopecia and loss of a breast, *Imbalanced Nutrition: Less Than Body Requirements* related to nausea and vomiting, *Risk for Injury* related to medication side effects, and *Deficient Knowledge* about cancer treatment and management of side effects. A thorough nursing assessment is needed to determine actual diagnoses.

REVIEW QUESTIONS

1. Which of the following is the hereditary material of cells?
   a. Protein in the ribosomes
   b. DNA in the chromosomes
   c. RNA in the nucleus
   d. Ribosomes in the cytoplasm

2. A patient asks, "How do malignant tumors differ from benign tumors?" Which of the following statements by the nurse are correct? **Select all that apply.**
   a. "Malignant tumors invade surrounding cells and tissues."
   b. "Malignant tumors are generally encapsulated."
   c. "Malignant tumors remain localized."
   d. "Cells in malignant tumors stop dividing prematurely."
   e. "Cells in malignant tumors lack contact inhibition."
   f. "Malignant tumors have defective cell communication."

3. A patient has received vinorelbine (Navelbine) on day 1 of treatment. The nadir will occur in about 10 days. The patient is at greatest risk for which of the following complications at day 10?
   a. Infection
   b. Hair loss
   c. Diarrhea
   d. Myalgia

4. A female patient is starting on doxorubicin (Adriamycin). Which of the following nursing interventions will be most helpful as she plans for hair loss?
   a. Obtain a prescription for a hair growth product.
   b. Massage her scalp to increase circulation and delay hair loss.
   c. Teach her to apply ice to her scalp to prevent hair loss.
   d. Help her choose a wig before her hair loss begins.

5. Which of the following nursing actions is best before administering pain medication for cancer pain?
   a. Assess the patient's anxiety level.
   b. Assess the patient's understanding of the side effects of pain medication.
   c. Determine the patient's pain tolerance.
   d. Assess the success of past pain management measures.

6. The nurse notes that a patient undergoing treatment for bone cancer is having trouble walking. For which oncological emergency should the patient be assessed?
   a. Tumor lysis syndrome
   b. Hypercalcemia
   c. Spinal cord compression
   d. Superior vena cava syndrome

REVIEW QUESTIONS—cont'd

7. A patient receiving radiation therapy has reddened skin over the treated area. How will the nurse know if nursing interventions have been effective?
   a. The patient will be able to describe a proper skin care regimen.
   b. The nurse will keep the skin clean and dry.
   c. The patient's skin will remain intact without breakdown or infection.
   d. The nurse will report the reddened area to the physician.

8. Which of the following patients will benefit from hospice care?
   a. A patient who has liver cancer and is expected to live 4 to 6 weeks
   b. A patient who is having multiple side effects from aggressive chemotherapy
   c. A patient who is trying to make a decision about whether to have surgery that could cure his cancer but may risk serious loss of function
   d. A patient who requires large doses of morphine to control pain related to his cancer and radiation treatment

9. A patient is receiving internal radiation therapy for a gynecological malignancy. The patient expresses feelings of isolation in her private room. What intervention would be best on the part of the nurse?
   a. Encourage the patient's significant other to stay overnight.
   b. Move the patient into a semiprivate room so she can have a roommate.
   c. Instruct the patient about the safety procedures for internal radiation therapy.
   d. Plan to spend more time in this patient's room once work is caught up.

References

American Cancer Society. (2008a). *Facts & figures 2008.* Atlanta: Author. Retrieved June 19, 2009, from www.cancer.org

American Cancer Society. (2008b). *Guidelines for early detection of cancer.* Atlanta: Author. Retrieved January 29, 2010, from http://www.cancer.org/docroot/ped/content/ped_2_3x_acs_cancer_detection_guidelines_36.asp

DavisPlus | For additional resources and information visit **http://davisplus.fadavis.com**

12

Nursing Care of Patients Having Surgery

LINDA S. WILLIAMS

KEY TERMS

adjunct (ADD-junkt)
anesthesia (AN-es-THEE-zee-uh)
anesthesiologist (an-es-THEE-zee-uhl-la-just)
aseptic (ah-SEP-tik)
atelectasis (AT-e-LEK-tah-sis)
debridement (da-breed-MAHNT)
dehiscence (dee-HISS-ents)
evisceration (E-VIS-sir-a-shun)
hematoma (HEE-muh-TOH-mah)
hypothermia (HY-poh-THUR-mee-ah)
induction (in-DUCK-shun)
intraoperative (IN-trah-AW-pruh-tiv)
perioperative (PER-ee-AW-pruh-tiv)
postoperative (post-AW-pruh-tiv)
preoperative (pre-AW-pruh-tiv)
purulent (PURE-u-lent)
serosanguineous (SEER-oh-SANG-gwin-ee-us)
surgeon (SURGE-un)

QUESTIONS TO GUIDE YOUR READING

1. What factors influence surgical outcomes?
2. What is your role in each perioperative phase?
3. What is your role in obtaining informed patient consent?
4. How would you enhance learning for the elderly preoperative patient?
5. What nursing interventions are used for common postoperative patient needs?
6. How will you know if your nursing interventions have been effective?
7. What are the signs and symptoms of common postoperative complications?
8. What are the criteria for ambulatory discharge?
9. What is the role of the home health nurse in caring for postoperative patients?

The Author Acknowledges the Contributions to this Chapter by Linda Kurpinski-Nabozny RN, BSN, and Suzanne Fox, RN.

Surgery is the use of instruments during an operation to treat injuries, diseases, and deformities. Surgical procedures are named according to (1) the involved body organ, part, or location and (2) the suffix that describes what is done during the procedure (Table 12.1). Physicians who perform surgery include **surgeons** or other physicians trained to do certain surgical procedures. Surgery is scheduled based on the urgency required for a successful outcome for the patient (Table 12.2). Surgery is performed for several reasons, examples of which are listed in Table 12.2.

TABLE 12.1 SURGICAL PROCEDURE SUFFIXES

Suffix	Meaning	Word-Building Examples
-ectomy	Removal by cutting	crani (skull) + ectomy = craniectomy appen (appendix) + ectomy = appendectomy
-orrhaphy	Suture of or repair	colo (colon) + orrhaphy = colorrhaphy herni (hernia) + orrhaphy = herniorrhaphy
-oscopy	Looking into	colon (intestine) + oscopy = colonoscopy gastr (stomach) + oscopy = gastroscopy
-ostomy	Formation of a permanent artificial opening	ureter + ostomy = ureterostomy colo (colon) + ostomy = colostomy
-otomy	Incision or cutting into	oust (bone) + otomy = osteotomy thoro (thorax) + otomy = thoracotomy
-plasty	Formation or repair	oto (ear) + plasty = otoplasty mamm (breast) + plasty = mammoplasty

TYPES OF SURGERY

Scope, robotic, and laser technologies continue to reduce the invasiveness of surgical procedures. Minimally invasive surgery is less damaging to tissues than traditional open incision surgery. This allows a faster and less painful recovery. An endoscope is used for minimally invasive surgery, also called keyhole surgery. Minimally invasive surgery includes laparoscopic surgery (abdominal and pelvic cavity) and thoracoscopic surgery (chest and thoracic cavity). The endoscope is a flexible tube with a light, camera, and suction attached. It is inserted through a small incision and projects an image on a screen for the surgeon to watch. Additional incisions are made for other instruments depending on the type of surgery.

Robotic surgery, which uses robots, includes minimally invasive surgery, remote surgery, and unmanned surgery. With remote surgery (telesurgery), the physician is not present in the same geographical location as the patient and uses robotics and telecommunication to perform the surgery.

The *da Vinci* is one type of surgical robot with three or four arms. One is a camera, two are robotic arms that act as the surgeon's hands, and the fourth arm moves obstructions out of the way (Fig. 12.1). As the surgeon moves his or her hands, the robotic arms (which are inside the patient's body) mimic the movements by cutting, suctioning, or suturing. Visit www.intuitivesurgical.com for more information and videos.

TABLE 12.2 SURGERY URGENCY LEVEL AND PURPOSES

Type	Definition	Examples
Urgency Level		
Emergency	Immediate surgery needed to save life or limb without delay	Ruptured aortic aneurysm or appendix, traumatic limb amputation, loss of extremity pulse from emboli
Urgent	Surgery needed within 24–30 hours	Fracture repair, infected gallbladder
Elective	Planned/scheduled, with no time requirements	Joint replacement, hernia repair, skin lesion removal
Optional	Surgery requested by the patient	Cosmetic surgery
Purposes of Surgery		
Aesthetic	Requested by patient for improvement	Blepharoplasty, breast augmentation
Diagnostic	To obtain tissue samples, make an incision, or use a scope to make a diagnosis	Biopsy
Exploratory	Confirmation or measurement of extent of condition	Exploratory laparotomy
Preventive	Removal of tissue before it causes a problem	Mole or polyp removal to prevent cancer
Curative	Removal of diseased or abnormal tissue	Inflamed appendix, tumor, benign cyst, hernia
Reconstructive	Correction of defects of body parts	Scar repair, total knee replacement, face lift, mammoplasty
Palliative	Alleviation of symptoms when disease cannot be cured	Rhizotomy (cuts nerve root to relieve pain), partial tumor removal to relieve pain or pressure; gastrostomy tube to provide tube feedings for swallowing problem; colostomy for incurable bowel obstruction

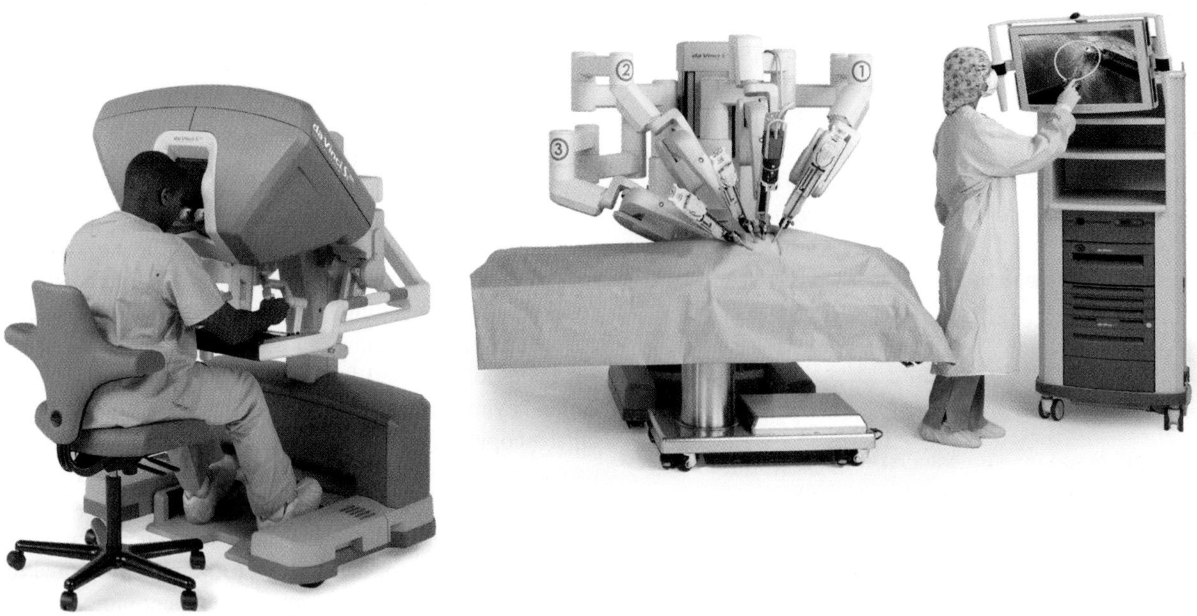

FIGURE 12.1 Surgeon using a da Vinci robotic surgery console and nurse at the vision cart. (Courtesy of Intuitive Surgical, Inc., Sunnyvale, CA.)

PHASES OF SURGERY

There are three phases in the surgical process: preoperative, intraoperative, and postoperative. These phases together are referred to as **perioperative**, which is the time before, during, and after surgery. Each of the perioperative surgical phases has a defined time frame in which specific events related to surgery occur (Table 12.3).

PREOPERATIVE PHASE

Your primary role as a licensed practical nurse/licensed vocational nurse (LPN/LVN) in the **preoperative** phase is to:

- Assist in data collection for developing the patient's plan of care.
- Reinforce explanations and instructions given to the patient and family by the physician and registered nurse (RN).
- Provide emotional and psychological support for patients and their families.

TABLE 12.3 PERIOPERATIVE SURGICAL PHASES

Perioperative	All three phases surrounding and during surgery
Preoperative	Begins with decision for surgery and ends with transfer to the operating room
Intraoperative	Begins with transfer to operating room and ends with admission to perianesthesia care unit (PACU)
Postoperative	Begins with admission to PACU and continues until recovery is complete

Patients' families experience anxiety during surgery. You can help reduce the family member's anxiety so that they are less anxious and able to assist the patient during recovery.

Other health team members assist in preparing the patient for surgery. The physician obtains a medical history, performs a physical examination, and orders diagnostic testing. RNs perform a baseline preoperative assessment, provide explanations and instructions, offer patients and families emotional and psychological support to ease anxiety, develop a plan of care, and then verify the patient's name, surgical site (along with the patient), allergies, and related information when the patient arrives in the surgical area.

Factors Influencing Surgical Outcomes

When preparing a patient for surgery and assisting in the development of a nursing care plan, the goal is to identify and implement actions that reduce surgical risk factors. Preoperative care focuses on helping the patient achieve the best possible surgical outcome by being in the healthiest possible condition for surgery.

Emotional Responses

The word *surgery* causes a common emotional reaction in patients and their families. You need to be aware of these reactions to assist the patient in coping with them. If any of the patient's fears are extreme, such as a fear of dying or not waking up after surgery, the physician should be informed.

Surgical patients may experience various fears related to **anesthesia** (reversible loss of sensation): possible brain damage, feeling sensation during surgery, feeling loss of control, or a fear of not waking up. The patient should discuss these concerns with the **anesthesiologist**. Listening to music or using guided imagery before surgery may reduce a patient's anxiety and help to calm the patient.

It is normal for patients to be concerned about pain. During surgery, the anesthesia provider gives medications to control pain. Nurses give prescribed analgesics for pain relief after surgery. Complementary techniques can also be used to help reduce pain, such as guided imagery or focused breathing.

Changes in body image may be a great fear for some patients. The thought of disfigurement, mutilation, bleeding, or having a scar causes great anxiety for some patients. Allow them to discuss these fears.

Age

Surgery can be a positive experience that promotes quality of life for many elderly patients. For healthy older patients, age alone does not mean that they are at greater surgical risk. Complications can occur, however, related to previous health status, immobilization occurring from surgery, normal aging changes reducing the effectiveness of deep breathing and coughing, and the effects of administered medications (Box 12.1, *Gerontological Issues*). Older patients may need a longer time to recover from anesthetic agents because of aging changes in drug metabolism and elimination.

Hydration and Nutrition

A normal fluid and electrolyte balance decreases complications. Patients should be well nourished to adequately heal and recover from surgery (Box 12.2, *Nutrition Notes*). Higher levels of protein (tissue repair and healing), vitamin C (collagen formation), and zinc (tissue growth, skin integrity, and cell-mediated immunity) are required. Patients who are obese or underweight may not heal as well and may have complications. Patients who are obese have more respiratory problems and wound healing difficulties, such as delayed healing and wound *dehiscence* (opening of the incision). Patients who are emaciated may have more infections and delayed wound healing because they lack the nutrients needed for tissue healing.

Smoking and Alcohol

Tobacco and alcohol use increases the surgical patient's risks. Smoking thickens and increases the amount of lung secretions and reduces the action of cilia that remove the secretions. Patients should be encouraged to avoid smoking for 24 hours before surgery or 3 to 4 weeks before surgery if they have a chronic lung disorder. Not smoking increases the action of the lungs' defense mechanisms and makes more hemoglobin available to carry oxygen during surgery. It also improves wound healing.

Long-term alcohol use may cause nutritional deficiencies and liver damage, which can create bleeding problems, fluid volume imbalances, and drug metabolism alterations. In addition, alcohol interacts with medications and should be avoided before surgery.

Diseases

Chronic disorders may increase the patient's surgical risk unless they are well controlled. A medical clearance for surgery may be needed from the patient's physician. For patients with diabetes, the stress of surgery can alter blood glucose levels. Patients with chronic lung disorders may be at risk for pulmonary complications from anesthesia.

Preadmission Surgical Patient Assessment

Nonemergent surgical patients have either a preadmission telephone or face-to-face interview with RNs in the preadmission testing (PAT) department. Patients have reduced anxiety and better understanding with prescreening. The interview process includes a health history, identification of risk factors, patient and family teaching, discharge planning, and necessary referrals to social work, support groups, and educational programs. Patients are asked if there have been any personal or family problems with anesthesia or malignant hyperthermia. Malignant hyperthermia is a rare hereditary muscle disease that can predispose the patient to a serious life-threatening reaction to certain anesthetic agents (discussed later).

Preoperative diagnostic testing is based on the patient's age, medical history, assessment findings, and institutional protocols (Table 12.4). A urine or serum pregnancy test as appropriate for female patients may be done to prevent fetal exposure to anesthetics. Health information and diagnostic testing results are reviewed by anesthesia providers. Abnormal test results are reported to the surgeon. Interventions are ordered for abnormalities.

Federal law says patients must be asked before surgery if they have a signed advance directive (e.g., health care durable power of attorney or living will) for their medical record (see Chapter 17). If there is no advance directive, written information on advance directives is provided.

Preoperative Teaching

Preoperative Routines

Preoperative teaching provides information about common surgical preparation procedures and routines:

- Date and time of admission and surgery
- Admission procedures, including arriving about 2 hours before surgery to allow preparation time
- Length of stay, items to bring and wear
- Recovery after surgery
- Family information, such as where to wait during surgery and who communicates patient's status to them
- Discharge criteria, including the need for a responsible adult to take the patient home after outpatient surgery.

Preoperative Instructions

To reduce the risk of aspiration during surgery, the anesthesiologist orders fluid and food restrictions. The minimal fasting time frame guidelines of the American Society of Anesthesiologists are listed in Box 12.2. However, patients may be instructed to stop fluid and food intake (NPO) after midnight the night before a morning surgery. Patients may brush their teeth or rinse their mouth without swallowing water. Cancellation of surgery can result if the patient has not been NPO as ordered.

Medications the patient is to take the morning of surgery, with an ounce of water, are explained. Special preparations,

Box 12.1

Gerontological Issues

Surgical Considerations for the Older Adult

Older adults usually have limited physiological reserve, resulting in decreased ability to compensate for changes that occur during surgery. The risk for hemorrhage, anemia, fluid/electrolyte imbalance, and infection are increased in older adults. Increased risk for complications is secondary to age-related loss of blood vessel elasticity and decreased cardiac, respiratory, and renal reserves. Nursing interventions should be aimed at these age-related changes before, during, and after the surgical procedure to help reduce complications.

Preoperatively

- Reassure the patient and family.
- Pad bony prominences to protect against pressure ulcers and muscle and bone discomfort.
- Teach what to expect before, during, and after surgery; diet changes, description and length of surgical procedure; activities in the recovery room; pain management; coughing and deep breathing exercises; procedures; and treatments (e.g., dressings, catheters).
- Ensure preoperative screening: blood work, radiographic studies, nutritional assessments, pulmonary function tests, electrocardiogram.

Intraoperatively

- Assess patient for hypothermia (cool temperature in operating room, medications that slow metabolism).
- Assess patient for hypoxia (older adult may exhibit restlessness).
- Assess patient for hemorrhage.
- Assess patient's output (urine, drainage, bleeding, emesis).

Postoperatively

Pain Control—Provide adequate pain relief so required postoperative activities, such as deep breathing, coughing, position changes, and exercise, can be performed more effectively.

Respiratory Function—Reduce respiratory complications by encouraging deep breathing and coughing:

- Perform after pain medication has begun to take effect to encourage deep breaths due to less pain. Assess the patient carefully when giving narcotics because they can cause respiratory depression.
- Use a pillow and instruct the patient to hold it firmly over abdominal or chest incisions to support the incision. Taking a deep breath increases chest expansion, as well as abdominal pressure, which may pull or stretch an incision.
- Older adults perform deep-breathing and coughing exercises better if the nurse performs the exercises with them. For example, say the following: "Let's take a deep breath in through the nose, hold it and count to three, then slowly blow it out completely through the mouth. When you blow the air out, shape your lips like they are going to whistle. Great, let's do it again."

Mobility—Encourage mobility through the following nursing actions and observations:

- Use pillows to support the patient's body alignment; assist the patient to ambulate as soon as possible after surgery; and regularly help the patient with passive or active range-of-motion exercises, along with flexion and extension exercises, for legs and feet.
- Monitor for unilateral swelling of the leg and calf or groin pain, which may indicate deep venous thrombosis, a risk related to venous pooling in the lower extremities. This risk is increased with postoperative inactivity.
- Assist the patient to change position at least every 2 hours. If patients lay in one position too long, pressure ulcers can develop. When tissues are compressed between bones and the bed surface, blood supply is reduced to the tissue and cells begin to die. This results in painful open wounds.

Bowel Function—Assess bowel sounds. It is common for patients to feel bloated after surgery. Increasing activity, such as walking—not just sitting in a chair—stimulates peristaltic action of the bowel. This helps expel flatus and reduce discomfort.

Urinary Function—Be aware of the following aspects of urinary function:

- Individuals often have difficulty emptying their bladder after surgery. Patients who are sleeping but restless should be evaluated for bladder distention. It is often difficult to void on a bed pan or in a urinal in a supine position.
- Older men with an enlarged prostate may have even greater difficulty voiding if they have received medications that have urinary retention side effects.
- Assisting patients to sit or stand to use urinals, use a bedside commode, or ambulate to the bathroom promotes bladder emptying and helps avoid the use of urinary catheters.
- Measure urine output that is voided or from a catheter. Note the color and odor of the urine. Older adults are prone to dehydration, and this provides an indication of their hydration status for intervention.

Delirium—Perform the following nursing actions to minimize delirium:

- Monitor level of consciousness routinely. Provide a calm environment and orient patients to their environment. Restraints should not be used because they can worsen delirium.
- Recognize that the presence of a urinary catheter can contribute to delirium, so methods to avoid the need for a catheter should be tried.

Box 12.2
Nutrition Notes

Screening and Nourishing the Preoperative Patient

Identifying and treating malnutrition before surgery may improve the patient's outcome. Unintended weight loss or a low serum albumin level should prompt further nutritional assessment. Before elective surgery, the patient may have time to correct some nutritional deficiencies. If patients are overweight they are often instructed to lose weight to reduce the risk of surgery. For anemia, an iron preparation can be administered. At least 2 to 3 weeks are required for objective evidence of the effectiveness of nutritional therapy. Before surgery on the gastrointestinal tract, a low-residue diet may be given for 2 to 3 days to minimize bowel contents.

Preoperative fasting time orders vary but the American Society of Anesthesiologists' guidelines (1999a) recommend a minimum of the following time frames before anesthesia:

- Clear liquids: 2 hours
- Breast milk: 4 hours
- Infant formula or a light meal: 6 hours
- A regular meal containing meat or fat: 8 hours.

Clinical judgment is required regardless of the guidelines, which do not apply to:

- Patients with gastromotility or metabolic disorders
- Those with potential airway problems
- Women in labor.

Many people take over-the-counter herbal products. The American Society of Anesthesiologists (1999b) issued a warning to consumers of herbal medicine to stop taking the products 2 to 3 weeks before scheduled surgery. Possible interactions include an unintended deepening of anesthesia and problems with bleeding and blood pressure.

TABLE 12.4 PREOPERATIVE DIAGNOSTIC TESTS

Diagnostic Test	Purpose
Chest x-ray	Detect pulmonary and cardiac abnormalities
Oxygen saturation	Obtain baseline level and detect abnormality
Serum Tests	
Arterial blood gases	Obtain baseline levels and detect pH and oxygenation abnormalities
Bleeding time	Detect prolonged bleeding problem
Blood urea nitrogen	Detect kidney problem
Creatinine	Detect kidney problem
Complete blood cell count	Detect anemia, infection, clotting problem
Electrolytes	Detect potassium, sodium, chloride imbalances
Fasting blood glucose	Detect abnormalities, monitor diabetes control
Pregnancy	Detect early, unknown pregnancy
Partial thromboplastin time	Detect clotting problem
International normalized ratio (INR), prothrombin time	Detect clotting problem, monitor warfarin therapy
Type and crossmatch	Identify blood type to match blood for possible transfusion
Urine Tests	
Pregnancy	Detect early, unknown pregnancy
Urinalysis	Detect infection, abnormalities

such as an enema, are also described. For abdominal or intestinal surgery, enemas are ordered to empty the bowel in order to reduce fecal contamination preoperatively and straining or distention postoperatively.

Instructions for postoperative care are given before surgery so the patient is alert when being taught and has time to learn. Patients should be told that active participation in postoperative care aids in their recovery. Teach patients how to report their pain level using a pain rating scale so that prompt pain relief can be provided (see Chapter 10). Pain rating scales include a 0 (none) to 10 (worst possible) rating scale, a color-based rating scale, or a scale using pictures of faces showing varying degrees of frowning or smiling that indicate a certain pain level. Pain relief methods are described, such as analgesic injections, an epidural catheter, or patient-controlled analgesia (PCA). Anticipated dressings, tubes, casts, or special equipment are also described. If needed, crutches are fitted to the patient, and their proper use is explained and demonstrated.

Postoperative exercises are taught to decrease complications. They include deep breathing and coughing, use of incentive spirometry, leg exercises, turning, and how to get out of bed. After an exercise is taught, the patient should perform a return demonstration so understanding and ability to perform the exercise correctly can be evaluated.

Deep breathing helps prevent the development of **atelectasis** (collapse of the lung caused by hypoventilation or mucous obstruction preventing some alveoli from opening and being fully ventilated) by expanding and ventilating the lungs. The patient is taught to sit up, exhale fully, take in a deep breath through the nose, hold the breath and count to three, and then exhale completely through the mouth. The patient is told to repeat this hourly while awake, in sets of five, for 24 to 48 hours postoperatively.

• WORD • BUILDING •

atelectasis: ateles—imperfect + ektasis—expansion

Incentive spirometry may also be ordered postoperatively to prevent atelectasis by increasing lung volume, alveoli expansion, and venous return (Fig. 12.2). All patients can benefit from incentive spirometry, especially the elderly and those at increased risk for lung complications. The spirometer stays at the patient's bedside for hourly use while awake (not on the window sill or in a drawer where it cannot be reached by the patient!). Offer the spirometer to the patient each hour to ensure that it is used. Teach patients to do the following:

- Sit upright, at 45 degrees minimum, if possible.
- Take two normal breaths. Place mouthpiece of spirometer in mouth.
- Inhale until target, designated by spirometer light or rising ball, is reached, and hold breath for 3 to 5 seconds.
- Exhale completely.
- Perform 10 sets of breaths each hour.

Coughing moves secretions to prevent pneumonia. Teach patients how to cough effectively if not contraindicated by the patient's condition (such as hernia repair or head injury) (Table 12.5). Give pain medication before asking the patient to cough and offer reassurance that coughing should not harm the incision. Splinting the incision with a pillow may be comforting. Several sets of coughing are performed every 1 to 2 hours while the patient is awake.

Leg exercises, if not contraindicated, improve circulation and help prevent complications related to stasis of blood, such as emboli formation. Instructions are to lie down, raise the leg, bend it at the knee, flex the foot, extend the leg, and lower it to the bed. Each leg is exercised in sets of five. Foot circles are also done every hour while awake. Teach the patient to raise a leg slightly off the bed with toes pointed. Draw a circle in the air with the great toe, rotating to the right four times, then to the left. Repeat this five times and then do the same with the other foot.

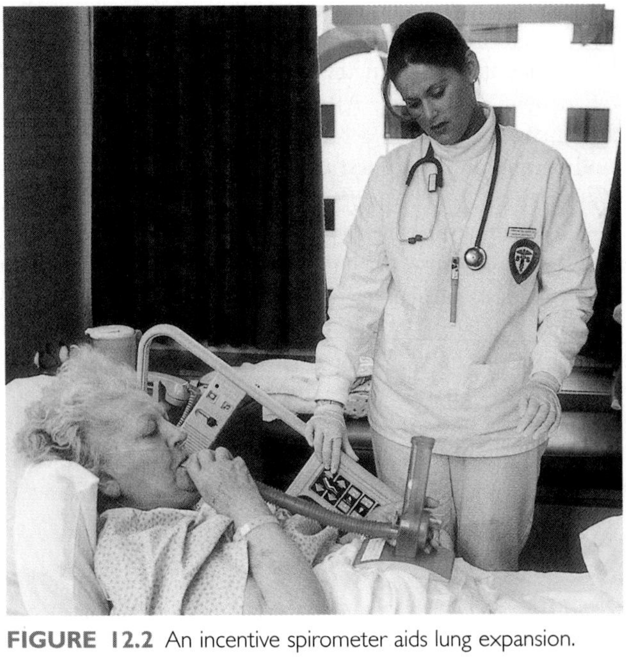

FIGURE 12.2 An incentive spirometer aids lung expansion.

TABLE 12.5 TEACHING PATIENTS COUGHING TECHNIQUES

Procedure	Rationale
Have patient sit up and lean forward.	Promotes lung expansion and ability to generate forceful cough.
Show patient how to splint incision with hands, pillow, or blanket.	Reduces incision pressure so it does not feel as if incision is opening.
Have patient inhale and exhale deeply three times through mouth.	Helps expand lungs.
Have patient take in deep breath and cough out the breath forcefully with three short coughs using diaphragmatic muscles. Take in quick deep breath through mouth, cough deeply, and deep breathe.	Generates forceful cough and expands lungs to help move secretions.

Patients are taught that turning from side to side in bed is aided by bending the leg that is to be on top and placing a pillow between the legs to support the top leg. They are told, unless contraindicated, to use the bed's side rail to pull themselves over to the side. To promote comfort, patients are encouraged to deep breathe while turning instead of holding their breath.

To make it easier for patients to get out of bed and to reduce strain on the incision, patients are instructed to turn to their side without pillows between their knees. Then they should place their hands flat against the bed and push up while swinging their legs out of bed and into a sitting position. Patients should be told to sit for a few minutes after changing position to avoid dizziness and falling. They should also deep breathe while sitting to promote lung expansion.

Nursing Process for Preoperative Patients

Data Collection

HEALTH HISTORY. Upon admission for surgery, patient data are collected (Table 12.6). Ensure that patients use their contact lenses, glasses, or hearing aids for accurate communication. Note the patient's emotional reaction to surgery. If the patient is anxious, explore the cause of the anxiety and allow the patient to express concerns. Anxiety is a feeling of apprehension or uneasiness resulting from the uncertainties and risks associated with surgery, whereas fear, a feeling of dread from a source known to the patient, is an extreme reaction to surgery.

Medications. All prescription and over-the-counter medications that the patient takes are reviewed, along with any herbal remedies or recreational drugs. As a result of this

TABLE 12.6 NURSING ASSESSMENT OF THE PREOPERATIVE PATIENT

Subjective Data: Health History Questions	
Demographic information	Name, age, marital status, occupation, roles?
Condition for which surgery is scheduled	Why are you having surgery?
Medical history	Any allergies, acute or chronic conditions, current medications, pain, or prior hospitalizations?
Surgical history	Any reactions or problems with anesthesia? Previous surgeries?
Tobacco use	How much do you smoke? Pack-year history (number of packs per day × number of years)?
Alcohol use	How often do you drink alcohol? How much?
Coping techniques	How do you usually cope with stressful situations? Support systems?
Family history	Hereditary conditions, diabetes, cardiovascular or anesthesia problems?
Female patients	Date of last menses and obstetrical information?
Physical Assessment	
Vital signs, oxygen saturation	
Height and weight	
Emotional status	Calm, anxious, tearful
Neurologic	Ability to follow instructions
Skin	Color, warmth, bruises, lesions, turgor, dryness, mucous membranes
Respiratory	Infection (cough; breath sounds); chronic obstructive pulmonary disease; respiratory rate, pattern, and effort; barrel chest
Cardiovascular	Angina, myocardial infarction, heart failure, hypertension, valvular heart disease, mitral valve prolapse, heart rate and rhythm, peripheral pulses, edema, jugular vein distention
Gastrointestinal	Bowel sounds, date of last bowel movement, abdominal distention, firmness, ostomy
Musculoskeletal	Deformities, weakness, decreased range of motion, crepitation, gait, artificial limbs, prostheses

review, the physician may need to order alterations in drug dosages and routes of administration. Medications such as warfarin (Coumadin), aspirin, or other NSAIDs may need to be stopped several days before surgery to avoid bleeding problems during surgery. Because herbal medicines can interfere with medications used during surgery or increase bleeding times, patients may be instructed to stop them 1 to 2 weeks before surgery.

Patients with diabetes who take insulin are usually instructed by the physician to either hold their insulin or take half of their normal dose of insulin the day of surgery. On the day of surgery, blood glucose monitoring may be done every 4 hours or as ordered to ensure that blood glucose levels are maintained within a desired range.

Patients on chronic oral steroid therapy cannot abruptly stop their medication even though they may be told to take nothing by mouth (NPO) before or after surgery. Serious complications, such as circulatory collapse, can develop if steroids are stopped abruptly. The physician should order a patient's steroid therapy to be given by a parenteral route if the patient is NPO, so that it is not interrupted. Make sure that the steroid therapy is ordered and continued for the patient via an alternate route.

Patients should be asked about the use of alcohol or drugs such as cocaine, marijuana, or opioids because they can interact with anesthesia or other medications. To obtain honest, accurate information, patients should be told of this potential interaction. Information and questions should be stated in a nonjudgmental manner. For example, you should ask, "How much alcohol do you drink daily or weekly?" instead of "Do you drink alcohol?" The first statement assumes that people drink alcohol. This allows the patient who does not drink to indicate none and the patient who does to state an amount rather than having to say yes and then give an amount upon further questioning. More accurate responses are given because this approach is viewed more positively by the patient who consumes alcohol. Another example would be to ask the patient, "What roles do drugs or alcohol play in your life?"

Physical Assessment

A physical assessment of body systems is performed. This information can highlight risk factors for surgery, determine the type of anesthesia to be used, and assist in planning interventions to reduce risk factors. A cough, cold, or fever is reported to the physician because surgery may be delayed until the patient recovers from an acute infection. Dentures, bridges, capped teeth, and loose teeth are documented because they can become dislodged during intubation (insertion of endotracheal breathing tube) for general anesthesia, causing complications.

Nursing Diagnoses, Planning, and Interventions

Anxiety or Fear Related to Potential Change in Body Image, Hospitalization, Pain, Loss of Control, and Uncertainties Surrounding Surgery

EXPECTED OUTCOME: Patient will state reduced anxiety or fear before surgery.

- Inform patients about procedures and surgical routines, *which helps reduce anxiety.*
- Allow patients to express their concerns *to allow inaccurate information to be corrected.*

- If patients express extreme anxiety or fear, inform the physician *because complications or even death could result. When fear is excessive, the physician may reschedule the surgery until the patient is better able to cope.*

Deficient Knowledge Related to Lack of Prior Experience with Surgical Routines and Procedures

EXPECTED OUTCOME: Patient will demonstrate understanding of surgical information and routines before surgery.

- Patient anxiety levels should be considered when providing explanations *because learning can be affected by high anxiety levels.*
- Identify knowledge deficiencies with the patient *so that he or she is motivated to learn.*
- Reinforce information provided before admission and new information to patients *to promote informed choice and increase self-care abilities. Teaching is caring in action and empowers patients to be a participant in their care.*
- Include the patient's family or caregivers in teaching sessions *so they can assist the patient through the surgical experience.*
- Use a variety of teaching methods (discussion, written materials and instructions, models, and videos) *to allow for different learning styles and to reinforce learning.*
- Individualize explanations *so the patient is not overwhelmed.*
- Use teaching methods that can be adapted to aging changes that may affect learning. *Box 12.3,* Gerontological Issues, *describes methods to provide a positive learning experience for the older patient.*
- Document teaching and patient understanding. *Documentation is essential as proof of what was explained and patient understanding.*

Evaluation

The goal of decreased anxiety is achieved if the patient states and demonstrates that anxiety is relieved. If the patient is able to learn during teaching sessions, anxiety is not a barrier to learning. The goal for correcting deficient knowledge is reached if the patient states understanding of the information presented and accurately performs return demonstrations of presented information.

Preoperative Consent

Before performing surgery, it is the physician's responsibility to obtain voluntary, written, informed consent from the patient. The consent gives legal permission for the surgery and has two purposes: It protects the patient from unauthorized procedures, and it protects the physician, anesthesiologist, hospital, and hospital employees from claims of performance of unauthorized procedures. A signed consent is needed for all invasive procedures, surgery, anesthesia, blood administration, and radiation or cobalt therapy. It is typically valid for 30 days after signing.

Box 12.3

Gerontological Issues

Considerations for Elderly Patient Teaching Sessions

Environmental Considerations

- Comfortable: anxiety free, quiet, appropriate temperature
- Correctly lit: small, intense lighting with nonglare, soft white light (not fluorescent)
- Private: no distractions, no background noise, turn off pagers

Presentation Considerations

- Assess readiness to learn.
- Assess comfort and safety needs.
- Use past experience and relate to new learning.
- Base learning on assessment data and current knowledge base.
- Use simple, understandable words and avoid medical jargon.
- Use legible audiovisual materials: large print, black print on white nonglare paper.
- If using colors, remember that older adults see red, orange, and yellow best; blue, violet, and green are more difficult to see.
- Perform ongoing assessment of energy level of patient.
- Answer questions as they occur.

Presenter Considerations

- Have a positive attitude and belief in self-care promotion for older adults.
- Earn trust by being viewed as a credible, positive role model.
- Maintain a professional appearance.
- Use knowledge of aging changes in presentation.
- Speak slowly in a low tone.
- Sit near patient for best visibility.
- Ensure that prostheses are in place, such as glasses, hearing aids.
- Allow patient increased response time, and use memory aids such as pictures or diagrams.
- Use touch appropriately to convey caring.
- Teach most important information first.
- Present one idea at a time.
- Provide instruction using multiple senses (vision and hearing).
- Provide repetition.
- Ask for feedback to ensure comprehension.
- Provide feedback and positive reinforcement.

Informed consent involves three elements:

1. The physician must explain in terms the patient understands about the diagnosis, the proposed treatment and who will perform it, the likely outcome, possible risks and complications of treatment, alternative treatments, and the prognosis without treatment. If the patient has questions before signing the consent, the physician must be contacted to provide further explanation to the patient. It is not within the nurse's scope of practice to provide this information.
2. The consent must be signed before analgesics or sedatives are given because patients must demonstrate to the witness that they are informed and understand the surgery.
3. Consent must be given voluntarily. No persuasion or threats can be used to influence the patient. The patient can withdraw consent at any time, even after the consent form has been signed.

To ensure that patients are truly informed before signing a consent form, in some institutions patients must take and pass a knowledge quiz, which can be given verbally. If they do not pass the quiz, then further explanation is needed by the physician. Also, in the surgical holding area, patients verbally reconsent. They are asked, "Do you still remember what you were told about your surgery?"

It is often your role to obtain and witness the patient's or authorized person's signature on the consent form (Fig. 12.3). As the patient's advocate, you must ensure that the person signing the consent form understands its meaning and has no further questions to be directed to the physician before it is signed, and that it is being signed voluntarily. If the patient is unable to read, the entire consent must be read to the patient before it is signed. Patients are unable to give consent if they are unconscious, are mentally incompetent, are minors, or have received analgesics or drugs that alter central nervous system function within time frames specified by agency policy. Consent may be obtained in any of these cases from parents, next of kin, or legal guardians as specified by law.

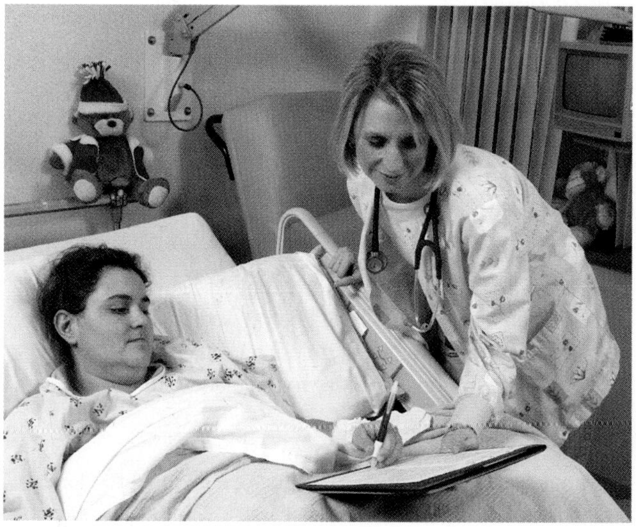

FIGURE 12.3 Nurse is witnessing signature of patient on surgical consent.

NURSING CARE TIP

Witnessing a Consent

Your signature as a witness on a consent form indicates that you observed the informed patient or patient's authorized representative voluntarily sign the consent form. It does not mean that you informed the patient about the surgical procedure; that is the responsibility of the physician.

In a medical emergency, the patient may not be able to give consent. In this case, the next of kin or legal guardian may give telephone consent, or a court order can be obtained. If time does not permit this, the physician documents the need for treatment in the chart as necessary to save the patient's life or avoid serious harm, according to state law and institutional policy.

Preparation for Surgery

Preoperative Preparation Checklist

A preoperative checklist is usually completed and signed by the nurse (per agency policy) before the patient is transported from the surgical unit to surgery (Fig. 12.4). The checklist provides guidance for preoperative preparation of the patient:

- An identification band is placed on the patient. A hospital gown is given to the patient to wear. Underwear is removed, depending on the type of surgery.
- Vital signs are taken and recorded as baseline information and to assess patient status.
- Makeup, nail polish, and artificial nails (if applicable) are removed to allow assessment of natural color and pulse oximetry for oxygenation status during surgery.
- Removal of hair pins, wigs, and jewelry prevents loss or injury. Rings, such as wedding rings, are taped in place if the patient does not want to take them off, except if the ring is on the operative side (arm or chest surgery), because edema may occur.
- Dentures, contact lenses, and prostheses are removed to prevent injury. Some patients are concerned about body image and do not want family members to see them without dentures or makeup. Remove dentures after the family goes to the waiting room and insert them before the family sees the patient postoperatively.

Pre-op Surgical Checklist **Client Name**

_____ I.D. BAND ON _______________

_____ NPO AS ORDERED

_____ PRE-OP TEACHING COMPLETED

_____ INFORMED CONSENT SIGNED

_____ HISTORY AND PHYSICAL ON CHART

_____ ALLERGIES

_____ LAB RESULTS

_____ CBC: HGB _____ HCT _____ WBC _____ PLATELETS _____

_____ POTASSIUM _______

_____ URINALYSIS _______

_____ PREGNANCY TEST SERUM _____ URINE _____

_____ PT _____ PTT _____ BLEEDING TIME _____

_____ TYPE AND SCREEN _____ CROSSMATCH _____-___ UNITS

_____ ECG ON CHART

_____ CHEST X-RAY REPORT ON CHART

_____ SHOWERED/BATHED

_____ HOSPITAL GOWN ON

_____ PREPS COMPLETED AS ORDERED

_____ ANTIEMBOLISM STOCKINGS

_____ JEWELRY TAPED/REMOVED: DISPOSITION _______

_____ VALUABLES: DISPOSITION _______________

_____ DENTURES, PROSTHESIS REMOVED

_____ HAIR PINS, WIGS, MAKE UP, NAIL POLISH, ONE ACRYLIC NAIL REMOVED

_____ CONTACT LENSES REMOVED

_____ VOIDED

_____ VITAL SIGNS: T _____ P _____ R _____ BP _____

_____ PRE-OP MEDICATIONS GIVEN _______________ SIDE RAILS UP _______

_____ IV STARTED _______________

_____ EYE GLASSES AND HEARING AID(S) TO OR

_____ OLD CHART TO OR

_____ X-RAYS TO OR

_____ FAMILY LOCATION _______________

_____ NEXT OF KIN _______________

CLIENT READY FOR SURGERY _______________

TIME _________ (NURSE SIGNATURE)

COMMENTS:

FIGURE 12.4 Sample preoperative checklist form.

- Glasses and hearing aids go with patients to surgery if they are unable to communicate without them. Label them with the patient's name and document where they go.
- All orders, diagnostic test results, consents, and history and physical (required on the chart) are reviewed for completion and documented on the checklist.
- Patient valuables are recorded and given to a family member or locked up per institutional policy by the nurse.
- Antiembolism devices are applied if ordered.
- Patients are asked to void before sedating preoperative medications are given, unless a urinary catheter is present, to prevent injury to the bladder during surgery.

Preoperative Medications

The final preparation before surgery is giving preoperative medications at the time ordered, usually 1 hour before, or on call to surgery (i.e., surgery calls to instruct that it is time to give the drugs) (Table 12.7). All medications administered are

TABLE 12.7 PREOPERATIVE MEDICATIONS

Class/Action	Examples	Route	Side Effects	Nursing Implications
Antianxiety and Sedative Hypnotics				
Sedation; anxiety reduction	Diazepam (Valium) Lorazepam (Ativan) Midazolam (Versed)	PO, IV PO, IV, IM IV, IM	Drowsiness, weakness, oversedation, respiratory depression	Contraindicated for acute narrow-angle glaucoma. Monitor respirations.
Anticholinergics				
Secretion reduction	Atropine sulfate Glycopyrrolate (Robinul) Scopolamine hydrobromide	IM Patch, PO	Dry mouth, headache, nausea	Contraindicated for acute narrow-angle glaucoma.
Antiemetics				
Control nausea and vomiting; may be effective into the postoperative period	Ondansetron (Zofran) Metoclopramide (Reglan) Promethazine hydrochloride (Phenergan)	IV PO, IV IM	Diarrhea, dizziness, drowsiness, headache	Redness, pain, or burning at the site of injection. Increased drowsiness with opioids. IV route can cause necrosis; dilute with 10 mL of normal saline; give through running IV line.
Alkalinizing Agents				
Increase gastric pH	Sodium citrate and citric acid (Bicitra)	Oral	Nausea, vomiting, diarrhea, stomach pain	Mix in 4 ounces of water or juice.
Antibiotics				
Prevention of postoperative infection	Variety of antibiotics used	IV	Review specific drug for side effects.	Give within 30–60 minutes of incision for best effect.
Histamine (H_2) Antagonists				
Reduction of acidic gastric secretions to prevent acid aspiration pneumonitis	Famotidine (Pepcid) Ranitidine (Zantac)	Oral, IV IV	Few side effects; dizziness, headache, diarrhea	Monitor creatinine clearance.
Opioids				
Bind to opioid receptors in the CNS to alter perception of pain and enhance postoperative pain relief	Morphine sulfate Fentanyl (Sublimaze, Duragesic) Meperidine (Demerol)	IM, IV PO, IV, IM IM	Respiratory depression, sedation, hypotension, constipation	Monitor vital signs, level of sedation, and respiratory status. Avoid meperidine use in elderly.

documented. The bed rails are raised for safety and the patient is instructed not to get up alone after medications are given.

Transfer to Surgery

When the surgery department is ready, the patient is transported to the surgical holding area on a gurney (Fig. 12.5). The patient's chart, inhaler medications for those with asthma, and glasses or hearing aids to aid communication are taken with the patient. The patient can be accompanied by family members.

During surgery, the family waits in the surgical waiting area, which is a communication center where the family is kept informed of the patient's status. The physician talks with the family when surgery is over. Families may be given beepers so that they can walk outside or to other areas of the hospital and still be reached.

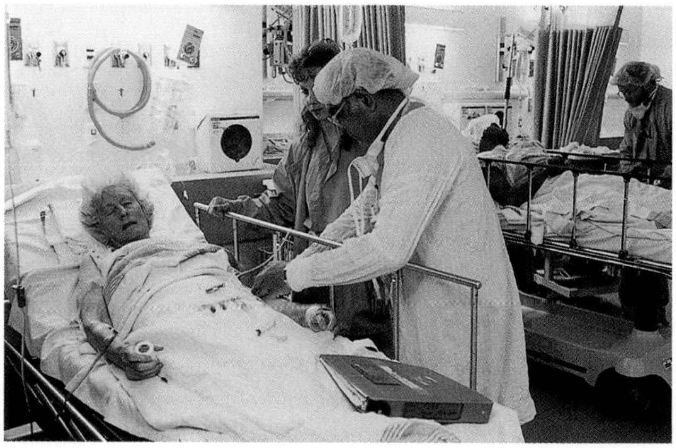

FIGURE 12.5 Surgical holding area.

After Transfer

After the patient goes to surgery, prepare the patient's room and necessary equipment so it is ready for the patient's return (Table 12.8).

INTRAOPERATIVE PHASE

When the patient is transferred to the operating table, the next phase of the perioperative period, the **intraoperative** phase, begins. Surgery may take place in a hospital operating room (OR) or free-standing ambulatory or outpatient surgical center (Figs. 12.6 and 12.7). Additionally, surgery is performed in

TABLE 12.8 POSTOPERATIVE PATIENT HOSPITAL ROOM PREPARATION

After patient transfer to surgery, prepare the patient's room for the patient's postoperative care needs on return from the perianesthesia care unit.

Preparation	Rationale
Bed	
Bed linens should be clean and are changed if used by patient before surgery.	Reduces contamination of surgical wound.
Place disposable, absorbent, waterproof pads on bottom sheet if drainage is expected.	Protects linen from wetness and soiling so a patient in pain does not have to be disturbed for linen change.
Apply lift sheet on bed of patient needing assistance with repositioning.	Makes lifting and turning easier for patient and nurse.
Have extra blankets available.	Patient may be cold.
Fanfold top cover to end of bed or to side of bed away from patient transfer side.	Readies bed to receive patient on transfer and allows covers to be easily pulled up over patient.
Obtain extra pillows as needed for positioning, elevating extremities, splinting during coughing.	Pillows help maintain position when patient is turned, or splint an incision during coughing, or elevate operative extremities for comfort and swelling reduction.
Equipment	
Have vital sign equipment available.	Promotes ability to promptly obtain vital signs.
Have intravenous (IV) pole/controller pump available.	Surgical patients have IV infusions postoperatively.
Have oxygen set up as needed.	After tracheostomy, patients wear humidified oxygen mask.
Prepare suction setup for tracheostomy, nasogastric tube, or drains as ordered.	Suction may be ordered related to surgical procedures: *Sterile suction:* tracheostomy *Nasogastric tube:* thoracic, abdominal, gastrointestinal surgery *T-tube:* cholecystectomy.
Have emesis basin at bedside.	Nausea or vomiting may occur, especially after movement during transfer.
Have tissues and washcloths in room.	Promotes comfort: washing face or a cool cloth on forehead.
Have urinal or bedpan available in room.	Patients may be unable to get out of bed for first voiding.
Obtain special equipment as indicated by the surgical procedure.	Institutional policy and physician orders may require specialized equipment. Examples: *Jaw surgery:* suction, wire cutters, tracheostomy tray *Tracheostomy:* suction, extra tracheostomy set, tracheostomy care supplies
Documentation Forms	
Place any agency postoperative documentation forms in room.	Promotes timely and accurate documentation of patient data.

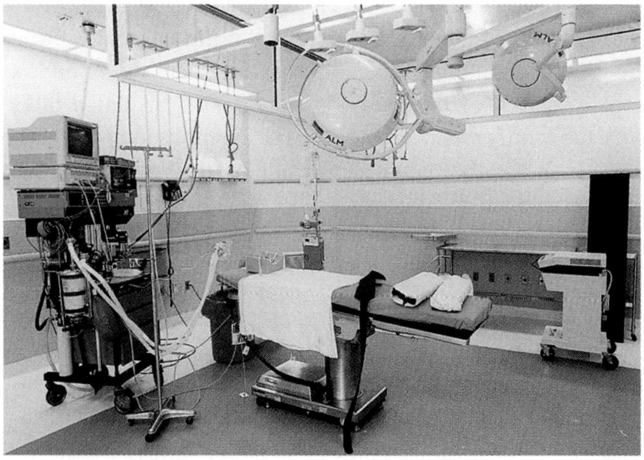

FIGURE 12.6 Operating room. Anesthesia equipment is on the left.

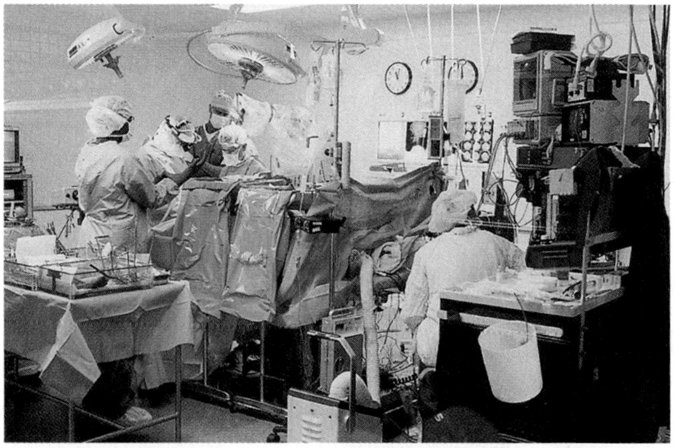

FIGURE 12.7 Operating room in use. Anesthesia equipment is on the right.

physician's offices, cardiac catheterization laboratories, radiology centers, emergency rooms, and specialized units that perform endoscopy procedures.

The OR team members must perform a sterile surgical hand scrub to reduce the amount of microorganisms on their hands and arms. Jewelry (e.g., watches, rings, bracelets) is also removed. Fingernails are kept short and clean. Artificial nails and nail polish may harbor microorganisms and therefore are recommended not to be worn. If nail polish is worn, it should not be chipped and should be removed and reapplied every 4 days. Gloves are then worn by the OR team to keep the surgical field sterile.

The OR is designed to enhance **aseptic** (elimination of microorganisms) technique. Clean and contaminated areas are separated. Special ventilation systems control dust and prevent air from flowing into the OR from hallways. The temperature and humidity in the room are controlled to discourage bacterial growth. Everyone entering the OR wears surgical scrubs, shoe covers, caps, masks, and goggles to protect the patient from infection and themselves from bloodborne pathogens. Traffic in and out of the OR is limited. Strong disinfectants are used to clean the OR after each surgical case, and instruments are sterilized.

Before the patient arrives in surgery, a nursing plan of care with intraoperative nursing diagnoses and expected outcomes is developed from preadmission assessment data (Box 12.4). Attention is given to the safety needs of the patient. A surgical case cart containing sterile instruments required for the patient's case is prepared ahead of time.

Health Care Team Members and Roles

Members of the health care team and their roles are as follows:

- *Physician* (medical doctor [MD], doctor of osteopathy [DO], oral surgeon, or podiatrist)
- *Surgical (first) assistant:* assists the physician and is another physician, a specially trained RN, or a physician's assistant
- *Anesthesiologist:* physician who specializes in administering anesthesia and supervises certified registered nurse anesthetists (CRNAs) in the operating room

Box 12.4

Intraoperative Nursing Diagnoses and Expected Outcome

- *Risk for Injury* related to perioperative positioning, chemicals, electrical equipment, and effect of being anesthetized
  Is free from injury.
- *Risk for Impaired Skin Integrity* related to chemicals, positioning, and immobility
  Skin integrity is maintained.
- *Risk for Deficient Fluid Volume* related to NPO status and blood loss
  Maintains blood pressure, pulse, and urine output within normal limits.
- *Risk for Infection* related to incision and invasive procedures
  Is free of symptoms of infection.
- *Pain* related to positioning, incision, and surgical procedure
  Reports pain is relieved to satisfactory level.

SAFETY TIP

The goal of the Surgical Care Improvement Project (SCIP), a national quality partnership, has been to improve the safety of surgical care by reducing postoperative complications by 25% by the year 2010. The partnership, developed by the Centers for Medicare and Medicaid Services (CMS) and the Centers for Disease Control and Prevention (CDC), includes more than 30 other national organizations.

Areas being examined by the SCIP include surgical site infections (SSIs), deep venous thrombosis (DVT), postoperative ventilator-related pneumonia, and adverse cardiac events. Methods for preventing SSIs include giving prophylactic antibiotics within 1 hour prior to incision time and controlling perioperative serum glucose during major cardiac procedures. DVT can be prevented by administering appropriate perioperative anticoagulants to those at risk. Postoperative pneumonia can be prevented by elevating the head of the bed by 30 or more degrees for major postoperative surgical patients on a ventilator. Avoiding adverse cardiac events includes giving beta blockers during the perioperative period to eligible major noncardiac surgical patients and to surgical patients who have coronary artery disease. Look for updates on the committee's work at www.medqic.org.

- *CRNA:* an RN trained and certified in administering anesthesia, usually at the master's degree level
- *RN:* circulates in the OR; roles include being patient's advocate, planning care, protecting patient safety, monitoring patient positioning, checking vital signs and patient assessment, reducing patient's anxiety, monitoring sterility during surgery, preparing skin before incision, managing equipment such as by making sponge counts, documenting the procedure, and aiding health team communications
- *Surgical (second assistant) technician:* assists physician (may be an RN, LPN/LVN, or surgical technologist)

Patient Arrival in Surgery

The holding area nurse greets the patient; verifies the patient's name, age, allergies, surgeon performing the surgery, informed consent, surgical procedure (right site, especially right or left when applicable), and medical history; answers questions; and alleviates anxiety. The patient is introduced to the anesthesiologist and CRNA, who also verify patient information and explain the type of anesthesia that is to be used. All surgical patients have intravenous (IV) fluids started. The patient may also receive prophylactic antibiotics.

SAFETY TIP

Follow the Joint Commission's Universal Protocol for Preventing Wrong Site, Wrong Procedure, Wrong Person Surgery. Conduct a preprocedure verification process to ensure that all relevant documents, information, and equipment are available. Implement a process to mark the surgical site and involve the patient in the marking process. Take a time out immediately before beginning the procedure to conduct a final assessment that the correct patient, site, and procedure have been identified (2010 National Patient Safety Goals, www.jointcommission.org).

Before entering the OR, the patient should be told what to expect:

- "The room may feel cool, but you can request extra blankets."
- "There is a lot of equipment in the room, including a table and large, bright overhead lights."
- "Several health care team members will introduce themselves to you."
- "Your physician will greet you and a safety checklist will be performed."

EVIDENCE-BASED PRACTICE

Clinical Question

Does the use of a surgical safety checklist to improve team communication and consistency of care reduce complications and deaths associated with surgery?

Evidence

Data were collected on surgical patient outcomes for 3733 patients who did not have the 19-item World Health Organization's Surgical Safety Checklist implemented and on 3955 patients who did (Haynes et al., 2009). Use of the checklist showed reductions in the rates of death and complications.

(To view the checklist, visit http://content.nejm.org/cgi/content/full/NEJMsa0810119#T1).

Implications for Nursing Practice

Participating in the use of a surgical safety checklist promotes patient safety during surgery.

REFERENCE

Haynes, A. B., Weiser, T. G., Berry, W. R., et al. (2009). A surgical safety checklist to reduce morbidity and mortality in a global population. *New England Journal of Medicine, 360*, 491–499.

The patient is assisted onto the operating table, and a safety strap is carefully applied.

Taking a "time-out" and using a surgical safety checklist requires all personnel to stop and verify correct patient information to prevent adverse events (see *Evidence-Based Practice* box). No procedure (conducted in any setting) should start unless all personnel involved in the patient's care have honored the "time-out."

Monitoring equipment is applied and readings recorded. Then the anesthesia provider begins administering anesthesia. When the anesthesia provider gives permission, the patient is carefully positioned to prevent pressure points that could cause tissue or nerve damage. Any needed tubes that are not already in place, such as a nasogastric tube or urinary catheter, are inserted by the RN.

Patient allergies are rechecked. If the patient requires body hair removal, hair should be removed with electric clippers or a depilatory. Shaving should be avoided because of the potential for microabrasions and colonization by microorganisms. Then a skin prepping solution that the patient is not allergic to, such as povidone-iodine, is used to cleanse the skin. (This may be done in preop holding or in surgery depending on the institution.) A large area surrounding the operative site is scrubbed to allow for extension of the incision. The scrub is completed in a circular motion from inside to outer edge. If an allergic reaction to the solution occurs, it can cause skin redness and blistering wherever the solution was used. After the skin is scrubbed, a sterile drape is applied with the incisional area left exposed.

SAFETY TIP

Improve the safety of using medications. Label all medications, medication containers (e.g., syringes, medicine cups, basins), or other solutions on and off the sterile field in perioperative and other procedural settings (2010 National Patient Safety Goals, www.jointcommission.org).

Anesthesia

Anesthesia is used during surgery to prevent pain and allow the procedure to be done safely. The type of anesthesia and the anesthetic agents are ordered by the anesthesia provider with input from the patient and physician (Box 12.5, *Cultural Considerations*).

There are two types of anesthesia: general and local (regional). General anesthesia causes the patient to lose sensation, consciousness, and reflexes. It acts directly on the central nervous system (Box 12.6). Local anesthesia blocks nerve impulses along the nerve where it is injected, resulting in the loss of sensation to a region of the body without the loss of consciousness.

Box 12.5

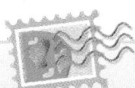

Cultural Considerations

Care of the Patient Having Surgery

Chinese people are more sensitive than non-Chinese people to the sedative effects of diazepam (Valium) and need lower doses and careful monitoring for adverse effects.

Box 12.6

Malignant Hyperthermia

Malignant hyperthermia is a rare hereditary muscular disease that can be triggered by some types of general anesthetic agents. A history of anesthetic problems in the patient or family members detects the potential for development of this condition so that precautions can be taken. A history of heat stroke increases the risk of malignant hyperthermia. A muscle biopsy diagnoses this problem. Patients with this condition can undergo surgery safely with careful planning and choice of anesthetic agents by the anesthesia provider.

In malignant hyperthermia, metabolism in the muscles is increased, which produces a very high fever and muscle rigidity, as well as tachycardia, tachypnea, hypertension, dysrhythmias, hyperkalemia, metabolic and respiratory acidosis, and cyanosis. Malignant hyperthermia is life threatening, so immediate treatment is required to prevent death. Surgery is stopped, and anesthesia discontinued immediately. Oxygen at 100% is given. The patient must be cooled with ice and infusions of iced solutions. Dantrolene sodium (Dantrium), a muscle relaxant that relieves the muscle spasms, is the most effective medication for malignant hyperthermia. Dantrolene sodium is kept readily available in the OR and given according to the treatment protocol of the Malignant Hyperthermia Association of the United States (www.mhaus.org).

General Anesthesia

General anesthesia is commonly given by IV or inhalation. It is chosen when patients are anxious or do not want local anesthesia, when the surgical procedure will take a long time and there is a need for muscle relaxation, or when the patient is unable to cooperate, as in head injury, muscle disorders, or impaired cognitive function.

INTRAVENOUS AGENTS. To begin most general anesthesia, the patient is induced (which means "to cause anesthesia") with a short-acting IV agent that provides a rapid, smooth **induction** (the period from when the anesthetic is first given until full anesthesia is reached). Because these agents last only a few minutes, they are used along with inhalation agents, which maintain anesthesia during surgery. After induction, the patient is intubated with an endotracheal (ET) tube to provide mechanical ventilation and anesthesia (Fig. 12.8).

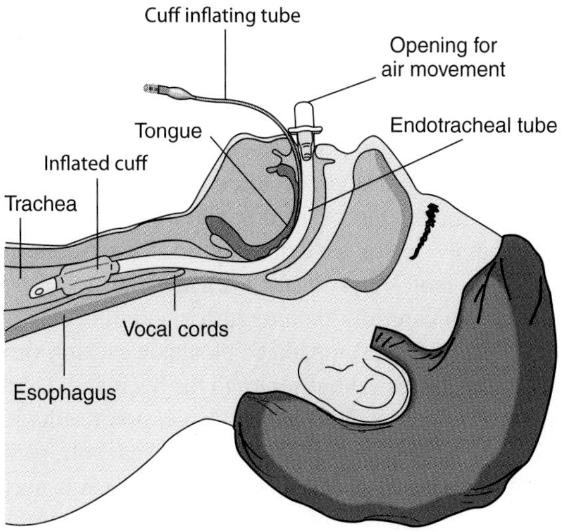
Cuff inflating tube
Opening for air movement
Endotracheal tube
Tongue
Inflated cuff
Trachea
Vocal cords
Esophagus

FIGURE 12.8 Endotracheal tube with cuff inflated.

INHALATION AGENTS. Maintenance of anesthesia is accomplished by using inhalation agents. These agents are delivered, controlled, and excreted through mechanical ventilation. Inhalation agents and the ET tube can be irritating to the respiratory tract. Complications that can occur from their use include laryngospasm (sudden violent contraction of the vocal cords), laryngeal edema, irritated throat, or injury to the vocal cords. When the tube is removed, the nurse should closely monitor the patient and be prepared to provide respiratory support and assist with reintubation if complications arise.

ADJUNCT AGENTS. An **adjunct** agent is a medication used along with the primary anesthetic agents. These medications can include opioids to control pain, muscle relaxers to avoid movement of muscles during surgery, antiemetics to control nausea or vomiting, and sedatives to supplement anesthesia.

Local (Regional) Anesthesia

Local anesthesia is selected for the patient who is not anxious, can tolerate the local agent, and is not required by the surgical procedure to be unconscious or relaxed. It is a good choice for some outpatient procedures. The anesthesia provider, or sometimes the physician, administers local anesthesia.

• WORD • BUILDING •
induction: inductio—to lead in

In topical administration, the agent is placed directly on the surgical area. Local infiltration is achieved by injecting the medication into the tissue where the incision is to be made. A regional block is done by injecting the local agent along a nerve that carries impulses in the region where anesthesia is desired. There are several types of regional blocks. A nerve block is the injection of a local agent into a nerve at a specific point. A Bier block is done by placing a tourniquet on an extremity to remove the blood and then injecting the local agent into the extremity. A field block is a series of injections surrounding the surgical area. A spinal or epidural block is injection of a local agent into an area around the spinal nerves.

SPINAL AND EPIDURAL BLOCKS. Injection of a local agent into the subarachnoid space produces spinal block (Fig. 12.9). Epidural block occurs when the local agent is injected into the epidural space. Spinal and epidural blocks are used mainly for lower extremity and lower abdominal surgery. Both motor and sensory function is blocked. The patient must be carefully monitored for complications. Hypotension results from sympathetic blockade causing vasodilation, which reduces venous return to the heart and therefore reduces cardiac output. Respiratory depression results if the block travels too far upward. As the block wears off, patients feel as if their legs are very heavy and numb. This is normal, and reassurance should be offered to the patient that this type of feeling does not last after the block wears off.

Complications. A postdural puncture headache results from leakage of cerebrospinal fluid (CSF) from the needle puncture hole in the dura that does not close when the needle is withdrawn. This reduces pressure on the spinal cord and brain, causing a headache. The use of a small-gauge (less than 25-gauge) spinal needle helps prevent headaches. Nausea, dizziness, tinnitus, and vision disturbances may also be present. The headache can worsen if standing or sitting. Postoperative orders usually include methods to help reduce the pain of a headache, including positioning the patient flat and forcing fluids.

If a spinal headache develops, it may be severe. Lying flat and prone (on abdomen) may help relieve the pain of the headache. Adequate fluid intake and analgesics may be ordered, and steroids may be helpful. If the headache lasts more than 24 hours, IV caffeine can be given that constricts cerebral blood vessels, or a blood patch treatment can be used to stop the CSF leakage. This sterile procedure can be done by the anesthesiologist at the bedside or in the perianesthesia care unit (PACU). To create a blood patch, approximately 10 mL of the patient's own blood is injected into the epidural space at the previous puncture site. The injected blood forms a clot that "patches" the dura hole to prevent further CSF leakage. Pain relief should occur quickly if the patch is successful. Blood patch treatment can be repeated.

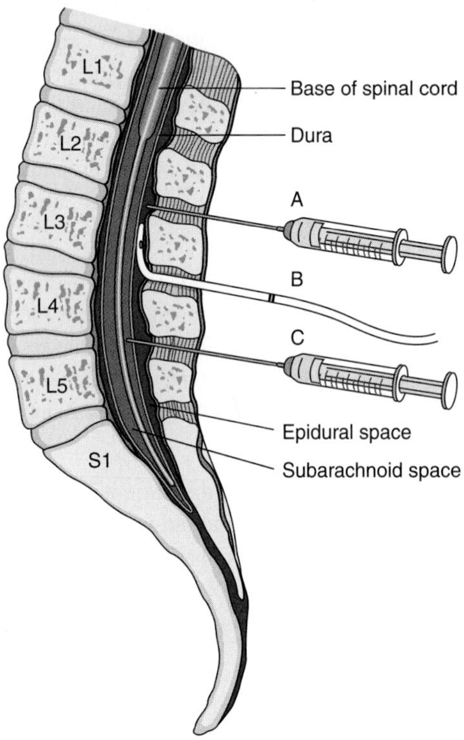

L1
L2
L3
L4
L5
S1
Base of spinal cord
Dura
A
B
C
Epidural space
Subarachnoid space

FIGURE 12.9 Injection of spinal anesthesia. (A) Epidural anesthesia. (B) Epidural catheter. (C) Spinal anesthesia.

Conscious Sedation

Conscious sedation (sometimes called twilight sleep) is purposeful, minimal sedation that does not cause the complete loss of consciousness during selected dental, diagnostic, or medical procedures. Patients still have control of their own airway. Medications such as sedatives, hypnotics, and opioids are given to produce conscious sedation. Selection of patients who are eligible for conscious sedation is based on the procedure, the patient's general health, patient preference, and physician preference. Examples of short procedures for which conscious sedation is used are dental procedures, endoscopy (esophagogastroduodenoscopy or colonoscopy), cardiac catheterization, cardioversion, and closed fracture reduction. During conscious sedation, patients are comfortable, respond purposefully, and maintain their own patent airway. Medications are ordered by the physician and usually administered by a specially trained registered nurse, as defined by agency and state scope of nursing practice.

A signed informed consent is obtained. Then an IV for medications and fluids is inserted before the procedure. Patient monitoring is done every 5 minutes to check vital signs, electrocardiogram, and oxygen saturation. Changes are reported to the physician. Oxygen may be given by nasal cannula or mask. Emergency equipment (e.g., airway suction, defibrillator, drugs) is on standby, according to advanced cardiac life support (ACLS) protocols.

After the procedure, the patient awakens easily and quickly. The patient is monitored every 15 to 30 minutes for response to the procedure and the drugs until the patient is fully awake and stable. The patient is ready for discharge when vital signs return to baseline and are stable, oral fluids are retained, he or she has voided (if applicable), and written and oral discharge teaching is given to both the patient and the responsible adult to whom the patient is being discharged. The responsible adult and the patient must sign the instructions. Instructions include the following: An adult must drive the patient home and provide a safe environment, and the patient must not and will not drive or operate heavy machinery or sign legal documents for 24 hours.

> **LEARNING TIP**
>
> In comparison with general anesthesia, conscious sedation:
>
> - Is less invasive.
> - Requires less medication.
> - Causes less depression of the cardiovascular and respiratory systems.
> - Allows the patient to more quickly return to a wakeful state.

Transfer from Surgery

When surgery is completed and anesthesia stopped, the patient is stabilized for transfer. After local anesthesia, the patient may return directly to a nursing unit. After general and spinal anesthesia, the patient goes to the PACU or, in some cases, an intensive care unit (ICU).

Patient safety, which is always a priority, is an important concern at this time. The patient is never left alone. Ensuring a patent airway and preventing falls and injury from uncontrolled movements are priorities. The anesthesia provider and OR nurses transfer the patient to the PACU and monitor the patient until the perianesthesia nurse is able to receive the report and assume care of the patient. This begins the final patient perioperative phase, the postoperative period.

> **SAFETY TIP**
>
> *Improve the effectiveness of communication among caregivers.* Implement a standardized approach for "handing off" communications, including an opportunity to ask and respond to questions (2010 National Patient Safety Goals, www.jointcommission.org).

POSTOPERATIVE PHASE

The **postoperative** phase begins when the patient is admitted to the PACU or a nursing unit and ends with the patient's postoperative evaluation in the physician's office. The family is updated on the patient's status by the surgeon as the patient is admitted to the PACU (Fig. 12.10).

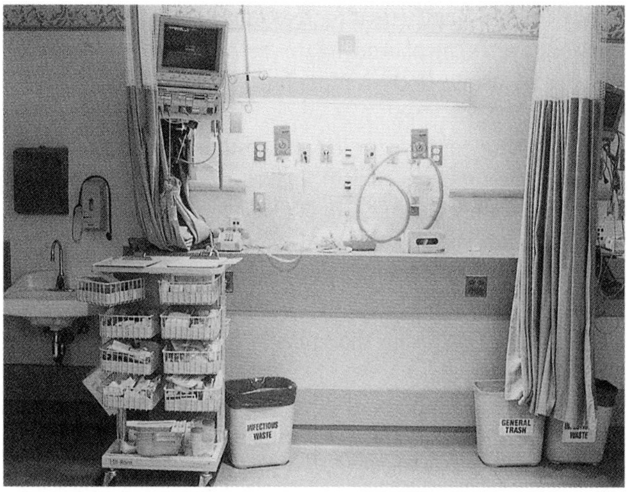
INFECTIOUS WASTE
GENERAL TRASH

FIGURE 12.10 Perianesthesia care unit (PACU).

Admission to the Perianesthesia Care Unit

The perianesthesia nurse's goal is to promote safe recovery from anesthesia. The nurse's role in the PACU begins by receiving a patient report from the OR nurse and anesthesia provider. When the patient is admitted to the PACU, an admission assessment is done. The priority areas of patient assessment are:

- Respiratory status and patency of airway
- Vital signs including SaO_2
- Level of consciousness and responsiveness
- Surgical site incision/dressing/drainage tubes
- Pain level and pain management.

Oxygen by nasal cannula or mask is given if the patient has had general anesthesia, or as ordered. Some patients who are still intubated may require mechanical ventilation. Continuous monitoring is done on all patients for ECG, pulse oximetry, and blood pressure measurements. The surgical site incision or dressing is assessed. Drainage and **hematoma** formation are documented and reported. The urinary catheter, drains, and nasogastric tubes or other equipment are checked for function and patency as applicable.

The patient's body temperature is measured on admission to the PACU. If the patient's temperature is below normal, a warming blanket is used. Body temperature may be decreased as a result of a cool OR environment, anesthesia, cool IV solutions, and incisional openings, which allow heat loss. Patient recovery is aided by avoiding a decrease in body temperature during surgery. Using forced warm air devices preoperatively to warm the patient, rather than warmed blankets, has been shown to maintain body temperature best upon arrival in the PACU. The

• **WORD • BUILDING •**
hematoma: heimatos—blood + oma—tumor

elderly (and infants) are at increased risk of **hypothermia**. Temperature is measured again before PACU discharge because a normal body temperature is usually one of the discharge criteria.

Shivering may occur from anesthesia or from being cold. It is important to control shivering because it increases oxygen consumption 400% to 500%. Meperidine (Demerol) is effective in relieving shivering when anesthesia is the cause. If the patient is cold, raising the body temperature is helpful to decrease shivering. It is important to provide supplemental O_2 during the episode of shivering and until the Sao_2 is normal.

The responsibilities of perianesthesia nurses are listed in Box 12.7. It is essential for nurses to wash their hands between patients in the PACU. Vital signs and assessment are done at least every 5 to 15 minutes, IV fluid infusion is maintained, and IV or PCA analgesics are given for pain as needed. Antiemetics are administered for nausea or vomiting. Deep breathing and coughing, if not contraindicated by the surgical procedure, are encouraged. Surgical procedures that prohibit coughing due to the increased pressure created include hernia repair; eye, ear, intracranial, and jaw surgery; and plastic surgery. If the patient is no longer NPO, ice chips or sips of water may be offered for a dry mouth when the patient is fully awake.

Nursing Process for Postoperative Patients in PACU

Postoperative complications may occur due to the surgical procedure, anesthesia, blood and fluid loss, immobility, unrelieved pain, or other diseases the patient may have. Nursing care focuses on preventing, detecting, and caring for these complications.

Box 12.7

Perianesthesia Nursing Responsibilities

- Airway maintenance
- Vital signs including Sao_2
- Respiratory assessment
- Neurologic assessment
- Surgical site status
- General assessment
- Patient safety
- Monitoring anesthetic effects
- Pain relief treatment
- Accurate intake and output
- Assessing PACU discharge readiness
- Documentation
- Transfer report to receiving nurse (name, allergies, procedure, type of anesthesia, status, complications, oxygen, dressing/drains/equipment, medications, postoperative orders, pertinent history, family, opportunity to ask questions)

Respiratory Function

DATA COLLECTION. Normal respiratory function can be altered in the immediate postoperative period by airway obstruction, hypoventilation, secretions, laryngospasm, or decreased swallowing and cough reflexes. Respiratory function assessment includes respiratory rate, depth, ease, and pattern. Breath sounds, chest symmetry, accessory muscle use, and sputum are also observed.

NURSING DIAGNOSES, PLANNING, AND IMPLEMENTATION

***Ineffective Breathing Pattern* Related to Anesthesia, Pain, and Analgesic/Sedative Medications**

EXPECTED OUTCOME: Patient will maintain normal Sao_2 levels at all times.

- Maintain oxygen therapy as ordered *to prevent hypoventilation, which can be an effect of anesthesia medications or analgesics, decreased level of consciousness, or an incision in the thorax causing painful respirations.*
- Encourage deep breathing *to expand the lungs.*
- Give analgesics carefully *to promote deep breathing but avoid respiratory depression.*
- Maintain CPAP/BiPap *to treat sleep apnea.* (Patients may bring their CPAP/BiPap machines with them.)
- Report respiratory depression to the anesthesiologist *to obtain prompt treatment.*

Ineffective Airway Clearance Related to Obstruction, Anesthesia Medications, and Secretions

EXPECTED OUTCOME: Patient will have a patent airway at all times.

- Ensure that patient maintains a patent airway *because airway obstruction may result when relaxed muscles allow the tongue to block the pharynx in patients with a decreased level of consciousness.*
- Use jaw-thrust method to manually open patient's airway *if patient has snoring respirations and has not completely emerged from anesthesia.*

Risk for Aspiration Related to Depressed Cough and Gag Reflexes and Reduced Level of Consciousness

EXPECTED OUTCOME: Patient will have clear lung sounds at all times.

- Position patients on their side, unless contraindicated, *to protect the airway until they are awake.*
- Have suction equipment always available *to clear secretions or emesis.*

EVALUATION. The goal for ineffective airway clearance and aspiration is achieved if the patient's airway remains patent and lung sounds remain clear. The goal for ineffective breathing pattern is met if the patient's respiratory rate is within normal limits, no dyspnea is reported, and arterial blood gases are within normal limits.

Cardiovascular Function

DATA COLLECTION. Alterations in cardiovascular function can include hypotension, dysrhythmias, and hypertension. Hypotension can be the result of blood and fluid volume loss or cardiac abnormalities. Shock can result from the significant blood and fluid volume loss or from sepsis (see Chapter 9). Dysrhythmias may occur from hypoxia, altered potassium or magnesium levels, hypothermia, pain, stress, or cardiac disease. New-onset hypertension can develop from pain, a full bladder, or respiratory distress.

Cardiovascular function assessment includes heart rate, blood pressure, ECG, and skin temperature, color, and moistness. Vital signs are compared with baseline readings to determine if they are normal. Tachycardia, hypotension, pale skin color, cool, clammy skin, and decreased urine output indicate hypovolemic shock, which requires reporting and prompt treatment.

NURSING DIAGNOSES, PLANNING, AND IMPLEMENTATION

Deficient Fluid Volume Related to Blood and Fluid Loss or NPO Status

EXPECTED OUTCOME: Patient will maintain blood pressure, pulse, and urine output within normal limits at all times.

- Check dressings and incisions for color and amount of drainage *to detect fluid loss.*
- Maintain IV fluids at ordered rate *to replace lost fluids but avoid fluid overload.*
- Monitor intake and output *to detect imbalances.*

EVALUATION. The goal for deficient fluid volume is met if vital signs and urine output are within normal limits.

NURSING CARE TIP

Tachycardia: An Early Warning Sign

Tachycardia is a compensatory mechanism designed to provide adequate delivery of oxygen in times of altered function. It is usually the earliest warning sign that an abnormality is occurring. It should be a red flag to assess the patient and ask yourself what this particular patient is likely to be experiencing that is compromising oxygenation, allowing you to begin prompt intervention.

PATIENT CONDITION	POSSIBLE CAUSES OF COMPROMISED OXYGENATION
Postoperative patient	Hemorrhage, respiratory depression, pain
Myocardial infarction patient	Cardiogenic shock, pain
Respiratory patient	Respiratory distress
Trauma patient	Hemorrhage, severe pain

Neurologic Function

Until its effects wear off, anesthesia can alter neurologic function. Patients may arrive in the PACU awake, arousable, or sleeping. Patients who are sleeping should become more alert during their stay in the PACU. As they emerge from anesthesia, they may become agitated or wild for a short time; this is called *emergence delirium.* During this time it is important to provide safety measures such as side rails and restraints—following restraint protocols—to protect IV lines and keep endotracheal tubes in place. Once resolved, the patient returns to a calm state and has no recollection of the episode. Movement, sensations, and perceptions may also be altered by anesthesia. Movement is the first function to return after spinal anesthesia.

For geriatric patients, it is important to review their history to understand if they have any cognitive or neurologic deficits. Confused patients may be agitated or frightened when they awaken. It is helpful to know how caregivers normally communicate with the patient. You should understand that the patient may not be able to report pain or follow commands. If possible, it may be helpful to have a familiar relative or caregiver with the patient in the PACU to calm him and help him communicate. You should watch for nonverbal pain cues such as moaning, grimacing, rubbing of an area, and restlessness because you recognize that a postoperative patient will have pain and require pain relief. If patients have limited movements or sensations before surgery, you should know this to obtain an accurate assessment of anesthetic effects.

DATA COLLECTION. A neurologic assessment includes level of consciousness; orientation to person, place, time, and event; pupil size and reaction to light; and motor and sensory function.

NURSING DIAGNOSES, PLANNING, AND IMPLEMENTATION

Disturbed Sensory Perception Related to Decreased Level of Consciousness, Amnesiac Effects of Anesthesia, or Spinal Anesthesia

EXPECTED OUTCOME: Patient will remain safe and be free from injury at all times.

- Verify patient data until patient is awake and can communicate *to prevent errors.*
- Maintain safety with side rails and extremities positioned in proper alignment and protected until patient is fully awake or extremity movement and sensation return following spinal anesthesia *to prevent injury.*
- Secure and observe tubes, dressings, and IVs *to prevent dislodgement.*
- Provide orientation explanations as patient awakens, and repeat them until amnesiac anesthesia effects have resolved. Examples of explanations include: "Mr. Smith, surgery is over; you are in the recovery room." "Your family is waiting for you and knows you are in the recovery room." "The doctor spoke with your family and told them how you are doing."

EVALUATION. The goal for disturbed sensory perception is met if the patient remains free from injury.

Pain

DATA COLLECTION. If the patient is awake, he or she is asked to rate the presence of pain using a scale, such as the 0-to-10 scale, a color scale, or pictures that rate pain. The location and character of the pain are documented. If the patient is not fully awake, vital signs and nonverbal indications of pain should be monitored. Nonverbal indications of pain can include abnormal vital signs, restlessness, moaning, grimacing, rubbing, or pulling at specific areas or equipment.

NURSING DIAGNOSES, PLANNING, AND IMPLEMENTATION

Pain Related to Tissue Damage (Mechanical [Incision])

EXPECTED OUTCOME: The patient will report that pain is relieved at a satisfactory level within 15 to 30 minutes of the pain report.

- Monitor the patient for pain, *because pain may result from surgical procedure, movement, deep breathing, anxiety, a full bladder, positioning during surgery, nasogastric tubes, catheters, IVs, ET tubes, or prior medical conditions, such as arthritis, cancer, or back pain.*
- Give IV opioid analgesics promptly *for their rapid onset.*
- Begin PCA as ordered, *because it is started in PACU.*
- Reposition the patient, provide warmth, and empty full bladder *to help alleviate pain.*
- Play music (e.g., nature sounds or classical music) in the PACU, dim lights, and reduce room noise *to help alleviate pain.*

EVALUATION. The goal for pain is met if the patient reports a satisfactory decrease in level of pain. For example, the patient reports pain of 10 on a scale of 0 to 10. You medicate the patient, and 30 minutes later the patient rates pain as 2 on a scale of 0 to 10. The patient indicates that 2 is an acceptable pain level, so the goal is achieved.

Family Visitation

Family visitation in the PACU has been shown to be helpful to patients and their families. Allowing family visitation varies by hospital. Patients and families should be educated about the expectations for family visitation to keep it safe for the patient. During visitation, remember that the confidentiality of all patients must be ensured according to HIPAA (Health Insurance Portability and Accountability Act of 1996). For example, some patients may not want the surgical procedure revealed to their spouse or any family members.

Discharge from the Perianesthesia Care Unit

The length of stay in the PACU if the patient remains stable is normally about 1 hour. A postanesthesia recovery scale is used to score the patient's readiness to be discharged. The scale rates categories such as respiration, oxygen saturation, level of consciousness, activity, and circulation. The anesthesiologist discharges the patient for transfer to a nursing unit, or home when discharge criteria are met (Box 12.8). The patient may be transferred to the ICU if patient status and/or frequent or invasive monitoring is needed.

Transfer to Nursing Unit

The perianesthesia nurse gives a report of the patient's condition to the unit nurse when the patient is transferred to the nursing unit. The patient is moved into bed on the nursing unit with assistance to prevent dislodging of IVs, tubes, drains, or dressings. After the patient is placed in bed, the following safety interventions are performed:

- The bed is placed in its lowest position, with the side rails raised.
- The nurse's call button is placed within easy patient reach and answered promptly.
- Patients are instructed that they should be assisted with ambulation when they get up.

When the patient gets up postoperatively, especially for the first time, he or she may be weak or dizzy. One or two health care workers should assist the patient and allow the patient to dangle before standing (Fig. 12.11). These precautions can help prevent falls.

Nursing Process for Postoperative Patients

A complete patient assessment is performed after transfer to the nursing unit. Respiratory status, vital signs (including temperature), level of consciousness, surgical site, dressings, and pain assessment are noted. IV site, patency, and

Box 12.8

Discharge Criteria for Perianesthesia Care Unit or Ambulatory Surgery

- Vital signs stable
- Patient awake or at baseline level of consciousness
- Drainage or bleeding not excessive
- Respiratory function not depressed
- Oxygen saturation above 90%

Additional Criteria for Ambulatory Surgery

- No nausea or vomiting
- No IV opioids within last 30 minutes
- Voided if required by surgical procedure or ordered
- Is ambulatory or has baseline mobility
- Understands discharge instructions
- Provides means of contact for follow-up telephone assessment
- Released to responsible adult

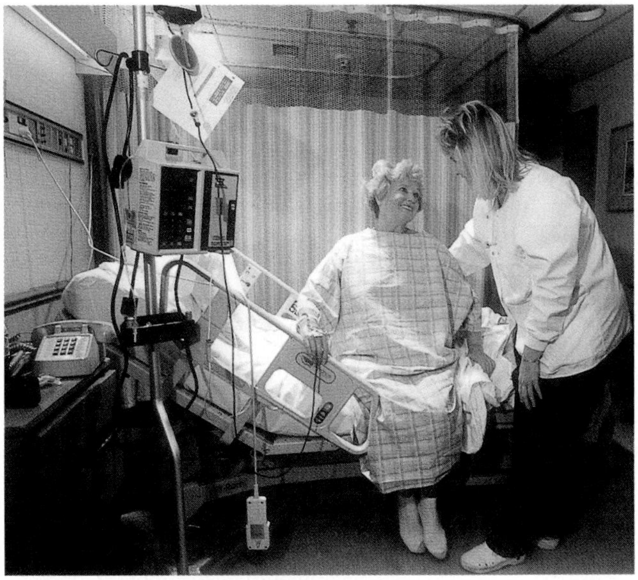

FIGURE 12.11 Postoperative patient dangling.

IV solution and infusion rate are assessed and monitored. Nasogastric tubes are hooked to suction or clamped as ordered. Drains and catheters are positioned to promote proper functioning.

After discharge from the PACU, interventions to promote recovery include monitoring for complications (respiratory depression, hemorrhage, and shock), providing postoperative care, educating patients and their significant others, making needed referrals, and providing home health care. See the *Nursing Care Plan for the Postoperative Patient.*

Respiratory Function

DATA COLLECTION. Regular monitoring of the patient's respiratory rate, depth, and effort and breath sounds as well as cough strength (if not contraindicated by the type of surgery, such as hernia repair or eye, ear, intracranial, jaw, or plastic surgery) should be done. Postoperative patients are at risk for developing atelectasis and pneumonia. They may have a weak cough as a result of being drowsy from anesthesia or analgesics. If fine crackles are heard in the lung bases, the patient should be encouraged to deep breathe or cough. Afterward you should listen again to see if the crackles have cleared. If the patient's airway is compromised, immediate action is taken to support the airway and the physician is notified.

NURSING DIAGNOSES, PLANNING, AND IMPLEMENTATION

Ineffective Breathing Pattern Related to Pain and Analgesic Medications

EXPECTED OUTCOME: Patient will maintain normal Sao_2 levels and normal arterial blood gases at all times.

- Encourage deep breathing *to expand the lungs.*
- Give analgesics as needed *to promote deep breathing so the patient does not guard against deep respirations or coughing, especially if incision is near the diaphragm.*

Ineffective Airway Clearance Related to Ineffective Cough and Secretion Retention

EXPECTED OUTCOME: Patient will have a patent airway and clear breath sounds at all times.

- Encourage deep breathing and coughing every hour while the patient is awake, especially through the first postoperative day, *to prevent mucous plugs that block bronchioles, causing alveoli to collapse and atelectasis or infection to develop from the stasis of mucus, resulting in pneumonia.*
- Place the incentive spirometer within patient's reach and encourage hourly use while awake *to prevent atelectasis.*
- Turn the patient at least every 2 hours *to help expand the lungs and move secretions.*
- Ambulate the patient as soon as possible *because immobility decreases movement of secretions.*

EVALUATION. If the patient's breath sounds are clear and arterial blood gases remain normal, the goals have been met.

Circulatory Function

DATA COLLECTION. Monitor the patient's circulatory status to detect and prevent hemorrhage, shock, and thrombophlebitis. Vital signs, Sao_2, and skin temperature, color, and moistness are monitored (per institutional policy) and compared with baseline data for abnormal trends. The incision or dressing is checked for drainage or hematoma formation. Drainage may leak down the patient's side and pool underneath the patient. While wearing gloves, feel underneath the patient or turn the patient to check for bleeding. Report any signs of hemorrhage or shock promptly.

The lower extremities of surgical patients are observed. Peripheral pulses and capillary refill are checked. Tenderness or pain in the calf may be the first indication of a deep venous thrombosis. Leg swelling, warmth, and redness, as well as fever, may also be present. Bilateral calf and thigh measurements are taken daily if thrombophlebitis is suspected or diagnosed.

NURSING DIAGNOSES, PLANNING, AND IMPLEMENTATION

Deficient Fluid Volume Related to Blood and Fluid Loss or NPO Status

EXPECTED OUTCOME: Patient will maintain blood pressure and pulse within normal limits at all times.

- Monitor dressings, incisions, drains, and tubes for color and amount of drainage and report bright red drainage or excessive drainage amounts immediately *to detect hemorrhage.*
- Monitor intake and output *to detect imbalances.*
- Maintain IV fluids at the ordered rate *to maintain fluid volume.*

NURSING CARE PLAN for the Postoperative Patient

Nursing Diagnosis: *Ineffective Airway Clearance* related to ineffective cough and secretion retention

Expected Outcomes: Patient will maintain a patent airway at all times. Breath sounds remain clear at all times.

Evaluation of Outcomes: Is patient able to clear own secretions? Are breath sounds clear?

Interventions	Rationale	Evaluation
Monitor breath sounds.	Abnormal breath sounds such as crackles or wheezes can indicate retained secretions.	Are breath sounds clear?
Encourage deep breathing and coughing and use of incentive spirometer hourly while awake.	Lung expansion helps prevent atelectasis and keeps lungs clear of secretions.	Does patient perform deep breathing and coughing and use incentive spirometer?
Ensure that patient's pain is relieved before activity.	Movement can cause or increase pain.	Does patient state pain is controlled before activity?
Encourage movement by turning every 2 hours and ambulating as able.	Movement promotes lung expansion and movement of secretions.	Is patient moving?

Nursing Diagnosis: *Pain* related to surgery, nausea, and vomiting

Expected Outcomes: Patient will report that pain management relieves pain satisfactorily within 30 minutes of report of pain. Patient will describe pain management plan by first postoperative day.

Evaluation of Outcomes: Does patient report satisfactory pain relief? Is patient able to describe pain management plan?

Intervention	Rationale	Evaluation
Explain pain relief interventions and set goals with patient for pain management.	Patients are partners in their pain management and need understanding of plan to collaborate on the goals.	Does patient understand plan and have a goal for acceptable pain level?
Assess pain using rating scale such as 0 to 10.	Self-report is the most reliable indicator of pain.	Does patient report pain using scale?
Provide analgesics prn.	Analgesics relieve pain.	Is patient's pain less after receiving medication?
Provide antiemetics prn.	Antiemetics relieve nausea and vomiting.	Is patient's nausea and vomiting less after receiving medication?
Position patient comfortably.	Incisions, drains, tubing, equipment, and bedrest can cause discomfort, which positioning can relieve.	Does patient report positioning is comfortable?
	GERIATRIC	
Prioritize assessment of cognitively impaired patients as high at beginning of shift and frequently throughout shift.	Cognitively impaired patients are vulnerable to undertreatment of pain and deserve excellence in pain relief management.	Is cognitively impaired patient assessed for pain first and at regular intervals?
When assessing pain speak clearly and slowly so elderly patient can hear.	If elderly patient does not hear or misunderstands, pain may not be reported accurately to ensure appropriate intervention is provided.	Does patient hear and report pain and relief accurately using pain scale?

NURSING CARE PLAN for the Postoperative Patient—cont'd

GERIATRIC

Assess elderly patients' pain level regularly, observing nonverbal pain cues (restlessness, grimacing, moaning), especially for those who are cognitively impaired.	The pain of elderly patients is often underreported and undertreated, especially if cognitively impaired, and noting nonverbal cues can aid in pain treatment.	Are nonverbal pain cues present in elderly patients, especially those who are cognitively impaired?

Nursing Diagnosis: *Risk for Infection* related to inadequate primary defenses from surgical wound

Expected Outcome: Patient will remain free from infection at all times.

Evaluation of Outcome: Does patient remain free from infection?

Intervention	Rationale	Evaluation
Observe incision for signs and symptoms of infection.	Redness, warmth, fever, and swelling indicate infection.	Are signs and symptoms of infection present?
Monitor drainage and maintain drains.	Drains remove fluid from the surgical site to prevent infection development.	Are drainage amount and color normal for procedure?
Maintain sterile technique for dressing changes.	Sterile technique reduces infection development.	Is incision free of signs and symptoms of infection?

Ineffective Peripheral Tissue Perfusion Related to Interruption of Blood Flow During Surgery, Dehydration, and Use of Leg Straps

EXPECTED OUTCOME: Patient will maintain normal tissue perfusion at all times.

- Encourage leg exercises hourly while the patient is awake *to prevent venous stasis and thrombosis.*
- Assist with early postoperative ambulation as ordered *to prevent thrombosis.*
- Apply thigh-length graduated compression stockings (if contraindicated, use knee-length stockings) or intermittent pneumatic compression as ordered *to help prevent stasis of blood.* Thigh-length stockings are more effective than knee-length stockings in reducing the risk of thrombophlebitis (Fig. 12.12).
- Give anticoagulants or plasma expanders such as dextran 40 and dextran 70 as ordered *to reduce clot formation.*
- Avoid pressure under the knee from pillows, rolled blankets, or prolonged bending of the knee and elevate legs *to help prevent venous stasis.*

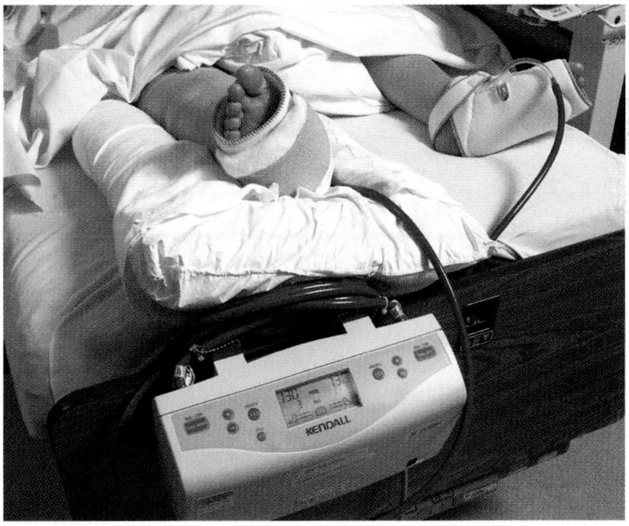
KENDALL

FIGURE 12.12 Postoperative patient wearing A-V Impulse System foot pump. The foot pump is used to prevent deep venous thrombosis, reduce pain and edema, and enhance arterial blood flow. (Courtesy of Kendall, Mansfield, MA.)

EVALUATION. The goal for deficient fluid volume is met if vital signs and urine output are within normal limits. The goal for ineffective tissue perfusion is met if tissue blood flow remains normal.

Postoperative Pain

Pain is common after surgery, although each patient's pain experience varies. In addition to incisional pain, painful muscle spasms can occur. Nausea and vomiting, ambulation, coughing, deep breathing, and anxiety can cause discomfort and increase postoperative pain. Unrelieved pain has negative physiological effects. It also impairs deep breathing and coughing and hinders early ambulation, which may increase complications, length of hospital stay, and health care costs. It is important for nurses to stay informed of advances in pain management and ensure that they make pain relief a priority in providing patient care to reduce suffering and promote a quicker recovery (see *Evidence-Based Practice* box; also see Chapter 10).

EVIDENCE-BASED PRACTICE

Clinical Question

Is single oral dose ibuprofen effective for moderate and severe postoperative pain in adults?

Evidence

Seventy-two randomized studies comparing ibuprofen and placebo analgesic effects were reviewed (Derry et al., 2009). Ibuprofen 200 mg or 400 mg was found to produce a high level of pain relief in about half of those with moderate or severe acute postoperative pain, which is good compared with other analgesics.

Implications for Nursing Practice

Ibuprofen can be effectively used for postoperative pain relief.

REFERENCE

Derry, C., Derry, S., Moore, R. A., et al. (2009). Single dose oral ibuprofen for acute postoperative pain in adults. *Cochrane Database of Systematic Reviews 2009, Issue 3* (Art. No. CD001548; DOI 10.1002/14651858.CD001548.pub2).

CRITICAL THINKING

Mrs. Owens

Mrs. Owens returned from a bowel resection 2 days ago. She is receiving 1000 mL of 0.9% normal saline solution over 10 hours on an IV controller pump.

1. As you monitor the patient, you understand that the IV pump rate would be set at what rate?
2. How many milliliters should you record as intake for 12 hours?

■ Intake for 12 hours:
- One 8-ounce (oz) cup of coffee
- 4 oz orange juice
- 6 oz tomato soup
- 3/4 cup gelatin
- Two cups of water
- 1200 mL of 0.9% normal saline solution IV

■ Output for 12 hours:
- 1700 mL of urine

Suggested answers at end of chapter.

DATA COLLECTION. If patients are not fully awake on transfer, vital signs and nonverbal indications of pain should be monitored (Box 12.9, *Gerontological Issues*). Nonverbal indicators of pain may include abnormal vital signs (usually elevated blood pressure, although hypotension can occur in some patients), restlessness, moaning, grimacing, and rubbing or pulling at specific body areas or equipment. Patients who are awake are asked the location of the pain, to rate the presence of pain, and to describe the pain quality, such as sharp, aching, throbbing, or burning, which is then documented.

NURSING DIAGNOSES, PLANNING, AND IMPLEMENTATION

Pain Related to Tissue Damage from Surgery, Muscle Spasms, Nausea, or Vomiting

EXPECTED OUTCOME: Patient will report pain relief at a satisfactory level using a pain rating scale within 30 minutes of pain report.

- Monitor pain using pain rating scale of 0 to 10 *to identify patient's needs.*
- Provide medications promptly as ordered *to relieve symptoms.*
- Understand appropriate timing intervals between IV to IM doses of analgesics *so that patients do not wait and suffer needlessly after an IV analgesic.* IV analgesics usually have a shorter duration than IM analgesics.
- Reposition patient *to promote comfort.*

EVALUATION. Thirty minutes after pain medication is given, patients are asked to rate their pain level. If patients are sleeping at this time, let them sleep. When they awaken, ask them to rate their pain level. The goal for pain is met when patients report a decreased level of pain that is satisfactory to them. If a patient does not report satisfactory pain relief and additional orders are needed, the physician should be promptly notified of the inadequate pain relief.

Box 12.9 Gerontological Issues

Postoperative Pain

Pain is not a normal part of aging. Careful assessment of older patients' unique aging changes, chronic diseases, and pain relief needs is required to appropriately treat their postoperative pain.

Cognitively impaired adults are at risk for undertreatment of their postoperative pain. Make these patients a priority to assess and provide pain relief at the start of your shift and throughout it. Pain rating scales are available for use with those who are cognitively impaired to determine if they are experiencing pain.

NURSING CARE TIP

- Anticipate the postoperative patient's pain by regularly assessing the pain level instead of waiting until the patient asks for the next dose of pain medication; this approach is essential to provide quality nursing care for pain relief.
- For the first dose of an IM analgesic, a patient in pain should not have to wait the ordered time interval of the IM dose after an intravenous analgesic dose is given (i.e., 3 hours if the IM order is morphine 10 mg IM every 3 hours prn). Having to wait while the IV analgesic is no longer effective can cause needless pain.
- The patient's ability to use PCA, the patient's response to the medication, and the relief obtained from it are monitored. If PCA is not effective or if side effects occur, the physician should be notified.
- Comfortable positioning, warming the patient, and relieving a patient's full bladder can also alleviate pain. Attention to environmental factors such as bright overhead lighting, excessive noise or visitors, and extreme room temperatures also helps promote comfort.
- Antiemetics should be given as ordered to relieve the discomfort of nausea and vomiting. If vomiting occurs, the patient should be turned onto one side to aid emesis removal and prevent aspiration.

CRITICAL THINKING

Mrs. Wood

■ Mrs. Wood, age 42, returns to the surgical unit after a hysterectomy. Her postoperative vital signs and assessment findings are normal. Mrs. Wood rates her pain level at 9, and the nurse notes that she moans occasionally, repeatedly moves her legs, and pulls at her covers near her abdominal incision. She is drowsy but repeatedly says it hurts. In the PACU, she received 10 mg of morphine IV 55 minutes ago. Morphine 5 to 10 mg IM is ordered every 3 hours as needed.

1. What nonverbal pain cues does Mrs. Wood display?
2. How should the nurse document Mrs. Wood's pain?
3. What action should the nurse take to relieve Mrs. Wood's pain?
4. When should the nurse next monitor Mrs. Wood's pain level?
5. If Mrs. Wood indicates that her pain is unrelieved after 30 minutes, what action should the nurse take?
6. The nurse is to give Mrs. Wood morphine 8 mg IM now. Morphine 10 mg/mL is available. How many milliliters will the nurse give?

Suggested answers at end of chapter.

Urinary Function

DATA COLLECTION. Monitor the patient's urinary status to ensure normal function is maintained after anesthesia administration. If the patient has a urinary catheter, the amount, color, and consistency of the urine are noted. Otherwise, watch for the patient's first postoperative voiding to prevent bladder distention. Patients should void within 8 hours of their last voiding. Patients having urinary or gynecological procedures may need to void within 4 to 6 hours to prevent increased pressure on the surgical site. Catheterization may be needed if the patient is unable to void. After outpatient surgery, patients may be required to void before being discharged.

If a patient reports the inability to void, the bladder is palpated for distention or a bladder volume measurement is done, which determines the amount of urine in the bladder. You should be aware that restlessness can be caused by discomfort from a full bladder. A distended bladder requires intervention to empty it. Efforts are made to promote voiding before inserting a urinary catheter because of the risk of infection.

The body's stress response to the surgical experience stimulates the sympathetic nervous system ("fight-or-flight" response), which saves fluid by reducing urine output. Therefore, initially urine output may be reduced and concentrated. Then it should gradually increase, becoming less concentrated and lighter in color.

NURSING DIAGNOSES, PLANNING, AND IMPLEMENTATION

Urinary Retention Related to Surgery, Pain, Anesthesia, Altered Positioning

EXPECTED OUTCOME: Patient will completely and regularly empty bladder.

- Measure and record output on postoperative patients, especially those undergoing major procedures or urological surgery, older patients, and those with an IV or urinary catheter *to detect urinary elimination problems.*
- Report urinary output of less than 30 mL in 1 hour from the urinary catheter *because this is typically the minimum acceptable output.*
- Recognize that patients who are voiding small amounts frequently (30 to 50 mL every 20 to 30 minutes) or who dribble may have retention overflow and may not be emptying their bladder. This is not normal and may require catheterization *to empty the bladder and prevent complications.*
- Assist patients to the bathroom or bedside commode, and allow men to stand or sit to urinate if possible *to promote voiding.*
- Warm bedpans *to prevent reflexive sphincter tightening.*
- Use techniques to promote voiding before catheterization for the patient who is unable to void (running water, pouring warm water over a female patient's

perineum, or drinking a hot beverage to stimulate voiding) *because catheterization increases the risk of infection.*

- Provide privacy after safety is ensured *to promote voiding.*
- Have patients place their feet solidly on the floor to relax the pelvic muscles *to aid voiding.*
- Notify the physician if the patient is uncomfortable, has a distended bladder, or has not voided within the specified time frame *to obtain treatment orders.*

EVALUATION. The goal for urinary retention is met if the patient is able to void without pain or complications.

Surgical Wound Care

An incision is a wound made by a physician with a sharp instrument such as a scalpel. A puncture wound has a small opening and is made to insert a tube or drain. Incisions are closed with sutures, staples (Fig. 12.13), or surgical glue, which is painless and produces less scarring. As the wound heals, sutures or staples are removed in 7 to 10 days, and Steri-Strips may be applied to continue supporting the wound as it heals.

Wounds can be clean or dirty. Clean wounds are surgical wounds that are not infected. Dirty (contaminated) wounds include accidental wounds or surgical incisions exposed to gastrointestinal (GI) contents or unsterile conditions. Infected wounds and dirty wounds contain microorganisms from trauma, ruptured organs, or infection. Necrotic and infected tissue is removed before infected wounds are closed. This is known as **debridement**.

WOUND HEALING. Wound healing occurs in phases (Table 12.9). Wounds can heal by first (primary) intention, second (secondary) intention, and third (tertiary) intention (Fig. 12.14). In first-intention healing, the edges of the wound are approximated with staples or sutures. This usually results in minimal scarring. To heal by second intention, the wound is usually left open and allowed to heal by granulation. Scarring is usually extensive with prolonged healing.

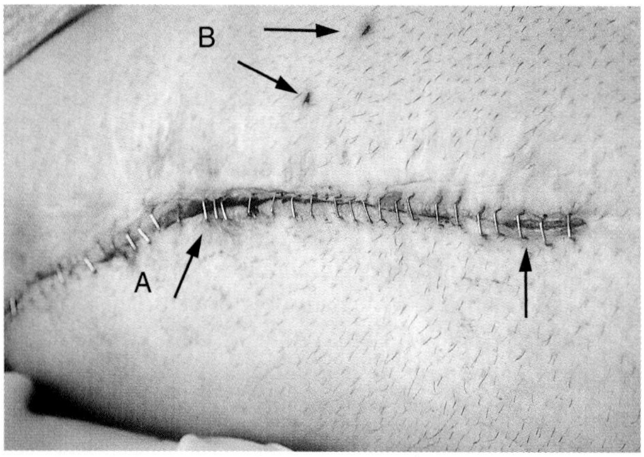
B
A

FIGURE 12.13 A stapled incision. (A) Note wound edges not approximated at arrows. (B) Arrows indicate puncture sites where drains were inserted.

TABLE 12.9 WOUND HEALING PHASES

Phase	Time Frame	Wound Healing	Patient Effect
I	Incision to 2nd postoperative day	Inflammatory response	Fever, malaise
II	Third to 14th postoperative day	Granulation tissue forms	Feeling better
III	3rd to 6th post-operative week	Collagen deposited	Raised scar formed
IV	Months to 1 year	Collagen deposited	Flat, thin scar

For healing by third intention, an infected wound is left open until there is no evidence of infection and the wound is then surgically closed.

WOUND COMPLICATIONS. Wound problems can include hematoma, infection, dehiscence, and evisceration. A hematoma occurs from bleeding in the wound and into the tissue around the wound. A clot forms from the bleeding. If the clot is large with swelling, the clot may need to be removed by the physician.

Infected wounds may be warm, reddened, and tender and have **purulent** drainage (pus). The drainage may have a foul odor. A fever and elevated white blood cell (WBC) count may be present. Antibiotics are used to treat the infection.

Dehiscence and evisceration are serious wound complications (Fig. 12.15). Wound **dehiscence** is the sudden bursting open of a wound's edges, which may be preceded by an increase in **serosanguineous** drainage. **Evisceration** is the viscera spilling out of the abdomen. Dehiscence and evisceration often occur with abdominal incisions in patients who are malnourished, obese, elderly, or who have poor wound healing. Supporting the wound during coughing and other activities that pull on the incision or applying an abdominal binder on patients who are at risk helps prevent dehiscence and evisceration. When evisceration occurs, the patient may have pain and vomiting and may report that "something let loose" or "gave way."

If dehiscence or evisceration occurs, place the patient in low Fowler's position with flexed knees. Cover the wound with sterile dressings or towels moistened with warm sterile normal saline. Notify the physician immediately of this surgical emergency. Apply gentle pressure over the wound and keep the patient still and calm. Monitor vital signs for evidence of shock (e.g., tachycardia, tachypnea, dyspnea, hypotension). IV fluids are infused as ordered. Prepare the patient for immediate surgery to close the wound.

• WORD • BUILDING •

serosanguineous: sero—whey + sanguineous—bloody
evisceration: e—out + viscera—body organs

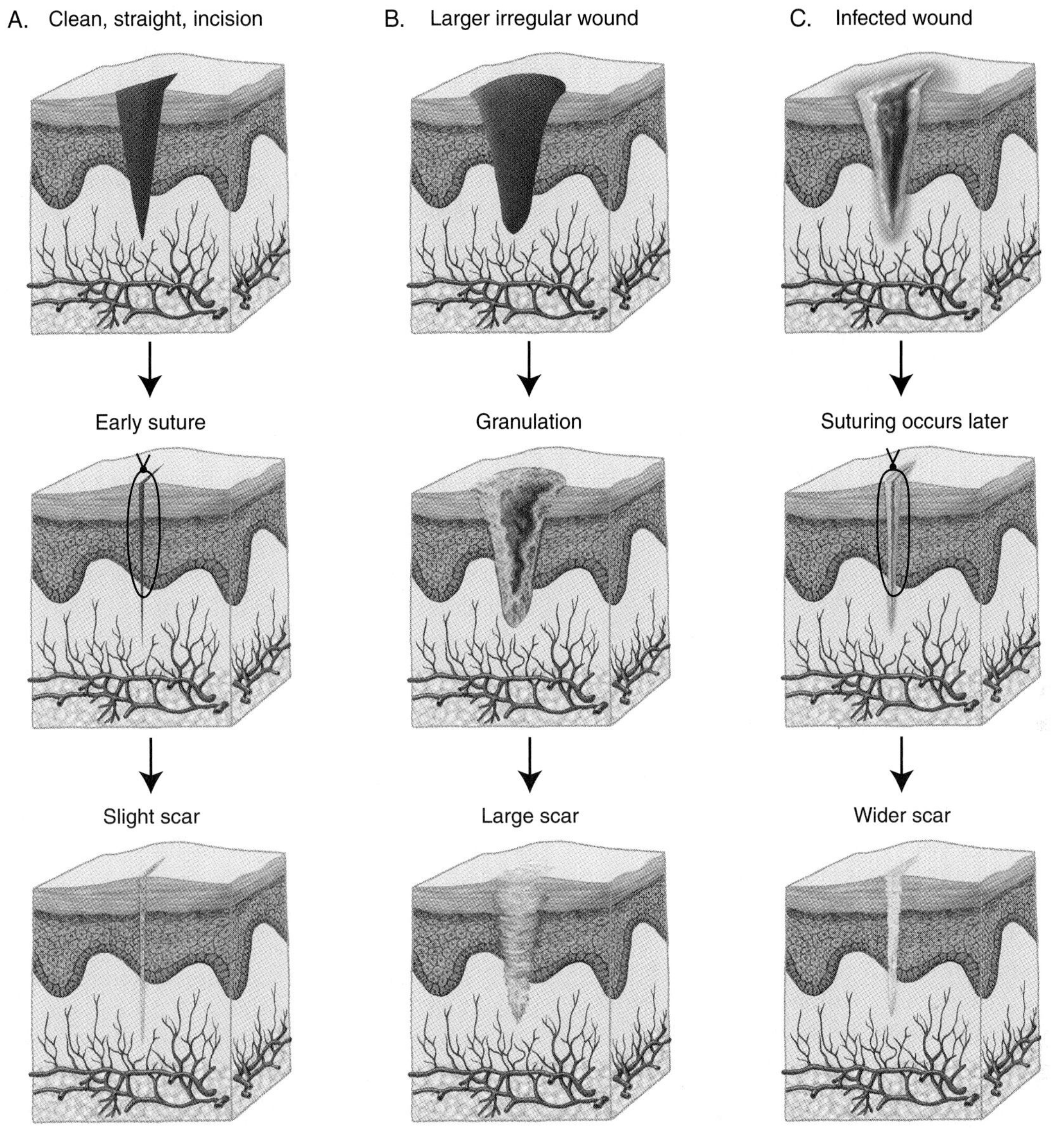
A. Clean, straight, incision
B. Larger irregular wound
C. Infected wound
Early suture
Granulation
Suturing occurs later
Slight scar
Large scar
Wider scar

FIGURE 12.14 Wound healing. (A) Primary intention. Wound healing occurs in a clean wound, such as a surgical wound, whose edges are approximated, typically with staples or sutures. Healing occurs quickly with slight scarring. (B) Secondary intention. Large irregular or infected wounds are left open to allow healing to occur from the inside out. Pressure ulcers or chronic wounds are often treated this way. Large scarring occurs with lengthy healing time. (C) Tertiary intention. Infected or contaminated wound is left open for a brief time period until wound is clean. Granulation tissue fills in for some wound healing and then edges are approximated and closed surgically. Wider scarring occurs.

For dehisced surgical incisions that resist healing, vacuum-assisted closure (VAC) aids in healing the incision (see Chapter 54). VAC applies negative pressure to wound edges. The device can also be used on other types of wounds.

DATA COLLECTION.

Drains. Drains are inserted into wounds during surgery to prevent accumulation of blood, lymph, or necrotic tissue in wounds that can lead to infection or delayed healing. Drains may work by gravity or suction. Penrose drains are soft, flat, drains that carry drainage from the wound. Moderate serosanguineous drainage is expected from a Penrose drain and may require frequent dressing changes. Examples of drains that use suction to gently enhance drainage include the Jackson-Pratt, Hemovac, and Mini-Snyder Hemovac (www.zimmer.com). These drains are closed systems that may require periodic emptying and reapplication of the suction by compressing the drain.

Output is recorded when the drainage is emptied. The amount of drainage expected varies with the type of surgery. Be alert for excessive amounts to report. Specialized drainage systems allow the autotransfusion of drainage containing blood back to the patient to maintain hemoglobin levels without the risks associated with blood transfusions, such as transfusion reactions or transmission of infections.

Dressings. Dressings protect the wound, absorb drainage, prevent contamination from body fluids, provide comfort,

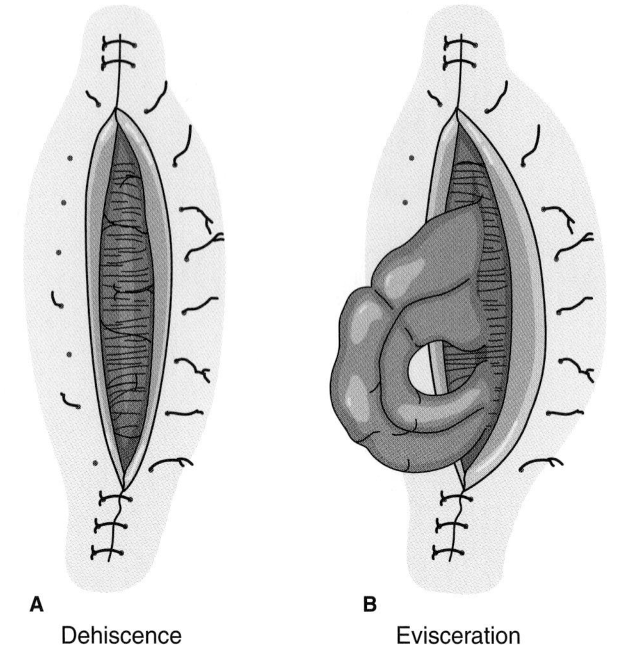
A
Dehiscence
B
Evisceration

FIGURE 12.15 (A) Wound dehiscence. (B) Wound evisceration.

and apply pressure to reduce swelling or bleeding as in a pressure dressing. The initial dressing is applied in surgery and then is usually removed by the physician approximately 24 hours postoperatively. If drainage appears on the initial dressing, reinforce it with another dressing, according to physician orders or institution policy.

After the initial dressing is removed, if the wound is dry and the edges intact (approximated), the physician may not order the dressing to be replaced. This allows easy observation of the wound and avoidance of applying tape to the skin. Draining wounds are dressed with several layers that are changed as needed. When the old dressing is removed, it should be done carefully to prevent dislodging of tubes or drains. The condition of the wound is documented with each dressing change. It is normal for the incision to be puffy and red from the inflammatory response. The surrounding skin should be the patient's normal color and temperature. Correct tape application over the dressing is done by gently laying the tape over the dressing and applying even pressure on each side of the wound. Pressure should not be applied on top of the wound by pulling on the tape from one side of the wound to the other side.

NURSING DIAGNOSES, PLANNING, AND IMPLEMENTATION

Impaired Skin Integrity Related to Surgical Incision

EXPECTED OUTCOME: Patient will regain skin integrity within [specify individualized realistic time frame].

- Monitor skin color and temperature and report changes *to detect need for treatment.*
- Monitor dressings and note drainage color, amount, and consistency. *Surgical wound drainage initially is sanguineous (red) and changes to serosanguineous (pink) and then serous (pale yellow) after a few hours to days.*
- Promptly report drainage that is bright red, remains sanguineous after a few hours, or is profuse to the physician *because the patient may be hemorrhaging.*
- Use standard precautions when changing dressings *to protect yourself.*

EVALUATION. The goal for impaired skin integrity is met if the patient's wound heals and skin integrity is regained without delayed healing or complications.

Gastrointestinal Function

Nutritional intake and bowel function can be affected by surgery and anesthesia. NPO status and a bowel preparation often occur preoperatively. After abdominal surgery, GI function is often impaired. A clinical trial is examining whether alvimopan 12 mg administered 30 to 90 minutes before surgery will result in earlier recovery of the functioning of the GI tract after partial small or large bowel resections.

DATA COLLECTION. After abdominal surgery, GI assessment should include monitoring vital signs, the return of flatus, the return of appetite, first bowel movement, any nausea or vomiting, or signs of ileus, such as distention, bloating, and cramps. The abdomen is documented to be soft or firm, and flat or distended. Abnormal findings are reported to the physician.

Traditionally after GI surgery, bowel sounds were monitored by the nurse and the patient was kept NPO until flatus and bowel sounds returned. No evidence exists to support this practice. Research about this practice shows that bowel sounds are not correlated with bowel motility and a patient's ability to safely drink and eat postoperatively. In fact, patients can be hydrated and fed early for nutrition to promote healing and faster recovery (see *Evidence-Based Practice* box). Monitoring bowel sounds has not been shown to be necessary to a positive patient outcome so traditional practice is changing to evidence-based practice.

After abdominal surgery, peristalsis and bowel sounds usually stop for 24 to 72 hours. Flatus is usually absent for 24 to 72 hours postoperatively. Flatus, bowel movements, and an appetite signal the return of GI function. Chewing gum after a colectomy can reduce time to flatus and first bowel movement. If a paralytic ileus develops, abdominal distention, absent bowel sounds, and pain may result. The patient's abdominal girth is measured if distention occurs. As ordered, a nasogastric tube can be used to decompress the GI tract until peristalsis returns. Drainage from the decompression tube is observed for amount, color, and consistency. Intake and output are measured. Removal of gastric secretions can cause electrolyte imbalances. Signs and symptoms of electrolyte imbalance can include new-onset confusion or weakness, which should be reported.

EVIDENCE-BASED PRACTICE

Clinical Question

Is early versus delayed oral intake of food and fluids after major abdominal gynecological surgery associated with complications?

Evidence

A Cochrane systematic review of randomized control trials of early versus delayed oral intake after major abdominal gynecological surgery showed early oral intake was associated with increased nausea (not vomiting), reduced time to bowel sound return, shorter time to first solid diet, and a shorter hospital stay (Charoenkwan, Phillipson, & Vutyavanich, 2007). No significant differences were seen in postoperative ileus, abdominal distention, time to flatus or passage of stool, nasogastric tube placement, fever, wound complications, and pneumonia.

Implications for Nursing Practice

Nurses can promote early feeding after major abdominal gynecological surgery as ordered. Monitoring for nausea should be done.

REFERENCE

Charoenkwan, K., Phillipson, G., & Vutyavanich, T. (2007). Early versus delayed oral fluids and food for reducing complications after major abdominal gynaecologic surgery. *Cochrane Database of Systematic Reviews 2007, Issue 4* (Art. No. CD004508; DOI 10.1002/14651858.CD004508.pub3).

NURSING DIAGNOSES, PLANNING, AND IMPLEMENTATION

Imbalanced Nutrition: Less Than Body Requirements Related to NPO, Pain, Nausea

EXPECTED OUTCOME: Patient will resume normal dietary intake and maintain weight within normal limits.

- Maintain IV fluids, total parenteral nutrition, or enteral feedings *until the patient resumes oral intake* (Box 12.10, *Nutrition Notes*).
- Try water and clear liquids at first as ordered, then advance the diet *to promote tolerance.*
- Give antiemetics as ordered *to control nausea and vomiting.*

Box 12.10

Nutrition Notes

Nourishing the Postoperative Patient

After surgery, intravenous 5% glucose in water is commonly prescribed. Two liters of this solution contain only 340 calories, which is insufficient to meet the patient's energy needs but enough to prevent ketosis from breakdown of adipose tissue. Previously well-nourished adults generally have nutrient reserves for 3 to 4 days of semistarvation. To prevent excessive muscle protein from being used for energy, adequate nourishment should be delivered to the patient within 3 days. (Citrotein and Enlive can be used to supplement clear liquid diets.)

To avoid abdominal distention, oral feedings traditionally have been delayed until peristalsis returns but scientific evidence supporting this practice is lacking. Researchers are beginning to test the practice. In some situations, delaying oral intake seems to offer no advantage in preventing complications over earlier resumption of feeding.

Patients usually progress from clear liquids to a regular diet as soon as possible. If "diet as tolerated" is prescribed, the patient should be asked what sounds good. Sometimes a full dinner when the patient doesn't feel well "turns off" the appetite.

After gastrointestinal surgery, oral food and fluids are deferred longer than with other surgeries to allow healing. When particular amounts are prescribed, those limits should be strictly implemented to preserve the suture lines.

After surgery on the mouth and throat, no red liquids are given so that bleeding can be seen and vomitus is not mistaken for blood.

Specific nutrients necessary for healing are:

- Vitamin C for collagen formation
- Vitamin K for blood clotting
- Zinc for tissue growth, skin integrity, and cell-mediated immunity
- Protein for controlling fluid balance and edema, for manufacturing antibodies and white blood cells, and for building scar tissue.

Constipation Related to Decreased Peristalsis, Immobility, Altered Diet, Opioid Side Effect

EXPECTED OUTCOME: The patient will return to normal bowel elimination patterns and report freedom from gas pains and constipation within 3 to 4 days postoperatively.

- Encourage early ambulation and exercise *to promote restoration of GI function.*
- Encourage ambulation, have patient lie prone, and pull the knees up to the chest if gas pains occur *to relieve the pain.*
- Monitor elimination and document *to detect problems.*
- Provide stool softeners or laxatives as ordered *to prevent constipation.*

EVALUATION. The goal for the *Imbalanced Nutrition: Less Than Body Requirements* nursing diagnosis is met if patients are able to maintain their baseline weight and resume a normal dietary intake. The goal for constipation is met if patients are free from discomfort and establish a regular bowel elimination pattern.

> **NURSING CARE TIP**
>
> Most IV solutions do not provide enough nutrients or calories to prevent malnutrition. The primary purpose of most IV fluids is to provide hydration. A 1000-mL IV solution containing 5% dextrose provides only about 170 calories. This does not meet an adult's daily caloric needs, especially if healing is occurring. You should ensure that early consideration of other nutritional methods is made to meet the patient's dietary needs.

Mobility

DATA COLLECTION. It is important for the patient to move as much as possible to prevent complications and promote healing. Pain, incisions, tubes, drains, dressings, and other equipment may make movement difficult. You should determine the patient's ability to move in bed, to get out of bed, and to walk. Pain levels that may interfere with movement are assessed. The patient's tolerance to activity is observed. Patient understanding of how to perform exercises is noted.

NURSING DIAGNOSES, PLANNING, AND IMPLEMENTATION

Impaired Physical Mobility Related to Surgery, Decreased Strength, and Movement Restriction

EXPECTED OUTCOME: Patient's goal will be to resume normal physical activity.

- Position patient in bed with pillows *to support the body in good alignment.*
- Turn at least every 2 hours, alternating from supine to side to side if not contraindicated, *to prevent complications.*
- Encourage patients to move themselves *to increase circulation and promote lung expansion.*
- If ambulation is not possible, encourage hourly exercises (deep breathing, range of motion of all joints, and isometric exercises of the abdominal, gluteal, and leg muscles) while awake *to prevent complications.*
- If patient cannot perform active range-of-motion exercises, perform passive joint range of motion *to prevent complications.*
- Raise the head of the bed slowly *to let the circulatory system adjust to the position change.*
- If patient reports dizziness or feeling faint, lower the head of the bed *to let the circulatory system adjust more slowly.*
- Dangle patient's feet on the side of the bed *to prepare for ambulation* (see Fig. 12.11).
- If dangling is tolerated, ambulate the patient. Before getting up, patient should pedal the feet to "wake up" the muscles controlling the arteries. To rise, patient should keep eyes forward and move slowly until feeling adjusted to being up. Usually the patient ambulates a short distance the first time and increases the distance as tolerated. One or two health care workers should assist the patient and use a gait (walking) belt for safety. Walkers with wheels and seats also may be used for support and for resting if the patient becomes dizzy or tired. If patient feels faint or dizzy or if vital signs change, help patient back to bed. A wheelchair may be needed for safe transport back to the room.

EVALUATION. The goal for impaired physical mobility is met if the patient can increase ambulation and resume normal activities.

Postoperative Patient Discharge

Discharge planning begins during preadmission testing and continues after admission to ensure that the patient is ready for a timely discharge. When the patient meets discharge criteria, the physician discharges the patient from either the ambulatory setting or the hospital.

Ambulatory Surgery

DISCHARGE CRITERIA. Usually, a patient can be considered a candidate for discharge 1 hour after surgery if the PACU discharge scoring system or clinical discharge criteria are met (see Box 12.8). Clinical discharge criteria include stable vital signs, no bleeding, no nausea or vomiting, and controlled pain that is not severe. Depending on the type of surgical procedure, such as urological, gynecological, or hernia surgery, the patient may be required to void before discharge. The patient also should be able to sit up without dizziness before discharge. Patients meeting discharge criteria are discharged by the physician and released to a responsible adult. Patients are not permitted to drive themselves home because of the effects of anesthesia and medications they have received.

DISCHARGE INSTRUCTIONS. Patients and their families are given written discharge instructions before discharge. Elderly patients should have a caregiver participate in the discharge instruction session to understand what observations to make and what to do if complications develop. The instruction form is signed by the patient or an authorized representative to indicate understanding. Prescriptions and a copy of the instructions, to provide a reference for later, are sent with the patient. The patient is encouraged to rest for 24 to 48 hours. The patient is to avoid operating machinery, driving, drinking alcoholic beverages, and making major decisions for 24 hours because the effects of undergoing surgery can alter energy levels and thinking ability. The physician orders any fluid, dietary, activity, or work restrictions.

Patients are taught wound care, medication information (including side effects), and signs and symptoms of complications to report to the physician. Phone numbers for the physician, surgical facility, and emergency care are provided. Patients are informed of the date for their follow-up visit to the physician and told to call and make an appointment.

Inpatient Surgery

DISCHARGE CRITERIA. The physician determines the patient's readiness for discharge from the hospital. Postoperative lengths of stay vary based on the surgical procedure and the patient's individual needs. Prior to discharge, a complete assessment of the patient is performed and documented.

DISCHARGE INSTRUCTIONS. All necessary teaching is completed before discharge (Fig. 12.16). Patients and their families or caregivers are given prescriptions and a copy of written instructions that are signed by the patient to indicate understanding before discharge. If more teaching or reinforcement is needed, a referral to a home health nurse can be requested.

The physician orders any fluid, dietary, activity, or work restrictions. Patients are taught wound care, medication information (including side effects), and signs and symptoms of complications to report to the physician. Patients are informed of the date for their follow-up visit to the physician.

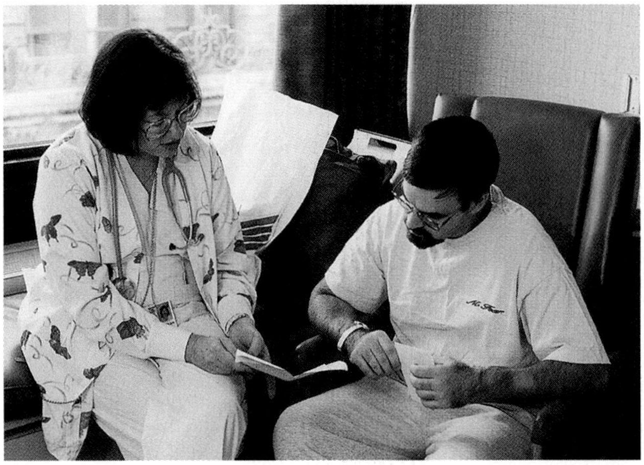

FIGURE 12.16 Nurse providing discharge teaching to patient.

Home Health Hints

A referral for a home health nurse to assist a patient in the recovery process is made when the patient needs the following:

- Continued assistance with skilled nursing interventions, such as wound care, IV medications, or ostomy care
- Additional teaching to be able to perform self-care, such as diabetic teaching for a patient with newly diagnosed diabetes or ostomy care
- Assessment of the recovery process
- Assistance because of weakness, lack of social support, or development of complications; care provided in the home is adapted to the patient's resources and environment to facilitate compliance.

It is helpful for caregivers to keep a notebook in the hospital and continue it at home. Treatments, medicines, observations, procedures, doctor and nurse visits, instructions, and therapies with dates and times can be recorded. This helps prevent confusion, prepares the next caregiver, and affords better organization of time and resources for everyone. It can also be nice to see who visited the patient.

Families of patients recovering from surgery should provide items to keep the patient occupied and comfortable: talking books, inspirational reading material, pictures, and their favorite pajamas, robe and slippers, and coverlet.

After a patient comes home from surgery, the home care nurse can help give direction to the family to prepare the room where the patient will be staying:

- It is helpful if the room can be on the same floor with the bathroom, kitchen, and living space.
- If an extended recovery period or illness is expected, the den or living room might be considered as the primary living space to provide room for equipment and make companionship easier. The patient can see activity in the home and be included in family activity. Also, caregivers can be more attentive to the patient's needs and save countless footsteps.

Reinforce any discharge instructions the patient and caregivers bring home with them. Although these instructions are reviewed by the surgeon and hospital nurses, frequently the patient and family are tired and anxious and can miss important details. If possible keep a copy of these instructions in the patient's home health folder in order to communicate to all members of the health care team.

Special equipment may be needed, including the following:

- For the patient on bedrest, a hospital bed with full side rails helps with a variety of position changes and better height for the caregiver.
- Draw sheets made of folded twin sheets are needed, as well as extra pillows for positioning.
- A bedside stand is needed for personal and toilet articles.
- A bedside commode can be placed near the bed if the patient cannot walk to the bathroom. A bedpan or urinal may be needed. A functional female urinal is easier to use than a bedpan.
- A flexible tube with a shower head that connects to the bathtub faucet is convenient and allows the patient more independence in bathing.
- Installation of grab bars and tub stools and skid-proofing of a shower or tub are important safety measures to help prevent falls.
- If the patient is eligible for insurance coverage for durable medical equipment, a physician's order must be obtained.

SUGGESTED ANSWERS TO

CRITICAL THINKING

■ *Mrs. Owens*

1. 100 mL per hour. IV pumps are always set to deliver the amount of milliliters per hour. Divide the total volume of 1000 mL by the total time of 10 hours = 100 mL per hour.
2. Intake = 2400 mL.

To calculate this:

Remember your conversions:

30 mL = 1 oz

1 cup = 8 oz (don't supersize the cup!)

Calculations:

1 8-oz cup of coffee = 1 × 8 × 30 = 240 mL

4 oz orange juice = 4 × 30 = 120 mL

6 oz tomato soup = 6 × 30 = 180 mL

3/4 cup gelatin = 3/4 × 8 × 30 = 180 mL

2 cups of water = 2 × 8 × 30 = 480 mL

1200 mL of 0.9 normal saline IV

The patient's output does not impact the intake total so it is not used for this calculation.

■ *Mrs. Wood*

1. Moaning occasionally, moving legs restlessly, and pulling covers near abdominal incision are nonverbal pain cues.
2. Document pain levels by actual observations: occasional moaning, restless leg movements, and pulling of covers near abdominal incision. By patient's statement: "It hurts." Because Mrs. Wood is too drowsy to use the pain scale, other data are used. When Mrs. Wood is more awake, explanation of the pain scale should be reinforced and used.
3. Review pain medication orders to determine if analgesics can be given. Noting that an IV analgesic was given 50 minutes ago and the IM analgesic is ordered every 3 hours, request that the physician or pharmacist be consulted to determine appropriate time intervals. The patient should not have to wait 3 hours to receive the next dose of pain medication. If the consultation indicates it is time to give the analgesic, verify that vital signs are still stable and then give the analgesic. Also consider other pain relief measures such as patient warmth, positioning, or environmental issues such as bright lighting, room temperature, and noise.
4. After administration of the analgesic, Mrs. Wood's pain level should be assessed in at least 30 minutes to determine pain relief. If Mrs. Wood is asleep, she should not be awakened unless it is necessary. Nonverbal cues should be observed and respirations counted and documented. If no indication of pain is noted, Mrs. Wood's pain level should be monitored at least hourly or as needed.
5. Document pain level on scale of 0 to 10 and have the physician notified of inadequate pain relief. The patient should not have to wait the 3-hour interval if in pain. Consider providing other pain relief measures while the physician is being notified.
6. Try unit analysis for solving mathematical calculations. It is easy to understand and our students say it is a helpful method.

Unit Analysis Method:

$$\frac{8\ \cancel{\text{milligrams}}}{} \left|\ \frac{1\ \text{milliliter}}{10\ \cancel{\text{milligrams}}}\right. = \frac{8}{10} = 0.8\ \text{milliliter}$$

REVIEW QUESTIONS

1. Which of the following nursing actions would reduce surgical risk factors for preoperative patients? **Select all that apply.**
   a. Playing music of patient's choice
   b. Avoiding discussion of fears
   c. Reinforcing pain control methods
   d. Showing use of incentive spirometer
   e. Monitoring blood glucose for a patient with diabetes
   f. Teaching to perform leg exercises hourly while awake

2. Which of the following is the patient care role for the LPN/LVN in the preoperative phase?
   a. Assisting in data collection
   b. Explaining the surgical procedure
   c. Obtaining preoperative orders
   d. Conducting the preoperative anesthesia interview

3. Which of the following is within the LPN/LVN's scope of practice related to the patient providing consent for surgery? **Select all that apply.**
   a. Witnessing minor patient's signature on the consent
   b. Providing informed consent
   c. Answering surgical procedure questions
   d. Requesting patient questions be referred to physician
   e. Witnessing the patient's signature on the consent
   f. Reading the consent to a patient prior to signing

4. When teaching the elderly preoperative patient, which of the following is a teaching strategy that improves learning?
   a. Sit near a window with bright sunlight.
   b. Use large black-on-white printed materials.
   c. Sit beside patient.
   d. Use blue and green colors for brochures.

5. Which of the following interventions would help prevent atelectasis in a postoperative patient? **Select all that apply.**
   a. Coughing and deep breathing
   b. Holding breath while moving
   c. Restricting fluids
   d. Leg exercises
   e. Pain control
   f. Ambulation

6. Which of the following would the nurse evaluate as indicating that interventions to prevent respiratory complications for the postoperative patient have been effective?
   a. Pain level "2"
   b. No abdominal distention
   c. Clear lung sounds
   d. Good appetite

7. Which of the following findings would the nurse recognize as being the earliest indicator of hemorrhage or shock that should be reported to the physician?
   a. Tachycardia
   b. Polyuria
   c. Nausea
   d. Fever

8. Which of the following criterion would a nurse use to determine patient readiness for discharge from ambulatory surgery?
   a. Ability to drive an automobile
   b. Ability to ambulate 50 feet
   c. Being pain free
   d. Absence of nausea or vomiting

9. What is the role of the home health nurse in caring for postoperative patients? **Fill in the blank.**
   Answer: ______________________________

References

American Society of Anesthesiologists. (1999a). Task force on preoperative fasting. Practice guidelines for preoperative fasting and the use of pharmacologic agents to reduce the risk of pulmonary aspiration: Application to healthy patients undergoing elective procedures. *Anesthesiology, 90,* 896. Retrieved July 27, 2009, from http://www.asahq.org/publicationsAndServices/NPO.pdf

American Society of Anesthesiologists. (1999b). Anesthesiologists warn: If you're taking herbal products, tell your doctor before surgery. Press release, May 26, 1999. Retrieved July 27, 2009, from http://www.asahq.org

Joint Commission. (2010). *2010 national patient safety goals.* Retrieved January 13, 2010, from http://www.jointcommission.org/patientsafety/nationalpatientsafetygoals

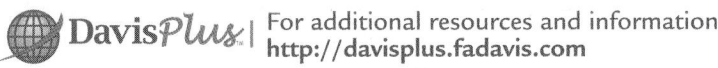

13 Nursing Care of Patients with Emergent Conditions and Disaster/Bioterrorism Response

ERIN MAZUR

KEY TERMS

abrasion (ah-BRAY-zhun)
amputation (am-pew-TAY-shun)
anaphylactic shock (an-uh-fah-LAK-tik SHAWK)
anaphylaxis (an-uh-fah-LAK-sis)
anthrax (AN-thracks)
asphyxia (as-FIX-ee-ah)
bioterrorism (BY-oh-TARE-UR-is-um)
botulism (BOTCH-uh-liz-um)
capillary refill (KAP-ih-lar-ee REE-fill)
cardiac tamponade (KAR-dee-ack tam-pon-AID)
cardiogenic shock (KAR-dee-oh-JEN-ick SHAWK)
distributive shock (dis-TRIB-u-tive SHAWK)
flail chest (FLAY-ul CHEST)
full-thickness burn (FUL-THICK-ness BERN)
gastric lavage (GAS-trick la-VAHJ)
heatstroke (HEET-strohk)
hypovolemic shock (HIGH-poh-voh-LEE-mick SHAWK)
laceration (lass-ur-A-shun)
obstructive shock (ub-STRUK-tive SHAWK)
partial-thickness burn (PARR-shul THICK-ness BERN)
plague (PLAYG)
shock (SHAWK)
smallpox (SMALL-pocks)
tetanus (TET-nus)
triage (TREE-ahj)

QUESTIONS TO GUIDE YOUR READING

1. What are the components of the primary survey?
2. What interventions would you use for a trauma victim?
3. What are the symptoms of inhalation injury?
4. What are the stages of hypothermia and hyperthermia?
5. What priorities of care are used for poison overdose?
6. What is your role in crisis situations and psychiatric emergencies?
7. What is your role in identifying a bioterrorist attack or disaster response?

The ability to recognize an emergent condition, prioritize, and provide quick assessments and interventions is essential in nursing. Upon arrival in the emergency department, most patients are triaged by a registered nurse (RN). During the triage process, the RN evaluates the patient's condition, asks appropriate questions related to the condition, and performs a rapid assessment of the patient to provide the appropriate level of care (Fig. 13.1). This chapter presents specific emergent conditions with application of the nursing process.

PRIMARY SURVEY

To recognize life-threatening conditions and determine priorities of care, an initial assessment of the patient's airway, breathing, circulation, and disability is conducted. This process is known as the primary survey. The components of the primary survey are listed in Table 13.1.

A—Airway

The airway is the most important component of the primary survey. The neck should not be hyperextended, flexed, or rotated until spinal injury is ruled out because any movement may worsen an existing cervical spine injury. During cardiopulmonary resuscitation (CPR) if there is a possible or known spinal injury, the jaw-thrust maneuver rather than the chin-lift maneuver must be used to avoid moving the head and neck (Fig. 13.2). The airway is inspected for obstruction, including loose teeth, foreign objects, bleeding, and vomitus. Next, any visible airway obstructions are removed using suction.

Airway adjuncts, such as nasopharyngeal or oropharyngeal airways, may be used to keep the airway open. When additional airway support and mechanical ventilation are required, advanced airway adjuncts, such as endotracheal intubation or cricothyroidotomy, may be performed by specially trained emergency personnel or physicians.

B—Breathing

After the airway is opened, the patient is assessed for spontaneous breathing and respiratory rate and depth. The nurse observes whether the patient's chest rises and falls spontaneously and auscultates for breath sounds bilaterally. If the patient is not breathing, interventions are performed before proceeding. The patient may be ventilated with a mouth-to-face mask or a bag-valve-face mask. Endotracheal intubation is the preferred method of maintaining an airway in an unconscious patient because it opens the airway and protects the lungs from aspiration (see Fig. 29.23).

C—Circulation

The carotid pulse is palpated for quality and rate. The skin is inspected for color and temperature. External bleeding is controlled by external pressure and elevation when possible. Any life-threatening conditions that may compromise circulation are assessed and interventions provided before proceeding.

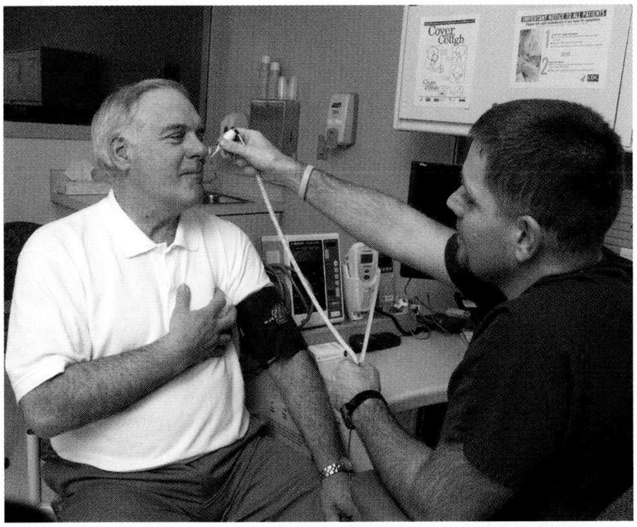

FIGURE 13.1 Triage nurse evaluating patient who has just arrived in the emergency department.

TABLE 13.1 COMPONENTS OF THE PRIMARY SURVEY

A	Airway
B	Breathing
C	Circulation
D	Disability/central nervous system

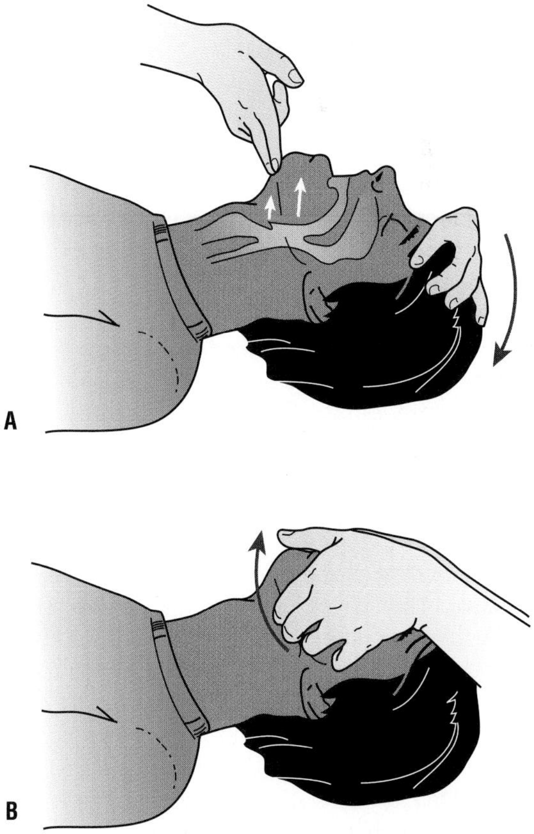

FIGURE 13.2 (A) Chin-lift maneuver is used to open the airway. (B) Jaw-thrust maneuver is used to open the airway if the patient may have a head or neck injury.

Other conditions that may compromise circulation include internal bleeding, shock resulting from hemorrhage, or major burns. Large-gauge intravenous (IV) cannulas (16 or 18 gauge) are initiated for fluid resuscitation. If the patient does not have a pulse, cardiopulmonary resuscitation must be initiated. If a pulse can be palpated, vital signs are taken and recorded.

D—Disability/Central Nervous System

To detect serious central nervous system injury, a brief neurologic assessment is conducted to determine the level of consciousness, which may range from alert (A) and responds to verbal stimuli (V) to responds to painful stimuli (P) or unresponsive (U). To assess response to painful stimuli, a painful stimulus is applied, such as rubbing the sternum, pressing a pen against the base of the nail, or applying periorbital pressure. The patient is observed for the response to the pain, and the response is recorded. Movement of all extremities is also assessed.

SECONDARY SURVEY

For victims of severe trauma, a secondary survey is conducted. This assessment identifies areas of medical or injury problems that are not immediately life threatening but require treatment (see *Evidence-Based Practice* box). Major body areas that may sustain serious injury, such as the head, spine, chest, abdomen, and musculoskeletal system, are quickly examined to detect additional injuries (Table 13.2). To adequately perform a head-to-toe assessment, the patient's clothing is removed. Each major body area is inspected and palpated for deformity, bruising, open wounds, bleeding, and pain.

EVIDENCE-BASED PRACTICE

Clinical Question

What are types and causes of medication errors in the emergency department (ED)?

Evidence

A 2006 study of 131 EDs looked at barriers to implementing the Joint Commission 2006 National Patient Safety Goals for medication safety and found barriers related to the complexity of the ED environment, such as residents in training, mixed-shift hours, and state designation as a trauma center (Juarez et al., 2009).

A study of medication errors reported in 496 EDs revealed that physicians were responsible for 24% of errors and nurses 54% (Pham et al., 2008). Most of the errors were during the administration phase and involved an improper dose or quantity caused by not following proper procedure/protocol, poor communication, distractions, emergencies, heavy workload, or computerized order entry.

Implications for Nursing Practice

Medication errors may result from the acute, crowded, and fast-paced nature of emergency care. Nurses and health care agencies need to be aware of the causes and types of medication errors and strive to take steps to prevent them.

REFERENCES

Juarez, A., Gacki-Smith, J., Bauer, M., et al. (2009). National patient safety goals. Barriers to emergency departments' adherence to four medication safety-related Joint Commission national patient safety goals. *Joint Commission Journal on Quality and Patient Safety, 35*(1), 49–59.

Pham, J. C., Story, J. L., Hicks, R. W., et al. (2008). National study on the frequency, types, causes, and consequences of voluntarily reported emergency department medication errors. *Journal of Emergency Medicine*, September 25, 2008, DOI:10.1016/j.jemermed.2008.02.060.

TABLE 13.2 COMPONENTS OF THE SECONDARY SURVEY

Head	Inspect for lacerations, bleeding from orifices. Check pupil size and response to light. Are pupils equal in size?
Chest	Auscultate for breath sounds in all lung fields. Inspect for lacerations, wounds, foreign bodies.
Abdomen	Auscultate for bowel sounds in all four quadrants. Palpate for areas of tenderness and rigidity. Inspect for lacerations, wounds, and foreign bodies.
Extremities	Inspect for lacerations, wounds, and foreign bodies. Inspect for injuries and deformities. Note areas of tenderness. Palpate for pulses. Evaluate temperature and capillary refill and compare the left to the right extremities.

SHOCK

Shock is a condition of acute peripheral circulatory failure, causing inadequate and progressively decreasing blood pressure and failing tissue perfusion (see Chapter 9). During the initial phases of shock, compensatory adjustments allow the body to adapt to the circulatory changes. Eventually, however, these compensatory mechanisms fail and cellular perfusion decreases, causing cell death.

There are four types of shock: hypovolemic, cardiogenic, obstructive, and distributive. **Hypovolemic shock** signs and symptoms are caused by a decrease in the circulating blood volume. **Cardiogenic shock** signs and symptoms result from cardiac failure. **Obstructive shock** caused by a blockage of blood flow in the cardiovascular circuit outside the heart results in signs and symptoms of reduced blood flow and oxygenation. **Distributive shock** caused by excessive dilation of the venules and arterioles causes signs and symptoms of decreased blood pressure. Therapeutic interventions for shock are listed in Box 13.1.

Box 13.1

Guiding Principles for Treating Shock

- Maintain an open airway and give oxygen as ordered.
- Control external bleeding by direct pressure.
- Keep the patient supine if possible.
- Accurately record vital signs.
- Give IV fluids as ordered.
- Give the patient nothing to eat or drink until surgery is ruled out.

ANAPHYLAXIS

Anaphylaxis is a severe allergic reaction. The reaction may occur suddenly after initial contact with an allergen or after any subsequent exposure. Signs and symptoms result from a massive release of chemical mediators from mast cells and basophils throughout the body (Box 13.2). Chemical mediators lead to vasodilation and capillary leakage, which results in hypotension and eventually vascular collapse.

NURSING CARE TIP

One of the increasing causes of anaphylactic shock is latex allergy reaction. This type of allergy is on the rise among health care workers as a result of repeated exposure to health care products made with latex, such as gloves. The use of latex-free products limits exposure and reduces the risk of developing this allergy.

Box 13.2

Signs and Symptoms of an Allergic Reaction

- Generalized itching and burning
- Urticaria (hives)
- Swelling of the lips and tongue
- Dyspnea
- Bronchospasm and wheezing
- Chest tightness and cough
- Anxiety
- Hypotension

• WORD • BUILDING •
anaphylaxis: an—without + phylaxis—protection

Pathophysiology

Anaphylactic shock is a form of distributive shock. There is no loss of blood, but excessive vasodilation occurs. Bronchi constrict, and air movement into the lungs becomes increasingly difficult. Increased fluid and mucus are secreted into the bronchial passages. Fluid in the air passages and constricted bronchi cause wheezing. The body is rapidly deprived of needed oxygen by this respiratory system reaction. Signs of severe anaphylaxis include hypotension due to vasodilation, decreased level of consciousness due to decreased oxygenation, and respiratory distress with stridor and cyanosis due to airway constriction and fluid.

Nursing Process for the Patient Experiencing Shock or Anaphylaxis

Data Collection

When monitoring a patient at risk for shock, be aware of the signs and symptoms common to all types of shock (Box 13.3). It is important to note the patient's initial level of consciousness and monitor the patient for any subsequent changes. A progressive decline in level of consciousness indicates an urgent need for intervention. Pulses indicate the strength of the heart's contractions. Because a pulse is an immediate indicator of the patient's condition, it should be taken frequently during any emergency condition. Changes in blood pressure may indicate changes in blood volume. Blood pressure changes can occur rapidly but usually not as swiftly as pulse changes.

Skin temperature and color changes may occur with shock. Severe blood loss activates the "fight-or-flight" response in the sympathetic nervous system, which causes the skin to become cool and clammy. This occurs when peripheral blood vessels constrict to shunt blood to vital organs. Skin color depends on the presence of circulating blood in the vessels of the skin. Pale, white, or ashen skin indicates insufficient circulation. In patients with deeply pigmented skin, color changes may be seen in the nailbeds, conjunctiva of the eye, or mucous membranes of the mouth.

Capillary refill is checked on nailbeds to evaluate arterial circulation to an extremity. The nailbed is compressed to produce blanching (lighter color change), released, and the seconds counted until color returns to the blanched area.

Box 13.3

Common Signs and Symptoms of Shock

- Restlessness and anxiety
- Weak, rapid, thready pulse
- Cold and clammy skin
- Pale skin color
- Shallow, rapid, labored breathing
- Gradually and steadily falling blood pressure
- Alteration in consciousness in severe shock state
- Thirst

Normally, nailbed color should return within 3 seconds after the pressure is released. Patients in shock may have delayed or absent capillary refill.

> **LEARNING TIP**
> Gently squeeze and release your own nailbed. Do you see the color change? Count the seconds until the color returns. That is your capillary refill time.

Nursing Diagnoses, Planning, and Implementation

Ineffective Tissue Perfusion (Cerebral and Other Organs) Related to Decreased Circulating Blood Volume Secondary to Internal and/or External Bleeding

EXPECTED OUTCOME: The patient's bleeding will be controlled to maintain vital signs within limits normal for the individual.

- Apply direct pressure to external bleeding site *to stop the flow of blood and allow normal coagulation to occur.*
- Elevate the bleeding limb and combine with direct pressure *to help stop venous bleeding.*
- When direct pressure and elevation do not control hemorrhage, pressure-point control should be attempted *to stop the bleeding* (Fig. 13.3). The chosen artery for pressure-point control must be proximal to the injury site and must be over a bony structure.
- Monitor vital signs continually, record, and report to the physician *to identify early changes in vital signs indicative of progressing shock.*
- Use a blanket *to help keep the patient from getting cold;* however, the patient also should not be allowed to overheat *because this causes peripheral blood vessels to dilate, which draws blood away from vital organs.*

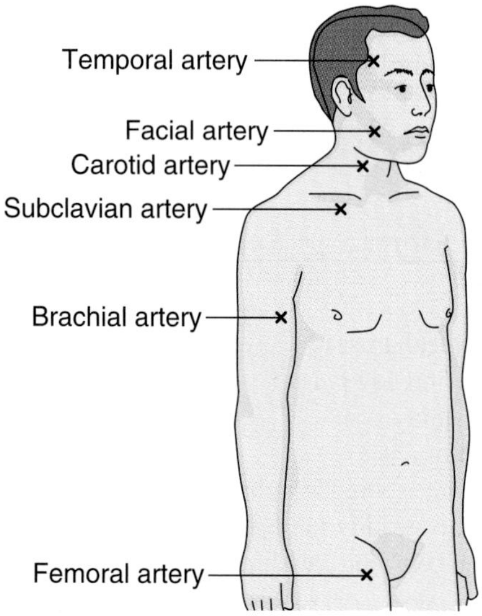
Temporal artery
Facial artery
Carotid artery
Subclavian artery
Brachial artery
Femoral artery

FIGURE 13.3 Arterial pressure points to control bleeding.

- Monitor IV fluids as ordered *to increase circulating volume* (IV fluid contraindicated in cardiogenic shock).

Ineffective Breathing Pattern Related to Airway Constriction

EXPECTED OUTCOME: The patient will maintain respiratory rate within normal limits and experience improved gas exchange in the lungs and normal arterial blood gases.

- Administer oxygen as ordered using appropriate method to deliver the maximum amount of oxygen needed *to maintain the pulse oximetry at 95% or greater.*
- Administer epinephrine (adrenaline) intramuscularly in the vastus lateralis muscle (preferred because it provides better absorption and works faster) with a 22-gauge, 1- to 1.5-inch needle or subcutaneously as ordered *to suppress the immune system.*
- Give antihistamines as second-line therapy as ordered *to control the allergic rash and pruritus.*
- Steroids are given in gradually tapered doses *to prevent return of symptoms.*

> **NURSING CARE TIP**
> Epinephrine should not be given IV for anaphylaxis (allergy symptoms with ABC involvement).

Evaluation

If interventions have been effective, the blood pressure will improve to within normal limits for the individual patient, and the patient will demonstrate a strong pulse; warm, dry skin; and be less anxious. The patient should show an immediate reversal of shock symptoms. Breathing becomes easy, and blood pressure and pulse return to the normal range. Breath sounds become clear, and hives and pruritus subside.

MAJOR TRAUMA

Major trauma was the fifth leading cause of death in the United States in 2005 according to the Centers for Disease Control and Prevention (CDC). It mainly affects persons under age 34 and over 70. Victims of major trauma may receive injury to an isolated vital organ or to multiple body systems.

Mechanism of Injury

When assessing a victim of major trauma, it is important to determine the mechanism of injury (Box 13.4, *Gerontological Issues*). Injuries are classified as either penetrating or blunt.

• WORD • BUILDING •

epinephrine: epi—on + nephros—kidney

adrenalin: ad—on + renes—kidney

Box 13.4

Gerontological Issues

Injuries and Older Adults

Older adults are at a high risk for falls that put them at risk for bruises, abrasions, cuts, and fractures. Nurses who initially assess older adults with injuries requiring treatment must ask questions and perform assessments that would identify if the patient is a victim of abuse or neglect.

Injuries Caused by Falls Versus Battery or Assault

Any unexplained bruises, burns, abrasions, cuts, fractures, evidence of old injuries or bruises, burns, and cuts that are in different stages of healing suggest abuse. The pattern of an injury can also suggest abuse—for example, cigarette burns in areas covered with clothing; bruises or friction burns in a ring around the neck, ankles, or wrists; welts, burns, or bruises in the outline of a hand or belt buckle; multiple similar injuries in an area, such as whip marks across the buttocks or back of the legs; defensive injury pattern of bruising; and trauma to the hands and forearms.

Injuries related to falls have a predictable injury pattern related to the history and report of the fall. When an older adult falls, there is bruising of the hands and knees caused when the person attempts to break the fall. Additional bruising or injuries to the front of the body, arms, and head could be caused by hitting furniture or other items during the fall. Skin tears on the arms are common with a fall. Often, a friend or family member sees the older adult starting to fall and tries to steady the person by grabbing the area, tearing the skin. Ask questions to be sure that the report of the fall incident is consistent with the presenting injuries.

Any form of abuse or suspicion of abuse must be reported to the state agency that investigates reports of suspected abuse. It is not the nurse's responsibility to prove that there has been abuse or neglect, only to report incidents or cases of possible abuse.

Penetrating—or open—injuries may be caused by any sharp object, such as broken glass or a knife, or by projectiles traveling at high speed, such as bullets or fragments from an explosion. In blunt—or closed—injuries, the skin surface is intact. An injury from blunt trauma usually extends beyond the point of impact to surrounding and underlying structures. For example, a blow to the chest may cause a fracture of several ribs that may, in turn, cause blunt trauma (such as a laceration or hematoma) to the spleen.

Damage caused by a gunshot wound and the trajectory of the bullet depends on the projectile mass, the type of tissue struck, the striking velocity, and the range. Entrance wounds are round or oval and may be surrounded by a rim of abrasion. Powder burns are visible if the firearm was discharged at close range. Documentation of these wounds should include a clear description of their appearance but should not include the words *entry* or *exit* because this is determined by trained experts. Patients with gunshot wounds near the level of the diaphragm should be evaluated for both abdominal and thoracic injuries.

Surface Trauma

Surface trauma includes any injury that does not break the skin (closed wound) and any open wound in which the skin surface is broken. Types of closed wounds include contusions (bruising) and hematomas (collection of blood under the skin). Types of open wounds include abrasions, punctures, lacerations, avulsions, and amputations.

Abrasions are a scraping away of the epidermal and dermal layers of the skin. They bleed very little but can be extremely painful because of inflamed nerve endings. Dirt may be ground into abrasions and can increase the risk of infection when large areas of skin are involved.

Puncture wounds result from sharp, narrow objects such as knives, nails, or high-velocity bullets. They can often be deceptive because the entrance wound may be small with little or no bleeding. It is difficult to estimate the extent of damage to underlying organs as a result. Puncture wounds usually do not bleed profusely unless they are located in the chest or abdomen.

Lacerations are open wounds resulting from snagging or tearing of tissue. Skin tissue may be partly or completely torn away. They vary in depth and may be irregular in shape. Lacerations can cause significant bleeding if blood vessels or arteries are involved.

Avulsions involve a full-thickness skin loss in which wound edges cannot be approximated. This type of injury is often seen in machine operators, or in lawn mower and power tool accidents.

An **amputation** is a partial or complete severing of a body part. In cases of complete amputation, the arteries usually spasm and retract into the tissue, resulting in less bleeding than does a partial amputation, in which the lacerated arteries continue to bleed.

If the patient has sustained an amputation, bleeding is controlled with direct pressure and elevation. A tourniquet is applied only as a last resort. If a tourniquet is needed, it should be made of wide material such as a blood pressure cuff, which is less damaging to nerves and blood vessels. A dressing is applied to the amputated extremity, which is referred to as the stump. The stump is covered with sterile saline–moistened gauze followed by dry gauze, which is held in place with an elastic bandage for pressure. Amputated parts are taken to the hospital with the patient for possible reattachment. At the hospital, the amputated part is rinsed with saline solution, wrapped in sterile gauze, and placed in a sealed plastic bag, which is then placed on ice (not covered with ice or in ice water). The goal is to keep the body part cool without causing further damage from cold ice.

For a patient impaled by an object, it is imperative that the object not be removed unless it is obstructing the airway. Removing an impaled object may cause additional trauma and uncontrollable internal bleeding. Impaled objects are never cut off, broken off, or shortened unless transportation to the emergency department is otherwise impossible. A bulky dressing is applied around the object to stabilize it and reduce motion.

Tetanus

Tetanus is a disease caused by the bacillus *Clostridium tetani,* which enters the body through an open wound. Tetanus causes seizures, muscle spasms, stiffness of the jaw, coma, and death. Tetanus vaccinations should begin at 2 months of age and be followed by a series of pediatric immunizations until age 15. Thereafter, booster vaccinations are recommended every 10 years in the absence of an open wound.

Head Trauma

Sharp blows to the head can cause shifting of intracranial contents and lead to brain tissue contusion. The pathophysiology of head trauma can be divided into two phases. The first phase is the initial injury that occurs at the time of the accident and cannot be reversed. The second phase involves intracerebral bleeding and edema from the initial injury, which causes increased intracranial pressure (ICP). Management of head trauma is directed at the second phase and involves decreasing ICP. Early and late signs and symptoms of ICP are listed in Box 13.5.

Spinal Trauma

Spinal cord injury most often results from motor vehicle crashes, sports injuries, falls, and assaults, with most cases occurring in men ages 16 to 30. The cervical spine is especially vulnerable to traumatic injury. Patients who have sustained severe multiple injuries should be suspected of having a spinal cord injury, especially when they have signs of head trauma. All trauma patients should be treated as though they have a spinal cord injury until proven otherwise. Moving a patient with a vertebral injury may cause displacement of the injured bones and may increase damage to the spinal cord. Patients should be moved only by qualified people. Stabilization of the neck and back with a cervical collar and backboard is essential until spinal cord injury is ruled out (Fig. 13.4).

Box 13.5

Signs and Symptoms of Increased Intracranial Pressure

Early Signs and Symptoms of Increased ICP

- Headache
- Nausea and vomiting
- Amnesia
- Altered level of consciousness
- Changes in speech
- Drowsiness

Late Signs and Symptoms of Increased ICP

- Dilated nonreactive pupils
- Unresponsiveness
- Abnormal posturing
- Widening pulse pressure
- Decreased pulse rate
- Changes in respiratory pattern

SAFETY TIP

Do not move a patient with suspected vertebral or spinal cord injury until sufficient qualified help is available to prevent further injury to the spinal cord.

Chest Trauma

Chest trauma can damage the heart and lungs and cause life-threatening injuries, including pericardial tamponade, hemothorax, tension pneumothorax, and **flail chest**. Potentially life-threatening injuries include pulmonary and myocardial contusion, aortic and tracheobronchial disruption, and diaphragmatic rupture.

Chest trauma can result in laceration of lung tissue and cause a change in the negative intrapleural pressure.

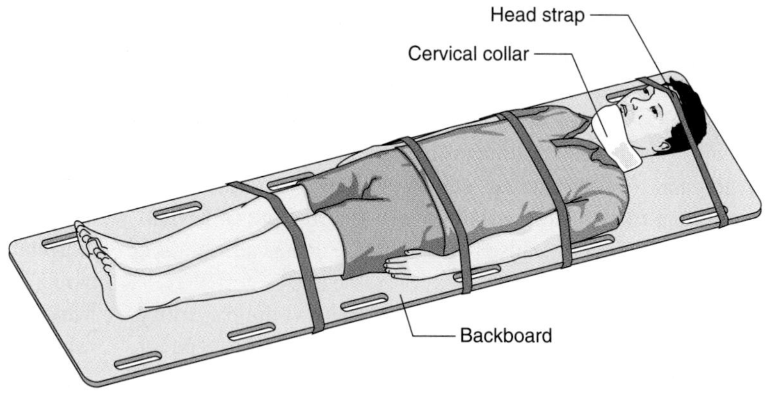
Head strap
Cervical collar
Backboard

FIGURE 13.4 Immobilization of a patient suspected of having a spinal cord injury using a backboard and cervical collar.

Air or blood leaking into the intrapleural space collapses the lung, resulting in a pneumothorax (air) or hemothorax (blood) and ineffective ventilation. In a tension pneumothorax, air is trapped in the pleural space during exhalation, resulting in increased pressure on the unaffected lung. The heart, great vessels, and trachea shift toward the unaffected side of the chest. As a result, blood flow to and from the heart is greatly reduced, causing a decrease in cardiac output. An uncorrected tension pneumothorax is fatal.

Chest trauma can also injure the heart and great vessels and reduce the amount of circulating blood volume. The heart may be bruised (myocardial contusion) or may sustain direct trauma. **Cardiac tamponade** occurs when blood accumulates in the pericardial sac and increases pressure around the heart. The increased pericardial pressure prevents the heart chambers from filling and contracting effectively. A patient with cardiac tamponade will have hypotension, tachycardia (rapid heart rate), and neck vein distention and requires immediate intervention to reduce the pressure in the pericardial sac and restore normal filling and contraction of the heart chambers.

Abdominal Trauma

The organs of the abdomen are vulnerable to injury because there is limited bony protection. Injury to organs such as the spleen and liver, which have a rich blood supply, can result in rapid loss of blood volume and hypovolemic shock. Abdominal organs may be injured as a result of severe blunt or penetrating trauma. If hypotension is present, intra-abdominal hemorrhage may exist. If the urinary bladder ruptures, urine leaks into the abdomen and blood may be detected at the urinary meatus or perineum. Penetrating trauma can cause lacerations to abdominal organs, resulting in rapid blood loss and hypovolemic shock.

Orthopedic Trauma

Fractured bones can result in blood loss, compromised circulation, infection, and immobility. Unstable pelvic fractures can cause injury to the genitourinary system or disrupt pelvic veins. Fractures of large bones such as the femur and tibia can cause significant blood loss. For example, a fractured femur can cause up to 1500 mL of blood loss, and a fractured tibia or humerus can cause up to 750 mL of blood loss. Joint dislocations can cause neurovascular compromise by applying pressure to the nerves and blood vessels. Delayed fracture reduction (realignment or setting) can cause avascular necrosis, which leads to death of the affected tissue and bone.

• WORD • BUILDING •

tachycardia: tachy—fast + cardia—heart condition

LEARNING TIP

If a limb is fractured, splint it as it lies to prevent further damage. If the distal circulation is severely compromised, the patient needs immediate medical intervention.

Nursing Process for the Patient Experiencing Trauma

Data Collection

The mechanism of injury is determined to identify the extent of injury. Loss of consciousness immediately after an injury indicates that a concussion has occurred. The Glasgow Coma Scale (GCS) is used to rate a patient's level of consciousness (Fig. 13.5). The highest score is 15, indicating that the patient is alert and needs only observation. Scores lower than 13 may indicate the need for immediate treatment. Morbidity and mortality are highest for patients with GCS scores of 8 or lower. Pupil size and reaction are monitored and recorded. Dilated or nonreactive pupils indicate increased ICP and a need for immediate intervention.

Spinal nerves are located in the spinal cord and transmit sensory impulses to the brain and motor impulses to the body. The higher a traumatic lesion is on the spinal column, the more extensive will be the loss of muscle and sensory function (Table 13.3). A spinal cord injury at the level of C5 or above interferes with diaphragm function and respiratory

GLASGOW COMA SCALE	
Areas of Response	**Points**
Eye Opening	
Eyes open spontaneously	4
Eyes open in response to voice	3
Eyes open in response to pain	2
No eye opening response	1
Best Verbal Response	
Oriented (e.g., to person, place, time)	5
Confused, speaks but is disoriented	4
Inappropriate, but comprehensible words	3
Incomprehensible sounds but no words are spoken	2
None	1
Best Motor Response	
Obeys command to move	6
Localizes painful stimulus	5
Withdraws from painful stimulus	4
Flexion, abnormal decorticate posturing	3
Extension, abnormal decerebrate posturing	2
No movement or posturing	1
Total Possible Points	**3–15**
Major Head Injury	**≤8**
Moderate Head Injury	**9–12**
Minor Head Injury	**13–15**

FIGURE 13.5 The Glasgow Coma Scale is used to determine level of consciousness.

TABLE 13.3 CORRELATING SPINAL INJURY WITH IMPAIRMENT OF MOTOR FUNCTION

Injury Level	Impairment
S3–S5 or above	Patient unable to tighten anus.
L4–L5 or above	Patient unable to flex foot and extend toes.
L2–L4 or above	Patient unable to extend and flex legs.
C5–C7 or above	Patient unable to extend and flex arms.

effort, which must be carefully assessed. The patient's level of muscle control and ability to feel each limb are noted and recorded.

Patients with major chest injuries can have dramatic symptoms, including classic signs of shock with cyanosis, dyspnea, and restlessness. The patient's breathing pattern and effectiveness of respirations are assessed. The rise and fall of the chest is observed, as well as symmetrical chest movement. Any bruising on the chest or upper abdomen is noted. Seat belts and restraint systems can cause significant bruising in high-impact crashes.

Vital signs are taken to detect tachycardia and hypotension from shock. The shape of the abdomen is observed to detect distention from intra-abdominal hemorrhage. Skin color, bruising, open wounds, and penetrating trauma are noted. The abdomen is auscultated for bowel sounds. The perineum is inspected for blood from the urethra.

Vital signs and pain level are assessed to detect orthopedic abnormalities. A respiratory assessment is done to detect a pulmonary embolism as a result of a long bone fracture. The injured extremity is inspected, and skin color and capillary refill time are noted. Skin integrity, protruding bone, or deformity is noted. Pulses distal to the injury are palpated to assess circulation to the area distal to the injury. Motor function and sensation are assessed to determine the extent of nerve injury.

Nursing Diagnoses, Planning, and Implementation

Acute Pain Related to Tissue Trauma

EXPECTED OUTCOME: The patient will experience relief after measures are provided to relieve pain as evidenced by verbal and nonverbal expressions of pain relief.

- Apply ice, elevate, and immobilize the affected area *to decrease swelling and relieve pain.*
- Provide analgesics as ordered *to relieve pain.*

Impaired Skin Integrity Related Tissue Trauma

EXPECTED OUTCOME: The patient will demonstrate healing of impaired tissue.

- Apply direct pressure to open wounds *to control bleeding.*
- Irrigate open wounds with sterile saline solution *to thoroughly remove dirt and debris and clean exposed tissue to prevent infection.*

Risk for Infection Related to Tissue Trauma

EXPECTED OUTCOME: The patient's wounds will remain free of infection.

- With open wounds, give tetanus immunization as ordered if it has been more than 5 years since one was last given *to prevent tetanus infection.*
- Give antibiotics as ordered *to prevent infection.*

Ineffective Cerebral Tissue Perfusion Related to Cerebral Edema

EXPECTED OUTCOME: The patient will maintain adequate cerebral homeostasis without cerebral edema as evidenced by a GCS score of 14 or greater.

- Give oxygen as ordered *to maintain adequate oxygenation of brain tissues and prevent cellular damage from hypoxia at the cerebral level.*
- If the patient has an altered level of consciousness or deteriorating respiratory effort, anticipate and assist with endotracheal intubation as needed *to provide respiratory support to patient.*
- Elevate the head of the patient's bed 15 to 30 degrees, if possible, *to reduce ICP.*
- Maintain the patient's head position at midline *to ensure unobstructed venous drainage to help reduce ICP.*
- Maintain intravenous access for fluids *to maintain hemodynamic stability and access for medications.*
- Monitor mannitol IV, an osmotic diuretic, or hypertonic saline (1.7% to 29.2%) as ordered *to decrease cerebral edema.*
- If the patient is agitated, provide calming measures *because agitation increases ICP.*

Ineffective Breathing Pattern Related to Neck Injury or Unstable Chest Wall Segment or Lung Collapse

EXPECTED OUTCOME: The patient will maintain effective respiratory rate and experience improved gas exchange in the lungs.

- If signs of respiratory distress are present, use the jaw-thrust or chin-lift maneuver, along with suction and airway adjuncts as needed *to maintain patency of the airway.*
- Maintain cervical collar and backboard *to prevent further injury.*
- Give oxygen as ordered *to improve tissue oxygenation.* Advanced adjunct airway equipment, including an endotracheal tube, must be readily available.
- Administer supplemental oxygen as ordered *to promote tissue oxygenation.*
- Maintain chest tube drainage system if inserted *to help expand lung.*

Ineffective Airway Clearance Related to Neck Injury

EXPECTED OUTCOME: The patient will maintain clear lung sounds.

- Suction the oropharynx and nasopharynx *to clear secretions and prevent aspiration of secretions into the airway.*

- If the patient vomits, log roll the patient onto one side and use suction as needed *to prevent aspiration of emesis.*

Impaired Physical Mobility Related to Neck Injury

EXPECTED OUTCOME: The patient will maintain movement of extremities normal for patient.

- Maintain neck immobility during initial treatment of a patient with head or neck trauma *to prevent serious injury until trauma damage is identified.*

Decreased Cardiac Output Related to Compression of Heart and Great Vessels

EXPECTED OUTCOME: The patient will maintain vital signs within baseline limits.

- Report unstable vital signs to physician *because patient may need immediate surgical intervention in the operating room.*
- Explain diagnostic testing to patients with stable vital signs if radiographic studies are ordered *to determine the extent of cardiac or pulmonary injury.*
- Monitor patient's vital signs and oxygen saturation continuously *to detect signs of shock.*

Deficient Fluid Volume Related to Hemorrhage or Abdominal Organ Injury

EXPECTED OUTCOME: The patient will maintain vital signs within baseline limits.

- Monitor for signs of shock *to detect hypovolemic shock.*
- Maintain IV fluids as ordered by 18- or 16-gauge IV cannulas *to restore circulating volume.*
- Assist with peritoneal lavage, if performed, *to detect intra-abdominal hemorrhage.*
- Maintain nasogastric tube, if ordered, *to decompress the stomach.*
- Cover abdominal wounds with a sterile dressing *to prevent infection.*
- If abdominal organs are exposed, cover with sterile saline-soaked dressings *to prevent tissue necrosis.*
- Assist with blood and blood product administration, as ordered and per agency policy, *to maintain circulating volume and improve tissue oxygenation.*

Impaired Physical Mobility Related to Bone Injury

EXPECTED OUTCOME: The patient will maintain movement of extremities normal for patient.

- Remove all jewelry before applying a splint *because the extremity may swell after injury.*
- Maintain extremity in a splint in the position found, unless distal circulation is severely compromised, and keep it immobilized if there is severe pain or deformity. *Splinting promotes comfort and prevents further damage to surrounding tissue by preventing movement of broken bone ends.*
- Immobilize the joints above and below the affected area using a folded towel or a pillow *to provide comfort and protection until the patient is evaluated by a physician.*
- Monitor skin color, temperature, distal pulses, capillary refill, movement, and sensation of the extremity after splint application *to detect abnormalities.*
- Elevate and ice extremity *to reduce edema and relieve pain.*

Evaluation

If interventions have been effective, the following results will be evident: A patient with trauma reports an acceptable pain level, and the patient's wound heals without infection; a patient with spinal injury maintains a regular rate, rhythm, and pattern of breathing, clear lung sounds, intactness of mobility, and GCS score of 14 to 15; a patient with chest trauma maintains an open airway and effective breathing pattern; a patient with abdominal trauma has effective circulating volume as evidenced by vital signs within normal limits; a patient with orthopedic trauma has strong and palpable pulses, normal blood pressure, normal skin color, skin that is warm and dry, capillary refill time of less than 3 seconds, pain controlled to a satisfactory level, and normal motor function and sensation in the extremity.

BURNS

The skin protects the body by preventing bacterial or viral invasion, enhancing temperature regulation, and conserving body fluids and electrolytes. These functions are impaired with a burn injury and can lead to multisystem alterations. Burn injuries are acutely painful and may be dramatic in appearance. Nursing care depends on the extent and depth of the burn injury and the presence of any associated factors, such as smoke inhalation, blunt trauma, or fractures. The more extensive the burn injury, the greater the potential for complications and mortality. The patient's age may contribute to the risk of mortality as well. Infants younger than age 2 and elderly patients older than age 60 have the highest mortality rates from major burns. (See Chapter 55 for more on burns.)

Assessment of the burn patient begins with the ABCDs of the primary survey. The history should include the mechanism and time of the injury and a description of the surrounding environment, including the presence of noxious chemicals and inhalation of smoke in an enclosed space. The greatest threat to life in a patient with a major burn injury is smoke or heat inhalation, which causes edema in the respiratory passages. Continuous assessment of respiratory status is essential when you observe burns or soot on the face, singed nasal hairs, a hoarse voice, coughing, or restlessness.

Burns of the face may swell rapidly and can compromise the airway. Facial burns are treated by elevating the head of the bed to 30 degrees to minimize edema. Oxygen is administered to the patient with potential pulmonary injury. Equipment for endotracheal intubation should be readily available. Because large fluid losses occur in burn injuries, an IV infusion with large-bore cannulas should be started. The patient's weight and the extent of the burn determine fluid resuscitation needs. The patient is kept warm because, when skin is lost, a burn victim cannot maintain body heat. IV opioids are administered for pain.

Burn depth is described as either partial thickness or full thickness (Fig. 13.6). **Partial-thickness burns** are either superficial (epidermis of the skin) or deep (entire epidermal layer and part of the dermis) (Fig. 13.7). **Full-thickness burns** involve all layers of the skin and subcutaneous tissue. Partial-thickness burns that involve a small area are cleaned with sterile saline solution, covered with a 1/8-inch layer of an anti-infective cream such as silver sulfadiazine (Silvadene, Flamazine), and covered with dry, bulky, fluffed dressings. Major full-thickness wounds are covered with dry, sterile dressings or linen. Patients with major burns are transferred to a specialized burn unit.

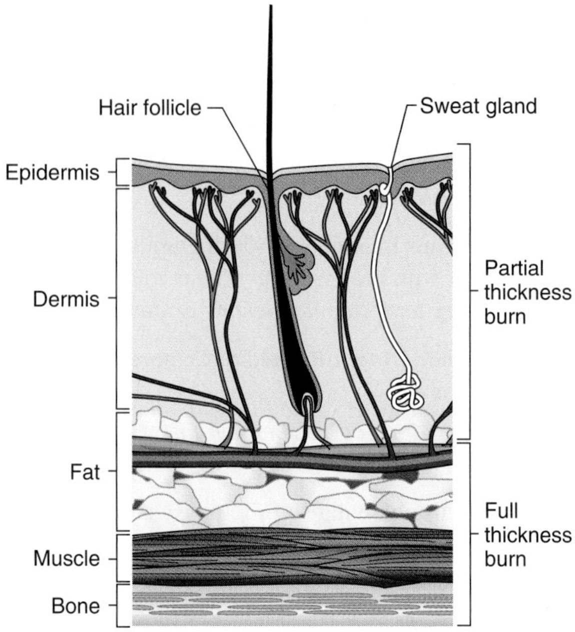
Hair follicle
Sweat gland
Epidermis
Dermis
Fat
Muscle
Bone
Partial thickness burn
Full thickness burn

FIGURE 13.6 Partial- and full-thickness burns and structures affected.

LEARNING TIP

Over-the-counter ointments, lotions, butter, and antiseptics are never used on a major burn because they may promote infection, retain heat, and cause more pain.

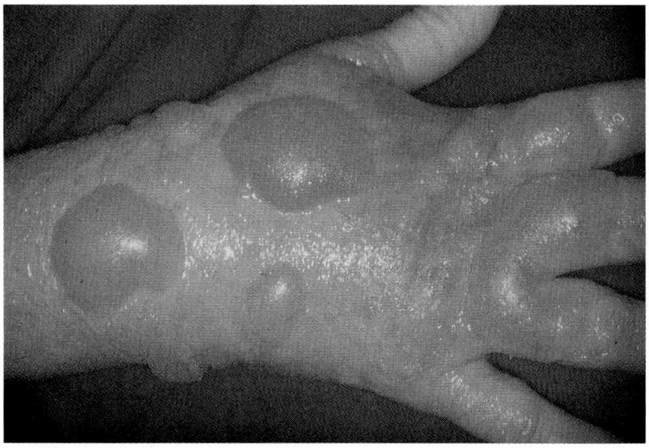

FIGURE 13.7 A blistered partial-thickness thermal burn.

CRITICAL THINKING

Mr. Smith

■ Mr. Smith is a 28-year-old man who was welding close to a natural gas line. The flame of the welder caused the gas line to explode, throwing Mr. Smith 50 feet. He landed on his back. He is brought to the emergency department by the rescue squad. Mr. Smith is awake, alert, and oriented. He has soot around his mouth and nose. He sustained deep partial-thickness burns to his neck, upper chest, and both forearms. He reports pain from his burns and also thoracic back and hip pain. His pulse rate is 100 beats per minute. His blood pressure is 160/90 mm Hg. His respiratory rate is 20 per minute.

1. What is the first priority of care for Mr. Smith?
2. Is Mr. Smith at risk for respiratory burns? Why?
3. Are Mr. Smith's vital signs within normal limits?
4. Would wet or dry dressings be preferable for his large areas of deep partial-thickness burns? Why?
5. Mr. Smith is wearing a neck chain and a wedding ring. Should they be removed immediately, or should you wait until Mr. Smith's wife arrives to take them? Why?
6. Mr. Smith continues to report hip and back pain. In reviewing his mechanism of injury, what other injuries could Mr. Smith have?

Suggested answers at end of chapter.

HYPOTHERMIA

Normally the body maintains its temperature in a narrow range on either side of 98.6°F (37°C) to allow chemical reactions to work most efficiently. Body heat escapes to the environment through conduction, convection, radiation, and evaporation. Heat loss is inversely proportional to body size and body fat. Fat insulates because it has less blood flow and consequently has less ability to vasodilate and lose heat.

Hypothermia occurs when the core body temperature falls below 95°F (35°C). As the core temperature falls below 95°F, the body is less able to regulate its temperature and generate body heat, causing progressive loss of body heat to occur.

Nursing Process for the Patient with Hypothermia

Data Collection

In cases of mild hypothermia (core temperature between 90° and 95°F [32.2° and 35°C]), the patient is usually alert, shivering, and may appear clumsy, apathetic, or irritable (Table 13.4). Hypoglycemia can occur because glucose and glycogen stores are depleted by long-term shivering. Respiratory rate, heart rate, and cardiac output decrease.

More severe hypothermia occurs between 85° and 90°F (29.4° and 32.2°C). Shivering stops and muscle activity decreases. Initially, fine muscle coordination ceases. Then, as core body temperature continues to drop, all muscle activity stops and the muscles become rigid. The patient becomes lethargic and less interested in fighting the cold environment. The patient's level of consciousness begins to markedly decrease at 89.6°F (32°C); the patient becomes lethargic and disoriented and begins to hallucinate. The pupils become dilated. As the core body temperature falls to 82°F (27.8°C), the patient becomes apneic, the pulse becomes slower and weaker, and cardiac dysrhythmias occur. The profoundly hypothermic patient has a core temperature of less than 80°F (26.7°C) and usually appears dead, with no obtainable vital signs. Determination of death should be made only after aggressive core rewarming to at least 90°F (32.2°C).

TABLE 13.4 DEFINING CHARACTERISTICS AND OUTCOME CRITERIA FOR HYPOTHERMIA

Core Body Temperature	Defining Characteristics
Below 95°F (35°C)	• Skin cold to touch • Lack of coordination • Slurred speech
Below 91.4°F (33°C)	• Cardiac dysrhythmias • Cyanosis
Below 89.6°F (32°C)	• Shivering replaced by muscle rigidity • Hypotension • Dilated pupils
Below 82.4°F (28°C)	• Absent deep tendon reflexes • Hypoventilation (3–4 breaths per minute) • Ventricular fibrillation possible
Below 80.6°F (27°C)	• Coma • Flaccid muscles • Fixed, dilated pupils • Ventricular fibrillation to cardiac standstill • Apnea

Outcome Criteria

- Core body temperature is greater than 95°F (35°C).
- Patient is alert and oriented.
- Cardiac dysrhythmias are absent.
- Acid-base balance is normal.
- Pupils react normally.

Nursing Diagnoses, Planning, and Implementation

Initial treatment of the hypothermic patient consists of rewarming the patient, stabilizing vital functions, and preventing further heat loss (see the *Nursing Care Plan for the Patient with Hypothermia*). The patient is removed from the cold environment. All wet clothing is removed to prevent further heat loss. The patient's core body temperature guides treatment. If body temperature is above 82.4°F (28°C), passive rewarming is preferred. The room temperature is set to 70° to 75°F (21.1° to 23.9°C). The patient is wrapped in warm, dry blankets. Heat loss from the head is reduced by covering the head with warm towels.

If core body temperature is below 82.4°F (28°C), active rewarming is needed. A heating blanket (carbon-fiber) and radiant heat lights are used. Warm, humidified oxygen is administered. Warm IV fluids are administered. Body temperature is constantly monitored using a rectal probe. Heated **gastric lavage**, heated peritoneal lavage, or cardiopulmonary bypass may be performed for profound hypothermia. Cardiac drugs are given sparingly because, as the body warms, peripheral vasodilation occurs. Drugs that were trapped in the peripheral circulation are then suddenly released during rewarming, leading to a bolus effect that may cause fatal dysrhythmias.

Evaluation

Desired outcome criteria for the patient with hypothermia is a core body temperature higher than 95°F (35°C), no cardiac dysrhythmias, pulse and blood pressure within normal limits, and an alert and oriented status.

FROSTBITE

The extremities are vulnerable to cold injury. Frostnip occurs when exposed parts of the body become very cold but not frozen. This condition usually is not painful. The skin becomes pale and blanched. Contact with a warm object such as someone's hand may be all that is needed to rewarm the part. During rewarming, the affected part may tingle and become red.

Frostbite occurs when body parts become frozen. The extremities are at increased risk because blood shunts away from them to maintain core body temperature. The affected tissue feels hard and frozen. Most frostbitten parts are white, yellow-white, or blue-white. When rewarmed, the skin appears deep red, hot, and dry to touch. The severity of a cold injury is determined by the duration of the exposure, the temperature to which the body part was exposed, and the wind velocity during exposure.

Interventions for frostbite include protecting the affected area from further trauma. To prevent additional damage, the frostbitten part is handled gently and never rubbed. The injured part is loosely covered with a dry, sterile dressing. The patient is not allowed to stand or walk on a frostbitten foot. The affected extremity is elevated to heart level to minimize edema and promote blood flow.

Nursing Care Plan for the Patient with Hypothermia

Nursing Diagnosis: *Hypothermia* related to exposure to cold environment

Expected Outcomes: The patient's body temperature and vital signs will be within normal limits.

Evaluation of Outcomes: Is patient's body temperature greater than 95°F (35°C)? Is patient alert and oriented? Is cardiac rhythm normal?

Intervention	Rationale	Evaluation
Monitor patient's core body temperature.	Abnormal body temperature can be detected and treated.	Is body temperature greater than 95°F (35°C)?
Monitor pulse and electrocardiogram (ECG) rhythm.	Cardiac dysrhythmias may occur at temperatures below 91.4°F (33°C).	Is pulse rate and ECG rhythm normal?
Monitor patient's level of consciousness.	Level of consciousness becomes markedly decreased at temperatures of 89.6°F (32°C).	Is the patient alert?
Institute rewarming passively or actively as ordered.	Rewarming is necessary to return body temperature to desirable range.	Is body core temperature rising to normal range?

HYPERTHERMIA

The body's heat-regulating mechanisms usually work very well, allowing people to tolerate significant temperature changes. The body's most efficient mechanisms for decreasing body heat are sweating and dilation of blood vessels in the skin. When blood vessels dilate, blood comes to the skin surface to increase the rate of radiation of heat from the body. However, when these mechanisms become overwhelmed, the consequences can be disastrous and irreversible. Those at greatest risk for heat illnesses include children, elderly people, and patients with cardiac disease.

Hyperthermia results when thermoregulation breaks down because of excess heat generation, an inability to dissipate heat, overwhelming environmental heat, or a combination of these factors. Unlike a fever, in which the thermal set point is elevated, in heat illness the thermal set point remains normal and hyperthermia occurs because of an inability to dissipate heat. Antipyretics are of no use in hyperthermia and may contribute to complications.

SAFETY TIP

Older adults are vulnerable to hyperthermia. In times of extreme summer temperatures, older people who live alone should be checked to make sure they are not experiencing hyperthermia. If they do not have fans or air conditioning available, they should be taken to a cooler environment.

Nursing Process for the Patient with Hyperthermia

Data Collection

Illness from heat exposure can take three forms: heat cramps, heat exhaustion, and heatstroke (Box 13.6). As heat illness progresses, circulating blood volume decreases, causing dehydration. Fluid intake is crucial in the prevention of heat illness.

HEAT CRAMPS. Heat cramps, the mildest form of heat illness, involve painful muscle spasms, usually in the legs or abdomen, that occur after strenuous exercise. Large amounts of salt and water can be lost as a result of excessive sweating, causing stressed muscles to spasm. With adequate rest and fluid replacement, the body adjusts the distribution of electrolytes and the cramps disappear.

HEAT EXHAUSTION. Heat exhaustion occurs when the body loses so much water and electrolytes through heavy sweating that hypovolemia occurs. Heat exhaustion is largely a manifestation of the strain placed on the cardiovascular system as it tries to maintain normothermia. Cerebral function is unimpaired, although the patient may show minor irritability and poor judgment. The ability to sweat remains. The skin is usually cold and clammy and the face gray. Sodium and water loss cause the patient to become dehydrated. The body temperature is usually normal or slightly elevated: from 100.4° to 102.2°F (38° to 39°C). The patient may report feeling dizzy, weak, or faint, with nausea or a headache. Vomiting and diarrhea may also be present.

HEATSTROKE. If symptoms of heat exhaustion are not treated, **heatstroke** can develop. Altered mental status and an

Box 13.6

Defining Characteristics and Outcome Criteria for Environmental Hyperthermia

Defining Characteristics

Early Signs

- Core body temperature 100.4° to 102.2°F (38° to 39°C)
- Diaphoresis
- Cool, clammy skin
- Dizziness
- Pulse rate greater than 100

Late Signs

- Increasing body core temperature of 106°F (41.1°C) or higher
- Hot, dry, flushed skin
- Altered mental status
- Coma or seizures possible
- Hypotension

Outcome Criteria

- Core body temperature less than 101°F (38.3°C)
- Patient alert and oriented
- Skin warm and dry to touch

inability to sweat are key symptoms in heatstroke. Some patients show confusion, irrational behavior, or psychosis; others develop seizures or go into a coma. Because the sweating mechanism has been overwhelmed, many heatstroke victims have hot, dry, flushed skin. The body temperature rises rapidly to 106°F (41.1°C) or higher, and level of consciousness decreases. If heatstroke is not treated, death results.

Patients with heatstroke are admitted to the intensive care unit because late complications can appear suddenly and require immediate management. Relatively common occurrences include seizures, cerebral ischemia, renal failure, late cardiac decompensation, and gastrointestinal bleeding. Long-term prognosis varies with the patient's previous state of health and length of time under heat stress.

Nursing Diagnoses, Planning, and Implementation

Hyperthermia Related to Exposure to Hot Environment

EXPECTED OUTCOME: The patient will maintain body temperature within normal limits.

- For heat cramps, remove the patient from the hot environment *to allow cooling to begin.*
- Have patient sit or lie down until muscle cramps subside *to prevent further injury.*
- Remove patient from the hot environment and undress patient *to allow patient to cool rapidly.*
- Mist-spray tepid water over the patient while maintaining a strong continual breeze from electric fans *because evaporative cooling is the most efficient method of cooling.*

Deficient Fluid Volume Related to Hypervolemia

EXPECTED OUTCOME: The patient will maintain blood pressure within normal limits of baseline.

- Give patient oral fluids, water, or a diluted (half-strength) balanced electrolyte solution if patient is fully alert *to replace lost fluids.*
- If patient is hypotensive, maintain IV fluids as ordered *to restore volume.*

Evaluation

Interventions have been successful if the hyperthermic patient has a core body temperature below 101°F (38.3°C), warm and dry skin, a strong pulse, blood pressure within normal limits, and is alert and oriented.

POISONING AND DRUG OVERDOSE

Poisons are introduced into the body by ingestion, inhalation, injection, absorption, or venomous bites. Poisons act by changing cellular metabolism, causing damage to structures, or disturbing function. Many toxins and poisons alter the patient's mental status, making it difficult to obtain an accurate history.

Nursing Process for the Patient with Ingested Poisoning

Data Collection

The primary nursing responsibility is to recognize that a poisoning has occurred and then try to determine the nature of the poison. The method of exposure is established so that removal or interruption of the toxin can begin. Most ingested poisons are drugs, but about one-third of poisonings are caused by cleaners, soaps, insecticides, acids, or alkalis. Many household plants are poisonous if they are accidentally ingested. Some plants cause local irritation of the skin, and others can affect the circulatory system, gastrointestinal tract, or central nervous system.

Empty medication bottles, scattered pills, and relevant chemicals should be examined by emergency medical personnel at the scene to help identify the poisonous substance. The patient's physical appearance also may give a clue to the type of substance ingested. Intravenous needle tracks, burns, erythema, and flushed skin may help identify the poison or toxic exposure.

Nursing Diagnoses, Planning, and Implementation

Risk for Injury Related to Absorption of Poisoning Agent

EXPECTED OUTCOME: The patient will maintain normal vital signs and be free of injury.

- Contact a poison control center *to access information concerning virtually all poisonous substances, available antidotes, and appropriate emergency treatment.*

> **NURSING CARE TIP**
> - Syrup of ipecac is no longer recommended for at-home treatment of accidental overdose because evidence shows that use of ipecac does not improve patient outcomes.
> - Gastric decontamination, activated charcoal, and gastric lavage are no longer routinely recommended and should be reserved for the most severe cases.

Evaluation

Interventions have been successful if the patient remains free from injury and has vital signs within normal limits.

Inhaled Poisons

Inhaled poisons include natural gas, pesticides, carbon monoxide, chlorine, and other gases. Carbon monoxide is odorless and can produce profound hypoxia by combining with hemoglobin molecules and displacing oxygen in red blood cells. The patient's carboxyhemoglobin level is monitored to direct appropriate therapy. Inhalation of chlorine is very irritating to the respiratory system and can produce airway obstruction and pulmonary edema.

When an inhalation injury occurs, the patient must be moved into fresh air and away from the toxin. Supplemental oxygen is given as ordered. A patient exposed to prolonged inhalation of a poison may experience lung damage. Respiratory status must be closely monitored to detect complications.

Injected Poisons

Injected poisons pose compelling problems because they are difficult to remove or dilute. Usually they result from drug overdose, but they can also result from the bites and stings of insects or animals. Local swelling and tissue destruction may occur at the injection site. All jewelry is removed because swelling may occur. A cold pack is applied to decrease local pain and swelling around the injection site. The identity of the injected drug or toxin must be established so that adverse effects can be anticipated and managed.

Insect Stings or Bites

Although insect stings or bites cause anaphylaxis in a small percentage of people, symptoms in most people are limited to localized pain, swelling, heat, and redness. Potentially dangerous stings or bites may come from bees, wasps, yellow jackets, hornets, certain ants, scorpions, and some spiders. Treatment involves applying ice to the site and elevating the affected part. Cellulitis can occur hours later and may require medical treatment.

When a patient has sustained a bee or wasp sting, examine the area for the stinger and remove it by gently scraping it off the skin. Tweezers or forceps are not used to remove the stinger because squeezing the stinger can inject more venom into the patient. Placing ice over the injury site may help slow the rate of toxin absorption.

Two types of spiders—the black widow and the brown recluse—can inflict serious and sometimes life-threatening bites. Both species are found throughout the United States. Antivenin for treating the toxic effects of both is available. Black widow spiders are glossy black and have a distinctive, bright red-orange marking in the shape of an hourglass on the abdomen. They are found in dry, dim places around buildings, in woodpiles, and among debris. Their venom is neurotoxic and causes systemic symptoms, including cramping of large muscle groups, dyspnea, weakness, sweating, nausea, vomiting, and rash. Death is uncommon, and symptoms typically subside in 48 hours.

The brown recluse spider is dull brown and has a dark violin-shaped mark on its back. It tends to live in dark areas, under rocks, in woodpiles, and in old abandoned buildings. The venom of the brown recluse causes severe local tissue damage. The area becomes red, swollen, and tender and develops a pale, mottled, cyanotic center. A large ulcer can develop within 48 hours if not treated promptly. Systemic symptoms include fever, chills, nausea, vomiting, arthralgia, and weakness.

Snakebites

Only a small percentage of snakebites are caused by poisonous snakes. The most prevalent poisonous snakes are the coral snake and the pit vipers, which include rattlesnakes, copperheads, and cottonmouth moccasins. Envenomation occurs when the snake's hollow fangs puncture the skin and inject venom, which is stored in sacs located at the back of the snake's head. A poisonous snakebite leaves two small puncture wounds with surrounding discoloration, swelling, and pain. Envenomation by any of the pit viper snakes produces burning pain at the site of the injury. Swelling and discoloration occur within 5 to 10 minutes after the bite.

Interventions are focused on decreasing the circulation of venom throughout the patient's system by keeping the patient calm and immobilizing the affected part. Venous tourniquets placed above and below the fang marks help limit the spread of venom through the veins of the extremity. The tourniquets should not stop arterial flow. The patient's pulse should be palpable below the tourniquets after they are applied. The site of the bite is cleaned with soap and water. The patient is kept calm until antivenin can be given. Medical treatment of the patient with a poisonous snakebite should be directed by an experienced toxicologist.

NEAR-DROWNING

Drowning is death from **asphyxia** (insufficient oxygen intake) after submersion in water. *Near-drowning* is used to describe submersion with at least temporary survival of the victim. Life-threatening complications of near-drowning are respiratory failure and ischemic neurologic injury from hypoxia and acidosis. When submersion occurs, conscious victims hold their breath until reflex inspiratory efforts override breath holding. As water is aspirated, laryngospasm occurs, producing severe hypoxia. In wet drowning, the laryngospasm is less prolonged and fluid enters the lungs after the vocal cords relax. In dry drowning, cold water causes laryngospasm and vagal stimulation, which leads to asphyxiation. Most successfully resuscitated victims experience dry drowning. Risk factors for drowning include inability to swim, diving accidents, use of alcohol and drugs prior to swimming, exhaustion, and hypothermia.

If a person survives submersion, acute respiratory failure may follow. The incidence of serious pulmonary complications is high in this group. Symptoms of impaired gas exchange (known as secondary near-drowning) may be delayed as long as 72 hours after the incident. Contaminants in the water can irritate the pulmonary system and cause inflammatory reactions and impaired surfactant functioning. Metabolic acidosis is usually present, leading to tissue anoxia and dysrhythmias.

Aggressive resuscitative efforts should be used on victims of cold-water drowning when submersion time is 1 hour or less. Hypothermia can decrease the metabolic needs of the brain and contribute to neurologic recovery even after prolonged submersion.

Nursing Process for the Near-Drowning Patient

Data Collection

Most near-drowning victims have mild dyspnea, a death-like appearance with blue or gray skin color, apnea or tachypnea (abnormally fast breathing), hypotension, slow heart rate (possibly less than 10 beats per minute), cold skin temperature, dilated pupils, hypothermia, and vomiting. Vital signs are assessed to detect abnormal readings. Respiratory rate and pattern are observed. Any dyspnea or signs of airway obstruction are noted. Skin color or cyanosis is noted. The patient's level of consciousness may be altered from anoxia.

Nursing Diagnoses, Planning, and Implementation

Ineffective Tissue Perfusion Related to Severe Anoxia

EXPECTED OUTCOME: The patient will maintain level of consciousness and vital signs within normal range, with clear breath sounds that are equal bilaterally.

- Conduct ABCDs of the primary survey, which always begin resuscitative efforts, *to determine patient's status.*
- Give supplemental oxygen as ordered *to increase tissue oxygenation.*
- Ensure that adjunct airway equipment is available *because endotracheal intubation and insertion of a nasogastric tube to decompress the stomach may be needed.*

• WORD • BUILDING •
tachypnea: tachy—fast + pnea—breathing

Evaluation

Factors that influence the outcome of near-drowning include the temperature of the water, length of time submerged, cleanliness of the water, and age of the victim. The younger the patient, the better the chance of survival. Interventions have been successful if the patient has normal respiratory rate and pattern and vital signs, is alert and oriented, and skin that is warm and dry to touch with a capillary refill time of less than 3 seconds.

PSYCHIATRIC EMERGENCIES

A psychiatric emergency occurs when a person no longer has the coping skills needed to maintain the usual level of functioning. The patient's moods, thoughts, or actions may be so disordered that the patient could harm self or others if the situation is not quickly controlled. If acute psychiatric episodes are not managed, they can result in life-threatening, suicidal, violent, or psychologically damaging behavior. If an emotional trauma is not managed successfully, a condition known as post-traumatic stress disorder may result, in which tension, anxiety, guilt, and fear concerning the traumatic event produce cognitive, affective, and behavioral responses to memories of the event long after the event has passed.

A crisis occurs when people enter a sudden state of emotional turmoil and are unable to resolve the situation with their own resources. Common emotional or behavioral manifestations of psychiatric crises include responses to stressful events, anxiety, depression, psychosis, and mania. Anxiety may range in severity from mild to a state of panic. Panic evolves into complete disorganization and loss of control. A patient in panic is terrified and needs external controls to avoid harm.

Depression is an affective disorder most commonly characterized by physical ailments and somatizations. Antidepressants and certain forms of therapy are used to restore the balance of brain neurochemicals and diminish the symptoms of depression.

Psychotic patients experience impaired thought processes and thought content characterized by hallucinations, delusions, ideas of reference, thought broadcasting, and thought insertion. Psychotic thinking and abnormal speech patterns interfere with the patient's attempt to communicate rationally.

Manic behavior is most commonly the result of manic-depressive (bipolar) disorder. Manic persons typically exhibit bizarre, extreme, and hyperactive behaviors. Manic persons are also at high risk for injuring themselves or others.

Nursing Process for the Patient with a Psychiatric Emergency

Data Collection

Causes of psychiatric emergency symptoms are varied and require thorough assessment of the patient's history and mental status. Information from the patient's medical history may produce possible organic causes contributing to the patient's presenting symptoms. Endocrine dysfunction, electrolyte abnormalities, and head trauma are examples of medical conditions that may cause changes in mental status. A medication history is obtained to determine compliance with medication regimens and any recent changes in medications. Information regarding recent use of alcohol or illicit drugs should be obtained because these substances can heighten psychiatric emergencies. A brief mental status examination is conducted. An assessment of the person's suicide risk is very important. The patient's appearance, behavior, cognitive function, thought content, and thought processes are noted. The nurse determines whether the patient is having problems concentrating, following instructions, or recalling his or her medical history.

Nursing Diagnoses, Planning, and Implementation

Anxiety Related to Situational Stress

EXPECTED OUTCOME: The patient will state reduced anxiety.

- Establish an atmosphere of trust *so the patient feels free to discuss problems.*
- Use active listening *to acknowledge patient's physical and emotional concerns.*
- Speak directly and truthfully to the patient *to gain patient trust,* and do not promise unachievable things.
- Trusted supportive members of the patient's family may be involved *to calm the person and encourage cooperation.*
- Do not allow bystanders or adversarial family members to visit the patient *because they could create further upset for the patient.*
- Speak compassionately with the patient, and refrain from laughing or joking, *to show respect for the patient.*

Risk for Injury Related to Impaired Judgment

EXPECTED OUTCOME: The patient will remain free from injury.

- Do not threaten, challenge, or argue with a disturbed patient *to prevent injury.*
- Make sure the environment is safe and that external sources of stimulation are reduced *to prevent injury.*
- Be firm but unthreatening *to help patient feel safe.*
- Administer antipsychotic medications as ordered, *to reduce psychosis,* and monitor the patient to determine their effect.
- Follow agency policy for use of physical restraint, if needed and ordered by physician, *to ensure patient safety.*
- Document need for restraints and monitor patient and check pulses and capillary refill after restraints have been applied *to prevent patient harm or restriction of circulation.*
- Administer haloperidol (Haldol) as ordered *if patient needs rapid tranquilization.*

Evaluation

Interventions are successful if the patient reports reduced anxiety and remains free from injury.

DISASTER RESPONSE

A *disaster* is defined as any event that overwhelms existing personnel, facilities, equipment, and capabilities of a responding agency, institution, or community. Potential sources of disaster include internal events such as fires and explosions; external events such as floods, storms, fires, earthquakes, and tornadoes; and created events such as motor vehicle accidents, plane crashes, and acts of terrorism.

External disasters involve a community-wide response of several different agencies, including emergency medical system (EMS) providers, fire agencies, law enforcement, and hospitals. These agencies work together to coordinate search, rescue, transportation, communication, and treatment of multiple victims. Hospitals serve as the major treatment area for victims of a disaster, referred to as *casualties* who have been injured. When a disaster occurs, the hospital activates its disaster plan, which outlines specific duties for each nursing unit and the staff for each nonnursing department as well. Typically, each nursing unit prepares for the influx of casualties by calling all available off-duty staff to report to work and by discharging noncritical patients. In a hospital disaster plan, each nursing unit is usually designated to receive specific types of casualties, such as major trauma, burns, medical, pediatric, or psychiatric. The emergency department serves as the triage and stabilization area for casualties. To facilitate the **triage** (sorting for the purpose of assigning priorities), stabilization, and transportation of numerous causalities, additional emergency department staff may be called in to work. In addition, the hospital disaster plan may require assigning one or more staff from each nursing unit and each nonnursing department to a specific area or task within the emergency department, such as triage, first aid, critical care, burn treatment area, family room, or transportation.

During a disaster, decision making and prioritization of patient care are guided by the resources and personnel available. Patients who are seriously injured and have the greatest chance of full recovery are treated first. Each hospital and agency involved in responding to a disaster follows a disaster response plan that outlines the roles and responsibilities of the staff and the procedures to follow when interacting with the media, families, other agencies, and casualties. Disaster drills are conducted on a regular basis to evaluate and rework plans. You should be familiar with your agency's disaster plans and policies and know your role and responsibilities during a disaster.

BIOTERRORISM

Public health and government leaders in the United States recognize the need for increased preparedness to detect and respond to acts of biological terrorism. The response to a **bioterrorism** attack is in many ways the same as the response to naturally occurring outbreaks of communicable disease. Both situations typically require early identification of ill or exposed persons, rapid implementation of preventive therapy, special infection control considerations, and collaboration or communication with the public health system.

During both bioterrorism attacks and naturally occurring outbreaks, nurses are faced with the challenge of identifying the disease in persons who are worried about potential exposure or who are ill with signs and symptoms similar to those of the outbreak disease. The nurse must have knowledge of the modes of transmission, incubation periods, and communicable periods of these diseases, as well as skill in both clinical evaluation and eliciting an appropriate and thorough history, including relevant occupational, social, and travel information.

Recognition of Potential Bioterrorism Agents

The CDC evaluates bacteria, viruses, and toxins thought to pose the greatest risk for use in a bioterrorism attack (see www.bt.cdc.gov and Table 13.5). Category A agents are thought to pose the highest immediate risk for use as biological weapons and category B agents the second highest risk. Category C agents are emerging threats that pose a potential, but not immediate, risk for use as biological weapons.

As in naturally occurring outbreaks, early recognition of a bioterrorism attack is critical for rapid implementation of preventive measures and treatment. Early recognition can be challenging, however, because patients presenting for medical care after exposure to a biological agent may initially have nonspecific symptoms. One of the most important lessons learned from the 2001 anthrax attack was that clinical illness caused by agents prepared as biological weapons may differ from typical natural infections.

TABLE 13.5 BIOLOGICAL WEAPONS RISK CATEGORIES

Category	Agent/Disease
A	Anthrax (*Bacillus anthracis*) Botulism (*Clostridium botulinum* toxin) Plague (*Yersinia pestis*) Smallpox (*Variola major*) Tularemia (*Francisella tularensis*) Viral hemorrhagic fevers (filoviruses; Ebola and arenaviruses; Lassa)
B	Brucellosis (*Brucella* species) Epsilon toxin of *Clostridium perfringens* Food safety threats (salmonella, *Escherichia, Shigella*) Glanders (*Burkholderia mallei*) Staphylococcal enterotoxin Psittacosis (*Chlamydia psittaci*) Q fever (*Coxiella burnetii*) Typhus fever (*Rickettsia prowazekii*) Viral encephalitis (alphaviruses) Water safety threats (*Vibrio cholerae, Cryptosporidium parvum*)
C	Emerging infectious diseases such as Nipah virus and hantavirus

Smallpox/Variola Major

Smallpox is caused by the variola virus, an orthopoxvirus unique to humans. This virus is not known to be transmitted by animals or insects. Smallpox was declared eradicated in 1980, three years after the last naturally occurring case was reported. Smallpox is stable and highly infectious in the aerosol form. The risk for a smallpox attack currently is considered low but not zero.

Classification/Variola Major

Smallpox has an average fatality rate of 30%. The incubation period is 7 to 17 days. Symptoms of the initial phase include the acute onset of high fever, malaise, headache, backache, and prostration. Other prominent symptoms include vomiting and abdominal pain. The characteristic rash occurs 2 to 3 days later, appearing first on the face and forearms. The rash progresses slowly, from macules to papules to vesicles and pustules and finally to scabs, with each stage lasting 1 to 2 days. The lesions are firm, discrete vesicles or pustules (4 to 6 mm in diameter) deeply embedded in the dermis. The patient remains febrile throughout the evolution of the rash, which may become painful as pustules enlarge. A second fever spike 5 to 8 days after onset of the rash may signify a secondary bacterial infection.

Pustules remain for 5 to 8 days, after which crusting occurs. Pustules are more concentrated on the face and distal limbs than on the trunk, and may involve the palms and soles. Scarring occurs with scab separation from destruction of sebaceous glands.

Complications of smallpox include fluid and electrolyte disturbances, extensive skin loss that resembles burns, bronchitis and pneumonitis, blindness from infection of the eye, arthritis, and encephalitis.

Diagnosis

A suspected case of smallpox is a public health emergency. Local and state health authorities, the hospital epidemiologist, and other members of a hospital response team for biological emergencies should be notified immediately if smallpox is suspected.

The differential diagnosis of smallpox includes other illnesses that can cause fever and a rash. Severe varicella (chickenpox) is the disease most likely to be confused with smallpox. However, familiarity with the clinical features of the two diseases, particularly the rash, should help differentiate them. Additional information that may be useful in differentiating smallpox from chickenpox includes a history of exposure to persons with chickenpox, a personal history of chickenpox, a history of vaccination against varicella or smallpox, and the clinical course of illness.

Infection Control and Postexposure Isolation

In the event of a limited outbreak, patients should be admitted to the hospital and confined to rooms that are under negative atmospheric pressure and equipped with high-efficiency particulate air (HEPA) filtration. Standard, contact, and airborne precautions, including use of gloves, gowns, and masks, should be strictly observed. Unvaccinated staff caring for patients suspected of having smallpox should wear fit-tested N95 or higher quality respirators. Patients should wear a surgical mask and be wrapped in a gown or sheet to cover the rash when they are not in a negative-airflow room.

All laundry and waste should be placed in biohazard bags and autoclaved before being laundered or incinerated. Surfaces that may be contaminated with smallpox virus can be decontaminated with disinfectants that are used for standard hospital infection control, such as hypochlorite and quaternary ammonia.

Anthrax

Anthrax is a disease caused by the spore-forming bacterium *Bacillus anthracis.* The organism is found worldwide in soil. Animals become infected through grazing in contaminated areas. Under natural conditions, humans contract the disease after close contact with infected animals or contaminated animal products such as hides, wool, or meat. On exposure to the tissues or blood of an animal or an infected human, the spores germinate.

Classification and Epidemiology

Anthrax occurs in three clinical forms in humans: inhalational, cutaneous, and gastrointestinal. In a biological attack, aerosol exposure to anthrax spores would be most likely. Before 2001, exposure to powdered anthrax spores in an envelope or package was not thought to be an efficient means of causing inhalational disease. However, exposure to anthrax spores sent through the U.S. mail in the 2001 anthrax attack resulted in cases of inhalational anthrax and cutaneous disease.

Cutaneous anthrax is the most likely way to develop anthrax. It results from inoculation of spores subcutaneously through a cut or abrasion. Gastrointestinal and oropharyngeal anthrax occur in rural parts of the world where anthrax is endemic. They result from ingestion of meat contaminated with spores.

Inhalational Anthrax

CLINICAL PRESENTATION AND DIAGNOSIS. Clinical symptoms develop rapidly after germination of anthrax spores. The incubation period for inhalational disease is most commonly reported as 1 to 6 days but may be prolonged by antibiotic administration.

Inhalational anthrax is a two-stage disease. The initial stage is a nonspecific, flu-like illness lasting from several hours to a few days. The early clinical presentation includes some combination of fever, myalgia, headache, cough, mild chest discomfort, weakness, abdominal pain, and chest pain. Profound malaise, fever, and drenching sweats are prominent symptoms, and nausea and vomiting are frequent. Classically, the initial stage is followed 1 to 3 days later, sometimes after brief improvement, by the rapidly progressive second stage, characterized by fever, dyspnea, diaphoresis, cyanosis, and shock.

There is no rapid screening test to diagnose inhalational anthrax in its early stages. In persons with a compatible clinical illness for whom there is a heightened suspicion of anthrax based on clinical and epidemiological data, the appropriate initial diagnostic tests are a chest x-ray or chest computed tomographic (CT) scan, or both, and culture and smear of peripheral blood. Pleural fluid and cerebrospinal fluid, as well as biopsy specimens taken from the pleura and lung, are also potentially useful for culture and other testing when disease is present in these sites, whereas sputum culture and Gram stain are unlikely to be useful.

THERAPEUTIC INTERVENTION. Early intravenous antibiotic treatment may improve survival in inhalational anthrax. Aggressive supportive care, including attention to fluid, electrolyte, and acid-base disturbances and drainage of pleural effusions, also play an important role in treatment. At present, intravenous ciprofloxacin or doxycycline plus one or two additional antimicrobials are recommended.

Cutaneous Anthrax

After an incubation period of approximately 7 days (range: 1 to 12 days), the primary lesion of cutaneous anthrax appears as a nondescript, painless, pruritic papule, usually on an exposed area such as the face, head, neck, or upper extremity. The papule enlarges and develops a central vesicle or bulla with surrounding brawny, nonpitting edema. The central vesicle enlarges and ulcerates over 1 to 2 days, becoming hemorrhagic, depressed, and necrotic and leading to a central black eschar. Satellite vesicles may be present. The eschar dries and falls off over the next 1 to 2 weeks. Tender regional lymphadenopathy, fever, chills, and fatigue may occur. Systemic disease has been reported to have a mortality of 20% if untreated.

INFECTION CONTROL. Person-to-person transmission of anthrax is not known to occur. Patients may be hospitalized in a standard hospital room with standard barrier isolation precautions. No treatment is necessary for persons who come in contact with the patient.

Plague

Plague is caused by the gram-negative coccobacillus *Yersinia pestis.* Under natural conditions, plague is transmitted to humans by the bite of an infectious flea and, less frequently, by direct contact with the infectious body fluids or tissues of an infected animal or by inhaling infectious droplets. Plague has a long history of use and development as a biological weapon. After a biological attack, primary pneumonic plague would be most likely.

Clinical Presentation

Plague is a severe febrile illness. Pneumonic plague, the most fatal form of the infection, can develop from inhalation of plague bacilli (primary pneumonic plague).

The incubation period for pneumonic plague is typically 2 to 4 days (range: 1 to 6 days). Presenting symptoms typically include the acute onset of malaise, high fever, chills, headache, chest discomfort, dyspnea, and cough concomitant with or followed rapidly by clinical sepsis. Hemoptysis is a classic sign that should suggest plague in the appropriate clinical context, but sputum may be watery or purulent. Gastrointestinal symptoms may be prominent with pneumonic plague; these include nausea, vomiting, diarrhea, and abdominal pain. A cervical bubo (swelling of the lymph nodes) is infrequently present. The disease is rapidly progressive, with increasing dyspnea, stridor, and cyanosis. Rapidly progressive respiratory failure and sepsis within 2 to 4 days of onset of illness is typical of pneumonic plague.

Diagnosis

During a confirmed outbreak of pneumonic plague after a biological attack, a presumptive diagnosis can be made on the basis of symptoms, especially if there is a high index of suspicion. However, other causes of severe pneumonia or rapidly progressive respiratory infection with or without sepsis should be considered.

Laboratory findings are consistent with the systemic inflammatory response syndrome. The leukocyte count is elevated and the differential shows a neutrophil predominance, including immature forms. Platelets may be normal or low. Coagulation abnormalities include prolongation of the international normalized ratio (INR), prothrombin time (PT), and partial thromboplastin time (PTT). Elevated liver function tests and abnormal renal function tests are seen with systemic disease.

Therapeutic Intervention

When plague is suspected, antibiotic treatment should begin before laboratory confirmation of the diagnosis.

Botulism

Botulism is a paralytic illness caused by a potent neurotoxin produced by *Clostridium botulinum,* an anaerobic, spore-forming bacterium. Natural forms of the disease are foodborne botulism, wound botulism, and infant botulism. Foodborne botulism results from ingestion of improperly processed foodstuffs containing preformed toxin produced by *C. botulinum.* Wound botulism results from production of botulinum toxin by *C. botulinum* organisms that contaminate wounds. Infant botulism results from the colonization of the intestinal tract of infants after ingestion of spores. Botulinum toxin has been developed as a biological weapon. An aerosol attack is considered the most likely use of botulinum toxin for bioterrorism.

Botulinum toxin is the most potent lethal toxin known. The estimated toxic dose of type A botulinum toxin is 0.001 mcg/kg of body weight. Botulinum toxin acts to block neurotransmission by binding to the presynaptic nerve terminal at the neuromuscular junction and preventing the release of acetylcholine, resulting in skeletal muscle weakness. The toxin is colorless, odorless, and presumably tasteless.

Clinical Presentation

The incubation period for foodborne botulism is 2 hours to 8 days; the typical incubation period is 12 to 72 hours. The incubation period for inhalational botulism has not been established. The neurologic features of botulism are similar. Although initial symptoms in foodborne botulism may include nausea, vomiting, abdominal cramps, and diarrhea, these symptoms are thought to result from other bacterial metabolites in contaminated food and may not occur in inhalational botulism.

The so-called classic triad of botulism summarizes the clinical presentation: an afebrile patient, symmetrical descending flaccid paralysis with prominent bulbar palsies, and a clear mentation. Patients typically present with difficulty seeing, speaking, or swallowing. Clinical hallmarks include ptosis, blurred vision, and the so-called four Ds: diplopia, dysarthria, dysphonia, and dysphagia.

Anticholinergic symptoms are common, including dry mouth, ileus, constipation, nausea and vomiting, urine retention, and mydriasis. Other symptoms include dizziness and sore throat. Sensory findings are not present, with the exception of circumoral and peripheral paresthesias secondary to hyperventilation resulting from anxiety. Botulinum toxin does not cross the blood-brain barrier. Cranial nerve dysfunction and facial nerve weakness may make communication difficult; these symptoms may be mistaken for lethargy and signs of central nervous system involvement.

Diagnosis

Treatment with botulinum antitoxin should begin based on the clinical diagnosis and should not await laboratory confirmation. For potential foodborne botulism, samples of stool, gastric aspirate, emesis, and suspect foods should also be submitted.

The possibility of a bioterrorism attack should be considered in any outbreak of botulism. A bioterrorism attack should especially be considered when a cluster of cases occurs, when an outbreak has a common geographical location but there is no common dietary exposure (suggestive of possible aerosol exposure), when there is an outbreak of an unusual botulinum toxin type, or when multiple simultaneous outbreaks occur. A careful dietary and travel history must be taken to help identify the source. Patients should be asked if they know of others with similar symptoms.

Therapeutic Intervention

The mainstay of treatment for botulism is supportive care, including intensive care, mechanical ventilation, and parenteral nutrition. Morbidity and mortality are usually from:

- Pulmonary aspiration secondary to loss of the gag reflex and dysphagia leading to inability to control secretions
- Respiratory failure secondary to inadequate tidal volume from diaphragmatic and accessory respiratory muscle paralysis
- Airway obstruction from pharyngeal and upper airway muscle paralysis.

Careful and frequent monitoring of the gag and cough reflexes, swallowing, oxygen saturation, vital capacity, and inspiratory force are critical. Airway intubation is indicated for inability to control secretions and impending respiratory failure. Secondary infections are common and should be sought in patients who develop fever.

Trivalent (ABE) equine antitoxin is available from the CDC through state and local health departments and should be administered as soon as possible after clinical diagnosis. Antitoxin can prevent progression of disease caused by subsequent binding of toxin, but does not reverse the effects of already bound toxin. For this reason, antitoxin is not useful if the patient is no longer showing progression of disease or is improving from maximum paralysis.

Transmissibility and Infection Control

Botulism is not transmitted from person to person. Botulinum toxin does not penetrate intact skin. Standard infection-control precautions are adequate. Clothes of persons exposed to an aerosol release of botulinum toxin should be removed and washed. Exposed persons should shower with soap and hot water. Exposed environmental surfaces can be decontaminated with 0.1% hypochlorite bleach solution.

SUGGESTED ANSWERS TO CRITICAL THINKING

■ *Mr. Smith*

1. The airway is the first priority because edema from inhalation burns can occlude the airway.
2. You know that Mr. Smith is at risk for respiratory burns because of the soot near his mouth and nose. He should be closely monitored. Assessment should include respiratory rate and pattern and the patient's ability to speak without a hoarse voice. Abnormal breathing sounds such as wheezing indicate partial upper airway occlusion.
3. The vital signs are within normal limits.
4. Deep partial-thickness burns should be covered with dry dressings. Because the skin can no longer protect the patient, wet dressings provide a medium for bacterial invasion. Wet dressings can also cause a decrease in body temperature because the skin can no longer maintain thermoregulation.
5. Jewelry should always be immediately removed before edema formation begins.
6. Mr. Smith was involved in an explosive incident and thrown 50 feet. He could have sustained fractures of the pelvis or back. He also may have internal organ injuries from blunt trauma.

REVIEW QUESTIONS

1. Which of the following assessments would the nurse include in a primary survey of a multisystem trauma victim? **Select all that apply.**
   a. Airway
   b. Breathing
   c. Circulation
   d. Chronic disability
   e. Vital signs
   f. Deformity

2. The nurse is caring for a trauma patient who is hemorrhaging from a puncture wound. Which of the following interventions should the nurse use to control the arterial bleeding?
   a. Pressure at the puncture site
   b. Application of a tourniquet
   c. Pressure-point massage
   d. Pressure dressing

3. Which of the following symptoms would alert the nurse to the potential for inhalation injury to a patient who was in a house fire?
   a. Peripheral edema
   b. Singed nasal hairs
   c. Jugular vein distention
   d. Increased capillary refill time

4. Which of the following actions should be taken first for a patient who is found with hyperthermia?
   a. Undress the patient.
   b. Use tepid water as a mist spray.
   c. Remove patient from the hot environment.
   d. Place patient in continual breeze from electric fans.

5. For which of the following should the nurse observe the patient who has inhaled chlorine? **Select all that apply.**
   a. Airway obstruction
   b. Sacral edema
   c. Increased capillary refill time
   d. Unequal pupils
   e. Dyspnea
   f. Pulmonary edema

6. When interacting with a psychotic patient, which of the following interventions is helpful to gain the patient's trust?
   a. Play along.
   b. Show respect.
   c. Avoid eye contact.
   d. Make promises.

REVIEW QUESTIONS—cont'd

7. Which of the following patients should be treated first in a disaster situation?
   a. A 10-year-old with a closed leg fracture that is painful
   b. A 32-year-old with slight bleeding from a hand laceration
   c. A 45-year-old with an open head injury, no pulse or respirations
   d. A 62-year-old reporting chest pain and shortness of breath

8. Which one of the following is an immediate threat to life during acute anaphylaxis?
   a. Hypotension
   b. Generalized itching
   c. Airway obstruction
   d. Tachycardia

9. The nurse is assessing a patient who is hypovolemic. Which of the following signs and symptoms indicate that the patient is experiencing profound shock?
   a. Sacral edema
   b. Jugular vein distention
   c. Decreasing blood pressure
   d. Palpable, bounding pulse

10. The nurse is to give penicillin G 500,000 units IM. The nurse has a 10-mL vial labeled "penicillin 400,000 units/mL." How many milliliters should the nurse give?
    Answer: ____________________ mL

DavisPlus | For additional resources and information visit http://davisplus.fadavis.com

unit THREE

UNDERSTANDING LIFE SPAN INFLUENCES ON HEALTH AND ILLNESS

14

Developmental Considerations in the Nursing Care of Adults

LINDA S. WILLIAMS

KEY TERMS

chronic illness (KRAW-nick ILL-ness)
developmental stage (deh-vell-up-MEN-tal STAYJ)
health (HELLTH)
hopelessness (HOHP-less-ness)
illness (ILL-ness)
powerlessness (POW-er-less-ness)
reminiscence (reh-meh-NISS-enss)
respite care (RESS-pit CARE)
spirituality (SPEER-ih-chu-AL-ih-tee)

QUESTIONS TO GUIDE YOUR READING

1. What are Erikson's eight stages of psychosocial development?
2. What are the effects of chronic illness?
3. What special needs do caregivers have?
4. What are health promotion methods?
5. What nursing interventions would you use in caring for a patient who is chronically ill?

HEALTH, WELLNESS, AND ILLNESS

Health is much more than just the absence of disease. Have you ever known someone with what appears to be a small health problem who considers himself unwell or disabled, or a person with major health problems who sees himself as well? Many things play a role in a person's perception of health. One is the ability to function or perform desired or necessary tasks such as activities of daily living (ADL). Another is the ability to fulfill one's roles, such as student, parent, or worker. The quality of one's life is another component of health. A person's ability to adapt to changes in physical, psychological, social, and spiritual aspects of life needs to be considered to plan health care. *Wellness* is a term used to describe a progression toward a higher level of functioning. Even though a person has a disabling illness, he or she may still be able to achieve a higher level of wellness.

> **NURSING CARE TIP**
>
> To foster understanding of how an ill patient, especially an older patient, was once healthy and active, ask family members to bring in photos showing the patient healthy at various ages or doing favorite activities. Displaying these photos in the patient's room allows caregivers to appreciate the patient in wellness roles.

The concept of illness is one of imbalance or disharmony with the environment. The physical causes of illness are most easily recognized, such as exercise that induces an asthma attack or a fall that causes a broken bone. But illness can also result from a psychological, sociological, cultural, or spiritual imbalance. After the loss of a spouse, for example, one may experience loneliness, depression, and a loss of balance in the social and psychological aspects of life.

A hospitalization may increase disharmony if cultural beliefs and practices are not understood or upheld by health care providers. A person faced with a terminal diagnosis may lose hope and direction in life, causing anxiety and despair. So rather than being exclusive concepts, **health** and **illness** are dynamic and ever-changing states of being. A health crisis such as a myocardial infarction (MI) overwhelms a patient's ability to maintain a normal level of wellness. Two months after the MI, however, the patient could be enjoying a higher level of wellness than before the MI if he or she has lost weight, is walking daily, and is eating a nutritious low-fat diet.

THE NURSE'S ROLE IN SUPPORTING AND PROMOTING WELLNESS

The goal of nursing care is to help patients achieve their highest possible level of wellness. To do this, the patient's strengths, assets, and resources, as well as weaknesses, liabilities, and disabilities are considered. Working together, the patient, family, and members of the health care team develop a plan of care that includes wellness goals and a plan of action to accomplish those goals. The plan of care focuses on six main areas:

- Mobilizing resources
- Providing a safe and adaptable environment
- Helping the patient learn about his or her health problem and treatment
- Performing and teaching the patient to perform health care procedures
- Anticipating problems and recognizing potential crises
- Evaluating the plan and progress toward the goals with the patient and family.

Nurses assume a variety of roles in promoting the health of their patients, such as advocate, caregiver, consultant, and educator.

DEVELOPMENTAL STAGES

Understanding the patient's **developmental stage** can help the nurse more accurately assess health and health practices. The developmental stages of life focus on the balance a person must achieve for high-level wellness within that stage. Erik Erikson (1980, 1993) described eight stages of psychosocial development (Table 14.1). These stages illustrate the acquisition of a sense of trust in self and others and a sense of personal worth. Each stage must be completed before accomplishing the next. The first five stages describe the development of the child and adolescent. The last three stages relate to young adulthood, middle adulthood, and late adulthood and are discussed next.

The Young Adult

Erikson's sixth developmental stage, from ages 18 to 40, addresses intimacy versus isolation. The young adult's task is to develop relationships with a spouse, family, or friends that are warm, affectionate, and developed through fondness, understanding, caring, or love. When this stage is not successfully resolved, the person typically experiences isolation from others. Physically, growth is usually completed by age 20. Socially, young adults begin to move away from their parents to start their own families. The young adult begins to develop a place in society through school, work, and social activities. This is the stage in which intimacy or closeness develops with partners and friends. Decisions to have a pet, to marry, and to have children show the desire for intimacy. Challenges to intimacy are tasks that must be overcome in this stage. Melding one's traditions and customs with the traditions and customs of a spouse, family, and friends is a major responsibility, as is the passing on of culture to children. Values and beliefs, which arise from a person's culture or conscience, serve as guidelines for behavior for the young adult.

TABLE 14.1 ERIC ERIKSON'S STAGES OF PSYCHOSOCIAL DEVELOPMENT

Stage	Age Range	Developmental Task
Infancy	Birth to 18 months	Trust versus mistrust
Toddler	18 months to 3 years	Autonomy versus shame and doubt
Preschool	3 to 5 years	Initiative versus guilt
School age	5 to 12 years	Industry versus inferiority
Adolescence	12 to 18 years	Identity versus role confusion
Young adulthood	18 to 40 years	Intimacy versus isolation
Middle adulthood	40 to 65 years	Generativity versus stagnation
Late adulthood	65 years to death	Integrity versus despair

Common Health Concerns

The lifestyle choices of young adults may place their health at risk. Health promotion for this age-group focuses on preventing or limiting risks through teaching. Young adults should understand the importance of diet and exercise in maintaining health for themselves and their children. Lifelong positive health practices help prevent long-term health complications. Maintaining an aerobic exercise program, a low-fat diet, and blood cholesterol below 200 mg/dL helps keep weight down and promotes cardiovascular health. Avoiding sun exposure and using sunscreen are important to avoid sunburn, permanent sun damage to the skin, and increased risk of skin cancer. Tobacco use started in the teen years is often carried on throughout young adulthood and is linked to chronic bronchitis, emphysema, and oral, throat, and lung cancer in later life. Additional preventive measures that may be taught at this stage include breast self-examination (BSE) for women and testicular self-examination (TSE) for men.

In the early part of young adulthood, the individual is in the workforce or is preparing for the work world with a college or vocational education. Being a novice in the work world and accepting new independence, freedom, and responsibilities can introduce stressors into the young adult's life. Overeating, alcohol use, drug use, cigarette smoking, and violence are risky lifestyle choices and poor coping mechanisms for stress. Young adults need to be aware of their individual stressors and be encouraged to develop positive coping mechanisms for stress. Exercise, support groups, music, and meditation are positive ways to cope with stress.

Although marriage commonly occurs during this phase, this group also has the highest rate of divorce. The blending of two people into a couple requires a lot of creative communication and loving care. When stressors overwhelm the couple's coping mechanisms or coping strategy, the relationship may be in trouble. Sometimes because of the high rate of divorce, couples choose to live together without being married. However, the avoidance of making a commitment may set these relationships up for failure.

If young adults are sexually active with multiple partners, they are at risk for sexually transmitted diseases. Safer sex guidelines and information on birth control should be available for the young adult.

Pregnancy is a common health occurrence for women in this age-group. Because research indicates that a mother's health practices directly affect the health of the developing fetus, nutrition, drug and alcohol use, physical health, and effective stress coping mechanisms are lifestyle issues that need to be discussed with every pregnant woman. Prenatal care should be encouraged and readily available to pregnant women.

CRITICAL THINKING

Mrs. Michaels

■ Mrs. Michaels, age 25, and her husband have been trying to start a family. Mrs. Michaels visits her physician, who confirms that she is pregnant. What information and health practices should Mrs. Michaels and her husband be taught during a prenatal health examination?

Suggested answers at end of chapter.

The Middle-Aged Adult

In the middle adult years, ages 40 to 65, the psychological developmental stage is developing generativity versus self-absorption. Generativity includes a sense of productivity and creativity, and is demonstrated by concern and support for others, along with a vision for future generations. Unresolved conflict may be seen as preoccupation with personal needs or self-absorption.

Physically, middle-aged adults start to notice signs of decreased endurance and intolerance for physical exercise if they have not maintained healthy lifestyle choices. Socially, their children are adolescents or young adults who need assistance with entering adulthood and launching their own careers and families. The term *empty nest* has been used to describe the middle-aged couple's home after their children have left.

This period is often complicated by the challenging demands of also caring for aging parents. Today's middle-aged adult generation has been labeled the *sandwich generation* because of the need to care for their children and their aging parents at the same time. Middle-aged adults look over their lives and assess accomplishments versus unrealized goals. Midlife crisis may occur as this self-inspection leads to a desire to change work, social, or family situations to try to meet unrealized goals. Planning for retirement by developing meaningful pastimes and interests outside of work and preparing for financial security is another important task during this stage.

Common Health Concerns

Unhealthy choices, such as smoking, use of alcohol or drugs, a sedentary lifestyle, a diet high in saturated fat, or overeating, often have serious consequences for middle adulthood. Hypertension and heart disease are major health concerns, as are chronic bronchitis, emphysema, and lung cancer. Cardiovascular disease and cancer cause most of the deaths in this age-group. However, middle adulthood is not too late to begin lifestyle changes that positively affect health, such as regular exercise, not smoking, healthful eating, weight reduction, and using positive stress-coping mechanisms. Helping adults in this age-group recognize the benefits of these positive lifestyle choices and empowering them to change is the major challenge for health care professionals.

The need for immunizations continues into adulthood. Adults at high risk for hepatitis B (health care workers, hemophiliacs, people on hemodialysis, intravenous drug users, and foreign travelers) should be vaccinated for hepatitis B if it was not done during childhood.

> **CRITICAL THINKING**
>
> ***Mr. Paul***
>
> ■ Mr. Paul, age 54, calls his primary care provider's office for the fourth time this month reporting severe indigestion and requesting a medication to fix it. He has refused to have an x-ray examination or other diagnostic tests because he "can't fit them" into his "busy schedule." Mr. Paul has his own insurance business. His wife quit her job to supervise their 15-year-old son, who was not going to school every day. The couple's twin daughters are both in college out of state.
>
> 1. What might be causing Mr. Paul to experience health problems?
> 2. What is affecting the developmental tasks Mr. Paul needs to perform?
>
> *Suggested answers at end of chapter.*

The Older Adult

The final developmental stage affects adults from age 65 until death. *Ageism* is a term that describes stereotypical misconceptions about older adults in society. Although they are the most diverse age group, common misconceptions about older people include that they are senile, disabled, and in nursing homes. However, more positive attitudes about aging are developing, in part as a result of the growing number of older adults. Advances in living conditions and health care have allowed more people to reach old age. People are living productive, fulfilling lives into their 80s, 90s, and even 100s. Older adults are likely to be found working in their gardens, hiking, exercising, or socializing (Fig. 14.1). Some older adults continue to work beyond typical retirement age or begin a rewarding second career after retiring.

Developmental work for older adults focuses on integrity versus despair. In this stage, older adults look back and evaluate what they have done with their lives. Integrity refers to accepting responsibility for one's life so far and reflecting on it in a positive way. Reaching this stage is a sign of maturity. Failing to reach this stage is an indication of unsuccessful completion of prior stages, causing feelings of despair that life has been lived in vain, and a fear of death. **Reminiscence** therapy may be one way to assist the older adult through this stage.

Aging is associated with role changes and transitions. Some roles, such as employee, son, or daughter, are lost because of retirement, death, or illness, causing sadness or

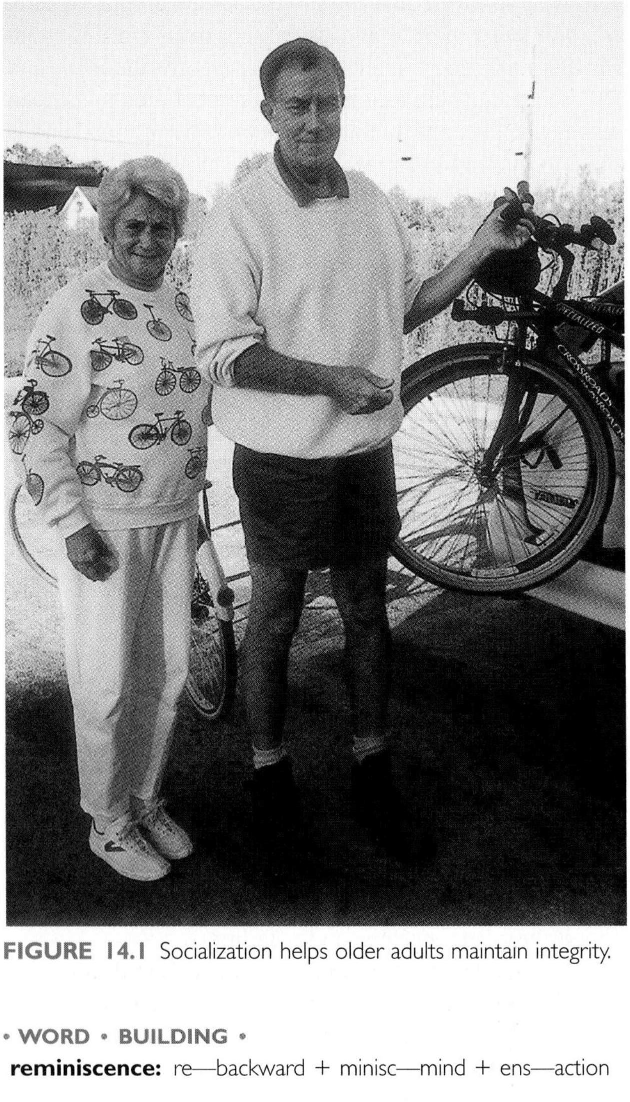

FIGURE 14.1 Socialization helps older adults maintain integrity.

• **WORD • BUILDING** •
reminiscence: re—backward + minisc—mind + ens—action

depression. New roles may arise, such as grandparent, volunteer, or widow/widower. With retirement, household management roles may need to change. If an older adult becomes ill and dependent and needs to be cared for by an adult child, the parent–child role may be reversed.

Health, relationships, lifestyle choices, and environment influence the diversity found in this age-group. Physical health is often a concern for older adults. Chronic health problems that require medication and treatment often require lifestyle changes or adaptations.

Life events such as decreased physical ability, retirement, illness, or death of a spouse are challenges that older adults face. The older adult's ability to cope with these stressors is essential for maintaining a sense of control. Coping with aging is influenced by the individual's cultural beliefs. Cultural viewpoints on the social role and value of aged community members affect the health of older adults. Sometimes the greatest loss for older adults is their lack of connection with the world and lack of being part of a greater purpose. However, being alone is not the same as being lonely. For most older adults, being by oneself for a time allows for reflection to better understand one's situation. Older adults who feel unwanted or unloved are more likely to develop anxiety, depression, and failure to thrive.

Common Health Concerns

The focus of care for the older adult is assistance in meeting physical, psychological, cultural, sociological, and spiritual needs. Promoting self-care and encouraging the use of community services for seniors is important. Most older adults continue to live in their own homes or apartments, but impairment in mobility and the ability to carry out instrumental activities of daily living (IADL), such as shopping for groceries, preparing meals, and cleaning and maintaining a home, threaten their independence. Having to ask or pay others to perform tasks that they formerly were able to do themselves is seen as a significant loss by many older adults. Adding the loss of a spouse, the death of friends, or the lack of social contacts further isolates an older person and can lead to depression and a feeling of **hopelessness**. The accumulation of losses can overwhelm an older adult's resources and coping mechanisms and is related to a high rate of suicide, especially for older men. Suicide is the ultimate expression of hopelessness.

Older adults need to be encouraged to remain active and to continue to pursue interests. Most communities have transportation services that operate to meet the needs of older adults. Senior centers offer diverse programs and services. Some senior groups are focused on community service; others mainly plan trips or sponsor activities such as dances or bowling leagues. Older adults also have opportunities to continue to work in areas of interest as volunteers. Schools, hospitals, nursing facilities, parks, museums, zoos, community theaters, and youth groups all welcome older adult volunteers. Colleges and universities offer discounted tuition for senior citizens, and there are Elderhostel programs across the country. Elderhostel offers thousands of educational travel programs, such as photography, Civil War history, nature survival, bird watching, and painting.

Chronic diseases can limit an older person's ability to be independent in self-care and activities of daily living. Hypertension is common in this age-group, as are heart disease and strokes. Managing blood pressure, losing weight, eating a low-fat diet, stopping tobacco use, enhancing effective stress-coping strategies, and exercising regularly decrease the potential for cardiovascular disease.

One of the most difficult tasks for the nurse in dealing with the older adult is to distinguish normal age-related changes from pathological changes. Changes in mobility and chronic pain may limit an older person's activity and impede an active lifestyle. Pain is not normal and should be investigated rather than being attributed to aging and ignored.

CRITICAL THINKING

Mr. Klein

■ Mr. Klein, age 82, visits his health care provider. He reports left hip pain. The health care provider replies, "It can be common to experience pain as you get older." Mr. Klein thinks a minute and says, "But my right hip doesn't hurt and it's as old as my left hip!"

1. What is occurring in this situation?
2. What actions could be taken to improve the quality of life for Mr. Klein?

Suggested answers at end of chapter.

Falls are a serious concern for older adults, resulting in decreased independence and death. Osteoporosis is a bone disease common among postmenopausal women and men over age 80, causing bone weakness and fracture risk. Falls and accidents can be prevented by in-home safety assessments and altering the home environment to ensure the safety of the older adult. Bathrooms should be equipped with grab bars and nonskid mats. Bath chairs or benches make getting into a bath or shower safer. Removing clutter, throw rugs, small furniture, and electrical cords decreases the risk of falls.

Hearing and vision loss can affect physical and psychological health in the older adult. Good sensory function is needed to protect oneself from accidents, social isolation, and limitations in self-care. One of the most dramatic losses for many older adults is not being able to safely drive a car. This is usually associated with a loss of independence. Sensory impairments can further isolate the patient. Impaired vision can be caused by decreased peripheral vision, macular degeneration, cataracts, or glaucoma. Many older adults continue to drive during the day but not at night because of night vision problems. Decreased hearing is also common in older adults. Loss of high-pitch discrimination and reduced ability to filter background noise causes older adults to hear the background noise more clearly than a one-to-one conversation when in a crowded room. Social stigmas related to memory changes such as forgetfulness, dementia, and senility are a serious worry for many older adults. They commonly confuse depression with senility and attempt to hide their symptoms rather than seek treatment.

CHRONIC ILLNESS

A major challenge facing health care providers is the management and prevention of chronic illness. A **chronic illness** is defined as an illness that is long lasting or that recurs. It usually interferes with the person's ability to perform activities of daily living. A chronic illness is never completely cured or prevented. The amount of disability a person has depends not only on the condition and its severity but also on the individual effects for that person. The degree of disability and altered lifestyle relate as much to the person's perception of the disease as to the disease itself. For example, both John F. Kennedy and Franklin D. Roosevelt would have been eligible for 100% disability benefits because of their chronic illnesses, but both managed to serve as presidents. The long-term effects of treatments such as radiation therapy can become chronic diseases in themselves. Radiation for a tumor can leave the person with persistent diarrhea that may cause malnourishment and exhaustion.

CRITICAL THINKING

Mrs. Riccardi

■ Mrs. Riccardi, age 87, lives alone in her small apartment. Her daughter and son are both retired and live in the same community. Mrs. Riccardi had a dizzy spell, so her daughter brought her to the hospital emergency department (ED). Upon admission, Mrs. Riccardi's blood pressure was 208/128 and she had blurred vision in the left eye that resolved after 1 hour in the ED. She was diagnosed with hypertension, which possibly contributed to a small stroke or transient ischemic attack (TIA). Mrs. Riccardi was started on metoprolol (Lopressor) 100 mg daily. She was discharged to her home with instructions to limit salt in her diet and to begin an exercise program. The plan of care addressed safety issues.

1. Why might Mrs. Riccardi be at increased risk of falling?
2. What nursing interventions would help promote Mrs. Riccardi's independence and safety?
3. The nurse is to give metoprolol 100 mg, and 50-milligram tablets are available. How many tablets should the nurse give?

Suggested answers at end of chapter.

When caring for those with chronic illnesses, the goal of nursing care is to maintain and improve the patient's quality of life. A chronic illness also affects the quality of life of the patient's family. Therefore, when planning patient care, consider the family's needs for adapting to the patient's chronic illness.

Fostering hope is an important intervention that should be a primary foundation of care planning for people who are chronically ill. A chronic illness may appear to be a hopeless situation if no cure is possible. If recovery from an illness is not possible, people might think that nothing can be done for the patient. However, whenever there is life, there is potential for growth in areas such as developmental tasks, health promotion, knowledge, or spirit. Individuals have developmental tasks to perform even as they cope with illness or prepare for a peaceful death.

Incidence of Chronic Illness

The incidence of chronic illness is rising for several reasons. First, people are living longer, in part because of better hygiene, nutrition, exercise, vaccinations, antibiotic development, and new treatment options. Fewer people are dying from acute diseases. As a result, a larger elderly population is living long enough to develop many chronic illnesses. Second, medical advances have resulted in reduced mortality from some chronic illnesses, so that patients live longer with these illnesses. Third, today's technology and modern lifestyles may contribute to the development of some chronic illnesses. Examples include a sedentary lifestyle; exposure to air and water pollution, chemicals, and carcinogens; substance abuse; and stress.

Some common chronic conditions include chronic sinusitis, arthritis, hypertension, orthopedic dysfunction, decreased hearing, heart disease, bronchitis, asthma, and diabetes. Preventive measures can be taught to help reduce the incidence of these conditions.

Types of Chronic Illnesses

Chronic illnesses have different causes (Box 14.1). These illnesses have varying degrees of severity and effect on length of life. A chronic illness can lead to development of other illnesses, such as hypertension, which then causes chronic renal failure. Chronic illnesses can begin at various ages, but with advancing age, the likelihood of developing a chronic illness increases, and many older adults have several chronic illnesses at once (Box 14.2).

Gerontological Influence

As people live longer, spouses or older family members are increasingly being called on to care for a chronically ill family member. Children of older adults who themselves are reaching their 60s are being expected to care for their parents. These older caregivers may have chronic illnesses of their own. A family in this situation is at great risk for ineffective coping or further development of health problems. Assessment of all members of the elderly family is essential to ensure that their health and coping needs are being met. *Healthy*

Box 14.1

Examples of Chronic Illnesses by Cause

Genetic

- Cystic fibrosis
- Huntington's disease
- Muscular dystrophy
- Sickle cell anemia

Congenital

- Heart defects
- Malabsorption syndromes
- Spina bifida

Acquired

- Acquired immunodeficiency syndrome (AIDS)
- Arthritis
- Cancer
- Chronic obstructive pulmonary disease
- Diabetes
- Head or spinal cord injury
- Multiple sclerosis

Box 14.2

Examples of Chronic Illnesses in the Older Adult

- Arthritis
- Cerebrovascular accident
- Chronic lung disease
- Diabetes
- Heart disease
- Hypertension
- Peripheral vascular disease
- Sensory losses: vision, hearing

People 2010, a national health promotion and disease prevention initiative, calls for public health surveillance and health promotion programs for people with disabilities and caregivers in all states and the District of Columbia. Visit www.healthypeople.gov for progress reports on this objective.

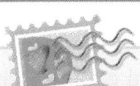

Older adults are very concerned about becoming dependent on others. They may become depressed and give up hope if they feel that they are a burden to others. Establishing short-term goals or self-care activities that allow them to participate or have small successes are important nursing actions that can increase their self-esteem (Box 14.3, *Cultural Considerations*).

Barriers to care for a chronically ill elderly patient include a lack of information about treatments, medications, or special diets and being unfamiliar with supportive services in the community such as meal programs or respite care. Develop an understanding of this information and share it, as well as a resource number for elderly patients and their families that they can call with questions.

Effects of Chronic Illness

When a patient lives with a chronic illness, many adjustments are usually needed. Lifelong routines and habits may need to be changed to cope with the illness. Treatment needs, such as going to therapy sessions, performing peritoneal dialysis exchanges, or monitoring blood glucose, can interrupt daily life and require adaptation into the daily routine.

Chronic Sorrow

Chronic sorrow is a normal response felt by those affected by a chronic illness. It is an intermittently occurring sadness in response to losses caused by a chronic illness. It can be felt by the patient or the patient's significant others. The nursing diagnosis *Risk for Chronic Sorrow* may apply to those with chronic illness. When this sadness occurs, nursing care should focus on active listening to understand the loss, and then offering appropriate comfort and support (see *Evidence-Based Practice* box). Providing information and assisting with coping strategies such as fostering support systems are great interventions to help those with chronic sorrow.

Spiritual Distress

Patients with chronic illness can experience spiritual distress when faced with the limitations of their illness. Maintaining patients' quality of life includes assisting with their spiritual needs. Religious and spiritual needs are important to most people whose lives have been disrupted by new challenges from chronic illness. Patients must be helped to find realistic hope and meaning in the illness. Interventions that address **spirituality** may need to be performed first to promote success in later nursing care.

Box 14.3

Cultural Considerations

Traditional Appalachians

Traditional Appalachians believe that disability is natural with aging and is inevitable. This belief discourages the use of rehabilitation as an option. Thus, to promote rehabilitation efforts among Appalachians, the nurse may need to stress self-help and a return to physical function.

EVIDENCE-BASED PRACTICE

Clinical Question

Is chronic sorrow, the reaction to personal losses in chronic illness, present in patients with a chronic illness?

Evidence

A study of people with chronic illness found they experienced repeated losses such as loss of bodily functions, relationships, autonomy, life imagined, roles, activities, identity, and uplifting emotions. Of 30 patients, 16 were found to be in a state of chronic sorrow due to these losses (Ahlstrom, 2007).

A study of patients with multiple sclerosis found 62% to be in a state of chronic sorrow due to losses experienced from their illness (Isaksson, Gunnarsson, & Ahlstrom, 2007).

Implications for Nursing Practice

Chronic sorrow exists in patients with chronic illness due to losses. Using active listening to understand a patient's losses can enhance communication and appropriate support to provide comfort, hope, encouragement of positive self-esteem, and relevant information to the patient experiencing chronic sorrow.

REFERENCES

Ahlstrom, G. (2007). Experiences of loss and chronic sorrow in persons with severe chronic illness. *Journal of Clinical Nursing, 16*(3A), 76–83.

Isaksson, A., Gunnarsson, L., & Ahlstrom, G. (2007). The presence and meaning of chronic sorrow in patients with multiple sclerosis. *Journal of Clinical Nursing, 16*(11c), 315–324.

Several factors may make one uncomfortable in caring for a patient's spiritual needs. These factors include a lack of training, a lack of understanding of one's own spiritual needs and beliefs, and not recognizing or believing that this is your role. Develop a comfortable approach in assessing and meeting patients' spiritual needs. Examine your own spiritual needs to define a personal spiritual view. By doing this, you will develop insight into others' spiritual needs and resources, as well as gain a greater understanding of issues surrounding your patients' spiritual needs.

Many people use spirituality to cope with chronic illness. It helps give them a sense of wholeness, hope, and peace during a time filled with uncertainty and anxiety. Spirituality plays an important role in empowering patients to handle their condition. It is a source of inner strength that allows the patient to experience a sense of unity. Hospital interventions may include use of a meditation room for quiet reflection or prayer, chaplain visits, or worship services. To help meet the patient's spiritual needs, assist the patient with transportation to the meditation room or worship services.

NURSING CARE TIP

Spiritual needs should not be thought of in only religious terms. Spirituality is feeling connected with a higher power. Everyone has spiritual needs that involve hope, peace, and wholeness. Spiritual care goes beyond simply asking the patient's religion. It involves assessing the patient's perceptions of spirituality and then devising ways to help meet the person's spiritual needs.

Accreditation agencies require the spiritual needs of patients to be addressed and documented by nurses. Nursing diagnoses related to spiritual needs may include *Spiritual Distress, Risk for Spiritual Distress, Readiness for Enhanced Spiritual Well-Being, Impaired Religiosity,* and *Risk for Impaired Religiosity.*

Powerlessness

A chronic illness can take an unknown course in relation to its seriousness and controllability. This leaves the patient vulnerable to the many phases of a chronic illness: the diagnosis, the instability phase, an acute illness or crisis, remissions, and a terminal phase. Treatments that the patient undergoes may be painful, frightening, and invasive. A patient who does not understand what is happening can feel overwhelmed and alone. This contributes to a feeling of **powerlessness** because the patient cannot control the outcome (Fig. 14.2). This lack of control throughout an illness influences the patient's reactions to the illness. The nursing diagnosis *Powerlessness* or *Risk for Powerlessness* may apply to chronically ill patients.

COPING. Patients can be helped to feel more in control of their illness if you remember to include them in their care; listen to their feelings, values, and goals; and explain all procedures before they occur. Avoid using complex medical language when talking with patients to increase their understanding and feeling of being included in their care instead of isolated. In addition, coping with a chronic illness can be aided if the patient develops a positive attitude toward the illness. This can be accomplished if the patient gains knowledge, uses a problem-solving approach, and becomes motivated to continue adapting to the illness.

Having a variety of coping techniques can be useful. Ask the patient's perception of the illness and coping techniques that the patient has previously used successfully. New coping resources may need to be added to help the patient effectively deal with the chronic illness. Support services in the community should be offered to the patient and family. To cope effectively, the patient should be helped to become comfortable with the newly defined person he or

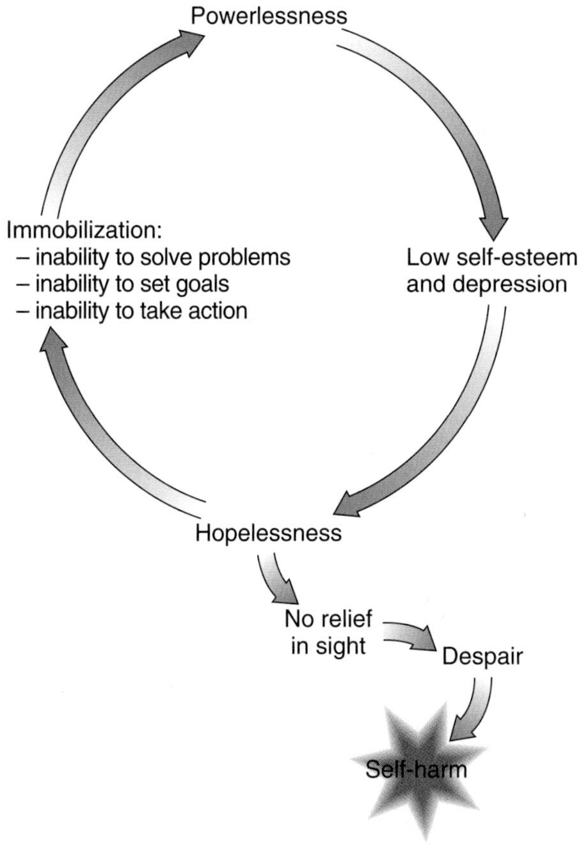
Powerlessness
Low self-esteem and depression
Hopelessness
No relief in sight
Despair
Self-harm
Immobilization:
– inability to solve problems
– inability to set goals
– inability to take action

FIGURE 14.2 Powerlessness–hopelessness cycle. (Modified from Miller, J. [2000]. *Coping with chronic illness: Overcoming powerlessness* [3rd ed., p. 526]. Philadelphia: F. A. Davis.)

she is to become. The nursing diagnoses *Ineffective Coping, Compromised Family Coping, Disabled Family Coping,* and *Readiness for Enhanced Family Coping* may apply to those dealing with chronic illness.

HOPE. Before coping resources can be used, hope must be established in the patient. False hope is not beneficial and should be replaced with realistic hope. Providing patients with accurate knowledge regarding their fears helps do this. Hope should not be directed toward a cure that may not be possible but rather at living a quality life with the functional capacity that the patient has. Over the course of the illness, hope needs to be maintained for both the patient and family. Periodically assess if the patient is maintaining hope. Many studies have shown that patients adapt better when hope is high. The nursing diagnoses *Readiness for Enhanced Hope* or *Hopelessness* may apply to chronically ill patients.

Many nursing interventions may increase hope. The use of humor helps patients be lighthearted and hopeful. Patients should be tactfully and sensitively encouraged to live each moment to the fullest and experience the joy of being alive. Awakening the senses to appreciate the environment can bring a feeling of hope and peace. Simple things, such as the smell of baking bread, the clean scent of the air after a rain, or the scent of pine trees, can make one appreciate the beauty of nature and inspire hope. Family members need to be encouraged to help foster hope for the patient. In doing this, family members may feel hopeful as well. During times of acute illness, the patient needs to maintain as much control as possible and be told that any loss of control related to treatments is usually temporary. This prevents a continual feeling of loss of power. The use of music or inspirational reading material can reduce stress and help the patient find meaning in life. This in turn fosters hope. Hopeful patients are empowered and no longer feel powerless.

Sexuality

Chronic illness can affect a patient's sexuality, which includes femininity and masculinity as well as sexual activity. Body image changes affect the way patients view themselves and are viewed by others. If patients have a negative body image perception, they may withdraw and become depressed. When interacting with patients, be aware of your facial expressions, nonverbal cues such as appearing hurried or keeping a distance, use of or lack of touch, and amount of time spent with the patient. When patients believe they have lost their femininity or masculinity, their self-worth decreases. Interventions to enhance sexuality should be used, such as obtaining a wig from the wig bank for patients undergoing chemotherapy.

There are many forms of sexual expression. Sexual intimacy can include touching, hugging, or sharing time together. Provide patients with the opportunity to discuss sexuality concerns or questions. Assume a professional and confidential approach to this topic, which is usually considered a private matter by patients. Chronically ill patients can be referred to sexuality counselors for information on ways to cope with sexual issues in relation to their illness. Support groups can also be helpful.

CRITICAL THINKING

Mr. Soloman

■ Mr. Soloman, age 88, lives in his own home with his wife of 60 years. He is in good health except for limited vision. He grows prize-winning tomatoes each year, plays golf weekly, and walks every day to the neighborhood stores. The employees know him and cheerfully assist him.

■ Mr. Soloman's wife was the homemaker, and now she is in the early stages of Alzheimer's disease. She cannot perform activities of daily living, so he has willingly assumed the caregiver role. They complement each other's limitations because she has good vision and is helpful when she is not confused.

■ Over time, Mr. Soloman's wife's health declines and she enters a long-term care facility. Mr. Soloman remains

continued

CRITICAL THINKING—cont'd

in his home alone, which concerns his family. They eventually convince him to move into senior housing. He is very reluctant to leave his home and does not actively participate in moving and selling his home. Mr. Soloman rarely leaves his apartment, sleeps 14 hours a day, and eats one daily meal. He tries to visit his wife by taking a bus but finds it difficult because of his limited vision, so he rarely sees her. A few months later, Mr. Soloman develops pneumonia and dies in his sleep.

1. Why do you think Mr. Soloman behaved the way he did after he moved?
2. What interventions could have been used to empower Mr. Soloman?
3. Why might Mr. Soloman have developed pneumonia and died?

Suggested answers at end of chapter.

Because sexuality is a part of a person's lifelong identity, make sure that elderly patients' sexuality is addressed in their plans of care. Patients in long-term care facilities should be given private time with their significant other, if appropriate. Grooming methods can increase a patient's self-esteem and sexual identity. Women may get their hair and nails done; men can be shaved or get a haircut. Older patients' sexuality needs should be met just as younger patients' are.

Roles

Chronically ill patients usually are faced with altering their accustomed roles in life. Common roles that may be affected for the adult patient include that of being a spouse, grandparent, parent, provider, homemaker, or friend. Not only must the patient deal with these role alterations, but the family must adapt to them as well. Family members may have to take on new roles themselves to compensate for roles the patient can no longer perform. The nursing diagnosis of *Ineffective Role Performance* should be included in the plan of care for the patient and family.

The patient is faced with giving up aspects of old roles at the same time that new roles related to being chronically ill need to be assumed. Grieving accompanies the loss of old roles. If a patient is no longer able to participate in social events such as golfing or being a committee member, grief work needs to occur to help the patient accept the loss and maintain dignity. With other roles, only certain aspects of the role may change. For example, in the parenting role, patients may still function as support systems for a child, although they can no longer be the disciplinarian. Whatever the role loss, the patient needs to be allowed to grieve the loss. The nursing diagnosis of *Grieving* may help in planning care for the patient.

New roles the patient may have to assume related to chronic illness include dependent, ongoing health care consumer, self-care agent, and chronically ill person. Patients need to learn how to cope with these new roles. They need to gather knowledge and be given understanding while they become familiar with these roles. For patients used to being independent before the illness, being dependent on others to meet activities of daily living can cause a loss in self-esteem. Navigating the complex health care and financial reimbursement systems can be overwhelming. Transportation needs and waiting times for medical appointments can be difficult for the patient who must deal with them on an ongoing basis. Becoming a self-care agent requires assuming responsibility for meeting one's own care needs. *Deficient Knowledge* and *Readiness for Enhanced Knowledge* are nursing diagnoses helpful for fostering learning for these new roles.

As patients live with chronic illness over time, they become experts on their own illness. However, today's health care system often tends to assume control over patients and does not respect the patient's own knowledge. Patients who are not given this respect take charge of caring for themselves by seeking knowledge and trying complementary healing methods. Being sensitive to the patient's knowledge and respecting it increases patients' self-esteem.

Family and Caregivers

Families are affected by the chronic illness of a family member in many ways. Most chronic illness care is provided in the home so that families become involved in the management of the illness (see the *Home Health Hints* box). Family members may have to take on new family roles or assume the role of caregiver. Decreased socialization, lost income, and increased medical expenses can increase family stress and tension. For more information, visit www.caregiver.org or contact Family Caregiver Alliance, 180 Montgomery St., Suite 1100, San Francisco, CA, 94104, (415) 434-3388 or (800) 445-8106.

Families must learn to cope with the stress of illness and its often unpredictable course. Most families develop ways to cope with the patient's illness the majority of the time and may become closer as a family unit. Families often deal with the illness on a day-by-day basis and take a passive approach to letting problems work themselves out. During times of exacerbation or crisis, however, the family may need coping assistance.

Patients are often concerned about being a burden to their families. It is important to determine both the family's and the patient's feelings about the care required by the patient. The family's ability to provide this care adequately must also be considered in care planning. If the family lacks the desire, skills, or resources to adequately care for the patient, alternative care options must be explored such as home health care, adult foster care, or long-term care.

Patients' caregivers often have certain ideas about the care that the patient should receive. This may come into conflict with the views of health care providers. Caregiver input into the patient's plan of care should be sought so that everyone has a clear understanding of goals and expectations for the patient's care.

Caregivers commonly experience depression, role strain, guilt, powerlessness, and grieving related to caregiving.

Home Health Hints

Self-Concept/Humor

- Home care nurses can strengthen a patient's self-care capacity by (1) saying "Let me assist you" instead of "Let me do this for you," (2) being a partner in caring instead of being a caregiver, and (3) empowering the patient instead of doing it all for him or her.
- The home health nurse has an opportunity to increase a patient's self-concept by emphasizing the patient's existing abilities, joys, and talents. This can be done by observing the home environment for clues: photographs, trophies, hobby paraphernalia, flowers, or homemade items. Each clue observed can be a springboard to discussing triumphs and losses. It can help the nurse understand how the patient copes, which will assist in planning care.
- Being attentive to any of the patient's efforts or accomplishments, such as number of steps taken, shaving without help, interest in a book or TV show, or decisions on fixing up the house or cleaning, provides opportunities to offer support and praise for accomplishments.
- Using humor can be helpful during a visit, unless the patient is distraught, anxious, or angry. Comics or jokes from magazines can be read. Humor can relieve the patient's and caregiver's stress and humanize the care that must be performed. Keep in mind, however, that humor may be irritating if it is taken as downplaying the seriousness of a situation.

Resources

- Encourage the family of bed-confined patients to purchase an inexpensive portable intercom (such as a nursery monitor) to give the caregiver freedom to move about the house and hear the patient if help is needed.
- When patients have the use of only one hand or arm, provide a sponge for personal grooming instead of a washcloth; it is easier to use and hold.
- The home health social worker should be informed of any patient concerns regarding cost of medicines or equipment. Many programs are available to assist chronically ill people to obtain resources.

Cardiopulmonary Resuscitation

- Always carry a pocket mask for cardiopulmonary resuscitation (CPR).
- Encourage discussion regarding advance directives with the patient and family/caregiver early in the care process. Decisions regarding resuscitation and the use of technology to prolong life are more difficult when the patient is in crisis.
- Refer families to community CPR classes as desired. Families can be empowered and the patient may feel more secure when families are taught CPR.
- Patients and families should be taught that if an ambulance is called they should turn on an outside light, open the door, and move furniture, if possible, to enable the emergency medical technicians to get to the patient more easily.

Being aware of this will help nurses detect indications that caregivers are in need of help in dealing with these feelings. Chronic-care coaches are available who can provide caregivers with insight, encouragement, and support for caring for someone who is chronically ill. Nursing diagnoses for caregivers include *Risk for Caregiver Role Strain* and *Caregiver Role Strain.*

RESPITE CARE. When caregivers are required to provide 24-hour care for a patient, they can experience burnout, fatigue, and stress, which, if extreme, might lead to patient abuse. Caregivers may not be able to leave patients alone even briefly because of wandering behaviors, confusion, or safety issues. They may not ever be able to get a normal night's sleep and suffer from sleep deprivation because of the patient's wandering or around-the-clock treatment needs.

Caregivers must be given periodic relief from their responsibilities of caregiving to reduce the stress of always having to be responsible. Everyone requires private time for reflection or pursuing favorite hobbies or interests. Caregivers may need to get away overnight or for a weekend simply to sleep soundly and be refreshed.

Respite care is designed to provide caregivers with a much-needed break from caregiving by providing someone else to assume the caregiver role. Be familiar with your community's respite care services and share that information with caregivers. Unfortunately, there are often not enough respite care services available to meet the needs of caregivers. Most respite care is provided by volunteers who receive training. As the number of chronically ill people grows, more respite care programs are being developed to promote the health of the caregiver and in turn the patient.

CRITICAL THINKING

Mrs. Burden

■ Mrs. Burden, age 64, is caring for her husband, who has Alzheimer's disease. He wanders. He gets up at night and in freezing winter weather is found walking down the street in only his pajamas. He tries to cook

continued

CRITICAL THINKING—cont'd

and burns the pans. He cannot express his needs. He disrobes frequently and is incontinent. Mrs. Burden quit her job to care for him. She no longer goes to lunch weekly with her friends. Her children live out of town. She places a chair and tin cans in front of the home's doors as an alarm in case her husband opens the doors while she tries to sleep.

1. What indicates that Mrs. Burden is experiencing stress related to caregiving?
2. What nursing diagnoses should be included in a plan of care for Mrs. Burden?
3. What nursing interventions would be beneficial for Mrs. Burden?

Suggested answers at end of chapter.

Finances

Managing a chronic illness can be expensive. Income can be lost if the patient is unable to work or caregivers are forced to stay home. Family savings can quickly be wiped out. If the patient is covered by insurance, it may not cover all of the patient's expenses or it may have caps on lifetime coverage amounts. Expenses may involve medications, medical equipment or supplies, therapy, acute care, and home care. Inadequate funds can place a strain on families. This can lead to the nursing diagnoses *Compromised Family Coping, Disabled Family Coping,* or *Readiness for Enhanced Family Coping.* Nurses may need to refer patients to a social worker or sources of financial aid to help them meet their financial needs.

Health Promotion

Health promotion is possible and necessary at all levels of age or disability. With the increase in the elderly population, it is essential to understand the role of health promotion for older adults who have chronic illness. Patients with chronic illness make daily lifestyle choices that affect their health. For example, the patient with chronic lung disease who smokes can make a choice to smoke or to quit smoking. Patients with degenerative joint disease can choose whether or not to keep their weight within ideal weight ranges to reduce wear and tear on their joints. Those with arthritis can reduce their fatigue levels by pacing their activities and scheduling daily rest periods.

Those with chronic illness consider health promotion important, so encourage health promotion efforts. Patients need to be helped to strive toward high-level wellness. This can be achieved by looking at the patient's strengths and weaknesses holistically to develop a plan of care. Determine the patient's risk factors to help plan methods of promoting health. Providing patients with knowledge to make informed decisions empowers them to take control of their lives and reach their greatest potential.

Nursing Care

Because of the nature of chronic illness, nurses should understand the unique needs of patients and families experiencing chronic illness. These needs differ from those of patients experiencing acute care as far as depth of knowledge needs and the compounding problems that are usually faced by the patient. Develop an understanding that the wishes of the patient must be respected even if you do not agree with them. Patients have the right to establish their own goals in partnership with the health care team.

Most chronic illness care occurs in the home and community rather than the acute care setting. Therefore, family members and caregivers, even more so than in acute care, must be assessed and included in the plan of care. As the numbers of those with chronic illness grow, community support for chronically ill people and their caregivers needs to continue to grow. Training programs for caregivers should be available and offered affordably.

A major focus of nursing care for the chronically ill is teaching. These patients and their families have tremendous educational needs if they are to learn to cope successfully with a long-term illness. The following are primary tasks that chronically ill patients need to perform:

- Be willing and able to carry out the medical regimen.
- Reorder time to meet demands caused by the illness, such as treatments, medication schedules, and pacing of activities.
- Understand and control symptoms.
- Prevent and manage crises.
- Adjust to changes in the disease over the course of time, whether positive or negative.
- Prevent social isolation as a result of physical limitations or an altered body image.
- Compensate for symptoms and limitations in order to be treated as normally as possible by others.

Explain individualized interventions to deal with these tasks during teaching sessions. Provide dignity and show respect to these patients (Box 14.4, *Patient Perspective*). Unique approaches are needed to positively assist chronically ill patients and their families on their long-term journey.

Box 14.4
Patient Perspective

Mr. Lyman

To the nurse caring for me:

- Don't call me "sweetie" or "honey." My name is Mr. Lyman. If I want you to call me by my first name, I'll tell you.
- Be polite!
- Don't give me a huge glass of water—give me a small glass and don't fill it full. Otherwise, when I drink it, it spills all down the front of me.
- When you leave my meal tray, make sure I can reach it. Then when you take it away, don't leave a bunch of stuff on my table. There is not much room on those little tables.
- Ask how I like my blankets. Don't just do them the way you do for anyone else.
- Make sure my call light is where I can reach it.
- Make sure my overhead light is working and that I can reach it.
- Keep a waste basket where I can reach it.
- Ask if I need anything before you leave the room.
- Try to talk quietly in the hallway, instead of being so loud.
- Thank you for preserving my dignity and showing me respect. I appreciate it!

SUGGESTED ANSWERS TO

CRITICAL THINKING

Mrs. Michael

Prenatal education information should be offered to Mrs. Michael and her husband. This education should include an overview of Mrs. Michael's health needs, what to expect during pregnancy, ways Mrs. Michael's husband can be supportive, and information on prenatal classes. Mrs. Michael's physical examination should include a vaginal examination, blood pressure, and blood work. It is important to be aware of any sexually transmitted diseases that may be transferred to the developing fetus or during birth. A rubella titer (a test for immunity to rubella or measles) is important because of potential birth defects if the mother has rubella while pregnant. Elevated blood glucose may be a sign of diabetes, and low red blood cell counts and low hemoglobin are related to anemia.

To prepare a woman for pregnancy, prenatal vitamins or vitamins with iron and folic acid (necessary for effective neural tube development in the first 3 months of pregnancy) are recommended. Because of the increased workload of the heart during pregnancy, blood pressure needs to be closely monitored. Eating a balanced diet, maintaining an exercise program, and continuing to develop effective and positive ways to deal with stress are very important for pregnant women. In preparation for pregnancy, Mrs. Michael also needs information on the negative effects that cigarette smoking, alcohol use, and drug use can have on the developing fetus.

Mr. Paul

1. Mr. Paul's physical health is being affected by poor diet choices, excessive stomach acid secretion or other gastrointestinal problems, and stress.
2. It is easy to recognize the psychological stress related to parenting skills when a child is in trouble. Decreased family income with increased family expenses (two children in college) can cause financial strains and more economic pressure on Mr. Paul's business. With family problems or health problems, Mr. Paul may be questioning why things are happening to him and his family, causing him spiritual distress.

Mr. Klein

1. Ageism, stereotypical misconceptions about older adults, is occurring. This can lead to the belief that pain is part of the aging process and, therefore, it is often not diagnosed and treated appropriately.
2. Gathering data to assist with the diagnosis of the cause of the pain and treatment for the pain would improve Mr. Klein's quality of life. Taking him seriously would also convey that Mr. Klein is a valued member of society and increase his self-esteem.

Mrs. Riccardi

1. Falls could be caused by environmental problems, such as throw rugs that may move or cause tripping, clutter, electrical cords in walking paths, lack of hand grips in the bathroom, or lack of nonskid mats in the

SUGGESTED ANSWERS TO—cont'd

shower or tub. Poor vision and altered depth perception can result in missing a stair step or obstacles. Weakness or orthostatic hypotension can cause an unsteady gait or fall.
2. It is important for the nurse to instruct the patient and family about home safety. Mrs. Riccardi may even benefit by using a cane or a walker if she is unsteady. Because Mrs. Riccardi lives alone, an emergency alert system, such as a small transmitter that is worn around the neck or wrist with a button that can be activated in emergencies, would be beneficial. When activated, the transmitter alerts an answering service to contact designated individuals to check on the patient. Safety with medications is also an important consideration. Patients who take medications that lower blood pressure must be aware of the potential for orthostatic hypotension. Orthostatic hypotension is a drop in blood pressure that happens when a person moves from a lying to sitting or sitting to standing position. It is often accompanied by dizziness or light-headedness. Some people may even faint, causing a fall.
3. Two tablets of 50 mg each.

■ *Mr. Soloman*

1. Mr. Soloman had lost control of his world and felt powerless. His environment, both home and outdoors, was shrinking. He had to give up his daily routines and interactions with others. His purpose in life was gone when he was no longer caring for his wife. He was separated from his loved one. His visual limitations made his new environment unfamiliar and frightening.
2. Options to keep him safely in his home could have been explored with his input. After the move, he should have been thoroughly oriented to his environment. He should have been asked to explain what he wanted his life to be like as he adapted to this new time in his life. Hobbies and interests should have been continued. Visual support services should have been contacted for ideas. Transportation should have been arranged to allow him to visit his wife and golf. It should have been determined whether phone calls to his wife were possible.
3. He was depressed and slept from a lack of interests. His lungs were at risk for pneumonia because of his long periods of immobility. He lost hope and gave up on living, which decreased his ability to fight the pneumonia.

■ *Mrs. Burden*

1. Mrs. Burden is at risk for sleep deprivation, fatigue, stress, and burnout.
2. Nursing diagnoses include *Disturbed Sleep Pattern, Fatigue, Social Isolation, Risk for Caregiver Role Strain,* and *Deficient Knowledge.*
3. Beneficial nursing interventions would include teaching about Alzheimer's, a chronic-care coach, respite care referral, alarm devices for wandering, and stress management techniques.

REVIEW QUESTIONS

1. The nurse is collecting data regarding a 68-year-old patient's developmental stage and finds that the patient is retired and that the patient's spouse died 4 months ago. The nurse identifies the patient as being in which of the following developmental stages?
   a. Generativity versus self-absorption
   b. Identity versus role confusion
   c. Integrity versus despair
   d. Intimacy versus isolation
2. The nurse is planning care for a patient with heart disease. Which of the following effects should the nurse consider is most likely to occur with a chronic illness when gathering further data collection?
   a. Hopefulness
   b. Increased socialization
   c. Powerfulness
   d. Spiritual distress

REVIEW QUESTIONS—cont'd

3. A 70-year-old man is the primary caregiver for his wife, who has moderately severe Alzheimer's disease. He becomes angry with her for spilling her dinner on the floor. He later feels guilty and begins to cry. The home health nurse is developing a plan of care. Which of the following would be an appropriate nursing diagnosis for the nurse to include?
   a. *Caregiver Role Strain*
   b. *Hopelessness*
   c. *Powerlessness*
   d. *Risk for Caregiver Role Strain*

4. A 64-year-old woman goes to a clinic for a yearly physical. She has a history of hypertension and osteoarthritis. In contributing to the plan of care, which of the following would be a priority intervention to promote wellness in this patient who has chronic illnesses?
   a. Demonstrating how to take a blood pressure
   b. Explaining hypertension and osteoarthritis
   c. Encouraging increased socialization
   d. Evaluating progress with the patient and family

5. The nurse is providing care for a chronically ill patient. Which of the following are appropriate nursing interventions for a chronically ill patient? **Select all that apply.**
   a. Limiting educational information
   b. Encouraging visits by family members
   c. Including family members in teaching sessions
   d. Setting the goals for the patient
   e. Limiting visits from friends
   f. Obtaining patient input on plan of care

6. Which of the following nursing interventions would be most appropriate for a patient with a chronic illness who is experiencing chronic sorrow? **Select all that apply.**
   a. Provide quiet time.
   b. Make time to listen.
   c. Share information.
   d. Limit interactions.
   e. Use active listening.
   f. Encourage hope.

7. The nurse would evaluate the patient with a chronic illness as responding positively to interventions for chronic sorrow if the patient stated which of the following?
   a. "I have nothing left to accomplish."
   b. "Maybe tomorrow will be a better day."
   c. "I should not keep hoping for a cure."
   d. "There is nothing I can do."

References

Erikson, E. H. (1980). *Identity and the life cycle.* New York: W.W. Norton & Company.

Erikson, E. H. (1993). *Childhood and society.* New York: W.W. Norton & Company.

15 Nursing Care of Older Adult Patients

MARYANNE PIETRANIEC-SHANNON

KEY TERMS

activities of daily living (ack-TIH-vih-tees of DAY-lee LIH-ving)
arrhythmias (uh-RITH-mee-yahs)
aspiration (AS-pi-RAY-shun)
constipation (KON-sti-PAY-shun)
contractures (kon-TRACK-churs)
delirium (del-LEER-ee-um)
dementia (dee-MEN-cha)
depression (dih-PRESH-shun)
edema (eh-DEE-muh)
expectorate (eck-SPEK-tuh-RAYT)
extrinsic factors (eks-TRIN-sick FAK-ters)
holistic (hoh-LISS-tick)
homeostasis (HOH-mee-oh-STAY-siss)
intrinsic factors (in-TRIN-sick FAK-ters)
nocturia (nock-TOO-ree-ah)
optimum level of functioning (OP-tih-mum LEV-uhl of FUNK-shun-ing)
osteoporosis (AWS-tee-oh-puh-ROH-siss)
perception (per-SEP-shun)
pressure ulcer (PRESH-ur ULL-sir)
range of motion (RAINJE of MOH-shun)
reality orientation (ree-AL-ih-tee OR-ee-en-TAY-shun)
sensory deprivation (SEN-suh-ree DEP-rih-VAY-shun)
sensory overload (SEN-suh-ree OH-ver-lohd)
urinary incontinence (YOUR-ih-NARE-ee in-KON-tih-nents)

QUESTIONS TO GUIDE YOUR READING

1. How would you define aging?
2. What basic physiological changes are associated with advancing age?
3. How would you describe the psychological and cognitive changes associated with advancing age?
4. What are the nursing implications for the physiological and psychological changes associated with advancing age?
5. What nursing practices promote safety for the older patient?

WHAT IS AGING?

Over time it is easy to see changes that occur in the human body. Both physical structures and body functions undergo changes and declines with advancing age. Although there is not one commonly accepted definition or theory to explain these declines, there is an understanding that aging is a universal and normal process that starts at conception and continues until death.

Older adults are increasing in number. In 2000, 34.7 million adults were older than age 65 and by 2030 this number is expected to be 71.5 million (U.S. Census Bureau, 2004). The fastest growing segment within this group is those older than age 85. Although this group accounted for 4.3 million people in 2000, it is expected to grow to more than 9.6 million by 2030. For current population data, visit www.census.gov.

In this chapter, *aging* is defined as a maturational process that creates the need for individual adaptation because of physical and psychological declines that occur throughout life. Even though aging truly begins at conception, the focus in this chapter is on the maturational process that is experienced after age 65 (older adult). People older than age 84 usually are the frailest, although chronological age should not be the basis for determining health issues. For some people, aging effects go unnoticed in their daily functioning; for others these effects cause varying degrees of impairment. Functional age (health, independence, and functional abilities) should be used as the basis of individual care needs. It is important to understand that most older adults function independently in the home and community. Many elders remain in the workforce by choice or financial necessity. With supportive, educative care as needed, these people are able to maintain their independent abilities. This chapter discusses aging changes and the resulting disabilities that may require more intensive nursing care than that required by older adults who are independent and healthy.

NURSING CARE TIP

Placing older adults into one category titled "old" overlooks aging as a unique experience. The concept of *functional age* recognizes that aging is individual and promotes individualized nursing assessment and development of plans of care for the older adult.

Although aging is universal, it remains a unique experience for each individual. Factors that contribute to this process can be grouped into two categories. **Intrinsic factors** focus on genetic theories of aging, such as the biological clock theory or programmed aging theory, and on some aspects of physiological theories of aging, such as wear-and-tear theory or stress adaptation theory. **Extrinsic factors** focus on environmental influences, such as pollutants, free-radical theory, and stress-adaptation theory.

Regardless of which factors have the greatest influence on this process of aging, **perception** and attitude also play key roles in how changes over time affect the individual. It is through the filter of perception and attitude that the individual identifies, defines, and adapts to the changes that occur in structure and function over time. These factors have implications not only for older patients but also for their families and the health care providers working with them.

PHYSIOLOGICAL CHANGES

Over time, cells change and do not function as efficiently as in earlier years (Table 15.1). Compared with cellular changes, the physical changes seen when looking at an older person are slight. Cellular decline in structure and function increases in severity and extent over time. Although the body works hard to maintain **homeostasis**, it is often unable to fully adapt to many of the declines that result from aging. Cells that die cannot regenerate themselves. As a result, structures are altered, and the body tries to adapt to make the revised structure meet functional demands.

Common Physical Changes in Older Patients and Their Implications for Nursing

Key Changes in the Muscular System

Some key age-related changes in the muscular system include the following:

- Decrease in muscle mass, so muscles look smaller
- Decrease in muscle tone, so muscles look less toned
- Slower muscle responses, so response time is increased
- Decrease in elasticity of tendons and ligaments, restricting movements.

NURSING IMPLICATIONS. Changes in the muscular system have implications for movement, strength, and endurance. Restricted movements are most commonly seen in the arms, legs, and neck of the older patient, who may have limited **range of motion** (ROM) in these areas. Because muscle response abilities are slowed, it will take longer for the older patient to move. This increased response time has implications for the older person's confidence in being able to perform routine tasks.

WORD BUILDING

homeostasis: homios—similar + stasis—standing

TABLE 15.1 PHYSIOLOGICAL CHANGES OF AGING

Body System	Aging Change	Effect of Change
Cardiovascular	Increased conduction time	Heart rate slows, unable to increase quickly
	Decreased cardiac output	Less oxygen delivered to tissues
	Decreased blood vessel elasticity	Increased blood pressure increases cardiac workload
	Irregular heartbeats	Poor heart oxygenation, decreased cardiac output, heart failure
	Dilated leg veins, less efficient valves	Varicose veins, fluid accumulation in tissues
Endocrine and Metabolism	Slowed basal metabolic rate	Possible weight gain
	Altered adrenal hormone production	Decreased ability to respond to stress
	Decreased insulin release	Hyperglycemia
Gastrointestinal	Reduced taste and smell	Appetite may be reduced
	Decreased saliva	Dry mouth, altered taste
	Decreased gag reflex, relaxation of lower esophageal sphincter	Increased aspiration risk
	Delayed gastric emptying	Reduced appetite
	Reduced liver enzymes	Reduced drug metabolism and detoxification
	Decreased peristalsis	Reduced appetite, constipation
Genitourinary	Kidney size decreases	Able to live with 10% renal function
	Decreased bladder size, tone, changes from pear to funnel shaped	Frequency of urination increased
	Weakened muscles	Incontinence
	Decreased ability to concentrate	Nocturia
	Less sodium saved	Risk for dehydration
	Reduced renal blood flow	Decreased renal clearance of all medications
Immunological	Decreased function	Increased infection and cancer risk
	Increased autoimmune response	Increased autoimmune diseases
Integumentary	Reduced cell replacement	Healing slower
	Water loss	Dryness of the skin
	Increased pigmentation	Aging spots
	Thinning of skin layers	Skin more fragile
	Decreased subcutaneous fat	Less insulation and protective cushioning
	Decreased sebaceous and sweat glands	Dryness and decreased temperature regulation
	Hard, dry nails	Brittle nails
	Thinning scalp hair	Baldness
	Decreased melanin	Gray hair
	Decreased skin elasticity	Wrinkle development
Musculoskeletal	Decreased muscle mass	Reduced strength
	Decreased muscle tone	Muscles look flabbier
	Decreased elasticity of tendons and ligaments	Movements are restricted
	Slowed muscle responses	Response time increased
	Bone thinning, softening	Decreasing bone density
	Joint stiffening	Decreased flexibility
	Vertebral disk water loss	Decreased height
Neurologic	Loss of brain cells	Able to maintain function with remaining cells
Central nervous system	Decreased brain blood flow	Short-term memory loss
	Decreased regulation of body temperature	Hypothermia, hyperthermia risk
	Decreased endorphins	Increased depression
Peripheral nervous system	Decreased sensation	Risk for injury, burns
	Increased reaction times	Slow response, injury risk
	Decreased motor coordination	Unsteady, fall risk
Respiratory	Decreased lung capacity	Dyspnea with activity
	Decreased cough and gag reflexes	Aspiration, infection risk
	Reduced lung tissue tone	Shallow, faster respirations
	Reduced lung emptying on exhalation	CO_2 retention
	Decreased fluid and ciliary action	Mucous obstruction, infection risk
Sensory	Lens less elastic	Decreased near and peripheral vision
Eye	Lens opaque, yellows	Cataracts
	Cornea more translucent	Blurry vision
	Smaller pupil	Decreased dark adaptation
	Decreased violet, blue, green color vision	See red, orange, yellow colors better
	Arcus senilis—milky lipid ring on iris edge that does not cover pupil	No effect on vision

TABLE 15.1 PHYSIOLOGICAL CHANGES OF AGING—cont'd

Body System	Aging Change	Effect of Change
Ear	Degeneration of auditory nerve	Lose high-frequency tones, deafness
	Excess bone impairs sound conduction	Deafness
Nose	Decreased smell	Decreased ability to smell substances such as smoke or gas, causing safety risk; appetite reduced
Sexuality	Availability of partner or privacy decreases	Lack of sexual expression, suppression of desires
Men	Slower sexual arousal time	Increased time needed for sexual stimulation
	Decreased erection, slower ejaculation	Psychologically causes concern
Women	Less vaginal lubrication	Painful intercourse
	Vaginal acidity reduced	Increased vaginal infection risk

Key Changes in the Skeletal System

Some key age-related changes in the skeletal system include the following:

- Eroding cartilage
- Exaggerated bony prominences
- Joint stiffening and decreased flexibility
- **Osteoporosis**, a thinning and softening of the bone
- Shortening in height caused by water loss in the intervertebral disks of the spinal column and flexion of the spine associated with the influence of gravity over time.

NURSING IMPLICATIONS. Because muscles and bones work together for movement, aging skeletal changes are most obvious when the older patient is moving. **Contractures** of the fingers and hands can limit the person's ability to perform self-care tasks called **activities of daily living** (ADL). It is important to assist the patient with ROM exercises if help is needed to prevent the long-term disabilities that contractures bring (Fig. 15.1). Performing ROM exercises in warm water helps the patient for whom movement is uncomfortable. If the person has arthritis, the administration of any prescribed anti-inflammatory medications should be timed so their action peaks when the exercises begin. Older patients on anti-inflammatory medicines should be monitored closely for gastrointestinal upset or bleeding and taught the symptoms of bleeding to report.

Decreased bone density is influenced by diet and weight-bearing exercise, so balanced diets rich in calcium and vitamin D and safe and sensible weight-bearing exercise programs should be promoted (see *Evidence-Based Practice* box).

Encourage patients to ambulate whenever possible wearing supportive, sensible shoes with nonskid soles. In addition to making sure the environment is safe for walking, sturdy assistive devices such as handrails, canes, or walkers should be encouraged as needed. Because of the decreasing density of older bones, fractures may not only result from falls; they may cause falls as well.

WORD BUILDING

osteoporosis: osteon—bone + poros—a passage + osis—condition

EVIDENCE-BASED PRACTICE

Clinical Question

What factors reduce falls in elderly residents in long-term care?

Evidence

A systematic reviews of 41 trials, which included 25,422 participants, revealed that vitamin D supplementation in nursing home residents is effective in reducing the rate of falls, but not the risk of falling (Cameron et al., 2010). Additionally, pharmacist review of medications may also reduce falls. Multifactorial interventions, when provided by a multidisciplinary team, were also shown to reduce the rate of falls.

Implications for Nursing Practice

Nurses can advocate for the use of vitamin D supplementation as appropriate, ensure that all residents have a pharmacist review of their medications, and participate in multidisciplinary teams to provide interventions to reduce falls for elderly residents.

REFERENCE

Cameron, I. D., Murray, G. R., Gillespie, L. D., et al. (2010). Interventions for preventing falls in older people in nursing care facilities and hospitals. *Cochrane Database of Systematic Reviews, Issue 1* (Art. No. CD005465; DOI 10.1002/14651858.CD005465.pub2).

SAFETY TIP

Implement a fall reduction program and evaluate the effectiveness of the program. Involve residents/patients and their families to promote patient safety. Identify patients at risk for falls. Evaluation may include a history of falls, medication review, alcohol use assessment, gait and balance screening, and use of assistive aids (2010 National Patient Safety Goals, www.jointcommission.org).

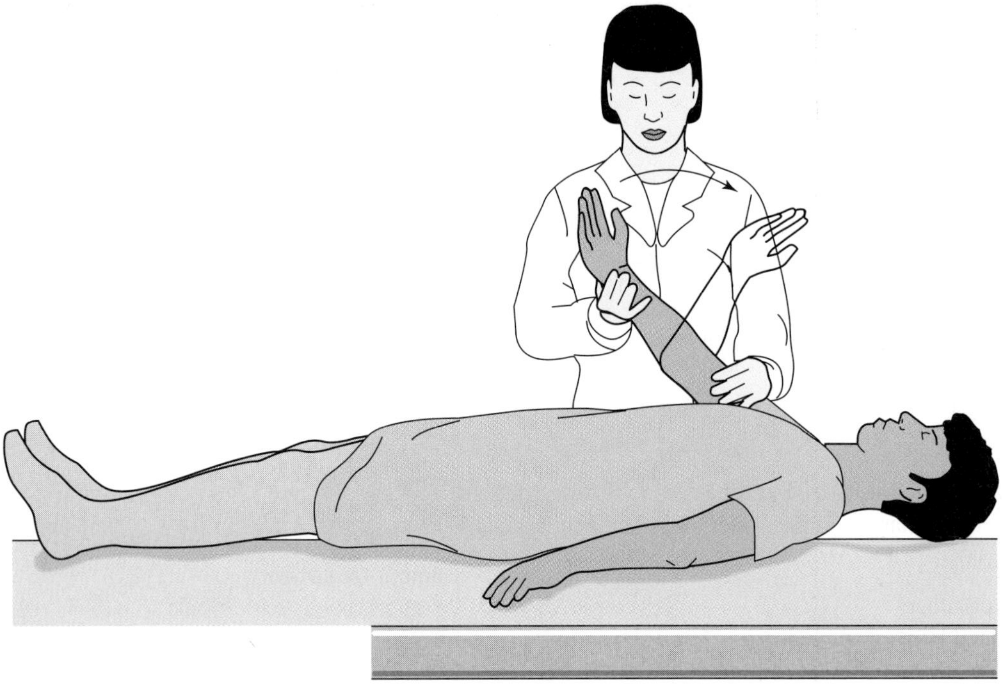

Figure 15.1 Nurse assists patient in range-of-motion exercises to prevent the development of contractures.

Key Changes in the Integumentary System

Some key age-related changes in the integumentary system include the following:

- Increased dryness of the skin
- Increased pigmentation, causing liver or aging spots
- Thinning of the skin layers, which makes the skin more fragile
- Decreased skin elasticity, causing wrinkles to develop
- Decreased subcutaneous fat layer, so older patients have less insulation and less protective cushioning
- Hardness and dryness of nails, making them more brittle
- Decrease in nail growth rate and strength
- Thinning of scalp hair, mainly in men
- Increased growth and coarseness of nose, ear, and facial hair
- Decrease in melanin, which result in gray hair
- Decreased sebaceous and sweat glands, which has implications for dryness and decreased temperature regulation.

NURSING IMPLICATIONS. The skin, which is the first line of defense against infection and injury, does not work as effectively in older patients (Fig. 15.2). In the older adult, skin injuries take longer to heal, and those longer healing times are usually complicated by the fact that many older patients have multiple chronic diseases, such as diabetes and circulatory ailments.

The older patient with limited mobility is especially prone to developing **pressure ulcers** (Fig. 15.3). These ulcers are caused by ischemia that results from continuous pressure on an area of the body. They usually develop over a bony prominence (e.g., ears, shoulders, elbows, tip of the

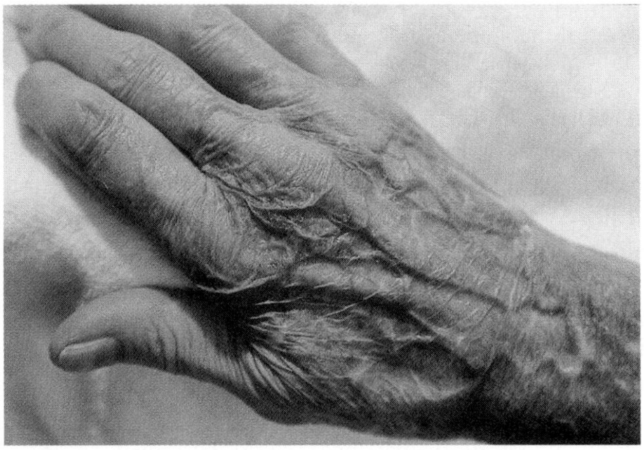

Figure 15.2 Thin, fragile skin of an older person.

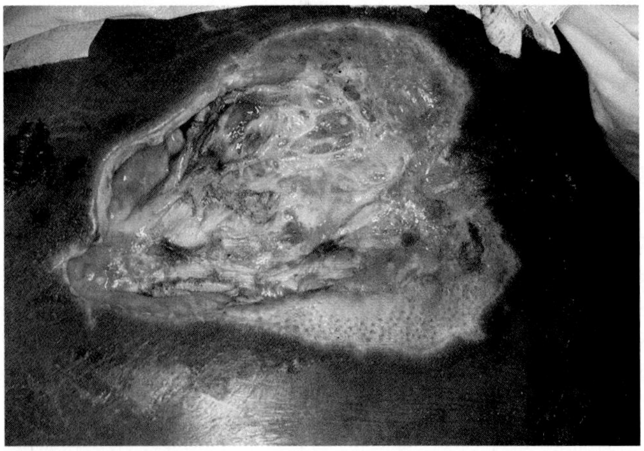

Figure 15.3 Pressure ulcer. (From Goldsmith, L. A., Lazarus, G. S., & Tharp, M. D. [1997]. *Adult and pediatric dermatology: A color guide to diagnosis and treatment* [p. 445]. Philadelphia: F. A. Davis.)

spine, pelvic bone ridges, knees, heels, or ankles). Ischemia from unrelieved pressure can begin to develop in 20 to 40 minutes. Early signs of pressure ulcer formation are warmth, redness, tenderness, and a burning sensation at the potential ulcer site. These potential ulcer sites are aggravated by lack of activity and the weight of the body. For this reason, it is especially important to take time to assess skin integrity daily, especially in high-risk areas of the body.

SAFETY TIP

Assess and periodically reassess each resident's risk for developing a pressure ulcer and take action to address any identified risks (2010 National Patient Safety Goals, www.jointcommission.org).

Skin care includes gently stimulating nonreddened intact skin sites with massage, using gentle bathing techniques, moisturizing with creams regularly, avoiding the use of hot water, refraining from overuse of a complete daily bath, and limiting the overuse of soap. If able, patients should be taught to shift their weight every 15 minutes when sitting. For immobile patients, consistent repositioning is essential. Ideally, use of pressure-relieving devices or repositioning every 30 minutes as able is the most beneficial for high-risk patients to help prevent pressure ulcer development (see Chapter 54). Keeping bed linens clean, dry, and wrinkle free also aids in the prevention of pressure ulcer formation.

As with care of the skin, nail care is important for older people. Soaking in warm water helps soften nails to ease in their trimming while encouraging blood flow to the peripheral areas of the body. Filing the nails with an emery board is safer than cutting the nails. To prevent accidental injury to the feet, patients should be instructed not to walk barefoot. Potential pressure points of the feet should be identified and closely monitored, and the patient should be referred to a podiatrist for treatment if there are any concerns. People with diabetes should assess their feet daily because they may have decreased sensation (neuropathy), causing lack of awareness of foot irritation or injury.

Key Changes in the Cardiovascular System

Some key age-related changes in the cardiovascular system include the following:

- Slowed heart rate
- Decreased cardiac output from less effective functioning of the heart and blood vessels, yielding less oxygen to body tissues
- Decreased elasticity of the blood vessels, so the circulatory system is less efficient
- Reduced ability of the heart to quickly increase its rate in response to an emergency because of thickening of the heart valves, left ventricle, and aorta (when rate does increase, the heart takes longer to return to resting rate)
- More **arrhythmias** (irregular heartbeats), which lead to poor oxygenation of the heart
- Commonly, a lack of classic symptoms of cardiac emergencies
- Increased peripheral vascular resistance in blood vessels, yielding increased blood pressure
- More visible superficial blood vessels of the legs
- Less efficient leg vein valves, creating the risk for an accumulation of excess fluids in the leg tissues.

NURSING IMPLICATIONS. Be a good observer when it comes to caring for older patients because many early symptoms related to circulatory problems are subtle. Cardiovascular disease, which is separate from the process of aging, accounts for half of all deaths in people older than age 65. Older adults must be educated about prevention practices that promote healthy circulation and encouraged to take prescribed medications as ordered. In addition to encouraging oral fluids to balance fluid output in older patients, the nurse must carefully monitor for the hazards of fluid overload in all older patients on intravenous therapy.

Special care should be taken to maintain good skin integrity and provide appropriate stimulation. If **edema** is present in the legs, they should be elevated to promote fluid return to the upper body; supportive, nonrestrictive stockings should be worn as ordered. Concerns regarding leg and foot circulation in the older patient must be identified and reported as early as possible so the primary care provider can order the appropriate arterial or venous therapy to address circulatory concerns before they become problems.

Because quick changes in body position can make the older patient feel weak and dizzy, it is important to stand next to older patients as they dangle their legs over the side of the bed before rising to stand. Changes in body position from lying to sitting to standing should occur gradually to accommodate the less efficient circulatory system seen in older patients. Older patients may find comfort in the security of an ambulatory belt or walker if they fear unsteadiness in an upright position. Because falls continue to rank as a leading cause of accidental death in older patients (and because a history of falls remains the key indicator to predict future falls), it is important for the nurse to identify fall risk to determine which older patient may be at greater risk so preventive measures can be documented in the care plan.

Key Changes in the Respiratory System

Some key age-related changes in the respiratory system include the following:

- Decreased lung capacity
- Weaker cough or gag reflex, increasing the risk of upper respiratory infection

WORD BUILDING

edema: oidema—swelling

- Reduced tone of lung tissue, so respirations increase to 16 to 25 per minute and are more shallow
- Reduced tone of the diaphragm muscle
- Less complete emptying of the lungs, with greater CO_2 retention
- Decreased blood flow to the lungs, contributing to cardiac arrhythmias.

NURSING IMPLICATIONS. Because the respiratory system is less efficient with advancing age, older patients have a decreased tolerance for activity. Nurses should, therefore, pace activities for older patients instead of letting them confine themselves to bed. The nurse should schedule rest periods to prevent overexertion; however, rest periods should not outnumber the activity sessions planned throughout the course of the patient's day.

Cough, marked fatigue, and confusion may be early signs of inadequate oxygen uptake. Respiratory rates greater than 25 per minute may be an early indication of a lower respiratory tract infection. Because overall muscle strength is reduced, the older patient performs the O_2–CO_2 exchange in the less efficient upper lobes of the lung instead of the larger lower lobes specifically designed for this purpose. Because lung recoil strength is decreased, mucus may be more difficult for the older patient to **expectorate** (cough up). This situation is compounded by the fact that older people also have less effective cough and gag reflexes, which creates greater potential for lung problems.

Because of the normal changes that take place in the respiratory system with aging, it is important to include coughing, deep breathing, and position changes in an exercise program designed to stimulate all lobes of the older patient's lungs. At the prevention level, encourage the older person to receive a pneumonia vaccination and an annual flu shot. This is important because influenza and pneumonia combine to be the fourth leading cause of death in people over age 65. Be aware that lifelong habits, such as smoking and respiratory pollutant exposure in employment settings, secondhand smoke, or paints and glues used in hobbies, are cumulative over time and can contribute to respiratory sensitivity for the older patient. Nurses can help prevent the spread of respiratory illnesses by getting flu shots themselves, washing hands between patients, not exposing patients to any nurses' illness, and using universal precautions.

Key Changes in the Gastrointestinal System

Some key age-related changes in the gastrointestinal system include the following:

- Changes in taste and smell, which affect the enjoyment of eating
- Decreased saliva production
- Decreased gag reflex and relaxation of lower esophageal sphincter, increasing the risk of **aspiration** (inhalation of oropharyngeal or gastric contents into the lower airways)
- Delayed gastric emptying
- No functional changes in the small intestine
- Decreased tone in the external sphincter
- Marked decline in liver enzymes, which affects drug metabolism and detoxification
- Decreased peristalsis from generalized weakness of muscle activity
- Alteration in bowel habits.

NURSING IMPLICATIONS. Many factors can alter appetite, ingestion, digestion, and absorption of nutrients in food, regardless of age. However, the structural and functional changes that occur with advancing age put the older patient at greater risk for not obtaining the nutrients needed to sustain a healthy body system (Box 15.1, *Nutrition Notes*).

Little can be done to change the physical alterations in the older body that make getting needed nutrients more difficult. Being knowledgeable and committed to providing the support needed to meet nutritional goals is important. Patients should be assisted with toileting before sitting down to eat. An appropriate amount of time must be provided for the older patient to accomplish the task of eating. If the patient needs help with eating, the nurse must be sensitive to the patient's pace while giving the patient as much control of the process as possible.

Additional forms of support recognize that, for some cultures, eating has a strong social component. Encourage the patient to eat out of bed and with others as much as possible, while respecting the patient's right of refusal to eat in a designated social setting. Some patients may not eat as well when seated next to agitated or confused residents in a common dining hall.

Offer continuing support by maintaining a calm and comfortable environment that aids digestion. Food combinations that enhance nutrient absorption should be offered together whenever possible (e.g., when a vitamin C food is taken with plant foods high in iron, vitamin C increases the iron absorption rate). Familiar seasonings can help stimulate a lagging appetite; ask family members to bring the patient's favorite seasonings in shakers so the patient can apply them as needed. Working with a dietitian may provide other ideas to promote healthful eating for older patients.

Although many older patients wear dentures or partial plates, it is important not to assume that all older people wear dentures. Tooth loss is not a normal change of aging because, with proper dental care, teeth can last a lifetime. If an older patient does have dentures, be aware that any significant change in body weight will affect the fit and comfort of the dentures and, therefore, affect nutritional intake. Because of this, it is important to conduct regular assessments of the mouth when assisting the older patient during oral care.

Medications may cause taste disturbances or problems with dry mouth that may also affect the older patient's ability to meet nutritional needs. Some medications create problems with bowel motility, resulting in **constipation**. Constipation

WORD BUILDING

expectorate: ex—out + pectus—breast

TABLE 15.2 NURSING CARE FOCUS ON SAFETY ALPHABET FOR OLDER PATIENTS

A is for ABILITIES	• Know your abilities. • Know patient's abilities. • Base nursing actions on your abilities. • Seek out assistance when needed.
B is for BODY MECHANICS AND ALIGNMENT	• Use proper body mechanics. • Use appropriate assistive devices. • Ensure patient is in proper body alignment.
C is for COMFORT	• Ensure physical and emotional comfort during care. • Use pain scale during each assessment.
D is for DELIBERATE MOVEMENTS	• Plan ahead and communicate plans to patient. • Demonstrate confidence during care. • Alert patient to planned movements by saying, "Moving on three. One, two, three." • Ensure patient assists with moves as able.
E is for ENVIRONMENT	• Always place call light within reach. • Keep environment uncluttered and safe. • Ask patient's permission before moving items. • Put items back as patient prefers.
F is for FALLS	• Remember that falls are a primary concern for older patients. • Use interventions to prevent falls: Assist patients with ambulation, use assistive devices, answer call lights promptly, provide accessible toileting facilities, use night-lights, avoid use of throw rugs.
G is for GIVING YOUR TIME	• Allow more time to perform actions. • Do not rush older patients. • Provide time for listening and observing, so concerns are addressed before becoming problems.
H is for HAND WASHING	• Use correct hand washing protocols to protect yourself and older patients. • Use standard precautions to protect yourself and older patients.

Home Health Hints

Home Visits

- Schedule therapy visits and nurse visits on the same day, if possible, to decrease the risk of fatiguing the older patient.
- Because many older patients keep their homes warm, wear layers of clothing, removing a layer as needed, rather than adjusting the heat in the home.
- Place cell phones and pagers on a silent mode, if possible, to avoid startling or confusing the older patient.
- Do not assume that the older patient will remember the health care nurses who come to the door. Each time, state your name and why you are there. Wear a large-letter photo name tag that is in clear view.
- To enhance the effectiveness of a visit, ask the older patient to talk in a quiet room of the home with the main caregiver invited in at the appropriate time. This may help the older patient stay more focused while ensuring privacy and fostering the person's ability to hear.
- Stressors in a patient's life, such as annoying visitors, chastisement by caregivers, and harassment by bill collectors, are often experienced firsthand by the home health nurse. Document and share those with the home care team, so a coordinated approach can be taken.

Home Environment

- Making a sign for the door of the home giving visitors instructions, such as ringing the doorbell several times, knocking loudly, or using another door, may be helpful to visitors of the older patient. Do not provide specific information that would put the older person at risk for victimization.
- Assess the older patient's environment for safety hazards on each visit, and promote safety. Patients can easily trip on a scatter rug or fall trying to navigate around furniture. Urge the patient and caregiver to pack away scatter rugs and unneeded furniture.
- If the home is two stories, help the patient and caregiver consider how to relocate the bedroom to the first floor. Stairs are difficult to manage, especially if patients have visual disturbances or use an assistive device.
- Assist patients in obtaining a medical alert device that can be worn around the neck and activated in case of falls or other emergencies.

Medications

- Assist patients and/or caregivers with obtaining and setting up a weekly pill dispenser. These can be purchased

Continued

Home Health Hints—cont'd

at the local pharmacy. For patients who are forgetful, a pill dispenser with a timer can be purchased. An audible or visual alarm will go off when it is time for them to take medications.

- It is important for the home health nurse to assess the patient's ability to follow instructions. During visits, check the medication dispenser to ensure that pills are being taken as prescribed. If there is a concern, inform the primary care provider.

Nutrition/Fluids

- One of the first signs of dehydration is tachycardia. Instruct the patient regarding adequate hydration.
- If the older patient has dentures, assess if they are worn for eating. If not, assess why they are not worn (e.g., sores, improper fit from weight loss) and discuss solutions.
- Check the refrigerator for outdated food. Many older patients are on a limited budget and have been taught not to waste food. These factors, along with a decreased sense of smell and taste, can increase the risk of food poisoning.
- Encourage the uses of spices and herbs, such as parsley, oregano, lemon, garlic, and basil, instead of salt and sugar. Suggest keeping pared apples and segments of oranges in the refrigerator for snacks.
- If a Meals on Wheels program is available, ask if the older patient would like to be placed on the service.
- Use a warming tray when feeding an older patient who takes a longer time to eat.
- When swallowing is difficult, freezing of liquids helps, so they can be eaten with a spoon or like a popsicle. Milkshakes, high-protein drinks, instant breakfast mix, or eggnog are thicker liquids that are easier to swallow.

Elimination

- If an older person wears perineal pads or adult briefs, ask how many are used in a 24-hour period to assess the degree of incontinency or amount of output. Have the patient keep a voiding diary to further assess the degree of incontinence.
- Suggest a bedside commode when a weakened older patient is on diuretics or has a history of falling or confusion. Placing it next to the bed at night helps reduce the risk of falls and eases caregiver burden.
- If the older patient reports constipation, review the diet and make suggestions regarding adequate fluid and fiber. A mixture of equal parts of applesauce, bran, and prune juice is often helpful to prevent or relieve constipation. Discourage the use of mineral oil because it will interfere with vitamin absorption.

Rest

- If the older patient seems fatigued early in the day, ask about sleeping patterns and things that disturb it, such as barking dogs, traffic noise, and visitors. Recommend ear plugs or changing rooms to obtain a good night's rest. Check medications for insomnia listed as a side effect and suggest dosing of these medications early in the day if appropriate. A 15- to 30-minute nap in the early afternoon can be helpful.

Infection Symptom

- One of the first signs of infection in the older patient is confusion.

Education

- Suggesting that limiting visitors or not allowing persons with colds to visit can be helpful in preventing illness in the older patient.
- When auscultating lungs, ask the older patient to take deep breaths slowly in and out through the mouth. This may stimulate coughing, which is an opportune time to teach deep-breathing and coughing exercises.
- When teaching, it is important to acknowledge the patient's knowledge and life experiences. When given a chance, patients tell how they have maintained their health over the years. Use open-ended scenarios for teaching, such as "What would you do if you fell and you were alone?"
- Teaching should occur with patients, not to them. The nurse is in the patient's home, which is a personal place. Patient dignity should always remain intact during home care visits and teaching sessions.

Lab Draws

- When drawing blood from the hand of an older patient, use the smallest needle possible and a butterfly device. Hold light pressure at the injection site for at least 2 minutes after the needle is removed.
- Do not use a bandage on the fragile skin of an older patient if the bleeding has stopped with pressure.

SUGGESTED ANSWERS TO

CRITICAL THINKING

■ *Mr. Jones*

1. Does he live alone? Does he have a fall history? If so, does he wear a safety device to signal for help? What type of night-light is used? How far is it to the bathroom? Does he take his bumetanide (Bumex) early in the day rather than at night? Does he void before going to bed? Does he anticipate needing to void 30 minutes after lying down?
2. Wood floors that are slippery when wet from incontinence are a safety hazard. Throw rugs may slide or cause tripping. An appropriate night-light should be available.
3. Nursing diagnoses include *Functional Urinary Incontinence* related to distance to bathroom; *Deficient Knowledge* related to safety, medication administration, and nocturia; and *Risk for Injury* related to slippery floors from incontinence, use of throw rugs, and inadequate lighting.
4. A teaching plan should include the following:
   - *Safety:* Place urinal at bedside to prevent incontinence on way to bathroom. Consider red night-light to improve vision and prevent falls. Use easily cleaned floor covering that is secure and absorbent to avoid falls. Consider the need for wearing a device that can send a signal for help.
   - *Medication administration:* Take diuretics early in the day to avoid having to get up frequently while sleeping at night.
   - *Nocturia:* Void before lying down. Anticipate need to void after lying down by reclining in chair for 30 minutes with legs elevated before going to bed and then void on way to bed.
5. Two 0.5-mg tablets.

REVIEW QUESTIONS

1. Which of the following does the nurse understand is considered the definition of aging in planning care for the older adult?
   a. A disease state that results in the death of a person's body cells all at once
   b. A condition that starts for all people when they reach the age of 65
   c. A maturational process with individual adaptations for physical and psychological changes over time
   d. A state of accelerating decline in body functioning directly related to a disease process

2. The nurse is collecting data on a patient who is 77 years old and says "I am shorter now." The nurse would recognize that which of the following commonly contributes to individuals becoming shorter with age?
   a. Contractures
   b. Bone degeneration in the legs
   c. Hyperextension of the cervical spine
   d. Water loss from the intervertebral disks of the spine

3. Which of the following is the best approach for the nurse to use with a cognitively alert older patient recently diagnosed with hypertension that would help encourage prescribed antihypertensive medication compliance?
   a. The nurse says "It is important that you take your blood pressure pill every day. Do you understand this?"
   b. The nurse explains the medication and gives the patient a grid to record daily when the pill is taken. The nurse then asks, "How do you see this working for you?"
   c. The nurse asks the patient "Do you have a relative or friend who can call you every day to remind you to take your BP pill? It is really important that you take it and as you get older it is harder to remember things."
   d. The nurse tells the patient, "If you don't take your blood pressure pill you will probably have a heart attack or a stroke, so you better figure out a way that you don't forget to take it everyday."

4. The nurse contributes to the plan of care for an older patient on bedrest based on the understanding that pressure ulcers occur at sites of ischemia and can begin to develop as early as which of the following time frames?
   a. 5 to 10 minutes
   b. 20 to 40 minutes
   c. 50 to 60 minutes
   d. 75 to 120 minutes

REVIEW QUESTIONS—cont'd

5. The nurse is planning care for an older patient at risk for aspiration. Which of the following does the nurse understand increases the older patient's risk for aspiration?
   a. Increased lung capacity
   b. Decreased lung capacity
   c. Decreased gag reflex
   d. Increased gag reflex

6. Which of the following actions could the nurse institute to help prevent constipation in the older adult patient? **Select all that apply.**
   a. Increase dietary fiber intake.
   b. Decrease water intake.
   c. Encourage participation in ADLs.
   d. Review medication effects.
   e. Increase daily exercise.
   f. Decrease fresh fruit intake.

References

Joint Commission. (2010). *2010 national patient safety goals.* Retrieved February 12, 2010, from http://www.jointcommission.org/patientsafety/nationalpatientsafetygoals

U.S. Census Bureau. (2004). *U.S. interim projections by age, sex, race, and Hispanic origin.* Retrieved October 1, 2009, from http://www.census.gov/population/www/projections/usinterimproj/natprojtab02a.pdf

DavisPlus | For additional resources and information visit **http://davisplus.fadavis.com**

16

Nursing Care of Patients at Home

KELLY McMANIGLE

KEY TERMS

autonomous (awe-TAH-nah-mus)
collaborative (cull-AB-rah-tiv)
respite (RES-pit)

QUESTIONS TO GUIDE YOUR READING

1. How has the history of home health nursing shaped the nursing care of today?
2. Who are the members of the home health team?
3. What needs to be included when documenting information about a home visit with a patient?
4. What are some of the differences between hospital-based nursing and home health nursing?
5. What are some steps the home health nurse can take to ensure infection control?

INTRODUCTION TO HOME HEALTH NURSING

Home health nursing is health care conducted in the home by qualified professionals. It is an important component of patient care. The Bureau of Labor Statistics (2010) indicates that there will be increased demand for licensed practical nurses (LPNs) and licensed vocational nurses (LVNs) in home care. This is due to the aging Baby Boomer population who will develop functional disabilities, patient preference for care in the home, and technological advances that are making complex care in the home cost effective. LPN/LVNs need to understand how care is received in the home because the home and hospital settings differ.

HISTORY OF HOME HEALTH NURSING

Home care is not a new concept. Nurses have been caring for patients in their homes for over a hundred years. In 1893, Lillian Wald set out to improve the New York community in which she lived. Health care was available only to those who could afford it. Because of limited access to health care and lack of education, the home environment that poor families and immigrants were living in was not conducive to health and wellness. With the help of fellow nurse Mary Brewster, Wald established the Henry Street Settlement in New York City. The services started by Wald and Brewster laid the groundwork for establishing home care as a nursing specialty. Because of Lillian Wald and the nurses who worked with her, families were able to receive care and education in their homes to maintain or improve their health (Friends of Mt. Hope Cemetery, n.d.).

During the early 20th century, nurses took the initiative to develop community programs to meet the needs of the patients in their care. Nurses in the 21st century can learn from this and be involved in improving the communities in which they live. Home health nurses focus not only on the patient but also on the patient's family and the community. In home health care, nursing care and its differences from medical care can be truly understood.

HOME HEALTH ELIGIBILITY

Home health care requires skilled nursing care and must be delivered by a licensed professional nurse. Physical therapy and occupational therapy may also be needed, independent of nursing. A patient who is receiving home health nursing is required to be home bound. If patients are able to drive, then it is felt they are able to transport themselves to health care services. Patients are allowed to attend special events, go to church, or go to medical appointments and still be considered home bound. If the nurse suspects a patient is driving daily, the nurse needs to reinforce eligibility for home health and suggest alternative options for health care to permit the patient to maintain independence. These options can include activities such as going to a clinic to have a blood pressure reading done, attending an outpatient physical therapy or occupational program, or having skilled needs (such as dressing changes) completed in a day surgery facility. If you have concerns about a patient, discuss them with the registered nurse (RN), who can work to assist the patient in receiving the needed care.

Home health services usually are ordered for care after discharge from the hospital when there is a need for skilled care in the home. Skilled care includes those skills that patients cannot complete alone and that require the interventions of a licensed health care professional (Box 16.1).

It is not uncommon, though, for a physician's office to request home health services after seeing a patient in the office. For example, a patient who is having difficulty

Box 16.1

Skilled Activities for the Home Health Nurse

According to the Centers for Medicare & Medicaid (n.d.), which is the agency responsible for establishing home health rules and guidelines, a visit is considered "skilled and necessary" when the patient cannot perform the needed skill, there is no family member available to perform it, and the patient's medical issues make it necessary to have a licensed professional nurse monitor and manage the situation. Examples of skilled activities include:

- Dressing changes
- Administration of IV medications
- Management and assessment of newly inserted feeding tubes and tracheostomies
- Management and assessment of a new colostomy or urostomy
- Foley insertion and maintenance
- Patient and family education
- Monitoring a patient's status following a change in medications or condition
- Blood draws (only if the patient is receiving other home health services; this is not covered as an independent skilled visit).

If a family member is present and able to perform the skill part of the time, the nurse can teach that person how to perform the skill. The nurse may still complete skilled visits to monitor patient progress and attend to the patient's needs when family members are not available. It is important to remember that a skill must be involved, as discussed earlier. If the patient can manage the care either independently or with help from a family member, the services of a home health nurse may not be required.

controlling blood glucose levels could benefit from having a nurse come to the home to assess how the patient is using a glucometer and what types of food are being purchased, to monitor the glucose level, and to teach the patient appropriate diabetic management. Another example would be patients who cannot easily get to the physician's office to have their blood pressure checked weekly. If the physician has changed the patient's medications, he or she might need to make sure the adjustment is improving the patient's health as demonstrated by stable blood pressure readings. These types of visits are usually short term with the goal of facilitating independent care by the patient and/or family.

SAFETY TIP

Accurately and completely reconcile medications across the continuum of care. Use a process for comparing the patient's current medications with medications ordered for the patient while under the care of the organization. When a patient is referred, transferred, or discharged to home, a complete and reconciled list of the patient's medications should be documented and communicated to the next provider of service, to the primary care provider, or to the original referring provider, as well as to the patient and family. The list should be explained to the patient and family (2010 National Patient Safety Goals, www.jointcommission.org).

THE HOME HEALTH CARE TEAM

The home care team consists of the physician, RN, LPN/LVN, home health aide, physical therapist, occupational therapist, speech therapist, social services, assisted living facility staff, and, of course, the patient. Home care is **collaborative**, and the LPN/LVN is an important part of the health care team. In others words, teamwork and communication play a large part in ensuring that patients and their families receive the care they need.

The Physician

The physician is the team leader. For a patient to receive home care, a physician's order is required. The physician works closely with the RN to determine what care the patient needs. Because the physician does not see the patient on a daily basis, he or she relies on the assessment findings of the nurse and communications with the home health agency staff.

The Registered Nurse

The RN is the case manager while the patient is receiving home health care. It is the RN who completes the initial assessment, establishes the plan of care (or treatment plan), and makes changes as needed. The frequency of nursing and home health visits is established during admission. After the initial assessment, a schedule is established and forwarded to the physician for approval (Box 16.2). If needed, visits can be increased or decreased based on how the patient is progressing.

The plan of care includes the number of skilled visits required; supplies and equipment needed to complete the care; other services that are required, such as a home health aide; and a nursing care plan that establishes goals for discharge. The plan of care or treatment plan is certified (ordered) for 60 days. At the end of this period, the patient is either discharged or services are extended or recertified for another 60 days.

The RN also works with the physician to adjust treatments such as wound care and medications. These adjustments are based on the nurse's assessment of the problem. Remember, the physician is relying on the home health team to be his or her eyes and ears in the home. The nurse's ability to expertly assess a situation is critical to the progress of the patient receiving home health services.

The LPN/LVN works closely with the RN collaboratively in order to help the patient reach the best possible health. The RN works closely with all members of the home care team so that the plan of care remains relevant to the patient's situation.

Box 16.2

Scheduling Home Health Care Visits

Home health care is ordered for a 60-day period. The start of care is considered the first day of the visit, with the end occurring on or before day 60. Skilled visits are usually projected during the start of care. Orders are written as follows:

- *Skilled nursing care:* 3 × wk × 3 weeks, 2 × wk × 3 weeks, 1 × wk × 2 weeks for skilled observation of vital signs and patient response to medication changes and home health aide services; 3 × wk × 8 weeks for assistance with personal care.
- *Skilled nursing care:* 7 × wk × 4 weeks, 4 × wk × 2 wk, 2 × wk × 2 weeks for wound observation and dressing changes, family education of wound care technique.

Included in the start-of-care orders are the supplies needed to complete the ordered skills, such as dressing supplies, urinary catheter supplies, or medical equipment. These need to be authorized and ordered by the physician. Including them with the start-of-care paperwork ensures all services are ordered by the physician. This function is completed by the registered nurse in conjunction with the physician.

Source: Adapted from Centers for Medicare & Medicaid Services (n.d.).

The Home Health Aide

The home health aide assists patients with performing activities of daily living (ADLs). This includes bathing, dressing, grooming, and toileting. The home health aide's frequency of visits is established based on the patient's acuity level and the help available in the home. Each case is different. One example would be an alert and oriented patient discharged home following spinal surgery who is widowed and has no assistance in the home. This patient might need frequent visits to ensure ADLs are met. Conversely, there is the patient who is discharged home after open heart surgery who has extensive family available to assist with personal care. Although this patient's acuity is higher, he or she has help available, thus requiring less frequent visits. During visits, the LPN/LVN can help determine if the frequency of visits needs to be adjusted. Findings can be discussed with the RN, who can contact the physician to adjust the plan of care.

The Physical Therapist

Physical therapists (PTs) work to help the patient regain strength and mobility. They teach the patient and family how to use assistive devices such as walkers and canes, and they develop exercise regimens that the patient can perform independently.

PTs work autonomously. They are responsible for developing a plan of care and visit frequency. The PT also works with medical supply companies to obtain needed equipment.

If the nurses believe a patient might benefit from PT services, such as if the patient is having trouble regaining stamina after surgery, they can recommend this service to the physician. The nurse can also reinforce the PT instructions during visits and check to make sure that the activities are being completed as prescribed.

The Occupational Therapist

Occupational therapists (OTs) also function autonomously. Similar to PTs, they establish their own treatment plan and visit frequencies. OT goals are to help the patient regain independence with ADLs and improve strength. They teach the patient how to use equipment that improves independence with daily activities.

Nurses can also identify a patient who might benefit from OT services. A patient who seems to be having a difficult time performing activities such as bathing, cooking, or cleaning would benefit from OT services. As with the PT, the nurse can review the OT's instructions with the patient to make sure they are understood.

The Speech Therapist

The services of a speech therapist (ST) are ordered for patients having trouble with swallowing or speaking. After assessing the patient, the speech therapist identifies a plan of care and visit frequencies. As with other such therapies, the nurse works closely with the ST and the patient to monitor understanding of instructions.

The Social Worker

Social services visits are usually completed in a shorter period of time. The social worker works closely with many community resources to help the patient obtain assistance for items such as obtaining a prescription card, setting up Meals on Wheels, assisting the family with long-term care placement if needed, identifying private agencies that offer **respite** care (short interval of rest or relief) and homemaker services, helping the patient create a living will, and helping the patient with financial assistive services.

Nurses who work in the patient's home are in a unique position to identify patients who would benefit from social services. The case manager (RN) can relay the concerns of the home care team to the physician and obtain an order for a social service visit.

CRITICAL THINKING

Mr. Rosa

■ Mr. Rosa, 75 years old, was just discharged from the hospital following an acute exacerbation of heart failure. You notice that he has little food in his house. It appears that the home has not been cleaned in several weeks and that the clothes he is wearing are torn and soiled. Talking with him, you learn that he lost his wife 6 months ago to cancer and has had a difficult time adjusting.

1. What are some community services that might be available to Mr. Rosa?
2. What information would be important to discuss with Mr. Rosa's physician?
3. Are there any other services that the home health agency can offer to assist Mr. Rosa?

Suggested answers at end of chapter.

Assisted Living Facilities

Home care may be provided in an assisted living facility (ALF) if the patient lives in such a facility. Because these homes are not considered skilled nursing facilities, the staff is not able to perform nursing skills. Many times the nurse visits several patients in the same location. Home health nurses need to understand the facility's policies when visiting a patient in assisted living.

Home health care for patients in assisted living can be ordered for wound care, blood glucose monitoring, blood pressure monitoring, urinary catheter insertion and maintenance, and patient education. If appropriate, communicate with staff regarding health care instructions (e.g., keep the dressing clean and dry).

TRANSITION FROM HOSPITAL-BASED NURSING TO HOME HEALTH CARE

When working in the hospital, the nurse has many resources available, including resource staff such as other nurses, physicians, respiratory therapists, and unit secretaries. Patients who enter the hospital are leaving behind the comfort of their own homes. They may be scared and isolated, not only trying to adjust to an illness, but also to a new environment. The opposite is true in home health nursing. In the patient's home, the nurse is the visitor. There are no resource staff to answer questions, and the surroundings are unfamiliar. This can be a difficult adjustment. As your confidence in being a home health nurse grows, so too will your comfort level with entering someone else's home.

It is important to remember that you have entered another person's home. Cultural issues need to be recognized and considered (Box 16.3, *Cultural Considerations*). Do not make quick judgments because the dishes are not done or the bed is not made. People have different values that may not always match yours. (See Chapter 4 for further information regarding cultural considerations.) If the home is in such a state that it poses a health or safety risk, then it might be necessary to inform the RN.

Resources are not always quickly available when working in a patient's home. As such, it is important to have a good understanding of nursing skills. Home health nursing requires an ability to adapt and remain flexible since the home environment, unlike the hospital environment, can be unknown. Because of this, it is necessary to assess both the patient and his or her home setting.

Consider the patient who has been referred to home health services after a fall at home and subsequent fracture of an arm. The referral was to start physical therapy services, not skilled nursing. During the initial assessment, the nurse notes that the patient is lethargic and has extremely low blood pressure readings upon standing. Further data gathering of the home environment leads the nurse to find that the patient's wife has not been administering the patient's heart medications appropriately. She has been giving too much. The home health nurse can contact the supervising RN, who can contact the physician to obtain the orders needed to assess the patient's blood levels of this medication.

This example demonstrates how nurses in the home need to evaluate the patient's case not just based on the referral diagnosis, but also on what can be occurring within the home that could have contributed to that diagnosis. This calls for remaining flexible and adapting to the patient's needs.

Families play a large part in your care of patients in the home. Do not be surprised to walk into a home and find several anxious family members with a list of questions they would like answered. They will be very involved in your visits. This can be very intimidating at first. When preparing for a visit, take the time to review and learn about an unfamiliar diagnosis or medication. Also be prepared for the unexpected. Carry extra common supplies such as various sizes of urinary catheters, sterile dressing gauze, different types of tape, and lots of alcohol wipes. This will help you feel more comfortable and assist with developing a trusting relationship with your patients and their families.

Because of the **autonomous**, or independent, nature of home health, most agencies require at least 1 year of medical-surgical nursing experience. This will ensure that you have gained the basic knowledge needed to work in home care. You will continue to learn as you work in the home setting. Home health agencies also hire nurses for specialty areas such as cardiac or wound care. Nurses with a specific specialty will usually work with patients who have diagnoses within their specialty. See Box 16.4 for a review of liability issues.

THE ROLE OF THE LPN/LVN IN HOME HEALTH

The nurse's role in home health is varied and complex. Tasks may be similar to those performed in the hospital setting, such as wound care or administration of IV medications (Fig. 16.1). The difference is the setting in which these skills are performed. Many factors need to be considered when assisting patients in the home (e.g., having the necessary supplies, infection control, patient education material, documenting, and personal and patient safety).

Box 16.3

Cultural Considerations

In the Hispanic culture, families may be large and their living spaces may be small. When you first enter such a home, you may have a feeling that the lack of space is unhealthy. It is important to realize, however, that this is part of the Hispanic culture. You must evaluate the overall home environment, not just its appearance. Chapter 4, *Cultural Influences on Nursing Care*, offers further discussion of transcultural nursing care.

Box 16.4

Liability Issues to Consider When Working in Home Health Care

When starting in home health care, review your state's nurse practice act and your scope of practice. The National Council of State Boards of Nursing (www.NCSBN.org) lists all the state boards of nursing Web sites. This is a very useful tool for any nurse.

Understanding your scope of practice will ensure that you complete care that follows your state's guidelines. When in patients' homes they might ask you to perform a skill or request something that is outside your scope of practice. It is important that you explain to them that it is outside your scope of practice but still address their concern by contacting your agency immediately to find out how to handle their request. It is important to address their request because it could indicate a change in the status of their health.

For example, if a patient asks you if it is okay to increase a medication, you should understand that as a nurse you cannot prescribe medications. So if you were to say it was okay, you would be altering the prescribed dose, and thus practicing outside your scope of practice since only a physician or nurse practitioner can prescribe medications.

Always discuss your concerns with your supervisor and review your agency's guidelines, policies, and procedures. Know what you can and cannot do before you start and never be afraid to question something that you feel or know violates your nurse practice act. Remember it is your license so follow your nurse practice act!

STEPS IN THE HOME HEALTH VISIT

Preparing for the Visit

A typical day for the home nurse consists of six to seven home visits. These visits typically last 30 to 45 minutes. Most agencies try to arrange visits in the same geographical location for convenience. If your visits are focused on a specialty, such as wound care, you might travel long distances to visit your patients, but then you would be assigned fewer than seven visits. Agencies allow for mileage reimbursement, so be sure to keep close track of mileage from house to house.

The night before your visit, develop a plan of action for how your visits will be structured. Sometimes you will need to be at a certain place at a particular time, so factor this into your planning. Each patient needs to be contacted. Give the patient a 1- to 2-hour window for your arrival time. Remember, you cannot always anticipate what is going to happen during a visit. It is better to give your patients a time range as opposed to an exact time. If you are unsure how to locate your patient's home, ask while you are arranging the visit time.

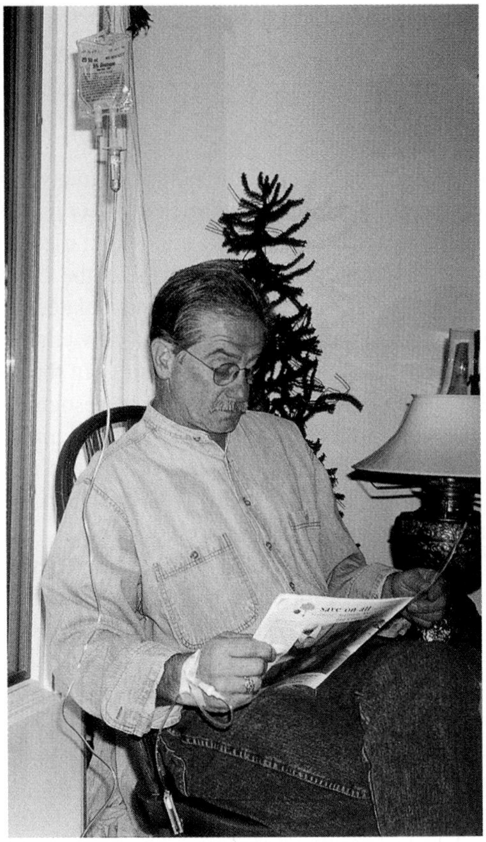

FIGURE 16.1 Patient receiving home IV therapy.

The agency will usually provide you with a form to use that reviews the patient's diagnosis, pertinent medical information, and reason for home health. Writing directions to the patient's home on these forms is an easy way to have the information close by. It is important for this process to be organized. If you have too many papers with information on them, it is difficult to manage both your time and the patient's needs, creating to frustration for all.

LEARNING TIP

Map sites on the Internet are a great place to find driving directions. (See http://maps.google.com or www.mapquest.com.) Simply type in starting and ending addresses to obtain detailed directions. Carry with you a map and cell phone—even the best of directions can be confusing once on the road.

If you are going to be late for any reason, inform the patient. Remember, these patients are home bound and anxious. Arriving late can interfere with developing an effective therapeutic relationship.

Safety Considerations

Home health nurses' travels can take them to dangerous areas. It is important to be vigilant about personal safety. Box 16.5 lists tips on how to protect yourself before, during, and after a home health visit.

Patient safety is of particular importance in the home. Stay alert to things in the home that can pose a hazard to the patient. Teaching the patient how to prevent injuries in the home is an essential intervention. Requesting a referral for physical or occupational therapy can help the patient build strength, teach the patient how to use assistive devices, and help them to maintain safety. Box 16.6, *Gerontological Issues,* offers some ideas for patient safety considerations in the home.

CRITICAL THINKING

Mrs. Ambani

■ Mrs. Ambani was referred to your home health agency following an appointment with her physician. During that visit, Mrs. Ambani was diagnosed as being anemic, resulting in dizziness, fatigue, and alterations in her blood pressure. The physician requested home health nurse visits for Mrs. Ambani to assess her safety and recommend appropriate safety devices.

1. What are some safety devices that would assist Mrs. Ambani?
2. What are some hazards in the home the nurse should look for?

Suggested answers at end of chapter.

Infection Control

Maintaining asepsis in the patient's home may be a challenge. The home health agency will review infection control policies and procedures during in-service orientation. In the hospital, everything is available for infection control. In the home, the nurse is responsible for bringing supplies, provided by the home health agency, for safe care. Periodically go through your equipment supply to make sure you have enough. It is always important to have extras of basic equipment, including:

- Personal protective equipment—disposable gowns, masks, goggles, and shoe covers
- Gloves, including latex-free gloves
- Biohazard bags and containers of various sizes
- Disposable underpads—can be used to provide a clean field for supplies; also used on the floor to place the home health bag on
- Antibacterial soap
- Sanitizing liquid

Box 16.5

Safety Guidelines for Home Health Nurses

In general, providing home health services is a safe occupation. Most communities recognize the importance of the role of home health nurses and are receptive to their visits. It is still important to understand how you can protect yourself in case an unsafe situation arises.

Here are some tips for maintaining safety when completing a home health visit:

- Always carry a map, whistle, and cell phone.
- Keep gas tank filled.
- Complete recommended maintenance on your car and have the tires checked regularly.
- If possible, park on the street or road in front of the house. This prevents someone from blocking you in the driveway.
- When entering a home, be aware of where the exit doors are and any windows that will allow safe evacuation from the home.
- Be aware of your outside surroundings. When leaving the home, have your supplies packed up and keys out, ready to open the car door.
- If lost in an unknown area, leave and go to a familiar place and contact the patient for directions. Call your agency if you are concerned about home safety.
- If you need to complete a visit at night, request an escort. Many communities will have a police officer accompany you to and from the home. Discuss this option with your supervisor.
- Never complete a visit if you feel concerned for your safety.

Box 16.6

Gerontological Issues

The elderly make up a significant proportion of home health patients. Because of changes in their health, many items in patients' homes can become potential safety hazards. The home health nurse should always assess the patient's safety in the home. Things to look for are:

- Overcrowded spaces
- Scatter/throw rugs
- Bathroom safety
- Adequate lighting
- Access to needed supplies
- Steps to enter the home
- Pets
- Electrical cords

- Disinfecting spray to clean equipment and bag after each visit
- Alcohol wipes for disinfecting thermometers and stethoscopes
- A small chemical spill kit.

An important infection control measure is hand hygiene. It is important to wash your hands with soap and water before and after completing your patient care. If water is not available, use sanitizing liquid. Do not wash your hands in the patient's kitchen sink; always ask to use the bathroom for washing your hands.

Documentation

Because of reimbursement guidelines, the nurse needs to document specific things during the visit. Home health agencies receive their income based on a prospective pay system (predetermined rate), not per-visit payments. On admission, the RN fills out information that is entered into a computer system. This information is called the Outcome and Assessment Information Set, or OASIS. This tool is used to generate information about the home health agency and patient outcomes. It is also used to help develop a plan of care that best meets the patient's problems. The LPN/LVN should be familiar with the general function of this form and its relevance to creating a plan of care.

In order for home health agencies to be reimbursed, they need to demonstrate that a skill was completed. Documenting information is based on the patient's plan of care and the corresponding skill that was completed at the visit. For example, the physician orders skilled nursing observation and medication management for a patient. In documenting the visit for this order, the nurse needs to state that this skill was completed. Documentation would include:

- Patient's response to medication—vital signs, level of consciousness, or other potential side effects
- Patient's current understanding of medication regimen and the action the nurse took to improve that understanding
- Patient's response to that education and any areas in which the patient might continue to need assistance.

Home health agencies, like hospitals, have different ways of documenting. The following items are typically included in all agencies' home health documentation:

- Nurse's arrival and departure times
- Assessment findings
- Vital signs
- A narrative note
- Patient's signature verifying that the nurse was present in the home.

The documentation flow sheet is returned to the agency within an identified time frame (usually within 24 hours of a visit). Some agencies have secure drop boxes to leave paperwork in after hours. When placing paperwork in the drop box, forms need to be neatly organized and attached together.

A folder with information is also kept at the patient's residence. It usually consists of relevant patient information and a communication form that all staff members complete at each visit. Similar to hospital charting, this documentation is important to ensure continuity of care. It is even more vital in the home setting because staff members might not cross paths for a verbal report.

Patient Education

A primary responsibility of nurses in home health is educating patients about their illness and ways to effectively manage that illness at home, hopefully decreasing the need for hospitalization. Most home health agencies have handouts to help reinforce the verbal instructions you provide. Many handouts are available from other sources as well, if needed.

> **LEARNING TIP**
>
> An easy way to make sure you always have the handouts you need is to organize them into a three-ringed binder. Always have plenty of these handouts when making a visit. Many times, family members who do not live with the patient request copies so that they can have them at home. You can organize the information in several different manners; for example, based on the diagnosis or alphabetically.

NURSING PROCESS FOR THE HOME HEALTH PATIENT

Data Collection

Monitor and document patient and family adjustment to change and illness. Perform a complete patient assessment during each visit. Assess the home environment for potential safety hazards and the need for devices to assist with care.

Nursing Diagnoses, Planning, and Implementation

Ineffective Self Health Management Related to Deficient Knowledge, Complexity of Medical Needs, and Limited Access to Social Support

EXPECTED OUTCOME: The patient will demonstrate changes in lifestyle needed to maintain health.

- Work with patient in developing both short- and long-term goals *to ensure patient's goals are being met.*

- Recognize small accomplishments positively *to reinforce patient's progress.*
- Educate patient on management of the health care regimen *to allow patient to carry out regimen.*
- Provide educational material in both written and verbal format *to promote understanding of complex issues.*
- Review plan of care with patient *to facilitate involvement and eventual independence.*
- Identify and work with social support systems *to meet patient's needs.*
- Help patient obtain needed supplies *to promote wellness.*
- Assess the home environment for hazards, and assist patient with making needed changes *to promote safety.*
- Assess the patient for changes in health status *to detect changes that can affect progress.*

Caregiver Role Strain Related to Management of a Chronic Illness and Lack of Understanding of Resources Available

EXPECTED OUTCOME: The caregiver will identify effective ways for dealing with the complexity of a chronic illness.

- Include caregiver in the plan of care *to help develop an understanding of the management of the illness.*
- Assist caregiver with identifying community resources available such as respite care, Meals on Wheels, and support groups *to meet patient's needs.*
- Enlist the help of a social worker *to facilitate contact with community resources.*
- Assess caregiver's expectations of the patient's health. *Misconceptions regarding progress can foster anger and frustration toward the patient.*
- Discuss ways to help caregiver deal effectively with feelings of anger and frustration *to allow dealing with the feelings and issues causing them.*
- Acknowledge the change in roles (for example, a child taking care of a parent) and the challenges associated with this change in family roles *to allow planning for the changes.*

Evaluation

The patient and caregiver will acknowledge acceptance and understanding of the change in health status. This is evidenced by involvement in the plan of care and participation with goal setting, use of community resources, maintenance of a safe home environment, and demonstration of ability to manage medical regimen.

OTHER TYPES OF HOME HEALTH NURSING

So far, this chapter has focused on home health care that is covered under the Medicare and Medicaid systems. The purpose of this version of home health is to assist the patient with managing health needs on an intermittent basis. Other types of home agency service work are also available for nurses, including private duty nursing and hospice nursing (see Chapter 17).

Private Duty Nursing

Private duty nursing consists of scheduled care to assist patients with personal and homemaking needs. These services have been called home companion services, homemaker services, and private duty care. Many of these services focus more on companionship and respite care. Families who are taking care of a patient with complex needs, such as a patient with Alzheimer's disease, may need time away from the home to complete personal tasks. Agencies can provide both licensed and unlicensed assistive personnel (UAP) to help the patient while the family is away. These services are considered an out-of-pocket expense and are not covered by Medicare and Medicaid.

Families can contract with an agency to have a staff member spend 2 to 3 hours a day in the home. The staff can complete homemaking tasks and companion tasks, such as arts and crafts or playing cards. Nurses can work in these agencies in the role of supervisor to unlicensed assistive personnel (UAP). Nurses also may be involved in helping a patient fill weekly medication dispensers. Many nurses enjoy this type of work because of the relationships that are formed with patients and families. They may be involved with the same family for months to years, as opposed to a few months, as is typical with Medicare home health patients.

SUMMARY OF HOME HEALTH NURSING

Home health nursing is a rewarding career path. Nurses who work in the home have the unique opportunity to assist patients during times of crisis and to experience the results of their interventions. Home health nursing will continue to grow in the 21st century, and the need for qualified professionals will offer many opportunities for the LPN/LVN. Thinking back on the impact that nurses like Lillian Wald had and her ability to change the lives of so many because of her willingness to meet those patients in their homes demonstrates the importance home health nurses have in the successful progression for patients from illness to health and wellness.

SUGGESTED ANSWERS TO CRITICAL THINKING

Mr. Rosa

1. The loss of Mr. Rosa's wife and his subsequent health problems have impacted his ability to properly care for himself. A proper diet is important for healing and maintenance of health. A referral to Meals on Wheels would be appropriate. This agency will deliver at least one healthy meal each weekday (usually lunch). The meal can be adapted to meet the patient's dietary guidelines.

   Many communities offer elder services to patients at a reduced cost to assist with housekeeping services. Helping the patient set up homemaker services will help him through this difficult time. Offering the patient information about grief counseling services in the community can be beneficial during this time. Once discharged from home health, the patient can begin attending counseling services. Other community resources to consider are neighborhood socials, church services if appropriate, and online communities that match the patient's values.
2. The physician needs to be contacted about the patient's withdrawn demeanor and lack of interest in self-care. Mr. Rosa may be experiencing a situational depression because of the recent loss of his wife and his own health problems. During this time the physician might decide to prescribe an antidepressant to help.
3. The nurse recognizes that Mr. Rosa needs extra help at this time. Consider a referral for social services to assist with community resources and grief counseling.

   Because heart failure is a chronic disease that can contribute to fatigue, an occupational therapist can work with the patient in developing energy-conserving techniques for completing activities of daily living. Also the services of a home health aide can help with personal care and provide additional emotional support.

Mrs. Ambani

1. Because anemia can cause extreme fatigue, it is important for Mrs. Ambani to have safety devices in the home to prevent falls. These devices can be obtained from a medical supply store and are usually covered by Medicare. Equipment to consider includes a bath stool for the shower so the patient can sit while bathing, a detachable shower head, handrails in the shower and hallways, a bedside commode, an over-the-toilet seat, a reacher to assist with obtaining objects at a distance, a medical alert device that can be worn at all times, and, if fatigue is severe enough, a motorized wheelchair.
2. The home has many hazards. Important things to assess for include scatter/throw rugs, overcrowded spaces, sharp edges along furniture, inadequate lighting, and stairs. Instruct the patient to keep frequently used kitchen appliances and foods on shelves that are easy to reach. The same is true for the bathroom and bedroom. Assist the patient with setting up a "command center" in the living room so that favorite items are kept in proximity and the patient does not have to get up so frequently.

REVIEW QUESTIONS

1. What impact did Lillian Wald have on the nursing profession?
   a. Allowed nurses to function as medical care providers.
   b. Demonstrated the impact nursing can have on patients' health and wellness.
   c. Made it possible for nurses to obtain prescription drugs for patients in the home.
   d. Developed the Henry Street Settlement in 1890.

2. Which of the following are members of the home health team? **Select all that apply.**
   a. LPN/LVN
   b. Physician
   c. Social worker
   d. Home health aide
   e. Lawyer
   f. Patient

3. A patient is being seen by home health nurses for monitoring of weight and vital signs and education about medication changes following an acute exacerbation of heart failure. Documentation for this visit needs to include which of the following?
   a. What the patient ate for breakfast
   b. How far the patient was able to ambulate while working with physical therapy
   c. Education about the role of the home health aide in assisting the patient with personal care
   d. Education about how to keep a log of daily weights and when to contact the physician about a potential problem

REVIEW QUESTIONS—cont'd

4. An LPN/LVN has started working for a local home health agency and is concerned about the transition to home health nursing after working in the hospital for 10 years. What are some recommendations that would ease this transition for the LPN/LVN?
   a. Explain that home health nursing is just like hospital nursing.
   b. Instruct the nurse to always be prepared, to keep paperwork organized, and spend some time the night before a visit to review patient health information to help gain confidence in the home.
   c. Allow an opportunity for exploring feelings and acknowledging that this is a hard transition.
   d. Let the nurse know it is not possible to completely adjust to home health nursing because of variability in the home.

5. What steps can the home health nurse take to ensure that a patient is not exposed to infectious materials in the home?
   a. Disinfect the home health bag after each patient visit with a germicidal spray supplied by the home health agency.
   b. Wash hands in the kitchen sink rather than the bathroom sink.
   c. Use the same red bag from patient to patient for disposing of soiled dressings.
   d. If a chemical spill occurs, contact the agency to send personnel to clean it up.

References

Bureau of Labor Statistics, U.S. Department of Labor. (2010). *Occupational outlook handbook, 2010–11 edition: Licensed practical and licensed vocational nurses.* Retrieved February 12, 2010, from http://www.bls.gov/oco/ocos102.htm

Centers for Medicare & Medicaid Services. (n.d.). *The home health agency manual.* Baltimore, MD: Author. Retrieved October 2, 2009, from http://www.cms.hhs.gov/manuals/pbm/ItemDetail.asp?ItemID=CMS021914

Friends of Mt. Hope Cemetery. (n.d.). *Famous women in Mt. Hope Cemetery: Lillian Wald (1867–1940).* Rochester, NY: Author. Retrieved September 16, 2009, from http://www.fomh.org/Data/Documents/Lillian_Wald.pdf

Joint Commission. (2010). *2010 national patient safety goals.* Retrieved January 13, 2010, from http://www.jointcommission.org/patientsafety/nationalpatientsafetygoals

DavisPlus | For additional resources and information visit **http://davisplus.fadavis.com**

17

Nursing Care of Patients at the End of Life

BETSY MURPHY

KEY TERMS

advance medical directive (ad-VANSE MED-ih-kuhl dur-EK-tiv)
advocate (ADD-vuh-ket)
artificial feeding (ART-ih-FISH-uhl FEE-ding)
artificial hydration (ART-ih-FISH-uhl hy-DRAY-shun)
do not resuscitate (DOO not re-SUSS-ih-TATE)
durable power of attorney (DUR-uh-buhl POW-ur OV uh-TUR-nee)
hospice (HOS-pis)
living will (LIH-ving WIL)
palliative (PAH-lee-uh-tiv)
postmortem care (pohst-MOR-tum KARE)

QUESTIONS TO GUIDE YOUR READING

1. Who is the patient who is approaching the end of life?
2. What are the necessary legal documents for patients with life-limiting illness?
3. What choices are available to patients at the end of life?
4. How do you communicate with dying patients and their families?
5. What physical changes are expected during the dying process?
6. What nursing interventions can you provide at the end of life?
7. What is postmortem care?
8. What nursing interventions can you implement for the grieving patient and family?
9. What is the role of the LPN/LVN in hospice care?

Mr. Moran, 89 years old, resides in a long-term care facility and has been losing weight and growing weaker for the past 6 months. Despite treatment for depression, he continues to grow weaker and more dependent on his caregivers. As you read this chapter, consider what decisions his family will face and what resources are available to them in their quest to provide appropriate care for him.

A GOOD DEATH

Despite our best efforts, there will become a time when all our patients will die. Death is the expected end to a life well lived. In America, only 10% of us will die suddenly. The remaining 90% will experience a gradual decline over a period of months or years.

In the 21st century, most Americans will die from chronic and acute illnesses, from diseases such as cancer, heart disease, stroke, and dementia. We have the technology to prolong life, but sometimes this longer life can carry with it profound disability and reduced quality of life. Our patients sometimes tell us that this is not what they intended for the last phase of their life. The challenge for nurses then is twofold: (1) to help identify patients with life-limiting illnesses early, so they and their families have the opportunity to define their goals of care, and (2) to help our patients communicate their wishes to health care providers, both orally and in writing, to ensure that their wishes are understood.

Perhaps the most important role for nurses is to give our patients support and validation as they move through the series of losses leading to a good death. Dying is, after all, the final phase of our growth and development. The developmental tasks associated with this phase involve reflecting on our lives, saying goodbye, saying, "I'm sorry," and saying, "I love you." The goal of having a "good death" is a valid goal.

In a 1999 study, a focus group of terminally ill patients defined what would constitute a good death for them. The results fit into five categories:

- Adequate pain and symptom management
- Ability to make their own decisions
- Dying that is not prolonged
- Minimal emotional and financial burden on their families
- Ability to use remaining time to strengthen their relationships with their loved ones (Singer, Martin, & Kelner, 1999).

This description of a good death helps nurses listen to what patients want and to focus on how best to help them achieve their goals. Nurses who choose to provide care for the dying will experience personal growth in their own lives. Facing the inevitability of our own mortality can force us to look more deeply at our beliefs, values, and priorities in life. This can result in a richer, more focused life.

IDENTIFYING IMPENDING DEATH

Although most Americans say that they want to die at home, almost 75% today die in facilities. Today, 20% die in long-term care facilities, but by the year 2020, it is estimated that 50% will die in these types of facilities. Some researchers have found that one-third to one-half of the patients who enter long-term care facilities die within a year. Nurses who are working in long-term care and assisted living facilities will find themselves in a position to both identify patients who are likely to die soon and also to support these patients' families in planning for a good death.

Death can be caused by disease, but some patients simply show weight loss and progressive weakness as indicators that they are in the final months of life. Research has shown that measuring progressive weight loss and increasing dependency can help identify patients who are dying. One research study showed that elderly patients in nursing homes who lose 10% of their body weight over 6 months have an 85% chance of dying in the next 6 months (Murden & Ainslie, 1994). Weight loss caused by depression or acute illness can sometimes be reversed with aggressive treatment. But if neither depression nor acute illness is the cause of the patient's decline, he or she may be entering the final months of life. Increasing symptoms also may be an indicator of decline. Half of long-term care patients have increased pain, increased shortness of breath, or both in their final month of life (Caprio et al., 2008).

Experience tells us that elderly patients with gradually increasing weakness and decreasing independence in activities of daily living (ADLs) are declining. Elderly patients who are having trouble swallowing and require treatment for aspiration pneumonia are likely to die within a year. Their decreased respiratory muscle strength, lack of lung elasticity, and poor immune response make recovery unlikely. Elderly patients with poor renal and cardiac functions are also at high risk for dying. The final truth is that for some patients with chronic illness, many treatments offer little benefit.

For most patients, the transition from treating an illness to allowing the patient to die is a gradual process. Figure 17.1 shows the evolving relationship between treatments intended to cure and treatments intended to comfort as the patient approaches the end of life. As curative therapies are reduced, comfort care, or **palliative**, measures are increased. This chapter explores some of the choices people need to make at the end of life, and the interventions you can use to help patients during this time.

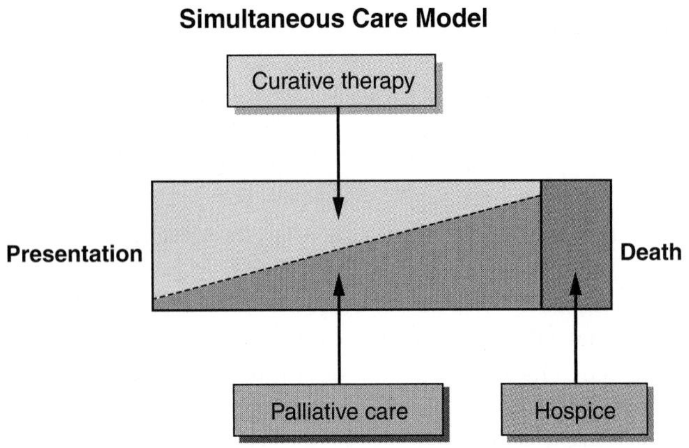
Simultaneous Care Model
Curative therapy
Presentation
Death
Palliative care
Hospice

FIGURE 17.1 The simultaneous care model. (From Emanuel, L. L., von Gunten, C. F., & Ferris, F. D. [Eds.]. [1999]. *The Education for Physicians on End-of-Life Care [EPEC] curriculum*. Chicago: The EPEC Project. Copyright Robert Wood Johnson Foundation.)

ADVANCE DIRECTIVES, LIVING WILLS, AND DURABLE MEDICAL POWER OF ATTORNEY

The Patient Self-Determination Act, which took effect in 1991, ensures that every patient has the right to accept or refuse any medical treatment that is offered. The act also requires health care professionals to ask patients entering a hospital if they have prepared **advance medical directives**. These include a **living will** and a **durable power of attorney** for health care. In preparing advance medical directives, patients are exercising their right to make their wishes known regarding specific medical treatments they would want—or not want—if they become unable to make decisions on their own. The directives require the signatures of two witnesses, neither of whom can be a family member or health care provider.

A living will is a document instructing physicians about a patient's preferences (such as to withhold or withdraw life-sustaining procedures) if the patient is unable to communicate, found to be permanently unconscious, and/or has been declared "terminal." A durable power of attorney for health care specifies who will speak for a patient when he or she cannot speak. Many states provide standard forms to use and may require the patient to have both a durable power of attorney for health care and a living will to ensure the patient's wishes are followed. An attorney, although not required, may be helpful for some families.

Encourage patients to not only fill out the necessary forms, but also to discuss their wishes with all family members. It is estimated that only about 15% of Americans have advance medical directives. Some patients are reluctant to complete them, concerned that they may change their minds about treatments in the future. It can be helpful to talk about advance care planning as a *process*. Patients can change their minds at any time about any treatment and write new advance directives. What matters most is that they get started and document their wishes today.

END-OF-LIFE CHOICES

Cardiopulmonary Resuscitation

During the 1960s, cardiopulmonary resuscitation (CPR) was developed as a method of rescuing healthy people who suffered a cardiac or respiratory arrest. Some of the early guidelines specified that CPR was not to be used in patients with terminal illnesses. It was intended for healthy patients with reversible conditions. Today, CPR has become standard in both hospitals and long-term care facilities. All patients receive CPR unless they have a **do not resuscitate** (DNR) order. There is also a perception that CPR can save most lives. The real statistics about CPR are presented in Table 17.1.

One reason for the low survival rates shown in Table 17.1 is that CPR must begin within 3 to 5 minutes of collapse. The most successful cases are ones in which CPR plus an automatic external defibrillator (called an AED) are used within 3 to 5 minutes of collapse. Medical researchers reviewed 113 studies on the use of CPR in hospitals over a 33-year period and found some additional reasons for the low survival rate (Saklayen, Liss, & Markert, 1995). They found that patients with the lowest chance of survival (less than a 2% chance) were those who (1) had more than one or two medical problems, (2) were unable to live independently, and (3) had a terminal illness. All patients living in long-term care and assisted living facilities are dependent and therefore will have a poor chance of survival after CPR. Patients with terminal illnesses would include those with cancer, dementia, or any progressive illness.

Some patients choose to have CPR because they fear that without CPR they will be deprived of treatments that will benefit them or alleviate their distress. Most patients do not realize that their chance of survival is statistically low and also that after CPR, if they survive, their quality of life may be diminished. A small number of patients erroneously believe that CPR is a procedure that may improve their overall medical condition. A helpful way of presenting the DNR option is to talk about three issues: (1) the statistics outlined above; (2) that the choice is really whether the patient will receive aggressive comfort care as he or she is dying a natural death or CPR, which may cause distress and will likely prove futile; and (3) even if elderly patients receive successful CPR, their quality of life afterward is usually greatly reduced, not improved.

TABLE 17.1 SUCCESS OF CARDIOPULMONARY RESUSCITATION IN SAVING LIVES

In hospital: all patients	10%–15% survival rate
In hospital: elderly patients	Less than 5% survival rate
Out of hospital: all patients	Less than 5% survival rate
Nursing home patients	1%–2% survival rate

Do Not Resuscitate Orders

A "No Code" or DNR order is written in a hospital or long-term care facility after collaboration with the patient, family, and health care provider, usually after it has been determined that the patient will not benefit from CPR. A DNR order simply means that CPR will not be done. Patients still must decide whether they want aggressive treatment of their underlying condition, up to but not including CPR, or whether they want only comfort measures without therapeutic treatment. Some hospitals offer several options:

- DNR/Comfort Care Only
- DNR/Full Therapeutic Support
- Full Code.

Outside the hospital, at home, or in most nursing facilities, patients will have fewer options for aggressive treatment. Patients can, however, choose to have a DNR order that will be recognized by emergency personnel. Many states have a "Durable DNR" document that, once signed, can be displayed in the patient's home to advise rescue personnel that the patient does not want CPR. These may also be called "out-of-hospital" or "prehospital" DNR orders.

Many people assume that their documented desire not to receive resuscitation in a living will is all that is needed. This is not correct. In states that have an out-of-hospital DNR policy, patients must also complete the durable DNR document or they will receive CPR regardless of their stated wishes.

Some patients fear that in choosing DNR status they will suffer and be alone at the time of their death. It is important to tell patients that DNR does not mean "do not treat." Even patients who have a DNR/Comfort Care Only order can receive oxygen, medications, and other comfort measures to aggressively manage their symptoms and ensure a comfortable death. All DNR orders and discussions with families should be documented on the patient's chart (Box 17.1, *Patient Perspective*).

CRITICAL THINKING

Mrs. Hart

■ Mrs. Hart has written a living will specifying her wishes should she become incapacitated. Because she has advanced disease, she tells you she would not want to be resuscitated if she has a cardiac arrest. She is currently hospitalized but will be discharged to her home in a few days. What documents does she need to have in place to ensure she will not receive resuscitation?

Suggested answers at end of chapter.

Box 17.1 Patient Perspective

Anna

My mom, Anna, was diagnosed with cardiomyopathy and congestive heart failure when she was 60 years old. At that time, she was still working and had just remarried. She thought she had many years left in life. She did not have an advance directive—why would she?

Two years later, as her disease progressed, she decided she did not ever want to "live on machines." So with the help of her doctor and our family, she wrote her living will and made her new husband her durable power of attorney for health care, with me as his backup person. Since she was still functioning really well with lots of medications and occasional hospitalizations, she chose a DNR status, but with full therapeutic, aggressive interventions. She even took a tour of Europe during this time in her life, knowing she would not be able to do it later.

By age 67, she had a lot less energy to do things, and her heart failure really cramped her lifestyle. But she still enjoyed life, and her goal was to see her oldest grandson, my son, graduate from high school. She considered a heart transplant, but her doctor told her she was too old to qualify. She did have a new kind of valve surgery that was supposed to make her feel better, but it didn't help much.

Three months after my son's graduation, she was hospitalized several times with progressively worse outcomes. She weighed barely 100 pounds and could not eat much. She was only 70 years old, and still looked and acted so young! Finally, she was in a semicoma in the hospital, and our family had to make the difficult decision to withdraw all therapeutic support. She was now a DNR, with comfort measures only. We were confident this would be what she wanted because we had talked about it with her.

She was discharged home with hospice care and died within a week. I moved in for her final days to help out, and between her husband and me, her hospice nurse (who was a godsend), and frequent visits from family and her minister, she was well cared for. We kept her comfortable with lots of attention and morphine. She was alert and able to converse much of the time. She ate what and when she wanted, which amounted to one-quarter of a cheese and tomato sandwich one day, but she enjoyed it! She could finally enjoy a glass of grapefruit juice, which she had been unable to have for years because it interacted with one of her heart medications.

At the end, she died with me holding her left hand and her husband holding her right. We were telling her we loved her. It was a good death.

Artificial Feeding and Hydration

Patients may no longer be able to eat or drink as a result of three conditions: an acute illness, a long illness with multiple medical problems, or simply the aging process. Otherwise healthy patients who are unable to eat while recovering from an acute illness will probably benefit from tube feeding. Patients who are declining either from multiple medical problems or the aging process probably will not.

In recent years, important research has been conducted to help guide the decision to insert a feeding tube. In 1999, a 30-year retrospective review of patients with dementia who received feeding tubes revealed the following: (1) Patients did not live longer than patients who were hand fed, (2) feeding tubes increased rather than decreased the risk of aspiration pneumonia, (3) feeding tubes did not prevent or reverse weight loss, and (4) they did not heal or prevent pressure ulcers (Finucane, Christmans, & Travis, 1999). As a result of this research, The Alzheimer's Association recommends that instead of a feeding tube, these patients receive an effective program of hand feeding. In contrast, patients with an acute stroke may recover faster if a feeding tube is placed soon after their stroke. It has long been known that although a feeding tube or total parenteral nutrition (TPN) is helpful for cancer patients who are losing weight from therapeutic treatments such as chemotherapy, it is not helpful for patients who are actively dying from cancer.

There are even some benefits to withholding **artificial feeding** and **artificial hydration** in the final weeks of life in actively dying patients. These benefits are:

- Fewer pharyngeal and lung secretions, which can reduce dyspnea
- Reduced swelling around tumors, which can reduce associated pain
- Less urination, resulting in dryer skin with less breakdown.

It has been theorized that as dehydration occurs, the body produces a form of endorphin that enhances comfort. As ketone levels rise from the breakdown of body fat, patients experience an anesthetic effect that creates a sense of well-being. Hospices have done comparative research studying patients who received IV hydration and those who did not to understand the effect of hydration on comfort (McCann, Hall, & Groth-Juncker, 1994). They asked both groups of patients about their discomfort in the days before their death. They discovered that both groups were comfortable and that both had only one complaint: having a dry mouth. Neither group reported feeling hunger or increased pain. Because both groups had dry mouths, it was speculated that the cause was the medications used at the end of life. When frequent mouth care was added to the care plan, patients no longer reported dry mouths.

The issue of feeding is emotionally very difficult for families. Often their loved one has been ill a long time. Bringing favorite foods may have been one of the ways they showed love and communicated caring. Families will need support in making decisions about feeding in three important ways:

- Identifying goals of care and evaluating whether artificial feeding will help meet those goals
- Weighing the benefits and burdens of feeding
- Finding new ways (besides feeding) to communicate their love such as skin care, mouth care, or reading to their loved one.

For a different perspective on artificial feeding, see Box 17.2, *Ethical Considerations.*

Hospitalization

A hospital is where patients go to receive aggressive medical treatment. The goal of care in a hospital is to improve the patient medically and transfer him or her to an appropriate level of care that will better meet individualized needs. There are burdens associated with hospitalization for elderly patients approaching the end of life. Elderly patients may actually decline more rapidly in a hospital setting. Research has shown that all elderly patients lose weight in a hospital and that patients with dementia lose weight and suffer irreversible cognitive decline with each hospitalization (Volicer, 2005). They enter a foreign environment and are cared for by health care workers who do not know them. Often the patients are restrained as they become agitated and fearful while away from where they call home. Patients who are frail and have poor immunity are also at risk. They often enter the hospital with one infection and are discharged with other infections that are resistant to antibiotics or caused by antibiotics, such as *Clostridium difficile.* There is evidence that antibiotic therapy does not prolong survival in those who are unable to communicate or unable to ambulate alone or with assistance.

Patients living in nursing facilities with end-stage dementia who have severe cognitive impairment will benefit from having a "do not hospitalize" order. This will maintain the patient in an environment that feels safe and preserves his or her chosen quality of life. Having hospice care in place (see next section) in the nursing home can help reduce hospitalizations.

Hospice Care

Many people think of **hospice** as a place. It is actually a service. The service is provided in private homes or independent and assisted living facilities. It can also be provided in hospitals and nursing homes when there is a signed contract between the hospice organization and the facility. To qualify for hospice, a patient must have an estimated prognosis of 6 months or less. Patients can receive hospice care longer than 6 months as long as their health continues to decline.

Some indicators of a 6-month or less prognosis (regardless of diagnosis) are 10% loss of weight in 6 months, functional decline, frequent hospital admissions, and recurrent infections. The goal of hospice care is holistic: to manage

Box 17.2
Ethical Considerations

Euthanasia

Karen has worked in a long-term care facility for the past 9 years. She works very hard in her job as an LPN to ensure that all of her patients receive the best care possible during their stay. Karen values life and has a special interest in palliative care and end-of-life issues.

Karen has been caring for Adam since he came to the hospice 5 years ago. Adam is a 28-year-old man who has been in a "waking coma" since a car accident. He has made no progress over the time he has been in care. Adam is married and both his wife and parents are actively involved in his care.

Adam occasionally makes indistinguishable sounds, his eyes are open but do not fix upon any object, and he can move his head from side to side, but otherwise he is unable to move. In addition, he has extensive limb contractures as well as chronic pressure ulcers. He can't swallow, so he has a gastric feeding tube. He is incontinent, so he wears an adult brief, and he has a urinary catheter. He suffers from frequent bouts of stomatitis, skin and urinary tract infections, and occasionally pneumonia.

Adam's wife believes that Adam will never fully recover or regain any meaningful control over his body and that keeping him alive is inconsistent with his previously held belief to live life to the fullest. She believes his tube feeding should be discontinued. If this happens, Adam will die from dehydration soon after. Adam's parents, in contrast, remain hopeful that Adam will eventually recover and regain some normal function. They are also firm believers in the value of human life, in any condition, and believe it would be wrong to let him die. As a result of the conflict, Adam's wife has petitioned the courts to have his tube feedings stopped. There is tension between the two parties, and they try to avoid each other as much as possible.

Eventually, Adam's wife wins her fight to have the feedings stopped. On the day that this is to happen, Karen is the LPN on duty, and it falls to her to discontinue the feeding and clamp the tubing. The tube is to be left intact in case it is needed to administer medications needed for comfort. Karen is aware that once the feeding is stopped, Adam will not be able to eat or drink by himself and he will die in the near future.

What are the important issues here? First, there are two opposing sides. Adam's wife insists that Adam has no viable future and would not have wanted to endure such a state for such a long time. She points out that there has been extensive neurologic damage that cannot be reversed, leading to her conclusion that Adam, as he was known, no longer exists. His parents maintain that life, in whatever form and at whatever cost, should be supported and protected.

- Who is right?
- What principles should guide Adam's care?
- What is Karen's primary obligation?
- Who is protecting Adam's rights?
- Should Karen stop the feeding?

Discussion and suggested answers at end of chapter.

symptoms such as pain and nausea, to provide emotional and spiritual counseling for the patient and family, and to support the patient in achieving his or her goals of care. Each patient is assigned a multidisciplinary hospice team (Table 17.2) to assist with care.

Most health insurance companies now provide a hospice benefit. Many are modeled after the Medicare hospice benefit. The Medicare benefit pays for both routine hospice care at home and for inpatient hospice care provided in a contracted hospital, skilled nursing facility, or freestanding hospice unit. Medications, medical supplies, oxygen, and medical equipment are also covered if they are related to the "terminal" diagnosis.

Hospice care can help a family take care of a patient at home, but hospice nurses do not routinely provide 24-hour in-home care. (A nurse is "on call" for in-home visits 24 hours a day.) Nurses and other team members make regular visits to support the patient and family. In times of medical crisis, short-term inpatient hospice services or 24-hour in-home continuous nursing care may be provided under some hospice benefits.

COMMUNICATING WITH PATIENTS AND THEIR LOVED ONES

Terminal illness is a family experience. Family is defined by the patient and may include blood relatives, friends, significant others, or partners. The primary role of the nurse is to facilitate a comfortable death that honors the choices of the patient and family. The nurse, therefore, becomes the **advocate**, assuring that patient and family wishes are communicated to other members of the health care team. In addition, the nurse is often the professional caregiver and educator of the nonprofessional caregivers and family.

To successfully work with dying patients and families, you must demonstrate empathy, unconditional positive regard, trustworthiness, and critical thinking. You are part of an interdisciplinary team. The team consists of the physician, nurse, social worker, chaplain, and others. Each discipline has expertise and can lend support to the others in providing care. As illustrated in the earlier section on end-of-life choices, patients and their loved ones need support

TABLE 17.2 THE HOSPICE TEAM

Physician	Works with the patient's primary physician, offering suggestions to improve care. Directs team activities and often will make visits to the patient's home.
Nurse	Makes routine home visits, assessing patient needs and implementing plan of care. Nurses are available 24 hours per day to make visits as needed.
Social worker	Provides emotional counseling and long-term planning, assists patients with insurance issues, and helps identify community resources.
Chaplain or minister	Provides spiritual counseling or coordinates care of spiritual issues with the patient's chosen spiritual counselor. May participate in funeral or memorial service.
Home health aide	Provides personal care, linen changes, light housekeeping.
Volunteers	Support caregivers by staying with the patient while they get out of the house. May also read to patient, run errands, etc.
Bereavement counselor	Provides counseling for family and significant others for 13 months after patient's death.

and evidence-based medical information to make good decisions. All members of the team can assist with this support.

Good communication requires that you take time to listen, answer questions honestly, help identify choices, and allow verbalization of fears. Eighty percent of communication is nonverbal, such as eye contact, body language, and tone of voice. Take time to identify your own communication barriers that will affect your ability to talk with families. Do you have fears about your own mortality or lack personal experience with death? Do you fear being blamed for decisions, or disagree with decisions that were made? These barriers will affect your ability to sit with patients and families in crisis, sustain eye contact, and support them in their process. Practice attentive listening with patients and families. Allow them to talk. Be silent, don't change the subject, and know that you do not need to have all the answers. Your role can be to help them reflect on what they are trying to communicate and to clarify their goals of care so you can better advocate for them.

Set the stage for communication by sitting down, to show you are not in a hurry (Fig. 17.2). Maintain eye contact, encourage patients to speak, repeat what they say to gain clarification, and reflect on its meaning. Some things to say to facilitate good communication include:

- "Do you feel like talking?"
- "Tell me more about your fears of…."
- Repeat back what you hear: "You mentioned you were upset by…."
- Reflect: "So are you saying that...?"
- "What does this mean to you?"
- "How can I help you?"

From the patient's perspective, many factors influence the content and quality of communication with you. Some patients are so afraid that they cannot hear what they have been told about their illness. It can be helpful to ask what the doctor has said in order to get baseline information about where they are in understanding their disease.

Patients may use denial as a mechanism to protect themselves from becoming overwhelmed by emotion. The denial is necessary to enable them to survive on a day-by-day basis. You do not need to correct their denial. Some patients remain in denial throughout the course of their illness. When patients in denial ask you a direct question about their condition, it can be an indicator that they are ready to hear the truth. It is essential that you always answer questions honestly and to the best of your knowledge. Dishonesty destroys trust and credibility.

Patients and their families may also feel angry. Allowing them to express their anger will validate it and enable them to progress emotionally. Comments like "It is okay to be angry with God and anybody else" will encourage them to continue to talk. Patients who fully understand their prognosis will express sadness and regret. Sitting with patients as they express sadness will allow them to share their feelings and give you an opportunity to offer emotional support.

THE DYING PROCESS

This section discusses the expected changes in the days and hours before death. Assessing patients for these changes, planning and implementing treatments, and evaluating patients' responses to interventions are all important. Nursing interventions are summarized in the *Nursing Care Plan for the Patient at the End of Life.*

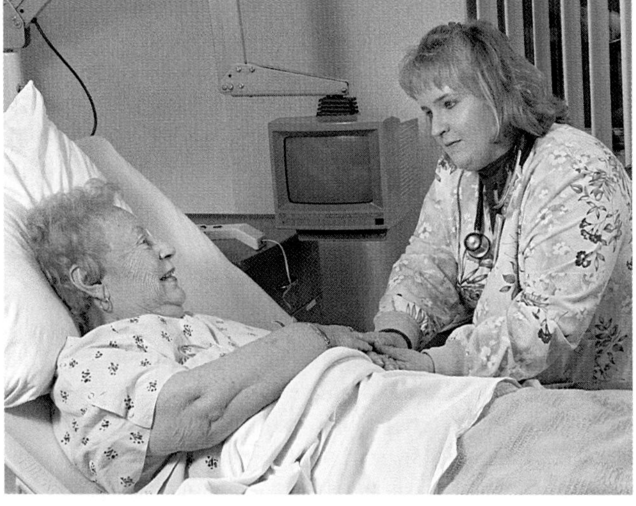

FIGURE 17.2 Nurses can be a comfort to patients and family members.

NURSING CARE PLAN for the Patient at the End of Life

Nursing Diagnosis: *Impaired Gas Exchange* related to dying heart and lungs as evidenced by dyspnea, change in respiratory rate, and Spo_2 less than 90%

Expected Outcomes: Patient will state that breathing is comfortable; respiratory rate is between 12 and 20 per minute; Spo_2 will be 90% or greater.

Evaluation of Outcomes: Is patient's breathing relaxed and rate between 12 and 20 per minute? Is Spo_2 90% or greater?

Interventions	Rationale	Evaluation
Monitor respiratory rate and effort.	Increased rate and effort indicate distress.	Is patient in distress? Are further interventions needed?
Administer diuretics or antibiotics as ordered.	Diuretics or antibiotics may be given to treat dyspnea and promote comfort, not to prolong life.	Do diuretics or antibiotics reduce dyspnea?
Explain to the family the rationale for medical interventions.	Blood transfusions may be given to improve oxygenation and reduce dyspnea; a thoracentesis may promote lung expansion. These are not intended to prolong life, but to promote comfort.	Are additional interventions needed and effective? Does family understand rationale for their use?
Plan activities to conserve energy.	Spacing rest with activity will help reduce oxygen consumption.	Can patient tolerate spaced activities?
Place patient in a recliner with pillows to 45 degrees.	An upright position allows lung expansion.	Does positioning reduce dyspnea?
Offer alternative comfort measures, such as massage and muscle relaxation.	Relaxation reduces anxiety and resulting dyspnea.	Are alternative measures effective?
Administer oxygen as ordered.	Oxygenation raises Spo_2 and reduces dyspnea.	Does oxygen raise Spo_2 and relieve dyspnea?
Place a fan in room if patient desires.	The feeling of breeze may reduce subjective feelings of dyspnea.	Does patient report increased comfort or appear more comfortable with fan on?
Administer low-dose morphine as ordered.	Morphine causes peripheral vasodilation, which can reduce pulmonary edema. It can also reduce anxiety.	Are respirations less labored after morphine?
Explain to patient and family that small dose of morphine will help to slow breathing, so patient feels more comfortable, and will work on the part of the brain that makes patient feel short of breath, reducing the sense of panic.	The informed patient and family will be able to cooperate and assist with keeping the patient comfortable.	Do patient and family understand reasons for care and feel secure that patient is receiving best possible care?

Continued

NURSING CARE PLAN for the Patient at the End of Life—cont'd

Nursing Diagnosis: *Ineffective Airway Clearance* related to excessive secretions and inability to swallow as evidenced by gurgling sound, "death rattle"

Expected Outcomes: The patient's airway will be free of secretions.

Evaluation of Outcomes: Is patient's breathing quiet and unlabored?

Interventions	Rationale	Evaluation
Adjust the patient's head to allow secretions to move down the throat.	This will help the patient swallow the secretions and decrease frightening noise.	Is breathing quieter?
Place a humidifier in the room.	Humidified air can liquefy secretions and help the patient cough.	Is patient able to cough up secretions?
If secretions are copious, administer hyoscyamine or scopolamine as ordered.	These anticholinergic medications can dry secretions.	Do medications help dry secretions?
Administer low-dose morphine as ordered.	Morphine has an anticholinergic action that can help dry secretions.	Does morphine help quiet breathing and help patient stay calm?
Suction patient as needed.	If secretions are not controlled by noninvasive measures, suctioning may be needed.	Is suctioning needed? Is it effective?
Explain to patient and family that, "Because he can no longer swallow saliva, it collects in the back of his throat. This medication will help reduce the secretions and reduce the feeling of shortness of breath."	The informed patient and family will be able to cooperate and assist with keeping the patient comfortable.	Do patient and family understand reasons for care and feel secure that patient is receiving best possible care?

Nursing Diagnosis: *Imbalanced Nutrition: Less Than Body Requirements* related to inability to swallow and lack of appetite as evidenced by refusing food, weight loss

Expected Outcomes: The patient will state satisfaction with amount and types of food offered. The patient will not aspirate food or fluid.

Evaluation of Outcomes: Does patient appear content with foods and fluids offered? Does he or she swallow without aspirating?

Interventions	Rationale	Evaluation
Let the patient choose when and what to eat. Do not force the patient to eat if he does not wish to.	The goal is no longer providing adequate nutrition, but keeping the patient comfortable.	Is the patient receiving the foods and fluids he wants?
Sit the patient upright to eat or drink.	This can help the patient swallow and prevent aspiration.	Does patient swallow effectively?

NURSING CARE PLAN for the Patient at the End of Life—cont'd

Interventions	Rationale	Evaluation
Explain to family, as needed, that, "He is afraid to swallow now because his swallowing is impaired and it causes him to choke. As he becomes dehydrated, his comfort will increase as the body produces endorphins and naturally occurring anesthesia."	The informed patient and family will be able to cooperate and assist with keeping the patient comfortable.	Do patient and family understand reasons for care and feel secure that patient is receiving best possible care?

Nursing Diagnosis: *Impaired Oral Mucous Membrane* related to dehydration, not eating, medication side effects

Expected Outcomes: The patient's mucous membranes will be clean and moist.

Evaluation of Outcomes: Are mucous membranes clean and moist? Does patient indicate that his mouth is moist?

Interventions	Rationale	Evaluation
If patient is alert, offer ice chips or sips of water.	These keep mucous membranes moist.	Does patient indicate mouth feels comfortable?
Provide frequent mouth care with sponge-tipped Toothettes.	This can keep mucous membranes moist when patient is not able to drink adequate fluids.	Is mouth clean and moist?
Apply lanolin to lips.	Lanolin keeps mouth and lips from becoming dry and crusty.	Are lips smooth and moist?

Nursing Diagnosis: *Impaired Comfort* (pain, terminal restlessness) related to disease process, dying process, medications

Expected Outcomes: The patient will state that he or she feels comfortable or, if unable to speak, will appear calm and peaceful, not restless or agitated.

Evaluation of Outcomes: Is patient comfortable, calm, and peaceful?

Interventions	Rationale	Evaluation
Assess for reversible causes of agitation: • Pain or other discomfort • Urine retention or fecal impaction • Medications that are no longer beneficial • $Spo_2 < 90\%$.	Often, agitation is a sign of discomfort. Identifying and removing the cause of the discomfort can help calm the patient.	Can causes be identified? Are they removed?

Continued

NURSING CARE PLAN for the Patient at the End of Life—cont'd

Reposition in bed at least every 2 hours and prn.	Repositioning frequently can promote comfort and relieve pressure on bony prominences. When other medical interventions are discontinued, the patient still needs to be repositioned regularly to prevent uncomfortable complications.	Does repositioning promote comfort?
If SpO_2 is low, administer oxygen as ordered.	Low SpO_2 causes dyspnea, which is not comfortable.	Is SpO_2 raised to 90%? Is patient's breathing unlabored?
Discuss with the physician discontinuing all uncomfortable procedures, such as blood draws and fingersticks for blood glucose.	Many procedures provide information to the staff but are not beneficial to the patient at the end of life. They should be discontinued.	Are any uncomfortable procedures still being carried out that are not absolutely necessary?
If the cause of the agitation cannot be determined, try medication for pain, dyspnea, or anxiety as ordered.	Medication may need to be administered based on objective observations if the patient is unable to communicate.	Does medication promote comfort?
Keep the patient safe with one-on-one monitoring and side rails up.	A fall would increase the patient's discomfort.	Is patient safety maintained?
Keep perineal area clean and dry, frequently checking adult briefs.	A wet brief is not comfortable. Unchanged briefs can also lead to skin breakdown, another source of discomfort.	Is patient clean and dry with intact skin?
Teach patient and family that "Restlessness can have many causes. It can be a sign of pain, bowel or bladder problems, or a medication issue. I will work with the health care provider to improve the situation."	The informed patient and family will be able to cooperate and assist with keeping the patient comfortable.	Do patient and family understand reasons for care and feel secure that patient is receiving best possible care?

Nursing Diagnosis: *Hypothermia* or *Hyperthermia* related to dying central nervous system and inability to regulate body temperature

Expected Outcomes: The patient's temperature will be maintained as close to normal as possible, and discomfort from temperature extremes will be managed.

Evaluation of Outcomes: Is temperature within normal limits (WNL)? If unable to control temperature, does patient appear comfortable?

Interventions	Rationale	Evaluation
Administer acetaminophen suppository as ordered.	Acetaminophen is an antipyretic. It is given by suppository if the patient cannot swallow.	Does acetaminophen reduce fever?

NURSING CARE PLAN for the Patient at the End of Life—cont'd

Keep the patient clean and dry. Change gown and bed linens as needed.	A fever can cause diaphoresis, and lying in damp sheets can be uncomfortable and cause skin breakdown.	Is patient kept dry and comfortable?
If the patient is cold, add blankets as needed. Do not use an electric blanket or heating pad.	Blankets will warm the patient without risking burns from electric heating devices.	Are blankets helpful?

Nursing Diagnosis: *Acute Confusion* related to neurologic changes

Expected Outcomes: The family will voice understanding that confusion is not uncommon and will show appropriate responses if it occurs.

Evaluation of Outcomes: Does the family respond appropriately to patient during times of confusion?

Interventions	Rationale	Evaluation
Assure families that some confusion is common.	If family is prepared, confusion will be less disturbing.	Is family informed? Do they verbalize understanding of what to expect?
Do not correct the patient but instead encourage the patient to talk about what is happening.	Sometimes patients talk about their fears in metaphor. Allowing them to express this fear will promote relaxation and decrease loneliness.	Is the patient less distressed after speaking?
Keep a dim light on in the room, and remind the person gently of who is present.	Being able to see clearly helps keep the patient oriented if he awakens during the night.	Is light on? Is patient able to orient himself when he awakens?
Explain to family that "Many patients don't make sense at times. It is as if they are in two worlds at the same time. The patient will be less distressed if you let him talk about what he is experiencing."	The family will be less distressed if they understand what is happening.	Does the family respond appropriately to the patient's confused statements?

Nursing Diagnosis: *Disturbed Sensory Perception* related to changes in neurologic function

Expected Outcomes: The patient will be treated as still present and respected, and not as though he is already gone.

Evaluation of Outcomes: Is communication respectful toward the patient?

Interventions	Rationale	Evaluation
When providing care, always speak as if the patient can hear you. When conversing with family members in the room, remember that the patient also can hear what you are saying.	Patients may be able to hear even when they appear to be nonresponsive. Always assume the patient can hear you.	Are caregivers and family members sensitive to the patient's presence when communicating?

Continued

NURSING CARE PLAN for the Patient at the End of Life—cont'd

When giving care, explain softly to the patient what you are doing and why.	Knowing what is happening can reduce anxiety and increase cooperation.	Does patient appear calm? Does he respond to your explanations?
Explain to family that "Hearing is the last sense to go. This can be a good time to say the things you have not been able to say. He may still hear you."	Continued communication can be comforting to both the patient and the family.	Is communication appropriate?

Nursing Diagnosis: *Anticipatory Grieving* related to impending death

Expected Outcomes: The patient and family will be able to openly communicate their feelings to each other and say goodbye.

Evaluation of Outcomes: Are patient and family able to communicate effectively and say goodbye to each other?

Interventions	Rationale	Evaluation
Be present with the patient. Just sit quietly and hold the patient's hand for a period of time.	This can help the patient feel less alone, especially if there are no family members present. Many patients fear dying alone.	Is someone present with the patient as much as possible?
Show appropriate concern.	This will promote trust and empower the family members to ask for what they need.	Is the family communicating openly with the providers?
Provide a quiet environment where each loved one can say goodbye in a way that will reflect their cultures and values.	These interactions will serve as valuable memories after the death and provide a feeling that each participant did what they needed to do for their loved one.	Do family members appear satisfied with their participation in the process?
Consult a minister or religious counselor of the family's choice.	A minister often has special skills and training in communicating with people during difficult times. Talking about an afterlife may also be comforting to the patient and family.	Does the family appear to benefit from the presence of a minister or religious counselor?
Ask about the family's cultural and religious beliefs, and allow time for prayers and ceremonies.	Providing a culturally familiar environment will reduce the patient's and family's anxieties and give them more control over the process.	Do family members feel free to carry out cultural and religious beliefs?

Educating caregivers about what to expect is essential. Caregivers who anticipate the expected changes and understand the rationale behind the interventions are more successful in their caregiving and have fewer regrets or concerns after the death. The *Nursing Care Plan* includes specific communications that may help caregivers understand what is happening and how they can help.

Eating and Drinking

As bodies move toward death, there is less desire for food and fluids. Patients are conserving energy and often do not feel hunger. The swallowing reflex can be impaired, increasing the risk of choking. Patients fear choking and may hold their mouth tightly closed when food or fluids are offered. This is normal, and the resulting dehydration will increase comfort due to endorphin production and rising ketone levels.

Changes in Breathing

About 50% to 70% of patients have dyspnea at the end of life. Patients who are alert may report dyspnea. Those who are not alert may have tachypnea (respiratory rate greater than 24 per minute), facial grimacing, and use of accessory muscles to breathe. Untreated dyspnea can lead to fear and agitation, leading to more dyspnea. Some patients also will have episodes of apnea in the days or hours before they die.

Dyspnea has many causes. Pneumonia, anemia, congestive heart failure, and pleural effusion can be successfully treated early in the course of illness. Dyspnea that occurs in the final hours of life is not treated by correcting the underlying condition, but can be effectively managed and controlled (see the *Nursing Care Plan for the Patient at the End of Life* and *Evidence-Based Practice* box).

Oral Secretions

Saliva that the patient is now unable to swallow may collect in the back of the throat, causing a sound sometimes called a *death rattle*. This can be disconcerting for the family. See the *Nursing Care Plan for the Patient at the End of Life* for interventions.

Temperature Changes

As the body loses its ability to control temperature, the patient may become diaphoretic or feel cold all the time. Some patients have experienced fevers as high as 105°F (40.5°C). As death approaches, the feet and legs may become cool, cyanotic, and mottled. This is often an indicator that death will occur within hours.

Bowel and Bladder Changes

Most patients will become incontinent of bowel and bladder during the course of the dying process. Urine output will decrease as dehydration occurs. Urine often will darken in color and have a strong odor.

Sleeping

In the final weeks of life, patients may be sleeping for most of the day. This is due to a change in metabolism. They also begin to emotionally detach from families as part of their preparation to leave.

Mental Status Changes

As patients progress, they often have episodes of confusion, possibly from electrolyte imbalance or medications. Some patients will say things like "I have to catch a train" or "I need my passport." This metaphorical communication is well documented in the hospice literature. It is almost like patients are living in two worlds (Callanan & Kelley, 1992).

EVIDENCE-BASED PRACTICE

Clinical Question

Are opioids (morphine) effective in controlling dyspnea? Do opioids compromise the respiratory system of patients with dyspnea?

Evidence

In a study of patients with both chronic obstructive pulmonary disease (COPD) and with cancer, participants who were administered opioids reported a beneficial effect in relieving the sensation of breathlessness. In addition, four studies measured arterial blood gases and nine studies measured oxygen saturation and the results demonstrated no important changes during treatment with opioids (Jennings et al., 2002).

In another study of elderly COPD patients with dyspnea at rest, despite optimal medical treatment, the authors concluded that oral sustained-release morphine can improve intractable breathlessness. Again, no evidence of respiratory depression was found. The authors call for larger studies to evaiuate the safety of morphine therapy but stress that oral sustained-release morphine could provide significant relief to severely ill patients with COPD (Abernathy et al., 2003).

Implications for Nursing Practice

Oral and parenteral opioids are effective for dyspnea and can be safely administered to patients with COPD and cancer.

REFERENCES

Abernathy, A. P., Currow, D. C., Frith, P., et al. (2003). Randomized, double blind placebo controlled crossover trial of sustained release morphine for the management of refractory dyspnea. *British Medical Journal, 327,* 523–526.

Jennings, A. L., Davies, A. N., Higgins, J. P., et al. (2002). A systematic review of the use of opioids in the management of dyspnea. *Thorax, 57,* 939–944.

Terminal Restlessness

Terminal restlessness is a syndrome observed in a significant number of patients with various diagnoses during the final days of life. The patient may be unable to concentrate or relax and may show nonpurposeful motor activities such as picking at the sheets. The patient may hallucinate or try to climb out of bed. Terminal restlessness can have many causes, including hypoxemia, metabolic abnormalities, and liver failure. Some physical causes may be reversible, so it is important to assess whether pain, urine retention, or fecal impaction may be the cause.

Restlessness also may be caused by medications. As kidney and liver functions decline, medication levels rise in the body and cause toxicity. Consult with the physician and pharmacist to determine if all the medications the patient is receiving are beneficial or necessary. Table 17.3 reviews medications that may be helpful at the end of life.

Unconsciousness

Most patients are unconscious for hours or days before they die. Before they lose consciousness, their ability to see may be diminished. Hearing is the final sense to be lost. It is important for you to remember as you are caring for the patient and conversing with the family that your patient likely hears everything you are saying. Encourage the family to continue talking to the patient.

TABLE 17.3 MEDICATIONS TO INCREASE COMFORT AT THE END OF LIFE

Medication Class/ Action	Examples	Route	Side Effects	Nursing Implications
Opioids				
Bind to opioid receptors to reduce pain and dyspnea.	morphine (MS, MS-IR, MS Contin)	IV, subcutaneously, PO, SL, rectal suppository	Constipation, dry mouth, respiratory depression	For pain and dyspnea. Must be given routinely to be effective.
	hydromorphone (Dilaudid)	IV, subcutaneously, PO, SL		Give routinely.
	fentanyl (Sublimaze, Actiq)	Patch, IV, SL		Give short-acting analgesia for 24–72 hours until fentanyl patch takes effect. Do not cut patches before application. Wear gloves when applying or removing patch because drug may be absorbed during handling. Do not apply heat over a patch. Heat increases drug absorption and may cause overdoses. Used patches may still contain drug. Dispose of used patches to prevent accidental exposure to others, especially children and pets.
Anxiolytics				
Depress central nervous system to reduce anxiety.	lorazepam (Ativan) alprazolam (Xanax) diazepam (Valium)	IV, PO, subcutaneously, SL	Dry mouth, unsteadiness. Assess for oversedation if used with opioids.	Not first-line drugs for treating dyspnea.
Neuroleptics				
Reduce severe agitation, terminal restlessness.	haloperidol (Haldol)	PO, IM	Tardive dyskinesia, pseudo-parkinsonism	Useful in treating anxiety or agitation when lorazepam ineffective.
Anticholinergics				
For treating excessive pharyngeal secretions	hyoscyamine (Cystospaz)	SL	Urine retention, dry mouth	Works faster than scopolamine patch.
	scopolamine (Transderm-Scop)	Patch		For early treatment of secretions. Place patch behind the ear. Consider if hyoscyamine ineffective.
	glycopyrrolate (Robinul)	Subcutaneously, PO		

CRITICAL THINKING

Mr. Johnson

■ Mr. Johnson is in the final hours of his life and has become increasingly short of breath throughout the day. With each inspiration, his respirations are moist and noisy. Currently, his respiratory rate is 30 per minute, and you notice he is using his accessory muscles to breathe.

1. What is the cause of his noisy breathing?
2. What can be done to lower his respiratory rate and decrease his dyspnea?

Suggested answers at end of chapter.

CARE AT THE TIME OF DEATH AND AFTERWARD

Death has occurred when you observe the absence of heartbeat and respirations. The skin becomes pale and waxen, the eyes may remain open, and pupils are fixed. Telling the family that the patient has died should be done with sensitivity, providing small amounts of information according to the family's level of understanding. Be sure to check and adhere to the policies in your setting and state regarding death pronouncement and organ donation. Document the general appearance of the body, including absent pulse and lung sounds. Your goal now is to provide a personal closure experience for the family.

After death has been pronounced, you will provide **postmortem care**. First, remove the tubes, medical supplies, and equipment. Bathing and dressing the patient and making him look presentable for the family shows respect. Some cultures dictate specific care of the body after death and who should provide that care (see Chapter 4 for more information). The nurse can assess and advocate for cultural practices requested by the family. Work toward providing a clean, peaceful impression of the deceased. Position the body in proper alignment, insert dentures, place dressings on leaking wounds, and use briefs as needed. Allow the family time with the body. Embalming is necessary within 12 hours. Do not remove the body from the room until the family is ready. Covering or uncovering the face at removal should be done according to the family's preference. Additional activities, such as contacting the physician or funeral home, should be carried out according to institution policy.

GRIEF

Grief is the emotional response to a loss. Loss is a daily experience in everyone's life. Loss can occur due to divorce, children leaving home, loss of job, loss of possessions, or other losses. People express grief in their own way according to their coping skills, life experiences, and cultural norms. In end-of-life care, grief is a process that begins before the patient's death and continues through a series of tasks that the survivors move through to resolve grief. Feelings associated with grief may include anger, frustration, regret, guilt, sadness, and many others. Although each person is different, the process commonly includes three general stages (Table 17.4).

Interventions for the grieving patient are addressed in the *Nursing Care Plan for the Patient at the End of Life*. The nursing process for the grieving family is addressed next.

Nursing Process for the Grieving Family

Data Collection

Some things to consider when assessing grief include the following:

- Where is the family in the grief process?
- Are family members experiencing physical problems, such as shortness of breath, sweating, skin color changes?

TABLE 17.4 STAGES OF GRIEF

Stage	Tasks	Characteristics
Stage 1		
Shock and disbelief	Acknowledge the reality of the loss. Recognize the loss.	Has difficulty with feelings of numbness, emotional outbursts, poor daily functioning, and avoidance.
Stage 2		
Experiencing the loss	Work through the pain by expressing and experiencing the feelings.	Anger, bargaining, depression. May feel guilt over not preventing the death or not providing enough care. May feel angry at loved one who has "left them behind." May experience insomnia, loss of appetite, apathy, lack of interest in daily life.
Stage 3		
Reintegration	Adjust to an environment without the deceased.	Finds hope in the future, participates in social events, feels more energetic.

- Is the stress of grieving worsening medical conditions?
- What support systems are available to the family?
- What interventions can I use to facilitate their grief process?

Nursing Diagnoses, Planning, and Implementation

Although many nursing diagnoses may be appropriate, the priority diagnosis is simply *Grieving.*

Grieving Related to Impending Death or Loss of Loved One

EXPECTED OUTCOME: The family will be able to express feelings of anger, guilt, or sadness. They will be able to think about the future and perform ADLs as needed.

- Simply be present. *Sitting with the bereaved, without having to have all the answers is very powerful. If you don't know what to say, just be silent.*
- Actively listen, letting the bereaved talk about the loved one and their feelings about the loss. Ask open-ended questions to encourage them to continue talking. *One of the greatest needs of the bereaved is to trust someone enough to share their pain.*
- Help family members identify their support systems (church, friends, family) and encourage them to use them. *Support systems can help in practical ways (meals, transportation) as well as lend emotional support.*
- Consider acknowledging the event by attending the memorial service or sending a card. *This simple act of caring is very important to families.*

Evaluation

Healing takes time. If interventions have been effective, however, the family will have the support to function effectively while they grieve.

THE NURSE AND LOSS

Working with dying patients triggers awareness of your own losses and fears about death and mortality. Adapting to the care of the dying requires that you explore and experience your personal feelings toward death. Unresolved losses from your past can resurface and affect your ability to care for dying patients. You may find that you continue to think about patients who have died long after the event. Emotionally continuing to care about deceased patients takes energy away from the daily care you are providing to current patients and your own family. Unresolved grief can lead to symptoms that resemble burnout, such as insomnia, headaches, and fatigue.

If you find yourself distancing and withdrawing from your dying patients, it is an indicator that you need to attend to caring for yourself. Some nurses may find counseling helpful to effectively process losses from the past and learn healthy ways to process future losses.

Both formal and informal support systems should be in place to support staff through multiple losses. Informal support can be one-on-one sharing of experiences with coworkers, peers, pastoral counselors, and physicians. Understanding and acknowledging your limitations, asking for help, and getting regular exercise and relaxation are important components. Some nurses find journal writing a helpful process, where writing down feelings allows you to release them. Formal support systems can be established in many different ways:

- Preplanned gatherings where nurses can express feelings in a safe environment
- Post-clinical debriefings after difficult deaths to alleviate anxiety and promote learning
- Ceremonies such as memorial services in facilities to allow both staff and residents to recognize and honor the loss of patients.

In addition, many employers offer free employee assistance programs that provide counseling.

REFLECTIONS ON MR. MORAN

Remember Mr. Moran from the beginning of the chapter? Clearly he is approaching the end of life. Determine what he and his family want to happen in the final months of his life and where he wants to be. What are the goals of care? If comfort is the goal, how can this best be achieved? If keeping him in his familiar and safe environment is the goal, then help his family weigh the benefits and burdens of CPR, hospitalization, artificial feeding, and artificial hydration.

Home Health Hints

- Allow time during your visit to sit quietly with the patient and caregiver. Sitting quietly lets the patient and caregiver know you are there to meet both physical and emotional needs.
- Encourage family involvement with care. Families need reassurance that they are not going to hurt the patient; take the time to teach them how to assist the patient with basic care.
- Prepare the family for what to expect as death approaches.
- When the patient is no longer conscious, encourage the family to continue to spend time at the bedside sharing personal thoughts and memories with the patient. For example, a spouse might talk about when they first met, or family members can play a favorite song.

ETHICAL CONSIDERATIONS DISCUSSION

Allowing someone to die, like abortion, generates huge controversy and debate. Each side of the argument can justify its stance using moral and ethical principles. Again, like abortion, religious and secular views may conflict. Both present strong but opposing arguments. Those supporting a peaceful death for Adam could state that respect for autonomy would mean that if Adam gave clear indication that he would not want to live in such a progressively worsening condition, his wishes for being allowed to die peacefully should be upheld, regardless of personal or public opinion. Conversely, the opposing side could argue that Adam's autonomy should be protected while he is incapable of making such choices. Therefore, his right to choose must be protected.

Karen chose to work in a facility where people often die, so she would be familiar with the process. The central question is whether she could actually participate in an act that would contribute to the death of a patient. Essentially, Karen must examine her own personal moral values to direct her actions. In this case, the ethical principles dictating the interaction between patient and nurse must be weighed carefully against what Karen holds dear. Karen also may want to distinguish between causing someone to die versus allowing someone to die of natural causes after stopping artificial feeding. Beneficence, nonmaleficence, and autonomy have their place in this scenario regardless of opposing sides. It is important to consider Adam's wishes if they are known. Sometimes the person who is the subject of the debate can be forgotten while groups argue about which approach is right.

In the end, the courts decided Adam's outcome. If Karen can't in good conscience discontinue his feeding, she may be able to ask for reassignment during this shift.

SUGGESTED ANSWERS TO

CRITICAL THINKING

■ *Mrs. Hart*

Mrs. Hart will need a DNR order in the hospital setting and, when she goes home, she will need an out-of-hospital, prehospital, or durable DNR, whatever is called for in her state of residence. In addition, her family members should be aware of her wishes.

■ *Mr. Johnson*

1. Mr. Johnson's noisy breathing may be caused by saliva collecting in the back of the throat, or by pulmonary edema.
2. Mr. Johnson may benefit from oxygen. Low-dose morphine will decrease his respiratory rate and improve his oxygenation. Morphine also has a drying effect on secretions. If morphine is unsuccessful, the addition of hyoscyamine may be helpful.

REVIEW QUESTIONS

1. A 94-year-old gentleman is admitted from home to the hospital with pneumonia. What factors would lead the nurse to believe he is nearing the end of his life?
   a. His abdomen is distended and his skin tone is yellow.
   b. He has a fever of 101.6°F (38.7°C) and a respiratory rate of 28 per minute.
   c. He has been having difficulty swallowing and is losing weight.
   d. He has crackles in his lung bases bilaterally.

2. What is a durable power of attorney for health care?
   a. A document that outlines a patient's wishes at the end of life
   b. A document that gives a patient a "do not resuscitate" status
   c. A document specifying the person who will make decisions for a patient once the document is signed
   d. A document specifying the person who will make decisions for a patient when the patient is no longer able to speak for himself

3. A patient's family member says, "I heard someone say my mother could have a 'good death.' What on earth is a good death?" Which response by the nurse is best?
   a. "Some things that can contribute to a good death are allowing patients to make their own decisions at the end of life and ensuring that they die comfortably."
   b. "In reality, no death is a good death, but we do our best to make sure patients are comfortable right up until they die."
   c. "Research has shown that patients can die good deaths if they are kept sedated so they don't really know what is happening during the last days until they die."
   d. "A good death occurs when the patient is kept alive as long as possible, so she can take care of all her unfinished business first."

REVIEW QUESTIONS—cont'd

4. A husband whose wife has just died cries, "What am I going to do? She is all I had." What is the best response the nurse can provide?
   a. "You are going to go on with your life. You still have your work and your children."
   b. "I am sorry you lost your wife, but I know she would not want you to be sad. You have to be strong for her."
   c. "I know how you feel. I lost my grandmother recently, and it was really hard."
   d. There is no need to say anything. Just be present and listen.

5. A dying patient has excessive secretions that are causing dyspnea. Which medication will best help dry the secretions and increase comfort?
   a. Haloperidol
   b. Scopolamine
   c. Acetaminophen
   d. Diazepam

6. Which of the following nursing interventions should the nurse provide at the end of life? **Select all that apply**.
   a. Position the patient to increase comfort and prevent complications.
   b. Provide comfort measures such as massage.
   c. Research experimental treatments that may help the patient find a cure.
   d. Administer medications to increase comfort.
   e. Teach the family CPR for use if the patient dies when the nurse is not present.
   f. Sit quietly with the patient and family.

7. A patient has just died, and his family is waiting to see him. What postmortem care is essential first?
   a. Document the time and circumstances of the death.
   b. Place identification on the body according to hospital policy.
   c. Clean the patient up and make him look peaceful.
   d. Cover the patient's body and face with a sheet.

8. The wife of a hospitalized patient who died an hour ago is crying and unwilling to leave the hospital room. The rest of the family is in the waiting room. The admitting department just called and wants to have the room cleaned for a new patient. Which action should the nurse take?
   a. Allow the wife to stay in the room as long as she likes.
   b. Call a taxicab for the wife and gently guide her out of the room.
   c. Sit with the wife for a few minutes, then take her to the waiting room.
   d. Tell the wife that you are sorry for her loss, but that another patient needs the room.

9. A patient who has been receiving hospice care for 3 months tells the LPN he has decided he wants to return to active treatment of his disease. What should the LPN do?
   a. Encourage the patient to discuss his desire with his physician.
   b. Tell the patient that he cannot change his goals once hospice care has been initiated.
   c. Check his medication supply for any leftover medications he was taking during treatment.
   d. Explain to the patient that since he is terminal, treatment will not help the course of his disease.

References

Callanan, M., & Kelley, P. (1992). *Final gifts: Understanding the special awareness, needs and communication of the dying.* New York: Bantam Books.

Caprio, A., Hanson, L., Munn, J., et al. (2008). Pain, dyspnea and the quality of dying in long term care. *Journal of the American Geriatrics Society, 56,* 683–688.

Finucane, T., Christmas, C., & Travis, K. (1999). Tube feeding in patients with advanced dementia: A review of the evidence. *Journal of the American Medical Association, 282,* 1365–1370.

McCann, R. M., Hall, W. J., & Groth-Juncker, A. (1994). Comfort care for terminally ill patients: The appropriate use of nutrition and hydration. *Journal of the American Medical Association, 272,* 1263–1266.

Murden, R. A., & Ainslie, N. K. (1994). Recent weight loss is related to short term mortality in nursing homes. *Journal of General Internal Medicine, 9,* 648–650.

Saklayen, M., Liss, H., & Markert, N. (1995). In-hospital cardiopulmonary resuscitation: Survival in one hospital and literature review. *Medicine, 74,* 163–175.

Singer, P. A., Martin, D. K., & Kelner, M. (1999). Quality end-of-life care: Patients' perspectives. *Journal of the American Medical Association, 281,* 163–168.

Volicer, L. (2005). *End of life care for people with dementia in residential settings.* Chicago: Alzheimer's Association National Office. Retrieved February 6, 2010, from http://www.alz.org/national/documents/endoflifelitreview.pdf

unit FOUR

UNDERSTANDING THE IMMUNE SYSTEM

18

Immune System Function, Assessment, and Therapeutic Measures

SHARON M. NOWAK AND
JANICE L. BRADFORD

KEY TERMS

active immunity (AK-tiv im-YOO-nih-tee)
anaphylactic (AN-uh-fih-LAK-tik)
antibody (AN-tih-baw-dee)
antigen (AN-tih-jen)
autoimmune (AW-toe-ih-mewn)
cell-mediated immunity (SELL mee-dee-ay-ted ih-MYOO-nih-tee)
humoral immunity (HYOO-mur-uhl ih-MYOO-nih-tee)
lymphocyte (LIM-fuh-site)
neutrophil (NEW-troh-fil)
passive immunity (PASS-iv ih-MYOO-nih-tee)
white blood cells (WYTE BLUHD SELLS)

QUESTIONS TO GUIDE YOUR READING

1. What type of immunity is obtained with a vaccine?
2. How does aging affect the immune system?
3. What subjective data are collected when caring for a patient with a disorder of the immune system?
4. What objective data are collected when caring for a patient with a disorder of the immune system?
5. What nursing care is provided for patients undergoing diagnostic tests for the immune system?
6. What common therapeutic measures are used for a patient with disorders of the immune system?

NORMAL IMMUNE ANATOMY AND PHYSIOLOGY

Immunity is defined as the ability to destroy pathogens or other foreign material and to prevent further cases of certain infectious diseases. Immunity is most often thought of in terms of the body's response to microorganisms such as bacteria, viruses, and fungi, all of which are foreign to the body. However, immunity also involves processes directed toward other cells or substances that are identified by the body, correctly or incorrectly, as foreign. Malignant cells are foreign in that they have mutated from normal form and are usually destroyed by the immune system after mutation and before they become malignant. Unfortunately, transplanted organs are usually perceived as foreign (cornea transplants and transplants from identical twins can be an exception to being perceived as foreign); rejection of a transplanted organ is an immune response. Occasionally, the immune system mistakenly reacts to self (autoimmune disease) or to a substance that should be tolerated (allergic reaction).

The immune system consists of lymphoid organs and tissues, **lymphocytes** and other **white blood cells**, and many chemicals involved in activation of our own cells for the destruction of foreign antigens (Fig. 18.1). The lymphatic system includes lymphatic vessels that help return tissue fluid to the circulatory system; lymph nodes and nodules, which are masses of lymphatic tissue that differ in size and location; the spleen, where macrophages phagocytize pathogens and B and T cells carry out immune functions; and the thymus,

• **WORD** • **BUILDING** •
lymphocyte: lympho—lymph + kytos—cell

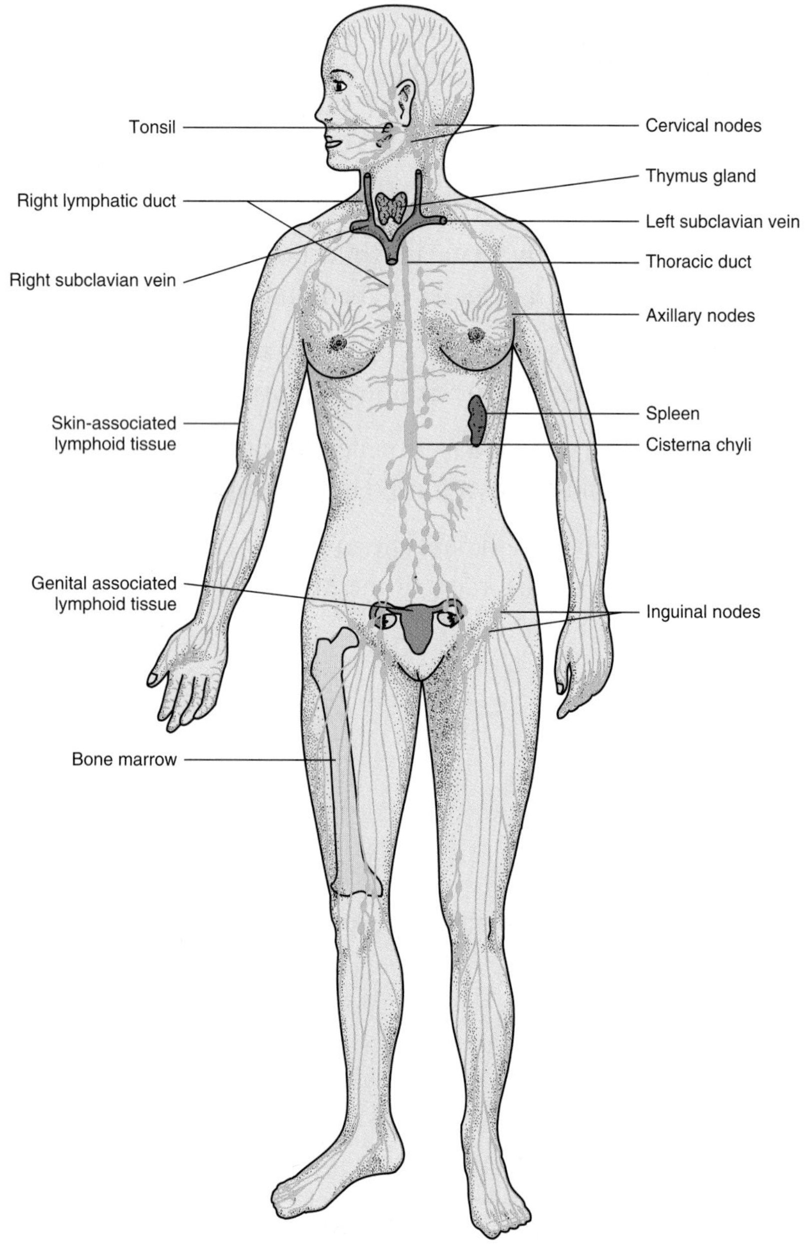
Tonsil
Right lymphatic duct
Right subclavian vein
Skin-associated lymphoid tissue
Genital associated lymphoid tissue
Bone marrow
Cervical nodes
Thymus gland
Left subclavian vein
Thoracic duct
Axillary nodes
Spleen
Cisterna chyli
Inguinal nodes

FIGURE 18.1 Immune system organs, lymph vessels, and major lymph nodes.

which functions primarily in childhood and atrophies with age. Lymph nodes are grouped along lymph vessels to destroy foreign material. Three major groups are the cervical, axillary, and inguinal nodes. Lymph nodules lack encapsulation and are smaller than nodes; lymph nodules are found under the surface of mucous membranes (e.g., tonsils).

Antigens

Antigens are chemical markers that identify cells or molecules. Examples of molecular antigens include bacterial toxins, plant pollens or proteins that trigger allergies, and the protein products of viral activity in cells. Human cells (except red blood cells [RBCs]) have their own self antigens—thousands of markers that identify the cell as belonging in the body. These are the major histocompatibility complex (MHC) antigens, also called human leukocyte antigens (HLAs), which are genetically determined. The MHC antigens of identical twins are identical. These MHC antigens serve as a comparison for cells of the immune system; the antigens of foreign cells do not "match" MHC antigens and may therefore be recognized as foreign and destroyed in one of several ways.

Lymphocytes

There are three types of lymphocytes: natural killer (NK) cells, thymus-derived lymphocytes (T cells), and bone marrow–derived lymphocytes (B cells), each with very different functions.

Natural Killer Cells

NK cells are found in the blood, red bone marrow, lymph nodes, and spleen and are able to destroy many kinds of infected body cells and tumor cells. NK cells attack any self-cell that displays abnormal plasma membrane proteins. After binding with an abnormal cell, NK cells release toxins in granules, either perforins or granzymes. Perforins create a hole in the plasma membrane of the attacked cell; the result is cytolysis. Granzymes induce apoptosis (self-destruction) of the target cell. Any released microbes are phagocytized by WBCs. The action of NK cells is considered a nonspecific resistance mechanism because it is effective against a variety of foreign antigens.

• WORD • BUILDING •

antigen: anti—against + gennan—to produce

T Cells and B Cells

The lymphocytes called T cells and B cells are involved in specific immune responses; that is, each cell is genetically programmed to respond to one kind of foreign antigen. It is estimated that the human immune system can respond to a billion or more different foreign antigens.

Both T cells and B cells arise in the red bone marrow. T cells then migrate to the thymus, where the thymic hormones bring about their maturation. Most T cells arise before puberty, but the process continues at a slower pace throughout life. From the thymus, T cells migrate to the lymph nodes and nodules and to the spleen. B cells mature in the bone marrow and migrate directly to lymphatic tissue. When activated during an immune response, some B cells become plasma cells that produce antibodies; others become memory cells.

Antibodies

Antibodies are also called immunoglobulins (Ig) or gamma globulins and are glycoproteins produced by plasma cells in response to foreign antigens. Antibodies do not themselves destroy foreign antigens, but rather become attached to such antigens to "label" them for destruction. Each **antibody** is specific for only one antigen, and B cells (those that become plasma cells) are capable of producing millions of different antibodies. There are five classes of human antibodies, designated by letter names: IgG, IgA, IgM, IgD, and IgE. Their functions are summarized in Table 18.1.

Mechanisms of Immunity

The two mechanisms of immunity are **cell-mediated immunity**, which involves T cells, and **humoral immunity**, which involves mainly B cells but is assisted by T cells. Although the mechanisms are different, invasion by a pathogen often triggers both.

The first step in the destruction of a foreign antigen is the recognition of it as foreign. When B cells in lymphatic tissue recognize and bind with foreign antigens, they become

TABLE 18.1 CLASSES OF ANTIBODIES

Immunoglobulin (Ig)	Location	Function
IgG	Blood, extracellular fluid, lymph	Crosses the placenta to provide passive immunity in newborns Provides long-term immunity following a vaccination or illness recovery
IgA	External secretions (e.g., tears, saliva)	Provides passive immunity for breastfed infants Found in secretions of all mucous membranes
IgM	Blood, lymph	Produced first during an infection (IgG production follows)
IgD	B cells	Are antigen-specific receptors on B lymphocytes
IgE	Mast cells or basophils	Important in allergic reactions Mast cells release histamine

Source: Scanlon, V., & Sanders, T. (2007). *Understanding human structure and function* (5th ed., p. 333). Philadelphia: F. A. Davis.

activated B cells. Their activation is greatly enhanced if the foreign antigen is presented to them by antigen-presenting cells called dendritic cells. T cells have foreign antigen recognition only if subjected to an antigen-presenting cell, such as a dendritic cell, macrophage, or B cell that has previously processed the antigen.

Cell-Mediated Immunity

This mechanism of immunity does not involve the production of antibodies, but it is effective against intracellular pathogens (such as viruses or fungi), malignant cells, and grafts of foreign tissue. The first step is the recognition of the foreign antigen by T cells, assisted by macrophages, followed by costimulation by a second signal, often cytokines.

The newly activated T cells divide many times and become specialized. Helper T cells (CD4) secrete cytokines to enhance T cells, B cells, and NK cells. Cytotoxic T cells (CD8) are able to lyse infected body cells, malignant cells, or transplanted tissues. They also release chemicals that activate phagocytes such as macrophages and **neutrophils**. Memory T cells remember the specific foreign antigen and quickly activate an immune response should the antigen reappear.

Humoral Immunity

Humoral immunity is also called *antibody-mediated immunity* and involves antibody production. Again, the first step is the recognition of the antigen as being foreign; this time by B cells. Helper T cells costimulate the activated B cells to proliferate and differentiate. Some B cells become plasma cells that produce antibodies specific for this particular antigen.

• **WORD** • **BUILDING** •
neutrophil: neutro—neuter + philein—to love

Other B cells become memory B cells that will remember this antigen and initiate a rapid response should it return. Humoral immunity is effective against extracellular pathogens, which are usually bacteria but can also be viral or fungal infections.

Although B cells are stationary, the antibodies produced by plasma cells circulate throughout the body. The antibodies bond to the antigen, forming an antigen-antibody complex. This immobilizes the bacteria; also, the antigen is now "labeled" for phagocytosis by macrophages or neutrophils. The antigen-antibody complex also activates the complement cascade.

Complement is a group of over 30 plasma proteins that circulate in the blood until activated by an antigen-antibody complex in the classic pathway. (There are two alternative pathways that initiate the complement cascade.) The activation of complement results in the formation of a protein complex that lyses the cell and brings about its death. Other complement proteins bind to foreign antigens and serve as further labels to attract macrophages.

ANTIBODY RESPONSES

The first exposure to a foreign antigen stimulates antibody production, but the antibodies are produced too slowly to prevent the disease. However, with time, the person accumulates antibodies and memory cells specific for that pathogen. On a second exposure to the antigen, the memory cells begin rapid production of large amounts of antibody, often enough to prevent a second occurrence of the illness (Fig. 18.2). This is the basis for the protection given by vaccines. A vaccine contains an antigen that is not pathogenic (e.g., bacterial capsules

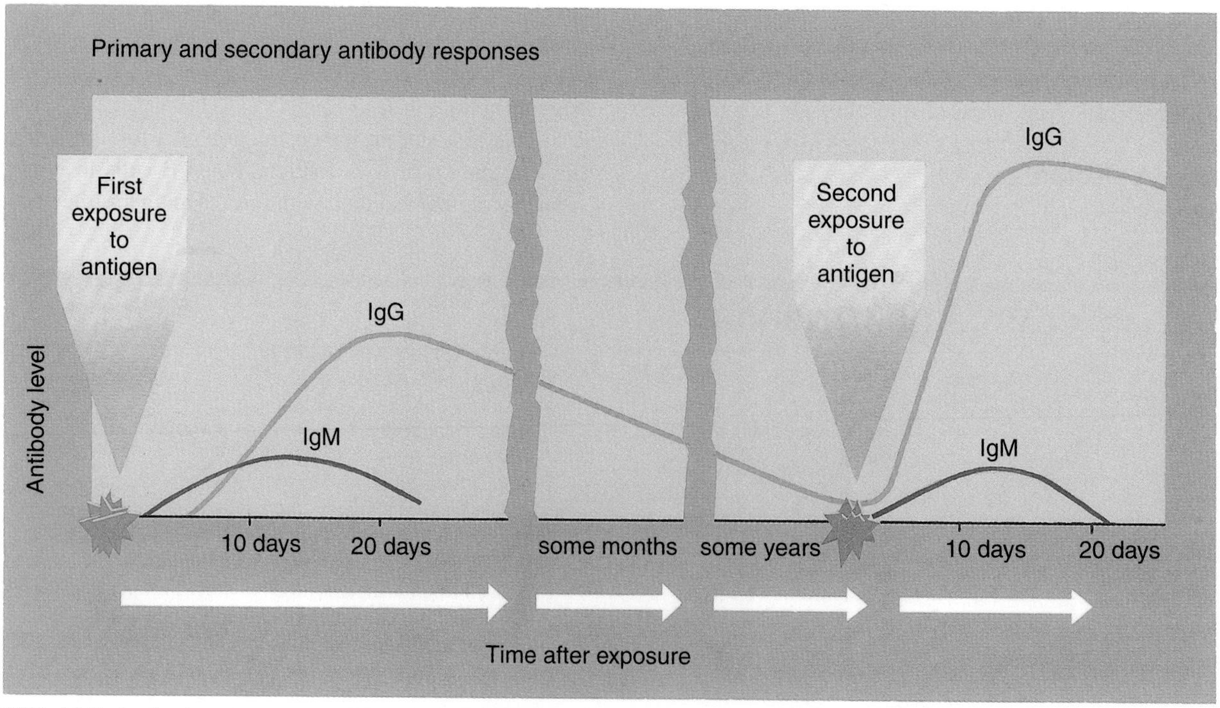
Primary and secondary antibody responses
First exposure to antigen
Second exposure to antigen
IgG
IgM
IgG
IgM
Antibody level
10 days
20 days
some months
some years
10 days
20 days
Time after exposure

FIGURE 18.2 Antibody responses to a first and then subsequent exposure to a pathogen. (From Scanlon, V., & Sanders, T. [2007]. *Essentials of anatomy and physiology* [5th ed., p. 335]. Philadelphia: F. A. Davis.)

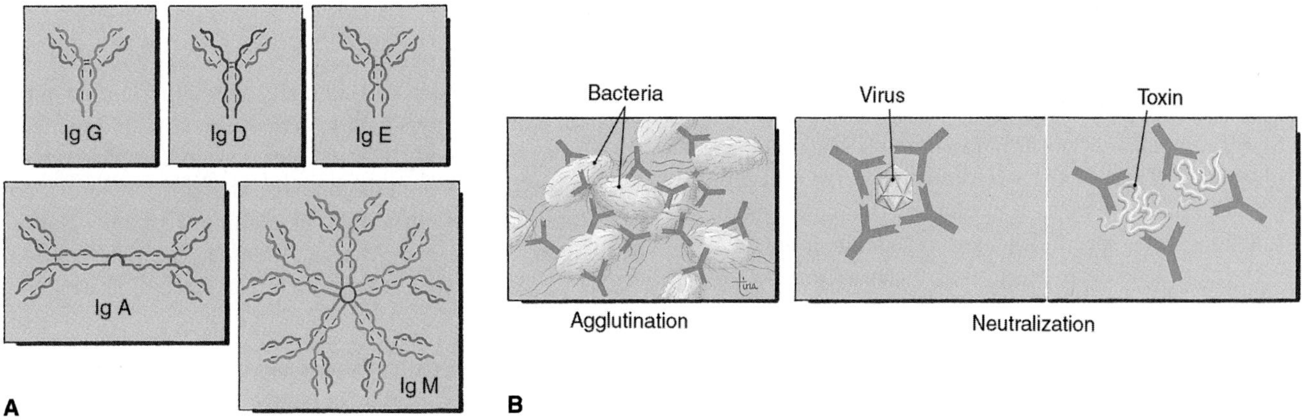
Ig G
Ig D
Ig E
Ig A
Ig M
A
Bacteria
Virus
Toxin
Agglutination
Neutralization
B

FIGURE 18.3 Antibodies. (A) Structure of the five classes of antibodies. (B) Antibody activity. (Adapted from Scanlon, V., & Sanders, T. [2007]. *Essentials of anatomy and physiology* [5th ed., p. 333]. Philadelphia: F. A. Davis.)

in the case of the pneumococcal vaccine). The vaccine stimulates the formation of antibodies and memory cells.

Antibodies also may neutralize viruses; that is, they attach to a virus and render it unable to enter a cell (Fig. 18.3). Viruses cannot reproduce outside of living cells, and those coated with antibodies are phagocytized by macrophages. Another aspect of our defenses against viruses is interferon, a chemical produced by cells infected with viruses. Although it does not help the infected cell, interferon protects surrounding cells by enabling them to resist viral replication.

Antibodies are also involved in allergic responses, in which the immune system responds to foreign but harmless antigens (an allergen), such as plant pollen. IgE antibodies bond to mast cells, which break down and release histamine and other chemicals that contribute to inflammation. **Anaphylactic** shock is an allergic reaction, but it is massive in nature. It is characterized by loss of plasma from capillaries (an effect of histamine) and a sudden drop in the intravascular blood volume and blood pressure.

TYPES OF IMMUNITY

Two categories of immunity are passive immunity and active immunity. In **passive immunity**, antibodies are not produced by the person but are obtained from another source. One form of *naturally* acquired passive immunity includes placental transmission of antibodies from mother to fetus and transmission of antibodies in breast milk. *Artificially* acquired passive immunity involves injection of preformed antibodies; this may help prevent disease after exposure to a pathogen such as the hepatitis B virus. Passive immunity is always temporary, in that antibodies from another source eventually break down.

Active immunity means that the person produces his or her own antibodies. An example of naturally acquired active immunity occurs when a person recovers from an infection and then has antibodies and memory cells specific for that pathogen. Artificially acquired active immunity occurs as the result of a vaccine that stimulates production of antibodies and memory cells. The duration of active immunity depends on the particular disease or vaccine; some confer lifelong immunity, but others do not.

Aging and the Immune System

The efficiency of the immune system decreases with age (Fig. 18.4). As such, older adults are more susceptible to infections and autoimmune disorders (Box 18.1, *Gerontological Issues*). The incidence of cancer is also higher; malignant cells that might once have been quickly destroyed by the immune system live and proliferate.

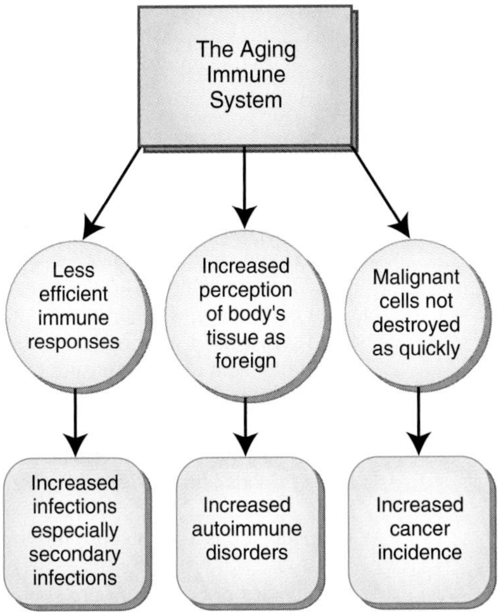
The Aging Immune System
Less efficient immune responses
Increased perception of body's tissue as foreign
Malignant cells not destroyed as quickly
Increased infections especially secondary infections
Increased autoimmune disorders
Increased cancer incidence

FIGURE 18.4 This concept map shows the effects the aging process has on the immune system.

• WORD • BUILDING •
anaphylactic: ana—up + phylaxis—protection

Box 18.1
Gerontological Issues

Significant changes occur in the immune system of the older adult. These changes are known as *immune senescence*, which refers to a decline in immune system function. Some specific changes include the following:

- Thymus gland decreases in size, increases production of immature T cells, and has a subsequent decline in response to antigens.
- Antibody response to foreign organisms decreases.

Immunizations to support the immune responses of older adults include the following:

- Influenza vaccine (plus H1N1 flu vaccine if recommended) yearly mid-October to mid-November, before influenza season
- Pneumococcal vaccine once after age 65
- Herpes zoster vaccine once after age 60
- Tetanus, diphtheria, and pertussis booster every 10 years.

NURSING ASSESSMENT OF THE IMMUNE SYSTEM

Disorders of the immune system can affect every system in the body so it is important to collect head-to-toe data as well as a patient history (Table 18.2).

History

Demographic Data

The patient's gender and ethnicity are important to note because some diseases tend to be associated with a particular gender or ethnicity. For instance, systemic lupus erythematosus (SLE), an autoimmune disorder, affects women up to eight times more than men. In addition, Hispanic, Native American, Asian, and African American women develop SLE two to three times more often than Caucasian women.

Health History

Assessment of the patient's past and present medical conditions should also include a family history. Many atopic (allergic) disorders, such as allergic rhinitis and asthma, and autoimmune disorders, such as ankylosing spondylitis, are thought to be either familial or have a genetic predisposition in certain ethnic or cultural groups (Box 18.2, *Cultural Considerations*). For example, 4 new genes have been identified that are strongly associated with SLE, and 10 others are possible risk factors.

Patients' previous surgeries may give clues about their previous health or current condition. For example, with thymus gland removal (thymectomy), T-cell production may be altered, which affects the cell-mediated immune response. Or if the spleen was removed (splenectomy), lymphocyte and plasma cell production may be altered, which affects the humoral immune response.

For current medications, include prescription drugs, over-the-counter drugs, and herbal preparations. Corticosteroids and immunosuppressants decrease the immune response, and some anti-infectives and antineoplastics depress the bone marrow. This results in decreased production of the cells made

TABLE 18.2 SUBJECTIVE DATA COLLECTION FOR THE IMMUNE SYSTEM

Category	Questions to Ask During the Health History	Rationale/Significance
Demographic Data	What is your age?	The immune system decreases in functional effectiveness as one ages, and a number of immune disorders tend to afflict individuals of particular age ranges.
	Where were you born? What is your ethnic or cultural background?	This information can aid in determining ethnic and cultural background influences. Some immune disorders tend to afflict individuals of particular cultural/ethnic groups more than others.
	Where have you lived? Where do you currently reside?	This information can aid in determining ethnic and cultural background as well as possible environmental influences.
History	Do you have allergies to any medications? Latex? Foods? Insects? Environmental allergens? If yes, have you had a recent exposure to any of these? Describe the reaction.	This information may lead to a direct cause of current symptoms and provides information regarding the status of the patient's immune system. Medication side effects are commonly inaccurately considered allergies by patients.
	Is anyone in your family allergic to medications? Latex? Foods? Insects? Environmental allergens?	If family members (especially immediate) have severe reactions to substances, the patient may be predisposed to immune reactions to the same antigen or in general.
	What medications are you currently taking?	Some medications can mask symptoms or immune responses, others can suppress immune responses.
	What illnesses or conditions are you currently being treated for? Have you been treated for?	May provide clues to patient's current condition or symptoms.

TABLE 18.2 SUBJECTIVE DATA COLLECTION FOR THE IMMUNE SYSTEM—cont'd

Category	Questions to Ask During the Health History	Rationale/Significance
	What surgeries have you had?	Have any immune organs been removed, therefore reducing immune function? May also provide indications about overall health.
	Have you ever had a blood transfusion? If so, why?	Antibodies to various antigen markers on the blood cells may have been formed. Additionally may provide indications to overall health.
	What is your occupation? Have you been exposed to hazardous chemicals, fumes, or radiation?	Many chemicals can produce local reactions, usually skin reactions or systemic immune reactions, and some can lead to bone marrow suppression in which all cell production is reduced.
	Do you engage in any form of risky behavior?	Risky behavior, such as intravenous drug usage and unprotected sex with multiple partners, increases a patient's chances of contracting the human immunodeficiency virus (HIV), which leads to a reduction in the immune system function.
	Describe your overall stress level and life stressors.	Stress is known to suppress the immune system and, over prolonged periods, can lead to a variety of illnesses.
	What do you do to cope with stress?	Not all coping behaviors and mechanisms are healthy; therefore, it is important to assess what the patient's coping behaviors are to see if the patient needs education.
	What sort of support systems do you have?	Support systems can buffer the day-to-day stress as well as during crisis.

Box 18.2

Cultural Considerations

The Navajo people have a high incidence of severe combined immunodeficiency syndrome (SCIDS), an immunodeficiency syndrome unrelated to acquired immunodeficiency syndrome (AIDS). SCIDS is a failure of the antibody response and cell-mediated immunity. Infants who survive initially are sent to tertiary care facilities. They must receive gamma globulin on a regular basis until a bone marrow transplant can be performed. Thus far, studies indicate that SCIDS is unique to the Navajo population.

in the bone marrow. Bone marrow depression of WBCs can alter cell-mediated and humoral immune responses. The herbal preparation licorice, which is sometimes used for its anti-inflammatory and expectorant effects, when taken with corticosteroids, increases the effects of the corticosteroids.

A patient's lifestyle may influence immune system function and should be assessed. Knowing a patient's dietary habits and supplemental vitamins gives insight into the potential reserve of the patient's immune system for fighting infection. Anaphylactic reactions can be caused by exposure to latex, which may be found in gloves and other medical products that health care workers and their patients touch. Be aware of this potentially life-threatening reaction, and know the agency's latex allergy protocol. Patients who are allergic to latex should wear a medical alert bracelet and carry an anaphylactic epinephrine kit.

The patient's life stressors, coping behaviors, and support systems should be explored. Stress (environmental, physical, and psychological) can depress immune system function. Coping behaviors are essential to keep stress within manageable limits to maintain optimum immune function. Support systems play an important role in coping with stress and should be encouraged and nurtured by nurses.

Current Problem

Use the WHAT'S UP? format to collect data about the current immune system problem. For immune disorders, ask the patient the following questions:

- Where is it? What part of the body is affected?
- How does it feel? Painful? Itching?
- Aggravating and alleviating factors?
- Timing: Was there exposure to a pathogen? Did you have a previous infection? Does it occur only in certain settings? Did you have chemotherapy or radiation therapy? How long have symptoms persisted?

- Severity. Does it affect activities of daily living (ADLs)? Work? Roles?
- Useful data for associated symptoms. Immunosuppression? Family history? Allergies?
- Perception of the patient of the problem. What do you think is wrong?

Common signs and symptoms present with immune disorders include fever, fatigue, joint pain, swollen glands, weight loss, and rash.

Physical Examination

Physical data collection begins by observing the patient's general appearance, color, posture, gait, facial expression, skin, and nailbeds (Table 18.3). Any cyanosis or erythema (redness) is noted. Rashes should be examined for size, shape, location, texture, drainage, and pruritus (itching). Visual and hearing changes can be associated with an immune disorder.

Adventitious lung sounds, such as wheezing, may indicate asthma or an allergic response. Crackles are often associ-

TABLE 18.3 OBJECTIVE DATA COLLECTION FOR THE IMMUNE SYSTEM

Category	Physical Examination Findings	Possible Abnormal Findings/Causes
Neurologic	Alertness and orientation	Confusion or lethargy are common in later stages of systemic lupus erythematosus (SLE) and acquired immunodeficiency syndrome (AIDS).
Skin	Warm, dry, smooth, supple, even coloring, nonpruritic	Rash, urticaria, pruritus, pustules are seen with many forms of allergic reactions. "Butterfly rash" (red rash over bridge of nose and cheek bones) is seen in 55%–85% of patients with SLE. Painless purple lesions are seen with Kaposi's sarcoma, which is associated with HIV and AIDS.
	Pink mucous membranes	Pale edematous mucous membranes along with rhinorrhea and "allergic shiners" (dark circles under the eyes) are seen with allergic rhinitis. Pale conjunctiva is associated with anemia. Periorbital edema may be indicative of hypothyroidism.
	Nail attached to nailbed	Onycholysis (nail detaches from nailbed) is seen in patient's with Hashimoto's thyroiditis.
Heart Sounds	Clear S_1 and S_2	Pericardial friction rub may be heard with rheumatoid arthritis or SLE because of inflammation of the connective tissue surrounding the heart (pericardium).
Lung Sounds	Clear throughout	Pleural effusion as evidenced by tachypnea with diminished sounds in bases may be seen in SLE or rheumatoid arthritis, or a pleural friction rub may occur in these patients. Crackles with a dry cough may be indicative of *Pneumocystis jiroveci* (formerly *carinii*) pneumonia (PCP).
Lymph Nodes	Nonpalpable and nontender	Enlarged lymph nodes that are painless, firm, and fixed are associated with cancerous lesions, whereas painful enlarged lymph nodes are associated with inflammation and infection.
Gastrointestinal	Appropriate appetite without nausea or vomiting	Anorexia, nausea, and vomiting may be associated with immune disorders.
	Regular pattern of brown, soft, formed stools	Diarrhea or diarrhea alternating with constipation is common in patients with irritable bowel syndrome (IBS).
Renal	An average of 30 mL per hour of clear, yellow/amber urine without presence of protein or pain	Urine output of less than 30 mL per hour, the presence of protein in urine, and edema are seen in patients with SLE or serum sickness. Transfusion reactions may cause hematuria, flank pain, or oliguria. Glomerulonephritis may cause hematuria, flank pain, or oliguria.
Musculoskeletal	Painless and nonswollen joints with full range of motion	Swollen, painful joints and limited joint range of motion are seen in rheumatoid arthritis.
	Overall strength, endurance and coordination appropriate for age and physical fitness	Decreased strength and coordination occur in patients with multiple sclerosis. Patients with myasthenia gravis lose strength and endurance with repetitive movements.

ated with upper respiratory infection. Lymph nodes should be inspected and then gently palpated (by the advanced practitioner). (See Fig. 18.1.) Normally, lymph nodes are not palpable in the adult. If enlarged, note the following characteristics: location, size, shape, tenderness, temperature, consistency, mobility, symmetry, pulsation, and if red streaks, redness, or edema are present.

LEARNING TIP

A normally functioning immune system is required to trigger an inflammatory response and production of the signs of inflammation or infection: fever, redness, pain, swelling, and warmth. If the immune system is suppressed or functioning abnormally, this normal inflammatory response may not occur. Thus, the patient may have only a low-grade fever with none of the other signs of inflammation or infection (redness, pain, swelling, and warmth).

Recognize patients with suppressed immune systems so that low-grade fevers are reported to the physician for prompt treatment. This may be the only sign of a life-threatening infection that develops because of the suppressed immune system.

CRITICAL THINKING

Mrs. Sims

■ Mrs. Sims is scheduled for a lymph node biopsy and is seen in preadmission testing before surgery. As the licensed practical nurse/licensed vocational nurse (LPN/LVN) prepares to draw blood specimens, he learns that Mrs. Sims is allergic to latex.

1. Why is this patient allergy information important?
2. What should the LPN/LVN do next?
3. What precautions should the LPN/LVN use for drawing the blood specimen?

Suggested answers at end of chapter.

If enlarged, the spleen may be palpable (by the advanced practitioner) in the left upper quadrant of the abdomen with disorders in which there is an overproduction or excessive destruction of red blood cells.

Renal impairment from an immune disorder causes a change in urinary output, flank pain, edema, weight gain, or elevated renal function studies.

A general neurologic assessment of muscle strength and coordination, changes, or abnormalities is made. Changes may be an indication of an immune-based disorder such as multiple sclerosis or myasthenia gravis.

DIAGNOSTIC TESTS FOR THE IMMUNE SYSTEM

Presenting signs and symptoms and the patient's history determine which tests and procedures may be ordered. Table 18.4 describes the most common blood tests for patients with allergic, autoimmune, or immune disorders. Table 18.5 presents common noninvasive and invasive procedures for immune disorders.

Gene Testing

With completion of the human genome mapping project, scientists are able to test for numerous diseases, predisposition to diseases, and enzyme deficiencies that can alter immune response.

TABLE 18.4 DIAGNOSTIC LABORATORY TESTS FOR IMMUNE SYSTEM

Test	Definition/Normal Value	Significance of Abnormal Findings
RBC Count	Number of RBCs per 1 mm of blood *Adult male:* 4.7–6.1 × 10^{12}/L *Adult female:* 4.2–5.4 × 10^{12}/L	Decreased in all forms of anemia, such as pernicious anemia that develops from the autoimmune form of gastritis or idiopathic autoimmune hemolytic anemia.
Differential	Each of these tests (MCV, MCH, MCHC, RDW) provides information about RBC size, shape, color, and intracellular structure. *Normal:*	Can help determine the cause of anemia. Pernicious anemia can develop because of the autoimmune form of gastritis.
• MCV	80–95 mm^3	
• MCH	27–31 pg	
• MCHC	32–36 g/dL	
• RDW	11.0%–14.5%	
WBC Count	Number of WBCs per 1 mm of blood *Adult:* 5–10 × 10^9/L	Increased with immunosuppression and infection.

Continued

TABLE 18.4 DIAGNOSTIC LABORATORY TESTS FOR IMMUNE SYSTEM—cont'd

Test	Definition/Normal Value	Significance of Abnormal Findings
Differential	Percentage of type of white blood cells in 1 mm of blood. Or the actual numbers of specific types of WBCs if an absolute count is performed. *Normal:* % — Absolute/mm^3	Eosinophils elevate with type I hypersensitivity reactions such as allergic rhinitis or anaphylaxis.
• Neutrophils	55–70 — 2500–8000	
• Lymphocytes	20–40 — 1000–4000	
• Monocytes	2–8 — 100–700	
• Eosinophils	1–4 — 50–500	
• Basophils	0.5–1.0 — 25–100	
Erythrocyte Sedimentation Rate (ESR)	A nonspecific test for generalized inflammation. Measures the red blood cell descent (in millimeters) in test tube after being in normal saline solution for 1 hr (Westergren method). *Male:* Up to 15 mm/hr *Female:* Up to 20 mm/hr	False negative may result if steroids or NSAIDs are being used when test is performed.
Rheumatoid Factor (RF or RA)	An abnormal protein found in serum when IgM reacts with an abnormal IgG; found in 80% of patients with rheumatoid arthritis and other autoimmune disorders. *Normal:* Negative	Increased in rheumatoid arthritis, SLE, leukemia, tuberculosis, older age, scleroderma, infectious mononucleosis.
Antinuclear Antibody (ANA)	Measures autoantibodies that attack the cell's nucleus. *Normal:* Negative	Most commonly present in SLE (greater than 95% sensitivity), leukemia, scleroderma, rheumatoid arthritis, and myasthenia gravis; many medications influence levels.
• Anti-DNA (ANA subset)	*Normal:* Less than 70 international units/mL *Borderline:* 70–200 international units/mL *Positive:* More than 200 international units/mL	Positive in 65%–80% of SLE patients.
Complement	Specific serum proteins that help mediate inflammation. Measures the amount of each of the components in the complement system. *Normal:*	Deficiencies of specific complement proteins are seen in SLE.
• Total	75–160 units/mL	
• C3	0.55–1.20 g/L	
• C4	0.2–0.5 g/L	
C-Reactive Protein (CRP)	An abnormal protein found in plasma during acute inflammatory processes; more sensitive than sedimentation rate. *Normal:* Less than 10 mg/L	Increased in rheumatoid arthritis, cancer, SLE. Suppressed by aspirin and steroids.
Radioallergosorbent test (RAST)	Patient serum is mixed with a specific allergen, incubated with radiolabeled anti-IgE antibodies, and then the total amount of the specific IgE antibodies is measured.	A viable alternative to skin testing if the patient does not have multiple allergies.
Enzyme-Linked Immunosorbent Assay (ELISA)	Patient's blood is tested for antibodies on HIV antigen test plates.	Positive results may indicate HIV infection, but results *must* be confirmed by another test, usually the Western blot.
Western Blot	A blood test to detect the presence of any of the four major HIV antigens. Is considered positive when at least two of the four antigens are detected. Used as a confirmation test.	If being used as the confirmation test, positive results indicate HIV infection. False positives do occur in patients who have autoimmune disease, leukemia, lymphoma, or syphilis, and in people with alcoholism.
Immunoglobulin Assay or Electrophoresis	Antibodies are made up of immunoglobulins, of which there are five different classes. *Normal (mg/dL):*	
• IgG	500–1500	Increased in all types of infections, liver disease, rheumatoid arthritis, dermatological disorders. Decreased in agammaglobulinemia, lymphoid aplasia, Bence-Jones proteinuria.
• IgM	50–300	Increased in malaria, infectious mononucleosis, SLE, rheumatoid arthritis. Decreased in lymphoid aplasia, chronic lymphoblastic leukemia.

TABLE 18.4 DIAGNOSTIC LABORATORY TESTS FOR IMMUNE SYSTEM—cont'd

Test	Definition/Normal Value	Significance of Abnormal Findings
• IgA	100–490	Increased during exercise, obstructive jaundice. Decreased in familial inheritance, immunosuppressive therapy, benzene exposure.
• IgE	Less than 100 international units/mL	Increased in allergic reactions, allergic infections.
• IgD	Less than 3 units/mL	Decreased in agammaglobulinemia.
CD4+ Count	CD4+ T lymphocytes are counted. *Percentage:* 60%–75% *Normal count:* 600–1500/mm^3	Increased in allergy-proven patients. Decreased in cancer, HIV and AIDS, and immunosuppression.
CD8+ Count	CD8+ T lymphocytes are counted. *Percentage:* 25%–30% *Normal count:* 300–1000/mm^3	Increased in viral infections. Decreased in SLE.
CD4+/CD8+ Ratio	Ratio of CD4+ and CD8+ absolute counts are determined. *Normal:* Greater than 1	As HIV/AIDS progresses, the CD4+/CD8+ ratio will become smaller as the CD4+ count decreases and the CD8+ count remains relatively unchanged.

AIDS = autoimmune deficiency syndrome; HIV = human immunodeficiency virus; MCH = mean corpuscular hemoglobin; MCHC = mean corpuscular hemoglobin concentration; MCV = mean corpuscular volume; NSAIDs = nonsteroidal anti-inflammatory drugs; RBC = red blood cell; RDW = red blood cell distribution width; SLE = systemic lupus erythematosus; WBC = white blood cell.

TABLE 18.5 DIAGNOSTIC PROCEDURES FOR THE IMMUNE SYSTEM

Procedure	Definition/Normal Finding (if applicable)	Significance of Abnormal Findings	Nursing Management (if applicable)
Noninvasive			
Chest X-Ray	Radiographic picture to determine size, shape, density of structures within the chest.	Pericarditis, pleuritis, pleural or pericardial effusions may occur with systemic lupus erythematosus (SLE) or rheumatoid arthritis. Arthritic changes may also be noted on x-ray.	None.
Gene Testing	A sample of DNA, which can be taken as an oral or nasal swab, is examined and mapped for a variety of genetic disorders.	Abnormal findings may confirm a certain diagnosis or indicate that the patient may develop symptoms or pass a disorder on to offspring.	Assess support systems and for possible counseling referral.
Noninvasive or Invasive			
Magnetic Resonance Imaging (MRI)	Can be noninvasive, but is invasive if an injected contrast dye is used. No radiation is used; magnetic fields are used. Various body planes can be examined. Better visualization of the central nervous system (CNS) than with the computed tomography scan.	Destructive bone and joint lesions. Brain lesions, tumors, abscesses, aneurysms, hematomas, and demyelinization of nerves can be visualized.	If dye is used, check for allergy; have patient's height and weight on record. Patients who weigh more than 300 lb, who are pregnant, who need continuous monitoring or intravenous equipment, who have implanted metal objects (bone pins, screws, pacemakers), or who are agitated or claustrophobic may not be eligible for MRI. Open MRI is available.

Continued

TABLE 18.5 DIAGNOSTIC PROCEDURES FOR THE IMMUNE SYSTEM—cont'd

Procedure	Definition/Normal Finding (if applicable)	Significance of Abnormal Findings	Nursing Management (if applicable)
Computed Tomography (CT) Scan	Can be noninvasive, but is invasive if an injected contrast dye is used.	See MRI above.	If dye is to be used, check for allergy; have patient's height and weight on record.
Invasive			
Biopsy (of Specific Organ in Question)	Used to confirm a diagnosis, determine a prognosis, or evaluate treatment. May be performed inpatient, outpatient, or in a physician's office. Specimen may be obtained through needle aspiration, incision, excision, or gavage and with or without endoscopy, fluoroscopy, stereotaxic, or needle localization.	Biopsy tissue is examined microscopically for diagnosis. Cancers, lymphomas, leukemias, transplant rejections are diagnosed in this manner.	Informed consent must be obtained before the procedure. Other preoperative and postoperative care is determined based on the specific organ biopsied. Most organs are quite vascular and there is a high risk for bleeding complications after the biopsy. Vital signs and site monitoring are important.
Skin Testing	Done if immune system is intact. Testing is done for *Candida,* tetanus, tuberculosis (purified protein derivative [PPD] test), or specific allergens such as medications, food, or environmental factors.	If erythema (redness) or induration (firmness) occurs at the site within a prescribed time frame, test is positive. Indicates patient has either been exposed to an organism, has an active infection, or has developed antibodies that stimulate an immune response.	Ask if patients have any allergies and the type of reaction or symptoms that occur.

THERAPEUTIC MEASURES FOR THE IMMUNE SYSTEM

Allergies

A medical alert bracelet or some sort of readily available identification of an allergy should be worn by the patient. It is important always to be aware of patient allergies. Allergies should be noted before giving any medications or foods. All allergies, including those to food, must be taken seriously (see *Evidence-Based Practice* box).

Food allergies create serious management problems and have caused numerous deaths from anaphylactic shock (Box 18.3, *Nutrition Notes*). The offending allergen may be present in extremely small amounts. Sometimes a food product is contaminated by a previous batch of food made with the same equipment. Occasionally, the allergen may enter the body not by ingestion but by inhalation or contact with skin or mucous membranes.

Epinephrine is the drug of choice for life-threatening anaphylactic reactions. If possible, treatment should begin immediately with administration of epinephrine until other medical care can be provided.

An EpiPen is commonly prescribed for patients with allergies to food or insect stings. It is a prepackaged, single-use device that allows the patient to self-inject a physician-ordered dose of epinephrine right through clothing. The patient must carry the EpiPen at all times when insect stings are possible. The expiration date of the EpiPen must be checked routinely and replaced as needed. The patient should be instructed that the EpiPen does not replace the need for immediate and continued medical attention because the duration of the single dose of epinephrine varies from 1 to 4 hours. Further, anaphylaxis can be biphasic, which means a relapse can occur hours after the initial improvement from the dose of epinephrine.

Immunotherapy

To help desensitize a patient with anaphylactic reactions or chronic allergic symptoms, immunotherapy involves preparing an extract of the allergen and injecting small amounts of it as a vaccine. Initially, the subcutaneous injections are given once or twice weekly with a very dilute preparation. Over a 3- to 6-month period, the concentration of the allergen in the vaccine is increased until the desired hyposensitivity is reached. Once the desired allergen concentration is reached, maintenance injections may be given every few weeks, usually for up to 3 to 5 years. It is important that the patient not miss a dose. If this happens, the allergen strength may need to be reduced.

EVIDENCE-BASED PRACTICE

Clinical Question

If a patient is allergic to shellfish, is the person allergic to iodine and therefore unable to tolerate iodine (Betadine, Povidone) being used on the skin?

Evidence

True hypersensitivity reactions to seafood, including shellfish, arise from the group of antigens called tropomyosins, which are proteins needed for muscle contraction. These reactions are not caused by iodine in the seafood (Beall, Mahan, & Blau, 2007).

Having an allergy to seafood does place a patient at higher risk of allergic reaction to the contrast media used in radiological tests, but it is basically the same risk as for a patient with any other type of allergy (UCSF Medical Center, Department of Radiology and Biomedical Imaging, n.d.).

Implications for Nursing Practice

Although nurses need to continue to ask patients about their allergies, there is no need to exchange the povidone-iodine solution found in procedural kits for a non-iodine–based bactericidal cleanser in patients with seafood allergies.

REFERENCES

Beall, J. W., Mahan, E. F., & Blau, A. B. (2007). Use of amiodarone in a patient with a shellfish allergy. *Southern Medical Journal, 100*(4), 405–406.

University of California San Francisco Medical Center, Department of Radiology & Biomedical Imaging. (n.d.). *Iodine allergy and contrast administration.* San Francisco: Author. Retrieved July 8, 2009, from http://www.radiology.ucsf.edu/patients/iodine_allergy

Box 18.3
Nutrition Notes

Respecting Food Allergies

Allergies to food can be fatal. An analysis of 13 anaphylactic reactions to food, 6 of which were fatal, identifies points along the critical path that had the potential to alter the outcome (Boch, Munoz-Furlong, & Sampson, 2001):

- In all cases, the patient was known to have asthma and to be allergic to some food.
- None of the patients was aware that the allergen was present in the foods consumed (candy, cookies, and pastry).
- Symptoms began soon after ingestion but in some cases abated before becoming severe.
- Of particular significance is the fact that *fewer than half the children had self-injectable epinephrine prescribed, and only one of the six children with a fatal reaction used a dose.*
- Mean time elapsed between ingestion of the allergenic food and a dose of epinephrine was 36 minutes in the survivors, all of whom had to have breathing tubes, and 93 minutes in the deceased.

Several recommendations came from this study:

- Epinephrine should be prescribed, kept available, and used for patients with IgE-mediated food allergies.
- Children and adolescents who have an allergic reaction to food should be observed for 3 to 4 hours after the reaction at a facility equipped to deal with anaphylaxis.
- Parents of such children should be taught to ensure an appropriate, rapid response by schools and other institutions (Sampson, Mendelson, & Rosen, 1992).

Analysis of 63 later cases of fatal anaphylaxis caused by food allergies confirm the original findings (Boch, Munoz-Furlong, & Sampson, 2007). More education at all levels—physicians, patients, families, school personnel, restaurateurs, and the public—is required to combat these potentially preventable tragedies. Food allergies deserve more respect.

When administering the allergen injection, it is important to understand that an anaphylactic reaction can occur. A physician and emergency equipment should be readily available. After the injection, the patient should be observed for about 20 to 30 minutes to detect a reaction. The patient and family should be taught that a reaction could occur up to 24 hours after the injection and how to respond if it does occur. Local inflammatory reactions are much more common than anaphylaxis and can be minimized by giving a histamine blocker before giving the vaccine.

Medications

Medications are one of the primary treatment options for immune disorders. General categories of these medications include epinephrine, corticosteroids, antihistamines, histamine (H_2) blockers, decongestants, mast cell stabilizers, antivirals, antibiotics, immunosuppressants, interferon, leukotriene antagonists, and hormone therapy. (See Chapter 19.)

Surgical Management

In some cases, splenectomy is needed to control symptoms of an immune disorder. It usually is done when other lines of treatment are not effective. A significant side effect of this surgery is the reduced ability of the immune system to fight infections.

Monoclonal Antibodies

Monoclonal antibodies can be produced against a variety of antigens. A monoclonal antibody is made by cloning one specific antibody and then growing unlimited amounts of it in tissue cultures. Many uses are being found for these antibodies, such as in dealing with transplant rejections.

Recombinant DNA Technology

Recombinant DNA technology combines genes from one organism with genes from another. This therapy is used to replace an abnormal or missing gene with the goal of producing a normal gene. The normal gene can then be injected into the patient in an attempt to cure the disorder if the patient's body reproduces the normal genes. T-lymphocyte–directed gene transfer for severe combined immune deficiency has been performed successfully. Along these same lines is the research regarding injection of stem cells, the precursors to all cells, into abnormal areas to produce normal cells. Studies continue in this area for possible uses of gene therapy. Since the completion of the mapping portion of the human genome project, new discoveries in this area occur daily. For additional up-to-date information on these topics, visit the National Institutes of Health at www.nhgri.nih.gov or www.ncbi.nlm.nih.gov/guide.

SUGGESTED ANSWERS TO

CRITICAL THINKING

■ *Mrs. Sims*

1. The patient may have an anaphylactic reaction if exposed to latex, which can result in death for some patients.
2. The LPN/LVN should follow the agency's latex allergy protocol, enter this information into the patient's medical record, notify surgery scheduling so latex precaution protocols can be planned for surgery, and have the patient's physician informed.
3. Following the agency's protocol, the nurse should wear nonlatex gloves and use nonlatex equipment to draw the specimens.

REVIEW QUESTIONS

1. The nurse who is teaching a patient about vaccines would be correct in teaching that a vaccine provides which of the following types of immunity?
   a. Naturally acquired passive immunity
   b. Artificially acquired passive immunity
   c. Naturally acquired active immunity
   d. Artificially acquired active immunity

2. Which of the following vaccines is recommended annually for the older patient?
   a. Influenza
   b. Pneumovax
   c. Diphtheria tetanus
   d. Polio

3. The nurse is assisting with data collection. Which of the following past surgeries found in the history may influence immune system dysfunction?
   a. Splenectomy
   b. Thyroidectomy
   c. Pneumonectomy
   d. Parathyroidectomy

4. During data collection, the patient reports tenderness in the cervical lymph nodes. The nurse recognizes that lymph nodes that are enlarged and tender usually indicate which of the following problems?
   a. Cancer
   b. Degeneration
   c. Inflammation
   d. Arthritis

REVIEW QUESTIONS—cont'd

5. The nurse is caring for a patient with suspected HIV. The nurse anticipates that which of the following is a confirmation test that will be ordered to test for HIV antibodies?
   a. Murex SUDS
   b. Western blot
   c. Enzyme-linked immunosorbent assay
   d. p24 antigen testing

6. Biaxin 200 mg oral suspension is ordered for a patient. The nurse has 125 mg/5 mL available. How many milliliters should the nurse give? **Fill in the blank.**
   Answer: _______ mL

References

Boch, S. A., Munoz-Furlong, A., & Sampson, H. A. (2001). Fatalities due to anaphylactic reactions to foods. *Journal of Allergy and Clinical Immunology, 107,* 191.

Boch, S. A., Munoz-Furlong, A., & Sampson, H. A. (2007). Further fatalities caused by anaphylactic reactions to food, 2001–2006 [Letter]. *Journal of Allergy and Clinical Immunology, 119,* 1016.

Sampson, A. A., Mendelson, I., & Rosen, J. P. (1992). Fatal and near-fatal anaphylactic reactions to food in children and adolescents. *New England Journal of Medicine, 327,* 380.

19

Nursing Care of Patients with Immune Disorders

SHARON M. NOWAK

KEY TERMS

anaphylaxis (AN-uh-fih-LAK-siss)
angioedema (AN-gee-oh-eh-DEE-mah)
ankylosing spondylitis (ANG-kih-LOH-sing SPON-da-LEYE-tiss)
histamine (HISS-tah-mean)
urticaria (UR-tih-KAIR-ee-ah)

QUESTIONS TO GUIDE YOUR READING

1. How would you explain the immunological mechanism for the four types of hypersensitivities?
2. How would you explain the pathophysiology of disorders of the immune system?
3. What are the etiologies, signs, and symptoms of immune system disorders?
4. What nursing care would you provide for patients undergoing tests for immune system disorders?
5. What is the current medical treatment for immune system disorders?
6. What data are collected when caring for patients with disorders of the immune system?
7. What factors alter or influence the self-recognition portion of the immune system?
8. What nursing care will you provide for patients with disorders of the immune system?
9. How will you know if your nursing interventions have been effective?

Disorders of the immune system can be divided into three categories. The first category is hypersensitivity reactions, which include conditions such as anaphylaxis, hemolytic transfusion reactions, measles, and transplant rejections. Autoimmune disorders (e.g., rheumatoid arthritis, ulcerative colitis, and multiple sclerosis) are the second category. The third category includes the immune deficiencies, such as hypogammaglobulinemia and acquired immunodeficiency syndrome (AIDS; see Chapter 20.)

HYPERSENSITIVITY REACTIONS

The immune system is an adaptive system that protects the body. However, sometimes this system can cause injury to the body because of its exaggerated response. One of these occasions is when a hypersensitivity reaction occurs. In 1963, Gell and Coombs developed a system of classifying hypersensitivity reactions as types I, II, III, and IV, according to the way the tissue is injured.

Type I

A type I reaction, an anaphylactic reaction, is an immediate reaction that occurs on exposure to a specific antigen (Fig. 19.1). The reaction can range from mild to severe and life threatening. The patient must have had previous exposure (sensitization) to the antigen. During this exposure, immunoglobulin E (IgE) antibodies are made and attach to mast cells throughout the body. When a subsequent exposure occurs, the antigen causes IgE to trigger mast cells to release their contents. One of the substances released is **histamine**, which causes vasodilation, changes in vascular permeability, an increase in mucous production, and contraction of various smooth muscles.

If the second antigen exposure is localized, the reaction is mild and remains local. However, if the exposure is systemic, the reaction is massive and widespread. Respiratory allergies, such as allergic rhinitis and allergic asthma, with associated disorders of atopic dermatitis, tend to be reactions of a larger scale. Anaphylaxis, urticaria, and angioedema are the severest forms of type I reactions.

A type I reaction occurs when the patient has a positive reaction to a scratch test. A scratch test is done to identify specific allergens to which a patient is reactive. Tiny amounts of a variety of common allergens are scratched onto the skin, which is then observed for indications of a reaction: redness, edema, and pruritus. If these indicators occur, it is considered to be a local reaction.

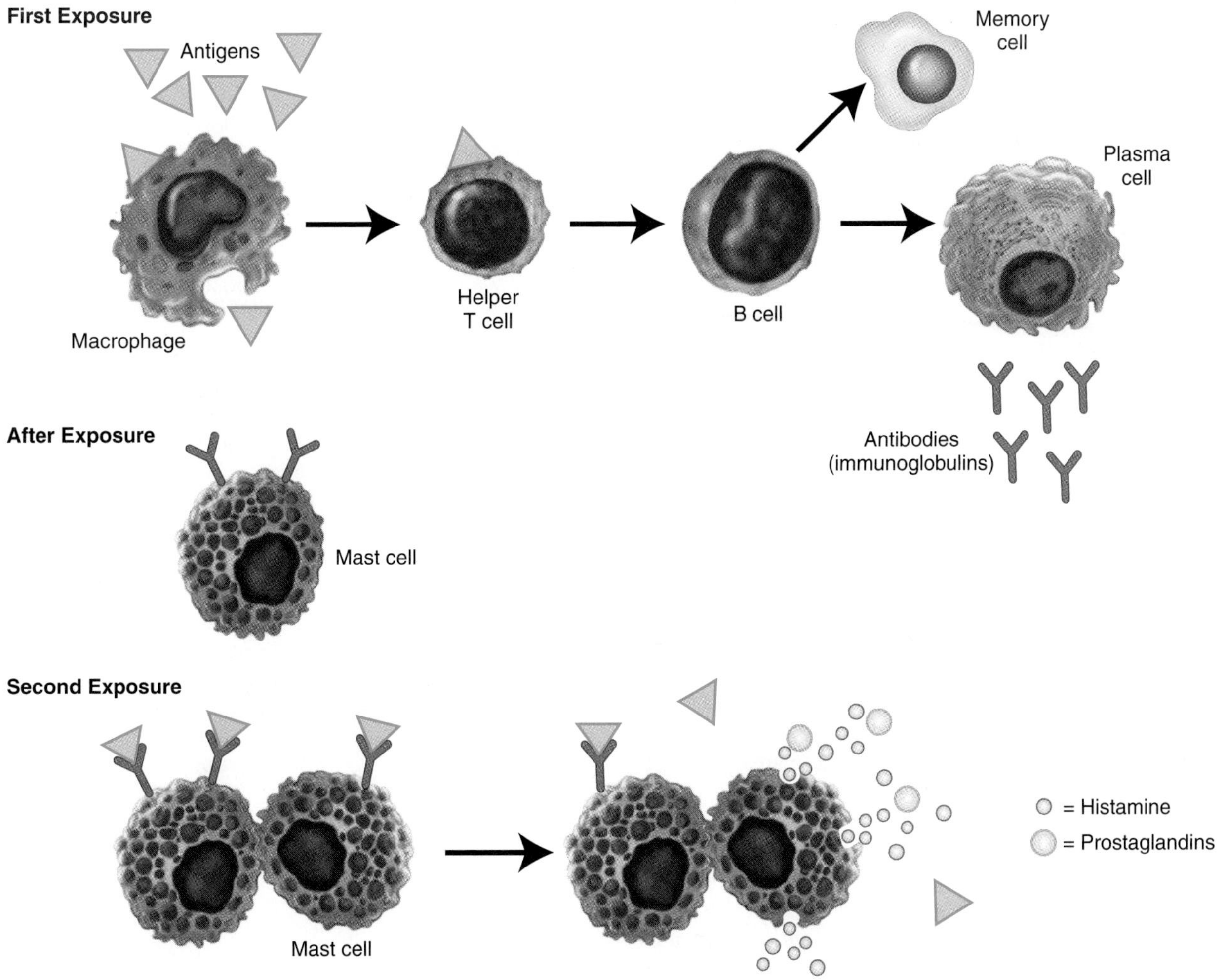
First Exposure
Antigens
Macrophage
Helper
T cell
B cell
Memory
cell
Plasma
cell
Antibodies
(immunoglobulins)
After Exposure
Mast cell
Second Exposure
Mast cell
= Histamine
= Prostaglandins

FIGURE 19.1 Type I hypersensitivity.

Allergic Rhinitis

Allergic rhinitis is the most common form of allergy. When symptoms occur throughout the year, it is called perennial allergic rhinitis. If the symptoms occur seasonally, it is called hay fever. The causative antigens are environmental and airborne.

PATHOPHYSIOLOGY. Allergic rhinitis is the result of an antigen-antibody reaction. Ciliary action decreases and mucous secretions increase. Vasodilation and local tissue edema occur.

SIGNS AND SYMPTOMS. Signs and symptoms vary in intensity and include sneezing, nasal itching, profuse watery rhinorrhea (runny nose), and itchy red eyes. The nasal mucosa is pale, cyanotic, and edematous. Frequently there are dark circles under the eyes, called allergic shiners, caused by venous congestion in the maxillary sinuses.

DIAGNOSTIC TESTS. Sometimes, skin testing is performed to identify the specific offending allergens to allow avoidance of the allergen. However, skin testing is expensive, does not always identify the allergen, and has limited usefulness for allergens that cannot be easily avoided once identified.

THERAPEUTIC MEASURES. Initial treatment involves eliminating the offending environmental stimuli. Antihistamines and nasal decongestants may be prescribed to relieve symptoms. If the symptoms are severe, corticosteroids also may be given via inhalation or nasal spray.

Rhinophototherapy uses light waves to reduce the hyperimmune response seen in this disorder. The treatment is usually done three times a week for 3 weeks and relieves symptoms such as sneezing, itching, and runny nose.

Immunotherapy, referred to as allergy shots, is reserved for patients with severe or debilitating symptoms (see Chapter 18). This therapy continues until the patient no longer has symptoms when exposed to the environmental antigen.

Atopic Dermatitis

Atopic dermatitis, often called eczema, is an inflammatory skin response.

PATHOPHYSIOLOGY. These skin lesions are not typical for a type I hypersensitivity reaction, and a specific antigen cannot usually be identified as the cause. However, the pathophysiology of atopic dermatitis is believed to be a type I hypersensitivity reaction, mediated by IgE antibodies, because it is commonly found in patients with allergic rhinitis or allergic asthma.

SIGNS AND SYMPTOMS. Initially there is pruritus, edema, and extremely dry skin, which is followed by eruptions of tiny vesicles (blisters); these eventually break open, crust over, and scale off. There is decreased sweating in these areas with the skin eventually thickening in the areas of dermatitis.

DIAGNOSTIC TESTS. There are no tests to confirm this diagnosis. A detailed history and physical examination are used to diagnose it and to exclude other diseases with similar symptoms. If an infection is present, culture and sensitivity tests may be ordered to determine the infecting organism and appropriate treatment.

THERAPEUTIC MEASURES. Treatment focuses on the symptoms of pruritus and dry and inflamed skin. Antipruritics are vital in reducing the itch-scratch cycle that predisposes the patient to lesion infections. Lukewarm soaks followed with application of emollients and oil-in-water lubricants such as Alpha Keri oil tend to be the most effective for dryness. Topical corticosteroids may be ordered for their anti-inflammatory properties. Topical calcineurin inhibitors also reduce the inflammatory response and relieve itching and rash when steroids are not effective. If skin lesions become infected, topical or systemic antibiotics are prescribed. For long-term management of symptoms, it is important to identify and eliminate the triggers of the hypersensitivity.

Anaphylaxis

Anaphylaxis is a severe systemic type I hypersensitivity reaction. Table 19.1 lists the numerous possible causes of anaphylaxis.

TABLE 19.1 SUBSTANCES THAT COMMONLY TRIGGER ANAPHYLACTIC REACTIONS

Antibiotics	Aminoglycosides
	Amphotericin B
	Cephalosporins
	Penicillins
	Sulfonamides
	Tetracyclines
Anesthetics,	Lidocaine
Antiarrhythmics	Procaine
Hormones	Adrenocorticotropic hormone
	Estradiol
	Insulin
	Vasopressin
Other Medications	Barbiturates
	Diazepam (Valium)
	Phenytoin (Dilantin)
	Protamine
	Salicylates
Diagnostic Agents	Contrast dyes
Medical Products	Latex rubber
Foods	Beans
	Chocolate
	Eggs
	Fruits (e.g., strawberries)
	Grains (e.g., wheat)
	Nuts
	Shellfish
Food Additives	Bisulfites
	Monosodium glutamate (MSG)
Proteins	Horse serum
	Rabbit serum
Venoms	Bees, wasps, hornets
	Fire ants
	Snakes
Pollens	Grass
	Ragweed

• WORD • BUILDING •

anaphylaxis: ana—up + phylaxis—protection

PATHOPHYSIOLOGY. IgE antibodies produced from previous antigen sensitization are attached to mast cells throughout the body. In this reaction, the antigen is introduced at a systemic level, which causes widespread release of histamine and other chemical mediators contained within the mast cells. The most profound complications of an anaphylactic reaction are respiratory and cardiac arrest. Immediate treatment is needed to prevent death.

SIGNS AND SYMPTOMS. Anaphylaxis produces sudden and life-threatening signs and symptoms (Table 19.2). Generalized smooth muscle spasms occur, causing bronchial narrowing and creating stridor, wheezing, dyspnea, and laryngeal edema, which can lead to respiratory arrest. Cramping, diarrhea, nausea, and vomiting also result from these spasms. Capillary permeability increases, allowing fluid to shift from the vessels to the interstitium. This causes hypotension, tachycardia, and an increase in respiratory symptoms. The blood volume in the vessels decreases while the blood vessels dilate, resulting in a further decrease in circulating blood volume. The dilation also causes diffuse erythema (redness) and warmth of the skin. Neurologic changes include apprehension, drowsiness, profound restlessness, headache, and possible seizures.

DIAGNOSTIC TESTS. There is no time for tests to be performed during an anaphylactic reaction other than those needed to guide symptom treatment, such as arterial blood gases or electrocardiogram (ECG) monitoring. Anaphylaxis is diagnosed based on physical assessment and history from the patient or significant other. After the patient's recovery, allergen testing may be considered for future prevention.

THERAPEUTIC MEASURES. Intravenous access is a priority for administration of intravenous epinephrine, vasopressor drugs (dopamine), and fluids to increase blood pressure. Oxygen therapy is started. If respiratory symptoms are severe, a tracheostomy or endotracheal intubation may be needed, with mechanical ventilation. Antihistamines and corticosteroids may also be given orally, by injection, or intravenously.

CRITICAL THINKING

Mrs. Barnes

■ Mrs. Barnes, a 32-year-old woman, was brought into the emergency room after having been stung multiple times by bees while gardening. She has numerous red welts over her body that she says are itchy. She is very anxious. Her temperature is 99.2°F (37.22°C), blood pressure is 102/58 mm Hg, pulse is 102 beats per minute, and respiratory rate is 26 per minute.

1. What might be causing Mrs. Barnes' symptoms?
2. What additional information is needed?
3. What should you do to help Mrs. Barnes?

Suggested answers at end of chapter.

TABLE 19.2 ANAPHYLAXIS SUMMARY

Signs and Symptoms	Generalized smooth-muscle spasms
	• Bronchial narrowing
	  • Stridor
	  • Wheezing
	  • Dyspnea
	  • Laryngeal edema
	• Abdominal cramping and diarrhea
	• Nausea and vomiting
	Increased capillary permeability
	• Fluid shifts from blood vessels to interstitium
	  • Hypotension
	  • Tachycardia
	  • Increased respiratory symptoms
	Blood vessels dilate
	• Further decreasing circulating volume
	• Diffuse erythema (redness)
	• Increased skin temperature
	Apprehension
	Drowsiness
	Profound restlessness
	Headache
	Possible seizures

Diagnostic Tests	Testing to guide treatment • Arterial blood gases • Electrocardiogram (ECG) monitoring History and physical exam After recovery—allergen testing for prevention
Therapeutic Measures	Intravenous (IV) access Epinephrine IV Vasopressive drugs IV (dopamine) Oxygen Antihistamines (oral, IV, injection) Corticosteroids (oral, IV, injection) If severe respiratory compromise: • Tracheostomy or endotracheal intubation • Mechanical ventilation
Complications	Respiratory and cardiac arrest
Priority Nursing Diagnoses	*Impaired Gas Exchange* *Anxiety* *Ineffective Health Maintenance*

Urticaria

PATHOPHYSIOLOGY AND ETIOLOGY. Urticaria (hives) is a type I hypersensitivity reaction. It is triggered by the antigen-stimulated reaction of IgE antibodies, which causes the release of mast cell contents, especially histamine. The causes of urticaria are numerous. In addition to medications and foods, cold, local heat, pressure, and stress can also cause urticaria. Many patients with underlying chronic conditions, such as systemic lupus erythematosus, lymphoma, hyperthyroidism, or cancer, are susceptible to urticaria.

SIGNS AND SYMPTOMS. The lesions of urticaria are raised, pruritic, nontender, and erythematous wheals on the skin. They tend to be concentrated on the trunk and proximal extremities.

DIAGNOSTIC TESTS. Diagnosis is based on physical examination and history.

THERAPEUTIC MEASURES. Treatment depends on the degree of symptoms. In the most severe cases, epinephrine may be given to quickly resolve the urticaria. Corticosteroids may be given orally, topically, or intravenously. Antihistamines and histamine (H_2) blockers may aid in resolution by blocking the release of histamine.

Angioedema

PATHOPHYSIOLOGY AND ETIOLOGY. Angioedema is a form of urticaria and has the same pathophysiology and etiology. However, angioedema affects submucosal and subcutaneous tissues rather than the skin.

SIGNS AND SYMPTOMS. Angioedema is painless and minimally pruritic, with dermal erythematous and subcutaneous eruptions. There is also skin and mucous membrane edema. The eruptions may last longer than with urticaria.

DIAGNOSTIC TESTS. A comprehensive history and physical examination confirm the diagnosis. Skin testing may be performed to determine the specific antigen.

THERAPEUTIC MEASURES. The most basic treatment involves avoiding the antigen. Symptoms may be relieved with antihistamines and corticosteroids. For long-term treatment, immunotherapy for allergen desensitization may be indicated.

Nursing Process for the Patient with a Type I Hypersensitivity Disorder

DATA COLLECTION. Gather information about the patient's signs and symptoms. Immediately report any sudden dyspnea, shortness of breath, anxiety, restlessness, or chest or back pain. Identify any allergies the patient may have as well as signs and symptoms that occur with exposure to the allergen. Perform a thorough skin assessment, and carefully document any lesions or rashes. Note any changes in rashes or lesions or signs of infection, such as redness, warmth, and drainage. Assess the patient's knowledge of disease process, causes, treatment plan, and self-care. Note responses to treatments.

NURSING DIAGNOSES, PLANNING, AND IMPLEMENTATION

Impaired Gas Exchange Related to Laryngeal Edema

EXPECTED OUTCOME: The patient will maintain clear lung fields and remain free of signs of respiratory distress at all times.

- Monitor respiratory rate, depth, and effort such as use of accessory muscles, nasal flaring, or abdominal breathing *to identify problems early.*
- Monitor the patient for restlessness, changes in mentation, level of consciousness, changes in voice, or dysphagia *to identify problems and intervene early.*
- Position the patient in a high-Fowler's or semi-Fowler's position *to improve ventilation and decrease upper airway edema.*

Anxiety Related to Dyspnea or Pruritus

EXPECTED OUTCOME: The patient will state that anxiety is controlled.

- Stay with the patient and speak calmly *to reduce fear or frustration.*
- Teach patient to visualize the absence of anxiety, itching, or dyspnea *to decrease anxiety.*
- Provide family with the information needed to distinguish between anxiety or panic and a serious physiological problem *so they can make informed decisions regarding obtaining emergency medical care.*

Risk for Impaired Skin Integrity Related to Effects of Allergic Reaction

EXPECTED OUTCOME: The patient's skin will remain intact.

- Assess and document skin and lesions *to provide a basis for interventions and evaluation.*
- Teach patient to keep fingernails short and clean *to minimize the damage or risk for infection if scratching does occur.*
- Teach patient to apply clean, white cotton clothing (socks, gloves/mittens, undershirt) over affected area, especially at bedtime, *to minimize scratching while allowing for air movement with minimal irritation from dyes.*
- Teach patient to use gentle rubbing or pressure instead of scratching *to minimize the amount of skin trauma.*

Ineffective Health Maintenance Related to Lack of Knowledge of Methods to Decrease Inflammation and Pruritus and Reduce Episodes of Inflammation

EXPECTED OUTCOME: The patient or caregiver will state understanding and follow the mutually agreed-on plan of care.

- Assess patient's knowledge of disease and its causes *to provide a basis for teaching and evaluation.*
- Assess patient's values and beliefs regarding plan of care *in order to have patient's values and beliefs correspond with the plan of care, thereby improving compliance.*
- Assess barriers to patient's ability to carry out plan of care, and plan interventions to decrease barriers *in order to improve the likelihood of the patient implementing the plan of care.*
- Discuss methods of avoiding the allergen with patient, such as wearing a mask when mowing the lawn or working outdoors, having heating ducts cleaned, covering heat registers with filters, and frequent home vacuuming and dusting *to promote an understanding of preventive methods and prevent allergen exposure and anaphylaxis.*
- Teach patient to wear medical alert identification for allergies *so prompt medical attention can be given if the patient is unable to give information.*

• WORD • BUILDING •

angioedema: angeion—vessel + oidema—swelling

- Explain need to obtain a prescription for an epinephrine pen, and teach patient how to use it if antigen is environmental (e.g., insect sting or foods). (See Chapter 18.)
- The teaching plan for atopic dermatitis includes signs and symptoms of infection, use of humidification during the winter months *to prevent dryness,* wearing cotton clothing *to minimize irritation,* and cool soaks *to decrease pruritus.*
- Teaching for urticaria includes stress management and relaxation techniques *to relieve urticaria* and to follow therapeutic regimen including prescribed medications and their correct usage *to reduce symptoms.*
- Document teaching and patient understanding.

EVALUATION. If interventions have been effective, there will be no signs of respiratory distress and lung fields will be clear. The patient's posture, facial expressions, gestures, and concentration will reflect no anxiety. The skin will remain intact. If there are lesions, they will be reduced and healing. The patient will express knowledge of disorder and treatment plan. The patient will verbalize no barriers to attaining treatment goals.

Type II

A type II hypersensitivity reaction involves the destruction of a cell or substance that has an antigen attached to its cell membrane, which is sensed by either immunoglobulin G (IgG) or immunoglobulin M (IgM) as being a foreign antigen (Fig. 19.2). When an antigen marker is sensed as foreign, an antibody attaches to the antigen on the cell membrane, causing lysis of the cell or accelerated phagocytosis (engulfing and ingestion). When a cell is foreign, such as a bacterium, this process is beneficial. However, sometimes antigens on the surface of a red blood cell (RBC) can be sensed as foreign for the different ABO blood types, which results in the RBC being destroyed.

Hemolytic Transfusion Reaction

PATHOPHYSIOLOGY. A hemolytic transfusion reaction is a type II hypersensitivity reaction in which incompatible surface antigens on RBCs are transfused. These antigens may be ABO or Rh incompatible. The recipient's antibodies attach to the foreign antigens on the transfused RBCs, causing rapid lysis of the RBC. The rapid RBC lysis results in a massive amount of cellular debris that occludes blood vessels throughout the body. This leads to ischemia and necrosis of tissue and organs and can be life threatening.

ETIOLOGY. Occasionally, antibodies form after a bacterial or viral infection. However, prior sensitization is usually from a previous blood transfusion or pregnancy. ABO and Rh blood type must be matched for transfusions. The ABO blood types are A, B, AB, and O (Fig. 19.3). People with blood type O are universal donors because they do not have A or B antigens. However, those with type O blood can receive only type O blood. People with type AB blood are universal recipients, because they do not make A or B antibodies. Those with blood types other than AB cannot receive AB blood because they have A or B antibodies.

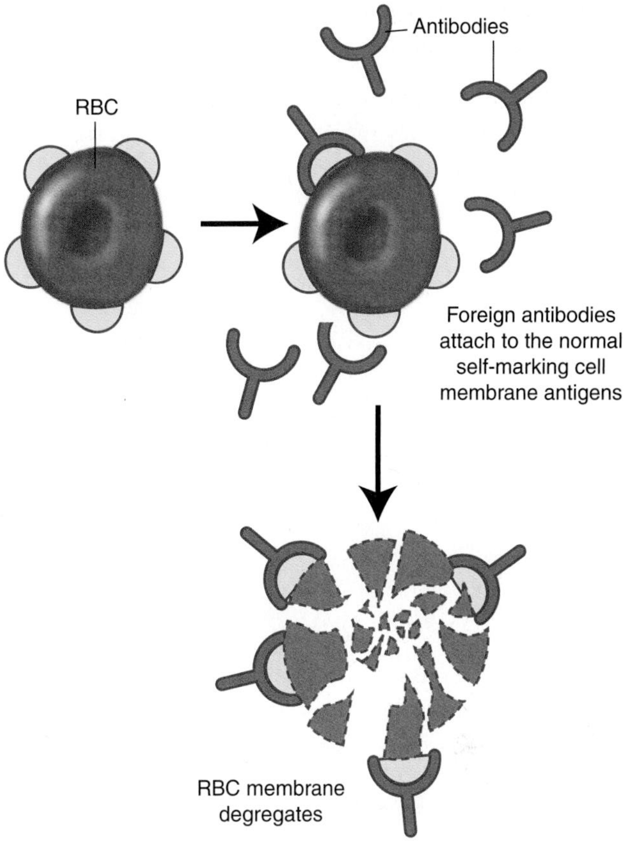
Antibodies
RBC
Foreign antibodies attach to the normal self-marking cell membrane antigens
RBC membrane degregates

FIGURE 19.2 Type II hypersensitivity.

Rh antigens are present in people who are Rh^+. A person who is Rh^+ has the D antigen, which is the strongest antigen of the 50 possible antigens. Rh antibodies are present in those who are Rh^- after a sensitizing event. A person who is Rh^- does not have the D antigen. Those who are Rh^+ can receive Rh^+ blood but those who are Rh^- cannot receive Rh^+ blood due to the formation of antibodies to the Rh^+ blood. If maternal and fetal blood Rh factors (RBC surface antigens) are different, the mother becomes sensitized by the fetal Rh type, which can affect future fetuses. For example, an Rh_0(D)-negative pregnant woman becomes sensitized by a Rh_0(D)-positive fetus. As a result, the blood cells of future Rh_0(D)-positive fetuses can be destroyed by maternal antibodies crossing the placenta.

> **CRITICAL THINKING**
>
> ***Blood Types***
>
> 1. Who is the universal ABO Rh recipient?
> 2. Who is the universal ABO Rh donor?
> 3. Can someone with an A Rh^- blood type safely receive O Rh^+ blood?
>
> *Suggested answers at end of chapter.*

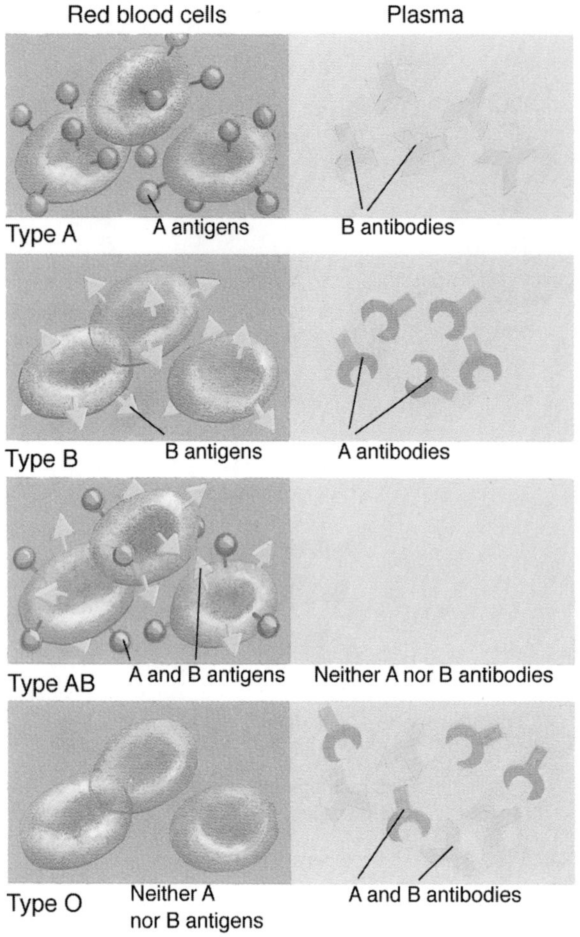
Red blood cells
Plasma
Type A
A antigens
B antibodies
Type B
B antigens
A antibodies
Type AB
A and B antigens
Neither A nor B antibodies
Type O
Neither A nor B antigens
A and B antibodies

FIGURE 19.3 ABO blood types. (From Venes, D. [Ed.]. [2009]. *Taber's cyclopedic medical dictionary* [21st ed., p. 287]. Philadelphia: F. A. Davis.)

SIGNS AND SYMPTOMS. A hemolytic transfusion reaction is usually accompanied by a rather sudden onset of low back (flank) or chest pain, hypotension, fever rising more than 1.8°F (1°C), chills, tachycardia, tachypnea, wheezing, dyspnea, urticaria, and anxiety (Table 19.3). The patient also may report a headache and nausea.

DIAGNOSTIC TESTS. The direct Coombs' test confirms this diagnosis. In the laboratory, a small amount of the patient's RBCs is washed to remove any unattached antibodies. Antihuman globulin is added to see if agglutination (clumping) of the RBCs results. If agglutination occurs, an immune reaction such as a hemolytic transfusion reaction is taking place.

THERAPEUTIC MEASURES. To prevent production of anti-Rh_0(D) antibodies, a Rh_0(D) immune globulin (RhoGAM) injection is given to Rh_0(D)-negative patients accidentally given Rh_0(D)-positive blood or exposed to Rh_0(D)-positive fetal blood by delivery, miscarriage, abortion, amniocentesis, or intra-abdominal trauma. When antibodies do not form, then a hemolytic reaction can be prevented.

If a reaction occurs, medications are given to treat the reaction such as those listed in Table 19.4.

TABLE 19.3 HEMOLYTIC TRANSFUSION REACTION SUMMARY

Signs and Symptoms	Low back or chest pain Hypotension Fever rising more than 1.8°F (1°C) Chills Tachycardia Tachypnea, wheezing, dyspnea Urticaria Anxiety Headache Nausea
Diagnostic Tests	Direct Coombs' test • Small amount of patient's RBCs are washed • Antihuman globulin is added • If agglutination (clumping) occurs, an immune reaction is occurring
Therapeutic Measures	Depends on severity of reaction and organs affected Antihistamines Corticosteroids Epinephrine Diuretics, to assist kidneys
Complications	If severe: shock, acute renal failure
Priority Nursing Diagnoses	*Fear* *Ineffective Tissue Perfusion* *Risk for Injury*

NURSING PROCESS FOR THE PATIENT EXPERIENCING A HEMOLYTIC TRANSFUSION REACTION.

Data Collection. Prevention of hemolytic reactions is crucial. Following strict institutional guidelines for blood transfusion administration helps ensure the patient's safety. After blood is released from the hospital blood bank, two nurses, designated per institutional policy, double-check specified data. At the bedside, transfusion guidelines include double-checking the patient's name and identification number on the chart, unit of blood, and patient's identification bracelet, as well as checking the patient's blood type in the chart, on the unit of blood, and paperwork with the unit of blood.

Agency policy is followed for taking vital signs during a blood transfusion. Minimally, vital signs are taken before the start of the blood transfusion, 15 minutes into the transfusion, and when the transfusion is completed. It takes only a small amount of blood to trigger a hemolytic transfusion reaction, so it is critical to stay with the patient at the bedside during the first 15 minutes of any blood transfusion. This enables detection of a blood transfusion reaction early for quick action to minimize cell destruction and complications, including death.

If symptoms of a reaction are noted, the blood transfusion is immediately stopped and agency policy for a suspected transfusion reaction is followed. A normal saline infusion with new tubing is started to keep the vein patent.

TABLE 19.4 MEDICATIONS USED IN HEMOLYTIC TRANSFUSION REACTIONS

Medication Class/Action	Examples	Route	Side Effects	Nursing Implications
Antihistamines				
Block histamine at $histamine_1$ receptors, thereby preventing or reversing the effects of histamine (capillary permeability, itching, and bronchospasms).	diphenhydramine (Benadryl)	PO	Significant drowsiness	Take with or without food. Avoid ethanol, CNS depressants, and OTC antihistamines. Avoid prolonged exposure to sunlight. Use caution with activities requiring mental alertness.
Corticosteroids				
Hormones with marked anti-inflammatory effects due to inhibition of prostaglandin synthesis and accumulation of macrophages and leukocytes at site.	dexamethasone (Decadron) hydrocortisone (Solu-Cortef) methylprednisone (Solu-Medrol) prednisolone (Delta-Cortef) prednisone (Deltasone) beclomethasone (Beconase)	IM, IV, PO	Burning, dryness, stinging, headache, edema, muscle wasting, thrombophlebitis, masking of infections, elevated blood glucose level, gastric irritation	Take PO with food. **Never** stop taking suddenly. Monitor weight. Assess for edema, shortness of breath, jugular vein distention, and signs and symptoms of congestive heart failure. Monitor blood glucose level. Monitor for evidence of GI bleeding.
Sympathomimetics				
Marked stimulation of alpha, $beta_1$, and $beta_2$ receptors, causing vasoconstriction, bronchodilation, and cardiac stimulation.	epinephrine (Adrenalin) (EpiPen)	IM, IV, subcutaneously, inhalation, topical	Disorientation, panic, anxiety, ventricular fibrillation, cerebral hemorrhage, decreased urine output, urine retention, angina	Use only 1:1000 solution for IV; 1:100 IV will cause death. Do not expose drug to heat, light, or air. Ophthalmic and nasal preparations may sting. May elevate blood glucose level.

The physician and blood bank are immediately notified. A nurse remains with the patient for reassurance and monitoring of symptoms and vital signs. If a blood incompatibility is suspected, the unused blood and blood tubing are returned to the blood bank for testing. A series of blood and urine specimens are collected and sent to the laboratory for analysis. The physician's orders are followed to treat the patient's symptoms.

SAFETY TIP

Every unit of blood, even of the same blood type, is unique and can trigger a blood transfusion reaction. Careful monitoring with every transfusion is necessary.

Nursing Diagnoses, Planning, and Implementation

Fear Related to Serious Threat to Health Status

EXPECTED OUTCOME: The patient will state reduced fear.

- Allow patients to express their concerns *to allow inaccurate information to be corrected.*
- Inform patients about procedures and treatments *to reduce fear.*
- Remain with patient and allow significant others to visit *to offer emotional support.*

Ineffective Tissue Perfusion, Cardiopulmonary and Peripheral, Related to Arterial/Venous Blood Flow Exchange Problems

EXPECTED OUTCOME: The patient will have adequate tissue perfusion as evidenced by palpable peripheral pulses, urinary output of 30 mL per hour, and no respiratory distress.

- Assess and maintain airway, and provide oxygen *to promote oxygenation.*

- Assess for pain and provide pain relief measures *to reduce pain.*
- Monitor vital signs and intake and output *to detect changes for prompt treatment.*
- Position patient with head elevated if short of breath *to aid breathing.*

Risk for Injury Related to Prolonged Shock Resulting in Multiple Organ Failure, Death

EXPECTED OUTCOME: The patient will remain free of injury at all times.

- Use two methods to identify patient before giving blood products *to prevent incorrect identification and administration of blood product.*
- Remain with patient during first 15 minutes of transfusion and then obtain vital signs *to detect signs of reaction.*
- Give medications such as epinephrine or steroids, as ordered, *to support affected tissues and organs.*
- Give diuretics as ordered *to assist kidney excretion of cellular debris from reaction.*

Deficient Knowledge Related to Lack of Exposure to Blood Transfusions

EXPECTED OUTCOME: The patient will state understanding of blood transfusion options.

- Encourage patient to discuss autologous (self) blood donation option with physician *to avoid a transfusion reaction.* This may be an option for patients having elective surgery.
- After a hemolytic transfusion reaction, explain to patients the importance of informing future health care providers about the reaction *to ensure that specific blood tests are performed for less common antibodies if the patient is ever typed for a blood transfusion again.*

EVALUATION. If interventions have been effective, the patient states reduced fear, shows normal organ and tissue function, and reports understanding of blood transfusion options to prevent transfusion reactions.

Type III

A type III hypersensitivity reaction involves immune complexes formed by antigens and antibodies, usually of the IgG type (Fig. 19.4). The patient is sensitized with an initial exposure to the antigen, and a reaction occurs with a later exposure. The reaction is localized and evolves over several hours, with symptoms ranging from a red, edematous skin lesion to hemorrhage and necrosis. The process involves formation of antigen-antibody complexes in the blood vessels as the antigen is absorbed through the vessel wall. Neutrophils are attracted to the area and release enzymes that ultimately lead to blood vessel damage.

Serum Sickness

PATHOPHYSIOLOGY AND ETIOLOGY. Serum sickness is a type III hypersensitivity immune reaction in which antigen-antibody complexes form and lodge in small vessels, which leads to inflammation, tissue damage, and necrosis. Serum sickness occurs occasionally after administration of penicillin or sulfonamide.

SIGNS AND SYMPTOMS. The signs and symptoms usually occur 7 to 10 days after the exposure. Most predominant is severe urticaria and angioedema. The patient may have a fever, malaise, muscle soreness, arthralgia, splenomegaly, and occasionally nausea, vomiting, and diarrhea. Lymphadenopathy may occur, especially in the lymph nodes closest to the antigen entry site.

DIAGNOSTIC TESTS. With serum sickness, there is often a slight elevation in the white blood cell count, sedimentation rate, and C-reactive protein. IgG and IgM immunoglobulins increase substantially, while the complement assay decreases.

THERAPEUTIC MEASURES. Because serum sickness tends to be self-limiting within about 10 days, treatment is focused on symptoms. Antipyretics may be given for fever and analgesics for arthralgia. Antihistamines and epinephrine may be given for urticaria and angioedema. If symptoms persist, corticosteroids may be ordered.

NURSING PROCESS FOR THE PATIENT WITH SERUM SICKNESS.

Data Collection. Symptoms are noted. Responses to prescribed medications are documented. The causative agent may be identified through the history-taking process and is important for the patient to determine to prevent a recurrence of the condition.

Nursing Diagnoses, Planning, and Implementation Pain Related to Muscle and Joint Soreness

EXPECTED OUTCOME: The patient will state pain is reduced to acceptable level within 30 minutes of report of pain.

- Monitor pain using a pain rating scale of 0 to 10 *to identify need for treatment.*
- Provide analgesics as ordered *to relieve symptoms.*

Risk for Deficient Fluid Volume Related to Fever and Gastrointestinal Fluid Loss

EXPECTED OUTCOME: The patient will maintain blood pressure, pulse, and urine output within normal limits.

- Observe for signs of hypovolemia, such as restlessness, weakness, muscle cramps, headaches, inability to concentrate, irritability, and postural hypotension *to detect deficiencies to report to the physician.*
- Monitor intake and output *to detect imbalances.*
- Provide antiemetics as ordered *to relieve nausea.*
- Encourage oral replacement therapy with hypotonic glucose-electrolyte solutions, such as sports replacement drinks or ginger ale, *because they*

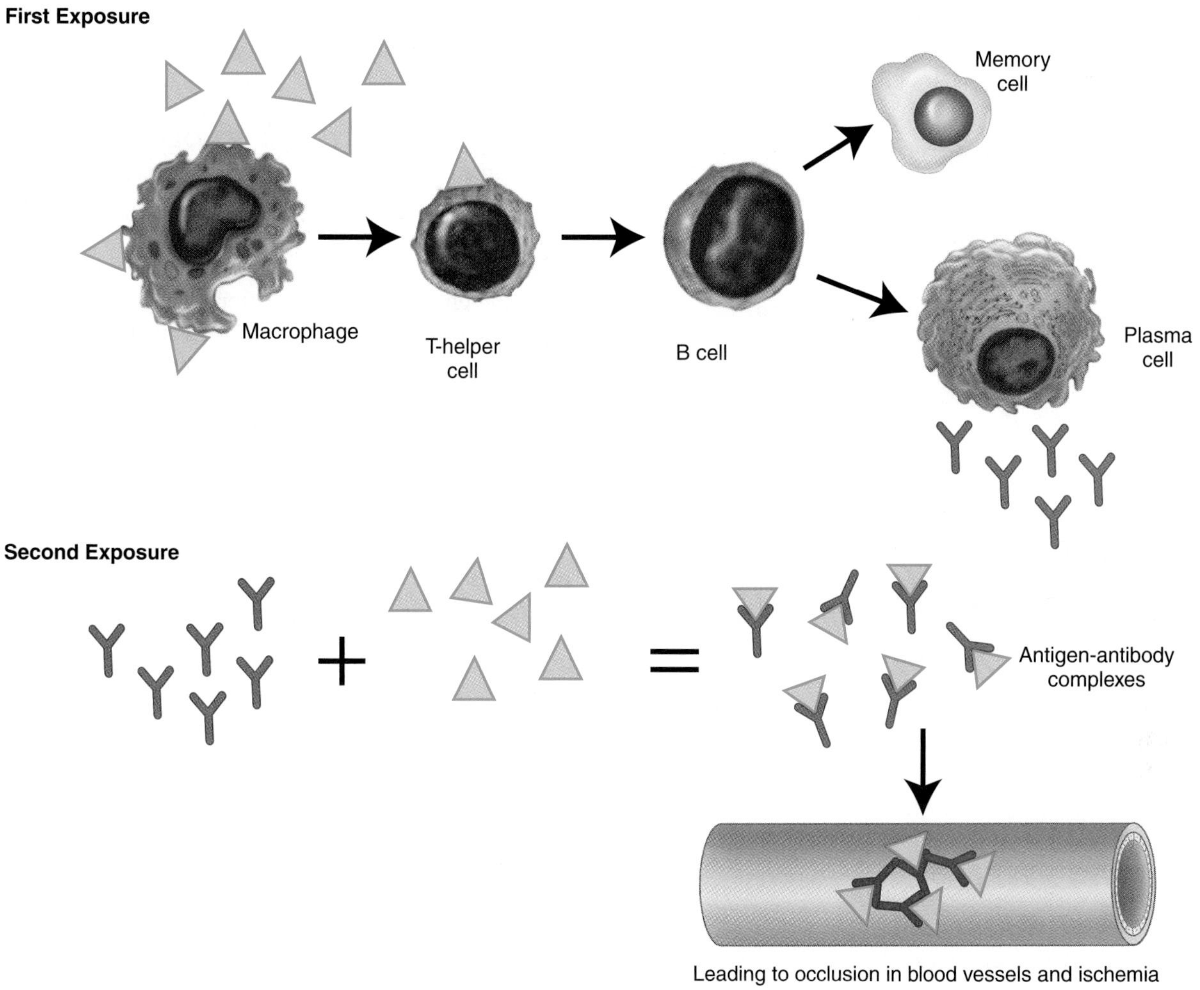
First Exposure
Memory cell
Macrophage
T-helper cell
B cell
Plasma cell
Second Exposure
Antigen-antibody complexes
Leading to occlusion in blood vessels and ischemia

FIGURE 19.4 Type III hypersensitivity.

increase fluid absorption and correct deficient fluid volume.

- Maintain IV fluids at ordered rate *to replace lost fluids, but avoid fluid overload.*

Evaluation. Goals are met if the patient reports less pain and if vital signs and urine output are within normal limits.

Type IV

A type IV hypersensitivity reaction, also called a delayed reaction, occurs when a sensitized T lymphocyte comes in contact with the particular antigen to which it is sensitized (Fig. 19.5). The resulting necrosis is caused by the actions of macrophages and the various T lymphocytes involved in the cell-mediated immune response.

Contact Dermatitis

PATHOPHYSIOLOGY. When a substance or chemical comes in contact with the skin, it is absorbed into the skin and binds with special skin proteins called haptens. With the first contact, there is no reaction or symptoms, but within 7 to 10 days, T memory cells are formed. Therefore, on subsequent exposures, the T memory cells quickly become activated T cells, which secrete the chemicals that may cause symptoms.

ETIOLOGY. Poison ivy and poison oak are the most common irritants causing this reaction. Latex rubber also may cause contact dermatitis and can trigger type I anaphylactic reactions.

Latex Allergy. Latex allergy is a serious problem for health care workers. Anaphylactic reactions to latex can be fatal. Exposure to latex for health care workers has increased dramatically since the implementation of universal precautions and the use of latex gloves began in 1987. Many times, latex gloves are worn when they are not needed, which increases exposure to the latex protein. Latex-free gloves are available for health care workers. For patients who are allergic to latex, special protocols are followed using latex-free equipment. For information about latex allergy, visit the American Academy of Allergy, Asthma, and Immunology at www.aaaai.org. Also visit the U.S. Food and Drug Administration at www.fda.gov.

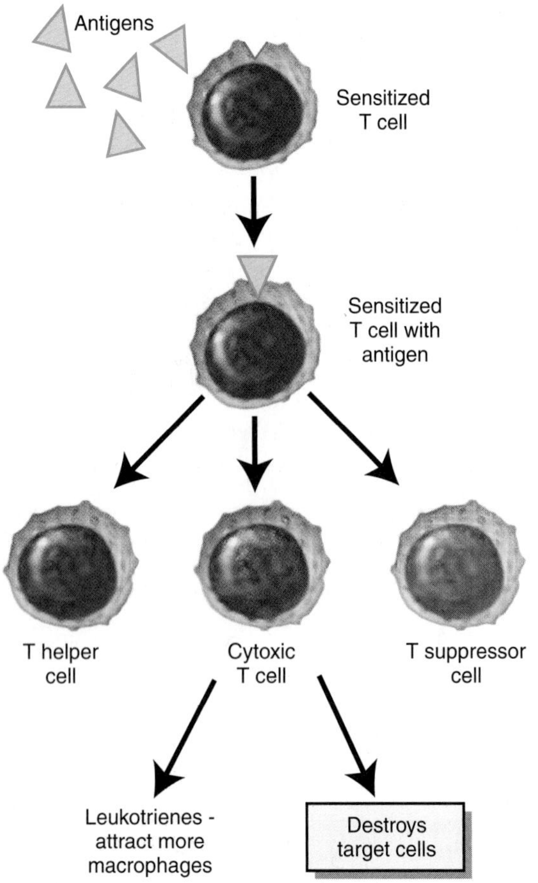
Antigens
Sensitized T cell
Sensitized T cell with antigen
T helper cell
Cytoxic T cell
T suppressor cell
Leukotrienes - attract more macrophages
Destroys target cells

FIGURE 19.5 Type IV hypersensitivity.

SIGNS AND SYMPTOMS. Within a number of hours of exposure, the area of contact becomes red and pruritic, with fragile vesicles. Secondary infections may develop. (See earlier discussion of atopic dermatitis.)

DIAGNOSTIC TESTS. Diagnosis is made by assessment of the skin and lesions and a detailed patient history.

THERAPEUTIC MEASURES. Treatment consists of controlling symptoms. Oral or topical antihistamines and topical drying agents may be used. Topical corticosteroids may be used and are most effective if sparingly applied after a bath or shower. If symptoms are severe, systemic corticosteroids may be prescribed. Tacrolimus (Protopic), an immunosuppressant, and pimecrolimus (Abreva), whose action is not clearly known, also may be prescribed when other treatments fail.

NURSING PROCESS FOR THE PATIENT WITH CONTACT DERMATITIS.

Data Collection. Symptoms are assessed for planning of interventions. Identification of the causative agent is noted in the patient's history. Patient recognition of the cause is important to prevent a recurrence of the condition. Special protocols are used for patients allergic to latex. Some facilities may prepare special latex-free kits containing common supplies nurses use to care for patients. Ensure that latex allergy protocols are followed if a patient has a latex allergy to prevent possible development of life-threatening anaphylaxis.

Nursing Diagnoses, Planning, and Implementation. See the *Nursing Care Plan for the Patient with Contact Dermatitis.*

Transplant Rejection

PATHOPHYSIOLOGY AND ETIOLOGY. Any form of transplanted living tissue is sensed as foreign material by the immune system. This is why lifelong immunosuppression is needed to help prevent transplant rejection, which can occur at any time. Lymphocytes become sensitized during an induction phase immediately after the tissue is transplanted. If immunosuppression is not effective, the sensitized lymphocytes invade the transplanted tissue and destroy it via the release of chemicals and macrophage activity, resulting in varying degrees of transplant rejection.

SIGNS AND SYMPTOMS. Various signs and symptoms occur depending on the transplanted tissue or organ involved and the severity of the rejection (Table 19.5). Signs and symptoms reflect failure of the organ or tissue, such as renal failure for a rejected kidney.

COMPLICATIONS. A total failure and loss of the transplanted tissue or organ can occur, or the tissue or organ can be damaged from immunological reactions and not function at full capacity. The greatest cause of death following a transplant is infection. Immunosuppression therapy, which is needed to prevent tissue rejection after the transplant, is a major contributory factor for severe infection development. Because the immune system is suppressed, it is unable to effectively fight infections.

DIAGNOSTIC TESTS. Biopsy, scans, blood tests, arteriography, and ultrasonography are some tests that may be performed to aid in diagnosing a transplant rejection.

THERAPEUTIC MEASURES. Depending on the type of transplant, the body's immunological system is prepared before surgery with medications, transfusions, or radiation to minimize the risk of rejection. After the transplant, lifelong immunosuppression is needed. If rejection occurs, medications may be used to attempt to reverse the rejection. Supportive care is provided based on the failing organ, such as hemodialysis if a kidney rejection occurs.

NURSING MANAGEMENT. Nursing care depends greatly on the type of transplant performed. Initially, the patient is in an intensive care unit under close observation and support. Observing for signs of rejection is a priority throughout the patient's hospitalization. Another consideration for nursing care is the psychological support of patient and family. Many patients wait on a transplant list a long time before a donor match is found. Once a matching donor is found, there is usually great elation. Yet if a donor's death made the transplant possible, the patient and family may be simultaneously feeling a profound sadness for the donor's family. Patients need time to verbalize feelings and understand that these feelings are normal and diminish with time. Also, the fear of transplant rejection is always present and must be discussed.

NURSING CARE PLAN for the Patient with Contact Dermatitis

Nursing Diagnosis: *Risk for Impaired Skin Integrity* related to effects of allergic reaction and pruritus

Expected Outcomes: The patient's skin will remain intact.

Evaluation of Outcomes: Is patient's skin intact? If not intact, is skin healing? Does patient express a plan for preventing impaired skin integrity?

Interventions	Rationale	Evaluation
Identify and document skin and lesions.	Provides a basis for intervention planning and evaluation of healing.	Are lesions present? Are lesions healing?
Teach patient to keep fingernails short and clean.	Short, clean nails cause less damage or infection if scratching occurs.	Does skin remain intact in spite of scratching?
Teach patient to apply clean, white cotton clothing (socks, gloves/mittens, undershirt) over affected area, especially at bedtime.	Cotton allows air movement. White cloth is less irritating than those with dyes. Scratching is decreased during sleep with the use of gloves/mittens or by covering affected area.	Are symptoms of skin irritation reduced?
Teach patient to use gentle rubbing or pressure instead of scratching.	Use of gentle rubbing or pressure instead of scratching causes less skin trauma.	Does skin remain intact in spite of itchy sensation?
Explain that tepid baking soda baths, colloidal oatmeal baths (e.g., Aveeno), and cool washcloths or cool baths reduce itching.	These items help dry the vesicle and minimize the pruritus.	Is itching reduced?

Nursing Diagnosis: *Ineffective Health Maintenance* related to lack of knowledge of methods to decrease inflammation and reduce episodes of inflammation

Expected Outcomes: The patient or caregiver will follow the mutually agreed-on plan of care.

Evaluation of Outcomes: Can patient express knowledge of etiology, signs and symptoms, and treatment plan? Does patient discuss any emotional, social, financial, or material blocks to attaining treatment goals?

Interventions	Rationale	Evaluation
Identify patient's knowledge of disease and causes.	Provides a basis for the teaching plan.	Does patient state baseline knowledge?
Ask patient's values and beliefs regarding plan of care.	Patients are more compliant if their belief system fits into plan of care.	Does patient's belief system work with plan of care?
Identify barriers to patient's ability to carry out plan of care and plan interventions to decrease barriers.	Barriers can prevent patient from carrying out plan of care.	Are barriers identified? Are solutions to barriers planned?
Teach patient to wear medical alert identification for allergen.	With allergen identification, prompt medical care can be given in case patient is unable to give information.	Does patient agree to use allergen identification?

Continued

NURSING CARE PLAN for the Patient with Contact Dermatitis—cont'd

Discuss methods of avoiding allergen with patient.	Understanding prevention methods can help prevent allergen exposure.	Can patient state methods to help prevent allergen exposure?
Teach patient to wash with a brown soap (e.g., Fels-Naptha) or, if unavailable, any soap when contact with the offending agent is suspected.	This removes offending agent.	Does patient state understanding of need to wash off agent with exposure?
Teach patient not to scratch skin.	Scratching can spread the dermatitis, as well as cause infection.	Does patient avoid scratching?

TABLE 19.5 TRANSPLANT REJECTION SUMMARY

Signs and Symptoms	Depends on: • Involved transplanted tissue or organ • Severity of reaction Reflect failure of the organ or tissue
Diagnostic Tests	Biopsy Scans Blood tests Arteriography Ultrasonography
Therapeutic Measures	Depends on type of transplant Preventive preoperative preparation with medications, transfusions, or radiation to minimize the risk of rejection
Complications	Total failure and loss of transplanted organ or tissue Cause of death is most commonly due to infection, with immunosuppression therapy a contributory factor
Priority Nursing Diagnoses	*Grieving* (actual or anticipatory) *Fear* *Deficient Knowledge* Other diagnoses depend on which organ is failing.

Education. Rejection can take place weeks, months, or years after a transplant (with decreasing risk). The patient and family need to be educated about specific signs and symptoms of rejection. Also, because infection is a major complication of long-term immunosuppressant medications, the patient and family need to know signs and symptoms of infection and when to notify the physician of problems. Steroid use may mask the symptoms of infection, so small indicators such as a low-grade fever should be promptly reported. Education regarding prescribed medications is a must because the long-term success of a transplant depends on compliance with immunosuppressant therapy. Avoidance of people with colds or infections is also important to reduce the immunosuppressed patient's risk of infection.

AUTOIMMUNE DISORDERS

In autoimmune disorders, the immune system no longer recognizes the body's normal cells as self. Instead, antigens on these normal body cells are recognized as foreign material, and the body launches an immune response to destroy them.

A number of factors either cause or influence this breakdown of self-recognition, including viral infections, drugs, and cross-reactive antibodies. Some microbes stimulate production of antibodies but are so closely related to normal cell antigens that the antibodies also attack some normal cells. Hormones also may influence this breakdown of self-recognition.

Some autoimmune disorders are discussed next, whereas others are discussed in chapters related to the body system most affected. Table 19.6 lists additional autoimmune disorders and the chapters in which they are discussed.

Pernicious Anemia

PATHOPHYSIOLOGY. Antibodies that destroy gastric parietal cells lead to decreased production of intrinsic factor. Other intrinsic factor antibodies (type I and type II) alter the binding sites, which ultimately decreases the ability of intrinsic factor to assist in the absorption of vitamin B_{12} in the ileum. Intrinsic factor plays a role in vitamin B_{12} absorption in the small bowel, so a vitamin B_{12} deficiency may result, causing decreased production of RBCs. Intrinsic factor is involved in most vitamin B_{12} absorption, but evidence has demonstrated that there is a route independent of intrinsic factor for some absorption of vitamin B_{12}. This has important treatment implications.

ETIOLOGY. There tends to be a familial tendency toward the autoimmune form of pernicious anemia. Causes of the

TABLE 19.6 AUTOIMMUNE DISORDERS

Disorder	Refer to
Idiopathic thrombocytopenic purpura	Chapter 28
Multiple sclerosis	Chapter 50
Myasthenia gravis	Chapter 50
Rheumatoid arthritis	Chapter 46
Ulcerative colitis	Chapter 34

acquired form of pernicious anemia (non–immune-related) include any type of gastric or small-bowel resections coupled with no or inadequate vitamin B_{12} or intrinsic factor replacement.

SIGNS AND SYMPTOMS. The patient experiences increasing weakness, loss of appetite, glossitis (inflammation or infection of the tongue), and pallor. Irritability, confusion, and numbness or tingling in the extremities (peripheral neuropathy) occur because the nervous system is affected.

DIAGNOSTIC TESTS. On microscopic examination of the patient's RBCs, macrocytic (enlarged cells) anemia is diagnosed. Macrocytic anemia and low vitamin B_{12} levels are indicators of pernicious anemia and folic acid deficiency. To determine if the diagnosis is pernicious anemia, intrinsic factor antibodies and parietal cell antibodies can be tested.

A Schilling test can be done but is used less today than in the past because it is a complicated test. For the Schilling test, radioactive vitamin B_{12} is administered to the patient. The patient's urine is then collected for 24 hours (48 hours for patients with renal disease), and the amount of radioactive vitamin B_{12} excreted in the urine is measured. If intrinsic factor is decreased, gastric absorption of vitamin B_{12} is also decreased, so that more vitamin B_{12} is excreted in the urine. Gastric secretion analysis is done to measure levels of hydrochloric acid (HCl) because low or absent HCl may indicate pernicious anemia.

Further studies such as radioimmunoassay (RIA) or enzyme-linked immunosorbent assay (ELISA) may be performed to confirm an autoimmune etiology and specify which antibody is present, type I or type II.

THERAPEUTIC MEASURES. Corticosteroids may correct the problem if it is immunologically caused. Otherwise, vitamin B_{12} therapy is needed, usually for life.

NURSING MANAGEMENT. Vitamin B_{12} is administered as ordered. Care related to fatigue and safety are important. Ambulation, frequent rest periods, and providing assistance with activities of daily living (ADLs) as indicated by the patient's activity tolerance are helpful for the patient with anemia.

Education. The patient and family need education regarding oral or parenteral medication therapy. If vitamin B_{12} injections are prescribed, the patient must understand that this is a lifelong need to prevent the return of symptoms. Patients should not miss injections, periodic vitamin B_{12} testing, or follow-up appointments.

Idiopathic Autoimmune Hemolytic Anemia

PATHOPHYSIOLOGY. In this disorder, autoantibodies, for no known reason, are produced that attach to RBCs and cause them to either lyse or agglutinate (clump). When lysis occurs, fragments of the destroyed RBCs circulate in the blood. If agglutination occurs, occlusions in the small blood vessels are followed by tissue ischemia.

SIGNS AND SYMPTOMS. Clinical manifestations vary from mild fatigue and pallor to severe hypotension, dyspnea, palpitations, and jaundice.

DIAGNOSTIC TESTS. The RBC count, hemoglobin (Hgb), and hematocrit (Hct) are low, and microscopic examination reveals fragmented RBCs. Lactate dehydrogenase (LDH) is elevated because of RBC destruction and tissue ischemia.

THERAPEUTIC MEASURES. Supportive measures such as supplemental oxygen may be started. Folic acid may be prescribed to increase production of RBCs. Immunosuppressant medications and corticosteroids may be useful in obtaining remission. In more severe cases, blood transfusions and erythrocytapheresis (a process whereby abnormal RBCs are removed and replaced with normal RBCs) may be instituted. For severe cases a splenectomy may be performed in an attempt to stop the destruction of RBCs.

NURSING MANAGEMENT. The patient's signs and symptoms should be monitored and reported as needed. Frequent rest periods should be planned into the patient's daily routine to prevent fatigue. Blood products are administered as ordered to replace RBCs.

Education. The patient and family are instructed on the medical regimen, and their understanding is verified.

Hashimoto's Thyroiditis

PATHOPHYSIOLOGY. Autoantibodies for thyroid-stimulating hormone (TSH) form in Hashimoto's thyroiditis. However, instead of inactivating TSH, the autoantibodies bind with hormone receptors on the thyroid gland and stimulate the thyroid gland to secrete thyroid hormones. The thyroid gland enlarges as a result of this overstimulation (hyperthyroidism). It becomes infiltrated with lymphocytes and phagocytes, causing inflammation and further enlargement. Then different autoantibodies appear that destroy thyroid cells, which slows secretion activity, causing hypothyroidism.

ETIOLOGY. The exact cause is unknown, although it occurs in females eight times more often than in males. It is also more common in people 30 to 50 years old and patients with Down syndrome and Turner's syndrome.

SIGNS AND SYMPTOMS. Initial signs and symptoms are those of hyperthyroidism, such as restlessness, tremors, chest pain, increased appetite, diarrhea, moist skin, heat intolerance, and weight loss.

These manifestations may go unrecognized and progress quickly into hypothyroidism. At this point, an enlarged thyroid gland (goiter) may be seen. Signs and symptoms may include fatigue, bradycardia, hypotension, dyspnea, anorexia, constipation, dry skin, weight gain, sensitivity to cold, facial puffiness, and a slowing of mental processes.

DIAGNOSTIC TESTS. Immunofluorescent assay, a test that detects antigens on cells using an antibody with a fluorescent tag, detects antithyroid antibodies. Serum TSH levels are elevated, while triiodothyronine (T_3) and thyroxine (T_4) levels are low. A thyroid scan is also done.

THERAPEUTIC MEASURES. Thyroid hormone replacement therapy of thyroxine is the primary means of treatment. Lifelong thyroid hormone therapy is needed.

NURSING MANAGEMENT. If the patient has a goiter, a soft diet may be needed for comfort. Frequent rest periods may be needed, as well as slowly increasing patient activity. Antiembolic stockings may help prevent venous stasis during the low-energy, decreased-activity phase. Daily weights and monitoring intake and output when cardiac status is compromised are important to detect abnormalities such as fluid retention. Because weight gain and facial puffiness alter patients' self-image, patients need an opportunity to verbalize their feelings to help them adjust to this disease process.

Education. Patients taking thyroid hormone replacement therapy should avoid foods high in iodine. The diet should also consist of large amounts of fiber to combat constipation. During the hyperthyroidism phase, a diet high in protein and carbohydrates encourages weight gain. Education regarding prescribed medications is also needed.

Lupus Erythematosus

PATHOPHYSIOLOGY. There are three types of lupus: discoid lupus erythematosus (DLE), drug-induced systemic lupus erythematosus, and systemic lupus erythematosus (SLE) (Table 19.7). The discoid type consists only of skin lesions. Drug-induced SLE develops after use of certain medications (Box 19.1). SLE is a chronic, inflammatory, multisystem disorder. The body develops antibodies against its own tissue. It is very unpredictable. See Box 19.2 for a list of flare triggers.

ETIOLOGY. SLE tends to develop in young women of childbearing years and is more common in the African American and Hispanic populations. First-degree relatives of lupus patients also have a greater tendency than the general population to develop SLE.

SIGNS AND SYMPTOMS. Clinical manifestations vary from mild to severe. See Table 19.7 and Figure 19.6.

THERAPEUTIC MEASURES. Medications used to treat lupus erythematosus are listed in Table 19.8. The human monoclonal antibody Benlysta has continued to have positive results through its phase III clinical trials and is the only medication that is specific for SLE. The next step will be for the clinical trial reports to be reviewed by the FDA for approval and release.

NURSING MANAGEMENT. It is vitally important for the patient and family to be aware of and avoid flare triggers. Fatigue during activities of daily living can be minimized through the use of a daily personal schedule. Additionally, the patient needs a minimum of 8 hours of sleep per night with naps as needed to combat fatigue. Because most patients with SLE develop transitory arthralgia, maintaining fitness and joint range of motion through a regular fitness program while decreasing activity during flares is vital. Warm baths may help with morning stiffness, and application of heat and cold compresses, splints, assistive devices, and physical therapy may help soreness. Eating a well-balanced diet will also influence the level of fatigue and the corticosteroid-induced weight gain, which also can affect joint soreness.

Education. Explain the signs of bleeding and of cardiac and vascular problems, such as myocardial infarction and thrombophlebitis. Encourage the use of a medical alert bracelet. Provide smoking cessation information to patients who smoke. Because renal disease is a major complication of SLE, patients must learn the signs of impending problems that need to be relayed to the physician immediately. These are such findings as facial puffiness and "foamy" urine or "coke-colored" urine indicative of proteinuria and hematuria, respectively. Explain that regular ophthalmic examinations are needed for early detection and treatment of the complications that antimalarials and corticosteroids can produce, such as retinal bleeding, glaucoma, and cataracts.

Finally, but most importantly, the patient's psychological state and support systems need to be addressed. The period from the onset of symptoms to the diagnosing of lupus is usually costly in terms of time, money, and emotions. Patients may face anger, frustration, and confusion prior to the diagnosis. For many, at diagnosis, there is a sense of relief that may quickly be replaced with feelings of anger, fear, depression, or grief. It is here when empathy, support, hope, and, most importantly, education for the patient, family, and significant others are vital for acquiring successful long-term coping skills. In addition, local support groups and educational and self-management programs available through the Lupus Foundation of America www.lupus.org can provide patients with avenues for attaining more specific knowledge and skills for coping and taking control of their lives.

TABLE 19.7 LUPUS ERYTHEMATOSUS SUMMARY

Signs and Symptoms	***Discoid***
	• Patchy, crusty, sharply defined skin plaques
	• Tend to occur on face or sun-exposed areas
	Drug-Induced
	• Pleuropericardial inflammation
	• Fever
	• Rash
	• Arthritis
	Systemic
	• Early symptoms are vague, then fatigue, fever
	• Dermatological:
	  • Butterfly rash (face), photosensitivity, mucosal ulcers, alopecia, pain, pruritus, bruising
	• Musculoskeletal:
	  • Arthralgia, arthritis
	• Hematologic:
	  • Anemia, leukocytopenia, elevated ESR, thrombocytopenia, false-positive VDRL
	• Cardiopulmonary:
	  • Pericarditis, myocarditis, myocardial infarction, vasculitis, pleurisy, valvular heart disease
	• Renal:
	  • Renal failure, urinary tract infections, fluid and electrolyte imbalances
	• Central nervous system:
	  • Cranial neuropathies, cognitive impairment, mental changes, seizures
	• Gastrointestinal:
	  • Anorexia, ascites, pancreatitis, intestinal vasculitis
	• Ophthalmological:
	  • Conjunctivitis, dry eyes, glaucoma, cataracts, retinal pigmentation

Diagnostic Tests	CBC
	Antinuclear antibody (ANA)
	Anti-Sm (a highly specific immunoglobulin for SLE)
	Anti-nDNA positive in 60%–80% of SLE patients
	Anti-Ro (SSA), an immunoglobulin, positive in 30% of SLE patients
	Anti-La (SSB), an immunoglobulin, positive in 15% of SLE patients
	Complement
	Estimated sedimentation rate (ESR) is nonspecific
	C-reactive protein (CRP) is nonspecific
	24-hour urine creatinine clearance
	If ruling out kidney involvement:
	  Urinalysis
	  Serum creatinine
	  Kidney biopsy

Therapeutic Measures	Symptomatic management Nonsteroidal anti-inflammatory drugs Immunosuppressants Corticosteroids Antimalarials Intravenous immunoglobulin
Complications	Osteonecrosis Renal failure Thrombocytopenia Emboli Myocarditis Vasculitis Mesenteric or intestinal vasculitis leading to obstruction, perforation, or infarction Sepsis
Priority Nursing Diagnoses	*Acute Pain* *Disturbed Body Image* *Fatigue* *Ineffective Health Maintenance*

CRITICAL THINKING

Mr. Ellis

■ Mr. Ellis is suffering from a flare of SLE. The physician has ordered Solu-Cortef 80 mg IM to be given every 8 hours. Solu-Cortef 125 mg per 2 mL is available. How many milliliters will the nurse administer per dose?
Suggested answer at end of chapter.

Box 19.1

Medications Associated with Triggering Lupus Erythematosus*

- Adalimumab
- Chlorpromazine
- Diltiazem
- Etanercept
- Hydralazine
- Infliximab
- Isoniazid
- Methyldopa
- Minocycline
- Nitrofurantoin
- Phenytoin
- Procainamide
- Quinidine
- Rifampin

*Information is inconclusive and contradictory regarding some medications.

Box 19.2

Common Lupus Erythematosus Flare Triggers

- Sunlight (reflected off water and snow, glass does not fully protect)
- Fluorescent and halogen lights
- Stress
- Emotional crisis
- Overwork
- Lack of rest
- Infection
- Surgery or injuries
- Hormones
- Pregnancy and after delivery (postpartum)
- Stopping medications suddenly
- Environmental sensitivities or allergies
- Immunizations
- Certain prescription drugs
- Some over-the-counter drugs, such as cough syrups

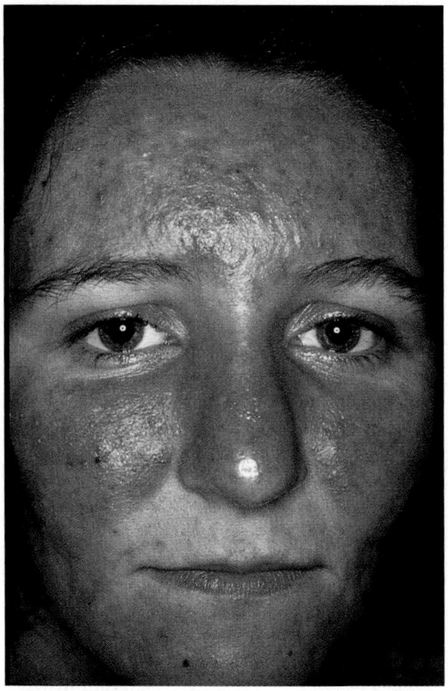

FIGURE 19.6 Lupus erythematosus: red papules and plaques in butterfly pattern on face. (From Goldsmith, L. A., Tharp, M., Lazarus, G., et al. [1997]. *Adult and pediatric dermatology* [p. 230]. Philadelphia: F. A. Davis.)

Ankylosing Spondylitis

PATHOPHYSIOLOGY. **Ankylosing spondylitis**, also called rheumatoid spondylitis, is a chronic progressive inflammatory disease primarily of the spine and sacroiliac area. It can also affect the large limb joints. The inflammatory process begins in the lower region of the back and progresses upward. A specific histocompatibility antigen (antigen that identifies self), human leukocyte antigen (HLA) B27, is formed that stimulates an immune response. It can result in complete fusion of the spine causing complete rigidity in the spine, a condition known as bamboo spine.

ETIOLOGY. There is strong evidence of a familial tendency, but no other specific causes are known. Ankylosing spondylitis tends to afflict men more than women and is usually diagnosed at ages 18 to 30.

SIGNS AND SYMPTOMS. Ankylosing spondylitis causes an insidious onset of lower back stiffness and pain, which is worse in the morning. As the disease progresses, the pain worsens and there are spasms of the back muscles. The normal curvature of the lower back (lordosis) flattens, and the curvature of the upper back increases (kyphosis). Patients may also experience fatigue, anorexia, and weight loss.

DIAGNOSTIC TESTS. Findings such as a positive family history, a positive HLA-B27 blood test, negative Rh, and

• **WORD • BUILDING** •

ankylosing spondylitis: anayle—stiff joint + osing—condition + spondyl—vertebrae + itis—inflammation

TABLE 19.8 MEDICATIONS USED TO TREAT LUPUS ERYTHEMATOSUS

Medication Class/ Action	Examples	Route	Side Effects	Nursing Implications
Nonsteroidal Anti-inflammatory Drugs (NSAIDs)				
Reduces inflammation.	ibuprofen (Motrin) indomethacin (Indocin) naproxen (Naprosyn)	PO	Gastric distress, headache, tinnitus, dizziness, rash, pruritus, fluid retention	Take with food. Avoid taking with ethyl alcohol. Protect from ultraviolet rays. Assess for abnormal bleeding.
Antimalarials				
Action is not clearly understood but can significantly help reduce inflammation, decreases platelet aggregation while lowering plasma lipid levels.	chloroquine (Aralen) hydroxychloroquine sulfate (Plaquenil)	PO PO	Gastric distress, anorexia, vomiting, diarrhea, headache, muscle weakness, alopecia, blurred vision, irritability, dry, itchy skin, rash	Administer before or after meals at the same time of day. Obtain a thorough assessment for a baseline, including an ophthalmic exam. May take weeks or months for effects to be noticed.
Corticosteroids				
Reduces inflammation and suppresses immune response.	dexamethasone (Decadron) methylprednisolone (Solu-Medrol) hydrocortisone (Solu-Cortef) prednisone (Deltasone)	PO, IV, IM PO, IV, IM, topical PO	Increased facial hair, acne, round "moon" face, mood changes, irritability, depression, increased appetite, increased weight, poor wound healing, headache, peptic ulcers, osteoporosis, steroid-induced diabetes	**Never** stop taking suddenly. Don't miss doses. Use measures to avoid infection. Take with food or milk. Monitor for weight gain >5 pounds, decreased urine output, pulse irregularities, increased blood pressure, edema, and temperature. May elevate blood sugar.
Immunosuppressants				
Target and damage autoantibody-producing cells.	azathioprine (Imuran) cyclosporine (Sandimmune) methotrexate (Rheumatrex)	PO PO, IV, PO, IM, IV	Gastric distress, nausea, vomiting, abdominal pain, oral ulcers, dark urine, pale stools, jaundice	Monitor joints for range of motion, edema, temperature, and erythema. Protect patients from those who may carry infections. Monitor CBC, renal and liver function tests. Give with food if gastrointestinal upset. Monitor for abnormal bleeding.

radiographs of the joints showing spinal changes and fusion (although these changes are a late finding) confirm a diagnosis of ankylosing spondylitis. There are no specific immunological tests to diagnose ankylosing spondylitis.

THERAPEUTIC MEASURES. Because there is no cure for ankylosing spondylitis, treatment consists of measures to minimize the symptoms. Analgesics for pain relief, anti-inflammatory agents to decrease joint inflammation, and physical therapy to maintain muscle strength and joint range of motion are used. Biological agents such as anti-TNF-alphas, such as etanercept (Enbrel) and infliximab (Remicade), have shown promising results in changing the disease progression. Surgery can be done to replace fused joints. For kyphosis, cervical or lumbar osteotomy can be performed. Physiotherapy and exercise can be beneficial in managing symptoms.

Research is looking at whether reducing starch in the diet reduces symptoms. *Klebsiella* bacteria, which is found in high levels in the feces of AS patients, requires starch to grow. *Klebsiella* may be a trigger for the disease.

NURSING MANAGEMENT. Nursing care focuses on patient education and administration and evaluation of prescribed medications (Box 19.3, *Patient Education*). Pain management, rest periods, assistance with ADLs, and exercise promotion are provided (see *Evidence-Based Practice* box).

CRITICAL THINKING

Mr. Beck

■ Mr. Beck, a truck driver who was recently diagnosed with ankylosing spondylitis, verbalizes concern about how this diagnosis will affect his ability to work.

1. How would the nurse answer his questions?
   a. "What is happening to me?"
   b. "Will I have to quit my job driving an interstate truck?"
   c. "Am I eventually going to have really bad pain?"
   d. "Am I eventually going to be dependent on someone?"
2. Mr. Beck plans to continue driving his truck and therefore has a need upon discharge for specific interventions that will help him maintain his independence. What will the nurse say to Mr. Beck on discharge about why each of the following instructions is important for him to follow?
   a. Perform range-of-motion exercises daily.
   b. Do not stay in one position too long. Stop and walk around often.
   c. Sleep on a firm mattress without a pillow.
   d. Maintain good posture, even when driving the truck.

Suggested answers at end of chapter.

Box 19.3

Patient Education
Ankylosing Spondylitis

Help reduce pain and stiffness by:
- Providing disease information
- Explaining proper posture and range-of-motion exercises
- Teaching to change positions frequently
- Urging to sleep on a mattress that is firm without a pillow.

EVIDENCE-BASED PRACTICE

Clinical Question
What is the effectiveness of physiotherapy interventions in the management of ankylosing spondylitis?

Evidence
A systematic review of 11 trials with a total of 763 participants looked at the benefits of physiotherapy and exercise to patients with ankylosing spondylitis (Dagfinrud, Hagen, & Kvien, 2007). Benefits were found to be improved movement in the spine, overall well-being, and/or improved physical functioning. Least benefit was from no therapy, progressing in benefit to individual home-based exercise, supervised group physiotherapy, and combined inpatient spa-exercise therapy followed by group physiotherapy, which was best.

Implications for Nursing Practice
Because physiotherapy or exercise is beneficial to patients with ankylosing spondylitis, nurses can teach and encourage patients to participate in these activities.

REFERENCE

Dagfinrud, H., Hagen, K. B., & Kvien, T. K. (2007). Physiotherapy interventions for ankylosing spondylitis. ***Cochrane Database of Systematic Reviews 2007, Issue 2*** **(Art. No. CD002822; DOI 10.1002/14651858.CD002822.pub3).**

IMMUNE DEFICIENCIES

Immune deficiencies occur when one or more components of the immune system are either completely absent or deficient in quantities sufficient to elicit or sustain an adequate immune response to combat an infectious agent.

Hypogammaglobulinemia

PATHOPHYSIOLOGY AND ETIOLOGY. This condition is either a hereditary congenital disorder or acquired after childhood from unknown causes. It is characterized by the absence or deficiency of one or more of the five classes of immunoglobulins (IgG, IgM, IgA, IgD, and IgE) from defective B-cell function. The lack of normal function of these antibodies makes the patient prone to infections. The congenital form of this disorder affects males. Patients usually have a normal life span.

SIGNS AND SYMPTOMS. The infant is usually asymptomatic until 6 months of age, when the maternal immunoglobulins are gone. At this time, the infant begins having many recurrent infections, especially from *Staphylococcus* and *Streptococcus* organisms.

DIAGNOSIS. Until an infant is 9 months old, diagnosis is extremely difficult. At 9 months of age, immunoelectrophoresis, which measures the level of each immunoglobulin, can be performed.

THERAPEUTIC MEASURES. Treatment is aimed at minimizing infections while increasing immune system function through injections of immunoglobulin. These injections mainly contain IgG, so fresh frozen plasma is given to replace IgM. IgA cannot be replaced, increasing the risk for frequent pulmonary infections.

NURSING MANAGEMENT. The infant is monitored for infections. Any break in the skin must be cleansed immediately and monitored for infection development. Genetic counseling may be recommended for parents.

Education. The family is educated about signs and symptoms of a variety of infections and the importance in seeking medical help immediately. They are taught that the infant should not be in crowds and that good nutrition, hydration, and hygiene are important in preventing infections.

Home Health Hints

Atopic Dermatitis

- Instruct patients with atopic dermatitis to use a skin moisturizer daily to help prevent dryness, which can lead to the complications of eczema. Avoid baby lotions or any lotion that contains perfumes, which can irritate the skin, and alcohol products, which can further dry the skin.
- Use of regular soaps can be drying to the skin. Urge the patient and family to use only soaps labeled for sensitive skin.
- Assist the patient with choosing an oatmeal bath product that can be helpful in relieving skin dryness.
- Use an ice pack on the irritated area to help relieve the itching of atopic dermatitis.
- Monitor for a rash, especially around the torso and abdomen. If rash develops, consider the laundry soap being used and encourage a mild soap, such as one of those used to wash baby clothes (e.g., Dreft).

Latex Allergy

- Always have on hand latex-free gloves.
- Use a latex-free silicone urinary catheter.

Transplants

- Teach patients who have had a transplant and are taking immune-suppressing medications to avoid public places such as malls and food stores to help prevent infection. If they do go out, let them know that they should wear a surgical mask to help prevent exposure to illness.
- Teach to take medications as prescribed, especially immunosuppressant medications for cardiac transplant patients.
- Prevent exposure for patients with cardiac transplants to people with illnesses such as colds or the flu.

SUGGESTED ANSWERS TO CRITICAL THINKING

■ *Mrs. Barnes*

1. Mrs. Barnes is most likely having an anaphylactic reaction to the bee stings with accompanying urticaria or even angioedema.
2. Further assessment might include identification of any previous allergies to food, medications, and environmental stimuli and what reactions occur with any allergies. Thorough respiratory assessment is needed, noting any adventitious sounds, in particular wheezing. Note any dysphagia or changes in her voice.
3. Therapeutic measures to implement include monitoring vital signs, staying with the patient, using semi-Fowler's to high-Fowler's position, giving oxygen at 2 to 3 liters per minute, and ensuring a patent intravenous access. Notify the RN and/or physician right away. Anticipate administration of antihistamines, epinephrine, and fluids.

SUGGESTED ANSWERS TO—cont'd

■ *Blood Types*

1. AB Rh^+.
2. O Rh^-.
3. No, they can safely receive only A Rh^- or O Rh^- blood.

■ *Mr. Ellis*

1.28 mL per dose.

■ *Mr. Beck*

1. a. "Human leukocyte antigen B27 is formed, stimulating a chronic immune (inflammatory) response specifically in the spine, sacroiliac area, and large peripheral joints. This leads to thickening of the joints, joint pain, and stiffness."
   b. "No, you shouldn't have to quit your job, but you may need to alter the way you drive your truck."
   c. "No, you may not eventually be in severe pain, with use of medications and exercise."
   d. "No, this disease may not affect your independence, with proper treatment and rehabilitation."
2. a. "Range-of-motion exercises will help maintain joint mobility and a full range of motion and prevent contractures from forming."
   b. "Again, this frequent movement prevents stiffness and joint pain and contractures of joints."
   c. "Sleeping on a firm mattress without a pillow keeps the spine in correct alignment, which in turn helps prevent progressive changes in spine alignment (kyphosis, scoliosis) that affect various major body systems (respiratory, etc.)."
   d. "Again, good posture will aid in preventing bone deformities."

REVIEW QUESTIONS

1. A patient asks the nurse how an allergy can develop to a medication that has been taken before without problems. Which of the following is the most appropriate for the nurse to respond?
   a. "It probably is due to your age, because as you age your body becomes more sensitive to environmental stimuli, which leads to hypersensitivities."
   b. "What have you eaten in the last 24 hours? Most medications are altered by food, thereby producing different effects in the body."
   c. "Viral illnesses and exposure to various chemicals and environmental substances can alter the immune system and its response to previously benign stimuli."
   d. "Patients who have autoimmune disorders such as lupus or arthritis tend to develop sensitivities to common medications."

2. A patient asks the nurse what ankylosing spondylitis is. Which of the following responses is appropriate?
   a. Chronic progressive inflammatory disease of large limb joints
   b. Autoantibodies that lyse RBCs
   c. Formation of antigen-antibody complexes leading to inflammation
   d. Production of IgE antibodies

3. Which of the following is a sign or symptom of pernicious anemia?
   a. Glossitis
   b. Itching
   c. Kyphosis
   d. Lower back spasms

4. What care would the nurse provide for a patient undergoing a Schilling test for pernicious anemia?
   a. Maintain on bedrest.
   b. Monitor vital signs.
   c. Collect 24-hour urine specimen.
   d. Maintain pressure dressing.

5. Which of the following interventions should the nurse anticipate will be included in the treatment plan for a patient with allergic rhinitis? **Select all that apply.**
   a. Antihistamines
   b. Avoiding environmental stimuli
   c. Immunotherapy
   d. Steroids
   e. Anticholinergics
   f. Decongestants

6. Which data are collected when caring for a patient with contact dermatitis?
   a. Date of gastric surgery
   b. Appearance of skin lesions
   c. Weight gain
   d. Appetite

REVIEW QUESTIONS—cont'd

7. A patient is admitted with an autoimmune disease and asks the nurse what autoimmune means. Which of the following would be the appropriate response by the nurse?
   a. "Immune cells produce too many antibodies."
   b. "Immune cells grow and multiply too rapidly."
   c. "Immune cells are not produced in sufficient amounts."
   d. "Immune cells are unable to distinguish between 'self' and 'not self.'"

8. A patient who has an allergy to penicillin is receiving preoperative medications, which include ranitidine (Zantac), metoclopramide (Reglan), and cefazolin (Ancef) intravenously. Fifteen minutes after the cefazolin is started, the patient reports an uneasy feeling, as well as feeling very warm. The nurse would appropriately recognize that the patient is experiencing anaphylaxis and perform which of the following? **Select all that apply.**
   a. Offer the patient ice water.
   b. Discontinue the IV.
   c. Stay with the patient.
   d. Turn off the IVPB (piggyback).
   e. Call for assistance.
   f. Monitor vital signs.

9. As a patient is being discharged after being diagnosed with SLE, the patient says that soon he is leaving on a 3-week tour of the Grand Canyon and going whitewater rafting. Which of the following patient statements conveys the patient's understanding of the plan of care?
   a. "As long as I wear sunscreen, I'll be fine in the sun."
   b. "I'll wear clothing on all exposed skin and use sunscreen."
   c. "If I develop a rash, I should avoid the sun."
   d. "I should avoid the sun in the morning."

Reference

Gell, P. G. H., & Coombs, R. R. A. (Eds.). (1963). *Clinical aspects of immunology*. Oxford, England: Blackwell.

20

Nursing Care of Patients with HIV Disease and AIDS

MARY DILLINGER

KEY TERMS

acquired immunodeficiency syndrome (uh-KWHY-erd im-yoo-noh-dee-FISH-en-see SIN-drohm)
cytomegalovirus (SY-tow-MEH-guh-low-vy-russ)
human immunodeficiency virus (HYOO-man im-yoo-noh-dee-FISH-en-see VY-rus)
Kaposi's sarcoma (ka-POE-sees sar-COH-mah)
personal protective equipment (PUR-sun-al pra-TEK-tiv ee-KWIP-mant)
Pneumocystis jiroveci pneumonia (new-moh-SISS-tiss yee-row-VET-zee new-MOH-nee-ah)

QUESTIONS TO GUIDE YOUR READING

1. What is human immunodeficiency virus (HIV) and how is it transmitted?
2. How is HIV diagnosed?
3. What is the prognosis for HIV and acquired immunodeficiency syndrome (AIDS)?
4. What would you include in a teaching plan to prevent HIV infection?
5. What prevention measures are used to decrease infection and opportunistic diseases for patients with HIV?
6. What would you include in a teaching plan for a patient with HIV receiving antiretroviral therapy?
7. What nursing care would you provide for patients with HIV/AIDS related to medications, coinfection prevention and maintaining nutritional status?

Acquired immunodeficiency syndrome (AIDS) is the late phase of a chronic immune function disorder caused by the **human immunodeficiency virus** (HIV). AIDS may develop after a long period of HIV infection and may eventually be fatal, if left untreated. The Centers for Disease Control and Prevention (CDC) specifies the criteria for determining when HIV infection has developed into AIDS (Box 20.1).

Not all HIV-infected people develop AIDS, largely because current treatments help to improve immune function and reduce the risk of opportunistic infections, which can be life threatening in these patients. Antiretroviral therapy, which was introduced in 1996, greatly reduced the death rate from AIDS. As a result, the number of people living today with HIV/AIDS is at its highest level ever.

Box 20.1

CDC Conditions in the AIDS Surveillance Case Definition

CD4+ T-lymphocyte count below 200/mm^3, or a CD4+ T-lymphocyte percentage under 14 of total lymphocytes, or the presence of one of the following specified clinical conditions:

- Candidiasis of bronchi, trachea, or lung
- Candidiasis, esophageal
- Cervical cancer, invasive
- Coccidioidomycosis, disseminated or extrapulmonary
- Cryptococcosis, extrapulmonary
- Cryptosporidiosis, chronic intestinal (greater than 1-month duration)
- Cytomegalovirus (CMV) disease (not including liver, spleen, or nodes)
- CMV retinitis with loss of vision
- Encephalopathy, HIV related
- Herpes simplex, chronic ulcers; or bronchitis, pneumonitis, or esophagitis
- Histoplasmosis, disseminated or extrapulmonary
- Isosporiasis, chronic intestinal (greater than 1-month duration)
- Kaposi's sarcoma
- Lymphoma, immunoblastic
- Lymphoma, Burkitt's
- Lymphoma of the brain, primary
- *Mycobacterium avium intracellulare* complex or *Mycobacterium kansasii,* disseminated or extrapulmonary
- *Mycobacterium* tuberculosis, any site (pulmonary or extrapulmonary)
- *Mycobacterium,* other species or unidentified species, disseminated or extrapulmonary
- *Pneumocystis jiroveci* (*carinii*) pneumonia
- Pneumonia, recurrent
- Progressive multifocal leukoencephalopathy
- Salmonella septicemia, recurrent
- Toxoplasmosis of brain
- Wasting syndrome

Source: Modified from Centers for Disease Control and Prevention. (1992). 1993 Revised classification system of HIV infection and expanded surveillance case definition for AIDS among adolescents and adults. *MMWR, 41*(RR17), 2.

LEARNING TIP

HIV disease is no longer characterized as a life-ending illness. With antiretroviral therapy, HIV disease is a chronic, sometimes progressive immune disorder.

NURSING CARE TIP

More than any other chronic disease in recent history, AIDS challenges nurses to call into play all of their physical, emotional, social, and spiritual care skills. As you care for patients who are HIV positive or have AIDS, it is important for you to understand current information. Being informed helps you to provide caring, competent, nonjudgmental care without fear (Table 20.1). Knowledge about HIV/AIDS and its treatment continues to evolve with new discoveries.

HISTORY AND INCIDENCE

The HIV epidemic was first reported by the CDC in June 1981. Cases of HIV infection and AIDS increased rapidly through the 1980s, followed by a decrease in the later 1990s. From 1981 through 2007, more than 980,000 people were estimated to have HIV/AIDS in the United States; of these, about 550,000 died (Table 20.2). In 2006, an estimated 56,300 people were newly infected in the United States, and the CDC estimated that 1 in 4 infected people were not aware of their status. In 2009, the CDC reported that every 9.5 minutes, someone in the United States is infected with HIV. The latest statistics can be found at www.cdc.gov.

Currently, HIV infections are increasing most rapidly in women and in men who have sex with men. Women account for 27% of HIV infections. In recent years in the United States, male-to-male sex has been the most likely cause of exposure to HIV (53%), followed by heterosexual contact (31%), and then by injection drug use (12%). African Americans are estimated to have an incidence rate seven times higher than that of Caucasians.

Although any age-group can be affected by HIV/AIDS, 57% of those diagnosed with it have been ages 25 to 44. Given the long latency period between infection with HIV and development of an AIDS-defining illness, most people diagnosed with HIV disease at age 30 or younger were probably infected

TABLE 20.1 STAYING CURRENT: HIV/AIDS INFORMATION RESOURCES

AIDS Education Global information System	www.aegis.com
AIDS information from U.S. Department of Health and Human Services (in English and Spanish)	www.aidsinfo.nih.gov (800)874-2571
AIDS worldwide	www.avert.org
AIDS drug fact sheets	www.aidsinfonet.org
Association of Nurses in AIDS Care	www.anacnet.org (800)260-6780
CDC (in English and Spanish)	(800)342–2437
CDC HIV and STD test site locator	www.hivtest.org (800)CDC-INFO
CDC National AIDS Hotline (TTY service)	www.cdc.gov/hiv (800)243–7889
CDC National Center for HIV/AIDS, Viral Hepatitis, STD, and TB Prevention	www.cdc.gov/nchstp/od/nchstp.html
CDC National Prevention Information Network	www.cdcnpin.org (800)458-5231
Gateway to federal domestic HIV/AIDS resources	www.AIDS.gov
HIV/AIDS Treatment Information Service (in English and Spanish)	www.hivatis.org (800)448–0440
National HIV/AIDS Clinicians' Consultation Center Post-Exposure Prophylaxis Hotline	www.nccc.ucsf.edu/Hotlines/PEPline.html (888)448-4911
National Library of Medicine	www.nlm.nih.gov (888)346-3656
The Body: HIV/AIDS Resource	www.thebody.com
World Health Organization: HIV/AIDS	www.who.int/hiv

TABLE 20.2 DATA FOR U.S. ADULTS/ADOLESCENTS WITH AIDS, 1981–2007

Gender		
Male	Declined from 92% to 73%	783,786
Female	Increased from 8% to 27%	189,566
Years of Age	***Estimate of AIDS Cases in 2007***	***Cumulative Estimate of AIDS Cases Through 2007***
12 or younger	28	9209
13–14	80	1169
15–24	2382	44,264
25–34	7567	322,370
35–44	12,701	396,851
45–54	9385	176,304
55–64	3020	52,409
65 and older	800	15,853
Ethnicity/Race		
Black	17,507	426,003
White	10,407	404,465
Hispanic	6,921	169,138
Asian/Pacific Islander	475	7,511
American Indian/Alaskan Native	158	3,492
Deceased	14,105	550,000
Estimated HIV/AIDS cases at end of 2007	1,200,000 24%–27% undiagnosed and unaware of their HIV infection and 44%–59% not in care	

Source: Centers for Disease Control and Prevention. (2007). *HIV/AIDS surveillance report* (Vol. 19). Retrieved February 10, 2010, from http://www.cdc.gov/hiv/topics/surveillance/basic.htm.

as adolescents. Older adults are increasingly contracting HIV. The number of infections in people over age 50 has doubled since 2004, and patients in this age-group must be educated about prevention. Although HIV/AIDS can occur in a person of any age, this chapter focuses on adults with HIV/AIDS.

PATHOPHYSIOLOGY

Infection with the HIV virus causes destruction of immune cells. Two subtypes of the HIV virus have been identified: HIV-1 and HIV-2. Both of these subtypes can cause AIDS. HIV-1 is found in Asia, Europe, and the Western Hemisphere. HIV-2 is found mainly in West Africa. Without a normally functioning immune system, infections and cancers may take over. AIDS is the result of this immunodeficiency.

HIV is a retrovirus (which only has ribonucleic acid [RNA] for genetic material). HIV is attracted to immune cells that have a surface-attaching site referred to as a CD4 receptor. Cells with CD4 receptors include lymphocytes (called CD4+ T lymphocytes, T4 lymphocytes, or helper T lymphocytes) and macrophages (in which HIV hides). HIV begins its infection by binding to the CD4 receptor of the host cell. The CD4+ T lymphocytes are the primary targets for HIV infection. Because CD4+ T lymphocytes orchestrate all immune functions, HIV's attack on these cells results in progressive impairment of the body's immune response. The CD4+ T lymphocytes do not function normally and are too busy replicating more HIV to perform their intended immune functions.

Recent understanding of how HIV fuses with the cell has been the focus of new treatments for preventing infection by blocking fusion of HIV with its host cell. After fusion with the host cell, the HIV viral particle is taken into a human cell and its covering is destroyed to expose its viral RNA. The retrovirus then uses an enzyme called reverse transcriptase to force the human cell to produce a new piece of deoxyribonucleic acid (DNA) from the viral RNA. The new DNA is integrated into the person's cellular DNA. As a result, the human cell creates more viral particles, which spread through the lymphoid system (Fig. 20.1). Inhibitors of reverse transcriptase were the first anti-HIV medications developed and are still an essential part of current treatment.

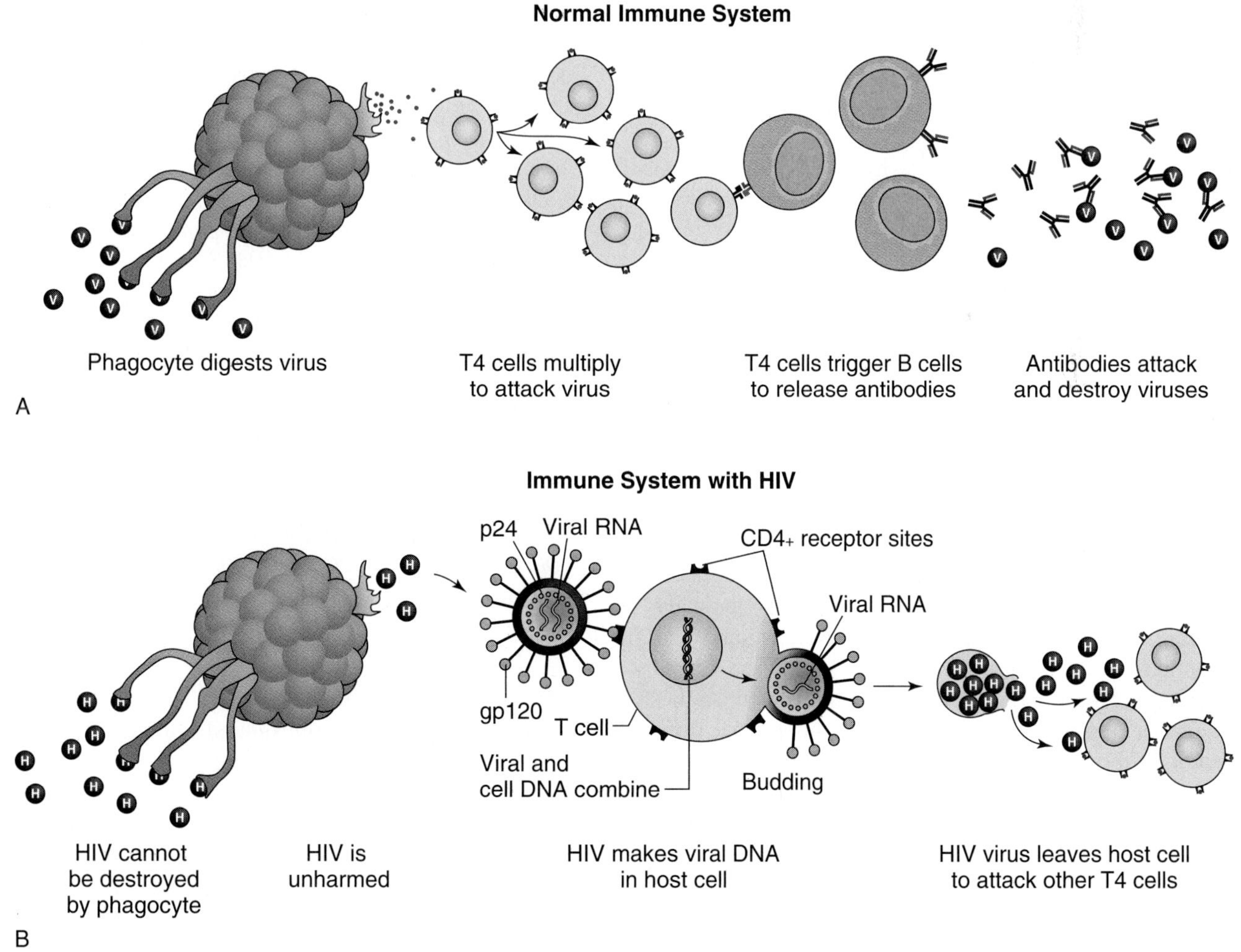
Normal Immune System
Phagocyte digests virus
T4 cells multiply to attack virus
T4 cells trigger B cells to release antibodies
Antibodies attack and destroy viruses
A
Immune System with HIV
p24
Viral RNA
CD4+ receptor sites
Viral RNA
gp120
T cell
Viral and cell DNA combine
Budding
HIV cannot be destroyed by phagocyte
HIV is unharmed
HIV makes viral DNA in host cell
HIV virus leaves host cell to attack other T4 cells
B

FIGURE 20.1 (A) Normal immune system. (B) HIV contains several proteins: gp 120 protein around it and viral RNA and p24 protein inside. The gp 120 proteins attach to CD4+ receptors of T lymphocytes; HIV enters the cell and makes viral DNA; the enslaved host cell produces new viruses that bud, which destroys the host cell's membrane, causing cellular death and allowing the virus to leave to attack other CD4+ T-lymphocyte cells.

Once the genetic material of HIV has been changed to DNA, the enzyme integrase integrates it into the genetic material of the host cell. The cell is then translated into viral proteins. Among these proteins is HIV protease, which is required to process other HIV proteins into their functional forms. Protease inhibitors, potent types of antiviral medications, act by blocking this critical step. Following development of the cell surface, the virus then buds from the cell and is released to infect another cell. The virus spreads throughout the body unless interrupted by treatment. HIV may persist in a latent state for many years. This makes it very difficult to eradicate or cure HIV. Because of this, currently, patients must remain on antiviral treatment for life. The ultimate challenge is to use knowledge of the HIV life cycle to develop treatments that will eradicate HIV from those who are infected and to create a vaccine that will prevent new infections in the future.

After a person has been infected with HIV, other immune system components form antibodies to fight the HIV. Detection of these antibodies via laboratory testing is the most common way HIV is diagnosed. HIV antibodies typically become present within 3 weeks to 3 months after infection. The time between infection and developing antibodies is called the "window period." Laboratory tests are available that detect the virus directly, rather than antibodies, but these are more costly for routine HIV testing.

LEARNING TIP

Being HIV positive means that the person has been infected with the HIV virus. It does not mean that the person has AIDS.

Progression

The initial infection is followed by a relatively symptom-free period called the clinical latency stage. The virus remains in the lymph nodes, liver, and spleen and reproduces. If the infection is untreated, CD4+ T lymphocytes gradually decrease. B lymphocytes also become dysfunctional and dysregulated by the events of HIV progression. B and T cells work together for a normal healthy immune system, so this may further impair the immune system. This period, from infection to the beginning of the symptomatic stage, varies for each person and averages 8 to 12 years. During this stage, the person is considered to be HIV infected. (Many are not aware of their HIV infection until they become symptomatic. They may unknowingly pass the virus on to others, and they do not have the benefit of antiviral treatments to maintain health.) During the early symptomatic stage of HIV disease, symptoms of the weakening immune system are seen. When the immune system is severely weakened, opportunistic infections and cancers may occur. When this occurs, the person is diagnosed with AIDS (see Box 20.1).

LEARNING TIP

Opportunistic diseases are referred to as opportunistic because a normal immune system would prevent them from occurring. With an impaired immune system, invading organisms have the "opportunity" to survive.

PREVENTION

Prevention and education are the best ways to manage the HIV/AIDS epidemic (see *Evidence-Based Practice* box). Education regarding the disease and its transmission should begin with the older school-age child and include the general population, including older adults (Box 20.2, *Gerontological Issues*).

EVIDENCE-BASED PRACTICE

Clinical Question

Does circumcision prevent heterosexual acquisition of HIV in men?

Evidence

Three large randomized controlled studies in Africa revealed strong evidence that male circumcision prevents men from acquiring HIV from heterosexual sex (Siegfried et al., 2009).

Implications for Nursing Practice

Understanding current evidence-based HIV prevention measures is important in providing care and education to patients.

REFERENCE

Siegfried, N., Muller, M., Deeks, J. J., & Volmink, J. (2009). Male circumcision for prevention of heterosexual acquisition of HIV in men. *Cochrane Database of Systematic Reviews 2009, Issue 2* (Art. No. CD003362; DOI 10.1002/14651858. CD003362.pub2).

Mode of Transmission

HIV is a fragile virus that is transmitted from person to person only through infected blood, sexual secretions, or, for an infant with an infected mother, through fetal transmission or via breast milk. HIV is not spread casually. It needs a portal of entry into the body, such as a tear in a mucous membrane, or nonintact skin, or access to the bloodstream or lymphatic tissue. Kissing, hugging, shaking hands, or sharing eating utensils, towels, or bathroom fixtures with an HIV-positive person does not transmit HIV. There is also no evidence that HIV can be transmitted through insect bites, tears, nasal secretions, saliva, sweat, sputum, emesis, urine, or feces unless blood is present. Even then the transmission risk is

Box 20.2

Gerontological Issues

In 2005, the CDC reported 15% of new cases and 24% of all persons living with HIV/AIDS are over the age of 50. Numbers will continue to rise as the older population increases, yet little attention has been given to this age-group. This may be due to an ageist view of the older adult and sexual activity. It is important to understand that HIV infection can occur at any age. Older adults should be asked about their sexual and drug use history and be given preventive education and information about products that reduce transmission of HIV and sexually transmitted diseases. At-risk people older than age 50 are less likely than younger at-risk adults to use condoms during sex or to be tested for HIV. In this age-group, condoms are often thought of as a birth control measure. The availability of treatments for erectile dysfunction has also contributed to the number of older adults who are sexually active.

HIV/AIDS is thought of as being a disease of young, sexually active people. Many older people remain sexually active, and may have multiple partners. Like their younger counterparts, older people are also contracting the virus through same-sex contact.

A decline in the older adult's immune system increases the risk for infection with HIV. Increased vaginal dryness and friability further increases an older woman's susceptibility to HIV infection. Because older adults are not usually taught HIV prevention, the rise in HIV infection among older adults is expected to continue. With AIDS death rates dropping as a result of more effective treatments, the number of older adults living with HIV will increase.

Symptoms of HIV in older adults may be confused with commonly perceived problems of aging, such as fatigue, decreased endurance, and altered cognitive status. The effect of HIV on the brain can be mistaken for Alzheimer's disease, delaying proper treatment.

considered very low. Blood transfusions before 1985 may have been a source for HIV transmission. However, since 1985, donated blood has been tested for HIV.

LEARNING TIP

A person infected with HIV can transmit HIV to others within a few days after initial infection and then throughout all stages of the disease. This is thought to be true even when antiretroviral treatment has driven the viral load below detectable levels.

Counseling

Early knowledge of HIV status aids in reducing the spread of HIV infection. The CDC revised their recommended guidelines for counseling and testing adults, adolescents, and pregnant women in 2006. The new guidelines recommend increased screening of people in health care settings, encouraging use of a verbal request to test with the ability to "opt out" also being verbal when declining the testing. However, written informed consent for testing is still the standard of care.

HIV test counseling should be done by trained workers to help the patient make an informed decision about testing. Education should also be provided that is culturally sensitive and fits the patient's personal risk situation. Post-test counseling is provided to help the patient understand the test results, assist with informing sexual partners and drug needle sharers, risk factor reduction, and care options, if needed.

Sexual Transmission

HIV is transmitted more easily to women than men. This is because the vagina has a greater amount of mucous membrane than the penis, and because an increased amount of virus is found in semen compared to the amount in vaginal secretions. Sexual acts that are the riskiest for transmission of HIV are those that promote contact between infected body fluids and mucous membranes or nonintact skin. These risky acts include anal sex and oral sex. Anal sex is the riskiest type of sexual act, for either gender, because it often results in tearing of the mucous membrane, which is then exposed to infected semen. The presence of a sexually transmitted infection (STI) can increase the risk of transmission due to the potential opening in the skin for HIV to enter through an STI-related lesion.

Safer Sex Practices

Abstaining from sexual intercourse is the only sure way to prevent sexual exposure to HIV. A long term, mutually monogamous sexual relationship is considered safe if both partners are not and will not become infected with HIV. Alternatives to sexual intercourse can be used that prevent exposure to blood and secretions, such as massage or masturbation. The benefits of limiting sexual partners should be explained. For vaginal or anal intercourse, the use of male or female condoms and safer sex techniques should be discussed (Box 20.3, *Patient Education*). Latex gloves protect hands during genital or anal contact. Dental dams (latex sheets) should be used as a barrier between the mouth and genitals or anus.

Parenteral Transmission

The best way to prevent parenteral transmission of HIV is to avoid injection drug use. Drug injection equipment should not be shared. If a person who uses injected drugs is unable or unwilling to stop sharing needles, he or she should be carefully taught how to clean the needle and syringe: To optimize the effectiveness of cleaning, soon after use the needle and syringe should be flushed with water until visibly

Box 20.3

Patient Education

Condom Use to Prevent HIV Transmission

Condoms should be:
- New for each sex act.
- Made of latex (polyurethane if allergic to latex) because other materials have large pores that allow HIV to pass.
- Nondamaged and within expiration date.
- Applied before partner is touched. (Tip of condom is held while unrolling over erect penis, allowing room at tip for semen collection.)
- Used with adequate amounts of only water-soluble lubricant. (Petroleum or oil-based lubricants such as petroleum jelly, cooking oil, shortening, or lotions can damage latex condoms.)
- Replaced if broken. (If ejaculation occurs before replacement, immediate use of a spermicide may give some protection.)
- Withdrawn from partner by holding condom against base of erect penis to avoid semen leakage.

clear of blood. Next, the syringe is filled with full-strength household bleach and shaken for 1 minute. The bleach is flushed through the needle and syringe and then both are rinsed with water. Additionally, sexual activity should be strongly discouraged when judgment is impaired from drug use because protective measures may not be used. There continues to be significant controversy regarding clean needle exchange programs for injection drug users, but they have been shown to decrease the risk of transmission of HIV and other bloodborne pathogens.

Autologous (one's own) blood transfusion, when possible, is the safest type of transfusion to prevent HIV infection. Screening of blood for HIV antibodies has been done on all donated blood in the United States since 1985. There is a reported 1 in 1.8 million units chance of HIV transmission from blood that is infected but has not yet had time to develop antibodies.

Perinatal Transmission

The U.S. Public Health Service guidelines for HIV screening of pregnant women recommend that voluntary HIV pretest counseling and testing be offered during prenatal care for all pregnant women (Branson et al., 2006). Pregnant women who know they are HIV positive can reduce the risk of perinatal HIV transmission to less than 4% by taking antiretroviral therapy (zidovudine [AZT, Retrovir]) during pregnancy, labor, and delivery. Every effort should be taken during labor and delivery to avoid any procedure such as a scalp monitor or episiotomy that increases the risk of exposure of the infant to the mother's blood. At the time of delivery, pregnant women who have not been tested for HIV or received prophylactic treatment should be offered testing for HIV. After delivery, the infant of a mother with HIV is given zidovudine (AZT, Retrovir) for 6 weeks.

Health Care Workers and HIV Prevention

The CDC has developed standard precautions to reduce the risk of HIV exposure, as well as other bloodborne pathogens (see Chapter 8). It is essential to understand and use these practices with all patients to protect yourself from exposure and transmission of HIV. If you are unsure of the appropriate **personal protective equipment** or isolation precautions to use, ask your instructor or the patient's nurse before providing care to the patient.

Needlesticks

Needlestick injury is a source of HIV transmission to health care workers. The Needlestick Safety and Prevention Act is designed to aid health care workers in preventing needlestick injuries. Careful use of needles—including not recapping used needles and using needless systems and other needle safety devices—can reduce needlestick injury. Consider an occupational exposure an urgent medical concern and seek medical care immediately. To prevent the risk of transmission of HIV after a needlestick or other form of exposure to patient body fluids, the CDC has developed postexposure prophylaxis guidelines (Panlilio et al., 2005). Know the protocol for the agency or hospital in which you are employed and follow that protocol.

If an exposure occurs, wash the exposure site with soap and water immediately. For mucous membrane exposure, flush with water, and then report to the closest emergency room immediately for further assessment and possible treatment.

SIGNS AND SYMPTOMS

Initially after HIV infection, the patient may have no symptoms or may develop mononucleosis-like symptoms (called an acute retroviral syndrome), such as extreme fatigue, headache, fever, lymphadenopathy (enlarged lymph nodes in two different sites other than inguinal nodes), diarrhea, or a sore throat (Fig. 20.2 and Table 20.3). Symptoms typically develop 6 to 12 weeks after HIV transmission and may last a few days to weeks. These symptoms are usually mild and not attributed to an HIV infection.

Each patient's response to HIV is unique. After an extended asymptomatic phase, untreated HIV infection usually progresses to a symptomatic stage when the virus has greatly impaired the immune system. The patient may have shortness of breath, fever, weight loss, fatigue, night sweats, persistent diarrhea, oral or vaginal candidiasis ulcers, dry skin, skin lesions, peripheral neuropathy, shingles (varicella zoster virus reactivation), seizures, or dementia. In the final stage of HIV infection, AIDS is diagnosed when the CD4+ T-lymphocyte count is below 200 or opportunistic infections

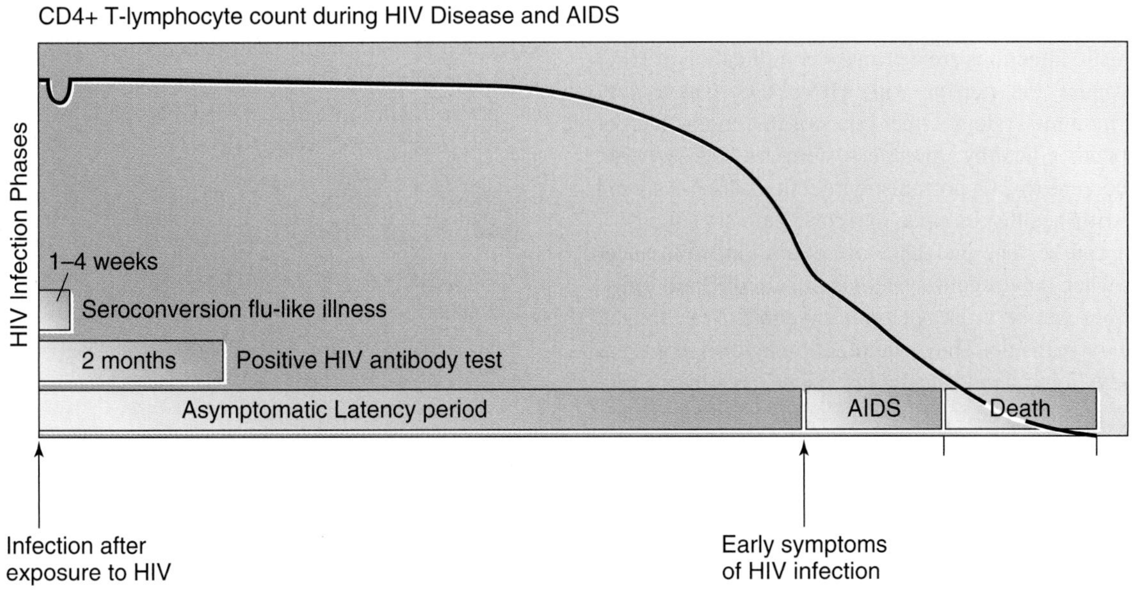
CD4+ T-lymphocyte count during HIV Disease and AIDS
HIV Infection Phases
1–4 weeks
Seroconversion flu-like illness
2 months
Positive HIV antibody test
Asymptomatic Latency period
AIDS
Death
Infection after exposure to HIV
Early symptoms of HIV infection

FIGURE 20.2 Typical phases of HIV infection, AIDS development, and CD4+ T-lymphocyte counts without treatment. Length of latency period varies but is usually many years. As CD4+ T-lymphocyte counts drop, symptoms, AIDS, opportunistic infections, and then death may result.

TABLE 20.3 HIV/AIDS SUMMARY

Signs and Symptoms	Initially vary; none or acute retroviral syndrome Asymptomatic phase Immune system impairment: dyspnea, fever, weight loss, fatigue, night sweats, persistent diarrhea, oral or vaginal candidiasis ulcers, dry skin, skin lesions, peripheral neuropathy, shingles, or dementia AIDS diagnosed when CD4+ T-lymphocyte count below 200 or opportunistic infections and diseases occur.
Diagnostic Tests	HIV antibody tests Complete blood cell count/lymphocyte count CD4+/CD8+ T-lymphocyte count Viral load testing Genotyping
Therapeutic Measures	Non-nucleoside reverse transcriptase inhibitors (NRTIs) Nucleoside/nucleotide reverse transcriptase inhibitors (NNRTIs) Protease inhibitors (PIs) Fusion inhibitors Integrase inhibitors
Complications	AIDS wasting syndrome Opportunistic infections and cancer AIDS dementia complex
Priority Nursing Diagnoses	*Ineffective Protection* *Acute* or *Chronic Pain* *Ineffective Coping* *Risk for Injury*

and diseases, with their specific signs and symptoms, occur (see Box 20.1).

COMPLICATIONS

Many complications are seen with HIV/AIDS that vary from patient to patient. Some of the common complications are discussed next.

AIDS Wasting Syndrome

AIDS wasting syndrome occurs in some patients with AIDS. The syndrome is defined by involuntary loss of more than 10% of baseline body weight plus chronic weakness or fever, or chronic diarrhea, for more than 30 days. Several factors contribute to this syndrome: decreased appetite, oral lesions, altered metabolism, malabsorption, gastrointestinal (GI) infections, diarrhea, medication side effects, and cognitive impairment. The progressive weight loss impairs the function of all body systems from malnourishment. Careful intervention, planning, and education of the patient when HIV is first diagnosed can help maintain body weight.

NURSING CARE TIP

AIDS wasting syndrome is challenging. Do not give up! Be creative in developing interventions to help increase the patient's appetite and calorie intake. Small, frequent meals are usually helpful.

Opportunistic Infection and Cancer

Opportunistic infections are a primary complication of HIV/AIDS because the person with HIV/AIDS has a very impaired immune system. Other types of infections that occur even with a healthy immune system are seen as well, such as tuberculosis. Opportunistic infections are not spread to those with healthy immune systems, but other types of infections can be. The incidence of certain kinds of cancer also rises when the immune system is impaired. Opportunistic infections can be viral, bacterial, mycobacterial, fungal, protozoal, or parasitic. They can affect many different areas of the body. Some opportunistic infections can now be prevented by prophylactic treatments. Common infections are discussed here.

Candida albicans

Candida albicans is a fungus normally found in the GI tract that does not infect a person with a healthy immune system. In AIDS, overgrowth of this fungus occurs as a result of the impaired immune system. Candidiasis of the mouth or esophagus is common in AIDS. Signs and symptoms of candidiasis include oral or esophageal pain, dysphagia, and yellow-white plaques that look like cottage cheese in the mouth and throat. Nutrition can be affected by oral or esophageal candidiasis. Recurrent vaginal candidiasis is more common in women with AIDS. Severe itching and a white discharge may occur.

Cytomegalovirus

Cytomegalovirus (CMV) is a viral infection that can affect many areas of the body. The eye is a common site (cytomegalovirus retinitis). Vision impairment ranges from little impairment to total blindness. Prompt diagnosis and treatment can minimize the loss of vision. A variety of symptoms are seen when other areas are involved, such as fever, fatigue, diarrhea, GI upset, and hepatitis.

Pneumocystis jiroveci Pneumonia

Pneumocystis jiroveci pneumonia (PCP, formerly *Pneumocystis carinii*) is caused by a fungus (formerly thought to be a protozoa) that produces shortness of breath, fever, nonproductive cough, and fatigue. PCP is the most common opportunistic infection in AIDS. To prevent PCP, oral trimethoprim-sulfamethoxazole (Septra) is given prophylactically. Other treatments for those who cannot tolerate Septra are available, including dapsone, atovaquone (Mepron), and pentamidine isethionate (Pentam) inhalation therapy to prevent PCP when CD4+ T-lymphocyte counts fall below 200/mm^3. PCP may be treated with oxygen, oral or intravenous trimethoprim-sulfamethoxazole, or parenteral pentamidine isethionate. Steroids may also be given to reduce lung inflammation.

Tuberculosis

Tuberculosis is a bacterial infection and may occur in up to 10% of those with AIDS. Symptoms include dyspnea, cough, chest pain, fever, night sweats, and weight loss. A purified protein derivative (PPD) skin test should be performed at least annually in patients with HIV infection. Induration of 5 mm or more is defined as a positive result in patients with HIV infection. (See Chapter 31.)

> **NURSING CARE TIP**
>
> When assessing the results of a PPD test, only the raised area (if present) is measured and recorded in millimeters. (If there is no induration, it is recorded as 0 mm.)

Other Viral Infections

Herpes simplex is a viral infection that may be found in the oral, genital, or rectal area of those with AIDS. Symptoms include blister-like lesions that rupture and leave ulcerations, fever, pain, or bleeding. Varicella zoster virus infection is usually the result of the virus being present from a prior episode of the chickenpox. The virus remains present in the nerve ganglia. With depressed immune function, the virus can cause shingles.

Neoplasms

Kaposi's sarcoma (KS) is the most common cancer associated with AIDS. Painless, small, purple-blue lesions develop on the skin. The lesions may scale, ulcerate, and bleed. They may occur anywhere on the body in patients with HIV. Antiretroviral therapy has greatly affected the incidence of KS, decreasing cases to 10% in 2009 of the number of cases seen in 1994. The incidence of non-Hodgkin's lymphoma has also decreased drastically with the use of antiretroviral therapy. Cervical neoplasia is more common in women with HIV.

AIDS Dementia Complex

HIV infection of the brain or other parts of the central nervous system results in AIDS dementia complex (ADC). Symptoms range from mild to severe and may include memory impairment, personality changes, hallucinations, leg weakness, loss of balance, and slower responses. ADC is a common complication of HIV/AIDS. When it occurs, safety is an important consideration for the patient and caregiver. The only treatment for ADC is optimal viral suppression from antiviral treatment.

DIAGNOSIS

Fingerstick blood, oral fluid, and urine and serum specimens are used for HIV testing. Rapid HIV testing provides results the same day. Home sample collection devices can be purchased; the sample is sent in for HIV testing, with the person calling for results, counseling, and referral if needed.

HIV Antibody Tests

After HIV infection, antibodies may not be formed for 3 weeks to 3 months or longer in some cases. The typical HIV antibody testing pattern is as follows:

- An enzyme-linked immunosorbent assay (ELISA) test is done to detect antibodies to HIV antigen in the patient's blood using test plates.
- If positive, the ELISA test is repeated because false positives may occur (0.1%).
- If the ELISA test is again positive, the Western blot test is done to detect the presence of antibodies to four major HIV antigens. The test is positive if two antibodies are present.
- If all test results are positive, the patient is HIV-antibody positive.
- If the test is negative, the patient is said to be in the window period or HIV negative.
- Other tests can be used, especially if initial test results are not conclusive. Testing directly for the virus is available but more costly.

Complete Blood Cell Count/Lymphocyte Count

Because patients with HIV are susceptible to leukopenia, lymphopenia, anemia, and thrombocytopenia related to HIV infection and as a complication of antiretroviral therapy, a complete blood cell count (CBC) including a lymphocyte count should be obtained. The CBC should be repeated at 3- to 4-month intervals or more often if there is a change in therapy or the patient's clinical course is unstable.

CD4+/CD8+ T-Lymphocyte Count

The count of CD4+ and CD8+ (cytotoxic cells) T lymphocytes is essential for evaluating the status of the immune system. In healthy adults, CD4+ levels average 500 to 1600 cells per mm^3. In HIV/AIDS, CD4+ cell levels drop but CD8+ cell levels do not. A low ratio of CD4+ cells to CD8+ cells is seen as HIV/AIDS progresses. It is recommended that CD4+/CD8+ T-lymphocyte counts be performed at 3-month intervals for most patients, especially those on antiretroviral therapy.

Viral Load Testing

Viral load testing measures the amount of HIV RNA in plasma and is extremely important for determining the risk of disease progression if left untreated, the risk of opportunistic infections, and the response to antiretroviral therapy. Combination antiretroviral regimens usually produce a 50% decrease in total-body HIV levels within just a few days. Viral loads should be performed 1 month after starting new treatments and at 3-month intervals thereafter. The goal on antiretroviral therapy is to obtain and maintain an ultra-sensitive undetectable viral load.

Genotyping

Genotyping measures resistance to currently available antiviral treatments. This information guides health care providers in choosing treatment regimens that will most likely be effective against that person's virus.

General Tests

Standard serological testing for syphilis is recommended annually in patients who are sexually active. Hepatitis A, B, and C serologies and liver chemistry panels are indicated in the early evaluation because of the high incidence of concurrent hepatitis co-infection for HIV-positive patients. Co-infections may influence the course of either the person's HIV or the co-infection. It may also affect the HIV treatment options.

THERAPEUTIC MEASURES

Because there is currently no cure for HIV/AIDS, the goal of therapy is to prevent or delay development of opportunistic diseases. In 2008, the federal *Guidelines for the Use of Antiretroviral Agents in HIV-1 Infected Adults and Adolescents* were updated (Panel on Antiretroviral Guidelines for Adults and Adolescents, 2008). They recommend that a patient with HIV be started on antiviral treatment when the CD4 count is less than 350 cells/mm^3 or the person has an AIDS-defining illness (Table 20.4). In addition, to increase life expectancy and treatment cost effectiveness, it may be recommended that patients be prophylactically treated for opportunistic infections, especially hepatitis A and hepatitis B viruses, herpes simplex virus, *Mycobacterium avium* complex, and *Pneumocystis jiroveci* pneumonia (Table 20.5). Other opportunistic infections are treated with appropriate medications if they occur.

Antiretroviral drugs that inhibit reproduction of the virus (but do not kill it) are used to treat HIV infection. These antiretroviral agents have been developed to act predominantly on processes specific to the viral particle to protect the integrity of the host cell. Strategies specifically aimed at interrupting the viral life cycle include the following:

- Preventing the virus from attaching to the CD4+ receptor of the T4 lymphocyte
- Interfering with "uncoating" of the virus within the cell, the first essential step in allowing the virus to integrate into the cell's DNA
- Inhibiting reverse transcriptase, a viral enzyme specific to retroviruses, which enables the virus to make a DNA copy from single-stranded viral RNA before integration into cellular DNA
- Blocking viral regulatory and transactivating proteins, which are involved in the transcription and translation of viral RNA proteins from proviral DNA as the virus goes from the quiet, integrated state to active replication
- Inhibiting protease, a viral enzyme responsible for the adherence of viral proteins both before proviral

TABLE 20.4 MEDICATIONS FOR HIV INFECTION

Medication Class/Action	Examples	Route	Side Effects	Nursing Implications
Non-Nucleoside Reverse Transcriptase Inhibitors (NNRTIs) Stop HIV from multiplying by preventing the reverse transcriptase enzyme from working.	delavirdine (Rescriptor)	PO: 400 mg tid. Take with/without food and a full glass of water. 100-mg tablet can be dissolved in 3 oz water and taken immediately. 200-mg tablet must be swallowed whole.	Rash, headache	Monitor WBC count, liver tests, especially with history of hepatitis B or C. Do not give within 1 hour of antacids or didanosine (ddI, Videx).
	efavirenz (Sustiva)	PO: 600 mg daily. Take on an empty stomach, preferably at bedtime.	Rash, vivid dreams, CNS symptoms False-positive cannabinoid test	Monitor for rash (especially during first month); may be severe and life threatening. Teach patient to report rash.
	nevirapine (Viramune)	PO: 200 mg daily for 7 days, then 200 mg bid. Take with/without food.	Rash	Monitor for rash (especially first month); may be life threatening and require stopping drug immediately. Teach patient to report rash immediately. Stevens-Johnson syndrome may occur. Monitor liver tests. For contraception, advise a nonhormonal contraceptive during therapy.
	etravirine, ETV (Intelence)	PO: Two 100-mg tablets bid following a meal. Tablets may be dispersed in water if patient has trouble swallowing.	Rash, nausea, headache, high blood pressure, ill feeling, abdominal pain, vomiting	Monitor for side effects. Teach patient to report side effects to care provider.
Nucleoside/ Nucleotide Reverse Transcriptase Inhibitors (NRTIs) Inhibit production of reverse transcriptase and viral replication.	lamivudine, (3TC) and zidovudine (AZT) (Combivir)	150 mg lamivudine and 300 mg zidovudine PO bid. Take with/without food.	Peripheral neuropathy	Monitor for peripheral neuropathy and report.
	emtricitabine, FTC (Emtriva)	PO: 200 mg daily. Take with/without food.	Minimal side effects Lactic acidosis rare	Monitor for symptoms of lactic acidosis.
	lamivudine, 3TC (Epivir)	PO: 150 mg bid or 300 mg daily. Take with/without food.	Peripheral neuropathy	Monitor for peripheral neuropathy and report.
	abacavir sulfate and lamivudine (Epzicom)	PO: abacavir 600 mg + lamivudine 300 mg (in 1 pill) daily. Take with/without food.	See abacavir, and lamivudine entries elsewhere in table.	See abacavir, and lamivudine entries elsewhere in table.
	(zidovudine) (Retrovir, AZT, ZDV)	PO: 300 mg bid. Take with/without food.	Nausea, vomiting, dizziness, decreased bone marrow function, liver and kidney toxicity	Monitor CBC for anemia. Use strategies to decrease nausea and vomiting. Monitor labs for kidney and liver function.
	abacavir + lamivudine + zidovudine (Trizivir)	PO: abacavir 600 mg + lamivudine 150 mg + zidovudine 300 mg bid Take with/without food.	See abacavir, lamivudine, and zidovudine entries elsewhere in table.	See abacavir, lamivudine, and zidovudine entries elsewhere in table.
	emtricitabine + tenofovir (Truvada)	PO: emtricitabine 200 mg + tenofovir 300 mg daily. Take with/without food.	See emtricitabine and tenofovir entries elsewhere in table.	See emtricitabine and tenofovir entries elsewhere in table.

TABLE 20.4 MEDICATIONS FOR HIV INFECTION—cont'd

Medication Class/Action	Examples	Route	Side Effects	Nursing Implications
	didanosine, ddI EC (Videx EC)	PO: 400 mg if patient is above 60 kg. Daily on an empty stomach. Must be swallowed whole. Also comes in 250 mg if patient less than 60 kg.	Peripheral neuropathy, pancreatitis, nausea, diarrhea	Monitor for peripheral neuropathy. Monitor CBC for bone marrow suppression.
	tenofovir (Viread)	PO: 300 mg daily Take with/without food.	Nausea, vomiting, diarrhea, headaches, flatulence.	Monitor for hepatomegaly with steatosis for lactic acidosis, which can be fatal, especially in women. Take 2 hours before or 1 hour after didanosine.
	stavudine, d4T (Zerit)	PO: 40 mg bid. Take with/without food.	Peripheral neuropathy, lactic acidosis (which can be fatal)	Monitor for peripheral neuropathy and report. Monitor liver function and report.
	abacavir sulfate (Ziagen)	PO: 300 mg or 300 mg bid daily. Take with/without food.	Fever, rash, nausea, vomiting, malaise or fatigue, loss of appetite, respiratory symptoms such as sore throat, cough, shortness of breath (hypersensitivity reaction, which can be fatal)	Flu-like symptoms indicate need to discontinue drug or life-threatening condition may develop. Report immediately.
Combined NRTIs + NNRTI Single tablet multiple-drug regimen.	efavirenz 600 mg + tenofovir 200 mg + 300 mg of Sustiva (Atripla)	PO: 1 tablet daily on an empty stomach, preferably at bedtime.	See efavirenz, tenofovir, and Sustiva entries elsewhere in table.	See efavirenz, tenofovir, and Sustiva entries elsewhere in table.
Protease Inhibitors (PIs) Bind to active site of HIV protease enzyme, which cuts reproduced HIV strands. Interrupt formation of mature viral particles and reduce viral replication. Rapid resistance develops if not taken as directed.	tipranavir (Aptivus)	PO: 500 mg + ritonavir 200 mg bid.	Diarrhea, nausea, vomiting, stomach pain, tiredness and headache	Monitor labs for cholesterol and triglycerides. Monitor for side effects. Educate patient to report any to care provider.
	indinavir (Crixivan)	PO: 400 mg every 8 hours on an empty stomach. One hour before or 2 hours after eating.	Nephrolithiasis, GI intolerance, headaches, asthenia, blurred vision, dizziness, rash, metallic taste, thrombocytopenia, alopecia, hemolytic anemia, hyperglycemia, lipodystrophy, elevated lipids.	Teach about importance of hydration (at least 48 oz of liquids in 24 hours). Manage GI symptoms. Monitor labs.
	lopinavir/ritonavir (Kaletra)	PO: 3 caps bid with food.	GI intolerance, asthenia, hyperglycemia, lipodystrophy, elevated lipids, elevated transaminases	Refrigerate caps. Manage GI symptoms. Monitor labs. Watch for increased bleeding in patients with hemophilia.
	fosamprenavir (Lexiva)	PO: 700 mg bid or 1400 mg with or without 100 or 200 mg Ritonavir daily. Take with/without food. Dose adjusted if used with Sustiva.	Skin rash, GI intolerance, headache, hyperglycemia, lipodystrophy, elevated lipids, elevated transaminases	Manage GI symptoms. Report rash. Watch for increased bleeding in patients with hemophilia. Should not be given if patient is allergic to sulfa.

Continued

TABLE 20.4 MEDICATIONS FOR HIV INFECTION—cont'd

Medication Class/Action	Examples	Route	Side Effects	Nursing Implications
	ritonavir (Norvir)	PO: 100 mg (6 caps) bid. Take with food. Dose is titrated up slowly. Mainly used in small doses to boost other PIs.	GI intolerance, paresthesias, hepatitis, pancreatitis, asthenia, taste perversion, elevated lipids, hyperglycemia, lipodystrophy	Manage GI symptoms. Monitor labs. Monitor side effects. Watch for bleeding episodes in patients with hemophilia.
	darunavir, DRV, or PRZ (Prezista)	PO: 800 mg + ritonavir 100 mg daily or 600 mg + ritonavir 100 mg bid. Dosing varies depending if treatment naive or experienced. Take with food.	Diarrhea, nausea, headache, common cold. Rash can be serious.	Monitor for side effects and potential drug interactions. Teach patient to report side effects to health care provider.
	atazanavir (Reyataz)	PO: 400 mg daily or 300 mg + ritonavir 100 mg daily. Take with food.	Indirect hyperbilirubinemia, hyperglycemia, lipodystrophy, headache, rash, stomach pain, vomiting, diarrhea, tingling in hands or feet or depression	Watch for jaundice and report. Monitor labs. Watch for bleeding episodes in patients with hemophilia.
	nelfinavir (Viracept)	PO: 1250 mg bid or 750 mg tid. Take with food.	Diarrhea, asthenia, hyperglycemia, lipodystrophy, elevated lipids, elevated transaminase	Manage diarrhea. Monitor labs. Watch for increased bleeding in hemophilia patients.
Fusion Inhibitors Blocks HIV-1 fusion with the CD4+ cell membrane to prevent cell entry.	enfuvirtide (Fuzeon), T20	Subcutaneously: 90 mg (1 mL) bid. Mix with 1.1 mL sterile water for injections. Rotate sites: upper arm, abdomen, upper thigh.	Local injection site reactions, hypersensitivity reaction (rash, fever, nausea, vomiting, chills, rigor, hypotension), diarrhea, nausea, fatigue, bacterial pneumonia	Teach subcutaneous injection technique and importance of injection site rotation. Use aseptic technique for administering injections. Teach if dizzy, do not drive.
Blocks the receptor called a CCR5 molecule. When this occurs HIV cannot infect that cell.	maraviroc (Selzentry)	PO: 150 mg bid or 300 mg bid or 600 mg bid. Take with/without food. There are multiple dosing schedules.	Cough, fever, upper respiratory infection, rash, sore muscles, abdominal pain, and dizziness. (May experience rash, jaundice, dark urine, vomiting, or abdominal pain from liver problems.)	Monitor for signs and symptoms of liver problems. Teach patient side effects and importance of reporting.
Integrase Inhibitor Blocks HIV from combining with its genetic code. When integration is blocked, HIV cannot make more copies of itself.	raltegravir, RAL (Isentress)	PO: 400 mg bid. Take with/without food.	Diarrhea, nausea, and headache	Encourage patient to report side effects and all other medications taken to health care provider.

CBC = complete blood count; CNS = central nervous system; GI = gastrointestinal.

TABLE 20.5 TREATMENT FOR AIDS-RELATED CONDITIONS

Opportunistic Infection/Complication	Treatment
Candidiasis	Nystatin, ketoconazole (Nizoral), fluconazole (Diflucan), amphotericin B (Fungizone)
Cytomegalovirus retinitis	Ganciclovir (Cytovene)
Hepatitis B virus	Hepatitis B virus vaccine when HIV infection diagnosed, unless already infected with hepatitis B
Hepatitis C virus	Interferon, lamivudine, tenofovir for infection; pegylated interferon and ribavirin
Herpes simplex, herpes zoster, varicella zoster	Acyclovir (Zovirax) therapy, valacyclovir, famciclovir, foscarnet
Influenza	Annual influenza vaccine
Mycobacterium avium complex	Azithromycin, clarithromycin, ethambutol
Pneumococcal pneumonia	Pneumococcal vaccine when HIV infection diagnosed
Pneumocystis jiroveci pneumonia	Trimethoprim-sulfamethoxazole (Bactrim, Septra), dapsone, atovaquone, pentamidine isethionate
Tuberculosis	PPD testing; drug therapy per CDC guidelines: pyrazinamide, isoniazid (Laniazid, Isotamine), ethambutol (Myambutol)
HIV wasting	*Patient education:* Eat frequent small meals of high-calorie and high-protein meals with snacks daily. Eat low-residue diet for diarrhea control. Control odors if they cause nausea. Develop easy meal plan: favorite foods, meal programs, frozen dinners, cold food to control nausea. Use antiemetics, appetite stimulants, and/or testosterone. Rest, listen to music. Numb painful oral sores with ice, popsicles, or topical analgesic; avoid spicy foods. Use artificial saliva for dry mouth. Use nutritional supplements. Use food stamps, community food pantries, or free meal programs as needed. Exercise to increase muscle mass. Take medications prescribed to treat HIV wasting.

integration and as the viral particles recombine into functional proteins needed for viral maturation
- Preventing viral assembly and budding out of the cell.

For more information, visit the Medscape quick reference guide to antiretrovirals at www.medscape.com.

Antiretroviral Therapy

Aggressive treatment with multiple-drug therapy, aimed at reducing the viral load to an undetectable amount, is the most effective line of treatment for HIV (see Table 20.4). "Cocktails" of multiple antiretroviral drugs (comprising antiretroviral therapy) have reduced viral loads in the bloodstream and increased CD4+ T lymphocyte counts, resulting in prolonged survival. Multiple-drug therapy, in use since 1996, has made monotherapy (using one drug) an outdated concept except for some cases involving pregnant women. Many combination drug regimens can be used. There are now five "classes" of HIV treatment available. Each class affects the virus in a different stage of its life cycle. Antiretroviral therapy usually combines at least three medications in at least two classes of treatment categories (see Table 20.4).

The major cause of drug resistance occurs when medications are not taken as directed. *Adherence* is the word used to describe taking medications exactly as directed. Another increasing potential cause of drug resistance is when an infected person with resistant virus exposes another infected person to the resistant virus through unprotected sexual exposure or drug use.

> **NURSING CARE TIP**
>
> **Medication Adherence Teaching**
>
> Teach patients that it is essential to take all medications as ordered. Missing just 10% of medication doses (1 out of 10) decreases effectiveness to about 80%, depending on the drug. This means that if a patient is taking three to seven pills each day, missing one to two pills a week will decrease the medications' effectiveness by 20%.

Many anti-HIV drugs have side effects. If they occur, the drug regimen may be changed or interventions may be used to help control the side effects. The patient should be taught to always report side effects immediately, especially rashes (such as with trimethoprim-sulfamethoxazole) and abdominal pain (such as with zidovudine [AZT, Retrovir]); they could be serious or even life threatening.

When someone with a very suppressed immune system (very low CD4/T-cell count) is started on antiretroviral therapy, the person may experience "immune reconstitution syndrome." The patient's immune system may be greatly improving, but the patient is feeling worse. This is because, when the patient's immune system was severely damaged, immune responses may have been too weak or absent to show the signs of infection. When immune function improves and the immune system begins to fight off infections that were already present in the body, such as *Pneumocystis jiroveci* pneumonia, symptoms can arise. This can be a very serious, sometimes fatal condition that may occur a few weeks after antiretroviral therapy starts. Educating the patient to immediately report any symptoms of opportunistic infections after starting therapy can allow for prompt diagnosis and treatment of the infection—and may save the person's life.

NURSING MANAGEMENT

Nursing Process for the Adult Patient with HIV/AIDS

Data Collection

Ongoing monitoring is important for the patient with HIV/AIDS to detect problems early. Health history information is obtained (Box 20.4). Determining the patient's understanding of HIV/AIDS information is necessary for planning and teaching. A physical examination provides data on the effects of HIV/AIDS and antiretroviral treatments. Monitoring the patient's level of pain is ongoing; however, many patients with HIV do not have pain related to their HIV. You should also check for signs and symptoms of opportunistic infections.

LEARNING TIP

Key points to remember:

- HIV and AIDS are disease labels, not people labels.
- Each person reacts to an HIV or AIDS diagnosis differently.
- It is not HIV that ultimately causes death; it is compromised immunity and the invasion of an opportunistic infection or disease that the patient's body is unable to successfully fight off, even with medical intervention.
- With today's current successful antiretroviral treatments, HIV has changed from being a life-ending infection to a chronic disease requiring constant management.

Nursing Diagnoses

Nursing care is individualized to the patient's presenting symptoms. Nursing diagnoses for HIV/AIDS may include:

- *Ineffective Protection* related to decreased immune function

Box 20.4

Data Collection: Health History Information for HIV/AIDS

- Demographic data: gender, age, marital status, occupation, residence
- Date of diagnosis of HIV/AIDS
- Past medical history and surgeries
- Current health status and concerns
- Allergies
- Medication history of antivirals used with reason for discontinuing
- Current medications, dose, and frequency (including over-the-counter medications and supplements)
- Immunizations
- Family history
- Height/weight: weight loss
- Infections/cancers (see Box 20.1, *CDC Conditions in the AIDS Surveillance Case Definition*)
- Sexually transmitted diseases and treatments
- Social history, sexual practices, risk behaviors, safe sex practices
- Needle and blood exposure, injection drug use, blood transfusions/treatment for hemophilia
- Tobacco use
- Drug and alcohol use
- Exercise and sleep
- Pets
- Occupational history
- Nutrition history
- Female: gynecological history, last Pap

- *Impaired Gas Exchange* related to respiratory infection
- *Acute* or *Chronic Pain* related to neuropathy, cancer, infection, or dyspnea
- *Fatigue* related to HIV infection and/or side effects of treatments
- *Risk for Injury* related to weakness, fatigue, sedation, neurologic impairment
- *Imbalanced Nutrition: Less Than Body Requirements* related to anorexia, nausea and vomiting, increased caloric need, diarrhea, dysphagia, oral lesions
- *Impaired Oral Mucous Membrane* related to decreased immune function
- *Diarrhea* related to infection, medications
- *Impaired Skin Integrity* related to infection, cancer, immobility, incontinence
- *Social Isolation* related to fear of disclosure of status, infection control, transmission of virus
- *Risk for Situational Low Self-Esteem* related to body image changes
- *Deficient Knowledge* related to lack of prior experience with HIV/AIDS and treatment
- *Anticipatory Grieving* related to loss of function or death

- *Disabled Family Coping* related to chronic, potentially progressive disease
- *Ineffective Coping* related to chronic progressive disease
- *Ineffective Sexuality Pattern* related to fear of disease transmission.

See the *Nursing Care Plan for the Patient with AIDS.*

Planning and Implementation

HIV/AIDS can affect every system of the body and every aspect of a person's life. Nurses have the opportunity to positively influence the patient's experience with HIV/AIDS by providing a nonjudgmental approach, empathy, and psychological support.

INEFFECTIVE PROTECTION. To reduce infection risk, the patient should be taught to wash hands frequently, especially before eating and after toileting; bathe regularly; avoid sharing personal grooming items (e.g., toothbrush, toothpaste, razor); wash toothbrush; and wash all dishes between uses (Table 20.6). In addition, the patient is taught signs of infection to report to the health care provider immediately (Box 20.5, *Patient Education*). Treatment of opportunistic infections is most effective when begun early.

IMPAIRED GAS EXCHANGE. If a patient develops a condition that interferes with respiration, the goal is to maintain oxygenation within normal limits and reduce dyspnea. PCP is a potential respiratory infection with AIDS (see Table 20.5). Monitoring the patient's vital signs, including respiratory rate, depth, rhythm, and oxygen saturation, is important. Medications and oxygen therapy are given as ordered. Positioning the patient for comfort is often done by raising the head of the bed. Assisting with activities helps reduce fatigue.

PAIN. Pain may occur from a variety of causes. Treatment is focused on the cause to achieve pain control and relief. Medications may be given as ordered. Timing medication administration before planned activities is helpful in increasing ability to function. Complementary therapy may be used by patients (see Chapter 5). Measures such as heat or cold, massage, and frequent position changes may be helpful.

FATIGUE. Some patients with HIV experience fatigue. Other causes of fatigue include infections, medications, anemia, dehydration, depression, and poor nutrition. The patient can help manage fatigue by alternating periods of activity and rest. Tasks that use more energy should be planned at times when the patient is most energetic. Helping a patient prioritize activities is important in planning the best use of the energy available.

IMBALANCED NUTRITION: LESS THAN BODY REQUIREMENTS. Maintaining general health and nutrition is important for a healthy immune system. For patients with HIV, maintaining nutrition is vital (Box 20.6, *Nutrition Notes*). Patients with AIDS may have difficulty maintaining adequate nutrition and preventing weight loss. Many factors interfere with nutrition in HIV/AIDS (e.g., anorexia, oral lesions, nausea and vomiting, diarrhea, or wasting syndrome). The cause needs to be identified for appropriate intervention planning.

The patient's baseline weight is obtained. Then ongoing monitoring of the patient's weight, calorie intake, and intake and output is done. A dietitian is consulted to help plan nutritious and affordable meals. The patient should be on a high-calorie, high-protein diet. Small, frequent meals may be helpful. Vitamins and/or nutritional supplements may be needed to maintain adequate nutrition. Antiemetics are used to control nausea and vomiting, if present. Medications that help stimulate appetite may be helpful. Easy-to-prepare meals are helpful when energy is limited. Creative interventions and resources may be needed to ensure the patient receives adequate nutrition (see Table 20.5). Along with adequate nutrition, exercise helps maintain muscle mass, promotes relaxation, aids sleep, and gives the person a sense of control and well-being. An effective exercise program includes exercises that increase strength, flexibility, and endurance. For many, becoming physically fit is a lifestyle change that requires dedication.

IMPAIRED ORAL MUCOUS MEMBRANE. Oral or esophageal candidiasis is more common in the late stage of AIDS. The painful lesions interfere with swallowing and nutrition. In patients with AIDS who smoke, there is an increased incidence of oral thrush (candidiasis). Therefore, patients should be encouraged to quit smoking. Antifungal medication is given. Mouth care is very important. A soft toothbrush promotes comfort. Viscous lidocaine can be given to decrease pain during eating.

DIARRHEA. Diarrhea may occur in the patient with HIV. Diarrhea can be caused by HIV infection, opportunistic infections, or antiretroviral treatments. An antimotility agent may be prescribed. Consulting the dietitian may be helpful in making dietary changes that reduce diarrhea (e.g., low-residue diet, no dairy products, no spicy foods, no caffeine or alcohol). Sitz baths may be soothing. Thorough cleansing of the anal area after each stool is a must. Ointments may be applied to protect and soothe the anal area from excoriation.

IMPAIRED SKIN INTEGRITY. Many skin conditions can occur with HIV infection. Medications can cause skin infections that can be life threatening and must be reported immediately. A dermatologist may need to be consulted to help diagnose and treat skin infections.

SOCIAL ISOLATION. Unfortunately, many patients with HIV/AIDS continue to face discrimination, rejection, and isolation. The Americans with Disabilities Act (ADA) makes discrimination toward patients with HIV illegal. Even relatives, friends, and others sometimes avoid or refuse to have anything to do with the person with HIV (Box 20.7, *Ethical Considerations*).

NURSING CARE PLAN for the Patient with AIDS

Nursing Diagnosis: *Ineffective Protection* related to immune disorder, inadequate nutrition, intravenous therapy, and possible invasive procedures

Expected Outcomes: The patient will remain free of nosocomial infections. Patient will describe measures to maintain skin integrity and avoid infections.

Evaluation of Outcomes: Is patient free of nosocomial infections? Can patient explain and demonstrate skin maintenance techniques?

Interventions	Rationale	Evaluation
Identify patient's risk factors, such as skin condition, laboratory results, portals of entry for infections, and presence of any infections.	Status of these assessment factors determines plan for care.	Does patient have intact skin or nonreddened, nonpurulent sites of interrupted integrity?
Caregivers should use standard precautions and strict aseptic technique for all patients and procedures.	Transmission of microorganisms can occur in both directions. Many patients with HIV are not aware of their HIV status.	Do all caregivers use standard precautions?
Instruct visitors about techniques to avoid transmission of infection, such as hand washing and not visiting when they have an infection. (Use extreme caution not to divulge the patient's HIV/AIDS status to visitors/family that may not be aware of it.) The nurse with an infection, especially respiratory infection, should not care for the patient with AIDS. (If must care for patient, wear a mask and explain why you are wearing it.)	The immune system is damaged by HIV. Ability to combat infections may be severely compromised. A minor infection for most people may kill a person who has AIDS.	Do those with infections avoid contact with patient until their infection is resolved? Do laboratory tests indicate that patient is so immunocompromised that reverse isolation may be necessary?
Promote skin integrity by frequent turning, optimum mobilization, use of protective mattress and chair pads, application of emollient to dry areas, and prompt treatment of any injuries.	Skin is the body's first line of defense.	Does patient's skin remain intact and infection free?
Teach strategies for skin care and avoidance of infection to patient.	Self-care offers a measure of control in a frequently uncontrollable situation.	Does patient satisfactorily explain or demonstrate good skin care and knowledge of how to avoid infection?

Nursing Diagnosis: *Risk for Injury* related to impaired mobility, weakness, fatigue, possible electrolyte imbalances, neurologic impairment, and sedative effects of pain medications

Expected Outcomes: The patient's care and mobility needs will be met without injury.

Evaluation of Outcomes: Does patient remain free from injury?

Interventions	Rationale	Evaluation
Identify patient's abilities and disabilities.	Particular disabilities may increase danger to patient.	Does patient have deficits?

NURSING CARE PLAN for the Patient with AIDS—cont'd

Look for potential hazards in environment (hospital or home) and eliminate as many hazards as possible.	Awareness of hazards is necessary to decrease occurrence of accidents and injuries.	Are there any hazards in the environment currently?
Instruct patient about how to avoid hazards (if cognitively and physically able to comply).	Patients can help avoid injury if they understand hazards.	Is patient effectively avoiding hazards, or is patient a danger to self?
Encourage self-care as much as is feasible without tiring patient.	Self-care promotes feelings of self-efficacy and can combat depression.	Does patient evidence satisfaction with self-care efforts?
Assist with care activities as needed.	Varying levels of assistance with care are necessary due to the potentially debilitating nature of disease.	Are patient's care and mobility needs being met satisfactorily without injury?
Institute safety measures as required, such as close observation, frequent reorientation, two staff members for ambulation, use of side rails, bed motion alarm, or room near nurse's station.	Protection of patient against inadvertent removal of tubes or equipment, falls, and other injuries may require extraordinary measures due to neurologic damage.	Are safety measures effective for patient? Does patient respond negatively to the protective measures? Can these be modified to be less offensive?

Nursing Diagnosis: *Ineffective Coping* related to potentially terminal disease and progressive debility

Expected Outcomes: The patient will show use of effective coping skills.

Evaluation of Outcome: Does patient show use of effective coping skills?

Interventions	Rationale	Evaluation
Establish and maintain open and trusting therapeutic relationship.	Effective communication is based on trust—*assurance of confidentiality is essential.*	Does patient talk about concerns with nurse?
Allow grieving to take place (keeping a journal has been effective for some patients who have AIDS).	AIDS brings about losses of health, strength, employment, and in many cases friends and threatens one's sense of security and reasonableness of life. Healthy grieving is a natural coping response.	Is grief being expressed? Is patient finishing things that matter to him or her?
Encourage patient to express feelings and concerns. Contact counselor, chaplain, or AIDS support worker if patient so desires.	Talking about feelings and concerns helps defuse anger, clarify needs, and relieve tension.	How are family members, friends, and support persons interacting with patient? How is patient responding to family members, friends, and support persons?
Provide patient with desired information or refer to others who can supply information.	Knowledge dispels unreasonable fears and helps patient prepare adequately to cope with stressors.	Does patient evidence enough understanding of disease to be able to cope effectively?
Ask if patient would like information about support group and arrange such.	Social support can help patient cope.	Does patient show satisfaction with coping resources?

Source: Linda Hopper Cook.

TABLE 20.6 PATIENT TEACHING: PREVENTING OPPORTUNISTIC INFECTIONS

Precaution Category	Reducing Exposure Risk	To Protect from
Environmental/ occupational	Consider risk for exposure to infectious agents from the following: health care setting, correctional facilities, homeless shelters.	Tuberculosis
	Child care settings: wash hands after diaper changing/body fluid contact.	CMV, cryptosporidiosis, hepatitis A, giardiasis
	Animal contact: exposure possible from veterinary work, pet stores, farms.	Cryptosporidiosis, toxoplasmosis, salmonellosis, campylobacteriosis
	Gardening/soil contact: avoid gardening/houseplant care/ bird-roosting site, soil, cleaning chicken coops. Wear gloves and mask and wash hands after soil contact.	Cryptosporidiosis, toxoplasmosis, histoplasmosis, coccidioidomycosis
Food/water	*General measures for home or restaurants include the following:* Food handlers should practice good hand washing and hygiene. Discard food past expiration date and dented or swollen cans. Maintain adequate refrigeration and cooking temperatures. Control insects and rodents to prevent food contamination. *Foods to avoid:* Raw/undercooked eggs and foods with raw eggs, such as hollandaise sauce, caesar dressing, mayonnaise, uncooked batters, ice cream, eggnog. Raw/undercooked poultry, meat, seafood. Unpasteurized milk/dairy products and fruit juice, raw seed sprouts. Soft cheeses, which may harbor bacteria: feta, Brie, Camembert, blue veined, queso fresco. Wash produce and avoid unwashed produce on salad bars. Avoid cross-contamination of foods with uncooked meat on food preparation surfaces. Cook meat until internal temperature is 180°F (82.2°C) for poultry, 165°F (73.8°C) for red meats, with no trace of pink.	Foodborne and waterborne infections caused by bacterial, viral, protozoal, or parasitic pathogens
	Foods to avoid or cook until steaming hot: leftovers, ready-to-eat, delicatessen foods, refrigerated pâtés, and meat spreads.	Cryptosporidiosis, giardiasis
	Water safety: Avoid public drinking fountains. Avoid drinking or swallowing water directly from lakes or rivers. Use safe water supply or boil water 1 minute when unsure. Avoid beverages made from tap water in public places in areas where water sources are known not to be safe. Drink bottled water purified from reverse osmosis, filtration through absolute 1-μm filter, or distillation (only safe methods) in areas where water sources are known not to be safe. For information, contact www.bottledwater.org. Bottled or canned carbonated soft drinks, commercially packaged nonrefrigerated beverages, pasteurized beverages, and beers are safe.	Hepatitis A, campylobacteriosis, *E. coli,* giardiasis, leptospirosis, norovirus, rotavirus, shigellosis
Sexual	Always use latex condom for every sex act.	STDs, herpes simplex virus, cytomegalovirus, human papillomavirus, resistant HIV strain
	Avoid oral-anal contact or use dental dams; use latex gloves for hand-anal contact; wash hands and genitals with warm soapy water after contact.	Intestinal infections: amebiasis, hepatitis A, cryptosporidiosis, shigellosis, campylobacteriosis, giardiasis
	Get hepatitis A vaccine.	Hepatitis A
	Get hepatitis B vaccine	Hepatitis B
Injection drug use	Get hepatitis A and B vaccines. Stop using injection drugs and enter substance abuse treatment. If unable to stop, never reuse or share syringes, needles, water, or drug preparation equipment. If shared, use bleach and water to clean equipment. Use sterile syringes from pharmacies or community syringe exchange programs and dispose of safely. Use clean water and equipment and new alcohol swab.	Hepatitis A, hepatitis B, hepatitis C, resistant HIV strain

TABLE 20.6 PATIENT TEACHING: PREVENTING OPPORTUNISTIC INFECTIONS—cont'd

Precaution Category	Reducing Exposure Risk	To Protect from
Pet-related	Avoid pet feces/diarrhea; seek veterinary treatment for pet's illness.	*Cryptosporidium, Salmonella, Campylobacter* spp. infection
	Counsel on pet contact risks but recognize emotional benefits of pets. Pets should have up-to-date immunizations.	.
	For new pet, avoid those younger than 6 months old (and cats younger than 1 year old); obtain pets from known sanitary source; avoid strays; wash hands after handling pets	
	Avoid exotic pets.	
	Cat ownership increases risk from litter box cleaning, scratches, bites, licking, fleas. If must clean litter box, wear mask and gloves and wash hands well afterward. Efforts should be made to keep cats indoors to avoid contact with infected prey.	Toxoplasmosis, *Bartonella* spp. infection, salmonellosis, campylobacteriosis
	Unhealthy birds may transmit infectious organisms.	*Cryptococcus neoformans, Mycobacterium avium, Histoplasma capsulatum* infection
	Avoid reptiles, turtles, chicks, and ducklings.	Salmonellosis
	Wear gloves for cleaning aquariums.	*Mycobacterium marinum* infection
Travel	Consult health care providers on travel to developing countries.	Opportunistic pathogens, foodborne and waterborne infections
	Traveler's diarrhea prophylaxis is not recommended. Carry supply of antimicrobial agent to take for diarrhea.	
	Consider prophylaxis for other types of exposures.	
	Avoid raw fruits, vegetables, raw/undercooked seafood or meat, tap water, ice from tap water, unpasteurized milk/dairy products, items from street vendors.	
	Safe items include steaming-hot foods, self-peeled fruits, bottled (especially carbonated) beverages, hot coffee/tea, beer, wine, and water boiled 1 minute.	
	Avoid soil/sand contact by wearing shoes, using beach towels.	

CMV = cytomegalovirus; STD = sexually transmitted disease.
Source: Data from U.S. Department of Health and Human Services (2001). *USPHS/IDSA guidelines for the prevention of opportunistic infections in persons infected with human immunodeficiency virus.* Washington, DC: Author. Retrieved February 10, 2010, from http://www.aidsinfo.nih.gov/Guidelines/GuidelineDetail.aspx?GuidelineID=13.

Misunderstanding and fear lead to misuse of infection control procedures and increase a patient's isolation. Being knowledgeable about the transmission of HIV allows interaction with the patient to reduce feelings of isolation. Providing patient education to reduce fear of HIV transmission also decreases isolation. Taking care to maintain confidentiality is essential. It is important to be aware that many patients with HIV do not share their diagnosis with family or friends who may visit when they are hospitalized.

RISK FOR SITUATIONAL LOW SELF-ESTEEM. Changes in self-esteem and self-concept occur from several of the effects of HIV infection. Patients often experience changes in their relationships with others and in day-to-day activities such as work. Major weight loss and changes in fat distribution from antiretroviral treatments, a condition called lipodystrophy, may cause dramatic changes in appearance that alter body image and reduce self-esteem. Nurses can assist patients in maintaining self-esteem and self-concept by ensuring a climate of acceptance and promoting a trusting relationship. Patients should be encouraged to express feelings, if ready, and to identify positive aspects of self. Receiving emotional and spiritual support can help improve the patient's self-esteem.

Stress impacts health. Having others to talk with and provide support is essential to stress management. Identifying and maintaining social networks is important. Patients should be taught a variety of relaxation strategies and techniques to reduce stress. Relaxation strategies can range from working on a favorite hobby to talking with friends. Relaxation techniques include progressive muscle relaxation and imagery to aid in relaxation. Stress management techniques are most effective when used every day, not just during times of stress.

DEFICIENT KNOWLEDGE. Extensive teaching is needed for patients to understand this chronic, potentially life-threatening disease that alters everything in their lives. (See also the *Prevention* section earlier in the chapter.) Teaching needs to be evaluated for understanding and done as the patient is ready. Adherence to treatment and medication regimens is essential to prevent resistance to treatment, and reduce the risk of disease progression.

CRITICAL THINKING

Zoe Sampson

■ Zoe, 22, is diagnosed as HIV positive. She is tearful and asks many questions.

1. How would you answer her questions?
   a. "Am I going to die?"
   b. "How is AIDS diagnosed?"
   c. "Can my boyfriend get it?"
2. What food and water safety methods would you teach her?
3. Years later, Zoe loses weight and becomes malnourished. What interventions can you use to promote adequate nutrition?

Suggested answers at end of chapter.

Box 20.5

Patient Education

Signs and Symptoms of Opportunistic Infections to Report

Teach patient to monitor temperature and to report the following symptoms to a health care provider immediately:

- New fever higher than 100°F (38.5°C) or a change in fever pattern if low-grade fevers are common
- Cough, shortness of breath, fever, or chest tightness, which may be signs of early pneumonia
- Signs of central nervous system infection, such as severe headache; stiff neck; visual changes; problems with balance, walking, or speech; weakness of an arm or leg; or changes in moods or memory
- Foul-smelling drainage or pus
- Cloudy or foul-smelling urine
- Signs of dehydration, such as a dry mouth, dark concentrated urine, or dizziness when standing
- Diarrhea lasting longer than 48 hours; more than six stools a day; watery, mucousy, or bloody stools
- Rashes (possible side effect of medication)
- Sore mouth or tongue, difficulty swallowing, white patches on tongue or back of mouth
- Worsening fatigue
- Change in vision and if floaters develop
- Unintended weight loss

MEDICATIONS. Nurses must stress during patient teaching that medication doses must not be missed. Using teaching aids to assist patients in remembering to take their medications is very important. Encourage the patient to take medications exactly as instructed. If a dose is missed, it should be taken as soon as possible unless it is very close to

Box 20.6

Nutrition Notes

Nourishing the Patient with HIV or AIDS

Nutrition has preventive and therapeutic functions for patients with HIV infections. Well-nourished people infected with the HIV virus are better able to resist opportunistic infections and tolerate the side effects of treatment. One study found that the use of a multivitamin supplement delayed the onset of advanced disease and the need for antiretroviral therapy in HIV-positive people (Fawzi et al., 2004).

For patients with AIDS, malnutrition is a major mediator and predictor of death. Diarrhea and malabsorption are probably the major nutrition-related problems for patients with AIDS. Carbohydrate malabsorption and steatorrhea are often associated with diarrhea, which also can occur as a side effect of antiretroviral medications. Dietary treatment involves identification of the cause of the diarrhea and a determination of which nutrients the patient cannot absorb.

Every effort should be made to feed the patient orally. The anorexia commonly seen in patients with AIDS might be resolved by changing the meal plan:

- Offer small, frequent feedings.
- Serve food cold or at room temperature.
- Alter seasonings.
- Add powdered milk to mashed potatoes or puddings to increase calories.
- Modify texture to accommodate chewing difficulty or oral lesions.

Box 20.7

Ethical Considerations

Caring for a Patient with AIDS

Ed Klees, 27, has AIDS and a lung infection. He wants to see his parents, whom he has not seen in 10 years. He does not want his parents to know about his disease because he feels that their rigid religious beliefs may push them toward disowning him. To prepare for their visit, Edward asks his nurse to answer his parents' questions about his illness by telling them he has leukemia or another rare disease that they would know nothing about. After visiting their ill son, Edward's parents approach the nurse and ask in a stern tone, "Does our son have AIDS?"

- How should the nurse respond?
- To whom does the nurse owe the greatest obligation, the patient or his family?
- What principles are in conflict?
- What virtues play a role in this situation?

Using the ethical decision-making model (see Chapter 3), determine several possible solutions for this situation.

the time of the next dose. Doses should not be doubled. Missing doses of medication could cause therapy failure because viral loads can increase and resistance can develop to current treatments. Strongly encourage the patient to consult the primary care provider with any questions or side effects promptly. Many of these medications can cause severe reactions.

FOOD AND WATER SAFETY. Food and water safety is vital to an immunocompromised patient. Bacterial, viral, protozoal, or parasitic pathogens can cause foodborne and waterborne infections. The patient must be taught methods to prevent foodborne and waterborne infections for all phases of handling (see Table 20.6). Kitchen counters and food preparation appliances (e.g., cutting boards, can openers) should be disinfected. Freezing does not kill bacteria in foods. Foods should not be thawed at room temperature. Dating and using the oldest foods first is helpful. If symptoms of foodborne or waterborne infection develop (e.g., diarrhea, nausea, vomiting, abdominal cramps, headache, fever), teach patient to report them immediately. In certain areas of the country, tap water is not safe to drink. Patients may need to be taught to boil water for drinking and making ice cubes or to drink bottled water.

RESOURCES. Financial resources may need to be addressed so that food and medications can be obtained. Treatment can be expensive, and the patient may be unable to work. However, with the new combination antiretroviral therapies, many people are now able to continue working longer. The Ryan White Comprehensive AIDS Resources Emergency (CARE) Act provides funding for some services and treatment-related needs. Knowledge of local resources and referrals to financial resources and support groups is very important.

COMMUNITY AND HOME HEALTH CARE. During the course of HIV infection, the patient will be mainly at home and in the community. Luckily, hospitalization is less frequently needed in the treated patient but may be needed intermittently for acute illness. If the disease progresses, the patient may need more care from caregivers and home health nurses. The home health nurse provides physical care, establishes a therapeutic relationship with AIDS patients and their significant others and family/friends, and coordinates care with other health care team members (see *Home Health Hints*).

Caregivers should be assessed for caregiver role strain. Support services should be identified, such as community AIDS organizations, Meals on Wheels, respite care services, community mental health, and Internet support groups. Respite care provides the caregiver time away from the caregiver role to reduce stress. When a patient is terminal, comfort care and emotional support for the family are essential. Hospice care may be used at this time.

Home Health Hints

- When providing patient care, wash hands frequently, follow standard precautions, and use plastic bags to contain soiled items or clothing.
- Teach patients with AIDS and their families how to properly clean and disinfect the home to prevent infections. The least expensive recommended disinfectant is a diluted bleach mixture that contains 1 part household bleach to 10 parts water. However, this solution must be mixed daily to be effective. Many spray-type disinfectants are available and may be easier for patients/families to use.
- Wearing gloves, clean body fluid spills with soap and water.
- Flush body fluids, solid waste, and contaminated solutions down toilet.
- Use disinfectant to (1) disinfect spill areas, (2) clean toilet seats and bathroom fixtures, and (3) clean inside the refrigerator to avoid mold growth.
- Rinse clothing and then wash separately from other clothes with 1 cup of bleach if soiled with blood, urine, feces, or semen.
- Patients with HIV/AIDS do not require separate sets of dishes or silverware. Dishes and silverware are washed in hot, soapy water and rinsed thoroughly or placed in dishwasher.
- Dispose of sharps (e.g., needles, razors) in a rigid labeled container (such as a tin can with a sealable lid). Add 1:10 bleach solution to disinfect. Tape the lid. Place in a bag and dispose of in the trash.
- Contaminated articles are disposed of by bagging in plastic and placing in the trash.
- Teach the family of a patient with AIDS which signs and symptoms to report to the physician or nurse immediately: fever; increased dyspnea; pain; change in sputum production; upper respiratory tract infection; pneumonia; respiratory distress syndrome; diarrhea five times a day or more for 5 days; uncontrolled weight loss greater than 10 pounds in the last month; persistent headaches; falling; seizures; mental status changes, including memory loss and personality changes; rashes and skin changes; difficulty swallowing; and problems with urination.

Evaluation

Patient goals are met if the patient remains free from infection and maintains the desired quality of life and activities as long as possible. If the disease progresses, goals are met if the patient's needs are met and the patient's dignity is maintained.

SUGGESTED ANSWERS TO

CRITICAL THINKING

■ *Zoe Sampson*

1. a. There currently is no cure for HIV/AIDS; however, medications are available that slow the disease's progression and make HIV a manageable chronic illness. Research continues to find improved treatments and search for a cure.
   b. AIDS is diagnosed when CD4+ T-lymphocyte counts are below 200 cells per microliter, or the CD4+ T-lymphocyte percentage is under 14 of total lymphocytes, and/or an opportunistic clinical disease, as defined by the CDC, is present in an HIV-infected person.
   c. Yes, your boyfriend could become infected through exposure to your blood or vaginal secretions. You need to learn about preventive measures and discuss them with him. If you have had unprotected sex, he should be tested.
2. Food handlers must maintain good hand washing and hygiene practices. Discard food past the expiration date and dented or swollen cans. Ensure adequate refrigeration and cooking. Control insects and rodents to prevent food contamination. Drink purified bottled water if you live in areas with unsafe drinking water. Use a safe water supply or boil water 1 minute when unsure. Avoid unpasteurized milk, other dairy products, and fruit juice and raw seed sprouts. Avoid raw and undercooked eggs, meats, and seafood.
3. Eat three high-calorie, high-protein meals and snacks daily. Eat a low-residue diet for diarrhea control. Develop an easy meal plan. Use antiemetics, if needed. Numb painful oral sores. Avoid spicy foods. Refer for food stamps/free meal programs if necessary. Engage in regular exercise.

REVIEW QUESTIONS

1. The nurse would evaluate the patient as understanding modes of HIV transmission if the patient stated that the modes of HIV transmission include which of the following?
   a. Saliva, tears, fecal-oral contamination
   b. Close physical contact involving skin surfaces, mosquito bites
   c. Sharing towels, sharing eating utensils, skin contact
   d. Unprotected sex with HIV-infected partner, contact with infected blood products

2. The nurse is teaching a patient about HIV testing. Place HIV diagnostic tests in the sequential order in which they are performed.
   a. Western blot test
   b. Enzyme-linked immunosorbent assay (ELISA) test
   c. Repeated ELISA test

3. A patient who is newly diagnosed with HIV infection asks what to expect for future health status. The best response for the nurse to give is based on the understanding that HIV disease and AIDS are characterized as which of the following?
   a. An acute disease
   b. A life-ending disease
   c. A chronically managed disease
   d. A disease with remissions and exacerbations

4. What should the nurse include in a teaching plan to prevent HIV infection? **Select all that apply.**
   a. Recapping of used needles by caregiver permitted.
   b. Abstain from sexual intercourse.
   c. Avoid injection drug use.
   d. Avoid use of male or female condoms.
   e. Plan for autologous blood transfusion.
   f. Test for HIV at time of labor.

5. Which of the following should the patient with HIV be taught to do to decrease risk of infections? **Select all that apply.**
   a. Wash hands before eating.
   b. Wash toothbrush.
   c. Reuse dishes.
   d. Buy prepared deli foods.
   e. Report signs of infection.
   f. May share razor with no visible blood.

REVIEW QUESTIONS—cont'd

6. The nurse would recognize that the patient needs further reinforcement of knowledge if the patient stated that one of the goals of antiretroviral therapy is which of the following?
   a. Reduce the viral load.
   b. Improve survival rates.
   c. Decrease CD4+ T lymphocytes.
   d. Delay the progression of HIV disease.
7. The nurse would recognize that the patient is having a reaction to delavirdine (Rescriptor) if which of the following occurred?
   a. Rash
   b. Edema
   c. Abdominal pain
   d. Blurred vision

References

Branson, B. M., Handsfield, H. H., Lampe, M. A., et al. (2006). Revised recommendations for HIV testing of adults, adolescents, and pregnant women in health care settings. *MMWR, 55*(RR), 1–17.

Fawzi, W. W., Msamanga, G. I., Spiegelman, D., et al. (2004). A randomized trial of multivitamin supplements and HIV disease progression and mortality. *New England Journal of Medicine, 351,* 23–32.

Panel on Antiretroviral Guidelines for Adults and Adolescents. (2008, November 3). *Guidelines for the use of antiretroviral agents in HIV-1-infected adults and adolescents.* Washington, DC: U.S. Department of Health and Human Services. Retrieved October 15, 2009, from http://aidsinfo.nih.gov/contentfiles/adultandAdolescentGL.pdf

Panlilio, A. L., Cardo, D. M., Grohskopf, L. A., et al. (2005). Updated U.S. Public Health Service guidelines for the management of occupational exposures of HIV and recommendations for postexposure prophylaxis. *MMWR, 54*(RR09), 1–17.

unit FIVE

UNDERSTANDING THE CARDIOVASCULAR SYSTEM

21 Cardiovascular System Function, Assessment, and Therapeutic Measures

LINDA S. WILLIAMS AND
JANICE L. BRADFORD

KEY TERMS

atherosclerosis (ATH-er-oh-skleh-ROH-siss)
bruit (brew-EE)
claudication (KLAW-dih-KAY-shun)
clubbing (KLUH-bing)
dysrhythmias (dis-RITH-mee-yahs)
Homans' sign (HOH-manz SYNE)
hypomagnesemia (HYE-poh-MAG-neh-SEE-mee-ah)
ischemic (iss-KEY-mick)
murmur (MUR-mur)
pericardial friction rub (PEAR-ih-KAR-dee-uhl FRIK-shun RUB)
poikilothermy (POY-kih-loh-THER-mee)
point of maximum impulse (POYNT OF MAKS-ih-muhm IM-puls)
preload (PREE-lohd)
pulse deficit (PULS DEF-ih-sit)
sternotomy (stir-NAW-tuh-mee)
thrill (THRILL)

QUESTIONS TO GUIDE YOUR READING

1. What is the normal anatomy of the cardiovascular system?
2. What is the normal function of the cardiovascular system?
3. What data should you collect when caring for a patient with a disorder of the cardiovascular system?
4. What diagnostic tests are commonly performed to diagnose disorders of the cardiovascular system?
5. What nursing care should you provide for patients undergoing each of the diagnostic tests?
6. What common therapeutic measures are used for patients with disorders of the cardiovascular system?
7. What preoperative and postoperative routines and procedures are used for cardiac surgery?

NORMAL CARDIOVASCULAR SYSTEM ANATOMY AND PHYSIOLOGY

The cardiovascular system consists of the heart, blood, and blood vessels (including arteries, capillaries, and veins). Its function is to pump and distribute the blood throughout the body.

Heart

Cardiac Location and Pericardial Membranes

The heart is located in the mediastinum, the area between the lungs in the thoracic cavity. It is enclosed by three membranes. The outermost is the fibrous pericardium, which forms a loose-fitting pericardial sac around the heart. The second, or middle, layer is the parietal pericardium, a serous membrane that lines the fibrous layer. The third and innermost layer, the visceral pericardium or epicardium, is a serous membrane on the surface of the heart muscle. Between the parietal and visceral layers is serous fluid, which prevents friction as the heart beats.

Cardiac Structure and Vessels

The walls of the four chambers of the heart are made of cardiac muscle (myocardium) and are lined with endocardium, which is smooth epithelial tissue that prevents abnormal clotting. The endocardium also covers the valves of the heart and continues into blood vessels as the lining. The coronary vessels include the arteries and capillaries that circulate oxygenated blood throughout the myocardium and the veins that return deoxygenated blood to the right atrium via the coronary sinus. The two main coronary arteries are the first branches of the ascending aorta, just outside the left ventricle (Fig. 21.1).

The upper chambers of the heart are the thin-walled right atrium and left atrium, which are separated by the interatrial septum. The lower chambers are the thicker walled right and left ventricles, which are separated by the interventricular septum. Each septum is made of myocardium that forms a common wall between the two chambers.

The right atrium receives deoxygenated blood from the upper body by way of the superior vena cava and from the lower body by way of the inferior vena cava (see Fig. 21.1). This blood flows from the right atrium through the tricuspid valve into the right ventricle. Backflow during ventricular systole (contraction and emptying) is prevented by the tricuspid, or right, atrioventricular (AV) valve (Fig. 21.2). The right ventricle pumps blood through the pulmonary semilunar valve to the lungs by way of the pulmonary artery. The pulmonary semilunar valve prevents backflow of blood into the right ventricle during ventricular diastole (relaxation and filling).

The left atrium receives oxygenated blood from the lungs by way of the four pulmonary veins. This blood flows through the mitral, or left, AV valve (also called the bicuspid valve) into the left ventricle. The mitral valve prevents backflow of blood into the left atrium during ventricular systole. The left ventricle pumps blood through the aortic semilunar valve to the body by way of the aorta. The aortic valve prevents backflow of blood into the left ventricle during ventricular diastole.

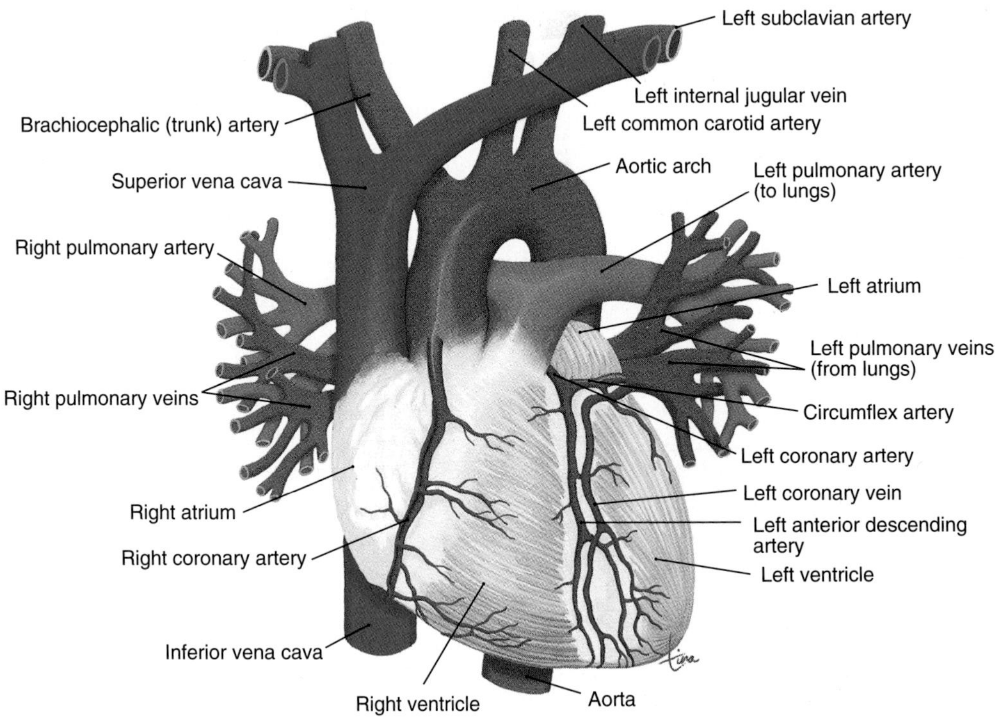
Left subclavian artery
Left internal jugular vein
Left common carotid artery
Brachiocephalic (trunk) artery
Aortic arch
Superior vena cava
Left pulmonary artery
(to lungs)
Right pulmonary artery
Left atrium
Left pulmonary veins
(from lungs)
Right pulmonary veins
Circumflex artery
Left coronary artery
Left coronary vein
Right atrium
Left anterior descending
artery
Right coronary artery
Left ventricle
Inferior vena cava
Right ventricle
Aorta

FIGURE 21.1 Anterior view of the heart and major blood vessels. (From Scanlon, V., & Sanders, T. [2007]. *Essentials of anatomy and physiology* [5th ed., p. 276]. Philadelphia: F. A. Davis, with permission.)

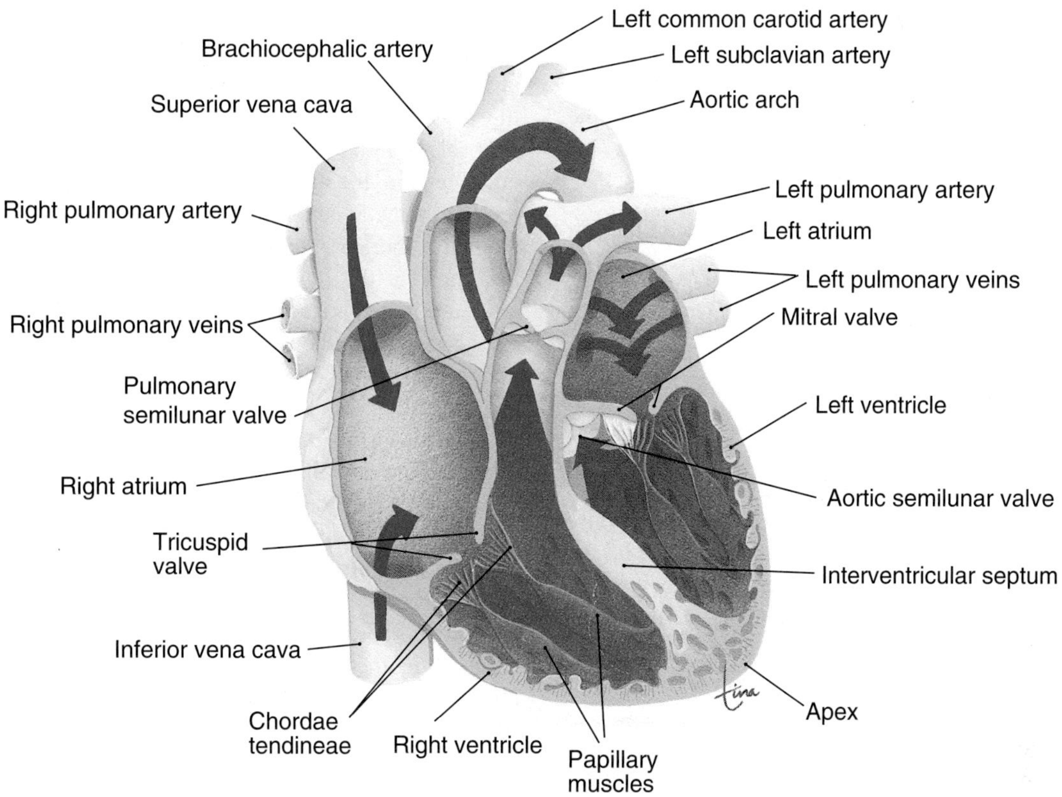
Left common carotid artery
Brachiocephalic artery
Left subclavian artery
Superior vena cava
Aortic arch
Left pulmonary artery
Right pulmonary artery
Left atrium
Left pulmonary veins
Right pulmonary veins
Mitral valve
Pulmonary semilunar valve
Left ventricle
Right atrium
Aortic semilunar valve
Tricuspid valve
Interventricular septum
Inferior vena cava
Apex
Chordae tendineae
Right ventricle
Papillary muscles

FIGURE 21.2 Frontal section of the heart showing internal structures and cardiac blood flow. (From Scanlon, V., & Sanders, T. [2007]. *Essentials of anatomy and physiology* [5th ed., p. 276]. Philadelphia: F. A. Davis, with permission.)

The tricuspid and mitral valves consist of three and two cusps, respectively. These cusps, or flaps, are connective tissue covered by endocardium and are anchored to the floor of the ventricle by the chordae tendineae and papillary muscles. The papillary muscles are columns of myocardium that contract along with the rest of the ventricular myocardium. This contraction pulls on the chordae tendineae and prevents hyperextension of the AV valves during ventricular systole (see Fig. 21.2).

Although each ventricle pumps the same amount of blood, the much thicker walls of the left ventricle pump with approximately five times the force of the right ventricle to distribute the blood throughout the body. This difference in force is reflected in the great difference between systemic and pulmonary blood pressure.

Cardiac Conduction Pathway and Cardiac Cycle

The cardiac conduction pathway is the pathway of electrical impulses that generates a heartbeat. The sinoatrial (SA) node in the wall of the right atrium is a specialized mass of cardiac muscle that depolarizes rhythmically and most rapidly, about 100 times per minute, and therefore initiates each heartbeat. (While at rest, parasympathetic fibers dominate and slow the SA node to about 75 bpm.) For this reason, the SA node is sometimes called the pacemaker, and a normal heartbeat is called a normal sinus rhythm. From the SA node, impulses travel to the AV node located in the lower interatrial septum, to the atrioventricular bundle (bundle of His) in the upper interventricular septum, to the right and left bundle branches in the septum, and to the Purkinje fibers in the rest of the ventricular myocardium. If the SA node becomes nonfunctional, the AV node can initiate each heartbeat, but at a slower rate of 40 to 60 beats per minute. The bundle of His is capable of generating the beat of the ventricles, but at the much slower rate of 20 to 35 beats per minute.

A cardiac cycle is the sequence of mechanical events that occurs during one heartbeat. Simply stated, the two atria contract simultaneously, followed by the simultaneous contraction of the two ventricles (a fraction of a second later). The contraction, or systole, of each set of chambers is followed by relaxation, or diastole, of the same set of chambers.

The atria in diastole continually receive blood from the veins. As pressure in the atria increases, the AV valves are forced open, causing most of the blood to flow passively into the ventricles. Atrial systole pumps the remaining blood into the ventricles, and then the atria relax. Ventricular systole follows. The pressure in the ventricles causes the AV valves to close and forces the semilunar valves to open. Blood is then pumped into the aorta and pulmonary artery. There is no passive blood flow. Any blood leaving the ventricles must be pumped. Toward the very end of ventricular systole, as the pressure drops, the blood tends to flow backward within the two exiting arteries. It is this backflow of blood that closes the semilunar valves. The ventricles and atria are then all in diastole; the atria continue to fill until pressure opens the AV valves again, and the cycle is repeated.

The events of the cardiac cycle create the normal heart sounds. The first of the two major sounds (the "lubb" of "lubb-dupp") is caused by the closure of the AV valves during ventricular systole. The second sound is created by the closure of the aortic and pulmonary semilunar valves.

Cardiac Output

Cardiac output is the amount of blood ejected from the left ventricle in 1 minute (the right ventricle pumps a similar amount). It is determined by multiplying stroke volume by heart rate. Stroke volume is the amount of blood ejected by a ventricle in one contraction and averages 60 to 80 mL/beat. With an average resting heart rate of 75 beats per minute, average resting cardiac output is 5 to 6 L (approximately the total blood volume of an individual that is pumped within 1 minute). During exercise, venous return increases and stretches the ventricular myocardium, which in response contracts more forcefully. This is known as Starling's law of the heart, and the result is an increase in stroke volume. More blood is pumped with each beat, and at the same time, the heart rate increases, causing cardiac output to increase by as much as four times the resting level, and even more for athletes.

The ejection fraction is a measure of ventricular efficiency and is usually about 60%. It is the stroke volume divided by total blood in the ventricle (also known as the end-diastolic volume, which is approximately 120 to 130 mL). Lower values indicate that the ventricle is not pumping as forcefully as normal and that more blood remains in the ventricle at the end of systole. The normal end-systolic volume is about 50 to 60 mL.

Regulation of Heart Rate

The heart generates its own electrical impulse, which begins at the SA node. The nervous system, however, can change the heart rate in response to environmental circumstances (Fig. 21.3). In the brain, the medulla contains the cardiovascular centers: the accelerator center and the inhibitory center. Sympathetic nerve impulses—along sympathetic nerves from the thoracic spinal cord to the SA node, AV node, and most of the myocardium—increase rate and force of contraction by releasing norepinephrine. Parasympathetic impulses—along the vagus nerve to the SA node, AV node, and atrial myocardium—decrease heart rate by releasing acetylcholine.

The information for changes necessary in the heart rate comes to the medulla from proprioceptors and from baroreceptors and chemoreceptors located in the internal carotid arteries and the aortic arch. The baroreceptors, specialized cells in the carotid and aortic sinuses, detect changes in blood pressure. The chemoreceptors are located in the carotid and aortic bodies and are cells specialized to detect changes in the oxygen content of the blood (as well as changes in carbon dioxide and hydrogen ion content). In response to either a drop in blood pressure or a decrease in blood oxygen level, the heart receives sympathetic impulses and beats faster in an attempt to provide sufficient oxygenation for tissues.

Hormones and the Heart

The hormone epinephrine, secreted by the adrenal medulla in stressful situations, is sympathomimetic in that it increases the heart rate and force of contraction and it dilates the

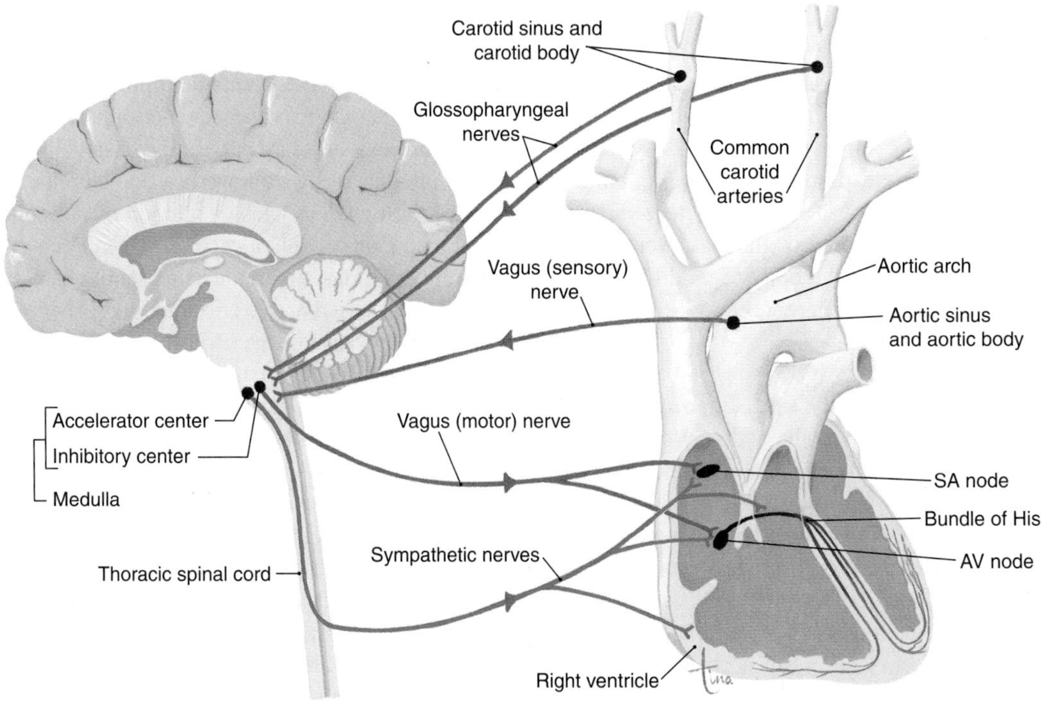

Carotid sinus and carotid body
Glossopharyngeal nerves
Common carotid arteries
Vagus (sensory) nerve
Aortic arch
Aortic sinus and aortic body
Accelerator center
Inhibitory center
Medulla
Vagus (motor) nerve
SA node
Bundle of His
AV node
Sympathetic nerves
Thoracic spinal cord
Right ventricle

FIGURE 21.3 Nervous system regulation of the heart. (From Scanlon, V., & Sanders, T. [2007]. *Essentials of anatomy and physiology* [5th ed., p. 285]. Philadelphia: F. A. Davis, with permission.)

coronary vessels. This in turn increases cardiac output and systolic blood pressure.

Aldosterone, a hormone produced by the adrenal cortex, is important for cardiac function because it helps regulate blood levels of sodium and potassium, both of which are needed for the electrical activity of the myocardium. The blood level of potassium is especially critical because even a small deficiency or excess impairs the rhythmic contractions of the heart.

The atria of the heart secrete a hormone of their own called atrial natriuretic peptide (ANP) or atrial natriuretic hormone (ANH). As its name suggests, ANP increases the excretion of sodium by the kidneys, by inhibiting secretion of aldosterone by the adrenal cortex. Atrial natriuretic peptide is secreted when a higher blood pressure or greater blood volume stretches the walls of the atria. The loss of sodium is accompanied by the loss of more water in urine, which decreases blood volume and therefore blood pressure as well.

Blood Vessels

Arteries and Veins

Arteries and arterioles carry blood from the heart to capillaries. Their walls are relatively thick and consist of three layers. Arteries carry blood under high pressure, and the outer layer of fibrous connective tissue prevents rupture of the artery. The middle layer of smooth muscle and elastic connective tissue contributes to the maintenance of normal blood pressure (BP), especially diastolic BP, by changing the diameter of the artery. The diameter of arteries is regulated primarily by the sympathetic division of the autonomic nervous system. By use of the smooth muscle, the arteries can also alter where the greatest volume of blood is directed. The inner layer or lining of the artery is simple squamous epithelium, called endothelium, which is very smooth to prevent abnormal clotting.

Veins and venules carry blood from capillaries to the heart. Their walls are relatively thin because they have less smooth muscle than arteries. (Veins do not have as important a role in the maintenance of BP as arteries.) Sympathetic impulses can bring about extensive constriction of veins, however, and this becomes important in situations such as severe hemorrhage. The lining of veins is, like arteries, endothelium that prevents abnormal clotting; at intervals it is folded into valves to prevent backflow of blood. Valves are most numerous in the veins of the extremities, especially the legs, where blood must return to the heart against the force of gravity.

Capillaries

Capillaries carry blood from arterioles to venules and form extensive networks in most tissues. The exceptions are cartilage, covering/lining epithelia, and the lens and cornea of the eye. Capillary walls, a continuation of the lining of arteries and veins, are one cell thick to permit the exchanges of gases, nutrients, and waste products between the blood and tissues (Fig. 21.4). Blood flow through a capillary network is regulated by a precapillary sphincter, a smooth muscle fiber ring that contracts or relaxes in response to tissue needs. In an active tissue such as exercising skeletal muscle, for example, the rapid oxygen uptake and carbon dioxide production cause dilation of the precapillary sphincters to increase blood flow. At the same time, precapillary sphincters in less active tissues constrict to reduce blood flow. This is important because the body does not have enough blood to fill all of the capillaries at once; the fixed volume must constantly be shunted or redirected to where it is needed most.

The blood pressure in capillaries is 30 to 35 mm Hg at the arterial end of the network, and it drops to about 15 mm Hg at the venous end. This pressure is low enough to prevent rupture of the capillaries but high enough to permit filtration. Tissue fluid is formed from the plasma in capillaries by the process of filtration. Because capillary blood pressure is higher than the pressure of the surrounding tissue fluid, plasma and dissolved materials such as nutrients are forced through the capillary walls to become tissue fluid. Some of this tissue fluid returns to the capillaries, and some is collected in lymph capillaries. Now called lymph, it too is returned to the blood by the system of lymph vessels. Should blood pressure within the capillaries increase, more tissue fluid than usual is formed, which is too much for the lymph vessels to collect. This may result in swelling, which is called edema.

Blood Pressure

Blood pressure is the force of the blood against the walls of the blood vessels and is measured in millimeters of mercury (mm Hg), systolic over diastolic. The normal range of systemic arterial pressure is less than 120/80 mm Hg. Blood pressure decreases in the arterioles and capillaries, and the systolic and diastolic pressures merge into one pressure. As blood enters the veins, BP decreases further and approaches zero as it flows into the right ventricle. As mentioned previously, the blood pressure in the capillaries is of great importance, and normal blood pressure is high enough to permit filtration for nourishment of tissues but low enough to prevent rupture.

The arterioles (and veins during increased sympathetic stimulation) are usually in a state of slight constriction that helps to maintain normal blood pressure, especially diastolic pressure. This is called peripheral resistance; it is regulated by the vasomotor center in the medulla, which generates impulses along sympathetic vasoconstrictor nerves to these vessels' smooth muscle. When the nerves carry more impulses per second to the smooth muscle, vasoconstriction increases and blood pressure rises; fewer impulses per second bring about vasodilation and lower blood pressure. The information for changes needed in the vessel diameter comes to the medulla from the baroreceptors and chemoreceptors located in the internal carotid arteries and aortic arch and also from proprioceptors.

Blood pressure is also affected by many other factors. If heart rate and force increase, blood pressure increases within limits. If the heart is beating very fast, the ventricles are not filled before they contract, cardiac output decreases,

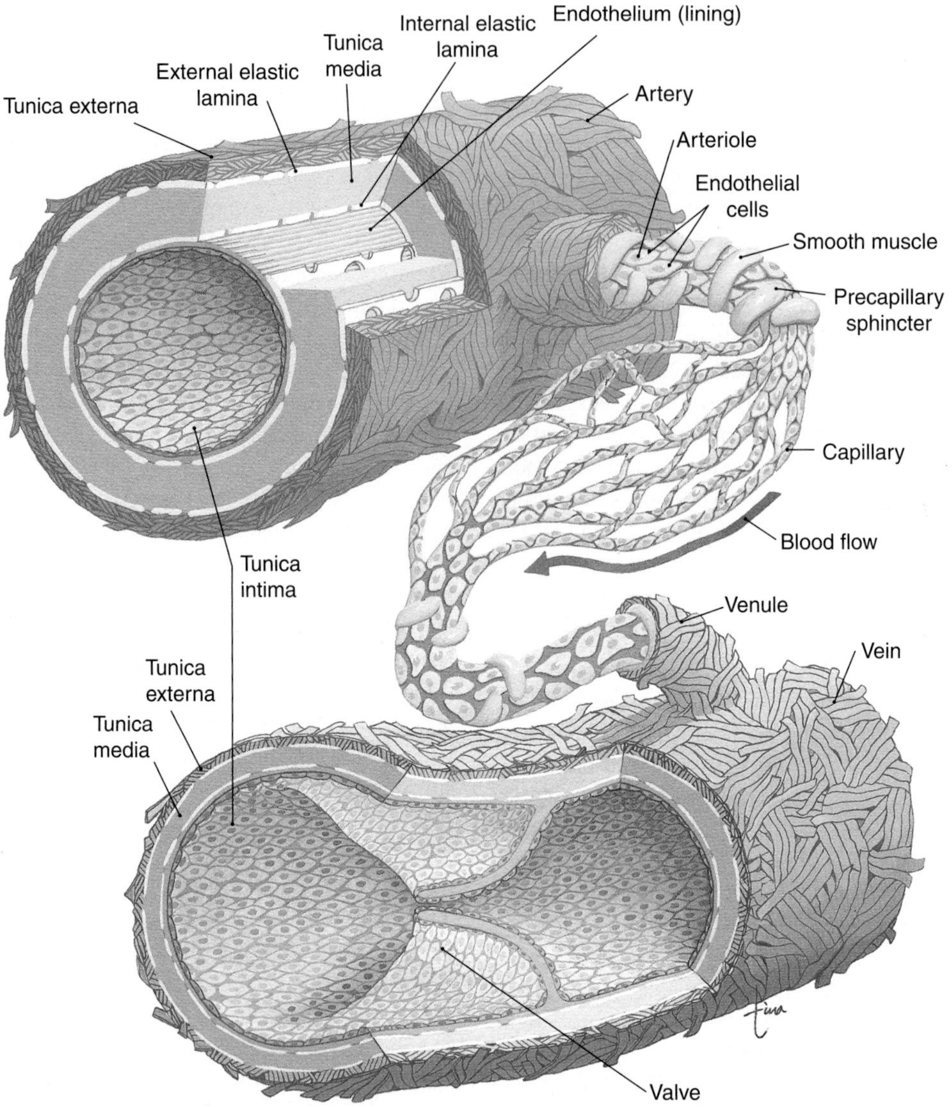
Endothelium (lining)
Internal elastic lamina
Tunica media
External elastic lamina
Tunica externa
Artery
Arteriole
Endothelial cells
Smooth muscle
Precapillary sphincter
Capillary
Blood flow
Tunica intima
Venule
Vein
Tunica externa
Tunica media
Valve

FIGURE 21.4 Structure of an artery, arteriole, capillary network, venule and vein. (From Scanlon, V., & Sanders, T. [2007]. *Essentials of anatomy and physiology* [5th ed., p. 293]. Philadelphia: F. A. Davis, with permission.)

and blood pressure drops. The strength of the heart's contractions depends on adequate venous return, which is the amount of blood that flows into the atria. Decreased venous return results in weaker contractions.

Venous return depends on several factors: constriction of the veins to reduce pooling, the skeletal muscle pumping to squeeze the deep veins of the legs, and the diaphragm's downward pressure during inhalation to compress the abdominal veins as the thoracic veins are decompressed. The valves in the veins prevent backflow of blood and thus contribute to the return of blood to the heart.

The elasticity of the large arteries also contributes to normal blood pressure. When the left ventricle contracts, the blood stretches the elastic walls of the large arteries, which absorb some of the force. When the left ventricle relaxes, the arterial walls recoil or snap back and put pressure on the blood. Normal elasticity, therefore, lowers systolic pressure, raises diastolic pressure, and maintains normal pulse pressure. Pulse pressure is the difference between the systolic and diastolic pressures. The usual ratio of systolic to diastolic to pulse pressure is 3:2:1.

Renin-Angiotensin-Aldosterone Mechanism

The kidneys are of great importance in the regulation of blood pressure. If blood flow through the kidneys decreases, renal filtration decreases and urinary output decreases to preserve blood volume. Decreased blood pressure stimulates the kidneys to secrete renin, which initiates the renin-angiotensin-aldosterone mechanism (Fig. 21.5). Renin splits the plasma protein angiotensinogen (from the liver) to form angiotensin I, which is changed to angiotensin II by a converting enzyme found primarily in lung tissue. Angiotensin II causes arteriole vasoconstriction and stimulates secretion of aldosterone, both of which raise blood pressure.

Aldosterone, secreted by the adrenal cortex, increases the reabsorption of sodium ions by the kidneys. Water follows the sodium back to the blood; this increases blood volume and blood pressure.

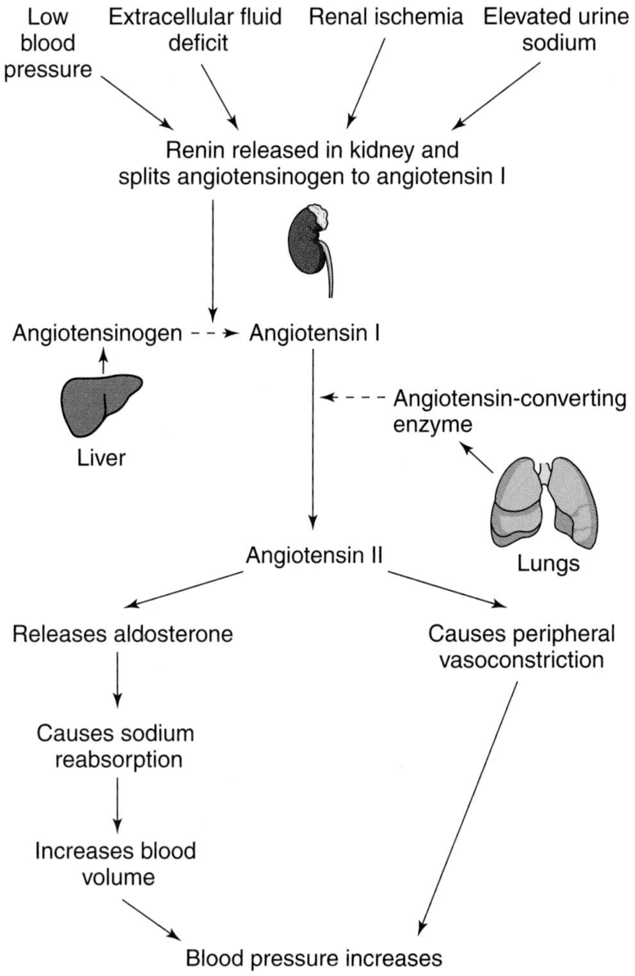
Low blood pressure
Extracellular fluid deficit
Renal ischemia
Elevated urine sodium
Renin released in kidney and splits angiotensinogen to angiotensin I
Angiotensinogen
Angiotensin I
Liver
Angiotensin-converting enzyme
Lungs
Angiotensin II
Releases aldosterone
Causes peripheral vasoconstriction
Causes sodium reabsorption
Increases blood volume
Blood pressure increases

FIGURE 21.5 The renin-angiotensin-aldosterone mechanism.

Other hormones that affect BP include those of the adrenal medulla, norepinephrine and epinephrine, which increase cardiac output and cause vasoconstriction in skin and viscera. Antidiuretic hormone (ADH), released from the posterior pituitary, directly increases water reabsorption by the kidneys, thus increasing blood volume and blood pressure. Atrial natriuretic peptide, secreted by the atria of the heart, inhibits aldosterone secretion and thereby increases renal excretion of sodium ions and water, which decreases blood volume and subsequently blood pressure.

Pathways of Circulation

The two pathways of circulation are pulmonary and systemic (see Fig. 21.2). Pulmonary circulation begins at the right ventricle, which pumps deoxygenated blood into the pulmonary artery. The pulmonary artery branches into two arteries, one to each lung. The pulmonary capillaries around the alveoli of the lungs are the site of gas exchange. Oxygenated blood returns to the left atrium by way of the pulmonary veins. The blood pressure in the pulmonary circulation is always low because the right ventricle pumps with only about one-fifth the force of the left ventricle. The pulmonary arterial pressure is approximately 20 to 25 over 8 to 10 mm Hg, and the pulmonary capillary pressure is lower still. This is important to prevent filtration in pulmonary capillaries, which keeps tissue fluid from accumulating in the alveoli of the lungs, causing pulmonary edema.

Systemic circulation begins in the left ventricle, which pumps oxygenated blood into the aorta, the many branches of which eventually give rise to capillaries within the tissues. Deoxygenated blood returns to the right atrium by way of the superior and inferior vena cava and the coronary sinus. The hepatic portal circulation is a special part of the systemic circulation in which blood from the capillaries of the digestive organs and spleen flows through the portal vein and into the capillaries (sinusoids) in the liver before returning to the heart. This pathway permits the liver to regulate the blood levels of nutrients such as glucose, amino acids, and iron and to remove potential toxins such as alcohol or medications from circulation.

Aging and the Cardiovascular System

The "aging" of blood vessels, especially arteries, is believed to begin in childhood, although the effects are not apparent until later in life (Fig. 21.6). **Atherosclerosis** is the deposition of lipids in the walls of arteries over a period of years. The deposited lipids can narrow the arteries' lumens and form rough surfaces that may stimulate intravascular clot formation. Atherosclerosis decreases blood flow to the affected organ: Cerebral flow can diminish by 20% and renal flow by 50% by age 80 (Tortora & Derrickson, 2005). With age, the heart muscle becomes less efficient, and maximum cardiac output and heart rate both decrease, although resting levels may be more than sufficient (Box 21.1, *Gerontological Issues*). Valves may become thickened by fibrosis, leading to heart murmur.

CARDIOVASCULAR DISEASE

In 2006, according to statistics of the American Heart Association (AHA), 80,000,000 people (one in three) had cardiovascular disease (CVD). It is the number one killer of people in the United States (AHA, 2009). In 2005, coronary heart disease was the single leading cause of death in America (AHA, 2009).

In women, the greatest cause of death is cardiovascular disease. The effect of cardiovascular disease and treatment for CVD in women have been understudied, but more attention is now being focused on these topics. A movement called Go Red for Women gives women encouragement and tools to prevent cardiovascular disease and live healthy. For more information on Go Red for Women, visit www.goredforwomen.org.

Lifestyle plays a major role in risk factors for cardiovascular disease. Smoking contributes to approximately one in five cardiovascular disease deaths. Eating two servings

• **WORD • BUILDING •**
atherosclerosis: athere—porridge + sklerosis—hardness

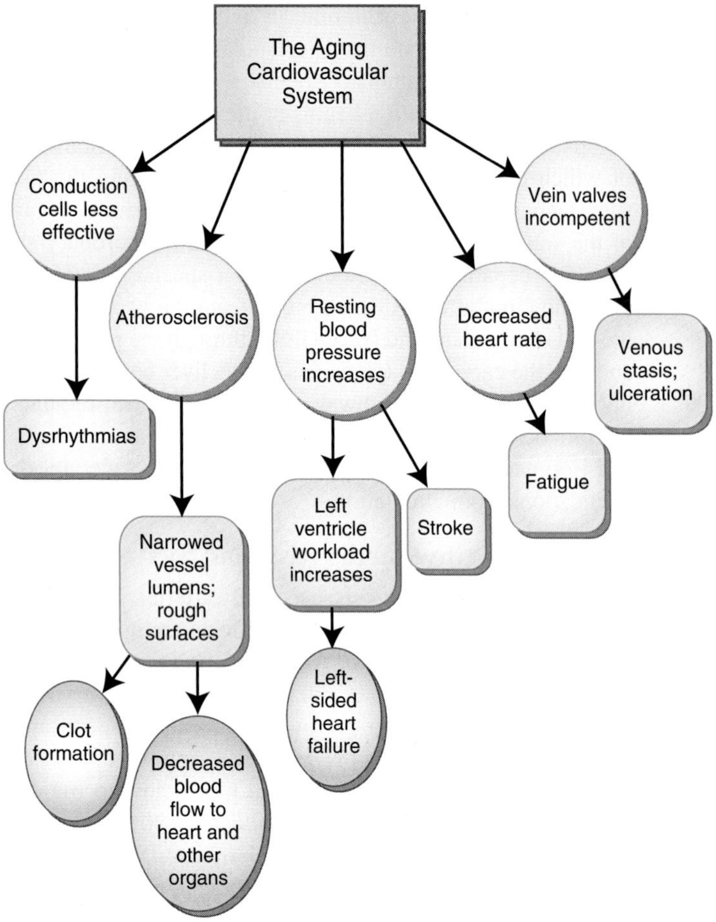
The Aging Cardiovascular System
Conduction cells less effective
Atherosclerosis
Resting blood pressure increases
Decreased heart rate
Vein valves incompetent
Venous stasis; ulceration
Dysrhythmias
Fatigue
Left ventricle workload increases
Stroke
Narrowed vessel lumens; rough surfaces
Left-sided heart failure
Clot formation
Decreased blood flow to heart and other organs

FIGURE 21.6 Aging and the cardiovascular system. This concept map shows the effects the aging process has on the cardiovascular system

weekly of oily fish such as tuna or salmon is recommended by the American Heart Association. Exercise promotion for all is essential, including children, because Americans continue to be sedentary and eat excess calories. For more information on cardiovascular disease statistics, visit www.americanheart.org.

NURSING ASSESSMENT OF THE CARDIOVASCULAR SYSTEM

Nursing assessment of the cardiovascular system includes a patient health history and physical examination (Box 21.2, *Gerontological Issues*). If the patient is experiencing an acute problem, focus on the most serious signs and symptoms and physical assessment data until the patient is stabilized (Table 21.1). An in-depth nursing assessment can be completed when the patient is stable.

Health History

To understand a patient's cardiovascular problems, ask about past and current symptoms, use of prescribed and over-the-counter medications, use of recreational drugs, surgeries, treatments, and such risk factors as diet, activity, tobacco use, and recent stressors. Assessment of symptoms includes asking questions in the WHAT'S UP? format: where it is, how it feels, aggravating and alleviating factors, timing, severity, useful data for associated symptoms, and perception by the patient of the problem.

The health history helps determine the cause of the symptom. For example, shortness of breath can be the result

Box 21.1

Gerontological Issues

The older adult is at increased risk for developing orthostatic hypotension, which could precipitate a fall. This is often due to a combination of age-related changes, immobility, chronic illnesses, and medications.

Box 21.2

Gerontological Issues

Older adults commonly have signs and symptoms that are not typical of a disorder, such as fatigue and nausea. The only symptom of myocardial infarction in an older patient may be dyspnea. Chest pain, a typical symptom, may not be present.

TABLE 21.1 ACUTE CARDIOVASCULAR DATA COLLECTION

History	Significance
Allergies	For medication administration, diagnostic dyes
Smoking history	Risk factor for cardiovascular disorders
Medications	Toxic levels; Influencing symptoms
Pain: location, radiation, description	Possible angina, myocardial infarction, thrombus, embolism
Dyspnea	Left-sided heart failure; pulmonary edema or embolism
Fatigue	Decreased cardiac output
Palpitations	Dysrhythmias
Dizziness	Dysrhythmias
Weight gain	Right-sided heart failure
Physical Examination	**Possible Abnormal Findings**
Vital signs	Bradycardia, tachycardia, hypotension, hypertension, tachypnea, apnea, shock
Heart rhythm	Dysrhythmias
Edema	Right-sided heart failure
Jugular venous distention	Right-sided heart failure
Breath sounds	Crackles, wheezes with left-sided heart failure
Cough, sputum	Acute heart failure—dry cough, pink frothy sputum

of heart failure or chronic obstructive pulmonary disease. With cardiovascular problems, the assessment focuses on the areas listed in Table 21.2.

Medical History

Previous medical records can provide objective patient data that can be supplemented with patient responses. Childhood illnesses that can lead to heart disease, such as rheumatic fever or scarlet fever, are noted. Other conditions noted include pulmonary disease, hypertension, kidney disease, cerebral vascular accident or brain attack, transient **ischemic** (restricted blood flow) attack, renal disease, anemia, streptococcal sore throat, congenital heart disease, thrombophlebitis, and alcoholism. Patient allergies, previous hospitalizations, and surgeries are documented. Baseline diagnostic tests are helpful for comparison with current tests. Functional limitations that are related to cardiovascular problems, such as difficulty performing activities of daily living (ADLs), walking, climbing stairs, or completing household tasks, are also assessed.

• WORD • BUILDING •

ischemic: ischein—hold back + haima—blood

TABLE 21.2 CARDIOVASCULAR HEALTH HISTORY

Question	Rationale
Pain: WHAT'S UP? Format	
Where is pain? Does it radiate?	Cardiac pain may radiate to shoulders, neck, jaw, arms, or back. Vascular disorders cause extremity pain.
How does it feel? Discomfort, burning, aching, indigestion, squeezing, pressure, tightness, heaviness, numbness in chest area? Fullness, heaviness, sharpness, throbbing in legs?	Pain can be associated with angina or myocardial infarction. The quality of pain varies. Venous pain is a fullness or heaviness. Arterial pain is sharp or throbbing.
Aggravating/alleviating factors that increase/relieve the pain?	Activity may cause or increase angina. Rest or medications may relieve angina. Leg activity pain, intermittent claudication, results from decreased perfusion that is aggravated by activity. Rest pain, from severe arterial occlusion, increases when lying. Dangling reduces the pain because blood flow is increased by gravity.
Timing of pain: onset, duration, frequency?	Pain may be continuous, intermittent, acute, or chronic. Arterial occlusion causes acute pain.
Severity of pain?	Rate pain on a scale of 0 to 10.
Useful data for associated symptoms?	Accompanying symptoms and their characteristics guide diagnosis and treatment.
Perception of patient about problem?	Patient's insight to problem is helpful in planning care.

Continued

TABLE 21.2 CARDIOVASCULAR HEALTH HISTORY—cont'd

Question	Rationale
Level of Consciousness (LOC)	
What is your name? What is the month? Year? Where are you now?	A lack of oxygen caused by cardiac disease can decrease LOC.
Dyspnea	
Are you short of breath? What increases your shortness of breath? What relieves your shortness of breath?	Dyspnea can be present with heart failure that reduces cardiac output, on exertion in angina pectoris or from a pulmonary embolus resulting from thrombophlebitis, heart failure, or dysrhythmias.
Palpitations	
Are you having palpitations or irregular heartbeat? Does your heart ever race, skip beats, or pound?	Palpitations can occur from dysrhythmias resulting from ischemia, electrolyte imbalance, or stress. Dizziness can be associated with dysrhythmias.
Fatigue	
Have you noticed a change in your energy level?	Fatigue occurs from reduced cardiac output resulting from heart failure.
Are you able to perform activities that you would like to?	Functional abilities can be limited from fatigue.
Edema	
Have you had any swelling in your feet, legs, or hands?	Right-sided heart failure can cause fluid accumulation in the tissues.
Have you gained weight?	Fluid retention causes weight gain.
Paresthesia/Paralysis	
Any numbness, tingling, or other abnormal sensations in extremities?	Numbness and tingling, pins and needles, and crawling sensations are paresthesia.
Can you move your extremity?	Paralysis is inability to move extremity. Reduced nerve conduction from decreased oxygen supply causes paresthesia and paralysis.

Medication

Medication use is noted. This includes prescription drugs, over-the-counter medications such as aspirin that can prolong clotting time, and recreational drugs. The medication history includes the patient's understanding of the medication and the medication name, dosage, reason for taking, last dose, and length of use.

Family History

A family history of cardiovascular conditions is assessed because many cardiac problems are hereditary. Health histories of close relatives, such as parents, siblings, and grandparents, are the most significant. For example, those who have had a parent die of sudden cardiac death before age 60 are at increased risk for sudden cardiac death.

Health Promotion

Risk factors such as diet, activity, tobacco use, and recent stressors for the patient are assessed in the health history. The patient's health promotion activities are noted, especially for risk factors that are modifiable through changes in lifestyle.

Physical Examination

The patient's general appearance is observed. The patient's level of consciousness, which is an indicator of oxygenation of the brain, is assessed. Height, weight, and vital signs are recorded.

Blood Pressure

Normal blood pressure is considered less than 120/80 (see Chapter 22). Readings in both arms are done for comparison. A difference in the readings is reported to the physician. The arm with the higher reading is used for ongoing measurements. If necessary, blood pressure may be measured in the leg using a larger blood pressure cuff. The reading in the leg is normally 10 mm Hg higher than in the arm (see *Evidence-Based Practice* box).

EVIDENCE-BASED PRACTICE

Clinical Question

Is self blood pressure (BP) measurement at home more accurate for hypertension control and predictive of the risk of cardiovascular events than office BP measurement?

Evidence

In a study of 325 patients, ambulatory and home BP were correlated with organ damage more closely than was office BP with a trend to better correlations with home BP (Gaborieau, Delarche, & Gosse, 2008). Home BP monitoring overcomes the "white coat effect" (increase in BP during an office visit) of traditional office BP measurement and allows more readings to be taken for evaluation for diagnosis (Pickering et al., 2008).

cont'd

Implications for Nursing Practice

Patients can effectively be taught to take BP at home. Teaching guidelines include using an oscillometric monitor that measures BP on the upper arm with proper cuff size; return demonstration of BP measurement; resting for 5 minutes in the seated position; then taking three consecutive readings in the morning and at night, over a period of 1 week. Monitors should be validated periodically.

REFERENCES

Gaborieau, V., Delarche, N., & Gosse, P. (2008). Ambulatory blood pressure monitoring versus self-measurement of blood pressure at home: Correlation with target organ damage. *Journal of Hypertension, 26*(10), 1919–1927.

Pickering, T., Miller, N., Ogedegbe, G., et al. (2008). Call to action on use and reimbursement for home blood pressure monitoring: A joint scientific statement from the American Heart Association, American Society of Hypertension, and Preventive Cardiovascular Nurses Association. *Journal of Cardiovascular Nursing, 23*(4), 299–323.

ORTHOSTATIC BLOOD PRESSURE. Measurements are taken with the patient lying, sitting, and standing to detect abnormal variations with postural changes. When the patient sits or stands, a drop in the systolic pressure of up to 15 mm Hg and either a drop or slight increase in the diastolic pressure of 3 to 10 mm Hg is normal. In response to the drop in blood pressure, the pulse increases 15 to 20 beats per minute to maintain cardiac output. Orthostatic hypotension (postural hypotension), is a drop in systolic blood pressure greater than 15 mm Hg, a drop or slight increase in the diastolic blood pressure greater than 10 mm Hg, and an increase in heart rate greater than 20 beats per minute in response to the drop in blood pressure. It indicates a problem that should be investigated by the physician (Box 21.3). The patient often reports light-headedness or syncope because the drop in blood pressure decreases the amount of oxygen-rich blood traveling to the brain. Factors that may cause orthostatic hypotension include fluid volume deficit, diuretics, analgesics, and pain.

NURSING CARE TIP

To effectively take a blood pressure reading:

- Use the correct cuff size.
- Allow the patient to be seated and relax for 5 minutes before the measurement.
- Determine the patient's baseline blood pressure by inflating the cuff and noting the reading when the radial pulse is no longer felt. Then, when taking blood pressure, inflate the cuff to 20 numbers above the obtained reading. (Overinflation may cause inaccurate reading.)
- Deflate the cuff slowly.

Box 21.3

Orthostatic Hypotension Assessment

To assess orthostatic hypotension:

1. Use correct size blood pressure cuff.
2. Explain procedure to patient; determine if patient can safely stand.
3. Have patient lie flat in bed at least 5 minutes prior to readings.
4. Patient should not eat or smoke 30 minutes before readings; patient should not talk during readings and should sit up with legs uncrossed while sitting.
5. Take patient's lying blood pressure and heart rate.
6. Assist patient to sitting position. Ask if dizzy or light-headed with each position change. If yes, ensure safety from fainting or falling. A gait or walking belt can be used. With any position change, if patient experiences additional symptoms with the dizziness and decreased blood pressure and increased heart rate, assist the patient to lie down, take blood pressure, and notify the physician. Consider the possible cause of the orthostatic hypotension (hemorrhaging, dehydration, diuretics) to plan patient care.
7. Wait 3 minutes, and then take patient's sitting blood pressure and heart rate. If patient is dizzy or light-headed, continue sitting position for 5 minutes if tolerated. Do not attempt to bring the patient to standing. Repeat sitting blood pressure. If blood pressure has increased and patient is no longer dizzy, assist patient to stand.
8. Assist patient to stand and take blood pressure and pulse immediately. Then take again in 3 minutes. If blood pressure drops and patient is dizzy or light-headed, do not attempt to ambulate patient.
9. Document all heart rate and blood pressure measurements, including extremity used and patient position when reading was obtained (e.g., right arm: lying 132/78 mm Hg, sitting 118/68 mm Hg, standing 110/60 mm Hg). Also document patient tolerance, symptoms, and nursing interventions if symptomatic.
10. Report abnormal findings to physician.

Pulses

The apical pulse is auscultated for 1 minute to assess rate and rhythm. Normal heart rate is 60 to 100 beats per minute. In athletic people, the heart rate is often slower, around 50 beats per minute, because the well-conditioned heart pumps more efficiently. Apical pulse rhythm is documented as regular or irregular. The apical rate can be compared with the radial rate to assess equality. If there are fewer radial beats than apical beats, a **pulse deficit** exists and should be reported to the physician.

Arterial pulses are palpated for volume and pressure quality. They are palpated bilaterally and compared for equality. A normal vessel feels soft and springy. A sclerotic vessel feels stiff. The quality of the pulses is described on a four-point scale as follows: 0 is absent; 1+ is weak, thready; 2+ is normal; and 3+ is bounding. An absent pulse is not palpable. A thready pulse is one that disappears when slight pressure is applied and returns when the pressure is removed. The normal pulse is easily palpable. The bounding pulse is strong and present even when slight pressure is applied. When the normal vessel is palpated, a tapping is felt. In the abnormal vessel that has a bulging or narrowed wall, a vibration is felt, which is called a **thrill**. When auscultating an abnormal vessel, a humming is heard that is caused by the turbulent blood flow through the vessel. This is referred to as a **bruit**.

> **SAFETY TIP**
>
> Anticipate potential drops in blood pressure with position changes. Orthostatic hypotension can be found in patients of any age but is most commonly found in the older patient. The blood pressure drop increases the risk of fainting and falling. Use fall precautions such as a walking belt or two-person assist for patients at risk of or with orthostatic hypotension.

Respirations

The rate and ease of respirations are observed. Breath sounds are auscultated. Sputum characteristics such as amount, color, and consistency are noted. Pink, frothy sputum is an indicator of acute heart failure. A dry cough can occur from the irritation caused by the lung congestion resulting from heart failure.

Inspection

During the health history, inspection begins by noting shortness of breath when the patient speaks or moves. The patient's skin is noted for oxygenation status through the color of skin, mucous membranes, lips, earlobes, and nailbeds. Pallor may indicate anemia or lack of arterial blood flow. Cyanosis shows an oxygen distribution deficiency. A reddish brown discoloration (rubor) found in the lower extremities occurs from decreased arterial blood flow. A brown discoloration and cyanosis when the extremity is dependent may be seen in the presence of venous blood flow problems. Hair distribution on the extremities is observed. Decreased hair distribution, thick, brittle nails, and shiny, taut, dry skin occur from reduced arterial blood flow. Venous blood return is assessed by inspecting extremities for varicose veins, stasis ulcers, or scars around the ankles and signs of thrombophlebitis such as swelling, redness, or a hard, tender vein.

The patient's internal and external jugular neck veins are observed for distention in a 45- to 90-degree upright position. Normally, in this position, the veins are not visible. Distention indicates an increase in the venous volume, often caused by right-sided heart failure.

Capillary refill time is 3 seconds or less and indicates arterial blood flow to the extremities. The patient's nailbed is briefly squeezed, causing blanching, and then released. The time that it takes for the color to return to the nailbed after release of the squeezing pressure is the capillary refill time. Longer times indicate anemia or a decrease in blood flow to the extremity.

Clubbing of the nailbeds occurs from oxygen deficiency over time. It is often caused by congenital heart defects or the long-term use of tobacco. The distal ends of the fingers and toes swell and appear clublike. With clubbing, the normal 160-degree angle formed between the base of the nail and the skin is lost, causing the nail to be flat (Fig. 21.7). Later, the nail base elevates, the angle exceeds 180 degrees, and the nail feels spongy when squeezed.

> **LEARNING TIP**
>
> Six P's characterize peripheral vascular disease:
>
> - Pain
> - Poikilothermia
> - Pulselessness
> - Pallor
> - Paralysis
> - Paresthesia (decreased sensation)

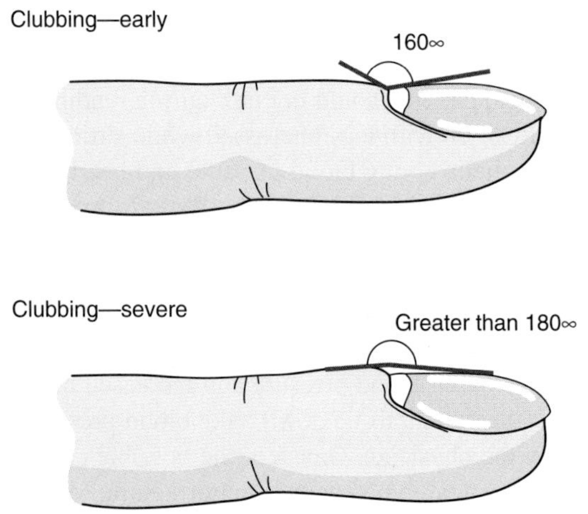
Clubbing—early
160∞
Clubbing—severe
Greater than 180∞

FIGURE 21.7 Clubbing of the fingers.

Palpation

In addition to palpating the arteries, the thorax can be palpated at the **point of maximum impulse** (PMI). The PMI is palpated by placing the right hand over the apex of the heart. If palpable, a thrust is felt when the ventricle contracts. An enlarged heart may shift the PMI to the left of the midclavicular line.

The temperature of the extremities is palpated bilaterally for comparison. Palpation begins proximally and moves distally along the extremity. In areas of decreased arterial blood flow, the ischemic area feels cooler than the rest of the body because it is blood that warms the body. In the absence of sufficient arterial blood flow, the area becomes the temperature of the environment (**poikilothermy**). A warm or hot extremity indicates a venous blood flow problem.

Edema is palpated in the lower extremities or dependent areas such as the sacrum for the supine patient (Fig. 21.8). Edema can occur from right-sided heart failure, gravity, or altered venous blood return. The nurse assesses the severity of the edema by pressing with a finger for 5 seconds over a bone, the medial malleolus or tibia, in the area of edema. If the finger imprint or indentation remains, the edema is pitting. Measuring the leg circumference is an accurate method for monitoring the edema.

Homans' sign is an assessment for venous thrombosis; however, in less than 50% of patients with thrombosis, the test is not positive. A positive Homans' sign is pain in the patient's calf or behind the knee when the foot is quickly dorsiflexed with the knee in a slightly flexed position (Fig. 21.9). Homans' sign should not be performed if a positive diagnosis of thrombosis has been made.

Auscultation

Normal heart sounds are produced by the closing of the heart valves. Sound in blood-flowing vessels is transmitted in the direction of the blood flow. The first heart sound (S_1) is heard at the beginning of systole as "lubb" when the tricuspid and mitral (AV) valves close (Fig. 21.10). The second heart sound (S_2) is heard at the start of diastole as "dupp" when the aortic and pulmonic semilunar valves close. The diaphragm of the stethoscope is used to hear the high-pitched sounds of S_1 and S_2. Normally, no other sounds are heard between S_1 and S_2. With the bell of the stethoscope placed at the apex, a third heart sound (S_3) or a fourth heart sound (S_4) may be heard. Having patients lean forward or lie on their left side can make the heart sounds easier to hear by bringing the area of the heart where the sound may be heard closer to the chest wall. The S_3 heart sound is normal for children and younger adults. It sounds like a gallop and is a low-pitched sound heard early in diastole. In older adults, S_3 may be heard with left-sided heart failure, fluid volume overload, and mitral valve regurgitation. The S_4 heart sound is also a low-pitched sound, similar to a gallop but heard late in diastole. It occurs with hypertension, coronary artery disease, and pulmonary stenosis.

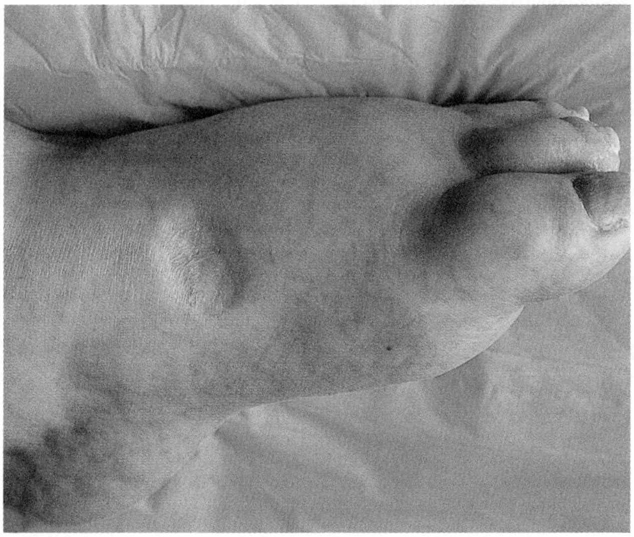

FIGURE 21.8 Pitting edema. Application of pressure over a bony area displaces the excess fluid, leaving an indentation or pit.

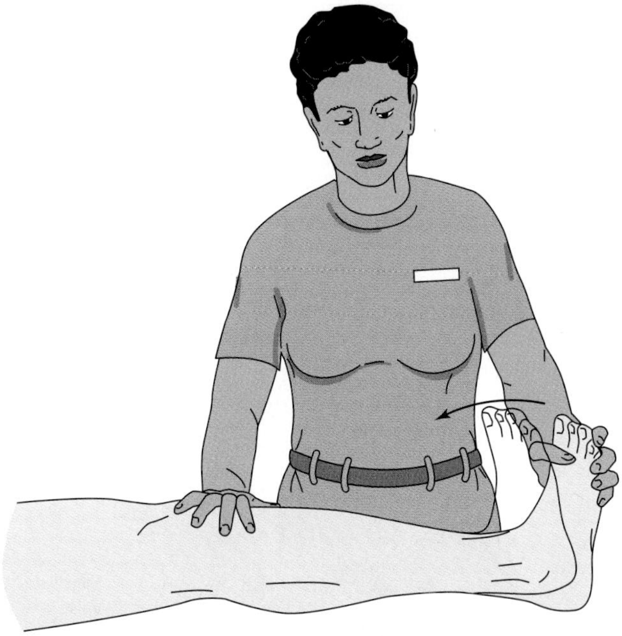

FIGURE 21.9 Assessment of Homans' sign for venous thrombosis. The foot is quickly dorsiflexed with the knee flexed. Calf or knee pain is noted. This assessment should not be performed if a positive diagnosis of thrombosis has been made.

• WORD • BUILDING •
poikilothermy: poikilos—varied + therme—heat

LEARNING TIP

This sentence can help you remember the heart's auscultation points:

All	(aortic)
People	(pulmonic)
Eat	(Erb's point)
Three	(tricuspid)
Meals	(mitral)

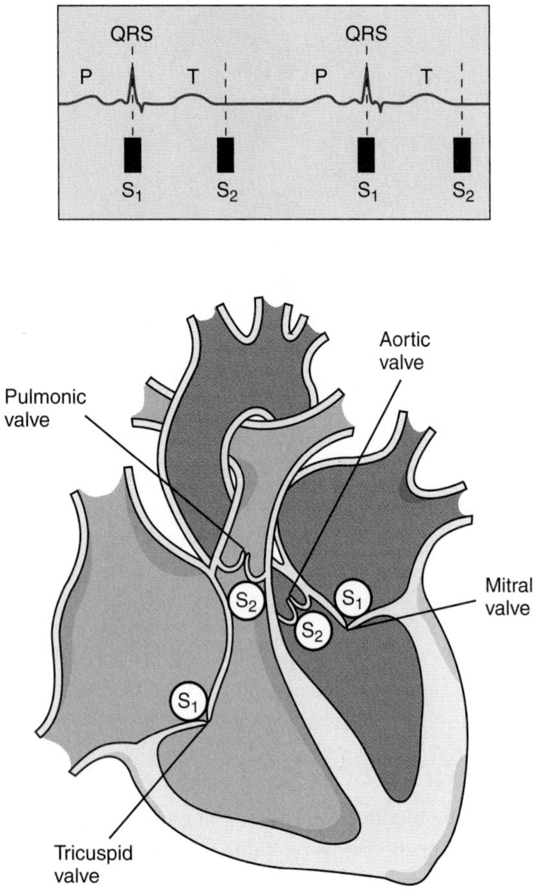
QRS
P
T
QRS
P
T
S1
S2
S1
S2
Pulmonic valve
Aortic valve
Mitral valve
Tricuspid valve
S2
S1
S2
S1

FIGURE 21.10 Heart sounds shown on electrocardiogram: S_1 is heard at the beginning of systole, and S_2 is heard at the beginning of diastole.

Murmurs are caused by a narrowed valve opening or a valve that does not close tightly. A **murmur** is a prolonged, swishing sound that ranges in intensity from faint to very loud.

A **pericardial friction rub** occurs from inflammation of the pericardium. The intensity of a rub can range from faint to loud enough to be audible without a stethoscope. A rub has a grating sound like sandpaper being rubbed together that occurs when the pericardial surfaces rub together during a heartbeat. (See the Learning Tip on pericardial friction rub in Chapter 23.) Having the patient sit and lean forward allows a rub to be heard more clearly. The rub is best heard to the left of the sternum using the diaphragm of the stethoscope. A pericardial friction rub may occur after a myocardial infarction or chest trauma.

CRITICAL THINKING

Mrs. Smith

■ Mrs. Smith, age 78, baseline weight 162 pounds, is admitted to the hospital with shortness of breath. Initial assessment findings are BP 152/88 mm Hg, pulse 104 beats per minute, respirations 26 per minute, temperature 99.4°F (37.2°C), shortness of breath at rest that increases with activity, ankles swollen, heart tones distant, nailbeds pale, no pain, has not eaten well for 2 weeks, 6-pound weight gain in 1 week, sleeps on three pillows, neck veins visible bilaterally. A diagnosis of acute myocardial infarction with heart failure is made by a physician.

1. Why might Mrs. Smith not be having chest pain with a diagnosis of acute MI?
2. How should swollen ankles be assessed to provide complete and measurable data?
3. What should be documented for the assessment performed on the swollen ankles and how should the assessment findings be documented?
4. How should the assessment findings be documented for the additional symptoms Mrs. Smith has?
5. What is Mrs. Smith's weight in kilograms?

Suggested answers at end of chapter.

DIAGNOSTIC TESTS FOR THE CARDIOVASCULAR SYSTEM

Diagnostic test results are combined with the health history and physical assessment to plan care for the patient (Table 21.3).

Noninvasive Studies

Chest X-Ray Examination

A chest x-ray examination shows the size, position, contour, and structures of the heart (Fig. 21.11). It can reveal heart enlargement, calcifications, fluid around the heart, heart failure, and placement of pacemaker leads and pulmonary artery catheters. Fluoroscopy uses a luminescent x-ray screen to guide cardiac catheter or pacemaker lead placement.

Computed Tomography Scan

Computed tomography (CT) scanning can be used to evaluate the heart, coronary arteries, pulmonary veins, aorta, pericardium, and cardiac masses. Areas with plaque or calcification (the body deposits calcium to harden plaques, which are not normally found in the coronary arteries) can be seen. Plaque indicates atherosclerosis.

Cardiac CT uses a contrast agent, so patient allergies and kidney function must be checked. To prevent contrast-induced nephropathy, patients have their glomerular filtration rate or creatinine level measured. Then if mild-to-moderate renal insufficiency is shown, patients should receive premedication and two post procedure doses with N-acetylcysteine (Mucomyst) and IV hydration with 0.45% sodium chloride hydration to help protect the kidneys.

TABLE 21.3 DIAGNOSTIC LABORATORY TESTS AND PROCEDURES FOR THE CARDIOVASCULAR SYSTEM

Procedure	Definition	Significance of Abnormal Findings	Nursing Management
Noninvasive			
Chest x-ray film	Anterior-posterior and left lateral views of chest taken to show heart size and contour and lungs.	Heart enlargement, calcifications, fluid around heart	Assess x-ray history and whether pregnant. Remove metal items. Teaching: no discomfort.
Computed tomography scan	Evaluates heart, coronary arteries, pulmonary veins, aorta, pericardium, cardiac masses.	Plaque or calcification indicates atherosclerosis.	Allergies and kidney function are checked if contrast used. If renal insufficiency N-acetylcysteine (Mucomyst) and IV hydration with 0.45% sodium chloride hydration given to protect kidneys.
Cardiac magnetic resonance imaging (MRI)/ angiography (MRA)	Provides three-dimensional image of heart. Dye given for MRA to visualize arteries.	Cardiac abnormalities	Assess for implants, pacemakers, metallic items, and claustrophobia. Give antianxiety medication as ordered before MRI. Assess allergies for dye. Teaching: must lie still in cylinder with loud, pounding sounds. Can talk to technician, listen to music.
Electrocardiogram (ECG)	Electrodes on skin carry electrical activity of heart from different views to show rhythm of heart, size of chambers, and heart damage.	Dysrhythmias, enlarged heart chamber size, myocardial ischemia or infarction, electrolyte imbalances	Teaching: no discomfort. Explain procedure.
Holter monitor	Recording of ECG for up to 48 hours to match abnormalities with symptoms recorded in patient's diary.	Dysrhythmias, infrequent myocardial ischemia	Apply electrodes and leads. Teaching: keep accurate diary; push event button for symptoms. No showers or baths. Return visit.
Echocardiogram	Sound waves bounce off heart to produce heart images and show blood flow.	Heart enlargement, coronary artery disease, valvular abnormalities, thickened cardiac walls or septum, pericardial effusion	May be done at bedside. Patient lies on left side. Teaching: no discomfort, gel applied.
Transesophageal echocardiogram	Probe with transducer on end inserted into esophagus. Provides clear images of heart as no lung or rib tissue crossed. Dye injected for blood flow study.	Heart enlargement, coronary artery disease, valvular abnormalities, thickened cardiac walls or septum, pericardial effusion	Monitor vital signs and oxygen saturation. Encourage patient to relax. Suction continually during procedure. Teaching: NPO 6 hours before test. Sedation and local throat anesthetic given.
Exercise stress test	Evaluates effects of exercise on heart and vascular circulation. ECG and vital signs are continuously monitored. Test stopped if symptoms develop.	Dysrhythmias, ischemia	Monitor vital signs and ECG before, during, and after test until stable. Teaching: explain procedure, wear walking shoes and comfortable clothes.
Plethysmography	Tested leg raised 30 degrees with patient supine. Pressure cuff inflated on the leg to distend the veins. Cuff is then rapidly deflated and venous volume changes measured with electrodes.	Thrombi detected by less venous volume.	Teaching: no discomfort. Explain procedure. Takes 30 to 45 minutes.
Pressure measurement	Blood pressures taken at several sites along extremity.	Shows area of occlusion or decreased blood flow at rest and with exercise.	Teaching: no discomfort. Explain procedure.
Doppler ultrasound	Sound waves bounce off moving blood producing recordings.	Decreased blood flow in peripheral vascular disease (PVD)	Teaching: explain procedure.

Continued

TABLE 21.3 DIAGNOSTIC LABORATORY TESTS AND PROCEDURES FOR THE CARDIOVASCULAR SYSTEM—cont'd

Procedure	Definition	Significance of Abnormal Findings	Nursing Management
Radioisotopes			
Thallium imaging	IV injection of thallium-201 to evaluate cardiac blood flow. With exercise, thallium given 1 minute before end of test to circulate thallium. Scan done within 10 minutes and repeated in 2 to 4 hours for comparison.	If thallium not delivered to cardiac cells by good blood flow then see "cold spots" that show ischemia initially or infarcted areas later.	Teaching: explain procedure, inform that radioactivity is small and gone within a few hours. Light meal only between scans.
Dipyridamole thallium imaging	Dipyridamole (Persantine) IV is a vasodilator given to increase blood flow to coronary arteries; test is same as thallium imaging.	If thallium not delivered to cardiac cells by good blood flow then see "cold spots" that show ischemia initially or infarcted areas later.	Teaching: explain procedure, instruct no caffeine or aminophylline 12 hours before. Same as thallium imaging.
Technetium pyrophosphate or technetium-99m sestamibi imaging	Radioisotope given IV. Scanned 1.5 to 2 hours later.	Areas of myocardial cell damage take up the radioisotope, which appears as hot spots.	Teaching: explain procedure, inform that radioactivity is small and gone within a few hours.
Multiple-gated acquisition (MUGA) scan	Technetium-99m pertechnetate is given IV. Serial studies are done over several hours. May be done at bedside.	Studies effects of drugs, recent myocardial infarction (MI), and congestive heart failure.	Teaching: explain procedure.
Positron emission tomography (PET)	Nitrogen-13 ammonia IV given and scanned for cardiac perfusion. Then fluoro-18-deoxyglucose IV given and scanned for cardiac metabolic function. Exercise may also be used.	In normal heart, scans match; in injured heart, they differ.	Patient's blood glucose must be 60 to 140 mg/dL for accuracy. Teaching: explain procedure. Must lie still during scan. If exercise used, NPO and no tobacco use.
Serum Tests			
Highly sensitive C-reactive protein (hs-CRP)	CRP level can indicate low-grade inflammation in coronary vessels. *CV disease risk:* Low = <1 mg/L Average = 1–3 mg/L High = > 3 mg/L	Elevated levels indicate MI risk.	No special care.
Homocysteine	Amino acid in the blood. *Normal:* 7–8 micromol/L	Elevated levels linked with higher risk of coronary artery disease (CAD) and PVD.	Encourage high-risk patients to have adequate intake of folic acid and vitamin B.
Creatine kinase (CK)	Heart, brain, skeletal muscle contain CK enzymes. *Normal male:* 5–55 units/mL *Normal female:* 5–25 units/mL	Damaged cells release CK. With MI, CK elevates in 6 hours and returns to baseline in 48–72 hours.	Avoid IM injections, and take baseline CK before inserting IVs to avoid elevating CK from muscle cell damage. Serial sampling done.
CK-MB	Heart muscle contains MB isoenzyme. *Normal:* 0–7 international units/L	Rises with MI in 6 hours and returns to baseline in 72 hours.	Same as CK.
Cardiac troponin I or T	Cardiac cell protein. *Normal:* Varies by lab; very low levels	Elevated levels sensitive indicator of MI. Levels elevated up to 7 days.	No special care.
Myoglobin	Protein found in cardiac cells; 99% indicative of MI. *Normal:* 0–85 ng/mL	Rises in 1 hour after MI and peaks in 4 to 12 hours, so must be drawn within 18 hours of chest pain onset.	No special care.
Magnesium	Electrolyte necessary to regulate heartbeat and blood pressure. *Normal:* 1.6 to 2.6 mg/dL	Hypomagnesemia may cause cardiac arrhythmias, hypertension, tachycardia.	No special care.

TABLE 21.3 DIAGNOSTIC LABORATORY TESTS AND PROCEDURES FOR THE CARDIOVASCULAR SYSTEM—cont'd

Procedure	Definition	Significance of Abnormal Findings	Nursing Management
Phospholipids	May elevate in cardiovascular disease. *Normal:* 125–380 mg/dL	CAD risk	Same as triglycerides.
Lipoproteins	Electrophoresis done to separate lipoproteins: VLDL, LDL, HDL. HDL protects against CAD *Normal lipoproteins:* 400–800 mg/dL *Desirable:* LDL less than HDL (values vary with age)	Elevated LDL increases CAD risk. LDL less than 100 desirable HDL greater than 60	Same as triglycerides.
Invasive			
Angiography	Dye injected into vessels to make them visible on x-rays. Coronary: coronary arteries via cardiac catheter. Peripheral: peripheral arteries or veins.	Assesses vessel patency, injury, or aneurysm.	Precare: Informed consent. NPO 4 to 18 hours before test. Assess allergies. Teaching: sedative and local anesthesia may be used; burning sensation from dye; monitored continuously. Postcare: Monitor vital signs, hemorrhage at the injection site, pulses.
Cardiac catheterization	Catheter inserted into heart for data on oxygen saturation and chamber pressures. Dye may be injected to visualize structures.	Cardiac disease	Precare: Same as angiography. Sensory teaching: table is hard; cool cleansing solution used; sting felt from local anesthetic; hear monitor beeping; feel pressure of catheter insertion; dye warm, burning feeling; headache; brief chest pain; hear camera; feel table move. Postcare: Monitor vital signs, circulation, mobility, sensation, catheter insertion site, for hemorrhage or hematoma every 15 minutes for 1 hour, then every 30 minutes to 1 hour. Apply insertion site pressure as needed. Immobilize extremity for several hours as ordered.
Hemodynamic monitoring	Diagnoses and guides treatment with continuous readings compared to normal for: *Right atrial pressure:* 2–6 mm Hg *Pulmonary artery systolic/diastolic:* 20–30/0–10 *Pulmonary artery wedge pressure:* 4–12 mm Hg *Cardiac output:* 4–8 L/min Svo_2: 60%–80%	Blood pressure, cardiac and pulmonary pressure abnormalities.	Informed consent signed. Continuous monitoring. Recording of readings and monitoring of insertion site for signs of infection.
Electrophysiological studies	Assesses heart's electrical system, with electrodes inserted into the right side of the heart.	Dysrhythmias	Consent is obtained. Patient is NPO 6 to 8 hours before the test.

Cardiac Magnetic Resonance Imaging and Angiography

Two- or three-dimensional still or moving images of the beating heart are produced with magnetic resonance imaging (MRI). Cardiac MRI is useful for identifying ischemia and heart damage as well as other conditions affecting the heart. Patients with pacemakers, defibrillators, cochlear implant, or brain aneurysm clips are not candidates for this test. For other types of metal or implants, the physician should be informed to determine if they will pose a problem during the test. An open MRI machine is available for those with claustrophobia or who are obese.

For magnetic resonance angiography, a non–iodine-based contrast, gadolinium-DTPA, may or may not be used to view the blood vessels.

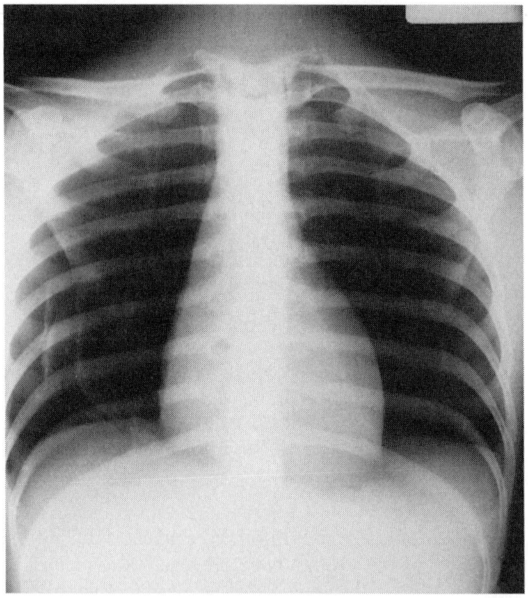

FIGURE 21.11 Normal chest x-ray film. Note white outline of heart borders in center. (From McKinnis, L. N. [1997]. *Fundamentals of orthopedic radiology* [p. 15]. Philadelphia: F. A. Davis.)

Visit www.radiologyinfo.org for more information on radiology tests.

Electrocardiogram

The electrocardiogram (ECG) records electrical activity of the heart in various views. Abnormalities related to conduction, rate, rhythm, heart chamber enlargement, myocardial ischemia, MI, and electrolyte imbalances may be reflected on an ECG. When an ECG is requested, information that aids in its interpretation is provided, including the patient's sex, age, height, weight, blood pressure, and cardiac medications. There is no special preparation for the ECG, which is painless.

To obtain an ECG, electrodes are placed on the skin to transmit electrical impulses to the ECG machine for recording. The electrical impulses from the heart appear as waves on graph paper. One view of the heart using a combination of the electrodes to obtain the view is called a lead. The standard 12-lead ECG, using a combination of the electrodes, provides 12 views of the heart. Eighteen-lead ECGs may also be done.

SIGNAL-AVERAGED ECG. The signal-averaged ECG is used to diagnose whether a patient is at risk of developing ventricular tachycardia and possible sudden death. A computer records low-level signals not detected by a regular ECG. These electrical signals, referred to as late potentials, occur at the end of the QRS wave and into the ST segment (see Chapter 25). Late potentials place the patient at risk for ventricular **dysrhythmias** (abnormal heart rhythms).

HOLTER MONITORING (AMBULATORY ELECTROCARDIOGRAM). A Holter monitor, which weighs 2 pounds, continuously records an ECG in one lead for up to 48 hours as a patient goes about his or her daily activities. The patient wears loose-fitting clothing and may only sponge bathe while wearing the monitor. The patient records a diary of activities and symptoms and pushes the event button if symptoms occur. Symptoms are documented for later correlation with the ECG recordings. Dysrhythmias or myocardial ischemia that occurs infrequently can be detected. Recordings are scanned by a computer and interpreted by a physician.

Echocardiogram

An echocardiogram is an ultrasound test that records the motion of the heart structures, including the valves, as well as the heart size, shape, and position. No preparation is required for a cardiac ultrasound. This test transmits ultrasonic sound waves across the chest wall (transthoracic) and through lung and rib tissue into the heart so that the returned echoes can be recorded on videotape as audio and visual information. An ECG is recorded at the same time for comparison purposes. Abnormalities that may be seen on the echocardiogram include heart enlargement, valvular abnormalities, thickened cardiac walls or septum, and pericardial effusion.

Exercise echocardiography diagnoses coronary artery disease during exercise-induced cardiac ischemia by detecting cardiac wall motion abnormalities. If the patient is unable to exercise, giving dobutamine for a dobutamine stress echocardiography simulates exercise while the echocardiogram is done.

Transesophageal Echocardiogram

A transesophageal echocardiogram (TEE) provides a clearer picture than transthoracic echocardiography. It produces images by using a transducer on a probe that is placed in the esophagus. The images are clearer because lung and rib tissue does not have to be penetrated by the sound waves. The physician controls the position of the probe and takes pictures as it travels within the esophagus. Patients take nothing by mouth (NPO) for about 6 hours before the test, receive a sedative, and have their throat locally anesthetized. After the procedure, patients remain NPO until the nurse has verified (by touching the back of the throat with a cotton tip swab) that their gag reflex has returned.

Exercise Stress Test

The exercise stress test measures cardiac function or peripheral vascular disease during a defined exercise protocol (Fig. 21.12). Before the test, patients are given an explanation of the test and told not to smoke, eat, or drink for 2 to 4 hours before the test. They are also instructed to wear comfortable walking shoes, a loose top, and for women a supportive bra. After the test, patients should rest and wait to eat. They should also avoid eating or drinking stimulants such as caffeine and temperature extremes such as going out into cold weather for a few hours after the test.

Cardiac Stress Test

The cardiac stress test simulates sympathetic nervous system (fight-or-flight) stimulation. It shows the heart's response to increased oxygen needs. Before the test, baseline vital signs are obtained. Then, while the patient exercises on a treadmill, on a stationary bicycle, or by climbing stairs,

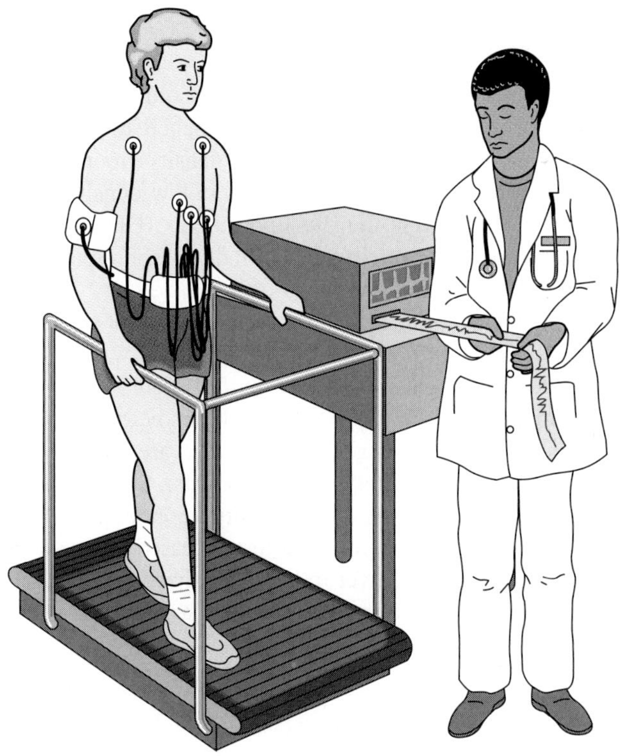

FIGURE 21.12 Performance of stress test.

vital signs, oxygen saturation, skin temperature, physical appearance, chest pain, and ECG are monitored to help ensure patient safety. The test is completed when the patient reaches his or her peak heart rate (patient's age subtracted from 220), experiences chest pain, is unable to exercise further, or develops vital sign or ECG changes. Vital signs and ECG continue to be monitored after the test until they return to baseline.

The cardiac stress test is used to evaluate coronary artery disease. It aids in diagnosing ischemic heart disease, the cause of chest pain and dysrhythmias. The functional capacity of the heart can also be measured after a cardiac event or to plan a physical fitness or rehabilitation program.

Peripheral Vascular Stress Test

In a peripheral vascular stress test, the patient walks for 5 minutes at 1.5 miles per hour on the treadmill. At certain intervals, pulse volume measurements are taken, including baseline resting, during the test, and final resting after the test. This test assesses response to activity. If intermittent **claudication** (pain in the legs with activity) occurs, the test is stopped.

Plethysmography

A plethysmography test measures blood volume and changes in blood flow to diagnose deep venous thrombosis and pulmonary emboli and to screen patients for peripheral vascular disease. The leg being tested is raised 30 degrees with the patient supine. A pressure cuff is then inflated on the leg to distend the veins. Blood flow is measured with electrodes, and the cuff is then rapidly deflated and venous volume changes are recorded. Thrombi are detected by reduction in venous volume.

Pressure Measurement

Pressure readings are done to assess areas of occlusion or narrowing in vessels. Blood pressure readings are taken at intervals along the extremity. Reduced readings are found in areas with blood flow problems.

Arterial Stiffness Index

Stiffness of the brachial artery is measured to determine arteriosclerosis and cardiovascular disease risk. The brachial artery correlates with the coronary arteries in regard to the extent of atherosclerosis. The arterial stiffness index (ASI) test is done with a device that has a blood pressure cuff hooked to a computer that maps the waveforms during the blood pressure reading.

Tilt Table Test

The tilt table test is used to help diagnose the cause of syncope (fainting spells). Heart rate and blood pressure are monitored during a change in position from lying down to standing up.

Doppler Ultrasound

In a Doppler ultrasound test, sound waves bounce off moving blood cells and return a sound frequency in relationship to the amount of blood flow. With decreased blood flow the sounds are reduced. This test requires no patient preparation, takes about 20 minutes to complete, and is painless.

Nuclear Radioisotope Imaging

For nuclear radioisotope imaging, small amounts of radioisotopes are given intravenously. The patient is then scanned with a gamma camera to produce a radionuclide image. Radiation exposure is similar to that of other x-ray examinations. These tests can provide information about myocardial ischemia or infarction, cardiac blood flow, and ventricle size and motion.

Thallium Imaging

Thallium-201, a radioactive analog of potassium, is used to detect impaired myocardial perfusion. It is injected intravenously (IV), and muscle cells absorb it. After 10 to 15 minutes, the heart is scanned to see where the thallium has concentrated. Four hours later the scan is repeated to look for changes. Healthy myocardial cells with good blood flow take up the thallium. Areas in which the thallium is not seen are referred to as cold spots and indicate ischemia or infarction. The patency of a coronary artery graft may also be assessed with this test. This test is used often because the short half-life of thallium results in lower radiation exposure.

Exercise testing may be combined with thallium injection to detect blood flow changes with activity and after rest. The patient exercises and about 2 minutes before stopping is given thallium. Scans are taken immediately and again in 2 to 4 hours. Cold spots on initial images indicate ischemia. If the cold spots are gone in later images, exercise-induced ischemia is present. If the cold spots are still present in later images, they show scarred areas.

If patients are unable to participate in exercise for the thallium stress test, dipyridamole (Persantine) or adenosine, coronary vasodilators, can be given. These drugs simulate the increased blood flow to healthy myocardial cells that occurs with exercise.

Technetium Pyrophosphate Scan

Technetium-99m pyrophosphate is injected for this test. Areas of ischemia or myocardial cell damage take up the radioisotope, and when scanned these areas appear as hot spots. Acute myocardial infarction size and location can be detected, but old MIs cannot be detected.

Technetium-99m Sestamibi

For this test, technetium-99m sestamibi is given IV and the patient is scanned 1.5 to 2 hours later. Areas of myocardial cell damage take up the radioisotope, and when scanned these areas appear as hot spots.

Multiple-Gated Acquisition Scan

In a multiple-gated acquisition (MUGA) scan, technetium-99m pertechnetate is injected IV and remains in the bloodstream; it is not taken up by myocardial cells. A camera follows the flow of the radioactivity, which shows ventricular function and wall motion and the ejection fraction of the heart.

Positron Emission Tomography

Positron emission tomography (PET) shows myocardial perfusion and viability with three-dimensional images. Nitrogen-13 ammonia is injected IV first and then scanned to show myocardial perfusion. Next, fluoro-18-deoxyglucose is given IV and then scanned to show myocardial metabolic function. If ischemia or heart damage is present, the two scans are different. For example, in ischemia of viable cells, blood flow is decreased but metabolism elevated. Treatment to increase blood flow improves cardiac function in this case. Before the test the patient's blood glucose should be in the normal range, and caffeine and tobacco should be avoided for 4 hours before the test.

> **SAFETY TIP**
>
> *Improve the accuracy of patient identification.* Use at least two patient identifiers (neither of which is the patient's location) whenever collecting laboratory samples or administering medications or blood products. Also use two identifiers to label sample collection containers in the presence of the patient.
>
> Just before the start of any invasive procedure, conduct a final, active communication verification process to confirm the correct patient, procedure, site, and availability of appropriate documents. Reestablish the patient's identity before starting the procedure (2010 National Patient Safety Goals, www.jointcommission.org).

Blood Studies

Blood Lipids

Lipids include triglycerides, cholesterol, and phospholipids. Lipoproteins carry these lipids attached to proteins. Triglycerides are found in very low-density lipoproteins (VLDLs). Cholesterol is mainly found in low-density lipoproteins (LDLs). High-density lipoproteins (HDLs) are a mixture of one-half protein and one-half phospholipids and cholesterol.

A lipid profile can screen for increased risk of coronary artery disease. For more information, visit www.nhlbi.nih.gov/guidelines/cholesterol/atglance.pdf. Patients must fast for 12 hours and avoid alcohol for 24 hours before the test. Water is not withheld. High levels of LDLs are linked to an increase in coronary artery disease because they circulate cholesterol in the arteries. High-density lipoproteins play a protective role against coronary artery disease because they carry cholesterol to the liver to be metabolized. Controlling lipids is very important in reducing coronary artery disease (Box 21.4, *Cultural Considerations*).

C-Reactive Protein

C-reactive protein is an acute phase protein that increases during the inflammatory process. A highly sensitive C-reactive protein (hs-CRP) test can predict heart attack risk. With elevated hs-CRP levels, nurses have the opportunity to help patients understand and reduce cardiac risk factors.

Homocysteine

Homocysteine is an amino acid in the blood that may damage the lining of arteries and promote blood clots. Elevated levels are associated with increased cardiovascular disease risk. Folic acid, vitamin B_6, and vitamin B_{12} break down homocysteine. Adequate dietary intake of green leafy vegetables and grains fortified with folic acid, as well as vitamin B, can help reduce homocysteine levels.

Cardiac Biomarkers

Proteins and enzymes released into the blood by damaged cardiac cells are known as cardiac biomarkers. These biomarkers help identify whether a patient is having or has had a recent myocardial infarction.

CREATINE KINASE. Creatine kinase (CK) is an enzyme found in the brain, skeletal muscle, and heart muscle. Isoenzymes of CK contained in these tissues are CK-BB (brain), CK-MM (skeletal muscle), and CK-MB (heart muscle). CK-MB helps diagnose a myocardial infarction because its level rises within 4 to 6 hours after cardiac cells are damaged, peaks in 12 to 18 hours, and returns to normal in 24 to 36 hours. Invasive procedures such as IV and intramuscular (IM) injections are avoided before drawing the first CK to prevent elevation in the CK levels from cell trauma caused by the procedure. Medications are often given IV rather than IM to prevent contributing to this elevation.

CARDIAC TROPONIN. Cardiac muscle contains proteins called troponin I and troponin T, which control the muscle fibers that contract or squeeze the heart muscle. They detect

Box 21.4

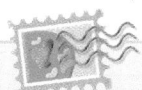

Cultural Considerations

Among French Canadians, familial chylomicronemia (hyperlipoproteinemia type I), an autosomal recessive disorder, occurs with the highest frequency worldwide. Familial chylomicronemia can lead to coronary thrombosis. Thus, the nurse can improve the health of French Canadians by encouraging early diagnostic workups for familial chylomicronemia and encouraging healthful lifestyles.

minor myocardial damage not detected by CK-MB to diagnose myocardial infarction. Levels elevate within 4 to 6 hours of damage. These levels peak in 10 to 24 hours and remain elevated for 10 to 14 days. Troponin T appears slightly earlier than troponin I and remains elevated longer after cardiac damage.

MYOGLOBIN. Myoglobin, a protein found in skeletal and cardiac muscle, is not site specific so it can only indicate that muscle damage has occurred. However, it rises before CK-MB or troponin so it can detect a myocardial infarction earlier for prompt treatment. Myoglobin levels elevate within 1 hour of an acute myocardial infarction. Peak levels are reached 4 to 12 hours after a myocardial infarction, and levels return to normal within 18 hours after the onset of chest pain.

Magnesium

Magnesium, an electrolyte, is important to many functions in the body. Among these is control of the heartbeat, and regulating blood pressure. A normal magnesium level is 1.6 to 2.6 mg/dL. **Hypomagnesemia**, a low level of magnesium in the blood, can cause cardiac arrhythmias, hypertension, and tachycardia. Many things can contribute to low magnesium levels including diuretic therapy, digitalis, some antibiotics, diabetes mellitus, and myocardial infarction.

SAFETY TIP

Improve the effectiveness of communication among caregivers. Provide critical results of tests or diagnostic procedures to responsible licensed caregiver within an established time frame so that the patient can be treated promptly (2010 National Patient Safety Goals, www.jointcommission.org).

• **WORD • BUILDING** •

hypomagnesemia: hypo—low + magnes—magnesium + emia—in blood

Invasive Studies

Angiography

Arteriography and venography are the two types of angiography (Fig. 21.13). Arteriography examines arteries. Venography studies veins. Angiography uses dye injected into the vascular system to visualize the vessels on radiographs. This test is used to assess blood clot formation, peripheral vascular disease (PVD), and test vessels for potential grafting use.

The patient must be assessed for allergies, give informed consent, be NPO for about 4 hours before the test, and be informed that the dye produces a hot, burning feeling when injected. After the procedure the patient is assessed for several hours. Vital signs, allergic reaction signs, hemorrhage at the injection site, and pulses are monitored.

Cardiac Catheterization

Cardiac catheterization allows the heart's anatomy and physiology to be studied. It is an invasive diagnostic procedure that measures pressures in the heart chambers, great blood vessels, and coronary arteries and provides information on cardiac output and oxygen saturation. Fluoroscopy, an x-ray procedure that produces real-time images of internal organs in motion on a video monitor, is used to guide the insertion of the catheter into the heart. Dye can be injected once the catheter is in place to visualize the heart chambers and vessels. This procedure is often done before heart surgery.

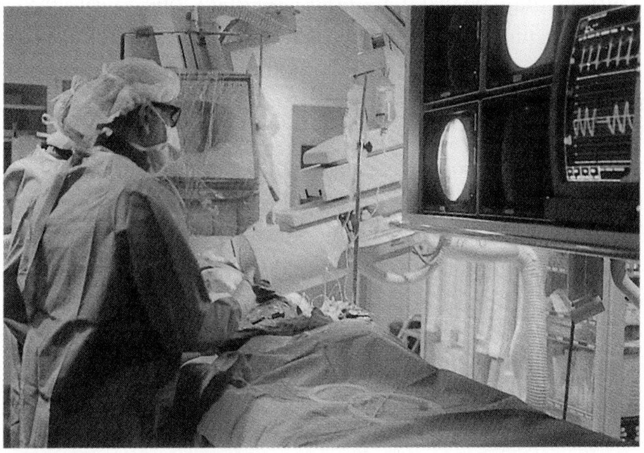

FIGURE 21.13 Coronary angiography and cardiac catheterization.

An informed consent must be obtained. The patient is assessed for allergies to iodine and dyes used in the procedure and kept NPO prior to the procedure. Patients should be told that during the test they will be awake and a warm, flushing sensation may be felt when the dye is injected; the room has a lot of equipment; a movable table is used; the patient's vital signs and ECG are monitored constantly; and the length of the procedure is 2 to 3 hours (see Fig. 21.13).

In right-sided catheterization, a catheter with or without a fiber-optic tip is inserted into the basilic or cephalic vein or the femoral vein and advanced into the vena cava. It is then moved through the right chambers of the heart and into the pulmonary artery. The catheter can be wedged momentarily in the artery by inflating the balloon at the tip of the catheter. This position provides the pulmonary artery wedge pressure (PAWP), which reflects pressures in the left side of the heart. Other pressures obtained with right-sided cardiac catheterization are right atrial pressure, which reflects central venous pressure, pulmonary artery systolic and diastolic pressures, cardiac output, and mixed venous oxygen saturation (Svo_2) if a fiber-optic catheter is used.

The left side of the heart can be directly assessed by inserting a catheter into the brachial or the femoral artery. It is advanced against the flow of blood into the aorta, through the aortic valve, and into the left ventricle. Coronary angiography, which visualizes the coronary arteries with dye, can be done with this approach. The catheter is inserted into the opening of the coronary arteries, the dye is injected, and x-ray films are taken. Coronary artery disease can be assessed with coronary angiography.

After the procedure the catheter is removed and firm pressure must be applied to the insertion site for several minutes to prevent hemorrhage or hematoma formation. A pressure dressing or sandbag may be applied to the site when bleeding is stopped and is removed after several hours. Vital signs are assessed according to the physician's orders and the institution's policies. During vital sign checks, the puncture site is assessed and peripheral pulses are verified. The patient is on bedrest. The extremity used for insertion is not moved or flexed for several hours after the procedure. For comfort, modified positioning and use of a pillow may be used without complications as ordered. Patients usually may eat and are instructed to drink fluids to help eliminate the dye from the body. If the patient is stable and no significant findings are found, the patient may be discharged.

Complications of cardiac catheterization can be allergic reaction, breaking of the catheter, hemorrhage, thrombus formation, emboli of air or blood, dysrhythmias, MI, cerebrovascular accident (CVA), and puncture of the heart chambers or lungs.

Hemodynamic Monitoring

Bedside monitoring can be done to monitor the pressures in the blood vessels or heart. A catheter attached to a transducer and monitor, called an arterial line, can be inserted into the radial or femoral artery to measure continuous arterial blood pressure.

Ongoing monitoring of cardiac pressures, cardiac output, and central venous pressure (CVP) can be done with either a central catheter or a pulmonary artery catheter. Central venous pressure is measured directly with a central catheter inserted into the vena cava via the brachial, femoral, subclavian, or jugular vein (Fig. 21.14). It is measured indirectly with the pulmonary artery catheter (Fig. 21.15). The right atrial pressure measurement obtained from the pulmonary artery catheter reflects the pressure in the vena cava. Central venous pressure measures **preload** (pressure stretching the ventricle of the heart from fluid returned to the heart) or fluid volume status; CVP readings used in fluid or diuretic therapy have been primarily replaced by pulmonary artery catheter measurements.

Electrophysiological Study

To study the heart's electrical system, one or more catheters with electrodes are inserted via the femoral vein into the right side of the heart. Two to three electrodes are inserted usually. The heart's electrical impulses are then recorded and pacing can also be done. Dysrhythmias can be triggered to help the physician diagnose why they are occurring. A consent is obtained and the patient is NPO 6 to 8 hours before the test.

THERAPEUTIC MEASURES FOR THE CARDIOVASCULAR SYSTEM

Exercise

A prescribed walking program helps promote blood flow by contracting the skeletal muscles and may reduce symptoms of peripheral vascular disease. For patients recovering from

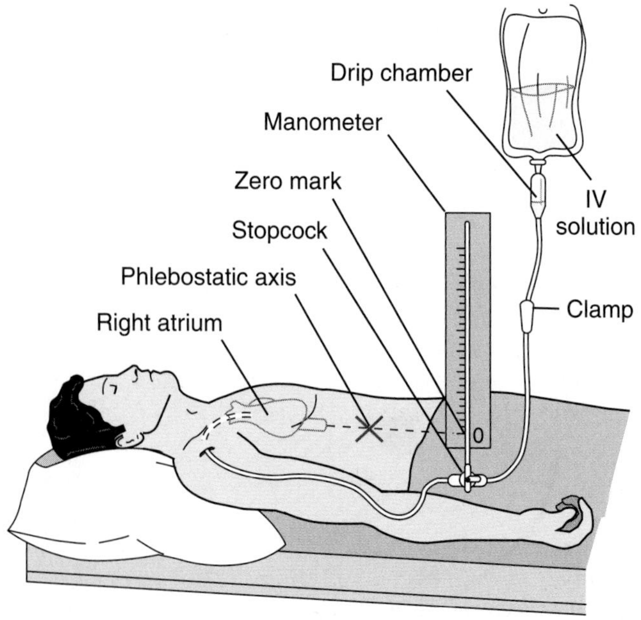
Drip chamber
Manometer
Zero mark
Stopcock
Phlebostatic axis
Right atrium
IV solution
Clamp
0

FIGURE 21.14 Central venous pressure measurement.

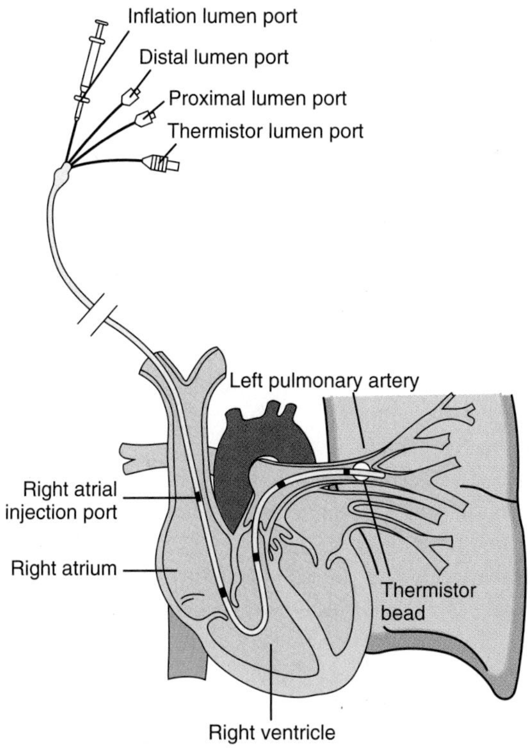
Inflation lumen port
Distal lumen port
Proximal lumen port
Thermistor lumen port
Left pulmonary artery
Right atrial injection port
Right atrium
Thermistor bead
Right ventricle
FIGURE 21.15 Pulmonary artery catheter and placement of the inflated balloon in the pulmonary artery.

cardiac surgery or a myocardial infarction, activity is gradually increased. Exercise is very important for optimum cardiac functioning. A cardiac rehabilitation program is usually prescribed, and individualized exercise goals are determined. After discharge from the hospital, exercise three times a week for 20 to 30 minutes is encouraged.

Smoking Cessation

Smoking causes vasoconstriction that can last up to 1 hour after the smoking of one cigarette. For patients with cardiac or vascular disease, blood flow is reduced, which can exacerbate symptoms. Patients should be encouraged to stop smoking and be provided with support information such as cessation programs and support groups. For more information on smoking cessation, visit www.americanheart.org.

Diet

Teaching the patient to eat a healthy, balanced diet is important to help reduce the risk for coronary artery disease. Weight reduction, if needed, is encouraged, as well as increasing physical activity. Eating at least five servings of fruits and vegetables daily, increasing fish intake, and eating poultry without skin are parts of a healthy diet.

Oxygen

Supplemental oxygen is administered to patients with chest pain to help ensure that the heart receives sufficient oxygen to function. Oxygen may be delivered via a nasal cannula or face mask. The patient must be taught safety precautions necessary for home use of oxygen if it is ordered, such as avoiding open flames and not smoking when the oxygen is in use.

Medications

The primary cardiovascular drugs are cardiac glycosides, vasodilators, antihypertensives, antidysrhythmics, antianginals, anticoagulants, and thrombolytics. They are discussed in further detail where the disorders they are used to treat are discussed (Box 21.5, *Nutrition Notes*).

Antiembolism Devices

Antiembolism devices improve arterial blood flow and venous return to prevent the formation of blood clots. They are used for patients with peripheral vascular disease, on bedrest, or after surgery or trauma.

Elastic Stockings

Antiembolism stockings apply pressure over the leg to promote the movement of fluid and prevent stasis of fluid. These stockings may be knee or thigh length. They must be applied correctly so that a tourniquet effect is not produced by the stockings. For ease in application, the stocking is turned inside out to the heel, the foot portion is placed on the patient up to the heel, and then the remaining stocking is pulled up over the leg. The tops of the stockings should be 1 to 2 inches below the bottom of the kneecap. They should not roll down or they will cause stasis rather than prevent it. Elderly patients may require assistance in applying the stockings if they have impaired manual dexterity.

Intermittent Pneumatic Compression Devices

An intermittent pneumatic compression device consists of plastic inflatable stockings that are filled intermittently with air by an attached motor (Fig. 21.16). This device simulates the contraction of the leg muscles, promoting fluid movement, which helps to prevent thrombosis development. The compartments in the stockings inflate to 35 to 55 mm Hg of pressure, beginning in the ankle compartment and progressing next to the calf compartment and finally the thigh compartment. The nurse should monitor the device for proper pressure inflation.

Lifestyle and Cardiac Care

To reduce risk factors or promote recovery from cardiovascular disease, lifestyle changes are often needed. Longstanding habits are difficult to change. Support groups can offer encouragement that is helpful in promoting a healthy lifestyle. Patients should be referred to community support groups as needed.

Patients recovering from cardiac disorders are often anxious about resuming sexual activity but are embarrassed to discuss it. This is an area that is often overlooked when caring for patients. Sexual counseling should be offered to patients and their partners. Patients often have misconceptions that are unfounded but interfere with resuming sexual activity. If patients have angina, nitroglycerin can be taken prophylactically before sexual activity. After a

Box 21.5

Nutrition Notes

CYP Enzymes and Fruit Juices

Cytochrome P450 (CYP450) is a superfamily of enzymes found mainly in the liver but also in the gastrointestinal tract, lungs, and kidneys. The isoenzyme CYP3A4, found in the small intestine, plays a major role in regulating the oral bioavailability of up to 70% of drugs, a function that may have evolved to protect the body from toxins. After uptake by the intestinal epithelial cells (enterocytes), many substances are metabolized by CYP3A4 or returned to the intestinal lumen by a transporter protein, P-glycoprotein (P-gp), thus limiting the amount of the substance available for absorption.

People show wide variation in the amount of CYP3A4 in the liver and the intestine due to genetic, physiological, and environmental factors with resulting differences in the severity of interactions.

The effect of grapefruit juice on drugs was discovered accidentally when the juice was used to mask the taste of a medication being tested. Grapefruit juice appears to inhibit intestinal CYP3A4 so that the oral bioavailability of affected drugs is increased dramatically, in some cases sufficient to cause drug toxicity or treatment failure. Even when intake of grapefruit juice is stopped, the increased bioavailability of the affected drugs continues for 72 hours until the intestine can manufacture more of the enzyme.

Applying this knowledge to clinical practice is complicated by the fact that even within a given class of drugs, not all are metabolized by CYP3A4. For instance, of calcium channel blockers given to manage hypertension and angina pectoris, grapefruit juice:

- Increases bioavailability of felodipine (Plendil), nisoldipine (Sular), and nicardipine (Cardene).
- Shows little interaction with nifedipine (Adalat) and amlodipine (Norvasc), presumably because they have a higher bioavailability compared with the first three (Dahan & Altman, 2004).

Likewise, differing effects with grapefruit juice are seen with statin drugs, given to lower cholesterol and prevent ischemic heart disease:

- Simvastatin (Zocor) and lovastatin (Altoprev) have greatly increased blood levels when given with grapefruit juice.
- Atorvastatin (Lipitor) showed a lesser effect than the previous two drugs.
- Pravastatin (Pravachol) showed no effect (Dahan & Altman, 2004) because pravastatin is not exclusively metabolized by CYP3A4 (Schmidt & Dalhoff, 2002).

A similar mechanism but a different isoenzyme is proposed to explain an interaction between warfarin (Coumadin) and cranberry juice. Warfarin is mainly metabolized by the cytochrome P450 isoenzyme CYP2C9, and cranberry juice contains flavonoids known to inhibit P450 enzymes. Bleeding problems and hemorrhage have been attributed to this interaction.

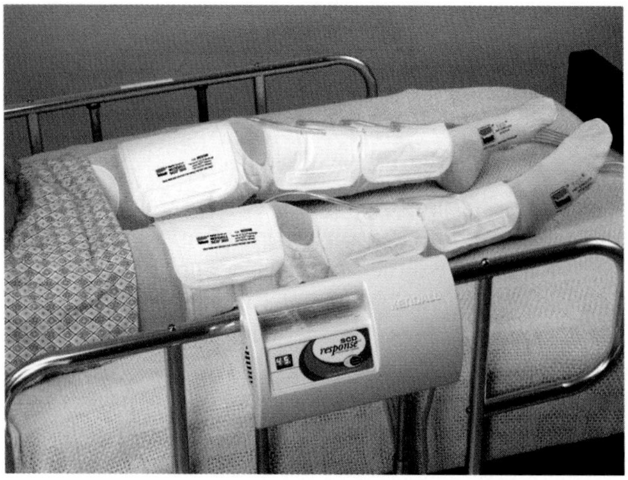
KENDALL
SCD
response

FIGURE 21.16 The Kendall SCD Response Compression system provides sequential personalized compression cycles that minimize stasis and maximize blood flow to prevent thrombosis and pulmonary embolus development. (Courtesy of Kendall, Mansfield, MA.)

myocardial infarction, sexual activity can be resumed in 1 to 2 months or when the patient can climb two flights of stairs without symptoms, as ordered by the physician. Patients should be given information to make an informed decision on when they are ready to resume this physical activity.

Cardiac Surgery

As heart disease symptoms increase in severity and frequency or the disease process worsens, cardiac surgery may be used as treatment.

Preparation for Surgery

A nursing assessment is important to provide baseline data that can be used for postoperative comparison and early discharge planning. In addition to routine admission testing, patients with chronic obstructive pulmonary disease (COPD) may have pulmonary function tests and baseline arterial blood gases (ABGs) done (Box 21.6). Patients with carotid bruits have carotid studies to determine the amount

Box 21.6

Routine Admission Testing

- Twelve-lead electrocardiogram (ECG)
- Chest x-ray exam
- Complete blood cell count (CBC)
- Coagulation studies
- Chemistry profile
- Crossmatched for blood

of occlusion in the carotid artery. If the occlusion is significant, a carotid endarterectomy, which removes the plaque on the lining of the blocked or diseased carotid artery, is performed, usually several weeks before having cardiac surgery.

Medications that may increase bleeding or reduce fluid volume may be ordered by the physician to be held before surgery. Drugs that increase bleeding include aspirin, often stopped 3 to 7 days preoperatively; warfarin (Coumadin), often stopped 4 to 5 days preoperatively; and heparin, usually stopped 4 hours preoperatively. During surgery, fluid volume and blood pressure may be decreased by blood loss or medications. Therefore, diuretics, which could further reduce fluid volume and blood pressure, are withheld up to 2 days before surgery. The patient usually takes nothing by mouth (NPO) 8 to 12 hours before surgery. Due to this, patients who are diabetic have insulin and oral hypoglycemic agents reduced or withheld the morning of surgery with blood glucose monitoring. The anesthesiologist assesses the patient before surgery and orders preoperative medications.

Patients recover more quickly and have less postoperative stress with thorough preoperative teaching. Explanations of expected procedures and care including pain management, endotracheal tube, methods of communicating, ventilator, chest tubes, coughing and deep breathing exercises, intravenous (IV) lines, urinary catheter, incision care, and various equipment alarms are provided to the patient and family. It should be emphasized that patients are not able to talk while the endotracheal tube is in place. Additionally, a preoperative family tour of the patient's postoperative unit and the waiting area helps prepare them for the surgical experience. A referral to pastoral care, if desired, can be comforting to the patient and family.

Cardiopulmonary Bypass

Cardiac surgeries may use a cardiopulmonary bypass pump in which blood is temporarily diverted away from the heart and lungs to the special pump (Fig. 21.17). This diversion allows for a bloodless and motionless surgical field while the function of the heart and lungs is maintained by the pump (Fig. 21.18).

Before going on the pump, the patient is anticoagulated with heparin until the partial thromboplastin time (PTT) is five to six times greater than normal. Immediately before the patient comes off the pump, the effects of the heparin are reversed with protamine sulfate (antidote for heparin). Heparin is absorbed and stored in organs and tissue and can be sporadically released hours after surgery. As a result, the patient may have excessive bleeding. The risk of an air embolism is minimized by priming the pump with lactated Ringer's solution. The priming solution increases circulating volume, which then results in a shifting of fluid into the interstitial tissue and edema formation. These fluid shifts can continue up to 6 hours after surgery and can cause hypotension.

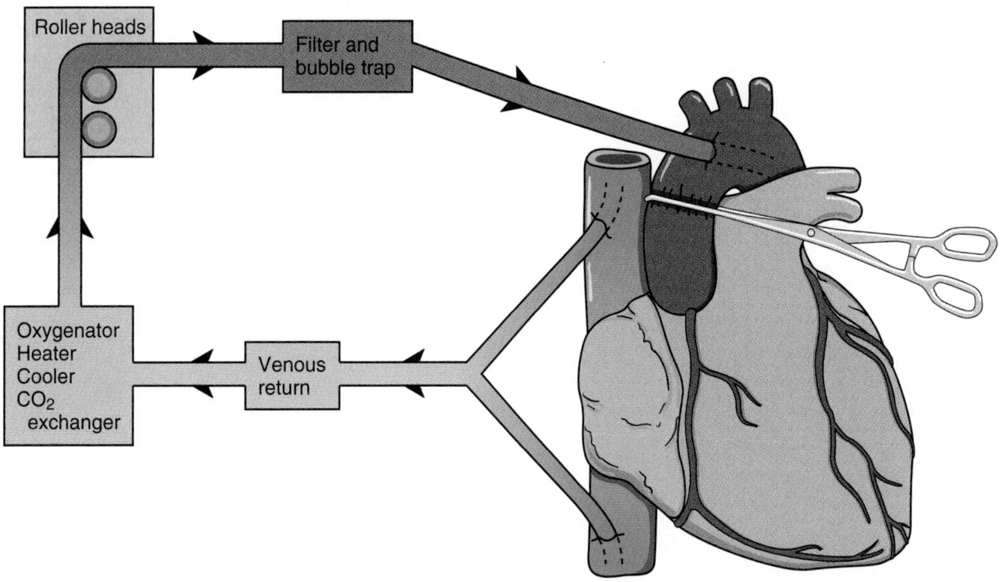
Roller heads
Filter and bubble trap
Oxygenator
Heater
Cooler
CO_2
exchanger
Venous return

FIGURE 21.17 Cardiopulmonary bypass pump components.

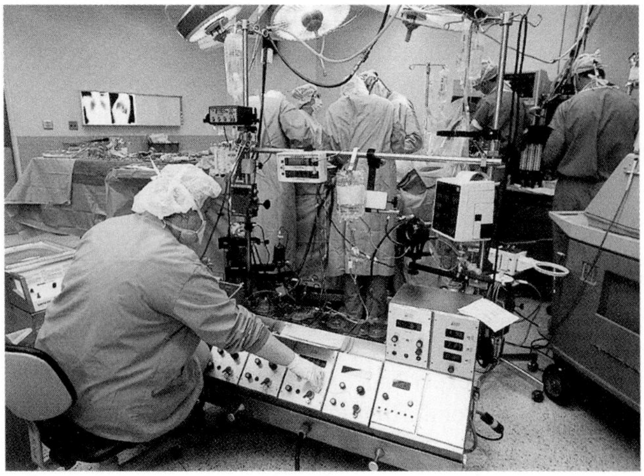

FIGURE 21.18 Cardiopulmonary bypass pump in use.

General Procedure for Cardiac Surgery

After the patient is placed on cardiopulmonary bypass (CPB), a cardioplegic solution is infused into the aortic root along with iced saline to cause cardiac standstill. When the surgery is completed, the patient's blood is warmed in the cardiopulmonary bypass circuit and the patient is slowly weaned from bypass. The heart starts beating again after it is warmed and defibrillated. Temporary pacing wires are attached to the heart before the cardiopulmonary bypass pump is discontinued, so an external temporary pacemaker can be used if bradycardia develops. Once the heart is beating, bypass is stopped. Mediastinal chest tubes are placed to drain remaining blood and fluid from the chest. The **sternotomy** is closed with wires through the sternum and then sutures for the layers of tissue and skin. While still under anesthesia, the patient is transferred to a cardiac care unit. A new trend is the use of cardiac universal beds (CUBs) where patients stay in the same room during their entire hospitalization. The nurse is able to provide care for all levels of recovery.

Minimally Invasive Cardiac Surgery

Less invasive forms of cardiac surgery are also being used. They include minimally invasive direct visualization coronary artery bypass (MIDCAB), which is a technique that is done without the use of cardiopulmonary bypass, and port-access coronary artery bypass, which combines peripheral cardiopulmonary bypass with minimally invasive heart access (see Chapter 24). Risk for complications associated with these surgeries are much lower than with the traditional procedure, and the recovery time is often weeks less.

• WORD • BUILDING •

sternotomy: stern—sternum + otomy—incision into

SUGGESTED ANSWERS TO

CRITICAL THINKING

■ *Mrs. Smith*

1. An older patient commonly does not experience typical disorder symptoms. Chest pain is often not present because of reduced nerve sensitivity with aging for a myocardial infarction. Dyspnea is the classic symptom of myocardial infarction in the older patient.
2. Inspect both legs to determine edematous areas. Determine location and severity of edema by pressing finger for 5 seconds over the medial malleolus and moving up the leg along the tibia until no edema is found. Assess bilaterally. Measure leg circumference.
3. Document location of edema and whether edema is nonpitting or pitting for both legs. Documentation should state "Bilateral pitting ankle edema" with leg circumference measurement number.
4. Additional symptoms should be documented as follows: Dyspnea at rest that increases with exertion, heart tones clear and distant, nailbeds pale, pain free, poor appetite for 2 weeks, 6-pound weight gain in 1 week, three-pillow orthopnea, bilateral jugular venous distention.
5. Unit analysis method:

162 pounds	1 kilogram	= 73.6 kilograms
	2.2 pounds	

REVIEW QUESTIONS

1. The mitral and tricuspid valves prevent backflow of blood from which of the following?
   a. Ventricles to atria when the ventricles contract
   b. Atria to ventricles when the ventricles relax
   c. Ventricles to atria when the atria contract
   d. Atria to ventricles when the atria contract

2. Which of the following describes the purpose of the endocardium of the heart?
   a. Covers the heart muscle and prevents friction.
   b. Supports the coronary blood vessels.
   c. Lines the chambers of the heart and prevents abnormal clotting.
   d. Prevents backflow of blood from atria to ventricles.

3. Which of the following is the function of the coronary arteries?
   a. Prevent abnormal clotting within the heart.
   b. Bring oxygenated blood to the myocardium.
   c. Carry deoxygenated blood to the lungs.
   d. Carry oxygenated blood to the lungs.

4. Where in the nervous system is the cardiac center found?
   a. Cerebrum
   b. Hypothalamus
   c. Spinal cord
   d. Medulla

5. Angiotensin II increases which of the following?
   a. Vasodilation and ADH secretion
   b. Vasoconstriction and aldosterone secretion
   c. Heart rate and vasodilation
   d. Heart rate and ADH secretion

6. The increase of resting blood pressure with age may contribute to which of the following?
   a. Dysrhythmias
   b. Thrombus formation
   c. Left-sided heart failure
   d. Peripheral edema

7. Which of the following is a modifiable cardiovascular risk factor that should be noted during patient data collection?
   a. Age
   b. Gender
   c. Ethnic origin
   d. Tobacco use

8. If it takes longer than 3 seconds for the color to return when assessing capillary refill, which of the following may be indicated?
   a. Decreased arterial flow to the extremity
   b. Increased arterial flow to the extremity
   c. Decreased venous flow from the extremity
   d. Increased venous flow from the extremity

9. Which of the following is an important safety intervention that should be used while assessing a patient for orthostatic hypotension?
   a. Reality orientation
   b. Gait or walking belt
   c. Liquids at bedside
   d. Standing patient quickly

10. In which area should the nurse assess a patient who is on bedrest for the presence of edema?
    a. Arms
    b. Ankles
    c. Sternum
    d. Sacrum

11. Which of the following should be included in patient teaching for a coronary angiography with femoral catheter insertion site? **Select all that apply.**
    a. Dye injection causes hot, flushing sensation.
    b. General anesthesia is administered.
    c. Claustrophobia may be experienced.
    d. Ambulation is not possible immediately after procedure.
    e. Allergies are assessed prior to testing.
    f. Firm pressure must be applied to the insertion site.

12. A high-fiber diet for cardiac patients is recommended for which of the following purposes?
    a. Increase absorption of nutrients.
    b. Reduce cardiac workload.
    c. Reduce edema development.
    d. Reduce appetite.

13. A patient is scheduled for vascular surgery. The patient is taking digoxin (Lanoxin), furosemide (Lasix), potassium, warfarin (Coumadin), and famotidine (Pepcid). Which medication may be stopped by the physician several days before surgery?
    a. Digoxin (Lanoxin)
    b. Furosemide (Lasix)
    c. Warfarin (Coumadin)
    d. Famotidine (Pepcid)

References

American Heart Association. (2009). *Heart disease and stroke statistics—2009 Update.* Dallas, TX: Author. Retrieved November 20, 2009, from http://www.americanheart.org/downloadable/heart/1240250946756LS-1982%20Heart%20and%20Stroke%20Update.042009.pdf

Dahan, A., & Altman, H. (2004). Food–drug interaction: Grapefruit juice augments drug bioavailability—Mechanism, extent and relevance. *European Journal of Clinical Nutrition, 58,* 1.

Joint Commission. (2010). *2010 national patient safety goals.* Retrieved January 13, 2010, from http://www.jointcommission.org/patientsafety/nationalpatientsafetygoals

Schmidt, L. E., & Dalhoff, K. (2002). Food–drug interactions. *Drugs, 62,* 1481.

Tortora, G. J., & Derrickson, B. H. (2005). *Principles of anatomy and physiology* (11th ed., p. 796). New York: John Wiley & Sons.

22

Nursing Care of Patients with Hypertension

LINDA S. WILLIAMS

KEY TERMS

cardiac output (KAR-dee-yak OWT-put)
diastolic blood pressure (dy-uh-STAH-lik BLUHD PREH-shure)
essential hypertension (ee-SEN-shul HY-per-TEN-shun)
hypertension (HY-per-TEN-shun)
hypertensive emergency (HY-per-TEN-siv ee-MUR-gehn-see)
hypertensive urgency (HY-per-TEN-siv UR-gehn-see)
hypertrophy (hy-PER-truh-fee)
isolated systolic hypertension (EYE-suh-lay-ted siss-TALL-lik HY-per-TEN-shun)
normotensive (nor-moe-TEN-siv)
peripheral vascular resistance (puh-RIFF-uh-ruhl VAS-kyoo-lar ree-ZIS-tense)
plaque (PLAK)
primary hypertension (PRY-mare-ee HY-per-TEN-shun)
secondary hypertension (SEK-un-DAR-ee HY-per-TEN-shun)
systolic blood pressure (siss-TALL-ik BLUHD PREH-shure)
viscosity (vis-KAW-sih-tee)

QUESTIONS TO GUIDE YOUR READING

1. How would you explain the pathophysiology of hypertension?
2. What are the causes and risk factors for hypertension?
3. What are the signs and symptoms of hypertension?
4. What current therapeutic measures are used for hypertension?
5. What are the classifications of hypertension in adults and recommendations for treatment?
6. How would you classify hypertensive emergency?
7. What are the common complications of hypertension?
8. What nursing care will you provide for patients with hypertension?
9. How will you know if your nursing interventions have been effective?

During 2005 and 2006, 29% of all U.S. adults age 18 or older had hypertension. The percentage of those with hypertension increases with age, from 7% in those ages 18 to 39 to 67% in those ages 60 or older (Ostchega et al., 2008). The highest occurrence was in non-Hispanic blacks at 41%, then non-Hispanic whites at 28%, followed by Mexican Americans at 22%. The prevalence of hypertension remains high despite effective treatments.

The *Seventh Report of the Joint National Committee on Prevention, Detection, Evaluation and Treatment of High Blood Pressure* (National Heart, Lung, and Blood Institute [NHLBI], 2004), called the JNC 7, redefined normal and abnormal blood pressures for adults ages 18 and older and established treatment guidelines for physicians, clinicians, nurses, and community programs to follow (Table 22.1). The NHLBI of the National Institutes of Health estimated that JNC 8 guidelines would be available in 2011 at www.nhlbi.nih.gov. It is important to stay current in this area to best serve your patients.

It is very important to take blood pressure readings correctly to prevent inaccurate readings. A normal blood pressure (BP) reading is one in which systolic pressure is below 120 mm Hg and diastolic pressure is below 80 mm Hg with the patient in a seated position and the arm supported at heart level (Box 22.1). Prehypertension is a **systolic blood pressure** of 120 to 139 mm Hg or a **diastolic blood pressure** of 80 to 89 mm Hg. **Hypertension**, also known as high blood pressure, is a condition in which the average of at least two or more readings on different dates is above prehypertension levels. For more information on hypertension, visit www.americanheart.org.

• WORD • BUILDING •

systolic: systole—concentration
diastolic: diastole—expansion
hypertension: hyper—excessive + tensio—tension

Box 22.1

Taking Accurate Blood Pressure Measurements

- Use auscultatory method with properly calibrated and validated blood pressure instrument.
- Seat patient quietly for at least 5 minutes in a chair (not on examination table) with feet on the floor and arm supported at heart level.
- Use appropriate-sized cuff in which cuff bladder encircles at least 80% of arm.
- Take at least two blood pressure measurements.
- Systolic blood pressure = first of two or more sounds heard.
- Diastolic blood pressure = disappearance of sounds.
- Provide patients, verbally and in writing, their specific BP reading.

Source: Adapted from NHLBI, 2004.

SAFETY TIP

Research studies show that stethoscopes used by all types of health care providers, such as nurses, physicians, paramedics, and emergency medical technicians, are contaminated with bacteria including methicillin-resistant *Staphylococcus aureus* (MRSA). With infection rates on the rise, keep your patients safe. Clean your stethoscope between *every* patient! (*See Evidence-Based Practice box.*)

TABLE 22.1 BLOOD PRESSURE CATEGORIES AND MEASURES*

Blood Pressure Category	Systolic Pressure (mm Hg)	Diastolic Pressure (mm Hg)	Recommended Follow-Up	Lifestyle Modification	Drug Therapy Without Other Indicators
Normal	Less than 120	Less than 80	2 years	Encourage	None
Pre-hypertension	120–139	80–89	1 year	Yes	None
Stage 1 hypertension	140–159	90–99	2 months	Yes	Thiazide-type diuretics. Consider ACEI, ARB, BB, CCB, or combination.
Stage 2 hypertension	160 or higher	100 or higher	1 month. For BP over 180/110 mm Hg, evaluate and seek treatment immediately; then 1 week as needed.	Yes	Two-drug combination (usually thiazide-type diuretic and ACEI or ARB, or BB or CCB).

*Treatment is based on highest BP category.
ACEI = angiotensin-converting enzyme inhibitor; ARB = angiotensin receptor blocker; BB = beta blocker; CCB = calcium channel blocker.
Source: Adapted from NHLBI, 2004.

EVIDENCE-BASED PRACTICE

Clinical Question

Are stethoscopes contaminated and what is the best way to decontaminate them?

Evidence

In a study comparing an ethanol-based cleanser (EBC) with isopropyl alcohol pads in reducing bacterial contamination of stethoscope diaphragms, 99 stethoscopes were cultured and all were positive for bacterial growth (Lecat et al., 2009). The use of either EBC or isopropyl alcohol reduced the bacteria count significantly.

Implications for Nursing Practice

Stethoscopes become contaminated with use. To protect patients from potential organism transmission and reduce infection, stethoscopes must be cleaned between every patient use by all health care providers. Stethoscopes should be cleaned as often as hands are washed using either EBC or isopropyl alcohol pads.

REFERENCE

Lecat, P., Cropp, E., McCord, G., & Haller, N. (2009). Ethanol-based cleanser versus isopropyl alcohol to decontaminate stethoscopes. *American Journal of Infection Control, 37*(3), 241–243.

PATHOPHYSIOLOGY OF HYPERTENSION

Normally the heart pumps blood through the body to meet the cells' needs for oxygen and nutrients. As it pumps, the heart forces blood through the blood vessels. The pressure exerted by blood on the walls of the blood vessels is measured as blood pressure. Blood pressure is determined by **cardiac output** (CO), **peripheral vascular resistance** (PVR; the ability of the vessels to stretch), the **viscosity** (thickness) of the blood, and the amount of circulating blood volume. Decreased stretching ability of blood vessels, increased blood viscosity, and/or increased fluid volume may cause an increase in blood pressure.

Several processes influence blood pressure. These processes include nervous system regulation, arterial baroreceptors and chemoreceptors, the renin-angiotensin-aldosterone mechanism, and the balance of body fluids. One way blood pressure is influenced is through adjustment of the CO, which is the amount of blood that the heart pumps each minute. The heart rate rises to increase CO in response to physical or emotional activities that increase the need for oxygen in the organs and tissues. PVR also influences blood pressure; it is the opposition that blood encounters as it flows through vessels. Anything causing blood vessels to become narrower increases PVR. Any time PVR is increased, more pressure is needed to push the blood through the vessels, so blood pressure increases as a result. If PVR is decreased, less pressure is needed. Increased arteriolar PVR is the main mechanism that elevates blood pressure in hypertension.

Factors that impair normal regulation of blood pressure may lead to hypertension. Many of these factors are not well understood. Sympathetic nervous system overstimulation, which causes vasoconstriction, can contribute to hypertension. Alterations in baroreceptors and chemoreceptors may also influence the development of hypertension. For example, baroreceptors may become less sensitive from prolonged increases in vessel pressure and subsequently fail to stimulate vasodilation through vessel stretching. Additionally, increases in hormones that cause sodium retention, such as aldosterone, lead to increased fluid retention. Changes in kidney function that alter the excretion of fluid also result in an increase in overall body fluid that may contribute to hypertension.

A study has shown that high blood pressure might be caused by the common virus cytomegalovirus (CMV) (Cheng et al., 2009). By age 40, most adults are infected with CMV, which is a herpes virus, although they remain asymptomatic until a weakened immune system occurs. CMV increases renin, an enzyme associated with high blood pressure, as well as angiotensin 11, a protein involved in high blood pressure. A vaccine for CMV or the use of antiviral medications may reduce cardiovascular disease and hypertension related to CMV infection.

Primary Hypertension

Primary, or **essential**, **hypertension** is the chronic elevation of blood pressure from an unknown cause.

Secondary Hypertension

Secondary hypertension has a known cause. In other words, it is a sign of another problem, such as a kidney abnormality, a tumor of the adrenal gland, or a congenital defect of the aorta. When the cause of secondary hypertension is treated before permanent structural changes occur, blood pressure usually returns to normal.

Isolated Systolic Hypertension

Isolated systolic hypertension (ISH) is a systolic pressure of 140 mm Hg or greater and a diastolic pressure of 90 mm Hg or less. This type of hypertension occurs mainly in the elderly, although it can occur at any age (Box 22.2, *Gerontological Issues*). People with a systolic pressure higher than 140 mm Hg and a diastolic pressure under 90 mm Hg found on two separate readings should be referred to a physician for further evaluation. Treatment of ISH is recommended to decrease cardiovascular disease, especially heart failure episodes and risk of stroke. Lifestyle modifications are usually tried first if the systolic elevation is not too severe. If lifestyle modifications fail to reduce the systolic pressure, antihypertensive medication is added.

• WORD • BUILDING •

viscosity: viscous—sticky

Box 22.2

Gerontological Issues

In the past, it was thought that diastolic pressure was the most important aspect of blood pressure to control. However, it is now known that after age 55, diastolic pressure falls while systolic pressure continues to rise with age. This means that it is important to control systolic blood pressure, not just diastolic pressure, in older adults to prevent heart disease and stroke. In fact, lowering diastolic blood pressure too much may be unhealthy.

Alcohol consumption in the elderly can aggravate age-related hypertension. Guided relaxation has been shown effective in reducing high blood pressure in older adults.

SIGNS AND SYMPTOMS OF HYPERTENSION

Often, hypertension causes no signs or symptoms other than elevated blood pressure readings. As a result, hypertension is referred to as the "silent killer." Patients with hypertension are often first diagnosed when seeking health care for reasons unrelated to hypertension. In a small number of cases, a patient with hypertension may report a headache, bloody nose, severe anxiety, or shortness of breath, although it is usually impossible for a patient to correlate the absence or presence of symptoms with the degree of blood pressure elevation (Table 22.2).

DIAGNOSIS OF HYPERTENSION

Diagnosis of hypertension considers a patient's risk factors for hypertension, a previous diagnosis of hypertension, presence of signs and symptoms, history of kidney or heart disease, and current use of medications. When the average seated blood pressure is above prehypertensive levels of 120 to 139 systolic or 80 to 89 diastolic on two or more occasions, then hypertension is diagnosed (see Table 22.1). Home blood pressure measurements obtained by the patient tend to be lower than the readings in the health care provider's office. They also are closer to the measurements recorded by 24-hour ambulatory monitors, which best indicate cardiovascular risk (Pickering et al., 2008).

The JNC 7 recommends that patients undergo various routine tests to identify damage to organs or blood vessels before beginning therapy for high blood pressure. Tests recommended by JNC 7 include electrocardiogram (ECG), blood glucose level, hematocrit, serum potassium and calcium levels, lipoprotein profile, high-density and low-density lipoprotein cholesterol (HDL-C and LDL-C, respectively), and triglyceride level. These tests help determine if target-organ damage has been caused by elevated blood pressure. An example of this is testing for kidney damage with a urinalysis or serum creatinine level.

RISK FACTORS FOR HYPERTENSION

A combination of genetic (nonmodifiable) and environmental (modifiable) risk factors is thought to be responsible for the development of hypertension, although the cause remains unknown. Nonmodifiable risk factors—those that cannot be changed—include a family history of hypertension, age, ethnicity, and diabetes mellitus. Modifiable risk factors—those that can be changed—include blood glucose level, activity level, smoking, salt and alcohol intake, and newly added insufficient sleep (less than 5 hours per night). Smoking cessation; reduced consumption of salt, caffeine, and alcohol; weight reduction; improved meal planning; increased physical activity; managing stress; and getting adequate sleep can all help to decrease blood pressure.

Nonmodifiable Risk Factors

Family History of Hypertension

Hypertension is more common among people with a family history of hypertension. Indeed, people with a family history

TABLE 22.2 HYPERTENSION SUMMARY

Signs and Symptoms	Often none Increased blood pressure Headache, bloody nose, severe anxiety, or shortness of breath
Diagnosis	Prehypertension is greater than systolic of 120 mm Hg and diastolic of 80 mm Hg. Hypertension is an average blood pressure, using two or more readings on different dates, greater than a systolic of 139 mm Hg and diastolic of 89 mm Hg.
Therapeutic Measures	Lifestyle modification Medications
Complications	Heart failure, myocardial infarction, stroke, renal failure
Priority Nursing Diagnoses	*Deficient Knowledge* *Ineffective Self Health Management*

have almost twice the risk of developing hypertension as those with no family history. People with a family history of hypertension should be encouraged to have their blood pressure checked regularly.

Age

People age differently because of their genetic and environmental risk factors and lifestyle habits. Thus, the results of the aging process may be reflected in wide variations of blood pressure among elderly people. As a person ages, **plaque** builds up in the arteries, and blood vessels become stiffer and less elastic, causing the heart to work harder to force blood through the vessels. These vessel changes increase the amount of work required by the heart to maintain blood flow into the circulation and, consequently, blood pressure increases.

Race and Ethnicity

Box 22.3 (*Cultural Considerations*) discusses hypertension among various ethnic groups.

Diabetes Mellitus

Many adults who have diabetes mellitus also have hypertension. The risk of developing hypertension with a family history of diabetes and obesity is greater than when there is no family history. Lifestyle modifications and adherence to therapy are crucial to prevent the heart attacks, strokes, blindness, and kidney failure associated with high blood glucose and blood pressure levels.

Modifiable Risk Factors

The JNC 7 suggests advising patients with hypertension to make lifestyle modifications. These modifications include weight reduction; adoption of the Dietary Approaches to Stop Hypertension (DASH) eating plan; moderation of dietary sodium, caffeine, and alcohol intake; increased physical activity; and smoking cessation (Box 22.4). Lifestyle modifications are often used with antihypertensive drugs to control hypertension and enhance drug effects (Box 22.5, *Nutrition Notes*).

Weight Reduction

There is a strong relationship between excess body weight and increased blood pressure. Weight reduction is one of the most important lifestyle modifications to lower blood pressure. The health care provider and dietitian should be consulted to help the patient develop a weight-reduction plan.

Meal Planning

SALT. High blood pressure is associated with a diet high in salt. Patients whose blood pressure can be lowered by restricting dietary sodium are called salt sensitive. This

Box 22.3

Cultural Considerations

Hypertension continues to be the most serious health problem affecting African Americans in the United States. These patients suffer higher mortality and morbidity rates related to hypertension and at an earlier age than all other ethnic groups. African Americans from lower socioeconomic backgrounds have higher blood pressure than African Americans from higher socioeconomic backgrounds. Additionally, African Americans are three to four times more likely to develop kidney failure related to hypertension than European Americans. Addressing obesity, high sodium intake, low potassium intake, and lack of physical activity is especially important for cardiovascular health in African Americans.

Hypertension among African Americans is usually caused by increased renin activity, resulting in greater sodium and fluid retention. Thus, African Americans respond better to diuretics such as furosemide (Lasix) and hydrochlorothiazide (HydroDIURIL) than to beta blockers such as propranolol (Inderal). Hypertension among European Americans is more often caused by chemical imbalances; thus, they respond better to beta blockers.

Chinese people are more sensitive than Caucasians to the effects of propranolol on heart rate and blood pressure, requiring only half the blood level of European Americans to achieve a therapeutic effect. Propranolol is eliminated from the bodies of many Chinese people at double the rate of European Americans. They are more likely to suffer fatigue as a side effect. Thus, the nurse must carefully monitor the Chinese patient for therapeutic and side effects.

Hypertension among Japanese Americans is primarily related to the high sodium content of the Japanese diet, stress, and a high rate of cigarette smoking.

High rates of hypertension among Koreans and Filipinos are due to the stress of immigration, salt preservatives in their foods, and the use of condiments high in sodium.

Box 22.4

Lifestyle Modifications for Hypertension

- Stop smoking.
- Limit alcohol intake.
- Decrease amount of salt intake.
- Obtain daily allowances of potassium and calcium.
- Reduce dietary saturated fat and cholesterol.
- Lose weight.
- Get regular aerobic exercise such as walking for 30 minutes.
- Get adequate sleep (more than 5 hours).

Also see Box 22.5, *Nutrition Notes.*

Source: Adapted from NHLBI, 2004.

sensitivity is particularly common among African Americans, elderly persons, and patients with diabetes and obesity. Patients with hypertension should be instructed not to add salt while cooking and/or table salt to their food. Processed foods and foods in which salt can be easily tasted (e.g., canned soups, ham, bacon, salted nuts) should also be avoided.

CAFFEINE. Intake of caffeine should be limited because it can increase aortic stiffness. This raises the risk of cardiovascular disease for those with high blood pressure.

POTASSIUM, MAGNESIUM, AND CALCIUM. The JNC 7 recommends a balanced diet that ensures adequate intake of potassium, magnesium, and calcium. Low levels of these nutrients can contribute to cardiovascular events. Foods rich in potassium include oranges, bananas, and broccoli. Magnesium is found in green vegetables such as spinach, nuts, seeds, and some whole grains. Milk, yogurt, and spinach are rich in calcium. Whenever possible, fresh or frozen foods should be selected rather than canned foods to increase intake of these nutrients.

Alcohol Consumption

The regular consumption of three or more drinks per day can increase the risk of hypertension and cause resistance to antihypertensive therapy. The nurse should counsel hypertensive patients who drink alcohol to consume no more than 1 oz of ethanol per day for men (two drinks) and no more than 1/2 oz per day for women (one drink). "One drink" is defined as 1.5 oz of 80-proof liquor, 12 oz of beer, or 5 oz of wine (NHLBI, 2004). Blood pressure may decrease or return to normal when alcohol consumption is modified.

Box 22.5

Nutrition Notes

Reducing Blood Pressure with Diet

The Dietary Approaches to Stop Hypertension (DASH) diet reduced blood pressure significantly in **normotensive** people and produced even greater reductions in hypertensive people in an 8-week trial. The DASH diet was especially effective for African Americans. Rather than emphasizing food restriction, the DASH diet increases the intake of certain commonly available, not specialty, foods. On a 2,000-calorie diet, a person following the DASH diet would consume the following:

Food Group	Number of Servings	Example of One Serving
Grains	7–8	• 1 slice of bread • ½ cup cooked cereal or pasta
Vegetables	4–5	• 1 cup raw leafy • ½ cup cooked, nonstarchy
Fruits	4–5	• 1 medium fresh • ½ cup canned or frozen • ¼ cup dried
Low-fat or nonfat dairy	2–3	• 8 ounces of milk • 1½ ounces of cheese
Lean meat, poultry, or fish	2 or fewer	• 3 ounces cooked
Fats and oils, preferably monounsaturated (canola, olive, peanut)	2½	• 1 teaspoonful
Nuts, seeds, legumes	4–5 weekly	• ⅓ cup of nuts • 2 tablespoonfuls of seeds • ½ cup cooked beans

Exercise

People with sedentary lifestyles have an increased risk of hypertension. Exercise helps prevent and control hypertension by reducing weight, decreasing peripheral resistance, and decreasing body fat. Anyone who is able should participate in regular aerobic physical activity, such as brisk walking, for at least 30 minutes daily on most days of the week. Patients with hypertension should be evaluated by a health care provider before starting an exercise program.

Smoking

Smoking is a major risk factor for cardiovascular disease. Blood pressure may increase because nicotine constricts the blood vessels. Nurses should counsel patients with hypertension to quit smoking to reduce overall cardiovascular risk. A referral to a smoking cessation program can be helpful in reaching this goal.

CRITICAL THINKING

Ms. Miller

■ Ms. Miller, age 54, visits a health clinic because she has a headache every morning. The nurse collects data on Ms. Miller and finds that she is an office manager, smokes a pack of cigarettes a day, eats fast food for lunch at her desk, has two adult children, is recently divorced, and has two to three alcoholic drinks every evening. Ms. Miller has been in good health and takes two aspirin tablets for her headaches daily.

1. What are Ms. Miller's risk factors for hypertension?
2. What is the most significant patient information identified? Why?
3. Why is hypertension referred to as the "silent killer"?
4. Why should Ms. Miller be told of the need for lifelong therapy if she is diagnosed with hypertension?

Suggested answers at end of chapter.

THERAPEUTIC MEASURES FOR HYPERTENSION

The JNC 7 provides guidelines for selecting therapy based on the patient's blood pressure, severity of blood pressure risk factors, and the presence of target-organ disease or cardiovascular disease. The no- or low-risk hypertensive patient's therapy begins with lifestyle modifications. If lifestyle modifications alone do not result in blood pressure reaching the target goal, then drug therapy is recommended. For patients with severe hypertension, high-risk factors, or target-organ disease, drug therapy is started immediately along with lifestyle modifications. Safe administration of medications is important, especially for the older person (Box 22.6, *Gerontological Issues*).

Box 22.6

Gerontological Issues

Managing Antihypertensive Therapy

For safety, teach older adults who take antihypertensive drugs to rise slowly to prevent the effects of orthostatic hypotension. Dizziness may increase the risk of falling.

Deficiencies in fluid volume can be a common problem for older adults as well, and diuretics can contribute to them. Careful monitoring of fluid balance is important to prevent dehydration.

Older adults may be more sensitive to medications, so monitor them carefully for adverse effects. Older patients may need lower dosages.

The goal of therapeutic intervention is a blood pressure lower than 140/90 mm Hg (lower than 130/80 mm Hg for those with diabetes, chronic kidney disease, or proteinuria of more than 1 g/day). For most patients with hypertension, initial drug therapy often involves thiazide-type diuretics (see *Evidence-Based Practice* box). If the response is inadequate to achieve the blood pressure goal, the dosage may be increased or a second drug from a different class may be added. Usually two, and sometimes three or four, medications for resistant hypertension are needed. Combination forms of medications are available.

Several types of medications are used to treat hypertension. See Table 22.3 for examples of these medications. At the American Society of Hypertension's Twenty-Third Annual Scientific Meeting and Exposition (called ASH 2008),

EVIDENCE-BASED PRACTICE

Clinical Question

For elevated blood pressure, what drug class should be used first?

Evidence

A systematic review of 24 random controlled trials comparing the effects of first-line drugs for hypertension showed that a low-dose thiazide diuretic reduces all morbidity and mortality outcomes, while other first-line drugs even at higher doses did not (Wright & Musini, 2009).

Implications for Nursing Practice

Understanding the effects of medication administered is beneficial for monitoring outcomes of treatment and providing patient teaching.

REFERENCE

Wright, J. M., & Musini, V. M. (2009). First-line drugs for hypertension. *Cochrane Database of Systematic Reviews 2009, Issue 3* (Art. No. CD001841; DOI 10.1002/14651858.CD001841.pub2).

TABLE 22.3 MEDICATIONS USED TO TREAT HYPERTENSION

Medication Class/Action	Examples	Route	Side Effects	Nursing Implications
Diuretics Increase urine output by inhibiting sodium and water reabsorption by the kidney. Several types.				Take with food to prevent GI upset. Monitor I&O and weight to determine fluid loss. Assess for improvement of edema in patients with HF and reduced BP in hypertension. Electrolyte imbalances may occur quickly. Teach patient to take during awake hours to prevent excessive urination during sleeping hours.
Thiazide and Thiazide-Like Diuretics Increase urine output by promoting sodium, chloride, and water excretion. No immediate effect. Most effective in normal renal function. Also causes loss of sodium potassium, magnesium. Calcium saved.	*Thiazide:* hydrochlorothiazide (HydroDIURIL) chlorothiazide (Diuril) *Thiazide-like:* chlorthalidone (Hygroton) indapamide (Lozol) metolazone (Zaroxolyn)	PO	Dizziness, fatigue, weakness, hypokalemia, hypercalcemia, nausea, vomiting, anorexia, hyperglycemia, rash	Blood glucose may increase in diabetics. Teach patient to wear sunscreen and protective clothing to prevent photosensitivity. Hypercalcemia could be hazardous to patient on digoxin.
Loop Diuretics Act on ascending loop of Henle in kidney to cause sodium and water loss. Also causes loss of potassium, magnesium, and calcium.	bumetanide (Bumex) furosemide (Lasix) torsemide (Demadex)	PO, IV, IM	Hyperkalemia, rash, nausea, hypoglycemia, tinnitus, rash, increased uric acid levels	Contraindicated if allergic to sulfonamides. Teach patient to use sunscreen to prevent photosensitivity. Take with food or milk to prevent GI upset.
Potassium-Sparing Diuretics Mild diuretic. Can be used as combination therapy. Promote sodium and water excretion and potassium retention by the kidney.	amiloride (Midamor) spironolactone (Aldactone)	PO	Hyperkalemia, headache, nausea, vomiting, anorexia, diarrhea, rash, itching	Avoid foods rich in potassium such as oranges, bananas, salt substitutes, dried fruits. Triamterene: Take after meals for GI upset; may turn urine blue.
Sympatholytics ***Beta Blockers*** Decrease sympathetic nervous system response, resulting in decreased blood pressure, heart rate, contractility, cardiac output, and renin activity.	atenolol (Tenormin) metoprolol (Lopressor) metoprolol, extended release (Toprol XL) nadolol (Corgard) propranolol (Inderal) propranolol, long acting (Inderal LA)	PO IV form available for atenolol, metoprolol, and propranolol	Orthostatic hypotension, decreased heart rate, diarrhea, nausea, vomiting, bronchospasm, blood dyscrasias, and HF	Daily I&O and weight. Check heart rate and blood pressure before administration. Teach patient not to stop drug abruptly to avoid rebound hypertension, angina, or dysrhythmias. **High alert:** IV vasoactive medications are inherently dangerous. Oral and parenteral doses of propranolol are not interchangeable; IV dose is 1/10 the oral dose. Patient harm or fatalities have occurred when switching from oral to IV route.

Alpha$_1$ Blockers				
Block effects of sympathetic nervous system on smooth muscle of blood vessels, resulting in vasodilation and decreased blood pressure.	prazosin (Minipress) terazosin (Hytrin)	PO	Hypotension, increased heart rate, nasal stuffiness, nausea, vomiting, diarrhea	Monitor for hypotension. Teach to make position changes slowly.
Combined Alpha and Beta Blockers				
Block alpha-adrenergic receptors, causing vasodilation and reduced blood pressure. Decrease sympathetic nervous system response, resulting in decreased heart rate and contractility.	carvedilol (Coreg) labetalol (Normodyne)	PO IV form available for labetalol	Dizziness, diarrhea, nausea, vomiting, tinnitus, bradycardia, postural hypotension, sexual dysfunction, high blood sugar	Daily I&O and weight. Assess heart rate before administration. Assess edema, neck vein distention, lung sounds. Teach patient not to stop drug abruptly.
Central Acting Alpha$_2$ Agonists				
Block effects of sympathetic nervous system centrally.	clonidine (Catapres) guanfacine HCl (Tenex) methyldopa (Aldomet)	PO Transdermal patch available for clonidine IV methyldopa	Drowsiness, sedation, headache, fatigue, nausea, vomiting, malaise, dry mouth, rash, postural hypotension, palpitations	Assess for edema and/or decreased BP. Suggest gum or hard candy for dry mouth. Teach not to stop drug abruptly.
Angiotensin-Converting Enzyme (ACE) Inhibitors				
Blocks production of angiotensin II, a potent vasoconstrictor. Reduces peripheral arterial resistance and blood pressure.	benazepril HCl (Lotensin) captopril (Capoten) enalapril (Vasotec) fosinopril (Monopril) lisinopril (Prinivil, Zestril) moexipril (Univasc) perindopril (Aceon) quinapril (Accupril) ramipril (Altace) trandolapril (Mavik)	PO Also: IV enalapril, SL captopril	Hypotension, increased heart rate, dyspnea, cough, angioedema	Monitor patient for edema with HF and decreased BP with hypertension. Teach patient that sensitivity to sunlight may occur. Advise against stopping drug abruptly.
Angiotensin II Receptor Antagonists (ARB)				
Block angiotensin II receptors causing vasodilation and reduction in blood pressure.	candesartan (Atacand) eprosartan (Teveten) irbesartan (Avapro) losartan (Cozaar) olmesartan (Benicar) telmisartan (Micardis) valsartan (Diovan)	PO	Dizziness, insomnia, diarrhea, cough	Monitor patient for edema with HF and decreased BP with hypertension. Teach patient sensitivity to sunlight may occur.

Continued

TABLE 22.3 MEDICATIONS USED TO TREAT HYPERTENSION—cont'd

Medication Class/Action	Examples	Route	Side Effects	Nursing Implications
Aldosterone Receptor Antagonist				
Blocks binding of aldosterone at receptor site to reduce sodium reabsorption and then blood pressure.	eplerenone (Inspra)	PO	Headache, dizziness, angina, hyperkalemia, increased creatinine	Monitor potassium before and during therapy.
Calcium Channel Blockers				
Prevent movement of extracellular calcium into the cell which vasodilates.	amlodipine (Norvasc) diltiazem (Cardizem) felodipine (Plendil) isradipine (DynaCirc) nicardipine HCl (Cardene, Cardene SR) nifedipine (Procardia) nisoldipine (Sular) verapamil (Calan SR, Isoptin SR)	PO IV form available for diltiazem, verapamil, nicardipine	Dysrhythmias, edema, headache, fatigue, drowsiness, flushing	Take pulse before administration. Assess for decreased BP, heart rate dysrhythmias, angina. May increase blood levels of digoxin.
Direct Vasodilators				
Relax smooth muscles of blood vessels, causing vasodilation and decreased blood pressure.	hydralazine (Apresoline) minoxidil (Loniten)	PO, IV, IM	Headache, nausea, hypotension or hypertension and changes in heart rhythm	Treat headache with acetaminophen. Monitor for increasing heart rate. Often given with diuretic to reduce edema resulting from water and sodium retention.

HF = heart failure; I&O = input and output; PO = oral; IV = intravenous; IM = intramuscular.

a study was presented that showed aspirin reduces blood pressure if taken at night rather than in the morning.

> **SAFETY TIP**
>
> Clonidine, an alpha-adrenergic agonist, and clonazepam, a benzodiazepine, have look-alike and sound-alike drug names. Be aware of drug names that look alike and sound alike to prevent errors involving these drugs.

The treatment plan of lifestyle modifications and medications is effective only when patients are motivated to accept the diagnosis of hypertension and include lifelong treatment in their daily routine. Empathy and trust can increase patient motivation. Patients should be instructed that antihypertensive therapy usually must be continued for the rest of their lives. Patients should be reminded that although they may be feeling better with the modifications and medications, the hypertension is still present even if it is well controlled. Patients should be told not to stop taking their medications unless instructed to do so by their primary care provider.

Antihypertensive medications can have unpleasant side effects. Patients should be told what these side effects are and to report them if they occur, so that medications can be altered if possible. Erectile dysfunction can be one of the side effects of these medications. Men may be reluctant to discuss this side effect and instead choose to stop the medication. The nurse should be proactive and inform men about this side effect so they will understand that, if it occurs and is reported, the primary care provider can make adjustments in the medication regimen.

> **LEARNING TIP**
>
> Walking for 30 minutes is an effective way to lower blood pressure, as is listening to 30 minutes of classical, Celtic, or raga music daily. Transcendental meditation has also been shown to help control high blood pressure.
>
> Here are additional, important lifestyle modifications arranged in an easy-to-remember mnemonic:
>
> L—Limit salt, caffeine, and alcohol.
> I—Include daily potassium and calcium.
> F—Fight fat and cholesterol.
> E—Exercise regularly (walking).
> S—Stay on your blood pressure regimen.
> T—Try to quit smoking.
> Y—Your medications are to be taken daily.
> L—Lose weight.
> E—End-stage complications will be avoided!

COMPLICATIONS OF HYPERTENSION

Common complications of hypertension include coronary artery disease, atherosclerosis, myocardial infarction (MI), heart failure (HF), stroke, and kidney or eye damage. The severity and duration of the increase in blood pressure determine the extent of the vascular changes causing organ damage. High blood pressure levels may also increase the size of the left ventricle, referred to as **hypertrophy**. Over time elevated blood pressure damages the small vessels of the heart, brain, kidneys, and retina. The results are a progressive functional impairment of these organs, known as target-organ disease.

SPECIAL CONSIDERATIONS

Blood pressure should be well controlled before the patient has any invasive procedure. Hypertensive patients are at greater risk for strokes, MI, HF, kidney failure, and pulmonary edema. These patients should be instructed to continue their blood pressure medications until the time of the procedure, unless otherwise directed by their primary care provider. Antihypertensive medications should be resumed as soon as possible after the procedure, as directed by the provider.

> **CRITICAL THINKING**
>
> ***Mrs. Bell***
>
> ■ Mrs. Bell, 80 years old, is seen in her physician's office. She lives a sedentary lifestyle alone in her own home with a bathroom down the hall from the bedroom. Mrs. Bell's son lives in the same city and visits her often. She has wood floors with throw rugs in the hall and a tile floor in the bathroom. She wears glasses and has a cataract. She has an unsteady gait and nocturia. She is 40 pounds overweight and has a 10-year history of hypertension for which she is taking chlorothiazide (Diuril) and propranolol (Inderal) when she remembers them.
>
> 1. What are Mrs. Bell's modifiable and nonmodifiable risk factors for hypertension?
> 2. Why is Mrs. Bell taking chlorothiazide and propranolol to treat her hypertension?
> 3. What teaching methods could be used to help ensure that Mrs. Bell will understand and follow her treatment plan?
> 4. Why should patient safety needs be addressed in the nursing care plan?
> 5. What safety interventions should the patient and family be taught?
>
> *continued*

CRITICAL THINKING—cont'd

6. Inderal 20 mg PO is ordered now because Mrs. Bell forgot to take her medication. The nurse has on hand Inderal 10-mg tablets. How many tablets should the nurse give?

Suggested answers at end of chapter.

HYPERTENSIVE EMERGENCY

Hypertensive emergency is a severe type of hypertension characterized by elevations in systolic blood pressure greater than 180 mm Hg and diastolic blood pressure greater than 120 mm Hg that are complicated by a risk for or progression of target-organ dysfunction (examples include MI, HF, and dissecting aortic aneurysm). Patients who are untreated, fail to comply with antihypertensive therapy, or stop their medication abruptly are at risk for hypertensive emergency.

These patients require immediate reduction of blood pressure to prevent or limit damage to target organs. Patients with hypertensive crises should be admitted to the critical care unit. In some cases, the blood pressure may need to be reduced by 25% within 1 hour to prevent organ damage. If the patient is stable, blood pressure is then decreased to 160/100 to 110 mm Hg in the next 2 to 6 hours. Gradual reduction of blood pressure is desired to prevent decreased blood flow to the kidneys, heart, and/or brain. An intravenous medication such as nitroprusside (Nipride) may be given to quickly reduce blood pressure during the crisis.

HYPERTENSIVE URGENCY

The JNC 7 considers **hypertensive urgency** to occur in situations when blood pressure is as elevated as in a hypertensive emergency but without progression of target-organ dysfunction. A patient with hypertensive urgency may have severe headaches, nosebleeds, shortness of breath, and severe anxiety. Patients with hypertensive urgency usually can be treated with combination oral medication and scheduled for a follow-up visit within several days.

NURSING PROCESS FOR THE PATIENT WITH HYPERTENSION

Data Collection

Data collection for a patient with hypertension includes the patient's health history, blood pressure measurements, medications, and physical assessment (Fig. 22.1). Determining what hypertensive patients and their families know about hypertension and associated risk factors is essential for planning patient and family education and subsequent lifelong lifestyle modification needs.

Nursing Diagnoses, Planning, Interventions, and Evaluation

Possible nursing diagnoses, planning, interventions, and evaluation must be agreed on by the patient and the health care team. See the *Nursing Care Plan for the Patient with Hypertension.*

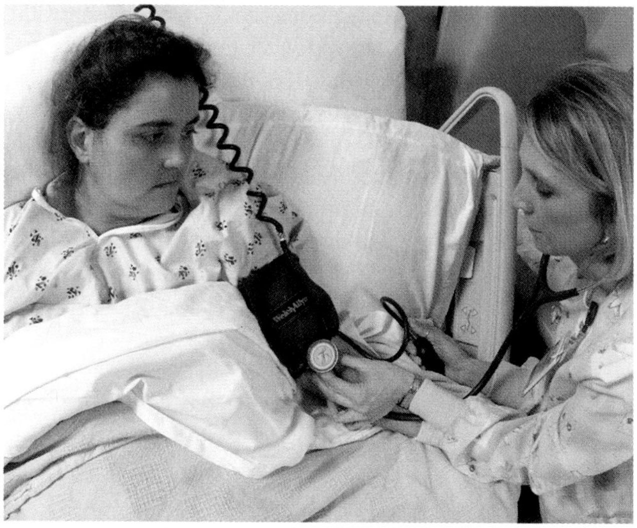

FIGURE 22.1 Nurse obtaining blood pressure measurement. Correct size cuff use is essential for accurate reading.

NURSING CARE PLAN for the Patient with Hypertension

Nursing Diagnosis: *Deficient Knowledge* related to disease process and treatment regimen

Expected Outcomes: The patient will verbalize knowledge of disease process and treatment regimen.

Evaluation of Outcomes: Is patient able to discuss and explain hypertension disease process, including its risk factors, complications, and treatment regimen?

Intervention	Rationale	Evaluation
Identify patient's readiness and ability to learn.	Patient must accept ownership of hypertension diagnosis and be able to receive and understand information given. Determine patient's preferred method of learning.	Does patient verbalize acceptance of hypertension diagnosis? Does patient demonstrate ability to read, write, and retain information?
Provide patient with information concerning disease process including risk factors, complications, and treatment regimen.	Patient will be more willing to participate in treatment regimen when able to understand need for changes in behavior.	Is patient able to participate in discussion concerning hypertension disease process including risk factors, complications, and treatment regimen?

Nursing Diagnosis: *Ineffective Self Health Management* related to complexity of therapy, cost of medications, lack of symptoms, side effects of medications, need to alter long-term lifestyle habits, normal blood pressure controlled by therapy

Expected Outcomes: The patient will verbalize ability and willingness to comply with treatment.

Evaluation of Outcomes: Is patient able to state how lifestyle will include therapy? Does patient identify and problem solve barriers for therapy?

Intervention	Rationale	Evaluation
Identify patient's modifiable risk factors and lifestyle modification needs.	Identifying risk factors is the first step in planning therapy. Patient must understand the relationship of these risk factors with hypertension and complication development.	Can patient state rationale for modifying risk factors to prevent complication development?
Identify factors that are barriers to patient complying with therapy.	Factors such as finances, transportation, aging changes, patient motivation, habits, and reading and educational level can be barriers for therapy.	Are barriers present for patient?

Continued

NURSING CARE PLAN for the Patient with Hypertension—cont'd

Intervention	Rationale	Evaluation
Develop plan to overcome barriers. Make referrals as needed.	Identified barriers can be overcome with planning and intervention, such as referral to support groups or for financial assistance or prescription delivery service, and instructions provided at level of patient's learning ability.	Have barriers been eliminated? Is patient willing to use referrals?
Assess ability to take medications daily: financially, obtaining refills, understanding directions.	Elderly patients may be on a fixed income, lack transportation, or lack ability to take several medications several times a day. Simplifying this process, to one medication if possible, can increase compliance.	Is patient able to obtain medications? Can patient self-administer medications accurately on daily basis?
Teach patient to take medications as prescribed and not to skip dosages.	Elderly patients may skip dosages to save money, reduce side effects, or reduce need to void.	Does patient take dosages as prescribed? Does patient express concern over cost, side effects, or frequent voiding?
Teach patient to change positions slowly to prevent falls.	Antihypertensive medications can cause hypotension, resulting in dizziness and weakness and possibly leading to falls.	Does patient understand how to change positions slowly? Does patient experience dizziness or weakness?

Home Health Hints

- Discuss medication usage with the patient, and count the number of remaining pills in the patient's pill bottles, if needed, to assess compliance. Remind the patient to get refills and keep medical appointments by writing them on a calendar.
- Monitor carefully for symptoms of congestive heart failure if the patient takes a beta blocker. This is a side effect that needs to be caught early and reported to the primary care provider.
- Instruct patients to take medication as prescribed even if they are feeling well or if side effects, which they should report, are present. Medication compliance can be a challenge for the elderly patient with hypertension. If medicines are too expensive for the patient, check with the primary care provider and pharmacist for less expensive alternatives.
- Encourage the patient to obtain a home blood pressure monitoring device. Instruct the patient or caregiver on proper use and logging the date, time, and reading obtained. The home health nurse should review the log on each visit.
- Teach the patient or caregiver to take the patient's pulse and to call the nurse if it is below 60 beats per minute or the parameters defined by the primary care provider or agency. Many antihypertensive medicines can cause bradycardia.
- Instruct patients to weigh themselves every morning after voiding, to wear the same amount of clothing each time, and to keep a log for the nurse to review.
- Advise patients who are leaving home for the weekend or holidays to refill medicines ahead of time to make sure they do not run out. The primary care provider can write a prescription for the patient to have for emergency refills.
- Assist the patient with meal planning. Since most patients eat fast foods occasionally, help them identify

Home Health Hints—cont'd

foods that are low in fat, sugar, and salt (e.g., chicken salads with low-fat dressing or fajitas without sour cream and guacamole).

- Discuss with the RN if the DASH (Dietary Approaches to Stop Hypertension) eating plan would be appropriate for the patient (see www.nhlbi.nih.gov/health/public/heart/hbp/dash/new_dash.pdf).
- Instruct patients and caregivers to avoid frozen dinners and deli meats because many are high in sodium.
- Teach patient to consult primary care provider about use of salt substitutes, which often contain potassium, because medication and electrolyte interactions can occur.
- Teach patients how to read food labels for fat and salt content. If patients are on a 2- to 3-g sodium diet, instruct them about eating breads or cereals that contain 200 mg or less of sodium per serving or canned vegetables that contain 150 mg of sodium per serving. Fresh vegetables are better, but cost and storage must be considered. Providing written suggestions for the caregiver who does the grocery shopping increases compliance with diet therapy.
- Provide the following suggestions to help a patient decrease or stop smoking: Use cinnamon mouthwash on arising; put away all ashtrays but one, and keep it in a place not normally used for smoking; find ways to keep hands busy at times when usually holding a cigarette, such as when drinking coffee or alcohol.
- Encourage patients to put "No Smoking" signs on their door to avoid passive smoking.
- Promote home exercise if cleared by primary care provider. Weights for exercising can be improvised using canned goods and bags of sugar. The amount of weight being used is easily identified for documentation by the labeling on the food item.

SUGGESTED ANSWERS TO CRITICAL THINKING

■ Ms. Miller

1. Risk factors include gender; age; smoking; a diet high in fat, salt, and calories; consumption of two to three alcoholic drinks per evening; and possibly her morning headaches.
2. Morning headaches. Ms. Miller may be experiencing an episode of hypertensive urgency and should be evaluated immediately by a health care provider.
3. "Silent killer" refers to the fact that there are often no signs or symptoms associated with hypertension.
4. Lifelong therapy is required because there is no cure for hypertension and complications need to be prevented.

■ Mrs. Bell

1. Nonmodifiable risk factors include age, gender, and history of hypertension. Modifiable risk factors include weight and compliance with antihypertensive therapy.
2. Thiazide diuretics are first-line drugs. Diuretics remove excess salt and water to decrease blood volume and lower blood pressure. Beta blockers stop the beta receptors from receiving the message from the brain for the heart to work harder. Therefore, the heart rate and blood pressure decrease.
3. Identify patient's reading level and primary language. Provide patient with written instructions in large letters about medications. Include family members and enlist their support in reinforcing the importance of adhering to the treatment plan.
4. Patient is 80 years old, makes frequent trips to the bathroom related to diuretics, has vision problems, and a side effect of propranolol is weakness and fatigue.
5. Make arrangements for a bedside commode to reduce the distance and urgency to get to the bathroom. Encourage the patient and family to place night-lights in the bedroom, hall, and bathroom. Explain that throw rugs increase the risk of falling and that wood or tile floors can be slippery when wet and hard if a fall occurs. Encourage removal of throw rugs, and suggest carpeting these areas if possible. Suggest the use of safety bars in the hall and bathroom for support or other walking aids as needed. If incontinence is a concern, suggest wearing an adult brief to prevent a wet, slippery floor. Suggest discussing with the physician an exercise program to increase strength, such as lifting small, lightweight objects (e.g., soup can), squeezing a rubber ball, or riding an exercise bike if able. These exercises can be done while sitting so they are not a fall-risk activity.
6. Unit analysis method:

$$\frac{20\text{ mg} \mid 1\text{ tablet}}{\quad \mid 10\text{ mg}} = 2\text{ tablets}$$

REVIEW QUESTIONS

1. Which of the following does the nurse understand is a cause of primary hypertension when planning care for a patient with hypertension?
   a. It is caused by a tumor of the adrenal gland.
   b. It is caused by renal artery stenosis.
   c. It is caused by coarctation of the aorta.
   d. The cause is unknown.

2. Which of the following is the most important lifestyle modification for the hypertensive patient who is obese?
   a. Reduce weight.
   b. Restrict salt intake.
   c. Increase potassium intake.
   d. Decrease alcohol intake.

3. Which of the following does the nurse understand is often the only sign of hypertension?
   a. Sacral edema
   b. Elevated blood pressure
   c. Tachycardia
   d. Jugular venous distention

4. Which of the following instructions would be included in dietary education for a patient with high blood pressure? **Select all that apply.**
   a. Canned fruit and vegetables are best to eat.
   b. Add salt to food during cooking and just before eating.
   c. Increase foods high in saturated fat.
   d. Choose fresh or frozen fruits and vegetables.
   e. Read food labels.
   f. Watch for potassium in salt substitutes.

5. For which of the following blood pressure readings should a 1-year follow-up visit be recommended?
   a. 108/66 mm Hg
   b. 116/76 mm Hg
   c. 138/84 mm Hg
   d. 142/90 mm Hg

6. During a health screening, a patient's blood pressure is confirmed by two nurses to be 210/120 mm Hg. Which of the following interventions should be recommended?
   a. The patient should take off work for the rest of the day and rest.
   b. The patient should rest quietly while the nurse calls 911 to request an ambulance.
   c. The patient should take two doses of blood pressure medication right now.
   d. The patient may return to work and have blood pressure rechecked in 2 days.

7. Which of the following would the nurse expect to find in a patient experiencing the complication of heart failure from hypertension?
   a. Abnormal hair growth pattern on face
   b. Distended jugular veins in semi-Fowler's position
   c. Pain in the right hand when writing
   d. Depression from taking blood pressure medication

8. The nurse should give which of the following instructions to a patient receiving a diuretic?
   a. Change positions slowly.
   b. Eliminate salt in your diet.
   c. Take your medication before bed.
   d. Empty your bladder after taking the first dose.

9. At a follow-up visit for a patient with hypertension, which of the following data best indicates that the patient's blood pressure therapy has been successful?
   a. Weight decreased by 3 pounds.
   b. Diary of dietary intake is within suggested diet.
   c. Blood pressure is less than 120/80 mm Hg.
   d. Patient reports walking 30 to 40 minutes daily.

References

Cheng, J., Ke, Q., Jin, Z., et al. (2009). Cytomegalovirus infection causes an increase of arterial blood pressure. *PLoS Pathogens* 5(5), e1000427 (doi:10.1371/journal.ppat.1000427).

National Heart, Lung, and Blood Institute. (2004). *The seventh report of the Joint National Committee on Prevention, Detection, Evaluation, and Treatment of High Blood Pressure*. Washington, DC: U.S. Department of Health and Human Services, National Institutes of Health. Retrieved August 12, 2009, from http://www.nhlbi.nih.gov/guidelines/hypertension/jnc7full.htm

Ostchega, Y., Yoon, S. S., Hughes, J., & Louis, T. (2008). *Hypertension awareness, treatment, and control—Continued disparities in adults: United States, 2005–2006* (NCHS Data Brief No. 3). Hyattsville, MD: National Center for Health Statistics. Retrieved February 18, 2010, from http://www.cdc.gov/nchs/data/databriefs/db03.pdf

Pickering, T. G., Miller, N. H., Ogedegbe, G., et al. (2008). Call to action on use and reimbursement for home blood pressure monitoring: Executive summary: A joint scientific statement from the American Heart Association, American Society of Hypertension, and Preventive Cardiovascular Nurses Association. *Hypertension, 52*(1), 1–9.

DavisPlus | For additional resources and information visit http://davisplus.fadavis.com

23 Nursing Care of Patients with Valvular, Inflammatory, and Infectious Cardiac or Venous Disorders

LINDA S. WILLIAMS

KEY TERMS

annuloplasty (AN-yoo-loh-PLAS-tee)
beta-hemolytic streptococci (BAY-tuh-HEE-moh-LIT-ick STREP-toh-KOCK-eye)
cardiac tamponade (KAR-dee-yak TAM-pon-AYD)
cardiomegaly (KAR-dee-oh-MEG-ah-lee)
cardiomyopathy (KAR-dee-oh-my-AH-pah-thee)
chorea (core-REE-ah)
commissurotomy (KOM-ih-shur-AHT-oh-mee)
Dressler's syndrome (DRESS-lers SIN-drohm)
emboli (EHM-boh-lye)
infective endocarditis (in-FEK-tive EN-doh-kar-DYE-tiss)
insufficiency (IN-suh-FISH-en-see)
international normalized ratio (IN-ter-NASH-uh-nul NOR-muh-lized RAY-she-oh)
murmur (MUR-mur)
myectomy (my-EK-tuh-mee)
myocarditis (MY-oh-kar-DYE-tiss)
pericardial effusion (PEAR-ih-KAR-dee-uhl ee-FYOO-zhun)
pericardial friction rub (PEAR-ih-KAR-dee-uhl FRICK-shun RUB)
pericardiectomy (PEAR-ih-kar-dee-EK-tuh-mee)
pericardiocentesis (PEAR-ih-KAR-dee-oh-sen-TEE-siss)
pericarditis (PEAR-ih-kar-DYE-tiss)
petechiae (peh-TEE-kee-eye)
regurgitation (ree-GUR-jih-TAY-shun)
rheumatic fever (roo-MAT-ick FEE-vur)
stenosis (steh-NOH-siss)
thrombophlebitis (THROM-boh-fleh-BYE-tiss)
valvotomy (val-VAW-tuh-mee)
valvuloplasty (VAL-vyoo-loh-PLASS-tee)

QUESTIONS TO GUIDE YOUR READING

1. What are the pathophysiology, etiology, signs and symptoms, and diagnostic tests for each of the valvular disorders?
2. What nursing care would you provide for a patient with a valvular disorder?
3. What are the differences between commissurotomy, annuloplasty, and valve replacement?
4. What postoperative complications can occur for the two types of cardiac valve replacements?
5. What are the pathophysiology, etiology, signs and symptoms, diagnostic tests, therapeutic measures, and nursing care for infective endocarditis, pericarditis, and myocarditis?
6. What are the pathophysiology, etiology, signs and symptoms, complications, diagnostic tests, therapeutic measures, and nursing care for dilated, hypertrophic, and restrictive cardiomyopathy?
7. What are the pathophysiology, etiology, signs and symptoms, complications, diagnostic tests, and therapeutic measures for thrombophlebitis?
8. What are the risk factors, prevention measures, and nursing care for thrombophlebitis?

CARDIAC VALVULAR DISORDERS

In the normal heart, blood flows in one direction because of the presence of heart valves. There are four valves in the heart: mitral, tricuspid, pulmonic, and aortic (see Fig. 21.2). The chordae tendineae and papillary muscles are attachment structures for both the mitral and tricuspid valves. They ensure that the valves close tightly. The pulmonic and aortic valves do not have these attachment structures.

Damage to the valves or their surrounding structures can result in abnormal valvular functioning (Fig. 23.1). The valves of the left side of the heart are most commonly affected and are discussed in this chapter. Forward blood flow can be hindered if the valve is narrowed, or stenosed, and does not open completely. If the valve does not close completely, blood backs up; this is referred to as **regurgitation** or **insufficiency**. The abnormal blood flow increases the workload of the heart and increases the pressures in the affected heart chamber.

Valvular damage may result from congenital defects, rheumatic fever, or infections. Congenital defects occur mainly in children, and rheumatic heart disease occurs mainly in adults. Prophylactic antibiotic therapy helps prevent rheumatic fever and subsequent rheumatic heart disease and valvular damage.

Rheumatic fever occurs as an autoimmune reaction to an upper respiratory (sore throat) group A **beta-hemolytic streptococci** infection. Two to 3 weeks after the streptococcal infection, rheumatic fever occurs. Although rheumatic fever can occur at any age, it typically occurs between ages 5 and 15. Signs and symptoms include polyarthritis, subcutaneous nodules, **chorea** (brief, rapid, uncontrolled movements), carditis, fever, arthralgia, and pneumonitis. Rheumatic fever and subsequent rheumatic heart disease and valvular damage can be prevented by detecting and treating streptococcal infections promptly with penicillin. A throat culture is used to diagnose a streptococcal infection at the time of the infection.

Valvular disorders are summarized in Table 23.1 and discussed in more detail in the following sections.

• WORD • BUILDING •
regurgitation: re—again + gurgitare—to flood
insufficiency: in—not + sufficiens—sufficient

Mitral Valve Prolapse

Pathophysiology

During ventricular systole, when pressure in the left ventricle rises, the flaps of the mitral valve normally remain closed and stay within the atrioventricular junction. In mitral valve prolapse (MVP), however, one or both flaps bulge backward into the left atrium (like a parachute) during systole. This can happen when one flap is too large or if a defect occurs in the chordae tendineae that secure the valve to the heart wall. If the bulging flaps do not fit together, blood can leak backward into the left atrium (mitral regurgitation). Increased pressure on the papillary muscles results in ischemia within the muscle, causing further dysfunction of the mitral valve.

Etiology

Mitral valve prolapse can be a hereditary collagen tissue disorder, although the cause is unknown. Infections that damage the mitral valve, ischemic heart disease, or cardiomyopathy may cause it. MVP is the most common form of valvular heart disease. It typically occurs in women, mainly from ages 15 to 30, who are thin and have slight chest deformities. Men older than age 50 commonly have more severe effects.

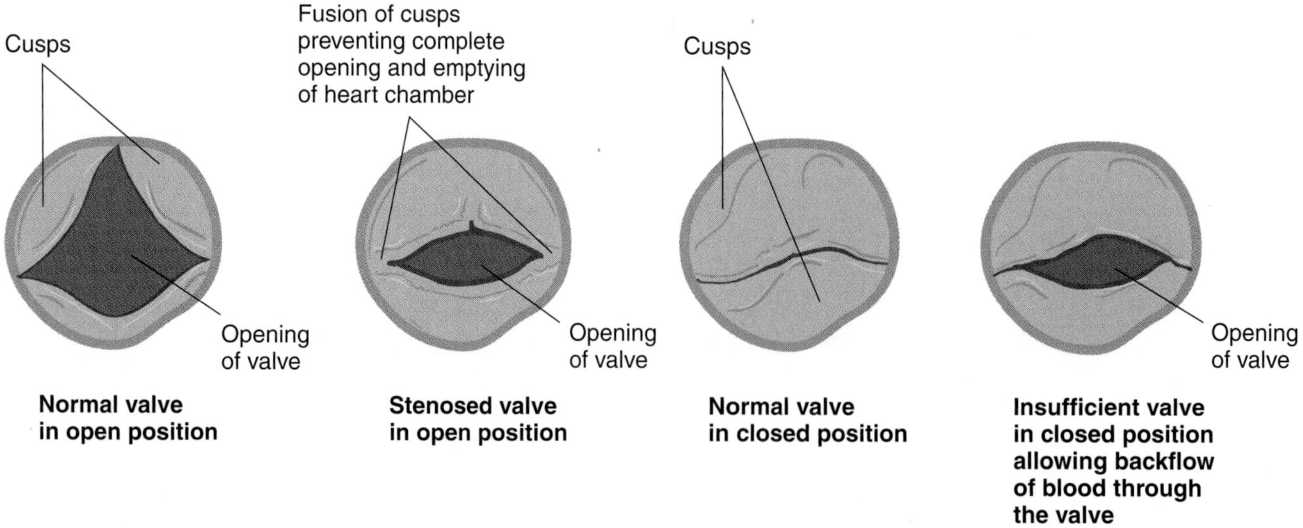
Cusps
Fusion of cusps preventing complete opening and emptying of heart chamber
Cusps
Opening of valve
Opening of valve
Opening of valve
Normal valve in open position
Stenosed valve in open position
Normal valve in closed position
Insufficient valve in closed position allowing backflow of blood through the valve

FIGURE 23.1 Openings of stenosed and insufficient valves compared with a normal valve.

TABLE 23.1 CARDIAC VALVULAR DISORDERS SUMMARY

Valve Disorder	Signs and Symptoms	Diagnostic Tests	Complications	Therapeutic Measures	Priority Nursing Diagnoses
Mitral valve prolapse	None Murmur Chest pain Palpitations Dizziness Syncope Fatigue Dyspnea	Echocardiography Cardiac catheterization	Emboli Infective endocarditis	None Beta blockers Antidysrhythmics Valvuloplasty Valve replacement	*Activity Intolerance* *Decreased Cardiac Output*
Mitral stenosis	None Murmur Chest pain Palpitations Fatigue Exertional dyspnea Cough Hemoptysis	ECG Chest x-ray Echocardiography Doppler ultrasound TEE Cardiac catheterization	Emboli Heart failure Anticoagulants	None PBV Valvuloplasty Valve replacement	*Activity Intolerance* *Decreased Cardiac Output*
Mitral regurgitation	None Murmur Chest pain Palpitations Fatigue Exertional dyspnea Cough Hemoptysis *Acute:* Pulmonary edema Shock	ECG Chest x-ray Echocardiography Doppler ultrasound TEE Cardiac MRI Cardiac catheterization	Emboli Heart failure	None ACEI Anticoagulants Valvuloplasty Valve replacement	*Activity Intolerance* *Decreased Cardiac Output*
Aortic stenosis	None Angina Murmur Syncope Heart failure	ECG Chest x-ray Echocardiography Serial echocardiogram Cardiac catheterization	Heart failure	Valve replacement	*Activity Intolerance* *Decreased Cardiac Output*
Aortic regurgitation	None Forceful pulse Murmur Chest pain Palpitations Fatigue Exertional dyspnea Corrigan's pulse Diaphoresis	ECG Chest x-ray Echocardiography Cardiac catheterization	Heart failure	Valve replacement Digitalis (Lanoxin) Diuretics Vasodilators	*Activity Intolerance* *Decreased Cardiac Output*

ACEI = angiotensin-converting enzyme inhibitor; ECG = electrocardiogram; TEE = transesophageal endoscopy; PBV = percutaneous balloon valvuloplasty.

Signs and Symptoms

Most patients with MVP do not have symptoms and prognosis is very good (see Table 23.1). MVP severity ranges from having a **murmur** to chordae tendineae rupture with mitral regurgitation. The murmur, which is best heard at the apex, begins midsystolic and becomes more intense until the end of systole. Symptoms may include atypical chest pain not related to exertion, dysrhythmias such as premature ventricular contractions (see Chapter 25) causing palpitations, dizziness or syncope, fatigue, dyspnea, or anxiety.

Complications

Rare complications include mitral regurgitation, dysrhythmias, heart failure, or infective endocarditis.

Diagnostic Tests

Auscultation for a click caused by the stress on the chordae tendineae or valve leaflets when they prolapse, or a murmur (if blood is leaking backward), is the first diagnostic step for MVP. Other diagnostic tests are used when MVP is suspected (Box 23.1). A normal electrocardiogram (ECG) is usually seen with MVP, although inverted (downward)

LEARNING TIP

The opening of a stenosed valve and an insufficient valve look very similar, and the results of extra blood building up in a chamber are the same (see Fig. 23.1). However, the problem is different. Remember what the defect is in each disorder to understand why the blood is building up in a chamber.

A valve that does not open fully (stenosed) does not allow a chamber to empty normally. Blood builds up in that chamber as a result. For example, mitral **stenosis** (valve narrowing) does not allow the left atrium to empty easily, so blood builds up in the left atrium.

A valve that does not close fully (insufficient) allows blood to flow back into the chamber that emptied. Blood builds up in that chamber as a result. For example, mitral insufficiency allows blood to backflow from the left ventricle into the left atrium after the left atrium has emptied, so blood builds up in the left atrium.

Box 23.2

Therapeutic Measures for Cardiac Valvular Disorders

Rheumatic fever prophylaxis
Prophylactic antibiotic therapy per high-risk infective endocarditis criteria
Anticoagulant therapy
Medication therapy
- Digitalis
- Diuretics
- Angiotensin-converting enzyme inhibitors
- Beta blockers
- Antidysrhythmics

Percutaneous balloon valvuloplasty
Surgery
- Valvuloplasty
- Closed commissurotomy
- Open commissurotomy
- Annuloplasty
- Valve replacement

T waves (indicating ischemia) may be seen (see Fig. 25.7). A two-dimensional echocardiogram can show valve abnormalities, and a Doppler echocardiogram identifies mitral regurgitation from MVP. For more severe cases, cardiac catheterization, an invasive test, can show the bulging flaps of the mitral valve on a coronary angiogram.

Therapeutic Measures

Unless patients have severe mitral regurgitation, MVP is a benign disorder. No treatment is needed unless symptoms are present (Box 23.2). The severity of MVP and symptoms produced determine the treatment used. A healthy lifestyle, including a good diet, exercise, stress management, and avoidance of stimulants and caffeine, can be important to prevent symptoms. Beta blockers reduce the heart rate and may help relieve chest pain. Aspirin or anticoagulants may be ordered to help prevent formation of blood clots on the valve. Surgical repair or replacement of the valve can be done for severe cases of MVP. (See Box 23.2 and the surgical interventions section later in the chapter.)

Box 23.1

Diagnostic Tests for Cardiac Valvular Disorders

- History and physical examination
- Electrocardiogram
- Chest x-ray examination
- Echocardiography
- Cardiac catheterization

CRITICAL THINKING

Mrs. Tepley

■ Mrs. Tepley, age 32, has mitral valve prolapse and reports palpitations whenever she experiences stress. She drinks three cups of coffee daily.

1. What might you hear when auscultating Mrs. Tepley's heart sounds?
2. Why does Mrs. Tepley experience palpitations?
3. What other information does Mrs. Tepley need to manage her MVP?

Suggested answers at end of chapter.

• WORD • BUILDING •
stenosis: stenos—narrow

Mitral Stenosis

Pathophysiology

Mitral stenosis results from thickening of the mitral valve flaps and shortening of the chordae tendineae, causing narrowing of the mitral valve opening. Older patients with mitral stenosis usually have calcification and fibrosis of the mitral valve flaps. The narrowed opening obstructs blood flow from the left atrium into the left ventricle. The left atrium enlarges to hold the extra blood volume caused by the obstruction. As a result of this increased blood volume, pressure rises in the left atrium. Pressures then rise in the pulmonary circulation and the right ventricle as blood volume backs up from the left atrium. The right ventricle dilates to handle the increased volume. Eventually the right ventricle fails from this excessive workload, reducing the blood volume delivered to the left ventricle and subsequently decreasing cardiac output.

Etiology

The major cause of mitral stenosis is rheumatic fever (which today is a rare complication of strep throat in the United States). Symptoms of the valvular damage often take two to four decades after the illness to appear. Because rheumatic fever is rare in developed nations, less mitral stenosis is being seen except in older adults exposed to rheumatic fever as children. Mitral stenosis is still a problem in underdeveloped areas where rheumatic fever still occurs. Less common causes include congenital defects of the mitral valve, tumors, rheumatoid arthritis, systemic lupus erythematosus, and calcium deposits.

Signs and Symptoms

Patients may be asymptomatic (see Table 23.1). A click or low-pitched murmur may be heard. The murmur is a rumbling sound over the apex during diastole and is more pronounced right before systole. Mild to more severe symptoms may occur. Pulmonary symptoms are most commonly seen. Exertional dyspnea (with activity), cough, hemoptysis (bloody sputum), and respiratory infections are the major symptoms. Fatigue, intolerance to activity, dizziness, or syncope result from decreased cardiac output. Edema of ankles and feet may be present. Palpitations from atrial flutter or fibrillation caused by atrial enlargement and chest pain from decreased cardiac output may be experienced.

Complications

Emboli can form from the stasis of blood in the left atrium and may cause stroke and seizures. Atrial fibrillation (a dysrhythmia) may develop from the enlargement of the left atrium (see Chapter 25). If the right ventricle fails, symptoms related to heart failure are seen (see Chapter 26). Pulmonary edema may develop from the backup of blood into the lungs.

Diagnostic Tests

Mitral stenosis is diagnosed with data from the patient history and physical examination and findings from diagnostic tests (see Box 23.1). The ECG shows enlargement of the left atrium and right ventricle and changes in the P waveform (see Fig. 25.2). Atrial flutter or fibrillation may be seen (see Chapter 25). A chest x-ray examination confirms enlargement of the affected heart chambers. Transthoracic two-dimensional color flow Doppler echocardiography and Doppler ultrasound are the noninvasive gold standard for evaluation of valvular disease. They show the narrowed mitral valve opening and decreased motion of the valve. Transesophageal echocardiography can be used if transthoracic images are not effective. CT scan and MRI may be done. A cardiac catheterization is typically done only if needed to validate unclear echocardiography results for preoperative evaluation or postprocedure for symptom recurrence.

Therapeutic Measures

No treatment is needed if symptoms are not present. Monitoring of the stenosis is done to provide invasive treatment if needed. Anticoagulants are given to patients at risk of development of emboli from stasis of blood in the atrium. Atrial fibrillation may develop and require treatment. For heart failure, symptoms are treated with medications (see Chapter 26).

For less severe cases, percutaneous balloon **valvuloplasty**, which uses a balloon to dilate the stenosed heart valve, is done in a cardiac catheterization laboratory (Fig. 23.2). Surgical treatment can include valvular repair (valvuloplasty) but mitral valve replacement is typically needed (Fig. 23.3). (See Box 23.2 and the surgical interventions section later in the chapter.)

Mitral Regurgitation

Pathophysiology

Mitral regurgitation, or insufficiency, is the incomplete closure of the mitral valve leaflets. It allows backflow of blood into the left atrium with each contraction of the left ventricle. This blood is then extra volume that is added to the incoming blood from the lungs. With chronic mitral regurgitation, the increase in blood volume dilates and increases pressure in the left atrium. In response to the extra blood volume delivered by the left atrium, the left ventricle compensates by dilating. If the compensatory mechanism of dilation is inadequate, pressures rise in the pulmonary circulation and then in the right ventricle as blood volume backs up from the left atrium. The left ventricle and eventually the right ventricle may fail from this increased strain.

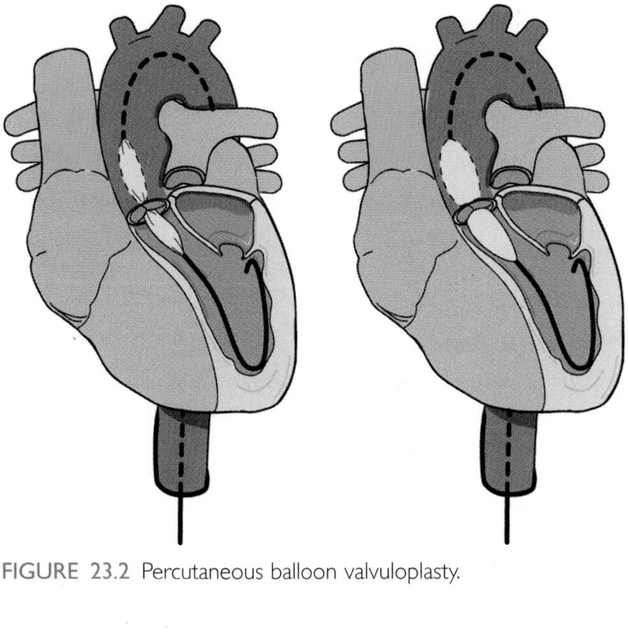

FIGURE 23.2 Percutaneous balloon valvuloplasty.

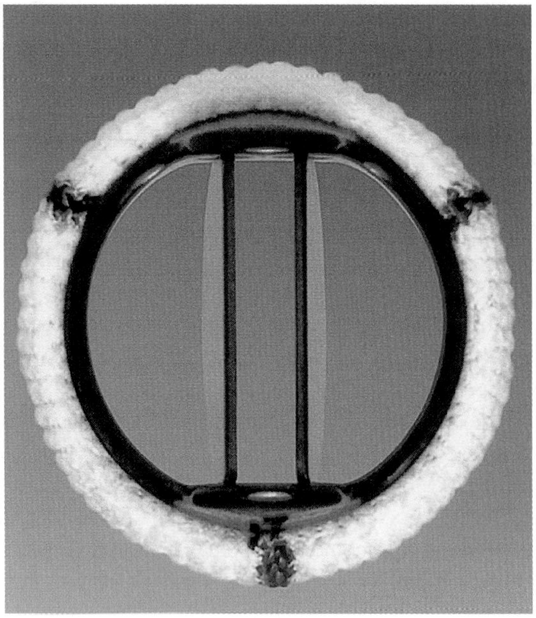

FIGURE 23.3 Valve prosthesis. An SJM Masters Series valve. (Courtesy of St. Jude Medical, Inc., St. Paul, MN.)

Etiology

Causes of mitral regurgitation include rheumatic heart disease, endocarditis, rupture or dysfunction of the chordae tendineae or papillary muscle, MVP, hypertension, myocardial infarction, cardiomyopathy, annulus calcification, aging, or congenital defects.

Signs and Symptoms

Initially, patients may be asymptomatic (see Table 23.1). Symptoms develop gradually and are similar to those of mitral stenosis. A murmur begins with S_1 (first heart sound) and continues during systole up to S_2 (second heart sound). Exertional dyspnea, fatigue, syncope, cough, and edema may occur. Palpitations and an irregular pulse due to atrial fibrillation may result. Weakness from decreased cardiac output occurs if the left ventricle begins to fail. If acute mitral regurgitation develops, such as in papillary muscle rupture following myocardial infarction, pulmonary edema and shock symptoms will be exhibited.

Complications

Atrial fibrillation may develop from the enlargement of the left atrium. Pulmonary hypertension or heart failure may occur (see Chapter 26). Endocarditis is a risk due to the damaged valve.

Diagnostic Tests

A patient history and physical examination are done. The ECG shows enlargement of the left atrium and left ventricle and changes in the P waveform (see Fig. 25.2). Atrial flutter or fibrillation may be seen. A chest x-ray examination confirms hypertrophy of the affected heart chambers. Two-dimensional or Doppler echocardiography shows left atrial enlargement and regurgitation of blood. Transesophageal echocardiography can also be used to identify causes. Cardiac MRI may be used for some people to determine treatment approaches. Cardiac catheterization further identifies regurgitation effects.

Therapeutic Measures

Without symptoms, there is no general medical treatment. Angiotensin-converting enzyme (ACE) inhibitors are often used to reduce afterload. If atrial fibrillation with rapid heart rate is present, it can be controlled with digitalis, calcium channel blockers, or beta blockers. Emboli occur less frequently, but anticoagulation is still prescribed. Symptoms of heart failure are treated with therapies for heart failure (see Chapter 26). When symptoms develop or surgery is indicated to prevent further left ventricular dysfunction, mitral valve repair or replacement is done (Fig. 23.4). For acute mitral regurgitation, emergency surgery may be needed. (See Box 23.2 and the section on surgical interventions later in the chapter.)

Aortic Stenosis

Pathophysiology

Blood flow from the left ventricle into the aorta is obstructed through the stenosed aortic valve. The opening of the aortic valve may be narrowed from thickening, scarring, calcification, or fusing of the valve's flaps. To compensate for the difficulty in ejecting blood into the aorta, the left ventricle contracts more forcefully. In chronic stenosis, the left ventricle hypertrophies to maintain normal cardiac output. With increased narrowing of the valve opening, the compensatory mechanisms are unable to continue and the left ventricle fails to move blood forward. This results in decreased cardiac output and heart failure.

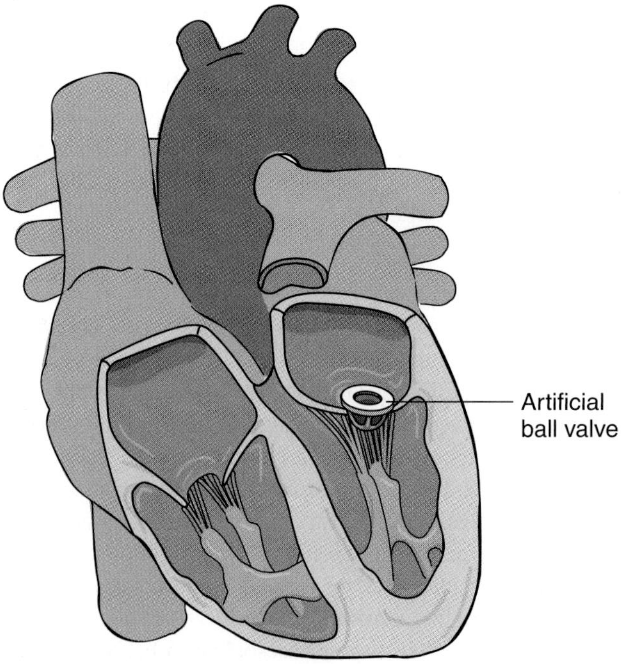
Artificial ball valve

FIGURE 23.4 Mitral valve replacement with ball valve prosthesis.

Etiology

The major causes of aortic stenosis are congenital defects or rheumatic heart disease. Calcification of the aortic valve can be related to aging and occurs after age 60. Mitral valve stenosis is also often present if rheumatic heart disease is the cause of aortic stenosis.

Signs and Symptoms

Many years or decades may pass before signs or symptoms of aortic stenosis are observed (see Table 23.1). When symptoms do occur, evaluation is essential because the disease can progress dramatically. If the mitral valve is also diseased, signs and symptoms may appear earlier.

Angina pectoris (chest pain) is a primary symptom that occurs as a result of the increased oxygen needs of the hypertrophied myocardium. The extra workload of the left ventricle and the hypertrophy of the cardiac muscle require more oxygen. Angina results if these oxygen needs are not met. In the young patient, angina indicates severe obstruction.

Other signs and symptoms include a murmur, syncope from dysrhythmias or decreased cardiac output, and heart failure signs and symptoms. The murmur is a systolic murmur that begins just after the first heart sound, increasing in intensity till midsystole, then decreasing and ending right before the second heart sound. Orthopnea, dyspnea on exertion, and fatigue are indicators of left ventricular failure. Progressive heart failure can result in pulmonary edema and right-sided heart failure.

Complications

Heart failure may occur (see Chapter 26). Life-threatening arrhythmias may occur. Endocarditis is a risk due to the damaged valve.

Diagnostic Tests

ECG usually shows enlargement of the left ventricle and left atrium. A chest x-ray examination confirms hypertrophy of the left ventricle and calcification of the aortic valve. Left atrial enlargement may be seen but occurs primarily when mitral stenosis is also present. Two-dimensional and Doppler echocardiography show thickening of the left ventricular wall, impaired movement of the aortic valve, and the severity of the disease. Serial echocardiography (e.g., annually or less often) may be recommended for those with moderate or severe disease. Cardiac catheterization will show elevated left ventricular pressure and decreased cardiac output.

Therapeutic Measures

Generally, the treatment of choice is valve replacement because of the risk of sudden death when severe symptoms are present. (See Box 23.2 and the section on surgical intervention later in the chapter.) Mechanical valves are often chosen for middle-aged adults and require lifelong anticoagulation. For older adults, biological valves are usually used as they do not require anticoagulation therapy and last about 12 years. Valvotomy is used only for those who are unable to have surgery. Heart failure symptoms are treated carefully. Medications that reduce the contractility of the heart and subsequently cardiac output are avoided to prevent further failure.

CRITICAL THINKING

Mrs. Pryor

■ Mrs. Pryor, age 72, has aortic stenosis and is admitted to the hospital with angina. She had an episode of syncope 2 days ago. She reports that she tires easily.

1. Mrs. Pryor asks what aortic stenosis is. What should you tell her and how will you document it?
2. Why might Mrs. Pryor be experiencing angina?
3. What nursing care related to safety needs is important to include in Mrs. Pryor's plan of care?
4. What nursing diagnoses and care are relevant for Mrs. Pryor's report of being tired?
5. Digoxin (Lanoxin) 0.25 mg is prescribed for Mrs. Pryor. It is time to give her digoxin and you have digoxin available in 0.125-mg tablets. How many tablets will you give?

Suggested answers at end of chapter.

Aortic Regurgitation

Pathophysiology

The aortic valve cusps may be scarred, thickened, or shortened in chronic aortic regurgitation. A backflow of blood from the aorta into the left ventricle occurs if the aortic valve cusps do not close completely. The left ventricle's blood volume increases with this backflow of blood that is in addition to the normal flow of blood from the left atrium. To handle the increased volume, the left ventricle compensates with dilation and hypertrophy to deliver a stronger contraction. This stronger contraction ejects more blood volume with each beat to maintain cardiac output. Over time the heart's contraction is not effective and the left ventricle fails, causing a cardiac output drop and pulmonary edema.

Etiology

Congenital defects, aging, rheumatic heart disease, syphilis, severe hypertension, and ankylosing spondylitis can cause aortic regurgitation. An acute cause of aortic regurgitation may be endocarditis or aortic dissection.

Signs and Symptoms

Symptoms may not become apparent for many years with chronic aortic regurgitation (see Table 23.1). Initially, the patient may report feeling a forceful heartbeat that is more pronounced when lying down. Also, palpitations and pounding in the head may be experienced. Then exertional dyspnea, fatigue, and worsening levels of dyspnea (orthopnea, paroxysmal nocturnal dyspnea) occur after years of progressive valvular dysfunction. A murmur is heard during diastolic after the second heart sound. The palpated pulse is forceful and then quickly collapses (Corrigan's pulse). The diastolic blood pressure decreases to widen the pulse pressure. This compensates for an increase in systolic blood pressure. Angina pectoris may occur late.

The angina is atypical, often happening at rest or at night along with diaphoresis, when a lower pulse rate results in delivery of less oxygen to the myocardium. Eventually heart failure symptoms develop if the left ventricle fails.

In acute dysfunction, profound symptoms of pulmonary distress, chest pain, and shock symptoms occur.

Complications

Endocarditis is a risk due to the damaged valve. Heart failure may occur (see Chapter 26).

Diagnostic Tests

The ECG shows left ventricle hypertrophy, ST-segment depression (see Fig. 25.10), and T-wave inversion (see Fig. 25.7) in some leads. A chest x-ray confirms hypertrophy of the left ventricle and aorta. With severe regurgitation, left atrial enlargement may also be seen. An echocardiogram, Doppler echocardiography, or transesophageal echocardiography show an enlarged left ventricle and severity of the aortic regurgitation. Cardiac catheterization reveals elevated left ventricular diastolic pressure and, with dye injection, shows the regurgitation of blood into the left ventricle.

Therapeutic Measures

Treatment with vasodilator therapy may be useful for some patients to reduce systolic blood pressure and subsequently cardiac workload until surgery is needed. Occasionally, surgical valve repair can be done but valve replacement is typically needed when symptoms develop. (See Box 23.2 and the surgical interventions section later in the chapter.)

Nursing Process for the Patient with a Cardiac Valvular Disorder

Data Collection

A history is obtained that includes information presented in Table 23.2. Vital signs are measured and recorded. Heart sounds are auscultated to detect murmurs. Any signs and symptoms of heart failure are noted (see Chapter 26).

TABLE 23.2 DATA COLLECTION FOR PATIENTS WITH CARDIAC VALVULAR DISORDERS

	Subjective Data
Health History	Infections (rheumatic fever, endocarditis, streptococcal or staphylococcal, syphilis)? Congenital defects? Cardiac disease (myocardial infarction, cardiomyopathy)?
Respiratory	Dyspnea at rest, on exertion, when lying, or that awakens patient? Cough or hemoptysis?
Cardiovascular	Palpitations, chest pain, dizziness, fatigue, activity intolerance?
Medications	
Knowledge of Condition	
Coping Skills	How does patient normally cope with stressors? Support System?
	Objective Data
Respiratory	Crackles, wheezes, tachypnea
Cardiovascular	Murmurs, extra heart sounds, dysrhythmias, edema, jugular venous distention, Corrigan's pulse, increased or decreased pulse pressure
Integumentary	Clubbing; cyanosis; diaphoresis; cold, clammy skin; pallor
Diagnostic Test Findings	

Nursing Diagnoses, Planning, Interventions, and Evaluation

The major nursing diagnoses for all valvular disorders are the same and include those for heart failure as well if heart failure symptoms are present. See the *Nursing Care Plan for the Patient with a Cardiac Valvular Disorder.*

Patient Education

Education, an important nursing intervention, promotes understanding of the valvular disorder, health maintenance, prevention of complications, and early recognition of symptoms, so medical care can be sought. For older adult patients, it is important to include caregivers or family members in teaching sessions to assist with understanding of the information being taught. Teaching is provided for medications the patient is taking. If the patient is on anticoagulants for atrial fibrillation or mechanical valve replacement, a medic alert identification should be used and monthly appointments to check international normalized ratio (INR)/prothrombin time (PT) values should be kept.

Information on endocarditis prevention is essential for patients with most valvular problems. Damaged cardiac valves are prone to developing infection from organisms such as *Streptococcus viridans* or *Staphylococcus epidermidis.* During invasive procedures in which bleeding is possible, these organisms can enter the circulation, attach to damaged valves, and multiply. Patients should discuss with their health care provider the American Heart Association guidelines for prophylactic antibiotics to prevent endocarditis (see the prevention section for endocarditis later in this chapter).

Cardiac Valvular Surgical Interventions

Surgical options include minimally invasive surgery using endoscopy or robotic surgery, or traditional open cardiac surgery. Cardiopulmonary bypass (CPB) is used with both options. Avoiding a sternotomy by using less invasive surgery leads to a quicker recovery and less pain and healing time.

Cardiac Valve Repairs

A balloon **valvotomy** opens a stenosed heart valve. A balloon catheter is inserted through the diseased valve and then inflated to open the stenosed valve leaflets. For mitral valve

NURSING CARE PLAN for the Patient with a Cardiac Valvular Disorder

Nursing Diagnosis: *Decreased Cardiac Output* related to valvular stenosis or insufficiency or heart failure

Expected Outcomes: The patient will have adequate cardiac output as evidenced by vital signs within normal limits (WNL), no dyspnea or fatigue at all times.

Evaluation of Outcomes: Are patient's vital signs WNL with no dyspnea or fatigue?

Interventions	Rationale	Evaluation
Assess vital signs, chest pain, and fatigue.	Vital signs, chest pain, and fatigue are indicators of cardiac output decline.	Are vital signs WNL with no chest pain or fatigue?
Give oxygen as ordered.	Supplemental oxygen provides more oxygen to the heart.	Is oxygen saturation WNL?
Provide bedrest or rest periods as ordered.	Cardiac workload and oxygen needs are reduced with rest.	Are vital signs WNL and no fatigue reported?
Elevate head of bed 45 degrees.	Venous return to heart is reduced and chest expansion improved.	Are vital signs WNL and respirations easy?
	GERIATRIC	
Assess for cardiac medication side effects and teach patient side effects to report.	Toxic side effects are more common owing to altered metabolism and excretion of medications in the older adult.	Are side effects present for medications patient is taking? Does patient understand side effects to report?

Nursing Diagnosis: *Activity Intolerance* related to decreased oxygen delivery from decreased cardiac output

Expected Outcomes: The patient will show normal changes in vital signs with less fatigue in response to activity.

Evaluation of Outcomes: Does patient have normal changes in vital signs with activity? Does patient report decreased fatigue with activity?

Interventions	Rationale	Evaluation
Assist as needed with activities of daily living (ADLs).	Energy is conserved with ADL assistance.	Are all ADLs completed? Are vital signs WNL with activity?
Provide rest and space activities.	Cardiac workload and oxygen needs are reduced with rest.	Is patient able to perform activities when allowed extra time?
	GERIATRIC	
Slow pace of care and allow patient extra time to perform activities.	Older patients can often perform activities if allowed time to slowly perform them and rest at intervals.	Does blood pressure remain WNL when changing position?
Ensure safety when mobilizing older patient.	Orthostatic hypertension is common in the older adult.	Does patient ambulate without injury?

valvoplasty the balloon catheter is inserted via the venous circulation into the right atrium. Then the catheter is threaded through a small hole pierced into the right atrial septum that emerges into the left atrium. The catheter is passed through the mitral valve and the inflation of the balloon within the mitral valve opens the stenosed valve flaps. Complications may include dysrhythmias, emboli, hemorrhage, and cardiac tamponade. A balloon valvuloplasty results in fewer complications than surgery.

A **commissurotomy** repairs a stenosed valve. The valve flaps that have adhered to each other and thus closed the opening between them, known as the commissure, are separated to enlarge the valve opening. The patient is placed on CPB (see Chapter 21) and an atriotomy (incision into the atrium) is made to expose the valve. The valve cusps are either incised with a knife or broken apart with a dilator. The atrium is sewn closed, CPB is discontinued, and surgery continues as described in Chapter 21. Commissurotomy is most commonly performed on the mitral valve. To see valve animations visit www.sjmprofessional.com/Resources/index.aspx.

Annuloplasty is the repair or reconstruction of the valve flaps or annulus. It may involve the use of prosthetic rings. The mitral valve is the most common valve repaired in this way. Sutures or a ring may be placed in the valve annulus to improve closure of the leaflets. Similar procedures are used on the tricuspid valve; however, the aortic valve is not readily repaired in this manner.

Heart Valve Replacement

Valves used for cardiac valve replacement may be either mechanical or biological. The three types of mechanical valves used are the caged ball, monoleaflet, and bileaflet (Fig. 23.5). Mechanical valves are durable but create turbulent blood flow. The turbulent flow can lead to clot formation, requiring lifelong anticoagulant therapy. Biological (tissue) valves come from three sources: xenograft (porcine [pig] and bovine [cow]) or allograft (human donor) (Box 23.3, *Cultural Considerations*). Allografts are available in limited numbers because they rely on donors. An autograft (Ross procedure) uses the patient's own pulmonary valve to replace the removed aortic valve; an allograft (human donor) pulmonary valve then replaces the patient's pulmonary valve. Visit www.lifenet.org for more information on allografts and www.sjm.com to view heart valves.

Tissue valves have a very low incidence of thrombus formation and do not require lifelong anticoagulant therapy, but do not last as long as mechanical valves. Selecting the type of valves to use depends on several factors. If anticoagulation is a concern, then biological valves may be preferred, especially for the older adult or women considering pregnancy.

• WORD • BUILDING •

commissurotomy: commissura—joining together + tome—incision

annuloplasty: annulus—ring + plasty—formed

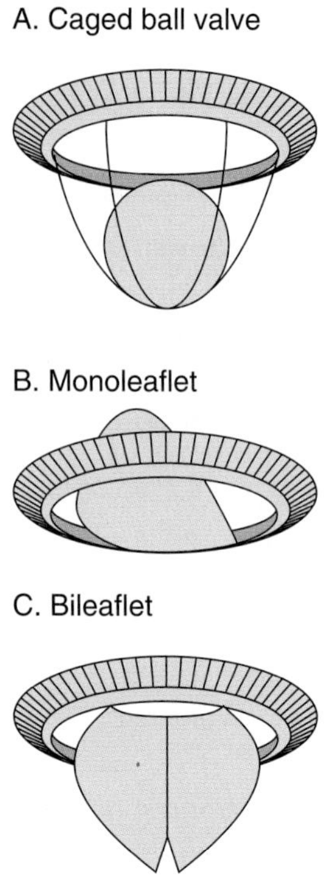
A. Caged ball valve
B. Monoleaflet
C. Bileaflet

FIGURE 23.5 Types of mechanical heart valves.

For mitral valve replacement (MVR), a left atriotomy is made after the patient is on CPB. For an aortic valve replacement (AVR), an incision is made above the right coronary artery in the aorta. Then in either valvular procedure, the diseased valve is excised and the new valve sutured in place. The incision is closed, and surgery then continues as described in Chapter 21.

VALVE REPLACEMENT COMPLICATIONS. In tissue valves, degenerative changes and calcification can occur, leading to valve failure. For mechanical valves, the most common complication is thrombus formation. An embolism can occur when thrombi form on the mechanical valve and then break off. Embolism rarely occurs with tissue valves and is prevented with anticoagulant therapy for mechanical valves. When the patient is on warfarin, ongoing monitoring of the international normalized ratio (INR) is important. The general target for INR with certain aortic valve replacements is 2.0 to 3.0, and 2.5 to 3.5 with mitral or aortic valve replacement along with thromboembolitic risks.

Other complications include anemia and endocarditis. Anemia is due to hemolysis of red blood cells (RBCs) as they come in contact with mechanical valve structures. In endocarditis, microorganisms tend to grow on the valve leaflets or the sewing ring of mechanical valves. These growths can make valves incompetent or break off to become emboli.

Nursing Process for the Preoperative Cardiac Surgery Patient

DATA COLLECTION. Baseline data collection is important for postoperative comparison and to begin discharge planning. Pain control needs and circulatory status are essential items.

Box 23.3

Cultural Considerations

Cardiac Valves

Because the pig is considered a dirty animal to religious Jews and Muslims, only bovine, synthetic, or human valves should be used for these patients. Because the cow is sacred among Hindus, only porcine, synthetic, or human valves should be used for Hindu patients.

Results of diagnostic laboratory tests, x-ray examinations, and other studies are reported if abnormal. Typing and crossmatching for ordered units of blood is done.

NURSING DIAGNOSES, PLANNING, INTERVENTIONS, AND EVALUATION. See the *Nursing Process for Preoperative Patients* section in Chapter 12.

Nursing Process for the Postoperative Cardiac Surgery Patient

After cardiac surgery, the patient goes to an intensive care unit (ICU) or cardiac universal bed unit (CUB). The patient is in ICU for about 1 to 2 days for close observation and cardiac monitoring and then transferred to a stepdown or general surgical unit for continued cardiac monitoring as recovery continues. In the CUB unit, the patient recovers in the same room until discharge, which avoids transfers to other units and increases continuity of care.

DATA COLLECTION. The patient is accompanied to ICU/CUB by the anesthesiologist, who gives the nurse a report of the procedure, complications, and hemodynamic and ventilatory management of the patient. The patient is connected to a cardiac monitor and mechanical ventilator. The mechanical ventilator is used for 4 to 24 hours. The patient is placed under a warming device, such as a light or blanket.

A head-to-toe assessment of the patient, including dressings, tubes, and IV lines, is performed. The patient may have several tubes that require monitoring including a chest tube, nasogastric tube, and a urinary catheter. Of importance are signs of awakening, shivering, pain, lung and heart sounds, and palpation of the entire chest and neck to detect crepitus (air in the subcutaneous tissue from opening the chest). Trends in the patient's cardiac output are monitored. Body temperature is continuously monitored until warming measures are discontinued, which occurs when the core body temperature nears 98.6°F (37°C). While patients are being rewarmed, they are assessed for shivering, which may be felt as a fine vibration at the mandibular angle of the jaw. Shivering greatly increases cardiac oxygen needs. Paralyzing agents given with narcotics eliminate shivering. Blood is drawn for a CBC, electrolytes, coagulation studies, and arterial blood gases.

After the initial transfer assessment, vital signs, oxygen saturation, and cardiac pressures are monitored and recorded every 15 to 30 minutes, with decreasing frequency as the patient stabilizes. Body temperature is monitored continuously while warming measures are used. The patient is warmed slowly to avoid peripheral vasodilation and onset of signs and symptoms of shock. Intake and output are measured and vital signs are checked. A 12-lead electrocardiogram (ECG) is done to detect perioperative myocardial infarction. A chest x-ray examination is done to check central line and endotracheal tube placement and to detect a pneumothorax or hemothorax, diaphragm elevation, or mediastinal widening from bleeding. At this point, the family may see the patient, and patient care is explained.

Awakening with many questions, strange auditory and tactile sensations, and the inability to speak are very frightening and frustrating to the patient. Keeping eye contact with the patient and using touch appropriately can be very soothing to the patient. If lip reading is unsuccessful, use simple closed-ended questions, nonverbal gestures, communication boards, and magic slates. Give explanations regarding procedures in simple terms.

After cardiac surgery, pain is monitored in relation to the patient's preoperative anginal or infarction-associated pain. Chest pain after surgery can be frightening for patients. Knowing that chest pain can occur from the surgical incision rather than the heart is important to the patient. Otherwise the patient may not associate surgical chest pain with the incision and instead think the pain is anginal or myocardial infarction pain.

NURSING DIAGNOSES, PLANNING, INTERVENTIONS, AND EVALUATION. Nursing diagnoses for postoperative cardiac surgery are discussed in the *Nursing Care Plan for the Postoperative Patient Undergoing Cardiac Surgery.* Additional general postoperative nursing care is discussed in Chapter 12.

INFLAMMATORY AND INFECTIOUS CARDIAC DISORDERS

The layers of the heart—the endocardium, pericardium, and myocardium (Fig. 23.6)—can become inflamed or infected, leading to endocarditis, pericarditis, and myocarditis, respectively.

Infective Endocarditis

Infective endocarditis (IE) is an infection of the endocardium that mostly occurs in hearts with artificial or damaged valves. Men develop infective endocarditis more often than

Nursing Care Plan for the Postoperative Patient Undergoing Cardiac Surgery

Nursing Diagnosis: *Pain* related to sternotomy, or pericarditis

Expected Outcomes: The patient will state pain is relieved or tolerable. Patient will be able to rest and perform respiratory treatments.

Evaluation of Outcomes: Does patient state pain is within acceptable levels? Is patient able to rest and perform respiratory therapies?

Interventions	Rationale	Evaluation
Ask about characteristics of pain with each episode.	A thorough description is needed to determine cause and plan actions.	Does patient describe pain on scale of 0 to 10?
Splint chest incision with all movement, including coughing and deep breathing.	Stabilizes sternum and incision to increase comfort.	Can patient splint chest incision independently?
Encourage patient to report pain even when pain is mild.	It is easier to keep pain under control when mild.	Does patient report pain when mild?
Turn, reposition every 2 hours.	Changes muscle position, relieving stiffness.	Is patient comfortable without stiffness?
Offer back rubs frequently.	Relaxes tense muscles retracted during operation.	Is patient able to rest comfortably?
Instruct patient to take a deep breath before movement and exhale slowly during movement.	Keeps muscles relaxed, minimizing tension with guarding and pain.	Can patient perform coughing and deep-breathing techniques as instructed?

Nursing Diagnosis: *Decreased Cardiac Output* related to myocardial depression, hypothermia, bleeding, unstable dysrhythmias, or hypoxemia

Expected Outcomes: The patient will remain free of major side effects of pharmacological support. The patient will maintain vital signs within normal limits (WNL), palpable peripheral pulses, urine output greater than 30 mL/hr, and normal sinus rhythm.

Evaluation of Outcomes: Is patient free of major side effects? Are vital signs WNL?

Interventions	Rationale	Evaluation
Monitor vital signs.	Trends reflect problems.	Are vital signs WNL?
Monitor peripheral circulation.	Mottling or weak pulses may indicate poor cardiac output (CO).	Do peripheral pulses remain strong with normal skin color, temperature, capillary refill?
Monitor intake and output.	Fluid deficit or excess can alter CO.	Does total intake equal output?
Listen to lung sounds and note character of sputum.	Wet lung sounds may indicate heart failure or pulmonary edema.	Are lungs clear?
Monitor temperature closely while rewarming the patient.	Febrile state increases heart rate and myocardial oxygen consumption.	Does temperature remain less than or equal to 98.6°F (37°C)?

Nursing Care Plan for the Postoperative Patient Undergoing Cardiac Surgery—cont'd

Monitor for shivering.	Shivering increases the blood pressure, decreasing CO and increasing risk for bleeding.	Is patient's shivering controlled?
Monitor chest tube drainage for increase or sudden decrease.	Drainage greater than 200 mL/hr may lead to hypovolemia and decreased CO.	Is patient free from cardiac tamponade and hypovolemia?
Monitor ECG.	Premature ventricular contractions and atrial fibrillation decrease CO.	Does patient remain in normal sinus rhythm or controlled dysrhythmia?
Monitor electrolytes.	Low calcium and magnesium and high potassium decrease contractility and CO.	Are electrolytes WNL?
Monitor arterial blood gases (ABGs).	Acidosis decreases heart function, and a low CO may lead to further acidosis.	Are ABGs WNL?

Nursing Diagnosis: *Risk for Infection* related to inadequate primary defenses from surgical wound

Expected Outcomes: The patient will remain free from infection.

Evaluation of Outcomes: Does patient remain free from infection?

Interventions	Rationale	Evaluation
Practice excellent hand hygiene and always cleanse stethoscope with ethanol-based cleanser or alcohol between patients.	Hands and stethoscopes carry infectious agents.	Are infectious preventive techniques used? Does patient remain free from infection?
Observe incision for signs and symptoms of infection.	Redness, warmth, fever, and swelling indicate infection.	Are signs and symptoms of infection present?
Monitor drainage and maintain drains.	Drains remove fluid from the surgical site to prevent infection development.	Are drainage amount and color normal for procedure? Are drains functioning?
Maintain sterile technique for dressing changes.	Sterile technique reduces infection development.	Is incision free of signs and symptoms of infection?
Monitor and report abnormal findings for temperature, lung sounds, sputum, and urine consistency.	Low-grade (immunosuppressed) or high-grade fever, crackles, yellow-green sputum color, or cloudy urine can indicate infection.	Is the patient's temperature WNL and are lung sounds, sputum, and urine clear?

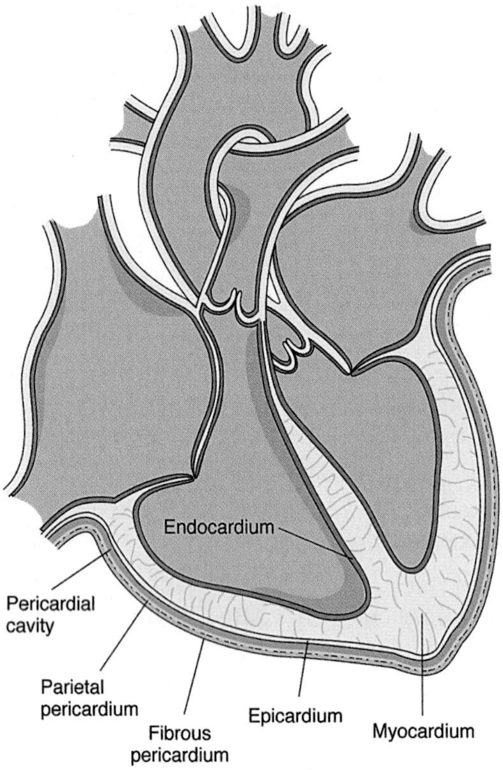
Endocardium
Pericardial cavity
Parietal pericardium
Fibrous pericardium
Epicardium
Myocardium

FIGURE 23.6 Layers of the heart.

women. Also, older adults have a higher incidence of infective endocarditis.

Pathophysiology

Cardiac defects result in turbulent blood flow that erodes the normally infection-resistant endocardium. Infective endocarditis begins when the invading organism (most commonly a bacteria, but possibly a fungi or other organism) attaches to eroded endocardium where platelets and fibrin deposits have formed a vegetative lesion. Then more platelets and fibrin cover the multiplying organism. This covering protects the microbes, reducing the ability to destroy them. Damage to valve leaflets occurs as the vegetations grow. As blood flows through the heart, these vegetations may break off and become **emboli**.

With bacteremia, bacteria attach mainly to the valves of the heart, although any heart endothelial surface can be infected. Damaged valves from conditions such as mitral valve prolapse with regurgitation, rheumatic heart disease, congenital defects, and valve replacements are especially prone to bacterial invasion. The mitral valve is the valve most commonly infected, with the aortic valve being the second most commonly infected. Heart failure may result from valve damage, especially of the aortic valve.

Etiology

Risk factors include:

- Compromised immune system
- Artificial heart valve
- Congenital or valvular heart disease
- History of endocarditis
- IV drug use
- Gingival gum disease.

Prevention

Dental disease may be a contributing factor to infective endocarditis, so daily oral care and regular dental care is an important preventive measure. For many years, patients with cardiac disease or prior endocarditis were taught that antibiotic therapy was recommended before dental or invasive procedures. In 2007, based on a review of the evidence, the American Heart Association released revised guidelines saying that fewer people require prophylaxis (Wilson et al., 2007). Only those with cardiac conditions associated with the highest risk of adverse outcomes from infective endocarditis (prosthetic cardiac valve or valve repair, history of infective endocarditis, some forms of congenital heart disease, or valvulopathy after cardiac transplantation) need prophylaxis before some types of dental procedures or respiratory tract, infected skin, skin structure, or musculoskeletal tissue procedures. Prophylaxis for procedures on the genitourinary or gastrointestinal tract is no longer recommended. Patients who were taught about former prophylaxis guidelines may be confused by these changes and need education about the new guidelines. For more information see www.americanheart.org/presenter.jhtml?identifier=3004539.

Signs and Symptoms

The onset of symptoms can be rapid or slow. Fever (99° to 103°F [37.2° to 39.4°C]) is a common sign, although the older adult may be afebrile (Table 23.3). Chills, aching muscles and joints, fatigue, dyspnea, cough, edema, and hematuria may occur. A new or different murmur is heard with valvular damage. Splinter hemorrhages may be seen in the distal nailbed (black or red-brown longitudinal short lines). **Petechiae** (tiny red or purple flat spots) resulting from microembolization of the vegetation may occur on mucous membranes, conjunctivae, or skin (Fig. 23.7). Janeway lesions (small, painless red-blue lesions on palms and soles) are an acute finding. Osler's nodes (small, painful nodes on fingers and toes) from cardiac emboli are a late finding (Fig. 23.8).

Complications

Vegetative emboli can be a major complication of infective endocarditis. If organ embolization occurs, signs and symptoms that reflect the organ that was affected by the emboli are seen. Brain emboli may produce changes in level of consciousness or stroke. Kidney emboli cause pain in the flank area, hematuria, or renal failure. Emboli in the spleen cause abdominal pain. Emboli in the small blood vessels can impair circulation in the extremities. Pulmonary emboli result in sudden dyspnea, cough, and chest pain.

• WORD • BUILDING •

petechiae: petecchia—skin spot

TABLE 23.3 INFECTIVE ENDOCARDITIS SUMMARY

Signs and Symptoms	Fever Chills Heart murmur Night sweats Fatigue Weight loss Weakness Aching in abdomen, joints, muscles, back Nailbed splinter hemorrhages Petechiae
Diagnostic Tests and Findings	Blood cultures Transesophageal echocardiography CBC Chest x-ray ECG
Therapeutic Measures	*Acute therapy:* IV antimicrobial medications such as penicillin, vancomycin, amphotericin B Antipyretics Rest Surgical valve replacement Prophylactic antibiotic therapy per high-risk infective endocarditis criteria
Complications	Emboli Heart failure Abscesses
Priority Nursing Diagnoses	*Activity Intolerance* related to reduced oxygen delivery from decreased cardiac output *Decreased Cardiac Output* related to impaired valvular function or heart failure *Ineffective Tissue Perfusion* related to emboli

CBC = complete blood count; ECG = electrocardiogram.

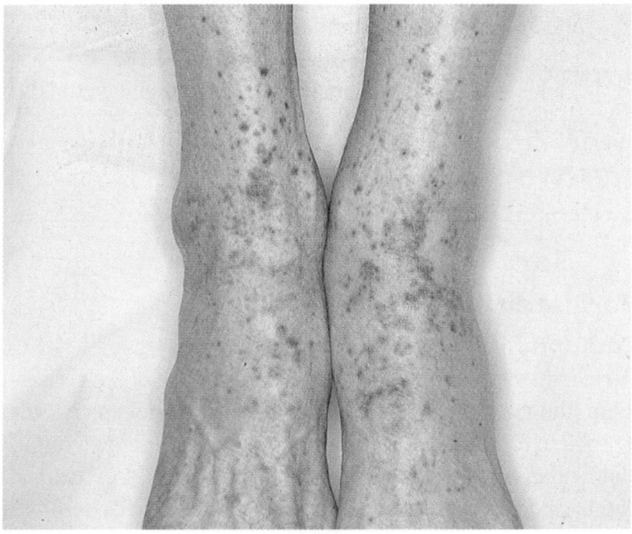

FIGURE 23.7 Petechiae. (From Goldsmith, L. [1997]. *Adult & pediatric dermatology* [p. 61]. Philadelphia: F. A. Davis.)

Heart structures can be damaged or destroyed by infective endocarditis. Stenosis (narrowing) or regurgitation (leakage) of a heart valve may also result. As the infection progresses and causes more damage to heart structures, heart failure may occur. Abscesses may also develop in the heart or other parts of the body.

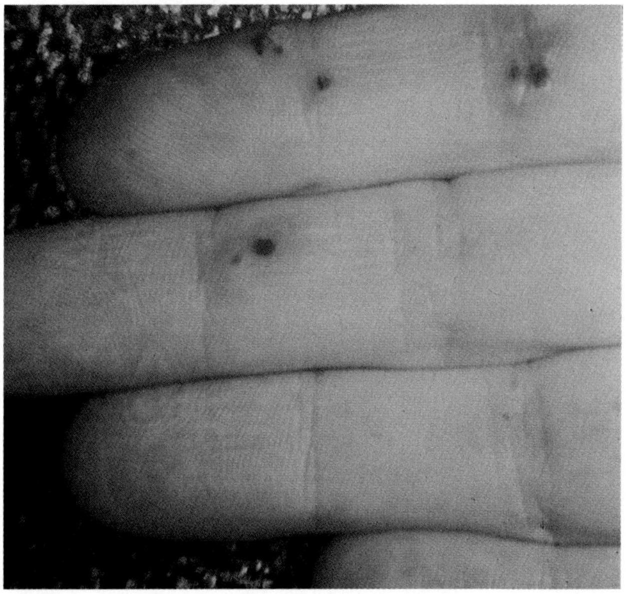

FIGURE 23.8 Osler's nodes. (From Goldsmith, L. [1997]. *Adult & pediatric dermatology* [p. 188]. Philadelphia: F. A. Davis.)

Diagnostic Tests

Table 23.3 lists diagnostic tests for infective endocarditis. Positive blood cultures identify the causative organism, and echocardiography shows cardiac effects.

Therapeutic Measures

Initial treatment begins with hospitalization. An antimicrobial drug is selected that will destroy the organism identified by the blood culture. For bacterial infections, penicillin (or vancomycin for those allergic to penicillin) is commonly used. These medications are given intravenously over a period of 4 to 6 weeks, often once a day. A lengthy course of high-dose antibiotics is needed to penetrate the vegetations to reach all of the microbes inside to kill them. Rest and supportive symptom care are also used. If afebrile and without complications, the patient is discharged to continue IV antibiotic therapy at home. The patient's response to the drug is monitored via the home care nurse and through laboratory testing. Changes in antibiotics may be made in response to side effects, allergies, organism resistance to the drug, or relapses.

Surgical replacement or repair of valves is usually required for patients with severely damaged heart valves, prosthetic valve infection, recurrent infection, multiple emboli from damaged valves, or heart failure. Antimicrobial therapy continues after surgery.

Nursing Process for the Patient with Infectious Endocarditis

DATA COLLECTION. A patient history is obtained that includes risk factors for IE and recent infections or invasive procedures (Table 23.4). Vital signs are measured and recorded, and heart sounds are auscultated to detect murmurs.

TABLE 23.4 DATA COLLECTION FOR PATIENTS WITH INFECTIVE ENDOCARDITIS

	Subjective Data
Health History	Infections (rheumatic fever, scarlet fever, previous endocarditis, streptococcal or staphylococcal, syphilis)? Cardiac disease (valvular surgery, congenital)? Childbirth? Invasive procedures (surgery, dental, catheterization, IV therapy, cystoscopy, gynecological)? Malaise? Anorexia?
Medications	Steroids, immunosuppressants, prolonged antibiotic therapy, IV drug use, alcohol use?
Respiratory	Dyspnea on exertion or orthopnea (when lying down)? Cough?
Cardiovascular	Palpitations, chest pain, fatigue, or activity intolerance?
Musculoskeletal	Weakness, arthralgia, myalgia?
Knowledge of Condition	Patient's understanding
	Objective Data
Fever, Diaphoresis	
Respiratory	Crackles, tachypnea
Cardiovascular	Murmurs, tachycardia, dysrhythmias, edema
Integumentary	Nailbed splinter hemorrhages; petechiae on lips, mouth, conjunctivae, feet, or antecubital area; paleness
Renal	Hematuria
Diagnostic Test Findings	Positive blood cultures, anemia, elevated WBC count, elevated ESR, ECG showing conduction problems, echocardiogram showing valvular dysfunction and vegetations, chest x-ray exam showing heart enlargement (cardiomegaly) and lung congestion

ECG = electrocardiogram; ESR = erythrocyte sedimentation rate; WBC = white blood cell.

Signs of heart failure and emboli are noted. The physician is notified immediately if circulatory impairment, such as cold skin, decreased capillary refill, cyanosis, or absent peripheral pulses in an extremity, or symptoms of organ-related emboli are detected.

NURSING DIAGNOSIS, PLANNING, IMPLEMENTATION, AND EVALUATION. See the *Nursing Care Plan for the Patient with Infective Endocarditis.* Teaching about the disease and its treatment provides patients and families with the ability to provide IV antibiotics at home and promotes health maintenance to prevent future infective endocarditis. Good hygiene including dental care is essential. Skin care includes bathing, using proper hand washing technique with soap, avoiding nail biting, not popping pimples or lancing boils, and washing and applying antibiotic ointment to cuts.

Brushing with a soft-bristle toothbrush (to prevent gum trauma) twice a day reduces the formation of plaque (which traps bacteria). Biannual dental cleaning (with prophylactic antibiotics for high risk) is important. Patients are taught to recognize symptoms (e.g., fever, chills, sweats), seek prompt medical care, and have blood cultures drawn before antibiotics are started. The patient's statement of understanding and a willingness to follow lifestyle changes support goal achievement.

CRITICAL THINKING

Mrs. Jones

■ Mrs. Jones, age 28, is admitted to the hospital with a fever of 100°F (37°C), chills, fatigue, anorexia, and pain in her joints. A physical assessment reveals splinter hemorrhages in left index finger nailbed and petechiae on her chest. She is diagnosed with a heart murmur and infective endocarditis.

1. Why is a heart murmur heard with endocarditis?
2. What do splinter hemorrhages look like?
3. What do petechiae indicate?
4. How would you document Mrs. Jones' data collection findings?
5. What type of medication would you expect to be ordered to treat the infection?
6. Why does Mrs. Jones have chills if her temperature is elevated?
7. What signs and symptoms might occur if the complications of heart failure develop?
8. Tylenol 650 mg q 6 hours for pain is ordered. It comes as 325-mg tablets. How many tablets would be given per dose?

Suggested answers at end of chapter.

Pericarditis

Pathophysiology and Etiology

Pericarditis is an acute or chronic inflammation of the pericardium (the sac surrounding the heart). The inflammation creates a problem for the heart as it tries to expand and fill. As a result, ventricular filling is reduced, which then decreases cardiac output and blood pressure. Acute pericarditis usually resolves in less than 6 weeks. Recurrence is possible. Acute pericarditis can be caused by a variety of factors, including the following:

- Infections: viruses, bacteria, fungi, or Lyme disease
- Drug reactions

• WORD • BUILDING •

pericarditis: peri—around + kardia—heart + itis—inflammation

Nursing Care Plan for the Patient with Infective Endocarditis

Nursing Diagnosis: *Decreased Cardiac Output* related to impaired valvular function or heart failure

Expected Outcome: The patient will have adequate cardiac output as evidenced by vital signs within normal limits (WNL), no dyspnea or fatigue at all times.

Evaluation of Outcomes: Are patient's vital signs WNL with no dyspnea or fatigue?

Interventions	Rationale	Evaluation
Assess vital signs, murmurs, dyspnea, and fatigue.	Vital signs, dyspnea, and fatigue are indicators of cardiac output decline.	Are vital signs WNL with no dyspnea or fatigue?
Give oxygen as ordered.	Supplemental oxygen provides more oxygen to the heart.	Is oxygen saturation WNL?
Provide bedrest or rest periods as ordered.	Cardiac workload and oxygen needs are reduced with rest.	Are vital signs WNL and no fatigue reported?
Elevate head of bed 45 degrees.	Venous return to heart is reduced and chest expansion improved.	Are vital signs WNL and respirations easy?

Nursing Diagnosis: *Activity Intolerance* related to reduced oxygen delivery from decreased cardiac output

Expected Outcomes: The patient will state less fatigue in response to activity.

Evaluation of Outcomes: Does patient report less fatigue? Is patient able to participate in desired activities?

Interventions	Rationale	Evaluation
Assist with activities of daily living (ADLs) prn.	Assistance conserves energy.	Are ADLs completed?
Provide rest and space activities.	Cardiac workload and oxygen needs are reduced with rest.	Does patient report less fatigue?

Nursing Diagnosis: *Deficient Diversional Activity* related to restricted mobility from prolonged intravenous therapy

Expected Outcomes: The patient will state diversional activities are satisfying.

Evaluation of Outcomes: Does patient participate in diversional activities? Does patient state satisfaction with activities?

Interventions	Rationale	Evaluation
Assess patient's preferred activities and hobbies.	Activity preference should be known to plan satisfactory diversional activities.	Are patient's preferred activities known?
Plan patient's schedule around relaxing and fun activities.	Self-esteem is fostered with increased patient control.	Does patient offer input into scheduled care? Is input followed?
Use pet therapy.	Individuals who interact with pets live longer and are healthier.	Does patient state enjoyment of pet therapy?
Provide a mix of physical, mental, and social activities on a rotating schedule.	Rotating stimulating activities and visitors will keep patient interested and avoid fatigue.	Does patient state satisfaction in activities with no fatigue?

- Connective tissue disorders: systemic lupus erythematosus, rheumatic fever, or rheumatoid arthritis
- Neoplastic disease
- Postpericardiotomy (e.g., after cardiac surgery)
- Postmyocardial infarction
- **Dressler's syndrome** (autoimmune response)
- Renal disease or uremia
- Trauma from chest injury or invasive thoracic procedures.

There are several forms of chronic pericarditis. Chronic constrictive pericarditis is the result of fibrous scarring of the pericardium. The heart becomes surrounded by a thickened, stiff sac that limits the stretching ability of the heart's chambers for filling. Heart failure may result. Chronic constrictive pericarditis results from neoplastic disease and metastasis, radiation, or tuberculosis.

Signs and Symptoms

Chest pain is the most common symptom of acute pericarditis (Table 23.5). The pain is located substernally and over the heart and may radiate to the clavicle, neck, left scapula, or epigastric area. Typically there is an intense, sharp, creaky, grating pain that increases with deep inspiration, coughing, moving of the trunk, or lying flat. For some the pain is not as intense and is instead a dull ache. The pain may be relieved by sitting up and leaning forward. Other symptoms depend on the cause of the pericarditis and may include orthopnea, low-grade fever, fatigue, cough, and edema.

A **pericardial friction rub**—a grating, scratchy, high-pitched sound—may be heard. The rub is a result of friction from the inflamed pericardial and epicardial layers rubbing together as the heart fills and contracts. Depending on the severity of the pericarditis, the rub may be faint when auscultated or loud enough to be audible without auscultation. The rub may be heard intermittently or continuously. It is usually heard over the lower left sternal border of the chest during each heartbeat. It is present in about 50% of those with pericarditis.

Chronic constrictive pericarditis produces dyspnea and signs and symptoms of right-sided heart failure and may also cause atrial fibrillation.

TABLE 23.5 PERICARDITIS SUMMARY

Signs and Symptoms	Chest pain Dyspnea Low-grade fever Cough Pericardial friction rub
Diagnostic Tests	Complete blood cell count Electrocardiogram Echocardiogram Magnetic resonance imaging Computed tomography
Therapeutic Measures	Anti-inflammatory medication Corticosteroids Pericardiocentesis Pericardial window
Complications	Pericardial effusion Cardiac tamponade
Priority Nursing Diagnoses	*Acute Pain* related to inflammation of pericardium *Anxiety* related to disease process *Decreased Cardiac Output* related to cardiac constriction

LEARNING TIP

To simulate the sound of a pericardial friction rub, hold the diaphragm of a stethoscope against the palm of one hand; listen through the stethoscope as you rub the index finger of the opposite hand over the knuckles of the hand holding the diaphragm. The sound you hear is similar to that of a pericardial friction rub.

Diagnostic Tests

Table 23.5 lists diagnostic tests for pericarditis. The electrocardiogram reveals ST-T wave elevation in all leads (see Fig. 25.11), which indicates cardiac injury. Echocardiogram results show **pericardial effusions** (buildup of fluid in pericardial space). Serum laboratory tests focus on causes of the pericarditis, such as an elevated white blood cell (WBC) count, indicating a bacterial or viral infection, or elevated blood urea nitrogen or creatinine levels, indicating uremia. Fluid obtained during **pericardiocentesis** (aspiration of fluid from pericardial sac) is examined to diagnose the cause. In chronic constrictive pericarditis, a computed tomography (CT) scan or magnetic resonance imaging (MRI) may show a thickened pericardium.

Therapeutic Measures

Mild cases may resolve without treatment. If the patient is unstable, prompt intervention is required, such as an emergency pericardiocentesis. The cause is determined so that appropriate treatment can be administered, such as antibiotics for bacterial infections. Bedrest is used to reduce the heart's workload during acute symptoms. Nonsteroidal anti-inflammatory drugs (NSAIDs) are given to resolve inflammation and reduce pain. Corticosteroids may be used when NSAIDs are not effective. Colchicine (Colsalide) may be given to reduce inflammation in more severe cases. Hemodialysis is used to treat uremic pericarditis.

Chronic effusive pericarditis can be treated with a pericardial window to allow continuous drainage of pericardial

• WORD • BUILDING •

pericardiocentesis: peri—around + kardia—heart + centesis—puncture fluid into the pleural space. A pericardial window is created surgically by removing a portion of the outer pericardial layer.

Chronic constrictive pericarditis is treated with **pericardiectomy**, which is the surgical removal of the entire tough, calcified pericardium. Pericardiectomy relieves constriction of the heart and allows normal filling of the ventricles.

Complications

A pericardial effusion is the most common complication of pericarditis. A rapidly developing effusion, such as one occurring from trauma, can produce symptoms with smaller amounts of fluid than slowly developing effusions, such as pericarditis from tuberculosis, with larger amounts of fluid. The increasing fluid presses on nearby tissue. Pressure on lung tissue can produce dyspnea, cough, and tachypnea. The heartbeat sounds distant. The body's compensatory mechanisms attempt to maintain blood pressure.

As the fluid accumulation grows, **cardiac tamponade**, another complication of pericarditis, can occur. Cardiac tamponade is a life-threatening compression of the heart by fluid accumulated in the pericardial sac. Cardiac output drops and, to compensate, the heart rate increases. Then blood pressure falls as compensatory mechanisms fail. The patient shows symptoms of decreased cardiac output, such as restlessness, confusion, tachycardia, and tachypnea. Jugular venous distention is present from increased venous pressure, and heart sounds are distant.

Cardiac tamponade requires immediate treatment with pericardiocentesis. The pericardium is punctured with a 16-gauge needle and excess fluid in the pericardial sac removed (Fig. 23.9). After the procedure, the patient is monitored for complications, such as dysrhythmias, laceration of a coronary artery, or laceration of the myocardium or pneumothorax.

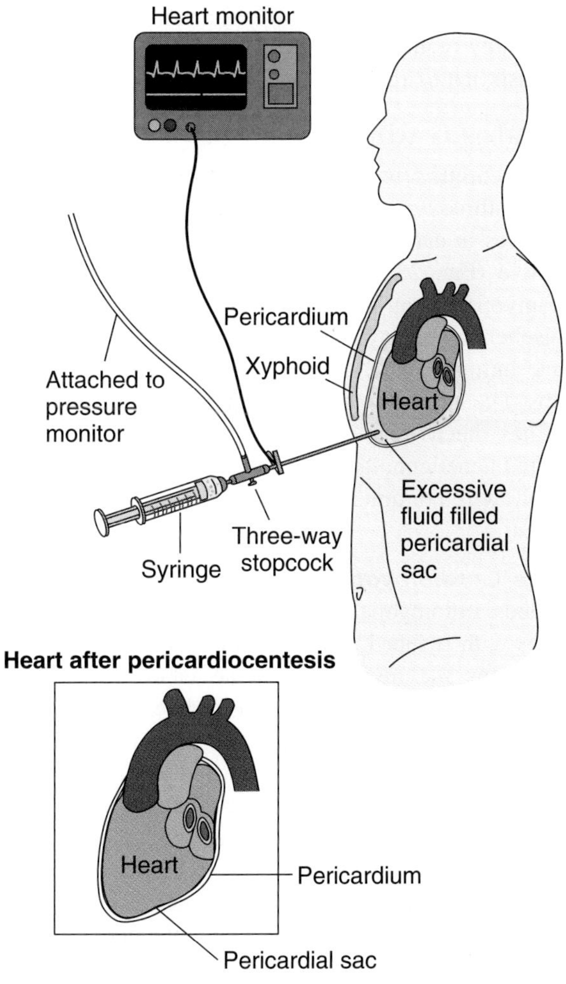
Heart monitor
Pericardium
Xyphoid
Heart
Attached to pressure monitor
Excessive fluid filled pericardial sac
Three-way stopcock
Syringe
Heart after pericardiocentesis
Heart
Pericardium
Pericardial sac

FIGURE 23.9 Pericardiocentesis.

• WORD • BUILDING •
cardiac tamponade: kardia—heart + tamponade—plug

Nursing Management

A patient history is obtained that includes any cardiac disease, recent infections, and current medications. Chest pain, pericardial friction rub, heart sounds, and signs of heart failure are noted. Vital signs are documented, noting fever and tachycardia.

Nursing care focuses on relieving the patient's pain and anxiety and maintaining normal cardiac function. Symptoms are monitored to detect complications. Pain, which may be severe, is relieved by giving NSAIDs or corticosteroids as ordered. Allowing the patient to assume a position of comfort by sitting up and leaning forward also relieves pain. Maintenance of normal cardiac function includes monitoring vital signs and observing for the presence of symptoms of cardiac tamponade or heart failure. The detection of these symptoms is immediately reported to the physician. Teaching the patient about pericarditis and its treatment relieves anxiety and allows a feeling of control by allowing the patient to make knowledgeable health care decisions.

Myocarditis

Pathophysiology and Etiology

In **myocarditis**, inflammation of the myocardium occurs. The amount of muscle destruction and necrosis that occurs as a result of myocarditis determines the extent of damage to the heart. The heart may enlarge in response to the damaged muscle fibers, although most cases of myocarditis are benign, with few signs or symptoms.

Myocarditis is a rare condition that most commonly develops following a viral infection. Other causes are bacteria, parasites, fungi, rickettsiae, spirochetes, medications, lead toxicity, autoimmune factors, human immunodeficiency virus (HIV), rheumatic fever, systemic lupus erythematosus, pericarditis or infective endocarditis, or cardiac transplant rejection.

• WORD • BUILDING •
myocarditis: myo—muscle + kardia—heart + itis—inflammation

Signs and Symptoms

Signs and symptoms of myocarditis vary from none to severe cardiac manifestations. Fatigue, fever, pharyngitis, malaise, dyspnea, palpitations, muscle aches, gastrointestinal (GI) discomfort, and enlarged lymph nodes may occur early from a viral infection. Cardiac manifestations such as chest pain or tachycardia may occur about 2 weeks after a viral infection. Occasionally, sudden death may occur.

Diagnostic Tests

A myocardial biopsy during the first 6 weeks of inflammation is the preferred diagnostic test for myocarditis, although it is positive only about 30% of the time. Echocardiogram and MRI are helpful. An electrocardiogram (ECG) shows dysrhythmias, commonly sinus tachycardia. Blood tests are done: CBC, viral antibodies, and enzyme levels that look for heart damage.

Therapeutic Measures

Treatment is aimed at the cause, if known, such as antibiotics for bacterial infections. Interventions to reduce the heart's workload during recovery are essential and include bedrest and limited activity. Exercise increases myocardial inflammation and mortality, and should be avoided until symptoms improve and inflammation is gone. The use of alcohol and tobacco should be avoided. Symptoms of heart failure are treated with medications such as beta blockers, ACE inhibitors, diuretics, or digoxin to reduce the heart's workload and oxygen needs. With myocarditis, the heart is sensitive to digoxin. The patient should be monitored closely for signs of digoxin toxicity, which may include anorexia, nausea, vomiting, bradycardia, dysrhythmias, or malaise.

Nursing Management

Recent illnesses, toxin exposure, cardiac diseases, activity tolerance, and current medications are documented. Vital signs and signs of heart failure, such as jugular venous distention, peripheral edema, crackles, and dyspnea are noted.

Nursing care is aimed at the patient's maintenance of normal cardiac function by monitoring vital signs and symptoms and administering medications as ordered. Interventions to reduce fatigue include providing assistance as needed, having frequent rest periods, and teaching energy conservation methods. Reducing the patient's anxiety and increasing the patient's knowledge can be achieved through teaching about the disease. Determining diversional activities with the patient for times when activity is restricted further reduces patient anxiety.

Cardiac Trauma

Two types of cardiac trauma can occur: nonpenetrating and penetrating. Nonpenetrating injuries, or contusions, occur from blunt trauma such as motor vehicle accidents or contact sports in which direct compression or force is applied to the upper torso. Contusions may vary from small bruises to hemorrhage.

There may be few or no external injuries indicating traumatic cardiac injury. The patient may be asymptomatic or exhibit signs and symptoms identical to a myocardial infarction. In severe contusions, laboratory results may show elevated creatine kinase MB (CK-MB) or troponin I levels.

If bleeding into the pericardial sac occurs, cardiac tamponade (compression of the heart from the blood collecting in the sac; see earlier discussion) may occur. If signs of shock occur, a pericardiocentesis must be performed. With its own pressure, the tamponade may seal the area of bleeding, so no cardiac decompensation occurs. In this case, only bedrest and observation are required. There are no long-term effects with most contusions. With severe contusions, however, scarring and necrosis of the myocardium may decrease cardiac output and increase the risk for cardiac rupture.

Penetrating traumas include an external injury to the chest, such as a stab or gunshot wound, or an internal injury, such as invasive lines that penetrate the cardiac muscle. Complications vary depending on the size, location, and cause of injury. Tamponade occurs from bleeding into the pericardial sac if the pericardium is sealed off by clot formation. A hemothorax develops if blood drains into the pleural space in the chest. A pneumothorax occurs if air collects in the pleural space. Signs and symptoms of hemorrhage and myocardial ischemia may be noted. Cardiac trauma treatment usually requires surgery to repair the damage so that hemostasis can be regained.

Cardiomyopathy

Cardiomyopathy is an enlargement of the heart muscle. There are three types of cardiac structure and function abnormalities in cardiomyopathy: dilated, hypertrophic, and restrictive (Fig. 23.10). A consequence of each type of cardiomyopathy can be heart failure (Fig. 23.11), myocardial ischemia, or myocardial infarction due to reduced cardiac output. There is currently no cure for cardiomyopathy. The greatest advancement for the cardiomyopathies has been seen in genetic research, which has identified genetic mutations that cause these diseases. This research will continue to lead to better diagnosis and treatment.

Dilated Cardiomyopathy

In dilated cardiomyopathy, the size of the ventricular cavity enlarges with reduced cardiac output. Contractile function decreases as the myocardial tissue is destroyed. Blood moves more slowly from the left ventricle, which often results in blood clot formation. Dilated cardiomyopathy is the most frequent type of cardiomyopathy and one of the most frequent causes of heart failure. Dilated cardiomyopathy may be caused by genetics, infectious myocarditis, hypertension, heart valve disorders, myocardial infarction, chronic alcohol or cocaine use, metals such as lead, elevated iron levels, HIV, thiamine or zinc deficiencies, cardiac

• WORD • BUILDING •

cardiomyopathy: kardia—heart + myo—muscle + pathy—disease

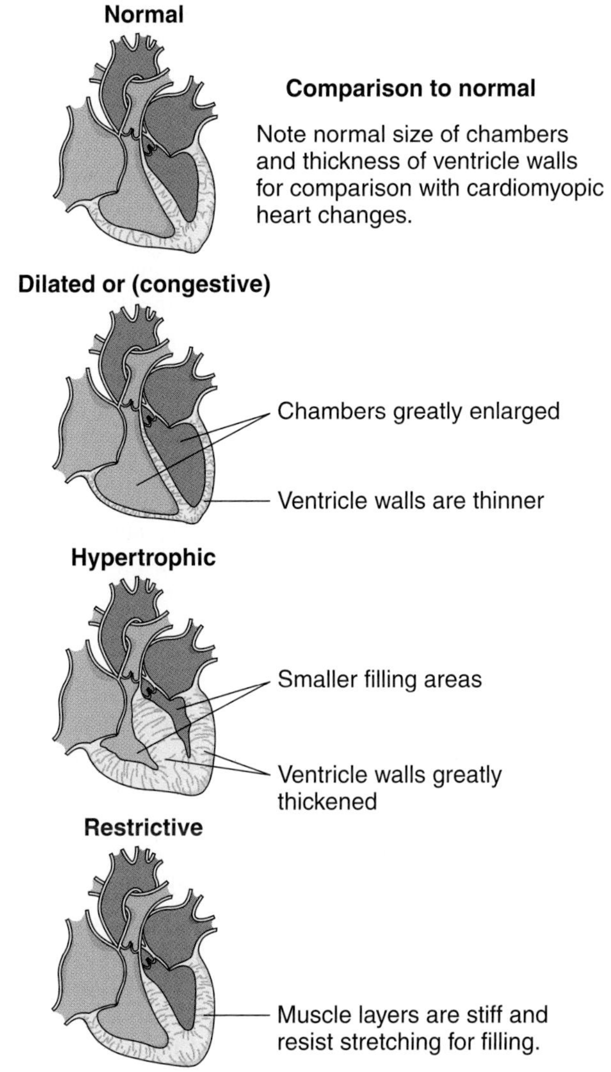
Normal
Comparison to normal
Note normal size of chambers and thickness of ventricle walls for comparison with cardiomyopic heart changes.
Dilated or (congestive)
Chambers greatly enlarged
Ventricle walls are thinner
Hypertrophic
Smaller filling areas
Ventricle walls greatly thickened
Restrictive
Muscle layers are stiff and resist stretching for filling.

FIGURE 23.10 Comparison of the normal heart structure with each type of cardiomyopic heart structure.

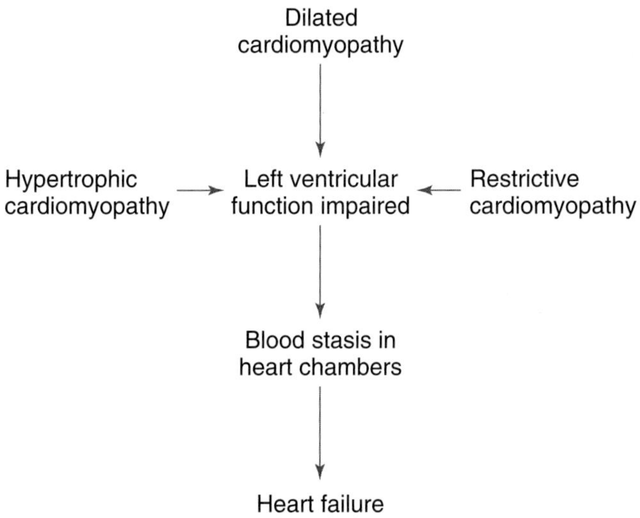
Dilated cardiomyopathy
Hypertrophic cardiomyopathy
Left ventricular function impaired
Restrictive cardiomyopathy
Blood stasis in heart chambers
Heart failure

FIGURE 23.11 Each type of cardiomyopathy can lead to heart failure.

infections, chemotherapy, neuromuscular disorders, or other causes.

Hypertrophic Cardiomyopathy

Hypertrophic cardiomyopathy is enlargement of the cardiac muscle wall, often of the septum and left ventricle. The hypertrophy may occur asymmetrically. It can be a hereditary disorder that is transmitted as a dominant trait. Hypertrophic cardiomyopathy causes the ventricular wall to be rigid, which decreases ventricular filling. If an enlarged septum obstructs the outflow of blood through the aortic valve, it is known as obstructive hypertrophic cardiomyopathy. Death can occur suddenly and is likely due to an abnormal heart rhythm.

Restrictive Cardiomyopathy

Restrictive cardiomyopathy impairs ventricular stretch and limits ventricular filling. Cardiac muscle stiffness is present with no ventricular dilation, although systolic emptying of the ventricle remains normal. Restrictive cardiomyopathy is the rarest form of cardiomyopathy. It may be caused by infiltrative diseases such as amyloidosis that deposit the protein amyloid within the myocardial cells, making the muscle stiff and resistant to stretching for easy ventricular filling. Treating the underlying cause may help reduce heart damage. Visit the American Heart Association at www.americanheart.org for more cardiac information.

Signs and Symptoms

Manifestations of cardiomyopathy depend on the type of abnormality. Most patients show varying degrees of signs and symptoms of heart failure (Table 23.6). With dilated cardiomyopathy, left ventricular and then right-sided heart failure with a poor prognosis are seen. Dyspnea on exertion, orthopnea, fatigue, and sometimes atrial fibrillation occur. In hypertrophic cardiomyopathy, exertional dyspnea related to the obstruction of cardiac output is the most common symptom. Angina is not common, but atypical chest pain that occurs at rest and is not relieved with nitrates may occur. With restrictive cardiomyopathy, heart failure symptoms result from the ventricles' inability to fill during diastole. Syncope, arrhythmias, and thrombi may occur.

Diagnostic Tests

Cardiomegaly is visible on a chest x-ray examination. Echocardiography shows muscle thickness and chamber size to differentiate between the types of cardiomyopathy. Changes related to enlarged chamber size, tachycardia, and dysrhythmias can be seen on the ECG. Cardiac catheterization and biopsy may be useful as well as cardiovascular magnetic resonance. Blood tests may be done to identify infections, elevated metal or iron levels.

• **WORD** • **BUILDING** •

cardiomegaly: kardia—heart + mega—large

TABLE 23.6 CARDIOMYOPATHY SUMMARY

Signs and Symptoms	Angina Arrhythmias Dyspnea Fatigue Syncope
Diagnostic Tests	Electrocardiogram Chest x-ray Cardiac catheterization Cardiac magnetic resonance imaging Echocardiography
Therapeutic Measures	Anticoagulants Antidysrhythmics *Dilated cardiomyopathy:* vasodilators, cardiac glycosides, biventricular pacing, ventricular assist device, heart transplant *Hypertrophic cardiomyopathy:* beta blockers, calcium channel blockers, myectomy, septal ablation *Restrictive cardiomyopathy:* vasodilators, heart transplant
Complication	Heart failure
Priority Nursing Diagnoses	*Decreased Cardiac Output* related to impaired myocardial function *Activity Intolerance* related to cardiac insufficiency *Anxiety* related to disease process

Therapeutic Measures

Treatment is palliative and aimed at managing heart failure and the underlying cause if known for both dilated and restrictive cardiomyopathies (see Chapter 26). In dilated cardiomyopathy, treatment focuses on the symptoms of heart failure seen. Angiotensin-converting enzyme (ACE) inhibitors, angiotensin II receptor blockers, beta blockers, diuretics, aldosterone antagonists, and digoxin may be given. Biventricular pacing and implantable defibrillators may be used. Therapy is not very useful for restrictive cardiomyopathy. Diuretics or nitrates may be used to relieve venous congestion that occurs due to heart failure. However, a fine balance is needed when using these drugs so that preload is not reduced too greatly, which would worsen symptoms. Anticoagulants are given to prevent emboli formation in patients with atrial fibrillation. Antidysrhythmics or cardioversion is used for dysrhythmias.

For obstructive hypertrophic cardiomyopathy, beta blockers (propranolol) and calcium channel blockers (Calan) are given to slow the heart rate to allow more filling time and lessen the strength of the heart's contraction. An antiarrhythmic agent such as disopyramide (Norpace) may be used. Patients must remain hydrated at all times to maintain cardiac output.

In obstructive hypertrophic cardiomyopathy, digoxin and vasodilators are avoided because they can increase the obstruction. Strenuous exercise and athletic sports are restricted to prevent sudden death. Lower levels of exercise may be allowed. For patients in whom medical therapy is not effective, atrioventricular (AV) sequential pacemakers, implantable automatic defibrillators, or invasive procedures are considered. For those without obstruction, fewer treatment options exist. Diuretics are used to reduce elevated pressures along with beta blockers and calcium channel blockers.

If medical therapy is not successful, surgery is considered. For hypertrophied muscle, surgery to remove part of the ventricular septum (**myectomy**) is done to allow greater outflow of blood. Another option especially for those who are not candidates for surgery is septal ablation. In septal ablation, alcohol is delivered via a catheter to necrose and reduce septal heart wall thickness.

For severe heart failure, primarily in those with dilated cardiomyopathy, a heart transplant may be the only hope for survival. A ventricular assist device may be used until a donor is found. Many patients die while waiting for a donor heart because donated organs are limited.

Nursing Management

A patient history is obtained that includes signs and symptoms and data collection related to family support systems because of the chronic nature of the disease. A physical assessment is done, noting vital signs and any signs or symptoms of heart failure.

Nursing care focuses on maintaining normal cardiac function, increasing activity tolerance, relieving anxiety, and educating the patient about the disease and its treatment. Patients with cardiomyopathy can be very ill. Careful monitoring is done to detect complications, such as heart failure, emboli, or dysrhythmias. The physician is immediately notified of problems. Home health care is often used for these patients to maintain their functional ability and reduce hospitalizations.

Maintenance of normal cardiac function includes monitoring vital signs and symptoms of heart failure. Increasing activity tolerance includes planning rest periods, scheduling activities in small amounts, avoiding tiring activities, and providing small meals that require less energy to digest than large meals. Patients are taught to avoid alcohol because it decreases cardiac function.

Reducing anxiety is important and can be accomplished by providing explanations for procedures, as well as educating the patient about the disease and its treatment. This may allow patients to feel in control of their lives by being able to make knowledgeable decisions about their health care. Methods to incorporate necessary lifestyle changes such as avoiding fatigue and scheduling rest periods can be helpful. Emotional support is greatly needed by these patients and their families because of the chronic nature of this disease (Box 23.4, *Patient Education*).

• WORD • BUILDING •

myectomy: myo—muscle + ectomy—cutting out

Box 23.4

Patient Education

Cardiomyopathy

Patients and families should understand the importance of:
- Medication compliance to prevent heart failure
- Having emergency telephone numbers readily available
- Cardiopulmonary resuscitation (CPR) training for family members
- The availability of hospice care and emotional support for families during the grieving process.

VENOUS DISORDERS

Thrombophlebitis

Thrombophlebitis is the formation of a clot and inflammation within a vein. The clot usually forms first and then inflammation occurs. Thrombophlebitis is the most common disorder of veins, with the legs being most often affected. Any superficial or deep vein in the body can be involved. Deep venous thrombosis (DVT) is the most serious form of thrombophlebitis because pulmonary emboli can result if the thrombus detaches. (See Chapter 28.)

Pathophysiology

A venous thrombus is made up of platelets, red blood cells, white blood cells, and fibrin. Platelets attach to a vein wall and then a tail forms as more blood cells and fibrin collect. As the tail grows, it drifts in the blood flowing past it. The turbulence of the blood flow can cause parts of the drifting thrombus to break off and become emboli that travel to the lungs.

Etiology

Three factors, Virchow's triangle, are involved in the formation of a thrombus: stasis of blood flow, damage to the lining of the vein wall, and increased blood coagulation (Table 23.7). Venous stasis occurs when blood flow is reduced, veins are dilated, muscle contractions are decreased, or vein valves are faulty. When the wall of a vein is damaged, it provides a site for a thrombus to form. Intravenous therapy and venipuncture cause trauma to the vein, and IV catheters in place longer than 48 to 72 hours increase the risk of inflammation and thrombus. Increased coagulation of the blood promotes thrombus formation. Patients on oral anticoagulants that are abruptly stopped experience increased clotting of the blood. Smoking, oral contraceptive use, and estrogen therapy also increase blood coagulation.

• WORD • BUILDING •

thrombophlebitis: thromb—lump (clot) + phleb—vein + itis—inflammation

Hematologic disorders can also lead to altered blood coagulation and increased risk of thrombus formation.

Prevention

Identification of risk factors for thrombosis (see Table 23.7) and patient education promote the use of interventions (discussed below) to prevent thrombosis (see *Evidence-Based Practice* box). Because the elderly are at increased risk for thrombus formation, a family member should be instructed along with the elderly person in techniques that may be difficult for the elderly person to perform. Dehydration, which is common in the elderly population, should be avoided to reduce thrombus risk.

EVIDENCE-BASED PRACTICE

Clinical Question

Are combined treatments more effective than single treatments in preventing deep venous thrombosis (DVT) and pulmonary embolism in high-risk patients?

Evidence

Eleven trials, six of them randomized controlled trials, were reviewed (Kakkos et al.). When compared with compression alone, combined prophylactic treatments were found to significantly decrease DVT and pulmonary embolism. When compared with pharmacological prophylaxis alone, combined treatments significantly decreased DVT.

Implications for Nursing Practice

The use of combined treatments for those at high risk for venous thromboembolism is more effective than a single treatment. Nurses can advocate for multiple treatment methods for these patients.

REFERENCE

Kakkos, S. K., Caprini, J. A., Geroulakos, G., et al. (2008). Combined intermittent pneumatic leg compression and pharmacological prophylaxis for prevention of venous thromboembolism in high-risk patients. *Cochrane Database of Systematic Reviews 2008, Issue 4* (Art. No. CD005258; DOI 10.1002/14651858.CD005258.pub2).

IMMOBILITY. People with sedentary jobs that require long periods of sitting, standing, or traveling long distances should change positions, perform knee and ankle flexion exercises, or walk at regular intervals to prevent stasis of blood. Patients on bedrest should have legs elevated above the level of the heart if possible and turn every 2 hours to prevent pooling of blood. Postoperatively or in times of bedrest, active or passive range-of-motion exercises should be done to increase blood flow. Postoperatively, early ambulation is a major

TABLE 23.7 PREDISPOSING CONDITIONS FOR THROMBOPHLEBITIS (VIRCHOW'S TRIANGLE)

Condition	Type	Example
Venous stasis	Reduction of blood flow	Shock, heart failure, myocardial infarction, atrial fibrillation
	Dilated veins	Vasodilators
	Decreased muscle contractions	Immobility, sitting for long periods as in traveling, fractured hip, paralysis, anesthesia, surgery, obesity, advanced age
	Faulty valves	Varicose veins, venous insufficiency
Venous wall injury		Venipuncture, venous cannulation at same site for >48 hours, venous catheterization, surgery, trauma, burns, fractures, dislocation, IV medications (potassium, chemotherapy drugs, antibiotics, IV hypertonic solutions), contrast agents, diabetes, cerebrovascular disease
Increased coagulation of blood		Anemia, malignancy, antithrombin III deficiency, oral contraceptives, estrogen therapy, smoking, discontinuance of anticoagulant therapy, dehydration, malnutrition, polycythemia, leukocytosis, thrombocytosis, sepsis, pregnancy

preventive technique for thrombosis. Patients' pain should be controlled to facilitate their ability to participate in early ambulation. Deep breathing aids in improving blood flow in the large thoracic veins. Smoking should be avoided because nicotine causes vasoconstriction.

PROPHYLACTIC ANTIEMBOLISM DEVICES. Patients with peripheral vascular disease, those on bedrest, and those who have had surgery or trauma may use antiembolism devices to improve blood flow. Knee- or thigh-length elastic stockings apply pressure to the leg. They must be applied correctly to avoid a tourniquet effect. Older patients with decreased manual dexterity may need assistance. The skin should be inspected daily for irritation under the stockings as ordered. Sequential compression devices (SCD) fill intermittently with air to move venous blood in the legs by simulating contraction of the leg muscles. They may be used in combination with elastic stockings. Research that compares the various preventive measures for DVT and rates of DVT in surgical patients has shown that the lowest incidence of DVT occurs with elastic stockings and SCDs used together.

PROPHYLACTIC MEDICATION. Low molecular weight heparin (LMWH) is given postoperatively to prevent thrombosis (Table 23.8). Anticoagulation tests are not monitored with LMWH due to the predictability of its dose-related response. Subcutaneous heparin may also be used postoperatively to prevent thrombosis. Platelet counts must be monitored with either LMWH or heparin to detect heparin-induced thrombocytopenia.

Oral anticoagulants such as warfarin (Coumadin) can be used in the high-risk patient to decrease thrombosis. The **international normalized ratio** (INR) measures the effectiveness of warfarin therapy using a standardized testing reagent. This means that INR can be used around the world with no variation in results as occurs with prothrombin time (PT) from lab to lab. INR is reported along with the PT. INR should be used; however, some practitioners still order PT, so a discussion of how to interpret the PT is presented in the following *Learning Tip* for your understanding.

INTRAVENOUS THERAPY. Monitoring of venous IV sites should be performed according to institutional policy time frames to detect signs of thrombophlebitis. Venous cannula sites should be changed regularly according to institutional guidelines (e.g., every 48 to 72 hours) to prevent thrombus formation.

LEARNING TIP

Before administering anticoagulants, laboratory values must be assessed to ensure patient safety. Normal and desired therapeutic INR values for the patient's disorder are provided on the laboratory report. These INR values do not require calculation of a therapeutic range because the values are given on the report. Compare the patient's INR value with the desired INR value to determine if it is safe to give the warfarin.

Although INR is the preferred test for warfarin effectiveness, you may still want to know how to calculate a therapeutic range for prothrombin time (PT). PT is measured in seconds. The normal value range gives the seconds required for a fibrin clot to form during the test. If a patient is on warfarin, the purpose is to increase the time (seconds) it takes the blood to clot. It is therefore expected that the PT will be elevated by warfarin therapy.

Because a therapy, warfarin, is being given, a PT range that safely considers the expected effects of the warfarin is needed. This is called the therapeutic range (i.e., a low and a high value). Warfarin's therapeutic range is 1.5 to 2 times the normal PT

range. To monitor the patient's therapeutic PT, compare the patient's result with the therapeutic range that you calculate. For example:
Patient's value on warfarin: 16 seconds (sec.)
Normal PT range: 9 to 12 seconds
To calculate therapeutic range, multiply

multiply	1.5	2
	× 9 sec.	× 12 sec.

The therapeutic range is: 13.5 sec. to 24 sec.

Compare the patient's value of 16 seconds with the therapeutic range of 13.5 to 24 seconds to determine that the patient is safely within the therapeutic range.

Signs and Symptoms

Up to 50% of patients have no symptoms with thrombophlebitis in the legs. For others, the symptoms vary according to the size and location of the thrombus (Table 23.9). If adequate collateral circulation is present near the involved area, symptoms may be reduced. For some patients a pulmonary embolus is the only evidence of a DVT.

SUPERFICIAL VEINS. Thrombophlebitis in a superficial vein may produce redness, warmth, swelling, and tenderness in the area around the site of the thrombus. The vein feels like a firm cord, which is referred to as induration. The saphenous vein is the most commonly affected vein in the leg. Varicosity of the vein is usually the cause. In the arm, IV therapy is the most common cause.

DEEP VEINS. In a deep venous thrombus of the leg (femoral vein), swelling, edema, pain, warmth, venous distention, and tenderness with palpation of the calf may be present in the affected leg. Obstruction of blood flow from the leg causes edema and varies with the location of the thrombus. An elevated temperature may also be present. Pain in the calf with sharp dorsiflexion of the foot, a classic indication known as a positive Homans' sign, is present in less than 50% of those with thrombophlebitis and is not specific to DVT. Once a DVT is positively diagnosed, it is important to avoid performing Homans' sign because it may cause the clot to become dislodged. Cyanosis and edema may occur if the large veins such as the vena cava are involved.

Complications

The most serious complication of deep venous thrombophlebitis is pulmonary embolism, which is a life-threatening emergency (see Chapter 28). Another complication, chronic

TABLE 23.8 ANTICOAGULANT MEDICATIONS

Medication Class/ Action	Examples	Route	Side Effects	Nursing Implications
Coumarin				
Inhibits liver synthesis of vitamin K dependent clotting factors: II, XII, IX, X.	warfarin (Coumadin)	PO	Hemorrhage or bleeding Risk increased with NSAIDs	Monitor INR/PT regularly. Acetaminophen (Tylenol) used instead of aspirin during therapy. Antidote: Vitamin K.
Heparins				
Bind to antithrombin III, which then inhibits fibrin formation.	heparin sodium	IV, subcutaneously	Bleeding, ecchymosis, severe hypotension	Do not give IM due to pain and hematoma. Monitor heparin anti-factor Xa or PTT: 1.5–2 times control. Monitor platelet count for decrease. Monitor for bleeding, and teach patient to report bleeding. Antidote: Protamine sulfate.
Low Molecular Weight Heparins (LMWHs)				
Bind with antithrombin III, inhibiting making of factor Xa and the formation of thrombin.	dalteparin sodium (Fragmin) enoxaparin (Lovenox) fondaparinux (Arixtra)	Subcutaneously	Bleeding rare. Contraindicated with renal failure due to increased bleeding risk.	Teach patient to give injection (prefilled syringes available), typically in abdomen. LMWH Xa monitored with renal insufficiency or obesity.
Thrombolytics				
Promote fibrinolysis to break down fibrin in blood clot.	rPA (Retavase, reteplase) TNK (TNKase, tenecteplase) tissue plasminogen activator (t-PA, alteplase)	IV	Hemorrhage	Minimize blood draws for 24 hours. Monitor for bleeding, Avoid ASA, NSAIDs.

TABLE 23.9 THROMBOPHLEBITIS SUMMARY

Signs and Symptoms	*Superficial veins:* redness, warmth, swelling, and tenderness *Deep veins:* swelling, edema, pain, warmth, venous distention, and tenderness
Diagnostic Tests	Venous duplex ultrasound Magnetic resonance venography
Therapeutic Measures	*Superficial veins:* warm, moist heat; analgesics; NSAIDs; compression stockings *Deep veins:* LMWH; heparin; warfarin; bedrest with extremity elevation above the level of the heart for 5–7 days; warm, moist heat; compression stocking therapy; thrombolytic therapy; thrombectomy; vena cava filter
Complications	Pulmonary embolism Chronic venous insufficiency Varicose veins Recurrent deep venous thrombosis
Priority Nursing Diagnoses	*Acute Pain* related to inflammation of vein *Impaired Skin Integrity* related to venous stasis *Anxiety* related to uncertain prognosis of disease

NSAID = nonsteroidal anti-inflammatory drugs.

venous insufficiency, results from damage to the valves in the vein and causes venous stasis. Signs and symptoms from venous insufficiency that may appear years after a thrombus include edema, pain, brownish discoloration and ulceration of the medial ankle, venous distention, and dependent cyanosis of the leg. This condition can be difficult to treat.

Therapeutic Measures

Diagnostic tests are done to guide treatment, with venous duplex ultrasound being the primary test used (see Table 23.9). The goals of treatment are to relieve pain and prevent pulmonary emboli, thrombus enlargement, and further thrombus development. Superficial thrombophlebitis is treated with warm, moist heat; analgesics; NSAIDs; and compression stockings.

Patients with a proximal DVT may be treated at home if they do not have pulmonary embolism, cardiovascular or pulmonary disease, obesity, or renal failure and are able to comply with follow-up care. LMWH is given subcutaneously daily or twice a day while oral warfarin is started (see Table 23.8). Both are taken until the INR is within therapeutic range (about 5 days); then the LMWH is stopped.

Traditional medical care for some DVTs involves a hospital stay. Treatment includes bedrest with leg elevation above heart level for 5 to 7 days; warm, moist heat; elastic stocking (initially on unaffected leg only until acute symptoms are gone on affected leg); and anticoagulants. An initial IV bolus of heparin and then a continuous heparin IV infusion is usually started for up to 10 days to prevent further enlargement of the thrombus and development of new thrombi; it has no effect on the existing clot, which the body dissolves over time. Daily heparin anti-factor Xa or PTTs are monitored to maintain therapeutic heparin levels. An oral anticoagulant, warfarin, is begun 4 to 5 days before the heparin is stopped. To monitor warfarin's effects, international normalized ratios (INRs) and prothrombin times (PT) are done daily, and adjustments in warfarin doses are made based on the results. Warfarin, an oral anticoagulant, takes 3 to 5 days to reach therapeutic levels. When the therapeutic INR goal is reached, the heparin is stopped. Warfarin is continued for several months. For second DVT episodes, lifelong warfarin therapy is used. Research continues to look at an oral thrombin inhibitor, which will have fewer side effects than warfarin.

An endovascular procedure using the Trellis Peripheral Infusion System is used to remove new-onset proximal (high in leg) blood clots. A catheter with two balloons is inserted into the vein and through the clot. The balloons are inflated. Then a thrombolytic medication is instilled into the clot through holes along the catheter between the two balloons. The balloons prevent the medication from being systemically absorbed and keep the clot material contained as it dissolves. A motor oscillates (moves) the catheter to disperse the medication along the clot to help dissolve it. Any clot material that remains is aspirated out of the vein through the catheter. To see this procedure, visit www.bacchusvascular.com/products/trellis/animation.html.

Early removal of the clot with this combined mechanical and pharmacological approach improves quality of life and reduces post-thrombotic syndrome (PTS) occurrence. PTS occurs after a DVT from damage to the vein valves and results in pain, swelling, and leg ulcers, which reduce quality of life. Little can be done for PTS, and treatment aims to prevent leg ulcers.

Other approaches are surgical treatment to prevent pulmonary emboli or chronic venous insufficiency when anticoagulant therapy cannot be used or the risk of pulmonary emboli is great. Venous thrombectomy removes the clot through a venous incision. In some cases, a vena cava filter is placed into the vena cava through the femoral or right internal jugular vein (Fig. 23.12). Once in place, it is opened and attaches to the vein wall. The filter traps clots traveling toward the lungs without hindering blood flow.

Nursing Process for the Patient with Thrombophlebitis

DATA COLLECTION. A patient history is obtained that includes recent IV therapy or use of contrast dyes, surgery, extremity trauma, childbirth, bedrest, recent long trip, cardiac disease, recent infections, and current medications. A physical assessment is done noting pain, fever, tenderness, positive Homans' sign, redness, warmth, swelling, edema, and a firm, cordlike vein in the affected extremity. Daily measurements are taken of bilateral thighs and calves and recorded to monitor swelling. Coagulation tests are monitored. Signs of a pulmonary embolism, such as dyspnea, tachycardia, tachypnea, blood-tinged sputum, chest pain, or changes in level of consciousness are immediately reported to the physician.

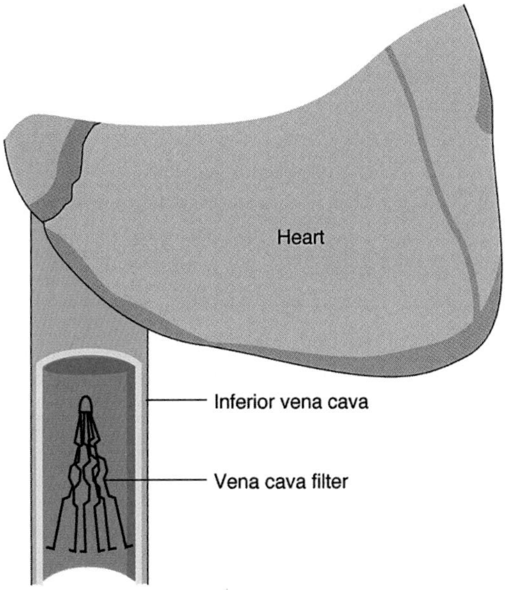
Heart
Inferior vena cava
Vena cava filter

FIGURE 23.12 Vena cava filter placed in the inferior vena cava to prevent emboli from reaching the lungs.

NURSING DIAGNOSES, PLANNING, INTERVENTIONS, AND EVALUATION. See the *Nursing Care Plan for the Patient with Thrombophlebitis,* for specific nursing interventions. Teaching the patient about the disease and treatment is important to reduce anxiety about complications and to enhance compliance with treatment to prevent complications (Box 23.5, *Patient Education*).

Box 23.5

Patient Education

Anticoagulant Therapy

Anticoagulants prolong the time it takes blood to clot, so it is important to prevent injury and to recognize and report signs of bleeding to the physician.

To Prevent Injury

- Wear shoes or slippers; avoid going barefoot.
- Use an electric razor to shave.
- Use a soft toothbrush.

Signs of Bleeding to Report to Physician

- Easy bruising
- Nosebleeds
- Bleeding that does not stop
- Blood in urine
- Blood in sputum
- Blood in stools or black stools

Additional Instructions

- Avoid use of aspirin/NSAIDs because they further prolong the time it takes for a clot to form.
- Have lab work done as prescribed by physician to monitor clotting time and medication dosage.

Home Health Hints

- On admission, measure the patient's midcalf area so you have a baseline size. Reassess measurements during each visit. Subtle changes in measurement can indicate a potential problem.
- Note whether pressure is being applied on the popliteal area or calf muscle when a patient with venous circulation problems is sitting in a recliner with the leg rest up. The angle of the recliner and the patient's height affect the position of the pressure. A small, flat pillow is placed underneath the knees and lower legs to open the angle and relieve the pressure.
- Report any abnormal findings following cardiovascular surgeries, because patients are at a high risk for thrombophlebitis. They also are at risk for incisional infection, pneumonia, and pulmonary emboli.
- Encourage the patient to move often because immobility can contribute to thrombophlebitis.
- If the patient is bed bound, instruct both the patient and caregiver on simple active and passive range-of-motion exercises. If necessary, consider involving occupational and physical therapists. Working collaboratively with therapy, an appropriate activity program can be planned.
- Assist patients to develop energy-conserving techniques by being observant of their lifestyles. For instance, notice the room and chair that the patient spends most of the day in. Trays and baskets can be used to hold items the patient may need or want, such as water, cup, medicines, tissues, a phone book, telephone, snacks, TV remote, reading material, paper, and pen. Other techniques to conserve energy are putting a carrying pouch on the front bar of a walker to carry items such as a portable phone or tissues and, if the house has stairs, putting a chair at the top and bottom of the stairs so the patient can rest.
- The caregiver should be the one to answer the door. When the patient is alone, a note can be placed on the door with instructions; however, the instructions should not convey that the patient is alone.

NURSING CARE PLAN for the Patient with Thrombophlebitis

Nursing Diagnosis: *Acute Pain* related to inflammation of vein

Expected Outcome: The patient will report satisfactory pain relief within 30 minutes of pain report.

Evaluation of Outcome: Does patient report satisfactory pain relief?

Interventions	Rationale	Evaluation
Assess pain using rating scale such as 0 to 10.	Self-report is the most reliable indicator of pain.	Does patient report pain using scale?
Provide analgesics and NSAIDs as ordered.	Pain is reduced when inflammation is decreased.	Is patient's rating of pain lower after medication?
Apply warm, moist soaks.	Heat relieves pain and vasodilates, which increases circulation to reduce swelling. Moist heat penetrates more deeply.	Does patient report increased comfort with warm, moist soaks? Is swelling reduced?
Maintain bedrest with leg elevation above heart level.	Elevation decreases swelling, which reduces pain.	Is swelling reduced?

Nursing Diagnosis: *Impaired Skin Integrity* related to venous stasis

Expected Outcome: The patient's skin will remain intact without edema at all times.

Evaluation of Outcome: Does patient's skin remain intact? Is edema present?

Interventions	Rationale	Evaluation
Observe skin for edema, skin color changes, and ulcers. Measure extremities.	Monitoring will detect signs of skin integrity impairment and extremity swelling.	Are skin changes seen? Do daily measurements show a change in swelling?
Elevate legs.	Elevation decreases swelling.	Is swelling reduced?
Fit and apply elastic stockings after edema reduced as ordered.	Elastic stockings are fitted after edema is reduced to avoid constriction. They increase venous blood flow to reduce swelling.	Is swelling reduced?
Teach patient to avoid crossing legs or wearing constricting clothes.	Crossing legs and constrictive clothes impair venous return.	Does patient state understanding of teaching?

SUGGESTED ANSWERS TO

CRITICAL THINKING

■ *Mrs. Tepley*

1. You might hear a murmur.
2. Stress and caffeine increase the occurrence of palpitations.
3. To help manage her condition, Mrs. Tepley needs a definition of MVP, stress management techniques, to know she should reduce caffeine intake (e.g., with decaffeinated coffee), and to understand symptoms of endocarditis to report to her physician.

■ *Mrs. Pryor*

1. In aortic stenosis, the valve is narrowed, which makes it more difficult for blood to leave the left ventricle and go into the aorta. This means there can be less blood flow to the body.

   Documentation: S: "What is aortic stenosis?"
   O: Listened attentively during explanation that in aortic stenosis the valve is narrowed making it more difficult for blood to leave left ventricle to go to aorta. This means there can be less blood flow to the body.
   A: Interested in learning more about diagnosis.
   P: Provide more information.
2. Angina results if the heart's oxygen needs are not met because of reduced cardiac output.
3. Nursing care should include fall precautions due to syncope and fatigue.
4. Diagnoses and care include the following: *Self-Care Deficits* related to fatigue, so plan for meeting ADL needs. *Activity Intolerance* related to fatigue, so plan rest periods between activity and monitor vital signs with activity.
5. You should give 2 tablets. Here is an example of how to solve this problem using the unit analysis method:

$$\frac{0.25 \text{ } \cancel{\text{milligrams}}}{} \left| \frac{1 \text{ tablet}}{0.125 \text{ } \cancel{\text{milligrams}}} \right. = 2 \text{ tablets}$$

■ *Mrs. Jones*

1. A heart murmur is heard from damaged heart valves.
2. Splinter hemorrhages appear as black or red lines in the nails.
3. Petechiae indicate that tiny pieces of a lesion on the endocardium or valves have broken off and become microemboli.
4. Subjective data collection findings might include patient statements such as "I have pain in my joints and am chilled" or "I am fatigued and have no appetite." Objective findings are as follows: temperature 100°F (37°C), red splinter hemorrhages in left index finger nailbed, many petechiae on chest.
5. Expected medications include IV antibiotics.
6. Removing blankets to decrease fever results in chills and shivering, which further increases body temperature from the heat generated by muscular activity during shivering. Therefore, Mrs. Jones should be kept covered to prevent chills.
7. For left-sided heart failure, crackles, wheezes, cough, or dyspnea might be seen. In right-sided heart failure, peripheral edema or jugular venous distention could be present.
8. Two tablets.

REVIEW QUESTIONS

1. Which of the following symptoms would the nurse identify as a priority to report for a patient with aortic stenosis?
   a. Angina
   b. Peripheral edema
   c. Headache
   d. Weight loss

2. The nurse is evaluating patient teaching for mitral valve prolapse. The patient shows understanding of the prognosis of MVP by stating which of the following?
   a. "The prognosis is poor."
   b. "There are often no symptoms."
   c. "Heart failure often occurs."
   d. "Symptoms quickly progress."

3. The nurse is evaluating patient preoperative teaching for a commissurotomy. The patient shows understanding of the purpose of this procedure by stating which of the following?
   a. "Fused valve flaps are separated to enlarge the valve opening."
   b. "A mechanical valve is inserted to replace a valve."
   c. "The valve flaps are repaired or reconstructed."
   d. "A biological valve is inserted to replace a valve."

REVIEW QUESTIONS—cont'd

4. The nurse is planning care for a patient having a cardiac valve replacement. With which type of valve will the patient be on anticoagulant therapy to prevent thrombus formation?
   a. Mechanical valve
   b. Porcine valve
   c. Allograft valve
   d. Bovine valve

5. The nurse evaluates the patient as understanding how to prevent rheumatic fever if the patient states that rheumatic fever can be prevented by treating streptococcal infections with which of the following?
   a. Penicillin
   b. Prednisone
   c. Cortisone
   d. Cyclosporine

6. The nurse is planning care for a patient with cardiomyopathy. For which of the following complications of cardiomyopathy should the nurse collect data?
   a. Thrombophlebitis
   b. Heart failure
   c. Rheumatic fever
   d. Pulmonary embolism

7. Which of the following signs and symptoms indicate to the nurse the presence of a deep venous thrombus in the patient's leg? **Select all that apply.**
   a. Calf swelling
   b. Crackles
   c. Jugular venous distention
   d. Positive Homans' sign
   e. Warmth
   f. Redness

8. The nurse is to give warfarin (Coumadin). Which of the following laboratory tests should the nurse review before giving the medication?
   a. International normalized ratio
   b. Partial thromboplastin time
   c. Plasma fibrinogen level
   d. Bleeding time

Reference

Wilson, W., Taubert, K. A., Gewitz, M., et al. (2007). Prevention of infective endocarditis: Guidelines from the American Heart Association. A guideline from the American Heart Association Rheumatic Fever, Endocarditis, and Kawasaki Disease Committee, Council on Cardiovascular Disease in the Young, and the Council on Clinical Cardiology, Council on Cardiovascular Surgery and Anesthesia, and the Quality of Care and Outcomes Research Interdisciplinary Working Group. *Circulation, 116,* 1736–1754.

24

Nursing Care of Patients with Occlusive Cardiovascular Disorders

MAUREEN McDONALD

KEY TERMS

acute coronary syndrome (ah-KYOOT KOR-uh-nare-ee sin-dr-OME)
anastomosed (an-AST-tah-most)
aneurysm (AN-yur-izm)
angina pectoris (an-JYE-nah PEK-tuh-riss)
arteriosclerosis (ar-TEER-ee-oh-skleh-ROH-siss)
atherosclerosis (ATH-er-oh-skleh-ROH-siss)
collateral circulation (kuh-LAH-tur-al SIR-kew-LAY-shun)
coronary artery disease (KOR-uh-nare-ee AR-tuh-ree dih-ZEEZ)
endarterectomy (en-DART-tur-eck-toe-me)
embolism (EM-buh-lizm)
high-density lipoprotein (HY DEN-sih-tee LIH-poh-PROH-teen)
hyperlipidemia (HY-pur-LIH-pih-DEE-mee-ah)
intermittent claudication (IN-tur-MIT-tent KLAW-dih-KAY-shun)
low-density lipoproteins (LOH DEN-sih-tee LIH-poh-PROH-teen)
lymphangitis (lim-FAN-jee-EYE-tiss)
myocardial infarction (MY-oh-KAR-dee-yuhl in-FARK-shun)
peripheral arterial disease (puh-RIFF-uh-ruhl ar-TEER-ee-uhl dih-ZEEZ)
plaque (PLAK)
Raynaud's disease (rah-NOHZ dih-ZEEZ)
thrombosis (throm-BOH-siss)
varicose veins (VAR-ih-kohz VAINS)
venous stasis ulcers (VEE-nus STAY-siss UL-sers)

QUESTIONS TO GUIDE YOUR READING

1. What are the etiologies, signs, symptoms, and therapeutic measures of coronary artery disease, angina pectoris, and myocardial infarction?
2. What data should you collect and what nursing care will you provide for patients with coronary artery disease, angina pectoris, or myocardial infarction?
3. What therapeutic measures are used to treat coronary artery disease, angina pectoris, and myocardial infarction?
4. What are the etiologies, signs, and symptoms for each of the peripheral vascular disorders?
5. What therapeutic measures are used to treat each peripheral vascular disorder?
6. What nursing care will you provide for patients with each peripheral vascular disorder?

Cardiovascular disorders are the leading cause of disability and death in the United States. Diseases of the heart and peripheral vessels can affect quality of life and alter the ability of the individual to perform tasks of everyday living. Many factors leading to cardiovascular diseases can be controlled or modified. Education is important in preventing and treating occlusive cardiovascular diseases.

In 2006, among adults ages 20 and older, the prevalence of coronary artery disease was 16,800,000 (American Heart Association, 2009). In that same year, 9,800,000 people had angina, with 500,000 new cases of stable angina and 150,000 cases of unstable angina occurring each year. One in three adults has cardiovascular disease (CVD). About every 25 seconds, an American will suffer a coronary event and about every minute someone will die from one. Two of three women develop CVD, which occurs on average about 6 years later than in men, often after menopause. The average age for a person having a first heart attack is 64.5 for men and 70.3 for women. Smoking lowers this age for both genders but more so for women. Because women typically have heart attacks at older ages than men they are more likely to die from heart attacks within a few weeks. Heart disease is the leading cause of death in African Americans, Hispanics, and American Indians (National Heart, Lung, and Blood Institute, 2008).

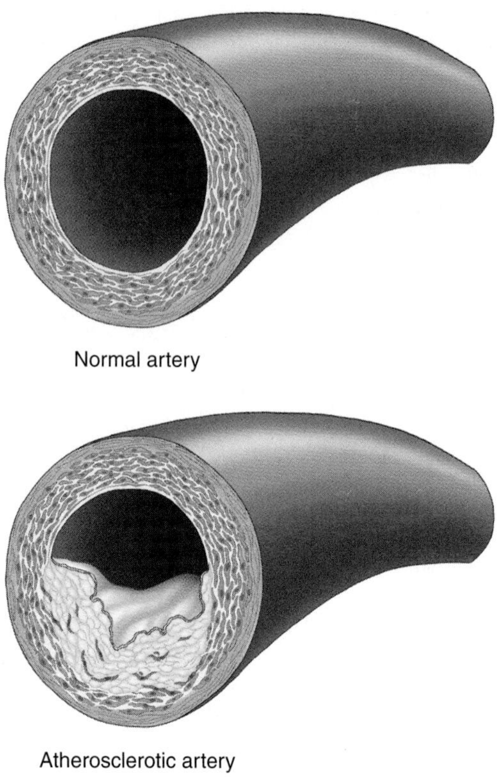
Normal artery
Atherosclerotic artery

FIGURE 24.1 (Top) Cross section of normal coronary artery. (Bottom) Coronary artery with atherosclerosis narrowing the lumen.

ARTERIOSCLEROSIS

Arteriosclerosis is a disorder characterized by thickening, loss of elasticity, and calcification of arterial walls. This condition is part of the aging process in which the intimal lining of the artery wall loses elasticity and weakens. This weakening is due to the high pressure that carries blood within arteries. Arteriosclerosis often develops with aging, hypertension, and diabetes.

ATHEROSCLEROSIS

Atherosclerosis is the formation of plaque within the arterial wall. Arteriosclerosis and atherosclerosis are conditions that may begin in early childhood and progress without symptoms through adult life.

Pathophysiology

Atherosclerosis is a multistep process that affects the inner lining of the artery (Fig. 24.1). First injury to the endothelial cells that line the walls of the arteries occurs, causing inflammation and immune reactions. Damage to the endothelium stimulates the growth of smooth muscle cells. These cells secrete collagen and fibrous proteins. Lipids, platelets, and other clotting factors accumulate. Scar tissue replaces some of the arterial wall.

An early indication of injury is a fatty streak on the lining of the artery. This buildup of fatty deposits is known as **plaque**. It is composed of smooth muscle cells, fibrous proteins, and cholesterol-laden foam cells. Plaque has irregular, jagged edges that allow blood cells and other material to adhere to the wall of the artery. The portion of the plaque that faces the bloodstream develops a fibrous cap, a firm shell that often contains calcium. Over time this buildup becomes calcified and hardened, causing turbulence that damages cells and increases the buildup within the vessel. Sometimes the plaque's fibrous cap tears or ruptures and a blood clot forms. This blood clot can completely block the coronary artery, or it may break loose and lodge within a smaller artery leading to the heart. The vessel may also become stenosed (narrowed) by plaque buildup. This buildup of plaque may cause partial or total occlusion of the artery resulting in reduced blood flow. The area distal to the occlusion may become ischemic as a result.

Etiology

Risk factors for atherosclerosis can be divided into two categories: those that can be modified and those that cannot. Nonmodifiable risk factors include:

- Age
- Gender

• WORD • BUILDING •
arteriosclerosis: arterio—artery + sklerosis—hardness

- Ethnicity
- Genetics: predisposition for **hyperlipidemia** (increased lipids in the blood including cholesterol and triglycerides).

Modifiable risk factors include:

- Diabetes mellitus
- Hypertension
- Smoking
- Obesity
- Sedentary lifestyle
- Increased serum homocysteine levels (an amino acid)
- Increased serum iron levels
- Infection
- Depression
- Hyperlipidemia
- Elevated apolipoprotein B
- Excessive alcohol intake.

Diagnostic Tests

Cholesterol and triglycerides are often elevated in patients with atherosclerosis (Table 24.1; also see Table 21.3). Total cholesterol levels above 200 mg/dL increase risk of myocardial infarction. **Low-density lipoproteins** (LDLs) increase coronary artery disease (CAD) risks, but **high-density lipoproteins** (HDL) are protective against CAD. A premature risk factor is a high Lp(a) cholesterol (a genetic variation of plasma LDL) level. Apolipoprotein B particles in LDL-type cholesterol are able to infiltrate the arterial wall, rapidly causing damage. People with a higher proportion of apolipoprotein B to apolipoprotein A are at a much higher risk for CVD. C-reactive protein (CRP) can indicate low-grade inflammation in coronary vessels and long-term heart disease risk. An elevated leukocyte count in women ages 50 to 79 increases the risk of CVD.

Blood glucose levels should also be checked because elevated levels may increase the risk for atherosclerosis.

TABLE 24.1 ATHEROSCLEROSIS SUMMARY

Diagnostic Tests	Cholesterol Triglycerides Arteriogram
Therapeutic Measures	Low-fat, low-cholesterol diet Smoking cessation Increased exercise—walk 30 minutes daily
Priority Nursing Diagnoses	*Deficient Knowledge* related to self-care and health promotion *Pain* related to reduced vascular or coronary artery blood flow

• WORD • BUILDING •
hyperlipidemia: hyper—above + lipos—fat + emia—blood

Radiological studies of the arteries can be performed to show narrowed or occluded vessels (see Chapter 21).

Therapeutic Measures

A healthy lifestyle, medications, and frequent checkups are helpful in controlling arteriosclerosis and atherosclerosis.

Diet

Because the formation of plaque within arteries is primarily caused by fatty deposits, an adherence to a low-fat diet is recommended (Box 24.1, *Nutrition Notes*). The American Heart Association (AHA) has posted complete guidelines and diets for decreasing fat and cholesterol intake at www.americanheart.org.

Smoking

The risk of developing CAD is two to six times higher in cigarette smokers than in nonsmokers. Risk is proportionate to the number of cigarettes smoked. Smoking contributes to a loss of HDLs. These proteins are the best cholesterol to have in the body to decrease the risk of cardiovascular disorders. Smoking also causes vasoconstriction, which leads to angina pectoris and cardiac dysrhythmias. The benefits of smoking cessation are dramatic and almost immediate. Education about the risks of smoking and effects of exposure to second-hand smoke should be presented to patients. The American Cancer Society has many programs to help patients quit smoking. Visit its website at www.cancer.org.

Exercise

Increased activity raises HDL levels. Increasing physical activity may also lower insulin resistance and facilitate weight loss. Over time, exercise also leads to the development of **collateral circulation**, which allows blood to flow around occluded sites. Before beginning an exercise program, patients should consult a physician.

Medications

Lowering lipid levels is the major treatment for atherosclerosis. When dietary control is not effective, medication is also used (Table 24.2). It may take 4 to 6 weeks before lipid levels respond to drug therapy. If one drug does not control lipids, another drug can be added.

CORONARY ARTERY DISEASE

Coronary artery disease is the term applied to obstruction of blood flow through the coronary arteries to the heart muscle cells, typically from atherosclerosis. Blood flow reduction resulting from CAD can cause angina and progress to **myocardial infarction** (MI, heart attack) or sudden death if blood flow is not restored.

Prevention

Risk factors for CAD are listed in Table 24.3. The guidelines for prevention of heart disease from the American Heart Association target the risk factors that have the potential for change. See the later section on therapeutic measures for

Box 24.1

Nutrition Notes

Controlling Blood Cholesterol with Diet

Two-thirds of the body's cholesterol is produced by the liver and intestines. Most people produce less cholesterol or increase its excretion in response to high levels of dietary cholesterol, but others respond weakly, a phenomenon that may be genetically based. Although only foods of animal origin contain cholesterol, some vegetable oil products contain trans fats, potent risk factors for cardiovascular disease.

The following actions may reduce LDL-cholesterol by the indicated percentages.

Recommendation	Possible LDL Reduction
Consuming less than 7% kcal as saturated fat (including less than 1% as trans fat)	8%–10%
Consuming less than 200 mg cholesterol daily	3%–5%
Consuming 5 to 10 g soluble fiber daily	3%–5%
Possibly consuming plant sterol/stanol-enriched foods, 2 g daily	6%–10%

Specific strategies to lower blood cholesterol include:

- Reducing saturated fat intake by
  - Using nonfat or low-fat dairy products (Milk fat contains more cholesterol-raising fatty acids than meat fat.)
  - Selecting lean meat, trimming fat from meat, rinsing browned ground beef, and skimming fat from meat juices for soup or gravy.
- Adding foods for which the U.S. Food and Drug Administration has approved health claims such as:
  - Foods rich in marine omega-3 fatty acids (herring, mackerel, rainbow trout, salmon, sardines, swordfish, and tuna)
  - Foods containing soluble fiber, particularly psyllium seed husk (e.g., Kellogg's Bran Buds)
  - Soy-containing foods if not contraindicated by patient history.
- Consuming foods containing plant sterols that bind with bile and cholesterol, increasing their excretion in the feces. They are found in table spreads (butter substitutes), juices, yogurts, and salad dressings and should be limited to prescribed amounts. They are contraindicated in a rare autosomal recessive disorder called sitosterolemia.

atherosclerosis. Low-dose aspirin, for women over age 64 and men, and anticoagulants are used to prevent the formation of a thrombus.

Angina Pectoris

Pathophysiology

When an increased workload is placed on the heart, as in exercise or strenuous activity, there is an increased demand for oxygen. Normally, when the heart needs more oxygen, the coronary arteries dilate to carry more blood. However, with CAD, the narrowed vessels are unable to dilate and supply the heart with this extra blood and oxygen. This inability to supply more blood and oxygen causes myocardial ischemia and **angina pectoris** (chest pain). Angina may also be caused by conditions other than CAD such as vasospasm, valvular heart disease, hypertension, or heart failure.

Types of Angina

Angina can be classified as stable (less serious) or unstable.

STABLE ANGINA. Stable angina is chest pain that occurs with moderate exertion in a pattern that is familiar to the patient. The pain is predictable and can usually be managed with nitroglycerin and rest. The pain of stable angina usually subsides when the activity is stopped.

VARIANT OR VASOSPASTIC ANGINA (PRINZMETAL'S ANGINA). This type of angina is caused by coronary artery spasms and is serious. The pattern of occurrence is often cyclical, with the pain presenting about the same time each day. The pain has a longer duration than stable angina, can occur with exercise or at rest and often occurs at night.

• WORD • BUILDING •

angina pectoris: angina—to choke + pectora—chest

LEARNING TIP

Angina pectoris is not a disease. It is the symptom of ischemia that results from a lack of oxygen and blood flow to the heart muscle. Ischemia = pain or angina.

Signs and Symptoms

Anginal pain manifests in several ways. Patients (especially men) often describe the pain as heaviness, tightness, squeezing, viselike, or crushing in the center of the chest or adjacent to the chest (Fig. 24.2). The pain can radiate down one or

TABLE 24.2 MEDICATIONS USED TO LOWER LIPID LEVELS

Medication Class/Action	Examples	Route	Side Effects	Nursing Implications
Statins				
First-line drugs to reduce low-density lipoprotein by reducing cholesterol synthesis.	atorvastatin (Lipitor) fluvastatin (Lescol XL) lovastatin (Mevacor) pravastatin (Pravachol) simvastatin (Zocor) rosuvastatin (Crestor)	PO	Impaired liver function, rhabdomyolysis (lethal breakdown of skeletal muscle)	Tell patient to take in the evening when cholesterol synthesis is highest. Teach patient to report any muscle pain. Monitor liver function studies.
Fibrates				
Reduce triglycerides.	fenofibrate (TriCor) clofibrate (Atromid-S) gemfibrozil (Lopid)	PO	Heartburn, gallstones	Tell patient to take 30 minutes before morning and evening meal. May increase the effects of anticoagulants and hypoglycemia.
Bile Acid Sequestrants				
Lower cholesterol by binding bile acids, so stored cholesterol is used to make more bile acids.	colestipol (Colestid) colesevelam HCl (Welchol, Sankyo) cholestyramine (Questran)	PO	Headache, heartburn, constipation, gas	Fruits and vegetables high in fiber should be added to diet to reduce constipation and other GI effects noted with bile acid sequestrants. May interfere with absorption of digoxin, thiazides, and beta blockers.
Niacin				
Prevents conversion of fats into very-low-density lipoproteins. Rarely used due to flushing.	niacin (Nicotinic acid) extended-release niacin (Niaspan)	PO PO	Gastritis, flushing Gout, flushing	Take aspirin 30 minutes prior to taking drug to reduce flushing.
Cholesterol Absorption Inhibitor				
Inhibits the absorption of cholesterol. Decreases LDLs and increases HDLs.	ezetimibe (Zetia)	PO	Headache, gastrointestinal disturbance. Should not be used in patients with liver impairment.	Tell patient to take with liquids and meals and to take other drugs 1 hour before or 4 hours after.
Combination Agent				
See each agent.	Vytorin (Zetia + Zocor)	PO	See each agent.	See each agent.

TABLE 24.3 RISK FACTORS FOR CORONARY ARTERY DISEASE

Risk Factors That Cannot Be Changed	
Heredity	Coronary artery disease (CAD) risk factors can run in families.
Ethnicity	African Americans have a higher incidence of atherosclerosis.
Gender	Men have more risk factors and higher incidence of CAD.
Age	Men have increased incidence after age 50. Women have increased incidence after menopause.
Risk Factors That Can Be Changed or Controlled	
Smoking	Causes vasoconstriction and increases myocardial oxygen demand. Decreases high-density lipoproteins.
Hypertension	Vasoconstriction increases myocardial oxygen demand.
Elevated serum cholesterol	Level above 240 mg/dL increases the risk of developing CAD.
Diabetes	Increases the risk of hypertension, obesity, and elevated blood lipids.
Obesity	Increases heart workload and risk of hypertension, diabetes, glucose intolerance, hyperlipidemia.
Stress	Increases heart workload and risk for hypertension.
Elevated serum homocysteine	Increases CAD risk. Foods that contain folic acid (fruits, green leafy vegetables) reduce homocysteine level.
Sedentary lifestyle	Increases obesity, hypertension, hyperlipidemia.
Excessive alcohol use	Raises blood pressure leading to heart failure. Increases triglycerides. Causes irregular heartbeats.

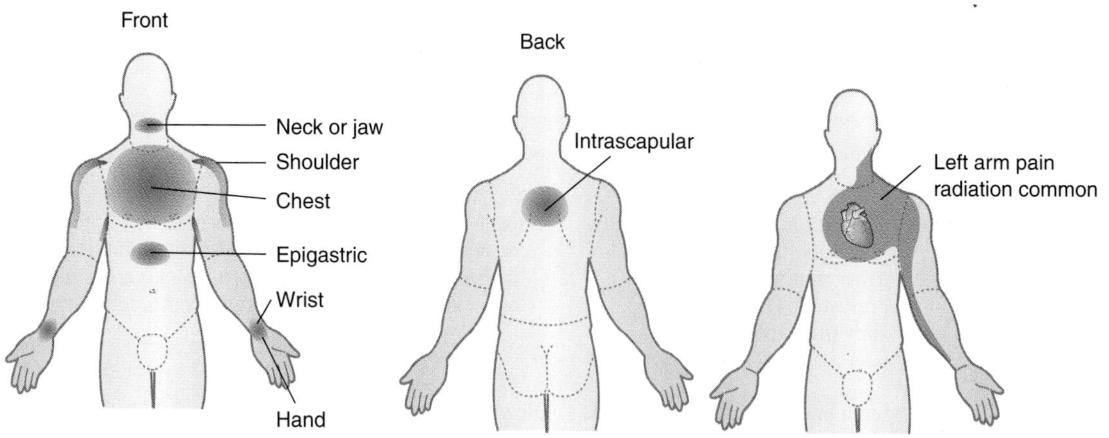
Front
Back
Neck or jaw
Shoulder
Chest
Epigastric
Wrist
Hand
Intrascapular
Left arm pain
radiation common

FIGURE 24.2 Common locations of anginal pain, which may vary in combination and intensity.

both arms, with pain in the left arm being more common, into the shoulder, neck, jaw, or back. Patients may also describe heaviness in their arms or a feeling of impending doom. During the episode of pain, the patient may be pale, diaphoretic, or dyspneic.

The pain is usually brought on by exertion and subsides with rest. It can be relieved with a vasodilator such as nitroglycerin. Episodes of chest pain may increase in frequency and severity over time. If patients do not heed this warning to stop their activity and rest, they may be at risk for myocardial infarction or sudden death. Any event that increases oxygen demand can cause an anginal attack. Most often, precipitating events include large meals, exercise, cold, stimulant drugs such as cocaine or amphetamines, stress, and emotional tension. Angina commonly occurs in the morning between 6:00 a.m. and noon when the patient arises and the workload of the heart increases.

Women may experience anginal pain as chest pain, jaw pain, or heartburn or have symptoms different than those thought of as being typical of angina. These symptoms include less severe pain, fatigue, nausea, and breathlessness. These atypical symptoms should be recognized as possibly being cardiac related so that treatment is sought. (See the *Women and Heart Health* section.)

Diagnostic Tests

Tests commonly done for CAD and angina include electrocardiogram, exercise electrocardiogram, graded exercise testing, stress echocardiography, chemical stress testing, radioisotope imaging, and coronary angiography (see Table 21.3).

Therapeutic Measures

Treatment for CAD and angina is directed at relieving and preventing anginal episodes that could lead to a myocardial infarction. The risk factors identified for the patient determine the course of treatment. Weight reduction; a low-fat, low-cholesterol diet; and stress reduction may help slow disease progression. The three major groups of medication used for angina are vasodilators (nitrates), calcium channel blockers, and beta blockers. Table 24.4 discusses these and other medications used to treat angina.

VASODILATORS. Nitroglycerin (NTG, a nitrate) is the drug of choice for acute anginal attacks. Nitrates dilate coronary arteries to increase oxygen to the myocardium, and dilate peripheral vessels so the heart does not have to work so hard to pump blood into them. NTG can be administered sublingually, orally, transdermally, intravenously, or as a lingual spray. When administered sublingually, NTG may relieve chest pain within 1 to 2 minutes (Box 24.2). AHA guidelines tell people to immediately call 911 after one tablet and 5 minutes if pain remains unrelieved and symptoms of a myocardial infarction are occurring.

Long-acting nitrates are used to prevent chest pain rather than to treat acute pain. They can be given orally, in ointment, or by transdermal patches. Always remove the prior ointment or patch before applying a new one. A problem with long-acting nitrates is the development of a tolerance to the drug. To prevent tolerance, the patch or ointment is usually removed at bedtime and reapplied in the morning, giving the patient an 8- to 12-hour nitrate-free period. Headaches may be experienced when nitrates are first begun. This side effect usually subsides after a week or two and can be relieved with aspirin.

CALCIUM CHANNEL BLOCKERS. Calcium is required for electrical excitability of cardiac cells and contraction of the myocardium and vascular smooth muscle. Calcium channel blockers relax vascular smooth muscle, which leads to decreased peripheral vascular resistance (afterload) and decreased myocardial oxygen demand. These drugs dilate main coronary arteries, increasing the myocardial oxygen supply. Amlodipine (Norvasc) and diltiazem (Cardizem) along with nitrates are used to treat variant (Prinzmetal's) angina. Calcium channel blockers are also used to decrease systolic and diastolic blood pressures and to slow the heart rate. These drugs are commonly given in conjunction with other vasodilators and beta blockers. Because these drugs are slow acting, they are ineffective in relieving acute anginal attacks. Side effects of calcium channel blockers are usually mild and include constipation, fluid retention, headache, and dizziness.

TABLE 24.4 MEDICATIONS USED TO TREAT ANGINA PECTORIS

Medication Class/Action	Examples	Route	Side Effects	Nursing Implications
Antiplatelets				
Inhibit platelet activation, adhesion, or procoagulant activity.	aspirin	PO	Increased risk of bleeding	Enteric coated may be given for daily dosing.
Statins *(See Table 24.2.)*				
Nitrates				
Vasodilate to reduce preload and afterload. Reduce oxygen consumption of myocardium.	nitroglycerin (Nitrostat, NitroQuick); nitroglycerin lingual spray (Nitrolingual Pumpspray) isosorbide dinitrate (Isordil)	SL, SL spray	Hypotension, headache, orthostatic hypotension, dizziness.	Document onset, type, radiation, location, and duration of chest pain. Take apical pulse and BP pre- and postadministration. Place SL tablet in buccal pouch to lessen burning sensation under tongue.
	isosorbide mononitrate (Imdur, ISMO)	PO, SL	Contraindicated in head trauma, hypotension, uncorrected hypovolemia	Do not shake aerosol canister before administration of lingual spray. Urge patient to rise slowly, especially with sublingual spray. If chest pain is not relieved, call physician or emergency medical assistance. Tablets should be replaced every 3 to 6 months. Check expiration date. Keep tablets in original bottle. Vasodilators become inactive when exposed to light, air, heat, and moisture. Tell patient burning or tingling sensation may be felt under the tongue with sublingual nitroglycerin. Tell patient to avoid alcohol.
	nitroglycerin (Transderm Nitro, Nitro-Bid) nitroglycerin patch (Nitro-Dur, Nitrek)	Transdermal		Remove old patch before placing new patch. Remove patch before MRI or defibrillation. Rotate application sites. Apply patch to clean, dry, hairless area. Remove at bedtime so tolerance does not develop.
Angiotensin-Converting Enzyme Inhibitors				
Block production of angiotensin II, a potent vasoconstrictor. Vasodilate and improve cardiac output and exercise tolerance.	captopril (Capoten) lisinopril (Prinivil, Zestril) ramipril (Altace) enalapril (Vasotec)	PO (captopril also SL)	Persistent dry cough may develop in 20% of patients. Hyperkalemia may develop in patients with diabetes mellitus or renal impairment.	If pulse is less than 60 beats per minute or systolic BP less than 90 mm Hg, notify physician. Give 1 hour before meals. Give captopril on empty stomach. *Teaching:* Take first doses at night to adjust to lower BP. Rise slowly. Check BP weekly. Report development of cough or other side effects.
Calcium Channel Blockers				
Dilate peripheral arteries, decrease myocardial contractility, depress conduction system, and decrease workload of the heart. In variant angina, reduce coronary artery spasm.	diltiazem (Cardizem, Dilacor XR) amlodipine (Norvasc) nicardipine (Cardene) felodipine (Plendil)	PO	Headache, peripheral edema, flushing, dizziness, atrioventricular blocks, nausea	If pulse less than 60 beats per minute or systolic BP less than 90 mm Hg, notify physician. Administer before meals and at bedtime.

Continued

TABLE 24.4 MEDICATIONS USED TO TREAT ANGINA PECTORIS—cont'd

Medication Class/Action	Examples	Route	Side Effects	Nursing Implications
Beta Blockers				
Decrease pulse, BP, and cardiac output and suppress renin activity. Decrease the risk of sudden death.	metoprolol (Lopressor, Toprol XL) atenolol (Tenormin)	PO, IV PO	Cold extremities, constipation, diarrhea, diaphoresis, dizziness, fatigue, and nausea. Abrupt withdrawal may result in diaphoresis, palpitations, headache, and tremors.	If pulse less than 60 beats per minute or systolic BP less than 90 mm Hg, notify physician. Instruct patient to rise slowly. Tell patient to avoid salt and alcohol. Beta blockers are contraindicated in asthma, heart block, bronchoconstriction.
Anti-Ischemic Agent				
Antianginal agent used as combination therapy for those not responding to other antianginal.	ranolazine (Ranexa)	PO	Prolongs QT interval on ECG. Dizziness, headache, nausea.	May not be as effective in women.

SAFETY TIP

Those who take nitrates should not use drugs such as sildenafil (Viagra), tadalafil (Cialis), or vardenafil (Levitra) for erectile dysfunction because these types of drugs dilate blood vessels and may cause a significant drop in blood pressure if used together.

Box 24.2

Key Points for Using Sublingual Nitroglycerin

- Carry nitroglycerin (NTG) at all times.
- Keep NTG tightly sealed in the original container and protected from heat, light, and moisture.
- Replace NTG at least every 6 months for maximum effect, or every 3 to 4 months if carried in a pocket next to body heat.
- Take NTG before an activity known to cause chest pain.
- Sit or lie down when taking NTG, if possible.
- Take one NTG tablet and repeat every 5 minutes up to three doses if pain is not relieved. If pain is unrelieved after one dose and other symptoms of myocardial infarction are present, call 911 for emergency medical care.
- Tingling should be felt under the tongue when NTG is used.
- NTG may cause a headache initially. Aspirin may relieve it.
- NTG may cause light-headedness. Rise slowly to prevent falls.

BETA BLOCKERS. Beta blockers decrease heart rate, lower blood pressure, and prevent release of renin. This results in decreased workload on the heart to help prevent anginal attacks. Because of these decreased effects, beta blockers should be used with caution in patients with any degree of heart failure because it may make heart failure worse. There are nonselective and selective types of beta-adrenergic blockers. People with asthma or chronic obstructive pulmonary disease (emphysema, bronchitis, and bronchiectasis) should avoid nonselective beta-adrenergic blockers because they cause bronchoconstriction. Metoprolol (Lopressor) and atenolol (Tenormin) are more cardioselective and can be used in patients with asthma and chronic obstructive pulmonary disease (COPD). Beta blockers are not effective for coronary artery spasms.

LEARNING TIP

To help you identify beta blockers, remember that their generic names end with *-olol.*

ANGIOTENSIN-CONVERTING ENZYME INHIBITORS. Angiotensin-converting enzyme inhibitors (ACEIs) block production of angiotensin II, which is a potent vasoconstrictor. This action reduces peripheral arterial resistance (vasodilation), which lowers blood pressure. ACEIs may cause retention of potassium in some patients. If a patient taking an ACEI develops a dry cough, the health care provider can be informed. The medication may then be changed.

STATINS. Cholesterol and inflammation in artery walls are involved in atherosclerosis development. Statins lower cholesterol levels by reducing cholesterol production in the liver (see Table 24.2). They also reduce inflammation and CRP levels, which improves patient outcomes in CAD. Statins are used to prevent and treat atherosclerosis and the disorders caused by it.

ANTIPLATELETS. Aspirin and clopidogrel (Plavix) are commonly used antiplatelets that help prevent cardiovascular events.

Nursing Process for the Patient with Atherosclerosis, Coronary Artery Disease, and Angina

Data Collection

A health history is obtained regarding the patient's risk for atherosclerosis and CAD. Data collected include nonmodifiable and modifiable risk factors. A history of chest pain, fatigue, or activity intolerance is noted. Allergies and current medications, including over-the-counter and prescription drugs are documented. Height, weight, and diet history are recorded.

Assess anginal pain by patient's description of pain: type, location, and pain radiation to other areas of the body. Note skin color and temperature. Note any factors that may make the pain worse or better. This will provide information to determine improvement or lack of improvement in pain. Ask how long the patient has had angina, triggering activities, and how the pain has been relieved in the past. Note the presence of dyspnea, labored respirations, diaphoresis, or nausea. Obtain vital signs, blood pressure, apical pulse, respiration, and oxygen saturation to provide a baseline of the patient status.

Nursing Diagnoses, Planning, and Implementation

Acute Pain Related to Reduced Coronary Artery Blood Flow and Increased Myocardial Oxygen Needs Causing an Imbalance Between Oxygen Supply and Demand

EXPECTED OUTCOME: The patient will report an absence of pain.

- Ensure vascular access is established. *Intravenous access may be necessary to use to administer drugs for pain relief.*
- Administer oxygen as ordered via nasal cannula *to increase oxygen availability to myocardium.*
- Obtain a 12-lead ECG as ordered *to determine ischemia or injury of the myocardium with evaluation of the ST segment.*
- Administer aspirin as prescribed *to decrease platelet aggregation.*
- Administer morphine as prescribed *to provide pain relief.*
- Administer sublingual nitroglycerin as ordered. Notify physician if pain is unrelieved after three doses of NTG or as prescribed, or if vital signs change. *Chest pain unrelieved by nitrates may represent unstable angina or myocardial infarction.*
- Remain with patient and reassess pain in 5 minutes after administration of medication. *A patient who has chest pain should never be left alone.*
- Notify physician of ECG changes. *ST-segment elevation may indicate a myocardial infarction.* (See Chapter 25.)
- Offer the patient assurance and emotional support *to decrease anxiety. Emotional support is important because patients and their families are often afraid that the patient may die.*
- Promote rest and decrease anxiety for the patient with chest pain *to help relieve stress and chest pain.*
- Document patient data in the medical record *to communicate patient's problem and outcome.*

Deficient Knowledge Related to Ineffective Management of Regimen for Atherosclerosis or Coronary Artery Disease

EXPECTED OUTCOME: The patient will report understanding and management of atherosclerosis and CAD.

- Identify cognitive or physical impairments *that would interfere with the patient's ability to learn desired information.*
- Include significant other as appropriate *to support patient during learning.*
- Collect data on patient's present understanding of atherosclerosis and CAD *to determine baseline knowledge.*
- Collect data on patient's readiness to learn and desired learning needs and feelings about incorporating lifestyle changes into daily routine *to prioritize teaching topics.*
- Determine cultural beliefs *because they may influence learning.*
- Provide for patient's physical comfort during teaching *to increase learning.*
- Use appropriate teaching tools *to meet individual learning needs, such as pamphlets, diagrams, or other written materials in simple language.*
- Use an interpreter as needed, and provide written materials in patient's native language *to facilitate understanding.*
- Explain pathophysiology of atherosclerosis and CAD, control of risk factors, and management of CAD symptoms *to promote understanding.*
- Explain action, side effects, and importance of taking medications as prescribed *to relieve pain and prevent complications.*
- Provide information about community resources *that can assist in making lifestyle changes, such as weight loss, smoking cessation, stress management, and exercise.*
- Teach patient to monitor blood pressure and heart rate as appropriate and to report chest pain or dyspnea, *which may point to the presence of complications from CAD.*

- Help patient plan how to incorporate information into daily life *to increase likelihood that change will occur.*
- Encourage questions and allow patient opportunity to verbalize new information and skills *to enhance learning.*
- Document teaching and evaluation of patient knowledge *to validate understanding.*

Evaluation

Interventions are successful if the patient is pain free and has an increased understanding of atherosclerosis and CAD and their management and states that he or she will modify risk factors of CAD.

ACUTE CORONARY SYNDROME

The term **acute coronary syndrome** (ACS) is used to encompass the continuum of coronary artery disease such as unstable angina pectoris and myocardial infarction.

Unstable Angina

Unstable angina occurs in patients with worsening CAD and is noted by its changing or unpredictable pattern. Rest does not decrease the chest pain of unstable angina. This pain may even occur when the patient is at rest. The episodes of chest pain with unstable angina increase in frequency and severity, placing the patient at risk for myocardial damage or sudden death. Symptoms of angina usually occur when an artery is narrowed by at least 60% to 70%.

Myocardial Infarction

A myocardial infarction (MI), or heart attack, results in the death of heart muscle. The affected myocardial cells in the heart are permanently destroyed. An MI occurs from a partial or complete blockage of a coronary artery, which decreases the blood supply to the cells of the heart supplied by the blocked coronary artery. The extent of the cardiac damage varies depending on the location and amount of blockage in the coronary artery. This is a potentially devastating condition. The ability of the heart to contract, relax, and propel blood throughout the body requires healthy cardiac muscle. Resulting depends on speed and effectiveness of treatment.

Myocardial infarction is identified by type. Non–ST-segment elevation myocardial infarction (NSTEMI) is also known as a non–Q-wave MI. An ST-segment elevation myocardial infarction (STEMI) is also known as a Q-wave MI and is the deadliest type because usually it is caused by a complete blockage of the artery. (See Chapter 25 for ST-segment definition.) With timely reperfusion, cell death may not occur, which reduces the permanent damage (reflected by a Q-wave appearance).

Those experiencing an MI are typically men over age 40 with atherosclerosis. Although MIs can occur at any age in men or women, women who smoke and use oral contraceptives are at greater risk.

Silent Ischemia

Silent ischemia occurs without pain and can carry great risk. The older adult and people with hypertension or diabetes are most often noted to have silent ischemia.

Sudden Cardiac Death

Sudden cardiac death is cardiac arrest triggered by lethal ventricular dysrhythmias or asystole from an abrupt occlusion of a coronary artery (see Chapter 25). Prompt treatment is required to prevent death.

Pathophysiology

Myocardial infarction does not happen immediately. Ischemic injury evolves over several hours before complete necrosis and infarction take place. The ischemic process affects the subendocardial layer, which is most sensitive to hypoxia. This process leads to depressed myocardial contractility. The body's attempt to compensate for decreased cardiac function triggers the sympathetic nervous system to increase the heart rate. The change in heart rate increases myocardial oxygen demand, further depressing the myocardium.

Prolonged ischemia can produce severe cellular damage and necrosis of cardiac muscle. Once necrosis takes place, the contractile function of the muscle is permanently lost. The heart has a zone of ischemia and injury around the necrotic area (Fig. 24.3). The zone of injury is next to the necrotic area and is susceptible to becoming necrosed. If treatment is initiated within the first hour of symptoms of the MI, the area of damage can be minimized. Around the injury zone is an area of ischemia and viable tissue. If the heart responds to treatment, this area can rebuild and maintain collateral circulation. If prolonged ischemia takes place, the size of the infarction can be quite large. The size of the infarction depends on how quickly the blood supply from the blocked artery can be restored.

The area affected by an MI depends on the coronary artery involved and the extent of occlusive coronary disease (Fig. 24.4). Being familiar with the anatomy of the heart and the area of the MI helps the nurse anticipate dysrhythmias, conduction disturbances, and heart failure, which are the major complications of MIs (Table 24.5).

The left coronary artery feeds the anterior wall of the heart, which also includes most of the left ventricle. An occlusion in this area causes an anterior wall MI. When the left ventricle is affected, there can be severe loss of left ventricular function, leading to severe changes in the hemodynamic status of the patient.

The right coronary artery (RCA) feeds the inferior wall and parts of the atrioventricular node and the sinoatrial node. An occlusion of the RCA leads to an inferior MI and abnormalities in impulse formation and conduction. Serious dysrhythmias can occur early in an inferior MI that may be life threatening.

The left circumflex coronary artery feeds the lateral wall of the heart and part of the posterior wall of the heart. A lesion in the circumflex leads to a lateral wall infarction of the left ventricle.

LEARNING TIP

To remember what coronary artery occlusion results in a specific MI location, use coast-to-coast U.S. location initials such as those given below. You can personalize the locations with initials of landmarks familiar to you.

Location	Coronary Artery	Resulting MI Location
Los Angeles	Left anterior descending	Anterior
Cedar Point	Circumflex	Posterior
Rhode Island	Right	Inferior

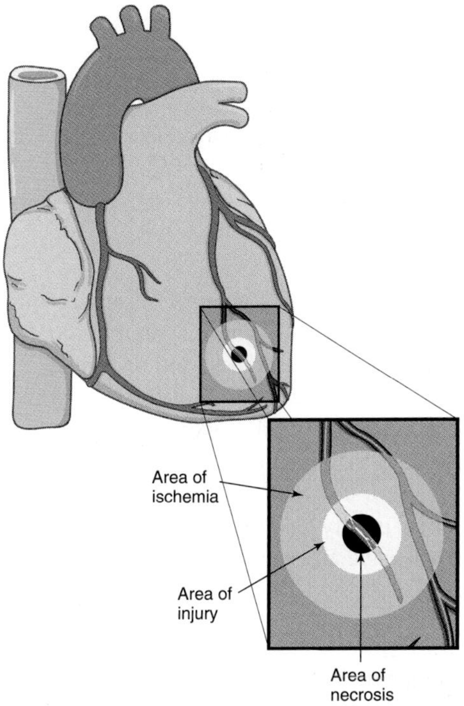
Area of ischemia
Area of injury
Area of necrosis

FIGURE 24.3 Myocardial infarction. Areas of ischemia, injury, and necrosis caused by a blockage in the left anterior coronary artery.

Signs and Symptoms

Chest pain is a classic symptom of an MI. The pain begins suddenly and continues without relief with rest or administration of NTG. The pain in the center of the chest is usually described as crushing, viselike, or as if an elephant is standing on the chest. The pain may radiate to the back, one or both arms and shoulders, neck, or jaw. The pain can imitate indigestion or a gallbladder attack with abdominal pain and vomiting. Other classic MI symptoms include shortness of breath, dizziness, nausea, and sweating (Table 24.6). When listening to lung sounds, crackles or wheezing may be heard. The pulse may be rapid or irregular, and an extra heart sound (referred to as S_3 or S_4) may be present. The presence of an extra heart sound can mean ventricular failure is imminent.

TIMELY SYMPTOM TREATMENT. People often deny or fail to recognize that they are having an MI because they experience atypical MI symptoms or their symptoms are similar to other mild conditions such as indigestion (Box 24.3, *Gerontological Issues*). Patients have reported that the symptoms of an MI that they experienced were not what they expected. If people expect to have the dramatic heart attack symptoms seen on television (which are usually not the same as those in real life) and they do not, they are likely to wait to seek treatment. People often wait 2 to 24 hours before seeking medical care, yet the first hour after symptom onset is crucial for administering the newer reperfusion treatments that restore blood flow, minimize tissue damage, and save lives. Patients should not drive themselves to the hospital if they are having chest pain. Emergency medical care (911 or local emergency services number) should be called.

Because so few patients arrive at the emergency room quickly enough to benefit from treatment, several agencies have educational programs to address this issue. People need to be educated that "time is muscle." As time passes during an MI, more muscle is lost. The National Heart, Lung, and Blood Institute (NHLBI) and the American

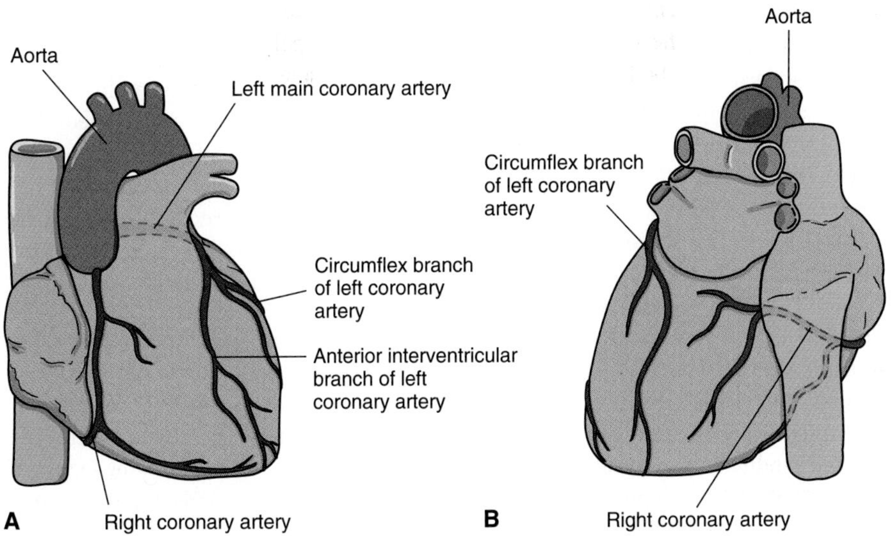
Aorta
Left main coronary artery
Circumflex branch of left coronary artery
Anterior interventricular branch of left coronary artery
A
Right coronary artery
Aorta
Circumflex branch of left coronary artery
B
Right coronary artery

FIGURE 24.4 Coronary arteries. (A) Anterior view. (B) Posterior view.

TABLE 24.5 COMPLICATIONS OF MYOCARDIAL INFARCTION

Complication	Types or Symptoms	Interventions
Dysrhythmias	Premature ventricular contractions, ventricular tachycardia, ventricular fibrillation, heart block	Continuous cardiac monitoring Protocols for treatment of dysrhythmias (see Chapter 25)
Cardiogenic shock	Decreased blood pressure; increased heart rate; diaphoresis; cold, clammy, gray skin	Immediate initiation of treatment to decrease infarct size, control pain and dysrhythmias Intra-aortic balloon pump Thrombolytic therapy Dopamine and dobutamine
Heart failure/pulmonary edema	Dizziness, orthopnea, weight gain, edema, enlarged liver, jugular venous distention, crackles	Correct underlying cause Relieve symptoms Increase cardiac contractility Administer furosemide (Lasix) and digoxin (Lanoxin)
Emboli	Dependent on location of emboli	Anticoagulants to prevent Supportive symptom treatment
Rupture of muscles or valves of the heart, septal rupture	Signs of cardiogenic shock, death	Mortality rate high Immediate treatment of MI to limit extent of damage
Pericarditis (inflammation of the heart muscle)	Chest pain, increased with movement, deep inspiration, or cough; pericardial friction rub (fine grating sound)	Relieved when sits up and leans forward Anti-inflammatory drugs (aspirin, indomethacin [Indocin])

Heart Association (AHA) have a campaign called "Act in Time to Heart Attack Signs." The purpose of this campaign is to educate people on the importance of recognizing heart attack symptoms, working with a physician to create a heart attack survival plan, and calling 911 as soon as symptoms begin. For more information, visit www.nhlbi.nih.gov/actintime, www.womenshealth.gov, and www.americanheart.org.

The National Heart Attack Alert Program (NHAAP) is another public education program developed by the NHLBI. The message of this program is symptom recognition and "60 minutes to treatment" to improve survival and reduce tissue damage. For more information, visit www.nhlbi.nih.gov/about/nhaap.

Women and Heart Health

Heart disease remains the leading cause of death in women in the United States. American women are six times more likely to die of heart disease than breast cancer. Heart disease kills more women than all cancers combined in the over-age-65 group. Ethnicity is also a factor among women. African American women are more likely than Caucasian women to develop heart disease. Women tend to have an acute myocardial infarction at an older age than men. Women also have a higher mortality rate and are more likely to have complications such as ventricular fibrillation and heart failure than men.

Women may have classic chest pain but they are also likely to have other symptoms as well that men do not typically have. Research is focusing on understanding women and cardiac disease. Atypical symptoms reported by women may include extreme fatigue, epigastric pain, jaw pain, indigestion, nausea and vomiting, dyspnea, shortness of breath, or cramping in the chest. A high percentage of women (more than 50%) noted prodromal symptoms a month before an acute MI. These symptoms included unusual fatigue, sleep disturbances, and shortness of breath. Less than 30% reported chest discomfort. Delay in seeking care has also been identified in women. Women also often do not associate their symptoms with a heart attack because they believe it is a male disease. Women with atypical symptoms usually delay treatment, and when treated have less aggressive management, which leads to increased mortality.

Diagnostic Tests

Patients with a strong familial history of MI should be considered at risk until an MI is ruled out. Indicators of an MI are patient history, ECG, and serum cardiac troponin I or T, myoglobin, and CK-MB levels. (See Chapter 21.) C-reactive protein levels are elevated in the presence of inflammation. Magnesium levels are also checked, especially for those on diuretic therapy. Before thrombolytic or heparin therapy, prothrombin time (PT) and partial thromboplastin time (PTT) are determined. The ECG usually shows the area that has infarcted, as well as the ischemic areas of the heart. Myocardial damage can be seen as ST-segment elevation, the presence of a Q wave, or T-wave abnormalities (Fig. 24.5). Serial ECGs are done to monitor changes indicating damage or ischemia.

Therapeutic Measures

Treatment should be sought within 5 minutes for any unrelieved chest pain. The American Heart Association recommends chewing one uncoated adult aspirin at the onset of chest pain. Delays in seeking care can limit treatment options and result in more cardiac damage (Box 24.4).

TABLE 24.6 MYOCARDIAL INFARCTION SUMMARY

Signs and Symptoms	***Classic*** Crushing, viselike chest pain with radiation to arm, shoulder, neck, jaw, or back Shortness of breath Dizziness Nausea Sweating ***Atypical*** Absence of chest pain Fatigue Cramping in chest Anxiety Feeling of impending doom Falling ***More Common in Women*** Epigastric or abdominal pain Chest discomfort, pressure, burning Arm, shoulder, neck, jaw, or back pain Discomfort/pain between shoulder blades Shortness of breath Fatigue Indigestion or gas pain Nausea or vomiting
Diagnostic Tests	ECG Serum cardiac troponin I or T Serum myoglobin Serum CK-MB CBC Serum magnesium and potassium Vital signs, oxygen saturation, intake and output
Therapeutic Measures	Medications Oxygen Morphine sulfate Nitrates Fab Four cardiac medications: aspirin, statin, ACEI, beta blocker Platelet aggregation inhibitors Thrombolytics Anticoagulants Antidysrhythmics Vasodilators Percutaneous coronary interventions and stents Myocardial revascularization–CABG Fluid restriction Daily weights Bedrest with bedside commode/bathroom privileges Low-sodium diet advanced to diet as tolerated; no caffeine Cardiac rehabilitation
Complications	Dysrhythmias Heart failure Cardiogenic shock Valvular insufficiency
Priority Nursing Diagnoses	*Acute Pain* *Anxiety* *Decreased Cardiac Output* *Deficient Knowledge*

Box 24.3
Gerontological Issues

With age the heart has decreased elasticity and decreased ability to respond to changes in pressure. This increases resistance to its pumping action and increases the workload of the myocardium. Older patients should be taught never to neglect symptoms of shortness of breath, fatigue, fast or slow heartbeats, or chest discomfort. Myocardial infarctions that can occur without the presence of pain, a silent MI, most often occur in the older adult or those with diabetes regardless of age. When pain is not present, the only symptom may be a sudden onset of shortness of breath or fainting, restlessness, or a fall. Atypical presentation of MI symptoms is normal in the older patient, especially in those older than age 85. Because the older adult has had more time to develop collateral circulation than younger people, they often do not have as many complications with an MI.

In the older adult, reperfusion therapies such as angioplasty and bypass surgery seem to be superior in improving quality of life without increasing mortality risk. Statin therapy has also shown to reduce mortality in those over age 80.

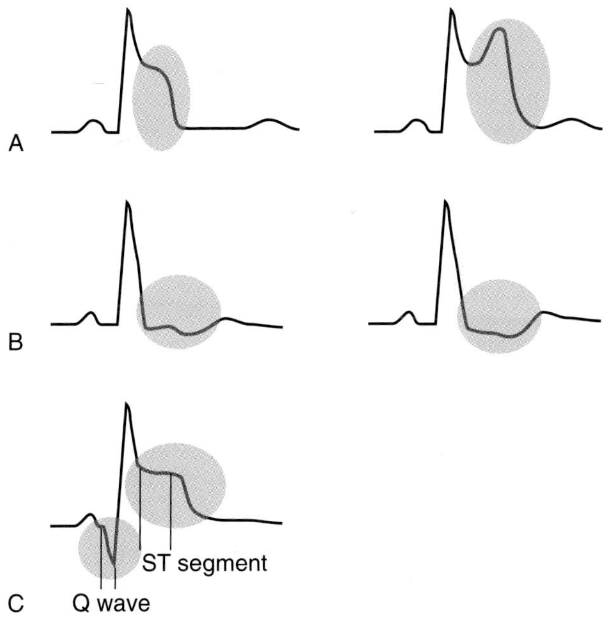
A
B
ST segment
C
Q wave

FIGURE 24.5 ECG changes during myocardial infarction. (A) Injury: ST-segment elevation. (B) Ischemia: ST-segment inversion. (C) Necrosis: large Q wave and ST-segment elevation.

Time until intervention is directly related to mortality. The AHA has a program titled "Mission: Lifeline" to improve care for STEMI patients (see www.americanheart.org). The goal is to restore blood flow to the heart muscle within 90 minutes or less of the patient's arrival at the emergency room door. This is

Box 24.4

Preventing Delays in Myocardial Infarction Treatment

- Understand symptoms and the "time is muscle" principle.
- Develop an action plan and rehearse it.
- Understand normal emotional responses of anxiety, denial, or embarrassment.
- Educate family to follow action plan.
- Establish protocols in workplaces for employees experiencing myocardial infarction.
- Establish emergency room policies that reduce delays, such as having equipment and medication readily available.

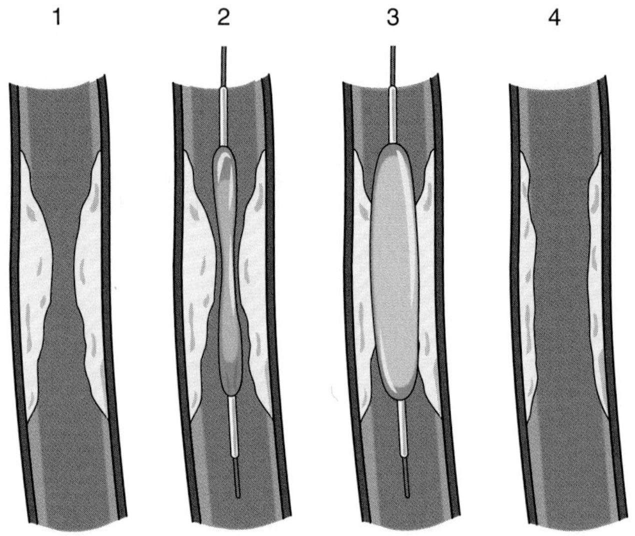
1
2
3
4

FIGURE 24.6 Percutaneous coronary intervention: Balloon angioplasty opens narrowed coronary arteries.

based on national guidelines developed by the American College of Cardiology and AHA for percutaneous coronary intervention (PCI) and is referred to as door-to-balloon time (see www.d2balliance.org). A reperfusion drug, when used, should be given within 30 minutes of the patient arriving at the emergency room door (door-to-needle time).

The presence of chest pain indicates a lack of oxygen to the myocardium. Patients reporting chest pain are treated as if they have an MI until proven otherwise through testing.

OXYGEN. Oxygen is administered immediately, usually at 2 L/min via nasal cannula. Oxygen therapy may be limited to the first 6 hours in stable patients. Too much oxygen can lead to systemic vasoconstriction, which may increase myocardial workload. Arterial blood gases (ABGs) are drawn to determine the patient's oxygen needs. Oxygen saturation should be monitored and kept above 94%. Oxygen can be administered via mask if higher concentrations are needed. Mechanical ventilation can be provided when indicated by ABGs.

PERCUTANEOUS CORONARY INTERVENTION. Percutaneous coronary intervention (PCI) is a variety of mechanical procedures used to increase blood flow and oxygen to the myocardium. Emergency PCI is being used frequently in the management of acute myocardial infarction with improved outcomes.

Balloon Angioplasty. In a cardiac catheterization laboratory, a catheter with a balloon tip is inserted, usually via the femoral artery, and advanced into the heart to open the blocked coronary artery (Fig. 24.6). Once the blocked artery is entered, the balloon on the catheter is inflated and the atherosclerotic plaque is compressed. The dilated vessel is able to deliver more oxygen-rich blood to the myocardium. Angioplasty can be done with or without the placement of stents.

Coronary Artery Stent. A coronary artery stent, placed during angioplasty, is used to prevent closure of a coronary artery from an atherosclerotic lesion. A stent is an expandable metal mesh tube that is implanted at the site of blockage in the coronary artery (Fig. 24.7). A stent provides support to a coronary artery wall at the area of stenosis to keep blood flowing through the artery. Complications associated with stent placement include **thrombosis** (formation of a blood clot inside a blood vessel), bleeding from anticoagulation, stent occlusion, or coronary artery dissection. Drug-eluting stents are coated with immunosuppressant medication that can be released at the implantation site to reduce the risk of restenosis. The medication is released over months to inhibit smooth muscle cell proliferation to reduce risk of restenosis. Plavix (clopidogrel bisulfate) is given for 1 year after stent placement to help prevent clot formation.

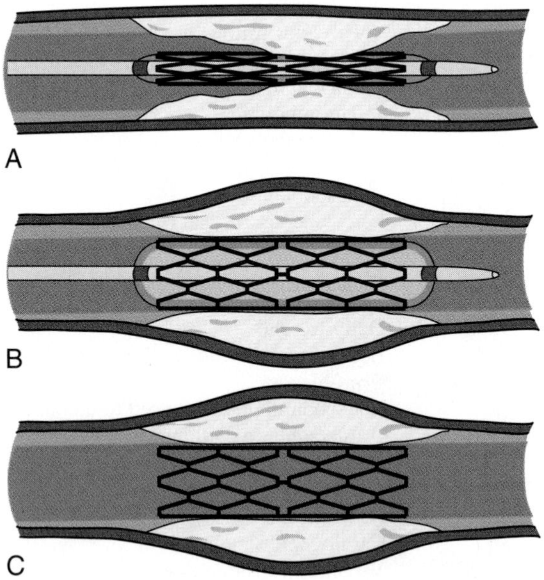
A
B
C

FIGURE 24.7 Insertion of a coronary artery stent: (A) A balloon catheter with a collapsed stent is advanced to the location of a coronary artery lesion. (B) The balloon is inflated, which expands the stent and compresses the lesion to increase the artery opening. (C) The balloon is then deflated and removed, leaving the expanded stent in place to prevent the artery from closing.

MEDICATION. For those with unstable angina, taking the "Fab Four" of cardiac drugs has been shown to be beneficial for heart health (NHLBI, 2008). The Fab Four include antiplatelets, statins, ACEIs, and beta blockers. A drug from each of these drug classes should be considered. When taken together, these drugs have a synergistic effect in fighting plaque, which means they have a greater positive result for the patient. Research has shown that not all eligible patients are prescribed each of these medications. Patient teaching can include the need to ask the health care provider about these drug classes to ensure they receive the ones for which they are eligible.

Table 24.7 summarizes pharmacological treatment of myocardial infarction. MONA is a mnemonic in the Advance Cardiac Life Support guidelines for remembering the medications to give in treating a suspected MI: morphine, oxygen, nitroglycerin, and aspirin.

TABLE 24.7 MEDICATIONS USED TO TREAT MYOCARDIAL INFARCTION

Medication Class/ Action	Examples	Route	Side Effects	Nursing Implications
Analgesics				
Opioid relieves pain. Reduces preload and afterload. Decreases anxiety.	morphine sulfate	IV	Respiratory depression, hypotension, and bradycardia. Use cautiously with COPD.	Monitor respirations, BP, and pulse before and after administration. Monitor vital signs for 10 minutes after IV administration.
Angiotensin-Converting Enzyme Inhibitors *(See Table 24.4.)*				
Anticoagulants				
Heparin Inhibits conversion of prothrombin to thrombin to prevent thrombus formation.	Heparin sodium	IV, subcutaneously	Bleeding Contraindicated in peptic ulcer disease, blood dyscrasias, recent eye surgery.	Dose regulated by heparin anti-factor Xa or activated partial thromboplastin time (aPTT). PTT Goal: 1.5–2.5 times control
Low Molecular Weight Heparin Antithrombotic. Prophylaxis of ischemic complications in unstable angina or NSTEMI with aspirin therapy.	dalteparin (Fragmin)	Subcutaneously	Bleeding, thrombocytopenia	Give deep subcutaneously while patient lying or sitting: Lift up fold of skin while giving injection around navel or outer thigh. Rotate sites. Periodic CBC and anti-factor Xa in renal failure.
Prophylaxis of ischemic complications in unstable angina or NSTEMI with aspirin therapy. STEMI treatment.	enoxaparin (Lovenox)	Subcutaneously IV bolus for acute STEMI under age 75	Bleeding, thrombocytopenia, anemia	Do not remove syringe air bubble. Given deep subcutaneously with patient lying: Lift up fold of skin while giving in anterolateral or posterolateral abdominal wall. Periodic CBC and anti-factor Xa in renal failure or obesity.
Antidysrhythmics				
Inhibit ventricular arrhythmias.	amiodarone (Cordarone, Pacerone)	IV, PO	Hypotension, bradycardia, dysrhythmias, slate blue skin discoloration, CNS disturbance, corneal microdeposits, photosensitivity	Contraindicated in AV block or pregnancy. Obtain baseline vital signs and ECG. Monitor for lung toxicity. Avoid grapefruit juice with oral form.
Antiplatelets				
Inhibit platelet activation, adhesion, or procoagulant activity.	Aspirin	PO Chewable if acute MI symptoms	Increased risk of bleeding, including hemorrhagic stroke. May cause diarrhea and other gastrointestinal distress.	Should be given as soon as ACS or MI is suspected. Enteric coated may be given daily. *Teaching:* Take with food. Report bleeding or bruising.
	Clopidogrel (Plavix)	PO		

Continued

TABLE 24.7 MEDICATIONS USED TO TREAT MYOCARDIAL INFARCTION—cont'd

Medication Class/ Action	Examples	Route	Side Effects	Nursing Implications
Glycoprotein 11b/111a inhibitors. Inhibit platelet aggregation. Used with PCI and stent.	eptifibatide (Integrilin) tirofiban (Aggrastat) abciximab (ReoPro)	IV	Bleeding, anemia, hypotension	Prevent injury for bleeding risk. Monitor vital signs and ECG.
Beta Blockers *(See Table 24.4.)*				
Nitrates				
Vasodilate to reduce preload and afterload. Reduce myocardial oxygen consumption. *(See Table 24.3 for other forms.)*	Nitroglycerin	IV	Hypotension, headache. Contraindicated in head trauma, hypotension, uncorrected hypovolemia	Document onset, type, radiation, location, and duration of chest pain. Monitor apical pulse and BP.
Statins *(See Table 24.2.)*				
Thrombolytics				
Dissolve blood clots in blood vessels or catheters, such as dialysis catheters.	alteplase (Activase, tissue plasminogen activator [t-PA]) reteplase (Retavase) tenecteplase (TNKase)	IV	Bleeding, stroke. Dysrhythmias may occur when blood flow is reestablished.	Most effective when given within 6 hours of coronary event. Goal is 30 minutes from arrival. Baseline INR, aPTT, platelet count, and fibrinogen levels checked. Avoid venipunctures for 24 hours after administration.
Additional Medications as Needed				
Antiemetics Anxiolytics Antacids Stool softeners	Specific for drugs given.	PO, IV	Drug specific	Control nausea, vomiting, anxiety, gastric upset, constipation.

ANALGESICS. Analgesics are given for relief of chest pain. Morphine sulfate is the most commonly used narcotic. It is usually given in increments of 2 to 8 mg intravenously every 5 to 15 minutes until pain is relieved. The patients should be monitored for hypotension, respiratory depression, oversedation, and morphine sensitivity. In addition to pain relief, morphine helps decrease anxiety, opens bronchioles, and increases peripheral blood pooling to decrease preload (blood returning to heart) and afterload (pressure within the aorta), which can help increase blood supply and oxygen to the myocardium.

VASODILATORS. NTG sublingually, topically, or by intravenous (IV) drip can be administered for vasodilation to supply more blood to the myocardium to reduce pain and the workload of the heart. In the acute phase, the IV route is usually used. Nitrates should not be given if the patient has a systolic blood pressure of less than 90 mm Hg, or 30 mm Hg or more below baseline, severe bradycardia less than 50 beats per minute, or if the patient has taken a phosphodiesterase inhibitor for erectile dysfunction. Catastrophic hypotension may result.

THROMBOLYTICS. Thrombolytic therapy is used to dissolve a blood clot that is occluding a coronary artery. (Note, however, that PCI has reduced the use of thrombolytics.) Thrombolytic therapy must be started within a specified time range from the onset of symptoms, usually within 1 to 6 hours, before necrosis results. The goal is to give thrombolytics within 30 minutes of arrival at the emergency room door.

Glycoprotein 11b/111a inhibitors [Eptifibatide (Integrilin), abciximab (ReoPro), tirofiban (Aggrastat)] may be used as an adjunct to thrombolysis or PCI in patients with unstable angina or non–ST-segment-elevation myocardial infarction. These drugs work by inhibiting platelet aggregation and are used along with aspirin or Plavix, and heparin.

ACTIVITY. Initially patients are kept on bedrest to decrease myocardial oxygen demand. A bedside commode for bowel movements is usually ordered to reduce straining. Then activity is advanced gradually as tolerated.

INTRA-AORTIC BALLOON PUMP. To support the ischemic heart, an intra-aortic balloon pump (IABP) may be used to increase circulation to the coronary arteries and reduce the work of the heart. (See Chapter 26.) While the heart is relaxed (diastole), the balloon is inflated, sending more blood into the coronary arteries. Just before the heart contracts (systole), the balloon deflates creating a suction effect that allows blood to flow past it with less resistance (decreased afterload) into the aorta.

GLUCOSE CONTROL. Guidelines for managing persistent hyperglycemia for critically ill patients include beginning treatment at no greater than 180 mg/dL with insulin infusions to maintain glucose within a range of 140 to 180 mg/dL (Moghissi et al., 2009). With IV infusions, frequent glucose monitoring is needed to prevent hypoglycemia.

DIET AND WEIGHT LOSS. During the acute phase of an MI, small, easily digested meals are served. Caffeine is restricted because it increases heart rate and causes vasoconstriction. Fluids may be restricted if the patient is in heart failure as well. Initially a low-sodium clear liquid diet may be ordered. Then a low-fat, low-cholesterol, and low-sodium diet may be ordered. If the patient is obese, weight loss can reduce cardiac workload. A dietitian can work with the patient and family to devise a weight-loss diet for the patient.

SMOKING. Patients are instructed on the hazards of smoking. Referral to a tobacco cessation program can be made. The nurse can help patients understand and accept lifestyle changes.

Coronary Artery Bypass Graft

Prior to PCI, coronary artery bypass graft (CABG) surgery was the only revascularization procedure available. It offers better long-term symptom relief and revascularization than PCI. AHA guidelines help determine which type of procedure would benefit the patient. During bypass surgery, a blood vessel from the leg or chest is used to reroute blood around a segment of a coronary artery that is narrowed by atherosclerosis. Significant occlusions in the coronary arteries are bypassed with vein or artery grafts (Fig. 24.8). One or more vessel bypasses can be performed during the procedure. The saphenous vein from the leg or an internal mammary artery from the chest wall is generally used.

While the sternotomy is made, the vein graft is being removed from the body. The graft is flushed with a heparinized solution to check for leaks, and then set aside for use during the surgery. The patient is then placed on cardiopulmonary bypass (CPB) (see Chapter 21). After cardiac standstill occurs, one end of the graft is **anastomosed** (joined) to the coronary artery distal to the occlusion, while the proximal end of the graft is anastomosed, usually to the ascending aorta.

Resecting the mammary arteries for grafting is more difficult and time consuming than resecting the saphenous vein, but their patency is longer. The proximal end of the artery is left attached to its origin, and the distal end is anastomosed to the coronary artery distal to the occlusion. See Box 24.5, *Patient Perspective*.

Minimally invasive direct visualization coronary artery bypass (MIDCAB) is a technique that is done without the use of cardiopulmonary bypass. Several small incisions (ports) are used to access the coronary artery instead of a sternotomy. This technique uses a thoracoscope. One- or two-vessel disease patients may use this technique.

Port-access coronary artery bypass combines peripheral cardiopulmonary bypass (CPB) with minimally invasive heart access. The advantage is that the heart is not beating during surgery. Several vessel repairs can be done and other areas of the heart, such as valves, can also be repaired with this technique.

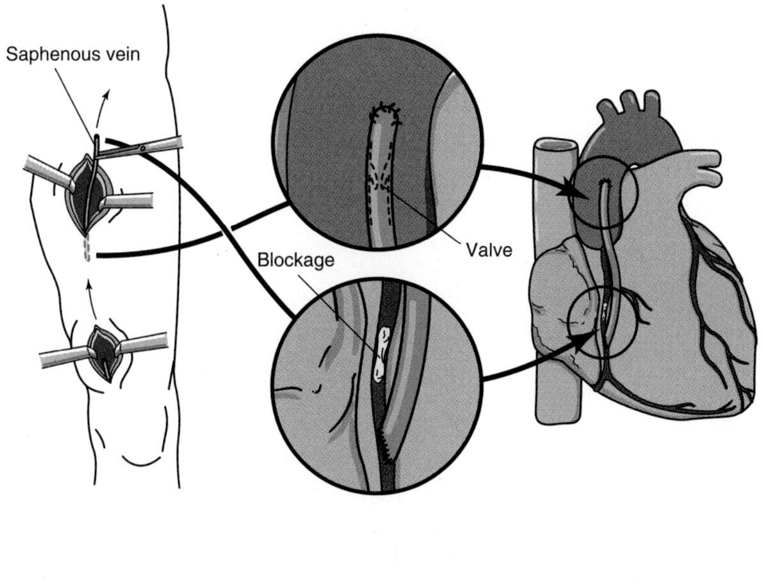
Saphenous vein
Blockage
Valve

FIGURE 24.8 Myocardial reperfusion by coronary artery bypass graft surgery.

CRITICAL THINKING

Mr. Jones

■ Mr. Jones is transferred to the critical care unit following a quadruple CABG. Preoperative vital signs were blood pressure 164/88 mm Hg, apical pulse 62 beats per minute and regular, respiratory rate 18 per minute, temperature 98.4°F (36.9°C). Data collection findings are blood pressure 100/56 mm Hg, apical pulse 105 beats per minute, and respiratory rate 28 per minute, irregular and shallow, temperature 99.8°F (37.7°C), lung sounds diminished with crackles in bilateral bases, pedal pulses weak bilaterally, chest and leg dressings dry and intact, and no urinary catheter. Mr. Jones is being monitored for first postoperative voiding.

1. Which findings may indicate pulmonary problems?
2. List four nursing interventions for the altered pulmonary status.
3. List three reasons why the apical pulse could be elevated.
4. Name two reasons why the blood pressure could be low.

Suggested answers at end of chapter.

Box 24.5

Patient Perspective

Keith: Coronary Artery Bypass Graft

I was 72 when I had coronary artery bypass surgery. I had some very minor symptoms, and a heart catheterization showed significant coronary artery blockage. I ended up having five bypass grafts performed. It was a long surgery. I felt disoriented for several days afterward—mostly while I was in the intensive care unit.

I have had a strange sensation in my legs at the incision sites ever since surgery, but not really pain! I also have experienced no depression, although post-op depression is common, and have assumed an attitude that I am in better condition than before surgery, so why should I worry?

I was provided with excellent care at home after discharge from the hospital. The nursing and rehab personnel were outstanding. I had a capable visiting nurse, physical therapist, or occupational therapist practically every day. Physical therapy was difficult at first, but shortly became routine and easy.

My experience during cardiac rehab was outstanding. I had three sessions per week for 12 weeks. I have always exercised a lot, so I had no problems attaining the exercise levels suggested. It was a very positive experience, and I enjoyed the association with others in the same situation. We even staged a graduation when we finished. I wore a tuxedo jacket with my gym shorts! Since completing my rehab, I have religiously maintained a minimum 40-minute exercise schedule three times per week. I do this because I want to stay healthy for a long time.

The only negative aspect I experienced was a minor stroke during surgery. As a result, my balance is not as good as I would like. I need to be more careful, particularly when running or bike riding. Perhaps this is just older age, but it started just after surgery, so that is the reason I assume it is due to the minor stroke.

The impact on my life and family has been minimal. The primary change is being more conscious of my diet and an emphasis on exercise. Otherwise, I live pretty much the same as before.

Nursing Process for the Patient Experiencing ACS or Acute Myocardial Infarction

DATA COLLECTION. A thorough history is obtained to identify risk factors that may contribute to a myocardial infarction. All patients admitted with chest pain are treated as having a possible MI until it has been ruled out. Continuous cardiac monitoring, serial ECGs, and laboratory values help identify life-threatening dysrhythmias and determine the degree of cardiac damage. Controlling chest pain immediately helps diminish anxiety and the negative physiological effects pain has on the body. Assessment for depression for those experiencing an MI is important to ensure appropriate referrals are made for treatment (see *Evidence-Based Practice* box).

EVIDENCE-BASED PRACTICE

Clinical Question

Does depression, stress, or other psychological stressors have an effect on patients with cardiovascular disease?

Evidence

A systematic review of several studies in the United States and Europe showed strong evidence that men and women of all ages with major depressive disorders are at risk for coronary heart disease (Green et al., 2009). Among the elderly, aging often predisposes older adults to decreased quality of life, increased risk of depression, and more difficulty in lifestyle modification (Arthur, 2006). Social connectedness and community participation have been shown to be inversely related to cardiovascular deaths. People who are socially isolated or depressed are at increased risk for acute myocardial infarction and cardiovascular death.

cont'd

Implications for Nursing Practice

Depression affects a patient's adherence to post-MI lifestyle changes and medication adherence. After an MI, patients should be screened for depression, anxiety, sleep disorders, and social isolation at regular intervals during hospitalization and cardiovascular rehabilitation.

REFERENCES

Arthur, H. (2006). Depression, isolation, social support and cardiovascular disease in older adults. *Journal of Cardiovascular Nursing, 21*(55), 52–57.

Green, L. A., Dickinson, W. P., Nease, D. E., et al. (2009). AAFP guideline for the detection and management of post-myocardial infarction depression. *Annals of Family Medicine, 7*(1), 71–79.

NURSING DIAGNOSES, PLANNING, IMPLEMENTATION, AND EVALUATION. See the *Nursing Care Plan for the Patient with Myocardial Infarction.* Also see the *Nursing Care Plan for the Patient Undergoing Cardiac Surgery* for additional nursing care.

NURSING CARE TIP

When caring for a patient after a coronary artery bypass graft (CABG), be sure to use infection-control procedures at all times to prevent surgical site infection. Surgical site infection following CABG (mediastinitis) is a "Never Event," which means that Medicare will not pay the hospital for care required for this condition.

Patient Education

Teaching about the therapeutic regimen includes information about the disease, medications, diet, activity, and rehabilitation needs that may require lifestyle changes. Diet, stress reduction, a regular exercise program, cessation of smoking if necessary, and following a medication schedule require extensive patient and family teaching. This disease can affect all aspects of a patient's lifestyle. Issues about family and job roles and sexual activities need to be addressed. Patients need time to understand information that has been presented and should be encouraged to express any questions, needs, or fears.

Cardiac Rehabilitation and Exercise

Cardiac rehabilitation begins when the patient's acute symptoms are relieved to improve cardiac function and quality of life. The first phase of rehabilitation occurs in the hospital. Activities for each hospital day, such as types and amounts of self-care and activity, are specified in protocols. Phase 2 occurs 4 to 6 weeks after discharge in an outpatient program and focuses on returning the patient to prior levels of activity and function. Phase 3 follows in which patients are encouraged to maintain optimum physical fitness and to continue healthy lifestyles that include exercising and losing weight to maintain an ideal body weight.

CRITICAL THINKING

Mrs. Sims

■ Mrs. Sims, age 43, is admitted to the intensive care unit with a diagnosis of atypical chest pain that radiates to her left shoulder and down her left arm. She has a history of midsternal chest cramping. Her pain increases with activity and decreases with rest. She smokes one and a half packs of cigarettes per day and is 50 pounds overweight. The cardiac monitor shows normal sinus rhythm without dysrhythmias. She has NTG sublingual ordered prn for chest pain.

One hour after admission, Mrs. Sims reports acute midsternal chest pain radiating to her left neck and jaw. The cardiac monitor shows sinus tachycardia with occasional premature ventricular contractions (PVCs). Her blood pressure is 100/70 mm Hg, respirations are 20 per minute and unlabored, and skin is warm and dry.

1. What actions should you take?
2. What is happening to Mrs. Sims?
3. How is angina differentiated from an MI?
4. What are four indicators of an MI?
5. What medical interventions can be used for an MI?
6. What education is indicated for Mrs. Sims?

Suggested answers at end of chapter.

PERIPHERAL VASCULAR SYSTEM

Peripheral vascular disease (PVD) may be either arterial or venous in origin. PVD is very common in people who are older or diabetic. It is important for the nurse to understand whether the origin of the problem is arterial or venous to prevent serious complications from occurring.

Arterial Thrombosis and Embolism

Pathophysiology

Acute arterial occlusions are often sudden and dramatic. Occlusions are most common in the lower extremity, but may occur in the upper extremity as well. A thrombus (blood clot) adheres to the vessel wall. Acute arterial thrombi occur where there is injury to an arterial wall, sluggish flow, or plaque formation secondary to atherosclerotic changes. Other causes of arterial thrombosis are polycythemia, dehydration,

Nursing Care Plan for the Patient with Myocardial Infarction

Nursing Diagnosis: *Acute Pain* related to decreased coronary blood flow causing myocardial ischemia

Expected Outcomes : The patient will exhibit signs of decreased pain. Patient will exhibit signs of relaxation.

Evaluation of Outcomes: Does patient state pain is reduced?

Interventions	Rationale	Evaluation
Monitor location, duration, intensity, and radiation of pain; use a scale of 0 to 10.	Identifies type and severity of pain.	What is pain level, location, duration, intensity, and radiation?
Monitor blood pressure, pulse, and respiration.	Vital signs may elevate with episodes of pain.	Are vital signs within normal limits?
Obtain ECG as ordered.	Identifies location of infarction or ischemia.	Is ECG normal?
Administer oxygen as ordered.	Helps prevent hypoxia.	Are ABGs within normal limits? Is oxygen saturation greater than 90%?
Instruct patient to report pain at first onset.	Helps control pain quickly to prevent further ischemia.	Does patient report pain?
Instruct patient to rest during pain.	Activity increases oxygen demand and can increase chest pain.	Does patient remain quiet and relaxed?
Remain with patient during chest pain until it is relieved.	Provides comfort and reassurance to decrease anxiety and fear.	Are anxiety and fear decreased?
Assist with alternative pain relief measures; related to positioning, diversional activities, relaxation techniques.	These measures help decrease painful stimuli, allowing the patient to focus on other things.	Does patient express relief and decreased stress?
Medicate as ordered.	Helps eliminate pain.	Is pain relieved?
	GERIATRIC	
Monitor and ensure that older patient's pain is relieved.	Pain is not an expected part of the aging process as many believe.	Does patient report pain is relieved?

Nursing Diagnosis: *Decreased Cardiac Output* related to ischemia or infarction, changes in heart rate and rhythm, and decreased contractility

Expected Outcomes: The patient will maintain adequate cardiac output and tissue perfusion. Patient will exhibit signs of improved cardiac output and tissue perfusion.

Evaluation of Outcomes: Does patient have heart rate greater than 60 and less than 100 beats per minute, blood pressure greater than 90/60 and less than 140/90 mm Hg, and urine output greater than 30 mL/hr?

Interventions	Rationale	Evaluation
Monitor blood pressure, heart rate, and urine output.	Indirect indicators of cardiac output.	Are indicators within normal limits?
Listen to lung sounds.	Crackles indicate heart failure.	Are lungs clear?

Nursing Care Plan for the Patient with Myocardial Infarction—cont'd

Monitor peripheral circulation, pulses, capillary refill, edema, color, and temperature.	Indicators of adequate tissue perfusion.	Does patient have strong peripheral pulses, capillary refill less than 3 seconds, no edema, warm skin, pink nailbeds?
Monitor ECG.	Identifies dysrhythmias.	Is patient's ECG within normal limits?
Administer medications as ordered by physician, such as vasodilators, beta blockers, calcium channel blockers, and cardiac glycosides.	Helps improve contractility, cardiac output, and tissue perfusion.	Does patient show signs of improved contractility, increased cardiac output, and tissue perfusion?
Promote and provide for adequate rest, quiet environment, bedrest; place in semi-Fowler's position.	Decreases cardiac workload and stress and allows for improved breathing.	Is patient relaxed?
	GERIATRIC	
Observe for atypical pain such as jaw pain or no pain with dyspnea or fatigue.	In acute MI older adults may have not had typical chest pain or have a silent MI.	Does patient have atypical symptoms of MI?
Observe patient carefully for side effects of medications.	Older patients are more likely to have medication toxicity owing to reduced renal and hepatic function.	Does patient exhibit toxic side effects of medications?

Nursing Diagnosis: *Fear* related to threat of death, changes in lifestyle, chest pain, and procedures

Expected Outcomes: The patient will verbalize reduced fear. Patient will demonstrate effective coping mechanisms.

Evaluation of Outcomes: Does patient verbalize reduced fear?

Interventions	Rationale	Evaluation
Assess level of fear and note nonverbal communication.	Controlling anxiety will reduce sympathetic activity that may intensify condition.	Does patient report fear or have signs of being fearful?
Ask the patient's usual coping pattern.	This allows building on patient's strengths.	What are patient's coping techniques?
Orient the patient and family to surroundings and equipment, oxygen, cardiac monitoring, IVs, and explain procedures.	Information may promote trust and reduce emotional stress.	Does patient state understanding of environment and equipment?
Assure patient he/she will be closely monitored.	Assurance of detection for prompt treatment of any complications will reduce fear.	Does patient state less fear due to continuous monitoring?
Allow patient to verbalize fear of dying.	Ventilation helps identify and reduce fear.	Is patient able to verbalize fears?

Continued

Nursing Care Plan for the Patient with Myocardial Infarction—cont'd

Interventions	Rationale	Evaluation
Provide diversional materials such as newspapers, music, and television.	Diversion can be relaxing and prevent feelings of isolation.	Does patient report that use of diversional activities reduces fear?
Offer family support.	Significant others often ignore their own needs, experience anxiety, and need support, including ongoing information and explanations, being allowed to stay with patient, and being involved in patient's care. Nurses need to help spouses or significant others meet their own needs, so they can better support the patient.	Does family verbalize ability to offer support to patient without anxiety?
	GERIATRIC	
Provide protective, safe environment with consistent caregivers.	Older adults adapt to change with more difficulty during illness than younger adults.	Is continuity of care provided? Does patient report less fear?

Nursing Diagnosis: *Activity Intolerance* related to imbalance between oxygen supply and demand, weakness, and fatigue

Expected Outcomes: The patient will tolerate progressive activity as evidenced by heart rate, blood pressure, pulse oximetry, and respiratory rate within normal limits (WNL).

Evaluation of Outcomes: Is patient's heart rate, blood pressure, pulse oximetry, and respiratory rate WNL with progressive activity?

Interventions	Rationale	Evaluation
Obtain patient's vital signs before activity.	Identifies baseline data comparison with activity.	What are vital signs?
Observe patient during and after activity and document abnormal responses to activity, including heart rate over 120 bpm or 20 beats over resting rate, systolic BP increased over 20 mm Hg during activity, chest pain, dizziness, skin color changes, diaphoresis, dyspnea, dysrhythmias, excessive fatigue, and ST-segment changes on ECG.	Observation allows detection of abnormal responses to stop activity.	Are vital signs WNL? Is activity tolerated without symptoms?
Position patient for comfort and ease in breathing.	Semi-Fowler's position is usually preferred by patients in respiratory distress. When patient is sitting upright in bed, supporting arms on pillows reduces cardiac workload by eliminating force of gravity on unsupported arms.	Is patient able to breathe easily?

Nursing Care Plan for the Patient with Myocardial Infarction—cont'd

Maintain progression of activities as ordered by physician or cardiac rehabilitation program. *Initial activities:* ADLs, dangle at bedside for 15 minutes, use commode with assistance *Progressive activities:* Out of bed to chair for 30 to 60 minutes, partial bath, range-of-motion exercises.	The patient should have increasing activity to condition the myocardium.	Is patient able to progress activity?
	GERIATRIC	
Slow the pace of care.	Allow patient extra time to complete activity to reduce cardiac demand and fatigue.	Is patient able to complete care without symptoms or fatigue?
Refer patient to cardiac rehabilitation as able.	Older adults benefit comparably to younger persons from exercise programs.	Does patient participate in cardiac rehab?
Encourage families to let patient be independent in activities.	Families may believe being sedentary is helpful to the patient.	Do family members encourage patient to be as active as able?

Nursing Care Plan for the Patient Undergoing Cardiac Surgery

Nursing Diagnosis: *Acute Pain* related to sternotomy, leg incisions, internal mammary artery resection, or pericarditis

Expected Outcomes: The patient will state pain is relieved or tolerable. Patient will be able to rest and perform respiratory treatments.

Evaluation of Outcomes: Does patient state pain is within acceptable levels? Is patient able to rest and perform respiratory therapies?

Interventions	Rationale	Evaluation
Assess characteristics of pain with each episode.	A thorough description is needed to determine cause and plan actions.	Does patient describe pain on scale of 0 to 10?
Encourage patient to report pain even when pain is mild.	It is easier to keep pain under control when mild.	Does patient report pain when mild?
Turn, reposition every 2 hours.	Changes muscle position, relieving stiffness.	Is patient comfortable without stiffness?
Offer back rubs frequently.	Relaxes tense muscles retracted during operation.	Is patient able to rest comfortably?

Continued

Nursing Care Plan for the Patient Undergoing Cardiac Surgery—cont'd

Teach patient "sternal precautions": • No pushing or pulling with arms. • Hug pillow for all movement, coughing, and deep breathing. • Do not use arms to raise yourself out of a chair. • No lifting over 5 to 10 lb. • Do not raise elbows higher than shoulders. • Bend elbows and lower head for grooming.	Stabilizes sternum and incision to increase comfort.	Does patient understand sternal precautions and use them?
Instruct patient to take a deep breath before movement and exhale slowly during movement.	Keeps muscles relaxed, minimizing tension with guarding and pain.	Can patient perform coughing and deep breathing techniques as instructed?

Nursing Diagnosis: *Decreased Cardiac Output* related to myocardial depression, hypothermia, bleeding, unstable dysrhythmias, or hypoxemia

Expected Outcomes: The patient will remain free of major side effects of pharmacological support. Patient will maintain vital signs within normal limits (WNL), palpable peripheral pulses, urine output greater than 30 mL/hr, and normal sinus rhythm.

Evaluation of Outcomes: Is patient free of major side effects? Are vital signs WNL?

Interventions	Rationale	Evaluation
Monitor vital signs.	Trends reflect problems.	Are vital signs WNL?
Check peripheral circulation.	Mottling or weak pulses may indicate poor cardiac output (CO).	Do peripheral pulses remain strong with normal skin color, temperature, capillary refill?
Monitor intake and output.	Fluid deficit or excess can alter CO.	Does total intake equal output?
Listen to lung sounds and note character of sputum.	Wet lung sounds may indicate heart failure or pulmonary edema.	Are lungs clear?
Note shivering.	Shivering increases the blood pressure, decreasing CO and increasing risk for bleeding.	Is patient's shivering controlled?
Monitor chest tube drainage for increase or sudden decrease.	Drainage more than 200 mL/hr may lead to hypovolemia and a decrease in CO.	Is patient free from cardiac tamponade and hypovolemia?
Monitor ECG.	Premature ventricular contractions and atrial fibrillation decrease CO.	Does patient remain in normal sinus rhythm or controlled dysrhythmia? (See Chapter 25.)
Monitor electrolytes.	Low calcium and magnesium and high potassium decrease contractility and CO.	Are electrolytes WNL?
Monitor ABGs.	Acidosis decreases heart function, and a low CO may lead to further acidosis.	Are ABGs WNL?

Nursing Care Plan for the Patient Undergoing Cardiac Surgery—cont'd

Nursing Diagnosis: *Risk for Infection* related to inadequate primary defenses from surgical wound

Expected Outcomes: The patient will remain free from infection.

Evaluation of Outcomes: Does patient remain free from infection?

Interventions	Rationale	Evaluation
Observe incision for signs and symptoms of infection.	Redness, warmth, fever, and swelling indicate infection.	Are signs and symptoms of infection present?
Monitor drainage and maintain drains.	Drains remove fluid from the surgical site to prevent infection development.	Are drainage amount and color normal for procedure? Are drains functioning?
Maintain sterile technique for dressing changes.	Sterile technique reduces infection development.	Is incision free of signs and symptoms of infection?
Monitor and report abnormal findings for temperature, lung sounds, sputum, and urine consistency.	Low-grade or high-grade fever, crackles, yellow-green sputum color, or cloudy urine can indicate infection.	Is the patient's temperature WNL and are lung sounds, sputum, and urine clear?
Encourage coughing and deep breathing and incentive spirometer use.	Lung infections can be prevented with lung expansion and secretion removal.	Does patient perform coughing and deep breathing and use incentive spirometer?

and repeated arterial needlesticks. If a thrombus breaks off and travels, it becomes an **embolism** that occludes an arterial vessel that is too small to allow it to pass. Some of the causes of an arterial embolism are dysrhythmias, prosthetic heart valves, and rheumatic heart disease.

Signs and Symptoms

Usually there is an abrupt onset of symptoms with acute arterial occlusion. If a patient also has chronic arterial insufficiency, the symptoms may not occur as rapidly because collateral circulation has developed and can supply some blood to the occluded area. Symptoms depend on the artery occluded, the tissue supplied by that artery, and whether collateral circulation is present.

The six clinical signs of acute arterial occlusion are known as the "six Ps": pain, pallor, pulselessness, paresthesia (numbness), paralysis, and poikilothermia (temperature). The patient experiences pain, numbness, and decreased movement in the extremity, which is pale and without pulses distal to the occlusion. The extremity feels cold because blood normally provides warmth. If treatment is not initiated immediately, ischemia occurs and can progress to tissue necrosis and gangrene development within hours.

Therapeutic Measures

Early treatment is necessary to protect and save the affected limb. Anticoagulant therapy is started immediately. Intravenous heparin is the treatment of choice to prevent further clotting. Heparin has no effect on existing clots. An initial IV bolus of heparin, usually 5000 international units, is given. An IV infusion is then started as ordered. The patient remains on heparin therapy for several days. Daily Heparin Xa or PTTs are monitored to maintain therapeutic heparin levels. After 3 to 7 days, warfarin (Coumadin) is added. Warfarin, an oral anticoagulant, takes 3 to 5 days to reach therapeutic levels. The heparin is continued until a therapeutic warfarin level is reached. To monitor warfarin's effects, international normalized ratios (INRs) and PTs are done daily, and adjustments in warfarin doses are made based on the results.

For patients with severe occlusions, especially if the risk of limb loss is imminent, surgery or thrombolytic agents are used to save the extremity. During an emergency embolectomy or thrombectomy, the artery is cut open, the emboli or thrombus is removed, and the vessel is sutured closed. Thrombolytic agents dissolve the thrombus or embolus.

Peripheral Arterial Disease

Peripheral arterial disease (PAD) is a disorder of the arterial circulation usually caused by chronic, progressive narrowing of arterial vessels that leads to obstruction or occlusion. PAD usually affects the lower extremities. Peripheral arterial disease is sometimes referred to as lower extremity arterial disease (LEAD). Atherosclerosis is the leading cause of occlusive disease. Peripheral arterial disease can be described as organic or functional. Organic disease is caused by structural changes from plaque or inflammation in the blood vessels. Functional disease is a short-term localized spasm in the blood vessel as noted in Raynaud's disease.

Pathophysiology

The purpose of the arterial system is to deliver oxygen-rich blood to the vascular beds. Anything that impedes this flow causes an imbalance in supply and demand for oxygen. Decreased nutrition, cellular waste accumulation, and the development of ischemia occur at the area distal to the obstruction. With the increased debris and sluggish flow, thrombosis and embolism become major problems.

> **CRITICAL THINKING**
>
> ***Mrs. May***
>
> ■ Mrs. May is admitted with severe rheumatoid arthritis, which has left her relatively immobile for 7 months. She is returning to her room following a whirlpool treatment when she suddenly reports severe pain in her left groin.
>
> 1. What is your first action?
> 2. After assessing Mrs. May, what action should be taken next?
> 3. What are the possible causes of these sudden symptoms?
> 4. How would you document Mrs. May's symptoms?
> 5. What immediate interventions are necessary?
> 6. What medical interventions would you anticipate?
> 7. What surgical procedure may need to be done if the risk of losing the limb is imminent?
>
> *Suggested answers at end of chapter.*

The body has several mechanisms that attempt to compensate for reduced blood flow, including peripheral vasodilation, anaerobic metabolism, and development of collateral circulation. However, these mechanisms are not intended to meet the ongoing blood supply needs of the body. It takes time for collateral circulation to develop, blood vessels eventually reach their limit of dilation, and anaerobic metabolism is only a very short-term compensatory mechanism. Eventually this lack of blood supply produces signs of ischemia that, if not corrected, result in ulceration, gangrene, and necrosis of the extremity; amputation of the limb may then become necessary.

Signs and Symptoms

Many people with PAD, especially women, have no symptoms. Symptoms often occur late in the course of PAD when diminished blood flow begins to produce changes in the extremities. Pain in the calves of the lower extremities associated with activity or exercise, called **intermittent claudication**, is a common symptom of arterial occlusive disease. When blood supply to the muscles is decreased, the muscles are unable to receive adequate oxygen and ischemia develops. As ischemia increases, the muscle develops a cramping-type pain that usually subsides when the activity is stopped. As PAD progresses, the pain is present even at rest, thus indicating severe arterial occlusion.

Skin color changes are associated with decreased blood supply. The extremity is pale when the leg is elevated. If the leg is in a dependent position, it becomes reddish purple or cyanotic. The extremity is cool to touch even in warm environments. There may be hair loss on the lower calf, ankle, and foot. Other findings include dry, flaky, scaly, pale, or mottled skin. The toenails may be thickened. As occlusion of the arteries progresses, arterial pulses become diminished or absent. Pulses should be palpated in both legs. The loss of circulation leads to tissue death and gangrene.

Diagnostic Tests

Noninvasive studies can be used to diagnose occlusive disorders. The ankle-brachial (ABI) blood pressure index is used to determine pressures in the upper and lower extremities. Normally, blood pressure readings in the thigh and calf are higher than those in the upper extremities. With the presence of arterial disease, these pressures are lower than the brachial pressure. Normally the ankle pressure is equal to or greater than the brachial pressure. When an occlusion occurs in the lower extremities, the pressures between the upper and lower extremities become unequal. After treadmill exercise, the ABI decreases in arterial insufficiency. A duplex ultrasound measures the velocity of the blood flow. Magnetic resonance imaging (MRI) can give definitive images of blood vessels and degrees of arterial closure. Plethysmography and angiography can also be used to evaluate arterial flow in lower extremities (see Chapter 21).

Therapeutic Measures

Conservative treatment is initiated with mild to moderate occlusive disease. This includes patients who experience pain on activity that ceases with rest. This type of patient usually receives medication for vasodilation and diet management if necessary. Surgical intervention is used for the patient who experiences pain at rest or who has leg ulcers that do not heal. Surgical treatment includes endarterectomy to remove atherosclerotic lesions or grafting to bypass the occluded area. (See the discussion of vascular surgery later in this chapter.)

DIET. The diet should aim to control atherosclerosis development. Teaching the patient to avoid red meats, fried foods, whole milk, and cheese is important. Avoiding high-cholesterol foods, such as organ meats, animal fats, and shellfish, helps lower lipid levels.

MEDICATIONS. Drug therapy is geared toward the symptoms and causes of the occlusive disease. The same drugs used to decrease cholesterol and lipid levels in atherosclerosis are used with occlusive disease. Vasodilators can be used, but their effectiveness is not the same for all patients. Pentoxifylline (Trental) or cilostazol (Pletal) is used for patients with occlusive disorders who experience intermittent claudication. This drug makes red blood cells more flexible to improve perfusion. The major side effect is gastrointestinal upset, so it should be taken with meals. Thrombolytic therapy is used when an occlusion is caused by a thrombus or an embolus.

INVASIVE THERAPIES. Percutaneous transluminal angioplasty (PTA) can be used to dilate a narrowed peripheral vessel, although it does not provide long-term results. It is similar to PCI, which was discussed earlier. Peripheral atherectomy is another invasive procedure used to remove plaque from atherosclerotic arteries. Intravascular stents can also be used to maintain patency of the artery. After stent placement, patients are given platelet aggregation inhibitors.

Raynaud's Disease

A vasoconstrictive response causing ischemia from exposure to cold and stress is known as **Raynaud's disease**. It occurs more often in women who live in cold climates. Raynaud's disease primarily affects the hands but also can occur in the feet, ears, or nose. To be diagnosed with Raynaud's disease, the patient must experience intermittent attacks of ischemia for at least 2 years.

Pathophysiology

Raynaud's disease is characterized by spasms of small arteries in the digits. These spasms prevent arterial blood from perfusing the fingertips and sometimes the toes. The spasms can occur unilaterally and in one or two digits, but most often they occur bilaterally and in all digits. Raynaud's disease may be seen with collagen diseases such as rheumatoid arthritis, scleroderma, and systemic lupus erythematosus. This disease can progress over time; the vessels remain constricted and the severe decrease in blood flow can lead to fingers becoming gangrenous and necrotic.

Signs and Symptoms

The hands, when exposed to cold, exhibit vascular spasms and a marked decrease in blood flow to the tissues. The resulting effect in the tissues is ischemic pain. After several minutes of ischemia, hyperemia occurs. Hyperemia is intense reddening of the hands from dilation of all the vessels of the hands. Pain becomes more intense at this time. Patients with Raynaud's disease go through various phases, which include blanching of the skin, pain, and reddening of the skin.

Therapeutic Measures

Conservative treatment is attempted first. The patient is instructed to keep the hands warm. Gloves should be worn when going outside, cleaning a refrigerator, or preparing cold foods. Patients are instructed in the importance of protecting the hands from injury and avoiding things that contribute to vasoconstriction, such as smoking, alcohol, and caffeine. Reducing stress levels can also help prevent vasoconstriction. Immersing the hands in warm water may decrease the vasospasm. Vasodilators are sometimes prescribed to help the patient avoid peripheral vasoconstriction. Nifedipine (Procardia), prazosin (Minipress), or topical nitroglycerin are examples of some of the drug agents used.

To treat Raynaud's disease surgically, the sympathetic reflex must be blocked. This is accomplished by interrupting the sympathetic nerve impulses from the spinal cord to the hand, a procedure known as a sympathectomy.

Nursing Management

Education is the primary goal for patients with Raynaud's disease. Teaching the patient to protect the hands is very important. Stressing the use of gloves in cold climates, reducing vasoconstrictive activity, and decreasing stress levels helps reduce the number and severity of attacks.

Thromboangiitis Obliterans (Buerger's Disease)

Buerger's disease is a recurring inflammation and thrombosis of small and medium arteries and veins of the hands and feet. It is associated with tobacco use, both cigarettes and smokeless tobacco. The cause is unknown, but it is thought to be an autoimmune disorder. It is most prevalent in young men between ages 25 and 40. It is increasing in women likely due to increased tobacco use by women.

Intermittent claudication and other symptoms of occlusive disease are common in patients with Buerger's disease. Other symptoms include numbness or decreased sensation and cool extremities. Lower extremities can be red or cyanotic when in a dependent position, and pulses may be diminished. Depending on the degree of ischemia, ulceration or gangrene may be present.

Because the primary contributing factor is smoking, there is an urgency in helping the patient to cease smoking and avoid second-hand smoke. The patient must be made aware of the effect smoking has on the body and that the disease will progress and further damage other vessels. There is no cure or effective treatment. The use of calcium channel blockers such as diltiazem (Cardizem) promotes vasodilation and may help with intermittent claudication. Surgery is not really effective. Supportive therapy and nursing care for Buerger's disease is used with the goal of reducing complications of ulceration, gangrene, and amputation. Careful inspection of the lower extremities for signs of breakdown is important, so early treatment can begin.

Nursing Process for the Patient with a Peripheral Arterial Disorder

DATA COLLECTION. Monitoring peripheral circulation is most important for patients with arterial occlusive disorders. Careful assessment of pulses, capillary refill, temperature, color, and presence of edema helps identify patients at risk for complications. Absent pulses are reported immediately to prevent limb loss. Skin that is shiny and hairless points to chronic diminished blood flow to the extremity. Laboratory blood testing is not necessary to test for peripheral arterial disease; but a lipid panel and serum glucose can identify diabetes, which is a significant risk factor for PAD. The presence of skin lesions and ulcerations is noted.

NURSING DIAGNOSES, PLANNING, IMPLEMENTATION, AND EVALUATION. See the *Nursing Care Plan for the Patient with a Peripheral Arterial Occlusive Disorder.*

Nursing Care Plan for the Patient with a Peripheral Arterial Occlusive Disorder

Nursing Diagnosis: *Acute Pain* related to impaired circulation to extremities causing intermittent or continuous pain

Expected Outcomes: The patient will report that pain is controlled at an acceptable level.

Evaluation of Outcomes: Does patient report relief from pain by nonpharmacological or pharmacological methods?

Interventions	Rationale	Evaluation
Note peripheral circulation, pulses, color, temperature, presence of edema, and skin breakdown.	Determines the degree of tissue perfusion and complications.	Does patient have pulses, warm skin, capillary refill less than 3 seconds, no evidence of skin breakdown?
Monitor for intermittent claudication or pain at rest.	Helps determine degree of occlusive disease. Pain at rest is an indicator that the arterial occlusion is becoming worse.	Does patient have pain during activity or at rest?
Administer medication as ordered:		Does patient show signs of increased circulation and relief of pain following administration of medications?
• Analgesics	Relieves chronic or acute pain.	
• Vasodilators	Increases blood flow to extremities.	
• Calcium channel blockers	Decrease vasospastic episodes.	
Encourage rest if pain is present.	Rest decreases muscle contraction and prevents further ischemia in extremities.	Is patient able to rest?
Position lower extremities below heart level.	Increases arterial flow to lower extremities.	Are pulses strong, capillary refill less than 3 seconds, extremities pink and warm?
Protect extremities from cold or trauma.	Extremities with decreased circulation have decreased sensation, which increases risk of injury.	Are extremities injury free?
Teach the patient importance and use of relaxation techniques.	Relaxation will decrease the stress response and vasoconstriction related to catecholamine release.	Does patient demonstrate use of relaxation techniques?

Nursing Diagnosis: *Ineffective Tissue Perfusion* related to interruption of arterial flow in arms and legs

Expected Outcomes: The patient will show signs of increased arterial blood flow and tissue perfusion.

Evaluation of Outcomes: Does patient have strong peripheral pulses, capillary refill less than 3 seconds, warm skin, absence of edema?

Interventions	Rationale	Evaluation
Check peripheral pulses, capillary refill, color, temperature, and presence of edema every 4 hours.	Indication of adequate tissue perfusion.	Are peripheral pulses strong, nailbeds pink, capillary refill less than 3 seconds with no edema noted?

Nursing Care Plan for the Patient with a Peripheral Arterial Occlusive Disorder—cont'd

Interventions	Rationale	Evaluation
Report absent or diminished pulses immediately.	Indication of inadequate tissue perfusion requiring immediate treatment.	Are peripheral pulses present and strong?
Check skin for intactness, healed areas, signs of ulceration or infection.	Chronic arterial occlusion leads to decreased blood flow, resulting in tissue damage and poor wound healing.	Is skin intact?
Place extremities lower than heart, feet on floor in sitting position, head of bed elevated on blocks.	Dependent position increases blood flow to the legs and feet.	Does patient have adequate tissue perfusion signs?
Avoid bending knees, pillows under knees, prolonged sitting, or crossing legs.	These activities impede blood flow to extremities.	Does patient exhibit understanding of improving blood flow?
Inspect lower extremities frequently. Clean feet with mild soap; dry carefully. Protect from injury.	Cleaning prevents trauma to feet, protecting feet from things that can lead to ulcerations.	Is patient free from trauma or breaks in skin of the lower extremities?
Encourage use of shoes that fit well.	Prevents irritation and tissue breakdown leading to ulcer.	Does patient verbalize shoes fit well?
Refer to progressive activity program.	Gradual progressive exercise promotes collateral circulation.	Does patient participate in exercise program?
Keep extremity warm using socks and blankets.	Prevents vasoconstriction and promotes comfort.	Are extremities warm?

Nursing Diagnosis: *Activity Intolerance* related to activity pain and diminished blood flow

Expected Outcomes: The patient will report that pain is relieved during desired activities.

Evaluation of Outcomes: Does patient participate in activities without pain?

Interventions	Rationale	Evaluation
Begin walking program: Start on flat surface. Walk 30 minutes per day.	Promotes collateral circulation without greatly increasing oxygen demand.	Does patient participate in walking program?
Walk every day, increasing the distance in small increments until experiencing claudication.	Walking through the pain will promote collateral circulation. Pain should subside with rest.	Does patient increase distance with claudication? Does pain stop with rest?
Walk one-half city block after pain begins per physician order. Stop and rest until pain subsides.		

Continued

Nursing Care Plan for the Patient with a Peripheral Arterial Occlusive Disorder—cont'd

Nursing Diagnosis: *Deficient Knowledge:* peripheral arterial disease related to complications, medications, or postoperative care

Expected Outcomes: The patient and family will verbalize self-care measures to control disease and prevent complications.

Evaluation of Outcomes: Do patient and family verbalize understanding of teaching?

Interventions	Rationale	Evaluation
Ask patient's and family's knowledge of the physiology of the disease, and treatment and preventive techniques.	This will determine educational topics.	What is patient's and family's baseline knowledge of peripheral artery disease (PAD)?
Describe peripheral arterial disease, symptoms, diagnosis, treatment, and complications to patient and family.	The patient should understand PAD to help control disorder.	Do patient and family verbalize understanding of PAD?
Teach healthy lifestyle and risk factor control: smoking cessation, low-fat diet, walking programs, hyperlipidemia, and diabetes and hypertension control.	Healthy lifestyle promotes circulation and decreases functional impairment and pain.	Is patient willing and able to incorporated healthy lifestyle into daily routine?
Explain daily foot care: • Inspect feet for ingrown toenails, redness, sores, or blisters, wash feet with warm soap and water, dry with gentle patting, lubricate skin to prevent cracking, wear clean socks.	Daily foot care and reporting problems promptly can help prevent complications of PAD.	Does patient state will perform daily foot care and verbalize understanding?
• Do not walk barefoot, and inspect inside of footwear for foreign objects before inserting foot.	Ulceration of the toes may follow trauma if foreign object is walked on, which can result in infection.	Does patient verbalize understanding of need to protect feet?
Explain prescribed drug treatment protocols.	Medication explanation can help patient comply with therapy.	Does patient verbalize understanding of medications?

Aneurysms

An **aneurysm** is a bulging, ballooning, or dilation at a weakened point of an artery. The artery diameter is often increased by 50%. The cause is unknown, but anything that weakens the artery wall or causes loss of elasticity in the artery can cause an aneurysm. Atherosclerosis, hypertension, smoking, trauma, and congenital abnormalities are risk factors for an aneurysm. Heredity may also play a role. Aneurysms can occur in any artery in the body but are common in the abdominal aorta, which is the focus of the rest of this discussion.

An abdominal aortic aneurysm (AAA) is often silent if it is less than 4 cm. Most people do not even know that they have an AAA. Men older than age 50 are at the highest risk of death from an AAA. The incidence of AAA increases with age. Survival improves with elective surgery rather than emergency surgery after the aneurysm ruptures.

Types of Aneurysms

The various types of aneurysms are shown in Figure 24.9. A fusiform aneurysm is the dilation of the entire circumference of the artery. A saccular aneurysm is one that bulges on only one side of the artery wall. A dissecting aneurysm occurs when a cavity is formed from a tear in the artery wall, usually the intimal (inner) layer. The layers of the artery are then separated as blood is pumped into the tear with each heartbeat, expanding the cavity, which is then prone to rupturing.

Signs and Symptoms

Aneurysms usually exhibit few if any symptoms (Table 24.8). As the AAA grows, symptoms may develop. Back or flank pain is the classic symptom; the pain is caused by the aneurysm pressing against nerves of the vertebrae. Depending on the location and size of the aneurysm, there may be reports of abdominal pain, a feeling of fullness, or nausea caused by pressure on the intestines. The pain may mimic pain associated with any abdominal or back disorder. Changing positions may temporarily relieve the symptoms. Because the symptoms are vague, they are often not associated with an AAA. There may be a pulsating mass in the abdomen caused by an AAA that is discovered only during routine physical or x-ray examination.

Severe, sudden back, flank, or abdominal pain and a pulsating abdominal mass can indicate that the aneurysm may be about to rupture. With rupture, the patient's blood pressure may drop and signs of shock may be present. Immediate surgery is needed for a ruptured AAA. The mortality rate is high with a ruptured aneurysm.

Diagnostic Tests

Computed tomography (CT) scan and abdominal ultrasound are the most common diagnostic tools used to confirm the presence of an aneurysm. Small aneurysms may be watched over time to see if they enlarge. Aortography can be performed when surgical intervention is considered to identify the size and exact location of the aneurysm.

Therapeutic Measures

Medical treatment consists of medication to maintain lower blood pressures because patients with aneurysms often have hypertension. If the blood pressure is allowed to get too high, it can cause the arterial wall to rupture. Surgical treatment—a bypass graft—is performed when the patient is experiencing pain or showing signs of circulatory compromise. An aneurysm that is larger than 5 cm requires surgery, because the risk of rupture is greatest when the aneurysm reaches 5 cm or greater.

An endovascular graft or a conventional open surgical repair may be done for an AAA. Endovascular grafting involves the transluminal placement (through the femoral artery) and attachment of a sutureless aortic endograft or stent-graft prosthesis at the site of the AAA. In the endograft procedure, a balloon catheter positions and opens the graft. The graft remains attached to the inner wall of the aorta when the catheter is withdrawn. Blood flow continues through the aorta, bypassing the aneurysm. Another method uses a stent-graft that opens to fit the diameter of the aorta to reduce pressure on the aneurysm. Endovascular surgery requires less hospitalization time and a quicker recovery.

TABLE 24.8 ANEURYSM SUMMARY

Signs and Symptoms	Back pain Flank pain Abdominal fullness Nausea Pulsating mass in abdomen Severe sudden back pain with rupture Shock from blood loss
Diagnostic Tests	Ultrasound Chest x-ray MRI CT scan Aortography
Therapeutic Measures	Observe for growth of aneurysm Maintain blood pressure Surgical repair and graft
Complications	Rupture Shock Hemorrhage
Priority Nursing Diagnoses	*Acute Pain* *Risk for Deficient Fluid Volume* *Risk for Ineffective Tissue Perfusion*

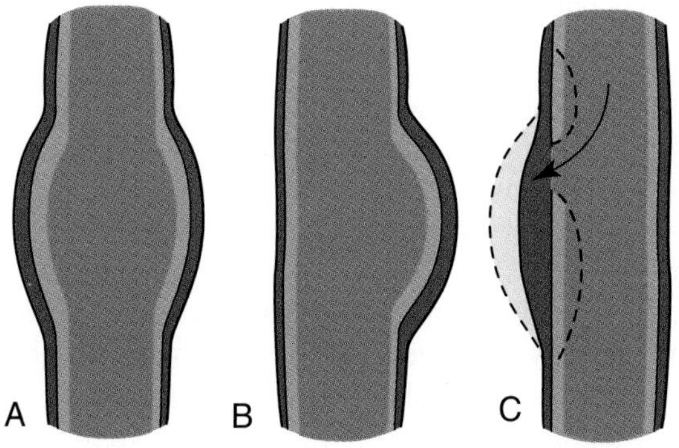
A
B
C

FIGURE 24.9 Types of aneurysms. (A) Fusiform. The entire circumference of the artery is dilated. (B) Saccular. One side of the artery is dilated. (C) Dissecting. A tear in the inner layer causes a cavity to form between the layers of the artery and fill with blood. The cavity expands with each heartbeat.

Nursing Process for the Patient with an Abdominal Aortic Aneurysm

DATA COLLECTION. Careful monitoring of a patient with an AAA is necessary. Patient understanding must be assessed so patients know their medications and the importance of taking antihypertensives as prescribed. Stress may be a risk factor that should be addressed. Lifting heavy objects can increase pressure within the artery and may be restricted even in the individual being treated with more conservative measures. Postoperatively, the patient should avoid lifting heavy objects (see *Home Health Hints*).

Home Health Hints

Cardiac

Both patients and caregivers can experience stress and frustration related to cardiovascular disease. Patients who have undergone open heart surgery may experience feelings of powerlessness, depression, and anger. The home health nurse can be instrumental in helping the family deal with these life-changing illnesses.

- Have a home health social worker visit a postsurgical cardiac patient. This can be useful to help the patient and family plan for lifestyle changes to reduce anxiety and environmental stress.
- Assess the ability of the patient caregiver to provide necessary care. The support and resources available to the caregiver should be explored to prevent caregiver role strain.
- Assist the caregiver to identify a plan to distribute the care workload among family members, if possible.
- Determine the need for caregiver respite care, especially over time. If respite care is needed, assist the caregiver in identifying respite care resources in the family or community.
- Teach the caregiver stress management techniques to use. This can include deep-breathing exercises, reading a book, meditation, massage therapy, guided imagery, exercise, socializing with friends, and/or working on a favorite hobby.
- After open heart surgery, many patients suffer from depression. If the patient appears withdrawn, offers limited eye contact during interaction, and seems uninterested with following through on postoperative instructions, discuss with the patient how he or she feels he/she has changed since having surgery. Report concerns to the patient's physicians; antidepressants might be helpful during this time. Also identify community resources that are available such as a support group and offer that information to your patient.
- Chest pain from esophageal reflux can mimic cardiovascular symptoms. Ask if the pain is related to consuming large meals, lying down, or bending over, or if it is relieved with antacids or food. Inform the physician of these findings.

Vascular

- Instruct the patient to stop and rest if pain develops in the lower extremities during exercise.
- Monitor peripheral pulses and capillary refill to ensure adequate tissue perfusion. Report absent pulses or sluggish capillary refill to the patient's physician.
- Instruct the patient to report changes in skin color, insect bites, and/or rashes to the physician. Patients with peripheral vascular disorders are at a high risk for developing lower extremity wounds that are often slow to heal.

NURSING DIAGNOSES, PLANNING, IMPLEMENTATION, AND EVALUATION. See the *Nursing Care Plan for the Patient After Vascular Surgery.*

Varicose Veins

Varicose veins are elongated, tortuous, dilated veins. The exact cause is unknown. The condition tends to be familial. Varicose veins are divided into primary and secondary varicosities.

Pathophysiology

Primary varicosities are believed to be caused by a structural defect in the vessel wall. Along with the defect, the dilation of the vessel can lead to incompetent venous valves. The valves help prevent blood from refluxing. If reflux occurs, it can cause further dilation of the vessel. The superficial veins are the vessels most often involved in primary varicosities.

Secondary varicosities are caused by an acquired or congenital pathological condition of the deep venous system. This produces dilation of collateral and superficial veins. As a result, there is an interference of blood return to the heart, which leads to stasis, or pooling, of the blood in the deep venous system. This increases the pressure within the system, pushing blood into the collateral vessels and producing varicosities in the superficial veins.

Etiology

A number of factors can lead to varicose veins. The wall defects have been identified as a familial tendency and may be inherited. Any factor that may contribute to increasing hydrostatic pressure within the leg, such as prolonged standing, pregnancy, and obesity, may promote venous dilation. Incompetent valves within the veins can cause blockage of blood flow and lead to dilated veins.

Signs and Symptoms

The most common manifestation is the disfigurement of the lower extremity with primary varicosities. There may be dull pain, especially after prolonged standing. This usually can be relieved by walking or elevating the extremity. With secondary varicosities, the pain and disfigurement may be more severe. Edema or ulceration can develop if circulation is severely compromised.

Therapeutic Measures

The primary goals are to improve circulation, relieve pain, and avoid complications. Treatment is usually not indicated if the problem is only cosmetic. Conservative treatment is geared to reduction of factors that contribute to varicose veins. Elastic compression stockings should be used as ordered. Injection sclerotherapy or lasers treat superficial varicosities. Minimally invasive ablation procedures include radio-frequency ablation (closure procedure) or endovenous laser treatment.

Venous Insufficiency

Venous insufficiency is a chronic condition. Damaged or aging valves within the veins interfere with blood return to the heart, causing pooling of blood in the lower extremities. Chronic venous insufficiency can lead to venous stasis ulcers.

Nursing Care Plan for the Patient After Vascular Surgery

Nursing Diagnosis: *Acute Pain* related to surgical incision and reperfusion of tissue

Expected Outcomes: The patient will state that the pain is relieved or is tolerable within 30 minutes of pain report. The patient will rest comfortably, perform respiratory treatments as necessary, and perform activities of daily living (ADLs).

Evaluation of Outcomes: Does patient state pain is relieved or acceptable? Is patient able to rest and participate in respiratory treatments and ADLs?

Interventions	Rationale	Evaluation
Ask severity of pain, as well as all other qualities.	Peripheral vascular surgery pain is usually mild, and severe pain may indicate reocclusion.	Does patient state pain is at a tolerable level with a patent vessel?
	Major vascular surgery pain is severe.	
	GERIATRIC	
Ask patient to rate pain after analgesic is given.	Pain relief is individualized.	Does patient state pain is controlled at a tolerable level?
Notify physician if pain is unrelieved.	Different analgesic may be needed to give relief.	Are patient's pain relief needs met?
Ensure that older patient's pain is relieved.	Pain is not a normal part of aging, and older patients need and are entitled to adequate pain relief.	Does patient rate pain as none or at a tolerable level using a scale of 0 to 10?
Use opioid pain medications cautiously. Consider reducing frail older patient's first opioid dose by 25% to 50%, and increase as safe and needed and as ordered.	Older patients are more susceptible to peak effects and duration of analgesia of opioids.	Are patient's vital signs and sedation levels within normal limits (WNL)?

Nursing Diagnosis: *Ineffective Tissue Perfusion* related to hypotension, hypothermia, emboli, vascular spasm, or reocclusion

Expected Outcomes: The patient will have palpable peripheral pulses: adequate capillary refill, and normal color, temperature, motor, and sensory function of extremities. The patient will have reactive pupils and baseline cognitive function.

Evaluation of Outcomes: Is patient's circulatory status within normal limits (WNL)? Does patient have reactive pupils and baseline cognitive function intact?

Interventions	Rationale	Evaluation
Monitor circulation, movement, and sensation to extremities every 1 to 4 hours.	Early detection of spasm or reocclusion minimizes risk of ischemia and necrosis.	Does graft or vessel remain patent?
Mark location of pulses on affected extremity.	Allows for quick location of pulses.	Are pulses located easily?

Nursing Care Plan for the Patient After Vascular Surgery—cont'd

Perform neurologic checks every 2 to 4 hours (carotid).	Allows early detection of complications.	Are major neurologic or circulatory problems detected?
Perform circulation or neurologic check between nurses when changing caregiver.	Subtle changes can be detected and new caregiver has baseline for comparison.	Is baseline assessment done?
Measure abdominal girth every shift (abdominal aortic surgery).	Increasing girth may indicate bleeding into abdomen.	Does abdominal girth remain unchanged?
Take temperature every 4 hours.	May indicate infection or hypothermia with need for further warming.	Does patient remain normothermic?
Monitor CBC as ordered.	RBC count, hemoglobin, and hematocrit decrease with insidious bleeding into abdomen or significant hematoma formations.	Is CBC WNL?
Avoid constricting measures on affected extremity: knee gatch of bed, adhesive tape, tight dressings.	Prevent further decrease in blood flow to compromised extremity.	Is blood flow to affected extremity maintained?

Venous Stasis Ulcers

PATHOPHYSIOLOGY. Venous stasis ulcers are the end result of chronic venous insufficiency. Dysfunctional valves in the venous system prevent or reduce venous blood return. As venous pressure increases, venous stasis occurs. Over time the congestion and decreased venous circulation lead to changes in the lower extremities. There may be edema and a brownish discoloration of the leg and foot, with the surrounding skin hardened and leathery in appearance. The brown color occurs when veins rupture, releasing red blood cells into the tissues; the red blood cells then break down and stain the tissue brown.

Stasis ulcers develop from the increased pressure and rupture of small veins. Signs of skin breakdown are most commonly seen at the medial malleolus of the ankle. Stasis ulcers are a serious complication of venous insufficiency that are difficult to cure and can affect the patient's quality of life.

THERAPEUTIC MEASURES. The focus of treatment is to decrease edema and heal skin ulcerations. Compression wraps such as elastic stockings or bandage wraps are necessary to decrease edema. Elastic wraps should be started at the foot, with greater tension applied there, and wrapped up the leg. Rewrapping the elastic bandage twice a day is necessary. It is important to ensure that the wraps are not too tight at the top, which prevents return of blood to the heart.

Bedrest and elevation of legs and feet above the heart are important to assist with drainage of lower extremities. Patients are advised not to keep legs dependent and to avoid long periods of standing or sitting to prevent increased pressure and pain. The foot of the bed should be elevated 5 to 6 inches. Additionally, patients should be encouraged to exercise and walk often during nonacute episodes. Patients should be taught not to cross their legs or wear constrictive clothing that would decrease venous blood return to the heart.

Skin ulcers are usually cultured and treated with topical antibiotics if needed. Wound care can be chronic and challenging. (See Chapter 54.) An Unna boot, which is a gauze dressing coated with zinc oxide, calamine, and glycerin, may be used to promote healing in severe ulcers. Zinc promotes wound healing and can be soothing. The Unna boot is applied snugly and provides compression therapy as well. It is changed every 2 to 7 days. Skin grafting may be necessary if ulcerations are severe or do not heal.

NURSING PROCESS FOR THE PATIENT WITH A VENOUS DISORDER.

Data Collection. Risk factors for varicose veins are identified. Symptoms and concerns about body image are noted. Leg appearance, presence of edema, and ulcerations are noted. Patient-coping skills are assessed to determine patient's ability to cope with chronic ulcers that may affect quality of life. Baseline knowledge of contributing factors for venous disorders is determined for teaching plans.

Nursing Diagnoses, Planning, and Implementation

Acute Pain related to edema and increased pressure

EXPECTED OUTCOME: The patient will report pain is at a tolerable level within 30 minutes of report of pain.

- Use rating scale such as 0 to 10 to identify pain level *to provide consistency in pain reporting.*
- Elevate legs above heart level (such as in a reclining chair) and avoid long periods of standing *to reduce pooling of fluid.*
- Apply compression therapy as ordered *to promote drainage and reduce edema.*
- Administer analgesics as prescribed *to provide pain relief.*

Impaired Tissue Integrity Related to Chronic Venous Congestion

EXPECTED OUTCOME: The patient will have intact tissue integrity.

- Assess and document size, shape, and depth of wound *to evaluate healing of wound over time.*
- Provide a comprehensive plan for wound care including methods of pressure relief from edema, treatments, and nutrition as ordered *to ensure that quality wound care is provided.*
- Provide wound care as ordered *to aid in wound healing.*

Ineffective Health Maintenance Related to Deficient Knowledge of Venous Disease

EXPECTED OUTCOME: The patient will report understanding and management of his or her venous disorder.

- Assess the patient's present understanding of the disease *to determine baseline knowledge.*
- Explain to patient how to control risk factors and prevention of varicose veins: weight reduction, elevation of the extremities, walking, and exercise *help increase muscle strength and contraction.*
- Explain that tight-fitting clothes at tops of legs or waist should not be worn *to prevent venous occlusion.*
- Encourage to wear support hose with varicose veins *to assist blood flow return to the heart.*
- Explain need to avoid heating devices *because of decreased sensitivity and risk of burns.*
- Encourage questions and allow the patient the opportunity to verbalize new information and skills *to enhance learning.*
- Document teaching and evaluation of patient knowledge *to communicate patient progress toward goal attainment.*

See also the *Nursing Care Plan for the Patient After Vascular Surgery.*

Evaluation. Interventions are successful if the patient reports understanding of venous disease and prevention and that pain is at an acceptable level.

Vascular Surgery

Vascular impairments requiring surgery may be acute or chronic and involve arteries, veins, or lymphatic vessels. When intermittent claudication becomes severe or disabling or when the limb is at risk for amputation, then surgical vascular grafting may be done.

Nursing Process for the Patient Undergoing Preoperative Vascular Surgery

DATA COLLECTION. A baseline assessment is important for postoperative comparison and discharge planning. Pain control needs and circulatory status are assessed. Diagnostic test (complete blood count [CBC], electrolytes, PT, PTT, and bleeding time) results are reviewed and typing and crossmatching of blood to be placed on hold is performed.

NURSING DIAGNOSES. The nursing diagnoses for preoperative vascular surgery may include:

- *Acute* or *Chronic Pain* related to ischemia of tissue distal to occlusion or aneurysm
- *Anxiety* related to unknown outcome, pain, powerlessness, or threat of death
- *Deficient Knowledge,* preoperative and postoperative procedures, related to unfamiliar process.

See Chapter 12 for further preoperative nursing process information.

Embolectomy and Thrombectomy

When an artery becomes completely occluded by an embolus or thrombus, it is considered a surgical emergency. Emergency embolectomy is the procedure of choice only if the affected extremity is viable. Surgical removal to restore blood flow and oxygenation to the tissue distal to the occlusion is imperative to decrease ischemia and necrosis.

Vascular Bypasses and Grafts

Vascular bypass surgery involves the use of either autografts, such as the patient's own saphenous vein, or a synthetic graft material. The graft is anastomosed to the artery proximal to the occlusion and tunneled past the occlusion, where the distal end of the graft is anastomosed to the artery (Fig. 24.10).The graft is assessed for hemostasis and function, and then the wound is sutured closed. Video-assisted aortofemoral bypass without laparotomy is a technique that is being used that reduces recovery time.

Repair of a diseased area of a blood vessel, such as an aortic abdominal aneurysm, is performed with resection of the diseased area and replacement with a graft (aortic aneurysmectomy). This is usually an elective procedure. However, if an aneurysm is dissecting or ruptures, it is a surgical emergency.

Endarterectomy

Arteriosclerotic plaques are dissected from the lining of the arterial wall and removed in a procedure called an **endarterectomy**. This is most commonly performed on the carotid artery but may be done on peripheral arterial vessels as well. To control blood flow, the artery is clamped on both sides of the occlusion, and an incision is made into the artery. The plaque within the artery is removed with forceps. The artery is irrigated to remove any further debris and then closed with

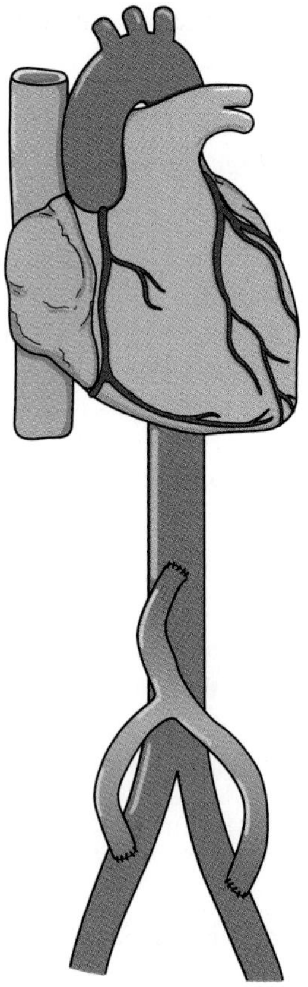

FIGURE 24.10 Aortofemoral bypass.

sutures. The clamps are removed, and the skin incision is closed. A drain may be placed to help prevent hematoma formation.

Angioplasty

Minimally invasive techniques can also be used to open plaque-blocked arteries. These techniques include balloon or laser angioplasty. A flexible laser-tipped catheter is inserted into an artery and advanced to the site of the blockage. The laser sends out pulsating beams of light, which vaporize the plaque. This procedure is used for patients with smaller occlusions in the distal superficial femoral, proximal popliteal, and common iliac arteries.

Stents

Stents are placed inside an artery to provide support to the artery walls and keep them open. Stents are placed in a procedure similar to PCI discussed earlier. Stents may also be used in combination with other procedures such as angioplasty.

Complications of Vascular Surgery

Bleeding and hemorrhage can occur with all vascular surgeries. Drainage can be expected with most surgeries. Drainage is usually small when peripheral vessels are involved. But with involvement of the great vessels, drainage is usually heavier and drains are often placed to prevent swelling and hematoma formation. If hemorrhage occurs, manual pressure is applied to the site of bleeding and the physician notified immediately. Extensive surgeries may also result in significant blood loss, leading to fluid volume deficit or shock.

Reocclusion is possible with any vascular surgery. If thrombi or emboli develop and block blood flow, a surgical emergency results. Loss of a pedal pulse may signify reocclusion and must be immediately reported to the physician. Blood flow needs to be reestablished within 4 to 6 hours to prevent risk of amputation of that extremity.

• WORD • BUILDING •

endarterectomy: end—inside + arter—artery + ectomy—excision

Postoperative Therapeutic Measures

Frequent assessments are ordered postoperatively. Neurovascular checks of extremities every 1 to 4 hours are usually ordered. The incisional area is monitored for hematoma formation. Abdominal girth measurements (for aortic aneurysm repair) are ordered. An increase in abdominal girth may indicate hemorrhage. Any abnormal change is reported immediately to the physician. A loss of a pulse can indicate that circulation has been impaired in the vessel. The patient's need to return to surgery is anticipated if signs of impaired circulation are found.

CBC, INR, PT, PTT, and electrolytes may be ordered daily. Intake and output monitoring may be initially ordered hourly, then every 4 to 8 hours. Imbalances in fluid status should be reported. IV crystalloid solutions, volume expanders, or blood may be ordered for fluid deficits.

Nursing Process for the Patient After Vascular Surgery

DATA COLLECTION. On transfer postoperatively to either the ICU or surgical unit, the patient is positioned comfortably and a head-to-toe assessment is performed and documented. Abnormal findings are reported to the physician. Once a patent airway is ensured, vital signs are monitored according to institutional policy or more frequently if they are unstable. The patient's pain level is rated on a scale of 0 to 10. All IVs and drains are monitored. Measurement of intake and output is usually done hourly. Laboratory tests are also monitored.

Initially, neurovascular checks are ordered every 15 minutes for the first 2 hours, then every 30 minutes for 1 to 3 hours, then hourly for aortic or extremity vascular surgery. Neurovascular checks include extremity movement and sensation, presence of numbness or tingling, pulses, temperature, color, and capillary refill (less than 3 seconds normally). Peripheral pulses are palpated, or assessed with Doppler ultrasound if not palpable, marked, and compared with the unaffected extremity to detect deficits. If a pulse is absent or weak or the extremity is cool or dusky, the physician is notified immediately. A return to surgery for an embolectomy or other procedure is anticipated.

NURSING DIAGNOSES, PLANNING, IMPLEMENTATION, AND EVALUATION. See the *Nursing Care Plan for the Patient After Vascular Surgery.*

NURSING CARE TIP

Neurovascular checks refer to the assessment of an extremity. (Neurologic checks refer to assessment of the central nervous system.) The following are areas to examine on an extremity when doing neurovascular checks. They are identified under the category for which they provide information:

Neurologic	Vascular
Movement	Pulses
Sensation	Capillary refill
Numbness	Color (nailbed or skin)
Tingling	Temperature

CRITICAL THINKING

Mr. Janeway

■ You are caring for Mr. Janeway, age 63, who has just returned from surgery after an embolectomy of the right lower leg. He has a history of insulin-dependent diabetes mellitus, hypertension, renal insufficiency, and a myocardial infarction 2 weeks ago. He is 6 feet tall and weighs 316 pounds.

1. What four priority areas of data collection should you be concerned about for Mr. Janeway?
2. What other information might you want to know regarding Mr. Janeway's medical history?
3. List three priority nursing diagnoses for Mr. Janeway.
4. State one outcome for each nursing diagnosis.
5. What nursing interventions are appropriate for each nursing diagnosis identified?

Suggested answers at end of chapter.

LYMPHATIC SYSTEM

The lymphatic system returns fluid from other tissues in the body to the bloodstream. It is a pumpless system with one-way valves that return the fluid to the heart. Any interruption in the flow of lymph results in edema.

Lymphangitis

Lymphangitis is a bacterial infection of the lymphatic channels. The infection can occur in the arms or legs and is commonly caused by *Staphylococcus* or *Streptococcus* bacteria. It is a serious infection that can cause sepsis and be fatal.

Signs and Symptoms

Symptoms include painful red streaks in the extremity. Fever and chills may be present. Lymph nodes in the area of infection can be enlarged and painful.

Therapeutic Measures

Therapy is initiated with a broad-spectrum antibiotic as the drug of choice. The use of heat on the extremity, as well as elevating it, can help improve circulation. Physicians may order the use of pneumatic pressure devices to help alleviate congestion.

Nursing Process for the Patient with Lymphangitis

DATA COLLECTION. Frequent monitoring of the affected area for edema and skin breakdown is needed to prevent complications from edema. The nurse monitors the size of the extremity and notifies the physician of any increase in size or possible spread of infection. Pain level and fever are monitored.

NURSING DIAGNOSES, PLANNING, AND IMPLEMENTATION

Acute Pain Related to Tissue Damage and Edema From Infection

EXPECTED OUTCOME: The patient will report an absence or acceptable level of pain within 30 minutes of reporting pain.

- Explain and have patient use pain rating *to report pain level for consistency.*
- Administer analgesics as prescribed *to provide pain relief.*
- Recheck pain level 30 to 60 minutes after analgesic given *to determine if pain relief has been obtained.*
- Position extremity *for comfort* and elevate *to reduce edema, which can cause pressure and pain.*

Risk for Excess Fluid Volume Related to Congested Lymph Nodes from Infection

EXPECTED OUTCOME: The patient will exhibit no evidence of edema.

- Apply heat on the extremity as ordered *to increase circulation and reduce edema.*
- Elevate extremity *to help improve circulation and prevent edema.*

EVALUATION. Interventions are successful if the patient reports pain is at an acceptable level and no edema is present.

SUGGESTED ANSWERS TO

CRITICAL THINKING

■ *Mr. Jones*

1. Irregular, respiratory rate 28 per minute and shallow, lung sounds diminished with crackles in bilateral bases.
2. Pain control, coughing and deep breathing, and incentive spirometer.
3. Pain, compensation for respiratory status, elevated temperature.
4. Hemorrhage, reduced cardiac output.

■ *Mrs. Sims*

1. Place on bedrest, administer oxygen via nasal cannula at 2 L/min, assess blood pressure and pulse, administer nitroglycerin sublingual as ordered, obtain ECG, and notify physician.
2. She may be having an anginal attack versus acute MI.
3. Nitroglycerin usually stops chest pain associated with angina. Rest may also alleviate chest pain. Neither nitroglycerin nor rest will relieve the pain of an acute MI.
4. Indicators of an MI include patient history, ECG changes with ST-segment elevation, elevated troponin I, and CK-MB elevation.
5. Medical interventions may include nitroglycerin drip, morphine, or anticoagulant therapy (heparin), and thrombolytic agents to dissolve the clot. A cardiac catheterization can determine which coronary artery is blocked. PCI or a coronary artery bypass graft may be done to reroute blood.
6. Educate Mrs. Sims about the risks of smoking and being overweight.

■ *Mrs. May*

1. Monitor the patient's left leg for color, temperature, capillary refill, and pulses: femoral, popliteal, dorsalis pedis, and posterior tibial. Compare findings with findings in the right leg.
2. If unable to palpate pulses, use a Doppler ultrasound that enhances sound to locate pulses.
3. The patient's symptoms could be caused by an embolism above left femoral artery.
4. To document finding, you would obtain more assessment data. A sample of SOAP charting for your additional findings is given:

   S: "I have a severe pain in my left groin that just started. It is at nine."

   O: Grimacing, moaning, and holding left upper leg. Left leg cool, color pale, nailbeds pale, capillary refill 10 seconds, unable to palpate pulses. Faint femoral and popliteal pulse, no dorsalis pedis or posterior tibial pulse heard with Doppler. Right leg warm, pink, capillary refill 3 seconds, with all pulses palpable.

   A: Ineffective tissue perfusion.

   P: Notify physician stat.
5. Immediate interventions include complete bedrest, protecting the leg, and notifying the physician.
6. Medical interventions could include medication for pain and use of an anticoagulant, such as heparin. If no pulses are present, a thrombolytic agent may be ordered. Surgery is possible.
7. Thrombolectomy or embolectomy may be necessary to save the limb.

■ *Mr. Janeway*

1. Priority areas for data collection include respiratory status, circulatory status of right leg and foot, vital signs, and pain level.
2. A medical history should include Mr. Janeway's usual blood sugar values, insulin dose, ambulation aids, gait, knowledge base regarding his various disease processes, and what led to this hospitalization.
3. Priority nursing diagnoses include (1) *Pain* related to surgery of right lower leg; (2) *Ineffective Tissue Perfusion* related to embolectomy of right lower leg, renal insufficiency; and (3) *Risk for Injury* related to leg surgery, diabetes, obesity.
4. Outcomes include (1) verbalizes relief of pain; (2) maintains adequate tissue perfusion as evidenced by palpable peripheral (pedal) pulses, warm and dry skin; and (3) remains free from injury.
5. Nursing interventions include the following: (1) Position (especially right leg) for comfort; keep the right leg slightly elevated; educate the patient regarding the need to ask for pain medication before pain is too severe; educate the patient regarding the need to take pain medication to minimize the negative physiological effects of pain; monitor pain on a pain scale; evaluate the effectiveness of medication using the same pain scale, report ineffective pain measures. (2) Check pedal pulses, surgical dressing, pedal sensation and movement, and color, initially and every hour; report changes; check capillary refill; monitor for pain in extremities; monitor for edema in extremities; keep leg elevated slightly. (3) Make sure the nursing call light is within reach; provide assistance with ambulation; use walking aids.

REVIEW QUESTIONS

1. Which of the following is a risk factor that can be controlled to prevent the development of cardiovascular disease?
   a. Family history of cardiovascular disease
   b. Hypertension
   c. Ethnicity
   d. Family history of diabetes mellitus

2. Which of these assessment findings is an atypical symptom of a myocardial infarction when chest pain is not present?
   a. Fatigue
   b. Dizziness
   c. Sweating
   d. Nausea

3. Which of the following is the purpose of CABG surgery?
   a. Cure coronary artery disease.
   b. Increase blood flow to the myocardium.
   c. Prevent spasms of the coronary arteries.
   d. Decrease blood flow to the coronary arteries.

4. Which of the following is a classic symptom of peripheral arterial occlusive disease?
   a. Angina
   b. Edema
   c. Intermittent claudication
   d. Stasis ulcers

5. Which of the following medications is used to treat intermittent claudication?
   a. Cholestyramine (Questran)
   b. Enoxaparin (Lovenox)
   c. Pentoxifylline (Trental)
   d. Ranolazine (Ranexa)

6. The nurse is caring for a patient who has peripheral arterial disease. Which of the following statements by the patient indicates understanding of how to manage the pain of peripheral arterial disease?
   a. "I will lie down frequently."
   b. "I will use a reclining chair."
   c. "I will sit with my legs down."
   d. "I will do knee flexion exercises."

References

American Heart Association (2009). *Heart disease and stroke statistics—2009 update.* Dallas, TX: Author. Retrieved November 20, 2009, from http://www.americanheart.org/downloadable/heart/1240250946756LS-1982%20Heart%20and%20Stroke%20Update.042009.pdf

Moghissi, E., Korytkowski, M., DiNardo, M., et al. (2009). American Association of Clinical Endocrinologists and American Diabetes Association consensus statement on inpatient glycemic control. *Endocrine Practice, 15*(4), 1–17.

National Heart, Lung, and Blood Institute. (2008). 4. Disease statistics. In *NHLBI factbook.* Retrieved November 20, 2009, from http://www.nhlbi.nih.gov/about/factbook/chapter4.htm

DavisPlus | For additional resources and information visit **http://davisplus.fadavis.com**

25

Nursing Care of Patients with Cardiac Dysrhythmias

LINDA S. WILLIAMS

KEY TERMS

ablation (uh-BLAY-shun)
atrial depolarization (AE-tree-uhl DEE-poh-lur-ih-ZAY-shun)
atrial systole (AE-tree-uhl SISS-tuh-lee)
atrioventricular node (AE-tree-oh-ven-TRICK-yoo-lur NOHD)
bigeminy (bye-JEM-ih-nee)
bradycardia (BRAY-dih-KAR-dee-yah)
bundle of His (BUN-duhl of HISS)
cardioversion (KAR-dee-oh-VER-zhun)
defibrillation (dee-FIB-ri-lay-shun)
dysrhythmia (dis-RITH-mee-yah)
electrocardiogram (ee-LECK-troh-KAR-dee-oh-GRAM)
fluoroscopy (fluh-RAHS-kuh-pee)
hyperkalemia (HIGH-per-kuh-LEE-mee-ah)
hypomagnesemia (HIGH-poh-MAG-nuh-ZEE-mee-ah)
isoelectric line (EYE-so-e-LECK-trick LINE)
multifocal (MUHL-tee-FOH-kuhl)
sinoatrial node (SIGH-noh-AY-tree-al NOHD)
trigeminy (try-JEM-i-nee)
unifocal (YOO-ni-FOH-cull)
ventricular diastole (ven-TRICK-yoo-lar dye-AS-tuh-lee)
ventricular repolarization (ven-TRICK-yoo-lar RE-pol-lahr-i-ZAY-shun)
ventricular systole (ven-TRICK-yoo-lar SIS-tuh-lee)
ventricular tachycardia (ven-TRICK-yoo-lar TACK-ee-KAR-dee-yah)

QUESTIONS TO GUIDE YOUR READING

1. How does electrical activity flow through the heart?
2. What are the six steps used for dysrhythmia interpretation?
3. What current medical treatments are used for each of the cardiac dysrhythmias?
4. What types of cardiac pacemakers and implantable cardioverter defibrillators are available and what are their uses?
5. What nursing care would you provide for patients with a dysrhythmia or implanted device?

CARDIAC CONDUCTION SYSTEM

The heart's electrical conduction system initiates an impulse whose purpose is to stimulate the mechanical cells of the heart to contract (Fig. 25.1). Electrical activity can be viewed on a cardiac monitor or recorded on an **electrocardiogram** (ECG) tracing. The activity seen on an ECG does not necessarily mean that the mechanical cells of the heart have contracted in response to the electrical impulse. The patient's blood pressure and pulses verify that cardiac contraction occurred.

Located in the upper posterior wall of the right atrium is the **sinoatrial** (SA) **node**. The SA node is the primary pacemaker of the heart because its inherent (built-in) rate is faster than those of the other conduction sites. It normally fires at a rate of 60 to 100 beats per minute (bpm). As a protective mechanism if the SA node slows or fails, other areas of the heart can initiate impulses to keep the heart beating. This mechanism is referred to as escape. The **atrioventricular** (AV) **node** has an inherent rate of 40 to 60 bpm. The body can usually function adequately with this rate. If the AV node is unable to initiate an impulse, then the ventricles can take over at 20 to 40 bpm. However, the ventricular rate of 20 to 40 bpm is not adequate to meet the body's oxygen needs, so the patient begins to show signs of inadequate cardiac output such as dyspnea, abnormal vital signs, and changes in level of consciousness. Treatment is usually needed to reestablish a normal heart rate as soon as possible.

After the SA node fires, the impulse spreads through the atria along internodal tracts to the AV node, stimulating the atria to contract. This is known as **atrial systole**. The atrial contraction propels blood out of the atria and into the relaxed ventricles during **ventricular diastole**. At the AV node, the impulse is briefly delayed. Next the impulse travels down the **bundle of His**, which divides into right and left bundle branches. From there the impulse quickly travels through the Purkinje fibers, stimulating both ventricles to contract upward from the apex of the heart pushing blood toward the arteries. This contraction is known as **ventricular systole**.

Cardiac Cycle

A cardiac cycle is the period from the beginning of one heartbeat to the beginning of the next. The cardiac cycle is the electrical representation of the impulse that stimulates contraction and relaxation of the atria and ventricles. Within the normal cardiac cycle, there is a P wave, a QRS complex, and a T wave (Fig. 25.2).

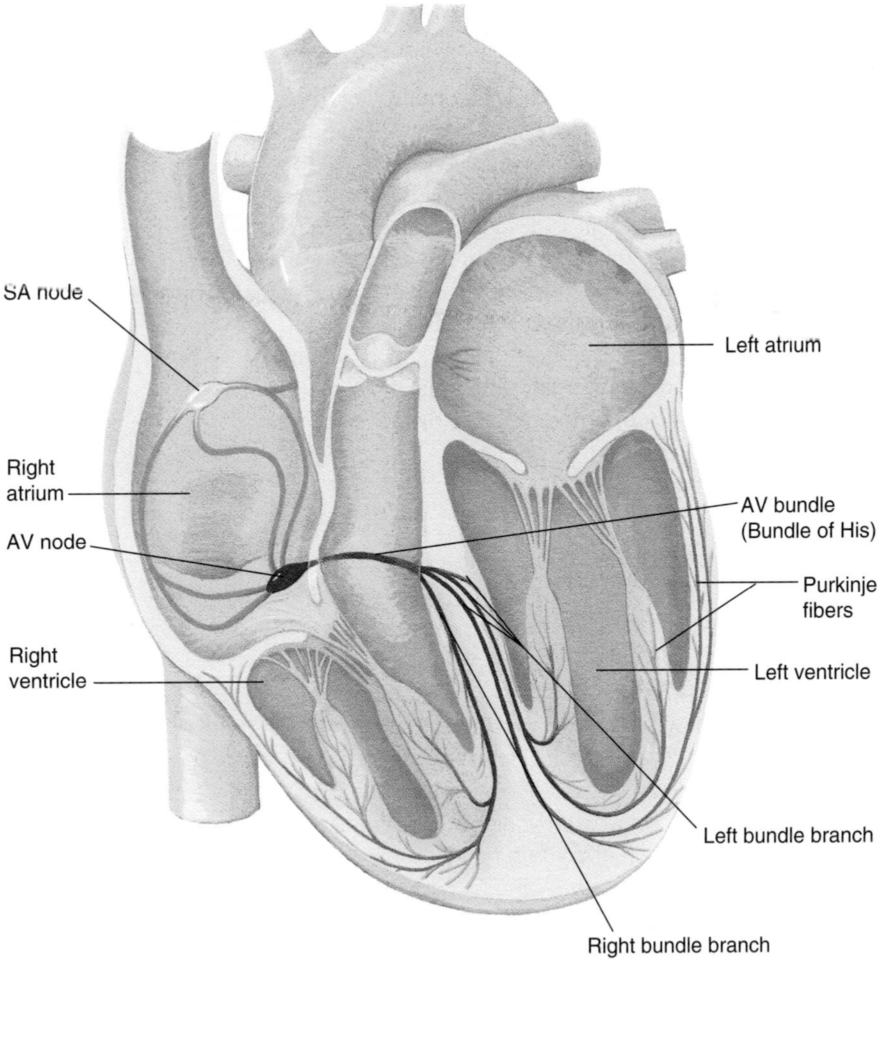
SA node
Left atrium
Right atrium
AV bundle (Bundle of His)
AV node
Purkinje fibers
Right ventricle
Left ventricle
Left bundle branch
Right bundle branch

FIGURE 25.1 Conduction pathway of the heart. (From Scanlon, V., & Sanders, T. [2007]. *Essentials of anatomy and physiology* [5th ed.]. Philadelphia: F. A. Davis Company.)

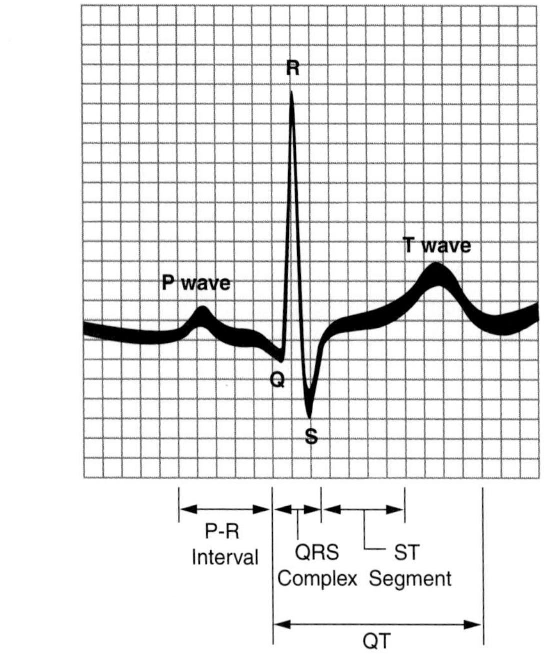
R
T wave
P wave
Q
S
P-R Interval
QRS Complex
ST Segment
QT

FIGURE 25.2 Components of the cardiac cycle. (From Scanlon, V., & Sanders, T. [2007]. *Essentials of anatomy and physiology* [5th ed.]. Philadelphia: F. A. Davis Company.)

ELECTROCARDIOGRAM

The electrical activity of the heart can be viewed with ongoing cardiac monitoring or by obtaining an ECG reflecting the activity at that moment. Electrodes placed on the patient allow different views of the heart to be seen. Each view of the heart is referred to as a lead. A 12-lead ECG provides 12 different views of the heart, whereas an 18-lead ECG shows 18 views. Waveforms may change in appearance in the different leads. For continuous monitoring of cardiac electrical activity, one lead providing a good view is used such as lead II or MCL_1.

Specialized training usually by physicians is required to interpret ECGs for normal and abnormal function. By learning characteristics of a normal heart rhythm and rules for common **dysrhythmias**, you will be able to report rhythm changes to your supervisor or the physician.

LEARNING TIP

Think of a 12- or 18-lead ECG as if you had a camera that you were using to take pictures or views of an object such as an apple. To obtain views that showed you all the sides of the apple—front, side, back, side—you would take a picture and then move the camera a little to get the view next to the one you had just taken. You would continue moving the camera until you had worked your way around the apple. This would then give you a complete view of the entire apple. This is what an ECG does for viewing the conduction system of the heart.

Electrocardiogram Graph Paper

The intervals of each of the components of a cardiac cycle can be measured on the ECG graph paper on which the rhythm is recorded. The graph paper is calibrated in a grid with small squares divided into heavy lined blocks of 25, five squares wide and five squares high (Fig. 25.3). Each small box is 0.04 seconds wide. There are five small squares, which equal 0.20 seconds of time, horizontally between two heavy vertical black lines (see Fig. 25.3). The height of waveforms (amplitude) is measured vertically. Measuring the amplitude is not necessary for basic dysrhythmia interpretation.

When the ECG does not detect electrical current or positive and negative electrical activity is equal, a straight line is produced. This **isoelectric line** occurs when there are no positive or negative electrical wave deflections. Cardiac cycle impulses (seen as waves), depending on the ECG lead, are either upright (positive) or downward (negative) from the isoelectric line on the ECG graph paper.

COMPONENTS OF A CARDIAC CYCLE

P Wave

The P wave is the first wave of the cardiac cycle and represents **atrial depolarization**. When the SA node fires, the electrical impulse spreads from the right to left atrium. The

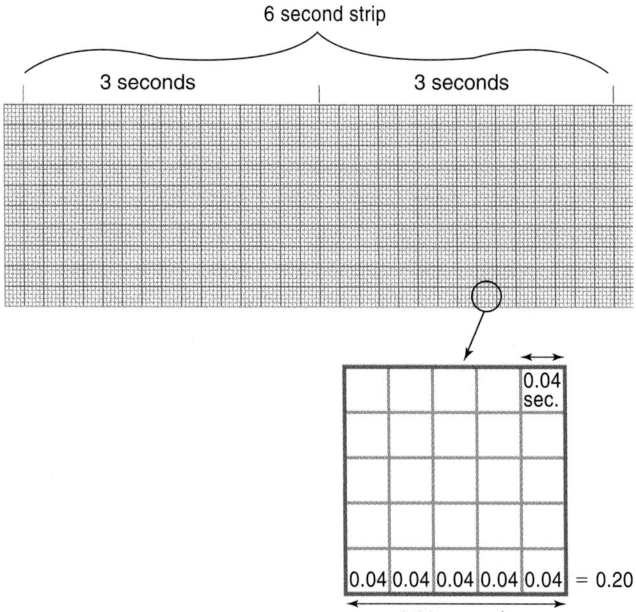
6 second strip
3 seconds
3 seconds
0.04 sec.
0.04 0.04 0.04 0.04 0.04 = 0.20
0.20 seconds

FIGURE 25.3 Electrocardiogram recording paper time intervals.

• WORD • BUILDING •

dysrhythmia: dys—difficult or abnormal + rhythm—rhythm

normal P wave appears rounded. Disorders that change atrial size cause alterations in P-wave shape and size.

LEARNING TIP

To make measuring waves easier:

- Identify the isoelectric line as you measure waveform tracings to help you determine the type of wave. Use a straight edge resting below the line to see any waves above the line; then rest the straight edge above the line to see any waves that fall below the line.
- Try to find a wave that begins on a line to make it visually easier to see the intervals (Fig. 25.4). If the wave starts or ends in the middle of a small box, count it as one-half of a box, which is 0.02 seconds.

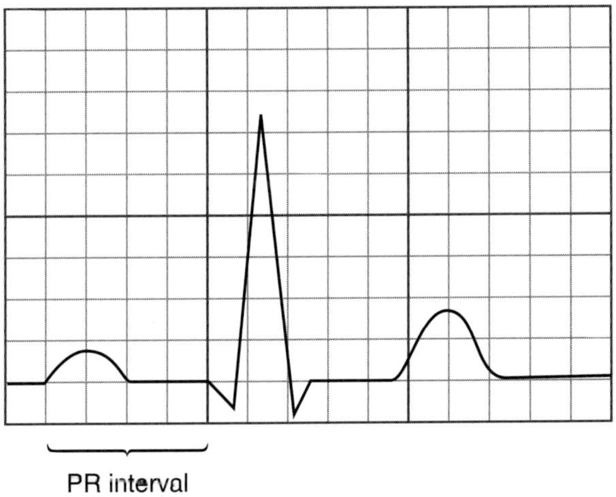
PR interval

FIGURE 25.4 PR interval.

PR Interval

The PR interval (PRI) represents the time it takes the electrical impulse to travel from the SA node to the AV node. The PRI starts at the beginning of the P wave and ends at the beginning of the QRS complex. Counting the number of small boxes horizontally that the interval covers determines the length of the PRI (see Fig. 25.4). The normal PRI is 0.12 to 0.20 seconds.

LEARNING TIP

To remember a normal PRI, think of normal respiratory rate and then add a decimal in front. A normal respiratory rate is 12 to 20 per minute, and a normal PRI is 0.12 to 0.20 seconds.

QRS Complex

The QRS complex represents ventricular depolarization and is composed of three waves: Q, R, and S. The Q wave is the first downward deflection after the P wave. The R wave is the first upward deflection after the P wave. The S wave is the first negative deflection after the R wave (see Fig. 25.2). The S wave ends when it returns to the isoelectric line (this is why locating the isoelectric line is helpful when first learning to identify waves). It is important to note that all three waves are not always present in every QRS complex. Even with absent waves, the QRS is still referred to as the QRS complex (Fig. 25.5). The QRS is larger than the P wave because the ventricles have more muscle mass.

QRS Interval

The QRS interval represents the time it takes for the electrical impulse to travel from the AV node rapidly through the ventricles. To measure the QRS interval, count the number of boxes from the wave that starts the QRS complex to the end of the wave that completes the QRS complex. For example, when a Q, R, and S are present, measure from the beginning of the Q wave to the end of the S wave (Fig. 25.6). If there is only an R present, measure from the beginning of the R to the end of the R. The normal QRS interval is usually considered to be less than or equal to 0.10 seconds.

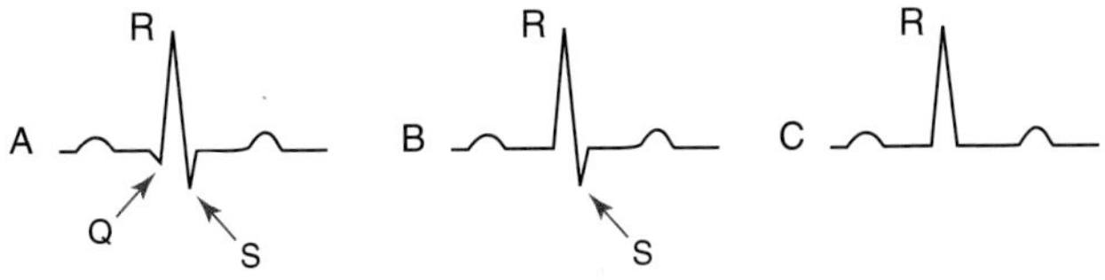
A
R
Q
S
B
R
S
C
R

FIGURE 25.5 (A) QRS complex with a Q wave. (B) QRS complex without a Q wave. (C) QRS complex without a Q or an S wave.

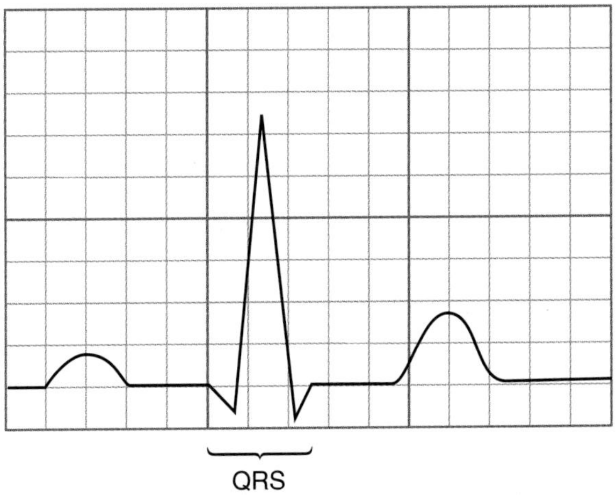
QRS

FIGURE 25.6 QRS interval. This QRS interval covers two and one-half boxes. Each full box is 0.04 seconds. One-half box is 0.02 seconds; $2.5 \times 0.04 = 0.10$ seconds.

T Wave

The T wave represents **ventricular repolarization**, the resting state of the heart, when the ventricles are filling with blood and preparing to receive the next impulse. In most leads, the T wave is an upward (positive) deflection, after the QRS complex, and ends with a return to the isoelectric line. An inverted (downward) T wave can indicate coronary ischemia (Fig. 25.7).

QT Interval

The QT interval measures the time from the start of the Q wave to the end of the T wave (see Fig. 25.2). This represents the time for ventricular depolarization and repolarization. Normal ranges, 0.34 to 0.43 seconds, vary based on gender, heart rate, and age (a QT chart for identifying normal values is used). Prolonged or shortened QT intervals can lead to ventricular dysrhythmias. Abnormal intervals may be due to genetic causes, heart conditions, electrolyte imbalances, or medications that can prolong the QT interval.

U Wave

The U wave is small and often not seen. It occurs shortly after the T wave. It is most prominent in patients with hypokalemia (low serum potassium level) (Fig. 25.8).

ST Segment

The ST segment reflects the time from completion of a contraction (depolarization) to recovery (repolarization) of myocardial muscle for the next impulse. The ST segment starts at the end of the QRS and ends at the beginning of the T wave (Fig. 25.9). The ST segment is examined for patients experiencing chest pain. If a patient has ischemia, the ST segment can be inverted or depressed (Fig. 25.10). With cardiac injury, the ST segment elevates from the isoelectric line (Fig. 25.11).

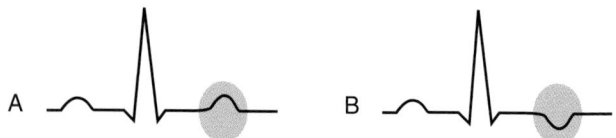
A
B

FIGURE 25.7 (A) T wave with positive deflection. (B) T wave with inverted, negative inflection, indicating ischemia.

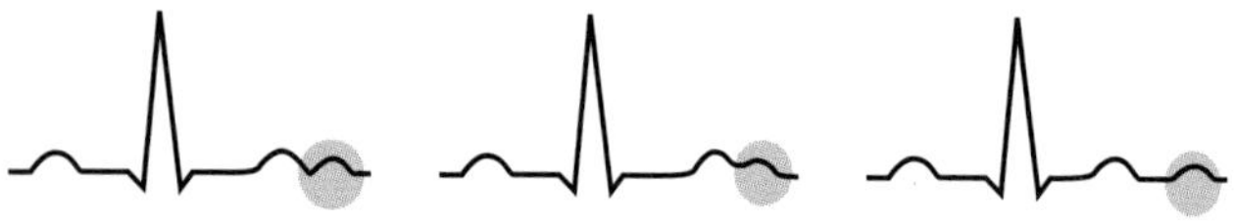

FIGURE 25.8 Various locations where U waves may appear.

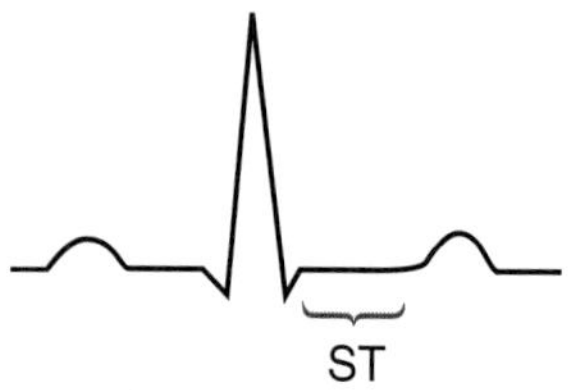
ST

FIGURE 25.9 ST segment.

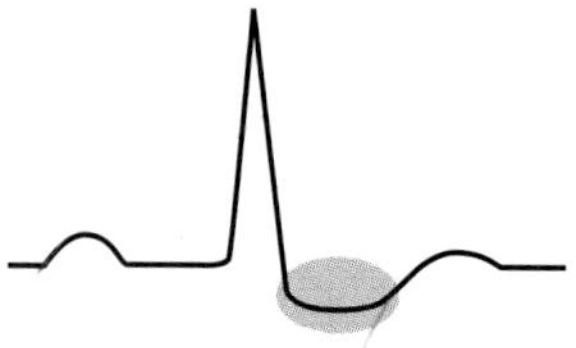

FIGURE 25.10 ST segment inverted or depressed.

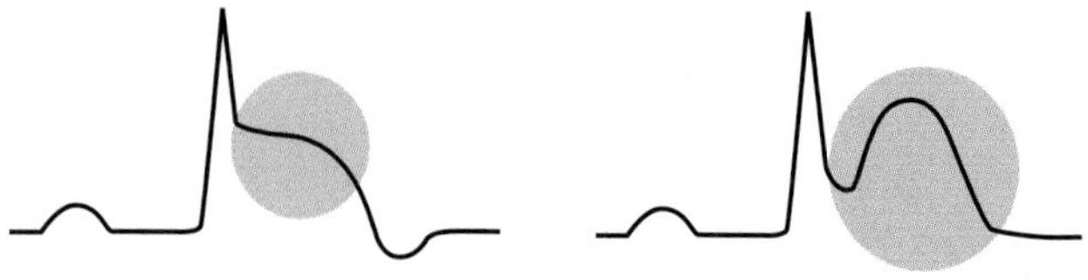

FIGURE 25.11 ST segment elevated.

INTERPRETATION OF CARDIAC RHYTHMS

Six-Step Process for Dysrhythmia Interpretation

An orderly, systematic method for interpreting ECG rhythms should be used to increase understanding of items to examine and ensure nothing is overlooked. Six steps are examined in this process (Table 25.1). Use the findings of the first five steps to identify the ECG rhythm according to the five rules for each dysrhythmia. Then measure the QT interval so that abnormalities can be reported to the physician. A 6-second ECG strip is used when interpreting rhythms. (See Fig. 25.3.)

TABLE 25.1 SIX-STEP PROCESS FOR DYSRHYTHMIA INTERPRETATION

After answering the questions listed here, you should be able to name the patient's dysrhythmia.

Step	Topic	Questions
1	Regularity of rhythm	Is the rhythm regular? Irregular? Is there a pattern to the irregularity?
2	Heart rate	What is the heart rate?
3	P waves	Is there one P wave in front of every QRS complex? Is the atrial rate the same as the ventricular rate? Are the P waves smooth, rounded, and upright?
4	PR interval	Is the PR interval normal and constant? Does the PR interval vary?
5	QRS interval	Is the QRS interval normal and constant? Do the QRS complexes all look alike?
6	QT interval	Is the QT interval normal?

Step 1. Regularity of the Rhythm

The regularity of the rhythm can be determined by looking at the R-to-R spacing on the ECG (Fig. 25.12). The same spacing between each R to R, with a rare variation of no greater than two small boxes, is seen in a normal rhythm. To determine the regularity of a rhythm, count the number of small boxes between each R wave, which normally should remain the same, or use a caliper (two-sided, movable metal instrument with sharp points) to measure the R-to-R spacing.

To use a caliper for measuring R waves, one point is placed on an R wave and the other point is placed in the same spot on the next R wave. Then, without changing the distance between the caliper points, march the caliper from R wave to R wave across the ECG tracing (also known as a strip) to see if R waves are regularly spaced. If the distance is the same, the rhythm is regular. If the distance varies, the rhythm is irregular. An irregular rhythm can be regularly irregular, which means it has a predictable pattern of irregularity, or irregularly irregular, without any pattern of irregularity.

LEARNING TIP

If a caliper is not available, a piece of paper can be placed on the ECG strip. A mark can be made on the paper at the top of one R wave and another mark made on the paper at the top of the next R wave. The marks on the paper can then be moved across the R-to-R intervals on the strip (as caliper points are) to determine rhythm regularity.

Step 2. Heart Rate

After rhythm regularity is determined, the heart rate is counted. One of the two following methods is used:

1. Count the number of small (0.04-seconds) boxes between two R waves and divide that number into 1500. This gives the beats per minute, because 1500 small boxes equals 1 minute (Fig. 25.13). This method is used only for regular rhythms and is very accurate.
2. Six-second method: The 6-second method is used for irregular rhythms. It may also be used when a rapid estimate of a regular rhythm is needed, although it is not the most accurate method for regular rhythms. At the top of ECG graph paper are vertical marks at 3-second intervals (see Fig. 25.3). Count the number of R waves in a 6-second strip and multiply the total by 10 (the number of 6-second time periods in a minute) to obtain the beats per minute (6 seconds $\times$ 10 = 60 seconds or 1 minute) (Fig. 25.14).

Step 3. P Waves

The P waves on the ECG strip are examined to see if (1) there is one P wave in front of every QRS, (2) the P waves are regular, and (3) the P waves all look alike. (See Fig. 25.12.) If all of the P waves meet these criteria, they are considered normal. If they do not, further examination of the strip is necessary to determine the dysrhythmia.

Step 4. PR Interval

All PR intervals are measured to determine whether they are normal and constant. If the PRI is found to vary, it is important to note whether there is a pattern to the variation.

Step 5. QRS Interval

The QRS intervals are measured to determine whether they are all within normal range. Abnormal QRS complexes require further examination.

Step 6. QT Interval

Finally, the QT interval is measured to ensure that it is not shortened or prolonged, which can lead to dysrhythmias. Abnormal QT intervals should be reported to the physician.

NORMAL SINUS RHYTHM

Description

Normal sinus rhythm is the normal cardiac rhythm (Fig. 25.15). It begins in the SA node and has complete, regular cardiac cycles at 60 to 100 bpm.

NORMAL SINUS RHYTHM RULES

1. Rhythm: regular
2. Heart rate: 60 to 100 bpm
3. P waves: rounded, upright, precede each QRS complex, alike
4. PR interval: 0.12 to 0.20 seconds
5. QRS interval: less than or equal to 0.10 seconds.

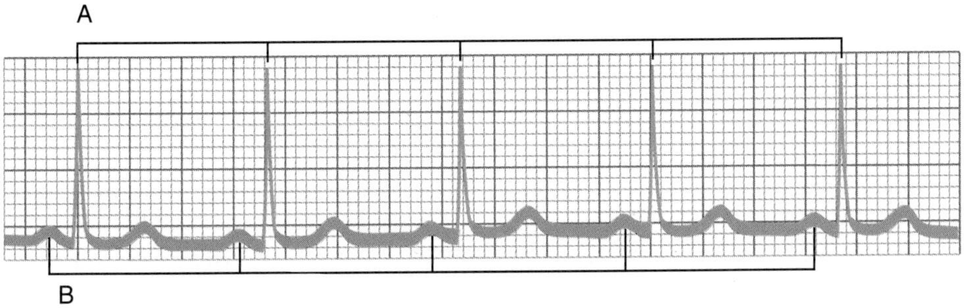
A
B

FIGURE 25.12 Normal cardiac waves are equal distances apart. (A) R to R waves. (B) P to P waves.

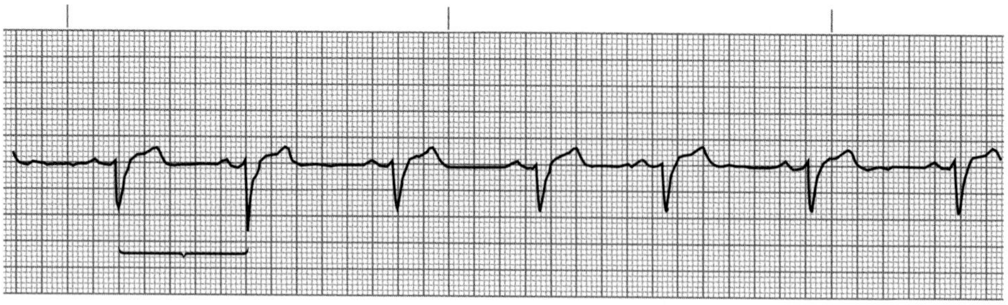

FIGURE 25.13 Heart rate regular. Count the small boxes between two of the R waves and divide into 1500: 1500/25 = 60 beats per minute. Alternatively, count the large boxes between two of the R waves and divide into 300: 300/5 = 60 beats per minute.

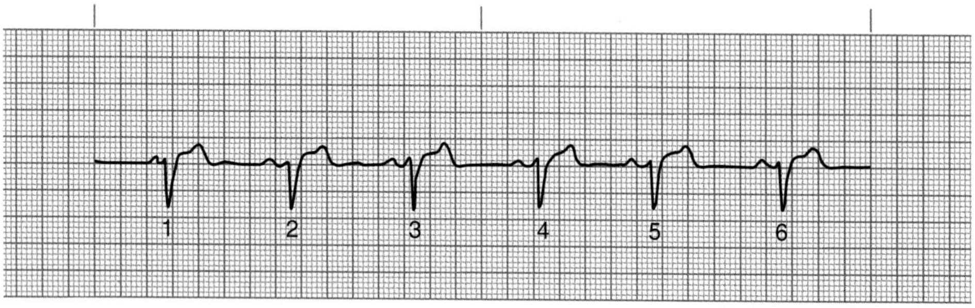
1
2
3
4
5
6

FIGURE 25.14 Heart rate irregular. Counting R waves in a 6-second strip. There are six R waves in this 6-second strip, and 6 × 10 = 60 beats per minute.

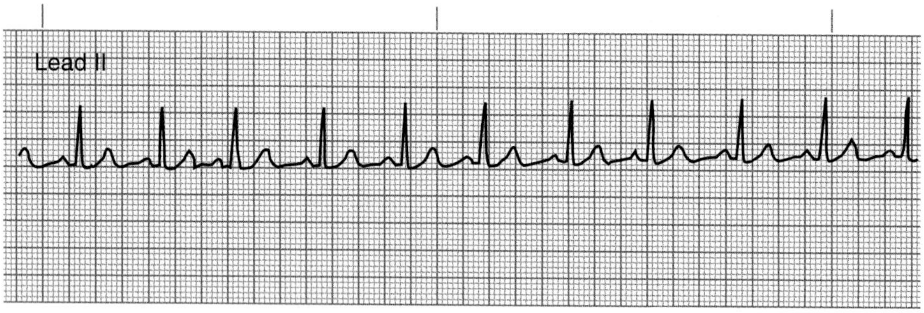
Lead II

FIGURE 25.15 Normal sinus rhythm.

DYSRHYTHMIAS

Two terms are used for rhythm disturbances: *arrhythmia* and *dysrhythmia.* An arrhythmia is an irregularity or loss of rhythm of the heartbeat, and a dysrhythmia is an abnormal, disordered, or disturbed rhythm. These two terms are used interchangeably, but *dysrhythmia* is the most accurate term for the discussion of abnormal rhythms. For more information about cardiac care for dysrhythmias, visit the American Heart Association Web site at www.americanheart.org.

Several mechanisms can cause irregularity or dysrhythmia. Two examples of these mechanisms are a disturbance in the formation of an impulse and a disturbance in the conduction of the impulse. When impulse formation is disturbed, the impulse may arise from the atria, the AV node, or the ventricles rather than the SA node. This disturbance can be seen as an increased or decreased heart rate, early or late beats, or atrial or ventricular fibrillation. With a disturbance in conduction there may be normal formation of the impulse, but it becomes blocked within the electrical conduction system, resulting in abnormal conduction (as in heart block or bundle branch blocks).

Dysrhythmias Originating in the Sinoatrial Node

Rhythms arising from the SA node are referred to as sinus rhythms. Disturbances in conduction from the SA node can cause irregular rhythms or abnormal heart rates. Dysrhythmias arising from the SA node are rarely dangerous. Patients, especially those with heart, lung, or kidney disease, who cannot tolerate a rapid or slow heart rate may require treatment.

> **LEARNING TIP**
>
> The origin and the type of a problem are used to name a dysrhythmia. Let's name a slow dysrhythmia that originates in the sinoatrial node. The origin is sinus and the type of problem (slow rate) is bradycardia = sinus bradycardia. The term *normal* is not used because there is a problem. So what would a fast dysrhythmia originating in the SA node be called? Yes, sinus tachycardia!

Sinus Bradycardia

Bradycardia is a slower than normal heart rate. Sinus bradycardia has the same cardiac cycle components as a normal sinus rhythm. The only difference between the two is a slower heart rate caused by fewer impulses originating from the SA node (Fig. 25.16). Do you see that the name *sinus bradycardia* tells you this difference? The name says the impulse is coming from the sinus node (sinus) but at a slower rate than normal (bradycardia). See, it is easy to understand what is happening in the dysrhythmia when you look at what the name tells you.

ETIOLOGY. Medications such as digoxin (Lanoxin), myocardial infarction (MI), and electrolyte imbalances can cause bradycardia. Well-conditioned athletes also can have slower heart rates because their hearts work more efficiently.

SINUS BRADYCARDIA RULES

1. Rhythm: regular
2. Heart rate: less than 60 bpm
3. P waves: smoothly rounded, precede each QRS complex, alike
4. PR interval: 0.12 to 0.20 seconds
5. QRS interval: less than or equal to 0.10 seconds.

• WORD • BUILDING •
bradycardia: bradys—slow + kardia—heart

SIGNS AND SYMPTOMS. Sinus bradycardia rarely produces symptoms unless it is so slow that it reduces cardiac output. Symptoms consist of fatigue or fainting episodes.

THERAPEUTIC MEASURES. Treatment is usually not required if the patient is asymptomatic. The patient is observed for symptoms, and the underlying cause is determined for correction. If bradycardia is due to a heart block dysrhythmia, insertion of a cardiac pacemaker may be required. If the patient is symptomatic, therapeutic interventions may include atropine, transcutaneous pacing, and dopamine or epinephrine while awaiting a pacemaker (Table 25.2). Medications are given IV for immediate effect. The treatments increase the heart rate for a short time until a cause can be determined and treated.

Sinus Tachycardia

Tachycardia is defined as a heart rate greater than 100 bpm. Sinus tachycardia has the same components as a normal sinus rhythm except the heart rate is faster (Fig. 25.17). More impulses originating from the SA node than normal cause this.

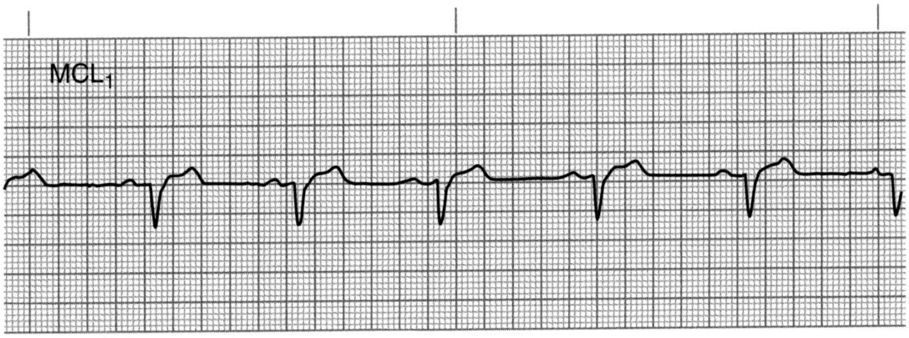
MCL$_1$

FIGURE 25.16 Sinus bradycardia.

TABLE 25.2 MEDICATIONS USED TO TREAT DYSRHYTHMIAS

Medication Class/ Action	Examples	Route	Side Effects	Nursing Implications
Anticoagulant Increases clotting time. Reduces risk of blood clots in atrial fibrillation.	warfarin (Coumadin)	Oral	Hemorrhage (increased with NSAIDs)	Monitor INR/PT regularly. Monitor for bruising. Acetaminophen (Tylenol) used instead of aspirin during therapy. Antidote: vitamin K.
Antidysrhythmics Inhibit ventricular dysrhythmias, atrial fibrillation, atrial flutter.	amiodarone (Cordarone, Pacerone)	Oral, IV	Bradycardia. *Significant toxicity:* pulmonary, dysthyroidism, slate blue skin discoloration, corneal deposits.	Contraindicated in AV block or pregnancy. Obtain baseline vital signs and ECG. Monitor for toxicity. Avoid grapefruit juice with oral form.

Continued

TABLE 25.2 MEDICATIONS USED TO TREAT DYSRHYTHMIAS—cont'd

Medication Class/ Action	Examples	Route	Side Effects	Nursing Implications
Inhibits atrial fibrillation, atrial flutter.	dronedarone (Multaq)	Oral	Creatinine elevation, diarrhea, nausea/ vomiting, rash, bradycardia, QT prolongation	Newer drug that has less toxicity than amiodarone. Contraindicated in heart failure.
Anticholinergic				
Increases heart rate. Treats symptomatic bradycardia, asystole.	atropine	IV	Dysrhythmia, hypotension, palpitation, tachycardia	Contraindicated in angle closure glaucoma.
Beta Blockers				
Decrease myocardial contractility. Controls rate in sinus tachycardia, PAC, atrial flutter, atrial fibrillation, PVC.	atenolol (Tenormin) metoprolol succinate (Lopressor, Toprol XL)	Oral Oral, IV	Dizziness, hypotension, bradycardia, heart blocks Contraindicated in bradycardia, heart block.	Check apical pulse and BP prior to giving. If pulse less than 60 bpm, BP less than 100 mm Hg systolic, notify physician. Instruct patient to rise slowly and not stop drug abruptly.
Calcium Channel Blocker				
Decreases myocardial contractility and depresses conduction system. Controls rate in sinus tachycardia, atrial flutter, and atrial fibrillation.	amlodipine (Norvasc)	Oral	Dysrhythmias, dizziness, AV blocks	Assess apical pulse and blood pressure. If BP less than 90 mm Hg systolic or apical rate less than 60 bpm, notify physician. Administer before meals and at bedtime.
Inotrope—Cardiac Glycoside (Positive Inotrope and Negative Chronotrope)				
Slows heart rate. Maintains sinus rhythm for sinus tachycardia, atrial flutter, atrial fibrillation.	Digoxin (Lanoxicaps, Lanoxin)	Oral, IV	Fatigue, nausea, vomiting, anorexia, headache, bradycardia, cardiac arrhythmias	Take apical pulse for 1 minute; if less than 60 bpm, notify physician. Therapeutic digoxin levels: 0.5–2 mg/mL. Monitor drug level and electrolytes (hypokalemia, hypomagnesemia, hypercalcemia increase toxicity).
Vasopressors				
Cardiac stimulation, vasoconstriction, bronchodilation. Treats asystole, ventricular tachycardia, ventricular fibrillation, symptomatic bradycardia.	epinephrine (Adrenalin)	IV, intraosseous	Tachycardia, dysrhythmia, hypertension, pulmonary edema	Contraindicated with nonselective beta blockers.
Vasoconstricts. Reduces urine volume. Single dose may replace dose of epinephrine. Treats pulseless ventricular tachycardia, ventricular fibrillation, asystole.	vasopressin (Pitressin)	IV	Dysrhythmia, asystole, hypertension	Avoid IV site extravasation because of risk of necrosis and gangrene.
Increases cardiac output and blood pressure. Treats bradycardia.	dopamine	IV infusion	Dysrhythmias	Monitor blood pressure.

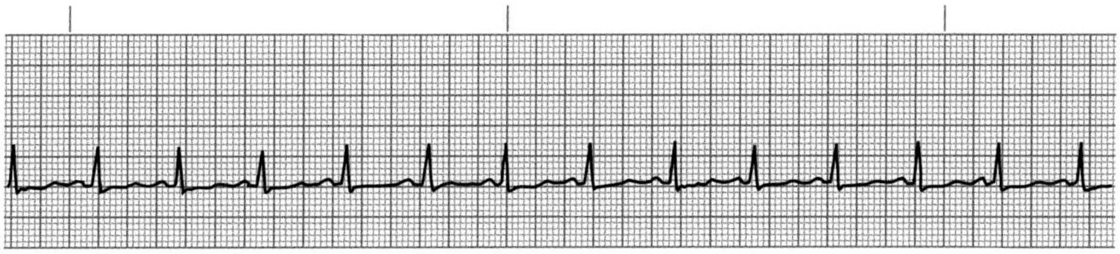

FIGURE 25.17 Sinus tachycardia.

ETIOLOGY. Sinus tachycardia causes include physical activity; hemorrhage; shock; medications such as epinephrine, atropine, or nitrates; dehydration; fever; MI; electrolyte imbalance; fear; and anxiety. Tachycardia occurs as a compensatory mechanism for hypoxia when more cardiac output is needed to deliver oxygen to organs and tissues.

SINUS TACHYCARDIA RULES

1. Rhythm: regular
2. Heart rate: 101 to 180 bpm
3. P waves: rounded, precede each QRS complex, alike
4. PR interval: 0.12 to 0.20 seconds
5. QRS interval: less than or equal to 0.10 seconds.

SIGNS AND SYMPTOMS. Sinus tachycardia may not produce symptoms. If the heart rate is very rapid and sustained for long periods, the patient may experience angina or dyspnea. Older patients may become symptomatic more rapidly than younger patients (Box 25.1, *Gerontological Issues*). Patients with MI may not tolerate a rapid heart rate and have more severe symptoms since cardiac workload is increased.

THERAPEUTIC MEASURES. Treatment depends on the cause and symptoms. Medications such as digoxin, calcium channel blockers, amlodipine (Norvasc), or beta blockers, metoprolol (Lopressor or Toprol), or atenolol (Tenormin) may be used to slow the heart rate (see Table 25.2). The treatment goal is to decrease the heart's workload and resolve the cause, which then usually corrects the tachycardia. For example, if the patient is hemorrhaging, immediate intervention is needed to stop the bleeding and restore normal blood volume. Once normal blood volume is restored, the heart rate should return to normal.

Box 25.1

Gerontological Issues

Dysrhythmia Risk

Factors that increase the risk of dysrhythmias in older adults include the following:

- Digitalis toxicity (most common)
- Hypokalemia
- Acute infection
- Hemorrhage
- Angina
- Coronary insufficiency or cardiomyopathy (exercise, stress)
- Thickness of the heart tissue
- Sleep apnea
- Hypothyroidism or hyperthyroidism.

Dysrhythmias that occur most often in older adults include the following:

- Atrial fibrillation (atria beating 400 to 700 times per minute)
- Sick sinus syndrome (alternating episodes of bradycardia, normal sinus rhythm, tachycardia, and periods of long sinus pause)
- Heart block (delayed or blocked impulses to the atria or ventricles)

Age-related effects of dysrhythmias include the following:

- Weakness
- Fatigue
- Forgetfulness
- Palpitations
- Dizziness
- Hypotension
- Bradycardia
- Syncope
- Dyspnea or shortness of breath
- Delayed capillary refill
- Diaphoresis
- Anxiety and fear
- Nausea and vomiting
- Stroke

Older adults are especially sensitive to changes in heart rate that increase the heart's workload. Whenever the heart works harder, as in tachycardia, the cardiac cells require more oxygen to function properly. Older patients have less ability to adapt to sudden changes or stressors, and they may not be able to tolerate tachycardia for very long. Any new-onset tachycardia in an older patient should be reported promptly.

LEARNING TIP

Tachycardia is often the first sign of hemorrhage. It is a compensatory mechanism to maintain cardiac output. If a patient develops sudden tachycardia, consider whether hemorrhage could be the cause, such as in postoperative patients, patients with gastrointestinal bleeding or cancer, or trauma patients. The bleeding may be external, or it may be internal and therefore not visible. Apply pressure to the site if the bleeding is obvious. Monitor the patient and report the tachycardia and any obvious bleeding promptly.

Dysrhythmias Originating in the Atria

As previously discussed, all areas of the heart can initiate an impulse. The SA node is the primary pacemaker, but if the atria initiate impulses faster than the SA node, they become the primary pacemaker. Atrial rhythms are usually faster than 100 bpm and can exceed 200 bpm. When an impulse originates outside the SA node, the P waves produced look different from the rounded P waves from the SA node (flatter, notched, or peaked), which indicates that the SA node is not controlling the heart rate. These atrial impulses travel to the ventricles to initiate a normal QRS complex after each P wave.

LEARNING TIP

- If a QRS complex measures less than or equal to 0.10 seconds and a dysrhythmia is present, the problem originated above the ventricles. This is known as a supraventricular (above the ventricle) dysrhythmia.
- Ventricular originating dysrhythmias produce wide QRS complexes that are greater than 0.10 seconds.

Premature Atrial Contractions

The term *premature* refers to an "early" beat. When the atria fire an impulse before the SA node fires, a premature beat results. If the underlying rhythm is sinus rhythm, the distance between R waves is the same except where the early beat occurs. When looking at the ECG strip, a shortened R-to-R interval is seen where the premature beat occurs. The R wave preceding the premature atrial contraction (PAC) and the PAC's R wave are close together, followed by a pause, with the next beat being regular (Fig. 25.18).

ETIOLOGY. Causes of PACs include hypoxia, cigarette smoking, stress, myocardial ischemia, enlarged atria in valvular disorders, medications (such as digoxin), electrolyte imbalances, atrial fibrillation onset, and heart failure.

PREMATURE ATRIAL CONTRACTIONS RULES

1. Rhythm: premature beat interrupts underlying rhythm where it occurs
2. Heart rate: depends on the underlying rhythm; if normal sinus rhythm (NSR), 60 to 100 bpm
3. P waves: early beat is abnormally shaped
4. PR interval: usually appears normal, but premature beat could have shortened or prolonged PR interval
5. QRS interval: less than or equal to 0.10 seconds (indicates normal conduction to ventricles).

SIGNS AND SYMPTOMS. Premature atrial contractions can occur in healthy individuals, as well as in the patient with a diseased heart. No symptoms are usually present. If many PACs occur in succession, the patient may report the sensation of palpitations.

THERAPEUTIC MEASURES. PACs are usually not dangerous, and often no treatment is required other than correcting the cause. Frequent PACs indicate atrial irritability, which may worsen into other atrial dysrhythmias. Beta blockers, metoprolol (Lopressor or Toprol) or atenolol (Tenormin) can be given to a patient having frequent PACs to slow the heart rate (see Table 25.2).

Atrial Flutter

In atrial flutter, the atria contract, or flutter, at a rate of 250 to 350 bpm. The very rapid P waves appear as flutter, or F waves, on ECG and appear in a saw-toothed pattern. Some of the impulses get through the AV node and reach the ventricles, resulting in normal QRS complexes. There can be from two to four F waves between QRS complexes. If impulses pass through the AV node at a consistent rate, the rhythm is regular (Fig. 25.19). The classic characteristics of atrial flutter are more than one P wave before a QRS complex, a saw-toothed pattern of P waves, and an atrial rate of 250 to 350 bpm.

ETIOLOGY. Causes of atrial flutter include rheumatic or ischemic heart diseases, congestive heart failure (CHF),

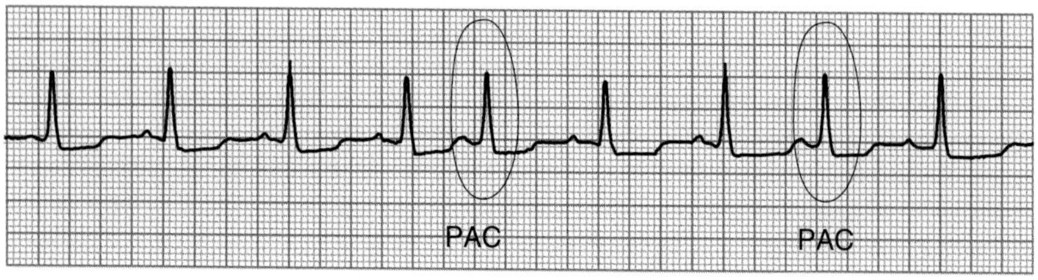
PAC
PAC

FIGURE 25.18 Premature atrial contractions (PACs).

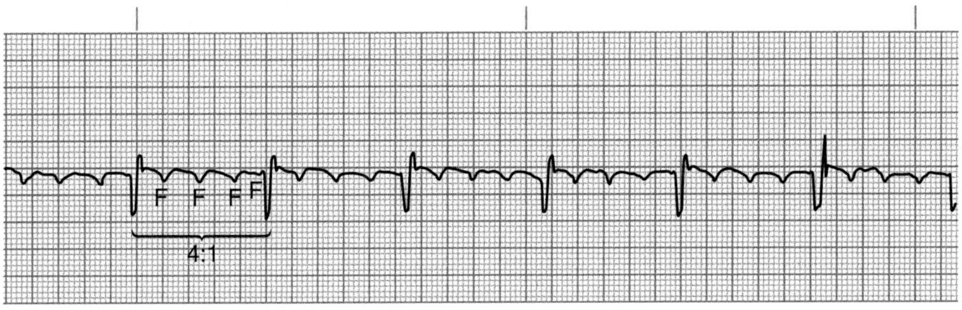
F F F F
4:1

FIGURE 25.19 Atrial flutter.

hypertension, pericarditis, pulmonary embolism, and post-operative coronary artery bypass surgery. Many medications can also cause this dysrhythmia.

ATRIAL FLUTTER RULES

1. Rhythm: atrial rhythm regular; ventricular rhythm regular or irregular depending on consistency of AV conduction of impulses
2. Heart rate: ventricular rate varies
3. P waves: flutter or F waves with saw-toothed pattern
4. PR interval: none measurable
5. QRS interval: less than or equal to 0.10 seconds.

SIGNS AND SYMPTOMS. The presence of symptoms in atrial flutter depends on the ventricular rate. If the ventricular rate is normal, usually no symptoms are present. If the rate is rapid, the patient may experience palpitations, angina, or dyspnea.

THERAPEUTIC MEASURES. The ventricular rate and cardiac output guide treatment. The goal is to control the ventricular rate with conversion to a normal sinus rhythm. For an unstable patient with a rapid ventricular rate, synchronized **cardioversion** (electrical shock) is used. Rapid atrial pacing may also stop the atrial flutter. Medications can be used to control the ventricular rate such as calcium channel blockers (see Table 25.2). Antiarrhythmic medications are used to convert atrial flutter. To terminate the atrial flutter in symptomatic patients, a radiofrequency catheter ablation (usually in the right atrium) may be done.

Atrial Fibrillation

In atrial fibrillation, the atrial rate is extremely rapid and chaotic. An atrial rate of 350 to 600 bpm can occur. However, the AV node blocks most of the impulses, so the ventricular rate is much lower than the atrial rate. There are no definable P waves because the atria are fibrillating, or quivering, rather than beating effectively. No P waves can be seen or measured. A wavy pattern is produced on the ECG. Because the atrial rate is so irregular and only a few of the atrial impulses are allowed to pass through the AV node, the R waves are irregular. The ventricular rate varies from normal to rapid.

Atrial fibrillation can be self-limiting, persistent, or permanent and doubles the risk of death. Stroke risk is increased due to thrombus formation in the atria from blood stasis caused by poor emptying of blood from the quivering atria (Fig. 25.20).

ETIOLOGY. A history of cigarette smoking raises the risk of developing atrial fibrillation even after quitting (Heeringa et al., 2008). Other causes of atrial fibrillation include aging (increases after age 60 and is the most common sustained dysrhythmia), rheumatic or ischemic heart diseases, heart failure, hypertension, pericarditis, pulmonary embolism, and postoperative coronary artery bypass surgery. Medications can also cause this dysrhythmia.

ATRIAL FIBRILLATION RULES

1. Rhythm: irregularly irregular
2. Heart rate: atrial rate not measurable; ventricular rate under 100 is controlled response; greater than 100 is rapid ventricular response
3. P waves: no identifiable P waves
4. PR interval: none can be measured because no P waves are seen
5. QRS interval: less than or equal to 0.10 seconds.

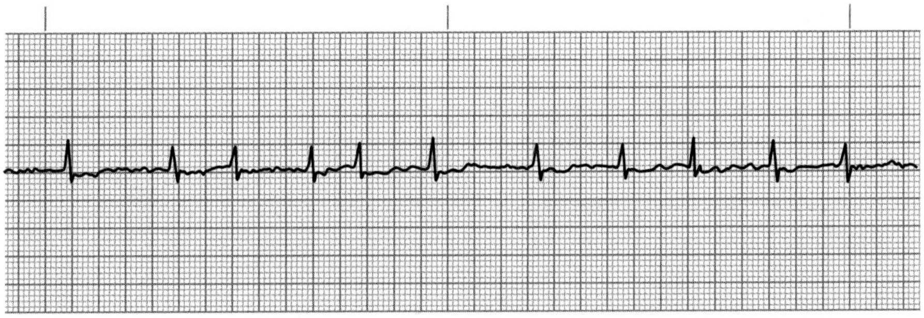

FIGURE 25.20 Atrial fibrillation.

LEARNING TIP

Atrial fibrillation is easy to identify based on its two classic characteristics: a lack of identifiable P waves and an irregularly irregular rhythm (R waves).

SIGNS AND SYMPTOMS. With atrial fibrillation, most patients feel the irregular rhythm. Many describe it as palpitations or a skipping heartbeat. When checking a patient's radial pulse, it may be faint because of a decreased stroke volume (volume of blood ejected with each contraction). If the ventricular rhythm is rapid and sustained, the patient can go into left heart failure.

THERAPEUTIC MEASURES. Treatment is based on the patient's stability. If the patient is unstable, cardioversion is done immediately to try to return the heart to normal sinus rhythm. If the patient is stable, medications to control the ventricular rate such as beta blockers, calcium channel blockers, or digoxin may be used (see Table 25.2). Medications may also be used to restore and maintain a normal sinus rhythm. These include amiodarone or dronedarone (which also control rate) or other rhythm control medications. Anticoagulant therapy (aspirin, warfarin [Coumadin]), which can be long term or lifelong, is given to reduce thrombi. The international normalized ratio (INR) and prothrombin time must be carefully monitored in patients taking warfarin. Chemical or electrical cardioversion may be performed to convert the rhythm after sufficient anticoagulation (about 3 weeks). If known, the underlying cause of the atrial fibrillation should also be treated.

For patients with atrial fibrillation who do not respond to medications or electrical cardioversion, procedures such as **ablation** (pulmonary vein isolation because most atrial fibrillation impulses arise from pulmonary veins) or device therapy may be performed. Surgery can be performed if other treatments fail.

• WORD • BUILDING •
ablation: ab—away from + lat—carry

Catheter Ablation. To isolate impulses coming from the pulmonary veins, catheter ablation may be used to cure atrial fibrillation. Intracardiac echocardiography maps the area of the heart requiring treatment. Then released energy such as radio-frequency waves create lesions on all four pulmonary veins that heal and scar to block pathways for future impulses. Postprocedural care is similar to postangioplasty or postcardiac catheterization care (see Chapter 21).

Device Therapy. Dual-chamber pacing for those with sinus node problems or biatrial pacing, as well as pacemaker recognition of atrial fibrillation, helps to prevent this dysrhythmia. Implantable atrial defibrillators (IADs) can deliver a shock activated by the physician or patient to end the atrial fibrillation and improve symptoms. It does not cure the condition. Because this is a planned event, medications for comfort can be taken by the patient before the shock.

Surgery. The Maze procedure is often done as minimally invasive robotic guided surgery. Incisions are made in the atria that create a "maze," or route, for electrical impulses to travel to the AV node. These impulses cannot go off course because scar tissue surrounds the incision sites. Variations of the Maze procedure include the use of radio-frequency, cryothermy, microwave, and laser energy. The left atrial appendage may be isolated or removed during surgery to prevent a source of blood clot formation and possibly eliminate the need for warfarin.

Future Treatments. Dabigatran (Pradaxa, Pradax) is a new anticoagulant with fewer side effects that could be used instead of warfarin therapy with U.S. Food and Drug Administration approval. Noninvasive x-ray beam ablation may also be used in the future.

Ventricular Dysrhythmias

Premature Ventricular Contractions

Premature ventricular contractions (PVCs) originate in the ventricles from an ectopic focus (a site other than the SA node). The ventricles are irritable and fire prematurely, before the SA node. When the ventricles fire first, the impulses are not conducted normally through the electrical pathway. This results in a wide (greater than 0.10 seconds), bizarre QRS complex on an ECG (Fig. 25.21).

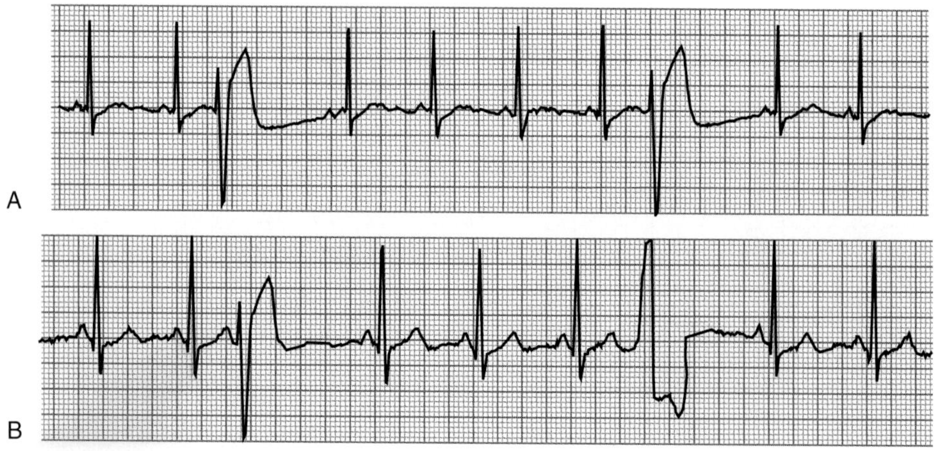
A
B

FIGURE 25.21 Premature ventricular contractions. (A) Unifocal PVCs arise from one area and look the same. (B) Multifocal PVCs arise from different foci and may look different.

PVCs can occur in different shapes. The shape of the PVC is referred to as unifocal (one focus) if all the PVCs look the same because they come from the same irritable ventricular area. **Multifocal** PVCs do not all look the same because they are originating from several irritable areas in the ventricle. There can be several repetitive cycles or patterns of PVCs:

- **Bigeminy** is a PVC that occurs every other beat (a normal beat and then a PVC) (Fig. 25.22).
- **Trigeminy** is a PVC that occurs every third beat (two normal beats and then a PVC).
- Quadrigeminy is a PVC that occurs every fourth beat (three normal beats and then a PVC).
- When two PVCs occur together, they are referred to as a couplet (pair).
- If three or more PVCs occur in a row, it is referred to as a run of PVCs or ventricular tachycardia.

ETIOLOGY. Use of caffeine or alcohol, anxiety, hypokalemia, cardiomyopathy, ischemia, and MI are common causes of PVCs.

PREMATURE VENTRICULAR CONTRACTION RULES

1. Rhythm: depends on the underlying rhythm; PVC usually interrupts rhythm
2. Heart rate: depends on underlying rhythm
3. P waves: absent before PVC QRS complex
4. PR interval: none for PVC
5. QRS interval: if PVC, is greater than 0.10 seconds; T wave is in the opposite direction of QRS complex (i.e., QRS upright, T downward; or QRS downward, T upright).

SIGNS AND SYMPTOMS. PVCs may be felt by the patient and are described as a skipped beat or palpitations. With frequent PVCs, cardiac output can be decreased, leading to fatigue, dizziness, or more severe dysrhythmias.

THERAPEUTIC MEASURES. Treatment depends on the type and number of PVCs and whether symptoms are produced. A few PVCs do not usually require treatment. However, if the PVCs are more than six per minute, regularly occurring, multifocal, falling on the T wave (known as "R-on-T phenomenon," which can trigger life-threatening dysrhythmias), or caused by an acute MI, they can be dangerous. Antidysrhythmic drugs that depress myocardial activity are used to treat PVCs such as amiodarone and beta blockers (see Table 25.2).

Ventricular Tachycardia

The occurrence of three or more PVCs in a row is referred to as **ventricular tachycardia** (VT) (Fig. 25.23). VT results from the continuous firing of an ectopic ventricular focus. During VT, the ventricles rather than the SA node become the pacemaker of the heart. The pathway of the ventricular impulses is different from normal conduction, producing a wide (greater than 0.10 seconds), bizarre QRS complex.

ETIOLOGY. Myocardial irritability, MI, and cardiomyopathy are common causes of VT. Respiratory acidosis, hypokalemia, digoxin toxicity, cardiac catheters, and pacing wires can also produce VT.

VENTRICULAR TACHYCARDIA RULES

1. Rhythm: usually regular, may have some irregularity
2. Heart rate: 150 to 250 ventricular bpm; slow VT is below 150 bpm
3. P waves: absent
4. PR interval: none
5. QRS interval: greater than 0.10 seconds.

SIGNS AND SYMPTOMS. The seriousness of ventricular tachycardia is determined by the duration of the dysrhythmia. Sustained VT compromises cardiac output. Patients are aware of a sudden onset of rapid heart rate and can experience

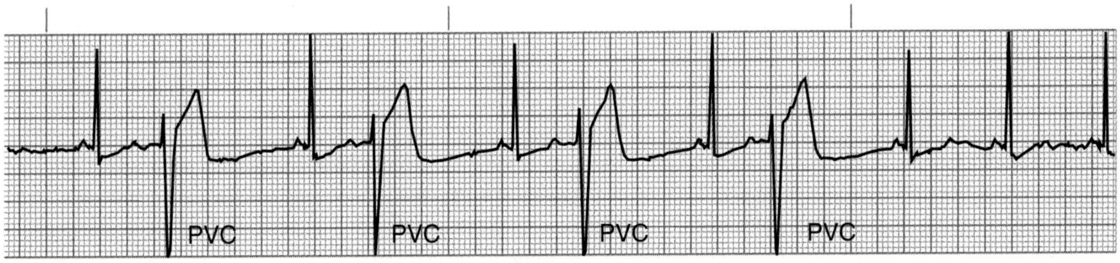
PVC
PVC
PVC
PVC

FIGURE 25.22 Bigeminal premature ventricular contractions.

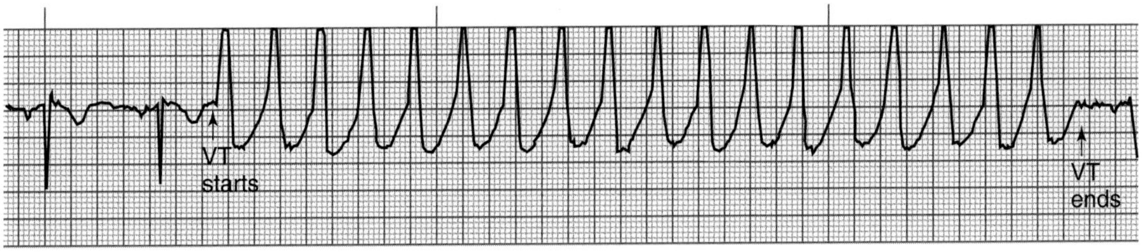
VT
starts
VT
ends

FIGURE 25.23 Ventricular tachycardia.

CRITICAL THINKING

Mrs. Mae

■ Mrs. Mae, age 70, is 5 days post-MI without complications. You assist her back to bed at 1400 hours after she ambulates. Her oxygen is on at 2 L/min via nasal cannula. Her vital signs are BP 126/78 mm Hg, apical pulse 82 bpm, R 18 per minute. She has no pain and says she feels good after walking. The cardiac monitor shows normal sinus rhythm. Five minutes later, you see that the monitor shows sinus rhythm with PVCs of less than six per minute. Her vital signs are now BP 132/84 mm Hg, apical pulse 92 bpm, irregular, and R 22 per minute. She reports no pain but says, "I can feel my heart skipping. It takes my breath away." You call the RN while staying with the patient for reassurance.

1. What should you do first?
2. What should you do regarding the dysrhythmia?
3. What might be some of the causes for this dysrhythmia?
4. What symptoms, if any, would you expect to be present?
5. What would you do if symptoms were present?
6. What type of orders would you anticipate from the physician?
7. How would you document your findings?

Suggested answers at end of chapter.

dyspnea, palpitations, and light-headedness. Angina commonly occurs. The severity of symptoms can increase rapidly if the left ventricle fails and complete cardiac arrest results.

THERAPEUTIC MEASURES. If the patient is pulseless or not breathing, cardiopulmonary resuscitation (CPR) and immediate defibrillation are required. Current advanced cardiac life support (ACLS) protocols for pulseless VT treatment should be followed (see www.circulationaha.org or http://circ.ahajournals.org/content/vol112/24_suppl). Medications may include epinephrine, vasopressin, and amiodarone (see Table 25.2).

If the patient is stable, medications may be tried first, such as amiodarone following ACLS protocols. Magnesium can be used to help stabilize ventricular muscle excitability if the patient's magnesium level is low.

CRITICAL THINKING

Mrs. Parker

■ You are caring for Mrs. Parker, age 66, on the cardiac medical unit. She had an MI and several episodes of ventricular tachycardia while she was in the ICU before transferring to your unit. At 1600 hours you find her unresponsive, with no palpable pulses and shallow respirations and in VT on the ECG. Vital signs are BP 80/40 mm Hg, P 150 bpm, R 6 per minute.

1. Why are there no palpable pulses?
2. What is occurring to the heart when it is in VT?
3. What action should you take?
4. How will you document your findings?

Suggested answers at end of chapter.

Ventricular Fibrillation

Ventricular fibrillation occurs when many ectopic ventricular foci fire at the same time. Ventricular activity is chaotic with no discernible waves (Fig. 25.24). The ventricle quivers and is unable to initiate a contraction. There is a complete loss of cardiac output. If this rhythm is not terminated immediately, death ensues.

ETIOLOGY. Hyperkalemia (elevated serum potassium), **hypomagnesemia** (low serum magnesium), electrocution, coronary artery disease, and MI are all possible causes of ventricular fibrillation. Placement of intracardiac catheters and cardiac pacing wires can also lead to ventricular irritability and then ventricular fibrillation.

VENTRICULAR FIBRILLATION RULES

1. Rhythm: chaotic and extremely irregular
2. Heart rate: not measurable
3. P waves: none
4. PR interval: none
5. QRS complex: none.

• WORD • BUILDING •

hyperkalemia: hyper—above + kalium—potassium + emia—blood

hypomagnesemia: hypo—below + magnes—magnesium + emia—blood

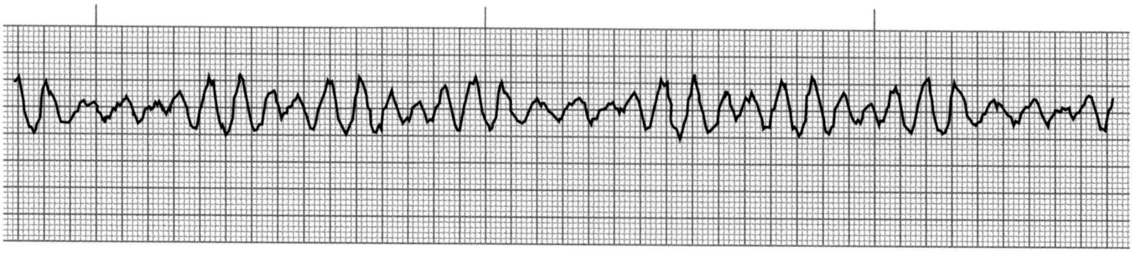

FIGURE 25.24 Ventricular fibrillation.

SIGNS AND SYMPTOMS. Patients experiencing ventricular fibrillation lose consciousness immediately. There are no heart sounds, peripheral pulses, or blood pressure. These are all indicative of circulatory collapse. Additionally, respiratory arrest, cyanosis, and pupil dilation occur.

THERAPEUTIC MEASURES. Immediate defibrillation is the best treatment for terminating ventricular fibrillation. Each minute that passes without defibrillation reduces survival. CPR is started until the defibrillator is available. Automatic external defibrillators (AEDs) provide quick access to easily used technology for defibrillation (see the later *Defibrillation* section). Endotracheal intubation and ventilation may support respiratory function. Medications are given according to ACLS protocols and may include epinephrine, vasopressin, amiodarone, and magnesium (see Table 25.2).

Asystole

Asystole (the silent heart) is the absence of electrical activity in the cardiac muscle. It is referred to as cardiac arrest. A straight line appears on an ECG strip (Fig. 25.25). Ventricular fibrillation usually precedes this rhythm and must be reversed immediately to help prevent asystole.

ETIOLOGY. Ventricular fibrillation and a loss of a majority of functional cardiac muscle due to an MI are common causes of asystole. Hyperkalemia is another cause of asystole.

ASYSTOLE RULES

1. Rhythm: none
2. Heart rate: none
3. P waves: none
4. PR interval: none
5. QRS interval: none.

SIGNS AND SYMPTOMS. Patients in asystole are unconscious and unresponsive. There are no heart sounds, peripheral pulses, blood pressure, or respirations.

THERAPEUTIC MEASURES. ACLS protocols for asystole are used. CPR is started immediately. Endotracheal intubation to support respirations is performed. Epinephrine, vasopressin, or atropine may be administered (see Table 25.2).

CARDIAC PACEMAKERS

Pacemakers can be temporary (epicardial, transcutaneous, transvenous) or permanent (Fig. 25.26). They are used to generate an impulse when the heart is beating too slowly or to override dysrhythmias.

CRITICAL THINKING

Mr. Peet

■ You are making rounds. When you enter Mr. Peet's room, you note that he is having difficulty breathing and is unresponsive.

1. What are your initial actions?
2. What should you do after assessing and finding no pulse or respirations?
3. What is your responsibility during a cardiac/respiratory arrest code?

Suggested answers at end of chapter.

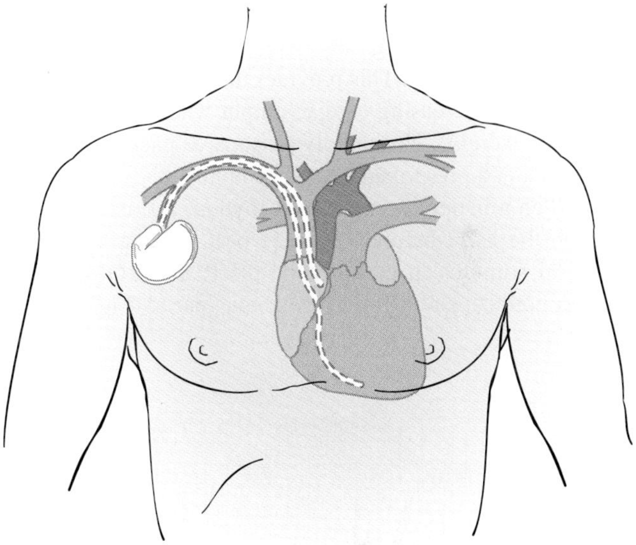

FIGURE 25.26 Dual-chamber permanent pacemaker.

Temporary pacemakers are used for bradycardias or tachycardias that do not respond to medications or cardioversion. They may also be used after an MI to allow the heart time to heal when the diseased myocardium is unable to respond to or is not receiving electrical conduction because of damage within the system. The temporary pacemaker becomes the electrical conduction system and stimulates the atria and ventricles to contract to maintain cardiac output. Temporary pacemakers can be inserted during valve or open heart surgery (epicardial) or in the cardiac catheterization

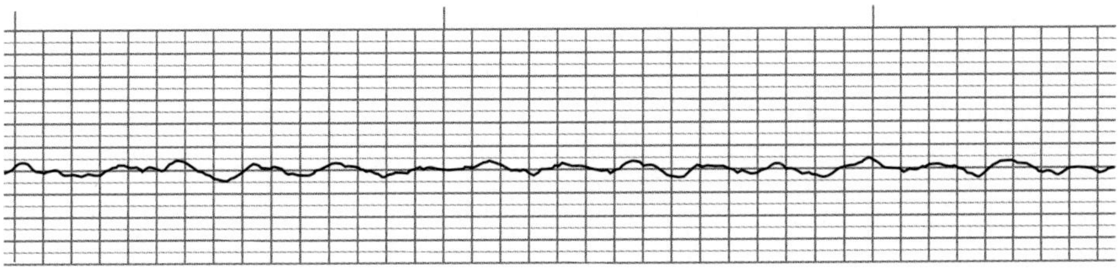

FIGURE 25.25 Asystole.

laboratory or critical care unit at the bedside (transvenous) as emergency treatment until surgery can be scheduled to insert a permanent pacemaker. Transcutaneous pacemakers are used in emergency situations because they are quick and easy to apply. Impulses are delivered to the heart through the skin from the external generator via electrodes that are attached to the chest and back.

Permanent pacemaker insertion is a surgical procedure in which **fluoroscopy**, a screen that shows an image similar to a radiograph, is used. The pacemaker generator is implanted subcutaneously and attached to leads (insulated conducting wires) that are inserted via a vein into the heart. The lead can then deliver the impulse directly to the heart wall. A single-lead pacemaker paces either the right atrium or right ventricle depending on its chamber placement. Dual-chamber pacemakers have two leads, with one in the right atrium and the other in the right ventricle. This allows pacing of both chambers. Activity-responsive pacemakers provide a rate range (e.g., 60 to 115 bpm) in response to a person's activity level. This provides the patient with greater flexibility for increasing cardiac output when needed, such as during exercise. Nonactivity responsive pacemakers are usually set at a prescribed rate of 72 bpm.

When a patient is in a paced rhythm, a small spike is seen on the ECG before the paced beat. This spike is the electrical stimulus. It can precede the P wave, QRS complex, or both depending on what is being paced (Fig. 25.27). Patients may have all paced beats (100% paced), a mixture of their own beats and paced beats, or all of their own beats. Pacemakers should not fire when patients have their own beats.

Problems that can occur with pacemakers include the following:

- Failure to sense the patient's own beat
- Failure to pace because of a malfunction of the pulse generator
- Failure to capture, which is a lack of depolarization.

Nursing Care for Patients with Pacemakers

Patients are placed on a cardiac monitor and rest for several hours after insertion of a pacemaker. The patient's apical pulse is monitored frequently to detect changes in the heart rhythm. Irregular heart rhythms or a rate slower than the pacemaker's set rate can indicate pacemaker malfunction. The dressing at the pacemaker insertion site is monitored every 2 to 4 hours for signs of bleeding. Any change in heart rhythm, reports of chest pain, or changes in vital signs must be reported immediately. Patients may have a sling on the operative side arm for 24 to 48 hours to help prevent dislodgement of the pacemaker lead from the cardiac wall. The patient may remain in the hospital for a short stay.

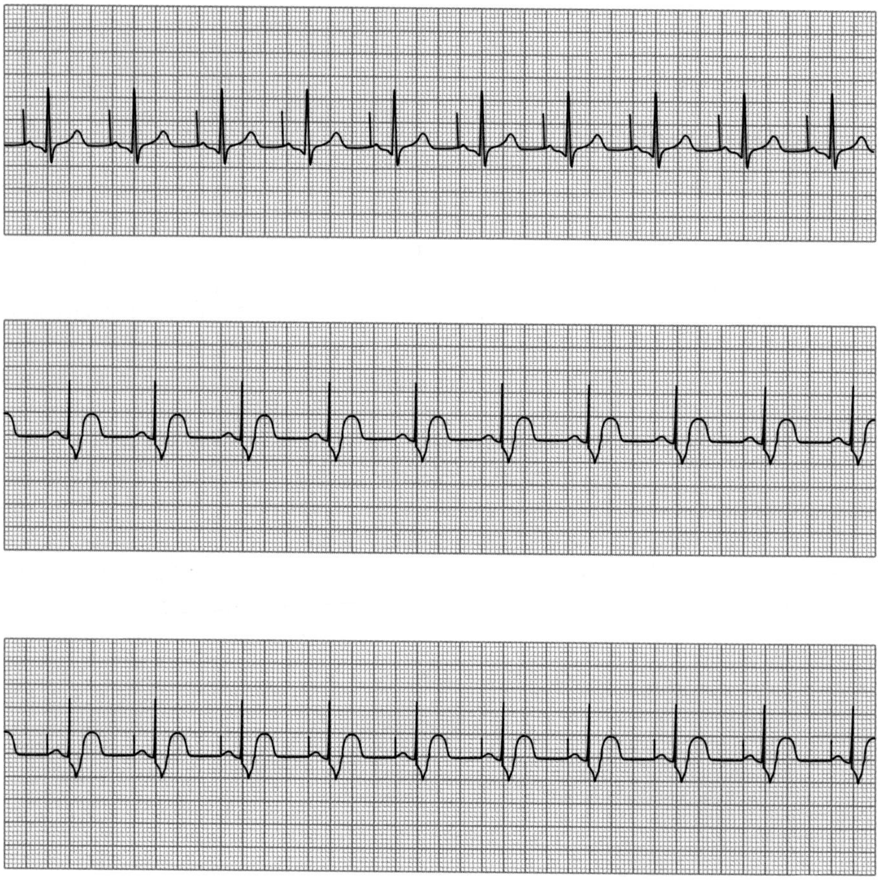

A

B

C

FIGURE 25.27 ECG tracings: (A) Atrial-only pacemaker (spike before P wave). (B) Ventricular-only pacemaker (spike before QRS). (C) AV sequential pacemaker that paces both atrial and ventricular chambers (spike before P and QRS).

Patients are educated about pacemaker care before discharge (see *Evidence-Based Practice* box). Teaching includes the following:

EVIDENCE-BASED PRACTICE

Clinical Question

What are the effects of a self-care program on the health-related quality of life (HRQL) of pacemaker patients?

Evidence

In a randomized study of 212 patients with pacemakers, those in the self-care program group had significantly better HRQL for experience of symptoms that decreased or disappeared after causing the need for a pacemaker (Malm, Karlsson, & Fridlund, 2007).

Implications for Nursing Practice

In the acute phase in the hospital, it is important to actively include pacemaker patients in a self-care program based on the nurse's assessment of the patient's learning needs.

REFERENCE

Malm, D., Karlsson, J., & Fridlund, B. (2007). Effects of a self-care program on the health-related quality of life of pacemaker patients: A nursing intervention study. *Canadian Journal of Cardiovascular Nursing, 17*(1), 15–26.

- Incision care. The patient should check the incision daily and report evidence of inflammation or infection (redness, swelling, warmth, tenderness, pain, fever, or discharge) to a physician. A hard ridge may form over the incision that will disappear with healing.
- Methods for taking a radial pulse. The patient should call a physician if the pulse is slower than the pacemaker's set rate.
- The patient should report symptoms of dizziness, fainting, irregular heartbeats, or palpitations.
- The patient should understand the importance of wearing medical alert jewelry and carrying a pacemaker information card.
- The patient should avoid radiation, magnetic fields (e.g., magnetic resonance imaging [MRI], industrial magnets), high voltage (e.g., power plant, arc welding, high-tension wires), antitheft devices, and large running motors (e.g., distributor coil of running engine).
- The patient will need to tell airport security about the pacemaker, because it may trigger metal detectors (they do not harm the pacemaker).
- Grounded appliances (usually includes microwave ovens) and office equipment are safe to use.
- The patient must avoid lifting more than 10 pounds, making major arm movements, or participating in contact sports for 6 weeks after surgery. Normal activity is usually resumed after 6 weeks.
- The patient must keep scheduled appointments with the physician. Periodic pacemaker checks will be done by the physician or over the telephone. Reprogramming of the pacemaker can be done by the physician if needed.

CRITICAL THINKING

Mr. Treacher

■ Mr. Treacher, age 58, underwent pacemaker placement 6 days ago and is being transferred to the medical floor. After transfer, his vital signs are BP 138/72 mm Hg, apical pulse 72 bpm, and 100% paced rhythm. Thirty minutes later, he says that he feels weak and tired. His vital signs are now BP 100/60 mm Hg, apical pulse 60 bpm, and irregular.

1. What is your first action?
2. What actions should be taken next?
3. What might be happening to Mr. Treacher?
4. What interventions should you anticipate next?

Suggested answers at end of chapter.

DEFIBRILLATION

Defibrillation is a lifesaving procedure used for pulseless ventricular tachycardia or ventricular fibrillation. It delivers an electrical shock to reset the heart's rhythm. Self-adhesive pads, conductive jelly, or saline pads are placed on the patient's chest to prevent electrical burns and promote conduction of the electrical charge. After the defibrillator is charged, the paddles are pressed firmly and evenly against the chest wall to prevent burns or electrical arcing (Fig. 25.28).

For safety, the person defibrillating must announce "Clear." The phrase "One. I'm clear. Two. You're clear. Three. All clear" is suggested. No one, including the person defibrillating, should touch the bed or patient during this time to avoid also being shocked. ACLS protocols specify guidelines for resuscitation.

After successful defibrillation, the patient is assessed for a pulse and adequate tissue perfusion. Vital signs, peripheral pulses, and level of consciousness should be noted. The patient is treated in the critical care unit after successful resuscitation.

Emotional support for an alert patient having experienced cardiac arrest and defibrillation is a very important

• WORD • BUILDING •

defibrillation: de—from + fibrillation—quivering fibers

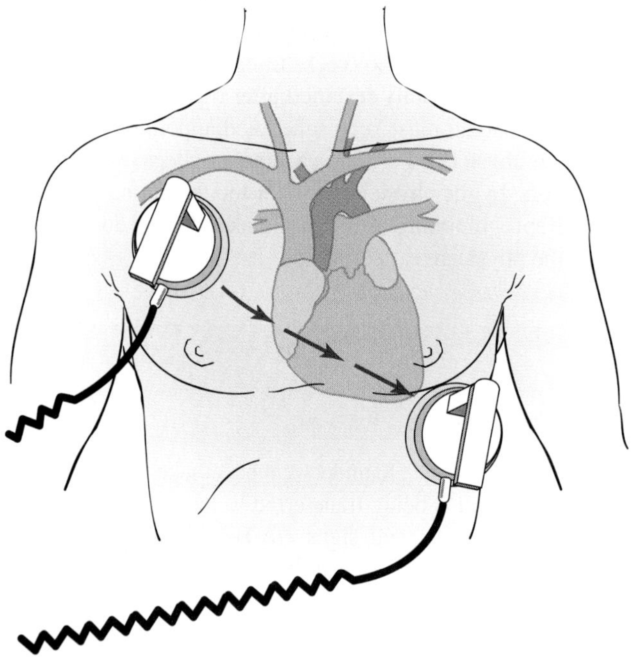

FIGURE 25.28 Placement of defibrillator paddles on chest.

aspect of nursing care. This can be an extremely frightening event for the patient. It is important to explain what happened to the patient and to listen and allow the patient to express any concerns. The patient is reassured that continuous monitoring is done in the critical care unit. Families also require emotional support during resuscitation of a loved one.

CARDIOVERSION

Cardioversion is performed with a defibrillator set in the synchronized mode. When the defibrillator is in the synchronized mode, it marks a highlighted area on the patient's R waves, which must be recognized to deliver a shock. When the discharge trigger is pressed, the shock is released when the machine senses it is safe to do so. The number of joules delivered with each shock usually ranges from 25 to 50. The procedure for delivering the shock is the same as for defibrillation.

Synchronized cardioversion is used for ventricular tachycardia with a pulse. Elective synchronized cardioversion is used for dysrhythmias such as atrial fibrillation, atrial flutter, and supraventricular tachycardia that are not responsive to drug therapy. The patient is given a sedative and monitored by anesthesia personnel during the procedure.

If cardioversion is successful, there should be a return to normal sinus rhythm. If the rhythm does not immediately convert, more cardioversion attempts can be made as determined by the physician. After the procedure, the patient is monitored for skin burns, rhythm disturbances, vital sign changes, respiratory problems, hypotension, and changes in the ST segment.

OTHER METHODS TO CORRECT DYSRHYTHMIAS

Automatic External Defibrillators

An AED is an external device that automatically analyzes rhythms and either automatically delivers or prompts operators to deliver an electrical shock if a shockable rhythm (ventricular fibrillation or VT) is detected (Fig. 25.29). Minimally trained laypersons or hospital and rescue personnel can use these devices with little risk of injury to the patient because the AED analyzes the rhythm rather than the operator. The patient is connected to the AED with adhesive sternal-apex pads attached to cables coming from the device. This connection allows hands-free defibrillation.

AEDs are found in public places such as shopping malls, airports, stadiums, casinos, golf courses, and airplanes for immediate access because defibrillation attempts must occur within minutes of cardiac arrest to increase chance of survival. AEDs are available for home use. They are recommended for people at high risk of sudden cardiac arrest, and for those at risk with rescue access that will take longer than 4 minutes such as those in rural areas, gated communities, or secured access buildings.

Implantable Cardioverter Defibrillator

An implantable cardioverter defibrillator (ICD) or a combination pacemaker/ICD is surgically placed during a minor procedure into the chest of a patient who experiences life-threatening dysrhythmias or is at risk for sudden cardiac death (Fig. 25.30). ICDs have decreased the number of deaths from these dysrhythmias by analyzing and treating these heart rhythms. When an abnormal rhythm is detected that could cause death (ventricular fibrillation), it automatically delivers an electrical shock. If the dysrhythmia does not convert on the initial shock, more shocks are delivered sequentially.

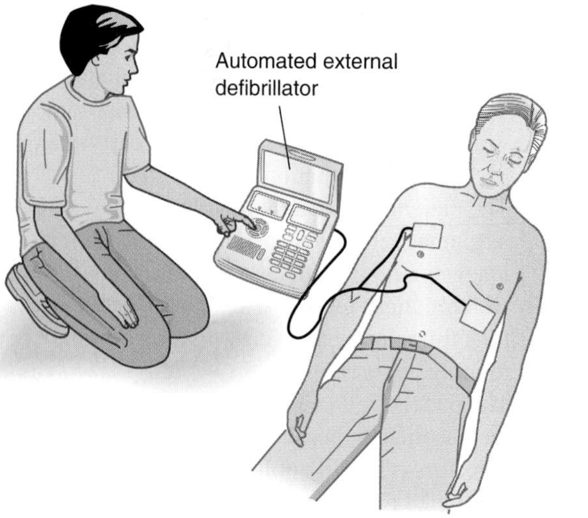
Automated external
defibrillator

FIGURE 25.29 Automatic external defibrillator.

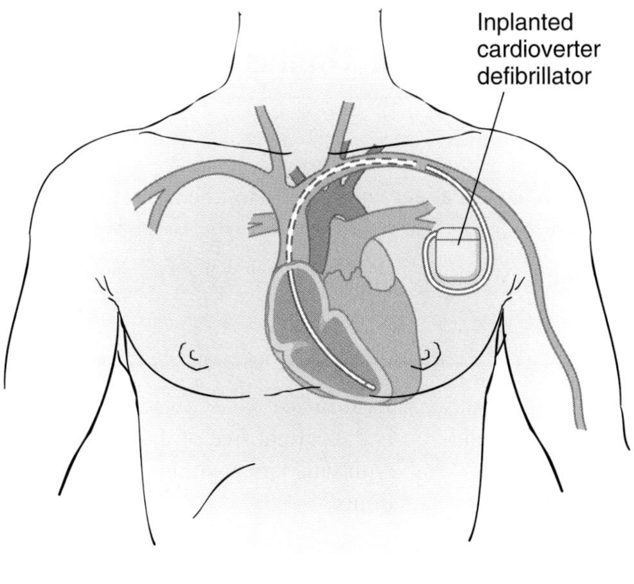
Inplanted
cardioverter
defibrillator

FIGURE 25.30 An implanted cardioverter defibrillator in place.

If the device detects VT, it cardioverts the rhythm using lower energy. ICDs also have antitachycardia pacing ability if a tachycardic rhythm is detected. Battery life depends on usage. A physician can tell when the battery is getting low and that the entire unit needs to be changed within a few months.

Patients with ICDs are extremely anxious about having another cardiac arrest and receiving shocks from the ICD. Defibrillator or cardioversion shocks may feel like a kick in the chest. Reinforcement of patient and family education is very important in preparing the patient for discharge. Those with ICDs should take precautions to prevent problems with the ICD by taking the following precautions:

- Avoid MRIs.
- Avoid metal detectors and standing near security gates or store entrances.
- Avoid equipment with strong electrical or magnetic fields (e.g., amusement rides, slot machines, remote-control toys, stereo speakers).
- Keep cell phones 6 inches from the ICD.

The nurse provides emotional support, answers all questions, and ensures that any misunderstood information is corrected before discharge.

NURSING PROCESS FOR THE PATIENT WITH DYSRHYTHMIAS

Data Collection

Monitoring the cardiac system, respiratory rate, breath sounds, and urinary output is important. Obtaining apical and radial pulses at frequent intervals helps detect dysrhythmias. Most dysrhythmias are not life threatening. Patients at risk for dysrhythmias require careful monitoring so that any dysrhythmias are detected and treated. A patient's report of dizziness, chest pain, or palpitations should always be reported to the physician.

Nursing Diagnoses, Planning, Implementation, and Evaluation

See the *Nursing Care Plan for the Patient with Dysrhythmias.*

To implement the plan of care, the patient and family should be included. Assist them in understanding the plan and the reasons for the prescribed interventions and allow them to express their needs and fears.

Family members should be taught CPR or given information on local CPR classes. This training gives the patient and family a sense of control and hope. In the event the patient requires CPR, the family can take action instead of simply standing by and feeling helpless. The patient will feel more secure in knowing that immediate help from family members is available at home until medical help arrives.

Home Health Hints

- A cell phone affords a home health nurse safety, convenience, and efficiency, especially if emergency help is needed, because some patients do not have phones.
- The nurse should have a pocket mask for CPR available at all times.
- Patients on beta blockers need to know how to take their pulse, because bradycardia is a major side effect. For pulse below 50 bpm, call the nurse or physician.
- Patients prone to dysrhythmias should avoid straining with bowel movements. If the patient reports straining, request a laxative or stool softener order from the physician.
- Advise patients who are leaving home for the weekend or holidays to refill medicines ahead of time. Also, the physician may write a prescription for patients to keep in their wallet for emergencies.
- Patients who come home with a pacemaker should be instructed to wear loose tops. Women should not wear tight bras.
- Symptoms of infection to watch for after a pacemaker is implanted are redness, swelling, warmth, and pain at the site.
- Instruct patients with a pacemaker to take their pulse once a day, in the morning, for a full minute. Assist them in setting up a log to record date, time, and pulse reading. Instruct them to call if the pulse varies outside parameters set by the physician.

NURSING CARE PLAN for the Patient with Dysrhythmias

Nursing Diagnosis: *Decreased Cardiac Output* related to dysrhythmias

Expected Outcomes: The patient's cardiac status will be stabilized. Patient will be able to tolerate activities of daily living (ADL).

Evaluation of Outcomes: There is an absence of dysrhythmias. Patient is able to perform ADLs without tachycardia, chest pain, or weakness.

Interventions	Rationale	Evaluation
Take apical and radial pulses every 2 to 4 hours.	Monitors for dysrhythmias, impending cardiac arrest, or shock.	Is the patient free of dysrhythmias with vital signs within normal limits?
Monitor blood pressure and urinary output.	Blood pressure, pulse, and urinary output are indicators of cardiac output.	
Monitor mental status every 2 to 4 hours.	Dizziness, confusion, and restlessness may indicate decreased cerebral blood flow.	Does patient show signs of decreased cerebral perfusion, such as confusion?
Listen to lung sounds every 2 to 4 hours.	Dysrhythmias can cause heart failure.	Are lungs clear with no report of dyspnea?
Administer O_2 as ordered.	Increases oxygenation to the heart and brain.	Is patient free of chest pain, confusion, and light-headedness?
Ensure that patient gets adequate rest and does not exceed activity tolerance.	Reduces dyspnea and decreases O_2 demand on the myocardium.	Does patient rest and tolerate activity without dyspnea or chest pain?
GERIATRIC		
Administer medications as ordered and observe for adverse reactions.	Older patients may have decreased renal and liver function that may lead to rapid development of toxicity.	Does patient have signs of toxicity?

Nursing Diagnosis: *Anxiety* related to situational crisis

Expected Outcomes: The patient will be able to effectively manage anxiety. Patient will report decreased anxiety.

Evaluation of Outcomes: Patient uses effective coping mechanisms to manage anxiety. Patient expresses decreased anxiety.

Interventions	Rationale	Evaluation
Ask about level of anxiety.	Establishes a baseline.	What is patient's level of anxiety?
Encourage patient and family to verbalize fears.	Helps correct and clarify their concerns.	What are patient's feelings or fears?
Explain procedures to patient and family.	Lack of knowledge increases anxiety. This knowledge will help with compliance of therapy.	Does patient express understanding of therapy with decreased anxiety?
Identify and reduce as many environmental stressors as possible.	Anxiety often results from lack of trust in the environment.	Can patient describe two situations that increase tension?

NURSING CARE PLAN for the Patient with Dysrhythmias—cont'd

Interventions	Rationale	Evaluation
Teach patient relaxation techniques to be performed every 4 to 6 hours, such as guided imagery, muscle relaxation, and meditation.	These measures can restore psychological and physical equilibrium and help decrease anxiety.	Is patient successful in demonstrating relaxation methods?
Medicate with antianxiety agents as ordered.	Aids the patient in decreasing anxiety.	Does patient show decreased anxiety?

SUGGESTED ANSWERS TO CRITICAL THINKING

■ *Mrs. Mae*

1. Assess the patient's vital signs and heart sounds; note symptoms; obtain an ECG per agency protocol.
2. Report the patient findings to the RN or physician.
3. Possible causes include hypokalemia or ischemia leading to irritability of the heart.
4. Symptoms might include light-headedness, feeling of heart skipping, chest pain, or fatigue.
5. To alleviate symptoms, elevate head of bed to comfort, monitor vital signs, and maintain oxygen at 2 L/min via nasal cannula per agency protocol. Remain with the patient to help alleviate anxiety. Notify the RN.
6. Orders might include ECG, oxygen, potassium, or electrolytes.
7. Documentation should include the following:

   1400: Ambulated 20 feet with one assist. Vital signs stable. Stated "Feel good. Pain zero."

   Tolerated well. Assisted to bed. Oxygen at 2 L/min via nasal cannula.

   1405: See ECG strip with intermittent PVCs. Vital signs: BP 132/84 mm Hg; apical 92 bpm, irregular; R 22 per minute.

   "Pain zero. I can feel my heart skipping, it takes my breath away." RN notified.

■ *Mrs. Parker*

1. A heart in VT has an ectopic focus that is initiating impulses. The heart is unable to maintain adequate cardiac output with such a rapid heart rate. The rapid and irregular heart rhythm does not allow the heart chambers time to adequately fill and empty, thereby reducing the blood volume with each beat. This in turn affects the peripheral circulation, causing the absence of palpable pulses.
2. In VT, one or more sites in the ventricle may be initiating impulses. The rapid rate of VT overrides the normal pacemaker of the heart. The rhythm can be regular or irregular. The inability of the heart to conduct impulses along normal pathways prevents the chambers from emptying and filling properly. This leads to a decreased cardiac output and can lead to cardiac arrest if the rhythm is not converted.
3. Call a code and begin CPR. Report findings to code team upon their arrival.
4. Documentation should include the following: 1600: Patient found in bed unresponsive to verbal and tactile stimuli. Respirations shallow. No palpable pulses. BP 80/40 mm Hg, P 150 bpm, R 6 per minute. Monitor shows VT (see strip). Code called from room. CPR started. Code team arrived at 1602. Report given to code team leader.

■ *Mr. Peet*

1. Initially you should assess responsiveness and the presence of a carotid pulse. Check for breathing.
2. Open the airway. Call for assistance or use the patient's phone to report a cardiac arrest. Initiate CPR until help arrives.
3. Once help or the code team arrives, the licensed practical nurse/licensed vocational nurse (LPN/LVN) reports the patient's status. The code team leader delegates responsibilities. Many facilities have protocols for each team member in a code. The LPN/LVN assists in the code as delegated by the RN in charge.

SUGGESTED ANSWERS TO—cont'd

■ *Mr. Treacher*

1. Your first actions should be to obtain an ECG per agency protocol and to notify the RN and physician.
2. You should keep the head of the bed elevated and administer oxygen at 2 L/min via nasal cannula per protocol. Turn the patient onto his side because this may help float the pacemaker wire to the chamber wall for better contact. Monitor the patient's ECG, vital signs, and symptoms, and remain with patient to provide emotional support.
3. Mr. Treacher could be experiencing pacemaker malfunction.
4. Interventions could include transfer to a step-down unit or intensive care unit (ICU), reprogramming of the pacemaker, or a return to surgery for manipulation or replacement of the pacemaker wires.

REVIEW QUESTIONS

1. Place the following in the correct sequence for normal electrical impulse movement through the cardiac conduction system.
   a. AV node
   b. SA node
   c. bundle of His
   d. Purkinje fibers
   e. Internodal tracts
   Sequence: ______________

2. Why is it most important for the nurse to use a systematic method for analyzing heart rhythm tracings?
   a. So abnormalities are not missed.
   b. To save time.
   c. To develop a routine for examining tracings.
   d. To increase memory of the analysis steps.

3. If a patient is in pulseless ventricular tachycardia, which of the following is the first choice of treatment?
   a. Synchronized cardioversion
   b. Pacemaker
   c. Defibrillation
   d. Antiarrhythmic medication

4. Which of the following instructions should the nurse give the patient regarding pacemaker care?
   a. "Avoid microwaves."
   b. "You may have an MRI."
   c. "Take your radial pulse daily."
   d. "You will need to be on bedrest for 48 hours."

5. The nurse is ambulating a patient who is recovering from an MI when the patient develops chest pain with an irregular pulse. What is the safest way to return the patient to bed?
   a. Ambulation to room with one assistant.
   b. With assistance by gurney.
   c. With assistance by a wheelchair.
   d. After completion of ambulation.

6. A patient has a radial pulse of 58 bpm. Which of the following is the appropriate term for documenting this rhythm?
   a. Normal
   b. Asystole
   c. Tachycardia
   d. Bradycardia

7. The nurse is to give a patient amiodarone 800 mg/day PO in two divided doses. The nurse has available 200-mg tablets. How many tablets should the nurse give for each dose? **Fill in the blank.**
   Answer: ________________ tablets

Reference

Heeringa, J., Kors, J. A., Hofman, A., et al. (2008). Cigarette smoking and risk of atrial fibrillation: The Rotterdam study. *American Heart Journal, 156,* 1163–1169.

26 Nursing Care of Patients with Heart Failure

KATHY BERCHEM AND
LINDA S. WILLIAMS

KEY TERMS

afterload (AFF-ter-lohd)
cor pulmonale (KOR PUL-mah-NAH-lee)
cyanosis (SYE-an-NOH-siss)
hepatomegaly (HEP-aa-toh-MEH-gah-lee)
orthopnea (or-THOP-knee-ah)
paroxysmal nocturnal dyspnea (PEAR-ox-IS-mul knock-TURN-al DISP-knee-ah)
peripheral vascular resistance (puh-RIFF-uh-ruhl VAS-kyoo-lar ree-ZIS-tense)
preload (PREE-lohd)
pulmonary edema (PULL-muh-NARE-ee eh-DEE-muh)
splenomegaly (SPLEE-noh-MEG-ah-lee)

QUESTIONS TO GUIDE YOUR READING

1. How would you describe the pathophysiology of left- and right-sided heart failure?
2. What is acute heart failure?
3. What are the causes of acute and chronic heart failure?
4. What are the signs and symptoms of acute and chronic heart failure?
5. What nursing care would you provide for diagnostic tests for heart failure?
6. What medical treatments are used for acute and chronic heart failure?
7. What nursing care would you provide for acute and chronic heart failure?
8. What would you include in your teaching plan for patients with heart failure and their families?

HEART FAILURE

Heart failure (HF) is a clinical syndrome that occurs as a result of the inability of the ventricle(s) to fill or pump enough blood to meet the body's oxygen and nutrient needs. It may cause dyspnea, fatigue, and fluid volume overload in the intravascular and interstitial spaces, resulting in reduced quality and length of life. Causes of heart failure are varied and may include coronary artery disease (most often), myocardial infarction, cardiomyopathy, heart valve problems, and hypertension. Any heart problem may potentially lead to heart failure. In the elderly, the most common cause of heart failure is cardiac ischemia. It may develop rapidly (acute), as with cardiogenic shock and pulmonary edema, or over time (chronic) as a result of another disorder, such as hypertension or pulmonary disease.

The incidence of heart failure is growing as the older adult population and patient survival rates increase. According to the American Heart Association (AHA), 5.7 million people have heart failure with more than 670,000 new cases each year. Heart failure is the most common reason for hospital admission in the older adult. The patient may experience many functional limitations and symptoms, and the mortality rate is high. Quality of life is often impaired. Readmission rates to hospitals soon after discharge for heart failure treatment are high and pose a challenge for health care providers. For more information, visit the AHA's website at www.americanheart.org.

Congestive Heart Failure

Congestive heart failure is an older term for heart failure. It is still used interchangeably by some to indicate heart failure in general. The newer term *heart failure* is preferred because volume overload or "congestion" either in the lungs or periphery is not present in everyone with heart failure or at all times (Hunt et al., 2005).

Pathophysiology

The heart is divided into two separate pumping systems, the right side of the heart and the left side of the heart. Proper cardiac functioning requires each ventricle to pump out equal amounts of blood over time. If the amount of blood returned to the heart becomes more than either ventricle can handle, the heart can no longer be an effective pump.

Conditions that cause heart failure may affect one or both of the heart's pumping systems. Therefore, heart failure can be classified as right-sided heart failure, left-sided heart failure, or biventricular heart failure. The left ventricle is typically the one to weaken first because it has the greatest workload pumping against the resistance in the aorta to eject blood. Because the right and left sides of the heart's pumping system work together in a closed system, failure of one side eventually leads to failure of the other side.

LEARNING TIP

To visualize and understand the effects of heart failure, trace the flow of blood backward from each ventricle. Along the backward path from the failing ventricle, congestion develops and produces the signs and symptoms seen in heart failure. If you understand the backward path of congestion, you can identify the signs and symptoms specifically associated with right- or left-sided heart failure.

LEARNING TIP

To understand heart failure, compare it to a dam in a river:

- In a river without a dam, the water flows freely; in the normal circulatory system, blood flows freely.
- In a river with a dam, the water is blocked by the dam and builds up behind it; in heart failure, the failing ventricle acts like a dam in the river, causing blood to back up behind it.
- When too much water builds up behind the dam, the riverbanks are flooded; in heart failure, if too much blood builds up behind the failing ventricle, the lungs (pulmonary edema) or peripheral tissues are flooded (peripheral edema).
- Heart failure can be the result of systolic (contractile) dysfunction, diastolic (relaxation) dysfunction, or a mixed systolic and diastolic dysfunction. Systolic dysfunction is a contractile problem in which the ventricle is unable to generate enough force to pump blood from the ventricle. Diastolic dysfunction is a problem with the ventricle's ability to relax and fill. Mixed systolic and diastolic dysfunction is a combination of the two defects.

Left-Sided Heart Failure

A certain amount of force must be generated by the left ventricle during a contraction to eject blood into the aorta through the aortic valve. This force is referred to as **afterload**. The pressure within the aorta and arteries influences the force needed to open the aortic valve to pump blood into the aorta. This pressure is called **peripheral vascular resistance** (PVR).

Hypertension is one of the major causes of left-sided heart failure because it increases the pressure within arteries. Increased pressure in the aorta makes the left ventricle work harder to pump blood into the aorta. Over time the strain caused by the increased workload causes the left ventricle to weaken and fail. Other conditions that can lead to left-sided heart failure are described in Table 26.1.

With left-sided heart failure, blood backs up from the left ventricle into the left atrium and then into the four pulmonary veins and lungs (Fig. 26.1). This increases pulmonary pressure, causing movement of fluid first into the interstitium and then the alveoli. Alveolar edema is more serious because it reduces gas exchange across the alveolar capillary membrane. Shortness of breath and cyanosis may result from the decreased oxygenation of the blood leaving the lungs. If the fluid buildup is severe, pulmonary edema occurs, which requires immediate medical treatment.

Right-Sided Heart Failure

Conditions causing right-sided heart failure increase the work of the right ventricle. They increase the amount of contractile force needed or they require pumping of excess blood volume (**preload**). Causes of right-sided heart failure are described in Table 26.2. The major cause of right-sided heart failure is left-sided heart failure. When the left side fails, fluid backs up into the lungs and pulmonary pressure is increased. The right ventricle must continually pump blood against this increased fluid and pressure in the pulmonary artery and lungs. Over time this additional strain eventually causes it to fail. When the right ventricle hypertrophies or fails because of increased pulmonary pressures, it is referred to as **cor pulmonale**.

TABLE 26.1 CAUSES OF LEFT-SIDED HEART FAILURE

Cause	Primary Effect on Left Ventricular Workload
Aortic stenosis	Increased volume to pump from restricted blood outflow
Cardiomyopathy	Increased workload from impaired contractility
Coarctation of the aorta	Restricted outflow and increased resistance from narrowing of aorta
Hypertension	Resistance increased from elevated pressure
Heart muscle infection	Increased workload from damaged myocardium
Myocardial infarction	Increased workload from impaired contractility
Mitral regurgitation	Increased volume to pump from backward blood flow

• WORD • BUILDING •
cor pulmonale: cor—heart + pulm—lung

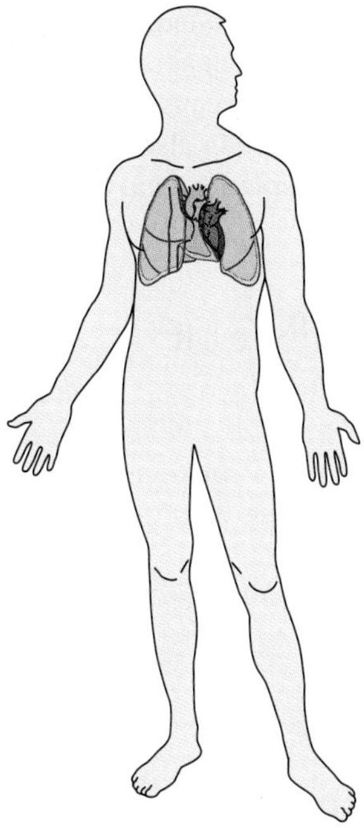

FIGURE 26.1 Left-sided heart failure. Shaded areas indicate areas of congestion from blood backup caused by the failing left side of the heart.

TABLE 26.2 CAUSES OF RIGHT-SIDED HEART FAILURE

Cause	Primary Effect on Right Ventricular Workload
Atrial septal defect	Left atrial blood flow into right atrium increases right ventricular volume to pump
Cor pulmonale	Resistance increased from elevated pressure
Left-sided heart failure	Resistance increased from backup of fluid and elevated pressures
Pulmonary hypertension	Resistance increased from elevated pressure
Pulmonary valve stenosis	Increased volume to pump from restricted right ventricular blood outflow

When the right ventricle fails, it does not empty normally and there is a backward buildup of blood in the systemic blood vessels. As the blood backs up from the right ventricle, right atrial and systemic venous blood volume increases. The jugular neck veins, which are not normally visible, become distended and can be seen when the person is in a 45-degree upright position. Edema may occur in the peripheral tissues, and the abdominal organs can become engorged (Fig. 26.2). Congestion in the gastrointestinal tract causes anorexia, nausea, and abdominal pain. As the failure progresses, blood pools in the hepatic veins and the liver becomes congested, known as **hepatomegaly**. Pain in the right upper quadrant of the abdomen and impaired liver function are caused by this liver congestion. Systemic venous congestion also leads to engorgement of the spleen, known as **splenomegaly**.

> **LEARNING TIP**
>
> To understand the signs and symptoms of left-sided versus right-sided heart failure, remember that left-sided signs and symptoms are found in the lungs. Left begins with L, as does Lung:
>
> Left = Lungs = L.
>
> Any signs and symptoms not related to the lungs (L) are caused by right-sided failure.

COMPENSATORY MECHANISMS TO MAINTAIN CARDIAC OUTPUT

Compensatory mechanisms help ensure that an adequate amount of blood is being pumped out of the heart. Although these mechanisms are designed to maintain cardiac output, they contribute to a cycle that instead of being helpful leads to further heart failure.

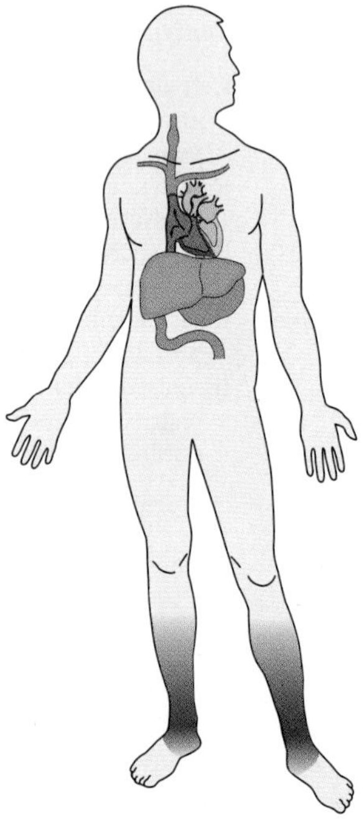

FIGURE 26.2 Right-sided heart failure. Shaded areas indicate areas of congestion from blood backup due to the failing right side of the heart.

• **WORD** • **BUILDING** •
hepatomegaly: hep—liver + mega—large
splenomegaly: splen—spleen + mega—large

When the sympathetic nervous system detects low cardiac output, it speeds up the heart rate by releasing epinephrine and norepinephrine. Although this raises cardiac output (cardiac output = heart rate = stroke volume), the increased heart rate also increases the oxygen needs of the heart. In response to low renal blood flow, the kidneys activate the renin-angiotensin-aldosterone system, and antidiuretic hormone is released from the pituitary gland to conserve water, causing decreased urine output. This adds to the fluid retention problem already found in heart failure.

Over time the heart responds to the increased workload by enlarging its chambers (dilation) and increasing its muscle mass (hypertrophy), referred to as remodeling. In dilation, the heart muscle fibers stretch to increase the force of myocardial contractions, which is known as the Frank-Starling phenomenon. In hypertrophy, the muscle mass of the heart increases, creating more contractile force. Both of these compensatory mechanisms temporarily improve patient symptoms, but also increase the heart's oxygen needs, which further contributes to heart failure. Additionally, the heart walls stiffen, which further reduces pumping ability.

PULMONARY EDEMA (ACUTE HEART FAILURE)

Pulmonary edema, also known as acute heart failure, is sudden severe fluid congestion in the alveoli of the lungs and is life threatening. Pulmonary edema occurs with an acute event such as a myocardial infarction (MI) or when the heart is severely stressed, causing the left ventricle to fail. Complications of pulmonary edema include dysrhythmias and cardiac arrest.

Pathophysiology

First, pressure rises in the lung's venous blood vessels as blood builds up. As pressures continue to rise, fluid moves into the interstitial spaces. Then, with continued pressure increases, fluid containing red blood cells leaks into the alveoli. Finally, the alveoli and airways become filled with fluid, reducing gas exchange and oxygen levels.

Signs and Symptoms

Signs and symptoms of pulmonary edema are listed in Table 26.3. Pink, frothy sputum is a classic symptom of pulmonary edema caused by the increased lung congestion and pressures that allow leaking of fluid into the alveoli. Compensatory mechanisms increase the heart rate and blood pressure; however, as pulmonary edema worsens, the blood pressure may fall.

Diagnostic Tests

Diagnostic studies are listed in Table 26.3. The congestion in the pulmonary system can be seen on x-ray examination. Arterial blood gases (ABGs) show a decrease in PaO_2 that

TABLE 26.3 ACUTE HEART FAILURE SUMMARY

Signs and Symptoms	Rapid respirations with accessory muscle use Severe dyspnea, orthopnea Crackles and wheezes Coughing Pink, frothy sputum Anxiety, restlessness Pale skin and mucous membranes Clammy, cold skin
Diagnostic Tests	Chest x-ray examination Arterial blood gases Electrocardiogram Hemodynamic monitoring
Therapeutic Measures	Oxygen via cannula, mask, or mechanical ventilation Positioning in high or semi-Fowler's position Bedrest IV drugs: morphine, diuretics, inotropic agents, vasodilators Frequent vital signs, urinary output Pulmonary pressures Daily weights Treatment of underlying cause
Priority Nursing Diagnoses	*Impaired Gas Exchange* *Decreased Cardiac Output* *Excess Fluid Volume*

continues as the edema worsens and an increase in $PaCO_2$, causing respiratory acidosis. The pulmonary artery catheter shows elevated pulmonary pressures and a decreased cardiac output.

Therapeutic Measures

Immediate treatment is needed to prevent patients from drowning in their own secretions (see Table 26.3). The goal of therapy is to reduce the workload of the left ventricle in order to improve cardiac output and reduce the patient's anxiety. Placing the patient in Fowler's position allows the lungs to expand more easily. Ask the patient what position provides him or her the most comfort in breathing. Oxygen is given, usually by mask to provide higher amounts. In severe cases of pulmonary edema, endotracheal intubation and mechanical ventilation may be necessary.

Medications are given intravenously to reduce anxiety, relax airways, and increase peripheral blood pooling to decrease preload (morphine); reduce fluid congestion; reduce preload; strengthen heart contractions; and reduce arterial pressure and sodium and water retention to relieve dyspnea.

Nursing Management

Supportive care based on symptoms is given. The patient is typically critically ill and in an intensive care unit. Psychosocial support is important because the patient will be anxious if alert.

CHRONIC HEART FAILURE

Signs and Symptoms

Chronic heart failure is a progressive disorder. Signs and symptoms may worsen over time (Table 26.4).

Fatigue and Weakness

Fatigue and weakness are the earliest symptoms of heart failure. They occur from the decreased amount of oxygen reaching the tissues. During the day the fatigue worsens, especially with activity.

Dyspnea

Dyspnea is a common symptom of left-sided heart failure. It is a result of the pulmonary congestion that impairs gas exchange between the alveoli and capillaries. Dyspnea stimulates compensatory mechanisms that produce short, rapid respirations. Dyspnea is classified in several ways:

- Exertional dyspnea is shortness of breath that increases with activity.
- **Orthopnea** is dyspnea that increases when lying flat. In an upright position, gravity holds fluid in the lower extremities. In a supine position, gravitational forces are removed, allowing fluid to move from the legs to the heart, which overwhelms the already congested pulmonary system. When orthopnea is present, two or more pillows are often used for sleeping. Documentation should state the number of pillows used. For example, use of three pillows would be "three-pillow orthopnea."
- **Paroxysmal nocturnal dyspnea** (PND) is sudden shortness of breath that occurs after lying flat for a time. PND results from excess fluid accumulation in the lungs. The sleeping person awakens with feelings of suffocation and anxiety. Relief is obtained by sitting upright for a short time, which reduces the amount of fluid returning to the heart.

Cough

A chronic, dry cough is common in heart failure. The coughing increases when lying down from increased irritation of the lung mucosa. This irritation is due to the increase in pulmonary congestion that occurs when gravity no longer keeps fluid in the legs and more fluid returns to the heart and lungs.

Crackles and Wheezes

Pulmonary congestion causes abnormal breath sounds such as crackles and wheezes. Crackles are produced from fluid buildup in the alveoli resulting from increased pressure in the pulmonary capillaries. Wheezes occur from bronchiolar constriction caused by the increased fluid.

Tachycardia

The sympathetic nervous system compensates for the decreased cardiac output in heart failure by releasing epinephrine and

• WORD • BUILDING •
orthopnea: orth—straight + pnea—to breathe

TABLE 26.4 CHRONIC HEART FAILURE SUMMARY

	Right-Sided Heart Failure	*Left-Sided Heart Failure*
Signs and Symptoms	Jugular venous distention Dependent peripheral edema Ascites Weight gain Splenomegaly Hepatomegaly GI pain, anorexia, nausea Fatigue, weakness Tachycardia Nocturia	Dyspnea on exertion Dry hacking cough, especially when supine Crackles, wheezing Orthopnea Paroxysmal nocturnal dyspnea (PND) Cheyne-Stokes respirations Cyanosis Tachypnea, tachycardia Nocturia
Diagnostic Tests	History and physical examination Electrocardiogram Chest x-ray 2D-echocardiography with Doppler Exercise stress test Coronary angiography Cardiac magnetic resonance imaging Nuclear imaging studies Cardiac catheterization Serum laboratory tests: CBC, BNP, electrolytes, BUN, creatinine, liver function tests, thyroid-stimulating hormone, fasting blood glucose, lipid profile, ferritin Arterial blood gases Urinalysis Sleep studies Hemodynamic monitoring	
Complications	Hepatomegaly Splenomegaly Pleural effusion Left ventricular thrombus and emboli Cardiogenic shock	
Therapeutic Measures	***Noninvasive*** Treat underlying cause Oxygen by cannula or mask Drug therapy (see Table 26.5) Individualized activity plan Dietary sodium restriction Fluid restriction Daily weights ***Invasive*** Pacemaker ICD Resynchronization therapy Mechanical assistive devices Intra-aortic balloon pump Left ventricular assist device Total artificial heart Surgery: CABG, valvuloplasty, heart valve replacement, cardiac transplant	
Priority Nursing Diagnoses	*Impaired Gas Exchange* *Decreased Cardiac Output* *Excess Fluid Volume*	

BNP = brain natriuretic peptide; BUN = blood urea nitrogen; CABG = coronary artery bypass graft; CBC = complete blood count; ICD = implantable cardioverter defibrillator.

norepinephrine to increase the heart rate. Normally, this is helpful because the increased heart rate increases the amount of blood ejected by the heart to maintain an adequate cardiac output. However, whenever the heart works faster, the heart itself also requires more oxygen, which the failing heart finds difficult to supply.

> **LEARNING TIP**
>
> To simulate the sound of crackles, open a piece of Velcro or rub hair together next to your ear. These sounds are similar to the sound of crackles heard with a stethoscope.

Chest Pain

Chest pain may occur from ischemia in the patient with heart failure. Decreased cardiac output results in decreased oxygen delivery to the heart itself via the coronary arteries. Compensatory mechanisms designed to maintain cardiac output increase the workload and oxygen needs of the heart and are counterproductive in heart failure. Tachycardia increases the oxygen needs of the heart. The kidneys compensate by retaining sodium and fluid, which increases the fluid volume returning to the heart (preload) and therefore the heart's workload and oxygen needs. Pain also increases oxygen requirements, adding further to the cycle of heart failure.

Cheyne-Stokes Respiration

A breathing pattern of shallow respirations building to deep breaths followed by a period of apnea characterizes Cheyne-Stokes breathing. The apneic period occurs because the deep breathing causes carbon dioxide levels to drop to a level that does not stimulate the respiratory center. This apnea may last up to 30 seconds and is then followed by the shallow to deeper respiratory pattern of Cheyne-Stokes as carbon dioxide levels rise again.

Edema

Edema occurs in heart failure as a result of (1) systemic blood vessel congestion and (2) sympathetic compensatory mechanisms that cause the kidneys to activate the renin-angiotensin-aldosterone system, in which antidiuretic hormone is released from the pituitary gland, causing sodium and water to be retained.

Systemic edema or pulmonary edema can occur in heart failure. The effect of backward buildup of pressure in the systemic blood vessels is seen with distention of the jugular veins, swelling of the legs and feet, sacral edema in the individual on bedrest, and increased fluid within the abdominal cavity and organs. An acute buildup of fluid in the lungs produces pulmonary edema.

Anemia

Many patients with heart failure are anemic due to decreased angiotensin-converting enzyme (ACE) action. The reduced ACE action decreases production of red blood cells.

Nocturia

Nocturia is an increase in urine output at night during sleep. After lying down, fluid in the lower legs returns to the circulatory system. Renal blood flow and filtration are increased, resulting in greater urine production and the need to urinate frequently during the night. Nocturia may occur up to six times per night, contributing to the patient's fatigue from lack of sleep.

> **NURSING CARE TIP**
>
> Patients often have to void shortly after going to bed. This is due to fluid in the legs returning to the heart and then the kidneys for filtering after a person lies down. To help patients get as much undisturbed rest as possible, teach them to recline with legs at or above heart level for at least 30 minutes before going to bed. Then they can void before going to bed, instead of soon after going to bed.

Cyanosis

The skin, nailbeds, or mucous membranes may appear blue, or cyanotic, from decreased oxygenation of the blood. **Cyanosis** is a late sign of heart failure. It is associated primarily with left-sided heart failure.

Altered Mental Status

Less cardiac output decreases the amount of oxygen delivered to the brain. As a result, restlessness, insomnia, confusion, and impaired memory may occur. A decrease in level of consciousness may occur.

Malnutrition

Several factors contribute to malnutrition in the person with chronic heart failure. Altered mental status, dyspnea, and fatigue interfere with the ability to eat. Anorexia and gastrointestinal (GI) upset occur from pressure exerted by excess fluid surrounding the GI structures. Absorption of food may also be impaired by this pressure.

> **CRITICAL THINKING**
>
> ***Mr. Shepard—Part 1***
>
> ■ Mr. Shepard, age 66, has a family history of cardiac disease. He has been hypertensive for 10 years and takes captopril (Capoten) daily. His baseline vital signs are BP 122/78 mm Hg, pulse 80 beats per minute (bpm), respirations 18 per minute, height 66 inches, and weight 170 lb. During a visit to his physician, he states that he has been short of breath during his daily 2-mile walk and has been using two pillows at night for sleep. As he talks, the physician notes that he has an intermittent dry cough.
>
> *Continued*

CRITICAL THINKING—cont'd

His physical examination shows BP 140/86 mm Hg, pulse 106 bpm, respiration 24 per minute, weight 178 lb, and bilateral crackles in the lung bases.

1. What signs and symptoms of heart failure does Mr. Shepard have?
2. Do the signs and symptoms reflect right- or left-sided heart failure?
3. Why are each of the signs and symptoms occurring?
4. Why is Mr. Shepard using two pillows for sleeping?

Suggested answers at end of chapter.

Complications of Heart Failure

Complications of heart failure are listed in Table 26.4. The liver and spleen enlarge from the fluid congestion, which causes impaired function, cellular death, and scarring. Pleural effusion, a leakage of fluid from the capillaries of the lung into the pleural space, can occur. The elevated pressures in the capillaries of the lung cause this leakage. Thrombosis and emboli can occur as a result of poor emptying of the ventricles, which leads to stasis of blood. Aspirin or anticoagulants are often prescribed to prevent thrombus formation in patients with heart failure. Cardiogenic shock, often caused by a myocardial infarction that damages the left ventricle, occurs when the left ventricle is unable to supply the tissues with enough oxygen and nutrients to meet their needs. Cardiogenic shock is a life-threatening condition that requires immediate treatment (see Chapter 9).

Diagnostic Tests

Diagnostic tests are done to identify the cause of heart failure and determine the degree of failure present (see Table 26.4):

- Serum laboratory tests can evaluate contributing factors for heart failure, such as elevated serum blood urea nitrogen (BUN) and serum creatinine from renal failure, elevated liver enzymes from liver damage, elevated ferritin with hemochromatosis (iron overload), and thyroid function tests.
- A serum B-type natriuretic peptide (BNP) or N-terminal proBNP (NT-proBNP) level may be obtained. Elevated levels indicate heart failure and severity; higher levels of this cardiac biomarker correlate with a worse prognosis. Brain natriuretic peptide is made by the heart to regulate blood volume to reduce cardiac workload. When the heart has to work harder over time, it releases more BNP.
- A chest x-ray examination shows the size, shape, and enlargement of the heart and congestion in the pulmonary vessels.
- Cardiac dysrhythmias that precipitate and contribute to heart failure are diagnosed with an electrocardiogram (ECG; see Chapters 21 and 25).
- Echocardiography may measure ventricular size, wall thickness, motion, and ejection fraction and assess valvular function.
- Exercise stress testing and nuclear imaging studies show activity tolerance, which is usually limited in heart failure.
- Cardiac magnetic resonance imaging shows both moving and still pictures of the heart and major blood vessels. Cardiac structure and function are analyzed to determine treatment for cardiac disease.
- Cardiac catheterization and angiography are used to detect underlying heart disease that may be the cause of heart failure.
- Sleep studies may be done because sleep apnea or breathing disorders can contribute to heart failure.
- Measurement of the pressure in the heart and lungs is done with hemodynamic monitoring to guide medical therapy.

CRITICAL THINKING

Mr. Shepard—Part 2

■ Mr. Shepard's chest x-ray examination shows an enlarged heart (cardiomegaly).

1. Why is Mr. Shepard's heart enlarged?
2. What is the significance of an enlarged heart?

Suggested answers at end of chapter.

Therapeutic Measures

The overall goal of medical treatment for chronic heart failure is to improve the heart's pumping ability and decrease the heart's oxygen demands. Treatment of heart failure focuses on (1) identifying and correcting the underlying cause, (2) increasing the strength of the heart's contraction, (3) maintaining optimum water and sodium balance, and (4) decreasing the heart's workload. Heart failure management requires a team approach that may involve physicians, case managers, nurses, dietitians, physical therapists, occupational therapists, pharmacists, social workers, and clergy. Heart failure critical pathways (treatment guidelines), as well as heart failure clinics, are being used to ensure quality-based outcomes while reducing treatment costs.

The severity of heart failure determines the individualized therapy selected. Noninvasive approaches are usually tried first. If noninvasive treatment is not effective, invasive approaches may be used. Often, multiple therapies are used in combination for optimum patient outcomes.

Oxygen Therapy

One of the major problems caused by heart failure is a reduction in oxygen delivered to the tissues. The signs and symptoms of this are fatigue, dyspnea, altered mental status, and cyanosis. Oxygen therapy may assist in supplying the oxygen needs of the tissues. In mild heart failure, oxygen may be delivered via nasal cannula. For more severe cases, arterial blood gas values guide oxygen delivery, either via masks that provide high concentrations of oxygen, or with mechanical ventilation.

Activity

Activity tolerance depends on the severity of heart failure signs and symptoms. Severe symptoms may require bedrest with restricted activity until treatment reduces the symptoms. For stable heart failure, a regular exercise program, such as one set up with referral to a cardiac rehabilitation program, has shown to improve cardiac function and reduce heart failure effects (see *Evidence-Based Practice* box).

EVIDENCE-BASED PRACTICE

Clinical Question

Do cardiovascular rehabilitation programs improve quality of life for heart failure patients?

Evidence

In a study of medically stable heart failure patients, exercise training was associated with modest but significant reductions in both all-cause mortality or hospitalization and cardiovascular mortality or heart failure hospitalization (O'Connor et al., 2009).

Cardiac rehabilitation has shown long-term benefits as well in a randomized controlled trial, with 1-month and 6-year evaluations (Mueller et al., 2007). Six years after participation in a residential cardiac rehabilitation program, patients with chronic heart failure had slightly better outcomes than control subjects, maintained exercise capacity, and engaged in activities that exceeded the minimal amount recommended by guidelines for cardiovascular health.

Implications for Nursing Practice

Cardiac rehabilitation programs for chronic heart failure patients have been shown to improve quality of life. Nurses should initiate referrals to cardiac rehabilitation programs and educate patients on their value toward overall cardiac health.

REFERENCES

Mueller, L., Myers, J., Kottman, W., et al. (2007). Exercise capacity, physical activity patterns and outcomes six years after cardiac rehabilitation in patients with heart failure. *Clinical Rehabilitation, 21*(10), 923–931.

O'Connor, C. M., Whelian, D. J., Lee, K. L., et al. (2009). Efficacy and safety of exercise training in patients with chronic heart failure: HF-ACTION randomized controlled trial. *Journal of the American Medical Association, 301*(14), 1439–1450.

Patients should be encouraged to stay as active as possible within the parameters the physician has prescribed. An individualized walking program that increases activity over time is often prescribed. Patients should be taught how to exercise safely without causing symptoms and to understand that overexertion can produce fatigue the next day.

Sodium and Weight Control

Dietary sodium is usually restricted to decrease fluid retention. Salt substitutes often use potassium in place of sodium, so the patient and physician should discuss their use. A normal weight range should be maintained. A dietary consult can include a plan for a low-sodium diet and weight reduction if needed.

NURSING CARE TIP

In severe heart failure with abdominal discomfort present, malnutrition is a concern. The patient can be anorexic, but the weight gain that occurs with fluid retention can mask the weight loss occurring from the anorexia. Monitor food intake to ensure that weight gain from fluid retention does not allow malnutrition to go undetected.

Drug Therapy

There is no cure for heart failure. Medications, however, can improve symptoms and quality of life. The American College of Cardiology Foundation/American Heart Association (ACC/AHA) 2009 guidelines recommend medication classes for the stages of heart failure development (Jessup et al., 2009). Stage A and B refers to people who are at risk of heart failure. Stage C applies to people with current or past symptoms of heart failure with structural heart disease. This includes most patients with heart failure. Stage D includes those with refractory heart failure, which requires extraordinary support or hospice care. Drug categories begin with angiotensin-converting enzyme inhibitors (ACEIs) or angiotensin receptor blockers (ARBs) for Stage A, then add beta blockers for Stage B, then diuretics for fluid retention, and consideration of aldosterone antagonists, digitalis, nitrates, and hydralazine (Apresoline) for Stage C (Table 26.5). Anticoagulants are also used on an individualized basis.

LEARNING TIP

To help you identify ACE inhibitors, remember that their generic names end with *-pril.*

ANGIOTENSIN-CONVERTING ENZYME INHIBITORS. ACEIs are considered the first-choice drug over angiotensin receptor blockers (ARBs). They are used for their vasodilation

TABLE 26.5 MEDICATIONS USED FOR HEART FAILURE

Medication Class/Action	Examples	Route	Side Effects	Nursing Implications
ACE Inhibitors				
First-line therapy to decrease afterload. Decrease cardiac hypertrophy.	captopril (Capoten) benazepril (Lotensin) enalapril (Vasotec) fosinopril (Monopril) lisinopril (Prinivil, Zestril) moexipril (Univasc) quinapril (Accupril) perindopril (Aceon) ramipril (Altace) trandolapril (Mavik)	PO (captopril also SL)	Cough, hypotension, rash, hyperkalemia, angioedema (dyspnea, facial swelling)	Check apical pulse and BP. If pulse less than 60 bpm or systolic BP less than 90 mm Hg, notify physician. Give 1 hour before meals. Give captopril and moexipril on empty stomach. *Teaching:* Take first doses at night to adjust to lower BP. Rise slowly. Check BP weekly. Report cough, or side effects.
Angiotensin II Receptor Inhibitors (ARBs)				
Block angiotensin II receptor blockers to prevent hypertension. May be used if ACE inhibitor not tolerated.	candesartan (Atacand) irbesartan (Avapro) losartan (Cozaar) valsartan (Diovan)	PO	Headache, dizziness, angioedema (dyspnea, facial swelling)	Check apical pulse and BP. If pulse below 60 bpm or systolic BP below 100 mm Hg, notify physician. *Teaching:* Rise slowly. Report rash, sore throat/mouth, fever, swelling, difficulty breathing, chest pain, or irregular heartbeat.
Beta-Adrenergic Blockers				
Reduce sympathetic nervous system input, cardiac remodeling; improve cardiac output to reduce symptoms, reduce disease progression and sudden death.	bisoprolol (Zebeta) carvedilol (Coreg) metoprolol succinate (Toprol XL)	PO	Dizziness, hypotension, hyperglycemia, fluid retention, diarrhea, bradycardia, heart blocks, impotence, bronchospasm (carvedilol)	Check apical pulse and BP. If pulse below 60 bpm or systolic or BP below 100 mm Hg, notify physician. *Teaching:* Take pulse daily and notify physician if below 60. Take BP biweekly. Rise slowly.
Loop Diuretics				
Decrease fluid overload. • Potassium wasting	bumetanide (Bumex) furosemide (Lasix) torsemide (Demadex)	PO, IV	Hypokalemia, hypochloremia, hypomagnesemia, hyponatremia, dehydration, hypotension	Check BP and pulse before giving. Monitor electrolyte levels (especially potassium and in those on digitalis) and fluid status (daily weight, intake, output, thirst, dry mouth, weakness, oliguria) throughout therapy. Administer per patient lifestyle (usually in a.m.) to avoid nocturia.
• Potassium sparing	spironolactone (Aldactone)	PO	Hyperkalemia, nausea, vomiting, anorexia, diarrhea, headache, clumsiness	Do not give potassium-sparing diuretic if hyperkalemic. Older patients are at higher risk for electrolyte imbalances. *Teaching:* Report signs of hyperkalemia: weakness, fatigue, confusion, dyspnea, arrhythmias, confusion.

TABLE 26.5 MEDICATIONS USED FOR HEART FAILURE

Thiazide Diuretics				
Decrease fluid overload. Potassium wasting	chlorothiazide (Diuril) hydrochlorothiazide (Hydro DIURIL, HCTZ, Microzide) metolazone (Zaroxolyn)	PO	Hypokalemia, dizziness, hypotension, photophobia	*Teaching:* Use of potassium supplements and, if on digitalis, increased risk of toxicity with hypokalemia. Monitor weight daily, and report 2- to 3-lb change over 1–2 days. Use sunscreen.
Inotropes—Cardiac Glycoside (Positive Inotrope and Negative Chronotrope)				
Increase force and contraction of myocardium, which increases cardiac output. Slow heart rate to reduce workload of heart and control atrial fibrillation, if present.	digoxin (Lanoxin)	PO, IV	Fatigue, nausea, vomiting, anorexia, headache, bradycardia, cardiac arrhythmias Toxicity: abdominal pain, anorexia, nausea, vomiting, visual changes (blurred, yellow-green halos, photophobia, diplopia), bradycardia, dysrhythmias	Take apical pulse for 1 minute; if below 60 bpm, notify physician. Older patients are more susceptible to toxicity. Periodically monitor drug level and electrolytes (hypokalemia, hypomagnesemia, and hypercalcemia make more susceptible to toxicity). *Teaching:* Take medication exactly as directed, at the same time each day. Take pulse before taking medication; if below 60 bpm hold and contact physician. Signs of digitalis toxicity.
Vasodilators				
Decrease afterload, which increases cardiac output and reduces cardiac workload. Used for patients who cannot take ACE inhibitors.	isosorbide dinitrate (Isorbid, Isordil) hydralazine (Apresoline) nitroglycerin	PO PO, IV SL, IV	Headache, dizziness, hypotension, tachycardia	Take blood pressure and pulse before giving. Notify physician if not within normal limits. *Teaching:* Rise slowly. Headache common initially, treated with aspirin.

ACE = angiotensin-converting enzyme.

effect, which lowers blood pressure and reduces workload on the heart. They also offer additional benefit by preventing remodeling, which is an effect that leads to progressive cardiac deterioration.

ANGIOTENSIN RECEPTOR BLOCKERS. ARBs are an alternative to ACEIs for inhibiting the renin-angiotensin-aldosterone system, thereby lowering blood pressure and workload on the heart. They should be used carefully if ACEIs are also used because hypotension, hyperkalemia, and renal dysfunction risks increase.

BETA-ADRENERGIC BLOCKERS. Initially the sympathetic nervous system (SNS) acts to compensate for heart failure. Long-term sympathetic effects, however, are not helpful in heart failure. Beta blockers block the adverse effects of the SNS. Improved cardiac output, reduced symptoms, reduced disease progression, and reduced sudden death are benefits of this therapy.

LEARNING TIP

To help you identify beta blockers, remember that their generic names end with -ol.

DIURETICS. Diuretics reduce fluid volume and decrease pulmonary venous pressure, which in turn decreases cardiac workload. Because they are given to help prevent edema, edema does not need to be present for their use. Diuretics act on various areas of the kidneys to promote the excretion of edema fluid. A combination of diuretics may be used to achieve the desired effect. Electrolytes (especially potassium levels to prevent hypokalemia) and fluid balance (to prevent dehydration) should be carefully monitored during therapy. Potassium supplements are often given with potassium-wasting diuretics.

NURSING CARE TIP

Always check potassium levels before giving a potassium-wasting diuretic such as the loop diuretics furosemide (Lasix), bumetanide (Bumex), or torsemide (Demadex) or before giving a potassium supplement, which the patient may be taking due to diuretic therapy. Do not give a diuretic if the potassium level is low or a potassium supplement if the potassium level is high.

ALDOSTERONE ANTAGONISTS. Spironolactone (Aldactone) blocks the effects of aldosterone, which causes the retention of sodium and fluid. Potassium must be monitored carefully, because spironolactone is a potassium-sparing agent and the risk of hyperkalemia increases if ACEIs or ARBs are also used.

INOTROPIC AGENTS. Inotropic drugs strengthen ventricular contraction to increase cardiac output. Inotropic agents include digitalis (digoxin), sympathomimetics (dobutamine), and phosphodiesterase inhibitors (milrinone). The sympathomimetics and phosphodiesterase inhibitors are usually used short term.

Digitalis. In addition to improving contraction strength, digitalis preparations decrease conduction time within the heart, which slows the heart rate to allow more complete emptying of the ventricles. Digitalis may increase myocardial oxygen needs, so it is used cautiously. Monitoring of serum drug levels is necessary to detect toxic levels of the drug. If toxic levels are present, the drug is stopped to allow digitalis levels to decrease over time.

CRITICAL THINKING

Mr. Shepard—Part 3

■ During Mr. Shepard's visit, the physician tells him to continue the ACE inhibitor, the diuretic, and a 2-g sodium diet.

1. Why is the ACE inhibitor continued?
2. Will the ACE inhibitor affect preload or afterload?
3. Why is the diuretic ordered?
4. Why is a 2-g sodium diet ordered?
5. What is the overall goal of the ordered treatment?

Suggested answers at end of chapter.

Pacemakers and Implantable Cardioverter Defibrillator

For patients at risk of sudden death, pacemakers and implantable cardioverter defibrillators (ICDs) are used along with medication therapy. They can pace the heart or deliver an electric countershock if a life-threatening rhythm occurs.

Cardiac Resynchronization Therapy

With heart failure, the ventricles do not always beat in normal synchrony with each other. This dyssynchrony results in less effective pumping by the ventricles and reduced stroke volume. Cardiac resynchronization therapy (CRT) restores normal contraction timing of the ventricles. It reduces symptoms and improves quality of life. A biventricular cardiac pacing system is used. An atrial lead senses or paces the atria as needed. A right and left ventricular lead stimulates the ventricles to synchronize their contractions in response to the atrial event. Left ventricular filling is then improved. CRT therapy is also available with an implantable cardioverter defibrillator (CRT-D). For more information and pictures of CRT devices, visit www.medtronic.com.

Mechanical Assistive Devices

Mechanical assistive devices can provide temporary support to patients in cardiogenic shock and act as a bridge to transplantation, destination therapy (long-term solution when other options are not available for the failing heart), or heart replacement. These devices increase the cardiac output of the patient. They include the intra-aortic balloon pump, ventricular assist devices, total artificial heart and implantable replacement heart. Technology in this area is continually changing. For current information and to see pictures of these devices, visit the following sites:

www.nlm.nih.gov
www.heartreplacement.com (AbioCor implantable replacement heart)
www.syncardia.com (CardioWest temporary total artificial heart)
www.thoratec.com (ventricular assist devices).

INTRA-AORTIC BALLOON PUMP. For acute care, an intra-aortic balloon pump (IABP) increases circulation to the coronary arteries and reduces the work of the heart. The IABP catheter is inserted into the femoral artery and positioned in the descending aortic arch (Fig. 26.3). It is attached to a computer that senses ventricular contraction and controls the balloon. While the heart is relaxed (diastole), the balloon is inflated, sending more blood into the coronary arteries. Just before the heart contracts (systole), the balloon deflates to allow blood to flow past it. The deflation of the balloon creates a suction effect, which allows the blood to flow past it with less resistance (decreased afterload) into the aorta. The IABP is inserted in a cardiac catheterization laboratory, critical care unit, or surgical suite and is used short term for several days.

VENTRICULAR ASSIST DEVICES. Ventricular assist devices (VADs) are implanted mechanical devices that assist cardiac pumping (Fig. 26.4). These devices maintain cardiac output and allow the failing ventricle to rest. VADs are used temporarily as a bridge to transplantation (while awaiting a donor heart), bridge to recovery (for hearts that potentially

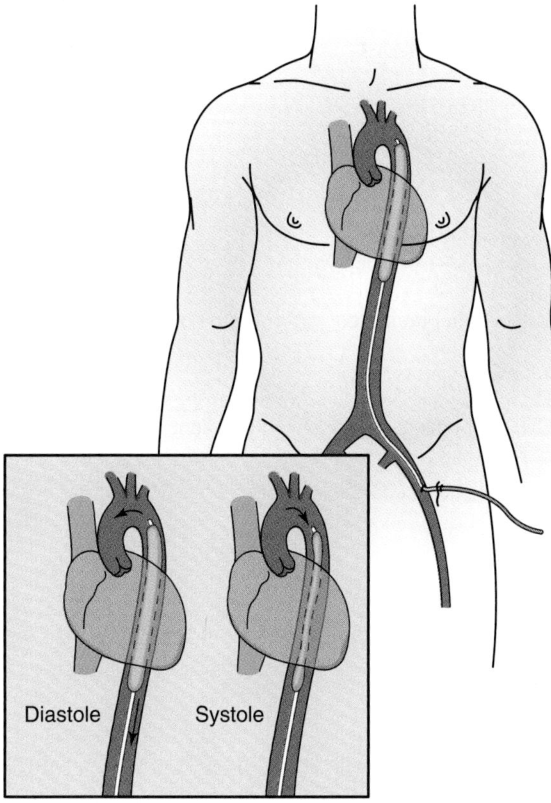
Diastole
Systole

FIGURE 26.3 Intra-aortic balloon pump.

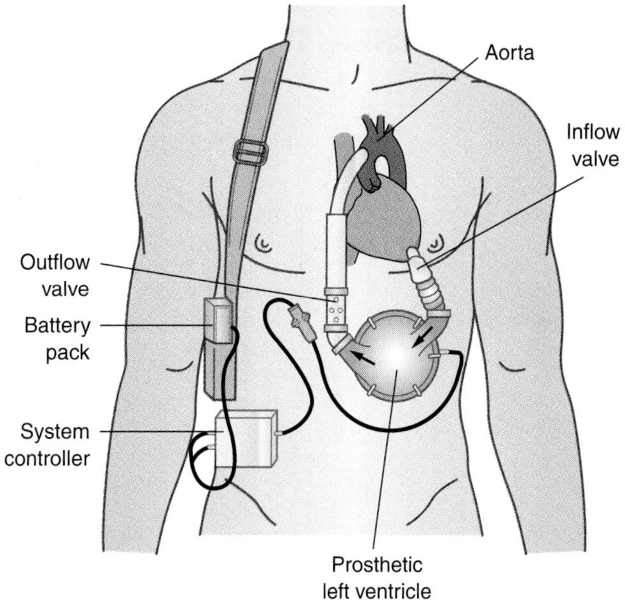
Aorta
Inflow valve
Outflow valve
Battery pack
System controller
Prosthetic left ventricle

FIGURE 26.4 Schematic of a left ventricular assist device.

can recover), or as destination therapy (long-term therapy) for those who are not candidates for heart transplant. They may also be referred to as left ventricular assist devices (LVADs) if used in the left ventricle only, right ventricular assist devices (RVADs) if used in the right ventricle only, or bi-VADs (biventricular assist devices) if used in both ventricles. VADs can pump blood directly from either the right atrium to the pulmonary artery (right ventricular failure) or the left atrium to the aorta (left ventricular failure). Two devices are used for biventricular failure. See www.thoratec.com for more information and a video clip.

Surgical Management

Heart failure causes may be treated surgically with coronary artery bypass for coronary artery disease or valve replacement for valvular disease (see Chapters 23 and 24). Once these conditions are treated, heart failure symptoms should resolve.

Surgical ventricular reconstruction (SVR) reduces left ventricular volume in heart failure patients. It is often done along with coronary artery bypass surgery. In 2009, the ongoing STICH trial reported that SVR showed no significant improvement over coronary artery bypass graft (CABG) surgery alone (Jones et al., 2009).

Nursing Process for the Patient with Chronic Heart Failure

Data Collection

While obtaining data for the patient with heart failure, focus on areas that might indicate the presence of heart failure (Table 26.6).

Nursing Diagnoses, Planning, Interventions, and Evaluation

See the *Nursing Care Plan for the Patient with Chronic Heart Failure,* for common nursing diagnoses.

The major focus of nursing care for chronic heart failure patients is to improve oxygenation and decrease the body's need for oxygen with rest, positioning, medications, fluid balance, and oxygen consumption control.

OXYGEN. Oxygen therapy is ordered by the physician and guided by blood gas analysis and patient symptoms. Before starting oxygen therapy, explain the therapy to the patient. For chronic heart failure, oxygen is administered at 2 to 6 L/min via nasal cannula. The effects of the oxygen should be monitored carefully. Oxygen should be used cautiously in all patients, so that their stimulus to breathe is not diminished (especially if the patient has chronic obstructive pulmonary disease [COPD]).

REST AND ACTIVITY. Reduction of the body's oxygen demands decreases the workload of the heart. A balance of rest and activity that does not produce signs or symptoms of oxygen deprivation is essential. The activity level of the patient is determined by the severity of the heart failure. During times of exertion, monitor the patient's vital signs and respiratory effort for oxygen deprivation. If activity intolerance develops, the activity should be stopped.

POSITIONING. Semi-Fowler's or high-Fowler's position makes breathing easier. In upright positions, the lungs are able to expand more fully and gravity decreases the amount of fluid returned to the heart, thereby reducing the heart's workload.

FLUID RETENTION. Monitoring daily weights for weight gain is important in detecting fluid retention. Edema usually is not observed until 5 to 10 pounds of extra fluid are present. A baseline weight should be obtained when heart

TABLE 26.6 NURSING DATA COLLECTION FOR THE PATIENT WITH CHRONIC HEART FAILURE

	Subjective Data
History	
Respiratory	Lung disease? How many flights of stairs can be climbed without dyspnea? How many pillows used for sleeping? Dyspnea at rest or that awakens from sleeping?
Cardiovascular	Any cardiac disease history: hypertension, myocardial infarction, valvular problem, anemia, dysrhythmias, palpitations? Chest pain: precipitating factors, severity, relieving factors? Can activities of daily living be performed? Can activities performed 6 months, 4 months, 2 months, 2 weeks ago still be done? Any dizziness (vertigo) or fainting (syncope)?
Fluid retention	Daily sodium intake? Weight gain? Are shoes tight? Do ankles swell?
Gastrointestinal	Is appetite good? Any nausea, vomiting, or abdominal pain?
Urinary	Decrease in daytime urine output? How often does patient go to the bathroom at night (nocturia)?
Neurologic	Any change in behavior?
Medications	
Knowledge of Condition	
Coping Skills	
	Objective Data
Respiratory	Tachypnea, crackles, wheezing, respiratory effort, dyspnea with exertion
Cardiovascular	Tachycardia, dysrhythmias, jugular venous distention, peripheral edema (degree of pitting)
Gastrointestinal	Abdominal distention, ascites, hepatomegaly, splenomegaly
Neurologic	Confusion, decreased level of consciousness, restlessness, impaired memory
Integumentary	Cold, clammy skin; pallor; cyanosis
General	Weight
Diagnostic Test Findings	

NURSING CARE PLAN for the Patient with Chronic Heart Failure

Nursing Diagnosis: *Activity Intolerance* related to fatigue caused by oxygen imbalance

Expected Outcomes: The patient will show increased activity tolerance with vital signs within normal limits (WNL) in response to activity.

Evaluation of Outcomes: Does the patient participate in activities and maintain vital signs WNL?

Interventions	Rationale	Evaluation
Provide rest, space activities, and conserve energy.	Myocardial oxygen need is decreased with rest and energy conservation.	Does patient participate in activity with minimal pulse rate or ECG changes?
Assist as needed with activities of daily living (ADLs).	Conserve energy by assisting with ADLs.	Are patient's ADLs met?
Teach use of assistive devices and lifestyle changes.	Assistive devices can overcome limitations to increase activity.	Does patient incorporate assistive devices into lifestyle changes?

NURSING CARE PLAN for the Patient with Chronic Heart Failure—cont'd

GERIATRIC

Increase time allowed to complete activities.	Independence and participation are increased if extra time is allowed for tasks.	Does patient report greater ability to complete activities with fewer symptoms?

Nursing Diagnosis: *Excess Fluid Volume* related to heart failure and the secondary reduction in renal blood flow for filtration

Expected Outcomes: The patient will remain free from edema and dyspnea, have clear lung sounds, and maintain baseline weight at all times.

Evaluation of Outcomes: Does patient have clear lung sounds with baseline weight maintained?

Interventions	Rationale	Evaluation
Monitor for edema, weight gain, jugular venous distention (JVD), lung crackles.	Excess fluid is indicated by edema, sudden weight gain, JVD, and crackles in the lungs.	Is edema, weight gain, JVD, or crackles present?
Monitor intake and output.	Intake and output will show imbalances.	Are intake and output balanced for 24 hours?
Administer diuretics.	Diuretics promote fluid excretion.	Is output increased and edema or dyspnea reduced?
Decrease sodium intake as ordered.	Sodium retains fluid.	Does patient restrict sodium intake?
Maintain fluid restriction as ordered.	Excess fluid intake contributes to edema.	Does patient restrict fluid intake?

Nursing Diagnosis: *Disturbed Sleep Pattern* related to nocturia and inability to lie down and sleep comfortably

Expected Outcomes The patient will awaken refreshed and be less fatigued during the day at all times.

Evaluation of Outcomes: Does patient wake up less frequently during the night and feel more refreshed with less fatigue during the day?

Interventions	Rationale	Evaluation
Identify barriers to sleep.	Anxiety, nocturia, diuretics, orthopnea, or paroxysmal nocturnal dyspnea can make sleep difficult.	Does patient identify sleep barriers?
Assist patient in identifying positions of comfort for sleeping.	Use of pillows or a recliner can decrease orthopnea.	Can patient identify a position of comfort?
Teach patient cause of dyspnea at night.	Anxiety about falling asleep and waking up short of breath is reduced.	Can patient explain cause of dyspnea?
Encourage patient to recline for 30 to 60 minutes before bedtime.	Reclining before bedtime redistributes fluid and increases voiding that can occur before going to sleep instead of after going to sleep.	Is patient awakened to void after going to bed less often?

GERIATRIC

Encourage patient to take diuretics early in the day.	Nocturia is reduced if diuretics are taken earlier in the day.	Does patient take diuretics early and report less nocturia?

failure is diagnosed. Daily weights should be measured on the same scale, at the same time of day, and with the same type of clothing worn to ensure accuracy. A good time to obtain a daily weight is in the morning after the bladder is emptied. Documentation of daily weights should include the date and time of the weight, the scale used, the clothing worn, and the weight measurement. A weight journal can be kept by the patient. Tell patients to report weight gains of 2 to 3 lb over 1 to 2 days.

OXYGEN CONSUMPTION. Increased oxygen consumption by the heart should be avoided. Tachycardia increases the oxygen needs of the heart and should be reported promptly to the physician for treatment. Older patients are especially vulnerable to the effects of tachycardia because of their decreased reserves. Constipation should be prevented because straining during defecation, known as Valsalva's maneuver, increases the heart's workload by increasing venous return to the heart. Stool softeners should be administered, as ordered, to prevent straining.

Patients should be taught methods of saving energy while performing activities of daily living (ADLs). Activities should be alternated with periods of rest. Fatigue should be avoided. A referral to occupational therapy and physical therapy can be helpful for developing techniques that allow the patient to conserve energy during self-care. Some suggestions for conserving energy include placing frequently used objects at waist level to avoid reaching overhead, planning bathing activities to include rest periods, and using Velcro fasteners to make dressing easier.

MEDICATIONS. Because heart failure is a progressive, chronic condition, patients may require lifetime medications. Combination drug therapy is often needed. Taking many pills each day can be challenging. Financial resources, compliance, and ongoing monitoring are issues that must be considered.

Diuretics require monitoring of the patient's potassium levels and blood pressure. To prevent hypokalemia, potassium supplements may be prescribed during diuretic therapy, and a diet with high-potassium foods is encouraged. If too much fluid is removed, the patient may become hypotensive, and orthostatic hypotension can develop. The patient may then be dizzy and at risk of falling. Caution the patient to change positions and rise slowly to prevent falls during diuretic therapy.

Before administration of a digitalis drug, which slows the heart rate, the patient's apical pulse should be counted for 1 minute. If the pulse is below 60 bpm, notify the physician to determine if the drug should be given. Some patients are given digitalis even if their heart rates are between 50 and 60 bpm, as long as their heart's conduction system is normal or if the rate is due to other medications such as a beta blocker. When giving digitalis, be aware that hypokalemia increases the heart's sensitivity to digitalis. A patient can become toxic on a normal dose of digitalis when hypokalemia is present. This is important to note because many people on digitalis also take diuretics, which may lower potassium levels. Monitoring for signs and symptoms of digitalis toxicity should be done routinely during patient assessment. Early signs and symptoms of digitalis toxicity are anorexia, nausea, and vomiting; bradycardia or other dysrhythmias; visual problems; and mental changes. The elderly are especially prone to the toxic effects of this drug and may exhibit confusion when levels are toxic.

Medications with vasodilating effects reduce the heart's workload by decreasing vascular pressure. Blood pressure is monitored when administering vasodilators.

Medication Teaching. Patients and their families are taught the purpose, side effects, and precautions for prescribed medications. Patients should understand the importance of taking their medication as prescribed, even if they do not have symptoms. A schedule should be developed so patients remember to take their medications. Teach them to report side effects to the physician. If dizziness occurs from drugs that reduce blood pressure, the drugs can be staggered so that they are not all taken at the same time. Patients taking digitalis or a beta blocker should be taught to take their pulse and to notify their physician if it is below 60 bpm or below the lower limit heart rate set by their physician. Patients on diuretics should be taught the following:

- Take drug during the day before 4 p.m. to decrease being awakened at night to void (if desired).
- Have a readily available and obstacle-free bathroom or commode to prevent incontinence and falls.
- Eat high-potassium foods if taking a potassium-wasting diuretic.
- Weigh yourself daily, and report weight gains of 2 to 3 lb over 1 to 2 days.

LOW-SODIUM DIET AND WEIGHT CONTROL. A dietician consult helps the patient and family understand the need for dietary compliance and ways to provide menus that are appealing and easy to use. Eating should remain pleasurable for the patient to avoid malnutrition. Discuss foods the patient likes and can still have rather than talking about only foods they cannot have. Patients are taught to read food labels to determine which foods are high and low in sodium content. They are also taught that salt substitutes may contain potassium. With this knowledge, patients can help design a daily meal plan using low-sodium foods that are appealing to them. Food preparers are taught not to salt food during cooking, and table salt should be eliminated. Spices, herbs, and lemon juice may be suggested to flavor unsalted foods.

For overweight patients, weight reduction may help eliminate the underlying cause of heart failure. Diet counseling and support should be given to the obese patient to encourage weight loss. The body mass index (BMI) and waist-to-hip ratio should guide weight loss.

If anorexia occurs in the later stages of heart failure, the patient's intake should be evaluated. Several small meals rather than three large meals will decrease the heart's workload. If the patient's nutritional needs are not being met, the physician should be informed for a referral to a dietitian.

EDUCATION. Chronic management of heart failure requires patient and family understanding of the disease process, management of home oxygen therapy, diet and weight control, need for immunizations such as the annual flu shot, and medications (see *Home Health Hints*). The patient and family must recognize the importance of each of these factors in order to foster a productive life for the patient with chronic heart failure. A discussion of heart failure and signs and symptoms to report to the physician using simple terms should be included in the teaching plan (Box 26.1, *Patient and Family Education*).

COPING. Living with a chronic illness can be frustrating for both patients and their families. An assessment of coping skills used by patients and their families can be used to develop a plan for coping with this current illness. Available support systems are explained to patients. Referrals to social workers, sexual counselors, telehealth management, and nurse-managed clinics can be helpful in providing resources that may make living with heart failure easier. Providing patients options for traveling can help maintain quality of life.

Understanding the chronic nature of heart failure is important for patients, families, and caregivers so they can positively deal with the emotions and feelings that can result. Nurse-managed heart failure clinics have been shown to decrease hospitalization rates and increase effective management of the therapeutic regimen.

NURSING CARE TIP

Provide written discharge instructions for all patients with heart failure and their caregivers. Instructions should focus on medications (stressing compliance), diet, activity level, follow-up appointments, daily weights, and to report or seek care for symptoms that worsen.

CRITICAL THINKING

Mr. Shepard—Part 4

■ The nurse meets with Mr. Shepard after the physician orders a continued ACE inhibitor, a diuretic, and a 2-g sodium diet.

1. What information should the nurse teach Mr. Shepard based on the prescribed treatment?
2. What types of foods should be included in Mr. Shepard's diet?
3. Why does the nurse instruct Mr. Shepard to weigh himself daily?
4. Why does the nurse tell Mr. Shepard to weigh himself at the same time of day, on the same scale, and wearing the same type of clothing?
5. What guidelines does the nurse teach Mr. Shepard to follow with reporting of weight gain?

Suggested answers at end of chapter.

Box 26.1

Patient and Family Education

Heart Failure Signs and Symptoms to Report to the Physician

- Shortness of breath
- Fatigue
- Dry cough
- Shortness of breath when lying down (orthopnea)
- Episodes of sudden awakening with shortness of breath (paroxysmal nocturnal dyspnea)
- Weight gain of 2 to 3 lb over 1 to 2 days
- Ankle or foot edema
- Nocturia
- Anorexia

CARDIAC TRANSPLANTATION

Cardiac transplantation is reserved for patients with end-stage cardiac disease. Guidelines for the selection of recipients and donors are applied to optimize survival (Box 26.2). Preoperative teaching is done once the recipient is accepted into the transplant program. For more information on heart transplantation, visit www.nhlbi.nih.gov/health/dci/Diseases/ht/ht_whatis.html.

Surgical Procedure

Once a donor heart is found, the recipient is notified, admitted to the hospital, and immediately prepared for surgery. The general procedures for this surgery are similar to

Box 26.2

Cardiac Transplant Guidelines

Donor Criteria

- Younger than age 40
- No significant cardiac or malignant disease
- No active infections
- No severe hypertension or diabetes mellitus
- Only about 20 lb difference in weight between donor and recipient

Recipient Criteria

- Consideration of physiological age
- Class IV cardiac disease (not treatable with other medical or surgical treatment, less than 6 to 12 months survival)
- No irreversible pulmonary hypertension
- No unresolved pulmonary infarcts
- No systemic disease limiting survival
- No drug addiction or peptic ulcer disease

those described in Chapter 21. Two types of cardiac transplant procedures are performed: orthotopic and heterotopic. In the orthotopic procedure, once the patient is on cardiopulmonary bypass (CPB), the recipient's diseased heart is removed, leaving the posterior wall of the atria, superior vena cava and inferior vena cava, and pulmonary vein (Fig. 26.5). The aorta and pulmonary artery are cut. The donor's atria, aorta, and pulmonary artery are then anastomosed to the recipient's atria, aorta, and pulmonary artery. The heterotopic procedure joins the donor heart and vessels to the recipient's heart and vessels without removing the recipient's heart. The donor heart rests in the right side of the chest.

Immunosuppressive therapy is required to prevent rejection of the transplanted heart. Medications such as cyclosporine (Neoral, Sandimmune), mycophenolate mofetil (CellCept), tacrolimus (Prograf), sirolimus (Rapamune), and Prednisone are used (Box 26.3, *Nutrition Notes*). It begins preoperatively with high loading doses of these medications. The risk for rejection is highest immediately after surgery and decreases with time but never goes away, so doses of immunosuppressive medication are also highest initially after surgery and decrease with time. Lifelong antirejection therapy is required and often involves the combination of three drugs to allow lower doses to help reduce side effects.

Complications

Heart transplantation complications may include those associated with cardiac surgery, as well as heart rejection, which is the major cause of death within the first year. To detect rejection, frequent biopsies of cardiac muscle or a newer blood test to detect activation of rejection genesis is done during the first year. If a biopsy shows damaged cells, indicating rejection, antirejection drug therapy may be changed.

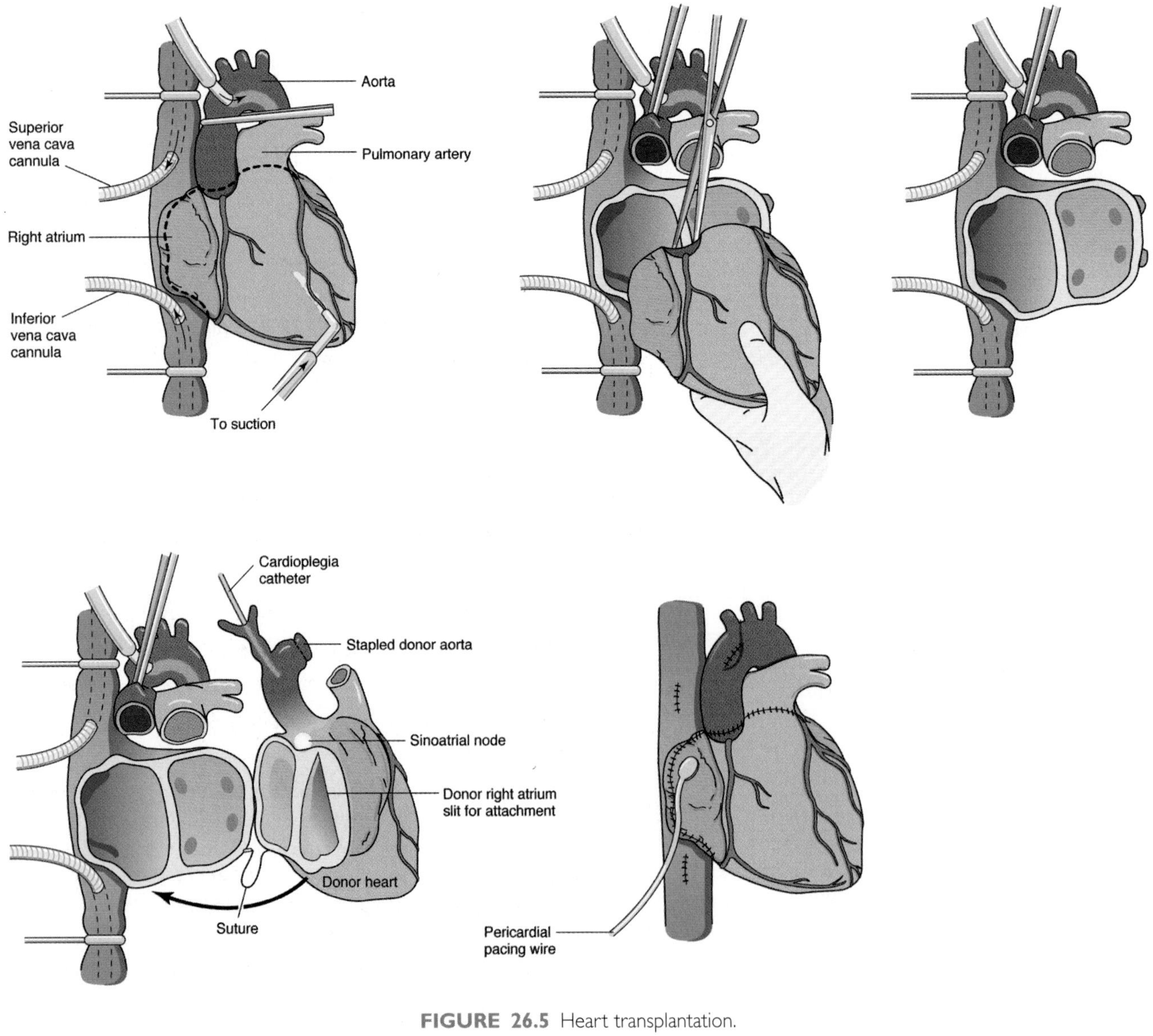
Aorta
Superior vena cava cannula
Pulmonary artery
Right atrium
Inferior vena cava cannula
To suction
Cardioplegia catheter
Stapled donor aorta
Sinoatrial node
Donor right atrium slit for attachment
Donor heart
Suture
Pericardial pacing wire

FIGURE 26.5 Heart transplantation.

Box 26.3

Nutrition Notes

Cyclosporine, an immunosuppressant used to prevent transplant rejection, is metabolized by intestinal CYP-3A4. Taking cyclosporine with grapefruit juice may cause elevated blood levels. St. John's wort, sold as a dietary supplement, has interacted with cyclosporine sufficiently to cause organ rejection.

In addition, as a result of immunosuppressive therapy, infection and cancer may occur. The medications used for immunosuppressive therapy also may cause adverse reactions such as increased cholesterol, diabetes, kidney disease, cataracts, or osteoporosis.

Therapeutic Measures

After cardiopulmonary bypass is stopped, the patient receives a diuretic to aid in excretion of excessive circulating fluid. Intake and output are monitored hourly, and the patient is observed for fluid overload. Lung sounds are monitored frequently for crackle, and weight and electrolyte levels are checked daily.

Postcardiotomy syndrome (PCS) may occur from days 2 to 5 after surgery and last a few weeks. Patients may arouse normally and be oriented but exhibit mild confusion or psychosis. Pupillary reaction and motor response are assessed. The safety of the patient is maintained with side rails up, bed in low position, and nursing call light within reach. The patient is given as much rest and as little sensory stimulation as possible. The family is kept informed and involved in the patient's recovery.

Sleeping is difficult because of postoperative pain and the continuous level of activity in the intensive care unit (ICU). Sleep is promoted in 90-minute intervals by dimming lights and decreasing all sensory stimulation near the patient. Additionally, listening to a favorite soothing tape recording with earphones or the use of ordered narcotics for pain may also help sedate and relax the patient.

Temperature is monitored every 4 hours and complete blood cell count (CBC) and white blood cell (WBC) results are monitored for indications of infection. If oral thrush (white patches) develops, an antifungal agent is ordered. A urine culture to diagnose a urinary tract infection is ordered if cloudy urine or urinary tract burning occurs.

Nursing Process for the Preoperative Cardiac Transplant Patient

General preoperative and postoperative surgical care is discussed in Chapter 12. Postoperative needs for the patient undergoing cardiac surgery are discussed next.

Nursing Process for the Postoperative Cardiac Transplant Patient

Data Collection

The patient is accompanied to the ICU by the anesthesiologist, who gives the nurse a report of the procedure, complications, and hemodynamic and ventilatory management of the patient. The patient is connected to a cardiac monitor and a mechanical ventilator for 4 to 24 hours. A temporary pacemaker is connected to the epicardial pacing wires if they were placed during surgery as a precaution to treat bradycardia and other dysrhythmias. The patient is placed under a warming device, such as a light or blanket. The chest tubes are monitored, the nasogastric tube is placed to suction, and the urinary catheter is placed for gravity drainage.

A head-to-toe assessment of the patient, including dressings, tubes, and IV lines, is performed. Of importance are signs of awakening, shivering, pain, lung and heart sounds, and palpation of the entire chest and neck to detect crepitus (air in the subcutaneous tissue from opening the chest). Blood is drawn for a CBC, electrolytes, coagulation studies, and arterial blood gases. Cardiac transplant patients may be in isolation for their own protection, depending on the agency's policy.

After the initial transfer assessment, vital signs, oxygen saturation, and cardiac pressures are monitored and recorded every 15 to 30 minutes, with decreasing frequency as the patient stabilizes. Body temperature is monitored continuously while warming measures are used. Intake and output are measured and vital signs are checked. An electrocardiogram (ECG) is done to detect perioperative myocardial infarction. A chest x-ray examination is done to check central line and endotracheal tube placement and to detect a pneumothorax or hemothorax, diaphragm elevation, or mediastinal widening from bleeding. At this point, the family may see the patient, and patient care is explained.

Nursing Diagnoses, Planning, Interventions, and Evaluation

Nursing diagnoses for postoperative cardiac surgery or transplant are discussed in the *Nursing Care Plan for the Postoperative Patient Undergoing Cardiac or Transplant Surgery.*

Coping with Cardiac Transplant

Cardiac transplant patients may have feelings of sadness and grief for the donor and his family. These feelings may be offset by great elation, relief, and hope after a long wait for the transplant. Patients should be told that these feelings are normal. They should be allowed to express their feelings when they are ready. Emotional support may be needed.

Transplant rejection is a possible complication of this surgery. Patients need to understand the importance of following instructions regarding medications and testing that are related to preventing or detecting rejection.

Cardiac transplant patients are followed in an exercise rehabilitation program that closely monitors their activity progression in relation to myocardial oxygen consumption and signs of activity intolerance. Most patients reach an activity level allowing them to participate in many recreational sports.

NURSING CARE PLAN for the Postoperative Patient Undergoing Cardiac or Transplant Surgery

Nursing Diagnosis: *Acute Pain* related to sternotomy, leg incisions, internal mammary artery resection, or pericarditis

Expected Outcomes: The patient will state pain is relieved or tolerable within 30 minutes of report of pain. Patient will be able to rest and perform respiratory treatments.

Evaluation of Outcomes: Does patient state pain is within acceptable levels? Is patient able to rest and perform respiratory treatments?

Interventions	Rationale	Evaluation
Obtain characteristics of pain with each episode.	A thorough description is needed to determine cause and plan actions.	Does patient describe pain on scale of 0 to 10?
Splint chest incision with all movement and coughing and deep breathing.	Stabilizes sternum and incision to increase comfort.	Can patient splint chest incision independently?
Encourage patient to report pain even when pain is mild.	It is easier to keep pain under control when mild.	Does patient report pain when mild?
Turn, reposition every 2 hours.	Changes muscle position, relieving stiffness.	Is patient comfortable without stiffness?
Offer back rubs frequently.	Relaxes tense muscles retracted during operation.	Is patient able to rest in comfort?
Instruct patient to take a deep breath before movement and exhale slowly during movement.	Keeps muscles relaxed, minimizing tension with guarding and pain.	Can patient perform coughing and deep-breathing techniques as instructed?
Explain that chest pain can occur from the surgical incision rather than the heart.	Chest pain after surgery can be frightening for patients because they may not associate surgical chest pain with the incision and instead think the pain is anginal or infarction pain.	Does patient state understanding of pain sources?

Nursing Diagnosis: *Decreased Cardiac Output* related to myocardial depression, hypothermia, bleeding, unstable dysrhythmias, or hypoxemia

Expected Outcomes: The patient will remain free of major side effects of pharmacological support. The patient will maintain vital signs within normal limits (WNL), palpable peripheral pulses, urine output greater than 30 mL/hr, and normal sinus rhythm post-transplant.

Evaluation of Outcomes: Is patient free of major side effects? Are vital signs WNL?

Interventions	Rationale	Evaluation
Monitor vital signs.	Trends reflect problems.	Are vital signs WNL?
Monitor peripheral circulation.	Mottling or weak pulses may indicate poor cardiac output (CO).	Do peripheral pulses remain strong with normal skin color, temperature, capillary refill?
Monitor intake and output.	Fluid deficit or excess can alter CO.	Does total intake equal output?
Listen to lung sounds and note character of sputum.	Crackles may indicate heart failure or pulmonary edema.	Are lungs clear?
Monitor temperature closely while rewarming the patient.	Febrile state increases heart rate and myocardial oxygen consumption.	Does temperature remain less than or equal to 98.6°F (37°C)?

NURSING CARE PLAN for the Postoperative Patient Undergoing Cardiac or Transplant Surgery—cont'd

Monitor for shivering.	Shivering increases the blood pressure, decreasing CO and increasing risk for bleeding.	Is patient's shivering controlled?
Monitor chest tube drainage for increase or sudden decrease.	Drainage =200 mL/hr may lead to hypovolemia and a decrease in CO.	Is patient free from cardiac tamponade and hypovolemia?
Monitor ECG.	Premature ventricular contractions and atrial fibrillation decrease CO.	Does patient remain in normal sinus rhythm or controlled dysrhythmia?
Monitor electrolytes.	Low calcium and magnesium and high potassium decrease contractility and CO.	Are electrolytes WNL?
Monitor arterial blood gases (ABGs).	Acidosis decreases heart function, and a low CO may lead to further acidosis.	Are ABGs WNL?

Nursing Diagnosis: *Risk for Infection* related to inadequate primary defenses from surgical wound or immunosuppression (transplants)

Expected Outcomes: The patient will remain free from infection post-transplant.

Evaluation of Outcomes: Does patient remain free from infection?

Interventions	Rationale	Evaluation
Observe incision for signs and symptoms of infection.	Redness, warmth, fever, and swelling indicate infection.	Are signs and symptoms of infection present?
Monitor drainage and maintain drains.	Drains remove fluid from the surgical site to prevent infection development.	Are drainage amount and color normal for procedure? Are drains functioning?
Maintain sterile technique for dressing changes.	Sterile technique reduces infection development.	Is incision free of signs and symptoms of infection?
Monitor and report abnormal findings for temperature, lung sounds, sputum, and urine consistency.	Low-grade (immunosuppressed) or high-grade fever, crackles, yellow-green sputum color, or cloudy urine can indicate infection.	Is the patient's temperature WNL and are lung sounds, sputum, and urine clear?
Encourage coughing and deep breathing and incentive spirometer use.	Lung infections can be prevented with lung expansion and secretion removal.	Does patient perform coughing and deep breathing and use incentive spirometer?

Nursing Diagnosis: *Deficient Knowledge* related to lack of prior experience with transplant

Expected Outcomes: The patient will demonstrate understanding of post-transplant care prior to discharge.

Evaluation of Outcomes: Does patient state understanding and ability to carry out post-transplant care?

Interventions	Rationale	Evaluation
Give information in small increments and use written materials and audiotapes.	Cardiac transplant patients commonly have memory deficits, cognitive dysfunction, and short attention spans resulting from long-term decreased cerebral perfusion.	Does patient state understanding of information?

Continued

NURSING CARE PLAN for the Postoperative Patient Undergoing Cardiac or Transplant Surgery—cont'd

Interventions	Rationale	Evaluation
Include families in teaching sessions and encourage them to promote self-care by the patient.	Family involvement in teaching sessions is important to promote understanding and retention.	Does family participate and state understanding of teaching sessions?
Address or refer sexual functioning questions with patients and their partners.	Patients usually have questions regarding sexual functioning. Referrals can be made to sexual counselors.	Does patient state that questions have been addressed?
Discharge teaching includes treatment, complications, activity, medications, and enhancing quality of life.	Patients need comprehensive information to comply with post-transplant care.	Does patient state understanding of discharge care?

CRITICAL THINKING

Mrs. Eden

■ Mrs. Eden, age 45, a single mother of two, is transferred to a surgical unit 5 days after a cardiac transplant. She is withdrawn and has a poor appetite. Her vital signs are stable. However, on ambulating to the bathroom, she is very weak, requiring two nurses to help her. Her respiratory rate increases from 20 to 32 per minute and is slightly labored, and her apical pulse increases from 88 to 103 mm Hg.

1. Is Mrs. Eden tolerating this activity? Why or why not?
2. List four reasons why Mrs. Eden has a poor appetite.
3. Give four nursing interventions for Mrs. Eden's poor appetite.
4. Give three reasons why Mrs. Eden is withdrawn.

Suggested answers at end of chapter.

Home Health Hints

- Some patients may not have a scale in their home. It may be necessary to assist them in obtaining one or to leave an agency scale in the home for daily weights.
- The most objective way to document edema is to use a tape measure (marked in centimeters) on the abdominal girth, thigh, calf, and ankle. Measure at the same place each visit, such as measuring the girth of the calf at a specified distance above the medial malleolus. Edema may be present if the patient's waistband is getting tighter or shoes and socks feel tighter.
- The sacrum, back, and sides of a bedridden patient should be checked to note edema. These are dependent areas in the bedridden patient, so fluid accumulates in these areas instead of the ankles.
- Blood drawn for potassium levels needs to be transported to the laboratory within 1 hour. Ice should not be put directly on the blood-draw tube because this can cause destruction of the cells and a false elevation in the potassium level.
- Blood drawn for digoxin (Lanoxin) levels should be taken to the lab within 2 to 3 hours.
- Patients should use no-salt-added canned vegetables. Patients on sodium-restricted diets who already have canned vegetables in their home can still use them even though they are not the low-sodium type. They should be instructed to pour off the liquid and rinse the vegetables before heating them for serving. The use of herbs and spices can help make them more flavorful.
- For the patient on a low-sodium diet, an effective diet teaching technique is to have the patient name the foods highest in sodium. Asking the patient to rename the list on each visit helps knowledge retention and compliance.
- If patients have a poor appetite, ask their caregiver if they eat well when eating with others. Anorexia could

Home Health Hints—cont'd

be a sign of loneliness and depression if they eat well with others instead of an effect of heart failure.

- Assist patients in taking medications at times that fit their lifestyle. A morning dose of a diuretic may limit what they can do for the next few hours. An afternoon dose might encourage compliance. Lack of compliance is a major factor in the rehospitalization of patients with heart failure. A dose of diuretic too late in the day may cause frequent awakenings during the night to void.
- The home health nurse should periodically check the contents of medicine bottles. If pills have been cut in half, ask about this. Often it is an attempt by the patient to "stretch" the medicine to decrease expenses. Find out about community or drug company programs that help purchase medicines for patients with financial need. Eligible Medicaid patients can apply for medication cards. The new Medicare Part D prescription program, as well as retail drug discount programs, may be helpful as well.
- Visual disturbances can occur from digitalis toxicity. If the patient sees halos around lights or red-green tinting on everything, report this to the physician.
- Troublesome side effects of an ACE inhibitor such as captopril (Capoten) are an intractable cough and hypotension. Note how the patient is coughing. Teach the patient to report the cough.
- Oxygen concentrators are widely used in home care. Instructions must be given on the proper use of the oxygen and safety precautions for oxygen use. Long tubing allows the patient ease in moving about the home. Patients need to be cautioned about keeping the tubing out of their way and not kinking it. If the patient also has chronic obstructive pulmonary disease (COPD), a note by the gauge should remind the patient not to let the flow exceed 2 L/min. Patients and caregivers should also be cautioned as to the explosive nature of oxygen and the danger of smoking in its presence.
- As the home health nurse becomes acquainted with the patient, it is easier to pick up on signs of oxygen deprivation and hypoxia, such as confusion, combativeness, or unusual expressions of anger.
- For patients with orthopnea, a foam wedge can be obtained from a medical equipment company to use under their head when sleeping instead of pillows.
- As patients with heart failure feel better, they may go back to the old habits that cause an increase in fluid. The home health nurse can help by providing information about the disease and help patients foster their own independence and ways of coping with the condition. Each home health visit is a teaching opportunity that empowers patients with a knowledge base to help them take control of their health.

SUGGESTED ANSWERS TO CRITICAL THINKING

■ *Mr. Shepard—Part 1*

1. Signs and symptoms of heart failure include shortness of breath, two-pillow orthopnea, dry cough, tachycardia (pulse 106 bpm), tachypnea (respiration 24 per minute), and bilateral crackles.
2. Left-sided heart failure is indicated by the findings.
3. *Shortness of breath:* fluid in the lungs impairs gas exchange; *orthopnea:* lying flat increases fluid accumulation in the lungs, causing dyspnea; *dry cough:* fluid in the lungs irritates the mucosal lining of the lungs; *tachycardia:* sympathetic compensation to increase cardiac output; *tachypnea:* sympathetic compensation to increase blood oxygenation; *bilateral crackles:* fluid trapped in the lungs.
4. The two pillows help prevent orthopnea by using a more upright position, which allows gravity to decrease fluid accumulation in the lungs.

■ *Mr. Shepard—Part 2*

1. Mr. Shepard's heart is enlarged to compensate for the strain caused by increased peripheral vascular resistance from hypertension in order to maintain an adequate cardiac output.
2. An enlarged heart requires more oxygen, which often cannot be supplied in heart failure.

■ *Mr. Shepard—Part 3*

1. The ACE inhibitor is needed for vasodilation to reduce peripheral vascular resistance and decrease the heart's workload, which in turn prevents cardiac remodeling and improves functioning.

SUGGESTED ANSWERS TO—cont'd

2 The ACE inhibitor will affect afterload.
3. The diuretic is ordered to decrease fluid volume, which reduces preload and decreases the heart's workload.
4. The low-sodium diet is ordered to reduce water retention, which decreases preload and decreases the heart's workload.
5. The goal is to decrease the heart's workload and increase its efficiency by reducing preload and peripheral vascular resistance and to decrease progression of chronic heart failure and improve survival.

■ *Mr. Shepard—Part 4*

1. After assessment of Mr. Shepard's knowledge base, medication teaching should be given on the ACE inhibitor and diuretic that includes their purpose, side effects, and precautions. A schedule for taking the medications can be planned. An explanation of the purpose of a low-sodium diet and menu planning based on Mr. Shepard's likes and dislikes should be done.
2. Low-sodium foods should be selected to prevent fluid retention, and high-potassium foods should be included to prevent hypokalemia from the diuretic if appropriate. Read food labels. Low-sodium foods include puffed rice, wheat cereals, fruits, chicken, beef, eggs, and potatoes. High-sodium foods include tomato juice, sauerkraut, softened water, buttermilk, cheese, smoked meats, canned tuna, canned soup, pickles, instant rice, and instant potatoes. High-potassium foods include salt substitutes, bran products, avocado, bananas, prunes, oranges, baked potato, sweet potato, spinach (cooked), chocolate, nuts, and molasses.
3. Daily weighing is necessary to detect a rapid weight gain that indicates fluid retention (2 lb in 24 hours) and to measure weight loss resulting from the diuretic.
4. These instructions ensure accuracy of the weight so that comparison to the baseline weight detects a weight gain or loss.
5. Weight increase reporting guidelines are as follows: increase of 2 to 3 lb in 1 to 2 days.

■ *Mrs. Eden*

1. No, Mrs. Eden is not tolerating this activity, as evidenced by her increased respiratory rate and apical rate.
2. Steroids, immunosuppressive therapy, depression, and fatigue could be causing her poor appetite.
3. Nursing interventions related to Mrs. Eden's poor appetite could include the following: offering small, frequent meals; having family bring favorite foods from home; allowing the patient to rest before meals; providing oral hygiene before meals; administering antiemetics before meals; giving a high-calorie meal at peak appetite.
4. Mrs. Eden could be withdrawn because of changes in her lifestyle as a result of her transplant, extreme fatigue, concerns regarding how she will raise her children, grieving for the donor, and fear that she will reject her new heart.

REVIEW QUESTIONS

1. A patient asks the nurse what heart failure is. Which of the following is the nurse's best response?
   a. "The heart pumps too much blood into the pulmonary veins."
   b. "The heart is unable to pump enough blood for the body's oxygen needs."
   c. "Heart failure is a buildup of blood in the aorta from the heart's left ventricle."
   d. "With a failing heart, the heart stops beating, so blood is not pumped out."

2. Which of the following does the nurse understand is a major cause of left-sided heart failure?
   a. Hypertension
   b. Congenital heart defects
   c. Pulmonary valve stenosis
   d. Septal defects

3. A patient who has been treated for heart failure is being discharged from the hospital on 20 mg furosemide (Lasix) daily. Which of the following statements by the patient would indicate understanding of instructions for this medication?
   a. "I will take the Lasix in the morning."
   b. "I will take the Lasix at bedtime."
   c. "I will drink lots of fluids with the Lasix."
   d. "I will take it with meals."

REVIEW QUESTIONS

4. The nurse is caring for a patient receiving bumetanide (Bumex) to reduce preload for heart failure. While assessing the patient the nurse notes the patient has less ankle edema and jugular venous distention than earlier. The next dose of bumetanide is scheduled in 1 hour. Which of the following actions should the nurse take next?
   a. Notify the physician.
   b. Hold the bumetanide.
   c. Give the bumetanide as scheduled.
   d. Give the bumetanide early.

5. Which of the following assessments should the nurse teach the patient to perform to monitor fluid status at home?
   a. Weigh daily.
   b. Weigh weekly.
   c. Weigh biweekly.
   d. Weigh monthly.

6. A 160-lb patient is to receive cyclosporine (Neoral) 12.5 mg/kg daily in two divided doses. How many milligrams will the patient receive with each dose? **Fill in the blank.**

Answer: ____________________ mg

References

Hunt, S. A., Abraham, W. T., Chin, M. H., et al. (2005). *ACC/AHA 2005 guideline update for the diagnosis and management of chronic heart failure in the adult.* American College of Cardiology Foundation and the American Heart Association. Retrieved November 20, 2009, from http://www.acc.org/qualityandscience/clinical/guidelines/failure/update/index.pdf

Jessup, M., Abraham, W. T., Casey, D. E., et al. (2009). 2009 focused update: ACCF/AHA guidelines for the diagnosis and management of heart failure in adults. *Circulation, 119,* 1977–2016.

Jones, R. H., Velazquez, E. J., Michler, R. E., et al. (2009). Coronary bypass surgery with or without surgical ventricular reconstruction. *New England Journal of Medicine, 360*(17), 1705–1717.

unit SIX

UNDERSTANDING THE HEMATOLOGIC AND LYMPHATIC SYSTEMS

27

Hematologic and Lymphatic System Function, Assessment, and Therapeutic Measures

JANICE L. BRADFORD AND
LUCY L. COLO

KEY TERMS

ecchymoses (ECK-ih-MOH-siss)
lymphedema (LIMPF-uh-DEE-mah)
petechiae (puh-TEE-kee-eye)
purpura (PURR-purr-uh)

QUESTIONS TO GUIDE YOUR READING

1. What are the components of blood?
2. What are the components of the lymphatic system?
3. How are changes in the blood or lymph systems manifested as disease processes?
4. What is the sequence of events in the process of blood clotting?
5. What data should you collect when caring for a patient with a disorder of the hematologic or lymphatic system?
6. What laboratory and diagnostic studies are used when evaluating the hematologic and lymphatic systems?
7. What nursing care should you provide for patients undergoing diagnostic tests of the hematologic or lymphatic systems?
8. What common therapeutic measures are used for patients with hematologic and lymphatic disorders?
9. What is the role of the licensed practical nurse/ licensed vocational nurse (LPN/LVN) in administering blood products?

NORMAL HEMATOLOGIC AND LYMPHATIC SYSTEM ANATOMY AND PHYSIOLOGY

Blood

The hematologic system includes the bone marrow, blood, and blood components. The lymphatic system includes the lymph nodes and nodules, which filter pathogens for destruction, and the lymph vessels, which return lymph to the blood.

The general functions of blood are transportation of oxygen, nutrients, and cellular waste products; regulation of body temperature, pH, and fluid balance; and transport of cells that offer the body protection. Specific aspects of these functions are discussed further with the particular part of the blood that is responsible for each.

A human body holds 4 to 6 L of blood; 46% to 63% is plasma and the remainder is formed elements. The blood cells are the red blood cells (RBCs or erythrocytes) and white blood cells (WBCs or leukocytes); platelets (thrombocytes) are cell fragments. All of these formed elements are produced by the red bone marrow (RBM), a hematopoietic (blood-producing) tissue found in flat bones, irregular bones, and the epiphyses of long bones. The red bone marrow contains the undifferentiated stem cells that are the precursor cells for all blood cells. Final maturation and differentiation of T lymphocytes occur in the thymus. Table 27.1 shows normal blood cell counts.

Plasma

Plasma is the liquid portion of the blood and is about 91% water. It is the transporting medium for nutrients, wastes, hormones, enzymes, electrolytes, and gases. Plasma proteins include clotting factors, albumin, and globulins. Clotting factors such as prothrombin and fibrinogen are synthesized by the liver and circulate until activated in the clotting mechanism. Albumin, also synthesized by the liver, helps maintain blood volume and blood pressure by pulling tissue fluid into the venous ends of the capillary networks. Alpha and beta globulins are synthesized by the liver to be carrier molecules for substances such as fats, and gamma globulins are the antibodies produced by lymphocytes.

Plasma is also important in maintaining body temperature because blood carries heat. The water of plasma is warmed by passage through active organs, such as the liver or skeletal muscles, and this heat is distributed as blood circulates throughout the body. This process may be visible in people with light skin. The flush of fever or vigorous exercise is caused by vasodilation in the dermis, allowing blood to circulate near the body surface and lose heat. A person in a cold environment may be pale, because vasoconstriction in the dermis keeps blood circulating in the core of the body, away from the body's surface, to preserve heat.

The normal pH range of blood is 7.35 to 7.45, which is slightly alkaline. Chemical buffer systems in the blood prevent sudden fluctuations in pH and contribute to the body's acid-base balance.

TABLE 27.1 REVIEW OF BLOOD CELL VALUES AND DISORDERS

Test	Normal Value	Significance of Abnormal Findings
Red Blood Cells		
Red blood cells (RBCs)	*Male:* 4.71–5.14 million/mm^3 *Female:* 4.2–4.87 million/mm^3	Increased in chronic hypoxia Decreased in anemia or blood loss
Hematocrit (cellular portion of blood)	*Male:* 43%–49% *Female:* 38%–44%	Increased in dehydration or chronic hypoxia Decreased in anemia or blood loss
Hemoglobin (reflects oxygen-carrying capacity of blood)	*Male:* 13.2–17.3 g/100 mL *Female:* 11.7–15.5 g/100 mL	Increased in chronic hypoxia Decreased in blood loss or anemia
Reticulocytes (number of circulating immature RBCs)	1.5%–2.5%	Increased in hypoxia or anemia Decreased in RBC maturation defect
White Blood Cells		
White blood cells (WBCs)	4500–11,000/mm^3	Increased in infection
Neutrophils	59%	Increased in infection
(Bands)	(3%)	
(Segments)	(56%)	
Eosinophils	2.7%	Increased in allergic response, some leukemias
Basophils	0.5%	Increased in hyperthyroidism, some bone marrow disorders, ulcerative colitis
Lymphocytes	34%	Increased in viral infections, chronic bacterial infection, some leukemias
Monocytes	4%	Increased in chronic inflammatory disorders, some leukemias
Platelets		
Thrombocytes/platelets	150,000–450,000/mm^3	Increased from trauma Decreased with blood disorders Increased risk of bleeding with low platelet count

Red Blood Cells

Mature RBCs are biconcave disks without nuclei; they carry oxygen bonded to the iron in hemoglobin (Hgb). Oxyhemoglobin is formed in the pulmonary capillaries where the hemoglobin combines with the oxygen in the lungs. Once hemoglobin gives up its oxygen to the cells of the body, it becomes reduced hemoglobin. The amount of hemoglobin in RBCs, the amount of iron in that hemoglobin, and the number of RBCs are the determining factors for the amount of oxygen the blood can carry. A lack of iron, hemoglobin, or RBCs can cause anemia, which results in symptoms such as shortness of breath and weakness.

The rate of RBC production by the red bone marrow is most influenced by the blood oxygen level. Hypoxia stimulates the kidneys to secrete erythropoietin, which increases the rate of RBC production and thus the oxygen-carrying capacity of the blood. At such times, immature RBCs (reticulocytes) may be found in greater abundance in peripheral blood. A reticulocyte becomes a mature RBC when it ejects its nucleus. This causes the characteristic biconcave disk shape. Reticulocytes usually remain in the red bone marrow until they mature; their presence in large numbers in peripheral blood indicates an insufficient amount of mature RBCs to meet the oxygen demands of the body.

Sufficient dietary intake of protein and iron to synthesize hemoglobin is also required for normal production of RBCs. The vitamins folic acid and vitamin B_{12} are needed for DNA synthesis in the stem cells of the red bone marrow. The continuous mitosis of these cells depends on their ability to produce new sets of chromosomes. Vitamin B_{12} is also called *extrinsic factor* because it comes from an extrinsic source: food. The parietal cells of the stomach lining produce intrinsic factor, which is a chemical that combines with vitamin B_{12} to promote its absorption in the small intestine.

RBCs live for about 120 days and then become fragile and are phagocytized by fixed macrophages in the liver, spleen, and red bone marrow. Iron is returned to the red bone marrow for synthesis of new hemoglobin or is stored in the liver. The heme portion of the hemoglobin is converted to bilirubin, a bile pigment that the liver excretes into bile for elimination in the feces. Diseases such as malaria and sickle cell anemia cause an accelerated destruction of RBCs. This hemoglobin release may cause the blood level of bilirubin to rise. When the bilirubin level is elevated, it discolors the sclerae, skin, and mucous membranes bright yellow to dark orange, depending on the bilirubin level. This condition is known as jaundice.

Each person has a hereditary blood type, which refers to the antigens present on the RBCs. The two most important type categories are the ABO group and the Rh factor. The ABO type (A, B, O, or AB) indicates the antigens present (or not present, as in the case of type O) on the RBCs. The plasma contains antibodies for antigens that are not present in the blood. These antibodies can interact with antigens in transfused blood if the donor's blood does not match the recipient's blood (Table 27.2). To be Rh-positive means that the D antigen is present on the RBCs; Rh-negative means that the antigen is not present. Rh-negative people do not have natural antibodies to the D antigen but will produce them if given Rh-positive blood.

TABLE 27.2 ABO BLOOD TYPES

Type	Antigens Present on RBCs	Antibodies Present in Plasma
A	A	Anti-B
B	B	Anti-A
AB	Both A and B	Neither anti-A nor anti-B
O	Neither A nor B	Both anti-A and anti-B

White Blood Cells

WBCs are larger than RBCs and have nuclei when mature. The granular WBCs (neutrophils, eosinophils, and basophils) are produced only in the red bone marrow. The agranular WBCs (lymphocytes and monocytes) are also produced in the red bone marrow; however, the T lymphocytes complete their development in the thymus. The T lymphocytes and B lymphocytes become activated, proliferate, and differentiate in the lymph nodes, spleen, and lymphatic nodules. Table 27.1 shows normal values and percentages for each type of WBC in a differential count. WBCs function in tissue fluid, as well as the blood, and all are involved in the immunity or inflammatory response to injury.

Monocytes become macrophages, which phagocytize pathogens and dead tissue; neutrophils are more numerous but phagocytize only pathogens. Eosinophils combat the effects of histamine, detoxify foreign proteins during allergic reactions, and respond to parasitic infections. Basophils release histamine as part of inflammatory reactions. There are two groups of lymphocytes: T cells and B cells. T cells may be helper, suppressor, killer, or memory T cells. B cells become plasma cells, which produce antibodies to foreign antigens and also become memory cells.

Platelets

Platelets are formed in the red bone marrow; they are fragments of large cells called megakaryocytes. Platelets are involved in all mechanisms of hemostasis: vascular spasm, platelet plugs, and chemical clotting.

When a blood vessel is damaged, platelets release serotonin, which promotes vasoconstriction of an artery or a vein. Such constriction makes the break smaller, perhaps small enough to be covered by a clot. Constriction also allows the clot to adhere and stop any continued bleeding because it has to cover a smaller area. Capillaries have no smooth muscle and cannot constrict but are so small that breaks can be closed by platelet plugs. Platelets become sticky, adhering to the rough edges of the broken capillary and to one another, eventually forming a platelet plug that stops the bleeding.

Platelets also produce platelet factors, chemicals whose release is stimulated by contact of blood with a rough surface such as a broken or damaged vessel lining. Platelet factors are needed for the first of the three stages of chemical clotting. In stage 1, platelet factors, clotting factors from the liver, tissue factor (thromboplastin), and calcium ions react to form prothrombinase (also called prothrombin activator). In stage 2, prothrombinase converts prothrombin (synthesized by the liver) into thrombin. In stage 3, thrombin converts soluble fibrinogen (also from the liver) into insoluble fibrin strands, which form the clot. Calcium ions are also required for stages 2 and 3.

Excessive clotting in the vascular system is prevented in several ways. The very smooth endothelial lining of blood vessels repels platelets so that they do not stick to intact vessel walls. Heparin produced by mast cells inhibits the clotting mechanism. And antithrombin (synthesized by the liver) inactivates excess thrombin to prevent the clotting mechanism from becoming a vicious cycle.

Lymphatic System

The lymphatic system consists of lymph, lymph vessels, lymph nodes and nodules, the spleen, and the thymus. Functions of the lymph system are to return tissue fluid to maintain blood volume and to protect the body against pathogens and other foreign material. (Immunity is covered in Unit 4.)

Lymphatic Vessels

Lymph is tissue fluid that has entered lymph capillaries. Lymph must be returned to the blood to maintain blood volume and blood pressure. Lymph capillaries are found in most tissue spaces; they anastomose, forming larger and larger lymph vessels, which have valves to prevent backflow of lymph. Lymph from areas below the diaphragm and the upper left quadrant enters the thoracic duct (in front of the vertebral column) and is returned to the blood in the left subclavian vein (Fig. 27.1). Lymph from the upper right quadrant enters the right lymphatic duct and is returned to the blood in the right subclavian vein.

Lymph Nodes and Nodules

Lymph nodes are masses of lymphatic tissue along the pathways of the lymph vessels. They house activated lymphocytes and monocytes. Nodes are scattered both superficially and deep. As lymph flows through the nodes, the WBCs enter the lymph. Foreign materials are phagocytized by fixed macrophages, and fixed plasma cells produce antibodies to foreign antigens. The major paired groups of lymph nodes are the cervical, axillary, and inguinal nodes. These nodes are located at the junctions of the head (cervical) and extremities (axillary and inguinal) with the trunk, where they are well situated to remove pathogens before the lymph is returned to the blood.

Lymph nodules are small masses of lymphatic tissue found just beneath the epithelium of all mucous membranes. They are often referred to as mucosa-associated lymphatic tissue (MALT). The body tracts lined with mucous membranes are those that have openings to the environment: the respiratory, digestive, urinary, and reproductive systems. Any natural body opening is a potential portal of entry for pathogens; any pathogens that penetrate the epithelium usually are destroyed by the macrophages in the lymph nodules. The tonsils, which protect the oral and nasal portions of the pharynx, are familiar examples of lymph nodules, although most lymph nodules do not have names.

Spleen

The spleen is located in the upper left quadrant of the abdominal cavity, just below the diaphragm, behind the stomach. The lower rib cage protects the spleen from mechanical injury. In the fetus, the spleen produces red blood cells, a function assumed by the red bone marrow after birth.

The spleen has several functions after birth. It contains B cells and T cells, which conduct immune responses. It also contains fixed macrophages that phagocytize pathogens and worn or defective blood cells and platelets. The heme unit from RBC destruction forms bilirubin. Bilirubin is sent to the liver by way of portal circulation for excretion in the bile. The spleen also stores up to one-third of the body's platelets.

The spleen is not considered a vital organ because other organs compensate for its functions if the spleen must be removed. However, a person without a spleen is somewhat more susceptible to certain bacterial infections, such as pneumonia and meningitis. The liver and red bone marrow remove worn RBCs from the circulation, and the many lymph nodes and nodules produce lymphocytes and monocytes and phagocytize pathogens (as does the liver).

Thymus

The thymus is located inferior to the thyroid gland and anterior to the trachea. With increasing age, the thymus atrophies; relatively little thymic tissue is found in adults. The thymus contains T lymphocytes, or T cells, that mature and proliferate. Thymic hormones contribute to the maturation of the T cells. (Immunity is covered in Unit 4.)

Aging and the Hematologic and Lymphatic Systems

Older adults undergo a number of changes in the hematologic and lymphatic systems (Fig. 27.2).

NURSING ASSESSMENT OF HEMATOLOGIC AND LYMPHATIC SYSTEMS

Health History

A thorough nursing assessment starts with an in-depth patient history (Table 27.3). Specific problems that might be seen in patients with hematologic disorders include abnormal bleeding, **petechiae** (small purplish hemorrhagic spots under the skin), **ecchymoses** (larger areas of discoloration from hemorrhage under the skin), and **purpura** (hemorrhage into the skin, mucous membranes, and organs), as well as fatigue, weakness, shortness of breath,

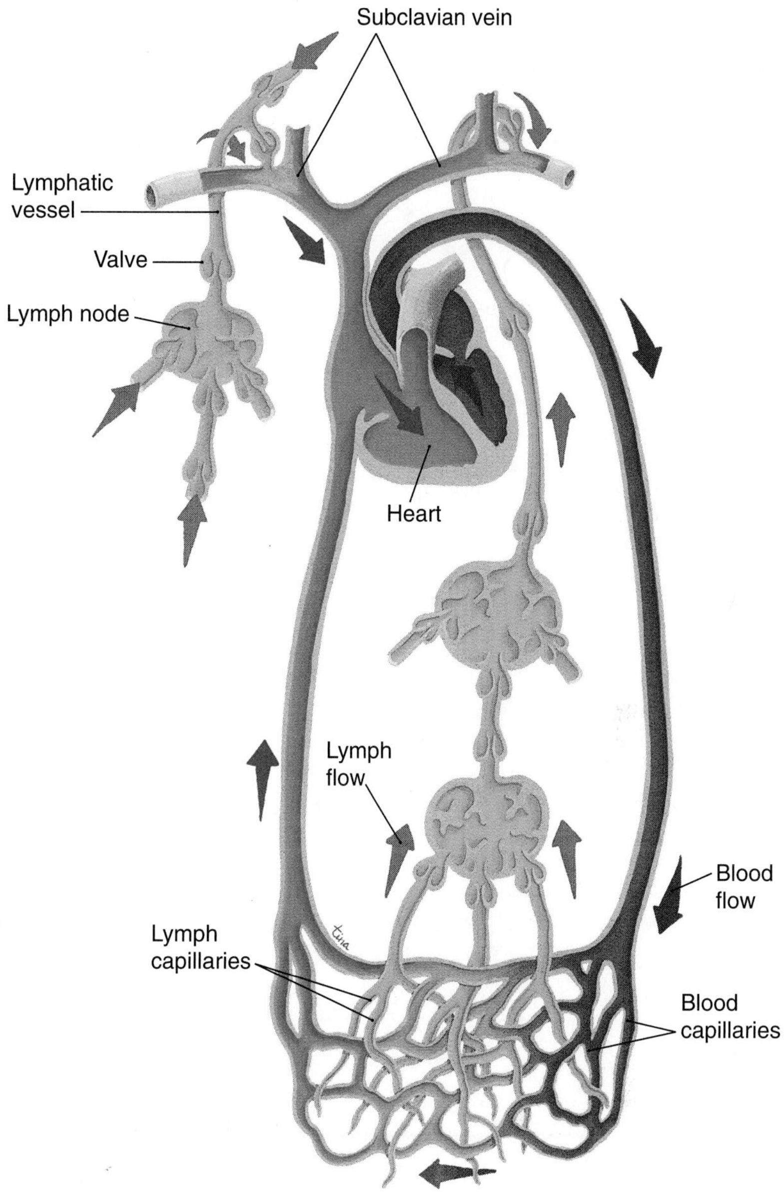
Subclavian vein
Lymphatic vessel
Valve
Lymph node
Heart
Lymph flow
Blood flow
Lymph capillaries
Blood capillaries

FIGURE 27.1 System of lymph vessels and major groups of lymph nodes. (From Scanlon, V., & Sanders, T. [2007]. *Essentials of anatomy and physiology* [5th ed.]. Philadelphia: F. A. Davis.)

and fever. Fatigue, malaise, and weight loss can accompany cancers of the lymphatic system.

Begin by obtaining the patient's biographical data, marital status, occupation, religion, age, sex, and ethnic background. This information can give you valuable clues to risk factors. For example, even though hemophilia almost always occurs in males, females may carry the gene. Sickle cell anemia occurs mostly in African Americans but also affects people of Mediterranean or Asian ancestry. Pernicious anemia occurs most often in people of northern European ancestry. By carefully collecting this information, you may be obtaining important clues that will help pinpoint a patient's problem. Finally, focus on collecting data about symptoms by using the WHAT'S UP? format presented in Chapter 1.

A complete review of past illnesses and family history is always indicated and can provide some valuable information. A social history is also useful. After developing good rapport with the patient, explore dietary and alcohol intake habits, any drug use or abuse, and sexual habits, all of which may cause changes in the hematologic system.

An occupational review can reveal exposure to some hazardous substances that can cause bone marrow dysfunction. Certain occupations, such as working in a paint factory, tool and dye processing, and even dry cleaning can be related to the formation of some hematologic cancers. Military history can also reveal sources of exposure that can help during the diagnostic phase for hematologic and lymphatic disorders.

Physical Examination

Hematologic and lymphatic disorders can involve almost every body system, so each system must be assessed. Signs and symptoms of hematologic and lymphatic disorders can

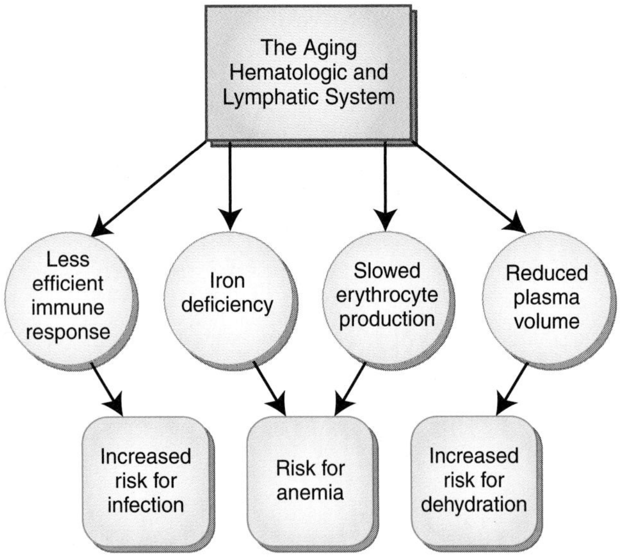
The Aging Hematologic and Lymphatic System
Less efficient immune response
Iron deficiency
Slowed erythrocyte production
Reduced plasma volume
Increased risk for infection
Risk for anemia
Increased risk for dehydration

FIGURE 27.2 Effects of aging on the hematologic and lymphatic systems.

be vague, such as shortness of breath or fatigue. A careful assessment will guide nursing care, but may also uncover important data that should be reported to the primary care provider. Table 27.4 reviews objective data that should be collected and possible interpretations of findings.

NURSING CARE TIP

If abdominal girth must be monitored for changes, use a marker to identify the site where you measure so it can be measured at the same spot each time.

DIAGNOSTIC TESTS FOR THE HEMATOLOGIC AND LYMPHATIC SYSTEMS

A number of diagnostic tests can help rule out or confirm a suspected diagnosis based on the analysis of the formed elements of the blood and the bone marrow. Specific studies include a complete blood cell count (CBC), coagulation studies, agglutination studies, bone marrow aspiration, lymphangiography, and needle biopsy.

Blood Tests

Examples of laboratory studies routinely done for patients with hematologic disorders include CBC, total hemoglobin

TABLE 27.3 SUBJECTIVE DATA COLLECTION FOR THE HEMATOLOGIC AND LYMPHATIC SYSTEMS

Category	Questions to Ask During the Health History	Rationale/Significance
Reason for Seeking Health Care	Why are you seeking health care?	Signs and symptoms of hematologic/lymphatic disorders may be nonspecific. Any body system can be involved.
Family History	How is the health of your blood relatives? Does anyone in your family have any blood-related diseases?	Some blood and immune disorders are hereditary.
Diet History	Describe your usual diet.	Dietary deficiencies can lead to anemia or altered immune responses.
Medications/Supplements	What medications do you take? What herbs or alternative therapies do you use? How much alcohol do you drink each day?	Herbs and drugs can cause adverse reactions in the blood and immune system. Excess alcohol intake can lead to folic acid–deficiency anemia.
Occupational/Exposure History	What is your occupational history? What is your military history?	Exposure to certain hazardous substances can lead to leukemias, other cancers, or anemias.
Fatigue	Have you noticed any change in your energy level?	Anemia and many cancers are associated with fatigue.
Bleeding Tendency	Have you experienced nosebleeds or any other unusual bleeding? Have you had bloody or black bowel movements?	Bleeding may indicate low platelet levels or a clotting factor deficiency.
Respiratory	Do you experience shortness of breath or faintness?	Red blood cells carry oxygen, so a reduced RBC count can cause dyspnea.
Integumentary	Have you noticed any changes in your skin?	Bleeding into the skin or mucous membranes can indicate a bleeding disorder.
Lymphadenopathy	Have you noticed swelling in your neck, armpits, or groin?	Swollen lymph nodes may indicate inflammation, infection, or some cancers.

TABLE 27.4 OBJECTIVE DATA COLLECTION FOR THE HEMATOLOGIC AND LYMPHATIC SYSTEMS

Category	Abnormal Findings	Possible Hematologic/Lymphatic Causes
Vital Signs	Fever	Poor immune function, infection
	Subnormal temperature	Possible overwhelming gram-negative infection
	Elevated heart rate	Blood loss
	Elevated respiratory rate	Decreased oxygen supply
Level of Consciousness	Decreased level	Hypoxia, fever, intracranial bleeding
Skin, Mucous Membranes	Pallor	Anemia
	Cyanosis	Poor oxygenation of RBCs
	Jaundice (yellow color)	Hemolysis, liver involvement
	Inflammation, redness, swelling, drainage	Poor immune function, infection
	Purpura, ecchymoses, petechiae	Bleeding disorder
	Dry or coarse skin	Some anemias
	Itching	Blood or lymph disorders, jaundice, liver involvement
Fingernails	Striations	Anemia
	Spoon-shaped nails	Anemia
	Clubbed fingers	Long-term hypoxia, anemia
Abdomen	High-pitched, tinkling bowel sounds	Intestinal obstruction
	Increasing abdominal girth	Ascites, bleeding
Neck, Axillae	Lymph nodes > 1 cm in size or tender nodes	**Lymphedema**, inflammation, some cancers
Sternum	Tenderness	Bone marrow "packed" with abnormal cells

concentration (Hgb), hematocrit level (Hct), and platelet level. (See normal values in Table 27.1.)

CRITICAL THINKING

Mrs. Brown

■ Mrs. Brown is on warfarin (Coumadin) therapy because of a blood clot in her leg. She has a PT drawn at the lab, and the result is 12 seconds. Will the physician most likely increase her daily dose of warfarin, decrease it, or leave it the same? (Use Table 27.5 to figure out the answer.)

Suggested answer at end of chapter.

Coagulation Tests

Coagulation tests include prothrombin time (PT), international normalized ratio (INR), partial thromboplastin time (PTT), thrombin clotting time (TCT), bleeding times, and the capillary fragility test (Table 27.5). Agglutination tests include ABO blood typing, Rh typing, crossmatching of blood samples, and direct antiglobulin tests (also known as Coombs' test).

Bone Marrow Biopsy

Biopsy information can be obtained through removal of a small amount of bone marrow with a needle. In most states this procedure must be performed by a physician. Aspiration of liquid and biopsy of the solid portion of the bone marrow are done to obtain a specimen that can be viewed under the microscope. Purposes of this test include the diagnosis of hematologic disorders; monitoring the course of treatment; discovery of other disorders, such as primary and metastatic tumors, infectious diseases, and certain granulomas; and isolation of bacteria and other pathogens by culture.

• WORD • BUILDING •

lymphedema: lymph—fluid found in lymphatic vessels + edema—swelling

LEARNING TIP

When a patient has a bacterial infection, the neutrophils, which are the most numerous of the white blood cells (WBCs), rise in number to help fight it. There are two forms of neutrophils: segmented (mature) and bands (immature). Initially, the number of segmented neutrophils rises. Then, as the infection becomes more severe, the number of immature bands begins to rise.

An easy way to remember this is that the WBCs are part of the body's defenses, just like the military is part of a country's defenses. When needed, sergeants who are fully trained or mature are called to assess the battle first. If they are unable to fight off the invading enemy, new recruits being trained in boot camp are called in to help.

So segmented neutrophils (called **S**egs) are like the **S**ergeants, fully mature and ready to fight. The **B**ands are like **B**oot camp recruits, immature and not fully trained. However, in an acute infection, bands are needed to keep the body from being overwhelmed by the infection and losing the battle.

Continued

LEARNING TIP—cont'd

As you look at the differential WBC count, if the segs are elevated but the bands are normal, the infection is probably new. If the bands are also elevated, the infection is worsening. The more elevated they are, the more severe the infection.

Lymphocytes fight viral infections and are elevated during a virus. A common pattern in the WBCs is produced for either a bacterial or viral infection. If the infection is acute bacterial:

Segs ↑ Bands ↑ Lymphocytes ↓

If the infection is viral:

Segs ↓ Bands ↓ Lymphocytes ↑

This can be remembered as the bone marrow producing the cells most needed during the time of viral infection and reducing production of those cells least needed. When the infection is resolved, all of the cells should return to their normal production levels.

An accurate bone marrow specimen in an adult can be obtained from the sternum, the spinous processes of the vertebrae, or the anterior or posterior iliac crest. Bone marrow biopsy is considered a minor surgical procedure, and is carried out under aseptic conditions. For iliac crest aspiration, the patient is placed comfortably on the side with the back slightly flexed. The posterior iliac crest is cleansed and covered with antiseptic solution. The skin, the subcutaneous tissue, and the periosteum are anesthetized using 1% or 2% lidocaine (Xylocaine). A 2- to 3-mm incision is made to facilitate penetration with a 14-gauge, 2- to 4-cm-long bone marrow needle. The incision is made to avoid introducing a skin plug into the marrow cavity, which can cause infection.

The nurse's role in bone marrow biopsy is multifaceted. You may need to help coordinate between the laboratory and the physician, establishing a time to do the procedure and determining who obtains the supplies, such as the disposable bone marrow aspiration tray and specialized needles, from the central supply department. Be sure to obtain an order for an analgesic, and administer it before the procedure. You may help position the patient before and during the procedure, help the patient maintain the needed position, and observe the aspiration site for bleeding and infection. You can also provide emotional support to the patient before, during, and after the procedure.

SAFETY TIP

For all surgical and nonsurgical invasive procedures, the intended procedure site should be marked. Before the start of any invasive procedure, a final verification process is conducted to confirm the correct procedure, for the correct patient, at the correct site. The patient is involved in the verification process when possible (2010 National Patient Safety Goals, www.jointcommission.org).

TABLE 27.5 COAGULATION STUDIES

Test	Normal Value	Significance of Abnormal Findings
Prothrombin time (PT) (affected by activity of clotting factors V, VII, X, prothrombin, and fibrinogen)	*Male:* 9.6–11.8 seconds *Female:* 9.5–11.3 seconds *Therapeutic range:* 1.5–2.0 times normal for patient on warfarin (Coumadin) therapy	Abnormalities in these values when the patient is not receiving anticoagulant therapy can indicate liver malfunction and bleeding tendency.
International normalized ratio (standardized test adopted by World Health Organization)	Less than 1.3 *Therapeutic range:* 2.0–3.0 for patient on warfarin (Coumadin) (3.0–4.5 for recurrent problems)	
Partial thromboplastin time (PTT) (affected by activity of clotting factors, prothrombin, and fibrinogen)	30–45 seconds *Therapeutic range:* 1.5–2.0 times normal for patient on heparin therapy	
Thrombin clotting time (TCT) (measures time for fibrin clot to form after addition of thrombin)	10–15 seconds *Therapeutic range:* 1.5–2.0 times normal for patient on heparin therapy	Prolonged TCT indicates fibrinogen deficiency.
Bleeding time (measures time for small puncture wound to stop bleeding)	2.5–9.5 minutes	Prolonged bleeding time indicates a platelet disorder.
Capillary fragility test	Fewer than 10 petechiae appearing in a 2-inch circle after application of a blood pressure cuff at 100 mm Hg for 5 minutes	Tests ability of capillaries to resist rupture under pressure. More than 10 petechiae could be related to fragile capillaries or thrombocytopenia.

Lymphangiography

Problems in the lymph system, such as lymphoma or metastatic cancers, can be evaluated using lymphangiography. This procedure involves injection of a dye into the lymphatic vessels of the hand or foot. Various x-ray views are then taken to determine lymph flow or blockages. X-ray examinations are repeated in 24 hours to assess lymph node involvement.

Following the procedure, the physician may order a pressure dressing and immobilization of the injected limb to prevent bleeding at the site. Continue to monitor the limb for swelling, circulatory status, and changes in sensation. Warn the patient that the skin, urine, or feces may be tinged blue from the dye for about 2 days.

Lymph Node Biopsy

If a lymph node is enlarged, it may be biopsied to determine whether the cause is infection or malignancy. A biopsy may be done with a needle aspiration or surgical incision. A small dressing or bandage is applied to the site. Following the procedure, review signs of bleeding and infection with the patient that should be reported to the physician.

THERAPEUTIC MEASURES FOR THE HEMATOLOGIC AND LYMPHATIC SYSTEMS

Blood Administration

Blood may be administered by a registered nurse (RN) or licensed practical nurse/licensed vocational nurse (LPN/LVN), depending on the state in which you practice. Some states require that only RNs administer blood. As an LPN/LVN, you may be called on to assist with proper identification procedures and monitoring of vital signs during the transfusion.

Table 27.6 lists blood components that may be ordered. The main goals are to administer them safely and to avoid mistakes. Make sure to use proper identifying information to ensure that the right patient is receiving the right blood products. In addition, it is important to note that some institutions require a special transfusion consent form to be completed and present in the patient's chart. A careful system most often used in health care institutions is outlined next.

Safety Steps

BASELINE DATA COLLECTION Before the blood transfusion, it is important to assess the patient's vital signs and history of transfusions or transfusion reactions. Vital signs provide baseline data. If the patient has had a reaction in the past, be sure to alert the physician and the lab before proceeding.

TABLE 27.6 BLOOD PRODUCTS

Product	Use
Packed red blood cells	Severe anemia or blood loss
Frozen red blood cells	Autotransfusion (blood taken from patient and saved for future surgery), prevention of febrile reactions
Platelets	Bleeding caused by thrombocytopenia
Albumin	Hypovolemia caused by hypoalbuminemia
Fresh frozen plasma	Provides clotting factors for bleeding disorders; occasionally used for volume replacement
Cryoprecipitates	Bleeding caused by specific missing clotting factors

IDENTIFICATION. Safety is the first priority. This includes checking and double checking the patient's identity. Great care is taken in the blood bank to match the donor's blood type with the recipient's blood type. After obtaining the unit of blood from the blood bank but before hanging the unit, two nurses (according to the state's guidelines) will perform the following tasks at the patient's bedside (Fig. 27.3). Do not take this identification step for granted because if you make an error and accidentally transfuse blood that does not match the patient's blood type, the result can be fatal.

- Ask the patient to state his or her name and birth date aloud if alert and able to speak.
- Use the patient's identification band to confirm the identity, and compare it with the information on the paperwork obtained from the blood bank.
- Examine the blood bag and verify that the patient information and any other information, such as the ABO type, Rh type, and unit number, all match.
- Finally, check the expiration date on the blood bag.

SAFETY TIP

Before starting a blood or blood component transfusion, use a two-person verification process to (1) match the blood or blood component to the order and (2) match the patient to the blood or blood component.

Note: If two people are not available, an automated identification technology (for example, bar coding) may be used in place of one of the people (2010 National Patient Safety Goals, www.jointcommission.org).

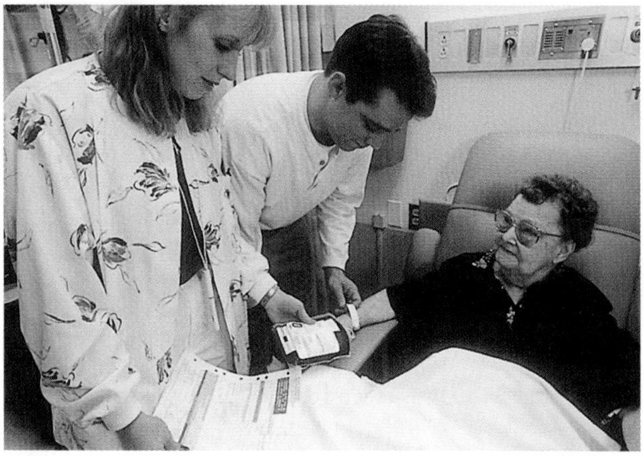

FIGURE 27.3 Two nurses check a patient's identification before administering a unit of blood.

Do not give the unit of blood if any of the information does not match. Notify the blood bank immediately of any discrepancies, and delay the transfusion until the differences have been resolved. Remember, there is no room for error when transfusing blood products.

FILTERING. Filters are used with blood administration tubing to prevent potentially harmful particles from entering the patient. Most often, the filter that comes with the transfusion tubing is sufficient for each unit of packed RBCs. In some situations, special filters may be needed to remove leukocytes or microaggregates. The blood bank can advise in these situations.

WASHED OR LEUKOCYTE-DEPLETED BLOOD. In some instances packed RBCs (PRBCs) are ordered as "washed" and often arrive from the blood bank in a special round bag. The washing process removes almost all of the plasma and can decrease the risk or severity of a febrile reaction. In addition, leukocyte filters may be used to completely remove all WBCs. This removal process is used in cases in which many transfusions are anticipated, because it decreases the chance of antigen sensitization. It can also reduce transmission of certain viruses, such as cytomegalovirus.

WARMED BLOOD. If the patient has had a severe bleeding episode and the nurses are helping to give replacement therapy through rapid, multiple transfusions, the physician may consider ordering a blood warmer. It works just as the name implies, warming the cold blood from the blood bank to the standard body temperature of 98.6°F (37.0°C). This warming helps prevent hypothermia, which can cause heart dysrhythmias, and shivering, which can destroy blood cells and platelets.

Administration

GUIDELINES. It is important to use the correct intravenous needle size to infuse blood. The best sizes are 18- or 20-gauge catheters to prevent the hemolysis of RBCs that can occur with smaller catheters. Make sure to use only normal saline solution to help dilute the blood and to flush the intravenous lines before and after the transfusions. Solutions that contain dextrose can cause red cells to lyse, and solutions with calcium can cause the blood product to clump, clot, or not infuse at all. Generally, 2 hours is a good time frame within which to transfuse each unit of packed cells. If it must transfuse more slowly because of the patient's condition, make sure the unit does not hang longer than 4 hours to prevent deterioration and bacterial proliferation.

MONITORING. Carefully monitor the patient's response to the transfusion to prevent complications or to detect and treat them quickly if they occur. Stay with the patient for the first 15 minutes of the blood transfusion to assess for any immediate reactions. The 15 minutes begins when the blood enters the vein. If saline solution is in the tubing, it may take several minutes before the blood reaches the patient. Check and document vital signs before starting the transfusion, after the blood has begun to infuse, and after the infusion is complete. Some institutions require vital sign monitoring every 15 to 30 minutes during the earliest part of the transfusion and then slightly less often for the duration of the infusion. Always follow institution guidelines. During the transfusion, assess the patient for signs and symptoms of transfusion reactions.

Complications

Quick detection of complications can be lifesaving. It is easy to think of transfusing blood components as a routine procedure because it is a common activity. Do not be fooled. It is a serious procedure that can be life threatening if errors occur. Complications include febrile reactions, hypersensitivities, hemolytic reactions, anaphylaxis, circulatory overload, and even death. Regular monitoring according to institution policy can help detect complications early when treatment can be most effective.

FEBRILE REACTION. By far the most common reaction is fever (febrile reaction). It occurs up to 2% of the time. The risk of a febrile reaction goes up with each unit of blood product given to the patient. Many times, febrile reactions occur after the transfusion is completed, but they can occur at any time. This is the reason for obtaining a set of baseline vital signs, including the patient's temperature. Once a febrile reaction begins, the most common signs are an increasing fever and shaking chills, which can be severe. Other symptoms may include headache and back pain. If febrile symptoms occur, stop the transfusion and notify the physician. Acetaminophen may be ordered. If a hemolytic reaction is not suspected, the physician may order the transfusion to continue once the patient is more comfortable. Make sure that the 4-hour hang rule is not violated. Future febrile reactions can usually be prevented by administering leukocyte-depleted blood as described previously.

URTICARIAL REACTION. Urticarial (hive) reactions are considered to be minor allergic reactions and are usually associated with antigens in the plasma accompanying the transfusion. There may be a fever, but the cardinal sign is the appearance of urticaria, a hive-like rash. On discovery of this reaction, stop the transfusion and notify the physician immediately. Expect that the patient will be given a dose of an antihistamine, such as diphenhydramine (Benadryl). If the transfusion is restarted, continue to monitor the patient closely. Again, make sure the 4-hour hang rule is not violated.

HEMOLYTIC REACTION. The most deadly and, fortunately, the rarest of the possible reactions is an acute hemolytic reaction. The cause of this reaction is transfusion of incompatible blood. The result is hemolysis (destruction) of RBCs. Usually, this type of serious reaction is noticed within minutes of starting the transfusion. The patient may report back pain, chest pain, chills, fever, shortness of breath, nausea, vomiting, or a feeling of impending doom. As the reaction progresses, the patient begins to show signs of shock, hypotension, oliguria, and decreased consciousness. Late signs and symptoms include those associated with disseminated intravascular coagulation: uncontrollable bleeding from many different sites at the same time, usually ending in death.

At the first sign of this type of reaction, immediately stop the transfusion and stay with the patient. Institute emergency procedures to notify the charge nurse, the physician, and the blood bank. Keep the vein open with normal saline using a new tubing set (ensuring that no more incompatible blood is administered) so that emergency drugs can be administered. High volumes of fluids are administered to decrease shock and hypotension, and high doses of diuretics are given to promote urine flow because the kidneys are the most likely organs to be damaged. Dialysis may be instituted.

ANAPHYLACTIC REACTION. Anaphylactic reactions are not common but may be seen more often in patients who have received many transfusions or have had many pregnancies. Usually, the source of the anaphylaxis is sensitization to immune globulins passed from the donor's unit of blood product. In this type of reaction, the very first milliliters of blood containing the allergens to pass into the patient's system may be enough to cause the patient to develop respiratory or cardiovascular collapse. Other more common symptoms include severe gastrointestinal cramping, instant vomiting, and uncontrollable diarrhea.

If the patient exhibits these signs and symptoms, stop the transfusion at once and stay with the patient. Have someone else notify the registered nurse and the physician, using institutional emergency procedures. Emergency resuscitation measures, including cardiopulmonary resuscitation if necessary, must be instituted until the code team arrives. Expect the patient to be intubated and receive oxygen, steroids, and other drugs as needed for life support. After the emergency has passed, this patient will likely need to receive transfusions from frozen, deglycerolized blood cells.

CIRCULATORY OVERLOAD. Circulatory overload is caused by rapid transfusion in a short period, particularly in older and debilitated patients. Usual signs and symptoms include chest pain, cough, frothy sputum, distended neck veins, crackles and wheezes in the lung fields, and increased heart rate. If symptoms occur, stop the transfusion and notify the physician. Anticipate administration of diuretics, which help get rid of the excess fluid. The transfusion may be restarted later at a slower rate (Box 27.1, *Gerontological Issues*).

Box 27.1

Gerontological Issues

Older patients have less cardiac and renal ability to adapt to changes in blood volume, so they have a much higher risk of fluid overload when receiving blood transfusions. Carefully monitor lung sounds and vital signs both before and during a transfusion. New onset of dyspnea, crackles, hypertension, or bounding pulse should be reported to the registered nurse or physician immediately.

SUGGESTED ANSWERS TO

CRITICAL THINKING

■ *Mrs. Brown*

The physician will most likely increase Mrs. Brown's warfarin dose. Note in Table 27.5 that the PT for a patient on warfarin should be 1.5 to 2.0 times normal. That is the reason the warfarin is ordered—to prolong the time it takes for blood to clot. If a normal PT is 9.5 to 11.3 seconds, a therapeutic PT for Mrs. Brown would be 14.25 seconds (9.5 × 1.5) to 22.6 (11.3 × 2.0). Her result of 12 seconds is not therapeutic.

REVIEW QUESTIONS

1. Clotting factors such as prothrombin are produced by which structure?
   a. Red bone marrow
   b. Liver
   c. Spleen
   d. Lymph nodes

2. Which of the following best describes the function of erythropoietin?
   a. Increases production of platelets to promote clotting.
   b. Decreases production of platelets to prevent abnormal clotting.
   c. Increases RBC production to correct hypoxia.
   d. Decreases RBC production to prevent hypoxia.

3. Why is the return of tissue fluid to the blood important?
   a. To maintain blood clotting
   b. To maintain blood volume
   c. To promote white blood cell formation
   d. To promote red blood cell formation

4. Which of the following is the portion of the blood in which cellular elements are suspended?
   a. Cytoplasm
   b. Platelets
   c. Plasma
   d. Hemoglobin

5. Which of the following actions should the nurse take when caring for a patient with a platelet count of 23,000/mm^3?
   a. Request an order for an anticoagulant.
   b. Protect the patient from injury.
   c. Encourage the patient to drink plenty of fluids.
   d. No action is necessary. This is a normal level.

6. A nurse is assessing a patient and finds small red-purple dots over most of his skin surfaces. The patient says that he has not noticed them before. Which action should the nurse take first?
   a. Report the findings immediately to the registered nurse or physician.
   b. Document the findings objectively in the medical record.
   c. Assist the patient to apply lotion.
   d. Administer an antihistamine as needed.

7. Which of the following checks should be done before starting a blood transfusion? **Select all that apply.**
   a. Ask the patient to state his or her name.
   b. Verify the correct room number.
   c. Check the patient's arm band.
   d. Check the identifying information on the unit of blood.
   e. Check the temperature of the blood.
   f. Check the expiration date on the unit of blood.

8. A nurse is monitoring a patient during a blood transfusion. After the blood has been hanging for 30 minutes, the patient's temperature rises from 98.6°F (37.0°C) at baseline to 101.0°F (38.3°C). The patient also experiences severe chills. Which action should the nurse take first?
   a. Document the vital signs in the medical record.
   b. Administer acetaminophen for the fever.
   c. Notify the physician of the change.
   d. Stop the transfusion and hang normal saline solution.

Reference

Joint Commission. (2010). *2010 national patient safety goals*. Retrieved January 13, 2010, from http://www.jointcommission.org/patientsafety/nationalpatientsafetygoals

28

Nursing Care of Patients with Hematologic and Lymphatic Disorders

LUCY L. COLO

KEY TERMS

anemia (uh-NEE-mee-yah)
aplastic (ay-PLAS-tik)
disseminated intravascular coagulation (dis-SEM-ih-NAY-ted IN-trah-VAS-kyoo-lar koh-AG-yoo-LAY-shun)
glossitis (gloss-SY-tiss)
hemarthrosis (HEEM-ar-THROH-sis)
hemolysis (hee-MAHL-eh-sis)
hemolytic (HEE-moh-LIT-ik)
hemophilia (HEE-moh-FILL-ee-ah)
idiopathic thrombocytopenic purpura (ID-ee-oh-PATH-ik THROMB-boh-SY-toh-PEE-nik PURR-purr-rah)
leukemia (loo-KEE-mee-ah)
lymphoma (lim-FOH-mah)
pancytopenia (PAN-sy-toh-PEE-nee-ah)
panmyelosis (PAN-my-eh-LOH-sis)
pathological fracture (PATH-uh-LAW-jik-uhl FRAK-chur)
phlebotomy (fleh-BAW-tuh-mee)
polycythemia (PAW-lee-sy-THEE-mee-ah)
splenectomy (spleh-NEK-tuh-mee)
splenomegaly (SPLEE-noh-MEG-ah-lee)
thrombocytopenia (THROM-boh-SY-toh-PEE-nee-ah)

QUESTIONS TO GUIDE YOUR READING

1. What is the pathophysiology of each of the hematologic and lymphatic disorders discussed in this chapter?
2. What are the etiologies, signs, and symptoms of each disorder?
3. What tests are useful for diagnosis of each of the disorders?
4. What are the current therapeutic measures for each disorder?
5. What data should you collect when caring for patients with disorders of the hematologic or lymphatic systems?
6. What nursing care will you provide for patients with hematologic disorders?
7. What nursing care will you provide for patients with lymphatic disorders?
8. How will you know if your nursing interventions have been effective?
9. What precautions should you institute to prevent bleeding in patients with clotting disorders?
10. What nursing care and teaching will you provide for patients undergoing a splenectomy?

HEMATOLOGIC DISORDERS

Patients with hematologic disorders have problems related to their blood. Some problems are caused by too many cells, others by too few or defective cells. When red blood cells (RBCs) are affected, oxygen transport is also affected, causing symptoms related to poor oxygenation. When white blood cells (WBCs) are affected, the patient is unable to effectively fight infections. If platelets or clotting factors are affected, bleeding disorders occur.

DISORDERS OF RED BLOOD CELLS

Anemias

The term **anemia** describes a condition in which there is a deficiency of RBCs, hemoglobin, or both, in the circulating blood. Because hemoglobin carries oxygen, this results in a reduced capacity to deliver oxygen to the tissues, producing symptoms such as weakness and shortness of breath, which lead the patient to seek medical help.

Pathophysiology

A decrease in the number of RBCs can be traced to three different conditions: (1) impaired production of RBCs, as in **aplastic** anemia and nutrition deficiencies; (2) increased destruction of RBCs, as in **hemolytic** or sickle cell anemia; or (3) massive or chronic blood loss. Some anemias are related to genetic problems in certain cultures (Box 28.1, *Cultural Considerations*). It is important to remember that the general term *anemia* refers to a symptom or a condition secondary to another problem and is not a diagnosis in itself. Different types of anemia are discussed later in this chapter.

Etiology

DIETARY DEFICIENCIES. Iron, folic acid, and vitamin B_{12} are all essential to the production of healthy RBCs. A deficiency of any of these nutrients can cause anemia. Pernicious anemia is associated with a lack of intrinsic factor in stomach secretions, which is necessary for absorption of vitamin B_{12}. See Box 28.2, *Nutrition Notes,* for more information.

HEMOLYSIS. Hemolysis is the destruction, or lysis, of RBCs. Destruction of RBCs leads to a type of anemia called hemolytic anemia. This may be a congenital disorder or it may be caused by exposure to certain toxins.

OTHER CAUSES. Thalassemia anemia is a hereditary anemia found in persons from Southeast Asia, Africa, Italy, and the Mediterranean islands. People with thalassemia do not synthesize hemoglobin normally. Those with chronic disease also develop anemia (Box 28.3, *Gerontological Issues*). Additional causes of anemia are discussed under the separate headings of aplastic and sickle cell anemias.

Signs and Symptoms

Symptoms of anemia include pallor, tachycardia, tachypnea, irritability, fatigue, and shortness of breath (Table 28.1). These symptoms occur because of the reduced number of functioning RBCs, with reduced ability to carry oxygen to tissues. In addition to these symptoms, the patient with pernicious (vitamin B_{12}) anemia may experience numbness of

• WORD • BUILDING •

anemia: a—not + emia—blood
aplastic: a—not + plastic—develop
hemolytic: heme—blood + lytic—break down
hemolysis: heme—blood + lysis—dissolution

Box 28.1

Cultural Considerations

In the past, Iranian cross-cousin marriages have resulted in an increased incidence of several forms of anemia and hemophilia. These marriages are now being addressed through genetic counseling and premarital screening for carriers.

A sex-linked genetic disease common in the Chinese is glucose-6-phosphate dehydrogenase (G6PD) deficiency, an enzyme deficiency affecting the person's red blood cells and resulting in anemia. Mediterranean G6PD deficiency is common, causing a hemolytic crisis when fava beans are eaten, when aspirin or certain other drugs are taken, or in acidotic or hypoxemic states. Mediterranean-type G6PD deficiency is an inherited disorder most fully expressed in males, with a carrier state in females.

Among Asian Indians, sickle cell disease is highly prevalent; the gene is detected in 16.5% of selected populations. Sickle cell anemia is the most common genetic disorder among African American populations. Sickle cell anemia is also found in individuals who live in areas where malaria is endemic, such as the Caribbean, the Middle East, the Mediterranean region, and Asia.

Box 28.2

Nutrition Notes

Understanding Common Nutritional Anemias

Nutritional deficiencies can produce some forms of anemia. Nutrients vital to the synthesis of red blood cells (RBCs) include iron, folic acid, and vitamin B_{12}. Even if the cause of the anemia is dietary, other therapies may be employed in addition to nutritional interventions.

Microcytic Anemia

Iron-deficiency anemia, the most common nutrient deficiency in the world, is characterized by smaller-than-normal RBCs. Insufficient intake of iron, excessive blood loss, or lack of stomach acid can lead to iron-deficiency anemia. Those at greatest risk of iron deficiency are women of childbearing age and young children. Even before obvious anemia is seen, cognitive abilities can be impaired.

The following are relatively good sources of iron that are commonly included in Western diets:

- Red meat
- Dark green leafy vegetables
- Dried fruits
- Enriched, fortified, or whole-grain products.

Techniques to enhance absorption of iron from nonmeat sources include the following:

- Consuming foods rich in vitamin C with iron-rich foods
- Stewing acidic foods such as tomatoes in iron cookware.

If iron supplements are given to treat iron deficiency, they should be continued for several months after hemoglobin and hematocrit levels return to normal to enable the body to rebuild iron stores.

Macrocytic Anemia

Folic acid or vitamin B_{12} deficiencies produce anemias characterized by larger-than-normal RBCs.

Folic acid aids in the formation of DNA and heme, the iron-containing portion of hemoglobin. Conditions that increase the metabolic rate increase the need for folic acid. Many drugs, including alcohol, anticonvulsants, and oral contraceptives, interfere with its absorption, metabolism, or excretion and can lead to anemia.

Good food sources of folic acid include the following:

- Liver
- Green leafy vegetables
- Legumes
- Enriched grain products.

Because folic acid markedly decreases the occurrence of fetal neural tube defects such as spina bifida, women capable of becoming pregnant are advised to consume 400 mcg of synthetic folic acid daily from fortified foods or supplements in addition to the folic acid furnished by a varied, balanced diet.

Vitamin B_{12} is essential for the manufacture of RBCs and for synthesis and maintenance of myelin, the fatty covering of nerves that facilitates rapid transmission of impulses. Vitamin B_{12} requires a highly specific protein-binding factor called intrinsic factor, secreted by glands in the stomach, to transport the vitamin to the ileum for absorption.

Vitamin B_{12} is found in foods from animal sources such as these:

- Meat
- Fish and shellfish
- Poultry
- Milk.

A healthy person eating these foods regularly is not at risk of vitamin B_{12} deficiency, but strict vegetarians are at risk. Because the deficiency in this case is dietary, a dietary supplement is the treatment.

Continued lack of vitamin B_{12} can cause irreparable nerve damage. Vitamin B_{12} deficiency should be considered in a person being evaluated for dementia.

the hands or feet and weakness because vitamin B_{12} is needed for normal neurologic function. Pernicious anemia is also associated with a sore, beefy red tongue. Patients with iron deficiency may have fissures at the corners of the mouth, an inflamed tongue (**glossitis**), and spoon-shaped fingernails.

• WORD • BUILDING •

glossitis: glos—tongue + itis—inflammation

Diagnostic Tests

A complete blood cell count (CBC) is done to determine the number of RBCs and WBCs per cubic millimeter. The size, color, and shape of the blood cells are determined by microscopic examination. Hemoglobin and hematocrit levels are below normal in anemia. Serum iron, ferritin, and total iron-binding capacity measurements are done to diagnose iron-deficiency anemia. Serum folate is measured if folic acid deficiency is suspected. A bone marrow biopsy and analysis may also be done.

Box 28.3

Gerontological Issues

Anemia of chronic disease is often diagnosed in an older patient who has an underlying medical condition that causes altered iron metabolism, deficiency of erythropoietin, or shortened life span of red blood cells. Unfortunately, anemia of chronic disease is often mistaken for iron-deficiency anemia. Nutritional deficiencies and blood loss are common causes of iron-deficiency anemia.

Patients with pernicious anemia have low gastric acid levels, and many have antibodies to intrinsic factor. Both abnormalities are associated with poor absorption of vitamin B_{12}. If blood loss is suspected, additional tests are done to determine the source of bleeding.

Therapeutic Measures

Treatment begins with elimination of contributing causes. Intake of the deficient nutrient can sometimes be increased in the diet or administered as a supplement (see Box 28.2, *Nutrition Notes*). Changing cooking habits, taking dietary supplements, decreasing alcohol intake, and controlling chronic diarrhea can help correct folic acid deficiency. If symptoms of anemia are acute, a blood transfusion may be needed.

Nursing Process for the Patient with Anemia

DATA COLLECTION. Monitor hemoglobin and hematocrit levels and other laboratory studies as ordered and report any downward trend. Monitor responses to therapy, the patient's fatigue level, and the patient's ability to ambulate safely and perform activities of daily living (ADLs). Monitor degree of dyspnea. Assess for pallor in the skin and conjunctivae.

NURSING DIAGNOSES, PLANNING, AND IMPLEMENTATION. Possible nursing diagnoses are listed next along with outcomes and interventions.

Activity Intolerance Related to Tissue Hypoxia and Dyspnea

EXPECTED OUTCOME: The patient will be able to tolerate activity as evidenced by the ability to complete ADLs with minimal assistance. The patient will have knowledge about conserving energy as evidenced by a verbal statement.

- Monitor vital signs to evaluate tolerance to activity. *The patient experiencing activity intolerance may have tachycardia, increased respiratory rate, and decreased blood pressure with activity.*
- If the pulse or respiratory rate increases more than 20% from baseline during activity, reduce the activity level. *This is evidence that the activity is too strenuous and can result in increased hypoxia and dyspnea.*
- Plan care to conserve energy after periods of activity. *Balancing activities and rest periods assists the patient to conserve energy.*
- Assist the patient with self-care activities as needed. *Assisting with ADLs helps to decrease the amount of energy expended by the patient.*
- Place articles within easy reach of the patient *to reduce physiological demands on the body.*
- Encourage the patient to limit visitors, telephone calls, and unnecessary interruptions *to conserve energy.*
- Administer oxygen as ordered to relieve dyspnea. *The patient with anemia does not have enough hemoglobin to carry oxygen to vital organs.*
- Assist with blood transfusion as ordered if hemoglobin levels are very low or symptoms are severe. *A blood transfusion is a quick way to raise hemoglobin levels and to correct severe symptoms.*

Imbalanced Nutrition: Less Than Body Requirements Related to Disease, Treatment, or Lack of Knowledge of Adequate Nutrition

EXPECTED OUTCOME: The patient will (1) have improved nutrition as evidenced by stable weight and stable hemoglobin

TABLE 28.1 CLINICAL MANIFESTATIONS OF ANEMIA

Body System	Mild (Hgb 10–14 g/dL)	Moderate (Hgb 6–10 g/dL)	Severe (Hgb less than 6 g/dL)
Skin	None	None	Pallor, jaundice, pruritus
Eyes	None	None	Jaundiced conjunctivae and sclerae, retinal hemorrhages, blurred vision
Mouth	None	None	Glossitis, smooth tongue
Cardiovascular	Palpitations	Increased palpitations	Tachycardia, increased pulse pressure, systolic murmurs, angina, congestive heart failure, myocardial infarction
Lungs	Exertional dyspnea	Significant dyspnea	Tachypnea, orthopnea, dyspnea at rest
Neurologic	None	None	Headache, vertigo, irritability, depression, impaired thought processes
Gastrointestinal	None	None	Anorexia, hepatomegaly, splenomegaly
Musculoskeletal	None	None	Bone pain
General	None	Fatigue	Sensitivity to cold, weight loss, lethargy

and hematocrit, and (2) will be able to appropriately select foods that will meet nutritional requirements.

- Consult a dietitian *to provide diet instruction if the anemia is caused by a dietary deficiency.*
- Teach the patient with folic acid deficiency that daily requirements can be met by including foods from each food group at every meal. *A balanced diet includes adequate amounts of folic acid.*
- Administer supplements as ordered *when dietary intake alone is not sufficient.*
- Instruct the patient to take the supplements as ordered by the physician. *The patient should not stop taking the medication until the physician advises him or her to do so.*
- Instruct the patient that vitamin B_{12} injections are given for lifetime with pernicious anemia *because it is a chronic disease.*
- Instruct the patient with iron deficiency about high-iron foods and the correct use of an iron supplement. *An iron supplement should be taken with vitamin C to enhance absorption.*
- Instruct the patient to notify the primary care provider of any side effects related to iron supplements *such as nausea, diarrhea, constipation, and dark stools.*
- Administer intramuscular iron injections by the Z-track method *to avoid staining the injection site.*
- Administer liquid supplements with a drinking straw *to avoid staining the teeth.*

Risk for Falls Related to Weakness and Dizziness

EXPECTED OUTCOMES: The patient will remain safe from injuries related to a fall.

- Assess the patient at risk for falls using a fall risk assessment tool *to determine risk.*
- Assist the patient to change positions slowly *to decrease dizziness and risk of falls.*
- Assist the patient with ambulation *to prevent a fall.*
- Protect the patient with pernicious anemia from injuries resulting from decreased sensation (e.g., take special care with heating pads and turning and positioning) *because the ability to sense pain may be impaired.*

Impaired Oral Mucous Membranes Related to Altered Dietary Status

EXPECTED OUTCOME: The patient will have intact oral mucous membranes.

- Monitor condition of oral mucous membranes *to detect changes.*
- Provide good oral hygiene *to keep the oral cavity clean and prevent infection.*
- Encourage soft, bland foods, *which are more tolerable until healing can occur.*
- Instruct the patient to use a soft toothbrush for oral care *because it is more gentle until the healing can occur.*

EVALUATION. When successfully treated, the patient should be able to tolerate a normal level of activity without shortness of breath or excess fatigue. The patient should be able to explain the correct treatment plan and therapeutic measures for long-term prevention of problems, including dietary choices and supplements as well as self-care measures. The patient will remain free from injury, and the oral mucosa will be intact.

Aplastic Anemia

PATHOPHYSIOLOGY. Aplastic anemia differs from other types of anemia in that the bone marrow becomes fatty and incapable of producing the needed numbers of RBCs. Also known as hypoplastic anemia, the cells that are produced are normal in size and shape, but there are not enough of them to sustain life. The resulting **pancytopenia** (reduced numbers of all formed elements from the bone marrow—RBCs, platelets, and WBCs) is the indicator that something is wrong with the bone marrow. Left untreated, aplastic anemia is almost always fatal.

ETIOLOGY. Aplastic anemia may be congenital—that is, the person is born with bone marrow incapable of producing the correct number of cells. Or it may be due to exposure to toxic substances such as industrial chemicals (e.g., benzenes and insecticides), chemotherapy medications, or use of cardiopulmonary bypass during surgery. Other causes include certain bacterial and viral infections, such as tuberculosis and hepatitis, or autoimmune disease.

SIGNS AND SYMPTOMS. The clinical features of aplastic anemia vary with the severity of the bone marrow failure. As with other anemias, early symptoms include progressive weakness, fatigue, pallor, shortness of breath, and headaches. As the disease progresses and the pancytopenia worsens, other symptoms, such as tachycardia and heart failure, may appear. Ecchymoses and petechiae appear on the skin surface because of the reduced platelet count (Fig. 28.1; also see Fig. 28.5). Blood may ooze from mucous membranes. Injection sites may progress from oozing to frank bleeding. Often, there is overt bleeding into vital organs. Infection occurs because of reduced WBCs. When aplastic anemia is left untreated, most patients die from infection or bleeding.

DIAGNOSTIC TESTS. The diagnosis of aplastic anemia begins with a CBC. Usually all values are very low, with the occasional exception of the RBC count, in part because of the longer life span of RBCs. Eventually the RBCs are also depleted. If the patient is having gross bleeding internally or externally, the RBC level can drop rapidly and dramatically. The most definitive test is a bone marrow biopsy. Because the bone marrow is essentially dead, the result is often described as a "dry tap," in which pale, fatty, yellow, fibrous bone marrow is extracted instead of the red, gelatinous bone

• WORD • BUILDING •

pancytopenia: pan—all + cyto—cell + penia—poverty

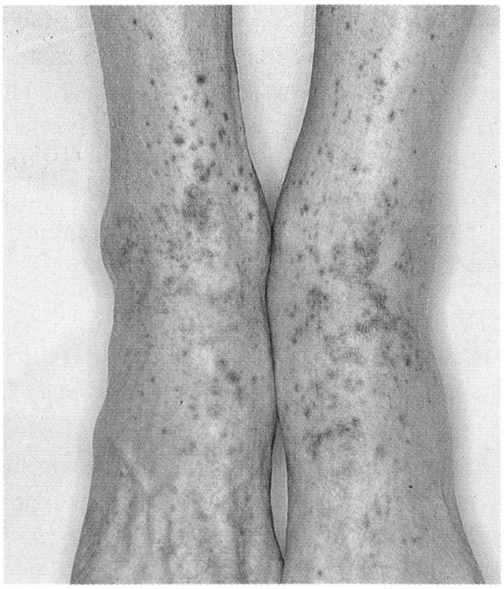

FIGURE 28.1 Petechiae on the skin from thrombocytopenia. (From Goldsmith, L. A., et al. [1997]. *Adult and pediatric dermatology* [p. 61]. Philadelphia: F. A. Davis, with permission.)

marrow normally seen. Not surprising, the more fatty and pale the marrow is, the more dysfunctional it is. Other diagnostic tests include total iron-binding capacity (TIBC) and serum iron level. It is common to find both of these levels elevated because the RBCs are not being produced and are using up the stores of iron in the production of hemoglobin.

THERAPEUTIC MEASURES. Early identification of the cause of the anemia and correction of the underlying problem are important to survival. Unfortunately, it is often difficult to determine the cause, and there is no way to reverse the damage already done. Aggressive supportive measures may be the only treatment. Most of these measures are aimed at prevention of infection and bleeding. Transfusions may be administered to replace deficient cells.

Today the most effective treatment for aplastic anemia is bone marrow transplantation (see Box 28.4, *Patient Perspective*). Another common therapy is the administration of steroids to stimulate production of cells in the weakened bone marrow. Immunosuppressant agents may be given if an autoimmune disorder is the underlying cause. Occasionally the administration of hormones may work to increase the viability of the marrow. Steroid or other treatments may be tried before attempting a bone marrow transplant.

In many treatment institutions, limited success is being obtained with the use of colony-stimulating factors, natural elements that can now be produced synthetically. (You can read more about these medications in Chapter 11.) For example, erythropoietin (Epogen) stimulates production of RBCs, and filgrastim (granulocyte colony stimulator [Neupogen]) stimulates production of WBCs. The major drawback to this type of therapy is the high cost. Many of the pharmaceutical manufacturers have patient access programs that help reduce the costs of these medications.

Box 28.4

Patient Perspective

Bone Marrow Transplant

In June 2002, I took my daughter to the doctor for her sports physical. Later that day, I received a call telling me to take her to the university hospital immediately because she had a serious life-threatening illness. I kept telling myself and my husband that our small-town hospital must have made some sort of error. As it turned out, they had not. My daughter was diagnosed with aplastic anemia and needed a bone marrow transplant. I became obsessed with the illness, poring over every tidbit of medical information I could find. Sometimes I found myself out in the car unable to remember where I was going; sometimes I had to pull over because my eyes were filled with tears and I could no longer see.

My daughter was 16 at the time of her illness, yet it is the parents who sign consent forms and make the choices in care. When the chemotherapy was started and running through the IV tubing, I felt like grabbing the tubing and pinching it off, yelling, "I need more time to think about this decision," but time was running out. Without a bone marrow transplant, she had about 8 months to live.

After transplantation, my daughter was in an isolation room for a month. I stayed with her every day, and at night I stayed at the inn that was attached to the hospital. If I was needed, I wanted to be no more than a minute away. I was one of the luckier parents because I had the financial means to manage this process. I thought about how horrible it would be if I had other children at home. Sometimes I would have such an urge to run away and escape from it all. I attended support groups that were held on the hospital unit. I got to know a lot of other parents with sick kids, and it became very upsetting to me at times. One day parents told me how well their child was doing; the next day I saw the child's room empty and thought he must have gone home, only to find out later that he had died during the night. I wondered if my daughter would be next.

I look at my daughter now, 4 years later, alive and perfectly healthy, and I tell myself that I made the right choices for her. But she tells me that if it happens again, she will not go through chemotherapy. I wonder, is chemo worse than death?

NURSING INTERVENTIONS. Nursing care of patients with symptoms related to reduced RBCs was presented earlier in the *Nursing Process for the Patient with Anemia* section. If the patient's platelet count is low (usually less than 20,000), the patient is placed on bleeding precautions (Box 28.5). If the WBC count is low, the patient must be protected from infection (Box 28.6).

Sickle Cell Anemia

PATHOPHYSIOLOGY. Sickle cell anemia is an inherited anemia in which the RBCs have a specific mutation that makes the hemoglobin in the red cells very sensitive to oxygen changes. Any time a decrease in the oxygen tension is sensed, the cells begin an observable physical change from their usual spherical shape to a sickle or crescent shape (Fig. 28.2). Sickled cells are very rigid and easily cracked and broken. The abnormal shape also causes the cells to become tangled in the blood vessels and organs. The result is congestion, clumping, and clotting.

As RBCs are broken, the cellular contents spill out into the general circulation. The resulting increase in the bilirubin level causes jaundice. Gallstones (cholelithiasis) may develop because of the increased amounts of bile pigments. The spleen and liver may enlarge because of the increase in retained cells and cellular materials.

Because the cells are fragile, the life span of the RBCs in patients with sickle cell anemia is significantly decreased. Normal red cells live about 120 days. Sickled cells survive only about 10 to 20 days, an 80% to 90% decrease in cell survival.

Box 28.5

Interventions to Prevent Bleeding in the Patient with Thrombocytopenia

- Use an electric razor instead of a safety razor for shaving.
- Use a soft toothbrush or gauze to clean the teeth. Avoid flossing.
- Avoid invasive procedures as much as possible, including enemas, douches, suppositories, and rectal temperatures.
- Avoid intramuscular injections.
- To avoid injury when checking blood pressure, pump cuff up only until pulse is obliterated.
- Avoid blood draws whenever possible. Use established access sites, or group specimen collections into once-daily draws.
- Maintain pressure on intravenous (IV), blood draw, and other puncture sites for 5 minutes.
- Encourage use of shoes or slippers when out of bed.
- Keep area clutter-free to prevent bumps and bruises.
- Avoid use of drugs that interfere with platelet function, such as aspirin products and nonsteroidal anti-inflammatory drugs (aspirin, ibuprofen, naproxen, and others).
- Administer stool softeners as ordered to prevent straining to have a bowel movement.
- Move and turn patient gently to avoid bruising.
- Instruct patient to blow nose very gently and only when necessary.
- Advise patient to consult with physician about whether sexual intercourse is safe.

Box 28.6

Interventions for the Patient at Risk for Infection

- Place the patient in a private room.
- Ensure that all staff and visitors wash hands before entering the room.
- Teach the patient to wash hands before and after using the toilet and before and after eating.
- Teach the patient and family to wash hands before touching each other.
- Prevent staff or visitors with known infections from entering the patient's room.
- Teach the patient to not handle flowers or plants brought into the room.
- Teach the patient to avoid raw fruits, vegetables, and milk products.
- Avoid use of indwelling urinary catheters and other invasive devices.
- Use strict aseptic technique if invasive procedures are needed.
- Use acetaminophen if an antipyretic is needed; aspirin can induce bleeding.

ETIOLOGY. Sickle cell disease is an autosomal recessive hereditary disorder. This means that if both parents pass on the abnormal hemoglobin, the child will have the disease. If only one parent passes on the abnormal hemoglobin, the child will have the sickle cell trait and will be able to pass the trait (or the disease if the other parent is also affected) on to his or her child.

In the United States, sickle cell anemia is most often found in those of African or Eastern Mediterranean heritage. Worldwide, many persons residing in Asia, the Caribbean, the Middle East, and Central America are affected. Nearly 10% of African Americans have the sickle cell trait; 1 of

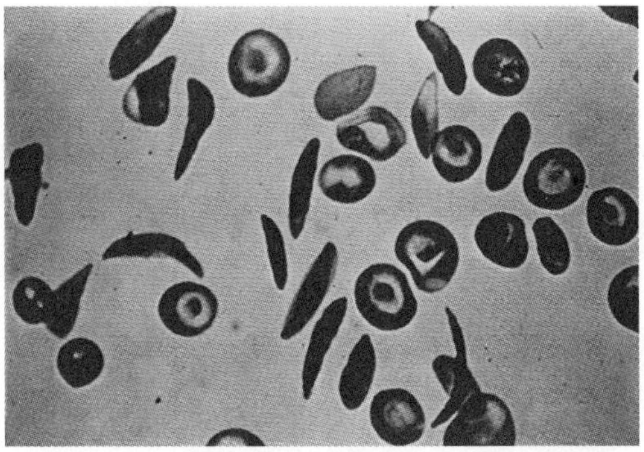

FIGURE 28.2 Sickled cells in sickle cell disease.

every 400 African American infants born has inherited the two sets of abnormal genes needed to have the disease. Symptoms do not appear in infants until after the age of 6 months because up to that age the infant is using hemoglobin manufactured during fetal life, which is not affected by the sickling process.

SIGNS AND SYMPTOMS. The sickling changes just described are a daily occurrence. The rapid return of the oxygen level to normal usually returns the cells to their normal shape.

Occasionally, the sickling process cannot be reversed and the problem continues unabated. This sudden and severe sickling is called a sickle cell crisis. As more and more sickling occurs, the blood becomes sluggish and does not flow easily. It tends to collect in the capillaries and veins of chest and abdominal organs, as well as joints and bones, and can cause infarction (tissue necrosis resulting from lack of blood supply). Tissue necrosis causes pain, fever, and swelling.

Any condition that leads to decreased oxygenation can contribute to the development of a sickle cell crisis. Some examples include pneumonia with hypoxia, exposure to cold, diabetic acidosis, and severe infection. Sickle cell anemia presents problems for the patient who needs surgery. Anesthesia and blood loss during surgery and postoperative dehydration can trigger a crisis.

Common symptoms produced during sickle cell crises include severe pain and swelling in the joints, especially of the elbows and knees, as the sickled cells impede circulation. Abdominal pain is common with swelling of the spleen and engorgement of the vital organs. Hypoxia occurs as fever and pain increase, causing the patient to breathe rapidly. A male patient may have a continuous, painful erection (priapism) from impaired blood flow through the penis. Symptoms of renal failure are common as circulation is slowed and the kidneys become clogged with cellular debris.

Repeated crises and infarctions lead to chronic manifestations such as hand-foot syndrome, an unequal growth of fingers and toes from infarction of the small bones in the hands and feet (Fig. 28.3). Additional manifestations of sickle cell disease are shown in Figure 28.4.

The patient with sickle cell anemia has impaired quality of life. Often, strenuous exercise or more exotic activities, such as scuba diving, are impossible because of the risk of crisis. Crises may occur without any apparent cause. In general, crises last from 4 to 6 days. They may occur in cycles close together for a time and then may become dormant for months to years. The cause of death in patients with sickle cell anemia is usually infection, stroke, or organ involvement.

DIAGNOSTIC TESTS. The most telling feature of sickle cell disease is a blood smear that shows sickle-shaped RBCs in circulation. The Sickledex test is a screening test that shows sickling of RBCs when oxygen tension is low. Hemoglobin electrophoresis is a test used to determine the presence of hemoglobin (Hgb) S, the abnormal form of hemoglobin. Also, there is a decreased amount of hemoglobin, a lowered RBC count, an elevated WBC count, and a decreased erythrocyte sedimentation rate.

THERAPEUTIC MEASURES. No cure is available for sickle cell anemia. Treatment is aimed at patient education to prevent crises and supportive care when crises occur. Some patients may be placed on low-dose oral penicillin to help prevent infections, decreasing the risk of crises.

During acute crises, the patient is admitted to the hospital for 5 to 7 days. The nurse can anticipate that the patient will require sedation and analgesia for severe pain and blood transfusions to replace the sickled red cells lost by their being caught, crushed, and destroyed. Oxygen therapy decreases the dyspnea caused by the anemia, and large amounts of oral and intravenous fluids are given to flush the kidneys of the by-products of the many broken cells' debris. Antibiotics are used to treat infection that may have triggered the crisis.

New treatments are being developed to treat sickle cell disease. Frequent blood transfusions, often monthly, are one of the newest treatment recommendations. However, frequent transfusions can cause high levels of iron to build up in the body. Deferasirox (Exjade) is a medication that may be given to decrease the excess iron levels. Hydroxyurea (Droxia) is a drug that has been shown to decrease crises, but it can cause life-threatening side effects; it should also be used with caution in women of childbearing years because of the risk of birth defects. Corticosteroids may reduce the need for analgesics and oxygen. Bone marrow transplantation is currently being investigated as a potential cure.

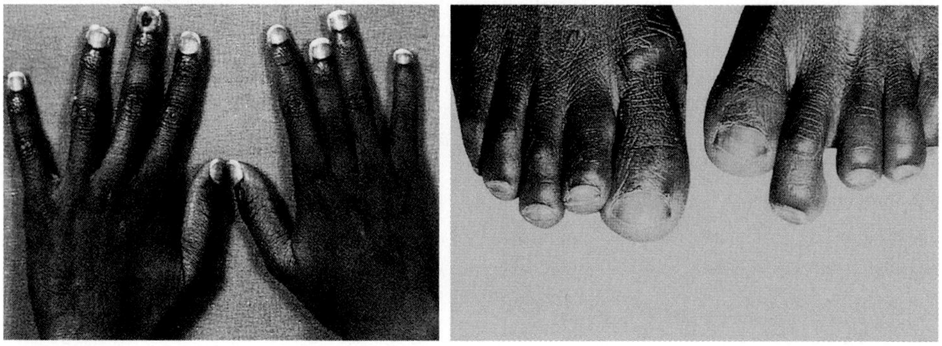

FIGURE 28.3 Hand-foot syndrome. Note different lengths of fingers and toes. (Courtesy of Sandoz Pharmaceutical Corp., East Hanover, NJ.)

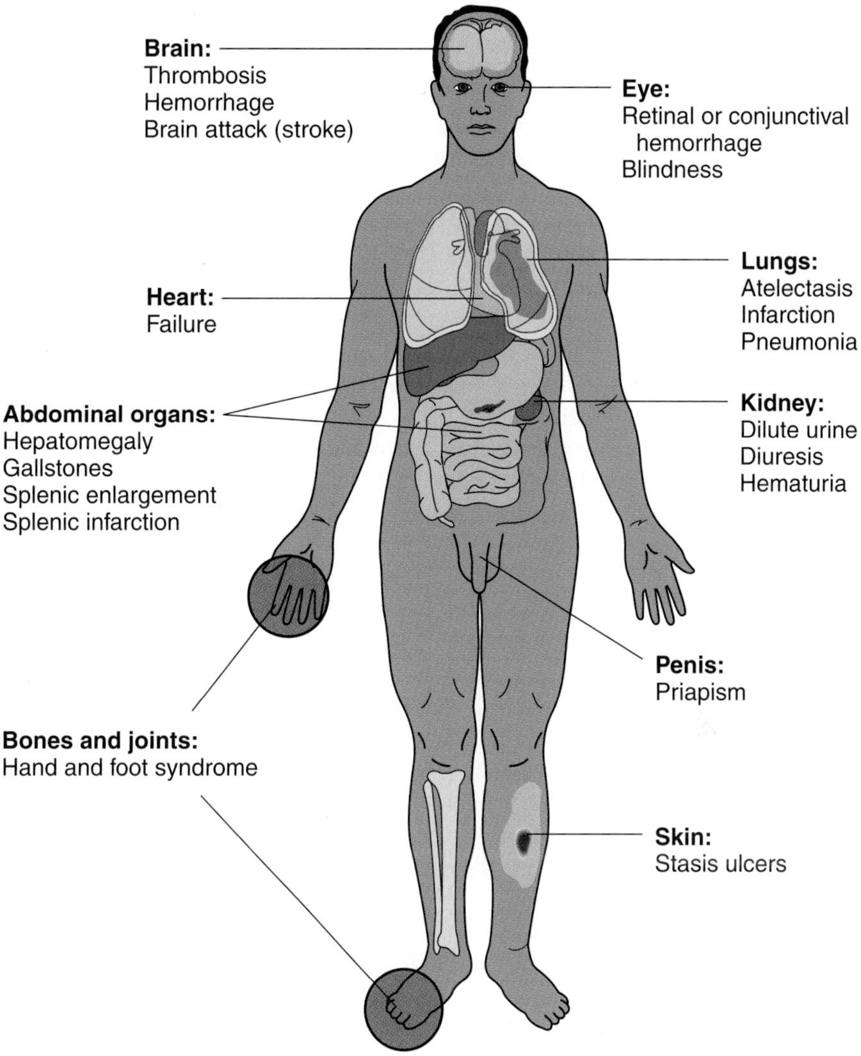
Brain:
Thrombosis
Hemorrhage
Brain attack (stroke)
Eye:
Retinal or conjunctival hemorrhage
Blindness
Lungs:
Atelectasis
Infarction
Pneumonia
Heart:
Failure
Kidney:
Dilute urine
Diuresis
Hematuria
Abdominal organs:
Hepatomegaly
Gallstones
Splenic enlargement
Splenic infarction
Penis:
Priapism
Bones and joints:
Hand and foot syndrome
Skin:
Stasis ulcers

FIGURE 28.4 Clinical manifestations of sickle cell anemia.

NURSING PROCESS FOR THE PATIENT WITH SICKLE CELL ANEMIA

Data Collection. In the patient in crisis, assess circulation in the extremities every 2 hours, including pulse oximetry, capillary refill, peripheral pulses, and temperature. Frequent pain assessment is also essential.

Nursing Diagnoses, Planning, and Implementation

Risk for Ineffective Tissue Perfusion Related to Sickled Cells and Infarction

EXPECTED OUTCOME: The patient will have adequate tissue perfusion as evidenced by the presence of peripheral pulses, warm extremities, urine output within normal limits, and a capillary refill time of less than 3 seconds.

- Encourage oral fluids, and assist the registered nurse (RN) to monitor intravenous (IV) fluids *to dilute and aid in elimination of cell debris.*
- Apply warm compresses as ordered to the painful areas, cover the patient with a blanket, and keep the room temperature above 72°F (~22°C) *to reduce the vasoconstricting effects of cold.*
- Avoid cold compresses *because they decrease circulation and increase the number of sickled cells caught in a painful area.*
- Avoid restrictive clothing and raising the knee gatch of the bed. *These can restrict circulation.*

Acute Pain Related to Tissue Infarction

EXPECTED OUTCOME: The patient will state pain is controlled at an acceptable level at all times.

- Administer opioid analgesics such as morphine as ordered *for acute pain.* (Analgesics may be given intravenously or by use of patient-controlled analgesia.)
- Administer acetaminophen (Tylenol) *to control fever.*
- Avoid giving aspirin *because it may increase acidosis, which can worsen the crisis.*
- Encourage bedrest during the acute phase of the crisis *to reduce oxygen demand.*

Evaluation. If nursing care has been effective, the patient will state that he or she is comfortable, and will not have signs of poor circulation.

PATIENT EDUCATION. During remission, teach the patient how to prevent acute episodes. Advise the patient to avoid tight-fitting clothing that restricts circulation. Also urge the patient to avoid strenuous exercise, which increases oxygen demand, and cold temperatures and smoking, which cause vasoconstriction. Alcoholic beverages can also trigger a crisis and should be avoided. Patients should never fly in unpressurized aircraft or undertake mountain climbing or other sports that can cause hypoxia. Encourage patients to get a pneumococcal vaccine and yearly flu vaccine. Encourage fluids to maintain hydration and reduce blood viscosity. Genetic counseling is important to prevent passing on the trait or disease to offspring. For more information, visit www.sicklecelldisease.org.

Polycythemia

Pathophysiology and Etiology

Polycythemia is really two separate disorders that are easily recognizable by similar characteristic changes in the RBC count. In both forms of polycythemia, the blood becomes so thick with an overabundance of RBCs that it closely resembles sludge. This thickness does not allow the blood to circulate easily. Laboratory tests show a hemoglobin level greater than 18 mg/dL, an RBC mass greater than 6 million, and a hematocrit of more than 55%.

Polycythemia vera (PV) is known as primary polycythemia. Its cause is unknown. In PV, the RBCs, platelets, and WBCs are all overproduced, and the bone marrow becomes packed with too many cells. As this overabundance of cells spills out into the general circulation, the organs become congested with cells and the tissues become packed with blood. The skin takes on a plethoric (dark, flushed) appearance from the buildup of red cells. The thick blood and excess platelets can cause thrombosis and occlusion of vessels. PV is usually found in patients over age 50.

In contrast, secondary polycythemia is the result of long-term hypoxia. Common coexisting conditions that may predispose a patient to secondary polycythemia include pulmonary diseases such as chronic obstructive pulmonary disease (COPD), cardiovascular problems such as chronic heart failure, living in high altitudes, and smoking. The body makes more RBCs in response to the low oxygenation associated with these conditions. Secondary polycythemia is a compensatory mechanism rather than an actual disorder.

Signs and Symptoms

A patient with PV commonly presents with hypertension, vision changes, headache, vertigo, dizziness, and ringing in the ears (tinnitus). Laboratory results show an increased level of all bone marrow components (RBCs, WBCs, platelets), which is called **panmyelosis**. The patient may have nosebleeds and bleeding gums, retinal hemorrhages, exertional dyspnea, and chest pain because of the increased pressure exerted by the excess cells. The patient usually has a dark, flushed complexion. Intense itching is related to excess mast cells (and, therefore, histamine) in the skin. Abdominal pain with an early feeling of fullness with meals occurs because of the enlarged liver and spleen. Nearly all of the symptoms in PV are due to the major problems of hypervolemia, hyperviscosity, and engorgement of capillary beds. Without treatment, patients with PV die of thrombosis or hemorrhage.

• WORD • BUILDING •
polycythemia: poly—many + cyt—cells + emia—in the blood

Diagnostic Tests

Diagnosis of PV is made based on a complete blood count and bone marrow aspiration. A low level of erythropoietin is present, caused by negative feedback to the kidneys, where erythropoietin is made.

Therapeutic Measures

Treatment of PV takes place in two stages. The first stage is to decrease the hyperviscosity problem. The most common first-line treatment is therapeutic **phlebotomy**. Phlebotomy involves withdrawal of blood, which is then discarded. From 350 to 500 mL of blood are removed each time on an every-other-day basis, with the goal being a hematocrit of about 45%. This reduces the RBC level, and the patient usually feels more comfortable quickly. Repeated phlebotomies eventually cause iron-deficiency anemia, which in turn stabilizes RBC production; phlebotomies can then be reduced to every 2 to 3 months. Low-dose aspirin may be ordered to reduce the risk of blood clots.

The problem that remains is the increased white blood cell and platelet counts because phlebotomy does very little to correct these overloads. Chemotherapeutic agents or radiation therapy, including radioactive phosphorus, may be used to suppress production of blood cells in some patients. Leukemia is a side effect of this therapy, so it is used only if the benefits outweigh the risks.

Nursing Management

Explain the phlebotomy procedure and reassure the patient that the treatment will relieve the most distressing symptoms. The procedure is the same as that used for donating blood. The patient should be active and ambulatory to help prevent thrombus formation. When bedrest is needed, passive and active range-of-motion exercises should be implemented. Monitor the patient for complications such as hypovolemia and bleeding. Advise the patient to report any signs or symptoms of bleeding immediately.

If the patient has more advanced manifestations, such as an enlarged liver or spleen, offer several small meals each day so the patient will be more comfortable while still receiving adequate nutrition. A dietitian can be consulted to discuss ways to maintain good nutrition. If the patient is on drug therapy, monitor CBC and platelet counts.

Patient Education

Instruct the patient to drink at least 3 L of water daily to reduce blood viscosity. Encourage smoking cessation, avoidance of tight or restrictive clothing, and elevation of feet when resting to prevent impairment of circulation. Use of support hose when active also promotes circulation. If anticoagulants or antiplatelet agents are ordered, instruct the patient about side effects to watch for and the importance of routine laboratory tests. Routine bleeding precautions are implemented (see Box 28.5). Warn the patient to stop activities at the first sign of chest pain. Instruct the patient to report chest pain, increased joint pain, decreased activity tolerance, or fever, as well as signs of iron-deficiency anemia, such as pallor, weight loss, and dyspnea.

HEMORRHAGIC DISORDERS

Disseminated Intravascular Coagulation

Pathophysiology

Disseminated intravascular coagulation (DIC) involves a series of events that result in hemorrhage.

As its name implies, this syndrome is a catastrophic, overwhelming state of accelerated clotting throughout the peripheral blood vessels. In a short period, all of the clotting factors and platelet supplies are exhausted and clots can no longer be formed. This results in bleeding from nearly every bodily route possible. DIC is not a disease; it is a syndrome that develops secondary to some other severe physical problem. Once this deadly syndrome develops, the progression of symptoms is rapid.

Massive clotting in blood vessels leads to organ and limb necrosis. Organs most often affected include the kidneys and the brain, but other blood-engorged organs, such as the lungs, the pituitary and adrenal glands, and the gastrointestinal mucosa, are commonly involved. DIC is usually acute in onset, although in some patients it becomes a chronic condition. The prognosis depends on early diagnosis and intervention and the severity of the hemorrhaging. DIC has a very high mortality rate.

Etiology

DIC can develop after any condition in which the body has sustained major trauma. The sources of trauma are varied and can include an overwhelming infection; obstetric complications such as abruptio placentae, amniotic fluid embolism, or a retained dead fetus; or cancer-related causes such as acute leukemia or lung cancer. Massive tissue necrosis found in severe crush or burn injuries may increase the risk of DIC. Tissue necrosis secondary to extensive abdominal surgery with leakage of the intestinal contents can also be related to DIC onset. Rarer causes of this condition have included heatstroke, shock, and poisonous snakebites, as well as fat embolism secondary to broken long bones.

Signs and Symptoms

Abnormal bleeding without a history of a serious hemorrhagic disorder is a cardinal sign of DIC. Early signs of bleeding include petechiae, ecchymoses (Fig. 28.5), and bleeding from venipuncture sites. Bleeding may progress to IV sites, skin tears, surgical sites, incisions, and the gastrointestinal tract and oral mucosa. Joints become painful and enlarged if bleeding into the joints occurs. All of these signs and symptoms may occur at the same time. Massive bleeding may also be accompanied by nausea, vomiting, dyspnea, oliguria, convulsions, coma, shock, major organ system failure, and severe muscle, back, and abdominal pain.

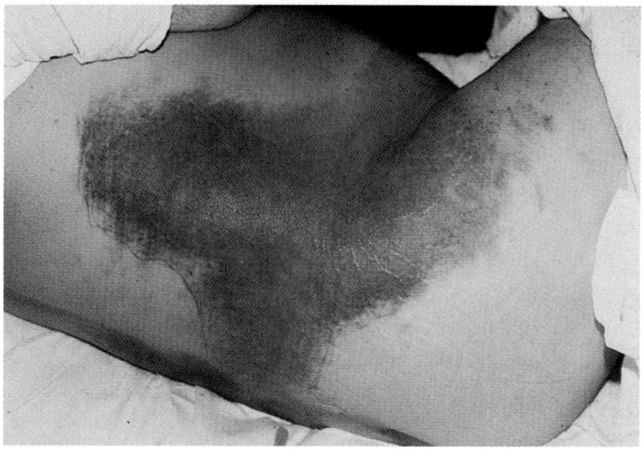

FIGURE 28.5 Extensive hemorrhage into the skin in DIC. Note how the area is outlined in pen so the nurse can assess if the area is spreading. (From Harmening, D. M. [1997]. *Clinical hematology and fundamentals of hemostasis* [3rd ed., p. 520]. Philadelphia: F. A. Davis, with permission.)

Diagnostic Tests

Initial laboratory findings in DIC include a prolonged prothrombin time (PT) and partial thromboplastin time (PTT), decreased platelet count, and increased evidence of fibrin degradation products (Table 28.2). A decrease in hemoglobin is the result of spilled hemoglobin from the increased numbers of broken red cells. Blood urea nitrogen (BUN) and serum creatinine levels may also be increased.

TABLE 28.2 LABORATORY ABNORMALITIES IN DISSEMINATED INTRAVASCULAR COAGULATION

Screening Test	Finding
Prothrombin time (PT)	Prolonged
Partial thromboplastin time (PTT)	Prolonged
Activated partial thromboplastin time (APTT)	Prolonged
Thrombin time (TT)	Prolonged
Fibrinogen	Reduced
Platelets	Reduced
Fibrin split products (FSP; also known as fibrin degradation products [FDP])	Elevated
Protamine sulfate	Strongly positive
Dimers (cross-linked fibrin fragments)	Elevated
Antithrombin III	Reduced
Factor assays (for factors V, VII, VIII, X, and XIII)	Reduced

Therapeutic Measures

Effective treatment of DIC depends on early recognition of the condition. Treatment is first aimed at correcting the underlying cause. Additional treatment consists of supportive interventions, including administration of blood, fresh frozen plasma, platelets, vitamin K, and the infusion of cryoprecipitate (containing clotting factors) to support hemostasis. Some health care organizations include the use of intravenous heparin to help prevent the initial microembolization, but this practice is controversial. Additional therapies are being investigated.

Nursing Management

Care of the patient with DIC is a nursing challenge. Early intervention requires early recognition and reporting of signs of bleeding. In addition to supportive care, focus on the prevention of further bleeding episodes. Care should be taken to avoid any trauma that might cause bleeding. Be careful not to dislodge clots from any site because another clot may not form and the patient will hemorrhage. See Box 28.5 for bleeding precautions.

Patient Education

Because a patient with DIC is often cared for in the intensive care unit, there are many opportunities for patient and family teaching. Explain all diagnostic tests to the patient if he or she is alert. If not, keep the family informed. A large part of family education is preparing the family for what the patient may look like in terms of bleeding and bruising, as well as specific equipment that may be in place, such as IV lines, a nasogastric (NG) tube, and an indwelling urinary catheter. It may be helpful to enlist the aid of social workers, chaplains, and other members of the health care team to help support the family.

CRITICAL THINKING

Mrs. Johns

■ Mrs. Johns is admitted to your unit with DIC following the difficult delivery of her new baby.

1. What data will you collect as you care for Mrs. Johns?
2. What treatment do you anticipate?
3. What concerns is Mrs. Johns likely to have?
4. Mrs. Johns is to receive IV fresh frozen plasma 300 mL over 30 minutes. How many milliliters per hour should be set on the IV controller?

Suggested answers at end of chapter.

Idiopathic Thrombocytopenic Purpura

Pathophysiology and Etiology

Acute **idiopathic thrombocytopenic purpura** (ITP) results from increased platelet destruction by the immune system. Any time platelet numbers are reduced, the risk for bleeding increases. Acute ITP usually affects children between ages 2 and 6, whereas chronic ITP mainly affects adults over age 60.

Acute ITP usually occurs after an acute viral illness such as rubella or chickenpox. It may also be drug induced or associated with pregnancy. ITP is generally thought to be related to an immune system dysfunction. Antibodies responsible for platelet destruction have been found in nearly all diagnosed patients.

Signs and Symptoms

ITP produces clinical changes that are common to all forms of **thrombocytopenia**: petechiae, ecchymoses, and bleeding from the mouth, nose, or gastrointestinal (GI) tract. Bleeding may occur in vital organs, such as the brain, which may prove fatal. In the acute type, onset may be sudden and without warning, causing easy bruising, nosebleeds, and bleeding gums. Onset of chronic ITP is usually insidious.

Diagnostic Tests

A platelet count of less than 20,000/mm^3 and a prolonged bleeding time suggest ITP. The greatly decreased platelet level places the patient at serious risk for hemorrhage. Examination of platelets under the microscope shows them to be small and immature. Anemia may be present if there has been a bleeding episode. If a bone marrow aspiration is performed, the results show an adequate amount of the precursor cells for platelets, the megakaryocytes. However, instead of the 7- to 10-day life span that platelets usually have, these immature platelets have a life span of just a few hours.

Therapeutic Measures

Most cases of acute ITP resolve spontaneously without treatment. Initial treatment, if needed, often involves the administration of steroids. The purpose of the steroids is to prolong the life of the platelets by decreasing immune activity. In acute situations, immune globulin may be given to quickly increase the blood count. Some physicians order the use of chemotherapeutic drugs. The spleen may be removed because it is the primary site of platelet destruction. Often the patient undergoing splenectomy has tried all other courses of treatment unsuccessfully and may be having bleeding episodes. Acute bleeding episodes are treated with transfusions of blood, platelets, and vitamin K.

Nursing Interventions

Care for the patient with ITP is the same as any patient with a bleeding disorder. See Box 28.5 for bleeding precautions. Teach the patient to watch for and report signs and symptoms of bruising and bleeding (Box 28.7, *Patient Education*). The patient should avoid trauma and restrict activity during severe episodes.

• WORD • BUILDING •

idiopathic thrombocytopenic purpura: idio—unknown + pathic—disease + thrombo—clot + cyto—cell + penic—lack + purpura—hemorrhage in the skin

thrombocytopenia: thrombocyte—platelet + penia—lack

Box 28.7

Patient Education

Signs and Symptoms of Bleeding

Notify your health care provider if the following occur:

- Easy bruising of skin
- Petechiae (small red spots on skin)
- Blood in urine
- Black tarry stools
- Bleeding from nose or gums
- Increase in vaginal bleeding
- New onset of painful joints

Hemophilia

Hemophilia is a group of hereditary bleeding disorders that result from a severe lack of specific clotting factors. The two most common are hemophilia A (classic hemophilia) and hemophilia B (Christmas disease). Von Willebrand's disease is another related bleeding disorder, but it represents a minority of cases and is not discussed in this chapter.

Pathophysiology

Recall that many different clotting factors make up the clotting mechanism. Hemophilia A accounts for 80% of all types of hemophilia and results from a deficiency of factor VIII. Hemophilia B is a factor IX deficiency; about 15% of people with hemophilia have this type. The severity and prognosis of hemophilia depend on the degree of deficiency of the specific clotting factors. Mild hemophilia has the best prognosis because it does not cause spontaneous bleeding and joint deformities like severe hemophilia can.

After an injury, the person with hemophilia forms a platelet plug (which differs from a clot) at the site of an injury as would normally be expected, but the clotting factor deficiency keeps the patient from forming a stable fibrin clot. Continued bleeding washes away the platelet plug that initially formed. Contrary to popular myths, people with hemophilia do not bleed "faster" and are not at risk from small scratches.

Etiology

Hemophilia A and B are inherited as X-linked recessive traits. This means that the female carrier (daughter of an affected father) has a 50% chance of transmitting the gene to each son or daughter. Daughters who receive the gene are carriers, and sons who receive the gene are born with hemophilia. It is technically possible for daughters to be affected with hemophilia, although it is very rare.

Signs and Symptoms

Bleeding occurs as a result of injury or, in severe cases, spontaneously (unprovoked by injury). Bleeding into the muscles and joints (**hemarthrosis**) is common. Severe and repeated episodes of joint hemorrhage cause joint deformities, especially in the elbows, knees, and ankles, which decrease the patient's range of motion and ability to walk.

In mild hemophilia, excessive bleeding is usually associated only with surgery or significant trauma. However, once a person with mild hemophilia begins to bleed, the bleeding can be just as serious as that of the patient with a more severe form.

The patient with moderate hemophilia has an occasional bout of spontaneous bleeding. In severe hemophilia, spontaneous bleeding occurs more frequently. It would be possible for the patient to develop hemarthrosis or bleeding into the brain without any precipitating trauma. Severe episodes can produce large subcutaneous and deep intramuscular hematomas. Major trauma can cause bleeding so severe that it becomes life threatening.

Another unfortunate problem related to hemophilia treatment is the frequent need to replace clotting factors and other blood products. Before 1986, blood banks and other centers did not routinely test for human immunodeficiency virus (HIV) antibodies. Depending on the patient's age and frequency of treatment, many patients may have been exposed to HIV or hepatitis. Blood banks and pharmacies have checked their blood supplies for the presence of HIV since 1986. Today, the plasma proteins are artificially created or thoroughly cleansed to prevent transmission of disease.

Diagnostic Tests

Laboratory data reveal a prolonged PTT. The various factor levels are measured to determine which is missing. Once the missing factor is identified, the type of hemophilia is determined and necessary treatments can be implemented. In some cases of mild hemophilia, a surgical procedure or trauma is the first time a bleeding problem is noticed.

Therapeutic Measures

Hemophilia is not curable. However, treatment advances have improved outcomes, and many patients can now live a normal life span. Treatment is aimed at preventing crippling deformities and at increasing life expectancy. Treatment involves stopping bleeding episodes by administering the missing clotting factors. Mild hemophilia A may be treated with injection or nasal inhalation of desmopressin (DDAVP, antidiuretic hormone), which can stimulate the body to release more clotting factors. More severe hemophilia A is treated with factor VIII; hemophilia B is treated with factor IX. Each is available in a freeze-dried powder that is reconstituted with water and administered intravenously. The newest treatment employs factors made using recombinant DNA technology without the use of any human blood products. Blood transfusions are uncommon but may be necessary after severe trauma or surgery.

Complications related to therapy usually occur when therapy is started too late. Minor trauma typically needs to

• WORD • BUILDING •

hemophilia: hemo—blood + philia—to love

hemarthrosis: hem—bleeding + arthr—joint + osis—condition be treated with at least 72 hours of added clotting factors; major traumas and surgeries may require up to 14 days of added factors to prevent sudden bleeding. Health care workers should pay careful attention to the patient who says that bleeding is starting even when no outward signs are evident. The patient usually knows from experience if bleeding is starting. If treatment is delayed at this time, the results can be disastrous. Some patients with severe disease are treated prophylactically to prevent bleeding.

Nursing Process for the Patient with Hemophilia

DATA COLLECTION. Because a major goal is prevention of bleeding episodes, assess the patient and family for knowledge of the disease and its treatment and understanding of preventive measures. Most patients care for themselves at home, starting their own IVs and administering treatment independently. Hospitalization is needed only for surgery or major trauma. During an acute episode of bleeding, the hemoglobin and hematocrit are carefully monitored. Factor VIII or IX levels are monitored to determine if factor replacement has reached adequate levels. Vital signs are monitored for falling blood pressure and rising pulse rate, which are signs of hypovolemic shock. All body systems are assessed for signs of bleeding (see Box 28.7). A pain assessment is done using the WHAT'S UP? format.

NURSING DIAGNOSES, PLANNING, AND IMPLEMENTATION

Acute Pain Related to Bleeding into Tissues

EXPECTED OUTCOMES: The patient's pain will be controlled as evidenced by verbalization that pain is relieved to a satisfactory level within [specify time frame depending on medication and route] of intervention.

- Have the patient report the location, intensity, and quality of the pain. *Assessment of the pain provides the caregiver with data that can be used to develop a treatment plan.*
- Administer opioids as prescribed, including patient-controlled analgesia. *Analgesics are the primary way to manage moderate to severe pain.*
- Avoid the administration of intramuscular injections *because of the risk of bleeding into the muscle, which would cause more pain.*
- Reassess the level of pain after administration of analgesia *to determine the effectiveness of the treatment ordered. IV medications will work almost immediately; oral medications may take 30 to 60 minutes.*
- Monitor sedation and respiratory status of the patient receiving opioids for pain. *Opioids depress the respiratory center of the brain.*

Risk for Bleeding Related to Factor Deficiencies

EXPECTED OUTCOMES: The patient will experience no signs or symptoms of bleeding. The patient will verbalize understanding of bleeding precautions.

- Instruct the patient on bleeding precautions (see Box 28.5). *Identification of signs of bleeding will promote early intervention to prevent injury.*
- Assist with administration of factor concentrates, fresh frozen plasma, cryoprecipitate, blood, or a combination of these as ordered *to treat acute episodes of bleeding.* See Chapter 27 for transfusion of blood products.
- Apply ice or pressure on bleeding sites *to help slow bleeding.*
- Avoid intramuscular, subcutaneous, or rectal medications. *These routes can cause bleeding into tissues.*
- Instruct the patient that preventive care will be needed if surgery or dental procedures are needed. *These invasive procedures can be life-threatening events for the patient with hemophilia.*

Risk for Ineffective Self Health Management Related to Knowledge Deficit

EXPECTED OUTCOME: The patient will be able to manage self-care requirements as evidenced by verbalization of understanding/demonstration of the treatment regimen.

- Assess knowledge base and determine readiness to learn and incorporate new information. *Each patient is unique in the way he or she learns new information.*
- Instruct the patient on ways to prevent bleeding and recognition of signs and symptoms of bleeding (see Boxes 28.5 and 28.7). *Identification of signs of bleeding will promote early intervention to prevent injury.*
- Instruct the patient to obtain emergency care in the event that bleeding occurs. *Intervention is critical for survival of an acute bleeding episode.*
- Instruct the patient to administer factor treatments at home. *Treatment can often be administered at home and can be given more promptly if a trip to the emergency department is not needed.*
- Instruct patients and families on the community services and hemophilia treatment centers available to the patient. *These centers are nationwide and coordinate care for patients with hemophilia.*
- Instruct the patient that the approach to care is multidisciplinary in nature and includes social services, dental, rehabilitation, nursing, financial, and medical needs. *These are all areas that impact the care of the patient with hemophilia.*

EVALUATION. If interventions have been effective, the patient will be comfortable and bleeding will be prevented or complications minimized. The patient and family will be able to state appropriate measures to prevent and treat bleeding episodes. The patient will be knowledgeable about the resources available to cope with the diagnosis of hemophilia.

DISORDERS OF WHITE BLOOD CELLS

Leukemia

The term *leukemia* literally means "white blood." It was first identified in 1845 when the blood of victims was examined and found to have an excess of "colorless" cells.

Pathophysiology

Leukemia is a malignant disease of the WBCs that affects all age groups. The immature WBCs (blast cells) generate in an explosive fashion in the bone marrow, lymph tissue, and spleen. The cells are abnormal and unable to effectively fight infection. So many abnormal cells develop and are dumped into the peripheral circulation that they tend to collect in the body tissues and organs, especially where circulation is sluggish. Areas especially prone to infiltration with immature WBCs are the oral mucosa, anus, sinuses, and lungs. At the time of diagnosis, these areas are often inflamed, painful, and infected. It is common for patients to be diagnosed only after experiencing an infection that does not clear up easily.

As the disease progresses, the bone marrow continues to produce large numbers of the useless cells; the peripheral circulation is filled with them, and the bone marrow is packed with blast cells. Because so many of the blood stem cells are being used to make defective white cells, production of most other normal cells is impossible. The patient becomes anemic because of the lack of RBC production, and bleeding becomes a problem as fewer and fewer platelets are manufactured. But most importantly, even though the WBC count is very high, there are few normal, mature, and active white cells with which to fight infection. Thus, the patient often begins to have raging infections that do not respond to antibiotics. Without treatment, leukemia leaves the patient unable to fight infection, unable to control bleeding, and in a downward spiral of fatigue and anorexia. Untreated leukemia is almost always fatal.

Classifications

Leukemias are classified as either acute or chronic and either lymphoid or myeloid. Symptoms of the acute leukemias begin suddenly and the patient is very sick, whereas chronic leukemias develop slowly and patients can be surprised by the diagnosis because they feel well. Lymphoid leukemias affect the lymphocytes. Myeloid leukemias originate in the stem cells of the bone marrow that develop into monocytes, granulocytes, erythrocytes, and platelets. The most common leukemias are discussed next.

ACUTE LEUKEMIAS. Acute lymphocytic leukemia (ALL) is the most common cancer in children and involves abnormal growth of the lymphocyte precursors (lymphoblasts). Acute myelogenous (myeloblastic) leukemia (AML) usually affects people over age 60 and has a poor prognosis. The patient with acute leukemia may present with sudden onset of high fever, abnormal bleeding from the mucous membranes, petechiae, ecchymoses, and easy bruising after minor trauma. Death usually results from infection.

CHRONIC LEUKEMIAS. Chronic lymphocytic leukemia (CLL) predominantly affects the B and T lymphocytes and usually occurs in adults. Chronic myelogenous leukemia (CML) is characterized by the Philadelphia chromosome and occurs most often in older adults.

Chronic leukemia usually develops in a three-phase process. The first, insidious phase is characterized by anemia and mild bleeding abnormalities. During this phase, the patient often feels well and is not even aware of being sick. After a time, generally years, the disease progresses to the accelerated and acute phases, in which the scenarios are similar to the events seen in acute leukemias. Chronic leukemia is almost always fatal; the average survival time is 3 to 5 years after onset of the chronic phase and 3 to 6 months after onset of the acute phase. With advances in treatments, however, it is not uncommon to encounter patients who have been living with chronic leukemia for 10 years or more.

Etiology

The cause of leukemia is unknown. Risk factors are thought to include certain viruses because remnants of viruses have been found in leukemic cells. Genetic and immunological factors are often involved. For example, persons with Down syndrome are more likely to develop leukemia. Other authorities point to exposure to radiation, in part because radiologists have been found to have a higher than average development of leukemia. Some patients have developed leukemia after being treated for another unrelated malignancy using radiation or chemotherapy. Researchers have noted the higher occurrence rate of leukemia in persons who lived through the Hiroshima and Nagasaki atomic bombings during World War II. Water polluted with benzenes and other chemicals may be a factor. There is no single clear-cut cause for the development of leukemia.

Signs and Symptoms

Symptoms are similar for all types of leukemia and include low-grade fever caused by infection and pallor, weakness, lethargy, shortness of breath, and malaise caused by anemia. These symptoms may be present weeks or months before the appearance of other symptoms. The patient also may have fatigue, tachycardia, palpitations, and abdominal pain. Sternal pain and rib tenderness may result from crowding of bone marrow. If the leukemia has invaded the central nervous system, the patient may experience confusion, headaches, and personality changes. During the acute phase the patient may have high fevers from infection. Ecchymosis or petechiae may result from thrombocytopenia.

Diagnostic Tests

Although a simple CBC often points toward the diagnosis, only bone marrow aspiration can show the degree of proliferation of the malignant WBCs and confirm the diagnosis of leukemia. The CBC also may show a decrease in the numbers of platelets, RBCs, and mature WBCs. A lumbar puncture helps determine if the central nervous system is involved.

Genetic analysis of the peripheral blood and bone marrow components may show the presence of the Philadelphia chromosome in patients with CML.

Therapeutic Measures

CHEMOTHERAPY. Systemic chemotherapy aims to eradicate the leukemic cells and induce a remission. Remission means that the bone marrow is free to produce normally occurring cells in normal proportions without production of the immature WBCs. The type of chemotherapy used varies with the type of leukemia and the level of involvement.

The overall goal of the initial treatments is to get the patient to a state of remission. Occasionally, partial remission is achieved when everything looks good except for an occasional leukemic cell seen in the bone marrow. Remission is not the same as cure.

There are four phases to the treatment of leukemia: induction, intensification, consolidation, and maintenance. Induction is the period in which an attempt to get the patient into remission is made. This first phase is difficult because chemotherapy is given in very high doses and on an aggressive timetable. Often the patient becomes quite ill from complications of the treatment. The patient may become depressed because the treatment seems worse than the disease at this stage. The nurse must help the patient deal with anemia, thrombocytopenia, and leukopenia, as well as other side effects (Table 28.3; also see Box 28.6 and Chapter 11).

If the first remission is accomplished, the other phases of treatment are begun. Intensification is similar to the initial induction phase, using the same drugs at even higher doses. The next phase, consolidation, is used to ensure that all leukemic cells have been eradicated from the body. Finally, the patient graduates to maintenance therapy in which the patient is kept free of leukemic cells and in remission for a period of years (and hopefully a lifetime). This requires years of continued chemotherapy treatments, often on a monthly basis. Radiation therapy may be used throughout this course of treatment to decrease the size of the liver or spleen or to decrease the numbers of leukemic cells in the central nervous system.

RADIATION THERAPY. Radiation therapy is sometimes used for initial treatment of leukemia. It may be directed at the entire body, or at specific areas where leukemic cells are collecting.

BONE MARROW TRANSPLANT. Bone marrow transplant (BMT) is sometimes used to treat leukemia. Preparation for BMT includes high-dose chemotherapy and/or total body irradiation. The goal is to destroy all of the patient's malignant bone marrow and then, at the last possible moment, replace it with a donor's clean and healthy bone marrow (allogenic transplant). Another type of bone marrow transplant, known as an autologous transplant, uses the patient's own diseased bone marrow, which is harvested, chemically treated and cleaned, stored, and later reinfused. Transplanted bone marrow is given to the patient like a blood transfusion; typically through a central line placed in the chest. Once infused into the bloodstream, the new marrow travels to the bones, where, ideally, it will begin to grow and function normally. Bone marrow transplants are being performed at more and more centers across the United States.

A new and promising treatment for leukemia is peripheral blood stem cell transplantation. Hematopoietic stem cells can be collected from the patient during remission and then reinfused at a later time. Donor stem cells are also sometimes used if a good match can be found.

OTHER THERAPIES. Biological therapies may be used to boost the patient's immune system. They may be used to help the body attack cancer cells, or to control side effects by boosting red cell or white cell production. Kinase inhibitors (the most common is mesylate [Gleevec]) may be used to inhibit abnormal proteins in leukemic cells in CML. By targeting just the cancer cells, the incidence of side effects is reduced.

TABLE 28.3 LEUKEMIA SUMMARY

Signs and Symptoms	Fever (related to infection) Pallor Weakness, malaise Tachycardia Dyspnea Bone pain Headaches, confusion
Diagnostic Tests	CBC Bone marrow aspiration Lumbar puncture
Therapeutic Measures	Chemotherapy Radiation therapy Bone marrow transplant
Priority Nursing Diagnoses	*Risk for Injury* (infection, bleeding) related to pancytopenia *Fatigue* related to decreased tissue oxygenation

Nursing Process for the Patient with Leukemia

The patient with leukemia is at risk for many problems, including fatigue, bleeding, infection, and other complications of the disease and its treatment. The patient must understand the disease process and treatment regimen in order to participate in self-care. See the *Nursing Care Plan for the Patient with Leukemia* for interventions to deal with these problems. Additional diagnoses include *Knowledge Deficit* and *Anxiety*. The following websites provide resources for patients and families with leukemia:

American Cancer Society, www.cancer.org
Leukemia and Lymphoma Society, www.leukemia.org
National Cancer Institute, www.nci.nih.gov.

Also see Chapter 11 for general care of the patient with cancer.

Nursing Care Plan for the Patient with Leukemia

Nursing Diagnosis: *Risk for Injury* (infection, bleeding) related to pancytopenia as evidenced by bleeding, bruising, petechiae, or fever

Expected Outcomes: The patient will be free from injury as evidenced by temperature within normal limits and no signs or symptoms of bleeding. Signs and symptoms of infection or bleeding will be reported promptly.

Evaluation of Outcomes: Is the patient free from infection and bleeding, or are problems reported so that quick intervention can prevent further complications?

Interventions	Rationale	Evaluation
Monitor vital signs every 4 hours and as needed.	Elevated temperature is a sign of infection. Falling blood pressure and elevated pulse rate may indicate sepsis or blood loss.	Are vital signs stable?
Monitor patient for swelling, redness, purulent drainage.	These are signs of infection and should be reported promptly.	Are signs of infection present?
Protect patient from sources of infection (see the *Evidence-Based Practice* box; also see Box 28.6).	Patient is at risk for infection because of ineffective WBCs.	Are precautions being observed to prevent infection?
Observe for tarry stools, petechiae, ecchymosis (see Box 28.7).	These are signs of bleeding and should be reported promptly.	Are signs of bleeding present?
Protect patient from injury that could cause bleeding (see Box 28.5).	Patient is at risk for bleeding because of reduced platelet count.	Are precautions being observed to prevent injury and bleeding?

Nursing Diagnosis: *Fatigue* related to decreased red cell count and oxygenation and effects of treatments as evidenced by patient statement of lack of energy, inability to participate in desired activities

Expected Outcomes: The patient's fatigue will be controlled at a level that is acceptable to the patient as evidenced by patient ability to participate in activities that are important to him or her.

Evaluation of Outcomes: Is patient able to identify and participate in activities that are important to him or her?

Interventions	Rationale	Evaluation
Assess fatigue using the WHAT'S UP? format.	A good assessment establishes a baseline and aids in planning.	Is fatigue present? To what degree?
Assist patient to identify activities that are important to him or her (e.g., activities of daily living [ADLs], attending a child's wedding, taking a trip). Assist in setting goals to work toward the desired activity.	If the patient cannot do everything he or she wishes, it may help to focus on the most important things.	Can patient identify important activities? What are they? How can the nurse assist the patient to reach activity goals?
Encourage a balanced diet. Contact dietitian as needed.	Poor nutrition contributes to fatigue.	Is patient eating a balanced diet? Is weight stable?

Continued

Nursing Care Plan for the Patient with Leukemia—cont'd

Interventions	Rationale	Evaluation
Allow periods of rest between activities.	Any activity (ADL, x-rays, even talking) can increase fatigue.	Is patient able to rest?
Ensure adequate sleep. Obtain order for sleeping aid if indicated.	Lack of sleep worsens fatigue.	Does patient state feeling rested on awakening? Is medication needed?
Provide for ADLs when patient is unable to do so independently.	Extreme fatigue may prevent the patient from participating in self-care.	Does patient need total assistance?

Nursing Diagnosis: *Impaired Oral Mucous Membranes* related to chemotherapy and pancytopenia as evidenced by bleeding, ulcerations, statement of pain, difficulty eating

Expected Outcomes: The patient's oral mucous membranes will remain intact as evidenced by pink, moist, smooth tissue without ulceration. The patient will be able to eat a balanced diet.

Evaluation of Outcomes: Are oral mucous membranes intact, without lesions? Is patient eating a balanced diet?

Interventions	Rationale	Evaluation
Assess mouth daily for redness, edema, and lesions.	Routine assessment helps identify problems early so treatment can be implemented.	Are mucous membranes intact?
Encourage adequate nutrition and fluids.	Poor nutrition and dehydration increase the risk of oral lesions.	Is patient eating and drinking?
Encourage patient to brush teeth after meals with a soft toothbrush. If irritation is severe or if the patient is at risk for bleeding, use swabs or sponge Toothettes instead of a toothbrush.	Brushing the teeth controls tooth and gum disease; a toothbrush may be too harsh if the patient is at risk for bleeding.	Is mouth care being provided after meals? Is mouth care irritating? Are alternative methods needed?
Avoid use of lemon-glycerin swabs for mouth care.	Lemon-glycerin swabs are drying to oral mucosa.	Are products used appropriate?
Obtain an order for a mouthwash containing diphenhydramine (Benadryl). Obtain an order for a topical anesthetic if mouth is very inflamed and painful.	Diphenhydramine reduces inflammation; anesthetics reduce pain.	Does mouthwash soothe pain?
Encourage the patient to avoid smoking, alcohol, acidic food or drinks, extremely hot or cold foods and drinks, and commercial mouthwash.	These things can be irritating to the mucosa.	Does patient state understanding of things to avoid?
GERIATRIC		
Advise patient to remove dentures for cleaning and at bedtime.	Dentures left in for long periods can impair circulation and increase risk of lesions.	Are oral mucous membranes intact?

EVIDENCE-BASED PRACTICE

Clinical Question

Is the use of protective isolation required for all patients with neutropenia after chemotherapy?

Evidence

The most current information related to protective or reverse isolation suggests that this type of isolation be considered for a limited group of patients being treated in specialty areas such as bone marrow transplant. Rooms with special airflow systems and filters are an important part of protecting patients at high risk for infection. "Patients receiving chemotherapy for solid tumors or lymphoproliferative diseases who become neutropenic have not been shown to benefit from reverse isolation the way that it is practiced in most hospital settings" (Srivdyalakshmi and Baumann, 2008, p. 628).

Implications for Nursing Practice

Isolation is unpleasant and lonely for patients. Question the use of protective isolation in rooms without special airflow systems and filters, and in patients receiving chemotherapy for solid tumors or lymphoproliferative diseases.

REFERENCE

Srivdyalakshmi, S., & Baumann, M.A. (2008). Reverse isolation for neutropenic patients. *Community Oncology,* 5(11), 628–632.

CRITICAL THINKING

Mr. Washington

■ Mr. Washington is on your unit undergoing initial treatment for leukemia. You enter his room and find it full of visitors.

1. What concerns do you have?
2. What do you do?

Suggested answers at end of chapter.

MULTIPLE MYELOMA

Multiple myeloma is a deadly cancer of the plasma cells in the bone marrow. When the disease is caught in its early stages, treatment can prolong life by 3 to 5 years. More important, early detection can decrease the amount of pain and disability due to bony destruction and **pathological fractures**. Unfortunately, almost half of patients die within the first 3 months after diagnosis because of the silent and deadly nature of the disease. Another 40% of patients die within 2 years after diagnosis. Because early diagnosis is not common, only 10% of patients can expect to live to the 5-year mark. Multiple myeloma most often affects men ages 50 to 70.

Pathophysiology

In this disorder, cancerous plasma cells in the bone marrow begin reproducing uncontrollably. These cells infiltrate bone tissue all over the body and produce hundreds of tumors that begin to devour the bone tissue. X-ray examination may show holes in the bones forming a Swiss cheese pattern (Fig. 28.6). As more and more of these holes are formed, the integrity of the bone is compromised and weakened. Multiple myeloma usually affects the bones of the skull, pelvis, ribs, and vertebrae.

As the disease progresses, plasma cells infiltrate the major organs, including the liver, spleen, lymph nodes, lungs, adrenal glands, kidneys, skin, and GI tract. Because the diagnosis is usually made only after widespread invasion of the bones is well under way, the prognosis for patients with this disease is poor. Although the overall result of the disease is the devastating destruction of the bone and widespread osteoporosis, death is often from sepsis.

Etiology

The cause of multiple myeloma is unknown, although it is being researched. Research suggests genetics may be one factor. People who work in rubber, leather, farming, and petroleum industries are more likely to develop multiple myeloma. Obesity, exposure to radiation, and long-term exposure to hair dyes also increase risk.

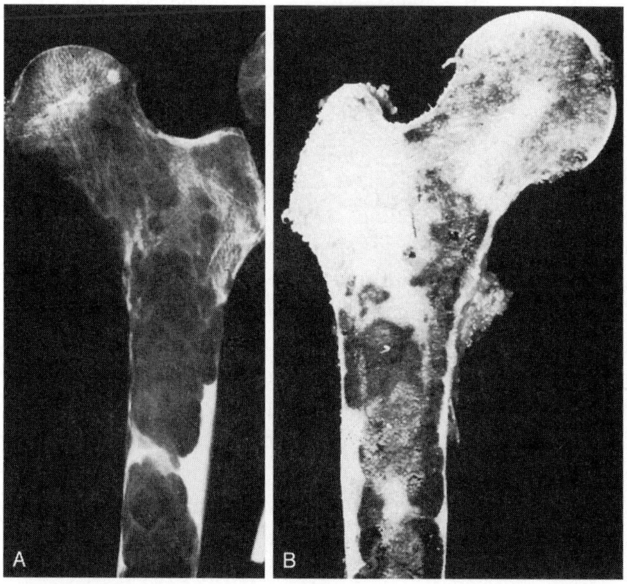
A
B

FIGURE 28.6 X-ray of bone destruction in multiple myeloma. (From Huether, S. E., & McCance, K. L. [1996]. *Understanding pathophysiology* [p. 548]. St. Louis: Mosby, with permission.)

Signs and Symptoms

Skeletal pain is the most common complaint. The patient may describe the pain as constant severe back pain that increases with exercise or movement or as pain in the ribs. Other signs and symptoms include achiness of the long bones, joint swelling and tenderness, low-grade fever, and general malaise. Sometimes there is evidence of early peripheral neuropathy secondary to vertebral collapse and mild spinal cord compression. The patient may be unable to feel the true temperature of bath water and be burned or may be unable to feel wounds and infections on the feet. In more severe cases of cord compression, the patient may lose control of bladder and bowels. This is a true oncological emergency. (See Chapter 11 for more on oncological emergencies.) Prompt emergency treatment is needed to keep the patient from becoming paralyzed.

Occasionally, patients have pathological fractures of the long bones. These are fractures that occur with no trauma, such as the person who breaks a leg just turning over in bed or breaks a rib while sneezing. In advanced disease there is anemia, weight loss, thoracic spinal deformities from multiple rib destruction, and a loss of height because of pathological fractures and compacting of the vertebrae.

Because calcium is mobilized from the bones and into the blood, the patient is at risk for hypercalcemia. Signs and symptoms of hypercalcemia include anorexia, nausea, vomiting, mental changes (especially confusion), seizures, weakness, and fatigue. Kidney stones may result as the excess calcium passes through the kidneys.

Patients are susceptible to infection because of compromised immune function. Pneumonia is a common finding in patients with multiple myeloma. They may develop anemia because of bone marrow dysfunction and reduced erythropoietin formation by diseased kidneys. Risk for bruising and bleeding occurs due to thrombocytopenia.

Patients often develop kidney failure because the filtering capacity of the kidney becomes blocked by calcium. Other factors include recurrent infections and deposits of myeloma cells in the kidneys.

Diagnostic Tests

A CBC shows moderate to severe anemia. The WBC count may show an increase in the number of white cells secondary to infection. Blood and urine studies are positive for M-type globulins (called Bence-Jones proteins when found in the urine) in 40% of patients. X-ray examinations or MRI may show changes in the lungs and diffuse osteoporosis in bones not already riddled with holes. Bone marrow biopsy is done to confirm the diagnosis and determine the stage of the disease.

Blood chemistries often show an increased amount of calcium in the blood. Hypercalciuria results when the calcium released out of the bones is flushed out in the urine. An intravenous pyelogram may be done to see how much calcium is collecting in the kidneys. A 24-hour urine collection is done to evaluate protein excretion.

C-reactive protein (CRP) is elevated in multiple myeloma; it is believed that the CRP actually promotes the cancer cells' proliferation and protects them from the effects of chemotherapy agents. Measurement of CRP helps determine prognosis. Elevated CRP levels are also associated with increased fatigue.

Therapeutic Measures

Long-term treatment of multiple myeloma consists of a two-pronged approach: (1) managing the disease and (2) managing the symptoms. To manage the disease, corticosteroids (prednisone or dexamethasone) and oral or intravenous chemotherapy agents are given. Another drug that is showing encouraging results for slowing progression of the disease is thalidomide. The goal of drug therapy is to suppress the plasma cell proliferation, which then helps decrease the amount and speed of bone destruction.

A new medication for multiple myeloma is bortezomib (Velcade). Bortezomib is a proteasome inhibitor that inhibits enzymes to disrupt cancer cell growth and survival.

Another option is high-dose chemotherapy combined with stem cell transplantation. Donor stem cells can be used or a patient's own peripheral stem cells can be removed and reinfused. These stem cells can then differentiate into new, healthy cells. Methods of cleaning the cells to prevent contamination with malignant cells are being researched.

The second approach is control of symptoms. The patient is monitored for signs and symptoms of hypercalcemia, hyperuricemia, dehydration, respiratory infection, renal problems, and pain. The physician may order the administration of intravenous bisphosphonate agents such as pamidronate (Aredia). This class of drugs inhibits bone resorption and is used to help keep serum calcium levels controlled. Oral compounds are also available to help keep the calcium within normal limits. The goal is to get the serum calcium level below 10 mg/dL. If hypercalcemia occurs, the physician will order an IV infusion of normal saline solution at a high rate, followed by regular administration of diuretics.

External beam irradiation may be given to especially painful areas of bone involvement. Fortunately, this treatment is quite effective, usually decreasing pain intensity in just a few days. The patient can expect to have a daily (or perhaps a twice-daily) therapy treatment over a course of 10 to 14 days that is delivered directly to the painful bony areas. Vigorous attention to administering pain medications during the early course of treatment greatly reduces the patient's pain levels.

The patient may need a laminectomy if vertebral collapse occurs. Because of demineralization of the bone, with resulting large amounts of calcium in the blood and urine, surgery for kidney stones and eventual dialysis for acute or chronic kidney failure may be needed.

Nursing Process for the Patient with Multiple Myeloma

The patient with multiple myeloma is at risk for many problems. In addition to those below, the diagnoses in the *Nursing Care Plan for the Patient with Leukemia* are appropriate.

Data Collection

Assess for fever or malaise, which can signal the onset of infection. Other conditions to be alert for include anemia, hypercalcemia, fractures, and renal complications. Monitor intake and output, and strain urine for stones. Elevated BUN and creatinine levels will alert you to possible renal failure. Report back pain, leg weakness, sensory loss, or loss of bowel or bladder function because these can indicate spinal cord compression. Monitor the patient for elevated CRP and low hemoglobin, which are associated with increased fatigue.

Nursing Diagnoses, Planning, and Implementation

Risk for Infection Related to Compromised Immune Function as Evidenced by Elevated Temperature or Other Symptoms Specific to Body System Affected

EXPECTED OUTCOME: Patient will remain free from infection as evidenced by temperature within normal limits and no signs or symptoms of infection.

- Intervene as appropriate *to reduce the risk of infection* (see Box 28.6).
- Encourage deep breathing, and keep patient active *to decrease the risk of respiratory complications.*

Risk for Injury: Fracture Related to Weakened Bones; Complications of Immobility; Complications Due to Hypercalcemia

EXPECTED OUTCOME: Patient will remain free from injury as evidenced by no fracture and no complications related to immobility or hypercalcemia.

- Keep the patient mobile. Consult physical and occupational therapy as needed. Bones in use are strongest, so the patient should remain up and moving as much as possible *to help stimulate calcium resorption and decrease demineralization.*
- Assist the patient with walking *to reduce the risk of pathological fractures of the long bones.*
- If the patient is unsteady, use a walker or a support belt *to reduce the risk of falls.*
- If the patient is bedridden, reposition him or her every 2 hours *to prevent complications related to immobility.*
- Use a lift sheet to move the patient gently in bed *to decrease the risk of skin damage and pathological fractures.*
- Provide passive range-of-motion exercises *to maintain mobility if the patient is unable to be independently mobile.*
- Administer fluids so that daily output is never less than 1500 mL *to flush kidneys and reduce the risk of kidney stones.*
- Teach the patient the importance of good hydration at all times *to minimize complications of hypercalcemia.* Depending on time of year and the type and level of patient activities, the patient may need to have an intake of more than 4 L daily.

Evaluation

If nursing care has been effective, the patient will be free of infection or infection will be recognized and treated promptly. The patient will avoid injury, with no fracture, skin breakdown, or complications related to hypercalcemia. See *Home Health Hints* at the end of this chapter for additional suggestions for patients being cared for at home.

LYMPHATIC DISORDERS

Lymphatic disorders include Hodgkin's disease and the non-Hodgkin's **lymphomas**. Because the spleen is part of the lymph system, this section also discusses splenectomy.

Hodgkin's Disease

Despite its name, Hodgkin's disease is a lymphoma, which is a cancer of the lymph system. Its distinguishing feature is the presence of Reed-Sternberg cells, which make it different from all the other forms of lymphoma. Hodgkin's disease is more prevalent in men than in women and occurs most often in young adults ages 15 to 40. After a decrease in incidence in persons ages 40 to 55, the incidence peaks again in adults older than age 55. Of all the lymphomas, Hodgkin's disease is the most curable type even when the disease is widely spread at the time of diagnosis.

Pathophysiology

Lymph nodes are made of tightly bound fibers and cells that serve as filtering devices for the body's immune system. Most often, Hodgkin's disease begins as a single changed lymph node, usually in the cervical lymph nodes of the neck. As the disease progresses, the cancer invades the lymph node chains node by node. The path of cancer infiltration is usually the same as the path of lymph fluid flow. Left untreated, other lymphoid tissues such as the spleen become infiltrated with Hodgkin's disease. The major organs eventually become involved. Common reports of patients with organ involvement may include shortness of breath, feelings of fullness, weakness, and malaise. These organ-related symptoms usually motivate the patient to seek medical help.

A tentative diagnosis of Hodgkin's disease is based on one or more painlessly enlarged nodes in the cervical, axillary, or inguinal areas. A biopsy of several of the enlarged nodes is performed to search for the presence of Reed-Sternberg cells, which confirms the diagnosis.

Etiology

The exact cause of Hodgkin's disease is unknown. A possible viral origin has been proposed; it is more common in people who have had mononucleosis. Sometimes it occurs in families, suggesting a genetic link. Patients with impaired

• WORD • BUILDING •

lymphoma: lymph—fluid found in lymphatic vessels + oma—tumor immune function, such as those with acquired immunodeficiency syndrome (AIDS) or those taking immunosuppressant drugs after organ transplant, are also at higher risk.

Signs and Symptoms

Painless swelling in one or more of the common lymph node chains is a usual presentation (Fig. 28.7). Swelling can range from barely perceptible to the size of a softball, occasionally even larger. The patient may report generalized pruritus. One other curious event, alcohol-induced pain, is occasionally present. With just a few sips of any type of alcohol-containing beverage (beer, wine, or liquor), the patient may describe intense pain at the site of disease. Because the lymph nodes in the upper chest and neck are often involved, the patient may have symptoms of obstruction, such as cough, dysphagia, or stridor.

Other common symptoms may include persistent low-grade fever, night sweats, fatigue, weight loss, and malaise. When these additional symptoms are present, the prognosis is worse. In older adults, enlarged lymph nodes might not be visible, so these secondary symptoms may be the only presenting symptoms. Other symptoms associated with late-stage disease include edema of the neck and face, possible jaundice, nerve pain, enlargement of the retroperitoneal nodes, and infiltration of the spleen; liver and bones may also be involved.

Diagnostic Tests and Staging

Diagnosis usually begins with a lymph node biopsy of the easiest lymph node to access. Lymph node biopsies are done to check for abnormal histiocyte proliferation, nodular fibrosis, and necrosis. Other tests include bone marrow biopsy and aspiration, liver and spleen biopsies, routine chest x-ray examination, abdominal computed tomography (CT) scan to check for disease in the liver and spleen, lung scan, and bone scan. Lymphangiography may be performed to view the flow of lymph in the lymph network. A gallium scan can also be done to view lymph tissue.

Hematologic tests (e.g., CBC) may show wide variability of red blood cells, indicating mild to severe anemia. The white blood cell (WBC) count is often abnormal and extreme (either very high or very low) because of bone marrow infiltration by disease.

- These same tests are used for staging the disease into one of four stages:
- Stage I disease is limited to a single lymph node or site or a single organ.
- Stage II disease occurs when two or more nodes are involved on the same side of the diaphragm.
- Stage III disease affects nodes on both sides of the diaphragm.
- Stage IV, the most serious form of the disease and the least curable, includes widely disseminated disease in both lymph nodes and other organs such as bone marrow or liver.

Therapeutic Measures

Appropriate therapy includes the use of radiation and chemotherapy and depends on the stage of the disease. Radiation therapy, administered on an outpatient basis over a 4- to 6-week period, can cure most patients with stage I or stage II disease. Combinations of chemotherapy and radiation therapy are used for patients with stage III and stage IV disease. Results vary depending on the location and the stage of disease. If the disease recurs after initial treatment, bone marrow or stem cell transplant may be considered.

Nursing Management

Most nursing interventions are aimed at symptom management. If the patient is experiencing pruritus or night sweats, nursing interventions are aimed at alleviation of discomfort. These may include changing the gown and bed linens several times a night and helping the patient remain clean and dry. Keeping the patient and family involved in the plan of care may relieve anxiety.

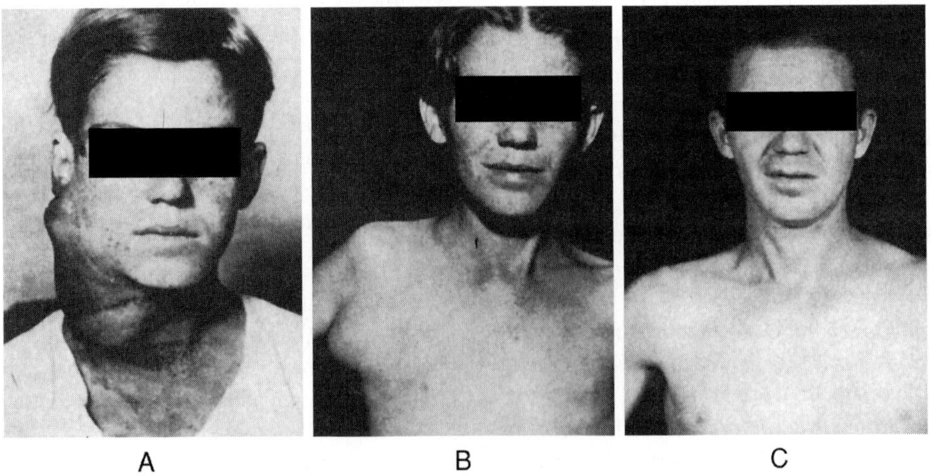

A B C

FIGURE 28.7 Cervical Hodgkin's disease. (A) Young boy with extensive cervical Hodgkin's disease. (B) Appearance several years later, when axillary manifestation developed. (C) Appearance 23 years after initial treatment with radiation. (From del Regato, J. A., Spjut, H. J., & Cox, J. D. [1985]. *Cancer: Diagnosis, treatment, and prognosis* [6th ed.]. St. Louis: Mosby, with permission.)

Later, nursing interventions are tailored to alleviate problems that arise secondary to chemotherapy and radiation therapy. See Chapter 11 for nursing interventions for these problems. Also see the *Nursing Care Plan for the Patient with Lymphoma.*

Patient Education

In addition to the teaching needs outlined above, make sure that the patient and the family know about local chapters of the American Cancer Society and the Leukemia and Lymphoma Society. Both of these organizations provide information, financial assistance, and counseling referral sources, which most patients find valuable. Another source for chemotherapy and radiation therapy information is the National Cancer Institute (NCI). The NCI can send as much information as the patient requests regarding all aspects of treatment at no charge. For more information about Hodgkin's lymphoma, visit www.cancer.org. Or visit the Leukemia and Lymphoma Society at www.leukemia.org or the National Cancer Institute at www.nci.nih.gov.

CRITICAL THINKING

Jeanine

■ Jeanine is a 60-year-old nurse diagnosed with stage II Hodgkin's disease. She wishes to continue working at her job on a respiratory unit at the local hospital while she undergoes treatment. What concerns do you have about this?

Suggested answers at end of chapter.

Nursing Care Plan for the Patient with Lymphoma

Nursing Diagnosis: *Activity Intolerance* related to fatigue and anemia as evidenced by inability to carry out activities of daily living (ADLs) without excessive fatigue or dyspnea

Expected Outcomes: The patient will have ADL needs met by self or caregiver as evidenced by patient statement

Evaluation of Outcomes: Is patient able to carry out ADLs or are ADL needs met by a caregiver?

Interventions	Rationale	Evaluation
Assess amount of activity that causes fatigue or dyspnea.	Assessment helps guide plan of care.	How much can patient do before becoming fatigued or dyspneic?
Assist patient with activities as needed.	The patient may need assistance with ADLs if fatigue is extreme.	Does the patient need assistance? Can family members assist?
Provide oxygen therapy as ordered.	Oxygen therapy can increase oxygen levels and activity tolerance.	Does patient tolerate activity better with oxygen therapy?
Instruct patient to space rest with activities.	Rest periods decrease oxygen needs and allow patient to conserve energy for next activity.	Is patient able to tolerate activity better after a rest period?

Nursing Diagnosis: *Risk for Infection* related to bone marrow involvement and side effects of treatment as evidenced by elevated temperature, redness, swelling, or other signs and symptoms based on infection site

Expected Outcomes: The patient will remain infection free as evidenced by temperature within normal limits and no signs or symptoms of infection.

Evaluation of Outcomes: Are signs and symptoms of infection absent? Is temperature within normal limits?

Interventions	Rationale	Evaluation
Assess patient for risk factors for infection.	The WBC count may be very high or very low, placing the patient at risk for infection.	Is the patient at risk? Are additional interventions indicated?

Continued

Nursing Care Plan for the Patient with Leukemia—cont'd

Interventions	Rationale	Evaluation
Monitor patient for signs and symptoms of infection, such as cough, fever, malaise, erythema, pain, or drainage and report immediately.	Early detection and treatment of infection provide the best results.	Are signs and symptoms of infection present?
Teach patient and significant other signs and symptoms of infection to watch for and report.	The patient must be involved in monitoring for infection when at home.	Does patient verbalize understanding of signs and symptoms of infection and importance of reporting?
Teach the patient to avoid exposure to others with influenza or other infections.	Exposure increases risk for infection, especially with compromised immune function.	Does patient verbalize understanding of sources of infection to avoid?
Teach patient proper hand washing and good oral and personal hygiene.	These activities reduce risk of infection.	Does patient demonstrate proper hand washing and hygiene?
Teach hand hygiene and infection risk reduction to family members.	Family caregivers can be sources of infection.	Do family members demonstrate appropriate hand washing and infection control measures?

Nursing Diagnosis: *Ineffective Coping* related to new diagnosis and potential lifestyle changes to accommodate treatments as evidenced by poor problem solving, lack of goal-directed behavior, statement of poor coping

Expected Outcomes: The patient will be able to cope effectively as evidenced by statement of ability to manage lifestyle changes and medical management of condition.

Evaluation of Outcomes: Does patient carry out self-care necessary to manage treatment?

Interventions	Rationale	Evaluation
Assess patient's level of distress related to uncertainty about the future, bothersome symptoms, changes in self-concept, and past coping mechanisms.	Obtaining information regarding past experiences helps the nurse identify and correct misconceptions. The nurse can support effective coping mechanisms that worked in the past.	Is patient able to identify sources of anxiety? Are past coping mechanisms effective?
Assess for signs of maladaptive behaviors that interfere with responsible health practices, such as missed appointments or failure to attend to symptoms.	Long-term survival depends on keeping the scheduled therapy appointments. The ability to manage and report symptoms early keeps the patient out of the hospital and in control of his or her own life.	Does the patient keep appointments? Does the patient participate in self-care activities and report symptoms promptly?
Assist the patient to identify support systems and resources. Refer to social worker or other community resources as needed.	Resources can assist with participation in treatment plan, home care, or financial assistance.	Are resources identified and helpful?
Refer patient and family to a cancer survivors' support group.	Others who have been through treatment themselves can be a good support for patients with cancer.	Does the patient state that the support group is helpful?

Non-Hodgkin's Lymphomas

All of the other types of lymphomas are clumped into a diverse classification known as the non-Hodgkin's lymphomas (NHLs). It is possible to sort these other types of lymphomas into different categories based on the degree of malignancy. Non-Hodgkin's lymphomas arise in the lymphoid tissues of the body, just as Hodgkin's disease does, but they differ in several ways (Table 28.4).

Pathophysiology

The most distinguishing difference is the absence of the Reed-Sternberg cells in non-Hodgkin's lymphomas. Instead, many of these lymphomas arise from the B cells and T cells. The B cells are involved in recognizing and destroying specific antigens. Cells specifically involved include the memory B cells and the plasma cells. The T cells also are involved in registering antigens, but there are many more kinds of T cells. These include the amplifier T cells, helper T cells, suppressor T cells, memory T cells, cytotoxic T cells, and delayed hypersensitivity T cells. An abnormality in any of these cells can result in a type of NHL. Most cases of NHL are of B-cell origin. Cancerous cells are found most commonly in the lymph nodes, but they can also be found in other lymph tissues such as the tonsils, thymus, or bone marrow.

Etiology

The cause of non-Hodgkin's lymphoma is unclear, but some viruses, such as the Epstein-Barr virus and herpesvirus, are thought to play a role in their development. *Helicobacter pylori,* the bacteria that causes ulcers, has been associated with non-Hodgkin's lymphoma. Genetics plays a role, as do immune problems such as AIDS. People working in farming, printing, medicine, electronics, and leather also have a higher risk for developing non-Hodgkin's lymphoma.

Signs and Symptoms

Clinical features of malignant lymphomas include enlarged, painless, rubbery nodes in the cervical and supraclavicular areas, axillae, and groin; enlarged tonsils and adenoids; and occasional symptoms of dyspnea and cough. As the disease progresses, the patient may report fatigue, malaise, weight loss, and night sweats similar to Hodgkin's disease. Non-Hodgkin's lymphoma usually progresses more rapidly than Hodgkin's disease.

Diagnostic Tests

Diagnosis is confirmed by histological evaluation of biopsied lymph nodes, tonsils, bone marrow, liver, bowel, skin, or other affected tissues. Other relevant tests include bone scans, chest x-rays, lymphangiography, liver and spleen scans, CT of the abdomen, MRI, PET scan, and intravenous pyelogram to determine the extent of the disease. Laboratory tests include a CBC (which often indicates anemia), serum uric acid level, and liver function studies. Serum calcium level may be elevated if bone lesions are present.

Therapeutic Measures

Treatment usually involves multimodal therapy, including the use of chemotherapy and radiation therapy in combination. Radiation therapy is given to affected areas in advanced stages of non-Hodgkin's lymphoma. Stem cell transplant may be tried in patients with advanced disease. Newer therapies include the use of monoclonal antibodies to target and destroy cancer cells, and interferon therapy to help boost the immune system to fight the cancer.

Nursing Management

You can provide emotional support by keeping the patient and family informed during the testing phase. Symptoms such as night sweats can be managed with frequent linen and gown changes. Help the patient maintain nutrition with attractively prepared meals. Spend time listening to the patient's concerns; involve the hospital chaplain in the patient's care if the patient desires. Refer the patient and family to the resources listed earlier for more information. See Table 28.5 and the *Nursing Care Plan for the Patient with Lymphoma* for more information.

TABLE 28.4 HODGKIN'S DISEASE VERSUS NON-HODGKIN'S LYMPHOMA

	Hodgkin's Disease	Non-Hodgkin's Lymphomas
Age	15–40 and over 55 years	Usually over 50 years
Incidence	Less common	More common
Prognosis	Good	Poorer
Reed-Sternberg cells	Present	Absent
Alcohol-induced pain	May be present	Absent

TABLE 28.5 LYMPHOMA SUMMARY

Signs and Symptoms	Swollen lymph nodes Fatigue Low-grade fever Night sweats
Diagnostic Tests	CBC Lymph node biopsy Lymphangiography CT scan
Therapeutic Measures	Chemotherapy Radiation Bone marrow or stem cell transplant
Priority Nursing Diagnoses	*Activity Intolerance* *Risk for Infection* *Risk for Ineffective Coping*

SPLENIC DISORDERS

The spleen is involved in a number of disorders, including cancers of the blood, lymph, and bone marrow; hereditary conditions such as sickle cell disease; and acquired problems such as idiopathic thrombocytopenia. Under normal circumstances, the spleen is not paid much attention; it generally performs its functions without much fanfare.

If the spleen enlarges markedly, the condition is referred to as **splenomegaly**. Other times, the spleen may or may not be enlarged, but the function is out of control so that too many RBCs and platelets are removed from the peripheral circulation. Sometimes the spleen is not able to perform its job because of bleeding into the pulp of the organ, which renders it useless. Bleeding into the spleen can occur from various illnesses or from trauma. Regardless of the nature of the malfunction, one treatment option may be splenectomy.

Splenectomy

Splenectomy is the surgical removal of the spleen. This is sometimes used to treat selective hematologic disorders and is also used, under different circumstances, to determine the stage of lymphomas. It may be done with traditional, open surgery or laparoscopically. Splenectomy is performed fairly often in the United States, but, like any surgery, it is not without risk.

Patient Education

Explain to patients that this surgery removes the spleen, usually under general anesthesia. Inform patients that they can live a normal life after the surgery but that they may be more prone to infection, and that they should receive the influenza vaccine each year, preferably in the early fall.

Preoperative Care

Before the surgery, ensure that the CBC and coagulation profile are completed and reported to the physician. Blood transfusion may be ordered to correct underlying anemia and to prepare for the loss of a great deal of blood stored in the spleen. Vitamin K is often ordered to correct clotting factor deficiencies.

Take the patient's vital signs, and perform a baseline respiratory assessment. Note especially any signs of respiratory infections such as fever, chills, crackles, wheezes, or cough. If any of these are noted, make sure that the physician is aware of them because surgery may need to be delayed. Teach the patient routine coughing and deep-breathing techniques to help prevent postoperative respiratory complications.

Postoperative Care

During the early postoperative period, watch carefully for bleeding, either external or internal. Be prepared to administer opioids for pain, usually on an around-the-clock schedule so the patient is comfortable enough to deep breathe, cough, and ambulate. After opioid administration, be sure to observe for side effects, which may include incomplete pain relief or hypoventilation. Monitor for fever every 4 hours, and expect a mild, low-grade, transient fever postoperatively. A persistent fever may indicate abscess or hematoma formation.

If the surgery was performed to decrease the numbers of cells being removed from the peripheral circulation, monitor the platelet count. Often the count begins to rise in just a few days, but it may take up to 2 weeks for the platelets to normalize.

Complications

A splenectomy can cause complications such as bleeding, pneumonia, and atelectasis. Respiratory problems occur because of the spleen's position close to the diaphragm. This placement requires the need for a high surgical incision that is very painful. Often the patient tries to restrict lung expansion after surgery to keep from hurting, but this splinting behavior may leave the patient at risk for pneumonia and respiratory problems. In addition, splenectomy patients are usually more vulnerable to infection, especially influenza, because the spleen's role in the immune response is no longer filled.

Other possible complications from splenectomy include the development of pancreatitis and fistula formation. This is due to the fact that the tail of the pancreas is very close to the spleen, and irritation may have occurred.

Another serious complication is overwhelming post-splenectomy infection (OPSI). The causative agents in OPSI include streptococci, *Neisseria* spp., and influenza bacteria (as opposed to a flu virus). OPSI can occur at any time from 1 week to 20 years after the splenectomy. Patients most at risk are those with poor immune function.

Early symptoms of OPSI include fever and malaise that seem unremarkable. However, the infection may progress within a few hours to sepsis and death. Unfortunately, OPSI has a mortality rate as high as 70%. Be sure to include the signs and symptoms of OPSI in pre-splenectomy patient education. Also, stress the need to promptly obtain medical attention for the patient at the first signs and symptoms of OPSI. The patient should be directed to continue to receive lifetime vaccinations against these bacteria.

• WORD • BUILDING •

splenomegaly: splen—spleen + megaly—large
splenectomy: splen—spleen + ectomy—excision

Home Health Hints

- Patients who are at risk for infection can place a sign on the front door of their homes to limit visitors or ask persons with colds to come back when they are well. The patient may appreciate the home nurse giving permission to be assertive in such circumstances.
- Teach patients with infection risk to avoid working with dirt or soil, to avoid manicures and pedicures, to avoid hot tubs or Jacuzzis, and to wash hands after contact with pets, fresh flowers, or plants.
- To prevent bruising, have the patient cut the feet off of white sport socks and wear them on the arms. They can be hidden under long-sleeve shirts and blouses and provide a cushion when doing housework.
- Teach patients with thrombocytopenia to avoid contact sports, and to consult with their physician about whether sexual intercourse is safe.
- Teach patients with thrombocytopenia to avoid over-the-counter medications unless approved by the physician. Many such agents contain aspirin or nonsteroidal anti-inflammatory drugs.
- Patients with sickle cell anemia usually have lower blood pressures. It is important to report even mild hypertension in these patients.
- If fatigue or nausea causes poor appetite, discuss eating smaller, more frequent meals. Ask the physician for an antiemetic order if needed.

SUGGESTED ANSWERS TO CRITICAL THINKING

■ *Mrs. Johns*

1. Monitor Mrs. Johns' vital signs and report falling blood pressure and rising pulse immediately. Inspect her skin for petechiae and ecchymoses. Outline ecchymotic areas with a marker to see if the area is increasing in size. Monitor urine for signs of blood. Test stools for occult blood. Monitor vaginal discharge for increasing bleeding. Report any changes promptly.
2. Anticipate assisting the RN with administration of blood or blood products. Instruct Mrs. Johns in the importance of preventing injury that could cause further bleeding. Other care will be supportive.
3. Mrs. Johns will be concerned for her new baby, who is most likely on another unit or already discharged home. Allow Mrs. Johns to talk about her concerns. Arrange visits with her family and baby if permitted by her condition and her physician.
4. $$\frac{300 \text{ mL}}{30 \text{ min}} \Bigg| \frac{60 \text{ min}}{1 \text{ hour}} = 600 \text{ mL per hour}$$

■ *Mr. Washington*

1. Because of his leukemia and his treatment, Mr. Washington is at risk for infection. If he develops an infection, he will have great difficulty getting over it. With so many visitors in the room, it is likely that one or more has a cold or virus. They may not be aware of the risk this poses to Mr. Washington. Mr. Washington is probably also fatigued because of his disease and treatment, and visiting requires energy.
2. You should kindly explain that while family visits are very important, Mr. Washington is very susceptible to catching colds or other illnesses and that it would be best to limit visitors to one or two at a time. Point out that persons with symptoms of colds or flu should not enter the room at all. Visits should also be brief to prevent overtiring the patient.

■ *Jeanine*

Jeanine will probably be fatigued from her disease, and fatigue may increase further as a side effect of treatment. Staff nursing jobs can be tiring even for healthy nurses. In addition, she will be around patients with respiratory diseases, many of whom are contagious. Because of the risk of infection secondary to the disease process and the treatment regimen, Jeanine might want to take a leave of absence during treatment or ask to be reassigned to an area that is less demanding and away from direct patient care until her treatments have been completed.

REVIEW QUESTIONS

1. Which assessment finding would the nurse expect to find in a patient who has anemia?
   a. Pain
   b. Dyspnea
   c. Vision changes
   d. Skin rash

2. Which of the following activities is contraindicated for the patient with sickle cell anemia?
   a. Riding in an elevator
   b. Taking a long car trip
   c. Running in a marathon
   d. Listening to a concert

3. Which explanation for bleeding should the nurse give to the family member of a patient with DIC?
   a. "He is bleeding because he does not have enough RBCs."
   b. "He is bleeding because his white cells are depleted."
   c. "He is bleeding because his blood pressure is so high that it forces blood from mucous membranes."
   d. "He is bleeding because his body's clotting factors have all been used up."

4. Which instruction will help the mother of a child with hemophilia prevent bleeding episodes?
   a. "Your son should avoid contact sports."
   b. "Your son will have to avoid all potentially irritating foods."
   c. "Your son must never shave."
   d. "Your son should always live near a major hospital system."

5. Which family member should not be permitted to visit a patient with newly diagnosed leukemia?
   a. The one who has a new baby at home
   b. The one who has a history of asthma
   c. The one who has received recent radiation treatment for cancer
   d. The one who has a runny nose

6. Which of the following nursing interventions is a priority for the patient with multiple myeloma found in the ribs and femur?
   a. Implement safety measures to prevent falls.
   b. Assist with all ADLs.
   c. Provide a high-protein, low-sodium diet.
   d. Institute neutropenic precautions.

7. Which of the following nursing interventions are appropriate for a patient with thrombocytopenia? **Select all that apply.**
   a. Avoid intramuscular injections.
   b. Keep visitors who are ill away from the patient.
   c. Encourage 4 L of fluid daily.
   d. Avoid use of aspirin and NSAIDs.
   e. Allow rest between activities.
   f. Encourage use of shoes or slippers.

8. A patient with hypercalcemia needs to drink at least 3 L of fluid per day. Today, he has had 1 measuring cup of coffee, 1 L of water, a can of soda that says it has 355 mL, and a half cup of juice. How many milliliters has he had so far today? **Fill in the blank.**

   Answer: __________ mL

9. Stage III Hodgkin's disease is defined as which of the following?
   a. Lymphatic involvement on both sides of the diaphragm
   b. Localized involvement of more than two adjacent or nonadjacent regions on one side of the diaphragm
   c. Diffuse involvement of one or more extralymphatic organs or tissues such as the bone marrow or liver
   d. Localized involvement of a single lymph node site, usually located in the cervical or supraclavicular area

10. Which circumstance places the patient at most risk for respiratory complications following a splenectomy?
    a. Disturbance of clotting factors
    b. Nothing by mouth (NPO) status
    c. Need for frequent dressing changes
    d. Location of surgical incision

unit SEVEN

UNDERSTANDING THE RESPIRATORY SYSTEM

29

Respiratory System Function, Assessment, and Therapeutic Measures

PAULA D. HOPPER AND
JANICE L. BRADFORD

KEY TERMS

adventitious (add-ven-TISH-uss)
apnea (AP-nee-ah)
crepitus (KREP-ih-tuss)
cyanosis (SY-uh-NOH-siss)
dyspnea (DISP-nee-ah)
respiratory excursion (RESS-prah-TOR-ee eks-KUR-zhun)
retraction (rih-TRAK-shun)
thoracentesis (THOR-uh-sen-TEE-siss)
tidaling (TY-dah-ling)
tracheostomy (TRAY-key-AW-stuh-mee)
tracheotomy (TRAY-key-AW-tuh-mee)

QUESTIONS TO GUIDE YOUR READING

1. What are the structures of the respiratory system, and what is the function of each?
2. How does aging affect the respiratory system?
3. What questions should you ask when you take a history from a patient with a respiratory problem?
4. What findings do you expect when you inspect, palpate, percuss, and auscultate the chest?
5. What common diagnostic tests are performed to diagnose disorders of the respiratory system?
6. What nursing care should you provide for patients undergoing each of the diagnostic tests?
7. What therapeutic measures can you use to help patients with respiratory disorders?

NORMAL RESPIRATORY SYSTEM ANATOMY AND PHYSIOLOGY

The respiratory system consists of the nose, nasal cavities, pharynx, larynx, trachea, bronchial tree, lungs, and respiratory muscles. The parts superior to the chest cavity are collectively called the upper respiratory system, and those within the chest cavity make up the lower respiratory system (Fig. 29.1). The alveoli of the lungs are the site of gas exchange between the air and the blood; the rest of the system moves air into and out of the lungs.

Nose and Nasal Cavities

The nose is made predominantly of bone and cartilage covered with muscle and epithelium. Hairs inside the nostrils block the entry of dust and other particles. The two nasal cavities are inside the skull and are separated by the nasal septum, which is made of the vomer, ethmoid, and septal cartilage. The nasal mucosa is ciliated epithelium that is highly vascular; it warms and moistens inhaled air. Dust and microorganisms become trapped on mucus produced by goblet cells and are swept backward and down into the pharynx by the cilia. See Table 29.1 for a summary of protective mechanisms in the respiratory system.

The paranasal sinuses are air cavities in the maxillae and the frontal, sphenoid, and ethmoid bones that open into the nasal cavities. They too are lined with ciliated epithelium. The mucus produced usually drains into the nasal cavities. The sinuses lessen the weight of the skull and provide resonance for the voice.

TABLE 29.1 PROTECTIVE MECHANISMS IN THE RESPIRATORY SYSTEM

Nasal hairs and turbinates	Trap dust and microorganisms.
Mucous membranes	Warm and moisten inhaled air; trap inhaled particles.
Cilia	Move particles toward pharynx to be swallowed or coughed out.
Irritant receptors in nose and airways	Trigger sneeze and cough to remove foreign debris.
Alveolar macrophages	Phagocytize foreign particles and bacteria.

Pharynx

The pharynx is posterior to the nasal and oral cavities. It has three parts: nasopharynx, oropharynx, and laryngopharynx. The nasopharynx is an air passage above the level of the soft palate. The soft palate and uvula rise to block the nasopharynx during swallowing. The eustachian tubes from the middle ear cavities open into the nasopharynx; the adenoid (pharyngeal tonsil) is a lymph nodule on its

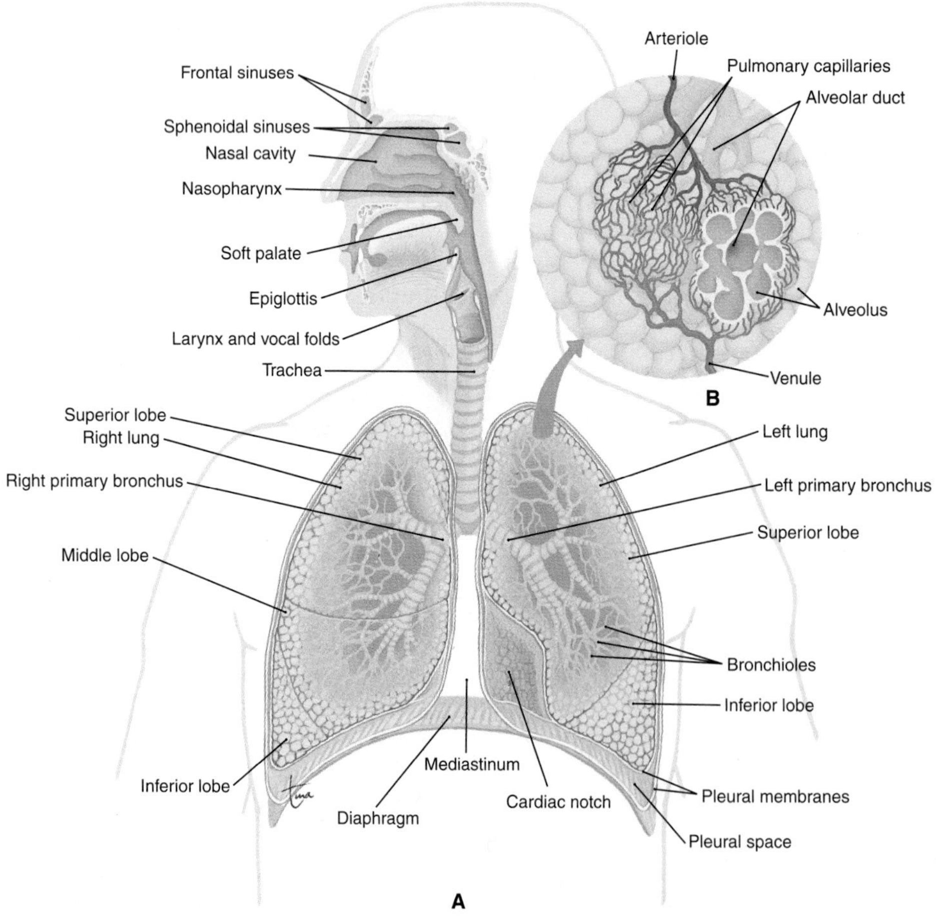
Frontal sinuses
Sphenoidal sinuses
Nasal cavity
Nasopharynx
Soft palate
Epiglottis
Larynx and vocal folds
Trachea
Superior lobe
Right lung
Right primary bronchus
Middle lobe
Inferior lobe
Diaphragm
Mediastinum
Cardiac notch
A
Arteriole
Pulmonary capillaries
Alveolar duct
Alveolus
Venule
B
Left lung
Left primary bronchus
Superior lobe
Bronchioles
Inferior lobe
Pleural membranes
Pleural space

FIGURE 29.1 Respiratory system, anterior view, with microscopic view of alveoli and pulmonary capillaries. (Modified from Scanlon, V. C., & Sanders, T. [2007]. *Essentials of anatomy and physiology* [5th ed.]. Philadelphia: F. A. Davis.)

posterior wall. The oropharynx is posterior to the oral cavity and is both an air and a food passage. The palatine tonsils are on the lateral walls. Together with the lingual tonsils on the base of the tongue and the adenoid, the palatine tonsils form a ring of lymphatic tissue around the pharynx and destroy pathogens that penetrate the mucosa. The laryngopharynx is both an air and a food passage; it opens anteriorly into the larynx and posteriorly into the esophagus.

Larynx

The larynx is the voice box and the airway between the pharynx and trachea. It is made of nine pieces of cartilage, yielding a firm yet flexible tissue that keeps the airway open. It is lined with ciliated epithelium. The thyroid cartilage, commonly called the Adam's apple, is the largest of these cartilage pieces and is palpable on the front of the neck. The epiglottis is the uppermost cartilage and covers the larynx like a flap when the larynx is elevated during swallowing. The vocal cords are on either side of the rima glottidis (the airway opening). When pulled together across the rima glottidis and vibrated by exhaled air, the vocal cords produce sounds that may be turned into speech. The vagus and accessory cranial nerves are the motor nerves to the larynx.

Trachea and Bronchial Tree

The trachea is a tube, 4 to 5 inches in length, that extends from the larynx to the primary bronchi. C-shaped pieces of cartilage in the wall keep the trachea open. The mucosa is ciliated epithelium; mucus with trapped dust and microorganisms is swept upward toward the pharynx and is usually swallowed.

The bronchial tree is the series of air passages within the lungs, a succession of progressively smaller tubes that terminate in the alveoli. The right and left primary bronchi are branches of the trachea. Each gives rise to secondary bronchi and then tertiary bronchi; their structure is like that of the trachea. The bronchioles, however, have no cartilage in the walls to maintain patency, and they may be closed completely by contraction of their smooth muscle.

Lungs and Pleural Membranes

The lungs occupy the chest cavity on either side of the heart, extending from the clavicles to the diaphragm. On the medial (mediastinal) surface of each lung is an indentation called the hilus, where the primary bronchus and the pulmonary artery and veins enter the lung.

The pleural membranes are the serous membranes of the thoracic cavity. The visceral pleura is the membrane that covers the lungs; the parietal pleura lines the chest cavity. A small amount of serous fluid between these membranes prevents friction and adheres the membranes together during breathing.

The functional units of the lung are the millions of alveoli, the air sacs that are the site of gas exchange. Both the alveoli and the surrounding alveolar capillaries are made of simple squamous epithelium; that is, their walls are only one cell in thickness to permit diffusion of gases (see Fig. 29.1).

Each alveolus is lined with a thin layer of tissue fluid that is essential for the diffusion of gases, but the surface tension of the fluid tends to make the walls of an alveolus stick together internally. Certain alveolar cells secrete pulmonary surfactant, a lipoprotein that mixes with the tissue fluid and decreases surface tension to permit inflation. Also in the alveoli are the alveolar macrophages, which phagocytize pathogens or fine dust particles and debris that have not been trapped and swept out by the cilia.

Between clusters of alveoli is elastic connective tissue that can recoil when stretched (during inhalation) and contributes significantly to normal exhalation. The recoil of this tissue ensures that normal exhalation during quiet breathing is a passive process that does not require the expenditure of energy.

Mechanism of Breathing

Ventilation is the term for the movement of air into and out of the alveoli. Air moves from high-pressure to low-pressure areas, some of which are created by the respiratory muscles that are controlled by the nervous system. The respiratory centers are in the medulla oblongata and pons. The main respiratory muscles are the diaphragm inferior to the lungs and the external and internal intercostal muscles between the ribs. Accessory muscles of respiration are used during exercise and times of respiratory distress; these include the sternocleidomastoid, scalene muscles, and abdominal musculature.

Pressures important to breathing include atmospheric pressure, intrapleural pressure, and intrapulmonic (alveolar) pressure. Atmospheric pressure is the pressure of the air around us, which at sea level is 760 mm Hg; atmospheric pressure decreases as altitude increases. Intrapleural pressure is in the potential pleural space between the pleural membranes. Serous fluid causes the two membranes to adhere to each other, and because the elastic lungs are always tending to collapse and pull the visceral pleura away from the parietal pleura, the pressure in this potential space is always below atmospheric pressure (about 756 mm Hg). This is called a negative pressure. Intrapulmonic (alveolar) pressure is the pressure inside the alveoli and bronchial tree. This pressure fluctuates below and above atmospheric pressure during each cycle of breathing.

Inhalation

Inhalation, also called inspiration, occurs when motor impulses from the medulla cause contraction of the respiratory muscles. Impulses along the phrenic nerves cause the dome-shaped diaphragm to contract and flatten downward. Impulses along the intercostal nerves cause the external intercostal muscles to pull the rib cage upward and outward, expanding the chest cavity in the anteroposterior dimension. This then expands the pleural membranes. Intrapleural pressure becomes even more negative, but the serous fluid keeps the membranes together and the lungs expand as well. As the lungs expand, alveolar pressure falls below atmospheric pressure and air enters the nose and respiratory passages. Entry of air continues until alveolar pressure equals atmospheric pressure; this is a normal inhalation. A deeper inhalation requires a more forceful contraction of the respiratory muscles (including accessory inspiratory muscles) to expand the chest cavity and lungs even further and permit the entry of more air.

Exhalation

Normal exhalation is a passive process that begins when motor impulses from the medulla decrease and the diaphragm and external intercostal muscles relax. The lungs are compressed as the chest cavity becomes smaller and the recoil of the elastic lung tissue compresses the alveoli. Alveolar pressure rises above atmospheric pressure, and air is forced out of the lungs until the two pressures are again equal. Under normal circumstances, energy is not required for exhalation (as it is for inhalation) because the elasticity of the lungs causes recoil and forces air out. A forced exhalation beyond the normal amount is an active process that requires contraction of the internal intercostal muscles to pull the rib cage downward and inward and contraction of the abdominal muscles to force the dome of the diaphragm upward, increasing compression of the lungs.

Transport of Gases in the Blood

Oxygen is carried in the blood by iron in the hemoglobin (Hgb) of red blood cells (RBCs). The iron-oxygen bond is formed in the lungs, where the partial pressure of oxygen (Po_2) is high. In tissues where the Po_2 is low, hemoglobin releases much of its oxygen.

Most carbon dioxide is carried in the blood in the form of bicarbonate ions in the plasma. These ions are formed when carbon dioxide enters RBCs and is converted to carbonic acid (H_2CO_3), which ionizes to bicarbonate ions (HCO_3^-) and hydrogen ions (H^+). The bicarbonate ions leave the RBCs for the plasma, and the remaining hydrogen ions are buffered by the hemoglobin in the RBCs. When the blood reaches the lungs, an area of lower partial pressure of carbon dioxide (Pco_2), these reactions are reversed—carbon dioxide is re-formed and diffuses into the alveoli to be exhaled.

Regulation of Respiration

Respiration is regulated by both nervous and chemical mechanisms. The medulla oblongata contains an inspiratory center and an expiratory center. The inspiratory center generates impulses that bring about contraction of the respiratory muscles, resulting in inhalation. When the impulses stop, exhalation occurs. If the lungs are overinflated, bronchi and bronchiole baroreceptors are stretched. The stretching inhibits the inspiratory center (and apneustic center) and exhalation follows. This protective mechanism is called the Hering-Breuer inflation reflex. In the pons, the apneustic center prolongs inhalation and the pneumotaxic center helps bring about exhalation. These centers provide a normal breathing rhythm, 12 to 20 breaths per minute with exhalation slightly longer than inhalation. When there is a need for more forceful exhalations, the inspiratory center activates the expiratory center, which brings about contraction of the internal intercostal muscles.

Normal breathing is essentially a reflex, but because the respiratory muscles are skeletal (or voluntary) muscles, it is possible to force changes. The cerebral cortex may override the medulla to permit voluntary changes in breathing, such as faster or slower breathing, holding one's breath, or singing. Eventually, the medulla resumes control and breathing is again a reflex.

Chemical regulation of respiration involves the blood levels of oxygen and carbon dioxide. Decreased blood oxygen is detected by chemoreceptors in the carotid body and aortic body; the response by the medulla is to increase respiration to take more air into the lungs. An increase in blood carbon dioxide or a decrease in pH is detected by central chemoreceptors in the medulla and peripheral chemoreceptors; the response is increased respiration to exhale more carbon dioxide, which raises the pH back toward normal.

Carbon dioxide is usually the major regulator of respiration because even small changes in its blood level change the pH. Fluctuations in the oxygen level have no effect on pH, and an adequate oxygen level in the blood can be maintained even if breathing ceases for a few minutes. Residual air in the lungs is a contributing factor, as is the fact that air contains much more oxygen than we typically use (exhaled air is 16% oxygen). Oxygen becomes the major regulator only when its blood level is very low, as may occur with severe, chronic pulmonary disease.

Respiration and Acid-Base Balance

Because of its role in regulating the amount of carbon dioxide in body fluids, the respiratory system is important in the maintenance of acid-base balance, measured by blood pH. Any decrease in the rate or efficiency of respiration permits excess carbon dioxide to accumulate in the blood. The resulting accumulation of excess hydrogen ions lowers pH. This is called respiratory acidosis and can occur as a consequence of pulmonary disease or any impairment of gas exchange in the lungs.

Respiratory alkalosis occurs when the rate of respiration increases, eliminating exhaled carbon dioxide very rapidly. Less carbon dioxide in the blood means that fewer hydrogen ions are formed and the pH rises. Although it is not a common condition, respiratory alkalosis may occur during states of anxiety and hyperventilation, or when acclimating to a high altitude, before RBC production increases to provide sufficient oxygenation of tissues.

The respiratory system may also help compensate for pH changes that are metabolic; that is, due to any cause other than respiratory. Metabolic acidosis occurs when the concentration of hydrogen ions in body fluids is above normal due to lowered HCO_3^- buffer. Common causes include kidney disease, uncontrolled diabetes mellitus, and severe diarrhea. Respiratory compensation involves an increase in the rate and depth of respiration to exhale more carbon dioxide, which decreases hydrogen ion formation and raises the pH toward normal. Metabolic alkalosis may be caused by over-ingestion of antacid medications or by vomiting acidic gastric contents. Respiratory compensation involves a decrease in the breathing rate to retain carbon dioxide in the body, increasing the formation of hydrogen ions, which lowers the pH toward normal.

Respiratory compensation for an ongoing metabolic pH imbalance (such as kidney failure) cannot be complete because the amount of carbon dioxide that may be exhaled or retained is limited. At most, respiratory compensation is only about 75% effective.

Acid-base balance is discussed further in Chapter 6.

Effects of Aging on the Respiratory System

See Figure 29.2 for the effects of aging on respiration.

NURSING ASSESSMENT OF THE RESPIRATORY SYSTEM

Health History

Many factors in a patient's personal and family history affect respiratory function. Questions to ask while assessing the patient with a history of respiratory dysfunction are presented in Table 29.2. If at any time while you are taking the history the patient relates a specific symptom, redirect the line of questioning to further assess that symptom. One such line of questioning, as presented in Chapter 1, is the WHAT'S UP? format. For example, if the patient reports shortness of breath, respond with the following questions (**W**here is it? doesn't apply to shortness of breath, so it may be skipped.):

- **H**ow does it feel? Does breathing feel tight, gasping, painful, suffocating?
- **A**ggravating and alleviating factors? How much activity causes the shortness of breath? Does anything else aggravate it? What do you do to lessen your shortness of breath?
- **T**iming? When did you first experience shortness of breath? Does it happen more at any particular time of day or year?
- **S**everity? Rate your shortness of breath on a scale of 0 to 10, with 0 being easy breathing and 10 being the worst shortness of breath you can imagine.
- **U**seful other data? Do you have any other symptoms that occur along with the shortness of breath?
- **P**atient's perception? What do you think is causing your shortness of breath?

Because smoking is such a major risk factor for many types of lung disease, it is essential to ask about smoking history and encourage the patient to quit (see the discussion of smoking cessation later in the chapter). Document the patient's smoking history in terms of pack-years. For example, if a patient has smoked two packs of cigarettes per day for 20 years, he has a 40 pack-year smoking history ($2 \times 20 = 40$ pack-years). It is also important to be aware of cultural influences on the patient's respiratory health (Box 29.1, *Cultural Considerations*).

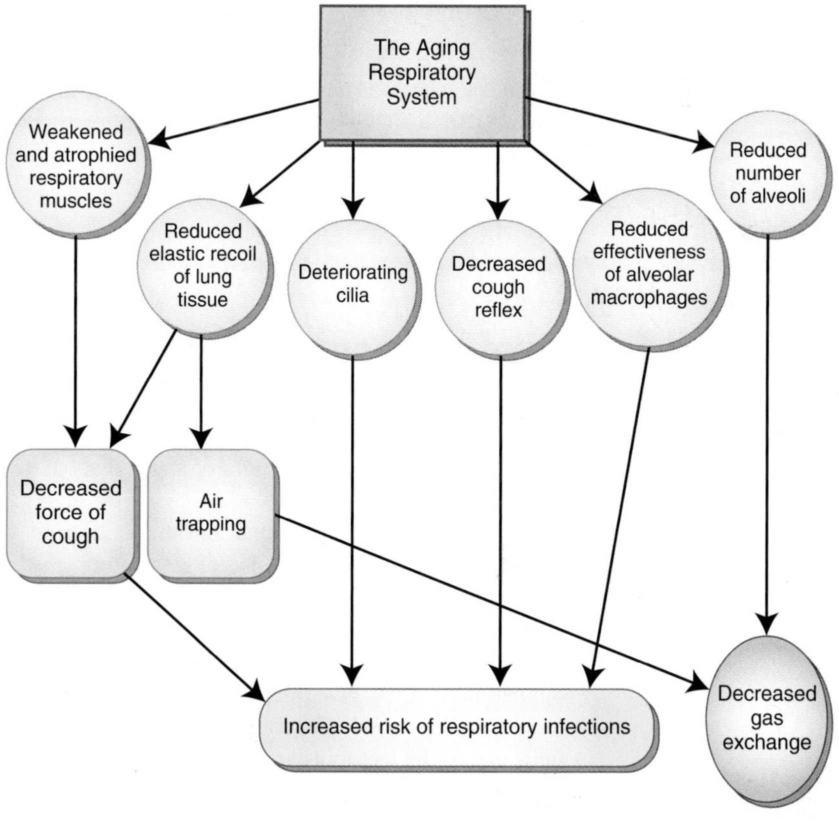
The Aging Respiratory System
Weakened and atrophied respiratory muscles
Reduced elastic recoil of lung tissue
Deteriorating cilia
Decreased cough reflex
Reduced effectiveness of alveolar macrophages
Reduced number of alveoli
Decreased force of cough
Air trapping
Increased risk of respiratory infections
Decreased gas exchange

FIGURE 29.2 Effects of aging on respiration.

TABLE 29.2 SUBJECTIVE DATA COLLECTION FOR THE RESPIRATORY SYSTEM

Category	Questions to Ask During the Health History	Rationale/Significance
Upper Respiratory Tract	Do you often have headaches or sinus tenderness?	These may indicate sinusitis.
	Do you often experience nosebleeds?	A history of nosebleeds may indicate an abnormality that can predispose to future nosebleeds.
	Has your voice changed?	A voice change may indicate a variety of disorders of the nose or throat, including cancer. Further investigation is needed.
Lower Respiratory Tract	Do you ever feel short of breath, like you can't get enough air?	Many respiratory and cardiac problems result in shortness of breath.
	Do you have a cough? Is it productive?	A cough indicates respiratory irritation or excessive secretions.
	What does the sputum look like?	Yellow, tan, or green sputum may accompany an infection. Blood in the sputum may occur with tuberculosis, pulmonary embolism, or cancer.
	Have you recently experienced night sweats, chills, or fever?	These are symptoms of tuberculosis.
	Do you ever feel confused, light-headed, or restless?	These symptoms might indicate a low Po_2, reducing oxygen to the brain.
	Have you had any chest surgeries?	This may reveal problem areas the patient has not yet mentioned.
Exposures	Do you have any allergies that cause respiratory symptoms? How do you treat them?	The patient may take over-the-counter medications for allergies that affect respiratory function or interact with prescribed medications.
	Do you smoke? How many packs per day? For how many years? Are you exposed to secondhand smoke?	Many respiratory disorders are caused or aggravated by exposure to tobacco smoke.
	Have you been exposed to airborne pollutants at home or work?	Pollutants such as asbestos, radon, coal dust, or chemicals can cause lung disease.
Treatments	Do you take any medications or use inhalers (prescribed or over-the-counter) for your respiratory problems?	Information about medications gives further information about disorders, severity, and treatment. You should also consider drug interactions and side effects.
	Do you use home oxygen or other home respiratory treatments?	This helps determine the severity of disease and the treatment.
Family History	Do any of your blood relatives have emphysema, asthma, or tuberculosis?	Some respiratory disorders have a hereditary tendency. Tuberculosis is contagious.

Box 29.1

Cultural Considerations

Pulmonary diseases associated with Japanese people include asthma related to dust mites in the straw mats that cover floors in Japanese homes, and air pollution from living in urban areas. Encourage patients who have straw mats and who wish to keep them to have them sterilized.

Patients from Poland, Ireland, or other countries where mining is a primary occupation may have an increased incidence of respiratory disease. It is essential for health care providers to carefully screen Polish and Irish immigrants for respiratory conditions.

Health care practitioners should be aware of variations among ethnic peoples of color when assessing for cyanosis. Cyanosis and decreased blood hemoglobin levels in darker-skinned individuals give the skin an ashen color instead of a bluish color. Thus, the nurse must examine the sclerae, conjunctivae, buccal mucosa, tongue, lips, nailbeds, and palms and soles of the feet to assess for lowered oxygen levels.

Box 29.1

Cultural Considerations—cont'd

Smoking is deeply ingrained in the Arab American culture. Offering cigarettes is a rite of Arab hospitality. Arab individuals may have difficulty stopping smoking because of these cultural rituals.

Strategies to increase the effectiveness of smoking cessation in African Americans include working with community and church groups in African American communities. Populations living in inner cities are at increased risk for respiratory diseases related to pollution.

Physical Examination

Inspection

Inspection begins during the nursing history and continues during the physical assessment. Start with the nose, observing for symmetry, swelling, or other abnormalities. Note whether the patient is short of breath while speaking or moving. If the patient feels very breathless, he or she may speak in short sentences.

Observe the patient for use of accessory muscles of breathing (Fig. 29.3). Use of the sternocleidomastoid muscles causes the shoulders to rise during labored inspiration. During forced expiration, the abdominal and intercostal muscles contract. The use of accessory muscles for breathing indicates respiratory distress. **Retraction** of the chest wall between the ribs can indicate serious distress. Retractions occur when airways are obstructed. When the patient inhales and air can't easily flow into the lungs, negative pressure in the chest pulls the soft tissue between the ribs inward.

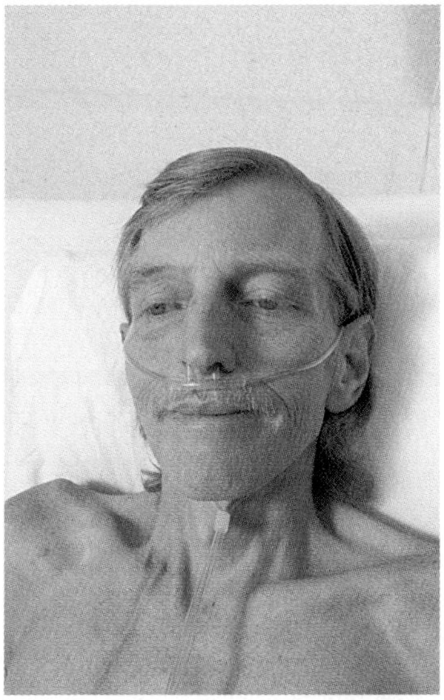

FIGURE 29.3 Accessory muscles of breathing. Note the prominent sternocleidomastoid muscles.

Note the color of the skin, lips, mucous membranes, and nailbeds. A bluish color is called **cyanosis** and is a late sign of oxygen deprivation. Observe the trachea and chest for symmetry. Count the number of respirations per minute, noting depth and rhythm. Irregular respirations, or periods of **apnea** (absence of respirations), can indicate a pathological condition and are described in Figure 29.4. Observe the shape of the chest. Normally the chest is about twice as wide (side to side) as it is deep (front to back). If it is more rounded, it is called a barrel chest, which is associated with trapped air in the lungs. See Table 29.3 for a summary of objective data.

Palpation

Palpate the frontal and maxillary sinuses if sinus inflammation is suspected (Fig. 29.5). Use your thumbs to palpate gently below the eyebrows and below each cheekbone. Tenderness may indicate sinus inflammation or infection.

Respiratory excursion can also be palpated. This is a rough measurement of chest expansion on inspiration. It is not necessary to palpate expansion on every patient, but it may be helpful if hypoventilation or asymmetry is suspected. Figure 29.6 illustrates how to palpate for respiratory excursion. You can palpate for **crepitus** (also called subcutaneous emphysema) if indicated. Crepitus feels like Rice Krispies under the skin when felt with the fingers. It occurs when air leaks into subcutaneous tissues because of pneumothorax or a leaking chest tube site. Palpation for crepitus is not done routinely, but rather when the possibility of an air leak exists.

Percussion

Percussion is done by the experienced nurse. It involves tapping on the anterior and posterior chest, in each intercostal space, and comparing sounds from side to side. A normal chest sounds resonant and is the same on both the right and left sides except over the heart. If other percussion notes are heard, they may indicate a pathological condition and should be reported.

Auscultation

Auscultation provides valuable information about respiratory status. Use the diaphragm of your stethoscope to listen to the anterior, lateral, and posterior chest during

• WORD • BUILDING •

cyanosis: cyan—dark blue + osis—condition

apnea: a—not + pnea—breath

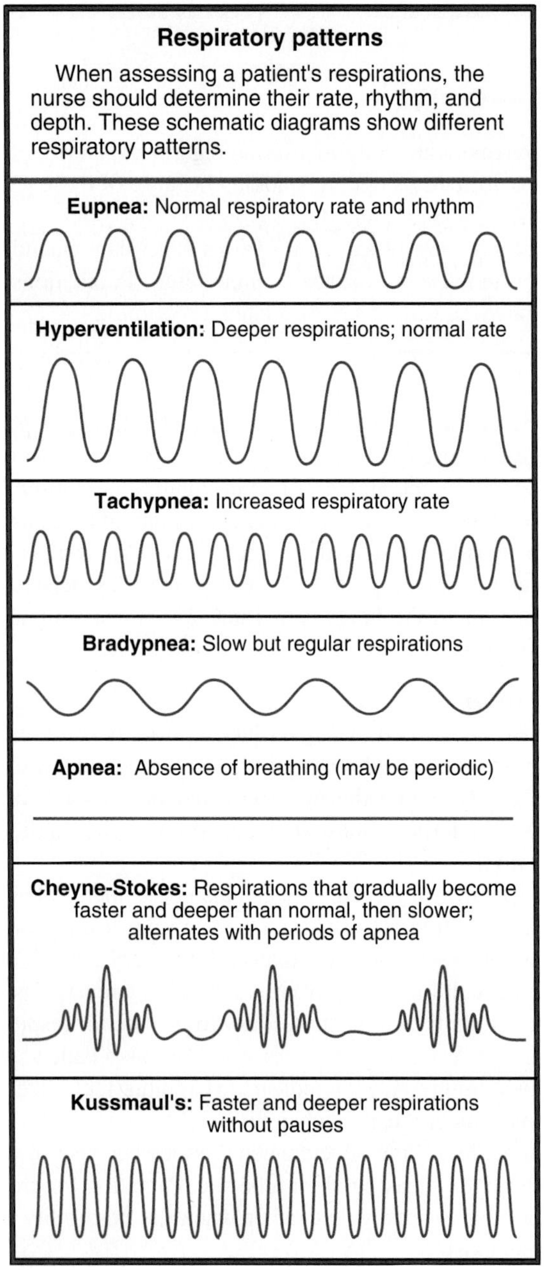
Respiratory patterns
When assessing a patient's respirations, the nurse should determine their rate, rhythm, and depth. These schematic diagrams show different respiratory patterns.
Eupnea: Normal respiratory rate and rhythm
Hyperventilation: Deeper respirations; normal rate
Tachypnea: Increased respiratory rate
Bradypnea: Slow but regular respirations
Apnea: Absence of breathing (may be periodic)
Cheyne-Stokes: Respirations that gradually become faster and deeper than normal, then slower; alternates with periods of apnea
Kussmaul's: Faster and deeper respirations without pauses

FIGURE 29.4 Abnormal respiratory patterns.

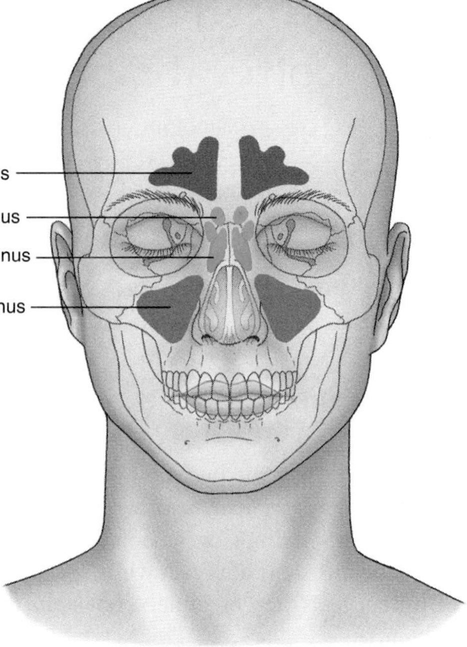
Frontal sinus
Ethmoid sinus
Sphenoid sinus
Maxillary sinus

FIGURE 29.5 Paranasal sinuses.

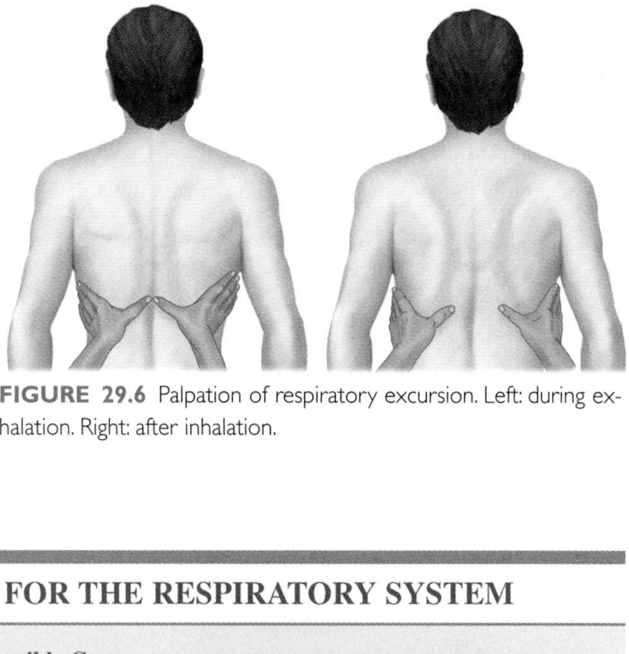

FIGURE 29.6 Palpation of respiratory excursion. Left: during exhalation. Right: after inhalation.

TABLE 29.3 OBJECTIVE DATA COLLECTION FOR THE RESPIRATORY SYSTEM

Category	Abnormal Findings	Possible Causes
Respiratory	Respiratory rate less than 12 per minute	Respiratory depression, possibly from opioid or sedative use
	Use of accessory muscles	Restrictive or obstructive disorders
	Barrel chest	Air trapping from obstructive disorder (COPD)
	Adventitious sounds	*See Table 29.4.*
	Cough	Airway irritation or secretions
	Sputum	Yellow, tan, or green sputum may indicate infection. Blood in sputum can indicate tuberculosis, cancer, or pulmonary embolism.
Integumentary	Cyanosis	Tissue hypoxia
	Nail clubbing	Chronic tissue hypoxia
Neurologic	Confusion	Lack of oxygen to the brain
Gastrointestinal	Weight loss	Dyspnea interfering with eating; use of calories for breathing

an entire inspiration and expiration at each interspace (Fig. 29.7). Auscultation of the posterior chest is easiest if the patient is sitting, but if necessary, it may be done with the patient in a side-lying position. Asking the patient to breathe deeply through the mouth can help enhance the sounds. Allow the patient to rest at intervals to prevent hyperventilation. Regular and frequent practice helps you learn to distinguish normal from abnormal breath sounds. Abnormal extra sounds (another term is **adventitious**) indicate a pathological condition and are described in Table 29.4.

LEARNING TIP

Listen to breath sounds on all your friends and family members. Assuming they are normal, this will give you a good baseline so when you hear an abnormal or adventitious sound on a patient, you will recognize it as "not normal"!

CRITICAL THINKING

Timothy

■ Timothy is a 16-year-old whose mother brought him to the emergency room because of an asthma attack. He says he feels short of breath, but when you listen to his lungs you hear no wheezing.

1. Does Timothy really need to be in the emergency room?
2. What should you do?
3. What do you think could be happening?

Suggested answers at end of chapter.

DIAGNOSTIC TESTS FOR THE RESPIRATORY SYSTEM

Laboratory Tests

Blood Tests

COMPLETE BLOOD COUNT. Measurement of red blood cells and hemoglobin can give information about the oxygen-carrying capacity of the blood. **Dyspnea** (shortness of breath) can be caused by a reduction in RBCs or hemoglobin. Elevated white blood cells indicate infection. See Table 29.5 for normal blood count values.

ARTERIAL BLOOD GAS ANALYSIS. Arterial blood gases (ABGs) are measured to determine the effectiveness of gas exchange. The "Pa" portion of the ABG results refers to the partial pressure of the gas in arterial blood. See Table 29.6 for a basic interpretation of ABGs. The blood sample is usually taken from the radial artery in the wrist by a physician or laboratory technician specially trained to do this. This can be painful for the patient. Place pressure on the site for 5 minutes after the test to prevent bleeding.

LEARNING TIP

If you remember that a normal blood pH is 7.35 to 7.45, then it is easy to remember that a normal $Paco_2$ is 35 to 45 mm Hg.

LEARNING TIP

Remember 50! If the Pao_2 falls below 50 and the $Paco_2$ is above 50, the patient is in trouble and the physician should be notified. This is a crude analysis, but it is helpful when a quick assessment is needed.

• WORD • BUILDING •
dyspnea: dys—bad + pnea—breathing

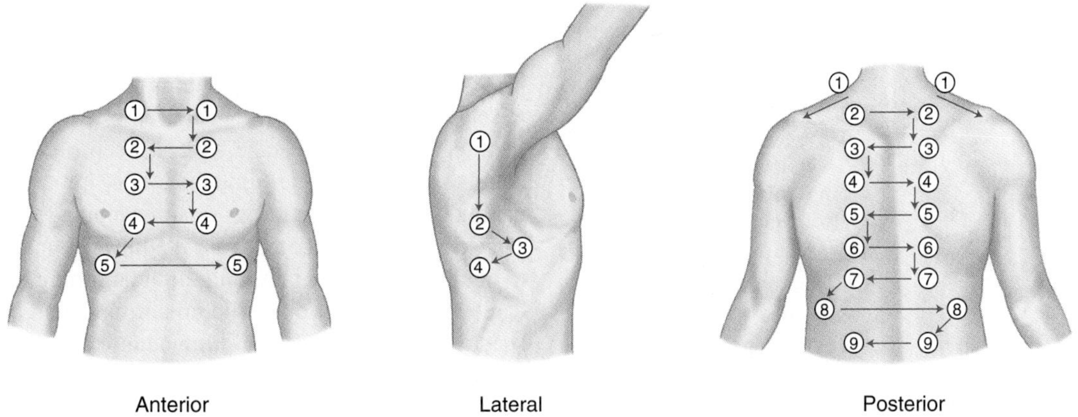
Anterior
Lateral
Posterior

FIGURE 29.7 Auscultation of the chest. Use a systematic approach to auscultate the chest, comparing sounds from side to side.

TABLE 29.4 ABNORMAL LUNG SOUNDS

Abnormal (Adventitious) Sound	Cause of Sound	Description	Associated Disorders
Coarse crackles (sometimes called rales)	Fluid in airways	Moist bubbling sound, heard on inspiration or expiration	Pulmonary edema, bronchitis, pneumonia
Fine crackles (rales)	Alveoli popping open on inspiration	Velcro being torn apart, heard at end of inspiration	Heart failure, atelectasis
Wheezes	Narrowed airways	Fine high-pitched violins mostly on expiration	Asthma
Stridor	Airway obstruction	Loud crowing noise heard without stethoscope	Obstruction from tumor or foreign body
Pleural friction rub	Inflamed pleura rubbing together	Sound of leather rubbing together; grating sound	Pleurisy, lung cancer, pneumonia, pleural irritation
Diminished	Decreased air movement	Faint lung sounds	Emphysema, hypoventilation, obesity, muscular chest wall
Absent	No air movement	No sounds heard	Pneumothorax, pneumectomy

TABLE 29.5 DIAGNOSTIC LABORATORY TESTS FOR THE RESPIRATORY SYSTEM

Test	Normal Values	Associated Conditions
Red Blood Cell Count	*Male:* 4.5–6.2 million cells/mm³ venous blood *Female:* 4.2–5.4 million cells/mm³ venous blood	↑ in chronic lung disease, dehydration ↓ in anemia, hemorrhage, overhydration with intravenous fluids
Hemoglobin	*Male:* 13.5–18 g/dL *Female:* 12–16 g/dL	Same as RBC count
White Blood Cell Count	5000–10,000 cells/mm³ venous blood	↑ in infection

TABLE 29.6 ARTERIAL BLOOD GAS ANALYSIS

	Normal Values	Interpretation
Pao_2	75–100 mm Hg	↑ in hyperventilation ↓ in impaired respiratory function
$Paco_2$	35–45 mm Hg	↑ in impaired gas exchange ↓ in hyperventilation
pH	7.35–7.45	↑ in respiratory alkalosis with low $Paco_2$ ↓ in respiratory acidosis with high $Paco_2$
HCO_3^-	22–26	↑ to buffer $Paco_2$ in acidosis ↓ to buffer $Paco_2$ in alkalosis
Oxygen saturation	95%–100%	↑ in hyperventilation ↓ in impaired respiratory function

D-DIMER. This blood test measures fibrin degradation products, which are present if there is a blood clot in the body. It helps diagnose the presence of a pulmonary embolism.

Sputum Culture and Sensitivity

A sputum culture identifies pathogens present in the sputum. The sensitivity test determines which antibiotics will be effective against those pathogens. To obtain a sputum specimen, first obtain a sterile container. Some institutions have special containers for sputum that help prevent transmission of infection to the health care worker (Fig. 29.8). Instruct the patient to take several deep breaths and then cough sputum into the container. It is important that the patient not simply spit saliva or sinus drainage into the cup. The specimen must come from the lungs. It may be easiest to obtain a specimen first thing in the morning (after mouth care) because secretions build up during the night. Send the specimen to the laboratory immediately. If the patient is unable to cough up sputum, extra fluids or a bedside humidifier may help. A respiratory therapist (RT) may be able to help obtain a specimen with a nebulized mist treatment or with a special suction catheter with a sputum trap. A physician's order may be needed for these procedures.

PATIENT CARE TIP

If the physician orders a "sputum for AFB," tuberculosis is suspected, which is caused by an acid-fast bacillus (AFB). Ask whether the patient should be placed in isolation while waiting for test results.

Throat Culture

A throat culture is done to determine the presence of viral or bacterial pathogens in the pharynx. Use a swab to reach into the pharynx (without touching the patient's mouth) and rub the red area or lesions. Use a tongue blade to help hold the tongue down while obtaining the culture. Warn the patient that a gag reflex may be triggered. Once the culture has been obtained, place it in a sterile tube with culture medium, according to package instructions. Send it immediately to the laboratory for analysis.

Nasal Samples

New tests are now available that use a nasopharyngeal swab or a nasal wash to identify flu or other respiratory viruses. To be accurate, it must be done in the first few days a person has symptoms. The sample may be obtained by swabbing the affected area in the nasal passages or pharynx, or by using a small amount of saline to wash out the nose, depending on the type of test ordered.

Oxygen Saturation

The oxygen saturation test (also called pulse oximetry, O_2 sat, or Spo_2) is a simple and noninvasive way to measure arterial oxygenation. A sensor is placed on the patient's finger or ear.

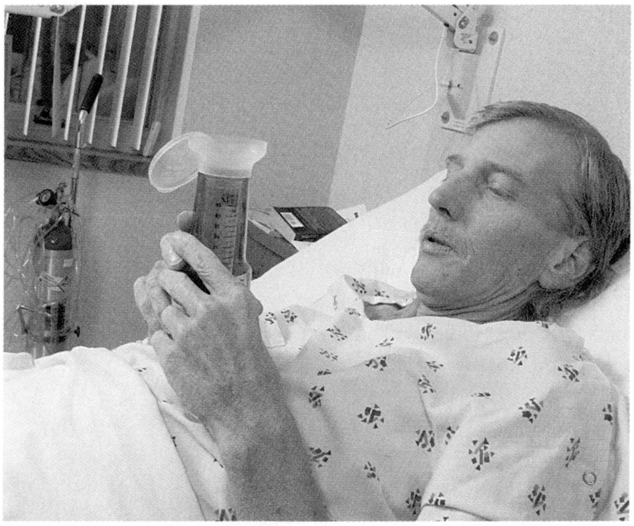

FIGURE 29.8 A special container that helps prevent transmission of infection is often used to collect sputum for culture.

The sensor measures the percentage of hemoglobin that is saturated with oxygen. Oxygen saturation can be measured at rest or while the patient is walking to determine the patient's exercise tolerance. It is also often done with and without supplemental oxygen to determine the patient's need for oxygen supplementation at home. See Table 29.6 for normal values. An Spo_2 value below 95% should be reported to the registered nurse (RN) or physician. If the Sao_2 is less than 75%, prepare for emergency intervention.

Oxygen saturations may be inaccurate in patients with low blood flow or decreased perfusion, patients who are moving, and patients who have smoke inhalation injury or carbon monoxide poisoning. Dark-skinned patients may have falsely high readings. Acrylic nails may need to be removed for accurate readings. Always correlate Spo_2 results with patient assessment findings.

Capnography

The process of measuring a person's exhaled carbon dioxide level is called capnography. It provides a continuous measurement of the patient's ventilation status. In the past, capnography was done primarily during surgery by an anesthetist. Now it is becoming more common in emergency departments and intensive care units; even emergency medical technicians are using it. It is most often used when patients are intubated. A special sensor is placed between the endotracheal tube and the ventilator to measure the exhaled carbon dioxide. Special nasal cannulas with sensors are also now available. Results from such sensors read out on a special monitor.

Other Tests

Chest X-Ray Examination

A chest x-ray examination may be ordered to help diagnose a variety of pulmonary disorders. Usually, posterior-anterior (PA) and side views (lateral) are taken. If a hospitalized patient is too ill to go to the radiology department, a portable chest x-ray machine can be used at the bedside to obtain a PA view.

Computed Tomography

A computed tomography (CT) scan combines x-ray and computer technology to produce multiple images of the chest or other body parts. A CT scan can show cancers, pneumonia, emphysema, and more. It may be used to obtain more information after an abnormal chest x-ray. A newer form of CT scanning, called a spiral CT scan, allows for faster imaging and more accurate results. This can be useful for evaluating trauma or blood vessel abnormalities in the chest. To prepare a patient for a CT scan, have the person remove dentures and all jewelry or other metal objects. Check orders to determine if the patient should receive nothing by mouth (NPO) prior to the procedure. Some patients receive contrast material during a CT scan. Be sure to notify the physician if the patient is allergic to contrast media.

Ventilation-Perfusion Scan

During a ventilation-perfusion scan (also called a lung scan or VQ scan), a radioactive substance is injected intravenously and a scan is done to view blood flow to the lungs (perfusion). Another radioactive substance is inhaled, and scanning shows how well oxygen is distributed in the lungs (ventilation). If an area of the lungs is well ventilated but has no blood supply, a pulmonary embolism is suspected. Chronic lung disease may cause poor ventilation and perfusion.

Pulmonary Function Studies

Pulmonary function studies are a series of tests done to determine lung volume, capacity, and flow rates. These are commonly used to help diagnose and monitor restrictive or obstructive lung disease. The patient is asked to use a special mouthpiece to blow into a cylinder that is connected to a computer. A computer printout is generated to show the results. See Table 29.7 for normal values. Some patients use handheld peak expiratory flow rate (PEFR) meters at home to monitor asthma symptoms. They might notice changes in PEFR before symptoms occur, allowing them to begin treatment before the problem becomes more serious.

Pulmonary Angiography

Pulmonary angiography involves an x-ray examination of the pulmonary vessels after intravenous (IV) administration of a radiopaque dye. A catheter is inserted into the femoral, brachial, or jugular vein and threaded through the heart to the pulmonary artery, where the dye is injected. Pulmonary angiography is used to help diagnose pulmonary embolism or other pulmonary vessel disorders. Patients receive nothing by mouth (NPO) for 4 to 8 hours before the procedure. Question the patient about allergies to x-ray dyes before scheduling the test. As with any procedure involving dye, inform the patient that the dye may cause a warm feeling when injected. Make sure a signed consent form is obtained before any invasive procedure is performed. Medications may be administered before or during the test for patient comfort.

After angiography, place the patient flat in bed for 3 to 8 hours to prevent bleeding from the injection site, as ordered by the physician. Monitor vital signs and observe the injection site for bleeding. A sandbag may be used to place pressure on the site. Encourage fluid intake to promote excretion of the dye.

Bronchoscopy

Bronchoscopy involves the use of a flexible endoscope to examine the larynx, trachea, and bronchial tree. Bronchoscopy can be used diagnostically for visualization or to obtain a biopsy specimen for examination. It can also be used therapeutically to remove an obstruction, foreign body, or thick secretions. Instruct the patient that he or she will be able to breathe through the nose and that oxygen can be administered through the tube if necessary. Be sure the patient has signed a consent form because this is an invasive procedure.

The patient is NPO for 6 to 8 hours before the procedure. Be prepared to administer a sedative and, commonly, an injection of atropine to dry excess secretions before the procedure. An anesthetic spray may be used to numb the throat. After the test, monitor vital signs and watch for signs of laryngeal edema. Sputum may be blood tinged. The patient is NPO until the gag reflex returns. Check for the gag reflex by touching the pharynx with a cotton swab. After the gag reflex returns, ask the patient to swallow a sip of water before offering foods or fluids. A sore throat may be relieved with lozenges once the patient is able to swallow.

THERAPEUTIC MEASURES FOR THE RESPIRATORY SYSTEM

Smoking Cessation

Probably the most important intervention for preventing and treating respiratory disease is smoking cessation. Many

TABLE 29.7 PULMONARY FUNCTION VALUES

Test	Definition	Normal Values*
Tidal volume (TV)	Air inspired and expired in one breath	400–600 mL at rest
Residual volume (RV)	Air remaining in lungs after maximum exhalation	1000–1500 mL
Functional residual capacity (FRC)	Air remaining in lungs after normal expiration	2300 mL
Inspiratory reserve	Amount of air beyond tidal volume that can be taken in with the deepest possible inhalation	2000–3000 mL
Expiratory reserve	Amount of air beyond tidal volume in the most forceful exhalation	1000–1500 mL
Forced vital capacity (FVC)	Maximum amount of air expired forcefully after maximum inspiration	3000–5000 mL
Forced expiratory volume in one second (FEV_1)	Amount of air expired in first second of forced exhalation, expressed as percent of FVC	65%–85% of the FVC
Peak expiratory flow rate (PEFR)	Maximum flow of air expired during FVC (this is a rate rather than a volume)	450 L/min

*Normal values are approximate. They are individualized based on patient's sex, height, and age.

respiratory disorders are caused or aggravated by smoking, and stopping can prevent disease from occurring or slow its progression significantly. Table 29.8 lists interventions to help patients stop smoking. Remind patients that if they have tried quitting before and failed, that does not mean that they will never be able to quit (see *Evidence-Based Practice* box). Many patients try several times before quitting successfully. Formal smoking cessation programs and support groups can be helpful.

EVIDENCE-BASED PRACTICE

Clinical Question

Can nurses make a difference in helping patients stop smoking?

Evidence

Thirty-one randomized trials comparing targeted nursing interventions to controls (usual care interventions) found that nursing intervention significantly increased the likelihood of patients quitting smoking (Rice & Stead, 2008). Nursing interventions were more effective in hospital settings, but less effective in outpatient settings.

Implications for Nursing Practice

Advice and support from nursing staff could increase people's success in quitting smoking, especially in a hospital setting.

REFERENCE

Rice, V. H., & Stead, L. F. (2008). Nursing interventions for smoking cessation. *Cochrane Database of Systematic Reviews 2008, Issue 1* (Art. No. CD001188; DOI 10.1002/14651858.CD001188.pub3).

Many Internet sites have information to help people stop smoking. Among these are the American Lung Association site at www.lungusa.org and the National Lung Health Education Program at www.nlhep.org. Or simply type "smoking cessation" into any search engine. The American Lung Association has a "Freedom from Smoking" online smoking cessation program that can be accessed at www.ffsonline.org. Alternatively, individuals can call 1-800-QUIT NOW to speak with a representative who will assist with cessation strategies.

Deep Breathing and Coughing

Effective coughing can keep the airways clear of secretions. An ineffective cough is exhausting and fails to bring up secretions. Instruct the patient to take two or three deep breaths, using the diaphragm. This helps get the air behind the secretions. After the third deep inhalation, tell the patient to hold the breath for a few seconds and then cough forcefully. This is repeated as necessary, usually every 1 to 2 hours. Good hydration can facilitate this process.

Huff Coughing

Patients with chronic obstructive pulmonary disease (COPD) typically have a weak cough and airways that collapse easily. Huff coughing may work better for them. To do this, instruct the patient to exhale deeply to remove as much trapped air as possible, then take a deep breath in to get air behind the secretions. Instead of closing the glottis to generate a forceful cough, the patient should keep the glottis and mouth open, and use the abdominal muscles to create a series of forced expirations, moving air and mucus up the bronchial tree. This creates "huff" sounds. Finally, the patient should take one more controlled inhalation and a final huff cough to expel the mucus.

Autogenic Drainage

Autogenic drainage is a variation on deep breathing and coughing that may be more effective for patients with thick secretions that are difficult to raise, such as those with cystic fibrosis or severe COPD. It is also gentler and less likely to cause declines in oxygen saturation or uncontrolled coughing

TABLE 29.8 INTERVENTIONS TO STOP SMOKING

Intervention	Rationale
Behavior modification	If the patient can identify situations associated with smoking, such as eating a meal or experiencing stress, then other healthier behaviors can be substituted, such as going for a walk.
Counseling	Counseling by a health care worker alone or in combination with other methods can greatly increase success.
Setting a quit date	The cold turkey (all-at-once) method is more effective than slow tapering, although the patient may choose to taper before the quit date.
Nicotine replacement therapy	Nicotine gum, patches, nasal sprays, lozenges, and inhalers can reduce withdrawal symptoms.
Drug therapy (bupropion [Zyban], varenicline [Chantix])	Bupropion may help reduce cravings. Varenicline attaches to nicotine receptors in the brain to block nicotine and reduce its pleasurable effects.
Acupuncture	Acupuncture may help curb the desire to smoke, but studies are not yet conclusive.
Hypnosis	Hypnosis is believed to help the person be open to the suggestion that smoking is undesirable.

than other methods. The patient is taught to sit upright and breathe in more deeply than usual, slowly through the nose, and then hold the breath for 2 to 4 seconds. When holding the breath, the patient should keep the glottis open, to prevent airway collapse. Exhaling is done as a quiet sigh, as if trying to steam up a mirror.

Using these breathing techniques, the patient is taught three phases:

1. *Unstick.* The patient breathes out completely and then takes a slow breath and exhales fully several times, suppressing the urge to cough. This loosens mucus in the lower airways.
2. *Collect.* The patient takes 10 to 20 slightly deeper breaths, exhaling normally, still suppressing the urge to cough. This helps move mucus up to the middle airways.
3. *Evacuate.* The patient takes 10 to 20 breaths and huff coughs to move the mucus up and out.

During the *unstick* and *collect* phases, airflow should be high enough to produce a rattle if secretions are present. This is a complex process that is typically taught by a respiratory therapist.

Breathing Exercises

Breathing exercises are essential for patients with chronic lung disease. Diaphragmatic and pursed-lip breathing increase the effectiveness of breathing and help reduce panic when dyspnea occurs.

Diaphragmatic Breathing

The diaphragm is the major muscle of breathing, but patients often use less efficient accessory muscles when they are short of breath. Conscious use of the diaphragm during breathing can be relaxing and conserve energy. With practice, the patient should be able to use diaphragmatic breathing all the time without thinking about it. Teach the patient to do the following:

1. Place one hand on the abdomen and the other on the chest.
2. Concentrate on pushing out the abdomen during inspiration and relaxing the abdomen on expiration. The chest should move very little.

Pursed-Lip Breathing

This technique can be used any time the patient feels short of breath. It helps keep airways open during exhalation, which promotes carbon dioxide excretion. It should be done with diaphragmatic breathing. Counting during breathing also distracts the patient, reducing panic. Teach the patient to do the following:

1. Inhale slowly through the nose to the count of two (using diaphragmatic breathing).
2. Exhale slowly through pursed lips to the count of four.

PATIENT CARE TIP

When teaching a patient to do pursed-lip breathing, try teaching them to "smell the roses" while inhaling slowly through the nose, and "blow out the candle" while exhaling. If you remind them not to let the wax splatter, then they'll blow slowly and gently!

Positioning

The patient who is short of breath should be positioned to conserve energy while allowing for maximum lung expansion. Most respiratory patients do not tolerate lying flat. The patient in bed can use Fowler's or semi-Fowler's position to keep abdominal contents from crowding the lungs. Some patients prefer to sit in a chair while leaning forward and placing their elbows on their knees or an over-bed table (Fig. 29.9).

Patients with unilateral (one-sided) lung disease can benefit from the "good lung down" lateral position. This is a side-lying position with the good lung in the dependent position. Gravity causes greater blood flow to the dependent, "good" lung, thereby increasing oxygen saturation. Some patients may also benefit from prone positioning.

PATIENT CARE TIP

Patients at home may choose to sleep in a recliner or La-Z-Boy type chair to keep their head elevated. Others may use a wedge under their mattress, or a hospital bed.

Oxygen Therapy

Oxygen therapy is ordered by the physician when the patient is unable to maintain oxygenation. Many patients are placed on supplemental oxygen when their oxygen saturation is less than 90% on room air. The physician's order should include the method of administration and the flow rate. A variety of delivery methods are described in the following sections. The role of the nurse in oxygen therapy includes monitoring the flow rate, ensuring that the cannula and tubing or other device remains properly placed, and monitoring the patient's response to treatment. If the patient becomes short of breath while on oxygen therapy, an RT, RN, or physician should be notified. Instruct the patient to avoid smoking, using electrical equipment, and performing other activities that can cause fire in the presence of oxygen. The RT is knowledgeable about oxygen therapy and is an excellent resource when questions arise.

PATIENT CARE TIP

If a patient suddenly becomes confused, check the oxygen delivery system. The patient may have taken off the cannula, or the tubing may be kinked or disconnected, resulting in hypoxia and confusion.

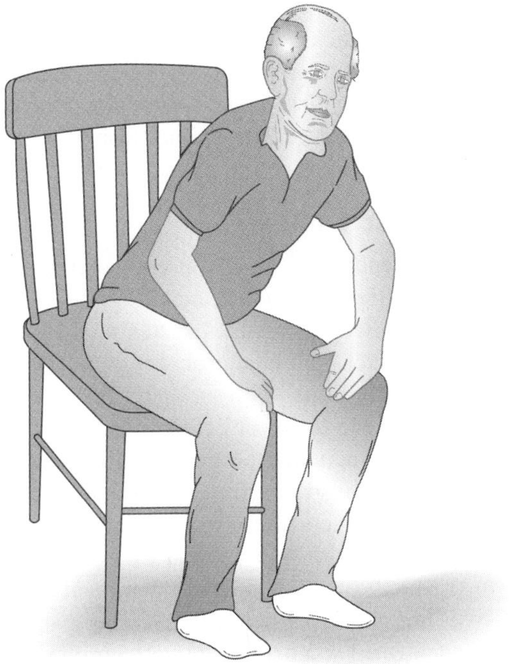

FIGURE 29.9 The tripod position may help reduce dyspnea.

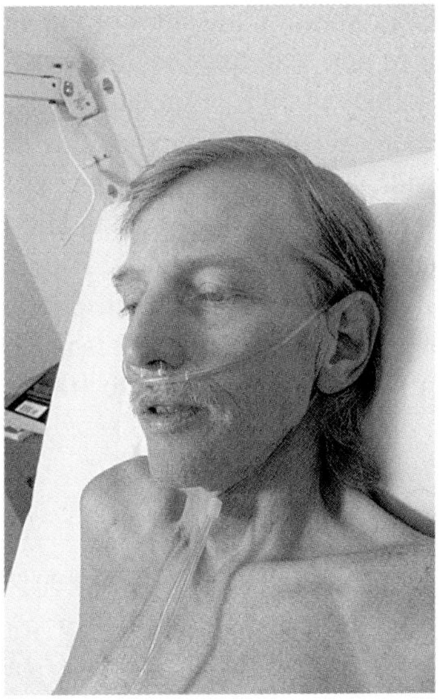

FIGURE 29.10 Nasal cannula for oxygen delivery.

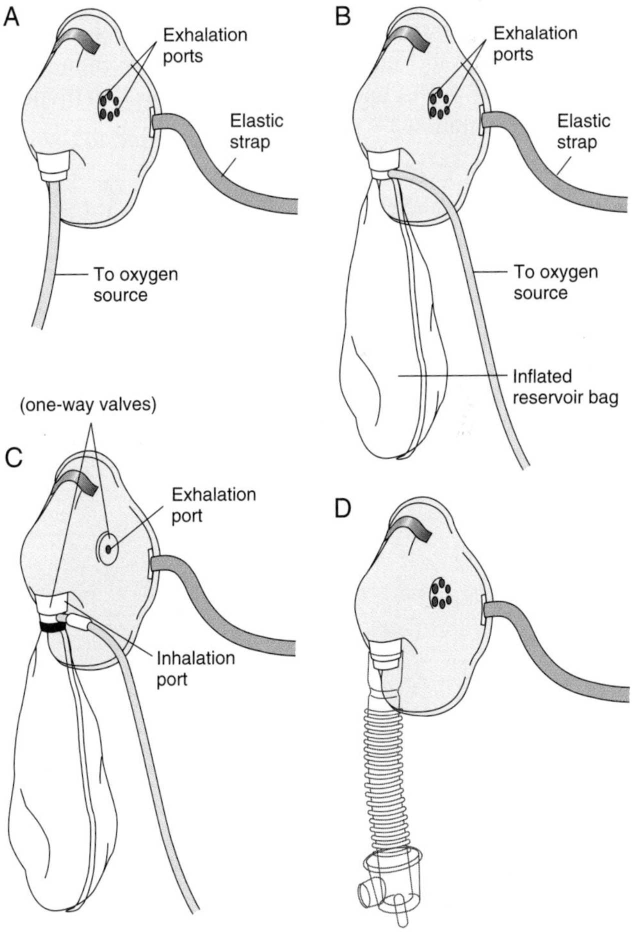
A
Exhalation ports
Elastic strap
To oxygen source
B
Exhalation ports
Elastic strap
To oxygen source
Inflated reservoir bag
(one-way valves)
C
Exhalation port
Inhalation port
D

FIGURE 29.11 Oxygen masks. (A) Simple mask. (B) Partial rebreather mask. (C) Nonrebreathing mask. (D) Venturi mask.

Low-Flow Devices

NASAL CANNULA. The nasal cannula is the most common method of oxygen administration. Oxygen is delivered through a flexible catheter that has two short nasal prongs (Fig. 29.10). For the nasal cannula to be most effective, the patient must breathe through his or her nose. The cannula allows the patient to eat and talk, and it is generally more comfortable than other methods of administration. If the nasal mucous membranes become dry, an RT can place a water source on the system to humidify the oxygen. Oxygen can be delivered at 1 to 6 L/min via a nasal cannula, according to the physician's order.

Masks. Masks are used when a higher oxygen concentration is needed (Fig. 29.11). A disadvantage of masks is that they make some patients feel claustrophobic. Also, a mask must be replaced by a cannula while the patient eats.

- *Simple face mask.* A rate of 5 to 10 L/min can deliver oxygen concentrations from 40% to 60% with a simple face mask.
- *Partial rebreather mask.* A partial rebreather mask uses a reservoir to capture some exhaled gas for

rebreathing. Vents on the sides of the mask allow room air to mix with oxygen. It can deliver oxygen concentrations of 50% or greater.

- *Nonrebreather mask.* A nonrebreather mask has one or both side vents closed to limit the mixing of room air with oxygen. The vents open to allow expiration but remain closed on inspiration. The reservoir bag has a valve to store oxygen for inspiration but does not allow entry of exhaled air. It is used to deliver oxygen concentrations of 70% to 100%.

> **PATIENT CARE TIP**
> When a patient is using a partial rebreather or nonrebreather mask, ensure that the reservoir bag is never allowed to collapse to less than half full.

High-Flow Devices

VENTURI MASK. A Venturi mask is used for the patient who requires precise percentages of oxygen, such as the patient with chronic lung disease with CO_2 retention. A combination of valves and specified flow rates determines oxygen concentration.

Transtracheal Catheter

A transtracheal catheter is a small tube that is surgically placed through the base of the neck directly into the trachea to deliver oxygen (Fig. 29.12). This is an attractive alternative for some patients who are on long-term oxygen therapy at home because it does not obstruct the nose or mouth and can be easily covered with a loose scarf or collar. The patient is taught to remove and clean the catheter two or three times a day to prevent mucus obstruction. Check institution policy and procedure for specific care instructions.

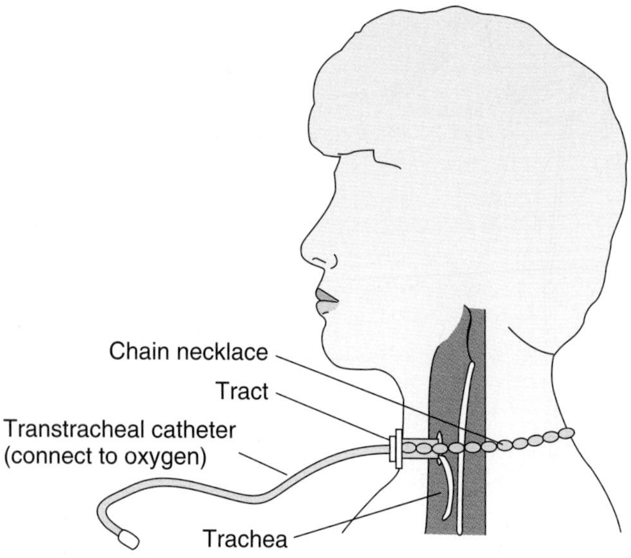
Chain necklace
Tract
Transtracheal catheter
(connect to oxygen)
Trachea

FIGURE 29.12 Transtracheal oxygen catheter.

Risks of Oxygen Therapy

Patients with chronic obstructive pulmonary disease usually have chronically high $Paco_2$ levels. Therefore, they depend on low Pao_2 levels to stimulate breathing, and high supplemental oxygen flow rates can depress respirations. Patients with COPD who retain CO_2 should be maintained on no more than 1 to 2 L of oxygen per minute. Occasionally, hospitalized patients require higher flow rates, but they must be carefully monitored and may require mechanical ventilation.

In addition, any patient can suffer lung damage from high oxygen concentrations delivered for more than 24 hours. If a patient exhibits symptoms of dry cough, chest pain, numbness in the extremities, lethargy, or nausea, the physician should be contacted. A Pao_2 greater than 100 mm Hg should also be reported.

Nebulized Mist Treatments

Nebulized mist treatments (NMTs) use a nebulizer to deliver medication directly into the lungs (Fig. 29.13). Such topical use of medication reduces systemic side effects. Bronchodilators such as albuterol or metaproterenol, mixed with normal saline solution and sometimes with supplemental oxygen, are most commonly administered. Other medications, including corticosteroids, mucolytics, and antibiotics, may also be given. An RT or a specially trained nurse administers the NMT. The patient uses a handheld reservoir with tubing and a mouthpiece to breathe in the medication. NMTs are commonly ordered every 4 to 6 hours and as needed. You may call for an NMT as needed (prn) when a patient with chronic pulmonary disease becomes acutely dyspneic. Some patients are taught to administer their own NMTs at home.

Metered-Dose Inhalers

Inhalers are another way to administer topical medication directly into the lungs, minimizing systemic side effects. Medications that can be inhaled include corticosteroids, bronchodilators, and mast cell inhibitors. Metered-dose inhalers (MDIs) use propellants to deliver medication. Figure 29.14 shows one way to use an MDI. Use of a spacer can increase the amount of medication that gets to the lungs (Fig. 29.15).

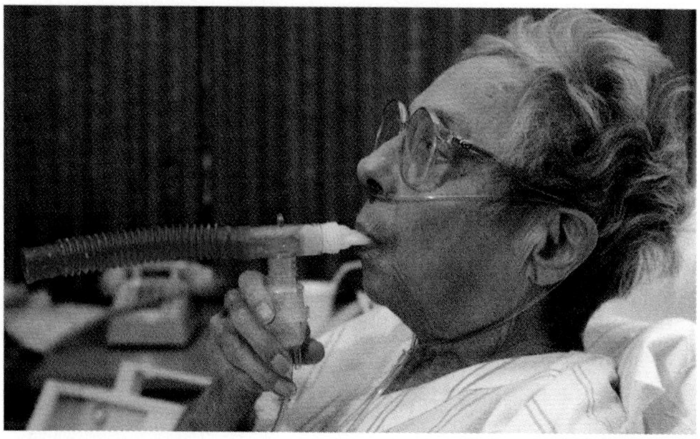

FIGURE 29.13 Patient receiving nebulized mist treatment.

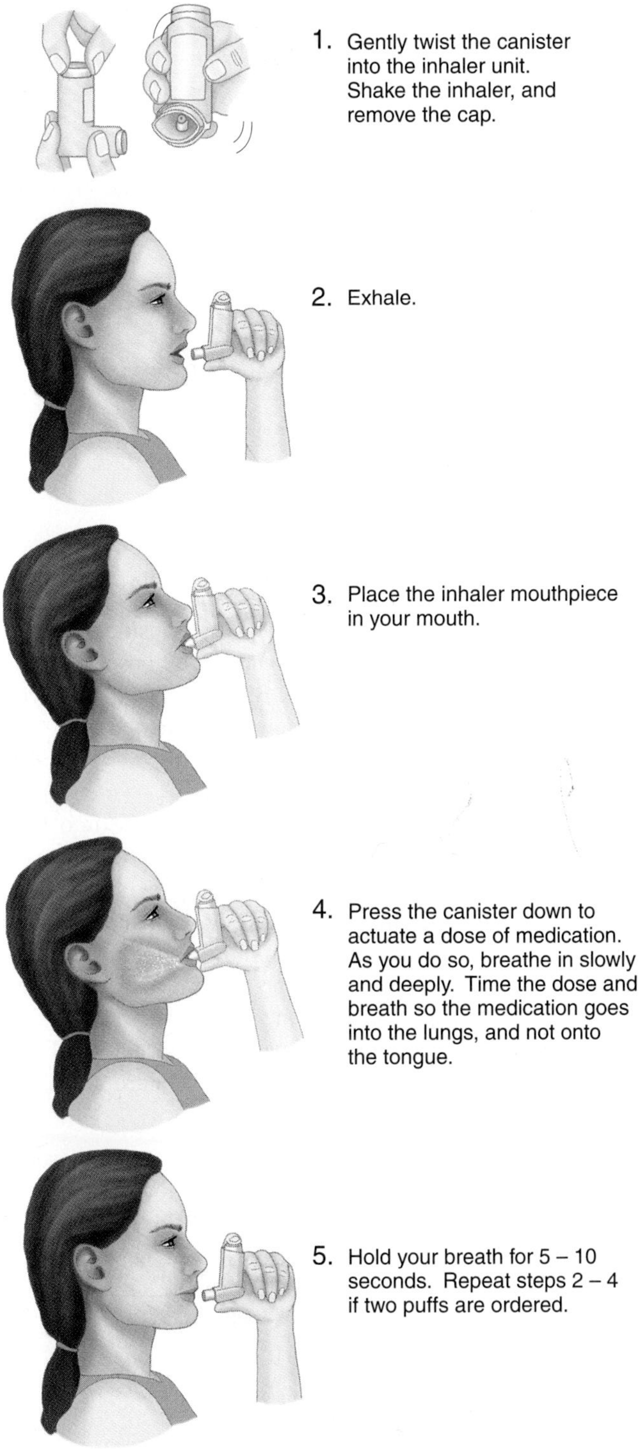
1. Gently twist the canister into the inhaler unit. Shake the inhaler, and remove the cap.
2. Exhale.
3. Place the inhaler mouthpiece in your mouth.
4. Press the canister down to actuate a dose of medication. As you do so, breathe in slowly and deeply. Time the dose and breath so the medication goes into the lungs, and not onto the tongue.
5. Hold your breath for 5 – 10 seconds. Repeat steps 2 – 4 if two puffs are ordered.

FIGURE 29.14 Instructions for use of a metered-dose inhaler. See package inserts for specific instructions because many types of inhalers are available.

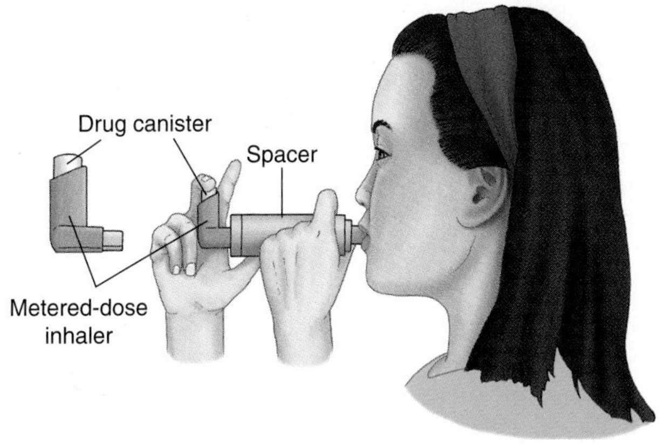
Drug canister
Spacer
Metered-dose inhaler

FIGURE 29.15 Use of a spacer increases the amount of medication that gets to the lungs.

Before December 31, 2008, many MDIs used a chlorofluorocarbon (CFC) as a propellant, but CFC damages the ozone, so new ways to deliver inhaled medications have been developed. Many new models of inhalers such as dry powder inhalers do not use any propellants, and some use an HFA (hydrofluoroalkane) propellant. With so many different types of inhalers, it is important to carefully read the instructions for use before assisting a patient.

The RT or nurse must carefully instruct the patient because improper use can reduce the effectiveness of the medication. It is also important to teach the patient to avoid overuse of adrenergic bronchodilator inhalers. Patients with chronic lung disease may tend to use extra puffs when they feel short of breath. Adrenergic bronchodilators, however, can cause severe rebound bronchoconstriction and even death when used too often.

Incentive Spirometry

Incentive spirometers (Fig. 29.16) are used to encourage deep breathing in patients at risk for collapse of lung tissue, a condition called atelectasis. These devices are commonly ordered for postoperative patients. Patients are instructed to use the spirometer 10 times each hour they are awake. Because a variety of spirometers are available, consult with an RT and read package inserts for specific directions for use.

Chest Physiotherapy

Chest physiotherapy (CPT), which includes postural drainage, percussion, and vibration, helps move secretions from deep inside the lungs (Fig. 29.17). It is indicated for the patient who has a weak or ineffective cough and is at risk for retaining secretions. Patients with COPD, cystic fibrosis, or bronchiectasis and patients on ventilators benefit from CPT.

CPT is performed by an RT or specially trained nurse. For postural drainage, the patient is placed in various positions (head down to help drain secretions) and turned periodically during the treatment so all lobes of the lungs are drained. The therapist uses cupped hands to strike the chest repeatedly (percussion), producing sound waves that are transmitted through the chest, loosening secretions. The therapist may also apply vibration to the patient's chest, using the hands or a vibrator, to loosen secretions. A nebulizer treatment should be given before CPT to humidify secretions. The patient is instructed to cough and deep breathe at intervals during and after the treatment.

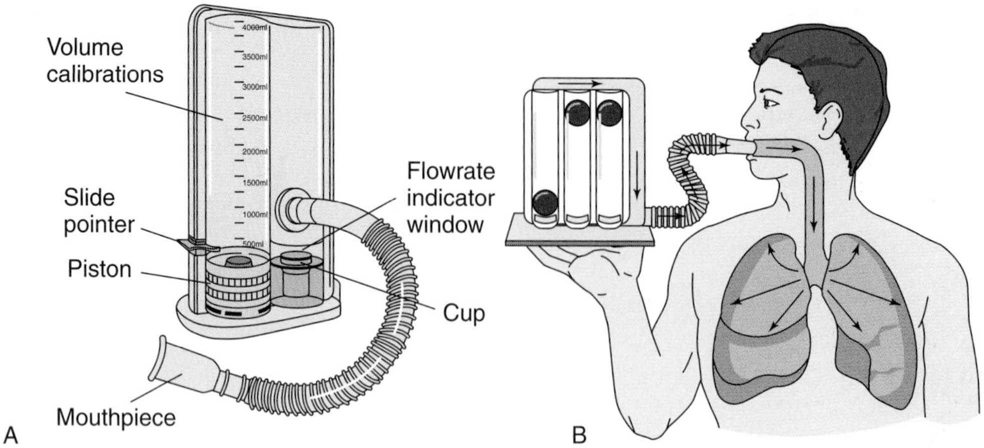
Volume calibrations
4000ml
3500ml
3000ml
2500ml
2000ml
1500ml
1000ml
500ml
Slide pointer
Piston
Flowrate indicator window
Cup
Mouthpiece
A
B

FIGURE 29.16 Incentive spirometers. (A) Voldyne volumetric deep-breathing exerciser. (B) Triflow II incentive breathing exerciser. (Modified from Barnes, T. A. [1991]. *Respiratory care principles* [p. 434]. Philadelphia: F. A. Davis.)

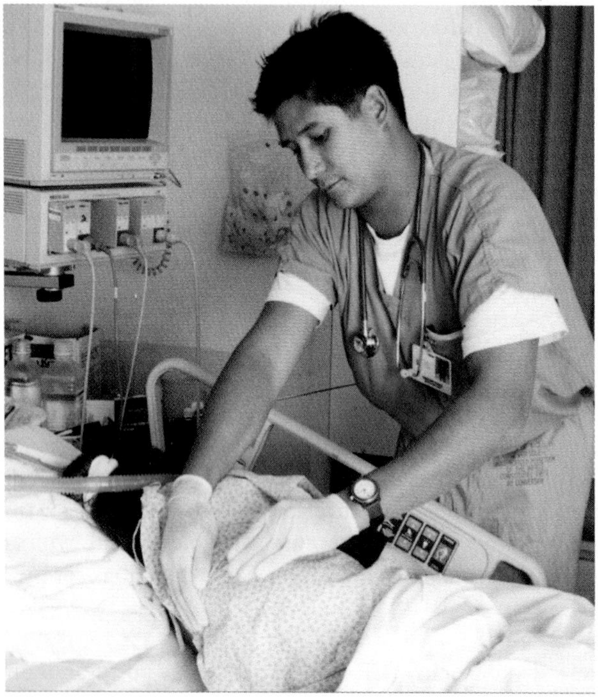

FIGURE 29.17 Patient receiving chest physiotherapy.

High-Frequency Chest Wall Oscillation Vest

The high-frequency chest wall oscillation vest (sometimes called "vest therapy") is an alternative to CPT. Because it does not require the presence of a therapist, it is less expensive over time. An inflatable vest is placed on the patient and a compressor generates pulses of air into the vest to vibrate the patient's chest. Like CPT, this helps loosen secretions so they can be expectorated. The patient must cough during and after the therapy for it to be effective.

Vibratory Positive Expiratory Pressure Device

Another alternative to chest physiotherapy is a small handheld device called a vibratory positive expiratory pressure (PEP) device. (One brand is the Flutter mucus clearance device shown in Fig. 29.18). When the patient blows into the mouthpiece, it makes a heavy steel ball inside bounce around in its chamber, which then sends vibrations back into the airways to help loosen mucus. Blowing into the device also creates positive pressure, which opens airways.

Thoracentesis

Thoracentesis involves the insertion of a needle into the pleural space. It is commonly done to aspirate fluid in patients with pleural effusion (fluid trapped in the pleural space). The procedure may be diagnostic, to determine the source of fluid, or therapeutic, to remove fluid and reduce respiratory distress. It may also be performed to aspirate blood or air or to inject medication.

When assisting a physician with a thoracentesis, first verify that the patient understands the procedure and that

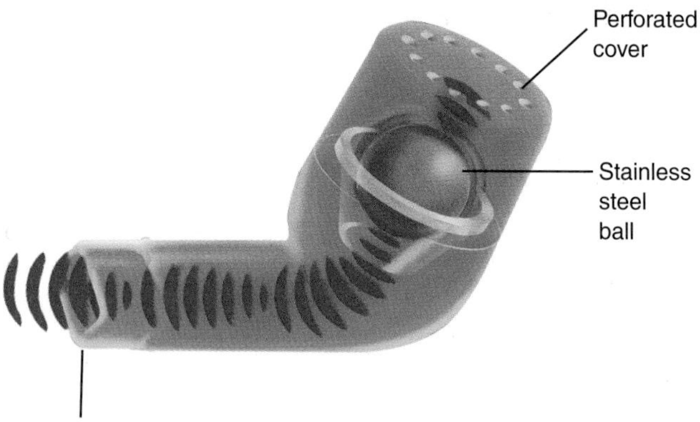
Perforated cover
Stainless steel ball
Mouthpiece

FIGURE 29.18 Flutter® mucus clearance device. When the patient blows into the mouthpiece, the stainless steel ball bounces up and down, causing airways to vibrate. This helps open airways and loosen mucus. Consult package instructions before use. (Courtesy of Axcan Scandipharm, Birmingham, AL.)

• WORD • BUILDING •

thoracentesis: thoraco—chest + centesis—puncture

written consent has been obtained if required by institution policy. Have the patient void before the procedure. The patient should be aware that a sensation of pressure may be felt, but that severe pain is rare. Administer an analgesic, if ordered, before the procedure. Obtain a special procedure tray that has the equipment needed by the physician. Place the patient in a sitting position, bending over a bedside table, or in a side-lying position if unable to sit. You can position yourself in front of the patient and encourage relaxation during the procedure. If you are asked to hand equipment to the physician, be sure to keep everything sterile.

The physician uses a local anesthetic before inserting a needle into the patient's back through the desired interspace. Specimens are withdrawn through the needle, labeled, and sent to the laboratory. If the thoracentesis is being done for therapeutic reasons, a sterile container is used to collect the remaining fluid. As much as 2 L can be removed, sometimes more, and the patient will usually report immediate reduction of dyspnea.

SAFETY TIP

Label all medications, medication containers, and other solutions on and off the sterile field (2010 National Patient Safety Goals, www.jointcommission.org).

After the procedure, the physician may apply a petroleum jelly dressing to prevent air leakage into the wound. Assess vital signs, breath sounds, and the puncture site according to the physician's orders (e.g., every 15 minutes times two, every 30 minutes times two, then every 4 hours for 24 hours). The patient is usually maintained on bedrest for 1 hour after the procedure. Label and send specimens to the laboratory as ordered. The physician may order a post-procedure x-ray examination to ensure that the lung was not punctured, causing a pneumothorax.

Chest Drainage

Continuous chest drainage involves insertion of one or two chest tubes by the physician into the pleural space to drain fluid or air. The tubes are connected to a chest drainage system that collects the fluid or allows escape of the air.

Indications

Chest tubes and a chest drainage system are used when fluid or air has collected in the pleural space. This can occur with a collapsed lung (pneumothorax), pleural effusion, penetrating chest injury, or during chest surgery. These conditions are covered in Chapter 31.

Chest Tube Insertion

The physician inserts drainage tubes through the chest wall into the pleural space either in surgery or at the bedside. If removal of air from around a collapsed lung is the goal, the tube is inserted into the upper anterior chest, in the second to fourth intercostal space. If removal of fluid is the goal, such as after an injury, the tube is inserted in the lower lateral chest, in the eighth or ninth intercostal space. If a patient has both air and fluid to drain, two tubes are inserted and may be joined with a Y connector before connecting to the tubing that leads to a drainage system.

You can assist the physician by obtaining a chest tube insertion tray and chest drainage system and preparing it according to the manufacturer's directions. Ensure that the patient understands the procedure and that written consent has been obtained according to institutional policy. Administer an analgesic as ordered, and help position the patient as directed by the physician. Chest tube insertion is often an emergency intervention, which necessitates preparing the patient quickly.

Once the tube has been inserted and the system is in place, ensure that each connection is securely taped with adhesive tape to prevent a break in the system. Petroleum jelly gauze and a sterile occlusive dressing are applied over the insertion site to prevent air leakage. If the dressing becomes soiled, do not change it; reinforce it with additional dressings, and notify the RN or physician. Some nurses may change chest tube dressings with special training.

Obtain two padded clamps to keep at the bedside. These are used for clamping the chest tube if the chest drainage system becomes accidentally disconnected from the tubing, for changing the drainage system, or for a trial period before chest tube removal. The tubes are never clamped for more than a few seconds, however, because this prevents air escape and can cause a buildup of air in the pleural space. This can create a tension pneumothorax, which is a life-threatening emergency (see Chapter 31).

Chest Drainage System

The drainage system has evolved from a set of glass bottles to a one-piece molded plastic system with chambers that correspond to the bottles. Some physicians, however, continue to use the bottle system. Studying the bottle system will help you understand the one-piece system (Fig. 29.19). One, two, or three bottles can be used. Study the picture as you read the following sections.

WATER SEAL BOTTLE OR CHAMBER. Each time the patient exhales, air trapped in the pleural space travels through the chest tube to the water seal bottle or chamber, under the water, and then bubbles up and out of the bottle. The water acts as a seal, allowing air to escape from the pleural space but preventing air from getting back in during the negative pressure of inspiration. Water in the tube fluctuates up with each inspiration and down with each expiration, as much as 5 to 10 cm. This is called **tidaling**. When the lung is reinflated, tidaling stops. If tidaling stops before the lung is reinflated, the tubing should be checked for a kink or occlusion. If constant bubbling occurs in the water seal chamber, the system should be checked immediately for leaks.

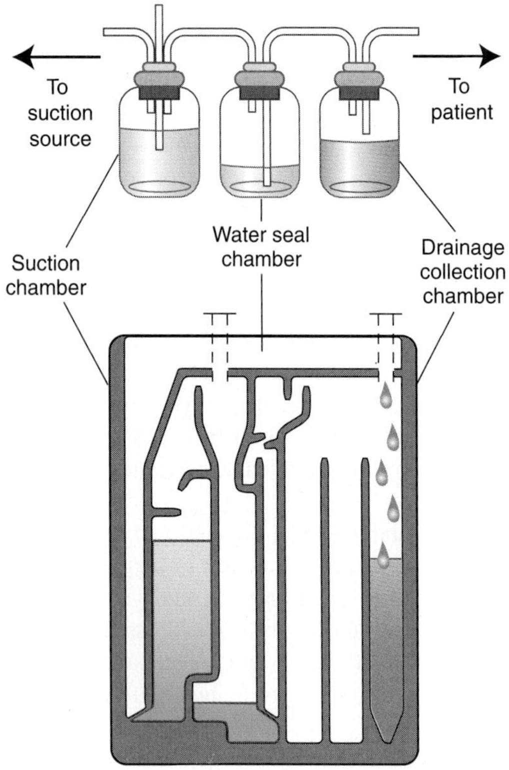
To suction source
To patient
Suction chamber
Water seal chamber
Drainage collection chamber

FIGURE 29.19 Pleur-Evac chest drainage system. (Courtesy of Deknatel Snowden Pencer, Inc., Tucker, GA.)

SUCTION BOTTLE OR CHAMBER. Sometimes a suction source is used to speed lung reinflation. A separate bottle with tubing attached to suction is used. The amount of suction depends on the level of water in the bottle, not the amount of suction set on the machine. (Look at the picture—some air is being suctioned from the atmosphere from the center straw, and some is being suctioned from the patient. The farther the straw is immersed in the water, the harder it will be for the suction to draw air from the atmosphere, and more will be suctioned from the patient.) The suction level is ordered by the physician and is almost always negative 20 cm of water. The suction should be turned on far enough to cause gentle bubbling in the suction bottle or chamber. Vigorous bubbling causes water evaporation, which alters the amount of suction. If water evaporates, more must be added to maintain the correct amount of suction. Some newer one-piece systems use special valves to eliminate the need for water.

DRAINAGE BOTTLE OR CHAMBER. Sometimes a third bottle is needed to catch fluid drained from the pleural space. Drainage may be from pleural effusion, chest trauma, or surgery. Sometimes a small amount of drainage occurs because of the insertion of the chest tube. The drainage chamber is not emptied to measure drainage. Rather the drainage level in the bottle or chamber is marked and timed each shift to monitor the amount. It is documented as output on the intake and output record. If drainage suddenly increases or becomes very bloody, notify the physician. If the drainage chamber fills up, either the chamber or the entire unit will need to be changed, depending on the type of system used.

Nursing Care of the Patient with a Chest Tube

Nursing care of a patient with a chest tube involves regular assessment of the patient and the drainage system. See Box 29.2 for specific assessment and care. If permitted by the physician, patients can be free to move around with the chest

Box 29.2

Care of the Patient with a Chest Drainage System

Assess the patient according to institution policy. Start with the patient and move toward the drainage system.

1. Observe respiratory rate, effort, and symmetry.
2. Assess shortness of breath, pain, anxiety, or other discomforts.
3. Auscultate lung sounds (lung sounds may initially be muffled or absent on the side of a collapsed lung but should gradually return to normal as the lung reinflates).
4. Confirm that dressing is intact; observe for drainage. If necessary, reinforce the dressing and notify the physician. Do not change the dressing unless specifically ordered to and trained to do so.
5. Palpate around insertion sites for crepitus.
6. Check all tubing for kinks, breaks, or broken connections. Verify that all connections are securely taped.
7. Ensure that there are no dependent loops of tubing. Excess tubing should be coiled on the bed.
8. Verify that drainage system is below level of patient's chest at all times.
9. Check drainage system or bottles for cracks or leaks.
10. Check water seal chamber for correct water level and for tidaling (unless lung reinflated). Add water if evaporation has decreased level. If continuous bubbling is present, check entire system for leaks and notify physician.
11. Check suction control chamber for gentle bubbling (or open to air). Confirm correct amount of water as ordered. Add water if needed.
12. Check and mark amount of drainage in collection chamber every 8 hours and prn or as ordered. Report any marked increase in bloody drainage. Record drainage as output.
13. Document findings.

Notify RN or physician if any of the following occur:

- *The patient suddenly reports increasing dyspnea.*
- *There is a change in the patient's assessment findings.*
- *The drainage chamber is full and needs to be changed.*

tube and drainage system. The drainage system must always be kept upright and below the level of the chest. If the patient must be transported, the drainage system is transported with the patient. Ask the physician if the patient can be safely transported without suction. If the answer is yes, the suction control chamber is then left open to allow air to escape. Tubing is not clamped for transport.

If a chest tube is accidentally pulled out before the pneumothorax is resolved, air can reenter the pleural space. Some physicians want an occlusive dressing placed over the site to prevent air from reentering. However, an occlusive dressing increases the risk of trapped air building up and placing pressure on the heart. Contact the RN or physician immediately if this occurs.

Stripping and Milking

In the past, it was routine to strip and milk the tubing from the patient toward the drainage system to dislodge clots and maintain patency. Stripping is done by holding the proximal end of the tubing and using the other hand to squeeze the tubing between two fingers while sliding the fingers toward the drainage system. This is repeated on small sections of tubing until all have been stripped. It is now known, however, that this process can create negative pressure at the openings in the tubing that are within the pleural space, which can suck lung tissue in and cause damage. Stripping should be done only if it is ordered by the physician, and even then only with specific instructions.

Milking is done by gently squeezing portions of tubing from the patient to the system without any sliding motion. This is somewhat safer for the patient but is still not done routinely. If tubing appears to be occluded, consult with the physician for specific orders.

CRITICAL THINKING

Miss Israel

■ Miss Israel has a chest tube in place for a spontaneous pneumothorax. You note that the water seal chamber is bubbling vigorously.

1. What could cause bubbling in the water seal chamber? What should you do?
2. You are totaling intake and output for your 8-hour shift. There is 240 mL of serous fluid in the drainage chamber of the drainage system at 10 p.m. At 2 p.m., there was 190 mL. How much output should you record?

Suggested answers at end of chapter.

Removal of Chest Tube

When the reason for the chest tube is resolved, the physician removes it and places petroleum jelly gauze and a sterile occlusive dressing over the site. Continue to watch for development of crepitus and to monitor the patient's respiratory status and dressing site.

Tracheostomy

A **tracheotomy** is a surgical opening through the base of the neck into the trachea. It is called a **tracheostomy** when it is more permanent and has a tube inserted into the opening to maintain patency (Fig. 29.20). The patient breathes through this opening, bypassing the upper airways. A tracheostomy is performed for a variety of reasons, such as in patients who have had a cancerous larynx removed, patients with airway obstruction caused by trauma or a tumor, patients who have difficulty clearing secretions from the airway, or patients who need prolonged mechanical ventilation.

The tracheostomy tube consists of three parts: an outer cannula, an inner cannula, and an obturator (Fig. 29.21). The obturator is a guide that is used only during insertion of the tube. After insertion, the obturator is immediately removed and kept at the bedside (commonly taped to the wall above the bed) for emergency use if the tracheostomy tube is accidentally removed. The outer cannula remains in place at all times and is secured by ties to prevent dislodging. The inner cannula is removed at intervals; usually every 8 hours and as needed for cleaning. Some newer tracheostomy tubes eliminate the need for an inner cannula.

The tube may be metal or plastic. Plastic tubes typically have disposable inner cannulas, which can be replaced rather than cleaned. Plastic tubes also may have balloon-like cuffs that are inflated to prevent air escape during mechanical ventilation. You know that the cuff is inflated if the small pilot balloon on the tubing used to inject air is inflated. Institution

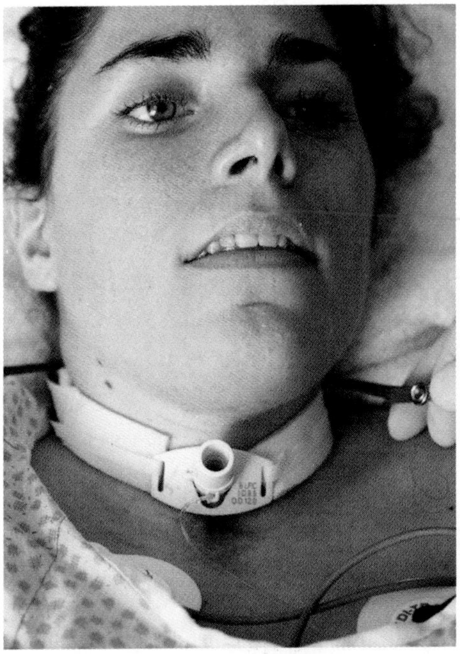

FIGURE 29.20 Patient with tracheostomy.

• **WORD • BUILDING •**

tracheotomy: trach—trachea + otomy—incision

tracheostomy: trache—trachea + ostomy—opening or mouth

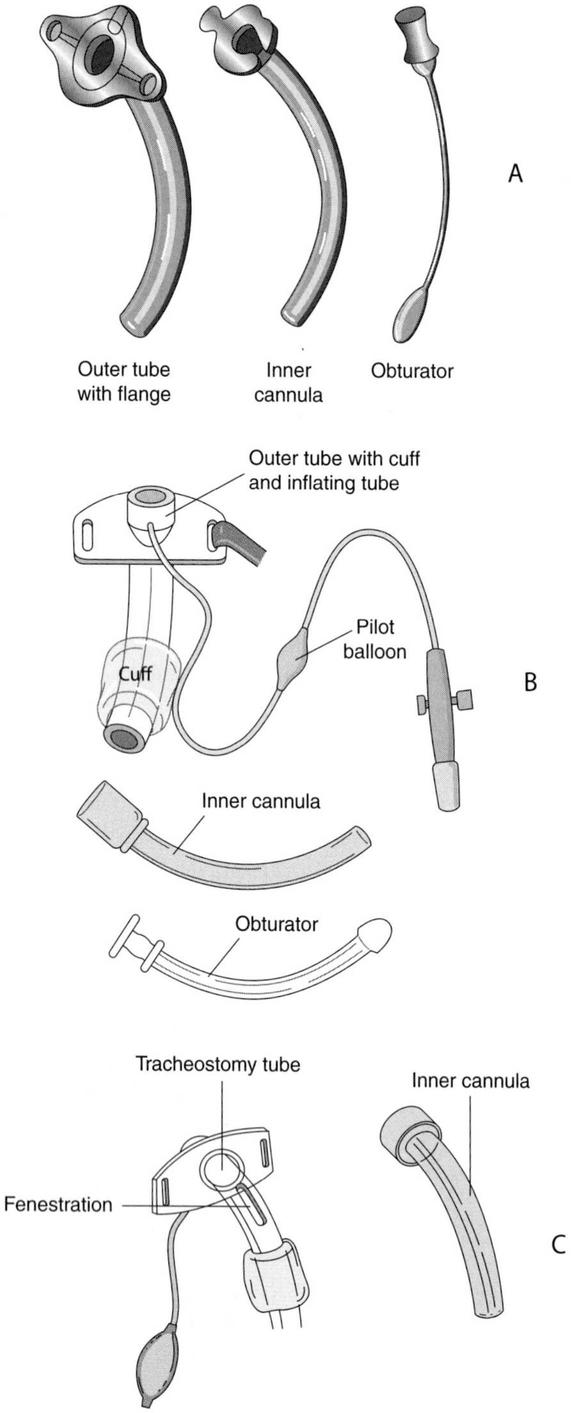

Outer tube with flange
Inner cannula
Obturator
A
Outer tube with cuff and inflating tube
Pilot balloon
Cuff
B
Inner cannula
Obturator
Tracheostomy tube
Inner cannula
Fenestration
C

FIGURE 29.21 Tracheostomy tube. (A) Metal tube. (B) Cuffed plastic tube. (C) Fenestrated tube.

Box 29.3

Tracheostomy Cleaning Procedure

1. Assemble equipment: tracheostomy care kit, new inner cannula (if disposable), sterile water or saline, hydrogen peroxide, suction equipment, personal protective equipment (gown, goggles, face shield) as indicated by patient's condition.
2. Put on personal protective equipment as necessary.
3. Explain the procedure to the patient.
4. If patient is receiving oxygen, keep mask intact as much as possible. If mask must be removed for care, replace immediately between each step of procedure.
5. Suction inner cannula if necessary. See Box 29.5, *Suctioning Procedure for the Patient with a Tracheostomy.*
6. Open and prepare the kit, keeping all equipment sterile. Fill one side of basin with half peroxide and half saline and the other with saline.
7. Don clean gloves.
8. Remove old tracheostomy dressing.
9. Remove inner cannula from tracheostomy tube and discard (if disposable) or place it in peroxide solution (if nondisposable).
10. Don sterile gloves.
11. Use brush and pipe cleaners to clean reusable inner cannula. Place in water or saline to rinse. Dry inside of cannula with pipe cleaner.
12. Reinsert new or cleaned inner cannula into tracheostomy tube.
13. Use cotton swab and sterile gauze with sterile peroxide and saline to clean around tracheostomy site. Rinse with saline to prevent skin irritation.
14. Replace ties or Velcro stabilizer. Remove old ties after new ties are securely in place.
15. Apply sterile tracheostomy dressing (drain sponge or "trach pants"). Use precut or folded dressing. (Cutting gauze creates fibers that can enter the tracheostomy.)

Note: A procedure manual should be consulted for more detailed instruction.

policy may dictate that cuffs be deflated routinely to prevent tissue damage. Box 29.3 lists the steps required for a routine tracheostomy cleaning.

Communication is problematic for the patient with a tracheostomy tube because air is diverted out the tube rather than past the vocal cords and out the mouth. Fenestrated tubes are tubes with openings (fenestra) in the cannula to allow air to flow up into the larynx for speaking (see Fig. 29.21). The patient can be taught to plug the opening of the tube while speaking to divert air through the fenestra. Another option is a valve such as the Passy-Muir tracheostomy speaking valve (Fig. 29.22). This is a special valve that allows air into the tracheostomy during inspiration but closes and redirects air up through the vocal cords and out the nose and mouth on expiration, allowing the patient to speak. For the valve to work, the tracheostomy tube must be small enough for air to flow around it or it must be fenestrated to allow air to flow up through the vocal cords. If cuffed, the cuff must be completely deflated. A patient with a tracheostomy tube in place due to laryngectomy surgery will not have vocal cords, and will not be able to plug the tube or talk. Laryngectomy is covered in Chapter 30.

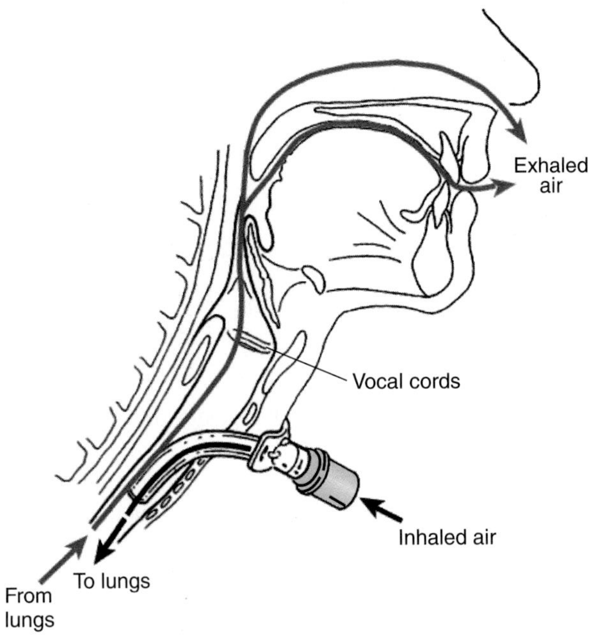
Exhaled air
Vocal cords
Inhaled air
To lungs
From lungs

FIGURE 29.22 The Passy-Muir tracheostomy speaking valve allows air into the tracheostomy during inspiration but closes and redirects air up through the vocal cords and out the nose and mouth on expiration, allowing the patient to speak. (Courtesy of Passy-Muir, Inc., Irvine, CA.)

Some tracheostomies are permanent. However, some patients can be weaned from the tracheostomy tube when their condition has improved enough to allow breathing without it. The physician may replace the tube with a smaller tube to prepare the patient for its removal. This allows a plug to be inserted into the tracheostomy tube at intervals to force the patient to breathe around the tube through the nose and mouth. When the tracheostomy tube has been removed, the opening may be taped shut and covered with gauze until it is healed. The gauze often becomes saturated with secretions and is changed as needed.

CRITICAL THINKING

Mr. Smith

■ Mr. Smith had a plastic, cuffed tracheostomy tube that was small enough to allow airflow around it for talking when the cuff was deflated. A friend stopped by for a chat and assisted Mr. Smith to plug his tracheostomy so he could talk. Mr. Smith's face turned dark red, and his expression showed extreme anxiety.

1. What happened?
2. How could you help prevent this in the future?
3. How would you document this occurrence?

Suggested answers at end of chapter.

Nursing Process for the Patient with a Tracheostomy

See the *Nursing Care Plan for the Patient with a Tracheostomy.*

Suctioning

Suctioning involves the use of a flexible catheter to remove secretions from the respiratory tract of a patient who is unable to cough effectively. This may be a patient with overwhelming secretions or a patient with a tracheostomy or endotracheal tube who is unable to clear the tube with coughing.

The procedures for suctioning are presented in Boxes 29.4 and 29.5. A procedure manual should be consulted for more detailed instruction. Remember that suctioning is both frightening and uncomfortable for a patient. Patients sometimes feel as though oxygen is being "vacuumed" from their lungs. Suctioning can cause hypoxia, vagal stimulation with resulting bradycardia, and even cardiac arrest. It is done only when necessary rather than on a routine basis. Coughing is the most effective way to clear secretions and should be encouraged if the patient is capable. Signs that suctioning is needed include crackles or wheezes heard with or without a stethoscope, or a dropping oxygen saturation value. Each step should be explained to the patient during suctioning even if he or she is unresponsive.

Intubation

Some patients are unable to breathe effectively and maintain adequate oxygenation because of airway obstruction or respiratory failure. These patients are intubated with a special endotracheal (ET) tube through the nose or mouth and into the trachea (Fig. 29.23). Patients in cardiopulmonary arrest are intubated during advanced cardiac life support, and patients undergoing general anesthesia during surgery are intubated and mechanically ventilated. Most intubated patients are also mechanically ventilated. Some patients have advance directives that indicate that they do not wish to be intubated. You should be familiar with the patient's wishes and bring them to the attention of the physician if necessary.

Because intubation can damage the vocal cords and surrounding tissues, it is usually a short-term intervention. Patients who need long-term ventilatory support have a tracheostomy tube placed.

Nursing Care for the Intubated Patient

Nursing care of the intubated patient includes regular assessment of the patient's respiratory status and tube placement. Lung sounds are auscultated bilaterally to ensure that the tube has not been displaced into one bronchus. The tube is carefully secured with tape or a Velcro holder to avoid dislodging. Oral tubes are repositioned and resecured to the opposite side of the mouth every 24 hours or according to institution policy to prevent tissue damage. An adhesive skin barrier should be applied under the tape to protect the skin. If the patient is alert, he or she is instructed to be careful not to pull on the tube. You may need to obtain an order for soft

NURSING CARE PLAN for the Patient with a Tracheostomy

Nursing Diagnosis: *Risk for Ineffective Airway Clearance* related to excessive secretions

Expected Outcome The patient's airway will be free of secretions as evidenced by no audible crackles or wheezes in airway and a clear inner cannula.

Evaluation of Outcome: Is airway free of secretions?

Intervention	Rationale	Evaluation
Assess lung sounds every 4 hours and prn.	Coarse crackles or wheezes may indicate secretions in airways.	Are coarse crackles or wheezes present?
Monitor oxygen saturation every 4 hours and prn.	Secretions may reduce gas exchange.	Is oxygen saturation less than 90%, indicating a problem?
Encourage patient to deep breathe and cough as able.	Patients may be able to clear own secretions without suctioning.	Is patient able to cough up secretions effectively?
Encourage fluids if not contraindicated.	Fluids help hydrate secretions, making them easier to cough up.	Is patient taking adequate fluids? Are secretions thin?
Provide a room humidifier if patient does not have humidified oxygen.	Humidification helps prevent drying of mucosa and secretions.	Are mucosa moist and secretions easily removed?
Encourage ambulation as able, or turn every 2 hours.	Movement helps mobilize secretions.	Is patient mobilized as much as possible?
Clean tracheostomy according to agency policy. (See Box 29.3, *Tracheostomy Cleaning Procedure.)*	Cleaning helps remove excess mucus and keeps airway clear.	Does cleaning help maintain an open airway?
Suction patient using sterile technique as needed. (See Box 29.5, *Suctioning Procedure for the Patient with a Tracheostomy.*) Suction only when necessary.	Suctioning clears secretions from airways. Unnecessary suctioning irritates airways.	Is suction necessary? Is airway free of secretions after suctioning?
Monitor and document amount, color, and character of secretions. Report change in secretions accompanied by fever.	Purulent sputum accompanied by fever may indicate pneumonia.	Is sputum clear or white and scant in amount? Is purulent sputum reported?

Nursing Diagnosis: *Risk for Infection* related to bypass of normal respiratory defense mechanisms and increased aspiration risk

Expected Outcome: The patient will be free of infection, as evidenced by vital signs within normal limits and clear secretions.

Evaluation of Outcome: Is patient free from symptoms of infection?

Intervention	Rationale	Evaluation
Monitor and report signs and symptoms of infection: fever, increased respiratory rate, purulent sputum, elevated white blood cell (WBC) count.	Early recognition and treatment of infection enhances outcome.	Are signs of infection present?
Use good hand washing practice.	Hand washing is important in preventing infection.	Do all caregivers use good hand washing technique?

NURSING CARE PLAN for the Patient with a Tracheostomy—cont'd

Intervention	Rationale	Evaluation
Protect tracheostomy opening from foreign material: food, sprays, powders.	Foreign materials in the tracheostomy may cause pneumonia.	Is tracheostomy adequately protected?
Use meticulous sterile technique for all tracheostomy care and suctioning.	Use of nonsterile technique may introduce microorganisms into the respiratory tract.	Is sterile technique used by all caregivers?
Encourage a well-balanced diet. Consult dietitian prn.	A well-balanced diet enhances immune function.	Is patient eating a balanced diet or receiving adequate supplementation?
Keep head of bed elevated 30 to 45 degrees.	Elevation helps reduce aspiration of gastric contents, which can lead to pneumonia.	Is head of bed elevated?
Consult with speech therapist and physician about whether to have cuff inflated or deflated on cuffed tube.	An inflated cuff can impair swallowing in some patients, and help prevent aspiration in others.	Is cuff properly inflated or deflated according to specific orders?

Nursing Diagnosis: *Impaired Verbal Communication* related to presence of tracheostomy tube

Expected Outcomes: The patient will use alternate methods of communication effectively. The patient will express satisfaction with ability to communicate needs.

Evaluation of Outcomes: Is patient able to use alternative methods to express needs? Does patient express satisfaction with ability to do so?

Intervention	Rationale	Evaluation
Take time to allow patient to communicate needs.	Patient may become frustrated if hurried.	Does patient feel he or she is given adequate time for communication of needs?
Watch for patient's nonverbal cues.	Gestures and facial expression can provide valuable cues.	Is the patient attempting to communicate with nonverbal cues?
Offer pen and paper or magic slate (if patient is literate).	The patient may be able to write out his or her needs/concerns.	Is patient able to write out needs?
Use picture board (available from speech therapy department).	The patient can point to a picture (water, toileting) that indicates his or her need.	Is patient able to point appropriately to needs?
Teach patient with fenestrated or small tracheostomy tube how to cover opening with a plug or clean finger in order to talk, or to use Passy-Muir valve, according to physician or speech therapy recommendations.	Covering opening or using valve diverts air into larynx and allows speech.	Is patient able to communicate in this manner?
Consult with speech therapist.	Speech therapist may have additional methods for communicating with patient.	Did speech therapist provide alternative communication techniques?

Continued

NURSING CARE PLAN for the Patient with a Tracheostomy—cont'd

Nursing Diagnosis: *Disturbed Body Image* related to presence of tracheostomy

Expected Outcomes: The patient will verbalize acceptance of tracheostomy. Patient will be willing to participate in tracheostomy care.

Evaluation of Outcomes: Does patient verbalize acceptance of tracheostomy? Does patient participate in learning to care for tracheostomy?

Intervention	Rationale	Evaluation
Assess patient's and family members' feelings about tracheostomy.	Assessment provides basis for care.	Are the patient's feelings within an expected range for such a change in body image? Are family members accepting?
Approach patient with an accepting attitude.	The patient will be aware of the nurse's nonverbal body language.	Does the patient indicate a feeling of acceptance from the nurse?
Allow patient opportunity to verbalize concerns about tracheostomy.	Verbalizing concerns helps the patient to sort out feelings and problem solve.	Does the patient verbalize feelings as needed? (*Note:* Some patients do not wish to share feelings and should not be forced to do so.)
Refer patient to support group if available.	The patient may benefit from talking with others with tracheostomies.	Is patient receptive to a support group referral?
Assist patient in finding attractive ways to conceal tracheostomy if desired.	Loose scarves or collars can help conceal and protect the tracheostomy.	Is patient satisfied with appearance of tracheostomy?

Nursing Diagnosis: *Deficient Knowledge* related to care of new tracheostomy

Expected Outcomes: The patient and significant other will verbalize understanding of self-care, demonstrate tracheostomy self-care procedures, and state resources for help after discharge.

Evaluation of Outcomes: Are patient and significant other able to verbalize self-care actions and rationale? Are patient and significant other able to correctly demonstrate care procedures? Is patient able to state how to obtain help after discharge?

Intervention	Rationale	Evaluation
Assess patient's and significant other's baseline knowledge of self-care.	Teaching should only be initiated if a knowledge deficit exists.	Does patient exhibit knowledge of self-care?
Instruct patient and significant other in the following (see text for specific instruction): • Tracheostomy cleaning • Deep breathing and coughing • Suctioning • Prevention of infection and symptoms to report to health care provider • Protection of tracheostomy from pollutants, water (no swimming, careful showering)	The patient will need to care for self after discharge.	Does patient verbalize understanding of self-care and demonstrate all procedures correctly?
Provide follow-up with home health nurse after discharge.	A home health nurse can provide reinforcement of instruction at home.	Is patient receptive to having a home health nurse assist?

Box 29.4

Oropharyngeal or Nasopharyngeal Suction Procedure

1. Gather equipment: sterile suction catheter, sterile gloves, sterile container (these items may be found in a single "cath and glove" kit); sterile water or saline, suction machine with tubing.
2. Explain procedure to patient.
3. Connect catheter to suction tubing, keeping catheter inside sterile sleeve. Turn on suction to level specified by institution policy (usually 80 to 120 mm Hg for wall suction).
4. Pour saline into sterile container.
5. Put on sterile gloves. Keep dominant hand and suction catheter sterile at all times.
6. Suction small amount of saline into catheter to rinse catheter and test suction.
7. Have patient take several deep breaths.
8. With thumb control uncovered to stop suction, insert suction catheter through mouth or nose into the trachea until resistance is met or patient coughs. Do not force the catheter.
9. Slowly withdraw catheter, suctioning intermittently while rotating it. The catheter should not be in the airway more than 10 to 15 seconds.
10. After allowing patient to rest, repeat steps 6 through 9 two more times if needed.

Note: A procedure manual should be consulted for more detailed instruction.

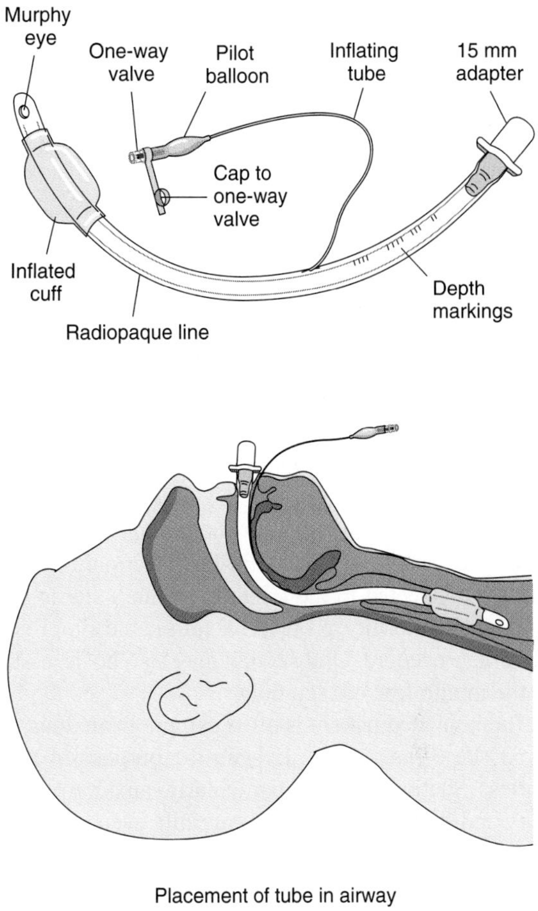
Murphy eye
One-way valve
Pilot balloon
Inflating tube
15 mm adapter
Cap to one-way valve
Inflated cuff
Depth markings
Radiopaque line
Placement of tube in airway

FIGURE 29.23 Endotracheal tube. (Modified from Barnes, T. A. [1991]. *Respiratory care principles* [p. 425]. Philadelphia: F. A. Davis.)

Box 29.5

Suctioning Procedure for the Patient with a Tracheostomy

1. Gather equipment: sterile suction catheter, sterile gloves, sterile container (these items may be found in a single "cath and glove" kit); sterile water or saline, suction machine with tubing, manual resuscitation bag.
2. Explain procedure to patient.
3. Connect catheter to suction tubing, keeping catheter inside sterile sleeve. Turn on suction to level specified by institution policy (usually 80 to 120 mm Hg for wall suction). Connect oxygen source to manual resuscitation bag.
4. Pour saline into sterile container.
5. Put on sterile gloves. Keep dominant hand sterile at all times.
6. Suction small amount of saline into catheter.
7. According to agency policy, oxygenate patient using manual resuscitation bag connected to oxygen source, using the nonsterile hand. If the patient is mechanically ventilated, use manual sigh.
8. With thumb control uncovered to stop suction, insert suction catheter through tracheostomy tube until patient coughs or resistance is met.
9. Slowly withdraw catheter, suctioning intermittently while rotating it. The catheter should not be in the airway more than 10 to 15 seconds.
10. Allow patient to rest.
11. Repeat steps 6 through 10 two more times if needed. Some older sources recommend instilling sterile saline into the tracheostomy to loosen secretions. This should be avoided. It is now known that this procedure is not effective and may actually cause a drop in the patient's Spo_2.

Note: A procedure manual should be consulted for more detailed instruction.

wrist restraints if absolutely necessary for the confused patient. Restraints can be avoided if a family member is available to sit with the patient. Many nursing interventions for the patient with a tracheostomy are also appropriate for the intubated patient. (See the *Nursing Care Plan for the Patient with a Tracheostomy.*)

Endotracheal tubes have a cuff (a balloon-like area around the tube) to help maintain proper placement and to prevent leakage of air around the tube. An RT usually inflates the cuff and maintains a specific cuff pressure and should be consulted for assistance with this activity.

Patients with ET tubes may need suctioning if they are unable to cough effectively. Visible secretions in the tube, crackles or wheezes heard with or without the stethoscope, or a drop in Sao_2 without another obvious cause are signs that suctioning is necessary. The ET tube suctioning procedure is sterile and is the same as suctioning a tracheostomy tube. Some institutions have in-line suctioning devices, which are connected to the ET tube within a sterile sleeve. This maintains sterility, protects the nurse, and simplifies the suctioning procedure. Oral suction may also be necessary to keep the mouth free of secretions.

The intubated patient is often extremely anxious, especially if she or he is alert. Explain the purpose of all care activities. Suctioning is a particularly anxiety-producing activity and should be explained carefully even if the patient is unresponsive.

Intubated patients are at risk of developing ventilator-associated pneumonia (VAP) because normal respiratory defense mechanisms are bypassed. Good hand washing and frequent mouth care to reduce risk of aspirating oral microorganisms can help prevent VAP. The head of the bed should also be kept elevated 30 to 45 degrees at all times.

Because the ET tube passes between the vocal cords, the patient is unable to speak. Provide paper and pencil or a picture board for communication. Yes/no questions can be answered by a nod or shake of the head.

Monitor arterial blood gas and oxygen saturation values and notify the physician of changes. If oxygen values drop or the patient becomes confused or agitated, the patient should be immediately assessed for a disconnected oxygen source or excessive secretions.

If the physician determines that the patient can breathe effectively without the tube, the tube will be removed. The patient will be slowly weaned from the ventilator first. Prior to tube removal, the patient's mouth and tube are suctioned and the cuff is deflated. After removal, the patient is observed closely for laryngeal edema or respiratory distress. The patient is maintained in high Fowler's position to maximize chest expansion.

Mechanical Ventilation

Ventilators are devices that provide ventilation (respirations) for patients who are unable to breathe effectively on their own (Fig. 29.24). Ventilators use positive pressure to push oxygenated air via a cuffed ET or tracheostomy tube into the lungs at preset intervals. Patients may need mechanical ventilation after some surgeries, after cardiac or respiratory arrest, for declining arterial blood gases related to worsening respiratory disease, or for neuromuscular disease or injury that affects the muscles of respiration.

Ventilator Modes

Ventilators can control ventilation or assist the patient's own respirations. See Table 29.9 for terms related to ventilator function. There are many types and models of ventilators. Consult with the respiratory care department for an explanation of a patient's ventilator and how to troubleshoot alarms that may sound.

Ventilator Alarms

Several types of alarms are found on ventilators. Low-pressure alarms sound if the ventilator senses reduced pressure in the system. This can be caused by disconnected tubing, leaks in tubing or around the ET tube, or an underinflated cuff. A low-pressure alarm may also sound if the patient has attempted to remove the tube.

High-pressure alarms sound for higher than normal resistance to airflow. This might occur if the patient needs to be suctioned; if the patient is biting on the tube, coughing, or trying to talk; if tubing is kinked or otherwise obstructed; or if worsening respiratory disease causes decreased lung compliance. In addition, the high-pressure alarm may be triggered if the patient is anxious and is unable to time his or her breaths with those of the ventilator. Water in the tubing might also cause a high-pressure alarm. Consult with the respiratory care department for guidance in draining the tubing.

A loss-of-power alarm may signal a power failure or a disconnected plug. Be aware of emergency power sources and be prepared to manually ventilate the patient if necessary. Volume and frequency alarms sound when tidal volume or number of breaths per minute fall outside preset parameters.

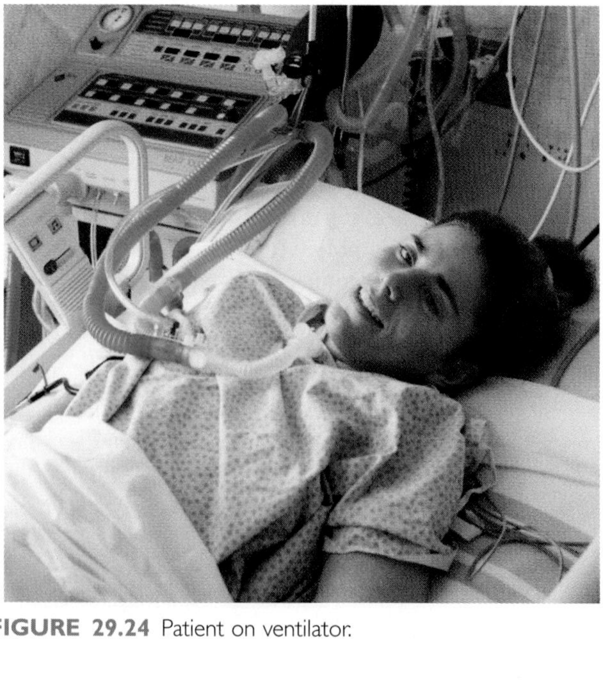

FIGURE 29.24 Patient on ventilator.

TABLE 29.9 VENTILATOR TERMINOLOGY

FIO_2	Fraction of inspired oxygen.
Tidal volume	Amount of air delivered with each breath.
Rate	Frequency of breaths delivered.
Assist control mode (AC; also called continuous mechanical ventilation, or CMV)	Ventilator delivers a breath each time patient begins to inspire. If patient does not breathe, the machine continues to deliver a preset number of breaths per minute.
Synchronized intermittent mandatory ventilation (SIMV)	Allows patient to breathe independently but delivers a minimum number of ventilations per minute as necessary. Synchronized to patient's own respiratory pattern.
Pressure support (PS)	Provides positive pressure on inspiration to decrease the work of breathing.
Continuous positive airway pressure (CPAP)	Provides positive pressure on inspiration and expiration to keep alveoli open in a spontaneously breathing patient.
Positive end-expiratory pressure (PEEP)	Provides positive pressure on expiration to help keep small airways open.

When an alarm sounds, always check the patient first. If the patient is stable, the machine may then be checked. Determine why the alarm is sounding and correct the problem quickly. If no cause can be found, disconnect the patient from the ventilator and call for help. Use a manual resuscitation bag until help arrives.

NURSING RESPONSIBILITIES. Before initiating mechanical ventilation, it is important for the health care team to be aware of any advance directives and consult with the patient and family, because many patients do not wish to be intubated and mechanically ventilated. Some patients accept mechanical ventilation if it is a temporary measure, but not if it might be a permanent intervention.

Until recently, ventilators were used only in intensive care units. Now ventilators are seen on medical-surgical units, in nursing homes, and even in patients' homes. It is important that a team approach be used when caring for a patient who is mechanically ventilated. The social worker; RT; physical, occupational, and speech therapists; dietitian; nurse; and physician all work together to provide the comprehensive care needed by the patient. Respiratory therapists usually take responsibility for routine monitoring and equipment maintenance. The nurse is responsible for monitoring the patient, ensuring that ventilator settings are maintained as prescribed, providing initial response to alarms, keeping tubing free from water accumulation, and keeping the patient's airway free from secretions. In addition, the nurse keeps a manual resuscitation bag at the bedside for emergencies.

Good nursing care is essential for preventing ventilator-associated complications, especially pneumonia. Keep the head of the bed at a 45-degree angle to reduce the risk of aspiration. Oral care including toothbrushing every 12 hours and the use of sponge Toothettes every 2 to 4 hours helps keep oral bacteria under control. Regular suctioning helps keep the airway clear (Lindgren & Ames, 2005). Good nutrition is also essential, and has been shown to be related to eventual successful weaning.

Patients who are mechanically ventilated are unable to talk and can become very uncomfortable and anxious with no easy way to communicate. See Box 29.6 for one nurse's tips for making ventilated patients feel more secure. These tips were developed after the author interviewed 12 patients who had been intubated. They shared their fears, anxieties, and physical discomforts.

Box 29.6

Tips for Caring for Patients Who Are Mechanically Ventilated

- Introduce yourself to the patient each time you enter the room. Make sure he or she can see you.
- Explain everything you are about to do.
- Check ventilator settings regularly.
- Give sedatives or antianxiety drugs as ordered. Request an order if necessary. Find out cause of unexplained anxiety (patient may be hypoxemic).
- Reassure the patient that anxiety is normal and that relaxing will help the ventilator to work with him or her.
- Assess for comfort and reposition at regular intervals. Be careful not to pull on the ventilator tubing. (Pulling hurts.)
- Suction quickly and smoothly, without jabbing. Avoid the use of saline with suctioning.
- Provide good oral care, moistening the lips with a cool washcloth and water-based lubricant. (Patients get thirsty.)
- Use restraints only as a last resort.
- Take the time to communicate with the patient. Talk to him or her, and provide a magic slate or pen and paper so the patient can "talk" to you. Make sure the call light is within reach at all times.
- Answer patient's call light and ventilator alarms promptly.

Source: Modified from Jablonski, R. A. S. (1995). If ventilator patients could talk. *RN, 58*(2), 32.

Noninvasive Positive-Pressure Ventilation

Noninvasive positive-pressure ventilation (NIPPV) is an alternative to intubation and mechanical ventilation for patients who are able to breathe on their own but are unable to maintain normal blood gases. Patients with severe respiratory disease, sleep apnea, or neuromuscular diseases such as amyotrophic lateral sclerosis (ALS) that weaken respiratory muscles can benefit from this treatment. Instead of the invasive endotracheal or tracheostomy tube, NIPPV uses an external mask-like device that fits over the nose or mouth and nose (Fig. 29.25). It can be successful in patients who are alert, able to cooperate, do not have excessive secretions, and are able to breathe on their own for periods of time. It can be used with or without supplemental oxygen. In an acutely ill patient, oxygen saturations are monitored.

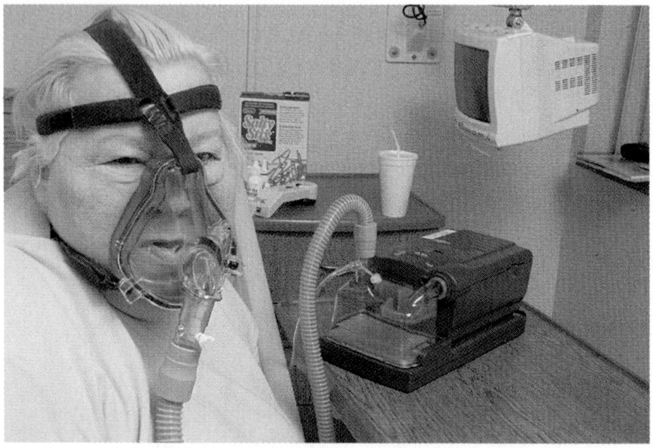

FIGURE 29.25 Noninvasive positive-pressure ventilation. Note round face from steroid use.

Two basic types of NIPPV are available: continuous positive airway pressure (CPAP) and bilevel positive airway pressure (BiPAP). With CPAP, the same amount of positive pressure is maintained throughout inspiration and expiration to prevent airway collapse. In BiPAP, a lower level of positive pressure is used on expiration.

Problems to be alert for in patients receiving NIPPV include skin irritation from the mask and gastric distention from swallowing air. Apply an adhesive skin barrier to the areas that come in contact with the mask to prevent irritation. To prevent gastric distention, place the patient in semi-Fowler's position and consult with the RT to adjust air delivery pressure if necessary. Topical saline or a special humidifier on the machine can reduce nose and mouth dryness. An air leak around the mask can cause air to blow in the patient's eyes, which can be irritating. If this happens, remove the mask and reposition it. Another problem is patient acceptance of NIPPV. Many patients do not like the tight mask covering their nose or mouth. Be patient in explaining the reason for this treatment and check the patient frequently to help control anxiety. Be sure to assess the patient's goals for therapy. Some patients may choose not to use NIPPV, but they must be fully aware of possible consequences.

Patients can use NIPPV nearly continuously, removing it to eat or use the bathroom. Other patients who are able to breathe effectively on their own during the day use it only when they are sleeping. Some use it for a few days until an acute exacerbation of disease is resolved, and others continue its use indefinitely at home.

SUGGESTED ANSWERS TO

CRITICAL THINKING

■ Timothy

1. There is no way to know whether Timothy needs to be in the emergency room without further assessment. Remember that shortness of breath is very subjective and must be evaluated before discharge.
2. Collect further data. Have Timothy rate his shortness of breath. Look at his color and use of accessory muscles. Check his vital signs, peak expiratory flow rate, and oxygen saturation.
3. If Timothy is having an asthma attack, one explanation for the absence of wheezing on auscultation is that he is not moving enough air to generate the wheezing sound. If his airways are extremely tight, breath sounds may be so diminished that wheezing is not heard. This is a bad sign rather than a good one. If you suspect that this is happening, call for help. The physician may want to begin treatment quickly before further evaluation is done.

■ Miss Israel

1. Bubbling in the water seal chamber indicates a leak in the system. Vigorous bubbling may indicate a large leak, and the physician should be contacted immediately. After you check the patient, check the entire system for cracks or leaks and correct any problems discovered.
2. 50 mL.

SUGGESTED ANSWERS TO—cont'd

■ *Mr. Smith*

1. Mr. Smith plugged his tracheostomy while the cuff was still inflated, so no air could get to his lungs. If the plug is not removed immediately, he will be totally unable to breathe. Whenever the plug is in place, air must be able to travel around the tracheostomy tube or through the opening of a fenestrated tube so the patient can breathe.
2. To prevent this from happening in the future, Mr. Smith should be taught how his tracheostomy tube works and how to care for it. He can be taught to check the pilot balloon if he is unsure.
3. "Answered call for help at 1230, found patient dark red in color, unable to breathe, trach plugged. Trach unplugged, respirations restored, vital signs stable. Patient stated he plugged trach so he could talk to his friend. Function of trach cuff explained to patient and friend. Both verbalize understanding to only plug trach when cuff is deflated or to call for nurse if unsure."

REVIEW QUESTIONS

1. During inhalation, which of the following muscle contractions takes place to enlarge the chest cavity from top to bottom?
   a. Diaphragm moves down.
   b. External intercostal muscles move down.
   c. Diaphragm moves up.
   d. Internal intercostal muscles move up.

2. Deteriorating cilia in the respiratory tract predispose the elderly to which of the following?
   a. Chronic hypoxia
   b. Pulmonary hypertension
   c. Respiratory infection
   d. Decreased ventilation

3. How should the nurse record smoking history on a patient who has smoked 2.5 packs of cigarettes per day for 10 years?
   a. Patient has smoked cigarettes for 10 years.
   b. Patient smokes 2.5 packs of cigarettes per day.
   c. Patient has a 12.5 pack-year smoking history.
   d. Patient has a 25 pack-year smoking history.

4. Which of the following terms is used to describe violin-like sounds heard on chest auscultation?
   a. Crackles
   b. Wheezes
   c. Friction rub
   d. Stridor

5. Which of the following is a normal value for oxygen saturation?
   a. Less than 60%
   b. 61% to 85%
   c. 86% to 95%
   d. More than 95%

6. Place the following steps in the correct sequential order for obtaining a sputum specimen for culture.
   a. Have the patient cough deeply from the lungs.
   b. Teach the patient to inhale deeply several times.
   c. Check the order for the test.
   d. Send the specimen immediately to the laboratory.
   e. Obtain the appropriate container.

7. Which instruction is correct when teaching a patient how to use a metered-dose inhaler?
   a. "Inhale deeply, place canister in mouth, depress top of canister, exhale."
   b. "Exhale, place canister in mouth, depress canister and inhale at the same time."
   c. "Cough, place canister in mouth, inhale deeply, cough again."
   d. "Exhale, depress canister, place in mouth, inhale deeply."

References

Joint Commission. (2010). *2010 national patient safety goals.* Retrieved January 13, 2010, from http://www.jointcommission.org/patientsafety/nationalpatientsafetygoals

Lindgren, V. A., & Ames, N. J. (2005). Caring for patients on mechanical ventilation. *American Journal of Nursing, 105,* 5.

30

Nursing Care of Patients with Upper Respiratory Tract Disorders

PAULA D. HOPPER

KEY TERMS

dysphagia (dis-FAY-jee-ah)
epistaxis (EP-iss-TAX-iss)
exudate (EKS-oo-dayt)
laryngectomee (lare-in-JEK-tuh-mee)
laryngitis (lare-in-JY-tiss)
myalgia (my-AL-jyah)
nasoseptoplasty (NAY-zoh-SEP-toh-plass-tee)
pharyngitis (fair-in-JY-tiss)
rhinitis (rye-NY-tiss)
rhinoplasty (RY-noh-plass-tee)
sinusitis (SY-nuss-EYE-tuss)

QUESTIONS TO GUIDE YOUR READING

1. What are the pathophysiologies of the disorders of the upper respiratory tract?
2. What are the etiologies, signs, and symptoms of disorders of the upper respiratory tract?
3. What are current therapeutic measures for disorders of the upper respiratory tract?
4. What nursing care should you provide for the patient with an upper respiratory disorder?
5. How will you know if your care has been effective?
6. What are the special needs of the patient who has undergone a laryngectomy?

Disorders of the upper respiratory tract include problems occurring in the nose, sinuses, pharynx, larynx, and trachea. Many of these problems are minor illnesses that can be cared for at home. Others can become serious if they are not recognized and treated in a timely manner.

DISORDERS OF THE NOSE AND SINUSES

Epistaxis

Pathophysiology

Epistaxis is more commonly known as a nosebleed. The nose can bleed either from the anterior or posterior region. Anterior bleeds are much more common and originate from a group of vessels called the Kiesselbach plexus. Anterior bleeds are easier to locate and treat than posterior bleeds. The blood vessels of the posterior nose are larger and bleeding can be severe and difficult to control.

Etiology

The most common cause of epistaxis is dry, cracked mucous membranes. Trauma, forceful nose blowing, nose picking, and increased pressure on fragile capillaries from hypertension are also factors. Anything that reduces the blood's ability to clot, such as hemophilia or leukemia, regular aspirin use, anticoagulant therapy, or chemotherapy can predispose a patient to nosebleeds. Cocaine use can also cause epistaxis.

Therapeutic Measures

Instruct a patient with a nosebleed to sit in a chair and lean forward slightly to avoid aspirating or swallowing blood. If the patient swallows blood, it will be difficult to assess the extent of bleeding, and it might cause nausea and vomiting. Be sure to wear gloves and follow standard precautions. Place pressure on the nares for 5 to 10 minutes to stop bleeding. However, avoid placing pressure on the nose if a fracture is suspected, to avoid further trauma. Ice packs to the nose and eye area may be used to constrict the bleeding vessels. Intranasal decongestants such as oxymetazoline (Afrin) are also vasoconstrictors and may help.

If first aid measures are ineffective in stopping bleeding, a physician may attempt more invasive treatment. Local application of a vasoconstrictive agent might be used to constrict the bleeding vessels. If the bleeding vessel can be located, the physician may cauterize it by use of an electrical cauterizing device or by application of silver nitrate.

Gauze may be used to pack the anterior or posterior nasal cavity. The anterior cavity is packed firmly but gently, usually with half-inch petroleum gauze. To pack the posterior cavity, the physician must use a catheter and string via the nose to draw the packing through the mouth and into the posterior nasal cavity (Fig. 30.1). The strings are then brought out the mouth and taped to the patient's face so they can be used 2 to 4 days later to remove the packing. Placement and removal of packing can be very uncomfortable for the patient. If there is time, administration of an analgesic before the procedure is helpful. Petroleum jelly on the packing helps prevent gauze from adhering to the nasal mucosa. If the packing is to remain in place for a prolonged period, it is coated with an antibiotic ointment to reduce the risk of infection, or oral antibiotics may be ordered.

Additional products such as compressed sponges and nasal tampons are also available to pack the nose. A nasal balloon catheter is a catheter with a balloon on the end (a specially made catheter, or a Foley urinary catheter) that is inflated after placing it near the bleeding vessels in the nasal cavity. The inflated balloon places pressure on the bleeding vessels to stop the bleeding.

If the patient has lost a significant amount of blood, IV fluid replacement or a transfusion may be needed. Nosebleeds rarely cause death because blood loss lowers blood pressure, which in turn slows the bleeding. Ultimately the cause of the epistaxis is determined and corrected if possible.

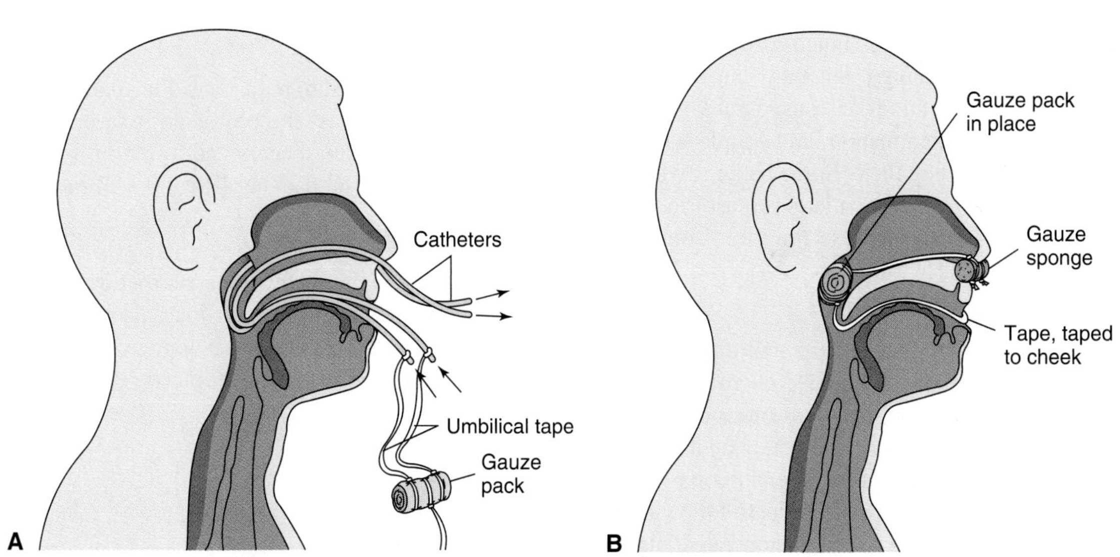
Catheters
Umbilical tape
Gauze pack
A
Gauze pack in place
Gauze sponge
Tape, taped to cheek
B

FIGURE 30.1 Nasal packing. (A) Catheters are used to pull packing into place. (B) Nasal packing in place.

Nursing Care for the Patient with Epistaxis

Monitor bleeding, noting the amount and color of drainage. Monitor vital signs and hemoglobin level for signs of excessive blood loss. If the patient swallows repeatedly, inspect the back of the throat for bleeding. If bleeding does not stop within 10 to 15 minutes, or if it worsens, notify a registered nurse (RN) or physician immediately.

If posterior packing has been used, monitor the patient for airway obstruction from slipped packing. Know how to remove the packing in case of emergency. Institute comfort measures, and maintain the placement of the strings that will be used to remove the packing. The packing will be removed by the physician. Once bleeding is controlled, caution the patient not to blow the nose for up to 48 hours and to avoid nose picking. The patient should also avoid bending over, which can increase pressure in the nose. If the cause of the bleeding is dryness, teach the patient to use nasal saline spray or a room humidifier.

> **CRITICAL THINKING**
>
> ***Mr. Jondahl***
>
> ■ Mr. Jondahl is brought to the emergency room with a nosebleed. His vital signs are BP 140/90 mm Hg, pulse 92 beats per minute, respirations 20 per minute. He states that he has never had a nosebleed before. He denies any history of coagulation disorders. His current medications include captopril (Capoten), furosemide (Lasix), and ibuprofen (Motrin). What are two areas you should assess further in trying to determine a cause? (*Hint:* If you are not familiar with Mr. Jondahl's medications, look them up.)
>
> *Suggested answers at end of chapter.*

Nasal Polyps

Pathophysiology and Etiology

Polyps are grapelike clusters of mucosa in the nasal passages. They are usually benign, but they can obstruct the nasal passages. Although the exact cause is unknown, they are related to chronic inflammation, and people with allergies are prone to developing them. Some patients with nasal polyps also have asthma and are allergic to aspirin. This is called *aspirin triad asthma* because the three components often occur together.

Therapeutic Measures

Control of allergy symptoms may help control polyp development. Oral antihistamines or nasal corticosteroid sprays can help control inflammation. If polyps obstruct breathing, they can be removed. This is done as an outpatient procedure under local anesthesia, using laser or endoscopic surgery. Patients are taught to avoid aspirin products following surgery because they increase the risk of postoperative bleeding and recurrence of the polyps.

Deviated Septum

Pathophysiology and Etiology

The septum dividing the nasal passages is slightly deviated in most adults. This may result from nasal trauma but often has no cause. Some septa may be so deviated that they block sinus drainage or interfere with breathing.

Signs and Symptoms

The patient may report a chronically stuffy nose or discomfort from blocked sinus drainage. Some patients have headaches and nosebleeds.

Therapeutic Interventions

Symptoms may be treated with decongestants, antihistamines, or intranasal cortisone sprays to reduce inflammation. However if the deviated septum is causing chronic discomfort, a **nasoseptoplasty** (sometimes called a submucous resection) can be done. This surgery involves making an incision through the mucous membrane covering the septum and revising or removing the deviated portion. Nasal packing is then placed to reduce bleeding. Typically, this is done as an outpatient surgical procedure under local anesthesia.

Nursing Care for the Patient after Nasoseptoplasty

After surgery, monitor vital signs and bleeding until the patient is stable. Excessive swallowing should alert you to check for blood running down the back of the throat. The patient will have nasal packing and a "mustache dressing" of folded gauze under the nose to catch drainage.

Most patients are discharged home once they are stable, so teaching is important. The patient should maintain a semi-Fowler's position as much as possible and avoid anything that might increase pressure and cause bleeding, such as sneezing, coughing, or straining to move the bowels.

Stool softeners and cough suppressants may be ordered by the physician if needed. Aspirin and related medications are avoided because they increase the risk of bleeding. Antibiotics may be ordered if packing is in place because of the risk of infection from nasal bacteria. The physician should be contacted for specific orders if the patient is on anticoagulant therapy at home.

Ice can be used to reduce swelling and bruising. Instruct the patient to contact the physician if fever, excessive pain, swelling, or bleeding occurs and to return in 24 to 48 hours for removal of nasal packing (Box 30.1, *Patient Education*).

Rhinoplasty

Rhinoplasty is the surgical reconstruction of the nose, usually for cosmetic purposes. It may also be done to correct deformity caused by trauma. Nursing care is similar to that for the patient after nasoseptoplasty, described previously and in Box 30.1.

• WORD • BUILDING •

nasoseptoplasty: naso—nose + septo—septum + plasty—to mold, as in plastic surgery

rhinoplasty: rhin—nose + plasty—to mold, as in plastic surgery

Box 30.1

Patient Education

Nasal Surgery

1. Your nose will feel stuffy and may drain. Change the moustache dressing as often as needed. Do *not* blow your nose. If you must sneeze, do so with your mouth open.
2. Drink plenty of fluids unless your physician advises otherwise.
3. Use a cool mist vaporizer to humidify air and prevent nasal drying.
4. Keep your head elevated on two pillows or sleep in a recliner chair.
5. Use an ice pack on your face to help reduce swelling.
6. Take pain medication as prescribed.
7. Call your physician if you have a fever higher than 101°F (38.3°C).
8. Return to see your physician as directed. Check hospital or surgeon policy for specific instructions.

Sinusitis

Pathophysiology and Etiology

Sinusitis is inflammation of the mucosa of one or more sinuses. It can be either acute or chronic. Chronic sinusitis is diagnosed if symptoms have existed for more than 2 months and are unresponsive to treatment. The maxillary and ethmoid sinuses are the most commonly affected. The inflammation is often the result of a bacterial infection and may follow a viral upper respiratory illness. Because the mucous lining of the nose and sinuses is continuous, nasal organisms easily travel to the sinuses. When the infected mucous lining of the sinuses swells, drainage is blocked. Bacteria that normally reside in the sinuses multiply in the retained secretions. The most common infecting organisms are *Streptococcus pneumoniae* and *Haemophilus influenzae.* Other causes of sinusitis include swelling caused by allergies, nasal polyps, fungal infection, or intubation with a nasotracheal or nasogastric tube.

Signs and Symptoms

The patient usually has pain over the region of the affected sinuses and purulent nasal discharge. If a maxillary sinus is affected, the patient will have pain over the cheek and upper teeth. In ethmoid sinusitis, pain occurs between and behind the eyes. Pain in the forehead typically indicates frontal sinusitis. Fever may be present in acute infection, with or without generalized fatigue and foul breath.

• WORD • BUILDING •
sinusitis: sinu—sinus + itis—inflammation

Complications

The patient who has received inadequate treatment, or who has not complied with treatment, is at risk for complications. Uncontrolled sinusitis may spread to surrounding areas, causing osteomyelitis, cellulitis of the orbit (infection of the soft tissues around the eye), abscess, or meningitis. Sinusitis can also trigger asthma symptoms.

Diagnostic Tests

Uncomplicated sinusitis may be diagnosed based on symptoms alone. If repeated episodes occur, x-ray examination, nasal endoscopy, computed tomography (CT) scan, or magnetic resonance imaging (MRI) may be done to confirm the diagnosis and determine the cause. Nasal discharge may be cultured to determine appropriate antibiotic therapy.

Therapeutic Measures

Treatment is aimed at relieving pain and promoting sinus drainage. Nasal irrigation with normal saline solution helps some sufferers of chronic sinusitis. Corticosteroids, usually via a nasal spray (such as fluticasone [Flonase]) reduce inflammation. Adrenergic nasal sprays such as oxymetazoline (Afrin) constrict blood vessels and therefore reduce swelling, but they should be used cautiously by patients with heart disease or hypertension because vasoconstriction increases blood pressure. Sprays may be used for up to 3 days; longer use may cause rebound congestion. Hot moist packs over the affected sinus for 1 to 2 hours twice a day may help decrease inflammation. Acetaminophen or ibuprofen is given for pain and fever. Opioids may be used if pain is severe. Expectorants such as guaifenesin (Robitussin, Mucinex), fluids, and a room humidifier can help loosen secretions. Antihistamines dry and thicken secretions and usually are avoided. Antibiotics are used only if bacterial infection is suspected, as in the patient with purulent drainage and fever. If conservative treatment does not relieve symptoms, the physician may surgically drain the affected sinus and irrigate it with normal saline or an antibiotic solution.

One such drainage procedure is the Caldwell-Luc procedure. The surgeon enters the maxillary sinus above the upper teeth, under the upper lip. The infected mucosa and bone are removed, and a new, larger opening is made to drain the sinus. Newer procedures, now more common, use nasal endoscopy to open and drain a chronically infected sinus.

Nursing Care for the Patient with Sinusitis

Patients with uncomplicated sinusitis are cared for at home. Instruct the patient to increase water intake to 8 to 10 glasses per day unless contraindicated. Excess water might be contraindicated in patients with fluid overload, such as those with cardiovascular or kidney disease. Pressure may be relieved if the patient maintains a semi-Fowler's position, as in a reclining chair. Explain the use of hot moist packs, analgesics, and prescribed medications. Instruct the patient to finish the antibiotic prescription even if he or she is feeling better before it is completed, and to call the primary care provider if pain becomes severe or if signs of complications such as a change in level of consciousness occur.

INFECTIOUS DISORDERS

Rhinitis/Common Cold

Pathophysiology and Etiology

Rhinitis (also called coryza) is inflammation of the nasal mucous membranes. The release of histamine and other substances causes vasodilation and edema. It may occur as a reaction to allergens (sometimes called hay fever) such as pollen, dust, molds, or some foods, or it may be caused by viral or bacterial infection. Viral rhinitis is another name for the common cold.

Signs and Symptoms

Common symptoms include nasal congestion, localized itching, sneezing, sore throat, and nasal discharge. Viral or bacterial rhinitis may also be accompanied by fever and malaise. Sometimes it is difficult to differentiate between a cold and the flu. See Table 30.1 for signs and symptoms of each.

Diagnostic Tests

If allergic rhinitis is suspected, skin testing may be done to determine the offending allergens. A blood test for IgE antibodies may also be done to determine if allergies are the cause.

Therapeutic Measures

Antihistamines help control allergy symptoms by inhibiting the histamine response. Severe allergies may be treated with desensitization (commonly called allergy shots).

Treatment of viral rhinitis is symptomatic. Because most colds are caused by viruses, antibiotics are not effective. In one study, however, researchers found that 60% of patients who visited their physician for cold symptoms received a prescription for an antibiotic (Mainous et al., 1996). This practice is not only expensive, it also increases the risk of developing antibiotic-resistant strains of bacteria. Explain to the patient that taking antibiotics for a viral infection is not only ineffective but potentially dangerous.

Acetaminophen can be used for generalized discomfort. Decongestants cause vasoconstriction, which reduces swelling and congestion. Any drugs that cause vasoconstriction should be used cautiously in patients with heart disease or hypertension. Cough syrups and cold medicines should be used with caution, because they do not treat the underlying cause of the cold, and often contain several drugs, many of which are not really needed. Teach the patient that rest and fluids are the most effective treatment (see the *Nursing Care Plan for the Patient with an Upper Respiratory Infection*).

Pharyngitis

Pathophysiology and Etiology

Pharyngitis, or inflammation of the pharynx, is usually related to bacterial or viral infection. It may also occur as a result of trauma to the tissues. The most common bacterial infection is caused by beta-hemolytic streptococci, commonly referred to as strep throat. If strep throat is not treated with antibiotics, it can lead to rheumatic fever, glomerulonephritis, or other serious complications.

Signs and Symptoms

The most common symptom of pharyngitis is a sore throat. Some patients may also experience **dysphagia** (difficulty swallowing). The throat appears red and swollen, and **exudate** (drainage or pus) may be present. Exudate usually signifies bacterial infection and may be accompanied by fever, chills, headache, and generalized malaise.

• WORD • BUILDING •

rhinitis: rhin—nose + itis—inflammation
pharyngitis: pharyng—pharynx + itis—inflammation
dysphagia: dys—bad + phagia—to swallow
exudate: to sweat out

TABLE 30.1 DIFFERENTIATING RESPIRATORY TRACT INFECTIONS

Signs and Symptoms	Cold	Influenza	Bacterial Infection
Onset	Slow	Sudden	Usually slow
Fever	None or low grade	Common, may exceed 101°F (38.3°C)	Common, may exceed 101°F (38.3°C)
Headache	Rare	Common	Less common
Muscle aches	Less common	Common, may be severe	Less common
Cough	Present	Present, usually dry	Present, may be dry or productive
Chest pain	Absent	Common	Common
Fatigue	Slight	Common, prolonged, may be severe	Common
Runny nose	Common	Less common	Less common
Sore throat	Common	Less common	Less common
Complications	Rare	Pneumonia	Pneumonia
Treatment	Rest and fluids	Rest and fluids, antiviral agents in some cases	Antibiotics

NURSING CARE PLAN for the Patient with an Upper Respiratory Infection

Nursing Diagnosis: *Impaired Comfort* related to infectious process

Expected Outcomes: The patient will be comfortable as evidenced by statement of increased comfort and ability to sleep at night.

Evaluation of Outcomes: Does the patient express comfort? Is the patient able to sleep?

Interventions	Rationale	Evaluation
Assess for cause of discomfort: malaise, muscle aches, fever.	Knowing cause of discomfort helps guide intervention.	Can interventions be directed toward specific symptoms?
Offer acetaminophen or NSAIDs as ordered.	Analgesics relieve pain. Antipyretics relieve fever, which may contribute to discomfort	Do analgesics/antipyretics relieve discomfort?
Offer throat lozenges, saltwater, or honey and lemon gargles as ordered for irritated throat.	Lozenges or gargles soothe irritated mucous membranes.	Do measures relieve throat irritation?
Encourage rest.	Physical stress increases need for sleep. Rest boosts immune function.	Is patient resting comfortably?

Nursing Diagnosis: *Hyperthermia* related to infectious process

Expected Outcomes: The patient will have a temperature lower than 103°F (39.4°C) and show no signs/symptoms of dehydration.

Evaluation of Outcomes: Is the patient's fever controlled at safe level? Is the patient well hydrated?

Interventions	Rationale	Evaluation
Monitor temperature daily; every 4 hours if fever present.	Screening helps detect temperature changes early.	Is patient febrile?
If patient begins chilling, recheck temperature when chilling subsides.	Chilling indicates rising temperature.	Is chilling present? Should temperature be checked more often?
Monitor for signs of dehydration: dry skin and mucous membranes, thirst, weakness, hypotension.	Fever causes loss of body fluids.	Are signs of dehydration present?
Encourage oral fluids if not contraindicated.	Fluids prevent or treat dehydration.	Is patient taking fluids well?
Administer antipyretic such as acetaminophen if fever is higher than 102ºF (39ºC) or for discomfort.	Antipyretics reduce fever. Fever enhances immune function, so should only be treated if very high, if patient has a history of febrile seizures, or if patient is uncomfortable.	Is fever higher than 102ºF (39ºC)? Are antipyretics indicated? Are they effective?

Continued

NURSING CARE PLAN for the Patient with an Upper Respiratory Infection—cont'd

Nursing Diagnosis: *Risk for Infection*: transmission to others related to presence of infectious disease

Expected Outcomes: Risk for infection of others will be reduced, as evidenced by the patient stating measures to prevent transmission and the patient taking precautions against spread.

Evaluation of Outcomes: Is transmission to others prevented?

Interventions	Rationale	Evaluation
Assess patient's understanding of infection transmission.	Understanding of mode of transmission is essential to prevention.	Does patient understand how infection is transmitted?
Based on patient's previous knowledge, teach patient and all caregivers the importance of good hand washing after contact with patient or patient's belongings, covering nose and mouth when coughing or sneezing, and not sharing eating or drinking utensils. See cough etiquette guidelines in Chapter 8.	The nurse should build on patient's previous understanding and not repeat information. Hand washing prevents spread of infection. Covering nose and mouth prevents spread of infectious droplets. Many infections are transmitted via contaminated objects.	Does patient take precautions to prevent spread of infection?

Diagnostic Tests

The physician may order a throat culture and sensitivity test (explained in Chapter 29) to identify the causative organism and determine which antibiotic will be effective.

Therapeutic Measures

If the pharyngitis is bacterial, antibiotics are ordered (see *Evidence-Based Practice* box). Acetaminophen or throat lozenges may be used to relieve discomfort. Saltwater gargles (half-teaspoon salt in a glass of warm water) or honey and lemon mixed with warm water help soothe inflamed tissues. Encourage fluids (if not contraindicated) and rest. (See the *Nursing Care Plan for the Patient with an Upper Respiratory Infection*.)

EVIDENCE-BASED PRACTICE

Clinical Question

Are antibiotics useful for sore throats?

Evidence

Twenty-seven research studies with 12,835 cases of sore throats were reviewed (Del Mar, Glasziou, & Spinks, 2006). Researchers found that antibiotics are often given for sore throat to prevent rheumatic fever, a serious but rare complication that affects the heart and joints. However, antibiotics can cause adverse reactions and communities can build resistance to them. This review found that antibiotics shorten the illness by about 16 hours and can reduce the chance of rheumatic fever where this complication is common.

Implications for Nursing Practice

Antibiotics are appropriate for sore throats caused by specific agents only. For patients with viral pharyngitis, discourage the use of antibiotics and encourage conservative measures. Teach all patients the dangers of inappropriate antibiotic use.

REFERENCE

Del Mar, C., Glasziou, P. P., & Spinks, A. (2006). Antibiotics for sore throat. *Cochrane Database of Systematic Reviews 2006, Issue 4* (Art. No. CD000023; DOI 10.1002/14651858.CD000023.pub3).

Laryngitis

Pathophysiology and Etiology

Laryngitis is an inflammation of the mucous membrane lining the larynx (voice box). It can be caused by irritation from smoking, alcohol, chemical exposure, gastroesophageal reflux disease (GERD), or a viral, fungal, or bacterial infection. It often follows an upper respiratory infection.

• WORD • BUILDING •

laryngitis: laryng—larynx + itis—inflammation

Signs and Symptoms
The most common symptom is hoarseness. Cough, dysphagia, or fever may also be present.

Diagnostic Tests
The physician may use a tiny mirror to view the larynx. If hoarseness persists for more than 2 weeks, a laryngoscopy and biopsy may be done to rule out cancer of the larynx.

Therapeutic Measures
Treatment includes rest, fluids, humidified air, and aspirin (in adults) or acetaminophen. Antibiotics are used if bacterial infection is present. Medication to control acid reflux is used if GERD is the cause. Encourage the patient to avoid speaking, which will help rest the voice. Also make sure the patient knows that whispering strains the voice even more than normal speech. Obtain a "magic slate" (from the speech therapy department) or paper and pen to help the patient communicate. Throat lozenges may help increase comfort. Help the patient to identify and avoid causative factors. (See the *Nursing Care Plan for the Patient with an Upper Respiratory Infection.*)

Tonsillitis/Adenoiditis

Pathophysiology and Etiology
The tonsils are masses of lymphoid tissue that lie on each side of the oropharynx. They filter microorganisms to protect the lungs from infection. Tonsillitis occurs when the filtering function becomes overwhelmed with a virus or bacteria and infection results. The adenoids, a mass of lymphoid tissue located at the back of the nasopharynx, can also become involved. Tonsillitis is more common in children, but it is more serious when it occurs in adults. Tonsillitis is usually viral, but bacteria that are commonly associated with tonsillitis include *Streptococcus* species, *Staphylococcus aureus, Haemophilus influenzae,* and *Pneumococcus* species.

Signs and Symptoms
Tonsillitis usually begins suddenly with a sore throat, fever, chills, and pain on swallowing. Generalized symptoms include headache, malaise, and **myalgia**. On examination, the tonsils appear red and swollen and may have yellow or white exudate on them. The patient's voice may sound like the patient has a hot potato in his or her mouth. If the adenoids are involved, the patient may mention snoring, a nasal obstruction, and a nasal tone to the voice.

Diagnostic Tests
A throat culture is done to discover the causative organism and determine effective treatment. A white blood cell count and differential can also help identify whether the infection is viral or bacterial. A chest x-ray may be done if respiratory symptoms are present.

Therapeutic Measures
Antibiotics are prescribed for bacterial infection. Acetaminophen, lozenges, and saline gargles help promote comfort. For care of the patient who is not having a tonsillectomy, see the *Nursing Care Plan for the Patient with an Upper Respiratory Infection.*

If tonsillitis becomes chronic, or if breathing or swallowing is affected, a tonsillectomy may be considered, although this is not a common procedure in an adult. An adenoidectomy may be performed at the same time. After the tonsillectomy, the patient is maintained in a semi-Fowler's position to reduce swelling and promote drainage. Monitor the patient for bleeding and airway patency, and provide comfort measures. Encourage fluids for hydration; cold fluids may help reduce pain and bleeding. Red-colored drinks are avoided because they interfere with observation for bleeding. A room humidifier helps prevent drying. Keep suction equipment available for emergencies.

> **CRITICAL THINKING**
>
> ***Mrs. Hiler***
>
> ■ You are caring for Mrs. Hiler after a tonsillectomy. She is sleeping, but you notice that she swallows every few seconds. She has an intravenous (IV) line of normal saline solution running at 100 mL per hour.
>
> 1. How do you respond?
> 2. How many drops per minute do you set on her IV if the tubing has a drop factor of 15?
>
> *Suggested answers at end of chapter.*

Influenza

Pathophysiology and Etiology
Influenza, commonly called the *flu,* is a viral infection of the respiratory tract. Many different flu viruses have been identified, and new strains appear each year. Influenza is the cause of millions of lost workdays each year. The elderly are at particular risk for complications and even death from influenza because of preexisting chronic disease and compromised immune function.

Influenza is easily transmitted via droplets from coughs and sneezes of infected people, or it may be transmitted by physical contact with a person or object that harbors the virus. The incubation period from time of exposure to onset of symptoms is 1 to 3 days.

Prevention
Yearly immunization is recommended for prevention of influenza. The Centers for Disease Control and Prevention (CDC) updates specific recommendations yearly based on research and availability of vaccine. Check the CDC Web site at www.cdc.gov for annual recommendations.

Although Medicare covers the cost of a flu shot, many elders do not get one. Stress to elderly people that they will not get the flu from the shot, because it does not contain any live virus. Once the shot has been administered, it takes about 2 weeks for antibodies to develop; it is then effective for about 4 months. Other important preventive measures include hand washing and avoidance of people with influenza.

• WORD • BUILDING •
myalgia: myo—muscle + algia—pain

SAFETY TIP

Reduce the risk of health care-associated infections by complying with either the Centers for Disease Control and Prevention (CDC) hand hygiene guidelines or the current World Health Organization (WHO) hand hygiene guidelines (2010 National Patient Safety Goals, www.jointcommission.org).

Signs and Symptoms

Symptoms of flu include abrupt onset of fever, chills, myalgia, sore throat, cough, general malaise, and headache. It can last for 2 to 5 days, with malaise lasting up to several weeks.

Complications

The most common complication of influenza is pneumonia, which may be caused by the same virus as the flu or by a secondary bacterial infection. This should be suspected if the patient has persistent fever and shortness of breath or if the lungs develop crackles or wheezes.

Diagnostic Tests

Viral cultures of throat or nasal swabbing can be done to identify influenza, but results may take 3 to 10 days. Rapid tests can identify the presence of flu virus in less than 15 minutes in an office setting, but are less reliable than cultures. Cultures may also be done to rule out bacterial infection. Once influenza has been identified in a geographical area, practitioners will test less often and will treat based on symptoms.

Therapeutic Measures

Treatment is primarily symptomatic. Acetaminophen is given for fever, headache, and myalgia. Aspirin is avoided in children because it increases the risk of Reye's syndrome. Rest and fluids are essential. Antibiotics are used only if a secondary bacterial infection is present.

Antiviral medications such as zanamivir (Relenza) and oseltamivir (Tamiflu) may reduce the severity and duration of symptoms if given within 48 hours of becoming ill. Antiviral agents may also be given prophylactically to high-risk people who have not been immunized, or to control outbreaks in high-risk situations, such as in long-term care facilities.

Nursing Care for the Patient with Influenza

Elderly or other high-risk patients may be hospitalized for treatment of influenza. These patients are closely monitored for complications. Assess lung sounds and vital signs every 4 hours, and monitor for dehydration. Report changes to an RN or a physician. Encourage rest and fluids (if not contraindicated), and provide comfort measures. Teach patients and families not to give aspirin to treat influenza symptoms in children under 18 because of the risk of Reye's syndrome. (See the *Nursing Care Plan for the Patient with an Upper Respiratory Infection.*)

For an excellent tutorial for you or your patients, visit www.nlm.nih.gov/medlineplus/tutorials/influenza/htm/index.htm.

CRITICAL THINKING

Mrs. Murdock

■ Mrs. Murdock is a 97-year-old resident of a long-term care facility who develops flu symptoms. She is lethargic, confused, and feverish. Because of her mental status changes, you want to send her to the hospital, but her son asks you to please keep her where she is. She has a history of chronic obstructive pulmonary disease (COPD) and diabetes.

1. How could Mrs. Murdock have caught the flu?
2. How could it have been prevented?
3. What can be done now to prevent her from developing complications that could lead to pneumonia or even death?
4. What other concerns do you have?

Suggested answers at end of chapter.

Other Viral Infections

In recent years, new viruses have become a worldwide concern. Several of these are described below. Continuous research is being conducted to learn more about the spread, prevention, and treatment of new viral infections.

Bird Flu

Avian influenza, more commonly known as bird flu, is an influenza virus that infects wild and domestic birds (often poultry), just as people get infected by the flu. Humans can contract it from contact with infected birds or their secretions or excrement. Transmission does not occur from eating infected poultry and eggs as long as they have been properly prepared and cooked. Eggs from infected poultry typically do not make it to stores. Transmission from human to human is rare, but is a potential concern.

Symptoms of bird flu are similar to the influenza symptoms described earlier, but complications can be more severe and deadly. Conventional vaccines are not effective in preventing bird flu. Oseltamivir (Tamiflu) may be useful in treatment, along with supportive measures.

SARS

Severe acute respiratory syndrome (SARS) is another newer virus that has influenza-like symptoms. High fever, body aches, and respiratory symptoms often progress to pneumonia. SARS first appeared in Asia in 2003. Transmission is believed to occur from close contact with a contaminated person or object, or through respiratory droplets when an ill person coughs or sneezes. Antiviral medications used to treat HIV infection are currently being researched for treatment of SARS.

H1N1 Flu

The H1N1 virus causes what is commonly known as the swine flu. It was first recognized in humans in 2009. It is called swine flu because the virus usually affects pigs, but it is also transmitted to humans, and from human to human. It cannot be contracted by eating cooked pork. Symptoms and prevention are similar to those for other types of flu. Antiviral agents may be used, but no agent is specific to swine flu.

West Nile Virus

West Nile virus is less deadly than some other flu viruses, but can still cause serious complications. West Nile virus is transmitted from birds to humans by mosquitoes and causes either no symptoms or flu-like symptoms. However, in a few people, especially the elderly, it can progress to encephalitis (inflammation of the brain) and meningitis (inflammation of the covering of the brain and spinal cord). Teach patients to prevent exposure by using mosquito repellant and to eliminate standing water where mosquitoes lay eggs. There is no specific treatment for West Nile virus. If patients develop complications, they are hospitalized for supportive care.

MALIGNANT DISORDERS

Cancer of the Larynx

Pathophysiology

Cancer of the larynx (the voice box) usually develops in the squamous cells of the mucosal epithelium. It is evaluated based on the tumor-node-metastasis (TNM) staging system described in Chapter 11. It is most often a primary cancer and can spread to the lungs, liver, or lymph nodes. The prognosis for a patient with laryngeal cancer is often poor because metastasis (spread) may occur before the patient seeks help.

Etiology

Risk factors for cancer of the larynx include a history of alcohol and tobacco use. Exposure to industrial chemicals, hardwood dust, chronic overuse of the voice, and a diet low in fruits and vegetables are also factors. Men are more likely to be affected than women.

Prevention

Prevention begins with education. You can help educate patients about the relationship between cancer of the larynx and use of alcohol and tobacco. It is also important to teach patients to seek help when symptoms first occur because a delayed diagnosis may mean metastasis of the cancer and a poor prognosis. Teach that any hoarseness that lasts longer than 2 weeks should be investigated by a physician.

Signs and Symptoms

The most common symptom is persistent hoarseness because the vocal cords are located in the larynx (Table 30.2). The patient may also have throat or ear pain, shortness of breath, a chronic cough, and difficulty swallowing. Stridor may indicate a tumor obstructing the airway. Late signs include weight loss and halitosis (foul breath).

Diagnostic Tests

The larynx can be examined with a laryngeal mirror. Laryngoscopic examination and biopsy are used to diagnose and determine the stage of laryngeal cancer. A CT scan, MRI, or other diagnostic tests may be done to determine the presence or extent of metastasis.

Therapeutic Measures

If laryngeal cancer is diagnosed early in the disease, it may be treatable with radiation therapy; this treatment can preserve the patient's voice. Chemotherapy may be used with radiation or surgery, but it is not usually used alone. New targeted chemotherapy attacks only certain cells in the body. Surgery may be done at any stage of the disease. The larynx will be either partially or completely removed (Fig. 30.2). If cancer has spread beyond the larynx, a radical neck dissection, which removes adjacent muscle, lymph nodes, and tissue, may be done. Surgery can be done using laser technology, endoscopy, or traditional methods.

After a partial laryngectomy, the patient may have a permanently hoarse voice. If a total laryngectomy is done, the patient will have a permanent tracheostomy (in this case called a laryngectomy) tube in place and no voice. Alternative methods of communication must be employed. A person who has had a total laryngectomy is sometimes referred to as a **laryngectomee**.

TABLE 30.2 LARYNGEAL CANCER SUMMARY

Signs and Symptoms	Hoarse voice Pain Cough Shortness of breath Difficulty swallowing Weight loss Foul breath
Diagnostic Tests	Examination with laryngeal mirror Laryngoscopy with biopsy Additional blood and radiographic studies to detect metastasis
Therapeutic Measures	Radiation therapy Chemotherapy (adjunct to radiation or surgery) Endoscopic laser surgery to destroy tumor Partial laryngectomy (preserves some voice) Radical neck dissection with total laryngectomy (loss of voice)
Nursing Diagnoses	*Risk for Ineffective Airway Clearance* *Acute Pain* *Impaired Verbal Communication* *Risk for Imbalanced Nutrition: Less Than Body Requirements*

• WORD • BUILDING •

laryngectomee: laryng—larynx + ectome—excision (person who has undergone laryngectomy)

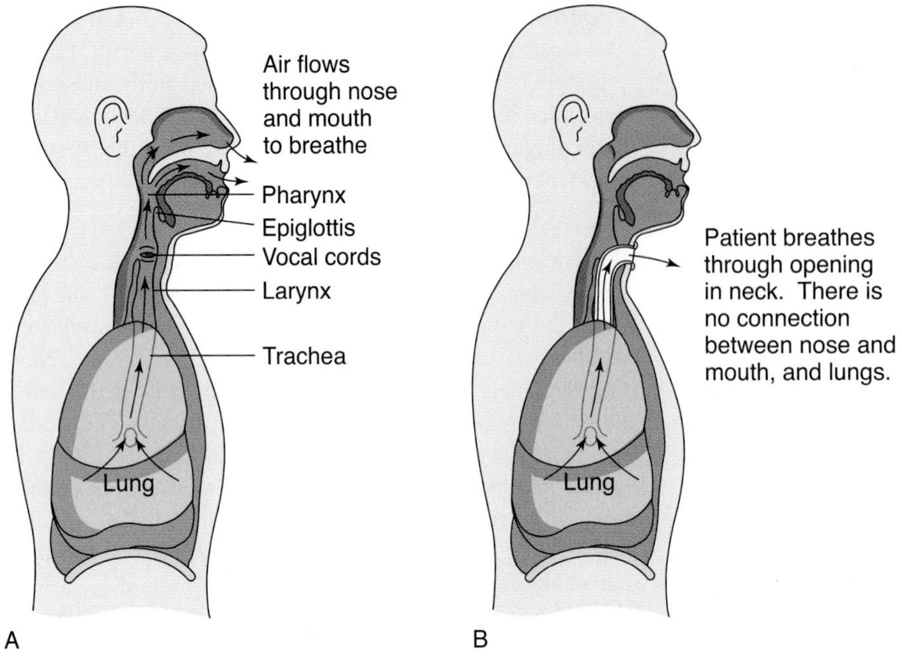
Air flows
through nose
and mouth
to breathe
Pharynx
Epiglottis
Vocal cords
Larynx
Trachea
Lung
A
Lung
B
Patient breathes
through opening
in neck. There is
no connection
between nose and
mouth, and lungs.

FIGURE 30.2 (A) Before laryngectomy. (B) After laryngectomy.

Several alternatives for long-term speech exist:

- Esophageal speech involves swallowing air and forming words as the air is regurgitated back up the esophagus.
- Electronic devices are available, which the patient places next to the neck or mouth. These devices use sound vibrations to help the patient form words. UltraVoice (UltraVoice Ltd.) is a new electronic device that is placed inside an upper denture or retainer, and the patient speaks into a small microphone (Fig. 30.3A).
- Another alternative is a tracheoesophageal puncture (TEP), such as the Blom-Singer voice prosthesis (InHealth Technologies), which uses a surgically implanted voice prosthesis that creates a valve between the trachea and esophagus. If the patient holds a finger over the laryngectomy, air is diverted into the esophagus and the patient forms words as the air exits the mouth (Fig. 30.3B).

All of these devices take time to adjust to, and the patient will need support after discharge to continue to develop communication skills.

> **LEARNING TIP**
>
> Did you or your child ever "burp the ABCs"? If not, ask most any child to demonstrate! This is the same idea as esophageal speech.

Nursing Process for the Patient Undergoing Total Laryngectomy

PREOPERATIVE CARE. In addition to routine preoperative teaching, the patient undergoing laryngectomy surgery must be prepared for the loss of ability to breathe through the mouth and nose and the loss of the ability to speak. Initial instruction in communication techniques should take place before surgery to prevent the patient from feeling panicky after surgery when he or she cannot communicate needs. A variety of techniques and devices are available. Consult a speech therapist before surgery to provide a picture board, magic slate, or paper and pencil. (See Chapter 49.) The patient is instructed to point to the picture that corresponds with the need or to write out his or her concern. A dietary consult is also important before surgery if the patient has been undernourished.

POSTOPERATIVE CARE

Data Collection. Collecting data about the patient's physical and psychosocial status, comfort, nutritional status, and ability to swallow is important both before and after surgery. After surgery, assessment of airway patency and respiratory function takes priority. Monitor lung sounds, oxygen saturation, and arterial blood gases. In addition, be sure to assess the patient's understanding of the disease process and self-care needs after surgery. It is important to evaluate the patient's support systems and ability to cope with the partial or total loss of voice after surgery. Continued alcohol and tobacco use will increase the patient's risk of recurrence.

Nursing Diagnoses, Planning, and Implementation
Risk for Ineffective Airway Clearance Related to Excessive Secretions and New Tracheostomy/Laryngectomy

EXPECTED OUTCOME: The patient will maintain a clear airway as evidenced by clear lung sounds and ability to cough up secretions.

- Monitor and record amount, color, and consistency of secretions; vital signs; oxygen saturation; lung sounds; and signs of respiratory distress. *Visible*

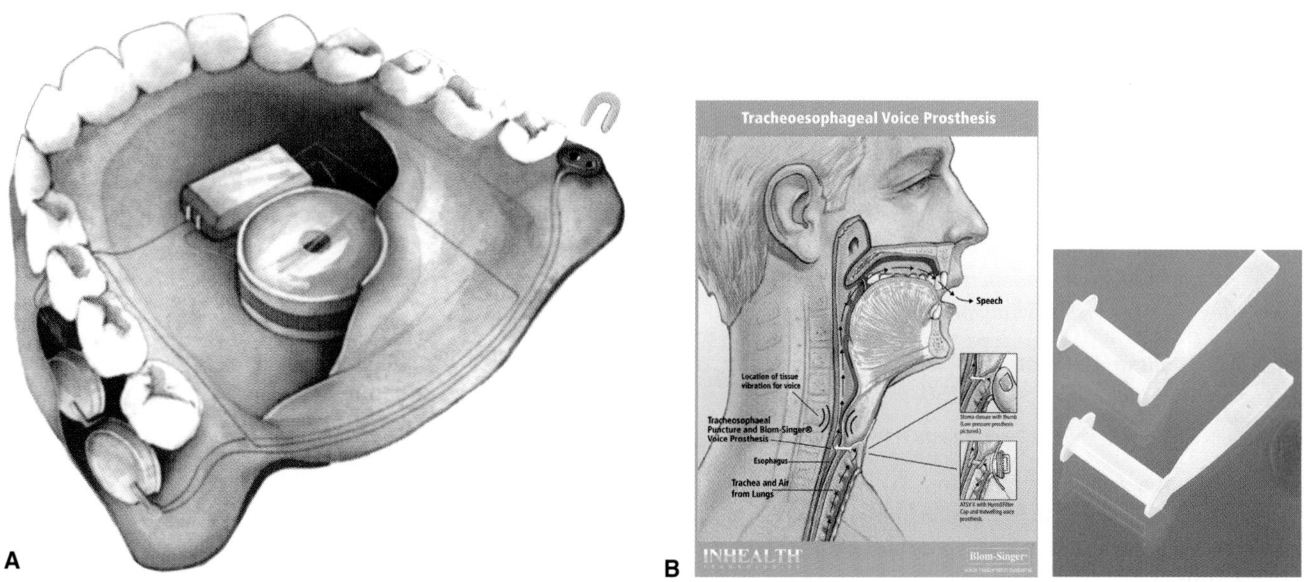
A
B
Tracheoesophageal Voice Prosthesis
Speech
Location of tissue vibration for voice
Tracheoesophaeal Puncture and Blom-Singer® Voice Prosthesis
Esophagus
Trachea and Air from Lungs
INHEALTH
Blom-Singer

FIGURE 30.3 Devices to aid speech in the laryngectomy patient. (A) UltraVoice is an electronic device placed inside a denture or retainer; the patient speaks into a small microphone. (Courtesy of UltraVoice Ltd.) (B) The Blom-Singer voice prosthesis diverts air into the esophagus and out the mouth to form tracheoesophageal speech. (Courtesy of InHealth Technologies, Carpinteria, CA.)

secretions, a drop in SpO_2, or an increase in crackles may indicate a need for suctioning. A change in amount or color of secretions, an increased temperature, or presence of adventitious sounds can indicate infection and should be reported to the physician immediately.

- Provide tracheostomy care and suctioning according to agency policy (see Chapter 29). *This keeps the airway clear.*
- Maintain strict sterile technique with tracheostomy care and suctioning. *Prevention of infection is essential, because the airway no longer has the protection of normal upper airway defense mechanisms.*
- Place the patient in semi-Fowler's position *to allow for lung expansion and more effective coughing.*
- Encourage the patient to deep breathe and cough every hour *to keep airway free of secretions.*
- Administer oxygen as ordered. A special tracheostomy collar may be used to provide oxygen and humidification. *Oxygen helps maintain oxygenation; humidification can help keep secretions mobile.*
- Avoid use of powders, sprays, or other airborne materials near the patient. *These can cause irritation or infection if they enter the laryngectomy.*

Acute Pain Related to Surgical Procedure

EXPECTED OUTCOME: The patient will state his or her pain level is acceptable.

- Assess pain level every 4 hours and prn. *A good assessment must guide treatment.*
- Assess sedation and respiratory status often. Opioids are given carefully *because they may reduce respiratory rate and cough reflex, which is vital to clearing the airway.*
- Include nonpharmacological pain control interventions (see Chapter 10). *Interventions such as distraction and relaxation may help with pain control and reduce (not eliminate) the need for opioids.*
- Administer analgesics as ordered, on an around-the-clock basis or via patient-controlled pump, for the first few days after surgery. If the liver has been damaged from previous alcohol use, dosages are adjusted by the physician. *The patient who is pain free will be better able to participate in care and take measures to prevent complications, such as coughing and ambulating.*

Impaired Verbal Communication Related to Loss of Vocal Cords

EXPECTED OUTCOME: The patient will be able to communicate his or her needs.

- Use a picture board or paper and pencil *so the patient can communicate without speaking.*
- Make sure the patient has a call light or bell nearby at all times. *Patients can become panicky if they have a need and no way to summon a nurse.*
- Work with the speech therapist and physician to provide the patient with a method of communication that best fits his or her needs (see Fig. 30.3). *Different patients prefer different long-term communication methods.*

Risk for Imbalanced Nutrition: Less Than Body Requirements Related to Absence of Oral Feeding Immediately Following Surgery and Possible Previous Alcohol Use or Abuse

EXPECTED OUTCOME: The patient's weight and serum albumin levels will be within normal limits for height and age.

- Monitor weight and albumin levels. *Weight loss or low albumin levels reflect inadequate nutrition.*

- Monitor parenteral nutrition or tube feedings after surgery until the neck has begun to heal and swallowing can be evaluated. *Nutrition must be maintained to support healing.*
- Consult a dietitian for nutrition guidance. If the patient has a history of alcohol abuse, he or she may have been undernourished before surgery. *You may need to advocate for the patient and ensure that he or she is receiving adequate calories for healing. A dietitian can assist with specific recommendations.*

Impaired Swallowing Related to Edema or Presence of Laryngectomy Tube

EXPECTED OUTCOME: The patient will be able to swallow safely.

- Consult a speech therapist to assist with a swallowing assessment and recommendations. *Speech therapists are trained to assess and treat swallowing disorders.*
- Assure the patient that aspiration will not occur *because there is no longer a connection between the mouth and the lungs.*
- Place the patient in high-Fowler's position *to make swallowing easier.*
- Stay with the patient during the first attempts *to eat to help alleviate anxiety.*

Grieving Related to Loss of Voice

EXPECTED OUTCOME: Patient will express feelings of loss and begin to plan for the future.

- Assess patient's feelings of loss. Inability to speak is a loss that cannot be overemphasized. *The patient may also be facing a career change if job-related exposure contributed to the disease or if loss of voice prevents his return to a previously held job.*
- Actively listen to the patient *to show your support and validate his feelings.*
- Assess and involve support systems. *Family support is important to the patient's long-term adjustment to his laryngectomy.*
- Contact the patient's clergy if he wishes. *A religious counselor can help with grief and spiritual distress.*

Disturbed Body Image Related to Change in Body Structure and Function

EXPECTED OUTCOME: The patient will verbalize acceptance of new laryngectomy and participate in self-care.

- Portray an accepting attitude. *Patients are very aware of nurses' nonverbal behavior, and looks of distaste can be very disturbing.*
- Allow the patient to share feelings if he or she indicates a need to do so. *This may help the patient to work through feelings about the changes to his or her body image.*
- With the patient's permission, contact a local support group that may have names of people who have had similar experiences who are willing to visit with the patient. *Such visitors can provide firsthand information and support.*
- Assist the patient to find ways to camouflage the change, such as scarves or necklines that conceal but do not obstruct the airway. *Camouflage can help the patient feel less conspicuous and also protect the airway.*

Evaluation. When evaluating the patient's progress toward goals, ask the following questions:

- Is the airway clear, without signs of infection?
- Does the patient verbalize an acceptable level of comfort?
- Do the patient and significant others demonstrate understanding of self-care at home or have referrals to continue learning self-care at home?
- Does the patient indicate satisfaction with the level and quality of communication?
- Are nutritional needs met, as evidenced by albumin levels greater than 3.0 and stable weight?
- Is the patient able to swallow if taking oral nutrition? Is the patient able to grieve appropriately?
- Does the patient have someone to talk to if he or she wishes?
- Does the patient show acceptance of the laryngectomy by learning to look at it and care for it?

Note that many of these evaluative criteria are long term and may not be seen while the patient is hospitalized, so follow-up by a home care nurse is essential.

Patient Education. After assessing the patient's readiness to learn, teach the patient self-care measures for his or her laryngectomy, including how to perform cleaning and suctioning. (See Chapter 29.) Involve the significant other or family whenever possible.

The patient must also be instructed to perform gentle range-of-motion exercises of the neck. Some patients may avoid extending the neck because of the location of the incision, causing muscle contracture and eventual inability to do so.

Referral to home nursing after discharge will provide assessment of the home environment, as well as follow-up instruction. A social service referral may be made for financial or psychosocial concerns if needed. Consult with the physician or check the local phone directory for laryngectomee support groups, and refer the patient to them if appropriate. The local branch of the American Cancer Society may also be able to provide information.

To find additional information for laryngectomees, visit the National Cancer Institute's website at www.cancer.gov. Many other websites can be found by using a search engine and searching the term "laryngectomy."

SUGGESTED ANSWERS TO CRITICAL THINKING

■ Mr. Jondahl

Consider the possibility of hypertension as a contributing factor. Mr. Jondahl's blood pressure is currently 140/90 mm Hg, which may be lower than normal for him because he has been bleeding. He is also on an antihypertensive drug and a diuretic. Explore the amount of ibuprofen being taken daily, because nonsteroidal anti-inflammatory drugs can interfere with platelet aggregation.

■ Mrs. Hiler

1. Mrs. Hiler may be swallowing blood. Examine the back of her throat with a flashlight. Check vital signs for evidence of impending shock. Notify a physician if bleeding is confirmed.
2. Use this formula to determine drops per minute:

$$\frac{100\text{ mL}}{1\text{ hour}} \times \frac{1\text{ hour}}{60\text{ minutes}} \times \frac{15\text{ gtt}}{1\text{ mL}} = 25\text{ gtt per minute}$$

■ Mrs. Murdock

1. Mrs. Murdock may have contracted the flu from a visitor or a staff person at the long-term care facility. She is susceptible because of her age and comorbid conditions (COPD, diabetes).
2. Mrs. Murdock's flu could probably have been prevented with a flu vaccination, but her son refused it because he believed it could cause her to get the flu. Good hand washing by staff and urging visitors not to visit when ill will also help.
3. If it is within 48 hours of symptom onset, a physician may prescribe an antiviral agent to help reduce her symptoms and shorten the course of her illness. In addition, you can provide fluids, acetaminophen, and comfort measures. You should also monitor her closely for evidence of bacterial infection or pneumonia, and report signs or symptoms immediately to the physician.
4. A major concern is that Mrs. Murdock could transmit the flu to other residents or staff. Hopefully, they have all been vaccinated. In addition, you must decide whether or not to send Mrs. Murdock to the hospital. Check her advance directives, and talk to her son about goals for her care. If needed, educate him about differences in long-term care and hospital care.

REVIEW QUESTIONS

1. Which is the best explanation by a nurse for why a physician did not prescribe antibiotics for influenza?
   a. "Most cases of influenza are caused by antibiotic-resistant bacteria."
   b. "Influenza is caused by viruses."
   c. "Antibiotics have too many serious side effects."
   d. "Antibiotics can interact with other medications used for influenza."

2. After a laryngectomy, which of the following assessments takes priority?
   a. Airway patency
   b. Nutritional status
   c. Lung sounds
   d. Patient acceptance of surgery

3. Which of the following responses is correct when a patient asks why her physician didn't order a new antiviral drug for flu symptoms that started 3 days ago?
   a. "Antiviral drugs are for AIDS, not the flu."
   b. "The side effects of the antiviral drugs are worse than having the flu."
   c. "Antiviral drugs are only for children."
   d. "These drugs work only if you start them within 48 hours after flu symptoms start."

4. Which of the following positions is recommended for a patient experiencing a nosebleed?
   a. Lying down with feet elevated
   b. Sitting up with neck fully extended
   c. Lying down with a small pillow under the head
   d. Sitting up leaning slightly forward

REVIEW QUESTIONS—cont'd

5. The nurse knows that the patient understands teaching related to prevention of influenza transmission when the patient demonstrates which behaviors? **Select all that apply**.
   a. Washing hands frequently
   b. Covering the nose and mouth during coughing or sneezing
   c. Taking acetaminophen as ordered
   d. Drinking extra fluids
   e. Avoiding sharing eating utensils with others
   f. Taking antibiotics until the entire prescription is finished
6. Which of the following communication methods will not work for the patient with a laryngectomy?
   a. Placing a finger over the stoma
   b. Providing a special valve that diverts air into the esophagus
   c. Obtaining a picture board
   d. Teaching the patient esophageal speech

References

Joint Commission. (2010). *2010 national patient safety goals.* Retrieved January 13, 2010, from http://www.jointcommission.org/patientsafety/nationalpatientsafetygoals

Mainous, A. G., Hueston, W. J., Clark, J. R., et al. (1996). Antibiotics and upper respiratory infection. *Journal of Family Practice, 42,* 4.

DavisPlus | For additional resources and information visit **http://davisplus.fadavis.com**

31

Nursing Care of Patients with Lower Respiratory Tract Disorders

PAULA D. HOPPER

KEY TERMS

anergy (AN-ur-jee)
antitussive (AN-tee-TUSS-iv)
atelectasis (AT-eh-LEK-tah-siss)
atypical (ay-TIP-ih-kuhl)
bleb (BLEB)
bronchiectasis (BRONG-key-EK-tah-siss)
bronchitis (brong-KY-tiss)
bronchodilator (BRONG-koh-DY-lay-ter)
bronchospasm (BRONG-koh-spazm)
bulla (BULL-ah)
compliance (kom-PLYE-ense)
ectopic (ek-TOP-ik)
emphysema (EM-fih-SEE-mah)
empyema (EM-pye-EE-mah)
exacerbation (egg-ZASS-ur-BAY-shun)
expectorant (eks-PEK-ta-rant)
exudate (EKS-yoo-dayt)
hemoptysis (hee-MOP-tih-siss)
hemothorax (HEE-moh-THOR-aks)
hypostatic (HYE-poh-STAH-tik)
induration (IN-dyoo-RAY-shun)
lobectomy (loh-BEK-tuh-mee)
mucolytic (MYOO-koh-LIT-ik)
paradoxical respiration (PEAR-uh-DOK-sih-kuhl RESS-per-AY-shun)
pleurodesis (PLOO-roh-DEE-siss)
pneumonectomy (NOO-moh-NEK-tuh-mee)
pneumothorax (NOO-moh-THOR-aks)
polycythemia (PAW-lee-sye-THEE-mee-ah)
status asthmaticus (STAT-us az-MAT-ih-kus)
tachypnea (TAK-ip-NEE-uh)
thoracotomy (THOR-ah-KOT-ah-mee)

QUESTIONS TO GUIDE YOUR READING

1. What is the pathophysiology of each of the disorders of the lower respiratory tract?
2. What are the etiologies, signs, and symptoms of each of the disorders?
3. What tests are useful for diagnosis of lower respiratory disorders?
4. What therapeutic measures are used for disorders of the lower respiratory tract?
5. What data should you collect when caring for patients with disorders of the lower respiratory tract?
6. What nursing care will you provide for patients with disorders of the lower respiratory tract?
7. What specific nursing care can you provide for patients experiencing impaired gas exchange, ineffective airway clearance, or ineffective breathing pattern?
8. How will you know if your nursing interventions have been effective?

Disorders of the lower respiratory tract include problems of the lower portion of the trachea, bronchi, bronchioles, and alveoli. These disorders may be related to infection, noninfectious alterations in function, neoplasm (cancer), or trauma. Any pathological condition of the lower respiratory tract can seriously impair carbon dioxide and oxygen exchange.

INFECTIOUS DISORDERS

Acute Bronchitis

Bronchitis is an inflammation of the bronchial tree, which includes the right and left bronchi, secondary bronchi, and bronchioles. When the mucous membranes lining the bronchial tree become irritated and inflamed, excessive mucus is produced. The result is congested airways. Acute bronchitis is usually an isolated episode. If it occurs more than 3 months out of the year for 2 consecutive years, chronic bronchitis is diagnosed. See the discussion of chronic bronchitis later in this chapter for more information that applies to both the acute and chronic forms.

Bronchiectasis

Pathophysiology

Bronchiectasis is a dilation of the bronchial airways (Fig. 31.1). The dilated areas become flabby and scarred. Bronchiectasis can remain localized or spread throughout the lungs. Secretions pool in these areas and are difficult to cough up. This creates an environment where bacteria can flourish, and infection is common.

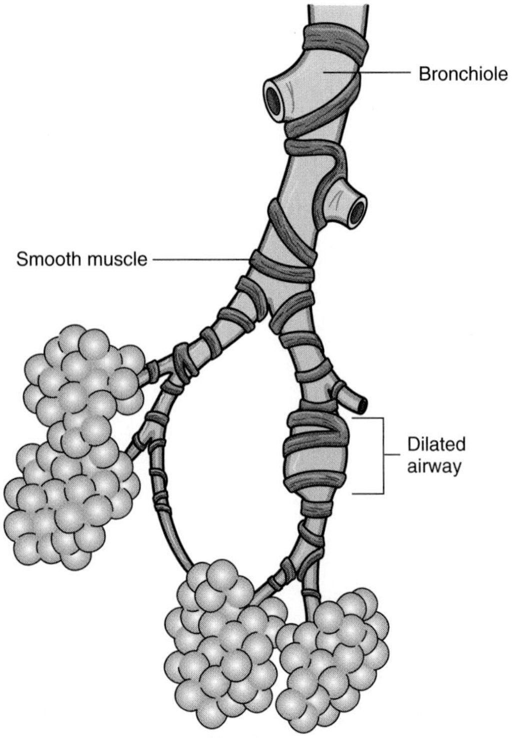
Bronchiole
Smooth muscle
Dilated airway
Alveolar sac

FIGURE 31.1 Bronchiectasis. Note dilated airway.

Etiology

Bronchiectasis usually occurs secondary to another chronic respiratory disorder, such as cystic fibrosis, asthma, tuberculosis, bronchitis, or exposure to a toxin. Airway obstruction from a tumor or foreign body can also be a predisposing factor. Infection and inflammation of the airways in these underlying disorders weakens the bronchial walls and reduces ciliary function. Airway obstruction from excessive secretions then predisposes the patient to development of bronchiectasis.

Signs and Symptoms

The patient with bronchiectasis has recurrent lower respiratory infections. Sputum is copious and purulent. The accompanying cough can produce as much as 200 mL of thick, foul-smelling sputum in a single episode of coughing. Interestingly, if the sputum is allowed to sit for a couple of hours, it will separate into a purulent bottom layer, a clear center layer, and a cloudy top layer. Extreme airway inflammation may cause sputum to be bloody. If bronchiectasis is widespread throughout the lungs, the patient may experience dyspnea even with minimal exertion. Wheezes and crackles may be auscultated. Fever is present during active infection. Cor pulmonale (right-sided heart failure; covered in Chapter 26) and clubbing of the fingers may develop with chronic disease.

Diagnostic Tests

A chest x-ray examination may be done, but it may not show early disease. A computed tomography (CT) scan provides a better view of the dilated airways. Bronchoscopy may be done if needed. Sputum cultures determine infecting organisms and guide antibiotic therapy. Additional testing may be done to determine the cause of bronchiectasis.

Therapeutic Measures

Treatment is aimed at keeping the airways clear of secretions, controlling infection, and correcting the underlying problem. Antibiotics may be used intermittently or for prolonged periods. Measures to prevent infection, including vaccinations for flu and pneumonia, should be implemented. **Bronchodilators** improve airway obstruction. **Mucolytic** agents and expectorants help loosen and mobilize secretions so they can be coughed up. Bronchitol, a form of mannitol, is an inhaled drug that is still being studied to promote mucus clearance. It is a sugar that draws fluid into the airways to help liquefy mucus. Inhaled beta-agonist bronchodilators help keep airways open. Chest physiotherapy or a high-frequency chest

• WORD • BUILDING •
bronchitis: bronch—airway + itis—inflammation
bronchiectasis: bronch—airway + ectasis—dilation or expansion

• WORD • BUILDING •
bronchodilator: broncho—airway + dilator—to expand
mucolytic: muco—mucus + lytic—break up

wall oscillation vest can help mobilize secretions. Oxygen is used if hypoxemia is present. Oral fluids are encouraged. If the affected area of the lung is localized and symptoms are severe, surgery may be considered to remove the diseased area. Lung transplant may be considered in severe cases.

NURSING CARE TIP

If your patient is coughing up a lot of sputum, line an emesis basin with a white tissue. This makes it easier to assess the color of the sputum, and also simplifies cleaning out the basin!

Pneumonia

Pneumonia is the cause of many hospital admissions each year and is a common cause of death from infection. Persons at risk for pneumonia are the very young, adults over age 65, and people who are immunocompromised, such as those with acquired immunodeficiency syndrome (AIDS), alcoholism, or another underlying illness. Pneumonia is categorized according to where it is acquired. For example, hospital-acquired pneumonia (HAP) is defined as pneumonia that develops at least 48 hours after a hospital admission. One type of HAP is ventilator-associated pneumonia, or VAP. Health care–associated pneumonia (HCAP) is pneumonia that develops in outpatient settings or nursing homes. Community-acquired pneumonia (CAP) develops in the community and is usually less serious than other forms. Each type of pneumonia may be caused by different organisms.

Pathophysiology

Pneumonia is an acute inflammation and/or infection of the lungs that occurs when an infectious agent enters and multiplies in the lungs of a susceptible person. Infectious particles can be transmitted by the cough of an infected individual, from contaminated respiratory therapy equipment, from infections in other parts of the body, or from aspiration of bacteria from the mouth, pharynx, or stomach. Organisms from the mouth and pharynx may be related to poor oral hygiene or may be present because of a cold or influenza virus. When pathogens enter the body of a healthy person, normal respiratory defense mechanisms and the immune system prevent the development of infection. In a person who is immunocompromised, however, even microorganisms that are normally present in the oropharynx can cause an infection.

When the microorganisms multiply, they release toxins that induce inflammation in the lung tissue, causing damage to mucous and alveolar membranes. This leads to the development of edema and **exudate**, which fills the alveoli and reduces the surface area available for exchange of carbon dioxide and oxygen. Some bacteria also cause necrosis of lung tissue.

• WORD • BUILDING •
exudate: to sweat out

Pneumonia may be confined to one lobe (lobar pneumonia), or it may be scattered throughout the lungs (bronchopneumonia). Bronchopneumonia occurs more often as a nosocomial (hospital-acquired) infection in hospitalized patients, the very young, or the very old, and can be quite serious. Patients may use terms such as walking pneumonia or double pneumonia. These are not medical terms, but it is helpful to understand them. *Walking pneumonia* refers to a mild infection that may not even keep the patient from working (or walking); *double* is a lay term for bilateral.

Etiology

Pneumonia has a variety of causes, as discussed next.

BACTERIAL PNEUMONIA. The most common cause of community-acquired bacterial pneumonias is *Streptococcus pneumoniae*, also called pneumococcal pneumonia. Other community-acquired infections are caused by *Staphylococcus aureus, Chlamydia trachomatis,* and *Mycoplasma pneumoniae.* Hospital-acquired pneumonias are often much more serious than CAP. They can be caused by *Escherichia coli, Haemophilus influenzae,* and *Klebsiella pneumoniae,* among others. Methicillin-resistant *Staphylococcus aureus* (MRSA), *Pseudomonas aeruginosa,* and other antibiotic-resistant pneumonias are especially difficult to treat.

VIRAL PNEUMONIA. Influenza viruses are the most common cause of viral pneumonia. The presence of viral pneumonia increases the patient's susceptibility to a secondary bacterial pneumonia. Generally, patients are less ill with viral pneumonia than with bacterial pneumonia, but they may be ill for a longer period because antibiotics are ineffective against viruses.

FUNGAL PNEUMONIA. *Candida* and *Aspergillus* are two types of fungi that can cause pneumonia. *Pneumocystis carinii* pneumonia (PCP) is caused by a fungus and typically causes pneumonia in patients with AIDS.

ASPIRATION PNEUMONIA. Some pneumonias are caused by aspiration of foreign substances. This most often occurs in patients with decreased levels of consciousness or an impaired cough or gag reflex. These conditions can occur with alcohol ingestion, stroke, general anesthesia, seizures, gastrointestinal reflux disease (GERD), or other serious illness. Aspiration pneumonia increases the risk for subsequent bacterial pneumonia.

VENTILATOR-ASSOCIATED PNEUMONIA. A type of aspiration pneumonia, ventilator-associated pneumonia (VAP), develops in patients who are intubated and mechanically ventilated. The endotracheal tube keeps the glottis open, so secretions can be easily aspirated into the lungs. A cuff on the tube is kept inflated to attempt to protect the lower airway, and suction can keep secretions under control, but risk of aspiration is still significant.

HYPOSTATIC PNEUMONIA. Patients who hypoventilate because of bedrest, immobility, or shallow respirations are at risk for **hypostatic** pneumonia. Secretions pool in dependent areas of the lungs and can lead to inflammation and infection.

CHEMICAL PNEUMONIA. Inhalation of toxic chemicals can cause inflammation and tissue damage, which can lead to chemical pneumonia. This increases the risk for subsequent bacterial infection.

CRITICAL THINKING

Mr. Smith

■ Mr. Smith is an 86-year-old man who was watching television when he couldn't sleep one night. After seeing a commercial for toilet cleaner, he decided his own toilet could use some attention. He used bleach and ammonia "to get it really clean." The combination created toxic fumes, which caused a severe chemical pneumonia. He was brought to the emergency room in acute respiratory distress.

1. As his nurse, what questions might you ask as you further assess the cause of his pneumonia?
2. What can you teach Mr. Smith related to prevention of similar episodes in the future?

Suggested answers at end of chapter.

Prevention

A vaccine is available to help prevent *Streptococcus pneumoniae* pneumonia in high-risk patients and people older than age 65. Usually only one dose is needed, but a second dose is recommended for people age 65 or over who received the first dose before age 65 and more than 5 years ago. Other high-risk people may also need a second dose (Centers for Disease Control and Prevention [CDC], 2009d). A yearly influenza vaccination is also recommended for high-risk individuals.

Nursing care plays an important role in the prevention of HAP. Regular coughing, deep breathing, and position changes for patients on bedrest or after surgery, prevention of aspiration for patients at risk, and good hand washing practices by both patients and health care personnel can help prevent many cases (Box 31.1, *Gerontological Issues*).

The risk of ventilator-associated pneumonia can be reduced with frequent mouth care and use of a special endotracheal tube that allows continuous suctioning of secretions above the inflated cuff. All patients should be positioned with the head of the bed elevated 30 to 45 degrees to help prevent aspiration. Medication to reduce gastric acid secretion and stress ulcers may help reduce aspiration, but may also increase bacterial growth.

• WORD • BUILDING •
hypostatic: hypo—below + static—standing

SAFETY TIP

To reduce the risk of health care–associated infections, comply with current World Health Organization (WHO) or Centers for Disease Control and Prevention (CDC) hand hygiene guidelines. CDC guidelines can be found at www.cdc.gov/handhygiene (2010 National Patient Safety Goals, www.jointcommission.org).

Box 31.1

Gerontological Issues

Advanced age is a significant risk factor for serious complications from respiratory infections such as influenza, pneumococcal pneumonia, and aspiration pneumonia. Therefore, it is recommended that people over age 65 and people with chronic disease have yearly influenza vaccines and pneumococcal vaccine with repeat dose as needed. Consistent oral care is also a significant nursing intervention to help prevent morbidity and mortality from aspiration pneumonia.

Signs and Symptoms

Patients with pneumonia present with fever, shaking, chills, chest pain, dyspnea, fatigue, and a productive cough. Sputum is purulent or may be rust colored or blood tinged. Crackles and wheezes may be heard on lung auscultation because of the exudate in the alveoli and airways.

Some bacterial and many viral pneumonias cause **atypical** symptoms. The patient may experience fatigue, sore throat, dry cough, or nausea and vomiting.

Elderly patients may not exhibit expected symptoms of pneumonia. New-onset confusion or lethargy in an older patient can indicate reduced oxygenation and should alert you to look for other symptoms or request evaluation by the primary care provider. New onset of fever or dyspnea should also cause suspicion of possible pneumonia in the elderly.

Complications

Complications from pneumonia most commonly occur in patients with other underlying chronic diseases. Pleurisy and pleural effusion (discussed later in this chapter) are two of the most common complications and generally resolve within 1 to 2 weeks. **Atelectasis** (collapsed alveoli) can occur as a result of trapped secretions and may be resolved by efforts to keep the airways clear, especially use of an incentive spirometer. Other complications result from spread of infection to other parts of the body, causing septicemia, meningitis, septic

• WORD • BUILDING •
atypical: a—not + typical—usual
atelectasis: atel—imperfect + ectasis—expansion

arthritis, pericarditis, or endocarditis. Treatment for each of these is antibiotics. Although antibiotics can greatly reduce the incidence of death related to pneumonia, it is still a common cause of death in the elderly.

Diagnostic Tests

A chest x-ray examination is done to identify the presence of pulmonary infiltrate, which is fluid leakage into the alveoli from inflammation (Fig. 31.2). In addition, sputum and blood cultures are obtained to identify the organism causing the pneumonia and determine appropriate treatment. If the patient is unable to produce a sputum specimen, a nebulized mist treatment may be ordered to promote sputum expectoration. If this is unsuccessful, nasotracheal suctioning or a bronchoscopy can be done to obtain a specimen from a very ill patient.

> **NURSING CARE TIP**
>
> Obtain culture specimens before antibiotics are started to avoid altering culture results. The best time to obtain a specimen is first thing in the morning, before breakfast. If the patient has eaten, be sure he has rinsed his mouth to keep food particles out of the specimen.

Therapeutic Measures

Broad-spectrum antibiotics are initiated as soon as cultures are sent to the lab, even if results are not completed. Once the culture and sensitivity report is available, antibiotic orders may change to more narrow-spectrum agents. Many patients can be treated with oral antibiotics as outpatients, but hospitalization and intravenous (IV) therapy may be necessary in the elderly or in individuals who are chronically or acutely ill. If the pneumonia is caused by a virus, rest and fluids are recommended. Occasionally, antiviral medications are used.

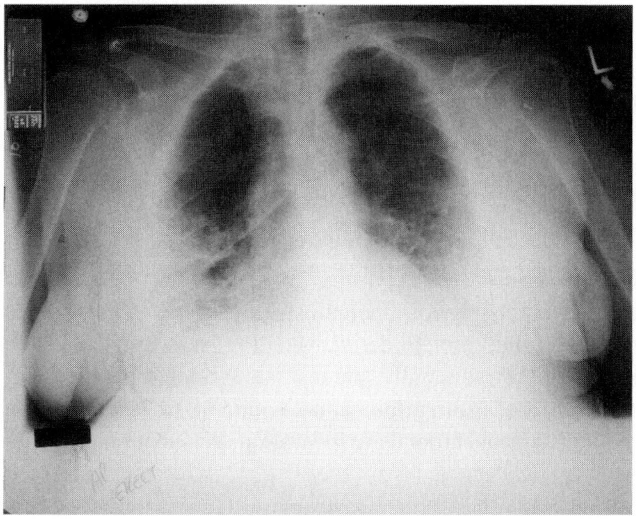

FIGURE 31.2 Chest x-ray examination showing infiltrates in pneumonia.

Expectorants, bronchodilators, and analgesics may be given for comfort and symptom relief. Nebulized mist treatments or metered-dose inhalers may be used to deliver bronchodilators. Supplemental oxygen via nasal cannula or mask is used as needed. (See Table 31.1 for a pneumonia summary.)

Tuberculosis

Pathophysiology and Etiology

Tuberculosis (TB) is an infectious disease caused by the bacterium *Mycobacterium tuberculosis.* TB primarily affects the lungs, although other areas, such as the kidneys, liver, brain, and bone, may be affected as well. *M. tuberculosis* is an acid-fast bacillus (AFB), which means that when it is stained in the laboratory and then washed with an acid, the stain remains, or stays "fast." *M. tuberculosis* can live in dark places in dried sputum for months, but a few hours in direct sunlight kills it. It is spread by inhalation of the tuberculosis bacilli from respiratory droplets (droplet nuclei) of an infected person.

Once the bacilli enter the lungs, they multiply and begin to disseminate to the lymph nodes and then to other parts of the body. The patient is then "infected" but may or may not go on to develop clinical (active) disease. TB infection without disease is called latent TB infection (LTBI). During this time the body develops immunity, which keeps the infection under control. If the lungs are involved, the immune system surrounds the infected area in the lung with neutrophils and alveolar macrophages. This process creates a lesion called a tubercle, which seals off the bacteria and prevents spread. Similar processes take place in other affected areas of the body. The bacteria within the tubercle die or become dormant, and the patient is no longer infectious. If the patient's immune system becomes compromised, however, some of

TABLE 31.1 PNEUMONIA SUMMARY

Signs and Symptoms	Fever, chills Chest pain Dyspnea Productive cough Crackles and wheezes
Diagnostic Tests	Chest x-ray Sputum cultures
Therapeutic Measures	Antibiotics Supplemental oxygen Bronchodilators, expectorants Rest, fluids
Complications	Pleurisy, pleural effusion Atelectasis
Priority Nursing Diagnoses	*Impaired Gas Exchange* *Ineffective Airway Clearance* *Activity Intolerance*

• **WORD • BUILDING** •
expectorant: ex—out of + pec—chest

the dormant bacteria can become active, causing active disease. Only 5% to 10% of infected people in the United States actually develop the disease, and even then it may not occur for many years (Box 31.2, *Gerontological Issues*).

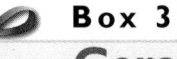

Risk Factors

Crowded or poorly ventilated living conditions place people at risk for becoming infected with tuberculosis. Although tuberculosis can infect any age group, the elderly are especially at risk. Elders may have contracted the disease many years before, but it can reactivate as the aging process diminishes immune function. AIDS, chronic alcohol abuse, and cancer chemotherapy can also compromise immune function and increase risk of activation. In the United States, tuberculosis is also prevalent among the urban poor and minority groups.

Before 1985, the incidence of TB in the United States was steadily decreasing. Since that time, it has increased in incidence, in part because of the prevalence of AIDS, the development of antibiotic-resistant strains of the TB bacillus, and ineffective treatment programs. One-third of the world's population is currently infected with TB (WHO, 2009).

Prevention

Clean, well-ventilated living areas are essential to the health of all people. If a hospitalized patient is known or suspected to have tuberculosis, he or she is placed in respiratory isolation to prevent spread to staff or other patients. Special negative-pressure isolation rooms are ventilated to the outside. Staff should wear special high-efficiency filtration masks when in the patient's room; a regular surgical mask is not effective against TB. Verify with the institution's infection control department that the masks provided are effective for use with TB patients. If the patient must travel through the hallway for tests or other activities, he or she must wear a mask. Additional protective barriers, such as gowns, gloves, or goggles, are used when contact with sputum is likely.

A vaccine against tuberculosis is available and is used in areas where TB is prevalent. It is safe, but its effectiveness has been questioned. It is not used routinely in the United States. Individuals who have had the vaccine will have a positive skin test for TB, so alternative methods for screening must be used.

Ultimately, prevention will come from adequate treatment of patients with TB. A current concern is the development of antibiotic-resistant strains of the tuberculosis bacillus, which can develop when patients are noncompliant with drug therapy. When antibiotics are taken intermittently or discontinued early, the more virulent (stronger) bacteria survive and multiply and become resistant to the drugs being used. This multi–drug-resistant TB (MDR-TB) can then be passed on to someone else. Some strains are resistant to nearly all antibiotics. They are called extensively drug resistant, or XDR-TB. It is therefore vital to teach all patients the importance of strict compliance with drug therapy. Patients who are at risk for noncompliance with drug therapy must have a visiting nurse or other health professional observe each dose of antibiotic taken. This is called directly observed therapy (DOT) or directly observed therapy–short course (DOTS). DOT transfers responsibility for making sure the drugs are taken from the patient to the health care worker. The World Health Organization reports the highest treatment success rates with DOT/DOTS.

In 2006, the World Health Organization launched a global plan to stop TB, with a goal of eliminating it by 2050. The six components of the plan include:

- Pursuing high-quality DOTS expansion
- Addressing TB in HIV infection, MDR-TB, and other challenges
- Contributing to health system strengthening
- Engaging all care providers
- Empowering people with TB, and communities
- Enabling and promoting research (WHO, 2009).

Signs and Symptoms

Active pulmonary tuberculosis is characterized by a chronic productive cough, blood-tinged sputum, and drenching night sweats. Chest pain, fatigue, poor appetite, weight loss, and a low-grade fever are common. If effective treatment is not initiated, a downhill course occurs, with pulmonary fibrosis, **hemoptysis**, and progressive weight loss.

Complications

Spread of the tuberculosis bacilli throughout the body can result in pleurisy, pericarditis, peritonitis, meningitis, bone and joint infections, genitourinary or gastrointestinal infection, or infection of many other organs.

Diagnostic Tests

Routine screening for tuberculosis infection is usually done with a purified protein derivative (PPD) skin test. The PPD is injected intradermally; the test is considered positive if a raised area of **induration** occurs within 48 to 72 hours. If a red area appears around the induration, this is not measured.

Box 31.2

Gerontological Issues

The age-related decline in immune system function can decrease the effectiveness of the tuberculosis antibodies in someone who previously had latent infection. The tuberculosis bacilli can be activated, causing active disease. Because of the risk of false negative tuberculin test results, a two-step test is recommended, with the second test done 1 to 3 weeks after the first. Decline in immune system function can also impact clinical manifestations of tuberculosis. Patients may exhibit fewer symptoms, making recognition difficult.

• WORD • BUILDING •

hemoptysis: hem—blood + ptysis—to spit

induration: in—in + durus—hard

The size of induration that indicates a positive test varies based on the individual's history (Table 31.2). A red area without induration is considered a negative result. A positive result indicates that a person has been exposed to TB; it does not mean that active TB disease is present.

Some health care institutions use a two-step process for baseline testing of employees and residents. If an individual has a negative PPD test, he or she is retested in 1 to 3 weeks. This is because someone who was exposed many years ago may not react to the first test. The first test acts as a "reminder" to the immune system to react. The second test will then be positive in the person with a past TB infection.

NURSING CARE TIP

You have probably had a PPD skin test so you can do your clinical practice for school. When you have it checked, the clinician should touch your arm. Just looking at it is not adequate to judge whether there is a raised area of induration.

In 2005, a new test was approved by the Food and Drug Administration (FDA) that provides an alternative to the PPD test. The QuantiFERON-TB Gold (QFT-G) test is a blood test that detects the cell-mediated immune response to TB bacteria in blood. Unlike the PPD skin test, the QFT-G is a simple blood test and is valid in individuals who have been vaccinated against TB.

A chest x-ray examination is used as a screening tool in someone with a known positive test. Final diagnosis is made based on sputum culture results.

NURSING CARE TIP

A *Candida* or mumps skin test may be ordered along with a PPD skin test. This does not mean the patient is being tested for *Candida* or mumps because everyone generally reacts to these. Rather the patient is being tested for **anergy**, or the inability of the immune system to react to an antigen. A positive *Candida* or mumps test means the immune system is intact, and the TB results are considered to be reliable.

The *Candida* or mumps test is administered in the same way as the PPD test. If more than one test is administered, use a permanent marker to identify which test is which, and clearly document (draw a picture) where each test was placed. Check institution policy; it may direct where the tests are administered—PPD in the right arm and *Candida* in the left, for example.

Therapeutic Measures

Treatment consists of specific antibiotic therapy. First-line drugs have the fewest adverse effects (Box 31.3). However, these drugs can be toxic to the liver and nervous system and have other side effects. Second-line drugs are more toxic and are reserved for cases that do not respond to first-line drug therapy. Generally, two or three antibiotics are given simultaneously to allow lower doses of each individual drug, reduce the incidence of serious side effects, and reduce the risk of developing resistant bacteria. Drugs must be taken for 6 to 9 months, or up to 2 years for MDR-TB. Because of the length of therapy and the incidence of side effects, compliance is often a problem.

TABLE 31.2 CLASSIFYING A TUBERCULIN SKIN TEST REACTION

Size of Induration	Considered Positive for
5 mm or more	HIV-infected persons
	Recent contacts of infectious TB cases
	Persons with fibrotic changes on chest radiograph consistent with prior TB
	Organ transplant recipients
	Those who are immunosuppressed for other reasons (taking equivalent of 15 mg/day or more of prednisone for 1 month or more), or those taking TNF-α antagonists
10 mm or more	Recent immigrants (within last 5 years) from high-prevalence countries
	Injection drug users
	Residents or employees of high-risk congregate settings (prisons, jails, long-term care facilities for the elderly, hospitals and other health care facilities, residential facilities for patients with AIDS, and homeless shelters)
	Mycobacteriology laboratory personnel
	Persons with clinical conditions previously mentioned
	Children younger than age 4
	Infants, children, or adolescents exposed to adults at high risk for TB disease
15 mm or more	People with no risk factors for TB

HIV = human immunodeficiency virus.
Source: Centers for Disease Control and Prevention. (2009). *Tuberculosis.* Retrieved June 17, 2009, from http://www.cdc.gov/tb/publications/LTBI/diagnosis.htm.

Box 31.3

Antibiotics Used to Treat Tuberculosis

First-Line Drugs

Isoniazid
Rifampin
Ethambutol
Pyrazinamide

Second-Line Drugs

Rifabutin
Rifapentine
Para-aminosalicylic acid
Streptomycin
Levofloxacin
Ethionamide
Amikacin
and others

Additional treatment is supportive. Rest and good nutrition are important for helping the patient's own immune system to work. Patients must be isolated until their sputum no longer contains TB bacteria.

Patients with latent TB infection do not need to be treated, but some health departments recommend treatment to reduce the risk of progression to active disease and subsequent spread to others.

The Centers for Disease Control and Prevention has an excellent website with lots of information about TB at www.cdc.gov. Simply type "tuberculosis" into the search window.

Nursing Process for the Patient with Tuberculosis

DATA COLLECTION. Perform a thorough history and head-to-toe physical examination, because TB can affect many systems. Focus on respiratory and psychosocial assessments. The severity of the disease determines the impact on the patient's lifestyle. It is also important to determine the patient's knowledge of the disease and treatment and his or her compliance with drug treatment.

NURSING DIAGNOSES, PLANNING, AND IMPLEMENTATION. Nursing interventions for impaired gas exchange, ineffective airway clearance, and activity intolerance are found in the *Nursing Care Plan for the Patient with a Lower Respiratory Tract Disorder*. Additional nursing diagnoses for the patient with TB follow.

Risk for Ineffective Self Health Management Related to Knowledge Deficit and Length of Treatment

EXPECTED OUTCOME: The patient will follow treatment regimen and infection will be resolved, as evidenced by negative cultures.

- Assess patient's and family's ability and intent to follow treatment regimen. *It is essential for patients to be diligent about taking their drugs in order to eradicate the infection and to prevent spread to others.*
- Teach patient and family that drugs must be taken as scheduled for the entire course (6 months or longer) or a drug-resistant form of disease may develop. *Patients may be more willing to comply if they understand the rationale for taking their medications.*
- Forewarn the patient that rifampin turns urine and other body fluids red. *This might frighten the patient and prevent her from taking the drugs if she is unprepared.*
- Teach patient to report side effects of medications. *If side effects can be managed, the patient is more likely to comply with therapy.*
- Request an order for a visiting nurse. *A visiting nurse can monitor compliance. Directly observed therapy (DOT) has been found to increase compliance with medications.*

Risk for Infection: Transmission to Others Related to Knowledge Deficit About how Infection is Spread, or Noncompliance with Control Measures

EXPECTED OUTCOME: The patient will verbalize understanding of and employ measures to prevent spreading infection.

- Assess patient's understanding of how TB is spread. *Teaching should build on patient's current knowledge.*
- Teach the patient how TB is spread and the importance of following measures to avoid spread. *The patient will be more likely to comply if he understands the rationale for his actions.*
- Teach the patient to use a tissue to cover the mouth and nose when coughing or sneezing. *TB is spread by droplet nuclei that can be contained with a tissue.*
- Teach patient to flush tissues down the toilet or dispose of carefully in the trash. *TB bacteria can live in dried sputum for months, so careful disposal is essential.*
- Teach all family members the importance of careful hand washing. *Hand washing is an important measure in preventing all kinds of infections.*
- Instruct the patient in the importance of compliance with follow-up sputum cultures. *Once sputum cultures are negative, the patient is no longer contagious.*

EVALUATION. If nursing care has been effective, the patient will understand his or her disease and the importance of taking care of himself or herself. The patient will take medications and receive follow-up care as ordered. He or she will take measures to protect others from catching TB. Additional evaluation is found in the *Nursing Care Plan for the Patient with a Lower Respiratory Tract Disorder*.

NURSING CARE PLAN for the Patient with a Lower Respiratory Tract Disorder

Note: The most commonly used nursing diagnoses related to respiratory disorders are presented in the following care plan. This is not a care plan for any one respiratory disorder. Rather, use it as a reference when one of the nursing diagnoses applies to the patient, based on a thorough respiratory assessment.

Nursing Diagnosis: *Impaired Gas Exchange* related to decreased ventilation or perfusion as evidenced by PaO_2 less than 80 mm Hg, $PaCo_2$ greater than 45 mm Hg, or Spo_2 less than 90%

Expected Outcomes: The patient will experience improved gas exchange, as evidenced by improving arterial blood gases or pulse oximetry and statement of acceptable level of dyspnea.

Evaluation of Outcomes: Are the patient's blood gases or Spo_2 improving? Does the patient state that dyspnea is gone or controlled at an acceptable level?

Interventions	Rationale	Evaluation
Assess lung sounds, respiratory rate and effort, use of accessory muscles.	Respiratory rate less than 12 per minute or more than 24 per minute or use of accessory muscles indicates distress. Diminished or adventitious lung sounds can lead to impaired gas exchange.	Are lung sounds clear and audible? Is respiratory rate 12 to 20 per minute and unlabored?
Observe skin and mucous membranes for cyanosis.	Cyanosis indicates poor oxygenation. Oral mucous membrane cyanosis indicates serious hypoxia.	Are skin and mucous membranes pink?
Assess degree of dyspnea on a scale of 0 to 10, with 0 = no dyspnea and 10 = worst dyspnea.	The patient's subjective report is the best measure of dyspnea; dyspnea indicates impaired gas exchange.	Is patient's degree of dyspnea within parameters that are acceptable to patient?
Monitor for confusion or changes in mental status.	Changes in mental status can signal impaired gas exchange.	Is patient alert and oriented? If not, could poor gas exchange be the reason?
Monitor arterial blood gas values and pulse oximetry as ordered.	Pao_2 less than 80 mm Hg, $PaCo_2$ greater than 45 mm Hg, or Spo_2 less than 90% indicate impaired gas exchange.	Are values within patient's baseline values?
Elevate head of bed or help patient to lean on over-bed table.	Upright positioning promotes lung expansion.	Did change of position relieve some distress?
Position with good lung dependent ("good lung down").	This position allows the healthier lung to be better perfused and increases gas exchange.	Is Spo_2 improved in this position?
Administer supplemental oxygen at less than 2 L/min unless ordered otherwise.	Supplemental oxygen decreases hypoxia. Rates more than 2 L/min may depress hypoxic drive.	Is oxygen placed properly on patient? Does it provide relief from dyspnea?
Place a fan in the patient's room.	The feeling of a breeze on the patient's face may make the patient feel he is getting more air.	Is a fan available to the patient and does it help?
Teach patient relaxation exercises.	Relaxation exercises decrease perceived dyspnea.	Does patient use relaxation effectively?

Continued

NURSING CARE PLAN for the Patient with a Lower Respiratory Tract Disorder—cont'd

For chronic disease, teach patient diaphragmatic and pursed-lip breathing. (See Chapter 29.)	Breathing exercises promote relaxation and increase CO_2 excretion.	Does patient use breathing exercises correctly? Do they help?
Encourage patient to stop smoking if patient is a current smoker.	Smoking is damaging to lungs and respiratory function.	Is patient receptive to smoking cessation? Are resources available?
For severe dyspnea, ask physician about an order for intravenous morphine sulfate.	Low doses of IV morphine cause peripheral vasodilation, which helps relieve pulmonary edema and anxiety.	Does morphine provide relief from dyspnea?

Nursing Diagnosis: *Ineffective Airway Clearance* related to excessive secretions as evidenced by crackles or wheezes, ineffective cough

Expected Outcomes: The patient will have improved airway clearance as evidenced by clear breath sounds and ability to cough up secretions.

Evaluation of Outcomes: Are the patient's breath sounds clear? Is the patient able to effectively cough up and expectorate secretions?

Interventions	Rationale	Evaluation
Assess lung sounds q4h and prn.	Crackles and wheezes may indicate excess secretions in airways.	Do lung sounds indicate retained secretions?
Monitor amount, color, and consistency of sputum.	Thick, purulent sputum indicates infection and should be reported to the physician.	Does sputum indicate infection?
Turn patient q2h or encourage to ambulate if able.	Movement mobilizes secretions.	Is patient mobile?
Encourage oral fluids; use cool steam room humidifier.	Hydration decreases viscosity of secretions and aids expectoration.	Is patient able to take oral fluids? Are secretions thin and easily expectorated?
Encourage patient to cough and deep breathe every hour and prn.	Controlled coughing following deep breaths is more effective in clearing airway.	Does patient cough and deep breathe effectively?
Administer expectorants or mucolytics as ordered.	Expectorants help liquefy secretions and trigger the cough reflex.	Are expectorants effective?
If patient is unable to cough up secretions, suction per institution policy.	Suctioning is necessary to remove secretions when the patient is unable to cough effectively.	Is suctioning necessary? Does it help remove secretions?
Obtain order for chest physiotherapy or flutter valve if indicated.	Chest physiotherapy helps mobilize secretions.	Is CPT effective and well tolerated by the patient?

NURSING CARE PLAN for the Patient with a Lower Respiratory Tract Disorder—cont'd

Nursing Diagnosis: *Ineffective Breathing Pattern* related to anxiety or pain as evidenced by respiratory rate less than 12 per minute or greater than 24 per minute, labored or shallow respirations, abnormal ABGs and Spo_2 values.

Expected Outcomes: The patient will maintain an effective breathing pattern as evidenced by respiratory rate between 12 and 20 per minute, even, and unlabored; and arterial blood gas and oxygen saturation results within patient's normal range.

Evaluation of Outcomes: Is the patient's respiratory rate within normal limits and unlabored? Does the patient's breathing pattern support normal blood gas and Spo_2 values?

Interventions	Rationale	Evaluation
Assess respiratory rate, depth, and effort q4h and prn.	Respirations less than 12 per minute or more than 20 per minute may indicate an ineffective pattern.	Is respiratory pattern ineffective?
Monitor blood gas and oxygen saturation values.	An ineffective breathing pattern will not maintain oxygenation.	Is breathing pattern adversely affecting oxygenation?
Determine and treat the cause of ineffective breathing pattern.	Pain or anxiety can cause a patient to change the breathing pattern.	Is a contributing factor identifiable and correctable?
Place patient in Fowler's or semi-Fowler's position.	This allows for maximum chest expansion.	Is the patient in a comfortable position that enables adequate expansion?
Teach patient to use diaphragmatic breathing, with a regular 2 second in, 4 second out pattern.	Breathing exercises promote relaxation and increase Co_2 excretion.	Is the patient able to demonstrate an effective breathing pattern?

Nursing Diagnosis: *Activity Intolerance* related to imbalance between oxygen supply and demand as evidenced by dyspnea or drop in Spo_2 with routine activity

Expected Outcomes: The patient will tolerate increasing activity level as appropriate based on prognosis, as evidenced by stable respiratory rate and Spo_2 with activity. The patient will receive assistance with self-care until he or she is able to carry out own ADLs and will space rest and activity in order to provide as much self-care as possible.

Evaluation of Outcomes: Are the patient's care needs met by self or caregiver?

Interventions	Rationale	Evaluation
Assess amount of activity the patient can tolerate without becoming short of breath.	Patients should be encouraged to do as much as they can for themselves, to avoid becoming deconditioned.	What is patient able to do?
Monitor vital signs and oxygen saturation with activities.	Respiratory rate will rise and Spo_2 will drop if activity is not tolerated.	Are vital signs and Spo_2 stable?
Allow patient to rest between activities. Bedrest may be needed during acute dyspnea.	Even talking or eating can be exhausting to a patient who is dyspneic.	Is patient able to catch his or her breath between activities?
Obtain bedside commode, shower chair, handheld showerhead, if needed.	Assistive devices can help the patient conserve energy.	Do assistive devices allow patient more independence?

Continued

NURSING CARE PLAN for the Patient with a Lower Respiratory Tract Disorder—cont'd

Interventions	Rationale	Evaluation
Obtain portable oxygen if patient is able to ambulate.	Portable oxygen may enable the patient to ambulate and prevent deconditioning.	Is patient able to ambulate and maintain Spo_2 within normal limits with portable oxygen?
Allow uninterrupted rest at night as much as possible.	Lack of sleep can contribute to activity intolerance.	Is patient able to sleep uninterrupted? Can interferences be delayed until morning?
Slowly increase activity as able.	Increasing activity helps maintain muscle tone and endurance.	Is patient able to increase a little each day? Is this a realistic goal for patient?
Refer patient with chronic lung disease to a pulmonary rehabilitation program.	Pulmonary rehabilitation programs can help patient increase exercise tolerance.	Is patient willing to participate in a rehabilitation program?

CRITICAL THINKING

Mr. Woo

■ Mr. Woo is being tested for tuberculosis. You check his skin tests and find that the PPD test in his left forearm is negative, with no redness or induration. You also find that the Candida test in his right forearm is negative, with no redness or induration.

1. How do you document these results?
2. How do you interpret them?

Suggested answers at end of chapter.

NURSING PROCESS FOR THE PATIENT WITH A LOWER RESPIRATORY INFECTION

Priority nursing diagnoses and interventions for patients with lower respiratory infections are presented in the *Nursing Care Plan for the Patient with a Lower Respiratory Tract Disorder.*

RESTRICTIVE DISORDERS

Restrictive disorders are those problems that limit the ability of the patient to expand his or her lungs and, therefore, inhale air. These are caused by a decrease in the **compliance** (or elasticity) of the lungs or chest wall. Restrictive disorders covered below include pleurisy, pleural effusion, empyema, pulmonary fibrosis, and atelectasis.

Pleurisy (Pleuritis)

Pathophysiology

Recall that the visceral and parietal pleurae are the membranes that surround the lungs. Between these membranes is a small amount of serous fluid that prevents friction as the pleurae slide over each other during inhalation and exhalation. If the membranes become inflamed for any reason, they do not slide as easily. Instead of sliding, one membrane may "catch" on the other, causing it to stretch as the patient attempts to take a breath. This causes the characteristic sharp pain on inspiration. The irritation causes an increase in the formation of pleural fluid, which in turn reduces friction and decreases pain.

Etiology

Pleurisy is usually related to another underlying respiratory disorder, such as pneumonia, tuberculosis, a tumor, or trauma. Nonrespiratory disorders such as pancreatitis or certain autoimmune disorders can also result in pleurisy.

Signs and Symptoms

Pleurisy causes a sharp pain in the chest on inspiration. Pain also occurs during coughing or sneezing. Breathing may be shallow and rapid because deep breathing increases pain. The patient may also exhibit fever, chills, and an elevated white blood cell count if the cause is infectious. A pleural friction rub is heard on auscultation.

Complications

As pleural membranes become more inflamed, serous fluid production increases, which may result in pleural effusion (see next section). If pleuritic pain is not controlled, patients have difficulty breathing deeply and coughing, which may lead to atelectasis. If infection goes untreated, empyema can result.

Diagnostic Tests

Diagnosis is based on signs and symptoms, including auscultation of a pleural friction rub. A chest x-ray examination or ultrasound and complete blood cell count (CBC) may be done. FVC (forced vital capacity) is reduced more than FEV_1 (forced expiratory volume in 1 second) since expansion is limited by the restrictive disorder; airways and FEV_1 may be normal. Additional testing is done to determine the underlying cause.

Therapeutic Measures

Treatment is aimed at correcting the underlying cause. Nonsteroidal anti-inflammatory drugs (NSAIDs) or opioids are given to control pain and facilitate deep breathing and coughing. The physician may perform a nerve block by injecting anesthetic near the intercostal nerves to block pain transmission.

Pleural Effusion

Pathophysiology

When excess fluid collects in the pleural space, it is called a pleural effusion. Fluid normally enters the pleural space from surrounding capillaries and is reabsorbed by the lymphatic system. When a pathological condition causes an increase in fluid production or inadequate reabsorption of fluid, excess fluid collects. A normal amount of pleural fluid around each lung is 1 to 15 mL. More than 25 mL of fluid is considered abnormal; as much as several liters of fluid can collect at one time. The effusion can be either transudative, forming a watery fluid from the capillaries, or exudative, with fluid containing white blood cells and protein from an inflammatory or infectious process.

Etiology

Like pleurisy, pleural effusion is generally caused by another lung disorder. It is a symptom rather than a disease. Transudative effusions may result from heart failure, liver disorders, or kidney disorders. Exudative effusions more commonly occur with lung cancer, infection, or inflammation.

Signs and Symptoms

Symptoms depend on the amount of fluid in the pleural space. The patient may or may not experience pleuritic pain. Increasing shortness of breath occurs because of the decreasing space for lung expansion. Cough and **tachypnea** may be present. A dull sound is heard when the affected area is percussed. Lung sounds are decreased or absent over the effusion, and a friction rub may be auscultated.

Diagnostic Tests

A chest x-ray examination is done to determine whether pleural effusion is present. If a thoracentesis is done, fluid samples are sent to the laboratory for culture and sensitivity and cytological examination. Further tests are done to determine the cause of the effusion.

Therapeutic Measures

Bedrest is recommended to enhance spontaneous resolution of the effusion. If symptoms are severe, a therapeutic thoracentesis is done to remove the excess fluid from the pleural space and relieve the patient of dyspnea. (Chapter 29 discusses how to assist with a thoracentesis.) The physician will use x-ray examinations and percussion, or sometimes ultrasound, to determine where to insert the needle to obtain the fluid. If the fluid accumulation is large or recurring, a chest tube might be placed to continuously drain the pleural space. Occasionally talc or another irritating agent will be instilled via the chest tube to cause the pleural membranes to adhere to each other, eliminating the pleural space and preventing future episodes of pleural effusion. Treatment of the underlying cause of the effusion is necessary to prevent recurrence.

• WORD • BUILDING •

tachypnea: tachy—rapid + pnea—breathing

Empyema

Empyema is the collection of pus in the pleural space. It is a pleural effusion that is infected. Empyema is usually a complication of pneumonia, tuberculosis, or lung abscess.

Symptoms, diagnosis, therapeutic measures, and nursing care are the same as the care of the patient with a pleural effusion, with an added emphasis on identifying and resolving the infection. A chest tube or surgery may be necessary to drain the area.

Pulmonary Fibrosis

Pathophysiology

Pulmonary fibrosis (PF), sometimes called interstitial lung disease, is a group of disorders that cause scarring and fibrosis of lung tissue. PF may evolve from injury to the alveoli, causing chronic inflammation; inflamed tissues are gradually replaced by fibrous connective tissue. Alveoli become thick and scarred, and gas exchange becomes difficult.

Etiology

Various factors are linked with pulmonary fibrosis, including heredity, exposure to certain viral illnesses, wood and metal dust exposure, medications, and smoking. It may also be associated with some autoimmune disorders such as lupus erythematosus or rheumatoid arthritis. Chronic GERD (gastroesophageal reflux disease) may play a role. Often PF is called idiopathic PF because no specific cause can be found.

Signs and Symptoms

Patients with PF experience progressive shortness of breath. Inspiratory crackles and chronic cough are present. Some experience flu-like symptoms. Fatigue is common, and clubbing of fingers may be present. Patients usually follow a downhill course.

Diagnostic Tests

A chest x-ray may show lung infiltrates. A CT scan may be done. Spirometry is done to verify that the condition is restrictive. Arterial blood gases (ABGs) may show reduced PaO_2. A bronchoscopy and lung biopsy can help rule out other causes of the patient's symptoms and can show inflammation and fibrosis. A blood test (ANA titer) may show whether an autoimmune process is involved.

Therapeutic Measures

Glucocorticoids (steroids) are used to reduce inflammation. Drugs to suppress the immune system may reduce autoimmune activity. Patients should be encouraged to stop smoking and to avoid secondhand smoke. Oxygen is used if needed to maintain oxygenation. Patients should receive flu and pneumococcal vaccines. Younger patients may be considered for a lung transplant. Pulmonary rehabilitation helps patients maintain optimum activity tolerance.

Atelectasis

Atelectasis is the collapse of alveoli. It most commonly occurs in postsurgical patients who do not cough and deep breathe effectively, although it can be caused by anything that causes hypoventilation. Areas of the lungs that are not well aerated become plugged with mucus, which prevents inflation of alveoli. As a result, alveoli collapse. Compression of lung tissue from effusion or a tumor can also cause atelectasis. The focus of nursing care is on prevention. Patients should be taught the importance of coughing and deep breathing whenever the risk for hypoventilation is present. Frequent position changes and ambulation are also helpful.

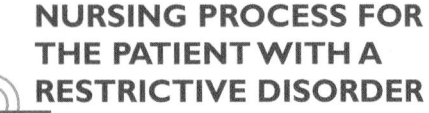

NURSING PROCESS FOR THE PATIENT WITH A RESTRICTIVE DISORDER

Data Collection

Perform a routine respiratory assessment. Monitor lung sounds for friction rub or decreasing breath sounds in any of the lobes. Assess pain level and vital signs. Be vigilant for an increase in dyspnea, tachypnea, changes in vital signs or pulse oximetry, or an increased white blood cell count or temperature.

Nursing Diagnoses, Planning, and Implementation

Priority nursing diagnoses are similar to those for other respiratory disorders and are addressed in the *Nursing Care Plan for the Patient with a Lower Respiratory Tract Disorder.* In addition, it is essential to address pain (see below), because pain can prevent the patient from breathing effectively.

Risk for Ineffective Breathing Pattern Related to Acute Pain

EXPECTED OUTCOME: The patient will be comfortable enough to breathe deeply and cough effectively and will have a respiratory rate of 12 to 20 per minute.

- Monitor respiratory rate and depth and pain location and level. *Some types of pain can cause shallow respirations, especially pleuritic pain.*
- Position patient for comfort. *Sometimes laying on the affected side for short periods will help reduce chest wall movement and pain.*
- Administer pain medication as ordered, preferably around the clock, to prevent pain from becoming severe. *Pain must be controlled so patient can breathe deeply and prevent further complications. NSAIDs or acetaminophen are usually tried first because they will not suppress cough and respirations.*
- If opioids are required to control pain, carefully monitor respirations and cough. *Opioids can suppress respirations and cough, which can further complicate the underlying disorder.*
- Teach patient the importance of effective deep breathing and coughing (see Chapter 29). *This can help prevent further complications, but may be difficult if associated with pain or suppressed by opioids.*
- Request an order for an incentive spirometer. *Incentive spirometry can help encourage the patient to breathe deeply.*

Evaluation

If interventions have been effective, the patient should report a decrease in dyspnea and anxiety. Pain will be controlled so that the patient is able to take deep breaths and cough effectively. Breath sounds will be clear and equal bilaterally, and the patient will be free of signs and symptoms of infection.

OBSTRUCTIVE DISORDERS

Chronic Obstructive Pulmonary Disease/ Chronic Airflow Limitation

Chronic obstructive pulmonary disease (COPD) is the fourth leading cause of death in the United States. More than 12 million adults have been diagnosed with COPD, and another 12 million likely have it but have not yet experienced symptoms or been diagnosed. COPD kills more than 120,000 Americans each year—one every 4 minutes (National Heart, Lung, and Blood Institute, n.d.). In the past, it was more common in men, but the incidence in women is rising because more women smoke now. The death rate from COPD in women nearly tripled between 1980 and 2000.

Pathophysiology

Chronic obstructive pulmonary disease is a group of pulmonary disorders characterized by difficulty exhaling because of airways that are narrowed or blocked by inflammation and mucus and because the loss of elastic fibers causes an increase in compliance. More effort is required for the weakened alveoli to push air out through obstructed airways (Fig. 31.3). Emphysema, chronic bronchitis, and asthma are disorders that limit airflow. A patient with COPD may have some degree of both emphysema and chronic bronchitis, although usually bronchitis is the dominant disorder. Asthma may also be present, but it differs somewhat because the airway limitation in asthma is usually reversible. A patient with asthma that is unremitting is treated as having COPD. Airflow limitation in emphysema and bronchitis is progressive and minimally reversible (Fig. 31.4).

COPD may also be referred to as chronic airflow limitation (CAL) or chronic obstructive lung disease (COLD). COPD develops slowly and may be present for many years before symptoms become evident, and it may be advanced

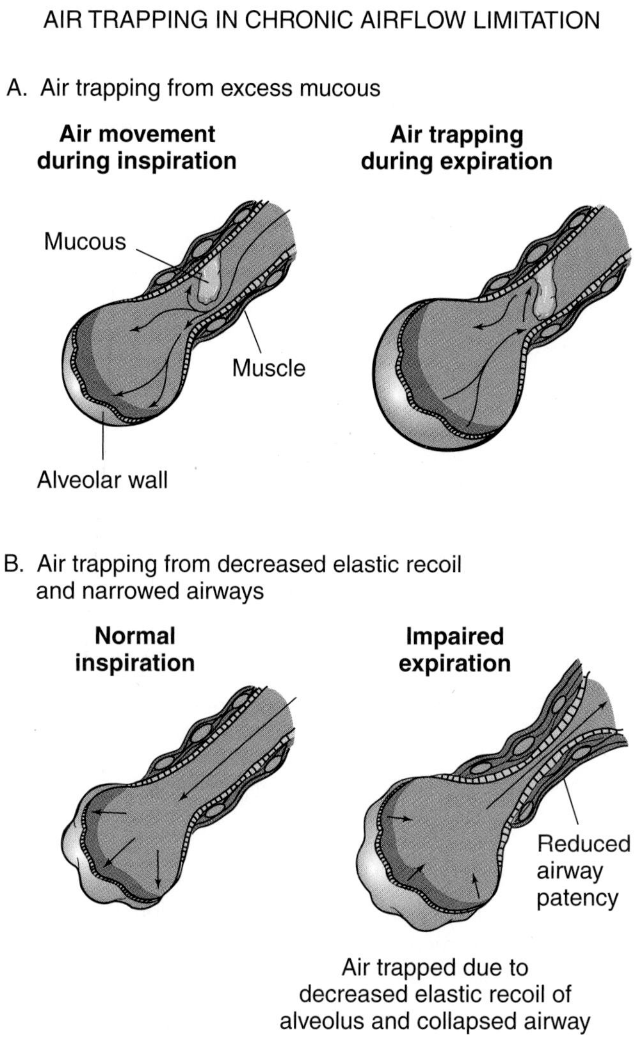
AIR TRAPPING IN CHRONIC AIRFLOW LIMITATION
A. Air trapping from excess mucous
Air movement during inspiration
Air trapping during expiration
Mucous
Muscle
Alveolar wall
B. Air trapping from decreased elastic recoil and narrowed airways
Normal inspiration
Impaired expiration
Reduced airway patency
Air trapped due to decreased elastic recoil of alveolus and collapsed airway

FIGURE 31.3 Air trapping in COPD.

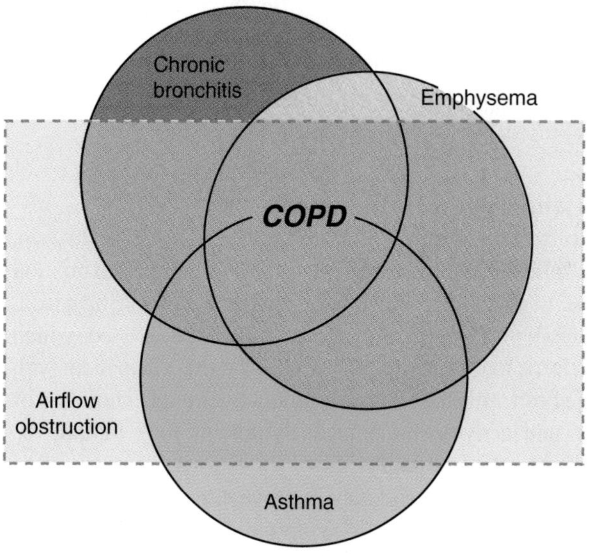
Chronic bronchitis
Emphysema
COPD
Airflow obstruction
Asthma

FIGURE 31.4 Chronic bronchitis and emphysema are the primary underlying disorders in COPD. Asthma also may play a role.

by the time the patient seeks treatment. It is characterized by periods of relative stability and **exacerbations** (acute worsening of symptoms), which may be triggered by respiratory infection or other stressors. (See Table 31.3 for a COPD summary.)

> **LEARNING TIP**
>
> Restrictive disorders cause difficulty with inhalation or air enteRing the lungs. Obstructive disorders are associated with difficulty exhaling or getting air Out.

CHRONIC BRONCHITIS PATHOPHYSIOLOGY. Chronic bronchitis is similar to acute bronchitis, with symptoms occurring for at least 3 months of the year for 2 consecutive years. Patients may have multiple exacerbations, each lasting 2 weeks or more. The bronchial tree becomes inflamed from inhaled irritants, and impaired ciliary function reduces the ability to remove the irritants. The mucus-producing glands in the airways become hypertrophied, producing excessive thick, tenacious mucus, which obstructs airways and traps air (Fig. 31.5A). These changes lead to chronic low-grade infection.

TABLE 31.3 COPD SUMMARY

Signs and Symptoms	Cough Chronic sputum production Dyspnea that occurs every day, worsens with exercise Activity intolerance Crackles, wheezes, diminished breath sounds Barrel chest Use of accessory muscles
Diagnostic Tests	Chest x-ray examination, CT scan Arterial blood gas analysis CBC Sputum analysis Spirometry α_1AT level if hereditary deficiency suspected
Therapeutic Measures	Smoking cessation Bronchodilators (PO, NMT, MDI) Corticosteroids, expectorants Flu and pneumonia vaccinations Supplemental oxygen Breathing exercises Chest physiotherapy Pulmonary rehabilitation
Priority Nursing Diagnoses	*Impaired Gas Exchange* *Ineffective Airway Clearance* *Activity Intolerance*

MDI = metered-dose inhaler; NMT = nebulized mist treatment; PO = by mouth.

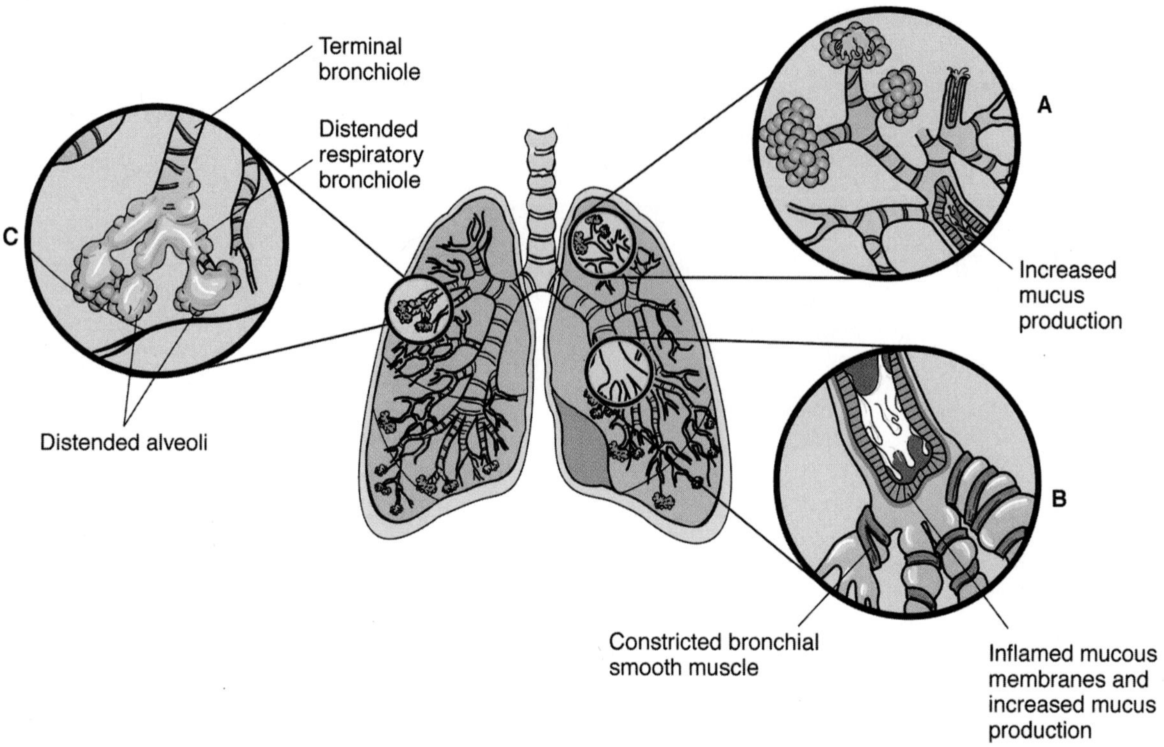
Terminal bronchiole
Distended respiratory bronchiole
C
Distended alveoli
A
Increased mucus production
B
Constricted bronchial smooth muscle
Inflamed mucous membranes and increased mucus production

FIGURE 31.5 (A) Chronic bronchitis. Note inflamed airways and excessive mucus. (B) Asthma. Note narrowed bronchial tubes and swollen mucous membranes. (C) Emphysema. Note distended respiratory bronchioles and alveoli.

EMPHYSEMA PATHOPHYSIOLOGY. Emphysema affects the respiratory bronchioles and alveoli distal to the terminal bronchioles, causing destruction of the alveolar walls and loss of elastic recoil (see Fig. 31.5C). This also causes damage to adjacent pulmonary capillaries. Because of the loss of elastic recoil, passive exhalation is impaired and air is trapped in the alveoli. The combination of destroyed alveoli and damaged capillaries causes reduced surface area for gas exchange. Emphysema can occur primarily in the respiratory bronchioles (centrilobular emphysema), with delayed alveolar damage, or in the respiratory bronchioles and alveoli (panlobular emphysema) (Fig. 31.6).

Etiology

Smoking is the single most important risk factor for COPD. Other factors include passive (secondhand) smoking, indoor and outdoor air pollution, and exposure to industrial chemicals. Some familial predisposition to chronic bronchitis has been demonstrated. A small number of individuals have an inherited deficiency of the enzyme alpha-antitrypsin (α_1AT), which causes a predisposition to the development of emphysema. Patients with this inherited tendency who also smoke have a very high risk of developing the disease. Children of smoking parents are at higher risk because of secondhand smoke exposure.

Prevention

Prevention is important because no cure for COPD is currently available. Avoidance of smoking and other inhaled irritants is vital, especially in those individuals with parents or siblings with COPD. According to the Global Initiative for Chronic Obstructive Lung Disease (GOLD) guidelines, "smoking cessation is the single most effective—and cost-effective—intervention to reduce the risk of developing COPD and slow its progression" (GOLD, 2009).

• WORD • BUILDING •
emphysema: to inflate

> **NURSING CARE TIP**
>
> This is a self-care tip. If you are a smoker, now is a good time to quit. COPD is deadly. Check Chapter 29 for ways to quit smoking. Good luck!

Signs and Symptoms

Classic symptoms of COPD are cough, sputum production, and dyspnea on exertion. Patients exhibit prolonged expiration because of obstructed air passages and reduced elastic recoil. Air trapping causes the lungs to become hyperinflated, which in turn leads to the classic barrel-shaped chest. The patient with chronic bronchitis has a chronic productive cough, shortness of breath, and activity intolerance. Symptoms may initially be worse in the winter months. Crackles and wheezing are often noted on auscultation and may improve after coughing.

The most characteristic symptom of emphysema is progressive shortness of breath, accompanied by activity intolerance. Use of accessory muscles is evident. Auscultation reveals diminished breath sounds. Remember that many patients have symptoms of both chronic bronchitis and emphysema.

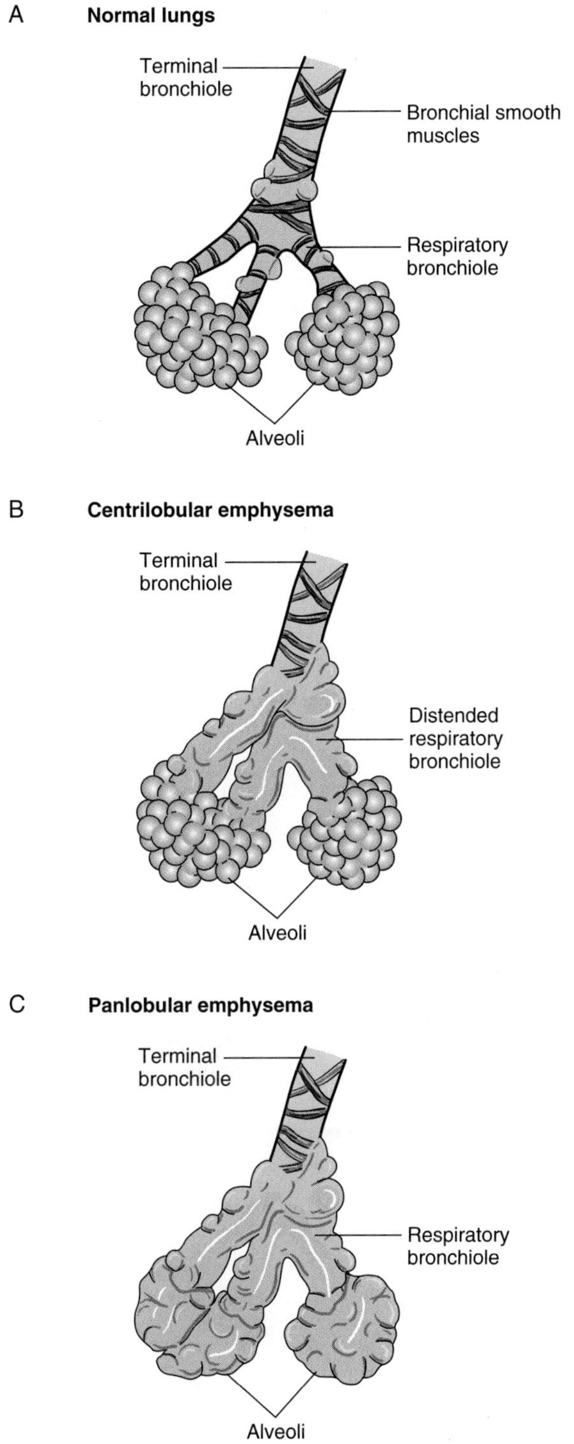
A
Normal lungs
Terminal bronchiole
Bronchial smooth muscles
Respiratory bronchiole
Alveoli
B
Centrilobular emphysema
Terminal bronchiole
Distended respiratory bronchiole
Alveoli
C
Panlobular emphysema
Terminal bronchiole
Respiratory bronchiole
Alveoli

FIGURE 31.6 Types of emphysema. (A) Normal lungs. (B) Centrilobular emphysema. (C) Panlobular emphysema.

Arterial blood gases (ABGs) may be checked during an acute exacerbation of COPD and show an increase in $PaCO_2$ and a low PaO_2. The patient develops **polycythemia** in response to chronic hypoxemia, which results in a ruddy skin color. Cyanosis may also be present.

• WORD • BUILDING •
polycythemia: poly—many + cyt—cells + emia—in the blood

In late stages of COPD, patients may lose weight and become malnourished. They have difficulty eating because of severe dyspnea, and the increased work of breathing expends more calories. Chronic hypoxemia causes release of certain chemicals that may also lead to weight loss. Patients use accessory muscles to breathe and tend to assume the classic tripod position to aid breathing.

Complications

Some patients with emphysema develop large air spaces within the lung tissue (**bullae**) or adjacent to the pleurae (**blebs**). These are like blisters that can rupture and cause the lung to collapse. Right-sided heart failure may develop because the heart has to work harder to pump blood to the diseased lungs. (See the section on cor pulmonale in Chapter 26.) Death usually results from respiratory infection or respiratory failure.

Diagnostic Tests

Information from spirometry, chest x-ray examination, and blood gas analysis is correlated with the history and physical examination to diagnose COPD. Spirometry is essential for diagnosis. Normally, the forced expiratory volume in 1 second (FEV_1) is about 70% to 80% of the forced vital capacity (FVC). In COPD, the FEV_1 is less than 70%. This is because the patient with airflow limitation is unable to forcefully exhale as much air in the first second as would normally be expected.

If lung function improves after administration of a bronchodilator, asthma is suspected rather than COPD. An α_1AT level is checked if deficiency is suspected, especially in patients with a family history of COPD. CBC, electrolytes, and sputum culture may also be assessed during exacerbations.

COPD is classified according to spirometry results and symptoms (Table 31.4).

Therapeutic Measures

The goals of COPD treatment, according to the GOLD guidelines, are as follows:

- Relieve symptoms.
- Prevent disease progression.
- Improve exercise tolerance.

TABLE 31.4 COPD STAGES

Stage I	*Mild COPD.* Mild airflow limitation, and sometimes, but not always, cough and sputum. Patient may not realize his lung function is abnormal.
Stage II	*Moderate COPD.* Airflow limitation worsening; patient begins to feel short of breath on exertion. Patient may seek medical help at this stage.
Stage III	*Severe COPD.* Increasing airflow limitation and shortness of breath. Patient experiences decreased quality of life.
Stage IV	*Very severe COPD.* Severe airflow limitation and significant reduction in quality of life; exacerbations may be life threatening.

Source: Adapted from Global Initiative for Chronic Obstructive Lung Disease, 2009.

- Improve health status.
- Prevent and treat complications.
- Prevent and treat exacerbations.
- Reduce mortality.
- Prevent or minimize side effects from treatment.

In addition, cessation of cigarette smoking should be included as a goal throughout any management program (GOLD, 2009).

SMOKING CESSATION. Even late in the disease process, stopping smoking can slow disease progression and prolong life. Exposure to other respiratory contaminants should also be minimized. Hair spray, body powder, and other household aerosols should be avoided. Figure 31.7 shows the benefit of smoking cessation and impact on the length of time to disability and death. Box 31.4, *Patient Perspective,* is a personal account from one woman who understood too late the importance of smoking cessation.

OXYGEN. Oxygen therapy is usually delayed until stage IV disease, and then is used to keep SpO_2 at or above 90%. It usually is ordered at a flow rate of 1 to 2 L/min. Higher flow rates may suppress the hypoxic drive in patients who are chronic CO_2 retainers, although this is uncommon. Higher flow rates may be used during acute exacerbations in a monitored setting. Patients with chronic oxygen saturation levels of 88% or less should be placed on oxygen at home.

MEDICATIONS. Medications commonly used include adrenergic and anticholinergic metered-dose inhalers (MDIs) or nebulized mist treatments (NMTs) to open airways, corticosteroid inhalers to control inflammation, and intermittently when needed, antibiotics. Much focus is now placed on a combination of long-acting adrenergic agents and corticosteroids (Advair, Symbicort) and a new long-acting anticholinergic agent (tiotropium [Spiriva]), all of which may reduce exacerbations and prolong survival. **Antitussive** agents should be avoided in patients with COPD because they need to be able to cough up secretions.

Oral theophylline bronchodilators are sometimes used, but have significant side effects so are avoided if possible. Oral corticosteroids may be used late in the disease to increase reduction in airway inflammation, but should ideally be reserved for acute exacerbations. A newer treatment is replacement of $\alpha 1AT$ in those patients who are deficient. See Table 31.5 for a more detailed list of medications used in the treatment of COPD.

Patients with COPD should also be assessed for depression. Depression is common with chronic illness and often

Box 31.4

Patient Perspective

Sarah

At age 17, I started the habit that would change my life. I started to smoke.

At first it was just a few cigarettes, but as time passed I smoked more and more until I reached two packs a day. This habit continued for 42 years. I disregarded all the warnings about what could happen. I was sure this would never happen to me.

Now at age 75, I must do three breathing treatments a day and carry an inhaler with me at all times. I have a cough that cannot be controlled. I can no longer ride a bike with my grandchildren, play badminton, or even bowl. My lungs won't let me. Going shopping is no longer fun—it's a chore. I have to walk slowly or I can't breathe.

All the things I enjoyed most I've given up because for 42 years I was a slave to cigarettes. If any of you smoke, stop now. Smell the coffee and roses without coughing.

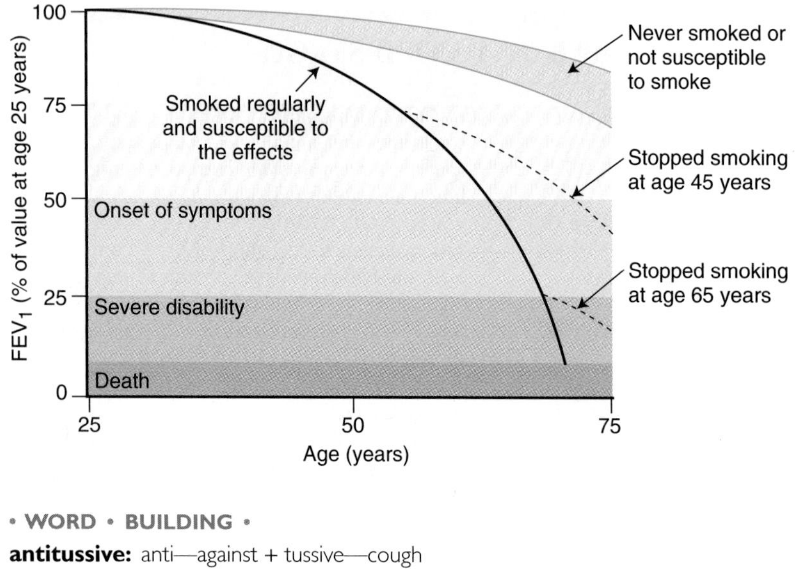
100
75
50
25
0
FEV1 (% of value at age 25 years)
Smoked regularly and susceptible to the effects
Never smoked or not susceptible to smoke
Stopped smoking at age 45 years
Stopped smoking at age 65 years
Onset of symptoms
Severe disability
Death
25
50
75
Age (years)

FIGURE 31.7 Fletcher and Peto chart. (Fletcher, C., & Peto, R. [1977]. The natural history of chronic airflow obstruction. *British Medical Journal, 1,* 1645–1648.)

• **WORD • BUILDING** •
antitussive: anti—against + tussive—cough

TABLE 31.5 SELECTED MEDICATIONS USED FOR LOWER RESPIRATORY TRACT DISORDERS

Drug Class/Action	Examples	Route	Side Effects	Nursing Implications
Adrenergic Bronchodilators				
Stimulate beta receptors to dilate bronchioles	albuterol (Ventolin-HFA, Proventil-HFA, ProAir-HFA) metaproterenol (Alupent, Metaprel) pirbuterol (Maxair)	PO, inhaled Inhaled	Increased heart rate, tremor, anxiety	Use with care in patients with cardiac disease. Overuse can cause rebound bronchospasm. Short acting; used as rescue inhalers.
Anticholinergic Agents				
Block parasympathetic response, causing bronchodilation	ipratropium (Atrovent) tiotropium (Spiriva)	Inhaled	Dry mouth	Anticholinergics should be avoided with narrow-angle glaucoma and prostatic hypertrophy. Tiotropium is a capsule that is placed in a device and activated before inhalation. Instruct patient not to swallow capsules.
Methylxanthines				
Relax bronchial smooth muscle to dilate airways	theophylline (Theo-24, Uniphyl) aminophylline	PO PO, IV	Tremor, anxiety, tachycardia, nausea, vomiting	Narrow therapeutic index; can become toxic. Therapeutic theophylline level 10–20 mcg/mL.
Corticosteroids				
Reduce inflammation in airways	methylprednisolone (Medrol, Solu-Medrol) prednisone triamcinolone acetonide (Azmacort) beclomethasone (Beclovent, QVAR) fluticasone (Flovent) budesonide (Pulmicort)	PO, IV PO Inhaled	Cushingoid side effects with prolonged use: moon face, sodium and water retention, buffalo hump, osteoporosis, hyperglycemia. Fewer side effects with inhaled route.	Must be used regularly to prevent symptoms. Never discontinue abruptly; must be tapered. Monitor blood glucose while on high doses. Rinse mouth following inhaler use to prevent local infection (candidiasis). If using glucocorticoid and adrenergic MDIs together, use adrenergic inhaler first to open airways.
Combination agents	albuterol and ipratropium (Combivent) fluticasone and salmeterol (Advair) budesonide and formoterol (Symbicort)	Inhaled	See individual agents. Upper respiratory infections, headache, sore throat.	See individual agents. Salmeterol and formoterol are long-acting beta agonists that are unsafe for use alone, but appear to be safer when used with inhaled corticosteroids. Use only as directed. Not for use as rescue inhalers.
Mast Cell Stabilizers				
Stabilize mast cells to reduce histamine release	cromolyn sodium (Intal) nedocromil (Tilade)	Inhaled	Few side effects.	Effective for allergic asthma. May be used prophylactically before exercise or allergen exposure.
Expectorants				
Liquefy secretions and stimulate cough	guaifenesin (Robitussin, Mucinex)	PO	Few side effects.	Encourage fluids.

Continued

TABLE 31.5 SELECTED MEDICATIONS USED FOR LOWER RESPIRATORY TRACT DISORDERS—cont'd

Drug Class/Action	Examples	Route	Side Effects	Nursing Implications
Antileukotrienes				
Inhibit leukotriene synthesis or activity, a mediator of inflammation in asthma	zafirlukast (Accolate) montelukast (Singulair) zileuton (Zyflo)	PO	Headache	Must be taken regularly to prevent symptoms. Monitor for elevation of liver enzymes.
Antitussives				
Suppress cough reflex	codeine dextromethorphan (DM suffix in cough preparations)	PO	Related to opioids; may be sedating at high doses.	Avoid giving to patient who has secretions that need to be expectorated.

Note: This table is an overview. A drug guide should be consulted for complete administration guidelines.
IV = intravenous; MDI = metered-dose inhaler; PO = by mouth.

goes undiagnosed. Patients may not report feeling depressed, but may experience more physical symptoms. Antidepressant medications, if indicated, can increase quality of life for COPD patients.

SUPPORTIVE CARE. A pneumococcal vaccination and yearly influenza vaccinations are recommended to reduce the risk of respiratory infection. Avoidance of crowds and exposure to people with respiratory infections is advised.

Good hydration and a cool mist humidifier help keep secretions loose. Chest physiotherapy may be used to help the patient remove excessive secretions. A dietitian consultation is helpful for the patient who is unable to maintain a desirable weight. Typically a high-protein, high-fat, low-carbohydrate diet is prescribed. Breathing exercises help improve oxygenation and reduce anxiety. (See Chapter 29.)

REHABILITATION. Pulmonary rehabilitation programs can help patients increase exercise tolerance and maintain a sense of well-being (Fig. 31.8). Patients exercise in a monitored environment and benefit from the support of other patients with similar problems. (See *Evidence-Based Practice box.*) Some groups of pulmonary rehabilitation patients have even formed harmonica clubs! Playing their harmonicas mimics pursed-lip breathing and may strengthen the diaphragm, the major muscle of breathing.

EVIDENCE-BASED PRACTICE

Clinical Question

Do pulmonary rehabilitation programs really help patients with COPD?

Evidence

A review of 31 research studies showed that pulmonary rehabilitation can help relieve dyspnea and fatigue, and improve emotional function and patients' sense of control over their conditions (Lacasse et al., 2006).

Implications for Nursing Practice

Request a referral to a pulmonary rehabilitation program for your patients who have COPD.

REFERENCE

Lacasse, Y., Goldstein, R., Lasserson, T. J., & Martin, S. (2006). Pulmonary rehabilitation for chronic obstructive pulmonary disease. *Cochrane Database of Systematic Reviews 2006, Issue 4* (Art. No. CD003793; DOI 10.1002/14651858.CD003793.pub2).

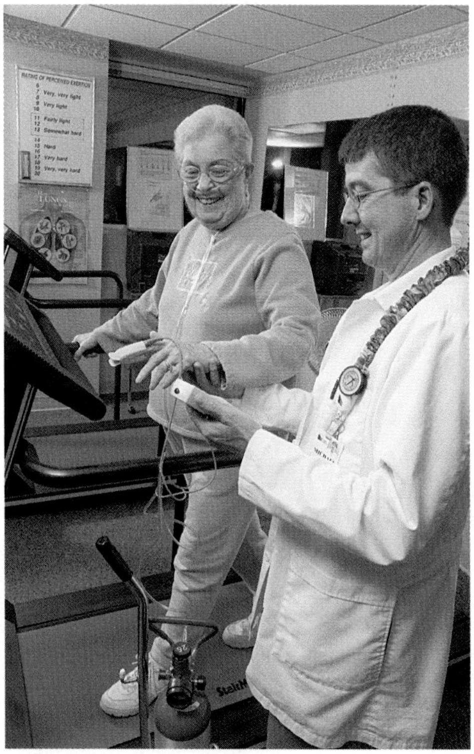

FIGURE 31.8 Patients build exercise tolerance in pulmonary rehabilitation programs. Note therapist monitoring oxygen saturation.

SURGERY. Surgical removal of some of the diseased lung tissue (called lung volume reduction surgery, or LVRS) increases the space available for good lung tissue to expand, reducing dyspnea and increasing exercise tolerance. This is a high-risk procedure, but it has allowed some patients to return to a more normal activity level and increase quality of life. It does not lead to longer survival in most patients. Surgery may also be performed to remove blebs in an attempt to prevent pneumothorax. Lung transplant may be an option in select patients.

ENDOBRONCHIAL VALVE. A new treatment is similar to lung reduction surgery, but without the surgery. It is a tiny one-way valve that is placed via bronchoscopy into an area of emphysematous lung, which causes the diseased area to collapse. This then allows the healthy lung tissue more space to expand. It has been shown to increase FEV_1 and exercise tolerance. Research is ongoing on this intervention.

MECHANICAL VENTILATION. If arterial blood gases worsen despite treatment, intubation and mechanical ventilation may be considered, depending on the patient's advance directive. Unfortunately, mechanical ventilation will not make a patient's disease better, and weaning may be difficult or impossible once it is initiated. Use of noninvasive positive-pressure ventilation (NIPPV; see Chapter 29) may be a good alternative for many patients.

END-OF-LIFE PLANNING. It is important to assess whether the patient has a living will or durable power of attorney for health care (DPOA; see Chapter 17). COPD is a progressive disease, and patients can increase the quality of their life and death by making decisions in advance. Patients should make decisions about whether they would want to be intubated and mechanically ventilated, or have CPR in event of a cardiac arrest. CPR is rarely successful in a patient with end-stage COPD. Patients should be made aware of palliative care options and assured they will be kept as comfortable as possible.

Research is ongoing to determine which treatments will alter long-term outcomes of the disease. Check the American Lung Association website for more information at www.lungusa.org.

Nursing Process for the Patient with COPD

See the *Nursing Process for the Patient with an Obstructive Disorder* section, following the section on cystic fibrosis, and the *Nursing Care Plan for the Patient with a Lower Respiratory Tract Disorder.* Priority nursing diagnoses for the patient with COPD include *Impaired Gas Exchange, Ineffective Airway Clearance,* and *Activity Intolerance.*

Asthma

The incidence of asthma is on the rise. More than 16 million adults and 6.7 million children in the United States have asthma (CDC, 2009a). It accounts for nearly a half-million hospitalizations each year. Asthma is more prevalent in African Americans than in whites. Asthma deaths are more common in lower socioeconomic groups, possibly because of less access to treatment or less compliance with treatment. With careful monitoring and treatment, however, patients with asthma can manage their symptoms and lead normal lives.

Pathophysiology

Asthma is characterized by inflammation and edema of the mucosal lining of the airways and spasm of the bronchial smooth muscles (**bronchospasm**). This causes narrowed airways and air trapping, which is why it is considered an obstructive disorder (see Fig. 31.5B). Inflammation occurs in part because things that trigger asthma (asthma triggers) cause release of inflammatory substances such as histamine and leukotrienes. Symptoms are intermittent and generally reversible, with periods of normal airway function. Some people develop chronic inflammation and permanent changes in their airways, called remodeling; this leads to a progressive loss of lung function.

About 50% of asthmatics develop the disorder in childhood, and some outgrow it. However, a significant number develop symptoms again later in life. Children with asthma should be counseled that smoking can increase the risk of recurrence in adulthood. Asthma may also complicate chronic bronchitis or emphysema.

Etiology

The tendency to develop asthma is inherited. The most common predisposing factor is the genetic tendency to be allergic to airborne allergens such as pollen or molds. Viral respiratory infections are also a contributing factor to asthma diagnosis and exacerbation. Tobacco smoke, air pollution, early use of antibiotics, and sensitization to house-dust mites and cockroaches have also been linked to asthma development.

Asthma Triggers

Once asthma develops, a number of things can trigger an acute attack. Exposure to allergens such as dust mites, cockroaches, certain medications, cat and dog dander, or pollen can trigger an attack. Other possible triggers include emotional upset, exercise, and gastroesophageal reflux disease (GERD). GERD can trigger an attack because stomach acid can reflux into the esophagus and then be aspirated, causing an exacerbation of symptoms. This occurs especially at night. GERD and its treatment are discussed in Chapter 33.

Prevention

Although asthma cannot be prevented at this time, research is ongoing to determine factors associated with its development. Some studies have suggested that the presence of older siblings in the home, early exposure to day care, certain infections, or a rural environment may be protective against asthma development in childhood. Appropriate control of childhood asthma may prevent more serious asthma in later years. Avoidance of smoking may reduce the risk of

• WORD • BUILDING •

bronchospasm: broncho—airway + spasm—convulsion, involuntary narrowing recurrence of asthma that started in childhood. To prevent acute attacks, it is important that the patient identify triggers of asthma symptoms and avoid them whenever possible. Monitoring of symptoms and compliance with prophylactic and maintenance therapy is also important.

Signs and Symptoms

Asthma symptoms are intermittent and are often referred to as "attacks," which may last from minutes to days. The patient reports chest tightness, dyspnea, coughing, and difficulty moving air in and out of the lungs. Once initial symptoms are controlled, airways may remain hypersensitive and prone to asthma symptoms for many weeks.

On examination, you will note an increased respiratory rate as the patient attempts to compensate for narrowed airways. Inspiratory and expiratory wheezing is heard because of turbulent airflow through swollen airways with thick secretions and may sometimes be audible even without a stethoscope. Air is trapped in the lungs, and expiration is prolonged. A cough is common and may produce thick, clear sputum. Use of accessory muscles to breathe is a sign that the attack is severe and warrants immediate attention.

Be aware that an absence of audible wheezing may not signal improvement but rather may be an ominous sign that the patient is not moving enough air to make any sound. If wheezing is not heard, use of accessory muscles and peak expiratory flow rate values must be carefully evaluated. Once treatment begins to be effective and the patient is moving more air, wheezing may become audible.

Asthma is classified according to frequency of symptoms (Table 31.6).

Complications

Status asthmaticus occurs if bronchospasm is not controlled and symptoms are prolonged. As the patient increases the respiratory rate to compensate for narrowed airways, a lot of carbon dioxide is blown off and respiratory alkalosis occurs. If the attack is not resolved and the patient begins to tire, the patient will no longer be able to compensate and $PaCO_2$ will rise, resulting in respiratory acidosis. This can lead to respiratory failure and death if untreated.

Diagnostic Tests

Diagnosis is based on the patient's report of symptoms, physical examination, and spirometry results. Peak expiratory flow rate and forced expiratory volume in 1 second (FEV_1) are reduced, especially during symptomatic periods. Asthma can be differentiated from COPD during spirometry testing by administering an adrenergic agonist (such as an albuterol inhaler) and then retesting. Asthma symptoms can generally be reversed with the medication, whereas COPD cannot. Allergy skin testing and increased serum IgE and eosinophil levels indicate allergic involvement and may help determine appropriate treatment. Arterial blood gasses may be evaluated during an acute attack.

On a long-term basis, asthma control can be evaluated using FEV_1 or peak flow measurements, frequency and severity of exacerbations and nighttime awakenings, and frequency of short-acting beta-agonist use.

Therapeutic Measures

Patients must learn to manage asthma at home. The better they can monitor and manage their symptoms, the fewer acute episodes and hospitalizations will be required.

TABLE 31.6 CLASSIFICATION OF ASTHMA FOR PATIENTS NOT CURRENTLY TAKING LONG-TERM CONTROL MEDICATIONS

	Symptoms	SABA Use	Activity	Lung Function
Intermittent	Asthma symptoms 2 days per week or less; nighttime awakenings twice a month or less.	SABA for symptom control 2 days a week or less.	No interference with normal activity.	Normal FEV_1 between exacerbations.
Mild persistent	Asthma symptoms more than twice a week, but not daily; nighttime awakenings 3 to 4 times per month.	SABA more than 2 days a week but not more than once daily.	Minor limitation of normal activity.	FEV_1 greater than 80% predicted. FEV_1/FVC normal.
Moderate persistent	Asthma symptoms every day; nighttime awakenings more than once a week but not every night.	SABA use daily.	Some activity limitation.	FEV_1 greater than 60% but less than 80% predicted. FEV_1/FVC reduced 5%.
Severe persistent	Symptoms throughout the day; nighttime symptoms often 7 times per week.	SABA several times daily.	Activity extremely limited.	FEV_1 less than 60% predicted. FEV_1/FVC reduced more than 5%.

SABA = short-acting beta agonist (such as albuterol).
Source: Adapted from the National Heart, Blood, and Lung Institute, Expert Panel Report 3. (2007, August 28). *Guidelines for the diagnosis and management of asthma.* Bethesda, MD: Author.

SELF-MONITORING. All patients benefit from learning to monitor their asthma symptoms and making treatment decisions accordingly. This can be done by carefully monitoring symptoms or by monitoring peak expiratory flow rate (PEFR) (Fig. 31.9). PEFR is a measurement, in liters per minutes, of the amount of air a patient can blow into a peak flow meter from fully inflated lungs. The patient determines his or her normal PEFR during symptom-free times. Readings can be charted to keep track of progress (Fig. 31.10). If symptoms worsen or PEFR begins to fall below the patient's personal norm, treatment that has been predetermined with the health care provider should be initiated (Fig. 31.11). If treatment does not improve PEFR to the expected degree, the patient is advised to go to the emergency room. PEFR results may indicate the onset of asthma before the patient experiences any obvious symptoms.

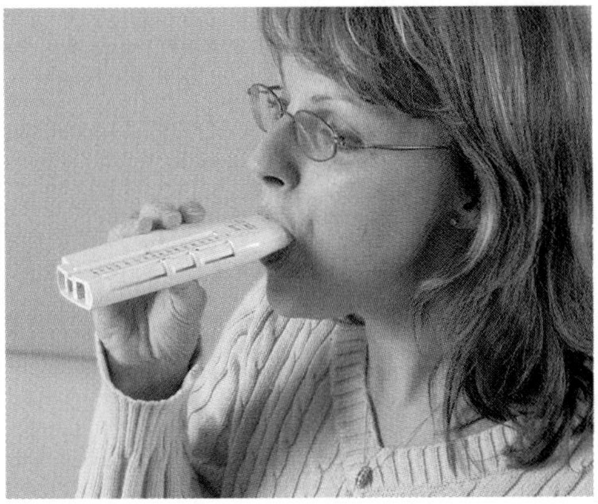

FIGURE 31.9 Patient with asthma using a peak flowmeter to monitor peak expiratory flow rate.

AVOIDANCE OF TRIGGERS. The patient is instructed to identify and avoid asthma triggers. If triggers cannot be avoided, the patient can use bronchodilator or mast cell stabilizer inhalers as prescribed before exposure. Inhalers can be especially useful before exercise. Recent studies have shown that a high-salt diet may worsen exercise-induced airway inflammation. Animal dander and foods that cause symptoms are best avoided when possible. Eliminating carpets and curtains in bedrooms, using vinyl mattress and pillow covers, and installing a portable or central air filter can reduce dust mite exposure. Maintenance of indoor humidity between 40% and 50% can reduce mold growth. If cold air triggers symptoms, the patient should keep the nose and mouth covered when outside in cold weather. Smoking and exposure to secondary smoke are strongly discouraged.

Aspirin and nonsteroidal anti-inflammatory drugs can cause asthma symptoms in some individuals. Beta-blocking medications (propranolol, metoprolol), used commonly for hypertension, block beta receptors in the lungs, preventing the sympathetic nervous system from promoting bronchodilation. These drugs should be avoided if they make symptoms worse.

MEDICATIONS. Medications for asthma treatment may be intermittent or continuous, depending on the persistence of symptoms. Inhaled medications are preferred, because they cause fewer adverse effects than oral or injected medications. See Table 31.5 for a summary of medications used in the treatment of lower respiratory disorders.

For patients with only intermittent symptoms, short-acting beta agonists (SABAs) such as albuterol are used to dilate bronchioles. They are administered via MDI when symptoms occur and are often called "rescue" inhalers.

Name

Green zone ______ Yellow zone ______ Red zone ______

Date														
	AM	PM	AM	PM	AM	PM	AM	PM	AM	PM	AM	PM	AM	PM
800														
750														
700														
650														
600														
550														
500														
450														
400														
350														
300														
250														
200														
150														
100														
Notes														

FIGURE 31.10 Peak flow chart. The green zone is 80% to 100% of the patient's normal peak flow rate. The yellow zone is 50% to 80% of normal. The red zone is less than 50% of normal. The patient works with the physician to determine which actions to take when readings fall in the yellow or red zones.

Asthma Action Plan for ____________________ Doctor's Name ____________ Date ____________

Doctor's Phone Number ____________ Hospital/ Emergency Room Phone Number ____________

GREEN ZONE: Doing Well

- No cough, wheeze, chest tightness, or shortness of breath during the day or night
- Can do usual activities

And, if a peak flow meter is used,
Peak flow: more than ____________
(80% or more of my best peak flow)

My best peak flow is: ____________

Take These Long-Term-Control medicines Each Day (include an anti-inflammatory)

Medicine	How much to take	When to take it

Before exercise ☐ ____________ ☐ 2 or ☐ 4 puffs 5 to 60 minutes before exercise

YELLOW ZONE: Asthma is Getting Worse

- Cough, wheeze, chest tightness, or shortness of breath, or
- Waking at night due to asthma, or
- Can do some, but not all, usual activities

-Or-

Peak flow: ______ to ______
(50% – 80% of my best peak flow)

First → **Add: Quick-Relief Medicine – and keep taking your GREEN ZONE medicine**

____________ (short-acting beta$_2$-antagonist) ☐ 2 or ☐ 4 puffs, every 20 minutes up to 1 hour ☐ Nebulizer, once

Second → **If your symptoms (and peak flow, if used) return to GREEN ZONE after 1 hour of above treatment**

☐ Take the quick-relief medicine every 4 hours for 1 to 2 days

☐ Double the dose of your inhaled steroid for ________(7-10) days

-Or-

If your symptoms (and peak flow, if used) do not return to GREEN ZONE after 1 hour of above treatment

☐ Take: ____________ (short-acting beta$_2$-antagonist) ☐ 2 or ☐ 4 puffs or ☐ Nebulizer

☐ Add: ____________ (oral steroid) mg/day For ________(3-10) days

☐ Call the doctor before/ ☐ within ______ hours after taking the oral steroid.

RED ZONE: Medical Alert!

- Very short of breath, or
- Quick-relief medicines have not helped, or
- Cannot do usual activities, or
- Symptoms are same or get worse after 24 hours in Yellow Zone

-Or-

Peak flow: less than ____________
(50% of my best peak flow)

Take this Medicine

☐ ____________ (short-acting beta$_2$-antagonist) ☐ 4 or ☐ 6 puffs or ☐ Nebulizer

☐ ____________ (oral steroid) mg

Then call your doctor NOW. Go to the hospital or call for an ambulance if:

✔ You are still in the red zone after 15 minutes AND
✔ You have not reached your doctor

DANGER SIGNS

- **Trouble walking and talking due to shortness of breath**
- **Lips or fingernails are blue**

✔ Take ☐ 4 or ☐ 6 puffs of your quick-relief medicine AND
✔ Go to the hospital or call for an ambulance (____________) NOW!

WHITE – PATIENT COPY YELLOW – WORK/SCHOOL COPY PINK – PROVIDER COPY

FIGURE 31.11 Asthma action plan.

They can also be administered preventively before exercise or other events that trigger asthma.

> **NURSING CARE TIP**
>
> If separate short-acting bronchodilator and corticosteroid inhalers are used at the same time, instruct the patient to use the bronchodilator first. This opens the airways and allows for better distribution of the corticosteroid in the lungs.

If the patient needs to use a rescue inhaler more than two times a week for symptoms, maintenance medications to prevent symptoms will likely be started. Inhaled corticosteroids such as fluticasone or budesonide are generally added first to control inflammation. Instruct the patient that corticosteroids must be used regularly to prevent symptoms and that they do not provide immediate symptom relief during an acute attack.

Long-acting beta-agonist bronchodilators (LABAs) such as salmeterol (Serevent) or formoterol (Foradil) can also help prevent symptoms by keeping airways dilated for up to 12 hours or more. Research in recent years, however, has questioned their safety and they are no longer recommended. If they are used, they should be used in combination with inhaled corticosteroids (Advair, Symbicort).

Mast cell stabilizers (cromolyn sodium, nedocromil) may help prevent symptoms, but are often not useful. Some patients use mast cell stabilizers 10 to 15 minutes before exposure to allergens or exercise to reduce symptoms.

If inhaled medications do not control symptoms, or if the patient has nocturnal symptoms, oral antileukotrienes may be added; theophylline bronchodilators are generally used as a last resort because of their many side effects. Immunotherapy (allergy shots) may be used for some patients with allergic asthma.

An acute asthma attack may be treated with an inhaled (MDI or NMT) or subcutaneous short-acting beta agonist (bronchodilator) or, rarely, intravenous aminophylline. Intravenous or oral corticosteroids (methylprednisolone, prednisone) are potent anti-inflammatory agents that are useful in an acute episode but are avoided for long-term therapy if possible because of their cushingoid side effects. (See the section on Cushing's syndrome in Chapter 39.) Corticosteroids must be tapered before discontinuing to prevent withdrawal symptoms. (See the section on addisonian crisis in Chapter 39.)

It is important for patients to understand the difference between long-acting maintenance medications and rescue medications and to use them appropriately. Oxygen is generally not necessary because many patients hyperventilate during an acute attack. If the attack is prolonged and the patient becomes cyanotic or PaO_2 levels begin to fall, oxygen therapy will be used.

> **NURSING CARE TIP**
>
> Instruct the patient to contact the health care provider if using more than two adrenergic MDI canisters per month. This has been associated with an increased risk of death.

Nursing Process for the Patient with Asthma

See the *Nursing Process for the Patient with an Obstructive Disorder* section, following the cystic fibrosis section in this chapter. Primary nursing diagnoses include *Impaired Gas Exchange, Ineffective Airway Clearance,* and *Anxiety.*

See Table 31.7 for an asthma summary.

Cystic Fibrosis

In the past, cystic fibrosis (CF) was thought to be just a childhood disease because most affected children did not survive past puberty. However, with new treatments, patients with CF are living longer and more productive lives. Some CF patients now marry, have careers, and live well into their 30s.

TABLE 31.7 ASTHMA SUMMARY

Signs and Symptoms	Chest tightness, dyspnea, cough Wheezing
Diagnostic Tests	Spirometry, before and after bronchodilator ABGs in acute attack
Therapeutic Measures	Identification and avoidance of triggers Inhaled corticosteroids Inhaled bronchodilators Oral bronchodilators and steroids if inhaled ineffective
Complications	Status asthmaticus
Priority Nursing Diagnoses	*Impaired Gas Exchange* *Ineffective Airway Clearance* *Anxiety*

Pathophysiology

CF is a disorder of the exocrine glands that affects primarily the lungs, gastrointestinal (GI) tract, and sweat glands. The disease varies in severity; some patients have no GI involvement. Abnormal sodium and chloride transport across cell membranes, causing thick, tenacious secretions, is responsible for many of the characteristic symptoms. Thick, sticky respiratory secretions that are difficult to remove cause airway obstruction, resulting in air trapping and frequent respiratory infections.

Similar abnormalities in the pancreas cause blocked ducts and retained digestive enzymes. These retained enzymes digest and destroy the exocrine pancreas. The absence of digestive enzymes in the intestines causes malabsorption of essential nutrients, frequent foul-smelling, fatty stools, and excess flatus.

Patients with CF secrete sweat that is high in sodium and chloride because these electrolytes are not reabsorbed as they pass through the sweat ducts.

Etiology

CF is a genetic disorder. Both parents must be carriers of the defective gene for CF to be present in a child. Patients with CF who marry are counseled on the risk of potential offspring having the disease.

Signs and Symptoms

Symptoms usually first appear in infancy or childhood, although a few individuals are not diagnosed until adulthood. Respiratory symptoms are often the first visible manifestation of the disease and range from chronic sinusitis to production of thick, tenacious sputum. Patients with CF are at risk for frequent respiratory infections, with coughing and purulent sputum. Finger clubbing is common. Late in the disease, hemoptysis may occur related to damaged blood vessels within the lungs. Over time, bouts of infection become more frequent, with eventual loss of lung function and respiratory failure. Antibiotic-resistant infections are a threat to life in these individuals.

Frequent foul-smelling stools result from the lack of enzymes in the small intestine. Inability to absorb fat-soluble vitamins and poor appetite due to respiratory disease result in malnutrition. Bowel obstruction, cirrhosis, cholecystitis, and cholelithiasis are associated findings. Chronic disease causes delayed sexual maturation in both males and females, and infertility is common.

Complications

Patients with CF are at risk for a variety of complications, including bronchiectasis, pneumothorax, cor pulmonale, and respiratory failure. Bowel obstructions can occur as a result of thick mucus binding with poorly digested fecal matter. Diabetes from pancreatic islet cell involvement may be present late in the disease. Death is usually the result of pulmonary complications, especially antibiotic-resistant infection.

Diagnostic Tests

Because so many different gene mutations can occur in CF, genetic testing may be used to confirm a suspicion of CF but not for screening. Testing can also help prospective parents determine if they are carriers. The standard diagnostic test is the sweat chloride test. If respiratory symptoms are TT by excessive amounts of sodium chloride in sweat, CF is diagnosed. You may recall public health campaigns that advise parents to kiss their babies and report any salty taste to their physicians. Genetic testing can be done on blood samples of newborns who have respiratory symptoms. Chest x-ray and spirometry also may be done.

Therapeutic Measures

Because there is no cure for CF, treatment is aimed at controlling infection and relieving symptoms. Removal of thick sputum is promoted with hydration, use of a vibratory positive expiratory pressure (PEP) device, chest physiotherapy, or high-frequency chest wall oscillation (the vest; see Chapter 29) up to four times a day. Regular exercise also helps mobilize secretions. A hot shower may be an easy occasional alternative to loosen secretions. Nebulized mist treatments using normal or hypertonic saline or mucolytic medications may be used before chest physiotherapy. An inhaled medication called dornase alpha (Pulmozyme) is an enzyme that breaks up and loosens mucous; it has been shown to reduce lung infections and improve lung function. Bronchitol, mentioned earlier in the section on bronchiectasis, is also being studied for CF. Inhaled beta-agonist bronchodilators help keep airways open. High doses of ibuprofen (Motrin) may slow lung deterioration. Breathing exercises, incentive spirometry, and effective coughing techniques such as autogenic drainage (see Chapter 29) are also helpful. Lung transplant is a potentially promising treatment.

Prevention of infection is vital to slowing progression of lung damage. Patients should receive a yearly flu vaccination. Antibiotics must be administered as soon as signs of infection occur. Prophylactic antibiotic therapy may be used. Some patients use inhaled antibiotics for chronic infection; others are on home intravenous antibiotic therapy. Antibiotic-resistant infections are a deadly threat to the patient with CF.

Pancreatic enzyme replacement (Pancrease, Viokase) helps reduce symptoms related to malabsorption and improve nutritional status. An increase in calorie requirements necessitates a high-calorie, nutrient-dense diet. For more information, visit the Cystic Fibrosis Foundation at www.cff.org.

Nursing Process for the Patient with Cystic Fibrosis

See the *Nursing Process for the Patient with an Obstructive Disorder* section next. Also, be sure to remember the special needs of the adolescent patient with this chronic, debilitating disease. Not only are normal physical growth and development delayed, but psychosocial development is also affected by repeated hospitalizations and the necessity of routine daily medication and treatments.

CRITICAL THINKING

Mr. Jenkins

■ Mr. Jenkins is a 36-year-old accountant with bronchiectasis secondary to cystic fibrosis. You enter his room during an episode of uncontrollable coughing and offer him support. You observe his sputum as you dispose of it—a whole Styrofoam coffee cup full of thick, bright yellow sputum; the smell makes you nauseated. Even after coughing, his lungs sound congested from retained secretions. You offer him mouth care before you leave his room.

1. What questions can you ask Mr. Jenkins to assess his cough?
2. What nursing diagnosis is most appropriate for Mr. Jenkins?
3. What nursing care can you provide to enhance secretion removal?
4. How would you document this episode of coughing?

Suggested answers at end of chapter.

NURSING PROCESS FOR THE PATIENT WITH AN OBSTRUCTIVE DISORDER

Data Collection

Perform a complete respiratory assessment as presented in Chapter 29. Frequency of assessment is dictated by the severity of the patient's condition. Note orientation and level of consciousness; poor gas exchange can cause confusion and lethargy. Assess respiratory rate and effort. Observe skin and mucous membranes for cyanosis. Auscultate lung sounds for adventitious sounds. Monitor cough and the color, viscosity, odor, and amount of sputum. Note exercise tolerance, and measure degree of dyspnea on a scale of 0 to 10. Monitor oxygen saturation or arterial blood gases. Careful documentation of findings allows you to monitor and report trends in the patient's progress.

Nursing Diagnoses, Planning, and Implementation

A number of nursing diagnoses are appropriate for the patient with an obstructive disorder. As always, choose diagnoses based on defining characteristics and the patient's individual assessment findings.

Priority nursing diagnoses for most chronic respiratory patients include *Impaired Gas Exchange, Ineffective Airway Clearance, Ineffective Breathing Pattern,* and *Activity Intolerance.* Interventions for these diagnoses are presented in the *Nursing Care Plan for the Patient with a Lower Respiratory Tract Disorder.* Related diagnoses are discussed next.

Imbalanced Nutrition: Less Than Body Requirements Related to Poor Appetite and Increased Calorie Expenditure as Evidenced by Weight Loss or Low Weight for Height

EXPECTED OUTCOME: The patient's weight will be stable at desired weight for height.

- Monitor food intake and weekly weight. *Regular monitoring can help identify nutrition problems before they are severe.*
- If the patient is too dyspneic to eat, schedule rest periods and bronchodilator treatments before meals. *Eating takes a lot of energy, and resting can help conserve energy before a meal. Bronchodilators can reduce dyspnea while eating.*
- Create a pleasant eating environment. *Unpleasant views or odors can spoil an appetite.*
- Provide smaller, more frequent meals of the patient's favorite foods. *Eating a lot at one time can fill up the stomach and reduce room for lung expansion.*
- Encourage family members to bring favorite foods from home for the hospitalized patient. *A large tray of unappetizing food may be more than a patient can handle and may spoil the appetite. Be sure to note sodium or other restrictions; although the patient with end-stage disease may be allowed a more lenient diet, excess sodium can cause fluid retention and increase dyspnea.*
- Consult a dietitian for liquid supplement recommendations. *A specialized supplement such as Pulmocare provides less carbon dioxide than other supplements when metabolized and may be used for patients with chronic respiratory disease.*
- See also Box 31.5, *Nutrition Notes.*

Anxiety Related to Acute Dyspnea as Evidenced by Statement of Anxiety, Tense Appearance, Tremors

EXPECTED OUTCOME: The patient will state that anxiety is controlled; appearance of tension and tremors will be absent. The patient will use techniques to control dyspnea and anxiety when they occur.

- Stay with a patient who is acutely dyspneic and anxious. *Feeling alone during episodes of dyspnea can increase anxiety.*
- Calmly remind the patient to breathe slowly in through the nose and out through pursed lips. *During acute episodes of dyspnea, the patient may forget that breathing exercises can help.*
- Teach relaxation exercises during times when anxiety is minimal, and remind the patient to use them during acute anxiety. *Relaxation exercises can help reduce muscle tension and distract the patient.*

Box 31.5
Nutrition Notes

Optimizing Nutrition in Patients with Respiratory Disease

Malnutrition and weight loss are common in patients with respiratory disease, worsening outcomes. The risk of chronic obstructive pulmonary disease (COPD)–related death doubles with weight loss. Nutrition support improves the likelihood of successful weaning in patients receiving mechanical ventilation.

Calorie requirements commonly are increased in patients with pulmonary disease. The caloric cost of breathing ranges from 36 to 72 calories each day in normal people, but it increases to 430 to 720 calories each day in patients with COPD. When caloric intake is inadequate, the body begins to break down muscle stores, including the respiratory and gastrointestinal muscles, which only worsens the problem.

Causes of inadequate food intake can include the following:

- Anorexia
- Shortness of breath
- Fatigue (too tired to eat)
- Pressure from the gastrointestinal tract impinging on the chest
- A combination of these problems.

Many patients with COPD have carbon dioxide retention and oxygen depletion. Because fat calories produce less carbon dioxide when metabolized than carbohydrate calories, diets with increased fat and decreased carbohydrate have been suggested, and special supplements for pulmonary patients have been designed and marketed. Medical opinion is not unanimous on the issue of distribution of calories, but it is important not to overfeed the patient. Excess intake can raise the demand for oxygen and the production of carbon dioxide beyond the patient's capacity to manage them.

For the patient with inadequate intake, useful dietary strategies include the following:

- Offer small, frequent feedings of nutrient-dense foods.
- Select foods that require little or no chewing.
- Include sources of the following vitamins:
  - A (fortified milk, carrots) for healthy epithelial tissue
  - C (citrus fruit, peppers) to prevent infections.
- Discourage gas-producing foods to lessen abdominal pressure on the diaphragm.

- Administer antianxiety medications as ordered. *Medications can reduce anxiety but can also depress respirations, so should be used with caution.*
- Contact RN to administer intravenous morphine. *Morphine helps acute dyspnea and anxiety in patients with end-stage disease.*

Evaluation

If interventions have been effective, the patient will learn techniques to make breathing as comfortable as possible, and will be able to cough up secretions and maintain a clear airway. He or she will be able to manage anxiety symptoms and complete activities of daily living (ADLs) or other desired activity without dyspnea. The patient's intake should be adequate to maintain a stable weight. If any of the patient's goals have not been met, the plan of care should be revised.

Patient Education

The patient must be aware of the contributing factors to the disease and eliminate them if at all possible. The patient who is a smoker should not simply be told to quit smoking; he or she should be referred to a smoking cessation program and be provided with medication, nicotine patches, or other resources and support as necessary to quit. (See Chapter 29.) Techniques for effective breathing and anxiety control should also be taught. A formal pulmonary rehabilitation program is an excellent resource for patient education.

CRITICAL THINKING

Mr. Franklin

■ Mr. Franklin is admitted to the respiratory unit with exacerbated COPD. He has a history of emphysema and now has an acute infection complicating his disease. His lung sounds are very diminished, and he is short of breath at rest, even on 2 L of oxygen per nasal cannula. You walk into his room when he puts on his call light and find him sitting on the bedside commode with a look of panic in his eyes. He is gasping for breath, his color is gray, and his respiratory rate is 36 per minute.

1. What do you do first?
2. What can you teach Mr. Franklin to prevent an acute dyspneic episode in the future?
3. How will you document this episode?

Suggested answers at end of chapter.

PULMONARY VASCULAR DISORDERS

Pulmonary Embolism

Pathophysiology

An embolism is a foreign object that travels through the bloodstream. It may be a blood clot, air, or fat. A pulmonary embolism (PE), sometimes called a pulmonary thromboembolism (PTE), is usually a blood clot that has traveled into a pulmonary artery (Fig. 31.12). Resulting obstruction of blood flow causes a ventilation-perfusion mismatch, which in this case means that an area of the lung is well ventilated with air but has no blood flow, or perfusion. Because reduced or no blood supply is available to pick up the oxygen in the affected portion of the lung, it becomes pulmonary "dead space," causing seriously impaired gas exchange.

Occasionally, damage occurs to a portion of the lung because of lack of oxygen. This is called lung infarction, and it is not common because oxygen is delivered to lung tissue not only from the pulmonary arteries but also via the bronchial arteries and the airways.

Etiology

Most pulmonary emboli originate in the deep veins of the lower extremities (deep venous thrombosis [DVT]). Some

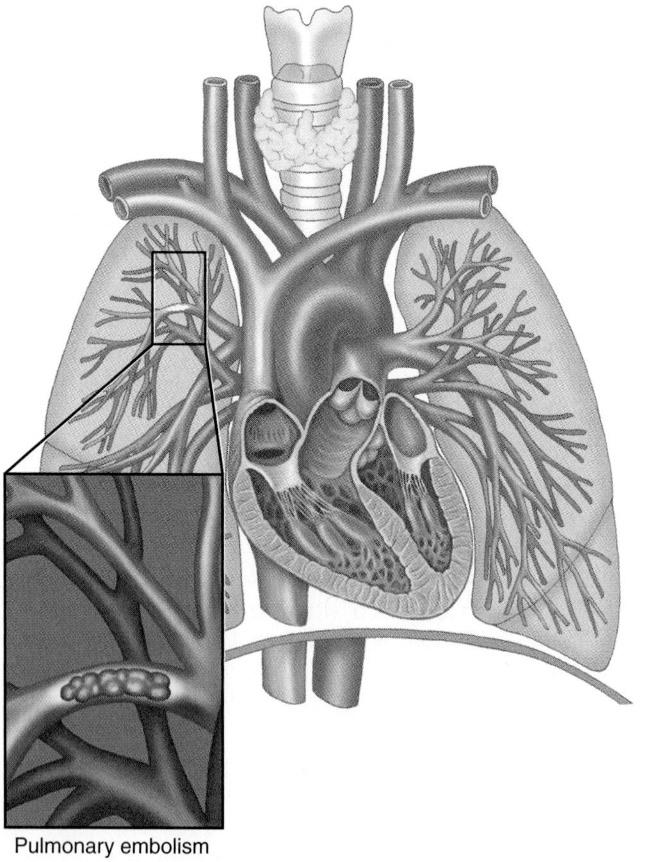
Pulmonary embolism

FIGURE 31.12 Pulmonary embolism.

risk factors of DVT, and therefore PE, include surgical procedures done under general anesthesia, heart failure, fractures of the lower extremities, immobility, obesity, oral contraceptive use, smoking, and a previous history of DVT or PE. Prolonged immobility on airline flights is also a risk factor. Less common causes of PE include fat emboli from compound fractures, amniotic fluid embolism during labor and delivery, and air embolism from entry of air into the bloodstream.

Prevention

Prevention of thrombi in the deep veins of the legs is the most important factor in the prevention of a pulmonary embolism. Regular ambulation is advised if the patient is able. If a patient is at risk for DVT or PE, low-dose subcutaneous heparin or enoxaparin, oral warfarin (Coumadin), or intermittent compression stockings are used to prevent thrombus formation. If a DVT is diagnosed, prompt treatment is essential to prevent PE.

Signs and Symptoms

The most common symptom of PE is a sudden onset of dyspnea for no apparent reason. The patient may be gasping for breath and appear anxious. Tachycardia, tachypnea, and cough may be present. Auscultation may reveal crackles or a friction rub. If lung infarction has occurred, hemoptysis and pleuritic chest pain may also be present. Some patients have no symptoms at all. Be alert to the presence of risk factors and obtain immediate assistance if the cause of dyspnea might be PE. Death can occur if treatment is not fast and effective.

Complications

High blood pressure within the pulmonary circulation (pulmonary hypertension) may result from arterial occlusion and lead to right ventricular failure. This occurs because the right ventricle is unable to push blood into the occluded artery. As a result, the contraction becomes weak, cardiac output falls, and the patient becomes hypotensive.

Diagnostic Tests

A spiral CT scan is a fast type of CT scan with contrast dye that is noninvasive and can diagnose PE quickly. If this is not available, a lung scan (ventilation-perfusion scan) is done to assess the degree of ventilation of lung tissue and the areas of blood perfusion. If an area is well ventilated but poorly perfused (i.e., a mismatch), PE is suspected.

A pulmonary angiogram is an invasive test that can outline the pulmonary vessels with a radiopaque dye injected via a cardiac catheter. It can show where blood flow is diminished or absent, suggesting an embolism.

Chest x-ray examination, electrocardiogram (ECG), arterial blood gas analysis, or magnetic resonance imaging (MRI) may also be done. However, many of these show changes only in the presence of a very large embolism or infarction.

A D-dimer blood test can be helpful to rule out PE. Results can be obtained in less than an hour. D-dimer is a fibrin fragment that is found in the blood after any thrombus formation. It can be present in a number of disorders, but if it is negative, PE can be eliminated as a possible cause of the patient's symptoms.

Therapeutic Measures

Thrombolytic agents, such as urokinase, tissue plasminogen activator (t-PA, Activase), or r-PA (Retavase) are used to dissolve the clot; heparin is used to prevent new clots from forming. Thrombolytics must be administered within 4 to 6 hours of the clot's occurrence and are associated with risk for hemorrhage.

In patients with life-threatening symptoms who cannot tolerate a thrombolytic agent, the clot may be removed with a cardiac catheter, or a surgical embolectomy can be performed. This is a rare procedure that is reserved for emergency situations.

Oxygen is administered even if Spo_2 is normal, because it may help dilate pulmonary vessels. Intubation and mechanical ventilation may be required in some cases.

Long-term use of anticoagulants follows initial treatment to prevent formation of additional clots. Initially, heparin, a potent anticoagulant medication, is administered via continuous intravenous infusion. Sometimes an intermittent IV or subcutaneous route is used. Heparin is never given intramuscularly because of the risk of hematoma development. Clotting studies (activated partial thromboplastin time [aPTT]) are monitored and maintained at 1.5 to 2 times the control value. Sometimes heparin therapy is initiated even before a diagnosis of PE is made. It is believed that it is safer to begin therapy and then stop if PE is not confirmed than to wait until all test results are available.

Warfarin sodium (Coumadin), an oral anticoagulant, is used for at least 3 to 6 months following PE to prevent recurrence. It can also be used for long-term prevention of repeated clots in patients who have risk factors that cannot be resolved. Warfarin therapy can begin 2 to 3 days after the heparin therapy begins. Because it has a slow onset of action, it may take several days for the full anticoagulant effect to occur. The patient will be on both anticoagulants for a time. Warfarin therapy is monitored regularly with prothrombin time (PT) or international normalized ratio (INR). See Chapter 23 for nursing care of patients on anticoagulant therapy.

If clots are a recurring problem, a filter may be placed into the inferior vena cava via the jugular or femoral vein. One filter that is commonly used is the Greenfield filter, which filters out clots traveling from the lower extremities toward the heart and lungs.

Nursing Process for the Patient with a Pulmonary Embolism

DATA COLLECTION. Assess the patient for respiratory distress, including respiratory rate and effort, cyanosis, confusion, and subjective feelings of dyspnea and anxiety. Auscultate lung sounds. Note sputum color and amount, watching especially for hemoptysis. Monitor arterial blood gases and oxygen saturation. Monitor heart sounds and peripheral edema for signs of heart failure. Contributing factors, such as calf pain, should be noted. Remember, any sudden onset of dyspnea should be taken seriously and reported quickly.

NURSING DIAGNOSES, PLANNING, AND IMPLEMENTATION. The priority nursing diagnosis for a patient with a pulmonary embolism is *Impaired Gas Exchange* (see the *Nursing Care Plan for the Patient with a Lower Respiratory Tract Disorder,* for interventions). Because of the impaired perfusion of the affected area of the lung, oxygen and carbon dioxide exchange are limited. Anxiety occurs related to dyspnea. Risk for injury related to anticoagulant therapy is a concern once treatment is initiated (also see Chapter 23).

Risk for Injury (Bleeding) Related to Anticoagulant Therapy

EXPECTED OUTCOME: The patient will remain safe as evidenced by absence of bleeding. The patient will verbalize understanding of self-care measures.

- Monitor coagulation studies and report results to the physician. *Anticoagulant therapy may be adjusted as often as every 6 hours based on laboratory results.*
- Protect the patient from injury *so that excessive bleeding does not occur.*
- Encourage the patient to wear shoes or slippers when ambulating *to protect from injury.*
- Teach patient to use a soft toothbrush and an electric razor *to prevent injury.*
- Avoid use of intramuscular (IM) injections. *An IM injection can result in hematoma in an anticoagulated patient.*
- Instruct the patient to report any signs of bleeding, such as hematuria or easy bruising. *Bleeding may be associated with excessively prolonged clotting and may require a change in anticoagulant dosing or administration of an antidote.*

EVALUATION. The patient should state that dyspnea and anxiety are resolved, and verbalize understanding of anticoagulant therapy and precautions.

(See Table 31.8 for a pulmonary embolism summary.)

Pulmonary Arterial Hypertension

Pathophysiology and Etiology

Idiopathic primary pulmonary arterial hypertension (IPAH) occurs when the arteries that carry deoxygenated blood from the heart to the lungs become narrowed as a result of changes in the lining and smooth muscle of the vessels. The result is elevated pressure in the pulmonary arteries, causing the right ventricle to work harder to push blood into them. Eventually the right ventricle fails (cor pulmonale). The reason for these vascular changes is not known. IPAH is more common in women between ages 20 and 40 and has a hereditary tendency.

TABLE 31.8 PULMONARY EMBOLISM SUMMARY

Signs and Symptoms	Sudden-onset dyspnea, tachypnea Tachycardia Hemoptysis Crackles History of blood clot
Diagnostic Tests	D-dimer CT scan Ventilation-perfusion lung scan Angiogram
Therapeutic Measures	Thrombolytic therapy Anticoagulants Oxygen
Complications	Pulmonary hypertension
Priority Nursing Diagnoses	*Impaired Gas Exchange* *Anxiety* *Risk for Injury* from anticoagulant therapy

Secondary pulmonary arterial hypertension (PAH) results from other disorders, such as coronary artery disease or mitral valve disease, both of which increase pressures in the left side of the heart. Liver disease, systemic lupus erythematosus, and scleroderma are also associated with PAH, as is capillary destruction related to alveolar damage in COPD. Right ventricular failure eventually occurs as the heart works to push blood against high pulmonary arterial pressures.

PAH has also been caused by use of the appetite suppressants fenfluramine (Fen-Phen) and dexfenfluramine. Both of these drugs have been removed from the U.S. market by the FDA.

Signs and Symptoms

The most common symptom is dyspnea; weakness and syncope are also common. Symptoms worsen over time. If heart failure is present, peripheral edema and distended jugular veins are seen. Angina may result from right ventricular ischemia. Death used to occur within 2 to 3 years of diagnosis, but newer treatments can extend life for up to 15 or 20 years.

Diagnostic Tests

Arterial blood gases commonly show hypoxemia and hypocapnia. Cardiac catheterization can be done to determine high pulmonary arterial pressures. An ECG may show right ventricular hypertrophy. A chest x-ray examination, spirometry, lung scan, and pulmonary angiogram may be done to determine underlying causes in secondary PAH.

Therapeutic Measures

No cure is available for pulmonary hypertension except for lung or heart-lung transplant. In secondary PAH, the underlying disorder is treated. Supportive care includes a low-sodium diet and diuretics to reduce blood volume (and therefore pressure), oxygen administration, and cardiac monitoring. Vasodilators such as calcium channel blockers are used to reduce pulmonary artery pressure. Warfarin may be used to prevent clotting. Epoprostenol (Flolan) is a vasodilator that may reverse some of the vascular changes and prolong survival, but has many serious side effects, and must be continuously administered IV via an implanted pump. Other drugs such as bosentan (Tracleer) block endothelin, a substance that causes blood vessels to constrict. Sildenafil (Viagra or Revatio) is also an effective vasodilator.

Nursing care is collaborative and focuses primarily on patient assessment. Fowler's or high-Fowler's position may help reduce dyspnea, and rest and comfort measures are helpful in treating fatigue and anxiety.

CHEST TRAUMA

Pneumothorax

The term **pneumothorax** literally means "air in the chest" and is used to describe conditions in which air has entered the pleural space outside the lungs. If the pneumothorax occurs without an associated injury, it is called a spontaneous pneumothorax. A secondary spontaneous pneumothorax may occur due to underlying lung disease. Traumatic pneumothorax results from a penetrating chest injury.

Pathophysiology and Etiology

Recall that the lungs are surrounded by the visceral and parietal pleurae. These membranes normally are separated only by a thin layer of pleural fluid. Each time a breath is taken in, the diaphragm descends, creating negative pressure in the thorax. This negative pressure pulls air into the lungs via the nose and mouth. If either the visceral pleura or the chest wall and parietal pleura are perforated, air will enter the pleural space, negative pressure will be lost, and the lung on the affected side will collapse (Fig. 31.13). Each time the patient takes a breath, the temporary increase in negative pressure will draw more air into the pleural space via the perforation. During expiration, air may or may not be able to escape through the perforation.

SPONTANEOUS PNEUMOTHORAX. If no injury is present, the pneumothorax is considered spontaneous. This occurs mostly in tall, thin individuals and in smokers. Patients who have had one spontaneous pneumothorax are at greater risk for a recurrence. Patients with underlying lung disease (especially emphysema) may have blister-like defects in lung tissue, called bullae or blebs, that can rupture, allowing air into the pleural space. Weakened lung tissue from lung cancer can also lead to pneumothorax.

TRAUMATIC PNEUMOTHORAX. Penetrating trauma to the chest wall and parietal pleura allows air to enter the pleural space. This can occur as a result of a knife or gunshot wound or from protruding broken ribs.

• WORD • BUILDING •

pneumothorax: pneumo—air + thorax—chest

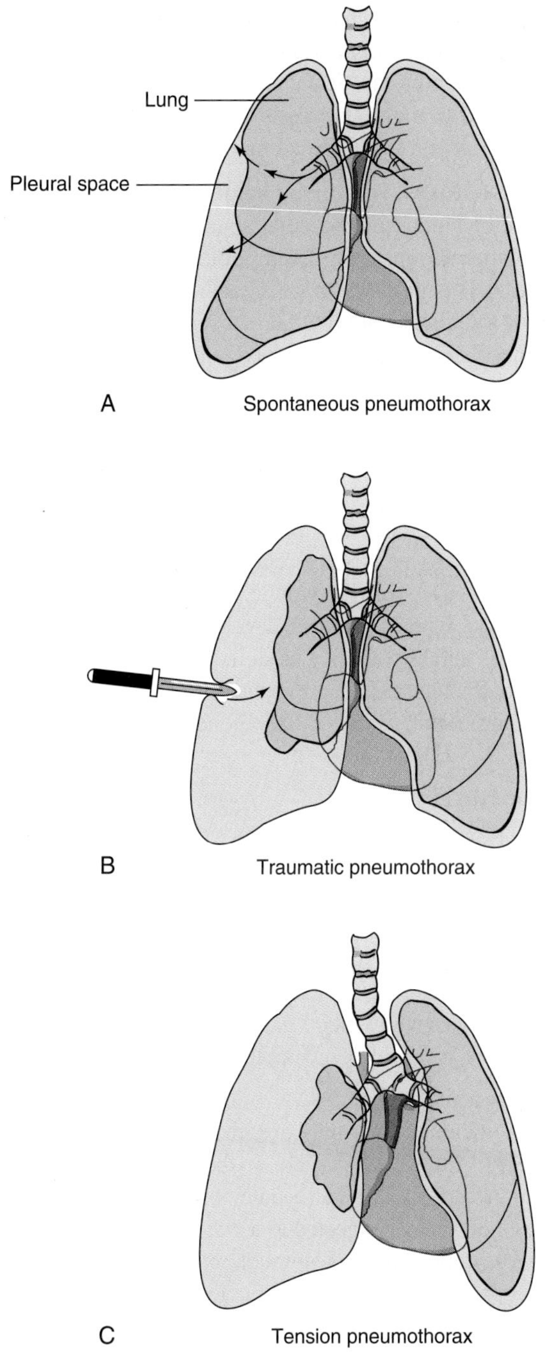
Lung
Pleural space
A
Spontaneous pneumothorax
B
Traumatic pneumothorax
C
Tension pneumothorax

FIGURE 31.13 Types of pneumothorax. (A) Spontaneous pneumothorax. (B) Traumatic pneumothorax. (C) Tension pneumothorax with mediastinal shift.

OPEN PNEUMOTHORAX. If air can enter and escape through the opening in the pleural space, it is considered an open pneumothorax.

CLOSED PNEUMOTHORAX. If air collects in the space and is unable to escape, a closed pneumothorax exists.

TENSION PNEUMOTHORAX. If a pneumothorax is closed, air, and therefore tension, builds up in the pleural space and is unable to escape. As tension increases, pressure is placed on the heart and great vessels, pushing them away from the affected side of the chest. This is called a mediastinal shift. When the heart and vessels are compressed, venous return to the heart is impaired, resulting in reduced cardiac output and symptoms of shock. Tension pneumothorax is often related to the high pressures present with mechanical ventilation. It is a life-threatening emergency.

HEMOTHORAX. The term **hemothorax** refers to the presence of blood in the pleural space. This can occur with or without accompanying pneumothorax (when they occur together it is called a hemopneumothorax) and is often the result of traumatic injury. Other causes include lung cancer, pulmonary embolism, and anticoagulant use.

Signs and Symptoms

Sudden dyspnea, chest pain, tachypnea, tachycardia, restlessness, and anxiety occur with pneumothorax. On examination, asymmetrical chest expansion on inspiration may be noted. Breath sounds may be absent or diminished on the affected side. In a "sucking" chest wound, air can be heard as it enters and leaves the wound.

If tension pneumothorax develops, the patient becomes hypoxemic and hypotensive as well. The trachea may deviate to the unaffected side. Heart sounds may be muffled. Bradycardia and shock occur if emergency intervention is not provided.

Diagnostic Tests

History, physical examination, ultrasound, chest x-ray examination, and CT scan can be used to diagnose pneumothorax. In the emergency department, bedside ultrasound can shorten the time required for diagnosis and intervention and avoid the wait for a chest x-ray to be completed. Chest x-ray examination may be done to monitor the resolution of the pneumothorax following treatment. Arterial blood gases and oxygen saturation are monitored as needed throughout the course of treatment.

Therapeutic Measures

A small pneumothorax may absorb with no treatment other than rest or high-flow oxygen, or the trapped air can be removed with a small-bore needle inserted into the pleural space. Chest tubes connected to a water seal drainage system are used to remove larger amounts of air or blood from the pleural space. See Chapter 29 for complete information about chest drainage. Smaller devices that have special one-way valves to allow air to escape but not reenter the chest may be used for some patients who are treated at home. Some injuries require surgical repair before the pneumothorax can be resolved. Oxygen and positioning help maintain oxygenation.

If the pneumothorax is recurrent, other treatments can be used to prevent additional episodes. Sterile talc or certain antibiotics (such as tetracycline) can be injected into the pleural space via thoracentesis, irritating the pleural membranes and making them stick together. This is called **pleurodesis**, or sclerosis, and prevents recurrent pneumothorax. Pleurodesis is painful; prepare the patient with an analgesic before the procedure.

• WORD • BUILDING •

hemothorax: hem—blood + thorax—chest
pleurodesis: pleur—pleural membrane + desis—binding

Nursing Care of the Patient with a Pneumothorax

Nursing care of the patient with a pneumothorax involves close monitoring of the condition. Frequent and thorough assessments should be done, including level of consciousness, skin and mucous membrane color, vital signs, oxygen saturation, respiratory rate and depth, and presence of dyspnea, chest pain, restlessness, or anxiety. Regular auscultation of lung sounds provides information about reinflation of the affected lung. Any signs of increasing or tension pneumothorax are reported to the physician immediately. See Chapter 29 for care of the patient with a chest tube and water seal drainage system.

See Table 31.9 for a pneumothorax summary.

Rib Fractures

Etiology and Signs and Symptoms

Chest trauma is often accompanied by fractured ribs. Uncontrolled coughing, especially in the presence of osteoporosis or cancer, can also fracture ribs. Falls are a common cause of broken ribs in the elderly. The fourth through ninth ribs are the most commonly affected. Broken ribs can be very painful, and often prevent the patient from breathing deeply or coughing effectively, which can result in atelectasis or pneumonia. Displaced ribs can also damage abdominal organs or lung tissue, causing pneumothorax.

Therapeutic Measures

In the past, elastic rib belts were used to stabilize the ribs while healing took place. These are no longer used because it restricts deep breathing. Pain control is the most important treatment. Keeping the patient comfortable allows coughing and deep breathing, which in turn prevents complications such as pneumonia and atelectasis. If traditional pain control measures such as NSAIDs or opioids are ineffective, intercostal nerve blocks may be used. Ribs generally heal in about 6 weeks.

TABLE 31.9 PNEUMOTHORAX SUMMARY

Signs and Symptoms	Sudden-onset dyspnea, chest pain, tachypnea Asymmetrical chest expansion Diminished or absent breath sounds on affected side
Diagnostic Tests	Ultrasound Chest x-ray, CT scan ABGs
Therapeutic Measures	Chest tube and water seal drainage Pleurodesis for recurrent pneumothorax
Complications	Tension pneumothorax Shock
Priority Nursing Diagnoses	*Impaired Gas Exchange* *Acute Pain* *Anxiety*

Flail Chest

Pathophysiology and Etiology

When multiple ribs are fractured, the structural support of the chest is impaired. As a result, the affected part of the chest collapses with the negative pressure of inspiration, and bulges with expiration. This is called **paradoxical respiration**, which may be ineffective in ventilating the lungs and result in hypoxia.

Signs and Symptoms

The patient with a flail chest exhibits chest movement that is opposite to that usually seen with respiration. The patient is dyspneic and anxious and may also be tachypneic and tachycardic.

Therapeutic Measures

Treatment includes supplemental oxygen and analgesics. Intubation and mechanical ventilation may be necessary, but are avoided if possible because of related risk for infection. If lung damage has occurred, treatment for pneumothorax may be needed. Surgical stabilization of the ribs may be done in some cases.

NURSING PROCESS FOR THE PATIENT WITH CHEST TRAUMA

The following nursing process is based on the stabilized patient. For emergency care of the trauma patient, see Chapter 13.

Data Collection

When caring for the patient following chest trauma, it is important to monitor respiratory status continuously. Report any sign of worsening status to the physician immediately, such as a change in vital signs, oxygen saturation, or lung sounds; change in respiratory rate; increase in dyspnea, chest pain, pallor, or cyanosis; development of tracheal deviation; or new onset of anxiety or restlessness. Monitor pain and condition of a chest wound, if present. Additional assessment may be necessary depending on the type of injury sustained.

Nursing Diagnoses, Planning, and Implementation

Priority nursing diagnoses for the patient with chest trauma include *Impaired Gas Exchange, Ineffective Breathing Pattern,* and *Acute Pain.* Additional diagnoses may be appropriate depending on the individual patient's assessment. See the *Nursing Care Plan for the Patient with a Lower Respiratory Tract Disorder* for interventions for *Impaired Gas Exchange* and *Ineffective Breathing Pattern*; see below for *Acute Pain.*

Acute Pain Related to Chest Trauma as Evidenced by Pain Rating

EXPECTED OUTCOME: The patient will state pain is controlled and will be able to cough and deep breathe effectively.

- Administer NSAIDs or opioids as ordered. *Pain must be controlled so the patient is able to breathe deeply and prevent atelectasis and pneumonia.*
- If opioids are used, monitor for depressed respirations and reduced cough reflex. *Depressed respirations and cough increase the risk of atelectasis and pneumonia.*
- Teach the patient to splint the chest with a pillow for coughing. *This may help reduce chest movement and pain during coughing.*

Evaluation

Are pain, anxiety, and dyspnea controlled? Are respiratory rate and SpO_2 within normal limits? Are vital signs stable? Frequent evaluation is essential, so that failure to progress can be quickly reported.

RESPIRATORY FAILURE

Acute Respiratory Failure

Pathophysiology

Acute respiratory failure is diagnosed when the patient is unable to maintain adequate blood gas values. Hypoxemia may result from inadequate ventilation (air movement in and out of lungs) or poor oxygenation (adequate ventilation but inability to get the oxygen into the blood and therefore the cells) or both. Hypercapnia and respiratory acidosis occur when the diseased lungs are unable to effectively eliminate carbon dioxide.

Etiology

An acute respiratory infection in a patient with chronic airway obstruction is often the precipitating factor in acute respiratory failure. Other causes include central nervous system disorders that affect the muscles of breathing, such as a stroke, spinal cord injury, or myasthenia gravis; inhalation of toxic substances; opioid overdose; and aspiration.

Prevention

Avoidance of respiratory infections in patients with chronic respiratory disease is important. Patients should be instructed to notify their physician immediately if sputum becomes purulent so treatment can be initiated.

Sedatives and narcotics should be used carefully or avoided in patients with chronic respiratory disease because these are respiratory depressants and can precipitate failure. Careful monitoring and early intervention are essential in patients at risk for respiratory failure.

Signs and Symptoms

The patient with impending respiratory failure may become restless, confused, agitated, or sleepy. Arterial blood gases show decreasing PaO_2 and pH and increasing $PaCO_2$, which lead to respiratory acidosis. The patient is cyanotic and dyspneic, and respiratory rate becomes rapid and deep in an effort to blow off excess CO_2.

Diagnostic Tests

Respiratory failure is diagnosed when PaO_2 falls below 60 mm Hg or $PaCO_2$ is elevated above 50 mm Hg. Some patients with chronic respiratory disease have adapted to impaired gas exchange. In these patients a drop in PaO_2 of 10 to 15 mm Hg is considered acute failure. Sputum cultures or chest x-ray examinations may be used to identify underlying respiratory problems. Additional tests may be done to determine nonpulmonary causes and guide treatment. Pulse oximetry is used to continuously monitor oxygen saturation. Patients cared for in intensive care units may have additional monitoring, including capnography (Chapter 29).

Therapeutic Measures

Carefully observe the patient and report significant findings to the physician immediately. It is easy to mistakenly treat symptoms of agitation or confusion with sedatives, which will speed the onset of respiratory failure. Oxygen therapy via nasal cannula or mask is provided. High-flow oxygen may be necessary to oxygenate the patient, but if the patient has a chronically high $PaCO_2$, the high flow can interfere with the hypoxic drive. (Remember the rule "Never give a chronic CO_2 retainer more than 2 liters of oxygen?" This is an exception to the rule.) If a flow rate greater than 1 to 2 L/min is necessary, mechanical ventilation via an endotracheal tube or noninvasive positive-pressure ventilation (NIPPV) may be required. Before invasive ventilation is undertaken, it is important to check the patient's advance directives.

Antibiotics or other treatments are ordered to correct the underlying cause of the failure. Bronchodilators promote ventilation and secretion removal. Interventions for ineffective airway clearance and impaired gas exchange are initiated. Suctioning is indicated if the patient is unable to cough effectively.

Acute Respiratory Distress Syndrome/ Acute Lung Injury

Acute respiratory distress syndrome (ARDS), also called adult respiratory distress syndrome, is a group of disorders that has diverse causes but similar pathophysiology, symptoms, and treatment.

Pathophysiology and Etiology

ARDS occurs because of acute lung injury (ALI). The most common cause of injury is widespread sepsis. Other causes include pneumonia, trauma, shock, narcotic overdose, inhalation of irritants, burns, pancreatitis, and aspiration. Each of these causes begins a chain of events leading to alveolocapillary damage and noncardiogenic pulmonary edema (pulmonary edema that is not caused by heart failure). ARDS usually affects patients without a previous history of lung disease.

The alveolocapillary membranes become inflamed and damaged either by direct contact with an inhaled irritant or by chemical mediators that are released when systemic injury occurs. The membranes become leaky, so that proteins, blood cells, and fluid move from the capillaries into the interstitial space and then into the alveoli. Surfactant, a substance that reduces surface tension in the alveoli, is reduced. Alveoli collapse (atelectasis) and fibrotic changes take place. These changes cause the lungs to become stiff, or less compliant, making the patient work very hard to inspire. Blood supply to the alveoli may be adequate, but collapsed, wet alveoli are unable to oxygenate it. In other areas of the lungs, vasoconstriction reduces the ability of the vessels to pick up oxygen from functioning alveoli. Tired respiratory muscles, in combination with edema and atelectasis, reduce gas exchange and result in hypoxia. As the condition progresses, atelectasis and edema worsen and the lungs may hemorrhage. A chest x-ray examination appears white because of the excessive fluid in the lungs. These changes explain some of the older names for what is now known as ARDS: wet lung, white lung, shock lung, and stiff lung.

Prevention

Early recognition and treatment of underlying disorders is important in prevention of ARDS. Good nursing care can help reduce aspiration and some types of pneumonia.

Signs and Symptoms

Initially the patient may experience dyspnea and an increase in respiratory rate. Respiratory alkalosis results from hyperventilation. Fine inspiratory crackles may be auscultated. As the condition worsens, breathing becomes more rapid and labored and the patient becomes cyanotic. When the patient is no longer able to oxygenate the blood and get rid of carbon dioxide, respiratory acidosis occurs. Oxygen therapy does not reverse the hypoxemia. If ARDS is not reversed, eventually hypoxemia leads to decreased cardiac output, shock, and death.

Complications

Complications that can result from ARDS include heart failure, pneumothorax related to mechanical ventilation, infection, and disseminated intravascular coagulation (DIC). The death rate for ARDS in the past was 100%. With newer treatments, it is now closer to 45% to 50%. Most patients who survive ARDS recover completely.

Diagnostic Tests

Diagnosis is made based on history of a causative injury, physical examination, chest x-ray examination, and blood gas analysis. An ECG is done to rule out a cardiac-related cause.

Therapeutic Measures

The patient with ARDS is cared for in an intensive care unit. Treatment begins with oxygen therapy that is adjusted based on repeated ABG results. Intubation and mechanical ventilation are necessary in most cases, with the use of positive end-expiratory pressure (PEEP) to keep the airways open. NIPPV may work for some patients. Diuretics may be used to reduce pulmonary edema, but care must be taken to prevent fluid depletion. IV fluids are administered if blood pressure or urine output is low. A pulmonary artery catheter may be used to monitor hemodynamic status. If infection or sepsis is the underlying cause, antibiotics are administered. Total parenteral nutrition (TPN) may be given to maintain nutritional status while the patient is acutely ill. Positioning the patient with the less involved lung in the dependent position ("good lung down") allows the better lung to be well perfused with blood and may increase Pao_2. Prone positioning has also been shown to increase oxygenation in patients with ARDS.

NURSING PROCESS FOR THE PATIENT EXPERIENCING RESPIRATORY FAILURE

Data Collection

Observe the patient's degree of dyspnea on a scale of 0 to 10 if the patient is able to participate. Respiratory rate, effort, and use of accessory muscles are noted. Arterial blood gases and oxygen saturation values are monitored as ordered. The presence of cyanosis is noted.

Monitor mental status, including restlessness, confusion, and level of consciousness, because reduced oxygenation can produce central nervous system (CNS) symptoms. Monitor symptoms of the underlying cause of respiratory failure. If the cause is infectious, monitor temperature and white blood cell counts; if the infection is respiratory in origin, monitor cough and sputum.

All assessment findings should be compared with earlier data. Even subtle changes in the assessment findings can be significant and should be reported.

Nursing Diagnoses, Planning, and Implementation

Priority nursing diagnoses include *Impaired Gas Exchange, Ineffective Airway Clearance,* and *Ineffective Breathing Pattern* (see the *Nursing Care Plan for the Patient with a Lower Respiratory Tract Disorder*). Related diagnoses include *Activity Intolerance, Anxiety, Disturbed Thought Processes,* and *Self-Care Deficit.*

NURSING CARE TIP

The "good lung down" position can help increase oxygenation in patients with lung disease. Gravity results in more blood in the dependent lung, where it can receive oxygen from the healthier lung tissue. If both lungs are diseased, the right lung down position may be beneficial, because the right lung has a larger surface area (Yeaw, 1992).

Evaluation

If interventions have been effective, the patient will state that dyspnea is controlled. Mental status will be normal for the patient. Airways will be kept clear at all times, and the patient's respiratory rate will be regular and within normal limits.

LUNG CANCER

Lung cancer is the leading cause of cancer death in the United States for both men and women. In 2005, the most recent year for which statistics are available, 107,416 men and 89,271 women were diagnosed with lung cancer, and 90,139 men and 69,078 women died from lung cancer (CDC, 2009c).

Pathophysiology

Lung cancers originate in the respiratory tract epithelium; most originate in the lining of the bronchi (Fig. 31.14). The four major types of lung cancer are identified by the type of cells that are affected. These include small cell lung cancer (SCLC), large cell carcinoma, adenocarcinoma, and squamous cell carcinoma. The latter three types are classified as non–small cell lung cancer (NSCLC).

About 20% of lung cancers are SCLC (sometimes called oat cell carcinoma). SCLC grows rapidly and often has metastasized by the time of diagnosis. It is usually caused by smoking and is most often found centrally, near the bronchi. The patient with small cell carcinoma has a poor prognosis, with survival time averaging less than 1 year.

The remaining 80% of lung cancers are classified as non–small cell. Large cell carcinoma is a rapidly growing cancer that can occur anywhere in the lungs. It metastasizes early in the disease, so these patients also have a poor prognosis.

Adenocarcinoma occurs more often in women, and most often in the peripheral lung fields. It is slow growing but often is not diagnosed until metastasis has occurred. It is less closely linked with smoking.

Squamous cell carcinoma is the most common form of NSCLC and usually originates in the lining of the bronchi; it metastasizes late in the disease. It is associated with a history of smoking. The prognosis for individuals with squamous cell carcinoma may be better than for some other lung cancers.

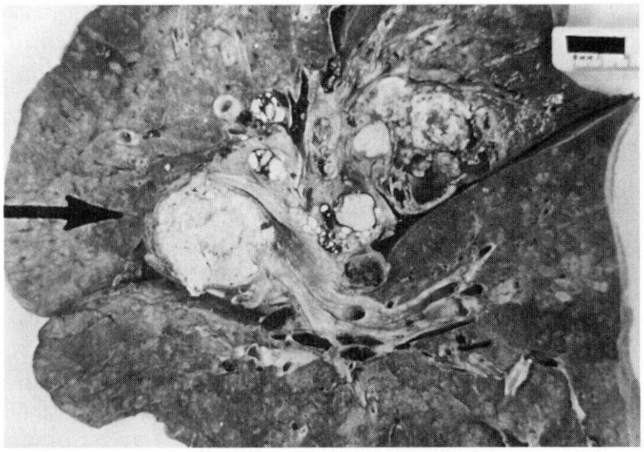

FIGURE 31.14 Lung cancer. The black arrow marks the tumor site. (Courtesy of Dinesh Patel, MD, Medical Oncology, Internal Medicine, Zanesville, OH.)

Etiology

Tobacco smoke causes nearly 90% of lung cancers. Cigarettes contain chemicals that cause DNA to mutate, creating changes in cells and development of tumors. Smokers are 10 to 20 times more likely to develop lung cancer or die from it than nonsmokers (CDC, 2009b). If a patient stops smoking, the risk of lung cancer decreases significantly. Unfortunately, even with all this information, 23.5% of men and 18.1% of women in the United States continue to smoke (American Heart Association, 2009).

Environmental tobacco smoke (ETS) has also been shown to cause lung cancer. A study by the American Cancer Society showed that women who were married to smokers but who had never smoked themselves were 20% more likely to die of lung cancer (Cardenas et al., 1997). Other factors that contribute to increased lung cancer risk are exposure to asbestos, radon, or arsenic; air pollution; diesel exhaust; and radiation. Genetic predisposition and a diet poor in fruits and vegetables may also be factors.

NURSING CARE TIP

Exposure to radon gas is a significant risk factor for lung cancer, and it can be found in homes. Check out www.epa.gov/radon/pubs/citguide.html for more information and to find out if radon is a concern in your area. Many local health departments and hardware stores have inexpensive radon test kits available for purchase.

Prevention

The single most important way to prevent lung cancer is to reduce smoking. Many programs educate schoolchildren about the dangers of smoking. Smoking cessation programs are available for people who desire to quit. Contact your local American Cancer Society chapter for smoking cessation programs that can be recommended to patients. See Chapter 29 for more information on smoking cessation.

Signs and Symptoms

Manifestations of lung cancer depend on the location of the tumor. Commonly, patients exhibit a persistent cough with sputum production. These symptoms may be ignored by the patient because they are also associated with smoking and other chronic respiratory disorders. Repeated respiratory infections may occur, producing thick, purulent sputum. Sputum may become bloody (hemoptysis). The patient may experience dyspnea. If the airway becomes obstructed by the tumor, wheezing or stridor may be heard. Late signs include chest pain, weight loss, anemia, and anorexia.

Complications

Pleural Effusion

Fifty percent of patients with lung cancer develop pleural effusion. Pleural fluid collects in the pleural space as a result of irritation or obstruction of lymphatic or venous drainage by the tumor (see earlier *Pleural Effusion* section).

Superior Vena Cava Syndrome

If the tumor obstructs the superior vena cava, blood flow is interrupted, causing distent ion of the jugular veins and swelling of the chest, face, and neck. Diuretics may help relieve the fluid buildup. Radiation may be used to shrink the obstruction.

Ectopic Hormone Production

Some lung cancers produce **ectopic** hormones that mimic the body's own hormones. Ectopic production of antidiuretic hormone (ADH) can produce syndrome of inappropriate ADH production (SIADH), which is associated with fluid retention. Ectopic production of adrenocorticotropic hormone (ACTH) can cause Cushing's syndrome. High calcium levels can be caused by ectopic secretion of a parathyroid-like hormone. These disorders are discussed in Chapter 39.

Atelectasis and Pneumonia

Atelectasis occurs when tumor growth prevents ventilation of areas of the lung. Patients with lung cancer also have a greater risk for pneumonia. (See earlier sections on both of these disorders.)

Metastasis

Common sites of lung cancer metastasis include the brain, bones, opposite lung, liver, adrenal gland, and lymph nodes.

Diagnostic Tests

A complete medical history and physical examination are done to look for symptoms and risk factors for lung cancer. A chest x-ray examination is done to identify a mass. However, all tumors may not show up on a radiograph. A CT or PET scan or MRI may be done to provide more specific information about the size and location of a tumor. Sputum is analyzed for abnormal cells. Brain and bone scans are done to find metastatic lesions.

Diagnosis is confirmed with a biopsy of the lesion. A biopsy specimen may be obtained via bronchoscopy, percutaneous biopsy (a needle through the skin guided by radiograph), or mediastinoscopy (placement of an endoscope into the mediastinum to look for changes in mediastinal lymph nodes).

Therapeutic Measures

Tumors are staged based on the tumor-node-metastasis (TNM) staging system. Staging helps determine appropriate treatment (Table 31.10). If NSCLC is localized and in an early stage, it may be cured with surgical removal of the tumor. This can be accomplished with a segmental or wedge

• WORD • BUILDING •
ectopic: displaced

resection, which removes only the affected lung segment. A **lobectomy** (removal of a lobe) or removal of an entire lung may be done in more advanced cases (Fig. 31.15). Chemotherapy or radiation may be done alone or in addition to surgery. Palliative surgery may be done to make a patient more comfortable.

Chemotherapy is the treatment of choice in SCLC, because usually it has metastasized by the time of diagnosis. Radiation may be used in combination with chemotherapy. Surgery is not usually indicated in SCLC; the goal of treatment may be palliation of symptoms rather than cure.

Radiation may be used to shrink a tumor to reduce symptoms in patients who are unable to undergo surgery. Both radiation and chemotherapy may be used before or after surgery as adjuvant treatments.

Newer therapies for lung cancer include targeted therapies, such as monoclonal antibodies, antiangiogenesis agents, and growth factor inhibitors. Targeted therapies attack the cancer cells and spare normal cells from damage. Vaccines and gene therapy are also being studied to treat lung cancer.

• WORD • BUILDING •
lobectomy: lobe—lobe (of lung) + ectomy—excision

TABLE 31.10 STAGES OF LUNG CANCER

Cancer Type	Stage	Characteristics
Non–small cell lung cancer	I	No metastasis to lymph nodes. Atelectasis or pneumonia may be present.
	II	Cancer has spread to local lymph nodes or chest wall.
	III	Cancer has invaded chest wall and mediastinum and usually has spread to lymph nodes.
	IV	Tumor has metastasized to distant organs and lymph nodes.
Small cell lung cancer	Limited	Cancer is limited to one side of the chest.
	Extensive	Cancer cells are found outside one side of the chest or in distant sites.

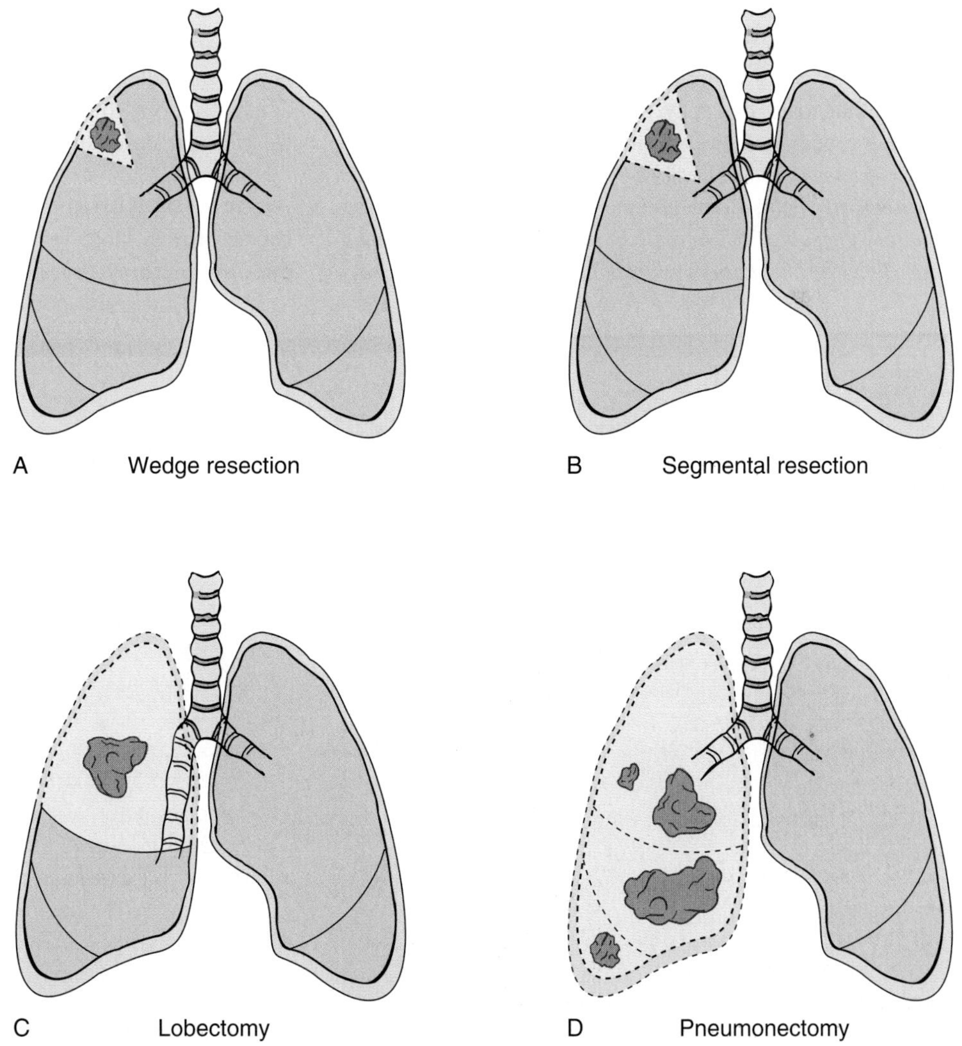
A Wedge resection
B Segmental resection
C Lobectomy
D Pneumonectomy

FIGURE 31.15 Types of surgeries for lung cancer. (A) Wedge resection. (B) Segmental resection. (C) Lobectomy. (D) Pneumonectomy.

For more information about cancer treatment and nursing care, see Chapter 11. For more on lung cancer, visit the American Cancer Society website at www.cancer.org.

NURSING PROCESS FOR THE PATIENT WITH LUNG CANCER

Data Collection

Perform a complete biopsychosocial assessment of the patient with lung cancer. Assess and document respiratory rate and depth, skin and mucous membrane color, lung sounds, oxygen saturation, cough, and sputum amount and character. Ask the patient to rate the degree of pain and dyspnea on appropriate scales. Ask about appetite and weight loss, as well as symptoms of other complications. Note activity tolerance and fatigue.

The patient will likely be grieving about his or her illness and its prognosis. Assessment of the patient's coping strategies and support systems will help you plan care for psychosocial needs (Box 31.6, *Ethical Considerations*). The presence of a living will or durable power of attorney and the desire for assistance with end-of-life planning should be noted (see Chapter 17).

Nursing Diagnoses, Planning, and Implementation

Possible diagnoses that may be experienced by the patient with lung cancer include *Impaired Gas Exchange*, *Ineffective Airway Clearance*, *Imbalanced Nutrition: Less Than Body Requirements*, *Pain*, *Constipation* related to opioid use, *Anticipatory Grieving*, and *Activity Intolerance*. See the *Nursing Care Plan for the Patient with a Lower Respiratory Tract Disorder* for care of patients with respiratory diagnoses. See Chapter 11 for interventions related to cancer diagnoses.

Evaluation

Carefully consider the patient's individual goals when evaluating care. Is the patient comfortable and free from unnecessary dyspnea? Is the airway clear, and is nutrition being maintained? Are medication side effects manageable? Have patients with terminal conditions come to terms with their impending death, and have they been able to do those things most important to them before their death?

See Table 31.11 for a lung cancer summary.

THORACIC SURGERY

A surgical incision made into the chest wall is called a **thoracotomy**. A thoracotomy may be performed for a number of reasons, including biopsy; removal of tumors, lesions, or foreign objects; to repair trauma following penetrating or crushing injuries; or to repair or revise structural problems.

Types of Thoracic Surgery

Pneumonectomy

A **pneumonectomy** is the surgical removal of a lung. This is usually done to treat lung cancer. It may also be used to treat severe cases of tuberculosis, bronchiectasis, or lung

• WORD • BUILDING •

thoracotomy: thora—chest + otomy—incision

pneumonectomy: pneum—lung + ectomy—excision

Box 31.6

Ethical Considerations

Truth Telling

Mr. David Hammill, 88 years old, is admitted to a room on the surgical unit following a thoracotomy. He has been diagnosed with a metastatic tumor of the lung but does not yet know the diagnosis. His son has power of attorney, so Dr. Lester told the son and family the diagnosis. Dr. Lester decided not to tell Mr. Hammill the diagnosis because he believes that Mr. Hammill would become upset and depressed. Dr. Lester has written an order saying that the patient should not be told his diagnosis.

Mr. Hammill has been asking the nurses, staff, and his family what the physician found in surgery and what the results of the pathology reports were. Dr. Lester has visited Mr. Hammill several times but has avoided talking about the diagnosis by saying that not all the laboratory tests are back yet. The family has been avoiding visiting the patient so that he will not ask them about the diagnosis. The family often asks the nurse when Mr. Hammill will be told his diagnosis. They believe the physician should tell him. Consider these questions:

- If the patient is continually asking for information, should the nurse tell him?
- What degree of "truth" is required?
- What about partial truths and white lies?
- Can it ever be beneficial to withhold the truth?
- Would it be different if the patient and family were not asking for information?
- What does paternalism mean, and why might the physician be taking such a position with this patient?
- Does the hospital have an ethics committee? Could such a committee help?
- What options are available to the nurse or for the nurse to suggest to the family?

Discussion and suggested answers at end of chapter.

TABLE 31.11 LUNG CANCER SUMMARY

Signs and Symptoms	Cough, hemoptysis Dyspnea, wheezing Repeat respiratory infections
Diagnostic Tests	Chest x-ray CT scan Biopsy
Therapeutic Measures	Surgery Chemotherapy Radiation Targeted therapies
Complications	Pleural effusion Superior vena cava syndrome Ectopic hormone production Atelectasis Metastasis
Priority Nursing Diagnoses	*Impaired Gas Exchange* *Ineffective Airway Clearance* *Activity Intolerance*

abscesses. Chest drainage is not usually used following a pneumonectomy because once the lung is removed, the air in the thoracic cavity is absorbed and the cavity fills with serosanguineous fluid. At about 6 months after surgery, the fluid is coagulated and the thoracic cavity is stabilized.

Lobectomy

Lobectomy is the surgical removal of one lobe. This also may be done for lung cancer, tuberculosis, or another localized problem.

Resection

Resection refers to removal of a smaller amount of lung tissue; that is, less than one lobe. A segmental resection is the removal of one segment of a lobe; a wedge resection is removal of a small wedge of lung tissue. See Fig. 31.15.

Video-Assisted Thoracoscopic Surgery

Video-assisted thoracoscopic surgery (VATS) is a newer technique that uses a specialized endoscope to perform surgery. It can be done with two or three small incisions, so is much less invasive than a traditional thoracotomy, which requires opening the chest. It can be used for biopsy, staging, or treatment of tumors.

Lung Transplantation

Lung transplant can benefit patients with a variety of serious pulmonary disorders, including pulmonary hypertension, emphysema, cystic fibrosis, and bronchiectasis. Either a single lung, both lungs, or heart and lungs have been successfully transplanted. Better criteria for selecting patients and donors, as well as advancements in surgical techniques, have improved outcomes for these patients.

NURSING PROCESS FOR THE PATIENT UNDERGOING THORACIC SURGERY

Preoperative Nursing Care

Work with the registered nurse to perform a thorough assessment before surgery, with a focus on the respiratory system. This gives a baseline against which to judge changes postoperatively. Routine preoperative teaching is done by the nurse in conjunction with the physician and health team. The patient should understand that he or she will wake up in an intensive care environment. If at all possible, it is helpful to have the patient and family tour the intensive care unit before the surgery to decrease anxiety postoperatively. Prepare the patient for waking up after surgery with an endotracheal tube connected to a ventilator, oxygen, chest tubes, intravenous fluids, cardiac monitor, Foley catheter, and possibly an epidural catheter for pain control. Let the patient know he or she will not be able to talk while the ET tube is in, and explain the use of the call light, picture board, or alternate communication techniques. Consult the surgeon for specific plans.

Advise the patient that position changes and early ambulation help prevent complications following surgery. Also instruct the patient in the use of an incentive spirometer and coughing and deep-breathing techniques.

Postoperative Nursing Care

Data Collection

Following thoracic surgery, patients initially are in an intensive care unit. Larger hospitals have special intensive care units specifically for surgical or thoracic patients. Here patients can be closely monitored for signs of complications. Frequent assessment of vital signs and hemodynamic stability; respiratory rate, depth, and effort; and lung sounds is performed. Remember that lung sounds are absent on the side of a pneumonectomy. An increase in pulse rate or a falling blood pressure may indicate internal bleeding and should be reported immediately. Oxygen saturation is monitored continuously. Often patients report an immediate improvement in breathing because the pulmonary blood supply is no longer being routed to diseased lung tissue.

Assessment for tracheal deviation alerts you to the possible complication of mediastinal shift. The trachea is normally positioned straight above the sternal notch. If the trachea deviates from the midline position, the surgeon should be notified immediately. Secretions are monitored and reported to the physician if they become thick, yellow or green, or foul smelling. Arterial blood gases are monitored closely. Chest tubes are usually present (except following pneumonectomy) and are monitored as explained in Chapter 29. Pain is assessed using a pain rating scale, and incision sites are monitored for redness, edema, or drainage. If the patient is mechanically ventilated, additional assessment of the endotracheal tube and ventilator settings will be needed.

Nursing Diagnoses, Planning, and Implementation

See the *Nursing Care Plan for the Patient with a Lower Respiratory Tract Disorder* for basic interventions. Following are some additional interventions specific to the patient following thoracic surgery.

Ineffective Airway Clearance Related to Presence of Ventilator, Inability to Cough, and Sedation, as Evidenced by Presence of Crackles and Wheezes, and High-Pressure Ventilator Alarm

EXPECTED OUTCOME: The patient will have a clear airway as evidenced by clear lung sounds and by absence of airway noise and high-pressure ventilator alarms.

- Suction according to agency policy. *The airway must remain free of secretions to prevent ventilator-associated pneumonia and dyspnea.*
- Once extubated, remind the patient to cough and deep breathe regularly. *This helps clear the airway.*
- Administer analgesics as ordered. *Postoperative pain must be controlled for the patient to be able to cough effectively.*

Impaired Gas Exchange Related to Surgical Intervention, Opioid Use, and Removal of Lung Tissue, as Evidenced by ABGs and by Spo_2 not within Normal Limits

EXPECTED OUTCOME: The patient's gas exchange value will be within acceptable limits as evidenced by Spo_2 of 90% or above.

- Monitor Spo_2. *Interventions should maintain Spo_2 at 90% or above.*
- Reposition patient every 1 to 2 hours. Consult surgeon for specific positioning orders. *Some surgeons want patients positioned with the operative side up, others with the operative side down. Fowler's position allows room for lung expansion and helps prevent aspiration.*
- Encourage use of an incentive spirometer as ordered following extubation *to encourage the patient to deep breathe and maximize oxygenation.*
- Monitor chest tube and water seal drainage system, if used. *This helps reexpand the lung and must remain intact at all times.*
- Administer oxygen and bronchodilators as ordered *to maintain oxygenation.*

Acute Pain Related to Surgical Procedure as Evidenced by Pain Rating

EXPECTED OUTCOME: The patient will be comfortable as evidenced by statement or indication that pain is controlled. If unable to communicate, objective signs of acute pain (increase in vital signs, restlessness) will be absent.

- Administer analgesics as ordered, around the clock. *Pain control is important for the patient to be able to ambulate and deep breathe and cough effectively.*
- Monitor respiratory rate and effort if not mechanically ventilated. *Opioids depress respirations.*
- Teach the patient to splint the incision while coughing. *This can stabilize the site and reduce pain, increasing the likelihood of effective coughing.*

Impaired Physical Mobility Related to Discomfort at Surgical Site as Evidenced by Inability or Unwillingness to Move

EXPECTED OUTCOME: The patient will maintain mobility as evidenced by ability to move arm and shoulder through range-of-motion exercises.

- Perform range-of-motion exercises, passively at first, then actively when the patient is able. *This helps prevent contracture of the arm and shoulder on the affected side.*
- Assist the patient to ambulate as tolerated on first or second postoperative day as ordered. *Ambulation helps maintain mobility and prevent postoperative complications.*

Risk for Infection Related to Intubation, Foley Catheterization, Surgical Incision, and Major Surgery

EXPECTED OUTCOME: The patient will be free of signs of infection as evidenced by clean and dry incision, temperature and WBC count within normal limits (WNL), clear sputum, and clear urine.

- Monitor temperature, WBC count, incision, sputum, and urine for signs of infection *so infection can be identified and treated quickly.*
- Use meticulous sterile technique for all invasive procedures: suctioning, dressing changes, catheter insertion. *This prevents introduction of pathogens.*
- Use standard infection control precautions, including careful hand washing, *because the patient is at increased risk for infection.*
- Monitor nutritional intake. Consult dietitian for recommendations. *Adequate nutrients are essential for wound healing and immune function.*
- Maintain head of bed at minimum 30 degrees elevation *to help prevent aspiration of gastric contents.*
- Provide frequent oral care *to reduce risk of aspiration of oral bacteria.*
- Assist with ventilator weaning and extubation as soon as possible. *Mechanical ventilation is associated with increased risk of pneumonia.*
- Request order to remove Foley catheter as soon as possible. *Foley catheter insertion is associated with risk of urinary tract infection (UTI).*

Evaluation

The patient's airway should remain clear, and secretions should be easily coughed up. The patient should report an acceptable comfort level and be able to cough, deep breathe, and ambulate without excessive discomfort. The patient's breathing should be unlabored, with a respiratory rate of 12 to 20 per minute. The patient's affected arm and shoulder should maintain full range of motion. Urine should be clear. Signs of infection should be absent.

Home Health Hints

- When a patient is using oxygen by nasal cannula, the area around the ears can become irritated or excoriated. A small sponge-type hair roller can be placed around the tubing to protect the ears. Avoid using gauze for this purpose. It can be abrasive and worsen the problem.
- When a home health patient has a metered-dose inhaler (MDI), the nurse should not assume he or she is using it correctly. The patient should be observed using it.
- When a patient requires more than one MDI, the canisters can be numbered in the order they are to be used.
- Read inhaler package inserts to find how many puffs are in an inhaler, and help the patient devise a system for keeping track of how many puffs are used so he does not run out. Manufacturers no longer recommend seeing if canisters float or sink in water to determine if they are empty because this method can be unreliable.
- To help the COPD patient conserve energy, he or she can be encouraged to sit on a stool when cooking at the stove or doing dishes. A shower stool can be obtained from a medical supply store. Personal care activities should be spaced throughout the day.
- Support bars, also obtained from a medical supply store, can be strategically placed in the shower area, on the walls along hallways, and in a passageway to the restroom. This can help the patient ambulate when fatigued and also help prevent falls.
- If the COPD patient is tempted to adjust his or her own oxygen flow rate, equipment suppliers can put on a locking flowmeter. Increasing the flow rate can reduce hypoxic drive and cause hypoventilation.
- Nebulizer parts should be cleaned at least three times a week, using warm water and a common home disinfectant solution for 30 minutes.
- COPD patients often have a difficult time eating. Not only do these patients have intolerance to activities but they also experience changes in their taste due to secretions and medications. Instruct the patient to rinse out his or her mouth prior to eating to help improve taste. Softer foods are often more palatable and require less energy to eat.
- When in the home it is important to not only assess your patient but also the primary caregiver. Many times he or she is experiencing caregiver role strain. Discuss options available and consider having a social worker consulted to assist with counseling and community resources. Contact the physician to discuss your concerns and ideas.

ETHICAL CONSIDERATIONS DISCUSSION

This is a difficult situation that provides an opportunity to examine autonomy, paternalism, and veracity. You can see that most of these principles have been placed on the "back burner" if not dismissed altogether in this situation.

Some elderly patients may not believe that they have a right to question a physician or be fully informed and will simply agree to whatever is suggested. Most families will express their needs, but there are some geographical areas where traditional physician–patient relationships follow a very paternalistic model, with the physician attempting to determine what is "best" for the patient.

Consider the principle of autonomy. You can see that respect for autonomy has been ignored in this situation. The patient was not given the opportunity to participate in his diagnosis and treatment plan, so he is no longer a participant in his own care. By disrespecting the patient's right to participate in his care, the physician has placed the patient in a precarious position. The patient is indicating that he would like to know his diagnosis. Most patients at this point need time to resolve life issues and prepare for death. This is a natural function, and by denying the patient this opportunity, not only is the team not maximizing benefit, they are causing harm.

Finally, what about veracity? Although telling partial truths may be justified in some cases, this decision must be weighed carefully. There is a danger for misinterpretation of facts when disclosure is less than full.

As a nurse, you must uphold your professional code of ethics and be an advocate for the patient. Insisting that a physician tell the patient can cause tension. However, protecting the autonomy of the patient is important. First approach the physician with your concerns. If he or she fails to understand the need for disclosure, then discuss the situation with your supervisor or ethics committee. Bad news is never welcome; however, in the case of terminal illness it provides the patient and family time to prepare for what is coming.

SUGGESTED ANSWERS TO CRITICAL THINKING

■ Mr. Smith

1. A complete respiratory history is taken as described in Chapter 29. An open-ended question such as "What happened to bring you to the hospital?" elicits information about the incident. In addition, questions to determine mental status and ability to make decisions and function safely on his own are appropriate. If any concerns arise, a social service consultation will be helpful for discharge planning.
2. Mr. Smith should be instructed to always read label warnings before using any cleaning products in the future and to never mix bleach and ammonia!

■ Mr. Woo

1. Document exactly what you see: "No redness or induration at either the PPD or *Candida* test sites." Date and time your entry, and sign.
2. Everyone has been exposed to, and should react to, *Candida* with some degree of redness and induration. The fact that Mr. Woo has no reaction at all may mean that his immune system is not working well—he is "anergic." Therefore, the fact that his PPD test shows no redness and swelling could just be because of his anergy even though he may be infected with TB. So, this is an unreliable test for him. Mr. Woo will need a chest x-ray and a sputum culture to be sure he is not infected.

■ Mr. Jenkins

1. Ask questions based on the WHAT'S UP? format:

Where (not applicable)

How does it feel? Does the coughing cause chest pain? Are you short of breath?

Aggravating and alleviating factors. What makes the cough worse? What seems to help? Do you use any techniques at home that are helpful?

Timing. How often do you cough during a day? Is it interfering with sleep and rest?

Severity. How bad is it on a scale of 0 to 10? How much sputum are you coughing up? Is it usually this color?

Useful other data. Are you experiencing any other symptoms with your cough (such as shortness of breath, nausea, loss of appetite)?

Patient's perception. Is it better or worse than usual today? How can I help? (The patient with long-standing disease often knows what will help but is hesitant to ask.)

2. The most appropriate nursing diagnosis is *Ineffective Airway Clearance* related to excessive secretions and ineffective cough.
3. Provide hydration with oral liquids and a room humidifier to liquefy secretions. Administer expectorants as ordered. Instruct the patient in coughing and deep-breathing exercises such as autogenic drainage to increase the effectiveness of his cough. Provide good oral care following expectoration of sputum to freshen the patient's mouth. Obtain an order for chest physiotherapy or a vibratory PEP device (Chapter 29) to help loosen and drain secretions.
4. "Patient expectorated 200 mL of bright yellow, foul-smelling sputum. Lungs have scattered crackles and wheezes throughout after coughing episode. Expectorant given; fluids encouraged. Mouth care provided."

■ Mr. Franklin

1. You need to do several things at once. You will begin by speaking in a calm voice and trying to help Mr. Franklin to calm himself by doing pursed-lip breathing. Assure him that you will help him and won't leave. At the same time, check his oxygen to make sure it is on the ordered number of liters and that his tubing is not kinked or disconnected. Grab the bedside table for him to lean on. Call for someone to page a respiratory therapist to do an NMT if ordered. Have someone bring a pulse oximeter to check his oxygen saturation. Also call for the registered nurse (RN) to administer IV morphine if ordered. All this should take about 1 minute! Once Mr. Franklin is a bit calmer, you can find out what happened. Did the exertion of moving to the bedside commode cause his dyspnea? Check his vital signs and lung sounds, and work with the RN to determine if this represents a change in Mr. Franklin's condition that should be reported to the physician.
2. Teach Mr. Franklin that he should probably stay on bedrest until his acute exacerbation is resolved. Once he is able to start moving around, he should call for help to get up. Review his controlled breathing exercises, which he can use during movement, and encourage rest between activities.

SUGGESTED ANSWERS TO—cont'd

3. "3:00: Patient up on BSC, RR 36 per minute and labored, color gray, appeared very apprehensive. O2 on at 2 L per min per NC, assisted to lean on over-bed table. Encouraged pursed-lip breathing. VS 146/64 mm Hg, 102 beats per minute, 36 per minute, Spo_2 82%. RT paged; administered PRN NMT. Breath sounds diminished, no cough. At 3:15, patient appears much calmer, RR 24 per minute and less labored, SpO_2 90%."

REVIEW QUESTIONS

1. A patient asks the nurse why he doesn't feel sick even though his TB test is positive. The nurse knows the patient has been diagnosed with LTBI. Which explanation is best to provide the patient?
   a. "TB often does not make people feel sick, but it is contagious nevertheless."
   b. "You have latent disease, which just stays in your system but won't ever make you sick."
   c. "You have TB infection, but not active disease. As long as your immune system stays strong, it can keep the infection from making you sick."
   d. "Even though you do not feel sick, the positive test shows that you have the disease and must be treated."

2. Which of the following assessment findings does the nurse expect in the patient with emphysema?
   a. Purulent sputum
   b. Diminished breath sounds
   c. Generalized edema
   d. Dull chest pain

3. A patient with shortness of breath is being tested for lung cancer. Which diagnostic test will be most conclusive?
   a. Chest x-ray
   b. MRI
   c. Sputum culture
   d. Biopsy

4. A patient with recurrent pneumothorax is scheduled to have pleurodesis done in one hour. Which nursing intervention should take priority at this time?
   a. Encourage fluids.
   b. Encourage coughing and deep breathing.
   c. Administer a prn analgesic as ordered.
   d. Administer a prn bronchodilator as ordered.

5. Which of the following assessment findings in the patient with pneumonia most indicates a need to remind the patient to cough and deep breathe?
   a. The patient reports chest pain.
   b. The patient has removed her oxygen.
   c. The patient develops coarse wheezes and crackles.
   d. The patient has a fever of 101°F (38.3°C).

6. A patient is admitted to the hospital with shortness of breath. The nurse notes increasing confusion and combativeness during the past hour. Which of the following actions is appropriate first?
   a. Assess the patient; check to see if the oxygen is flowing correctly.
   b. Page the physician stat.
   c. Put up the patient's side rails and apply soft restraints.
   d. Administer an intramuscular sedative.

7. Which of the following interventions is most appropriate for the patient with an ineffective breathing pattern?
   a. Encourage the patient to cough and deep breathe.
   b. Teach the patient controlled diaphragmatic breathing.
   c. Encourage oral fluids.
   d. Allow the patient to rest between activities.

8. A patient with end-stage COPD has a nursing diagnosis of *Impaired Gas Exchange.* Which assessment finding shows that interventions have been effective?
   a. The patient's Spo_2 is 97% on 2 liters of oxygen.
   b. The patient appears comfortable.
   c. The patient is coughing up copious white sputum.
   d. The patient is able to move in bed without difficulty.

References

American Heart Association. (2009). Cigarette smoking statistics. Retrieved November 20, 2009, from http://www.americanheart.org/presenter.jhtml?identifier=4559

Cardenas, V. M., Thun, M. J., Austin, H., et al. (1997). Environmental tobacco smoke and lung cancer mortality in the American Cancer Society's Cancer Prevention Study II. *Cancer Causes Control, 8,* 57–64.

Centers for Disease Control and Prevention. (2009a). Asthma. Updated May 15, 2009. Retrieved June 14, 2009, from http://www.cdc.gov/nchs/FASTATS/asthma.htm

Centers for Disease Control and Prevention. (2009b). *Lung cancer.* Retrieved June 17, 2009, from http://www.cdc.gov/cancer/lung/basic_info/risk_factors.htm

Centers for Disease Control and Prevention (2009c). *Lung cancer statistics.* Retrieved June 17, 2009, from http://www.cdc.gov/cancer/lung/statistics/index.htm

Centers for Disease Control and Prevention. (2009d). *Pneumococcal polysaccharide vaccine.* Retrieved June 13, 2009, from http://www.cdc.gov/vaccines/pubs/VIS/downloads/vis-ppv.pdf.

Global Initiative for Chronic Obstructive Lung Disease. (2009). Pocket guide to COPD diagnosis, management, and prevention. Retrieved November 20, 2009, from http://www.goldcopd.org/Guidelineitem.asp?l1=2&l2=1&intId=2002

Joint Commission. (2010). *2010 national patient safety goals.* Retrieved January 13, 2010, from http://www.jointcommission.org/patientsafety/nationalpatientsafetygoals

National Heart, Lung, and Blood Institute. (n.d.). *Take the first step to breathing better. Learn more about COPD.* Retrieved November 20, 2009, from http://www.nhlbi.nih.gov/health/public/lung/copd/index.htm

World Health Organization. (2009). *Global tuberculosis control: Epidemiology, strategy, financing.* Retrieved November 20, 2009, from http://www.who.int/tb/publications/global_report/2009/en/index.html

Yeaw, E. (1992). How position affects oxygenation: Good lung down? *American Journal of Nursing, 92,* 26.

unit EIGHT

UNDERSTANDING THE GASTROINTESTINAL, HEPATOBILIARY, AND PANCREATIC SYSTEMS

32 Gastrointestinal, Hepatobiliary, and Pancreatic Systems Function, Assessment, and Therapeutic Measures

LAZETTE V. NOWICKI,
LINDA S. WILLIAMS, AND
JANICE L. BRADFORD

KEY TERMS

basal cell secretion test (BAY-zuhl SELL seh-KREE-shun TEST)
bowel sounds (bough-UL SOWNDS)
caput medusae (KAP-ut meh-DOO-see)
carcinoembryonic antigen (KAR-sin-oh-EM-bree-aw-nick AN-tih-jen)
colonoscopy (KOH-lun-AW-skuh-pee)
endoscopy (EN-daw-skuh-pee)
esophagogastroduodenoscopy (ee-SOFF-ah-go-GAS-troh-doo-AW-den-AW-skuh-pee)
esophagoscopy (ee-SOFF-ah-GAW-skuh-pee)
fluoroscope (FLOOR-oh-skohp)
gastric acid stimulation test (GAS-trick AS-id STIM-yoo-LAY-shun TEST)
gastric analysis (GAS-trick ah-NAL-ih-siss)
gastroscopy (gas-STRAW-skuh-pee)
gastrostomy (gas-STRAW-stoh-mee)
gavage (gah-VAZH)
icterus (ICK-tur-us)
impaction (im-PACK-shun)
jaundice (JAWN-diss)
lavage (lah-VAZH)
lower gastrointestinal series (LOH-er GAS-troh-in-TESS-tih-null SEER-ees)
occult blood test (uh-KULT BLUHD TEST)
peripheral parenteral nutrition (puh-RIFF-uh-ruhl par-EN-teh-ruhl new-TRISH-un)
peristalsis (pear-ih-STALL-sis)
proctosigmoidoscopy (PROCK-toh-SIG-moy-DAWS-kuh-pee)
retrograde cholangiopancreatography (RET-roh-grayd koh-LAN-jee-oh-PAN-kree-ah-TOG-rah-fee)
spider angioma (SPY-der AN-jee-OH-mah)
steatorrhea (STEE-ah-toh-REE-ah)
striae (STREYE-ee)
upper gastrointestinal series (UH-pur GAS-troh-in-TES-tih-nuhl SEER-ees)

QUESTIONS TO GUIDE YOUR READING

1. What are the structures of the gastrointestinal tract and of the accessory glands: liver, gallbladder, and pancreas?
2. What are the functions of each organ of the gastrointestinal tract and of the accessory glands: liver, gallbladder, and pancreas?
3. How does age affect the gastrointestinal tract and accessory glands?
4. Which data should you collect when caring for a patient with a disorder of the gastrointestinal system, liver, gallbladder, or pancreas? Differentiate normal and abnormal findings.
5. What techniques are used in a physical examination of the abdomen conducted for a patient with possible gastrointestinal system, liver, gallbladder, or pancreas disease?
6. How would you prepare, teach, and provide follow-up care for patients having various diagnostic tests of the gastrointestinal tract?
7. What types of nasogastric tubes are available and what are their uses?
8. What nursing care is provided for insertion and maintenance of nasogastric tubes?
9. What therapeutic measures are used for patients with gastrointestinal disease?

NORMAL GASTROINTESTINAL, HEPATOBILIARY, AND PANCREATIC SYSTEMS ANATOMY AND PHYSIOLOGY

The gastrointestinal (GI) tract (or alimentary tube) is part of the digestive system (Fig. 32.1). It extends from the mouth to the anus and consists of the oral cavity, pharynx, esophagus, stomach, small intestine, and large intestine (or colon). Digestion begins in the oral cavity and continues in the stomach and small intestine. Most absorption of nutrients takes place in the small intestine. The large intestine is where the majority of water is reabsorbed from digested food. Indigestible material, mainly cellulose, is then eliminated from the large intestine.

Oral Cavity and Pharynx

The boundaries of the oral cavity are the hard and soft palates superiorly, the cheeks laterally, and the floor of the mouth inferiorly. Within the oral cavity are the teeth and tongue and the openings of the ducts of the salivary glands.

The teeth begin mechanical digestion, the physical breakup of food into smaller pieces to create more surface area for the chemical digestion brought about by enzymes. The roots of the teeth are in sockets in the jawbones (the mandible and maxillae). The gums, or gingiva, cover the jawbones and surround the bases of the crowns (tops) of the teeth. The tooth sockets are lined with a periodontal membrane (ligament) of dense fibrous connective tissue that cements the roots of the teeth.

The tongue is made of skeletal muscle innervated by the hypoglossal nerve (12th cranial nerve). The papillae on the upper surface of the tongue contain taste buds, innervated by the facial and glossopharyngeal nerves (7th and 9th cranial nerves). The tongue is important for chewing because it keeps food between the teeth. Elevation of the tongue is the first step in swallowing.

The three pairs of salivary glands are the parotid, submandibular, and sublingual glands. Their ducts carry saliva to the oral cavity. The presence of anything in the mouth increases the rate of secretion; this is a parasympathetic response mediated by the facial and glossopharyngeal nerves. Saliva is mostly water, which is used to dissolve food for tasting and moisten the food for swallowing. The only digestive enzyme in saliva that functions in the mouth is amylase, which digests starch to maltose. Usually, however, food does not remain in the mouth long enough for amylase to have any significant effect. There is also lingual lipase, however being activated by acidic pH, it begins its action in the stomach.

The pharynx is a muscular tube that acts as a passageway for food exiting the oral cavity and entering the esophagus. When a mass of food is pushed backward by the tongue, the constrictor muscles of the pharynx contract as part of the swallowing reflex. This reflex is regulated by the medulla and pons. The uvula closes off the nasopharynx while the epiglottis closes the opening to the larynx.

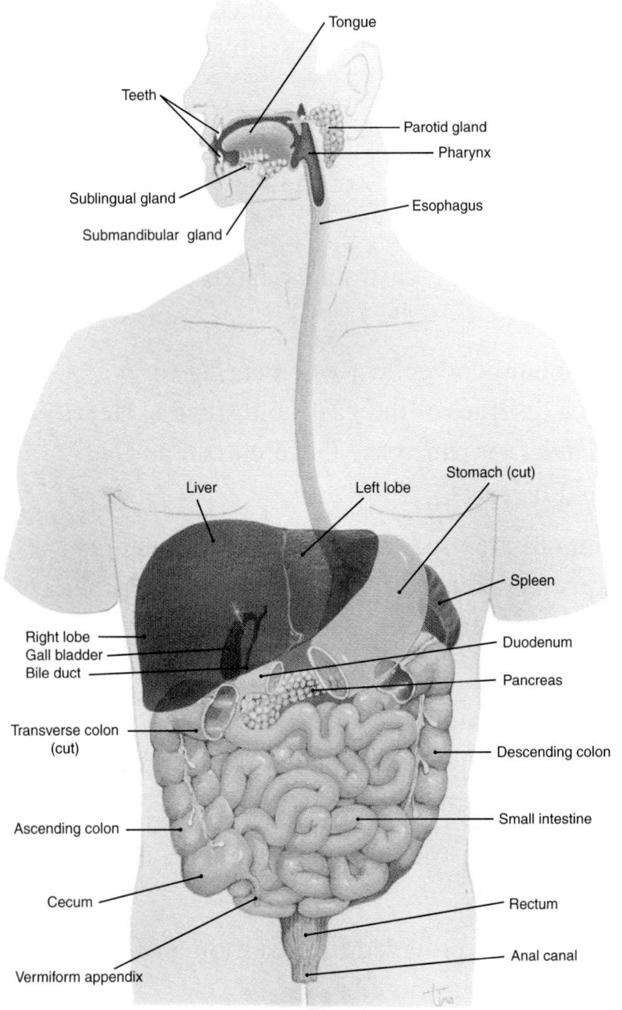
Tongue
Teeth
Parotid gland
Pharynx
Sublingual gland
Submandibular gland
Esophagus
Liver
Left lobe
Stomach (cut)
Spleen
Right lobe
Gall bladder
Bile duct
Duodenum
Pancreas
Transverse colon (cut)
Descending colon
Ascending colon
Small intestine
Cecum
Rectum
Anal canal
Vermiform appendix

FIGURE 32.1 Anterior view of the digestive system. (From Scanlon, V. C., & Sanders, T. [2007]. *Essentials of anatomy and physiology* [5th ed.]. Philadelphia: F. A. Davis, with permission.)

Esophagus

The esophagus is about 10 inches long and carries food from the pharynx to the stomach. No digestion takes place in the esophagus. **Peristalsis** (rhythmic contraction of muscles) of the muscle layer in the wall of the esophagus propels food down to the stomach and through the gastrointestinal tract. At the junction with the stomach, the lumen of the esophagus is surrounded by the lower esophageal sphincter (LES; also cardiac sphincter, gastroesophageal sphincter, or esophageal sphincter), a circular smooth muscle. The LES relaxes to permit food to enter the stomach and then contracts to prevent the backflow of stomach contents. Incomplete closure of the LES may allow gastric juice to splash up into the esophagus.

• WORD • BUILDING •

peristalsis: peri—around + stellein—to place

Stomach

The stomach is in the upper left abdominal quadrant, to the left of the liver and in front of the spleen. It is a J-shaped, saclike organ that extends from the esophagus to the duodenum of the small intestine. Some digestion takes place in the stomach; mainly it serves as a reservoir for food so that digestion may take place gradually.

The parts of the stomach are shown in Figure 32.2. The LES provides the opening from the esophagus to the stomach. The fundus forms the upper curve of the stomach. The body of the stomach is the large, central portion, bounded laterally by the greater curvature and medially by the lesser curvature. The pylorus is adjacent to the duodenum, and the pyloric sphincter surrounds the junction of the two organs.

When the stomach is empty, the mucosa has folds called rugae. The rugae flatten out as the stomach fills and permit expansion of the lining. The mucosa contains gastric pits, the glands of the stomach that produce gastric juice. Gastric juice is mostly water and contains mucus, pepsinogen, hydrochloric acid, gastric lipase, and intrinsic factor. Mucus helps form a bolus and protects the mucosal lining. Pepsinogen is an inactive enzyme that activates to pepsin by hydrochloric acid; pepsin begins the digestion of proteins to polypeptides. Hydrochloric acid creates the pH of 1 to 2 that is necessary for pepsin to function and to kill most microorganisms that enter the stomach; it also denatures (breaks down structure) proteins. Gastric lipase helps digest triglycerides. Intrinsic factor aids in the absorption of vitamin B_{12}.

Gastric juice is secreted at the sight or smell of food; this is a parasympathetic response. The presence of food in the stomach stimulates the secretion of the hormone gastrin by the gastric mucosa. Gastrin increases the secretion of gastric juice.

The stomach wall has three layers of smooth muscle: circular, longitudinal, and oblique. These provide for very efficient mechanical digestion to change food to a thick liquid called chyme. The pyloric sphincter contracts when the stomach is churning food and relaxes at intervals to allow small amounts of chyme to pass into the duodenum, then contracts again to prevent the backflow of intestinal contents into the stomach. Carbohydrates are most readily digested by the stomach, followed by proteins and fats.

Small Intestine

The small intestine is about 1 inch in diameter and approximately 20 feet long. Within the abdominal cavity, the coils of the small intestine are encircled by the colon. The small intestine extends from the stomach to the cecum of the colon. The duodenum is the first 10 inches and contains the hepatopancreatic ampulla (ampulla of Vater), the entrance of the common bile duct and the pancreatic duct. The jejunum is about 8 feet long, and the ileum is about 11 feet in length.

Digestion is completed in the small intestine, and the end products of digestion are absorbed into the blood and lymph. Bile from the liver and enzymes from the pancreas function in the small intestine (Table 32.1). When chyme enters the duodenum, the intestinal mucosa produces the enzymes sucrase, maltase, and lactase, which complete the digestion of disaccharides to monosaccharides; the peptidases, which complete the digestion of proteins to amino acids; and the nucleosidases and phosphatases, completing nucleotide digestion.

The absorption of nutrients requires a large surface area, and the small intestine has extensive folds for this purpose. The circular folds (plicae circulares) are macroscopic folds of the mucosa and submucosa. Villi are folds of the mucosa, and microvilli are microscopic folds of the cell membranes on the free surface of the intestinal epithelial cells. Within each villus is a capillary network and a lymph capillary called a lacteal. Water-soluble nutrients (monosaccharides,

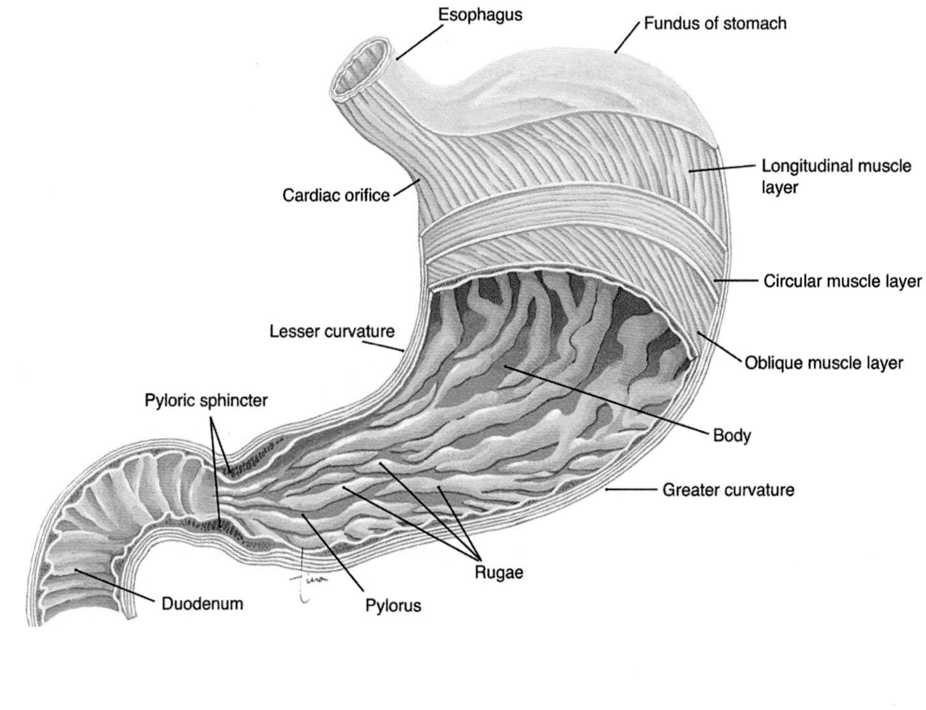
Esophagus
Fundus of stomach
Longitudinal muscle layer
Cardiac orifice
Circular muscle layer
Lesser curvature
Oblique muscle layer
Pyloric sphincter
Body
Greater curvature
Rugae
Duodenum
Pylorus

FIGURE 32.2 Stomach: anterior view and partial section. (From Scanlon, V.C., & Sanders, T. [2007]. *Essentials of anatomy and physiology* [5th ed.]. Philadelphia: F. A. Davis, with permission.)

TABLE 32.1 DIGESTIVE SECRETIONS

Organ	Enzyme or Other Secretion	Function	Site of Action
Salivary glands	Amylase	Converts starch to maltose	Oral cavity
Stomach	Pepsin	Converts proteins to polypeptides	Stomach
	Hydrochloric acid	Changes pepsinogen to pepsin	
		Maintains pH of 1–2	
		Destroys pathogens	
Liver	Bile salts	Emulsify fats	Small intestine
Pancreas	Amylase	Converts starch to maltose	Small intestine
	Lipase	Converts emulsified fats to fatty acids and glycerol	
	Trypsin	Converts polypeptides to peptides	
Small intestine	Peptidases	Convert peptides to amino acids	Small intestine
	Sucrase, maltase, lactase	Convert disaccharides to monosaccharides	

amino acids, minerals, water-soluble vitamins) are absorbed into the blood in the capillary networks. Fat-soluble vitamins and fatty acids and glycerol are absorbed into the lymph in the lacteals.

Large Intestine

The large intestine extends from the ileum of the small intestine to the anus. It is about 5 feet long and 2.5 inches in diameter. The cecum is the first part, and at its junction with the ileum is the ileocecal valve, which prevents backflow of colon contents into the small intestine. Attached to the cecum is the small, dead-end appendix.

The other parts of the colon are the ascending, transverse, and descending colon, which encircle the small intestine; the sigmoid colon, which turns medially and downward; the rectum, which is about 6 inches long; and the anal canal, the last inch of which surrounds the anus (clinically, the terminal end of the colon is usually referred to as the rectum).

Although no digestion takes place in the colon, its functions are important. The colon temporarily stores and then eliminates indigestible material. The mucosa absorbs significant amounts of water and minerals, as well as the vitamins produced by the normal bacterial flora.

Elimination of feces is accomplished by the defecation reflex, a spinal cord reflex over which voluntary control may be exerted. When peristalsis propels feces into the rectum, receptors in the smooth muscle layer detect the stretching and generate impulses to the spinal cord. The returning motor impulses cause contraction of the smooth muscle of the rectum and relaxation of the internal anal sphincter, which surrounds the anus. Surrounding the internal sphincter is the external anal sphincter, which is made of skeletal muscle and may be voluntarily contracted to prevent defecation.

The liver, gallbladder, and pancreas are called accessory organs of digestion because they produce or store digestive secretions but are not sites of the digestive process. Mechanical and chemical digestion of ingested foods take place throughout parts of the GI tract.

Liver

The liver fills the right side and center of the upper abdominal cavity just below the diaphragm. Its right lobe is larger than the left lobe.

The blood supply of the liver differs from that of other organs. The liver receives oxygenated blood by way of the hepatic artery. By way of the portal vein, blood from the abdominal digestive organs and the spleen is brought to the liver before being returned to the heart. This special pathway is called hepatic portal circulation and permits the liver to regulate blood levels of nutrients or to remove potentially toxic substances such as alcohol from the blood before the blood circulates to the rest of the body.

The only digestive function of the liver is the production of bile by the hepatocytes (liver cells). Bile flows through small bile ducts, converges into larger ones, and leaves the liver by way of the common hepatic duct (Fig. 32.3). The common hepatic duct joins the cystic duct of the gallbladder to form the common bile duct, which carries bile to the duodenum.

Bile is mostly water and bile salts. Its excretory function is to carry bilirubin and excess cholesterol to the intestines for elimination in feces. The digestive function of bile is accomplished via bile salts, which emulsify fats in the small intestine. Emulsification is a type of mechanical digestion in which large fat globules are broken into smaller globules but are not chemically changed. Production of bile is stimulated by the hormone secretin, which is produced by the duodenum when acidic chyme enters the small intestine.

Functions of the Liver

The liver is involved in a great variety of metabolic functions, most of which involve the synthesis of specific enzymes. For the sake of simplicity, these functions can be grouped into categories.

CARBOHYDRATE METABOLISM. The liver regulates the blood glucose level by storing excess glucose as glycogen and changing glycogen back to glucose when the blood glucose level is low. The liver also changes other monosaccharides

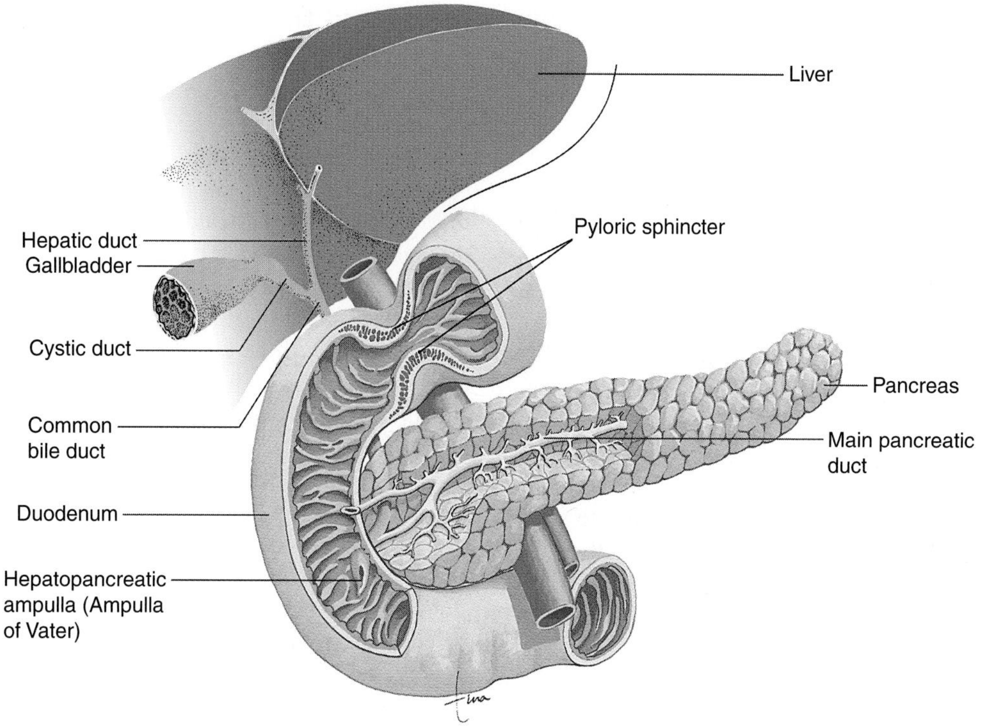
Liver
Pyloric sphincter
Hepatic duct
Gallbladder
Cystic duct
Pancreas
Common
bile duct
Main pancreatic
duct
Duodenum
Hepatopancreatic
ampulla (Ampulla
of Vater)

FIGURE 32.3 The liver, gallbladder, pancreas, and duodenum.

such as fructose and galactose to glucose, which is more readily used by cells for energy production.

AMINO ACID METABOLISM. The liver regulates the blood levels of amino acids based on tissue needs for protein synthesis. Of the 20 amino acids needed for the production of human proteins, the liver is able to synthesize 12, called the nonessential amino acids, by the process of transamination. The other 8 amino acids, which the liver cannot synthesize, are called the essential amino acids. Essential amino acids are required in the diet.

Excess amino acids (those not needed for protein synthesis) undergo the process of deamination in the liver; the amino group is removed and the remaining carbon chain is converted to a simple carbohydrate that is used for energy production or converted to fat for energy storage. The amino groups are converted to urea, a nitrogenous waste product that is removed from the blood by the kidneys and excreted in urine.

LIPID METABOLISM. The liver forms lipoproteins for the transport of lipids in the blood to other tissues. The liver also synthesizes cholesterol and excretes excess cholesterol into bile to be eliminated in feces.

The liver is also the main site of the process called beta oxidation, in which fatty acid molecules are split into two-carbon acetyl groups. These acetyl groups may be used by the liver to produce energy, or they may be combined to form ketones to be transported to other cells for energy production.

SYNTHESIS OF PLASMA PROTEINS. The liver synthesizes albumin, clotting factors, and globulins. Albumin, the most abundant plasma protein, helps maintain blood volume by pulling tissue fluid into capillaries. Clotting factors produced by the liver include prothrombin and fibrinogen, which circulate in the blood until needed for chemical clotting. The globulins synthesized by the liver become part of lipoproteins or act as carriers for other molecules in the blood.

PHAGOCYTOSIS BY KUPFFER CELLS. The fixed macrophages of the liver are called Kupffer cells (or stellate reticuloendothelial cells). They phagocytize worn erythrocytes, leukocytes, and some bacteria that circulate through the liver. Many of the bacteria that enter the liver come from the colon, after being absorbed along with water. Portal circulation brings this blood to the liver before entering circulation throughout the remainder of the body. These bacteria are normal flora of the colon but would be harmful elsewhere.

FORMATION OF BILIRUBIN. Hepatocytes form bilirubin from the heme portion of hemoglobin removed from worn erythrocytes. The liver also removes bilirubin from the blood collected from the spleen and red bone marrow and excretes it into bile to be eliminated in feces.

STORAGE. The liver stores the minerals iron and copper; the fat-soluble vitamins A, D, E, and K; and the water-soluble vitamin B_{12}.

DETOXIFICATION. The liver synthesizes enzymes that alter harmful substances to less harmful ones. Alcohol and medications are examples of potentially toxic chemicals.

The liver also converts ammonia from protein metabolism to urea, a less toxic substance.

ACTIVATION OF VITAMIN D. The skin, kidneys, and liver each perform a different role in providing the body with activated vitamin D.

Gallbladder

The gallbladder is a muscular sac about 3 to 4 inches long located on the undersurface of the liver. Bile in the common hepatic duct from the liver flows through the cystic duct (see Fig. 32.3) into the gallbladder, which stores bile until it is needed in the small intestine. The gallbladder also concentrates bile by absorbing water.

When fatty foods or partially digested proteins enter the duodenum, the duodenal mucosa secretes the hormone cholecystokinin. One function of cholecystokinin is to stimulate contraction of the smooth muscle of the wall of the gallbladder. Contraction of the gallbladder forces bile into the cystic duct, then into the common bile duct, which empties into the duodenum.

Pancreas

The pancreas is about 6 inches long and is located posterior to the greater curvature of the stomach (see Fig. 32.3). The digestive secretions of the pancreas are produced by exocrine glands called acini. The small ducts of these glands unite to form larger ducts and finally converge into the pancreatic duct, which joins the common bile duct to enter the duodenum at the hepatopancreatic ampulla. The accessory duct has a direct line from the pancreas into the duodenum.

The pancreatic digestive enzymes are involved in the digestion of all four of the organic molecule categories. The enzyme pancreatic amylase digests starch to maltose. Pancreatic lipase converts emulsified fats to fatty acids and monoglycerides. Trypsinogen is an inactive enzyme that is changed to active trypsin in the duodenum. Trypsin digests polypeptides to shorter chains of amino acids. Pancreatic juice also contains proteolytic enzymes: chymotrypsin, carboxypeptidase, and elastase. Ribonuclease and deoxyribonuclease, for the digestion of RNA and DNA, respectively, are contributed by the pancreas as well.

The pancreas also produces a bicarbonate juice, which is alkaline because of its high sodium bicarbonate content. The function of bicarbonate juice is to neutralize the hydrochloric acid in gastric juice as it enters the duodenum from the stomach. The pH of duodenal chyme is raised to about 7.5, which prevents corrosive damage to the mucosa and creates the optimal pH for intestinal enzyme action.

Secretion of pancreatic juice is stimulated by the hormones of the duodenal mucosa. Secretin stimulates the production of bicarbonate pancreatic juice, and cholecystokinin stimulates secretion of the pancreatic enzyme juice.

Aging and the Gastrointestinal, Hepatobiliary, and Pancreatic Systems

Many changes occur in the aging gastrointestinal (GI) system (Fig. 32.4). The sense of taste becomes less acute, and the likelihood of developing periodontal disease and oral cancer increases. If teeth have been lost, an older person may experience difficulties with chewing. Secretions throughout the GI tract are reduced, and the effectiveness of peristalsis diminishes because of loss of muscle elasticity and slowed motility. Indigestion may become more common, especially if the LES loses its tone, and peptic ulcers are more common. In the colon, diverticula may form. Constipation may be a problem, as may hemorrhoids. The risk of colon cancer also increases with age.

The liver usually continues to function well into old age, unless damaged by pathogens such as the hepatitis viruses or by toxins such as alcohol (Box 32.1, *Gerontological Issues*). There is a greater tendency for gallstones to form, sometimes necessitating removal of the gallbladder. In the absence of specific pathological conditions, the pancreas usually functions well, although acute pancreatitis of unknown cause is somewhat more common in the elderly.

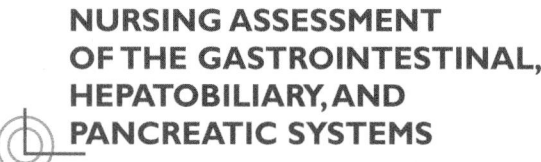

NURSING ASSESSMENT OF THE GASTROINTESTINAL, HEPATOBILIARY, AND PANCREATIC SYSTEMS

Health History

Assessment of current signs and symptoms includes asking the WHAT'S UP? questions as presented in Chapter 1 (Tables 32.2 and 32.3). Demographic data is obtained, including travel history, which may help in diagnosing the cause of GI symptoms such as diarrhea.

Ask the patient about any nausea, vomiting, or abdominal distention. Information about the timing or other common triggers of episodes of nausea or vomiting may help the practitioner identify their cause. Such information may also help determine appropriate treatment for any future nausea or vomiting. Abdominal distention in the presence of nausea and vomiting may indicate intestinal obstruction. Patients with liver, gallbladder, or pancreatic disease may also report feeling bloated, having gas or belching frequently, or right upper quadrant (RUQ) tenderness.

Question the patient about any observed changes in bowel elimination. Diarrhea may be caused by irritation of the bowel. Constipation may indicate decreased water intake or excessive water loss. Observe the patient's stool for evidence of bacteria (a foul smell), fat (stool floats on the water surface and appears greasy), pus, blood, or mucus. Patients with liver or gallbladder disease may have pale or clay-colored stools.

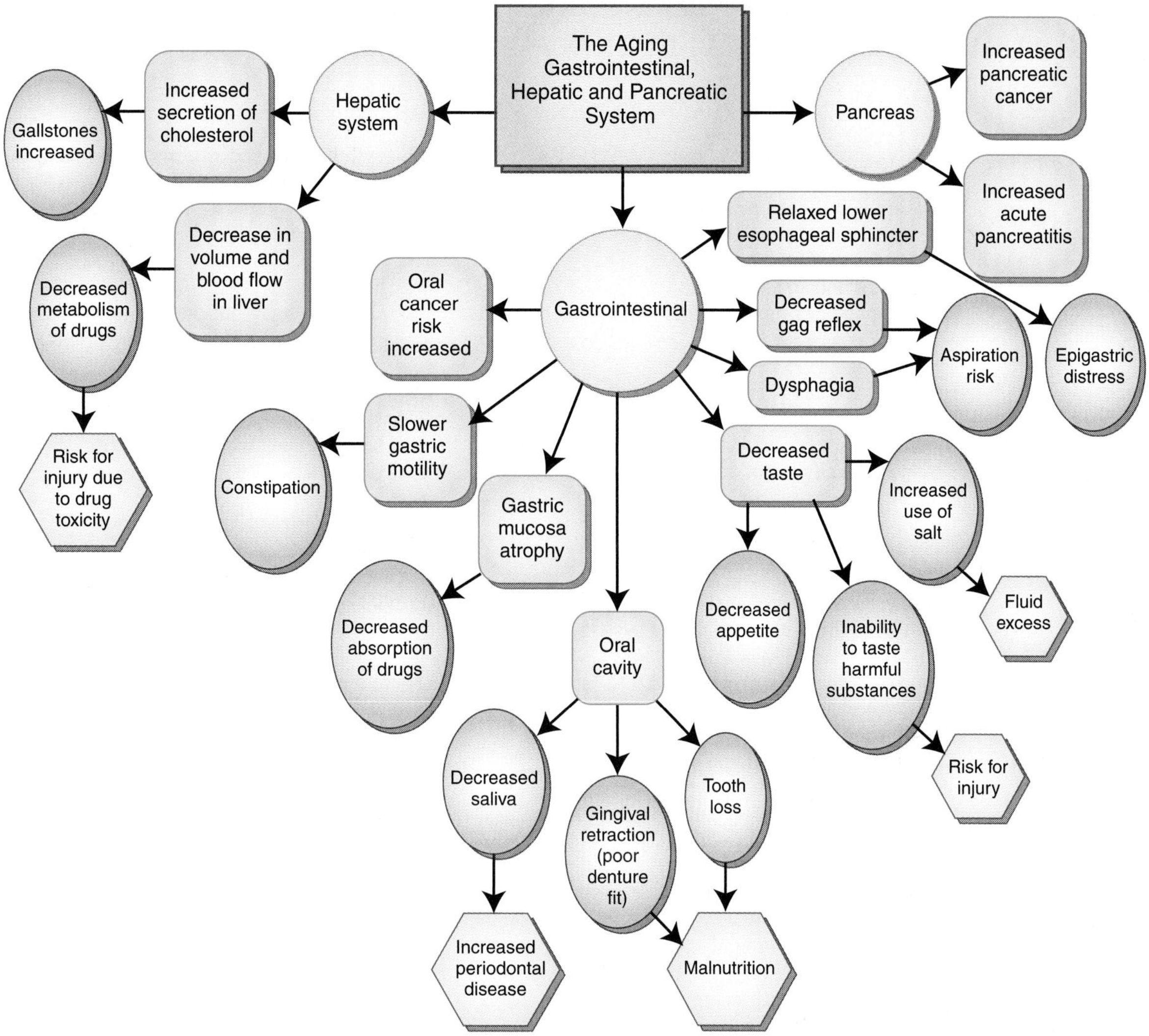
The Aging Gastrointestinal, Hepatic and Pancreatic System
Hepatic system
Increased secretion of cholesterol
Gallstones increased
Decrease in volume and blood flow in liver
Decreased metabolism of drugs
Risk for injury due to drug toxicity
Pancreas
Increased pancreatic cancer
Increased acute pancreatitis
Gastrointestinal
Relaxed lower esophageal sphincter
Epigastric distress
Oral cancer risk increased
Decreased gag reflex
Aspiration risk
Dysphagia
Slower gastric motility
Constipation
Gastric mucosa atrophy
Decreased absorption of drugs
Decreased taste
Increased use of salt
Fluid excess
Decreased appetite
Inability to taste harmful substances
Risk for injury
Oral cavity
Decreased saliva
Increased periodontal disease
Gingival retraction (poor denture fit)
Tooth loss
Malnutrition

FIGURE 32.4 Aging and its effects on the gastrointestinal, hepatic, and pancreatic systems is shown on this concept map.

> **Box 32.1**
> ## Gerontological Issues
> With increasing age, the liver decreases in volume, mass, and blood flow. These changes are significant because the liver acts to metabolize many drugs. If a patient has impaired liver function, toxic levels of a drug may be present in the blood. It is important to assess liver function tests and perform a medication review to determine those that are metabolized by the liver. Older adults may require reduced doses of many drugs.

Determine if the patient has had any recent blood transfusions or blood products, dental procedures, body piercing or tattooing, or intravenous injection with a potentially contaminated needle. These procedures cause a break in the skin that can become an entry point for hepatitis virus (type B or C) as well as other pathogens.

Ask about the patient's usual work activities and work setting. Document exposure to chemicals such as paint fumes, industrial dyes, acids, farm pesticides, or other liver-toxic substances.

Investigate the patient's activities other than work. Document reports of fatigue along with information about when the fatigue occurs. Ask the patient about stressors such as financial concerns, problems dealing with the health care environment, and any family or personal problems. Attempt to determine what coping mechanisms the patient usually employs to deal with stressors.

Medications

The patient is asked about medication use such as nonsteroidal anti-inflammatory drugs (NSAIDs), aspirin, vitamins, laxatives, enemas, or antacids. Heavy use of medications that can cause irritation and bleeding in the GI tract, such as NSAIDs or aspirin, should be carefully noted. Older patients with arthritis often use these types of medications for pain control. The patient's knowledge of the side effects of these medications should be assessed to identify important teaching

TABLE 32.2 SUBJECTIVE DATA COLLECTION FOR THE GASTROINTESTINAL SYSTEM

Category	Questions to Ask During the Health History	Rationale/Significance
Health History	Identify current symptoms using the WHAT'S UP format.	This will help you adequately assess the patient's current problem.
	What are your bowel patterns? How often do you usually have a bowel movement?	Changes in bowel habits could indicate new disease process.
	What is the color? Consistency?	
	Diarrhea or constipation?	
	Have you had any blood in your stool or on the toilet tissue?	Blood in stool may indicate hemorrhoids, early sign of cancer, or inflammatory diseases such as ulcerative colitis.
	Have you had any change in appetite?	Appetite changes can be common with gastrointestinal disorders.
	Nausea and/or vomiting?	
	Bloating? Excess gas?	Can be associated with GI disorders.
	Do you have any history of gastrointestinal illnesses or surgeries?	Patient may have a recurring problem.
	Do you smoke?	Nicotine can irritate the GI mucosa. Smoking is related to esophagitis, ulcers, and GI cancers such as esophagus and mouth cancer.
Medications	What medications are you currently taking?	Provides baseline information about patient.
	How do the drugs relate to the GI system?	
	Are they working? How do you know?	
	Have you recently taken any NSAIDs, aspirin, anticoagulants, or steroids?	These medications can cause gastric upset and/or bleeding.
	Do you routinely take laxatives? Fiber?	Patient may have dependency on laxatives.
	Are you taking or have you recently taken antibiotics?	Diarrhea due to *Clostridium difficile* can be caused by recent antibiotic use.
Nutrition	Describe your usual diet. Tell me what you ate yesterday for the entire day.	Provides information about your patient's nutritional status. Older adults may be on a fixed income and unable to afford adequate nutrition.
	Do you have any food allergies?	These may interfere with proper nutrition.
	Do you have indigestion, dysphagia, heartburn, nausea, vomiting, diarrhea, constipation, flatulence, or bowel incontinence?	If patient has any of these symptoms, use the WHAT'S UP format to gather more specific information.
	Have you had a change in appetite?	
	Have you had a change in weight—gain or loss?	
	Are there any foods that you cannot eat?	
Family History	Do you have a family history of any gastrointestinal disorders such as cancer?	Some diseases are thought to be hereditary.
Cultural Influences	Are there any cultural considerations I should be aware of regarding your food intake or care?	Many societies use herbs, vitamins, or home remedies to care for disorders.

TABLE 32.3 SUBJECTIVE DATA COLLECTION FOR THE HEPATOBILIARY AND PANCREATIC SYSTEMS

Category	Questions to Ask During the Health History	Rationale/Significance
Health History	Do you have abdominal pain? (Use WHAT'S UP? format to further identify.) Do any foods cause pain?	Pain can be associated with disease of the liver, gallbladder, or pancreas. Fatty foods can cause pain related to gallbladder disease.
	What do your stools look like?	Clay-colored stools indicate liver or gallbladder disease. Black stools may indicate bleeding, which can be related to liver disease. Fatty stools occur with pancreatic disease.
	Does your abdomen feel distended or full?	Fluid in the abdomen, or ascites, occurs with liver disease.
	How much alcohol do you drink each day?	Excess alcohol intake is associated with liver disease and pancreatitis.
	Do you bruise or bleed easily?	Bleeding is associated with liver disease, because clotting factors are made in the liver.

TABLE 32.3 SUBJECTIVE DATA COLLECTION FOR THE HEPATOBILIARY AND PANCREATIC SYSTEMS—cont'd

Category	Questions to Ask During the Health History	Rationale/Significance
	Have you had any recent blood transfusions or blood products, dental procedures, body piercing or tattooing, or intravenous injection with a potentially contaminated needle?	Breaks in skin may be the route of entry for hepatitis (type B or C) or other pathogens.
Nutrition	Have you experienced nausea and vomiting?	These are generalized symptoms that may be associated with disease of the liver, gallbladder, or pancreas.
	Has your appetite or weight changed?	Anorexia and weight loss accompany many liver, gallbladder, and pancreatic disorders.
Family History	Does anyone in your family have liver, gallbladder, or pancreatic disease or alcoholism?	These disorders tend to run in families.
Medications	Do you use any over-the-counter drugs or herbal remedies?	Many drugs and herbs are toxic to the liver.

needs. Older patients may use laxatives regularly and develop a dependence on them. Teaching may be needed on normal bowel patterns and laxative use. Also ask the patient what medications are being taken with or without a physician's prescription, such as acetaminophen, which can be hepatotoxic. Many people do not consider it necessary to report over-the-counter preparations and herbal, natural, or other nonprescription products and must be asked specifically about them.

CLOSTRIDIUM DIFFICILE. Question the patient about recent hospitalizations or antibiotic use. Hospitalization or recent antibiotic use is a risk factor for *Clostridium difficile*. Taking probiotics when on antibiotics, if not immunocompromised, can help reduce this risk. With antibiotic use, a decrease in normal flora can result, allowing an overgrowth of *C. difficile*. The toxins produced by *C. difficile* can cause diarrhea, colitis, toxic megacolon, dehydration, colonic perforation, and sometimes death. Nurses should monitor patients closely for signs of *C. difficile* infection such as diarrhea, nausea, anorexia, and abdominal tenderness or pain. These symptoms should be reported to the physician because this infection can be fatal.

LEARNING TIP

Consider *C. difficile* infection if the patient has diarrhea associated with recent antibiotic use or hospitalization. Educate patients to report its occurrence. Protect everyone by practicing excellent hand hygiene and by following strict isolation procedures. *C. difficile* can be carried on your hands, nails, rings, or shoes.

At home, remove your shoes and uniform in an area where their contact with other items is prevented and bathe and launder your uniform separately from your family's laundry.

CRITICAL THINKING

Mrs. Todd

■ Mrs. Todd, age 74, has arthritis and takes eight aspirin daily for pain control. She is scheduled for an esophagogastroduodenoscopy (EGD) for suspected GI bleeding causing unexplained anemia.

1. What is a likely cause of the GI bleeding?
2. What could you do to help prevent future bleeding episodes for Mrs. Todd?
3. What nursing care will need to be completed before the test and after the test?

Suggested answers at end of chapter.

Nutritional Assessment

A diet history should include usual foods and fluids, allergies, appetite patterns, swallowing difficulty, and use of nutritional and herbal supplements. A food diary can be used to provide more detailed information. Older patients may be on fixed incomes, which may limit their food budget and result in meal skipping or purchasing of inexpensive foods. The older patient's daily food intake should be explored, especially if malnutrition, financial limitations, or living alone is noted.

Also explored during a nutritional assessment are patterns of gastric acid reflux, indigestion, heartburn, nausea, vomiting, diarrhea, constipation, flatulence, and bowel incontinence, all of which may interfere with proper nutrition (Box 32.2, *Gerontological Issues*). Acid reflux can be assessed by asking patients if they experience reflux with a bile taste or awaken with an unpleasant taste in their mouth.

Patients with disease of the liver, pancreas, or gallbladder commonly have changes in appetite such as anorexia or alterations in eating preferences. Ask the patient about any abnormal weight loss or unexpected weight gain and changes

Box 32.2

Gerontological Issues

A complete bowel history should be obtained for older adults before beginning a bowel program. A bowel history includes the following:

- Normal bowel evacuation pattern
- Characteristics of stool
- Presence of any bleeding or mucus with the stool
- Use of products and medications to stimulate or slow bowel function
- Report of usual diet
- Amount of fluids—number and size of beverages, glasses per day (beverages containing caffeine, such as coffee, tea, and sodas, do not count as fluids because of the diuretic effect of caffeine)
- Exercise and physical activity
- Rituals and practices related to bowel function.

in food tolerance, including the type or amount of offending foods. For example, patients with gallbladder disease may report that they feel nauseated or bloated after eating fried or greasy foods. Ask if the patient smokes, ingests alcohol, or uses other recreational drugs. If the patient acknowledges alcohol or other drug use, record the type, frequency, and amount used.

Family History

Family history of close relatives with conditions that may influence the patient's GI status is noted. Some GI problems such as colon cancer are thought to be hereditary. The patient's history should note whether there is a family history of liver, pancreas, or gallbladder diseases, such as diabetes mellitus, alcoholism, cancer, heart disease, or bleeding tendencies. These diseases tend to run in families.

Cultural Influences

Many cultures have special dietary practices and restrictions (Box 32.3, *Cultural Considerations*). See Box 32.4, *Cultural Considerations,* for assessment questions. Understanding these cultural influences, respecting them, and assisting the patient to maintain desired cultural practices are important for nutritional maintenance.

Physical Examination

Table 32.4 summarizes findings from the objective assessment of the gastrointestinal, hepatobiliary, and pancreatic systems discussed next.

Height, Weight, and Body Mass Index

The patient's height and weight are obtained for planning care. It is compared to the patient's ideal body weight obtained using current reference charts. Body mass index (BMI) is calculated to measure body fat and used with waist-to-hip ratio measurements to determine patient's health risk factors (Table 32.5). Excess waist circumferences (for women, more than 35 inches; for men, more

Box 32.3

Cultural Considerations

Most societies of the world use various foods and herbs for maintaining health. With increased attention to herbal therapies in the United States, the National Institutes of Health is studying 40 foods that are thought to fight disease. Among them are garlic, carrots, soy, cranberry juice, licorice, and green tea. Green tea has been used in Japan and China for centuries as a means of maintaining health and preventing disease.

African Americans

Obesity is seen as positive among many African Americans. They often view individuals who are thin as "not having enough meat on their bones." One needs to have adequate meat on his or her bones so that when an illness occurs, one can afford to lose weight. Many African American diets are high in animal fat and fried foods and low in fiber, fruits, and vegetables.

Appalachians

The diet of some Appalachians is deficient in vitamin A, iron, and calcium. The nurse working with this population needs to do a dietary assessment and teach patients food selections that include adequate vitamin A, iron, and calcium.

Arabs

Many Arabs eat food only with their right hand because it is regarded as the clean hand. The left hand, commonly used for toileting, is considered unclean. Thus, the nurse should feed the Arab

Box 32.3

Cultural Considerations—cont'd

patient with the right hand regardless of the nurse's dominant handedness. Additionally, some may not drink beverages with their meals because some consider it unhealthy to eat and drink at the same meal. Likewise, mixing hot and cold foods may be seen as unhealthy.

Muslim Arabs may refuse to eat meat that is not halal (slaughtered and prepared in a ritual manner). Because Muslim Arabs are prohibited from ingesting alcohol or eating pork, they may refuse medication that includes alcohol, such as mouthwashes, toothpaste, alcohol-based syrups and elixirs, and products derived from pigs, such as insulin, gelatin-coated capsules, and skin grafts. However, if no substitute is available, Muslims are permitted to use these preparations.

The condition of the alimentary tract has priority over all other body parts in the Arab's perception of health. Gastrointestinal problems are the most common reason Arab Americans seek care.

Asian Indians

Among Asian Indians, nutritional deficiencies are patterned from the region of emigration. For example, beriberi (thiamine deficiency) is found in people emigrating from rice-growing areas. Pellagra (niacin deficiency), causing skin and mental disorders and diarrhea, is found in people emigrating from maize-millet areas. Thorough milling of rice, washing rice before cooking, and allowing the cooked rice to remain overnight before consumption the following day result in the loss of thiamine.

Asian Indians use chili, which may make it difficult for them to eat food that is tasteless, or the use of chili may cause problems with upper gastrointestinal conditions.

The commitment to the sacred cow concept encourages dairy and milk use by Hindus. However, lactose intolerance affects more than 10% of adults. The adequacy or inadequacy of the ability to digest lactose may be due to genetic differences among Asian Indians.

Goiter is prevalent among some Asian Indian immigrants as a result of an iodine deficiency in food and water from their homeland. Fluorosis occurs in other parts of India from drinking water high in fluoride. Osteomalacia is prevalent where diets are deficient in calcium and vitamin D. Endemic dropsy is prevalent among Asian Indians emigrating from West Bengal, resulting from the use of mustard oil for cooking. The nurse needs to be aware of these conditions and their causes when working with Hindus and Asian Indians and teach patients prevention.

Brazilians

Brazilians experience an increase in gastrointestinal distress when they first come to the United States, partially because many have a lactose intolerance and partially because of different methods of milk pasteurization. The nurse can assist with identifying alternative food sources for Brazilian patients to obtain needed calcium in their diet.

Jews

Among Jews, the laws regarding food are commonly referred to as the laws of Kashrut, or the laws of what foods are permissible in accordance with the religious law. The term *kosher* means "fit for eating"; it is not a brand or form of cooking.

Foods are divided into those that are permitted (clean) and forbidden (unclean). The kosher slaughter of animals prevents undue cruelty to the animal and ensures the animal's health for its consumer. Care must be taken that all blood is drained from the animal before eating it.

Among the more conservative and Orthodox Jews, dairy products and meat may not be mixed together, whether in cooking, serving, or eating. This involves separating the utensils used to prepare foods and the plates used to serve them. To avoid mixing foods, religious Jews have two sets of dishes, pots, and utensils: one set for dairy products and one for meat.

Cheeseburgers, meat lasagna, and grated cheese on meatballs and spaghetti are not acceptable. Milk cannot be used in coffee if served with a meat meal. Nondairy creamers can be used as long as they do not contain sodium caseinate, which is derived from milk.

Fish, eggs, vegetables, and fruits are considered neutral and may be used with either dairy or meat dishes. A "U" with a circle around it or a "K" is used on food products to indicate kosher.

Continued

Box 32.3

Cultural Considerations—cont'd

When working in a Jewish person's home, the nurse should not bring food into the house without knowing whether the patient is kosher. If the patient is kosher, do not use any cooking items, dishes, or silverware without knowing which are used for meat and which are used for dairy. It is important for the nurse to understand the dietary laws so as not to offend the patient. The nurse should advocate for kosher meals if they are requested and plan medication times accordingly.

Although liberal Jews decide for themselves which dietary laws, if any, they follow, many still avoid pork and pork products out of a sense of tradition and symbolism. It would be insensitive to serve pork products to Jewish patients unless they specifically request them.

Kosher meals are available in hospitals and long-term care facilities. Even though the organization may not have a kosher kitchen, frozen kosher meals can be obtained from several organizations, most of which are located in large cities with large Jewish populations. The address and telephone number of the kosher kitchen closest to your organization can be obtained by calling the nearest Jewish synagogue. Kosher meals arrive on paper plates with plastic utensils sealed in plastic. The nurse should not unwrap the utensils if the patient is able to do so or change the foodstuffs to another serving dish. Determining a patient's dietary preferences and practices regarding dietary laws should be done during the admission assessment.

Mexican Americans

Good health to Mexican Americans, which is largely a part of "God's will," can be maintained by dietary practices that keep the body in balance. To provide culturally competent care, the nurse must be aware of the hot-and-cold theory of disease when offering health teaching. Many diseases are thought to be caused by a disruption in the hot-and-cold balance theory of the body. Thus, by eating foods of the opposite variety, one may either cure or prevent specific hot-and-cold illnesses and conditions.

Examples of hot disease conditions include infection, diarrhea, sore throats, stomach ulcers, liver conditions, kidney problems, gastrointestinal upsets, and febrile conditions. Foods that are considered "cold" are therefore viewed as remedies for hot illness conditions. Cold foods include fresh fruits and vegetables, dairy products, barley water, fish, chicken, goat meat, and dried fruits. However, significant differences are seen in terms of what are considered hot and cold foods and illnesses among Mexican American families depending on their native region in Mexico.

Examples of cold illness conditions include cancer, malaria, earaches, arthritis and related conditions, pneumonia and other pulmonary conditions, headaches, menstrual cramping, and musculoskeletal conditions. Hot substances used to treat these conditions typically include cheeses, liquor, beef, pork, spicy foods, eggs, grains other than barley, vitamins, tobacco, and onions.

than 40 inches) place people at greater risk for diabetes and cardiovascular disease. Also the location of excess fat, mainly around the waist, increases the risk of health problems even with a normal BMI.

Oral Cavity

Gastrointestinal assessment begins with the oral cavity. The lips are examined for lesions, abnormal color, and symmetry. With a penlight and tongue blade, the oral cavity is inspected for inflammation, tenderness, ulcers, swelling, bleeding, and discolorations. Any odor of the patient's breath is noted. A foul odor may indicate infection or poor oral care. The tongue should be pink with a rough texture and assessed for signs of dehydration such as dryness, cracks, or furrows. The patient's gums should be pink without swelling, redness, or irregularities. The teeth or dentures are examined for loose, broken, or absent teeth and the fit of the dentures or dental work. Ill-fitting dentures can affect the patient's nutritional intake and obstruct the airway. Loose teeth can become dislodged and aspirated into the airway. Broken teeth can be a source of pain and contribute to poor nutritional intake.

The patient's knowledge of dental and oral care is assessed. The ability of the patient to perform oral care is noted and included in the plan of care if there are deficits. Oral health is very important to a person's overall health and well-being.

Abdomen

Be prepared to assist with a thorough physical assessment of the patient. Instead of following the usual inspect-palpate-percuss-auscultate (IPPA) format, assess the abdomen starting with inspection, then auscultation, percussion, and palpation. This is to prevent palpation from changing other assessment findings.

Box 32.4

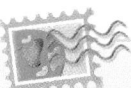

Cultural Considerations

Questions to ask when performing a cultural nutritional assessment:

- What types of your cultural foods are available in your community?
- What are your preferred foods over foods available and eaten?
- Which foods do you most commonly consume?
- How and where are your foods chosen and purchased?
- Who prepares the food in your household?
- Who purchases the food in your household?
- How is your food stored for future use?
- How is your food prepared before being eaten?
- How is any uneaten food discarded?
- What foods do you eat to maintain your health?
- What foods do you avoid to maintain your health?
- What foods do you eat when you are ill?
- What foods do you avoid when you are ill?

TABLE 32.4 OBJECTIVE DATA COLLECTION FOR THE GASTROINTESTINAL, HEPATOBILIARY, AND PANCREATIC SYSTEMS

Category	Physical Examination Findings	Possible Abnormal Findings/Causes
Height, Weight, and Body Mass Index (BMI)	Normal height, weight and body mass index	Decreases in height, weight, and BMI could indicate inadequate nutrition or malabsorption problems. Current weight loss could indicate new onset of a disease such as cancer.
Oral Cavity	Moist, pink oral mucosa, without lesions, inflammation, tenderness, or discolorations.	Foul odor may indicate infection or poor oral hygiene.
	Pink, rough tongue.	Dry tongue with cracked furrows could indicate dehydration possibly due to vomiting or diarrhea.
	Teeth should be intact. Dentures should fit properly.	Broken teeth or ill-fitting dentures can contribute to inadequate nutrition.
Abdomen *Inspection*	Abdomen contour should be flat, rounded, or convex.	Irregularities in contour such as bulging or masses may be due to distention, tumors, hernia, or previous surgeries.
	Shape should be symmetrical.	Any scars, dressings, appliances such as an ostomy should be noted. Indicate what the stoma looks like.
	Skin color should be consistent with overall skin tone. No visible scars or discolorations.	Scars may be present if the patient has had previous surgeries or injuries. Striae are present if the skin has been stretched (i.e., with pregnancy or weight gain). Bruising could be related to injury or altered liver function. Note any caput medusae or spider angiomas. Jaundice color may indicate liver or gallbladder disease.
Auscultation	Soft bowel sounds should be heard in all quadrants every 5–15 seconds.	Hyperactive sounds are heard with increased motility such as diarrhea. Hypoactive sounds are associated with decreased motility such as abdominal surgery, paralytic ileus, or bowel obstruction.
	Circulatory sounds should be absent.	A humming sound may be heard over the liver in patients with chronic liver failure.
Percussion	Completed by physician or nurse practitioner.	
Palpation	No pain, muscle tension, rigidity, or masses should be felt on light palpation. The abdomen should feel soft. Abdominal girth should be appropriate for patient without increasing. Deep palpation is done by the advanced practitioner.	Muscle tension, rigidity, or pain may occur in many abdominal disorders. Patients with ascites from liver disease may have an increased girth that increases as the disease worsens.
Anus	No lumps, rashes, scars, erythema, bleeding, fissures, or hemorrhoids.	Hemorrhoids may be present. Patients with diarrhea may have skin breakdown or rash.

TABLE 32.5 CALCULATING BODY MASS INDEX AND WAIST-TO-HIP RATIO MEASUREMENT

To calculate body mass index:	*Formulas:* *Pounds and inches:* weight (lb) / [height (in.)]^2 × 703 Step 1. Multiply height (in inches) by height. Step 2. Divide weight (in pounds) by Step 1 answer. Step 3. Multiply Step 2 answer by 703. *Kilograms and meters:* weight (kg) / [height (m)]^2 Step 1. Multiply height (in meters) by height. Step 2. Divide weight (in kilograms) by Step 1 answer.
Findings	Below 18.5: underweight 18.5–24.9: normal 25–29.9: overweight 30 and over: obese
To obtain waist measurement:	Step 1. Place measuring tape around bare waist at top of the iliac crest. Step 2. Pull snugly around the waist. Step 3. Read measurement at end expiration.
To obtain waist-to-hip ratio (WHR) measurement (preferred method for patients who are overweight and obese who are predominantly muscular):	Step 1. Place measuring tape at the level of the top of the iliac crest. Step 2. Pull snugly around the waist. Step 3. Read measurement at end expiration. Step 4. Place measuring tape around hip at widest part and read measurement. Step 5. Waist measurement is divided by hip measurement.
Findings/risk for health complications:	Female: ≤ 0.8—low risk; > 0.85—high risk Male: ≤ 0.95—low risk; > 1.0—high risk

*Preferred method for patients who are overweight or obese and who are predominantly muscular.

INSPECTION. To inspect the abdomen, patients are placed in a supine position with their arms at their sides. The abdomen is visually inspected to note the condition of the skin and the contour. The contour may be rounded, flat, concave, or distended, depending on the patient's body type. Abdominal pulsatile masses are noted. Such masses may be visible in thin persons or they may indicate an abdominal aortic aneurysm. Irregularities in contour may be due to distention, tumors, hernia, or previous surgeries. Also note any wounds, tubes, or ostomy devices including type and location.

Inspect the patient's skin for scars, **striae** (commonly called stretch marks; light silver-colored or thin red lines on the abdomen), bruising, **caput medusae** (bluish purple swollen vein pattern extending out from the navel), and **spider angiomas** (thin reddish purple vein lines close to the skin surface). Note any petechiae. The patient's abdomen is observed for any visible masses, visible movement or peristalsis, or **jaundice** (also called **icterus**; a yellowing of the skin and the sclerae of the eyes).

Jaundice is a cardinal symptom of liver or gallbladder disease and red blood cell disorders. Old red blood cells are cleared from the circulatory system by phagocytes in the spleen, liver, lymph nodes, and bone marrow. In the process, the compound heme (part of hemoglobin) is split into iron and another substance that is metabolized to bilirubin. The liver is then responsible for converting bilirubin to a water-soluble compound that can be excreted in bile. If the liver is unable to convert or conjugate bilirubin to a water-soluble compound or if bile drainage is obstructed, serum bilirubin is elevated and pigments are deposited in body tissues.

When serum bilirubin levels elevate, the patient's skin color changes to yellow. The yellow color varies from pale yellow to a striking golden orange. The color intensity is directly related to the amount of elevation of the serum bilirubin. Jaundice can be seen in nearly every body tissue and fluid where there is any amount of albumin (Box 32.5, *Cultural Considerations*). Pigment may occasionally be seen in cerebrospinal fluid or joint fluid. Pigment is not seen in saliva or tears. Urine becomes dark, and if bile flow to the bowel is obstructed, stools will be a light clay color. Describe any abnormal finding completely in the patient's record, and report your findings promptly.

The perianal and anal areas are inspected. Inspect the area for color, rashes, scars, fissures, external hemorrhoids, or skin breakdown. Describe any abnormal findings.

AUSCULTATION. When auscultating the patient's abdomen, the upper right quadrant is auscultated first (Fig. 32.5). Then a clockwise direction is followed to listen to the other quadrants. The stethoscope is pressed lightly on the abdomen to listen for bowel sounds, which are soft clicks and gurgles that may be heard every 5 to 15 seconds, occurring irregularly 5 to 30 times per minute. Bowel sounds at this rate are considered normal.

• WORD • BUILDING •

caput medusae: caput—head + medusae—Medusa's snaky locks
jaundice: jaune—yellow

Box 32.5

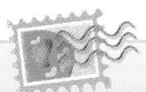

Cultural Considerations

The nurse should be aware of the variations among people of color when assessing for jaundice. To assess for jaundice in a patient with dark skin, look at the sclerae, conjunctivae, palms of hands, soles of feet, and in the buccal mucosa for patches of bilirubin pigment.

Bowel sounds are produced when peristalsis moves air and fluid through the GI tract, and they are categorized as normal, hyperactive, hypoactive, or absent. Hyperactive bowel sounds are usually rapid, high pitched, and loud and may occur with hunger or gastroenteritis. Hypoactive bowel sounds are bowel sounds that are infrequent and can occur in patients with a paralytic ileus or following abdominal surgery. Bowel sounds are considered absent if no sounds are auscultated after listening to all four quadrants for 2 to 5 minutes in each quadrant. However, this timing is an area for further research because, in practice, auscultation for this amount of time is rarely done. With a bowel obstruction, a high-pitched tinkling sound that is proximal to the obstruction and absent distal to the obstruction may be heard. Abnormal or absent bowel sounds are important findings and should be documented and reported to the physician.

Note the presence of any vascular sounds or bruits (swooshing sounds), which are normally not present, are heard with the stethoscope over the aorta. Patients with chronic liver failure may have a humming sound over their liver. This finding usually indicates overloaded venous circulation in the liver.

PERCUSSION. Percussion produces a sound that identifies the density of the organs beneath the area being percussed and is performed by the physician or advanced nurse practitioner. Percussion is used to detect fluid, air, and masses in the abdomen and to identify size and location of abdominal organs (especially the liver and spleen). Tympanic high-pitched sounds indicate the presence of air, and dull thuds indicate fluid or solid organs.

LEARNING TIP

In a complete bowel obstruction, air and fluid are propelled forward by peristalsis proximal to the obstruction. This produces proximal high-pitched bowel sounds when the air and fluid create turbulence as they hit the obstruction and are unable to pass. Absent bowel sounds are heard distal to the obstruction. If a patient has a nasogastric (NG) tube for suction, turn off the suction before listening for bowel sounds.

PALPATION. Light palpation of the abdomen concludes the physical assessment. If the patient is having pain, that area should be palpated last. Using the same quadrant approach as previously mentioned (see Fig. 32.5), lightly depress the abdomen not more than 0.5 to 1.0 inch during

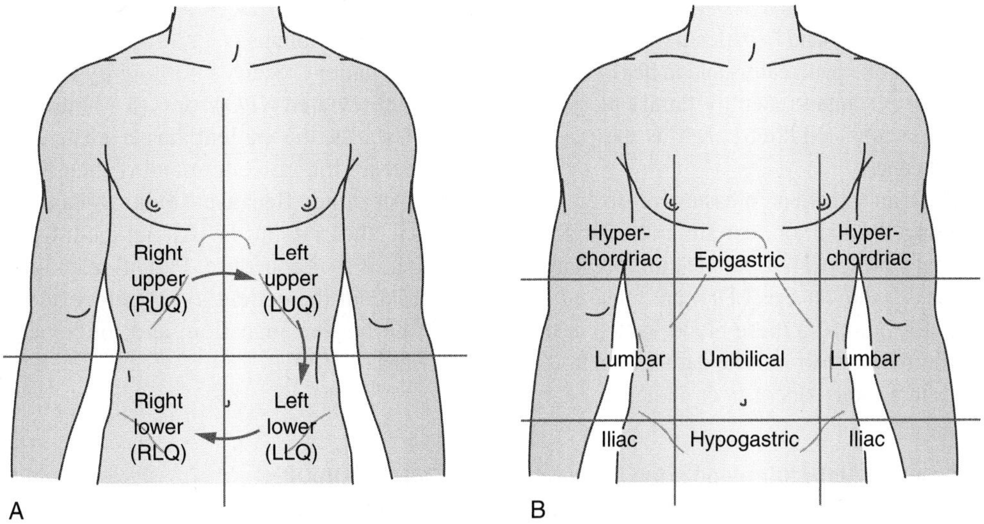
Right upper (RUQ)
Left upper (LUQ)
Right lower (RLQ)
Left lower (LLQ)
A
Hyper-chondriac
Epigastric
Hyper-chondriac
Lumbar
Umbilical
Lumbar
Iliac
Hypogastric
Iliac
B

FIGURE 32.5 (A) Abdominal quadrants are auscultated from the right upper quadrant in a clockwise manner. (B) Nine abdominal regions.

the palpation using the fingerpads. Note any muscle tension, rigidity, masses, or expressions of pain. Deep palpation of the abdomen is done only by physicians and highly skilled nurses such as nurse practitioners.

Abdominal girth is measured by placing a tape measure around the patient's abdomen at the iliac crest. A mark can be made at the measurement site so that measurements obtained by others are made at the same location for comparison. Abdominal girth is increased in patients with distention or conditions such as ascites (accumulation of fluid in the peritoneal cavity). When abdominal girth is abnormal, daily measurements should be obtained and recorded to monitor changes.

The advanced nurse practitioner or physician performs all other types of palpation. The liver is not normally palpable, but if enlarged, it may be felt below the right lower rib cage. Rebound tenderness is determined by pressing down on the abdomen a few inches and quickly releasing the pressure. If the patient feels a sharp pain during this procedure, appendicitis may be indicated.

DIAGNOSTIC STUDIES OF THE GASTROINTESTINAL, HEPATOBILIARY, AND PANCREATIC SYSTEMS

Use standard precautions when obtaining specimens of body fluids, substances, or blood. Practicing good hand hygiene before and after the procedure, wearing gloves, and using goggles (in case of splashing) are important.

Laboratory Tests

The complete blood cell count (CBC) reveals if anemia or infection is present (Tables 32.6 and 32.7). Anemia may occur with GI bleeding or cancer. Electrolyte imbalances often occur with GI illness as a result of vomiting, diarrhea, malabsorption, or use of GI suction. **Carcinoembryonic antigen** (CEA) and carbohydrate antigen 19-9 are markers used to monitor GI cancer treatment effectiveness and detect recurrence. These markers are also found in patients with cirrhosis, hepatic disease, and alcoholic pancreatitis and in heavy smokers. Genetic testing can be done to identify family members at risk of developing serious conditions such as the polyps associated with colon cancer.

Bilirubin level is an excellent measure of liver and gallbladder functioning. In addition, certain enzymes such as alanine aminotransferase (ALT), aspartate aminotransferase (AST), and lactic dehydrogenase (LDH) are released by damaged liver cells. Elevations in these blood values in the absence of known trauma or heart muscle damage such as a heart attack are excellent indicators of liver damage.

Stool Tests

Stool samples can be tested for **occult blood** (blood not seen by the naked eye). A series of three tests is usually done to increase the chances of detecting blood. False-positive occult blood results can occur with bleeding gums following a dental procedure; ingestion of red meat within 3 days before testing; ingestion of fish, turnips, or horseradish; and use of drugs, including anticoagulants, aspirin, colchicine, iron preparations in large doses, NSAIDs, and steroids.

Stool is collected to detect intestinal infections caused by parasites and their ova (eggs). The test usually requires a series of three stool specimens collected every second or third day. The stool specimen is collected using a tongue blade, placed in a container with a preservative, and sent immediately to the laboratory. The stool must be examined within 30 minutes of collection. False-negative results can occur as a result of urine in the specimen or if the specimen is not fresh.

Stool cultures (sterile collection technique) are done to determine the presence of pathogenic organisms in the GI tract. Stool can also be examined for lipids (fat). Excessive secretion of fecal fats (**steatorrhea**) may occur in various digestive and absorptive disorders. The stools are collected for 72 hours and stored on ice if necessary before being sent to the laboratory.

Radiographic Tests

Flat Plate of the Abdomen

A flat plate of the abdomen is an x-ray examination giving an anterior-to-posterior view (see Table 32.8). Radiographs visualize abdominal organs and can detect such abnormalities as tumors, obstructions, and strictures. For an x-ray examination, the patient should be dressed in a hospital gown and all metal such as zippers, belts, or jewelry should be removed. Pregnant patients or those thought to be pregnant should avoid x-ray examinations.

Upper Gastrointestinal Series (Barium Swallow)

An **upper gastrointestinal series** (UGI series) is an x-ray examination of the esophagus, stomach, duodenum, and jejunum using an oral liquid radiopaque contrast medium (barium) and a **fluoroscope** (an x-ray source and fluorescent screen that the patient is placed between) to outline the contours of the organs. A UGI series is used to detect such things as strictures, ulcers, tumors, polyps, hiatal hernias, and motility problems.

The patient receives nothing by mouth (*non per os* in Latin, abbreviated NPO) for 6 to 8 hours before the procedure. Usually the patient has a clear liquid supper the night before the procedure and is then NPO until the procedure is done. Because smoking can stimulate gastric motility, the patient is discouraged from smoking the morning of the procedure. Patient teaching includes information about the patient's diet before and after the procedure, the barium ingestion, and the appearance of stools afterward.

• WORD • BUILDING •

steatorrhea: steato—fat + rrhea—flow
fluoroscope: fluor—a flowing + skopeîn—to look at

TABLE 32.6 COMMON LABORATORY TESTS USED TO ASSESS GASTROINTESTINAL FUNCTION

Test	Definition	Normal Range	Significance of Abnormal Findings
Carcinoembryonic Antigen			
	Blood test to detect protein that is usually found in fetal gut tissue.	Less than 5 nanograms/mL (nonsmokers)	Increased values indicate possible colorectal cancer, other cancers, or inflammatory bowel disease.
Complete Blood Cell Count			
Red blood cell count	Blood test to determine size, shape, color, and intracellular structure of red blood cells.	*Women:* 4.2–5.2 million/mm^3 *Men:* 4.5–6.2 million/mm^3	Decreased values indicate possible anemia or hemorrhage.
Hemoglobin	Blood test to determine the amount of hemoglobin in circulation. Hemoglobin reflects oxygen-carrying capacity of blood.	*Women:* 12–16 g/dL *Men:* 14–18 g/dL	Increased values indicate possible hemoconcentration, caused by dehydration. Decreased levels can indicate anemia, hemorrhage, or hemodilution, as with cirrhosis.
Hematocrit	Measures the percentage of the total blood volume that is made up of RBCs.	*Women:* 38%–46% *Men:* 42%–54%	Same as hemoglobin.
Electrolytes			
Calcium	Blood test used to determine serum calcium level.	8.0–10.5 mg/dL	Decreased values indicate possible malabsorption.
Chloride	Blood test used to determine serum chloride level.	98–107 mEq/L	Decreased values indicate possible malabsorption.
Potassium	Blood test used to determine serum potassium level.	3.5–5.0 mEq/L	Decreased values indicate possible GI suction, diarrhea, vomiting, intestinal fistulas.
Sodium	Blood test used to determine serum sodium level.	135–145 mEq/L	Decreased values indicate possible malabsorption and diarrhea.
Fecal Analysis			
Stool for occult blood	Normally minimal quantities of blood are passed into the GI tract. Stool sample is taken to determine if blood is present in the stool.	Negative	Presence indicates possible peptic ulcer, cancer of the colon, ulcerative colitis.
Stool for ova and parasites	Stool sample to determine if pathogenic bacteria or parasites are present in the stool.	Negative	Presence indicates infection.
Stool cultures	Same as above.	No unusual growth	Presence of pathogens may indicate *Shigella, Salmonella, Staphylococcus aureus,* or *Bacillus cereus* infections.
Stool for lipids (fecal fat)	Test that measures the fat content in the stool. Used to confirm diagnosis of steatorrhea.	2–5 g per 24 hours (normal diet)	Increased values indicate possible malabsorption syndrome or Crohn's disease; increased in pancreatic disease.

TABLE 32.7 COMMON LABORATORY TESTS FOR HEPATOBILIARY AND PANCREATIC SYSTEMS DISORDERS

Test	Definition	Normal Range	Significance of Abnormal Findings
Blood			
Alanine aminotransferase (ALT)	Blood test to determine serum ALT levels. ALT is found mainly in the liver. With liver injury or disease, ALT is released into bloodstream.	5–35 international unit/dL	↑ in chronic liver failure and hepatitis
Albumin	Blood test to measure serum protein level.	3.1–4.3 g/dL	↓ in liver disease
Amylase	Blood test to determine serum level used to detect and monitor pancreatitis.	53–123 unit/L	↑ in pancreatitis, gallstones
Ammonia	Blood test to determine serum levels. Ammonia is a by-product of protein catabolism.	12–55 mol/L	↑ in chronic liver failure, hepatitis
Aspartate aminotransferase (AST)	Enzyme found in highly metabolic tissues such as the liver. AST is released into bloodstream when cells lyse.	8–20 unit/L	↑ in chronic liver failure, viral hepatitis, acute pancreatitis
Bilirubin	Serum blood test used to evaluate liver function.		
• Total serum bilirubin	Sum of the conjugated and unconjugated bilirubin.	0.1–1.0 mg/dL	↑ in liver and gallbladder disease with red blood cell destruction
• Conjugated (direct) bilirubin	Bilirubin that is conjugated in the liver (joined with glucuronide).	0.0–0.4 mg/dL	↑ with gallstones, gallbladder obstruction, extensive liver metastasis
• Unconjugated (indirect) bilirubin	Bilirubin in the bloodstream that has not yet passed through the liver.	0.1–1.0 mg/dL	↑ with red blood cell destruction or liver disease such as hepatitis or cirrhosis
Calcium	Blood test to determine serum level.	9–10.5 mg/dL	↓ with acute pancreatitis, liver disease, or malabsorption
Cholesterol	Blood test to determine serum level.	150–200 mg/dL	↑ in pancreatitis, gallbladder disease ↓ may indicate severe liver disease Patient should fast 12–14 hours before test.
Lactic dehydrogenase (LDH)	Blood test to determine level of this intracellular enzyme, which is released with injury or disease.	110–250 international unit/L	↑ in liver disease
Lipase	Blood test to determine serum levels to detect and monitor pancreatitis.	0–110 unit/L	↑ in acute pancreatitis. ↑ in acute cholecystitis.
Potassium	Blood test to determine serum levels. Major cation in the cell.	3.5–5.0 mEq/L	↓ with diarrhea, intestinal fistulas, vomiting, suctioning
Prothrombin time	Blood test used to determine adequacy of clotting mechanism. Used to monitor anticoagulation therapy with warfarin (Coumadin).	11–13.5 sec	↑ in liver disease, vitamin K deficiency
Urine amylase	Urinalysis examination used to assist in making diagnosis of pancreatitis.	Depends on test	↑ in acute pancreatitis
Urine bilirubin	Urinalysis exam used to measure predominantly conjugated bilirubin.	Negative	↑ in chronic liver failure, hepatitis, biliary obstruction. Used primarily for screening purposes.
Urobilinogen	Included in a routine urinalysis to support the diagnosis of hemolysis.	0.3–1.0 Ehrlich unit in 2 hr	↑ with destruction of red blood cells, hepatitis, chronic liver failure, obstructive jaundice

TABLE 32.8 DIAGNOSTIC PROCEDURES FOR THE GASTROINTESTINAL SYSTEM

Procedure	Definition/Normal Finding	Significance of Abnormal Findings	Nursing Management
Noninvasive			
Radiologic flat plate of abdomen	X-ray of abdomen showing an anterior to posterior view.	Stool or gas may be detected as with constipation or bowel obstruction.	No preparation needed.
Upper GI series	X-ray examination of esophagus, stomach, duodenum, and jejunum using oral liquid radiopaque contrast medium. Fluoroscope outlines contours of the organs. Normal finding should show normal anatomical structures.	Used to detect strictures, ulcers, tumors, polyps, hiatal hernias, and motility problems.	Clear liquid diet night before procedure. NPO for 6–8 hours before test. No smoking the morning of procedure. Provide increased fluids and laxative after procedure.
Lower GI series (barium enema)	Colon is filled with barium and x-rays taken to visualize position, movements, and filling of colon. Normal finding would be no polyps, inflammation, diverticula, stenosis, or tumors.	Tumors, diverticula, stenosis, obstructions, inflammation, ulcerative colitis, and polyps can be detected.	Patient is placed on low-residue or clear liquid diet for 2 days before test. Laxatives, bowel cleansing solutions, and enemas may be given the evening before the test. Bowel needs to be adequately cleaned for adequate visualization during the test. Encourage fluids and possibly laxatives to clear barium from colon.
Computed tomography (CT)	Uses a beam of radiation to allow three-dimensional visualization of abdominal structures. Diluted oral barium or other contrast media may be used to distinguish normal bowel from abnormal masses. Normal finding is no masses.	May show abnormal masses.	Clear liquid diet the morning of the test. If a contrast medium will be used, note allergies to contrast media. Consent form is needed. NPO for 2 to 4 hours before procedure.
Ultrasonography	High-frequency sound waves are passed through the abdomen to view soft-tissue structures.	Abnormal soft tissue structures.	NPO after midnight.
Invasive			
Nuclear scanning (cholescintigraphy, di-isopropyl iminodiacetic acid scintigraphy [DISIDA], hepatobiliary imino-diacetic acid [HIDA] scan, or iminodiacetic acid [IDA])	Involves injecting patient with a small amount of intravenous radioactive isotope. Serial images of gallbladder, bile duct, and duodenum are recorded. Normal finding is no evidence of biliary disease, obstruction, or ejection problems.	Confirms any biliary disease, ejection problem, or obstruction.	Fast for 2–6 hours before procedure. May be given cholecystokinin.
Angiography	Contrast medium is injected to identify abnormalities of vascular structure and function, observe masses, and note bleeding sites. A normal finding is no evidence of abnormal vasculature or masses.	Neoplasms of liver, gallbladder, or pancreas. May indicate abnormal vasculature.	Ask if allergies to contrast media or iodine. NPO for 2–8 hours before test. Stop medications that interfere with clotting about 1 week before exam. Assess for bleeding and hematoma formation after exam.
Endoscopy	Uses a tube and fiber-optic system (endoscope) or a capsule for observing the inside of a hollow organ or cavity. With endoscope, physician can remove polyps, take biopsy specimens, or coagulate bleeding sites.	Strictures, polyps, tumors, bleeding.	Consent form is signed for endoscope procedure.

Continued

TABLE 32.8 DIAGNOSTIC PROCEDURES FOR THE GASTROINTESTINAL SYSTEM—cont'd

Procedure	Definition/Normal Finding	Significance of Abnormal Findings	Nursing Management
Esophagogastroduodenoscopy (EGD)	Endoscopy that visualizes esophagus, stomach, and duodenum. Biopsy or cytology specimens can be obtained. Normal findings indicate all normal structures without inflammation, bleeding, or cancer.	Abnormalities such as inflammation, cancer, bleeding, injury, and infection can be detected.	See endoscopy. May use a preoperative checklist. NPO for 8–12 hours. May need to premedicate to relax patient. Monitor vital signs and prevent aspiration after procedure. Monitor for pain, bleeding, fever, and dysphagia after procedure.
Endoscopic retrograde cholangiopancreatography (ERCP)	Endoscopy that permits physician to visualize liver, gallbladder, and pancreas. May use contrast medium. Endoscope is passed through esophagus to duodenum, where dye is injected that outlines pancreatic and bile ducts. Normal findings indicate all normal structures without inflammation, bleeding, or cancer.	Liver, gallbladder, or pancreas disease.	See endoscopy and EGD. NPO after 8 p.m. the night before exam. Check prothrombin time before procedure. Monitor for pain, fever, chills, which could indicate infection. Monitor for onset of pancreatitis.
Proctosigmoidoscopy	Examination of distal sigmoid colon, rectum, and anal canal using a rigid or flexible endoscope (sigmoidoscope). Normal finding would be no ulcerations, punctures, laceration, tumors, hemorrhoids, polyps, fissures, or fistulas.	Ulcerations, punctures, lacerations, tumors, hemorrhoids, polyps, fissures, fistulas, early malignancies, and abscesses can be detected.	Clear liquid diet for 24 hours before exam. Laxative the night before exam. Enemas the morning of exam.
Colonoscopy	Visualization of lining of the large intestine to identify abnormalities through a flexible endoscope, inserted rectally. Biopsy specimen may be obtained or polyps removed. Normal finding would show a normal colon without signs of inflammation, ulcers, polyps, or cancer.	Colon cancer, polyps, inflammation.	Clear liquid diet for 24 hours before exam. Bowel preparation the night before exam. Possibly enemas the evening before exam and morning of exam. Patient will receive conscious sedation during exam. Monitor for complications, such as hemorrhage and severe pain. Explain that cramping may last several hours after test, and blood may be present in stool if specimen was taken.
Endoscopic ultrasonography	Performed with endoscope using sound waves.	Tumors in various GI structures and organs.	Similar to endoscopy.
Analysis • Basal cell secretion test	Measures secretions in the stomach. For basal cell secretion test, nasogastric tube is inserted and contents of stomach suctioned out through tube using a syringe. Stomach contents are collected at intervals.	Diagnosis of duodenal ulcer, gastric carcinoma, pyloric or duodenal obstruction, and pernicious anemia are made.	Patient should avoid drugs that could interfere with gastric acid secretion, such as cholinergics and antacids. Patient is NPO after midnight the night before test.
• Gastric acid stimulation test	Measures amount of gastric acid for 1 hour after subcutaneous injection of a histamine.		

TABLE 32.8 DIAGNOSTIC PROCEDURES FOR THE GASTROINTESTINAL SYSTEM—cont'd

Procedure	Definition/Normal Finding	Significance of Abnormal Findings	Nursing Management
• Percutaneous liver biopsy	Usually a needle inserted through skin and into liver to withdraw a small sample for examination. Normal finding would be negative for cancer, cirrhosis, hepatitis, or other liver diseases.	May identify cancer, cirrhosis, hepatitis, or other causes of liver disease.	Signed consent needed. Ensure laboratory tests such as CBC and coagulation studies have been ordered and reviewed. NPO for 6–8 hours before procedure. Rest for several hours after procedure; restricted activity 1 day. Monitor biopsy site pressure dressing for bleeding. Monitor vital signs after procedure. Coughing and straining avoided after the procedure. Medicate for pain.

During the procedure, the patient drinks thick, chalky barium while standing in front of a fluoroscopic tube. X-ray films are taken in various positions and at specific intervals to visualize the outline of the organs and to note the passage of the barium through the GI tract. The patient should understand that the procedure may take several hours depending on the rate at which the barium moves through the patient's gastrointestinal tract.

A laxative is usually ordered after the procedure to expel the barium and prevent constipation or a barium **impaction** (impassable mass of stone-like feces). The patient is instructed to drink 12 eight-oz glasses of water per day for several days to prevent dehydration, which can lead to constipation. The abdomen is assessed for distention and bowel sounds. The stool is monitored to determine whether the barium has been completely eliminated. Initially, the barium causes the patient's stool to be white, but it should return to its normal color within 3 days. Constipation with distention indicates a barium impaction.

Lower Gastrointestinal Series

The **lower gastrointestinal series** (barium enema) is performed to visualize the position, movements, and filling of the colon. Tumors, diverticula, stenosis, obstructions, inflammation, ulcerative colitis, and polyps can be detected. The patient is placed on a low-residue or clear liquid diet for 2 days before the test to empty the bowel. Laxatives, bowel-cleansing solutions (such as GoLYTELY), and enemas may be administered the evening before the test. GoLYTELY is chilled and drunk full strength with no ice, 8 oz every 10 minutes for a total of 4 L. Drinking this solution can be unpleasant for the patient. Inform the patient that a watery diarrhea will begin in about 1 hour and continue for up to 5 hours as the bowel is cleared. This is necessary for adequate visualization during the procedure. Inadequate bowel preparation may result in poor test results or test cancellation (Fig. 32.6). The patient either receives a clear liquid diet the morning of the test or is NPO after midnight the night before. The area around the rectum should be clean before the patient is sent for the procedure. If the patient has active inflammatory disease of the colon or suspected perforation or obstruction, a barium enema is contraindicated. Active GI bleeding may also prohibit the use of laxatives and enemas.

During the procedure, barium is instilled rectally and x-ray films are taken with or without fluoroscopy. The patient may experience some abdominal cramping and an urge to have a bowel movement during the procedure. The patient is told to take slow, deep breaths and to tighten the anal sphincter. The rate of flow of the barium is slowed until the cramping diminishes. The procedure takes about 15 minutes, and the patient is allowed to use the bathroom immediately after the procedure.

The patient's stools are monitored after the procedure to note if all the barium is passed, as with the UGI series. Constipation development is monitored. The patient is encouraged to drink at least one 8-oz glass of liquid per hour for the next 24 waking hours to help remove the barium. Laxatives may be ordered to help clear the barium from the colon. The patient is told to report any abdominal pain, bloating, or absence of stool, all of which could indicate constipation or bowel obstruction, as well as any rectal bleeding.

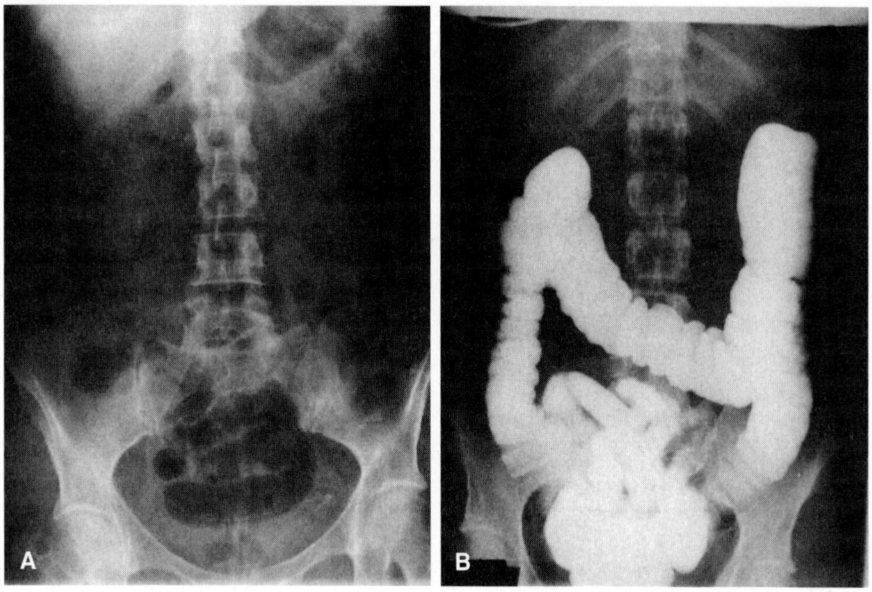
A
B

FIGURE 32.6 (A) An image of a patient who was poorly prepared for a barium enema. (B) An image of a patient who was adequately prepared for a barium enema. (Courtesy Dr. Russell Tobe.)

CRITICAL THINKING

Mrs. Pearl

■ Mrs. Pearl is a 95-year-old woman undergoing a lower GI series for abdominal pain. As her nurse, what concerns might you have for Mrs. Pearl as she undergoes this test? How can you address them?
Suggested answers at end of chapter.

Computed Tomography

Computed tomography (CT) uses a beam of radiation to allow three-dimensional visualization of abdominal structures. Diluted oral barium or other contrast media may be used to distinguish normal bowel from abnormal masses. The patient may have a clear liquid diet the morning of the test. If a contrast medium is to be used, any allergies to iodine or contrast media are noted, a consent form is signed, and the patient is NPO for 2 to 4 hours before the procedure.

CT colography is a CT scan of the abdomen or colon. It does not require sedation but has the same prep as a colonoscopy. It diagnoses many major problems of the colon and is used for those who have a higher risk with invasive procedures.

Nuclear Scanning

Nuclear scanning involves injecting a patient with a small amount of radioactive isotope. The scan may be called a cholescintigraphic, DISIDA, HIDA, or IDA scan, depending on the radioactive isotope and exact procedure that is used. Prior to the procedure, the patient fasts and does not chew gum for at least 2 to 6 hours. After the injection, the isotope is secreted into the bile and goes anywhere the bile goes. Visualization of these areas occurs about 60 minutes after the IV injection. The scanning camera (like a Geiger counter) traces the path of the isotope as it travels through the bile ducts, gallbladder, and intestines. Serial images are recorded. A patient may be given a fatty meal or cholecystokinin to stimulate emptying of the gallbladder. Any biliary disease, ejection problem, or obstruction can be confirmed with this examination. The test takes about 2 hours.

Angiography

Angiography may be ordered for patients with symptoms of arterial occlusive disease of the hepatic, biliary, and pancreatic arterial vessels. This test is used to evaluate suspected neoplasms in these organs. Medications that might cause bleeding, such as aspirin, NSAIDs, or anticoagulants, are stopped per physician order about 1 week prior to the procedure. A contrast medium is injected to identify abnormalities of vascular structure and function and masses and to show bleeding sites. Prior to the procedure, the patient usually is NPO for 2 to 8 hours. The injection of contrast medium is done about 1 hour before the examination. Radiographs are taken about every 20 minutes for 1 hour or until the structures are readily viewed. The radiopaque material is iodine based, so ask the patient about any allergies to iodine. Following the procedure, observe for bleeding at the puncture site. Patients with liver disease may have clotting disorders and should be assessed for bleeding or hematomas at the site. Monitor pulses distal to the insertion site.

Liver Scan

A liver scan involves injecting a slightly radioactive medium that is taken up by the liver. An instrument is passed over the liver that records the amount of material taken up by the liver and forms a composite "picture" of the liver. The physician may be able to determine tumors, masses, and abnormal size and patterns of blood vessels. The procedure takes a short time.

Endoscopy

Endoscopy uses a tube and a fiber-optic system (endoscope) or a tiny capsule for observing the inside of a hollow organ or cavity. In addition to viewing the structures with the endoscope, the physician can also remove polyps, take biopsy specimens, or coagulate bleeding sites that are identified. A consent form must be signed for any endoscope procedure.

Esophagogastroduodenoscopy

Esophagogastroduodenoscopy (EGD) visualizes the esophagus (**esophagoscopy**), the stomach (**gastroscopy**), and the duodenum. Abnormalities such as inflammation, cancer, bleeding, injury, and infection can be seen.

The procedure is explained to the patient. Because this is an invasive procedure, patients may be asked to sign an operative consent form, and a preoperative checklist may be necessary, depending on institution policy. To prevent aspiration of stomach contents into the lungs if vomiting occurs, the patient is NPO for 8 to 12 hours before the procedure. Sedatives such as diazepam (Valium) or midazolam (Versed) may be given before the procedure to help relax the patient. The patient may be given atropine sulfate to dry secretions in the mouth. A local anesthetic in spray or gargle form is administered just before the scope is inserted to inhibit the gag reflex.

The patient is placed on the left side, and the flexible fiber-optic endoscope tube is passed orally down the GI tract (Fig. 32.7). Photographs or videotapes of the procedure can be made. Biopsy or cytology specimens can be obtained.

After the procedure, vital signs are checked as ordered. Patients are placed on one side to prevent aspiration while sedation and the local anesthetic wear off. Patients are NPO until the gag reflex returns (usually within 4 hours). Patients are assessed for signs of perforation, which include bleeding, fever, and dysphagia. Midesophageal perforation can cause referred substernal or epigastric pain. Blood loss secondary to perforation can lead to hematoma formation, which in turn can result in cyanosis and referred back pain. Distal esophageal perforation may result in shoulder pain, dyspnea, or symptoms similar to those of a perforated ulcer. The patient may have a sore throat for a few days.

Capsule endoscopy makes use of a capsule with a microchip in it that is swallowed. As the capsule moves through the GI tract, pictures are taken along the way of the stomach and small intestine to diagnose conditions such as bleeding, tumors, or Crohn's disease. It is most helpful in the small intestine, which is difficult to scope due to its length and twists. Advances in this technology are focusing on the power supply and performing treatments as with an endoscope.

Endoscopic Retrograde Cholangiopancreatography

Endoscopic **retrograde cholangiopancreatography** (ERCP) permits the physician to visualize the liver, gallbladder, and pancreas (Fig. 32.8). The procedure allows both direct viewing and use of contrast medium. An endoscope is passed through the esophagus to the duodenum, where dye is injected that outlines the pancreatic and bile ducts.

The patient is prepared for an ERCP in the same manner as for an EGD, with nothing by mouth after 8 p.m. the night before the examination. In addition, the patient is asked about allergies to iodine. Ensure that any ordered laboratory studies, such as a prothrombin time, have been done before the procedure and that the patient has removed dentures. Follow-up care is similar to that for an EGD. In addition, the nurse is alert to patient reports of increased right upper quadrant pain, fever, or chills, which may indicate infection. Hypotension, tachycardia or rapid heart rate, increasing RUQ pain, nausea, or vomiting may indicate perforation or the onset of pancreatitis. Report such findings immediately.

Lower Gastrointestinal Endoscopy

PROCTOSIGMOIDOSCOPY. Proctosigmoidoscopy is the examination of the distal sigmoid colon, the rectum, and the anal canal using a flexible endoscope (sigmoidoscope). Ulcerations, punctures, lacerations, tumors, hemorrhoids,

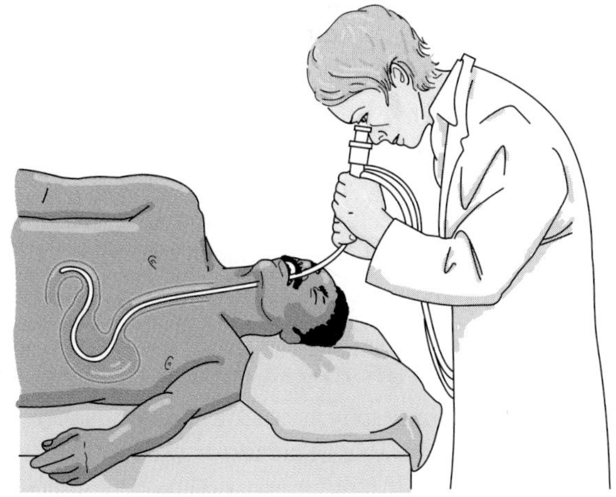

FIGURE 32.7 Gastroscopy.

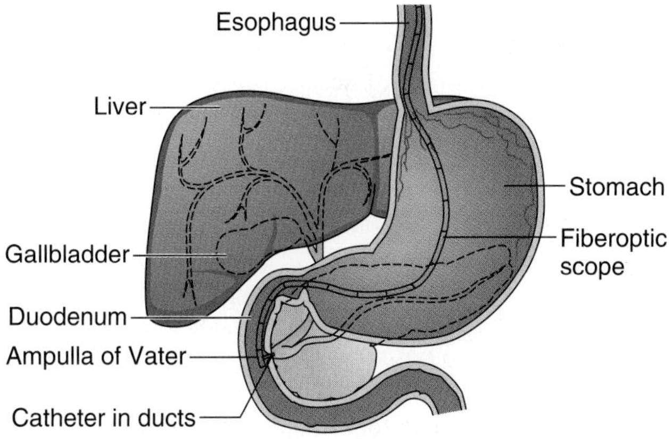
Esophagus
Liver
Stomach
Fiberoptic scope
Gallbladder
Duodenum
Ampulla of Vater
Catheter in ducts

FIGURE 32.8 Endoscopic retrograde cholangiopancreatography. (Modified from Watson, J., & Jaffe, S. [1995]. *Nurse's manual of laboratory and diagnostic tests* [2nd ed., p. 525]. Philadelphia: F. A. Davis, with permission.)

polyps, fissures, fistulas, and abscesses can be detected. Malignancies at an early stage can be detected, so an examination for patients age 50 and older is recommended every 5 years.

Proctosigmoidoscopy requires the lower bowel to be cleaned out. The patient usually receives a clear liquid diet 24 hours before the test and a laxative the night before the test. The morning of the procedure a warm tap-water enema or sodium biphosphate (Fleet) enema may be given. Bowel preparation may not be ordered for patients with bleeding or severe diarrhea.

The patient is positioned in a left lateral knee-to-chest position, which allows the sigmoid colon to straighten by gravity. A rigid proctoscope is used to visualize the rectum. A flexible scope is then used to permit visualization above the rectosigmoid junction. Patients are told they may feel pressure as though they are going to have a bowel movement. During the procedure, one or more small pieces of intestinal tissue may be removed (biopsy specimens). Rectal or sigmoid polyps are removed with a snare. An electrocoagulating current is used to cauterize sites to prevent or stop bleeding. Specimens are labeled and sent to the pathology laboratory immediately for examination.

After the procedure, the patient is allowed to rest for a few minutes in the supine position to avoid orthostatic hypotension when standing. Pain and flatus may occur from instilled air. The patient is observed for signs of perforation such as bleeding, pain, and fever.

COLONOSCOPY. Colonoscopy provides visualization of the lining of the large intestine to identify abnormalities through a flexible endoscope, which is inserted rectally. A biopsy specimen may be obtained or polyps removed during the colonoscopy.

The patient receives a clear liquid diet 24 hours before the test and is NPO after midnight before the procedure. A bowel preparation solution is given the night before the procedure such as a laxative, suppository (bisacodyl [Dulcolax]), or enema.

> **SAFETY TIP**
>
> Older patients may experience fatigue and weakness during bowel preparation and may be unable to complete it. Monitor the patient for distress. Consult the physician if you note any patient distress during bowel preparation. Observe the patient often because defecation urgency, especially in unfamiliar surroundings, may create a fall risk.

Conscious sedation, for example, midazolam (Versed), is used to relax and ease pain during the procedure. The patient is positioned on the left side with the knees bent. A small amount of air is instilled into the colon to help the physician visualize the bowel. The air causes pressure and may be uncomfortable for the patient. The patient is encouraged to relax and take slow deep breaths through the nose and out the mouth. Vital signs are monitored throughout the procedure to watch for a vasovagal response, which can lead to hypotension and bradycardia.

After the procedure, the patient is monitored until stable. Complications such as hemorrhage or severe pain are reported. When giving the patient discharge instructions, explain that flatus and cramping will occur for several hours after the test, that blood may be present in the stool if a biopsy specimen was taken, and to report problems to the physician.

Gastric Analysis

Gastric analysis measures the secretions in the stomach. Diagnoses of duodenal ulcer, gastric carcinoma, pyloric or duodenal obstruction, and pernicious anemia are made with this test. A diagnosis of pernicious anemia is ruled out by the finding of acid. A diagnosis of gastric carcinoma may be made by the presence of cancer cells in the gastric secretions. The two gastric analysis tests performed are the **basal cell secretion test** and the **gastric acid stimulation test**.

Before the basal cell secretion test, the patient should avoid taking any drugs that could interfere with gastric acid secretion, such as cholinergics and antacids. The patient is NPO after midnight the night before the test. For the procedure, a nasogastric (NG) tube is inserted and the contents of the stomach are suctioned out through the tube using a syringe. The NG tube is connected to wall suction, and stomach contents are collected every 15 minutes for 1 hour. The specimens are labeled according to the time they were collected and the order in which they were obtained. The gastric acid is tested for pH using indicator paper or a pH meter. The amount of gastric acid is also measured. Too much hydrochloric acid may indicate a peptic ulcer; too little could be a sign of cancer or pernicious anemia.

The gastric acid stimulation test measures the amount of gastric acid for 1 hour after subcutaneous injection of a histamine drug. If abnormal results occur, radiographic tests or endoscopy can be done to determine the cause.

Ultrasonography

In ultrasonography, high-frequency sound waves travel through the abdomen to allow the physician to view soft-tissue structures. The sound waves reflect varying images based on the density of the soft tissues in the abdomen. The patient is NPO after midnight the night before the test. A clear gel is applied to the abdomen and to the transducer on the sonograph. The gel improves the conduction of sound waves and thus improves the images obtained. The transducer is placed on the skin and moved over the abdomen while the technician views the sonograph screen and takes periodic pictures. The procedure takes about half an hour and requires no follow-up care.

Endoscopic Ultrasonography

Endoscopic ultrasonography is performed through an endoscope using sound waves. This test is used to detect tumors in various GI structures and organs. Preprocedure and postprocedure care are similar to those for endoscopic care. During the test the patient must lie still while a transducer with gel is moved back and forth over the abdomen to produce images.

Percutaneous Liver Biopsy

If less invasive tests do not aid in diagnosis of liver disease, a liver biopsy can be done. This type of biopsy can identify cancer, cirrhosis, hepatitis, or other causes of liver disease. The physician generally inserts a needle through the skin and into the liver to withdraw a small sample for examination. This procedure places the patient at risk for bleeding because the liver is highly vascular and because many patients with liver disease have reduced clotting ability.

Before the biopsy, ensure that the patient understands the procedure and that a consent has been signed if required by institution policy. You should also ensure that laboratory tests, such as a complete blood cell count and coagulation studies, have been completed and reviewed as ordered. The patient may be ordered NPO for 6 to 8 hours before the procedure. Baseline vital signs are taken, and a sedative is given if ordered.

During the procedure the nurse assists the physician to position the patient on his or her back or left side and assists the patient to hold very still while the needle is being introduced. The physician may also ask the patient to exhale and hold his or her breath during the needle insertion.

After the biopsy, the patient should remain on bedrest for 24 hours. The patient lies on the right side for the first 2 hours with a small pillow or rolled towel under the biopsy site to provide pressure and prevent bleeding. Vital signs and the site are monitored for signs of bleeding. The patient is advised to avoid coughing or straining. Analgesics are offered for comfort if ordered.

> **CRITICAL THINKING**
>
> ***Mr. Wozynski***
>
> ■ Mr. Wozynski is admitted with chronic liver failure and jaundice. What specific laboratory value can you expect to be elevated related to his jaundice? Mr. Wozynski's physician orders a liver biopsy. Why is it important for you to check Mr. Wozynski's laboratory reports before the procedure?
>
> *Suggested answers at end of chapter.*

THERAPEUTIC MEASURES FOR THE GASTROINTESTINAL, HEPATOBILIARY, AND PANCREATIC SYSTEMS

Gastrointestinal Intubation

Gastrointestinal intubation is the placement of a tube within the GI tract for therapeutic or diagnostic purposes (Fig. 32.9). When the GI tube is inserted orally into the stomach it is an orogastric tube. When it goes from the nares into the stomach, it is referred to as a nasogastric tube. A variety of tubes are available, each designed for specific purposes (Table 32.9). Orogastric tubes reduce sinus infection risk because they do not block normal drainage of the sinuses as can nasal tubes. Nasogastric tubes are inserted for a variety of reasons:

- To remove gas and fluids from the stomach (decompression)
- To diagnose GI motility and to obtain gastric secretions for analysis
- To relieve and treat obstructions or bleeding within the GI tract
- To provide a means for nutrition (**gavage** feeding), hydration, and medication when the oral route is not possible or is contraindicated
- To promote healing after esophageal, gastric, or intestinal surgery by preventing distention of the GI tract and strain on the suture lines
- To remove toxic substances (**lavage**) that have been ingested either accidentally or intentionally and to provide for irrigation.

Feeding tubes include nasogastric, esophagostomy, **gastrostomy**, or jejunostomy tubes (see Fig. 32.9). Nasogastric tubes are usually temporary and short term. Esophagostomy, gastrostomy, or jejunostomy tubes are generally used for longer term nutrition delivery.

Provide emotional support and explanations to the patient and significant others to facilitate the process of tube insertion and maintenance. Assessing tube placement is essential to prevent complications or death from incorrect tube placement. Nasogastric tube placement must be assessed after insertion and then intermittently to ensure that it is in the correct position and not in the lungs (most common), esophagus, pleural space, or brain. Box 32.6 lists the nursing care steps for insertion and maintenance of nasogastric tubes.

Gastrostomy or jejunostomy tube placement is verified by comparing current exposed length with documented exposed length at insertion. The tube may not be in the desired position if the current and insertion exposed tube lengths are different, so the physician should be consulted before using the tube.

Tube Feeding

A tube feeding supplies patients with nutrition when oral intake is not possible. Feedings can be given to the patient as a supplement or to provide the patient's total nutritional needs. If the esophagus and stomach need to be bypassed, tube feedings are delivered directly into the duodenum or proximal jejunum. Reasons for administering tube feedings include inability to swallow, severe burns or trauma to the face or jaw, debilitation, mental retardation, and oropharyngeal or esophageal paralysis. Research shows that patients may benefit from either oral or tube feeding within 24 hours postoperatively from GI surgery (see *Evidence-Based Practice box*). Complications associated with tube feeding are presented in Table 32.10.

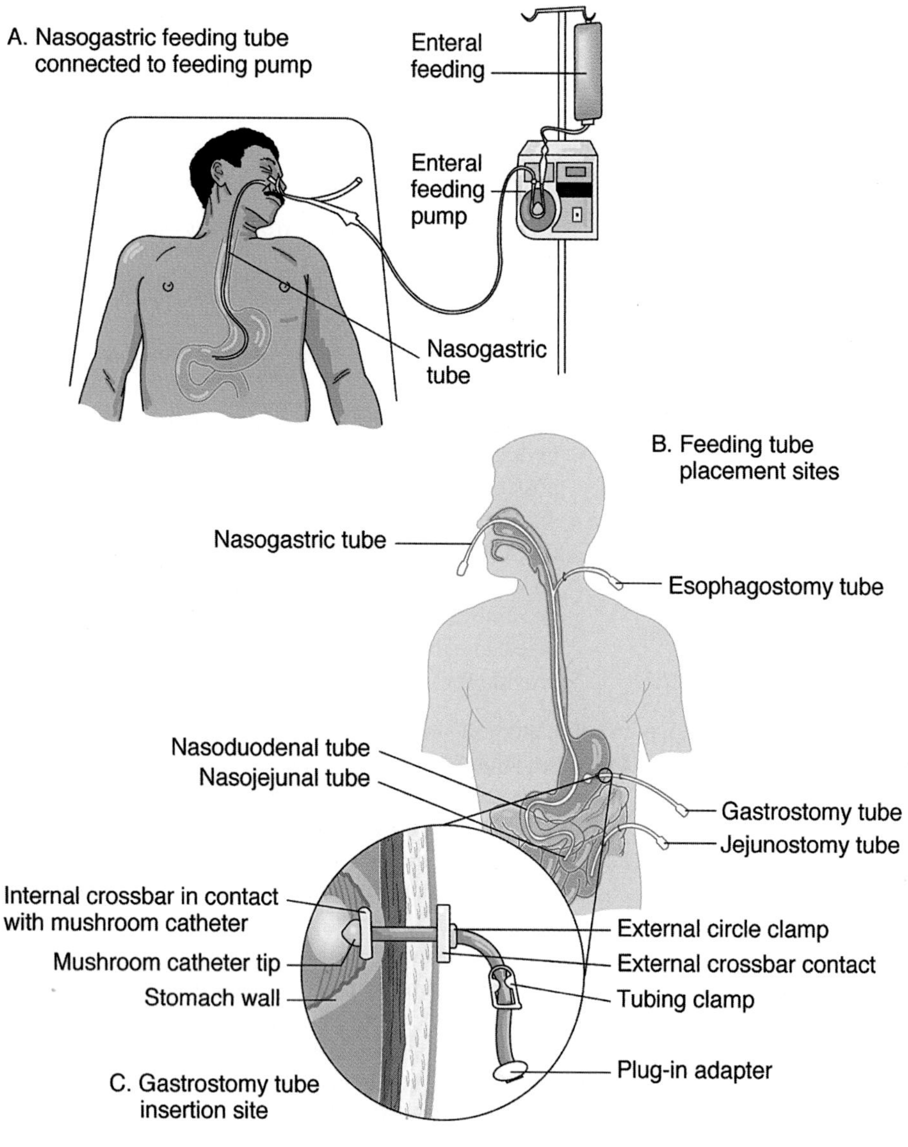
A. Nasogastric feeding tube connected to feeding pump
Enteral feeding
Enteral feeding pump
Nasogastric tube
B. Feeding tube placement sites
Nasogastric tube
Esophagostomy tube
Nasoduodenal tube
Nasojejunal tube
Gastrostomy tube
Jejunostomy tube
Internal crossbar in contact with mushroom catheter
Mushroom catheter tip
Stomach wall
C. Gastrostomy tube insertion site
External circle clamp
External crossbar contact
Tubing clamp
Plug-in adapter

FIGURE 32.9 Feeding tubes. (A) Nasogastric tube connected to tube feeding pump. (B) Feeding tube placement sites (esophagostomy, nasointestinal, gastrostomy, and jejunostomy). (C) Gastrostomy tube insertion site.

TABLE 32.9 GASTRIC TUBES

Tube	Uses and Description	Nursing Considerations
Levin tube	Single lumen. May be used for gastric decompression, irrigation, lavage, and feeding.	Tube is not vented. Avoid use with continuous suction to prevent injury to stomach lining.
Salem sump tube	Double lumen, "pigtail" acts as an air vent and prevents excess suction, which could damage stomach lining. Air vent must not be plugged off. Used for decompression, irrigations, and lavage.	May be used with continuous suction because of air vent.
Weighted, flexible feeding tubes with stylets	Small-bore tube for tube feeding only. Less injury. Remains in place for extended periods.	Suction collapses tube. Use 10-mL syringe or greater because smaller syringe creates too much pressure, possible rupture of tube. Inject 30 mL of air with a 60-mL syringe immediately before withdrawing fluid to make it easier to withdraw.

Box 32.6

Nursing Care for Insertion and Maintenance of Nasogastric Tubes

1. Explain the procedure and reason for the tube to the patient. Explain how the patient can help by swallowing when instructed to do so, if able.
2. Assist patient into high Fowler's position (right side-lying as an alternative) as able.
3. Measure tube for correct insertion length:
   - Hold insertion end of tube from nose tip to earlobe to xiphoid process.
   - Mark tube with tape at this point.
4. Select naris that is straightest and from which patient breaths easiest, because tube is inserted more easily in a straight naris.
5. Lubricate tube with water-soluble lubricant before insertion.
6. Insert tube as follows:
   - As tube is inserted, aim it along the floor of the naris and laterally. Rotate tube gently if resistance is met.
   - Encourage patient to swallow to advance the tube. Drinking water with a straw or ice chips facilitates the swallowing process, if patient is able.
   - If patient is unconscious, flex patient's head to bring chin toward chest to help prevent tube from passing into the trachea.
   - Observe for coiling of the tube in patient's mouth.
   - To assist in assessing correct placement, insert tube to level of carina tracheae and listen for air at end of tube. If air is present, remove tube. If no air is heard, advance tube to stomach.
   - If at any time the patient begins to cough uncontrollably, becomes cyanotic, or begins to have any respiratory distress, remove the tube, allow rest time, and then reattempt insertion.
7. After tube is inserted to premeasured length, confirm gastric placement per institutional policy with the following methods:
   - Flexible feeding tubes need x-ray confirmation.
   - Document length of exposed tube from tube end to naris for ongoing verification of placement.
   - Aspirate for gastric contents with a 30- or 60-mL catheter-tipped syringe:
     - Gastric fluid—green with sediment; colorless and clear with off-white or tan mucus; brown if digested blood is present.
     - Esophageal contents—scant fluid, aspirate is unreliable for confirmation.
     - Intestinal fluid—light to dark golden yellow to brownish green.
     - Lung secretions—off-white or tan mucus.
     - Pleural fluid (with stylet perforation)—watery, straw colored, may be blood-tinged from perforation.
   - For fasting patients, can measure pH of secretions to rule out lung or small bowel placement:
     - Gastric pH range is acidic (1–5).
     - Lung and intestinal secretions are alkaline with pH greater than 6.
   - If any doubts about gastric placement exist, notify physician for x-ray order to confirm tube placement.
   - Do not use auscultation of an air bolus to verify placement because it is not a reliable or safe practice.
8. Secure tube in place with tape so that pressure is not put on the naris. Provide daily skin care to taped area to prevent skin breakdown. Slipknot a rubber band around tube and pin rubber band to patient's gown.
9. If suction is ordered, low intermittent suction is used with nonvented tubes (Levin); vented tubes (Salem) may have continuous low suction.
10. If patient is NPO, provide frequent care to keep oral mucous membranes moist (do not use lemon/glycerin swabs because they damage tooth enamel and are drying when a moist oral cavity is needed to remain healthy). When suction is used, prevent excessive intake of ice chips, if ordered, because electrolyte imbalances may result when water is suctioned out along with electrolytes. Normal saline solution instead of water can be made into ice chips to help prevent imbalances.
11. Gastric placement is periodically confirmed, especially before instilling anything into the tube:
    - Review any recent chest or abdominal x-ray report with tube status.
    - Measure exposed tube from end of tube to naris and compare to original insertion measurement to verify tube has not moved from original position. If it has, do not use the tube until repositioned or confirmation of placement has been verified.
    - Bolus feeding/medications—4 hours after last feeding, verify tube measurement.
    - Continuous feeding—note tolerance. If tolerating, along with verified tube measurement and any confirming x-ray reports, continue feeding.
    - For patients at high risk of dislodgement or tube movement (e.g., those who are vomiting or have severe coughing), consider x-ray examination.
12. The tube is flushed at intervals, every 2 to 4 hours, to maintain patency. When tube feedings are administered, residual feeding amounts are checked at specified intervals (hourly when begun, every 4 hours thereafter) to ensure feeding is being absorbed.
13. With a nasogastric tube, record accurate intake and output, including tube feeding, irrigation solution instilled (use normal saline solution to prevent electrolyte imbalance), and drainage or vomitus.

EVIDENCE-BASED PRACTICE

Clinical Question

Does early (24-hour) postoperative enteral nutrition result in fewer complications in patients undergoing gastrointestinal surgery?

Evidence

Thirteen randomized controlled trials, with a total of 1173 patients, compared early feeding within 24 hours postoperatively with no feeding in patients undergoing gastrointestinal surgery (Andersen, Lewis, & Thomas, 2006). Effects indicate that earlier feeding may reduce the risk of postsurgical complications, although the results were not statistically significant. There does not appear to be an advantage to keeping patients NPO postoperatively until bowel function returns.

Implications for Nursing Practice

If ordered, nutrition can be provided to patients early after gastrointestinal surgery, which may improve their recovery with fewer complications.

REFERENCE

Andersen, H. K., Lewis, S. J., & Thomas, S. (2006). Early enteral nutrition within 24h of colorectal surgery versus later commencement of feeding for postoperative complications. *Cochrane Database of Systematic Reviews 2006, Issue 4* (Art. No. CD004080; DOI 10.1002/14651858.CD004080.pub2).

Tube Feeding Formulas

Tube feeding formulas are chosen by the physician based on the patient's nutritional needs, the consistency of the formula, the size and location of the tube, the method of delivery, and the convenience for the patient at home. Commercially prepared formulas are composed of protein, carbohydrates, and fats. When patients receive tube feeding, their daily water needs in addition to any water supplied by the feeding should be considered. Dietitians can help calculate the patient's water needs. The water used to flush the tube or administer medications can be considered as satisfying part of the patient's daily total water needs. Dehydration can occur if the patient's water needs are not met.

Method of Feeding Delivery

Feedings are administered either by gravity or by a controlled pump that delivers continuous volume through the feeding tube. Gravity feedings are placed above the level of the stomach and dripped in by gravity slowly or given as a bolus feeding over a few minutes. Intermittent feedings are defined as either being delivered by a pump that runs continuously throughout the day and is discontinued each night or as a 4- to 6-hour volume of feeding given over 20 to 30 minutes. Intermittent feedings via a pump allow the stomach to rest at night and more closely simulate normal eating and nutrient absorption patterns. A continuous feeding administered 24 hours a day through a pump allows for small amounts to be given over a long period. Pumps are set at the specified rate to control the speed of the feeding being delivered to the patient.

TABLE 32.10 COMMON MECHANICAL, GASTROINTESTINAL, AND METABOLIC COMPLICATIONS OF TUBE-FED PATIENTS AND PREVENTION STRATEGIES

Complication	Prevention Strategies
Mechanical	
Tube irritation	Consider oral tubes and avoid nasal tubes due to sinus infection risk. Oral tubes also help prevent ventilator-associated pneumonia.
	Consider using a smaller or softer tube.
	Lubricate tube before insertion.
	Make sure tube is secured in place.
Tube obstruction	Flush tube after use.
	Do not mix medications with tube-feeding formula.
	Use liquid medications if available.
	Crush other medications thoroughly (if not contraindicated).
	Use infusion pump to maintain constant flow (see Fig. 32.9).
Aspiration and regurgitation	Feeding should not be started until tube placement is radiographically confirmed.
	Avoid use of blue dye to detect aspiration because it has not been shown predictive and dye can be absorbed in critically ill patients, who then turn blue and can die.
	Elevate head of patient's bed 30 degrees or more at all times.
	Discontinue feeding at least 30–60 minutes before treatments requiring head to be lowered (e.g., chest percussion).
	If patient has an endotracheal tube in place, keep cuff inflated during feeding.
Tube displacement	Place a black mark at the point where tube, when properly placed, exits the nostril. Measure exposed length for future placement verification.
	Replace tube and obtain physician's order to confirm with x-ray imaging.

TABLE 32.10 COMMON MECHANICAL, GASTROINTESTINAL, AND METABOLIC COMPLICATIONS OF TUBE-FED PATIENTS AND PREVENTION STRATEGIES

Complication	Prevention Strategies
Gastrointestinal	
Cramping, distention, bloating, gas pains, nausea, vomiting, diarrhea*	Practice good personal hygiene when handling any feeding product. Bring formula to room temperature before feeding. Initiate and increase amount of formula gradually. Change to a lactose-free formula. Decrease fat content of formula. Administer drug therapy as ordered (e.g., Lactinex, kaolin-pectin, Lomotil). Change to formula with a lower osmolality. Change to formula with a different fiber content. Evaluate diarrhea-causing medications patient may be receiving (e.g., antibiotics, digitalis preparations).
Metabolic	
Dehydration	Note patient's fluid requirements before treatment. Monitor hydration status. Provide adequate daily water.
Overhydration	Note patient's fluid requirements before treatment. Monitor hydration status.
Hyperglycemia	Initiate feeding at a slow rate. Monitor blood glucose. Use hyperglycemic medication if needed. Select a low-carbohydrate formula.
Hypernatremia	Note patient's fluid and electrolyte status before treatment. Provide adequate fluids.
Hyponatremia	Note patient's fluid and electrolyte status before treatment. Restrict fluids. Supplement feeding with rehydration solution and saline. Diuretic therapy may be beneficial.
Hypophosphatemia	Monitor serum level. Replenish phosphorus before refeeding.
Hypercapnia	Select a low-carbohydrate, high-fat formula.
Hypokalemia	Monitor potassium level. Supplement feeding with potassium if needed.
Hyperkalemia	Reduce potassium intake. Monitor potassium level.

* The most commonly cited complication of tube feeding is diarrhea.
Source: Modified from Lutz, C. A., & Przytulski, K. R. (2010). *Nutrition & diet therapy: Evidence-based applications* (5th ed.). Philadelphia: F. A. Davis.

When feedings are administered, patients must be positioned in a sitting or high-Fowler's position to reduce the risk of aspiration. Monitor the rate carefully to avoid administering feedings too rapidly, and watch for signs that the feeding is not being absorbed. Abdominal distention, patient report of a feeling of fullness, and nausea or vomiting are indicators that the feeding is not being absorbed and should be stopped to prevent aspiration. A residual check to see how much feeding, if any, has not been absorbed is done hourly when the feeding is initiated, then every 4 hours or before giving any medications or adding more feeding for infusion. If there is more than 100 mL or the amount specified by the agency or physician, the feeding should be stopped to prevent vomiting or aspiration and the physician notified. Continuous or intermittent feedings reduce the risk of aspiration, distention, nausea, vomiting, and diarrhea.

If medications are administered during tube feeding, understand possible drug–nutrient interactions. Some medications cannot be given with certain substances. Other medications, such as enteric-coated or sustained-release medications, should not be crushed. Liquid medications should be used when possible to reduce clogging of the tube. Pharmacists and dietitians should be consulted for special considerations.

Gastrointestinal Decompression

Gastrointestinal decompression may be necessary when the stomach or small intestine becomes filled with air or fluid. Swallowed air and GI secretions enter the stomach and intestines and collect there if they are not propelled through the GI tract by peristalsis. Accumulating air or fluid causes distention, a feeling of fullness, and possibly pain in the abdomen. Gastric distention may occur after major abdominal

SAFETY TIP

Incorrect connection of enteral feeding equipment is a hazard to patient safety. An enteral feeding incorrectly connected and administered through a nonenteral system (such as an intravenous line, peritoneal dialysis catheter, oxygen tubing, or tracheostomy tube cuff) can result in patient injury or death. Luer connections require extra caution. Equipment redesigns have been undertaken to make these types of faulty connections less possible. Nurses must be vigilant to ensure that they understand the appropriate use of the equipment and all tubing connections being made to prevent harmful errors:

- Avoid rigging connections that may impair designed safety features.
- Package together all parts needed for enteral feeding within the agency to avoid improper equipment being selected and connected.
- Label or color-code feeding tubes and connectors within the institution.
- Verify the solution's label (a 3-in-1 parenteral nutrition solution looks similar to enteral nutrition).
- Label enteral bags with large words such as "ALERT! For Enteral Use Only."
- Use adequate room lighting when working with equipment.
- Route tubes/catheters with different purposes in standardized directions (IV lines routed toward the patient's head; enteric lines routed toward the feet).
- If disconnection occurs, only staff familiar with the equipment should make a reconnection.
- During a reconnection, always trace the lines back to their origins and then ensure that they are secure.
- During the handoff process, trace all tubes to their origin and check connections.

CRITICAL THINKING

Mrs. Wood

■ Mrs. Wood is receiving a tube feeding because of dysphagia, the cause of which is being investigated. Mrs. Wood is not receiving any medications. You note that Mrs. Wood's tongue is bright red with deep furrows. She states her mouth is very dry. Her skin remains tented when skin turgor is checked.

1. What do Mrs. Wood's assessment findings indicate?
2. How would you document your assessment findings?
3. Why might Mrs. Wood be exhibiting this condition?
4. What actions could you take for this condition?
5. How would you record the total of Mrs. Wood's 8-hour intake, which is tube feeding at 50 mL per hour?

Suggested answers at end of chapter.

surgery. Ambulating or turning the patient frequently can help prevent this. However, when GI decompression is necessary, a nasogastric tube or occasionally a nasointestinal tube may be inserted and suction applied. Nasointestinal tubes are more difficult and slower to place and may be uncomfortable, so they are not used often. The tube remains in place until full peristaltic activity (active bowel sounds and passage of flatus) has returned. The diet is then progressed as ordered and tolerated by the patient.

Total Parenteral Nutrition

Total parenteral nutrition (TPN; also known as intravenous hyperalimentation) is a method of supplying nutrients to the patient by an intravenous (IV) route. TPN solutions usually contain dextrose (sugar), amino acids (protein), vitamins, minerals, and fat (intralipid) emulsions. TPN solutions are designed to improve the patient's nutritional status, achieve weight gain, and enhance the healing process. Patients with conditions such as burns, trauma, cancer, acquired immunodeficiency syndrome (AIDS), malnutrition, anorexia nervosa, or fever and those undergoing major surgery may need TPN.

Usually, registered nurses are responsible for administering TPN. A filter must be used with TPN solutions and possibly lipid solutions. TPN is started slowly to give the pancreas time to adjust to increasing insulin production for the high amounts of glucose in the TPN. The TPN rate is increased until the ordered rate, as tolerated by the patient, is reached. When TPN is discontinued, the patient might be gradually weaned to allow the pancreas to adjust to decreasing glucose levels. The patient, if ordered, is fed before the TPN is stopped to help prevent hypoglycemia. Signs of hypoglycemia include weakness, shakiness, sweating, and confusion.

It is important to monitor glucose levels as ordered and to look for signs of hyperglycemia in the patient receiving TPN. Refer to agency policy for obtaining glucose levels when a hyperglycemic reaction is suspected in the patient receiving TPN.

During TPN administration, the following laboratory values, as ordered, are usually monitored:

- Complete blood cell count (CBC)
- Albumin
- Glucose
- Electrolytes

- Platelet count
- Prothrombin time (PT).

TPN can be irritating to the peripheral veins because it is five or six times more concentrated than blood. Therefore, TPN dextrose more than 12% is administered through a central venous catheter into a large vein such as the subclavian or internal jugular (see Fig. 7.7). The volume in the large vein dilutes the TPN solution, so it is less irritating.

Peripheral Parenteral Nutrition

Peripheral parenteral nutrition (PPN) is a method of supplying nutrients to the patient by an IV route that is not a central vein. PPN is used for less than 10 days when the patient does not need more than 2000 calories daily. PPN solutions can contain a mixture of dextrose (of less than 12%), amino acids, and lipids, in addition to electrolytes or water, which can be found in routine IV solutions. The all-in-one PPN system mixes dextrose, amino acids, and lipids all in one container, which causes less vein irritation.

NURSING CARE TIP

Patients with any of the following may need to be considered for TPN or PPN:

- Any significant weight loss (10% or more of healthy weight)
- A decrease of oral food intake for more than 3 days
- Any significant sign of protein loss: serum albumin levels below 3.2 g/dL
- Muscle wasting
- Decreased tissue healing
- Persistent vomiting and diarrhea.

LEARNING TIP

- Patients may respond to TPN with an elevated serum glucose level, even though they do not have diabetes. This is due to the high concentration of glucose used in TPN. These elevated serum glucose levels do not usually indicate that the patient who does not have diabetes has acquired the disease. After the TPN is discontinued, the serum glucose levels should return to baseline or normal levels.
- Regular insulin is given, as ordered, to control hyperglycemia during TPN therapy. The insulin is ordered on a sliding scale (regular insulin given based on blood glucose levels measured at ordered intervals over 24 hours) or as an additive to the TPN solution, or both.
- Administration of insulin according to a sliding scale requires a current blood glucose level. Based on the obtained glucose level, if it is elevated, specified regular insulin units may be ordered. Usually blood glucose is measured before meals, but for a patient who is not eating, as with most patients receiving TPN, there is no mealtime. Instead, specified time intervals are ordered (typically every 6 hours).
- Insulin given on a sliding scale is always regular insulin. Can you figure out why? Regular insulin is rapid acting, which is what is needed to treat the current blood glucose level that was obtained to determine what insulin coverage was needed, if any.

Home Health Hints

- Be familiar with community nutritional support services: the Women, Infants, and Children (WIC) program, elderly nutrition sites, Meals on Wheels, school food programs, and government surplus food programs.
- Observe patient's food preparation facilities to ensure the patient's nutritional needs can be met. Some older patients may have outdated or spoiled food in their refrigerators or cupboards because they are unable to see dates or mold growing on foods.
- Ensure that patients are able to use appliances to heat food safely. Patients with limited vision may not see gas flames and can ignite their clothing. Confused patients might try to heat foods in cardboard containers. If the patient is able to obtain and learn to use a microwave, it may be a safer cooking appliance than a stove.
- A feeding tube can be prevented from kinking by slipping a split straw lengthwise around the area that tends to kink and lightly taping over the split in the straw.
- Wire coat hangers make good hooks for enteral feeding solution bags. They can be bent and hung over doorways or closet bars.

SUGGESTED ANSWERS TO CRITICAL THINKING

■ *Mrs. Todd*

1. Daily aspirin use is the most likely cause of her bleeding.
2. Medication teaching including side effects can help Mrs. Todd prevent future bleeding episodes. Assessment of pain relief needs and consultation with the physician will also help.
3. See Table 32.8.

■ *Mrs. Pearl*

Mrs. Pearl is at risk for dehydration and electrolyte loss as a result of the laxative and enema preparation and NPO status. This risk is increased because of her age. Her fluid and electrolyte status should be monitored closely.

Mrs. Pearl will likely have a concern about "making it" to the bathroom during the preparation and should have a bedside commode placed within easy reach. Her call light should be answered promptly. If enemas are ordered "until clear," Mrs. Pearl will be at greater risk for fluid and electrolyte loss. If more than two or three enemas are required, the physician should be notified.

Older patients can become very fatigued during testing and test preparation. Mrs. Pearl should be allowed plenty of rest before and after the test. She may also have a concern about being able to hold the barium in her bowel during the test without having an "accident." She should be assured that the barium is held in with a balloon that is on the end of the enema catheter and that bathrooms are nearby.

■ *Mr. Wozynski*

You can expect to find that Mr. Wozynski's serum bilirubin is elevated because his liver is unable to convert or conjugate bilirubin into a water-soluble compound that can be eliminated in feces. Mr. Wozynski is at risk for bleeding because the liver is highly vascular and prone to bleed when a biopsy specimen is taken. In addition, he may not be manufacturing the necessary amount of prothrombin needed for blood clotting and is less likely to stop bleeding once the biopsy has been performed. It will be especially important to check his coagulation studies and report any elevations to the physician before the biopsy.

■ *Mrs. Wood*

1. Assessment of Mrs. Wood indicates dehydration.
2. Document as follows: "0800 'Mouth very dry.' Tongue bright red with deep furrows, tented turgor. Tube feeding infusing (include solution and rate). Physician notified. K. Ohno, LVN."
3. Mrs. Wood's daily water needs are not being met. She is not receiving medications that would incidentally provide water during their administration.
4. Consult a dietitian and/or physician to review Mrs. Wood's daily water needs. Divide the water needs over 24 hours and ensure that water is administered. Ensure tubing is flushed per agency policy, and calculate water used toward daily water needs. Monitor intake and output. Continue assessing Mrs. Wood's signs and symptoms, and report abnormal findings.
5. 50 mL × 8 hours = 400 mL.

REVIEW QUESTIONS

1. The nurse is collecting data on a patient with a ruptured appendix that is painful. Where would the nurse expect the patient's pain to be located?
   a. Right upper quadrant
   b. Right lower quadrant
   c. Left upper quadrant
   d. Left lower quadrant

2. Which of the following is a function of the liver?
   a. Synthesis of plasma proteins
   b. Elimination of carbohydrates
   c. Concentration of bile
   d. Secretion of cholecystokinin

3. The nurse is contributing to the plan of care for a 78-year-old patient's elimination needs. Which of the following should the nurse recommend to reduce complications from the aging change of slowed motility?
   a. Decrease ambulation.
   b. Decrease fluid intake.
   c. Increase dairy products.
   d. Increase dietary fiber.

4. The nurse is listening to a patient's bowel sounds. The nurse understands that bowel sounds heard at an irregular rate every 5 to 15 seconds should be documented as which of the following?
   a. Normal
   b. Hyperactive
   c. Hypoactive
   d. Abnormal

REVIEW QUESTIONS—cont'd

5. Which of the following best describes the technique of palpation?
   a. Firmly place hands on abdomen, depressing tissues 1 to 2 inches.
   b. Randomly feel the patient's abdomen with fingertips.
   c. Lightly depress the abdomen 0.5 to 1 inch.
   d. Light palpation is completed by an experienced practitioner.

6. The nurse is contributing to the plan of care for a patient who is to have a lower GI series. Which of the following measures should the nurse recommend be included in the plan of care?
   a. Have the patient cough and deep breathe hourly while awake.
   b. Encourage fluids.
   c. Check for return of a gag reflex.
   d. Keep the patient in semi-Fowler's position.

7. A patient is admitted with an order for a sump tube (Salem sump). The nurse knows this tube is used for which of the following purposes? **Select all that apply**.
   a. Supplemental feeding
   b. Decompression
   c. Irrigation
   d. Lavage
   e. Gavage
   f. Parenteral nutrition

8. The nurse assisted with the insertion of a flexible feeding tube into a patient. Which of the following actions should the nurse take to confirm tube placement?
   a. Aspirate gastric contents for green-colored fluid.
   b. Measure the pH of secretions from tube.
   c. Obtain x-ray to check placement.
   d. Look in the back of the mouth for a coiled tube.

9. The nurse is caring for a patient who is receiving a TPN infusion. Blood glucose monitoring every 6 hours is ordered to detect which of the following complications?
   a. Hyponatremia
   b. Hyperkalemia
   c. Hypocalcemia
   d. Hyperglycemia

DavisPlus | For additional resources and information visit http://davisplus.fadavis.com

33

Nursing Care of Patients with Upper Gastrointestinal Disorders

LAZETTE V. NOWICKI

KEY TERMS

anorexia (AN-uh-REK-see-ah)
anorexia nervosa (AN-uh-REK-see-ah nur-VOH-sah)
aphthous stomatitis (AF-thus STOH-mah-TY-tiss)
bariatric (BEAR-ry-AT-trick)
bulimia nervosa (buh-LEE-mee-ah ner-VOH-sah)
gastrectomy (gast-TREK-tuh-mee)
gastritis (gas-TRY-tiss)
gastroduodenostomy (GAS-troh-DOO-oh-den-AW-stuh-mee)
gastrojejunostomy (GAS-troh-JAY-joo-NAW-stuh-mee)
gastroplasty (GAS-troh-PLAS-tee)
Helicobacter pylori (HEH-lih-koh-back-tur PIE-lore-ee)
hiatal hernia (hy-YAY-tuhl HER-nee-ah)
obesity (oh-BEE-sih-tee)
peptic ulcer disease (PEP-tick UL-sir dih-ZEEZ)
Roux-en-Y (roo-ehn-WHY)
steatorrhea (STEE-ah-toh-REE-ah)
stomatitis (STOH-mah-TY-tiss)

QUESTIONS TO GUIDE YOUR READING

1. What are anorexia, anorexia nervosa, and bulimia nervosa and their therapeutic measures and nursing care?
2. What is obesity, and what medical, surgical, and nursing management is used to treat it?
3. What nursing care would you give to a patient with stomatitis?
4. How would you care for patients with acute or chronic gastritis?
5. How would you explain the pathophysiology, signs and symptoms, and diagnostic testing for hiatal hernia, peptic ulcer disease, gastric bleeding, and gastric cancer?
6. What current pharmacological treatments are used for peptic ulcer disease?
7. What nursing care would you provide for patients with hiatal hernia, peptic ulcer disease, gastric bleeding, and gastric cancer?

NAUSEA AND VOMITING

Nausea is the subjective feeling of the urge to vomit. Vomiting is the act of expelling stomach contents from the body through the esophagus and mouth. Nausea and vomiting are common occurrences that most people experience at some time. Vomiting is a protective function to rid the body of harmful substances from the gastrointestinal (GI) tract. This reflex is controlled by the vomiting center of the brain. It is a complex process. Many stimuli and conditions that are directly related to the GI tract or independent of it can trigger nausea and vomiting. Viral GI infection and other infections, motion sickness, stress, pregnancy, medications (narcotics), myocardial infarction, uremia, and other conditions may cause nausea and vomiting.

Therapeutic Measures

Nausea and vomiting may be self-limited and require no intervention. If it is prolonged, however, dehydration and electrolyte imbalances can occur. The loss of hydrochloric acid from the stomach can result in metabolic alkalosis. Emesis that looks like coffee grounds (dark brown) occurs from bleeding in the stomach.

Protection of the airway during vomiting is a priority to prevent aspiration. Those at risk of aspiration are persons who are unconscious, older, and experiencing gag reflex impairments. Place these types of persons on their side when they begin to vomit. This allows the gastric contents to be expelled from the mouth rather than pooling at the back of the throat and being aspirated.

If the cause of vomiting is known, it is treated. Various medications can be given to control nausea and vomiting (e.g., diphenhydramine [Benadryl], metoclopramide [Reglan], promethazine [Phenergan], prochlorperazine [Compazine], ondansetron [Zofran], scopolamine [Transderm Scop], thiethylperazine [Torecan], and trimethobenzamide [Tigan]). Ginger used with antiemetic medications may help ease nausea (*see Evidence-Based Practice box*). For severe or prolonged vomiting, IV fluids and possibly nutrition need to be provided. Occasionally, a nasogastric (NG) tube with suction may be ordered to decompress the stomach. After the vomiting is resolved, clear liquids are started, with water being preferred. If liquids are tolerated, crackers or dry toast may be tolerated as well.

EVIDENCE-BASED PRACTICE

Clinical Question

Does ginger help alleviate nausea?

Evidence

A placebo-controlled, double-blind study with 644 cancer patients evaluated the use of ginger for nausea. The patients were divided into four groups that received placebos, 0.5 gram of ginger, 1 gram of ginger, or 1.5 grams of ginger along with antiemetics. Results indicated that nausea was reduced by up to 40% when using a ginger supplement along with antiemetic medication (Ryan et al., 2009). Another study demonstrated that ginger was more effective than vitamin B_{12} at relieving nausea in pregnant women (Chaiyakunapruk et al., 2006). Another study performed a meta-analysis of the literature looking at the effectiveness of ginger and relieving nausea. The meta-analysis demonstrated that a fixed dose of at least 1 g of ginger is more effective than a placebo for the prevention of postoperative nausea and vomiting and postoperative vomiting (Chittumma, Kaewkiattikun, & Wiriyasiriwach, 2007).

Implications for Nursing Practice

Research shows that ginger can be an effective aid in relieving nausea in cancer patients receiving chemotherapy and in pregnant patients and postoperative patients.

REFERENCES

Chaiyakunapruk, N., Kitikannakorn, N., Nathisuwan, S., et al. (2006). The efficacy of ginger for the prevention of postoperative nausea and vomiting: a meta-analysis. *American Journal of Obstetrics and Gynecology 194*(1), 95–99.

Chittumma, P., Kaewkiattikun, K., & Wiriyasiriwach, B. (2007). Comparison of the effectiveness of ginger and vitamin B_6 for treatment of nausea and vomiting in early pregnancy: A randomized double-blind controlled trial. *Journal of the Medical Association of Thailand, 90*(1), 15–20.

Ryan, J. L., Heckler, C., Dakhil, S. R., et al. (2009). Ginger for chemotherapy-related nausea in cancer patients. *Journal of Clinical Oncology, 27,* 15s.

Nursing Process for the Patient with Nausea and Vomiting

Data Collection

The characteristics of the episodes of the nausea and vomiting are noted. Medical conditions, medications, and treatments are documented to aid in diagnosing the cause. Signs of early fluid deficit, such as weakness, headache, muscle cramps, restlessness, inability to concentrate, and postural hypotension, are reported for treatment. Later signs include confusion, oliguria, cold clammy skin, and chest or abdominal pain.

Nursing Diagnoses, Planning, and Implementation

Nausea Related to Various Causes

EXPECTED OUTCOME: Patient will report no nausea or relief from nausea within 30 minutes of reporting nausea.

- Provide quiet, odor-free, visually clean environment *to avoid triggering stimuli.*
- Give antiemetics as ordered *to relieve nausea.*
- Provide frequent oral care *to remove emesis taste and enhance patient comfort.*
- Teach patient to avoid triggering fluids or foods *to prevent nausea and vomiting.*

Risk for Aspiration Related to Decreased Gag Reflex or Unconsciousness

EXPECTED OUTCOME: Patient's airway and lung sounds will remain clear at all times.

- Identify patients who are nauseated and at risk of aspiration *to plan preventive care.*
- Turn patient onto side if nauseated and vomiting *to protect airway and prevent aspiration.*

Deficient Fluid Volume

EXPECTED OUTCOME: Patient's vital signs will remain within normal limits.

- Monitor for early signs of hypovolemia in patient with vomiting *to allow treatment and prevent complications.*
- Obtain daily weight on same scale, at same time of day, with same type of clothing *to detect fluid losses.* (A 1-pound weight loss reflects a fluid loss of 500 mL.)
- Monitor intake and output and vital signs including orthostatic blood pressure per shift or daily or more frequently as patient's condition indicates *to report changes for prompt treatment.*
- Provide fluids as ordered to hydrate patient. *IV fluids allow the GI tract to rest. Slightly chilled sports replacement drinks or ginger ale may be given in small frequent amounts.*
- Monitor older adults for excess fluid volume during treatment of deficient fluid volume *to prevent and detect fluid overload, which may occur quickly in the older adult.*

Evaluation

The patient's goals are met if nausea is not present, lung sounds remain clear, and vital signs remain within normal limits.

EATING DISORDERS

Anorexia

Anorexia, which is a lack of appetite, is a common symptom of many diseases and can be caused by noxious food odors, certain drugs (as an intended or side effect), emotional stress, fear, psychological problems, and infections. Prolonged anorexia with an inadequate nutritional intake can lead to serious electrolyte imbalances, which in turn can lead to cardiac dysrhythmias. Although eating is the preferred method of weight gain, other measures such as tube feedings and intravenous infusion can be used. Ask patients what causes them to lose their appetite and what improves it to plan their care. Nursing actions for the patient with anorexia include documenting accurate intake and output; monitoring vital signs, electrolytes, and electrocardiograms; and monitoring the rate of the intravenous infusion and tube feeding.

Anorexia Nervosa

Anorexia nervosa is an eating disorder recognized by the American Psychiatric Association (Box 33.1). This disease most commonly occurs in females between ages 12 and 18 who are from the middle and upper classes of Western culture. Males account for less than 10% of those with anorexia nervosa. Young women with low self-esteem seem to be at highest risk. Anorexia nervosa is thought to be psychological in origin. Patients may have a phobia about weight gain, be afraid of a loss of control, and be mistrusting.

Signs and Symptoms

Early signs and symptoms of anorexia nervosa include severe weight loss, low self-esteem, compulsive dieting, and an altered body image (patients imagine themselves as fat, although they are within or below normal weight range). As the disease progresses, additional symptoms appear, including amenorrhea in females, electrolyte imbalance, cardiac dysrhythmias, constipation, dry skin, lanugo (downy hair covering body), bradycardia, hypothermia, hypotension, muscle wasting, and facial puffiness. Often patients with anorexia nervosa deny the existence of any problem. They may develop bizarre food rituals and sometimes weigh themselves several times a day. Anorexia nervosa sometimes overlaps with bulimia nervosa (compulsive eating with self-induced vomiting).

Complications

Chronic poor nutritional health takes its toll on the body. Complications from starvation occur as the body tries to conserve energy. Pulse and blood pressure fall. Heart and kidney failure are a risk. Osteoporosis and muscle loss occur. Vitamin and electrolyte imbalances result. Diabetes may develop with a high morbidity.

Box 33.1

Diagnostic Criteria for Anorexia Nervosa

1. Refusal to maintain body weight over a minimum normal weight for age and height.
2. Intense fear of gaining weight or becoming fat, even though underweight.
3. Disturbance in the way in which one's body weight, shape, or size is experienced.
4. In postmenarchal females, the absence of at least three consecutive menstrual cycles when otherwise expected to occur.

Therapeutic Measures

Treating this disorder is complex and requires a multidisciplinary approach. Patients often do not see the need for medical intervention. They do not usually seek help on their own and are often resistant to treatment. When treatment is sought, often through a concerned person's urgings, a medical and psychological workup is necessary. Nutritional status is also evaluated to determine the urgency of intervention. Establishing a trusting relationship, which can be difficult, is a key element in initiating treatment. Early treatment results in a better prognosis.

Often the most important initial intervention for anorexia nervosa is the restoration of nutritional health; up to 18% of anorexia patients eventually die as a result of starvation and complications from it. For those who are underweight with severe weight loss, life-threatening electrolyte imbalances and dysrhythmias or other symptoms, nutrition is supplied by intravenous infusions containing electrolytes. Oral food supplements may also need to be given. Restoring normal weight is a long, slow process. Gains may be small with setbacks along the way. Praise and rewards for small achievements in weight gains (not food intake) are positive reinforcements that aid recovery. Programs that treat eating disorders are often set up on a reward system, with privileges being increased as progress occurs.

The patient's damaged self-image and self-esteem are underlying causes of the disorder that must be addressed in conjunction with the nutritional aspect. Psychotherapy and behavior modification that includes participation of the patient's significant others are included in treatment of anorexia nervosa. The altered body image is the main focus of therapy. Educating the patient on normal body weight can be helpful. Individual or group therapy is used. Family counseling may be used since childhood events often create the negative self-image. During treatment, a support system is vital to success.

Bulimia Nervosa

Bulimia nervosa is compulsive eating with self-induced vomiting, which is commonly known as binge-purge. A high percentage of patients with bulimia are young women.

The patient with bulimia typically eats massive amounts of food at one sitting and then purges the food by intentionally inducing vomiting so weight is not gained. Laxatives are also sometimes used by the bulimic patient to purge the body of food to avoid weight gain. Excessive exercise may also be used to control weight.

Signs and Symptoms

Patients with bulimia nervosa exhibit many of the same signs and symptoms as patients with anorexia nervosa, with a few exceptions. Bulimic patients often have enamel erosion of the front teeth and staining caused by the acid content of the emesis. They also spend a great deal of time locked in the bathroom vomiting, especially after meals. Electrolyte imbalances occur from dehydration. The loss of potassium and sodium may result in dysrhythmias, heart failure, and death. As the electrolyte imbalance worsens, metabolic alkalosis develops as a result of the loss of gastric acid in the stomach contents. Signs and symptoms of metabolic alkalosis include hypokalemia and hypocalcemia. Laxative use results in irregular bowel movements.

Therapeutic Measures

The treatment for bulimia nervosa is essentially the same as for the patient with anorexia nervosa.

Nursing Process for the Patient with an Eating Disorder

Caring for patients with eating disorders is challenging. Gaining the patient's genuine cooperation by using therapeutic communication and setting realistic, mutual goals is important for establishing trust and preventing relapse. To work with patients with an eating disorder, a therapeutic relationship must be developed to facilitate effective interactions. Empathy, acceptance of the patient, trust, warmth, and being nonjudgmental are important.

Data Collection

Data is collected related to inadequate nutrition. Note changes in weight (15% or more below expected weight), poor skin turgor, poor muscle tone, lanugo, amenorrhea, electrolyte imbalances, and hypothermia. Data collection findings may also include a normal weight, enamel erosion of front teeth, and metabolic alkalosis for the patient with bulimia. Note abnormal diagnostic studies such as anemia, electrolyte imbalances, altered endocrine studies, and electrocardiographic (ECG) changes.

Nursing Diagnoses, Planning, and Implementation

Imbalanced Nutrition: Less Than Body Requirements Related to Inadequate Food Intake, Self-Induced Vomiting, and/or Chronic/Excessive Laxative Use

EXPECTED OUTCOME: The patient will establish dietary pattern and gain weight toward desired individual weight range.

- Monitor patient's weight *to determine baseline and monitor patient's progress toward goal.*
- Monitor vital signs and laboratory studies *to detect changes in cardiac function related to electrolyte imbalances.*
- Promote consistent approach *to enhance acceptance by patient and to build trust.*
- Promote pleasant eating environment and record intake *to enhance patient intake.*
- Provide six small meals and snacks *to prevent gastric dilation.*

Disturbed Body Image Related to Psychosocial or Cognitive/Perceptual Changes

EXPECTED OUTCOME: The patient will verbalize satisfaction with body appearance.

- Assess and document patient's verbal and nonverbal responses to own body *to provide baseline understanding of patient's perceptions of body image.*

- Listen to patient and acknowledge reality of concerns regarding treatment and progress *to establish therapeutic relationship.*
- Monitor frequency of negative statements about self *to determine if interventions are helping patient.*
- Assist with referrals to social services or counseling *to help patient overcome psychosocial issues.*
- Provide care in a nonjudgmental manner *to maintain the patient's dignity.*
- Use positive praise when patient verbalizes positive comments about own body.
- Encourage patient to verbalize consequences of eating disorder that have influenced self-concept *to help patient realize the negative impact of the eating disorder.*

Evaluation

The patient's goals are met if the patient gains weight toward expected weight goal and if the patient verbalizes satisfaction with body appearance and increases the number of positive statements about own appearance.

OBESITY

Several methods can be used to diagnose a patient as overweight or obese, although there is no one definitive measure of either. Factors such as age, body frame size, and gender can influence these measurements:

- *Height-weight chart:* Weight 10% to 20% above ideal body weight is overweight; 20% or more above ideal body weight is **obesity**.
- *Waist-to-hip ratio:* Waist-to-hip ratio is waist measurement divided by hip measurement.
- *Body mass index (BMI):* BMI, calculated using height-to-weight ratios, is one of the best methods for defining obesity (see Table 32.5 and Fig. 33.1).

Obesity is caused by a caloric intake that exceeds energy expenditure. Only a small percentage of obesity is associated with a metabolic or endocrine abnormality within the body. Health risks can result from being overweight. Diseases associated with obesity are called comorbidities and include, but are not limited to, atherosclerosis, heart disease, diabetes mellitus, hypertension, sleep apnea, osteoarthritis, decreased mobility, lack of self-esteem, and depression.

Obesity that interferes with activities of daily living, such as breathing or walking, is known as morbid obesity. Morbid obesity refers to people whose BMI is above 40, which is about 100 lb overweight for men and about 80 lb overweight for women. Surgery can be an option for people whose BMI is above 40 or for people whose BMI is between 35 and 40 and who have life-threatening obesity-related diseases such as severe sleep apnea or heart disease. For more information, visit the websites of the National Heart, Lung, and Blood Institute (www.nhlbisupport.com/bmi) or the American Obesity Association (www.obesity.org). For information about surgery for obesity, finding a surgeon, chat rooms, and more, visit (www.obesityhelp.com).

People who are overweight are at increased risk for developing other diseases. These can include hypertension, type 2 diabetes, heart disease, degenerative joint disease, sleep apnea, and gallbladder disease. When combined with a high-fat diet, there is also an increased risk of breast, colon, rectum, and prostate cancer. For more information, visit the

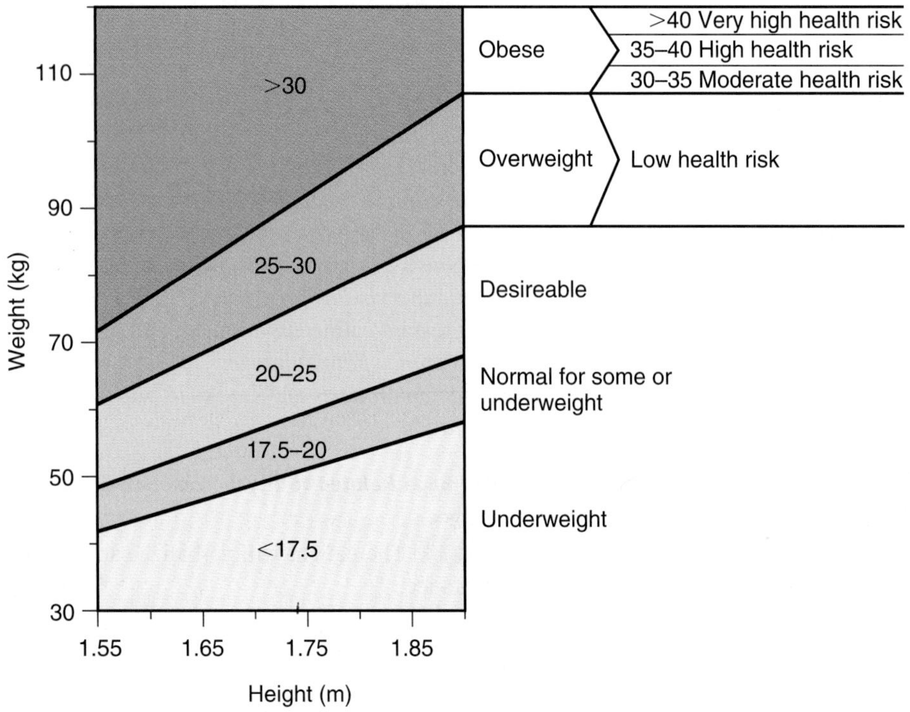
>40 Very high health risk
35–40 High health risk
30–35 Moderate health risk
Obese
Overweight
Low health risk
Desireable
Normal for some or underweight
Underweight
>30
25–30
20–25
17.5–20
<17.5
Weight (kg)
110
90
70
50
30
1.55
1.65
1.75
1.85
Height (m)

FIGURE 33.1 Body mass index ranges and associated level of health risk with obesity.

Centers for Disease Control and Prevention at www.cdc.gov/nccdphp/dnpa/obesity/defining.htm.

Therapeutic Measures

Initial treatment for obesity is weight loss through exercise and calorie restriction. For weight loss to occur, the patient must want to cooperate and have sustained motivation. Support groups such as Take Off Pounds Sensibly (TOPS) and Weight Watchers can help patients be successful. Behavior modification methods that provide rewards for successful weight loss are often included in a weight loss plan. Short-term use of medications that suppress appetite or block fat absorption may also be used. The patient should receive education regarding a healthy and balanced diet.

Surgical Management

Patients who do not respond to medical methods of weight loss or whose BMI is 40 or above may have surgery to reduce their weight if they meet established criteria for the surgery (Box 33.2, *Patient Perspective*). Established criteria for surgery may include gross obesity for 5 years, failure to reduce weight with other forms of therapy, body weight 100% above ideal weight, absence of other medical conditions, psychiatric and social stability, and presence of a high-risk condition that weight loss would relieve.

Surgical techniques produce weight loss by restriction (limiting how much the stomach can hold) or malabsorption (decreased calorie and nutrient absorption) (Box 33.3, *Nutrition Notes*). The field of obesity surgery is called bariatric surgery and is designed to treat severe obesity. The word **bariatric** comes from the Greek word *baros,* which means "weight." For a complete list of surgical obesity centers and surgical procedures, visit the American Society for Bariatric Surgeons at www.asbs.org. Examples of some bariatric surgeries are discussed next.

Restrictive Surgery

Restrictive bariatric surgery limits the size of the stomach (Fig. 33.2). Examples of this type of surgery are laparoscopic adjustable gastric banding and vertical banded **gastroplasty** (VBG). Laparoscopic adjustable gastric banding helps achieve weight loss by limiting intake, reducing appetite, and slowing digestion. The surgeon places an adjustable inflatable ring around the upper portion of the stomach. This creates a small pouch that limits the amount of food the patient can ingest. The band is adjustable, allowing for a larger or smaller pouch. The surgery is performed laparoscopically, which helps reduce the risks of open surgeries. Because no portion of the stomach or intestine is removed, malabsorption issues are avoided. Weight loss with the gastric band procedure is slower compared to other procedures. However, the procedure is reversible.

VBG also creates a pouch that limits food intake and creates a feeling of fullness. A small stomach pouch is made with a staple line and a mesh band. A circular window made

• **WORD** • **BUILDING** •

gastroplasty: gastro—stomach + plasty—repair

Box 33.2

Patient Perspective

Curtis

I am 47, with eight children. For many years, I experienced weight control problems. By the time I was in high school, I weighed 250 pounds, and the weight just kept building from there. I had tried many weight control programs, including some medications that now have been removed from the market.

When I was about 38, I began to look into weight loss surgeries such as the Roux-en-Y. Many of the older techniques were dangerous and risky. Even the newer procedures are major procedures with many risks.

I had spoken to many people who had bariatric surgery. Many pointed out the psychological aspect, talking about how differently people treated you after weight loss, and how some couples ended up divorcing. This was a very scary aspect to me.

However, after much research and after reaching a weight of about 380 pounds, I arranged to have the surgery done. I had my surgery at a facility that did only bariatric surgery. I felt very comfortable through the whole process. This included all the presurgical testing, including psychological evaluation and counseling.

One of the nice features was that the facility itself was patient friendly, with large chairs, etc. When I had the surgery I had a rough first 24 hours spent in the CCU (critical care unit). The nursing staff was very professional and understanding. The care was very personal and responsive to my needs. The staff was very courteous and made me comfortable.

I think that understanding the medical field you are working in is very important to this feeling of patient comfort. Several of my nurses had gone through the procedure themselves. This really helped them to know what I was experiencing. Nurses should be well informed about the procedures.

It has been 6+ years now and I have continued to keep my weight down around 230 to 250 pounds, which is a loss of approximately 120 pounds. My health has improved a good deal. I would do it again, even though at about day 21 I would have said "never again."

As nursing professionals, it is very important to treat everyone as a human being and with much respect regardless of their socioeconomic status or medical needs. If patients are treated with respect and caring, it is a step for them in the right direction. I believe it is not only kind but helps in the healing and recovery processes as well. I was treated with a great deal of kindness and respect during my procedure and I greatly appreciated this. Thanks to all the professional nurses out there who do a great job.

Box 33.3
Nutrition Notes

Supplying Nutrition in Upper Gastrointestinal Conditions

Obesity

Candidates for bariatric surgery should be carefully selected. The procedure should be viewed as one tool to assist with weight control, along with behavioral changes. It is not done to permit overeating. After the first year, due to stretching of the pouch or intestinal adaptation, much of the effect of the surgery can be negated, and the lost weight may be regained.

Intake is rigidly controlled immediately after the surgery and during rehabilitation. Long-term dietary strategies include the following:

- Eating three to six small balanced meals daily
- Chewing thoroughly and eating slowly
- Drinking most fluids between meals
- Taking vitamin and mineral supplements as prescribed.

Potential complications of these surgeries include nausea, vomiting, bloating, heartburn, staple disruption, obstruction, dumping syndrome, and osteoporosis.

Gastroesophageal Reflux and Hiatal Hernia

Thorough chewing and correct timing of intake is helpful in controlling symptoms:

- Six small meals
- Liquids
  - ½ cup liquid with meals
  - Other liquids ½ hour before or 1½ hours after meals
- No food within 3 hours of bedtime

Avoiding certain substances can alleviate symptoms:

- Those that relax the sphincter:
  - Fatty foods
  - Chocolate
  - Peppermint and spearmint
  - Caffeine
- Those that stimulate gastric secretions:
  - Decaffeinated coffee
  - Pepper
- Those that may be irritating:
  - Citrus juices
  - Tomato juice.

Postprandial Hypotension

This refers to a drop in systolic blood pressure of 20 mm Hg or more within 75 to 120 minutes after the beginning of a meal, most often resulting in dizziness and fatigue but also weakness, light-headedness, disturbed speech, and vision changes.

Normally, the body compensates for the increased blood flow to the digestive tract following meals, but in the elderly, the mechanisms maintaining adequate circulation to the rest of the body become less effective. Most at risk are people with neurologic, cardiovascular, or renal diseases. Complications include a higher incidence of coronary events, stroke, and total mortality.

To prevent postprandial hypotension, a person should:

- Limit carbohydrate intake.
- Eat frequent small meals.
- Lie in a semirecumbent position for 90 minutes after eating.
- Avoid excessive exercise for 2 hours after meals.
- Schedule antihypertensive medications between rather than just before meals.

Special dietary additives or medications to delay gastric emptying are sometimes prescribed.

Dumping Syndrome

The recommended meal pattern for patients with dumping syndrome includes six small meals per day that are high in protein and low in simple sugars; fluids between rather than with meals; and reclining for 30 minutes after meals. Supplementation with the vitamins B_{12} and D, folic acid, and the minerals calcium and iron may be necessary to prevent deficiencies.

Gastric Cancer

If a patient has a poor prognosis following a total gastrectomy for cancer, dietary interventions should focus on symptoms the patient wishes to control. An overly restricted diet that causes the patient discomfort or distress is inappropriate.

---

with staples allows the band to be placed around the pouch. The band restricts and slows food flow from the stomach pouch. As the small pouch fills, there is a feeling of fullness even with small meals. There is little malabsorption of food with this procedure, and it is technically easier to perform than gastric bypass surgery. If a reversal is needed, it is easier to reverse the VBG than the gastric bypass. About 30% of patients who have had VBG achieve normal weight.

Combination Surgery

The **Roux-en-Y** gastric bypass combines restrictive and malabsorptive surgery (see Fig. 33.2). In the first part of this two-step surgery, a small stomach pouch the size of a thumb is created with staples. This small pouch causes a quick satisfactory feeling of fullness during a meal, which is the key to the success of this procedure. Next, a Y-shaped section of the small intestine is attached to the pouch to allow food to bypass the lower stomach and duodenum. Digestive

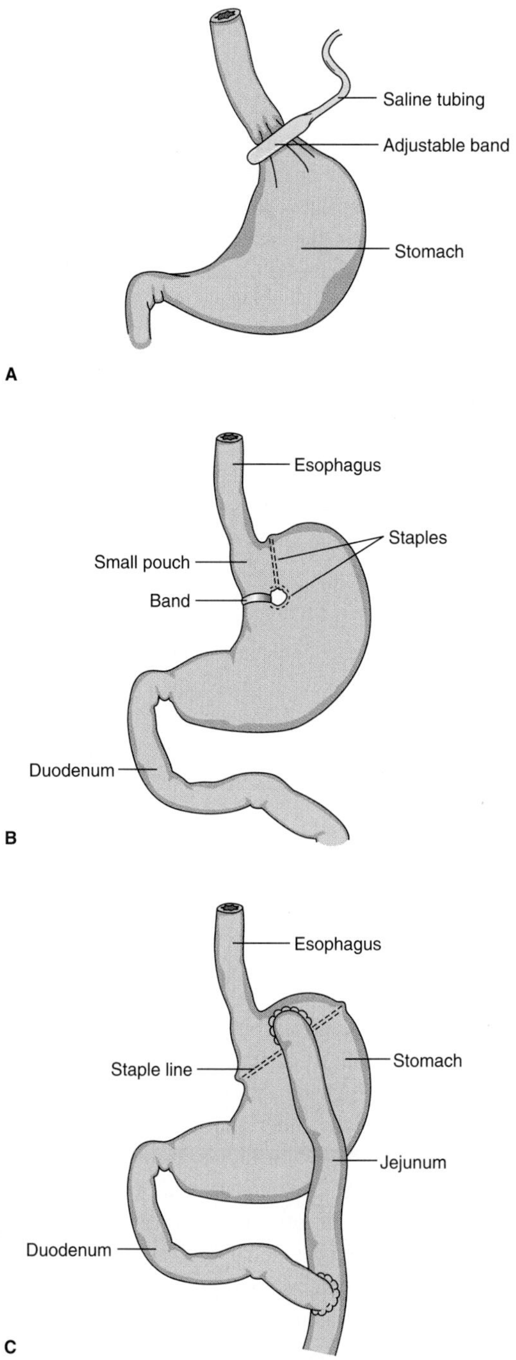
Saline tubing
Adjustable band
Stomach
A
Esophagus
Small pouch
Staples
Band
Duodenum
B
Esophagus
Staple line
Stomach
Jejunum
Duodenum
C

FIGURE 33.2 (A) Adjustable gastric band. Using laparoscopic technique, the surgeon loops a band around the upper portion of the stomach and tightens it by filling the band's liner with adjustable amounts of saline solution. The procedure requires no cutting or stapling of stomach or intestine. (B) Vertical banded gastroplasty for gastric bypass. A small stomach pouch is made with a staple line and a mesh band. A circular window made with staples allows the band to be placed around the pouch. (C) Roux-en-Y gastric bypass. A staple line creates a small pouch at the top of the stomach, which is then attached to the jejunum. Food bypasses most of the stomach and the duodenum and goes into the jejunum.

juice flow is maintained, and food enters the jejunum within 10 minutes of eating. There is little malabsorption of food. This procedure has also been performed laparoscopically.

Complications of Gastric Restrictive Surgeries

A common side effect of restrictive surgery is vomiting caused by overeating or by not chewing food well. Severe side effects of VBG include erosion of the gastric tissue surrounding the band, breakdown of the staple line, and leaking of the stomach secretions into the abdomen. Leaking of the stomach secretions can lead to peritonitis, a very serious infection of the peritoneum that requires emergency surgery. Infection or death from any of these complications can occur.

> **NURSING CARE TIP**
>
> When caring for a patient after bariatric surgery for laparoscopic gastric bypass, gastroenterostomy, or laparoscopic gastric restrictive surgery, be sure to use infection control procedures at all times to prevent surgical site infection. Surgical site infection following these bariatric surgeries is a Medicare-designated "never event"—hospitals will not be paid by Medicare for the care required for this condition.

Postoperative Care

Postoperative bariatric patients require care similar to that for most types of gastric surgeries. (See the *Nursing Process for the Patient Having Gastric Surgery* section later in this chapter.) The bariatric diet, however, is very different. Most patients will have an NG tube in place after surgery. It is important to keep the head of the bed elevated to ensure adequate lung expansion. Patients are started on a clear liquid diet because of the small stomach pouch that has been created. Only a small amount of fluid, 30 mL, is allowed at a time. Then the diet progresses to full liquids, pureed foods, and, finally, at about 6 weeks after surgery, regular foods as tolerated. Patients will need to be taught to restrict the amount of food ingested at one time. The patient will also have increased protein requirements following surgery.

Bariatric patients will need long-term follow-up. Many patients experience significant weight loss by 6 to 8 months after surgery. This can lead to a large amount of flabby skin. It is recommended that they wait at least 1 full year before having reconstructive surgery to remove the excess skin.

Nursing Process for the Patient Who Is Obese

Data Collection

Data collection for the patient with obesity should include measurements of height, weight, and BMI. Information about eating patterns and exercise patterns should be obtained. The nurse should determine if any problems exist for the patient related to excess weight such as physical limitations, social interaction issues, and personal issues (e.g., changes in sexuality or financial status). The nurse should complete a complete physical assessment noting any abnormalities. Assessment should include any areas in which the patient has expressed concerns or problems. Persons who are overweight have an increased risk for other diseases. The nurse should assess for signs and symptoms of these diseases.

Nursing Diagnoses, Planning, and Implementation

Imbalanced Nutrition: More Than Body Requirements Related to Caloric Intake Greater than Metabolic Needs and/or Decreased Activity Level

EXPECTED OUTCOMES: The patient will achieve and maintain weight loss to specified weight.

- Establish desired weight goal and monitor weight *to track progress toward goal.*
- Modify eating habits and patterns *to lose weight and then maintain weight loss.*
- Establish and maintain increased activity pattern *to lose weight and then maintain weight loss.*
- In collaboration with a dietician, implement eating plan for patient *to safely reduce weight and maintain adequate protein intake.*
- Discuss realistic weight loss goals of 1 to 2 lb/week *to achieve lasting weight loss effects.*
- Discuss emotions, events, and patterns of eating *to help patient identify when she or he is eating to satisfy an emotional need versus a physiological hunger.*
- In collaboration with physician, establish increased activity pattern *to promote weight loss.*
- Provide preoperative instructions if surgical interventions are planned *to help patient understand the procedure.*

Evaluation

The patient's goals are met if the patient maintains progressive weight loss to specified weight goal and safely progresses through the perioperative period if a surgical intervention is completed.

NURSING CARE TIP

For the patient who is obese, it is often necessary to have on hand special equipment for patient care. Some items you may need include:

- Larger hospital bed, wheelchair, or walker
- Patient lifting devices
- Extra pillows to ease breathing
- Larger hospital gowns
- Larger blood pressure cuff.

ORAL HEALTH AND DENTAL CARE

Good oral health care is important to overall health. Nutrition can be affected if oral problems interfere with eating and drinking. Respiratory illness and cardiac disease are associated with pathogens in the mouth. Regular mechanical oral hygiene is needed to remove plaque and prevent infections. Functional limitations may interfere with self-care for oral hygiene especially for older adults (Box 33.4, *Gerontological Issues*). Regular dental care is also important in the prevention of infections (Box 33.5). Providing oral hygiene using oral

Box 33.4

Gerontological Issues

Nurses can positively impact older patients' outcomes by providing mechanical oral hygiene. Studies have shown that because mechanical oral care removes plaque, it helped to prevent pneumonia and pneumonia-related death in elderly clients who were either hospitalized or in an extended care facility.

Box 33.5

Common Concerns in Oral Health and Dental Care

Oral care is important throughout life and has been found to have a link to cardiac health. The importance of daily and ongoing oral care should be considered for all patients, especially older adults.

Patients who have artificial joints or some heart conditions who must undergo a dental procedure need to take prophylactic antibiotics prior to some dental procedures to prevent bacteria entry and bacterial endocarditis. The dentist should be informed of the patient's history so that appropriate antibiotics can be prescribed.

Xerostomia (Dry Mouth)

As people age, it is not unusual for them to experience a condition known as xerostomia (dry mouth). Also, some medications and radiation treatment of the head and neck areas can cause xerostomia. Xerostomia can lead to rampant tooth decay in older adults, putting their dentition at risk. Before any radiation therapy of the head or neck area, a thorough oral examination and any needed restorative dental procedures should be completed.

Although water is used as a common substitute for saliva, it does not contain the necessary compounds, such as lubricants, to protect the teeth. Therefore, an artificial saliva substitute should be considered, such as OralBalance gel, Salivart solution, or Salix lozenges.

Box 33.5

Common Concerns in Oral Health and Dental Care—cont'd

Dentures

It is helpful to have a person's name implanted into their dentures to avoid lost or mixed up dentures, especially when the person lives in an extended care facility. This service can be requested when the dentures are made, and the dentist will place a small identity tag in the acrylic of the denture with the person's name on it.

Those with complete dentures still need to be routinely screened by a dentist or dental hygienist for proper denture fit, sore areas, oral cancer detection, and oral fungal infections.

Gingival Recession

As people age, it is not unusual for their gingivae (gums) to recede or shrink, exposing the root surfaces of the teeth. This can lead to root sensitivity, tooth decay, or both.

To protect the teeth from tooth decay as a result of dry mouth or gingival recession, a fluoride gel or rinse is strongly recommended. Over-the-counter products include Act rinse and Gel-Kam.

Gingivitis

As people get older, the gingivae have a greater tendency to bleed, a condition known as gingivitis. If the supporting tissues in the sockets of the teeth become inflamed, bone loss occurs, resulting in a condition known as periodontitis (pyorrhea). Periodontitis can lead to tooth mobility or loss.

Good oral hygiene habits cannot be overemphasized in the prevention of gum disease. Flossing every day is very important. If the patient is unable to floss due to arthritis or other conditions, an electric toothbrush or a Waterpik device is helpful in providing oral hygiene.

Candida Albicans Infection (Yeast Infection)

Older adults are susceptible to oral yeast infections (caused by *Candida albicans*) due to certain medications, systemic conditions, or chemotherapy. Nystatin (Mycostatin, Nadostine) as an oral rinse treats this infection.

Angular Cheilosis

A condition known as angular cheilosis (red, raw corners of the mouth) develops more often in older adults. It may be from infection, deficiency of riboflavin (vitamin B_2), or loss of facial profile due to worn dentures or not wearing dentures. Depending on the cause, it is treated with anti-infective medications, vitamins, or new dentures.

Source: *Contributed by Dr. Ralph Kluk and Dr. Cheryl Kluk.*

chlorhexidine gluconate (germicidal) mouthwash has been shown to be effective in preventing pneumonia in long-term care residents as well as reducing ventilator-associated pneumonia in cardiac surgery patients. This is an easy and inexpensive way to promote patient health.

Aging changes as well as disease and treatment can result in oral inflammation and infection. Those who are immunosuppressed (i.e., with AIDS) or undergoing chemotherapy or who have vitamin deficiencies are more at risk. Candidiasis is a common oral infection that is often treated with nystatin oral swish and swallow. During data collection, especially in these higher risk patients, the nurse should note any oral signs of inflammation or infection requiring prompt treatment. This is important to preserve oral comfort and nutrition.

ORAL INFLAMMATORY DISORDERS

Stomatitis

Stomatitis is the general term for inflammation of the oral cavity. There are many causes of stomatitis, such as an infection or a systemic disease. The most common types of stomatitis are **aphthous stomatitis** (canker sores) and herpes simplex virus type 1 infection (also known as cold sores or fever blisters).

Aphthous Stomatitis (Canker Sores)

Aphthous stomatitis appears as small, white, painful ulcers on the inner cheeks, lips, tongue, gums, palate, or pharynx and typically lasts for several days to 2 weeks. Self-induced trauma such as biting the lips and cheeks can cause these ulcers to develop, as can stress or exposure to irritating foods. Application of topical tetracycline several times a day usually shortens the healing time. A topical anesthetic such as benzocaine or lidocaine provides pain relief and makes it possible to eat with minimal pain.

Herpes Simplex Virus Type 1 Infection

Herpes simplex virus type 1 (HSV-1) infection may appear as painful cold sores or fever blisters on the face, lips, perioral area, cheeks, nose, or conjunctivae. These lesions recur over time but last only for a few days each time. The onset can be provoked by fever or stress, among other things. Acyclovir ointment can be used to ease the pain, but it does not cure the lesions. Oral acyclovir may reduce recurrences. These lesions are infectious, and standard precautions should be used when ointment is applied or oral care is given.

ORAL CANCER

Pathophysiology and Etiology

Oral cancer can occur anywhere in the mouth or throat. If detected early enough, it is curable. Oral cancer is found most commonly in patients who use alcohol or any form of

• WORD • BUILDING •
stomatitis: stoma—mouth + itis—inflammation

tobacco. The highest incidence of oral cancer is found in the pharynx (throat), with the lowest incidence being on the lips.

Signs and Symptoms

Any oral sore that does not heal in 2 weeks should be assessed by the patient's physician. Cancerous ulcers are often painless but may become tender as the cancer progresses. In the later stages, the patient may report difficulty chewing, swallowing, or speaking or may have swollen cervical lymph glands.

Diagnostic Tests

Biopsy specimens are taken to determine the presence of cancer.

Therapeutic Measures

Oral cancer treatment varies depending on the individualized diagnosis. Radiation, chemotherapy, and surgery are used alone or in combination to treat oral cancer. Radical or modified neck dissection is often performed since this type of cancer frequently has metastasized to cervical lymph nodes by the time it is diagnosed (Fig. 33.3). The tumor is removed along with lymph nodes, muscles, blood vessels, glands, and part of the thyroid, depending on the extent of the cancer. Drains are inserted into the incision to prevent fluid accumulation. A tracheostomy is usually performed to protect the airway and prevent obstruction.

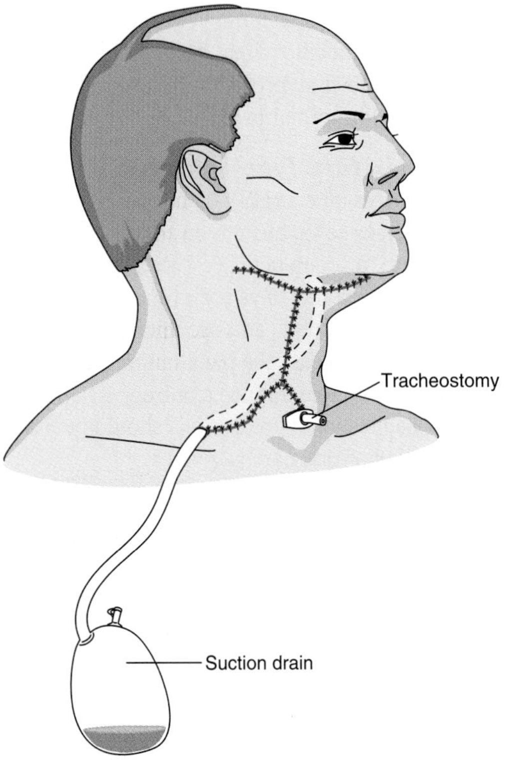
Tracheostomy
Suction drain

FIGURE 33.3 Radical neck dissection with tracheostomy tube and drains inserted.

Nursing Care

For the patient undergoing surgery, preoperative and postoperative nursing care are discussed in Chapter 12. Preoperatively, issues that are addressed in planning care include the use of alcohol or tobacco. Referrals to cessation programs and support groups should be offered. Preoperative teaching also includes how the patient will communicate if a tracheostomy is placed. Postoperatively, major concerns are airway patency, communication, and nutritional needs. Nursing care for the patient with a tracheostomy is discussed in Chapter 29. The airway must be monitored and secretions controlled to prevent aspiration. Determining that the methods the patient is using for communication are satisfactory is evaluated. Tube feedings (discussed in Chapter 32) are usually given to meet the patient's nutritional needs because swallowing is difficult.

ESOPHAGEAL CANCER

Pathophysiology and Etiology

As with oral cancer, esophageal cancer is associated with the use of tobacco or alcohol. Esophageal cancer is usually detected late because of its location near many lymph nodes that allow it to metastasize. As the cancer progresses, obstruction of the esophagus can occur, with possible perforation or fistula development that may cause aspiration. The appearance of signs and symptoms usually means that the cancer is in the late stages.

Signs and Symptoms

Signs and symptoms may include progressive dysphasia (difficulty swallowing), a feeling of fullness, pain in the chest area after eating, foul breath, or regurgitation of foods if there is an obstruction.

Diagnostic Tests

Diagnosis of esophageal cancer is usually made by esophagogastroduodenoscopy (EGD) and biopsy. Mediastinoscopy (endoscopic examination of mediastinum) is used to determine whether the cancer has spread to the lymph nodes and surrounding structures.

Therapeutic Measures

Treatment for esophageal cancer includes radiation, chemotherapy, and surgery alone or in combination. Surgical procedures include esophageal resection (esophagectomy), resection of the esophagus and anastomosis to the remaining part of the stomach (esophagogastrostomy), Dacron esophageal replacement, or use of a section of colon to replace the esophagus (esophagoenterostomy). If the tumor is inoperable, esophageal dilation or stent placement can be done to relieve dysphagia and allow food to pass through the esophagus.

Nursing Process for the Patient with Esophageal Cancer

The patient with esophageal cancer may undergo various forms of treatment: chemotherapy, radiation, or surgery. Nursing care is provided based on the effects of the therapies (see Chapters 11 and 12).

Data Collection

Patient data are collected for risk factors of esophageal cancer, pain, dysphagia, and nutritional status.

Nursing Diagnoses, Planning, and Implementation

Pain Related to Tumor and Pressure Exerted on Surrounding Tissues

EXPECTED OUTCOME: Patient will state a reduction of pain to acceptable level or total relief of pain within 30 minutes of report of pain.

- Assess pain level using pain rating scale *to identify pain level.*
- Provide pain medications as ordered *to provide pain relief.*

Risk for Deficient Fluid Volume Related to Decreased Intake

EXPECTED OUTCOME: Patient's vital signs will remain within normal limits and intake and output will be balanced for 24 hours at all times.

- Assess fluid intake and swallowing ability with fluids *to plan care.*
- Obtain daily weights *to detect changes in fluid volume.*
- Provide fluids as able to swallow *to ensure adequate intake.*
- Monitor intravenous infusion as ordered *to prevent hypovolemia.*
- Monitor vital signs and report abnormal findings *for prompt treatment.*

Imbalanced Nutrition: Less Than Body Requirements Related to Dysphagia

EXPECTED OUTCOME: Patient will maintain weight within normal limits for body frame, and laboratory values such as albumin, electrolytes, and lymphocytes will be within normal limits.

- Obtain patient height and weight, and weigh weekly *to monitor changes during care.*
- Identify patient's ability to swallow and eat food *to determine plan of care.*
- Provide oral care frequently *to refresh mouth and encourage desire to eat.*
- Provide nutrition as ordered in form patient is able to tolerate (liquid supplements, tube feedings, total parenteral nutrition, etc.) *to maintain adequate nutrition.*

Evaluation

The goals are met if the patient reports pain is relieved and fluid volume and nutritional needs are met.

HIATAL HERNIA

Pathophysiology

The esophagus passes through an opening in the diaphragm called the hiatus. A **hiatal hernia** is a condition in which the lower part of the esophagus and stomach slides up through the hiatus of the diaphragm into the thorax (Fig. 33.4). A sliding hiatal hernia is the most common type in which the stomach slides up into the thoracic cavity when a patient is supine and then usually goes back into the abdominal cavity when the patient stands upright. Hiatal hernia occurs most commonly in women and those who are older than age 60, obese, or pregnant. People with hiatal hernia often have gastroesophageal reflux disease (GERD) as well (discussed later).

Signs and Symptoms

A small hernia may not produce any discomfort or require treatment. However, a large hernia can cause pain, heartburn, a feeling of fullness, or reflux, which can injure the esophagus with possible ulceration and bleeding.

Diagnostic Tests

Hiatal hernias are diagnosed by x-ray studies and fluoroscopy.

Therapeutic Measures

Medical treatment for symptomatic hiatal hernia includes taking antacids; eating small meals that pass easily through the esophagus; not reclining for 1 hour after eating; elevating

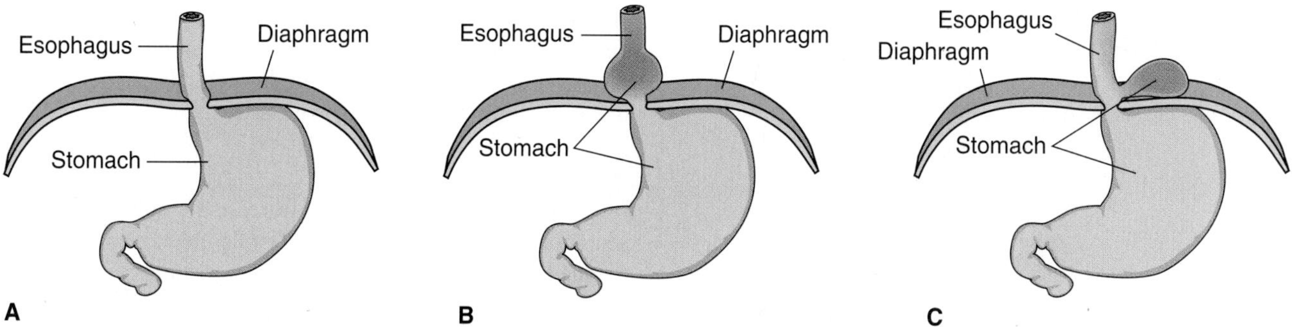

Esophagus
Diaphragm
Stomach
A
Esophagus
Diaphragm
Stomach
B
Esophagus
Diaphragm
Stomach
C

FIGURE 33.4 Hiatal hernia. (A) Normal esophagus and stomach. (B) Sliding hiatal hernia. (C) Rolling hiatal hernia.

the head of the bed 6 to 12 inches to prevent reflux; and avoiding bedtime snacks, spicy foods, alcohol, caffeine, and smoking (see Box 33.3, *Nutrition Notes*). If the patient is overweight, weight loss is recommended.

Surgical Management

Surgical procedures can be done to prevent the herniated portion of the stomach from moving upward through the hiatus. Fundoplication, in which the stomach fundus is wrapped around the lower part of the esophagus, is the most common surgical procedure performed (Fig. 33.5).

Nursing Care

Teaching the patient interventions to reduce symptoms of hiatal hernia is included in the plan of care. If the patient undergoes surgery, general postoperative nursing care is provided. In addition, following fundoplication, patients are assessed for dysphagia during their first postoperative meal. If dysphagia occurs, the physician should be notified because the repair may be too tight, causing obstruction of the passage of food.

GASTROESOPHAGEAL REFLUX DISEASE

Pathophysiology

Gastroesophageal reflux disease (GERD) is a condition in which gastric secretions reflux into the esophagus. The esophagus can be damaged by acidic gastric secretions and exposure to digestive enzymes. GERD is caused primarily by conditions that affect the ability of the lower esophageal sphincter to close tightly, such as hiatal hernia.

Signs and Symptoms

Signs and symptoms of GERD include heartburn, regurgitation, dysphagia, and bleeding (Table 33.1). Aspiration is a concern. Scar tissue can develop from the inflammation.

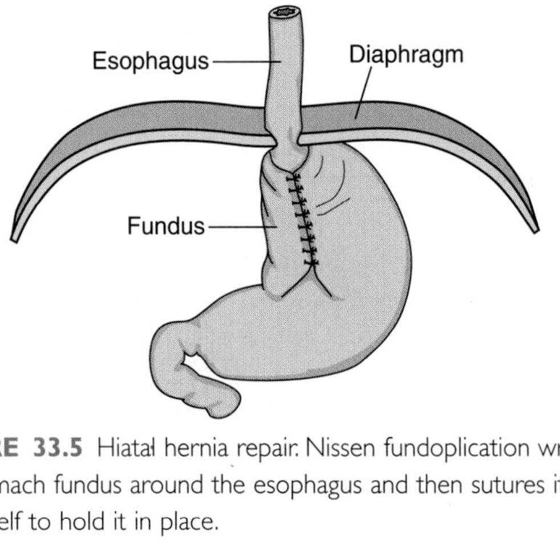

Esophagus
Diaphragm
Fundus

FIGURE 33.5 Hiatal hernia repair. Nissen fundoplication wraps the stomach fundus around the esophagus and then sutures it onto itself to hold it in place.

TABLE 33.1 GERD SUMMARY

Signs and Symptoms	***Heartburn*** Regurgitation Dysphagia Bleeding
Diagnostic Tests	X-ray studies Endoscopy Fluoroscopy
Therapeutic Measures	Medications to decrease acid, improve gastric emptying, and function of lower esophageal sphincter: antacids, histamine (H_2) receptor antagonists, proton pump inhibitors, cytoprotective agents (sucralfate), and cholinergic drugs Controlling symptoms Low-fat, high-protein diet Avoiding triggers Raising head of bed on 4- to 6-inch blocks Instructing patient to drink fluids between meals rather than with meals
Complications	Esophagitis Barrett's syndrome Respiratory symptoms
Priority Nursing Diagnoses	*Acute Pain* *Deficient Knowledge*

Diagnostic Tests

Diagnostic tests include a barium swallow, esophagoscopy, or pH monitoring of the normally alkaline esophagus. GERD often occurs in older people.

Complications

Complications of GERD can result in esophagitis (inflammation of the esophagus) due to acid reflux. Over time this can lead to changes in the epithelium of the esophagus and lead to Barrett's esophagus. This is a precancerous lesion that puts the patient at risk of developing esophageal cancer. Barrett's tissue can be removed during a 30-minute outpatient endoscopic procedure using radio-frequency ablation (the BARRx system). Normal tissue returns, and the risk of cancer is reduced. Respiratory complications such as bronchospasm, laryngospasm, and aspiration pneumonia can also occur owing to aspiration of gastric contents. There is the potential for asthma, chronic bronchitis, or pneumonia due to the aspiration of gastric contents.

Therapeutic Measures

Interventions for GERD aim to decrease the reflux of gastric secretions into the esophagus. Lifestyle changes are recommended along with medications. Obese patients are encouraged to lose weight. A low-fat, high-protein diet is recommended because fat causes decreased functioning of the lower esophageal sphincter. See Box 33.3 (*Nutritional Notes*) for additional things to avoid. Patient teaching includes eating small meals often during the day, drinking fluids between meals instead of with meals, avoiding late evening meals and snacking, and limiting fluid intake 2 to 3 hours before bedtime. Medications may include nonprescription antacids for mild symptoms (Mylanta, Tums, Gaviscon). Histamine (H_2) receptor antagonists (acid reducers) that are available in nonprescription and prescription strengths are used for mild to moderate symptoms (cimetidine [Tagamet], famotidine [Pepcid], ranitidine HCl [Zantac], nizatidine [Axid]). Proton pump inhibitors (PPIs) reduce acid in the stomach and are used for frequent, severe symptoms and Barrett's esophagus, a precancerous condition (esomeprazole [Nexium], lansoprazole [Prevacid], omeprazole [Prilosec], pantoprazole [Protonix], rabeprazole [AcipHex]). Prokinetic agents (metoclopramide [Reglan, Maxolon]), which are not used as a first choice because of side effects, improve gastric emptying and function of the lower esophageal sphincter (see Table 33.4). If surgery is necessary to alleviate symptoms, a fundoplication can be done.

A newer minimally invasive procedure, Esophy X, uses an endoscope to tighten the lower esophageal sphincter, which aids in improving or eliminating gastroesophageal reflux with good success. Other endoscopic procedures that use radio-frequency waves, such as the Stretta, can be done. The radio-frequency waves are injected into the lower esophageal sphincter muscle to form collagen contraction, which leads to a barrier against reflux. Other procedures have used injection or implantation of foreign material. These procedures have had limited success.

Nursing Process for the Patient with GERD

Data Collection

Assessment of the patient with GERD includes evaluation of reports of heartburn. The onset, duration, characteristics, and precipitating or relieving factors are noted.

Nursing Diagnoses, Planning, and Implementation

Acute Pain Related to Inflammation of Esophageal Tissues

EXPECTED OUTCOME: The patient will state a reduction of pain to an acceptable level or total relief of pain within 30 minutes of report of pain.

- Identify factors that increase pain *to develop teaching plan.*
- Monitor pain level using pain rating scale *to identify pain level.*
- Instruct patient regarding factors that aggravate pain *to enhance management of condition.*
- Instruct patient to sleep with head of bed elevated 4 to 6 inches, eat small meals, and avoid lying down for 2 hours after eating *to prevent reflux of gastric contents into esophagus.*
- Instruct patient to avoid smoking and alcohol *because they decrease functioning of the lower esophageal sphincter.*
- Instruct patient to avoid foods that cause discomfort *to avoid pain.*
- Review medication schedule and teach patient to take medications even if symptoms are relieved *because the underlying pathology still exists.*
- Provide pain medications on routine schedule, especially postoperatively, *to provide optimum pain relief and control.*

Evaluation

The goals are met if the patient is able to manage medications, pain is controlled, and symptoms are relieved.

MALLORY-WEISS TEAR

Pathophysiology

A Mallory-Weiss tear (MWT) is a longitudinal tear in the mucous membrane of the esophagus at the stomach junction (gastric cardia). These tears occur from a sudden powerful or prolonged force due to coughing, vomiting, seizures, prolapse of the stomach into the esophagus, or cardiopulmonary resuscitation (CPR). Hiatal hernia is present in most patients with MWTs.

Signs and Symptoms

Bleeding may result from the tear. Up to 15% of GI bleeding is caused by MWTs. Symptoms include bright red, bloody emesis or bloody or tarry stools.

Diagnostic Tests

The tear can be diagnosed with an esophagogastroduodenoscopy (EGD). Hemoglobin and hematocrit are checked to determine amount of bleeding.

Therapeutic Measures

The tears usually self-heal without intervention in several days and bleeding stops within a few hours. It is rare to have it happen again. Medications such as a PPI and an antiemetic may be given. Alcohol use should be avoided. Up to 75% of those with MWT use alcohol excessively. Rarely, excessive bleeding may occur, resulting in shock and/or the need for a blood transfusion. Bleeding is treated with injection of epinephrine to constrict the blood vessel, and during endoscopy, endoclips can be placed to stop the bleeding. The prognosis for MWTs is good. The condition is seen in men more often than in women.

Nursing Care

Monitoring the patient for signs of bleeding and reporting them to prevent complications from hemorrhage are the focus of nursing care. If excessive bleeding occurs, shock symptoms may occur and require prompt intervention. Teaching about medications and the avoidance of alcohol use is also done. See the section on gastric bleeding later in the chapter for more information.

ESOPHAGEAL VARICES

Esophageal varices are dilated blood vessels in the esophagus (see Chapter 35). Their rupture can precipitate a life-threatening event. Varices develop from portal hypertension. This occurs when pressure rises in the portal vein from blocked blood flow in the liver. This is often due to cirrhosis of the liver.

GASTRITIS

Gastritis is inflammation of the stomach mucosa and can be acute or chronic. Causes are listed in Box 33.6.

Acute Gastritis

Pathophysiology

Gastritis results when the protective mucosal barrier is broken down and allows autodigestion from hydrochloric acid and pepsin to occur. This results in edema of the tissue and possible hemorrhage. With severe gastritis, the gastric mucosa can become gangrenous and perforate, which can lead to peritonitis (infection of the peritoneum). Scarring may also occur, resulting in pyloric obstruction.

Box 33.6

Causes of Gastritis

Diet
- Alcohol
- Spicy foods

Microorganisms
- *Helicobacter pylori*
- *Salmonella*

Medications
- Aspirin
- Nonsteroidal anti-inflammatory drugs
- Corticosteroids
- Digitalis
- Chemotherapy drugs

Stress
- Physiological
- Psychological

Trauma

Other Factors
- Reflux of bile
- Smoking
- Radiation
- Nasogastric suctioning

Endoscopic procedures

• WORD • BUILDING •

gastritis: gastr—stomach + itis—inflammation

Signs and Symptoms

The major symptom of gastritis is abdominal pain, which is often accompanied by nausea and anorexia. The patient may also experience abdominal tenderness, a feeling of fullness, reflux, belching, and hematemesis. If the cause of the gastritis is contaminated food, symptoms including diarrhea usually start within 5 to 6 hours.

Therapeutic Measures

Treatment of gastritis is removal of the irritating substance and provision of a bland diet of liquids and soft foods along with antacids. Medication therapy may include phenothiazines to control vomiting and antacids and/or histamine receptor antagonists to control pain. With a bland diet, the patient usually recovers in a short period of time.

Chronic Gastritis

Chronic gastritis occurs over time and is classified as type A or type B.

Type A

Type A chronic gastritis is often referred to as autoimmune gastritis and occurs in the fundus (body of stomach). Chronic gastritis type A is diagnosed by endoscopy, upper GI x-ray examination, and gastric aspirate analysis (see Chapter 32). Type A gastritis is often asymptomatic. Patients with type A gastritis usually do not secrete enough intrinsic factor from their stomach cells and as a result have difficulty absorbing vitamin B_{12}, which leads to pernicious anemia (discussed later).

Type B

Type B chronic gastritis affects the antrum and pylorus (lower end of the stomach near the duodenum) and is associated with ***Helicobacter pylori*** bacterial infection. Type B is the most common type of chronic gastritis. Signs and symptoms include poor appetite, heartburn after eating, belching, a sour taste in the mouth, and nausea and vomiting. Type B gastritis can also be diagnosed by endoscopy, upper GI x-ray examination, and gastric aspirate analysis. *H. pylori* infection is treated with antibiotics.

PEPTIC ULCER DISEASE

Pathophysiology

Peptic ulcer disease (PUD) is a condition in which the lining of the stomach, pylorus, duodenum, or the esophagus is eroded, usually from infection with *H. pylori.* The erosion may extend into the muscular layers or the peritoneum. Peptic ulcers occur in the portions of the gastrointestinal tract that are exposed to hydrochloric acid and pepsin. The erosion is due to an increase in the concentration or activity of hydrochloric acid and pepsin. The damaged mucosa is unable to secrete enough mucus to act as a barrier against the hydrochloric acid. Some individuals have more rapid gastric emptying, which, combined with hypersecretion of acid, creates a large amount of acid moving into the duodenum. As a result, peptic ulcers occur more often in the duodenum. Ulcers are named by their location: esophageal, gastric, or duodenal. Duodenal ulcers are more common than gastric ulcers.

Etiology

Until 1982, the cause of peptic ulcers was poorly understood and thought to be related to stress, diet, and alcohol or caffeine ingestion. However, research results have found that PUD is primarily caused by infection with the gram-negative bacterium *Helicobacter pylori* (*H. pylori*). This bacterium is responsible for 80% of gastric ulcers and more than 90% of duodenal ulcers. Two-thirds of all people are infected with *H. pylori,* and it is most common in those who are elderly, Hispanic, African American, or in lower socioeconomic groups in the United States. The discovery of *H. pylori* has led to changes in treating and curing peptic ulcers. It is not known how *H. pylori* is transmitted, although the oral-oral or fecal-oral route is likely. Contaminated water may also play a role. Vaccines to prevent peptic ulcers are being developed.

LEARNING TIP

Most peptic ulcers are caused by an infection (*H. pylori*) that can be cured with antibiotics.

Risk factors that contribute to peptic ulcer disease include smoking, chewing tobacco, stress, caffeine use, and medications such as steroids, aspirin, and nonsteroidal anti-inflammatory drugs (NSAIDs). Peptic ulcer development is influenced by smoking because it increases the harmful effects of *H. pylori,* alters protective mechanisms, and decreases gastric blood flow. For more information on *H. pylori,* visit www.cdc.gov or call 1-888-MY-ULCER (1-888-698-5237).

Signs and Symptoms

Symptoms vary with the location of the ulcer (Table 33.2). Symptoms, including pain, may not be experienced with gastric or duodenal ulcers until complications such as hemorrhage, obstruction, or perforation develop. If pain does occur, patients with gastric ulcers commonly experience a burning and gnawing pain in the high left epigastric region. Pain may increase with food ingestion or 1 to 2 hours after a meal. Duodenal ulcers produce cramping or burning pain in the midepigastric or upper abdominal area. The pain occurs 2 to 4 hours after meals or in the middle of the night. This intermittent pain may be relieved by the ingestion of food or antacids. Anorexia and nausea and vomiting may also occur with either ulcer location. Bleeding may occur with massive hemorrhaging or slow oozing. Patients often have low hematocrit and hemoglobin levels, and gastric or fecal occult blood may be found, depending on where the ulcers are located.

Complications

Major complications can result from PUD. These include bleeding, perforation, and obstruction. Bleeding can occur in varying degrees from occult blood in stool and emesis to massive bright red bleeding. Hemorrhage tends to occur more often with gastric ulcers in older adults. The patient may experience signs and symptoms of shock. Treatment includes stopping the bleeding, replacing fluid and electrolytes, and possibly administering vasopressin to stop the bleeding.

Diagnostic Tests

H. pylori can be diagnosed with several tests. The urea breath test is performed by having the patient drink carbon-labeled urea. The urea is metabolized rapidly if *H. pylori* is present, allowing the carbon to be absorbed and measured in exhaled carbon dioxide. An IgG antibody detection test for *H. pylori* identifies whether the patient is infected with *H. pylori.* These are both noninvasive detection tests. Biopsy specimens for the *Campylobacter*-like organism (CLO) biopsy urease test and a histological examination can be obtained during esophagogastroduodenoscopy (EGD). Biopsy is the most conclusive test for *H. pylori.* Cultures of the biopsy specimen may also be done to determine antimicrobial susceptibility.

Peptic ulcers are diagnosed on the basis of symptoms, upper GI series (barium swallow), and EGD. Endoscopy allows direct visualization of the ulcer and mucosal tissues.

Therapeutic Measures

Several treatment options are used to cure *H. pylori* without recurrence (Table 33.3). The first antibiotic treatment for ulcer disease caused by *H. pylori* was approved by the Food and Drug Administration (FDA) in 1996. For better effectiveness, triple therapy with two antibiotics to decrease resistance of the bacteria and a proton pump inhibitor or H_2 antagonist is used. Treatment lasting 14 days has better eradication rates than 10-day treatments. Bismuth subsalicylate (Pepto-Bismol) may also be used for its antibacterial effects. Proton pump inhibitors are powerful agents that stop the final step of gastric acid secretion to reduce mucosa erosion and aid in healing ulcers (Table 33.4). H_2 antagonists block H_2 receptors to decrease acid secretion, although not as powerfully as gastric acid pump inhibitors. A bland diet may also be recommended, and foods known to cause discomfort to the patient, such as spicy foods, carbonated drinks, and caffeine, should be avoided until the ulcer heals. Alcohol should also be avoided during the healing period. Endoscopy can be used to view the degree of healing of the ulcer.

TABLE 33.2 PEPTIC ULCER DISEASE SUMMARY

Signs and Symptoms	Gastric ulcer	Intermittent high left epigastric or upper abdominal burning or gnawing pain, increased 1–2 hours after meals or with food Variable pain pattern possibly made worse by food Antacids ineffective Can lead to gastric cancer Patient may be malnourished Hematemesis more common than melena
	Duodenal ulcer	Intermittent midepigastric or upper abdominal burning or cramping pain, increased 2–4 hours after meals or in the middle of the night Relieved by food or antacids Patient usually well nourished Melena more common than hematemesis Anorexia Nausea and vomiting Bleeding (stomach secretions or stool positive for occult blood)
Diagnostic Tests	*H. pylori*	Urea breath test IgG antibody detection test for *H. pylori* Biopsy Culture
	Peptic ulcer	Upper GI series (barium swallow) Esophagogastroduodenoscopy
Therapeutic Measures	Antibiotics Proton pump inhibitors H_2 antagonists Bismuth subsalicylate Sucralfate (Carafate) Antacids Bland diet Avoiding irritants, such as smoking, caffeine, alcohol, trigger foods	
Complications	Bleeding Perforation Obstruction	
Priority Nursing Diagnoses	*Acute Pain* *Risk for Injury* *Deficient Knowledge*	

TABLE 33.3 MEDICATION REGIMEN OPTIONS FOR *H. PYLORI* INFECTION

Type of Therapy	Included in Therapy	Examples of Therapy Options
Triple therapy*	Two antibiotics + proton pump inhibitor	Amoxicillin (Amoxil) + clarithromycin (Biaxin) + omeprazole (Prilosec) Amoxicillin (Amoxil) + clarithromycin (Biaxin) + lansoprazole (Prevacid) (available as Prevpac, combined for convenience)
Dual therapy	Antibiotic + proton pump inhibitor	Clarithromycin (Biaxin) + omeprazole (Prilosec) Amoxicillin (Amoxil) + lansoprazole (Prevacid)
	Antibiotic + H_2 antagonist	Clarithromycin (Biaxin) + H_2 antagonist
Other therapy	Two antibiotics + bismuth subsalicylate + H_2 antagonist	Metronidazole (Flagyl) + tetracycline + bismuth subsalicylate (Pepto-Bismol) + H_2 antagonist

*Triple therapy has the best eradication rate.

SUGGESTED ANSWERS TO—cont'd

NG tube in a patient who has had gastric surgery. Repositioning the NG tube could damage the surgical suture line.

c. Next check the suction equipment for ordered settings and to ensure that it is turned on. The suction setting normally is ordered to be on low. A whistling sound is heard when the tube is disconnected from the suction setup. The seals should be tight on the suction canister. When the tubing is hooked to suction, gastric contents should start moving into the suction canister. It is important to make sure equipment is functioning properly to ensure patient safety.

d. Check the nasogastric tube for clogs only if the physician orders aspiration or irrigation to be done. The tube is gently aspirated with a 60-mL catheter-tipped syringe. If the tube remains clogged, it is gently flushed as ordered with 10 to 20 mL of sterile normal saline.

e. After the gastric distention has been relieved, Mr. Wong's pain level is reassessed to determine if he needs pain medication. Considering that he is less than 1 day postoperative, he probably needs it.

2. Necessary equipment includes stethoscope, 60-mL catheter-tipped syringe, gloves, goggles, and normal saline for irrigation.

3.

$$\frac{1000 \text{ mL} \times 10 \text{ drops/mL}}{(60 \times 8) = 480 \text{ min}}$$

$$= \frac{10{,}000 \text{ drops}}{480 \text{ min}} = 21 \text{ drops/min}$$

■ *Mrs. Lindsay*

Although there are many variations, the following is an example of a 1-day meal plan for Mrs. Lindsay:

Breakfast: one egg, any style; ½ orange; one glass milk

Snack: one slice toast with apple butter, jelly, or jam

Lunch: 2 oz ham, ½ cup cottage cheese, four asparagus spears

Snack: ½ serving chicken salad on bed of lettuce

Dinner: 2 oz broiled fish, ½ serving corn, ½ serving broccoli

Snack: ½ cup yogurt or sherbet

REVIEW QUESTIONS

1. The nurse is planning care for a patient with an eating disorder. The patient is 40 kg and 68 inches tall. Serum laboratory data: potassium 2.6 mEq/dL, sodium 126 mEq/dL, chloride 95 mEq/dL, calcium 10.8 mg/dL. The nurse understands that which of the following is the most important intervention for this patient?
   a. Weigh the patient daily at the same time.
   b. Maintain IV of dextrose and electrolytes.
   c. Praise intake of any type of food.
   d. Document intake and output.

2. In planning care for patients, the nurse understands that which of the following patients are considered obese?
   a. A 25-year-old woman with body weight 5% above ideal body weight
   b. A 45-year-old man with waist-to-hip ratio measurement of 0.5
   c. A 50-year-old man with body mass index of 31
   d. A 16-year-old girl with anorexia nervosa weighing 98 pounds

3. A patient is diagnosed with aphthous stomatitis (canker sore). Which of the following actions would be appropriate?
   a. Tell patient to avoid brushing teeth until the sore has healed.
   b. Encourage patient to use a mouthwash four times a day.
   c. Apply acyclovir ointment to ease the pain of the lesion.
   d. Teach patient to apply topical tetracycline several times a day to sore.

4. The nurse is caring for a patient with gastritis. Which of the following interventions would be appropriate for a patient with acute gastritis?
   a. Monitor patient for bloody diarrhea.
   b. Explain that aspirin rarely causes gastritis.
   c. Administer phenothiazine to control vomiting.
   d. Encourage a regular diet during the acute phase of gastritis.

REVIEW QUESTIONS—cont'd

5. The nurse is planning a teaching session for a patient with a peptic ulcer. Which of the following would the nurse include in the teaching plan as the primary cause of peptic ulcers?
   a. Eating spicy foods
   b. A stressful life
   c. A bacterial infection
   d. Excessive caffeine intake

6. After a teaching session for a patient with a peptic ulcer, the nurse would evaluate the patient as understanding the teaching if the patient stated that the purpose of H_2 antagonists is which of the following?
   a. Neutralize gastric acid.
   b. Form a protective paste.
   c. Determine gastric pH levels.
   d. Inhibit secretion of gastric acid.

7. A patient who has just returned from surgery after a total gastrectomy begins to vomit bright red blood. Which of the following is a priority action for the nurse to take?
   a. Increase the IV rate.
   b. Take blood pressure.
   c. Place patient onto side.
   d. Administer oxygen.

8. For the patient with dumping syndrome, which of these foods would the nurse instruct the patient to avoid?
   a. Spinach and avocado salad
   b. Coffee and glazed doughnut
   c. Sausage and liver
   d. Creamed chipped beef

9. To deliver 1000 mL of 5% dextrose in 0.45 normal saline (at 150 mL per hour using 10 drop tubings), the nurse would monitor the IV infusion at how many drops per minute? **Fill in the blank.**

Answer: ________________ drops per minute

34 Nursing Care of Patients with Lower Gastrointestinal Disorders

LAZETTE V. NOWICKI

KEY TERMS

appendicitis (uh-PEN-dih-SYE-tiss)
colectomy (koh-LEK-tuh-me)
colitis (koh-LYE-tiss)
colostomy (kuh-LAW-stuh-mee)
constipation (KON-stih-PAY-shun)
diarrhea (DYE-uh-REE-ah)
diverticulitis (DYE-ver-tik-yoo-LYE-tiss)
diverticulosis (DYE-ver-tik-yoo-LOH-siss)
enteritis (en-tur-EYE-tiss)
fissures (FISH-ers)
fistulas (FIST-yoo-lahs)
hematochezia (HEM-uh-toh-KEE-zee-uh)
hemorrhoids (HEM-uh-royds)
hernia (HER-nee-uh)
ileostomy (ILL-ee-AW-stuh-mee)
impaction (im-PAK-shun)
intussusception (IN-tuh-suh-SEP-shun)
megacolon (MEG-ah-KOH-lun)
melena (muh-LEE-nah)
obstipation (OB-stih-PAY-shun)
peristomal (PEAR-ih-STOH-muhl)
peritonitis (pear-ih-toh-NYE-tiss)
stoma (STOH-mah)
volvulus (VOL-view-luss)

QUESTIONS TO GUIDE YOUR READING

1. What are the causes, signs, and symptoms of constipation and diarrhea?
2. What nursing care and teaching do patients with constipation or diarrhea require?
3. What medical treatment, nursing care, and teaching are appropriate for patients with inflammatory and infectious disorders of the lower gastrointestinal tract?
4. How would you describe Crohn's disease, ulcerative colitis, irritable bowel syndrome, and the nursing care for these conditions?
5. What nursing care is practiced for an abdominal hernia?
6. What nursing care and teaching do patients with absorption disorders require?
7. What are the causes, signs and symptoms, therapeutic measures, and nursing care of intestinal obstruction?
8. What therapeutic measures and nursing care are provided for lower gastrointestinal bleeding?
9. What are the causes, signs and symptoms, therapeutic measures, and nursing care of colon cancer?
10. What nursing care and teaching does a patient with an ostomy require?

The lower gastrointestinal (GI) system includes the small and large intestines, rectum, and anus.

PROBLEMS OF ELIMINATION

Constipation

Pathophysiology

Constipation occurs when the fecal mass is held in the rectal cavity for a period of time that is not usual for the patient. While the feces are held for a prolonged time in the rectum, more water is absorbed. This makes the feces drier, harder, more difficult and sometimes painful to pass.

If a patient repeatedly ignores the urge to have a bowel movement (laxation), the musculature and rectal mucous membrane become insensitive to the presence of feces. Eventually a stronger stimulus is needed to produce the peristaltic rush required for defecation. Prolonged constipation is called **obstipation**.

Etiology

There are many causes of constipation. Medications such as narcotics, tranquilizers, and antacids with aluminum decrease motility of the large intestine and may contribute to constipation. Rectal or anal conditions such as hemorrhoids or fissures may lead to a delay in defecation because of the associated pain. Metabolic or neurologic conditions such as diabetes mellitus, multiple sclerosis, lupus erythematosus, or scleroderma may interfere with normal bowel innervation and function. Colon cancer may cause an obstruction that prevents normal bowel function and leads to constipation. Low intake of dietary fiber and fluids decreases the bulk of the feces and causes constipation. Decreased mobility, weakness, and fatigue, especially in the elderly, reduce the strength of the muscles used for defecation, increasing the likelihood of constipation. Chronic laxative use can also contribute to constipation because the laxative overrides the bowel's ability to recognize the urge to defecate.

Prevention

Regular exercise and a diet high in fiber and fluids are the best preventive measures for constipation. Laxatives should be used only occasionally to prevent dependence and complications.

Signs and Symptoms

Abdominal pain and distention, indigestion, rectal pressure, a sensation of incomplete emptying, and intestinal rumbling are indications of constipation (Table 34.1). The patient may also report headache, fatigue, decreased appetite, straining at stool, and elimination of hard, dry stool.

Complications

A variety of problems can result from constipation. Fecal **impaction** may result when the fecal mass is so dry it cannot be passed. Pressure on the colon mucosa from a mass of stool may cause ulcers to develop. Often, small amounts of liquid stool ooze around the fecal mass and cause incontinence of liquid stools. The incontinence may be treated with an antidiarrheal medication, which will worsen the constipation if a thorough assessment is not performed to rule out impaction. Straining to have a bowel movement (Valsalva's maneuver) can result in cardiac, neurologic, and respiratory complications. If the patient has a history of heart failure, hypertension, or recent myocardial infarction, straining can lead to cardiac rupture and death. Grossly dilated loops of the colon, known as **megacolon**, can occur proximal to the dry fecal mass and obstruct the colon. Abdominal distention occurs, and in severe cases, loops of bowel can be palpated through the abdominal wall.

Chronic laxative abuse can lead to colonic mucosal atrophy, muscle thickening, and fibrosis. These conditions can result in perforation of the colon and necessitate an emergency **colectomy**.

TABLE 34.1 CONSTIPATION SUMMARY

Signs and Symptoms	Abdominal distention Indigestion Rectal pressure Feeling of incomplete emptying Straining at stool Hard, dry stool Intestinal rumbling
Diagnostic Tests	History Physical examination
Therapeutic Measures	High-fiber diet 2–3 L fluid daily Strengthening of abdominal muscles Exercise Bulk-forming agents Stool softeners
Priority Nursing Diagnoses	*Constipation* *Deficient Knowledge*

Diagnostic Tests

Constipation is usually self-diagnosed or diagnosed by history and physical examination. If complications are suspected, a radiographic examination, sigmoidoscopy, and stool testing for occult blood may be needed.

Therapeutic Measures

Treatment of constipation depends on the cause. Fiber should be added to the diet, and exercises to strengthen abdominal muscles should be done. Behavior changes, such as setting a daily defecation time, appropriately responding to the urge to defecate, and drinking 8 oz of warm water every morning and 2 to 3 L of water every day,

• WORD • BUILDING •

megacolon: mega—large + colon—colon

colectomy: col—pertaining to colon + ectomy—surgical excision if not contraindicated for other reasons, can help establish a more normal bowel pattern. Chronic laxative use should be discontinued. Bulk-forming agents such as psyllium (Metamucil) or stool softeners such as docusate sodium (Colace) should be used instead of laxatives. Enemas and rectal suppositories are used only in extreme cases and are discontinued when an acute episode is resolved. Methylnaltrexone (Relistor) given subcutaneously treats opioid-induced constipation for patients receiving palliative care when other laxatives have not been effective. It does not treat other forms of constipation.

Nursing Process for the Patient with Constipation

DATA COLLECTION. The patient may feel self-conscious or embarrassed when interviewed about bowel habits and history. Consideration should be given to the patient's feelings by postponing the discussion until rapport has been established. Data gathered in privacy should include the onset and duration of constipation, past elimination pattern, current elimination pattern, occupation, lifestyle (stress, exercise, nutrition), history of laxative or enema use, medical-surgical history, and current medications being taken. Color, consistency, and any odor of the stool, as well as any intestinal symptoms, are also important.

After the interview, the patient's abdomen is inspected and palpated for distention and symmetry. Inspection of the perianal area may reveal fissures, external hemorrhoids, or irritation.

NURSING DIAGNOSES, PLANNING, AND IMPLEMENTATION

Constipation Related to Irregular Defecation Habits

EXPECTED OUTCOME: The patient will maintain passage of soft, formed stool every 1 to 3 days without straining.

- Assess normal pattern of defecation, diet and fluid intake, medications, surgeries, and use of laxatives *to help identify factors contributing to constipation.*
- Determine patient's access to the bathroom and ability to use the toilet *to ensure barriers to safe toileting, such as unsafe obstructing furniture arrangements or clutter, are removed.*
- Set a specific time for defecation, such as after a meal, *to facilitate the urge reflex.*
- Place feet on a footstool *to promote flexion of the hips, which aids defecation.*
- Provide a high-fiber, high-residue diet including fresh fruits, vegetables, and whole grains with 2 g of bran added to cereal daily for constipation caused by decreased motility and muscle tone or a low-fiber diet *to significantly increase bowel movements and decrease the number of laxatives, enemas, or stool softeners required* (Box 34.1, *Nutrition Notes*).
- Increase fluid if not contraindicated to 2 to 3 L per day *to aid in ability to discontinue laxative use.*
- Increase activity through a daily walking program and abdominal exercises designed to improve the muscle tone *to improve peristalsis and promote more spontaneous defecation.*

Box 34.1

Nutrition Notes

Treating Constipation with Food Formula

Constipation may be successfully treated with 1 to 2 oz of the following mixture taken with the evening meal:

1 cup applesauce,
1 cup All-Bran cereal, and
½ cup 100% prune juice.

Mixture may be stored in the refrigerator for 5 days and then should be discarded. In all cases of constipation, especially when increased fiber is given, adequate fluid intake is essential.

CRITICAL THINKING

Mrs. Burns

■ Mrs. Burns is a 93-year-old resident in an assisted living facility. You see on her chart that she has not had a bowel movement in 5 days. What action would you take?
Suggested answers at end of chapter.

Deficient Knowledge Related to Practices to Prevent Constipation

EXPECTED OUTCOME: The patient will state understanding and ability to carry out preventive measures for constipation.

- Teach factors leading to constipation, such as a low-fiber diet, and preventive interventions such as increasing fiber or fluid intake. *Prevention of constipation may be as simple as correcting the contributing factors.*
- Explain the physiology of defecation and the importance of responding to the urge to defecate when it occurs *to help prevent constipation.*
- Assure the patient that having a daily bowel movement is not always necessary *to provide education and reassurance.*
- Explain that regular laxative use may increase motility and pressure in the bowel and cause further complications *to promote understanding and use of other preventive measures.*

EVALUATION. The plan has been effective if the patient has established a regular bowel function pattern (Table 34.2), verbalizes understanding of self-care measures, and expresses satisfaction with the outcomes.

TABLE 34.2 CRITERIA FOR REGULAR BOWEL FUNCTION

1. A regular time for defecation is routine.
2. A regular exercise program is followed.
3. Laxative use is avoided.
4. Water consumption is 2–3 L per day.
5. High-fiber and high-residue foods are added to the diet.
6. Consistency of stools reported is soft and formed.
7. Frequency of stools is every 1 to 3 days.

Diarrhea

Diarrhea occurs when fecal matter passes through the intestine rapidly, resulting in decreased absorption of water, electrolytes, and nutrients and causing frequent, watery stools. Classification and severity of diarrhea are based on the number of unformed stools in 24 hours.

Pathophysiology and Etiology

The most common cause of acute diarrhea is a bacterial or viral infection. Bacteria (normal flora) are normally found in the intestines. If these bacteria grow out of control or if bacteria or viruses are ingested in contaminated food or water, infection results. Some bacteria release toxins that irritate the intestinal mucosa, causing an inflammatory response and an increase in mucus production. Hyperperistalsis occurs, which lasts until the irritants have been excreted. The most common infectious agents are *Escherichia coli, Campylobacter jejuni, Shigella* spp., *Clostridium difficile, Giardia* spp., and *Salmonella* spp.

Poor tolerance or allergies to certain foods may cause diarrhea. Foods that most commonly cause diarrhea are additives (such as nutmeg or sorbitol), caffeine, milk products, meats, wheat, and potatoes. Acute diarrhea usually resolves in 7 to 14 days.

Chronic diarrhea may result from inflammatory disease, osmotic agents, excessive secretion of electrolytes, or increased intestinal motility. Inflammatory diseases such as Crohn's disease or ulcerative colitis (discussed later) may impair absorption, resulting in frequent, watery stools. Osmotic diarrhea results from ingestion of laxatives or other agents that prevent absorption of water or nutrients in the intestine. Additional causes of malabsorption include surgical resection or disease of certain areas of the intestinal tract, such as the terminal ileum or pylorus. Radiation therapy for cancer also may induce a malabsorption syndrome. Enteral tube feedings commonly result in diarrhea, especially when malnutrition has caused edema in the gut wall, which decreases absorption.

Increased secretion of water and electrolytes by the intestinal mucosa associated with certain hormonal disorders results in high-volume fecal output. An irritable bowel or a neurologic disorder may cause increased motility problems. Also, as described earlier, diarrhea can indicate fecal impaction.

Prevention

To prevent diarrhea, proper handling, storage, and refrigeration of all fresh foods helps to minimize contact with infectious agents. Milk and milk products must be kept refrigerated and protected. Hand washing and cleaning of the kitchen and the food preparation and serving items are extremely important. Also enteral feedings should be given using full-strength formula rather than diluting the formula. This reduces the risk of contaminating the formula.

Signs and Symptoms

Initial diarrhea stools are foul smelling and may have undigested food particles and mucus (Table 34.3). The stools may also contain blood or pus. Diarrhea resulting from food poisoning usually has an explosive onset and may be accompanied by nausea and vomiting. Abdominal cramping, distention, anorexia, intestinal rumbling, and thirst are common. Fever indicates infection. Weakness and dehydration from fluid loss may occur (Box 34.2, *Gerontological Issues*).

Diagnostic Tests

The diagnosis of diarrhea is determined by the onset and progression of the condition, presence of fever, laboratory examinations, and visual inspection of the stool for bacteria, pus, or blood. Diarrhea mixed with red blood cells and mucus is associated with cholera, typhoid, typhus, large-bowel cancer, or amebiasis. Diarrhea mixed with white blood cells and mucus is associated with shigellosis, intestinal tuberculosis, salmonellosis, regional enteritis, or ulcerative colitis. Bulky, frothy stool is seen in celiac disease. Pasty stools usually have a high fat content and may be associated with common bile duct obstruction and celiac disease. A "butter stool" appearance is seen in patients with cystic fibrosis.

TABLE 34.3 DIARRHEA SUMMARY

Signs and Symptoms	Frequent, watery stools Abdominal cramping Distention Anorexia Intestinal rumbling
Diagnostic Tests	History Laboratory examinations of stool
Therapeutic Measures	Replacement of fluids and electrolytes Antidiarrheal medications Antimicrobials Lactinex
Priority Nursing Diagnoses	*Diarrhea* *Deficient Fluid Volume* *Deficient Knowledge*

• WORD • BUILDING •

diarrhea: dia—through + rhea—to flow

Box 34.2

Gerontological Issues

Diarrhea can cause older people to quickly become dehydrated and hypokalemic because both fluid and potassium are lost in stools. The signs and symptoms of hypokalemia include muscle weakness, hypotension, anorexia, paresthesia, and drowsiness. It can also cause cardiac dysrhythmias, such as atrial and ventricular tachycardia, premature ventricular contraction, and ventricular fibrillation, which can be fatal.

If the older person has decreased mobility, quick access to the bathroom is important. Because of poor muscle control, older patients may be incontinent. This might embarrass patients or cause them to hurry, which increases chances of patients falling and causing other problems such as fracture, dislocation, or hematoma. Also, because older patients' skin is more sensitive resulting from poor turgor and a reduction in subcutaneous fat layers, perirectal skin excoriation can occur secondary to the acidity and digestive enzyme content of diarrheal stools.

Therapeutic Measures

Replacing fluids and electrolytes is the first priority. This can be done by increasing oral fluid intake and using solutions with glucose and electrolytes if ordered by the physician. Intravenous fluid replacement may be necessary for rapid hydration, especially in the very young or very old. An elimination diet can be tried to identify foods that may contribute to diarrhea. Foods known to cause diarrhea are eliminated to see if a change in bowel function occurs. Each food item is then added back into the diet, one at a time, to see which ones cause diarrhea.

If the patient has three or more watery stools per day, motility of the intestines can be decreased with the use of drugs, such as diphenoxylate (Lomotil), difenoxin HCl (Motofen), and loperamide (Imodium). If diarrhea is thought to be caused by antibiotics that change the normal flora of the bowel, a *Lactobacillus* granule dietary supplement (Lactinex) may be used to restore the normal flora. Antimicrobial agents are prescribed if infectious agents have been documented.

Nursing Process for the Patient with Diarrhea

DATA COLLECTION. Observation of the patient's behaviors and symptoms assists in identifying the cause of diarrhea. Ask the patient to describe any symptoms, when they started, and how long they have been present. Questions should include "Is there any abdominal pain, urgency, or cramping?" and "What time of the day does it happen?" Stool consistency, color, odor, and frequency are documented.

Assess for symptoms of dehydration, such as tachycardia, hypotension, decreased skin turgor, weakness, thready pulse, dry mucous membranes, and oliguria. Obtain the patient's height and weight to establish a baseline. Abnormal laboratory studies that may indicate dehydration include increased serum osmolality, increased specific gravity of urine, and increased hematocrit. Decreased serum potassium may result from intestinal loss of potassium.

Inspect the abdomen for distention. The patient's usual dietary habits and any changes or recent exposure to contaminated food or water are assessed. Determine if medications such as antibiotics or laxatives contributed to the diarrhea. If the patient has traveled recently, discover the geographical location and whether exposure to an infected person or someone with similar symptoms occurred.

Data are collected on the patient's coping mechanisms for use if the patient needs to express concerns or anxiety regarding incontinence of liquid stools and embarrassment.

NURSING DIAGNOSES, PLANNING, AND IMPLEMENTATION

Diarrhea Related to Infection or Possible Ingestion of Irritating Foods

EXPECTED OUTCOME: The patient will maintain formed, soft stool every 1 to 3 days.

- Obtain history including medications regarding diarrhea episode *to help identify cause.*
- Monitor and record stool characteristics, amount, and frequency *to plan care.*
- Ensure hand washing by patient, family, and health care staff *to prevent the spread of infection.*
- Identify potentially infected persons or contaminated foods *to prevent the spread of infection.*
- Consider private patient room *to prevent infection transmission.*
- Maintain nothing by mouth (NPO) as ordered *to promote bowel rest.*
- Give antidiarrheal medications as ordered. *Controlling diarrhea controls comfort and fluid balance.*
- Keep skin clean, dry, and protected with a moisture barrier, such as petrolatum or medicated ointment, after each bowel movement or use a fecal incontinence appliance to protect perianal skin from contact with liquid stools and their enzymes (see *Evidence-Based Practice* box).
- Provide clear liquids, such as water, juices, bouillon, and gelatin, with progression to a low-residue diet when the acute diarrhea phase is over (Box 34.3, *Nutrition Notes*).
- Limit caffeine intake *because it stimulates intestinal motility.*

Risk for Deficient Fluid Volume Related to Frequent Passage of Stools and Insufficient Fluid Intake

EXPECTED OUTCOME: The patient will maintain a stable weight and vital signs and urine output will remain within normal limits at all times.

- Record intake and output (including diarrheal stools) *to determine fluid balance.*
- Weigh patient daily *to determine fluid loss.*

EVIDENCE-BASED PRACTICE

Clinical Question

Can an indwelling fecal incontinence device be safely used for patients with diarrhea or fecal incontinence?

Evidence

A prospective single-arm study looked at 42 patients with diarrhea and/or fecal incontinence (Padmanabhan et al., 2007). The Flexi-Seal Management System was used. The system consists of a soft silicone tube with a silicone low-pressure balloon at the end. The tube is inserted into the rectum, the balloon inflated and the system is connected to a collection bag. Ninety-two percent of the patients in the study either maintained the baseline skin integrity or improved the skin integrity. Rectal mucosa remained healthy in select patients who had endoscopy before and after the system.

Implications for Nursing Practice

The Flexi-Seal Management System may be used in the hospital setting for patients with diarrhea and fecal incontinence. The system seems to be tolerated well by patients, skin remains intact, and rectal mucosa remains healthy. More studies are needed to determine clinical and economic outcomes with the device.

REFERENCE

Padmanabhan, A., Stern, M., Wishin, J., et al. (2007). Clinical evaluation of a flexible fecal incontinence management system. *American Journal of Critical Care, 16*(4), 384–393.

Box 34.3 Nutrition Notes

Deciding When to Refer an Adult with Diarrhea for Medical Care

Most instances of diarrhea in healthy adults are self-limiting and resolve without treatment. Indications for medical consultation include the following:

- Large volumes of stool
- Severe abdominal pain
- Bloody stools
- Protracted duration
- Systemic symptoms such as fever or prostration
- Medical conditions for which fasting, dehydration, or infectious disease are hazardous.

Healthy adults at minimal risk of electrolyte imbalance may institute self-treatment as follows:

- *For the first 12 hours:* Water or oral rehydration solutions at room temperature. Easily absorbed fluids maintain hydration. Hot or cold liquids are more likely to stimulate peristalsis.
- *For the second 12 hours:* Clear liquids, no caffeine or extremes of temperature. If more than 5% of body weight is lost, seek medical attention.
- *For the third 12 hours:* Full liquids. Experiment with milk in case temporary lactose intolerance has developed as a result of intestinal inflammation.
- *For the fourth 12 hours:* Soft diet. Include applesauce or banana for pectin and also rice, pasta, and bread without fat (digested by enzymes usually unaffected in gastroenteritis).
- *By the 48th hour:* Regular diet. If diarrhea has not resolved and regular diet is not tolerated, seek medical treatment.

- Maintain intravenous fluid replacement as ordered *to maintain fluid balance if output is greater than intake.*
- Encourage fluids when acute diarrhea subsides *to maintain fluid balance.*
- Teach patient signs and symptoms of dehydration to report *to allow prompt treatment.*

EVALUATION. Goals have been met if frequency of diarrheal stools is decreased and balance of fluid and electrolytes is achieved.

INFLAMMATORY AND INFECTIOUS DISORDERS

Many diseases of the lower GI tract are a result of inflammation in the bowel. Sometimes the inflamed areas become infected, resulting in a worsening of symptoms and necessitating antimicrobial therapy.

Appendicitis

Pathophysiology

Appendicitis is the inflammation of the appendix, the small, finger-like appendage attached to the cecum of the large intestine (see Fig. 32.1). Because of the small size of the appendix, obstruction may occur, making it susceptible to infection. The resulting inflammatory process causes an increase in intraluminal pressure of the appendix.

Signs and Symptoms

Signs and symptoms of appendicitis include fever, increased white blood cells, and generalized pain in the upper abdomen. Within hours of onset the pain usually becomes localized to the right lower quadrant at McBurney's point, midway between the umbilicus and the right iliac crest (Fig. 34.1). This is one of the classic symptoms of appendicitis. Nausea, vomiting, and anorexia are also usually present.

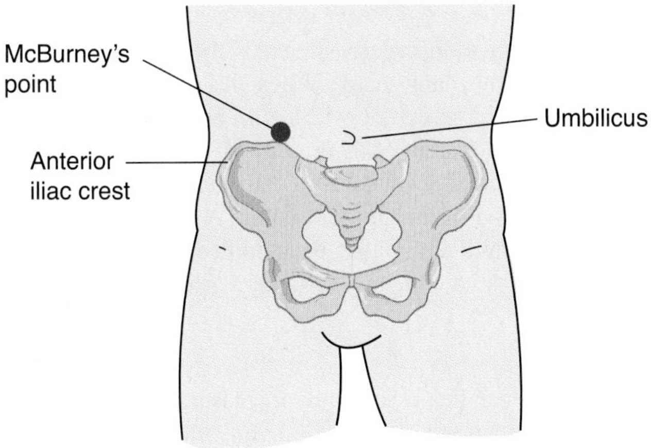
McBurney's point
Umbilicus
Anterior iliac crest

FIGURE 34.1 Pain at McBurney's point is a symptom of appendicitis.

Physical examination reveals slight abdominal muscular rigidity (guarding), normal bowel sounds, and local rebound tenderness (intensification of pain when pressure is released after palpation) in the right lower quadrant of the abdomen. Sometimes there is pain in the right lower quadrant when the left lower quadrant is palpated (Rovsing's sign). The patient may keep the right leg flexed for comfort and experience increased pain if the leg is straightened.

Diagnostic Tests

A complete blood cell count (CBC) reveals elevated leukocyte and neutrophil counts. An ultrasound or computed tomography (CT) scan reveals an enlargement in the area of the cecum.

Therapeutic Measures

The patient is kept NPO and surgery is done immediately unless there is evidence of perforation or peritonitis. Ice to the site of pain and keeping the patient in a semi-Fowler's position may help reduce pain while the diagnosis is being made. The patient is often readied for an appendectomy by emergency department staff.

Laxatives and enemas are avoided because they may trigger or complicate a rupture. The use of a heating pad on the abdomen is avoided because the warmth may increase inflammation and risk of rupture. If the appendix has ruptured, intravenous fluids and antibiotic therapy are started to treat infection and peritonitis. Surgery may or may not be done right away. If infection is present a tube to drain the infection may be inserted into the abdomen by a radiologist. Surgery may then be delayed for up to several weeks while the infection is resolved.

After surgery, the diet is advanced as ordered and tolerated. If the appendix has ruptured, the patient may have an orogastric or nasogastric tube to decompress the stomach. Vital signs and abdominal data are collected to monitor for signs and symptoms of peritonitis. Pain control to promote early ambulation, coughing, deep breathing, and movement help prevent respiratory complications.

Complications

Perforation, abscess of the appendix, and peritonitis are major complications of appendicitis. With perforation, the pain is severe and temperature is elevated to at least 100°F (37.7°C). An abscess is a localized collection of pus separated from the peritoneal cavity by the omentum or small bowel. This is usually treated with parenteral antibiotics and surgical drainage. An appendectomy is done about 6 weeks later.

Peritonitis

Peritonitis is inflammation of the peritoneum that occurs from a variety of causes. It is a serious condition that can be life threatening.

Pathophysiology and Etiology

Trauma, ischemia, or tumor perforation in any abdominal organ causes leakage of the organ's contents into the peritoneal cavity. The most common cause of peritonitis is a ruptured appendix, but it may also occur after perforation of a peptic ulcer, gangrenous gallbladder, intestinal diverticula, incarcerated hernia, or gangrenous small bowel. It may also be a complication of peritoneal dialysis. Peritonitis results from the inflammation or infection that is caused by the leakage. The tissues become edematous and begin leaking fluid containing increasing amounts of blood, protein, cellular debris, and white blood cells. Initially, the intestinal tract responds with hypermotility, but this is soon followed by paralysis (paralytic ileus).

Signs and Symptoms

Generalized abdominal pain evolves into localized pain at the site of the perforation or leakage. The area of the abdomen that is affected is extremely tender and aggravated by movement. Rebound tenderness and abdominal rigidity are present. Decreased peristalsis results in nausea and vomiting. Infection causes fever, increased white blood cells, and an elevated pulse.

Diagnostic Tests

Rapid diagnosis is essential in preventing complications. Tests include an abdominal x-ray or CT scan to show distention or perforation; white blood cell count that is significantly elevated; paracentesis and laboratory studies to identify a causative organism; or exploratory surgery to identify the cause.

Therapeutic Measures

The patient is NPO because of impaired peristalsis. Fluid and electrolyte replacement is crucial to correct hypovolemia and prevent or treat shock. Abdominal distention is relieved through insertion of an orogastric (or nasogastric) tube with low intermittent suction. Antibiotics are used to treat or prevent sepsis. Depending on the cause of the peritonitis, surgery may be performed to excise, drain, or repair the cause. An ostomy may be formed to divert feces, allowing resolution of the infection. After surgery, the patient

• WORD • BUILDING •

peritonitis: periton—pertaining to peritoneum + itis—inflammation usually has a wound drain, a nasogastric (NG) tube, and a urinary catheter. Pain control is essential to overall recovery. Severely compromised patients may receive total parenteral nutrition (TPN) to meet nutritional needs for increased immune function and healing.

Complications

Complications of peritonitis are intestinal obstruction (discussed later), hypovolemia caused by the shift of fluid into the abdomen, and septicemia from bacteria entering the bloodstream. Shock and ultimately death may result. Wound dehiscence or evisceration can occur if the patient has had abdominal surgery.

Diverticulosis and Diverticulitis

Pathophysiology

A diverticulum is a herniation or outpouching of the bowel mucous membrane caused by increased pressure within the colon and weakness in the bowel wall. **Diverticulosis** is a condition in which multiple diverticula are present without evidence of inflammation (Fig. 34.2). Many people have diverticulosis without knowing it because it develops gradually. When food and bacteria are trapped in a diverticulum, inflammation and infection develop. This is called **diverticulitis**.

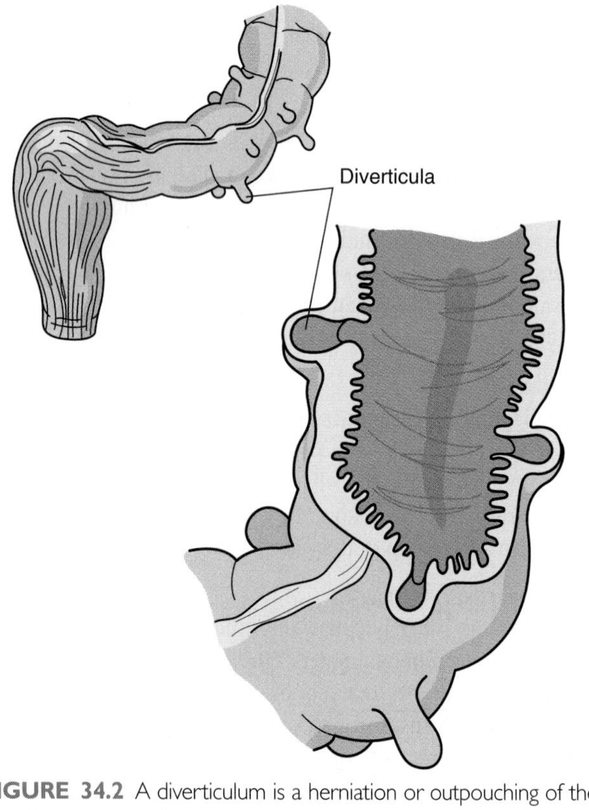
Diverticula

FIGURE 34.2 A diverticulum is a herniation or outpouching of the bowel mucous membrane. Having multiple diverticula is a condition called diverticulosis. If they become inflamed or infected, the condition is called diverticulitis.

• WORD • BUILDING •

diverticulosis: diverticul—blind pouch + osis—condition
diverticulitis: diverticul—blind pouch + itis—inflammation

Etiology

Chronic constipation usually precedes the development of diverticulosis by many years. When the patient is chronically constipated, pressure within the bowel is increased, leading to development of diverticula. A major cause of the disease is a decreased intake of dietary fiber. Diverticulosis is most common in the sigmoid colon. A small percentage of patients with diverticulosis develop diverticulitis. People older than age 60 are the most common group to experience diverticulitis.

Prevention

Diverticulitis can be prevented by increasing dietary fiber to prevent constipation and onset of diverticulosis.

Signs and Symptoms

The patient with diverticulosis is generally asymptomatic. When diverticulitis is present, the patient exhibits bowel changes, possibly alternating between constipation and diarrhea (Table 34.4). Steady or crampy pain in the left lower quadrant of the abdomen is the most common symptom. As the condition worsens, bleeding may occur, along with weakness, fever, fatigue, and anemia. Guarding and rebound tenderness may be present. If an abscess develops, the diverticulum may rupture, leading to peritonitis (Box 34.4, *Gerontological Issues*).

Diagnostic Tests

Diverticulosis is confirmed with sigmoidoscopy, colonoscopy, or barium enema. The diverticula and specific areas of inflammation can be seen during a colonoscopy or sigmoidoscopy. If an abscess is suspected, a CT scan may be done. Barium enema may show irregular narrowing of the colon and thickened muscle walls. A stool specimen may show occult blood. An abdominal x-ray examination may be done to identify a perforated diverticulum.

TABLE 34.4 SYMPTOMS ASSOCIATED WITH DIVERTICULITIS

W—Where is the pain?	Usually in the left lower quadrant
H—How does it feel? (Describe quality)	Tender, crampy
A—Aggravating and alleviating factors	Constipation and low-fiber diet may aggravate; treatment of constipation may alleviate
T—Timing (onset, duration, frequency)	Gradual onset, intermittent, gradual increase in frequency of pain events
S—Severity (0–10)	Usually 5–7
U—Useful other data/ associated symptoms	Intermittent rectal bleeding; straining at stool; constipation alternating with diarrhea; elevated white blood cells and sedimentation rate; elevated temperature and pulse rate; and pus, mucus, and blood in stool
P—Patient's perception	Fear of cancer diagnosis

Box 34.4

Gerontological Issues

With age-related weakness in the intestinal wall, about half of people in the United States and virtually all those older than age 80 have diverticular disease (Johns Hopkins Medicine, 2008). Clinical manifestation of this condition may include abdominal pain, rectal bleeding, nausea, and vomiting. Patients may not notice the abdominal pain until infection is present. Many times the symptoms are not reported early because patients fear it may be cancer. Blood in the stool, which can be an indication of diverticulitis, may not be seen by the older adult due to impaired vision.

Therapeutic Measures

Diverticulosis is managed by preventing constipation. With acute diverticulitis, the patient may be hospitalized for administration of intravenous antibiotics and pain control. A nasogastric tube, intravenous fluids, and NPO status may be ordered until pain, nausea or vomiting, fever, and inflammation decrease. When the acute period is over, a progressive diet is started. Whether or not perforation occurs, surgical resection with anastomosis or a temporary colostomy (discussed later) may be done to allow the inflammation to subside and the diseased portion of the colon to rest.

Dietary considerations for a patient with diverticulosis (without evidence of inflammation) include foods that are soft but high in fiber, such as prunes, raisins, and peas. Unprocessed bran can be added to soups, cereals, and salads to give added bulk to the diet. Fiber should be increased in the diet slowly to prevent excess gas and cramping. Some health care providers recommend avoiding nuts or foods with small seeds that can get caught in diverticula, such as tomatoes and raspberries, but this has not been shown to prevent diverticulitis. If the patient is overweight, he or she is encouraged to lose weight.

Nursing Process for the Patient with an Inflammatory or Infectious Disorder

Data Collection

Assessment of pain is essential for patients with inflammation or infection. Monitor the patient closely and notify the physician immediately if pain increases, especially if associated with abdominal rigidity. Increased pain may indicate that the bowel has ruptured and peritonitis is developing. Abdominal distention is monitored and recorded. With diverticulitis, a firm mass may be palpated in the sigmoid area.

Vital signs are monitored for fever or signs of septic shock. Intake and output are monitored and recorded accurately so that appropriate fluid replacement therapy is ordered. Monitoring for reduced urinary output, dropping blood pressure, and rising pulse rate can show fluid volume imbalance. If a fever is noted, the patient may be developing sepsis. All symptoms are reported to the physician promptly.

Nursing Diagnoses, Planning, and Implementation

Acute Pain Related to Inflammatory Process

EXPECTED OUTCOME: The patient will report pain is at an acceptable level within 30 minutes of report of pain.

- Have patient rate pain on objective scale such as 0 to 10 *to determine pain level.*
- Give analgesics or antispasmodic drugs as ordered *to relieve pain.*
- Use position changes, diversion, and relaxation exercises to help relieve pain. *Semi-Fowler's position may reduce tension on the abdomen.*
- Provide frequent mouth care if an NG tube is in place *to increase comfort.*

Risk for Deficient Fluid Volume Related to Diarrhea or Fluid Shifting from the Circulation to the Peritoneal Cavity

EXPECTED OUTCOME: The patient will maintain vital signs and urine output within normal limits at all times.

- Record intake and output *to determine fluid balance.*
- Weigh patient daily *to determine fluid loss.*
- Monitor vital signs and urine output and report changes *to detect changes from within normal limits.*
- Maintain intravenous fluid replacement as ordered *to maintain fluid balance if output is greater than intake.*

For constipation related to a low-fiber diet, see the earlier section on constipation.

Evaluation

The goals are met if the patient reports that pain is controlled, vital signs and urinary output are stable, and patient has regular, comfortable bowel elimination.

INFLAMMATORY BOWEL DISEASE

Crohn's Disease (Regional Enteritis)

Pathophysiology

Crohn's disease, also known as regional **enteritis** or granulomatous enteritis, is an inflammatory bowel disease (IBD) that can involve any part of the GI tract but most commonly affects the terminal portion of the ileum, or first part of the large intestine. The inflammation extends through the intestinal mucosa, which leads to the formation of abscesses, **fistulas** (abnormal connections between structures), and fissures (unnatural tracts or ulcers). The inflamed areas from Crohn's disease can alternate with areas of healthy tissue so the inflamed areas are referred to as being "skip lesions" (because

• WORD • BUILDING •

enteritis: entero—intestine + itis—inflammation

they are not continuous lesions along the intestine). As the disease progresses, obstruction occurs because the intestinal lumen narrows with inflamed mucosa and scar tissue.

Etiology

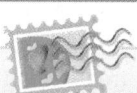

Although the exact cause of Crohn's disease has not been identified, it tends to occur within families. Other possible influences are autoimmune processes and infectious agents. Crohn's disease is most often diagnosed between the ages of 15 and 30 and occurs more often in women than men. Smoking increases the risk for Crohn's disease. The patient experiences periods of remissions and exacerbations. Physical or psychological stress may trigger exacerbations (Box 34.5, *Cultural Considerations*).

Signs and Symptoms

Crampy abdominal pains (unrelieved by defecation), weight loss, fever, and diarrhea occur. Because the crampy pains occur after eating, the patient often does not eat in order to avoid the pain. A lack of eating and poor absorption of nutrients results in weight loss and malnutrition. Chronic diarrhea contributes to fluid deficit and electrolyte imbalance. The inflamed intestine may perforate, leading to the formation of intra-abdominal or anal fissures, abscesses, or fistulas. Symptoms outside the GI tract, such as arthritis, skin lesions, and inflammatory disorders of the eyes, and abnormalities of liver function may also occur.

Complications

In addition to malnutrition, the development of fissures, abscesses, strictures, or fistulas is the most common complication of Crohn's disease. Fistulas may include enterovaginal (small bowel to vagina), enterovesical (small bowel to bladder), enterocutaneous (small bowel to skin), enteroentero (small bowel to small bowel), or enterocolonic (small bowel to colon) (Fig. 34.3). Fistulas communicating with organs that then drain externally can cause tremendous skin irritation, as well as increased risk of developing infections. Fistulas are corrected surgically.

Diagnostic Tests

Laboratory testing is to done to look for anemia, infection, liver function, low albumin due to poor absorption of protein, and stool infections or occult blood.

Endoscopy (colonoscopy and sigmoidoscopy), with multiple biopsies of the diseased colon and terminal ileum, is used to diagnose Crohn's disease. Other endoscopic tests include capsule endoscopy (swallowed camera the size of a pill), ultrasound to help identify fistulas and areas of bleeding, and double balloon enteroscopy, which provides views of the inside of tissue folds. Crohn's disease is confirmed by granulomas in the biopsy specimen.

Radiology tests include multiphase CT enterography and magnetic resonance enterography (MRE), which provide detailed images of the intestines. MRE does not use radiation.

Therapeutic Measures

Management of Crohn's disease is aimed at achieving remission and maintaining it because there is no cure. Symptoms are controlled by reducing the intestinal inflammation that is the underlying cause of the symptoms. Medications are available today that offer better control of the disease than in the past.

The classes of medications used to achieve these goals are aminosalicylates, antibiotics, biologics, corticosteroids, and immunomodulators (Table 34.5). Treatment is individualized. Aminosalicylates reduce inflammation and have various formulations to be delivered to specific sites in the intestines. They do not prevent acute episodes. Biologics selectively target agents in the inflammatory process to block their action and effects. Corticosteroids are used during an acute inflammation, then tapered and discontinued. Budesonide (Entocort EC), an anti-inflammatory synthetic corticosteroid, acts locally rather than affecting the whole body. Immunomodulators modify the immune system to decrease inflammation. They may be used with steroids to treat acute episodes because they have a longer onset of action. Traditionally, corticosteroids, then azathioprine, then infliximab, which inhibits tumor necrosis factor, a primary cause of the inflammation, are given. In a research study, the monoclonal antibody infliximab was shown to be more effective than azathioprine used alone (Mayo Clinic, 2008).

Antibiotics are helpful in Crohn's disease as long-term therapy and when fistulas are present. Antidiarrheal medications such as diphenoxylate with atropine (Lomotil) or loperamide (Imodium) are used. Bulk-forming laxatives may help reduce loose stools and subsequently skin irritation.

As complications develop, surgery may be indicated for obstruction, stricture, fistula, abscess, excessive bleeding, perforation, toxic megacolon (loss of muscle tone and dilation in colon), or symptoms that do not respond to treatment. Surgery does not cure Crohn's disease because it can recur elsewhere in the GI tract. Surgical procedures include strictureplasty to widen areas of stricture, resection of the affected area with anastomosis, colectomy with ileorectal anastomosis, or

Box 34.5

Cultural Considerations

Ulcerative colitis and Crohn's disease are more common in Caucasians, persons of Jewish descent, and upper middle class urban populations. The incidence of Crohn's disease is increasing rapidly in western Europe and North America. These findings support possible hereditary or environmental risk factors for inflammatory bowel disease.

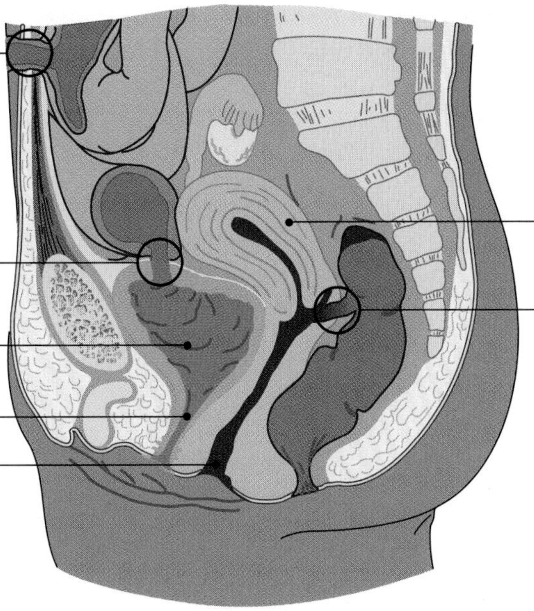
Enterocutaneous fistula
Enterovesicular fistula
Urinary bladder
Urethra
Vagina
Uterus
Enterovaginal fistula

FIGURE 34.3 Fistulas are a common complication of Crohn's disease.

TABLE 34.5 MEDICATIONS FOR CROHN'S DISEASE AND/OR ULCERATIVE COLITIS

Medication/Action	Examples	Route	Side Effects	Nursing Implications
Aminosalicylates				
Decrease intestinal inflammation.	sulfasalazine (Azulfidine)	PO, rectal	Headache, nausea, anorexia, rash, fever	Contraindicated in sulfa allergy. Some patients do not tolerate sulfasalazine but can tolerate other drugs in this class.
	mesalamine (Asacol, Canasa, Pentasa, Rowasa)	PO, rectal based on drug	Abdominal pain, diarrhea, nausea, hair loss, headache, dizziness	Monitor for signs of reduced kidney function.
	olsalazine (Dipentum)	PO	Diarrhea, headache, rash, fatigue	Take with food.
	balsalazide (Colazal)	PO	Headaches, abdominal pain	Continue drugs even if feeling better to maintain remission.
Antibiotics				
In Crohn's disease, reduce intestinal bacteria.	metronidazole (Flagyl)	PO, IV	Headache, N/V, diarrhea, anorexia, metallic taste, dark urine, tingling of hands or feet	Avoid alcohol and sun. Interferes with oral contraceptives, warfarin.
	ciprofloxacin (Cipro)	PO, IV	Headache, N/V, diarrhea, rash, abdominal pain, muscle or tendon pain	Do not give with antacids, calcium, iron, zinc. Avoid sun. Interferes with oral contraceptives, warfarin.
Biologics				
Selectively target inflammatory agents to interfere with inflammatory response.	infliximab (Remicade) adalimumab (Humira) certolizumab pegol (Cimzia)	IV Subcutaneously	Headache, chills, fever, hypotension, dyspnea, hives, nausea, rash, sore throat, lymphoma	TB test should be done before therapy begins. Monitor for infections, bone marrow suppression, CNS disorder.

Continued

TABLE 34.5 MEDICATIONS FOR CROHN'S DISEASE AND/OR ULCERATIVE COLITIS—cont'd

Medication/Action	Examples	Route	Side Effects	Nursing Implications
Corticosteroids				
Decrease inflammation and suppress immune system. May be used with aminosalicylates.	prednisone (Deltasone)	PO	Hypertension, moon face, infection, mood swings, weight gain, osteoporosis	Teach patient not to stop taking medication abruptly.
	methylprednisolone (Medrol, Solu-Medrol)	PO, IV		
	hydrocortisone (Cortenema)	Enema		Patient should lie on left side for 30 minutes and retain enema for 1 hour if not all night.
Anti-Inflammatory Synthetic Corticosteroid				
Reduce inflammation locally for Crohn's disease.	budesonide (Entocort EC)	PO	Fewer steroid side effects (e.g., moon face and acne)	Grapefruit juice should be avoided. Take in morning. Swallow whole.
Immunomodulators				
Immunosuppression to reduce inflammation.	azathioprine (Imuran)	PO	Headache, N/V, diarrhea, malaise	Report symptoms of infection when taking any immunomodulators.
	6-mercaptopurine (6-MP, Purinethol)	PO	Headache, N/V, diarrhea, malaise	Monitor for infection.
	cyclosporine (Sandimmune, Neoral)	PO	Infections, headache, hypertension	Blood pressure and renal function are monitored.
	tacrolimus (Prograf)	PO, topically	Infections, headache, hypertension	Blood pressure and renal function are monitored.
	methotrexate (MTX, Mexate, Rheumatrex)	IM	Bone marrow depression, infections, rash, nausea, diarrhea, stomatitis	Monitor for infections.

CNS = central nervous system; N/V = nausea and vomiting; TB = tuberculosis.

proctocolectomy (rectum and colon) with ileostomy. See details regarding intestinal ostomies later in this chapter. A Kock pouch is not recommended for those with Crohn's disease because the disease may affect the pouch.

A healthy diet is important in overall health but there is no special diet for Crohn's disease. A dietitian referral is important for nutritional support. Malnutrition is a concern if the small intestine is affected and nutrients are not absorbed properly. Folic acid and vitamin B_{12} supplements may be needed. Calcium intake may be decreased and osteoporosis is a concern. Calcium 1500 mg daily and vitamin D supplements are considered. Foods that increase symptoms should be avoided. Enteral feedings may be required and can be done at night through a gastrostomy tube (G tube) or feeding tube. For acute flare-ups, total parenteral nutrition (TPN) may be used to rest the GI tract. Adequate fluid intake is essential to prevent dehydration if diarrhea is present.

Nursing Process for the Patient with Crohn's Disease

Because of the similarities between Crohn's disease and ulcerative colitis, the nursing processes for both are discussed together in the *Nursing Process for the Patient with Inflammatory Bowel Disease* section below.

Ulcerative Colitis

Pathophysiology

Ulcerative **colitis** is similar to Crohn's disease. Crohn's disease, however, can occur anywhere in the gastrointestinal system, whereas ulcerative colitis occurs in the large colon and rectum. Multiple ulcerations and diffuse inflammation occur in the superficial mucosa and submucosa of the colon. The lesions spread in a continuous pattern throughout the large intestine and usually involve the rectum. The patient with ulcerative colitis has increased risk of developing colorectal cancer.

Etiology

Several theories exist to explain the cause of ulcerative colitis. These include infection, allergy, and autoimmune response. Environmental agents such as pesticides, tobacco, radiation, and food additives may precipitate an exacerbation. Diet or psychological stress may trigger or worsen an attack of symptoms. Ulcerative colitis usually begins between ages 15 and 40.

• WORD • BUILDING •

colitis: col—pertaining to colon + itis—inflammation

Signs and Symptoms

Abdominal pain, diarrhea, rectal bleeding, and fecal urgency are common symptoms of ulcerative colitis (Table 34.6). Anorexia, weight loss, cramping, vomiting, fever, and dehydration associated with passing 5 to 20 liquid stools a day may also occur. Along with the potential for fluid and electrolyte imbalance, calcium is lost. Anemia often develops as a result of rectal bleeding. Serum albumin level may be low because of malabsorption. Like Crohn's disease, arthritis, skin lesions, inflammatory disorders of the eyes, and abnormalities of liver function may also occur. Symptoms are usually intermittent, with remissions lasting from months to years.

Complications

Malnutrition occurs less often with ulcerative colitis than with Crohn's disease. Other complications include the potential for hemorrhage during an acute phase, bowel obstruction, perforation, and peritonitis. The risk for colon cancer is also increased in patients with ulcerative colitis.

Diagnostic Tests

Examination of stool specimens is done to rule out the presence of any bacterial or amebic organisms. The stool is positive for blood in the presence of ulcerative colitis. Anemia is often present because of blood loss. Electrolytes may be depleted from chronic diarrhea. There is a protein loss because of liver dysfunction and malabsorption. Endoscopy is used. Biopsy specimens taken during sigmoidoscopy and colonoscopy typically show abnormal cells. Leukocyte scintigraphy, a noninvasive imaging test, uses the patient's white blood cells tagged with a radioactive material to detect infection and inflammation in the colon.

TABLE 34.6 INFLAMMATORY BOWEL DISEASE SUMMARY

Signs and Symptoms	Abdominal pain or cramping Weight loss Diarrhea Fluid and electrolyte imbalance Fissures, fistulas, abscesses Arthritis and skin lesions Inflammatory eye disorders Abnormal liver function
Diagnostic Tests	Endoscopy with biopsy Barium enema Laboratory examination Stool examination Absent bowel sounds
Therapeutic Measures	Medications: anti-inflammatories, antidiarrheal, antibiotics, immunosuppressants, corticosteroids Surgery if necessary Avoidance of offending foods Elemental formula or TPN if required
Priority Nursing Diagnoses	*Constipation* *Diarrhea* *Deficient Fluid Volume* *Deficient Knowledge*

Therapeutic Measures

Diet and lifestyle changes and then medications are used for treatment. Foods that cause gas or diarrhea should be avoided. Because the offending foods may be different for each patient, foods are tried in small amounts if they are thought to cause symptoms. In general, high-fiber foods, caffeine, spicy foods, and milk products are avoided. Total parenteral nutrition may be needed to meet nutritional needs during acute exacerbations. Diarrhea may increase the need for fluids to prevent dehydration.

Many of the medication classes used with Crohn's disease are used for ulcerative colitis (see Table 34.5).

Surgery is considered for excessive bleeding, severe symptoms, perforation, or toxic megacolon. Because ulcerative colitis usually involves the entire large intestine, surgery removes the entire colon and rectum. An ileoanal pouch (restorative proctocolectomy) or proctocolectomy with ileostomy (discussed later) are the procedures done. Surgery cures ulcerative colitis if the colon is removed.

An ileoanal pouch does not require an ostomy bag to be worn, and is the more common surgery performed. Because the anus and sphincter are saved, stool still passes through the anus. The rectum and colon are removed and the end of the ileum, which is made into a J-shaped pouch, is attached to the anus. A temporary ileostomy is created to allow the pouch to heal. After about 12 weeks, the ileostomy is closed. Several bowel movements per day occur. The stool is of soft consistency. Surgical complications can include a bowel obstruction, or an inflammation of the pouch (pouchitis), which is treated with antibiotics.

Nursing Process for the Patient with Inflammatory Bowel Disease

Data Collection

A history obtained from the patient should include identification of symptoms, including the onset, duration, frequency, and severity. Ask if there has been any correlation between exacerbations of symptoms related to dietary changes or stress. Determine the presence of any food allergies or intolerances that may increase diarrhea. Also, note the daily and weekly intake of caffeine, nicotine, and alcohol because all these stimulate the bowel and can cause cramping and diarrhea.

Assess the patient for nutritional status and signs of dehydration. Ten to 20 pounds can be lost in a 2-month period. Perianal skin should be assessed for irritation and excoriation.

Assessment of emotional status, coping skills, and verbal and nonverbal behaviors is essential. The patient may withdraw from family and friends because of frequent bowel movements. Anxiety, sleep disturbances, depression, and denial can be problems. If surgery involving an ileostomy is planned, the patient is at risk for body image problems.

Nursing Diagnoses, Planning, and Implementation

Acute Pain Related to Increased Peristalsis and Cramping

EXPECTED OUTCOME: The patient will state pain is relieved or at an acceptable level within 30 minutes of report of pain.

- Have patient rate pain on objective scale such as 0 to 10 *to determine pain level.*
- Document the character of the pain (dull, cramping, burning) and ask whether the pain is associated with meals or other activities *to plan care.*
- Give analgesics and medications *to relieve cramping, as prescribed.*

Diarrhea Related to the Inflammatory Process

EXPECTED OUTCOME: The patient will maintain formed, soft stool every 1 to 3 days.

- Document characteristics of stools, including color, consistency, amount, frequency, and odor *to plan care.*
- Ensure patient has quick access to the bathroom or provide a bedside commode *to prevent incontinence.*
- Administer antidiarrheal medication as prescribed. *Controlling diarrhea controls comfort and fluid balance.*
- Encourage bedrest *to decrease peristalsis.*
- Keep the environment clean and odor free *to help alleviate anxiety.*
- Teach the patient to avoid high-fiber foods such as whole grains and raw fruits and vegetables, as well as caffeine, alcohol, and nicotine *because they stimulate intestinal motility.*

Risk for Deficient Fluid Volume Related to Diarrhea and Insufficient Fluid Intake

EXPECTED OUTCOME: The patient will maintain vital signs and urine output within normal limits at all times.

- Weigh patient daily *to determine fluid loss.*
- Record intake and output (including diarrhea stools) *to determine fluid balance.*
- Document and report signs of deficient fluid volume to the physician *to allow treatment.*
- Maintain IV fluids as ordered *to maintain fluid balance.*
- Encourage fluids when acute diarrhea subsides *to maintain fluid balance.*
- Teach patient signs and symptoms of dehydration to report *to allow prompt treatment.*

> **CRITICAL THINKING**
>
> ***Judy Moore***
>
> ■ Judy Moore is an 18-year-old college student who has just been diagnosed with Crohn's disease.
>
> 1. What questions can you ask Judy to identify her symptoms?
> 2. What nursing diagnoses would be relevant for Judy's condition?
> 3. What can you do to help her adapt to this disease?
> 4. If Judy's condition were to worsen what manifestations would be exhibited?
>
> *Suggested answers at end of chapter.*

Anxiety Related to Symptoms and Frequency of Stools and Treatment

EXPECTED OUTCOME: The patient will report anxiety is reduced.

- Answer questions, talk in a calm, confident manner, and actively listen to the patient *to reduce anxiety, which aggravates symptoms of inflammatory bowel disease.*

Impaired Skin Integrity Related to Frequent Loose Stools

EXPECTED OUTCOME: The patient's skin will remain intact at all times.

- Keep perianal skin clean, dry, and protected with a moisture barrier, such as petrolatum or medicated ointment, after each bowel movement *to protect perianal skin from contact with liquid stools and their enzymes.*
- Provide sitz baths that may be comforting and helpful in keeping skin clean *to prevent excoriation.*

Imbalanced Nutrition: Less Than Body Requirements Related to Malabsorption

EXPECTED OUTCOME: The patient will maintain weight within normal range for height and age.

- Weigh weekly *to detect weight loss.*
- Give special liquid (elemental) formula that is absorbed in the upper bowel as ordered *to allow the colon to rest.*
- Maintain TPN as ordered to provide nourishment *if the patient is unable to tolerate oral intake.*

See the *Nursing Care Plan for the Patient with Inflammatory Bowel Disease.*

Evaluation

Goals have been met if pain is relieved, frequency of diarrhea stools is decreased, fluid and electrolyte balance is

NURSING CARE PLAN for the Patient with Inflammatory Bowel Disease

Nursing Diagnosis: *Ineffective Coping* related to inflammatory bowel disease

Expected Outcomes: The patient will identify strategies that promote effective coping.

Evaluation of Outcomes: Is the patient able to state strategies for effective coping?

Interventions	Rationale	Evaluation
Ask knowledge of Crohn's disease or ulcerative colitis.	Many people have little knowledge of a disease unless they know someone who has it. Inaccurate information must be corrected.	Does the patient verbalize information about ulcerative colitis and its effects on the body?
Encourage the patient to express feelings about the disease and how it may affect his or her life.	Expressing feelings about the disease and its perceived effect enables the patient to identify and talk about concerns. Once identified, these concerns can then be addressed by the health care team.	Does the patient talk about feelings regarding the potential impact of the disease on his or her life?
Determine whether the patient would like to speak with a person of similar age from the Crohn's and Colitis Foundation of America.	Speaking with someone close in age with the same disease lets the patient know that he or she is not the only person having to cope with this disorder. It can also help him or her learn some strategies for effectively coping with the disease.	Does the patient show an interest in speaking with someone with the same disease?
Identify strategies for effective coping that are acceptable to the patient.	Talking about concerns and possible solutions is a positive step. Coping strategies identified with the patient are more likely to be implemented.	Is the patient able to identify strategies for effective coping that he or she believes will work?

achieved, anxiety is reduced, skin is intact, and weight is within normal range for height and age.

IRRITABLE BOWEL SYNDROME

Pathophysiology

Irritable bowel syndrome (IBS) is not a disease but rather a functional problem. The colon mucosa is not damaged by the condition and there is no increased risk of colorectal cancer. IBS is a disorder of altered intestinal motility in which the colon does not contract in a normal pattern. Instead it contracts in a disorderly way that can be violent and last for long times or, at times, it may not contract at all. The abnormal contractions lead to changes in bowel patterns. Thus, the disorder may be classified as IBS with diarrhea, IBS with constipation, or IBS with mixed diarrhea and constipation. Additionally, patients experience increased abdominal discomfort or pain. Localized prolonged contractions may cause stool to be retained for a long time, causing it to become hardened as water is absorbed from it. Bloating may also occur as air is unable to be expelled. Mucus may be seen in the stool, although this is not abnormal and does not typically cause a problem. Symptoms may be exacerbated by psychological stress or food intolerances. The nerves in the bowel are overly sensitive in people with IBS. At times of stress in daily living, abnormal contractions may result.

Etiology

There is a hereditary tendency for IBS. IBS is more common in women than men and in those who are young to middle aged. Flare-ups can be caused by other illnesses, infections, or the menstrual cycle.

Signs and Symptoms

IBS is characterized by reports of gas, bloating, constipation, diarrhea, or alternating constipation and diarrhea. The patient also has feelings of abdominal bloating, with or without visible abdominal distention. Other symptoms include the rectal passage of mucus, a feeling of incomplete evacuation, abdominal pain, depression, anxiety, and palpitations.

Diagnostic Tests

Diagnosis of IBS is made based on history and physical examination along with stool examination, colonoscopy, and sigmoidoscopy to rule out other disorders. Avoiding milk products for a time may be advised to rule out lactose intolerance.

Therapeutic Measures

IBS is a chronic condition, but symptoms can generally be controlled through lifestyle, diet, stress management, and medication. A high-fiber and high-bran diet (psyllium [Metamucil] or methylcellulose [Citrucel]) may help to form softer, larger stools but may increase other symptoms in some people. Foods that cause distress or gas formation are avoided such as fresh fruits or vegetables, spices, milk, coffee, carbonated drinks, and alcohol. Eating smaller, frequent meals can be helpful in reducing bowel contractions. Stress management, behavioral therapy (biofeedback, hypnosis, psychotherapy), and exercise are helpful in relaxing the bowel as well as contributing to overall health. Patients can keep a diary of foods eaten, stressors, and symptoms. This can help health practitioners identify flare-up triggers.

Various medications are used depending on the type of IBS. Antidepressants are given to block the brain's perception of abdominal pain. For IBS with constipation, selective serotonin reuptake inhibitors (SSRIs) such as paroxetine HCl (Paxil) are given. Tricyclic antidepressants (such as amitriptyline HCl [Elavil]) are used for IBS with diarrhea because they tend to cause constipation. Antispasmodics such as hyoscyamine (Levbid) or dicyclomine (Bentyl) are used in IBS for diarrhea to relieve the painful colon spasms.

For women in whom treatment for IBS with constipation has not been successful, lubiprostone (Amitiza) may be used. It is a chloride channel activator that increases fluid secretion in the small intestine to help pass stool.

Nursing Process for the Patient with IBS

Data Collection

Height, weight, and data are collected on the symptoms including pain that the patient experiences. Timing of the symptoms, food and fluid intake, elimination patterns, effects on self-esteem, socialization, and personal and family roles are explored since IBS is a significant cause of missed work and school and also causes social withdrawal and embarrassment for people with it. Knowledge of the syndrome and its treatment are determined. Readiness for managing the syndrome is determined to plan care.

Nursing Diagnoses, Planning, and Implementation

Constipation Related to Irregular Motility of GI Tract

EXPECTED OUTCOME: The patient will maintain passage of soft, formed stool every 1 to 3 days without straining.

- Assess normal pattern of defecation, diet and fluid intake, and medications *to help identify factors contributing to constipation for planning care.*
- Increase fluid intake, if not contraindicated, to 2 to 3 L per day *to prevent hard stools.*
- Teach patient about the benefits of increasing fiber and bran in the diet *to promote soft, larger stools that are easier to pass.*
- Give medication as ordered *to control symptoms.*

Diarrhea Related to Irregular Motility of GI Tract

EXPECTED OUTCOME: The patient will maintain formed, soft stool every 1 to 3 days.

- Obtain history including medications regarding diarrhea episodes *to help identify cause.*
- Monitor and record stool characteristics, amount, and frequency *to plan care.*
- Give antidiarrheal medications as ordered. *Controlling diarrhea controls comfort and fluid balance.*
- Limit caffeine intake *because it stimulates intestinal motility.*
- Keep skin clean, dry, and protected with a moisture barrier, such as petrolatum or medicated ointment, after each bowel movement *to protect perianal skin from contact with liquid stools and their enzymes.*

Readiness for Enhanced Self Health Management Related to Desire to Manage Symptoms of IBS

EXPECTED OUTCOME: The patient will state understanding and ability to carry out preventive measures to control symptoms prior to discharge.

- Explain IBS including symptoms, aggravating factors, and treatments *to promote understanding, which will aid ability to follow therapeutic regimen.*
- Encourage use of food diary documenting foods eaten and timing of symptom occurrence *to identify food triggers for symptoms including lactose intolerance.*
- Consult registered dietitian and share food diary *to allow identification of food connection with symptoms and meal planning to prevent symptoms.*
- If lactose intolerant, teach patient to avoid dairy products and substitute yogurt *to reduce symptoms.*

Evaluation

The plan has been effective if the patient has regular bowel function pattern, verbalizes understanding of self-care measures, and expresses satisfaction with the outcomes.

ABDOMINAL HERNIAS

Pathophysiology and Etiology

A **hernia** is an abnormal protrusion of an organ or structure through a weakness or tear in the wall of the cavity normally containing it, which in this case is the abdominal wall. Hernias are caused by a weakness in the abdominal wall along with increased intra-abdominal pressure, such as the pressure from coughing, straining, and heavy lifting. Obesity, pregnancy, and poor wound healing are also risk factors. The hernial sac is formed by the peritoneum protruding through the weakened muscle wall. Contents of the hernia can be small or large intestine or the omentum. Indirect hernias are caused by a defect of structural closure. Direct hernias are acquired and arise from a weakness in the abdominal wall, usually at old incisional sites.

Figure 34.4 illustrates the many types of hernias. Inguinal hernias are located in the groin where the spermatic cord in males or the round ligament in females emerges from the abdominal wall. This common hernia is an example of an indirect hernia and is usually seen in males.

Umbilical hernias are seen most often in obese women and in children. They are caused by a failure of the umbilical orifice to close. Ventral (incisional) hernias usually result from a weakness in the abdominal wall following abdominal surgery, especially in the obese patient, if a drainage system was used, the patient experienced poor wound healing, or the patient received inadequate nutrition.

Prevention

Congenital defects cannot be prevented. However, reducing strain on abdominal muscles is helpful. Those who do heavy lifting, tugging, or pushing should wear a support binder or avoid the lifting. A healthy lifestyle of maintaining normal weight, not smoking, and eating high-fiber foods is recommended.

Signs and Symptoms

Unless complications occur, few symptoms are associated with hernias. An abnormal bulging can be seen in the affected area of the abdomen, especially when straining or coughing. The patient may have some discomfort due to tension on tissues around the hernia. The herniation may disappear when the patient lies down. If the intestinal mass easily returns to the abdominal cavity or can be manually placed back in the abdominal cavity, it is called a reducible hernia. When adhesions or edema occur between the sac and its contents, the hernia becomes irreducible or incarcerated.

Complications

An incarcerated hernia may become strangulated if the blood and intestinal flow are completely cut off in the trapped loop of bowel. Strangulated hernias do not develop in adults very often. Incarceration leads to an intestinal obstruction and possibly gangrene and bowel perforation. Symptoms are pain at the site of the strangulation, nausea and vomiting, and colicky abdominal pain.

Therapeutic Measures

Hernias are diagnosed by physical examination. Treatment options include no treatment, observing the hernia, using short-term support devices, or surgery to cure the hernia. A supportive truss or brief applies pressure to keep the reduced hernia in place. Emergency surgery is needed for strangulation or the threat of bowel obstruction. Surgical repair is recommended for inguinal hernias. Surgical procedures include herniorrhaphy (open hernia repair) or hernioplasty (open or laparoscopically). Herniorrhaphy involves making an incision in the abdominal wall, replacing the contents of the hernial sac, sewing the weakened tissue, and closing the opening. Hernioplasty involves replacing the hernia into the abdomen and reinforcing the weakened muscle wall with wire, fascia, or mesh. Bowel resection or a temporary colostomy may be necessary if the hernia is strangulated.

Nursing Care

The patient is instructed to avoid activities that increase intra-abdominal pressure, such as lifting heavy objects. The patient is taught to recognize signs of incarceration or strangulation and the importance of notifying the physician immediately. If a support truss or brief has been ordered, the patient is taught to apply it before arising from bed each morning while the hernia is not protruding. Special attention should be paid to maintenance of skin integrity beneath the truss.

Postoperative Care

Care following inguinal hernia repair is generally similar to any abdominal postoperative care (see Chapter 12). Patients can perform deep breathing to keep lungs clear postoperatively but should avoid coughing. Coughing increases abdominal

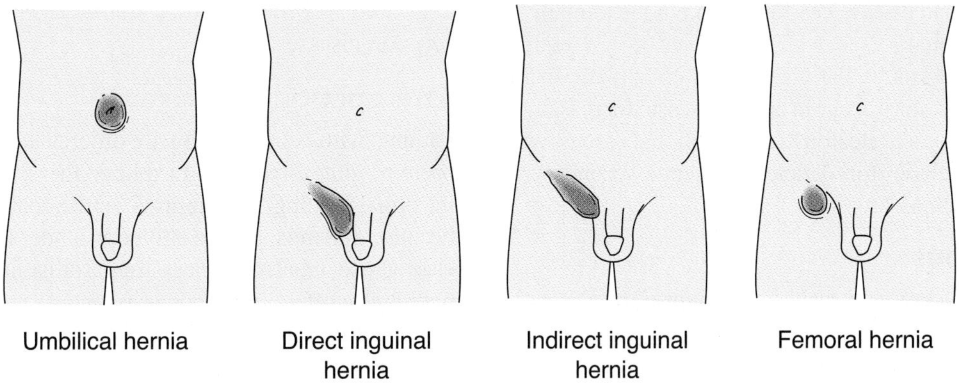
Umbilical hernia
Direct inguinal hernia
Indirect inguinal hernia
Femoral hernia

FIGURE 34.4 Types of hernias.

pressure and could affect the hernia repair. The male patient may experience swelling of the scrotum. Ice packs and elevation of the scrotum may be ordered to reduce the swelling. Because most patients are discharged the same day of surgery, they are taught to change the dressing and report difficulty urinating, bleeding, and signs and symptoms of infection, such as redness, incisional drainage, fever, or severe pain. The patient is also instructed to avoid lifting, driving, or sexual activities for 2 to 6 weeks as specified by the physician. Most patients can return to nonstrenuous work within 2 weeks.

ABSORPTION DISORDERS

The process of digestion reduces nutrients to a liquid form that can be absorbed through intestinal mucosa into the portal bloodstream. More than 8000 mL of liquid with nutrients and electrolytes is absorbed, mostly proximal to the ileocecal valve.

Pathophysiology and Etiology

Malabsorption occurs when the GI system is unable to absorb one or more of the major nutrients (carbohydrates, fats, or proteins). Some causes of malabsorption are ileal dysfunction, jejunal diverticula, parasitic disease, celiac disease, enzyme deficiency, and inflammatory bowel diseases such as Crohn's disease and ulcerative colitis. The primary malabsorption disorders are celiac disease and lactose intolerance.

In celiac disease, a sensitivity to gluten is thought to cause malabsorption of protein. Gluten is a protein found in wheat, barley, and rye. Oats may become contaminated with gluten in the milling process of these other grains (Box 34.6, *Nutrition Notes*).

A deficiency in lactase, an enzyme that breaks down lactose (milk sugar), causes lactose intolerance. When lactose is not digested, a high concentration of it occurs in the intestines, causing an osmotic retention of water in the colon and watery stools (Box 34.7, *Nutrition Notes*).

Box 34.6

Nutrition Notes

Treating Celiac Disease

Celiac disease, or gluten-sensitive enteropathy, is classically diagnosed in infants after gluten-containing foods are introduced to the diet. Now the peak age of diagnosis is the fourth and fifth decades, suggesting the disease goes undetected for many years. Adults with celiac disease may present with anemia or have the disease discovered through endoscopy for symptoms not suggestive of celiac disease. A prior diagnosis of irritable bowel syndrome is common (Green & Jabri, 2006).

The etiology is considered to be multifactorial involving a combination of:

- Genetic predisposition
- Ingestion of gluten
- An autoimmune response that produces chronic inflammation of the small intestine.

Definitive diagnosis is made with a biopsy of the small intestine. In all cases, the patient should consume a gluten-containing diet until the diagnostic testing has been completed.

Treatment requires permanent elimination of wheat, rye, and barley from the diet. Although gluten free, oats can pick up gluten from other grains during milling and may have to be avoided also. Careful selection of prepared foods is mandatory because of the widespread use of these grains as thickeners. If a patient with celiac disease ingests gluten, damage to the intestine continues even in the absence of symptoms. Instruction from and follow-up by a dietitian are indicated to ensure adequate nutritional intake despite the many dietary limitations.

Signs and Symptoms

Weight loss, weakness, and general malaise resulting from malnutrition are associated with malabsorption disorders. Lactose intolerance causes abdominal cramping, excessive gas, and loose stools after eating milk products. Signs and symptoms of celiac disease can range from none to many in various body systems (see www.csaceliacs.org). Frequent loose, bulky, foul stools that are gray in color with an increased fat content may occur in celiac disease. Increased fat in the stool is named steatorrhea. Nutritional issues with celiac disease include iron-deficiency anemia secondary to poor iron absorption.

Complications

Vitamin K deficiency and resulting hypoprothrombinemia can increase the risk of bleeding. Calcium deficiency can be severe enough to cause bone pain and neuromuscular hyperirritability, including tetany. Folic acid, vitamin B_{12}, and iron deficiencies can result in glossitis, stomatitis, anemia, and dry, rough skin.

Diagnostic Tests

See Table 34.7 for diagnostic studies used to identify malabsorption diseases.

Therapeutic Measures

Patients with celiac disease are ordered a high-calorie, high-protein, gluten-free diet to relieve the symptoms, promote intestinal healing, and improve nutritional status. However, because gluten is used as a filler or binder in many products, even those labeled "wheat free," diligence in identifying potentially offending foods is essential.

Lactose intolerance is treated by removing foods from the diet that contain lactose, such as milk and milk products.

Box 34.7

Nutrition Notes

Managing Lactose Intolerance

About 70% of the world's population has some degree of lactose intolerance that may be hereditary or secondary to other conditions of the small intestine. An episode of diarrhea sometimes results in temporary lactose intolerance.

Patients with lactose intolerance control the condition through trial and error because the degree of intolerance varies greatly from person to person. Moderate amounts of many lactose-containing foods can be digested when taken with a mixed meal. A dietitian's services may be advised to begin dietary management after diagnosis.

Label reading is mandatory. Ingredients to avoid include milk, milk solids, lactose, and whey. Low-lactose foods (up to 2 g per serving) include sherbet, cheese aged longer than 90 days, processed cheese, and milk treated with lactase enzyme.

In cheese making, the whey containing most of the lactose is removed, so that hard, ripened cheeses such as blue, brick, Brie, Camembert, Cheddar, Colby, Edam, Gouda, Monterey, Muenster, Parmesan, Provolone, and Swiss are classified as low lactose. Some brands of yogurt, a high-lactose food, may be tolerated because they contain bacterial lactase.

Lactaid, an over-the-counter natural enzyme, is available as chewable tablets or as liquid that is added to milk. Milk treated with Lactaid is slightly sweeter than regular milk because the milk sugar, lactose, is broken down into glucose and galactose by the enzyme.

Long-term monitoring is necessary. A lactose-restricted diet may be low in calcium, riboflavin, and vitamin D.

Some fermented milk products, such as cheese and yogurt, may be lower in lactose and better tolerated. Lactaid is an over-the-counter lactase substitute that can be taken when milk products cannot be avoided. It can be added to milk in liquid form or taken as a tablet before eating foods containing lactose. Lactaid digests about 70% of the lactose in foods, making them more tolerable.

Nursing Care

Nursing care involves monitoring fluid and electrolyte balance, nutritional status, and skin integrity. Recording daily weight and intake and output helps determine if fluid loss is occurring. Intake of electrolyte-rich fluids is encouraged to replace losses. Antidiarrheal agents are given if ordered. Electrolyte levels, especially potassium, are monitored as ordered. The patient is instructed in dietary limitations. Nutritional supplements may be ordered if needed. Perianal skin is kept clean and dry, and barrier ointments are used as needed to protect the skin from excoriation.

INTESTINAL OBSTRUCTION

Intestinal obstructions occur when the flow of intestinal contents is blocked. The two types of intestinal obstruction are mechanical and nonmechanical, both of which can be either partial or complete.

Mechanical obstruction occurs when a blockage occurs within the intestine from conditions causing pressure on the intestinal walls such as adhesions, twisting of the bowel, or strangulated hernia. Nonmechanical obstruction occurs when peristalsis is impaired and the intestinal contents cannot be propelled through the bowel. Nonmechanical obstruction is seen following abdominal surgeries, trauma, mesenteric ischemia, or infection. The severity of the obstruction depends on the area of bowel affected, the amount of occlusion within the lumen, and the amount of disturbance in the blood flow to the bowel (Table 34.8).

TABLE 34.7 DIAGNOSTIC TESTS FOR DISORDERS OF MALABSORPTION

Diagnostic Test	Test Result and Associated Malabsorption Syndrome
Hemoglobin and hematocrit	Decreased if anemia is present.
Mean corpuscular volume	Decreased values are found with malabsorption of vitamin B_{12}.
Upper GI series	Thickening of the intestinal mucosa, narrowed mucosa of the terminal ileum, or a change in fecal transit time are indicative of malabsorption syndrome.
D-xylose absorption test	Decreased excretion of xylose after 5 hours is indicative of malabsorption.
Sudan stain for fecal fat	Malabsorption can be distinguished from maldigestion if this test shows abnormally large numbers of fat droplets.
72-hour stool collection for fat	Stool fat greater than 5 g per 24 hours after ingestion of 80 g of fat in 2 days implies a fat digestion disorder.
Biopsy	Shows flattened mucosa and loss of villi with celiac disease

TABLE 34.8 BOWEL OBSTRUCTION SUMMARY

Signs and Symptoms	Abdominal pain Blood and mucus from rectum Feces and flatus cease Visible peristaltic waves in thin person Possible fecal vomiting Bowel sounds high pitched, tinkling, or absent Abdominal distention Fluid and electrolyte imbalance
Diagnostic Tests	Abdominal x-ray examination CT scan CBC and electrolytes
Therapeutic Measures	NPO status Frequent mouth care Nasogastric tube Fluid and electrolyte replacement Medications: antibiotics, antiemetics, analgesics Surgery
Priority Nursing Diagnoses	*Pain* *Deficient Fluid Volume* *Risk for Electrolyte Imbalance* *Risk for Dysfunctional Gastrointestinal Motility*

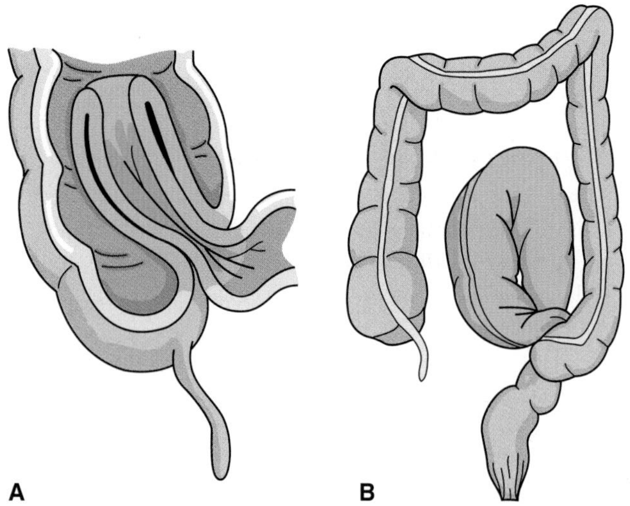
A
B

FIGURE 34.5 Mechanical bowel obstructions. (A) Intussusception. (B) Volvulus.

Box 34.8

Causes of Nonmechanical Obstruction

- Abdominal surgery and trauma
- Pneumonia
- Spinal injuries
- Hypokalemia
- Myocardial infarction
- Peritonitis
- Vascular insufficiency

Small-Bowel Obstruction

Pathophysiology

When obstruction occurs in the small bowel, a collection of intestinal contents, gas, and fluid occurs proximal to the obstruction. The distention that results stimulates gastric secretion but decreases the absorption of fluids. As distention worsens, the intraluminal pressure causes a decrease in venous and arterial capillary pressure, resulting in edema, necrosis, and eventually perforation of the intestinal wall.

Etiology

Following abdominal surgery, loops of intestine may adhere to areas in the abdomen that are not healed. This may cause a kink in the bowel that occludes the intestinal flow. These adhesions, or bands of scar tissue, are the most common cause of small-bowel obstruction and are usually acquired from previous abdominal surgery or inflammation. Hernias and neoplasms are the next most common causes, followed by inflammatory bowel disease, foreign bodies, strictures, volvulus, and intussusception. A **volvulus** occurs when the bowel twists, occluding the lumen of the intestine. **Intussusception** occurs when peristalsis causes the intestine to telescope into itself (Fig. 34.5). These conditions are mechanical obstructions. Paralytic, or adynamic, ileus is a nonmechanical obstruction that occurs when the intestinal peristalsis decreases or stops because of a vascular or neuromuscular pathological condition. Box 34.8 lists causes of nonmechanical obstructions.

Signs and Symptoms

The patient initially reports wavelike abdominal pain and vomiting. Initially, flatus and feces that are low in the bowel and blood and mucus may be passed, but this stops as the obstruction becomes worse. The symptoms progress as the obstruction worsens or becomes complete. As the obstruction becomes more extreme, peristaltic waves reverse, propelling the intestinal contents toward the mouth, eventually leading to fecal vomiting. Peristaltic waves may be visible in a thin person. Pain and abdominal distention are present. Pain that is sharp and sustained may indicate perforation. In mechanical obstructions, high-pitched, tinkling bowel sounds are heard proximal to the obstruction and are absent distal to it. If the obstruction is nonmechanical, there is an absence of bowel sounds.

Loss of fluid and electrolytes leads to dehydration, with its associated symptoms of extreme thirst, drowsiness, aching, and general malaise. The lower in the gastrointestinal tract the obstruction is, the greater the abdominal distention.

• WORD • BUILDING •
intussusception: intus—within + suscept—to receive

An uncorrected obstruction can lead to shock and possibly death.

Diagnostic Tests

Dilated loops of bowel are evident in radiographic studies and CT scans. If strangulation or perforation occurs, leukocytosis is evident. Hemoglobin and hematocrit levels are elevated if the patient is dehydrated, and serum electrolyte levels are decreased.

Therapeutic Measures

In most cases, the patient is kept NPO and the bowel is decompressed using a nasogastric (or, rarely, a tungsten-weighted intestinal) tube, which relieves symptoms and may resolve the obstruction. An IV solution with electrolytes is initiated to correct the fluid and electrolyte imbalance. Sometimes IV antibiotics are begun. Complete mechanical obstruction requires surgical intervention, such as removal of tumors, release of adhesions, or bowel resection with anastomosis.

Large-Bowel Obstruction

Pathophysiology

Obstruction in the large bowel is less common and not usually as dramatic as small-bowel obstruction. Dehydration occurs more slowly because of the colon's ability to absorb fluid and distend well beyond its normal full capacity. If the blood supply to the colon is cut off, the patient's life is in jeopardy because of bowel strangulation and necrosis.

Etiology

Most large-bowel obstructions occur in the sigmoid colon and are caused by carcinoma, inflammatory bowel disease, diverticulitis, or benign tumors. Impaction of stool may also cause obstruction.

Signs and Symptoms

Symptoms of large-bowel obstruction develop slowly and depend on the location of the obstruction. If the obstruction is in the rectum or sigmoid, the only symptom may be constipation. As the loops of bowel distend, the patient may report crampy lower abdominal pain and abdominal distention. Vomiting, if it occurs, is a late sign and may be fecal. High-pitched tinkling bowel sounds may be heard. A localized tender area and mass may be felt on palpation. Large-bowel obstructions, if not diagnosed and treated, can lead to gangrene, perforation, and peritonitis (discussed earlier).

Therapeutic Measures

Radiological examination reveals a distended colon. If impaction is present, enemas and manual disimpaction may be effective. Other mechanical blockages may require surgical intervention.

Surgical resection of the obstructed colon may be necessary. A temporary colostomy may be indicated to allow the bowel to rest and heal. Sometimes an ileoanal anastomosis is done. A patient who is a poor surgical risk may have a cecostomy (an opening from the cecum to the abdominal wall) to allow diversion of stool.

Nursing Process for the Patient with a Bowel Obstruction

DATA COLLECTION. Each quadrant of the abdomen is auscultated for bowel sounds to identify the location of the obstruction. The abdomen is palpated for distention, firmness, and tenderness. The amount and character of stool, if any, are documented. Pain is assessed using the institution's pain scale and described according to location and character, such as crampy or wavelike. Vital signs are monitored for signs of infection or shock. Daily weight and intake and output are monitored. Skin turgor is assessed for fluid deficit. If a nasogastric or nasointestinal tube is in place, the amount, color, and character of drainage are documented.

NURSING DIAGNOSES, PLANNING, AND IMPLEMENTATION

Acute Pain Related to Abdominal Distention

EXPECTED OUTCOME: The patient will state pain is relieved or at an acceptable level within 30 minutes of report of pain.

- Assess pain level using rating scale *to consistently communicate patient level.*
- Give medications ordered for pain cautiously *because they may mask symptoms of perforation and decrease intestinal motility.*
- Position patient in semi-Fowler's position *to reduce tension on the abdomen.*
- Provide frequent mouth care *to promote comfort.*

Risk for Deficient Fluid Volume Related to Vomiting

EXPECTED OUTCOME: The patient will maintain vital signs and urine output within normal limits at all times.

- Accurately monitor intake and output *to identify fluid deficit.*
- Maintain fluid replacement as ordered *to prevent dehydration.*

Risk for Electrolyte Imbalance Related to Suctioning

EXPECTED OUTCOME: The patient will maintain vital signs and urine output within normal limits at all times.

- Monitor electrolyte values *to identify imbalances.*
- Monitor vital signs, and watch for signs of electrolyte imbalances such as weakness accompanied by low potassium levels *to identify imbalances for prompt treatment.*
- Give ice chips sparingly if ordered by the physician. *Melted ice increases electrolyte and hydrochloric acid removal when suctioned from the stomach, and electrolyte imbalance and metabolic alkalosis occur.*

Risk for Dysfunctional Gastrointestinal Motility

EXPECTED OUTCOME: The patient will maintain passage of flatus and stool.

- Monitor GI function for presence of flatus and bowel movements *to detect problems.*

- Maintain orogastric, nasogastric, or nasointestinal tube on low intermittent suction as ordered *to relieve discomfort from distention.*
- Maintain NPO status *to rest the bowel and promote comfort.*

EVALUATION. Goals are met if the patient states that pain is controlled, fluid is balanced, electrolytes are within normal limits, and GI motility is normal.

CRITICAL THINKING

Mrs. Loos

■ Mrs. Loos is admitted for abdominal pain. She has a history of abdominal surgery. You find her abdomen distended, firm, and tender to touch. She states that she feels nauseated.

1. How would you know if Mrs. Loos could be developing a small-bowel obstruction?
2. Is she at risk for developing an obstruction?
3. If she is at risk, what data should you collect?
4. What do you expect to find if things are normal?
5. How will you determine if an obstruction is developing?
6. What will you do if the patient's assessment has changed?
7. How will you document your findings?
8. After treatment is started, how will you know the patient is improving, getting worse, or developing complications as a result of the treatments?

Suggested answers at end of chapter.

ANORECTAL PROBLEMS

Hemorrhoids

Hemorrhoids are enlarged veins within the anal tissue. They are caused by an increase in pressure in the veins, often from increased intra-abdominal pressure. Internal hemorrhoids occur above the internal sphincter, and external hemorrhoids occur below the external sphincter. Most hemorrhoids are caused by straining during bowel movements. They are common during pregnancy. Prolonged sitting or standing, obesity, and chronic constipation also contribute to hemorrhoids. Portal hypertension related to liver disease may also be a factor.

Internal hemorrhoids are usually not painful unless they prolapse. They may bleed during bowel movements. External hemorrhoids cause itching and pain when inflamed and filled with blood (thrombosed). Inflammation and edema occur with thrombosis, causing severe pain and possibly infarction of the skin and mucosa over the hemorrhoid.

Treatment is aimed at preventing constipation, avoiding straining during defecation, maintaining good personal hygiene, and making lifestyle changes to relieve hemorrhoid symptoms and discomfort. Increased fluid intake and stool softeners can be used to reduce the need for straining. Daily sitz baths increase circulation to the area and aid in comfort and healing. Prolonged standing and sitting are avoided. Astringents, such as witch hazel, can be used for symptom relief. Anti-inflammatory medications may be tried, such as steroid creams or suppositories. Alternating ice and heat helps relieve edema and pain if hemorrhoids are thrombosed.

If hemorrhoids are prolapsed and are no longer reduced by palliative measures, more aggressive measures may be used. Rubber band ligation uses rubber bands placed around a hemorrhoid until the tissue dies from lack of blood supply and sloughs off into the stool. Surgical hemorrhoidectomy involves surgical removal of hemorrhoids, and is only used for large or severe hemorrhoids.

Patient education includes prevention and self-care. The patient should be instructed to consume a high-fiber diet and 2 to 3 L of fluid a day to promote regular bowel movements. The effects and side effects, proper dosage, and frequency of local or topical medications should be explained.

If the patient has surgery, analgesics should be given as needed because the many nerve endings in the anal canal can cause severe pain. Comfort measures such as a side-lying position and fresh ice packs should also be used to relieve pain. After the first postoperative day, sitz baths may be ordered. Unfortunately, a side effect of opioid analgesics is constipation, which needs to be avoided, especially in the immediate postoperative period. Because the first bowel movement can be painful and anxiety provoking, stool softeners are given and analgesics administered before the first bowel movement.

Anal Fissures

Anal **fissures** are cracks or ulcers in the lining of the anal canal. They are most commonly associated with constipation and stretching of the anus with passage of hard stool, although Crohn's disease or other factors may also play a role. The patient may experience bright red bleeding. Pain may be so severe that the patient delays defecation, leading to further constipation and worsening symptoms. Treatment of anal fissures involves measures to ensure soft stools to allow fissures time to heal. Sitz baths may be used to promote circulation to the area to aid in healing. Anesthetic suppositories and nonopioid analgesics may be ordered for comfort. If conservative measures are not helpful, surgical excision of the fissure may be needed.

Anorectal Abscess

An anorectal abscess is a collection of pus in the rectal area. Common causative organisms include *Escherichia coli, Proteus* spp., staphylococci, or streptococci. Symptoms include pain, redness and swelling, fever, and sometimes drainage. Abscesses are treated with antibiotics and surgical incision and drainage of pus. The area may be left open to drain, with gauze packing placed to assist with drainage and healing.

Nursing Care

Nursing care includes dressing or packing changes as ordered. Sitz baths are used to keep the area clean and promote healing, especially after bowel movements. The patient is instructed in the importance of keeping the area clean and dry. Other postoperative care is similar to care following hemorrhoidectomy.

LOWER GASTROINTESTINAL BLEEDING

Etiology

Major causes of lower gastrointestinal bleeding are diverticulitis, polyps (growths in the colon), anal fissures, hemorrhoids, inflammatory bowel disease, and cancer.

Signs and Symptoms

Bleeding from the GI tract is seen in the stool. When blood has been in the GI tract for more than 8 hours and has come in contact with hydrochloric acid, it causes **melena**, or black and tarry stools. The presence of melena indicates bleeding above or in the small bowel. Bleeding from the colon or rectum is usually bright red (**hematochezia**).

Significant blood loss causes hypotension, light-headedness, nausea, and diaphoresis. The patient may be pale and have cool skin. The onset of tachycardia and worsening hypotension indicate hypovolemic shock and should be reported to the physician immediately.

Diagnostic Tests

A thorough history is necessary to determine underlying disorders that may be causing the bleeding. Decreased hemoglobin and hematocrit levels result from blood loss. Blood urea nitrogen (BUN) may be elevated as a result of breakdown of proteins in the blood by the GI tract. Stool can be tested for occult blood if it is not evident on inspection. Digital examination, colonoscopy, or sigmoidoscopy may be done by the physician.

Therapeutic Measures

Treatment involves correction of the cause of the bleeding: surgery to correct diverticulosis, to correct inflammatory bowel disease, or to resect cancer may be considered.

Nursing Care

Stools are checked for the presence and amount of blood. Vital signs are monitored for signs of shock. Decreasing blood pressure and rising heart rate are reported to the physician immediately. The patient is prepared for diagnostic tests, and nursing care for the underlying disorder is provided.

• WORD • BUILDING •
hematochezia: hemat—blood + chezia—in stool

COLORECTAL CANCER

Pathophysiology and Etiology

Colorectal cancer is one of the most common types of internal cancer in the United States. It originates in the epithelial lining of the colon or rectum and can occur anywhere in the large intestine. People with a personal or family history of ulcerative colitis, colon cancer, or polyps of the rectum or large intestine are at higher risk for developing cancer. Colorectal cancer has also been linked with previous gallbladder removal and dietary carcinogens. A major causative factor is lack of fiber in the diet, which prolongs fecal transit time and in turn prolongs exposure to possible carcinogens. Also, bacterial flora is believed to be altered by excess fat, which converts steroids into compounds having carcinogenic properties. Lifestyle factors such as obesity, smoking, alcohol intake, and a large amount of red meat in the diet increase the risk of colon cancer.

Signs and Symptoms

Manifestations of colorectal cancer vary according to the type of tumor and the location (Fig. 34.6). A change in bowel habits is the most common symptom (Table 34.9). Blood or mucus in stools may occur. Although all tumors cause varying degrees of obstruction, those in the descending colon and rectum generally do not cause anemia, weight loss, nausea, or vomiting.

Complications

Complications include bleeding, complete obstruction of the colon, perforation, anastomosis leaking leading to peritonitis, and extension of the tumor to adjacent organs. Colorectal cancer can metastasize to the lymphatic system and liver.

If the patient has an anastomotic leak, the location of the leak determines the effects that are seen. The patient may need to be NPO for up to 4 weeks to rest the GI tract and prevent more leakage and also receive high-dose antibiotic therapy such as ciprofloxacin (Cipro) or metronidazole (Flagyl). Ongoing monitoring includes WBCs, sedimentation rate, and fever. The patient will likely go home with special home care needs. A peripherally inserted central catheter (PICC) line is placed to continue the antibiotic therapy.

Diagnostic Tests

Although screening for colorectal cancer in those over age 50 is the best prevention, screening rates could be higher. Screening guidelines can be found in Chapter 11 or on the American Cancer Society's website at www.cancer.org.

Home screening for blood in the stool can be done with a home colon cancer test kit. Immunological tests look for small amounts of blood. If blood is found, a physician should be contacted for follow-up. Most colorectal cancers are identified by biopsy done at the time of endoscopy (proctosigmoidoscopy, sigmoidoscopy, or colonoscopy). A CT scan can perform a virtual colonoscopy to view the inside of the colon. The carcinoembryonic antigen (CEA) blood test

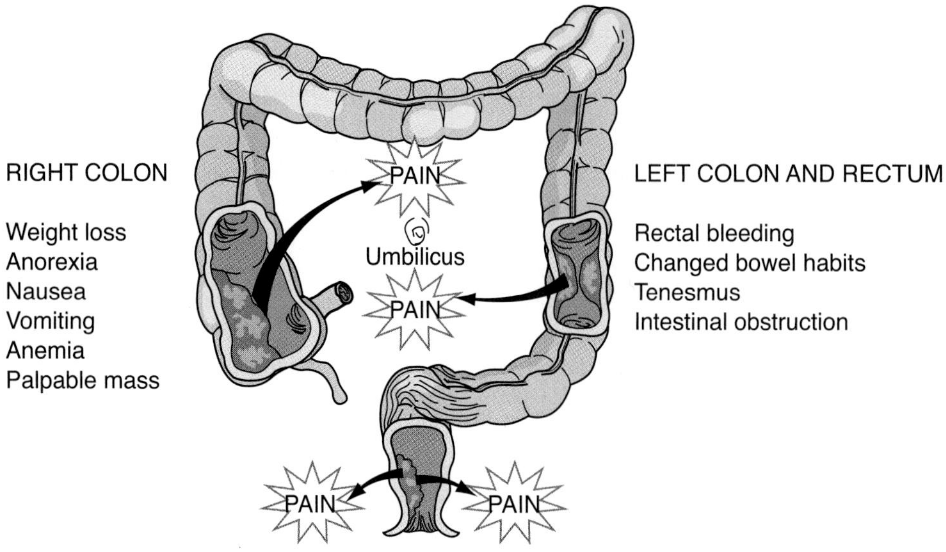
RIGHT COLON
Weight loss
Anorexia
Nausea
Vomiting
Anemia
Palpable mass
PAIN
Umbilicus
PAIN
PAIN
PAIN
LEFT COLON AND RECTUM
Rectal bleeding
Changed bowel habits
Tenesmus
Intestinal obstruction

FIGURE 34.6 Symptoms of carcinoma of the colon. Pain usually radiates toward the umbilicus or perianal area. (Modified from Black, J. M., & Matassarin-Jacobs, E. [1997]. *Medical-surgical nursing* [5th ed., p. 1810]. Philadelphia: W. B. Saunders, with permission.)

TABLE 34.9 COLON CANCER SUMMARY

Signs and Symptoms	Change in bowel habits Blood or mucus in stools Abdominal or rectal pain Weight loss Anemia Obstruction
Diagnostic Tests	Colonoscopy with biopsy Sigmoidoscopy with biopsy Proctosigmoidoscopy Barium enema Abdominal and rectal examination Fecal occult blood
Therapeutic Measures	Surgery, possibly colostomy Radiation Chemotherapy and/or radiation Medications: analgesics TPN as needed Support and education
Priority Nursing Diagnoses	*Acute Pain* *Fear* *Imbalanced Nutrition*

is used to assess response to treatment of GI cancer. CEA is present when epithelial cells rapidly divide and provides an early warning that the cancer has returned.

Therapeutic Measures

Small localized tumors may be excised and treated during endoscopy or laparoscopy. These procedures can also be used as palliative care for patients with advanced tumors who cannot tolerate major surgery. If a tumor is causing obstruction, a stent can be placed to keep the colon open for bowel function until surgery.

Surgery is performed to either resect larger tumors and anastomose the remaining bowel or create a fecal diversion by forming an ostomy. A variety of surgical procedures can be done depending on the location and extent of the cancer (Table 34.10 and Fig. 34.7). Medical management can include radiation therapy, chemotherapy, and monoclonal antibody therapy. When used, along with surgery, increased survival rates have been demonstrated.

Monoclonal antibody therapy uses antibodies that are made in a laboratory and work like normal antibodies do. They can enhance immune system function, interfere with the cancer cell's growth, or even carry treatment such as drugs or radiation to cancer cells. The antibody is designed to attach to cancer cells to flag them for the immune system so they can be destroyed. Bevacizumab (Avastin) blocks the making of new blood vessels to deprive cancer cells of nourishment. Cetuximab (Erbitux) blocks the cell's growth signal to stop it from growing.

Nursing Process for the Patient with Colorectal Cancer

Data Collection

Risk factors for colorectal cancer are identified by asking questions about the patient's personal and family history: Is there a history of inflammatory bowel disease? What were the patient's dietary habits? What foods were usually eaten, and how much fluid was usually consumed? Prior to diagnosis, did the patient experience constipation or diarrhea? Has there been a change in bowel habits? Has mucus or blood been noted in the stools? What social habits does the patient have? Did the patient smoke, drink alcoholic beverages, exercise? Has there been a recent weight loss? If so, how much and over what period of time? Does the patient admit to unusual fatigue or insomnia? Stool should be checked for mucus or blood.

TABLE 34.10 INTESTINAL SURGERIES

Types of Intestinal Surgery	Definition	Effect on Stool Elimination
Laparoscopic-assisted colectomy	Affected part of colon and nearby lymph nodes removed with laparoscope through smaller incisions.	Anastomosed ends. Stool is passed via rectum and anus.
Open colectomy	Affected part of colon and nearby lymph nodes removed through traditional incision.	Anastomosed ends. Stool is passed via rectum and anus.
Ileocolectomy	Right side of colon and diseased portion of ileum removed.	Anastomosed ends. Stool is passed via rectum and anus.
Hemicolectomy	Right or left side of colon removed.	Right: Colon attached to small intestine. Left: Anastomosed ends. Stool is passed via rectum and anus.
Total colectomy	Entire colon removed; rectum and anus remain.	Ileorectal anastomosis. Stool is passed via rectum and anus.
Total proctocolectomy	Entire colon, rectum, and sometimes anus removed.	Ileostomy. If anus left, ileal pouch-anal anastomosis and stool is passed via anus.
Rectal Cancer		
Local transanal resection Cancer in lower area of rectum Transanal endoscopic microsurgery Cancer higher in rectum	No incision. Rectal cancer removed through anus.	Anastomosed ends. Stool is passed via anus.
Lower anterior resection Cancer in upper 2/3 of rectum	Affected part of colon and nearby lymph nodes removed through traditional incision.	Anastomosed ends. Stool is passed via rectum and anus.
Abdominoperineal resection Cancer in lower 1/3 of rectum	Sigmoid colon, rectum, anus removed.	End colostomy. Stool passed via ostomy.
Proctectomy Cancer in lower 2/3 of rectum	Rectum removed.	Colo-anal anastomosis. Stool passed via anus.

If the patient has surgery, postoperative assessment includes monitoring vital signs and the return of flatus and bowel movements. Lung sounds are monitored for response to coughing and deep breathing and early ambulation. Dressings are observed for drainage. Large amounts of drainage or bleeding are reported. If a drain is inserted in the perineal wound, moderate amounts of serosanguineous (light pink) drainage are expected. If the patient has an ostomy, it is monitored (see ostomy section below).

Nursing Diagnoses, Planning, and Implementation

Acute Pain Related to Tissue Compression from the Tumor

EXPECTED OUTCOME: The patient will report pain relieved or at an acceptable level.

- Have patient identify pain using a rating scale *to identify pain level consistently.*
- Administer analgesics as prescribed postoperatively *to relieve pain.*

Fear Related to Serious Threat to Well-Being

EXPECTED OUTCOME: The patient will state fear is reduced after information is given related to patient's condition.

- Assist patient in identifying fears *to develop plan for reducing fears.*
- Set aside time to allow the patient who so desires to talk, cry, or ask questions about the diagnosis and planned surgery *to help reduce fear.*
- Answer questions accurately *to provide a trusting relationship.*

Imbalanced Nutrition: Less Than Body Requirements Related to Nausea and Anorexia

EXPECTED OUTCOME: The patient will maintain normal weight for height and age.

- Give antiemetics as ordered *to relieve nausea.*
- Identify foods patients like and provide them *to stimulate appetite.*
- Give total parenteral nutrition as ordered *to provide depleted vitamins, minerals, and nutrients if the patient has been anorexic for any length of time or has had a significant weight loss.*
- Provide the patient with a high-protein, high-calorie diet, as ordered, that is low in residue *to decrease excessive peristalsis and minimize cramping.*

Evaluation

Expected outcomes are that the patient verbalizes control of pain and less fear and attains an optimum level of nutrition.

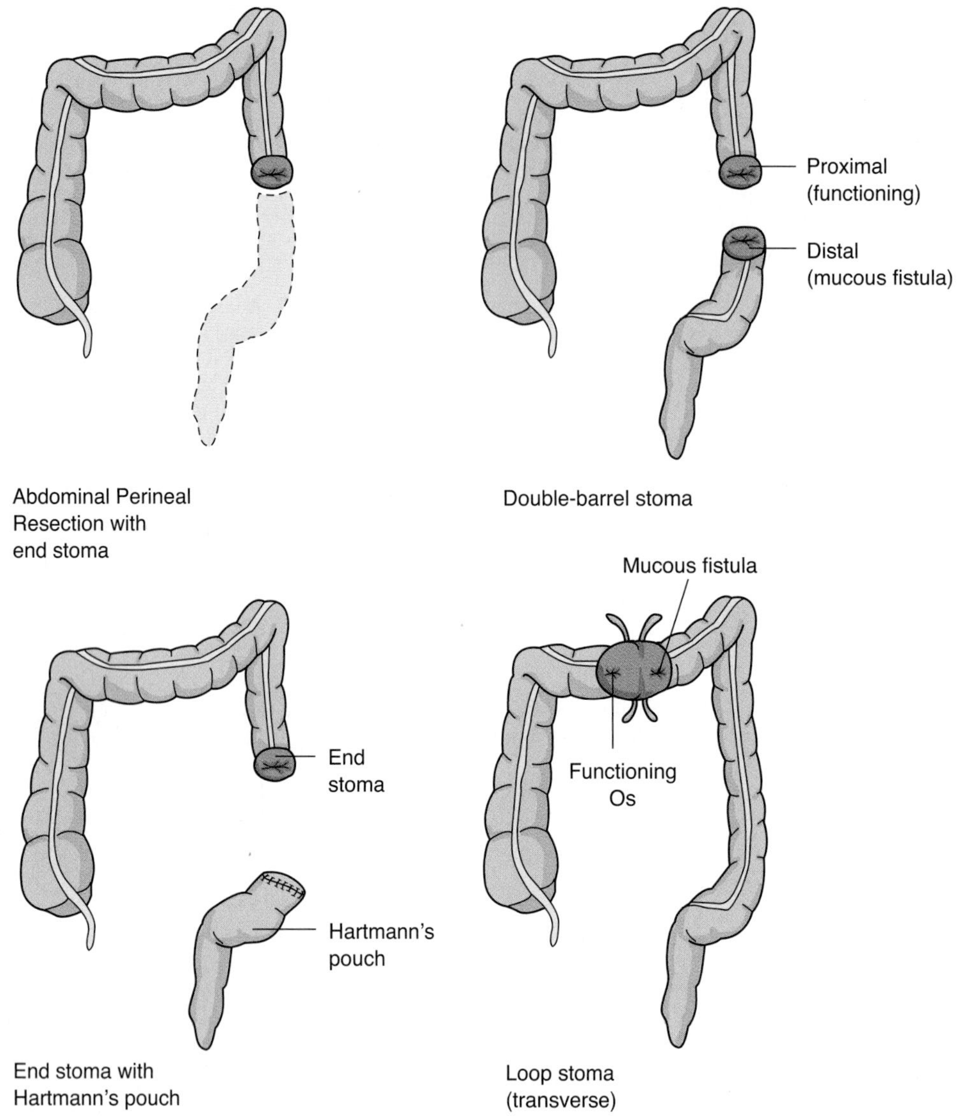
Proximal
(functioning)
Distal
(mucous fistula)
Abdominal Perineal
Resection with
end stoma
Double-barrel stoma
Mucous fistula
End
stoma
Functioning
Os
Hartmann's
pouch
End stoma with
Hartmann's pouch
Loop stoma
(transverse)

FIGURE 34.7 Types of stomas.

OSTOMY AND CONTINENT OSTOMY MANAGEMENT

An ostomy is a surgically created opening (traditional abdominal incision or laparoscopic) that diverts stool or urine to the outside of the body through an opening on the abdomen called a **stoma**. A stoma is the portion of bowel that is sutured onto the abdomen. A continent ostomy uses an internal reservoir to collect stool. The types of abdominal ostomies include ileostomy, colostomy, and urostomy. (Urinary ostomies are discussed in Chapter 37.) The stomas can be end, loop, or double barrel (see Fig. 34.7).

Ileostomy

An **ileostomy** is an end stoma formed by bringing the terminal ileum out to the abdominal wall following a total proctocolectomy. Two types of ileostomies can be formed: a conventional ileostomy and a continent ileostomy, such as a Kock pouch (sometimes called a Koch pouch) or Barnett's continent internal reservoir, which is a modification of a Kock pouch (Fig. 34.8). A conventional ileostomy has a small stoma in the right lower quadrant that requires a pouch at all times because of the continuous flow of liquid effluent.

Continent ileostomies are formed by taking a portion of the terminal ileum to construct an internal reservoir with a nipple valve. A stoma is created and the patient is taught to insert a catheter into the stoma three or four times a day to empty the reservoir. A continent ileostomy surgical procedure takes longer and requires additional instruction for the patient to be able to do self-care. It is important for the patient to empty the pouch routinely to prevent pouch rupture. Complications can occur, especially for the Kock pouch, such as valve slippage or leaking, pouch rupture, or pouchitis. Corrective surgery may be required.

• WORD • BUILDING •
ileostomy: ileo—pertaining to ileum + stoma—mouth or opening

LEARNING TIP

As stool travels through the colon, water is absorbed and the stool becomes firmer. Therefore, an ileostomy produces the most liquid effluent, followed by an ascending colostomy. A descending or sigmoid colostomy produces the firmest stool. Those with an ileostomy are at increased risk for dehydration due to greater water loss.

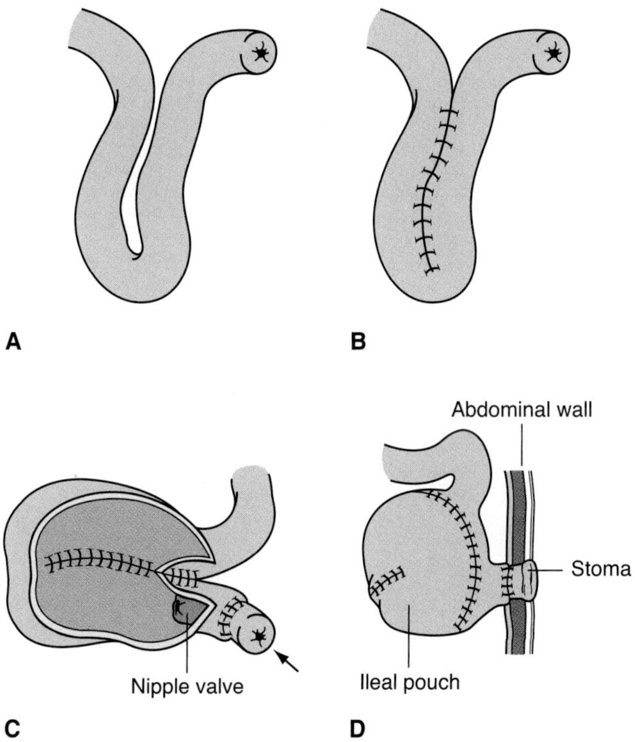
A
B
Abdominal wall
Stoma
Nipple valve
Ileal pouch
C
D

FIGURE 34.8 Surgical formation of continent ileostomy (Kock pouch). (A) Loop of terminal ileum. (B) Both limbs of ileum are brought together and sutured into a U shape. (C) Pouch created with nipple valve. (D) Pouch sutured to abdominal wall.

An ileoanal anastomosis connects the ileum to the anus and avoids the need for a stoma (Fig. 34.9). This is usually a two-step procedure. During the first surgery, the diseased bowel is removed. A reservoir (named by its shape: J [most common], S, W, or H pouch) is then formed from part of the ileum and connected to the anus. A temporary ileostomy is also formed to divert stool while the reservoir heals. After about 3 months, the temporary ileostomy is reversed and the patient can have bowel movements from the anus. Problems with perianal skin irritation resulting from frequent liquid stools may occur. An ileorectal anastomosis can also be performed, but this may not be a curative procedure for a patient with ulcerative colitis because the rectum may still be diseased.

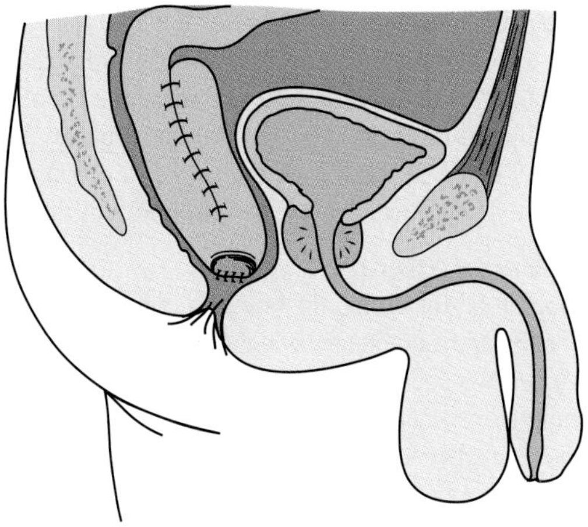

FIGURE 34.9 Ileal J pouch-anal anastomosis. The two-loop ileal pouch is simple to construct, provides adequate storage capacity, and is evacuated spontaneously and fully.

Colostomy

A **colostomy** is named according to where in the bowel it is formed: It may be an ascending, transverse, descending, or sigmoid colostomy. The type of effluent is dependent on the location of the bowel used (Table 34.11).

End Stoma

An end stoma is formed when the proximal end of the bowel is brought to the outside abdominal wall. If an AP resection is done, the rectum is removed and the proximal sigmoid or descending colon is brought out as a stoma. Another procedure that may be done involves removing the segment of diseased or injured bowel and using the proximal portion to form the stoma. The remaining limb of bowel is sutured closed and left in the peritoneal cavity so that the rectum is intact. This is called a Hartmann's pouch, or mucous fistula, and may be permanent or temporary depending on the diagnosis. Because the rectum is intact, the patient may feel the urge to defecate. This is normal because the colon continues to produce mucus. As the rectal stump fills with mucus, the sphincter is triggered and alerts the patient as if it were stool.

TABLE 34.11 LOCATION OF STOMA AND TYPE OF EFFLUENT

Location of Stoma	Type of Effluent
Ileostomy	Liquid to mushy
Cecostomy, ascending colostomy	Liquid to mushy, foul odor
Right transverse colostomy	Mushy to semiformed
Left transverse colostomy	Semiformed, soft
Descending or sigmoid colostomy	Soft to hard formed

• WORD • BUILDING •

colostomy: colo—pertaining to colon + stoma—mouth or opening

Loop Stoma

To create a loop stoma, a loop of bowel, usually the transverse colon, is pulled to the outside abdominal wall and a bridge is slipped under the loop to hold it in place. An incisional slit is made in the top of the exposed colon to allow stool to exit. The entire loop of bowel is not cut through.

Double-Barrel Stoma

With a double-barrel stoma, the bowel is completely dissected and both ends of the colon are brought to the outside abdominal wall to form two separate stomas. The proximal stoma is the functioning stoma that expels stool. The distal stoma is called a mucous fistula because mucus produced by the bowel passes from it. A double-barrel stoma is often temporary, allowing the bowel to rest during healing after trauma or surgery.

Preoperative Care

A wound ostomy continence nurse (WOCN) should be consulted before surgery. The WOCN can help prepare the patient both emotionally and physically for the surgery. In addition, the WOCN has expertise in selecting the stoma site for the surgeon to ensure that it is easy to sit with it, care for it, and wear clothing over it. This involves observing the abdomen as the patient assumes different positions and noting how clothing is worn, such as where the belt rides. The site for the stoma can then be chosen so it is visible to the patient for self-care, avoids skin or fat folds, and is where clothing will not interfere with the appliance. Properly planned stoma placement can prevent agony over discomfort when sitting, inability to perform self-care, and uncomfortable, leaking, or poorly fitting appliances postoperatively.

Routine preoperative instruction, including the importance of coughing and deep breathing, splinting, and early ambulation, is provided. Orders for cleansing of the bowel are performed to reduce the risk for infection following surgery. Unless the patient has chronic diarrhea related to IBD, an oral agent to cleanse the bowel is given. Oral and intravenous antibiotics are given as ordered.

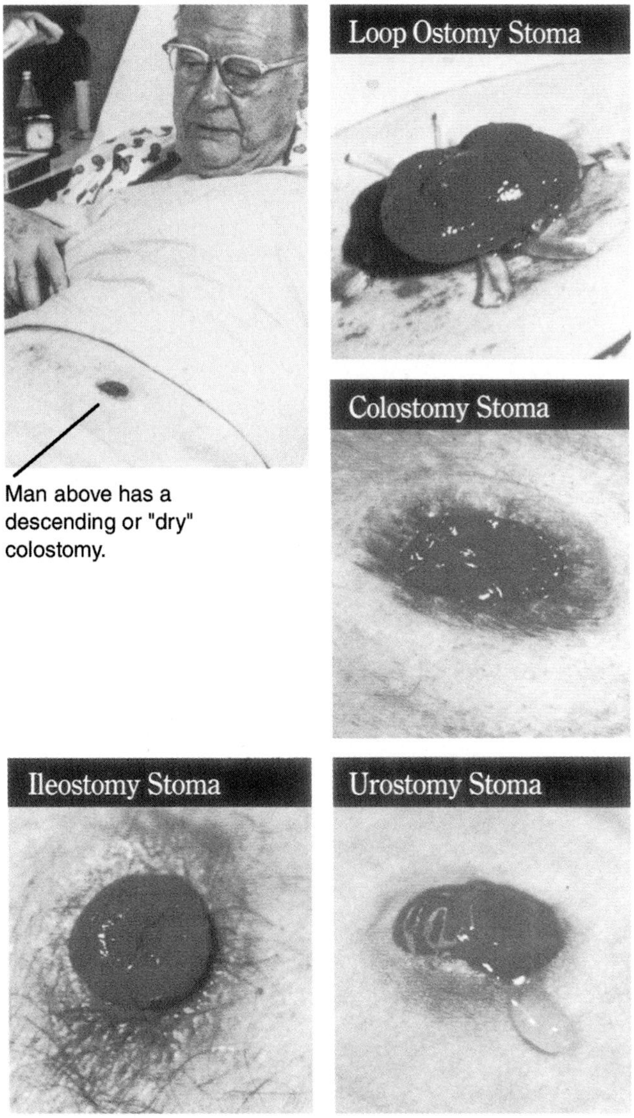
Loop Ostomy Stoma
Man above has a descending or "dry" colostomy.
Colostomy Stoma
Ileostomy Stoma
Urostomy Stoma

FIGURE 34.10 Types of stomas. Note moist, pink to red appearance of healthy stoma. (Reproduced with permission of Hollister Inc., Libertyville, IL.)

Nursing Process for the Patient with a New or Established Ostomy or Continent Ostomy

Data Collection

For a patient with a new ostomy, in addition to routine postoperative assessment, a stoma should be inspected at least every 8 hours. The stoma should be pink to red, moist (similar to the inside of the mouth), and well attached to the surrounding skin (Fig. 34.10). A bluish stoma indicates inadequate blood supply; a black stoma indicates necrosis. Either complication should be reported to the physician immediately for treatment, which may require that the patient return to surgery. Note edema of stoma. The stoma size gradually decreases over the first few weeks following surgery.

For both new and established ostomies, skin is assessed for irritation around the pouch and under the pouch each time it is changed. Ostomy discharge (effluent) is monitored and documented. Unexpected changes, such as liquid stool from a descending ostomy, are reported. For the patient with a continent ostomy pouch, assessing that regular emptying of the pouch is done is important to prevent rupture and leakage. The characteristics of the stool are noted for any type of continent ostomy so that problems can be reported.

Nursing Diagnoses, Planning, and Implementation

See the *Nursing Care Plan for the Patient with an Intestinal Ostomy* and Table 34.12.

Deficient Knowledge Related to Ostomy

EXPECTED OUTCOME: Patient will demonstrate how to care for ostomy.

- Determine patient readiness and ability to learn and perform self-care. *The patient experiencing pain, nausea, or vomiting is not likely to be ready to look at the ostomy or learn about ostomy care.*

NURSING CARE PLAN for the Patient with an Intestinal Ostomy

Nursing Diagnosis: *Disturbed Body Image* related to new ostomy

Expected Outcomes: The patient will verbalize acceptance of intestinal ostomy before discharge.

Evaluation of Outcomes: Is the patient able to verbalize acceptance of the ostomy?

Interventions	Rationale	Evaluation
Ask about knowledge of self-care of ostomies.	Many people have misconceptions regarding ostomies. Identification of misconceptions and "hearsay" knowledge is important to clarify or correct.	Does the patient verbalize appropriate knowledge of ostomy care?
Encourage patient to verbalize feelings about the stoma.	Allowing the patient to express his or her feelings provides opportunity to identify and verbalize concerns, which then can be addressed by health care providers.	Does the patient discuss his or her feelings regarding the stoma with the nurse or significant other?
Explain the normal characteristics of the stoma before the patient's first look.	Helping the patient understand what to expect will help relieve anxiety. Being available to answer questions immediately also relieves anxiety.	Does the patient look at the stoma without hesitation?
Demonstrate ostomy appliance change and daily care and encourage patient participation.	When the patient observes and participates in self-care, his or her self-concept improves.	Is the patient participating in self-care? Has the patient performed return demonstration of appliance change and emptying of pouch?

TABLE 34.12 SUMMARY OF RECOVERY FROM INTESTINAL SURGERY

Intestinal Surgery	Elimination Needs	Discharge Teaching Needs	Possible Psychological Needs
Total colectomy	Normal or continent anal passage	Continent ostomy care. Soft diet until first doctor visit. Monitor for constipation and report.	Chronic sorrow related to inflammatory bowel disease (IBD)
Hemicolectomy (right or left) or ileocolectomy	Normal, no appliance needed	Avoid stress to abdomen: heavy lifting, sit-ups. Soft diet until first doctor visit. Monitor for constipation and report.	Fear of cancer Chronic sorrow related to IBD
Partial colectomy	Normal, no appliance needed	Monitor for constipation.	Fear of cancer
Abdominoperineal resection	Pouch	Ostomy care.	Fear of cancer Body image changes
Proctosigmoidectomy	Normal, no appliance needed	Soft diet until first doctor visit. Monitor for constipation and report.	Fear of cancer
Total proctocolectomy	Continent anal passage or pouch	Continent ostomy care. Soft diet until first doctor visit. Monitor for constipation and report.	Chronic sorrow related to IBD

- Provide special instructions or a specific type of ostomy appliance for patients with special needs, such as blindness, deafness, language barrier, severe arthritis, or other physical conditions that limit ability to perform self-care, *so they will be able to perform self-care.*
- Include caregiver in teaching if the patient is not ready or able to learn. *With short hospital stays, time for teaching is limited and must begin soon after surgery.*
- Ensure referral to home care nurse is made *to continue teaching in the patient's home.*
- Consult a WOCN or equipment supplier if needed *for suggestions for appliances to identify appliances suited to individual patient's needs.* Figure 34.11 shows types of appliances.
- Explain how to change appliance (Fig. 34.12) *to promote self-care.*
  - Demonstrate how to apply appliance using moldable or traditional skin barrier to promote self-care. *Moldable (able to change shape) skin barrier does not require measuring a pattern or cutting and does not leave a gap around the stoma.*
- For the traditional skin barrier:
  - Fit the traditional skin barrier over the stoma on the skin with no gaps around the base of the stoma *to prevent skin contact with stool.*
  - Measure stoma initially with each appliance change *because the stoma will be edematous until it shrinks over time.*
  - Trace a stoma pattern, if using a nonmoldable barrier, *to teach the patient proper size and shape because most stomas are not round.*
- Change appliance every 3 days or every 10 to 14 days depending on the type of appliance *to reduce skin shearing from frequent removal.*

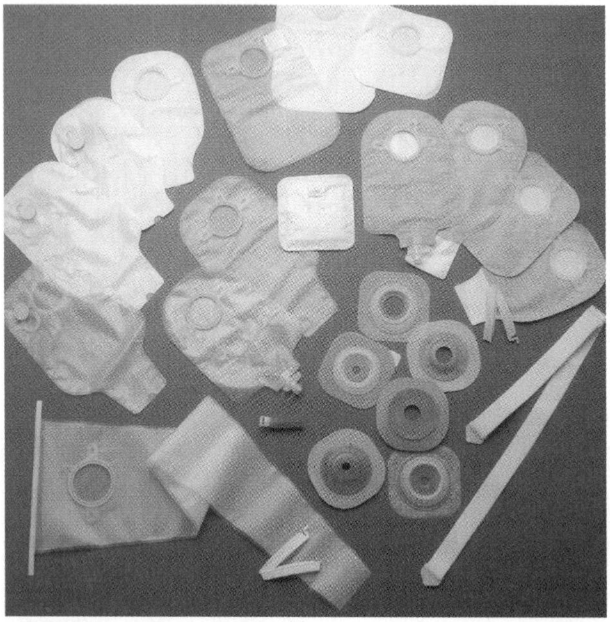

FIGURE 34.11 Appliances used for ostomies. The long sleeve at the lower left of the photograph is used to drain the bowel following irrigation. (Reproduced with permission of Hollister Inc., Libertyville, IL.)

Preparation of the Stomahesive Wafer with Sur-Fit Flange

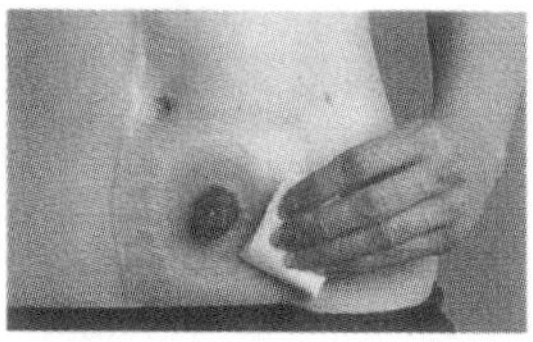

1. Cleanse the peristomal area with water and pat thoroughly dry. Measure your stoma size with the measuring guide provided and trace the proper opening on the white paper backing of the Stomahesive® disc.

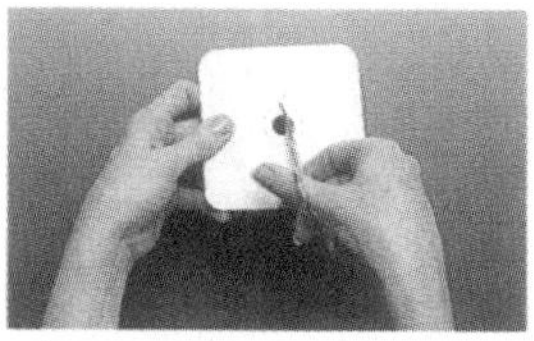

2. Leaving the white paper backing of the wafer in place, cut a hole in the wafer to the same shape and size as the base of the stoma. The best result is usually obtained by cutting from the reverse side of the wafer, using curved, short-bladed scissors.

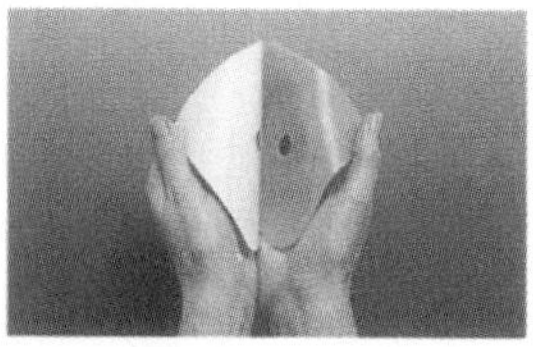

3. Peel the white paper backing from the wafer just prior to application.

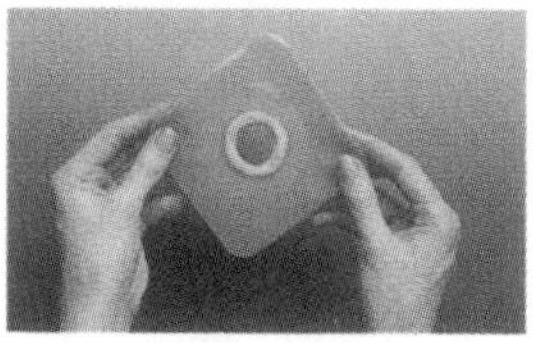

4. Gaps between the wafer and the base of the stoma may be further protected by applying Stomahesive® Paste to the wafer.

Application of the Stomahesive Wafer with Sur-Fit Flange

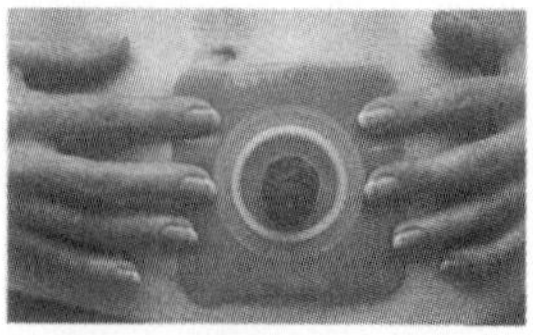

5. Center the enlarged hole over the stoma, place on abdomen, and apply light pressure.

FIGURE 34.12 Preparation to apply an ostomy appliance. (Courtesy ConvaTec, a Bristol-Myers Squibb Company, Princeton, NJ, with permission.)

- Change appliance immediately if leakage occurs *to avoid* ***peristomal*** *skin irritation.*
- Use an open-ended or drainable pouch for all colostomies or ileostomies, especially during the first 8 weeks after surgery *to facilitate emptying and comfort.*
  - Explain to the patient who has a left-sided (descending or sigmoid) colostomy that the bowel can be regulated either by diet or regular irrigation of the stoma. After bowel regulation has been achieved, the patient may use a closed-end pouch or a stoma cap.
- Explain daily care and hygiene:
  - Empty pouch when it is one-third to one-half full. The amount of effluent and the frequency of emptying depend on the location of the stoma in the bowel. *If the pouch is allowed to get more than half full of stool, the weight of the effluent will pull on the pouch and weaken the seal of the skin barrier.*
  - Empty pouch and then clean inside of the tail of the pouch before the clamp is replaced *to help control odor.* If a two-piece system is used, the pouch can be taken off, washed out, and replaced.
  - Place spray deodorants or chlorophyll tablets in the pouch *to control odor.* Chlorophyll is more effective if taken by mouth.
  - Bathe or shower with the appliance in place but check seal and retape or change it if it is loosening. Water will not harm stoma or leak into stoma.
- Explain dietary considerations:
  - Identify foods that contribute to odor and gas. If foods that are known to cause odor or gas are eaten, the patient should know to empty the pouch of flatus more often and to be aware that more odor is probable.
  - Identify foods that contribute to and control diarrhea and what to do for constipation. A list of foods that may contribute to ileostomy blockage must be given to the ileostomy patient (Box 34.9 and Box 34.10, *Nutrition Notes*).
- Explain colostomy irrigation if patient is interested:
  - Explain that colostomy irrigation is done *to regulate bowel movements at a regular time.* Candidates for irrigation are those with more formed stool (descending or sigmoid portion of colon).
  - Show how to perform irrigation (similar to an enema), with special equipment used to instill fluid into the bowel via the stoma. *Because a stoma does not have a sphincter, specially designed tubing with a cone at the end is used to irrigate the ostomy. The cone prevents the fluid that is being instilled from flowing back out of the stoma.*

• WORD • BUILDING •
peristomal: peri—surrounding + stoma—mouth or opening

Box 34.9

Foods That Can Cause Ileostomy Blockage

Cole slaw
Celery
Corn, popcorn
Coconut
Mushrooms
Nuts
Chinese vegetables

Green leafy vegetables:
- Spinach
- Collards
- Mustards

Foods with nondigestible peels:
- Apples
- Grapes
- Potatoes

Dried fruits:
- Raisins
- Figs
- Apricots

Meats with casings:
- Sausage
- Hot dogs
- Bologna

Readiness for Enhanced Self Health Management Related to Difficulty Carrying Out Self-Care Measures

EXPECTED OUTCOME: Patient will demonstrate ability to perform self-care measures.

- Identify financial ability to obtain supplies. *The cost and availability of ostomy supplies is problematic for many patients. Most insurers, including Medicare, pay for ostomy supplies, although some limit the type of appliance and number allowed per month. Each state-funded Medicaid system is different. The type of appliance needed to eliminate leakage may not always be covered, requiring the patient to either pay the difference or wear what the insurance company will provide. If the patient has no insurance, costs can be high. Some patients find they have to choose whether to purchase ostomy appliances or prescriptions with their limited funds. Fortunately, the pouches in most two-piece systems can be washed out and reused to save money (see* Home Health Hints*).*

Box 34.10
Nutrition Notes

Anticipating Dietary Management of Ostomies

Ostomy patients receive a soft diet initially, progressing to a general diet as the surgeon prescribes. Stringy, high-fiber foods are initially avoided until a definite tolerance has been demonstrated and then are best tried in small amounts, one at a time. Stringy, high-fiber foods include:

- Celery, cabbage, coleslaw, sauerkraut, spinach, peas, corn
- Coconut, dried fruit, pineapple, membranes on citrus fruits
- Popcorn, nuts, seeds, skins of fruits and vegetables.

Some patients avoid fish, eggs, beer, and carbonated beverages because they produce excessive odor. Dietary restrictions are usually based on individual tolerance.

Certain foods may be therapeutic because they thicken the stool, including:

- Cheese
- Creamy peanut butter
- Marshmallows
- Pasta
- Pretzels
- White bread
- White rice (Willcutts, Scarano, & Eddins, 2005).

Patients with ostomies should be encouraged to do the following:

- Eat at regular intervals.
- Chew food well to avoid blockage at the stoma site.
- Drink adequate amounts of fluid.
- Avoid foods that produce excessive gas, loose stools, offensive odors, and undesirable bulk.
- Avoid excessive weight gain.

Home Health Hints

- Patients with ostomies may be able to have some of their supplies covered by insurance. The home health nurse can work with the medical supply store to assist the patient in receiving the needed equipment. Most companies will deliver supplies to the patient's home.
- Foods such as broccoli, cauliflower, brussels sprouts, and cabbage can cause increased malodorous gas production. Encourage the patient with a colostomy to eat these in moderation. Offer alternative choices, such as green leafy vegetables, carrots, and cucumbers.
- If the patient requires a stool for occult blood test, deliver a collection hat before you visit to assist with obtaining the specimen. Plan to deliver the specimen to the laboratory the day it is collected.
- Dietary instruction is important for home health patients with lower GI disorders. Give instructions both verbally and in writing. Written format allows the patient to have the information available for review and to assist with creating a shopping list.

Sexual Dysfunction Related to Body Image Change or Erectile Dysfunction

EXPECTED OUTCOME: Patient will discuss satisfying acceptable sexual practices for self and partner.

- Identify if male patient who had an AP resection is experiencing erectile dysfunction. *This impotence may be transient, depending on the severity of nerve damage or edema associated with the surgery.*
- Ensure consultation with urologist is made *to treat erectile dysfunction if present.*
- Encourage patients to discuss any concerns regarding sexuality with his or her sexual partner. *This may help them work through any fears or embarrassment.*
- Explain that attractive pouch covers can be purchased and worn *to help disguise the pouch and its contents.*
- Encourage personal hygiene and emptying ostomy bag before sexual encounters *to decrease odors and enhance experience*
- Refer to sex counselor *who can suggest alternative sexual positions to increase satisfaction for partners.*

Risk for Injury Related to Skin and Stomal Complications

EXPECTED OUTCOME: The patient will remain free from injury with intact skin, red, moist stoma, and functioning ostomy.

- Identify allergies *to prevent complications because allergic dermatitis from sensitivity to the adhesive may develop.*
- Consult WOCN for complications associated with care of the ostomy. *A WOCN has had specialized instruction in caring for the stoma and peristomal skin and has a wealth of information to offer.*
- Use a skin barrier such as Stomahesive *to prevent peristomal skin irritation. The skin around the stoma may become irritated if the opening in the skin barrier around the stoma is cut too large and exposes skin to the GI effluent. Prolonged contact with effluent can lead to a reaction similar to a chemical burn.*
- Remove tape and adhesive only when necessary *to prevent skin shearing from frequent removal.*
- Leave pouches on for several days unless leakage occurs *to prevent skin shearing from frequent removal.*
- Monitor for peristomal hernia *to detect hernias that may develop around the stoma as a result of weakened abdominal muscles and cause leakage by the change in body contours associated with the hernia.*

- Use a more flexible ostomy appliance if peristomal hernia is present *to fit body contours better.*
- Monitor for and report stomal prolapse, especially in older adults. *Weakened abdominal muscles contribute to the falling down (or out) of the intestinal mucosa, which can make pouching difficult.*
- Monitor stoma color and immediately report dusky or blue color, *which occurs when there is circulatory compromise. This may arise as a result of vascular collapse, blockage in the mesentery of the intestines, or edema in the intestine from obstruction proximal to the stoma. Usually, necrotic tissue occurs only at the very end of the stoma and will eventually slough off, revealing viable mucosa.*
- Explain signs and symptoms of an ileostomy blockage: absent stool, abdominal cramping, edematous stoma, and stoma color that is pale or dusky *to detect it for treatment.*
- Have patient consider what was eaten in the past 24 hours if blockage occurs *because certain foods are considered to cause stomal blockage (see Box 34.9).*
- Have the patient get into a tub of warm water (not too hot or cold), get into a knee-to-chest position, and sip on warm liquid, such as coffee, tea, bouillon, broth, or hot chocolate for an ileostomy blockage. *If the blockage is partial, relief will occur fairly soon after these measures are taken.*
- Explain to patient that if no relief is obtained, medical treatment should be sought. *For a complete blockage, an ileostomy lavage must be performed by a physician or WOCN.*

Evaluation

The plan of care has been effective if the patient is able to accept the change in body image, competently care for the ostomy (or caregiver will), carry out self-care, is satisfied with sexual practices, and describes self-care measures to prevent or treat complications.

Rehabilitative Needs

Ensuring that the patient is becoming comfortable with self-care, is able to perform the ostomy appliance change, and is able to return to work or civic activities as before are the goals of care. The patient can generally perform any activity he or she was able to do before the ostomy including swimming. Several support resources are available (Box 34.11).

Box 34.11

Resources and Support Groups

American Cancer Society
www.cancer.org
(800)227-2345

Celiac Sprue Association
www.csaceliacs.org
(877)272-4272

Crohn's and Colitis Foundation of America, Inc.
www.ccfa.org
(800)932-2423

International Foundation for Functional Gastrointestinal Disorders
http://aboutgerd.org
(888)964-2001

National Institute of Diabetes and Digestive and Kidney Diseases
www2.niddk.nih.gov

United Ostomy Associations of America, Inc.
www.uoaa.org
(800)826-0826

Wound, Ostomy and Continence Nurses Society
www.wocn.org
(888)224-WOCN (9626)

SUGGESTED ANSWERS TO

CRITICAL THINKING

■ *Mrs. Burns*

You need to assess the situation before intervening. First, ask Mrs. Burns or her caregivers if she had a bowel movement that was inadvertently not charted. Next, ask Mrs. Burns if she feels constipated or if she has abdominal discomfort. Assess Mrs. Burns' abdomen for distention and presence or absence of bowel sounds. A digital examination may be necessary to determine if a fecal impaction is present. If simple constipation appears to be the problem, the medical record should be checked for as-needed laxative or enema orders. Once Mrs. Burns has had a bowel movement, laxatives should be discontinued and preventive measures such as regular fluids, fiber, and exercise should be instituted.

■ *Judy Morrow*

1. Characteristics of pain: location, quality, intensity, precipitating factors, relieving factors.

Characteristics of bowel elimination: frequency, characteristic of stool, amount, color, consistency.

Nutritional status: Weight loss, appetite, daily food intake, food likes/dislikes, irritating foods, fluid intake.

Anxiety and coping skills: Support systems, usual coping methods.

SUGGESTED ANSWERS TO—cont'd

2. *Acute Pain* related to increased peristalsis and cramping

Diarrhea related to inflammatory process

Risk for Deficient Fluid Volume related to diarrhea and insufficient fluid intake

Anxiety related to symptoms and frequency of stools and treatment

Impaired Skin Integrity related to frequent loose stools

Imbalanced Nutrition, Less Than Body Requirements related to malabsorption

Ineffective Coping related to frequency of stools.

3. You need to further assess how Judy perceives that Crohn's disease will affect her lifestyle. What does she know about Crohn's disease? What is she concerned about? How has Crohn's disease affected her ability to sleep, what she eats, her participation in sports, and her relationships with other people?

   Convey a caring manner to Judy by being accepting of her, listening actively to her concerns, and helping her to find acceptable ways of resolving them. Provide her with information that she needs about Crohn's disease. Arrange to have a well-adapted person of approximately the same age from the Crohn's and Colitis Foundation of America meet with her to share coping strategies with her.
4. Increased frequency of stools leading to fluid volume deficit and possibly shock symptoms; bleeding leading to anemia and hypovolemia and possibly shock symptoms.

■ *Mrs. Loos*

1. The first consideration is to be aware of whether the patient is at risk for a small-bowel obstruction. After abdominal surgery, loops of intestine may adhere to areas in the abdomen that are not healed, causing a kink in the bowel that occludes the intestinal flow.
2. Yes, due to her history of abdominal surgery she is at risk of adhesion development that can cause obstruction. If assessment findings confirm this possibility, the physician should be contacted. Because of the nausea and the potential obstruction, withhold food and oral fluids until the physician can be contacted.
3. Begin by asking the WHAT'S UP? questions, including exactly where the pain is occurring, how it feels, if there is anything that aggravates or alleviates the pain, when it started, how bad it is on a scale of 0 to 10, whether there are associated symptoms, and if Mrs. Loos has some insight regarding the cause of her problem. Then, in this order, inspect, auscultate, and palpate (prevents palpation from changing other assessment findings). Inspect her abdomen to note distention. Listen for bowel sounds for 5 minutes in each quadrant. Lightly palpate her abdomen noting tenderness or rigidity. Ask when her last bowel movement was.
4. Bowel sounds normal in all quadrants, abdomen flat, soft with no tenderness, flatus present.
5. Abnormal bowel sounds; either absent for a nonmechanical obstruction or for a mechanical obstruction, high-pitched, tinkling bowel sounds proximal to the obstruction and absent distal to it; pain; abdominal distention.
6. Discuss findings with registered nurse or physician. Prepare for new orders such as an NG tube, NPO status, and pain management.
7. When documenting, answer the questions what, why, when, where, how, who (either explicitly or implicitly by professional knowledge, in narrative or flow sheet format) for completeness.

What = Patient is experiencing large, firm, tender to touch abdomen with nausea (additional assessment data should be included).

Why = Unknown, physician notified

When = Current date and time

Where = Abdomen

How = Unknown

Who = J. Morgan, LPN

8. If improving, symptoms will be resolving: no nausea, abdomen soft, bowel sounds present in all quadrants, flatus present, and bowel movements normal. If condition is worsening or complications are developing, symptoms will not improve and fecal vomiting and shock may occur.

REVIEW QUESTIONS

1. The nurse is collecting data on a patient admitted with a history of severe diarrhea. Findings include cool, pale skin, red tongue with furrows, blood pressure 102/74 mm Hg, pulse 106 beats per minute, respirations 20 per minute, temperature 99.9°F (37.7°C). Which of the following actions should the nurse take now?
   a. Report findings to registered nurse.
   b. Give acetaminophen (Tylenol) as ordered.
   c. Obtain bedside commode.
   d. Apply warm blankets.

2. Which of the following statements about laxative use would the nurse include in the teaching plan to promote patient understanding?
   a. "Laxatives may be used as needed."
   b. "Regular laxative use can be harmful."
   c. "Daily use of laxatives prevents constipation."
   d. "Laxative use has no complications."

3. Which of the following interventions should the nurse include in the plan of care for a patient after an appendectomy to prevent respiratory complications? **Select all that apply**.
   a. Pain control
   b. Early ambulation
   c. Bedrest
   d. Coughing, deep breathing
   e. Ankle exercises
   f. Incentive spirometer

4. Which of the following foods would the nurse teach the patient with ulcerative colitis to avoid?
   a. Fresh fruits
   b. White bread
   c. Sweet dessert
   d. Meat

5. Following a teaching session, which of the following statements would indicate to the nurse that the patient understood the teaching for postoperative care to prevent respiratory complications after a hernia repair?
   a. "I will cough every hour while awake."
   b. "I will deep breathe four times daily."
   c. "I will cough and deep breathe every hour."
   d. "I will deep breathe every hour while awake."

6. The nurse would evaluate the patient as understanding teaching for celiac disease if the patient selected which of the following foods to eat?
   a. Fresh fruit and oatmeal with milk
   b. Tomato juice and waffles
   c. Hard boiled egg, bacon, and blueberries
   d. Banana, cream of wheat cereal, and coffee

7. The nurse is caring for a patient with a small-bowel obstruction. The patient is NPO with an orogastric tube providing low intermittent suction. Which of the following ongoing data would be a priority for the nurse to monitor and collect? **Select all that apply**.
   a. Intake and output
   b. Pain level
   c. Bowel sounds
   d. Pulse rate
   e. Temperature
   f. Edema

8. The nurse is caring for a patient who has a sudden onset of diarrhea. Which of the following terms should the nurse use to document the patient's black, tarry stool?
   a. Melena
   b. Hematochezia
   c. Hematemesis
   d. Steatorrhea

9. Which of the following of the patient's dietary habits does the nurse understand may increase the risk for development of colon cancer?
   a. High-fat, low-fiber intake
   b. High intake of milk and milk products
   c. Low-meat and protein intake
   d. Low-fat, high-carbohydrate intake

10. The nurse is caring for a 1-day postoperative patient who has a new end colostomy. Which of the following findings regarding the stoma would be a priority for the nurse to report?
    a. Dusky color
    b. Mucus drainage
    c. Slight bleeding with touch
    d. Round shape

11. A patient with Crohn's disease is to receive sulfasalazine (Azulfidine), 500 mg oral suspension qid. The oral suspension is available as 250 mg/5 mL. How many milliliters should the nurse give for the 0800 dose?
    a. 5 mL
    b. 10 mL
    c. 20 mL
    d. 50 mL

References

Green, P. H., & Jabri, B. (2006). Celiac disease. *Annual Review of Medicine*, *57*, 207–221.

Johns Hopkins Medicine (2008). *When diverticulosis leads to diverticulitis.* Retrieved November 20, 2009, from http://www.johnshopkinshealthalerts.com/reports/digestive_health/861-1.html

Mayo Clinic. (2008, October 8). *Mayo Clinic collaborates to advance Crohn's treatment. Outlook for Crohn's disease improves due to new therapies.* Retrieved August 2, 2009, from http://www.mayoclinic.org/news2008-rst/5014.html

Willcutts, K., Scarano, K., & Eddins, C.W. (2005). Ostomies and fistulas: a collaborative approach. *Practical Gastroenterology, 29*(11), 63.

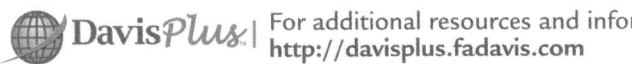

35 Nursing Care of Patients with Liver, Pancreatic, and Gallbladder Disorders

ELAINE KENNEDY

KEY TERMS

ascites (ah-SYE-teez)
asterixis (AS-tur-IK-siss)
cholecystitis (KOH-lee-siss-TYE-tiss)
choledocholithiasis (koh-LED-oh-koh-lih-THIGH-ah-siss)
cholelithiasis (KOH-lee-lih-THIGH-ah-siss)
cirrhosis (sih-ROH-siss)
colic (KAW-lick)
encephalopathy (en-SEF-uh-LAW-pah-thee)
extracorporeal shock-wave lithotripsy (EKS-trah-kor-POR-ee-uhl SHAWK-WAYV LITH-oh-TRIP-see)
fetor hepaticus (FEE-tur heh-PAT-tih-kuss)
hepatitis (HEP-uh-TYE-tiss)
hepatorenal syndrome (heh-PAT-oh-REE-nuhl SIN-drohm)
laparoscopy (LAP-uh-ROSS-kuh-pee)
pancreatectomy (PAN-kree-uh-TEK-tuh-mee)
portal hypertension (POR-tuhl HYE-per-TEN-shun)
T-tube (TEE-toob)
transjugular intrahepatic portosystemic shunt (TRANZ-jug-you-lur in-trah-heh-PAT-tik por-toe-siss-TEM-ik SHUNT)
varices (VAR-i-seez)

QUESTIONS TO GUIDE YOUR READING

1. How would you explain the causes, risk factors, and pathophysiology of the various types of liver disease?
2. What current therapeutic measures are used for patients with liver disease?
3. What nursing care should you provide for the patient experiencing a liver disorder?
4. What are the causes, risk factors, and pathophysiology of the various pancreatic disorders?
5. What current therapeutic measures are used for patients with pancreatic disorders?
6. What nursing care would you provide for a patient with a pancreatic disorder?
7. What are the causes, risk factors, and pathophysiology of gallbladder disorders?
8. What current therapeutic measures are used for patients with gallbladder disorders?
9. What nursing care would you provide for the patient with a gallbladder disorder?

The liver has many functions that are essential to life. When the liver is healthy, it has the amazing ability to grow back after it is damaged. Many types of diseases can affect the liver. Usually the damage occurs over time, but it can occur acutely (acute liver failure). First inflammation occurs, then over time, if the inflammation continues, scar tissue (fibrosis) replaces healthy liver cells. If the scarring becomes severe, the damage is irreversible and progressive, which is termed cirrhosis. Over time, chronic liver failure can result from cirrhosis.

DISORDERS OF THE LIVER

Hepatitis

Hepatitis is an inflammation of the liver, resulting from viral or bacterial infection, drugs, alcohol, or chemicals toxic to the liver, and some metabolic or vascular disorders. Viral hepatitis is common and discussed below. Symptoms of hepatitis range from nearly no symptoms to life-threatening symptoms due to death of liver tissue.

> **SAFETY TIP**
>
> Acetaminophen (Tylenol) can be toxic to the liver. It should be used carefully and patients educated about its safe use. When medications containing acetaminophen are administered, the total daily dose of acetaminophen should be calculated so that the maximum recommended daily dose is not exceeded. See www.tylenol.com for more safety information.

Pathophysiology and Etiology

Viral hepatitis is usually caused by one of six viruses:

- Hepatitis A virus (HAV)
- Hepatitis B virus (HBV)
- Hepatitis C virus (HCV)
- Hepatitis D virus (HDV)
- Hepatitis E virus (HEV)
- Hepatitis G virus (HGV).

The viral agents vary by mode of transmission, incubation period, symptoms, diagnostic tests, and preventive vaccines (Table 35.1). The infecting organism causes inflammation of the liver, with resulting damage to liver cells and loss of liver function. If damage involves the bile canaliculi, obstructive jaundice will occur. If complications do not occur, cells regenerate and normal liver function eventually resumes.

There are an estimated 85,000 new hepatitis A, B, and C infections in the United States each year (CDC, 2009). The incidence of all types of viral hepatitis is at a historic low. HAV is the most common cause of hepatitis and has a low mortality rate. However, HBV is more common among some groups, including health care workers and intravenous drug users.

• WORD • BUILDING •
hepatitis: hepat—liver + itis—inflammation

Hepatitis G virus (also known as GB virus C) is an RNA virus that was identified in 1995. Not much is known about it. Because it is a bloodborne infection, transmission may occur with transfusions, hemodialysis, IV drug use, sexual contact, and mother to newborn. Those with HBV and HCV are often co-infected with HGV. Those with HIV who are also infected with HGV have an increased survival rate. It is not clear how serious an illness hepatitis G is or if it causes long-term liver damage. However, it is thought to cause a mild illness.

Prevention

The hepatitis viruses are very resistant to a wide range of anti-infective measures, such as drying, heat, ultraviolet light exposure, freezing, and bleach and other disinfectants. At least 30 minutes in boiling water is required to destroy them. The best methods for preventing the transmission of the hepatitis viruses are careful attention to cleanliness and the use of vaccines to HAV and HBV or the use of immune globulin (IG) after exposure. IG can be given up to 2 weeks after exposure to HAV; up to 1 week with a repeated injection in 1 month after HBV exposure. Health care workers must use standard precautions at all times to prevent transmission. Infection control precautions should reflect the usual mode of transmission of the particular hepatitis virus.

Permanent, active immunity is acquired from the body's own antibodies in response to an actual viral infection. The active immunity is to the specific virus to which the body has developed antibodies. Immune globulin provides temporary, passive, nonspecific immunity to hepatitis. A vaccine for HAV and HBV is available that provides permanent, active immunity. Health care workers are strongly encouraged (and often required by employers as a condition of employment) to be vaccinated for HBV.

Public health measures such as health education programs, licensing and supervision of public facilities, screening of blood donors, and careful screening of food handlers are general measures to prevent the transmission of hepatitis viruses.

> **SAFETY TIP**
>
> Protect yourself! Reduce the risk of health care–associated infections. Comply with current Centers for Disease Control and Prevention (http://www.cdc.gov) hand hygiene guidelines and standard precautions (2010 National Patient Safety Goals, www.jointcommission.org).

Signs and Symptoms

Hepatitis usually shows a typical pattern of loss of liver function, which generally occurs in three stages:

1. The prodromal (preicteric [prejaundice]) stage occurs about 2 weeks after exposure to the hepatitis virus and lasts about 1 week. The patient

TABLE 35.1 COMPARISON OF TYPES OF VIRAL HEPATITIS

	Hepatitis A Virus	Hepatitis B Virus	Hepatitis C Virus	Hepatitis D Virus	Hepatitis E Virus
Mode of transmission	Oral-fecal contamination of water, shellfish, eating utensils, or equipment	Blood or body fluids such as saliva, semen, and breast milk; equipment contaminated by blood	Blood transfusions, IV drug use Rarer: unprotected sex	Blood or body fluids as with HBV Strongly linked as a co-infection with HBV	Usually contaminated water
Incubation period	3–7 weeks	2–5 months	1 week to months	Same as HBV	2–9 weeks
Symptoms	Early (prodromal): fatigue, anorexia, malaise, nausea, or vomiting Icteric: jaundice, pale stools, amber or dark urine, RUQ pain	Early (prodromal): 1–2 months of fatigue, malaise, anorexia, low-grade fever, nausea, headache, abdominal pain, muscle aches May have no early symptoms Icteric: jaundice, rashes	Same as HBV, usually less severe	Similar to HAV and to HBV but more severe	Similar to HAV
Diagnostic tests	**Anti-HAV IgM** Acute infection **Anti-HAV IgG** Recovery and immunity to virus	**HBsAg** Surface antigen of virus Disappears by month 5 Continued presence: chronic or carrier state **Anti-HBs IgM** Antibody to surface antigen Acute illness and infectiousness Protective, immunity **Anti-HBc IgM** Antibody to core antigen during acute illness and recovery **HBeAg** Active viral replication **Anti-HBe** Lower infectivity but still possible	**Anti-HCV** Antibody to virus several weeks after exposure Does not provide immunity **HCV EIA** If positive, RIBA to confirm **HCV RIBA** If positive with elevated ALT, diagnosis of HCV **HCV-RNA** Presence of replicating virus **Liver biopsy** Shows liver damage **HCV genotype (1-6)** Guides treatment type	**HDV-RNA** Presence of replicating virus **HDAg** Acute infection	**Anti-HEV** Acute infection
Preventive vaccine	Immune globulin; hepatitis A vaccine	Hepatitis B immune globulin (HBIG); hepatitis B vaccine	None	None	None
Groups at risk	Individuals in military or day care Travelers to endemic areas	Correctional facility employees, health care workers, IV drug users, men who have sex with men, transplant or hemodialysis patients	Same as HBV	Same as HBV	Travelers to endemic areas

Anti = antibody; ALT = alanine aminotransferase; EIA = enzyme-linked immunosorbent assay (ELISA-2); IV = intravenous; RUQ = right upper quadrant; RIBA: recombinant immunoblot assay.

reports flu-like symptoms of malaise, headache, anorexia, low-grade fever, possibly dull right upper quadrant (RUQ) pain, nausea, vomiting, and diarrhea or constipation
2. With the appearance of jaundice (see Chapter 32), the icteric stage begins. It occurs about 5 to 10 days after the prodromal stage and lasts 2 to 6 weeks. The patient continues to have prodromal symptoms. Dark urine can be present due to increased bilirubin. The liver is usually enlarged and tender on examination.
3. The convalescent stage (posticteric) begins when the patient starts feeling better. It can last from 2 to 6 weeks. Recovery varies and depends on the type of hepatitis. Full recovery is measured by the return to normal of all liver function tests and may take as long as 1 year. The effects of hepatitis can be considered reversible if the patient complies with a medical regimen of adequate rest, good nutrition, and abstinence from alcohol or other liver-toxic agents for at least 1 year after liver function laboratory values return to normal.

Complications

Hepatitis may lead to fulminant (sudden, severe), acute or chronic liver failure. Chronic infection can develop in those with HBV or HCV. Some people become asymptomatic carriers of HBV or HCV and they never have an active illness. However, they can infect others and have a greater risk of developing cancer of the liver.

Diagnostic Tests

Serum liver enzymes are elevated (Table 35.2). Serum bilirubin may be elevated. In patients with severe hepatitis, prothrombin time may be prolonged. Serological tests can determine the specific virus causing the hepatitis via viral antigens and also identify the presence of antibodies to the virus (see Table 35.1). Abdominal x-ray examination may show an enlarged liver. Liver biopsy is done to assess liver damage and healing.

LEARNING TIP

Understanding Hepatitis C Diagnostic Test Results

Recovery from hepatitis C infection	Positive ELISA-2 Positive RIBA-2 Negative RNA Normal ALT
Hepatitis C carrier	Positive ELISA-2 Positive RIBA-2 Positive RNA Normal liver enzyme readings
Chronic hepatitis C infection	Positive ELISA-2 Positive RIBA-2 Elevated ALT levels

Therapeutic Measures

Treatment goals are to identify the cause of hepatitis, monitor liver status, and provide symptom relief and supportive care. To promote healing, limited activity with bathroom privileges and adequate nutrition are ordered. As the patient

TABLE 35.2 LABORATORY TESTS FOR LIVER FUNCTION IN HEPATITIS AND CIRRHOSIS

Test	Normal Value	Significance of Abnormal Findings
Indicate Liver Damage		
Alanine amino-transferase (ALT)	*Male:* 10–40 units/L *Female:* 7–35 units/L	Most specific enzyme for liver damage. Released with death of liver cells.
Aspartate aminotransferase (AST)	*Male:* 15–40 units/L *Female:* 13–55 units/L	Enzyme found in liver and heart; released and elevates 10 times or greater than normal with death of liver cells.
Alkaline phosphatase (ALP)	*Male:* 35–142 units/L *Female:* 25–125 units/L	Enzyme found in liver and bone; released and elevates greatly with severe liver damage.
Measures Functioning of Liver		
Albumin	3.4–4.8 g/dL	Decreased because of impaired protein synthesis; edema and ascites may result.
Ammonia	15–45 mcg/dL	Increased because liver cannot metabolize protein end product; contributes to hepatic encephalopathy.
Bilirubin	0.3–1.2 mg/dL	Increased because the liver is unable to use it to produce bile.
Prothrombin time (PT)	11–13.5 seconds	Prolonged. Liver can no longer make prothrombin; patient bleeds easily.

improves, activity may be increased as tolerated. Patients are restricted from using any alcohol or drugs that are known to be toxic to the liver (Box 35.1).

Currently, there are no specific drugs or other medical therapies for hepatitis. To prevent chronic hepatitis C infection, interferon therapy (peginterferon alpha-2b [Peg-Intron] or interferon alpha-2a [Pegasys]) may be used with an antiviral medication (oral ribavirin [Rebetol]). To manage chronic hepatitis B, the antivirals adefovir (Hepsera) or lamivudine (Epivir) may be used. New medications are being researched to treat hepatitis C that may be used along with other drugs to attack the virus at various parts (as in HIV treatment). Visit www.hepfi.org for information on these drugs.

Box 35.1

Common Causes of Hepatic Inflammation

Medications

- Acetaminophen (Tylenol)
- Acetylsalicylic acid (aspirin)
- Allopurinol (Zyloprim)
- Captopril (Capoten)
- Carbamazepine (Tegretol)
- Diazepam (Valium)
- Erythromycin estolate (Ilosone)
- Estrogen
- Halothane (Fluothane)
- Isoniazid (INH)
- Methotrexate (Trexall)
- Methyldopa (Aldomet)
- Oral contraceptives
- Phenobarbital (Luminal)
- Phenytoin (Dilantin)
- Sulfonamides
- Tetracycline (Sumycin)

Metabolic Disorders

- Alpha-1 antitrypsin deficiency
- Hemochromatosis (iron buildup)
- Wilson's disease (copper buildup)

Toxins

- Ethyl alcohol
- Carbon tetrachloride
- Cholecystographic dyes
- Kava-containing products (herb)
- Poisonous wild mushrooms
- Trichloroethylene
- Toluene

Vascular Disorders

- Budd-Chiari syndrome (hepatic vein occlusion)
- Heart failure
- Shock

Viruses

- Cytomegalovirus
- Epstein-Barr
- Hepatitis A, B, C, D, E
- Herpes
- Yellow fever

Nursing Process for the Patient with Hepatitis

DATA COLLECTION. Identify the patient for subjective data such as malaise, fatigue, pruritus (itching), nausea, anorexia, and RUQ abdominal pain. Objective data, such as baseline weight, vomiting, pale stools, dark-colored (tea-colored) urine, and jaundice, are recorded. The patient's vital signs are taken, and a low-grade fever or any abnormal bruising or bleeding is reported immediately. Identify the patient for knowledge of disease process and how to prevent spread of the disease.

NURSING DIAGNOSES, PLANNING, AND IMPLEMENTATION

Pain Related to Inflammation and Enlargement of the Liver

EXPECTED OUTCOME: The patient will state that pain level is acceptable.

- Monitor pain level on 10-point scale, including WHAT'S UP? questions *to determine treatment needs.*
- Give analgesics as ordered *to control pain.* Lower doses may be needed for a patient with liver dysfunction. Acetaminophen usually is avoided *due to risk of liver toxicity.*
- Encourage nondrug pain relief, such as distraction, imagery, and relaxation *to supplement and possibly decrease need for analgesics.*

Imbalanced Nutrition, Less Than Body Requirements Related to Anorexia, Nausea, or Vomiting

EXPECTED OUTCOME: The patient's weight will be stable and appropriate for height.

- Monitor weight and nutritional intake *to determine treatment needs.*
- Provide a high-calorie, high-protein, high-complex-carbohydrate, low-fat diet *to provide a well-rounded, nutritious diet for healing.*
- Administer antiemetic drugs as ordered *to reduce nausea and increase appetite.*
- Provide frequent, smaller meals *because these may be tolerated better than larger meals.*
- Place the patient in an upright or sitting position for meals *to decrease abdominal discomfort.*
- Serve meals in a quiet environment without unpleasant noise or odors *to increase intake by making eating as pleasant as possible.*
- Teach patient to avoid alcohol and vitamin supplements unless specifically prescribed by the physician *to prevent further damage to liver because alcohol and some vitamins are metabolized by the liver.*

Risk for Impaired Skin Integrity Related to Itching Secondary to Bilirubin Pigment Deposits in Skin

EXPECTED OUTCOME: The patient's skin will remain intact and free from secondary infection.

- Administer antihistamines as ordered *to decrease itching.*
- Encourage the patient not to scratch, but to press firmly on the itchy area. *Scratching can damage skin and increase risk for infection.*
- Encourage the patient to keep fingernails trimmed short *so that vigorous scratching does not tear the skin.*
- Maintain room temperature at a comfortable level *to decrease perspiration, which may increase itching.*

Risk for Ineffective Self Health Management Related to Lack of Knowledge of Hepatitis and its Transmission and Treatment

EXPECTED OUTCOME: The patient will state how to self-manage the treatment regimen for viral hepatitis and how to prevent spread of the disease.

- Determine patient's knowledge of hepatitis *to guide teaching.*
- Teach patient how hepatitis affects the body and the importance of adequate rest and proper nutrition *to promote recovery.*
- Teach the importance of avoiding alcohol and other liver-toxic drugs *to prevent further damage to liver.*
- Teach patient how to prevent spreading virus to others: hand washing after toileting, using soap and hot water to clean eating utensils, cookware, and food preparation surfaces, practicing safer sex (abstinence, condoms, monogamy), and not sharing needles *because hepatitis is contagious.* (See *Home Health Hints.*)

Home Health Hints

- For patients with hepatitis, home health nurses are concerned with proper treatment and patient education to prevent transmission in the community.
- If possible, the patient with hepatitis should have a separate bedroom and bathroom. The person cleaning the bathroom should wear disposable gloves or rubber gloves and then clean the gloves with a 10% bleach solution. The family is advised to use liquid soap instead of bar soap.
- Contaminated linens used by a patient with hepatitis should be washed separately from household laundry and in hot water. One cup of bleach should be added with the detergent to each load. Rubber gloves should be worn to wash the patient's laundry.
- A patient with abdominal ascites needs a hospital bed at home so the patient can be positioned to aid in breathing. A physician's order must be obtained for insurance coverage.
- Measure abdominal girth of the patient with ascites at each visit and record in the nurse's notes. The patient should weigh on the same scale, first thing in the morning, and record the weight so the nurse can document the findings.

EVALUATION. Management of the patient with hepatitis has been successful if the patient reports pain is satisfactorily relieved; body weight is maintained within 2 lb of pre-illness weight; skin has no breaks, cuts, or tears, or secondary infections; patient can define disease; and patient follows transmission precautions and treatment.

For more information, visit Hepatitis Foundation International at www.hepfi.org, www.cdc.gov, or the American Liver Foundation at www.liverfoundation.org.

CRITICAL THINKING

Carl Young

■ Carl Young, 23, has returned from being a missionary in Africa. He reports that during his time there he sustained a serious laceration that required sutures. Carl also mentions his fondness for seafood and that he has had several "feasts" that have included raw oysters. Carl states that since his return he has lost nearly 8 pounds, is nauseated, has frequent headaches, tires easily, and is very irritable.

1. What information might lead you to suspect hepatitis A? Hepatitis B?
2. What precautions should be instituted for Carl until a diagnosis is made?
3. What nursing actions might you implement to help Carl improve his nutrition?
4. What medications should Carl avoid?
5. What information should be included in a discharge teaching plan for Carl?

Suggested answers at end of chapter.

Acute Liver Failure

Acute liver failure (ALF) is a rare but serious condition that can develop rapidly, sometimes in just 2 days. When the liver is severely damaged, its many functions are impaired. The outcome of the disease may be decided within 48 to 72 hours of diagnosis. Possible outcomes are liver recovery, need for liver transplantation, and death. Acetaminophen (Tylenol) overdose is the most common cause of ALF. See Box 35.1 for other possible causes. Box 35.2 (*Patient Education*)

Box 35.2

Patient Education

Liver Failure Prevention

Ways to avoid hepatitis and cirrhosis that can lead to liver failure include the following:

- Wash hands after using the bathroom and before handling food.
- Do not share personal grooming items (especially toothbrushes or razors).
- Obtain hepatitis A and B vaccine.
- Eat a balanced diet.
- Avoid or drink alcohol in moderation.
- Use acetaminophen (Tylenol) safely.
- Avoid exposure to blood.
- Use condoms for safer sex.
- Ensure sanitary conditions and equipment when obtaining a body piercing or tattoo.
- Do not share intravenous needles.

teaches patients ways to prevent liver damage and possible liver failure.

Initial symptoms of liver failure—fatigue, GI upset, and diarrhea—are vague and make detection difficult. As the condition worsens, symptoms become more severe: jaundice, hepatic encephalopathy, bleeding, and abdominal distention. The patient may suddenly lapse into an extremely serious illness, starting with confusion and progressing to coma. In a matter of hours, on x-ray, the liver shows a rapid reduction in size, a typical sign of onset of ALF. In addition, there is a sudden elevation of liver enzymes, alanine aminotransferase (ALT), aspartate aminotransferase (AST), and bilirubin. Prothrombin time is elevated, with marked elevation being an ominous sign. Potassium and blood glucose levels drop.

Medical treatment is directed toward stopping and reversing the damage to the liver. An attempt is made to put the liver completely at rest. The patient is on bedrest. All drugs are discontinued, since they are metabolized by the liver. Dialysis may be ordered if the liver damage results from an overdose of a hepatotoxic substance. A high-calorie, low-sodium, low-protein diet is given. Lactulose, neomycin, magnesium citrate, or sorbitol may be given to decrease ammonia levels (see later section on hepatic encephalopathy). The patient needs intensive amounts of supportive care. If a liver transplant is needed, an otherwise healthy patient may be a priority organ recipient, depending on age and whether the patient is alcohol dependent.

Nursing Process for the Patient with Acute Liver Failure

Nursing care of the patient with acute liver failure is essentially the same as for the patient with cirrhosis, which is discussed next.

Cirrhosis

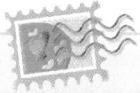

Cirrhosis is the progressive, irreversible replacement of healthy liver tissue with scar tissue. It is caused by chronic liver diseases. In 2006, chronic liver disease/cirrhosis was the 12th leading cause of death in the U.S. population (Heron et al., 2009). It occurs more commonly among men than women (Box 35.3, *Cultural Considerations*). There are a variety of causes of cirrhosis (see Box 35.1). Chronic alcohol use is the most common cause of cirrhosis in the United States.

Pathophysiology

Healthy liver cells exposed to toxins become inflamed. Then the liver cells are infiltrated with fat and white blood cells and are replaced by fibrotic tissue. The liver makes some repairs. But if the damage continues over many years, and more and more liver cells are replaced with fatty tissue and scar tissue,

• WORD • BUILDING •

cirrhosis: cirrh—orange yellow + osis—condition

Box 35.3

Cultural Considerations

The incidence of liver disease is more common among Mexican Americans. Risk factors include working in occupations such as mining, factories using chemicals, and farming using pesticides. Additionally, the use of alcohol is increased in men, and cigarette smoking is common.

Egyptian Americans may suffer from schistosomiasis, known as bilharziasis in Egypt. Schistosomiasis can lead to cirrhosis, liver failure, portal hypertension, esophageal varices, bladder cancer, and renal failure. Thus, the nurse may need to screen newer Egyptian American immigrants for this disease.

Alcohol use and abuse is common among African American communities. For many it is a socially accepted behavior and carries little or no stigma. The mortality rate from cirrhosis of the liver among African Americans is nearly twice that of European Americans. The nurse needs to provide counseling, teaching the detrimental effects of alcohol, and work with African American churches and community leaders to help prevent the detrimental effects of alcohol abuse.

cirrhosis can develop. Liver regeneration continues abnormally, disrupting the lobes of the liver and creating nodules. The liver becomes hardened and lumpy. Early in the disease, the liver is enlarged, firm, and hard from the inflammatory process. Blood flow through the liver becomes impaired due to the nodules, resulting in portal venous hypertension. Later, the liver shrinks and is covered with gray connective tissue. As the disease progresses, liver function is impaired and after many years cirrhosis can lead to chronic liver failure.

Signs and Symptoms

Initially, symptoms are not usually seen with cirrhosis. As liver function becomes impaired, symptoms may begin to be seen. They include anorexia, nausea, vomiting, weight loss, and fatigue, which is due to decreased metabolic function of the liver. Jaundice may be present. The patient's skin may be dry from bile products deposited in the skin. The patient may report severe pruritus (itching). The liver may be enlarged, firm, and tender. Laboratory values reflect progressive loss of liver function. As cirrhosis progresses, signs and symptoms of increasing loss of liver function and complications related to the increasing loss of function develop. Figure 35.1 shows signs and symptoms of cirrhosis. (See Table 35.3.)

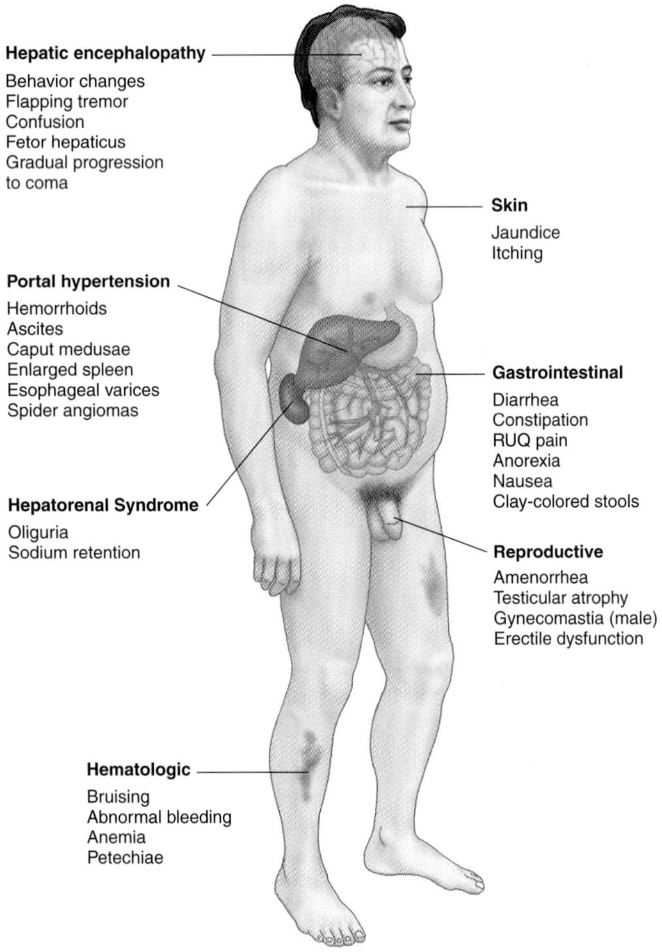
Hepatic encephalopathy
Behavior changes
Flapping tremor
Confusion
Fetor hepaticus
Gradual progression to coma
Skin
Jaundice
Itching
Portal hypertension
Hemorrhoids
Ascites
Caput medusae
Enlarged spleen
Esophageal varices
Spider angiomas
Gastrointestinal
Diarrhea
Constipation
RUQ pain
Anorexia
Nausea
Clay-colored stools
Hepatorenal Syndrome
Oliguria
Sodium retention
Reproductive
Amenorrhea
Testicular atrophy
Gynecomastia (male)
Erectile dysfunction
Hematologic
Bruising
Abnormal bleeding
Anemia
Petechiae

FIGURE 35.1 Signs and symptoms of cirrhosis.

TABLE 35.3 CIRRHOSIS SUMMARY

Signs and Symptoms	Anorexia, nausea Dull RUQ pain Bruising Jaundice Ascites
Diagnostic Tests	Elevated ALT, AST, ALP, ammonia, bilirubin, PT Decreased albumin Liver biopsy
Therapeutic Measures	Prevent disease progression and treat complications.
Complications	***C:*** Clotting defects ***H:*** Hepatorenal syndrome ***E:*** Encephalopathy ***A:*** Ascites ***P:*** Portal hypertension
Priority Nursing Diagnoses	*Pain* *Excess or Deficient Fluid Volume* *Imbalanced Nutrition*

Complications

Complications of cirrhosis include blood clotting defects, portal hypertension, ascites, hepatic encephalopathy, and hepatorenal syndrome.

CLOTTING DEFECTS. Blood clotting defects may develop because of impaired prothrombin and fibrinogen production in the liver. Further, the absence of bile salts prevents the absorption of fat-soluble vitamin K, which is essential for some blood clotting factors. Patients with cirrhosis have a tendency to bruise easily and may develop disseminated intravascular coagulation (DIC) or hemorrhage.

PORTAL HYPERTENSION. Portal hypertension is persistent blood pressure elevation in the portal circulation of the abdomen. Liver damage causes a blockage of blood flow in the portal vein. Increased resistance from delayed drainage causes enlargement of the visible abdominal veins around the umbilicus (called caput medusae), rectal hemorrhoids, enlarged spleen (splenomegaly), and esophageal **varices** (dilated veins) (Fig. 35.2).

The most serious result of portal hypertension is bleeding esophageal varices. The walls of the esophageal veins are thin and tear easily. Varices usually develop from the fundus of the stomach upward and may extend into the upper esophagus. The blood-filled, thin-walled varices may tear easily from sudden excessive pressure, such as the intra-abdominal pressure that results from coughing, lifting, or straining, causing severe bleeding.

ASCITES. Ascites is an accumulation of serous fluid in the abdominal cavity. The fluid accumulates from portal

• WORD • BUILDING •
encephalopathy: encephalo—brain + pathy—disease

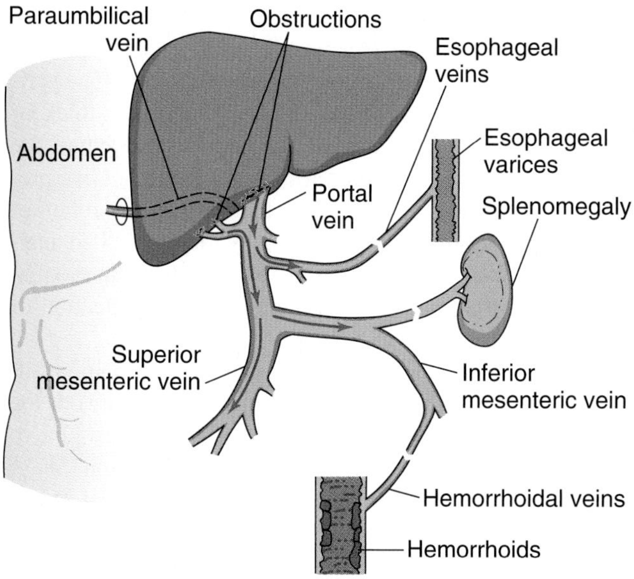
Paraumbilical vein
Obstructions
Esophageal veins
Esophageal varices
Abdomen
Portal vein
Splenomegaly
Superior mesenteric vein
Inferior mesenteric vein
Hemorrhoidal veins
Hemorrhoids

FIGURE 35.2 Portal hypertension. Obstruction of normal blood flow through the liver causes blood to back up into the venous system, leading to esophageal varices, splenomegaly, hemorrhoids, and caput medusae.

hypertension, and low production of albumin by the failing liver and aldosterone accumulation. An insufficient amount of albumin causes plasma to seep into the abdominal cavity. The kidneys respond to the decreased circulating blood volume by saving sodium and water. The accumulated fluid causes a markedly enlarged abdomen. The fluid may cause severe respiratory distress as a result of elevation of the diaphragm.

HEPATIC ENCEPHALOPATHY. Hepatic **encephalopathy** is caused by elevated ammonia, a by-product of protein metabolism, which disrupts mental status. The damaged liver is unable to make the ammonia water soluble for excretion in the urine. Signs and symptoms of hepatic encephalopathy include progressive confusion; **asterixis**, or flapping tremors in the hands caused by toxins at peripheral nerves; and **fetor hepaticus**, or foul breath caused by metabolic end products related to sulfur.

Stages of hepatic encephalopathy and signs and symptoms of the stages are:

- *Early:* The patient exhibits subtle changes in personality, fatigue, drowsiness, and changes in handwriting (the best assessment for the early stage).
- *Stuporous and confused:* The patient is often belligerent and irritable and develops asterixis, muscle twitching, hyperventilation, and marked confusion.
- *Comatose:* The patient gradually loses consciousness and becomes comatose.

With treatment, if ammonia levels decrease, the patient gradually regains consciousness. Hepatic encephalopathy represents end-stage liver failure and has a mortality rate as high as 90% once coma begins.

HEPATORENAL SYNDROME. Hepatorenal syndrome is a secondary failure of the kidneys in some patients with cirrhosis. Symptoms of hepatorenal syndrome include oliguria without detectable kidney damage, reduced glomerular filtration rate (GFR) with essentially no urine output or less than 200 mL per day, and nearly total sodium retention. Hepatorenal syndrome is considered an ominous sign.

LEARNING TIP

For complications of cirrhosis, remember the pneumonic CHEAP:
C: Clotting defects
H: Hepatorenal syndrome
E: Encephalopathy
A: Ascites
P: Portal hypertension

Diagnostic Tests

Tests that show liver damage and functioning of the liver are shown in Table 35.2. Abdominal radiographs of patients with cirrhosis may show ascites and enlargement of the liver. An abdominal ultrasound may show liver enlargement early in cirrhosis or a small liver later in the disease. An esophagogastroscopy may be done to detect bleeding and treat esophageal varices that are bleeding (see below). A liver biopsy may be done to determine the extent and nature of the liver damage (see Chapter 32).

NURSING CARE TIP

Patients with cirrhosis undergoing a liver biopsy need careful observation for bleeding after the procedure due to possible impaired clotting.

Therapeutic Measures

Interventions for cirrhosis are to prevent advancement of the disease and treat complications.

ASCITES. Ascites is treated with diuretics such as spironolactone (Aldactone) or furosemide (Lasix), sodium and fluid restriction (800 to 1000 mL/day), and albumin

• WORD • BUILDING •
asterixis: a—not + sterixis—fixed position
fetor hepaticus: fetor—offensive odor + hepat—liver + icas—related to

• WORD • BUILDING •
hepatorenal syndrome: hepato—liver + renal—kidneys + syndrome—group of symptoms

infusions for severe ascites. Paracentesis can be done to remove accumulated fluid from the peritoneal cavity when the fluid is compromising the patient's breathing, causing abdominal discomfort, or posing a threat of ruptured umbilical hernia. If large amounts of fluid are removed, albumin may be given to replace lost proteins to prevent fluid shifting.

Ascites may be treated by the placement of a shunt, called a **transjugular intrahepatic portosystemic shunt** (TIPS), under fluoroscopy (Fig. 35.3). Access to place the shunt is gained through the jugular vein. A stent is placed to connect the portal vein to the hepatic vein, in the middle of the liver. This reduces portal pressure by allowing blood to bypass the liver and be carried to the heart. It reduces fluid accumulation and aids in reducing the risk of bleeding.

ESOPHAGEAL VARICES. The medical goals for managing bleeding from esophageal varices are to stop the bleeding immediately, maintain normal clotting, and treat infection. Bleeding varices can be treated with the synthetic hormone octreotide (Sandostatin) IV, which may vasoconstrict, and therapeutic endoscopy for ligation (banding) or sclerotherapy to close the varices. Vitamin K, which is often deficient in liver disease, is given to assist with the clotting process. Antibiotics are given, sometimes prophylactically, because bacterial infection is either a precursor to bleeding varices or commonly occurs with varices.

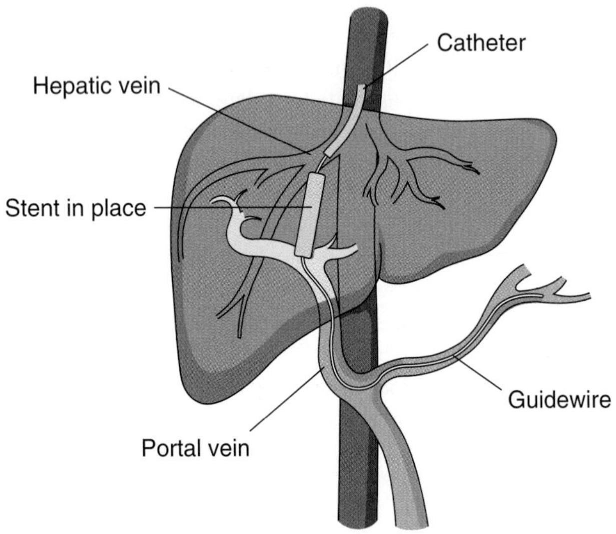
Catheter
Hepatic vein
Stent in place
Guidewire
Portal vein

FIGURE 35.3 Transjugular intrahepatic portosystemic shunt. A stent is placed to shunt blood from the portal vein to the hepatic vein and systemic circulation to divert blood flow around the diseased liver.

transjugular intrahepatic portosystemic shunt: trans—across + jugular—jugular vein + intra—within + hepatic—liver + porto—portal (liver circulation) + systemic—systemic (circulation) + shunt—to divert

Banding of varices with rubber bands during endoscopy is done to stop the bleeding (Fig. 35.4). Sclerotherapy is another method of treatment during endoscopy. The varices are injected with a sclerosing agent that causes thickening and closing of the dilated vessels. Postprocedure the patient may report chest pain for up to 72 hours. Give prescribed analgesics, and monitor the patient for relief of pain. Report severe pain unrelieved by the prescribed analgesic immediately because the patient may have an esophageal perforation or ulceration, which is a complication of sclerotherapy.

In emergency cases when other methods are not available, temporary tamponade (application of pressure) of the bleeding varices may be done with a multilumen esophagogastric tube that has a balloon on the end for inflation (Sengstaken-Blakemore tube or Minnesota tube). Complications of esophagogastric tamponade may include aspiration, erosion of the mucosa, perforation, and suffocation, so it is not often used.

HEPATIC ENCEPHALOPATHY. Lactulose may be given by mouth, nasogastric tube, or enema (depending on how alert the patient is) to make the colon contents more acidic. This creates an insoluble form of ammonia that is then excreted in the stool. Neomycin, an intestinal antibiotic, occasionally may be given to reduce colonic bacteria that change ammonium to ammonia. Hepatic encephalopathy is also treated by restricting dietary protein during acute episodes to reduce ammonia production (Box 35.4, *Nutrition Notes*).

Nursing Process for the Patient with Acute Liver Failure and Cirrhosis

DATA COLLECTION. A complete history and physical assessment are done. Be alert to subjective symptoms of liver dysfunction, such as abdominal pain, anorexia, nausea, severe itching, and dull, aching RUQ pain. Note objective evidence of liver problems, such as jaundice, light-colored

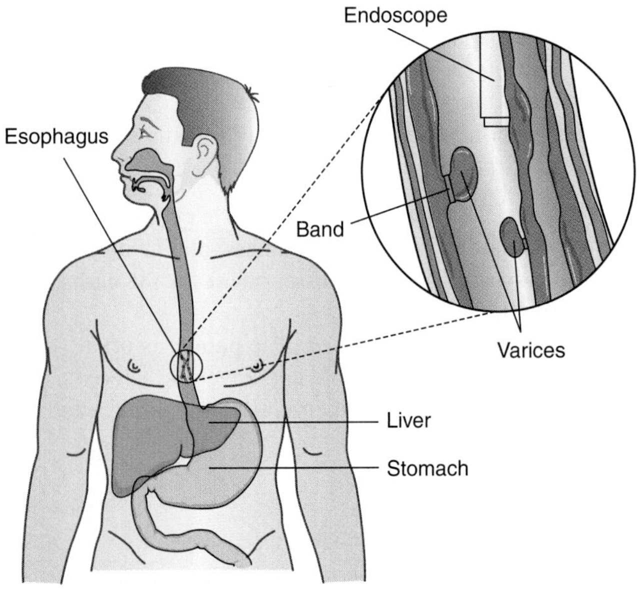
Endoscope
Esophagus
Band
Varices
Liver
Stomach

FIGURE 35.4 Variceal banding.

Box 35.4

Nutrition Notes

Supplying Nutrients to Patients with Liver Disease

A registered dietitian may modify the diet daily for patients with liver disease. Usually these patients suffer from severe anorexia, often displaying their best appetites for breakfast. For early or mild disease, protein is encouraged to support healing; later in liver disease, protein may be restricted. For esophageal varices, foods are soft, in addition to other restrictions.

For liver failure, the following dietary considerations are necessary:

- Protein is restricted according to the person's ability to metabolize it.
- Complete protein foods are selected to provide all the essential amino acids.
- Homogenized milk and eggs are offered because the fat is already emulsified, requiring less bile for digestion.
- Adequate carbohydrates are given to prevent the use of tissue protein for energy.
- Fluid and sodium are likely to be restricted if ascites is present.

Hepatic encephalopathy is associated with increased serum levels of ammonia and aromatic amino acids. Early research suggested a benefit to altering the ratio of aromatic to branched-chain amino acids but later findings have not been clearly supportive. Although administering branched-chain amino acids may benefit some patients, their routine use is not recommended. However special enteral feeding formulas (e.g., Hepatic-Aid II and Travasorb-Hepatic) containing branched-chain amino acids are available.

stools, ascites, ecchymosis (bruising) of the skin, GI bleeding, and any evidence of alterations in thought processes, such as confusion, disorientation, or inability to make decisions.

NURSING DIAGNOSES, PLANNING, AND IMPLEMENTATION. Common nursing diagnoses for cirrhosis include the following.

Excess Fluid Volume Related to Portal Hypertension (Ascites)

EXPECTED OUTCOME: Fluid volume will be controlled as evidenced by stable weight and abdominal girth within normal limits for the patient.

- Weigh the patient on admission and daily *to measure fluid retention.*
- Measure and record the patient's abdominal girth (circumference) daily *to monitor ascites.* Mark the place where you measured *so the same site will always be measured during subsequent assessments.*
- Report any weight gain or increase in girth promptly *so treatment can be ordered and complications minimized.*
- Check the patient's vital signs every 4 hours; report changes and any evidence of difficulty breathing or changes in mental status promptly *to detect fluid overload.*
- Maintain a low-sodium diet and order fluid restrictions *to reduce fluid retention.*
- Administer ordered diuretics as scheduled *to reduce fluid volume.*
- If intravenous fluids or albumin have been ordered, assist in careful monitoring of the rate of infusion *to prevent or detect fluid overload.*

Imbalanced Nutrition: Less Than Body Requirements Related to Anorexia and Impaired Metabolism of Needed Nutrients

EXPECTED OUTCOME: The patient's (dry) weight will be within normal limits for height.

- Monitor weight; report unexpected (nonfluid) weight loss *so timely intervention can be implemented.*
- Monitor serum prealbumin, total protein, vitamin, and mineral levels *because these may be better indicators of nutrition if accurate weights are complicated by fluid overload.*
- Monitor the patient's diet to ensure that any ordered protein restriction is carried out *to assist in reducing ammonia levels.*
- Offer frequent mouth care *to increase comfort and make food more palatable.*
- Make sure that odors and other unpleasant stimuli are eliminated *to prevent further worsening of appetite.*
- Offer the patient frequent, small, high-calorie meals *to reduce feeling of fullness that can occur with larger meals.*
- Administer vitamins or supplements as ordered *to correct deficiencies.*

Pain Related to Abdominal Pressure

EXPECTED OUTCOME: The patient will state pain level is acceptable.

- Monitor pain level using a 10-point scale and WHAT'S UP? questions *to guide treatment.*
- Give analgesics as ordered to control pain. *Lower doses may be needed for the patient with liver dysfunction. Acetaminophen usually is avoided due to risk of liver toxicity.*
- Encourage nondrug pain relief activities, such as distraction, imagery, and relaxation *to possibly decrease the need for analgesics.*

Risk for Disturbed Thought Processes Related to Elevated Ammonia Levels

EXPECTED OUTCOME: The patient will remain alert and oriented to person, place, and time.

- Assess the patient's level of consciousness and orientation often *to allow prompt treatment.*
- Assess neuromuscular function by asking the patient to hold his or her arms out straight in front and steady. *If asterixis, or liver flap, is present, the patient's hands will unwillingly dip and return to the horizontal position in a flapping motion due to elevated ammonia.*
- Look for changes in the patient's handwriting *because changes can indicate altered neuromuscular function.*
- Give lactulose, neomycin, magnesium citrate, or sorbitol as scheduled *to decrease serum ammonia levels.*
- Be aware that lactulose causes loose stools, and do not withhold the medication when the patient develops diarrhea. *Loose stools are a sign that the medication is working, not a reason to withhold it.*
- Question giving medications such as sedatives, opioids, and tranquilizers *because these may increase the serum ammonia levels and depress level of consciousness (LOC).*
- Reorient the patient to time and place frequently *to reinforce reality.*
- Give simple, clear explanations of care, and give the patient time to understand the explanation *because short, simple explanations are easier to process.*
- Provide a safe environment for the confused or unsteady patient *to prevent injury.*

Risk for Ineffective Breathing Pattern Related to Excess Fluid in the Abdomen

EXPECTED OUTCOME: The patient's respirations will be even and unlabored, 16 to 20 per minute.

- Assess the patient's respiratory rate, rhythm, chest movement, skin color, and oxygen saturation frequently *to determine if breathing pattern is effective.*
- Assist the patient to use an incentive spirometer and to cough gently every 2 to 4 hours *to encourage deep breathing and keep airways clear.*
- Elevate the head of the patient's bed *so that the patient's lungs have maximum room for expansion.*
- Administer analgesics carefully, as ordered, if pain is causing shallow respirations. *Reducing pain with breathing allows for a more effective breathing pattern.*
- Reposition the patient at least every 2 hours *to ventilate all areas of the lungs.*
- Assist with treatments to decrease ascites as ordered *to increase room for lung expansion.*

Risk for Deficient Fluid Volume Related to Bleeding Esophageal Varices or Gastrointestinal Bleeding Secondary to Clotting Dysfunction

EXPECTED OUTCOME: Fluid volume will remain within normal limits without bleeding as evidenced by no signs and symptoms of bleeding, and vital signs within normal limits for the patient.

- Monitor gastric secretions, stool, and urine at least every 8 hours, and report any signs of bleeding. *Early identification of bleeding is essential to prompt treatment.*
- Monitor blood clotting laboratory studies such as prothrombin time and report any abnormal values *to identify risk for bleeding.*
- Caution the patient to use a soft-bristle toothbrush and an electric rather than straight razor *to avoid injury and bleeding.*
- Avoid suctioning the patient if possible *because suctioning can cause varices to bleed.*
- Use a small-gauge needle for injections and apply direct pressure to all puncture sites *to avoid bleeding.*
- Teach the patient to avoid hot, spicy, or irritating foods *because these may irritate the esophageal mucosa and increase risk of bleeding.*
- Instruct the patient to avoid forceful coughing or nose blowing, straining, vomiting, or gagging if at all possible. Administer medications as ordered to prevent their occurrence. *These can increase pressure and risk of bleeding varices.*

Risk for Infection Related to Impaired Immune Function

EXPECTED OUTCOME: The patient will be free from infection as evidenced by white blood cell count within normal limit, afebrile.

- Monitor for signs of infection and report promptly *so treatment can begin.*
- Be aware that the earliest warning signs of infection may be subtle changes in the patient's behavior, such as sudden restlessness, an increase in confusion, or irritability. *Early recognition is essential to prompt treatment.*
- Carefully evaluate laboratory studies such as the white blood cell count. *The white blood cell count may not elevate or may elevate slowly because the white cell activity is impaired.*
- Teach the patient careful hand washing and avoidance of people who are ill *to prevent exposure to infection.*

EVALUATION. Nursing care has been effective if the patient is alert and oriented and has no signs of fluid retention, a stable weight appropriate for height, no abdominal pain greater than 2 on a 10-point scale, a respiratory rate between 16 and 20 respirations per minute with no cyanosis or changes in level of consciousness, no bleeding, no infection, no injuries, and an accurate knowledge of cirrhosis and proper disease management requirements.

PATIENT EDUCATION. Teach patients how cirrhosis is affecting their bodies. In particular, patients need to know about portal system hypertension and hepatic encephalopathy. In addition, teach:

- How to observe for and report any confusion, tremors, or personality changes
- The importance of adequate rest and avoidance of strenuous activity
- The need for a diet high in calories, low in sodium, and high in protein if hepatic encephalopathy has not developed
- The need to avoid opioids, sedatives, and tranquilizers
- The need to promptly report any bleeding; any sign of low potassium, such as muscle cramps, nausea, or vomiting caused by diuretics; changes in mental status, such as confusion or personality changes; changes in weight; and any increase in current symptoms
- The importance of avoiding alcohol
- The importance of frequent follow-up care and laboratory studies.

CRITICAL THINKING

Mrs. Conner

■ Mrs. Conner, a 76-year-old retired businesswoman, has lived alone for the past 20 years, since the death of her husband. She has a long history of poor nutritional habits but does not consume alcohol. She is admitted with cirrhosis.

1. What risk factors does Mrs. Conner have for cirrhosis?
2. What symptoms would you expect Mrs. Conner to exhibit with early cirrhosis?
3. What values do you expect to see for serum albumin? Prothrombin time?
4. What are the two greatest concerns with portal hypertension?
5. What is the usual treatment for ascites?

Suggested answers at end of chapter.

Liver Transplantation

The patient with end-stage liver failure from cirrhosis, hepatitis, biliary disease, metabolic disorders, or hepatic vein obstruction who is not responding to treatment may be evaluated for a liver transplant. Usually, patients who have cancer are not considered for liver transplantation because the drugs used to suppress tissue rejection by the immune system can cause the cancer cells to grow at an increased rate. The patient will be evaluated for emotional and physical stability and must accept that he or she will be on daily medications for life (Box 35.5, *Cultural Considerations*).

After the surgical implantation of a donor liver, the patient must be closely observed for evidence of donor organ rejection. The patient will be in intensive care until stable enough to be transferred to a medical unit. The patient will be on drugs such as cyclosporine (cyclosporin A), tacrolimus (Protopic), azathioprine (Imuran), prednisone (Deltasone), and mycophenolate mofetil (CellCept) to suppress immune system responses and prevent tissue rejection. Observe the patient for the following signs of impending rejection:

- Pulse greater than 100 beats per minute
- Temperature greater than 101°F (38°C)
- Reports of RUQ pain
- Increased jaundice
- Decrease in bile from the T-tube or change in bile color.

In addition, laboratory studies may show increased serum transaminases (ALT and AST), serum bilirubin, alkaline phosphatase, and prothrombin time. Symptoms of acute tissue rejection usually develop between the 4th and 10th postoperative days. The patient who has received an organ transplant needs extended medical follow-up. Teach the patient to promptly report to the physician any symptoms of infection, bleeding episodes, or RUQ pain (Box 35.6, *Ethical Considerations*).

Cancer of the Liver

Cancer of the liver usually results from metastasis from a primary cancer at a distant location. The liver is a likely area of involvement if cancer originated in the esophagus, lungs, breast, stomach, colon, pancreas, kidney, bladder, or skin. For some patients, liver cancer is the primary tumor site. Patients with a history of chronic hepatitis B, hepatitis C, nutritional deficiencies, heavy alcohol use or smoking, and exposure to hepatotoxins have an increased risk for cancer of the liver.

Symptoms of cancer of the liver include encephalopathy, abnormal bleeding, jaundice, and ascites. Laboratory tests show elevated serum alkaline phosphatase. Radiologic examinations may include abdominal radiographs or radioisotope scans, which show tumor growth. Liver cancer is definitively diagnosed with a positive needle biopsy combined with an ultrasound exam of the liver. Most patients with liver cancer die within 6 months of diagnosis.

Rarely, liver cancer can be surgically removed if it is localized or in a removable lobe. Care of the postsurgical patient is similar to other abdominal surgery patients. If surgery is not an option, the patient may receive chemotherapeutic drugs by injection directly into the affected lobe of the liver or into the hepatic artery. Intra-arterial injection

Box 35.5

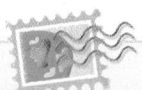

Cultural Considerations

Jewish law addresses organ transplantation from the perspectives of the recipient, the living donor, the cadaver donor, and the dying donor. If a recipient's life can be prolonged without considerable risk, transplant is ordained. For a living donor to be approved, the risk to the life of the donor must be considered. One is not obligated to donate a part of himself or herself unless the risk is small. The use of a cadaver for transplant is usually approved if it is saving a life. The nurse may need to help the Jewish patient contact a rabbi when making a decision regarding organ donation or transplantation.

Box 35.6

Ethical Considerations

Organ Transplantation

Despite widespread public and medical acceptance of organ transplantation as a highly beneficial procedure, ethical questions remain. Many people are involved in the process: the donor, the donor's family, nursing and medical personnel, the recipient, the recipient's family, and society due to the use of tax dollars or increased insurance premiums. These people or groups may have conflicting rights.

Most institutions involved in the transplant process have detailed procedures to help deal with the ethical and legal issues involved in transplantation.

One of the most difficult ethical issues involved in organ transplantation is the selection of recipients; this can be considered under the principles of justice or fairness. Because there are fewer organs than needed, potential ethical dilemmas can arise. Should someone receive an organ due to being rich, famous, or knowing the right people? The national organ recipient list attempts to list and rank all persons who need organs in a nondiscriminatory manner. Some of the important criteria include need, length of time on the list, potential for survival, prior organ transplantation, value to the community, and tissue compatibility.

Nurses working with organ transplantation need to be sensitive to the potential for bias. Most people who are seeking organ transplantations are desperately ill or near death. They, and their families, can be very easily manipulated or can be very manipulating. On the other side, the families of potential organ donors are usually emotionally distraught because of the sudden and traumatic loss of a loved one. As a rule, neither the donor nor the donor's family should play any part in the selection of a recipient. Nurses must avoid making statements or giving nonverbal indications of approval or disapproval of potential recipients.

of chemotherapy drugs has the advantage of being less toxic to the rest of the body. (See Chapter 11 for care of patients with cancer.)

DISORDERS OF THE PANCREAS

Pancreatitis

Pancreatitis, inflammation of the pancreas, may be either acute or chronic. The two forms of pancreatitis have different courses and are considered two different disorders.

Acute Pancreatitis

Pathophysiology

Inflammation of the pancreas appears to be caused by a process called autodigestion. Recall that the pancreas normally secretes digestive enzymes. For reasons not fully understood, pancreatic enzymes can be activated while they are still in the pancreas and begin to digest the pancreas. In addition, large amounts of enzymes are released by inflamed cells. As the pancreas digests itself, chemical cascades occur. Trypsin destroys pancreatic tissue and causes vasodilation. As capillary permeability increases, fluid is lost to the retroperitoneal space, causing shock. In addition, trypsin appears to set off another chain of events that causes the conversion of prothrombin to thrombin, so that clots form. The patient may develop disseminated intravascular coagulation (DIC). (See Chapter 28.)

Etiology

Pancreatitis is most commonly associated with excessive alcohol consumption. Alcohol appears to act directly on the acinar cells of the pancreas and the pancreatic ducts to irritate and inflame the structures. Biliary disease such as cholelithiasis (gallstones) or cholangitis (inflammation of the bile ducts) may also trigger pancreatitis. Gallstones may plug the pancreatic duct and cause inflammation from excessive fluid pressure on sensitive ducts. The irritant effect of bile itself may cause inflammation. Blunt trauma to the abdomen or infection may trigger the process by causing ischemia, inflammation, and activation of the pancreatic enzymes. Drugs such as thiazide diuretics (HydroDIURIL), estrogen, opioids, corticosteroids, and excessive serum calcium from hyperparathyroidism are less common causes of pancreatitis.

Elderly patients and patients with a first diagnosis of pancreatitis have a higher mortality rate. In addition, patients who have pancreatitis associated with biliary disease have a higher mortality rate than patients with alcohol-related pancreatitis.

Prevention

Caution patients who drink alcohol to stop. Patients with biliary disease need to seek medical treatment for these conditions so that pancreatitis does not develop as a complication. Monitor patients, especially the elderly, for any abdominal complaints when they are placed on medications that are associated with pancreatitis (Box 35.7, *Cultural Considerations*).

Signs and Symptoms

Patients with acute pancreatitis are very ill, with dull abdominal pain, guarding, a rigid abdomen, hypotension or shock, and respiratory distress from accumulation of fluid in the retroperitoneal space. The abdominal pain usually is located in the midline just below the sternum, with radiation to the spine, back, and flank. The location and degree of pain indicate the area of the pancreas involved and to some extent the amount of involvement. Respirations are likely to be shallow as the patient attempts to splint painful areas. Eating makes the pain worse.

The patient may have a low-grade fever, dry mucous membranes, and tachycardia. If the primary cause is biliary, the patient may report nausea and vomiting, and jaundice may be evident. The islets of Langerhans in the terminal one-third of the pancreas are usually not impaired.

Complications

It may be useful to think of acute pancreatitis as a chemical burn to the organ. As with other severe burns, death is likely to occur from secondary causes. From the onset of symptoms, cardiovascular, pulmonary (including acute respiratory distress syndrome), and renal failure are the most likely causes of death. Hemorrhage, peripheral vascular collapse, and infection are also major concerns for patients with pancreatitis. A purplish discoloration of the flanks (Turner's sign) or a purplish discoloration around the umbilicus (Cullen's sign) may occur with extensive hemorrhagic destruction of the pancreas.

Diagnostic Tests

Serum amylase (normal: 80 to 180 units/dL) and serum lipase (normal: 0 to 160 units/L) may be elevated to 5 to 40 times normal. The levels usually begin to drop within 72 hours. Urine amylase elevates and stays elevated for a longer period of time. Glucose, bilirubin, alkaline phosphatase, lactic dehydrogenase, ALT, AST, cholesterol, and potassium are all elevated. Decreases are seen in serum albumin, calcium, sodium, and magnesium.

X-ray examination may show pleural effusion from local inflammatory reaction to pancreatic enzymes, pulmonary infiltrates, or a change in the size of the pancreas. Computed tomography and ultrasonography can provide more complete information about the pancreas and surrounding tissues.

Therapeutic Measures

Resting the pancreas is essential to reduce autodigestion. The patient usually is ordered to have nothing by mouth (NPO), although research suggests that patients may experience fewer complications if enteral feeding is maintained (see *Evidence-Based Practice* box). The patient may have a nasogastric tube inserted and attached to low suction to empty gastric contents and gas. A histamine (H_2) antagonist such as famotidine (Pepcid) may help decrease acid stimulation of pancreatic secretions. See Table 35.4 for a summary of medications. If NPO therapy is prolonged or if the patient is malnourished, the patient will need total parenteral nutrition (TPN) (Box 35.8, *Nutrition Notes*). As the patient recovers, a clear liquid diet is ordered, which is advanced as tolerated to low fat.

Pain relief is essential and opioids such as morphine or hydromorphone (Dilaudid) are ordered for pain. Pain and anxiety increase pancreatic secretion by stimulating the autonomic nervous system.

The patient may be given antianxiety agents to decrease oxygen demand. Supplemental oxygen may be required if abdominal pressure, pleural effusion, or acidosis cause impaired gas exchange or an ineffective breathing pattern.

A Foley catheter may be inserted to provide accurate output measurements and to assess need for fluid replacement. Strict intake and output must be documented. Intravenous

Box 35.7

Cultural Considerations

Pancreatic disease is more common among Mexican Americans and Chinese Americans. Risk factors include working in occupations such as mining, factories using chemicals, and farming using pesticides and also the high use of alcohol and cigarette smoking.

EVIDENCE-BASED PRACTICE

Clinical Question

Does the use of enteral nutrition have outcomes similar to parenteral nutrition in patients with acute pancreatitis?

Evidence

A review of five randomized clinical trials using both enteral and parenteral nutrition for patients with acute pancreatitis showed no difference in mortality between patients receiving enteral versus parenteral nutritional support (McClave et al., 2006). The incidence of complications attributed to the method of nutritional support, for example, sepsis, hyperglycemia, and catheter-related infections, was higher in patients receiving parenteral nutrition. Although the incidence of complications was greater in number, in some instances the increases were not statistically significant. All the studies found that enteral support was less costly than parenteral support, with slightly longer lengths of stay for the patients with parenteral support.

Implications for Nursing Practice

Enteral nutrition is a cost-effective method with fewer complications for providing nutritional support to patients with acute pancreatitis. Being informed about options for nourishment allows nurses to advocate for patient nourishment to promote healing.

REFERENCE

McClave, S. A., Chang, W. K., Dhaliwal, R., & Heyland, D.K. (2006). Nutrition support in acute pancreatitis: A systematic review of the literature. *Journal of Parenteral and Enteral Nutrition, 30*(2), 143–156.

TABLE 35.4 MEDICATIONS USED FOR LIVER, GALLBLADDER, OR PANCREATIC DISORDERS

Medication Class/Action	Examples	Route	Side Effects	Nursing Implications
Antiemetics				
Reduce nausea	prochlorperazine (Compazine)	PO, IM, rectal	Extrapyramidal (parkinsonian) symptoms	Contraindicated in glaucoma or prostatic hypertrophy. Give antacids 2 hours before or after.
	metoclopramide (Reglan)	IV, PO, IM	Dry mouth, constipation, drowsiness, extrapyramidal symptoms	Monitor for extrapyramidal symptoms. Monitor for extrapyramidal symptoms. Administer 30 minutes before meals.
	promethazine (Phenergan)	PO, IM, IV, rectal	Dizziness, drowsiness, constipation, extrapyramidal symptoms, urine retention	For IV, dilute in minimum of 10 mL of fluid and administer in free-flowing IV to prevent vein irritation. May be additive when used with opioids. Monitor I&O, sedation, urine retention.
	odansetron (Zofran)	PO, SL, IM, IV	Headache	Monitor for hypersensitivity.
Antihistamines				
Reduce itching	diphenhydramine (Benadryl)	PO, IM, IV, topical	Drowsiness, dry mouth, confusion in elderly	If using topical preparation, do not apply to open skin.
Anticholinergics				
Decrease GI secretions	propantheline bromide (Pro-Banthine)	PO	Constipation, dry mouth, urine retention, tachycardia	Contraindicated in glaucoma or prostatic hypertrophy.
	dicyclomine hydrochloride (Bentyl)	PO, IM		
Bile Acid Sequestrants				
Bind with circulating bile acids for excretion in the stool to relieve itching.	cholestyramine (Questran, LoCholest) colestipol (Colestid)	PO	GI upset, constipation, headache	Give 4–6 hr before or 1 hr after other medications.

TABLE 35.4 MEDICATIONS USED FOR LIVER, GALLBLADDER, OR PANCREATIC DISORDERS—cont'd

Medication Class/Action	Examples	Route	Side Effects	Nursing Implications
Bile Acid Agents				
Prevent or dissolve (noncalcified) cholesterol gallstones	ursodiol (Actigall) chenodiol (Chenix)	PO	GI upset, diarrhea, constipation, headache, dizziness, back pain, flu/cold symptoms	Give with a full glass of water. Aluminum antacids may reduce absorption.
Histamine (H_2) antagonists				
Lock histamine receptors in acid, producing cells to inhibit gastric acid secretion	famotidine (Pepcid) ranitidine (Zantac)	PO, IV PO, IV, IM	Confusion, drowsiness, dizziness	If ordered once a day, give at bedtime. Smoking may interfere with action.
Proton Pump Inhibitors				
Inhibit proton pump to reduce gastric acid production	rabeprazole (AcipHex) esomeprazole (Nexium) lansoprazole (Prevacid) omeprazole (Prilosec) pantoprazole (Protonix)	PO, IV	Headache, diarrhea, abdominal pain	Monitor bowel sounds, liver function (AST, ALT)
Pancreatic Supplements				
Replace pancreatic digestive enzymes: lipase, protease, amylase	pancrelipase (Cotazym, Creon Pancrease, Ultrase, Viokase)	PO	GI upset, diarrhea, constipation, greasy stool, bloating	Give with meals. Teach not to hold medication in mouth because it may irritate inside of mouth.

Box 35.8
Nutrition Notes

Nourishing the Patient with Pancreatitis

For acute pancreatitis, the patient may be given ice chips made with electrolyte solutions to minimize gastric secretions and subsequent electrolyte loss through a nasogastric tube. Eighty percent of patients with acute pancreatitis have mild cases and relatively benign courses.

Mild pancreatitis may be treated with:

- Nothing by mouth to avoid stimulating the pancreas
- Intravenous fluids
- Clear liquids after pain has been controlled for 24 hours
- Nasojejunal feedings only if needed
- Soft to general diet over 3 or 4 days if satisfactory progress.

Patients with severe pancreatitis display an intense systemic inflammatory response and often develop multiple organ failure. Because mortality and morbidity rates are directly related to protein metabolism, improving nutrition is a high priority that requires constant monitoring and adjusting.

Initial dietary treatment for severe pancreatitis is similar to that in mild cases, individualized according to the patient's response. The goal of nutritional support is to meet the elevated metabolic demands as much as possible without stimulating pancreatic secretion and self-digestion. In general, both TPN and jejunal nutrition avoid stimulating pancreatic secretions. The more distally the feeding enters the gut, the less it stimulates pancreatic secretions.

In chronic pancreatitis, the dietary prescription may include:

- Six small meals per day, beginning with clear liquids and progressing to a high-carbohydrate, low-fat diet
- Medium-chain triglyceride (MCT) oil added to foods because it is absorbed without pancreatic lipase or bile
- Pharmaceutical preparations of pancreatic enzymes.

For both acute and chronic pancreatitis, antioxidant supplements (selenium, methionine, and vitamins A, C, and E) may reduce inflammation and pain (Raimondo & Scolapio, 2006).

When monitoring progress, an increase in serum amylase levels may necessitate the return to a more restricted diet.

fluids may be needed to maintain fluid volume. Blood or blood products may also be ordered if the patient has significant blood loss from hemorrhage.

Additional typical drug orders include electrolytes such as calcium and magnesium to replace losses, short-acting insulin to combat hyperglycemia, and antibiotics to treat sepsis. (See Table 35.5.)

Surgery may be needed for debriding necrotic tissue. Abscesses or pseudocysts may need to be drained.

CRITICAL THINKING

Mrs. Samuels

■ Mrs. Samuels, an 85-year-old retired librarian, is admitted to the nursing unit from the emergency department with severe midepigastric pain that radiates to her back. On admission, she is noted to have guarding of the abdomen, and her abdomen is full and tense. Her medical record documents that she had an endoscopic retrograde cholangiopancreatograph (ERCP) 2 days ago for recurrent episodes of RUQ abdominal pain. She has no history of excessive alcohol intake.

1. What is the most common cause of acute pancreatitis? Does Mrs. Samuels fit the description?
2. Why do patients such as Mrs. Samuels have difficulty breathing?
3. Why is Mrs. Samuels at risk for hemorrhage?
4. What laboratory test is most likely to be abnormal in early acute pancreatitis?
5. Why are opioids commonly ordered for acute pancreatitis?
6. Why does the physician usually order a histamine antagonist?

Suggested answers at end of chapter.

TABLE 35.5 PANCREATITIS SUMMARY

Signs and Symptoms	Midline abdominal pain Low-grade fever Nausea and vomiting
Diagnostic Tests	Elevated serum amylase and lipase
Therapeutic Measures	Pain control NPO NG suction IV fluids, TPN, enteral nutrition
Complications	Hemorrhage, shock, infection
Priority Nursing Diagnoses	*Pain* *Imbalanced Nutrition* *Risk for Ineffective Breathing Pattern*

Chronic Pancreatitis

Chronic pancreatitis is continuing pancreatic cellular damage and decreased pancreatic enzyme functioning usually following repeated occasions of acute pancreatitis.

Pathophysiology

Chronic pancreatitis is a continuous, progressive disease that replaces functioning pancreatic tissue with fibrotic tissue as a result of inflammation. Pancreatic ducts become obstructed, dilated, and finally atrophied. The acinar, or enzyme-producing, cells of the pancreas ulcerate in response to inflammation. The ulceration causes further tissue damage and tissue death, and it may cause cystic sacs filled with pancreatic enzymes to form on the surface of the pancreas. The pancreas becomes smaller and hardened, and progressively smaller amounts of pancreatic enzymes are produced.

Etiology and Incidence

The major cause of chronic pancreatitis in men is excessive alcohol ingestion that causes repeated attacks of acute pancreatitis. The major cause in women is chronic obstructive biliary disease that leads to persistent inflammation of the pancreatic ducts. Other conditions known to cause chronic pancreatitis are prolonged malnutrition, cancer of the pancreas or duodenum, and prolonged use of enteral feedings, which can cause atrophy of the pancreas. The usual age for chronic pancreatitis to develop is between ages 45 and 60. The patient's mean life span is 25 years after the diagnosis of chronic pancreatitis is made. Death is often not related to pancreatic failure.

Prevention

Advise patients with acute pancreatitis from excessive alcohol ingestion that abstinence could prevent recurrence of the pancreatitis and prevent the possibility of chronic pancreatitis. Advise all patients with obstructive biliary disease to seek medical treatment for their condition to prevent the progression from acute to chronic pancreatitis. Carefully monitor patients who are unable to feed themselves for nutritionally adequate diets. Monitor routine laboratory values. Report any trend toward reduced functioning of the pancreas.

Signs and Symptoms

The signs and symptoms of chronic pancreatitis are less severe than acute pancreatitis but more long term. The patient's history will show a pattern of remissions and exacerbations over a period of years. The patient will report epigastric or LUQ pain, weight loss, and anorexia. Malabsorption and fat intolerance occur late in the disease. Usually the islets of Langerhans function until late stages of the disease; diabetes mellitus is a late-occurring symptom.

Complications

A variety of complications can result from chronic pancreatitis. Abscesses and fistulas may develop when cysts filled with pancreatic enzymes burst into the abdominal cavity, causing severe inflammation and tissue necrosis. Pleural effusion may develop from inflammation just under the diaphragm.

Pancreatic enzymes are essential for normal absorption of nutrients from the intestines. Malabsorption syndrome with fatty stools and diarrhea may develop in response to the limited amount of pancreatic enzymes produced. In addition, biliary obstruction may further complicate fat absorption. As the terminal third of the pancreas becomes involved and the islets of Langerhans are destroyed, the patient exhibits symptoms of insulin-dependent diabetes mellitus (discussed in Chapter 40).

Diagnostic Tests

Serum amylase and serum lipase levels are only elevated in acute disease. In chronic pancreatitis, enzymes will be normal or below normal. Fecal fat analysis shows higher than normal amounts of fat. Both computed tomography and ultrasonography show characteristic pancreatic structural changes such as masses, calcification of ducts, cysts, and change in pancreatic size. Endoscopic retrograde cholangiopancreatography (ERCP) can locate specific obstructions and detect ductal leaks.

Therapeutic Measures

Treatment is aimed at promoting comfort and maintaining adequate nutrition. Pain is managed with analgesics. Nutrition is maintained with the careful replacement of pancreatic enzymes and specially prepared nutritional supplements. Surgery may be necessary to treat biliary disease, repair fistulas, drain cysts, or repair other damage.

Nursing Process for the Patient with Pancreatitis

See the *Nursing Care Plan for the Patient with Acute and Chronic Pancreatitis.*

Cancer of the Pancreas

Cancer of the pancreas is the fourth leading cause of cancer death in men in the United States and the fifth leading cause in women, killing more than 30,000 people each year. Nearly 32,000 new cases of cancer of the pancreas are diagnosed yearly (American Cancer Society, 2009); it most often affects people between ages 65 and 79. About 70% of cancers of the pancreas occur in the head of the pancreas. About 30% are located in the body and tail of the pancreas.

Pathophysiology

Most primary tumors of the pancreas are ductal adenocarcinomas and occur in the exocrine parts of the pancreas. The tumors in the head and body of the pancreas tend to be large. Cancer of the pancreas spreads rapidly by direct extension to the stomach, gallbladder, and duodenum. Cancer located in the body of the pancreas usually spreads further and more rapidly than do masses in the head. Cancer of the pancreas may spread by the lymphatic and vascular systems to distant organs and lymph nodes.

Etiology

The cause of cancer of the pancreas is not known. Cancer of the pancreas has been associated with chemical carcinogens such as high-fat diets and cigarette smoking, diabetes mellitus, excessive alcohol intake, exposure to chemicals such as coke and benzidine, and chronic pancreatitis. It may also occur as a result of metastasis from a primary cancer of the lung, breast, kidney, or thyroid gland or malignant melanomas of the skin.

Signs and Symptoms

The patient with cancer of the pancreas usually experiences vague symptoms early in the disease process. Weight loss, pain, anorexia, nausea, vomiting, and weakness are among the early symptoms. Detection is often difficult because of the nonspecific symptoms identified by the patient. The patient may report abdominal pain that is worse at night. The pain is described as gnawing or boring, and it radiates to the back. The pain may be lessened by a side-lying position with the knees drawn up to the chest or by bending over when walking. The pain becomes increasingly severe and unrelenting as the cancer grows.

The patient may report a bloated feeling or fullness after eating. If the cancer obstructs the bile duct, the patient may have jaundice, dark urine, pruritus, and light-colored stools. The patient often reports fatigue and depression. The patient's health history may include a recent diagnosis of diabetes mellitus.

Complications

Complications may occur before or after surgical treatment. Preoperative complications include malnutrition, spread of the cancer, and gastric or duodenal obstruction. Postoperative complications include infection, breakdown of the surgical site, fistula formation, diabetes mellitus, and malabsorption syndrome. If the patient has had chemotherapy or radiation therapy, complications specific to those therapies may also occur.

Thrombophlebitis is a common complication of cancer of the pancreas. As the tumor grows, by-products of the tumor growth appear to increase the levels of thromboplastic (clotting) factors in the blood, making clotting easier. The potential for thrombophlebitis increases if the patient is confined to bed or has surgery.

Diagnostic Tests

Serum alkaline phosphatase, glucose, and bilirubin levels may be elevated. Amylase and lipase are elevated if the cancer has caused a secondary pancreatitis. Blood coagulation tests, such as clotting time, may be done. Carcinoembryonic antigen (CEA) may be ordered to confirm the presence of cancer (normal: less than 5 nanograms/mL).

Abdominal radiographs may be ordered to determine the size of the pancreas and the presence of masses. Computed tomography and ultrasonography may be done to more precisely locate any masses in the pancreas. ERCP can be used to visualize the common ducts and to take tissue samples for microscopic analysis. Pancreatic biopsy is necessary for definitive diagnosis of pancreatic cancer. A tissue sample may be obtained by needle aspiration during ultrasonography. This procedure may cause seeding of the tumor along the needle pathway.

NURSING CARE PLAN for the Patient with Acute and Chronic Pancreatitis

Nursing Diagnosis: *Pain* related to edema and inflammation

Expected Outcome: The patient will state pain level is less than 2 on a scale of 0 to 10 within 30 minutes of pain report.

Evaluation of Outcome: Does patient state pain level is less than 2 on a pain scale of 0 to 10?

Interventions	Rationale	Evaluation
Assess the patient every 2 hours for pain by:	Intense pain is likely to occur with acute pancreatitis.	Does patient state that pain is less than 2 on a pain scale of 0 to 10, where 0 = no pain and 10 = worst possible pain?
• Asking the patient to rate pain on a scale of 0 to 10.	A pain scale allows for a consistent and individual evaluation of pain.	
• Observing the patient for pain behaviors such as grimacing, irritability, reluctance to move, or inability to lie quietly.	Observation of pain behaviors, such as reluctance to move, shallow respirations, grimacing, or irritability, may be a reliable indicator of pain. However, the patient in pain may have no observable pain behaviors.	Does patient exhibit pain behaviors that differ from his or her report of pain?
Administer analgesics as ordered, before pain becomes severe.	Analgesics are most effective if given before pain becomes too great.	Are analgesics effective?
Assist the patient to a position of comfort, usually high Fowler's or leaning forward slightly.	An upright position keeps abdominal organs from pressing against the inflamed pancreas.	Does positioning promote comfort?
Keep the environment free from excessive stimuli.	Quiet, restful, anxiety-free atmosphere permits the patient to relax and may decrease pain perception.	Does patient state atmosphere is relaxing?
Teach the patient alternative pain control strategies such as guided imagery and relaxation techniques.	Successful use of pain control strategies may decrease the amount of analgesics needed and give the patient a greater sense of control.	Are alternative strategies effective?

Nursing Diagnosis: *Imbalanced Nutrition: Less Than Body Requirements* related to pain, medical restrictions (NPO), and treatment (suction)

Expected Outcome: The patient will experience improved nutrition as evidenced by stable weight and serum albumin level greater than 3.5 g/L.

Evaluation of Outcome: Is weight stable? Is serum albumin level greater than 3.5 g/L?

Interventions	Rationale	Evaluation
Assess the patient's nutritional status by:		
• Weighing the patient every other day.	A loss of 1 lb of body weight occurs when the body uses 3500 calories more than is taken in.	Has patient lost less than 5% of total baseline body weight?
• Monitoring serum albumin levels as ordered.	Serum albumin of 3.5–5.5 g/L indicates normal protein metabolism in the absence of liver or renal disease.	Is patient's albumin level above 3.5 g/dL?

NURSING CARE PLAN for the Patient with Acute and Chronic Pancreatitis—cont'd

• Observing for nausea or vomiting.	Nausea, vomiting, and pain are risk factors for inadequate intake.	Does nausea need to be treated to prevent vomiting? Is intake adequate?
• Monitoring blood sugar at least every 6 hr if the patient is on TPN.	Patients on TPN are more likely to have high blood glucose.	Is blood sugar normal?
• Observing for diarrhea, bloating, or steatorrhea (fatty stools).	Diarrhea, bloating, or fatty stools may indicate malabsorption syndrome.	Are stools normal?
Report steatorrhea immediately.	Steatorrhea (fatty stools) may indicate that the enzyme replacement doses are not meeting the patient's needs.	
Administer nutritional supplements, including pancreatic enzymes, as ordered.	Provides adequate nutrition.	Does patient take any supplements?
Teach the patient to avoid alcohol.	Alcohol may trigger another episode of pancreatitis.	Does patient verbalize understanding of importance of avoiding alcohol? Is follow-up support for alcohol avoidance provided?
Teach the patient and family the signs and symptoms of diabetes mellitus.	Patients with pancreatitis are at great risk for developing diabetes mellitus.	Does patient verbalize signs and symptoms of diabetes to report?
Teach the patient and family to self-monitor for symptoms of malabsorption syndrome, such as fatty stools, weight loss, dry skin, or bleeding.	Absence of pancreatic enzymes causes problems with digestion of fats, carbohydrates, and proteins.	Does patient verbalize understanding of symptoms of malabsorption to report?

Nursing Diagnosis: *Risk for Ineffective Breathing Pattern* related to abdominal pressure and pain

Expected Outcome: The patient will have an effective breathing pattern as evidenced by unlabored respirations, 16–20 per minute, SaO_2 95% or greater at all times.

Evaluation of Outcome: Are respirations unlabored, 16–20 per minute, SaO_2 95% or greater?

Interventions	Rationale	Evaluation
Assess the patient's breathing patterns: • Observe respirations for depth, regularity, and rate. • Observe respiratory effort. • Observe for evidence of respiratory distress, such as use of accessory muscles, use of intercostal muscles, SaO_2 less than 95%, and rapid or difficult breathing.	Abdominal pressure from inflammation and tissue damage under the diaphragm may cause the patient to take shallow, rapid respirations, which can tire the patient.	Are patient's respirations 16–20 per minute, unlabored, and regular? Is patient alert and oriented? Has there been a change in the level of patient's arousal? Does patient exhibit signs of distress?

Continued

NURSING CARE PLAN for the Patient with Acute and Chronic Pancreatitis—cont'd

Administer oxygen as ordered.	Oxygen can decrease the amount of effort the patient must expend to breathe.	Does oxygen help patient breathe easier?
Place the patient in an upright or slightly forward-leaning position.	Relieves pressure on the diaphragm.	Is positioning effective?
Prepare the patient's food by opening cartons and lids and cut food into bite-size portions.	Decreases the demand for oxygen.	Does patient accept assistance with food preparation?
Teach the patient to move slowly and to take frequent rests.	Helps decrease the demand for oxygen.	Does patient tolerate activity?

Nursing Diagnosis: *Risk for Injury* related to hemorrhage or fluid and electrolyte imbalances

Expected Outcome: The patient will experience no injury during illness.

Evaluation of Outcome: Is there evidence of injury? Are signs and symptoms of impending injury recognized and reported early?

Interventions	Rationale	Evaluation
Monitor sodium, potassium, calcium, and magnesium levels daily.	Electrolyte levels can become imbalanced in pancreatitis.	Do laboratory studies show that patient's electrolytes are within acceptable ranges?
Evaluate neuromuscular status by checking Chvostek's/Trousseau's signs.	These are signs of calcium depletion (see Chapter 6).	Are signs of calcium depletion present?
Monitor the patient's hematocrit, hemoglobin, and blood clotting times frequently.	Destruction of the pancreas can result in hemorrhage.	Does patient have any abnormal bruising, bleeding gums, or pink urine?
Observe abdomen and flanks for Cullen's and Turner's signs.	These are signs of hemorrhage.	Are signs of hemorrhage present?
Weigh the patient daily.	To monitor fluid balance.	Is weight stable?
Measure and record intake and output every shift.	To monitor fluid balance.	Is urinary output greater than 30 mL/hr?
Observe for nausea and vomiting.	Vomiting can contribute to fluid loss.	Does nausea need to be treated to prevent vomiting?
Report any drop in blood pressure greater than 5% of the patient's baseline.	May indicate severe fluid loss.	Are vital signs stable? Is patient's blood pressure within 5% of baseline?
Teach the patient to report any weakness or muscle twitching.	May indicate electrolyte imbalance.	Does patient verbalize understanding of signs and symptoms of electrolyte imbalance to report?

Therapeutic Measures

Medical treatment depends on the staging of the cancer. If diagnosed early, treatment may be aimed at cure. If the patient's cancer has progressed to distant involvement of other organ structures and lymph nodes, treatment is directed at easing symptoms and making the patient more comfortable.

Surgery is usually done. When the tumor is located at the head of the pancreas, the Whipple procedure is done to remove the head of the pancreas, the lower portion of the common bile duct, most of the duodenum, and possibly parts of the stomach nearby (Fig. 35.5). Potential postoperative problems after the Whipple procedure include failure of the suture lines to hold, causing leakage of pancreatic enzymes and bile into the abdomen; pneumonia or atelectasis from shallow breathing because the incision line is directly under the diaphragm; paralytic ileus; gastric retention or ulceration; wound infection; fistula formation; unstable diabetes mellitus; and renal failure.

For tumors in the body and tail of the pancreas, a distal **pancreatectomy** is done.

Relief of biliary obstruction can sometimes be accomplished by implanting a stent or plastic tube in the common bile duct during an endoscopic procedure. Pain can be reduced by surgical removal of a portion of the greater splanchnic nerve.

Before or after surgery, radiation therapy is used to shrink or destroy the tumor. Intraoperative radiation therapy can be used during surgery when the tumor is exposed to deliver high doses of radiation directly to the tumor while sparing other tissue. Chemotherapy is used for metastatic disease and with radiation therapy to prevent metastasis. In some instances, either radiation therapy or chemotherapy may be used for relief of symptoms if the cancer has become too widespread for surgery. (See Chapter 11 for care of the patient undergoing radiation or chemotherapy.)

Nursing Process for the Patient with Pancreatic Cancer

DATA COLLECTION. Observe the patient with cancer of the pancreas for evidence of malnutrition and fluid imbalance, including weight loss, inelastic skin turgor, vomiting, fatty stools, and reports of anorexia or nausea. Review laboratory tests, especially blood glucose, liver function studies, and clotting studies. Evaluate the patient every 2 to 4 hours for pain. Observe the skin for bruising, scaling, and yellowing, and question the patient about itching. Evaluate the patient's mental status for evidence of depression.

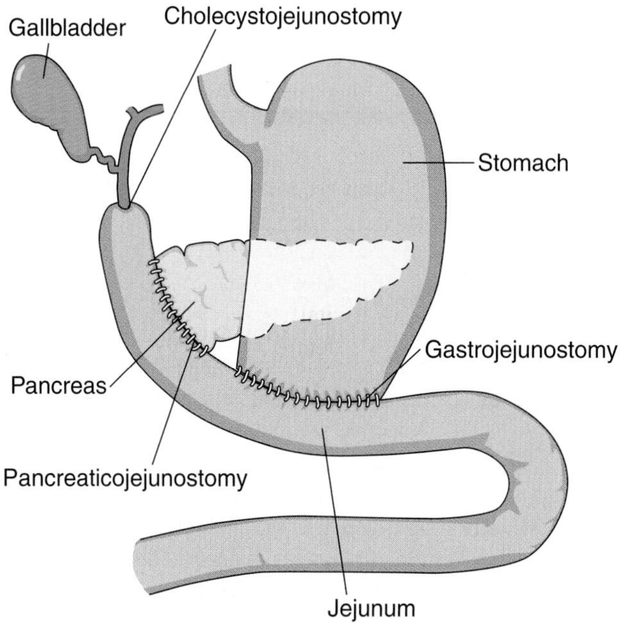
Gallbladder
Cholecystojejunostomy
Stomach
Gastrojejunostomy
Pancreas
Pancreaticojejunostomy
Jejunum

FIGURE 35.5 Pancreatoduodenectomy (Whipple procedure) for cancer of the head of the pancreas.

• **WORD • BUILDING •**
pancreatectomy: pancreat—pancreas + ectomy—excision

NURSING DIAGNOSES, PLANNING, AND IMPLEMENTATION. The patient with cancer of the pancreas will have numerous problems. Interventions for *Imbalanced Nutrition: Less Than Body Requirements* related to inability to digest food, anorexia, nausea, and vomiting, and *Pain* related to pancreatic tumor or surgical incision are the same as for patients with pancreatitis and are found in the *Nursing Care Plan for the Patient with Acute and Chronic Pancreatitis.* Other care is listed below. Additional interventions for patients with cancer, including psychosocial interventions, can be found in Chapter 11.

Risk for Deficient Fluid Volume

EXPECTED OUTCOME: The patient will have adequate fluid volume as evidenced by stable vital signs, elastic skin turgor, and moist mucous membranes.

- Monitor the patient's intake and output carefully. *Low intake increases risk of deficient fluid volume; low output is a sign of deficient fluid.*
- Monitor vital signs. *Tachycardia, tachypnea, and low blood pressure may indicate excessive fluid loss.*
- Monitor laboratory values, especially serum sodium, potassium, calcium, and chloride levels. Report abnormal values. *If electrolyte values are low, the physician may order intravenous replacement solutions.*
- Report low serum albumin level (normal is 3.4 to 4.8 g/dL) and assist with monitoring intravenous albumin therapy if ordered. *Low albumin places the patient at risk for fluid imbalances.*
- Carefully observe the patient for signs of blood loss *that may indicate abnormal bleeding:*
  - Bruising, bleeding gums, or pink-tinged urine
  - Cullen's sign (bluish discolorations around the umbilicus)
  - Turner's sign (bluish discolorations on the flanks)
  - Bleeding at incision and drain sites and in drainage tubing.
- Teach the patient to use a soft-bristle toothbrush and electric razor rather than a straight razor *to reduce risk of injury and bleeding.*
- Administer vitamin K as ordered *to replace deficiency and to reduce risk for bleeding.*

Risk for Impaired Tissue Integrity Related to Itching and to Leaking around Drainage Tubes

EXPECTED OUTCOME: The patient's skin will remain intact.

- Assess the patient for any reports of itching *because scratching can cause a break in the skin.*
- Help the patient keep fingernails short *to reduce damage to skin with scratching.*
- Provide frequent skin care with products free of soap or alcohol *to prevent further dryness and itching.*

- Protect skin around drains with skin-protective barrier products and ostomy bags *to prevent skin damage.*
- Apply products such as calamine lotion as ordered *to decrease itching.*
- Exercise special care of any drains *to prevent unnecessary tension that may cause sutures to give way.*
- Keep all drains patent, and keep drainage tubing and bags free from kinks *to prevent fluid leakage onto the skin.*
- Place the patient in semi-Fowler's position *to help with gravity drainage and reduce risk of fluid leakage.*

EVALUATION. The plan of care for the patient with pancreatic cancer is successful if the patient maintains body weight within 5% of normal body weight and experiences no nausea or vomiting; states that pain remains at 2 or less on a pain scale of 0 to 10; has urinary output greater than 30 mL/hr, elastic skin turgor, moist mucous membranes, pulse and blood pressure within 10% of patient's baseline, no sudden, excessive abdominal pain or rigidity, and incisions heal at the expected rate; demonstrates the appropriate self-care procedures for tubes, drains, dressings, and medication administration; and states the signs and symptoms of complications that are to be reported immediately.

PATIENT EDUCATION. Teach the patient and family self-care measures such as blood glucose monitoring, insulin administration, signs and symptoms of hyperglycemia and hypoglycemia (see Chapter 40), and the regimen for pancreatic enzyme replacement. Instruct the patient on how to manage dressing changes if he or she is to be discharged with tubes or drains. Patient and family should know the signs and symptoms of hemorrhage, gastric ulceration, infection, and fistula formation. A patient being cared for at home should have a referral for hospice care or home nursing care.

For more information, visit the National Pancreas Foundation at www.pancreasfoundation.org.

DISORDERS OF THE GALLBLADDER

Cholecystitis, Cholelithiasis, and Choledocholithiasis

Gallstones and inflammations of the gallbladder and common bile duct are the most common disorders of the biliary system.

Pathophysiology

Cholecystitis is an acute or chronic inflammation of the gallbladder. It is most often a response to obstruction of the common bile duct resulting in edema and inflammation. Often bacteria invade the bile and add to the inflammation and irritation of the gallbladder. Chronic cholecystitis may be the result of repeated attacks of acute cholecystitis or chronic irritation from gallstones. The gallbladder becomes fibrotic and thickened and does not empty easily or completely.

Cholelithiasis is the formation of gallstones in the gallbladder that are most often composed of cholesterol in the United States. **Choledocholithiasis** refers to gallstones in the common bile duct. Although the exact cause of gallstones is unknown, one theory suggests that cholesterol may supersaturate the bile in the gallbladder. After a time, the supersaturated bile crystallizes and begins to form stones. Another type of gallstone is a pigment stone. Pigment stones appear to be composed of calcium bilirubinate, which occurs when free bilirubin combines with calcium.

Etiology and Incidence

CHOLELITHIASIS. Pooling, or stasis, of bile within the gallbladder appears to contribute to the formation of stones. Stasis may be caused by a decreased gallbladder emptying rate or a partial obstruction in the common duct. Pregnancy, with a growing fetus, may also contribute to biliary stasis. Excessive cholesterol intake combined with a sedentary lifestyle is linked with an increased incidence of cholelithiasis.

Some low-fat diets have been linked to cholelithiasis because the diet appears to free cholesterol from body tissues; the cholesterol then crystallizes in the gallbladder before it is excreted. Fasting can contribute to cholelithiasis because the gallbladder is less active, and bile becomes concentrated. Further, a family history of cholelithiasis, obesity, diabetes mellitus, pregnancy, some hemolytic blood disorders, and bowel disorders such as Crohn's disease have also been linked to a higher incidence of cholelithiasis.

CHOLECYSTITIS. Cholelithiasis is responsible for most cases of cholecystitis, or inflammation of the gallbladder. Women between ages 20 and 50 are about three times more likely to have gallstones than men; especially women with multiple pregnancies, women who are pregnant, or women who are using birth control pills. After age 50, the rate of gallstones is about the same for men and women (Box 35.9, *Cultural Considerations*). The incidence of gallstones increases with age.

Signs and Symptoms

Signs and symptoms of cholecystitis and cholelithiasis are similar. Subjective symptoms include epigastric pain, RUQ tenderness, nausea, and indigestion, especially after eating foods high in fat. Objective symptoms include evidence of inflammation, such as an elevated temperature, pulse, and respirations; vomiting; and jaundice. The patient may have a positive Murphy's sign, which is the inability to take a deep breath when an examiner's fingers are pressed below the liver margin. Family history of either cholecystitis or cholelithiasis,

• WORD • BUILDING •
cholecystitis: chole—bile + cyst—bladder + itis—inflammation

• WORD • BUILDING •
cholelithiasis: chole—bile + lith—stone + iasis—condition
choledocholithiasis: chole—bile + docho—duct + lith—stone + iasis—condition

Box 35.9

Cultural Considerations

Gallbladder disease is more common among Mexican Americans. Risk factors include working in occupations such as mining, factories using chemicals, and farming using pesticides. The disease has a lower incidence in blacks in Africa and in blacks living in the Western world. Native Americans have an increased incidence of pancreatic and gallbladder disease. It is unknown how much increased dietary risk factors may contribute to gallbladder disease. The nurse can positively affect the nutritional status of at-risk patients by teaching food preparation practices that use less fat.

dietary habits such as high fat intake or a recent low-fat diet, and reports of flatulence (gas), eructation (belching), nausea, vomiting, or abdominal discomfort after a high-fat meal are common evidence of a gallbladder disorder.

CHOLELITHIASIS. The epigastric pain caused by cholelithiasis may also be called biliary **colic**. The pain is a steady, aching, severe pain in the epigastrium and RUQ that may radiate back to behind the right scapula or to the right shoulder. The pain usually begins suddenly after a fatty meal and lasts for 1 to 3 hours. If the pain is caused by a stone in the common bile duct (choledocholithiasis), the pain may last until the stone has passed into the duodenum. Jaundice is more commonly present with acute choledocholithiasis because the common bile duct is blocked or inflamed.

CHOLECYSTITIS. The biliary colic caused by cholecystitis typically lasts 4 to 6 hours. The pain is made worse with movement such as breathing. The patient usually has nausea, vomiting, and a low-grade fever with the pain. Heartburn, indigestion, and flatulence are more common with chronic cholecystitis. Patients often report repeated attacks of acute cholecystitis symptoms (Table 35.6).

CRITICAL THINKING

Donna Stewart

■ Donna Stewart, a 23-year-old woman, is diagnosed with possible acute cholecystitis. She is 5 feet, 6 inches tall and weighs 138 pounds. She is 4 months pregnant. Her physician wishes to delay surgery until her inflammation has subsided.

1. What risk factors does Donna have for cholecystitis?
2. What diagnostic tests might be ordered to confirm Donna's diagnosis of cholecystitis?
3. What considerations should be weighed when scheduling diagnostic tests?
4. What medications can you anticipate that the physician will order for Donna?
5. What type of diet will Donna need to eat after discharge?
6. If the diagnosis of cholecystitis is confirmed, what type of surgical treatment might be ordered?

Suggested answers at end of chapter.

TABLE 35.6 SYMPTOMS OF GALLBLADDER DISORDERS

	Acute Cholecystitis	Chronic Cholecystitis	Cholelithiasis and Choledocholithiasis
Biliary colic	Lasts 4–6 hr Worse with movement	Only during acute attack	Sudden onset
Jaundice	Present (if common bile duct is inflamed or blocked)	Present	Lasts 1–3 hr Radiates to right scapula or shoulder
Low-grade fever	Present	Present	Present
Nausea, vomiting	Present	Only during acute attack	Present
Repeated attacks		Present	
Heartburn, indigestion, and flatulence		Present	
Complications	Cholangitis Necrosis or perforation Fistulas	Empyema Fistulas Adenocarcinoma	Acute pancreatitis

• WORD • BUILDING •
colic: colic—spasm

Complications

Complications of cholecystitis include cholangitis (inflammation of the bile ducts), necrosis or perforation of the gallbladder, empyema (a collection of purulent drainage in the gallbladder), fistulas, and adenocarcinoma of the gallbladder. A major complication of choledocholithiasis is acute pancreatitis if the pancreatic duct is obstructed.

Diagnostic Tests

An ultrasound of the gallbladder is the classic test done to detect stones, inflamed walls of the gallbladder, and dilated ducts. An ERCP can be done to directly visualize the pancreatic ducts and bile ducts to determine the presence of stones in the common duct and allows the ability to remove stones from the common duct. Further examination may include a radionuclide scan, such as a hepatobiliary iminodiacetic acid (HIDA) scan. For this procedure, the patient will be given an IV injection of a radioactive isotope that is metabolized by the liver and excreted in the bile. The scanning camera then traces the path of the isotope as it travels through the bile ducts, gallbladder, and intestines to identify blockages.

The patient may have an elevated white blood cell count (normal: 5000 to 10,000 cells/mm^3). If direct bilirubin is elevated (normal: 0.3 to 1.2 mg/dL) its cause is likely obstruction in the biliary or liver areas. Serum amylase and lipase may be elevated if the pancreas is involved or if there is a stone in the common duct.

Therapeutic Measures

Treatment of an acute episode of cholecystitis centers on pain control, prevention of infection, and maintenance of fluid and electrolyte balance. Pain control is achieved with analgesics. For itching relief if the patient is jaundiced from bile acid deposits in the skin, colestipol (Colestid) or cholestyramine (Questran, LoCholest) is given. These drugs bind with the circulating bile acids for excretion in the stool. If the patient has nausea and vomiting, an antiemetic may be ordered (see Table 35.4). Patients are placed on high-protein, low-fat diets after the nausea and vomiting subside (Box 35.10, *Nutrition Notes*).

SURGERY. Treatment for cholelithiasis typically involves surgical removal of the gallbladder. The surgical procedure done most often is cholecystectomy via **laparoscopy**. A laparoscopic cholecystectomy is done with a laparoscope through four small puncture wounds in the abdomen. Patients are usually discharged in 24 hours or less and recovery time is reduced with laparoscopic surgery.

For large stones or an infected gallbladder, a traditional open cholecystectomy may be required. A **T-tube** may be inserted into the common duct to ensure that bile drainage is not obstructed (Fig. 35.6). T-tube drainage ranges from 500 to 1000 mL the first day and decreases to 200 mL by the third day. The patient with a traditional cholecystectomy has incisional pain that creates difficulty with coughing and deep breathing postoperatively because deep breathing causes the diaphragm to press on the operative site. Patients are hospitalized for 2 to 3 days with a traditional cholecystectomy.

EXTRACORPOREAL SHOCK-WAVE LITHOTRIPSY (ESWL). Extracorporeal shock-wave lithotripsy is done less frequently now due to the availability of laparoscopic cholecystectomy. It uses shock waves to destroy stones in the gallbladder or biliary ducts. Patients who have few cholesterol stones that are not calcified are the most likely candidates for ESWL. After ESWL, the patient is usually put on a course of oral dissolution drugs to ensure complete removal of all stones and stone fragments.

MEDICATION. Dissolution of small noncalcified stones (less than 2 centimeters) with the bile acid drugs ursodiol (Actigall) or chenodiol (Chenix) may be used for a few patients who are poor surgical risks. Treatment with the dissolution drugs may take months to years and stones may return.

Box 35.10

Nutrition Notes

Modifying the Diet for Patients with Gallbladder Disease

During an acute attack of cholecystitis, a full liquid diet with minimal fat is usually allowed. For treatment of chronic cholecystitis, the patient is instructed to do the following:

- Correct obesity.
- Avoid troublesome and gas-forming foods.
- Decrease dietary fat each day by (1) selecting skim-milk dairy products, (2) limiting fats or oils to 3 tsp, and (3) consuming no more than 6 oz of very lean meat.

Cholelithiasis has been associated with a long overnight fast that permits concentrated bile to remain in the gallbladder for an extended period. Eating a light bedtime snack or drinking two glasses of water on arising if breakfast is delayed alter this risk factor.

Foods are introduced after cholecystectomy as for other surgical procedures. Later in convalescence, balanced meals should be well tolerated because bile enters the duodenum continuously. Patients who become nauseated and suffered pain after eating certain foods preoperatively, however, may continue to avoid them postoperatively because of the association.

• WORD • BUILDING •
laparoscopy: laparo—pertaining to flank + scopy—to examine

• WORD • BUILDING •
extracorporeal shock-wave lithotripsy: extra—outside + tripsy—rub or crush

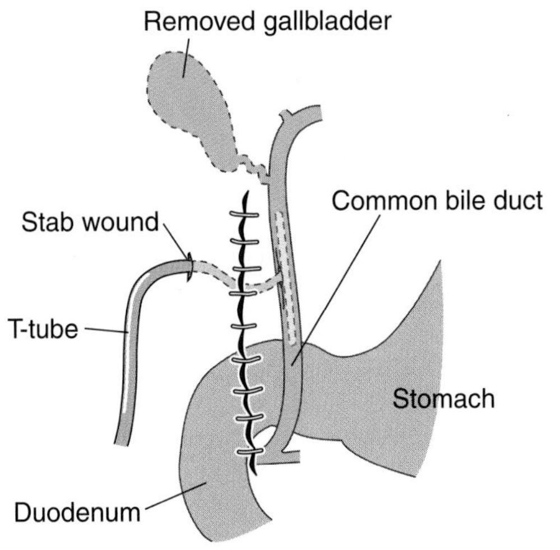
Removed gallbladder
Stab wound
Common bile duct
T-tube
Stomach
Duodenum

FIGURE 35.6 T-tube. A T-tube is used to drain bile after a cholecystectomy until swelling of the duct subsides.

Nursing Process of the Patient with a Gallbladder Disorder

DATA COLLECTION. Monitor the patient frequently for pain, using the WHAT'S UP? questions. Take the patient's vital signs, particularly the temperature and pulse, frequently to monitor for signs of infection. Weigh the patient and inspect mucous membranes, skin turgor, and urinary output for signs of dehydration. Measure intake and output, including any emesis or drainage from nasogastric tubes or T-tubes. Observe stools and urine for color and consistency. Obstruction of bile flow may result in stools that are clay colored or have a foul, greasy appearance or urine that is dark amber or tea colored. Report either new finding immediately. Evaluate laboratory studies for elevation in the white blood cell count or abnormalities in electrolytes or serum bilirubin levels.

NURSING DIAGNOSES, PLANNING, AND IMPLEMENTATION. Common nursing diagnoses for the patient with cholecystitis include pain and risk for deficient fluid volume. Additional nursing diagnoses for the patient with cholelithiasis who has a surgical procedure include risk for impaired skin integrity related to surgical incision and T-tube drainage, and risk for ineffective breathing pattern related to abdominal incision.

Acute Pain Related to Biliary Colic

EXPECTED OUTCOME: The patient will rate pain as 2 or less on a 10-point scale.

- Assess the patient frequently for pain *to guide treatment.*
- Administer analgesics as ordered *to reduce pain.*
- Administer antispasmodics or anticholinergics as ordered *for biliary colic.*
- Assist patient with positioning *to assume whatever position provides the most comfort.*

Risk for Deficient Fluid Volume Related to Anorexia, Nausea, Vomiting, or Excessive Tube Drainage

EXPECTED OUTCOME: The patient will have adequate fluid volume as evidenced by stable vital signs, elastic skin turgor, and moist mucous membranes at all times.

- Monitor intake and output, daily weights, and skin turgor *to monitor fluid balance.*
- Monitor T-tube drainage. Carefully observe the T-tube drainage unit to prevent kinking of the tubing. *Pressure in the biliary drainage system from poor drainage may greatly increase the patient's pain and the risk for infection.*
- Give antiemetics as needed *to control nausea and vomiting.*
- Assist with administration of intravenous fluids and electrolytes as ordered while the patient is on restricted oral intake *to maintain hydration.*

Risk for Impaired Skin Integrity Related to Surgical Incision and T-tube Drainage

EXPECTED OUTCOME: The patient's skin will remain intact at all times.

- Inspect the patient's skin and the sclerae of the eyes for jaundice, and report jaundice or pruritus, *to provide treatment to reduce itching injury to skin.*
- Inspect the cholecystectomy incision for excessive drainage or evidence of infection such as redness, edema, or warmth, *which can irritate and break down skin.*
- Change dressings frequently *to protect the skin around the incision site from irritating drainage.*
- Protect the skin with a skin barrier product or bag such as those used with colostomies if bile is leaking around the T-tube site. An enterostomal therapist (if available) can be consulted for the best choice of dressing. *A skin barrier can protect skin from breakdown due to contact with bile.*

Risk for Ineffective Breathing Pattern Related to Abdominal Incision

EXPECTED OUTCOME: The patient will have effective breathing pattern as evidenced by a respiratory rate of 16 to 20 per minute, even, unlabored, depth within normal limits at all times.

- Monitor respiratory rate, depth, and effort, and ability to cough effectively. *The high abdominal incision can cause pain with deep breathing and coughing.*
- After surgery, encourage the patient to cough and deep breathe at every encounter. Instruct the patient in the proper techniques before surgery and give the opportunity to practice. *Deep breathing and coughing after any surgical procedure helps prevent atelectasis and respiratory tract infections.*

- If the patient is reluctant to cough because of pain, evaluate the pain medication regimen *so pain is controlled.*
- Assist the patient with splinting when coughing *to make coughing less painful.*
- Encourage the patient to walk as soon as able *to help mobilize secretions.*

EVALUATION. The plan of care for a patient with cholecystitis or cholelithiasis is successful if the patient reports pain not greater than 2 on a pain scale of 0 to 10, or pain that is tolerable, no weight loss, excessive thirst, urinary output greater than 50 mL/hour; has moist mucous membranes, elastic skin turgor, intact skin with no warmth, redness, swelling, or purulent drainage at the wound site; no jaundice or itching; clear breath sounds; and a normal white blood cell count. (See Table 35.7.)

PATIENT EDUCATION. Discharge education focuses on diet. Patients are put on high-protein, low-fat diets. Encourage obese patients to lose weight. After a cholecystectomy, fat should be slowly reintroduced into the diet. Once the duodenum becomes accustomed to a constant infusion of bile, the patient's individual tolerance for fat becomes the only restriction for diet.

TABLE 35.7 CHOLECYSTITIS SUMMARY

Signs and Symptoms	Epigastric/RUQ pain, especially after a fatty meal Elevated temperature, pulse, respirations Jaundice if common bile duct blocked
Diagnostic Tests	Ultrasound ERCP Radionuclide scan (HIDA) WBC count elevated
Therapeutic Measures	Pain control Laparoscopic or open cholecystectomy Extracorporeal shock-wave lithotripsy Medications (see Table 35.4) Low-fat diet
Priority Nursing Diagnoses	*Pain* *Risk for Deficient Fluid Volume* *Risk for Ineffective Breathing Pattern* *Risk for Impaired Skin Integrity*

SUGGESTED ANSWERS TO CRITICAL THINKING

■ *Carl Young*

1. Foreign travel within the past 2 months, fatigue, nausea, and irritability suggest hepatitis A virus. Recent possible exposure to materials contaminated with blood or body fluids and fatigue, headache, and nausea suggest hepatitis B virus.
2. Careful hand washing and standard precautions when handling any body fluids or feces should be instituted.
3. The nurse should plan to give an antiemetic if Carl is nauseated. Larger meals should be given early in the day, with Carl in an upright or sitting position. The nurse should also ensure that the environment is free of noxious stimulants such as unpleasant odors. The diet should be high calorie, high protein, high carbohydrate, and low fat.
4. Any medication that is known to be hepatotoxic, such as acetaminophen, aspirin, and diazepam (Valium), should be avoided.
5. Carl should be reminded that cleanliness, especially with food preparation, is essential. He should also be reminded that frequent hand washing is crucial. Carl needs to know that alcohol and other liver-toxic substances should be avoided.

■ *Mrs. Conner*

1. Mrs. Conner has a history of poor nutrition that puts her at risk, as does her age.
2. Mrs. Conner may report that she has malaise, nausea, weight loss, a change in bowel habits, and dull, aching RUQ pain.
3. Serum albumin level may be less than 3.2 g/dL. Her prothrombin time will probably be greater than 25 seconds.
4. Esophageal varices and ascites are the two greatest concerns for the patient with portal hypertension.
5. The physician will usually order diuretics, a sodium-restricted diet, and possibly intravenous albumin infusions.

■ *Mrs. Samuels*

1. The most common cause of acute pancreatitis is excessive alcohol intake. Mrs. Samuels denies alcohol consumption, but she does have the risk factor of having had a recent ERCP, which may have dislodged a gallstone or irritated the pancreatic duct.
2. Respiratory distress may result from excess fluid accumulation in the retroperitoneal space and from shallow respirations that seek to decrease pressure

SUGGESTED ANSWERS TO—cont'd

from the diaphragm on the inflamed pancreas and surrounding tissues.

3. Pancreatitis is similar to a chemical burn and may cause erosion of major blood vessels in surrounding tissue.
4. Serum amylase may be elevated as much as 40 times more than normal early in acute pancreatitis.
5. Opioids are ordered because pain is intense, and pain with anxiety stimulates the autonomic nervous system, which may stimulate greater production of pancreatic enzymes.
6. Stomach acid stimulates the production of pancreatic enzymes. Histamine antagonists decrease stomach acidity.

■ *Donna Stewart*

1. Some low-fat diets have been linked to the development of cholesterol gallstones, which then irritate the gallbladder and cause inflammation.
2. Donna's physician might order a white blood cell count, which will be elevated if she has cholecystitis. In addition, the physician may order an ultrasound or radionuclide scan to visualize the gallbladder and its contents and the common bile duct.
3. Donna is 4 months pregnant. Radionuclide scans should be cleared with her obstetrical care provider before being scheduled.
4. You can anticipate that the physician will order an antibiotic and an analgesic.
5. Donna will need to eat a low-fat diet after discharge. Eventually she may be able to add more fats to her diet as her body adjusts.
6. If the diagnosis is confirmed, Donna will probably have a laparoscopic cholecystectomy unless her surgeon decides that she needs a traditional cholecystectomy.

REVIEW QUESTIONS

1. Which of the following conditions most places a patient with cirrhosis at risk for bleeding?
   a. Encephalopathy
   b. Low vitamin K
   c. Elevated liver enzymes
   d. Hepatorenal syndrome

2. The nurse is caring for a patient with cirrhosis. The nurse would cautiously use sedatives for the patient based on which of the following?
   a. The liver's ability to synthesize protein is altered.
   b. Sedatives may increase the risk of jaundice.
   c. Sedatives are potentially toxic to the cirrhosis patient.
   d. Sedatives promote the conversion of ammonia to ammonium ion.

3. Which clinical manifestations of acute hepatitis A would the nurse expect a patient to report?
   a. Brown urine and anorexia
   b. Malaise, lighter colored stools, and pruritus
   c. Headache, nausea, and flu-like symptoms
   d. Abdominal pain and jaundice

4. The nurse is caring for a patient with chronic pancreatitis. The nurse would expect an elevation in which of the following laboratory tests?
   a. Serum bilirubin
   b. Serum calcium
   c. Serum albumin
   d. Serum amylase

5. A patient with acute pancreatitis is NPO and has been receiving only IV hydration. Which laboratory result indicates the need to consult the dietitian for nutritional support?
   a. Potassium 4.2 mEq/L
   b. Sodium 130 mEq/L
   c. Fasting glucose 82 mg/dL
   d. Serum albumin 2.9 g/dL

6. In planning care for the newly admitted patient with acute pancreatitis, which patient outcome should receive highest priority?
   a. Patient expresses satisfaction with pain control.
   b. Patient verbalizes understanding of medications for home.
   c. Patient increases activity tolerance.
   d. Patient maintains normal bowel function.

REVIEW QUESTIONS—cont'd

7. The nurse is collecting data for a patient who develops jaundice and dark, amber-colored urine. The nurse recognizes that which of the following is most likely the cause?
   a. Encephalopathy
   b. Pancreatitis
   c. Bile duct obstruction
   d. Cholecystitis

8. The nurse reinforces teaching for a patient after a cholecystectomy on a low-fat diet. The nurse will know that the patient understands the diet if which of the following menu items is selected?
   a. Roast chicken, rice, gelatin dessert
   b. Cream of chicken soup, milk, gelatin dessert
   c. Meat loaf, mashed potatoes with small amount of gravy, green beans
   d. Turkey and cheese sandwich on whole-grain bread, apple, milk

9. The nurse is caring for a patient who had an open cholecystectomy 24 hours ago. Which of the following actions should the nurse take to assist the patient to maintain an effective breathing pattern? **Select all that apply**.
   a. Place in a supine position.
   b. Provide analgesics for pain relief.
   c. Encourage coughing and deep breathing.
   d. Monitor bowel sounds.
   e. Assist with splinting during coughing.
   f. Maintain bedrest for 48 hours after surgery.

10. The nurse is to administer promethazine 12.5 mg IM and has 50 mg/mL on hand. How many mL should be drawn up? **Fill in the blank.**

Answer: _____________ mL

References

American Cancer Society. (2009). *Estimated new cancer cases and deaths by sex, United States, 2009*. Retrieved May 29, 2009, from http://www.cancer.org/docroot/MED/content/downloads/MED_1_1x_CFF2004_page10.asp

Centers for Disease Control and Prevention. (2009). *Viral hepatitis*. Retrieved November 23, 2009, from http://www.cdc.gov/ncidod/diseases/hepatitis/resource/dz_burden02.htm

Heron, M., Hoyert, D., Murphy, S., et al. (2009). Deaths: Final data for 2006. *National Vital Statistics Reports*, 57(14). Hyattsville, MD: National Center for Health Statistics. Retrieved June 23, 2009, from http://www.cdc.gov/nchs/data/nvsr/nvsr57/nvsr57_14.pdf

Joint Commission. (2010). *2010 national patient safety goals*. Retrieved January 13, 2010, from http://www.jointcommission.org/patientsafety/nationalpatientsafetygoals

Raimondo, M., & Scolapio, J. S. (2006). Nutrition in pancreatic disorders. In M. E. Shils et al. (Eds.). *Modern nutrition in health and disease* (10th ed.). Philadelphia: Lippincott Williams & Wilkins.

unit NINE

UNDERSTANDING THE URINARY SYSTEM

36 Urinary System Function, Assessment, and Therapeutic Measures

MAUREEN McDONALD
AND JANICE L. BRADFORD

KEY TERMS

cystoscopy (sist-TAW-skuh-pee)
dysuria (diss-YOO-ree-ah)
hematuria (HEE-muh-TOOR-ee-ah)
incontinence (inn-CON-tin-ense)
nephrotoxic (NEF-row-TOCKS-sick)
nocturia (knock-TOO-ree-ah)
percutaneous (PURR-kyoo-TAY-nee-us)
pyelogram (PIE-eh-loh-gram)
uremia (yoo-REE-mee-ah)
pinocytosis (PIE-noh-sye-TOE-siss)

QUESTIONS TO GUIDE YOUR READING

1. What is the normal anatomy of the urinary system?
2. What is the normal function of the urinary system?
3. What are the effects of aging on the urinary system?
4. What data should you collect when caring for a patient with a disorder of the urinary system?
5. How do you collect a midstream, clean-catch urine specimen and 24-hour creatinine clearance specimen?
6. What is the preparation and postprocedure care for diagnostic tests of the urinary system?
7. What nursing care is given for patients with incontinence?
8. Which nursing actions can be taken to decrease the risk of infection in catheterized patients?

NORMAL URINARY SYSTEM ANATOMY AND PHYSIOLOGY

The urinary system consists of two kidneys, two ureters, the urinary bladder, and the urethra. The kidneys form urine, and the rest of the system eliminates urine. The purpose of urine formation is the removal of potentially toxic waste products from the blood; however, the kidneys have other equally important functions as well:

- Regulation of the blood volume, composition, and pressure by the excretion or conservation of water
- Regulation of the electrolyte balance of the blood by the excretion or conservation of minerals
- Regulation of the acid-base balance of the blood by the excretion or conservation of ions such as hydrogen or bicarbonate
- Regulation of all of the above in tissue fluid
- Production of erythropoietin, which then stimulates erythrocyte production in the bone marrow
- Activation of vitamin D.

The process of urine formation thus helps maintain the normal composition, volume, and pH of blood and tissue fluid.

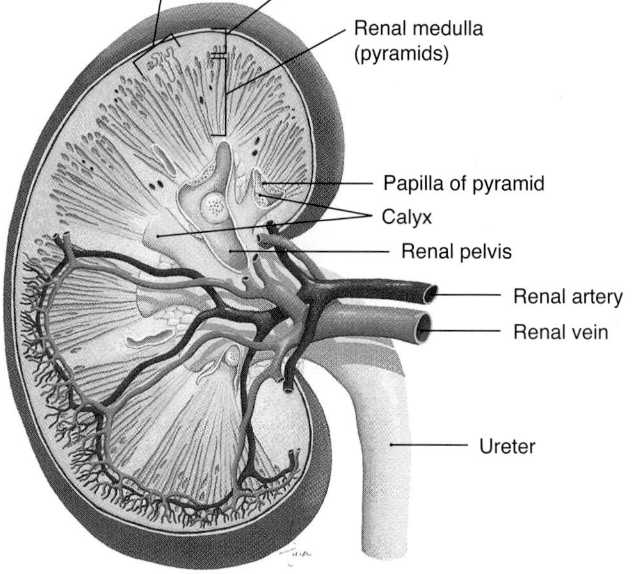
Nephron
Renal cortex
Renal medulla
(pyramids)
Papilla of pyramid
Calyx
Renal pelvis
Renal artery
Renal vein
Ureter

FIGURE 36.1 Frontal section of the right kidney. (From Scanlon, V., & Sanders, T. [2007]. *Essentials of anatomy and physiology* [5th ed., p. 422]. Philadelphia: F. A. Davis, with permission.)

Kidneys

The two kidneys are located in the upper abdominal cavity behind the peritoneum on each side of the vertebral column. The upper portions of both kidneys rest on the lower surface of the diaphragm and are enclosed and protected by the lower rib cage. The kidneys are cushioned by surrounding adipose tissue, which is in turn covered by a fibrous connective membrane called the renal fascia; both help hold the kidneys in place. On the medial side of each kidney is an indentation called the hilus, where the renal artery enters and the renal vein and ureter emerge. The renal artery is a branch of the abdominal aorta, and the renal vein returns blood to the inferior vena cava. The ureter carries urine from the kidney to the urinary bladder.

Internal Structure of the Kidney

A frontal section of the kidney shows three distinct areas (Fig. 36.1). The outermost area is the renal cortex, which contains the parts of the nephrons called renal corpuscles and convoluted tubules. The middle area is the renal medulla, which contains loops of Henle and collecting tubules. The renal medulla consists of wedge-shaped pieces called renal pyramids; the apex, or papilla, of each pyramid points medially. The third area is a cavity called the renal pelvis; it is formed by the expansion of the ureter within the kidney at the hilus. Funnel-shaped extensions of the renal pelvis, called calyces, enclose the papillae of the renal pyramids. Urine flows from the pyramids into the calyces, then to the renal pelvis, and finally into the ureter.

Nephron

The nephron is the structural and functional unit of the kidney. Urine is formed in the approximately 1 million nephrons in each kidney. The two major parts of a nephron are the renal corpuscle and the renal tubule; these and their subdivisions and blood vessels are shown in Figure 36.2.

A renal corpuscle consists of a glomerulus surrounded by a Bowman's (glomerular) capsule. The glomerulus is a capillary network that arises from an afferent arteriole and empties into an efferent arteriole. The diameter of the efferent arteriole is smaller than that of the afferent arteriole, which helps maintain a fairly high blood pressure in the glomerulus. Bowman's capsule is the expanded end of a renal tubule; it encloses the glomerulus. The inner layer of Bowman's capsule has pores and is highly permeable; the outer layer has no pores and is not permeable. The space between the inner and outer layers contains renal filtrate, the fluid that is formed from the blood in the glomerulus and that will eventually become urine.

The renal tubule continues from Bowman's capsule and consists of the proximal convoluted tubule, the loop of Henle, and the distal convoluted tubule. The distal convoluted tubules from several nephrons empty into a collecting tubule. Several collecting tubules then unite to form a papillary duct that empties urine into a calyx of the renal pelvis. All parts of the renal tubule are surrounded by the peritubular capillaries, which arise from the efferent arteriole and receive the materials reabsorbed by the renal tubules.

Blood Vessels of the Kidney

The pathway of blood flow through the kidney is an essential part of the process of urine formation. Blood from the abdominal aorta enters the renal artery, which branches extensively within the kidney into smaller arteries. The smallest arteries give rise to afferent arterioles in the renal cortex.

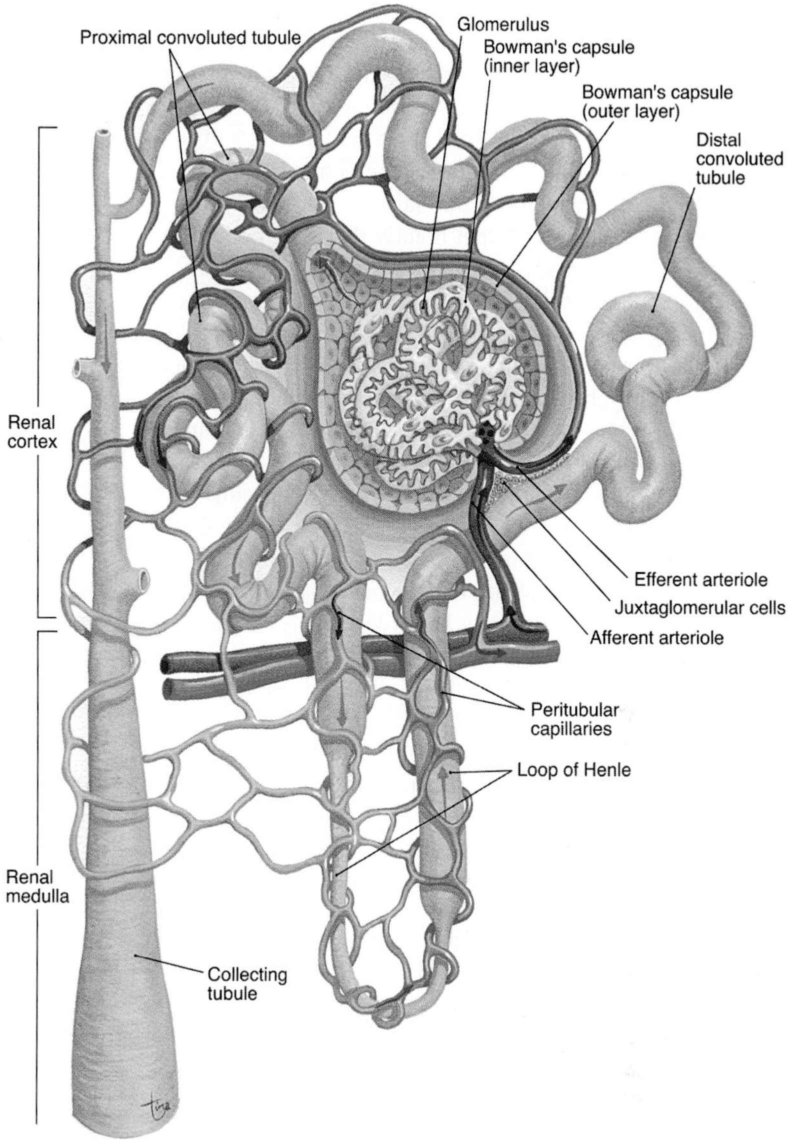
Proximal convoluted tubule
Glomerulus
Bowman's capsule (inner layer)
Bowman's capsule (outer layer)
Distal convoluted tubule
Renal cortex
Efferent arteriole
Juxtaglomerular cells
Afferent arteriole
Peritubular capillaries
Loop of Henle
Renal medulla
Collecting tubule

FIGURE 36.2 A nephron and its associated blood vessels. (From Scanlon, V., & Sanders, T. [2007]. *Essentials of anatomy and physiology* [5th ed., p. 423]. Philadelphia: F. A. Davis, with permission.)

From the afferent arterioles, blood flows into the glomeruli (capillaries), to efferent arterioles, to peritubular capillaries, to veins in the kidney, to the renal vein, and finally to the inferior vena cava. In this pathway are two sets of capillaries; that is, two sites of exchanges between the blood and the surrounding tissues (in this case, the parts of the nephrons). The exchanges that take place in the capillaries of the kidneys form urine from blood plasma.

Formation of Urine

The formation of urine involves three major processes: glomerular filtration in the renal corpuscles, tubular reabsorption, and tubular secretion.

Glomerular Filtration

Filtration is the process by which blood pressure forces plasma and dissolved materials out of capillaries. In glomerular filtration, blood pressure forces plasma, dissolved substances, and small proteins out of the glomeruli and into Bowman's capsules. This fluid is then called renal filtrate.

The blood pressure in the glomeruli is relatively high—about 55 mm Hg. With opposing pressures, a net filtration pressure of 10 mm Hg results. Still, the capsule is permeable, so that about 20% of the blood that enters glomeruli becomes renal filtrate. The larger proteins and blood cells are too large to be forced out of the glomeruli, so they stay in the blood. Waste products such as urea and ammonia are dissolved in plasma, so they pass to the renal filtrate, as do dissolved nutrients and minerals. Renal filtrate is similar to blood plasma except it has far less protein and no blood cells.

The glomerular filtration rate (GFR) is the amount of renal filtrate formed by the kidneys in 1 minute. It averages 105 to 125 mL/min. The GFR may change if the rate of blood flow through the kidney changes. If blood flow increases, GFR increases, more filtrate is formed, and urinary output increases. If blood flow decreases, GFR decreases, less filtrate is formed, and urinary output decreases.

Tubular Reabsorption

Tubular reabsorption is the recovery of useful materials from the renal filtrate and their return to the blood in the peritubular capillaries. About 99% of the renal filtrate's water is reabsorbed, and normal urine output is 1000 to 2000 mL per 24 hours. The largest percentage of reabsorption takes place in the proximal convoluted tubules, whose cells have microvilli that greatly increase their surface area. The mechanisms of reabsorption are active transport, osmosis, diffusion, facilitated diffusion, and **pinocytosis**.

Active transport requires energy either in the form of adenosine triphosphate (ATP) or from stored energy provided in concentration gradients. The cells of the renal tubule use energy to transport useful materials such as glucose, amino acids, vitamins, and ions back to the blood. Many of these substances have a threshold level of reabsorption—that is, a limit to how much the renal tubules can remove from the filtrate. The level of a substance in the renal filtrate is directly related to its blood level. If the blood level of a substance such as glucose is normal, the filtrate level is normal, the threshold level cannot be exceeded, and no glucose appears in the urine.

The reabsorption of water by osmosis follows the reabsorption of minerals, especially sodium. The conservation of water is very important to maintain normal blood volume and blood pressure. The hormones that influence the reabsorption of water or minerals are summarized in Table 36.1.

Simple diffusion is a passive transport mechanism whereby small solutes move down their concentration gradient through the phospholipid bilayer of the cell membrane. Facilitated diffusion involves a membrane protein that assists in diffusion to transport solutes that are either highly polar or charged.

TABLE 36.1 EFFECTS OF HORMONES ON THE KIDNEYS

Hormone (Gland)	Function
Aldosterone (adrenal cortex)	Promotes reabsorption of sodium ions from the filtrate to the blood and excretion of potassium ions into the filtrate. Water is reabsorbed following the reabsorption of sodium.
Antidiuretic hormone (posterior pituitary)	Promotes reabsorption of water from the filtrate to the blood.
Atrial natriuretic hormone (atria of heart)	Decreases reabsorption of sodium ions, which remain in the filtrate. More sodium and water are eliminated in urine.
Parathyroid hormone (parathyroid glands)	Promotes reabsorption of calcium ions from filtrate to blood and excretion of phosphate ions into filtrate.

Source: Scanlon, V., & Sanders, T. (2007). *Essentials of anatomy and physiology* (5th ed., p. 428). Philadelphia: F. A. Davis, with permission.

Small proteins in the filtrate are reabsorbed by pinocytosis. The proteins become attached to the membranes of the tubule cells and are engulfed and digested. Normally, all proteins in the filtrate are reabsorbed and none are found in urine.

Tubular Secretion

In tubular secretion, substances are actively secreted from the blood in the peritubular capillaries into the filtrate in the renal tubules. Waste products, such as ammonium ion and creatinine, excess water-soluble vitamins, some potassium ions, and the metabolic products of medications may be secreted into the filtrate to be eliminated in urine. Hydrogen ions may be secreted by the tubule cells to help maintain the normal pH of the blood.

In summary, tubular reabsorption conserves useful materials, tubular secretion may add unwanted substances to the filtrate, and most waste products simply remain in the filtrate and are excreted in urine.

The Kidneys and Acid-Base Balance

Other than exhalation of carbon dioxide by the respiratory system, the kidneys are the organs most responsible for maintaining the normal pH range of blood and tissue fluid. They have the greatest ability to compensate for or correct the pH changes that are part of normal body metabolism or the result of disease.

At its simplest, this function of the kidneys may be described as follows. If body fluids are becoming too acidic, the kidneys secrete more hydrogen ions into the renal filtrate and return more bicarbonate ions back to the blood. This helps raise the pH of the blood back to normal. In the opposite situation, when body fluids become too alkaline, the kidneys return hydrogen ions to the blood and excrete bicarbonate ions in urine. This helps lower the pH of the blood back to normal.

Other Functions of the Kidneys

The kidney has some additional functions that are not related to the formation of urine and maintaining acid-base balance. These include the secretion of renin, activation of vitamin D, and production of erythropoietin. The production of renin does influence urine formation and is considered first.

When blood pressure decreases, the juxtaglomerular cells in the walls of the afferent arterioles secrete the enzyme renin. Renin then initiates the renin-angiotensin-aldosterone mechanism, which results in the formation of angiotensin II. Angiotensin II stimulates vasoconstriction and increases the secretion of aldosterone, both of which help raise blood pressure.

Vitamin D exists in several structural forms, which are converted to calcitriol, the most active form, by the kidneys. Vitamin D is important for the efficient absorption of calcium and phosphate from food in the small intestine.

Erythropoietin is a hormone secreted by the kidneys during states of hypoxia; it stimulates the red bone marrow to increase the rate of red blood cell (RBC) production. With more RBCs in circulation, the oxygen-carrying capacity of the blood is greater and the hypoxic state may be corrected.

Elimination of Urine

The ureters, urinary bladder, and urethra do not change the composition or volume of urine but are responsible for its elimination.

Ureters

The ureters are behind the peritoneum of the dorsal abdominal cavity. Each ureter extends from the hilus of a kidney to the lower, posterior side of the urinary bladder. The smooth muscle in the wall of the ureter contracts in peristaltic waves to propel urine toward the urinary bladder. As the bladder fills, it expands and compresses the lower ends of the ureters to prevent backflow of urine.

Urinary Bladder

The urinary bladder is a muscular sac inside the peritoneum and behind the pubic bones. In women, the bladder is inferior to the uterus; in men, the bladder is superior to the prostate gland. The functions of the bladder are the temporary storage of urine and its elimination.

Urethra

The urethra carries urine from the bladder to the exterior. Within its wall, near the bladder, is an involuntary, internal urethral sphincter. Inferior to that is the external urethral sphincter, which is made of skeletal muscle and is under voluntary control.

In women, the urethra is 1.0 to 1.5 inches long and is anterior to the vagina. In men, the urethra is 7 to 8 inches long and extends through the prostate gland and penis. The male urethra carries semen as well as urine.

Urination Reflex

Urination (micturition) is a spinal cord reflex over which voluntary control may be exerted. The stimulus is the stretching of the detrusor muscle as urine accumulates in the bladder. Sensory impulses travel to the sacral spinal cord, and motor impulses return along parasympathetic nerves to the detrusor muscle, causing contraction. At the same time, the internal urethral sphincter relaxes. If the external urethral sphincter is voluntarily relaxed, urine flows into the urethra and the bladder is emptied.

Characteristics of Urine

Amount

Normal urinary output is 1000 to 2000 mL per 24 hours. Any changes in fluid intake or other fluid output (such as sweating) change this volume.

Color

The color of urine is often referred to as straw or amber. Dilute urine is a lighter color (straw) than is concentrated urine. Freshly voided urine is clear. Cloudy urine may indicate an infection.

Specific Gravity

Specific gravity is a measure of the dissolved materials in urine. The specific gravity of urine is 1.002 to 1.035. (The specific gravity of distilled water is 1.000.) The higher the specific gravity, the more dissolved material is present. Specific gravity of urine is a measure of the concentrating ability of the kidneys. They must excrete the waste products that are constantly formed in as little water as possible.

pH

The pH range of urine is 4.6 to 8.0, with an average of 6.0. Diet has the greatest influence on urine pH. A vegetarian diet results in more alkaline urine; a high-protein diet results in more acidic urine.

Constituents

Urine is about 95% water, which is the solvent for waste products and salts. Nitrogenous wastes include urea, creatinine, and uric acid. Urea is formed by liver cells when excess amino acids are deaminated (metabolized) to be used for energy production. Creatinine comes from the metabolism of creatine phosphate, an energy source in muscles. Uric acid comes from the metabolism of nucleic acids—that is, the breakdown of DNA and RNA. Other solutes, such as enzymes and hormones, are present in small quantities.

Aging and the Urinary System

With age, the number of nephrons in the kidneys decreases, often to half the original number by age 70 or 80 (Fig. 36.3). The GFR also decreases. This results in part from arteriosclerosis and diminished renal blood flow. The urinary bladder decreases in size, and the tone of the detrusor muscle decreases. This may result in the need to urinate more often or in residual urine in the bladder after voiding. Elderly people are also more subject to infections of the urinary tract, and the changes of aging may influence medication therapy for elderly people (Box 36.1, *Gerontological Issues*).

NURSING ASSESSMENT OF THE URINARY SYSTEM

Health History

Table 36.2 describes questions to ask for a health history. Any symptoms should be further assessed using the WHAT'S UP? format found in Chapter 1.

If the patient has impaired kidney function or is in kidney failure, a complete head-to-toe assessment is needed because urinary disease and kidney failure (renal failure) affect every system of the body (see Chapter 37).

Physical Examination

Table 36.2 lists objective data that should be collected. The nurse first inspects the skin for color, texture, edema, or swelling. A patient with chronic renal failure may have a yellow or gray cast to the skin. The presence of crystals on the skin is called uremic frost and is a late sign of waste

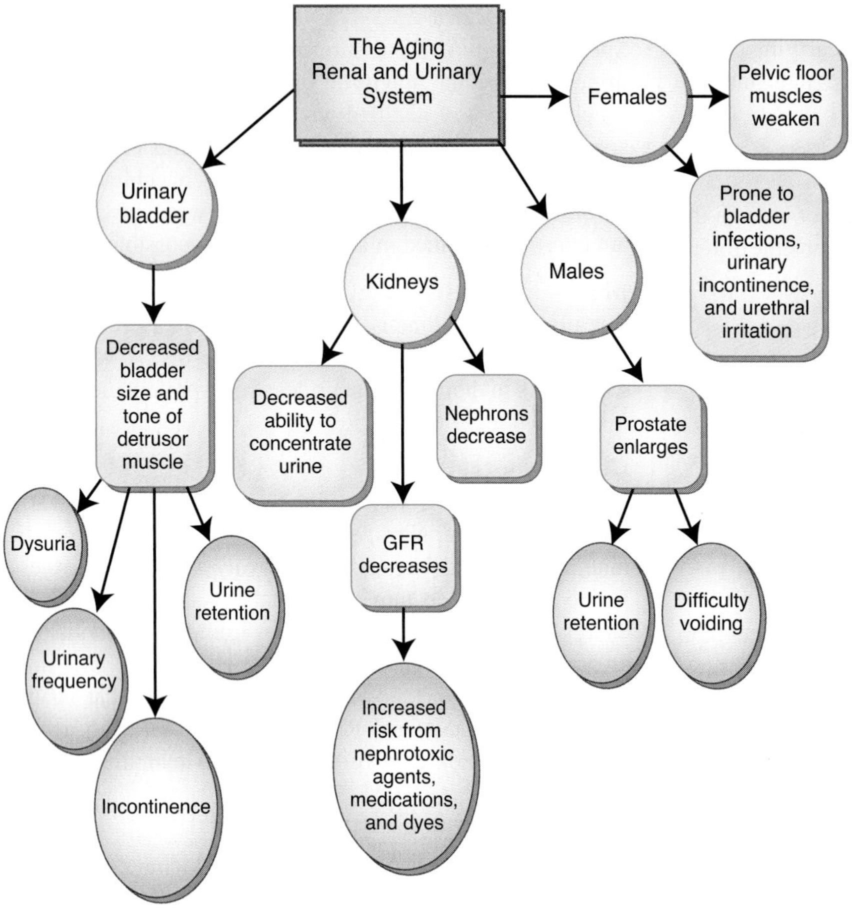
The Aging Renal and Urinary System
Urinary bladder
Kidneys
Males
Females
Pelvic floor muscles weaken
Prone to bladder infections, urinary incontinence, and urethral irritation
Decreased bladder size and tone of detrusor muscle
Decreased ability to concentrate urine
Nephrons decrease
Prostate enlarges
Dysuria
Urine retention
GFR decreases
Urine retention
Difficulty voiding
Urinary frequency
Incontinence
Increased risk from nephrotoxic agents, medications, and dyes

FIGURE 36.3 Aging and the urinary system. This concept map shows effects of the aging process on the urinary system.

Box 36.1

Gerontological Issues

Age-Related Renal Changes

Certain changes typically occur in the renal system as people age. They include the following:

- The renal mass becomes smaller.
- Renal flow decreases by 50%, with subsequent decreased glomerular filtration rate.
- Tubular function and the exchange of substances decrease.
- Bladder muscles weaken and bladder capacity decreases, leading to increased frequency and **nocturia** (awakening from sleep at night to urinate).
- The voiding reflex is delayed.

Also, keep in mind that most drugs are excreted through the kidneys. Consequently, dehydration—which the older adult is prone to having—and changes in renal function become a serious consideration for older adults who need drug therapy. Decreased renal function could slow the excretion of some drugs, keeping them in the body longer. This can increase the risk of adverse drug reactions, such as toxicity and overdose. It is important to monitor kidney function (such as creatinine and blood urea nitrogen levels) in an older person receiving drug therapy.

products building up in the blood (**uremia**). When the waste products are not filtered by the kidneys or with treatment, they can come out through the skin and look like a coating of frost.

• WORD • BUILDING •

nocturia: nox—night + uria—urine
uremia: ur—urine + emia—blood

Assess for difficulty with cognition, mobility, or manual dexterity. Problems in these areas may be reflected in the ability to toilet self.

Most assessment of the urinary system is done using indirect measures. Assessment of vital signs, lung sounds, edema, daily weights, characteristics of the urine, and intake and output can provide valuable data related to urinary function. The nurse often collects urine specimens for analysis.

TABLE 36.2 DATA COLLECTION FOR THE URINARY SYSTEM

Health History

Category	Questions to Ask	Rationale/Significance
Age	How old are you?	Aging is associated with a gradual loss of nephrons and decreased urine-concentrating ability and bladder capacity.
Gender	Male or female?	Men are at risk for prostate problems. Women have a high incidence of incontinence.
Ethnicity	What is your ethnic origin?	African American men over age 40 have a higher incidence of prostate and bladder cancer; those between ages 25 and 35 have an increased incidence of testicular cancer.
	Do you prefer to speak in a language other than English?	Language barriers may exist for gathering data.
Occupation	What type of work do you do?	Renal cancers may occur with occupational exposure to nephrotoxic chemicals, such as phenol and ethylene glycol.
	Have you had any exposure to chemicals in your present or past jobs or hobbies?	Some occupations and hobbies are related to a higher incidence of bladder tumors.
	Has your job affected your health, if so how?	Stress may predispose to hypertension and cardiovascular disease.
Health habits	Do you use alcohol, caffeine, tobacco, or recreational drugs?	Alcohol can irritate the bladder and increase urinary output. Tobacco use increases risk of renal cancer.
Medical history	Have you been diagnosed with any of the following: • Beta-hemolytic streptococci • Cancer • Diabetes • Glomerulonephritis • Gout • Heart disease • Hyperlipidemia • Hypertension • Lupus erythematosus • Polycystic kidney disease • Renal stones • Sickle cell disease • Systemic infections • Urinary tract infection	Diabetes is the most common cause of chronic kidney disease worldwide, and hypertension is a significant risk factor. Systemic diseases such as gout, lupus, sickle cell disease, coronary artery disease, and atherosclerosis increase the risk of renal disease. Streptococcal infection may precede renal disease.
	Do you have any history of falls, motor vehicle accidents, or other trauma?	Risk of renal damage secondary to infection, abscess formation, and strictures.
	How many children do you have?	Increased parity may affect pelvic floor muscles, which can lead to stress incontinence.
Family history of urinary disorders	Is there a family history of hypertension, diabetes, kidney stones, polycystic kidney disease, or other kidney or urinary problems?	Hereditary tendency for some renal conditions.
Current medications, over-the-counter medications, or herb use	What prescription or over-the-counter medications are you taking?	Nephrotoxic drugs increase risk for renal failure.
	What herbs or minerals are you taking?	Herbs with aristolochic acid may be renal toxic.
	Do you have any allergies to antibiotics, contrast media, or dyes?	Allergies and contrast media can lead to renal disease.

Continued

TABLE 36.2 DATA COLLECTION FOR THE URINARY SYSTEM—cont'd

Category	Questions to Ask	Rationale/Significance
Renal/urinary problems	Have you experienced any of the following?: • Pain, burning with urination • Blood in urine • Use of urinary catheter • Kidney or bladder surgery	Painful voiding may indicate an infection. **Hematuria** may indicate an infection or cancer.
	Have you noticed changes in your urination patterns?: • Urgency, frequency • Difficulty starting stream of urine • Nocturia • Incontinence	Urgency with diminished amounts of urine suggests urinary retention. Difficulty starting urination may indicate a prostate obstruction. Nocturia occurs with nephrotic syndrome, diabetes, heart failure.
	Have you had changes in the color, odor, clarity, or amount of urine?	Cloudy urine or foul odor indicates possible infection; decreased amount may indicate renal disease; increased amount may indicate diabetes or inability to concentrate urine.
	Have you had any pain in the costovertebral angle (the area formed by the rib cage and the vertebral column)?	Renal calculus (stone) may produce dull ache in kidney area or colicky pain radiating to genital area or leg on affected side.
	Have you noticed any swelling of your lower legs or around your eyes in the morning?	Edema occurs with fluid retention; periorbital edema is noted around the eyes in the morning.
New onset of symptoms	Have you noticed any of the following symptoms?: • Fatigue • Shortness of breath • Fever or chills • Nausea, vomiting, anorexia • Blurred vision • Headache • Lethargy • Confusion • Itchy skin • Metallic taste • Bone or joint problems	Fatigue and shortness of breath may be from anemia because erythropoietin is produced in the kidney. Fever occurs with urinary tract infections. Uremic toxins may produce many symptoms in multiple body systems. Metallic taste may be due to electrolyte imbalances. Bone and joint problems may be due to problems with calcium and vitamin D metabolism.
	Have you had pain in your back, lower abdomen, or perineum? Pain over the bladder? Leg pain?	May indicate infection, obstruction, or inflammation of the urinary system. Kidney pain: dull, aching, steady, flank area. Ureteral pain begins in the costovertebral angle radiating into lower abdomen and groin. Bladder pain felt over symphysis pubis. Back or leg pain may be due to prostrate or metastasis of cancer.
Diet and fluid intake	Describe your appetite, fluid intake, and nutritional status. Have you noticed any changes in weight over the last year? Are you able to shop and cook for yourself?	Anorexia occurs with renal disease. Large intake of protein or dairy products may lead to kidney stone formation. The person who is obese is at greater risk for renal ischemia from fluid losses and dehydration. Inability to take care of shopping and cooking can have a direct effect on diet.
Objective Assessment		
Category	**Possible Abnormal Findings**	**Possible Causes**
Vital signs: • Blood pressure	Hypertension	Hypertension is related to renal disease and fluid volume overload.
• Pulse	Orthostatic hypotension	Orthostatic hypotension may be due to dehydration.
• Respiratory rate	Irregular heart rate	Hyperkalemia causes arrhythmias.
• Temperature	Fever	Infection elevates temperature.

• WORD • BUILDING •

hematuria: hemat—blood + uria—urine

TABLE 36.2 DATA COLLECTION FOR THE URINARY SYSTEM—cont'd

Category	Possible Abnormal Findings	Possible Causes
Cognitive function and neurologic status	Confusion Lethargy Insomnia	Changes in level of consciousness may be due to changes in electrolytes and fluid balance.
	Diminished deep tendon reflexes Hyperesthesia Paresthesias Peripheral neuropathy	Increased levels of altered fluid balance, urea, creatinine, ammonia levels, and parathyroid hormone may interfere with nerve function and contribute to neuropathies.
Skin, hair, and nail assessment	Skin pallor, color, yellow gray cast	Pallor may be due to anemia.
	Dry skin Excoriations	Scratching from dry skin, pruritus may lead to excoriations.
	Changes in turgor	Dehydration is associated with oliguria.
	Bruising	Thrombocytopenia.
	Distal portion of nailbeds white	Distal portion of nailbeds turn white with renal failure.
	Capillary refill less than 3 seconds	Increased capillary refill may result from poor blood flow to the extremity or anemia.
	Impetigo—a streptococcal infection of the skin	Streptococcal infections may precede glomerulonephritis.
Eyes	Conjunctival pallor	Anemia
	Corneal calcification	Corneal calcification results from phosphate retention
	Retinal arteriosclerotic changes	Retinal changes in blood vessels result from prolonged hypertension or diabetes.
	Blurred vision	Retinitis pigmentosa may accompany hereditary nephropathies.
Ears, nose, and throat	Deafness	High-frequency deafness may accompany hereditary nephritis.
	Strep throat	Acute glomerulonephritis may be accompanied by pharyngitis or group A beta-hemolytic streptococcal infections.
Cardiovascular	Hypertension	Causes renal disease; can result from alterations of sodium and renal secretion of vasoconstrictors.
	Friction rub	Friction rub may occur with uremia.
	Cardiac enlargement of the left ventricle	Occurs from hypertension, increased fluid volume.
	Angina or chest pain	Angina may occur from chronic anemia.
	Distended neck veins, pericardial effusion, heart failure, pulmonary edema	Results from increased fluid volume.
	Dysrhythmias	Dysrhythmias may occur as a result of imbalances of potassium, magnesium, and calcium.
	Edema	Edema occurs from decreased serum albumin.
Respiratory	Shortness of breath Tachypnea Rales	Shortness of breath, tachypnea, and rales result from fluid volume overload.
	Acid-base disturbances Kussmaul's respirations	Metabolic acidosis occurs early in renal disease and causes Kussmaul's respirations.
Hematologic	Anemia Bruising	Result from decreased erythropoietin production in the kidneys.
	Bleeding tendencies	All blood cells are defective in renal disease.
Gastrointestinal	Weight changes Malnutrition	Nausea and changes in taste may lead to diminished appetite.
	Gastroparesis Gastritis	Metabolic and hormonal changes in renal disease lead to GI upset, malnutrition, and decreased nutrient intake.
	Metallic taste Foul urine odor to breath	Urea buildup causes metallic taste in the mouth or foul breath odor.
	Constipation Diarrhea	Alterations in elimination occur with renal disease.
Genitourinary	Nocturia	Kidneys lose concentrating ability.
	Hematuria	Blood in the urine may indicate urinary infection, irritation, obstruction, or cancer.

Continued

TABLE 36.2 DATA COLLECTION FOR THE URINARY SYSTEM—cont'd

Category	Possible Abnormal Findings	Possible Causes
	Dysuria	Dysuria is a sign of urinary tract infection or interstitial cystitis.
	Anuria	Less than 100 mL of urine in 24 hours seen in acute renal disease, end-stage renal disease, bilateral ureteral obstruction.
	Oliguria	Urine output of 100–400 mL in 24 hours with severe dehydration, shock, transfusion reactions, end-stage renal disease.
	Polyuria	Occurs with diabetes, diabetes insipidus, and chronic renal failure.
	Interrupted urine stream, dribbling, urine retention	Urine flow difficulty may be due to prostate problems.
	Incontinence	Incontinence may be a sign of urological disorders or neurologic disease.
	Cloudy urine, foul odor	Cloudy, foul-smelling urine may indicate a urinary tract infection.
	Perineal pain	Occurs with infection, foreign body in urinary tract, urethritis, pyelonephritis, and renal colic or stone.
Musculoskeletal	Muscle weakness Bone and joint problems Gait disturbances Osteoporosis Fractures	Vitamin D synthesis decreases with the increase of parathyroid hormone causing changes in the calcium-phosphorus ratio and hyperparathyroidism. Bone and mineral disease occurs from low calcium level, high phosphorus level, and inability to activate vitamin D.
Endocrine system	Hypertension	Renin produced in the kidney activates angiotensin II, which is a potent vasoconstrictor that elevates blood pressure.
	Hyperglycemia	Renal disease inhibits kidney's ability to break down insulin.

Vital Signs

If renal disease is suspected, blood pressure should be assessed and documented while the patient is lying, sitting, and standing. An increase in blood pressure is common with renal disease. A drop in blood pressure accompanied by a rise in pulse rate as the patient rises to a sitting or standing position is called orthostatic, or postural, hypotension and may indicate fluid deficit (see Chapter 21). A rapid respiratory rate may indicate fluid retention in the lungs.

Lung Sounds

If the patient retains more fluid than the heart can effectively pump, fluid may build up in the lungs. This is manifested as crackles (popping sounds heard on inspiration and sometimes on expiration). Wheezes may also be present. New-onset crackles and wheezes should be reported to a physician (see Chapter 29).

Edema

Fluid retention may be manifested as edema (excess fluid in tissues). The nurse assesses and documents the degree and location of edema (see Chapter 21). Edema may be generalized in renal disease.

Daily Weights

Weight is the single best indicator of fluid balance in the body. Patients with renal disease often have fluid imbalances. The patient should be weighed at the same time each day, in the same or similar clothing, and with the same scale. The nurse looks for trends in weight gain or loss. If the patient's weight is steadily increasing, fluid retention is suspected and should be reported. A patient undergoing diuresis is expected to have decreasing weight.

Intake and Output

The intake and output of all patients with renal disease should be carefully measured with each voiding. The nurse measures and records all liquids taken in, including oral, intravenous, irrigation, tube feeding, and other fluids. Output includes urine, emesis, nasogastric effluent, wound drainage if it is copious, and any other drainage.

Intake and output totals are analyzed and recorded every 8 or 12 hours or more often for unstable patients. As with daily weights, the nurse notes trends in retention or loss of fluid to report to the physician. Accurate documentation is vital because the physician may base medication and intravenous fluid orders on intake and output results.

CRITICAL THINKING

Mr. Nolan

■ It is the end of the shift. As you empty Mr. Nolan's indwelling catheter bag, you find that it has only 50 mL of concentrated urine in it. What do you do?
Suggested answers at end of chapter.

DIAGNOSTIC TESTS FOR THE URINARY SYSTEM

Laboratory Tests

Urine Tests

URINALYSIS. A urinalysis (urine analysis) is a commonly performed diagnostic test for the renal system. Urinalysis is an invaluable tool in the diagnosis of kidney disease and other systemic diseases that may affect the kidneys. The results of the urinalysis give information regarding kidney function and various body functions. Table 36.3 lists normal and abnormal findings on a urinalysis.

A routine urinalysis specimen may be collected at any time of day; however, the first morning specimen is best. First morning specimens are usually concentrated and more likely to contain abnormal constituents if they are present. The specimen should be examined within 1 hour of collection. Urine that cannot be examined promptly should be refrigerated. Urine standing at room temperature longer than 2 hours has more bacteria present, changes in pH, and hemolysis of RBCs. Urine collected for cytology should not be a first morning specimen due to changes in epithelial cells in urine held overnight. Random specimens are used for cytology.

If an order is written to collect a midstream, clean-catch urine specimen for urinalysis, the nurse has the patient wash the perineum using soap and water or a special towelette from a midstream, clean-catch urine collection kit. Women should be directed to wash from the front to the back of the perineum. They are told to separate the labia with one hand and keep them separated while washing and collecting the specimen to decrease the risk of contaminating the specimen. The patient is instructed to start urinating into the toilet, then move the collection container under the urine stream, and then finish urinating into the toilet. If the female patient is menstruating, this should be specified on the laboratory form. A tampon may be used to

TABLE 36.3 URINALYSIS RESULTS

Test	Normal Results	Significance of Abnormal Results
Color of urine	Pale yellow to amber	Dark-amber urine suggests dehydration. Yellow-brown to green urine indicates excessive bilirubin. Dark, smoky color suggests hematuria. Orange-red or orange-brown color caused by phenazopyridine (Pyridium). Cloudiness of freshly voided urine indicates infection. Nearly colorless urine is seen with a large fluid intake, renal disease, or diabetes insipidus.
Odor of urine	Aromatic	With infection, urine becomes foul smelling. In diabetic ketoacidosis, urine has a fruity odor. Urine that has been standing for a while develops a strong ammonia smell.
pH	4.6–8.0	pH is greatly affected by food eaten. pH below 4.6 is seen with metabolic and respiratory acidosis. pH above 8.0 is seen when urine has been standing or with infection because bacteria decompose urea to form ammonia.
Specific gravity	1.002–1.035	Low specific gravity indicates excessive fluid intake or diabetes insipidus. High specific gravity is seen with dehydration. Specific gravity fixed at 1.010 indicates kidney dysfunction. The specific gravity of glomerular filtrate is 1.010.
Protein	0–18 mg/dL 0–150 mg/24 hr	Persistent proteinuria is seen with renal disease from damage to the glomerulus. As a general rule, protein in the urine is a significant sign of renal problems. Intermittent protein in urine can result from strenuous exercise, dehydration, or fever. Vaginal secretions may contaminate urine and give a positive reading.
Glucose	None	Glucose in urine indicates diabetes mellitus, excessive glucose intake, or low renal threshold for glucose reabsorption.
Ketones	None	Ketones in urine indicate diabetes mellitus with ketonuria or starvation from breakdown of body fats into ketones. Can also be seen with carbohydrate-free diets, severe diarrhea, dehydration, and vomiting.

Continued

TABLE 36.3 URINALYSIS RESULTS—cont'd

Test	Normal Results	Significance of Abnormal Results
Bilirubin	None	Bilirubin in urine indicates liver disorders causing jaundice. Bilirubin may appear in the urine before jaundice is visible.
Nitrite	Negative	Nitrites in urine indicate infection. Bacteria in urine convert nitrate to nitrite, which gives a positive reading.
Leukocyte esterase	Negative	Positive leukocyte esterase in urine indicates infection in urine. It determines the presence of an enzyme released by WBCs in the urine.
Red blood cells	0–4/hpf	Blood in urine may be caused by kidney stones, infection, cancer, renal disease, or trauma.
White blood cells	0–5/hpf	WBCs in urine indicate infection or inflammation in the urinary tract.
Casts	None to occasional hyaline cast	Casts are formed when abnormal urine contents settle into molds of the renal tubules and may be made of protein, WBCs, RBCs, or bacteria. A few hyaline casts may be found in normal urine. The presence of casts usually indicates renal damage or infection.

hpf = high-power field; RBC = red blood cells; WBC = white blood cells.

prevent contamination of the specimen. The uncircumcised male patient should be directed to retract the foreskin with one hand and keep it retracted while cleansing and voiding. At least 10 mL of urine should be collected.

If a urinalysis is ordered for a patient with a urinary catheter, the nurse obtains the urine specimen. This specimen is considered sterile because it is going directly from the bladder into the urinary catheter tubing. To obtain the specimen, wear clean gloves and use an alcohol swab to clean the sample port on the catheter tubing. Insert a needleless system syringe (usually 10 mL) into the port and withdraw urine from the tubing into the syringe. Then empty the urine from the syringe into a collection container and safely dispose of the syringe.

Composite urine specimens are collected over a period of time that may range from 2 to 24 hours. These specimens are usually used to examine the urine for specific components such as glucose, electrolytes, protein, 17-ketosteroids, catecholamines, creatinine, and minerals. These specimens may need refrigeration or may have preservatives added to the collection container.

The patient is instructed to urinate and discard this specimen. The time is noted and is the start time of the test. All subsequent voiding is saved in the container for the designated time period. At the end of the time frame, the patient is asked to void and this is the last amount added to the container. Reminding the patient to save all of the urine is critical for accurate results. Incomplete collections do not result in accurate results.

Renal Function Tests

A number of blood and urine tests reflect kidney function (Table 36.4). If the kidneys are not functioning adequately, the serum test results will be elevated. These tests are useful because they provide information about the severity of a patient's kidney disease and also the patient's response to any treatments or medications being used. In this way, clinical progress can be monitored. Renal function tests may still be within the normal range until the glomerular filtration rate is less than 50% of normal. The most accurate way to assess kidney function is to use several tests and analyze the results together.

Diagnostic Procedures

Table 36.5 summarizes diagnostic procedures for the urinary system.

> **LEARNING TIP**
>
> A handy approximation to determine kidney function is to equate the creatinine clearance result to percentage of renal function. For example, creatinine clearance of
>
> - 100 mL per minute = 100% renal function
> - 30 mL per minute = 30% renal function
> - 5 mL per minute = 5% renal function.

Radiological Studies

With all contrast studies, the patient should be questioned for allergies to contrast media before the test. Contrast media may be **nephrotoxic** and can worsen impaired renal function. When contrast media are used, metformin hydrochloride (Glucophage) must not be given before and for 48 hours after administration of contrast media. Severe lactic acidosis as well as renal failure may occur.

To prevent contrast media–induced nephropathy, patients have a GFR or creatinine level done. Then, if mild-to-moderate renal insufficiency is shown, patients should receive premedication and two postprocedure doses with *N*-acetylcysteine (Mucomyst) and IV hydration with 0.45% sodium chloride hydration to help protect the kidneys.

TABLE 36.4 DIAGNOSTIC LABORATORY TESTS FOR THE URINARY SYSTEM

Test	Definition/Normal Value	Significance of Abnormal Findings
Urine Studies		
Residual urine	Looks at the amount of urine left in the bladder after voiding. *Reference value:* Less than 50 mL (increases with age)	Bladder ultrasound equipment may be used to determine amount of urine remaining after voiding. Increased residual volume may occur in urethral strictures, sphincter impairment, or neurogenic bladder.
Urinalysis	Used to establish baseline information, confirm or establish a diagnosis, or determine if further testing needs to be done.	May be used to monitor progress of an existing condition or plan a program of care.
Urine culture	Determines number of bacteria in urine and identifies organism causing urinary tract infection. Sensitivity test also may be ordered to determine most effective antibiotic against offending bacteria. *Reference value:* Negative if less than 10,000/mL of urine Positive if 100,000 or more/mL of urine. An amount less than 100,000 may result from contamination during specimen collection.	Urine should be collected before antibiotic treatment starts to avoid altering results. Midstream, clean-catch system is used to obtain voided specimens. Catheterized specimen may be ordered to avoid risk of contamination from vagina if female patient is menstruating or patient is incontinent.
Urine specific gravity	Evaluates the concentration of urine. *Reference value:* 1.002–1.035	Low specific gravity may occur in patients with diabetes insipidus, glomerulonephritis, or severe renal damage. High specific gravity may occur from diabetes mellitus, high urine glucose level, nephrosis, congestive heart failure, or dehydration.
Quantitative test for protein	A 12- or 24-hour urine collection is obtained to measure protein. *Reference values:* Less than 150 mg/24 hours (conventional units) Less than 0.15 g/24 hours (SI units)	Persistent proteinuria is usually seen with glomerular renal disease.
Creatinine clearance	Measures amount of creatinine cleared from blood in a specified time by comparing amount of creatinine in blood with creatinine in urine. An excellent indicator of renal function. *Reference value:* 85–135 mL/min	Creatinine clearance is computed in the laboratory and is expressed in volume of blood that is cleared of creatinine in 1 minute. Minimum creatinine clearance of 10 mL per minute is needed to live without dialysis. To carry out the test, urine is collected for a 24-hour period, and a sample for serum creatinine is collected sometime during the 24 hours. The following procedure should be followed: 1. At start of test, patient is directed to void and discard that urine. 2. Urine is collected for 24 hours in a large container provided by the laboratory. The container is kept refrigerated. 3. Twenty-four hours after test started, patient is instructed to void again. This urine is added to the collection container. 4. Laboratory collects serum creatinine during this 24-hour period.
Urine cytology	Microscopic examination of urine to detect atypical epithelial cells shed from the surface of the urinary tract.	Used to screen people at high risk for cancer in the urinary system. Atypical cells indicate need for further testing.
Bladder tumor antigen (a bladder cancer marker)	Measurement of a protein produced by bladder tumor cells. *Reference value:* Less than 14 units/mL	No special preparation needed. A single voided specimen collected before noon is taken directly to the laboratory.

Continued

TABLE 36.4 DIAGNOSTIC LABORATORY TESTS FOR THE URINARY SYSTEM—cont'd

Test	Definition/Normal Value	Significance of Abnormal Findings
NMP22 (a bladder cancer marker)	Measurement of a protein deposited into urine during nuclear disruption (apoptosis) of bladder cells. *Reference value:* Less than 10 units/mL	No special preparation needed. A single voided specimen collected before noon is taken directly to the laboratory.
Blood Chemistry Studies—Kidney Function		
Blood urea nitrogen (BUN)	Urea is a waste product of protein metabolism that is excreted by the kidneys. *Reference value:* 8–20 mg/dL	Not as sensitive an indicator of kidney function as creatinine level because BUN is affected by increased protein intake, dehydration, and other factors in the body. Elevated level: kidney disease, shock, severe heart failure, dehydration, high-protein diet, gastrointestinal bleeding, steroid use.
Serum creatinine	Creatinine is a waste product from muscle metabolism and is released into the bloodstream at a steady rate. *Reference value:* 0.6–1.5 mg/dL	Very good indicator of kidney function. The higher the creatinine level, the more impaired the kidney function. More than 1.5 mg/dL indicates kidney dysfunction.
BUN-to-creatinine ratio	Evaluates hydration status. *Reference value:* About 10:1	An elevated ratio occurs in hypovolemia. A normal ratio with an elevated BUN and creatinine occurs in intrinsic renal disease.
Cystatin C (Cys C)	Proteinase inhibitor produced by all cells with chromosomes and genetic material at their center at a constant rate, filtered out of blood by the glomerulus, and reabsorbed by tubular epithelial cells. *Reference values:* 0.53–0.95 mg/dL In young adults, less than 0.70 mg/mL (0.9 micromol/mL) In elderly adults, less than 0.85 mg/mL (3.5 micromol/mL)	Cystatin C is a sensitive marker that reflects glomerular filtration rate independent of body weight and height. Cystatin C level increases with impaired renal function.
Uric acid	Uric acid is an end product of purine metabolism and the breakdown of body proteins. Uric acid is not as diagnostic as creatinine because many factors can cause an elevated uric acid level. *Reference value:* 2–7 mg/dL	Elevated uric acid level can be caused by kidney disease, gout (patients with gout metabolize uric acid abnormally), malnutrition, leukemia, use of thiazide diuretics (because of impaired uric acid clearance by the kidney).
Blood Chemistry Studies		
Sodium (Na^+)	Extracellular electrolyte regulating blood volume. *Reference value:* 135–145 mEq/L	Remains within normal range until late stages of renal disease. Decreases with fluid retention (dilutional effect).
Potassium (K^+)	Intracellular electrolyte excreted by kidneys. *Reference value:* 3.5–5.5 mEq/L	In renal disease, K^+ is one of the first electrolytes to become abnormal. Level greater than 6 mEq/L can lead to muscle weakness and cardiac arrhythmias.
Calcium (Ca^{2+})	Main mineral in bone and aids in muscle contraction, neurotransmission, and blood clotting. *Reference values:* 4.5–5.5 mEq/L and 9–11 mg/dL	In renal disease decreased reabsorption of calcium leads to bone and mineral disease.
Phosphorus	Mineral found in bone, teeth, bloodstream, cells. Many functions. *Reference values:* 2.8–4.5 mg/dL and 0.95–1.45 mmol/L	Phosphorus balance is inversely related to calcium balance. Elevated in renal disease.
Bicarbonate (HCO_3^-)	An alkaline that indicates status of acid-base system. *Reference value:* 22–28 mEq/L	Most patients with renal disease have metabolic acidosis and low serum HCO_3^- levels
Magnesium	Found in bone and intracellularly and excreted by the kidney. *Reference value:* 1.3–2.1 mEq/L	Elevated in chronic renal disease. Symptoms of elevated magnesium level include lethargy, nausea, vomiting, and slurred speech.
Serum albumin	Plasma protein maintaining oncotic pressure in vascular system. *Reference value:* 3.5–5.0 g/dL	Low level occurs in nephrotic syndrome and renal disease and leads to edema.

TABLE 36.5 DIAGNOSTIC PROCEDURES FOR THE URINARY SYSTEM

Procedure	Definition	Uses and Possible Abnormal Findings	Nursing Management
Noninvasive			
Renal ultrasound or ultrasonography	High-frequency sound waves image the kidneys, ureters, and bladder or map the kidneys before a biopsy is done.	Congenital disorders of the kidney, abscesses, hydronephrosis, kidney stones or tumors, kidney enlargement, structural changes with chronic infection	No special preparation or aftercare. No known complications. No radiation exposure.
Bladder ultrasound	Portable ultrasound instrument computes bladder volume from 12 cross-sectional readings.	Residual urine volume, bladder wall thickness, bladder calculi, tumors, diverticula	Determines postresidual voiding accurately to reduce catheterizations for bladder distention.
Kidney-ureter-bladder x-ray study	X-ray (flat plate) of size, shape, and position of the kidneys, ureters, and bladder.	Renal calculi, kidney size, masses in the kidney	Usually, no special care is needed. If done as preliminary study, bowel prep may be done.
Computed tomographic (CT) scan	A radiological procedure in which a computer constructs images of the area scanned from a series of tomograms or cross-sectional slices. Contrast media may be given.	Evaluation of kidneys, ureters, bladder, abdominal and pelvic organs for kidney size, tumors, cysts, abscesses, malignant masses, metastases, lymph node enlargement; nonfunctioning kidneys, renal stones, obstructions, infections	*Precare:* NPO 4 hours before procedure. Check allergies and BUN and creatinine levels before patient receives contrast media. Withhold metformin before and for 48 hours after contrast is given. *Postcare:* Encourage fluids after test to remove contrast media.
Magnetic resonance imaging (MRI)	Computer-generated films produced by interaction of radio waves and magnetic fields of kidneys, bladder, prostate, testes, and retroperitoneum.	Staging of cancers of the kidney, bladder, and prostate	MRI is contraindicated if patient has metallic objects in the body, surgical clips, or pacemakers. Metal objects, jewelry, and clothing with metal clips must be removed. Patients with claustrophobia may need to be sedated or use open MRI. Contrast media may be used.
Invasive			
Intravenous **pyelogram** (IVP)	X-ray examination of renal tissue, calyces, pelvises, ureters, and bladder after intravenous injection of contrast media or dye. Radiographs taken at frequent intervals to see dye filling the renal pelvis and going down the ureters into the bladder (see Fig. 36.4).	Abnormal size or shape of kidneys, absent kidneys, polycystic kidney disease, tumors, hydronephrosis, renovascular hypertension	*Precare:* NPO 8 hours before procedure. Enemas may be given the evening before the test to empty the colon. Check allergies and BUN and creatinine levels before patient receives contrast media. Explain warm, flushing sensation up arm and sometimes all over the body when the dye is injected. Strange taste may occur as well. *Postcare:* Encourage fluids to remove contrast media. Monitor urine output.

Continued

• WORD • BUILDING •

pyelogram: pyelo—pelvis of the kidney + gram—radiograph

TABLE 36.5 DIAGNOSTIC PROCEDURES FOR THE URINARY SYSTEM—cont'd

Procedure	Definition	Uses and Possible Abnormal Findings	Nursing Management
Renal angiography or arteriogram	Visualizes renal blood vessels. Femoral artery is pierced with a needle, and a catheter is threaded upward through femoral and iliac arteries into the aorta and then the renal artery. Contrast agent is injected to make renal arterial supply visible on x-ray examination.	Hypervascular tumors, renal cysts, renal artery stenosis, renal artery aneurysms, pyelonephritis, obstructions, renal infarction, renal trauma evaluation	*Precare:* NPO 4–8 hours before procedure. Check allergies and BUN and creatinine levels before patient receives contrast media. Enemas may be given the evening before the test. *Postcare:* Bedrest up to 12 hours to prevent bleeding at injection site. Check distal pulses in leg every 30–60 minutes. Instruct patient not to bend leg or raise head of bed more than 45 degrees. Monitor vital signs, dressing, and pulses in leg frequently.
Nephrotomogram	Series of x-rays using intravenous contrast media taken from different angles to create a three-dimensional image of the kidney.	Renal cysts, tumors, areas of nonperfusion, renal fractures or lacerations following renal trauma	Monitor fluid intake and output before and after test. Prepare patient as for an IVP, checking allergies to contrast media and BUN and creatinine levels. Encourage fluids after test.
Renal scan	Nuclear scan, in which radioactive substance (a radioisotope) injected into bloodstream is detected by a special camera (gamma camera) similar to an x-ray machine. Radioactive isotope that is rapidly excreted by the kidneys is injected intravenously. Radiation detectors (cameras) placed over the kidney monitor the radioactive material in the kidney. As isotope passes through kidneys and into urine, kidneys "light up."	Renovascular hypertension diagnosis; kidney function; renal blood flow; glomerular filtration rate; tubular function; excretion of urine; kidney size and shape; abscesses, cysts, and tumors, which may appear as cold spots because of nonfunctioning kidney tissue; determination of vascular supply to the kidneys in patients with renal trauma, dissecting aneurysm, and other disorders affecting blood flow to the kidneys	Assesses kidneys' ability to perfuse blood and secrete urine. Usually, no special preparation needed. Determine if any of patient's medications will interfere with test, such as nonsteroidal anti-inflammatory drugs or antihypertensives. Patient may be asked to drink two glasses of water before test. Level of radiation is very low and produces no side effects. Pregnant and nursing mothers are advised to be cautious.
Renal biopsy	Laboratory analysis of renal tissue ***Percutaneous:*** local anesthetic, needle through skin *Open:* surgical incision. CT scan or ultrasound done first to locate kidney for biopsy.	Microscopic examination of kidney tissue for diagnosis or treatment of renal disorder, benign and malignant masses, causes of renal disease, renal transplant rejection, lupus	*Precare:* Before biopsy, patient is NPO for 6 to 8 hours. Mild sedative is given. No anticoagulants, CBC, coagulation studies. *During:* Prone position, with sandbag under the abdomen, for biopsy through flank area. Patient instructed to hold breath while needle is inserted to prevent kidney from moving. *Postcare:* May remain in prone position. Bandage is applied, and patient is maintained on bedrest for 24 hours or more.

• WORD • BUILDING •
percutaneous: per—through + cutaneous—skin

TABLE 36.5 DIAGNOSTIC PROCEDURES FOR THE URINARY SYSTEM—cont'd

Procedure	Definition	Uses and Possible Abnormal Findings	Nursing Management
			Monitor vital signs, urine, bleeding for 24 hours because kidney is highly vascular. Grossly bloody urine, falling blood pressure, and rising pulse are signs of bleeding and are reported immediately. Encourage fluids. No heavy lifting for 2 weeks. Notify physician of flank pain, hematuria, light-headedness, or fainting.
Cystoscopy and pyelogram (C&P)	Minor surgical procedure with lighted fiber-optic cystoscope *Diagnostic:* Inspect inside of bladder, collect urine specimen from either kidney, take x-rays (pyelogram) or biopsy growths. *Therapeutic:* Remove small bladder tumors, stones from bladder/ureters, dilation of ureters.	Urinary calculi, infection, vesicoureteral reflux, enlarged prostate, bladder tumors, urethral strictures, polyps, congenital abnormalities	*Precare:* Surgical preparation. *Postcare:* Measure urine to detect retention from swelling of urinary meatus. Encourage fluid intake. Expect dysuria for 24 hours and initial voidings to be blood tinged. *Complications:* Urinary tract infection, urine retention, bladder perforation.
Cystogram or voiding cystourethrogram	X-ray of bladder and lower urinary tract with contrast media or radioisotope instilled into bladder via catheter or cystoscope to evaluate bladder filling and emptying.	Incomplete bladder emptying, distention, reflux, obstruction to urine outflow	No special prep. After the scan, may be slight dysuria and pink urine for 1–2 days. Bright red urine, fever, or persistent discomfort should be reported to physician.

Renal Ultrasound

Ultrasonography is a noninvasive study using sound waves to examine the anatomy of the urinary tract. Ultrasound has no contraindications and requires no contrast media and no preparation.

Renal Biopsy

A renal biopsy may be done to diagnose or gain more information about kidney disease. A small section of the renal cortex is obtained percutaneously or with a small flank incision. Patients with bleeding tendencies, uncontrolled hypertension, or a solitary kidney generally do not undergo renal biopsy.

Nursing Process for Diagnostic Tests of the Urinary System Assessment

The patient is assessed for baseline understanding of and comfort with testing procedures to plan teaching sessions. Possible contraindications to testing, such as a renal function test and the use of dyes or an MRI if the patient has metal in the body, are assessed and reported.

• WORD • BUILDING •

cystoscopy: cysto—bladder + scopy—to examine

Nursing Diagnoses, Planning, and Implementation

Anxiety Related to Unfamiliar Environment, Procedure, Diagnostic Test, Health Status, or Severity of Disease

EXPECTED OUTCOME: The patient will have reduced anxiety concerning health status or severity of disease before procedure or test.

- Assess patient for signs and symptoms of anxiety: verbalization, tenseness, tachycardia, elevated blood pressure, facial pallor, and self-focused behaviors. *A high level of fear will interfere with teaching and learning and also diminish cooperation during testing.*
- Examine patient's health beliefs *to provide insight into patient behaviors that may affect outcome.*
- Acknowledge patient's anxiety and the perceived threat of the situation *to facilitate communication and trust.*
- Maintain a calm, supportive, and confident environment and manner when interacting with patient *to reduce anxiety.*

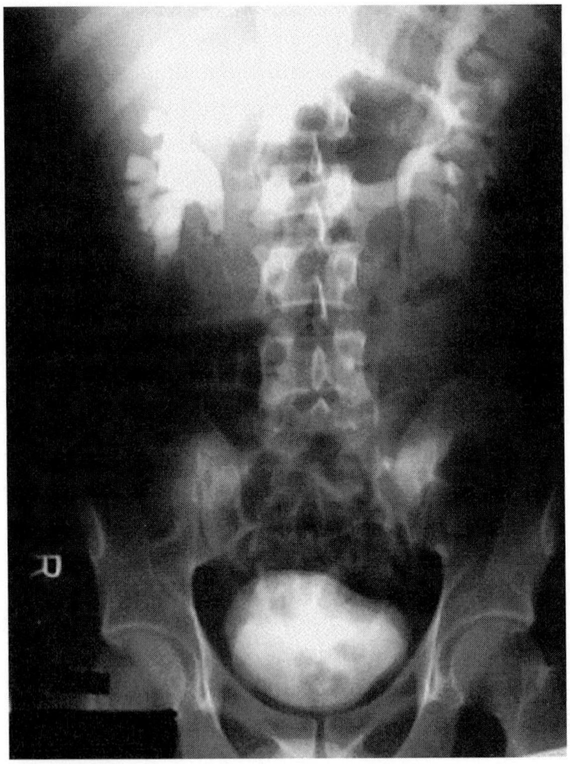
R

FIGURE 36.4 Intravenous pyelogram x-ray.

- Encourage patient to verbalize feelings, concerns, or specific stressors *to provide a baseline of information to develop an individualized teaching plan.*
- Provide patient with access to timely information regarding outcome of diagnostic testing *to facilitate trust and promote comfort.*
- Engage support from patient's family throughout diagnostic testing *for patient's coping.*
- Instruct patient in relaxation techniques and facilitate their use *to reduce anxiety.*
- Respond to patient call signals as soon as possible *to reduce anxiety.*
- Reinforce explanations and correct misconceptions the patient has about diagnostic tests or disease condition *to facilitate trust and promote comfort.*

Acute Pain Related to Infection, Edema, Obstruction, or Bleeding Along the Urinary Tract or to Invasive Diagnostic Tests

EXPECTED OUTCOME: The patient will report a decrease in discomfort or pain within 30 minutes of report of discomfort or pain.

- Assess location and level of pain, **dysuria**, burning on urination, or abdominal or flank pain *to provide baseline data to evaluate progression of pain and effectiveness of treatment plan.*
- Provide comfort measures *to relieve pain.*
- Provide analgesics and antispasmodics as prescribed *for pain relief.*
- Report severe pain to primary care provider. *Severe pain may indicate complications are present or the need for a change in pain control medications.*

Impaired Urinary Elimination Related to Complications from Diagnostic Tests of the Urinary System

EXPECTED OUTCOME: The patient will maintain urine output greater than 30 mL per hour in the postprocedure period.

- Encourage fluid intake after renal diagnostic testing *to facilitate dye or contrast removal from the body.*
- Monitor fluid intake and output closely *to ensure adequate renal function.*
- Monitor serum creatinine level *to assess for complications from diagnostic testing.*
- Observe patient for hypersensitivity reactions to contrast media or injectable materials *to help prevent renal complications.*
- Assess patient for pruritus, rashes, breathing difficulties, generalized edema, or urinary retention *to detect possible reaction symptoms.*

Deficient Knowledge Related to Unfamiliar Environment, Procedure, Diagnostic Test, and Health Status

EXPECTED OUTCOME: The patient will report understanding of the environment, procedure, or diagnostic test before the procedure.

- Assess patient's understanding of the procedure *to provide a baseline for teaching.*
- Introduce staff who will be caring for the patient. *Familiarity with staff will decrease anxiety.*
- Include family members or significant others in orientation and teaching sessions *to encourage their support of the patient.*
- Orient patient to the environment, equipment, and routines *to increase understanding.*
- Explain all activities that will take place in the diagnostic area and afterward *to reduce fear and promote cooperation during testing.*
- Provide information at the patient's level *to promote understanding.*
- Reinforce physician's explanations and correct misconceptions about the diagnostic test or procedure *to help alleviate anxiety.*
- Explain that patient may have to drink increased fluids after the test and that patient's intake and output will be closely monitored. *Increased fluids help rid the patient of the contrast media after the procedure.*
- Provide information about self-care following procedure or diagnostic test *to facilitate the patient in self-care.*

Evaluation

If interventions have been effective, the patient will report reduced anxiety, maintain urine output greater than 30 mL per hour, and a decrease in pain and increased understanding of the procedure.

THERAPEUTIC MEASURES FOR THE URINARY SYSTEM

Management of Urinary Incontinence

Urinary **incontinence** is defined as the involuntary leakage of urine and is very common. There are several types of incontinence. The incidence is rising and affects both men and women. Urinary incontinence is often underdiagnosed and underreported because many patients are too embarrassed to talk about the problem.

Most patients do not seek treatment until the problem profoundly affects quality of life. At times, urinary incontinence can be prevented by patient teaching or physician intervention. Incontinence that cannot be treated is managed by the use of padding and absorptive products worn by the patient. With all kinds of incontinence, the nurse or patient should keep a voiding diary for at least several days to determine when incontinence occurs and to look for any predisposing events. The patient should be referred to a urologist specializing in the area of incontinence or a continence clinic for a careful examination to determine the cause and identify potential medical or surgical treatment.

Stress Incontinence

Stress incontinence is the involuntary loss of less than 50 mL of urine associated with increasing abdominal pressure during coughing, sneezing, laughing, or other physical activities. Stress incontinence is commonly seen in women after childbirth and after menopause. In men, stress incontinence is associated with prostatectomy and radiation.

Urge Incontinence

Urge incontinence is the involuntary loss of urine associated with an abrupt and strong desire to void. The patient typically reports being "unable to make it to the bathroom in time." Urge incontinence is the most common type of urinary incontinence in older adults. Patients with stress incontinence or urge incontinence can be taught Kegel exercises to increase perineal muscle tone (Box 36.2, *Patient Education*).

Functional Incontinence

Functional incontinence is the inability to reach the toilet because of environmental barriers, physical limitations, loss of memory, or disorientation. People with functional incontinence are often dependent on others and have no other urinary problems. This is a common cause of incontinence in the elderly who are institutionalized.

Overflow Incontinence

Overflow incontinence is the involuntary loss of urine associated with overdistention of the bladder. It occurs with acute or chronic urinary distention with dribbling of urine. The bladder is unable to empty normally despite frequent urine loss. Spinal cord injuries or an enlarged prostate may cause this type of incontinence.

Box 36.2

Patient Education

Kegel Exercises

Kegel exercises decrease incontinence by strengthening the pubococcygeal muscle, which supports the pelvic organs. By increasing the tone of this muscle, the patient has an increased ability to tighten the muscle that encircles the urinary meatus and stop the flow of urine. These exercises can also help prevent uterine prolapse, enhance sensation during sexual intercourse, and hasten postpartum healing. It may be used by the older male patient to control dribbling.

1. Establish awareness of pelvic muscle function by instructing the patient to "pull in" the muscles in the perineum as if to control urination or defecation. The muscles of the buttocks, inner thigh, and abdomen are not used to do Kegel exercises.
2. To help identify the correct muscles to tighten, ask the patient to tighten the muscles that control urination. It can be helpful to use an analogy of an elevator: start squeezing at the bottom floor and then squeeze upward to the top floor.
3. Instruct the patient to tighten the pelvic muscles for 10 seconds, followed by at least 10 seconds of relaxation.
4. Advise the patient to perform these exercises 30 to 80 times per day. Help devise cues to remind the patient to perform the exercises, such as stopping the stream of urine 10 times each time the patient urinates.

Source: Adapted from Agency for Healthcare Research and Quality. (2007). *Prevention of fecal and urinary incontinence in adults* (AHCPR Pub No 08-E003). Rockville, MD: Author. Retrieved July 28, 2009, from http://www.ahrq.gov/clinic/tp/fuiadtp.htm.

Total Incontinence

Total incontinence is a continuous and unpredictable loss of urine. It usually results from surgery, trauma, or a malformation of the ureter. Bladder training has been tried and proven ineffective. Often the patient with total incontinence is neurologically impaired. In these situations, the nurse's priority is to keep the patient clean and dry using absorptive products. For the male patient, an external condom catheter can be effective in some situations.

Nursing Process for the Patient with Stress or Urge Incontinence

The medical diagnoses of stress and urge incontinence are also nursing diagnoses. Many nursing interventions can help to improve these types of incontinence. See the *Nursing Care Plan for the Patient with Stress or Urge Incontinence* and the *Nursing Care Plan for the Patient with Functional Incontinence.*

NURSING CARE PLAN for the Patient with Stress or Urge Incontinence

Nursing Diagnosis: *Stress Incontinence* or *Urge Incontinence* related to decreased tone of perineal muscles

Expected Outcomes: The patient will be continent of urine and will state three actions that can be taken to decrease incidence of stress or urge incontinence.

Evaluation of Outcomes: Is the patient continent? Is the patient able to state three actions that can be taken to decrease the incidence of stress or urge incontinence?

Interventions	Rationale	Evaluation
	STRESS INCONTINENCE OR URGE INCONTINENCE	
Ask about the history of incontinence. Have patient keep a voiding journal.	A journal helps identify the severity and timing of incontinence.	Does patient complete the voiding journal?
Instruct patient on how to perform Kegel exercises (see Box 36.2).	Kegel exercises increase perineal muscle tone and help prevent incontinence.	Does patient explain how to perform Kegel exercises?
Work with the patient to incorporate Kegel exercises into normal activities of daily living (e.g., do 10 pelvic muscle contractions during each voiding).	An excellent time to perform Kegel exercises is when voiding because the correct muscles are used.	Does patient perform Kegel exercises when voiding or at other cued times during the day?
Encourage patient to drink at least 2000 mL of fluid per day, preferably 3000 mL per day unless medical reason for fluid restriction.	Concentrated urine is irritating to the urinary tract and can increase the incidence of urge incontinence and dribbling.	Is urine dilute?
Encourage patient to avoid alcohol and caffeine.	Alcohol serves as a diuretic. Caffeine is irritating to the urinary tract.	Does patient explain the need to avoid alcohol and fluids containing caffeine?
Discuss use of and provide small adhesive peripads to wear in underclothing.	Peripads provide protection in case of incontinence.	Does patient have and use peripads if desired?
Refer patient to a continence clinic or to a physician specializing in incontinence.	Specialists in the area of incontinence can use medical or surgical interventions to decrease incontinence.	Does patient understand what resources are available to further assist with treatment of incontinence?
Refer patient to supportive and educational groups such as Help for Incontinent People (HIP).	Support groups can help patients deal with the embarrassment of incontinence and learn methods and resources to prevent incontinence.	Does patient know the names and addresses of support groups to help with incontinence?
	URGE INCONTINENCE	
Teach patient to void at frequent intervals (every 2 hours), and then gradually increase the length of time between voidings.	By emptying the bladder at frequent intervals, the incidence of urge incontinence can be decreased.	Does patient follow a frequent voiding schedule?
Teach urge inhibition techniques (distraction), such as counting back from 100 by sevens and relaxation breathing.	These distraction techniques can help patients reach the bathroom in time to prevent incontinence.	Do distraction techniques help patient prevent incontinence?

NURSING CARE PLAN for the Patient with Functional Incontinence

Nursing Diagnosis: *Functional Urinary Incontinence* related to interference with rapid voiding

Expected Outcomes: The patient will be continent of urine and will state three measures to increase continence.

Evaluation of Outcomes: Is the patient continent of urine? Is the patient able to state three measures to increase continence?

Interventions	Rationale	Evaluation
Ask about the history of incontinence. Keep a voiding log of when patient is incontinent.	A voiding log helps demonstrate when incontinence is most likely to occur and can help determine the cause of incontinence.	Does the patient cooperate so that a voiding log can be kept?
Determine any acute causes of incontinence, including new onset of urinary tract infection, constipation or impaction, medication effect, or poor fluid intake.	These may be readily treatable causes of incontinence.	Does the patient have any easily treatable causes of incontinence?
Determine if clothing is inhibiting timely voiding. If needed, Velcro fasteners or sweat shirts and sweat pants might be appropriate.	Clothing can be difficult to remove for the elderly, resulting in voiding before the clothing can be removed. Clothing can be modified so that it comes off quickly.	Does the patient have easy-to-remove clothing?
Determine if there are any obstacles to reaching appropriate urine receptacle, such as poor lighting, busy bathroom, lack of assistive devices.	Obstacles can make it impossible for the patient to reach the voiding receptacle in time to prevent incontinence.	Does the patient have ready access to a voiding receptacle?
Provide appropriate urinary receptacles, such as a three-in-one commode, female or male urinal, or no-spill urinal.	Assistive devices can be helpful for the patient to increase continence.	Does the patient need and have access to an appropriate assistive device?
Initiate a voiding schedule of every 2 hours, or base schedule on voiding log. Always assist patient to the toilet when patient first awakens and before sleep. Use prompted voiding techniques, including checking patient regularly, providing positive reinforcement if dry, prompting patient to toilet, praising patient after toileting, and returning patient to toilet in a specified time.	Frequent scheduled voiding using prompting techniques can increase continence.	Does the patient receive help to do bladder training with prompted voiding?
Teach patient to set up schedule of voiding using environmental cues such as meals, bedtime, and television shows.	Environmental cues help the patient remember when it is time to void.	Can the patient indicate cues throughout the day that prompt voiding?

Management of Urine Retention

Urinary retention is the inability to empty the bladder completely during attempts to void. Urine retention can be caused by many factors. It can be acute, with a sudden onset of retention and no urine output, or chronic, with a slower onset of retention of urine and some urine being expelled. Acute retention often results from surgery and is caused by anesthesia, medications, or local trauma to the urinary structures. Acute retention can be a medical emergency causing extreme pain, a large bladder, and the possibility of bladder rupture or acute renal failure. Chronic urine retention may be related to an enlarged prostate gland, diabetes, pregnancy, a medication effect, strictures, or other causes of obstruction of the urinary tract.

Gentle palpation and percussion of the bladder may be done by the licensed practical nurse/licensed vocational nurse (LPN/LVN) if urine retention is suspected. If the patient has a feeling of fullness but is unable to urinate, the nurse gently palpates the suprapubic area for a full bladder or performs a bladder scan. Normally, the bladder is not palpable. If the bladder is percussed, it sounds dull over a fluid-filled bladder and may extend up to and beyond the umbilicus.

A bladder scan assesses the volume of urine in the bladder (Fig 36.5). Sound waves estimate the amount of urine in the bladder. It is painless, noninvasive, and requires no patient preparation. The nurse performs this scan at the bedside. It helps guide the need for catheterization, thereby reducing unnecessary catheterizations and associated risks. The bladder scan may be used instead of catheterization (the gold standard for determining urine retention) after the patient urinates to determine the amount of urine remaining in the bladder. Normally the bladder contains less than 50 mL after urination. A residual volume of 150 to 200 mL of urine indicates a need for treatment for urine retention. Bladder scanning may also be used as a tool for incontinent patients to plan their care.

Urinary Catheters

Indwelling Catheters

Indwelling urinary catheters may be inserted into hospitalized patients for various justifiable reasons, such as shock, heart failure, or urinary tract obstruction. As a general rule, catheters should be avoided if possible because of the high risk of urinary tract infections. Urinary incontinence is not a justification for insertion of a catheter. Urinary catheters result in infection of the urinary tract in many patients, especially the longer these catheters are in place. The incidence of infection is decreased when intermittent straight catheterization is used instead of an indwelling urinary catheter.

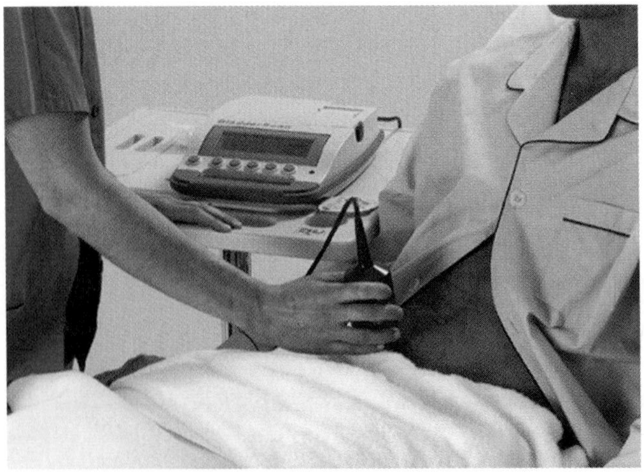

FIGURE 36.5 A bladder scan can be used to determine the volume of urine in a patient's bladder.

With an indwelling catheter, bacteria enter the bladder mainly in one of two ways: (1) through the outlet at the end of the drainage bag contaminating the urine, which is then inadvertently drained back into the bladder, or (2) around the catheter up the urethra and into the bladder. Routine perineal care during the daily bath is sufficient to minimize infection from an indwelling urinary catheter (see *Evidence-Based Practice* box). Box 36.3 outlines steps that should be followed to decrease infection in the patient with an indwelling catheter. (See also *Home Health Hints*.)

After an uncircumcised male is catheterized, the foreskin must be properly repositioned over the glans penis and not left retracted to prevent injury. If left retracted, subse-

EVIDENCE-BASED PRACTICE

Clinical Question

Does the practice of daily meatal cleansing decrease the incidence of urinary tract infections (UTIs) in patients with indwelling urinary catheters?

Evidence

Catheter care and meatal cleansing with antimicrobials or antiseptic soap have not shown a reduction in catheter-related UTIs (Leaver, 2007; Wilson, 2009). Indeed, any regimen of daily routine meatal care has been associated with increased risk of bacteriuria. The most important intervention is to avoid catheter insertion when possible and limit the length of time a catheter remains in place (Leaver, 2007).

Implications for Nursing Practice

Normal daily genital hygiene with soap and water is sufficient to achieve meatal cleanliness. Avoid vigorous and specific regimens because they may lead to meatal trauma from catheter manipulation.

REFERENCES

Leaver, R. (2007). The evidence for urethral meatal cleansing. *Nursing Standard, 21*(41), 39–42.

Robinson, J. (2009). Urinary catheterization: Assessing the best options for patients. *Nursing Standard, 23*(29), 40–45.

Wilson, M., Wilde, M., Webb, M., et al. (2009). Nursing interventions to reduce the risk of catheter associated urinary tract infection. Part 2: Staff education, monitoring, and care techniques. *Journal of Wound Ostomy and Continence Nursing, 36*(2), 137–154.

Box 36.3

Guidelines for Care of the Patient with an Indwelling Catheter

1. Maintain a closed system. Do not separate the catheter from the tubing of the bag. Instead, collect specimens and irrigate through the specimen port in the tubing.
2. Keep the catheter securely taped or fastened to the patient's leg. This decreases traction on the catheter and the back-and-forth movement of the catheter that can help bacteria enter the bladder.
3. Encourage fluid consumption to naturally irrigate the catheter, if fluids are not contraindicated because of heart or kidney disease.
4. Use good aseptic technique when emptying the drainage bag by washing hands, wearing clean gloves, and using a container designated for a single patient to collect the urine.
5. Wash the perineum with soap and water once a day and again if there is any bowel incontinence.
6. Keep the tubing coiled on the bed and positioned to allow free urine flow. Keep the catheter bag below the level of the bladder at all times.
7. Do not clamp catheters. Clamping a catheter results in obstruction and increases risk of infection. Periodic clamping has not been found to be effective in bladder retraining.
8. Remove indwelling catheters as soon as possible.

Home Health Hints

- The home health nurse should always have a sterile specimen container available. This provides a quick way to get a specimen to the physician's office without the nurse having to obtain the container, saving time and money.
- When catheters become plugged and irrigation fails, families can be taught to take the catheter out. A syringe for removing water from the balloon should be left in the home for this purpose. The family is instructed to avoid cutting the valve stem.
- The family should contact the nurse to reinsert the catheter, but in the meantime, the patient's bed or chair can be padded with towels or diapers. Plastic bags can be used to line the mattress. The family must be instructed to notify the nurse immediately if the catheter is plugged or has been removed.
- Not all homes have adequate lighting, which is a must for inserting a catheter. If lighting is inadequate, a caregiver can be asked to hold a flashlight while the nurse inserts the catheter. The nurse should always have a flashlight available. Having two catheters and catheter trays is also wise in case of a defect or contamination.
- Urine bags can be used safely for up to 4 weeks. Instruct the patient or family to cleanse the bag daily with a 1:10 bleach solution to decrease bacteria.
- To encourage fluid intake, urge patient and family to keep a large container of water (1 to 2 quarts) next to the place the patient usually sits. The goal is to drink 2 quarts of water by the end of each day, unless contraindicated by other medical problems. This also simplifies measuring intake. A sports bottle helps to keep water at hand while moving about the home.

quent swelling may make it impossible to pull the foreskin over the glans penis later. This can then cause ischemia of the glans penis, which is an emergency. A physician must be notified immediately and may need to perform an emergency circumcision if the foreskin cannot be properly positioned. Always make sure that the foreskin is positioned properly following catheterization or perineal care.

Intermittent Catheterization

For the patient who is unable to void, the best intervention is intermittent catheterization. A postoperative patient or a patient with a neurologic disorder or urine retention may benefit from intermittent catheterization. It reduces the risk of infection as long as the bladder is not allowed to overfill. A full bladder stretches the muscle fibers, which in turn reduces circulation to the bladder and increases the risk of infection.

Intermittent catheterization involves the use of a straight plastic or rubber catheter that is inserted into the urethra about every 3 hours to empty the bladder. Once the bladder is empty, the catheter is removed. Patients may be taught to do intermittent self-catheterization (ISC) at home. Patients doing ISC may be taught to wash and reuse the same catheter repeatedly when they are in their own environment. In the hospital, however, sterile technique is used.

Suprapubic Catheter

After some surgeries of the urinary tract and in some long-term situations, a suprapubic catheter may be used. This is an indwelling catheter that is inserted through an incision in the lower abdomen directly into the bladder.

Nursing care of a suprapubic catheter involves keeping the area clean and dry, changing the dressing when the site is new, and keeping the catheter taped to prevent tension. A skin barrier such as Stomahesive may help protect the skin from urine leakage. All other care is the same as for any indwelling catheter.

Box 36.4 lists resources related to the urinary system and its disorders.

Box 36.4

Resources

National Kidney Foundation
www.kidney.org
800-622-9010

National Institute of Diabetes and Digestive and Kidney Diseases
www2.niddk.nih.gov
301-496-3583

Kidney & Urology Foundation of America
www.kidneyurology.org
800-633-6628

Organ Procurement and Transplantation Network
www.optn.org

The Nephron Information Center
www.nephron.com

SUGGESTED ANSWERS TO CRITICAL THINKING

■ *Mr. Nolan*

You should realize that 50 mL of concentrated urine for 8 to 12 hours is not adequate or normal. Further investigation is needed to determine the cause and seriousness of the problem. Some items to assess follow:

1. Consider Mr. Nolan's diagnosis. Is he in renal failure? Is he severely dehydrated and retaining water?
2. Ask if anyone emptied Mr. Nolan's bag earlier in the shift.
3. Look at the trends in Mr. Nolan's intake and output record. Has his output been decreasing? Is this a change?
4. Has Mr. Nolan been taking in enough fluids?
5. Look at trends in daily weights. Is Mr. Nolan's weight increasing? Is this an expected finding?
6. Listen to Mr. Nolan's lung sounds. Check for edema. Do findings indicate fluid retention?
7. Palpate Mr. Nolan's bladder. Is it distended? Maybe the catheter is blocked.
8. If a problem is identified, the physician should be contacted.

REVIEW QUESTIONS

1. Where is urine formed?
   a. Nephrons
   b. Ureters
   c. Urethra
   d. Bladder

2. Which of the following are functions of the kidney? **Select all that apply**.
   a. Maintaining acid-base balance
   b. Removal of waste products
   c. Regulation of the blood volume
   d. Regulation of electrolytes
   e. Removal of CO_2
   f. Production of erythropoietin

3. A home health nurse visits a patient who is 82 years old, uses a cane, and is not incontinent. Which of the following interventions should be included in the plan of care, based on an understanding of normal age-related changes of the urinary system, to promote patient safety?
   a. Encourage fluids after 6 p.m.
   b. Limit fluids to 1000 mL per day.
   c. Provide a night-light in the bathroom.
   d. Provide adult briefs to prevent dribbling.

4. Which of the following is the most accurate assessment of fluid balance in the patient with renal failure?
   a. Voiding pattern
   b. Daily weight
   c. Laboratory studies
   d. Skin turgor

REVIEW QUESTIONS—cont'd

5. Which of the following should be included in patient teaching for collecting a midstream clean-catch urine specimen for culture and sensitivity?
   a. A second voided specimen is preferred.
   b. A 24-hour urine specimen is needed.
   c. As soon as the urine starts to flow, it should be collected in a sterile container.
   d. Women should keep the labia separated while voiding.

6. Which of the following care should the nurse provide following an intravenous pyelogram test? **Select all that apply**.
   a. Maintain NPO.
   b. Encourage fluids.
   c. Check gag reflex.
   d. Measure urine output.
   e. Position patient prone.
   f. Maintain bedrest for 24 hours.

7. A patient is experiencing stress incontinence with frequent involuntary loss of urine. Which of the following directions would be most appropriate when teaching the patient how to perform Kegel exercises?
   a. "Tighten your rectum at frequent intervals throughout the day."
   b. "Keep your abdominal muscles tightened; do this every time you stand up."
   c. "Do at least 20 sit-ups per day."
   d. "When urinating, stop and start the stream of urine by tightening the perineal muscles."

8. Which of the following is the most important nursing action for the nurse to take to prevent urinary tract infection in the catheterized patient?
   a. Force fluids to 4000 mL every 24 hours.
   b. Empty the Foley bag every 4 hours around the clock.
   c. Maintain a closed catheter system.
   d. Wash the perineum every 8 hours.

9. What is the patient's total output as recorded during the 7-3 shift?
   8 a.m. voided 165 mL
   11:30 a.m. voided 450 mL
   1 p.m. emesis 42 mL
   3 p.m. voided 255 mL
   Answer: ______________ mL

37

Nursing Care of Patients with Disorders of the Urinary System

MAUREEN McDONALD

KEY TERMS

anuria (an-YOO-ree-ah)
azotemia (AH-zoh-TEE-mee-ah)
calculi (KAL-kyoo-lye)
cystitis (siss-TYE-tiss)
glomerulonephritis (gloh-MURR-yoo-loh-neh-FRY-tiss)
hemodialysis (HEE-moh-dye-AH-lih-siss)
hydronephrosis (HYE-droh-neh-FROH-siss)
nephrectomy (neh-FREK-tuh-mee)
nephrolithotomy (NEH-froh-lih-THAW-tuh-mee)
nephropathy (neh-FROP-uh-thee)
nephrosclerosis (NEH-froh-skleh-ROH-siss)
nephrostomy (neh-FRAW-stoh-mee)
nephrotoxin (NEH-froh-TOK-sin)
oliguria (AW-lih-GYOO-ree-ah)
peritoneal dialysis (PEAR-ih-toh-NEE-uhl dye-AL-ih-siss)
polyuria (PAW-lee-YOOR-ee-ah)
pyelonephritis (PYE-eh-loh-neh-FRY-tiss)
stent (STENT)
uremia (yoo-REE-mee-ah)
urethritis (YOO-reh-THRYE-tiss)
urethroplasty (yoo-REE-throw-PLAS-tee)
urosepsis (YOO-roh-SEP-siss)

QUESTIONS TO GUIDE YOUR READING

1. What are the predisposing causes, symptoms, laboratory abnormalities, and treatment of urinary tract infections?
2. What are the predisposing causes, symptoms, treatment, and teaching for kidney stones?
3. What are risk factors and symptoms of cancer of the bladder and cancer of the kidneys?
4. How do you provide care for a patient with an ileal conduit or continent reservoir?
5. How would you explain the pathophysiology and nursing care for diabetic nephropathy, nephrosclerosis, hydronephrosis, and glomerulonephritis?
6. What are the symptoms for patients with acute kidney injury or chronic kidney disease?
7. What nursing care is provided to patients with acute kidney injury or chronic kidney disease?
8. What nursing care is provided for a vascular blood access site?
9. What nursing care is provided to patients on hemodialysis or peritoneal dialysis?

Disorders of the urinary tract include a variety of problems involving the kidneys, ureters, bladder, and urethra. These problems may arise from infection, obstructions, cancer, hereditary disorders, and metabolic, traumatic, or chronic diseases. Some may lead to chronic kidney disease if not treated or controlled. Infection may be found in three different anatomical parts of the urinary tract: the urethra, resulting in urethritis; the bladder, with a diagnosis of cystitis; or the kidneys, with a diagnosis of pyelonephritis.

URINARY TRACT INFECTIONS

Urinary tract infection (UTI), a general term, refers to invasion of the urinary tract by bacteria. Normally, the urinary tract is sterile above the urethra. UTI is the second most common bacterial disease and causes more than 100,000 people to be hospitalized each year. In the hospital, UTIs are the most common hospital-acquired infection. They are described by their location in the urinary tract. Lower urinary tract infections include urethritis, prostatitis, and cystitis. Upper urinary tract infections include pyelonephritis and ureteritis. Infections may result in chronic kidney disease, sepsis, or damage to the kidney.

Predisposing Factors for Urinary Tract Infections

UTIs are caused most often by an ascending infection, starting at the external urinary meatus and progressing toward the bladder and kidneys. Most UTIs are caused by the bacterium *Escherichia coli,* which is commonly found in feces. Predisposing factors for UTI include the following:

- Stasis of urine in the bladder can result from obstruction, such as a clamped catheter or simply from not voiding frequently enough. Urine overdistends the bladder, decreasing the blood supply to the wall of the bladder, which keeps white blood cells (WBCs) from fighting contamination that may have entered the bladder. The standing urine then serves as a culture medium for bacterial growth. Incomplete emptying of the bladder prevents flushing out of the bacteria and allows bacteria to ascend to higher structures.
- Contamination in the perineal and urethral areas can be from fecal soiling, from sexual intercourse in which bacteria are massaged into the urinary meatus, or from infection in the area, such as vaginitis, epididymitis, or prostatitis.
- Instrumentation or having instruments or tubes inserted into the urinary meatus can cause infection. The most common cause of instrumentation infection is urinary catheterization. Bacteria ascend around or within the catheter, causing infection. Within 48 hours of catheter insertion, bacterial colonization begins. Many patients develop a UTI within 2 weeks of placement of an indwelling catheter.
- Faulty valves that do not maintain one-way flow can cause reflux of urine from the urethra to the bladder or the bladder to the ureter. Reflux can be congenital or it may be acquired as a result of previous infections.
- Previous UTIs are thought to provide a reservoir of persistent bacteria that cause reinfection.
- Women are more susceptible to UTIs than men due to the short length of the female urethra and its proximity to the anus and vagina. Pregnant women may have asymptomatic bacteruria. Untreated, 40% to 50% will develop pyelonephritis. Pregnant women may be prone to infection with group B streptococci. Most commonly, infection occurs in the second and third trimesters.
- Older adults have an increased incidence of UTIs due to diminished immune response, diabetes, and neurogenic bladder. Aging increases the risk of lower UTIs and may also mask the symptoms. UTI is the most common cause of acute bacterial sepsis in patients over age 65. Older men are predisposed to infection because an enlarged prostate obstructs urine flow. In older women, the decline in estrogen can contribute to the risk of UTI.

> **NURSING CARE TIP**
>
> When caring for a patient at risk for a catheter-related UTI, limit the use of urinary catheters, use infection control procedures at all times, and discontinue the use of the catheter as soon as possible. Catheter-related UTI is a "never event." Hospitals will not be paid by Medicare for the costs of care provided if this condition occurs.

Signs and Symptoms

UTIs are characterized by common symptoms of dysuria, urgency, frequency, incontinence, nocturia, hematuria, back pain, and cloudy, foul-smelling urine (Table 37.1). In the elderly, the most common presenting symptom of UTI is generalized fatigue. The elderly may experience atypical symptoms or present with a change in cognitive functioning, especially noted in patients without dementia. A decline in mental status and fever in any patient with an indwelling catheter meet the diagnostic criteria for a UTI.

Types of UTIs

Urethritis

Urethritis is inflammation of the urethra that may result from a chemical irritant, bacterial infection, trauma, or exposure to a sexually transmitted disease. Post-traumatic urethritis can

• WORD • BUILDING •

urethritis: urethr—urethra (canal that discharges urine from bladder) + itis—inflammation

TABLE 37.1 URINARY TRACT INFECTION (URETHRITIS, CYSTITIS, PYELONEPHRITIS) SUMMARY

Signs and Symptoms	Urinary urgency, frequency, dysuria Flank pain, fever, chills, costovertebral tenderness Cloudy urine with casts, bacteria, and WBCs Urine positive for nitrites
Diagnostic Tests	Urinalysis culture greater than 100,000 bacteria Elevated WBCs Elevated sedimentation rate Increased neutrophils
Therapeutic Measures	Antibiotic therapy sensitive to organism cultured from urine Force fluids
Complications	Pyelonephritis Urosepsis Chronic kidney disease
Priority Nursing Diagnoses	*Pain* *Impaired Urinary Elimination: Frequency* *Ineffective Health Maintenance*

occur with intermittent catheterization or instrumentation of the urethra. Bubble bath and bath salts are common urethral irritants and should not be used by anyone with a history of UTIs. Urethritis can also be caused by spermicidal agents. Gonorrhea and chlamydiosis are sexually transmitted diseases that can cause urethritis in men. It is common to have some degree of urethritis in association with bladder or prostatic infections.

Symptoms of urethritis include urinary frequency, urgency, and dysuria. The male patient may have discharge from the penis. A urinalysis or urine culture is done to diagnose urethritis.

The treatment of urethritis is removal of the cause if the cause is a chemical irritant. If urethritis is caused by bacteria, an antibiotic is prescribed based on the results of a culture. Possible organisms include gram-negative rods, gram-positive cocci, and *Chlamydia.* Phenazopyridine (Pyridium), a urinary analgesic, is often used to treat dysuria. The patient should be forewarned that urine will turn orange while taking phenazopyridine. If urethritis is sexually transmitted, it is important that the sexual partner also be treated.

Cystitis

Cystitis is inflammation and infection of the bladder wall. It can be caused by bacteria, viruses, fungi, or parasites. Fungal infections can occur during long-term antibiotic therapy. About 90% of UTIs are caused by *Escherichia coli.* In most cases, the causative organisms first grow in the perineal area and then ascend into the bladder. Catheters are the most common predisposing factor for UTIs in the hospital setting.

Symptoms include dysuria, frequency, urgency, and cloudy urine. Cystitis acquired outside the hospital is diagnosed with a routine urinalysis collected as a midstream, clean-catch specimen. Changes seen in the urinalysis include cloudy urine and the presence of WBCs, bacteria, and sometimes red blood cells (RBCs) in the specimen. Nitrites are usually positive. Some laboratories also examine for leukocyte esterase, which is positive if infection is present in the urine. In complicated UTIs, such as one acquired in the hospital or a repeat infection, a urine culture and sensitivity should be done. Hospital-acquired UTIs are often caused by bacteria that are resistant to the usual antibiotics used for UTIs. A sensitivity test can identify which antibiotics will be effective against the offending organism.

Treatment of uncomplicated cystitis is most often a combination of sulfa medication, such as sulfamethoxazole and trimethoprim (Bactrim, Septra). Complicated cystitis is often treated with ciprofloxacin (Cipro). Other antibiotics may be prescribed depending on the results of the urine culture and sensitivity. Estrogen used as an intravaginal cream may prevent recurrent UTIs in postmenopausal women. The patient is told to finish all prescribed medications, force fluids unless contraindicated, and return for a follow-up urinalysis or culture after the antibiotic course is complete to ensure that the infection is gone.

Pyelonephritis

PATHOPHYSIOLOGY. Pyelonephritis is infection of the renal pelvis, tubules, and interstitial tissue of one or both kidneys. Pyelonephritis usually begins with colonization and infection of the lower urinary tract by means of the ascending urethral route. A preexisting condition is usually present, such as obstruction, strictures, stones, or vesicoureteral reflux. Risk factors include urological surgery, lymphatic infection, urinary stasis, and decreased immunity. Acute pyelonephritis begins in the renal medulla and spreads to the adjacent cortex.

Pathophysiology includes formation of small abscesses throughout the kidney and gross enlargement of the kidney. On occasion, kidney infection is caused by bacteria spreading from a distant site through the bloodstream and entering the kidney through the glomerulus. Urosepsis is a systemic infection arising from a source within the urinary system. Prompt diagnosis and treatment are essential to prevent septic shock and death. Urosepsis can occur in the elderly or persons susceptible to infection.

SIGNS AND SYMPTOMS. Symptoms include fatigue, urgency, frequency, dysuria, flank pain, fever, and chills. Costovertebral tenderness on the right or left side (tenderness posteriorly at angle where rib and vertebrae join when struck gently with heel of examiner's closed fist), which is associated with renal disease, is noted. The urine is cloudy with increased WBCs, bacteria, casts, RBCs, and positive nitrites. In contrast to cystitis, the patient with pyelonephritis

• WORD • BUILDING •
cystitis: cyst—closed sac containing fluid + itis—inflammation

• WORD • BUILDING •
pyelonephritis: pyelo—pelvis + nephr—kidney + itis—inflammation

is much sicker and shows signs of systemic disease. In acutely ill patients, blood cultures may be obtained.

DIAGNOSTIC TESTS. Several tests are helpful to differentiate pyelonephritis from cystitis. With kidney infection, the urinalysis will show casts. Casts are microscopic particles formed in the kidney from abnormal constituents in the urine such as WBCs, RBCs, or pus. The urine specimen will have more than 100,000 colonies of bacteria per milliliter. The presence of casts always indicates a problem in the kidneys. The complete blood cell (CBC) count will show an elevated WBC count. There will also be an increase in sedimentation rate.

THERAPEUTIC MEASURES. Treatment of pyelonephritis includes administration of antibiotics based on the results of the culture and sensitivity (Table 37.2). With severe gram-negative infections, the patient is hospitalized for intravenous (IV) antibiotics. The patient with acute pyelonephritis generally heals completely after treatment and has no lasting kidney damage. Men who have recurrent UTIs require a 6-week regimen of antibiotic therapy.

TABLE 37.2 MEDICATIONS USED TO TREAT URINARY TRACT INFECTIONS

Medication Class/Action	Example	Route	Side Effects	Nursing Considerations
Antibiotics				
Effective against *Escherichia coli, Klebsiella, Serratia*	aztreonam (Azactam)	IV	Headache, diarrhea, nausea, blurred vision	Contraindicated in patients allergic to penicillins and cephalosporins or if creatinine clearance is less than 30 mL/min. Check BUN and creatinine before administration.
Effective against *E. coli* and *Enterococcus faecalis*	fosfomycin (Monurol)	PO	Headache, diarrhea, nausea	Dissolve packet in 3–4 oz of cold water.
Effective against *E. coli,* enterococci, *Staphylococcus aureus, Klebsiella,* and *Enterobacter.*	nitrofurantoin (Macrobid)	PO	Headache, anorexia, diarrhea, nausea	Give with food or milk and full glass of water. Avoid antacids.
Fluoroquinolones				
Effective against *E. coli, Klebsiella, Pseudomonas,* and other organisms.	ciprofloxacin (Cipro) levofloxacin (Levaquin)	PO IV	Nausea, headache, diarrhea, photosensitivity, increased risk of tendinitis and tendon rupture	Absorption may be decreased if given within 2 hr of aluminum antacids. Give with large amounts of water. Teach to avoid sunlight and report tendon aches promptly.
Sulfonamides				
Effective against *E. coli* and *Pseudomonas.* Used for uncomplicated UTIs.	trimethoprim-sulfamethoxazole (Bactrim, Septra)	PO	Photosensitivity, GI upset, hemolytic anemia, rash Severe hypersensitivity erythema multiforme or exfoliative dermatitis (Stephens-Johnson syndrome)	Teach to avoid sunlight. Give with large amounts of water. Contraindicated in severe renal or liver disease.
Urinary Antiseptic				
Antibacterial action in the urine; not systemic. Effective against *E. coli, Klebsiella,* and other gram-negative organisms.	cinoxacin (Cinobac)	PO	Photosensitivity, GI upset, rash	Teach to avoid sunlight. Encourage fluids. May discolor urine. Absorption may be decreased if given within 2 hr of aluminum or magnesium antacids.
Urinary Antiseptic, Anti-Infective				
Effective against gram-negative and gram-positive organisms, *E. coli.*	methenamine (Mandelamine)	PO	Nausea, vomiting, rash	Do not use with sulfa drugs because may cause crystalluria.
Urinary Analgesic				
Topical analgesic. Relieves pain urgency and frequency associated with UTI.	phenazopyridine (Pyridium)	PO	GI upset, rash, and blue to purple skin discoloration Nephrotoxic and hepatotoxic	Urine color changes to red-orange. Avoid in renal insufficiency. Changes urine glucose testing.

COMPLICATIONS. Repeated kidney infections can result in scarring and loss of kidney function, leading to chronic kidney disease. Septicemia may occur from bacteria invading the bloodstream. When septicemia results from a urinary cause, it is called **urosepsis**. In the elderly, urosepsis can be the cause of new-onset confusion. The elderly or immunocompromised patient may develop septic shock from infection in the urinary tract that has invaded the bloodstream, which may result in death.

Nursing Process for the Patient with a Urinary Tract Infection

Data Collection

It is important to listen to the patient's concerns about the diagnosis. The patient is asked about pain on urination, flank pain, or general symptoms of infection, such as fever, chills, and malaise. The patient's usual pattern of voiding is assessed. Urinary frequency, burning, or pain on urination is noted. Assess the patient for pain in the lower abdomen, flank, or costovertebral angle. The presence of a catheter, recent instrumentation, surgery, or other predisposing factor is determined. The urine is examined for volume, color, concentration, cloudiness, blood, or foul odor. Urinalysis and culture results are examined.

Nursing Diagnoses, Planning, and Implementation

Acute Pain Related to Inflammation of the Urethra, Bladder, and Other Urinary Structures

EXPECTED OUTCOME: The patient will report relief from pain and discomfort.

- Encourage fluids at 2 to 3 L per day *to flush bacteria from urinary tract and promote renal blood flow.*
- Give antimicrobial therapy as ordered *to relieve pain and discomfort from inflammation and infection.*
- Teach patient to finish all prescribed medications *to prevent recurrent infection.*
- Give antispasmodic agents as ordered *to relieve bladder irritability and pain.*
- Administer antipyretics *to relieve fever, pain, and discomfort.*
- Encourage voiding every 3 hours *to empty the bladder, lower bacterial counts, reduce stasis, and prevent reinfection.*
- Teach patient to avoid cola, coffee, tea, and alcohol *because they are urinary irritants.*
- Suggest consuming cranberry juice or capsules *to prevent bacteria from sticking on the walls of the bladder* (see *Evidence-Based Practice* box).
- Apply heat to suprapubic area *to relieve discomfort.*
- Instruct patient to empty bladder as soon as urge is felt and after sexual intercourse *to flush bacteria out of the body.*

• WORD • BUILDING •

urosepsis: uro—urine + sepsis—infection in the blood

EVIDENCE-BASED PRACTICE

Clinical Question

Do cranberries prevent urinary tract infection (UTI)?

Evidence

A systematic review of 10 studies with 1049 participants compared the use of cranberries to prevent UTI with placebo, juice or water (Jepson & Craig, 2007). It was found that cranberry juice or capsules may prevent recurrent infections in women. Cranberries contain a substance that can prevent bacteria from sticking on the walls of the bladder.

Implications for Nursing Practice

Teach women that cranberry products might help prevent recurrent UTI.

REFERENCE

Jepson, R. G., & Craig, J. C. (2007). Cranberries for preventing urinary tract infections. *Cochrane Database of Systematic Reviews 2007, Issue 3* (Art. No. CD001321; DOI 10.1002/14651858.CD001321.pub4).

- Avoid substances such as bubble bath and scented toilet paper, *which can be irritating.*
- Teach patient to practice good perineal hygiene and to wipe front to back *to reduce risk of reinfection.*
- Teach patient to wear cotton underwear *to reduce perineal moisture.*

Impaired Urinary Elimination Related to Frequency, Nocturia, Dysuria, and Incontinence

EXPECTED OUTCOME: The patient will return to previous voiding patterns.

- Monitor urinary elimination, including frequency, consistency, volume, and color, *to identify signs and symptoms of UTI.*
- Administer antimicrobial drugs as ordered *to eliminate symptoms produced by microbial growth.*
- Teach patient to recognize signs and symptoms of UTI *to monitor effectiveness of treatment and detect recurrence.*
- Encourage adequate fluids *to prevent infection and dehydration.*
- Encourage women to void after sexual intercourse *to flush bacteria out of the urethra.*

Risk for Injury Related to Sepsis, Kidney Disease, or Kidney Injury

EXPECTED OUTCOME: The patient will be free from injury due to sepsis or recurrent infection.

- Administer antimicrobial drugs as prescribed *to prevent recurrent infection or complications.*
- Teach signs and symptoms of UTI *so patient can detect recurrence or complications.*

- Monitor patient for signs and symptoms of bacteriuria and bacteremia such as fever, chills, recurrent pain.
- Explain need for follow-up urine culture and imaging studies *when indicated by recurrent symptoms.*
- Monitor intake and output *to ensure adequate intake and normal output.*
- Teach need for adequate fluid intake *to prevent dehydration and renal impairment.*

Evaluation

The outcomes have been met if the patient verbalizes relief of pain and discomfort, returns to previous voiding patterns, and is free from injury related to sepsis, chronic kidney disease, or recurrent infection.

CRITICAL THINKING

Mrs. Milan

■ Mrs. Milan is a 25-year-old woman who recently had a 3-day weekend getaway with her husband. On Monday she notices that she has symptoms of dysuria, frequency, and urgency. She visits her family practitioner and is diagnosed with a UTI. She is placed on an antibiotic.

1. What do you think could have predisposed Mrs. Milan to developing a UTI?
2. What should Mrs. Milan be taught to prevent further occurrences of a UTI?
3. What urinalysis findings would you expect for Mrs. Milan?
4. What should you include in her teaching plan based on her therapeutic regimen?

Suggested answers at end of chapter.

Patient Education

It is very important that patients be advised to take all of the prescribed antibiotic until it is gone. Commonly, patients take medication for several days, until symptoms are gone, and then they stop. Stopping the antibiotic too early allows the infection to continue. It may become chronic and resistant to antibiotics as a result.

Patients who have one UTI commonly develop repeat infections. It is important that such patients receive health teaching to prevent repeated infections of the urinary tract (Box 37.1, *Patient Education*, and Box 37.2, *Nutrition Notes*).

Box 37.1

Patient Education

Preventing Urinary Tract Infection

1. Void frequently—at least every 3 hours while awake.
2. Drink up to 3000 mL of fluid a day if there are no fluid restrictions from the physician. Preferably drink water.
3. Drink one glass of cranberry juice (10 oz) per day.
4. Take showers; avoid tub baths.
5. Wipe perineum from the front to the back after toileting.
6. Urinate after sexual intercourse.
7. Avoid bubble bath and bath salts, perfumed feminine hygiene products, synthetic underwear, and constricting clothing such as tight jeans.
8. Take medication prescribed for urinary tract infection (UTI) until it is all gone.
9. If UTI is associated with another source of infection, such as vaginitis or prostatitis, ensure that both infections are treated.

Box 37.2

Nutrition Notes

Urinary Tract Infections

An effective intervention for urinary tract infection (UTI) is increasing fluid intake, both for its flushing effect and to excrete urinary drugs. Instructions to increase fluid intake should specify amounts to consume or the amount of urine to be produced. Patients have developed electrolyte imbalances by overenthusiastically forcing fluids.

Verifying anecdotal evidence of the effect of cranberry juice in preventing UTI, certain compounds have been identified in cranberries that prevent *Escherichia coli* from adhering to cells in the urinary tract. Cranberry juice has been useful in preventing UTI, and daily intake of 8 to 16 oz of cranberry juice (at least 30% concentration) is recommended for patients with indwelling catheters to prevent UTI.

UROLOGICAL OBSTRUCTIONS

Obstruction of urine flow in the urinary tract is always a significant problem. Urinary tract obstruction is an interference with the flow of urine at any location along the urinary system. The obstruction of urine flow causes dilation and thinning of the renal tubules with eventual atrophy of renal tissues. When urine does not drain normally from the kidney, local compensation occurs initially. The area decompensates and damage occurs, moving the pressure along the continuum of the renal system. The resulting backup of urine and pressure causes dilation and thinning of renal tissue. Renal blood flow is compromised. Eventually renal tissue is destroyed by the compression. The causes of urological obstructions include strictures, stones, and tumors.

Urethral Strictures

A urethral stricture is a narrowing of the lumen of the urethra caused by scar tissue. Urethral strictures are becoming more prevalent due to the rising incidence of sexually transmitted diseases. Increasingly in young adults, gonococcal and chlamydial infections may result in urethral strictures. Most strictures are acquired from injury or infection. Strictures from urethral injury tend to be localized to the area where the injury occurred. Some strictures are a result of trauma from insertion of catheters or surgical instruments. Strictures also may be caused by trauma from straddle injuries, a result of direct application of force to the perineal area, as well as untreated gonorrhea and congenital abnormalities.

The patient with a urethral stricture has a diminished urinary stream and is prone to develop UTIs because of obstruction of urine flow. Urethral strictures are often seen in elderly men. The problem becomes more apparent when attempts to insert a urinary catheter are unsuccessful because of the narrowed lumen.

Initially the treatment of a urethral stricture is mechanical dilation by a urologist, who inserts instruments to stretch open the urethra and then inserts a urinary catheter. If the stricture continues to be a problem after dilation, the area can be surgically repaired (**urethroplasty**).

The dilation process is often done at the bedside when the patient is awake. This is a painful experience for the patient, and it is helpful and caring to encourage the urologist to order pain medication before the procedure. The nursing diagnosis of *Acute Pain* is very relevant. An indwelling catheter is typically inserted after the dilation, so the nursing diagnosis of *Risk for Infection* is also present. Patients need teaching about how to prevent UTIs (see Box 37.1, *Patient Education*).

Renal Calculi

Renal **calculi** (kidney stones; one stone is a *calculus*) are hard, usually small stones that form somewhere in the renal structures. The stones are masses of crystals and protein that form when the urine becomes supersaturated with a salt capable of forming solid crystals. Symptoms occur when the stones become impacted in the urinary tract. When stones are found in the kidneys, the condition is called nephrolithiasis (Fig. 37.1).

Pathophysiology

Normally, substances dissolved in urine, including urinary salts, are diluted and readily excreted from the body. Calculi are formed when urinary salts are concentrated enough to settle out; the salts often collect and deposit around a nucleus. Substances that can serve as a nucleus include pus, blood, dead tissue, a catheter, and crystals. Stones usually grow on the papillae or in the renal tubules, calyces, or renal pelvis. Stones may also form in the ureter or bladder. Stones less than 5 mm are readily passed in the urine. The following are common urinary salts that make up renal calculi, which are arranged in order of commonness:

1. Calcium oxalate
2. Calcium phosphate
3. Magnesium ammonia
4. Uric acid
5. Cystine.

Most renal calculi contain calcium, either as calcium oxalate or calcium phosphate, but it is also possible to have combination stones (Table 37.3).

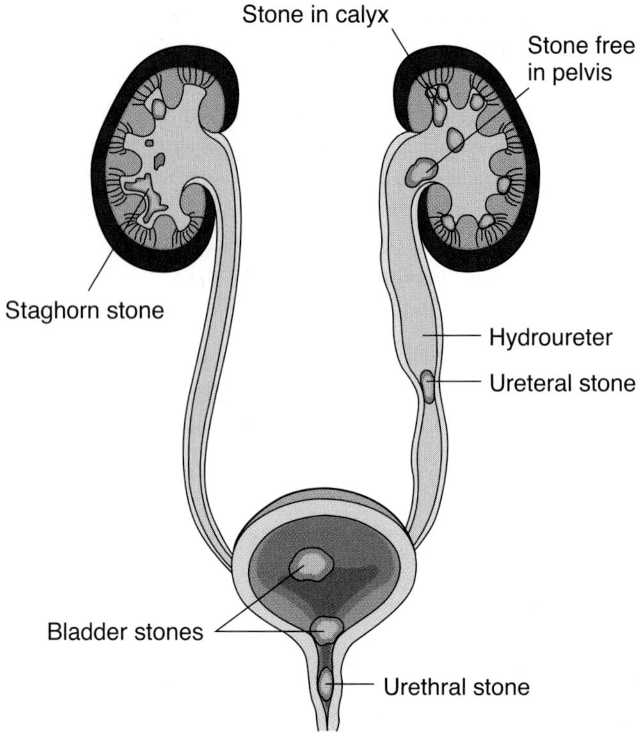

Stone in calyx
Stone free in pelvis
Staghorn stone
Hydroureter
Ureteral stone
Bladder stones
Urethral stone

FIGURE 37.1 Location of calculi in the urinary tract.

Etiology

Causes of calculi formation include a family history of stones, chronic dehydration (causing more concentrated urinary salts), and infection, because the latter provides a nucleus for stone formation. Additional contributing causes of calcium stones include dietary factors (Box 37.3, *Nutrition Notes*) and medications (Table 37.4). Excessive amounts of calcium in the water in some geographical areas may also be a factor. Immobility causes stone formation because of the resulting urinary stasis; in addition, calcium leaves the unstressed bones during immobility, so more calcium is in the blood, which is then filtered through the kidneys. Stones are more common in men than women. The risk peaks between ages 30 and 50.

Signs and Symptoms

Symptoms of renal calculi include excruciating flank pain and renal colic. When a stone is lodged in the ureter, it is common to have pain radiate down to the genitalia. The pain results when the stone prevents urine from draining. Additional

• WORD • BUILDING •
urethroplasty: urethro—urethra + plasty—surgical repair

TABLE 37.3 OVERVIEW OF RENAL CALCULI

Type of Stone	Features	Possible Causes	Interventions
Calcium oxalate, calcium phosphate, or mixture	Accounts for two-thirds of stones Small, rough, and hard Shaped like needles Colors vary from gray to white	Excessive calcium Excessive urea Hyperparathyroidism, Cushing's disease, immobility, osteolysis from tumors of the breast, lung	Force fluids. Restrict protein and sodium in the diet. Administer hydrochlorothiazide. Treat hyperparathyroidism. Cellulose sodium phosphate (Calcibind) may prevent calcium stones by binding calcium from food in the GI system.
Struvite—magnesium ammonium phosphate	Second most common type of stone Calculi crumble easily Stones have a yellow color	Infection by urea splitting microbes, usually *Proteus*. May cause abscess formation in the kidney.	Force fluids. Decrease urine pH. Administer antibiotics.
Uric acid stones	Dye enhancement needed for x-ray visualization Small Color varies from yellow to red Hard	Gout High uric acid levels Decreased fluid intake	Force fluids. Administer sodium citrate to alkalinize urine. Administer allopurinol to reduce urinary uric acid levels. Low-purine diet. Avoid shellfish, anchovies, asparagus, organ meats, and mushrooms.
Cystine stones	Small, smooth calculi Smooth, waxy stones	Cystine-containing crystals appear in the urine	Force fluids. Use low-protein diet; urine is alkalinized. Give penicillamine to decrease amount of cystine in urine.
Triamterene	Type of stone recently identified	Triamterene ingestion	Withhold triamterene (Dyrenium) from at-risk patients.

TABLE 37.4 MEDICATIONS AFFECTING STONE FORMATION

Acetazolamide (Diamox)	Decreases urinary citrates and increases uric acid concentration in urine.
Adrenocorticosteroids	Increases urinary calcium.
Allopurinol	Used to prevent uric acid calculi. May cause the rarer xanthine calculi.
Antacids such as magnesium trisilicate (Gaviscon)	May cause rare silicon-based calculi. Phosphate binding nonabsorbable antacids can increase urinary calcium.
Aspirin	Increases urinary uric acid levels in patients with hyperuricemia.
Chemotherapeutic agents and external radiation	May cause cellular breakdown and cause acute hyperuricemia.
Hydrochlorothiazide (used to prevent calcium calculi)	May cause uric acid calculi by increasing urinary uric acid levels.
Furosemide (Lasix)	May cause hyperuricemia.
Vitamin C in large doses	Increases oxalate excretion in urine.
Vitamin D	Increases calcium and oxalate excretion in urine.

Box 37.3

Nutrition Notes

Renal Calculi

Concentrated urine enhances the formation of crystals so sufficient fluid should be consumed to produce 2000 mL of urine per day. About 3000 mL or 13 cups of water per day are needed to produce this amount of urine.

About 80% of kidney stones are composed of calcium oxalate, which led to early prescriptions for low-calcium diets, but it was later found that a high-calcium intake binds dietary oxalate in the gastrointestinal tract and prevents its absorption, thereby reducing urinary oxalate formation. If a low-oxalate diet is prescribed, foods such as beets, rhubarb, spinach, cocoa, and instant coffee may be restricted.

Uric acid kidney stones can be a complication of gout, which is a disorder of purine metabolism. Purines are end products of digestion of certain proteins and are present in some medications. High-purine foods include organ meats, anchovies, herring, sardines in oil, meat extracts, consommé, and gravies. Low-purine foods include fruits, milk, cheese, eggs, refined grains, sugars, coffee, tea, carbonated beverages, tapioca, yeast, and vegetables (except asparagus, beans, cauliflower, mushrooms, peas, and spinach).

symptoms include hematuria from irritation by the stone, dysuria, frequency, urgency, and enuresis. The patient also may have costovertebral tenderness. Some people develop nausea, vomiting, and diarrhea because of the proximity of the gastrointestinal structures. Table 37.5 summarizes the discussion of renal calculi.

Prevention

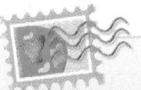

The patient may be advised to avoid foods that increase the risk of recurrent calculus development. Box 37.3 (*Nutrition Notes*) discusses foods that may contribute to calculi (see also Box 37.4, *Cultural Considerations*). Encourage fluid intake to prevent dehydration. Consult with the physician and dietitian to determine which foods should be avoided, depending on the type of stone found. Encourage the patient to walk, which promotes the excretion of stones and reduces bone calcium resorption (release).

TABLE 37.5 RENAL CALCULI SUMMARY

Signs and Symptoms	Costovertebral angle pain
	Groin pain
	Renal colic
	Flank pain radiating to genitalia
	Hematuria
	Anuria
	Restlessness
	Pallor
	Temperature
	Diminished or absent bowel sounds with ileus
Diagnostic Tests	Urinalysis
	Crystals and urine pH
	24-hour renal creatinine clearance
	BUN
	Creatinine
	KUB—reveals most calculi
	Retrograde pyelography
	Ultrasound
Therapeutic Measures	Treat pain to prevent shock
	Chemolysis—stone dissolution using infusions of chemicals to dissolve stone
	Surgery—lithotripsy
	Nephrolithotomy
	Pyelolithotomy
	Percutaneous nephrostomy tube
Complications	Shock
	Sepsis
	Hydronephrosis
	Hydroureter
	Chronic kidney disease
Priority Nursing Diagnoses	*Acute Pain*
	Risk for Infection
	Deficient Knowledge

Complications

The presence of renal calculi increases the risk for UTIs because of obstruction of the free flow of urine. Untreated obstruction of a stone in a ureter or the urethra can also result in retention of urine and damage to the kidney. This process is called **hydronephrosis** (discussed later).

Diagnostic Tests

The diagnosis of renal calculi may be made initially by doing a kidney-ureter-bladder (KUB; flat plate of the abdomen) examination or an intravenous pyelogram. Both of these tests will identify the anatomical location of the stone. Renal ultrasound may be done to identify a stone in the renal pelvis, calyx, or ureter. Urinalysis may indicate gross or microscopic hematuria and could indicate abrasion of the urinary tract. The presence of crystals or urinary pH may indicate calculus type.

Therapeutic Measures

Renal calculi are treated medically if possible. Most stones are flushed out of the body during urination. Patients can pass stones in the urine if they are 5 mm or smaller; larger stones do not pass. Patients who develop severe renal colic are admitted to the hospital. Intravenous fluids are given to hydrate the patient and help flush the stone out of the body. All urine is strained to detect passage of stones, and pain medication such as morphine is given. If the patient is unable to pass the stone and infection, impaired renal function, or severe pain continues, intervention is needed. The solubility of stone-forming substances can be changed by altering the pH of the urine. Calcium stones may be treated with thiazide diuretics and allopurinol (Aloprim, Zyloprim). Surgical removal may be required for large stones, obstructions, or intractable pain.

• WORD • BUILDING •

hydronephrosis: hydro—pertaining to water + nephrosis—degenerative change in kidney

Box 37.4

Cultural Considerations

Recurrent Calculus Development

Filipino immigrants are at high risk for developing renal stones, hyperuricemia, and gout. A shift from a traditional Filipino diet to a U.S. diet increases the occurrence of hyperuricemia, with some older Filipinos developing gout. The nurse may need to assist Filipino patients to identify food choices that will help prevent these conditions.

Caucasians have the highest incidence of kidney stones, followed by Mexican Americans. African Americans have the lowest risk. Prevalence of stones is increased in the south and lowest in the Western part of the United States.

urine instead of functioning kidneys. Sometimes, in a matter of hours, the blood vessels and renal tubules can be damaged extensively.

If the onset of obstruction is gradual, the patient initially may be asymptomatic. Patients commonly develop UTIs because of the obstruction of urine flow and may have symptoms of frequency, urgency, and dysuria. As the disease progresses, flank and back pain may occur. Eventually the patient develops symptoms of chronic kidney disease (discussed later).

Treatment of hydronephrosis always involves relieving the obstruction. Initial removal of the obstruction may be done by insertion of an indwelling urinary catheter. Long-term correction depends on the cause and includes treatments and surgeries to relieve obstruction from strictures, stones, tumor, or an enlarged prostate. At times, the obstruction cannot be relieved because a stone is too large or removal of tumor growth would result in the patient's death. In these situations, **stents**, which are tiny tubes, may be placed inside the ureters during a cystoscopy and pyelogram (C&P) to hold the ureters open, or a **nephrostomy** tube may be inserted directly into the kidney pelvis to drain urine. A nephrostomy tube exits through an incision in the flank area and allows urine to drain into a collecting bag, so that function of the kidney can be maintained. Figure 37.4 shows a stent in place in a ureter and a nephrostomy tube.

Complications associated with hydronephrosis include increased incidence of UTIs because of obstruction of urine flow and kidney failure from unrelieved pressure on the kidneys.

Intake and output are carefully measured. Urine retention can worsen the condition and must be recognized and reported promptly. If the patient has a nephrostomy tube, ensure that it is draining adequately and prevent kinking or clamping of the tube. Kinking of the tube results in continuation of the hydronephrosis, and the resulting pressure will destroy kidney function. If both a nephrostomy tube and urinary catheter are present, output from each should be measured and documented separately.

• WORD • BUILDING •

nephrostomy: nephr—pertaining to the kidney + ostomy—surgically formed artificial opening to the outside

TUMORS OF THE RENAL SYSTEM

Cancer of the Bladder

Cancer of the bladder is the most common kind of cancer of the urinary tract. It is most common in men ages 50 to 70, and is more common in Caucasians than in African Americans. The incidence of bladder cancer has been rising in the United States, and the American Cancer Society estimated that more than 70,000 new cases of bladder cancer occurred in 2009. The chance of having bladder cancer is about 1 in 27 for men and 1 in 85 for women. Bladder cancer is rare in people younger than age 40.

Pathophysiology

Cancer of the bladder often starts as a benign growth on the bladder wall that undergoes cancerous changes. Most bladder cancers begin in the inner lining of the bladder called the urothelium. They are called transition cell cancers. They come in a variety of forms and can behave in different ways. Some occur as small wartlike growths on the inside of the bladder. Others form large tumors that grow into the muscle wall of the bladder and require surgical removal. If the cancer affects only the inner lining of the bladder, it is known as a superficial cancer. If it has spread to the muscle wall, it is called an invasive cancer. Common sites for metastasis include the liver, bones, and lungs.

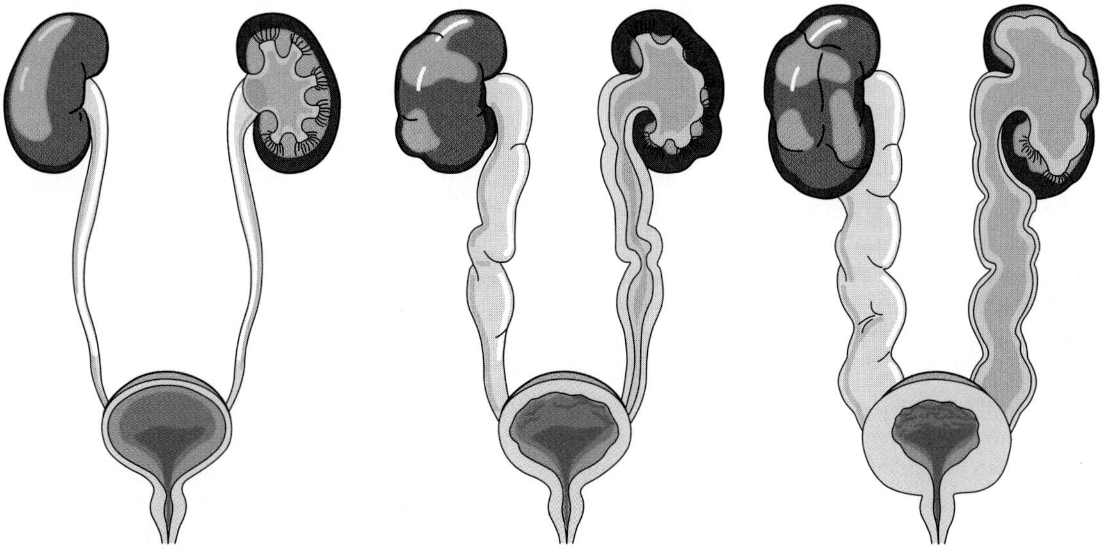

FIGURE 37.3 Hydronephrosis. Progressive thickening of bladder wall and dilation of ureters and kidneys results from obstruction of urine flow.

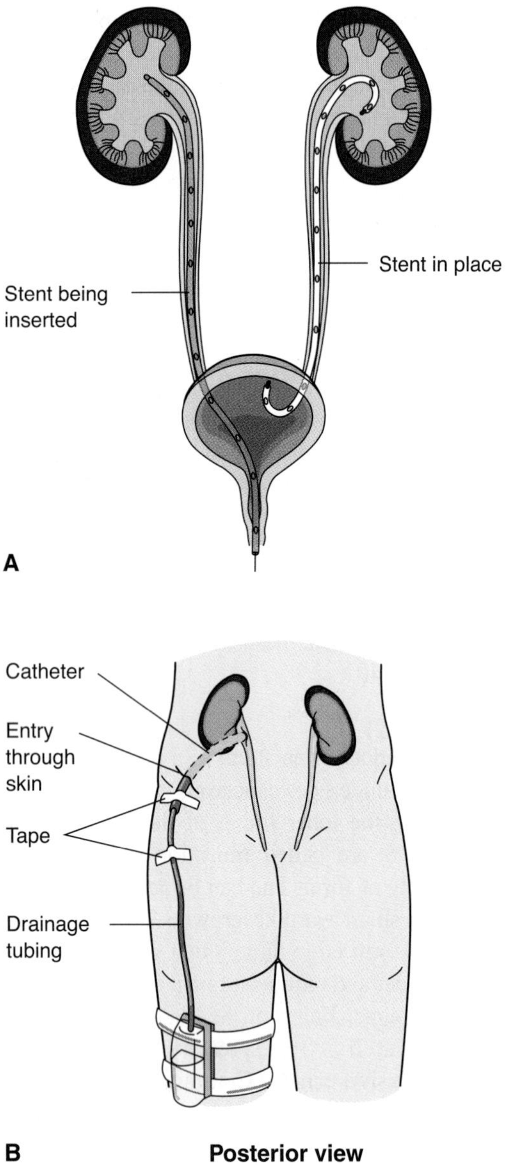
Stent being inserted
Stent in place
A
Catheter
Entry through skin
Tape
Drainage tubing
B
Posterior view

FIGURE 37.4 (A) Ureteral stents. (B) Nephrostomy tube inserted into renal pelvis; catheter exits through an incision on flank.

Etiology

There is a strong correlation between cigarette smoking and bladder cancer. Smokers get bladder cancer twice as often as people who do not smoke. Specific chemicals that cause bladder cancer have been found in cigarette smoke. The more cigarettes smoked, the greater the risk. The lung absorbs the chemicals from tobacco. These chemicals are then passed via the bloodstream to the kidneys and collected in the urine. From there, they accumulate in the urine and damage the cells that line the bladder. Exposure to industrial pollution such as aniline dyes, benzidine and naphthylamine, leather finishings, metal machinery, and petroleum processing products also increases the incidence. It can take about 25 years after exposure to chemicals for bladder cancer to develop. Cancer may also arise from the prostate, colon, and rectum in men and the lower reproductive tract in women. Bladder cancer is often diagnosed at a later stage in women.

Signs and Symptoms

Cancer of the bladder usually causes painless hematuria. The patient may notice that the urine is darker or more reddish in color than usual. Blood in the urine is one of the American Cancer Society's seven warning signs of cancer. Initially the bleeding is intermittent, which often causes the patient to delay seeking treatment. As the disease progresses, the patient develops frank hematuria, bladder irritability, urine retention from clots obstructing the urethra, and fistula formation (an opening between the bladder and an adjoining structure such as the vagina or bowel). Other common signs and symptoms of bladder cancer include pelvic pain, pain in the lower back, painful urination, changes in bladder habits, and inability to void.

Diagnostic Tests

Routine urinalysis can detect evidence of bladder cancer. A urine test for the enzyme telomerase has been found to be 90% accurate in detecting bladder cancer in early and late stages. Urine for cytology can be obtained to determine if cancer cells are present in the urine. Urine culture should also be done. Symptoms of bladder infection may be similar to those of bladder cancer. Diagnosis of bladder cancer may also be made with cystoscopy and transurethral biopsy. An intravenous pyelogram (IVP) also may be done.

Therapeutic Measures

Treatment depends on the type and severity of the bladder cancer. For small, confined tumors, chemotherapeutic agents are instilled into the bladder through a urinary catheter, allowed to dwell, and then removed along with the catheter. Systemic chemotherapy is also used and can be helpful to prolong life when other treatments are no longer indicated. The bacille Calmette-Guérin (BCG) vaccine may be instilled into the bladder to prevent recurring tumors.

Photodynamic therapy, in which drugs are given that make tumors sensitive to light, may be used. When light is applied to the tumor area, cancer cells are killed.

Surgical treatment of bladder cancer includes a number of procedures. A cystoscopy and pyelogram with fulguration (destruction of tissue with electrical current) may be done to burn off cancerous tissue. An alternate method is use of a laser to destroy tumor tissue. Advances in surgical techniques involve robotic and laparoscopic techniques. If the bladder requires removal, robotic laparoscopic radical cystectomy with urinary diversion is an option. In this procedure, robotic surgical equipment, which imitates surgical movements guided by the surgeon, allows more precision, steadiness, and maneuverability than manual surgery, as well as the use of small openings rather than larger incisions into the abdomen. Recovery time is reduced as a result.

INCONTINENT URINARY DIVERSION. If the patient has a potentially curable disease with significant bladder involvement, complete removal of the bladder and creation of a urinary diversion may be done. A urinary diversion means that urine leaves the body in a different manner. A common incontinent surgery for urinary diversion is called an ileal conduit, an involved surgery in which a 6- to 8-inch section of the ileum or colon is removed and used as a conduit for urine. The remaining portions of the bowel are stitched back together. The surgeon is careful to keep the blood and neurologic supply intact to the section of bowel that has been removed. The isolated section of bowel is closed off on one end, the ureters are stitched into it, and the other end is brought out as a stoma on the abdomen that almost continuously drains urine (Fig. 37.5). The urine from an ileal conduit contains mucus because it comes through the ileum, which normally secretes mucus. The patient must wear an ostomy appliance at all times over the stoma to collect urine. Box 37.5 explains how to apply an appliance to an ileal conduit stoma.

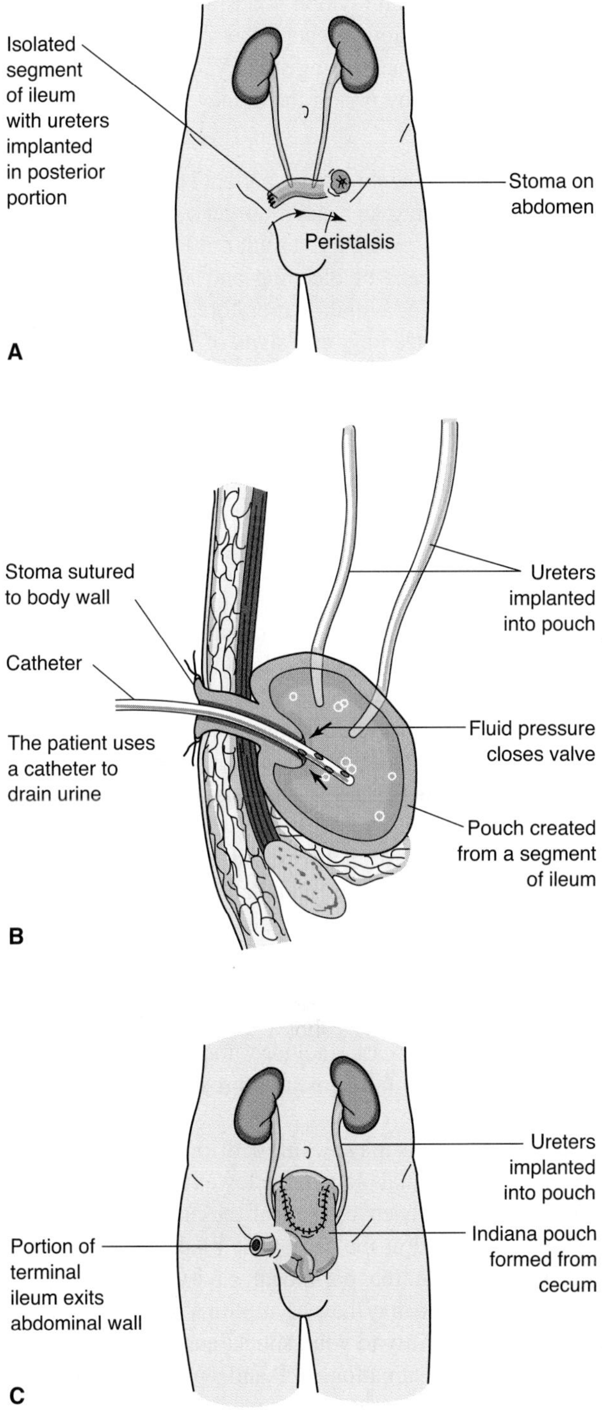
Isolated segment of ileum with ureters implanted in posterior portion
Stoma on abdomen
Peristalsis
A
Stoma sutured to body wall
Catheter
The patient uses a catheter to drain urine
Ureters implanted into pouch
Fluid pressure closes valve
Pouch created from a segment of ileum
B
Ureters implanted into pouch
Indiana pouch formed from cecum
Portion of terminal ileum exits abdominal wall
C

FIGURE 37.5 Urinary diversion surgery. (A) Ileal conduit. (B) Kock pouch. (C) Indiana pouch.

CONTINENT URINARY DIVERSION. Continent urinary diversion surgeries are being done for patient convenience. One version is the Kock pouch (continent internal ileal reservoir), which is created from a segment of ileum that has been made into a reservoir for urine (see Fig. 37.5B). The ureters are implanted into the side of the reservoir. A special nipple valve is constructed and is the passageway through which the patient inserts a catheter at 4- to 6-hour intervals to drain urine. Another version of this surgery is the Indiana pouch (see Fig. 37.5C). A reservoir is created using a portion of the ascending colon and terminal ileum, making a larger pouch than the Kock pouch. Additional versions of this type of surgery use other parts of the bowel and include the Mainz pouch or Florida pouch.

Box 37.5

Application of a Disposable Pouch to an Ileal Conduit

1. Gather all supplies: a washcloth, towels, and water; a pouch to apply with a Stomahesive flange; and wicks such as gauze to absorb continually flowing urine. Wear clean gloves.
2. Empty the old pouch.
3. Gently remove soiled pouch by pushing down on skin while lifting up on the flange. Discard soiled pouch and flange.
4. Place a towel around the stoma to catch urine.
5. Mold or cut an opening in the flange that is only 1/16 to 1/8 inch larger than the stoma. Once stomal shrinkage is complete, a presized pouch can be used that fits the stoma.
6. Remove paper backing from the Stomahesive and set the flange to one side.
7. Clean the skin around the stoma with water. Pat dry. Immediately wrap the stoma in wicks to absorb urine. Otherwise urine will leak onto the skin, and the flange will not adhere.
8. Center the flange over the stoma, remove the wick, and immediately apply the flange. Then snap the pouch onto the flange. *Note:* The flange and pouch may be snapped together before application to the stoma.
9. Use the heat of your hand to compress the flange to ensure a good seal.
10. Ensure that the bottom of the pouch is closed off, or connect to a urinary catheter bag at night or if patient is in bed most of the time.

ORTHOTOPIC BLADDER SUBSTITUTION. This surgery involves formation of an orthotopic bladder using a section of the intestine to make a neobladder (neo = new) and implanting both the ureters and the urethra into the neobladder. Various types of orthotopic bladder substitution surgery include the Studer pouch, hemi-Kock pouch, and ileal W-neobladder. After this surgery, the patient can void through the urethra, although incontinence may be a problem and intermittent catheterization may be needed.

Nursing Care

Nursing care of the postoperative patient is similar to care following any major surgical procedure. (See Chapter 11.) Specific postoperative care should be aimed at preventing complications of shock, atelectasis, pneumonia, deep venous thrombosis, and paralytic ileus. It is important to ensure adequate urinary output and to detect and report any obstruction of urine drainage early to prevent complications. The skin around the stoma will require special care to prevent skin breakdown. The patient needs to be taught how to care for the urinary diversion after surgery, either by frequent draining with a catheter or by wearing an appliance. Be sensitive to the patient's anxiety about caring for the urinary diversion.

Body image disturbance may occur because of the change in body function. A consultation with a nurse who specializes in wound, ostomy, and continence care (WOC nurse; sometimes referred to as an enterostomal therapy nurse, which was the original name for this specialty) or an ostomy support group may be helpful both before and after surgery.

Cancer of the Kidney

Pathophysiology and Etiology

Cancer of the kidney is among the 10 most common cancers in both men and women. The American Cancer Society estimated about 57,760 new cases of kidney cancer occurred in 2009. The lifetime risk of kidney cancer is 1 in 75. Risk factors include smoking, obesity, hypertension, years of kidney dialysis, and exposure to radiation, asbestos, and industrial pollution. Most patients are between ages 50 and 70. During the last 35 years, there has been an increased incidence in renal cell cancer, with an increase of 43% since 1973. This is probably due to the use of CT scans and ultrasound evaluation of the abdomen. More than 50% of tumors are found incidentally. Men have twice the incidence of women. Often the cancer has metastasized before it is diagnosed because the kidney has such a large volume of circulating blood, which increases the risk of tumor spread. In addition, the disease has few early symptoms.

Signs and Symptoms

The three classic symptoms of kidney cancer are hematuria, dull pain in the flank area, and a mass in the area. Often, symptoms of kidney cancer do not occur until the tumor invades surrounding tissue. Less specific symptoms include fever, weight loss, night sweats, hypertension, anemia, polycythemia, swelling in the legs, fatigue, anorexia, and constipation. Symptoms of metastasis may be the first evidence of kidney cancer and include weight loss, cough, bone fractures, liver abnormalities, and increasing weakness.

Diagnostic Tests

A number of diagnostic tests will be done, including an IVP, cystoscopy and pyelogram, ultrasound examination of the kidneys, computed tomography (CT) scans of the abdomen, and magnetic resonance imaging (MRI). A definitive diagnosis is made with a renal biopsy.

Therapeutic Measures

Surgery is the commonly used treatment for cancer of the kidney. A radical **nephrectomy** removes the entire kidney along with the adrenal gland and other surrounding structures, including fascia, fat, and lymph nodes, in the area. Radiation therapy, immunotherapy, or chemotherapy may be used after the surgery. In nephron-sparing surgery, only the tumor is removed and the healthy part of the kidney is saved.

Nursing Care

Nursing care of the nephrectomy patient is similar to postoperative care following any major surgery. (See Chapter 11.) Because the kidney is highly vascular, it is essential that the nurse watch for onset of bleeding and any signs of hypovolemic shock. Urine output is monitored. Changes in urine amount or color, bleeding, and signs of infection are reported. The patient should be assessed for shortness of breath or diminished breath sounds on the affected side. Surgically induced or spontaneous pneumothorax may occasionally occur after a nephrectomy.

RENAL SYSTEM TRAUMA

Renal trauma is the most common injury to the urinary system. The kidneys are highly vascular and have a lot of mobility, so they are vulnerable to vascular and tissue damage. The many causes of trauma to the kidney, ureters, and bladder include motor vehicle accidents, sports injuries, falls, gunshot wounds, and stabbing. Young men are at greatest risk for renal system trauma.

Patient assessment includes a history of the injury and inspection of the abdomen and flank for asymmetry and bruising or swelling of the flank area. Flank pain and hematuria may be present. Diagnostic tests include urinalysis, IVP, ultrasound, CT, and MRI. Treatment depends on the extent of the injury and ranges from bedrest to surgical intervention. Nursing care includes measuring intake and output, monitoring vital signs, and providing IV fluids and pain relief.

Bladder trauma may occur with pelvic fractures and multiple trauma from a blow to the lower abdomen when the bladder is full. The weakest part of the bladder wall, which is the dome located at the top of the bladder, may rupture. Urine leaks out of the peritoneal cavity and around the bowel. The patient may have symptoms of hematuria, abdominal pain, inability to void, shock, and pelvic hematoma noted on rectal examination. IVP and x-ray of the abdomen

• WORD • BUILDING •

nephrectomy: nephr—kidney + ectomy—excision

may be done. A urinary or suprapubic catheter should be in place until the bladder heals.

POLYCYSTIC KIDNEY DISEASE

Polycystic kidney disease is a hereditary disorder that can result in chronic kidney disease. The disease affects men and women equally. Polycystic kidney disease is characterized by formation of multiple cysts in the kidney that can eventually replace normal kidney structures. The cysts are grapelike and contain serous fluid, blood, or urine. The patient typically first shows signs of the disease in adulthood. The initial symptoms include a dull heaviness in the flank or lumbar region and hematuria. Other symptoms include hypertension and UTIs. People with inherited polycystic kidney disease may also experience aneurysms in the brain and diverticulosis in the colon. As the disease progresses, the patient develops symptoms of chronic kidney disease (discussed later). The renal cysts are usually diagnosed with ultrasound imaging. Ultrasound uses no dyes or radiation, so it is safe for all patients, including pregnant women. Often there is a strong family history of polycystic kidney disease.

There is no treatment to stop the progression of polycystic kidney disease. Complications such as UTIs are treated as needed. Headaches that are severe due to hypertension or seem to feel different might be caused by aneurysms in the brain. A patient with severe or recurring headache should see a physician. As the disease progresses, treatment for hypertension and eventual chronic kidney disease may be needed. Because polycystic disease is hereditary, patients should be counseled about the risks of children inheriting it.

CHRONIC RENAL DISEASES

Diabetic Nephropathy

Diabetic **nephropathy** is the most common cause of chronic kidney disease. It is a long-term complication of diabetes mellitus in which the effects of diabetes result in damage to the small blood vessels in the kidneys. Microalbuminuria may be detected within 5 years of the onset of type 1 diabetes and 10 to 15 years after the onset of type 2 diabetes. Renal damage appears about 15 to 20 years after onset of type 1 diabetes, but it may also be a complication of type 2 diabetes. Risk factors for development of diabetic nephropathy include hypertension, genetic predisposition, smoking, and chronic hyperglycemia. Careful control of blood glucose levels reduces the risk of nephropathy in patients with diabetes.

• WORD • BUILDING •
nephropathy: nephro—pertaining to the kidney + pathy—disease

Pathophysiology

Multiple factors contribute to diabetic nephropathy. It begins with increased osmotic pressure from hyperglycemia, increased diuresis and compensatory cell growth and expansion, and increased glomerular filtration rate. Widespread atherosclerotic changes occur in the blood vessels of patients with diabetes, decreasing the blood supply to the kidney. Abnormal thickening of glomerular capillaries damages the glomerulus, allowing protein to leak into urine. Patients with diabetes also commonly develop pyelonephritis and renal scarring. Another complication of diabetes, neurogenic bladder, causes incomplete bladder emptying. This results in urine retention, which can cause infection or obstruction of urine, further damaging the kidneys.

Initially, patients lose only small amounts of protein in their urine (microalbuminuria); this disease can be detected only with careful watching by the physician, using frequent examinations of the urine. As the disease progresses, high-output chronic kidney disease (nonoliguria) can develop, in which a large amount of diluted urine is excreted without the usual amounts of waste products dissolved in the urine. The patient can lose large amounts of protein in the urine and may develop nephrotic syndrome, which causes massive edema because of low levels of albumin in the blood. As renal function decreases, the patient needs smaller doses of insulin because the kidney normally degrades insulin. Because the kidney is no longer able to break down insulin and excrete it, small doses of insulin circulate in the body for long periods.

Symptoms

The progression of nephropathy is marked by microalbuminuria advancing to proteinuria. Hypertension accelerates the renal damage. As diabetic nephropathy progresses, urine output decreases, toxic wastes accumulate, and the patient develops chronic kidney disease. For symptoms, see the discussion of chronic kidney disease in a later section.

Complications

Patients with diabetic nephropathy often have a guarded prognosis because they are vulnerable to all the complications of long-term diabetes in addition to kidney disease. The risk of cardiovascular disease is significant with the progression of protein spilling in the urine.

Diagnostic Tests

Diabetic nephropathy is diagnosed by carefully watching the patient with diabetes for onset of protein spillage or microalbuminuria in the urine, which is an early sign of the disease. Serum creatinine levels and 24-hour creatinine clearance tests are then done to confirm the presence and extent of diabetic nephropathy.

Therapeutic Measures

In the early stages of diabetic nephropathy, strict control of blood glucose levels and blood pressure can help slow the progress of the disease and reduce symptoms. Angiotensin-converting enzyme (ACE) inhibitors or angiotensin II receptor blockers (ARBs) may be given to slow the decline of the glomerular filtration rate and microalbuminuria. As the disease progresses, the patient needs dialysis to maintain life. Unfortunately, other complications related to diabetes cause patients to tolerate dialysis less well than patients with chronic kidney disease from other causes. Kidney or kidney-pancreas transplant, when available, is the treatment of choice for the patient with diabetic nephropathy and often improves the patient's chance for a healthier life.

Nephrotic Syndrome

Nephrotic syndrome is the excretion of 3.5 g or more of protein in the urine per day. Nephrotic syndrome may occur as a result of other disease processes. In nephrotic syndrome, large amounts of protein are lost in the urine from increased glomerular membrane permeability. As a result, serum albumin and total serum protein are decreased. Normally, albumin and other serum proteins maintain fluid within the vascular space. When levels of these proteins are low, fluid leaks from the blood vessels into tissues, resulting in edema. With very low levels of protein, ascites and massive widespread edema (anasarca) occur. In response to the low protein levels, the liver produces lipoproteins. As a result, serum cholesterol, low-density lipoproteins, and triglyceride levels are elevated. Urine may appear foamy from lipoproteinemia. Loss of immunoglobulins may lead to increased susceptibility to infection. Elevated blood pressure readings are noted.

Treatment is focused on the cause and symptoms of nephrotic syndrome. To control edema, sodium intake is restricted. A low to moderate protein intake is ordered to prevent buildup of nitrogen wastes (which result from protein metabolism) from impaired kidney function. Protein intake is based on the severity of urinary protein loss. Diuretics may be used. Lipid-lowering drugs may be tried. Anticoagulants are given for thrombosis. In some cases, corticosteroids may be used.

Complications of nephrotic syndrome include impaired immune function, nutritional imbalances, and most importantly increased blood coagulation. Nursing care focuses on the edema and preventing infection. For edema, daily weights, careful measurements of intake and output, and abdominal girth measurements are performed and documented. Edematous tissue must be protected from injury. Preventing malnutrition is challenging but important in maintaining normal body functions.

Nephrosclerosis

Hypertension damages the kidneys by causing sclerotic changes in the small arteries and arterioles, such as arteriosclerosis with thickening and hardening of the renal blood vessels (**nephrosclerosis**). Arteriosclerotic changes in the kidney blood vessels result in a decreased blood supply to the kidney (ischemia of the kidney) and can eventually destroy the kidney. The remaining nephrons try to compensate with vasodilation to increase blood flow to the glomeruli. This results in increased glomerular pressure and filtration, which thickens the blood vessels. High pressure in the kidneys causes the vessels to weaken and hemorrhage. Large areas of the kidney become damaged. Symptoms of nephrosclerosis include proteinuria, hyaline casts in the urine, and, as it progresses, symptoms of chronic kidney disease.

The treatment for nephrosclerosis is to reduce blood pressure and treat the hypertension. The patient is placed on antihypertensive medications or, if already on these, changed to stronger antihypertensive medications. The patient is placed on a low-sodium diet. Dialysis may be used to maintain life.

The prognosis is often poor because by the time the patient has developed nephrosclerosis, there is widespread arteriosclerosis throughout the body. Arteriosclerosis makes the patient prone to myocardial infarctions or cerebrovascular accidents.

The major nursing diagnosis that is relevant when the patient develops nephrosclerosis is *Ineffective Health Maintenance.* The priority is to help the patient learn as much about the control of hypertension as possible. The patient should also be taught the symptoms of chronic kidney disease. Once the patient has lost renal function, the nursing care plan for chronic kidney disease is appropriate.

> **CRITICAL THINKING**
>
> ***Mr. Stevens***
>
> ■ Mr. Stevens is a 35-year-old African American man admitted to the intensive care unit with uncontrolled hypertension. His blood pressure is controlled by intravenous medication. His laboratory tests show protein and hyaline casts in the urine. He is diagnosed with nephrosclerosis.
>
> 1. What data should the nurse collect as part of the morning evaluation of the patient's condition?
> 2. What other renal function tests are appropriate for the nurse to check?
> 3. What teaching does Mr. Stevens need when his condition is more stable?
>
> *Suggested answers at end of chapter.*

GLOMERULONEPHRITIS

Pathophysiology

Glomerulonephritis is an inflammatory disease of the glomerulus. It can be caused by a variety of factors including immunological abnormalities, toxins, vascular disorders, and systemic diseases. Inflammation occurs as a result of the

• WORD • BUILDING •
nephrosclerosis: nephro—pertaining to the kidney + sclerosis—hardening

• WORD • BUILDING •
glomerulonephritis: glomerulo—glomerulus + nephr—kidney + itis—inflammation

deposition of antigen-antibody complexes in the basement membrane of the glomerulus or from antibodies that specifically attack the basement membrane. The resulting immune reaction in the glomerulus causes inflammation, which in turn causes the glomerulus to be more porous, allowing proteins, white blood cells, and red blood cells to leak into the urine.

Etiology

Acute Poststreptococcal Glomerulonephritis

Glomerulonephritis is most commonly associated with a group A beta-hemolytic streptococcal infection following a streptococcal infection of the throat or skin. This is the most common cause in children and young adults. Antibodies form complexes with the streptococcal antigen and are deposited in the basement membrane of the glomerulus, inducing damage from inflammation. Damaged glomeruli become unable to filter blood correctly, and protein leaks into the urine. Edema, oliguria, and hypertension result. Glomerulonephritis typically develops about 6 to 10 days after the preceding infection. The disease has an abrupt onset. Other kinds of bacteria and viruses can also be the offending infectious agent.

Goodpasture's Syndrome

Occasionally glomerulonephritis is caused by an autoimmune response, in which the person for unknown reasons forms antibodies against his or her own glomerular basement membrane. Glomerulonephritis caused by an autoimmune response usually progresses rapidly and often leads to chronic kidney disease.

Chronic Glomerulonephritis

Chronic glomerulonephritis occurs over years as a result of glomerular inflammatory disease. There may be no history of renal disease before the diagnosis. Often, proteinuria and hematuria may have been noted previously before the diagnosis. Lupus erythematosus and insulin-dependent diabetes mellitus may precede chronic glomerular injury. It is often discovered during an examination for another concern. Ultrasound, CT scan, or renal biopsy is used to diagnose the cause.

Symptoms

Symptoms of glomerulonephritis include fluid overload with oliguria, hypertension, electrolyte imbalances, and edema (Table 37.6). Edema may begin around the eyes (periorbital edema) and face and progress to the abdomen (ascites), lungs (pleural effusion), and extremities. Flank pain may be present. Blood urea nitrogen (BUN) and creatinine levels may be elevated. Urinalysis shows red blood cells, white blood cells, albumin, and casts. The urine is dark or cola colored from old red blood cells and may be foamy because of proteinuria.

Complications

The prognosis is good for acute glomerulonephritis acquired in childhood, and most children recover completely. Adults who develop glomerulonephritis may recover renal function or progress to chronic glomerulonephritis. Some patients develop rapidly progressive glomerulonephritis, which can quickly lead to acute renal injury. Chronic glomerulonephritis is a slow process characterized by hypertension, gradual loss of renal function, and eventual chronic kidney disease.

TABLE 37.6 GLOMERULONEPHRITIS SUMMARY

Signs and Symptoms	Fluid volume overload Hypertension Electrolyte imbalances Edema Periorbital edema Flank pain
Diagnostic Tests	Urinalysis shows red cells, WBCs, protein, and casts Urine dark or cola colored Foamy urine from protein Creatinine, urea level elevated Renal biopsy
Therapeutic Measures	Treatment is symptomatic Nonsteroidal anti-inflammatory drugs Steroids Antibiotics prophylactically to prevent further kidney damage
Complications	Chronic kidney disease
Priority Nursing Diagnoses	*Fluid Volume Excess* *Decreased Tissue Perfusion*

Diagnostic Tests

Glomerulonephritis is diagnosed with urinalysis, which shows protein, casts, or RBCs and elevated serum levels of nitrogenous wastes (creatinine, urea). Hypertension may be present. Kidney ultrasound, x-ray, or biopsy may be done to determine abnormal kidney shape, size, blood flow, inflammation, or scarring of the glomeruli.

Therapeutic Measures

Most cases of acute glomerulonephritis resolve spontaneously in about a week, but some progress to chronic kidney disease. Treatment is primarily symptomatic. Sodium and fluid restrictions may be ordered along with diuretics to treat fluid retention. Medications may be given to control hypertension. If associated with a streptococcal infection, antibiotics are given to treat any remaining infection. If fluid overload is severe, dialysis may be done.

Nursing Care

Nursing care for a patient with glomerulonephritis focuses on symptom relief. Vital signs are monitored because the patient may be critically ill. During the acute phase, rest is encouraged. Edema is controlled with fluid and sodium intake restrictions. Protein intake may be limited if the kidneys are not filtering protein waste products (as seen by increased serum BUN and creatinine levels). Other care is discussed in the next section on chronic kidney disease. Teaching the patient about preventing glomerulonephritis is important. Antibiotics for diagnosed streptococcal throat infections should be taken for prevention.

ACUTE KIDNEY INJURY OR CHRONIC KIDNEY DISEASE

Kidney disease is diagnosed when the kidneys are no longer functioning adequately to maintain normal body processes. This results in dysfunction in almost all other parts of the body as a result of imbalances in fluid, electrolytes, and calcium levels, as well as impaired RBC formation and decreased elimination of waste products. It can be acute (acute kidney injury) with sudden onset of symptoms, or it can be chronic (chronic kidney disease), occurring gradually over time. For more information on kidneys, visit the American Kidney Fund at www.kidneyfund.org, the National Kidney Foundation at www.kidney.org, and the American Association of Kidney Patients at www.aakp.org.

Acute Kidney Injury

Acute kidney injury is the sudden (hours to days) loss of the kidneys' ability to clear waste products and regulate fluid and electrolyte balance. Rapid accumulation of toxic wastes from protein metabolism in the blood (**azotemia**) occurs. In azotemia, the serum urea level (measured by BUN) and creatinine level are elevated. Most types of acute kidney injury are reversible if diagnosed and treated early; however, acute kidney injury can lead to chronic kidney disease. It often is associated with a urine output of less than 30 mL/hr or 400 mL/day. It may be caused by hypotension, dehydration, vascular obstruction, glomerular disease, or acute tubular necrosis, in which the tubules are damaged after administration of diagnostic contrast media.

> **NURSING CARE TIP**
>
> To protect patients' kidneys, be aware of the following:
>
> - The patient's renal function status. Serum BUN and creatinine levels will tell you this.
> - Nephrotoxic substances:
>   - Diagnostic contrast media (dyes) in the presence of dehydration or renal impairment
>   - Medications—IV aminoglycosides (gentamicin [Garamycin], tobramycin [Tobrex], amikacin [Amikin], cisplatin [Platinol])
>   - Chemicals—arsenic, carbon tetrachloride, lead, mercuric chloride.
> - Preventive measures:
>   - Before administering nephrotoxic dyes or medications, check serum BUN and creatinine levels.
>   - With contrast media (dye) tests, encourage fluids before and after to dilute and flush, flush, flush the dye away!
>
> Make sure peak and trough drug levels of nephrotoxic drugs are obtained on an ongoing basis per institutional policy.

• WORD • BUILDING •

azotemia: azo—nitrogenous waste products + temia—blood

Pathophysiology

In acute kidney injury, rapid damage to the kidney causes waste products to accumulate in the bloodstream, resulting in signs and symptoms. The patient becomes oliguric, with urine output decreasing to less than 20 mL/h. Treatment is directed toward correcting the cause, supporting the patient with dialysis, and preventing complications that may lead to permanent damage. Many patients with acute kidney injury recover completely. About 50% of patients with intrarenal acute kidney injury die from complications, such as infection, pneumonia, or septicemia.

Acute kidney injury can progress through four stages, with an intrarenal cause taking a longer recovery time because there is actual renal damage. Once an event causes acute kidney injury in the initial phase, symptoms occur in hours to days.

OLIGURIC PHASE. In the oliguric phase, less than 400 mL of urine is produced in 24 hours. Fifty percent of those with acute kidney injury experience this phase, which occurs from 24 hours to 7 days after the initial phase. This phase can last up to 2 weeks to several months. Prognosis for renal recovery is decreased the longer this phase lasts.

In the oliguric phase, fluid is retained, electrolytes become imbalanced, and waste products are not excreted as urine output decreases. Signs of fluid overload arise. Serum potassium rises while sodium is lost in the urine, creating a normal or low serum sodium level. The longer this phase lasts, the more effects are seen. These may include metabolic acidosis from reduced hydrogen ion excretion and sodium bicarbonate levels, increased phosphate and decreased calcium levels, abnormal blood cells (RBC, WBC, platelets), neurologic effects ranging from confusion to seizures to coma, and finally effects on all body systems as is seen in chronic renal failure (discussed later).

DIURETIC PHASE. As the kidneys begin to excrete waste products again, 1 to 3 L/day of urine is produced. Osmotic diuresis occurs from the elevated waste products (urea), which the body is attempting to eliminate. The kidneys are not yet able to concentrate urine and so dehydration and hypotension are a concern. It is important for the nurse to monitor for hypovolemia, hyponatremia, and hypotension in this phase. Serum BUN and creatinine levels are high until the end of this phase, when they begin to return to normal. This phase may last 1 to 3 weeks.

RECOVERY PHASE. In this final phase, recovery begins as the glomerular filtration rate rises. Waste product levels (BUN, creatinine) decrease greatly within the first 2 weeks of this phase. However, recovery can take up to 1 year.

Those who do recover usually do so without complications. Older adults are more at risk for reduced recovery of renal function. In those who do not recover renal function, chronic kidney disease occurs.

Etiology

Acute kidney injury is often classified as prerenal, intrarenal, or postrenal. These categories relate to the causes leading to the injury. Each category is associated with the location of the cause in the kidney. Understanding the cause can point to the direction of treatment plans helpful to the patient.

PRERENAL INJURY. Prerenal (before the kidney) injury is associated with a decrease or interruption of blood supply to the kidneys. This cause accounts for 55% to 60% of all cases of acute kidney injury. Causes may include decreased blood pressure from dehydration, blood loss, shock, or trauma to or blockage in the arteries that carry blood to the kidneys. When the nephrons receive an inadequate blood supply, they are unable to make urine, and waste products are not adequately removed. Use of nonsteroidal anti-inflammatory drugs (NSAIDs) and cyclooxygenase-2 (COX) inhibitors can also lead to prerenal injury. These drugs impair the autoregulatory responses of the kidney by blocking prostaglandin, which is needed for renal perfusion.

Prerenal injury can be diagnosed by evaluating possible causes. If dehydration is the cause, then an IV fluid challenge may be given. With increased IV fluid, more blood flows to the kidneys for filtering, which increases urine output and waste product filtering. An arteriogram of the renal arteries is helpful to determine if the blood supply to the kidneys is decreased or blocked; angioplasty may be used to open the blockage. Serum creatinine increases and creatinine clearance decreases. Urinalysis may be helpful in determining the cause as well.

INTRARENAL INJURY. Intrarenal (inside the kidney) injury occurs when there is damage to the nephrons inside the kidney. The most common causes are ischemia, reduced blood flow, and toxins. Other causes are infectious processes leading to glomerulonephritis, trauma to the kidney, exposure to **nephrotoxins**, allergic reactions to radiographic dyes, and severe muscle injury, which releases substances that are harmful to the kidneys.

A number of substances can be toxic to the kidneys (nephrotoxic) when they enter the body (Table 37.7). Kidney damage is most likely to occur when these substances enter the body in high concentrations or when preexisting kidney damage is present for some other reason. Environmental nephrotoxins, such as insecticides and lead paint, may be ingested by children. Many commonly administered medications can be nephrotoxic. Aminoglycosides are nephrotoxic antibiotics; when they are administered, blood levels of the drugs are carefully monitored to avoid toxic levels.

• WORD • BUILDING •

nephrotoxin: nephro—kidney + toxin—poison

TABLE 37.7 COMMON NEPHROTOXINS

Antibiotics	Aminoglycosides Amphotericin B Cephalosporins Sulfonamides Tetracyclines
Analgesics	Acetaminophen Nonsteroidal anti-inflammatory drugs Salicylates
Other Drugs	ACE inhibitors Amphetamines Cisplatin Dextran Heroin Interleukin-2 Mannitol
Heavy Metals	Arsenic Copper Gold Lead Lithium Mercury
Contrast Dyes	Contrast media used for diagnostic testing such as intravenous pyelograms, cardiac catheterizations
Organic Solvents	Gasoline Glycols Kerosene Tetrachloroethylene Turpentine

ACE = angiotensin-converting enzyme.

Contrast media used during tests such as intravenous pyelograms and CT scans can cause kidney damage when the patient is dehydrated or has preexisting renal damage. The medium can precipitate out in the tubules, damaging the kidney. It is important for the patient to be adequately hydrated before and after any diagnostic test using a contrast medium to decrease the incidence of toxicity.

POSTRENAL INJURY. Postrenal (after the kidney) injury is associated with an obstruction that blocks the flow of urine out of the body. Only 5% of acute kidney injuries are classified as postrenal. In this case, the blood supply to the kidneys and nephron function initially may be normal, but urine is unable to drain out of the kidney, resulting in the backup of urine and impaired nephron function. Common causes are kidney stones, tumors of the ureters or bladder, and an enlarged prostate that blocks the flow of urine.

Diagnosis of causes can be done with x-ray examination of the kidneys, ureters, and bladder. Cystoscopy will show tumors, stones, or prostate enlargement. Renal ultrasound can measure kidney size, detect tumors and blockages, and reveal cystic disease. Surgical intervention may be needed to correct the problem.

Therapeutic Measures

Acute kidney injury is treated by relieving the cause. Prevention of permanent damage is the goal of treatment. Signs and symptoms are managed as they develop, and supportive care is given. Treatment may include restoring fluid and electrolyte balance, discontinuing nephrotoxic drugs that may have caused the problem, bypassing urinary tract obstructions with catheters, or using short-term continuous renal replacement therapy to filter blood and restore potassium and other electrolytes to normal. Some symptoms, such as anemia, may not have time to develop in the patient with acute kidney injury as they do in chronic kidney disease. The care of the patient with acute kidney injury is similar to care of the patient with chronic kidney disease, as explained in the next section.

CONTINUOUS RENAL REPLACEMENT THERAPY. Continuous renal replacement therapy (CRRT) is used to remove fluid and solutes in a controlled, continuous manner in unstable patients with acute kidney injury. Unstable patients may not be able to tolerate the rapid fluid shifts that occur in hemodialysis, so CRRT provides an alternative therapy that results in less dramatic fluid shifting. CRRT can be used with **hemodialysis**, which is needed if severe symptoms of **uremia** (hyperkalemia) are present. CRRT is not as complex as hemodialysis and can be done for more than a month, if needed, via temporary vascular access.

During CRRT, a permeable hemofilter is attached to the vascular access. Blood flows through the hemofilter and excess fluids and solutes move into a collection bag. The remaining blood returns to the patient via the venous access. If desired, replacement fluid and electrolytes can be given through the vascular access. Monitoring intake and output, fluid and electrolytes, daily weights, hourly vital signs, and vascular access is important.

Chronic Kidney Disease

Chronic kidney disease affects about 290,000 people in the United States. Incidence is on the rise. This disease is a progressive, irreversible deterioration in renal function in which the body is unable to maintain metabolic, fluid, and electrolyte balance. It occurs with a gradual decrease in the function of the kidneys over time. The result is nitrogenous waste products in the blood and uremia. Chronic kidney disease affects every body system (Table 37.8).

Pathophysiology

When a large proportion of the body's nephrons are damaged or destroyed, acute kidney injury or chronic kidney disease occurs. As the nephrons die off, the undamaged ones increase their work capacity and take over the work previously done by the dead ones, so the patient may experience significant kidney damage without showing symptoms.

Chronic kidney disease is a progressive disease process. In the early, or silent, stage (decreased renal reserve), the patient is usually without symptoms, even though up to 50% of nephron function may have been lost. This stage is often not diagnosed.

The renal insufficiency stage occurs when the patient has lost 75% of nephron function and some signs of mild kidney disease are present. Anemia and the inability to concentrate urine may occur. BUN and creatinine levels are slightly elevated. These patients are at risk for further damage caused by infection, dehydration, drugs, heart failure, and use of diagnostic x-ray dyes. The goal of care is to

• WORD • BUILDING •

hemodialysis: hemo—blood + dialysis—passage of a solute through a membrane

uremia: ur—urea + emia—in the blood

TABLE 37.8 CHRONIC KIDNEY DISEASE SUMMARY

Signs and Symptoms	Decreased urine output Acute kidney injury symptoms appear rapidly Fatigue Nausea and vomiting Shortness of breath Platelet dysfunction
Diagnostic Tests	Urinalysis Elevated BUN, creatinine levels Urine sodium level less than 10 mEq/L Acidosis Anemia Electrolyte abnormalities Elevated potassium, magnesium levels Hypertension Pericarditis Platelet dysfunction Dialysis
Therapeutic Measures	Transplant Diet Dialysis
Complications	Headache Uremic encephalopathy—lethargy, coma, seizures Hypertension Accelerated atherosclerosis Heart failure Pulmonary edema Uremic pericarditis Anorexia, nausea, and vomiting Impotence Anemia Dry itchy skin, ecchymosis, and subcutaneous bruises Osteomalacia Osteoporosis
Priority Nursing Diagnoses	*Fluid Volume Excess* *Electrolyte Imbalance* *Imbalanced Nutrition: Less Than Body Requirements* *Sexual Dysfunction* *Urinary Retention* *Anxiety* *Infection* *Noncompliance* *Ineffective Coping*

prevent further damage, if possible, by control of blood glucose levels and blood pressure.

End-stage renal disease (ESRD) occurs when 90% of the nephrons are lost. Patients at this stage experience chronic and persistent abnormal kidney function. BUN and creatinine levels are always elevated. These patients may make urine but not filter out the waste products, or urine production may cease. Dialysis or a kidney transplant is required to survive.

Uremia (urea in the blood) is present in chronic kidney disease. Patients eventually develop problems in all body systems (Table 37.9). If left untreated, the patient with uremia dies, often within weeks.

Etiology

The causes of chronic kidney disease are numerous. The most common include diabetes mellitus resulting in diabetic nephropathy, chronic high blood pressure causing nephrosclerosis, glomerulonephritis, and autoimmune diseases. Diabetes and hypertension account for close to 70% of all chronic kidney disease.

Symptoms of Kidney Disease

Patients in either acute kidney injury or chronic kidney disease have multiple symptoms. Figure 37.6 illustrates symptoms and some of the more common ones are explained next.

Disturbance in Water Balance

Disturbances in the removal and regulation of water balance in the body occur with signs of fluid accumulation. An early symptom is edema (swelling) of the extremities, sacral area, and abdomen. Patients may report shortness of breath. Crackles and wheezes (signs of fluid accumulation) may be present on auscultation of the lungs. Blood vessels in the neck may be distended, and the patient may be hypertensive. These patients may produce a large amount of dilute urine (**polyuria**), small amounts of urine (oliguria), or no urine (anuria).

Disturbance in Electrolyte Balance

As kidney function decreases, the kidneys lose their ability to absorb and excrete electrolytes. Important electrolytes are sodium, potassium, and magnesium. When the kidneys are unable to maintain normal amounts of electrolytes in the blood, these substances accumulate at high levels and may be life threatening.

• WORD • BUILDING •
polyuria: poly—much + uria—urine

TABLE 37.9 EFFECTS OF CHRONIC KIDNEY DISEASE ON BODY SYSTEMS

Body System	Disease Process
Cardiovascular	Hypertension due to fluid overload and accelerated arteriosclerosis
	Congestive heart failure/pulmonary edema due to fluid overload, increased pulmonary permeability, left ventricular failure
	Angina due to coronary artery disease, anemia
	Dysrhythmias due to electrolyte imbalance, coronary artery disease
	Edema due to fluid overload and a decrease in osmotic pressure
	Pericarditis due to presence of waste products in the pericardial sac
Gastrointestinal	Stomatitis due to fluid restriction, presence of waste products in the mouth, secondary infections
	Anorexia, nausea, vomiting due to uremia
	Gastritis/gastrointestinal bleeding due to urea decomposition in gastrointestinal tract releasing ammonia that irritates and ulcerates the stomach or bowel; patient is also under stress, increasing ulcer formation, and may have platelet dysfunction
	Constipation due to electrolyte imbalances, decrease in fluid intake, decrease in activity, phosphate binders
	Diarrhea, hypermotility due to electrolyte imbalance
Hematopoietic	Anemia due to impaired synthesis of erythropoietin, a substance needed by the bone marrow to stimulate formation of RBCs; also due to decreased life span of RBCs from uremia and interference in folic acid action
	Bleeding tendency due to abnormal platelet function from effects of uremia
	Prone to infection due to a decrease in immune system function from uremia; renal patients can rapidly become septic and die from septic shock
Integumentary	Dry, itchy, inflamed skin due to calcium-phosphate deposits in the skin
	Pale yellow skin color due to urobilins, which give urine its yellow color.
	Skin will have an odor of urine because skin is an organ of excretion and the body attempts to remove toxins
	Decreased function of oil and sweat glands
Neurologic	Confusion due to uremic encephalopathy from an increase in urea and metabolic acids
	Peripheral neuropathy due to effects of waste products on neurologic system
	Cerebrovascular accidents due to accelerated atherosclerosis
Pulmonary	Pleurisy/pleural effusion due to waste products in the pleural space causing inflammation with pleurisy pain and collection of fluid resulting in effusion
Reproductive	Loss of libido, impotence, amenorrhea, infertility due to a decrease in hormone production
Skeletal	Bone and mineral disease due to hyperphosphatemia and hypocalcemia

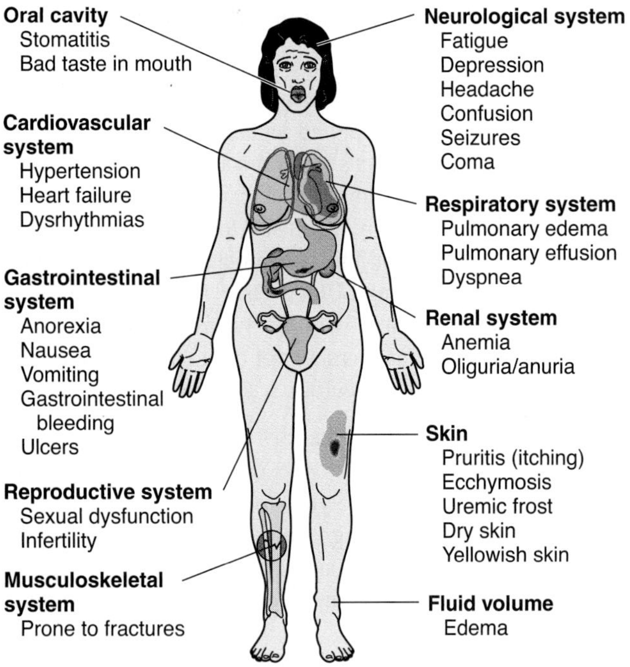
Oral cavity
Stomatitis
Bad taste in mouth
Cardiovascular system
Hypertension
Heart failure
Dysrhythmias
Gastrointestinal system
Anorexia
Nausea
Vomiting
Gastrointestinal bleeding
Ulcers
Reproductive system
Sexual dysfunction
Infertility
Musculoskeletal system
Prone to fractures
Neurological system
Fatigue
Depression
Headache
Confusion
Seizures
Coma
Respiratory system
Pulmonary edema
Pulmonary effusion
Dyspnea
Renal system
Anemia
Oliguria/anuria
Skin
Pruritis (itching)
Ecchymosis
Uremic frost
Dry skin
Yellowish skin
Fluid volume
Edema

FIGURE 37.6 Symptoms of chronic kidney disease.

When the kidneys are unable to regulate sodium levels adequately, the patient may show signs of hypernatremia (excessive sodium in the blood), which causes water retention, edema, and hypertension. Hyponatremia (too little sodium) may occur when too much sodium is lost. This can occur when the patient has experienced prolonged episodes of vomiting or diarrhea or is urinating large amounts of diluted urine. Patients with hyponatremia may show signs of confusion. The sodium may be normal or low due to being diluted from excess fluid.

Hyperkalemia (potassium level exceeding 5 mEq/L) may be life threatening if the level goes above 7 mEq/L. The patient may have dysrhythmias and cardiac arrest if the potassium level is too high. Patients with hyperkalemia report muscle weakness, abdominal cramping, and diarrhea. The nurse may identify that the patient is confused or disinterested in care. These patients should be placed on a cardiac monitor and observed for cardiac dysrhythmias.

A high potassium level in the patient with chronic kidney disease may be caused by a diet high in potassium-rich foods, injuries, or blood transfusions. Monitoring daily laboratory values, restricting potassium intake, and reporting abnormalities are important. Intravenous insulin, glucose, or calcium gluconate may be used as a temporary measure to drive excess potassium into the cells. Sodium polystyrene sulfonate (Kayexalate) may be given either orally or as a retention enema; it causes potassium to be eliminated through the stool. The definitive treatment for hyperkalemia is hemodialysis, which removes potassium from the body. Dietary education is extremely important. The patient is instructed to avoid foods that are high in potassium (Box 37.6).

Calcium levels decrease because the kidneys are unable to produce the hormone that activates vitamin D, the vitamin needed for calcium absorption. Hypocalcemia exists when the calcium level falls below 8.5 mg/dL. Also associated with a low calcium level is hyperphosphatemia, a phosphorus level above 5 mg/dL. These imbalances cause the bones to release calcium, increasing the risk of fractures. These patients should ambulate regularly to prevent further calcium loss from the bone. Many patients who are on dialysis develop hypercalcemia due to hyperparathyroidism (excess release of parathyroid hormone). Cinacalcet (Sensipar) reduces excess levels of parathyroid hormone, which reduces calcium levels.

Phosphates are also found in some foods. Medication to bind phosphate is given to patients with high phosphate levels. Sevelamer hydrochloride (Renagel) is the commonly ordered phosphate binder. These medications must be given to the patient with meals so they can bind with phosphates and be eliminated in the stool. High phosphorus levels may cause severe itching, and patients may have open sores from scratching, placing them at risk for infections. Patients also may have muscle cramps and aches.

Box 37.6

Foods High in Potassium

- Citrus fruits and juices
- Bananas
- Raisins
- Lima beans
- Tomato products
- Salt substitutes
- Potatoes, sweet and white
- Excessive dairy products
- Excessive meats
- Chocolate

Disturbance of Removal of Waste Products

With azotemia, the patient may show signs of weakness and fatigue, confusion, seizures, twitching movements of extremities (asterixis), nausea, vomiting, and lack of appetite and may report a metallic or bad taste in the mouth. There may be a smell of urine on the patient's breath. The patient may have yellowish pale skin and report itching due to urea crystals on the skin. Dialysis to remove excessive waste products in the blood is the only treatment for the underlying causes of these symptoms.

Disturbance in Maintaining Acid-Base Balance

Hydrogen ion excretion is affected, causing a disturbance in the acid-base balance that results in metabolic acidosis. Patients may report headache, fatigue, weakness, nausea, vomiting, and lack of appetite. As metabolic acidosis progresses, the patient shows signs of lethargy, stupor, and coma. Respirations become fast and deep as the lungs attempt to blow off carbon dioxide to correct the acidosis (Kussmaul's respirations). See Chapter 6 for a more detailed discussion of acid-base balance.

Disturbance in Hematologic Function

This change is seen mainly in chronic kidney disease, which causes disturbances in blood cells over time. Usually, with treatment, there is no time for this to occur in acute kidney injury. Damaged kidneys do not produce adequate erythropoietin, the hormone that stimulates RBC production. Nutritional deficiencies and blood loss during dialysis also contribute to anemia. Regular injections of epoetin (Epogen, Procrit), a synthetic form of erythropoietin, help restore RBC production and prevent anemia. A common side effect of erythropoietin is development of hypertension.

Impaired white blood cell and immune functions contribute to an increased risk for infection. The patient should be protected from potential sources of infection.

Impaired platelet function creates a risk for bleeding. The patient should be protected from injury, and signs of bleeding, such as blood in stool or emesis, are reported.

Therapeutic Measures for Kidney Disease

Kidney insufficiency and early kidney disease are treated based on symptoms with a restricted diet and fluid intake, medications, and careful monitoring for onset of serious problems that warrant initiation of dialysis. In later stages, dialysis is necessary to replace lost kidney function. A kidney transplant, when available, may return the patient to a nearly normal state of health.

Diet

Dietary recommendations are individualized by the dietitian and physician based on the patient's needs. Calories are high to maintain weight and energy needs. Protein is usually restricted to limit nitrogen intake but may be increased for a patient on dialysis because protein is lost during the dialysis process. Sodium is restricted to minimize sodium and fluid retention. Potassium is restricted, especially later in the disease when the kidneys are unable to eliminate it. Calcium is increased or supplemented because of poor absorption related to faulty vitamin D activation. Phosphorus is restricted because of high blood levels related to hypocalcemia. Saturated fat and cholesterol are restricted for patients with hyperlipidemia. Fluids are restricted to prevent overload. Most patients are given iron, folic acid, vitamins, and minerals to supplement the restricted diet (Box 37.7, *Nutrition Notes*).

Box 37.7

Nutrition Notes

Understanding Dietary Changes in Renal Disease

Patients with impaired renal function require careful coordination of diet with current physiological status, which may change frequently, necessitating the services of a dietitian who specializes in renal treatment. Six national meal-planning systems were developed for renal insufficiency with/without diabetes, hemodialysis with/without diabetes, and peritoneal dialysis with/without diabetes. The following principles are offered as general guidelines:

- Maintaining caloric intake is essential to avoid catabolism of tissue for energy.* Simple carbohydrates and monounsaturated and polyunsaturated fats are given freely because their end products, carbon dioxide and water, are less likely than protein to tax the kidney. Patients with diabetes and uremia may receive more sugar than usual because treatment of the uremia may take precedence over the diabetes; however, patients with type IV hypertriglyceridemia may have to limit carbohydrates.
- Protein may be restricted when the patient's kidneys are failing but increased when the patient is treated with dialysis to compensate for losses in the dialysate. Sometimes proteins of high biological value (e.g., eggs, meat, and dairy products) are prescribed because they are more easily converted to body protein than those of low biological value. In other situations, vegetarian diets may be given, with the plant proteins carefully selected to manage potassium and phosphorus serum levels.
- Sodium may be restricted, depending on blood pressure, edema, and laboratory findings.
- Potassium may be restricted for patients with oliguria. Salt substitutes are often potassium compounds that are to be avoided. Potassium content in foods varies with processing and preparation methods so patients should choose from prescribed foods only.
- Fluid restriction may be altered daily according to output. Renal insufficiency patients may receive 500 mL plus the amount of the previous day's output.

In short, renal diets are individualized for the patient's current condition. Nurses should not expect various patients to be served the same meals or even the same patient to require the same restrictions from one day to the next.

*A special oral supplement such as ReNeph LP/HC (low protein, high calorie) from Ross Laboratories may be prescribed for patients who are unable to eat enough food. Nepro (Abbott Laboratories) is a specially formulated oral supplement to meet the altered nutrition needs of patients on dialysis. Nepro blends carbohydrates to maintain steady glucose levels and increase albumin levels.

Source: Lutz, C. A., & Przytulski, K. R. (2010). *Nutrition and diet therapy* (5th ed.). Philadelphia: F. A. Davis.

Because restrictions are complex, the diet may be a source of frustration for patients. The nurse should assist the patient to identify foods that are palatable yet within the diet plan. The dietitian should be consulted for instruction and assistance.

Medications

Early in the disease, diuretics are given to increase output, and ACE inhibitors, calcium channel blockers, or beta blockers may be used to control hypertension. Phosphate binders are given with meals to reduce phosphate levels. Calcium and vitamin D supplements are used to raise calcium levels. Both the active and storage forms of vitamin D should be considered because evidence shows they decrease fractures, cancer, and infection rates and improve cardiac function (Wesseling-Perry & Salusky, 2009). Agents to lower potassium levels are used if needed. All drug therapy is closely monitored because diseased kidneys are unable to effectively remove medications from the body. The patient with diabetes needs less insulin because one of the functions of the kidneys is to break down insulin. Since it is not being broken down, it remains in the body longer, and therefore less is needed as the kidney disease progresses.

Dialysis

Dialysis is started when the patient develops symptoms of severe fluid overload, high potassium levels, acidosis, pericarditis, vomiting, lethargy, fatigue, or symptoms of uremia that are life threatening. Both peritoneal dialysis and hemodialysis involve the movement and diffusion of particles from an area of high concentration to an area of low concentration through a semipermeable membrane. Substances move from blood through the semipermeable membrane into the dialysate. Fluid and electrolyte imbalances can be corrected with dialysis. Dialysis can also be used to treat drug overdoses.

HEMODIALYSIS. Hemodialysis involves the use of an artificial kidney to remove waste products and excess water from the patient's blood. During the dialysis procedure, the patient's blood and the dialyzing solution flow in opposite directions through the dialyzer across an enclosed semipermeable membrane. The dialysate contains electrolytes and water in a balanced mix that resembles blood plasma. On the other side is the patient's blood with metabolic waste products, excess water, and electrolytes. The waste products from the patient's blood move into the dialysate by diffusion through the membrane because of the difference in their concentrations. The dialysate solution carries the waste products away, and the cleansed blood is returned to the patient's body through another tube (Fig. 37.7). A hemodialysis treatment takes 3 to 4 hours and is done three or four times a week. Hemodialysis is done at a hemodialysis center (Fig. 37.8) or in the hospital if the patient develops a complication and needs hospitalization.

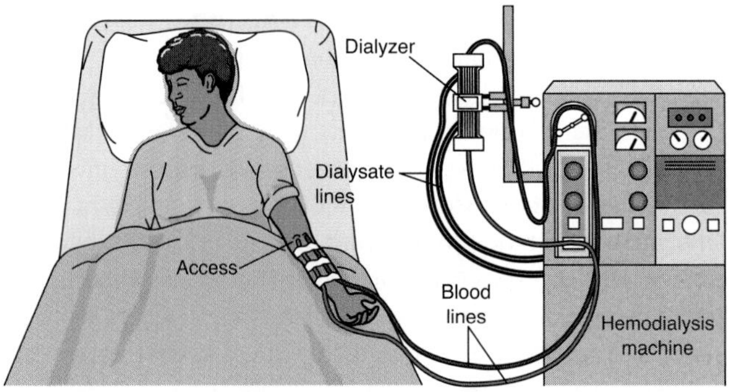
Dialyzer
Dialysate lines
Access
Blood lines
Hemodialysis machine
FIGURE 37.7 Hemodialysis.

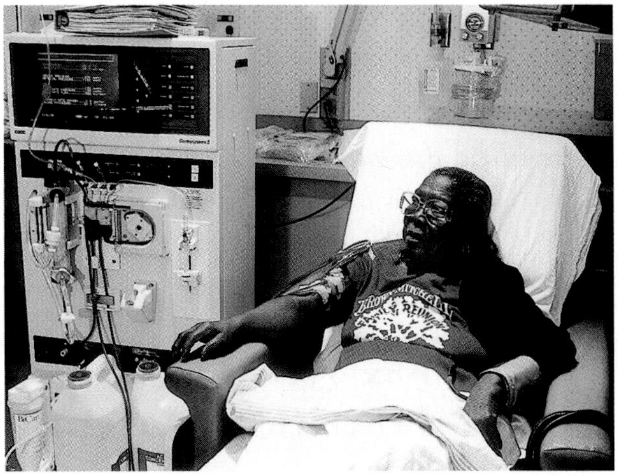
FIGURE 37.8 Patient undergoing hemodialysis at dialysis center.

Hemodialysis provides a rapid and efficient way to remove waste products from the blood. It is also an excellent means to correct excessive fluid-overloaded states such as occur in heart failure.

Hemodialysis is not without side effects. Following a treatment, the patient normally feels weak and fatigued, sometimes even too tired to eat. Sudden drops in blood pressure may cause the patient to become weak, dizzy, and nauseated. Cardiac dysrhythmias and angina may occur. Fluid and electrolyte levels drop rapidly and cause the patient to feel lethargic and have muscle cramps. Patients are given large amounts of heparin, an anticoagulant, to keep the blood from clotting while it is in the artificial kidney; this may cause bleeding from the puncture sites, gastrointestinal tract, nose, or other sites if injury occurs. Box 37.8 reviews nursing care for patients having hemodialysis.

Vascular Access. Hemodialysis requires a permanent way to access the bloodstream for blood removal and return to the body during dialysis. Typical permanent vascular access options are an arteriovenous (AV) fistula (considered to be the gold standard) or a vascular access graft. Fistulas or grafts are placed in the arm when possible.

Box 37.8

Nursing Care of the Patient Receiving Hemodialysis

1. Consult with the physician about medications to hold before hemodialysis. Some medications, such as antihypertensives, can be harmful when they become effective during dialysis and can reduce blood pressure to dangerously low levels. Other medications are water soluble and will be dialyzed out of the body, and thus are not effective.
2. Ensure that the patient is weighed both before dialysis in the morning and after dialysis to document weight loss as a result of fluid removal.
3. If the patient has laboratory tests ordered and blood needs to be drawn, coordinate this process with the dialysis nurse, who can obtain the blood samples and save the patient unnecessary needlesticks.
4. Try to get morning care done early and breakfast given before dialysis. After dialysis, patients are often exhausted and need rest.
5. When the patient returns from dialysis, weigh the patient, assess the access site for bleeding, and make sure the vital signs are stable. Administer medications that were held if not contraindicated and vital signs are stable.
6. Protect the patient's dialysis access as outlined in Box 37.9, *Care of Blood Access Graft or Fistula.*

NURSING CARE TIP

It is important to save the veins of patients with chronic kidney disease for possible future fistula creation. The non-dominant patient arm should not be used for IVs, blood draws, or blood pressure to avoid damage to the veins because it will likely be the arm used for the fistula. Early consultation with a nephrologist can identify which veins to protect.

Early referral to a nephrologist can allow for the establishment of vascular access so that it is matured before the need for dialysis. If this does not occur, then a temporary access is used until a fistula or graft is placed or usable. A central venous catheter with two or three ports (the third port can be used for medications by trained staff) is placed in the subclavian vein, the jugular vein, or the femoral vein for temporary access. Central catheters cannot be used long term because of the risk of infection. The LifeSite Hemodialysis Access system is an implantable port system for blood access. Two systems are implanted for hemodialysis. No maturation time is required. This system can be used longer than can temporary access catheters.

An AV fistula is made by sewing a vein and artery together under the skin (Fig. 37.9). AV fistulas may take 2 to 6 months to mature.

An arteriovenous graft (AV graft) uses a tube of synthetic material to attach to an artery and a vein. Needles are inserted into the graft to access the patient's blood. Traditional graft material is not self-sealing and requires time for tissue growth to serve as a plug for the hole that the needle makes before it can be used. This may take 1 to 2 weeks. The Vectra vascular access graft is self-sealing and does not require tissue growth so it can be used almost immediately after surgical implantation. This self-sealing property also decreases postdialysis bleeding time and reduces the time required for the dialysis session.

Vascular Access Care. Arteriovenous fistulas and grafts are regularly checked for patency by palpating for a thrill (a tremor) and auscultating for a bruit (swishing sound) at the site of the graft or fistula. Any decrease or cessation of bruit or thrill indicates occlusion. If a thrill or bruit is diminished or not present, the physician is notified immediately by the nurse. Special care of the access site must be taken because this is the patient's only way to eliminate waste products (Box 37.9). It is important for the site to be carefully monitored per institution policy to detect any clotting or problems. Early detection of clotting allows the surgeon an opportunity to save the access by performing a declotting procedure rather than a total revision.

Postoperative Care. Initially, neurovascular checks are performed hourly for vascular surgery. Neurovascular checks

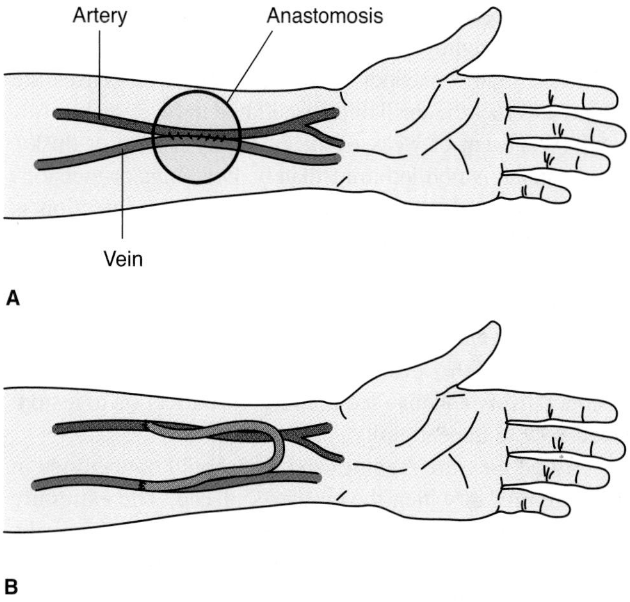
Artery
Anastomosis
Vein
A
B

FIGURE 37.9 Hemodialysis access sites. (A) Arteriovenous fistula. (B) Arteriovenous graft.

Box 37.9

Care of Blood Access Fistula or Graft

These dialysis access sites should not be utilized for any purpose other than dialysis.

1. Watch for signs of bleeding or infection at the site.
2. Listen for a bruit at the site by placing the diaphragm of a stethoscope gently on the site. A bruit is a swishing sound made as the blood passes through the access site.
3. Gently palpate the site for a thrill, which is a buzzing or pulsing feeling that indicates good blood flow through the access site.
4. Do not take blood pressure, use a tourniquet, draw blood, or start any intravenous lines in the affected arm. Injections should be avoided if possible.
5. Many hospitals have the patient wear a red arm bracelet to signify that the arm should be protected. A sign above the bed may also be used.
6. Teach the patient to keep the site clean and not to bump or cut it.
7. Teach the patient not to lift heavy objects or carry a purse on the access arm.
8. Teach the patient to avoid wearing constrictive clothing or jewelry over the site.
9. Teach the patient to avoid prolonged bending or sleeping on the arm with an access.
10. Notify the physician if signs of bleeding, reduced circulation, or infection occur in the access extremity: coldness, numbness, weakness, redness, fever, drainage, or swelling.

include extremity movement and sensation, presence of numbness or tingling, pulses, temperature, color, and capillary refill (less than 3 seconds normally). Peripheral pulses are palpated to feel the thrill and auscultated to hear the bruit. If a pulse is absent or weak or the extremity is cool or dusky, the physician is notified immediately. Dressings or incisions are checked, and any drainage, hematoma, or infection is documented and reported as needed. Vascular surgery pain is usually mild. Severe pain may indicate an occlusion of the graft. Arteriovenous grafts can cause distal ischemia or "steal syndrome" because too much of the arterial blood is being "stolen" from the distal extremity. This is usually seen postoperatively and may require surgical correction to restore blood flow to the extremity.

Blood pressure readings and IVs should not be done in the extremity in which the access is placed. The extremity with the vascular access should be elevated postoperatively. Range-of-motion exercises should be encouraged. Patients are taught care of the access (see Box 37.9).

PERITONEAL DIALYSIS. Peritoneal dialysis provides continuous dialysis treatment and is done by the patient or family in the home. The peritoneal membrane is used as a semipermeable membrane across which excess wastes and fluids move from blood in peritoneal vessels into a dialysate solution that has been instilled into the peritoneal cavity. A peritoneal catheter is placed into the patient's peritoneal space between the two layers of the peritoneum below the waistline. This catheter is used to perform an exchange. The exchange process has three steps: filling, dwell time, and draining.

The fill step involves instilling a bag of sterile dialyzing solution (dialysate) into the patient's peritoneal cavity through the catheter. The amount of solution is usually 1500 to 2000 mL. The solution is left to dwell in the abdomen for several hours, allowing time for the waste products from the blood to pass through the peritoneal membrane into the dialysate solution (Fig. 37.10).

The solution is then drained out of the body and discarded. This process is repeated three or four times a day and is continuous for the patient. Several different treatment plans use this exchange process. The treatment plan that best suits the patient's needs is determined by the patient and the dialysis team.

Continuous ambulatory peritoneal dialysis (CAPD) is the most commonly used treatment plan. Usually three exchanges are done during the day and one before bedtime. Other treatment plans allow for the use of a computerized machine called a cycler to regulate the exchanges during sleeping hours. Sometimes medications are added to the dialyzing solutions, such as heparin to prevent clotting of the catheter, insulin for the patient with diabetes, or antibiotics if there is infection.

Patient and family education is extremely important for peritoneal dialysis to be successful. The patient must be taught and be able to demonstrate that he or she is able to do a successful exchange. Sterile technique while performing the exchanges is imperative and the exchanges should be done in a clean environment. A major complication is peritonitis (infection of the peritoneum), which can be life threatening. The major cause of peritonitis is poor technique when connecting the bag of dialyzing solution to the peritoneal catheter. The first sign of peritonitis is usually abdominal pain. (See Chapter 34 for additional signs and symptoms of peritonitis.) If any symptoms of peritonitis occur, the patient must contact the physician immediately so antibiotic treatment can begin. The patient should be taught to care for the exit site (the site where the catheter comes out of the abdomen) and the need to inspect both the site and the dialysate solution for any signs of infection.

Dietary education is also important. A dietitian can assist the patient in making appropriate choices for adequate calories, protein, and potassium intake. The peritoneal dialysis patient typically has fewer dietary and fluid restrictions than the patient on hemodialysis because

• WORD • BUILDING •

peritoneal dialysis: peritoneal—peritoneum + dialysis—passage of a solution through a membrane

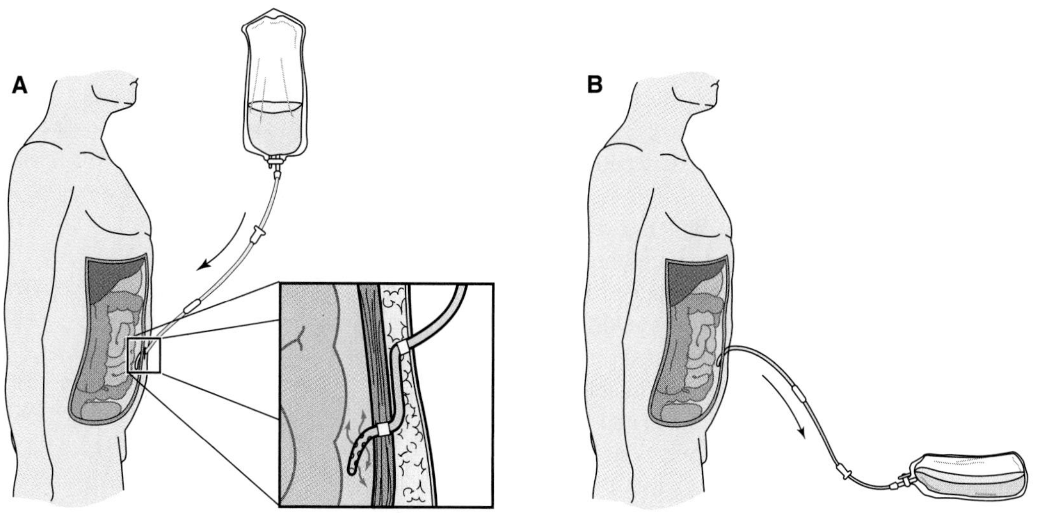
A
B

FIGURE 37.10 (A) Peritoneal dialysis works inside the body. Dialysis solution flows through a tube into the abdominal cavity, where it collects waste products from the blood. (B) Periodically the used dialysis solution is drained from the abdominal cavity, carrying away waste products and excess water from the blood.

peritoneal dialysis is continuous and maintains serum waste levels. Proteins are lost through the peritoneal membrane into the dialysate fluid, so increased dietary protein is needed. This loss increases with peritonitis, which further increases permeability.

LEARNING TIP

Differences between hemodialysis (HD), peritoneal dialysis (PD), and continuous renal replacement therapy (CRRT) include the following:

- **Patient access:** HD requires vascular access. PD requires insertion of a catheter into the peritoneal cavity. CRRT requires temporary vascular access such as a central line.
- **Equipment:** HD requires a specialized complex dialyzer. PD and CRRT do not require the specialized dialyzer, although machines are available for these therapies.
- **Training:** HD requires a skilled HD nurse. CRRT can be done by a non-HD nurse in a critical care setting. PD can be done by the patient.
- **Timing:** HD is intermittent. PD and CRRT are continuous.
- **Solute removal:** HD and PD use the principles of osmosis and diffusion, which require a dialysate solution. CRRT uses convection, so no dialysate is needed.
- **Cardiovascular effects:** HD may cause hypotension, which is a risk in the unstable patient. PD and CRRT have few cardiovascular effects. CRRT can be used for the unstable patient.

CRITICAL THINKING

Ms. Jackson

■ Ms. Jackson is a single, 56-year-old woman with a 20-year history of type 1 diabetes, hypertension, hyperlipidemia, chronic anemia, and a total knee replacement. She has been diagnosed with chronic kidney disease (CKD). She was admitted to a medical unit for treatment of shortness of breath and CKD. Treatment will include hemodialysis. She has had increasing shortness of breath, has pitting edema, urine output of about 375 mL/day, and is having premature ventricular contractions (PVCs) as seen on the cardiac monitor. Her admitting laboratory values are Na 131, K 6, Cl 97, Ca 10, iron (Fe) 64, WBC 4000, RBC 3.12, Hgb 10.1, Hct 32, creatinine 7, BUN 30. Her blood glucose level yesterday was 7 a.m., 154 mg/dL; noon, 122 mg/dL; 5 p.m., 188 mg/dL. She has sliding-scale insulin ordered. She is having an echocardiogram and chest x-ray done. She is having a two-tailed subclavian catheter placed for blood access. She is withdrawn and quiet.

1. What would be the first thing the nurse would address after getting the report?
2. What do Ms. Jackson's physical symptoms indicate and the laboratory values reflect?
3. What should the nurse say to Ms. Jackson related to her withdrawn behavior?
4. What should the nurse identify related to Ms. Jackson's understanding of self-care?
5. What teaching is needed for the diagnostic tests?
6. What care is required for the blood access?
7. What type of insulin is used for sliding-scale insulin coverage? Why?

Suggested answers at end of chapter.

Kidney Transplantation

Kidney transplantation is another treatment for chronic kidney disease and is extremely successful. An advantage of transplant compared to dialysis is that it reverses many of the physiological changes. The patient is also not dependent on dialysis and dietary restrictions.

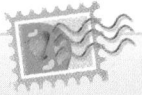

A kidney transplant is a procedure in which a donor kidney is placed in the abdomen of a patient with chronic kidney disease (Fig. 37.11). This healthy transplanted kidney functions as a normal kidney does. The donated kidney can come from a family member, a living, nonrelated donor, or a cadaver donor. Tissue and blood types must match so the body's immune system does not reject the donated kidney. Patients receive drugs to help prevent rejection; they usually must be taken for the rest of the patient's life. Sometimes even with these drugs, the body rejects the kidney and the patient must go back on dialysis (Box 37.10, *Cultural Considerations,* and Box 37.11, *Patient Perspective*).

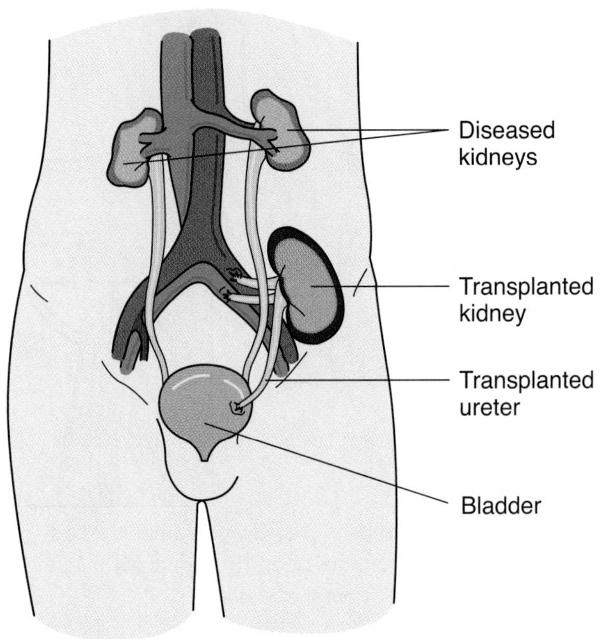
Diseased kidneys
Transplanted kidney
Transplanted ureter
Bladder

FIGURE 37.11 A transplanted kidney is placed in the abdomen. The patient's kidneys are usually left in place.

Nursing Process for the Patient with Kidney Disease

Data Collection

Kidney disease progressively affects all body systems. If acute kidney injury is short term, fewer effects may be seen because some effects will not develop. In chronic kidney disease, more effects are seen because the disease has time to progress. Data should be collected for signs and symptoms in all body systems. Family history of kidney disease and patient history of health problems such as hypertension, diabetes, systemic erythematous lupus, or urinary disorders are noted in the history. Also noted are medications the patient takes because they may be nephrotoxic and require adjustments. Recent changes in weight are documented.

Signs and symptoms vary depending on the severity of chronic kidney disease and its cause. Common signs are hypertension, abnormal laboratory values (creatinine, BUN), or changes in urine. See signs and symptoms section for other effects.

Nursing Diagnosis, Planning, Intervention, and Evaluation

See the *Nursing Care Plan for the Patient with Chronic Kidney Disease.*

Box 37.10

Cultural Considerations

Because many Vietnamese people believe that the body must be kept intact, even after death, they may object to removal of body parts or organ donation. Jewish law views organ transplantation from the recipient, the living donor, the cadaver donor, and the dying donor differently (see Box 35.5).

Box 37.11

Patient Perspective

Kidney Transplantation: Pat

My experience with a kidney transplant spans three decades, but my overall renal illness experience also spans several years of illness and dialysis before the transplant. I think the biggest changes I have seen over the years are the involvement of patients in their own care options, as well as increased technical advances that allow transplantation to be much more successful. Some of the feelings one experiences before transplantation are fear, uncertainty, and—if awaiting a donor—the guilt of knowing someone must die before you can live.

More than 30 years ago, there were no support groups and no one to talk to except family and doctors. Today, there are many support mechanisms in place for

Box 37.11

Patient Perspective—cont'd

patients and families both before and after transplantation. As a nurse, you can help patients by knowing these support resources for referral. After a transplant, it is wonderful to feel better, almost immediately. However, as wonderful as transplantation is, the side effects of the antirejection medications may be immediately felt, while other problems take years to develop. Unfortunately, no one escapes the side effects of the medications. I have had breast cancer, osteoarthritis, cataracts, ulcers, skin cancer, anemia, weight gain, and other side effects of prednisone and Imuran (azathioprine). However, I can assure you that this is much better than the alternative of dialysis.

NURSING CARE PLAN for the Patient with Chronic Kidney Disease

Nursing Diagnosis: *Excess Fluid Volume* related to kidney's inability to excrete water

Expected Outcomes: Fluid volume will be stable as evidenced by stable weight, absence of edema, lung sounds clear, and blood pressure within the patient's normal parameters.

Evaluation of Outcomes: Is weight stable? Is edema absent? Are lungs clear? Is blood pressure within the patient's normal parameters?

Interventions	Rationale	Evaluation
Monitor weight daily at same time; report gain of greater than 2 pounds.	Those retaining fluid will have weight gain.	Is weight stable? Should physician be notified of change?
Monitor intake and output.	This reveals degree of fluid retention.	Is output less than intake? Is this a change?
Monitor and report shortness of breath, tachycardia, crackles in lungs, frothy sputum, heart irregularities, hypotension, cold clammy skin.	These are symptoms of heart failure that may accompany fluid overload.	Are symptoms of heart failure present?
Watch for new onset of jugular vein distention with patient's head raised to 30- to 45-degree angle.	Fluid overload causes right-sided heart failure resulting in distended jugular veins.	Are jugular veins distended? Is this a new finding?
Monitor vital signs, including orthostatic blood pressure.	Blood pressure changes reflect fluid volume.	Is blood pressure increased?
Monitor for edema.	Edema is a symptom of fluid overload.	Is edema present? Is this a change?
Monitor activity tolerance.	Reduced activity tolerance may indicate heart failure related to fluid retention.	Is patient's tolerance of activity stable? Worsening?
Monitor serum protein and albumin levels.	Low serum protein and albumin levels contribute to edema.	Are levels within normal limits?
Maintain sodium and fluid restrictions (often 600 mL plus the previous day's urine output) as ordered. Develop a plan with specific allotted amounts of fluid at each meal and for medications. Teach patient importance of each.	For those on dialysis, fluid intake is adjusted so that weight gains are no more than 1–3 kg between dialysis sessions.	Does patient understand and maintain sodium and fluid restriction?

Continued

NURSING CARE PLAN for the Patient with Chronic Kidney Disease—cont'd

Nursing Diagnosis: *Impaired Skin Integrity* related to dryness, excess fluid, crystal deposits

Expected Outcome: The patient will maintain intact skin.

Evaluation of Outcome: Does patient report no itching or dryness? Is patient's skin intact?

Interventions	Rationale	Evaluation
Observe skin for open areas and signs of infection.	Detects early signs of problems.	Is skin intact?
Bathe with tepid water, oils, or oatmeal.	Bathe regularly to reduce crystals with nondrying items to reduce itching and dryness and promote comfort.	Does patient report no itching or skin dryness?
Apply lotion to skin after bathing.	Lotion is used for itching to reduce dry skin.	Is skin dry?

Nursing Diagnosis: *Activity Intolerance* related to anemia secondary to impaired synthesis of erythropoietin by the kidneys

Expected Outcome: The patient will be able to perform activities important to him or her.

Evaluation of Outcome: Does patient state satisfaction with level of activity tolerance?

Interventions	Rationale	Evaluation
Assess for pale mucous membranes and skin color, dyspnea, chest pain.	These are signs and symptoms of anemia.	Does patient exhibit symptoms of anemia?
Monitor hemoglobin (Hgb), hematocrit (Hct).	Low hemoglobin and hematocrit indicate anemia.	Are Hgb and Hct within normal limits?
Watch for signs of bleeding.	Bleeding will worsen anemia.	Are signs of bleeding present?
Administer erythropoietin as ordered.	Erythropoietin stimulates production of red blood cells by bone marrow.	Are Hgb and Hct rising with use of erythropoietin?
Assist with blood transfusion as needed.		
Have patient space activities with rest periods.	Rest periods decrease demand for oxygen.	Is patient able to tolerate activities with rest periods?

Nursing Diagnosis: *Risk for Injury* related to bleeding tendency from platelet dysfunction and use of heparin during dialysis, and from tendency for gastrointestinal bleeding

Expected Outcome: The patient will not experience bleeding. If bleeding occurs, it will be recognized and stopped quickly.

Evaluation of Outcome: Are signs and symptoms of bleeding absent or recognized and reported quickly?

Interventions	Rationale	Evaluation
Observe for and report blood in stool or emesis, easy bruising, bleeding from mucous membranes or puncture sites, and report immediately if present.	Bleeding must be recognized quickly to prevent complications.	Does patient have signs of bleeding?

NURSING CARE PLAN for the Patient with Chronic Kidney Disease—cont'd

Monitor Hgb, Hct, clotting studies, and platelets, and report results.	Declining Hgb and Hct indicate blood loss. Declining platelet count or rising clotting times indicate increased risk of bleeding.	Are lab results stable?
Monitor vital signs.	Falling blood pressure and rising pulse may indicate volume deficit from bleeding.	Are vital signs stable?
Avoid giving injections if possible.	Injections can cause bleeding into tissue.	Can medications be given by another route?
If bleeding, apply gentle pressure to site if possible.	Pressure promotes hemostasis.	Does pressure stop bleeding?
Teach patient to prevent injury to self and symptoms of bleeding to report.	Injury can cause bleeding. Understanding symptoms of bleeding promotes early reporting.	Does patient verbalize understanding of need to prevent injury and report bleeding?
Protect patient from injury if confusion or seizures occur.	Waste product accumulation or hyponatremia puts patient at risk of altered mental status or seizures.	Does patient require protection, such as seizure precautions? Is patient free from injury?

Nursing Diagnosis: *Risk for Infection* related to impaired immune system function

Expected Outcomes: The patient will not develop infection as evidenced by WBCs and temperature within normal limits, no signs and symptoms of infection.

Evaluation of Outcomes: Are WBCs and temperature within normal limits?

Interventions	Rationale	Evaluation
Monitor for signs and symptoms of infection, and report promptly to physician.	Early recognition of infection and prompt treatment help prevent complications.	Does patient have signs or symptoms of infection?
Protect patient from any source of infection, including infected roommates, visitors, or caregivers.	Exposure to pathogens increases risk for infection.	Does anyone in contact with the patient have an infection?
Maintain skin integrity.	Intact skin protects against infection.	Is skin intact?
Caregivers and patient practice good hand washing technique.	Hand washing helps control spread of infection.	Is good hand washing being practiced?
Culture any suspected site of infection as ordered by physician.	A culture identifies pathogens and guides treatment.	Is a culture needed?
Consult with physician about influenza and pneumonia vaccines.	Patients with impaired immune function are at risk for influenza and pneumonia.	Has the patient been vaccinated?
Teach patient and family signs and symptoms of infection to report to physician.	Early reporting of symptoms allows for prompt treatment.	Do patient and family verbalize understanding of symptoms to report?

NURSING CARE PLAN for the Patient with Chronic Kidney Disease—cont'd

Nursing Diagnosis: *Imbalanced Nutrition: Less Than Body Requirements* related to restricted diet, anorexia, nausea, and vomiting, and stomatitis secondary to effect of excessive urea on the gastrointestinal system

Expected Outcomes: The patient will maintain ideal weight, and serum protein and albumin levels will be within normal limits.

Evaluation of Outcomes: Are weight and lab values at desired levels?

Interventions	Rationale	Evaluation
Monitor weekly weight and serum protein and albumin levels.	Weight and laboratory results provide information about nutrition status.	Are weight and laboratory values stable?
Consult dietitian for low-protein diet planning and teaching.	Low-protein diets decrease formation of waste products (urea, creatinine).	Does patient understand low-protein diet?
Initiate a calorie count—consult dietitian for assistance.	A calorie count can provide information about the adequacy of the patient's diet.	Is patient receiving adequate calories?
Provide frequent oral care.	Oral care enhances appetite and reduces urine taste in mouth.	Does oral care enhance appetite?
Offer frequent small feedings and dietary supplements.	Smaller feedings are better tolerated and reduce risk of nausea.	Does patient tolerate small feedings?
Offer medications ordered for nausea before meals.	Nausea reduces appetite and must be controlled.	Are antiemetics effective?
Ensure bowel movement daily or according to patient's usual pattern.	Constipation can interfere with appetite.	Are patient's bowels functioning normally for him or her?

SUGGESTED ANSWERS TO

CRITICAL THINKING

■ *Mrs. Milan*

1. Sexual intercourse can be a predisposing factor to UTI, especially if the patient does not urinate after intercourse.
2. Mrs. Milan should be cautioned to always urinate after intercourse. (See also Box 37.1, *Patient Education*).
3. The urinalysis will show WBCs, bacteria, RBCs, and positive nitrites.
4. Teaching should include the need to take all of the medication until it is gone even if she feels better. The reason for this is to ensure the infection is completely resolved so it does not return due to some remaining bacteria. She should return for a urine culture after the therapy is complete.

■ *Mr. Stevens*

1. Weight, intake and output, blood pressure, and laboratory tests should be assessed as part of the morning evaluation.
2. BUN, serum creatinine, and potassium levels should also be checked.
3. Mr. Stevens should be taught that he needs to take antihypertensive medications, keep his follow-up visits to his physician, follow a low-sodium diet, and restrict fluids if ordered.

SUGGESTED ANSWERS TO—cont'd

■ *Ms. Jackson*

1. Collect data related to Ms. Jackson's breathing and respiratory status first. Then address the cardiovascular system to see how she is tolerating the dysrhythmia. Obtain Ms. Jackson's weight and intake and output to monitor fluid balance.
2. Shortness of breath and pitting edema related to fluid overload; urine output 375 mL/day is due to chronic kidney disease; PVCs are due to elevated K. Na is low due to dilutional effect of excess fluid. K is retained due to chronic kidney disease. WBC low due to chronic kidney disease. RBC, Hgb, Hct low due to anemia. Creatinine and BUN are not excreted and are elevated due to chronic kidney disease. Blood glucose is elevated due to diabetes.
3. Therapeutic conversation suggestions: "Ms. Jackson, would you like to talk about your diagnosis?" "How do you feel about your diagnosis?" "Do you have questions or concerns?" "What are your usual coping methods?" Provide explanations for procedures and interventions.
4. Determine Ms. Jackson's understanding of what chronic kidney disease is, how it is treated, how to follow the renal diet and fluid restrictions, and the action and importance of medications. Identify barriers to self-care and her support systems.
5. Teaching includes that the chest x-ray and echocardiogram require no preparation and are not painful.
6. A two-tail subclavian blood access is dedicated for hemodialysis. It is not used for any other purpose. Monitoring includes observing the site for signs of infection: redness, warmth, swelling, tenderness, drainage, and fever.
7. Regular insulin because it is rapid acting. Sliding-scale insulin is used to treat a current blood glucose. A rapid-acting insulin will affect a current blood glucose, so only rapid-acting insulin is used.

REVIEW QUESTIONS

1. When teaching a patient about preventing urinary tract infections, which of the following information should the nurse include? **Select all that apply**.
   a. Void frequently.
   b. Drink large amounts of citrus juices.
   c. Eat large amounts of vegetables.
   d. Wash the perineum every 8 hours.
   e. Void after sexual intercourse.
   f. Avoid drinking cranberry juice.

2. A patient is admitted to the hospital with a diagnosis of a kidney stone. Which of the following interventions should be included in the plan of care?
   a. Restrict fluids.
   b. Strain all urine.
   c. Increase calcium intake.
   d. Maintain bedrest.

3. The nurse is taking a history on a patient with a diagnosis of bladder cancer. Which of the following would the nurse expect to find in the patient's history?
   a. Tobacco use
   b. Vegetarian diet
   c. Caffeine use
   d. Alcohol use

4. While changing the pouch at the stoma site of an ileal conduit, the nurse notes the stoma is constantly spilling urine. Which of the following actions should the nurse take?
   a. Notify the physician of the constant spillage.
   b. Continue changing the pouch.
   c. Remove the overflow of urine with a straight catheter.
   d. Irrigate the stoma with a sterile solution of normal saline.

5. The nurse is caring for a patient with glomerulonephritis. Which of the following interventions would the nurse recommend be included in the patient's plan of care?
   a. Increase fluid intake.
   b. Decrease sodium intake.
   c. Increase potassium intake.
   d. Decrease carbohydrate intake.

REVIEW QUESTIONS—cont'd

6. The nurse is caring for a postoperative patient who is receiving 0.9% normal saline IV at 125 mL/hour, morphine for pain control, and gentamicin (Garamycin) IVPB every 8 hours for 24 hours. The patient is allergic to iodine. Morning labs are WBC 8500, Hgb 12.4 g/dL, creatinine 2.2 mg/dL. Which of these findings is a priority for the nurse to report to the RN?
   a. WBC
   b. IV rate of 125 mL/hour
   c. Allergies
   d. Creatinine level

7. A patient with chronic kidney disease who is on hemodialysis asks for a snack in the afternoon. The patient's potassium level remains high. Which of the following foods could be given? **Select all that apply**.
   a. Banana
   b. Gelatin dessert
   c. Clear carbonated beverage
   d. Cranberry juice

8. How should the nurse assess the patency of a new right arm AV fistula?
   a. Auscultate the right brachial pulse.
   b. Auscultate and palpate the right radial pulse.
   c. Measure blood pressure in the right arm.
   d. Palpate for thrill and auscultate bruit over the fistula.

9. A patient is returning to the medical unit after a dialysis session. The nurse notes bleeding from the patient's vascular access in the left arm. Which of the following is the nurse's first action?
   a. Call the physician.
   b. Notify the dialysis nurse.
   c. Apply pressure to site.
   d. Take patient's blood pressure.

10. A patient is to receive 1600 mg of Renagel (sevelamer) orally with meals. Renagel 400-mg tablets are available. How many tablets should the nurse give?
    Answer: ________________tablets

Reference

Wesseling-Perry, K., & Salusky, I. (2009, July). Is replacement therapy with nutritional and active forms of vitamin D required in chronic kidney disease mineral and bone disorder? *Current Opinion in Nephrology and Hypertension, 18*(4), 308–314.

DavisPlus | For additional resources and information visit **http://davisplus.fadavis.com**

unit TEN

UNDERSTANDING THE ENDOCRINE SYSTEM

38

Endocrine System Function and Assessment

PAULA D. HOPPER
AND JANICE L. BRADFORD

KEY TERMS

affect (AF-feckt)
exophthalmos (EKS-off-THAL-mus)

QUESTIONS TO GUIDE YOUR READING

1. What are the glands of the endocrine system?
2. What is the function of each of the hormones in the endocrine system?
3. What are the effects of aging on endocrine system function?
4. What data should you collect when caring for a patient with a disorder of the endocrine system?
5. What nursing care should you provide for patients undergoing testing for an endocrine disorder?

NORMAL ENDOCRINE SYSTEM ANATOMY AND PHYSIOLOGY

The endocrine system consists of the endocrine (ductless) glands, which secrete chemicals called hormones. Unlike other organ systems, the glands of the endocrine system are anatomically separate (Fig. 38.1). Their hormones are involved in the composition and volume of interstitial fluid; all aspects of metabolism, energy balance, and growth/development; contraction of smooth and cardiac muscle; glandular secretion; reproduction; and the establishment of circadian rhythms. Each hormone is secreted in response to a particular and specific stimulus, is circulated by the blood throughout the body, and exerts its effects on certain target cells that have receptors for that hormone. The effects of the hormone often reverse the stimulus and ultimately lead to decreased secretion of the hormone. This is called a negative feedback system; many hormone secretions are regulated this way. Some hormones are secreted in response to hormones from other endocrine glands.

Pituitary Gland

The pituitary gland, called the hypophysis, is suspended by a short stalk from the hypothalamus in the brain. The two major regions are the posterior pituitary (neurohypophysis) and anterior pituitary (adenohypophysis).

Posterior Pituitary Gland

The posterior pituitary gland stores antidiuretic hormone (ADH; sometimes called arginine vasopressin or vasopressin) and oxytocin, which are actually produced by the hypothalamus. Their release is stimulated by nerve impulses from the hypothalamus.

Antidiuretic hormone increases the amount of water reabsorbed by the kidney tubules, which decreases urine output. The water is reabsorbed back into the blood, thereby maintaining normal blood volume and normal blood pressure. The stimulus for secretion of ADH is a decrease in the water content of the body—that is, dehydration. When body water is lost and not replaced, specialized cells in the hypothalamus called osmoreceptors detect the elevated blood osmotic pressure (increased concentration) and transmit impulses to the

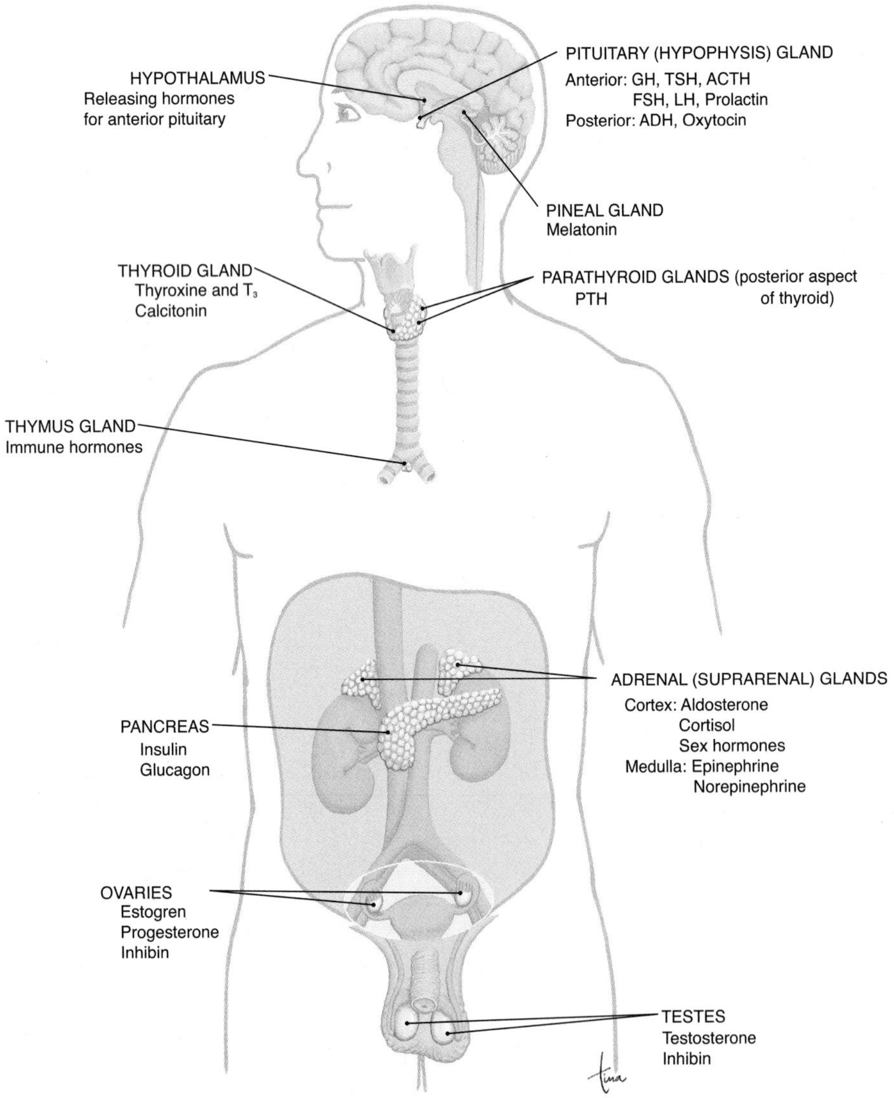
HYPOTHALAMUS
Releasing hormones for anterior pituitary
PITUITARY (HYPOPHYSIS) GLAND
Anterior: GH, TSH, ACTH FSH, LH, Prolactin
Posterior: ADH, Oxytocin
PINEAL GLAND
Melatonin
THYROID GLAND
Thyroxine and T_3
Calcitonin
PARATHYROID GLANDS (posterior aspect of thyroid)
PTH
THYMUS GLAND
Immune hormones
ADRENAL (SUPRARENAL) GLANDS
Cortex: Aldosterone
Cortisol
Sex hormones
Medulla: Epinephrine
Norepinephrine
PANCREAS
Insulin
Glucagon
OVARIES
Estogren
Progesterone
Inhibin
TESTES
Testosterone
Inhibin

FIGURE 38.1 Glands of the endocrine system. (From Scanlon, V., & Sanders, T. [2007]. *Essentials of anatomy and physiology* [5th ed.]. Philadelphia: F. A. Davis, with permission.)

posterior pituitary to secrete ADH to prevent the further loss of water in urine. In cases of great fluid loss, as in severe hemorrhage, the large amount of ADH secreted is especially important because it causes arteriole vasoconstriction, which increases blood pressure to homeostatic levels.

Oxytocin causes contraction of the smooth muscle in the uterus and mammary glands. At the end of pregnancy, stretching of the cervix generates sensory impulses to the hypothalamus, which then transmits impulses to the posterior pituitary for the release of oxytocin. Oxytocin causes strong contractions of the myometrium to bring about delivery of the baby and the placenta. This is an example of a positive feedback mechanism. During breastfeeding, the baby's sucking generates sensory impulses from the mother's nipple to the hypothalamus. The subsequent release of oxytocin causes contraction of the smooth muscle cells around the mammary ducts. This release of milk is called milk ejection (or letdown).

Anterior Pituitary Gland

The anterior pituitary gland secretes its hormones in response to releasing hormones from the hypothalamus. The anterior pituitary synthesizes and secretes growth hormone, thyroid-stimulating hormone, adrenocorticotropic hormone, prolactin, follicle-stimulating hormone, and luteinizing hormone.

Growth hormone (GH, or somatotropin) increases cell division in tissues capable of mitosis, which is one of the ways it is involved in growth. It also increases the transport of amino acids into cells and their use in protein synthesis. Growth hormone also increases the release of fat from adipose tissue and the use of fats for energy production; this is important even after growth in height has ceased. The secretion of GH is regulated by growth hormone–releasing hormone (GHRH) and by growth hormone–inhibiting hormone (GHIH, or somatostatin), both from the hypothalamus. GHRH is produced during hypoglycemia or when there is a high blood level of amino acids (to be turned into protein). GHIH is secreted during hyperglycemia, when carbohydrates are available for energy production and the mobilization of fat is not needed.

Thyroid-stimulating hormone (TSH, or thyrotropin) has only one target organ: the thyroid gland. TSH stimulates growth of the thyroid and the secretion of two of its hormones, thyroxine (T_4) and triiodothyronine (T_3). Secretion of TSH is stimulated by thyrotropin-releasing hormone (TRH) from the hypothalamus when the metabolic rate decreases and there is a need for thyroxine.

Adrenocorticotropic hormone (ACTH) stimulates secretion of cortisol and related hormones from the adrenal cortex. Corticotropin-releasing hormone (CRH) from the hypothalamus stimulates the release of ACTH. CRH is produced during any type of physiological stress situation, such as injury, disease, exercise, or hypoglycemia.

Prolactin initiates and maintains milk production by the mammary glands. The hypothalamus produces both prolactin-releasing hormone (PRH) and prolactin-inhibiting hormone (PIH). Prolactin is not secreted in high enough levels to produce milk until pregnancy is over and the levels of estrogen and progesterone (from the placenta) have dropped. The action of a nursing infant reduces PIH, thus the prolactin level rises.

Follicle-stimulating hormone (FSH) is a gonadotropic hormone; that is, its target organs are the ovaries or testes. In women, FSH initiates growth of ova in ovarian follicles and secretion of estrogen by the cells of those follicles. In men, FSH initiates sperm production in the seminiferous tubules of the testes. FSH is secreted in response to gonadotropin-releasing hormone (GnRH) from the hypothalamus. Another hormone called inhibin (from the ovaries or testes) decreases the secretion of FSH.

Luteinizing hormone (LH) is another gonadotropic hormone whose secretion is increased by GnRH from the hypothalamus. In women, LH causes ovulation and stimulates the ruptured ovarian follicle to become the corpus luteum and begin secreting progesterone, as well as estrogen. In men, LH stimulates the secretion of testosterone by the interstitial cells of the testes.

Thyroid Gland

The thyroid gland consists of two lobes connected by a middle piece called the isthmus; the gland is located on the front and sides of the trachea just below the larynx. Three hormones are produced by the thyroid gland. The T_4 and T_3 hormones are produced in the thyroid follicles, require iodine (T_4 has four iodine atoms, T_3 has three iodine atoms), and have the same functions. Calcitonin is the third hormone produced by the thyroid gland; it is produced by parafollicular cells.

The T_4 and T_3 hormones increase energy production and protein synthesis. They increase cellular respiration of glucose and fatty acids, which increases the metabolic rate—that is, energy and heat production. These hormones are the most important daily regulators of metabolic rate. Their activity is reflected in the functioning of the heart, brain, muscles, and virtually all other organs. They are essential for normal physical growth, mental development, and reproductive maturation.

The direct stimulus for secretion of T_4 and T_3 is TSH from the anterior pituitary. The sequence of events is as follows: A decrease in the metabolic rate (energy production) is detected by the hypothalamus, which secrets TRH. TRH stimulates the anterior pituitary to secrete TSH, which stimulates the thyroid to increase secretion of T_4 and T_3, which increase energy production to raise the metabolic rate. As the metabolic rate rises, negative feedback decreases the secretion of TRH from the hypothalamus until the metabolic rate decreases again.

The third thyroid hormone, calcitonin, targets bone tissue and therefore is especially important during childhood when bone growth is accelerated. Calcitonin inhibits resorption of calcium and phosphate by osteoclasts, thereby lowering the blood levels of these minerals and retaining them in bones. This one function of calcitonin has two important results: the maintenance of normal blood levels of calcium and phosphate and the maintenance of a strong, stable bone matrix.

The stimulus for secretion of calcitonin is hypercalcemia (a high blood calcium level). When the blood calcium level rises, increased calcitonin ensures that no more will be removed from bones until need for blood calcium returns.

> **LEARNING TIP**
>
> An easy way to remember the function of calcitonin is to remember calciTONin TONes down serum calcium.

Parathyroid Glands

There are usually four parathyroid glands, two on the back of each lobe of the thyroid gland. The hormone they produce is called parathyroid hormone (PTH), which is an antagonist to calcitonin; it maintains normal blood levels of calcium and phosphate. Besides bone, the target organs of PTH are the small intestine and kidneys.

PTH increases resorption of calcium and phosphate from the bones to the blood, which raises their blood levels. Absorption of calcium and phosphate from food in the small intestine is also increased by PTH through its action of activating vitamin D (calcitriol) in the kidneys. PTH also increases the resorption of calcium by the kidneys and the excretion of phosphate (more than is obtained from bones). Therefore, the overall effect of PTH is to raise the blood calcium level and lower the blood phosphate level.

Secretion of PTH is stimulated by hypocalcemia (a low blood calcium level) and inhibited by hypercalcemia. In adults, PTH is probably the most important regulator of the blood calcium level. Calcium ion delivery through the blood is essential for normal excitability of neurons and muscle cells and for the process of blood clotting.

Adrenal Glands

The two adrenal (also called suprarenal) glands are located one on top of each kidney. Each adrenal gland consists of an inner adrenal medulla and an outer adrenal cortex.

Adrenal Medulla

The cells of the adrenal medulla are called chromaffin cells. They secrete epinephrine and norepinephrine, which are collectively called catecholamines and are sympathomimetic (mimicking the sympathetic nervous system). Secretion of both hormones is stimulated by sympathetic impulses from the hypothalamus in stressful situations. The functions of the catecholamines mimic and prolong those of the sympathetic nervous system, which enable the person to respond physiologically to stress situations.

Of the two hormones, epinephrine is secreted in larger amounts (about four times that of norepinephrine) and has many effects. It increases the heart rate and force of contraction and therefore blood pressure, stimulates vasoconstriction in skin and most viscera, stimulates vasodilation in skeletal muscles, dilates the bronchioles, decreases peristalsis, stimulates the liver to convert glycogen to glucose, increases the use of fats for energy, and increases the rate of cell respiration. The most significant function of norepinephrine is to cause vasoconstriction in the skin and most abdominal viscera, thereby raising blood pressure.

Adrenal Cortex

The adrenal cortex secretes three types of steroid hormones: mineralocorticoids, glucocorticoids, and gonadocorticoids.

> **LEARNING TIP**
>
> An easy way to remember the hormones of the adrenal cortex is to remember salt, sugar, and sex. Mineralocorticoids promote salt retention, glucocorticoids affect sugar (carbohydrate) metabolism, and gonadocorticoids are sex hormones.

Aldosterone is the most abundant of the mineralocorticoids, and its target organs are the kidneys. Aldosterone increases the reabsorption of sodium ions and the excretion of potassium ions by the kidney tubules. This means that sodium ions are returned to the blood and potassium ions are eliminated in urine. This function of aldosterone has important consequences. As sodium ions are reabsorbed, hydrogen ions may be excreted in exchange. This is one mechanism to prevent the accumulation of hydrogen ions that would lead to acidosis. Also, as sodium ions are reabsorbed, water and negative ions such as bicarbonate follow and are thus returned to the blood. Although the reabsorption of water is an indirect effect of aldosterone, it is important for maintaining normal blood volume and blood pressure.

Aldosterone secretion can be stimulated in several ways: a low blood sodium level, a high blood potassium level, or loss of blood or dehydration that lowers blood pressure. Low blood pressure activates the renin-angiotensin mechanism of the kidneys, which culminates in the formation of angiotensin II. One function of angiotensin II is to increase secretion of aldosterone. The hormone called atrial natriuretic peptide (ANP), secreted by the atria of the heart when blood pressure or blood volume rises, seems to inhibit secretion of aldosterone (and renin) and thereby promotes elimination of sodium ions and water by the kidneys.

Cortisol is the most abundant of the glucocorticoids and has many target tissues. Cortisol stimulates gluconeogenesis (the conversion of triglycerides, lactic acid, and some amino acids to glucose) in the liver. It also increases lipolysis and protein breakdown to liberate fatty acids and amino acids, respectively, for gluconeogenesis. The goal is to increase capabilities of energy production. By providing these secondary energy sources to most cells, cortisol ensures that whatever glucose is present will be available for the brain (the glucose-sparing effect).

Cortisol also has an anti-inflammatory effect because it blocks the effects of histamine and stabilizes the lysosomes in cells. Normal cortisol secretion seems to limit the inflammation process to what is useful for tissue repair and to prevent excessive tissue destruction. Excess cortisol has damaging effects, however: it raises blood glucose levels, decreases the immune response, and delays healing of damaged tissue.

The direct stimulus for cortisol secretion is ACTH from the anterior pituitary gland. Cortisol is also a "stress" hormone, and any type of physiological stress (injury, disease, malnutrition) stimulates the hypothalamus to secrete CRH. CRH increases the secretion of ACTH by the anterior pituitary, which increases cortisol secretion by the adrenal cortex.

The gonadocorticoids are small amounts of male androgens, which in females are converted to estrogens. Their function is not known with certainty, although they may contribute to the growth spurt that often occurs just before puberty and to the libido (sex drive) in adult women.

Pancreas

The pancreas extends from the curve of the duodenum to the spleen. The endocrine portions of the pancreas are called islets of Langerhans (pancreatic islets); they contain alpha cells, which produce glucagon, and beta cells, which produce insulin. Delta cells in the islets secrete somatostatin, which inhibits secretion of both insulin and glucagon.

The functions of glucagon are all related to energy production. Glucagon stimulates the liver to catabolize glycogen to glucose (glycogenolysis) and to increase gluconeogenesis to use fats and excess amino acids for energy production. The overall effect, therefore, is to raise the blood glucose level for cellular uptake and respiration.

The secretion of glucagon is stimulated by hypoglycemia, a low blood glucose level. Such a state may occur during physiological stress situations such as exercise or simply being between meals.

Insulin increases the transport of glucose from the blood into cells by increasing the permeability of cell membranes to glucose (brain and liver cells, however, are not dependent on insulin for glucose intake). Inside cells, glucose is broken down in cellular respiration to release energy. The liver and muscles are also stimulated by insulin to change glucose to glycogen (glycogenesis) to be stored for later use. Insulin also enables cells to take in fatty acids and amino acids to use in the synthesis of lipids and proteins (not energy production). Insulin, therefore, decreases the blood glucose level by increasing the use of glucose for energy, promoting the storage of excess glucose, and decreasing energy production from other food sources.

Secretion of insulin is stimulated by hyperglycemia, a high blood glucose level. This state occurs after meals, especially those high in carbohydrates. It should be apparent that insulin and glucagon function as antagonists and that normal secretion of both hormones ensures a blood glucose level that fluctuates within normal limits. Table 38.1 reviews endocrine hormone function.

TABLE 38.1 REVIEW OF ENDOCRINE FUNCTION

Hormone	Function(s)	Regulation of Secretion
Hormones of the Posterior Pituitary Gland		
Antidiuretic hormone (ADH or vasopressin)	Increases water reabsorption by the kidney tubules (water returns to the blood) Decreases sweating Causes vasoconstriction (in large amounts)	Decreased water content in the body stimulates secretion Alcohol inhibits secretion
Oxytocin	Promotes contraction of myometrium of uterus (labor)	Nerve impulses from hypothalamus, the result of stretching of cervix or stimulation of nipple
	Promotes release of milk from mammary glands	Secretion from placenta at the end of gestation—stimulus unknown
Hormones of the Anterior Pituitary Gland		
Growth hormone (GH)	Increases rate of mitosis Increases amino acid transport into cells Increases rate of protein synthesis Increases use of fats for energy	GHRH (hypothalamus) stimulates secretion GHIH—somatostatin (hypothalamus) inhibits secretion
Thyroid-stimulating hormone (TSH)	Increases secretion of thyroxine and T_3 by thyroid gland	TRH (hypothalamus)
Adrenocorticotropic hormone (ACTH)	Increases secretion of cortisol by the adrenal cortex	CRH (hypothalamus)

Continued

TABLE 38.1 REVIEW OF ENDOCRINE FUNCTION—cont'd

Hormone	Function(s)	Regulation of Secretion
Prolactin	Stimulates milk production by the mammary glands	PRH (hypothalamus) stimulates secretion PIH (hypothalamus) inhibits secretion
Follicle-stimulating hormone (FSH)	*In women:* Initiates growth of ova in ovarian follicles Increases secretion of estrogen by follicle cells	GnRH (hypothalamus) stimulates secretion Inhibin (ovaries or testes) inhibits secretion
	In men: Initiates sperm production in the testes	GnRH (hypothalamus)
Luteinizing hormone (LH)	*In women:* Causes ovulation Causes the ruptured ovarian follicle to become the corpus luteum Increases secretion of progesterone by the corpus luteum	
	In men: Increases secretion of testosterone by the interstitial cells of the testes	GnRH (hypothalamus)
Hormones of the Thyroid Gland		
Thyroxine and triiodothyronine (T_4 and T_3)	Increase energy production from all food types Increase rate of protein synthesis	TSH (anterior pituitary)
Calcitonin	Decreases the reabsorption of calcium and phosphate from bones to blood	Hypercalcemia
Hormones of the Parathyroid Glands		
Parathyroid hormone (PTH)	Increases the reabsorption of calcium and phosphate from bone to blood Increases absorption of calcium and phosphate by the small intestine Increases the reabsorption of calcium and the excretion of phosphate by the kidneys; activates vitamin D	Hypocalcemia stimulates secretion Hypercalcemia inhibits secretion
Hormones of the Adrenal Medulla		
Epinephrine	Increases heart rate and force of contraction Dilates bronchioles Decreases peristalsis Increases conversion of glycogen in glucose in the liver Causes vasodilation in skeletal muscles Causes vasoconstriction in skin and viscera Increases use of fats for energy Increases the rate of cell respiration	Sympathetic impulses from the hypothalamus in stress situations
Norepinephrine	Causes vasoconstriction in skin, viscera, and skeletal muscles	
Hormones of the Pancreas		
Glucagon (alpha cells)	Increases conversion of glycogen to glucose in the liver Increases the use of excess amino acids and fats for energy	Hypoglycemia
Insulin (beta cells)	Increases glucose transport into cells and the use of glucose for energy production Increases the conversion of excess glucose to glycogen in the liver and muscles Increases amino acid and fatty acid transport into cells, and their use in synthesis reactions	Hyperglycemia
Somatostatin (delta cells)	Decreases secretion of insulin and glucagon. Slows absorption of nutrients.	Rising levels of insulin and glucagon

TABLE 38.1 REVIEW OF ENDOCRINE FUNCTION—cont'd

Hormone	Function(s)	Regulation of Secretion
Hormones of the Adrenal Cortex		
Aldosterone	Increases reabsorption of Na^+ ions by the kidneys to the blood Increases excretion of K^+ ions by the kidneys in urine	Low blood Na^+ level Low blood volume or blood pressure High blood K^+ level
Cortisol	Increases use of fats and excess amino acids for energy Decreases use of glucose for energy (except for the brain) Increases conversion of glucose to glycogen in the liver Anti-inflammatory effect: stabilizes lysosomes and blocks the effects of histamine	ACTH (anterior pituitary) during physiological stress

K^+ = potassium; Na^+ = sodium.
Source: Adapted from Scanlon, V. C., & Sanders, T. (2007). *Essentials of anatomy and physiology* (5th ed.). Philadelphia: F. A. Davis.

Aging and the Endocrine System

Most of the endocrine glands decrease their secretions with age, but normal aging usually does not lead to serious hormone deficiencies or illness (Fig. 38.2). Unless specific pathological conditions develop, the endocrine system usually continues to function adequately in old age.

NURSING ASSESSMENT OF THE ENDOCRINE SYSTEM

Health History

When performing a health history, a number of questions can be asked to determine whether an endocrine problem exists. Often, however, you might be aware of a history of an endocrine disorder, such as diabetes or hypothyroidism. When a disorder exists or is suspected, you can do more focused data collection. Assessment of individual disorders is provided in Chapters 39 and 40. Table 38.2 offers general questions that can help you identify new problem areas. If the data reveal abnormalities, they should be reported to a registered nurse or physician.

NURSING CARE TIP

Some patients call diabetes mellitus "sugar." So instead of asking if anyone in their family has diabetes, you may need to ask if anyone has "sugar."

Physical Examination

The physical examination starts with height, weight, and vital signs. Compare findings with the patient's baseline assessment if available. Table 38.3 includes common endocrine-related causes of physical examination abnormalities.

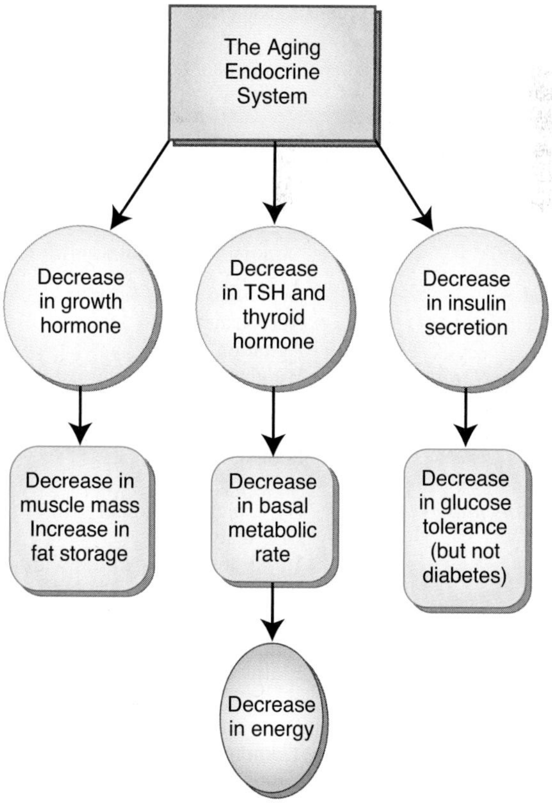

The Aging Endocrine System
Decrease in growth hormone
Decrease in TSH and thyroid hormone
Decrease in insulin secretion
Decrease in muscle mass Increase in fat storage
Decrease in basal metabolic rate
Decrease in glucose tolerance (but not diabetes)
Decrease in energy

FIGURE 38.2 Effects of aging.

TABLE 38.2 SUBJECTIVE DATA COLLECTION FOR THE ENDOCRINE SYSTEM

Category	Questions to Ask During the Health History	Rationale
Neuromuscular	Have you noticed muscle spasms or twitching?	These symptoms may be associated with excessive antidiuretic hormone secretion (SIADH) or calcium depletion resulting from hypoparathyroidism.
	Do you have numbness, tingling, or pain in your feet, legs, or hands?	These may be associated with neuropathy resulting from diabetes mellitus. Numbness and tingling may also indicate hypocalcemia related to hypoparathyroidism.
Nutrition/Fluid Balance	Have you gained or lost weight without trying?	Actual weight gain may be associated with hypothyroidism. Weight gain due to water retention may result from Cushing's syndrome or SIADH. Weight loss may result from uncontrolled diabetes or hyperthyroidism. Weight loss due to dehydration may be related to Addison's disease.
	Have you noticed excessive thirst or urination?	Excessive thirst and urination are classic symptoms of diabetes mellitus and diabetes insipidus.
	Have you noticed a change in your energy level?	Lack of energy may be associated with uncontrolled diabetes, hypothyroidism, hyperthyroidism, Addison's disease, or pituitary disorders.
Metabolic	Do you generally tolerate changes in environmental temperature?	Hypothyroidism can cause cold intolerance. Hyperthyroidism can cause heat intolerance.
Mood/Memory	Have you noticed a change in your mood or memory?	Mental function may be dull with hypothyroidism. Mood swings may occur with Cushing's syndrome. Agitation or confusion may result from hypoglycemia in a person with diabetes.
Family History	Does anyone in your family have a thyroid problem, diabetes, or another endocrine disorder?	Some disorders are hereditary.

SIADH = syndrome of inappropriate antidiuretic hormone.

TABLE 38.3 ENDOCRINE-RELATED CAUSES OF ABNORMAL PHYSICAL EXAMINATION FINDINGS

Category	Abnormal Examination Finding	Possible Causes
Mood	Depressed mood or affect	Hypothyroidism
	Nervousness	Hyperthyroidism, pheochromocytoma
	Agitation	Low blood glucose level
Nutrition/Fluid Balance	Weight gain	Decreased metabolic rate in hypothyroidism, fluid excess
	Weight loss	Increased metabolic rate in hyperthyroidism; uncontrolled diabetes, dehydration
	Poor skin turgor	Dehydration due to water loss in Addison's disease, diabetes mellitus, diabetes insipidus
Integumentary	Hyperpigmentation of skin	Addison's disease
	Dry, scaly skin	Hypothyroidism
	Dusky lower extremities with weak peripheral pulses	Circulatory changes in diabetes mellitus
Vital Signs	Change in pulse or temperature	Elevated due to increased metabolic rate in hyperthyroidism Decreased due to slowed metabolic rate in hypothyroidism
	Elevated blood pressure	Increased catecholamine release in pheochromocytoma or fluid retention in Cushing's syndrome
	Decreased blood pressure	Sodium and water loss in Addison's disease
Neuromuscular	Tremor	Hyperthyroidism, hypoglycemia, or pheochromocytoma
Head and Neck	Exophthalmos (bulging eyes)	Fat deposits and edema behind the eyes in Graves' disease
	Fat pads on neck and shoulders ("buffalo hump"), round "moon" face	Accumulation of fat in Cushing's syndrome
	Enlarged thyroid gland	Excessive stimulation by TSH in hypothyroidism or hyperthyroidism

Inspection

Observe the patient for mood and **affect** (emotional tone) throughout the physical assessment. Inspect the neck for thyroid enlargement. Look for eyes that bulge (**exophthalmos**). Note posture, body fat, and presence of tremor. Observe skin and hair texture and moisture. Note the presence of a moonlike face or "buffalo hump" on the upper back. Observe the lower extremities for skin and color changes that might indicate circulatory impairment. See Table 38.3 for rationales for these observations.

Palpation

The thyroid gland is the only palpable endocrine gland. The licensed practical nurse/licensed vocational nurse (LPN/LVN) may assist a physician or nurse practitioner to palpate the thyroid gland. The practitioner stands behind or in front of the seated patient and palpates the gland while the patient swallows a sip of water (Fig. 38.3). You can assist with positioning the patient, providing water, and instructing the patient to take a sip of water and hold it in his or her mouth until told to swallow. The thyroid gland should never be palpated in a patient with uncontrolled hyperthyroidism because this can stimulate secretion of additional thyroid hormone.

Palpate all peripheral pulses. The posterior tibial and dorsalis pedis pulses may be diminished in patients with circulatory impairment. Palpate skin turgor by gently pinching a small piece of skin. The sternum is a good place to check. If a "tent" of skin remains in place, the patient may be dehydrated as a result of water loss, as in ADH deficiency.

Auscultation and Percussion

Auscultation and percussion are not usually part of an endocrine assessment.

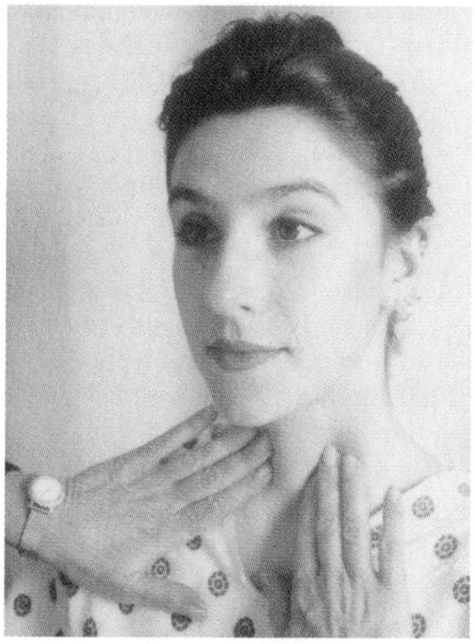

FIGURE 38.3 Thyroid palpation. (From Dillon, P. M. [2007]. *Nursing health assessment: A critical thinking approach* [2nd ed.]. Philadelphia: F. A. Davis, with permission.)

• WORD • BUILDING •
exophthalmos: exo—outward + ophthalmos—relating to the eye

DIAGNOSTIC TESTS FOR THE ENDOCRINE SYSTEM

Hormone Tests

Serum Hormone Levels

Many hormones can be measured from a simple blood specimen. This is useful in diagnosing hypofunctioning or hyperfunctioning gland states. See Table 38.4 for some commonly measured hormones.

Stimulation Tests

Stimulation tests may also help determine endocrine gland function. For this type of test, a substance is injected to stimulate a gland. The hormone secreted by that gland is then measured in the blood to determine how well it responded to the stimulation. For example, in a TRH stimulation test, TRH is injected. If the pituitary gland responds appropriately, TSH is secreted. If the thyroid gland responds appropriately to the TSH, T_3 and T_4 levels rise. Failure of TRH to stimulate TSH and thyroid hormone indicates a pituitary or thyroid condition. Further studies might be done to determine the cause.

Suppression Tests

Suppression tests are the opposite of stimulating tests. For this type of test, a substance is injected that is expected to suppress a hormone's release. For example, if dexamethasone (a steroid hormone) is injected, cortisol release from the adrenal cortex is expected to be suppressed via a negative feedback mechanism. If the cortisol level is not suppressed, adrenal cortex dysfunction is suspected.

CRITICAL THINKING

Ms. Hackworth

■ Ms. Hackworth is tired all the time, and the nurse practitioner (NP) orders a TSH level drawn. The result is higher than normal.

1. You make the call to have Ms. Hackworth come in to the clinic for further evaluation, and she asks, "If my thyroid level is high, then why am I so tired?" How should you respond?
2. After further testing, the NP places Ms. Hackworth on levothyroxine (Synthroid) 50 mcg daily. Her pharmacist supplies Synthroid 0.05 mg. Is her dose correct?

Suggested answers at end of chapter.

Urine Tests

Sometimes it is helpful to measure the amount of hormone or hormone by-product excreted in the urine during a 24-hour period. Examples are cortisol and vanillylmandelic acid, a product of catecholamine metabolism.

TABLE 38.4 COMMON ENDOCRINE-RELATED LABORATORY TESTS

Test	Normal Values*	Significance of Abnormal Findings
Thyroid Tests		
Thyroid-stimulating hormone	0.4–4.2 microinternational units/mL	↑ in primary hypothyroidism ↓ in primary hyperthyroidism
Triiodothyronine (T_3), total	70–204 ng/dL	↓ in hypothyroidism ↑ in hyperthyroidism
Triiodothyronine (T_3), free	260–480 pg/dL	
Thyroxine (T_4), total	*Male:* 4.6–10.5 mcg/dL *Female:* 5.5–11 mcg/dL	↓ in hypothyroidism ↑ in hyperthyroidism
Thyroxine (T_4), free	0.8–1.5 ng/dL	
Parathyroid Tests		
Parathyroid hormone	8–24 pg/mL	↑ in primary hyperparathyroidism ↓ in primary hypoparathyroidism, parathyroid trauma during thyroid surgery
Calcium, blood	8.2–10.2 mg/100 mL *Over age 90:* 8.2–9.6 mg/dL	↑ in some cancers, hyperparathyroidism ↓ in hypothyroidism
Phosphorus	2.5–4.5 mg/dL	↑ in hypoparathyroidism ↓ in hyperparathyroidism
Pituitary Tests		
Growth hormone	*Male:* 0–5 ng/mL *Female:* 0–10 ng/mL	↑ in acromegaly ↓ in small stature
Antidiuretic hormone (vasopressin)	0–4.7 pg/mL	↑ in SIADH ↓ in diabetes insipidus
Urine specific gravity	1.001–1.029	↓ in diabetes insipidus
Adrenocorticotropic hormone (ACTH)	9–52 pg/mL in a.m. *Women on oral contraceptives:* 5–29 pg/mL	↑ in Addison's disease ↓ in Cushing's syndrome, long-term corticosteroid therapy
Adrenal Tests		
Aldosterone	*Supine:* 3–16 ng/dL *Upright:* 7–30 ng/dL	↑ in heart failure, COPD, hypovolemia ↓ in Addison's disease, hypoaldosteronism
Cortisol	5–25 mcg/dL at 8 a.m. 3–16 mcg/dL at 4 p.m.	↑ in Cushing's syndrome, stress ↓ in Addison's disease, steroid withdrawal
Vanillylmandelic acid (VMA; urine test)	1.4–6.5 mg/24 hr	↑ in pheochromocytoma
Pancreas Tests		
Fasting plasma glucose (FPG)	70–100 mg/dL	↑ in stress, Cushing's syndrome 101–125 mg/dL = pre-diabetes 126 mg/dL or greater = diabetes mellitus ↓ in hypoglycemia, Addison's disease
Fructosamine (glycated albumin)	174–286 micromol/L *Diabetes:* *Controlled:* 210–421 micromol/L *Uncontrolled:* 268-870 micromol/L	↑ in poor diabetes control ↓ in severe hypoproteinemia
Ketones, blood and urine	Negative	Positive in acidosis, fasting or starvation, diabetic ketoacidosis
Oral glucose tolerance test	Blood glucose level less than 140 mg/dL at 2 hr	140–199 mg/dL at 2 hr = pre-diabetes 200 mg/dL or greater at 2 hr = diabetes mellitus
Glycosylated hemoglobin	4%–6%	↑ in poor diabetes control

SIADH = syndrome of inappropriate antidiuretic hormone.
*All normal values are for a fasting test.

To collect a 24-hour urine specimen, you must obtain a special urine container from the laboratory. It is usually an opaque container that protects the specimen from light; it may have preservative in it. Check with the laboratory to find out whether the specimen needs to be kept on ice during the test and whether the patient needs to be on a special diet before or during the test. Follow these steps to collect the urine:

1. If the specimen needs to be on ice, fill a bath basin with ice and place the container in the basin. Refill the ice every few hours to keep the specimen cold.
2. Instruct the patient how to do the test, place a sign on the toilet with the start and stop time of the test, and remind all staff to save the urine.
3. Ask the patient to urinate and discard the urine. The time of this first discarded voiding is considered the start of the test.
4. Save all urine from the start time forward for 24 hours. Have the patient void into a urinal or other collector, and then carefully pour it into the specimen container.
5. At the end of the 24-hour period, ask the patient to urinate, and pour this final urine into the specimen container.
6. Label the entire collection and send it to the laboratory.

If the patient is incontinent or otherwise unable to participate in the test, a catheter may need to be inserted. If the patient already has an indwelling catheter, a new bag and tubing should be attached before the start of the test. The laboratory should be consulted to determine the need for a preservative or ice. Preservative can be added to the catheter bag if necessary. If ice is needed, the bag should be kept in a basin of ice rather than hanging on the side of the bed. If the specimen must be protected from light, the bag can be covered with dark plastic or foil.

> **CRITICAL THINKING**
>
> ***Mrs. Trombley***
>
> ■ Mrs. Trombley is having a 24-hour urine test done. You begin the test at 0600, and it progresses well until you learn that the nursing assistant helped her up to void in the toilet at noon, forgetting to save her urine.
>
> 1. What do you do?
> 2. How can you prevent this from happening again?
> 3. How would you document this incident?
>
> *Suggested answers at end of chapter.*

Other Laboratory Tests

Some laboratory tests may indirectly reflect the function of an endocrine gland. For example, a serum calcium level helps indicate PTH or calcitonin secretion, and a blood glucose level reflects insulin secretion.

Nuclear Scanning

Thyroid Scan

A thyroid scan may be done to determine the presence of tumors or nodules. For this test, a radioactive material is injected or radioactive iodine is taken orally. The material is taken up by the thyroid gland. After a specified time, the thyroid gland is scanned with a scintillation camera. The scan will show hot spots (nodules), which are not malignant, or cold spots (areas that do not take up the radioactivity), which indicate malignancy. Cold spots can then be biopsied to confirm a diagnosis. Because such a small amount of radioactive material is used, the risk to the patient is minimal. The patient should be aware that the test takes approximately 30 minutes to complete.

Radioactive Iodine Uptake

A radioactive iodine uptake test is similar to a thyroid scan and is done to evaluate thyroid function. Several scans are taken over a 24-hour period after administration of radioactive iodine. The amount of iodine taken up by the thyroid indicates the activity of the gland. This is especially helpful in diagnosing hyperthyroidism.

PET Scan

Positron emission tomography (PET) scanning is another type of scan that can be done to differentiate between benign and malignant endocrine tumors. PET scans are helpful because they can show metabolic changes in organs or tissues.

Radiographic Tests

A computed tomography (CT) scan or magnetic resonance imaging (MRI) may be done to locate a tumor or identify hypertrophy of a gland.

Ultrasound

Ultrasound may be done of the thyroid or parathyroid glands to determine if they are enlarged or to find masses.

Biopsy

Biopsy is done to obtain tissue to examine for possible cancerous cells. The thyroid gland can be biopsied either by needle aspiration under local anesthesia or using a surgical incision.

SUGGESTED ANSWERS TO

CRITICAL THINKING

■ *Ms. Hackworth*

1. "It's not your thyroid hormone that is high, it's your thyroid-stimulating hormone. That means your pituitary gland has to work extra hard to try to stimulate your thyroid gland."
2.

$$\frac{50\ mcg}{} \Big| \frac{1\ mg}{1000\ mcg} = 0.05\ mg$$

■ *Mrs. Trombley*

1. The specimen must include all urine for a 24-hour period. Restart the test from noon.
2. To prevent this from happening again, try placing an incontinence pad or other large item directly over the toilet as a reminder to the patient. Be sure there is a sign posted above the toilet or on the toilet handle, and communicate with the nursing assistants why the urine needs to be saved.
3. "Patient voided in toilet at 1200. 24-hour urine test restarted; importance of saving urine explained to patient and staff. RN notified." Note that it is not appropriate to "blame" the nursing assistant for making a mistake.

REVIEW QUESTIONS

1. Which hormones are secreted by the posterior pituitary gland? **Select all that apply**.
   a. Antidiuretic hormone
   b. Thyroid-stimulating hormone
   c. Growth hormone
   d. Luteinizing hormone
   e. Oxytocin
   f. Calcitonin

2. What are the functions of T_4 and T_3?
   a. Retention of salt and water
   b. Maintenance of blood sugar
   c. Maintenance of blood pressure
   d. Regulation of energy production

3. Which hormone maintains strong bones?
   a. ADH
   b. Insulin
   c. Calcitonin
   d. TRH

4. The nurse is doing an admission assessment on a new resident to an extended care facility. The patient's face and shoulders seem to have a lot of fat, but the patient's arms and legs are thin. Excess of which hormone might be involved?
   a. Cortisol
   b. ADH
   c. Insulin
   d. Epinephrine

5. When explaining a thyroid scan to a patient, which of the following statements is correct?
   a. "You will take a special pill, and then an ultrasound will be taken of your neck."
   b. "You will receive an injection of radioactive material, and then a special camera will take pictures of your thyroid gland."
   c. "You will be placed into a special machine, and x-rays will be taken of your neck. It may be noisy."
   d. "You will be given a special drink, and then magnetic energy is used to visualize the thyroid area."

DavisPlus | For additional resources and information visit http://davisplus.fadavis.com

39 Nursing Care of Patients with Endocrine Disorders

PAULA D. HOPPER

KEY TERMS

amenorrhea (ay-MEN-uh-REE-ah)
ectopic (ek-TOP-ik)
euthyroid (yoo-THY-royd)
goitrogenic (GOY-troh-JEN-ik)
goitrogens (GOY-troh-jenz)
hyperplasia (HEYE-per-PLAY-zee-ah)
hypophysectomy (HEYE-pah-fi-SEK-tuh-mee)
myxedema (MIK-suh-DEE-mah)
nephrogenic (NEFF-roh-JEN-ik)
nocturia (nok-TYOO-ree-ah)
osmolality (ahs-moh-LAL-i-tee)
pheochromocytoma (FEE-oh-KROH-moh-sigh-TOH-mah)
polydipsia (PAH-lee-DIP-see-ah)
polyuria (PAH-lee-YOO-ree-ah)
psychogenic (SEYE-koh-JEN-ik)
tetany (TET-uh-nee)

QUESTIONS TO GUIDE YOUR READING

1. What disorders are caused by variations in the hormones of the pituitary, thyroid, parathyroid, and adrenal glands?
2. How would you explain the pathophysiology of each of the endocrine disorders presented?
3. What are the etiologies, signs, and symptoms of each of the endocrine disorders?
4. What current therapeutic measures are used for each of the selected endocrine disorders?
5. What data would you collect when caring for patients with each of the endocrine disorders discussed?
6. What nursing care would you provide for patients with each of the disorders?
7. How will you know if your nursing interventions have been effective?

The endocrine system is subject to a variety of disorders. Although the causes vary, the pathophysiology usually involves either too little or too much hormone activity. Insufficient hormone activity may be the result of hypofunction of an endocrine gland or insensitivity of the target tissue to its hormone. Excessive hormone activity may be the result of a hyperactive gland, **ectopic** hormone production, or self-administration of too much replacement hormone (Table 39.1). If you can remember the function of each hormone in the body, understanding the problems involved with an altered amount of each hormone becomes easier.

Most endocrine disorders are either primary or secondary. A primary disorder is a problem within the gland that is out of balance. Secondary disorders are caused by problems outside the gland, such as an imbalance in a tropic hormone, certain drugs, trauma, surgery, or a problem in the feedback mechanism. For example, if the thyroid gland is diseased and causing hypothyroidism, it would be considered a primary problem. Sometimes hypothyroidism is caused by not enough thyroid-stimulating hormone from the pituitary gland, even though the thyroid gland is healthy. This would be considered a secondary problem.

LEARNING TIP

If you can remember what each hormone does in the body, it will be easier to remember what results from imbalances of that hormone. Most symptoms of hormone hyperactivity are the opposite of symptoms of that hormone's hypoactivity.

PITUITARY DISORDERS

Pituitary disorders often involve several hormone imbalances at once, caused by general hypopituitarism or hyperpituitarism. Problems involving all of the pituitary hormones at once, however, are rare. For simplicity, imbalances are considered separately here.

TABLE 39.1 CAUSES OF ENDOCRINE PROBLEMS

Insufficient hormone activity	Gland hypofunction Lack of tropic or stimulating hormone Target tissue insensitivity to hormone
Excess hormone activity	Gland hyperfunction Excess tropic or stimulating hormone Ectopic hormone production Self-administration of too much replacement hormone

• WORD • BUILDING •

ectopic: ec—away from normal + topic—place

Disorders Related to Antidiuretic Hormone Imbalance

Antidiuretic hormone (ADH; also called arginine vasopressin [AVP]) is synthesized in the hypothalamus and stored and secreted by the posterior pituitary gland. A decrease in ADH activity results in diabetes insipidus (DI). An increase in ADH activity is called syndrome of inappropriate antidiuretic hormone (SIADH). Table 39.2 compares DI and SIADH. Note how symptoms of too little ADH (water loss) are the opposite of symptoms of too much ADH (water retention).

Diabetes Insipidus

PATHOPHYSIOLOGY. Diabetes insipidus is caused by a deficiency of ADH. Recall that ADH is responsible for reabsorption of water by the distal tubules and collecting ducts in the kidneys. If ADH is lacking, adequate reabsorption of water is prevented, leading to diuresis. In **nephrogenic** diabetes insipidus, there is enough ADH but the kidneys do not respond to it. Patients can urinate from 3 to 15 L per day. This leads to increased serum **osmolality** (concentrated blood) and dehydration. The increased osmolality and decreased blood pressure normally trigger ADH secretion, which causes water retention and dilutes the blood; in patients with DI, this does not happen. Increased osmolality also leads to extreme thirst, which usually causes the patient to drink enough fluids to maintain fluid balance. In an unconscious patient or a patient with a defective thirst mechanism, however, dehydration may quickly occur if the problem is not recognized and corrected. For more information, check out the Nephrogenic Diabetes Insipidus Foundation at www.ndif.org.

ETIOLOGY. Diabetes insipidus has a variety of causes. Tumors, trauma, or other problems in the hypothalamus or pituitary gland can lead to decreased production or release of ADH. Surgery in the area of the pituitary and certain drugs, such as glucocorticoids or alcohol, may also cause DI. Occasionally, the cause is **psychogenic**, which means the patient drinks large quantities of water in the absence of true disease. Nephrogenic DI occurs mostly in males and may be inherited or acquired. It is diagnosed when the kidneys do not respond to ADH. It can be triggered by certain drugs or neoplasms, or by damage to the kidneys from pyelonephritis, polycystic disease, or other causes.

SIGNS AND SYMPTOMS. The patient with DI urinates frequently (**polyuria**), and nighttime urination (**nocturia**) is present. This results in high serum osmolality and low urine osmolality. Urine specific gravity is decreased, making the urine diluted and light in color.

• WORD • BUILDING •

nephrogenic: nephro—kidney + genic—to produce
psychogenic: psycho—related to the mind + genic—to produce
polyuria: poly—much + uria—urine
nocturia: noct—night + uria—urine

TABLE 39.2 ANTIDIURETIC HORMONE DISORDERS SUMMARY

	Insufficient ADH	Excess ADH
Disorder	Diabetes insipidus	SIADH
Signs and Symptoms	Polyuria, polydipsia, dehydration, dilute urine	Fluid retention, weight gain, concentrated urine
Diagnostic Tests	Urine specific gravity, urine and plasma osmolality, water deprivation test	Serum and urine sodium and osmolality; water load test
Therapeutic Measures	Synthetic ADH replacement	Treat cause
Priority Nursing Diagnoses	*Deficient Fluid Volume* *Risk for Ineffective Self Health Management*	*Excess Fluid Volume* *Risk for Ineffective Self Health Management*

The patient experiences extreme thirst (**polydipsia**), and consumes large volumes of water. Often patients crave ice-cold water. If urine output exceeds fluid intake, dehydration occurs, with characteristic symptoms of hypotension, poor skin turgor, and weakness. Hypovolemic shock occurs if fluid balance is not restored. Dehydration and electrolyte imbalances result in a decrease in level of consciousness and death if the problem is not corrected.

The patient with DI may develop an enlarged bladder and kidney damage from constantly trying to "hold" too much urine.

DIAGNOSTIC TESTS. Diagnosis is based initially on a history of risk factors and reported symptoms. Urine specific gravity will be less than 1.001 (normal: 1.001 to 1.029), and can be monitored by laboratory tests or by using reagent strips at the bedside. Plasma and urine osmolality are measured and compared to each other. The actual amount of sodium in the blood may be normal, but it appears elevated in relation to the decreased amount of water. Computed tomography (CT) scanning or magnetic resonance imaging (MRI) may show a pituitary tumor.

A water-deprivation test may be done. For this test, the patient is deprived of water for up to 6 hours. Body weight and urine osmolality are tested hourly. If the urine continues to be diluted, even though the patient is not drinking and is losing weight as a result of volume depletion, DI is suspected. In the second stage of the test, the patient receives an injection of ADH, with a final urine test done 1 hour later. If the DI is nephrogenic, the kidneys will not respond to the injected ADH.

ADH levels can be measured in plasma or urine following administration of hypertonic saline or fluid restriction. The normal response would be elevated ADH; if it is not elevated, DI is suspected. The urine glucose level may also be checked to rule out diabetes mellitus.

THERAPEUTIC MEASURES. Hypotonic intravenous (IV) fluids such as 0.45% saline solution may be ordered to replace intravascular volume without adding excessive sodium. IV fluids are especially important if the patient is unable to take oral fluids.

• WORD • BUILDING •
polydipsia: poly—much + dipsia—thirst

Medical treatment of DI involves replacement of ADH. In acute cases, vasopressin, a synthetic form of ADH, is given by the intravenous or subcutaneous route, along with IV fluid replacement. In patients who require long-term therapy, synthetic ADH (desmopressin, or DDAVP) in the form of a nasal spray is used, usually twice a day. Other drugs, such as chlorpropamide (Diabinese), help the kidneys respond better to ADH. Thiazide diuretics may decrease urine flow in the absence of ADH (even though they usually are used to increase urine output!). If a pituitary tumor is involved, treatment usually involves removal of the pituitary gland (**hypophysectomy**).

NURSING PROCESS FOR THE PATIENT WITH DIABETES INSIPIDUS.

Data Collection. When collecting data for a patient with DI, pay special attention to fluid balance. Daily weights are the most reliable method for monitoring the amount of fluid that is being lost. Taking accurate intake and output (I&O) measurements is also helpful. Skin turgor will be poor and mucous membranes will be dry and sticky if the patient is becoming dehydrated. Monitor skin integrity because dehydration increases risk of breakdown. Monitor vital signs for signs of shock. Use a reagent strip (dipstick) or urimeter to measure urine specific gravities. Monitor serum electrolytes and osmolality as ordered, and watch for changes in level of consciousness. Assess the patient's understanding of his or her disease and treatment. Once treatment is initiated, continue to monitor fluid balance, being especially alert to signs of fluid overload.

Nursing Diagnoses, Planning, and Implementation

Deficient Fluid Volume Related to Failure of Regulatory Mechanisms

EXPECTED OUTCOME: The patient's fluid balance will be maintained as evidenced by urine specific gravity between 1.001 and 1.029, skin turgor within normal limits, and stable daily weight.

- Monitor daily weight, I&O, vital signs, and urine specific gravity. *Decreased weight, output greater than intake, low blood pressure, elevated pulse rate, and high urine specific gravity may all indicate fluid deficit.*

• WORD • BUILDING •
hypophysectomy: hypophysis—pituitary + ectomy—surgical removal

- Monitor patient for restlessness or weakness. *These may indicate early fluid deficit.*
- Provide free access to oral fluids if the DI is not psychogenic. If the patient's thirst mechanism is not intact, give the patient fluids every hour. *Oral fluids are essential to replace the excess lost in diuresis. If the patient is alert with an intact thirst mechanism, the patient can usually manage this independently.*
- Encourage the patient to participate in maintaining intake and output records, monitoring weight, and checking urine specific gravity, if able. *This involves the patient and helps prepare him or her for self-monitoring at home.*
- Report a significant drop in blood pressure and a rising pulse to the registered nurse or physician *because these may be signs of hypovolemic shock.*

Risk for Ineffective Self Health Management Related to Deficient Knowledge

EXPECTED OUTCOME: The patient will manage condition effectively as evidenced by statement and demonstration of understanding of medication administration and self-monitoring of disease.

- Assess patient's understanding of his or her disease process and treatment. *Teaching should build on baseline knowledge.*
- Teach the patient about DI. *The patient will have to self-medicate and monitor his or her disease at home.* Include:
  - Basic pathophysiology of the disease
  - How to administer medications and monitor their effectiveness
  - How to measure urine specific gravity and the significance of results
  - Signs and symptoms of dehydration and fluid overload to report.
- Stress the importance of monitoring daily weight: losses or gains of greater than 2 pounds in a day should be reported to the physician. *Weight loss or gain can indicate fluid imbalance and the need for a change in medication regimen.*
- Advise the patient to wear identification, such as a medical alert bracelet, that identifies the disorder. *Faster treatment can be initiated if emergency personnel are aware of a DI diagnosis.*

Evaluation. If treatment has been effective, signs of dehydration will be absent and weight and vital signs will be stable. The patient should be able to explain what is happening in the disease and symptoms to report and also demonstrate how to manage self-care.

Syndrome of Inappropriate Antidiuretic Hormone

PATHOPHYSIOLOGY. Syndrome of inappropriate antidiuretic hormone (SIADH) results from too much ADH in the body. This causes excess water to be reabsorbed by the kidney tubules and collecting ducts, leading to decreased urine output and fluid overload. As fluid builds up in the bloodstream, osmolality decreases and the blood becomes diluted. Normally, a decreased serum osmolality inhibits release of ADH. In SIADH, however, ADH continues to be released, adding to the fluid overload.

ETIOLOGY. Certain cancers such as pancreatic cancer or some types of lung cancer may be ectopic sites of production of an ADH-like substance. Drugs such as certain antidepressants, chemotherapy, or general anesthetic agents may increase ADH secretion. Neurologic problems such as central nervous system (CNS) infections or a brain tumor affecting pituitary function may also cause SIADH. It may also be a complication of diabetes insipidus treatment.

SIGNS AND SYMPTOMS. Symptoms of SIADH include symptoms of fluid overload, such as weight gain (usually without edema) and dilutional hyponatremia (Box 39.1). The actual amount of sodium in the blood may be normal, but appear to be low because of the diluting effect of the retained fluid. Serum osmolality is less than 275 mOsm/kg. The urine is concentrated because water is not being excreted. Muscle cramps and weakness may occur because of electrolyte imbalance. Because the osmolality of the blood is low, fluid may leak out of the vessels and cause brain swelling. If untreated, this results in lethargy, confusion, seizures, coma, and death.

DIAGNOSTIC TESTS. Serum and urine sodium levels and osmolality are measured. Serum ADH is high. Additional testing may be done to diagnose and locate an ADH-secreting tumor. Occasionally, a water load test may be done, which involves administering a specific amount of water, then measuring blood and urine sodium and osmolality hourly for 6 hours. The patient with SIADH retains the water instead of excreting it. This test can cause an unsafe fluid overload, so is not done unless necessary for diagnosis.

THERAPEUTIC MEASURES. Treatment is aimed at eliminating the cause. If a tumor is secreting ADH, surgical removal may be indicated. Symptoms may be alleviated by restricting fluids to 800 to 1000 mL per 24 hours. Hypertonic saline fluids may be administered intravenously, and oral salt may be encouraged to maintain the serum sodium level. If the cause is inoperable cancer, drugs such as furosemide (Lasix) and demeclocycline (Declomycin) may be used to block the action of ADH in the kidney.

> **LEARNING TIP**
>
> Remember "a pint's a pound the world around." So each time a patient gains 1 pound of fluid, it is equal to approximately 1 pint or 480 mL!

Box 39.1

Manifestations of Dilutional Hyponatremia

- Bounding pulse
- Elevated or normal blood pressure
- Muscle weakness
- Headache
- Personality changes
- Nausea
- Diarrhea
- Convulsions
- Coma

NURSING PROCESS FOR THE PATIENT WITH SYNDROME OF INAPPROPRIATE ANTIDIURETIC HORMONE.

Data Collection. Excess fluid volume with hyponatremia is the primary concern for the patient with SIADH. To monitor fluid balance, assess vital signs, weight, I&O, urine specific gravity, skin turgor, and edema. Auscultate lung sounds for crackles, a sign of fluid overload. Determine the patient's ability to maintain a fluid restriction. Assess level of consciousness and neuromuscular function. Monitor laboratory tests, including serum sodium level, as ordered by the physician. Assess the patient's understanding of the disease process and treatment.

Nursing Diagnoses, Planning, and Implementation

Excess Fluid Volume Related to Compromised Regulatory Mechanism as Evidenced by Weight Gain, Imbalanced I&O, Low Serum Sodium, or Crackles

EXPECTED OUTCOME: The patient's fluid balance will be maintained as evidenced by weight, I&O, and serum sodium within normal limits, lungs clear.

- Monitor daily weight, I&O, vital signs, lung sounds, and laboratory values. *Increased weight, intake greater than output, elevated blood pressure, bounding pulse, crackles, and low serum sodium may all indicate fluid overload.*
- Maintain fluid restriction *to reduce serum dilution and normalize serum sodium.*
- Offer small amounts of fluids high in sodium, such as broth, cola, or tomato juice, as ordered. *These may help correct dilutional hyponatremia.*
- Offer hard candy *to reduce sensation of thirst.*
- Provide ice chips (count as half the volume of fluid; that is, 100 mL of ice chips equal approximately 50 mL of water). *Ice chips take longer to consume than water, and may be more satisfying to some patients.*
- Provide calibrated cups *to help the patient maintain the restriction independently if able.*
- Allow the patient to participate in planning the types and times of fluid intake. *Fluid restrictions are not pleasant for patients; patients who feel in control may be more likely to comply with restriction.*
- Report a change in level of consciousness immediately, and monitor the patient for seizures. *These are signs of serious fluid imbalance.*

Risk for Ineffective Self Health Management Related to Knowledge Deficit

EXPECTED OUTCOME: The patient will have requisite knowledge to be able to manage self care as evidenced by a statement or demonstration of self-care activities.

- Assess patient's understanding of his or her disease process and treatment. *Teaching should build on baseline knowledge.*
- Explain self-care measures as needed to the patient, including fluid restriction, monitoring of fluid balance, and medications. *The patient must understand the treatment to manage it at home.*
- Instruct the patient to report any weight gain greater than 2 pounds in 1 day, a change in urine output, or acute thirst. *These are signs of fluid overload or risk for overload.*
- Encourage use of medical alert bracelet or other identification *so emergency personnel will have information if needed.*

Evaluation. Weight should stabilize at the pre-illness level once treatment is begun. Serum sodium level should be within normal limits. Patients should be able to verbalize the cause of their symptoms and demonstrate self-care, including ability to maintain a fluid restriction if necessary.

CRITICAL THINKING

Mrs. Jackson

■ You are caring for Mrs. Jackson, a 78-year-old woman who has just returned to your unit following hip surgery. During the next 2 days, you notice that her weight increases from 118 to 124 pounds and she seems lethargic, but the nurse's report didn't indicate concern about it. You check her ankles and sacrum for edema but find none. In the afternoon, her son rushes out of the room and tells you she is becoming confused, adding that this is not like her at all.

1. What assessment should you do?
2. What do you suspect?
3. What should be your next steps?
4. Based on her weight gain, about how much water is Mrs. Jackson retaining?

Suggested answers at end of chapter.

Disorders Related to Growth Hormone Imbalance

Growth hormone (GH), also called somatotropin, is responsible for normal growth of bones, cartilage, and soft tissue. GH is synthesized and secreted by the anterior pituitary gland. An excess or deficiency of GH may be related to a more generalized problem with the pituitary gland or hypothalamus. A deficit of GH results in short stature if not corrected in childhood, and a variety of problems in adulthood. Excess GH results in gigantism (Fig. 39.1) or acromegaly.

Growth Hormone Deficiency

PATHOPHYSIOLOGY. When growth hormone is deficient in childhood, a condition called short stature occurs. In the past this was referred to as dwarfism (see Fig. 39.1). A deficiency of GH in adults does not affect growth, but in recent years it has been found to have important functions even during adulthood.

ETIOLOGY. Growth hormone deficiency may be due to tumors, surgery, or trauma to the pituitary or hypothalamus. It may also be deficient in some cases of neglect or severe emotional stress. Malnutrition is the most common cause worldwide. Sometimes the cause is not known (Box 39.2, *Cultural Considerations*).

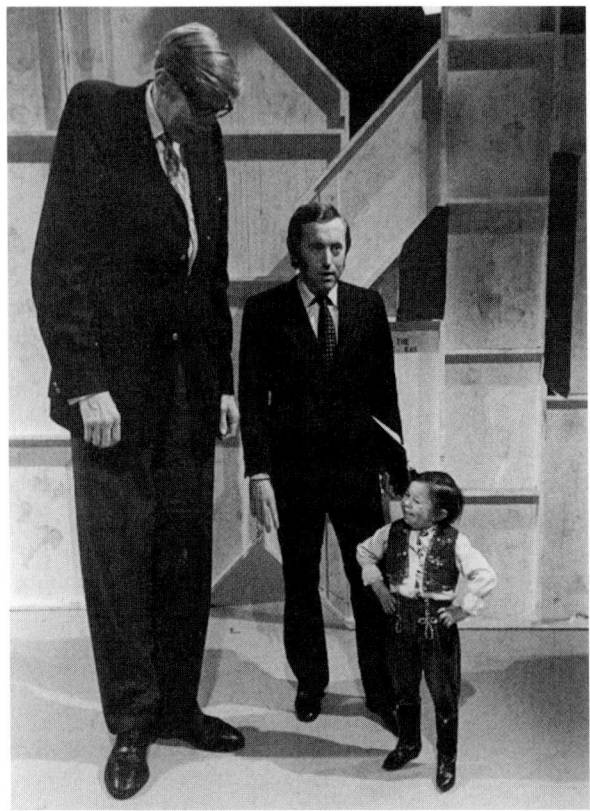

FIGURE 39.1 Gigantism and dwarfism. (From Tamparo, C. D., and Lewis, M. A. [2000]. *Diseases of the human body* [3rd ed., p. 247]. Philadelphia: F. A. Davis, with permission.)

SIGNS AND SYMPTOMS. Children may grow to only 3 to 4 feet in height but have normal body proportions. Sexual maturation may be slowed, related to involvement of additional pituitary hormones. Short stature in children is sometimes accompanied by mental retardation.

In adults, symptoms of GH deficiency include fatigue, weakness, excess body fat, decreased muscle and bone mass, sexual dysfunction, high cholesterol, and increased risk for cardiovascular and cerebrovascular disease. Headaches, mental slowness, and psychological disturbances may also occur. All of these signs and symptoms can lead to decreased quality of life.

DIAGNOSTIC TESTS. Growth hormone levels in the blood can be measured by a routine laboratory test, but the results may be unreliable because GH is not evenly secreted over the course of a day. A more reliable test is a growth hormone stimulation test that measures GH in response to induced hypoglycemia. An MRI can help determine the presence of a tumor; radiographic studies may be used to determine bone age. Genetic testing may also be done.

THERAPEUTIC MEASURES. Treatment of GH deficiency is administration of growth hormone. In the past, GH was derived from human pituitary glands, so treatment was expensive and risky. Now GH (somatotropin [Humatrope]) can be made in a laboratory using recombinant DNA technology, so it is more readily available to those who need it. It is administered by subcutaneous injection. Surgery may be indicated if a tumor is the cause.

NURSING PROCESS FOR THE PATIENT WITH GROWTH HORMONE DEFICIENCY.

Data Collection. Assessment of the adult with GH deficiency includes mental status, ability to cope with the effects of the disorder, and understanding of the treatment plan. Also assess for signs of cardiovascular disease and other complications of the disorder.

Nursing Diagnoses, Planning, and Implementation. If the problem has been present since childhood, most related problems will not be new to the patient. The priority for the nurse, then, is to approach the patient with respect while assessing current problems that may need attention. Nursing diagnoses in the adult with GH deficiency will depend on assessed needs. These may include diagnoses such as *Risk for Ineffective Self Health Management* (see below), *Fatigue*, *Knowledge Deficit*, *Imbalanced Nutrition*, *Risk for Injury*, or *Risk for Spiritual Distress*.

An excellent resource for people with short stature is the Little People of America organization, found at www.lpaonline.org.

Risk for Ineffective Self Health Management Related to Knowledge Deficit

EXPECTED OUTCOME: The patient will have requisite knowledge to be able to manage self care as evidenced by statement and demonstration of self-care activities.

Box 39.2

Cultural Considerations

Dwarfism, mostly related to a limited gene pool, often occurs among Amish communities. Ellis–van Creveld syndrome is prevalent among the Amish of Lancaster County, Pennsylvania. This syndrome is characterized by short stature and an extra digit on each hand, with some affected people having a congenital heart defect and nervous system involvement resulting in a degree of mental disability.

- Assess patient's understanding of his or her disease process and treatment. *Teaching should build on baseline knowledge.*
- Explain and demonstrate self-care measures as needed to the patient, including administration of GH injections. *The patient must understand the treatment in order to participate.*
- Help the patient explore the meaning of the disorder. *Talking about the disorder may help the nurse and patient identify needs that can be addressed.*

Evaluation. Nursing care has been effective if the patient is able to demonstrate self-administration of GH and describe plans for related self-care activities.

CRITICAL THINKING

Adoption

■ Three siblings were adopted to a loving home after having been in several foster homes. After a year in their new home, each child suddenly grew 6 to 8 inches. What do you think happened?

Suggested answers at end of chapter.

Acromegaly

Acromegaly is a rare excess of GH that affects adults, usually in their 30s or 40s. If a GH excess occurs in children, the condition results in gigantism.

PATHOPHYSIOLOGY. Acromegaly occurs as a result of oversecretion of GH in an adult. Bones increase in size, leading to enlargement of facial features, hands, and feet. Long bones grow in width but not length because the epiphyseal disks are closed. Subcutaneous connective tissue increases, causing a fleshy appearance. Internal organs and glands enlarge. Impaired tolerance of carbohydrates leads to elevated blood glucose.

ETIOLOGY. Excess secretion of growth hormone can be caused by pituitary **hyperplasia**, a benign pituitary tumor, or excess of GH-releasing hormone due to hypothalamic dysfunction. Sometimes tumors in other parts of the body secrete ectopic GH or GH-RH.

SIGNS AND SYMPTOMS. Often the first symptom noticed is a change in ring or shoe size. The nose, jaw, brow, hands, and feet enlarge (Fig. 39.2). The teeth may be displaced, causing difficulty chewing, or dentures may no longer fit. The tongue becomes thick, causing difficulty in speaking and swallowing (dysphagia). The patient may develop sleep apnea. Vertebral changes may lead to kyphosis. Visual disturbances may occur because of tumor pressure on the optic nerve. Headaches may result from tumor pressure on the brain. Diabetes mellitus may develop because GH increases blood glucose and causes an increased workload for the pancreas. (See Chapter 40.) Osteoporosis and arthritis may occur. Erectile dysfunction may occur in men and **amenorrhea** in women. With treatment, soft tissues reduce in size, but bone growth is permanent.

DIAGNOSTIC TESTS. Serum growth hormone levels are measured, and radiographs show abnormal bone growth. Growth hormone may also be measured following a large dose of oral glucose. Normally, glucose suppresses GH release. If it continues to be released even after a glucose

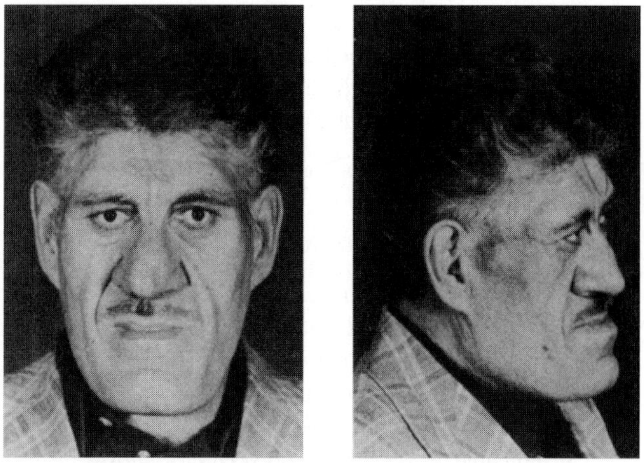

FIGURE 39.2 Patient with acromegaly. (From Martin, J. B., Reichlin, S., & Brown, G. M. [1977]. *Clinical neuroendocrinology* [p. 353]. Philadelphia: F. A. Davis, with permission.)

• WORD • BUILDING •
hyperplasia: hyper—excessive + plasia—formation or deviation

• WORD • BUILDING •
amenorrhea: a—not + men—month + orrhea—flow

load, acromegaly is suspected. A CT scan or an MRI is done to locate a pituitary tumor.

THERAPEUTIC MEASURES. Treatment is aimed at the cause. Lanreotide (Somatuline Depot) or octreotide (Sandostatin) are injectable medications that mimic the body's natural somatostatin, and will decrease GH levels. Bromocriptine (Parlodel) is a pill that can lower GH. Pegvisomant (Somavert) blocks the effect of GH on receptor sites.

Hypophysectomy or radiation may be indicated if a tumor is the cause. If the pituitary is removed, lifelong replacement of thyroid hormone, corticosteroids, and sex hormones is important to maintain homeostasis.

NURSING PROCESS FOR THE PATIENT WITH ACROMEGALY.

Data Collection. The nurse caring for the patient with acromegaly is concerned with the patient's response to the disease. Assess safety in relation to impaired eyesight, chewing, swallowing, and sleep apnea. Monitor serum glucose levels for onset of diabetes mellitus. Assess knowledge and acceptance of the disease. If hypophysectomy is planned, assess the patient for anxiety related to the surgery and perform a preoperative baseline neurological assessment.

Nursing Diagnoses, Planning, and Implementation

Disturbed Body Image Related to Changes in Appearance as Evidenced by Patient Statement of Distress

EXPECTED OUTCOME: The patient will be able to accept new body image as evidenced by expression of feelings of acceptance of self. (This may occur over a long period of time.)

- Approach patient with an attitude of acceptance and caring *to help develop trusting nurse-patient relationship.*
- Acknowledge patient's feelings of anger or depression related to body image changes. *Most changes will be permanent and may be distressing to patient.*
- Provide information about support groups. *A support group can help the patient feel less alone.*

Risk for Injury Related to Poor Eyesight, Sleep Apnea, Dysphagia

EXPECTED OUTCOME: The patient will not experience injury.

- Assess for increased risk of injury. *An accurate assessment will guide interventions.*
- Maintain safe, uncluttered environment *to prevent injury from falls related to poor eyesight.*
- Request swallowing evaluation from speech therapy if indicated. *A speech therapist can diagnose swallowing problems and make recommendations.*
- Observe for sleep apnea and discuss with physician if indicated. *Sleep apnea, if present, will require sleep studies and treatment.*

  Additional nursing diagnoses are identified if diabetes mellitus or other problems exist.

Patient Education. Teach the patient and significant others about the disease and treatment. If the patient is having a hypophysectomy, be sure he or she understands that some symptoms will be relieved but that bone growth and visual changes may not reverse. Stress the need for lifelong hormone replacement after surgery. See the section on care of the patient undergoing hypophysectomy later in this chapter.

Evaluation. The patient who is effectively treated will have some soft tissues return to normal size. The patient will be safe and free from injury. The patient should be able to accurately describe self-care requirements, and show beginning acceptance of changes.

Pituitary Tumors

Most tumors of the pituitary gland are benign adenomas. However, even benign tumors in the brain can cause many symptoms, including visual disturbances, symptoms of increased pressure in the brain, and symptoms related to hormone imbalances, as described earlier. Treatment for pituitary tumors is usually hypophysectomy (surgical removal of the pituitary gland). Radiation may also be used, either alone or as an adjunct to surgery.

Nursing Care of the Patient Undergoing Hypophysectomy

Removal of the pituitary gland is called hypophysectomy. The procedure is most often done using minimally invasive endoscopic surgery, via the nose or a small incision just under the upper lip. This allows access through the sphenoid sinus to the pituitary gland, without disturbing brain tissue. Figure 39.3 shows the transsphenoidal approach to the gland through the upper lip. Some large tumors may need removal via transfrontal craniotomy (entry through the frontal bone of the skull).

PREOPERATIVE CARE. Make sure the patient understands the physician's explanation of surgery. Perform and document

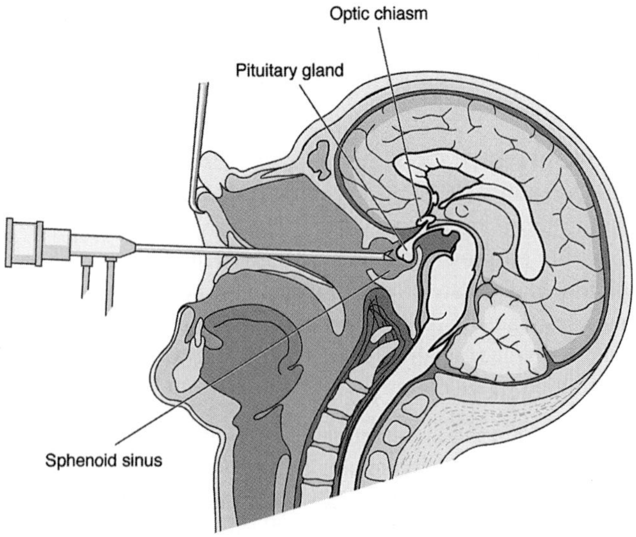
Optic chiasm
Pituitary gland
Sphenoid sinus

FIGURE 39.3 Transsphenoidal approach to pituitary gland for hypophysectomy.

a baseline neurologic assessment. Prepare the patient for what to expect following surgery. Explain that it will be important after surgery to avoid any actions that increase pressure on the surgical site, such as coughing, sneezing, nose blowing, straining to move bowels, or bending from the waist. Because coughing can raise intracranial pressure and is therefore contraindicated, instruct the patient in deep-breathing exercises or use of an incentive spirometer. Patients can usually expect to stay in the hospital about 1 day.

POSTOPERATIVE CARE. Although complications are rare, perform routine neurologic assessments to monitor the patient for neurologic damage. Also be sure to check urine for specific gravity because diabetes insipidus can occur following pituitary surgery. If a patient has had transsphenoidal surgery, he will have nasal packing and a "mustache dressing," which is placed under the nose to collect drips. These are left in place and not removed unless ordered by the physician. Monitor the dressing for signs of cerebrospinal fluid (CSF) leakage. CSF contains glucose, so glucose testing strips can be used to determine if drainage is actually CSF or just nasal discharge. Remind the patient to avoid any actions that increase pressure on the surgical site. The patient is placed on hormone replacement therapy following hypophysectomy. Pituitary hormones are difficult to replace, so target hormones are generally given. These may include thyroid hormone, glucocorticoids, intranasal desmopressin, and sex hormones.

PATIENT EDUCATION. Instruct the patient prior to discharge according to agency guidelines. These usually include instructions to prevent increased pressure on the surgical site, as well as instructions on how to administer the hormones and side effects to report. Give the patient these instructions:

- Expect a small amount of bloody or mucous drainage from your nose.
- If you must blow your nose, do so very gently. Blowing can injure the surgical site and cause bleeding or spinal fluid leakage.
- Take stool softeners as needed to prevent straining for bowel movements.
- Take antitussives as directed to prevent coughing.
- If an upper lip incision was used, wait until the incision line is healed to brush teeth with a toothbrush. Floss and mouth rinses can be used instead.
- Take all medications as prescribed. You will be on hormone therapy to replace the hormones made by your pituitary gland.
- Call immediately if you develop a fever; if you have more than a small amount of blood drainage from the incision site; if you have clear drainage; if you feel very thirsty or urinate more than usual (a sign of diabetes insipidus); or any other symptoms that concern you.

DISORDERS OF THE THYROID GLAND

Triiodothyronine (T_3) and thyroxine (T_4) are thyroid hormones secreted by the thyroid gland. These hormones may be collectively referred to as thyroid hormone (TH). Deficient secretion of TH results in hypothyroidism; excess TH results in hyperthyroidism. For more information on disorders of the thyroid gland, visit the American Thyroid Association at www.thyroid.org.

Hypothyroidism

Hypothyroidism occurs primarily in women over 50 years old. If hypothyroidism occurs in an infant, severe problems with growth and development occur. This is why all babies born in the United States are tested for hypothyroidism at birth.

Pathophysiology

Primary hypothyroidism occurs when the thyroid gland fails to produce enough TH even though enough thyroid-stimulating hormone (TSH) is being secreted by the pituitary gland. The pituitary responds to the low level of TH by producing more TSH. Secondary hypothyroidism is caused by low levels of TSH, which fail to stimulate release of TH. Tertiary hypothyroidism results from inadequate release of thyrotropin-releasing hormone (TRH), secreted by the hypothalamus. Most cases of hypothyroidism are primary (Table 39.3).

Because thyroid hormones are responsible for metabolism, low levels of these hormones result in a slowed metabolic rate, which causes many of the characteristic symptoms of hypothyroidism. Other symptoms are related to **myxedema**, which refers to a nonpitting type of edema that occurs in connective tissues throughout the body.

Etiology

Primary hypothyroidism may be a result of a congenital defect, inflammation of the thyroid gland, or iodine deficiency. Hashimoto's thyroiditis is an autoimmune disorder that eventually destroys thyroid tissue, leading to hypothyroidism. Secondary or tertiary hypothyroidism may be caused by a pituitary or hypothalamic lesion or by postpartum pituitary

TABLE 39.3 THYROID HORMONE ABNORMALITIES

	Hyperthyroidism	Hypothyroidism
Primary	↑ TH ↓ TSH	↓ TH ↑ TSH
Secondary (pituitary cause)	↑ TH ↑ TSH	↓ TH ↓ TSH

• WORD • BUILDING •
myxedema: myx—mucus + edema—swelling

necrosis, a rare disorder in which the pituitary is destroyed following pregnancy and delivery. Treatment of hyperthyroidism, whether with medication or thyroidectomy, can lead to secondary hypothyroidism. Peripheral resistance to TH may also occur.

Signs and Symptoms

Manifestations are related to the reduced metabolic rate and include fatigue, weight gain, bradycardia, constipation, mental dullness, feeling cold, shortness of breath, decreased sweating, and dry skin and hair (Box 39.3, *Patient Perspective,* and Table 39.4). Heart failure may occur because of decreased pumping strength of the heart. Altered fat metabolism causes hyperlipidemia, which can lead to cardiovascular disease. In advanced disease, myxedema develops.

Complications

If the metabolic rate drops so low that it becomes life threatening, the result is myxedema coma. This usually occurs in patients with long-standing, untreated hypothyroidism and can be triggered by stress, such as infection, trauma, or exposure to cold. The patient becomes hypothermic, with a temperature less than 95°F (35°C) and a decreased respiratory rate. Depressed mental function and lethargy may occur. Blood glucose drops. Cardiac output drops, which in turn can reduce perfusion of kidneys. Nonpitting edema of the face, hands, and feet may develop. Death can occur as a result of respiratory failure. If you note changes in mental status or vital signs, the physician should be contacted immediately. Treatment of myxedema coma involves intubation and mechanical ventilation. The patient is slowly rewarmed with blankets. Intravenous levothyroxine (Synthroid) is given, and any underlying cause is treated.

Diagnostic Tests

The levels of T_3 and T_4 are low, and the level of TSH may be high or low, depending on the cause. If the pituitary is functioning normally, TSH is elevated in an attempt to stimulate an increase in TH. Serum cholesterol and triglycerides are elevated. Antibodies are usually present in autoimmune disease.

Therapeutic Measures

Primary hypothyroidism is easily treated with oral thyroid replacement hormone. Most patients now take synthetic thyroid hormone (levothyroxine [Synthroid]). Doses are started low and are slowly increased to prevent symptoms of hyperthyroidism or cardiac complications.

Nursing Process for the Patient with Hypothyroidism

See the *Nursing Care Plan for the Patient with Hypothyroidism.*

Box 39.3

Patient Perspective

Mary

When I turned 40-something, I began to notice a few changes in my body. I seemed to be easily fatigued, but I attributed that to moving our family across country and all the adjustments that needed to be made. I also noticed weight gain, most notably around my waist. Again, I thought, "Well, I *am* 40-something," but it seemed no matter how much I exercised and watched what I ate, I couldn't lose weight. Worse, I was gaining! One day a friend of mine pointed out that I always seemed tired. Each time she called to do something, my reply was always the same, "I'd love to, but not today. I'm just so tired."

Things started to get worse; I began losing hair by the handfuls each time I shampooed. It was so bad that every time I went to my hair stylist she had to reassure me that I wasn't going bald. However, my hair just didn't seem as full as it once did. I began to notice dry skin (I thought it was just our hard water) and constipation (I thought I had irritable bowel syndrome). Finally, I went to the doctor for a physical, including laboratory test, which included a TSH and free T_4. The diagnosis came back: I had hypothyroidism and was started on Synthroid. I noticed the effect on my energy almost immediately. Now I am able to exercise effectively. I have lost nearly all the weight I gained and my husband no longer complains about having to clean out the drain in our shower every time I wash my hair. I am thankful for the diagnosis and treatment because I feel like myself again.

TABLE 39.4 SYMPTOMS OF THYROID DISORDERS

	Hypothyroidism	Hyperthyroidism
Cardiovascular	Bradycardia, decreased cardiac output, cool skin, cold intolerance	Tachycardia, palpitations, increased cardiac output, warm skin, heat intolerance
Neurologic	Lethargy, slowed movements, memory loss, confusion	Fatigue, restlessness, hyperactive reflexes, tremor, insomnia, emotional instability
Pulmonary	Dyspnea, hypoventilation	Dyspnea
Integumentary	Cool, dry skin; brittle, dry hair	Diaphoresis; warm, moist skin; fine, soft hair
Gastrointestinal	Decreased appetite, weight gain, constipation, increased serum lipid levels	Increased appetite, weight loss, frequent stools, decreased serum lipid levels
Reproductive	Decreased libido, erectile dysfunction	Decreased libido, erectile dysfunction, amenorrhea

NURSING CARE PLAN for the Patient with Hypothyroidism

Nursing Diagnosis: *Activity Intolerance* related to fatigue as evidenced by inability to carry out daily activities

Expected Outcomes: The patient will be able to tolerate activity as evidenced by (1) reports of lessening fatigue after treatment initiated and (2) the ability to carry out usual activities of daily living (ADLs).

Evaluation of Outcomes: (1) Does patient report lessening fatigue? (2) Is patient able to carry out ADLs?

Interventions	Rationale	Evaluation
Assess level of fatigue.	Assessment guides nursing care.	What is patient's fatigue level?
Assist patient with self-care activities.	Patients with fatigue may have difficulty carrying out activities independently.	Are patient's self-care needs being met? Is assistance needed?
Allow for rest between activities.	Rest periods will enable patient to conserve energy for activities.	Does patient state rest is adequate?
Slowly increase patient's activities as medication begins to be effective.	As thyroid replacement therapy becomes effective, patient's fatigue will subside.	Does patient tolerate increases in activity?
	GERIATRIC	
When getting elderly patients up, watch for orthostatic hypotension.	Orthostatic hypotension is common in elderly and may cause falls.	Does patient's blood pressure drop when changing positions?

Nursing Diagnosis: *Constipation* related to slowed gastrointestinal motility as evidenced by passage of hard, dry stools

Expected Outcomes: Constipation will be resolved as evidenced by soft, formed stool passed at patient's pre-illness frequency.

Evaluation of Outcomes: Are bowels moving according to patient's pre-illness pattern?

Interventions	Rationale	Evaluation
Monitor and record bowel movements.	A record helps determine if a problem exists.	Does record show a problem?
Help patient follow usual pre-illness pattern (e.g., after morning coffee).	A schedule allows bowel movement to occur before stool becomes hard and dry.	Is patient able to identify and implement usual self-care for bowels?
Increase fluids to eight 8-ounce glasses of water daily if cardiovascular status is stable.	Adequate fluid intake helps prevent hard, dry stools.	Does patient take adequate fluids?
Add fiber to diet: fresh fruit, vegetables, bran.	Fiber helps increase the number of bowel movements.	Does patient tolerate fiber? Is it effective?
Encourage regular ambulation.	Activity increases peristalsis.	Is patient able to ambulate or engage in other activity?
Use bedside commode or bathroom rather than bedpan.	The sitting position aids in evacuation.	Is sitting position effective?
Obtain physician order for stool softener if needed.	Soft stools are passed more easily.	Is stool softener needed? Effective?
If stool is impacted, break up stool digitally and gently remove.	Breaking up stool eases evacuation.	Is stool impacted? Is digital disimpaction effective?
Avoid use of enemas.	Enemas can cause fluid and electrolyte imbalances and can damage mucosa.	Does patient understand need to avoid enemas?

NURSING CARE PLAN for the Patient with Hypothyroidism—cont'd

Nursing Diagnosis: *Risk for Impaired Skin Integrity* related to dry skin, inactivity

Expected Outcomes: The patient's skin will remain intact as evidenced by soft moist skin without lesions

Evaluation of Outcomes: Is skin soft, moist, and intact?

Interventions	Rationale	Evaluation
Assess skin daily for breakdown and risk for breakdown.	Skin lesions are more effectively treated when identified early.	Is breakdown present? Is patient at risk?
Avoid use of soap on dry areas. Try bath oil.	Soap is drying to skin.	Does use of bath oil help?
Use nondrying lotion following bath.	Lotion helps trap moisture in skin. Some lotions contain alcohol, however, which is drying.	Does patient state relief with use of lotion?
Encourage/assist with position changes at least every 2 hours.	Changing position enhances circulation to the skin, promoting healing and preventing breakdown.	Does patient change position at least every 2 hours? Are pressure areas prevented?

Nursing Diagnosis: *Imbalanced Nutrition: More Than Body Requirements* related to decreased metabolic rate, as evidenced by weight gain

Expected Outcomes: (1) Nutrition will be balanced as evidenced by return to patient's pre-illness weight. (2) The patient will verbalize understanding of dietary recommendations.

Evaluation of Outcomes: (1) Is patient approaching pre-illness weight? (2) Is patient able to explain dietary recommendations and how they will be implemented?

Interventions	Rationale	Evaluation
Weigh weekly and record.	Weekly weights record progress without the frustration of daily fluctuations.	Is patient losing or maintaining weight?
Consult dietitian for therapeutic diet until hypothyroidism is controlled.	The dietitian can provide food choices for gradual weight loss if necessary.	Does patient verbalize understanding of and ability to follow diet?
Encourage regular exercise within limits of fatigue.	Exercise promotes weight control.	Does patient verbalize understanding of and ability to follow exercise plan?
Counsel patient that weight should normalize once hypothyroidism is controlled.	Thyroid replacement hormone increases the metabolic rate, allowing return to normal weight.	Does patient verbalize understanding of instruction?
	GERIATRIC	
Allow patient to help determine acceptable diet modifications.	Older patients may have long-standing dietary habits that are hard to change.	Is patient satisfied with weight loss plan?

Patient Education

Instruct the patient in the importance of consistent use of thyroid replacement medication and regular blood tests to monitor TSH. The patient needs to be aware that too much thyroid hormone will cause symptoms of hyperthyroidism. Such symptoms should be reported to the physician immediately. In addition, if the patient is experiencing mental status changes, discuss the need to avoid driving or operating machinery until symptoms are resolved.

> **CRITICAL THINKING**
>
> ***Mrs. Maino***
>
> ■ Mrs. Maino is a 59-year-old woman who is tired all the time and has gained 16 pounds during the past year. Laboratory results show low T_3 and T_4 and elevated TSH levels. Her physician prescribes levothyroxine PO.
>
> 1. Why is Mrs. Maino's TSH elevated?
> 2. What will happen to Mrs. Maino's caloric requirements as she begins treatment? Why?
> 3. Why should you teach Mrs. Maino to check her pulse?
>
> *Suggested answers at end of chapter.*

Hyperthyroidism

Hyperthyroidism is most often diagnosed in young women. Graves' disease, which is one cause of hyperthyroidism, is more common in young women. Multinodular goiter is more common in older women.

Pathophysiology

Hyperthyroidism results in excessive amounts of circulating thyroid hormone (thyrotoxicosis). Primary hyperthyroidism occurs when a problem within the thyroid gland causes excess hormone release. Secondary hyperthyroidism occurs because of excess TSH release from the pituitary, causing overstimulation of the thyroid gland; tertiary hyperthyroidism is caused by excess TRH from the hypothalamus. A high level of thyroid hormone increases the metabolic rate. It also increases the number of beta-adrenergic receptor sites in the body, which enhances the activity of norepinephrine. The resulting fight-or-flight response is the cause of many of the symptoms of hyperthyroidism.

Etiology

A variety of disorders can cause hyperthyroidism. Graves' disease is the most common cause; it is an autoimmune disorder in which thyroid-stimulating antibodies cause the thyroid gland to make too much thyroid hormone.

Other causes include thyroid nodules that secrete excess thyroid hormone (multinodular goiter and toxic adenoma), inflammation of the thyroid (thyroiditis), or a thyroid tumor. A pituitary tumor can secrete excess TSH, which overstimulates the thyroid gland. Patients taking thyroid hormone for hypothyroidism may take too much. Each of these problems can cause excess circulating TH and symptoms of hyperthyroidism.

Radiation exposure may predispose a patient to develop hyperthyroidism. Heredity may also play a role in autoimmune hyperthyroidism. Women who smoke nearly double their risk of Graves' disease.

Signs and Symptoms

Many signs and symptoms are related to the hypermetabolic state, such as heat intolerance, increased appetite with weight loss, and increased frequency of bowel movements. Nervousness, tremor, tachycardia, and palpitations are caused by the increase in sympathetic nervous system activity and may be more common in younger patients. Heart failure can occur because of tachycardia and the resulting inefficient pumping of the heart. See additional signs and symptoms in Table 39.4. If treatment is not begun, the patient may become manic or psychotic. Additional signs that occur only with Graves' disease include thickening of the skin on the anterior legs and exophthalmos (bulging of the eyes; Fig. 39.4) caused by swelling of the tissues behind the eyes. Other eye changes include photophobia and blurred or double vision.

Elderly patients may not have the typical signs and symptoms of hyperthyroidism, so be especially alert for this. These patients may present with heart failure, atrial fibrillation, fatigue, apathy, and depression.

Complications

THYROTOXIC CRISIS. Thyrotoxic crisis (sometimes called thyroid storm) is a severe hyperthyroid state that can occur in hyperthyroid people who are untreated or who develop another illness or stressor. It also may occur after thyroid surgery in patients who have been inadequately prepared with antithyroid medication. Thyrotoxic crisis can result in death in as little as 2 hours if untreated. Symptoms include

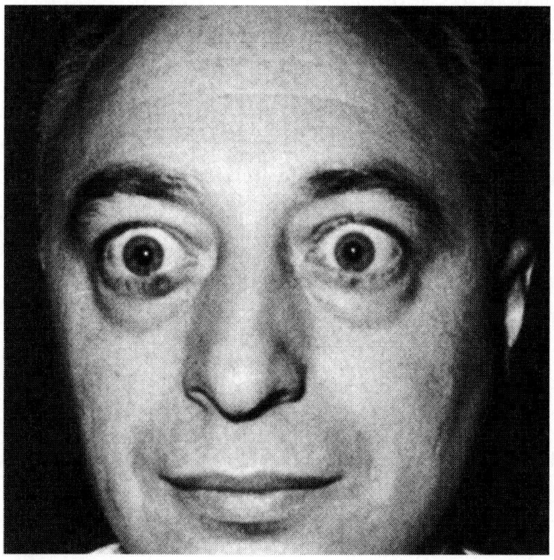

FIGURE 39.4 Exophthalmos caused by Graves' disease. (From Tamparo, C. D., & Lewis, M. A. [2005]. *Diseases of the human body* [4th ed., p. 339]. Philadelphia: F. A. Davis, with permission.)

tachycardia, high fever, hypertension (with eventual heart failure and hypotension), dehydration, restlessness, and delirium or coma.

If thyrotoxic crisis occurs, treatment is first directed toward relieving the life-threatening symptoms. Acetaminophen is given for the fever. Aspirin is avoided because it binds with the same serum protein as T_4, freeing additional T_4 into the circulation. Intravenous fluids and a cooling blanket may be ordered to cool the patient. A beta-adrenergic blocker, such as propranolol, is given for tachycardia and symptom control. Oxygen is administered and the head of the bed is elevated because the high metabolic rate requires more oxygen. Once symptoms are controlled and the patient is safe, the underlying thyroid problem is treated.

HYPOTHYROIDISM. Another complication of hyperthyroidism can be hypothyroidism. This can occur as a result of long-term disease or as a result of treatment. Patients with a history of hyperthyroidism should be monitored for recurrent hyperthyroidism or the onset of hypothyroidism.

Diagnostic Tests

Serum levels of T_3 and T_4 are elevated. TSH is low in primary hyperthyroidism or high if the cause is pituitary. A radioactive iodine uptake test or a thyroid scan can be done to determine hyperactivity of the gland or to locate a nodule or tumor. The thyroid gland may be enlarged; palpation of the thyroid in a patient suspected to be hyperthyroid should only be performed by a physician. TSI (thyroid-stimulating immunoglobulin) is present in Graves' disease.

Therapeutic Measures

Several medications can be used to treat hyperthyroidism. Propylthiouracil (PTU) and methimazole (Tapazole) inhibit the synthesis of TH, but they may take several months to be effective, and must be continued for 12 to 18 months. Propranolol (Inderal) is a beta-blocking medication that relieves the sympathetic nervous system symptoms. High doses of oral iodine suppress the release of thyroid hormone.

Radioactive iodine (^{131}I or RAI) may be used to destroy a portion of the thyroid gland. The patient takes one oral dose of RAI. Dietary iodine normally goes to the thyroid gland, where it is used to make thyroid hormone. When RAI is given, the radioactivity destroys some of the cells that make thyroid hormone.

Sometimes medications alone control hyperthyroidism. If this does not occur, surgery is planned. If surgery is the treatment chosen, antithyroid medications are given to calm the thyroid before surgery. They help slow the heart rate and reduce other symptoms, making surgery safer. Iodine also reduces the vascularity of the thyroid gland, decreasing the risk of bleeding during surgery. Adequate preparation of the patient is important because a **euthyroid** state helps prevent a postoperative thyrotoxic crisis.

Thyroidectomy can be done with a traditional, open approach, or with newer minimally invasive techniques that use a combination of a tiny incision and an endoscope. Patients can usually go home the same day, and have a faster recovery time with minimally invasive surgery. The surgeon may choose to leave some of the thyroid gland intact, to continue to secrete some hormone. Following surgery, the patient will likely be hypothyroid and will require thyroid replacement hormone (levothyroxine [Synthroid]). Nursing care of the patient undergoing a thyroidectomy is discussed later in this chapter.

If vision is impaired from exophthalmos, surgical orbital decompression can be done. Current endoscopic techniques have made this a safer option than in the past.

• WORD • BUILDING •

euthyroid: eu—normal, healthy + thyroid

Nursing Process for the Patient with Hyperthyroidism

DATA COLLECTION. Monitor the patient with hyperthyroidism closely until normal thyroid activity is restored. Monitor vital signs and report any increases in pulse or blood pressure to the registered nurse or physician. Monitor lung sounds because crackles can indicate heart failure. Assess level of anxiety and ability to cope with symptoms. Monitor weight, bowel function, and ability to sleep. Assess eyes for risk for injury caused by exophthalmos, and note degree of muscle weakness. Never palpate the thyroid gland of a patient with hyperthyroidism because palpation can stimulate release of thyroid hormone and precipitate a thyrotoxic crisis.

NURSING DIAGNOSES, PLANNING, AND IMPLEMENTATION

Hyperthermia Related to Hypermetabolic State as Evidenced by Elevated Temperature

EXPECTED OUTCOME: The patient's body temperature will be within normal limits.

- Monitor temperature. *Temperature may be elevated due to hypermetabolic state.*
- Administer acetaminophen as ordered (avoid aspirin) to reduce temperature. *Aspirin can cause an increase in circulating thyroid hormone.*
- Apply cooling blanket as ordered. *External cooling may be needed if acetaminophen is not effective.*
- If a cooling blanket is needed, set it to 1 to 2 degrees below the current temperature, and wrap the extremities with towels to prevent shivering, *which can further increase temperature.*
- Offer fluids *to replace fluids lost through diaphoresis.*

Diarrhea Related to an Increase in Peristalsis as Evidenced by Frequent Loose Stools

EXPECTED OUTCOME: The patient will maintain fluid and electrolyte balance.

- Provide a low-fiber diet. *Fiber can increase peristalsis and stools.*
- Provide small, frequent meals of bland foods (bananas, rice, applesauce) *that are less likely to worsen diarrhea.*

- Monitor electrolytes, especially sodium and potassium. *Diarrhea can cause electrolyte loss.*
- Monitor for dehydration. *Diarrhea causes fluid loss.*
- Keep skin clean and dry; apply barrier cream to protect *skin from injury from stool.*

Imbalanced Nutrition: Less Than Body Requirements Related to Increased Metabolism

EXPECTED OUTCOME: The patient will have balanced nutrition as evidenced by stable weight in proportion to height.

- Determine healthy weight for height, *so the expected outcome is realistic for the patient.*
- Monitor weight weekly *to make sure interventions are working.*
- Consult dietician for high-calorie diet with six meals per day *to meet caloric requirements.*

Disturbed Sleep Pattern Related to Sympathetic Stimulation as Evidenced by Difficulty Sleeping and not Feeling Rested on Awakening

EXPECTED OUTCOME: The patient will have improved sleep as evidenced by stating feeling rested upon awakening.

- Provide a quiet, restful environment *to assist the patient to fall asleep.*
- Ask the patient if music or earplugs are desired *to mask environmental noise.*
- Administer propranolol or sedative as ordered *to reduce sympathetic stimulation and calm patient.*

Anxiety Related to Sympathetic Stimulation as Evidenced by Patient Statement

EXPECTED OUTCOME: The patient will experience reduced anxiety as evidenced by patient statement that anxiety is controlled.

- Provide the patient with accurate information about the disorder and treatment, and explain that proper treatment will correct symptoms. *Fear of the unknown can produce anxiety.*
- Administer propranolol or antianxiety agent as ordered *to reduce sympathetic stimulation and calm patient.*
- Offer massage, music, or other relaxation techniques preferred by the patient. *These may promote relaxation.*

Risk for Injury Related to Hypermetabolic State and Eye Involvement

EXPECTED OUTCOME: The patient will remain safe and without injury.

- Report changes in vital signs to RN or physician. *Prompt treatment can reduce complications.*
- Administer lubricating saline eyedrops as ordered to *protect eyes from drying.*
- Advise use of dark, tight-fitting glasses *to protect eyes from light and injury.*
- Gently tape eyes shut with nonallergic tape for sleeping. *Exophthalmos may prevent the patient from fully closing the eyes.*
- Elevate the head of the bed *to reduce edema behind the eyes.*
- Provide a low-sodium diet. *This may decrease edema behind the eyes.*
- Teach patient to notify the physician immediately if eye pain or vision changes occur. *These can be signs of pressure from edema on optic nerve, which can cause permanent damage if not corrected.*

PATIENT EDUCATION. Teach the patient about the disease and symptoms of hyperthyroidism or hypothyroidism to report. Also teach the patient how to take medications and the importance of routine follow-up laboratory testing.

EVALUATION. If the plan of care is effective, the patient will remain free from complications or injury. Eyes will be comfortable and free from injury. Body temperature will be kept within normal limits. Diarrhea will be controlled, and complications of diarrhea such as skin breakdown and dehydration avoided. The patient's weight should remain stable. The patient should report that he or she is rested on awakening and that anxiety is controlled.

Nursing Care of the Patient Receiving Radioactive Iodine

If radioactive iodine is used, it is usually given orally in one dose. If the dose is high, such as for the patient with thyroid cancer, the patient is hospitalized. Patients receiving lower doses may be treated as outpatients. You should limit time spent with the patient and maintain a safe distance when providing direct care (see Chapter 11). Pregnant caregivers should avoid caring for patients receiving radioactive iodine. Urine, vomitus, and other body secretions are contaminated and should be disposed of according to hospital policy. Flush the toilet twice following disposal of contaminated material. The radiation safety officer and hospital policy should be consulted for specific precautions.

At home, the patient is instructed to avoid close contact with family members for about a week and to use careful hand washing after urinating. Oral contact with others should be avoided, and eating utensils should be washed thoroughly with soap and water. Hospital teaching protocols should be used for specific patient teaching. If the treatment is being administered for hyperthyroidism, inform the patient that symptoms will subside in about 6 to 8 weeks.

Side effects are rare, and may include a sore throat, dry mouth or eyes, and nausea. Sore throat is easily treated with acetaminophen, and nausea can be reduced by taking the dose on an empty stomach. Dry eyes can be relieved with moisturizing eye drops. Encourage the patient to drink plenty of fluids to help remove the RAI from the body. In addition, the patient should be aware of symptoms of hypothyroidism to be reported because hypothyroidism can occur up to 15 years after the treatment.

Goiter

Pathophysiology and Etiology

Enlargement of the thyroid gland is called a goiter. The thyroid gland may enlarge in response to increased TSH levels, or sometimes in response to the autoimmune process that occurs in Graves' disease. TSH is elevated in response to low TH, iodine deficiency, pregnancy, or viral, genetic, or other conditions. When a goiter is caused by iodine deficiency or other environmental factors, it is called an endemic goiter.

Some foods and medications are **goitrogens**. These substances interfere with the body's use of iodine and include such foods as turnips, cabbage, broccoli, horseradish, cauliflower, and carrots (Box 39.4, *Nutrition Notes*). Some **goitrogenic** medications include propylthiouracil, sulfonamides, lithium, and salicylates (aspirin).

A goiter may be associated with a hyperthyroid, hypothyroid, or euthyroid state. Goiter that occurs with hyperthyroidism is sometimes called a toxic goiter. Once the cause of the goiter is removed, the gland usually returns to normal size.

Signs and Symptoms

The thyroid gland is enlarged, and swelling may be apparent at the base of the neck (Fig. 39.5). Alternatively, the gland may enlarge posteriorly, which can interfere with swallowing or breathing. The patient may have a full sensation in the neck. Symptoms of hypothyroidism or hyperthyroidism may be present.

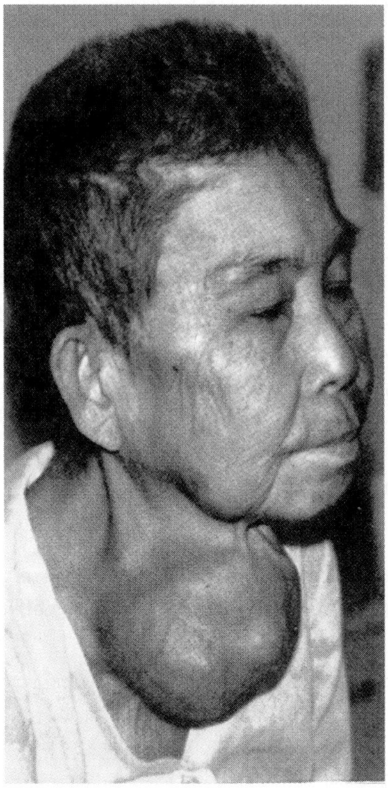

FIGURE 39.5 Patient with unusually large goiter.

Box 39.4

Nutrition Notes

Iodine Deficiency

Inland areas of all continents have iodine-poor soils. People in developing countries with only local food sources are still subject to endemic goiter; however, addition of iodine to table salt has significantly reduced the occurrence of endemic goiter in developed countries.

Vegetables in the cabbage family contain goitrogens, substances that block the body's absorption or utilization of iodine, but the risk is small. At higher risk of iodine deficiency are strict vegetarians who consume sea salt, which contains virtually no iodine, rather than iodized salt.

Iodine Excess

Saltwater fish, shellfish, and seaweed are naturally high in iodine so that iodine toxicity from seaweed has occurred in Japan. Excessive iodine can be manifested as either hyperthyroidism or hypothyroidism, sometimes producing "iodine goiter."

• WORD • BUILDING •

goitrogenic: goitro—goiter + genic—producing

Diagnostic Tests

Serum TSH, T_3, and T_4 levels are measured to determine thyroid function. Ultrasound or a thyroid scan may be done to determine the cause or evaluate the size of the gland.

Therapeutic Measures

Treatment is aimed at the cause. If goitrogens are suspected, the patient is given a list of foods to be avoided. If iodine deficiency is a problem, it is added to the diet with supplements or iodized salt. Hypothyroidism or hyperthyroidism is treated if indicated. Levothyroxine (Synthroid) may be given to reduce TSH levels via negative feedback. Radioactive iodine therapy or thyroidectomy may be needed to treat hyperthyroid symptoms or if the enlarged gland is interfering with breathing or swallowing.

Nursing Care

Be careful to assess the effect of the goiter on breathing and swallowing. Stridor, a whistling sound, may be heard if the airway is obstructed. Stridor is an ominous sign and should be reported to the physician immediately. If the patient experiences difficulty swallowing, notify the physician and collaborate with the dietitian to provide soft foods that are easy to swallow. A swallowing study might be ordered, which can assist a speech pathologist or other expert to make specific recommendations for safe swallowing.

Cancer of the Thyroid Gland

Although thyroid cancer is rare, it is the most common cancer of the endocrine system. Women are affected more often than

Box 39.5

Cultural Considerations

Because of the Chernobyl nuclear disaster in Russia in 1986, Russian immigrants are at exceptionally high risk for developing pituitary, thyroid, and parathyroid disorders and cancers. The proximity of Estonia, Latvia, Lithuania, Poland, and other Eastern European countries to Russia places immigrants and long-term visitors from these countries at risk as well. The nurse needs to be alert for endocrine disorders among these populations and assist patients to arrange genetic counseling for those who desire it.

men. Most tumors of the thyroid gland are not malignant. See Chapter 11 for cancer pathophysiology.

Etiology

Thyroid hyperplasia may lead to thyroid cancer. Other causes include exposure to radiation (Box 39.5, *Cultural Considerations*), iodine deficiency, and prolonged exposure to goitrogens. The tendency to develop some forms of thyroid cancer is inherited.

Signs and Symptoms

A hard, painless nodule may be palpable on the thyroid gland. Difficulty breathing or swallowing, persistent cough, or changes in the voice may occur if the tumor is near the esophagus and trachea. Most patients with cancer of the thyroid have normal TH levels.

Diagnostic Tests

A thyroid scan shows a "cold" nodule. This is because malignant tumors of the thyroid do not take up the radioactive iodine administered for the scan. A "hot" nodule indicates a benign tumor. A fine-needle aspiration biopsy confirms the diagnosis.

Therapeutic Measures

A partial or total thyroidectomy may be done. Chemotherapy, radioactive iodine therapy, or external beam radiation may also be used, alone or following surgery.

Nursing Care

Nursing care is determined by the symptoms the patient is experiencing. See Chapter 11 for care of the patient with cancer.

Nursing Process for the Patient Undergoing Thyroidectomy

Patients may undergo thyroidectomy for cancer of the thyroid, hyperthyroidism, or a goiter that is causing dyspnea or dysphagia. See Chapter 12 for general care of a patient having surgery.

A total thyroidectomy is usually performed if cancer is present. After a total thyroidectomy, lifelong replacement hormone must be taken. A subtotal (partial) thyroidectomy may be done for hyperthyroidism, leaving a portion of the thyroid gland to secrete TH.

Preoperative Care

Before undergoing a thyroidectomy, the patient should be in a euthyroid state. This is accomplished with the use of antithyroid medication. A saturated solution of potassium iodide (SSKI) may also be administered to decrease the size and vascularity of the gland, reducing the risk of bleeding during surgery.

Do a baseline assessment of vital signs and voice quality, so you can compare findings postoperatively. Explain what the patient can expect before, during, and after surgery and clarify misconceptions. Preoperative teaching should include how to perform gentle range-of-motion exercises of the neck, how to support the neck during position changes, and how to use an incentive spirometer after surgery. See Chapter 12 for routine preoperative care.

Postoperative Care

DATA COLLECTION. Monitor vital signs, oxygen saturation, drain (if present), and dressing every 15 minutes initially, progressing to every 4 hours, as ordered. Decreased blood pressure with increased pulse should alert you to the possibility of shock related to blood loss. Tachycardia and fever, along with mental status changes, may indicate thyrotoxic crisis. Check the back of the neck for pooling of blood. Because of the location of the surgery, observe for signs of respiratory distress, including an increase in respiratory rate, dyspnea, or stridor. Ask the patient to speak to detect hoarseness of the voice, which may indicate trauma to the recurrent laryngeal nerve. Monitor the patient's serum calcium levels and watch for evidence of tetany (discussed later in this chapter). Report abnormal findings to the RN or physician immediately.

NURSING DIAGNOSES, PLANNING, AND IMPLEMENTATION

Risk for Ineffective Airway Clearance Due to Edema at Surgical Site

EXPECTED OUTCOME: The patient will maintain a clear airway as evidenced by easy breathing without stridor.

- Notify physician about respiratory distress immediately; keep a tracheostomy set at the bedside.
  Although not common, a tracheostomy may be needed in an emergency if edema obstructs the airway.

- Maintain patient in semi-Fowler's position *to help reduce edema and promote comfort.*
- Monitor neck dressing. *If the dressing seems to get tighter, it may be a sign that the patient's neck is swelling, which could impair the airway.*
- Use room humidifier or humidified oxygen *to keep airways and secretions moist.*
- Remind the patient to do coughing and deep-breathing exercises every hour. *This keeps the airway clear of secretions.*
- Have suction equipment available *in case patient is unable to cough up secretions effectively.*
- Encourage the patient to use the incentive spirometer *to assist with deep breathing.*
- Assess the patient's swallowing and gag reflexes before offering clear liquids *to guard against aspiration.*

Risk for Injury (Tetany, Thyrotoxic Crisis) Related to Surgical Procedure

EXPECTED OUTCOME: Complications will be recognized and treated quickly.

- Monitor patient for muscle spasms or numbness or tingling around the mouth, and report immediately if they occur. *These are symptoms of tetany that must be treated immediately. Tetany is most likely to occur 24 to 72 hours postoperatively.*
- Monitor vital signs often, and report changes immediately. *Elevated vital signs may be signs of thyrotoxic crisis, which is most likely to occur up to 18 hours postoperatively.*

Acute Pain Related to Surgical Procedure as Evidenced by Patient Pain Rating

EXPECTED OUTCOME: The patient's pain will be controlled as evidenced by patient stating pain rating is acceptable.

- Administer acetaminophen or opioids as ordered. Avoid aspirin products. *Aspirin binds to the same protein as thyroid hormone and can precipitate a thyrotoxic crisis.*
- Use pillows or sandbags to support the patient's head. *Unexpected movement may be painful.*

Risk for Ineffective Self Health Management Related to Knowledge Deficit

EXPECTED OUTCOME: The patient will be able to effectively manage self care needs as evidenced by (1) verbalizing understanding of follow-up care, (2) weight stabilizes at appropriate weight for height, and (3) thyroid hormone levels are within normal limits.

- Teach the patient to do gentle range-of-motion exercises, avoiding hyperextension of the neck, which can cause strain on the incision line. *Avoidance of neck movement due to pain can result in contracture.*
- Consult dietitian to assist the patient with potential dietary changes needed following surgery. *With correction of metabolic alterations, dietary needs may be significantly altered.*
- Teach the patient the importance of follow-up care *to avoid complications:*
  - How to administer replacement hormone if indicated.
  - How to change the dressing and to report bleeding or signs of infection at the site.
  - Importance of immediately reporting unusual irritability, fever, or palpitations.
  - Importance of follow-up lab work for thyroid function and medication adjustment.

EVALUATION. If the plan has been effective, complications caused by surgery will not occur or will be recognized and reported early. Pain will be prevented or controlled, and the patient will demonstrate understanding of dietary modifications and postoperative self-care.

Complications

THYROTOXIC CRISIS. Thyrotoxic crisis can result from manipulation of the thyroid gland during surgery, with the subsequent release of large amounts of thyroid hormone. This is a rare complication because the use of antithyroid drugs before surgery has become routine. For more information on thyrotoxic crisis, see the section on hyperthyroidism earlier in this chapter.

TETANY. Tetany is caused by low calcium levels and is characterized by tingling in the fingers and perioral area (around the mouth), muscle spasms, twitching, and cardiac dysrhythmias. Muscle spasms in the larynx can lead to respiratory obstruction. Watch carefully for symptoms of tetany and report them immediately if they occur because if the problem is not recognized quickly, death can result.

Tetany can occur if the parathyroid glands are accidentally removed during thyroid surgery. Because of the proximity of the parathyroid glands to the thyroid, it is sometimes difficult for the surgeon to avoid them. In the absence of parathyroid hormone, serum calcium levels drop and tetany results. Intravenous calcium gluconate is given to treat acute tetany.

DISORDERS OF THE PARATHYROID GLANDS

Recall that the parathyroid glands secrete parathyroid hormone (PTH) in response to low serum calcium levels. PTH raises serum calcium levels by promoting calcium movement from bones to blood, by increasing absorption of dietary calcium, and by increasing resorption of calcium by the kidneys. Decreased PTH activity is called hypoparathyroidism. Increased PTH activity is called hyperparathyroidism.

Hypoparathyroidism

Pathophysiology

A decrease in PTH causes a decrease in bone resorption of calcium, a decrease in calcium absorption by the GI tract, and decreased resorption in the kidneys. This means that calcium stays in the bones instead of being moved into the blood, and more calcium is excreted from the body. The result is a decreased serum calcium level, called hypocalcemia. As calcium levels fall, phosphate levels rise.

Etiology

The most common causes of hypoparathyroidism are heredity and the accidental removal of the parathyroid glands during thyroidectomy or other neck surgeries. Hypoparathyroidism also occurs following purposeful removal of the parathyroid glands for hyperparathyroidism or cancer. Another cause is hypomagnesemia, which impairs secretion of PTH. Hypomagnesemia can occur with chronic alcoholism or certain nutritional problems.

Signs and Symptoms

Calcium plays an important role in nerve cell stability. Hypocalcemia causes neuromuscular irritability. In acute cases, tetany may occur, with numbness and tingling of the fingers and perioral area, muscle spasms, and twitching (Table 39.5). Positive Chvostek's and Trousseau's signs are early indications of tetany. To check Chvostek's sign, tap on the patient's facial nerve just in front of the ear. Spasm of the face is a positive result, indicating hypocalcemia. To elicit Trousseau's sign, place a sphygmomanometer on the patient's arm and pump it to above the patient's systolic pressure. Spasm of the thumb and fingers occurs within 3 minutes if the patient has hypocalcemia. See Figures 6.4 and 6.5 in Chapter 6 for illustrations of these tests.

Chronic hypocalcemia can lead to lethargy; calcifications in the brain, leading to psychosis; cataracts; and convulsions. Bone changes may be evident on x-ray examination. Electrocardiogram (ECG) changes and heart failure can develop because of the importance of calcium to cardiac function. Death can result from laryngospasm if treatment is not provided.

Diagnostic Tests

Chvostek's and Trousseau's signs are present. Laboratory studies show decreased serum calcium and PTH levels and increased serum phosphate. An ECG is done to evaluate cardiac function. Radiographs show bone changes.

Therapeutic Measures

Acute cases of hypoparathyroidism are treated with intravenous calcium gluconate. Long-term treatment includes a high-calcium diet (Box 39.6), with oral calcium and vitamin D supplements. Thiazide diuretics may also be used because they reduce the amount of calcium excreted in the urine. Magnesium is given if hypomagnesemia is present.

Nursing Process for the Patient with Hypoparathyroidism

DATA COLLECTION. The patient at risk for hypoparathyroidism should be closely monitored for symptoms of tetany. If you suspect tetany, check for Chvostek's and Trousseau's signs. Monitor respirations closely for stridor, a sign of laryngospasm.

NURSING DIAGNOSES, PLANNING, AND IMPLEMENTATION

Risk for Injury Related to Hypocalcemia and Tetany

EXPECTED OUTCOME: The patient will remain free from injury; signs of tetany will be recognized and treated quickly.

- Monitor patient for signs of tetany, and report immediately to RN or physician *so treatment can begin quickly.*
- Make sure a tracheostomy set, endotracheal tube, and intravenous calcium are available *for emergency use if laryngospasm occurs.*
- Consult a dietitian for high-calcium diet teaching. *The patient may need a lifelong high-calcium diet.*
- Teach the patient about the importance of long-term diet and medication therapy and follow-up laboratory testing. *The patient needs to understand self-care for follow-up at home.*

EVALUATION. Injury is prevented through early recognition and reporting of signs and symptoms of tetany. The patient should be able to describe correct treatment and self-care measures for home.

Hyperparathyroidism

Pathophysiology

Overactivity of one or more of the parathyroid glands causes an increase in PTH, with a subsequent increase in the serum calcium level (hypercalcemia). This is achieved through

TABLE 39.5 PARATHYROID DISORDERS SUMMARY

	Insufficient PTH	Excess PTH
Disorder	Hypoparathyroidism	Hyperparathyroidism
Signs and Symptoms	Hypocalcemia, neuromuscular irritability, tetany, positive Chvostek's and Trousseau's signs	Hypercalcemia, fatigue, pathological fractures
Diagnostic Tests	Serum PTH, calcium, and phosphate	Serum PTH, calcium, and phosphate
Therapeutic Measures	Calcium and vitamin D replacement; high-calcium, low-phosphorus diet	Calcitonin, parathyroidectomy
Priority Nursing Diagnoses	*Risk for Injury* related to tetany	*Risk for Injury* related to bone demineralization

Box 39.6

Dietary Sources of Calcium

- Milk
- Cheeses
- Yogurt
- Sardines
- Oysters
- Salmon
- Cauliflower
- Green leafy vegetables

See Chapter 6, Table 6.3, for a more detailed list.

movement of calcium out of the bones and into the blood, absorption in the small intestine, and reabsorption by the kidneys. PTH also promotes phosphate excretion by the kidneys.

Etiology

Hyperparathyroidism is usually the result of hyperplasia or a benign tumor of the parathyroid glands, or it may be hereditary. Some cancers can also make a substance that mimics PTH and causes hypercalcemia. Secondary hyperparathyroidism occurs when the parathyroids secrete excessive PTH in response to low serum calcium levels. Serum calcium may be reduced in kidney disease because of the kidneys' failure to activate vitamin D, which is necessary for absorption of calcium in the small intestine.

Signs and Symptoms

Signs and symptoms of hyperparathyroidism are caused primarily by the increase in serum calcium level, although many patients are asymptomatic. Symptoms include fatigue, depression, confusion, increased urination, anorexia, nausea, vomiting, kidney stones, and cardiac dysrhythmias. The increased serum calcium level also causes gastrin secretion, resulting in abdominal pain and peptic ulcers. Because calcium is being removed from bones, bone and joint pain and pathological fractures can occur (see *Evidence-Based Practice* box). With severe hypercalcemia, the result may be coma and cardiac arrest.

EVIDENCE-BASED PRACTICE

Clinical Question

Do elevated parathyroid hormone (PTH) levels contribute to bone loss in older adults?

Evidence

In a study of 302 residents of a state veterans home, researchers found that furosemide (Lasix), a drug used commonly in older adults, was associated with increased PTH levels (Drinka et al., 2007). Calcium supplementation and increased serum vitamin D levels were associated with reduced PTH levels.

Implications for Nursing Practice

If you care for residents who take furosemide, ask the medical care provider about calcium and vitamin D supplementation.

REFERENCE

Drinka, P., Krause, P., Nest, L., & Goodman, B. (2007). Determinants of parathyroid hormone levels in nursing home residents. *Journal of the American Medical Directors Association, 8*(5), 328–331.

Diagnostic Tests

Laboratory studies include serum calcium, phosphate, and PTH levels. Radiographs or bone density testing may show decreased bone density. A 24-hour urine test might be used to test how much calcium is being excreted in the urine. Nuclear scanning or ultrasound may be used to help locate the parathyroid glands if surgical removal is planned.

Therapeutic Measures

In acute situations, intravenous normal saline is given to hydrate the patient and lower the calcium level by dilution; furosemide (Lasix) is given to increase renal excretion of calcium. For longer term care, the patient is monitored for bone changes and decline in renal function. Oral calcium and vitamin D supplements are prescribed. Alendronate (Fosamax) or calcitonin may be given to prevent calcium release from bones. Estrogen therapy might be used in women, although side effects must be considered.

If hypercalcemia is severe or if the patient is at risk for bone or kidney complications, surgery to remove the diseased parathyroid glands (parathyroidectomy) is performed. If possible, some parathyroid tissue is left intact to continue to secrete PTH. Minimally invasive radio-guided parathyroidectomy can be done under local anesthesia through a small incision.

Preoperative and postoperative care is similar to that of the patient undergoing thyroid surgery, with special attention paid to calcium and PTH levels. The patient will likely continue to be on calcium and vitamin D supplements following surgery.

Nursing Process for the Patient with Hyperparathyroidism

DATA COLLECTION. Assess the patient for symptoms related to hypercalcemia, including muscle weakness, lethargy, bone pain, anorexia, nausea, vomiting, behavioral changes, and renal insufficiency. Monitor serum calcium levels as ordered.

NURSING DIAGNOSES, PLANNING, AND IMPLEMENTATION. Nursing diagnoses depend on assessment findings. Risk for injury usually takes priority.

Risk for Injury (Fracture, Complications of Hypercalcemia) Related to Calcium Imbalance

EXPECTED OUTCOME: The patient will remain free from injury.

- Monitor patient for and report signs or symptoms of calcium imbalance promptly. *Prompt treatment can prevent serious complications.*
- Encourage oral fluids *to prevent dehydration and kidney stones and help excrete calcium.*
- Encourage strengthening and weight-bearing exercises *to help keep calcium in the bones.*
- Provide a safe environment for ambulation; assist the patient with ambulation if needed. *A fall could result in fracture if bones are demineralized.*
- Encourage smoking cessation. *Smoking causes bone loss.*
- Teach patient symptoms to report and use of long-term medications *so patient can manage self-care at home.*

EVALUATION. If the plan is effective, symptoms of hypercalcemia will be recognized and reported quickly, and complications and injury will be prevented.

DISORDERS OF THE ADRENAL GLANDS

Adrenal disorders may involve the adrenal medulla or the adrenal cortex. A rare tumor of the adrenal medulla, called a **pheochromocytoma**, causes hypersecretion of epinephrine and norepinephrine. Hyposecretion of epinephrine is rare and generally causes no symptoms. Hypersecretion of cortisol from the adrenal cortex results in Cushing's syndrome. Hypofunction of the adrenal cortex results in Addison's disease.

Pheochromocytoma

Pathophysiology

A pheochromocytoma is an uncommon tumor that arises from the chromaffin cells of the adrenal medulla. Occasionally, a pheochromocytoma occurs outside the adrenal gland, in the chest or abdomen. The tumor autonomously secretes catecholamines (epinephrine and norepinephrine) in excessive amounts. Ninety percent of pheochromocytomas are benign.

Etiology

The cause of pheochromocytoma is unknown. About 5% of cases are hereditary.

Signs and Symptoms

Because norepinephrine is the fight-or-flight hormone, patients with a pheochromocytoma have exaggerated fight-or-flight symptoms. These might be fairly constant, or occur in sporadic "attacks." Manifestations include hypertension, tachycardia (with heart rate greater than 100 beats per minute), palpitations, tremor, diaphoresis, feeling of apprehension, and severe pounding headache. Nausea and vomiting are occasionally present. Blood glucose may increase because catecholamines inhibit insulin release from the pancreas. Constipation may occur because catecholamines relax the bowel. The most prominent characteristic is intermittent unstable hypertension. Diastolic pressure may be greater than 115 mm Hg. If hypertension and tachycardia are not controlled, the patient is at risk for stroke, heart attack and failure, vision changes, seizures, psychosis, and organ damage. It is estimated that about 0.1% of cases of hypertension are caused by a pheochromocytoma.

• WORD • BUILDING •

pheochromocytoma: pheo—dark + chromo—color + cyt—cell + oma—tumor

Diagnostic Tests

Patients with a suspected pheochromocytoma will have a 24-hour urine test for metanephrines and vanillylmandelic acid (VMA). These are end products of catecholamine metabolism. A blood test for metanephrines may also be done. The patient should avoid caffeine and medications for 2 days before and during the test. Check institution policy for other dietary restrictions. If results are elevated, a CT scan or an MRI is done to locate the tumor.

Therapeutic Measures

Treatment for pheochromocytoma is surgical removal of one or both adrenal glands. Newer laparoscopic techniques make surgery safer than in the past. The patient must be stabilized before surgery. Alpha-blocking medications such as phenoxybenzamine (Dibenzyline) dilate blood vessels to control acute hypertension. Beta-blocking medication may be added to block beta-adrenergic receptors in the heart and lungs, reducing other fight-or-flight symptoms.

After surgery, the patient is at risk for hypotension, hypertension, and hypoglycemia. Monitor vital signs and blood glucose and report variations from normal. If both adrenal glands have been entirely removed, the patient will require lifelong replacement hormones. (See section on adrenalectomy later in this chapter.)

Nursing Process for the Patient with Pheochromocytoma

DATA COLLECTION. Monitor vital signs frequently, and report elevations promptly.

NURSING DIAGNOSES, PLANNING, AND IMPLEMENTATION

Risk for Injury Related to Hypertensive Crisis

EXPECTED OUTCOME: The patient will be free from injury related to hypertension.

- Monitor vital signs and report elevated pulse and blood pressure promptly. *Prompt treatment helps prevent complications.*
- Approach the patient calmly and maintain a quiet environment. *Stress may precipitate a hypertensive episode.*
- Administer alpha and beta blockers as ordered *to control symptoms.*
- Teach the patient how the medications will reduce symptoms, and the importance of avoiding foods and beverages containing caffeine, *so the patient can participate in self-care.*

- If patient has surgery, continue careful monitoring *because manipulation of tumor can increase catecholamine release.*

EVALUATION. If interventions have been effective, the patient's vital signs will be within normal limits, and complications will be avoided.

Adrenocortical Insufficiency/Addison's Disease

Adrenocortical insufficiency (AI) is the insufficient production of the hormones of the adrenal cortex. Primary AI is called Addison's disease.

Pathophysiology

Adrenal insufficiency is associated with reduced levels of cortisol, aldosterone, or both hormones. A deficiency in androgens may also exist. In primary disease, ACTH levels from the pituitary can be elevated in an attempt to stimulate the adrenal cortex to synthesize more hormone. In secondary disease, deficient ACTH fails to stimulate adrenal steroid synthesis. In most cases, the adrenal glands are atrophied, small, and misshapen and are unable to produce adequate amounts of hormone.

Etiology

Addison's disease is thought to be autoimmune; that is, the gland destroys itself in response to conditions such as tuberculosis, fungal infection, infection related to acquired immunodeficiency syndrome (AIDS), or metastatic cancer. It may also be associated with other autoimmune diseases, such as Hashimoto's thyroiditis. Bilateral adrenalectomy also results in adrenal insufficiency.

Secondary AI may be caused by dysfunction of the pituitary or hypothalamus. In addition, prolonged use of corticosteroid drugs may depress ACTH and corticotropin-releasing hormone production, which in turn reduces steroid hormone production. A patient receiving long-term corticosteroid therapy is particularly at risk for AI if the drugs are abruptly discontinued. Because the pituitary has been suppressed for a prolonged period, it may take up to a year before ACTH is produced normally again.

> **NURSING CARE TIP**
>
> Always taper corticosteroid therapy slowly to avoid adrenal crisis.

Signs and Symptoms

The most significant sign of Addison's disease is hypotension. This is related to the lack of aldosterone. Remember that aldosterone causes sodium and water retention in the kidney and potassium loss. If aldosterone is deficient, sodium and water are lost and hypotension and tachycardia result. Low cortisol levels cause hypoglycemia, weakness, fatigue, weight loss, confusion, and psychosis. In primary AI, increased ACTH may produce hyperpigmentation of the skin, causing the patient to have a tanned or bronze appearance. Anorexia, nausea, and vomiting may also occur, possibly as the result of electrolyte imbalances. Women may have decreased body hair because of low androgen levels. Patients may report craving salt.

Complications

If a patient is exposed to stress, such as infection, trauma, or psychological pressure, the body may be unable to respond normally with secretion of cortisol and an adrenal crisis can occur. Loss of large amounts of sodium and water and the resulting fluid volume deficit cause profound hypotension, dehydration, and tachycardia. Potassium retention can cause cardiac dysrhythmias. Hypoglycemia may be severe. Coma and death result if treatment is not initiated. Treatment of adrenal crisis involves rapidly restoring fluid volume and cortisol levels. Intravenous fluids (containing glucose) and large doses of IV glucocorticoids are administered. Electrolytes are replaced as needed. The cause of the crisis should be identified and treated.

Diagnostic Tests

Serum and urine cortisol levels are measured. Blood glucose is low. Blood urea nitrogen (BUN) and hematocrit levels may appear to be elevated because of dehydration. An ACTH stimulation test may help determine whether the adrenal glands are functioning. Serum sodium and potassium levels are monitored. A CT scan or an MRI may be done to evaluate the size of the adrenal glands or to locate a pituitary tumor in secondary disease.

Therapeutic Measures

Long-term treatment consists of replacement of glucocorticoids (hydrocortisone) and mineralocorticoids (fludrocortisone). Some patients also receive androgen therapy. Patients will need hormone replacement therapy for the rest of their lives. Hormones are given in divided doses, with two-thirds of the daily dose given in the morning and one-third in the evening to mimic the body's own diurnal rhythm. Remember that steroid hormones are our natural stress hormones and so are naturally elevated during times of stress. Therefore, during times of stress or illness, doses need to be increased to two to three times normal. The patient may also be placed on a high-sodium diet.

Nursing Process for the Patient with Addison's Disease

DATA COLLECTION. The patient with Addison's disease should be assessed for understanding of and compliance with the treatment regimen. Monitor vital signs and daily weights or intake and output to track fluid status. Monitor serum glucose levels and symptoms of hyperkalemia and hyponatremia. Report changes in mental status. If the patient is in crisis, monitor vital signs closely and report any signs of fluid volume deficit such as orthostatic hypotension or poor skin turgor to the physician immediately.

NURSING DIAGNOSES, PLANNING, AND IMPLEMENTATION

Risk for Deficient Fluid Volume Related to Deficient Adrenal Cortical Hormones

EXPECTED OUTCOME: The patient's fluid volume will be stable as evidenced by stable weights and vital signs, and skin turgor within normal limits.

- Monitor vital signs, and report change promptly. *Hypotension and tachycardia indicate hypovolemia.*
- Monitor fluid status and report changes promptly *so treatment can begin.*
- Administer steroid replacements as ordered *to maintain fluid and electrolyte balance.*

Risk for Ineffective Self Health Management Related to Deficient Knowledge about Self-Care of Addison's Disease

EXPECTED OUTCOME: The patient will verbalize understanding of self-monitoring and self-medication at home.

- Assess patient's understanding of his or her disease process and treatment. *Teaching should build on baseline knowledge.*
- Teach the patient the importance of hormone replacement as ordered. *The patient who does not secrete endogenous adrenocortical hormones must rely on replacements.*
- Help the patient identify the causes and symptoms of stress, and explain the need to increase medication dosage during times of stress or illness according to the physician's instructions. *Because these hormones are normally increased during times of stress, it is important that the patient understand how to increase the dose during stress to prevent adrenal crisis.*
- Advise patient he or she may need to increase salt intake in hot weather *because of fluid and salt losses.*
- Recommend medical alert identification. *A patient in adrenal crisis may not be able to provide a medical history to emergency personnel, and identification can prevent delay of treatment.*
- If ordered by the physician, teach the patient and significant other how to use an emergency intramuscular (IM) hydrocortisone injection kit. *IM medication may be needed during stress or times when the patient is unable to take oral medications.*

EVALUATION. If nursing care is effective, the patient's fluid status will be stable, and the patient and family will be able to carry out proper self-care of Addison's disease.

Cushing's Syndrome

Cushing's syndrome is caused by exposure to excess cortisol. This can occur because of an adrenal problem, a pituitary problem, or from treatment with exogenous corticosteroids. See Table 39.6 for a comparison of adrenal insufficiency and Cushing's syndrome.

Pathophysiology

Recall that cortisol, aldosterone, and androgens are the three steroid hormones secreted by the adrenal cortex. Cortisol is essential for survival and is normally secreted in a diurnal rhythm, with levels increasing in the early morning. Secretion is increased during times of stress. In Cushing's syndrome, cortisol is hypersecreted without regard to stress or time of day. When levels of cortisol are very high, effects related to excess aldosterone and androgens are also seen.

> **LEARNING TIP**
>
> Remember from Chapter 38, an easy way to remember the hormones of the adrenal cortex is to think salt, sugar, and sex. Aldosterone promotes salt retention, cortisol affects sugar (carbohydrate) metabolism, and androgens are sex hormones.

Etiology

Cushing's syndrome can be caused by the hypersecretion of ACTH by the pituitary. This is most often the result of a benign pituitary adenoma. Sometimes ACTH is produced by a tumor in the lungs or other organs. The high levels of ACTH cause adrenal hyperplasia, which in turn increases production and release of cortisol. A problem within the adrenal gland, such as an adrenal adenoma or carcinoma can also produce excess cortisol.

TABLE 39.6 ADRENAL CORTEX HORMONE SUMMARY

	Hypofunction	Hyperfunction
Disorder	Adrenocortical insufficiency, Addison's disease	Cushing's syndrome
Signs and Symptoms	Sodium and water loss, hypotension, hypoglycemia, fatigue	Weight gain, sodium and water retention, hyperglycemia, buffalo hump, moon face
Diagnostic Tests	Serum and urine cortisol	Serum and urine cortisol
Therapeutic Measures	Glucocorticoid and mineralocorticoid replacement	Alter steroid therapy dose or schedule; surgery if tumor
Priority Nursing Diagnoses	*Risk for Deficient Fluid Volume*	*Risk for Excess Fluid Volume, Unstable Blood Glucose Level, Infection*

The most common cause of Cushing's syndrome is prolonged use of glucocorticoid medication (e.g., prednisone) for chronic inflammatory disorders such as rheumatoid arthritis, chronic obstructive pulmonary disease, and Crohn's disease. The use of smaller doses of glucocorticoids (in inhalers for asthma) or topical creams does not usually cause a problem.

Signs and Symptoms

Most signs and symptoms of Cushing's syndrome are related to excess cortisol levels. Weight gain, central obesity with thin arms and legs, fat pads on the upper back (buffalo hump), and a round, moon-shaped face result from deposits of adipose tissue at these sites (Fig. 39.6). Cortisol also causes insulin resistance and stimulates gluconeogenesis, which results in glucose intolerance. Some patients develop secondary diabetes mellitus (see Chapter 40). Muscle wasting and thin skin with purple striae occur as a result of cortisol's catabolic effect on tissues. Catabolic effects on bone lead to osteoporosis, pathological fractures, and back pain from compression fractures of the vertebrae. Because cortisol has anti-inflammatory and immunosuppressive actions, the patient is at risk for infection. Hyperpigmentation of the skin may occur. About half of patients develop mental status changes, from irritability to psychosis (sometimes referred to as steroid psychosis). Sodium and water retention are related to the mineralocorticoid effect. As sodium is retained, potassium is lost in the urine, causing hypokalemia. (See Chapter 6 to review these electrolyte imbalances.) Androgen effects include acne, growth of facial hair, and amenorrhea in women.

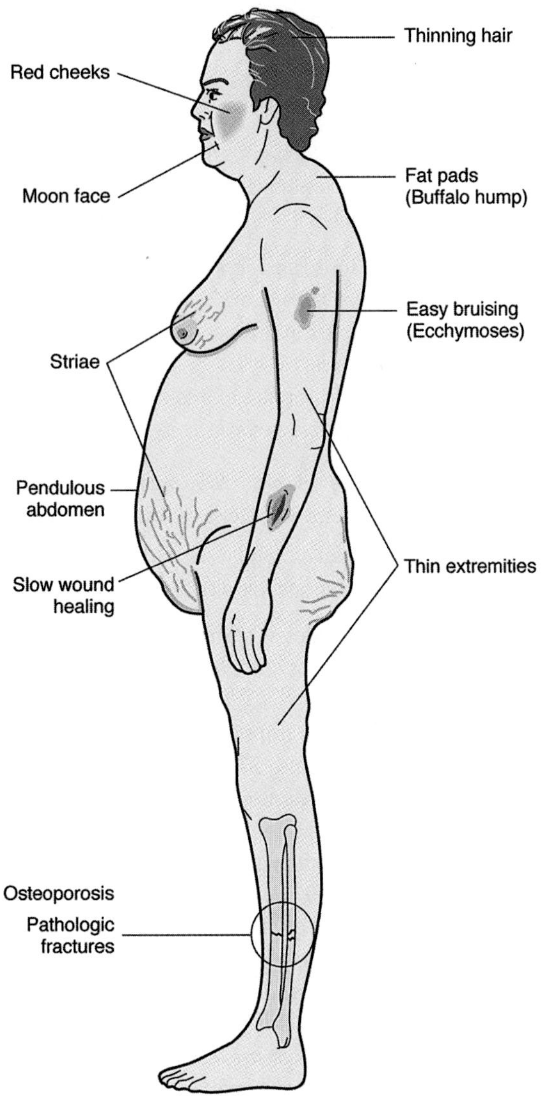

Thinning hair
Red cheeks
Moon face
Fat pads
(Buffalo hump)
Easy bruising
(Ecchymoses)
Striae
Pendulous
abdomen
Thin extremities
Slow wound
healing
Osteoporosis
Pathologic
fractures

FIGURE 39.6 Physical manifestations seen in Cushing's syndrome.

Diagnostic Tests

Suspicion of Cushing's syndrome may initially be based on a cushingoid appearance and history of taking steroid medication. Plasma and urine cortisol and plasma ACTH are measured. A 24-hour urine test for cortisol may be collected. Levels of cortisol in the saliva may also be measured. A dexamethasone suppression test may be done. Serum potassium is measured. Additional tests to locate the cause of excess endogenous cortisol may be done.

Therapeutic Measures

If a pituitary or ACTH-secreting tumor is present, surgical removal or radiation therapy to the pituitary gland may be employed. If the adrenals are the primary cause of the problem, radiation or removal of the adrenal gland or glands may be performed. Drugs such as ketoconazole can be used to block production of adrenal steroids.

If the cause of Cushing's syndrome is administration of steroid medication, a lower dose, an every-other-day schedule, or once-a-day dosing in the morning may reduce side effects. Usually steroids are prescribed as a last resort for chronic disorders that are unresponsive to other treatment. The patient and physician must weigh the risks and benefits of continuing the medication. The physician may order a high-potassium, low-sodium, high-protein diet. Potassium supplements may be ordered. If the patient has high blood sugar, appropriate therapy for diabetes is instituted. (See Chapter 40.)

Nursing Process for the Patient with Cushing's Syndrome

DATA COLLECTION. When caring for the patient with Cushing's syndrome, assess the patient's medication history. Monitor vital signs and complications related to fluid and sodium excess. Auscultate the lungs for crackles, and assess extremities for edema. Assess skin integrity, and monitor capillary glucose as ordered by the physician. Watch for signs of infection.

NURSING DIAGNOSES, PLANNING, AND IMPLEMENTATION

Risk for Excess Fluid Volume Related to Sodium and Water Retention

EXPECTED OUTCOME: The patient's fluid volume will be stable as evidenced by stable daily weights.

- Monitor daily weights and report changes promptly *so treatment can begin.*
- Teach the patient ordered dietary modifications. *A low-sodium, high-potassium diet may help keep electrolytes in balance.*

Risk for Impaired Skin Integrity Due to Thin, Fragile Skin

EXPECTED OUTCOME: The patient's skin will remain intact.

- Observe skin, and monitor for breakdown with every position change. *Early recognition and treatment of a problem can prevent further breakdown.*
- Assist patient to change positions at least every 2 hours *to prevent pressure ulcers.*
- Use a lift sheet to move patient in bed *to prevent friction and shear.*
- Avoid harsh soaps and hot water. *These can dry skin and increase risk for injury.*
- Use moisturizing cream *to keep skin from drying.*
- Secure IVs and dressings without tape whenever possible. *Removal of tape can tear fragile skin.*
- Consider a specialty pressure-reducing mattress if the patient is very thin or unable to move *to reduce the risk of pressure ulcer.*
- Consult a dietitian if nutritional status is poor. *Poor nutrition further increases risk for skin breakdown and poor healing.*

Risk for Infection Related to Immune Suppression

EXPECTED OUTCOME: The patient will be infection free as evidenced by a white blood cell (WBC) count and temperature within normal limits.

- Monitor patient for signs of infection and report promptly *so treatment can begin.*
- Use good hand washing technique before and after patient care. *Hand washing is important in reducing exposure to pathogens.*
- Instruct the patient in good hand washing and in the importance of avoiding others who are ill. *A patient with an impaired immune system is more likely to contract illness from others.*
- Consult a dietitian if nutritional status is poor. *Poor nutrition further impairs immune function.*
- Encourage flu and pneumonia vaccinations *to help prevent illness in event of exposure.*

Risk for Unstable Blood Glucose Level Related to Impaired Glucose Tolerance

EXPECTED OUTCOME: The patient's blood glucose level will remain within normal limits.

- If glucose intolerance occurs, be prepared to administer insulin *because oral hypoglycemics are not usually effective.*
- Refer the patient and family to diabetes education classes *because diabetes is a complex disease that requires knowledge of self-care.*
- See Chapter 40 for care of the patient with diabetes.

Disturbed Body Image Related to Cushingoid Appearance as Evidenced by Patient Statement of Distress

EXPECTED OUTCOME: The patient will express feelings of acceptance of self.

- Approach patient with an attitude of acceptance and caring *to help develop trusting nurse-patient relationship.*
- Provide an opportunity for patient to verbalize feelings. *Expressing feelings may help reduce anxiety.*

EVALUATION. If care has been effective, complications of fluid overload will be recognized and treated early. The patient will have intact skin and be free from signs of infection. The patient will demonstrate skill in self-care of diabetes if indicated, and will verbalize acceptance of self in spite of changes in appearance.

Nursing Care of the Patient Undergoing Adrenalectomy

Preoperative Care

Monitor the patient for electrolyte imbalance and hyperglycemia. Abnormalities must be corrected before surgery. To prevent adrenal crisis, glucocorticoids are administered because removal of the adrenals causes a sudden drop in adrenal hormones. Prepare the patient for adrenalectomy or hypophysectomy, depending on which surgery will be performed.

Postoperative Care

See care of the patient undergoing hypophysectomy earlier in this chapter. Following adrenalectomy, the patient receives routine postoperative care. In addition, the patient is closely monitored for changes in fluid and electrolyte balance and adrenal crisis. Patients who undergo bilateral adrenalectomy must take replacement glucocorticoid and mineralocorticoid hormones for the remainder of their life. If only one adrenal gland is removed, the remaining gland should eventually produce enough hormone to enable the patient to discontinue replacement hormone.

See Table 39.7 for a summary of endocrine disorders and Table 39.8 for a summary of medications used for endocrine disorders.

TABLE 39.7 SUMMARY OF ENDOCRINE DISORDERS

Hormone	Hypofunction	Hyperfunction
Antidiuretic hormone	Diabetes insipidus—water loss	SIADH—water retention
Growth hormone	Short stature	Acromegaly, gigantism—bone and tissue overgrowth
Thyroid hormone	Hypothyroidism—slow metabolism	Hyperthyroidism—increased metabolism
Epinephrine	Rare	Pheochromocytoma—hypertension
Parathyroid hormone	Hypoparathyroidism—low serum calcium, tetany	Hyperparathyroidism—high calcium, weakness
Cortisol	Addison's disease—sodium and water loss	Cushing's syndrome—sodium and water retention, hyperglycemia; see text

TABLE 39.8 MEDICATIONS USED FOR ENDOCRINE DISORDERS

Medication Class	Examples/Action	Route	Side Effects	Nursing Implications
Medications for ADH disorders	vasopressin (Pitressin): replaces antidiuretic hormone (ADH)	IM, IV, subcutaneously	Water retention, hyponatremia	Check daily weights and urine specific gravity. Do not give demeclocycline with dairy products or antacids.
	desmopressin (DDAVP): replaces ADH	PO, IV, Intranasal (by rhinal tube)		
	demeclocycline (Declomycin): reduces ADH release	PO	Photosensitivity, allergy, water loss	
Medications for growth hormone disorders	bromocriptine (Parlodel): reduces growth hormone (GH) release	PO	Dizziness, hypotension, nausea	Monitor blood pressure, serum GH.
	octreotide (Sandostatin): suppresses GH	Subcutaneously, IM, IV	Uncommon: dizziness, nausea, constipation	Teach patient self-administration.
	somatropin (Humatrope): replaces GH	Subcutaneously, IM	Insulin resistance, hypothyroidism	Monitor growth; teach patient self-administration.
Medications for thyroid disorders	levothyroxine (Synthroid): replaces T_3 and T_4	PO, IM, IV	Tachycardia, insomnia, nervousness, weight loss	Monitor vital signs and thyroid lab results.
	propylthiouracil (PTU): inhibits synthesis of thyroid hormones	PO	Nausea, vomiting, agranulocytosis; has been associated with liver failure	Monitor WBC and differential, thyroid function, liver function.
	methimazole (Tapazole): inhibits synthesis of thyroid hormones	PO	Rash, agranulocytosis	
Medications for parathyroid disorders	calcium gluconate: replaces calcium	PO, IV	Dysrhythmia, cardiac arrest, constipation	Monitor vital signs and electrocardiogram during IV therapy. Do not take PO calcium with other medications.
	alendronate (Fosamax): inhibits resorption of bone; keeps calcium in bones	PO	Abdominal pain, constipation, diarrhea, nausea	Do not take with calcium supplements or caffeine.
Medications for adrenal disorders	phenoxybenzamine (Dibenzyline): blocks action of epinephrine at alpha receptors in pheochromocytoma	PO	Orthostatic hypotension	Monitor vital signs.
	hydrocortisone: replaces cortisol in adrenal insufficiency	PO, IV	Cushing's effects	Teach patient to take with food and not to discontinue abruptly.
	fludrocortisone (Florinef): replaces aldosterone in adrenal insufficiency	PO	Fluid retention, heart failure, hypokalemia	Monitor daily weights, vital signs, and serum potassium.

CRITICAL THINKING

Mrs. Tercini

■ Mrs. Tercini is a 62-year-old woman admitted to your unit in addisonian crisis. She is lethargic, with a blood pressure of 86/58 mm Hg, pulse 112, and respirations 18. While interviewing her daughter, you learn that Mrs. Tercini has a history of Cushing's syndrome treated with bilateral adrenalectomy 25 years ago. She has been taking 150 mcg fludrocortisone (Florinef) and 200 mg hydrocortisone daily ever since. Three days ago she developed the flu.

1. Why is an adrenalectomy done to treat Cushing's syndrome?
2. What is the most effective schedule for Mrs. Tercini's medication?
3. What precipitated this addisonian crisis?
4. Why is Mrs. Tercini's blood pressure low?
5. How could this crisis have been prevented?
6. Fludrocortisone is available as 0.1-mg tablets. How many should you administer?

Suggested answers at end of chapter.

SUGGESTED ANSWERS TO CRITICAL THINKING

■ *Mrs. Jackson*

1. Assess mental status and level of consciousness. Assess edema, lung sounds, and vital signs. Check intake and output during the past 2 days. Check recent lab work to see if her serum sodium is low. You also check a book on the unit and recall that anesthetics are possible causes of SIADH. Opioids, which Mrs. Jackson is likely taking following surgery, can also cause confusion.
2. Her weight gain is most likely caused by fluid retention, which can be a result of heart failure or SIADH, among other things.
3. Notify the registered nurse of your findings and suspicions. Be prepared to place Mrs. Jackson on a fluid restriction. Reassure her son that the physician is being notified of the changes he noted.
4. Remember "a pint's a pound." A pint is 2 cups for 480 mL.

$$\frac{6 \text{ pounds} \quad 480 \text{ mL}}{1 \text{ pound}} = 2880 \text{ mL or almost 3 liters}$$

■ *Adoption*

The children's growth hormone secretion was probably suppressed because of psychosocial stress. Once they felt secure in a loving environment, growth hormone levels returned to normal.

■ *Mrs. Maino*

1. Mrs. Maino's TSH is elevated because her pituitary gland is working overtime to try to stimulate the underactive thyroid gland.
2. Mrs. Maino's metabolism has been slow, so she has been burning fewer calories. When she starts on thyroid replacement hormone, her metabolic rate will return to normal and she will need more calories. Intake of calories should be balanced with the possible need for weight loss.
3. If Mrs. Maino receives too much thyroid hormone, she will have symptoms of hyperthyroidism, including an increased pulse rate. She should know how to check her pulse and to call her physician if it is elevated.

■ *Mrs. Tercini*

1. Cushing's syndrome is caused by too much cortisol. The adrenal cortex is responsible for secreting cortisol.
2. Mrs. Tercini should take two-thirds of her daily dose of hydrocortisone and fludrocortisone in the morning and one-third in the evening, or as ordered. This most closely mimics the body's natural corticosteroid secretion.
3. The flu probably triggered this crisis. Illness is a stressor, and normally the body secretes steroids during stress. Because Mrs. Tercini's body is unable to produce steroids, she experiences symptoms of hypoadrenalism during stressful times.
4. Mrs. Tercini's blood pressure is low because she has insufficient circulating mineralocorticoids. Without aldosterone, sodium and water are lost and blood pressure drops.
5. Mrs. Tercini should have taken extra medication when she became ill.
6. $$\frac{150 \text{ mcg}}{1000 \text{ mcg}} \Big| \frac{1 \text{ mg}}{0.1 \text{ mg}} \Big| \frac{1 \text{ tab}}{} = 1.5 \text{ tablets}$$

REVIEW QUESTIONS

1. Which disorder results from too much cortisol secretion in the body?
   a. Addison's disease
   b. Hypothyroidism
   c. Cushing's syndrome
   d. Pheochromocytoma

2. A patient with SIADH asks the nurse why he has gained 10 pounds. Which response is best?
   a. "SIADH causes an increase in appetite. As soon as you are effectively treated, the weight should drop back to normal for you."
   b. "You are retaining a lot of sodium and potassium, and that causes you to gain a lot of water weight."
   c. "You have too much of a hormone in your system that causes you to retain water. The extra 10 pounds is likely water weight."
   d. "Your kidneys are not working correctly, so they can't get rid of extra water from your system."

3. Which assessment finding should the nurse expect to see in the patient with uncontrolled diabetes insipidus? **Select all that apply**.
   a. Edema
   b. Polyuria
   c. Heat intolerance
   d. Diarrhea
   e. Polydipsia
   f. Dehydration

4. Which of the following instructions should the nurse provide to the patient who is being discharged after a thyroidectomy?
   a. "You must take your thyroid replacement every day just as the physician prescribed."
   b. "You must weigh yourself daily and report any gain or loss of more than 1 pound."
   c. "You will need to return to the physician's office for a weekly blood pressure check."
   d. "You will need to restrict your sodium and potassium intake."

5. Which of the following nursing assessments is most important in the patient with hyperthyroidism and risk for thyrotoxic crisis?
   a. Intake and output
   b. Breath sounds
   c. Bowel sounds
   d. Vital signs

6. Which action by the nurse is most important following hypophysectomy?
   a. Performing a routine neurologic assessment
   b. Encouraging the patient to cough and deep breathe
   c. Monitoring for tracheal edema
   d. Assisting with use of an incentive spirometer

7. Which of the following statements by the patient with hypothyroidism indicates to the nurse that the plan of care has been effective?
   a. "I feel so much better now that my energy is returning."
   b. "I'm really glad the diarrhea has stopped."
   c. "I'm so glad I won't have to take medication for very long."
   d. "My fingers aren't tingling any more."

DavisPlus | For additional resources and information visit http://davisplus.fadavis.com

40

Nursing Care of Patients with Disorders of the Endocrine Pancreas

PAULA D. HOPPER

KEY TERMS

diabetes mellitus (DYE-ah-BEE-tis mel-EYE-tus)
endogenous (en-DAW-jen-uss)
gastroparesis (GASS-troh-puh-REE-sus)
glycosuria (GLY-kos-YOO-ree-ah)
hyperglycemia (HY-per-glye-SEE-mee-ah)
hypoglycemia (HY-poh-glye-SEE-mee-ah)
ketoacidosis (KEE-toh-as-ih-DOH-sis)
Kussmaul's respirations (KOOS-mahlz RESS-per-AY-shuns)
nephropathy (neh-FROP-uh-thee)
neuropathy (new-RAW-puh-thee)
nocturia (nok-TYOO-ree-ah)
polydipsia (PAH-lee-DIP-see-ah)
polyphagia (PAW-lee-FAY-jee-ah)
polyuria (PAH-lee-YOO-ree-ah)
postprandial (POHST-PRAN-dee-uhl)
preprandial (PREE-PRAN-dee-uhl)
retinopathy (RET-ih-NAW-puh-thee)

QUESTIONS TO GUIDE YOUR READING

1. What are the pathophysiologies of type 1 and type 2 diabetes mellitus?
2. What are the risk factors for type 1 and type 2 diabetes mellitus?
3. What are the signs and symptoms of diabetes mellitus?
4. What are the causes, signs and symptoms, and treatment of high and low blood glucose levels?
5. Why are persons with diabetes prone to complications such as heart disease, blindness, and kidney failure? How can you help your patients prevent these complications?
6. What diagnostic tests are used to diagnose and monitor diabetes mellitus and its complications?
7. What therapeutic measures help patients with diabetes control their blood glucose levels?
8. How do the different insulins and oral hypoglycemic agents lower blood glucose levels? What should you know when administering these medications?
9. How would you apply the nursing process to care of the patient with diabetes mellitus?
10. What measures can be taken to increase the safety of the patient with diabetes who is undergoing surgery?
11. What is reactive hypoglycemia? How is it diagnosed and treated?

DIABETES MELLITUS

Diabetes mellitus (be careful not to confuse this with diabetes insipidus) is a group of metabolic diseases in which defects in insulin secretion or action result in elevated blood glucose (**hyperglycemia**). According to the latest Centers for Disease Control and Prevention (CDC) data, approximately 23.6 million people in the United States have diabetes mellitus; 10.7% of Americans ages 20 or older, and 34.1% of Americans ages 60 or older have diabetes. Approximately 5.7 million people have diabetes and don't know it. The direct and indirect cost (such as lost work time) of diabetes in the United States is about $174 billion per year. The incidence of diabetes mellitus varies by race and ethnicity. In the United States, Hispanic, African American, Native American, and Asian American populations have a higher rate of diabetes than non-Hispanic white ethnic groups (CDC, 2007).

Diabetes is a serious disease that can cause complications such as blindness, kidney failure, heart attacks, and strokes. It is a leading cause of lower limb amputations in the United States. With good education and self-care, patients with diabetes can prevent or delay these complications and lead full, productive lives. Nurses play a major role in helping patients learn to care for themselves effectively.

Pathophysiology

Body tissues, and the cells that compose them, use glucose for energy. Glucose is a simple sugar provided by the foods we eat. When carbohydrates are eaten they are digested into sugars, including glucose, which is then absorbed into the bloodstream. Carbohydrates provide most of the glucose used by the body; proteins and fats can indirectly provide smaller amounts of glucose. Glucose is able to enter the cells only with the help of insulin, a hormone produced by the beta cells in the islets of Langerhans of the pancreas (Fig. 40.1). When insulin comes in contact with the cell membrane, it combines with a receptor that allows activation of special glucose transporters in the membrane (Fig. 40.2). By helping glucose enter the body's cells, insulin lowers the glucose level in the blood. Insulin also helps the body store excess glucose in the liver in the form of glycogen.

Another hormone, glucagon, is produced by the alpha cells in the islets of Langerhans. Glucagon raises the blood glucose when needed by releasing stored glucose from the liver and muscles. Insulin and glucagon work together to keep the blood glucose at a constant level.

Diabetes results from deficient production of insulin by the beta cells in the pancreas, or from inability of the body's cells to use insulin. When glucose is unable to enter body cells, it stays in the bloodstream; hyperglycemia results, and the cells are denied their energy source. Abnormal glucagon secretion may also play a role in type 2 diabetes.

• WORD • BUILDING •

diabetes mellitus: diabetes—passing through + mellitus—sweet

hyperglycemia: hyper—excessive + glyc—glucose + emia—in the blood

Types and Causes

Type 1 Diabetes Mellitus

Type 1 diabetes (formerly called juvenile diabetes mellitus, insulin-dependent diabetes mellitus, or IDDM) is caused by destruction of the beta cells in the islets of Langerhans of the pancreas. When the beta cells are destroyed, they are unable to produce insulin. Insulin must then be injected for the body to use food for energy. See Box 40.1, *Patient Perspective,* for Dave's story about having type 1 diabetes. Only 5% to 10% of people with diabetes have type 1 diabetes.

It is believed that the pancreas may attack itself following certain viral infections or administration of certain drugs. This is called an autoimmune response. Almost 90% of patients newly diagnosed with type 1 diabetes have islet cell antibodies in their blood. These antibodies might be present for years before actual symptoms of diabetes develop. About 10% of people with type 1 diabetes cases also have a genetic predisposition to its development. The patient with type 1 diabetes is most often young and thin and is prone to develop ketoacidosis when blood glucose is elevated. Diabetic ketoacidosis is discussed later in this chapter. See Table 40.1 for a comparison of type 1 and type 2 diabetes. Research studies are ongoing to try to find ways to prevent type 1 diabetes once antibodies have been detected.

LATENT AUTOIMMUNE DIABETES OF ADULTHOOD (LADA). LADA is a variation of type 1 diabetes that has recently been identified. Some patients who were initially diagnosed with type 2 diabetes were later found to have islet cell and insulin antibodies (which are usually associated with type 1), and their blood glucose levels were not controlled with oral medications. However, beta cell destruction tended to occur more slowly than with type 1 diabetes. This is possibly because of differences in the antibodies or the individual's response to the antibodies. Some experts distinguish patients with LADA as either thin or obese because the disorder has slightly different characteristics depending on the patient's body fat.

Type 2 Diabetes Mellitus

Ninety to 95% of people with diabetes have type 2 diabetes mellitus (formerly called adult-onset diabetes mellitus, non–insulin-dependent diabetes mellitus, or NIDDM). In type 2 diabetes mellitus, tissues are resistant to insulin. Insulin is still made by the pancreas, but in inadequate amounts. Sometimes the amount of insulin is normal or even high, but because the tissues are resistant to it, hyperglycemia results. As the disease advances, the pancreas eventually wears out and insulin production decreases. When this occurs, the patient will likely require insulin injections. Simply using insulin, however, does not make the person a type 1 diabetic. He or she is a type 2 diabetic who needs insulin to control the blood glucose level.

Heredity is responsible for up to 90% of cases of type 2 diabetes. Obesity is also a major contributing factor. Often the patient with a new diagnosis of type 2 diabetes is obese, relates a family history of diabetes, and has had a recent life stressor such as the death of a family member, illness, or loss of a job.

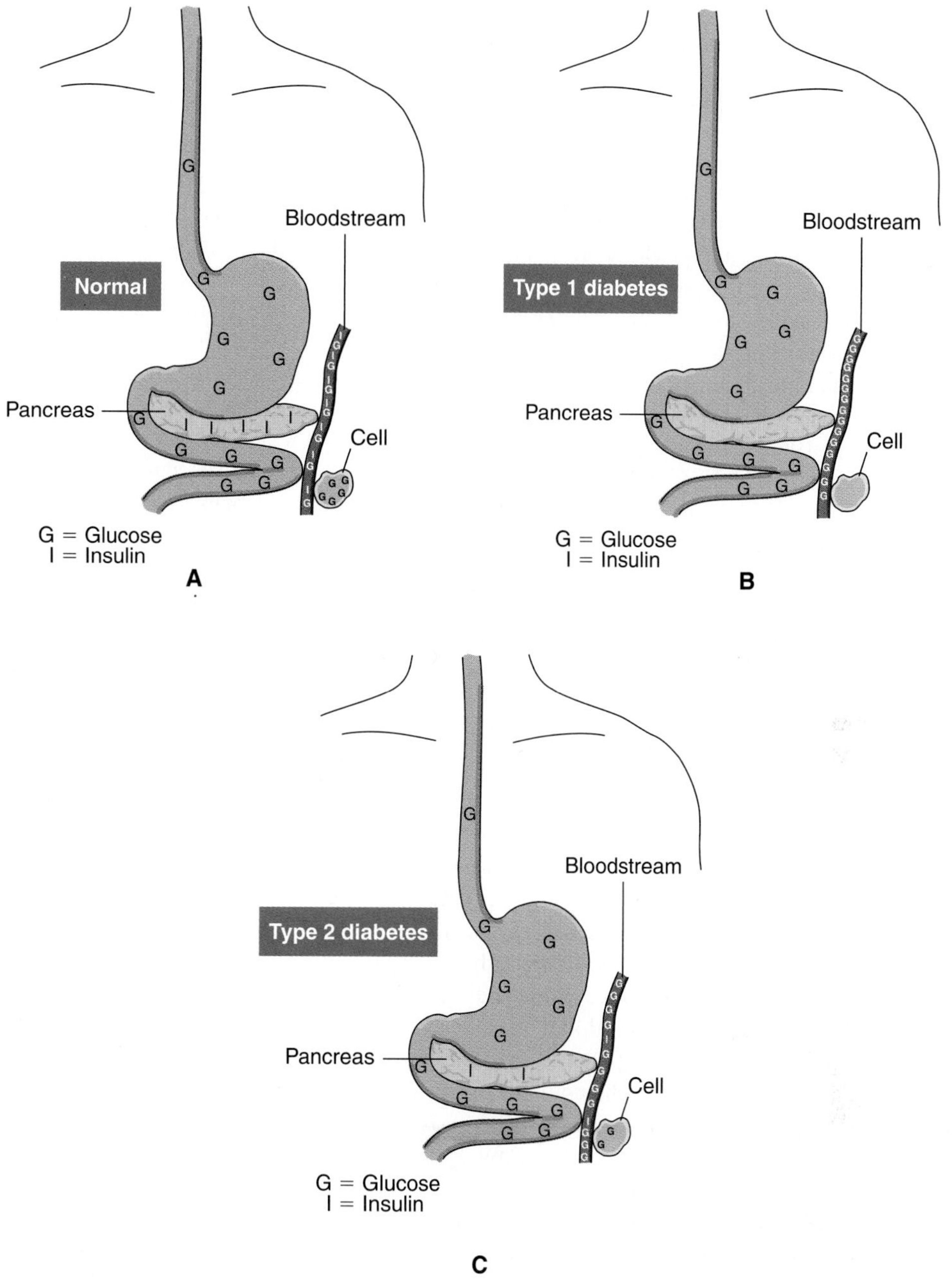

Normal
Bloodstream
Pancreas
Cell
G = Glucose
I = Insulin
A
Type 1 diabetes
Bloodstream
Pancreas
Cell
G = Glucose
I = Insulin
B
Type 2 diabetes
Bloodstream
Pancreas
Cell
G = Glucose
I = Insulin
C

FIGURE 40.1 Maintenance of blood glucose levels. (A) Normal physiology: Foods (especially carbohydrates) are broken down into glucose, which is absorbed into the bloodstream for transport to the cells. Insulin, produced by the beta cells of the islets of Langerhans in the pancreas, is needed to "open the door" to the cells, allowing the glucose to enter. (B) In type 1 diabetes mellitus, the pancreas does not produce insulin. Because glucose is unable to enter the cells, it builds up in the bloodstream, causing hyperglycemia. (C) In type 2 diabetes mellitus, insulin production is reduced and/or cells are resistant to insulin. Less glucose enters the cell, and hyperglycemia results.

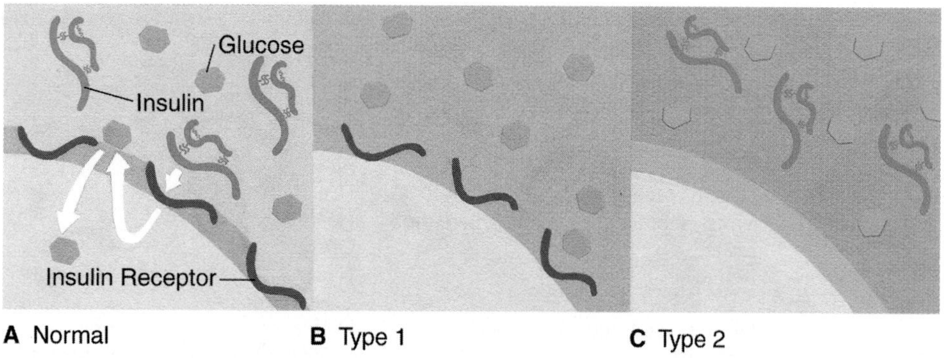

Glucose
Insulin
Insulin Receptor
A Normal
B Type 1
C Type 2

FIGURE 40.2 (A) Cell membrane in normal state, with insulin receptors and insulin to regulate glucose intake. (B) Cell membrane in type 1 diabetes: insulin not present, glucose remains outside of cell. (C) Cell membrane in type 2 diabetes: without insulin receptors, glucose remains outside cell. (From Scanlon, V. C., & Sanders, T. [2007]. *Essentials of anatomy and physiology* [5th ed.]. Philadelphia: F. A. Davis, with permission.)

Box 40.1

Patient Perspective

Dave

I was diagnosed with type 1 diabetes mellitus at age 3 years. I remember being left in a children's ward of the hospital with the nuns (who were nurses) in their habits and looking into the parking lot as my parents got in the car and drove away. I remember the fear and horror of being left alone. Later, I remember my doctor teaching my mother and me about the diet and monitoring my urine for glucose and ketones. This was all we had in those days (the early 1960s). I was supposed to test my urine before meals and at bedtime, just like we monitor blood glucose today. Every time I saw my doctor he would review and change my treatment based on the results. Insulin then was extracted from pig and cow cadavers.

I remember my life being pretty normal except at holidays. When my brothers and sisters were getting Halloween candy and Christmas candy canes, I felt odd and left out. My mom was really tough and observant and I had to be sneaky to get away with stealing a treat or two left momentarily unobserved by those around me. I was thrilled when sugarless candy became available around age 10 or so and I could have my own candies to hoard for myself.

Hypoglycemic reactions were always a trauma-filled event at our house. They came at unexpected times, and my mom sometimes blamed herself. I can honestly say that my mom deserves more credit than I have ever given her for my good fortune with my diabetes. She did not have glucometers, glycohemoglobin tests, or even diabetes specialists and educators; she just had the desire of a mother who did everything she could to make sure I had and did everything right as far as she knew.

In my late teens I took everything my doctor and my mom had done for me and trashed them. I lived with reckless abandon: I did what I wanted, ate what I wanted, and didn't even think about the disease I lived with until I was about 30. I worked hard those years in construction, and the physical activity probably delayed the complications that might otherwise have occurred.

At age 35, I began to experience the inevitable effects of long-term hyperglycemia. I developed diabetic retinopathy, the leading cause of adult-onset blindness in the United States. My vision was restored in my left eye with laser surgery. It would take another surgery (vitrectomy) to bring the vision in my right eye back to the 20/60 it is now from the 20/2000 it was before the surgery.

About that time I was referred to an endocrinologist who specialized in diabetes, and my treatment took a remarkable turn for the better. The endocrinologist began to aggressively change my medications, insulin regimen, exercise program, and diagnostic testing, all with the purpose of controlling blood glucose and preventing the onset and advancement of diabetic complications. This aggressive plan of action was taught to me by a registered nurse certified diabetes educator who worked with my doctor. I must also give enormous credit to the office staff nurses who were an integral part of the team, supporting me throughout the whole experience. The doctors and nurses made my education both understandable and pertinent. They basically put the ball in my court, and then it was up to me to take control of my own life. My wife was more than supportive throughout this time period too, and sacrificed much for the new array of medications and doctor's appointments that took a huge chunk out of our family finances.

I have mentioned briefly those involved in my life with diabetes. I take no credit for any of the results though; I believe it was God who made these choices available and miraculously reversed the effects of disease in my body. To the amazement of medical professionals, He continues to bless me with good health. It is because of all I have gone through with diabetes that I have recently completed my nursing degree and hope to become a diabetes educator myself.

TABLE 40.1 COMPARISON OF TYPE 1 AND TYPE 2 DIABETES

	Type 1	Type 2
Onset	Rapid	Slow
Age at onset	Usually younger than 40	Usually older than 40
Risk factors	Virus, autoimmune response, heredity	Heredity, obesity
Usual body type	Lean	Obese
High blood glucose complication	Ketoacidosis	Hyperosmolar hyperglycemia; may develop ketoacidosis
Treatment	Diet, exercise; must have insulin to survive	Diet, exercise; may need oral hypoglycemics or insulin to control blood glucose level

TYPE 2 DIABETES IN YOUTH. More and more children and adolescents are developing type 2 diabetes, which in the past only occurred in adults. This is related to increasing obesity and decreasing activity levels in children today. Many experts are concerned about the growing number of obese children in the United States because of their increased risk for diabetes, heart disease, and other obesity-related problems.

Gestational Diabetes

Gestational diabetes mellitus (GDM) may develop during pregnancy, especially in women with risk factors for type 2 diabetes. The extra metabolic demands of pregnancy trigger the onset of diabetes. Blood glucose usually returns to normal after delivery, but the mother has an increased risk for type 2 diabetes in the future. If the mother with GDM is overweight, she should be counseled that weight loss and exercise will decrease her risk of later developing diabetes. Mothers with GDM require specialized care and should be referred to an expert in this area.

Prediabetes

Prediabetes refers to blood glucose levels that are above normal but do not meet the criteria for diagnosing diabetes (Fig. 40.3). Prediabetes usually occurs before the onset of type 2 diabetes. It is diagnosed by evaluating fasting blood glucose levels, glucose tolerance tests (see tests of diabetes below), or HbA_{1c}. Those with prediabetes may be able to prevent the onset of diabetes with weight loss and exercise.

Other Types of Diabetes

Secondary diabetes may develop as a result of another chronic illness that damages the islet cells, such as pancreatitis or cystic fibrosis. Prolonged use of some drugs, such as steroid hormones, phenytoin (Dilantin), thiazide diuretics, and thyroid hormone, may also impair insulin action and raise blood glucose. Maturity-onset diabetes of the young (MODY) is an inherited defect in insulin secretion that usually occurs in individuals under the age of 25. Less common causes include pancreatic trauma and other endocrine disorders.

Metabolic Syndrome

A newer finding is the link between prediabetes and a condition called metabolic syndrome or cardiometabolic syndrome. According to the American Heart Association and the National Heart, Lung, and Blood Institute, metabolic syndrome is diagnosed when at least three of the following criteria are met (National Institutes of Health, 2001):

- Elevated waist circumference (greater than 40 inches in men, 35 inches in women)
- Triglyceride level 150 mg/dL or higher
- High-density lipoprotein (HDL) ("good") cholesterol lower than 40 mg/dL for men and lower than 50 mg/dL for women
- Blood pressure 130/85 mm Hg or higher
- Fasting glucose level 110 mg/dL or higher.

Other risk factors include physical inactivity, aging, hormonal imbalance, and genetic predisposition. Hispanic Americans are at higher risk than Caucasians. A major factor is the growing obesity epidemic in the United States.

Any patient who fits this profile should be monitored closely for the onset of type 2 diabetes and heart disease. Patients should be counseled on the importance of a diet low in saturated fats and cholesterol, weight loss, physical activity, and control of blood pressure and cholesterol levels.

Signs and Symptoms

Classic symptoms of diabetes mellitus include **polydipsia** (excessive thirst), **polyuria** (excessive urination), and **polyphagia** (excessive hunger). The large amount of glucose in the blood causes an increase in serum concentration, or osmolality. The renal tubules are unable to reabsorb all the

• WORD • BUILDING •

polydipsia: poly—many or much + dipsia—thirst
polyuria: poly—many or much + uria—urine
polyphagia: poly—many or much + phagia—to eat

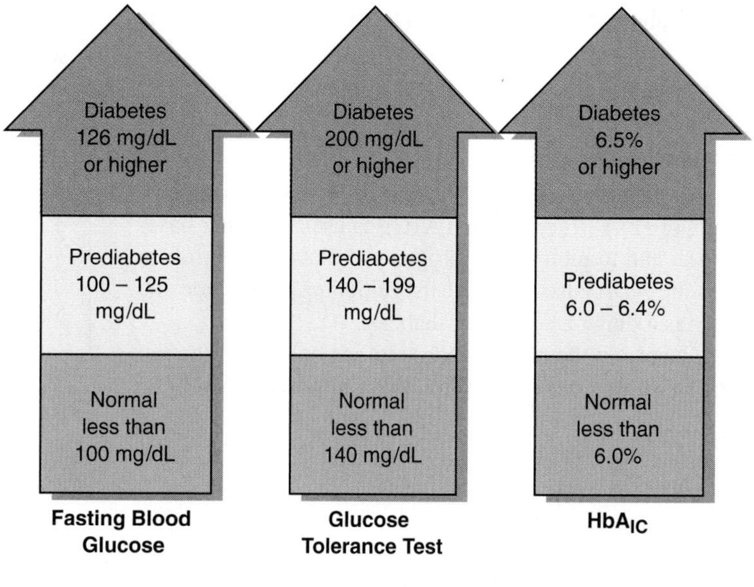

Diabetes 126 mg/dL or higher
Prediabetes 100 – 125 mg/dL
Normal less than 100 mg/dL
Fasting Blood Glucose
Diabetes 200 mg/dL or higher
Prediabetes 140 – 199 mg/dL
Normal less than 140 mg/dL
Glucose Tolerance Test
Diabetes 6.5% or higher
Prediabetes 6.0 – 6.4%
Normal less than 6.0%
HbA1C

FIGURE 40.3 Prediabetes is the period between normal blood glucose levels and levels that are diagnostic for diabetes. Tests used to determine whether a patient has normal blood glucose levels, high-risk prediabetes, or diabetes include the fasting glucose level, glucose tolerance, and HbA_{1c} tests.

excess glucose that is filtered by the glomeruli, and **glycosuria** results. Large amounts of body water are required to excrete this glucose, causing polyuria, **nocturia** (nighttime urination) and dehydration. The increased osmolality and dehydration cause polydipsia. Because glucose is unable to enter the cells, the cells starve, causing hunger. High blood glucose may also cause fatigue, blurred vision, abdominal pain, and headaches. Ketones may build up in the blood and urine of patients with type 1 diabetes or late in the course of type 2 diabetes (**ketoacidosis**).

> **LEARNING TIP**
>
> Remember the classic symptoms of diabetes by the **three Ps:** polydipsia, polyuria, and polyphagia.

Diagnostic Tests

Fasting Plasma Glucose Level

Diagnosis of diabetes mellitus is based on plasma glucose levels measured by a laboratory. According to the American Diabetes Association (ADA, 2009), a normal plasma glucose level is less than 100 mg/dL. When the fasting plasma glucose (drawn after at least 8 hours without eating) is 126 mg/dL or greater, diabetes is diagnosed. A second test may be required if the first test is not clearly diagnostic. If the fasting plasma glucose is between 100 and 125 mg/dL, the patient has impaired fasting glucose (IFG).

Casual Plasma Glucose

Sometimes it is not feasible to check a fasting plasma glucose. A casual plasma glucose (CPG) is checked without regard to the last meal. Diabetes is diagnosed if the CPG is 200 mg/dL or greater, with symptoms of diabetes.

Oral Glucose Tolerance Test

Another test to diagnose diabetes is the oral glucose tolerance test (OGTT). An OGTT measures blood glucose at intervals after the patient drinks a concentrated carbohydrate drink. Diabetes is diagnosed when the blood glucose level is 200 mg/dL or greater after 2 hours. A result between 140 and 199 mg/dL at 2 hours leads to a diagnosis of impaired glucose tolerance (IGT).

Glycohemoglobin

The glycohemoglobin test (also called glycosylated hemoglobin, or HbA_{1c} [hemoglobin A1C]) is used to gather baseline data and to monitor the progress of diabetes control. In 2009, the ADA also changed its guidelines to include the HbA_{1c} as a diagnostic test for diabetes.

Glucose in the blood attaches to hemoglobin in the red blood cells. Red blood cells live about 3 months. When the glucose that is attached to the hemoglobin is measured, it reflects the average blood glucose level for the previous 2 to 3 months. This is a helpful measurement when blood glucose levels fluctuate, and a single measurement would be misleading. It also assists in determining the degree of effectiveness of a patient's treatment plan. A normal HbA_{1c} is 4% to 6%. An HbA_{1c} of 6.5% or higher is diagnostic for diabetes. An HbA_{1c} between 6% and 6.5% indicates high risk for developing diabetes.

Newer methods allow this test to be done in a physician's office while the patient waits. See Table 40.2 for average blood glucose levels based on HbA_{1c} results.

Glycohemoglobin testing might be inaccurate in some people, such as those with anemia. These patients may instead be tested for glycated serum protein (also called fructosamine), which is a similar test that indicates glucose levels over a period of 1 to 2 weeks instead of 3 months.

Estimated Average Glucose

Some practitioners are using a new calculation to convert HbA_{1c} results to estimated average glucose (eAG) numbers, which may be more meaningful to patients. The formula is

$$28.7 \times HbA_{1c} - 46.7 = eAG$$

Here is an example for a patient whose HbA_{1c} is 8.6:

$$28.7 \times 8.6 - 46.7 = 200.12, \text{ which can be rounded to } 200 \text{ mg/dL}$$

Additional Tests

Because diabetes affects so many body systems, additional tests recommended for baseline data include a lipid profile, serum creatinine and urine microalbumin levels to monitor kidney function, urinalysis, and electrocardiogram.

> **CRITICAL THINKING**
>
> ***Mr. McMillan***
>
> ■ Mr. McMillan is a 50-year-old patient brought into the emergency department with extreme fatigue and dehydration. After the physician sees him, you ask Mr. McMillan some additional questions. Based on the patient's answers, you request that the physician add a glucose level to the laboratory tests ordered. The result is 1400 mg/dL.
>
> 1. What questions would you ask Mr. McMillan if you suspected diabetes?
> 2. Why was Mr. McMillan fatigued?
> 3. Why was he dehydrated?
>
> *Suggested answers at end of chapter.*

Prevention

Although there is currently no known way to prevent type 1 diabetes, there are ways to prevent type 2 diabetes. Research studies have shown that patients at risk for diabetes, even those who already have IGT or IFG, can prevent or delay the

• WORD • BUILDING •

glycosuria: glyc—glucose + uria—urine
nocturia: noc—by night + uria—urine
ketoacidosis: keto—ketones + acid—acidic + osis—condition

TABLE 40.2 CORRELATION BETWEEN HBA_{1C} AND MEAN FASTING PLASMA GLUCOSE

HbA_{1c} (%)	Fasting Plasma Glucose (mg/dL)
Less than 6	Less than 135
7	170
8	205
9	240
10	275
11	310
12	345

Source: American Diabetes Association. (2006). Your A1C results: What do they mean? *Clinical Diabetes, 24*(1), 9.

onset of diabetes with weight loss and regular exercise. Losing as little as 5% to 10% of body weight through a half hour of exercise 5 days a week, and reducing fat and calories can reduce the risk of diabetes by 58% (Diabetes Prevention Program Research Group, 2002). The study also showed that using the diabetes medication metformin can delay onset of diabetes. Patients at risk should have their plasma glucose level checked regularly.

Therapeutic Measures

The only cure for diabetes is a pancreas (or islet cell) transplant. However, diabetes can be controlled. Treatment begins with diet and exercise. Insulin is added in patients with type 1 diabetes and insulin or oral hypoglycemic medication as needed in those with type 2 diabetes. Blood glucose monitoring and education are also important to good diabetes control.

To monitor the effectiveness of treatment, patients should have regular health care follow-up visits. See Box 40.2 for a summary of the diabetes goals and recommendations proposed by the ADA for 2009.

Goals of Treatment

The ADA recommends that patients maintain a **preprandial** (premeal) plasma glucose level of 70 to 130 mg/dL, peak **postprandial** glucose less than 180 mg/dL, and glycohemoglobin level of less than 7% to prevent or delay complications of diabetes. Because of the risk for cardiovascular disease, they also recommend maintaining blood pressure of less than 130/80 mm Hg (ADA, 2009). All goals may be adjusted in individual circumstances. For example, the patient who is unable to feel symptoms of **hypoglycemia** (low blood glucose) might have a higher preprandial glucose goal to prevent undetected hypoglycemic episodes.

Box 40.2

Summary of Diabetes Goals and Recommendations

Capillary plasma glucose should be measured at least three times a day for patients using multiple insulin injections. Blood pressure should be measured at every office visit. Serum creatinine and urine microalbumin should be assessed yearly. Target levels* are:

• HbA_{1c} (every 3–6 months)	Less than 7%
• Preprandial capillary glucose	70–130 mg/dL
• Peak postprandial capillary glucose	Less than 180 mg/dL
• Blood pressure	Less than 130/80 mm Hg

Blood lipids should be measured at least yearly. Target levels are:

Low-density lipoproteins	Less than 100 mg/dL Less than 70 mg/dL in patients with cardiovascular disease (CVD)
Triglycerides	Less than 150 mg/dL
High-density lipoproteins	Greater than 40 mg/dL (men) Greater than 50 mg/dL (women)

Patient should receive:

- Yearly flu vaccine for all patients age 6 months and older
- One lifetime pneumococcal vaccine for patients older than age 2 years, with revaccination for patients older than age 64 if first vaccine was more than 5 years earlier
- Aspirin therapy, 75–162 mg/day, if older than age 30
- Statin therapy if history of CVD or if older than age 40 with CVD risk factors
- Smoking cessation counseling
- Yearly comprehensive foot examination
- Dilated comprehensive eye examination within 5 years of onset of type 1 diabetes, or at diagnosis of type 2 diabetes, and every year thereafter.

* Target levels for blood glucose are different in hospitalized patients.

Source: Adapted from American Diabetes Association. (2009). Clinical practice recommendations 2009. *Diabetes Care, 32*(Suppl 1).

• WORD • BUILDING •

preprandial: pre—before + prandial—meal
postprandial: post—after + prandial—meal
hypoglycemia: hypo—deficient + glyc—glucose + emia—in the blood

Medical Nutrition Therapy

The goal of medical nutrition therapy (MNT) is to achieve and maintain blood glucose and lipid levels as near to normal as possible to prevent long-term complications. For some, especially those with type 2 diabetes, weight loss and cholesterol and blood pressure control may be additional goals of nutrition therapy.

Because the patient with diabetes has a limited amount of insulin, either **endogenous** (from within the body) or injected, it is important to eat an amount of food that will not exceed the insulin's ability to carry it into the cells. This requires a meal plan that includes consistent amounts of carbohydrates, proteins, and fats each day. Because carbohydrates contribute most to the blood glucose level, it is most important that the amount of carbohydrates consumed is consistent from one day to the next. If a patient eats a small amount of carbohydrate one day and a large amount the next, the blood glucose will fluctuate, leading to complications. It is possible to relax nutrition restrictions somewhat if the patient is willing to test blood glucose frequently at home and adjust treatment accordingly. This requires in-depth instruction by a diabetes educator.

The ADA recommends a complete assessment by a specially trained dietitian and an individualized nutrition therapy plan and teaching. Various meal plans are available, as shown in Box 40.3, *Nutrition Notes.* Because diabetes increases the risk of high serum cholesterol and triglycerides, all plans limit fat intake. Patients who use fat replacers (in foods such as fat-free baked goods or ice cream) should be aware that they still have food value and calories, so they cannot be considered "free" foods. Most plans also encourage the use of complex carbohydrates such as whole grains, pastas, vegetables, and fruits. Simple sugars, which may raise blood glucose more than complex carbohydrates (they have a higher glycemic index), are used less but are not prohibited as they were in the past. Sodium intake is limited in individuals with hypertension. Protein is limited in patients with any degree of kidney impairment. Any meal plan should be chosen to fit the patient's lifestyle and food preferences. Patient preferences based on

Box 40.3

Nutrition Notes

Nutrition is integral to the management of diabetes. The goals of nutritional care for persons with diabetes are control of blood glucose and prevention of complications. No single approach is suitable for everyone.

Overall goals and strategies differ by type of diabetes. In general, patients with

- type 1 diabetes need to prevent wide swings in blood glucose levels through careful timing of meals and snacks in relation to insulin therapy and activity.
- type 2 diabetes use diet modifications with medication as needed to maintain near-normal glucose, blood pressure, and lipid levels and to lose weight as needed.

People with diabetes usually benefit from eating on a regular basis (every 4 to 5 hours while awake). Evidence has shown that the use of sucrose (table sugar) as part of the meal plan does not impair blood glucose control in individuals with type 1 and type 2 diabetes.

A certified diabetes educator can devise a meal plan based on the patient's abilities and commitment. Several meal-planning approaches are described below. The education of the patient with diabetes is a process that may take months, and should not be expected to be accomplished in a single visit or with a paper handout.

Using MyPyramid

The U.S. Department of Agriculture has developed a basic educational tool called MyPyramid that can be adapted for a first-level meal plan for the newly diagnosed person with diabetes. The physician or diabetes educator can select the calorie level appropriate for the patient and common household measures are used as guidelines. Foods chosen from the MyPyramid guide should be divided into three or more equal meals. Carbohydrate-containing foods are especially important to distribute evenly throughout the day. A patient can use online tracking at www.mypyramidtracker.gov.

Using ADA Exchange Lists

The ADA Exchange Lists, published jointly by the American Dietetic Association and the American Diabetes Association, have been used for many years. This system is composed of six lists of foods plus a "free food" list. Foods in each list contain similar energy nutrients (carbohydrate, protein, and fat). For example, green peas are on the starch list rather than the vegetable list because they are closer in composition to a slice of bread than to green beans.

Individual food items within an exchange list are essentially equal to each other in nutrient composition and can thus be exchanged or "swapped" for each other. Exchanges were designed to be approximately equal in nutrients, not in volume; therefore, portion sizes vary widely. For instance, one fruit exchange is equal to 1¼ cups of whole strawberries but to only three dates.

To correctly use this method of meal planning, for each meal patients must choose the prescribed number of items from each appropriate list: starch, fruit, milk, vegetable, meat, and fat.

A specific meal plan should be given to the patient with the exchange lists. A meal plan is a food guide that shows the number of choices or exchanges the patient should eat at each meal and snack, based on the total daily calories prescribed.

• WORD • BUILDING •

endogenous: endo—within + genous—to produce

Box 40.3

Nutrition Notes—cont'd

A meal plan based on exchange lists allows patients a variety of food choices yet requires minimal calculation. Even experienced users of the exchange list system should be advised to weigh or measure their portions several times per week to avoid portion inflation.

Using Carbohydrate Counting

Because carbohydrate is the energy nutrient that has the greatest influence on blood glucose levels, the amount and timing of carbohydrate intake directly affect diabetes control. Only carbohydrates are counted but patients are counseled to eat about the same amount of protein each day and to choose low-fat foods. Reading labels is mandatory; some fat-free products are higher in carbohydrate than the items they replace.

Carbohydrate counting classifies all carbohydrates together, whether from starch, fruit, or milk (see Table 40.3). This method offers more flexible food choices within a day's meal plan than the exchange list system and may achieve better control of blood glucose.

Despite those advantages, however, carbohydrate counting may entail the following:

- Weighing and measuring food
- Keeping food records
- Monitoring blood glucose before and after eating
- Controlling body weight.

Knowledge of carbohydrate counting is often a prerequisite to consideration of insulin pump therapy.

Using the Glycemic Index

All carbohydrates are not metabolized identically. Foods containing equal amounts of carbohydrate impact blood glucose levels differently. The glycemic index is a classification of foods according to the speed and degree of change in blood glucose levels. The standard is commonly set with glucose given a value of 100; other foods are then compared to glucose. For example, a sweet potato has a glycemic index of 54, and peanuts have a glycemic index of 14. Use of the glycemic index is not recommended for diabetes care at this time.

Source: Lutz, C. A., & Przytulski, K. R. (2010). *Nutrition and diet therapy* (5th ed.). Philadelphia: F. A. Davis.

Box 40.4

Cultural Considerations

The "standard" diabetic diet may need significant adjustment for patients not of the dominant U.S. culture. Giving such a patient the typical food exchange list may prove unhelpful because it does not include the patient's usual foods. The patient may be labeled noncompliant when, in reality, the health care worker has been culturally insensitive. Helping the patient choose a meal plan that fits the appropriate cultural preference is important.

Some helpful websites include www.diabetes.org/espanol and www.eatright.org.

EVIDENCE-BASED PRACTICE

Clinical Question

Does culturally appropriate health teaching affect outcomes in patients with diabetes?

Evidence

Eleven research studies were reviewed and showed improvement in knowledge level and HbA_{1c} scores at 3 and 6 months after culturally appropriate education (Hawthorne et al., 2008).

Implications for Nursing Practice

Nurses must take cultural background into account when providing education about diabetes self-care to their patients.

REFERENCE

Hawthorne, K., Robles, Y., Cannings, J. R., & Edwards, A. G. K. (2008). Culturally appropriate health education for type 2 diabetes mellitus in ethnic minority groups. *Cochrane Database of Systematic Reviews 2008, Issue 3* (Art. No. CD006424; DOI 10.1002/14651858.CD006424.pub2).

ethnic background should also be considered (Box 40.4, *Cultural Considerations,* and see *Evidence-Based Practice* box).

Many patients now use a carbohydrate counting method, which allows some degree of freedom for the patient who is able to learn to read labels and monitor carbohydrate intake (Table 40.3). If the patient carefully counts carbohydrates, other foods do not need to be as tightly controlled, as long as general recommendations such as low fat or low sodium, are followed. The success of MNT is evaluated by monitoring glucose levels, HbA_{1c}, lipids, weight, blood pressure, and kidney function.

Exercise

Exercise is an important factor in controlling blood glucose and lipid levels. Exercise lowers blood glucose, both immediately and for approximately 24 to 48 hours after the exercise. Insulin is not needed for glucose to enter exercising muscle cells. Exercise also improves blood lipid levels and circulation, which is important for the person with diabetes, who already has an increased risk of cardiovascular disease. Patients are instructed to exercise on a regular basis, ideally 30 minutes on most days of the week, to keep blood glucose levels stable and promote health.

Some patients with complications of diabetes must be careful in their exercise choices. For example, a patient with retinopathy should not do anything that causes straining. (See the *Long-Term Complications* section later in this chapter.) A patient with neuropathy or foot problems should limit weight-bearing exercise. A physician or exercise physiologist should be consulted for an individualized exercise plan.

Persons with diabetes should always carry a quick source of sugar when exercising in case the blood glucose drops too low. Individuals on intermediate-acting insulin are taught to avoid exercising at the time of day when their blood glucose is at its lowest point (i.e., when insulin or medication is peaking) and to have a carbohydrate snack before exercising if blood glucose is less than 100 mg/dL. Exercising at similar times each day also helps prevent blood glucose fluctuations.

Patients should be cautioned to avoid exercise when their glucose level is higher than 250 mg/dL and ketones are present in the urine or if glucose is more than 300 mg/dL without ketones. This indicates that insufficient insulin is available and glycogen may be released during exercise, further increasing the serum glucose.

Medication

INJECTED INSULIN. The person with type 1 diabetes has no endogenous insulin and therefore must administer insulin daily. At this time, insulin cannot be taken by mouth because it is a protein and is therefore digested. Insulin is typically given subcutaneously, although fast-acting insulin may be ordered via the intramuscular or intravenous route in urgent situations. Several types of insulin are available with various schedules by which it may be given. The type and schedule are determined by the physician, in collaboration with the patient, based on the patient's lifestyle and willingness to spend time on injections. In general, the more frequent the injections, the better the glucose control.

Insulin injections should be given in a different subcutaneous site each time to avoid injury to the tissues. A sample rotation chart is shown in Figure 40.4. Because each area absorbs insulin at a slightly different rate, it is advisable to use one area for a week, then move on to the next area. Within that area, each injection should be spaced at least 1 inch from the previous injection. Some experts recommend using primarily the torso (abdomen and buttocks) to provide more uniform absorption. Aspirating for blood before injection and rubbing the site following injection are not recommended with insulin injections.

Patients who desire tighter control of blood glucose levels and a more flexible lifestyle may choose to use an insulin pump (Fig. 40.5). This is a small device that delivers subcutaneous insulin via a tiny catheter continuously in small (basal) amounts. The patient can then add a bolus of insulin with the push of a button before meals or snacks. This provides insulin levels that are more normal, like those of a person without diabetes. A pump typically is worn on

TABLE 40.3 EXAMPLE OF CARBOHYDRATE COUNTING

Meal	Prescribed Carbohydrate Exchanges	Carbohydrate Selected*
Breakfast	3	¾ cup dry cereal 8 ounces skim milk ½ cup unsweetened orange juice
Lunch	3	8 oz regular cola 1 cup melon 1 slice whole-wheat bread
Dinner	3	½ cup cooked potato ½ cup corn ½ cup regular ice cream
Snack	1	8 ounces skim milk

* Additional proteins and fats are added in moderate amounts, but need not be counted. Each item selected is approximately 15 grams carbohydrate or 1 carb exchange.

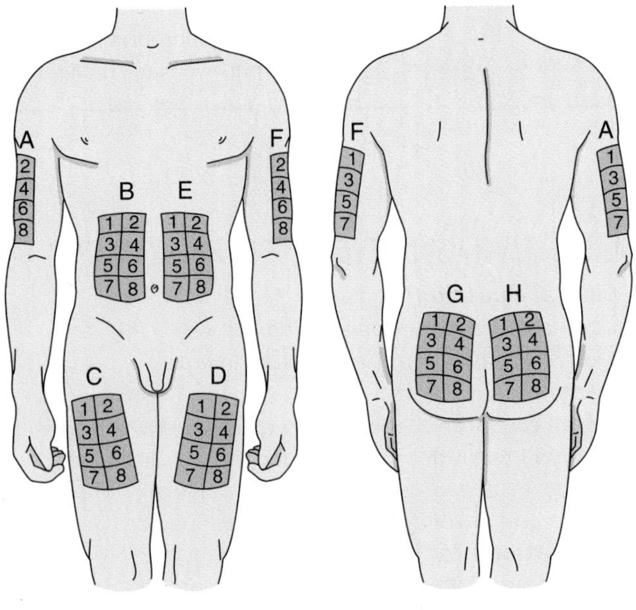
A
B
E
F
C
D
G
H
1 2
3 4
5 6
7 8
2 4 6 8
1 3 5 7

Rotation sites for injection of insulin.

FIGURE 40.4 Sample insulin rotation chart.

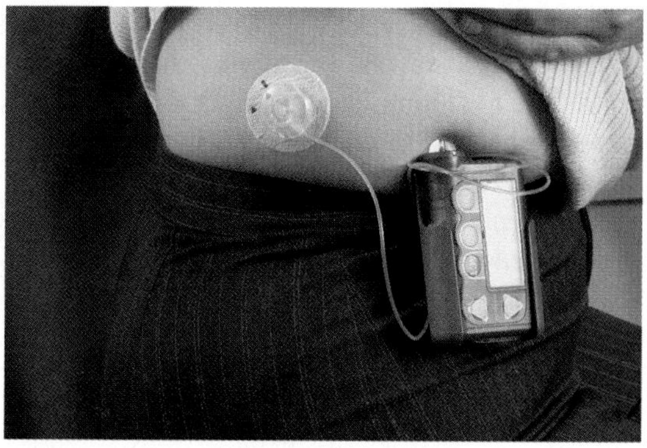

FIGURE 40.5 Patient wearing insulin pump.

the abdomen or buttocks. Some models receive input from continuous glucose monitors.

Insulin is synthetically produced in a laboratory and is either identical to human insulin, or one or two amino acids different (called insulin analogs). In the past, insulin was derived from cows and pigs; this is no longer available in the United States, but may be available from other countries. Be careful to check the source when preparing insulin for injection (especially if you work in home care, where patients could purchase their insulin online from another country), because insulins from different sources may act slightly differently. Some people may be allergic to beef or pork preparations or may refuse them based on cultural practices.

Once insulin is injected, a period elapses before it begins to lower blood glucose. This time is called the *onset of action.* The *peak action* occurs when the insulin is working at its hardest and the blood glucose is at its lowest point. It is during this peak time that the patient is most at risk for an episode of low blood glucose. *Duration of action* is the length of time the insulin works before it is used up. Onset, peak, and duration are determined by whether the insulin is short, intermediate, or long acting (Table 40.4). It is important for the individual with diabetes and the nurse to be aware of the onset, peak, and duration of any insulin given. This assists in making decisions such as when to give insulin in relation to meals, when to exercise, and when to be alert to low blood glucose symptoms.

In the past, most patients with diabetes used an injection of intermediate-acting insulin before breakfast and possibly a second injection before supper. Many patients are now choosing to take more frequent injections of short-acting insulin before meals or a combination of short- and intermediate-acting or long-acting insulins to achieve better, "tighter" control. These patients are often taught to adjust their insulin dose based on blood glucose level and the amount of carbohydrates eaten. Although patients who choose tight control have to be more cautious about risk for hypoglycemia, it can significantly reduce the risk of long-term complications.

One regimen that is becoming more common because it mimics normal insulin secretion is sometimes called "basal-bolus" insulin. This consists of an injection of a basal insulin (such as Lantus) once a day, often at bedtime, to provide a constant small amount of insulin in the bloodstream. Then an injection of very short-acting insulin is given before meals to mimic the extra insulin that is secreted normally with meals.

When two insulins need to be given at the same time, they can often be mixed together to prevent having to give more than one injection (Box 40.5). Preset mixtures of intermediate- and short-acting insulins are available for patients who have trouble learning to mix insulins.

LEARNING TIP

The Evens-and-Odds Rule: To remember the onset, peak, and duration of intermediate-acting insulin, think evens—2, 12, and 24 hours. To remember short-acting insulin, think odds—1, 3, and 5 hours. These times are not exact, but they are a great memory booster when you need to think fast.

NURSING CARE TIP

When mixing insulins, remember clear to cloudy. Always draw up the clear insulin first. This involves injecting air into the cloudy vial first. This is because if the clear is drawn up last, the vial may be contaminated by the cloudy insulin, altering the action of the clear insulin. If cloudy insulin is unknowingly contaminated by clear insulin, the clear will become cloudy and its effect will be diminished. *Note:* Glargine (Lantus) and detemir (Levemir) insulins cannot be mixed with other insulins.

TABLE 40.4 ONSET, PEAK, AND DURATION OF INSULINS

Insulin Type	Example	Sample Brand Names	Onset	Peak	Duration
Very short acting	Insulin lispro	Humalog	5–15 min	30–90 min	5 hr or less
	Insulin aspart	NovoLog	10–20 min	1–3 hr	3–5 hr
	Insulin glulisine	Apidra	15–20 min	30–90 min	6 hr
Short acting	Regular	Humulin R, Novolin R	30 min	2–5 hr	5–8 hr
Intermediate acting	NPH	Humulin N, Novolin N	1–2 hr	6–12 hr	18–26 hr
Basal	Insulin glargine	Lantus AE	1–2 hr	No peak	Up to 24 hr
	Insulin detemir	Levemir	1 hr	No peak	Up to 24 hr

Note: A variety of premixed formulas are also available.

Box 40.5

How to Mix Insulins

1. Assemble equipment: insulins, syringe large enough to hold the entire insulin dose, alcohol swab, physician's order.
2. Check physician's order to confirm correct insulin types and doses of regular (clear) and an intermediate-acting (cloudy) insulin.
3. Roll the bottle of cloudy insulin to mix. Do not shake, because this will cause bubbles.
4. Wipe tops of both vials with alcohol swab.
5. Draw up and inject an amount of air equal to the dose of intermediate-acting insulin into the cloudy vial. Remove syringe from vial.
6. Draw up and inject an amount of air equal to the dose of short-acting insulin into the clear vial.
7. Draw up the correct amount of clear insulin. Double-check amount with another nurse if this is the institution's policy.
8. Remove the syringe and insert into the cloudy vial. Carefully draw up the correct amount of insulin. If too much insulin is accidentally drawn into the syringe, the syringe must be discarded and the process repeated. Double-check again with another nurse according to institution policy.

Note: Some insulins cannot be mixed. Check a drug reference before mixing.

During times of stress or illness, some patients who usually take the same insulin doses every day are placed on "sliding-scale" insulin. This involves determining each dose of short-acting insulin based on blood glucose results, usually before meals and at bedtime. For example, a sliding-scale order might read "For blood glucose less than 200, no insulin; 201 to 250, 2 units regular insulin; 251 to 300, 4 units regular insulin; 301 to 350, 6 units regular insulin; greater than 350, call physician." Actual amounts vary from patient to patient.

INHALED INSULIN. A new short-acting human insulin that was inhaled, Exubera, was approved by the Food and Drug Administration (FDA) in January 2006. Unfortunately, it was removed from the market in 2007 because it never became popular. Research continues on inhalation and other alternate routes for insulin administration.

PROBLEMS REQUIRING INSULIN ADJUSTMENT. Two problems that can occur with glucose control are the Somogyi effect and the dawn phenomenon. The Somogyi effect may be at fault when the patient's blood glucose seems to be rising in spite of increasing insulin doses. If insulin levels are too high, the blood glucose may drop too low, stimulating release of counterregulatory hormones (epinephrine, glucagon, corticosteroids, growth hormone), which then elevate the blood glucose. The low glucose levels often occur during the night, and the patient may report night sweats or morning headaches. The high morning glucose is then interpreted as hyperglycemia, and the insulin dose may be further increased, compounding the problem.

The dawn phenomenon is thought to occur because of the natural release of growth hormone and cortisol during the early morning hours. This causes hyperglycemia on arising in the morning.

The patient might be asked to monitor blood glucose between 2 a.m. and 4 a.m. in addition to bedtime and morning testing to assess whether the Somogyi effect or the dawn phenomenon is occurring. Correction of the Somogyi effect involves reducing the insulin dose. The dawn phenomenon is treated with careful adjustment of meals and insulin so that insulin is peaking when the blood glucose is highest.

CRITICAL THINKING

Mrs. Evans

■ Mrs. Evans is a 68-year-old woman with type 2 diabetes who resides in an assisted living facility. She is on 42 units of NPH insulin every morning.

1. If Mrs. Evans eats her breakfast at 8:00 every morning, when should she take her insulin?
2. At what time of day should she be alert for symptoms of low blood glucose?
3. What could happen if Mrs. Evans has a busy day and misses her lunch?

Suggested answers at end of chapter.

ORAL HYPOGLYCEMIC MEDICATION. The patient with type 2 diabetes may be able to control blood glucose levels with medical nutrition therapy and exercise alone. If needed, oral hypoglycemic medication or insulin will also be prescribed. Oral hypoglycemics are not insulin pills, but rather work in ways such as stimulating the pancreas to produce more insulin, or making the tissues more sensitive to insulin. Remember that if insulin is ingested, it is digested, because it is a protein. Because most oral hypoglycemic agents depend on at least a partially functioning pancreas, most are not useful for patients with type 1 diabetes. See Table 40.5 for a list of commonly used oral hypoglycemic agents and their mechanisms of action.

Most insulins and oral hypoglycemics should be administered before meals. Care should be taken to prevent passage of more than 30 minutes between medication administration and the meal because this may result in a hypoglycemic episode. Some must be taken with, rather than before, meals. Check individual drugs for specific timing.

If the blood glucose level is not controlled with an oral hypoglycemic agent, insulin may be needed for the person

TABLE 40.5 ORAL HYPOGLYCEMIC AGENTS

Medication Class/Action	Examples	Side Effects	Nursing Implications
Absorption Delayers			
Alpha-glucosidase inhibitors (AGIs) Lower postprandial glucose by reducing rate of carbohydrate digestion and absorption.	acarbose (Precose), miglitol (Glyset)	Flatulence, bloating	Give at start of each meal. No weight gain or hypoglycemia risk. Multiple dosing less convenient. If used in combination with another drug and hypoglycemia occurs, treat with milk or glucose tablets, not table sugar.
DPP-4 inhibitor Inhibits DPP-4, an enzyme that breaks incretins. Incretins are hormones secreted by the GI system in response to food; they reduce glucagon secretion and increase insulin synthesis and release.	sitagliptin (Januvia)	Upper respiratory infection, headache; hypoglycemia when administered in combination with a sulfonylurea	Administer once a day. Only works when blood glucose is high, so does not cause hypoglycemia when used alone. Watch for allergic reactions.
Insulin Sensitizers			
Biguanide Decreases glucose production by liver; increases glucose uptake by muscle.	metformin (Glucophage, Glucophage XR, Fortamet, Riomet, Glumetza)	Nausea, diarrhea, decreased appetite; less likely to cause hypoglycemia than other agents	Give with meals. May enhance weight loss. Withhold if patient is having tests involving contrast dye. Contraindicated in renal and hepatic disease and heart failure. Monitor serum creatinine level. Notify physician of early symptoms of lactic acidosis: hyperventilation, myalgia, malaise.
Thiazolidinediones (glitazones) Reduce insulin resistance in muscles. Improve blood lipids; may lower blood pressure and improve cardiovascular risk.	pioglitazone (Actos), rosiglitazone (Avandia)	Nausea, weight gain, and fluid retention	Give with meal. Work well with obese patients. Avoid with liver disease; monitor liver enzymes. Monitor for heart failure. May alter effectiveness of some birth control pills.
Insulin Stimulators			
Sulfonylureas Stimulate insulin secretion by pancreas, increase insulin receptor sensitivity.	glipizide (Glucotrol) glimepiride (Amaryl) glyburide (Micronase, Diabeta)	Hypoglycemia, weight gain, possible increased risk of cardiovascular disease	Monitor patient for hypoglycemia. Teach patient to avoid alcohol.
Combination Agents			
	metformin and glyburide (Glucovance) metformin and rosiglitazone (Avandamet) glipizide and metformin (Metaglip)	See individual agents.	See individual agents.

with type 2 diabetes. This does not mean the person has type 1 diabetes. Insulin may be needed to control blood glucose but, unlike in the person with type 1 diabetes, insulin is not needed to sustain life.

OTHER DIABETES MEDICATIONS. A novel medication is exenatide (Byetta), an injectable drug that was first isolated in the saliva of the Gila monster! It is an "incretin mimetic," meaning it mimics natural incretins in the body. Incretins are hormones secreted by the gastrointestinal (GI) tract that stimulate insulin release in response to nutrients in the intestine. Byetta works in conjunction with oral hypoglycemic agents, and stimulates insulin secretion, lowers production of glucagon, slows gastric emptying, and promotes weight loss.

Another newer drug, pramlintide (Symlin), is an injectable agent that is used with insulin. It is a synthetic analog of amylin, a naturally occurring hormone that reduces glucose levels following meals. It may also promote weight loss in individuals who are overweight. Patients using Symlin have an increased risk of hypoglycemia.

Self-Monitoring of Blood Glucose

The ability to test blood glucose levels at home has been a major advance in diabetes care. Blood glucose can be better controlled because of the availability of monitoring at any time, in any place. A variety of blood glucose monitors are on the market at reasonable prices; one example is shown in Fig. 40.6. Most of the cost involved in monitoring is in the test strips that must be used. Health insurance programs sometimes cover this cost.

Self-monitoring of blood glucose (SMBG) usually is done before meals and at bedtime by the person on insulin who wants to maintain tight control of blood glucose. Less frequent schedules may be prescribed for patients who are unable or unwilling to test four times a day or for patients not on insulin. Some may test before breakfast and supper, and some may vary testing times from day to day. Patients are also often recommended to periodically test 2 hours after meals.

New devices are available that continuously monitor glucose via a small catheter inserted into the abdomen. The device records the glucose level every 5 minutes on a monitor that is worn like a pager on a belt. It can be set to alarm if the blood glucose level drops too low.

The diabetes provider should be consulted for desirable blood glucose ranges because these may differ for each patient. The ADA recommends a preprandial goal of 70 to 130 mg/dL for most patients. Patients who are prone to insulin reactions (hypoglycemia) or small children or the elderly may have higher goal ranges, such as 100 to 150 mg/dL. Lower blood glucose levels for these populations could increase the risk of hypoglycemia.

An important aspect of blood glucose monitoring is the interpretation of results. Monitoring is useless if the results are not used to improve blood glucose control. The patient should be instructed to keep a diary of blood glucose levels (Fig. 40.7). Some patients have computer software that graphs results. The patient may be taught by a diabetes educator to interpret the trends in the results, or the diary may be taken on a regular basis to the health care provider for interpretation and adjustment of the treatment plan.

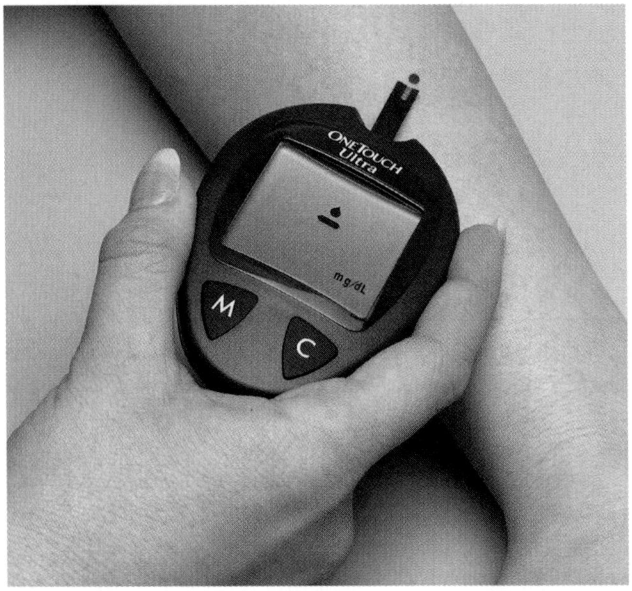
ONETOUCH Ultra
mg/dL
M
C

FIGURE 40.6 OneTouch Ultra glucose monitor. (Courtesy Life Scan.)

Urine Glucose and Ketone Monitoring

Urine also may be tested for glucose and for ketones. Urine glucose testing was done routinely before the development of SMBG. A variety of dipsticks and tape products are available for urine testing. If glucose appears in the urine, the patient is warned that the blood glucose is elevated, but the actual level is unknown. Most people have glucose in their urine when their blood glucose is more than about 180 mg/dL. It is difficult to base treatment on urine glucose levels, and so routine urine testing for glucose is no longer recommended.

Urine should be tested for ketones during acute illness or stress, when blood glucose levels are consistently above 300 mg/dL, during pregnancy, or when symptoms of ketoacidosis are present. If ketones are present, the patient knows an insulin deficiency is present and should notify the physician. Patients with type 1 diabetes are most at risk for developing ketoacidosis; however, it is wise for the patient with type 2 diabetes to test for ketones if risk factors are present.

See Table 40.6 for a review of diabetes symptoms, diagnosis, and treatment.

Transplant

If the patient is determined to be an appropriate candidate, a pancreas transplant may be considered. This is especially beneficial in the patient with kidney disease, who can receive both a kidney and pancreas transplant at the same time. Another promising treatment is the implantation of pancreatic islet cells.

Acute Complications of Diabetes

A person with diabetes is at risk for a variety of complications. Acute complications related to high and low blood glucose levels are treatable and can often be prevented with appropriate care.

Hyperglycemia

When calories eaten exceed insulin available or glucose used, high blood glucose (hyperglycemia) occurs. A common cause of hyperglycemia is eating more than the meal plan prescribes. Another major cause is stress. Stress causes the release of counterregulatory hormones, including epinephrine, cortisol, growth hormone, and glucagon. These hormones all increase the blood glucose level. In a person without diabetes, this is an adaptive function. However, the patient with diabetes is unable to compensate for the increased blood glucose with increased insulin secretion, and hyperglycemia results.

Patients must be able to recognize signs and symptoms of high blood glucose levels and know what to do if they occur (Table 40.7). For many patients, these are similar to the symptoms they experienced when they were first diagnosed with diabetes. Chronic high blood glucose levels can lead to long-term complications (discussed later in this chapter).

Day		Breakfast	Lunch	Supper	Bedtime	Urine Ketones	Notes
Sunday	Time	7:00	11:30	6:00	11:00		
	Glucose	186	108	116	142		
	Insulin	38N, 6R		16N, 2R			
Monday	Time	7:30	12:00	6:00	10:45	6:00-neg	Ate cake at Betty's party at 3 pm-oops!
	Glucose	171	97	302	180		
	Insulin	38N, 6R		16N, 2R			
Tuesday	Time						
	Glucose						
	Insulin						
Wednesday	Time						
	Glucose						
	Insulin						
Thursday	Time						
	Glucose						
	Insulin						
Friday	Time						
	Glucose						
	Insulin						
Saturday	Time						
	Glucose						
	Insulin						

FIGURE 40.7 Sample diary of blood glucose results and insulin use.

TABLE 40.6 DIABETES SUMMARY

Signs and Symptoms	Polyuria Polydipsia Polyphagia Fatigue Blurred vision Headache Abdominal pain
Diagnostic Tests	Fasting plasma glucose HbA_{1c} (glycosylated hemoglobin) Oral glucose tolerance test Additional testing for complications
Therapeutic Measures	Nutrition therapy Exercise Insulin Oral hypoglycemic medication Self-monitoring of blood glucose levels Education
Complications	Hypoglycemia, hyperglycemia Diabetic ketoacidosis, hyperosmolar hyperglycemia Long-term complications
Priority Nursing Diagnosis	*Risk for Unstable Blood Glucose Level*

Hypoglycemia

Low blood glucose, or hypoglycemia, occurs when there is not enough glucose available in relation to circulating insulin. This is sometimes referred to as an insulin reaction. Hypoglycemia is usually defined as a blood glucose level below 50 mg/dL, although patients may feel symptoms at higher or lower levels. Occasionally, symptoms occur as a result of a rapid drop in blood glucose, even though the actual glucose level is normal or high. Causes of hypoglycemia may include skipping a meal, exercising more than usual, or accidentally administering too much insulin. An occasional hypoglycemic episode, treated promptly, should not lead to chronic complications. Repeated or extremely low blood glucose levels can cause neurologic damage because there is not enough glucose for brain function. It is therefore important to teach patients how to prevent and treat low blood glucose (see Table 40.7).

Symptoms of low blood glucose include hunger, sweating, pallor, tremor, palpitations, and headache. These symptoms are caused by activation of the sympathetic nervous system. As hypoglycemia progresses, the brain is deprived of glucose (called neuroglycopenia) and neurologic symptoms such as irritability, confusion, seizures, and coma may occur.

CRITICAL THINKING

Jeff

■ Jeff is a 16-year-old who is having trouble with repeated insulin reactions. He says he has not had this trouble before, and it is interfering with his new job. What questions might you ask as you do your assessment to help him figure out how to prevent future reactions?

Suggested answers at end of chapter.

TABLE 40.7 COMPARISON OF HIGH AND LOW BLOOD GLUCOSE LEVELS

	Hyperglycemia	Hypoglycemia
Causes	Overeating Stress Illness Too little insulin or medication	Undereating, skipping a meal Too much insulin or medication Exercise
Symptoms	Polyuria Polydipsia Polyphagia Blurred vision Headache Lethargy Abdominal pain Ketonuria Coma	Hunger Sweating Tremor Blurred vision Headache Irritability Confusion Seizures Coma
Treatment	Confirm hyperglycemia with glucose meter; if glucose level exceeds 300 mg/dL, check urine for ketones and increase fluid intake. Assess cause of hyperglycemia, and teach prevention. Return to prescribed treatment plan if applicable. Call physician for medication adjustment if indicated or if blood glucose exceeds 180 mg/dL for 2 days. Call physician if patient is ill or vomiting.	Confirm hypoglycemia with glucose meter (if able). Administer 15 g fast-acting carbohydrate. Recheck glucose in 15 minutes. If still low, readminister carbohydrate. Continue cycle of checking glucose and administering fast sugar until hypoglycemia subsides. If symptoms worsen, call physician or emergency help. Administer glucagon subcutaneously or dextrose 50% IV if ordered. Assess cause of hypoglycemia, and teach prevention.

If you find someone with symptoms of altered blood glucose but are unable to identify whether it is high or low, do a blood glucose test. However, if the patient has neurologic symptoms, treat for low blood glucose immediately. The blood glucose may then be checked and further treatment provided as indicated.

To treat low blood glucose, administer a "fast sugar"—15 to 20 grams of carbohydrate that will enter the bloodstream quickly (Box 40.6). This may be 4 oz of orange juice, commercially available glucose tablets, or another quickly available source of sugar. If the patient is not alert or is unable to safely swallow, subcutaneous glucagon can be given. If the patient is hospitalized, intravenous 50% dextrose can be administered by the RN. Recheck the blood glucose in 15 minutes. If it does not return to at least 70 mg/dL, repeat the procedure every 15 minutes until 70 mg/dL is reached—even if the patient is feeling better. Do not overtreat hypoglycemia with too much sugar because this may cause hyperglycemia and rebound hypoglycemia.

Box 40.6

Fast Sugars

- 4 oz orange juice
- 6 oz regular (not diet) soda
- Miniature box of raisins
- Commercial glucose tablets
- 6–8 Life Savers (hard candies)

NURSING CARE TIP

Avoid the temptation to add sugar to orange juice to treat hypoglycemia. Also be sure to avoid giving a fast sugar that has fat in it—this will slow down its digestion and delay recovery of the blood glucose level.

Once the hypoglycemic episode is resolved, the patient should eat a complex carbohydrate to prevent recurrence, unless the next meal is within a half hour. If symptoms worsen instead of improve, call 911, or contact a hospitalized patient's physician. Check hospital or agency policy for the specific protocol for treating hypoglycemic episodes.

Some elderly patients with poor autonomic nervous system function or patients taking beta-adrenergic–blocking medication such as propranolol or atenolol (which block the sympathetic response) may not feel the symptoms of hypoglycemia. These patients should check glucose levels more often and keep the levels in a safe range to prevent hypoglycemic episodes.

Those with diabetes should be instructed to keep a fast sugar in their purse or pocket at all times. Fast sugars may also be stored in bedside tables, cars, and desks at work.

Diabetic Ketoacidosis

PATHOPHYSIOLOGY. Diabetic ketoacidosis (DKA) occurs when blood glucose levels become very high and insulin is deficient. This most commonly occurs in people with type 1 diabetes, but it may occur in type 2 diabetes when insulin deficiency exists. DKA symptoms are often the reason a person with undiagnosed type 1 diabetes first seeks help. It may also be the result of stress or illness in a person with previously diagnosed type 1 (or rarely, type 2) diabetes. When there is insufficient insulin to allow glucose into cells, the cells starve. The body then breaks down fat to be used for energy. The fat breakdown releases an acid substance called ketones. As ketones build up in the blood, ketoacidosis occurs.

The body attempts to compensate for acidosis by deepening respirations, thereby blowing off excess carbon dioxide. (See the section on metabolic acidosis in Chapter 6.) The deep, sighing respiratory pattern is called **Kussmaul's respirations**. The expired air has a fruity odor caused by the ketones and may be mistaken for alcohol. Some nurses have likened the odor to Juicy Fruit chewing gum.

With such high blood glucose and the accompanying polyuria, the body becomes dehydrated very quickly. Tachycardia, hypotension, and shock can result. Acidosis also causes potassium to leave the cells and accumulate in the blood (hyperkalemia). Potassium is then lost in large amounts in the urine, which can lead to hypokalemia. The combination of dehydration, potassium imbalance, and acidosis causes the patient to develop flu-like symptoms, including abdominal pain and vomiting. The patient loses consciousness and death occurs if DKA is not treated. The mortality rate for DKA can be up to 10%.

THERAPEUTIC MEASURES. Treatment includes IV fluids, IV insulin, and blood glucose monitoring, often initially in an intensive care unit (ICU) setting. Glucose is added to the IV when the blood glucose drops to about 180 mg/dL to avoid hypoglycemia. Potassium should also be monitored closely, since it is essential to have normal levels for cardiac function. Arterial blood gases help monitor acidosis. The cause of the DKA should be identified and treated.

Prevention of ketoacidosis involves careful monitoring of blood glucose levels at home. Teach patients to use a urine dipstick to check for ketones (Ketostix) if blood glucose rises above 300 mg/dL. If ketones are present, the patient should drink water and recheck with the next urination. If ketones are still present, the physician should be notified. Instruct patients to never stop their insulin without a physician's supervision.

Hyperosmolar Hyperglycemia

PATHOPHYSIOLOGY. Hyperosmolar hyperglycemia (also called hyperosmolar hyperglycemic nonketotic syndrome, or HHNK) occurs mainly in type 2 diabetes, when blood glucose levels are high as a result of stress or illness. Because the person with type 2 diabetes has some insulin production, cells do not starve and DKA usually does not occur. Hyperosmolar hyperglycemia occurs more often in the elderly.

As the blood glucose level rises (hyperglycemia), polyuria causes profound dehydration, producing the hyperosmolar (concentrated) state. Blood glucose may rise as high as 1500 mg/dL, and electrolyte imbalances occur. Because ketoacidosis is not present, the patient may not feel as physically ill as the patient with DKA and may delay seeking treatment. Symptoms of hyperosmolar hyperglycemia develop slowly and include extreme thirst, lethargy, and mental confusion. Shock, coma, and death occur if it is left untreated. The mortality rate for hyperosmolar hyperglycemia is between 10% and 20%.

THERAPEUTIC MEASURES. Treatment includes IV fluids and insulin, and glucose monitoring. Electrolytes are closely monitored. The cause of hyperosmolar hyperglycemia should be identified and treated. Hyperosmolar hyperglycemia can be prevented with careful monitoring of glucose levels at home. Instruct patients to drink plenty of fluids if blood glucose levels are beginning to rise, especially in times of stress and illness. They should also know when to call their physician with high blood glucose results.

> **NURSING CARE TIP**
>
> Government insurers (Medicare and Medicaid) consider diabetic ketoacidosis, hyperosmolar hyperglycemia, and hypoglycemic coma to be preventable problems and will no longer pay hospitals for the extra expense of caring for patients who develop these conditions after they are in the hospital. You can help control costs by being vigilant for signs and symptoms of these complications and reporting them promptly. The website that lists additional hospital-acquired conditions is www.cms.hhs.gov/HospitalAcqCond/06_Hospital-Acquired_Conditions.asp.

Long-Term Complications

Over time, chronic hyperglycemia causes a variety of serious complications in persons with diabetes. These involve the circulatory system, eyes, kidneys, skin, and nerves. Most of the complications involve either the large blood vessels in the body (macrovascular complications) or the tiny blood vessels, such as those in the eyes or kidneys (microvascular complications). The Diabetes Control and Complications Trial (DCCT), a large classic research study completed in 1993, showed that individuals with type 1 diabetes who maintain tight control of blood glucose experience fewer long-term microvascular complications than individuals who take traditional care of their diabetes (Diabetes Control and Complications Trial Research Group, 1993). Similarly, the United Kingdom Prospective Diabetes Study (UKPDS), completed in 1998, showed that individuals with type 2 diabetes who maintain an HbA_{1c} below 7% can significantly reduce complications. In fact, for every percentage of decrease in HbA_{1c}, there were 25% fewer deaths from diabetes-related complications (U.K. Prospective

Diabetes Study Group, 1998). Unfortunately, tight control can be accompanied by an increased risk of hypoglycemia, and even tight control does not guarantee the prevention of all long-term complications.

Macrovascular Complications

CIRCULATORY SYSTEM. People with diabetes develop atherosclerosis and arteriosclerosis faster than the general population. They are more likely to have hypertension and elevated low-density lipoprotein (LDL) cholesterol and triglyceride levels. High blood glucose also may affect platelet function, leading to increased clotting. These problems lead to a higher incidence of strokes, heart attacks, and poor circulation in the feet and legs. The risk of cardiovascular disease and strokes is two to four times more common in persons with diabetes than in the general population.

Control of blood glucose, blood pressure, and cholesterol levels is vital to help prevent these deadly complications. Patients should also avoid smoking, maintain normal weight, and exercise regularly. All patients should be evaluated for treatment with aspirin or other antiplatelet medication, angiotensin-converting enzyme (ACE) inhibitor therapy, and statin therapy for control of blood lipids.

Microvascular Complications

EYES. Small blood vessels can become diseased, eventually leading to retinopathy in most patients with diabetes. **Retinopathy** involves damage to the tiny blood vessels that supply the eye. Small hemorrhages occur, which can cause blindness if not corrected. Diabetes is the leading cause of blindness in adults in the United States, causing 12,000 to 24,000 new cases each year (CDC, 2007). Newer laser surgery techniques may help improve vision after hemorrhages occur. Diabetes is also associated with a high incidence of cataracts. Patients with diabetes should have a yearly dilated eye examination.

KIDNEYS. Nephropathy is caused by damage to the tiny blood vessels within the kidneys. Up to 40% of patients with diabetes develop some degree of nephropathy. Native Americans, Hispanics, and African Americans have the highest risk. A primary risk factor for diabetic nephropathy is poor control of blood glucose. If nephropathy occurs, the kidneys are unable to remove waste products and excess fluid from the blood. Diabetes is the leading cause of end-stage renal (kidney) disease (ESRD) in the United States. When the kidneys have lost most of their function, patients may have their blood cleansed artificially by either hemodialysis or peritoneal dialysis. (See Chapter 37.) The only cure for ESRD is a kidney transplant.

Patients should be taught the importance of blood glucose control to prevent or delay kidney disease. ACE inhibitor and angiotensin receptor blocker (ARB) medications have been shown to slow the development of kidney problems in patients with diabetes. Patients who have both diabetes and hypertension should be placed on an ACE inhibitor or ARB. Routine urine tests are done to check for microalbuminuria (tiny amounts of protein in the urine) or microalbumin-to-creatinine ratios. If microalbuminuria occurs, a low-protein diet may help delay further development of nephropathy. A trained renal dietitian should work with the patient and physician to determine the best diet for the patient.

Nerve Complications

Another complication of diabetes is **neuropathy**, which is damage to nerves as a result of chronic hyperglycemia. Neuropathy can cause numbness and pain in the extremities, erectile dysfunction (impotence) in men, sexual dysfunction in women, **gastroparesis** (delayed stomach emptying), and other problems. Unfortunately, pain caused by neuropathy is difficult to treat with traditional analgesics. Some antidepressant and anticonvulsant drugs may be helpful, and in some cases local injections of anesthetics may be used. A newer drug, pregabalin (Lyrica), reduces painful nerve impulses and was recently approved by the FDA specifically for nerve pain. Improved control of blood glucose levels may also help.

Infection

Persons with diabetes are prone to infection for several reasons. If injuries occur, healing may be slow because of impaired circulation. There may not be enough blood supply to heal the wound or fight an infection. For the same reason, it may be difficult for IV antibiotics to reach an infected site, and topical antibiotics may be preferable. In the presence of hyperglycemia, white blood cells become sluggish and ineffective, further reducing the body's ability to fight infection.

The incidence of periodontal (gum) disease, caused by bacteria in plaque, is also increased in individuals with diabetes. Patients must be taught to maintain good oral hygiene and make regular visits to the dentist.

Foot Complications

The combination of vascular disease, neuropathy, and risk for infection makes patients with diabetes prone to foot problems. Consider the patient who has no feeling in his or her feet because of neuropathy. If the patient steps on a tack, it may not be felt right away. Vascular disease will prevent a good blood supply from preventing infection and promoting healing. If infection sets in, it is slow to resolve and may progress to necrosis and gangrene. Pressure points on the feet may also break down (Fig. 40.8). One woman had a Bic pen in her shoe all day and did not realize it! Neuropathy can also lead to deformities of the feet, further increasing the risk of injuries.

For these reasons, diabetes is the leading cause of nontraumatic amputation of the lower extremities in the United States (CDC, 2007). Teach patients to protect their feet at all

• WORD • BUILDING •

retinopathy: retino—nervous tissue of the eye + pathy—illness
neuropathy: neuro—nervous system + pathy—illness

• WORD • BUILDING •

nephropathy: nephro—of the kidney + pathy—illness
gastroparesis: gastro—stomach + paresis—partial paralysis

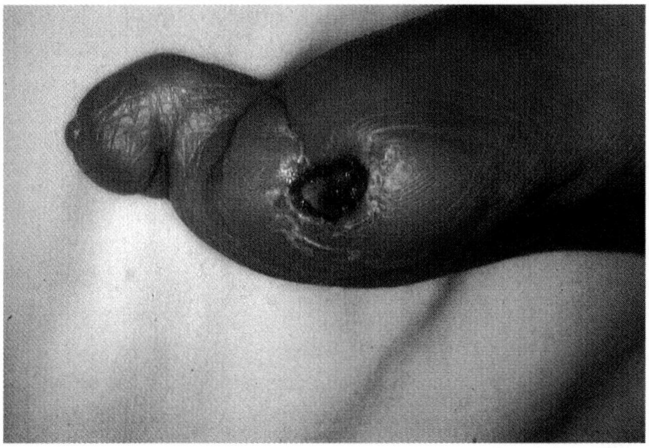

FIGURE 40.8 Diabetic foot ulcer at site of amputated toe. (From Goldsmith, L. A., Lazarus, G. S., & Tharp, M. D. [1997]. *Adult and pediatric dermatology* [p. 438]. Philadelphia: F. A. Davis, with permission.)

times by wearing well-fitting shoes and by washing, drying, and inspecting their feet daily (Box 40.7). If any sores are noted, the patient should not delay in seeking treatment. During routine visits to the physician, teach the patient to be sure to remove shoes and socks so feet can be thoroughly examined. The physician or diabetes specialist can test sensation in the feet with tiny filaments. Loss of protective sensation is an early risk factor for amputation, so any reduction in sensation is a warning sign that extra care must be taken. A podiatrist (foot doctor) can be consulted if problems occur. Specialized wound treatment centers have new healing techniques that have prevented many amputations (Box 40.8, *Ethical Considerations*).

NURSING CARE TIP

Encourage patients to wear white or light-colored socks. One woman did not know she had a wound on her foot till she saw blood coming through her white cotton socks!

CRITICAL THINKING

Mr. Jones

■ Mr. Jones is a 54-year-old banker with type 2 diabetes admitted to your unit with a tiny red area on his right heel. His admitting blood glucose is 360 mg/dL. The lesion is so small you wonder what the fuss is about. While doing his assessment, you find that he wore a new pair of shoes to work all day about a month ago and has been avoiding seeing his physician about the resulting red area. He is placed on IV antibiotics, and within 3 days the red area has broken open and has yellow drainage. He is sent home with topical antibiotics and crutches, to be followed by a visiting nurse. The wound takes 6 months to fully heal.

1. List three risk factors for foot problems.
2. Why did the sore take so long to heal?
3. Why do you think crutches are necessary?
4. Why might topical antibiotics work better than IV antibiotics?
5. The nurse documents the following description of Mr. Jones' wound: "Small red open area on heel, with yellow drainage on dressing." What is wrong with this charting? How can you improve it?

Suggested answers at end of chapter.

Box 40.7

Foot Care Tips

- Wash and dry feet every day. Use warm (not hot) water to avoid burns.
- Apply lotion that does not contain alcohol, avoiding areas between toes.
- Inspect feet for sores or red areas daily (have a family member help if necessary).
- Report any abnormalities immediately.
- Wear leather shoes and white or light-colored cotton socks.
- Never go barefoot.
- Avoid garters and tight socks.
- Avoid crossing legs.
- Cut toenails to natural shape of nail—not into corners.
- See a podiatrist for calluses or problem toenails (avoid "bathroom surgery").
- Have feet checked at least once a year, preferably three to four times a year, for loss of sensation.

Special Considerations for the Patient Undergoing Surgery

Surgery is a stressor. The counterregulatory hormones released during stress cause the blood glucose to rise, even if the patient has been fasting. High blood glucose levels interfere with immune function and healing, and can promote an environment conducive to infection. Some research studies have shown that tight blood glucose control during hospitalization and surgery can significantly reduce complications. Other studies have shown that tight control increases the risk of hypoglycemia and death. In 2009, the ADA and American Association of Clinical Endocrinologists determined that glucose levels in critically ill hospitalized patients should be maintained between 140 and 180 mg/dL, preferably with the use of IV insulin (Moghissi et al., 2009). See the *Nursing Care Plan for the*

Box 40.8

Ethical Considerations

Refusal of Treatment

Mr. Mann is 55 years old and has had diabetes for more than 20 years. He has not managed his diabetes well and has subsequently suffered many complications. Mr. Mann does not regularly test his blood glucose level, so he does not always get the appropriate amount of insulin. In addition, he does not eat properly. He picks up fast food during his lunch break and he binges on various snack foods before he eats his dinner, or sometimes instead of eating his dinner.

Mr. Mann is now dealing with long-term complications of diabetes and is seeking health care because of a neglected leg ulcer. He tried to treat it at home with over-the-counter remedies, but it did not improve, and it is now infected. Part of his foot is gangrenous, and an amputation is recommended. The first time the surgery is mentioned, Mr. Mann becomes outraged and refuses to discuss it. He says he is "not going to leave this earth without all his parts." After further discussions with Mr. Mann, it is clear that he understands the consequences of his condition. He is more annoyed by the drainage from the ulcer than worried about the progressive gangrene. This is a complex case. Questions that should be asked may include these:

- Does Mr. Mann really understand his current situation and likely consequences?
- Can or should Mr. Mann be treated without his permission?
- Can Mr. Mann exercise his autonomy or should a legal guardian be appointed?
- Does disagreement with the medical establishment in itself denote incompetence?
- Does the level of risk if treatment is refused make any difference in the health professional's response?
- What if Mr. Mann's refusal is based on religious or cultural beliefs?
- Should his wishes be supported at all costs?
- What are the nurse's responsibilities?
- How does the application of ethical theory help to sort out the critical elements of this case?

Patient with Diabetes Mellitus, for goals for patients who are not critically ill.

Check with the physician for actual insulin orders. Often patients are placed on intravenous infusions of glucose and insulin during and immediately after surgery, in place of longer acting insulins. Monitor blood glucose levels every 2 to 4 hours or as ordered, and monitor carefully for signs and symptoms of hypoglycemia or hyperglycemia. If a patient uses a pump at home, check with a diabetes resource nurse to determine if the patient can continue to use it during hospitalization.

Patients who were not previously on insulin may be placed on insulin during surgery and postoperatively. They can generally return to their presurgical treatment plan after the stress of surgery is past.

Nursing Process for the Patient with Diabetes Mellitus

Data Collection

A complete nursing history and physical examination should be carried out because diabetes affects every body system. Some areas on which to focus are shown in Table 40.8. It is especially important to assess each patient's knowledge of diabetes and its care so that appropriate teaching can be done.

Nursing Diagnoses, Planning, and Implementation

Because diabetes affects so many different areas, nearly any nursing diagnosis may be appropriate. It is important to assess each patient as an individual and choose diagnoses based on assessment findings. See the *Nursing Care Plan for the Patient with Diabetes Mellitus* for an example of the diagnosis *Risk for Unstable Blood Glucose Level.* The actual presence of the defining characteristics should be confirmed with the patient before choosing any nursing diagnosis.

Once diagnoses have been identified, planning takes place. This should be done with the patient and family. Diabetes affects not only the person with the disease, but the entire family as well. The desired outcomes for the plan of care are for the patient to be knowledgeable about and able to care for his or her disease and to prevent complications. Consult the dietitian, social worker, certified diabetes educator (CDE), home care nurse, outpatient education programs, and other resources as needed (*Home Health Hints*).

Evaluation

The best indicator of the success of a care plan for diabetes is controlled blood glucose and glycohemoglobin within target levels. The patient should also be without symptoms of hypoglycemia or hyperglycemia and be able to state what to do if they do occur. Long-term complications should be minimized. Another important indicator is the patient's statement of satisfaction and comfort with the plan and his or her ability to carry it out on a daily basis.

Diabetes Self-Management Education

The individual with diabetes must receive diabetes self-management education (DSME) if at all possible. No amount of care from a physician or nurse can replace the self-care required of the person with diabetes. The involvement of family or significant others is also important for the successful treatment and well-being of the person with diabetes.

If the patient is hospitalized at diagnosis, the initial instruction is done in the hospital. However, hospital stays are so short, you cannot waste any time. Begin assessing baseline knowledge and teaching as soon as the patient is feeling physically well enough to learn. Depending on your state nurse practice act, this may be the responsibility of the primary

NURSING CARE PLAN for the Patient with Diabetes Mellitus

Nursing Diagnosis: *Risk for Unstable Blood Glucose Level*

Expected Outcomes: The patient will maintain at all times:
- HbA_{1c} less than 7%
- Premeal glucose 70–130 mg/dL
- Postmeal glucose no higher than 180 mg/dL.

Critically ill, hospitalized patient treated with insulin will maintain:
- All blood glucose measurements between 140 and 180 mg/dL.

Non-critically ill, hospitalized patient treated with insulin will maintain:
- Premeal glucose less than 140 mg/dL
- Random glucose less than 180 mg/dL.

(Verify individual goals with physician.)

Evaluation of Outcomes: Are blood glucose levels within predetermined parameters? Does patient show understanding of diabetes self-care?

Interventions	Rationale	Evaluation
Assess knowledge of diabetes self-care.	Teaching should be initiated only if a knowledge deficit exists.	Does patient exhibit knowledge of diabetes self-care?
Assist patient to collaborate with health care provider to determine appropriate blood glucose levels and action to be taken if glucose levels are too high or too low.	Appropriate blood glucose levels may be different for each patient. The patient should know what blood glucose levels require notification of the health care provider.	Does patient state appropriate blood glucose levels and action to take if glucose is high or low?
Teach patient to assess glucose levels before meals and at bedtime or as ordered by health care provider. Ensure that patient knows how to obtain glucose monitor and instruction for home use.	Good blood glucose control depends on knowledge of glucose levels and trends.	Does patient demonstrate correct use of glucose monitor or state how monitor and instruction will be obtained?
In a hospitalized patient who is NPO or on continuous feeding, check glucose level every 4–6 hours around the clock. Check patient on insulin drip every 1–2 hours.	Regular blood glucose monitoring is needed for scale insulin administration and maintaining glucose levels within safe parameters.	Is blood glucose monitoring carried out on an appropriate schedule?
Teach patient how to administer insulin or oral hypoglycemic agent after evaluating blood glucose. Ensure that meals are timed appropriately with medications. Replace any uneaten foods to prevent hypoglycemia.	If most medications are taken without food to supply calories, hypoglycemia can occur. Check individual medication for specific instructions.	Does patient state appropriate meal and medication schedule?
Teach technique for administering insulin if indicated.	The patient and family will be administering insulin independently at home.	Does patient demonstrate correct injection technique?

Continued

NURSING CARE PLAN for the Patient with Diabetes Mellitus—cont'd

Interventions	Rationale	Evaluation
Observe for symptoms of hypoglycemia and hyperglycemia, and treat as needed. Teach causes, prevention, recognition, and treatment of hypoglycemia and hyperglycemia.	If the patient has a good understanding of hypoglycemia and hyperglycemia, most episodes can be prevented. If hypoglycemia or hyperglycemia does occur, prompt treatment is essential to prevent complications.	Does patient state causes, prevention, symptoms, and treatment of hypoglycemia? Does patient carry fast sugar at all times?
Administer 15–20 g glucose or carbohydrate if blood glucose level falls below 70 mg/dL, or according to institution hypoglycemia guidelines.	A "fast sugar" provides prompt treatment of hypoglycemia to prevent complications.	Does "fast sugar" resolve hypoglycemic episode? If not, repeat.
Contact RN or physician if blood glucose is above 180 mg/dL.	Glucose levels over 180 mg/dL are associated with poor outcomes.	Are glucose levels within safe range?
Consult with dietician for nutrition therapy instruction.	The dietitian is trained to provide in-depth meal plan instruction.	Is patient able to state plan for obtaining appropriate meals?
Teach patient on insulin to eat additional complex (not fast-acting) carbohydrate before exercise if glucose is less than 100 mg/dL.	Exercise can further lower blood glucose.	Does patient state appropriate plan for eating additional carbohydrate?
Consult with social worker or case manager as needed.	Some patients may not have the resources or support to carry out effective self-care.	Does patient state availability of adequate resources for self-care at home?
Provide patient with information regarding comprehensive diabetes education. Remind patient that only survival skills have been taught during initial instruction.	Instruction provided in the hospital usually is not comprehensive. Outpatient diabetes classes can provide additional self-care and health promotion information.	Does patient state plan for obtaining further diabetes education after discharge?
Assist patient to obtain medical alert card or tag that identifies diabetes.	If the patient is ever unresponsive for any reason, the health care provider would need to be aware of diabetes condition.	Does patient state plan to carry or wear identification at all times?
	GERIATRIC	
Assess ability to see and manipulate syringe, glucose monitor, and other equipment. Obtain assistive devices as needed.	The older adult patient may have poor eyesight or other sensory deficits.	Is patient able to manipulate equipment to safely care for self?

Home Health Hints

- Patients with newly diagnosed diabetes may be anxious and overwhelmed. Instruction may need to be repeated several times before they understand.
- Some home glucose monitoring devices have a memory that the nurse can access during the visit. It gives the date, time, and blood glucose result. This is a good indication of compliance with self-monitoring performed by patient or caregiver.
- Assist your patients in obtaining the necessary supplies to manage their diabetes. Many medical supply companies can deliver these supplies to the home. Work with your agency to identify reliable companies in your area.
- Remember to call the patient the day before performing a venipuncture for a fasting blood glucose and remind him or her not to eat after midnight.
- Older patients tend to skip meals. Assist them to identify easy but nutritious meals, such as frozen dinners that are low in sodium. Another option is Meals-on-Wheels, which is able to deliver meals that are tailored to special diets.
- Prefilled syringes should be stored in the refrigerator flat or with needles pointing up. This prevents crystals from settling and clogging the needles. Allow syringes to come to room temperature before injecting.
- Patients can discard used syringes and needles in a hard plastic container such as a Clorox bottle with a screw top if red needle boxes are not available.
- If the patient has a visual or dexterity problem, suggest a syringe magnifier (check with the pharmacy) or a prefilled insulin pen.
- Help the patient learn to use a mirror to look at the bottom of the feet or have a family member examine the patient's feet. The patient should remove shoes and socks at each physician visit for a thorough foot inspection. Catching a "red spot" early is the goal.
- Instruct the patient on the importance of wearing comfortable shoes. The patient should avoid sandals, high heels, flip flops, or ill-fitting shoes. If necessary, the physician can request a podiatry consult. A podiatrist can arrange for the patient to be measured and fitted with special shoes that properly fit his or her feet. Special shoes may be covered by Medicare.
- The patient should keep a pair of nonskid slippers at the bedside. If the patient needs to get up in the night to use the restroom, putting on secure slippers can help prevent the possibility of stepping on something and causing a foot injury.
- Due to decreased skin sensation in some persons with diabetes, hot water heaters should be set below 120°F (48.8°C).
- Even if patients have had diabetes for many years, observe them preparing and injecting their insulin. This provides an opportunity to praise good technique or correct bad habits.
- Diabetic patients with vision problems can become isolated and depressed. Assist your patient with obtaining vision aids that can help improve social outlets. Many communities have stores that specialize in low-vision products, such as a magnifier that attaches to a computer. This can help them gain some independence and facilitate communication with family and friends via e-mail, or they can join an online support group to share experiences and discuss feelings with others who have similar physical ailments.

TABLE 40.8 DATA COLLECTION FOR THE PATIENT WITH DIABETES MELLITUS

Subjective Data	• Age and symptoms at onset • Understanding of diabetes (type 1 or type 2) and self-care • Current treatment plan (medication, nutrition therapy, exercise) and adherence to plan • Frequency of blood glucose self-monitoring, and pattern of blood glucose levels (check diary if patient has kept one) • History of diabetes-related complications • Involvement of family or other support systems
Objective Data	• Vital signs • Height, weight, body mass index • Skin: integrity, turgor, condition of injection sites • Feet: pulses, color, temperature, skin integrity, pressure points, sensation • Laboratory results: blood glucose, HbA_{1c}, creatinine, lipid profile, albuminuria, urine and serum ketones

or registered nurse, although aspects of the instruction may be delegated to the LPN/LVN. Some hospitals have a certified diabetes educator (CDE) who provides classroom or bedside instruction. The dietitian should be contacted to provide nutrition instruction.

Most hospitals have policies or management plans describing the instruction to be provided by the nurse. Generally this encompasses "survival skills," which include the basic information the patient needs initially to survive at home. Survival skills include medication administration, glucose monitoring, meal plan basics, and what to do if high or low blood glucose levels occur. A variety of helpful aids, such as pamphlets and videos, are available. Diabetes equipment suppliers provide kits that are full of samples and information. These are a significant help when you are teaching a patient. Also advise the patient to purchase a medical alert bracelet or necklace.

It is difficult to know how to operate and teach glucose monitoring with the variety of glucose monitors available. Many drugstores and medical supply stores not only sell the monitors but also provide training for the patient and family. You can obtain this information by calling local medical suppliers or by contacting the diabetes educator or discharge planner at your institution.

After discharge, the patient should be referred to outpatient diabetes classes for further instruction. If classes are unavailable or if the patient is unable to leave home, a referral to a visiting nurse should be made. It is usually advisable to have a nurse present for the patient's first insulin injection at home. The ADA recommends that DSME include information about the following:

- Disease process and treatment options
- Nutritional management
- Incorporating physical activity into lifestyle
- Using medications safely
- Monitoring blood glucose and using results
- Preventing, detecting, and treating acute complications
- Preventing, detecting, and treating chronic complications
- Personal strategies for psychosocial adjustment
- Personal strategies for health promotion and behavior change (Funnell et al., 2009).

Two websites that might be helpful to both you and your patients are www.diabetes.org and www.lifeclinic.com/focus/diabetes/resources.asp.

Because many people with diabetes are elderly, it is important to be aware of their special needs (Box 40.9, *Gerontological Issues*).

> **Box 40.9**
> ## Gerontological Issues
> Diabetes care can be a challenge for many older adults. Syringe magnifiers and talking glucose meters are available for those with impaired vision. Family members may be taught to draw up a week's supply of insulin for the patient to store in the refrigerator. Family members should also be able to recognize signs and symptoms of hypo- and hyperglycemia. Home meal programs may help ensure an adequate diet. Older adults should also have an emergency call system in their home and regular contact with family members or other support people.

REACTIVE HYPOGLYCEMIA

Reactive hypoglycemia occurs when the blood glucose drops below a normal level, usually below 70 mg/dL. Hypoglycemia is most often a complication of diabetes treatment, but at times it may occur without the presence of diabetes. It may be a warning sign of impending diabetes.

Pathophysiology and Etiology

Low blood glucose may occur as an overreaction of the pancreas to eating. The pancreas senses the blood glucose level rising and produces more insulin than is necessary for the use of that glucose. As a result, the blood glucose drops to below normal. It may be due to abnormally low levels of glucagon, or alternatively, it may be due to high levels of insulin. Some experts believe that this is a rare condition and that many "hypoglycemic" episodes are due to activation of the sympathetic nervous system for other reasons, without true hypoglycemia.

Signs and Symptoms

Low blood glucose causes release of epinephrine, which in turn causes the blood glucose to rise. Epinephrine release causes a fight-or-flight reaction, which may produce shaking, sweating, and palpitations. Headache, chills, and confusion may also occur. Symptoms are the same as those described earlier related to hypoglycemia in diabetes.

Diagnosis

Diagnosis is often based on a 5-hour glucose tolerance test, with below-normal readings between 2 and 5 hours. However, with the availability of home glucose monitors, it is now preferable for patients to monitor blood glucose levels at home. Readings should be taken in the morning on arising, 2 hours after each meal, at bedtime, and during symptoms of hypoglycemia. These results may then be taken to the physician for interpretation.

Therapeutic Measures

Treatment includes frequent small meals and avoidance of fasting. Simple sugars are avoided because they may aggravate symptoms. High-fiber foods, complex carbohydrates, and proteins are recommended. See Table 40.9 for a sample diet.

TABLE 40.9 SAMPLE MEAL PLAN FOR HYPOGLYCEMIC DIET

Exchange Group	Sample Menu
Morning	
1 fruit	1/2 cup unsweetened orange juice
1 starch	3/4 cup whole-grain cereal
1 meat	1 oz low-fat cheese or meat
1/2 skim milk	1/2 cup skim milk
Free	Decaffeinated coffee
Midmorning	
1 meat	1 tbsp peanut butter
1 starch	4 whole-grain crackers
Noon	
Chef salad:	
2–4 meat	2–4 oz lean meat
1 vegetable	Lettuce, tomatoes
1 fat	Dressing
1 fruit	1 small piece fresh fruit
1 skim milk	1 cup skim milk
1 starch	2 breadsticks (4 × 1/2 in.)
Midafternoon	
1 meat	1 oz low-fat cheese
1 starch	4 whole-grain crackers
Evening	
2–4 meat	2–4 oz lean meat
1 starch	1/2 cup potato or pasta
1 vegetable	1/2 cup vegetable
1 fat	Lettuce salad with dressing
1 fruit	1 piece fresh fruit
Free	Decaffeinated coffee or tea
Bedtime	
1 starch and 1 meat	1/2 sandwich (1 slice whole-grain bread and 1 oz lean meat)
1 vegetable	Fresh vegetables
Free	Decaffeinated beverage

ETHICAL CONSIDERATIONS DISCUSSION

The principles of autonomy, nonmaleficence, and beneficence come into play in this case. Preservation of the patient's autonomy regardless of personal feelings or even mounting evidence is paramount. The only exceptions are when the patient is not making decisions based on sound and accurate information (does he really know what to expect should he refuse treatment?) or when the patient can be considered not of sound mind. In this case, there is no evidence that Mr. Mann is not of sound mind. We all make decisions that may appear to others to be unwise, but it is a basic human right to make such decisions.

The principles of "do good" and "do no harm" have significant application in this case. If the patient's wishes are upheld, the respect for autonomy means that the patient's integrity and humanity have been respected. If the patient's wishes are overridden and he is forcibly subjected to treatment "for his own good," then the patient is harmed at a fundamental level because there has been infringement of basic human rights. The role of the patient as an active participant in treatment planning must be protected. If the patient is forced to have the treatment against his will, the outcome for the patient's foot may be good but his basic rights have been violated.

SUGGESTED ANSWERS TO CRITICAL THINKING

■ *Mr. McMillan*

1. "Have you been eating or drinking more than usual? Have you been urinating more than usual? Do you get up at night to urinate? How is your appetite? Does anyone in your family have diabetes?"
2. Fatigue occurs because the glucose is unable to enter the cells without insulin, so they are starving.
3. Mr. McMillan is dehydrated because he is losing excessive amounts of urine as his kidneys lose excess glucose.

■ *Mrs. Evans*

1. Mrs. Evans should take her insulin no earlier than 7:30 a.m., 30 minutes before eating.
2. She should be alert for low blood glucose at midafternoon to just before supper. Although her insulin peaks between 1:30 and 7:30 p.m., her chances of having a hypoglycemic episode are slim once she has eaten her supper.
3. If she misses a meal, her blood glucose will drop further, increasing her risk of a hypoglycemic episode.

■ *Jeff*

What kind of new job is it? What schedule is he working? Is it more physically strenuous than his previous job? Does it interfere with his usual meal schedule? What other changes has he experienced in his life that may have affected his blood glucose?

■ *Mr. Jones*

1. Poor circulation, neuropathy, and slow wound healing place Mr. Jones at risk for problems.
2. Circulation to the foot may be poor, and white blood cells are sluggish if the blood glucose is high.
3. Any pressure on the foot while walking may further impair circulation. He should not bear weight on the affected foot.
4. If circulation to the area is poor, IV antibiotics may not reach the sore.
5. "Small red open area on right posterior heel, 1 cm × 1.5 cm, 2 mm deep, 2-cm area of yellow drainage on dressing." In addition, many agencies are now taking instant photos of wounds to include in the chart. If no camera is available, a drawing of the size and shape is helpful.

REVIEW QUESTIONS

1. Which of the following is the best definition of diabetes mellitus?
   a. It is a disease in which high blood glucose results from defective insulin secretion or action.
   b. It is a disease that causes polyuria and polydipsia.
   c. It is a disease characterized by macrovascular and microvascular complications.
   d. It is a complex disease of protein and fat metabolism.

2. Which of the following is a risk factor for type 2 diabetes mellitus?
   a. Cardiovascular disease
   b. Obesity
   c. Age younger than 40 years
   d. Virus exposure

3. Diabetes is diagnosed when the fasting blood glucose is greater than ____ mg/dL.

4. Which of the following symptoms is most commonly associated with hyperglycemia?
   a. Tremor
   b. Flank pain
   c. Sweating
   d. Polyuria

5. Protein in the urine is a sign of which long-term complication of diabetes?
   a. Nephropathy
   b. Neuropathy
   c. Retinopathy
   d. Gastroparesis

REVIEW QUESTIONS—cont'd

6. What is the best way for patients to avoid long-term complications of diabetes?
   a. See the doctor for a complete checkup every 6 months.
   b. Check feet daily.
   c. Maintain premeal blood glucose levels under 130 mg/dL.
   d. Follow a strict meal plan for diabetes.

7. Which breakfast menu is most appropriate for a patient with diabetes?
   a. Two eggs, two strips bacon, orange juice, coffee
   b. Oatmeal with artificial sweetener, whole-grain toast, tea
   c. One half grapefruit, cranberry juice, bagel with sugar-free jelly
   d. One slice whole-grain toast with peanut butter, skim milk, orange juice

8. Place the steps for mixing insulin in correct sequential order.
   a. Draw up cloudy insulin.
   b. Draw up clear insulin.
   c. Roll cloudy vial.
   d. Inject air into cloudy insulin.
   e. Inject air into clear insulin.
   f. Clean vial tops with alcohol.

9. For which of the following blood glucose results would the nurse administer a fast sugar?
   a. 48
   b. 80
   c. 126
   d. 223

10. A patient who is preparing for surgery asks the nurse why his physician took him off his oral hypoglycemic and placed him on sliding-scale insulin. Which response by the nurse is best?
    a. "It helps us maintain better control of your blood glucose during surgery. You will most likely be back on your pills before you go home."
    b. "The stress of surgery often exacerbates diabetes. We will teach you how to give insulin before you go home."
    c. "Oral hypoglycemics are ineffective during times of stress. Insulin is the only way to keep your blood glucose under control."
    d. "The oral agents must not be controlling your blood glucose any longer. I will check and see which insulin you will be going home on."

11. Which meal plan is best for the patient with reactive hypoglycemia?
    a. High-carbohydrate meals
    b. Small, frequent meals
    c. Avoidance of fats and proteins
    d. Three medium to large meals daily

References

American Diabetes Association. (2009). Standards of medical care in diabetes—2009. *Diabetes Care, 32*(Suppl 1), S13–S61.

Centers for Disease Control and Prevention. (2007). *National diabetes fact sheet.* Retrieved June 2, 2009, from http://www.cdc.gov/diabetes/pubs/estimates07.htm

Diabetes Control and Complications Trial Research Group. (1993). The effect of intensive treatment of diabetes on the development and progression of long-term complications in insulin-dependent diabetes mellitus. *New England Journal of Medicine, 329,* 14.

Diabetes Prevention Program Research Group. (2002). Reduction in the incidence of type 2 diabetes with lifestyle modification or metformin. *New England Journal of Medicine, 346*(6), 393–403.

Funnell, M. M., Brown, T. L., Childs, B. P., et al. (2009). National standards for diabetes self-management education. *Diabetes Care, 32*(Suppl 1), S87–S94.

Moghissi, E. S., Korytkowski, M. T., DiNardo, M., et al. (2009). American Association of Clinical Endocrinologists and American Diabetes Association consensus statement on inpatient glycemic control. *Endocrine Practice, 15*(4), 1–17.

National Institutes of Health. (2001). *National cholesterol education program: ATP III guidelines at-a-glance quick desk reference* (NIH Publication No. 01-3305). Retrieved June 2, 2009, from http://www.nhlbi.nih.gov/guidelines/cholesterol/atglance.pdf

U.K. Prospective Diabetes Study Group. (1998). Intensive blood-glucose control with sulphonylureas or insulin compared with conventional treatment and risk of complications in patients with type 2 diabetes. *Lancet, 352,* 837.

unit ELEVEN

UNDERSTANDING THE GENITOURINARY AND REPRODUCTIVE SYSTEM

41 Genitourinary and Reproductive System Function and Assessment

LAURA L. McCULLY
AND JANICE L. BRADFORD

KEY TERMS

adnexa (ad-NECK-sah)
bimanual (by-MAN-yoo-uhl)
circumcised (SIR-kum-sized)
colposcopy (kul-PAHS-koh-pee)
conization (KOH-ni-ZAY-shun)
culdoscopy (kul-DOSS-kuh-pee)
curet (kyoo-RET)
cystic (SISS-tik)
ejaculation (ee-JACK-yoo-LAY-shun)
epispadias (EP-ih-SPAY-dee-ahz)
erection (ee-RECK-shun)
gravida (GRAV-vid-ah)
gynecomastia (JY-neh-koh-MASS-tee-ah)
hydrocele (HEYE-droh-seel)
hypospadias (HY-poh-SPAY-dee-ahz)
hysterosalpingogram (HISS-tur-oh-SAL-pinj-oh-gram)
hysteroscopy (HISS-tur-AW-skoh-pee)
insufflation (in-suff-LAY-shun)
libido (lih-BEE-doh)
mammography (mah-MAW-grah-fee)
menarche (meh-NAR-kee)
menopause (MEN-oh-pawz)
orgasm (OR-gazm)
para (PAR-ah)
salpingoscopy (SAL-ping-JOSS-koh-pee)
transillumination (TRANS-ih-loo-mih-NAY-shun)
varicocele (VAR-ih-koh-seel)

QUESTIONS TO GUIDE YOUR READING

1. What is the normal anatomy of the reproductive system?
2. What are the normal functions of the reproductive system?
3. What are the effects of aging on the reproductive system?
4. What data should you collect when caring for a patient with a disorder of the reproductive system?
5. Which diagnostic tests are commonly performed to diagnose disorders of the reproductive system?
6. What nursing care should you provide for patients undergoing each of the diagnostic tests?

NORMAL GENITOURINARY AND REPRODUCTIVE SYSTEM ANATOMY AND PHYSIOLOGY

The male and female reproductive systems produce gametes (sperm and egg cells [ova]) and facilitate the union of gametes in fertilization following sexual intercourse. Ideally, the uterus provides the site for the developing embryo/fetus until birth.

Female Reproductive System

The female reproductive system consists of paired ovaries and fallopian tubes, a single uterus and vagina, and external genitalia (Fig. 41.1). The mammary glands may be considered accessory organs to the system.

Ovaries

The ovaries are a pair of oval structures, about 5 cm long and 2.5 cm wide, located on either side of the uterus in the pelvic cavity (Fig. 41.2). The ovarian ligament extends from the medial side of the ovary to the uterine wall, and the broad ligament of the uterus is a fold of the peritoneum that also attaches to the ovaries. These ligaments help keep the ovaries in place.

The ovaries produce egg cells by the process of meiosis, more specifically called oogenesis, which begins fetally and continues through puberty, then ends at menopause, usually occurring between the ages of 45 and 55. This process is cyclical in that usually one mature ovum is produced and released every 28 days and is under hormonal control (covered in the section on the menstrual cycle). The follicles of the ovary produce the hormone estrogen and later, as the corpus luteum, secrete progesterone as well.

Fallopian Tubes

Each fallopian, or uterine, tube is about 10 cm long. The lateral end with its fringe-like fimbriae approaches but does not touch the ovary, and the medial end attaches and opens into the uterus. The fallopian tube is lined with ciliated epithelium; in the wall is smooth muscle. The sweeping of the cilia and the peristaltic contractions of the smooth muscle usually ensure that the ovum (called a *zygote* after fertilization) will reach the uterus. Fertilization usually takes place within the fallopian tube, and the zygote is swept into the uterus within 4 to 5 days.

Uterus

The uterus is a muscular organ about 8 cm long and 5 cm wide. It is superior to the urinary bladder and medial to the ovaries in the pelvic cavity. Ligaments help keep the uterus in place, tilted forward over the top of the bladder. During pregnancy the uterus increases greatly in size and contains the placenta, which nourishes the embryo (later called the fetus). It expels the infant near the end of gestation.

The fundus of the uterus is the upper portion above where the fallopian tubes enter laterally. The body is the large central portion. The cervix is the narrow, inferior portion, which opens into the vagina. The uterus is divided into

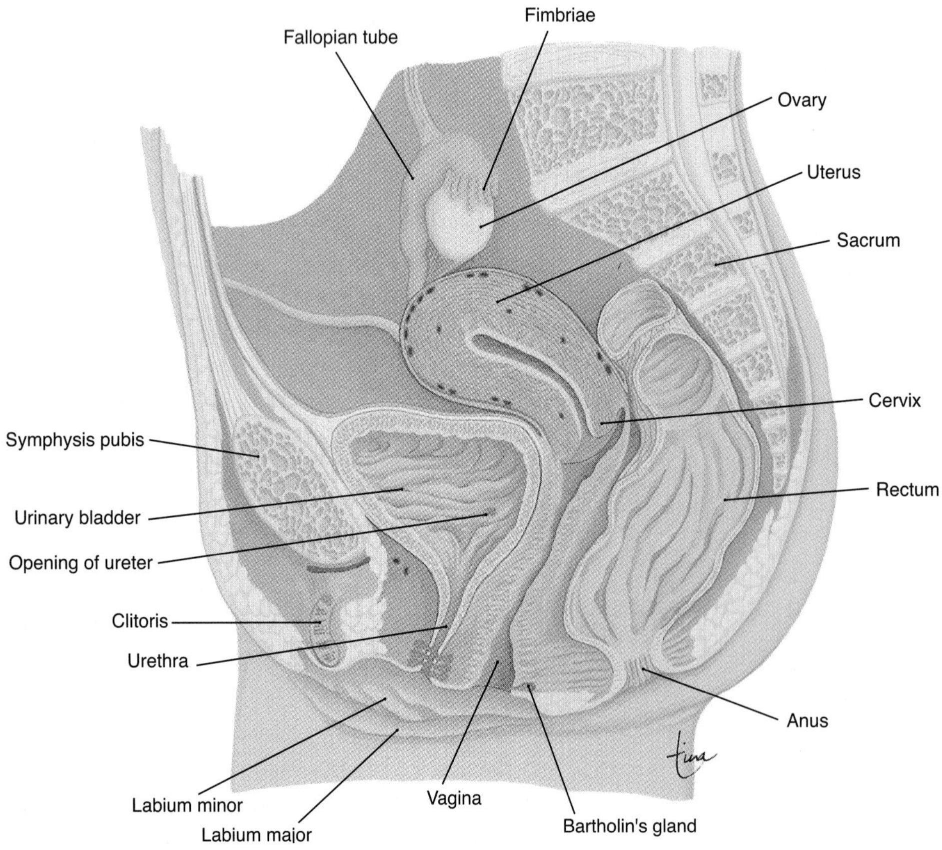
Fimbriae
Fallopian tube
Ovary
Uterus
Sacrum
Cervix
Rectum
Symphysis pubis
Urinary bladder
Opening of ureter
Clitoris
Urethra
Anus
Labium minor
Labium major
Vagina
Bartholin's gland

FIGURE 41.1 Female reproductive system in a midsagittal section. (From Scanlon, V. C., & Sanders, T. [2007]. *Essentials of anatomy and physiology* [5th ed.]. Philadelphia: F. A. Davis, with permission.)

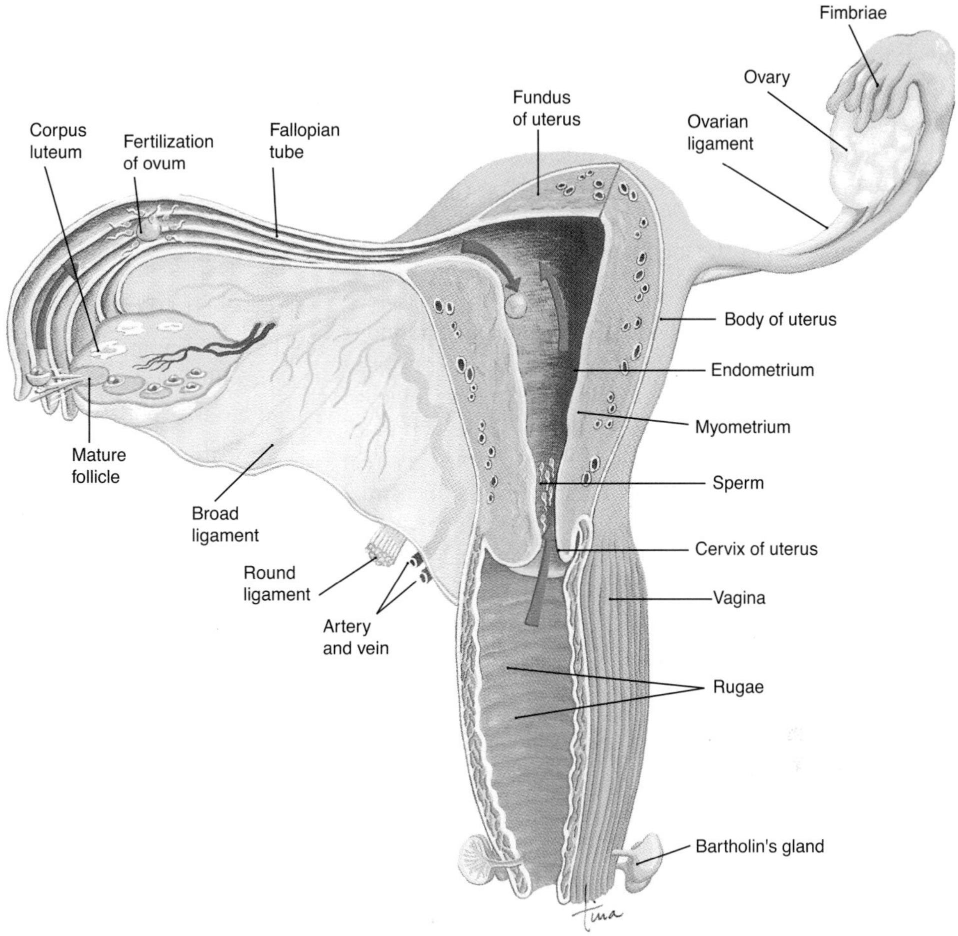
Fimbriae
Ovary
Fundus
of uterus
Ovarian
ligament
Corpus
luteum
Fertilization
of ovum
Fallopian
tube
Body of uterus
Endometrium
Myometrium
Mature
follicle
Sperm
Broad
ligament
Cervix of uterus
Round
ligament
Vagina
Artery
and vein
Rugae
Bartholin's gland

FIGURE 41.2 Female reproductive system in an anterior view and a longitudinal section. (From Scanlon, V. C., & Sanders, T. [2007]. *Essentials of anatomy and physiology* [5th ed.]. Philadelphia: F. A. Davis, with permission.)

three layers. The external layer of the uterine wall is the perimetrium, a fold of the visceral peritoneum. The myometrium is the middle, smooth muscle layer. During pregnancy the myometrial cells increase in size to accommodate the growing fetus, and during labor and delivery, oxytocin causes coordinated contractions of this middle layer to expel the fetus.

The lining of the uterus is called the endometrium, and it is a highly vascular mucous membrane, part of which is lost and regenerated with each menstrual cycle. During pregnancy, the endometrium helps in forming the maternal side of the placenta.

Vagina

The vagina is a muscular tube about 7 to 10 cm long that extends from the cervix to the vaginal orifice in the perineum. It is between the urethra and the rectum. The functions of the vagina are to receive sperm from the penis during sexual intercourse, to serve as the exit for menstrual blood flow, and to serve as the birth canal at the end of pregnancy.

After puberty, the vaginal mucosa is relatively resistant to infection. The normal bacterial flora of the vagina creates an acidic pH, which retards microbial growth. Prior to puberty, the hymen, a fold of mucous membrane, provides mechanical protection.

External Genitals

Also called the vulva, the female external genital structures are the clitoris, mons pubis, labia majora and minora, and Bartholin's glands. The clitoris is a small mass of erectile tissue, approximately 6 mm long, anterior to the urethral orifice. Its function is sensory; it responds to sexual stimulation, and its vascular sinuses become filled with blood.

The mons pubis is a pad of fat over the pubic bones that is covered with skin and pubic hair. Extending posteriorly from the mons are the lateral labia majora and the medial labia minora; these are paired folds of skin. The area between the labia minora is the vestibule; it contains the openings of the urethra and vagina. The labia cover these openings and prevent drying of their mucous membranes. Bartholin's glands, also called vestibular glands, are within the floor and at the base of the vestibule. Their ducts open into the mucosa at the vaginal orifice. Their secretion keeps the mucosa moist and lubricates the vagina during sexual intercourse.

Mammary Glands

Enclosed within the breasts and surrounded by adipose tissue, the mammary glands produce milk after pregnancy. The milk enters the lactiferous ducts, which converge at the nipple. The skin around the nipple is a pigmented area called the areola. The formation of milk occurs secondary to hormonal influence. During pregnancy, high levels of estrogen and progesterone prepare the glands for milk production. Prolactin from the anterior pituitary causes the production of milk after pregnancy. The sucking of the infant on the nipple stimulates the release of oxytocin from the posterior pituitary gland, which in turn stimulates the release of milk as well as contraction of the uterine muscle.

The Menstrual Cycle

The menstrual cycle depends on follicle-stimulating hormone (FSH) and luteinizing hormone (LH) from the anterior pituitary gland, estrogen from the ovaries and ovarian follicles, and progesterone from the corpus luteum. These hormones bring about changes in the ovaries and uterus. The ovarian cycle may be described in terms of three phases: menstrual phase, follicular phase, and luteal phase.

The menstrual phase involves the loss of the endometrium during menstruation, which may last 2 to 8 days, with an average duration of 5 days. At this time, secretion of FSH is increasing and several ovarian follicles, each with a potential ovum, begin to develop. Table 41.1 includes a summary of these hormones.

During the follicular phase, FSH stimulates growth of ovarian follicles and secretion of estrogen by the follicle cells. The secretion of LH also increases, but more slowly. FSH and estrogen promote the growth and maturation of the ovum, and estrogen stimulates the growth of blood vessels to regenerate the endometrium. This phase ends with ovulation, when a sharp increase in LH causes rupture of a mature ovarian follicle and an egg is released.

During the luteal phase, LH causes the ruptured follicle to become the corpus luteum, which begins to secrete progesterone in addition to estrogen. Progesterone stimulates further growth of blood vessels in the endometrium and promotes the storage of nutrients such as glycogen. As progesterone secretion increases, LH secretion decreases, and if the ovum is not fertilized, the secretion of progesterone also begins to decrease. Without progesterone, the endometrium cannot be maintained and begins to slough off in menstruation. FSH secretion begins to increase (as estrogen and progesterone decrease), and the cycle begins again. Although an average cycle is 28 days, cycles of 23 to 35 days may also be considered normal.

Male Reproductive System

The male reproductive system consists of the testes and a series of ducts and glands. Sperm are produced in the testes and are transported through the reproductive ducts: epididymis, ductus deferens, ejaculatory duct, and urethra (Fig. 41.3). The reproductive glands are the seminal vesicles, prostate gland, and bulbourethral glands, all of which produce secretions that become part of semen.

Testes

The testes are located in the scrotum between the upper thighs, where the temperature is slightly lower than body temperature, which is necessary for the production of viable sperm. Each testis is about 5 cm long and 3 cm wide and contains the seminiferous tubules in which spermatogenesis (meiosis) takes place. In contrast to oogenesis, once started at puberty, spermatogenesis is a constant rather than cyclical process and usually continues throughout life. Also in the testes are specialized cells that produce the hormones testosterone and inhibin. Spermatogenesis is initiated by FSH from the anterior pituitary. LH from the anterior pituitary stimulates the secretion of testosterone, which contributes to the maturation of sperm. The secretion of inhibin is stimulated by testosterone; inhibin decreases the secretion of FSH, which helps keep the rate of spermatogenesis fairly constant. The functions of these hormones are summarized in Table 41.2.

TABLE 41.1 HORMONES OF FEMALE REPRODUCTION

Hormone	Secreted By	Functions
Follicle-stimulating hormone	Anterior pituitary	Initiates development of ovarian follicles Stimulates secretion of estrogen by follicle cells
Luteinizing hormone	Anterior pituitary	Causes ovulation Converts ruptured ovarian follicle into corpus luteum Stimulates secretion of progesterone by corpus luteum
Estrogen	Ovary (follicle) Placenta	Promotes maturation of ovarian follicles Promotes growth of blood vessels in endometrium Initiates development of secondary sex characteristics Promotes growth of duct system of mammary glands
Progesterone	Ovary (corpus luteum) Placenta	Promotes further growth of blood vessels in endometrium Inhibits contractions of the myometrium during pregnancy Promotes growth of secretory cells of mammary glands
Inhibin	Ovary (corpus luteum)	Decreases secretion of FSH toward end of cycle
Prolactin	Anterior pituitary	Promotes production of milk after birth
Oxytocin	Posterior pituitary	Promotes release of milk

Source: Scanlon, V. C., & Sanders, T. (2007). *Essentials of anatomy and physiology* (5th ed.). Philadelphia: F. A. Davis, with permission.

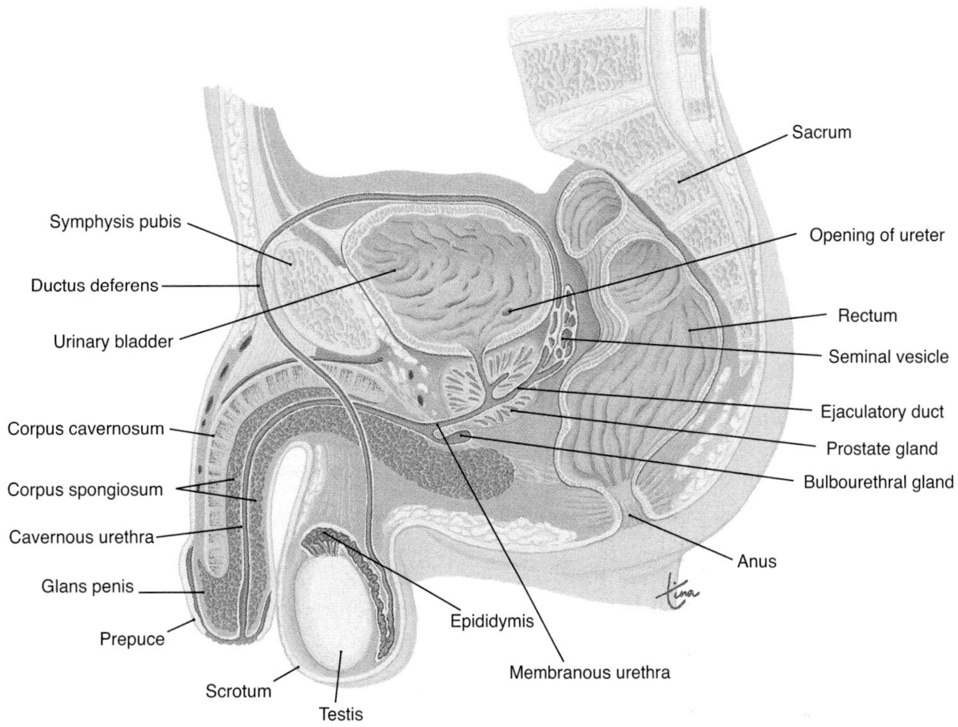
Sacrum
Symphysis pubis
Opening of ureter
Ductus deferens
Rectum
Urinary bladder
Seminal vesicle
Ejaculatory duct
Corpus cavernosum
Prostate gland
Bulbourethral gland
Corpus spongiosum
Cavernous urethra
Anus
Glans penis
Epididymis
Prepuce
Membranous urethra
Scrotum
Testis

FIGURE 41.3 Male reproductive system in a midsagittal section. (From Scanlon, V. C., & Sanders, T. [2007]. *Essentials of anatomy and physiology* [5th ed.]. Philadelphia: F. A. Davis, with permission.)

The head of the sperm cell contains 23 chromosomes, and has an acrosome on the tip that contains enzymes to digest the membrane of the egg cell during fertilization. Attached to the head is a midpiece with high numbers of mitochondria, and attached to the midpiece is a flagellum, which provides motility. Sperm from all the seminiferous tubules of a testis pass through tubules leading to the epididymis.

Epididymis, Ductus Deferens, and Ejaculatory Ducts

The epididymis is a tube about 6 meters long that is coiled on the posterior side of a testis. Smooth muscle within its wall propels sperm from the testes into the ductus deferens.

Also called the vas deferens, the ductus deferens extends from the epididymis in the scrotum to the ejaculatory duct within the pelvic cavity. Exterior to the body, the ductus deferens is contained within the spermatic cord, a connective tissue sheath. Testicular blood vessels and nerves share the spermatic cord; and the cord opens into the abdominopelvic wall at the inguinal canal. Within the pelvic cavity, the ductus deferens loops over the ureter and extends down the posterior side of the urinary bladder to join the ejaculatory duct.

Each of the two ejaculatory ducts receives sperm from the ductus deferens and the secretion of the seminal vesicle on its own side. Both ejaculatory ducts propel sperm and seminal secretions through the urethra.

Seminal Vesicles, Prostate Gland, and Bulbourethral Glands

The paired seminal vesicles are posterior to the urinary bladder. Their secretion is alkaline and contains fructose, prostaglandins, and clotting proteins. The alkalinity neutralizes the urethra and the acidic environment of the female reproductive tract. The fructose is used for adenosine triphosphate (ATP) production, the prostaglandins enhance motility, and the clotting proteins coagulate the semen after ejaculation. The duct of a seminal vesicle joins the ductus deferens laterally to form the ejaculatory duct.

TABLE 41.2 HORMONES OF MALE REPRODUCTION

Hormone	Secreted By	Functions
Follicle-stimulating hormone	Anterior pituitary	Initiates production of sperm in the testes
Luteinizing hormone	Anterior pituitary	Stimulates secretion of testosterone by the testes
Testosterone	Testes	Promotes maturation of sperm Initiates development of male secondary sex characteristics
Inhibin	Testes	Decreases secretion of FSH to maintain a constant rate of spermatogenesis

Source: Scanlon, V. C., & Sanders, T. (2007). *Essentials of anatomy and physiology* (5th ed.). Philadelphia: F. A. Davis, with permission.

The prostate surrounds the first 2 to 3 cm of the urethra as it emerges from the urinary bladder. The secretion of the prostate is alkaline and contributes to sperm motility. The bulbourethral glands are located below the prostate gland and empty into the urethra. Their alkaline secretion coats the interior of the urethra just before ejaculation, which neutralizes any acidic urine that might be present.

The alkaline secretions of the male reproductive glands work to ensure that many sperm remain viable in the acidic environment of the vagina. The normal bacterial flora of the vagina create the acidic pH, but the pH of semen is about 7.4 and permits sperm to remain motile.

Urethra and Penis

The urethra is the last of the male reproductive ducts, and its longest portion is within the penis. The penis is an external genital organ; its distal end is called the glans penis and when uncircumcised is covered with a fold of skin called the prepuce, or foreskin. Within the penis are three layers of erectile or cavernous tissue. Each consists of a framework of smooth muscle and connective tissue that contains blood sinuses, which are large, irregular vascular channels.

When blood flow through these sinuses is minimal, the penis is flaccid (soft). Sexual stimulation causes the arterioles of the penis to dilate; the sinuses fill with blood, and the penis becomes erect and firm. This is brought about by parasympathetic impulses. The culmination of sexual stimulation is **ejaculation** (the expelling of semen from the urethra with force), which is brought about by peristalsis of the reproductive ducts and contraction of the prostate gland.

Aging and the Reproductive System

For women, there is a definite end to reproductive capability; this is called **menopause** and is defined as having occurred when menses have ceased for 12 months. Menopause usually occurs between the ages of 45 and 55. Estrogen secretion decreases, and ovulation and menstrual cycles become irregular and finally cease. The decrease in estrogen has other effects as well. See Figure 41.4 for a concept map on the effects of aging.

For most men, testosterone secretion continues throughout life, as does sperm production, although both diminish with advancing age. Perhaps the most common reproductive problem for older men is enlargement of the prostate gland, called benign prostatic hyperplasia.

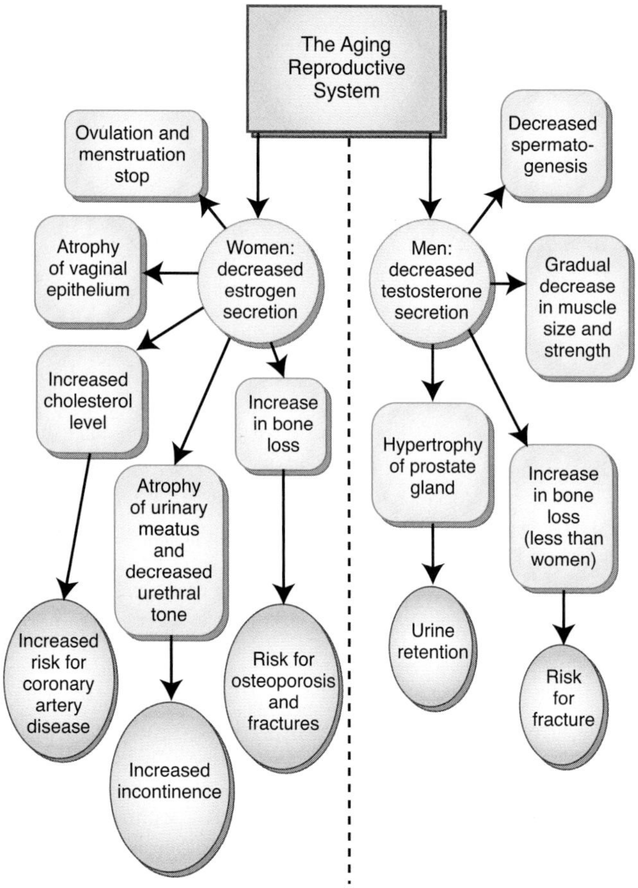

The Aging Reproductive System
Ovulation and menstruation stop
Atrophy of vaginal epithelium
Women: decreased estrogen secretion
Increased cholesterol level
Increase in bone loss
Atrophy of urinary meatus and decreased urethral tone
Increased risk for coronary artery disease
Risk for osteoporosis and fractures
Increased incontinence
Decreased spermato-genesis
Men: decreased testosterone secretion
Gradual decrease in muscle size and strength
Hypertrophy of prostate gland
Increase in bone loss (less than women)
Urine retention
Risk for fracture

FIGURE 41.4 Aging and the reproductive system. This concept map shows the effects the aging process has on the reproductive system.

FEMALE REPRODUCTIVE SYSTEM DATA COLLECTION

Collecting data related to a women's reproductive health can seem challenging because of the complex relationship of physical and psychosocial factors. Hormones not only affect a multitude of body functions, they also can influence moods and mental functioning. Reproduction involves not only physical processes, but also relationships, role identification, and self-esteem issues.

Normal Function Baselines

Knowing about expected functioning of the reproductive system is the nurse's best preparation for data collection. Regular, relatively pain-free shedding of an appropriate amount of the endometrial lining of the uterus is expected from puberty through midlife or later. Intercourse is normally expected to be free of pain and infection, to occur when desired by both partners, to be satisfying, and generally to result in pregnancy within a few months (unless precautions are taken). A pregnancy is expected to last approximately 40 weeks and to produce a healthy child. Physical and psychological sexual characteristics and function including **libido** (sexual desire) are expected to be adequately maintained by hormones. Sexual functioning, desire, and fertility are expected to change throughout the process of aging. Although individuals may vary somewhat from these expected descriptions, these serve as a baseline for collecting data related to possible disorders. Chapter 42 further defines specific female reproductive system disorders.

• WORD • BUILDING •

menopause: men—month + pause—stop

Much of what happens in female reproductive system disorders occurs inside the body and may not show external signs. Skill in asking appropriate questions, documenting patient statements, and describing observations is essential. Descriptions of symptoms should be thorough and follow the WHAT'S UP? format described in Chapter 1. Because many signs and symptoms of reproductive system disorders occur in a cyclic fashion, you or the provider may ask the patient to keep an accurate written record of occurrences, noting times and dates to identify patterns.

Health History

Subjective data related to the female reproductive system includes general personal information as well as menstrual, obstetrical, gynecological, sexual, family, and psychosocial histories. See Table 41.3 for specific data to collect.

> **NURSING CARE TIP**
>
> It is helpful to have women retain a monthly calendar of their menstrual cycle, and bring it to any appointment during which discussion of the cycle may take place.

An obstetrical history includes number of pregnancies, pregnancy outcomes, and complications. These are generally documented using abbreviations of Latin words: G = number of pregnancies (from the Latin word **gravida**); P = births, whether alive or stillborn (regardless of number of fetuses) after 20 weeks' gestation (from the Latin word **para**); A = abortions, whether spontaneous or therapeutic (from the Latin word *abortus*; a spontaneous abortion is sometimes called a miscarriage). Roman numerals follow the letters to specify the number of each. For example, three pregnancies—twins, one single birth, and one spontaneous abortion—are recorded as GIII, PII, AI. This may also be written as G3P2A1. Some hospitals use additional notations such as number of premature or full-term births, number of living children, and number of therapeutic abortions. Be sure to follow your institution's documentation policy.

> **LEARNING TIP**
>
> Remember the word *gravida* by thinking of gravity and that a woman typically is heavier when pregnant.

You will also want to ask about any tests, surgeries, or treatments done on the reproductive organs and excretory system. Medications the patient is taking (for whatever reasons), height-to-weight ratio, and marked changes in weight may also provide significant data for diagnostic and care planning purposes related to reproductive system disorders.

> **LEARNING TIP**
>
> There are many things to remember when asking health history questions. Making up an index card for your pocket or purchasing a prepared one from a medical bookstore can provide a handy reference.

Many nurses feel awkward asking reproductive history questions, and patients may also feel some uneasiness with this line of questioning. A matter-of-fact attitude, an assurance of confidentiality, and an adequate explanation about why the information is needed tend to encourage patient comfort and cooperation.

Breast Examination

Palpation

Palpation is the most important technique for breast examination because it can be used to identify alterations from normal consistency, to confirm the presence of lumps, and to locate areas of tenderness. Even mammograms are not sensitive enough to detect a small percentage of masses that can be felt by the patient or health care provider.

Breast Self-Examination

Self-palpation during breast self-examination (BSE), if done regularly and thoroughly, may be even more sensitive than physician or nurse palpation because the patient becomes so familiar with her own breasts that she is more likely to notice subtle changes that an infrequently visited health practitioner might overlook. Because recent studies of BSE have failed to show a reduction in cancer deaths, some practitioners are now simply urging women to be familiar with their breasts and report changes, rather than teaching them to do monthly examinations. Other providers, however, continue to teach and recommend monthly BSE because they have seen it make a significant difference for many women.

See Table 41.4 for additional objective data to collect.

Patient Education

If BSE is to be done monthly, a good time to perform it is 1 week following menses, when edema and swelling of normal breast tissue structures is at a minimum. For women who no longer have a regular menstrual period, any regular monthly schedule is fine. Although most women's breasts are not exactly the same size, marked differences between the breasts or a change in the size of one breast should be checked with a health care provider. Puckering or dimpling of skin, asymmetrical movement, and different pointing position of the

TABLE 41.3 SUBJECTIVE DATA COLLECTION FOR THE FEMALE REPRODUCTIVE SYSTEM

Category	Questions to Ask During the Health History	Rationale/Significance
Personal History	Have you ever been diagnosed or treated for any health problems?	Data may reveal general state of health, knowledge/practice of health promotion behaviors, meaning of health, expectations related to care.
	Have you had any recent weight changes? What type of change (if any)?	Weight changes may reflect physical or psychological pathology.
	Are you experiencing pain? (Use WHAT'S UP? questions if patient reports pain.)	Subjective indication of pain may indicate a variety of disorders.
	Do you have any allergies? (Agent/type of reaction?)	Allergy status should always be assessed to guide possible intervention should treatment be needed.
	Are you using any medications? (Include prescription, over-the-counter, and herbal remedies.) How much/how often do you take the medication?	May lead to health issues not yet revealed, and may guide possible interventions should treatment be needed.
	Do you smoke, consume caffeine, drink alcohol, or use recreational drugs? How much/how often?	Recreational behaviors may indicate risk of health disorders. Smoking increases risk of coagulation disorders with use of contraceptives containing estrogen.
	Do you exercise? What type of exercise do you do? How often?	Exercise is recognized as an activity that improves health status, in general, and for many disorders.
	How many hours of sleep do you get in a 24-hour period of time? Do you feel you get enough rest?	May indicate state of health or lead to discussion of social issues that lead to stress and, ultimately, physical disorders.
	Do you feel under stress? How do you deal with stress?	May indicate social issues that may lead to physical disorders.
	Have you been hit, kicked, slapped, or made to do anything sexually against your will since your last visit?	Abuse screening should be considered during all primary care visits; may indicate need for intervention or guide care.
Menstrual History	At what age did you begin menstruating (**menarche**)? How often do you menstruate and how long do your periods last? How heavy is your flow?	May reveal abnormalities of cycle and lead to a diagnosis of benign/malignant tumors, endometriosis, pregnancy, anemia, endocrine disorders.
	At what age did you enter menopause (if applicable)? If menopausal, has bone density screening been done? What is your calcium/vitamin D intake?	May determine need for bone density screening and teaching related to calcium and vitamin D supplementation.
Obstetric/Gynecological History	How many pregnancies and deliveries have you had? Were they full term or preterm? Were your deliveries vaginal or by cesarean section? Did you have any complications following your deliveries?	May indicate health of reproductive system, knowledge/meaning of health maintenance practice, and risk for disease.
	Have you had previous treatment/surgery on your reproductive organs?	May indicate past health issues related to the reproductive organs and need for current evaluation related to issues.
	Have you had any itching of your perineum or have you noted any vaginal discharge (describe)?	Subjective report of itching or discharge may indicate disorder of inflammation or lead to diagnosis of sexually transmitted disease.
	When was your last Pap/pelvic exam? What were the results?	May reflect meaning of health and guide current care.
	Do you do BSE? How often? Have you noticed any breast changes? When was your last mammogram (if applicable)?	If changes have been noted by the patient, they should be evaluated by the primary care provider for the possible pathology.

• WORD • BUILDING •

menarche: men—month + arche—beginning

TABLE 41.3 SUBJECTIVE DATA COLLECTION FOR THE FEMALE REPRODUCTIVE SYSTEM—cont'd

Category	Questions to Ask During the Health History	Rationale/Significance
	Did you breastfeed? How long?	Breastfeeding may offer some protection against breast cancer. If patient currently breastfeeding, may help guide care and diagnosis.
Sexual History	Are you sexually active? How many partners do you have? Of what gender? What is your lifetime number of partners? Is your sexual activity satisfying?	May indicate risk of sexually transmitted diseases, risk of unintended pregnancy, and indicate state of sexual satisfaction/intimacy.
	At what age did you become sexually active?	Early onset of sexual activity increases risk of cervical cancer.
	What contraceptive method(s) do you use (if sexually active with a male)? How do you use them?	May reflect meaning of health, high-risk health behaviors, and risk for unintended pregnancy or sexually transmitted disease.
	How long have you used this method?	Asking length of use of a particular method allows assessment of need for replacement as in an intrauterine device, or need for a bone density exam.
	Have you ever been diagnosed with a sexually transmitted disease? If so, when, what type, and how was it treated? That you are aware, was treatment successful?	May indicate high-risk sexual behavior patterns or potential for active disease and, therefore, indicate need for diagnostic testing and treatment.
Family History	Do you have a family history of cardiovascular problems, cancer, osteoporosis, diabetes, thyroid abnormalities?	May indicate underlying cause of or risk for sexual/physical abnormalities of the reproductive system.
Psychosocial History	Are you married or in a significant relationship? Is the relationship satisfying? Are you employed? Where?	Relevant to determine financial, social, and emotional support.

TABLE 41.4 OBJECTIVE DATA COLLECTION FOR THE FEMALE REPRODUCTIVE SYSTEM

Category	Physical Examination Findings	Possible Abnormal Findings/Causes
Clinical Breast Examination	Observe and palpate for presence of swelling, lumps, skin changes, nipple exudate.	Changes may indicate breast cancer, fibrocystic breast disease.
External Genitalia (mons pubis, clitoris, labia majora/minora, Bartholin's glands)	Observe for color, symmetry, hair distribution, lesions, swelling or exudate.	Changes may indicate vulvular cancer, developmental abnormalities, infection, or injury.
Vagina	Observe for shape, bulges, color changes, lesions, exudate.	Changes may indicate infection, structural abnormalities, or injury.
Internal Genitalia (uterus/cervix, fallopian tubes, ovaries) (exam performed by trained personnel)	Palpate for tenderness, size, shape, mobility. Observe for color, lesions, exudate, bleeding.	Changes may indicate infection, structural abnormalities, cervical cancer, polyps, endometriosis, fibroid/malignant tumors, pregnancy, or injury.
Perineum	Observe for lesions, shape.	Abnormalities may indicate infection, structural abnormalities, or injury.
Anus	Observe for shape, color changes, lesions.	Abnormalities can indicate hemorrhoids or injury.
Inguinal Nodes	Palpate for swelling, tenderness.	May indicate infectious process or regional malignancy.

Note: A female physical examination typically is done by a physician or other trained provider.

nipples should also be reported. Whether the breasts are examined in parallel lines, a spiral formation, or a wedge pattern is not important. It is important, however, for the examination to be methodical and cover all areas of the breast, including the tail of Spence, which extends into the axilla (Fig. 41.5).

NURSING CARE TIP

Some women do BSE the day their telephone bill arrives each month because it is a dependable monthly reminder.

CRITICAL THINKING

Jilli

■ Jilli, age 24, states, "Why should I do breast exams at my age? I probably won't get breast cancer until I'm older, if I get it at all."

1. What should your response to Jilli include?
2. Why would this be a good time to provide education about health maintenance?

Suggested answers at end of chapter.

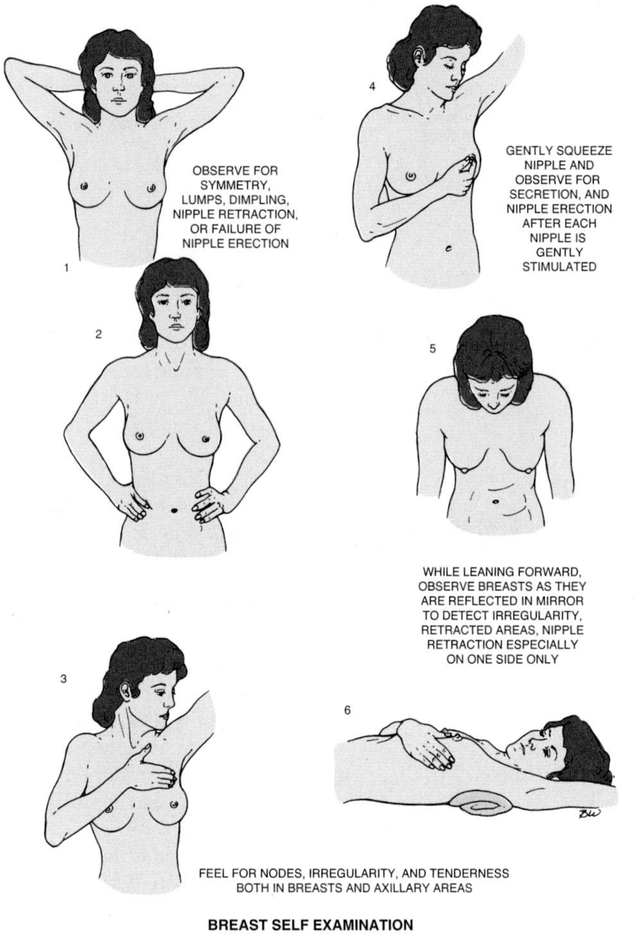
1
OBSERVE FOR SYMMETRY, LUMPS, DIMPLING, NIPPLE RETRACTION, OR FAILURE OF NIPPLE ERECTION
2
3
4
GENTLY SQUEEZE NIPPLE AND OBSERVE FOR SECRETION, AND NIPPLE ERECTION AFTER EACH NIPPLE IS GENTLY STIMULATED
5
WHILE LEANING FORWARD, OBSERVE BREASTS AS THEY ARE REFLECTED IN MIRROR TO DETECT IRREGULARITY, RETRACTED AREAS, NIPPLE RETRACTION ESPECIALLY ON ONE SIDE ONLY
6
FEEL FOR NODES, IRREGULARITY, AND TENDERNESS BOTH IN BREASTS AND AXILLARY AREAS
BREAST SELF EXAMINATION

FIGURE 41.5 Breast self-examination. (From Venes, D. J. [Ed.]. *Taber's cyclopedic medical dictionary* [21st ed., p 310]. Philadelphia: F. A. Davis, with permission.)

Diagnostic Tests of the Breasts

Ultrasound and Mammography

Further assessment of the breast can be done by methods other than BSE. Ultrasound examination is done by bouncing high-frequency sound waves off the tissues within the breast to determine the density of the tissues and to map the breast structures (Fig. 41.6). This is mainly useful for distinguishing fluid-filled (**cystic**) lumps from solid tumors but may also be used to guide a needle for fine-needle aspiration of cystic fluid or core needle biopsies.

Mammography is a radiographic (x-ray) examination of the breasts. A special machine is used that spreads and flattens the breast tissue to a thin layer to more effectively show benign and malignant growths, which might be hidden by breast structures on typical chest examination (Fig. 41.7). Generally, at least two radiographs are taken of each breast, with the machine compressing the breast top to bottom and side to side to give comparison views from more than one angle. If suspicious or unclear spots are seen, additional views may be taken. New digital technology is now available that may be more effective in detecting cancers in younger women and women who have dense breasts. The actual procedure is the same for a digital mammogram, but the image is computerized, allowing the radiologist to look more closely at problem areas.

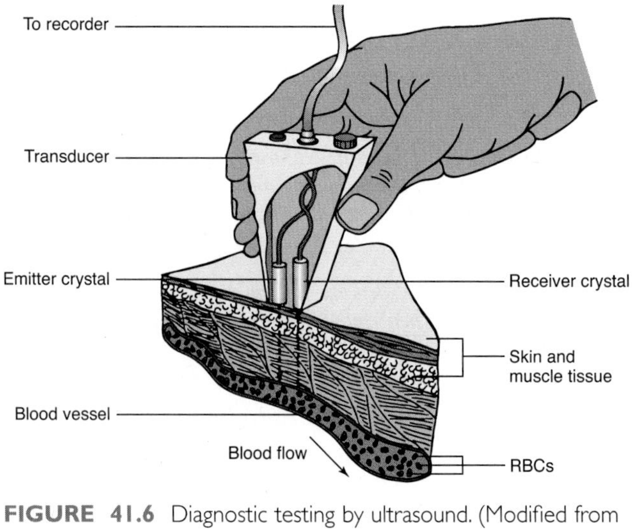
To recorder
Transducer
Emitter crystal
Receiver crystal
Skin and muscle tissue
Blood vessel
Blood flow
RBCs

FIGURE 41.6 Diagnostic testing by ultrasound. (Modified from Cavanaugh, B. M. [2003]. *Nurse's manual of laboratory and diagnostic tests* [4th ed.]. Philadelphia: F. A. Davis, with permission.)

• **WORD • BUILDING** •
cystic: baglike
mammography: mammo—breast + graphy—recording

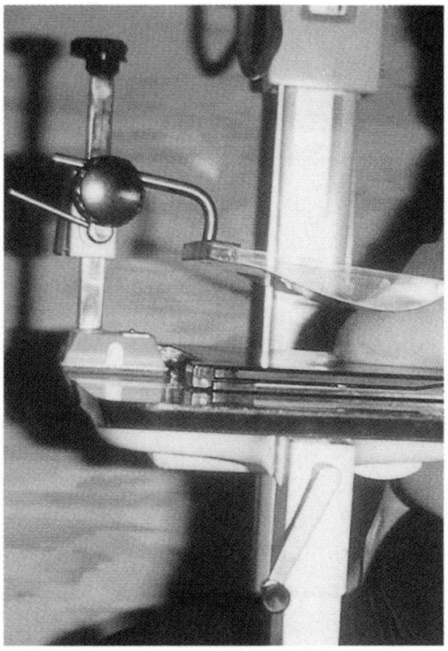

FIGURE 41.7 Mammogram machine. (Photo courtesy of Dinesh Patel, MD, Medical Oncology, Internal Medicine, Zanesville, OH.)

The American Cancer Society (2009) recommends the following for women:

- A screening mammogram at age 40 and yearly thereafter
- A clinical breast exam every 3 years during the 20s and 30s, then yearly at age 40 and thereafter
- Optional breast self-examination starting in the 20s
- MRI and mammogram every year for women at high risk of breast cancer.

PATIENT EDUCATION. Patients preparing for mammography should be advised to bathe and not to apply deodorant, powder, or any other substance to the upper body because these may cause false shadows on the test. They should be instructed that if a shadow is seen on a mammogram, further testing will be done to determine the reason for the shadow.

Thermography, Tomography, and Magnetic Resonance Imaging

Several other methods for diagnosis of breast disorders are available, but are not commonly used. Thermography is a method of mapping the breast using photographic paper, which records temperature variations throughout the tissue in different colors. Computerized tomography (CT) takes very precise x-ray pictures of the breast, layer by layer, as it would look if it were in thin slices, and stores these pictures on a computer. This allows for precise measurement of the position of tumors without the displacement caused by flattening the breast for a mammogram. Tomography, however, is much more expensive than mammography, so it is not a practical method to use for general screening of all women to detect possible breast cancers. Magnetic resonance imaging (MRI) uses radio-frequency radiation and magnetic fields to map the breast tissue. The equipment needed for this method is also expensive, and it is unavailable in some areas.

PATIENT EDUCATION. Ask patients preparing for MRI whether they have any metal inside their bodies, such as orthopedic wires, metal sutures, or artificial joint replacements. If they do, the procedure may be contraindicated because of the strong magnets used with MRI.

Biopsy

If suspicious lesions are found in the breast by any of these assessment methods, the lesion may be further assessed using one of the other methods and then a biopsy performed to confirm the diagnosis. This procedure involves removing a small portion of tissue, fluid, or cells from the breast or lymph nodes for microscopic examination. This may be done by surgically removing a portion of tissue or by aspirating fluid or cells through a needle that is placed into the lump or lesion.

Needle biopsies are often done with local anesthetic and may take place in a clinic or physician's office. More extensive biopsies may require a general anesthetic. A frozen section examination may be done in the laboratory by moistening and rapidly freezing a section of tissue, slicing it very thinly, and immediately examining it by microscope. This allows for diagnosis to be made during the course of an operation, so that the patient is spared an additional later operation for removal of cancerous tissue.

NURSING CARE. As with any surgical intervention, be prepared to set out the sterile equipment and supplies needed for the procedure and ensure that a signed consent has been obtained after the risks and benefits of the procedure have been explained to the patient by the provider. Following the biopsy, assess the patient for excessive bleeding and instruct about signs or symptoms to report. It is important that biopsy samples be clearly labeled, packaged appropriately for transport to laboratory facilities, and delivered promptly. Consult the laboratory for information about the transport container and whether a cell fixative is required in the container.

Assessment of the patient's psychological condition during breast diagnosis procedures is essential. Most women know someone who has had breast cancer. Although breast cancer screening procedures can seem routine to health care workers, they may be a cause of much anxiety for patients and their families. An understanding and calm nurse who can explain the procedures can help the assessment phase to be less traumatic.

SAFETY TIP

Use at least two patient identifiers when providing care, treatment, and services. Label containers used for blood and other specimens in the presence of the patient (2010 National Patient Safety Goals, www.jointcommission.org).

Bone Health Assessment

Bone health assessment is important for women of all ages. The discussion of calcium intake is an integral component of the health assessment. Teaching women early about the importance of good calcium and vitamin D intake will be of benefit later in life. Women of childbearing age produce estrogen, which helps prevent bone loss and works with calcium and other minerals to build bone. As women age and approach menopause, estrogen production slowly decreases, which decreases the processes of building and remodeling bone. Once a woman reaches menopause, her body is producing very little estrogen and therefore does not have the added benefit of bone protection. In fact, the body tends to break down more bone than it rebuilds. At this point in a woman's life, dietary calcium and vitamin D requirements increase unless the woman is on hormone replacement therapy. See Table 41.5 for recommendations for calcium and vitamin D intake from the National Institutes of Health (NIH) Office of Dietary Supplements. The National Osteoporosis Foundation (NOF; www.nof.org) sets their requirements even higher than the NIH. See Chapter 6 for the calcium content of selected foods.

Diagnostic Tests of the Bones

In addition to recommending increasing the dietary intake of calcium and vitamin D, menopausal women older than age 50 who are not on hormone replacement therapy should be assessed for bone loss. The NOF recommends bone density testing for all postmenopausal women over age 65 and for younger postmenopausal women ages 50 to 65 if they are at high risk (see Chapter 46).

The best test for bone density is a dual energy x-ray absorptiometry (DEXA) scan, which measures bone density at the hip or spine. This is a specialized x-ray that takes only 5 to 10 minutes to complete. A quantitative computed tomography (QCT) scan can also be done to determine bone density. Pharmacies or other outpatient facilities may offer tests of peripheral locations such as the heel. These are less sensitive but may still provide useful information that can be followed up with more extensive testing.

TABLE 41.5 ADULT CALCIUM AND VITAMIN D RECOMMENDATIONS

Adult Women and Men	Calcium (Daily)	Vitamin D (Daily)
Ages 19 to 50	1000 mg	200 international units
Ages 51 to 70	1200 mg	400 international units
Age 71 and older	1200 mg	600 international units
Pregnant and Breastfeeding Women	**Calcium (Daily)**	**Vitamin D (Daily)**
Ages 14 to 18	1300 mg	200 international units
Age 19 and older	1000 mg	200 international units

Source: From Office of Dietary Supplements, National Institutes of Health, Bethesda, MD. Retrieved April 27, 2009, from http://ods.od.nih.gov.

Additional Diagnostic Tests of the Female Reproductive System

Many tests are used to assess reproductive system function; this is currently an area of rapid change. The names of the individual procedures may also vary among institutions or according to particular methods used (e.g., a salpingoscopy is also called a falloposcopy, and a laparoscopy is the same as a peritoneoscopy). For this reason, this chapter is limited to general descriptions of categories of medical and surgical assessment procedures rather than an attempt to name all tests.

Hormone Tests

Hormone tests are commonly used to assess endocrine system function as it relates to reproduction. These tests may be used to measure potential fertility, to find reasons for abnormal menses, to assess hormone-producing tumors, and to determine whether treatments to adjust hormone levels have been effective. Several hormones may be assessed at any one time. Some hormone tests are time specific, so the samples can be rendered useless if not gathered within a certain time range.

NURSING CARE. Consult institution policy for specific instructions for each test. Explain the procedure to the patient and provide support. Women who are undergoing hormone tests may feel embarrassed, worried about their femininity and potential fertility, and depressed because of repeated tests, often with little positive result. Some may fear loss of their spouse's love (and perhaps the relationship) if they are diagnosed with alterations in hormone levels or function that lead to infertility.

Pelvic Examination

The pelvic examination allows visual inspection of the vagina and cervix, as well as sampling of mucus, discharge, cells, and exudates. Palpation of portions of the reproductive system and some treatments may also be done as part of the procedure (Fig. 41.8).

NURSING CARE. Be prepared to assist the health care provider with the examination. Explain the procedure as you set out the supplies. Vaginal specula range from tiny virginal sizes to extra large. The appropriate size is related to the size and shape of the woman's (or child's) pelvis and whether or not she has had children. For a small child, a nasal speculum may be used. A small amount of surgical lubricant should be placed near but not on the speculum (because some tests may be affected by water or lubricant). If reusable equipment is being used, be sure it has been sterilized between patients. Two clean gloves for the examiner should be placed nearby, and a light should be adjusted to illuminate the area. Other equipment may be set out according to the tests or treatments that will be carried out during the pelvic examination.

Instruct the patient to empty her bladder before the examination, remove her underclothing, and change into a gown. Instruct the patient to lie either on her back with her

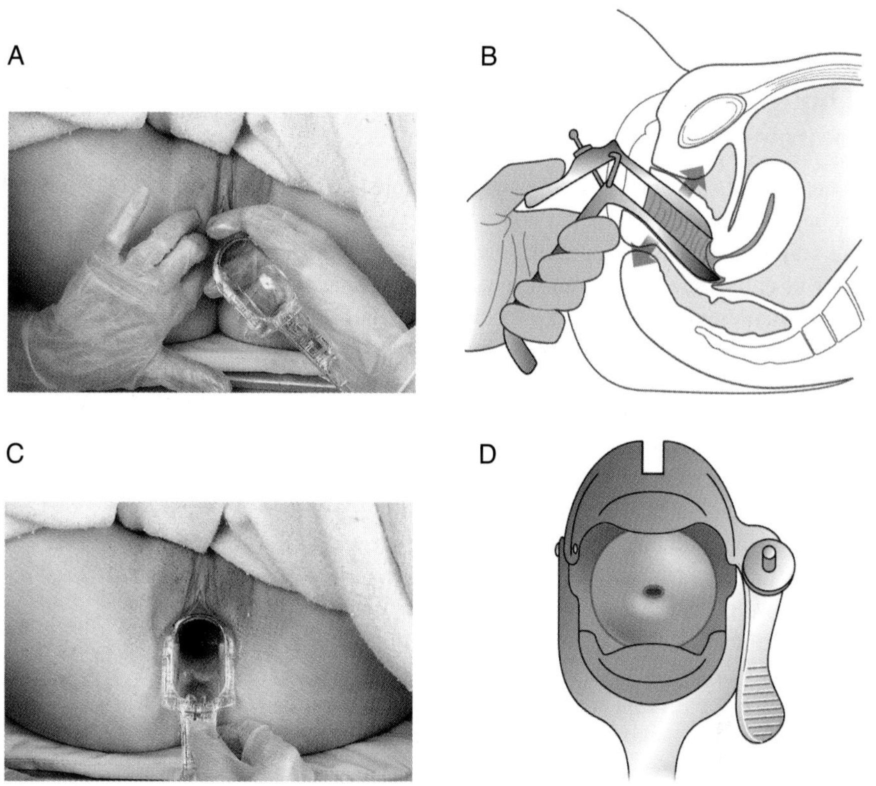
A
B
C
D

FIGURE 41.8 Pelvic exam with pap smear (From Dillon, P. M. [2007]. *Nursing health assessment: A critical thinking case studies approach* [2nd ed.]. Philadelphia: F. A. Davis, with permission.)

arms resting down at her sides (to aid relaxation of abdominal muscles) or in a side-lying position, according to the health care provider's preference. Provide a sheet large enough to cover her even while her legs are spread during the exam.

Bimanual Palpation

Because much of the reproductive system is not visible even with a speculum, **bimanual** palpation is often done during a pelvic examination. One hand is placed on the abdomen and the other gloved hand is inserted deeply into the vagina. The uterus and **adnexa** are moved about between the two hands to feel the size, shape, and consistency of the uterus and adnexa and to check for any abnormal growths.

NURSING CARE. Explain the procedure, and support the patient. Some women may be fearful, embarrassed, or tense and may find the procedure uncomfortable (Box 41.1). Active relaxation strategies may decrease discomfort.

Cytology

Cytology is the study of cells taken as tissue samples. Cells required for microscopic examination can be removed from the reproductive system in several ways. During a Papanicolaou (Pap) smear, one or more small samples of cells are gently scraped away from the surface of the cervical canal using a small wooden spatula, tiny cylindrical brush, and/or long cotton-tipped applicator. They are then smeared or rolled onto microscope slides and sprayed with a fixative to preserve them for viewing, or placed into a fixative solution for later preparation and viewing in a laboratory. Cells may also be collected by **conization**, which involves removing a small cone-shaped sample from the cervical canal, or by punch biopsy, which removes a small core of cells. Endometrial biopsy specimens are samples of cells taken from the lining of the uterus by scraping with a small spoon-shaped tool called a **curet**, which is inserted through the cervix. Small biopsy specimens may also be taken by cutting or removing a suspicious lesion. Cells may be observed for changes indicative of hormonal secretion, cellular maturation, or abnormalities such as are seen with viral growths and cancerous or precancerous conditions.

NURSING CARE. Add appropriate sample collection materials and fixatives to the pelvic examination supplies according to the type of cytological examination being done. For a Pap smear, this may include one or two clear glass slides, fixative spray, cytobrush and/or wooden cervical spatula, and transport box for the slides. In some settings, or for larger cell samples in most settings, a sterile collection container that includes a preservative solution may be used. Consult the procedure manual or health care provider

• WORD • BUILDING •
bimanual: bi—two + manual—hands
adnexa: ad—together + nexa—to tie (usually refers to ovaries and tubes)

• WORD • BUILDING •
conization: coniz—cone-forming + ation—process

Box 41.1

Thoughts from a Sexual Assault Nurse Examiner

When patients come in to see me, they are in crisis. They are unsure how or what to feel and whom to trust. They are very apprehensive. As patients give me the history of their assaults, they begin to trust me. They see someone who is interested in them and who believes them. By the time I actually start the head-to-toe physical examination, they know they are safe. Often, when I am performing the physical examination, I start small talk and take an interest in their lives that has nothing to do with the assault. When they are discharged from my care, they are more animated, talkative, and sometimes smiling.

The patient I remember the most was a child whose father was molesting her when her mother went to work. She was about 6 years old. When she came to the hospital, she wasn't talking to anybody, let alone a nurse in a scary hospital at midnight. I spent 4 hours with this child. We colored, played, and talked about her brothers. By the end of the night, she allowed me to examine her. And she trusted me enough to let the physician come in and look at her. Unfortunately, in her young life, she had a reason to be scared. Her life became much worse before it got better. Her father tried to kill her mother and himself as a result of this.

So many of us have grown up with pop culture television and we think of forensic examiners as professionals working with dead people. In fact, forensic nursing is caring for patients as it applies to the law. As a sexual assault nurse examiner, I care for people who have experienced interpersonal violence. I care for this special population of patients through the nursing process. I not only care for their physical trauma but also for their spiritual needs; lastly, I collect evidence for the prosecution of a crime. I advocate for their safety needs, and I help provide for their physical needs. I provide a bridge to the legal and mental health systems.

I began forensic nursing 8 years ago when the concept was still new. We were navigating uncharted waters and were unsure what the end result would bring. What we quickly learned is, when you deliver good nursing care to patients, the end result can be a positive change in their lives, and that is the reward of the job: making a positive difference in patients' lives, giving them some tools to help in their recovery process. Having the patient and family look at you and say "thank you for helping me" is what we all went into nursing for.

Becoming a sexual assault nurse examiner has made me become a more empathetic person, a more compassionate nurse, and a better citizen of my community.

concerning specific types of instruments to put out for biopsies and Pap smears. Cells die and degrade rapidly once removed from the patient, so they must be packaged securely for transport to laboratory facilities. Always label specimens carefully.

Prepare the patient by explaining the procedure and providing support. The woman may be fearful of cancer or other abnormality. Removal of the sample may cause pain, bleeding, swelling, or, later, inflammation, so the patient is monitored after the procedure and alerted to watch for and report these complications if they occur. After the procedure, document the woman's status on the chart and record that the sample was sent to the laboratory.

CRITICAL THINKING

Reproductive Assessment

■ How might the age of the patient change your approach, plans, and teaching for patients who have disorders of the reproductive system? Consider your approach, plans, and teaching for each of the following scenarios:

1. A 2-year-old child is brought into the clinic by her mother because she has a foul-smelling discharge coming from her perineal area and a slight yellowish discharge from her vagina.
2. A 19-year-old woman comes to the physician's office where you work to obtain a renewal of her yearly birth control pill prescription. Your employer enforces regular checks for cervical changes by renewing the prescription only after a Pap smear is done. As you start setting out the Pap smear materials, your patient expresses some reluctance to have it done today because she is so sore already.
3. Your 56-year-old patient comes in to "get things checked out" because she hurts every time that she and her husband have intercourse.

Suggested answers at end of chapter.

Swabs and Smears

Swabs and smears are done to determine which microorganisms are causing infection, and consequently which antibiotics should be used.

NURSING CARE. If infection is suspected, add sample collection materials, including swabs, slides, and sterile saline in site-specific receptacles, and a gonorrhea/*Chlamydia* collection kit, to the pelvic examination equipment. It is important to place samples of discharge or exudate into culture media that support growth. Clear media are required for some and charcoal media for others, so both types should be set out.

Viral Swabs Require a Special Collection Kit. *Chlamydia* samples are especially difficult to transport to laboratories, and special kits are available for this pathogen. Some microorganisms, such as yeasts and *Trichomonas*, can be identified well from smears on slides. Wet mounts are smears of discharge spread onto a slide. These must be taken to the microscope immediately after they are obtained. Sodium chloride and potassium hydroxide are dropped onto individual wet-mount slides before they dry to aid in identification of some microorganisms. Support the patient, who may be anxious about possible sexually transmitted diseases and effects on relationships.

Sonography

Ultrasound assessment (also called sonography) may be done to determine size, shape, development, and density of structures associated with the female reproductive system, as well as fetal measurements and some types of prenatal diagnoses. This procedure is especially useful for differentiating cysts from solid tumors and for locating ectopic pregnancies and intrauterine devices. Ultrasound may also be used to guide needles for obtaining samples of fluid or cells. Either external or vaginal transducers may be used to send and receive the signals for this procedure. Vaginal transducers are placed in a plastic sheath before insertion into the vagina. A full bladder may be required for some ultrasound tests.

NURSING CARE. Explain the procedure and support the patient. The pressure of the transducer on the skin or in the vagina may be painful if the adjacent structures are inflamed or swollen, or if the bladder is very full.

Radiographic Procedures

Several radiographic procedures may be used for diagnosis of reproductive system problems. Computed tomographic (CT) scanning and MRI are used to locate tumors of the reproductive system. Structures of the female reproductive system may also be outlined by taking x-ray pictures of cavities that have been filled with a radiopaque substance. During a **hysterosalpingogram**, dye is injected into the uterus until it comes out the ends of the fallopian tubes. This test is useful for identifying congenital abnormalities in the shape or structure of the uterus and blockages of the fallopian tubes.

NURSING CARE. Prepare the patient for this test according to the radiology department policy and the physician's orders, which may include a laxative, suppository, or enema. Ensure that the patient understands the procedure and that appropriate consents are signed as required. Ask about allergies to dye or iodine. Notify the supervisor immediately if the patient reports an allergy. After the procedure, assess for nausea, light-headedness, and signs of allergic reaction, and promote comfort, because some cramping may occur. Discharge teaching should include signs of infection and advice that the x-ray dye may stain clothing. Provide a perineal pad following the procedure and advise the patient to wear a perineal pad until vaginal drainage stops.

• WORD • BUILDING •

hysterosalpingogram: hystero—womb + salpingo—tube + gram—record

NURSING CARE TIP

No one is really allergic to iodine—iodine is an essential element in our bodies. But some people may be allergic to dyes that contain iodine.
It is still important to ask about iodine allergy, because that is how some women identify an allergy to dye.

Endoscopic Examinations

Several types of endoscopic examinations are done to visually inspect internal areas to diagnose (and sometimes treat) reproductive system disorders. The names of the tests vary according to the area inspected, but all generally make use of a fiber-optic light and lens system, which is inserted through a tube called a cannula into a small incision. A laparoscopy is done to view the abdominal cavity and is useful for identifying problems such as endometriosis (Fig. 41.9). A **salpingoscopy** is performed to see the inside of the fallopian tubes and a **hysteroscopy** to see the inside of the uterus. A binocular microscope is used with an endoscope that is introduced into the vagina to closely study lesions of the cervix during a **colposcopy**. During **culdoscopy**, an endoscope is introduced into the vagina and through a small incision in the vagina into the cul-de-sac of Douglas, a cavity behind the uterus, in order to observe for abnormalities in this region (Fig. 41.10).

NURSING CARE. Preoperatively the patient is prepared for an endoscopic examination according to institutional protocol. This generally involves asking the patient whether she has fasted as instructed, assessing vital signs, recording the time of last voiding, helping the patient into an operating room gown, and ensuring that the consent form has been signed. General anesthesia may be given for some endoscopic procedures. Explain what to expect and provide support for the woman. She may be anxious about possible disorders.

Postoperatively, provide comfort measures. These procedures produce almost no blood loss. The woman may experience pain in the neck, shoulders, and upper back if carbon dioxide (CO_2) gas was pumped into the body

• WORD • BUILDING •

salpingoscopy: salpingo—tube + scopy—looking
hysteroscopy: hystero—womb + scopy—looking
colposcopy: colpo—vagina + scopy—looking
culdoscopy: culdo—cul de sac + scopy—looking

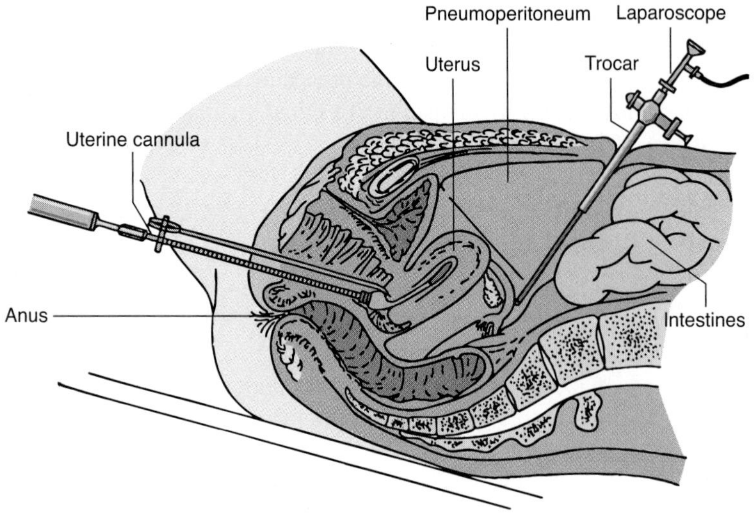
Pneumoperitoneum
Laparoscope
Uterus
Trocar
Uterine cannula
Anus
Intestines

FIGURE 41.9 Laparoscopy. (Modified from Cavanaugh, B. M. [2003]. *Nurse's manual of laboratory and diagnostic tests* [4th ed.]. Philadelphia: F. A. Davis, with permission.)

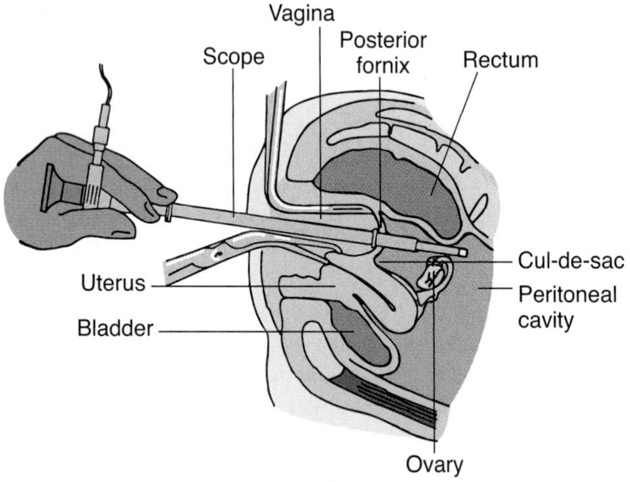
Vagina
Scope
Posterior fornix
Rectum
Cul-de-sac
Uterus
Peritoneal cavity
Bladder
Ovary

FIGURE 41.10 Culdoscopy. (Modified from Cavanaugh, B. M. [2003]. *Nurse's manual of laboratory and diagnostic tests* [4th ed.]. Philadelphia: F. A. Davis, with permission.)

compartment being examined. This is called **insufflation**, and is done to increase the distance between structures, so that it is easier for the physician to visualize structures and diagnose possible disorders. The CO_2 remaining after completion of the examination travels to the highest level of the body before being absorbed, so lying flat for a few hours after the examination may decrease discomfort. If incisions were made through the abdominal wall for insertion of the endoscope and for insufflation, these are tiny and a Band-Aid or small dressing is applied.

PATIENT EDUCATION. Advise the patient to observe the incision sites for redness, bleeding, or drainage, seeking evaluation by the physician promptly if these should occur or otherwise seeing the physician approximately 1 week later for suture removal (according to physician preference). If the endoscopic procedure was done transvaginally, provide a perineal pad following the procedure and advise the patient to wear a pad until the drainage stops. Also instruct the patient to report any bright bleeding after the operative day, and to report any fever or foul-smelling discharge.

Further detail about some specific forms of the tests that have been described in this chapter are included with the disorders to which they apply in Chapters 42 and 43. Also see Table 41.6.

• WORD • BUILDING •
insufflation: in—in + suffl—to blow + ation—process

MALE REPRODUCTIVE SYSTEM DATA COLLECTION

As with the female reproductive system, the male reproductive system is a complex interaction of both physical and psychosocial factors. Unlike women, however, men may find it much more difficult in our society to talk about or admit to having problems related to reproductive health. From toilet training through adulthood, men are expected to have behaviors associated with maleness. Unfortunately, by the time some boys reach manhood, their male identity may be defined by the successful functioning of their sex organs.

One of the important first steps in obtaining a male reproductive assessment is to provide a comfortable, nonjudgmental, confidential atmosphere for discussion. This means you must first be knowledgeable and comfortable with sexual issues. While it may be challenging to ask questions about **erection** or ejaculation history, such questions may allow men to talk about difficulties they are experiencing. Be open and straightforward with all questions and answers. It may be necessary at times to use more commonly expressed sexual words instead of medical terminology. You will discover that many men do not know the function of their prostate gland or the difference

TABLE 41.6 DIAGNOSTIC PROCEDURES FOR THE FEMALE REPRODUCTIVE SYSTEM

Procedure	Definition/Normal Finding	Significance of Abnormal Findings	Nursing Management
Noninvasive			
Breast self-examination (BSE), clinical breast examination (CBE)	Assessment of breast tissue by patient (BSE) or health care provider (CBE) through inspection and palpation	Abnormal physical exam may indicate pathology and does indicate need for further assessment.	Educate about appropriate technique and witness a return demonstration of BSE. Education about BSE may be demonstrated during CBE.
Ultrasound/sonography	High-frequency sound waves bounce off tissue to map tissue structure and determine tissue density. Also may be used to guide biopsy procedure.	May help to determine abnormal lesions, abnormalities of tissue structure, or presence of abnormal fluid volume.	Follow institutional guidelines for patient preparation and support, which may be determined by testing goals.
Mammography	Radiographic examination of tissue. X-ray may be used with dye contrast injected into body before procedure.	May help to determine abnormal lesions or abnormalities of normal tissue structure.	Educate patient not to apply lotions/powders or deodorant prior to test. If dye is used, inquire about past allergic reaction to dye and/or observe for allergic response.
Thermography, computed tomography (CT), magnetic resonance imaging (MRI)	Precise pictures of tissue using temperature (thermography), x-ray (computed tomography), or radio-frequency (MRI)	May help to determine abnormal lesions or abnormalities of normal tissue structure.	Ask patients about presence of metal or wire inside their bodies before MRI because the procedure may then be contraindicated.
Hormonal tests	Assessment of endocrine function related to reproduction	Abnormal hormone levels may reflect fertility potential, determine reasons for abnormal menses, identify hormone-producing tumors, or evaluate hormone replacement.	Explain procedure to patient and provide support.
Invasive			
Pelvic examination, bimanual examination	Inspection and palpation of external/internal reproductive organs by health care provider	Abnormal physical examination may detect pathology or may indicate need for further testing.	Explain procedure to patient and provide support. Consult institutional policies for specific instructions.
Biopsy, cytology, swabs, smears	Obtainment of body cells/tissue through aspiration or excision or by swabbing/scrapping of tissue/exudate	May diagnose pathology or infection.	Explain procedure to patient and provide support. Consult institutional policies for specific instructions.
Endoscopy, laparoscopy	Use of fiber-optic light and lens system to inspect internal structures	May help to determine abnormal lesions or abnormalities of normal tissue structure. Tissue biopsies may be taken during procedure.	Explain procedure to patient and provide support. Observe for postprocedure complications.

between ejaculation and **orgasm**. Use the assessment as an opportunity to teach men the facts about their own sexual functioning.

Health History

Some basic questions to ask a male patient during a reproductive assessment are found in Table 41.7. As mentioned earlier, a professional, matter-of-fact attitude, along with an explanation as to why the questions are necessary, can put both you and the patient at ease while collecting data.

Physical Examination

The physical examination is generally performed by a physician or provider trained in physical assessments. The examination begins with the patient's general appearance. He is observed for male patterns of hair growth on the head, face, chest, arms, and legs. Normal male pubic hair pattern is in an upside-down triangular shape, with hair growth up toward the umbilicus. The patient's height and muscle mass are noted. Men are commonly taller than 5 feet, 6 inches tall, weigh more than 135 pounds, and have shoulders that

TABLE 41.7 SUBJECTIVE DATA COLLECTION FOR THE MALE REPRODUCTIVE SYSTEM AND SEXUAL HEALTH

Category	Questions to Ask During the Health History	Rationale/Significance
Medication	Are you using any medications? (Include prescription, over-the-counter, and herbal remedies.) How much/how often? (For medications that affect sexual desire, erection, or ejaculation, see Chapter 43.)	Loss of sexual desire, erection, ejaculation, orgasm, or fertility can occur as a result of some medication use.
Family History	Do you have a family history of genetically transmitted diseases (e.g., heart problems, hypertension, diabetes, cancer)? Did your mother use DES during pregnancy?	These conditions put men at high risk for circulation problems that interfere with erections, or congenital anomalies of reproductive organs.
Personal Habits and Health Promotion Behaviors	Do you smoke, consume caffeine, drink alcohol, use recreational drugs, or use steroids? How much/how often? Do you use hot tubs, engage in long-distance drives, or ride a bike? How much/how often? Do you use contraceptives? What type of contraceptives do you use? How do you use them? Do you do TSE? Have you noticed any changes in your testicles or other reproductive organs?	These habits may lead to decreased blood flow to penis, loss of erection; decreased testosterone (male hormone) interferes with erection and fertility; excessive heat decreases sperm production. Data will reveal knowledge/practice of health promotion behaviors, meaning of health, as well as history of changes or abnormalities.
Personal Health History	Did you have mumps during adolescence or have you recently had an infection or fever?	Some infectious processes may lead to decreased sperm production.
Mental Health	Are you experiencing stress? How do you deal with stress? Are you having problems with a sexual partner? Have you ever or are you experiencing performance anxiety or depression?	Decreased sexual desire and ability to have an erection may result from mental and/or emotional stress.
Circulatory/Respiratory	Have you ever been diagnosed with or treated for heart problems/surgery, high blood pressure, sickle cell disease, lung disease, or sleep apnea?	Decreased circulation can lead to inability to have usable erection; decreased respiratory function can result in activity intolerance, loss of erection.
Gastrointestinal	Have you ever been diagnosed or treated for liver infection/disease or bowel problems?	Liver infections/disease can lead to decreased testosterone and increased estrogen production, and loss of erection; gastrointestinal/bowel problems can lead to pain, loss of desire; surgery may result in loss of blood flow or innervation.
Musculoskeletal	Do you have painful joints, pelvic/lower back pain, or nerve damage?	Pain, loss of desire; limited movement/positions, loss of erection, ejaculation, and orgasm may result from musculoskeletal problems.
Neurologic	Have you ever experienced a stroke or suffered from multiple sclerosis, Parkinson's disease, or other neurologic disorders?	Limited movement/positions, loss of sensations, and loss of control can result from neurologic problems.
Metabolic/Endocrine	Have you ever suffered from diabetes, obesity, or thyroid problems?	Diabetes mellitus can result in circulation problems, retrograde ejaculation, nerve damage; obesity can result in decreased male hormones, excess female hormones.
Genitourinary	Have you ever been diagnosed with a congenital deformity of the penis/testicles, suffered from prostate problems, or experienced erection/ejaculation problems? Have you ever been diagnosed with a sexually transmitted disease? When, what type, and how was it treated? That you are aware, was treatment successful? Do you have any lesions, pain, discharge, or swelling of the reproductive organs? Have you noticed any abnormalities/changes in size, shape, or color of your external reproductive organs? (Describe)	Difficulty with erection, penetration problems, retrograde ejaculation, or infertility may be associated with genitourinary abnormalities, stress, or medication use. Lesions, pain, discharge, swelling, or other abnormalities of the external reproductive organs may indicate infection, structural abnormalities such as varicocele, or other disease processes such as cancer.

TABLE 41.7 SUBJECTIVE DATA COLLECTION FOR THE MALE REPRODUCTIVE SYSTEM AND SEXUAL HEALTH—cont'd

	For patients younger than age 40: "Do you practice monthly testicular self-examinations?"	Men younger than age 40 should be encouraged to perform monthly testicular examinations as a cancer prevention measure.
	For patients older than age 40: "When was the last time you had a prostate examination?"	A digital rectal examination (DRE) should be a regular part of a man's routine physical after age 41. Prostate cancer is treatable when detected early.
Sexual Practices	Are you sexually active? How many partners do you have? Of what gender? How often do you have intercourse (including positions, timing with female ovulation cycle if heterosexual)? Is the amount/type of sexual activity satisfying? Do you masturbate or use lubricants?	Some sexual practices can lead to a decrease in quality and quantity of sperm that reach the female egg.

DES = diethylstilbestrol.

are broader than their hips. The presence of excess breast tissue may indicate **gynecomastia,** from an excess of female hormones. Abnormal findings in either hair patterns or muscle mass often indicate a hormone imbalance.

The penis, scrotum, and testes (testicles) are examined by observation and palpation. On observation, the penis is normally flaccid (soft) and hanging straight down. The size can vary greatly and should not be a concern unless it is unusually small (microphallus) or edematous. The left testis typically hangs slightly lower in the scrotum than the right.

The penis is examined for warts, sores (evidence of sexually transmitted diseases), swelling, curves, or lumps along the shaft. The examiner also makes sure the urethral opening is at the tip of the penis and not on the underside of the shaft (**hypospadias**) or on the dorsum of the shaft (**epispadias**). If the man is not **circumcised** (surgical removal of the foreskin), the foreskin should be pulled back carefully and the glans inspected for signs of inflammation or foul-smelling discharge. The provider should be sure to replace the foreskin in the forward position after the examination is completed.

The scrotum and testes are carefully examined and palpated. Both testes should be present and a normal size (approximately 2 cm to 4 cm). The testes are egg shaped and should feel smooth and rubbery when lightly palpated between the thumb and fingers. The epididymis can be felt along the top edge and posterior section of each testis. The testes and scrotum are palpated for any lumps, cysts, or tumors. If a fluid-filled mass (**hydrocele**) is found, further evaluation should be done.

A simple noninvasive test called **transillumination** is used to determine if the mass is fluid filled or solid. With the room lights out, a flashlight is held behind the scrotum. If the mass is fluid, a red glow appears; if it is solid, it appears opaque. Each spermatic cord (made up of veins, arteries, lymphatics, nerves, and the vas deferens) is palpated and should feel firm and threadlike. If a condition called a **varicocele** is present, the area feels like a bag of worms. A varicocele, which is swelling of the veins of the spermatic cord, is one of the most common problems associated with male infertility.

The male patient is also examined for inguinal hernias by pressing up through the scrotum into each of the inguinal rings while asking him to cough or bear down. Each side is examined separately while he is in the standing position. A hernia feels like a pulsation against the examiner's fingertips.

A digital rectal examination (DRE) may be done by an experienced practitioner. During DRE, the prostate gland is palpated by inserting a gloved, lubricated finger into the rectum while the man is in a knee-to-chest position. The entire posterior lobe of the gland can be felt this way. The gland should feel slightly firm and without any lumps. If the prostate gland feels very hard or soft, enlarged, or contains any lumps, a rectal ultrasound with needle biopsy is often ordered. A swollen, painful prostate generally indicates that an infection is present.

Remind all men older than age 40 that unless they have had a complete removal of the prostate gland, they still need a DRE every year. Many men are under the impression that any prostate surgery means the gland has been completely removed. When simple surgery is performed, prostate tissue is left in the body and will begin to regrow over time. This prostatic tissue can become cancerous and needs to be monitored with a yearly DRE.

See Table 41.8 for a summary of objective data to collect for the male reproductive system.

• WORD • BUILDING •

gynecomastia: gyneco—female + mastia—breast
hypospadias: hypo—under + spadias—span, to draw
epispadias: epi—upon + spadias—span, to draw
circumcised: circum—around + cised—cut
hydrocele: hydro—water + cele—hernia

• WORD • BUILDING •

transillumination: trans—across + illumin—light + ation—process
varicocele: varico—twisted vein + cele—swelling

TABLE 41.8 OBJECTIVE DATA COLLECTION FOR THE MALE REPRODUCTIVE SYSTEM

Category	Physical Examination Findings	Possible Abnormal Findings/Causes
Clinical Breast Examination	Observe and palpate for presence of swelling, lumps, skin changes, nipple exudates.	Changes may indicate breast cancer, though rare in males.
Glans of Penis	Observe for lesions, exudate, tenderness. Observe for placement of the urethra. If foreskin is present, attempt to reduce to observe for lesions, exudate, inflammation.	Lesions, exudate, tenderness can indicate presence of infective or disease process, injury. Epispadias/hypospadias may be noted when observing for placement of the urethra.
Shaft of Penis	Observe for lesions, tenderness, shape.	Lesions, exudate, tenderness can indicate presence of infectious or disease process, injury. Irregularity of shape may indicate structural abnormalities/disease.
Scrotum	Visualize and palpate for swelling, pain, lesions.	Inguinal herniation may be noted. Swelling may occur with heart or renal failure, local inflammation, injury.
Testes	Palpate for descent, pain, lesions, size, shape, consistency. Palpate for lesions/swelling of epididymitis.	Absence of palpated testes may indicate non-descent. Testicular lesion can indicate testicular cancer. Swelling, pain can indicate infectious process.
Spermatic Cord	Palpate for swelling, size, consistency, pain	Presence of swelling, pain can indicate infection or varicocele.
Inguinal Ring (exam performed by trained personnel)	Palpate for bulge, pain.	Bulge, pain may indicate inguinal hernia.
Inguinal Lymph Nodes	Palpate for swelling, pain.	Swelling, pain may indicate infectious process or regional malignancy.
Digital Rectal Exam: DRE (exam performed by trained personnel)	Observe external rectum for lesions, exudate. Palpate for pain, swelling, penile exudate.	Pain, swelling, exudate may indicate benign changes, infectious process, cancer, or injury.

Note: A male physical examination is typically done by a physician or other trained provider.

Testicular Self-Examination

All men after puberty should do a monthly testicular self-examination (TSE) to detect any tumors or other changes in the scrotum. See Box 41.2 for instructions that can be used to teach a man how to examine his testicles. Also see Figure 41.11.

CRITICAL THINKING

Tony

■ Tony is a 20-year-old who reports a "bump" on his right testicle. He comes into the health clinic and asks if he can take any medication for his "disease."

1. What would be the best action?
2. What should your health assessment include?

Suggested answers at end of chapter.

Breast Self-Examination

Although breast cancer in men is rare, it can occur. Men, like women, should be familiar with their breasts and report changes.

Box 41.2

Guidelines for Monthly Testicular Self-Examination

A testicular self-examination is easiest during or right after a warm shower or bath, when the scrotum is relaxed and the testicles are hanging low. Choose 1 day a month to always do the examination.

1. Raise the penis up out of the way and look for any difference in size or shape of each side of the scrotum (sac). The left side usually hangs a little lower than the right.
2. Using both hands, hold the scrotum in the palms. Begin, one at a time, to gently roll each testicle between the thumb and first three fingers, feeling for any lumps or hard spots.
3. Identify the parts. The testicles should feel round, smooth, and egg shaped. The epididymis along the top and back side should feel soft and a little bit tender. The spermatic cord is a tube that runs from the epididymis and usually feels firm, smooth, and movable.
4. See your physician immediately if you feel any lumps or unusual changes.

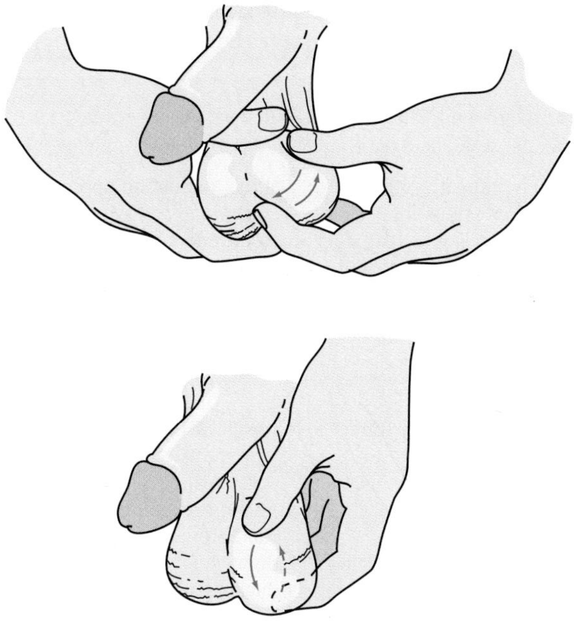

FIGURE 41.11 Testicular self-examination.

Diagnostic Tests of the Male Reproductive System

Ultrasound

An ultrasound may be done to diagnose or evaluate a variety of male reproductive or genitourinary problems. A transrectal ultrasound may be done to diagnose prostate cancer. For this procedure, a rectal probe transducer is inserted into the rectum and sound waves are used to evaluate the prostate gland.

Pelvic or scrotal ultrasound helps evaluate and locate masses. Ultrasound may also be done to guide a needle during a fine-needle biopsy.

NURSING CARE. Explain the procedure to the patient. An enema may be ordered before the procedure. No special aftercare is needed.

Cystourethroscopy

A cystourethroscopy may be done to evaluate the degree of obstruction by an enlarged prostate gland. For this procedure, a Foley catheter is inserted and a dye is injected into the bladder. Radiographs are taken with the dye in the bladder and while voiding after the catheter has been removed.

NURSING CARE. The procedure is explained to the patient, and possible allergic reaction to dyes is assessed and communicated to the physician as necessary. The patient is instructed to void before the procedure. A sedative or analgesic may be ordered to help the patient relax during the procedure.

After the procedure, intake and output are measured for 24 hours and alteration from the patient's normal pattern or absence of urination is reported to the physician. Fluids are encouraged to promote excretion of the dye.

Laboratory Tests

PROSTATE-SPECIFIC ANTIGEN. Prostate-specific antigen (PSA) is a glycoprotein produced by prostate cells. The normal value of PSA is less than 4 ng/L. An elevated level indicates prostatic hypertrophy or cancer.

PROSTATIC ACID PHOSPHATASE. Prostatic acid phosphatase (PAP) is an enzyme that normally affects metabolism of prostate cancer cells. The normal value of PAP is less than 3 ng/mL. An elevated level indicates prostate cancer.

OTHER TESTS. If prostate cancer is suspected or diagnosed, additional tests may be done. Acid phosphatase may be elevated in metastatic prostate cancer. Alkaline phosphatase and serum calcium levels may be elevated if metastasis to the bone has occurred. See Table 41.9 for a summary of diagnostic procedures.

Tests for Infertility

Various hormone levels may be measured, including FSH, LH, testosterone, and adrenocorticotropic hormone (ACTH) to help determine causes of infertility in male patients.

Semen analysis may be done to provide information about causes of infertility or to evaluate whether a vasectomy has been effective. Semen may be analyzed for sperm count, motility, and shape. Other tests determine whether the semen contains adequate nutrients to support sperm, whether antibodies to the sperm are present, and the ability of the sperm to penetrate an ovum.

NURSING CARE. The patient is instructed to refrain from ejaculation for 3 days before collecting the semen sample to avoid altering findings. Generally, specimens are collected on three separate occasions over a period of 4 to 6 days. Masturbation and ejaculation directly into a sterile container are recommended to avoid loss of semen. Condoms and lubricants should be avoided. The sample should be taken to the laboratory within 1 hour of collection. Additional tests of the male reproductive system are discussed in Chapter 43.

TABLE 41.9 DIAGNOSTIC PROCEDURES FOR THE MALE REPRODUCTIVE SYSTEM

Procedure	Definition/Normal Finding	Significance of Abnormal Findings	Nursing Management
Noninvasive			
Testicular self-examination (TSE)	Palpation of testes by patient.	Abnormalities may indicate pathology and require further evaluation.	Instruct patient on appropriate technique and witness a return demonstration.
Ultrasound	High-frequency sound waves bounce off tissue to map tissue structure and determine tissue density. Also may be used to guide biopsy procedure.	May help to determine abnormal lesions, abnormalities of tissue structure, or presence of abnormal fluid volume.	Follow institutional guidelines for patient preparation and support.
Hormonal tests, antigen level testing	Blood test to measure hormone or antigen levels.	Abnormal hormone levels may reflect fertility potential. Abnormal antigen levels may indicate pathology.	Consult institutional policies for specific instructions for each test. Explain procedure to patient and provide support.
Invasive			
Digital rectal examination	Palpation of internal reproductive organs, especially prostate gland, through rectum.	Abnormal physical exam may indicate pathology and indicates need for further testing.	Educate patient about procedure and provide support.
Cystourethroscopy	Insertion of a Foley catheter and dye into the bladder to evaluate for obstruction (usually an enlarged prostate) by radiography.	Obstruction may cause difficulty with urination.	Educate patient about the procedure and postprocedure care. Instruct patient to void before procedure. Measure intake and output for 24 hours following procedure. Observe for allergic reaction.

SUGGESTED ANSWERS TO CRITICAL THINKING

■ *Jilli*

1. The answer should include basic breast health statistics and risks, as well as proper assessment practice and techniques as discussed in this chapter. She should be informed that while monthly BSE is not absolutely necessary, knowing her breasts and reporting changes is essential. Technique should be demonstrated and a return demonstration received during the visit. The patient should also verbalize understanding of risks related to breast health and proper BSE technique to verify teaching was effective.
2. Questions about breast health and self-assessment practices provide an opportunity for the nurse to educate a patient about health facts and technique. Patient questions can also be a cue to patient readiness and willingness to learn.

■ *Reproductive Assessment*

1. Calm fears. Explain simply. Allow the parent to stay with the child if appropriate. Consider whether it is possible that the child has been abused. (If so, evidence needs to be collected and a report filed with the appropriate child protection authorities. Check with your supervisor if you believe this is a possibility.) Place a nasal speculum out for examination. Place a forceps out for removal of a possible foreign body (not uncommon at this age). Teach the child that this is a normal part of the body that is to be protected and taken care of.
2. Assess knowledge and maturity. Set out supplies for a Pap smear and for swabs and smears. Teach while getting supplies ready. Explain that vaginal soreness usually needs to be treated and that the physician must know more about the problem to do so effectively. Explain that inflammations can interfere with Pap smear results, so it may have to be repeated later

SUGGESTED ANSWERS TO—cont'd

after treatment. Explain culture and sensitivity testing. Teach about risk reduction and inform that oral contraceptives do not offer a barrier against sexually transmitted diseases.

3. Try to put the woman at ease through general conversation. Set out supplies for a Pap smear (if needed) and for swabs and smears. Teach while getting supplies ready. Discuss aging and the effects of decreased estrogen in general and specifically on vaginal tissues. Inform her that there are several ways to deal with problems resulting from decreased estrogen, such as oral hormonal replacements, water-soluble vaginal lubricants, vaginal creams, estrogen patches, and estrogen receptor modulator medication.

■ *Tony*

1. Palpable scrotal changes can result from a variety of reproductive and/or genitourinary abnormalities. Before Tony's question can be answered, a complete history needs to be obtained and a clinical exam of the genitalia performed.
2. The history should explore:
   - If TSEs are regularly performed and if changes have been noted.
   - If Tony is sexually active and has, recently or in the past, been knowingly exposed to a sexually transmitted disease.
   - If there has been pain associated with the "bump" or exudate noted from the penis.

The assessment, done by a physician or primary care provider should include:

- Visual inspection of the size, shape, symmetry, and color of the scrotum and its contents.
- Palpation to assess for abnormalities and pain.
- Cultures to rule out sexually transmitted diseases.
- An inguinal exam to rule out herniation.

Ultimately, based on the patient's report, a testicular tumor should be ruled out.

REVIEW QUESTIONS

1. Which male reproductive duct carries sperm into the abdominal cavity?
   a. Urethra
   b. Epididymis
   c. Ductus deferens
   d. Ejaculatory duct

2. Which of the following is the usual site of fertilization?
   a. Ovary
   b. Uterus
   c. Vagina
   d. Fallopian tube

3. Which procedure is most helpful in distinguishing a fluid-filled mass from a solid mass of the breast?
   a. BSE
   b. Mammogram
   c. Clinical breast examination
   d. Ultrasound

4. Which of the following items should be set up in preparation for a Pap smear? **Select all that apply.**
   a. 50-mL syringe
   b. Vaginal speculum
   c. Lubricant
   d. Clean gloves
   e. Slides and fixative spray

5. When obtaining the history of a 17-year-old male during a sports physical, what important screening practice should be discussed?
   a. Yearly DRE
   b. Monthly TSE
   c. Yearly PSA
   d. Bimonthly bimanual examination

REVIEW QUESTIONS—cont'd

6. A patient has just had a laparoscopy to investigate the causes of her infertility. Why should the nurse instruct her to lie flat in the bed for a few hours?
   a. She could rupture her abdominal incision.
   b. Her blood pressure will be extremely low because of blood loss.
   c. The carbon dioxide left over from the test will travel upward and cause pain.
   d. Her uterus needs to be at the same level as her heart to prevent excessive swelling.

7. A 66-year-old woman is seen in an outpatient clinic for routine care. What teaching should the nurse provide related to bone health?
   a. "You should be taking in at least 1200 mg of calcium and 400 international units of vitamin D a day to protect your bones."
   b. "The benefit of eating red meat outweighs the risk as you age. You should eat 6 ounces three times a week."
   c. "Your bones are protected by the calcium you ate in your younger years; increasing intake now will not help your bones."
   d. "You can easily protect your bones by drinking milk twice a day."

References

American Cancer Society. (2009). *Overview: Breast cancer. How is breast cancer found?* Retrieved November 20, 2009, from http://www.cancer.org/docroot/CRI/content/CRI_2_2_3X_How_is_breast_cancer_found_5.asp?sitearea=

Joint Commission. (2010). *2010 national patient safety goals.* Retrieved January 13, 2010, from http://www.jointcommission.org/patientsafety/nationalpatientsafetygoals

42 Nursing Care of Female Patients with Reproductive System Disorders

LAURA L. McCULLY
AND DEBRA PERRY-PHILO

KEY TERMS

agenesis (ay-JEN-uh-sis)
amenorrhea (AY-men-oh-REE-ah)
anteflexion (AN-tee-FLEK-shun)
anteversion (AN-tee-VER-zhun)
augmentation (AWG-men-TAY-shun)
colporrhaphy (kohl-POOR-ah-fee)
contraceptive (KON-truh-SEP-tiv)
cryotherapy (KRY-oh-THER-uh-pee)
culdocentesis (KUL-doh-sen-TEE-sis)
culdotomy (kul-DOT-uh-mee)
cystocele (SIS-toh-seel)
dermoid (DER-moyd)
dilation and curettage (DIL-AY-shun and kyoor-e-TAHZH)
dysmenorrhea (DIS-men-oh-REE-ah)
dyspareunia (DIS-puh-ROO-nee-ah)
dysplasia (dis-PLAY-zee-ah)
fibrocystic (FIGH-broh-SIS-tik)
hypertrophy (high-PER-truh-fee)
hypoplasia (HEYE-poh-PLAY-zee-ah)
hysterectomy (HISS-tuh-RECK-tuh-mee)
hysterotomy (HISS-tuh-RAH-tuh-mee)
imperforate (im-PER-foh-rate)
in vitro fertilization (in-VEE-troh FER-ti-li-ZAY-shun)
laparotomy (LAP-uh-RAH-tuh-mee)
leiomyoma (LYE-oh-my-OH-mah)
lumpectomy (lump-EK-tuh-mee)
mammoplasty (MAM-oh-PLAS-tee)
marsupialization (mar-SOO-pee-al-i-ZAY-shun)
mastalgia (mass-TAL-jee-ah)
mastectomy (mass-TECK-tuh-mee)
mastitis (mass-TIGH-tis)
mastopexy (MAS-toh-PEKS-ee)
myomectomy (MY-oh-MECK-tuh-mee)
panhysterectomy (PAN-hiss-tuh-RECK-tuh-mee)
perimenopausal (PER-ee-MEN-oh-PAWS-uhl)
phytoestrogens (FY-toh-ES-troh-jenz)
postcoital (post-KOH-i-tal)
rectocele (RECK-toh-seel)
retroflexion (RET-roh-FLEK-shun)
retrograde (RET-roh-grayd)
retroversion (RET-roh-VER-zhun)
salpingo-oophorectomy (sal-PINJ-oh-ah-fuh-RECK-tuh-mee)
teratoma (ter-uh-TOH-muh)
vaginitis (VAJ-in-EYE-tis)
vaginosis (VAJ-in-OH-sis)

QUESTIONS TO GUIDE YOUR READING

1. How would you explain the pathophysiology of each of the disorders of the female reproductive system?
2. What are the etiologies, signs, and symptoms of each disorder?
3. What care would you provide for patients undergoing tests for each disorder?
4. What is the current therapeutic management for each disorder?
5. What data should you collect when caring for patients with disorders of the female reproductive system?
6. What nursing care will you provide for patients with each of the disorders?
7. How will you know if your nursing interventions have been effective?
8. How do the different forms of contraceptives available vary in effectiveness?

Reproductive system disorders can be frightening, irritating, frustrating, embarrassing, and in some cases fatal. They involve not just body parts but also roles, relationships, and sense of identity and purpose in life. Nurses can play an important role in helping women with these disorders. Women's health is an area where much research is being done. The Nurses' Health Study, conducted at Harvard Medical School, is a large ongoing study on many topics related to women's health. You can learn about it at www.nurseshealthstudy.org.

BREAST DISORDERS

Benign Breast Disorders

Much has been done in recent years to educate the general public concerning breast cancer. It is the most commonly diagnosed cancer in women (Centers for Disease Control and Prevention [CDC], 2009). Heightened awareness of the risks of breast cancer, however, sometimes results in excessive anxiety among women with benign breast conditions. The following section covers benign, or noncancerous, breast disorders.

Cyclic Breast Discomfort

PATHOPHYSIOLOGY, ETIOLOGIES, AND SIGNS AND SYMPTOMS. The most common breast symptoms result from cyclic variations in hormone levels. Swelling, tenderness, and sometimes pain (**mastalgia**) can be related to hormone-mediated changes within the breast tissues that prepare them for their potential role of breastfeeding.

TREATMENT. If persistent or severe, these symptoms can be treated with oral contraceptives that modify hormone levels or nonsteroidal anti-inflammatory drugs (NSAIDs) to control pain. Explaining that cyclic discomfort is temporary and not from a disease process helps to reduce fears.

Fibrocystic Breast Disease

Fibrocystic breast disease is common in women between the ages of 30 and 50. Many refer to it as simply "fibrocystic breast changes."

PATHOPHYSIOLOGY, ETIOLOGIES, AND SIGNS AND SYMPTOMS. Overresponsiveness of cells in the breasts to hormonal stimulation (especially estrogen) may cause long-term changes resulting in replacement of normal tissue with fibrous tissue, overdevelopment of cells, and blockage of ducts so that cysts form around trapped fluid. This makes the breasts feel somewhat hard and lumpy, and sometimes painful. These changes often occur during the reproductive years, and can respond to hormonal variations during the menstrual cycle. Fibrocystic changes usually subside with menopause.

DIAGNOSIS AND TREATMENT. Fibrocystic breast changes can be identified on palpation. A mammogram or ultrasound may be done to assist in diagnosis. A biopsy may be done to rule out cancer. Treatment for fibrocystic breast changes is based on patient symptoms. Often, no treatment is necessary. Analgesics, primarily NSAIDs, may help reduce discomfort. Herbal remedies, such as evening primrose oil, or supplemental vitamin therapy may offer symptomatic relief, but these therapies remain controversial. Limitation of dietary fat and caffeine and addition of oral contraceptive use may help control hormonal changes that result in discomfort.

Although **fibrocystic** changes are not cancerous, more frequent mammography or ultrasound may be advised because fibrocystic changes may make it more difficult to feel early cancerous lumps during breast self-examination (BSE). Some types of breast cysts are associated with a higher cancer risk. Needle aspiration may be used to treat cystic lesions.

Mastitis

PATHOPHYSIOLOGY, ETIOLOGIES, AND SIGNS AND SYMPTOMS. Breast infection with inflammation (**mastitis**) occurs as a result of injury and introduction of bacteria into the breast. This condition most commonly occurs while breastfeeding. The breast becomes swollen, hot, red, and painful and can form an abscess.

TREATMENT. Mastitis can be treated either with antibiotics or by incision and drainage (I&D) of the abscessed area. NSAIDs, warm packs, and breast supports are often used to control pain and swelling.

NURSING CARE AND PATIENT EDUCATION. You can assist with an I&D by setting out the equipment: a wrapped sterile sharp-pointed scalpel blade, a blade handle, clean gloves, and dressing materials. A dressing may be applied over the I&D site to absorb drainage.

Patient teaching should include instructions to wash hands carefully to prevent the spread of infection. If the patient is breastfeeding, it is often continued to promote drainage of the breast, mother-infant bonding, and infant nutrition. The infant is often already colonized with the bacteria so further exposure is not thought to be detrimental.

NURSING CARE TIP

To help prevent mastitis in a breastfeeding mother, recommend frequent changes in feeding positions to empty all portions of the breast, as well as good hygiene techniques such as hand washing when handling the breasts.

• WORD • BUILDING •
mastalgia: mast—breast + algia—pain

• WORD • BUILDING •
fibrocystic: fibro—fibrous + cystic—saclike
mastitis: mast—breast + itis—inflammation

Malignant Breast Disorders

Pathophysiology and Etiology

Breast cancer is an abnormal growth of breast cells. It can arise from the milk-producing glands, the ductal system, or the fatty and connective tissues of the breast.

Research has identified factors that increase the risk of breast cancer: increasing age; personal or family history of breast, ovarian, or prostate cancer; a high-fat diet; high alcohol intake; treatment with estrogens (especially when used without progestins); early menarche; late menopause; and first pregnancy after age 25.

Signs and Symptoms

A lump or thickening of breast tissue, or a change in the shape or contour of a breast can indicate breast cancer. A tumor can also cause dimpling of the overlying skin or retraction of the nipple. Clear or bloody nipple discharge can occur. Swelling, tenderness, or discoloration of the breast may indicate inflammatory breast cancer, a rare but deadly form. Breast symptoms have many causes, but all should be investigated by a health care provider.

Prevention

Breast cancer risk can be reduced by exercising moderation in fat and alcohol consumption and using non-hormonal methods for birth control and menopausal symptoms. Breastfeeding may also reduce risk, even in women who have late first pregnancies (see *Evidence-Based Practice* box). However, many factors cannot be controlled, so the importance of early detection cannot be overemphasized. Recent research has discovered genes (BRCA1 and BRCA2) that are linked with susceptibility to breast cancer. These findings offer the possibility of very early identification of women at the most risk of developing breast cancer (and also ovarian cancer for those with BRCA1). These women can then be monitored closely for breast changes, and receive early treatment if cancer develops.

> ### EVIDENCE-BASED PRACTICE
>
> **Clinical Question**
>
> Does breastfeeding reduce risk of breast cancer?
>
> **Evidence**
>
> A systematic review of 31 research studies was undertaken (Yang & Jacobsen, 2008). Eleven found that breastfeeding significantly reduces breast cancer risk, and 13 studies found a reduced risk only with extended lactation. The authors conclude that more information is needed.
>
> **Implications for Nursing Practice**
>
> There are many reasons to advise women to breastfeed their babies. Possible protection against breast cancer is one reason.
>
> REFERENCE
>
> **Yang, L., & Jacobsen, K. H. (2008). A systematic review of the association between breastfeeding and breast cancer. *Journal of Women's Health, 17*(10), 1635–1645.**

Diagnostic Tests

Breast self-examination (BSE) and clinical breast examinations play an important role in cancer identification. Cancerous growths tend to be harder, less mobile, less painful, more irregularly shaped, and have less clearly defined borders than benign growths. The prognosis is good for women who have breast cancers removed in the early stages but gets worse when treatment begins during later stages of the disease process. Teaching and encouraging regular use of BSE and appropriate use of mammography can save lives. See Chapter 41 for more about BSE and for explanations about diagnostic tests used to assist in determining whether tumors of the breast are malignant.

Staging

The spread (metastasis) of cancerous cells from the primary site to other areas of the body by way of the blood or lymph is denoted by staging classifications 0 to IV (see Chapter 11). Lower numbers indicate less cancer spread.

Therapeutic Measures

The five main treatment options for breast cancer are surgery, radiation therapy, chemotherapy, hormone therapy, and targeted therapy. These options may be used separately or in combination depending on the condition of the patient and the stage of the disease. Patients may also choose complementary and holistic therapies. Immunotherapy is a new and promising field of breast cancer treatment that uses the body's immune system to fight cancer. A number of immunotherapies are currently being studied, including the use of vaccines.

SURGERY. A **lumpectomy** removes just the tumor and a margin around it. A **mastectomy** may be partial (removing only part of the breast), simple (removing the breast tissue of one or both breasts), or radical (removing breast tissue, underlying muscle, and surrounding lymph nodes). The amount of tissue removed varies depending on the size, nature, and invasiveness of the cancer. Surgical practice has shifted from radical mastectomies to more breast-conserving surgeries with the addition of radiation therapy, resulting in survival rates similar to those for radical mastectomy. Surgeries to remove cancerous breast tissue can be disfiguring and have profound effects on a patient's body image and self-esteem.

RADIATION THERAPY. Radiation can be administered externally or internally to attack the rapidly dividing cells of a tumor. Although radiation affects all rapidly dividing cells in its path, including healthy cells, radiation to an area of the breast just surrounding the tumor bed reduces the incidence

• WORD • BUILDING •

lumpectomy: lump + ectomy—excision

mastectomy: mast—breast + ec—away + tomy—cutting

of side effects. It is usually used after surgery to reduce the risk of cancer recurrence or spread.

CHEMOTHERAPY. Chemotherapy kills all rapidly dividing cells, not just breast cancer cells, which leads to many side effects. This therapy may be used alone or in combination with other therapies. Newer chemotherapy options use higher doses over a shorter treatment period to reduce side effects (see Chapter 11).

HORMONE THERAPY. Hormone therapy may be used to deprive cancer cells of hormones that stimulate their growth. Because breast cancer cells are often estrogen sensitive, this may be accomplished by decreasing circulating estrogen levels with drugs or by blocking the use of estrogen by cancer cells. Interference with estrogen levels, however, may produce menopausal symptoms and increase the risk of osteoporosis and heart disease. Table 42.1 lists estrogen antagonists.

TARGETED THERAPIES. Targeted therapies attack specific molecular agents or pathways involved in the development of cancer. Some targeted therapies are given to intensify positive body responses (e.g., stimulate the immune system) or to decrease negative body responses. Examples include biological response modifiers such as interferons, tumor necrosis factor, interleukins, and various experimental immunotherapy formulations. Two drugs that target the protein HER2, which is found in larger than normal amounts on the surface of breast cancer cells, are trastuzumab (Herceptin) and lapatinib

TABLE 42.1 MEDICATIONS FOR DISORDERS RELATED TO HORMONAL ALTERATIONS (BREAST DISORDERS, MENSTRUAL DISORDERS, MENOPAUSE)

Medication Class/Action	Examples	Route	Side Effects	Nursing Implications
Oral Contraceptives/HRT				
Interfere with gonadotropin-releasing hormone, luteinizing hormone (LH), and follicle-stimulating hormone (FSH) release; maintain stable hormonal levels, relax uterus, limit endometrial proliferation, promote vasomotor stability, prevent bone loss.	**Progesterone and estrogen** norethindrone/levonorgestrel/ medroxyprogesterone and ethinyl estradiol/ conjugated estrogens (*Birth control:* Ortho-Novum, Alesse) (*Menopause:* Prempro)	PO, topical patch	Hypertension, breakthrough bleeding, amenorrhea, headache, increased risk of gallbladder/ liver disease and thromboembolitic disorders secondary to hypercoagulation, glucose intolerance, decreased breast milk production, depression	Educate patient regarding use and side effects. (See "ACHES" side effects presented later in this chapter.) Smoking increases risk of blood clots; advise to stop smoking while on these medications.
	Estrogen only conjugated estrogens (Premarin) estrogen derivatives (Estrace, Climara, Vagifem)	PO, topical patch, vaginal		
	Progesterone only norethindrone/medroxyprogesterone (Micronor, Provera)	PO		
	Estrogen and testosterone esterone/methyltestosterone (Estratest)	PO		
NSAIDs				
Inhibit prostaglandin synthesis, therefore interrupt pain receptors and produce anti-inflammatory effect.	ibuprofen (Motrin, Nuprin, Advil) naproxen (Aleve) ketoprofen (Orudis) ketorolac (Toradol)	PO, IV, IM	Peptic ulcer or GI perforations, GI bleeding, bleeding tendency, rash, pruritus, liver/renal dysfunction	Avoid with aspirin allergy; administer with milk or food, caution about side effects, use during pregnancy, or use when on anticoagulant therapy.
Antineoplastic Medications (Estrogen Antagonists)				
Act as estrogen antagonists to inhibit growth of estrogen-dependent tumors.	tamoxifen (Nolvadex) anastrozole (Arimidex) toremifene (Fareston) exemestane (Aromasin) letrozole (Femara) fulvestrant (Faslodex)	PO	Vasomotor changes, menstrual changes, increased vaginal discharge, endometrial hyperplasia/ polyps, rash, bone pain, retinopathy (with high doses)	Report vaginal bleeding, leg cramps, shortness of breath, weakness. Promote use of nonhormonal contraceptives during use. Smoking increases the patient's risk of blood clots; advise patients to stop smoking during use.

(Tykerb). Another drug, bevacizumab (Avastin), works by blocking the growth of new blood vessels that cancer cells depend on to grow and function. Targeted therapy is an area of much research and is likely to expand greatly during the next few years.

Alternative therapies are also available for many cancers. See Chapter 5 for information about helping patients evaluate alternative and complementary therapies. The American Cancer Society and cancer treatment centers also have people who can answer questions about experimental and alternative therapies and discuss research findings. For more information about breast cancer, visit the American Cancer Society at www.cancer.org or www.breastcancer.org. Also visit Susan G. Komen for the Cure at ww5.komen.org.

Nursing Care

See the *Nursing Care Plan for the Patient Undergoing a Mastectomy.* In addition to the diagnoses covered, the patient will need diagnoses for postoperative pain. See Chapters 10 and 12, respectively, for additional interventions for pain and postoperative patients.

CRITICAL THINKING

Julie

■ Julie, age 32, reports pain and grapelike "lumps" in her breasts, and her nurse practitioner diagnoses fibrocystic changes.

1. What questions would you ask to further assess Julie's symptoms?
2. What might you teach Julie to help her control her symptoms?

Suggested answers at end of chapter.

NURSING CARE PLAN for the Patient Undergoing a Mastectomy

Nursing Diagnosis: *Anxiety* related to uncertainty about diagnosis, prognosis, and treatments

Expected Outcomes: The patient will verbalize and demonstrate a decrease in anxiety.

Evaluation of Outcomes: Does the patient report a decrease in anxiety following education and explanation of the procedure? Do patient's vital signs, verbal, and nonverbal behavior suggest a decrease in anxiety?

Interventions	Rationale	Evaluation
Assess vital signs and observe verbal and nonverbal behavior.	An increase in blood pressure, pulse, and respirations as well as observation of mild to severe agitation may indicate anxiety.	Are the patient's vital signs within normal range for the patient? Is verbal and nonverbal behavior consistent with anxiety?
Assess patient's current knowledge of the procedure and level of anxiety related to the procedure. Teach patient what to expect about the surgical experience based on patient's understanding, concerns, and willingness to learn. Support the physician's explanations, answer questions, and refer to knowledgeable sources.	Knowledge dispels unreasonable fears and helps patient to prepare to cope with stressors.	Does patient express satisfaction with amount and type of information? Does patient evidence adequate understanding of the procedure as well as understanding of what to expect afterward?

NURSING CARE PLAN for the Patient Undergoing a Mastectomy—cont'd

Nursing Diagnosis: *Risk for Ineffective Breathing Pattern* related to pain with chest movement

Expected Outcomes: The patient will have an effective breathing pattern with clear lung sounds and SpO_2 of 95% or above.

Evaluation of Outcomes: Are respirations regular, easy, and unlabored? Are respiratory rate and oxygen saturation within a normal range for the patient? Are lung sounds clear?

Interventions	Rationale	Evaluation
Assess patient's vital signs, oxygen saturation, pain level, and lung sounds.	Pain contributes to shallow breathing, which can affect vital signs, SpO_2, and lung sounds.	Are the patient's vital signs and oxygen saturation within normal range for the patient? Does patient report pain at an acceptable level? Are lung sounds clear?
Medicate to relieve pain as necessary.	Pain may inhibit deep breathing efforts.	Does patient evidence pain or guarding during chest movement?
Encourage deep breathing and coughing each hour.	This helps to loosen secretions and to prevent atelectasis, pneumonia, and inadequate oxygenation of tissues.	Does chest sound clear? Are skin color and oxygen saturation adequate?
Encourage use of an incentive spirometer each hour when awake.	To encourage deep breathing	Does patient use spirometer correctly?

Nursing Diagnosis: *Risk for Ineffective Tissue Perfusion* related to damage to blood and lymph vessels and tension at surgical incision site

Expected Outcomes: The patient's incision will heal by primary intention without excessive bleeding or swelling.

Evaluation of Outcomes: Are edges of the incision well approximated, with scant bleeding/serous drainage, and mild edema/erythema?

Interventions	Rationale	Evaluation
Monitor vital signs and oxygen saturation according to agency policy and as necessary.	Vital signs and oxygen saturation affect tissue perfusion and oxygenation.	Are vital signs and SpO_2 stable and within normal range?
Avoid use of the affected arm for blood pressures, venipunctures, and injections.	Restrictive and invasive procedures might further compromise tissue integrity of the affected arm.	Is the arm protected?
Assess incision for bleeding, amount and color of drainage, and swelling. Empty drain device prn.	Excessive bleeding or swelling can compromise tissue perfusion.	Does incisional area look swollen, smooth, or shiny? Are drainage amount and color appropriate?
Measure circumference of arms daily and compare. Report changes.	Swelling causes an increase in circumference and impairs circulation.	Is affected arm larger than unaffected arm?
Elevate affected arm if swelling occurs.	Gravity aids fluid return to the heart.	Does elevation reduce swelling?
Place items where patient can easily reach them.	Excessive movement of the arm may exert tension on incision and increase bleeding.	Can patient reach items without abducting the arm more than 90 degrees?

NURSING CARE PLAN for the Patient Undergoing a Mastectomy—cont'd

Interventions	Rationale	Evaluation
Encourage post-mastectomy exercises of the affected arm according to agency policy.	Appropriate exercise promotes circulation, preserves muscle and joint function, and increases self-care ability.	Is patient moving the arm appropriately and gradually increasing range of motion and self-care ability?
Teach postoperative self-care and signs and symptoms of ineffective healing to report.	Early assessment and intervention help prevent the development of serious complications.	Does patient demonstrate and verbalize understanding of appropriate postoperative self-care?

Nursing Diagnosis: *Risk for Ineffective Coping* related to cancer threat and body image disturbance

Expected Outcomes: The patient will verbalize ability to cope and will seek help and support appropriately.

Evaluation of Outcomes: Does patient take an interest in care of condition? Does patient ask appropriate questions related to care and verbalize appropriate concerns?

Interventions	Rationale	Evaluation
Observe patient's interest in self-care, ability to problem solve, and level of family or other support.	Poor self-care, problem-solving skills, and lack of support may indicate a risk for ineffective coping.	Does patient solve problems appropriately? Are family members or other support persons present? Is patient taking an active interest in her personal appearance?
Use therapeutic communication and listening skills to allow patient to share concerns.	Loss of a breast disturbs many aspects of body image, and cancer threatens one's sense of security and reasonableness of life.	Is patient able to share concerns?
Help patient remember previous successes in coping and strategies used.	Memory of prior success can encourage hope for future success.	Does patient possess appropriate coping strategies?
Provide accurate information according to agency policy.	Fear of the unknown can increase anxiety and reduce coping.	Does patient relate understanding of follow-up treatment?
Refer to appropriate agencies for further support as needed (e.g., American Cancer Society, Reach for Recovery, local support groups).	Social support can assist individuals to meet their needs while developing effective coping skills and strategies.	Does patient have resources to call on as needed?

See Table 42.2 for a breast cancer summary.

Breast Modification Surgeries

Mammoplasty is surgical modification of the breast. This may be done to restore a normal shape after removal of cancerous tissues. Many women, however, undergo mammoplasty electively to reduce or increase the size or to improve the shape of their breasts. Because nurses are very aware of the dangers involved with surgery, psychosocial issues may seem to be a trivial reason to voluntarily assume such risks to life and health. However, body image is an important component of quality of life. Patients' informed decisions should be respected if they choose this surgery. It is essential that you present a caring and nonjudgmental attitude.

• WORD • BUILDING •
mammoplasty: mamm(o)—breast + plasty—to mold

Breast Reduction and Mastopexy

Generally, in breast reduction operations the nipple is separated from the surrounding tissue except for a small section with the blood vessels and nerves that supply it (Fig. 42.1).

TABLE 42.2 BREAST CANCER SUMMARY

Signs and Symptoms	Swelling, tenderness, pain, redness Palpable lumps Leakage of fluid/blood from nipple Changes in contour of skin of breast/nipple
Diagnostic Tests and Findings	BSE/CBE Mammography Excisional/fine-needle biopsy
Therapeutic Measures	Lumpectomy/mastectomy/breast reconstruction Radiation Chemotherapy Hormone therapy Targeted therapy
Complications	Metastasis Significant treatment side effects Profound negative effect on patient's self-image.
Priority Nursing Diagnoses	*Anxiety* *Risk for Ineffective Breathing Pattern* *Risk for Ineffective Tissue Perfusion* *Risk for Ineffective Coping*

BSE = breast self-examination; CBE = clinical breast examination.

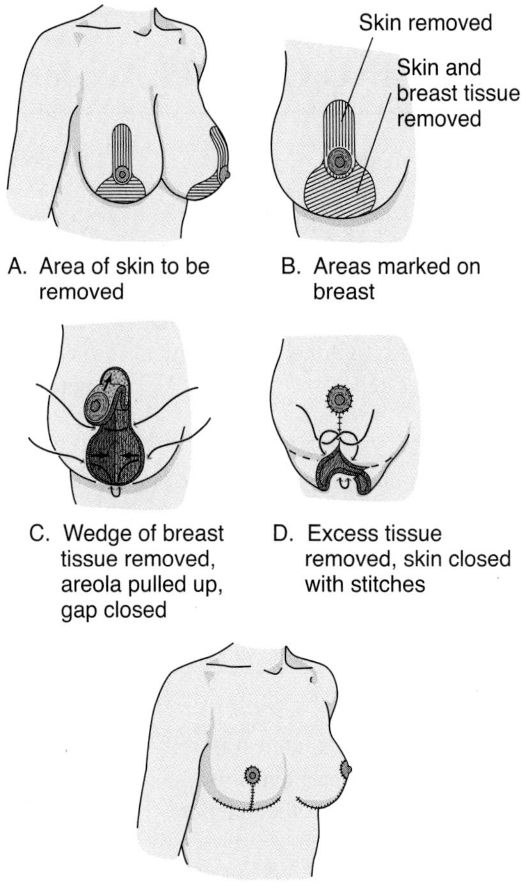
Skin removed
Skin and breast tissue removed
A. Area of skin to be removed
B. Areas marked on breast
C. Wedge of breast tissue removed, areola pulled up, gap closed
D. Excess tissue removed, skin closed with stitches
E. Post-operative appearance

FIGURE 42.1 Breast reduction. (Modified from Love, S. M. [2000]. *Dr. Susan Love's breast book* [3rd ed.]. Cambridge, MA: Perseus Publishing, with permission.)

A large wedge of tissue is removed from the bottom of the breast, the edges are sewn together, and the nipple is reimplanted in a higher position. This not only decreases the overall size of the breast, which may help with back, neck, and head pain, but it also corrects excessive sagging—a common problem for women with large breasts.

A **mastopexy** involves the removal of some skin and fat with subsequent resuturing so that the breast tissues are held higher on the chest to correct sagging breasts. This procedure usually does not remove as much tissue as a breast reduction.

Augmentation and Reconstruction Mammoplasty

Augmentation is a surgery to increase the size of the breasts. An implant—either a bag containing saline solution or silicone gel or a transplanted portion of the patient's own body tissues from another area—is inserted through an incision and positioned either under or over the pectoral muscles (Fig. 42.2).

For reconstructive mammoplasty, use of the patient's own tissues is generally safer than use of artificial implants because no foreign material is introduced into the body. For situations in which significant amounts of tissue are needed for reconstruction, a portion of tissue may be moved from one area of the body to another as a pedicle graft. Pedicle literally means "little foot" because the graft remains attached to a stalk (containing the blood vessels and nerves) somewhat resembling a little leg with a foot (the graft) attached.

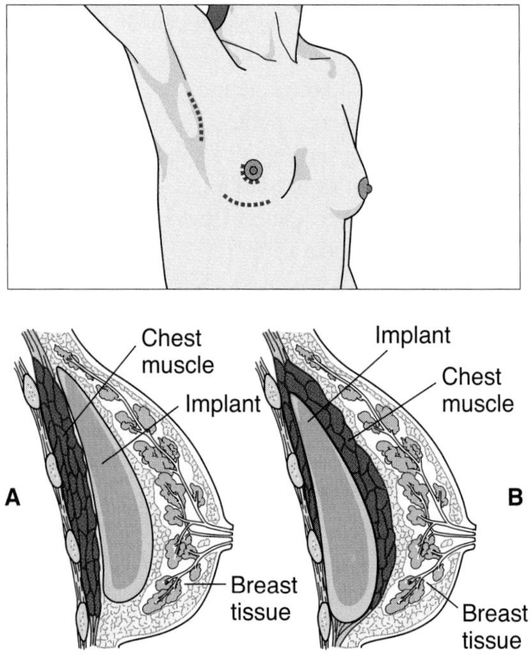
Chest muscle
Implant
A
Breast tissue
Implant
Chest muscle
B
Breast tissue

FIGURE 42.2 Breast implants. (A) Implant over muscle. (B) Implant under muscle. (Modified from Love, S. M. [2000]. *Dr. Susan Love's breast book* [3rd ed.]. Cambridge, MA: Perseus Publishing, with permission.)

• **WORD • BUILDING** •
mastopexy: masto—breast + pexy—fixation

Figure 42.3 shows two options for mastectomy graft repair—using the latissimus dorsi muscle and overlying tissue on the side of the chest or using the rectus abdominis muscle of the abdomen with its overlying tissue. For both of these procedures, a portion of muscle is separated from its usual attachment. Tissues overlying a part of the muscle are excised and left attached to the muscle. This segment of tissue is then pulled under the skin and superficial layers to an incision at the mastectomy site. There it is brought to the surface and attached to reconstruct a breast shape. Tissue from the buttock area or the abdomen may also be grafted onto a mastectomy site without a pedicle.

Complications

Any surgery may be complicated by infection or impaired healing. The use of silicone implants has been less than satisfactory for many women. Some women have experienced hardening of breast tissues and others have developed serious autoimmune disease problems after receiving silicone gel implants. Although actual etiologies of all the problems are uncertain, many surgeries have been undertaken recently to remove silicone implants, and saline implants are now more common.

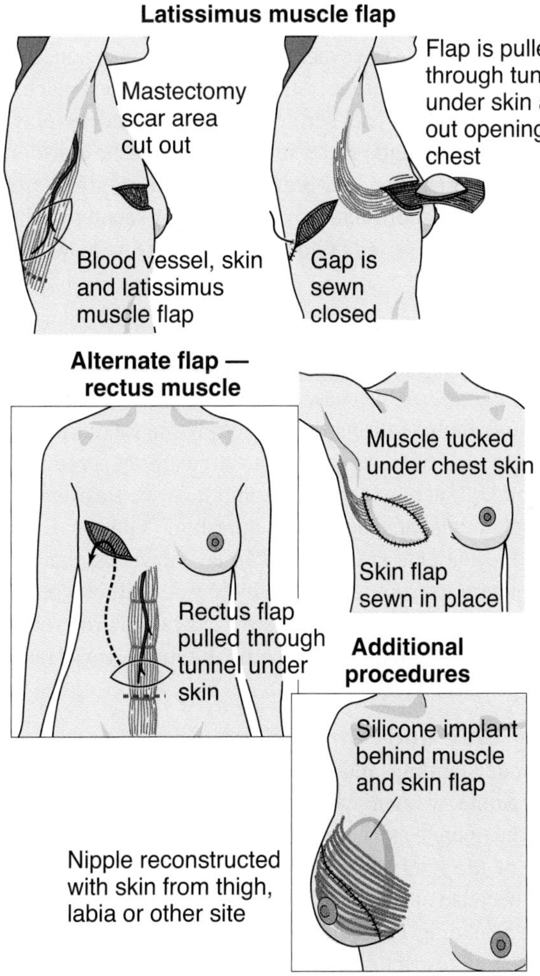
Latissimus muscle flap
Mastectomy scar area cut out
Flap is pulled through tunnel under skin and out opening in chest
Blood vessel, skin and latissimus muscle flap
Gap is sewn closed
Alternate flap — rectus muscle
Muscle tucked under chest skin
Skin flap sewn in place
Rectus flap pulled through tunnel under skin
Additional procedures
Silicone implant behind muscle and skin flap
Nipple reconstructed with skin from thigh, labia or other site

FIGURE 42.3 Mastectomy reconstruction. (Modified from Love, S. M. [2000]. *Dr. Susan Love's breast book* [3rd ed.]. Cambridge, MA: Perseus Publishing, with permission.)

Nursing Care and Patient Education

Carefully assess the healing process when changing dressings and explain to the patient how to assess healing, because not all tissues successfully attach at the new site. Failure of attachment can require surgical revision. Signs of poor attachment include unnatural color of the incision, graft, or surrounding tissues; swelling; drainage; gaping incision lines; and sloughing of the graft or edges of the site.

MENSTRUAL DISORDERS

Flow and Cycle Disorders

Pathophysiology, Etiologies, and Signs and Symptoms

There are many types of menstrual abnormalities (Table 42.3). Causes can include stress, pregnancy, hormonal imbalances, metabolic imbalances (such as obesity, anorexia nervosa, and loss of too much body fat through excessive exercise), tumors (both benign and malignant), infections, organ diseases (such as liver, kidney, or thyroid disease), blood or bone marrow abnormalities, and the presence of foreign bodies in the uterus (such as intrauterine devices). Menstrual abnormalities can be distressing and can result in anemia, persistent fatigue, and sexual dysfunction. Establishment of a comfortable and open professional relationship between a woman and her health provider is essential for communication about such concerns.

TABLE 42.3 MENSTRUAL FLOW DISORDERS

Disorder	Description
Amenorrhea	Menses absent for more than 6 months or three of previous cycles Called primary amenorrhea when menarche has not occurred by age 17 Called secondary amenorrhea when menses are absent after menarche
Hypermenorrhea	Menses lasting longer than 7 days
Hypomenorrhea	Less than the expected amount of menstrual bleeding
Menometrorrhagia (also called metro-menorrhagia)	Overly long, heavy, and irregular menses
Menorrhagia	Passing more than 80 mL of blood per menses
Oligomenorrhea	Menstrual cycles of more than 35 days
Polymenorrhea (also called metrorrhagia)	Menses more frequently than 21-day intervals

Diagnostic Tests

Appropriate testing to determine the cause of menstrual abnormalities can involve a thorough medical history and physical examination. Papanicolaou (Pap) smear, cervical and vaginal cultures, laparoscopy, ultrasound, pregnancy testing, urine testing, and extensive blood testing may be done to screen for any of the disorders that can influence the menstrual cycle and flow. Generally, health care providers initially test to rule out the most likely causes and then begin to test for less common disorders until the cause of the disorder is identified.

Therapeutic Measures

Medical treatment of menstrual disorders often involves manipulation of hormone levels. Surgical treatment of menstrual disorders can involve **dilation and curettage** (D&C), laser ablation of endometrial tissue, and **hysterectomy**. During D&C the cervix is first dilated (opened wider) and then a curet—a sharp, spoonlike instrument—is inserted through the cervix and used to scoop out the inner lining of the uterus. Laser ablation involves targeted burning of endometrial tissue so that scar tissue forms that does not bleed. Hysterectomy (removal of the uterus), a last-resort treatment, is described later in this chapter.

Nursing Care

The only accurate way to estimate menstrual flow is to weigh used sanitary pads (sealed in a biohazard bag) and then subtract the weight of the original pads. A 1-g increase in pad weight equals approximately 1 mL of blood loss. Simply counting numbers of pads used is much less accurate, since women may change pads at different intervals. You may have to rely on a woman's report of blood loss. Be sure to document "patient estimate" after the quote.

Dysmenorrhea

Pathophysiology, Etiologies, and Signs and Symptoms

Painful menstruation, or **dysmenorrhea**, is a common problem in women. Primary dysmenorrhea (menstrual cramps) is not pathological and is thought to be caused mainly by the action of endogenous prostaglandins that stimulate uterine contractions, producing cramping pain. Secondary dysmenorrhea is caused by a reproductive tract disorder such as endometriosis, pelvic infection, retroversion of the uterus, or fibroid tumors.

Diagnostic Tests

Hormonal tests such as estrogen and progesterone levels may be evaluated for primary dysmenorrhea. Additional tests such as laparoscopic examination, biopsies, or cultures may be required for investigation of secondary dysmenorrhea.

• WORD • BUILDING •

dilation and curettage: dilat(e)—to widen + ation—the process of + curet—scoop + tage—doing

hysterectomy: hyster—womb + ec—away + tomy—cutting

dysmenorrhea: dys—painful + men(o)—month + rrhea—flow

Therapeutic Measures

Primary dysmenorrhea can be treated with drugs that inhibit prostaglandin synthesis, such as aspirin and nonsteroidal anti-inflammatory drugs (NSAIDs). Correction of secondary causes of dysmenorrhea may include such measures as hormonal adjustment, usually with oral contraceptives or hormone replacement therapy (HRT), dilation and curettage, or other surgical or medical intervention based on the cause.

Nursing Care and Patient Education

Several nonprescription preparations are available for treatment of dysmenorrhea, but women should be advised to read the labels carefully because aspirin and NSAIDs (the main component of many of the drugs) can be bought less expensively. Other added drugs in these compounds, such as diuretics, may not be necessary. If dysmenorrhea is related to uterine retroversion, assuming a knee-to-chest position may relieve the discomfort. Sudden development of dysmenorrhea in a woman with no previous menstrual discomfort should always be investigated.

Premenstrual Syndrome

Pathophysiology, Etiologies, and Signs and Symptoms

Premenstrual syndrome (PMS) is a recurrent problem for many women. While the exact cause is not understood, ovarian hormones, aldosterone, and neurotransmitters such as monoamine oxidase and serotonin are believed to play a role. Symptoms include water retention; headaches; discomfort of joints, muscles, and breasts; changes in affect, concentration, and coordination; and sensory changes. Few women find PMS serious enough to interfere with work or relationships.

Therapeutic Measures

A variety of drugs have been given to combat PMS with varying degrees of success. Some commonly used PMS medications include drugs that affect prostaglandin production, hormonal balance, and neurotransmitter production and reuptake (such as antidepressants), as well as diuretics and supplements of calcium, magnesium, vitamin E, and vitamin B_6. Patients should be warned, however, that dosages of vitamins should not be increased without professional advice because vitamins are medications (as well as nutrients) and high doses of some vitamins can lead to physiological damage.

Nursing Care and Patient Education

Being understanding and nonjudgmental is especially important. Some women who suffer from severe PMS may have been treated as if they are psychologically impaired because of the interaction of hormones and neurotransmitters and because of outdated ideas concerning PMS. You can help by providing educational materials on lifestyle measures, such as restriction of alcohol, caffeine, nicotine, salt, and simple sugars; participation in regular exercise; and development of stress management skills that may help to reduce symptoms.

Endometriosis

Pathophysiology, Etiologies, and Signs and Symptoms

Endometriosis is a condition in which functioning endometrial tissue is located outside the uterus (Fig. 42.4). Several theories have been proposed to explain development of endometriosis, including faulty developmental differentiation of cells, transport of endometrial cells via blood and lymph to other parts of the body, and **retrograde** menstruation—a backward leakage of blood and tissue into the fallopian tubes during the menstrual period.

Endometriotic cells grow in areas of sufficient blood supply, extending into tissues such as intestinal walls, ovaries, and other abdominal structures. On a cyclic basis, mediated by ovarian hormones, these cells build up and slough just as they would in the uterus, but the sloughing and bleeding occur in the enclosed abdominal cavity or into the tissues that they have invaded. The buildup of the blood and cells can result in pain, swelling, damage to abdominal organs and structures, scar tissue development, and infertility.

Therapeutic Measures

Surgical intervention may be required, especially if scar tissue develops into tight bands that strangulate sections of bowel or ureters. Reduction of estrogen and prevention of ovulation either with medications or by surgical removal of the ovaries can be very effective but result in infertility and menopausal symptoms. Analgesics may be required for pain.

Nursing Care and Patient Education

The severity and persistence of the pain of endometriosis may lead to reliance on pain medication, so it is important to teach patients alternative pain relief strategies such as relaxation exercises and application of heat to the abdomen or back.

Menopause

Pathophysiology and Signs and Symptoms

Menopause is the permanent cessation of menstrual cycles resulting from decreased hormone production. This is a natural part of aging, but related uncomfortable symptoms and conditions can occur. The climacteric (perimenopause) is the period of gradual decline in hormone production before the permanent end of menses and may last from a few months to several years. **Perimenopausal** physical symptoms vary widely and may include erratic menses, atrophy of urogenital tissues with a marked decrease in the amount of natural lubrication, a pH shift toward alkalinity (encouraging yeast overgrowth), and vasomotor instability (resulting in hot flashes and night sweats).

Estrogen protects women against several disease processes; the risk of heart disease and osteoporosis increases with declining estrogen production. Mental changes may also occur because of the complex interplay of reproductive hormones and neurotransmitters. It is important to acknowledge symptoms such as irritability, anxiety, insomnia, memory problems, and mild depression as a normal, temporary result of hormonal changes, so that perimenopausal women do not doubt their sanity.

Therapeutic Measures

Hormone replacement therapy (HRT) is a controversial prevention and treatment for perimenopausal symptoms. Hormone replacement (see Table 42.1 for examples) may be prescribed for severe symptoms, and can be administered orally, vaginally, or transdermally. The National Heart, Lung, and Blood Institute (NHLBI) of the National Institutes of Health (NIH) conducted a major research project to study the risks and benefits of combined estrogen and progestin therapy for healthy women (NIH, 2002). The project was halted in July 2002, three years early, because of very worrisome results. Positive findings included a one-third reduction in hip fractures, a 24% decrease in total fractures, and a 37% decrease in colorectal cancer with HRT. Disturbing findings, however, included a 26% increase in breast cancer, a 41% increase in strokes, a 29% increase in heart attacks, doubling of venous thromboembolism rates, and an overall 22% increase in cardiovascular disease. It is uncertain what to make of these data because there was no difference in total mortality when comparing women treated with HRT and those given a placebo. Long-term results will continue to be examined, but for now, the risks of HRT have been deemed too great to continue the study.

As a result of this study and others, HRT is now used only for treating menopausal symptoms, not disease prevention. HRT is prescribed at the lowest dose for treating the symptoms and for the shortest possible length of time. The NHLBI continues to research these issues. Stay updated on the latest findings at www.nhlbi.nih.gov/whi/whi_faq.htm.

Dietary changes to include **phytoestrogens**, which are present in foods and herbs such as soy, tofu, flax seeds, black cohosh, and dong quai, may provide some of the benefits of estrogen replacement without HRT. However, even phytoestrogens are not without risk. Women should discuss

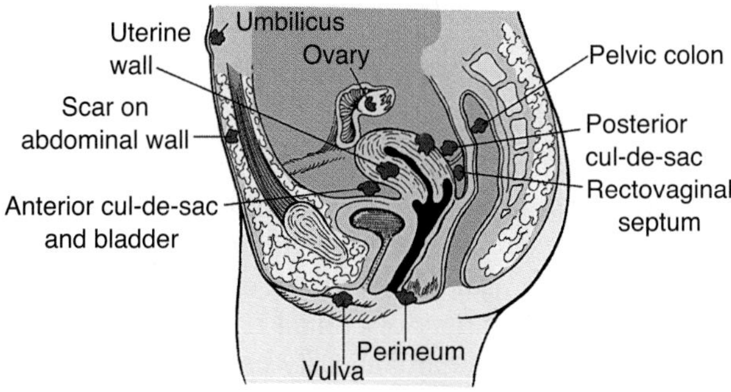

Uterine wall
Umbilicus
Ovary
Pelvic colon
Scar on abdominal wall
Posterior cul-de-sac
Rectovaginal septum
Anterior cul-de-sac and bladder
Perineum
Vulva

FIGURE 42.4 Possible sites of endometriosis.

• WORD • BUILDING •
retrograde: retro—backward + grade—step

• WORD • BUILDING •
perimenopausal: peri—around + men(o)—month + pausal—stopping
phytoestrogens: phyto—plant + estrogens—hormones

food and herb supplements with their primary care providers before using them.

Prevention of osteoporosis begins in early adulthood, long before perimenopause. Fair-skinned, Caucasian women are at greatest risk for bone loss. Throughout life, adequate intake of calcium and vitamin D (preferably from foods) and regular weight-bearing exercise help to maximize bone mass. At menopause, some women may receive HRT or intensive treatment with bone-building medications to slow bone loss.

Complications

It is important to note that resumption of vaginal bleeding after menstruation has finally ceased can be a sign of an endometrial cell disorder caused by either benign changes, such as polyps, or malignant changes of internal reproductive organs. Any bleeding that occurs following previous cessation should always be investigated.

Nursing Care and Patient Education

Teach perimenopausal women that they can plan ahead for hot flashes by dressing in layers of clothing that may be removed. Not allowing hot flashes to interrupt activities is an important strategy, as is engaging in satisfying and calming activities that contribute to a sense of serenity. Vaginal symptoms can be treated with a water-soluble moisture restorer or lubricant, or with an estrogen cream (following prescription directions). Eating a healthy diet that is light in caffeine, sugar, and alcohol can help women better control their bodies and minds. Looking forward to new challenges rather than toward the past may help to counteract hormone-related depressive tendencies. It is important to remind perimenopausal women that they may still be fertile even after several months of **amenorrhea**. To prevent conception, they need to continue to practice birth control until they receive confirmation from their primary care provider that menopause is complete.

See Table 42.4 for a summary of menstrual disorders.

CRITICAL THINKING

Lola

■ Lola, age 53, has been experiencing menopausal hot flashes during the afternoons as she works in her office.

1. What treatments can you suggest to help with her symptoms?
2. If she considers HRT, what information should you share with her?

Suggested answers at end of chapter.

• WORD • BUILDING •

amenorrhea: a—without + men(o)—month + rrhea—flow

TABLE 42.4 MENSTRUAL DISORDERS SUMMARY

Signs and Symptoms	Increase or decrease in menstrual flow Increased pain with menses or generalized abdominal pain Fluid retention Headaches Breast pain/lesions/swelling Mood changes
Diagnostic Tests	Hormone levels Pregnancy test Pap smear Cervical/vaginal cultures Urine testing Ultrasound Laparoscopy Biopsy
Therapeutic Measures	Medication to stabilize hormone levels NSAIDs D&C, laser ablation, hysterectomy Treatment of underlying causes Vitamin/mineral supplements Diuretics/SSRIs/dietary changes
Priority Nursing Diagnoses	*Deficient Fluid Volume* related to increased bleeding *Pain* related to uterine cramping *Deficient Knowledge* related to self-care measures

D&C = dilation and curettage; NSAIDs = nonsteroidal anti-inflammatory drugs; SSRIs = serotonin reuptake inhibitors.

IRRITATIONS AND INFLAMMATIONS OF THE VAGINA AND VULVA

Various causative agents can irritate the vulva and the vagina. Signs and symptoms are often similar, but there are some differences in the discharge produced in response to the disorders. Table 42.5 lists common vaginal irritations and inflammations that are not generally sexually transmitted. See Chapter 44 for information on sexually transmitted diseases.

Pathophysiology, Etiologies, and Signs and Symptoms

The normal vaginal environment is a balanced ecosystem with a pH of less than 4.2 as a result of lactic acid and hydrogen peroxide production by cells in the vagina. This acidic pH protects against the growth of many pathogenic microorganisms. A variety of normal resident microorganisms coexist relatively harmoniously unless the ecological balance is destroyed. Candidiasis, bacterial **vaginosis**, and

• WORD • BUILDING •

vaginosis: vagin—vagina + osis—condition

TABLE 42.5 COMMON VAGINAL IRRITATIONS AND INFLAMMATIONS

Disorder and Etiology	Signs and Symptoms	Discharge/ Examination	Diagnostic Tests	Usual Treatment
Candidiasis: *Candida albicans, glabrata,* or *tropicalis* overgrowth	Burning, itching, redness of vulva; burning on urination	White, cottage cheese appearance	Wet-mount slides (yeasts look like tiny, budding tree branches); may be cultured	Antifungal agents (drugs mostly ending in *-azole*)
Bacterial vaginosis: *Gardnerella vaginalis, Mycoplasma,* or anaerobe overgrowth	None or vulvar or vaginal irritation	White or gray, homogeneous, foul-smelling discharge; pH higher than 4.5	Wet-mount slides show "clue cells" or release fishy odor when potassium hydroxide is applied	Antibiotics
Trichomoniasis: *Trichomonas vaginalis* (may be transmitted by inanimate objects or sexually)	Itching, irritation, foul odor, redness, dysuria	Discharge may be frothy; pH higher than 4.5; "strawberry cervix" resulting from petechiae	Wet-mount slides treated with normal saline show motile cells with flagella (like tiny whips); may also be cultured	Metronidazole
Cytolytic vaginosis: *Lactobacilli* overgrowth, stress, some medications	Burning, irritation, pain with intercourse	Nonodorous, thick, white, pasty, or dry and flaking	Lower than normal pH as tested with pH indicator tape (or litmus strip); may be cultured	Depends on cause; alkaline douches may be prescribed
Contact vulvovaginitis: contact with allergens or irritating chemicals such as contraceptive creams or bubble baths	Itching, burning, redness	Generally no change from normal discharge, though may be increased	History and physical information, recent contact with chemicals	Avoidance of the offending substance; warm sitz baths or application of hydrocortisone cream
Atrophic vaginitis: estrogen levels too low to support estrogen-sensitive vaginal tissues	Vulvovaginal irritation, dryness, dyspareunia, increased tendency for resident microbe overgrowth	May have little or increased discharge; discharge may be watery, yellow, or green; may be blood tinged	Maturation index may be determined during Pap test to identify atrophic cellular changes, but diagnosis is usually by history and physical information	HRT (oral, patch, or vulvovaginal cream) or water-soluble lubricant replacing vaginal lubricants

cytolytic **vaginitis** are all instances of overgrowth of normally present, nonpathogenic microorganisms. Trichomoniasis also is included here because it can be transmitted nonsexually (on fomites, such as toilet seats), as well as sexually, and it grows well when the vaginal environment is disturbed.

Several conditions can predispose patients to an overgrowth of resident microbes: poor nutrition (especially diets high in simple sugars), inconsistent control of blood glucose levels in patients with diabetes, stress, pregnancy, marked hormonal fluctuations, pH changes, prolonged overheating of the genital area with little aeration (as happens with sitting still for long periods in restrictive clothing), and changes in the balance of vaginal flora types because of antibiotic treatment or douching. Patients who have a compromised immune system may experience frequent overgrowth of resident microbes, and, conversely, vaginal infections can make women more susceptible to infection with sexually transmitted diseases, such as gonorrhea and human immunodeficiency virus (HIV). Frequent and persistent yeast infections may be one sign of HIV. Vaginosis (overgrowth) and vaginitis (inflammation) can sometimes produce irritation and inflammation in the male sexual partner as well and may lead to urethritis, excoriation, and penile inflammation or lesions. A variety of anti-infective medications are used for these disorders (Table 42.6). If the male partner is not also treated, he may reactivate the problem for the woman. Therefore, several types of medication come in "partner packs" for both partners to use.

• WORD • BUILDING •

vaginitis: vagin—vagina + itis—inflammation

Nursing Care and Education of the Patient Undergoing Diagnostic Testing

The patient may feel embarrassed to talk about what is bothering her. A safe question to begin with for most patients is "Hello. What can I write on your chart as the reason for your

TABLE 42.6 MEDICATIONS FOR IRRITATIONS AND INFLAMMATIONS OF THE VAGINA AND VULVA

Medication Class/Action	Examples	Route	Side Effects	Nursing Implications
Antibiotics				
Inhibit bacterial protein synthesis.	clindamycin (Cleocin)	Intravaginal, PO	Candidiasis, pruritus, rash, hypersensitivity, abdominal pain Overgrowth of other infectious organisms	Educate on correct use. Use as directed even if symptoms cease. Report change in symptoms.
Antifungals				
Believed to bind to sterol in fungal cell membrane, thereby altering cell permeability	fluconazole (Diflucan) miconazole (Monistat) terconazole (Terazol) clotrimazole (Gyne-Lotrimin)	PO Topical to external genitalia; intravaginal	Pruritus, rash, hypersensitivity, abdominal pain	Education on correct use; use as directed even if symptoms cease. Report side effects.
Antiprotozoal				
Enters cells of microorganisms that contain nitroreductase, interferes with DNA synthesis and causes cell death	metronidazole (Flagyl)	PO, vaginal cream	Dizziness, weakness, insomnia, abdominal cramping, anorexia, nausea/diarrhea/emesis, vaginal dryness, overgrowth of other infectious organisms, metallic taste	Teach patient to avoid alcohol use while on medication and for 48 hours after completion. Concurrent use of alcohol and metronidazole will induce severe nausea and vomiting. Use medication as directed, even if symptoms cease. Take with meals. Treat partner.

visit today?" If embarrassment is evident, a comment that you need to know a bit about what materials to put out for examination purposes often defuses an uncomfortable situation. As you set up materials for a pelvic examination, swabs, and cultures, you can explain that some information is needed to determine how to treat the problem. (See Chapter 41.) Often this is a good time to ask about vaginal discharge or other signs and symptoms using the WHAT'S UP? format (Chapter 1). Allow the patient privacy while she changes into a gown. Return to the room if requested as a chaperone, assistant, and support for the woman.

NURSING CARE TIP

If any wet-mount slides are made, these must be taken to the laboratory immediately while still wet. Use standard precautions to transport samples. Although samples may be taken for culture, the health care provider may prescribe medication before the results return because such irritations are so uncomfortable.

Nursing Care and Education of the Patient Undergoing Treatment

Vaginal inflammations and infections may require oral medication or local application of medication in cream, suppository, or medicated douche form. You may apply this for patients who cannot do so themselves, or you may teach patients to self-administer. Anatomically, the vagina slopes back toward the sacrum for about the length of an adult finger (although it can stretch longer). Application is easiest when the patient is lying down ready to sleep because vaginal medications tend to run out when the patient stands or sits. Medicated douches may be administered to a hospitalized patient sitting on a bedpan in bed in semi-Fowler's position. Patients may self-administer while sitting on a toilet. Most vaginal medications come with an applicator that either injects a dose of creamy medication or pushes a firmer, shaped dose of medication off the end of the tube when the plunger is depressed. Consult the instructions supplied with the medication. Instruct patients to use all the medication as prescribed and to wear an absorbent pad to prevent possible staining of clothing.

TOXIC SHOCK SYNDROME

Pathophysiology, Etiologies, and Signs and Symptoms

Toxic shock syndrome (TSS), first identified in 1978, is mainly associated with superabsorbent tampon use during menstruation but can also occur with use of nasal packings, or in other individuals with no specific risk factors. It is a severe systemic infection with strains of *Staphylococcus aureus* that produce an epidermal toxin. The effect of the toxin on the liver, kidneys, and circulatory system makes TSS a life-threatening condition. A streptococcal infection can cause a similar syndrome.

Individuals with TSS may experience a sudden high fever with sore throat, headache, dizziness, confusion, redness of the palms and soles of the feet, rash, blisters, and petechiae, followed by peeling of the skin. Muscle pain and weakness, and gastrointestinal upset also have been reported. Signs and symptoms of TSS should be reported to a health care provider immediately.

Prevention

Tampon makers have removed the highly absorbent fibers that were most often associated with the syndrome from their product lines, and TSS is now rare. Women can also reduce their risk of developing TSS by substituting sanitary pads for tampons at least part of the time, such as at night; changing tampons every 4 hours; washing hands carefully before inserting anything into the vagina; not leaving female barrier contraceptives in place for longer than needed; and not using tampons or female barrier contraceptives in the first 12 weeks after giving birth.

Nursing Care and Patient Education

All menstruating women should be taught measures to prevent TSS. They should also be taught to recognize symptoms of TSS because early identification and treatment can save lives.

DISORDERS RELATED TO THE DEVELOPMENT OF THE GENITAL ORGANS

Pathophysiology, Etiologies, and Signs and Symptoms

Several types of congenital malformations of the reproductive organs can affect the health of female patients. Genetic or environmental factors during pregnancy may cause these, and they may require medical or surgical treatment at some point in life. **Agenesis** of structures means that they never developed. **Hypoplasia** of reproductive tract portions means that they are underdeveloped. **Imperforate** means that expected openings do not exist. Blind pouches exist where cavities should meet but do not. The uterus can form in several different configurations, including a double uterus.

Many malformations are discovered during childhood or early adolescence, but some are identified when patients seek medical help because of dysmenorrhea, **dyspareunia** (pain with intercourse), infertility, repeated spontaneous abortions (miscarriages), or preterm labor during pregnancy.

Diagnostic Tests

Procedures such as ultrasonography, hysterosalpingography, computed tomography (CT), magnetic resonance imaging (MRI), and endoscopy may be used to determine the type and extent of developmental defects.

Therapeutic Measures

Some defects can be repaired surgically; others cannot. Depending on the type and location of the defect, surgeries may be done by endoscopy or by surgical incision. Postoperatively the absence of hormone-producing tissue may be overcome by hormone replacements.

Nursing Care and Patient Education

Patients who have these problems may struggle with self-esteem issues, such as feeling that they are somehow incomplete or have been cheated of something they desire. You can show that you are willing to listen if and when the patient wishes to talk, while allowing her as much privacy as she desires.

DISPLACEMENT DISORDERS

Pathophysiology and Etiologies

The pelvic organs are suspended in the pelvis by ligaments and supported by muscles and fascia. The pubococcygeal muscle runs from the pubis to the coccyx and supplies support from below. Pregnancies (especially those producing large babies) and rapid or traumatic deliveries may result in stretching and injury of the supporting structures, which can cause displacement of the uterus, vagina, bladder, or bowel from a normal position.

The observation that some children have defective muscular support of the pelvic organs and that prolapse is more prevalent in some families seems to suggest that congenital defects and genetic inheritance may also influence displacement disorders even without pregnancy. Scarring from sexually transmitted diseases also may cause some displacement of the pelvic organs. Aging generally increases the problem because the effects of gravity over time contribute to stretching, and lower estrogen levels weaken estrogen-dependent supportive tissues. Chronic constipation, obesity, and lack of exercise also worsen these problems.

• WORD • BUILDING •

agenesis: a—without + genesis—production
hypoplasia: hypo—little + plasia—shape (or form)

• WORD • BUILDING •

imperforate: im—not + perforate—pierced
dyspareunia: dys—painful or abnormal + pareunia—mating

Diagnostic Tests

Ultrasonography, hysterosalpingography, computed tomography (CT), magnetic resonance imaging (MRI), and endoscopy may be used to determine the type and extent of displacement disorders.

Therapeutic Measures

A pessary is a supportive (usually ring-shaped) device that is placed in the proximal end of the vagina to help support the pelvic organs. A pessary is usually removed daily at bedtime for cleaning, but some types are designed to remain in the vagina for months at a time. When pessary use is begun, it is important that the woman return to the physician for a recheck after an initial period of use to determine whether it is causing pressure damage to tissues. Because the pessary is a foreign object in the vagina, increased vaginal discharge may be expected. Discharge should not be pink, bloody, or purulent.

Nursing Care and Patient Education

Teach patients to eat a healthy diet to avoid obesity and constipation, and how to do Kegel exercises to keep the pubococcygeal muscle strong and able to support the organs in the pelvic cavity. One way to do Kegel exercises follows:

1. To find the pubococcygeal muscle, tighten while urinating so that the flow of urine stops.
2. Squeeze the muscle that stopped urinary flow tightly, holding for 10 seconds, and totally relaxing the muscle afterward. Repeat 15 times per day.
3. Practice controlling the muscle by contracting and relaxing it to move the pelvic floor upward and downward very slowly. Thinking of an elevator helps some women. Repeat this 15 times per day.

> **NURSING CARE TIP**
>
> Teach women to do Kegel exercises while waiting in lines to use otherwise wasted time to promote their health. Another suggestion is to plan specific times of day or activities that would include Kegel exercises, such as while in a car or working at a computer. Kegel exercises can be done anywhere and are not apparent to anyone watching.

Cystocele

Pathophysiology, Etiologies, and Signs and Symptoms

Cystocele occurs when the bladder sags into the vaginal space because of inadequate support (Fig. 42.5A). A feeling of pelvic pressure and stress incontinence are common with this condition.

Therapeutic Measures

Kegel exercises or the use of a pessary may help. If these measures are ineffective, anterior **colporrhaphy**, which is a

• WORD • BUILDING •
cystocele: cysto—bag (bladder) + cele—hernia
colporrhaphy: colpo—vagina + rrhaphy—suture

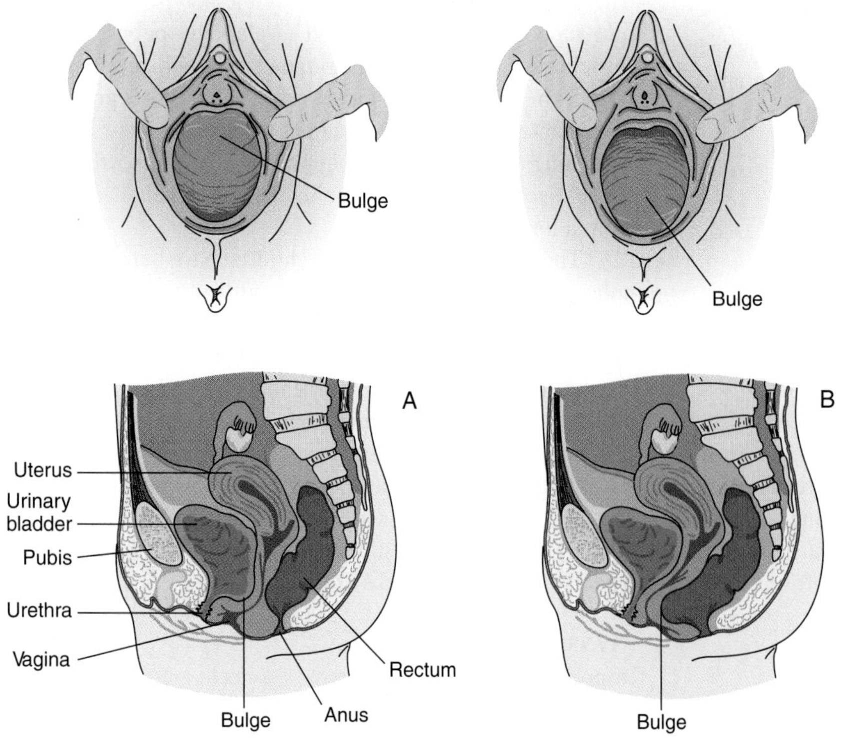
Bulge
Bulge
A
B
Uterus
Urinary bladder
Pubis
Urethra
Vagina
Rectum
Bulge
Anus
Bulge

FIGURE 42.5 (A) Cystocele. (B) Rectocele.

surgical repair of the anterior portion of the vagina, may be needed. Another possible surgical treatment involves resuspending the bladder.

Rectocele

Pathophysiology, Etiologies, and Signs and Symptoms

Rectocele occurs when a portion of the rectum sags into the vagina because of inadequate support (see Fig. 42.5B). A feeling of pelvic pressure, as well as fecal incontinence, constipation, and hemorrhoids, may result.

Therapeutic Measures

Kegel exercises may help strengthen the supporting muscles. The patient should maintain bowel regularity with a high-fiber diet to avoid further discomfort and sagging from bowel overdistention. Posterior colporrhaphy may be necessary to correct this problem.

Uterine Position Disorders

Pathophysiology, Etiologies, and Signs and Symptoms

The most common variations in position of the uterus are **anteversion**, **anteflexion**, **retroversion**, and **retroflexion** (Fig. 42.6). In anteversion, the uterus lies too far forward, and in retroversion, it lies too far backward. In anteflexion, the upper portion of the uterus bends forward, and in retroflexion, it bends backward.

Symptoms that may result from these uterine displacements include painful menstruation and intercourse, infertility, and repeated spontaneous abortion.

Therapeutic Measures

A pessary may correct some positional problems. If infertility or recurrent spontaneous abortion is involved or the condition is very painful, surgery to correct the condition may be necessary.

Uterine Prolapse

Pathophysiology, Etiologies, and Signs and Symptoms

Uterine prolapse occurs when the uterus sags into the vagina (Fig. 42.7). The amount of sagging can vary and may increase over time as a result of the effects of gravity, poor pelvic support, and excessive lifting or straining. In first-degree prolapse, less than half the uterus sags into the vagina. In second-degree prolapse, the entire uterus sags into the vagina. In third-degree prolapse, the uterus sags outside the body.

• WORD • BUILDING •

rectocele: recto—rectum + cele—hernia
anteversion: ante—front + version—turning
anteflexion: ante—front + flexion—bending
retroversion: retro—back + version—turning
retroflexion: retro—back + flexion—bending

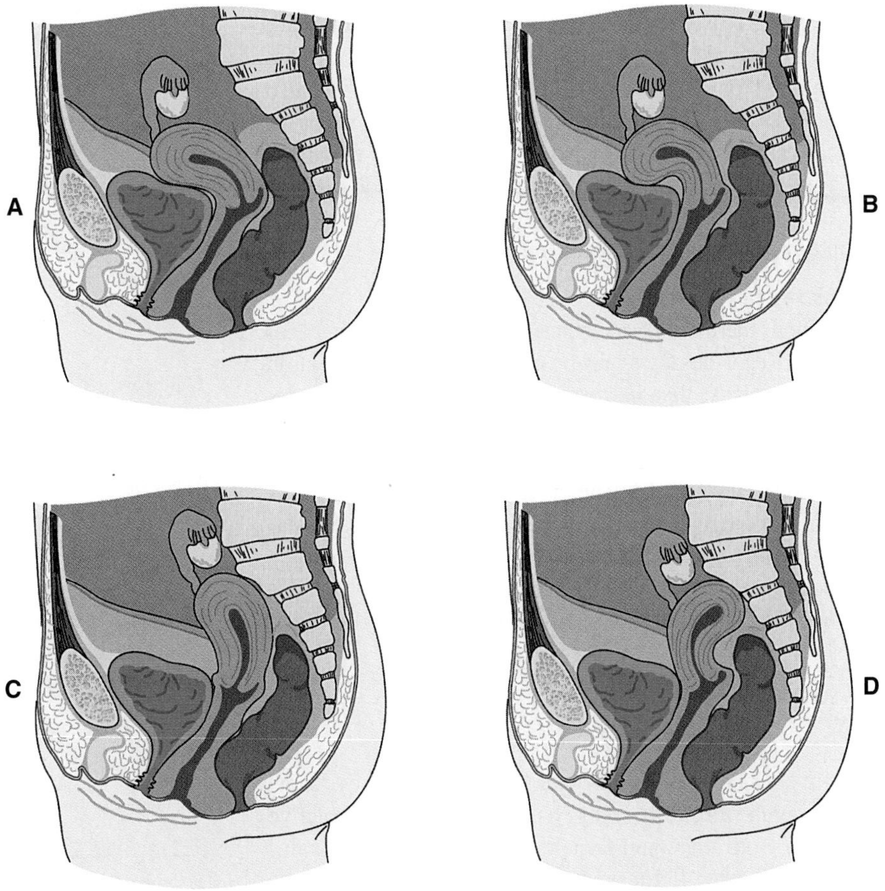
A
B
C
D

FIGURE 42.6 Uterine positions. (A) Anteversion. (B) Anteflexion. (C) Retroversion. (D) Retroflexion.

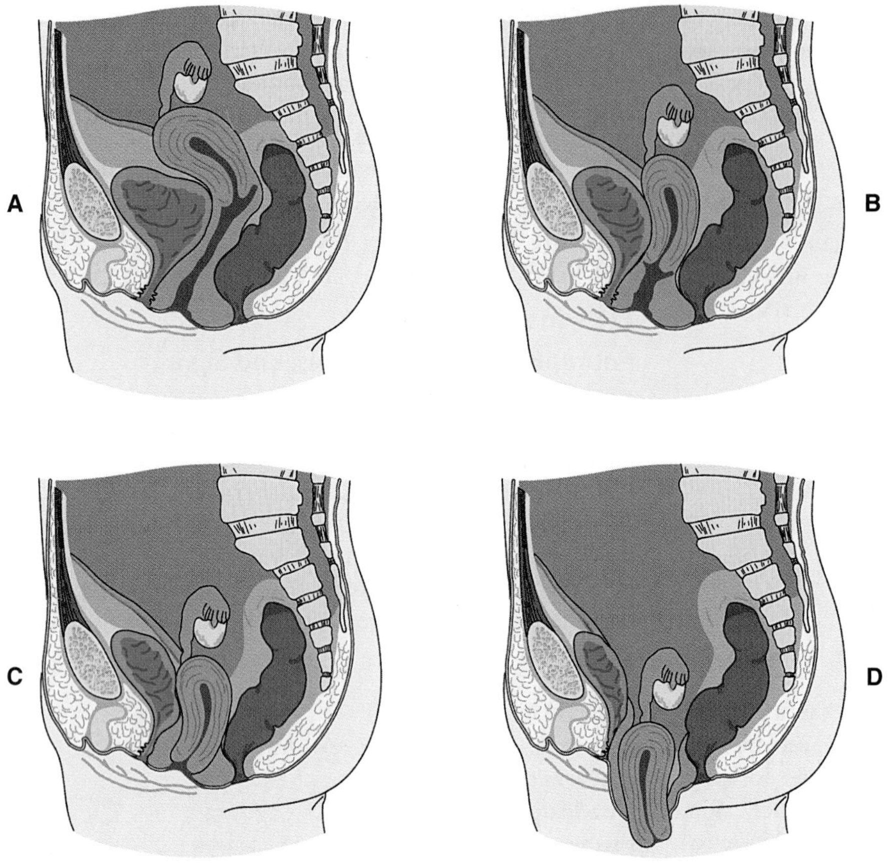
A
B
C
D

FIGURE 42.7 Uterine prolapse. (A) Normal uterus. (B) First-degree prolapse: descent within the vagina. (C) Second-degree prolapse. (D) Third-degree prolapse: vagina is completely everted.

Uterine prolapse can be very uncomfortable, resulting in back pain, pelvic pain, pain with intercourse (or inability to have intercourse), urinary incontinence, constipation, and development of hemorrhoids. Pressure on the uterus also may compromise circulation, resulting in tissue necrosis. Vaginal vault prolapse may also occur in women who have had a hysterectomy, so that the vagina turns inside out and sags downward with similar signs and symptoms. This condition typically requires surgical resuspension.

Therapeutic Measures

Some minor uterine displacements may be treated with use of a pessary. Kegel exercises may be more effective in prevention of uterine prolapse than in treatment because, once the tissues become stretched sufficiently for the uterus to sag into the vagina, the continued weight of the uterus prevents adequate contraction of the muscles. Surgery may be done to correct this problem. Although the uterus may be resuspended by shortening the muscles and fascia, hysterectomy is the more common treatment unless further childbearing is desired.

See Table 42.7 for a summary of displacement disorders.

FERTILITY DISORDERS

Infertility is a complicated problem with many causes. Some couples with infertility may have multiple reproductive problems. Both male and female partners should be examined. (See Chapter 43 for greater detail on male reproductive

TABLE 42.7 DISPLACEMENT DISORDERS OF THE GENITAL ORGANS SUMMARY

Signs and Symptoms	Pain with menses or sexual intercourse Infertility Spontaneous abortion or preterm labor Prolapse of uterus, bladder, or rectum into vagina or outside of body
Diagnostic Tests and Findings	Physical examination Ultrasound Hysterosalpingography CT or MRI scan Endoscopy
Therapeutic Measures	Kegel exercises Surgery Hormone supplements
Priority Nursing Diagnoses	*Acute* or *Chronic Pain* related to structural abnormality or surgery *Urinary Incontinence* or *Constipation* related to structural abnormalities *Sexual Dysfunction* related to disturbance in self-concept *Grief* related to absence or loss of reproductive status

CT = computed tomography; MRI = magnetic resonance imaging.

system disorders.) Often the woman sees the health care provider first and may be given a specimen container and advised to give the container to her partner for provision of a semen sample for analysis. See Table 42.8 for a summary of fertility disorders and diagnostic tests.

Nursing Care and Education of the Patient Undergoing Fertility Testing

An understanding attitude is very important because infertility can be a cause of low self-esteem, as well as relationship problems. Patients who have been undergoing diagnostic testing or treatment for infertility can become very discouraged with the process and the expense, especially if it has been ineffective. Having to plan your sexual activity around a health care provider's directions can compromise feelings of spontaneity, enjoyment, and privacy. Extensive questioning by nurses can aggravate the situation, but avoiding conversation may convey a lack of caring. A friendly, "Which test shall I help you get ready for today?" may well be enough to get the needed information. Many women undergoing infertility testing are very well informed about the test they will be having and can tell you so that you know which equipment to prepare.

On the first infertility investigation visit, the nurse may teach or give a handout to the patient about keeping a precise record of her oral temperatures with a basal thermometer each morning on awakening, before any other activity. The first day of her menses is day 1 on the temperature chart. Changing levels of hormones result in slight temperature changes, which can be used to identify when ovulation seems to be occurring and when particular hormone levels should be tested. Because many factors can influence temperature and cycles, explain that it may take a few months of recording to clearly identify her own pattern.

You may assist with office procedures such as endometrial biopsy, which may be done during a pelvic examination 2 or 3 days before menses is expected. A pregnancy test should be done before this procedure to avoid interfering with a pregnancy. The woman may receive pain medication and paracervical block anesthesia for the procedure. Assess pulse and blood pressure. A vasovagal reaction treatment kit containing epinephrine (or atropine, according to the health care provider's choice), a tourniquet, and a syringe should be available for injection if a vasovagal reflex occurs during the procedure. Vasovagal reflex is a reflex stimulation of the vagal nerve that can happen when the cervix, larynx, or trachea is manipulated and results in slowing of the heart rate and decreased cardiac output, so that the blood pressure drops markedly.

Therapeutic Measures

Treatment of infertility is designed to ensure that an adequate amount of sperm and an ovum can be in proximity in the most conducive environment for fertilization. Removal

TABLE 42.8 FERTILITY DISORDERS

Disorder	Pathophysiology/Etiology	Diagnostic Tests
Male	Possible anatomic abnormalities, hormonal imbalances, genetic defects, inflammatory conditions, immune system disorders, difficulties with sexual function, psychological factors, or exogenous influences such as drug use, radiation or chemical exposure, trauma, and excessive testicular temperatures (may occur with prolonged hot tub use or tight clothing)	Semen analysis of number, condition, and movement of the sperm and composition of seminal fluid
Female		
• Ovulation	Possible anatomic and physiological abnormalities of ovaries; hormonal imbalances related to hypothalamus, thyroid, or adrenal glands; polycystic ovary syndrome	Basal body temperature charting, midluteal serum progesterone blood levels, luteinizing hormone levels, blood or urine testing, ultrasound monitoring of a follicle for evidence of release of ovum, endometrial biopsy, observation of male hair distribution, other hormone testing as indicated
• Tubal	Possible obstruction of the fallopian tubes resulting from anatomic variations, scarring, or adhesions; prior surgeries; inflammatory processes involving other abdominal tissues	Hysterosalpingography (see Chapter 41), laparoscopy
• Uterine	Possible abnormalities in shape or blockages within the uterus (rare cause of infertility but a potential cause of pregnancy loss before maturity), menstrual disorders involving the endometrium	Hysteroscopy (see Chapter 41), removal of tissue samples using curet or endoscope
• Other Sources	Possible reproductive environmental factors such as destructive antigen-antibody responses, inappropriate pH of seminal fluid for maximal sperm motility, or substances in female partner's genital tract fluids that disable sperm	Postcoital test: Couple is advised to have intercourse when luteinizing hormone and estrogen levels are high, then a specimen of cervical mucus is taken from the woman 2–12 hours later for analysis of reproductive environment

of barriers such as scar tissue may require surgery. Depending on the results of blood tests and the **postcoital** test (described in Table 42.8), adjustments of environmental factors may involve such actions as sperm washing to avoid destructive antigen-antibody responses, changing the pH of the seminal fluid to encourage sperm motility, treating the female partner to prevent substances in her genital tract fluids from disabling the sperm, or adjusting her hormone levels. The number of sperm or ova available may be increased through use of such fertility drugs as clomiphene citrate or various hormone preparations. Infertility treatments are quite complicated and expensive and change periodically as a result of ongoing research. In-depth coverage of these treatments is beyond the scope of this book.

Various methods can be used to bring the gametes into proximity. If the problem involves inability to get the sperm close enough to the ovum (as may happen with ejaculatory problems), the physician may use intrauterine insemination (IUI) to place a semen sample from the male partner closer to the ovum via a small catheter. **In vitro fertilization** (IVF) involves bringing ova and sperm together outside the bodies of the participants. Ova may be harvested using a long needle or an endoscope after hormonal preparation of the woman. Sperm may be obtained through masturbation; intercourse with a nonlubricated, nonspermicidal condom; or electrical stimulation of ejaculation for patients with spinal cord injuries. Once fertilized, the ova are implanted in the woman's uterus.

For those whose sperm is unable to successfully penetrate the ovum, procedures involving gamete micromanipulation may be done. Under a microscope, an ovum from the female partner is partially opened by removing a portion of the outer covering to facilitate sperm penetration, or sperm may be injected into the ovum. This fertilized ovum is then reinserted into the woman's body.

When measures to improve the chances of conception using the partners' own gametes are unsuccessful, gametes from donors may be used. Artificial insemination by injecting another man's sperm into the woman's genital tract is the simplest of the donor procedures. Ova also may be harvested from a donor woman and used for in vitro fertilization using the male partner's sperm if possible. Both of these procedures allow for genetic inheritance from one member of the couple. If genetic inheritance is not possible or desirable (as with familial disease carriers), both donor sperm and ova may be used for in vitro fertilization to be transferred into the female patient. Surrogacy is a situation in which an embryo from one couple is placed into a "host" mother for growth of a baby for the couple, and is a topic of much ethical debate.

• WORD • BUILDING •

postcoital: post—after + coital—pertaining to intercourse

in vitro fertilization: in—inside + vitro—glass + fertiliz—fruitful + ation—process

Nursing Care and Education of the Patient Undergoing Treatment

Patients who are undergoing infertility treatment may experience many upsetting and distressing feelings. Feelings of inadequacy, frustration, depression, and anger are common. If the infertility was caused by something the patient perceives as avoidable, such as sexually transmitted disease, guilt feelings may add to the psychological discomfort. Any or all of the previously described tests may be completed and some repeated many times without success in identifying an underlying etiology for infertility, and may result in repeated disappointments. Some patients cling to the hope that new tests and treatments are being developed that may help them, whereas others feel that they are being used as "guinea pigs" for development of new strategies. The beginning of menses may signal a time of mourning for these couples. Depression may result after failed IVF attempts. Strained relationships may develop between marriage partners, especially if there is disagreement about the value of testing or the importance of having children.

In IVF, usually more than the desired number of embryos is implanted because it is expected that not all will survive and because this is more cost effective with less physical risk for the mother. However, this requires heart-wrenching decisions of whether to "reduce" (abort) extra pregnancies or to risk having more than the desired number of children at once as a result of the fertility treatments.

Offer a listening ear while being careful not to give advice about treatment modalities. Researchers and practitioners are engaging in ongoing debate as to the value of particular procedures; consequently, strategies may vary widely from one health care provider to another. Encourage open communication among the patient, the health care provider, and the patient's significant other, and encourage decision making that is informed and based on the patient's values.

Many varieties of assistive reproductive technology are available, and the number is increasing with research. Most of the procedures are known by their acronyms. For example, *GIFT* means "gamete intrafallopian transfer" (gametes are placed together in the fallopian tube with the hope that fertilization will occur). *ZIFT* means "zygote intrafallopian transfer" (fertilization of gametes occurs outside of the body; the conceptus is then placed into a woman's fallopian tube to make the journey to the uterus). Acronyms can be useful shortcuts but can be confusing to patients. Most nurses probably do not need to know all acronyms or infertility treatments unless they work in a gynecologist's office or infertility clinic.

REPRODUCTIVE LIFE PLANNING

Reproductive life planning is a more comprehensive term than *contraception* and implies reasoned decisions related to pregnancy timing and whether or not to have children. Nurses can contribute to the overall health and quality of life for women and families by assisting them to find the information they need to make wise choices.

Many different types of birth control are available, and several additional types are in developmental and testing stages. General categories of agents are discussed in this section. General knowledge of how the different types of contraceptives work can assist the nurse in answering patients' questions or helping patients find additional information. The World Health Organization has put together a helpful publication called "Medical Eligibility Criteria for Contraceptive Use" (WHO, 2009). This publication assigns an eligibility category of 1 to 4 to each contraceptive. Assignment of a contraceptive method to category 1 means there is no restriction for the use of that specific method, whereas assignment to category 4 means that the method poses an unacceptable health risk. *Note:* The material in this section is not intended to be a substitute for discussions with a health care provider or for information supplied with individual products.

No numerical statements of effectiveness are included here because several different sets of statistics are currently in use. Methods are introduced in the order of usual effectiveness from most to least effective (with the exception that experimental methods are discussed at the end regardless of their efficacy). Consult your clinic or health care provider for an approved, current comparison list of methods for distribution.

For some patients, the distinction of whether a birth control method actually prevents conception or only interferes with implantation or maintenance of a pregnancy is an important factor in their decision. If a patient believes life begins at conception, any action other than prevention of conception would be considered equivalent to abortion.

Oral Contraceptives

Oral **contraceptive** medications are among the most widely used forms of birth control in North America. Most contain an estrogen and a progestin in combination, although some (mini-pills) contain only a progestin. Some work to prevent conception by inhibiting ovulation or changing the environment of the reproductive tract so that activity of the sperm is inhibited. Others do not prevent conception, but make implantation less likely and hasten the breakdown of the corpus luteum so that pregnancy-sustaining hormones are not produced. Many of the adverse effects that occurred in the past have been overcome by adjustment of dosage levels.

Oral contraceptives may also be used in some instances to regulate irregular menses, to decrease dysmenorrhea, or to decrease the symptoms associated with endometriosis or cyclic breast changes. There is much debate about whether hormonal contraceptive agents may offer some protection against some sexually transmitted diseases (STDs) based on lower statistical rates of STDs among oral contraceptive users. However, cellular changes of the cervix seen with hormonal contraceptive use actually tend to be associated with higher rates of some sexually transmitted diseases. Unless some specific mechanism of prevention is demonstrated by research, it seems irresponsible to suggest that oral contraceptives alone offer protection against anything other than pregnancy. Therefore, women should still be advised about the risks of contracting sexually transmitted diseases while taking an oral contraceptive.

Advantages, Disadvantages, Side Effects, and Risks

Oral contraceptives are very effective. Improvement of dysmenorrhea, endometriosis, increased regularity of menses, and decrease in menstrual flow may occur; however, some women experience menstrual changes such as amenorrhea, irregular or prolonged menses, and intermenstrual spotting.

Oral contraceptives require a great deal of commitment because irregular use decreases their effectiveness. To encourage regular use, oral contraceptives are generally dispensed in containers labeled with the days of the week, and some companies include unmedicated pills in the package to be taken during the time of hormone cessation for menses, so that the woman only has to remember to take a daily pill, instead of timing the taking of the pills with her cycle. Some oral contraceptives are now available to be taken continuously. Women should speak to their care providers to determine which method is best for them.

Some women experience side effects such as acne, fluid retention, headaches, breast swelling and discomfort, midcycle bleeding, and sometimes depression. Use of an oral contraceptive also has some risks. Higher rates of blood clot formation, strokes, high blood pressure, heart attacks, and worsening of diabetes are rare occurrences with some hormonal contraceptives and are generally related to additional preexisting risk factors. Women who smoke or have diabetes, high blood pressure, heart disease, or a history of thrombophlebitis should receive counseling about the risks of oral contraceptives and education about alternative methods of contraception.

Oral contraceptives decrease the risk of endometrial and ovarian cancer, but there is debate about risk of breast cancer, and cervical **dysplasia** (cell changes that may become cancerous) sometimes occurs among oral contraceptive users. Women should definitely be advised to have regular annual (or more frequent if abnormalities develop) Pap smears while taking oral contraceptives.

Many medications can alter the effectiveness of oral contraceptives, and women should be warned to always alert health care providers and pharmacists that they are using oral contraceptives whenever a new medication is to be started or a regular medication is discontinued. Use of hormonal contraceptives increases the risk of vitamin B deficiencies, so a healthy diet with good sources of B vitamins is advisable.

• WORD • BUILDING •
contraceptive: contra—against + ceptive—taking in (conceiving)

• WORD • BUILDING •
dysplasia: dys—painful or abnormal + plasia—shape or form

LEARNING TIP

Side effects of oral contraceptives can be serious. Teach your patient to watch for "ACHES," and to contact her primary care provider immediately if they occur. ACHES stands for:
Abdominal pain
Chest pain
Headache
Eye pain
Severe leg pain

Contraceptive Implants and Depot Medications

Contraceptive implants are small permeable tubes surgically implanted through a small incision under the skin; they slowly release hormones for long-term contraception. Implants have been used with varying success; examples include etonogestrel implant (Implanon) and nomegestrol acetate (Uniplant).

Medroxyprogesterone acetate (Depo-Provera) is a contraceptive agent available in a slow-release (depot) form that can be injected intramuscularly. Medication is continuously released for 3 months.

Advantages, Disadvantages, Side Effects, and Risks

The main advantage of depot medications and implants is that the woman does not have to remember to take daily medication. Disadvantages are that the medications may not be immediately effective, so another method may be necessary for 1 to 2 weeks after the initial injection, and that fertility may not return for several months to 1 year after discontinuation.

Alterations in menstrual flow, especially amenorrhea, are the most commonly noted side effects with both depot medications and implants. Weight gain of 5 to 10 pounds is also common, which can lead to discontinuation of use. Other side effects and risks are similar to those encountered with oral contraceptives that contain progesterone only.

Estrogen-Progestogen Contraceptive Ring

A newer method is an estrogen-progestogen contraceptive ring (NuvaRing). It works in much the same manner as other hormonal contraceptives by slowly releasing hormones. The user inserts the ring into the vagina around the cervix, similar to a diaphragm. The ring is left in place for 3 weeks and then removed for 1 week in order for menses to occur.

Advantages, Disadvantages, Side Effects, and Risks

Not having to remember daily medication can be an advantage to the contraceptive ring, but failing to remove it at the right time may disrupt the regularity of the menstrual cycles. With consistent use, it is very effective in preventing pregnancy. Because it does not provide a barrier over the cervix, there is less risk of infection than with a diaphragm or cervical cap. A common side effect is an increase in normal vaginal discharge. Other side effects and risks are similar to other low-dose hormonal contraceptives.

Transdermal Contraceptive Patch

A transdermal patch is now available that contains norelgestromin and ethinyl estradiol (Ortho Evra). This patch is placed on the abdomen, upper arm, or buttock following a menstrual period and left in place for 1 week. A new patch is placed on the body each week for 3 weeks. After 3 weeks, the patch is removed and not replaced for 1 week in order for menses to occur.

Advantages, Disadvantages, Side Effects, and Risks

The contraceptive patch has been found to be similar to oral contraceptives in effectiveness, side effects, and risks, without having to remember to take a pill each day. Bathing, swimming, and other activities can continue because the patch will remain where placed.

Barrier Methods

Barrier methods of birth control are less effective in preventing pregnancy than most of the previously mentioned methods when used alone. Barriers are intended to prevent sperm from reaching the ovum. There are several forms of barrier contraceptives. Used in combination, the effectiveness of barrier methods and spermicidal preparations comes close to that of oral contraceptives. Spermicidal preparations may be purchased without a prescription.

Condoms

Condoms are to be used once and then discarded into an appropriate waste receptacle. They should be stored in a cool, dry place before use and should not be stored tightly pressed because heat and continued pressure can weaken them. Storage in a wallet or glove compartment is not advisable. Petroleum-based substances, such as Vaseline, can also weaken condoms, so use of water-soluble lubricants (preferably spermicides) should be advised.

ADVANTAGES, DISADVANTAGES, SIDE EFFECTS, AND RISKS OF MALE CONDOMS. Male condoms have long been used for contraception because they are a relatively inexpensive, totally reversible method that men can control at the time of intercourse. They provide some barrier protection against transmission of sexually transmitted disease organisms as well. An electron microscopic study of a sample of nonlubricated latex condoms, however, found that most of those viewed had surface abnormalities, including cracking and melted areas. Patients should be informed that barrier methods can reduce risk but do not absolutely prevent transmission of STDs, especially in areas of contact not covered by the barrier.

The main disadvantages of condom use are interruption of foreplay for application, decreased sensation, and the possibility of slippage or breakage during intercourse. These disadvantages may be overcome by incorporating application of the condom by the female partner as a part of foreplay; using thinner, lubricated, or textured condoms to increase sensation; using the correct size condom with a reservoir or application that leaves about a half-inch at the tip of the condom loose enough to serve as a reservoir for semen (Fig. 42.8); and removal from the vagina before relaxation of the erection.

ADVANTAGES, DISADVANTAGES, SIDE EFFECTS, AND RISKS OF FEMALE CONDOMS. Female condoms are a more recent innovation that allows female initiation of contraception, as well as some barrier protection against infection with sexually transmitted diseases. Coverage of the labia by the condom may provide more of a barrier than male condoms (Fig. 42.9). Disadvantages are similar to those of male condoms; they are also more expensive than male condoms.

Diaphragms and Cervical Caps

Diaphragms and cervical caps work in the same manner as condoms by blocking the entry of sperm through the cervix (Fig. 42.10). The barrier effect is enhanced by simultaneous use of a spermicide. Application of a spermicide to the edge of the device, and placement of a small amount in the cup before use, increases effectiveness.

ADVANTAGES, DISADVANTAGES, SIDE EFFECTS, AND RISKS. These methods are relatively inexpensive, are female initiated, and work without systemic medication. Diaphragms and cervical caps require initial fitting and a prescription to buy them, may need to be refitted after childbirth and the loss or gain of weight, and can last for years. These devices should be replaced periodically based on manufacturer recommendations or whenever there is any evidence of hardening, cracking, or thin spots. They need to be washed with soap and water, dried, and stored in a case away from heat and sunlight between uses.

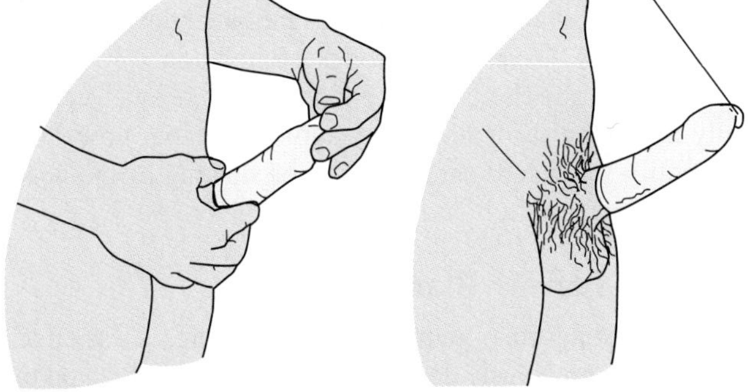
Half inch of
space at tip

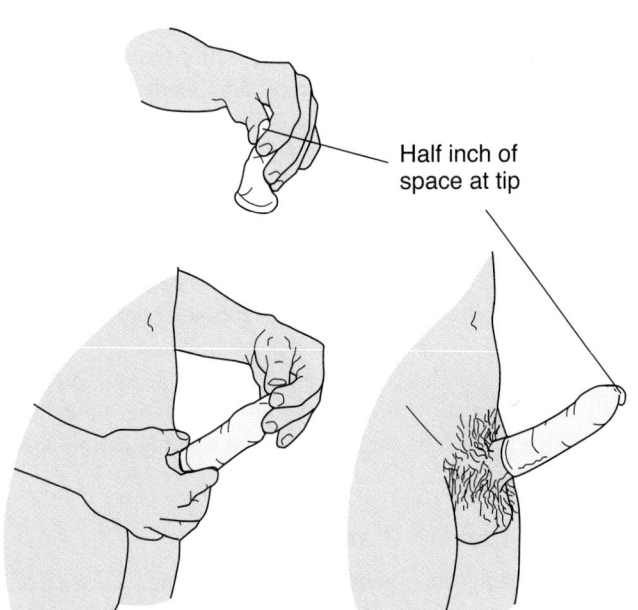

FIGURE 42.8 Correct application of a condom.

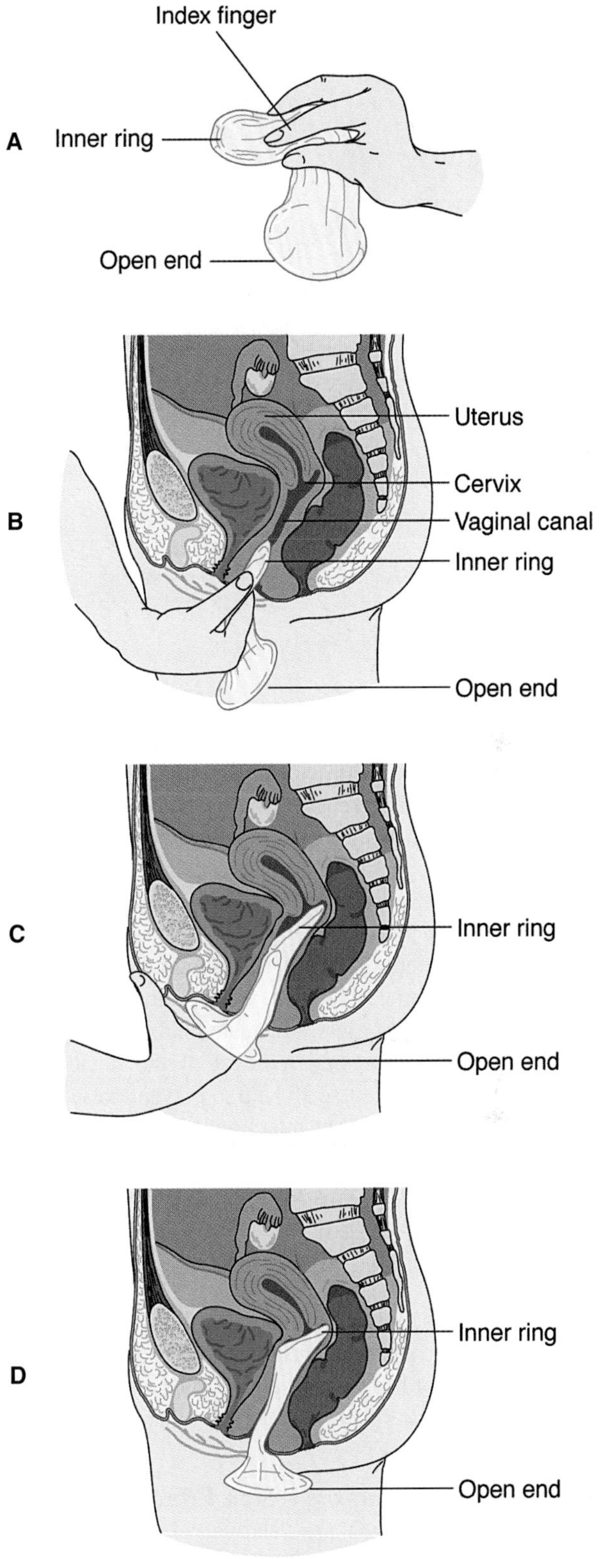
Index finger
A
Inner ring
Open end
B
Uterus
Cervix
Vaginal canal
Inner ring
Open end
C
Inner ring
Open end
D
Inner ring
Open end

FIGURE 42.9 Female condom application. (A) Inner ring is squeezed for insertion. (B) Sheath is inserted similar to a tampon. (C) Inner ring is pushed up as far as it can go with index finger. (D) Condom in place.

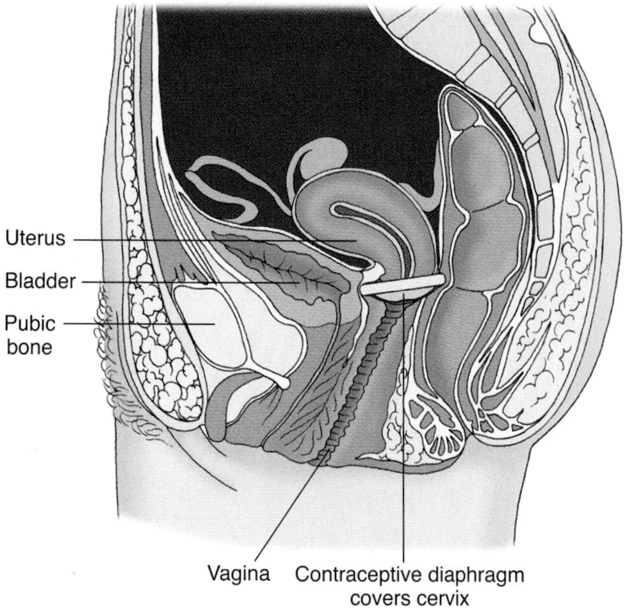
Uterus
Bladder
Pubic bone
Vagina
Contraceptive diaphragm covers cervix

FIGURE 42.10 Contraceptive diaphragm.

Women and their partners can experience irritation or allergic reaction to the spermicide or the contraceptive device material, which would require changing birth control methods. These types of methods require that the device be inserted before intercourse and left in place for several hours after intercourse. (See package inserts for specific recommendations.) An increase in incidence of urinary tract infection has been reported with use of the diaphragm, and risk of toxic shock syndrome increases with prolonged uninterrupted use of cervical barriers. Adequate fluid intake, voiding shortly after intercourse, and removal of the device 6 to 8 hours following intercourse all help to prevent these potential problems. If urinary tract infections are recurrent using the diaphragm, changing to a cervical cap may decrease the occurrence because there is less pressure against the bladder through the anterior vagina.

Spermicides

Spermicidal agents may be used alone, although use in combination with a barrier method is much more effective. They come in a variety of forms, such as creams, gels, foams, and suppositories, which kill or disable sperm so that fertilization does not occur.

Advantages, Disadvantages, Side Effects, and Risks

Spermicidal preparations are relatively inexpensive and can be male or female initiated. They do not produce systemic effects, and no hormones are involved. However, they are less effective alone than with the previously described barrier methods. Spermicides require application before each act of intercourse and are considered by some patients to be somewhat messy. Many contain the same ingredient—nonoxynol 9. If genital irritation or a rash occurs with a spermicide, the patient should read labels carefully to avoid future contact with the same ingredient.

Intrauterine Devices

The presence of a foreign object in the uterus is thought to alter the environment, so that implantation is less likely to occur. Intrauterine devices (IUDs) are generally made from a form of plastic and may contain copper wire (such as the ParaGard) or a supply of a progestin (for example, Mirena) that is slowly released into the system to further alter the uterine environment, so that fertilization or implantation is hindered.

Advantages, Disadvantages, Side Effects, and Risks

The main advantage of an IUD is continued contraception without the necessity of remembering to take medication and without the side effects associated with medications. The other advantage is the long-term use of these devices. The ParaGard is effective for 10 years and the Mirena is effective for 5 years. Mirena may help lighten and potentially eliminate menstrual bleeding in women who have a history of anemia or heavy menstrual flow.

Disadvantages are changes in menstrual bleeding, cramping, and increased risk of pelvic inflammatory disease (PID). Rarely, an IUD has caused a uterine perforation. New research and changes in the medical eligibility criteria set up by the World Health Organization has shown that IUDs can be used by women who have never been pregnant because the advantages far outweigh the theoretical or proven risks. IUDs should be avoided in women with uterine abnormalities, those with PID, and those who have current STDs. Expulsion or displacement of the IUD can occur, so women should be taught to feel for the presence of the external string before intercourse.

Insertion Procedure

Insertion of an IUD typically is done in a physician's office with a nurse assisting. Usually this is done during the first 7 days of the menstrual cycle because the cervix is slightly dilated at this time. If you are assisting with this procedure, you will need to put out a vasovagal reaction treatment kit, an IUD insertion kit containing one or more uterine "sounds," a tenaculum (a special long forceps) for grasping the cervix, long scissors for string cutting, and the IUD package.

The IUD is generally inserted into the cervix through a tube that comes packaged with the IUD, which temporarily holds the IUD flat or folded for insertion. When the IUD is pushed out the end of the tube, it springs into a shape that helps to keep it inside the uterus. One potential danger of IUD insertion is vasovagal reflex stimulation (previously described in association with endometrial biopsy). Periodically assess pulse or blood pressure during the procedure and notify the health care provider of slowing of the heart rate or a decrease in blood pressure.

Natural Family Planning

Periodic abstinence, or natural family planning, is less effective than the previously described methods. It is a method by which couples control their fertility by restricting intercourse to "safe periods" during which risk of conception is low. Many signs may be assessed to determine "safe" days, including temperature changes, cervical consistency and mucus changes, calendar timing, and awareness of symptoms of fertility.

Slight body temperature changes can indicate ovulation. During the first half of the menstrual cycle, the temperature remains low, with a marked drop just before ovulation occurs. With ovulation the temperature rises and stays higher for the last half of the cycle. Women who use this assessment method should use a basal body temperature thermometer when they awaken, before doing anything else, and record it on a chart.

Cervical consistency and mucus changes may also help pinpoint ovulation. As hormone levels change, the consistency of cervical mucus changes. As ovulation approaches, there is an increase in the amount of mucus and the mucus becomes more clear, thin, slippery, and stretchable than at other times of the month. Around the time of ovulation, the cervix becomes softer to touch and more open than at other times of the cycle.

Following the calendar can work fairly well if a woman's menstrual periods are regular, but becoming aware of her pattern may take time. Symptoms such as breast tenderness and midcycle discomfort (*mittelschmerz*) may also help identify ovulation. Users of this method should be advised to abstain from intercourse for approximately 3 days before ovulation and 3 to 4 days after because the sperm and ovum can survive for a long period in the female genital tract.

Advantages and Disadvantages

The advantages of this method are that it requires no expense or medication, and it is the only birth control method presently approved by the Catholic Church. The disadvantages are that it requires the cooperation of both partners and may interfere with spontaneity of sexual expression. It is generally not very effective as a means of birth control. It may be difficult to accurately identify ovulation times because infectious and inflammatory processes can affect temperature readings, infections and feminine hygiene products can affect cervical mucus, and irregularity of flow and symptoms may make prediction difficult.

Less Effective Methods

Coitus Interruptus

Coitus interruptus involves removal of the penis from the vagina before ejaculation occurs.

ADVANTAGES, DISADVANTAGES, AND RISKS. Although this method requires no expense or preparation, it is not very effective. Excellent control of ejaculation is required, and even the small amount of sperm that may be present in pre-ejaculatory fluid can result in pregnancy.

Postcoital Douching

The intended purpose of postcoital douching is to wash sperm out of the reproductive tract or to kill or immobilize sperm that the douche solution contacts.

ADVANTAGES, DISADVANTAGES, AND RISKS. This is relatively inexpensive and female initiated, but it is not very effective. Sperm move very rapidly once deposited, and douching may actually push the sperm upward.

Lactational Amenorrhea Method (Breastfeeding)

Breastfeeding is sometimes used as a method of birth control because the high blood levels of prolactin that occur with breastfeeding may suppress ovulation. This may be effective in the first 6 months after delivery and requires "full or nearly full" breastfeeding, and that the woman has not experienced her first postpartum menses (any bleeding after 56 days postpartum).

ADVANTAGES, DISADVANTAGES, AND RISKS. This method costs nothing but is not very effective. Prolactin levels can vary widely, and ovulation may resume at any time without any noticeable signs, resulting in pregnancy before even experiencing a menstrual period after the birth.

Ongoing Research: Future Possibilities for Contraceptive Choices

Many researchers have tried to develop effective and reversible male contraceptives. When taken orally a plant called *Tripterygium*, used in Chinese herbal medicine, yields substances that can limit numbers and mobility of sperm, but it also has active ingredients that suppress immunity somewhat, so further investigation is necessary. Reversible injection procedures to block the seminal vas deferens are also being investigated, as are reversible injection procedures to block the fallopian tubes. Reversible birth control vaccines are also being investigated for both men and women with the goal of causing an immune response to occur at some vital point in the process of conception.

Some questions related to contraceptive vaccines include the unknown long-term repercussions of stimulating the body to respond with immunity to itself and whether governments could use vaccines as a means to control populations without individuals' consent. Another frightening possibility is that with further removal of the threat of pregnancy, even fewer people would use barrier methods and STDs would increase even more dramatically.

CRITICAL THINKING

Jessica

■ You have just observed a patient who appears to be about 13 years old announce loudly at the clinic reception desk that she is "ready to be a responsible adult" and would like some birth control.

1. What information should be gathered from her?
2. What do you think she needs to know before making a decision?
3. How can contraceptive teaching capitalize on her desire to be a responsible adult?

Suggested answers at end of chapter.

Sterilization

Permanent sterilization can be accomplished by either interrupting the fallopian tubes or vas deferens (by vasectomy, as discussed in Chapter 43) or by removing the uterus and suturing the proximal end of the vagina closed. Tubal interruption may be done by tying a suture or placing a ring or clip around each fallopian tube, by coagulating a section of the tubes, or by surgically removing a portion of the tube and suturing the ends. These procedures are usually done by laparoscope in an outpatient setting, as an additional procedure performed during a cesarean section, or within a few days following a vaginal delivery. A new nonsurgical procedure (Essure) uses an endoscope to implant a tiny insert into each fallopian tube to block patency.

Advantages, Disadvantages, Side Effects, and Risks

Although sterilization is not absolutely certain to be permanent, the failure rate is low and has been decreasing recently with newer surgical methods. After vasectomy, men must return to the physician's office to supply at least two semen samples to ensure no sperm are present. Reversal is sometimes requested at a later time to reestablish fertility. This requires microsurgery with anesthesia and has a poor success rate.

Patient Education

Patients should be advised by their surgeon about the complications of the surgery and reversal before they sign a consent form for sterilization. If any uncertainty about the surgery is evident, the physician should be notified promptly.

PREGNANCY TERMINATION

Termination of pregnancy (abortion) is a difficult topic. Discussions about it are often highly charged with emotion. Both pro-life and pro-choice advocates argue on the basis of human rights—the former based on rights of the fetus and the latter on rights of the mother—because of the humanity of each party. There are very few people on either side of the philosophical argument, however, who would describe abortion as a healthy medical intervention. Most agree that abortion is a problematic solution to a difficult situation. There are instances in which carrying a pregnancy to term threatens the life of the mother. There are also many more instances in which a pregnancy is inconvenient or undesired.

Therapeutic Abortion for Ectopic Pregnancy

An ectopic pregnancy is the implantation of a fertilized ovum in an area other than the uterus. This can occur because of an abnormally shaped uterus or fallopian tubes that are obstructed as a result of abnormal development, scarring from STDs or other inflammatory processes, or for unknown reasons. This is a life-threatening situation for the mother, and currently a therapeutic abortion is the only treatment.

Therapeutic Abortion for Prenatal Abnormalities

Development of a variety of prenatal testing methods has introduced the possibility of knowing many things about a baby before birth. Prenatal testing may be done using ultrasound, samples of fluid taken from the amniotic sac or the placental villi, or blood samples from the mother. From these tests, several genetic diseases and congenital deformities can be identified. After anomalies are diagnosed, some patients choose to abort the baby. This is a very difficult decision to consider even in instances in which the baby has a fatal defect that will not allow it to live outside the uterus. It is important to provide information about alternatives to abortion and possible treatments for their child when a patient has a serious prenatal diagnosis. No one should feel pressured to make the decision quickly to abort, but legal requirements and increasing risk for the mother may limit the time to decide. Abortion because of fetal abnormality may result in much grieving and guilt for the patient and her family.

Methods of Abortion

Several methods are available. The method is determined primarily by the length of the gestation and the goal of inflicting as little trauma to the mother's reproductive system as possible while still inducing pregnancy loss. Time periods for the different abortion methods and the allowable reasons for legal abortion vary according to the laws of the state, province, or country.

Chemical Agents

Two types of postcoital medications are available. One is an emergency contraceptive known as Plan B, sometimes called the "morning after" pill. Treatment consists of postcoital administration of sufficient estrogen/progestin (levonorgestrel) to prevent ovulation and possibly to prevent fertilization if ovulation has already occurred. The drug also prevents a fertilized ovum from implanting in the uterine lining. If a fertilized ovum has already implanted when the patient takes the drug, the pregnancy will not be terminated. For this reason, some scientists disagree about whether Plan B is a form of contraception or a form of abortion.

Plan B is available at pharmacies without a prescription to women over age 18. Typically, it is used after unexpected, unprotected sexual intercourse (as with sexual assault) or with unexpected risk of conception (as with condom failure). For the medication to be effective, the initial dose typically is given within 72 hours after intercourse and preferably within the first 24 hours. Because no advance planning is required before intercourse, Plan B can be misused as a casual form of birth control. Patients who use it in this way will need education about more appropriate birth control methods.

Side effects of Plan B may include nausea, vomiting, headaches, and breast tenderness.

Another type of postcoital medication prevents the binding of progestins at their receptors, which causes a chemically induced abortion up to the 10th week of pregnancy. Called mifepristone (also known as RU-486 and marketed under the name Mifeprex), this drug is a progestin antagonist. It must be used within 49 days after the first day of the woman's last period. Nausea and cramping may accompany expulsion of the uterine contents.

There is much debate about whether mifepristone should be used at all or only within specific guidelines. The U.S. Food and Drug Administration approved mifepristone in 2000 in an accelerated drug-approval process, but legislative bills have been repeatedly introduced to stipulate prescribing regulations for health care providers. Undoubtedly mifepristone, as well as methotrexate (a chemotherapy medication) and misoprostol (a medication to prevent stomach ulcers), all of which can stimulate abortion, will continue to be the subject of much debate.

Abortion Methods for Early Pregnancy

Early in a pregnancy (during approximately the first 13 weeks) there are three primary means of pregnancy termination: menstrual extraction, vacuum aspiration, and D&C. Menstrual extraction is removal of the endometrial lining by manual suction and can be done during the first 7 weeks following the last menstrual period (LMP). This can be done without anesthesia and without cervical dilation by inserting a small cannula into the cervix and aspirating with a large syringe. Vacuum aspiration is a similar process that is used from confirmation of pregnancy through the first 13 weeks. It requires cervical dilation and usually is done with local anesthesia. The patient returns home 1 to 4 hours after the procedure. D&C also may be used during the first 13 weeks. In this procedure, the cervix is dilated and the uterine contents are scooped away with a curet. This is done as an outpatient procedure under general, regional, or local anesthesia.

Abortion Methods for Later Pregnancy

During the second trimester, the fetus is much larger, so more dilation is required. A dilation and evacuation (D&E) may be performed in much the same manner as a D&C. Generally, dried laminaria (a type of seaweed) or some other absorbent substance is placed inside the cervical canal. This absorbs fluid and swells, thus gradually dilating the cervix. Prostaglandin may be administered either by suppository into the vagina or by injection into the amniotic sac; this usually induces uterine contractions and results in delivery a few hours later. Unfortunately, a live fetus too premature to survive may be born by this method and continue to breathe for a time until death.

An induction with either a saline or urea injection may be used for pregnancies beyond 16 weeks. A portion of amniotic fluid is removed and replaced with concentrated saline or urea solution, which kills the fetus and stimulates contractions. Sometimes saline and prostaglandins are used in combination to terminate a pregnancy.

Hysterotomy involves removal of the uterine contents through an abdominal incision in the same manner as a cesarean section. This procedure is rarely done for pregnancy termination.

• WORD • BUILDING •

hysterotomy: hystero—womb + tomy—cutting

Risks and Complications

Abortion involves risks. Some are the same risks inherent in childbirth, such as possible hemorrhage or introduction of infection, but there are additional risks related to the interruption of natural processes and the aggressiveness with which the products of conception are removed during abortion. During an uncomplicated childbirth, the uterine lining is not scraped or forcefully emptied by suction. Natural hormonal preparation for term childbirth contributes to uterine contraction after the birth, which decreases blood loss, but no such preparation occurs for abortion. Artificial dilation of the cervix may cause injury, as may introduction of the instruments used for abortion. Injured tissues can become sites for growth of microorganisms. Finally, the possibility of infertility as a result of complications related to abortion, although relatively uncommon, is a risk.

Some possible physical complications following therapeutic abortion are injuries to the uterus or cervix, excessive bleeding, infection, retention of some products of conception, and possible failure of abortion. Rarely, second-trimester abortions can be complicated by amniotic fluid embolism, in which amniotic fluid is absorbed into the uterine circulation because of disruption of placental attachments with instruments. Amniotic fluid in the mother's circulatory system can result in circulatory collapse and disseminated intravascular coagulation (DIC). DIC is a serious derangement of the body's blood clotting controls and, although rare, can be fatal.

Nursing Care and Patient Education

Care after abortion is very important. Patients rarely stay overnight, and complications can occur after they are discharged. Patients should be carefully assessed after the procedure for signs of bleeding. Instruct that bleeding should not exceed that of a heavy period, that the passage of clots larger than a quarter may be a sign of complications, and that the discharge should not become foul smelling. Patients should be given a phone number to call 24 hours per day, 7 days per week if fever, chills, excessive bleeding, or foul-smelling discharge occur. The patient should be advised to abstain from sexual intercourse for the time specified by the health care provider (usually about 3 weeks).

A grief response may occur after a pregnancy termination, even if the baby was definitely unwanted and the patient does not have strong beliefs against abortion. There is much debate about frequency of post-abortion syndrome or whether such a condition exists. However, loss and trauma have occurred in any case, and reorganization of the self takes time. Availability of psychological counseling for women after abortion is very important. Women should be given a number to call if they experience psychological discomfort. The need for birth control should be assessed.

Ethical Issues

Ethically, an individual nurse should not be required to assist in any treatment that demands that he or she act in a way that contradicts personal moral beliefs. This would violate the nurse's rights. However, there is also an ethical duty to provide care to patients for whom the nurse is responsible. Therefore, it is wise for nurses who have moral objections to abortion to carefully choose their work setting. For example, choosing to work in day surgery in a hospital that performs abortions and refusing to care for abortion patients is not a legitimate option (Box 42.1, *Ethical Considerations*). One way that nurses can positively influence the abortion situation is by teaching about family planning, which may lower the number of requests for abortions. Another way might be to become involved with agencies that help pregnant women find viable alternatives to abortion.

TUMORS OF THE REPRODUCTIVE SYSTEM

Benign Growths

Fibroid Tumors

PATHOPHYSIOLOGY, ETIOLOGIES, AND SIGNS AND SYMPTOMS. Fibroid tumors, or **leiomyomas** (plural form is leiomyomata), are benign tumors made up of endometrial cells that have implanted on or within the walls of the uterus. These can grow very large and may cause pain or menstrual disorders, exert pressure on the bladder or bowel, cause necrosis because of pressure on the blood supply to tissues, and interfere with fertility. Although the exact cause is unknown, heredity and hormones play a role.

THERAPEUTIC MEASURES. Because fibroid tumors are estrogen sensitive, medical treatment may involve hormone suppression. Surgical treatment may involve myomectomy or hysterectomy. **Myomectomy** is removal of only the fibroid tumor and may be chosen to preserve fertility. Myomectomy may be done surgically through an abdominal or vaginal incision or with a laser introduced through a laparoscope. Hysterectomy may be necessary for very large fibroids or those that cause severe bleeding or discomfort.

Polyps

PATHOPHYSIOLOGY, ETIOLOGY, AND SIGNS AND SYMPTOMS. Polyps are benign growths that grow inside the uterus or on the cervix and may bleed after intercourse

• WORD • BUILDING •

leiomyoma: leio—smooth + myom(a)—fibroid

myomectomy: myom(a)—fibroid + ec—away + tomy—cutting

Box 42.1

Ethical Considerations

Abortion

The famous case of *Roe v. Wade* (1973) changed the legal status of therapeutic abortion in the United States but added a great deal of confusion to its ethical and moral status. A careful reading of the *Roe v. Wade* decision reveals that the court made no decision about the ethics or morality of elective (therapeutic) abortion. Rather, the court said that according to the U.S. Constitution, all people, including women, have a right to determine what they can do with their bodies (right to self-determination) and a right to privacy. Therefore, during the first trimester, a woman and her physician may decide to terminate a pregnancy without interference from the state. During the second trimester, the state may regulate the circumstances under which an abortion may occur to protect the woman's health. Once the fetus is viable, the state may also prohibit abortion. Although a woman may have a right to obtain an abortion, there is not a right to require the death of the fetus should a viable fetus be identified after the abortion procedure. Pro-choice groups put the right to self-determination and privacy central to their concerns. Pro-life groups generally believe that abortion is fundamentally killing and therefore wrong.

The fetus is the central issue in this debate. Is the fetus considered a person with individual rights separate from those of the woman who is pregnant? Another central question asks when human life begins. Is abortion at any stage of pregnancy morally acceptable? Each fertilized egg contains the essential genetic material for the development of a unique individual. However, many fertilized eggs never successfully implant in the uterus in the natural process of conception. Does such a factor make the timing of the procedure a critical element? Related to this problem is the status of frozen embryos created through in vitro fertilization. They too contain the essential, unique genetic material for the development of a human being. If every embryo should be respected as potential human life, what moral obligation do we have toward those embryos? What about embryos left in freezers unclaimed? Should we implant them into childless women? Should we use cells that are otherwise scheduled to be destroyed to instead treat disease or further the understanding of genetic disorders?

The issues around abortion are huge, and there are no easy answers. Many resources can provide information and guidance to the public about the variables. However, health care workers are not only members of the public, they are the people on the front line interacting with and serving women who are having these procedures. Anyone who decides to work in an abortion clinic or a unit where terminations occur is expected to be fully prepared to participate in treatments and procedures. The fundamental question of the morality of such procedures has no bearing in such a facility. Each nurse must examine his or her own beliefs before choosing to work in a facility that carries out abortions.

or between menstrual cycles. They are generally teardrop shaped and are attached by a stalk. Polyps develop most often after the age of 42. The cause is unknown, but estrogen plays a role in their development.

THERAPEUTIC MEASURES. Polyps are generally removed vaginally or transcervically by separating the stalk from the uterus and then stopping the bleeding by use of chemical, electrical, or laser cautery. Removal of polyps in the vagina can be done without anesthetic in a physician's office. Removal of polyps transcervically requires cervical dilation and is more likely to be done in a hospital with anesthesia.

Reproductive System Cysts

PATHOPHYSIOLOGY, ETIOLOGIES, AND SIGNS AND SYMPTOMS. Several types of cysts can affect women's health. Cysts of the ovaries can develop associated with incomplete ovulation, **hypertrophy** of the corpus luteum after ovulation, or inflammation of the ovary. Most ovarian cysts eventually will shrink spontaneously and merely cause discomfort for a time. Chocolate cysts are formed when endometrial cells bleed into an enclosed space, as occurs with endometriosis. They are called chocolate cysts because they are filled with old blood that has become chocolate colored. Cystoadenomas are benign growths that can sometimes undergo cellular transformation and become cancerous. Any pelvic mass in a postmenopausal woman should be investigated for malignancy.

THERAPEUTIC MEASURES. Most cysts are not surgically removed, but excessive size, interference with fertility, and high cancer potential may make needle drainage, biopsy, laparoscopic surgery, or **laparotomy** advisable. If cysts are painful, application of heat to the abdomen or back may help promote comfort.

Polycystic Ovary Syndrome

PATHOPHYSIOLOGY AND ETIOLOGY. Polycystic ovary syndrome (PCOS) is a complex abnormality of endocrine balance of unknown etiology. Multiple cysts on the ovaries are a sign that was discovered early and for which the disease was named, but they are not present in all cases. There seem to be strong genetic links with such family history as too much or too little hair (especially for women), severe acne, diabetes, irregular menses, and infertility. Many of the symptoms of PCOS are a result of insulin resistance with excessive levels of insulin in the blood, which in turn stimulates secretion of androgens.

SIGNS AND SYMPTOMS. Women with PCOS often have infertility, obesity, and menstrual disturbances. They also may have masculinization because of the excess androgen secretion. They have an increased risk of diabetes mellitus, elevated blood pressure, coronary artery disease, and endometrial cancer.

• WORD • BUILDING •

hypertrophy: hyper—too much + trophy—nourishment (growth)
laparotomy: laparo(o)—abdominal wall + tomy—cutting

DIAGNOSTIC TESTS. Diagnostic tests can include blood tests to rule out other causes of endocrine abnormality, tests to determine whether ovulation is occurring (such as midluteal progesterone levels and basal body temperature graphing), endometrial biopsies to determine the level of proliferation and to check for endometrial cancer, and blood tests to determine lipid levels and glucose tolerance.

THERAPEUTIC MEASURES. Medical treatments can involve blood pressure medications, lipid control medications, and oral hypoglycemic agents such as metformin (Glucophage). Diet and exercise may be recommended for weight reduction, control of lipid levels, and cardiac health. Oral contraceptives may be used to normalize hormone levels and protect the endometrium for those not desiring to conceive. Ovulation-inducing medication may be used for women who desire to conceive; treatment with metformin also may prompt ovulation.

If masculinization is a problem, antiandrogen medication such as spironolactone (Aldactone) may be prescribed. In severe cases, gonadotropin-releasing hormone (GnRH) agonists may be used to produce medical suppression of the ovaries, with results similar to removal of the ovaries. This is followed 6 months later with an estrogen-progestin combination to protect the bones from osteoporosis.

Bartholin's Cysts

PATHOPHYSIOLOGY, ETIOLOGY, AND SIGNS AND SYMPTOMS. Bartholin's cysts are actually infected Bartholin's glands at either side of the vaginal opening that occur due to obstruction of the glands. Excessive swelling of Bartholin's glands results in pain with sitting and with intercourse.

THERAPEUTIC MEASURES. Incision and drainage may alleviate the discomfort. If Bartholin's cyst formation occurs often, **marsupialization**—the surgical formation of a pouch around an opening made into a gland to facilitate drainage—may be needed. Sitz baths may be ordered to cleanse the area and to promote comfort and healing.

Dermoid Cysts

PATHOPHYSIOLOGY, ETIOLOGY, AND SIGNS AND SYMPTOMS. Rarely and for unknown reasons, a **dermoid** cyst (also called a cystic **teratoma**) may develop from a germinal cell of an ovary. This cell divides and differentiates into various tissue types such as skin, teeth, bones, hair, and even extremities in a disordered arrangement. This type of cyst may grow quite large and may occur on both ovaries at the same time.

THERAPEUTIC MEASURES. Dermoid cysts are removed by laparoscopy or laparotomy. If the cyst contains glandular tissue that is secreting hormones, adjustment of hormone

• WORD • BUILDING •

marsupialization: marsupial—pouch + ization—process of making
dermoid: derm—skin + oid—form
teratoma: terat—monster + oma—growth

levels to normal may take some time. Although most teratomas are benign, some are malignant, especially in postmenopausal women, so a biopsy is generally done on the tissue.

NURSING CARE AND PATIENT EDUCATION. Growth of a dermoid cyst can be a frightening experience for a woman. Reassurance that this is a disordered group of cells identical to the other cells in her body, rather than a deformed baby, is important.

Malignant Disorders

It is sometimes difficult to distinguish benign growths from malignant growths without biopsy results, and some benign growths can become cancerous. Malignancies can occur in all parts of the reproductive system and can occur at all ages. Although reproductive system cancers are more common in older age groups, ovarian tumors can occur even in young children. Both male and female children of women who were given diethylstilbestrol (DES) in the past to prevent premature delivery in high-risk pregnancies have experienced a high incidence of developmental defects and cancers of the reproductive organs.

This section presents a general overview of the most common cancers. If investigated and treated early enough, cure is often possible.

> **LEARNING TIP**
>
> "Three C" changes that may indicate cancer are changes in color, contour, and consistency of a tissue.

Vulvar Cancer

PATHOPHYSIOLOGY, ETIOLOGIES, AND SIGNS AND SYMPTOMS. Although vulvar cancer is not common, alertness to changes in visible parts of the reproductive system such as the vulva can result in early diagnosis, requirement of less drastic treatment, and end with more positive results. Persistent itching of the vulva or appearance of white or red patches, rough areas, skin ulcers, or wartlike growths should not be ignored; these can be signs of precancerous or cancerous changes. Risk factors for development of vulvar cancer are an STD of any type, precancerous or cancerous changes of the anus or any of the genitalia, immune system depression, and smoking.

DIAGNOSTIC TESTS. Regular Pap smears and physical examinations can identify lesions. Biopsy of suspicious lesions is necessary to diagnose vulvar cancer.

THERAPEUTIC MEASURES. If discovered early, vulvar cancer may be treated with removal or destruction of cancerous cells. If not diagnosed early, it may require surgical removal of the entire vulva and associated lymph nodes (a radical vulvectomy) with subsequent skin grafting from other areas of the body for repair.

Cervical Cancer

PATHOPHYSIOLOGY, ETIOLOGIES, AND SIGNS AND SYMPTOMS. Changes in the cells of the cervix (called cervical intraepithelial neoplasia [CIN]) can progress to cervical cancer. Dysplastic cells (those with dysplasia) are generally less differentiated or less ordered than expected for their cell type.

Some identified risk factors for development of cervical cancer include starting sexual activity at an early age, having multiple sexual partners, having several pregnancies, smoking, and being infected with human papillomavirus or herpes simplex virus type II (HSV-II). Use of oral contraceptives may also increase a woman's risk of developing cervical cancer, although some of the increase in incidence may be because women using oral contraceptives may not be using barrier protection against STDs. Although some women experience slight spotting or serosanguineous discharge with cervical cancer, many are asymptomatic until the cancer is widespread.

DIAGNOSTIC TESTS. Pap smears are the best method of screening for cervical cancer currently available, but some work is being done on self-tests that women can collect. A Pap smear determines the degree of cellular change, or dysplasia. Ranking systems vary, but Pap smear results are usually presented in categories that range from no atypical cells seen to invasive cancer evident (0 to IV). This procedure has significantly reduced the incidence of invasive cervical cancer over the years since its introduction because cellular changes can be identified early enough for treatment to begin before the cells become cancerous. Schiller's test may be done if a patient has an abnormal Pap smear. This involves painting the cervix with iodine. Dysplastic cells stain differently than normal ones. Biopsy is done to confirm a cancer diagnosis. Recommendations for frequency of screening vary, but most recommend that Pap smears begin at either age 21 or with the start of sexual activity and be done yearly unless abnormalities develop. After a period of normal Pap smears, some health care providers advocate longer intervals for low-risk people.

THERAPEUTIC MEASURES. Treatments for preinvasive neoplasia include **cryotherapy** (freezing), laser therapy (burning), and surgical removal of the involved area with a loop excision instrument or by conization (Fig. 42.11). All of these procedures are done through the vagina, so there are no external incisions. After any of these treatments, the patient is advised not to douche, use tampons, or have intercourse for approximately 2 weeks to allow healing to take place. She should be advised to report immediately if fever, bloody vaginal discharge, or foul-smelling vaginal discharge occurs. For invasive cancers, hysterectomy, radiation implant, or chemotherapy may be done.

• WORD • BUILDING •

cryotherapy: cryo—cold + therapy—treatment

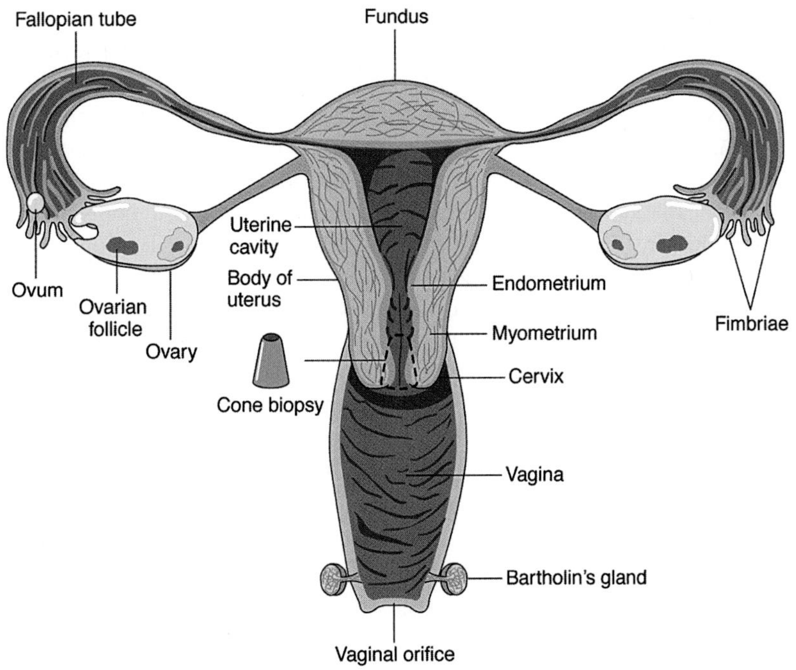
Fallopian tube
Fundus
Uterine cavity
Body of uterus
Endometrium
Myometrium
Cervix
Ovum
Ovarian follicle
Ovary
Cone biopsy
Fimbriae
Vagina
Bartholin's gland
Vaginal orifice

FIGURE 42.11 Conization.

PREVENTION. In 2006, a vaccination to help protect against HPV types 6, 11, 16, and 18 was introduced, known as Gardasil (human papillomavirus vaccine). Although there are many high-risk types of HPV, types 16 and 18 cause 70% of cervical cancers. The vaccination is for women ages 9 to 26, regardless of sexually activity status or exposure to HPV. The vaccination consists of three injections over a 6-month period. The vaccination is still being studied for its longevity. More research is being done and more vaccinations may be available in the future for women of all ages.

Endometrial Cancer

PATHOPHYSIOLOGY, ETIOLOGIES, AND SIGNS AND SYMPTOMS. Endometrial cancer is the most common type of uterine cancer. Most develop in response to relative estrogen excess. Abrupt changes in bleeding patterns, especially bleeding in a menopausal woman, may indicate endometrial cancer development. Estrogen excess can develop for many reasons. Estrogen levels fluctuate widely in the perimenopausal period. Obesity results in increased estrogen production that is not balanced by progestins. Estrogen replacement therapy for menopausal symptoms without the addition of progestins also has been associated with an increase in endometrial cancer, but addition of a progestin may decrease the risk of endometrial cancer to less than that of untreated women. Alcohol consumption may increase the risk of endometrial cancer by interfering with estrogen metabolism, but this is still a matter of debate. Some endometrial cancer is unexplained by any currently known risk factors.

DIAGNOSTIC TESTS. Diagnosis is generally done by endometrial biopsy, but MRI may be used to evaluate invasiveness and involvement of lymph nodes.

THERAPEUTIC MEASURES. Depending on the stage of endometrial cancer and metastasis, treatment with hysterectomy, radiation, or chemotherapy may be used.

Ovarian Cancer

PATHOPHYSIOLOGY, ETIOLOGIES, AND SIGNS AND SYMPTOMS. Ovarian cancer is an especially insidious killer because cellular changes in the ovaries often are asymptomatic until the cancer is advanced. Little is known about what prompts these cells to undergo malignant changes. Risk factors are not definitely identified, but some proposed factors include low fertility and number of children, late menopause, a family history of reproductive or colon cancers, and a diet rich in animal fats. Use of hormonal contraception may help prevent ovarian cancer because it results in less ovulation during a woman's lifetime.

DIAGNOSTIC TESTS. Identification of abnormal growths on the ovaries may begin with bimanual examination, so it is important for women, especially in the older age-groups, to continue to have regular pelvic examinations even if they are not sexually active and even if they have had a hysterectomy. Various blood tests measuring tumor marker substances, ultrasonography, CT scanning, and MRI may also be used to assist in diagnosis.

THERAPEUTIC MEASURES. Treatment may involve surgical removal of the ovaries by laparoscopy or laparotomy. Sometimes the ovaries are removed to prevent the disease in women who have a high familial risk. Radiation and combination chemotherapy may also be used.

Nursing Care and Education of Patients with Malignant Disorders

Radiation therapy for cancers of the reproductive system may involve the placement of radioactive implants into the patient's body for 24 to 72 hours. Prevent inappropriate radiation of the patient's other body parts by such actions as maintaining patency of a urinary catheter to avoid unnecessary exposure of the bladder. Follow institutional guidelines for radiation precautions. A foul-smelling vaginal discharge is expected after radiation by implant because of tissue destruction caused by the radiation; document the amount and character of the discharge. Chemotherapy treatments often cause severe nausea, as well as anorexia and sores of the mouth, vagina, and anus. See Chapter 11 for care of patients receiving radiation or chemotherapy.

See Table 42.9 for a summary of tumors of the reproductive system.

GYNECOLOGICAL SURGERY

Endoscopic Surgeries

Many of the surgeries performed on the reproductive system can be done using an endoscope. The endoscopes used contain not only magnifying lenses and a light source but may also include tiny tools for performing surgery, for removal of small areas of diseased tissue and samples, for suction, and for cauterization of bleeding vessels. Because endoscopic surgeries require tiny incisions (usually less than 1 inch long), there is less tissue disruption and very little bleeding when compared with traditional surgical techniques. Smaller incisions also present less risk of infection than traditional methods, and recuperation is generally more rapid with fewer complications.

Overall the danger to the patient is generally low for endoscopic surgeries; however, not all surgical situations may be satisfactorily handled in this way. The size of the cannula restricts the size of tissues that can be removed, unless they can be divided into smaller sections and then pulled out through the cannula. If affected areas are widespread, the endoscope may not be able to reach all sites. Traditional surgery still may have to be done when endoscopic surgery has been ineffective, and this can be frustrating to patients. However, information gained through the prior endoscopic surgery may decrease the time required for the traditional surgery.

Laparoscopies are the most common type of endoscopic surgical procedure employed for women's reproductive system surgeries. This method can be used for access to the abdominal cavity and the anterior portions of the reproductive organs. Tubal ligations, tubal repairs, removal of ectopic pregnancy implantations, removal of small tumors, removal of endometriotic tissue, and aspiration of fluid-filled cysts can all be done by this method.

The newest method of surgery, which is minimally invasive, is known as the daVinci surgical system. This method is robot and computer assisted and allows the surgeon to make a small number of 1- to 2-cm incisions to gain access and 3-D visualization into the pelvic cavity. Gynecologically, this method can be used for hysterectomy and myomectomy. The benefits of this method versus other surgical methods are that the hospital stay is shorter and the patient experiences less pain and scarring, less risk of infection, less blood loss, fewer transfusions, faster recoveries, and quicker return to normal activities.

Culdoscopies may be done to access the area at the back of the uterus. A **culdotomy**, which is an incision into the upper posterior portion of the vagina, is necessary to insert the cannula. A **culdocentesis**, which is the removal of fluid from the cul-de-sac of Douglas, may be done during a culdoscopy. Aftercare is much the same as for a laparoscopy. The patient should be informed that a small amount of vaginal spotting may be expected from the incision but that heavy, purulent, or foul-smelling discharge should be reported because it could indicate infection.

Colposcopies typically are used to screen, diagnose, or treat problems of the cervix. The binocular microscope attached to the scope cannula, which is introduced into the

TABLE 42.9 TUMORS OF THE REPRODUCTIVE SYSTEM SUMMARY

Signs and Symptoms	Menstrual pain/dysfunction Infertility Constipation Vaginal bleeding Abdominal/perineal pain/swelling Androgen characteristics Obesity Diabetes Coronary artery disease
Diagnostic Tests and Findings	Physical examination Laparoscopy Ultrasound CT or MRI scan Biopsy Hormone levels
Therapeutic Measures	Surgery Chemical/electrical/laser cautery Oral contraceptives and medications Incision/drainage/marsupialization Chemotherapy Radiation therapy
Priority Nursing Diagnoses	*Acute* or *Chronic Pain* related to lesion/surgery *Urinary Incontinence* or *Constipation* related to lesion or surgery *Disturbed Body Image* related to body structure abnormality *Sexual Dysfunction* related to disturbance in self-concept

CT = computed tomography; MRI = magnetic resonance imaging.

• WORD • BUILDING •

culdotomy: culdo—cul-de-sac + tomy—cutting

culdocentesis: culdo—cul-de-sac + centesis—puncturing

vagina, allows the physician to examine dysplastic cells while they are still in their normal place and to treat cervical dysplasia as previously described. Hysteroscopy may be used to treat problems within the uterus. Removal of polyps and other growths, modification of congenital malformations such as septa (walls of tissue where there should be none), and laser ablation of endometrial tissue may all be done during hysteroscopy. The endoscope may be inserted further into the fallopian tubes to perform a salpingoscopy, allowing surgical or laser opening of blocked tubes.

Nursing Care and Patient Education

Postoperative care involves careful assessment for signs of possible excessive internal bleeding, including assessment of vital signs, skin color and temperature, and pain. Women may experience pain because of carbon dioxide insufflation, which makes the internal organs easier to visualize and manipulate. Measures to reduce the related discomfort while the carbon dioxide is absorbed include instructing the patient to lie flat for a few hours, massaging the back and shoulders, and administering pain medication. Instruction about signs of complications to report, medications, and when and where to go for suture removal complete the discharge teaching.

Hysterectomy

Removal of the uterus (hysterectomy) may be done for a variety of reasons, including abnormally heavy or painful menstruation, large fibroid or other benign tumors, severe uterine prolapse, and cancer of the uterus. It should not be done merely as a sterilization procedure because the risks involved in hysterectomy are much greater than the risks associated with tubal ligation. The surgery can be done through an abdominal incision, vaginally, laparoscopically, or with the daVinci robotic method. The vagina is left intact and the proximal end (which had been attached to the uterus) is sutured, forming a blind pouch. Although less vaginal lubrication is present after hysterectomy, nerve routes are maintained and satisfactory sexual intercourse is expected to continue.

The uterus alone may be removed, and in some cases the fallopian tubes and ovaries may also be removed—a procedure called total abdominal hysterectomy with bilateral **salpingo-oophorectomy** (TAH-BSO), or **panhysterectomy**. If the ovaries are removed, the woman undergoes immediate menopause and may suffer from symptoms associated with menopause, including the increased risks of cardiovascular disease and osteoporosis. If removal of the ovaries was usually done because of the presence of estrogen-dependent cancer, estrogen replacement is not usually feasible, and extra care, comfort, and explanation from nurses is needed.

See the *Nursing Care Plan for the Patient Undergoing Hysterectomy.* In addition to the nursing diagnoses covered, also assess for anxiety related to surgery, body image disturbance, and for ineffective coping. See Chapters 10 and 12, respectively, for additional interventions for pain and postoperative patients.

• WORD • BUILDING •

salpingo-oophorectomy: salpingo—tubal + oophor—ovary + ec—from + tomy—cutting

panhysterectomy: pan—all + hyster—uterus + ec—from + tomy—cutting

NURSING CARE PLAN for the Patient Undergoing Hysterectomy

Nursing Diagnosis: *Risk for Ineffective Tissue Perfusion* related to surgical incision and removal of the uterus (and possibly the ovaries)

Expected Outcomes: The patient's incision(s) will heal by primary intention without excessive bleeding.

Evaluation of Outcomes: Is dressing dry and intact and/or does perineal pad show less than 3-cm stain every hour? Are edges of the incision well approximated, with scant bleeding/serous drainage, and mild edema/erythema (if applicable)?

Interventions	Rationale	Evaluation
Monitor vital signs and oxygen saturation according to hospital policy and as necessary.	Vital signs and oxygen saturation reflect tissue perfusion status.	Are vital signs stable and within normal range?
Assess for bleeding or other discharge on perineal pad and on abdominal dressing (if applicable).	Excessive bleeding may compromise tissue perfusion and slow healing.	Is pad or dressing dry?

NURSING CARE PLAN for the Patient Undergoing Hysterectomy—cont'd

Interventions	Rationale	Evaluation
	Vaginal discharge gives clues to healing of incision at the proximal end of the vagina.	Is discharge foul smelling?
Assess wound healing (if applicable) twice a day and report any evidence of infection or inadequate healing promptly.	Early treatment of inadequate wound healing decreases postoperative complications.	Is incision area swollen, reddened, or draining purulent material?
Teach patient to report changes in incision site or excessive bleeding.	Patients are discharged quickly and should know what to monitor at home.	Does patient verbalize understanding of instruction?

Nursing Diagnosis: *Risk for Urinary Retention* related to manipulation of the bladder and ureters during surgery, anticholinergic drugs, fluid intake changes, and fear of pain

Expected Outcomes: The patient will void 30 mL/hr or more without difficulty.

Evaluation of Outcomes: Is patient able to void and effectively empty bladder when voiding? Is patient voiding at least 30 mL/hr?

Interventions	Rationale	Evaluation
Assess urinary output after surgery. Report to RN or physician if less than 30 mL/hr or unable to void.	Inadequate urinary output can be an evidence of dehydration, low glomerular perfusion, kidney dysfunction, damage to ureter, or urinary retention.	Is output greater than 30 mL/hour? Is patient able to void without discomfort?
Assess bladder fullness using Doppler monitoring or scratch test (listening with a stethoscope, lightly scratch abdomen as you move downward from xiphoid until you hear change in sound indicating top of the bladder).	Urine retention can cause infection and damage to kidneys, ureters, and bladder. The scratch test and Doppler monitoring cause less discomfort and pressure than palpation of the abdominal incision area.	Does patient feel she is emptying fully when voiding? Does Doppler or scratch test indicate residual urine after voiding?
Medicate for pain on a fixed schedule for operative day and first postoperative day (unless patient declines).	Maintenance of a consistent blood level of medication in the immediate postoperative period provides relief of pain and promotes voiding without fear of discomfort.	Does patient state that she is comfortable?

NURSING CARE PLAN for the Patient Undergoing Hysterectomy—cont'd

Nursing Diagnosis: *Risk for Constipation* related to manipulation of the bowel during surgery, use of opioid analgesics and anticholinergic drugs, diet changes, less exercise than usual, and fear of pain when passing stool

Expected Outcomes: The patient will pass soft, formed stool without excessive gas discomfort by third postoperative day.

Evaluation of Outcomes: Are bowel sounds active in all four quadrants? Is patient passing gas without difficulty? Is patient able to have a soft, formed bowel movement within 3 days of surgery?

Interventions	Rationale	Evaluation
Assess for active bowel sounds in all four abdominal quadrants before giving anything orally.	Manipulation of the bowel during surgery and anesthetics or other medications can interfere with bowel function.	Are bowel sounds within normal limits?
Encourage high fluid intake, and graduate diet toward a high-fiber, regular diet as soon as patient is able to tolerate it (or physician orders prescribe).	Adequate fluid and fiber in the diet softens the stool for easy passage.	Is patient able to tolerate fluids and high-fiber foods?
Encourage adequate exercise.	Reasonable exercise promotes peristalsis and relieves gas discomfort.	Has patient dangled at bedside the day of surgery and then walked increasing amounts each following day?
Assess quantity and quality of pain. Control pain with analgesics, especially before administering suppository or enema.	The presence of pain may inhibit defecation.	Is pain controlled? Does patient express concern about pain with bowel movement?
Administer stool softeners, laxatives, suppositories, or enemas as ordered (check bowel protocol or standing orders).	Soft stool is easier to pass.	Has patient passed soft, formed stool by the third day after surgery?

SUGGESTED ANSWERS TO CRITICAL THINKING

■ *Julie*

1. Questions to further assess Julie's symptoms should include the following: How long have you been noticing the lumps? Do you do BSEs? Has there been a change in the characteristics of the lumps? Are the lumps mobile or fixed? Have you noticed any breast skin or nipple changes? Have you noticed any leakage of fluid or blood from your breasts? Are you breastfeeding or have you recently delivered an infant? Have you had a fever? Are the pain and lumps related to your menstrual cycle? Is there anything that makes the symptoms better or worse?
2. You can teach Julie to continue to do BSE, since she is the best person to detect changes. Teach her that limiting fat and caffeine in her diet may help reduce symptoms. Reinforce any information or treatments provided by the nurse practitioner.

■ *Lola*

1. Interventions that may help control Lola's discomfort related to hot flashes include possible inclusion of HRT therapy, inclusion of phytoestrogens in her diet (with primary provider direction), limiting caffeinated foods or beverages, dressing in layers so that some may be removed as needed, and lowering the thermostat as needed.

SUGGESTED ANSWERS TO—cont'd

2. Information that should be shared with Lola concerning HRT therapy includes the risks as well as benefits according to most recent studies. Risks include increased risk of stroke, cardiovascular disease, breast cancer, and thromboembolism. Benefits include symptomatic relief and decreased risk of complications from osteoporosis.

■ *Jessica*

1. Some important information from Jessica would include her true age (laws vary concerning birth control for minors), her intentions, her family situation, whether she is already sexually active, and what information she wants.
2. She needs to know that being sexually active involves more risks than just pregnancy. Discussion of STDs is vital. Early sexual activity may also be associated with abuse and psychological suffering. The choices of birth control should be explained, including the risks, effectiveness, disadvantages, and advantages of each method. Follow clinic protocol to determine your role in teaching the patient.
3. Potential scenarios can be presented for her "responsible" consideration, such as these: What would she do if contraceptive failure resulted in a pregnancy? How would she feel if she contracted an incurable or permanently damaging sexually transmitted disease that she might pass on to someone else? How would she react to a breakup with her partner after she has engaged in sexual intercourse? Ask about her goals and plans in life. Counseling that evidences concern for the individual at this stage may do a lot to postpone sexual activity until the patient is more mature. It is important for her to realize that choosing to delay sexual activity at this time may be the most responsible and health-promoting life decision she can make.

REVIEW QUESTIONS

1. A patient who is breastfeeding her baby says "My doctor said I have mastalgia. What does that mean?" Which response by the nurse is best?
   a. "That means you may have an infection in your breasts."
   b. "Mastalgia is just the normal discomfort that is associated with breastfeeding."
   c. "The word mastalgia just means breast pain; it can occur with monthly cycles of hormone levels."
   d. "Mastalgia is the medical term for fibrocystic breast disease. It is important to have it treated promptly."

2. Which response by the nurse is most appropriate when a 60-year-old woman who has been menopausal for several years relates that she has begun having vaginal bleeding again?
   a. "Don't be concerned—it is perfectly normal."
   b. "Try taking some ibuprofen. That may reduce the bleeding."
   c. "You should see a physician to have that checked as soon as possible."
   d. "Give it time—bleeding after menopause usually goes away within a month."

3. During an endometrial biopsy, for which of the following signs and symptoms of vasovagal response should the nurse observe?
   a. Pain in the chest and abdomen
   b. Cramping and diaphoresis
   c. High blood pressure and tachycardia
   d. Bradycardia and falling blood pressure

4. Which of the following medications can be used to treat vasovagal response during gynecological procedures?
   a. Atropine
   b. Morphine
   c. Epinephrine
   d. Norepinephrine

5. The nurse is discharging a patient with endometriosis from an office visit. The patient says her medication helps but does not relieve all her discomfort. What other measures can the nurse recommend?
   a. "Check with the health food store. There are several herbal remedies that can be very effective."
   b. "Try using the relaxation exercises you learned in your childbirth classes. A warm compress to your abdomen might also help."
   c. "You can double up on your pain medication on occasion, but you shouldn't do it on a regular basis."
   d. "If the medications aren't effective, then it is time to talk to the physician about a hysterectomy."

REVIEW QUESTIONS—cont'd

6. The nurse enters the room of a patient who is 1 day postoperative left-sided mastectomy and notes a phlebotomist taking blood from her left antecubital space. What should the nurse do first?
   a. Nothing; the nurse is not the phlebotomist's supervisor.
   b. Nothing; blood pressures should be avoided in the affected arm, but blood draws are safe.
   c. Stop the phlebotomist and point out that needlesticks must be avoided in the affected arm.
   d. Notify the physician.

7. Following a panhysterectomy, what should the nurse teach the patient to expect?
   a. Heavy bleeding for a week
   b. Symptoms of menopause
   c. Painful intercourse for approximately 6 months
   d. Monthly cramping but no menstrual flow

8. A patient who has just returned from an abdominal panhysterectomy is at risk for impaired urinary elimination. At least how many milliliters should be in her catheter bag 8 hours postoperatively? **Fill in the blank.**

Answer: __________ mL

9. Which of the following is the least effective form of contraception?
   a. Douching
   b. Condom with spermicide
   c. Diaphragm with spermicide
   d. Oral contraceptive medication

References

Centers for Disease Control and Prevention. (2009). *Breast cancer statistics.* Retrieved November 20, 2009, from http://www.cdc.gov/cancer/breast/statistics

National Institutes of Health. (2002). *NHLBI stops trial of estrogen plus progestin due to increased breast cancer risk, lack of overall benefit.* Retrieved November 20, 2009, from http://www.nhlbi.nih.gov/new/press/02-07-09.htm

World Health Organization. (2009). *Medical eligibility criteria for contraceptive use* (4th ed.). Retrieved November 20, 2009, from http://whqlibdoc.who.int/publications/2009/9789241563888_eng.pdf

DavisPlus | For additional resources and information visit http://davisplus.fadavis.com

43

Nursing Care of Male Patients with Genitourinary Disorders

PAULA D. HOPPER
AND DEBRA PERRY-PHILO

KEY TERMS

cryptorchidism (kript-OR-ki-dizm)
epididymitis (EP-i-DID-i-MY-tis)
erectile dysfunction (e-REK-tile dis-FUNK-shun)
hydrocele (HEYE-droh-seel)
orchiectomy (or-ki-EK-toh-mee)
orchitis (or-KIGH-tis)
paraphimosis (PAR-uh-fih-MOH-sis)
phimosis (fih-MOH-sis)
priapism (PRY-uh-pizm)
prostatectomy (PRAHS-tah-TEK-tuh-mee)
prostatitis (PRAHS-tuh-TIGH-tis)
retrograde (RET-roh-GRAYD)
suprapubic (SOO-pruh-PEW-bik)
tamponade (TAM-pon-AYD)
urodynamic (YOO-roh-dye-NAM-ik)
vasectomy (va-SEK-tuh-mee)

QUESTIONS TO GUIDE YOUR READING

1. How would you explain the pathophysiologies associated with male genitourinary and reproductive disorders?
2. What are the etiologies, signs and symptoms, and treatments of prostate disorders?
3. What nursing care will be provided to patients with male genitourinary or reproductive disorders?
4. What are the disorders of the testicles and penis, and how do they impact sexual function?
5. What are some physical and emotional causes of erectile dysfunction?
6. What is the nurse's role in helping men cope with the loss of sexual function?
7. Which disorders of the male reproductive system interfere with fertility?
8. What treatment options are available for male infertility?

Problems affecting the male genitals and urinary system typically are difficult areas for both the patient and the nurse to deal with because of the sexual nature of the male anatomy. Nurses need to realize that sexuality is a natural part of each of us as human beings and should not be avoided when we provide care to patients. Often the nurse is an ideal person to provide important sexual health care teaching. If the patient is approached in a confident, confidential manner, discussions about sexual health can be positive learning experiences for both the patient and the nurse.

Some good general health guidelines for men can be found at the Agency for Healthcare Research and Quality's Put Prevention into Practice website at http://www.ahrq.gov/ppip/healthymen.htm.

PROSTATE DISORDERS

The prostate gland sits at the base of the bladder and wraps around the upper part of the male urethra like a doughnut. The primary purpose of the prostate is to provide alkaline secretions to semen and to aid in ejaculation. The prostate does not contain any hormones; however, many men fear that prostate problems and treatment will cause problems with their erections or their "nature" (sexual activities).

Prostatitis

Pathophysiology

Prostatitis, or inflammation of the prostate gland, can occur any time after puberty. The problem may be chronic or a single, acute episode. The inflammation causes the prostate gland to swell, resulting in pain, especially when standing. It eventually may lead to difficulty in passing urine as a result of an inward squeezing on the urethra that causes a mild obstruction.

Etiology

According to the National Institutes of Health, there are four basic types of prostatitis: (1) acute bacterial, (2) chronic bacterial, (3) chronic prostatitis/chronic pelvic pain syndrome, and (4) asymptomatic inflammatory prostatitis (McNaughton-Collins et al., 2007). Bacterial prostatitis is most common in older men. It results in edema and inflammation of all or part of the prostate gland.

Any bacteria that can cause a urinary tract infection can also cause infectious prostatitis. Common bacteria are organisms such as *Escherichia coli* and *Staphylococcus aureus*. Sexually transmitted infections can also cause prostatitis. The prostate gland may become infected in the following ways:

- Bacteria ascending the urethra
- Infected urine refluxing from the bladder into the prostatic ducts
- Bacteria in the blood or lymph supply to the gland
- Surgical instrumentation or other forms of urethral trauma.

• WORD • BUILDING •

prostatitis: prostat—prostate gland + itis—inflammation

Prevention

Ways to avert prostatitis are regular and complete emptying of the bladder to prevent urinary tract infection (UTI), avoiding excess alcohol (more than 2 to 3 oz per day—alcohol is a bladder irritant), and avoiding high-risk sexual practices, such as multiple partners.

Signs and Symptoms

The most common symptoms are those that occur with any UTI: reports of urgency, frequency, hesitancy, and dysuria. Because of the location and function of the prostate gland, the patient may report low-back, perineal, and postejaculation pain. He may also have a fever and chills.

Complications

One complication of acute bacterial prostatitis is urinary retention. If the prostate is extremely swollen, the bladder cannot be completely emptied. Another complication may be a temporary problem with erections. Ascending infections, prostatic abscess, epididymitis, and prostatic calculi (stones) are some of the more serious and rare complications of prostatitis.

Diagnostic Tests

Initial diagnosis is based on symptoms. The first test performed is a careful, gentle, digital rectal examination (DRE) of the prostate. The prostate gland is examined by the health care provider by insertion of a gloved finger into the rectum. The examiner may find a warm, irregular, swollen, and painful prostate gland. A urine culture generally is positive for bacteria. The examiner may also gently massage the prostate gland and order an expressed prostate secretion (EPS) test that reveals bacteria and a large number of white blood cells. Cystoscopy also may be done.

Therapeutic Measures

Acute bacterial prostatitis is usually treated with antibiotic therapy. The preferred treatment is trimethoprim and sulfamethoxazole (Bactrim) for 30 days. Other antibiotics, including the fluoroquinolones (ciprofloxacin, ofloxacin, levofloxacin), may be used for chronic prostatitis (Table 43.1).

Other forms of treatment may include anti-inflammatory agents, stool softeners, warm sitz baths, prostatic massage, and dietary changes such as decreasing spicy foods and alcohol. Alpha-adrenergic blockers such as alfuzosin (Uroxatral) can help relax the bladder neck and reduce the pain on urination. Patients should avoid alpha-adrenergic agonist medications, which can cause urine retention. In some cases, prostate surgery is needed to remove the obstruction.

Nursing Process for the Patient with Prostatitis

DATA COLLECTION. Begin the assessment by asking the patient to describe signs and symptoms that indicate evidence of a UTI, such as sudden fever, chills, and reports of urgency, frequency, hesitancy, dysuria, and nocturia. The patient may also have pain in the lower back, the perineum, or after ejaculating. Ask the patient if he has ever had a UTI or prostate infection in the past. Care must be taken to assess

TABLE 43.1 MEDICATION USED TO TREAT DISORDERS OF THE MALE REPRODUCTIVE ORGANS

Medication Class	Medication/Action	Route	Side Effects	Nursing Implications
Medications Used for Cancer of the Male Reproductive System				
Testosterone suppressing/ blocking agents	leuprolide (Lupron) *Initially stimulates and then inhibits follicle-stimulating and luteinizing hormones (FSH and LH) to suppress testosterone.*	Subcutaneously, IM	GI upset, insomnia, sexual dysfunction, tremor, bone pain, constipation, gynecomastia, CNS disturbance, photosensitivity *Serious:* elevated liver enzymes, arrhythmias, MI	Store drug at room temperature and protect from light. Instruct patient that signs and symptoms may increase initially. Monitor for side effects.
	goserelin (Zoladex) *Analogue to luteinizing-releasing hormone; works on pituitary to decrease FSH to decrease sex hormones.*	Subcutaneous implant	GI upset, CNS disturbance, bone pain, sexual dysfunction, skin disorders, gynecomastia *Serious:* arrhythmias, hypertension, urinary obstruction, spinal cord compression	Inject into upper abdominal wall. Do not aspirate syringe. Teach patient that medication may increase testosterone initially and thus also increase signs and symptoms.
	flutamide (Eulexin) *Inhibits androgen uptake and/or binding in tissues.*	PO	GI upset, fatigue, sexual dysfunction, incontinence, constipation, rash, photosensitivity, gynecomastia *Serious:* hypertension, hepatotoxicity, blood dyscrasias	Instruct patient that urine color changes to amber/ yellow-green. Teach patient to avoid excess exposure to sun and to promptly report side effects. Monitor hepatic function tests.
Medications Commonly Used for BPH				
Alpha-adrenergic antagonists and alpha-reductase inhibitors	tamsulosin (Flomax) terazosin (Hytrin) alfuzosin (Uroxatral) doxazosin (Cardura) *Alpha-adrenergic antagonists. Relax smooth muscle; produce vasodilatation.*	PO	GI upset, dry mouth, CNS disturbance, visual disturbance, palpitations, urinary urgency, sexual dysfunction *Serious:* profound hypotension	Warn patient dizziness may occur with onset of use. Urge him to report side effects. Monitor blood pressure/ pulse. Tell patient not to crush or chew tablets. Caution against driving or use of heavy machinery.
	finasteride (Proscar) dutasteride (Avodart) *Alpha reductase inhibitors. Inhibit enzyme responsible for formation of potent androgen from testosterone.*	PO	Sexual dysfunction, gynecomastia, decreased volume of ejaculation	Do not chew or crush tablets. Obtain baseline PSA and DRE before use. Instruct patient on side effects. Caution with liver dysfunction.
Medications Commonly Used for Erectile Dysfunction				
Vasodilators, smooth muscle relaxers, hormone replacement	sildenafil (Viagra) tadalafil (Cialis) vardenafil (Levitra) *Relaxes smooth muscle; produces vasodilation.*	PO	GI upset, dizziness, headache, visual disturbance, hearing loss, flushing, rash *Rare but serious:* prolonged erection, arrhythmias, MI, stroke	Take about 1 hour before sexual activity (may be taken ½ to 4 hours before). Assess cardiovascular status before use; may be contraindicated. Avoid use when taking nitroglycerin preparations. If erection lasts more than 4 hours, seek emergency care.
	alprostadil (Caverject injection or Muse suppository) prostaglandin E1 *Relaxes smooth muscle; produces vasodilation.*	Intracavernosal injection, intraurethral suppository	Flu-like symptoms, diarrhea, penile pain/fibrosis, urethral burning/bleeding, prolonged erection, CNS disturbance, flushing *Serious:* hypotension, seizures, heart rate disturbance	Monitor vital signs. Inform patient erection should occur in 2 to 5 minutes and not last more than 4 hours. Instruct patient to report side effects immediately.

TABLE 43.1 MEDICATION USED TO TREAT DISORDERS OF THE MALE REPRODUCTIVE ORGANS—cont'd

Medication Class	Medication/Action	Route	Side Effects	Nursing Implications
	Yohimbine *Herbal vasodilator*	PO	GI upset, tremors, CNS disturbance, insomnia, tachycardia *Serious:* hypertension *or* severe hypotension, arrhythmias, cardiac failure	Assess for other medical conditions before use. Monitor blood pressure and renal and hepatic function.
	testosterone transdermal (Testoderm, Androderm) testosterone cypionate (Depo-testosterone injection) *Testosterone replacement; produces androgen effects.*	Transdermal patch, gel, IM	Gynecomastia, acne, nausea, insomnia, edema, male pattern baldness, itching, erythema, skin irritation, bladder irritability	Rule out cancer before use. Monitor hepatic function. Instruct patient to report side effects, prolonged erection or difficulty urinating.

CNS = central nervous system; GI = gastrointestinal; MI = myocardial infarction.

urinary retention resulting from obstruction. Obtain a urine culture and assist with collection of the EPS specimen, if requested, as part of the patient assessment.

NURSING DIAGNOSES, PLANNING, AND IMPLEMENTATION. The nursing diagnoses and interventions for patients with prostatitis are discussed next.

Urinary Retention Related to Obstruction as Evidenced by Residual Urine in Bladder After Voiding

EXPECTED OUTCOME: The patient will be able to void effectively as evidenced by residual urine of less than 25% of bladder capacity.

- Evaluate patient's medications for urinary retention as a side effect. *Many medications, especially those with anticholinergic effects, can cause urinary retention.*
- If suspicion of urine retention is present, determine residual urine volume by catheterizing patient (according to physician order) or obtaining a bladder ultrasound immediately after voiding. *Incomplete emptying of the bladder may lead to increased discomfort or ascending infection.*
- Have the patient complete a bladder log including patterns of elimination and urine loss, as well as volume/type of fluid consumed for 3 to 7 days. *This will provide for an objective verification of intake and output volumes and aid in determination of urinary retention.*
- Educate patient about avoidance of risk factors for urine retention (e.g., alpha-adrenergic agonists, anticholinergic agents, overfilling of the bladder). *These are modifiable variables that may limit retention of urine.*
- Report urine retention to RN or physician. *Catheterization may be needed to empty bladder and prevent complications.*

Risk for Ineffective Self-Health Management Related to Knowledge Deficit About Cause, Treatment, and Prevention of Prostatitis

EXPECTED OUTCOME: The patient will verbalize understanding of disorder and demonstrate appropriate self-care.

- Determine patient's current knowledge and understanding about cause and treatment of prostatitis. *This will allow for additional and/or correct information to be provided about the disorder for appropriate understanding.*
- Provide patient with additional and/or correct information about the cause and treatment of prostatitis. *This will allow the patient to have a full understanding of the etiology and care related to the disorder and increase likelihood of patient compliance.*
- Teach avoidance of risk factors such as urinary catheterization, poor hygiene, risky sexual practices, and excessive intake of bladder irritants such as alcohol, caffeine, or citrus juices. *Avoiding risk factors is important to resolving or preventing prostatitis.*
- Encourage the patient to wash his hands and sitz bath equipment before and after each treatment *to prevent infection.*
- Encourage the patient to empty his bladder every 2 to 3 hours even if he does not feel the urge to urinate. *An overstretched bladder increases risk of infection.*

- Encourage fluids such as water and cranberry juice up to 2500 to 3000 mL/day unless contraindicated by heart failure or other chronic illness. *Fluids help flush the bladder and prevent infection.*
- Include patient's partner in care. *Some treatment options may also include treatment of the partner (e.g., sexually transmitted diseases such as gonorrhea, chlamydiosis, or trichomoniasis; see Chapter 44).*
- Encourage use of antibiotics as directed, and advise patient to take complete course of medication *in order to best treat infection and prevent development of antibiotic-resistant bacteria.*

Acute Pain Related to Swelling and Irritation of the Prostate Gland as Evidenced by Pain Rating

EXPECTED OUTCOME: The patient's pain will be controlled as evidenced by patient statement that comfort is at an acceptable level.

- Use a culturally appropriate pain scale to help patient identify comfort level. *This will aid in understanding comfort level as defined by the patient and aid in guiding appropriate interventions.*
- Encourage appropriate use of anti-inflammatory medication as ordered. *This will decrease inflammation and promote comfort.*
- Encourage use of comfort measures such as warm sitz baths, sitting on a pillow, or prostatic massage, as needed, *to decrease swelling and promote comfort.*
- Teach patient to avoid spicy and acidic foods, alcohol, and caffeine. *These can exacerbate symptoms.*
- Consult physician about need for stool softeners. *Firm stool will further irritate the prostate during defecation and increase discomfort.*

Anxiety Related to Sexual Concerns as Evidenced by Patient Statement

EXPECTED OUTCOME: The patient will identify presence of anxiety and verbalize concerns about sexuality.

- Identify source of concern related to sexual activity and meaning assigned to disorder as described by patient. *This will help in guiding appropriate interventions related to etiology of concern.*
- Explore coping skills previously used by patient to relieve anxiety; reinforce these skills and explore other outlets for stress management. *Coping mechanisms that have been helpful in the past may aid patient in dealing with current stressors that result in anxiety.*
- Encourage patient to discuss possible complications and questions about sexual practices with his health care provider. *In some cases, sexual intercourse is encouraged as a means of relieving prostatic congestion; in other situations, it may be contraindicated.*

EVALUATION. A clean urine culture with absence of all symptoms of prostatitis is the desired outcome. If interventions have been effective, the patient will have an acceptable comfort level, understand the cause and treatment plan, and verbalize concerns related to the disorder. Prevention of chronic prostatitis can generally be achieved with patient education.

Benign Prostatic Hyperplasia

Enlargement of the prostate gland is a normal process in older men. It begins around age 50 and exists in 75% of men older than age 70. Benign prostatic hyperplasia (BPH) is a nonmalignant growth of the prostate that gradually causes urinary obstruction. According to current studies, BPH does not increase a man's risk of developing cancer of the prostate.

Pathophysiology

There is a slow increase in the number of cells in the prostate gland, generally the result of aging and the male hormone dihydrotestosterone. As the size of the prostate gland increases, it begins to compress or squeeze the urethra. Narrowing of the urethra means that the bladder must work harder to expel the urine. More effort and a longer time is needed to empty the bladder. Eventually the narrowing causes obstruction and may lead to urine retention or eventually distention of the kidney with urine (hydronephrosis).

It is the location of the enlargement, not the amount, that causes the problem. A small growth in the prostate gland closest to the urethra may cause more problems with urination than a growth the size of an orange in the outer portion of the gland.

Etiology

There is no known cause of BPH other than normal aging. Some men think they may have caused the problem by certain sexual practices; however, there is no scientific proof of that at this time. Some factors that are being investigated in research studies are high-fat diet and ethnic background.

Prevention

Because there is no known cause, there is no proven method to prevent enlargement of the prostate gland. Many new treatments are aimed at slowing down the enlargement process. One such treatment that is being researched is the herbal supplement saw palmetto.

Signs and Symptoms

Symptoms of BPH are usually identified in two ways: problems related to obstruction or problems related to irritation. Symptoms related to obstruction include a decrease in the size or force of the urinary stream, difficulty in starting a stream, dribbling after urination is complete, urinary retention, and a feeling that the bladder is not empty. The patient may also experience overflow incontinence or an interrupted stream, where the urine stops midstream and then starts again.

Symptoms related to irritation include nocturia, dysuria, and urgency. A prostatic symptom index score sheet has been developed, and health care providers use this questionnaire with older patients to assess symptoms and determine treatment options.

Complications

When BPH is untreated and obstruction is prolonged, serious complications may occur. Urine that sits in the bladder for too long can back up into the kidneys, causing hydronephrosis, renal insufficiency, or **urosepsis**; it can also damage the bladder walls, leading to bladder dysfunction, recurrent UTIs, or calculi (stones). Acute urine retention with total inability to urinate can occur; this is a medical emergency that requires catheterization.

Diagnostic Tests

The first step is a medical history, including specific questions about the patient's symptoms. A DRE of the prostate is then conducted by the health care provider to assess for enlargement and whether the gland is hard, lumpy, or "boggy." Primary tests include urinalysis and blood work. BUN (blood urea nitrogen), serum creatinine, and prostate-specific antigen (PSA) levels may be elevated. Secondary tests include **urodynamic** flow studies, which may show a decreased urine flow rate. Transrectal ultrasound of the prostate and cystoscopy may reflect structural abnormalities.

Therapeutic Measures

If the patient has no symptoms or mild symptoms, the most current medical approach is "watchful waiting." The health care provider watches for any increase in symptoms that suggest the urethra is becoming obstructed. Treatment of symptoms may include use of a catheter (indwelling or intermittent), encouraging oral fluids, and antibiotics for UTI.

Conservative medical treatment includes the use of medication to either relax the smooth muscles of the prostate and bladder neck or block the male hormone to prevent or shrink tissue growth. Alpha-adrenergic antagonists, such as tamsulosin (Flomax), are medications that relax the smooth muscles. These medications are also used to treat high blood pressure; therefore, patients need to work closely with their health care providers to avoid overdose or the negative side effects of postural hypotension (see Table 43.1).

The most commonly used medications to block the action of the male hormone in the prostate gland are finasteride (Proscar) and dutasteride (Avodart). These medications must be taken on a long-term, continuous basis to achieve results. Conservative measures are used initially unless the patient is experiencing recurring infections, repeated gross hematuria, bladder or kidney damage, evidence of cancer, or unsatisfactory lifestyle changes.

Nonsurgical invasive treatments, some of which are experimental, are available in some areas of the country in addition to surgical options. These include transurethral microwave therapy (TUMT), which involves heat applied directly to the gland to inhibit growth, and transurethral needle ablation (TUNA), which uses radio waves to destroy part of the gland. Prostatic stents may be used to open the passageway for urine to flow more freely.

Surgical Treatment

Because so many other treatments are available now, surgery is not needed as often. When symptoms are severe enough to require surgery, several types are available, as described next.

TRANSURETHRAL RESECTION OF THE PROSTATE. Called TURP, this is the surgical treatment used most often to relieve obstruction caused by an enlarged prostate (Fig. 43.1). Several other transurethral options also exist. Transurethral incision of the prostate (TUIP) uses surgical incisions into the gland to relieve obstruction. Transurethral ultrasound-guided laser-induced prostatectomy (TULIP) uses a laser to relieve obstruction.

For TURP, the patient is anesthetized and the surgery is performed using an instrument called a resectoscope. The resectoscope is inserted into the urethra and the prostate gland is "chipped" away a piece at a time. Special surgical instruments are used to "vaporize" or "microwave" the pieces and cut down on the amount of bleeding during surgery. During routine TURP, the "chips" are flushed out using an irrigating solution and are sent to the laboratory to be analyzed for possible evidence of cancer. The prostate gland is not completely removed but peeled away like the rind of an orange. The prostatic tissue that remains eventually grows back and can cause obstruction again at a later time. Patients need to be reminded to continue having yearly prostate examinations.

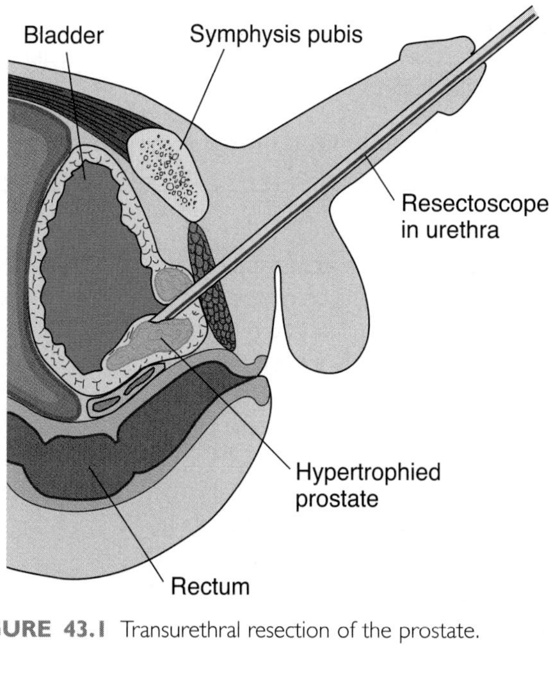
Bladder
Symphysis pubis
Resectoscope in urethra
Hypertrophied prostate
Rectum

FIGURE 43.1 Transurethral resection of the prostate.

• **WORD • BUILDING** •
urosepsis: uro—urine + sepsis—systemic infection
urodynamic: uro—urine + dynamic—force

As the tissue is removed during TURP, bleeding occurs. A Foley catheter is left in place with 30 to 60 mL of sterile water inflating the balloon. The balloon is overfilled and may be secured tightly to the leg or abdomen to **tamponade** (compress) the prostate area and stop the bleeding. Irrigation solution generally flows continuously (Fig. 43.2); manual irrigation may be done for the first 24 hours to help maintain catheter patency by removing clots and chips. The Foley catheter is removed after the danger of hemorrhage has passed.

You may need to save "serial urines" after the Foley catheter has been removed. To do this, each time the patient urinates or the catheter bag is emptied, save a sample of urine in a transparent cup. Place it in a safe place, such as on a shelf in the bathroom. With each subsequent urination, place the new cup to the right of the previous cup. When five or six cups are lined up, you can start over at the left side, replacing the oldest cup with the newest one. This allows the nurse or physician to examine the urine for progressively less blood with each void.

Complications associated with prostate surgery depend on the type and extent of the procedure performed. The main medical complications include clot formation, bladder spasms, and infection. Less common complications may be urinary incontinence, hemorrhage, and erectile dysfunction (see the *Nursing Care Plan for the Postsurgical Patient Having Transurethral Resection of the Prostate for Benign Prostatic Hyperplasia*).

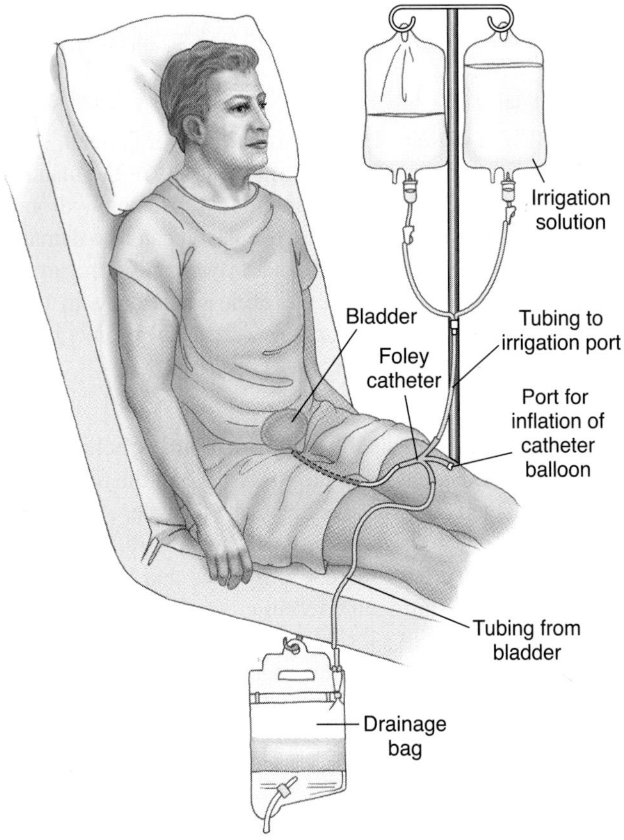
Irrigation solution
Bladder
Foley catheter
Tubing to irrigation port
Port for inflation of catheter balloon
Tubing from bladder
Drainage bag

FIGURE 43.2 Bladder irrigation.

NURSING CARE PLAN for the Postsurgical Patient Having Transurethral Resection of the Prostate for Benign Prostatic Hyperplasia

Nursing Diagnosis: *Risk for Bleeding* related to surgical intervention as evidenced by presence of blood in urine

Expected Outcomes: The patient's bleeding will be minimal, as evidenced by urine becoming progressively more clear.

Evaluation of Outcomes: Is urine clearing? Is bleeding reported promptly?

Interventions	Rationale	Evaluation
Closely monitor urinary output in terms of amount, color, and presence of clots at least every hour for the first 24 to 48 hr postoperatively. Monitor serial urines.	Careful monitoring and reporting of changes can help prevent major complications.	Is urine becoming progressively less bloody and more clear with each void?
Explain to patient that some bloody urine is normal after a TURP, as long as it does not suddenly get much worse. Also explain that a little blood mixed with irrigating fluid in a Foley bag may look worse than it actually is.	Seeing the catheter bag filled with bloody drainage may be upsetting to a patient or his family.	Is patient aware of what to expect in Foley bag?

NURSING CARE PLAN for the Postsurgical Patient Having Transurethral Resection of the Prostate for Benign Prostatic Hyperplasia—cont'd

Interventions	Rationale	Evaluation
Encourage patient to drink up to 2500 mL/day (unless contraindicated by other medical conditions) of water, noncitrus juices, and other noncaffeinated, nonalcoholic beverages.	Increasing urine flow can help flush blood from bladder.	Is patient drinking adequate amounts?
Teach patient to avoid constipation (suggest stool softener, fluids, prune juice) and heavy lifting.	These can increase pressure in the abdomen and increase risk of bleeding.	Does patient verbalize understanding of instructions?
Advise patient to lie down if urine becomes bright red or has large clots.	Activity can increase bleeding.	Does patient reduce activity if bleeding increases?
Teach patient to avoid aspirin and NSAIDs until risk of bleeding is over.	Aspirin and NSAIDs inhibit platelet function and increase risk of bleeding.	Does patient verbalize understanding?

Nursing Diagnosis: *Acute Pain* related to bladder spasms, obstruction, or surgical process as evidenced by patient pain rating

Expected Outcomes: The patient's pain will be controlled as evidenced by lower pain rating

Evaluation of Outcomes: Does patient state that pain is decreased to acceptable level?

Interventions	Rationale	Evaluation
Monitor pain every 2 to 4 hr for first 48 hr and within 30 minutes of any intervention.	A pain scale is the most accurate measure of pain.	Does patient verbalize pain as increasing or decreasing on the scale?
Monitor for signs of pain related to bladder spasms, obstruction, or surgical process, such as facial grimaces, irrigation solution that does not flow into bladder, urinating around catheter, multiple clots.	Relief of mechanical cause of pain promotes comfort, rest, and healing.	Is patient free from signs of pain related to bladder spasms, obstruction, or surgical process?
Give prescribed medication (analgesics, antispasmodics such as B&O suppository) and monitor response.	B&O suppositories relieve bladder spasms.	Does patient state relief when medications are given?
Irrigate catheter as ordered.	Irrigation promotes removal of clots to reduce spasms and pain.	Does irrigating solution flow in and out easily? Are clots being removed?
Educate patient regarding nonpharmacologic methods to control pain such as relaxation and deep-breathing techniques.	Relaxation calms spasms and relieves pain. Nonpharmacologic measures should be used with, not in place of, medication.	Is patient able to relax?

Continued

NURSING CARE PLAN for the Postsurgical Patient Having Transurethral Resection of the Prostate for Benign Prostatic Hyperplasia—cont'd

Nursing Diagnosis: *Urge Urinary Incontinence* related to poor sphincter control as evidenced by inability to control urination

Expected Outcomes: The patient will be able to prevent incontinence.

Evaluation of Outcomes: Is incontinence prevented?

Interventions	Rationale	Evaluation
Teach Kegel (pelvic floor) exercises (see Chapter 42)—to be practiced every time patient urinates and throughout the day.	Kegels strengthen muscle tone to hold urine after catheter is removed.	Is patient able to start and stop urine stream?
Discuss use of condom catheter or penile pads.	These can keep patient dry until incontinence can be controlled.	Does patient indicate an informed choice of incontinence products?
Instruct patient to continue drinking 2000 to 4000 mL of noncaffeinated, nonalcoholic beverages each day.	Adequate nonirritating fluid intake is important for healing and preventing UTI.	Does patient drink adequate fluids even though he dribbles?
Encourage patient to discuss long-term (longer than 6 months) incontinence problems with physician.	Patient may need to learn self-catheterization or try medication.	Does patient verbalize understanding of what to do if incontinence continues?
Refer patient to national incontinence support group if indicated.	Support groups can provide information and emotional support.	Does patient show interest in a support group?

Nursing Diagnosis: *Risk for Ineffective Self Health Management* related to lack of knowledge of postoperative restrictions and care

Expected Outcomes: The patient will avoid activities that increase intra-abdominal pressure resulting in excessive bleeding. The patient will verbalize understanding of how to prevent postoperative infection.

Evaluation of Outcomes: Does patient verbalize understanding of how to prevent bleeding? Is infection prevented?

Interventions	Rationale	Evaluation
Teach patient to avoid lifting heavy objects (more than 10 lb), stair climbing, driving, strenuous exercise, constipation, straining during bowel movements, and sexual activities until approved by physician (about 6 weeks).	Heavy lifting or straining can disrupt the healing process and result in tissue damage or excess bleeding.	Does patient verbalize understanding of reasons for limitation of heavy lifting and straining?
Instruct patient on proper catheter care using verbal, written, and demonstration techniques (some patients are sent home before catheter is removed). Include the following information: • Keep catheter bag secured to abdomen or thigh and keep bag below bladder.	Urinary tract infections are extremely dangerous and can cause death following genitourinary surgery in an elderly patient.	Can patient give a return demonstration of proper catheter care? Is patient free from signs and symptoms of infection?

NURSING CARE PLAN for the Postsurgical Patient Having Transurethral Resection of the Prostate for Benign Prostatic Hyperplasia—cont'd

Interventions	Rationale	Evaluation
• Wash catheter/meatus junction with soap and water once daily. • Use clean technique to change from leg bag to night drainage bag. • Report signs and symptoms of UTI to physician immediately. • Encourage oral fluids.		
Teach all patients to report bleeding that is not stopped with resting; fever; swelling; or difficulty urinating to physician promptly.	These are signs of complications that may require prompt medical intervention.	Does patient verbalize understanding of signs and symptoms to report?

Nursing Diagnosis: *Anxiety* related to concerns over loss of sexual functioning following prostate surgery as evidenced by patient statement

Expected Outcomes The patient will verbalize normal sexual changes that happen after prostate surgery. The patient will identify available support systems if needed.

Evaluation of Outcomes: Is patient able to verbalize understanding of expected body function following prostate surgery? Does the patient access support systems?

Interventions	Rationale	Evaluation
Explain to patient that he will probably have retrograde ejaculation into bladder after surgery. It is not harmful and semen will come out when he urinates.	Removal of the prostate gland often results in retrograde ejaculation.	Does patient understand what will happen when he ejaculates?
Instruct patient to talk with urologist if erection problems occur.	Urologists who specialize in treatment of erectile dysfunction can provide information and treatment.	Is patient aware of local support services?

B&O = belladonna and opium; NSAIDs = nonsteroidal anti-inflammatory drugs; TURP = transurethral resection of the prostate; UTI = urinary tract infection.

Retrograde ejaculation is a common side effect of prostate surgery. When any of the prostate gland is removed, there is a decrease in the amount of semen produced and a part of the ejaculatory ducts may be removed. This results in less semen being pushed outside the body, and instead it "falls back" into the bladder. This causes no harm; the semen is simply passed during the next urination.

It is important to understand that erection, ejaculation, and orgasm are all separate actions. Erection means the penis becomes hard, ejaculation is the release of semen, and orgasm is felt as pulsations along the urethra. Unless additional problems are present, the patient continues to have erections and orgasmic sensations but decreased or no ejaculation.

RADICAL PROSTATECTOMY. When the prostate gland is very large, is causing obstruction, or is cancerous, a radical prostatectomy may be performed to remove the entire prostate gland.

• WORD • BUILDING •
retrograde: retro—backward + grade—step

• WORD • BUILDING •
prostatectomy: prostat—prostate gland + ectomy—excision

Open Prostatectomy. Several approaches may be taken during traditional radical surgery (Fig. 43.3). In the **suprapubic** approach, an incision is made through the lower abdomen into the bladder. The gland is removed, and the urethra is reattached to the bladder. The retropubic approach is similar except there is no incision into the bladder. A perineal prostatectomy involves making an incision between the scrotum and anus to remove the gland. This procedure is rarely done because of the increased risk of contamination of the incision (close to the rectum), and risk of urinary incontinence, erectile dysfunction, or injury to the rectum.

An open prostatectomy means a longer hospital stay compared with other BPH surgeries. A suprapubic catheter and care for an abdominal incision increase the length of stay and risk for complications. Follow-up home care for wound and catheter care is important for these patients.

Minimally Invasive Prostatectomy. Newer techniques use laparoscopy and tiny robot arms to perform radical prostatectomy through five small "porthole" incisions in the abdomen. The surgeon makes all the decisions about the surgery while guiding the robotic arms. The robotic arms allow more precision and maneuverability, especially in small areas. Because robotic surgery is so much less invasive, patients experience better results with less postoperative bleeding and incontinence and shorter hospital stays.

Nursing Process for the Patient with BPH Who Undergoes a TURP Procedure

DATA COLLECTION. Begin by asking the patient if he has ever had treatment or surgery for prostate trouble. Assess amount and type of fluid intake per day and whether the patient has noticed any of the symptoms of BPH. Monitor output, and, if he is not catheterized, ensure that urine retention is being managed appropriately.

• WORD • BUILDING •
suprapubic: supra—above + pubic—pubic bone

NURSING DIAGNOSES, PLANNING, AND INTERVENTIONS. Nursing diagnoses for patients with mild or no symptoms are directed at knowledge deficits related to prevention of UTIs, knowing when to report an increase in symptoms to the health care provider, and taking medication exactly as the health care provider orders. Instruct patients to report changes in urinary output or difficulty voiding. Advise the patient to keep a log book of intake and output and difficulty voiding. Ensure that patients scheduled for prostate surgery understand what to expect after surgery.

For nursing care of the patient following TURP, see the *Nursing Care Plan for the Postsurgical Patient Having Transurethral Resection of the Prostate for Benign Prostatic Hyperplasia*. In addition, each patient experiences individual responses and needs. Care plans must be individualized, keeping in mind that the majority of these patients are elderly and have secondary medical problems such as cardiovascular disease.

EVALUATION. A patient should be discharged home with a minimum of bladder discomfort, light pink to clear urine, no evidence of UTI, and knowledge related to self-care at home. Home care nursing may be required if the patient lives alone or does not have the capacity to provide for meals, toileting, or transportation for the follow-up visit. Table 43.2 provides a summary of BPH.

Cancer of the Prostate

Cancer of the prostate is the most common cancer in American men. Most prostate cancers grow very slowly and often do not cause a major threat to health or life. Many treatment options are available, and the prognosis is often very good.

Pathophysiology

Prostate cancer depends on testosterone to grow. The cancer cells are usually slow growing and begin in the posterior (back) or lateral (side) part of the gland. The cancer spreads

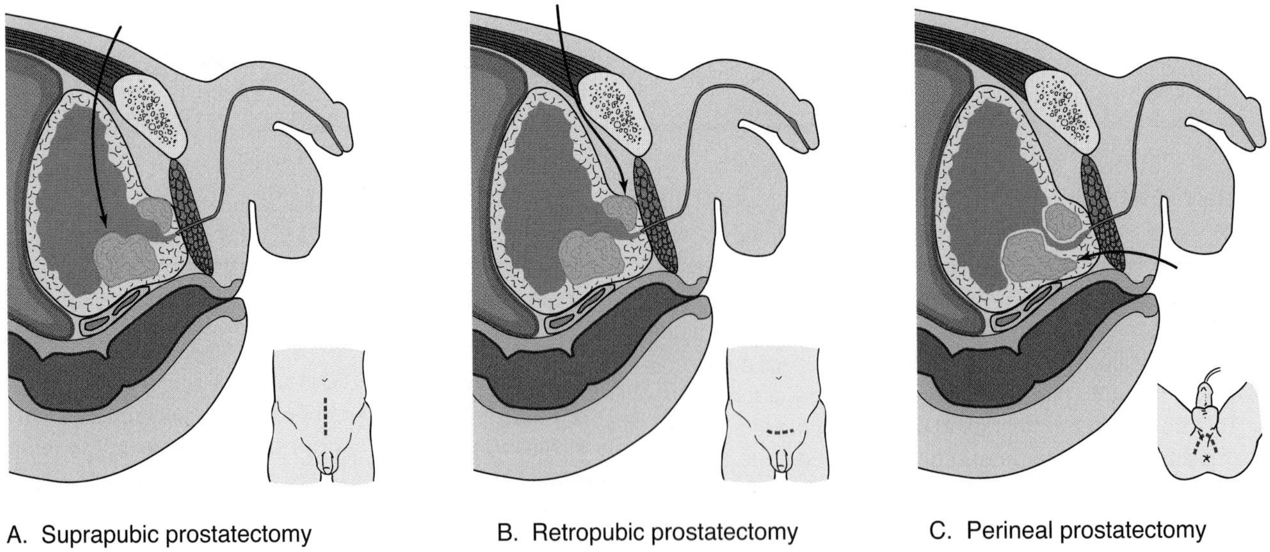
A. Suprapubic prostatectomy
B. Retropubic prostatectomy
C. Perineal prostatectomy

FIGURE 43.3 (A) Suprapubic prostatectomy. (B) Retropubic prostatectomy. (C) Perineal prostatectomy.

TABLE 43.2 BENIGN PROSTATIC HYPERPLASIA (BPH) SUMMARY

Signs and Symptoms	**Related to obstruction:** Decrease in size/force of stream, difficulty in starting stream, dribbling, interrupted stream, urinary retention, overflow incontinence **Related to irritation:** Nocturia, dysuria, urgency
Diagnostic Tests	**Primary:** DRE, urinalysis, BUN, serum creatinine, prostate-specific antigen (PSA) **Secondary:** Urodynamic flow studies, transrectal ultrasound, cystoscopy
Therapeutic Measures	**Conservative:** Alpha-blockers, testosterone blockers **Nonsurgical:** Transurethral microwave antenna (TUMA), prostatic balloon, prostatic stents **Transurethral:** Transurethral incision of the prostate (TUIP), transurethral ultrasound-guided laser-induced prostatectomy (TULIP), transurethral resection of the prostate (TURP) **Radical prostatectomy:** Suprapubic, retropubic, perineal, laparoscopic, or robotic resection
Complications	Ascending or localized infection Injury to surrounding tissues during surgery Impaired sexual function related to tissue injury
Priority Nursing Diagnoses	*Impaired Urinary Elimination* related to obstruction

CRITICAL THINKING

Mr. Atkinson

■ Mr. Atkinson is a 68-year-old African American farmer with an enlarged prostate. He lives on a 75-acre farm with his wife and one son. He is scheduled for a TURP in 6 weeks.

1. Mr. Atkinson is currently taking terazosin (Hytrin), and his physician wants him to increase his dose from 2 to 5 mg daily until surgery. He has a bottle at home of 2-mg tablets. How should you instruct him to take his medication? What side effect should he be advised to watch for?
2. What postoperative instructions should he be given in light of his occupation?
3. What should you tell him if he asks about how the surgery will affect his "nature" (sexual activities)?

Suggested answers at end of chapter.

by one of three routes. If it spreads by local invasion, it will move into the bladder, seminal vesicles, or peritoneum. The cancer may also spread through the lymph system to the pelvic nodes and may travel as far as the supraclavicular nodes. The third route is through the vascular system to bone, lung, and liver. Prostate cancer is staged or graded based on the growth or spread.

Etiology

Age is the primary risk factor. Prostate cancer is found most often in men older than age 65 and is rare in men younger than age 40. Other risk factors are higher levels of testosterone, high-fat diet, and immediate family history.

Prostate cancer rates are highest in African American men and lowest in American Indian and Native Alaskan men (American Cancer Society, 2009). Occupational exposure to cadmium (e.g., welding, electroplating, alkaline battery manufacturing) has been identified as an added risk factor.

Signs and Symptoms

Symptoms are rare in the early stage of prostate cancer. Later stages include symptoms of urinary obstruction, hematuria, and urinary retention. In the advanced (metastatic) stage, symptoms may be pain in the back or hip from metastasis to the bone, anemia, weakness, weight loss, and overall tiredness.

Complications

Early complications of prostate cancer are related to bladder problems, such as difficulty urinating, and bladder or kidney infection. Erectile dysfunction can occur as a result of the cancer or its treatment (see *Evidence-Based Practice* box).

EVIDENCE-BASED PRACTICE

Clinical Question

What interventions are available for men with sexual dysfunction following treatment for prostate cancer?

Evidence

Two Cochrane reviews have looked at treatments for erectile dysfunction. The first found that focused group therapy was as effective as local injection or vacuum devices, and that group therapy combined with drug therapy (sildenafil [Viagra]), was more effective than drug therapy alone (Melnik, Soares, & Nasello, 2007). The second found that PDE5 inhibitors (such as sildenafil [Viagra] and tadalafil [Cialis]) are effective following treatment for prostate cancer (Miles et al., 2007).

Implications for Nursing Practice

Nurses can play a role in assessing men's knowledge of interventions for erectile dysfunction related to treatment for prostate cancer. Although specific intervention is beyond the scope of practice of the LPN/LVN, it is appropriate to advise men that medications, local injections, vacuum devices, and group therapy have all been shown to help, and refer them to their physicians for further assistance.

Continued

cont'd

REFERENCES

Melnik, T., Soares, B., & Nasello, A. G. (2007). Psychosocial interventions for erectile dysfunction. *Cochrane Database of Systematic Reviews 2007, Issue 3* (Art. No. CD004825; DOI: 10.1002/14651858.CD004825.pub2).

Miles, C. L., Candy, B., Jones, L., et al. (2007). Interventions for sexual dysfunction following treatments for cancer. *Cochrane Database of Systematic Reviews 2007, Issue 4* (Art. No. CD005540; DOI: 10.1002/14651858.CD005540.pub2).

If the cancer metastasizes, the patient may develop problems such as pain, bone fractures, weight loss, and depression; eventually death can occur if treatment is not successful.

Diagnostic Tests

A routine DRE of the prostate is the first test; often the examiner finds a hard lump or hardened lobe. Blood tests looking for high levels of prostate-specific antigen (PSA) or prostatic acid phosphatase (PAP) may be done. When there is a palpable tumor, the health care provider may order a transrectal ultrasound and biopsy to help confirm the diagnosis. Bone scans and other tests may be ordered to determine if the cancer has spread outside the prostate gland.

In the past, the PSA test was used to screen men for prostate cancer, but more recently, the American Cancer Society withdrew this recommendation because routine screening has not been found to save lives. Instead, many slow-growing, noninvasive cancers were discovered and treated. Although aggressive cancers require treatment, many prostate cancers are not aggressive, and the treatment may be worse than the disease. Patients with elevated PSA levels may now have additional testing to determine how aggressive the cancer is, so that appropriate treatment decisions can be made.

Therapeutic Measures

Prostate cancer in the early stages may be treated with testosterone-suppressing medications, such as leuprolide (Lupron) or goserelin (Zoladex), or drugs that block testosterone's action on the prostate gland, such as bicalutamide (Casodex). Surgery, such as TURP or radical prostatectomy, or a combination of medication and radiation therapy may be done. In later stages, the treatment is usually a radical prostatectomy, radiation therapy, or implantation of radioactive "seeds" into the prostate (brachytherapy). A new vaccine, sipuleucel-T (Provenge), that will slow the growth and aggressiveness of some prostate cancers is currently being tested.

Metastatic prostate cancer treatment involves relief of symptoms or blocking testosterone by bilateral **orchiectomy**, administration of antiandrogen (flutamide [Eulexin]), or use of agents such as leuprolide and goserelin. Sometimes chemotherapy is used to help relieve symptoms resulting from spread of the cancer.

Unfortunately, any therapy that reduces androgen activity in a man can cause side effects, such as hot flashes, breast tenderness and growth, osteoporosis, and loss of muscle mass. These in turn can cause significant concerns with body image.

Brachytherapy, external-beam radiation therapy, and radical prostatectomy combinations are showing favorable results in the treatment of advanced cancer. Gene therapy and immune-based interventions are other new medical treatment options under investigation. Nontraditional prostate cancer prevention using vitamin E and selenium was being investigated, but has been shown to be ineffective, and may even increase risk.

RADICAL PROSTATECTOMY. A radical prostatectomy (described earlier in this chapter) is done for patients with cancer of the prostate or when the gland is too large to resect using a less invasive method.

The patient returns from surgery with a large indwelling catheter in the urethra and may also have a suprapubic catheter. A drain is often placed to remove fluids from the abdominal cavity and allow the wound to heal from the inside outward. Special care must be taken to keep the incision and drain sites clean and dry. Dressings should be changed according to institution policy using sterile technique.

Radical prostatectomy has more complications associated with it than any other treatment option. The major complications are hemorrhage, infection, loss of urinary control, and erectile dysfunction.

Patient Education

All men older than age 40 should be encouraged to have a yearly DRE of the prostate. Prevention and early detection are the best ways to fight prostate cancer.

PENILE DISORDERS

Problems of the penis, aside from those caused by sexually transmitted diseases, are fairly rare but may cause great concern and worry for the patient. Many men have difficulty seeking help for such a personal problem. It is important to be sensitive when assessing or providing care for these patients.

Peyronie's Disease

Peyronie's disease gives the penis a curved or crooked look when it is erect. Fibrous bands or plaques form mainly on the dorsal (top) part of the layer of tissue that surrounds one of the corpora cavernosa of the penis. The plaque may be caused by injury or inflammation of the penile tissue, or it may come and go spontaneously. If the plaque is thick enough, it can cause curvature, painful erection, difficulty in vaginal penetration, and erectile dysfunction. When conservative treatments such as oral vitamin E, colchicine, or potassium aminobenzoate do

• WORD • BUILDING •
orchiectomy: orchi—testicles + ectomy—excision

not work, surgery may be needed to remove the plaque. Another option is injections into the scar tissue to break it down. Patients need to be reassured that the problem is not life threatening and can be treated.

Priapism

Priapism is a painful erection that lasts longer than 4 hours. If not relieved, it can become a medical emergency. The small veins in the corpora cavernosa spasm, so blood cannot drain back out of the penis as it should. When the blood cannot drain, penile tissue does not get oxygen, and permanent tissue damage may result. There may be a complete loss of erection ability after the priapism episode. Prolonged priapism can also prevent the patient from passing urine, which can lead to painful bladder and kidney problems. Some causes of priapism are sickle cell anemia, leukemia, widespread cancer, spinal cord injury or tumors, and use of medications to manage erectile dysfunction (such as sildenafil [Viagra]) or recreational drugs such as crack cocaine. Treatment in the emergency department may include ice packs, sedatives, analgesics, injection of medications directly into the penis to relax the vein spasms, needle aspiration, and irrigation of the corpora. Surgery to implant a shunt that reroutes blood flow can also be done.

Phimosis and Paraphimosis

Phimosis is the term used to describe a condition in which the foreskin of an uncircumcised male becomes so tight that it is difficult or impossible to pull back away from the head of the penis. It may make it impossible to clean the area underneath. Smegma, a cottage cheese–like secretion made by the glands of the foreskin, becomes trapped under the foreskin and is an excellent place for the growth of bacterial and yeast infections. Treatment usually begins with antibiotics and warm soaks to the area. The physician may cut a small slit in the foreskin to relieve the pressure and treat the infection. A full circumcision may be recommended if the problem continues or if a condom catheter is necessary for urine drainage. Phimosis is generally prevented by teaching uncircumcised males to pull the foreskin back carefully, wash with mild soap and water daily, and replace the foreskin to its normal position.

Paraphimosis occurs when the uncircumcised foreskin is pulled back, during intercourse or bathing, and not immediately replaced in a forward position. This causes constriction of the dorsal veins, which leads to edema and pain. Moderate to severe paraphimosis is a medical emergency and requires immediate care by a physician. The longer the problem continues, the greater the risk of circulation problems and possible gangrene. Prevention through daily cleaning and replacing the foreskin in its normal place is important.

• WORD • BUILDING •

priapism: priap—phallus + ism—condition of
phimosis: phimo—muzzling + osis—condition
paraphimosis: para—abnormal + phimo—muzzling + osis—condition

Cancer of the Penis

Cancer of the penis has been found in men who were not circumcised as infants or have acquired the human papillomavirus (HPV). The tumor is typically a squamous cell carcinoma, and may look like a small round raised wart, induration, or red area. This form of cancer may be spread to a sexual partner. Several research studies have found a link between cancer of the penis and cancer of the uterine cervix. Cancer of the penis may be treated with minor surgery, such as a circumcision or laser removal of the growth. If the cancer has spread, sections of the penis may require surgical removal, radiation, or chemotherapy. Penile reconstruction can be done if necessary following surgery. Finding and treating any lesion in its earliest stages is an important part of patient education, as is education about circumcision of infants as a preventive measure.

TESTICULAR DISORDERS

Cryptorchidism

Cryptorchidism (undescended testicles) is a congenital condition in which an infant boy is born with one or both of his testicles not in the scrotum. The testicles normally drop down (descend) into the scrotum in the last 1 to 2 months before the boy is born. Often, undescended testicles descend into the scrotum on their own by the time the boy reaches age 2. If they do not descend by that time, surgery should be done to correct the problem. Testicles that are not brought down into the scrotum decrease a man's chances of producing a child, because excessive body heat damages sperm production in the testicles. Also, the risk of testicular cancer is higher if the condition is not corrected before the child reaches his teen years.

If normal male sex characteristics do not develop during puberty because the testosterone level is too low, extra testosterone may be given. Testosterone can be administered by daily pill, by long-term injection, or by patch.

Hydrocele

A **hydrocele** is a collection of fluid in the scrotal sac. Hydroceles are not dangerous and generally do not cause pain. Their cause is not known, and they can happen at any point during the lifetime. No treatment is necessary unless the hydrocele is so large that it causes discomfort or embarrassment or is a threat to the blood supply to the testicles. If treatment is needed, the health care provider can aspirate or surgically drain the fluid.

Varicocele

A varicocele is a condition sometimes called varicose veins of the scrotum. The main blood supply to the testicles travels

• WORD • BUILDING •

cryptorchidism: crypt—hidden + orchid—testicle + ism—condition
hydrocele: hydro—water + cele—swelling

along the spermatic cord. The veins become dilated, and when the man is standing, the area in the scrotum begins to feel like a "bag of worms." The patient may report a pulling sensation, a dull ache, or scrotal pain. The sensations are most often felt when standing up. Most varicoceles occur on the left side because of the way the scrotal vein enters at a sharp angle from the left renal vein.

A varicocele is often not discovered until a couple is unable to conceive. It is believed that the varicose veins may increase the temperature of the testicles and cause damage to the sperm. The most successful treatment is surgical repair of the varicose veins.

Epididymitis

The epididymis is a small tube along the back of the testicles where sperm is matured for its last 10 to 12 days before it is ready to be ejaculated. **Epididymitis** is inflammation or infection of the epididymis that can be caused by bacteria, viruses, parasites, chemicals, or trauma. Risk factors include sexual or nonsexual contact, sexually transmitted disease (STD), a complication of some urological procedures, or reflux (backflow) of urine. The problem also may be associated with prostate infections and is usually painful, with the scrotal skin being tender, red, and warm to the touch.

Epididymitis is treated with antibiotics; the partner is also treated if it was sexually transmitted. Depending on the severity of the pain, the patient may be placed on bedrest with the scrotum elevated, possibly on ice packs, and given analgesics. The pain and tenderness usually go away in about a week, although the swelling may last for several weeks. Complications include chronic epididymitis, abscess formation, and sterility.

Orchitis

Orchitis is a rare inflammation or infection of the testicles. The problem may be caused by trauma or infection from epididymitis, UTI, STD, or systemic diseases such as influenza, infectious mononucleosis, tuberculosis, gout, pneumonia, or mumps (after puberty). The patient has swollen, extremely tender testicles, red scrotal skin, and a fever. Interventions are basically the same as for epididymitis and include bedrest, scrotal support, antibiotics, and medication to relieve pain and fever. Complications such as sterility as a result of orchitis caused by mumps can be prevented by giving boys the mumps vaccine at an early age.

Cancer of the Testicles

Pathophysiology and Etiology

Cancer of the testicles is the most common cancer in men between ages 15 and 34 in the United States. The etiology of testicular cancer is unknown. Some of the known risk factors are cryptorchidism, family history, white race, and high socioeconomic status. Some older studies showed a link between a mother's use of DES (diethylstilbestrol, an estrogen preparation once used to prevent spontaneous abortion) while pregnant, but current research has not shown this risk to be significant. The tumors are mostly a germ cell type of cancer formed during normal embryo development.

Prevention

The best prevention is early detection with a monthly testicular self-examination (TSE). The American Cancer Society does not necessarily recommend monthly TSE for all men, because not enough studies have been done to show that it reduces death. However, men should be aware of what is normal for them, so they can recognize changes if they occur. The TSE procedure is simple and easy to learn, and it makes sense to teach it to all men until more data are available. See Chapter 41 for instructions on TSE.

Signs and Symptoms

Early warning signs of cancer may include a small, usually painless lump on the side or front of a testicle. The patient may also notice that the scrotum is swollen and feels heavy. Late symptoms of back pain, shortness of breath, difficulty swallowing, breast enlargement, and changes in vision or mental status indicate metastasis of the cancer.

Complications

Emotional complications can range from fear of cancer and death to feelings of loss of masculine body image and sexual function. Physical complications may involve dealing with pain and the effects of metastasis to areas such as the lungs, abdomen, or lymph nodes. Other less common areas of cancer spread are the liver, brain, and bone.

Diagnostic Tests

When a lump is found, several laboratory and radiographic tests are done. An ultrasound of the testicles is done first, to differentiate a possible tumor from a hydrocele or other noncancerous condition. Blood is drawn to look for tumor markers. An example of a tumor marker for testicular cancer is human chorionic gonadotropin (HCG). A surgical biopsy or removal of the testicle is done to determine the stage of the tumor. If cancer is confirmed, a chest x-ray examination is done to look for spread to the lungs. A scan of the lymph nodes, liver, brain, and bones also may be ordered.

Testicular tumors may be staged or classified in several ways. The simplest way to stage a testicular tumor is as follows:

- Stage I—tumor only in the testicles
- Stage II—tumor spread to abdominal lymph nodes
- Stage III—tumor spread past lymph nodes, usually to the lungs, liver, bones, and/or brain.

Therapeutic Measures

Intervention depends on the stage of the cancer. All treatment begins with complete removal of the cancerous testicles, spermatic cord, and local lymph nodes. Based on the stage of the cancer, radiation or chemotherapy may be done in addition to surgery. If the cancer is found in the beginning stages, the chances for complete recovery are very good. All patients should have regular follow-up testing.

• WORD • BUILDING •

epididymitis: epididymis + itis—inflammation
orchitis: orch—testicle + itis—inflammation
vasectomy: vas—vas deferens + ectomy—excision

Nursing Care

Nursing care is directed first at prevention, by teaching young men to practice monthly testicular self-examination and to see their health care provider if they notice any changes. If a diagnosis of cancer has been made, provide emotional support for the patient. If the patient wants to have children, he should be encouraged to make deposits in a sperm bank before any surgery or treatment is started. The patient and his partner may have many questions about sexual activities as they go through treatment. Encourage them to talk with their health care provider or a sex therapist about ways to express love and tenderness toward one another. Helping patients deal with pain and the side effects of chemotherapy or radiation therapy are also important nursing interventions for these men. See Chapter 11 for care of the patient with cancer.

> **CRITICAL THINKING**
>
> ***Mr. Cunningham***
>
> ■ Mr. Cunningham is a 23-year-old college student engaged to be married next spring. While taking a shower one day, he discovers a lump on his left testicle.
>
> 1. What should he do?
> 2. What are the treatment options if Mr. Cunningham has testicular cancer?
> 3. How can you help Mr. Cunningham cope with the diagnosis?
>
> *Suggested answers at end of chapter.*

SEXUAL FUNCTIONING

Vasectomy

A **vasectomy** uses tiny clamps or cauterization to seal off the vas deferens to prevent sperm from reaching the outside of the body (Fig. 43.4). This 15- to 30-minute surgery is done through a small puncture in the upper part of the scrotum. It is performed as a permanent birth control method for men. The patient should carefully discuss the surgery with his physician, so there is a clear understanding of the results following the procedure.

Following the procedure, the testicles continue to produce the male hormone testosterone and sperm. The prostate gland, along with the seminal vesicles, still ejaculates semen, but the semen does not contain sperm. There should be no major change in the way the ejaculate looks or feels following the procedure. The patient should be encouraged to continue using another birth control method for about 3 months after surgery to be sure there are no sperm left in the tract above the surgical site. A semen sample should be sent to be evaluated for the absence of sperm before the procedure is considered successful. Sperm continue to be produced in the testicles but are absorbed by the body.

Vasectomy Reversal

Sometimes a man may decide he wants to have more children and asks to have a vasectomy reversed. The surgical procedure to reverse a vasectomy is called a vasovasostomy. Using microscopic instruments, the surgeon reconnects the vas deferens. If this is not possible, the surgeon may reconnect the vas deferens to the epididymis. During the surgery the physician

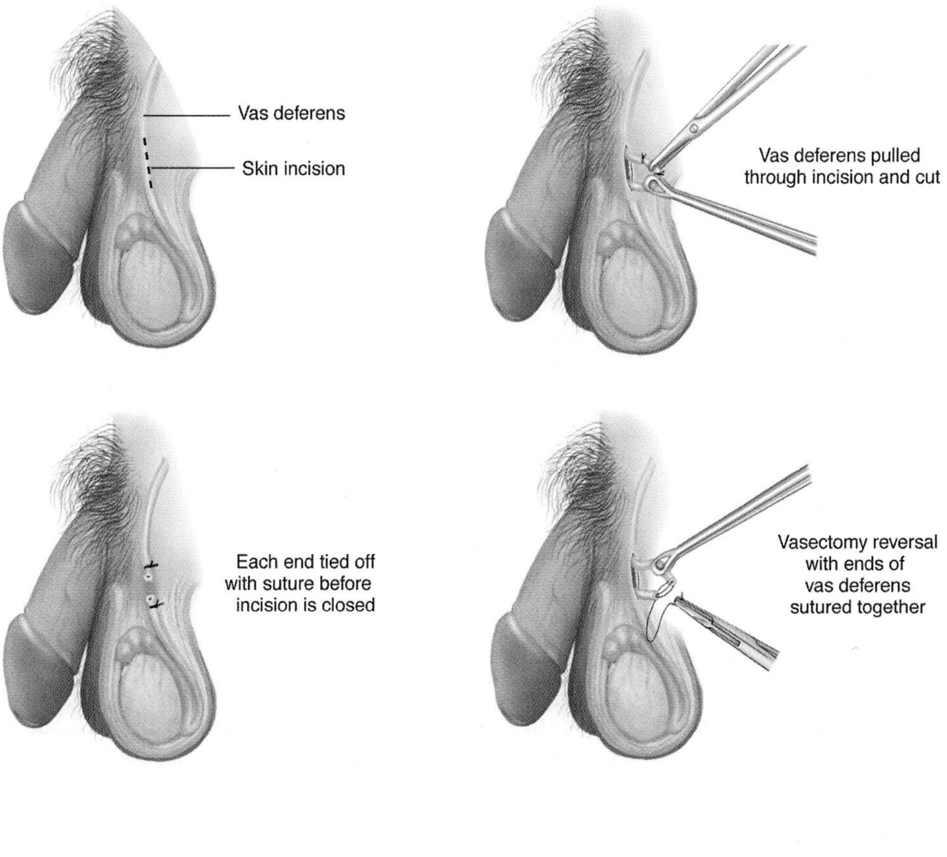
Vas deferens
Skin incision
Vas deferens pulled through incision and cut
Each end tied off with suture before incision is closed
Vasectomy reversal with ends of vas deferens sutured together

FIGURE 43.4 Vasectomy and reversal.

typically tries to determine whether the testicles are still producing good sperm. Vasectomy reversal is more successful if it is done soon after the vasectomy. Success rates drop as the period of time between vasectomy and reversal grows longer.

Erectile Dysfunction

A problem getting or keeping an erection can happen at any age and has been a concern of men and their partners for centuries. It is a unique problem because it affects not only the man but his partner as well. Most men experience a temporary erection problem at some time during their lives. It is often caused by stress, illness, fatigue, or an excessive use of alcohol or drugs. When the problem becomes persistent, it is time to seek medical help.

Before the 1980s, 90% of men who went to their physicians for help were told the problem was emotional, not physical. As a result of improved testing methods, however, researchers now believe that 80% to 90% of erection problems have a physical cause.

Pathophysiology

The term *impotence* means powerlessness. This term is being replaced with the more accurate term **erectile dysfunction** (ED), which describes a physical condition. Erectile dysfunction means that a man cannot obtain or keep a usable erection that is firm enough and long-lasting enough for satisfactory sexual intercourse. For a man to have a usable erection, several conditions must be met:

1. *Circulatory system.* The blood supply coming into the penis from the arteries must be sufficient to fill the corpus cavernosa (spongy erectile tissue inside the penis), causing the penis to become rigid. The veins in the penis must then be able to constrict to trap the blood in the corporal bodies to keep the penis erect. The most common cause of erectile dysfunction is failure in the circulatory system.
2. *Nervous system.* Both the sympathetic and parasympathetic nerves are involved in the erection, ejaculation, orgasm, and resting phases of the penile response cycle. There are many nerve receptors and transmitters in the spinal cord and the penis that must be intact for a usable erection. Spinal cord injury is the most common neurologic cause of erectile dysfunction.
3. *Hormonal system.* There are three basic male hormones involved with an erection. The most important hormone, testosterone, affects a man's sex drive and desire. Luteinizing hormone stimulates testosterone production, and prolactin in large amounts may block testosterone.
4. *Limbic system.* This is the center in the brain that affects how we feel emotionally. It works with our five senses to stimulate the desire for sex.

All of these systems can be influenced by physical, emotional, and chemical factors. A good assessment is important to determine the cause of erectile dysfunction.

Etiology

Erectile dysfunction has many psychological and physical causes. It can also be caused by many medications and chemicals that interfere with desire, blood supply, or nerve transmission (Table 43.3). The most common types of medications that cause problems are those prescribed for high blood pressure and cardiovascular disease.

Diagnostic Tests

In the first step of the assessment process, the health care provider obtains a history, including medical-surgical history; use of medications, including any substance abuse; lifestyle patterns; and sexual history. During physical examination, the provider looks for evidence of genital disorders, hormonal imbalance (such as hair patterns or enlarged breasts), surgical interventions, decreased circulation, and lack of nerve sensation. Blood tests evaluate glucose levels; testosterone; evidence of liver, heart, or kidney disorders; signs of infection; or blood disorders. Some physicians may use intracorporeal injection of vasoactive medications that can create an erection to test the blood flow in the penis.

TABLE 43.3 CAUSES OF ERECTILE DYSFUNCTION

Psychological	Stress Anxiety Depression Fatigue
Urological	Peyronie's disease Kidney failure Treatment for prostate disease
Endocrine	Low testosterone levels Diabetes mellitus
Cardiovascular	Heart disease Atherosclerosis Metabolic syndrome Stroke
Neurologic	Spinal cord injury Parkinson's disease Multiple sclerosis
Lifestyle	Tobacco use Alcohol use Drug use (marijuana, cocaine, others) Excessive caffeine use
Medications*	Antianxiety agents Antidepressants Antihistamines Antineoplastic agents Angiotensin-converting enzyme inhibitors Beta blockers Diuretics Estrogens Histamine (H_2) antagonists Muscle relaxants Nonsteroidal anti-inflammatory drugs Opioids Drugs for Parkinson's disease

* *Note:* Not all drugs in a category cause erectile dysfunction.

A psychosocial evaluation may be recommended to rule out any relational or emotional problems that may contribute to erectile dysfunction or affect the treatment outcome.

A second level of testing may involve the use of sophisticated vascular flow studies to locate areas where either the blood vessels are narrowed or the veins allow the blood to drain out of the penis too rapidly. Another area of testing may monitor erections during sleep. A healthy man typically has erections every 60 to 70 minutes while he sleeps. Absence of erections during sleep indicates a physical cause for erectile dysfunction. Because of the expense of vascular flow studies and sleep studies, they are used on a limited basis.

Therapeutic Measures

One of the most important treatment options begins with the couple being able to share intimate communication. No matter what is causing the problem, if the patient and his partner are not touching, talking, and sharing feelings with one another, treatment options are going to have limited success.

When the problem has clearly been identified as psychological, counseling therapy is the treatment of choice. If long-term therapy has been tried with only limited success, the addition of oral medication or even intracorporeal injection therapy may be added to provide a boost in confidence and self-esteem. Medical treatment for physical erection problems begins with conservative, nonsurgical treatment and then progresses to surgical options if needed. See Table 43.1 for additional information on medications.

MEDICATION CHANGES. Sometimes all that is needed to correct the problem is a change in medication. It is important for the patient to talk with the health care provider before stopping any medication. Some men have stopped taking their blood pressure medication and risked a stroke or heart attack because it interfered with their sexual activity.

ORAL MEDICATIONS. Oral medications (sildenafil [Viagra], tadalafil [Cialis], and vardenafil [Levitra]) are now the first line of therapy used to treat erectile dysfunction. These medications cause the arterioles and cavernous tissue to relax, allowing more blood to flow into the penis in response to sexual stimulation. The pill is usually taken 30 to 60 minutes before anticipated sexual intercourse. Men using nitrate medication (antianginal agents) should avoid using the pills because of risk for severe low blood pressure.

HORMONE TREATMENT. If the testosterone level is low, replacement hormone may be needed. The health care provider should first examine the patient carefully for any evidence of prostate cancer because testosterone replacement can cause the cancer to grow and spread. Testosterone replacement can be given by IM injection, topical gel, or transdermal patch.

HERBAL REMEDIES. Several herbal remedies may be effective, including yohimbine, DHEA, ginseng, ginkgo, and others. Herbal remedies have side effects, just like prescription medications, and should not be taken without a physician's recommendation.

INJECTED MEDICATION. After careful evaluation, a patient or his partner may be taught how to inject a medication into the penis using a 26- or 27-gauge needle on a tuberculin syringe or a prefilled autoinjector. The injections are nearly painless and produce a natural erection in 10 to 15 minutes. The most serious side effect is priapism, which requires immediate reversal in a physician's office or emergency room.

TRANSURETHRAL SUPPOSITORY. To facilitate medication dispersion and absorption, a patient may choose to use a suppository. The patient is instructed to urinate before use of the suppository. A tiny pellet (microsuppository) is inserted into the urethra using a specialized single-dose applicator. The medication usually begins to work in 5 to 10 minutes, and the effects last for about 30 to 60 minutes.

OTHER NONSURGICAL TREATMENTS.

Sexual Devices and Techniques. A variety of mechanical sexual aids can be considered by patients who do not want or cannot afford expensive medical treatment. Men should be encouraged to talk with a health care provider or qualified sex therapist before trying these alternatives.

Suction devices are another nonsurgical treatment option. This is an external cylinder vacuum device that fits over the penis and draws the blood up into the corporeal bodies, causing an erection. A penile ring is then slipped onto the base of the penis. Once the cylinder is removed, sexual intercourse can begin. Special care must be taken to remove the penile ring within 15 to 20 minutes to prevent tissue damage.

SURGICAL TREATMENTS.

Penile Implants (Prostheses). Penile implants are a pair of solid or fluid-filled chambers that are surgically placed into the corporeal bodies in the penis to produce an erection. There are two basic types of implants—noninflatable and inflatable (Fig. 43.5).

Vascular Surgery If a younger man has an erection problem caused by poor blood flow into the penis or from blood leaking out of the penis, rapidly causing the loss of the erection, corrective surgery may be performed. A bypass graft may be done to increase blood flow into the penis or to go around a blockage (as occurs, for example, with Peyronie's disease).

Nursing Process for the Patient with Erectile Dysfunction

DATA COLLECTION. Your role as a nurse may vary based on your work setting. It is always appropriate to ask a man if he has any concerns related to sexual health. It may open the door for him to talk further. It is important to provide privacy and ensure confidentiality. Ask history questions about possible psychosocial causes, including use of medications, street drugs, alcohol, or nicotine. If a problem is identified, alert the health care provider, who will continue a more thorough assessment.

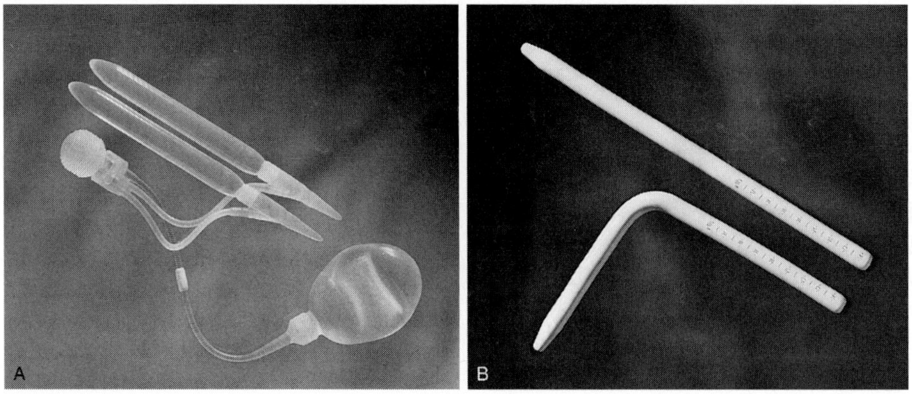
A
B

FIGURE 43.5 Penile implants. (A) Inflatable penile implant. Inflatable cylinders are implanted in the penis, the small hydraulic pump in the scrotum, and the fluid-filled reservoir in the lower abdomen. Sterile radiopaque saline from the reservoir fills the cylinders to provide an erection. (B) Malleable penile implant. Malleable rods are implanted into the penis. The penis is always firm, but the rods can be bent close to the body when erection is not desired. (Alpha-1 implant [A] and Acu-Form implant [B] photographs courtesy Mentor Urology, Santa Barbara, CA.)

NURSING DIAGNOSES, PLANNING, AND IMPLEMENTATION

Ineffective Self Health Management Related to Knowledge Deficit of Cause and Treatment of Sexual Dysfunction

EXPECTED OUTCOME: The patient will verbalize understanding of the cause and treatment options for erectile dysfunction.

- Determine patient and partner's current knowledge and understanding about cause and treatment of the disorder. *This will allow for additional and/or correct information to be provided about sexual dysfunction for appropriate understanding.*
- Provide patient and partner with additional and/or correct information about cause and treatment of disorder. *This will allow the patient to have a full understanding of the etiology and care related to the disorder, and increase likelihood of patient compliance and success of treatment.*
- Refer patient and partner (as appropriate) for medical treatment, psychological treatment, or counseling. *An individualized treatment plan (determined by the etiology) is needed to move toward restoration of sexual functioning.*

EVALUATION. The best indicator of a positive outcome is restoration of erectile function with a verbal account of understanding the disorder and satisfaction with the treatment process. Sometimes the physical problem is easier to correct than the emotional scars that the problem has created. It is important to evaluate both the physiological and emotional outcomes of treatment.

PATIENT EDUCATION. The nurse plays an important role in public education related to erectile dysfunction. Men need to know that they are not alone with their problem. More than 30 million men in the United States experience ongoing problems with erections. Usually, the cause is physical, and help is available through health care providers who specialize in treating erectile dysfunction.

See Table 43.4 for a summary of male sexual dysfunction.

TABLE 43.4 MALE SEXUAL DYSFUNCTION SUMMARY

Signs and Symptoms	Report of problems with obtaining and keeping an erection Reported dissatisfaction with sexual performance
Diagnostic Tests	Primary: History and physical Secondary: Vascular flow evaluation, sleep studies
Therapeutic Measures	Counseling Medication to increase blood flow to the penis Surgical implants or repair of structural disorders
Priority Nursing Diagnosis	*Ineffective Self-Health Management* related to knowledge deficit about cause and treatment of sexual dysfunction

CRITICAL THINKING

Mr. Kittle

■ Mr. Kittle presents to the clinic saying that he is not able to sustain an erection long enough for sexual intercourse that is satisfactory for himself and his partner.

1. You have never had a patient tell you his sexual problems, and you feel a little uncomfortable. How should you respond?
2. What will your assessment include?
3. What treatment options might be offered?

Suggested answers at end of chapter.

Infertility

A growing number of couples in the United States are having difficulty conceiving children. Several factors can interfere with a man's ability to father a child.

Physiology

A number of conditions must be present in the man for conception to occur. Endocrine function, autonomic nervous system function, and male reproductive structures must all be functioning properly. Normal healthy sperm in a concentration of at least 20 million per milliliter of semen are needed.

Etiology

The factors related to infertility are divided into three general categories: pretesticular, testicular, and post-testicular.

PRETESTICULAR (ENDOCRINE) FACTORS. The first factor involves the proper functioning of the hypothalamus, the pituitary gland, and the testicles. These endocrine functions are complex and are a rare cause of infertility. Examples of endocrine causes might be pituitary or adrenal tumors, thyroid problems, or uncontrolled diabetes.

TESTICULAR FACTORS. The two most common causes of male infertility are varicoceles (40% to 50%) and idiopathic causes (40%). It is believed that a varicocele lowers the sperm count by raising the blood flow and temperature in the testicles. Sperm cannot live if the temperature is too high or too low.

Congenital anomalies such as Klinefelter's syndrome (a chromosomal defect) or cryptorchidism result in absent or damaged testicles. Certain disease or inflammatory processes may cause damage to the storage area (epididymitis) or to the testicles themselves (mumps orchitis). Any high fever or viral infection can interfere with the production of sperm for up to 3 months.

Medications, radiation, substance abuse, environmental hazards, and lifestyle practices have all been identified as possible factors that can interfere with spermatogenesis (sperm production). Excessive use of hot tubs and saunas, wearing tight jeans, and long-haul truck driving have all been identified as raising the temperature level in the scrotum to the extent that sperm production is decreased.

POST-TESTICULAR FACTORS. The most common factor in post-testicular infertility is the result of surgery or injury along the pathway from the testicles to the outside of the man's body. Examples of surgical causes are vasectomy, bladder neck reconstruction, pelvic lymph node removal, or any surgery that causes retrograde ejaculation. Congenital anomalies and various types of infections may also cause infertility problems.

Prevention

Prevention involves possible lifestyle changes to avoid excessive heat to the scrotum, substance abuse, exposure to toxins, and environmental hazards. Problems related to medication or infections should be discussed with the health care provider.

Signs and Symptoms

A couple is considered infertile if they have been unsuccessful at becoming pregnant after at least 1 year of unprotected intercourse. If pregnancy has occurred during the year but there was no delivery, the problem usually is considered a female rather than a male factor.

Diagnosis

Diagnosis begins with a detailed history and physical examination that looks for known male causes of infertility.

HISTORY. Initial assessment includes frequency of intercourse, timing (according to ovulation cycle), use of contraceptives, problems with premature ejaculation, and erection problems. Use of hot tubs or saunas; tight jeans; use of nicotine, caffeine, alcohol, or marijuana; and the desire for children on the part of the man are all assessed. High stress, long periods of sitting, and exposure to environmental toxins are determined. The patient also may be questioned about STDs, endocrine problems, congenital urinary problems, serious illnesses or groin injuries, cancer, and treatment with chemotherapy or radiation.

PHYSICAL EXAMINATION. The examiner (usually a primary care practitioner) will observe for normal hair pattern and growth, muscle development, size of testicles, and any evidence of a varicocele or hydrocele.

DIAGNOSTIC TESTS. Analysis is done on several semen specimens to see if they contain the right amount and type of healthy sperm needed for a pregnancy. Infection should be ruled out. Several other tests may be done, including hormone tests, genetic testing, ultrasound, and others, depending on the level of desire and the financial resources of the couple. Many insurance companies do not pay for testing or treatment for infertility.

Therapeutic Measures

Treatment may be as simple as making a change in sexual or lifestyle practices. Surgery to correct a varicocele or obstruction may be done. If the couple is able to handle the emotional and financial strain, they may try a variety of in vitro fertilization (IVF) procedures. IVF is very costly, and success rates vary. Another option that may be presented to the couple is adoption.

You can play an important role in the emotional support a couple needs during infertility studies. It is important that the couple feel comfortable in communicating their feelings and frustrations with one another and their health care provider. You may need to be the communication link, explaining various tests and related costs. It also may help them to talk with other couples or attend a support group designed for couples experiencing infertility. For more information, visit www.nlm.nih.gov/medlineplus/infertility.html.

SUGGESTED ANSWERS TO CRITICAL THINKING

■ *Mr. Atkinson*

1.

$$\frac{5\text{ mg} \mid 1\text{ tablet}}{\mid 2\text{ mg}} = 2.5\text{ tablets}$$

Mr. Atkinson should be alert for signs of hypotension, such as dizziness or light-headedness on arising. He should not drive until effects and side effects of the medication are known.

2. Mr. Atkinson should be instructed not to lift anything heavier than 10 lb for the first 6 weeks, and he will not be able to plow or drive for the first 6 weeks. It is important that his son understand his father's limitations and how important it is for him or someone else to help out with the farm chores.
3. Mr. Atkinson will notice a change in his ejaculation (either very little ejaculate or none at all). If he could have an erection before surgery, the chances are very good that he will continue to be able to have intercourse; however, he will not ejaculate.

■ *Mr. Cunningham*

1. Mr. Cunningham should be encouraged to see his health care provider immediately for an evaluation to rule out testicular cancer.
2. Depending on the stage of the cancer, he will have the cancerous testicle, cord, and lymph nodes removed. He may need chemotherapy or radiation treatments as well.
3. Mr. Cunningham should be encouraged to make deposits at a certified sperm bank before any treatments. It is also important to include his future wife and his family in the decision-making process and encourage them to share their feelings and concerns with one another. Cancer support groups may also be helpful to Mr. Cunningham.

■ *Mr. Kittle*

1. It is okay to "pretend" here! Act like you are perfectly comfortable, and that you hear this sort of thing every day. (Of course, you would never pretend to know something you don't—it is always okay to say you don't know.) Have a matter-of-fact communication style. If you get nervous and forget what questions you should ask, start with something general like "Can you tell me more about your symptoms?"
2. Begin a psychosocial assessment to identify presence of stress, fear, depression, fatigue or problems with interpersonal relationships; also ask about medication, alcohol, and nicotine use. Assure him you will alert the health care provider to follow up with further assessment.
3. While oral medications such as sildenafil (Viagra) are the most common treatment, other options will depend on the cause. A complete workup and recommendations will be carried out by the physician or other health care provider.

REVIEW QUESTIONS

1. A patient with benign prostatic hyperplasia expresses concern that he has cancer. Which response by the nurse is best?
   a. "Don't worry; prostatic hyperplasia is not the same thing as cancer."
   b. "Since it is called benign, you don't have to worry about it. No treatment should be necessary; you will just need to have it watched."
   c. "Hyperplasia means your prostate is growing too many cells. They are not cancerous, but they could interfere with your ability to urinate, so it is important to have it treated."
   d. "You are correct, it is a form of cancer, but it is very slow growing and very treatable. Your doctor will recommend treatments for you."
2. Which of the following is the most commonly used surgical treatment for BPH?
   a. TUIP
   b. TUMA
   c. TURP
   d. TULIP
3. A patient who is 1 day post–transurethral resection of the prostate says he is having pain in his bladder, and the nurse notices urine leakage around his catheter. Which of the following responses by the nurse is best?
   a. "Bladder spasms are common after your surgery. Take some deep breaths while I get a B&O suppository."
   b. "You should not be experiencing spasms. I will notify the RN right away."
   c. "Spasms can be very painful. Would you like an injection of Demerol?"
   d. "Your catheter is leaking; we will need to replace it right away."

REVIEW QUESTIONS

4. A nurse working in a nursing home notes that it is difficult but not impossible to retract the foreskin for washing on an older gentleman. Which action is correct?
   a. Avoid retracting the foreskin for cleaning to prevent paraphimosis. The penis secretes an antibacterial substance that is self-cleaning.
   b. Gently retract the foreskin for cleaning, then replace it and notify the physician.
   c. Retract the foreskin for cleaning, and leave it retracted to prevent infection.
   d. Retract the foreskin and leave it retracted until the physician can evaluate it.

5. Which of the following is the most common cause of erectile dysfunction?
   a. Endocrine problems
   b. Circulatory problems
   c. Nervous system problems
   d. Excessive alcohol use

6. A patient is admitted to a medical unit for complications of diabetes. The nurse asks if he is satisfied with his level of sexual functioning, and he becomes tearful. Which initial response by the nurse is best?
   a. "You seem upset with my question. Are you having a problem you would like to talk about?"
   b. "Impotence is common with diabetes. Don't let it worry you."
   c. "What kind of sexual dysfunction are you experiencing?"
   d. "I am sorry you are having problems with your sexual functioning. Would you like a referral to a sex therapist?"

7. What are common complications of varicocele? **Select all that apply.**
   a. Infertility
   b. Infection
   c. Erectile dysfunction
   d. Pain
   e. Priapism
   f. Cancer

8. Which of the following should the nurse anticipate teaching about when caring for a man with infertility?
   a. Penile implants
   b. Prostatectomy
   c. TURP
   d. Decrease in nicotine and alcohol use

References

American Cancer Society (2009). *Cancer incidence and mortality rates by site, race, and ethnicity, US, 2001–2005.* Retrieved November 20, 2009, from http://www.cancer.org/docroot/MED/content/downloads/MED_1_1x_CFF2009_Incidence_Mortality_Site_Race_Ethn.asp

McNaughton-Collins, M., Joyce, G. F., Wise, M., & Pontari, M. A. (2007). Prostatitis. *In* M. S. Litwin & C. S. Saigal (Eds.). *Urologic diseases in America* (NIH Publication No. 07–5512, p. 11). U.S. Department of Health and Human Services, Public Health Service, National Institutes of Health, National Institute of Diabetes and Digestive and Kidney Diseases. Washington, DC: U.S. Government Publishing Office.

44

Nursing Care of Patients with Sexually Transmitted Diseases

LAURA L. McCULLY
AND DEBRA PERRY-PHILO

KEY TERMS

cervicitis (SIR-vih-SY-tiss)
chancre (SHANK-er)
condylomata acuminata (KON-dih-LOH-mah-tah ah-KYOOM-in-AH-tah)
condylomatous (KON-dih-LOH-mah-tus)
conjunctivitis (kon-JUNK-tih-VY-tis)
cytotoxic (SY-toh-TOK-sick)
electrocautery (ee-LEK-troh-CAW-tur-ee)
electrocoagulated (ee-LEK-troh-coh-AG-yoo-LAY-ted)
endometritis (EN-doh-meh-TRY-tiss)
epidemiological (EP-ih-DEE-mee-ah-LAH-jih-kuhl)
gummas (GUH-mahs)
hepatosplenomegaly (heh-PAT-oh-SPLEH-noh-MEG-ah-lee)
herpetic (her-PET-ick)
lymphadenopathy (lim-FAHD-deh-NAW-puh-thee)
mucopurulent cervicitis (MYOO-koh-PYOOR-uh-lent SIR-vih-SY-tiss)
ophthalmia neonatorum (off-THAL-mee-ah NEE-oh-nuh-TOR-uhm)
proctitis (prok-TY-tiss)
puerperal (pyoo-UR-pur-uhl)
sacral radiculopathy (SAY-krul ra-DIK-yoo-LAW-puh-thee)
salpingitis (SAL-pin-JY-tiss)
serological (SEAR-uh-LAW-jih-kuhl)
urethritis (YOO-reh-THRY-tiss)
verrucous (veh-ROO-kuss)
vesicular (veh-SIK-yoo-lur)
vulvovaginitis (VUL-voh-VAJ-ih-NY-tiss)

QUESTIONS TO GUIDE YOUR READING

1. What pathogens are involved with each of the common sexually transmitted diseases (STDs)?
2. What are the signs and symptoms of each of the common STDs?
3. What teaching can you provide to promote prevention of STDs?
4. What are the current treatment options for common STDs?
5. What nursing care will you provide for patients with STDs?
6. How will you know if your nursing interventions have been effective?

Sexually transmitted diseases (STDs) are infections that can be transmitted through intimate contact with the genitals, mouth, or rectum of another individual. Some STDs can also be spread by other routes such as blood or body fluids. A nurse's best protection against catching diseases from blood and body fluids of infected patients is the strict practice of standard precautions and maintaining his or her own healthy, intact skin.

Physically, STDs can cause tremendous suffering through pain, scarring of genitourinary structures, damage to other body organs, infertility, birth defects, nervous system damage, development of cancer, and even death of infected patients and sometimes their children. Psychologically and socially, these diseases also have profound effects on individuals, families, and relationships. Guilt about passing on an incurable disease to a loved one or feelings of betrayal because of being infected as a result of someone else's choices are some of the emotional consequences of STDs.

Changing social values have been associated with increasing incidence of almost all types of sexually transmitted diseases, including some previously rare diseases related to anal intercourse. Coexistence of more than one STD in an individual is also occurring more often. Many diseases and syndromes are associated with sexually transmitted diseases; the more common ones are discussed here. Human immunodeficiency virus (HIV) and acquired immunodeficiency syndrome (AIDS) are discussed separately in Chapter 20.

Symptoms, diagnostic techniques, and treatment regimens vary for different geographical areas, depending on availability of equipment for diagnosis and health care provider preferences. As an introduction for practical/vocational nurses, general overviews are presented in this chapter.

One of the most important ways you can help those who experience STDs is by being kind, nonjudgmental, and sensitive to the patient's communication. Maintaining an open posture and eye contact that is appropriate for the patient's culture relays a sense of openness and willingness to talk and preserves the possibility of continuing health promotion with these individuals in the future.

DISORDERS AND SYNDROMES RELATED TO SEXUALLY TRANSMITTED DISEASES

Vulvovaginitis

Vulvovaginitis is an inflammation of the vulva and vagina and can be asymptomatic or involve redness, itching, burning, excoriation, pain, swelling of the vagina and labia, and discharge. A variety of sexually and nonsexually transmitted infectious agents can cause vulvovaginitis. The odor, consistency, and color of the discharge vary with the different microbes involved. Nonsexually transmitted vaginitis, vulvovaginitis, and vaginosis are described in Chapter 42. Some microorganisms may be acquired either by sexual or nonsexual routes, so they are also mentioned in this chapter. Bartholin's glands can develop abscesses as a result of infection with nonsexually transmitted microbes or STDs such as gonorrhea and chlamydia.

• WORD • BUILDING •
vulvovaginitis: vulvo—vulva + vagin—vagina + itis—inflammation

> **SAFETY TIP**
> Observe standard precautions and careful hand washing to avoid contact with infectious organisms. Go to www.cdc.gov and type in "hand hygiene" for complete guidelines.

Urethritis

Both STDs and nonsexually transmitted microorganisms can cause **urethritis** in men and women. In men, inflammation of the urethra, prostate, and epididymis can result in difficult, painful, and frequent urination and a urethral discharge, which may be clear, cloudy, or yellow. Female partners of men with urethritis may also suffer from urethritis, and they may also develop **mucopurulent cervicitis** (MPC) and a variety of other symptoms of the particular infection. Some causative agents for urethritis include *Neisseria gonorrhoeae, Chlamydia trachomatis, Ureaplasma urealyticum, Trichomonas vaginalis, Candida albicans,* and herpes simplex. Often this disease category is divided into gonococcal urethritis caused by *N. gonorrhoeae* (GU) and nongonococcal urethritis (NGU).

Mucopurulent Cervicitis

MPC is an inflammation of the cervix that may produce a mucopurulent yellow exudate on the cervix or may have no noticeable symptoms. MPC during pregnancy can result in **conjunctivitis** and pneumonia in newborn infants, as well as **puerperal** infection of the mother. MPC can be caused by such organisms as *C. trachomatis*, *N. gonorrhoeae*, *T. vaginalis*, *C. albicans*, and herpes simplex. MPC may spread to become pelvic inflammatory disease (PID).

Proctitis and Enteritis

Proctitis is inflammation of the rectum and anus that may be due to either nonsexually transmitted microbes or to STDs. This is especially prevalent among those who practice both

• WORD • BUILDING •
urethritis: ureth—urethra + itis—inflammation
mucopurulent cervicitis: muco—involving mucus + purulent—involving pus + cervic—cervix + itis—inflammation
conjunctivitis: conjunctiv(a)—lining of the eyelids and sclera of the eye + itis—inflammation
puerperal: childbirth
proctitis: proc—anus + itis—inflammation

heterosexual and homosexual anal intercourse. Enteritis, which is inflammation of the lining of the intestine, may occur as a result of contamination during anal intercourse. Infection with *Campylobacter* species, *Shigella* species, and *Giardia lamblia* can be a problem for homosexual men. Care of patients who have gastrointestinal disorders is discussed in Unit 8.

Genital Ulcers

Genital ulcers are formed when papules or macules erode and leave often painful raw, pitted, or excoriated areas on or around the genitals. Not all genital ulcers are caused by STDs—injury, some non-STD viruses, some types of drug reactions, radiation, and some forms of cancer can also produce genital ulcers. STDs that can produce genital ulcers include syphilis, herpes, and HIV. Genital ulcers from one type of disease may increase the risk of infection with other STDs during sexual activity because the open areas present an easy portal of entry for the infecting organism.

Cellular Changes

Cellular changes can also be caused by STDs, including **condylomatous** (wart-like) growths and dysplasia or neoplasia, which may result in precancerous or cancerous conditions. Herpes viruses, HIV, and human papillomavirus (HPV) have all been linked to the development of cancer.

Pelvic Inflammatory Disease

Pathophysiology and Etiology

Pelvic inflammatory disease (PID) is an infection of the upper genital tract that can cause chronic pelvic pain due to inflammation. The primary sources of infection include *C. trachomatis* and *N. gonorrhoeae,* but it may result from any organism that is associated with a sexually transmitted infection. These organisms can invade the endocervical canal, resulting in **cervicitis**, and move upward resulting in infection of the endometrium (**endometritis**), fallopian tubes (**salpingitis**), and pelvic cavity. The chronic inflammation results in extensive scarring and adhesions, which can cause infertility and increase the risk of ectopic pregnancy. Increased risk for PID occurs with a history of multiple sexual partners, STDs, substance abuse, frequent vaginal douching, and intrauterine device (IUD) contraceptive use.

Signs and Symptoms

Some women with PID are asymptomatic or have minimal symptoms. Other women present with lower abdominal pain and tenderness, purulent vaginal discharge or vaginal bleeding, pain with sexual intercourse, fever, nausea and vomiting, and pain with urination. Findings during physical examination include adnexal tenderness upon palpation, and pain in the uterus and cervix when moved during a bimanual examination.

Diagnostic Tests

Laboratory tests may reveal positive culture of causative organism(s) and leukocytosis. Urinary tract infection may need to be ruled out.

Therapeutic Measures

With serious infection, hospitalization and intravenous antibiotics may be indicated. Intravenous therapy can be changed to oral therapy after 48 hours if status improves. Outpatient therapy with oral antibiotics is used with minor infections. Laparoscopic surgery may be done to release adhesions and reduce complications. Testing and treatment for other STDs should be considered for both the patient and her partner. Education on the cause of the infection and prevention of future episodes is essential.

• WORD • BUILDING •

condylomatous: condyl—rounded projection + oma(t)—growth + ous—like

cervicitis: cervic—cervix + itis—inflammation

endometritis: endo—inside + metr—womb + itis—inflammation

salpingitis: salping—tube + itis—inflammation

SEXUALLY TRANSMITTED INFECTIONS

Chlamydia

Etiology and Signs and Symptoms

Chlamydia is the most commonly diagnosed STD in the United States (see Table 44.1 for a summary of this and other common STDs). It can be transmitted sexually and by blood and body fluid contact. There are several different strains of the bacteria *C. trachomatis.* Chlamydia is often asymptomatic (a "silent" STD) in women, but it can cause urethritis, MPC, and conjunctivitis. Fitz-Hugh–Curtis syndrome, a surface inflammation of the liver, can also be caused by *C. trachomatis.* This inflammation can cause nausea, vomiting, and sharp pain at the base of the ribs that sometimes refers to the right shoulder and arm. Chlamydia is a frequent cause of pelvic inflammatory disease (PID) and infertility, and it increases the risk of ectopic pregnancy. The infection can be passed from mother to baby during birth, resulting in neonatal pneumonia and conjunctivitis. It also increases the risk of HIV infection.

Lymphogranuloma venereum (LGV) is also caused by some strains of *C. trachomatis* but is more commonly seen in tropical climates or among people who emigrated from tropical areas. This disease also causes urethritis and proctitis, and it inflames lymph nodes that drain the pelvic area, resulting in draining sores and fistula development. Scarring from this disease can complicate vaginal deliveries.

Diagnostic Tests

Several tests for chlamydia are available. Samples are gathered in a special collection tube to send to a laboratory for culture. Culturing is difficult and expensive and generally requires 2 to 6 days for results. A newer type of testing, called nucleic acid amplification testing (NAT or NAAT), identifies the presence of chlamydial DNA or RNA in urine, cervical, or urethral specimens. Because this disease is so common, it is wise to set out an unopened *Chlamydia* collection kit within easy reach of the health care provider for each pelvic examination.

TABLE 44.1 COMMON SEXUALLY TRANSMITTED DISEASES SUMMARY

	Chlamydia	Gonorrhea	Syphilis	Trichomoniasis	Herpes Simplex	Condylomata (HPV)
Signs and Symptoms	Conjunctivitis; in men, urethritis, epididymitis, prostatitis; in women, MPC, urethritis	In men, urethritis, penile discharge, epididymitis, prostatitis; in women, MPC, urethritis, abnormal menses	Primary syphilis, chancre; secondary syphilis, flu-like symptoms, rashes, condylomatous growths	Genital redness, swelling, itching, burning, foul discharge; in men, urethritis, prostatitis; in women, "strawberry cervix"	Vesicles/ulcerations in mouth, genitals; flu-like symptoms, lymphadenopathy, urethritis, cystitis, MPC	Fleshy tumors, primarily on genitalia
Diagnostic Tests	NAT culture	NAT culture	VDRL, ELISA, RPR, FTA-ABS	Microscopic examination	Culture, Western blot	Colposcope examination biopsy, visualization of lesions
Therapeutic Measures	Antibiotics (see Table 44.1)	Antibiotics (see Table 44.12)	Penicillin	Metronidazole	Antiviral medication (see Table 44.2)	Wart removal, interferon therapy
Complications	Fitz-Hugh–Curtis syndrome, increased susceptibility to HIV infection; PID, infertility, transmission to baby at birth; co-infection with gonorrhea	PID, disseminated gonococcal infection, Fitz-Hugh–Curtis syndrome, transmission to baby at birth, co-infection with chlamydia	Tertiary syphilis, gumma damage to heart, circulatory system, nervous system; transmission to fetus during pregnancy	Preterm delivery, infertility, increased risk of HIV transmission	Lifelong infection, disseminated infection, nervous system invasion, increased risk of cervical cancer, transmission to baby at birth	Cancers of the reproductive organs and anus, including cervical cancer; transmission to fetus during pregnancy

ELISA = enzyme-linked immunosorbent assay; FTA-ABS fluorescent treponemal antibody absorption; HPV = human papillomavirus; MPC = mucopurulent cervicitis; NAT = nucleic acid amplification testing; PID = pelvic inflammatory disease; RPR = rapid plasmin reagin; VDRL = Venereal Disease Research Laboratory.

Therapeutic Measures

Antibiotics are typically given to treat chlamydia in adults (Table 44.2). Erythromycin or azithromycin is used during pregnancy, because other antibiotics may pose a risk to the fetus. Use of an ophthalmic ointment or solution containing silver nitrate, erythromycin, or tetracycline is recommended as treatment of the neonate shortly after birth for the prevention of conjunctivitis. This is done regardless of whether or not the mother is diagnosed with chlamydia, because asymptomatic or undiagnosed chlamydia is common, and this simple treatment can prevent serious complications later. Institutional policies and state regulations determine the type of eye preparation to be used and whether administration of the medications requires specific consent of the parents.

Gonorrhea

Etiology and Signs and Symptoms

According to the Centers for Disease Control and Prevention (CDC, 2007), 355,991 new cases of gonorrhea were reported to the CDC in 2007 (the most recently available statistics). It is caused by the bacterium *N. gonorrhoeae* and may be transmitted vaginally, rectally, orally, or via contact with other mucous membranes, or through contact with blood and body fluids. It can produce a variety of signs and symptoms. Men may be asymptomatic or may have urethritis with a yellow urethral discharge. Women who have gonorrhea may have either no noticeable symptoms or have a sore throat, MPC, urethritis, or abnormal menstrual symptoms such as bleeding between periods. Many cases of PID are caused by gonorrhea. Intercourse with an infected partner during menstruation may be especially risky for development of PID because removal of the cervical mucous barrier can promote the growth of the gonococcus in the higher reproductive tract. Gonorrhea can also cause Fitz-Hugh–Curtis syndrome. Fever, nausea, vomiting, and lower abdominal pain may be present. Gonorrhea may also infect the throat and the rectum and may cause disseminated gonococcal infection, resulting in inflammation of the joints, skin, meninges, and lining of the heart.

TABLE 44.2 MEDICATIONS USED TO TREAT SEXUALLY TRANSMITTED DISEASES

Medication Class	Examples/Action	Route	Side Effects	Nursing Implications
Chlamydia				
Antibiotics	*Macrolides:* erythromycin azithromycin *Inhibit bacterial protein synthesis.*	PO, IV	Abdominal pain, cramping, GI upset, rash, overgrowth of nonsusceptible bacteria	Administer on empty stomach. Do not administer with antacids. Use caution with hepatic disorders.
	Tetracyclines: doxycycline *Inhibits protein synthesis by binding to ribosomes.* amoxicillin *Binds to bacterial cell wall, causing cell death.*	PO, IV	GI upset, anorexia, dysphagia, photosensitivity, rash, urticaria, increased pigmentation, may increase anticoagulation	Do not administer during pregnancy due to bone/teeth effects. Do not give with antacids or dairy products. Administer on empty stomach. Avoid unnecessary exposure to sunlight.
	Fluoroquinolones: ofloxacin levofloxacin *Inhibit cell wall synthesis.*	PO, IV	GI upset, dizziness, headache, CNS disturbances, flatulence, rash, photosensitivity *Rare but serious:* tendon rupture	Safety under age 18 not established. Do not administer with antacids. Use caution with other medications and with renal, hepatic, or CNS disorders.
Gonorrhea				
Antibiotics	*Cephalosporins:* ceftriaxone cefixime *Inhibit cell wall synthesis.*	PO, IM, IV	GI upset, CNS disturbance, rash, pruritus, elevated liver enzymes, pain at injection site	Use caution with penicillin allergies or renal or hepatic dysfunction. Avoid excess sun exposure.

TABLE 44.2 MEDICATIONS USED TO TREAT SEXUALLY TRANSMITTED DISEASES—cont'd

Medication Class	Examples/Action	Route	Side Effects	Nursing Implications
Syphilis				
Antibiotics	*Penicillin:* penicillin G *Inhibits cell wall synthesis.* *Tetracyclines:* tetracycline doxycycline *(see information above)*	PO, IM, IV (tetracycline not available IV)	GI upset, CNS disturbance, rash, itching, fever, chills, pain at injection site, allergy	Administer deep IM or slow IV. Apply ice packs to injection site as needed. Administer PO on empty stomach. Instruct patient to report fever/rash. Avoid tetracycline in children and pregnant women.
Trichomoniasis				
Amebicides/ antiprotozoals	metronidazole *Bind to DNA to inhibit synthesis and cause cell death.*	PO, IV	GI upset, anorexia, headache, metallic taste or dry mouth, dysuria *Rare but serious:* Seizures and peripheral neuropathy, ECG changes	Administer with food. Avoid alcohol; abstain for a minimum of 48 hr following treatment to prevent severe flu-like reaction. Treat partner as well as patient.
Herpes				
Antivirals	acyclovir valacyclovir famciclovir *Inhibit DNA synthesis.*	PO, IV, topical	GI upset, CNS disturbance, rash, urticaria, elevated liver enzyme/BUN levels	Use systemic preparations cautiously with CNS, hepatic, or renal disorders. Infuse IV slowly. Maintain hydration. Caution patient that viral transmission can still occur during treatment.
Genital Warts				
Antimitotics and acidic agents	Podophyllin/trichloroacetic acid (TCA)/ bichloracetic acid (BCA)	Topical application to wart(s)	Local pain, burning, inflammation, erosion, itching	Instruct patient to return for repeated applications as needed. Avoid medication contact with eyes or tissue surrounding lesion.
Antimitotic agent	podofilox solution (Condylox)	Topical solution	Local pain, burning, inflammation, erosion, itching	Can be applied by patient at home with cotton-tipped applicator. Instruct patient to apply to warts only and allow to dry completely, or as ordered by provider.
Antiviral/immune response modifier	imiquimod (Aldara)	Topical (cream)	Local irritation, pain, itching, burning, swelling	Can be applied by patient at home. Instruct patient to apply thin film to clean dry skin at bedtime, as ordered by provider. May take up to 16 weeks to completely clear warts.

CNS = central nervous system; GI = gastrointestinal.

Newborns born to mothers who have gonorrhea can develop **ophthalmia neonatorum**, which involves inflammation of the conjunctivae and deeper parts of the eye and can, ultimately, result in blindness. The newborn may also experience a gonorrheal infection at other sites following birth. Abscesses may develop where fetal scalp monitors were attached during labor, and infection of the nose, lungs, and rectum may occur.

Diagnostic Tests

Diagnosis is done by microscopic examination of smears and cultures of the discharge or identification of bacterial DNA (nucleic acid testing) in the urine. More than one test may be done to verify the diagnosis.

Therapeutic Measures

Development of antibiotic resistance by *N. gonorrhoeae* and co-infection with other microorganisms, such as *C. trachomatis,* is making treatment more complicated. Cephalosporin antibiotics are recommended for the treatment of gonorrhea (see Table 44.2). It is also recommended that the patient be treated for chlamydia because co-infection is common. Ophthalmia neonatorum may be prevented by use of antibiotic eye preparations that contain silver nitrate, erythromycin, or tetracycline. It is recommended, as with prophylactic treatment of chlamydial conjunctivitis, that all infants be treated shortly after birth regardless of diagnostic status of the mother. The treatment is simple, and may prevent a devastating outcome for the newborn. Institutional policies and state regulations determine the type of eye drops to be used and whether administration of the drops requires specific consent of the parents.

CRITICAL THINKING

Mrs. Miller

■ Mrs. Miller delivered an infant boy 1 hour ago. The nurse is currently applying erythromycin ointment to the infant's eyes bilaterally. Mrs. Miller asks if the medication is necessary.

1. How will you respond?
2. Should all infants receive prophylactic eye treatment at birth?

Suggested answers at end of chapter.

Syphilis

Pathophysiology, Etiology, and Signs and Symptoms

Syphilis is an ancient disease that has not disappeared, although it is overshadowed by more commonly occurring diseases such as chlamydia. It occurs in stages. The primary stage of syphilis begins with the entry of the *Treponema pallidum* spirochete through the skin or mucous membranes. Between 3 and 90 days later, a papule develops at the site of entry, then sloughs off, leaving a painless, red, ulcerated area called a **chancre** (Fig. 44.1). Chancres may also develop in other areas of the body at this time. Chancre formation typically is the only symptom of this stage of syphilis. The chancre eventually heals, but the spirochete remains active in the infected individual and can be passed on to others.

Secondary syphilis begins 2 to 8 weeks later and affects the body more generally, causing such problems as flu-like symptoms, joint pain, hair loss, skin rashes (primarily on the soles of the hands and feet), mouth sores, and condylomatous growths in moist areas of the body.

Serious damage can occur if syphilis is untreated in the early stages. About 15% of infected individuals will progress to the tertiary (or late) stage, up to 10 to 20 years later. At this stage, it can involve any organ system of the body. The spirochete may form **gummas**, which are tumors of a rubbery consistency that can break down and ulcerate, leaving holes in body tissues. The gummas can damage the heart, circulatory system, and nervous system (called neurosyphilis). Ulceration of gummas can destroy areas of vital tissue and lead to mental and physical disability or early death.

Syphilis can be passed on to the unborn children of women who carry the spirochete, resulting in **hepatosplenomegaly**, increase in bilirubin, destruction of red blood cells, birth defects (especially of the face), **lymphadenopathy**, and a baby who can transmit the spirochete

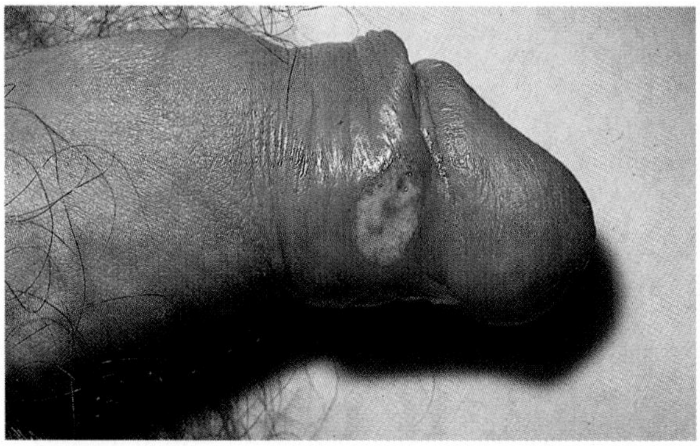

FIGURE 44.1 Syphilis chancre. (From Reeves, J. R. T., & Maibach, H. [1991]. *Clinical dermatology illustrated: A regional approach* [p. 88]. Philadelphia: F. A. Davis.)

• WORD • BUILDING •

ophthalmia neonatorum: ophthalmia—eye disease + neonatorum—of the newborn

• WORD • BUILDING •

chancre: hard ulceration

gummas: from the word meaning "rubber"—rubbery tumors

hepatosplenomegaly: hepato—liver + spleno—spleen + megaly—enlargement

lymphadenopathy: lymph—lymph nodes + adeno—node + pathy—disorder through nasal drainage. If left untreated, syphilis during pregnancy may cause lesions in various organs of the unborn baby and result in higher rates of spontaneous abortion, stillbirth, and premature birth.

Diagnostic Tests

Several tests for syphilis exist, and a combination may be used for accurate diagnosis. Cultures may be done but are difficult to grow. **Serological** (blood) tests include the Venereal Disease Research Laboratory (VDRL) test, the rapid plasma reagin (RPR) test, and the automated reagin test (ART). These tests indirectly check for syphilis by detecting the presence of antibodies that the body forms in response to treponema and, unfortunately, in response to some other disorders, so false-positive results can occur. Diagnosis of neurosyphilis is even more difficult because some testing of cerebrospinal fluid may result in false-negative results. Treponemal enzyme-linked immunosorbent assay (ELISA), fluorescent treponemal antibody absorption (FTA-ABS), and polymerase chain reaction (PCR) tests for treponemal DNA are some newer methods that reduce the risk of false results.

Therapeutic Measures

Penicillin G is the treatment of choice for patients diagnosed with syphilis (see Table 44.2). For those who are allergic to penicillin, doxycycline and tetracycline are treatment options. When HIV and syphilis are diagnosed in the same individual, symptoms of neurosyphilis are more likely to occur.

Trichomoniasis

Pathophysiology and Etiology

Trichomoniasis is generally a sexually transmitted disease, but it may be transmitted through nonsexual contact with infected articles because it can survive for a long time outside the body. Carriers of *Trichomonas vaginalis* may be asymptomatic for several years until changes in vaginal or urethral conditions encourage an outbreak of the disease. A decrease in resident bacteria, injuries to the vaginal tissues, and development of lesions from other STDs or from some forms of cancer can activate the organism.

Signs and Symptoms

Symptoms include redness, swelling, itching, and burning of the genital area; pain with intercourse and voiding; and a frothy, foul-smelling discharge. Men with trichomonal infection can develop prostatitis and infertility. Men who are also infected with HIV are more likely to transmit HIV to others, and women with *Trichomonas vaginalis* are more susceptible to HIV infection if exposed. Women who are pregnant risk preterm delivery and low birth weight babies.

• WORD • BUILDING •

serological: sero—blood + logical—science

Diagnostic Tests

Visualization of the cervix during pelvic examination shows a characteristic "strawberry cervix." When wet-mount slides of the discharge are viewed under a microscope, the organisms can be identified by their motility and whip-like flagella. Trichomoniasis may produce abnormal Papanicolaou (Pap) smear readings, which require that more frequent Pap smears be done to provide adequate surveillance of cellular changes.

Therapeutic Measures

The drug treatment of choice is metronidazole (see Table 44.2). Some strains of *Trichomonas* may exhibit resistance to this medication, but generally succumb to high doses of the drug. Because some people carry the organism without symptoms, sexual partners should also be treated regardless of symptoms.

CRITICAL THINKING

Kerri

■ Kerri presents to the health clinic with a report of generalized redness, swelling, itching, and burning of her external genitalia. Following history, physical, and microscopic examination, trichomoniasis is diagnosed. Kerri is upset, stating she has been in a monogamous relationship for 2 years.

1. What should your response to Kerri include?
2. Kerri is placed on metronidazole (Flagyl), but you are not comfortable with the dose prescribed, so you look it up. You find that she should receive 7.5 mg/kg every 6 hours. Kerri weighs 140 pounds. What should her dose be every 6 hours?
3. What teaching should you provide for Kerri?

Suggested answers at end of chapter.

Herpes

Pathophysiology, Etiology, and Signs and Symptoms

Herpes infection is caused by the herpes simplex virus types 1 and 2 (HSV-1 and HSV-2). Herpes viruses have an affinity for tissues of the skin and nervous system and can lie dormant in nervous system tissues and then reactivate periodically when the body undergoes stress, fever, or immune system compromise. Both HSV-1 and HSV-2 can cause "fever blisters" of the mouth (Fig. 44.2), as well as genital lesions. However, HSV-1 is more frequently associated with oral lesions and HSV-2 with genital lesions.

Genital HSV-2 outbreaks are more severe than genital HSV-1 outbreaks. After infection, vesicles develop, spontaneously rupture, and produce painful ulceration of the underlying skin tissues. Asymptomatic latent periods are generally

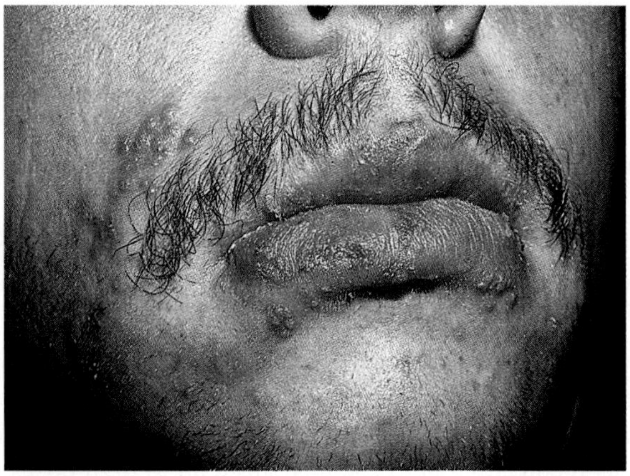

FIGURE 44.2 Herpes simplex. (From Reeves, J. R. T., & Maibach, H. [1991]. *Clinical dermatology illustrated: A regional approach* [p. 64]. Philadelphia: F. A. Davis.)

interspersed between the **vesicular** outbreaks. Although not as common, the virus may still be transmitted even during latent periods.

An initial outbreak following infection with the herpes virus occurs 2 days to 2 weeks after exposure and may produce a flu-like condition. Urethritis, cystitis, and MPC with vaginal discharge may also be evident. Infection of the spinal nerve roots by HSV may result in **sacral radiculopathy** (damage of the sacral spinal nerves), causing retention of urine and feces. Although rare, disseminated herpes infection can result in inflammation of the spinal cord, meninges, nerve pathways, and lymph nodes. Urethral strictures and increased risk for development of cervical cancer in women are also consequences of herpes.

It is estimated that one in five of all pregnant women carry herpes, although most of their babies do not develop **herpetic** disease. If infected, the baby's skin, eyes, mucous membranes, and nervous system may be involved and death from disseminated herpes infection is possible. The greatest risk of herpes transmission from mother to child during pregnancy occurs if the mother has an active genital lesion at the time of delivery. If an active genital lesion is present when a woman is close to the time of delivery, a cesarean section is likely to be performed. However, an active lesion at any time during pregnancy poses a risk for transmission.

Diagnostic Tests

Testing for HSV requires special viral collection kits for swabbed or scraped specimens from lesions. Follow the directions on the viral collection kit as well as institutional policies. Blood tests are improving; for example, the Western blot assay can determine whether the person has HSV-1 or HSV-2 antibodies.

Therapeutic Measures

There is currently no known cure for herpes infection, although antiviral medications may be given to decrease the severity of symptoms (see Table 44.2). Acyclovir treatment late in pregnancy reduces the frequency of cesarean sections among women who have recurrent genital herpes by diminishing the frequency of recurrences at term. See the *Nursing Care Plan for the Patient with Genital Herpes.*

Genital Warts

Signs and Symptoms

Condylomata acuminata (genital warts) is a common sexually transmitted viral disease, and its incidence is increasing rapidly. Infection with human papillomavirus (HPV) produces the condylomata—soft, raised, **verrucous** fleshy tumors, which may also have finger-like projections and resemble cauliflower (Fig. 44.3). Lesions most commonly develop on the external genitalia and perineum, as well as on the internal vaginal wall and cervix in women. However, lesions can also develop on other areas of the body after contact with the virus. Some people remain asymptomatic, but can still transmit the infection.

More than 100 types of HPV have been identified, and several have been closely linked to the development of cancers of the reproductive organs and anus in both males and females. The latent period from the time of exposure to development of the warts can be as long as 3 years.

HPV can be passed on from a pregnant woman to her fetus, resulting in the growth of genital warts on the baby, HPV infection of the baby's respiratory tract, and a possible future increased risk of cancer development. HPV infection

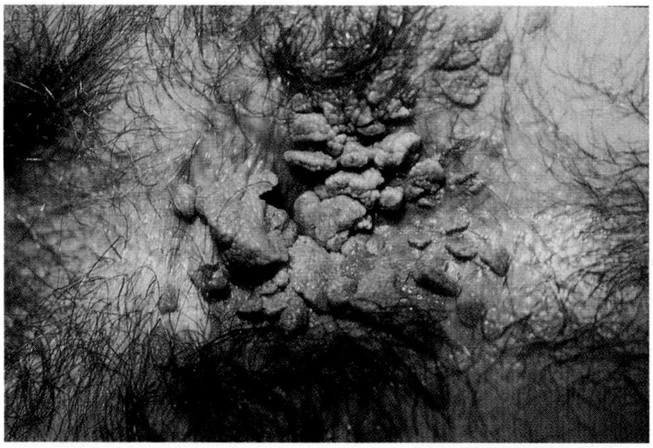

FIGURE 44.3 Condylomata, commonly known as genital warts. (From Lemone, P., & Burke, K. M. [1996]. *Medical-surgical nursing: Critical thinking in client care* [p. 2079]. Menlo Park, CA: Addison-Wesley, with permission.)

• WORD • BUILDING •

vesicular: vesicul—blister + ar—type

sacral radiculopathy: sacral—sacrum + radiculo—root + pathy—disorder or disease

herpetic: herpet—herpes + ic—pertaining to

• WORD • BUILDING •

condylomata acuminata: condyl—rounded projection + oma—growth + ta—pluralizes the word (singular form is condyloma) + acuminata—genital growths

verrucous: verruc—wart + ous—like

NURSING CARE PLAN for the Patient with Genital Herpes

Nursing Diagnosis: *Acute Pain* related to inflammation and skin lesions as evidenced by patient pain rating

Expected Outcomes: The patient will experience relief as evidenced by a decrease in pain rating to a level that is acceptable to patient; patient will rest and move well.

Evaluation of Outcomes: Does patient state relief of pain level is acceptable?

Interventions	Rationale	Evaluation
Assess pain using the WHAT'S UP? format.	Assessment of the characteristic of the pain assists the nurse in providing appropriate relief measures.	Can patient describe the pain characteristics?
Recommend pain relief measures appropriate to the type and location of the pain (both alternative measures, such as heat, ice, and change of position, and medication may be offered).	Not all types of pain respond well to the same treatment.	Does patient express satisfactory relief of pain? Does patient move and rest without evidence of pain?
Document results of pain relief measures.	Documentation alerts other caregivers about what works and does not work, thus providing more consistent, effective pain relief.	Have you gained sufficient information from patient to document results?
Instruct patient about self-care for pain and STD treatment at home.	Most STDs are treated at home.	Does patient verbalize understanding of self-care measures?

Nursing Diagnosis: *Risk for Infection*, transmission to others, related to lack of knowledge about transmission, symptoms, and treatment

Expected Outcomes: The patient will verbalize understanding of measures to prevent transmission to others.

Evaluation of Outcomes: Does patient verbalize understanding of transmission prevention? Does patient practice preventive behaviors?

Interventions	Rationale	Evaluation
Assess patient's understanding of transmission, symptoms, complications, and treatment of STDs.	New instruction should be based on patient's previous knowledge.	Is patient's current understanding accurate? What teaching is needed?
Assess whether patient is engaging in high-risk behaviors.	If patient is continuing to engage in high-risk behaviors, the risk for infection of others is high.	Is patient protecting self and others appropriately?
Use standard precautions and strict aseptic technique for all procedures involving blood and body fluids.	The health team, in addition to other patient contacts, must be protected.	Are standard precautions observed?
Instruct patient in appropriate strategies to reduce risk of infecting others: • Abstinence • Monogamy (if no active infection) • Use of barrier methods and spermicides • Adherence to treatment regimen.	These measures may help prevent transmission of infection to others.	Does patient verbalize understanding of methods to prevent transmission and intent to practice them?

Continued

NURSING CARE PLAN for the Patient with Genital Herpes—cont'd

Interventions	Rationale	Evaluation
Teach patient signs and symptoms of STDs to report immediately.	Prompt treatment of patient and partners further reduces risk of transmission of infection.	Does patient verbalize understanding of signs and symptoms to report?

Nursing Diagnosis: *Fear* related to diagnosis of an incurable illness and effects on sexual relationships and reproduction as evidenced by patient statement

Expected Outcomes: The patient will verbalize realistic and accurate information about disease process and relate control of excessive fear.

Evaluation of Outcomes: Does patient relate accurate knowledge? Is fear manageable?

Interventions	Rationale	Evaluation
Assess patient's fears.	Fear is a normal response and may be appropriate.	What does patient fear?
If fear is based on misconceptions, provide factual information.	When fear is based on misconceptions, they should be corrected.	Are fears based on factual information?
Allow patient to verbalize feelings. Be empathetic, but do not offer false hope.	Sharing fears may help patient gain insight into dealing with them.	Is patient able to verbalize feelings?
Explain all procedures and treatments.	Unfamiliar procedures or treatments may contribute to fear.	Does patient understand procedures and treatments?
Help patient identify support systems and coping strategies that have worked in the past.	Methods that have worked for patient before are likely to be helpful again.	Does patient have effective coping skills and support systems?

during pregnancy can cause particularly difficult problems. Genital warts tend to grow more rapidly in pregnant women and to bleed more easily with injury than in nonpregnant women.

Diagnostic Tests

Diagnosis may be made by applying dilute acetic acid (vinegar) to the skin of the external genital area, vagina, cervix, and anus and then closely examining with a colposcope the areas that turn a lighter color. Biopsy specimens of the suspicious areas can be sent for further study of the cells. Other tests to diagnose HPV include an antigen test and the Southern and dot blot tests, which use radioactive probes. Cancerous changes stimulated by this virus may be identified on Pap smears.

Therapeutic Measures

There is currently no known cure for papillomavirus infection. The warts may be treated by freezing, burning, or chemically destroying them or by manipulating the patient's immune system to attack the virus. Cryotherapy (freezing) of the warts may be done by touching each wart with a cryoprobe or a liquid nitrogen–soaked swab. Warts may also be burned or **electrocoagulated** with an **electrocautery** or a laser. Heat causes the proteins to coagulate, resulting in death of the wart tissue. Several topical agents are also available (see Table 44.2).

Some treatment options are not appropriate for use during pregnancy because of their **cytotoxic** effects, which might damage the fetus, but cryosurgery and laser destruction of the wart tissue can be done during pregnancy. All treatments may require multiple applications and generally result in a great deal of discomfort as the warts degenerate, ulcerate, and slough over a long period. Wart removal does not cure the infection, and new wart growth can occur after treatment.

Various types of immunotherapy have been used against HPV. Interferons are proteins produced by the body that can inhibit viral growth. Several types of interferons have been used to combat HPV. These substances may be applied topically, injected into the condyloma, or administered systemically. Interferons can produce side effects of flu-like

• WORD • BUILDING •

electrocoagulated: electro—electrical + coagul—curdled or hardened + ated—process completed
electrocautery: electro—electrical + cautery—branding iron
cytotoxic: cyto—cell + toxic—poison

symptoms, a drop in the number of white blood cells, and changes in liver function. Systemic interferon treatment, however, may offer the advantage of being able to attack warts all over the body at the same time, rather than individually as with topical treatments, thus speeding the process of treatment.

Research to develop vaccines against HPV strains is ongoing, but the multitude of varieties makes this difficult. The Gardasil vaccine was introduced in 2006 for the prevention of four types of HPV. Gardasil protects against the low-risk types of HPV, 6 and 11, which cause 90% of genital warts. Gardasil also protects against high-risk types of HPV, types 16 and 18, which are known to cause 70% of cervical cancers. Women ages 9 through 26 receive three doses of the vaccine, starting with the initial dose, then again at 2 and 6 months after the initial dose. The vaccine does not prevent many of the other types of both high-risk and low-risk HPV.

Home Care

Patients who have genital warts (condylomata acuminata) burned off need to recuperate at home. Multiple areas may be treated. If the burns are near the urethra or rectum, the patient may need a Foley catheter inserted to avoid contamination and irritation of the lesions after treatment. Also, the patient is instructed to increase dietary roughage and fluids to prevent constipation. Consult the health care provider for orders on care of the burns. Use sterile technique for dressing changes, and premedicate the patient for pain control as needed for dressing changes.

Hepatitis B

Pathophysiology and Etiology

Hepatitis B is an infection of the liver caused by the hepatitis B virus (HBV). There are several hepatitis viruses, but this section deals only with hepatitis B virus, which is generally considered within the STD category because it can be transmitted through sexual contact with blood and body fluids. During pregnancy, hepatitis B virus may be transmitted to the unborn baby, which can result in acute hepatitis and the possibility of becoming a chronic carrier of HBV. (See Chapter 35 for a full discussion on hepatitis.)

Prevention

Prevention is better than treatment and may be accomplished by using HBV vaccine. This is especially recommended for health care workers who come in contact with blood and body fluids. Standard precautions should be used when contact with any body fluids is expected. All infants now receive HBV vaccine at birth before discharge from the hospital, again at 1 to 2 months, and a final dose at age 24 weeks or older.

Infants whose mothers are HBV-positive will receive HBV immune globulin and HBV vaccine within 12 hours of birth. After two additional doses of the vaccine, these infants should be tested for the hepatitis B surface antigen (CDC, 2009).

Signs and Symptoms

Early signs of hepatitis are loss of appetite, rashes, malaise, muscle and joint pain, headaches, nausea, and vomiting. Because the virus affects the liver, the urine may darken and the stool color may lighten (as a result of changes in bile excretion), liver enzymes may rise, and jaundice may appear. Enlargement of the spleen, enlargement and tenderness of the liver, necrosis of liver cells, cirrhosis, coma, and death may follow if the disease is severe. Chronic asymptomatic carrier status may follow hepatitis virus infection, with an increased risk of liver cancer.

Diagnostic Tests

Diagnosis of hepatitis is generally made using a variety of blood tests based on antigen and antibody responses. A blood test for liver enzymes and liver biopsy may be done to determine extent of liver damage.

Therapeutic Measures

If a person is aware of being exposed to HBV, hepatitis B immune globulin can be injected within 24 hours to provide passive immunity. Supportive medical care with avoidance of drugs that require liver metabolism may help the patient through the active stage of the disease. Interferon-alpha therapy and antiviral agents are also available for patients with chronic hepatitis B. In severe cases, liver transplant may be needed.

Genital Parasites

Etiology and Signs and Symptoms

Genital parasites are not a true STD, but they may be transmitted during close body contact. The two most commonly seen parasites are pubic lice (*Phthirus pubis,* commonly called "crabs" because of the shape of the lice) and scabies (*Sarcoptes scabiei*). These parasites cause itching, redness, and, for scabies, tracks under the skin where the females burrow to lay their eggs.

Diagnostic Tests

History, physical examination, and direct visualization or magnified view of the parasites aid in diagnosis.

Therapeutic Measures

Parasites are treated with topical insecticides such as permethrin (Elimite, Acticin, for scabies) or malathion (Ovide, for pubic lice). Advise the patient to refer to package inserts for application instructions and precautions to avoid reinfection.

REPORTING OF SEXUALLY TRANSMITTED DISEASES

The nurse may be required to facilitate the reporting and public health follow-up of STDs by filling in patient information on an STD reporting form and placing the form in the patient's chart for completion by the health care provider. The requirements for reporting STDs may vary for different states, provinces, and countries. In some areas, laboratories are also required to submit a report form for positive reportable STD results. Laboratory reports that are not followed by a health care provider's report may result in investigation by an STD investigator. Generally, the report form has spaces for listing of sexual contacts that should be notified of possible STD exposure. Depending on the laws of the state, province, or country, health care providers may notify identified sexual contacts or patients may do so themselves. Contacts may also be notified by a public health authority that they have been listed as a sexual contact by an anonymous person who has tested positive for an STD.

NURSING PROCESS FOR SEXUALLY TRANSMITTED DISEASES

Data Collection

STDs are usually assessed, diagnosed, and treated in health care providers' offices and in clinics. It is important to evaluate the patient's reason for seeking health care with every outpatient visit. Sometimes patients visit clinics or health care providers' offices for stated reasons other than STDs, yet their real concern is an STD.

If a patient presents with signs and symptoms that could lead to an STD diagnosis, inquire about whether he or she currently has any irritation, pain, lesions, or discharge in the genital region. Explaining to the patient the need to know what examination supplies to prepare for an appropriate assessment may allow him or her to share concerns and true reasons for the visit. Establishing rapport and conveying acceptance may also facilitate communication. Often the nurse is present during the examination to assist the health care provider and to serve as a chaperone or patient support person.

STDs may also be discovered in hospitalized patients. Nurses are often the ones who bathe and provide perineal care to patients. It is important to be aware of signs and symptoms in older adults as well as younger people (Box 44.1, *Gerontological Issues*). Unusual discharge, redness, blisters, swollen areas, ulcers, and evidence of parasites in the genital area may be observed during patient care. STD awareness can also sensitize you to the possible significance of patient reports of persistent pelvic pain, dysuria, discharges, and rectal soreness. Such problems should be accurately documented and reported, so that further investigation and possible treatment can take place.

NURSING CARE TIP

Neighbors, friends, or family members may seek information from you because they know nurses are educated about health issues. Such questions may be stated in indirect terms, such as "I have a friend who is having a problem. . . ." You can provide accurate information and stress the importance of diagnosis and treatment to prevent the serious consequences of untreated STDs, without asking probing or embarrassing questions.

Box 44.1

Gerontological Issues

Older adults retain interest in and are capable of engaging in sex. Do not assume that because an older adult is single or widowed that he or she is not sexually active.

Older adults who have enjoyed active and fulfilling sex lives with a previous spouse or partner may seek that in new relationships. Older adults who engage in high-risk sexual behaviors (multiple partners, genital-anal sex, no use of barriers during sexual intercourse) are also at risk for sexually transmitted diseases.

Nursing Diagnoses, Planning, and Implementation

Acute Pain Related to Inflammation or Skin Lesions as Evidenced by Patient's Pain Rating

EXPECTED OUTCOME: The patient will express that pain relief is at an acceptable level.

- Assess pain using an appropriate scale. *This will aid in providing appropriate relief measures.*
- Recommend pain relief measures appropriate to the type and location of the pain (see Chapter 10 and consult with primary care provider). *Pain from STDs can vary from local discomfort to severe pain. Treatment may involve interventions ranging from topical applications to opioids and should be tailored to meet the assessment findings.*
- Document results of pain relief measures. *This will communicate to others effective pain interventions.*
- Instruct patient about self-care for pain and STD treatment *to promote resolution of infectious process and related symptoms.*

Risk for Infection Transmission to Others (Related to High-Risk Behaviors)

EXPECTED OUTCOME: The patient will verbalize understanding of measures to prevent transmission to others.

- Assess whether patient is engaging in high-risk behaviors *to determine risk of transmission to others.*
- Assess patient's understanding of symptoms, complications, treatment, and transmission of STDs. *This will allow for additional, appropriate information to be given.*
- Use standard precautions and strict aseptic technique for all procedures involving blood and body fluids *to limit risk of transmission of infectious organism to health care members.*
- Instruct patient in appropriate strategies to reduce risk of infecting others, such as abstinence, monogamy, use of barrier and spermicidal contraceptives, and adherence to the treatment regimen *in order to reduce the risk of disease transmission.*

- Consult with primary care provider for specific strategies for risk reduction based on infecting organism. *Ways to prevent infection differ based on infecting organism.*
- Explain importance of follow-up evaluation *in order to affirm that treatment was successful.*

Ineffective Sexuality Pattern Related to Infection and Risk for Transmission of Infectious Organism

EXPECTED OUTCOME: The patient will describe acceptable, alternative sexual practices and safer sex practices.

- Provide privacy and be verbally and nonverbally nonjudgmental when allowing patient and patient's partner to express concerns about sexual practice. *Treatment success rates are generally higher when a rapport is established with the health care provider and the partner is included in the decision-making process.*
- When teaching patients, the terms *safe sex* and *STD prevention* are misnomers. *You should more accurately refer to information about barrier methods as safer sex practices, which may decrease the risk of (but not absolutely prevent) transmission of STDs* (Table 44.3).
- Discuss alternative means of sexual expression, as appropriate, *because this may allow for intimacy when the desired sexual expression is not recommended.*
- Support realistic expectations about treatment and outcomes. *Unrealistic expectations may lead to additional undesired issues related to sexuality pattern.*

Fear Related to Diagnosis of Possible Incurable Illness as Evidenced by Patient Statement

EXPECTED OUTCOME: The patient will verbalize realistic and accurate information about the disease process and relate that fear is at an acceptable level.

- Assess patient's fears *because understanding the basis for fear will aid in implementing coping strategies.*
- If fear is based on misconceptions, provide factual information. *Knowledge may decrease fear.*
- Allow patient to verbalize feelings, while being empathetic. *Sharing fears may help patient gain insight into dealing with issues of concern.*
- Explain all procedures and treatments. *Unfamiliar practices may increase fear.*
- Help patient identify support systems and coping strategies that have worked in the past. *These may be helpful in dealing with current fears.*

TABLE 44.3 BARRIER METHODS FOR SAFER SEX

Barrier	Related Information
Male condoms	• Latex condoms are less likely than other types to break during intercourse. • Lubrication decreases the chance of breakage during use. Only water-soluble lubricants should be used, because substances such as petroleum jelly (Vaseline) may weaken the condom. • Condoms should never be inflated to test them; doing so can weaken them. • Condoms should be applied only when the penis is erect. • Condoms should have a reservoir tip or should be applied while holding about ½ inch of tip flat between the fingertips to allow room for ejaculate; otherwise, the condom might break. • The penis should be withdrawn after ejaculation and before the erection begins to subside while holding the condom securely around the penis to avoid spillage. • Condoms should never be reused and should be discarded properly after use so that others will not come in contact with contents.
Female condoms	• Female condoms should be applied before any penetration occurs; even preejaculation fluid can contain microorganisms. • Lubrication decreases the chance of breakage during use, but only water-soluble lubricants should be used, because substances such as petroleum jelly (Vaseline) may weaken the condom. • Female condoms should never be reused and should be discarded properly after use so that others will not come in contact with contents.
Cervical caps or diaphragms	• These may provide some protection for the cervix only. They are not effective barriers against STDs.
Rubber gloves, rubber dental dams, split (opened) male condoms	• These may provide some barrier protection for manual and oral sex. Although some groups suggest that male condoms may be split down one side and opened or rubber dental dam material may be taped over areas that have lesions to avoid direct contact with blood and body fluid, especially during sadomasochistic sexual activity, this very high-risk behavior is not recommended.
Double condoms	• Anal intercourse is a very high-risk activity for transmission of many types of STDs, as well as many intestinal organisms, and is not recommended. Homosexual networks advise wearing double condoms and using water-soluble lubricants, preferably containing nonoxynol-9, to decrease risk somewhat if engaging in this type of sexual activity.

Readiness for Enhanced Self Health Management Related to Lack of Knowledge About STDs as Evidenced by Patient Requesting Information

EXPECTED OUTCOME: The patient will verbalize correct understanding related to STD prevention.

- Assess the patient's health beliefs and correct misconceptions. *Many myths about sexual activity are sincerely believed by some patients* (Table 44.4).
- Explain the importance of patients knowing the sexual and lifestyle history of any potential partner before sexual activity has occurred. *Having a sexual relationship with someone is the* **epidemiological** *equivalent of engaging in sexual activity with all of that person's previous partners.*
- Provide pamphlets or other reading materials *to reinforce teaching.*
- Explain that abstinence or lifelong monogamy of both sexual partners in a relationship is the only sure prevention against STDs. *These practices eliminate risk of exposure.*
- Educate the patient that consumption of alcohol or other psychoactive drugs can reduce inhibitions and may result in unintended sexual encounters, which can transmit STDs. *Avoiding or limiting alcohol and other drug consumption when with potential partners may help prevent STD infection from occurring.*

• WORD • BUILDING •
epidemiological: epi—on + demio—people + logical—study of

Evaluation

Goals have been met if the patient is able to state that pain is controlled at an acceptable level; verbalizes understanding of transmission prevention and practices preventive behaviors; describes acceptable, alternative sexual practices and safer sexual practices; and relates accurate information and reduction in fear.

For more information on STDs, visit www.cdc.gov/std/healthcomm/fact_sheets.htm and www.ashastd.org.

CRITICAL THINKING

Stephanie

■ As you seat a young woman in an examining room of the clinic where you work, she comments, "I am new to this area and I've heard that there are three guys in this town who have syphilis and are spreading it around. Is that true?"

1. What are some concerns this question might reflect?
2. You find out that Stephanie knows very little about syphilis. List in outline form a teaching plan that includes the information that is important for Stephanie to know about syphilis.

Suggested answers at end of chapter.

TABLE 44.4 COMMON MYTHS ABOUT SEXUALLY TRANSMITTED DISEASES

Myth	Factual Data
People who have STDs are easily identifiable.	Inspection of the potential partner's genitals before sexual activity may decrease the risk (if one does not participate in sexual activity with a person who has visible lesions), but: • Not all people who are infected have visible symptoms. • There is no standard personality or physical profile for people who can be infected with STDs—anyone can be and may be infected.
Avoiding persons who have a history of engaging in casual sex, intravenous drug use, homosexual activity, bisexual activity, or a previous sexual relationship with persons who engage in these high-risk practices effectively protects one from infection with STDs.	Avoiding people with these types of history may decrease risk, but: • Not everyone is honest when responding to questions about sexual history. • Not everyone is aware of their previous partners' histories or the histories of others with whom their previous partners have had sexual relationships. • Asking these kinds of questions is difficult and may be postponed at times until emotional factors complicate such communication.
STDs never happen the first time.	Only one contact with one microorganism is needed for infection.
Intact genital skin is impervious to the pathogens (and gentle sexual activity does no harm).	Intact skin is the body's first line of defense, but: • Some microorganisms can be transmitted without a noticeable tissue injury. • Minor injuries can occur during many types of sexual activity, including vaginal intercourse.
Condoms prevent the spread of all STDs.	Condoms can greatly decrease the risk of STDs, but: • Condoms can have tiny channels in the latex or other material that can allow microorganisms to pass through. • Condoms can break, slip off, or be applied improperly. • Petroleum-based lubricants may weaken latex condoms. • Condoms do not provide a barrier for any area other than the penis and most of the vagina or anus. Some STDs may still be transmitted by contact with surrounding uncovered tissues.

TABLE 44.4 COMMON MYTHS ABOUT SEXUALLY TRANSMITTED DISEASES—cont'd

Myth	Factual Data
The female condom prevents all transmissions of STDs.	It does cover more surface area, but it may have problems similar to male condoms (see previous entry).
Manual, oral, and anal stimulation cannot transmit STDs.	Contact of hands to genitals can allow for transmission of microorganisms through breaks in the skin. Oral sex can transmit some STD-causing microorganisms. Anal intercourse is a very high-risk activity for transmission of STDs because anal tissues are easily injured and the gastrointestinal tract can be a reservoir for many microorganisms.
Nonoxynol-9 spermicide kills all STD germs.	Nonoxynol-9 can reduce the risk of transmission of STDs, but: • Nonoxynol-9 is not guaranteed to kill all microorganisms.
People get AIDS only by homosexual sexual activity or by blood transfusion.	Homosexual activity may result in a higher incidence of transmission of HIV, but: • HIV can be transmitted during heterosexual activity.
A woman cannot transmit HIV to a man.	
A man cannot transmit HIV to a woman.	• Gender does not protect a person from being infected with HIV.
Sexual activity during menstruation is less likely to result in STDs.	Sexual activity during menstruation is more likely to result in transmission of some microorganisms that cause STDs because of the vulnerability of the lining of the uterus caused by sloughing of the outer layers of cells and because blood and cellular debris may serve as a nutritious medium for growth of microorganisms.
Lesbian sexual activity cannot transmit STDs.	Transmission of microorganisms can occur by contact with mouth, anus, genital tissues, or fomites (inanimate objects, such as vibrators and other sex paraphernalia) that have been contaminated with microorganisms from an infected person—regardless of the original source of the infection.
Those who have not been infected after sexual activity with several people are naturally immune to STDs.	There is no known natural immunity to STDs. The person may not yet have had contact with someone who has an active STD.
Those who have had an STD and have been cured of it by taking medicine are now immune to that disease.	Infection that has been eradicated by medication does not confer immunity.
People can be certified free of all STDs by having a blood test and taking a simple medication if an infection is present.	Testing of those who suspect they may have contracted an STD and treatment (if possible) may decrease the spread of STDs, but: • No one test identifies all STDs. Some are identified by examination, and not all infected people show symptoms. • Some STDs do not show positive test results for long periods yet may be transmitted by the person while the tests are still negative. • People may be infected with more than one agent at a time, and each must be treated (if possible). One STD may obscure the symptoms of other concurrent STDs, so that one or more types may go unnoticed and untreated or may not be evident until other STDs have been treated. • There are no known cures for some STDs.
Oral contraceptive pills give protection against STDs.	Oral contraceptives are not antibiotics—they provide only some protection against conception. Use of a barrier method with spermicide along with the oral contraceptive can decrease risk of STDs and pregnancy.

SUGGESTED ANSWERS TO

CRITICAL THINKING

■ *Mrs. Miller*

1. You can educate Mrs. Miller about the possibility of neonatal infections from *C. trachomatis* or *N. gonorrhoeae,* especially of the eyes. Institutional and governmental policies related to treatment should be explained. Care should be taken to explain to Mrs. Miller that treatment is widely used, so as not to make her feel she has a condition she has not been told about.
2. Because the benefits of prophylactic eye treatment of the neonate for *C. trachomatis* and *N. gonorrhoeae* exposure are generally seen as greater than the risks, it is recommended by governmental agencies and supported by most institutional policies to treat all newborns, regardless of known exposure, shortly after birth.

SUGGESTED ANSWERS TO—cont'd

■ *Kerri*

1. Explain to Kerri the fact that trichomoniasis is generally considered to be an STD, but that the organism that causes the disorder can be transmitted through infected articles (during nonsexual contact), can survive a long time outside the body, and that one can be asymptomatic for many years following exposure to the organism before an outbreak occurs.
2.

7.5 mg	1 kg	140 pounds	= 477 mg
1 kg	2.2 pounds		

Her dose will probably be rounded to 500 mg every 6 hours.

3. Teach Kerri that it is possible that her partner could have an undiagnosed infection, and that it is possible to become infected during a monogamous relationship. Treatment should be provided to Kerri's partner regardless of symptoms. Also, reinfection may occur if both partners are not treated. Be sure to tell her that she should abstain from alcohol while on metronidazole and for at least 48 hours following its completion. Patients who drink alcohol while taking it are *very* likely to vomit.

■ *Stephanie*

1. Concerns might include (a) a wish to speak with a health care worker, (b) uncertainty about whether patient information will be kept confidential (give assurance that if you knew about anyone with syphilis, it would be your professional responsibility to keep it confidential), (c) fear that she might have become infected through heterosexual contact, (d) a desire to protect herself by avoiding those who have syphilis, and (e) a desire for information about syphilis and its transmission routes.
2. The teaching plan might include information about (a) the spirochete that causes syphilis, (b) signs and symptoms, (c) diagnostic tests, (d) means of transmission, (e) strategies for risk reduction, (f) treatment, (g) research, and (h) rights and responsibilities of those who have the disease.

REVIEW QUESTIONS

1. Which of the following pathogens causes syphilis?
   a. *Treponema pallidum*
   b. *Chlamydia trachomatis*
   c. Human papillomavirus
   d. Human immunodeficiency virus

2. What signs and symptoms of STDs should nurses assess for in all patients? **Select all that apply.**
   a. Itching
   b. Discharge
   c. Dysuria
   d. Genital ulcers
   e. Genital warts
   f. Rectal pain

3. A young woman is seen at a walk-in clinic and is diagnosed with an STD. She says, "How could I have an STD? I only have sex with my boyfriend. I don't sleep around!" Which of the following responses by the nurse is best?
   a. "You are right, that should have kept you safe. There just are no guarantees."
   b. "If your boyfriend is not infected, then it is apparent that you have had sex with someone else."
   c. "You or your boyfriend could be infected from past sexual encounters. He should also be tested at this time for STDs."
   d. "Even lifelong monogamy cannot prevent many STDs."

4. A home care nurse is preparing to change a dressing on a patient who had genital warts removed the previous day. Which intervention should be completed first?
   a. Clean the wounds.
   b. Remove the old dressing.
   c. Assess for drainage.
   d. Administer an analgesic.

5. An older man is admitted to the hospital with mental status changes. As the nurse begins the shift assessment, the patient begins to cry and says his doctor thinks his problems stem from an untreated syphilis infection when he was in the military as a young man. Which response by the nurse is best?
   a. "Why didn't you have it treated when it occurred?"
   b. "What's done is done; it's unfortunate that treatment is too late now."
   c. "That must be upsetting for you. Do you want to talk about it?"
   d. "Don't cry; I am sure there is treatment that can help now."

REVIEW QUESTIONS—cont'd

6. A nurse has completed instruction related to STD risk reduction with a 17-year-old woman. Which statement by the patient indicates that teaching has been effective?
   a. "I should avoid drinking alcohol when I will be in situations with potential sex partners."
   b. "If I make sure my partners wear condoms, I will be protected from STDs."
   c. "Use of a barrier method of birth control will prevent infection with an STD."
   d. "As long as I know my partner well, I am safe."

References

Centers for Disease Control and Prevention. (2007). *Sexually transmitted diseases surveillance, 2007: Gonorrhea*. Retrieved July 10, 2009, from http://www.cdc.gov/std/stats07/gonorrhea.htm

Centers for Disease Control for Prevention. (2009). *Recommended immunization schedule for persons aged 0 through 6 years, United States, 2009*. Retrieved July 10, 2009, from http://www.cdc.gov/vaccines/recs/schedules/downloads/child/2009/09_0-6yrs_schedule_pr.pdf

unit TWELVE

UNDERSTANDING THE MUSCULOSKELETAL SYSTEM

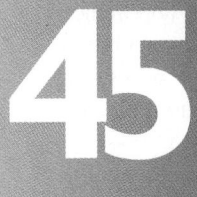

45 Musculoskeletal System Function and Assessment

KELLY McMANIGLE AND
JANICE L. BRADFORD

KEY TERMS

arthrocentesis (AR-throw-sen-TEE-siss)
arthroscopy (ar-THROSS-scuh-pee)
articular (ar-TIK-yoo-lar)
bone (BOWN)
bursae (BURR-sah)
crepitation (crep-ih-TAY-shun)
gout (GOWT)
hemarthrosis (heem-ar-THROW-siss)
joint (JOYNT)
muscle (MUH-suhl)
resorption (ree-SORP-shun)
synovitis (sin-oh-VY-tiss)
vertebrae (VER-teh-bray)

QUESTIONS TO GUIDE YOUR READING

1. What is the normal anatomy and function of the musculoskeletal system?
2. What areas are included in a nursing assessment of the musculoskeletal system?
3. What areas are reviewed when performing a neurovascular assessment?
4. How would you describe diagnostic tests for musculoskeletal problems?
5. What nursing care would you provide for each musculoskeletal diagnostic test?

NORMAL MUSCULOSKELETAL SYSTEM ANATOMY AND PHYSIOLOGY

The skeletal and muscular systems may be considered one system because they work together to enable the body to move. The skeleton is the framework that supports the body and to which the voluntary **muscles** are attached. The skeletal framework includes the **joints**, or articulations, between **bones.** Contraction of a muscle pulls a bone and changes the angle of a joint. It is important to remember that movement would not be possible without the proper functioning of the nervous, cardiovascular, and respiratory systems. Voluntary muscles require nerve impulses to contract, a continuous supply of blood provided by the circulatory system, and oxygen provided by the respiratory system.

SKELETAL SYSTEM TISSUES AND THEIR FUNCTIONS

The tissues that make up the skeletal system are bone tissue; cartilage, which covers most joint surfaces; and fibrous connective tissue, which forms the ligaments that connect one bone to another and also form part of the structure of joints. The tissues of the muscular system are skeletal (also called striated, voluntary) muscle; fibrous connective tissue, which forms the tendons that connect muscle to bone; and the fasciae, the strong membranes that enclose individual muscles.

Besides its role in movement, the skeleton has other functions. It protects organs and tissues from mechanical injury. For example, the brain is protected by the skull and the heart and lungs are protected by the rib cage. Flat and irregular bones as well as the ends of long bones contain and protect the red bone marrow, the hematopoietic (blood-forming) tissue. The bones are also a storage site for excess calcium, which may undergo **resorption** (process of osteoclasts breaking down bone) from bones to maintain a normal blood calcium level. Calcium in the blood is needed for blood clotting and for the proper functioning of nerves and muscles.

Although the primary function of the muscular system is to move or stabilize the skeleton, the voluntary muscles collectively contribute significantly to heat production, which maintains normal body temperature. Heat is one of the energy products of cellular respiration, the process that produces adenosine triphosphate (ATP), the direct energy source for muscle contraction. Another important function of the muscular system is that it aids in returning blood from the legs through muscular compression on the leg veins.

Bone Tissue and Bone Growth

Bone tissue is composed of bone cells, called osteocytes, within a strong nonliving matrix made of calcium salts and the protein collagen. In compact bone, the osteocytes and matrix are in precise arrangements called osteons (or haversian systems). Compact bone is very dense and, to the unaided eye, appears solid. In spongy bone, the arrangement of cells and matrix is less precise, giving the bone a spongy appearance. Compact bone forms the diaphyses (shafts) of the long bones, covers the spongy bone of the epiphyses of long bones, and covers the spongy bone that forms the bulk of short, flat, and irregular bones.

A living bone is covered by a fibrous connective tissue membrane called the periosteum, which is the anchor for tendons and ligaments as the collagen fibers of all these structures merge to form connections of great strength. This membrane also contains the blood vessels that enter the bone itself (most bone is highly vascular) and bone-producing cells called osteoblasts that are activated to initiate repair when bone is damaged.

The growth of bone from fetal life until a person attains final adult height depends on many factors. Proper nutrition (particularly vitamins and minerals) provides the raw material to produce bone matrix, which is comprised of calcium, phosphorus, and protein. Vitamin D is essential for the efficient absorption of calcium and phosphorus from food in the small intestine. Vitamins A and C do not become part of bone but are needed for production of bone matrix (a process called ossification). Hormones directly needed for growth include growth hormone (GH) from the anterior pituitary gland, thyroxine from the thyroid gland, and insulin from the pancreas. Growth hormone increases mitosis and protein synthesis in growing bones; thyroxine stimulates osteoblasts and also increases energy production from food. Insulin is essential for the efficient use of glucose to provide energy. If a child is lacking any of these hormones, growth is much slower and the child does not reach his or her genetic potential for height.

Bone is not a fixed tissue, even when growth in height has ceased. Calcium and phosphate are constantly being removed and replaced (usually the rates are equal) to maintain normal blood levels of these minerals. Parathyroid hormone secreted by the parathyroid glands increases the removal of calcium and phosphate from bones; the hormone calcitonin from the thyroid gland promotes the retention of calcium in bones, although its greatest effects may be during childhood.

Osteoblasts produce bone matrix during normal growth to replace matrix lost during normal turnover and to repair fractures. Other cells called osteoclasts resorb bone matrix when more calcium is needed in the blood and during normal growth and fracture repair when excess bone must be removed as bones change shape.

The sex hormones, estrogen from the ovaries or testosterone from the testes, are important for retention of calcium in adult bones. For women after menopause, more calcium may be removed from bones than is replaced, leading to a thinning of bone tissue and the possibility of spontaneous fractures.

Structure of the Skeleton

The 206 bones of the human skeleton are in two divisions: the axial skeleton and the appendicular skeleton. The axial skeleton consists of the skull, hyoid, vertebral column, and rib cage; all are flat or irregular bones and contain red bone marrow (hematopoietic tissue). The appendicular skeleton consists of the bones of the limbs and the shoulder and pelvic girdles, by which the limbs attach to the axial skeleton (Fig. 45.1).

The long bones of the limbs are those of the arm, forearm, hand, and fingers and those of the thigh, leg, foot, and toes. All long bones have the same general structure: a central diaphysis, or shaft, with two ends called epiphyses. The diaphyses of long bones contain yellow bone marrow, which is mostly adipose—that is, stored energy; the epiphyses enclose red bone marrow. The bones of the wrist and ankle are short bones (except for the calcaneus, which is an irregular bone). The scapula is considered a flat bone, and the pelvic girdle is made of irregular bones. These bones contain red bone marrow.

Skull

The skull consists of 8 cranial bones and 14 facial bones and also contains the 3 auditory bones found in each middle ear cavity. The cranial bones that enclose and protect the brain are frontal, two parietal, two temporal, occipital, sphenoid, and ethmoid (Fig. 45.2). All of the joints between the cranial bones and those between most of the facial bones are immovable joints called sutures (comprised of dense collagenous connective tissue). The mandible is the only movable facial bone. It articulates with the temporal bone of the skull to form a combined hinge and planar joint

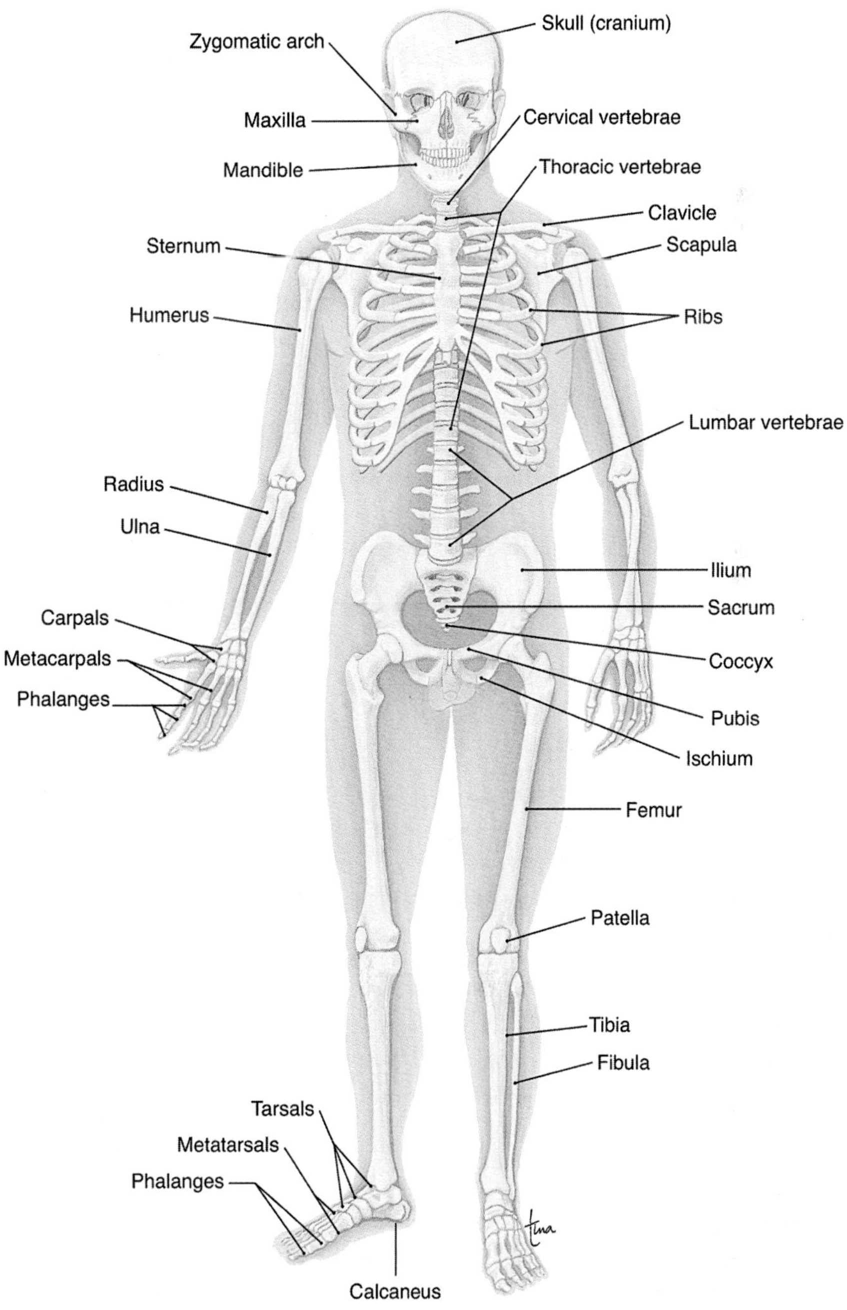

Skull (cranium)
Zygomatic arch
Maxilla
Cervical vertebrae
Mandible
Thoracic vertebrae
Clavicle
Sternum
Scapula
Humerus
Ribs
Lumbar vertebrae
Radius
Ulna
Ilium
Sacrum
Carpals
Metacarpals
Coccyx
Phalanges
Pubis
Ischium
Femur
Patella
Tibia
Fibula
Tarsals
Metatarsals
Phalanges
Calcaneus

FIGURE 45.1 The full skeleton in anterior view. (Modified from Scanlon, V. C., & Sanders, T. [2007]. *Anatomy and physiology* [5th ed.]. Philadelphia: F. A. Davis, with permission.)

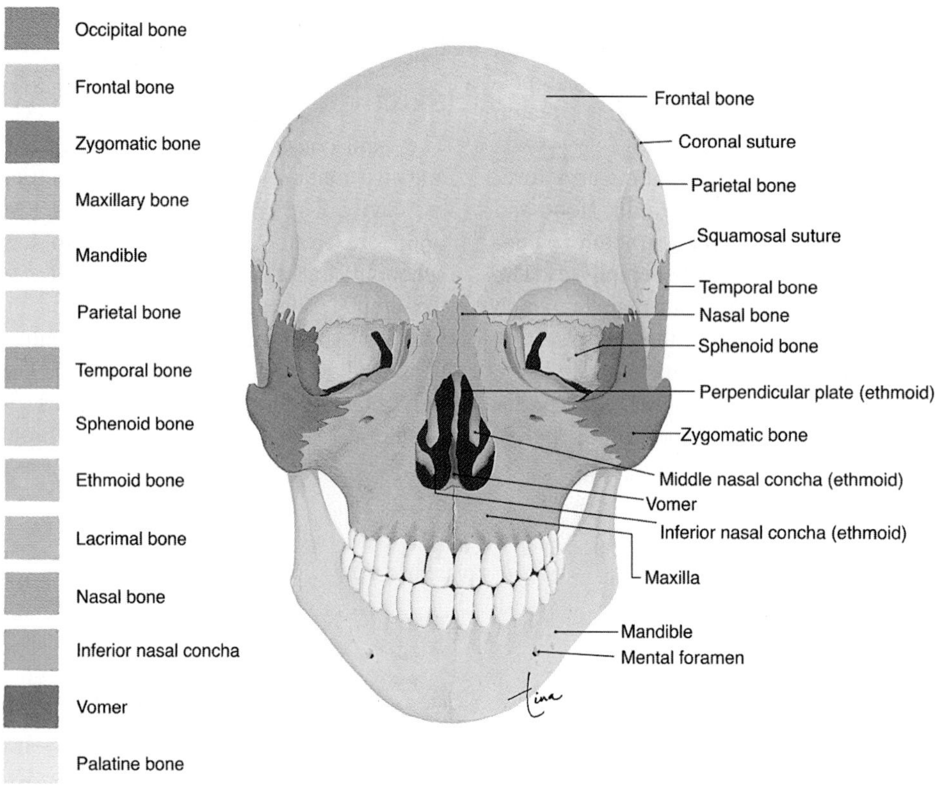
Occipital bone
Frontal bone
Zygomatic bone
Maxillary bone
Mandible
Parietal bone
Temporal bone
Sphenoid bone
Ethmoid bone
Lacrimal bone
Nasal bone
Inferior nasal concha
Vomer
Palatine bone
Frontal bone
Coronal suture
Parietal bone
Squamosal suture
Temporal bone
Nasal bone
Sphenoid bone
Perpendicular plate (ethmoid)
Zygomatic bone
Middle nasal concha (ethmoid)
Vomer
Inferior nasal concha (ethmoid)
Maxilla
Mandible
Mental foramen

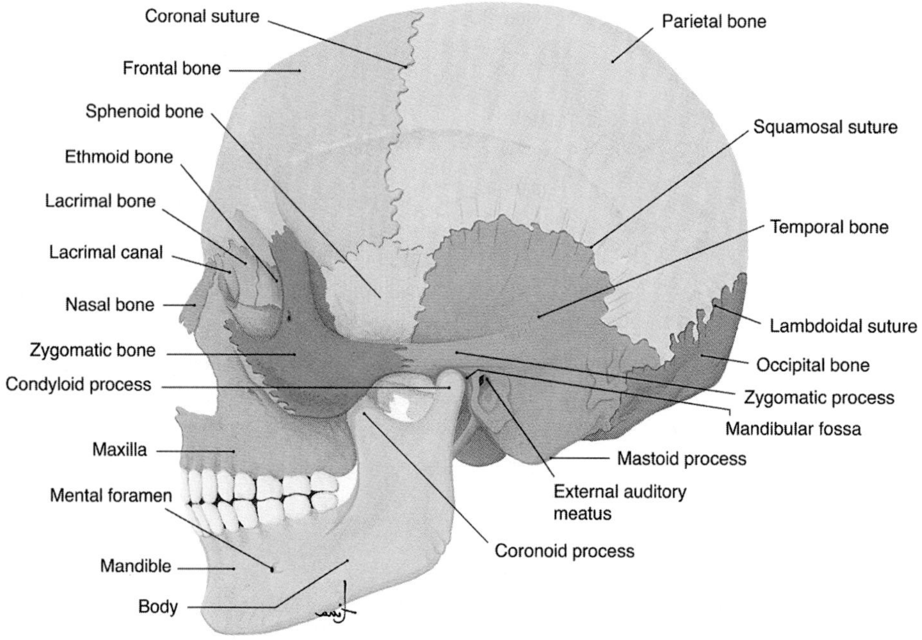
Coronal suture
Frontal bone
Sphenoid bone
Ethmoid bone
Lacrimal bone
Lacrimal canal
Nasal bone
Zygomatic bone
Condyloid process
Maxilla
Mental foramen
Mandible
Body
Parietal bone
Squamosal suture
Temporal bone
Lambdoidal suture
Occipital bone
Zygomatic process
Mandibular fossa
Mastoid process
External auditory meatus
Coronoid process

FIGURE 45.2 Anterior (upper) and lateral (lower) views of the skull. (Modified from Scanlon, V. C., & Sanders, T. [2007]. *Anatomy and physiology* [5th ed.]. Philadelphia: F. A. Davis, with permission.)

called the temporomandibular joint (Table 45.1). The maxillae are the upper jaw bones, which also form the front of the hard palate (part of the roof of the mouth). The rest of the facial bones are shown in Figure 45.2.

Vertebral Column

The vertebral column (or spinal column) is made of individual bones called **vertebrae** (see Fig. 45.1). From top to bottom there are 7 cervical vertebrae, 12 thoracic, 5 lumbar, 5 sacral (fused into 1 sacrum), and 4 or 5 coccygeal (fused into 1 coccyx).

The first cervical vertebra, called the atlas, articulates with the occipital bone of the skull and forms a pivot joint with the axis, the second cervical vertebra. The thoracic vertebrae articulate with the posterior ends of the ribs. The lumbar vertebrae are the largest and strongest. The sacrum

TABLE 45.1 JOINTS OF THE APPENDICULAR SKELETON

Type of Joint and Description	Examples
Symphysis—disk of fibrous cartilage between bones	Between vertebrae Between pubic bones
Ball and socket—movement in all planes	Scapula and humerus (shoulder) Pelvic bone and femur (hip)
Hinge—movement in one plane	Humerus and ulna (elbow) Femur and tibia (knee) Between phalanges (fingers and toes)
Combined hinge and planar	Temporal bone and mandible (lower jaw)
Pivot—rotation	Atlas and axis (neck) Radius and ulna (distal to elbow)
Gliding—side-to-side movement	Between carpals (wrist)
Saddle—movement in several planes	Carpometacarpal of thumb

Source: Modified from Scanlon, V. C., & Sanders, T. (2007). *Essentials of anatomy and physiology* (5th ed., p. 120). Philadelphia: F. A. Davis, with permission.

permits the articulation of the two hip bones (os coxae) at the sacroiliac joints. The coccyx serves as an attachment point for some muscles of the perineum.

The vertebrae as a unit form a flexible backbone that supports the trunk and head and contains and protects the spinal cord. Openings, or intervertebral foramina, between the vertebrae allow for the exit of spinal nerves and entry of blood vessels. The joints between vertebrae are symphysis joints in which a disk of fibrous cartilage serves as a cushion and permits slight movement.

Rib Cage

The rib cage consists of 12 pairs of ribs and the sternum. All of the ribs connect posteriorly with the thoracic vertebrae. The 7 pairs of true ribs articulate directly with the sternum by means of costal cartilages; the 3 pairs of false ribs join indirectly with the sternum, and the inferior 2 pairs of floating ribs do not connect to the sternum at all.

The rib cage protects the heart and lungs, as well as upper abdominal organs such as the liver and spleen, from mechanical injury. During breathing, the flexible rib cage is pulled upward and outward by the external intercostal muscles to expand the chest cavity and bring about inhalation.

Appendicular Skeleton

The bones of the appendicular skeleton are shown in Figure 45.1. The important joints of the appendicular skeleton are summarized in Table 45.1.

Structure of Synovial Joints

All freely movable joints (this excludes amphiarthroses and synarthroses) are synovial joints in that they share similarities of structure (Fig. 45.3). On the joint surface of each bone is the articular cartilage, which provides a smooth surface. The joint capsule is similar to a sleeve. It is made of fibrous connective tissue and forms a strong sheath that encloses the joint. Lining the joint capsule is the synovial membrane, which secretes synovial fluid into the joint cavity. Synovial fluid is a mixture of hyaluronic acid, proteins, fat, and cells that provides a slippery consistency that prevents friction as the bones move.

Many synovial joints also have **bursae,** which are small sacs of synovial fluid between the joint and structures of friction that cross over the joint. Bursae lessen wear and tear in areas of friction.

MUSCLE STRUCTURE AND ARRANGEMENTS

One muscle is made of thousands of skeletal muscle cells (fibers), which are specialized for contraction. When a muscle contracts, it shortens and pulls on a bone. Each muscle fiber receives its own motor nerve ending, and the numbers of fibers that contract depend on the job the muscle has to do. Muscles are anchored to bones by tendons, which are made of fibrous connective tissue. A muscle usually has at least two tendons, each attached to a different bone. The more stationary muscle attachment is called its origin; the more movable attachment is the insertion. The muscle itself crosses the joint formed by the two bones to which it is attached, and when the muscle contracts, it pulls on the insertion and moves the bone in a specific direction. The muscle causing this particular action is termed the agonist.

The approximately 700 muscles in the body are arranged to bring about a variety of movements (Fig. 45.4). The general

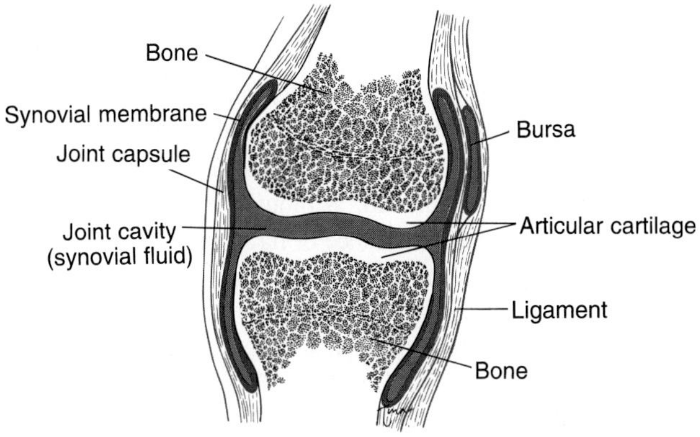
Bone
Synovial membrane
Joint capsule
Joint cavity
(synovial fluid)
Bursa
Articular cartilage
Ligament
Bone

FIGURE 45.3 Longitudinal section through a typical synovial joint. (Modified from Scanlon, V. T., & Sanders, T. [2007]. *Workbook for essentials of anatomy and physiology* [5th ed.]. Philadelphia: F. A. Davis, with permission.)

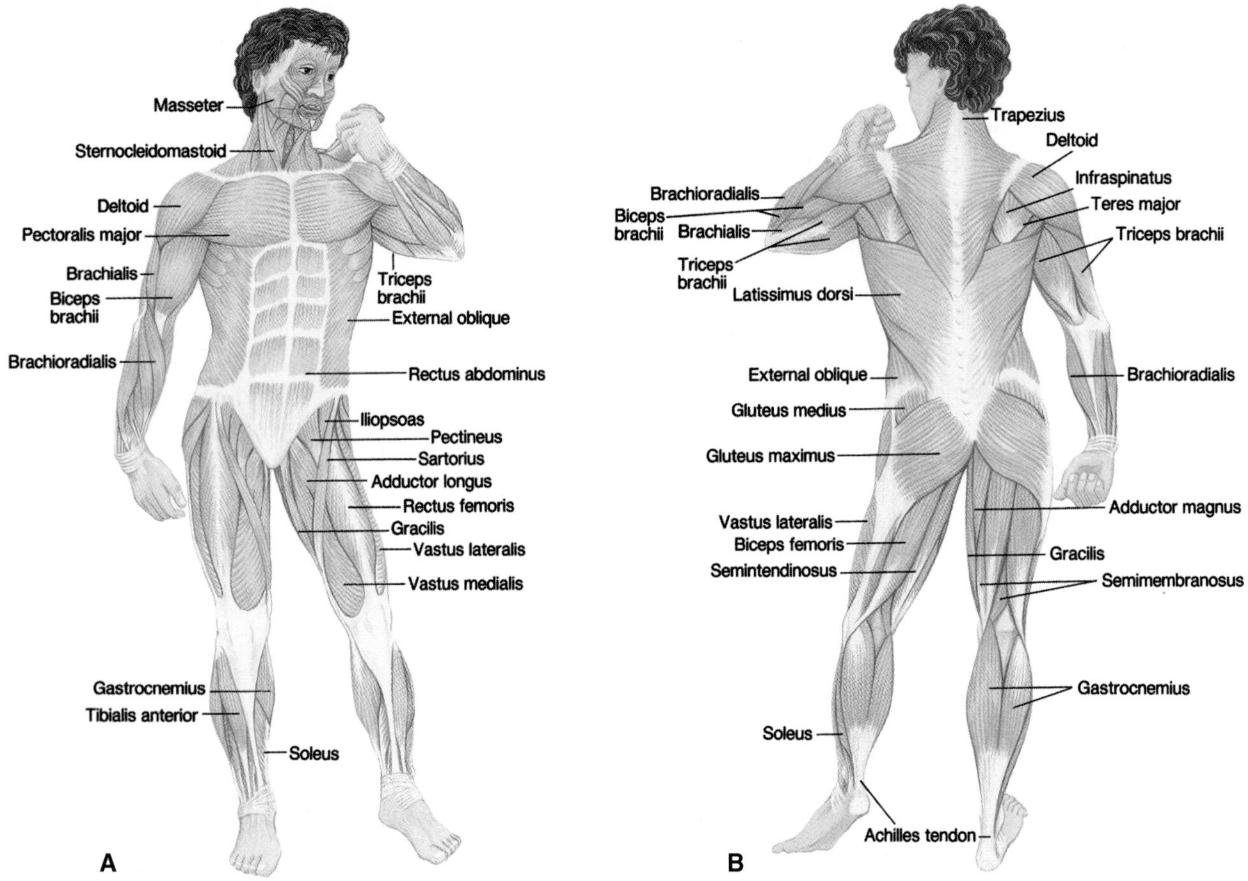
Masseter
Sternocleidomastoid
Deltoid
Pectoralis major
Brachialis
Biceps brachii
Brachioradialis
Triceps brachii
External oblique
Rectus abdominus
Iliopsoas
Pectineus
Sartorius
Adductor longus
Rectus femoris
Gracilis
Vastus lateralis
Vastus medialis
Gastrocnemius
Tibialis anterior
Soleus
A
Trapezius
Deltoid
Infraspinatus
Teres major
Triceps brachii
Brachioradialis
Biceps brachii
Brachialis
Triceps brachii
Latissimus dorsi
External oblique
Gluteus medius
Gluteus maximus
Brachioradialis
Adductor magnus
Vastus lateralis
Biceps femoris
Semintendinosus
Gracilis
Semimembranosus
Gastrocnemius
Soleus
Achilles tendon
B

FIGURE 45.4 Major muscles. (A) Anterior view. (B) Posterior view. (Modified from Scanlon, V. C., & Sanders, T. [2007]. *Essentials of anatomy and physiology* [5th ed.]. Philadelphia: F. A. Davis, with permission.)

types of arrangements are the agonist with opposing antagonists and the cooperative synergists.

Antagonistic muscles have opposite functions; such arrangements are needed because muscles can only pull, not push. If the biceps brachii, for example, flexes the forearm, an antagonist, the triceps brachii, is needed to extend the forearm. Other examples of antagonists are the quadriceps femoris and hamstring groups, the pectoralis major and the latissimus dorsi, and the tibialis anterior and gastrocnemius.

Synergistic muscles have similar functions or work together to perform a particular function. The brachioradialis is a synergist to the biceps brachii for flexion of the forearm; the sartorius is a synergist to the quadriceps group for flexion of the thigh. Synergists are needed to provide slight differences in angles when joints are moved. Without synergism we would be unable to maintain our balance or have the fine motor control needed to do such movements as writing or talking.

ROLE OF THE NERVOUS SYSTEM

Skeletal muscles are voluntary muscles in that consciously controlled nerve impulses cause contraction. Such nerve impulses originate in the motor areas of the frontal lobes of the cerebral cortex. The coordination of voluntary movement is a function of the cerebellum. Neurons in the central nervous system (CNS) regulate muscle tone, the state of slight contraction usually present in muscles. Good muscle tone is important for posture and coordination.

Neuromuscular Junction

Each of the thousands of fibers in a muscle has its own motor nerve ending; the neuromuscular junction is the termination of the motor neuron at the muscle fiber (see Fig. 50.2A). The motor neuron's axon terminal ends in an enlarged distal tip, the synaptic end bulb. It contains vesicles of the neurotransmitter acetylcholine. The membrane of the muscle fiber, called the sarcolemma, contains receptor sites for acetylcholine. The synaptic cleft is the minute space between the end bulb and the sarcolemma. The inactivating enzyme acetylcholinesterase is available in the synaptic cleft.

When a nerve impulse arrives at the end bulb, it causes the release of acetylcholine, which diffuses across the synaptic cleft and bonds to the acetylcholine receptors on the sarcolemma. This makes the sarcolemma permeable to sodium ions, which rush into the cell and generate an electrical impulse (an action potential) along the entire sarcolemma. This electrical change triggers a series of reactions in the internal units of contraction called sarcomeres. Put simply, filaments of the protein actin slide over filaments of the protein myosin, and the sarcomere shortens. All of the thousands of sarcomeres in a muscle fiber shorten, and the entire cell contracts. If a muscle has little work to do, few of its many muscle fibers contract, but if the muscle has more work to do, more of its muscle fibers contract.

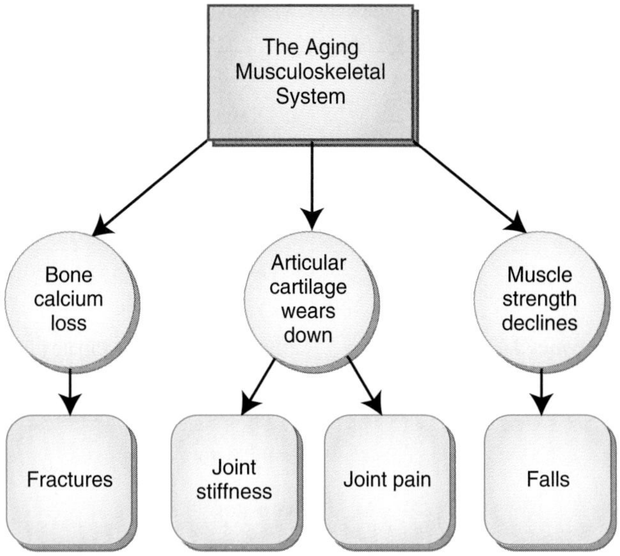
The Aging Musculoskeletal System
Bone calcium loss
Articular cartilage wears down
Muscle strength declines
Fractures
Joint stiffness
Joint pain
Falls

FIGURE 45.5 Aging and the musculoskeletal system. This concept map shows the effects the aging process has on the musculoskeletal system.

AGING AND THE MUSCULOSKELETAL SYSTEM

The amount of calcium in bones depends on several factors (Fig. 45.5). Good nutrition is certainly one factor, but age is another, especially for women. One function of estrogen or testosterone is the maintenance of a strong bone matrix. For women after menopause, bone matrix loses more calcium than is replaced. Calcium loss can lead to weakened bones that may result in bone fractures. Weight-bearing joints are also subject to damage after many years. Often the articular cartilage wears down and becomes rough, leading to pain and stiffness.

Muscle strength declines with age as the process of protein synthesis decreases. Such loss of strength need not be exaggerated because aging muscles benefit from regular exercise, which has been shown to increase strength and reduce falls and accidents (Box 45.1, *Gerontological Issues,* and see *Evidence-Based Practice* box).

EVIDENCE-BASED PRACTICE

Clinical Question

What are risk factors for falls in older people with dementia or cognitive impairments?

Evidence

Six prospective studies of varied design were reviewed (Härlein et al., 2009). Eight risk factors for falls in older people were found: disease-specific motor impairments, behavioral disturbances, impaired vision, dementia (by type and severity), functional impairments, history of falls, use of neuroleptics, and low bone-mineral density. The common risk factors of motor impairment and behavioral disturbances placed patients with dementia at high risk of falling.

Implications for Nursing Practice

Recognizing risk factors that place patients with dementia at higher risk for falling is important in planning interventions to help prevent falls.

REFERENCE

Härlein, J., Dassen, T., Halfens, R., & Heinze, C. (2009). Fall risk factors in older people with dementia or cognitive impairment: A systematic review. *Journal of Advanced Nursing, 65*(5), 922–933.

Box 45.1 Gerontological Issues

Age-Related Changes in the Older Adult

Age-related changes can lead to impaired mobility, an increased risk of falls, and pain. Common age-related musculoskeletal changes include the following:

- Decreased muscle mass and strength
- Decreased number of muscle cells, and replacement by fibrous connective tissue
- Decreased elasticity of ligaments, tendons, and cartilage, resulting in weaker bones
- Decreased intervertebral spaces from loss of water, causing a loss of height
- Altered posture and gait (a wider stance and smaller steps in men, and a narrow stance and waddling gait in women).

NURSING ASSESSMENT OF THE MUSCULOSKELETAL SYSTEM

The initial assessment begins with a history that includes the effects the condition is having on the patient's life. It then proceeds to a physical and psychosocial assessment (Table 45.2). Frequent neurovascular assessments may be needed if there is a risk of circulation impairment, such as might happen if the patient has a fracture or has had musculoskeletal surgery (Table 45.3).

TABLE 45.2 DATA COLLECTION FOR THE MUSCULOSKELETAL SYSTEM

Category	Questions to Ask During the Health History	Rationale/Significance
Subjective Data Collection		
Demographic	Age, gender, socioeconomic status	Increased age, being female, and lower socioeconomic status increase risk of musculoskeletal injury/problems.
	Occupation	Enables nurse to begin planning for discharge teaching if the patient has to alter his or her employment.
Previous Health History	Activities patient participates in	Provides information regarding the level of activity the patient had before the concern.
	Risk factors for musculoskeletal problems	Smoking and a sedentary lifestyle are risk factors for musculoskeletal problems.
	Family history	Some musculoskeletal conditions have genetic and familial tendencies.
	Diet history	Dietary intake such as calcium and vitamin D influences some musculoskeletal disorders.
History of Injury or Present Concern	Allergies	Prevents exposure to medication or compounds used in diagnostic tests, treatments, and therapies.
	History of the injury (if there was one)	Provides information that helps in the diagnosis of the problem, as well as making you aware of possible complications of the injury.
	Pain (use pain assessment scale)	Provides information about severity of the condition and effectiveness of the treatment and therapy.
Psychosocial Assessment	Determine if deformities, changes in body image, self-concept, socialization, or employment are present.	The patient may need assistance with strategies to cope with the stress of a possible chronic musculoskeletal condition.
	Determine coping skills.	Some musculoskeletal conditions require lifestyle alterations that can cause increased stress and difficulties in coping.
Objective Data Collection		
Physical Examination	Inspect, palpate, and observe range of motion (ROM) of affected areas.	Altered gait, tone, size, shape, posture, contractures, deformities, ROM, pain, and effects on activities of daily living (ADLs) can be determined.
	Assess color, warmth, circulation, and movement of affected areas.	Nerve function, sensation, movement, weakness, and the potential development of compartment syndrome can be determined.
	Palpate all pulses below involved area.	Alterations may indicate altered vascular integrity (and therefore tissue integrity) of affected area or demonstrate developing compartment syndrome.

TABLE 45.3 NEUROVASCULAR DATA COLLECTION

Monitor	Report
Color	Pallor, cyanosis, redness, or discoloration
Temperature	Unusual coolness or warmth
Pain	Pain that is worse on passive motion; pain that no longer responds to analgesics
Movement	Alterations in movement
Sensation	Alterations in feeling; tingling or paresthesias
Pulses	Diminished or absent distal pulses
Capillary refill	Nailbed that does not blanch in 3–5 seconds

Health History

The patient's history should include the following:

- For an injury, how and when it happened
- Occupation and activities, including sports and other physical activities
- Risk factors for musculoskeletal problems and family history of musculoskeletal problems (to detect hereditary problems)
- Current health status, including ongoing or chronic medical conditions (such as heart disease, diabetes, lung conditions)
- Diet history (including whether calcium and vitamin D intake are adequate to ensure

proper bone and muscle maintenance and repair)
- Information specific to the patient's musculoskeletal problems.

Patients with musculoskeletal problems frequently report pain or related stiffness and tenderness as a major concern. The pain may be acute or chronic and may limit the patient in everyday life. Assessment includes previous diagnoses, pain severity, medications, treatments, and procedures the patient uses to alleviate the pain. The WHAT'S UP? model can be used to assess the patient's pain (see Chapter 1).

Physical Examination

Three areas of musculoskeletal data collection are important: inspection, palpation, and range of motion (ROM). If the patient can walk, inspect posture and gait, noting poor posture or alterations in movement, such as limping. Note the use of mobility aids, such as a cane or walker. Document other gross deformities, such as unequal limbs, malalignment, or contractures. Spinal deformities are especially significant because they can compromise breathing and balance. Inspect the joints and muscles of the arms, hands, legs, and feet for deformity, redness, swelling, or **crepitation** (grating sound as joint or bone moves). Also note the patient's general nutritional status (e.g., normal, obese, emaciated).

After inspection, gently palpate for warmth and tenderness in the areas of swelling, and areas where the patient reported pain (being careful to minimize the pain this may cause). For example, reddened joints should be palpated for **synovitis** (swollen synovial tissue within the joint) or the presence of bony nodes. In some cases, joints and muscles may seem healthy but are tender when palpated.

Next, assess joint mobility. Stabilize the body area proximal to the joint being moved. Observe the patient's range of motion (ROM) for performing independent activities of daily living. Pay particular attention to the hands and observe movement in finger joints. For a quick and easy assessment of range of motion in the hands, ask the patient to touch each finger, one by one, to the thumb (known as opposition) and then to make a fist.

Also assess the size, shape, strength, and tone of muscles. Evaluate bilateral muscle strength by asking the patient to grip your hands. This enables you to feel the strength and equality. Pushing an extremity against your hand provides a general indication of muscle strength. More specific evaluation is performed by a physical therapist (PT) or an occupational therapist (OT). Using a scale of 0 to 5 (0 paralysis and 5 moving a muscle against resistance), the PT or OT measures the strength of each muscle group and rates it as a fraction. For example, 5/5 means that the patient reached 5 out of a possible 5 on the muscle strength scale.

• WORD • BUILDING •
synovitis: synovia—joint + itis—inflammation

Psychosocial Data Collection

Deformities resulting from arthritis or other musculoskeletal disorders can affect a patient's body image and self-concept and result in social withdrawal (see Chapter 46). Chronic pain may keep the patient from working or socializing. Data collection should include questions related to the psychological effects of the musculoskeletal disorder.

Patients may experience a tremendous amount of psychological stress resulting from the withdrawal from friends and family, pain, and loss of income. Assess the patient's ability to cope, asking what coping strategies have been used in the past for other life stressors and support systems for the patient. As needed, consult the appropriate member of the health care team (social work, clergy, support groups) to ensure that the patient's psychosocial needs are being met.

CRITICAL THINKING

Mr. O'Donnell

■ Mr. O'Donnell, age 80, is brought to the emergency department with a fractured left hip. He is positioned for comfort while you collect data.

1. What information should you obtain in Mr. O'Donnell's history?
2. What should be assessed in Mr. O'Donnell's physical examination?

Suggested answers at end of chapter.

DIAGNOSTIC TESTS FOR THE MUSCULOSKELETAL SYSTEM

Diagnosis of musculoskeletal problems is assisted by laboratory tests and diagnostic imaging (Tables 45.4 and 45.5). Specific tests for connective tissue diseases are described in Chapter 46.

Laboratory Tests

Calcium and Phosphorus

Bone disorders commonly cause changes in calcium and phosphorus (or phosphate) levels. In a healthy person, calcium and phosphorus have an inverse relationship. This means that when serum calcium increases, serum phosphorus decreases, and vice versa. Some disorders, however, cause an increase in both values or a decrease in both values. Calcium and phosphorous levels are regulated by calcitonin from the thyroid gland and parathyroid hormone from the parathyroid glands. When these glands are not functioning properly, alterations in calcium and phosphorous levels can occur.

Serum calcium tends to decrease in patients with osteoporosis or in people who consume inadequate amounts

TABLE 45.4 DIAGNOSTIC LABORATORY TESTS FOR THE MUSCULOSKELETAL SYSTEM

Test	Normal Value	Significance of Abnormal Findings
Calcium	8.5–10.5 mg/dL	Hypercalcemia—may be related to metastatic bone disease or extended immobilization. Hypocalcemia—may be due to poor dietary intake. Can ultimately lead to rickets in a child or osteomalacia (bone softening) or osteoporosis in the elderly.
Phosphorus	2.6–4.5 mg/dL	Usually evaluated with serum calcium. A number of disorders can be associated with high or low serum phosphorus.
Alkaline phosphatase (ALP)	*Male:* 45–115 units/L *Female:* 30–100 units/L	ALP increases may indicate bone abnormality (examples: Paget's disease, metastatic bone cancer). ALP is increased when new bone is formed.
Myoglobin	50–120 mcg/mL	Increased myoglobin can indicate MI or skeletal muscle destruction.
Creatine kinase (CK)	*Male:* 60–400 units/L *Female:* 40–150 units/L	IM injections can cause increase in CK.
Isoenzyme CK3 (MM)	95%–100%	High levels indicate need for further testing for muscle disease. Can be used as a screening test for malignant hyperthermia. Will be increased in rhabdomyolysis.
Uric acid	*Male:* 4.4–7.6 mg/dL *Female:* 2.3–6.6 mg/dL	Elevated serum levels indicate gout.

TABLE 45.5 DIAGNOSTIC PROCEDURES FOR THE MUSCULOSKELETAL SYSTEM

Procedure	Definition	Significance of Abnormal Findings	Nursing Management (if applicable)
Noninvasive			
Standard X-Rays	Visualization of skeletal abnormality or deformity. Can also be used to visualize dense or inflamed tissues and joints.	Aids in treatment plan and provides additional information for care. Example: Broken ribs demand increased attention to respiratory system.	Inform patient of what to expect during ordered procedures.
Computed Tomography	Radiographic "slices" of bone or soft tissue. Provides a better image.		Check for allergies to contrast medium. Patient should have nothing by mouth (NPO) for 4 hours before test.
Magnetic Resonance Imaging (MRI)	Electromagnets provide a three-dimensional visualization of the area. Produces the best image available.		
Ultrasonography	Visualizes bone or soft tissue using sound waves.		Inform the patient that the jelly-like conducting substance will feel cold when applied.
Nerve Conduction Studies	Electromyography (EMG) is the electrical testing of nerves and muscles.	Alterations usually indicate a problem with the nerves or the muscles.	Explain that there may be some discomfort during nerve and muscle stimulation as well as when the needles are inserted (if needed).

TABLE 45.5 DIAGNOSTIC PROCEDURES FOR THE MUSCULOSKELETAL SYSTEM—cont'd

Procedure	Definition	Significance of Abnormal Findings	Nursing Management (if applicable)
Invasive			
Arthrography	Air or a contrast medium is injected into a synovial joint which is then x-rayed.	Aids in the diagnosis of joint abnormalities.	Inform patient that the test is uncomfortable during injection. Joint swelling is common after the procedure. Apply ice and elevate limb. Discourage physical activity for 12 to 24 hours after procedure.
Myelogram	Visualizes the spine and spinal cord after injection of a contrast medium.		Assess for headache and nausea post-procedure. Maximum head raise is 45 degrees for at least 3 hours post-procedure (or as ordered).
Nuclear Medicine Scans	A radioisotope is injected to help visualize bone and other soft tissue abnormalities.	Finding a "hot spot" usually indicates metastases or bone infection.	Inform patient that the test is not dangerous. Inform patient that the test may take up to 90 minutes.
Gallium/Thallium Scans	A radioactive element is injected that migrates to bone, brain, breast, and inflammatory tissue.		Check if your facility recommends that children and pregnant women stay a few feet away from the patient for the first 48 hr.
Arthroscopy	Provides direct visualization of a joint and its capsule using an instrument inserted into the joint space.		Assess color, warmth, circulation, and movement often. Monitor patient for complications. Apply ice, and keep limb elevated to minimize swelling (if ordered).
Arthrocentesis	Involves the withdrawal of synovial fluid from a joint space. Used for analysis of synovial fluid or reduction of excess fluid pressure.		Monitor patient for infection, inflammation, or hemarthrosis.
Bone or Muscle Biopsy	Involves needle aspiration (closed) or surgical extraction (open) of bone or muscle tissue.		Monitor site of biopsy for bleeding. Provide normal wound care for open biopsy. Perform neurovascular assessments as needed.

of calcium in their diets. Serum calcium levels increase in patients with bone cancer, particularly those with metastatic disease.

Alkaline Phosphatase

Alkaline phosphatase (ALP) is an enzyme that increases when bone or liver tissue is damaged. In metabolic bone diseases and bone cancer, ALP increases to reflect osteoblast (bone-forming cell) activity.

Myoglobin

Myoglobin is a protein found in striated (skeletal or cardiac) muscle. It is what causes the red color of muscle. When skeletal or cardiac muscle is damaged, myoglobin levels rise in the blood.

Muscle Enzymes

When muscle tissue is damaged, a number of serum enzymes are released into the bloodstream, including skeletal muscle creatine kinase (CK-MM [CK3]), aldolase (ALD), aspartate aminotransferase (AST), and lactate dehydrogenase (LDH). These enzymes increase in certain muscle diseases such as muscular dystrophy, polymyositis, and dermatomyositis.

Uric Acid

Uric acid is normally found in blood. Gout can occur when there is precipitation of uric acid crystals on tendons, articular cartilage of joints, and in other tissues. **Gout** is a type of arthritis. Patients with gout often report joint pain, especially in the great toe or knee.

LEARNING TIP

Rhabdomyolysis is a very serious and potentially fatal condition associated with muscle destruction due to such things as injury (especially crushing), high fever, convulsions, or prolonged muscle compression (such as from lying in a coma). The patient can have creatine kinase (CK) levels greater than five times normal. If the patient suffered muscle destruction, look at the CK, myoglobin, and serum potassium levels to assess for rhabdomyolysis; the three laboratory values will be elevated due to their release from the damaged muscle cells.

Radiographic Tests

SAFETY TIP

For any radiographic test requiring injection or instillation of a medication or contrast solution, it is important for the nurse to assess for allergies or untoward responses resulting from previous examinations or exposures. Many of the contrast mediums used have alternate substances available in case of allergies. If the patient is unable to do so, then it is the nurse's responsibility to inform the technologist of the allergies or previous adverse responses experienced by the patient.

Standard X-Rays

An x-ray examination can determine bone density, texture, changes in alignment and bone relationship, erosion, swelling, and intactness. In addition, x-ray examinations can be useful in identifying certain soft tissue damage (e.g., ligaments and tendons) because of alterations in bone position and spacing. Patients should be informed that they will have to lie still during the examination and that the x-ray table will be cold and hard.

Computed Tomography

Tomograms are radiographs that focus on a particular slice of bone or soft tissue, such as ligaments and tendons. Computed tomography (CT) is especially helpful for diagnosing problems of the joints or vertebral column (Fig. 45.6). It may be used with or without a contrast medium (similar to a dye), which is given orally or intravenously. Often, a CT scan is ordered when x-rays are inconclusive for injury despite continued symptoms; such as with pelvic fractures or following severe trauma.

Inform patients that they must lie completely still during the test and that they will be surrounded by the scanner during the test. Headphones are worn for communication with the technician and to listen to soothing music of the patient's choice.

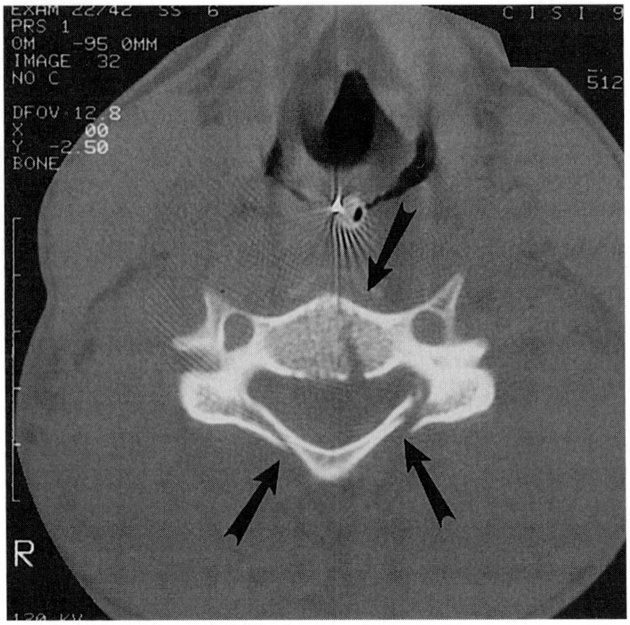
PRS 1
OM -95 0MM
IMAGE 32
NO C
512
R

FIGURE 45.6 Computed tomography scan of fifth cervical vertebra showing a burst fracture of the vertebral body (top arrow) and both laminae (bottom arrows). (From McKinnis, L. N. [2005]. *Fundamentals of musculoskeletal imaging* [2nd ed., p. 164]. Philadelphia: F. A. Davis, with permission.)

Bone Density Screening

A bone density test measures both bone strength and weight-bearing abilities. A special x-ray process, dual-energy x-ray absorptiometry (DEXA), is used to measure bone density. Osteoporosis, a disorder characterized by bone loss that exceeds bone formation, can lead to less dense and more porous bone structure. A decrease in bone density can lead to fractures.

Arthrography

An x-ray examination of any synovial joint can be performed for patients with suspected joint trauma. The most common joints tested are the knee and shoulder.

Myelogram

During a myelogram, a contrast medium is injected into the subarachnoid space so that the spine and spinal cord can be visualized. Inform patients that they may be positioned head down for a short period to allow the contrast medium to flow up to the level of the neck. This test is usually reserved for those patients unable to have a CT or MRI or for complicated spinal surgery revisions

Other Diagnostic Tests

Magnetic Resonance Imaging

Magnetic resonance imaging (MRI), with or without contrast media, is a commonly performed test to diagnose musculoskeletal problems, especially those involving soft tissue (Fig. 45.7). MRI is more accurate than CT for

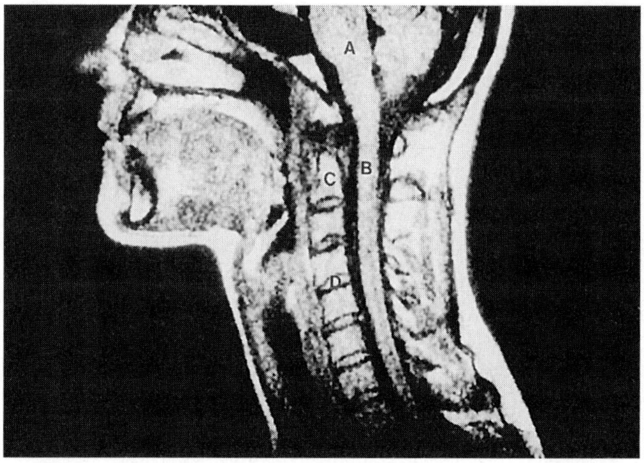
A
B
C
D

FIGURE 45.7 Magnetic resonance image of a normal cervical spine. (A) Cerebellum. (B) Spinal cord. (C) Marrow of C2 vertebral body. (D) C4-5 intervertebral disk. (From McKinnis, L. N. [1997]. *Fundamentals of orthopedic radiology* [p. 26]. Philadelphia: F. A. Davis, with permission.)

diagnosing many problems of the vertebral column. If the patient has had previous spinal surgery, a contrast medium is used.

The image is produced by interaction of magnetic fields and radio waves. For very large patients or those who are claustrophobic, the open MRI can offer a comfortable alternative to the traditional machine (Box 45.2, *Patient Perspective*).

The use of an electromagnet in the machine requires the removal of anything metal or with metal components, such as body piercings, from the patient's body. Pacemakers, surgical clips, and any other internally implanted metal device or apparatus are contraindications for MRI.

SAFETY TIP

Check with the facility where the MRI will take place for all contraindications for metal implants within a person's body to prevent injury to the patient.

Nuclear Medicine Scans

Several tests are performed using radioactive material to help visualize bone and other tissues. A bone scan allows visualization of the entire skeleton. The patient is injected with a radioisotope 2 to 3 hours before the scan. The radioisotope is attracted to bone and therefore travels to bone tissue. If the bone scan is ordered to assess for bone infection (osteomyelitis), a picture will be taken immediately after the first injection. Then a second series is done 2 to 3 hours later, once the radioisotope has collected in the bone.

For an accurate test, the patient must be able to lie still for up to 90 minutes during scanning. Patients who are elderly, restless, agitated, or in pain may therefore find this test uncomfortable. Sedatives or analgesics may have to be administered before or during the procedure. Patients need to be instructed to remove all jewelry before testing.

The physician looks for "hot spots," which indicate areas where the radioactive substance is concentrated. These hot spots indicate abnormal bone metabolism, a sign of bone disease.

Box 45.2

Patient Perspective

Emily: Undergoing an MRI

The nurse told me that the MRI scanner could cause feelings of claustrophobia. I am not claustrophobic, but I decided to keep my eyes closed during the test to be sure to prevent these feelings. I shut my eyes and imagined myself walking on my favorite beach. The cool air that was blowing in the machine I imagined to be the wind blowing. That air really is essential in keeping you cool and the claustrophobic feeling away. I had on headphones through which music was playing. I focused on the music as I "walked on the beach." Through the headphones the technician kept me informed of how much longer the test would be. This really helped. I knew that I had to be very still for the test, so I gave myself pep talks: "Only 10 more minutes. Lie still and this will be over soon."

Then, halfway through the MRI, I accidentally opened my eyes for an instant. "Uh, oh." I quickly shut them again with a feeling of panic rising. The wall of the MRI machine was only inches from my face! I quickly told myself I could get through this and focused on calming myself down by "going back to the beach." Before I knew it, the test was over and I was told that because I held so still it was a great test that went more quickly than usual. I sure was glad to hear that! My personal coping techniques really helped me through the MRI so that I could complete the test. Providing information to your patients on what to expect during the test, as well as coping methods to use, can help them successfully complete an MRI.

LEARNING TIP

Hot spots are created because increased circulation occurs in abnormal bone areas, resulting in increased amounts of the radioactive substance being transported to the abnormal area by the circulation.

Gallium/Thallium Scans

A gallium or thallium scan is similar to a bone scan but is more specific and sensitive as a diagnostic test. Gallium not only migrates to bone but also to brain and breast tissues and is therefore used to diagnose problems in these tissues as well.

Traditionally used for heart problems, thallium is now used for evaluation of bone cancers. Thallium is best for detecting osteosarcoma. Like the bone scan, these scans are not harmful to the patient.

Arthroscopy

An arthroscope allows the surgeon to directly visualize a joint. The knee and shoulder are the joints most often evaluated. Because **arthroscopy** is an invasive procedure performed under local or light general anesthesia, the patient is treated as a surgical candidate.

Arthroscopy is done in same-day surgery settings. The surgeon makes several small incisions and distends the joint with injected saline. The scope is inserted and the joint is visualized from different angles. The joint is moved through range of motion, so tears, defects, or other soft tissue damage can be assessed and/or repaired through the scope using special instrumentation. Depending on the extent of the procedure, a bulky or small dressing wrapped with an elastic bandage may be applied.

The nurse in the postanesthesia care unit (PACU) assesses the neurovascular status of the surgical limb frequently (see Table 45.3). If the patient had a diagnostic arthroscopy and no surgical repair, the PACU nurse encourages the patient to exercise the leg, including straight-leg raises. A mild analgesic usually relieves pain, and the patient returns to regular activities in 24 to 48 hours. If a surgical repair was performed, the patient may have activity restriction and need a stronger analgesic, such as oxycodone with acetaminophen (Tylox, Percocet).

Although complications are not common, monitor and teach the patient to watch for and report to the physician the following:

- Thrombophlebitis (blood clot and vein inflammation)
- Infection (fever or warmth, pain, redness, swelling at surgical site)
- Increased joint pain.

If a repair was done during the surgery, the patient is seen by the physician in 1 week to check for complications and progress. The patient may need crutches for the first week to limit weight bearing, depending on the surgical procedure performed. Physical or occupational therapy may be ordered (see *Home Health Hints*).

• WORD • BUILDING •

arthroscopy: arthro—joint + scopy—to examine

Home Health Hints

- When visiting a patient at home, the nurse needs to determine if the patient is homebound. Patients are considered homebound if (1) they are bedbound or require maximum assistance to ambulate while using a walker or to transfer, (2) they can ambulate with only moderate assistance while using a cane to negotiate uneven surfaces, or (3) they can leave home only for periods of relatively short duration or when in need of medical treatment. If it is determined that the patient is not homebound, then services such as physical and occupational therapy can be performed in an outpatient setting.
- When testing strength, extend two or three fingers and ask the patient to squeeze the fingers. Deficits in arm strength can be easily detected using this simple method.
- Observe patients moving around a room or bed. If they are clumsy or have involuntary movement, make efforts during that visit and later visits to protect them from potential injury. Research has shown that pain or fear of falling may prevent a patient from moving and functioning to maximum potential.
- Use sand or cat box filler on icy steps to increase traction, preventing slips and falls.

CRITICAL THINKING

Mrs. Gardenio

■ Mrs. Gardenio was walking down the street when, without warning, she suddenly fell to the ground with extreme pain in her left leg. She was taken to the hospital, where it was determined that the greater trochanter of her left femur was fractured.

1. What information should you obtain from Mrs. Gardenio?
2. What possible condition may be the cause of her fracture?
3. What tests may be performed to identify the condition creating her problem?

Suggested answers at end of chapter.

Bone or Muscle Biopsy

Bone or muscle tissue can be surgically extracted for microscopic examination to confirm cancer, infection (bone biopsy), inflammation, or damage (muscle biopsy). Muscle can also be biopsied to diagnose malignant hyperthermia, a genetic disorder (see Chapter 12). Two techniques are used to retrieve muscle tissue: a needle (closed) biopsy or an incisional (open) biopsy.

A closed biopsy can be performed in the patient's room or special procedures area. After local or general anesthesia, the physician inserts a long needle into the tissue for extraction of a sample.

The open biopsy is performed in the operating suite under general anesthesia. A small incision is made and a section of bone or muscle is removed. A sterile pressure dressing is applied because bone is highly vascular.

The nurse inspects the biopsy site for bleeding, swelling, and hematoma formation. Increased pain that is unresponsive to analgesic medication may indicate bleeding in the soft tissue. The area is not moved for 8 to 12 hours to prevent bleeding. Vital signs and neurovascular assessments are monitored (see Table 45.3).

CRITICAL THINKING

Mr. Jablonski

■ Mr. Jablonski, age 45, comes to emergency with extreme pain in his lower back. The pain radiates down his right buttock and down the back of his leg to his knee. He tells you that he hurt his back picking up a box in the warehouse where he works.

1. What other information should you obtain from Mr. Jablonski?
2. What is a probable cause of Mr. Jablonski's pain?
3. What tests, procedures, and treatments may be done for Mr. Jablonski's condition?
4. How might this injury impact Mr. Jablonski's life?
5. Mr. Jablonski is to receive morphine 10 mg by intramuscular injection. You have available morphine 15 mg/mL. How many milliliters will you give?

Suggested answers at end of chapter.

Ultrasonography

Sound waves are used to detect osteomyelitis (bone infection), soft tissue disorders, traumatic joint injuries, and surgical hardware placement. The technologist applies a jelly-like conducting substance over the area to be tested. A transducer is moved over the area while the ultrasound machine records the images.

Arthrocentesis

Arthrocentesis is a diagnostic or therapeutic procedure in which synovial fluid is aspirated from a joint for analysis or to relieve pressure (pain) from effusion. This fluid buildup often occurs secondary to an inflammatory process such as bursitis. Analysis of the synovial fluid can also aid in the diagnosis of noninflammatory conditions, septic arthritis, crystal detection, and **hemarthrosis** (blood in the joint cavity). In addition, the removal of fluid will decrease pain and improve mobility.

Using aseptic technique, the physician provides local anesthetic and then uses a needle to aspirate the contents of the joint space. The fluid can then be sent to the lab to evaluate for infection and/or inflammation. If required, the physician will also instill medications such as a corticosteroid, an anti-inflammatory, or an antibiotic. The site is covered with a sterile dressing to prevent infection.

Nursing considerations following the test include monitoring the injection site for increased bruising, bleeding, redness, and warmth.

Nerve Conduction Studies

Electromyography (EMG) measures a muscle's electrical impulses. This aids in the diagnosis of muscle diseases or nerve damage, which may follow a traumatic injury. An indication of nerve damage is limited return of muscle function following injury resolution. Inform the patient what will occur, and instruct the patient to not apply lotions before the test and to remove all jewelry. Occasionally, slight discomfort and bruising occurs at the site where the study occurred. Warm compresses or mild analgesics can be offered for pain relief (see Table 45.5).

SUGGESTED ANSWERS TO

CRITICAL THINKING

■ *Mr. O'Donnell*

1. Determine if Mr. O'Donnell has any allergies, how and when the injury occurred, if he has had any previous surgeries, what medications he takes, his medical history, and any past problems with anesthesia (in Mr. O'Donnell or his family).
2. Inspect his left leg in comparison to his right leg, including limb length, deformity, pain, loss of range of motion, edema, and ecchymosis. Perform neurovascular checks, including movement, sensation (numbness/tingling), presence of pulses, skin temperature, color, and capillary refill.

■ *Mrs. Gardenio*

1. Assess Mrs. Gardenio's age, her diet (does she have a low-calcium or vitamin D–deficient diet?), what she was doing at the time of the break, whether anything like this has happened before, whether anything

SUGGESTED ANSWERS TO—cont'd

similar has happened to any of her relatives, her pain level, when she ate last, her medications, her medical history, whether she smokes, and whether she has any allergies.

2. Mrs. Gardenio may have osteoporosis that has resulted in a pathological fracture from decreased bone density. This is common in postmenopausal women.
3. X-ray examinations, bone scans, bone density tests, and laboratory tests such as serum calcium, phosphorus, acid phosphatase, thyroid, and vitamin D levels are tests that might be performed.

■ *Mr. Jablonski*

1. Determine what occurred, when it occurred, how it happened, if the pain was immediate, where exactly the pain is, whether anything makes it better or worse, if any kind of treatment was started, what kind of job Mr. O'Donnell has, whether he has had any back problems in the past, what medications he is on, and whether he has any allergies.
2. Mr. Jablonski may have ruptured a vertebral disk, which can happen with improper lifting or trying to lift something too heavy.
3. Testing might include x-ray examination, MRI, bone scan, CT scan, or myelogram. Conservative treatment will be attempted first, but ultimately a diskectomy may be needed.
4. Many back injuries result in lifelong chronic pain. Depending on the severity of the injury and the effectiveness of therapy, Mr. Jablonski may have to limit his physical and social activities. He may also have to find another type of employment.
5. Unit analysis method:

$$\frac{10\ \cancel{\text{mg}}}{} \Bigg| \frac{1\ \text{mL}}{15\ \cancel{\text{mg}}} = \frac{10}{15} = 0.67\ \text{mL}$$

REVIEW QUESTIONS

1. Which of the following is the function of synovial fluid in joints?
   a. Exchange nutrients.
   b. Prevent friction.
   c. Absorb water.
   d. Wear away rough surfaces.

2. A patient has been diagnosed with a musculoskeletal disease that causes decreased bone density. Which assessment questions are most appropriate by the nurse? **Select all that apply.**
   a. "Do you have any broken bones?"
   b. "Has your doctor informed you not to exercise so you will not break a bone?"
   c. "What forms of physical activity are you able to participate in?"
   d. "Do any of your spouse's relatives have problems with their bones?"
   e. "Do you exercise regularly?"
   f. "What is typically included in your daily diet?"

3. Which of the following assessments is included in neurovascular checks of the lower extremities?
   a. Radial pulses
   b. Checking for clubbing
   c. Biceps reflex
   d. Pedal pulses

4. A patient is scheduled for an MRI of the pelvis. Which of the following would the nurse do if during data collection the nurse found out that the patient had had a previous surgery for heart problems?
   a. Ask if there is any metal in the patient's body.
   b. Order a chest x-ray to identify metal objects.
   c. Cancel the MRI.
   d. Inform the physician.

5. A patient has undergone an arthroscopy. Two hours after the procedure, the patient's pedal pulses are diminished from the previous assessment. What should the nurse do?
   a. Take vital signs.
   b. Notify the physician.
   c. Perform neurovascular assessment in 30 minutes.
   d. Change the dressing and rewrap the elastic wrap.

46

Nursing Care of Patients with Musculoskeletal and Connective Tissue Disorders

KELLY ANN MORRIS AND
LINDA S. WILLIAMS

KEY TERMS

arthritis (ar-THRYE-tiss)
arthroplasty (AR-throw-PLAS-tee)
avascular necrosis (a-VAS-cue-lar neh-KROW-siss)
fasciotomy (fash-ee-OTT-oh-mee)
hemipelvectomy (heh-mee-pell-VEC-tuh-mee)
hyperuricemia (HYE-purr-yoor-eh-SEE-mee-ah)
osteogenesis imperfecta (AWS-TEE-oh-geh-nih-siss im-purr-FEC-tah)
osteomyelitis (AWS-tee-oh-my-eh-LEYE-tiss)
osteosarcoma (AWS-tee-oh-sar-KOH-mah)
polymyositis (PAW-lee-my-oh-SYE-tiss)
replantation (ree-plan-TAY-shun)
scleroderma (SKLER-uh-DER-mah)
synovitis (sin-oh-VYE-tiss)
vasculitis (VAS-kyoo-LYE-tiss)

QUESTIONS TO GUIDE YOUR READING

1. What are the pathophysiology, signs and symptoms, and complications of fractures?
2. Which nursing interventions are appropriate when caring for a patient in a cast or traction?
3. What are the causes of, prevention measures, and nursing care for osteomyelitis?
4. What are the risk factors, pathophysiology, treatment, and nursing care for osteoporosis?
5. What is the pathophysiology, signs and symptoms, treatment, and nursing care for Paget's disease?
6. What are the pathophysiology, treatment, and nursing care for gout?
7. Which nursing interventions are appropriate when caring for patients with systemic lupus erythematosus, scleroderma, and polymyositis?
8. How would the care for osteoarthritis and rheumatoid arthritis be differentiated?
9. What would be included when preparing a plan of care for the patient with a fractured hip or undergoing a total joint replacement?
10. What patient education would be included for a patient with a lower extremity amputation and prosthesis?

BONE AND SOFT TISSUE DISORDERS

The musculoskeletal system is the second largest system in the body. A variety of injuries and diseases can affect bone, soft tissue, or both. Common problems are discussed in this section.

Strains

A strain is a soft tissue injury that occurs when a muscle or tendon is excessively stretched. Causes of strains include falls, excessive exercise, and lifting heavy items without using proper body mechanics. Back and ankle injuries are common. Strains can be mild, moderate, or severe. A mild strain causes minimal inflammation; swelling and tenderness are present. A moderate strain involves partial tearing of the muscle or tendon fibers. Pain and inability to move the affected body part result. The most severe strain occurs when a muscle or tendon is ruptured, with separation of muscle from muscle, tendon from muscle, or tendon from bone. Severe pain and disability result from this injury.

RICE is an acronym for rest, ice, compression, and elevation. These four components are the basis of therapy for strain injuries. Immediately after a strain, the injured area should be **R**ested to protect it. **I**ce should be applied to decrease pain, swelling, and inflammation. Applying an elastic bandage for **C**ompression and **E**levating the affected area (if appropriate) provide support and minimize swelling. Once inflammation subsides, heat application (15 to 30 minutes four times a day) brings increased blood flow to the injured area for healing. Activity is limited (depending on the severity of the injury, casting may even be required for immobilization) until the soft tissue heals, and anti-inflammatory drugs are prescribed. Muscle relaxants may also be used. Exercise may begin as early as 2 to 5 days after the injury depending on the severity of the injury; in some cases, it may take 1 to 3 weeks of immobility before exercise can begin. For more severe strains, surgery to repair the tear or rupture may be needed. These procedures are done on an ambulatory, same-day-surgery basis.

Sprains

A sprain is excessive stretching of one or more ligaments that usually results from twisting movements during a sports activity, exercise, or fall. Like strains, sprains also vary in severity. A mild sprain involves tearing of just a few ligament fibers and causes tenderness. In a moderate sprain, more fibers are torn but the stability of the joint is not affected. A moderate sprain is uncomfortable, especially with activity. A severe sprain causes instability of the joint and usually requires surgical intervention for tissue repair or grafting. Pain and inflammation prevent mobility.

For mild sprains, RICE is used for several days until swelling and pain diminish. Anti-inflammatory drugs are also used to decrease inflammation and control pain. Moderate sprains may need immobilization with a brace or cast until healing occurs.

Dislocations

Dislocations are a common injury in which the ends of the bones are forced from their normal position. They are usually caused by trauma as in falls or contact sports or by a disease such as rheumatoid arthritis. Any joint, large or small, may become dislocated. Severe pain along with lost range of motion of the joint and joint deformity occurs. Immediate medical treatment is required to preserve function. Splint the extremity as it is found, apply ice, and seek help. Do not move the extremity because blood vessels, muscles, and nerves could be damaged.

> **NURSING CARE TIP**
>
> For patients with disease processes that could result in a dislocation or fracture, careful moving is essential. It is important to use lift sheets when moving a patient rather than pulling on the patient's arms to avoid injury. Always follow institutional policy for moving patients to avoid patient injury and liability for a patient's injury.

Bursitis

Bursae (fluid-filled sacs) cushion tendons during movement to prevent friction between the bone and tendon. Several joints have bursae (shoulder, elbow, hip, knee, ankle, heel). Inflammation of a bursa, called bursitis, occurs from arthritis, gout, repetitive movement, or sleeping on one's side, which compresses the shoulder bursa. Prevention is key because bursitis may become harder to cure over time. To protect the bursae and prevent compression, teach patients to stretch and strengthen muscles, move frequently, avoid repetitive movements for long periods, use cushioned seats, and avoid leaning on the elbows.

Symptoms of bursitis include achy pain, stiffness, or burning pain over the joint area that worsens with activity. Usually pain decreases in about a week. The condition can become chronic if it lasts more than 6 months. Treatment includes resting the joint, application of ice 20 minutes several times per day until joint warmth is gone, then switching to heat, elevating the joint, ultrasound, massage, nonsteroidal anti-inflammatory drugs (NSAIDs), or physical therapy.

Rotator Cuff Injury

Short tendons that are connected to muscles around the shoulder form the rotator cuff. The cuff covers the top, front, and back of the shoulder. Muscle contraction causes these tendons to tighten and move or rotate the shoulder. Various injuries can occur. The top tendon of the cuff (supraspinatus tendon) and bursa may become impinged in the narrow space under the acromion bone. This causes inflammation when the arm is repeatedly moved forward, and pain results. This is known as chronic impingement syndrome. Over time the tendon may finally tear from the bone.

Symptoms of rotator cuff injury include shoulder aching, increased pain with lifting the arm, pain that is greater at night, weakness, and sometimes limited range of motion. Magnetic resonance imaging (MRI) is used to diagnose rotator cuff injury. For minor injury, resting the shoulder, NSAIDs, ice, and physical therapy are recommended. For a more severe injury, arthroscopic and/or small-incision surgery may be needed to relieve the impingement or repair the tear. A sling or special brace is worn after surgery. Physical therapy for rehabilitation after surgery is used.

Carpal Tunnel Syndrome

Pathophysiology

Carpal tunnel syndrome results in the compression of the median nerve within the carpal tunnel when swelling in the tunnel occurs. This swelling can result from edema, trauma, rheumatoid arthritis, or repetitive hand movements (repetitive motion injury) as used in some occupations such as typing or cash register operation.

Signs and Symptoms

Carpal tunnel syndrome usually results in slow-onset finger, hand, and arm pain and numbness. Painful tingling and paresthesias may also be present. Eventually, fine motor deficits and then muscle weakness may develop.

Diagnostic Tests

Diagnosis is based on signs and symptoms, along with the patient's history. A positive Phalen's test (numbness with wrist flexion) is indicative of carpal tunnel syndrome. Electromyography (EMG) can also be used to detect nerve abnormalities.

Therapeutic Measures

Medical treatment focuses on relieving the inflammation and resting the wrist. A splint is often ordered for the patient to wear. Medications to reduce pain and inflammation are ordered, such as aspirin and NSAIDs. Cortisone may be injected into the carpal tunnel to decrease pain and inflammation.

For some patients, surgery may be necessary. The surgeon may use an open incision or may perform an endoscopy. The median nerve is released from compression during the surgery, thus correcting the problem of the nerve and the surrounding area becoming inflamed. Physiotherapy helps in the recovery of function.

Nursing Care

Educate the patient on methods to prevent carpal tunnel syndrome, such as frequent short breaks during the workday, interspersing ongoing tasks with repetitive movements throughout the day, and using ergonomically appropriate devices to minimize the pressure placed in the area of the wrist.

Provide pain relief as ordered, and if surgery is performed, provide routine preoperative and postoperative care. Postoperatively, elevate the patient's hand and instruct the patient on use of a splint as ordered for up to 2 weeks. Lifting is restricted for several weeks. The patient is taught to report signs and symptoms of neurovascular compromise, such as numbness and tingling, coolness, lack of pulse, pale skin or nailbeds, or limited movement. The patient may need family assistance with activities of daily living (ADLs).

Fractures

A fracture is a break in a bone and can occur at any age and in any bone. Some fractures are minor and are treated on an ambulatory basis; others are more complex and require surgical intervention with hospitalization and rehabilitation.

Pathophysiology

Bone is a dynamic, changing tissue. When it is broken, the body immediately begins to repair the injury (Fig. 46.1). For an adult, within 48 to 72 hours after the injury, a hematoma (blood clot) forms at the fracture site because bone has a rich blood supply. Various cells that begin the healing process are attracted to the damaged bone. In about a week or so, a non-bony union called a callus develops and can be seen on x-ray examination. As healing continues, osteoclasts (bone-destroying cells) resorb any necrotic bone, and osteoblasts (bone-building cells) make new bone as a replacement. This process is referred to as bone remodeling. Young, healthy adult bone completely heals in about 6 weeks; however, it can take up to a year before the whole process of remodeling is complete. An older person takes longer to heal, and children tend to heal more quickly.

Adequate nutrition that includes vitamins, minerals, and protein is essential to heal fractures and keep the musculoskeletal system healthy (see Chapter 45).

Etiology and Types

The major reason for a fracture is trauma from a fall, an accident (usually motor vehicle), or a crushing injury. Bone disease (such as osteoporosis and metastatic bone cancer), malnutrition, and regular drinking of carbonated beverages with added phosphoric acid (which may interfere with calcium absorption) can lead to fractures as can various drugs (e.g., certain drugs used to treat human immunodeficiency [HIV] and endometriosis) that as a side effect cause a decrease in bone density. Fractures resulting from any of these diseases are referred to as pathological fractures. One of the most common types of fracture is the hip fracture, which occurs most frequently in middle-aged and older adult women who have osteoporosis (irreversible bone loss).

Fractures can be classified in several ways, including the extent of the fracture, the extent of the associated soft tissue damage, and the configuration of the bone after it breaks. In a complete fracture, the bone is broken into two separate pieces. Complete fractures have the potential to be life threatening because sharp bone fragments can sever blood vessels and nerves. In an incomplete fracture, the bone does not divide into two pieces. In a displaced fracture, the bone sections are out of alignment.

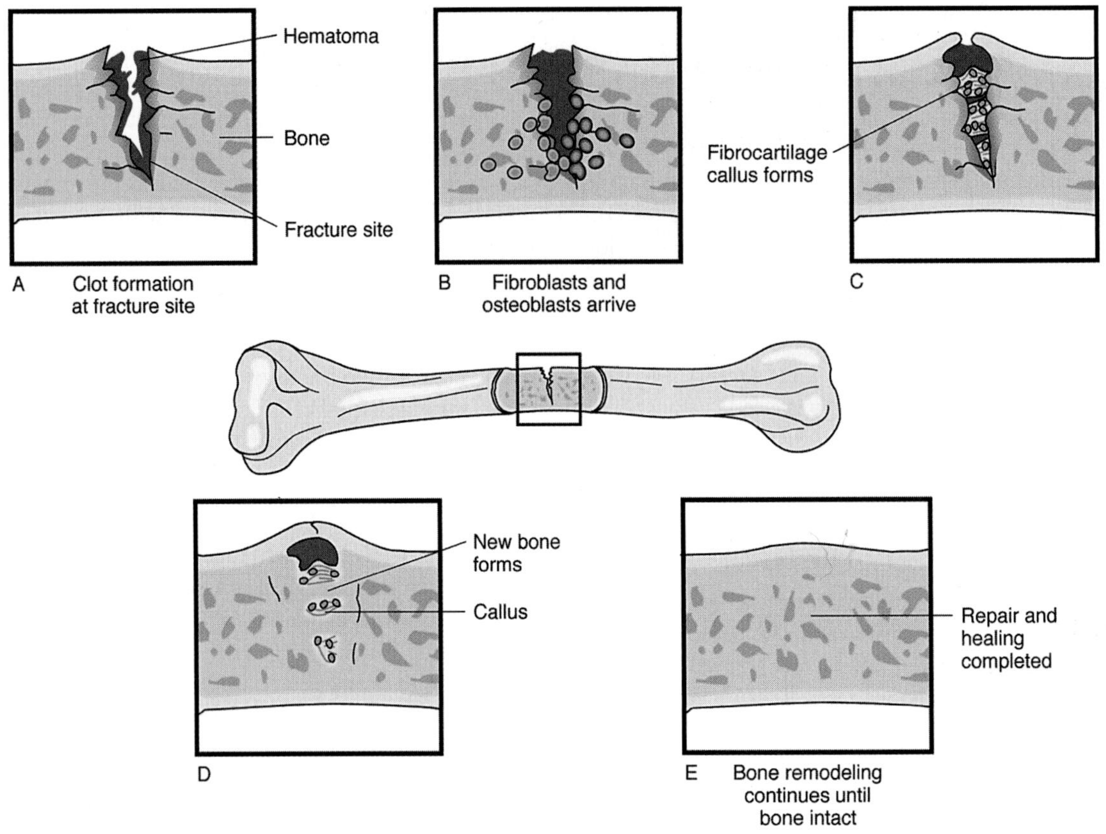
Hematoma
Bone
Fracture site
A Clot formation at fracture site
B Fibroblasts and osteoblasts arrive
Fibrocartilage callus forms
C
New bone forms
Callus
D
Repair and healing completed
E Bone remodeling continues until bone intact

FIGURE 46.1 Fracture healing phases.

A fracture can also be classified as open or closed. In an open (or compound) fracture, the bone breaks the skin. In a closed fracture, the bone does not disrupt the skin. Open fractures are more likely to become infected than closed fractures.

Another way to describe a fracture is by the way the bone breaks, such as in a spiral or oblique fashion (Fig. 46.2). These fractures may be open or closed, complete or incomplete. Table 46.1 describes the types of fractures.

Signs and Symptoms

This section focuses on fractures of upper and lower extremities. If the patient sustains a hairline (microscopic) fracture, the signs and symptoms are not readily observable. The patient may report tenderness over the site of the injury or more severe pain when moving the affected part of the body. The patient with a hip fracture usually experiences pain either in the groin area (the hip is a deep joint) or at the back of the knee (referred pain). If the fracture is complete, the limb is often shortened because of contraction of the muscles pulling on the bone sections.

In addition to pain, patients with more complex fractures experience limb rotation or deformity and shortening of the limb (if a limb bone is broken). Range of motion is decreased. If the affected part is moved, a continuous grating sound (crepitation) caused by bone fragments rubbing on each other may be heard. The extremity should not be moved (to try and reposition the bone alignment) if crepitation is present.

Inspect the skin for intactness. A patient with a closed fracture may have ecchymosis (bruising) over the fractured bone from bleeding into the soft underlying tissue. Ecchymosis may not develop for several days after the injury. Swelling may also be present and can impair blood flow, causing marked neurovascular compromise. In an open fracture, one or more bone ends pierce the skin, causing a wound, thus increasing the possibility of infection.

Diagnostic Tests

An x-ray examination usually visualizes bone fractures, showing bone malalignment or disruption. Computed tomography may be needed to help detect fractures of complex areas, such as the hip and pelvis. Magnetic resonance imaging is useful in determining the extent of associated soft tissue damage.

For patients with moderate to severe bleeding, a hemoglobin and hematocrit level is obtained. If soft tissue damage is extensive, the erythrocyte sedimentation rate (ESR) usually is elevated, indicating the expected inflammatory response. The physician may order a serum calcium level to determine baseline values because bone repair requires a sufficient amount of calcium and other minerals.

Emergency Treatment

A patient with a suspected fracture often has injuries elsewhere in the body. Observe the patient for respiratory distress, bleeding, and head or spine injury. If any of these

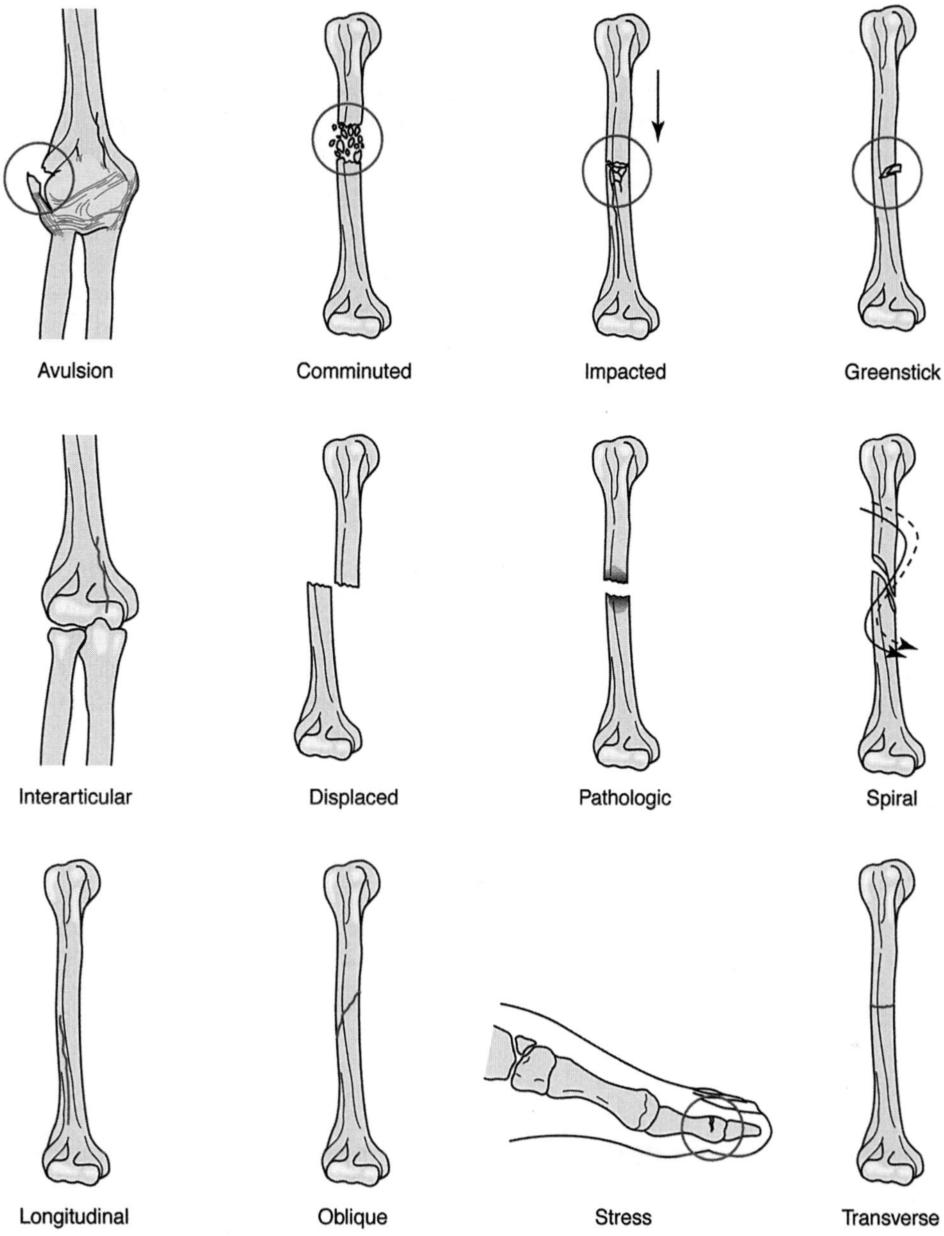
Avulsion
Comminuted
Impacted
Greenstick
Interarticular
Displaced
Pathologic
Spiral
Longitudinal
Oblique
Stress
Transverse

FIGURE 46.2 Types of fractures.

TABLE 46.1 TYPES OF FRACTURES

Fracture Type	Description
Avulsion	Piece of bone is torn away from the main bone while still attached to a ligament or tendon.
Comminuted	Bone splintered or shattered into numerous fragments. Often occurs in crushing injuries.
Impacted	Bone is forcibly pushed together, resulting in bone being pushed into bone.
Greenstick	Bone is bent and fractures on the outer arc of the bend. Often seen in children.
Interarticular	Fracture involves bones within a joint.
Displaced	Bone pieces are out of normal alignment. One or more pieces may be out of alignment.
Pathological (also called neoplastic)	Caused when bone is weakened either by pressure from a tumor or an actual tumor within the bone.
Spiral	Fracture curves around the shaft of the bone.
Longitudinal	Fracture occurs along the length of the bone.
Oblique	Fracture occurs diagonally or at an oblique angle across the bone.
Stress	Results in the bone being fractured across one cortex. This is an incomplete fracture.
Transverse	Bone fractured horizontally.
Depressed	Bone pushed inward. Often seen with skull and facial fractures.

problems occurs, emergency treatment is provided before concern is given to extremity or other fractures.

Treatment depends on the type and extent of the injury. Emergency treatment is essential to prevent possible life-threatening complications. Box 46.1 describes the emergency interventions for the patient with an extremity fracture.

LEARNING TIP

For emergency care of a suspected fracture, do not try to reposition the limb. Remember: Splint it as it lies. Also, ensure that the limb is secured above and below the break to minimize movement and bone grating.

Fracture Management

The goals of fracture management are reduction, or realignment, of bone ends; immobilization of the fractured bone (with bandages, casts, traction, or a fixation device); prevention of deformity or further injury; preservation or restoration of function; promotion of early healing; and pain relief.

CLOSED REDUCTION. Closed reduction is the most common treatment for simple fractures. While manually pulling on the bone (limb), the physician manipulates the bone ends into realignment. Analgesia and/or conscious sedation is typically used before the procedure. An x-ray examination is done to confirm that the bone ends are aligned before the area is immobilized.

Box 46.1

Urgent Management of Fractures

1. Immediately immobilize affected limb. If movement is required before splinting, support limb above and below fracture.
2. Unless there is bleeding, apply splints and padding above and below the fracture site, directly over the clothing. If bleeding is present, visualization may be needed before pressure can be applied where bleeding is originating. Keep patient covered to preserve body heat.
3. If the fractured extremity is a leg bone, the unaffected extremity can be used as a splint by bandaging both legs together. An arm can be bandaged to the chest or put into a sling to minimize further tissue damage.
4. Assess color, warmth, circulation, and movement (CWCM) of the limb distal to the fracture.
5. For an open fracture, the protruding bone should be covered with a clean (sterile preferred) dressing.
6. Do not attempt to straighten or realign a fractured extremity. Move the affected limb as little as necessary.
7. Transport to an emergency department as soon as possible.

BANDAGES AND SPLINTS. For some areas of the body, such as the clavicle or wrist, an elastic or muslin bandage or a splint may be used to immobilize the bone during the healing phase. Splints can be used when the fracture has some associated soft tissue damage that needs care or if there is an expectation of swelling. It is important for the splint to be well padded, thereby preventing skin breakdown or unnecessary pressure. Perform neurovascular assessments hourly (or as ordered) to monitor adequate blood flow to the area until the concern for swelling has passed, then typically every 2 to 4 hours (see Chapter 45).

CASTS. Casts provide a strong support for fractured bones, thereby aiding in early mobility and decreased pain. They are also used to correct deformities and to support weak joints while restricting movement. The type of cast used depends on the reason the cast is applied. For more extensive fractures or for weight-bearing areas, a rigid and durable cast is used for immobilization. Once the need for the cast is resolved (e.g., when bone healing is complete), the cast is removed.

Several types of materials are used for casts, including the traditional plaster of Paris (anhydrous calcium sulfate) and a variety of synthetic products such as fiberglass. Plaster is used for large casts and for weight-bearing areas. Because of a chemical reaction that occurs when the plaster is wet, the cast feels hot when applied for about 30 minutes and then feels cool, taking anywhere from 24 to 72 hours to completely dry. The cast is dry when it feels hard and firm, is odorless, and is shiny white. Keep the wet cast open to air, and turn the patient about every 2 hours to expose all sides of the cast to the air to aid in drying and to prevent mold growth. A wet cast should be handled with the palms of the hand ("palming the cast") to prevent indentations or a change in the shape of the cast (Fig. 46.3). This prevents the possibility of pressure points forming inside the cast. Unlike plaster of Paris, synthetic material casts such as fiberglass harden quickly and dry in less than 2 hours.

A casted limb is elevated for 24 to 48 hours, and ice can be applied over the injury to reduce swelling. Observe the cast for dryness, tightness, drainage, and odor. A serious complication of a cast being too tight is compartment syndrome (discussed later). If the cast becomes too tight, the physician orders it to be cut (bivalved) with a cast cutter to relieve pressure and prevent pressure necrosis of the underlying skin (Fig. 46.4). If a wound is present or an odor is detected, a window opening into the cast is created to treat the underlying skin problem, often an infected area. The cast window should always be taped in place when wound care is not being provided to prevent the skin from "popping up" through the window and developing pressure points and

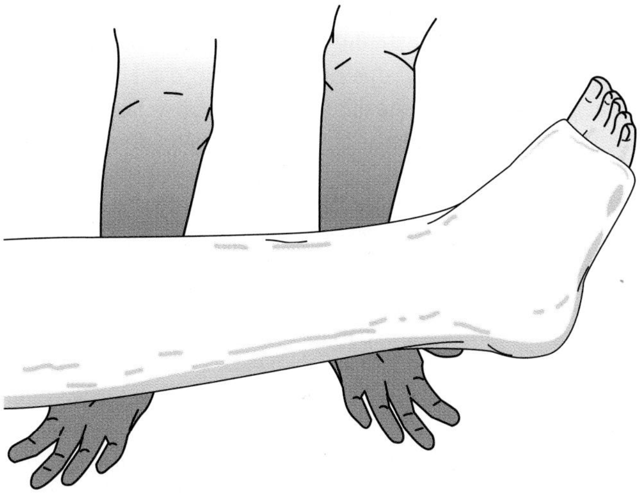

FIGURE 46.3 A wet plaster cast is moved with the palms of the hand to prevent making indentations in the plaster that could become pressure points.

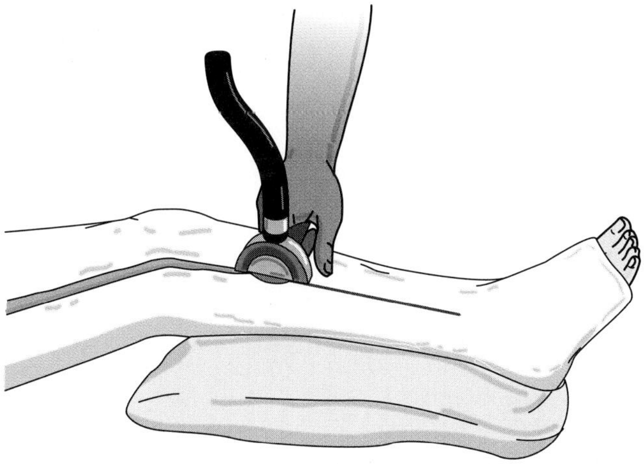

FIGURE 46.4 Bivalving a cast with a cast saw.

ischemia. Box 46.2 describes nursing interventions for a patient with a cast.

TRACTION. As a general definition, traction is the application of a pulling force to a part of the body to provide fracture reduction (positioning bone fragments in correct alignment), reduce movement, or relieve pain. Although still used in certain situations, improvements in surgical techniques and orthopedic devices have greatly decreased the use of traction.

Traction is classified as either continuous or intermittent. Continuous traction is required for fracture management. Intermittent traction, although not commonly used, may be used for patients with muscle spasm. Traction also can be performed manually for short periods of time (e.g., to maintain traction on a leg when removing Buck's traction for skin assessment or skin care).

The most common types of traction are either skin or skeletal. Skin traction typically involves the use of a Velcro

Box 46.2

Nursing Interventions for a Patient with a Cast

1. Assess color, warmth, circulation, and movement (CWCM) every 1 to 2 hours for 24 hours and then qid and prn.
   a. Assess cast for tightness (ask patient) and for rough or frayed edges (can interfere with skin integrity).
   b. Make sure patient can move (wiggle) all digits distal to the cast.
2. With newly applied casts (wet):
   a. Never grasp a wet cast to hold or move it, and do not place it on any surface that can cause an indentation. Use only the palms of the hands, because finger pressure on a wet cast can cause pressure points on the inside surface.
   b. Make sure patient is turned every 1 to 2 hours to prevent flattening of cast surface during drying.
   c. With hip spicas or any cast with an abductor bar, do not use bar to move limb or to help with turns.
   d. Inform patient that plaster casts give off heat when drying. Make sure cast air dries (may require 24 to 72 hours for complete drying). Do not cover cast or use drying aids such as blow dryers. Place cast on absorbent surfaces, not plasticized pillows.
   e. Protect skin integrity by ensuring rough edges of cast are properly covered.
   f. Make sure patient knows to keep cast dry during bathing by covering with plastic and preventing water from seeping into cast ends.
   g. Synthetic casts (e.g., fiberglass) can be exposed to water (e.g., for hydrotherapy) as needed but require complete drying afterward.
3. Maintain tissue integrity within the cast.
   a. When assessing CWCM, assess visible skin for signs of impaired integrity.
   b. Cast edges can be smoothed and covered with stockinettes or gauze and tape (make sure there are no tape allergies) to prevent rubbing of skin.
   c. Monitor for signs and symptoms of infection, such as foul odor, heat, redness, and pain.
   d. Do not use skin products on affected limb.
   e. Monitor visible blood on the surface of the cast. Outline area with a pen to observe for increasing size. Shadowing of blood not quite reaching the surface of the cast is fairly common but also should be circled and monitored.
   f. Never place any object inside the cast, and instruct patient not to do so. Explain the risk of skin damage.

boot (Buck's traction), sling (Russell's traction or knee sling), belt (pelvic), or halter, which is secured around a part of the body (Fig. 46.5). This type of traction does not promote bone alignment or healing but is used instead for relief of painful muscle spasms that often accompany fractures. Buck's traction is indicated for patients with hip fractures and is commonly applied to prevent further trauma while the patient waits for surgery. Occasionally, the patient's physical condition or inflammation around the fracture prohibits early surgical intervention, thus warranting application of skin (Buck's) traction. When traction is being applied to the skin, the amount of weight that can be applied is restricted. The weight applied usually is between 5 and 10 lb (2.2 to 4.5 kg).

Skeletal traction, also called balanced suspension, involves the use of pins (Steinmann), screws, wires (Kirschner), or tongs (Gardner-Wells, Crutchfield), which are surgically inserted into the bone for the purpose of alignment while the fracture heals (Fig. 46.6). From 20 to 40 lb (9 to 18 kg) of weight is usually applied for skeletal traction, as ordered.

Balanced suspension maintains traction while allowing the patient some mobility in bed. A Thomas (or T) splint with Pearson's attachment can be used to provide balanced suspension for the lower extremity. The patient's leg rests on a suspended sheepskin-covered splint (see Fig 46.6). Balanced traction methods require countertraction to ensure the patient does not move toward the pull and therefore minimize the effectiveness of the traction. Usually the patient's weight and elevating the foot of the bed provide the needed countertraction. An overbed frame with a trapeze bar allows the patient to move while in bed (see Fig. 46.6).

Traction must be maintained at all times when used for fracture alignment. Caring for the patient in traction includes monitoring neurovascular status frequently for impaired blood flow, checking the equipment to ensure proper functioning, and monitoring skin condition for pressure points or irritation from equipment. All knots, ropes, weights, and pulleys are inspected every 8 to 12 hours for any loosening and intactness. For active patients, the frequency of the traction checks may be increased.

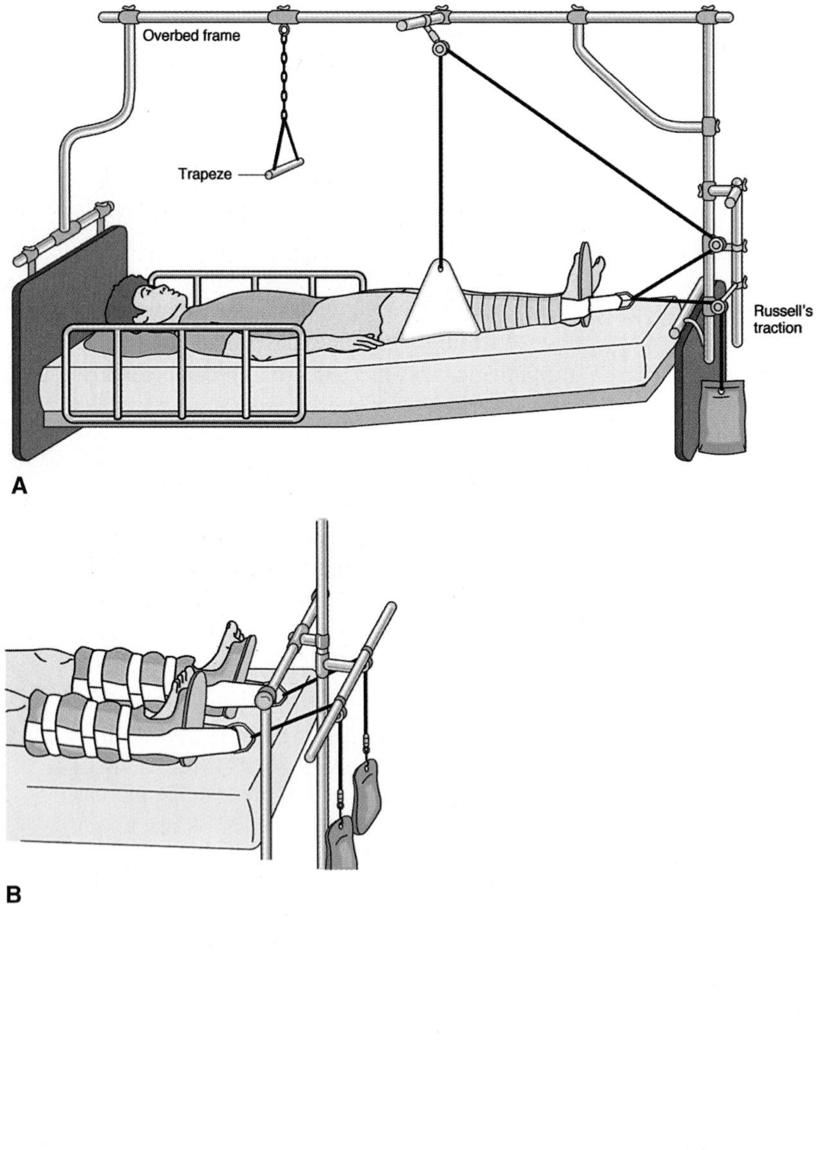
Overbed frame
Trapeze
Russell's traction
A
B

FIGURE 46.5 Types of skin traction. (A) Russell's traction. (B) Buck's (boot) traction.

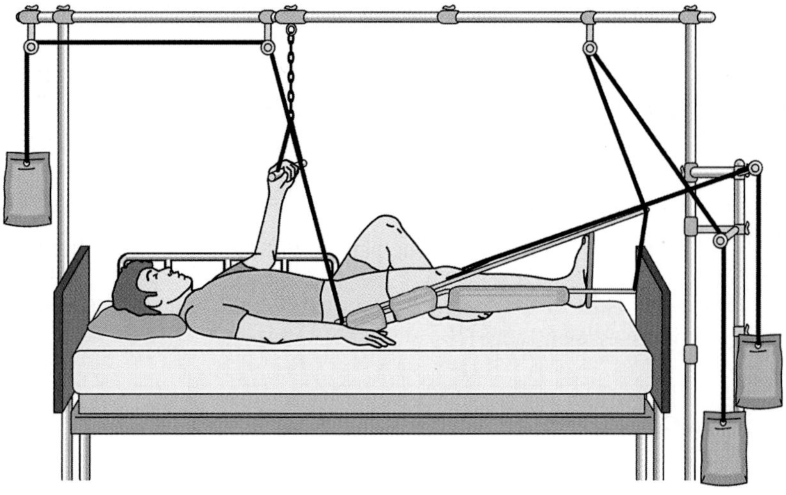

FIGURE 46.6 Balanced suspension and skeletal traction for femur fracture.

Weights are to hang unobstructed and should never touch the floor or be removed or lifted while traction is in use. The patient's feet should not rest against the end of the bed. It is important that the traction not be inhibited by any form of friction or impedance. Assistance should be obtained to reposition the patient in bed to prevent lifting injuries, especially with heavy weights in use.

For patients in skeletal traction, pin sites are observed for redness, drainage, odor, swelling, and excessive warmth. Clear, odorless drainage is expected. Follow agency policy or physician's order for pin site care.

Patients are in traction may be immobilized for an extended period and often experience problems associated with immobility. Use of the trapeze bar helps promote independence for patients and prevents complications of immobility through movement while in traction. For example, pressure ulcers on heels are common among older adult patients in traction. Unfortunately, loss of bone density is also a complication of immobility, which may create an additional impairment for normal healing.

Another common concern is the person's psychosocial health. Ensure that the patient does not become socially isolated because of the need for extended bedrest.

OPEN REDUCTION WITH INTERNAL FIXATION. One of the most common indications for this surgical procedure is a fractured hip. Hip fractures involve the proximal femur and affect older adults more than any other age group. Open reduction with internal fixation (ORIF) of the hip allows early mobilization while the bone is healing.

As the name implies, the bone ends are realigned (reduced) by direct visualization through a surgical incision (open reduction). The bone ends are held in place by internal fixation devices such as metal plates and screws or by a prosthesis with a femoral component similar to that used for total joint replacement (Fig. 46.7). For hip surgery, the internal fixation device is not removed after the fracture heals. For ankle or long-bone surgery, the hardware may be removed after healing because of loosening or pain (see the *Nursing Care Plan for the Patient After Open Reduction with Internal Fixation of the Hip*).

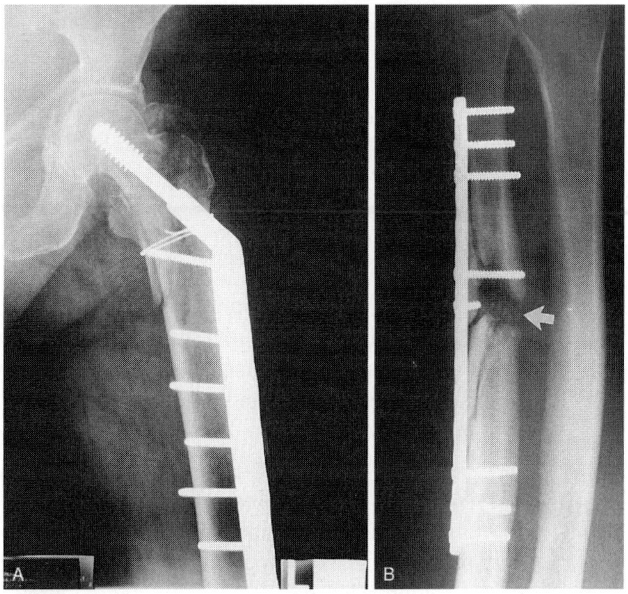
A
B

FIGURE 46.7 Internal fixation. (A) Intertrochanteric fracture of the hip with fracture fixation via a side plate and screw combination device. (B) Side plate and screw fixation of radial fracture. (From McKinnis, L. N. [1997]. *Fundamentals of orthopedic radiology.* Philadelphia: F. A. Davis, with permission.)

NURSING CARE PLAN for the Patient After Open Reduction with Internal Fixation of the Hip

Nursing Diagnosis: *Pain* related to surgical wound

Expected Outcomes: The patient will state that pain relief is satisfactory.

Evaluation of Outcomes: Does patient state that pain is absent or at a tolerable level (pain rated 0 to 2 on pain assessment scale)?

Intervention	Rationale	Evaluation
Give analgesics as needed; anticipate need for pain relief.	Analgesics relieve pain, especially if given before pain is severe.	Does patient state pain is relieved?
Give analgesics before activity (e.g., session with physical therapist).	Increased activity can cause pain.	Is patient restless or agitated during activity?
Use nondrug pain relief measures, such as distraction, guided imagery, other relaxation techniques.	Analgesic therapy is enhanced with complementary pain relief measures.	Does patient report pain relief is enhanced with music or relaxation?
Use fracture bedpan.	Fracture bedpans are more comfortable and easier to position for patients.	Is patient able to use fracture pan with comfort?

Nursing Diagnosis: *Impaired Physical Mobility* related to hip precautions and surgical pain

Expected Outcomes: The patient will maintain desired level of activity.

Evaluation of Outcomes: Does patient maintain activity desired?

Intervention	Rationale	Evaluation
Reinforce transfer and ambulation techniques.	Activity is restricted due to hip precautions and weight-bearing limitations.	Does patient transfer and ambulate as instructed by physical therapist?
Place overhead frame with trapeze bar on bed; teach patient how to use it.	Patient mobility is increased and pain decreased with use of trapeze bar for movement.	Does patient use trapeze bar for movement in bed with less pain?
Monitor patient for and take measures to prevent complications of immobility: • Turn patient every 2 hours and check skin. • Keep heels off bed. • Teach patient to deep breathe and cough every 2 hours. • Teach use of incentive spirometer.	Immobility complications can occur if preventive measures are not used.	Does patient experience complications of immobility?
Apply thigh-high elastic stockings or sequential compression device to unaffected limb as ordered. Give anticoagulants as ordered. Get patient out of bed as soon as ordered. Ambulate patient as early as possible. Remind patient to practice leg exercises.	These precautions and activities help prevent blood clots.	Is patient free from blood clots?

EXTERNAL FIXATION. An alternative treatment for some fractures is external fixation. This treatment is used when bone damage is severe, as in crushed or splintered fractures, or if the bone has numerous fractures. After the fracture is reduced, the physician surgically inserts pins into the bone. The pins are held in place by an external metal frame to prevent bone movement (Fig. 46.8). External fixation is ideal for the patient who has an open fracture with soft tissue damage that needs to be treated at the same time. Like the patient in skeletal traction, the patient with this device is at risk for complications of skeletal pins, which include pin reaction, compromised circulation, and infection. Pin sites are observed often for evidence of infection. Pin site care varies from facility to facility. The overriding principle is to ensure that strict aseptic technique is always maintained because the pin is a pathway for microorganisms to directly enter bone tissue and cause osteomyelitis (see the *Nursing Care Plan for the Patient with External Fixation of the Lower Extremity*).

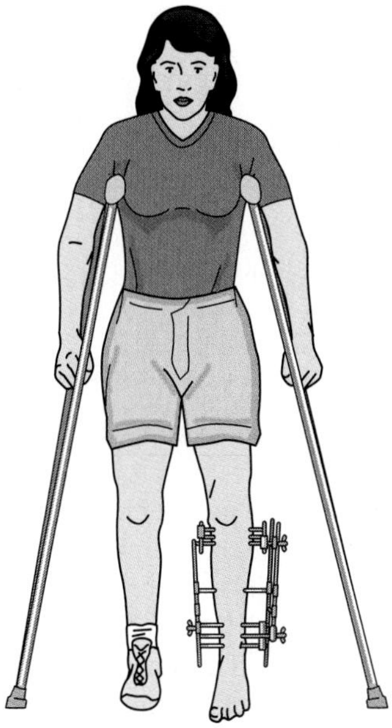

FIGURE 46.8 External fixation for complex fractures and wound care.

NURSING CARE PLAN for the Patient with External Fixation of the Lower Extremity

Nursing Diagnosis: *Risk for Infection* related to skin integrity impairment

Expected Outcomes: The patient does not develop an infection.

Evaluation of Outcomes: Does patient remain free from infection?

Interventions	Rationale	Evaluation
Inspect dressings, wounds, pin sites for signs and symptoms of infection.	Signs and symptoms of infection include warmth, redness, heat, swelling, drainage, pain.	Are any wounds infected?
Monitor color of and measure wound drainage.	Wound drainage color and amount can indicate severity of infection.	Does wound have large amount of purulent drainage?
Change dressings or provide wound and pin care per facility policy using aseptic technique.	Use of aseptic technique minimizes chance of infection. Pin wound sites should be free of crusting, which promotes infections because of decreased skin integrity.	Are pin sites clean with no crusting?
Monitor vital signs frequently.	Alterations in vital signs can indicate infection.	Are vital signs within baseline findings?

Nursing Diagnosis: *Impaired Physical Mobility* related to the external fixation (EF) device

Expected Outcomes: The patient will maintain desired level of mobility/activity.

Evaluation of Outcomes: Has patient maintained desired level of mobility and activity?

Continued

NURSING CARE PLAN for the Patient with External Fixation of the Lower Extremity—cont'd

Interventions	Rationale	Evaluation
Reinforce transfer and ambulation techniques.	Depending on severity of fracture and size of EF device, there may be special needs to transfer and ambulate.	Does patient transfer and ambulate as instructed?
Place overhead frame and trapeze bar on bed. Teach patient how to use them.	Patient mobility is increased and pain decreased with use of trapeze bar for movement.	Does patient use overhead frame and trapeze bar for movement with less pain?
Teach patient how to move limb using EF device.	Providing patient with instruction on moving the extremity promotes independence and minimizes pain.	Does patient move the extremity using EF device?
Assess patient for and take measures to prevent complications of immobility. Promote early ambulation to minimize complications.	Immobility complications can occur if preventive measures are not used.	Does patient have any complications of immobility?
Include other disciplines such as the physiotherapist in promoting and teaching about ambulation.	EF devices allow for earlier ambulation. Physiotherapy can provide initial or reinforce the education needed to promote ambulation (e.g., with crutch walking).	Has patient used information learned from other disciplines to aid ambulation?

Nursing Diagnosis: *Disturbed Body Image* related to external fixation device

Expected Outcomes: The patient will not experience disturbed body image while EF device is in place.

Evaluation of Outcomes: Does patient experience disturbed body image resulting from EF device?

Interventions	Rationale	Evaluation
If possible, explain to patient preoperatively what EF device will look like.	Preparing patient for what to expect postoperatively increases likelihood of acceptance and minimizes the unknown.	Was patient able to verbalize why device is to be used and what device will look like?
Reinforce the idea that the EF device will decrease discomfort and allow for earlier ambulation.	Promoting early ambulation and increased comfort enhance acceptance.	Did patient understand benefit of EF device allowing for early ambulation and increased comfort?
Provide psychological support and an environment of acceptance.	Accepting the patient and allowing for discussion of concerns promote a sense of well-being and acceptance of EF device.	Did patient feel comfortable expressing concerns related to body image?

CRITICAL THINKING

Mrs. Heinrick

■ Mrs. Heinrick, a care center resident, was found lying on her left side, moaning and holding her left leg at 10 a.m. She cried out with any movement, and said she fell and broke her leg. The supervisor notified paramedics and Dr. Jones. Vital signs are blood pressure 150/84 mm Hg, pulse 100 beats per minute, and respirations 20 per minute. Her left leg is noticeably shorter than her right leg. The LPN remained with Mrs. Heinrick and instructed her not to move until help arrived. The LPN got blankets and a pillow for her head. The paramedics took Mrs. Heinrick to nearby Grace Hospital, where she was diagnosed as having an incomplete femoral neck (hip) fracture. Dr. Jones ordered 5 pounds of Buck's traction.

Later, Mrs. Heinrick is restless and picking at her bedcovers when the nurse arrives to assess her at the beginning of the nurse's shift.

1. How should the licensed practical nurse (LPN) document the incident of Mrs. Heinrick's fall at the care center?
2. What is the purpose of Buck's traction for Mrs. Heinrick?
3. What are the nursing responsibilities while caring for Mrs. Heinrick?
4. What might explain Mrs. Heinrick's restlessness?

Suggested answers at end of chapter.

CRITICAL THINKING

Tommy Martin

■ Tommy, age 18, was in a motor vehicle accident that resulted in a fractured pelvis and femur. He is going to require skeletal traction for several weeks.

1. Identify three nursing diagnoses related to Tommy's physical or emotional well-being.
2. What are nursing interventions for these diagnoses?
3. How can the constipating effects of opioids be balanced with the benefits of pain relief to manage bowel elimination? (See Chapter 10.)

Suggested answers at end of chapter.

NONUNION MODALITIES. Although most bones heal properly with the correct treatment, some patients experience malunion (malalignment of healed bone) or nonunion (delayed or no healing). A number of variables influence how a bone heals, including age, nutritional status, and the presence of other diseases that alter the healing process, such as diabetes mellitus.

Several methods for treating nonunion are available, including electrical bone stimulation and bone grafting. For selected patients, bone stimulation may be effective in promoting healing; the exact mechanism of action is not known. Bone grafting involves adding packed bone to the fracture site in an attempt to facilitate healing. Bone-stimulating compounds such as OsteoSet, Pro Osteon, or Allomatrix may be used to promote bone growth. These compounds are used during surgical procedures as glue, cement, or filler.

Another fracture healing method is low-intensity pulsed ultrasound (also called Exogen therapy). Ultrasound treatment has provided excellent results for slow-healing fractures, as well as for new fractures. The patient applies the treatment for about 20 minutes each day.

NURSING CARE TIP

When moving a limb that has an external fixation device, grasp the device and lift, raise, or move the limb as needed. By grasping the device, there is less movement of the healing bone and therefore less trauma to the healing site and less pain with movement. Care must be taken not to loosen any fasteners holding the pins in place.

Complications of Fractures

Monitor the patient for possible complications, and implement interventions to prevent them. The most common complications include impaired neurovascular status, hemorrhage, infection, and thromboembolitic complications. Although they do not occur often, acute compartment syndrome and fat embolism syndrome (more common with fractures of long bones) can be life-threatening complications of fractures.

NEUROVASCULAR STATUS. Neurovascular checks are done to detect abnormalities. Decreased or absent pulses, cool skin temperature, and dusky color indicate circulation alterations. Numbness and tingling, decreased sensation, and mobility indicate neurologic alterations. These findings should be reported to the physician promptly.

HEMORRHAGE. Bone is highly vascular, and damage to or surgery on bone (particularly the large long bones of the extremities) can cause bleeding. Assess for bleeding and monitor vital signs carefully. Hypovolemic shock may result from severe hemorrhage (see Chapter 9).

INFECTION. Trauma predisposes the body to infection, especially when the skin, the body's first line of defense, is disrupted. Wound infections, pin site infections, drainage tube infections, and osteomyelitis (bone infection) are common. Hospital-acquired infections, such as pneumonia or urinary tract infection, can occur in patients who are immobilized for extensive periods while their fractures heal.

THROMBOEMBOLITIC COMPLICATIONS. Deep venous thrombosis or pulmonary embolus (PE) (see Chapter 31) can develop in patients who are immobile because of trauma or surgery. Thromboembolitic complications are the most common problems of lower extremity surgery or trauma and the most fatal complication of musculoskeletal surgery, particularly in the older adult. Leg exercises, early ambulation, and anticoagulant therapy, usually using low molecular weight heparin, such as fondaparinux (Arixtra), dalteparin (Fragmin) or enoxaparin (Lovenox), help prevent these problems.

ACUTE COMPARTMENT SYNDROME. Compartments are sheaths of fibrous tissue that support and partition nerves, muscles, and blood vessels, primarily in the extremities (Fig. 46.9). Each extremity has several compartments. Acute compartment syndrome is a serious problem in which pressure in one or more limb compartments increases, causing massive circulation impairment to the area. An external device such as a cast or bulky dressing can increase pressure when there is tissue swelling or compression in the area. The early symptom of acute compartment syndrome is the patient's report of severe, increasing pain that is not relieved with opioids and occurs more in active movements than passive movements. Decreased sensation follows before ischemia becomes severe. In severe acute compartment syndrome, the patient has the six *P*s:

- Pain (severe, unrelenting, and increased with passive stretching)
- Paresthesia (painful tingling or burning)
- Paralysis (late symptom)
- Pallor (but there may be warmth or redness over the area)
- Pulselessness (late and ominous sign)
- Poikilothermia (temperature matches environment; i.e., the extremity is cool to touch).

Relief of pressure is the goal. It may be accomplished by removing the source of pressure, such as by bivalving a cast, or by performing a **fasciotomy**, which is an incision into the fascia that encloses the compartment. This incision allows the compartment tissue to expand and relieves the pressure. If more than one compartment has increased pressure, multiple fasciotomies are required. These surgical wounds remain open until the pressure decreases. Then they are closed and may require skin grafting. If this condition continues without pressure relief, tissue necrosis, infection, extremity contracture, or renal failure may result. Renal failure is a potentially fatal complication of acute compartment syndrome.

CRITICAL THINKING

Mr. Andrews

■ Mr. Andrews has suffered an incomplete fracture of his right femur. He has a cast on from his groin to the middle of his foot. An hour ago he received 10 mg of morphine intravenously (IV), and he is reporting continued and increasing pain.

1. What data should be gathered now?
2. What might be happening with Mr. Andrews?
3. What interventions may be needed?

Suggested answers at end of chapter.

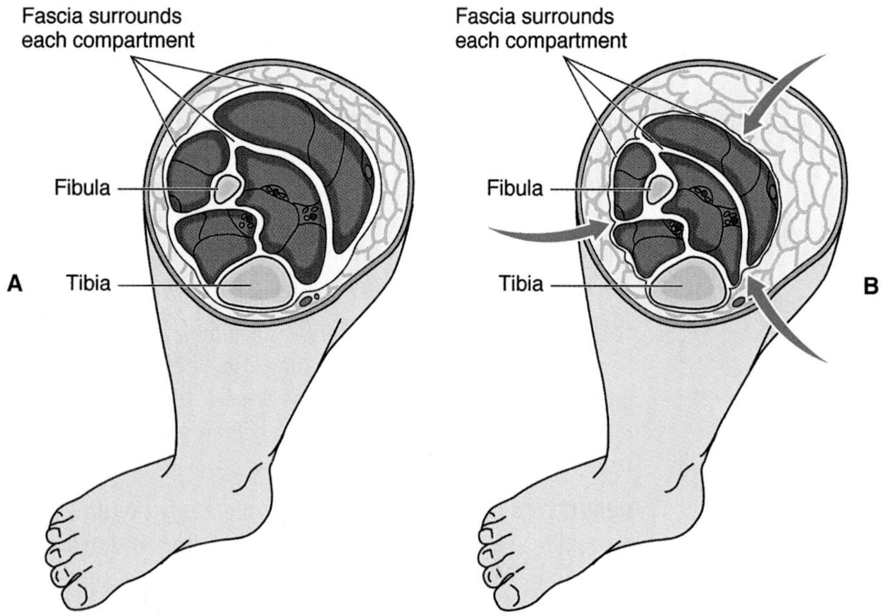
Fascia surrounds each compartment
Fibula
A
Tibia
Fascia surrounds each compartment
Fibula
Tibia
B

FIGURE 46.9 (A) Lower leg compartments. Each compartment contains muscles, an artery, a vein, and a nerve. (B) Compartment syndrome. Increased pressure in a compartment compresses structures within the compartment.

• **WORD • BUILDING** •
fasciotomy: fascia—fibrous tissue + otomy—opening into

FAT EMBOLISM SYNDROME. Fat embolism syndrome is another serious complication of fractures in which small fat globules are released from yellow bone marrow into the bloodstream. The globules then travel to the lung fields, causing respiratory distress. This process most often occurs when long bones (especially the femoral shaft) are fractured or when the patient has multiple fractures. The older adult patient with a fractured hip is also at a high risk for fat embolism syndrome. This condition can occur up to 72 hours after the initial injury.

The earliest manifestation of fat embolism syndrome is altered mental status resulting from a low arterial oxygen level. The patient then experiences tachycardia, tachypnea, fever, high blood pressure, and severe respiratory distress (shortness of breath). Most patients also have a measles-like rash, called petechiae, over the upper body. Even when aggressively treated, patients with fat embolism syndrome commonly die from the pulmonary edema that typically develops. Note early signs and symptoms of fat embolism syndrome, and report them to the physician immediately. If a fat embolism is suspected, the following actions should be taken:

- Promote oxygenation by administering oxygen at 2 L/min via nasal cannula.
- Place the patient in high-Fowler's position or raise the head of the bed as tolerated.
- Maintain bedrest, and minimize movement of the extremity.
- Prepare patient for a chest x-ray examination or lung scan.
- Prepare patient for arterial blood gas (ABG) determination.
- Administer intravenous fluids as ordered.
- Administer corticosteroids as ordered.
- Provide emotional support and calm environment.

Nursing Process for the Patient with a Fracture

Caring for the patient with a fracture requires coordinated teamwork with other health team members.

DATA COLLECTION. The most important aspect of monitoring the patient with a fracture is frequent checking of neurovascular status (circulation, sensation, mobility) distal to the fracture site (see Chapter 45). As mentioned earlier, acute compartment syndrome is a potentially limb- or life-threatening complication that results when blood flow is impaired.

Pain is managed by both medications and complementary therapies. Bone pain can be excruciating and must be treated aggressively. For the patient who cannot report pain, such as a patient who is cognitively impaired or comatose, ensure that pain relief is maintained by regularly scheduled analgesic administration.

NURSING DIAGNOSES, PLANNING, AND IMPLEMENTATION. Determination of the appropriate nursing diagnosis depends on the type of fracture. See the *Nursing Care Plan for the Patient After Open Reduction with Internal Fixation of the Hip.*

Acute Pain Related to Fractured Bone

EXPECTED OUTCOME: The patient will report relief from pain using a pain assessment scale.

- Provide analgesics and anti-inflammatories as ordered *to relieve pain and swelling.*
- Ensure proper positioning and alignment *to promote pain relief and future functioning.*
- Assess for compartment syndrome if patient has a cast in place *to prevent neurovascular complications.*
- Apply ice as ordered *to decrease swelling and pain.*
- Teach alternative measure of pain relief *to maximize means to relieve pain.*

Impaired Physical Mobility Related to Bone Fracture

EXPECTED OUTCOME: The patient will demonstrate increased mobility.

- Encourage independence *to promote mobility.*
- Utilize other disciplines such as occupational and physiotherapy *to encourage and promote patient mobility.*
- Provide equipment and resources such as crutches and wheelchairs *to improve mobility.*

Risk For Peripheral Neurovascular Dysfunction Related to Increased Tissue Volume or Restrictive Envelope

EXPECTED OUTCOME: The patient will maintain peripheral pulses, warm skin, sensation, and ability to move extremity.

- Assess often for compartment syndrome *to promote prompt reporting.*
- Assess for swelling of affected limb (especially if patient has a cast or tight dressing) *to detect complications.*
- Keep limb elevated above heart *to minimize edema.*
- Administer anti-inflammatory agents as ordered *to reduce pain and swelling.*
- Monitor for increasing pain even after analgesic administration *to detect complications.*

NURSING CARE TIP

A patient who is confused or comatose may not be able to report pain, which can be problematic because the most reliable indicator of pain is the patient's report. Nonverbal indicators (e.g., grimacing, restlessness, elevated blood pressure and heart rate) are not reliable for pain assessment and should not be used to assume the absence of pain. Prevent pain by anticipating it and treating it in advance. This can be done by recognizing causes of pain and understanding

Continued

NURSING CARE TIP—cont'd

that the effects of mild but repetitive pain (as in turning several times a day) can adversely affect the patient (e.g., by leading to exhaustion). Causes of pain include conditions or diseases (such as fractures, trauma, or cancer), procedures (such as surgery, turning, or wound care), and biomedical devices (such as orthopedic fixation devices, wound drains, urinary catheters, nasogastric tubes, and chest tubes).

With few patients being medicated before painful procedures, some of which may be done several times a day (turning), patients who are confused or comatose are at greater risk for lack of pain relief. To keep patients comfortable, provide analgesics as ordered before painful procedures and on a regular basis when pain is assumed to be present. For anticipated pain, use the acronym APP (assume pain present).

Use pain assessment tools designed for those who are cognitively impaired to ensure that their pain is adequately relieved. The **P**ain Assessment **IN A**dvanced **D**ementia (PAINAD) tool, for example, was developed for this purpose. Share pain research findings with institution administrators to establish policies that support proactive pain management for all patients.

EVALUATION. The outcome is met if the patient reports or demonstrates that pain is within tolerable levels on a pain assessment scale, demonstrates increased physical mobility, and maintains peripheral pulses, warm skin, sensation, and ability to move extremity.

PATIENT EDUCATION. If the patient has a cast, review appropriate instructions for cast care (see Box 46.2). Health teaching is also important for care of the extremity after cast removal (Box 46.3). If the patient has a wound, teach patient and caregiver how to assess and dress the wound, including pin care if needed, and when to report changes, such as signs and symptoms of infection.

Teach the importance of adequate protein, calories, vitamins, and minerals in healing. Unless otherwise contraindicated, milkshakes and instant breakfast preparations are good sources of additional protein and calories, as well as a source of calcium.

Osteomyelitis

Osteomyelitis is an infection of bone that can be either acute or chronic. A bone infection lasting less than 4 weeks is considered acute; one that lasts more than 4 weeks is chronic.

Box 46.3

Extremity Care Following Cast Removal

- Make sure skin is properly cleansed. Soak rather than rub skin to remove dry scales.
- The extremity likely will be weak, with decreased range of motion (ROM). Move it gently, and provide analgesics prn.
- When extremity is not in use, provide support with pillows or orthotic device until strength and movement return.
- Make sure active and passive ROM are performed as recommended by physical therapist and as patient tolerance will allow.
- Lower extremity swelling can be prevented with elastic support stockings.

Pathophysiology

Regardless of the type of osteomyelitis, the infection results from invasion of bacteria into bone and surrounding soft tissues. Inflammation occurs, followed by ischemia (decreased blood flow) (Fig. 46.10). Bone tissue then becomes necrotic (dies), which retards healing and causes more infection, often as a bone abscess.

Pathogens enter bone in several ways. Direct inoculation means that an injury to the body allows the offending microbes direct access to bone tissue. An open fracture is an example of that process. Contiguous spread occurs when surrounding soft tissue becomes infected. An example is the patient with cellulitis whose infection then spreads to underlying bone. In hematogenous spread, an infection beginning in another part of the body migrates to bone. For instance, a patient with a total hip replacement may acquire osteomyelitis from a urinary tract infection.

Etiology

Penetrating trauma leads to acute osteomyelitis by direct inoculation. The most common pathogens causing osteomyelitis are *Pseudomonas aeruginosa, Staphylococcus aureus,* and *Proteus.* The leading cause of contiguous spread is a slow-healing foot ulcer in the patient who has diabetes mellitus or peripheral vascular disease. Multiple organisms may be present in the wound and subsequently the bone. Hematogenous spread results from bacteremia (infection of the blood), underlying disease, or nonpenetrating trauma. Long-term intravenous catheters are primary sources of infection.

Signs and Symptoms

The patient with acute osteomyelitis has fever, as well as local signs of inflammation, such as tenderness, redness, heat, pain, and swelling. Pain (particularly over the area of infection), may be the only apparent complaint. Ulceration,

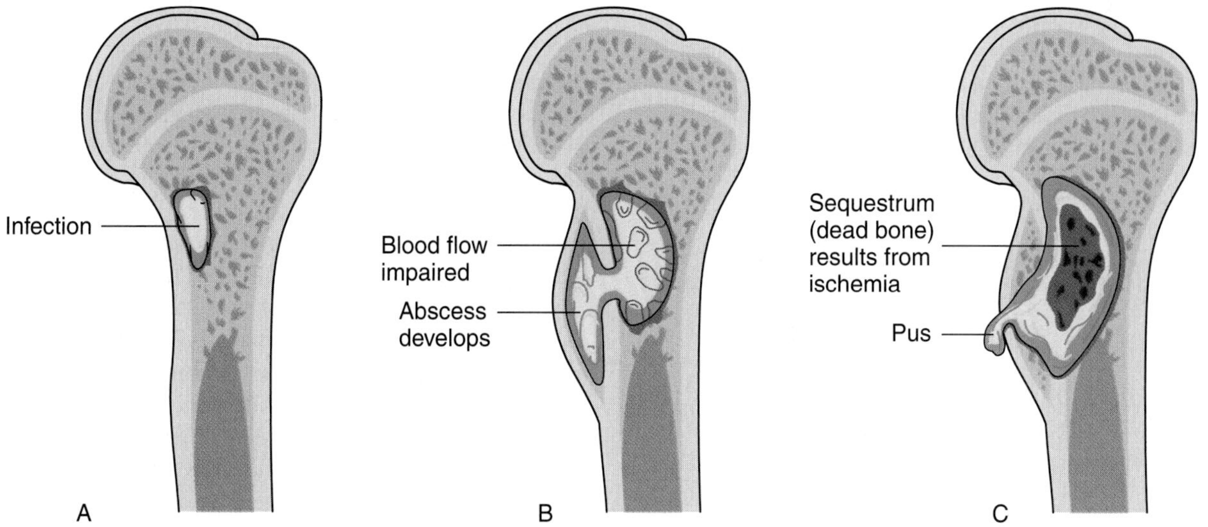
Infection
Blood flow impaired
Abscess develops
Sequestrum (dead bone) results from ischemia
Pus
A
B
C

FIGURE 46.10 Sequence of osteomyelitis development. (A) Infection begins. (B) Blood flow is blocked in the area of infection. An abscess with pus forms. (C) Bone dies within the infection site, and pus formation continues.

drainage, and localized pain are typical signs and symptoms of chronic osteomyelitis.

Diagnostic Tests

The patient with osteomyelitis typically has an elevated leukocyte (white blood cell) count, an elevated ESR, and positive bone biopsy for infection. Some patients also have a positive blood culture. MRIs, x-ray examinations, and computed tomography (CT) scans can show areas of infection.

Therapeutic Measures

Long-term antibiotic therapy is the treatment of choice for patients with bone infection. Infection in bone tissue is difficult to resolve and may require weeks to months of medication. Antibiotic therapy alone may not resolve the infection. Patients with chronic osteomyelitis may require surgery to remove necrotic bone tissue or replace it with healthy bone tissue. Amputations are reserved for patients who have massive infections that have not responded to one or more of the conventional treatments.

Nursing Care

Patients often administer their intravenous antibiotics at home rather than have a costly stay in a hospital. Teach the patient and caregiver about the side effects, toxicity, interactions, and precautions for antibiotic therapy. A home care nurse may be needed to assist the patient.

If a soft tissue wound is present, ensure that sterile technique is used for dressing changes. The home health nurse may teach the patient and family how to perform dressing changes, the importance of hand washing prior to dressing changes, and how to avoid the spread of pathogens.

Osteoporosis

Osteoporosis (porous bone) is a metabolic disorder in which there is low bone mass and deterioration of bone structure, resulting in fragile bones that are prone to fracture. The spine, wrist, and hip are most commonly involved although all bones can be affected.

Prevalence

More than 10 million people have osteoporosis, and 34 million more have low bone mass (National Osteoporosis Foundation, 2009). Both women (8 million) and men (2 million) develop osteoporosis, although it is often thought that only women are affected. Women are at greatest risk because their bones are smaller than men's bones. Osteoporosis can occur at any age, but older adults are most affected. As the American population ages, the incidence and costs of osteoporosis will rise. After age 50, about one in two women, and one in four men will have a fracture due to osteoporosis. This is significant because hip or vertebral fractures are associated with reduced quality of life, increased disability, and increased risk of death, especially within the year after the fracture.

Pathophysiology

Bone is living tissue that is resorbing (breaking down) old bone tissue (osteoclast cells) and constantly building new bone tissue (osteoblast cells). Normally, this bone remodeling process is balanced. An imbalance results in osteoporosis. Bone density (mass) peaks between ages 30 and 35. After these peak years, the rate of bone breakdown exceeds the rate of bone buildup. For postmenopausal women, decreased estrogen appears to slow the absorption of calcium, leading to increased bone loss.

Trabecular (cancellous) bone is lost first, followed by a loss of cortical (compact) bone. The result is irreversible bone loss that makes the inside of bones porous and, hence, weaker. As a result, more than 2 million fractures from osteoporosis occurred in 2005, including 547,000 vertebral fractures, 397,000 wrist fractures, and 297,000 hip fractures (National Osteoporosis Foundation, 2009).

Types and Risk Factors

Osteoporosis is either primary or secondary. Primary osteoporosis is the most common and is not associated with another disease or health problem. Risk factors for primary osteoporosis include the following:

- Aging
- Female gender
- Caucasian, Asian, or Hispanic/Latino heritage (although risk exists for all ethnicities)
- History of fractures
- Family history of osteoporosis or fractures
- Small boned, petite body build
- Postmenopausal status (because less estrogen is available to protect bone)
- Low testosterone and estrogen in men
- Low calcium intake
- Low vitamin D intake (to absorb calcium)
- Excessive caffeine, protein, sodium intake (impairs calcium retention)
- Sedentary lifestyle
- Excessive alcohol consumption
- Cigarette smoking

For a personal bone-risk survey, visit www.niams.nih.gov/Health_Info/Bone/Optool/index.asp.

Secondary osteoporosis results from an associated medical condition or procedure, such as hyperparathyroidism; renal dialysis; drug therapy with steroids, certain antiseizure drugs, sleeping medications, aluminum-containing antacids, hormones for endometriosis, or cancer drugs; and prolonged immobility, such as that seen with patients who have a spinal cord injury.

Prevention

To protect against osteoporosis, practicing good health and nutritional habits that build bone is especially important through age 30, before bone mass begins to decrease. These habits should include consuming recommended amounts of calcium (800 mg/day for ages 3 to 8, and 1300 mg/day for ages 9 to 17) and vitamin D; performing weight-bearing and muscle-strengthening exercises, especially in childhood; avoiding alcohol; and not smoking.

Signs and Symptoms

Most people do not realize they have osteoporosis until they fracture a bone falling, sustaining a mild bump, or sneezing. With vertebral compression fractures, a decrease in height (up to 6 inches), severe back pain, and the classic "dowager's hump," or kyphosis of the spine, is present as the spine begins to collapse. The patient may be embarrassed by the change in body image and may have curtailed social activities. Some patients have difficulty finding clothes that fit comfortably.

General effects of the disease go beyond the obvious bone deformities. Quality of life can be impacted. Acute or chronic pain may occur. Physiological effects can include decreased respiratory capacity due to spinal deformities. It can be difficult to expand the lungs because of curvature of the spine or painful vertebral fractures. This can increase fatigue and the risk of pneumonia. Osteoporosis can be associated with chronic obstructive pulmonary disease (COPD) due to limited activity related to dyspnea and corticosteroid therapy (which breaks down bone). Gastric function can be decreased due to decreased activity from pain and fear of falling. GI upset may occur from medications.

Functional abilities (activities of daily living and instrumental activities of daily living) may be limited, which increases the patient's dependence. Emotional effects can relate to body image changes, depression, or anxiety from fear of breaking a bone including during intimacy. Socialization may be reduced because of activity limitations or fear of injury. Because these effects are interrelated, the whole person, not just the disease, needs to be assessed and treated to improve quality of life.

Diagnostic Tests

Dual-energy x-ray absorptiometry (DEXA) is the standard screening tool to measure bone density (Box 46.4, *Gerontological Issues*). This noninvasive scan is a low-dose x-ray and takes about 5 minutes to perform while the patient lies on a table. A DEXA scan identifies low bone density before a fracture occurs and provides a baseline comparison for future tests to detect bone loss and fracture risk. It also helps guide treatment decisions.

Serum calcium and vitamin D levels may be decreased, and serum phosphorus may be increased. With severe bone loss, alkaline phosphatase levels may be elevated, confirming bone damage.

Therapeutic Measures

There is no cure for osteoporosis, but it can be treated. The cornerstone of treatment for osteoporosis is medication and modifying risk factors to prevent bone loss.

MEDICATION. Supplements and medication are used for prevention or treatment. These include calcium supplements, vitamin D, antiresorptive drugs, and bone-forming drugs.

Calcium is important to prevent bone loss. If serum calcium falls below normal levels, the parathyroid glands stimulate bone to release calcium into the bloodstream. The result is demineralized bone. Therefore, calcium

Box 46.4

Gerontological Issues

Bone mineral density testing can be helpful in assessing the risk of fractures for residents in extended care. Testing bone mineral density and providing treatment for osteoporosis can reduce the risk of hip fractures.

supplements to maintain normal levels are important. The patient should be taught to drink plenty of fluids to prevent calcium-based urinary stones. Vitamin D supplementation, to aid calcium absorption, also may be needed, especially for patients who have reduced exposure to sunlight (residents of extended care facilities or northern geographical areas, for example) or who cannot metabolize vitamin D.

Antiresorptive Medications. Bisphosphonates are used to prevent or slow the progress of osteoporosis. They bind to bone and suppress osteoclast activity to prevent or reduce the breakdown process. They include alendronate (Fosamax, Fosamax Plus D), ibandronate (Boniva), risedronate (Actonel), and zoledronic acid (Reclast). Bisphosphonates have been shown to be effective for at least 10 years. However, over time bone loss still continues. Bone remodeling is a two-part process, and blocking one part may eventually impair the other part.

Side effects of bisphosphonates include bone, muscle, or joint pain; GI upset; gastric ulcers; and rarely osteonecrosis (bone death) of the jaw. Teach the patient specifically how to take each medication to reduce side effects. Typically, the tablet or solution form is taken in the morning after awakening on an empty stomach. It is followed by a full glass of water (only water) with nothing else to eat or drink for up to 1 hour. The patient should not lie down for at least 30 minutes to 1 hour after taking the drug.

Calcitonin (Fortical, Miacalcin) is a synthetic thyroid hormone and treats osteoporosis by decreasing bone loss. It is used for women who have been menopausal for 5 years.

Raloxifene (Evista) is a selective estrogen receptor modulator (SERM) that increases bone mass by 2% to 3% each year. SERM drugs are designed to mimic estrogen in some parts of the body while blocking its effects elsewhere.

Estrogen therapy may be used to prevent the bone loss that occurs with menopause as estrogen levels fall. However, other treatments should be considered first due to risk factors associated with estrogen therapy.

Anabolic (Bone-Forming) Medications. Teriparatide (Forteo) is used for men and women at great risk for fracture. Teriparatide increases bone mass by increasing the action and number of osteoblasts to form bone. It should not be taken for more than 2 years.

DIET. Increasing calcium and vitamin D intake are the main dietary considerations. Generally, calcium intake should be 1000 mg/day for those ages 18 to 49 and 1200 mg for those over age 50. Teach patients which foods are high in calcium, such as dairy products (yogurt and skim milk may have low levels) and dark green, leafy vegetables.

Currently, recommendations for vitamin D intake are 400 international units for those ages 50 to 60 and 600 international units for those over age 70 or in areas with reduced sunlight. Research is being done to see if higher levels would be more effective. If the patient consumes excessive amounts of caffeine or alcohol, teach about the need to avoid these substances.

EXERCISE. Exercise in childhood is essential in preventing osteoporosis. Weight-bearing exercise, especially walking, stimulates bone building. The patient should wear well-supporting, nonskid shoes at all times and avoid uneven surfaces that could contribute to falls. Resistance exercise such as weight training is also beneficial (Box 46.5, *Gerontological Issues*).

Fall Prevention

Osteoporotic bone may cause a pathological fracture, in which the hip breaks before the fall. For other patients, a fall can cause a hip or other fracture. Therefore, fall prevention programs in hospitals and extended care facilities are important.

In collaboration with the physical or occupational therapist, case manager, or discharge planner, assess the patient's home environment. Patient and family are taught how to create a hazard-free environment, such as avoiding scatter rugs and slippery floors. Walking paths in the home must be kept free of clutter to prevent falls. If needed, a walker or cane provides additional support.

Nursing Care

Nursing care for osteoporosis focuses on education for prevention, providing pain relief and support for symptoms, and medication teaching. For more information, visit the National Osteoporosis Foundation at www.nof.org.

Paget's Disease

Paget's disease, also called osteitis deformans, is a metabolic bone disease affecting normal bone remodeling (synchronized breakdown of older bone and formation of new bone). When unsynchronized remodeling occurs, there is increased breakdown and formation of bone that results in enlarged, abnormally formed, and brittle bone. This can weaken the bone, causing deformities, bone pain and fractures, and osteoarthritis. Paget's disease affects mainly older adults and men.

Box 46.5

Gerontological Issues

Falls become more common as people age. Exercise is one way of reducing falls in older adults. It should focus on at least two of these components: strength, balance, flexibility, and endurance. Exercise can be done in supervised groups or individually, or in tai chi classes (Gillespie et al., 2009).

Pathophysiology

Three phases occur: active, mixed, and inactive. In the active phase, an increase in osteoclasts (cells that break down bone) causes massive bone deformity and destruction. Osteoblasts (bone-building cells) then form new bone during the mixed phase. However, the resulting structure is disorganized. Finally, when osteoblastic activity exceeds the osteoclastic activity, the inactive phase occurs. The newly formed bone becomes sclerotic with increased vascularity. Paget's disease can affect one or several bones (whereas osteoporosis affects all bones). The most common areas involved are the spine, femur, skull, and pelvis.

Etiology

The cause of Paget's disease is not known, but it tends to run in families. Certain genes have been found to be associated with Paget's disease. It may be the result of a latent viral infection contracted in young adulthood for those susceptible to it.

Signs and Symptoms

Most patients with Paget's disease have no obvious symptoms, particularly when the disorder is confined to one bone. Pain is a major symptom in many. Other symptoms vary based on the bone affected. They can include limping, joint stiffness, and a pinched nerve with numbness and tingling. With skull involvement, headache and vision or hearing impairments may occur. Other conditions, such as heart failure, can occur with severe Paget's disease.

Diagnostic Tests

Diagnosis is made with x-rays. Radiographs of pagetic bone show punched-out areas that indicate increased bone resorption. The overall mass of bone may be enlarged. Bone scans can show how widespread the disorder is. An increased serum alkaline phosphatase (ALP) level occurs due to osteoblast activity (normal in males is 35 to 142 units/L and in females is 25 to 125 units/L). Those who have parents or siblings with Paget's disease may have ALP testing annually after age 40 to see if they have inherited the disease. Rarely, a bone biopsy is done.

Therapeutic Measures

There is no cure for Paget's disease, but medications can control it. Medications are used to relieve pain and promote quality of life. For mild disease, NSAIDs are given for pain control. Bisphosphonates (discussed earlier in the *Osteoporosis* section) may be given to reduce bone resorption and include alendronate (Fosamax), etidronate (Didronel), ibandronate (Boniva), pamidronate (Aredia), risedronate (Actonel), tiludronate (Skelid), and zoledronic acid (Reclast). Calcitonin (Fortical, Miacalcin) is a synthetic thyroid hormone that decreases bone loss.

If therapy is effective, serum or urine bone markers (products of bone remodeling) decrease. Resorption markers include C-telopeptide, N-telopeptide, and pyridinium cross-links. Formation markers include ALP, procollagen type 1 *N*-terminal propeptide, and osteocalcin.

Exercise is important in controlling pain and maintaining bone health and joint mobility. For uncontrolled pain or arthritis, surgery—such as joint replacement—may be done.

Nursing Care

Nursing care for Paget's disease focuses on providing pain relief and support for symptoms. Teaching about the disease, medications, and other therapies is provided. For more information, visit the Paget Foundation at www.paget.org.

Bone Cancer

Bone tumors may be benign or malignant. Malignant tumors may be either primary (originating in the bone) or metastatic, originating from another location and migrating to bone. Primary bone tumors tend to develop in people younger than age 30 and account for only a small percentage of bone cancers. Metastatic lesions are much more common and most often affect older adults. The pathophysiology depends on the type of bone cancer. The cause of bone cancer is not known.

Primary Malignant Tumors

Osteosarcoma, or osteogenic sarcoma, is the most common primary malignant bone tumor as well as being the most fatal bone tumor. It is a fairly large tumor that typically metastasizes to the lung within 2 years of diagnosis and treatment. This type of cancer usually affects young people between ages 10 and 25, and boys are twice as likely to develop the disease. Long bones of the legs and arms are most often the sites of origin (particularly around the knees), but osteosarcoma can be found in other bones. More than 50% of osteosarcomas occur in the distal femur in young men. The disease itself is relatively rare, with an occurrence rate of about 2 per million people.

Pain and swelling in an arm or leg that worsens with exercise or at night are some of the manifestations of osteosarcoma. A lump in the area or an unexplained limp also may be cause for further investigation. X-rays, bone biopsy, CT scan, bone scan, and MRI are some of the diagnostic tests that can be performed to help diagnose the malignancy. Older patients with Paget's disease also may develop these lesions. Chemotherapy and surgical excision of the affected bone with bone grafting or amputation of the affected limb are the treatments most commonly used for osteosarcomas.

Ewing's sarcoma is the most malignant bone tumor. In addition to local pain and swelling, systemic signs and symptoms, including low-grade fever, leukocytosis, and anemia, are common. The pelvis and legs are most often affected in children and young men.

Patients with a *chondrosarcoma* (cancer of cartilaginous cells) have a better prognosis than those with the previously described types of bone cancer. This type of cancer occurs in middle-aged and older people.

• WORD • BUILDING •

osteosarcoma: osteo—bone + sarc—flesh + oma—tumor

METASTATIC BONE DISEASE. Primary malignant tumors that occur in the prostate, breast, lung, and thyroid gland are called bone-seeking cancers because they migrate to bone more than any other primary cancer. Once cancer has metastasized, multiple bone sites are typically seen. Pathological fractures and severe pain are major concerns in managing metastatic disease. (See Chapter 11.)

Signs and Symptoms

Primary tumors cause local swelling and pain at the site. A tender, palpable mass is often present. Metastatic disease is not as visible, but the patient reports diffuse severe pain, eventually leading to marked disability.

Diagnostic Tests

Diagnosis of bone cancer is made by x-ray, CT scan, bone scan, bone biopsy, or MRI. (See Chapter 45.)

The patient with metastatic disease has an elevated ALP level and possibly an elevated ESR, indicating secondary tissue inflammation.

Therapeutic Measures

Management of bone cancer depends on the type and extent of the tumor. The treatment of primary bone tumors is usually surgery, often combined with chemotherapy or radiation. The surgeon attempts to salvage the limb and performs a resection of the tumor. For patients with Ewing's sarcoma or early osteosarcoma, external radiation may be the treatment of choice to reduce tumor size and pain.

Care of the postoperative patient is similar to that for any patient undergoing musculoskeletal surgery. Monitoring the neurovascular status of the operative limb is a vital nursing intervention (see Chapter 45). Other general postoperative care is discussed in Chapter 12.

For metastatic bone disease, surgery is not appropriate. External radiation is given, primarily for palliation. The radiation is directed toward the most painful sites in an attempt to shrink them and provide more comfort for the patient.

Nursing Care

Nursing care for the patient with bone cancer is not unlike that for patients with any other type of cancer. Help the patient adjust to the diagnosis, and refer the patient to resources such as the American Cancer Society and its various support groups. Chapter 10 describes the nursing care associated with chemotherapy and radiation therapy. For more information, visit the American Cancer Society at www.cancer.org.

CONNECTIVE TISSUE DISORDERS

Connective tissue disorders comprise a group of more than 100 diseases in which the major signs and symptoms result from joint involvement. Some connective tissue diseases affect only one part of the body; others affect many body organs and systems. Several disorders are discussed here, including gout, systemic lupus erythematosus, scleroderma, osteogenesis imperfecta, polymyositis, muscular dystrophy, osteoarthritis, and rheumatoid arthritis.

Gout

Gout is an easily treated systemic connective tissue disorder. Men, especially those middle aged and older, are more often affected than women. Patients with gout are seldom hospitalized for their disease.

Pathophysiology

Uric acid is a waste product resulting from the breakdown of proteins (purines) in the body. Urate crystals are formed because of excessive uric acid buildup (**hyperuricemia**) and are deposited in joints and other connective tissues, causing severe inflammation. When an "attack" of gout occurs, the patient has severe pain and inflammation in one or more small joints, usually the great toe. The inflammation may resolve in several days, with or without treatment. Months or years may pass between attacks, and the patient may have no signs or symptoms of joint inflammation between episodes. Urate deposits (tophi) may appear under the skin (Fig. 46.11) or in the kidneys or urinary system, causing stone (calculi) formation (see Chapter 37).

Etiology and Types

The causes and types of gout are well known. Primary gout is the most common and is caused by an inherited problem with purine metabolism. Uric acid production is greater than the kidneys' ability to excrete it. Therefore, the amount of uric acid in the blood increases. About 25% of patients have a family history of primary gout. Acute attacks of gout may be triggered by stress, alcohol consumption, illness, trauma, dieting, or certain medications.

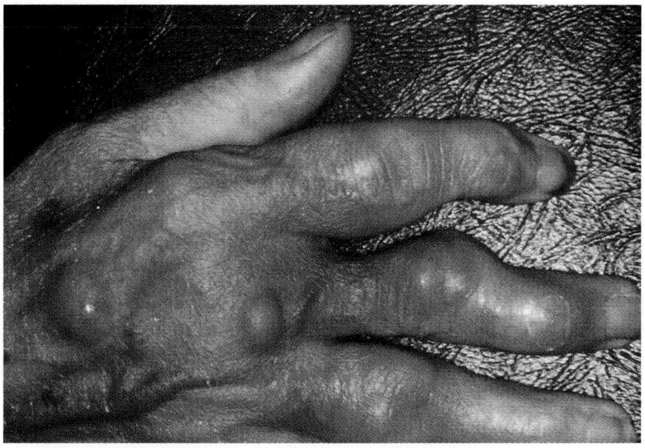

FIGURE 46.11 Gout: subcutaneous nontender lesions near joints. (From Goldsmith, L. A., Lazarus, G. S., Tharp, M. D., et al. [1997]. *Adult and pediatric dermatology* [p. 405]. Philadelphia: F. A. Davis, with permission.)

• WORD • BUILDING •
hyperuricemia: hyper—excessive + uric—uric acid + emia—in blood

Patients with secondary gout also experience hyperuricemia, but the increase is the result of another health problem, such as renal insufficiency, or medications, such as diuretic therapy and certain chemotherapeutic agents.

Signs and Symptoms

ACUTE GOUT. Patients with acute gout have one or more severely inflamed joints due to the uric acid crystals, usually small joints, often in the joint of the great toe. The joint is swollen, red, hot, and usually too painful to be touched.

CHRONIC GOUT. Patients with chronic gout may not have obvious signs and symptoms. Tophi are not commonly seen today because management of patients with gout has improved. If they are present, they tend to appear most often in the outer ear. Renal stones develop in about 20% of patients with gout. Various diagnostic tests may be needed to determine stone formation.

Diagnostic Tests

Diagnosis of gout is based on an elevated serum uric acid level. Joint fluid aspiration analysis can identify uric acid crystals in the synovial fluid, further confirming the diagnosis of gout.

Therapeutic Measures

MEDICATION. Drug therapy is the first-line treatment for primary gout. Treatment for secondary gout involves management or removal of the underlying cause. When a patient has an acute gout episode, the physician usually prescribes either colchicine or an NSAID to reduce the inflammatory response to urate crystals. The patient usually takes these medications until joint inflammation subsides.

Uricosuric agents (medications used to decrease uric acid) are the drug of choice to decrease serum uric acid levels. Febuxostat (Uloric) and allopurinol (Zyloprim) decrease uric acid production. The patient must take these drugs every day to keep the uric acid level within the normal range. Probenecid (Benemid) may also be used temporarily to increase renal excretion of uric acid. The patient's serum uric acid level is monitored periodically.

DIET. For a patient with gout, certain foods should be avoided or consumed in moderation (Box 46.6). The patient should avoid all forms of aspirin and diuretics because they can trigger an attack. Increasing daily fluid intake is also important to help prevent kidney stones. The patient also should avoid alcohol (especially beer), because this too can provoke an attack.

Box 46.6

Health Promotion for Patients with Gout

- Avoid high-purine (protein) foods, such as organ meats, shellfish, and oily fish (e.g., sardines).
- Avoid alcohol.
- Drink plenty of fluids, especially water.
- Avoid all forms of aspirin and drugs containing aspirin.
- Avoid diuretics.
- Avoid excessive physical or emotional stress.

Systemic Lupus Erythematosus

The word *lupus* comes from the Latin word for "wolf" and was originally associated with leg ulcers. However, it became associated with facial ulcers, and the butterfly facial rash that patients with lupus may develop is one of the most defining characteristics of lupus. The rash is red, and thus the word *erythematosus,* meaning "reddened," was added to describe the disease.

Most patients with lupus have the systemic type, but a small percentage have the type that affects only the skin, a condition called discoid lupus erythematosus. Discoid lupus is not life threatening; systemic lupus erythematosus (SLE) can be life threatening because it is a progressive, systemic inflammatory disease that can cause major body organ and system failure. Although this definition seems similar to the definition of rheumatoid arthritis, one distinct difference exists. Patients with SLE typically have more body organ involvement earlier in their disease than patients with rheumatoid arthritis.

Pathophysiology

SLE is an autoimmune disease characterized by spontaneous remissions and exacerbations. The body's immune system normally produces antibodies to fight invaders such as bacteria, viruses, and other materials foreign to the body. In SLE, the body does not recognize itself and begins to produce antibodies directed at the foreign "self." These antibodies attack the self antigens and form immune complexes. Production of abnormal antibodies (antinuclear antibodies [ANAs]), immune complex formation, and complement system activation results in autoimmune effects on the patient's healthy connective tissue. Many of the manifestations result from recurring injuries to the patient's vascular system. The immune complexes that result lodge in the blood and organs, leading to inflammation, damage, and possibly death.

The cause of SLE is unknown, but the disorder tends to occur in families. Identified chromosomal markers indicate a genetic link. Environmental factors also may play a critical role in development of SLE. Infections, high stress levels, various hormones and drugs (especially antibiotics such as sulfa and penicillin), and ultraviolet (UV) light have all been linked to triggering SLE. Exacerbation of symptoms often occurs before the start of menstruation and during pregnancy, demonstrating the link hormones have in triggering SLE.

African Americans, Hispanics, Native Americans, and Asians are two to three times more likely to develop SLE than others. Lupus most often affects women between ages

15 and 40 and at a rate 10 to 15 times more often than for men. Women represent 90% of all cases of SLE.

With improved therapy, the mortality rate for patients with SLE has improved greatly during the past 30 years. The leading causes of death are kidney failure, heart failure, and central nervous system involvement.

Signs and Symptoms

Unfortunately, there is no classic description of patients with SLE. Some patients have a very mild form of the disease in which only the skin and joints are affected. Others have devastating effects on multiple body systems at the same time.

The classic feature of lupus is the characteristic raised, reddened butterfly rash found over the bridge of the nose that extends to both cheeks, although only half of patients develop it (Fig. 46.12). The rash is usually dry and may itch. It commonly is photosensitive, tends to worsen during an exacerbation, and can be triggered by exposure to ultraviolet light or by physical stressors, such as pregnancy or infection. Instead of the butterfly rash, some patients have discoid (coinlike) skin lesions on other parts of the body. During flare-ups, a fever develops that can rise to more than 100°F (38°C). Fatigue, arthralgia or arthritis, myalgia, malaise, weight loss, mucosal ulcers, and alopecia are some other possible signs and symptoms of SLE (Table 46.2).

Diagnostic Tests

Skin lesions can be biopsied and examined microscopically for signs of inflammation. Patients with suspected SLE are evaluated using the same immunologically based laboratory tests that are used to assess patients with rheumatoid arthritis. These tests include ESR (to detect systemic inflammation) and ANA titers (to detect the presence of abnormal antibodies). There are also two subtypes of ANA: anti-DNA and anti-sm antibodies, which are found only in patients with SLE and can be useful in confirming a diagnosis of SLE. A blood test involving serine/arginine-rich (SR) proteins also may aid in diagnosis of SLE. Patients with SLE make antibodies against SR proteins (which are important in cell division). Seventy percent of SLE patients react positively to these anti-SR antibodies. This new diagnostic tool should help in identifying SLE patients who do not produce some of the other antibodies looked for in the diagnosis of SLE. Although no laboratory test confirms a diagnosis of SLE, the results of immunological tests may support the diagnosis.

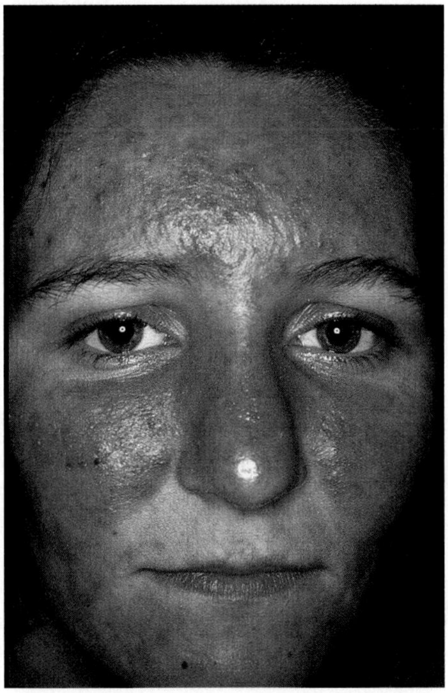

FIGURE 46.12 Lupus erythematosus: red papules and plaques in butterfly pattern on face. (From Goldsmith, L. A., Lazarus, G. S., Tharp, M. D., et al. [1997]. *Adult and pediatric dermatology* [p. 230]. Philadelphia: F. A. Davis, with permission.)

TABLE 46.2 MANIFESTATIONS OF SYSTEMIC LUPUS ERYTHEMATOSUS

Body System	Manifestations
Central nervous system	Headache, epilepsy, psychoses Peripheral or sensory neuropathies Personality changes, mild alterations in cognition
Cardiovascular system	Inflammation of pericardium (pericarditis) Alteration in circulation, particularly to digits (Raynaud's phenomenon)
Pulmonary system	Pleural effusions
Renal system	Inflammation of kidney Glomerulonephritis
Gastrointestinal system	Peritonitis
Musculoskeletal system	Arthralgias (due to inflammation), especially of the hands, wrists, and knees Myalgias
Skin	Butterfly rash across bridge of nose Rash that is reddened and raised
Constitutional signs and symptoms	Increased temperature Malaise, tiredness Weight loss

Therapeutic Measures

Treatment of SLE focuses on decreasing inflammation and preventing life-threatening organ damage. At present, the therapy of choice includes medications to treat the symptoms or the body systems affected. Research is ongoing regarding the possible cause of SLE. Researchers have found the general location of a gene that is believed to predispose a person to lupus. Identifying the genetic cause of lupus will enable researchers to develop new methods of therapy, including gene therapy. Prevention of exacerbations (flares) is important, and therefore taking preventive measures is suggested. Minimizing exposure to the sun and wearing sunscreens helps those patients who are photosensitive. Regular exercise and keeping immunizations up to date are also helpful.

MEDICATION. Medications are prescribed according to the patient's needs. NSAIDs, acetaminophen, corticosteroids, antimalarials (chloroquine [Aralen], hydroxychloroquine [Plaquenil]), immunomodulating drugs, and anticoagulants all may be part of the medication regimen. Topical cortisone preparations may help reduce skin inflammation and promote fading of skin lesions.

Patients who experience joint inflammation are usually placed on an NSAID. Patients with organ or major body system involvement are given more potent drugs that suppress the immune process, including oral steroids such as prednisone or immunomodulating agents such as azathioprine (Imuran) or cyclophosphamide (Cytoxan). These drugs have serious side effects, and patients receiving them are monitored very carefully. In addition to monitoring for a variety of side effects, patients must be taught to avoid people with infections because they are immunocompromised while taking any of these medications.

Nursing Process for the Patient with Systemic Lupus Erythematosus

DATA COLLECTION. Determine the extent and severity of signs and symptoms, such as pain, fatigue, skin lesions, and fever. Individualize the plan of care because every patient with SLE is unique.

NURSING DIAGNOSES, PLANNING, AND IMPLEMENTATION. See the nursing process sections on osteoarthritis and rheumatoid arthritis for:

- *Acute Pain* related to joint swelling
- *Chronic Sorrow* related to loss of health, role changes, and having a chronic disease
- *Fatigue* related to chronic disease process
- *Disturbed Body Image* related to alterations in skin integrity
- *Self-Care Deficits.*

Ineffective Coping Related to Chronic Disease Condition and Alteration in Body Integrity

EXPECTED OUTCOME: The patient will make appropriate decisions related to personal life and condition.

- Assess patient's coping pattern and ability *to assist in determining patient's coping needs.*
- Provide support and reassurance to patient *to let patient know someone is there to help.*
- Assist in problem solving when needed, without taking over, *to help and improve self-confidence.*
- Encourage inclusion of support systems and resources *to utilize all avenues available to help.*
- Include input from other disciplines, such as social work and clergy, *to ensure all alternatives are considered.*

Risk For Impaired Skin Integrity Related to Disease Condition and Increased Susceptibility to UV Light

EXPECTED OUTCOME: The patient will maintain skin integrity.

- Teach importance of protecting self from UV light (decrease sun exposure, wear sunscreen and appropriate clothing) *to minimize flare-ups.*
- Ensure good hygiene *to help minimize infections and promote skin integrity.*
- Apply topical creams and ointments as ordered *to help with inflammation and discomfort.*

EVALUATION. The outcome is met if patient makes appropriate decisions related to personal life and condition and if skin integrity is maintained.

PATIENT EDUCATION. Teach the patient about skin care and ways to prevent disease exacerbations. Skin care includes use of a mild soap, patting the skin dry, using lotion, avoiding drying agents, protecting from sunlight with sun block (SPF 30) and protective clothing and hats, and avoiding tanning beds. Exercise can prevent muscle weakness and fatigue. The patient should be encouraged to be vaccinated against specific infections. Methods of stress reduction should be identified and utilized.

The Arthritis Foundation and the Lupus Foundation are national organizations that can provide information, assistance, and community support groups for patients diagnosed with lupus. For more information, visit the Arthritis Foundation at http://arthritis.org and the Lupus Foundation of America at www.lupus.org.

Scleroderma

The term **scleroderma** is Greek in origin meaning "hard skin." It is similar to SLE in that it can affect multiple organs and other connective tissues. Scleroderma is not as common as SLE but has a higher mortality rate. There are two types of scleroderma: localized and systemic. As the name implies, systemic scleroderma can affect any part of the body. Among other names for systemic scleroderma are diffuse and progressive systemic scleroderma; however, because scleroderma is not necessarily progressive, this term is not encouraged. What is more frequently seen is the term *systemic sclerosis* (SSc).

Pathophysiology

Scleroderma is characterized by inflammation that ultimately develops into fibrosis (scarring) and then sclerosis (hardening) of tissues. The disease is an autoimmune response to the body's normal tissues. As in some of the other systemic connective tissue diseases, abnormal antibodies damage healthy tissue, resulting in inflammation, which then triggers overproduction of collagen, which is deposited in the skin. The collagen produced is insoluble and, when deposited in the skin, causes inflammation. Edema in the

• WORD • BUILDING •

scleroderma: sclero—hardening + derma—skin

skin ultimately results in loss of elasticity and tissue function. The same process can occur internally, affecting blood vessels and organs.

SSc affects about 300,000 Americans, women three to four times more often than men. It can occur at any age but usually develops between ages 25 and 55. The disease tends to progress rapidly and does not respond well to treatment. Spontaneous remissions and exacerbations can occur. There is a relationship between scleroderma and Raynaud's syndrome. About 95% of patients with scleroderma have Raynaud's phenomenon.

Signs and Symptoms

Although arthritis and fatigue are commonly seen, the most obvious sign of SSc is manifested at first by pitting edema, starting in the upper extremities. The skin is taut, shiny, and without wrinkles. The swelling is replaced by tightening, hardening, and thickening of skin tissue. The skin then loses its elasticity, range of motion is decreased, and skin ulcers may appear. As the disease progresses, the patient loses range of motion and the affected area becomes contracted.

The same pathophysiological process affects certain body systems, especially the kidneys, lungs, heart, and gastrointestinal tract. If any of these systems are affected, the corresponding signs and symptoms are present. For example, gastrointestinal tract involvement usually manifests as esophagitis, dysphagia (difficulty swallowing), and decreased intestinal peristalsis caused by decreased smooth muscle elasticity.

The prognosis is thought to be worse when the patient has CREST syndrome, a group of signs and symptoms occurring at the same time:

Calcinosis (calcium deposits)
Raynaud's phenomenon (severe vasospasms of the small vessels in the hands and feet)
Esophageal dysmotility (decreased activity)
Sclerodactyly (scleroderma of the finger digits)
Telangiectasia (spiderlike skin lesions).

Diagnostic Tests

The patient's clinical history and physical manifestations (particularly the sclerotic changes that occur in the skin) aid in the diagnosis of scleroderma. Biopsies of the skin, laboratory tests (ANA, and most recently anti–Scl-70 antibodies and anticentromere antibodies [ACA]), pulmonary function tests, and electrocardiographic (ECG) or x-ray examinations (including esophageal studies) are used to determine the severity of organ involvement or if other diagnostic testing is not helpful in diagnosing this condition.

Therapeutic Measures

The goal of medical management is to slow disease progression. Systemic steroids, such as prednisone, and immunosuppressant drugs are used in large doses and in combination during a flare-up of SSc.

Other care approaches are directed toward symptom management. Skin-protective measures can help minimize the chance of ulcerations or irritation. For example, teach the patient to use mild soaps and lotions to moisturize the skin.

If the patient has esophageal involvement, small, frequent, bland meals are better tolerated than large, spicy ones. Difficulty swallowing may necessitate cutting the food into smaller, more manageable portions or providing food that is pureed. (Thicker liquids are easier to swallow than thin liquids.) Medications to treat esophageal reflux, such as antacids and histamine blockers, may be prescribed.

Patients with Raynaud's phenomenon or other types of **vasculitis** usually experience severe pain when small blood vessels constrict. Joints may also be painful. Pain management is a priority in the care of patients with SSc. A bed cradle or footboard keeps bed covers away from skin. Socks and gloves may keep the fingers and toes warm, thus diminishing pain. Minimizing exposure to cold and avoiding stressful situations, stopping smoking, and taking certain medications, such as calcium channel blockers, antiadrenergic agents, and angiotensin-converting enzyme (ACE) inhibitors, can all help promote circulation or minimize the likelihood of an attack. Research has suggested that antioxidant therapy may provide another approach to treating SSc.

Rehabilitative therapy may be needed to help the patient be as independent as possible with activities of daily living and mobility. Collaborate with other members of the interdisciplinary team to individualize care.

Osteogenesis Imperfecta

Osteogenesis imperfecta is a rare inheritable disease that is also called fragilitas ossium or brittle bones disease. It is a congenital abnormality characterized by skeletal bone fragility. The fragility predisposes the person to pathological fractures and bone deformities. In addition, there is connective tissue involvement that can cause changes or abnormalities in the eyes, ears, joints, skin, and teeth.

Pathophysiology

In osteogenesis imperfecta, osteoblasts and fibroblasts synthesize collagen abnormally, resulting in fragile bones, multiple fractures (especially of the long bones), bone deformities (resulting from improper healing and weak callus formation along with thinner, smaller, and shorter bones), fragile and discolored teeth, loose joints, and thin, easily damaged skin. There are four types of osteogenesis imperfecta classified according to severity and characteristics, with type 1 being the most common and least severe form of the condition.

Signs and Symptoms

People with osteogenesis imperfecta exhibit many variations in signs and symptoms. Some of the symptoms common to all types include:

- Fragile bones (easily broken or bent)
- Triangular-shaped face

• WORD • BUILDING •
vasculitis: vascul—blood vessel + itis—inflammation

- Potential hearing loss
- Scoliosis (spine curvature), which may create respiratory problems
- Loose joints
- Alterations in muscle tone or development
- Blue, purple, or gray tint to sclerae
- Brittle or discolored teeth
- Smooth, thin skin.

Types II, III, and IV also include:

- Decreased height (may only grow to 3 feet tall)
- Barrel-shaped rib cage.

Diagnosis

Diagnosis may be based on clinical features. Most often, diagnosis is made because of frequent fractures without an apparent cause, usually in an infant or child. Most patients with osteogenesis imperfecta can have 40 to 100 fractures by the time they reach puberty, depending on the type of osteogenesis imperfecta they have. It is also not uncommon for babies with type II to be born with fractures and to either be born dead or die shortly after birth. The only test currently available is a biopsy of the skin assessing the collagen fibers. The test can take weeks to get results and is not definitive.

Therapeutic Measures and Nursing Care

There is no treatment for osteogenesis imperfecta. Interventions include treating fractures and trying to minimize bone deformities. Splints, casts, and braces are used to aid in healing the fractures and maintaining structure and function. Medications such as pamidronate (Aredia), a bone resorption inhibitor, are being tried to see if bone density can be increased, fractures decreased, mobility improved, and pain decreased. Gene therapy is also being suggested; however, this form of therapy will not be available soon.

Nursing care requires careful handling of the patient with the understanding that fractures will occur despite taking great care. It is important to teach the family and for the nurse to understand that it is not necessarily something that they did that caused a fracture; rather, it is the pathological process causing the breaks. The Osteogenesis Imperfecta Foundation (www.oif.org) is an excellent resource for patients, family, and the health care team.

Polymyositis

Polymyositis is a disease with an unknown cause that results in diffuse inflammation of skeletal muscle, leading to weakness, atrophy, and degeneration. When a rash is present with muscle inflammation, the disease is called dermatomyositis. The disease is progressive; however, remissions and exacerbations are common. Women are affected more than men, especially in their middle-aged years.

The shoulder and pelvic girdle muscles (proximal muscles) are most commonly affected. The patient may have associated conditions, such as arthritis, fatigue, and possibly Raynaud's phenomenon (spasms and constriction of small vessels in the hands and feet). Patients with dermatomyositis also have the classic heliotrope (lilac) rash and periorbital (around the eyes) swelling. Malignant tumors occur in patients with these diseases more often than in the rest of the population.

Patients are treated symptomatically, using an interdisciplinary approach, to maintain optimum function. The drug of choice is high doses of prednisone. Side effects, such as immunosuppression, can occur with prednisone.

• WORD • BUILDING •

polymyositis: poly—many + myo—muscle + itis—inflammation

Muscular Dystrophy

Muscular dystrophy (MD) is a group of nine disorders resulting in loss of muscle tissue and progressive muscle weakness. A number of disorders are diagnosed in childhood (e.g., Duchenne's MD is most common in children); however, other forms of MD, such as myotonic MD, are most common in adults. People with MD are now living longer into adulthood as a result of advances in treatment.

Pathophysiology and Etiology

MD has a genetic origin. However, the exact cause is unknown. Skeletal (voluntary) muscle fibers degenerate and atrophy. This loss of muscle tissue results in muscle weakness and wasting. Muscle tissue is replaced by connective tissue. These changes in muscle tissue result in increasing disability and deformity. Life expectancy after diagnosis depends on the type of MD as well as the speed and severity of progression. Involvement of the heart and lungs also influences the life expectancy. In some forms of MD, young adulthood (mid to late 20s) is the average life expectancy.

Signs and Symptoms

Signs and symptoms usually become apparent in childhood. Difficulty walking and muscle weakness in the arms, legs, and trunk are indicators of MD. People with MD may have difficulty raising their arms above their heads or climbing stairs. Other signs and symptoms include frequent falls, developmental delays involving muscle skills, drooping eyelids (ptosis), drooling, intellectual retardation (only in some types of MD), contractures, and skeletal deformities.

Diagnostic Tests

An increase in serum creatinine phosphokinase (CPK) caused by muscle atrophy is present in MD. Electromyography (EMG) and muscle biopsy can be used for diagnosis. Lactic dehydrogenase (LDH) and the isoenzymes, myoglobin (urine or serum), creatinine (urine or serum), CPK isoenzymes, and aspartate aminotransferase (AST) levels may also be altered in patients with MD. Tests for gene mutations are also available for some of the various types of MD.

Therapeutic Measures

Goals include supportive care and prevention of complications. Treatment regimens focus on controlling symptoms and maximizing quality of life. Keeping the patient as active as possible is a priority in planning care. Exercise programs (e.g., range of motion, physical therapy) help prevent muscle tightness, contractures, and atrophy. Splints and braces provide support during activities of daily living. Surgery may be done to correct deformities. The potential benefit of gene therapy is currently being investigated.

Nursing Process for the Patient with Muscular Dystrophy

DATA COLLECTION. Assess for muscle weakness, noting what areas of the body are affected and the severity of the weakness. Asking the patient and family what activities can be done with and without assistance helps determine the plan of care.

NURSING DIAGNOSES, PLANNING, AND IMPLEMENTATION

Impaired Physical Mobility Related to Muscle Weakness

EXPECTED OUTCOME: The patient's mobility will increase or be maintained for as long as possible.

- Provide assistive devices (e.g., braces, splints, wheelchair) *to assist with mobility.*
- Provide active and passive range-of-motion exercises and other physical therapy *to prevent contractures and improve muscle strength.*
- Encourage the patient to do as much as possible *to increase independence and help maintain muscle function.*
- Include disciplines such as physiotherapy and occupational therapy *to provide equipment and devices that will help with independence and mobility.*

Ineffective Breathing Pattern Related to Muscle Weakness

EXPECTED OUTCOME: The patient will demonstrate normal respiratory function and normal oxygen saturation.

- Monitor respiratory function (rate and effort) every 4 hours *to detect changes.*
- Monitor oxygen saturation and keep above 90% *to promote oxygenation.*
- Administer oxygen at 2 L/min or as ordered *to keep oxygen saturation above 90%.*
- Position patient *to increase respiratory efficiency.*
- Teach patient about lung function studies *to prepare patient.*
- Teach patient to minimize chances of infection (e.g., stay away from crowds) and to ensure early attention to respiratory alterations *to obtain prompt treatment.*

EVALUATION. The outcome is met if the patient improves or maintains physical mobility and the patient's oxygen saturation level is normal.

PATIENT EDUCATION. The patient and family need to understand the importance of physical therapy in maintaining function and preventing complications. National organizations and support groups provide information, resources, and emotional support. Family members need to encourage the patient to have activity and rest periods. As with any neuromuscular condition, the patient needs to avoid exposure to the cold and persons with infections. For more information on muscular dystrophy, visit www.mdausa.org or www.mdac.ca.

Osteoarthritis

Osteoarthritis (OA) is the most common type of connective tissue disorder, affecting more than 20 million people in the United States. The term **arthritis** means inflammation of the joint, but OA is not a primary inflammatory process. Therefore, some health care providers may refer to this disorder as *degenerative joint disease.* This term better reflects its pathophysiology.

Pathophysiology

OA occurs when the articular cartilage and bone ends of joints slowly deteriorate (Table 46.3). The joint space narrows, bone spurs develop, and the joint may become

TABLE 46.3 OSTEOARTHRITIS AND RHEUMATOID ARTHRITIS SUMMARY

	Osteoarthritis	Rheumatoid Arthritis
Pathophysiology	Articular cartilage and bone ends deteriorate. Joint is inflamed.	Inflammatory cells cause synovitis. Synovium becomes thick and fluid accumulates, causing swelling and pain. Joint becomes deformed.
Etiology	*Primary (idiopathic):* • Cause unknown. • Risk factors include age, obesity, activities causing joint stress. *Secondary:* • Causes include trauma, sepsis, congenital abnormalities, metabolic disorders (Paget's disease), rheumatoid arthritis.	Autoimmune disease. Can occur at any age (including juvenile rheumatoid arthritis). Cause unknown. Familial history possible.

Continued

• WORD • BUILDING •
arthritis: arthr(on)—joint + itis—inflammation

TABLE 46.3 OSTEOARTHRITIS AND RHEUMATOID ARTHRITIS SUMMARY—cont'd

	Osteoarthritis	Rheumatoid Arthritis
Signs and Symptoms	Joint pain and stiffness. Pain increases with activity and decreases with rest. Nodes on joints of fingers (Heberden's nodes, Bouchard's nodes).	Symptoms vary according to disease process. *Early symptoms:* • Bilateral and symmetrical joint inflammation • Redness, warmth, swelling, stiffness, pain • Stiffness after resting (morning stiffness) • Activity decreases pain and stiffness • Low-grade fever, weakness, fatigue, anorexia (mild weight loss) • Organ system involvement. *Late symptoms:* • Joint deformity • Secondary osteoporosis.
Therapeutic Measures	Medication • Nonsteroidal anti-inflammatory drugs (NSAIDs) • Acetaminophen • Muscle relaxants. Balanced rest and exercise. Splinting of joint to promote rest. Heat and cold. Diet for weight loss. Complementary therapies. Surgery for total joint replacement.	Medication • NSAIDs • Biological response modifier • Prednisone • Disease-modifying antirheumatic drug (DMARD) • T-cell modulators. Heat and cold. Balanced rest and activity. Surgery for total joint replacement.
Priority Nursing Diagnoses	*Chronic Pain* *Impaired Physical Mobility* *Disturbed Body Image*	*Chronic Pain* *Self-Care Deficits* *Ineffective Health Maintenance*

somewhat inflamed. The repair process is not able to overcome the rapid loss of cartilage and bone, eventually resulting in joint deformities, pain, and immobility, leading to the patient's functional decline. Weight-bearing joints (hips and knees), hands, and the vertebral column are most often affected (Fig. 46.13).

Etiology and Types

The most common type of OA is primary (idiopathic) osteoarthritis. The cause of OA is unknown, but several risk factors have been identified. Aging, obesity, and physical activities that create mechanical stress on joints are major risks. Each of these factors causes prolonged or excessive wear and tear on synovial joints. Most people over age 60 have some degree of symptomatic joint degeneration. Native Americans are affected more often than other groups, but the reason for this is unknown.

Patients with secondary OA develop joint degeneration as a result of trauma, sepsis, congenital anomalies, certain metabolic diseases (such as Paget's disease), or systemic inflammatory connective tissue disorders such as rheumatoid arthritis.

Signs and Symptoms

The patient usually seeks medical attention when joint pain and stiffness become severe or the patient has problems with everyday activities. One or more joints may be affected, most commonly in the hands, hips, knees, spine, and feet. Joint pain intensifies after physical activity but lessens following rest. If the vertebral column is involved, the patient reports radiating pain and muscle spasms in the extremity innervated by the area affected.

About half of patients with OA have bony nodes on the joints of their fingers, called Heberden's and Bouchard's nodes. Women tend to have them more often than men, and they may or may not be painful. The nodes have a familial tendency and often are a cosmetic concern to female patients.

Diagnostic Tests

X-ray examinations are useful in outlining joint structure and detecting bone changes. A CT scan or MRI may be used to diagnose various joint involvement. Analysis of synovial fluid can aid in the diagnosis of OA while ruling out other pathological conditions of the joint.

Therapeutic Measures

There is no cure for OA. Management centers on pain control, which is accomplished by drug therapy, other pain relief measures, or ultimately surgery (see *Evidence-Based Practice* box). An interdisciplinary approach is needed to prevent decreased mobility and preserve joint function.

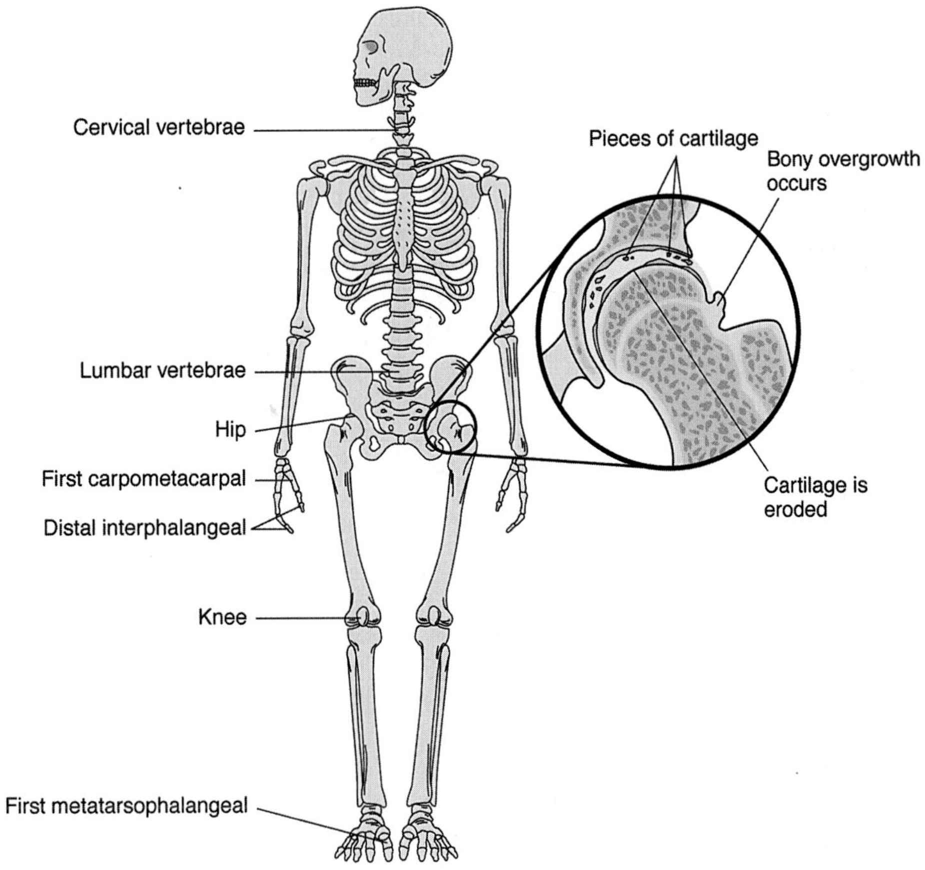
Cervical vertebrae
Lumbar vertebrae
Hip
First carpometacarpal
Distal interphalangeal
Knee
First metatarsophalangeal
Pieces of cartilage
Bony overgrowth occurs
Cartilage is eroded

FIGURE 46.13 Common joints affected by osteoarthritis and the changes that result in the joint.

EVIDENCE-BASED PRACTICE

Clinical Question

Does acetaminophen control osteoarthritis pain more effectively than a placebo?

Evidence

In a review of seven randomized controlled trials, acetaminophen provided statistically more pain reduction than a placebo (Towheed et al., 2006). Patients who took acetaminophen had less pain with movement, rest, sleeping, and overall generalized pain. Pain decreased by 4 points more on a scale of 0 to 100 when using acetaminophen.

Implications for Nursing Practice

Acetaminophen can be helpful in reducing the pain of osteoarthritis. Nurses should address common side effects and the maximum daily dose during patient education (Schofield, 2008).

REFERENCES

Schofield, P. (2008). Pain management in osteoarthritis. *Practice Nurse, 35*(6), 20–25.

Towheed, T., Maxwell, L., Judd, M., et al. (2006). Acetaminophen for osteoarthritis. *Cochrane Database of Systematic Reviews 2006, Issue 1* (Art. No. CD004257; DOI 10.1002/14651858.CD004257pub2).

Synvisc is injected directly into osteoarthritic knees and acts like healthy, cushioning synovial fluid. Pain is relieved and flexibility restored when the knee joint is again lubricated and cushioned. For more information about this therapy, visit www.synvisc.com.

CRITICAL THINKING

Mr. Dennis

■ Mr. Dennis is 59 years old, overweight, and a carpenter who visits his physician because of knee and wrist pain. He has noticed that it is becoming increasingly difficult to climb a ladder or use a hammer. The physician suspects osteoarthritis.

1. What data collection questions should be included in a patient history?
2. What risk factors does the patient have?
3. What other signs and symptoms might he have?

Suggested answers at end of chapter.

MEDICATION. Drug therapy is commonly used to reduce pain in patients with OA. Often, it is combined with other pain-reducing therapies. The most commonly used drugs are

NSAIDs (Table 46.4). These drugs have analgesic and anti-inflammatory effects. Common side effects include gastrointestinal distress and bleeding, which can be severe; and sodium and fluid retention. They also may increase the risk of cardiovascular events, such as myocardial infarction or stroke. Older adult patients taking NSAIDs on a routine basis should be carefully monitored for congestive heart failure and high blood pressure from fluid retention. Topical creams such as capsaicin (ArthriCare) also may be ordered and applied to the joints.

TABLE 46.4 COMMON DRUGS USED TO TREAT CONNECTIVE TISSUE DISEASES: OSTEOARTHRITIS, RHEUMATOID ARTHRITIS, AND OTHERS

Medication Class/Action	Examples	Route	Side Effects	Nursing Implications
Biological Response Modifiers				
Interleukin-1 inhibitors that reduce inflammation and cartilage degradation.	anakinra (Kineret)	Subcutaneously	Increased risk of infection, bruising, nausea, diarrhea	Monitor neutrophils.
Corticosteroids				
Reduce inflammation and swelling.	prednisone (Deltasone, Orasone)	PO	Weight gain, fat deposits, edema, hypertension, infection, fractures, poor wound healing, GI bleeding, depression, mood swings	Take daily weight. Monitor I&O. Assess for infection. Give with food/milk. Recommend patient obtain medic alert ID. Not used for osteoarthritis.
Disease-Modifying Antirheumatic Drugs (DMARDs)				
For rheumatoid arthritis, ankylosing spondylitis, lupus. Reduce symptoms, prevent joint damage, and preserve joint function by suppressing immune or inflammatory systems.				Slow-acting drugs may take months for effect. Other drugs used to control symptoms until effective. Effect ends when drug stopped.
Pyrimidine synthesis inhibitors	leflunomide (Arava)	PO	Diarrhea, nausea, respiratory infection, hypertension	Screen for tuberculosis before starting. Monitor BP, CBC, liver function. Teach patient to report rash promptly.
Gold preparations	auranofin (Ridaura) aurothioglucose (Solganal)	PO IM	Gold toxicity: blood dyscrasias	Lab testing for gold toxicity effect recommended.
Immunosuppressives	azathioprine (Imuran) cyclophosphamide (Cytoxan) cyclosporine (Sandimmune, Neoral) leflunomide (Arava; rheumatoid arthritis only) methotrexate (Mexate) d-penicillamine (Cuprimine, Depen).	PO IV, PO PO PO PO, IM PO	Infection	Protect from infection. Monitor for infections.
Tumor necrosis factor inhibitors	adalimumab (Humira) etanercept (Enbrel)	Subcutaneously	Infection, headache, sinus pain, nausea	Screen for tuberculosis.
Antimalarials	chloroquine (Aralen)	PO, IM	GI upset, dizziness, headache	Report vision problems.
	hydroxychloroquine (Plaquenil)	PO		Promote safety due to dizziness.

TABLE 46.4 COMMON DRUGS USED TO TREAT CONNECTIVE TISSUE DISEASES: OSTEOARTHRITIS, RHEUMATOID ARTHRITIS, AND OTHERS—cont'd

Medication Class/Action	Examples	Route	Side Effects	Nursing Implications
Nonsteroidal Anti-Inflammatory Drugs (NSAIDs)				
Block activity of enzyme cyclooxygenase (COX-1, COX-2), which makes prostaglandins that produce inflammation, fever, pain; support platelets; and protect stomach lining (COX-1 only).	acetylsalicylic acid (aspirin) diclofenac sodium (Voltaren) diflunisal (Dolobid) etodolac (Lodine; osteoarthritis only) fenoprofen (Nalfon) flurbiprofen (Ansaid) ibuprofen (Motrin) indomethacin (Indocin) ketoprofen (Orudis) naproxen (Aleve, Naprosyn) oxaprozin (Daypro) piroxicam (Feldene) nabumetone (Relafen) sulindac (Clinoril) tolmetin (Tolectin)	PO	Varies with drug: nausea, vomiting, GI bleeding, diarrhea, constipation, anorexia, rash, dizziness, headache, drowsiness, edema	Teach risk of GI bleeding. Those with asthma at higher risk for allergic reaction.
T-Cell Modulators				
Reduce activation of T cells in the inflammatory process.	abatacept (Orencia)	IV	Headache, nausea, respiratory infections	Screen for tuberculosis. Use silicone-free syringe only. Infused over 30 minutes. Monitor for serious infections.

REST AND EXERCISE. Joint pain from OA tends to decrease with rest; therefore, pain is less severe in the morning. Activities should be scheduled at this time. A severely inflamed joint may be splinted by the occupational or physical therapist to promote rest to a selected joint. However, rest must be balanced with exercise to prevent muscle atrophy from disuse. Exercise has been identified as a means to maintain general health and weight, range of motion, and muscle strength, while decreasing anxiety and depression. To minimize muscle atrophy and to stabilize and protect arthritic joints, patients should be encouraged to perform exercises to strengthen their quadriceps if they have OA of the knee.

Joints should always be placed in their functional position—that is, a position that does not lead to contractures. For example, only a small pillow should be placed under the head when sleeping to prevent excessive neck flexion.

HEAT AND COLD. The patient with OA usually prefers heat therapy unless the joint is acutely inflamed. Hot packs, warm compresses, warm showers, moist heating pads, and paraffin dips provide sources of heat. Cold therapy minimizes inflammation while altering cutaneous pain receptors, thereby decreasing pain. Cold packs should be applied for no longer than 20 minutes at a time.

DIET. Obese or overweight patients benefit from losing weight to decrease stress on weight-bearing joints and thereby reduce pain. If the patient is on medications that can alter fluid volumes (corticosteroids), a diet low in sodium may be appropriate.

COMPLEMENTARY THERAPIES. The popularity of complementary therapies to reduce pain and stress has grown tremendously. Imagery, music therapy, acupressure, acupuncture, and other holistic modalities that foster the mind-body-spirit connection work well for many people.

SURGERY. If the patient's pain is not managed successfully, a total joint replacement (TJR) may be indicated. TJR is the most common type of **arthroplasty** (see later section on musculoskeletal surgery).

Nursing Process for the Patient with Osteoarthritis

DATA COLLECTION. The patient's report of pain is assessed and the joints observed for signs of inflammation or deformity. Also assessed are function, alterations in activities of daily living (ADLs), and mobility (Box 46.7, *Gerontological Issues*).

• **WORD • BUILDING** •
arthroplasty: arthro—joint + plasty—creation of

Box 46.7

Gerontological Issues

Osteoarthritis (OA) affects millions of Americans. Because of the large number of people with this condition, it is recommended that nurses check for OA even when it is not the admitting diagnosis to help identify functional deficits and treatment needs.

OA treatment focuses on pain management and functional ability. In addition, interventions that have been shown to help a hospitalized older adult patient after discharge include:

- Identifying a social support system
- Teaching medication side effects as well as interactions that may cause bleeding
- Encouraging participation in occupational and physical therapy
- Referring to a nutritionist for weight loss if indicated
- Referring for cognitive-behavioral therapy for pain management and coping as prescribed.

NURSING DIAGNOSES, PLANNING, IMPLEMENTATION, AND EVALUATION

Chronic Pain Related to Chronic Inflammatory Disease

EXPECTED OUTCOME: The patient will state that pain is within tolerable levels on a pain assessment scale of 0 to 10.

- Ask patient to rate pain on a scale of 0 to 10 *to determine level of pain and need for pain relief.*
- Provide analgesics as ordered *to help alleviate painful sensations.*
- Collaborate with interdisciplinary team such as pain clinic *to explore alternative pain relief measures.*
- Consider alternative methods of therapy such as guided imagery, distraction, acupuncture, and biofeedback *to use all possible methods of pain control.*

Activity Intolerance Related to Pain

EXPECTED OUTCOME: The patient will participate in ADLs as tolerated.

- Encourage as much independence as possible *to promote activity.*
- Assist with ADLs as needed *to ensure that patient does not become exhausted.*
- Provide pain relief measures before activity *to enable an increase in activity level.*
- Ensure nursing interventions are performed in "groups" *to minimize patient exertion.*
- Collaborate with interdisciplinary team (e.g., occupational therapy, home care physiotherapy) *to utilize their resources and knowledge.*

Chronic Sorrow Related to Altered Body Image, Altered Role, Pain, and Ongoing Losses

EXPECTED OUTCOME: The patient will verbalize improvement in feelings of sorrow.

- Allow time to discuss feelings and anticipate trigger events *to ensure the patient is aware of what may increase feelings of sorrow.*
- Encourage use of interdisciplinary team such as social worker, psychologist, clergy, or spiritual adviser *to provide alternate methods of dealing with sorrow.*
- Encourage use of support groups *to enable the patient to discuss concerns with others experiencing the same problems.*

Disturbed Body Image Related to Changes in Joint Function and Structure

EXPECTED OUTCOME: The patient will demonstrate acceptance of changes in body image.

- Encourage patient to discuss feelings and concerns *so patient knows that nurse understands what patient is experiencing.*
- Provide information and clarify misconceptions *to ensure that patient is aware of expected problems and concerns.*
- Encourage socialization *to improve the patient's perceptions of how he or she appears to others.*

Impaired Physical Mobility Related to Altered Joint Function and Pain

EXPECTED OUTCOME: The patient will demonstrate improved physical mobility.

- Administer analgesics and anti-inflammatory agents as ordered *to improve joint function and decrease pain.*
- Encourage active range-of-motion exercises *to prevent or minimize further alteration in joint function.*
- Ensure proper positioning and alignment *to promote joint function and decrease pain.*
- Use interdisciplinary team such as physiotherapy and occupational therapy *to utilize resources and knowledge from other sources.*

Self-care Deficit Related to Chronic Degenerative Joint Disease

EXPECTED OUTCOME: The patient will be able to provide own self-care.

- Encourage independence *to decrease feelings of despair about being unable to care for self.*
- Assist when necessary *to minimize frustration when patient cannot perform self-care.*
- Teach patient about assistive devices to help with activities of daily living *to promote self-care.*
- Collaborate with interdisciplinary team such as home care, occupational therapy, or physiotherapy *to acquire assistive devices and use alternate resources.*

EVALUATION. The outcomes are met if patient reports pain is within tolerable levels on a pain assessment scale of 0 to 10, is able to participate in ADLs, verbalizes improvement in feelings of sorrow, demonstrates acceptance of changes in body image, demonstrates improved physical mobility, and is able to provide own self-care.

PATIENT EDUCATION. A vital function of each member of the health care team is health teaching. The patient with OA is seldom admitted to the hospital for treatment of OA unless surgery is scheduled. However, many patients with OA are admitted for other reasons, and their arthritis needs must also be considered in the comprehensive plan of care. Most patients residing in extended care facilities also have OA, which can affect their participation in recreational activities, as well as activities of daily living.

In any setting, including the home, patients can be taught ways to protect their joints and conserve energy. Nurses need to teach patients and their families how to promote health. For information on educational materials and self-help courses, visit the Arthritis Foundation at www.arthritis.org.

Rheumatoid Arthritis

Rheumatoid arthritis (RA) is a chronic, progressive, systemic inflammatory disease that destroys synovial joints and other connective tissues, including major organs. It affects women three times more often than men and Native Americans more often than other ethnic groups. RA can occur at any age. When it occurs in children it is called juvenile RA (JRA). The peak onset of RA is ages 30 to 60, and it affects 1% to 3% of the U.S. population. Etiology is still unknown; however, there are indications that genetic predisposition and the environment play a role in triggering development.

Pathophysiology

Inflammatory cells and chemicals cause synovitis, an inflammation of the synovium (the lining of the joint capsule). As the inflammation progresses, the synovium becomes thick and fluid accumulation causes joint swelling and pain. A destructive pannus (new synovial tissue growth infiltrated with inflammatory cells) erodes the joint cartilage and eventually destroys the bone within the joint (Fig. 46.14). Ultimately the pannus is converted to bony tissue, resulting in loss of mobility. Joint deformity and bone loss are common in late RA (see Table 46.3).

Synovial joints are not the only connective tissues involved in RA. Any connective tissue may be affected, including blood vessels, nerves, kidneys, pericardium, lungs, and subcutaneous tissue. The result of body system involvement is malfunction or failure of the organ or system. Death can occur if the disease does not respond to treatment.

Many patients experience spontaneous remissions and exacerbations (flare-ups) of RA. Symptoms may disappear without treatment for months or years. Then the disease may flare up just as unpredictably. Exacerbations usually occur when the patient has physical or emotional stress, such as surgery or infection.

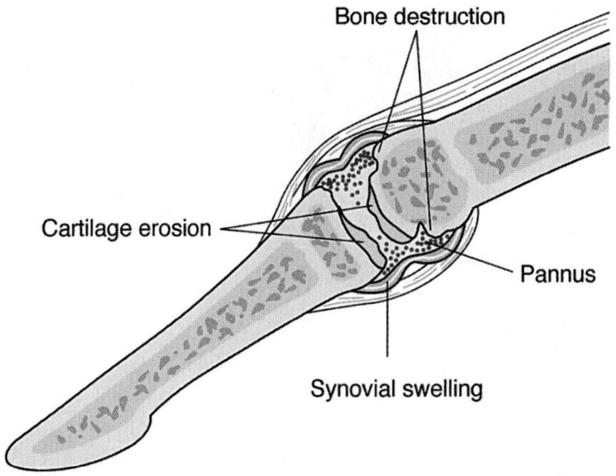
Bone destruction
Cartilage erosion
Pannus
Synovial swelling

FIGURE 46.14 Rheumatoid arthritis.

Etiology

The exact cause of RA is unknown. An autoimmune response occurs that affects the synovial membrane of the joints; it is unknown what triggers the initial response. Antibodies (called rheumatoid factor) are often found in patients with RA. It is suggested that these antibodies join with other antibodies and form antibody complexes. These complexes lodge in synovium and other connective tissues, causing local and systemic inflammation, and may be responsible for the destructive changes of RA in body tissues.

The origin of the rheumatoid factor is not clear, but a genetic predisposition is likely. RA affects people with a family history of the disease two to three times more often than the rest of the population.

Signs and Symptoms

Signs and symptoms vary because the disease progresses differently in patterns and rates from person to person. In general, the signs and symptoms can be divided into early and late manifestations.

The typical pattern of joint inflammation is bilateral and symmetrical. The disease usually begins in the upper extremities and progresses to other joints over many years (Fig. 46.15). Affected joints are slightly reddened, warm, swollen, stiff, and painful. The patient with RA often has morning stiffness lasting for up to an hour, and those with severe disease may report experiencing stiffness all day. Generally, activity decreases pain and stiffness.

Because of the systemic nature of RA, the patient may have a low-grade fever, malaise, depression, lymphadenopathy, weakness, fatigue, anorexia, and weight loss. As the disease worsens, major organs or body systems are affected. Joint deformities occur as a late symptom, and secondary osteoporosis (bone loss) can lead to fractures.

Several associated syndromes are seen in some patients with rheumatoid arthritis. For example, Sjögren's syndrome is an inflammation of tear ducts (causing dry eyes) and salivary glands (causing dry mouth). Felty's syndrome is less common and is characterized by an enlarged liver and spleen and leukopenia (decreased white blood cell count).

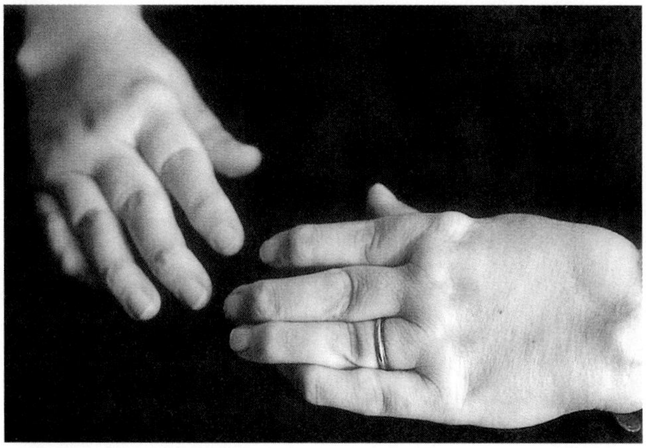

FIGURE 46.15 Joint abnormalities in hands of patient with rheumatoid arthritis.

Diagnostic Tests

No specific diagnostic test confirms RA, but several laboratory tests help support the diagnosis. An increase in white blood cells and platelets is typical, unless the patient has Felty's syndrome. A group of immunological tests are usually performed, and typical findings for patients with RA include the following:

- Presence of rheumatoid factor (RF) in serum
- Decreased red blood cell (RBC) count
- Decreased C4 complement
- Increased erythrocyte sedimentation rate (ESR)
- Positive antinuclear antibody (ANA) test
- Positive C-reactive protein (CRP) test.

RF can indicate the aggressiveness of the disease. However, it is not specific to RA and can also be found in systemic lupus erythematosus, connective tissue disease, and myositis. The ESR is also obtained to evaluate the effectiveness of treatment. If the disease responds to treatment, the ESR decreases. The higher the ESR, the more active the disease process.

> **LEARNING TIP**
>
> The erythrocyte sedimentation rate (ESR) test is a general screening test for inflammation. It measures the amount of time it takes for RBCs to settle to the bottom of a test tube. In the presence of inflammation, RBCs settle faster in the tube. Therefore, the ESR increases with the presence of inflammation.

X-ray examination and MRI detect joint damage and bone loss, especially in the vertebral column. A bone or joint scan assesses the extent of joint involvement throughout the body. For some patients, an arthrocentesis may be performed; the synovial fluid is cloudy, milky, or dark yellow with inflammatory cells present.

Therapeutic Measures

Like patients with osteoarthritis, patients with RA experience chronic joint pain. Pain can interfere with mobility or the ability to perform ADLs. Drug therapy is often needed to relieve or reduce pain as well as to slow the progression of the disease. Treatment for RA includes disease-modifying antirheumatic drugs (DMARDs), which can prevent joint destruction, deformity, and disability with early single or combination drug use; NSAIDs; and corticosteroids (see Table 46.4). Many of these medications have potentially serious side effects, such as severe infection, that must be monitored carefully.

Complementary therapies that may help decrease inflammation or pain include capsaicin cream, fish oil, magnetic therapy, and antioxidants such as vitamin C, vitamin E, and beta carotene (see Chapter 5).

HEAT AND COLD. Heat applications or hot showers help decrease joint stiffness and make exercise easier for the patient. For acutely inflamed, or "hot," joints, cold applications are preferred. As for patients with osteoarthritis, a program that balances rest and exercise later in the day is most beneficial for the patient.

SURGERY. If nonsurgical approaches are not effective in relieving arthritic pain, the patient may have a total joint replacement (discussed later). In general, patients with RA who have surgery are not as successful when compared with patients with osteoarthritis. The presence of a systemic disease predisposes patients with RA to more postoperative complications.

Nursing Process for the Patient with Rheumatoid Arthritis

DATA COLLECTION. A thorough history and physical examination are needed for the patient with RA because the disease can involve every system of the body. In addition to assessing physical signs and symptoms, assess the patient for psychosocial, functional, and vocational needs.

After having the disease for approximately 15 years, fewer than half of RA patients are totally independent in their activities of daily living. These limitations may place a burden on family members, who must be included in the care of the patient with RA. Many patients with the disease are young or middle aged. RA can impair their ability to work, depending on the type of job they have. The health care team assesses the patient's work skills to determine the need for changes in the workplace or a need to train for a new type of work.

NURSING DIAGNOSES, PLANNING, AND IMPLEMENTATION

Acute Pain Related to Chronic Disease Process

EXPECTED OUTCOME: The patient will report relief from pain within 30 minutes of pain relief intervention.

- Ask patient to rate pain on a scale of 0 to 10 *to determine level of pain and need for pain relief.*
- Provide analgesics as ordered *to relieve pain.*

- Ensure proper positioning and alignment *to minimize discomfort and promote pain relief.*
- Teach alternative measure of pain relief *to maximize means to relieve pain.*
- Encourage maintenance of normal weight *to prevent excess wear and tear on joints.*

Disturbed Body Image Related to Changes Resulting From Disease Process

EXPECTED OUTCOME: The patient will come to accept alterations in body.

- Encourage patient to discuss feelings and concerns *to provide the nurse with an understanding of what the patient is experiencing.*
- Provide information and clarify misconceptions *to ensure that the patient is aware of the expected problems and concerns.*
- Encourage socialization *to improve on the patient's perceptions of how he or she "looks" to others.*
- Encourage sharing with support groups *so that the patient discusses his or her concerns with others experiencing the same problems.*

Fatigue Related to Chronic Pain and Suffering and Difficulty with Mobilization

EXPECTED OUTCOME: The patient will have decreased episodes of fatigue.

- Ensure regular rest periods throughout the day *to not overexert the patient.*
- Assist as required *to minimize the amount of energy the patient needs to use.*
- Teach patient the need to delegate *to avoid overexertion.*
- Teach energy conservation techniques *to reduce workload.*

Self-care Deficit Related to Chronic Degenerative Disease Process

EXPECTED OUTCOME: The patient will be able to provide own self-care.

- Encourage independence *to decrease feelings of despair about being unable to care for self.*
- Assist when necessary *to minimize frustration when patient is unable to perform self-care function.*
- Teach patient about assistive devices *to help with activities of daily living and promote self-care.*
- Collaborate with interdisciplinary team such as home care and occupational or physical therapy *to acquire assistive devices and use alternate resources.*

Impaired Physical Mobility Related to Chronic Inflammation of Joints

EXPECTED OUTCOME: The patient will have improved physical mobility.

- Administer analgesics and anti-inflammatory agents *to reduce pain and increase mobility.*
- Administer heat and cold therapy *to aid in joint function and movement.*
- Encourage continued mobilization *to minimize complications of immobility.*
- Collaborate with other disciplines *to help with maintaining mobility.*

EVALUATION. The outcomes are met if the patient reports pain is within acceptable levels on a pain assessment scale of 0 to 10, demonstrates acceptance of changes in body image, has decreased episodes of fatigue, is able to provide own self-care, and demonstrates improved physical mobility.

CRITICAL THINKING

Mrs. Summers

■ Mrs. Summers is a 48-year-old nurse who has had upper extremity joint pain and swelling for about 4 years. She was recently diagnosed with rheumatoid arthritis (RA) but has no systemic involvement other than extreme fatigue at this time. She is concerned that she will have to give up providing direct patient care on a busy medical unit in the local hospital.

1. What questions might the nurse ask her at this time about her illness?
2. What should the nurse teach her about pain management?

Suggested answers at end of chapter.

PATIENT EDUCATION. The patient with RA needs extensive patient education regarding the disease process, medication management, and the comprehensive plan of care. Many fads and myths published in popular tabloids are available, and some publicized "cures" can actually be harmful to the patient.

In collaboration with health team members, help the patient plan a daily schedule that balances rest and exercise. Child care responsibilities and other day-to-day activities need to be scheduled. A vocational counselor may be necessary for job training if the patient needs to pursue a different occupation. Patients who are unable to work may be able to qualify for disability benefits through the federal Social Security program.

Inform the patient about community resources. For example, the local chapter of the Arthritis Foundation (www.arthritis.org) provides support groups, information, and other resources for patients with RA and other types of connective tissue disorders.

MUSCULOSKELETAL SURGERY

Some health problems cannot be managed conservatively and require surgery. Other disorders are initially treated medically but may need surgery if treatment is unsuccessful. The most common surgeries are discussed here.

Total Joint Replacement

Total joint replacement (TJR) is most often performed for patients who have some type of connective tissue disease in which their joints become severely deteriorated. TJR may also be done for patients on long-term steroid therapy, such as patients with SLE or asthma. Long-term use of steroids, trauma, and complications of joint replacement can cause **avascular necrosis**, a condition in which bone tissue dies (usually the femoral head) as a result of impaired blood supply. Advanced avascular necrosis is very painful and usually does not respond to conservative pain relief measures. The primary goal of TJR is to relieve severe chronic pain and improve ability to carry out ADLs when no other treatment is successful.

The most common surgeries are the total hip replacement and total knee replacement surgeries, although any synovial joint can be replaced. Another term used for joint replacement is *arthroplasty*. The replacement devices, sometimes referred to as prostheses, are made of metal, ceramic, plastic, or a combination of these materials. Some prostheses are held in place by cement. Others are secured by the patient's bone as it grafts and connects to the prosthesis. Bone substitutes, also called biologics, are being used more often when the amount of available bone is insufficient to provide a good base of support for the replacement devices. Bone glues and fillers such as OsteoSet or Pro Osteon and bone stimulants such as Allomatrix help in providing better support for the prosthetics used.

Total Hip Replacement

A total hip replacement (THR) uses a two-piece device consisting of an acetabular cup that is inserted into the pelvic acetabulum and a femoral component that is inserted into the femur to replace the femoral head and neck (Fig. 46.16). The average life span of a cemented total hip replacement is about 10 years. Noncemented prostheses used in younger patients may last longer.

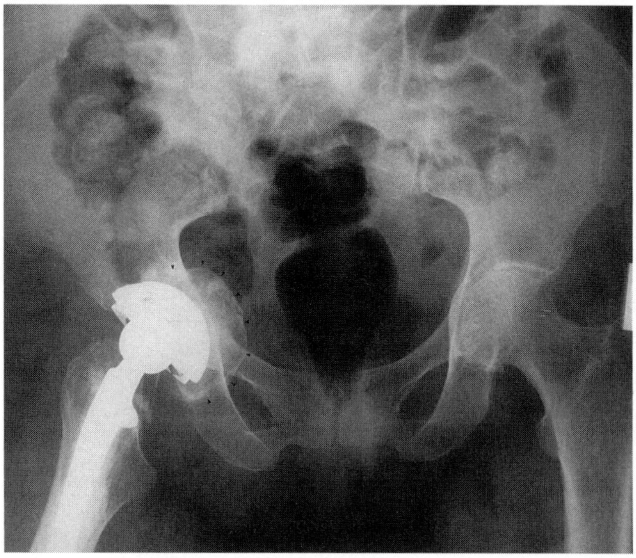

FIGURE 46.16 Total hip arthroplasty of arthritic right hip. (From McKinnis, L. N. [1997]. *Fundamentals of orthopedic radiology.* Philadelphia: F. A. Davis, with permission.)

PREOPERATIVE CARE. Total joint surgery is an elective procedure and scheduled far enough in advance to allow ample time for preoperative teaching and screening. A case manager (registered nurse or social worker) may be assigned to assess the patient's needs and the support systems that are available postoperatively. It is important for the patient to have a caregiver who can assist the patient after surgery.

In addition to the normal preparations for preoperative care (see Chapter 12), the orthopedic patient requires some preoperative baseline assessments. The nurse assesses the neurovascular status (circulation, sensation, mobility) of the extremity to be operated on as well as the patient's level of pain preoperatively. Preoperative mobility can also be assessed to help determine the effectiveness of the surgery postoperatively. The patient may require an IV to be started because the surgeon frequently orders a prophylactic antibiotic preoperatively to minimize the chance of an infection (especially osteomyelitis) developing. The patient is taught about the surgery and what to expect postoperatively. Some patients are scheduled to meet with the physical therapist to learn postoperative exercises and how to ambulate with a walker or crutches. Some institutions have total joint education programs, which provide a series of educational sessions designed to make the recovery process smoother and more effective for the patient.

Depending on the amount of blood loss during surgery, some patients receive postoperative blood transfusions. Because total joint surgery is an elective procedure, the physician may order autologous blood donation by the patient. The patient donates blood before surgery per guidelines (e.g., time frames specified, hemoglobin levels normal), which is then available for reinfusion postoperatively as needed. This predeposited blood donation is cost effective and reassures patients who are concerned about receiving blood from other donors.

Patients are often admitted to the hospital the morning of surgery. The patient's length of stay varies but is about 2 to 5 days, depending on the patient's age and progress. Some hospitals have joint camp programs where a group of patients undergoing joint replacements are admitted on the same day, undergo their surgery, and then recover together during activities such as physical therapy with each other for support. Patients have been known to recover more easily in this type of supportive environment and are typically discharged in about 3 days.

POSTOPERATIVE CARE. Care for the patient having a total hip replacement is interdisciplinary. The patient usually gets out of bed and into a chair the night of surgery or early

• WORD • BUILDING •

avascular necrosis: a—without + vascular—blood + necrosis—death the next day. Ensure that the patient does not adduct or hyperflex the surgical hip during transfer to the chair. The chair should have a straight back and be high enough to prevent excessive flexion. The toilet seat should also be raised for the same purpose. Permitted amounts of weight bearing depend on the type of prosthesis used. In general, weight bearing as tolerated or full weight bearing is used for cemented prostheses. If an uncemented device is used, the patient may be restricted to toe-touch, or partial weight bearing, or featherweight bearing.

Because patients undergoing total hip replacement are in chronic pain preoperatively, some patients report that they have less pain postoperatively than they had before surgery. Initially, pain typically is managed by epidural analgesia, patient-controlled analgesia (PCA), or injections with analgesics. After the first postoperative day, the patient usually progresses to an oral analgesic. Proper positioning also helps minimize surgical discomfort.

Early ambulation helps prevent postoperative complications such as atelectasis and deep venous thrombosis (DVT). The physical therapist works with the patient for ambulation with a walker or crutches. Crutches are reserved for young patients. After 4 to 6 weeks, the patient progresses to a cane. The patient does not need an ambulatory device if there is no limping.

Because of restrictions in hip flexion, patients are instructed not to bend forward to tie shoes or put on pants. The occupational therapist provides adaptive or assistive devices, such as dressing sticks and long-handled shoe horns, to assist the patient in being independent in activities of daily living.

In addition to providing the general postoperative care that all patients undergoing general or epidural anesthesia require, plan and implement interventions to help prevent the following common complications of total hip replacement (see Chapter 12).

Hip Dislocation. The most common postoperative complication for the patient having a total hip replacement is subluxation (partial dislocation) or total dislocation. Dislocation occurs when the femoral component becomes dislodged from the acetabular cup. Often, if a dislocation occurs, there is an audible "pop" followed by immediate pain in the affected hip. In addition to pain, the patient experiences shortening of the surgical leg and possibly rotation of the surgical leg. If any of these signs and symptoms occur, notify the surgeon immediately and keep the patient in bed. Additional analgesics may be ordered until the patient can be taken to the operating room. Under anesthesia, the surgeon manipulates the hip back into alignment and immobilizes the leg until healing occurs.

Prevention of dislocation is a major nursing responsibility. Correct positioning of the surgical leg is critical. The primary goals are to prevent hip adduction (across the body's midline) and hyperflexion (bending forward more than 90 degrees). To accomplish these goals, place the patient returning from the postanesthetic care unit (PACU) in a supine position with the head slightly elevated. A trapezoid-shaped abduction pillow (sometimes called a triangular pillow), splint, wedge, or regular bed pillows may be used between the legs to prevent adduction. The patient can be turned to the side specified by the physician (even the operative side if the patient is comfortable enough), with hip adduction avoided. The patient is turned with the abductor pillow or three regular pillows (one proximal and two distal) in place between the legs. When turning, it is important to turn the hip and legs simultaneously to minimize the chance of dislocation. Support for the leg and abductor pillow is also required when the patient is turned on his or her side to decrease the chance of dislocation.

To prevent hyperflexion, some surgeons initially allow the patient to sit at no more than a 60-degree angle in a reclining chair. The patient's position is progressed to 90 degrees, the maximum allowed to prevent hyperflexion (Fig. 46.17). While the patient is on bedrest, the use of a fracture (also called a slipper) pan is recommended when helping the patient with toileting needs to minimize discomfort and to prevent the possibility of dislocation.

Skin Breakdown. Because most patients having total joint replacements are older, skin breakdown is a major part of postoperative care. Turning the patient at least every 2 hours (more often if high risk) and keeping the heels off the bed are the key nursing interventions to prevent pressure ulcers.

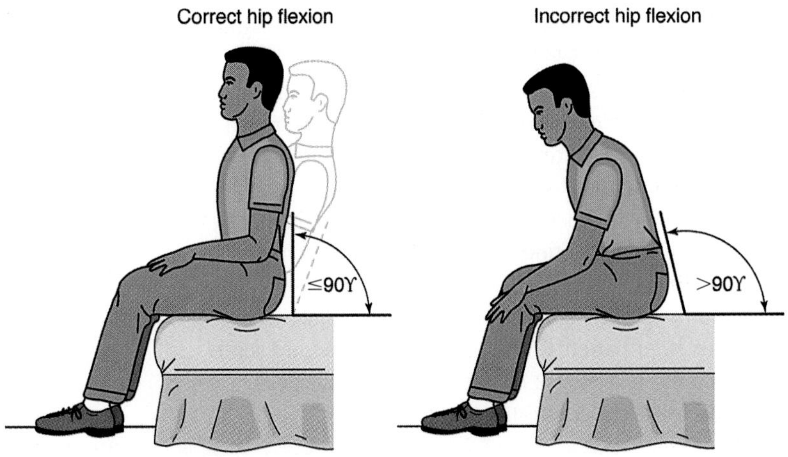
Correct hip flexion
Incorrect hip flexion
≤90Y
>90Y

FIGURE 46.17 Hip flexion after total hip replacement should be 90 degrees or less to prevent dislocation.

Heels, elbows, and the sacrum are vulnerable and can break down in 24 hours. A reddened area that does not blanch is a stage 1 pressure ulcer and must be treated aggressively to prevent progression to other stages. Prophylactic application of DuoDERM dressings and the use of heel protectors help to decrease the chance of skin breakdown of the heels.

Patients who are incontinent must be kept clean and dry. Assisting the patient to use the toilet every 2 hours and using a protective barrier cream also help prevent skin problems related to incontinence. Adequate diet and hydration are also important to prevent skin breakdown. Box 46.8 describes additional nursing interventions that meet the needs of postoperative patients recovering from total hip replacement.

Infection. Orthopedic surgery patients are at an increased risk for infection because of the nature of the surgery and because the patients are often older adults with an already increased risk for postoperative complications. In addition to the preoperative prophylactic intravenous antibiotic, the surgeon can administer antibiotics intraoperatively, and may continue antibiotics for 24 hours postoperatively.

Depending on the institution's policies, the surgeon may or may not remove the initial dressing. Regardless of who removes the dressing, meticulous aseptic care of the surgical wound is important to minimize the chance of infection. Care of the incision, as well as exit sites for drains, needs to be performed aseptically. When doing dressing changes, observe the incision routinely for signs and symptoms of infection (redness, swelling, warmth, odor, pain, or yellow, green, or brown-tinged drainage). Monitor temperature carefully. An older patient may not experience a fever but may appear confused.

Infection may not occur during the patient's hospital stay but can occur 1 or more years later. If this late infection does not respond to antibiotics, the prosthesis may be removed and replaced. To prevent infection, antibiotics are often instilled directly into the wound during surgery as beads, as part of the cement mixture, or as an irrigating solution.

Box 46.8

Nursing Interventions Following Total Hip Replacement

- Make sure that the hip is not allowed to become adducted. May use triangular (abductor) pillow or pillows.
- Turning patient requires abduction to be maintained. Turn patient as a whole, not allowing hip or legs to fall forward or backward. Use pillows to support raised limb.
- Monitor for skin integrity of the opposite heel, which often is used to help mobilize in bed and so is prone to friction and pressure sores. Apply protective devices for heels.
- Make sure limb remains in abduction when moving patient out of bed.
- Prevent postoperative pneumonia by encouraging deep breathing and coughing and use of incentive spirometer.
- Pain control is of utmost importance. Provide regularly scheduled analgesics, and make sure breakthrough analgesia is provided as needed. Decreased pain allows for earlier mobilization and fewer complications of immobility.
- Monitor level of consciousness and orientation. Many older patients have alterations in mental status after surgery because of anesthetics, analgesics, blood loss, and environmental changes.

CRITICAL THINKING

Mrs. Jacobs

■ Mrs. Jacobs' is 78 years old and had a left total hip replacement 3 days ago. When changing her dressing, the nurse notices a purulent discharge. Cefaclor (Ceclor) 500 mg PO q8hr is ordered. It is available as a 375-mg/5-mL suspension. How many milliliters should Mrs. Jacobs be given?

Suggested answers at end of chapter.

Bleeding. Like any surgical wound, some bleeding is expected. In joint replacement surgery, up to two-thirds of the blood loss can occur postoperatively. The patient may have a surgical drain (e.g., Hemovac or Jackson-Pratt) that is emptied every 8 to 12 hours or as required for the first day or two although the use of drains has decreased. Monitor the dressing for signs of bleeding and reinforce the dressing if needed. On the second or third postoperative day, the patient's hemoglobin and hematocrit may decrease to the point that blood transfusion is needed. The patient may receive the preoperatively donated autologous blood or may receive salvaged operative or postoperative blood. Using a cell saver (sometimes called an orthopat, which stands for orthopedic patient autotransfusion) during surgery, about 50% of blood that is lost can be recovered and saved for reinfusion into the same patient. Postoperatively, blood can be replaced by collecting shed blood via suction into a reservoir, then filtering and reinfusing it within 6 hours of collection. Monitoring for blood loss and signs of shock is an important nursing consideration.

Neurovascular Compromise. For any musculoskeletal surgery or injury, frequent neurovascular checks for circulation (color, warmth, pulses), sensation, and movement are performed distal to the surgical procedure or injury (and compared to the unaffected side) when vital signs are checked. The procedure and significance of these assessments are described in Chapter 45.

Thromboembolitic Complications. Patients having hip surgery are at greatest risk for DVT or pulmonary embolus. Older adult patients are especially at risk because of compromised circulation. Obese patients and those with a history of thromboembolitic problems are also at an exceptionally high risk for potentially fatal problems.

Thigh-high elastic stockings and sequential compression devices may be used while the patient is hospitalized (see Chapter 12). The surgeon orders an anticoagulant medication to help prevent clot formation, including subcutaneous low molecular weight heparin (such as fondaparinux [Arixtra], enoxaparin [Lovenox], dalteparin [Fragmin]) or oral warfarin (Coumadin). Occasionally, heparin is still used, and if so, it is important to monitor for heparin-induced thrombocytopenia, which can occur as early as 3 days after the start of heparin therapy. The ordered daily dosage of these drugs is determined by coagulation studies. Partial thromboplastin times are monitored for patients on heparin. International normalized ratio (INR) reported with prothrombin time is monitored when giving warfarin.

NURSING CARE TIP

When giving medications such as enoxaparin or dalteparin, follow manufacturer's instructions for administration. The air bubble should not be removed from the prefilled syringe before administration to ensure the whole dose is given.

Because most DVTs occur in the lower extremities, leg exercises are started in the immediate postoperative period and continued until the patient is fully ambulatory. The physical therapist teaches the patient how to perform foot and ankle exercises such as heel pumping, foot circles, and straight-leg raises (SLRs). The patient also performs quadriceps-setting exercises (quad sets) by straightening the legs and pushing the back of the knees toward the bed. Remind the patient to do several sets of these exercises each day to improve muscle tone and to help prevent blood clots in the leg.

If the patient is medically stable, he or she is discharged home for rehabilitation or to a subacute care unit, rehabilitation unit, or nursing home for short-term rehabilitation, lasting a week or less. The rehabilitation program that began in the hospital continues after discharge until the patient is independent in ambulation and self-care.

Before hospital discharge, the interdisciplinary team provides patient education for home care, including hip precautions that need to be used until the surgeon reevaluates the patient at the 6- to 8-week follow-up visit (Box 46.9).

Total Knee Replacement

The knee is the second most commonly replaced joint. It requires three components for total replacement: a femoral component, a tibial component, and a patellar button (Fig. 46.18). For patients who do not yet need a total replacement, partial knee resurfacing is available.

Box 46.9

Educating the Patient After Total Hip Replacement

Follow these safety measures to prevent hip dislocation:

- Keep legs abducted (away from center of body) with pillows.
- Sleep with pillows between legs until physician states otherwise.
- Bend at the waist (hip) no more than 90 degrees.
- Get up from a sitting position by pushing straight up off of the chair or bed without leaning forward.
- Use a walker, if desired, to assist walking.
- Physiotherapy and occupational therapy can provide equipment that aids in putting on socks and shoes.
- Sexual activity can be started when tolerated, provided hip safety measures are followed.

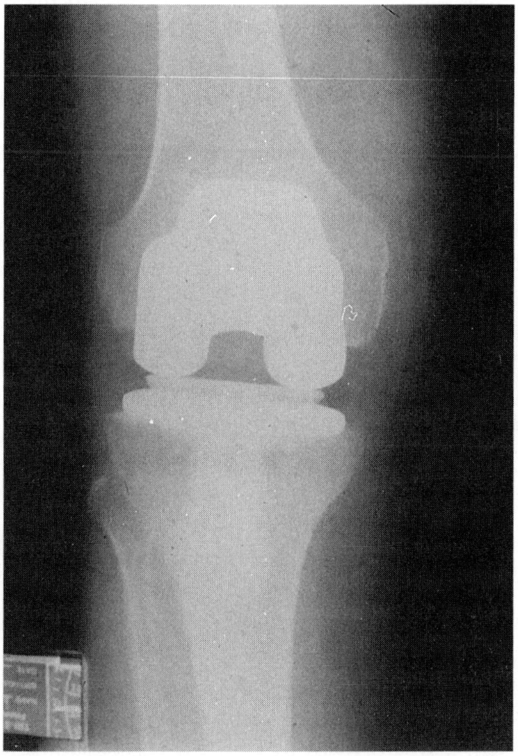

FIGURE 46.18 Knee joint replacement. (From Richardson, J. K., & Iglarsh, Z. A. [1994]. *Clinical orthopaedic physical therapy* [p. 651]. Philadelphia: W. B. Saunders, with permission.)

Care for the patient with a total knee replacement is similar to that required for a patient with a hip replacement except that dislocation and, therefore, preventive positioning are not a concern. Postoperatively, a bulky dressing and a surgical drain are usually in place. Once again, it is important to monitor for bleeding along with the usual postoperative interventions. Although precautions to prevent dislocation are not applicable for the patient with a knee replacement, other medical complications described for total hip replacement, such as DVT, may be seen in the patient undergoing knee replacement (see Box 46.8).

Postoperatively, a continuous passive motion (CPM) machine may be used for the operative leg. This motorized machine has a flexible extremity rest (for either the leg or arm) that glides back and forth on a track (Fig. 46.19). The CPM machine is set at the degree of flexion and speed ordered by the physician and usually is begun in the PACU. The machine can be applied by a nurse, physical therapist, or technician and is used either intermittently up to 8 to 12 hours a day or continuously while the patient is in bed. The purpose of CPM is to keep the knee joint mobile. Nursing care associated with the use of the machine is summarized in Box 46.10. A postoperative knee splint may be worn until the patient can do straight leg raises, indicating that leg strength has returned.

Amputation

Simply defined, an amputation is the removal of a body part, which can be as limited as removing part of a finger or as devastating as removing nearly half the body. Amputations may be *surgical* as a result of disease or *traumatic* as a result of an accident. Surgical amputations are the most common type and are most often scheduled as elective surgery.

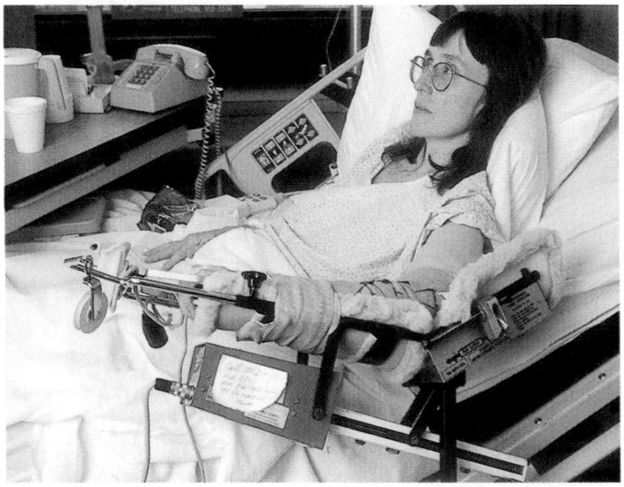

FIGURE 46.19 A continuous passive motion machine can be used following knee or elbow (as shown here) joint replacement to increase joint mobility and enhance recovery. The CPM machine slowly moves along the track at the set degree of flexion and speed.

Box 46.10

Application of a Continuous Passive Motion (CPM) Machine

- Position joint (knee) over flexion point of machine.
- Padding (e.g., sheepskin) is particularly important at proximal end near gluteal fold.
- Ensure speed and angle settings are correct and monitored according to facility policy. A minimum of every shift is required.
- The patient is provided the controls to stop the machine prn unless he or she is mentally incompetent to do so. If unable to self-monitor, ensure patient is checked frequently.
- Assess how well patient tolerates the speed and angle of movement.
- Speed and angle adjustments are determined by agency policy, physiotherapist, or the physician.
- Ideal utilization is three times a day for at least 1 hour per session, or as ordered.

Surgical Amputation

The main indication for surgical amputations is ischemia from peripheral vascular disease in the older adult. The rate of lower extremity amputation is much higher in the diabetic patient than in the nondiabetic patient (see discussion of diabetes in Chapter 40). Surgical amputations may also be done for bone tumors, thermal injuries (frostbite, electric shock), crushing injuries, congenital problems, or infections.

Traumatic Amputation

Traumatic amputations occur from accidents, often in young and middle-aged adults. Industrial machinery, motor vehicles, lawn mowers, chain saws, and snow blowers are common causes of accidental amputation.

Because in these patients the amputated part is usually healthy, attempts at **replantation** may occur. One of the most common replantations is one or more fingers. The current recommendation for prehospital care of the severed body part is to wrap it in a cool, slightly moist cloth and place it in a sealed plastic bag. The bag may be submerged in cold water until the body part is transported to the hospital.

The surgical procedure is performed by specialists who operate using a microscope. Nerves, vessels, and muscle must be reattached. These procedures are generally performed at large tertiary care centers that have specialty practitioners and equipment for replantation.

• WORD • BUILDING •

replantation: re—again + plant—to plant + ation—process

Levels of Amputation

The most common surgical amputation is part of the lower extremity. The loss of any or all of the small toes presents little problem. However, the loss of the great toe is more important because balance and gait are affected. Midfoot amputations are preferred over below-the-knee amputations for peripheral vascular disease. For the Syme amputation, the surgeon removes most of the foot but leaves the ankle intact for ambulation and weight bearing.

If the lower leg is amputated, a below-the-knee amputation is preferred over an above-the-knee amputation to preserve joint function. The higher the level of amputation, the more energy required for ambulation. Hip disarticulation (removal through the hip joint) and **hemipelvectomy** (removal through part of the pelvis) are reserved for young patients who have cancer or severe trauma. Rarely, a hemicorporectomy (hemipelvectomy plus a translumbar amputation) is performed as a last resort for young patients with cancer. This radical surgery removes nearly half of the body and requires both bowel and urinary diversion surgeries (ostomies) as well.

Upper extremity amputations are usually more significant than lower extremity amputations and more often result from trauma. The arms and hands are necessary for performing activities of daily living. Early replacement with a prosthesis is crucial for the patient with an upper extremity amputation.

Preoperative Care

Patients who are scheduled for elective amputations have the advantage of time for preoperative teaching, prosthesis fitting, and adjustment to the loss of part of their bodies. Preoperative teaching is started in the surgeon's office. Postoperative and rehabilitative care is reviewed with the patient and family or significant other. Those patients experiencing a traumatic amputation have no opportunity to prepare for the significant changes that will result from the accident. Preoperative care will not only involve physical needs being met, but significant psychological and emotional concerns also have to be addressed (this also continues postoperatively).

Preoperatively, the patient should be referred to a certified prosthetist-orthotist to begin plans for replacing the removed body part with a prosthesis.

Disturbed Body Image is a common nursing diagnosis for the patient having an amputation. If possible, it is helpful for the preoperative patient to meet with a rehabilitated amputee. Assess the patient's reaction to having an amputation with the expectation that the patient will experience many of the stages of loss and grieving. Support systems and coping mechanisms are identified that can help the patient through the surgery and postoperative period. Ensure that appropriate support is provided by other disciplines such as social work and clergy.

Postoperative Care

In addition to the general postoperative care described here, plan and implement interventions to help prevent postoperative complications, including hemorrhage and infection (see Chapter 12).

PREVENTION OF HEMORRHAGE AND INFECTION. When a patient loses part of the body, because of either surgery or trauma, blood vessels are severed or damaged. The patient returns from surgery with a large pressure dressing that is secured with an elastic wrap. Assess the closest proximal pulse between the heart and the amputated body part for strength and compare findings with the nonsurgical extremity. Assess the bulky dressing for bloody drainage. If blood is on the dressing when the patient is admitted to the PACU or the surgical unit, circle, date, and time the area of drainage and closely monitor for enlargement. If bleeding continues, the surgeon is notified immediately. A tourniquet should be readily available in case severe hemorrhage occurs.

After the dressing is removed, observe for adequate perfusion to the skin flap at the end of the residual limb, referred to as the stump. The skin should be pink in a light-skinned patient and not discolored (lighter or darker than other skin pigmentation) in a dark-skinned patient. The residual limb should be warm but not hot.

Infection of the wound can be problematic, especially if the infection enters the bone (**osteomyelitis**). Inspect the wound for intense redness or drainage. Localized infections usually do not cause an increase in body temperature. If temperature is elevated, it could indicate a serious wound infection, a systemic infection, or some other type of infection. Traumatic amputations are at risk for developing infection due to the nature of the injury and the likelihood of exposure to environmental pathogens from the source of the amputation.

PAIN CONTROL. In addition to the usual incisional pain that is expected following a surgical procedure, phantom limb pain occurs in as many as 80% of all amputees (surgical or traumatic). The patient reports severe pain where the removed body part was located. The pain may be described as either intense burning, a crushing sensation, or cramping.

Phantom limb pain can be triggered by touching the residual limb, feeling fatigued, or experiencing emotional stress. It is reported that phantom limb pain can also be triggered by pressure or changes in the weather. Although it occurs most often in the immediate postoperative period, phantom limb pain may occur at any time during the first

• WORD • BUILDING •

hemipelvectomy: hemi—half + pelv—pelvis + ectomy—removal of

• WORD • BUILDING •

osteomyelitis: osteo—bone + myel—bone marrow + itis—inflammation postoperative year or sometimes even years after the amputation. The pain may be mild to severe. The cause is not clear.

Never doubt that a patient is experiencing phantom limb pain. Treat the pain aggressively with medication and complementary therapies. The surgeon prescribes medication based on the type of pain sensation the patient experiences. For example, anticonvulsants, such as phenytoin (Dilantin), are used for knifelike pain. Beta-blocking agents, such as propranolol (Inderal), are appropriate for burning sensations, and gabapentin (Neurontin) or amitriptyline (Elavil) can be used for nerve pain. To complement traditional therapy, a number of alternative therapies may be useful, including biofeedback, massage, imagery, hypnosis, acupuncture, acupressure, and distraction.

MOBILITY AND AMBULATION. To reduce surgical swelling, cold application may be ordered. Alternately, the residual limb may be elevated on a pillow for 24 hours or less. Continued use of a pillow for elevation can lead to flexion contractures, especially for patients with a below-the-knee or above-the-knee amputation. If the hip becomes contracted, using a prosthesis will not be possible because the patient will not be able to walk. Check the limb periodically to ensure that it lies completely flat on the bed. The patient should avoid positions of flexion such as sitting for long periods. If the patient is able, lying prone (on the stomach) for 30 minutes four times daily helps prevent contracture.

Postoperative care after amputation is interdisciplinary, often requiring an extensive rehabilitation program in a subacute unit, an extended care facility, or on an ambulatory basis. The physical therapist teaches the patient muscle-strengthening exercises that help with ambulation and transfers and prevent flexion contractures. A trapeze bar on an overhead bed frame aids in strengthening the arms and helps the patient move around in bed.

PROSTHESIS CARE. The residual limb must be prepared for wearing the prosthesis. A temporary prosthesis may be worn until the swelling subsides.

The residual limb is wrapped at least every 8 hours using an elastic wrap (such as an Ace wrap) in a figure-of-eight fashion (Fig. 46.20). It is important to perform neurovascular checks and assess the residual limb for infection and alterations in tissue integrity at each rewrapping. Begin with the most distal portion and proceed proximally until the bandage is secured to the most proximal joint. The bandage should be tighter at the distal end.

The prosthesis requires special care, which the patient should be taught:

- Clean the prosthesis socket with mild soap and water and then dry it.
- Clean inserts and liners regularly.

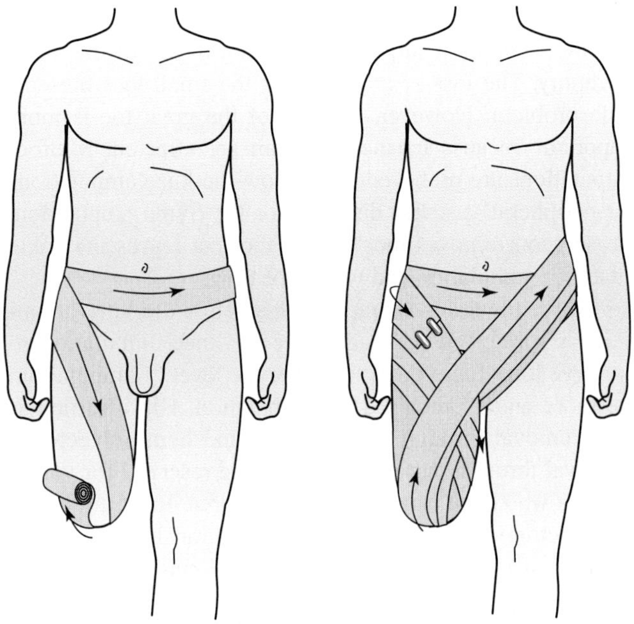

FIGURE 46.20 Application of elastic wraps on an above-the-knee amputation helps mold the stump for a prosthesis.

- Use garters to keep socks in place.
- Grease parts as instructed.
- Replace shoes when they wear out with same height and type of shoe.

LIFESTYLE ADAPTATION. The patient may feel that life will be markedly changed as a result of the amputation. If the discharge planner or case manager thinks it is needed, a job analysis may be conducted by a vocational analyst or specialized case manager. With technological advances in prostheses, most patients who worked before surgery are able to return to their jobs after surgery. Many patients with amputations are able to bowl, ski, hike, and continue with all of the recreational hobbies that they were able to do before surgery.

A supportive family or significant other is vital to help the patient adjust to body image change. Consider the need for a sexual counselor or psychologist if indicated. For any patient with an amputation, help the patient set realistic expectations.

For the patient who is not a candidate for a prosthesis, home adaptations for a wheelchair may be needed. The patient must have access to toileting facilities and areas necessary for self-care. Structural changes in the living environment may be needed before the patient can be discharged from rehabilitation.

A small percentage of amputees return to their extended care environment without prostheses. These patients need rehabilitation to ensure that they can be as independent as possible.

Home Health Hints

- If equipment or modifications to the home are needed following hospitalization for an orthopedic problem, it is best if they can be arranged or obtained before discharge.
- Physical and occupational therapy are often ordered for the orthopedic patient discharged from the hospital to help with ambulation, activities of daily living, and obtaining and use of assistive devices: raised toilet seats, handheld reachers, walkers, canes, wheelchairs, and hand rails.
- Physical and/or occupational therapy can also be ordered to help the patient regain strength following surgery. The home health nurse can work with the therapist to educate the patient on the prescribed exercises.
- Patients who use walkers can get pressure ulcers on their palms. One way to relieve the pressure is to wear padded cycling gloves that leave the fingers free.
- A patient on crutches can use the crutch to prop a casted leg or foot.
- Research has shown that pain or fear of falling may prevent a patient from moving and functioning to maximum potential. Encourage patients to wear flat, sturdy, rubber-soled shoes to prevent slipping, tripping, or turning an ankle.
- Encourage the patient to dispose of all throw rugs, unnecessary furniture, and other possible fall hazards in the home.
- The risk of deep venous thrombosis (DVT) after hip or knee surgery is highest by the fifth postoperative day, and the risk persists for up to 12 weeks. Be alert for such signs as warmth, redness, edema, Homans' sign, and protective behavior of the affected leg.
- Patients who are having a difficult time putting on antiembolism stockings can be instructed on an easy way of slipping them on. Using a plastic grocery bag, instruct the patient to tie a knot on the closed end. Slip the bag over the foot, and then put the stocking on over the bag. Once the stocking is on over the heel, the patient or caregiver can pull the bag out using the knot that was tied.
- Many times the patient is discharged home still requiring medication injections to prevent DVT formation. The nurse needs to educate the patient on how to administer the injection. If the patient cannot do this and no one is available to teach him or her, the home health nurse can make visits in order to administer the injection.
- Instruct the patient with rheumatoid arthritis to rest during acute inflammations and to stop activity if pain develops.
- Home health nurses frequently remove staples and sutures. Always have several of each type of removal device on hand. Remember staples, scissors, or other items that are "sharp" need to be disposed of in a biohazard container.

SUGGESTED ANSWERS TO

CRITICAL THINKING

■ *Mrs. Heinrick*

1. When documenting, answer (either explicitly or implicitly by professional knowledge, in narrative or flowsheet format) what, why, when, where, who, and how for completeness.

   What = Patient found on the floor lying on her left side, moaning and holding her leg, crying out with any movement.

   Why = Fell

   When = Date/Time: 10 a.m.

   Where = Day room

   Who = Mrs. Heinrick (patient)

   How = Unknown; was not witnessed.

   DATE 1000 Found on floor in day room lying on left side, moaning and holding left leg, crying out with any movement. Stated, "I fell. I think my leg is broken." Supervisor immediately notified, and paramedics and Dr. Jones called. Vital signs BP 150/84 mm Hg, P 100 bpm, R 20 per minute. Left leg shorter than right. Remained with patient and instructed not to move until paramedics arrived. Blankets applied and pillow placed under head for comfort. 1030 Taken by ambulance to Grace Hospital. I. Smith, LPN

2. The purpose of the traction is to reduce the muscle spasms that often accompany fractures and to increase comfort.

SUGGESTED ANSWERS TO—cont'd

3. Nursing responsibilities include the following:
   a. Check neurovascular status frequently.
   b. Check equipment, including rope, pulleys, knots, and weights at least every shift.
   c. Do not allow the weights to rest on the floor.
   d. Do not allow the traction to be impeded in any way.
   e. Monitor the patient's skin often for areas of potential breakdown.
   f. Remove and rewrap the elastic bandages, maintaining the traction, at least every shift. Provide skin care during this time.
   g. Monitor area of the fracture for bruising and increased diameter of the limb.
   h. Monitor for pain (using pain assessment scale) frequently.
   i. Turn and position regularly.
4. The restlessness is most likely the result of pain. She may be unable to state that she is in pain. Evaluate behaviors such as restlessness and other nonverbal cues to evaluate pain management needs. She may also be experiencing shock as a result of blood loss from the fracture. Monitor vital signs, and check the area of the fracture for increased signs of bruising or swelling.

■ *Tommy Martin*

1. Possible nursing diagnoses may include:
   a. *Pain* related to injury and immobility
   b. *Risk for Social Isolation* related to extended need for immobilization
   c. Potential complications of inactivity: *Constipation*, *Impaired Skin Integrity* related to extended need for traction
   d. *Deficient Diversional Activity* related to extended need for bedrest.
2. Nursing interventions may include:
   a. Monitor pain level, provide analgesics as ordered, assess pain relief. Assess position for comfort. Provide backrubs prn.
   b. To address social isolation, encourage Tommy's friends to come visit, have an occupational therapist assess Tommy's needs, and alternate visits from family.
   c. To avoid complications of inactivity, ensure Tommy's diet includes fiber and adequate hydration (1.5 to 2 L/day); give stool softener, especially if on opioids as ordered; monitor daily defecation; ensure Tommy does the exercises recommended by occupational and physical therapists; reposition him every 2 to 3 hours; have trapeze bar set up for Tommy to use; use skin assessment tool to determine risk for skin breakdown; assess for pressure points and signs and symptoms of skin breakdown.
   d. To alleviate boredom, encourage Tommy to listen to music; encourage visitors; and ensure access to hobbies, videos, books, magazines, and comics.
3. Because opioids are an essential part of pain management and can cause constipation when used long term, planning is necessary to prevent it. Monitor daily bowel movements. Give medications to prevent constipation as ordered such as stool softeners, laxatives, or opioid antagonists like methylnaltrexone. Be proactive in ensuring normal elimination. Report lack of bowel movements promptly for intervention. Reduce opioid dosage and move to nonopioids promptly as pain relief allows.

■ *Mr. Andrews*

1. Data collection should include the following:
   a. Perform a neurovascular check.
   b. Perform a further pain assessment.
   c. Asking Mr. Andrews to flex the muscles in his limb to see if the pain worsens.
   d. Take his vital signs.
   e. Check for the six *P*s: pain, paresthesia, paralysis, pallor, pulselessness, and poikilothermia.
2. He might be experiencing compartment syndrome.
3. Interventions may include the need for a bivalved cast or a possible fasciotomy.

■ *Mr. Dennis*

1. a. "What is your typical day on the job like?"
   b. "Do certain activities increase joint pain?"
   c. "When is your pain worse—after activity or after rest?"
   d. "How long have you experienced joint pain?"
   e. "What relieves the joint pain?"
2. Risk factors include that he is overweight, is in late middle age, and has a physically demanding job.
3. Other signs and symptoms may include bony nodules on his fingers (such as Heberden's nodes) and secondary inflammation causing joint swelling.

■ *Mrs. Summers*

1. Ask:
   a. The nature of her pain
   b. If it is worse after activity or rest
   c. If she experiences joint stiffness and, if so, when.

SUGGESTED ANSWERS TO—cont'd

Follow the WHAT'S UP? method of pain assessment.

2. Teach her to do the following:
   a. Balance rest with exercise.
   b. Use ice for very hot, swollen joints.
   c. Use heat to decrease stiffness.

■ ***Mrs. Jacobs***

Unit analysis method:

$$\frac{500\ \cancel{mg}}{} \Big| \frac{5\ mL}{375\ \cancel{mg}} = 6.7\ mL$$

REVIEW QUESTIONS

1. The nurse is caring for a patient who just had a plaster cast applied. Which action should the nurse take to facilitate cast drying?
   a. Cover the cast with blankets to provide extra warmth.
   b. Turn the patient every 2 hours.
   c. Increase the room temperature.
   d. Apply a heating pad.

2. Which of the following nursing interventions would be appropriate to properly care for external fixation pins inserted into a patient's leg?
   a. Do not touch the pins.
   b. Follow agency protocol for pin care.
   c. Cleanse with hydrogen peroxide qid.
   d. Loosen the screws holding the pins during cleaning.

3. Which of the following actions can the nurse take to help prevent osteomyelitis for a patient with an open fracture? **Select all that apply.**
   a. Wash hands prior to dressing changes.
   b. Wear a protective gown.
   c. Wear a mask.
   d. Wear goggles.
   e. Wear sterile gloves to apply new dressing.

4. A patient is postmenopausal, has osteoporosis, has lost 2 inches of height, is thin, and has never exercised regularly. Which of these interventions should be included in the plan of care to prevent further bone loss?
   a. Decrease participation in ADLs.
   b. Decrease weight-bearing activities.
   c. Encourage regular exercise.
   d. Encourage weight gain.

5. A priority nursing diagnosis for the patient with Paget's disease includes which of the following?
   a. *Pain*
   b. *Deficient Knowledge*
   c. *Excess Fluid Volume*
   d. *Deficient Fluid Volume*

6. Which of the following lab values would the nurse expect to be elevated in the patient with gout?
   a. WBC
   b. RBC
   c. Uric acid
   d. Ammonia

7. A butterfly rash is a classic symptom of which of the following disorders?
   a. Lupus
   b. Paget's disease
   c. Rheumatoid arthritis
   d. Osteosarcoma

8. A patient with osteoarthritis who had a right total knee replacement tells the nurse that the other knee is becoming painful. Which of the following is the most appropriate instruction to help the patient preserve function of the left knee?
   a. Reduce dietary purines.
   b. Maintain ideal body weight.
   c. Maintain normal uric acid levels.
   d. Begin a jogging program.

9. A patient is scheduled for a right total hip replacement. The nurse should include which of the following postoperative leg positions in the preoperative teaching plan?
   a. Maintain legs in adduction.
   b. Maintain legs in abduction.
   c. Maintain internal leg rotation.
   d. Maintain more than 90-degree hip flexion.

10. Following amputation, which of these assessments should the nurse consider a priority to monitor for potential postoperative amputation complications?
    a. Sacral edema
    b. Level of consciousness
    c. Stump dressings
    d. Blood sugars

REVIEW QUESTIONS—cont'd

11. Which of the following findings would indicate a complication of a left fibula fracture?
    a. The patient has an increased red blood cell count.
    b. The patient has a decreased temperature.
    c. The patient has a decreased lymphocyte count.
    d. The patient has an absent left pedal pulse.

12. A patient who has a 36-hour-old fractured femur had morphine 5 mg intramuscularly 1 hour ago and is now reporting severe unrelieved pain. Which nursing action is most appropriate?
    a. Give analgesic.
    b. Adjust the traction.
    c. Bivalve the cast.
    d. Notify the physician.

13. A patient who had a total knee replacement is to receive Toradol 15 mg intramuscularly every 6 hours as needed for pain. The Toradol comes as 30 mg/mL. How many milliliters should the nurse give?
    Answer: ________ mL

References

Gillespie, L. D., Robertson, M. C., Gillespie, W. J., et al. (2009). Interventions for preventing falls in older people living in the community. *Cochrane Database of Systematic Reviews, Issue 2* (Art. No. CD007146; DOI 10.1002/14651858.CD007146.pub2).

National Osteoporosis Foundation. (2009). Retrieved November 21, 2009, from http://www.nof.org

unit THIRTEEN

UNDERSTANDING THE NEUROLOGIC SYSTEM

47 Neurologic System Function, Assessment, and Therapeutic Measures

DEBORAH L. WEAVER AND
JANICE L. BRADFORD

KEY TERMS

anisocoria (an-ih-suh-KOR-ee-ah)
aphasia (ah-FAY-zee-ah)
cerebrovascular (sur-EE-broh-VASS-kyoo-lur)
contractures (kon-TRAK-churs)
decerebrate (dee-SER-eh-brayt)
decorticate (dee-KOR-tih-kayt)
dysarthria (diss-AR-three-ah)
dysphagia (diss-FAYJ-ee-ah)
electroencephalogram (ee-LEK-troh-en-SEFF-uh-loh-gram)
myelogram (MY-eh-loh-gram)
nystagmus (nih-STAG-mus)
paresis (puh-REE-sis)
paresthesia (PAR-es-THEE-zee-ah)
subarachnoid (SUB-uh-RAK-noyd)

QUESTIONS TO GUIDE YOUR READING

1. What is the normal anatomy of the nervous system?
2. What are the normal functions of the nervous system?
3. What are the effects of aging on the nervous system?
4. What data should you collect when caring for a patient with a disorder of the nervous system?
5. What diagnostic tests are commonly performed to diagnose disorders of the nervous system?
6. What nursing care should you provide for patients undergoing each of the diagnostic tests for disorders of the nervous system?
7. What common therapeutic measures are used for patients with disorders of the nervous system?

NORMAL NEUROLOGIC SYSTEM ANATOMY AND PHYSIOLOGY

The nervous system has two divisions: the central nervous system (CNS), which consists of the brain and spinal cord, and the peripheral nervous system (PNS), which includes the nerves of the autonomic nervous system (ANS). Electrical impulses are transmitted through the nervous system to permit sensory and motor activity. Some actions are reflexive or occur without conscious thought, while others are the result of gathering, organizing, and processing data for immediate and future use.

Nerve Tissue

Nerve tissue consists of neurons and specialized supporting cells called neuroglia. There are many kinds of neurons (nerve cells or nerve fibers); however, they all have the same general structure (Fig. 47.1). The cell body contains the nucleus and is essential for the continued life of the neuron. All neuron cell bodies are found in the brain, spinal cord, or within the trunk of the body. A neuron has one axon that transmits impulses away from the cell body and may have one or many dendrites that carry impulses toward the cell body. The cell membrane of the dendrites, cell body, and axon transmits the electrical nerve impulse.

In the PNS, axons are wrapped in specialized neuroglial cells called Schwann cells (neurolemmocytes). The concentric layers of cell membrane of a Schwann cell's plasma membrane form the myelin sheath. Myelin is a phospholipid that electrically insulates neurons from one another. The spaces between adjacent Schwann cells along an axon are called nodes of Ranvier (neurofibril nodes). Only the nodes of the neuron cell membrane depolarize

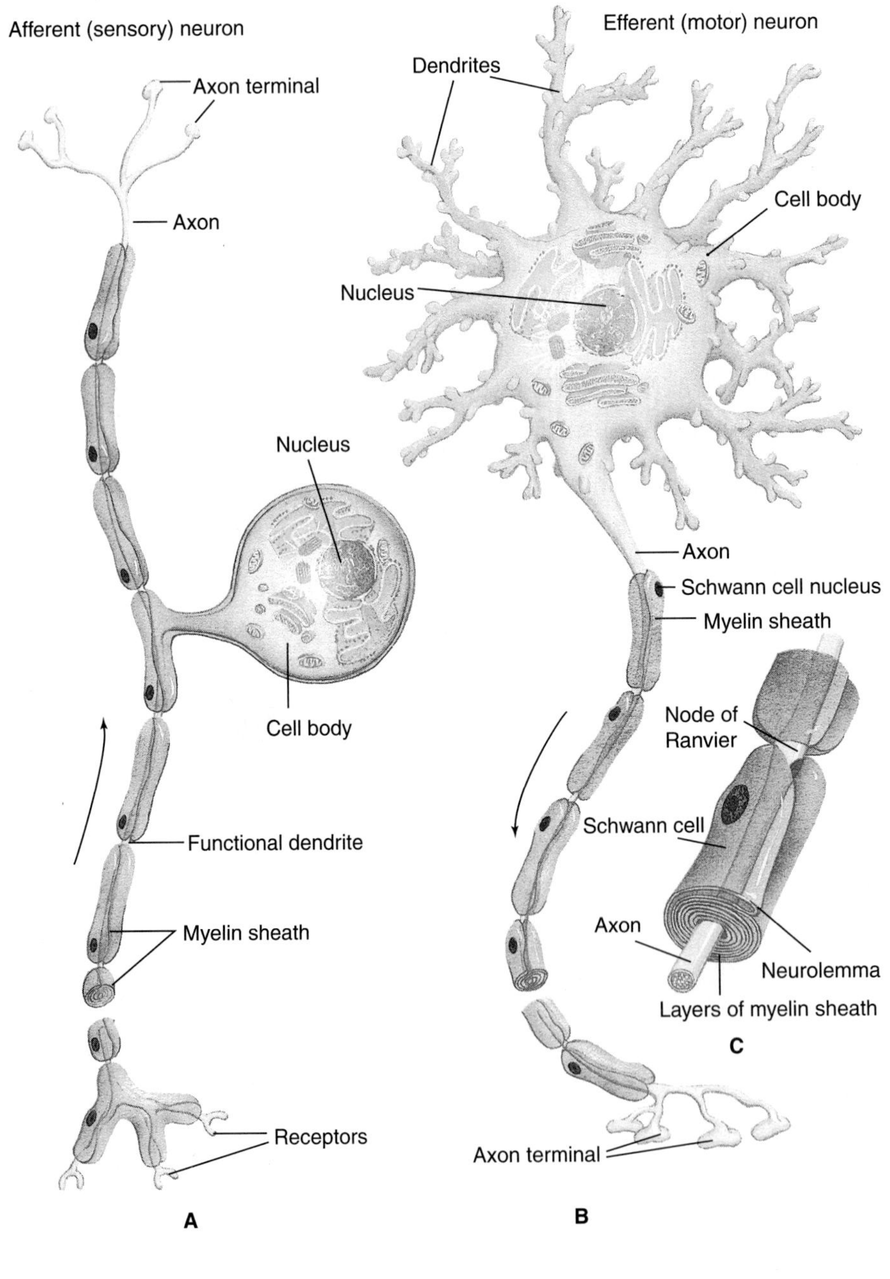
Afferent (sensory) neuron
Axon terminal
Axon
Nucleus
Cell body
Functional dendrite
Myelin sheath
Receptors
A
Efferent (motor) neuron
Dendrites
Cell body
Nucleus
Axon
Schwann cell nucleus
Myelin sheath
Node of Ranvier
Schwann cell
Axon
Neurolemma
Layers of myelin sheath
C
Axon terminal
B

FIGURE 47.1 Structure of sensory and motor neurons. (From Scanlon, V. C., & Sanders, T. [2007]. *Essentials of anatomy and physiology* [5th ed., p. 167]. Philadelphia: F. A. Davis, with permission.)

when an electrical impulse is transmitted, which makes impulse conduction rapid. The nuclei and cytoplasm of Schwann cells are on the external edge of the myelin sheath and form the neurolemma. If a peripheral nerve is severed and reattached, the individual axons may regrow through the tunnels provided by the neurolemma. In the CNS, the myelin sheaths (but not a neurolemma) are formed by oligodendrocytes, another type of neuroglial cell. See Table 47.1 for the names and functions of the other CNS neuroglial cells.

Synapses

When the axon of a neuron must transmit an impulse to the dendrite or cell body of another neuron, the impulse must cross a small gap called a synapse. An electrical impulse is incapable of crossing this microscopic space, so when the impulses reach the synapses, impulse transmission becomes chemical. The end of the axon (the presynaptic neuron) is called the synaptic end bulb and contains a chemical neurotransmitter that is released into the synapse by the arrival of the electrical impulse. The neurotransmitter diffuses across the synapse and combines with specific receptor sites on the postsynaptic membrane (Fig. 47.2). At excitatory synapses, the neurotransmitter makes the postsynaptic membrane more permeable to sodium ions, which rush into the cell, initiating an electrical impulse on the membrane of the postsynaptic neuron. The neurotransmitter is then inactivated to prevent continuous impulses. Each neurotransmitter also has a designated inactivator. For example, the neurotransmitter acetylcholine is inactivated by the chemical called acetylcholinesterase.

Some synapses are inhibitory synapses in that the neurotransmitter makes the postsynaptic membrane more permeable to potassium ions, which leave the cell and make the membrane resistant to the electrical charge required for an impulse. Thus, the electrical impulse is stopped. Inhibitory synapses are important for events such as slowing the heart rate or balancing the excitatory impulses transmitted

TABLE 47.1 NEUROGLIA

Name	Function
Oligodendrocytes	• Produce the myelin sheath to electrically insulate neurons of the CNS.
Microglia	• Capable of movement and phagocytosis of pathogens and damaged tissue.
Astrocytes	• Contribute to the blood-brain barrier, which prevents potentially toxic waste products in the blood from diffusing out into brain tissue. • Disadvantage: Some useful medications cannot cross the blood-brain barrier, which becomes important during brain infection, inflammation, or other disease.
Ependyma	• Line the ventricles of the brain. • Many of the cells are ciliated. • Involved in production and circulation of cerebrospinal fluid.

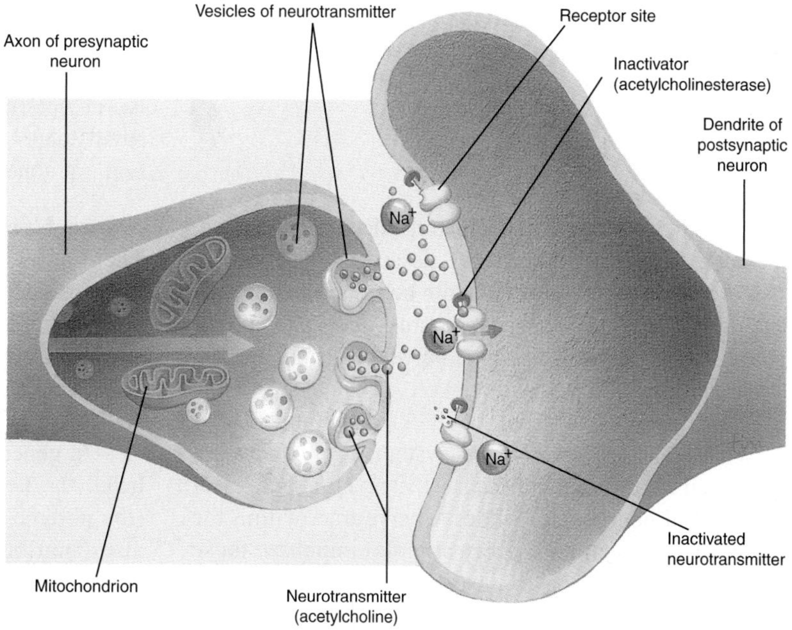

Vesicles of neurotransmitter
Receptor site
Axon of presynaptic neuron
Inactivator (acetylcholinesterase)
Dendrite of postsynaptic neuron
Na+
Na+
Na+
Inactivated neurotransmitter
Mitochondrion
Neurotransmitter (acetylcholine)

FIGURE 47.2 Structure of a synapse, and the effect of a neurotransmitter such as acetylcholine. (From Scanlon, V. C., & Sanders, T. [2007]. *Essentials of anatomy and physiology* [5th ed. p. 169]. Philadelphia: F. A. Davis, with permission.)

to skeletal muscles, which prevents excessive contraction and is important for coordination.

At chemical synapses, impulse transmission is one way only because the neurotransmitter is released only by the presynaptic neuron; the impulse cannot go backward. This is important for the normal activity of the functional types of neurons. The relative complexity of synapses also makes them a potential target for the actions of medications.

Types of Neurons

A useful classification of neurons is according to their function: a neuron is sensory, motor, or an interneuron. Sensory (afferent) neurons transmit impulses from receptors to the central nervous system. Receptors are specialized to detect external or internal changes and then generate electrical impulses. Sensory neurons, which form receptors in the skin, skeletal muscles, and joints, are called somatic. Those sensory neurons which form receptors in internal organs are called visceral sensory neurons. Motor (efferent) neurons transmit impulses from the CNS to effectors—that is, muscles and glands. Motor neurons to skeletal muscle are called somatic; those to smooth muscle, cardiac muscle, and glands are called visceral. Sensory and motor neurons make up the PNS. Visceral motor neurons form the ANS, a specialized part of the PNS. Interneurons are found entirely within the CNS and are specialized to transmit sensory or motor impulses or to integrate these functions. Such integration of impulses is involved in thinking and learning.

> **LEARNING TIP**
>
> To remember the difference between afferent and efferent, try these clues:
>
> - Afferent: A is for affect or sense.
> - Efferent: E is for effect (action).
> - Or, think of the alphabet—A before E: You have to feel or sense (afferent) a stimulus before you can take action (efferent).

Nerves and Nerve Tracts

A nerve is a group of peripheral axons, dendrites, or both, with blood vessels and connective tissue. Most peripheral nerves are mixed; that is, they contain both sensory and motor neurons. Some, however, are not mixed. An example of a purely sensory nerve is the optic nerve for vision, and the autonomic nerves are purely motor nerves.

A nerve tract is a group of thickly myelinated neurons within the central nervous system; such tracts are often called white matter because the myelin sheaths of the individual neurons are white. A nerve tract within the spinal cord carries either sensory or motor impulses; those within the brain may have sensory, motor, or integrative functions.

Nerve Impulses

A nerve impulse, which may also be called an action potential, is an electrical change brought about by the movement of ions across the neuron cell membrane. When a neuron is not carrying an impulse, it is in a state of polarization with a positive charge outside the membrane and a relatively negative charge inside the membrane. Sodium ions are more abundant outside the cell, and potassium and negative ions are more abundant inside the cell. A stimulus makes the membrane very permeable to sodium ions, which rush into the cell, making the inside positive and the outside relatively negative. This reversal of charges is called depolarization and spreads from the point of the stimulus along the entire neuron membrane.

Immediately following depolarization, the membrane becomes very permeable to potassium ions, which rush out of the cell. This is called repolarization and restores the positive charge outside and the negative charge inside. The sodium and potassium pumps return the sodium ions back outside and the potassium ions inside, and the neuron is polarized again and ready to respond to another stimulus. A neuron is capable of transmitting hundreds of impulses per second, and at speeds of more than 100 meters per second.

Spinal Cord

The spinal cord transmits impulses to and from the brain and is the integrating center for the spinal cord reflexes. The spinal cord is within the vertebral canal formed by the vertebrae and extends from the foramen magnum of the occipital bone to the intervertebral disk between the first and second lumbar vertebrae. The spinal nerves emerge from the intervertebral foramina.

In cross section, the spinal cord is oval shaped; internally it has an H-shaped mass of gray matter surrounded by white matter (Fig. 47.3). The gray matter is where the cell bodies of motor neurons and interneurons are located. The white matter is formed by the myelinated axons. These nerve fibers are arranged in tracts based on their functions; ascending tracts transmit sensory impulses to the brain, and descending tracts transmit motor impulses from the brain to motor neurons. The central canal of the spinal cord is a small tunnel that is continuous with the ventricles of the brain; it contains cerebrospinal fluid (CSF).

Spinal Nerves

There are 31 pairs of spinal nerves, named according to their respective vertebrae: 8 cervical pairs, 12 thoracic pairs, 5 lumbar pairs, 5 sacral pairs, and 1 very small coccygeal pair. These nerves are often referred to by letter and number: the second cervical nerve is C2, the tenth thoracic is T10, and so on.

In general, the cervical nerves supply the back of the head; the neck, shoulders, and arms; and the diaphragm (the phrenic nerves). The first and second thoracic nerves also contribute to peripheral nerves in the arms. The remaining thoracic nerves supply the trunk of the body. The lumbar and sacral nerves supply the hips, pelvic cavity,

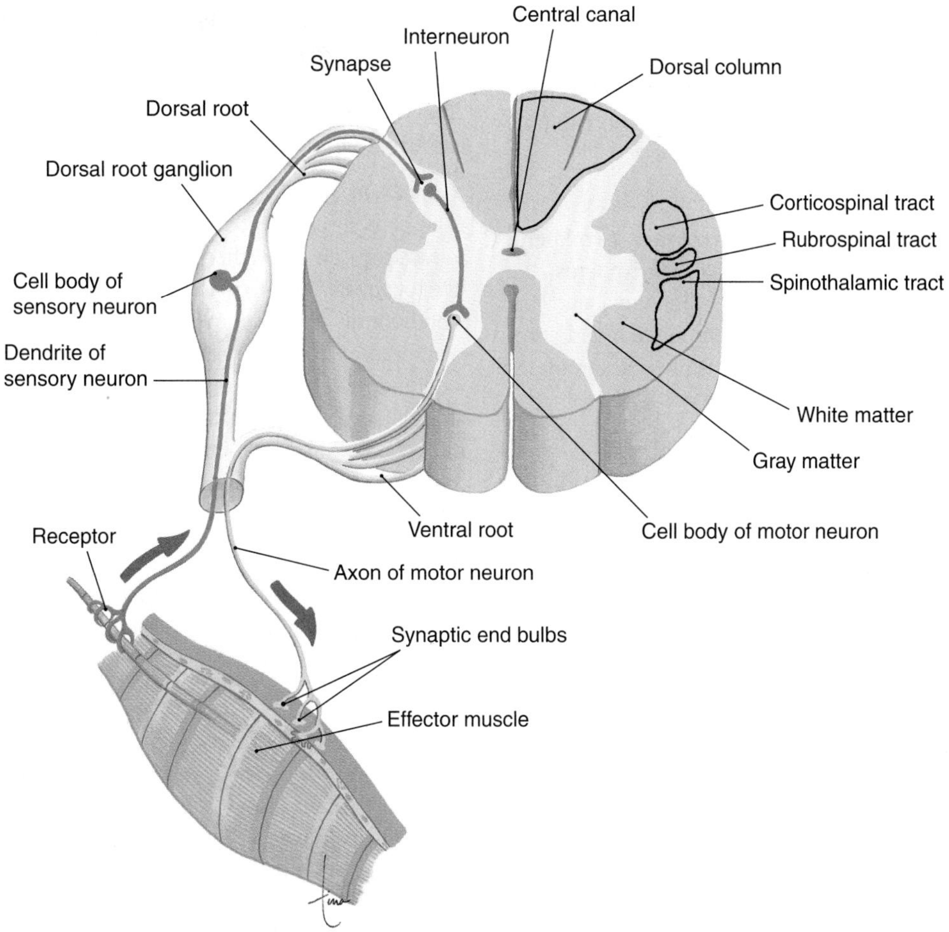
Central canal
Interneuron
Synapse
Dorsal column
Dorsal root
Dorsal root ganglion
Corticospinal tract
Rubrospinal tract
Cell body of sensory neuron
Spinothalamic tract
Dendrite of sensory neuron
White matter
Gray matter
Receptor
Ventral root
Cell body of motor neuron
Axon of motor neuron
Synaptic end bulbs
Effector muscle

FIGURE 47.3 Spinal cord in cross section, with nerve roots and meninges. (From Scanlon, V. C., & Sanders, T. [2007]. *Essentials of anatomy and physiology* [5th ed., p. 170]. Philadelphia: F. A. Davis, with permission.)

and legs. The small coccygeal pair (Co1) supplies the area around the coccyx.

Neurons entering or leaving the spinal cord are referred to as nerve roots. The nerve root carrying the impulses to the spinal cord is referred to as the dorsal root and is made of sensory neurons. The dorsal root ganglion is an enlargement of this root that contains the cell bodies of these sensory neurons. Impulses carried away from the spinal cord to the muscles or glands are carried by the ventral root or motor root. These cell bodies form the gray matter of the spinal cord. When these two nerve roots merge, they form a mixed nerve.

Spinal Cord Reflexes

A reflex is an involuntary, predictable response to a stimulus, an automatic reaction triggered by a specific change. Spinal cord reflexes are those that do not depend directly on the brain, although the brain may inhibit or enhance them.

A reflex arc is the pathway nerve impulses travel when a reflex is elicited. There are five parts:

1. Receptors detect a change (the stimulus) and generate impulses.
2. Sensory neurons transmit impulses from receptors to the central nervous system (CNS).
3. The CNS contains one or more synapses and the interneurons that may be part of the pathway.
4. Motor neurons transmit impulses from the CNS to an effector.
5. The effector performs its characteristic action.

The spinal cord reflexes include stretch reflexes and flexor reflexes. In a stretch reflex, a muscle that is stretched automatically contracts; an example is the familiar patellar, or knee-jerk, reflex, but all skeletal muscles have such a reflex. The purpose of these reflexes is to keep us upright (because gravity exerts a constant pull on the body) without our having to think about it. They also avoid possible injury from overstretching a muscle. Flexor reflexes may also be called withdrawal reflexes; the stimulus is something painful and the response is to pull away from it. Again, this occurs without the need for conscious thought; the brain is not directly involved.

The clinical testing of certain spinal cord reflexes provides a way to assess the functioning of their reflex arcs. For example, if the patellar reflex were absent, the problem might be in the quadriceps femoris muscle, the femoral nerve, or the spinal cord itself. If the reflex is present, it indicates that all parts of the reflex arc are functioning normally.

Brain

The brain consists of many parts that function as an integrated whole. The major parts are the medulla, pons, and midbrain (the brainstem); the cerebellum; the hypothalamus and thalamus; and the cerebrum (Fig. 47.4).

Ventricles

The ventricles are four cavities within the brain: two lateral ventricles are located within the cerebral hemispheres, the third ventricle lies midline within the thalamus, and the fourth ventricle is midline between the brainstem and cerebellum. Cerebrospinal fluid is formed within, and circulates through the four ventricles.

Medulla Oblongata

The medulla is just above the spinal cord and extends to the pons. It regulates our most vital functions. Within the medulla are cardiac centers that regulate heart rate, respiratory centers that regulate breathing, and vasomotor centers that regulate the diameter of blood vessels and therefore blood pressure. Also in the medulla are reflex centers for coughing, sneezing, swallowing, and vomiting.

Pons

The pons is anterior to the cerebellum and superior to the medulla. Within the pons are two respiratory centers that work with those in the medulla to produce a normal breathing rhythm.

Midbrain

The midbrain extends from the pons to the hypothalamus and encloses the cerebral aqueduct, a tunnel that connects the third and fourth ventricles. Primarily a reflex center, the midbrain regulates visual reflexes (coordinated movement of the eyes), auditory reflexes (turning the ear toward a sound), and righting reflexes that keep the head upright and contribute to balance.

Cerebellum

The cerebellum is posterior to the medulla and pons, separated from them by the fourth ventricle; it is overlapped by the occipital lobes of the cerebrum. The functions of the cerebellum are concerned with the involuntary aspects of voluntary movement: coordination, the appropriate direction and endpoint of movements, and the maintenance of posture and balance or equilibrium. For the maintenance of balance, the cerebellum (and midbrain) uses sensory information provided by the receptors in the inner ear that detect movement and changes in position of the head.

Hypothalamus

The hypothalamus is located above the pituitary gland and below the thalamus. It has many diverse functions:

- Production of antidiuretic hormone (ADH) and oxytocin; these hormones are then stored in the posterior pituitary gland. ADH increases the reabsorption of water by the kidneys and thus helps maintain blood volume. Oxytocin causes contractions of the myometrium of the uterus to bring about labor and delivery.
- Production of releasing hormones that stimulate secretion of the hormones of the anterior pituitary gland. An example is growth hormone–releasing

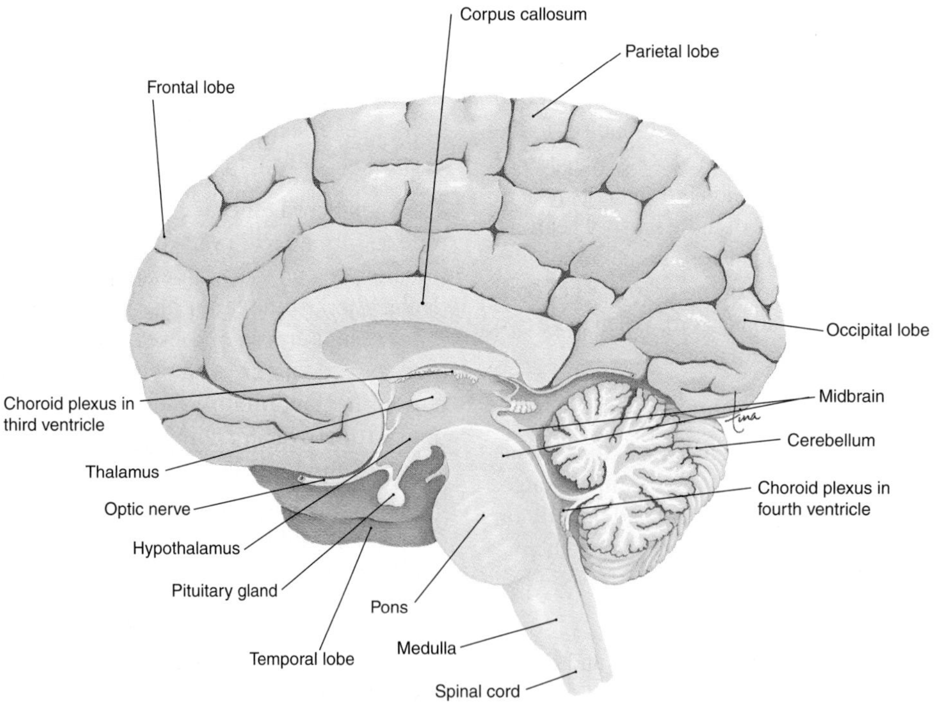
Corpus callosum
Parietal lobe
Frontal lobe
Occipital lobe
Choroid plexus in third ventricle
Midbrain
Cerebellum
Thalamus
Choroid plexus in fourth ventricle
Optic nerve
Hypothalamus
Pituitary gland
Pons
Temporal lobe
Medulla
Spinal cord

FIGURE 47.4 The brain's midsagittal section; medial surface of the right cerebral hemisphere. (From Scanlon, V. C., & Sanders, T. [2007]. *Essentials of anatomy and physiology* [5th ed., p. 177]. Philadelphia: F. A. Davis, with permission.)

hormone (GHRH), which stimulates the anterior pituitary to secrete growth hormone.
- Regulation of body temperature by promoting responses such as shivering in a cold environment or sweating in a warm environment.
- Regulation of food and fluid intake; the hypothalamus is believed to respond to changes in blood nutrient levels and hormones to bring about feelings of hunger or fullness.
- Integration of the functioning of the autonomic nervous system (discussed in a later section).
- Stimulation of visceral responses in emotional situations, such as an increased heart rate with anger or fear. The neurologic basis of emotions is not well understood, but the hypothalamus brings about physiological changes by way of the autonomic nervous system.

Thalamus

The thalamus is above the hypothalamus and below the cerebrum; its functions are primarily concerned with sensation. Sensory pathways to the brain (except olfaction) converge in the thalamus, which begins to integrate sensations, permitting more rapid interpretation by the cerebrum. The thalamus is also capable of suppressing minor sensations, which permits the cerebrum to concentrate on more important sensations with less distraction.

Cerebrum

The two cerebral hemispheres form the largest part of the human brain. The right and left hemispheres are connected by the corpus callosum, a band of about 300 million nerve fibers that transfers information from one hemisphere to the other.

The cerebral cortex is the surface of the cerebrum; it is gray matter that consists mainly of the cell bodies of neurons. The cerebral cortex is folded extensively into convolutions (or gyri) that create more surface area for neurons. The grooves between the folds are called fissures (deeper) or sulci (shallower). Interior to the gray matter is white matter, myelinated axons that connect the parts of the cerebral cortex to one another and the cerebrum to other parts of the brain. The cerebral cortex is divided into lobes, whose functions have been extensively mapped.

The frontal lobes contain the motor areas that generate the impulses that bring about voluntary movement. Each motor area controls movement on the opposite side of the body. Also in the frontal lobe, usually only the left lobe, is Broca's motor speech area, which controls the movements involved in speaking.

The parietal lobes contain the general sensory areas for the cutaneous senses, conscious muscle sense (proprioception), and taste (gustation). This is where these sensations are felt and interpreted.

The temporal lobes contain sensory areas for hearing and olfaction (smell). Also in the temporal and parietal lobes, usually only on the left side, is Wernicke's area where comprehension of speech occurs.

The occipital lobes contain the visual areas that receive impulses from the retinas of the eyes. Perception and interpretation of sight occur here.

In all lobes of the cerebral cortex are association areas that enable us to learn, remember, and think; they also help form our individual personalities. These are complex behaviors requiring integration of several cerebral and lower brain areas.

Deep within the white matter of the cerebral hemispheres are masses of gray matter called the basal ganglia. Their functions are concerned with certain subconscious aspects of voluntary movement: regulation of muscle tone, inhibiting tremor, and use of accessory movements such as arm swinging when walking.

Meninges and Cerebrospinal Fluid

The meninges are the three layers of connective tissue that cover the central nervous system. The outermost is the dura mater, made of thick, fibrous connective tissue. The middle layer is called the arachnoid mater, which has a weblike appearance; the inner layer is the pia mater, a very thin connective tissue on the surface of the brain and spinal cord. Between the arachnoid mater and the pia mater is the **subarachnoid** space, where cerebrospinal fluid circulates.

Each of the four ventricles of the brain contains a choroid plexus, a capillary network where surrounding ependymal cells form cerebrospinal fluid from blood plasma. This is a continuous process, and the cerebrospinal fluid then circulates from the ventricles to the central canal of the spinal cord and to the subarachnoid space around the brain and spinal cord. From the cranial subarachnoid space, cerebrospinal fluid is reabsorbed back to the blood through arachnoid villi that project into the cranial venous sinuses between the two layers of the cranial dura mater. The rate of reabsorption normally equals the rate of production.

As the tissue fluid of the CNS, cerebrospinal fluid permits the exchanges of nutrients and wastes between the blood and CNS neurons. It also acts as a cushion or shock absorber for the CNS. The pressure and constituents of cerebrospinal fluid may be determined by means of a lumbar puncture (spinal tap) and may be helpful in the diagnosis of diseases such as meningitis.

Cranial Nerves

The 12 pairs of cranial nerves emerge from the brainstem, with the exception of pair one, which originates from the temporal lobe and pair two from the occipital lobe. Some are purely sensory nerves, whereas others are mixed nerves. The impulses for sight, smell, hearing, taste, and

• WORD • BUILDING •

subarachnoid: sub—below + arachnoid—middle layer of the meninges equilibrium are all carried by cranial nerves to their respective sensory areas in the brain. Other cranial nerves carry motor impulses to muscles of the face, neck, shoulders, and tongue, or to glands. Cranial nerves III, VII, IX, and X contain axons of both the somatic and autonomic nervous systems. The functions of all the cranial nerves are summarized in Table 47.2.

LEARNING TIP

The cranial nerves are easier to remember when a mnemonic device is used:

On	Olfactory
Old	Optic
Olympus'	Oculomotor
Mountain	Trochlear
Top	Trigeminal
A	Abducens
Finn	Facial
And	Acoustic
German	Glossopharyngeal
Viewed	Vagal
Some	Spinal Accessory
Hops	Hypoglossal

Autonomic Nervous System

The ANS is part of the peripheral nervous system in that it consists of the motor portions of some cranial and spinal nerves. These are the visceral motor neurons to visceral effectors—that is, smooth muscle, cardiac muscle, and glands. The ANS has two divisions: sympathetic and parasympathetic. These two divisions often function in opposition to each other, and their activity is integrated by the hypothalamus.

An autonomic nerve pathway from the CNS to a visceral effector consists of two motor neurons that synapse in a ganglion outside the CNS (Fig. 47.5). The first neuron is called the preganglionic neuron and runs from the CNS to the ganglion. The second neuron is called the postganglionic neuron and runs from the ganglion to the visceral effector. The ganglia are actually cell body collections of the postganglionic neurons.

Sympathetic Division

The cell bodies of the sympathetic preganglionic neurons are in the thoracic and some of the lumbar segments of the spinal cord. The axons of these neurons extend to the sympathetic ganglia, most of which are in two chains just lateral to the spinal column. Within the ganglia are the synapses between the preganglionic and postganglionic neurons; the axons of the postganglionic neurons then go to the visceral effectors. One preganglionic neuron often synapses with many postganglionic neurons to many effectors; thus permitting widespread responses in many organs.

TABLE 47.2 CRANIAL NERVES

Number	Name	Function
I	Olfactory	• Sense of smell
II	Optic	• Sense of sight
III	Oculomotor	• Movement of eyeball • Constriction of pupil for bright light or near vision
IV	Trochlear	• Movement of eyeball
V	Trigeminal	• Sensation in face, scalp, and teeth • Contraction of chewing muscles
VI	Abducens	• Movement of eyeball
VII	Facial	• Sense of taste • Contraction of facial muscles • Secretion of saliva
VIII	Vestibulocochlear	• Sense of hearing • Sense of equilibrium
IX	Glossopharyngeal	• Sense of taste • Secretion of saliva • Sensory input for cardiac, respiratory, and blood pressure reflexes • Contraction of pharynx
X	Vagus	• Sensory input in cardiac, respiratory, and blood pressure reflexes • Sensory and motor input to larynx (speaking) • Decreased heart rate • Contraction of alimentary tube (peristalsis) • Increased digestive secretions
XI	Accessory	• Contraction of neck and shoulder muscles • Motor input to larynx (speaking)
XII	Hypoglossal	• Movement of the tongue

The sympathetic division is dominant in stressful situations such as fear, anger, anxiety, and exercise, and the responses it brings about involve preparedness for physical activity, whether or not it is actually needed. (Table 47.3 summarizes both ANS divisions.) The heart rate increases, vasodilation in skeletal muscles supplies them with more oxygen, the bronchioles dilate to take in more air, and the liver changes glycogen to glucose to provide energy. Relatively less important activities such as digestion are slowed, and vasoconstriction in the skin and viscera permits greater blood flow to more vital organs such as the brain, heart, and muscles.

The neurotransmitters of the sympathetic division are acetylcholine and norepinephrine. Acetylcholine is released by sympathetic preganglionic neurons; its inactivator is acetylcholinesterase. Norepinephrine is released by most sympathetic postganglionic neurons at the synapses with the effector cells; its inactivator is catechol-*O*-methyltransferase (COMT) or monoamine oxidase (MAO).

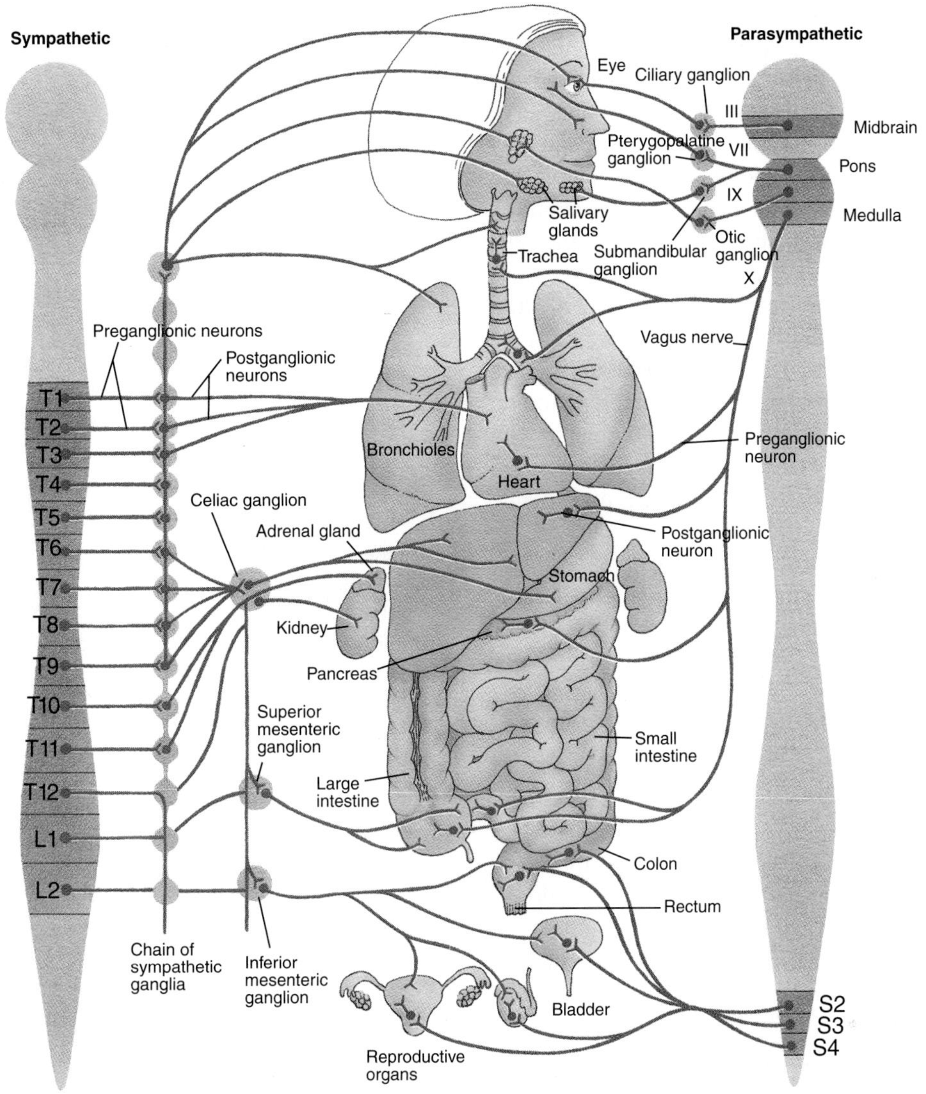
Sympathetic
Parasympathetic
Eye
Ciliary ganglion
III
Midbrain
Pterygopalatine ganglion
VII
Pons
IX
Salivary glands
Otic ganglion
Medulla
Trachea
Submandibular ganglion
X
Preganglionic neurons
Postganglionic neurons
Vagus nerve
T1
T2
T3
T4
T5
T6
T7
T8
T9
T10
T11
T12
L1
L2
Bronchioles
Heart
Preganglionic neuron
Celiac ganglion
Adrenal gland
Postganglionic neuron
Stomach
Kidney
Pancreas
Superior mesenteric ganglion
Small intestine
Large intestine
Colon
Rectum
Chain of sympathetic ganglia
Inferior mesenteric ganglion
Bladder
Reproductive organs
S2
S3
S4

FIGURE 47.5 Autonomic nervous system (From Scanlon, V.C., & Sanders, T. [2007]. *Essentials of anatomy and physiology* [5th ed., p. 190]. Philadelphia: F. A. Davis, with permission.)

TABLE 47.3 FUNCTIONS OF THE AUTONOMIC NERVOUS SYSTEM

Organ	Sympathetic Response	Parasympathetic Response
Heart (cardiac muscle)	Increase rate	Decrease rate (to normal)
Bronchioles (smooth muscle)	Dilate	Constrict (to normal)
Iris (smooth muscle)	Pupil dilates	Pupil constricts (to normal)
Salivary glands	Decrease secretion	Increase secretion (to normal)
Stomach and intestines (smooth muscle)	Decrease peristalsis	Increase peristalsis for normal digestion
Stomach and intestines (glands)	Decrease secretion	Increase secretion for normal digestion
Internal anal sphincter	Contract to prevent defecation	Relax to permit defection
Urinary bladder (smooth muscle)	Relax to prevent urination	Contract for normal urination
Internal urethral sphincter	Contract to prevent urination	Relax to permit urination
Liver	Change glycogen to glucose	None
Sweat glands	Increase secretion	None
Blood vessels in skin and viscera (smooth muscle)	Constrict	None
Blood vessels in skeletal muscle (smooth muscle)	Dilate	None
Adrenal glands	Increase secretion of epinephrine and norepinephrine	None

Source: From Scanlon, V. C., & Sanders, T. (2007). *Essentials of anatomy and physiology* (5th ed., p. 191). Philadelphia: F. A. Davis, with permission.

Parasympathetic Division

The cell bodies of the parasympathetic preganglionic neurons are in the brainstem and the sacral segments of the spinal cord. The axons of these neurons are in cranial nerve pairs III, VII, IX, and X and in some sacral nerves, and they extend to the parasympathetic ganglia. These ganglia are close to or actually in the visceral effector and contain the postganglionic cell bodies, with very short axons to the cells of the visceral effector. One preganglionic neuron synapses with just a few postganglionic neurons to only one effector, permitting localized responses.

The parasympathetic division dominates during relaxed, nonstressful situations to promote normal functioning of several organ systems. Digestion proceeds normally, with increased secretions and peristalsis; defecation and urination may occur, and the heart beats at a normal resting rate (see Table 47.3).

Acetylcholine is the neurotransmitter at all parasympathetic synapses, both preganglionic and postganglionic; it is inactivated by acetylcholinesterase.

CRITICAL THINKING

Mrs. Stevens

■ Mrs. Stevens receives albuterol treatments for her chronic obstructive pulmonary disease. The medication opens her airways effectively, but after her treatments, she often reports that her heart is racing. What part of the peripheral nervous system do you think this medication affects?

Suggested answers at end of chapter.

Aging and the Nervous System

With age, the brain loses neurons, but this is only a small percentage of the total and is not the usual cause of mental impairment in the elderly; far more common causes of mental changes include depression, malnutrition, hypotension, and the side effects of medications. Some forgetfulness is to be expected as is a decreased ability for problem solving (Fig. 47.6).

LEARNING TIP

Sympathetic—S is for STRESS RESPONSE: The sympathetic response is often referred to as the fight-or-flight response. When you think of the sympathetic nervous system, think about getting away from a man-eating lion. You need dilated pupils to see the path better, copious production of sweat to lose heat through evaporation, increased rate and force of heartbeat to ensure that enough blood gets to the extremities so you can run faster, dilated bronchioles to get more oxygen to your muscles, decreased digestion so you won't get hungry while you are trying to get away from the lion, decreased urine output so you won't have to stop for the restroom, and increased mental alertness so you are always aware of where the lion is.

Parasympathetic—P is for PEACEFUL: The parasympathetic nervous system brings the body back to balance and rest. It is sometimes referred to as the rest-and-digest response. Think, "I just got away from a man-eating lion. Now my body can go back to normal and start digesting and urinating again!"

This is a great way to remember the responses, rather than an accurate description of the exact physiology involved.

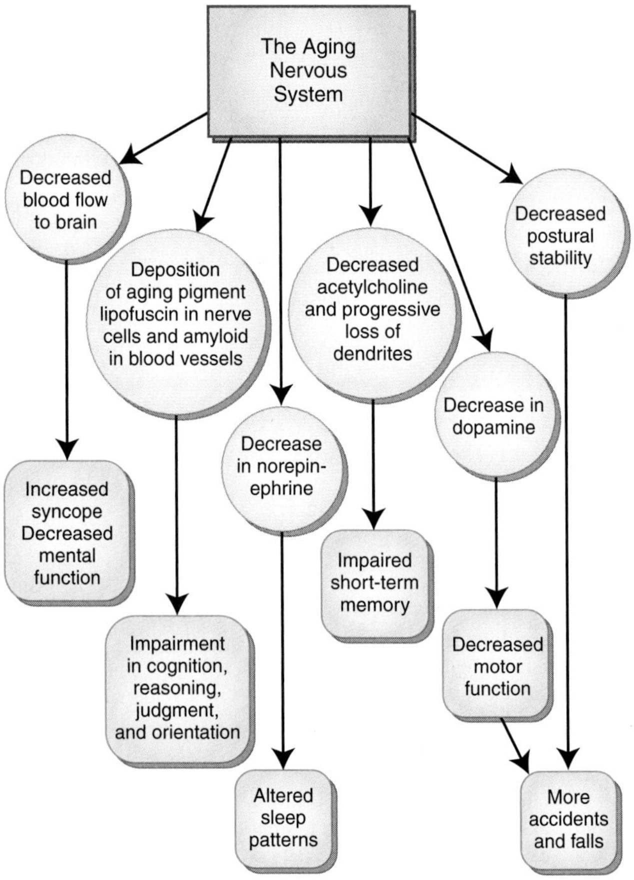

The Aging Nervous System
Decreased blood flow to brain
Deposition of aging pigment lipofuscin in nerve cells and amyloid in blood vessels
Decreased acetylcholine and progressive loss of dendrites
Decreased postural stability
Decrease in dopamine
Decrease in norepinephrine
Increased syncope Decreased mental function
Impaired short-term memory
Impairment in cognition, reasoning, judgment, and orientation
Decreased motor function
Altered sleep patterns
More accidents and falls

FIGURE 47.6 Aging and the neurologic system. This concept map shows the effects the aging process has on the neurologic system.

NURSING ASSESSMENT OF THE NEUROLOGIC SYSTEM

The focus of a nursing neurologic assessment is to establish the present function of the patient's neurologic system and to detect changes from previous assessments. A complete neurologic assessment, intended to determine the existence of neurologic disease, is typically performed by a physician or nurse practitioner. A baseline neurologic assessment should be performed on every patient admission (Box 47.1). In addition to providing valuable information about the current functioning of the patient's neurologic system, the assessment provides baseline data for comparison purposes. This is especially important if the patient has chronic neurologic deficits on admission.

Consider a patient admitted for surgery, who has had a previous **cerebrovascular** accident resulting in **paresis** of the right arm. A complete neurologic assessment would document that the right arm is weaker than the left. If during the postoperative course you assess that both arms are equal in strength, you would want to notify the physician so the patient could be further assessed for possible causes of weakening of the left arm.

The results of the baseline assessment are invaluable in planning and implementing safe care. For example, patients who have a history of seizure activity need careful monitoring, and all staff members who interact with such patients should be aware of how to respond to a seizure. Patients with **dysphagia** (difficulty swallowing) may need to have restrictions placed on the types of food or fluids they can have. This information must be consistently communicated to all staff involved in the patient's care.

The patient's admitting diagnosis, the presence of any chronic neurologic disorders, and the current functioning of the patient's neurologic system all influence how often neurologic assessments should be done. Orders for neurologic assessments may vary from every 15 minutes for an acutely ill or injured patient, to every 8 hours for a patient who is close to being discharged, to every 24 hours for a resident living in long-term care. It is always appropriate to assess a patient more often than ordered, based on observed changes in the patient's condition, and to communicate the findings of those assessments to the primary care provider. The changes noted while assessing the patient may indicate changes in the central nervous system. Rapid detection and intervention may mean the difference between chronic dysfunction and recovery or even between life and death for the patient.

Box 47.1

Basic Neurologic Assessment

1. Assess level of consciousness (patient's response to verbal or tactile stimulation) and orientation.
2. Obtain vital signs (specifically blood pressure, pulse, and respirations).
3. Check pupillary response to light.
4. Assess strength and equality of hand grip and movement of extremities.
5. Determine ability to sense touch or pain in extremities.

• WORD • BUILDING •

cerebrovascular: cerebro—brain + vascular—vessels
paresis: partial paralysis
dysphagia: dys—difficult + phagia—eating

Health History

To understand the patient's neurologic status, ask about past and current symptoms, use of prescription and over-the-counter medications, use of recreational drugs, past surgeries, treatments, and risk factors such as family history, diet, exercise, sedentary lifestyle, caffeine intake, and recent stressors. Assessment of symptoms, as with other body systems, includes asking the WHAT'S UP? questions.

You should also obtain a history of the patient's general health and then focus on any neurologic symptoms. Symptoms of neurologic disorders vary in type, location, and intensity. It is important to remember that some neurologic disorders can affect the patient's ability to think, remember, speak, or interpret stimuli. It may be necessary to question significant others about duration and severity of symptoms. Some patients may not be able to recognize their own neurologic deficits. In such cases, the significant other usually initiates contact with the health care system and provides the medical and social history. See Table 47.4 for sample questions to ask if the patient has a change in mental status.

In addition to questioning the patient, the nurse observes the patient during the health history. Is he or she shifting positions and exhibiting signs of discomfort? Is the patient able to change position and move about easily? Is he or she able to carry on a coherent conversation?

Physical Examination

The physical examination begins when you first meet the patient and make an overall evaluation of the patient's mental and physical status. The neurologic system is assessed using inspection, palpation, and percussion (with a reflex hammer). When conducting the mental status and cognitive portions of the examination, be aware that fatigue, illness, or medications can alter findings. When interpreting neurologic findings be sure to consider the patient's age, educational background, and cultural background.

Level of Consciousness

Level of consciousness exists along a continuum from full wakefulness, alertness, and cooperation to unresponsiveness to any form of external stimuli. A fully conscious patient responds to questions spontaneously. As consciousness becomes impaired, a patient may show irritability, a shortened attention span, or an inability to cooperate. The level of

TABLE 47.4 COLLECTION OF DATA RELATING TO MENTAL STATUS

Category	Questions to Ask During the Health History	Rationale/Significance
Mental Status	• What is your name? What is the month? Year? Where are you now?	• Disorientation is often an initial sign of a neurologic disorder.
Intellectual Function	• Subtract 7 from 100, then 7 from that answer, and so on (serial 7s).	• Most people with intact neurologic function can complete serial 7s in about 90 seconds.
Thought Content	• What would you do if you smelled smoke? • Where would you put milk?	• Assessment of the patient's ability to interpret information and act appropriately is an important safety issue and activity of daily living.
Perception	• Show patient pencil and pen and ask what each is.	• Agnosia (inability to interpret or recognize familiar objects) can occur in stroke and brain lesions.
Language Ability	• Read the following sentence: ____.	• Different types of aphasia can result from injury to different parts of the brain.
Memory	• Repeat these four or five words: ____. Repeat them again in 5 minutes.	• Impaired memory can be affected by both delirium and dementia. Delirium can cause impaired immediate and short-term memory, whereas dementia not only affects immediate and short-term memory but also the ability to learn new information. It also may be related to stroke.
Pain	• On a scale of 0 to 10 with 0 as no pain and 10 as the worst you have ever had, what is your pain level?	• Pain perception may be altered or impaired by spinal injury, medications, alcohol, stress, and level of consciousness. Some spinal injuries may be critical but the patient will not report pain.

consciousness should be the first thing assessed during a neurologic examination because the information obtained can be used to modify the remainder of the examination if necessary. Keep in mind that a decrease in the level of consciousness can be caused by problems such as hypoxia, hypoglycemia, or intoxication, not just dysfunction of the neurologic system.

Many health care institutions use the Glasgow Coma Scale (GCS), which is an international scale used to assess level of consciousness (LOC) and document findings (Table 47.5). The GCS is based on simple and clearly defined aspects of patient responses that provide for consistent assessment data. It is used to evaluate patients who have a potential for rapid deterioration in consciousness. The GCS assesses three parameters of consciousness: (1) eye opening, (2) verbal response, and (3) motor response. When assessing LOC, consider the patient's physical ability to respond, taking into consideration trauma, medical condition, and medications. For example, a patient who cannot open his or her eyes because of facial trauma may still have an intact neurologic system.

Motor response is scored in the GCS based on following commands, responding to pain, or displaying abnormal postures. Abnormal postures includes **decorticate** and **decerebrate**. In decorticate, or flexion, posturing, the patient's arms are flexed at the elbow, the hands are raised toward the chest, and the legs are extended (Fig. 47.7A). This posture indicates significant impairment of cerebral functioning. In decerebrate, or extension, posturing, both the arms and legs are extended and the arms are internally rotated (Fig. 47.7B). This abnormal posturing indicates damage in the area of the brainstem.

The total possible score on the GCS ranges from 3 to 15. A score of less than 7 indicates a comatose patient and a score of 15 indicates the patient is fully alert and oriented. When used to score the effects of a head injury, a score of 13 or 14 indicates mild head injury, 9 to 12 indicates moderate injury, and any score of 8 or below indicates severe head injury. For all categories of the GCS, the type of painful stimuli required to elicit a response should be documented. Deterioration in the patient's condition (i.e., a lowering of the GCS score) should be reported to the physician promptly. See *Evidence-Based Practice* box.

TABLE 47.5 GLASGOW COMA SCALE

Eye opening	Spontaneous	4
	To verbal stimulus	3
	To painful stimulus	2
	No response	1
Verbal response	Normal conversation	5
	Confused conversation	4
	Inappropriate words	3
	Incomprehensible sounds	2
	No response	1
Motor response	Obeys commands	6
	Localizes pain	5
	Withdraws from pain*	4
	Abnormal flexion	3
	Abnormal extension	2
	No response	1

* To elicit pain, place pressure on a nailbed or on the trapezius muscle. Be sure to apply the stimulus long enough to elicit a response.

Note: This scale is for adults only. Criteria specific to children should be used.

• WORD • BUILDING •

decorticate: de—down + corticate—cerebral cortex

decerebrate: de—down + cerebrate—cerebrum

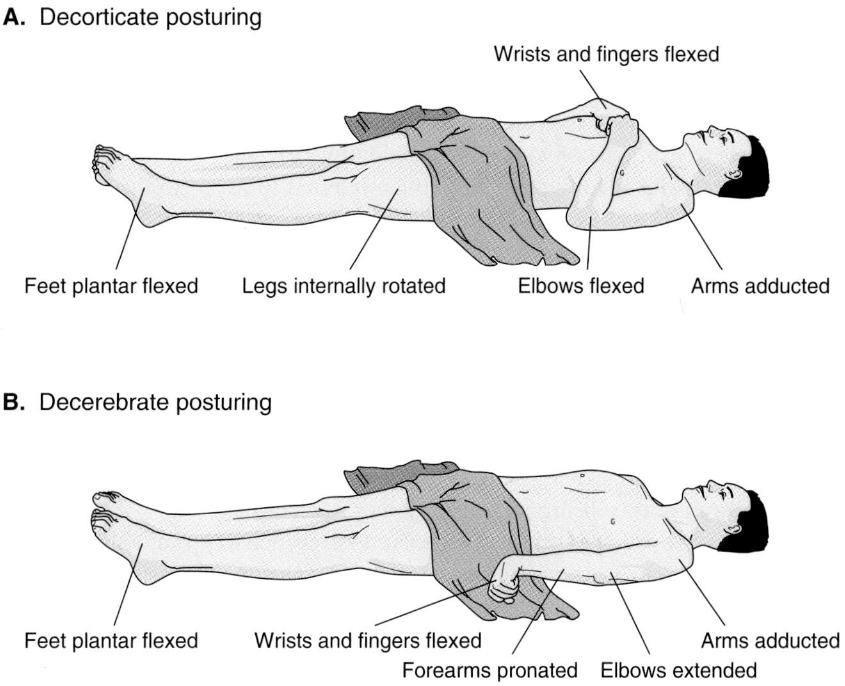
A. Decorticate posturing
Wrists and fingers flexed
Feet plantar flexed
Legs internally rotated
Elbows flexed
Arms adducted
B. Decerebrate posturing
Feet plantar flexed
Wrists and fingers flexed
Arms adducted
Forearms pronated
Elbows extended

FIGURE 47.7 Abnormal posturing. (A) Decorticate posturing. (B) Decerebrate posturing.

EVIDENCE-BASED PRACTICE

Clinical Question

Is the Glasgow Coma Scale (GCS) the best tool for neurologic assessment?

Evidence

A summary of evidence compiled by Zachary Munn in 2007 and submitted to the Joanna Briggs Institute confirms the validity and reliability of this scale when used to assess current neurologic status. The GCS has been shown to have a high inter-rater reliability with experienced staff and adds no extra cost to the care of the patient. A limitation of this scale is that if one of the three components cannot be measured, the resulting score is of no use. Contrary to popular assumptions, alcohol ingestion is not shown to have a significant effect on the GCS score.

Implications for Nursing Practice

Use the GCS whenever a patient is at risk for neurologic changes. Be sure to keep a copy of the scale in your pocket or on your clipboard for easy reference.

REFERENCE

Munn, Z. (2007, October 19). Neurologic assessment: Glasgow Coma Scale. *Evidence summaries—Joanna Briggs Institute*, Adelaide. Retrieved July 25, 2009 from http://proquest.umi.com/pqdweb?did=1451744661&Fmt=3&=clientId=30337&RQT=309&VName=PQD.

Mental Status

Mental status can be affected not only by the aging process but by a variety of neurologic disorders and injuries. A traumatic brain injury can result in memory impairment, delayed amnesia, affective (mood) disorders, and dementia. To assess for cognitive impairment, the Mini-Mental State Examination (MMSE) or Confusion Assessment Method can be used. The Confusion Assessment Method uses the following criteria to help diagnose delirium (Waszynski, 2007):

- Acute onset and fluctuating course
- Inattention
- Disorganized thinking
- Altered level of consciousness.

Find more about the Confusion Assessment Method at the Hartford Institute for Geriatric Nursing, http://consultgerirn.org, an excellent collaborative website that provides best practice information related to older adults. A change in mental status should be taken seriously, especially when the patient takes multiple medicines or has had a recent change in medicines. A primary cause of delirium and acute states of confusion is adverse effects from medications.

When you assess cognitive function, you are evaluating the patient's thinking capacity. You want to determine the length of attention span, ability to concentrate, judgment, memory, orientation, perception, problem-solving ability, and motor function.

You can learn a great deal about a patient's mental capacities and emotional state by simply interacting with the patient. Behavior, mood, hygiene, grooming, and choice of dress reveal pertinent information about mental status. Mental status examinations can be performed to determine patients' cognitive functioning, thought processes, and perceptions by observing the patient's verbal and nonverbal responses to questions and specific requests. Table 47.4 includes some ways to assess these areas.

Orientation refers to the patient's ability to comprehend himself or herself in relation to person, location (place), and time. A patient who is fully oriented is often referred to as "oriented times three." Typical questions include "What is your name? Where are you? What day is it?" (Keep in mind that we all forget the date from time to time!) You can also ask if the person knows what season it is (spring, fall, etc.). A resident of a long-term care facility who says he is "at home" may consider the facility his home and is not necessarily disoriented. Be sure your question is appropriate to the patient's age, culture, living conditions, lifestyle, and medical condition. If the patient is unable to speak because of a stroke (expressive **aphasia**) or being intubated, do not rule out the possibility that the patient is oriented. Give expressively aphasic patients yes-or-no questions such as "Are you in a grocery store? Are you in a bowling alley? Are you in a hospital?" Patients may be able to answer with a shake of the head, eye blinks, or hand squeezes as instructed.

Examination of the Eyes

Examination of the pupils is an important part of the neurologic assessment and cranial nerve evaluation. The size of the pupils at rest is documented. Many institutions use a millimeter gauge for measuring pupils (Fig. 47.8). This allows an objective description of the size. If the patient's pupils are unusually large or small, you should determine if the patient has had any medications that might affect pupil size. If the patient's pupils are unequal in size (**anisocoria**), without a correlating diagnosis or symptoms, ask the patient or significant others if the patient normally has unequal pupils. Anisocoria may be congenital; it can also be caused by cataract surgery. Development of unequal pupils in a patient who previously had equal pupils is an emergency and should be reported to the physician immediately. Any deviation from the normal round shape of the pupils is documented.

Once the resting size of the pupils has been noted, the next step is to assess their response to light. In a darkened room, a light source (such as a flashlight) is directed at the pupil from the lateral aspect of the eye. This allows the examiner to see the direct and the consensual response to the light. A consensual response means that when one pupil is exposed to direct light, the other pupil also constricts. Absence of a consensual response may indicate a pathological condition in the area of the optic chiasm. Typically, the speed of the reaction to light is described as brisk, sluggish, or absent. Differences in the speed or size of constriction between the two pupils should be reported to the practitioner.

Accommodation is the process of visual focusing from far to near. To evaluate for accommodation, have the patient focus on an object at a distant point and then refocus on the object at a near point. Pupils should constrict with the adjustment to the near object and the eyes should converge. Upon completion of the assessment of the pupils, document your findings. PERRLA is a commonly used abbreviation to note that pupils are equal, round, and reactive to light and accommodation.

You will also evaluate for range of motion and for smoothness and coordination of movements. Eyes that move in the same direction in a coordinated manner are said to have a conjugate gaze. Conversely, a dysconjugate gaze is movement of the eyes in different directions. Some patients may be unable to move one or both eyes in a specific direction; this is called ophthalmoplegia. It is often documented as "limited extraocular movements." Always document what the limitation is (e.g., "Patient is unable to look laterally with left eye"). This allows colleagues to compare their findings with yours and detect any changes.

Nystagmus is involuntary movement of the eyes. Nystagmus varies in the speed of the movement and the direction. Horizontal nystagmus is the most common. Common causes of nystagmus are phenytoin (Dilantin) toxicity and injury to the brainstem.

Examination of Muscle Function

Examine muscle groups systematically in the upper extremities and then the lower extremities, comparing right to left. Compare muscle groups for symmetry of size and strength. Keep in mind the patient's age and general physical condition when evaluating muscle strength. You would not expect the same amount of strength from a 75-year-old woman as from a 20-year-old man. If the patient has chronic neurologic deficits, ask if the results of the assessment are different from his or her usual level of function.

Many health care providers use a 5-point scale to document muscle strength. A score of 5 describes a patient who is able to move the extremity against gravity and the resistance of the examiner, displaying normal muscle strength. If the examiner is able to provide more resistance than the patient can overcome with active movement, the score is 4. If the patient can move the extremity only against gravity, but not

• WORD • BUILDING •

aphasia: a—absence + phasia—speech

anisocoria: aniso—unequal + coria—pupil

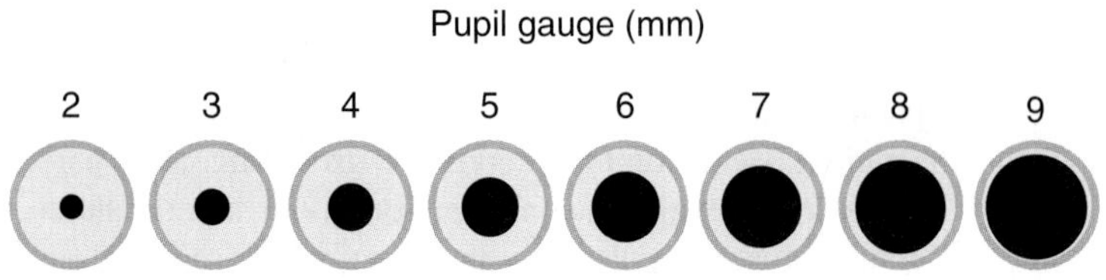
Pupil gauge (mm)
2
3
4
5
6
7
8
9

FIGURE 47.8 Assessment of pupil size.

resistance, the score is 3. If gravity must be eliminated by having the examiner support the extremity to allow the patient to move the extremity, the score is 2. A score of 1 is given if there is no active movement of the extremity, but a minimum muscular contraction can be palpated. If the examiner is unable to detect any muscular function, a score of 0 is given.

To test the deltoid muscles, ask the patient to raise his or her arms at the shoulder. Have the patient resist as you push down on the upper arms. The biceps are tested by having the patient flex the arm at the elbow and bring the palm toward the face, then resist as you attempt to straighten the arm by pulling on the forearm. With the arm similarly flexed, ask the patient to straighten the arm while you resist the movement.

Hand grasps are tested by having the patient squeeze your fingers. Remember to cross your index and middle fingers to prevent the patient from hurting your fingers. If the patient does not release the grasp when told to, it is a reflex grasp, not a response to command. A reflex palmar grasp may indicate a pathological condition of the frontal lobe.

Assess for arm drift by asking the patient to hold both arms straight in front with the palms upward while keeping the eyes closed. A downward drift of the arm, or rotation so that the palm is down, indicates impairment of the opposite side of the brain. If a pathological condition is present, arm drift may be apparent before differences in muscle strength can be detected.

Assessment of leg muscle strength begins with the iliopsoas muscle. Place your hand on the patient's thigh and ask the patient to raise the leg, flexing at the hip. Hip adductors are tested by having the patient bring his or her legs together against your hands. The hip abductors and gluteus medius and minimus are tested by having the patient move the legs apart against resistance. Hip extension by the gluteus maximus is tested by placing the hand under the thigh and having the patient push down with the leg. The quadriceps femoris extends the knee and is tested by having the patient attempt to straighten the leg at the knee. The hamstrings are responsible for knee flexion and are evaluated by having the patient attempt to keep the heel of the foot against the bed or chair rung. Dorsiflexion is tested by having the patient pull the toes toward the head against resistance. Plantar flexion is tested by having the patient push against the examiner's hand with the ball of the foot.

Babinski's reflex is tested by firmly stroking the sole of the foot. Normal response is flexion of the great toe. If the great toe extends and the other toes fan out, neurologic dysfunction should be suspected if the patient is more than 6 months old. Deep tendon reflexes are not usually part of a routine nursing assessment. The patient's gait should be assessed to detect any neurologic dysfunction and also to assess ability to ambulate safely. Patients who stagger, weave, or bump into objects may need assistance with walking.

Romberg's test is performed by having the patient stand with feet together and eyes closed. Be sure to stand close to the patient, especially if he or she is an older adult, to prevent falling. A negative Romberg's test means that the patient experiences minimal swaying for up to 20 seconds. A patient who experiences swaying or who leans to one side is said to have a positive Romberg's test. A positive Romberg's test may be seen in cerebellar dysfunction.

> **SAFETY TIP**
>
> A positive Romberg's test in an older adult is expected as a result of normal aging changes in the cerebellum. Be sure to protect the patient with a positive result from falls. A gait belt may be helpful when assisting the patient with ambulation.

Examination of Cranial Nerves

The cranial nerves are usually not examined in depth during a routine bedside neurologic assessment. Testing requires a patient who is able to cooperate with the examiner. Table 47.6 provides basic testing techniques that provide a superficial assessment of cranial nerve function.

Summary of Examination Findings

In all cases, the findings of the neurologic examination should be correlated with the remainder of the physical examination findings. A decreased level of consciousness, coupled with a decreased oxygen saturation on pulse oximetry, point to hypoxia as a cause. Correlation of vital signs with neurologic signs is particularly important. Bradycardia, increasing systolic blood pressure with widening pulse pressure, and irregular respirations, commonly referred to as Cushing's triad, are late indications of increasing intracranial pressure. These findings, in conjunction with a unilateral dilated pupil, may indicate impending herniation of the brain (discussed further in Chapter 48).

> **CRITICAL THINKING**
>
> ***Tim Thompson***
>
> ■ You are caring for Tim, a 78-year-old man admitted with heart problems. As you enter his room with his afternoon medications, you find Tim confused. He thinks he is at home, that the year is 1968, and he does not understand who you are or why you are there. He recognizes his wife, who is at his bedside, and he knows his own name.
>
> 1. How would you describe and document his mental status?
> 2. What additional data do you need to decide how to proceed?
> 3. What may have contributed to his confusion?
>
> *Suggested answers at end of chapter.*

TABLE 47.6 COLLECTION OF DATA RELATED TO CRANIAL NERVE FUNCTION

Nerve	Test
Olfactory nerve	Ask patient to identify common scents, such as cinnamon and coffee.
Optic nerve	Ask patient to read something or tell how many fingers you are holding up.
Oculomotor nerve	Check pupils for reaction to light and accommodation.
Oculomotor, trochlear, and abducens nerves	Ask patient to follow your finger while moving it in front of his or her eyes in the positions of a clock: 1, 3, 5, 7, 9, and 11 o'clock.
Trigeminal nerve	Ask patient to identify touch on different parts of the face with eyes closed.
Facial nerve	Ask patient to frown, smile, wrinkle forehead; check for symmetry.
Vestibulocochlear nerve	Have patient identify whisper close to each ear. Observe gait for balance.
Glossopharyngeal and vagus nerves	Watch for uvula and palate to rise when patient says "ahh." Touch back of throat with cotton-tipped applicator to elicit gag reflex.
Spinal accessory nerve	Ask the patient to turn head and shrug the shoulders against resistance.
Hypoglossal nerve	Ask the patient to stick out the tongue and move it from side to side.

DIAGNOSTIC TESTS FOR THE NEUROLOGIC SYSTEM

Laboratory Tests

Specific diagnostic blood tests do not exist for neurologic disorders. However, depending on the history and physical examination, the practitioner may include laboratory tests to look for underlying causes of symptoms: thyroid hormone levels, vitamin B_{12}, complete blood count, electrolytes, creatine kinase and isoenzymes (CK), VDRL test (for syphilis), liver function, and renal function. Measurement of erythrocyte sedimentation rate (ESR) and white blood cell (WBC) count may indicate an infection, such as meningitis. Hormone levels, such as prolactin or cortisol, may indicate dysfunction of the pituitary gland related to a brain tumor. Anticholinesterase testing and antibody titers are useful in diagnosing myasthenia gravis (MG). Research is ongoing to develop a blood test for Alzheimer's disease.

Lumbar Puncture

Cerebrospinal fluid (CSF) may be obtained via lumbar puncture and evaluated for glucose and protein levels, the presence of bacteria and white blood cells, levels of immunoglobulin, antibodies, and culture and sensitivity. During lumbar puncture, the physician anesthetizes the area and then inserts a needle into the spinal canal to draw off a sample of CSF. Typically, the lumbar puncture needle is placed at the level of L3–4 or L4–5 in an adult. Because the spinal cord ends at the L1 level, this placement prevents damage to the cord by the needle. If there is any difficulty inserting the needle, the procedure may be done under fluoroscopy to help guide needle placement. CSF samples should be sent to the laboratory immediately after the procedure.

Nursing Care

Make sure that informed consent has been obtained before the procedure. Assist the patient into a side-lying position with his or her back as close to the edge of the bed nearest the practitioner as possible. Depending on the patient's condition, you may need to help the patient flex the knees up to the chest (Fig. 47.9). This position maximizes the space between vertebrae, which makes it easier for the practitioner to insert the needle. An alternative position is to have the patient sit with the back perpendicular to the edge of the bed. Leaning over a bedside table may help the patient maintain the position. During the procedure, you may be asked to assist the physician with equipment handling.

After the lumbar puncture is completed, instruct the patient to remain on bedrest with the head of the bed flat for 6 to 8 hours, as ordered by the physician, and to increase oral intake of fluids. Keeping the head flat decreases the likelihood of leakage of CSF from the puncture site, which can result in a severe headache. Increasing fluid intake promotes replacement of the fluid that was removed. Label and send the specimens to the laboratory as ordered. Assess the puncture site for swelling or drainage of CSF and report any leakage to the health care provider. Assess the movement and sensation to the lower extremities frequently for the first 4 hours after the procedure. Assess the patient for headache and, if needed, obtain an order for an analgesic.

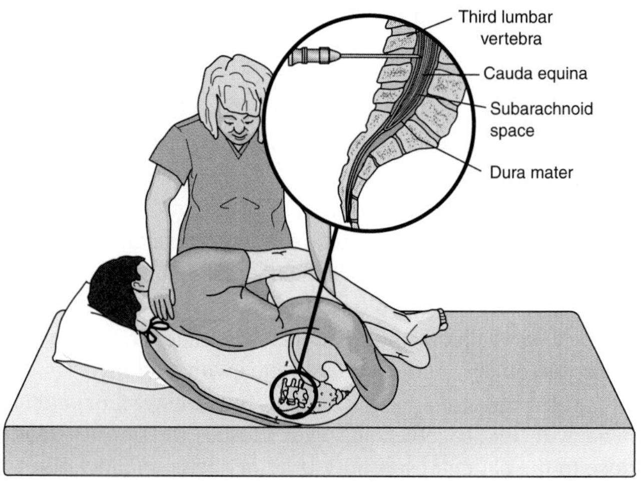
Third lumbar vertebra
Cauda equina
Subarachnoid space
Dura mater
FIGURE 47.9 Position for lumbar puncture.

> **NURSING CARE TIP**
>
> The idea of a needle being introduced into the spinal canal is frightening to many people. Give simple, clear directions to the patient; help the patient maintain his or her position; and provide emotional support throughout the procedure.

X-Ray Examination

Spinal x-ray examinations are done to determine the status of individual vertebrae and their relationship to one another. If the patient experiences pain with certain movements, he or she may be asked to flex and extend the area of the spine being examined while the radiographs are taken. This allows detection of abnormal movement of the vertebrae. If the patient may have sustained trauma to the spine, particularly the cervical spine, radiographs are taken before the immobilizing devices are removed. Skull radiographs may be taken to detect skull fractures or foreign bodies. No special nursing care is required.

Computed Tomography

A computed tomography (CT) scan is used for diagnosing neurologic disorders of the brain or spine. Some of the disorders that can be detected by CT are hemorrhage, altered ventricle size, cerebral atrophy, tumors, skull fractures, and abscesses. CT is used when MRI is contraindicated because of metal aneurysm clips or other metal implants.

The scan may be performed with or without radiopaque contrast material to enhance the clarity of the images. If contrast material is used, a series of images is filmed, and then the contrast material is given intravenously and another series of images is filmed. The patient should be questioned about any allergies to contrast material, iodine, or shellfish. The blood urea nitrogen (BUN) and creatinine levels should be checked before contrast material is administered because it is excreted through the kidneys. Patients with elevated BUN and creatinine levels or known renal disease may be unable to tolerate the contrast material. Contrast material is most commonly used if a tumor is suspected or following surgery in the area to be scanned. CT scans are commonly used in emergency evaluations because they can be done quickly, an important consideration if the patient is ventilated or unstable.

> **NURSING CARE TIP**
>
> No one is really allergic to iodine—iodine is an essential element in the body. However, many patients are allergic to dyes. Because patients might confuse the two, it is still important to ask about an iodine allergy.

Nursing Care

During the CT scan, the patient must lie still on a movable table. Noncontrast scans take about 10 minutes; contrast scans take 20 to 30 minutes. Patients who are receiving dye should be warned that they may feel a sensation of warmth following the injection; warmth in the groin area may make them feel as though they have been incontinent of urine. Nausea, diaphoresis, itching, or difficulty breathing may indicate allergy to the dye and should be reported immediately to the physician or nurse practitioner. Sedation may be required for patients who are agitated or disoriented. Patients who are in pain may need pain medication before the examination.

Magnetic Resonance Imaging

Magnetic resonance imaging (MRI) uses magnetic energy to provide a more detailed picture of soft tissue than a CT scan provides. It is not as useful when looking for bony abnormalities. MRI is used for diagnosis of degenerative diseases such as multiple sclerosis, arteriovenous malformations, small tumors, hemorrhages, and cerebral and spinal cord edema. An MRI of the mediastinal cavity will determine if the thymus gland is enlarged and facilitate diagnosis of myasthenia gravis. It is a longer procedure and may be difficult for unstable, disoriented, or ventilated patients. As with a CT scan, the MRI can be done with or without contrast material. Some facilities have the capability to perform magnetic resonance angiograms (MRAs). This test allows visualization of blood vessels and assessment of blood flow without being as invasive as a traditional angiogram.

Nursing Care

Because of the magnetic fields being used, restrictions are placed on patients undergoing an MRI and the health care personnel who work in the MRI facility. People with pacemakers or any type of metallic prosthesis cannot undergo MRI or be in the room when one is performed. This is because the magnetic field is so strong that it could dislodge the prosthesis or pacemaker. Those who may have accidentally acquired metallic foreign bodies (e.g., metal slivers in the eye or shrapnel that was not removed) may need an x-ray examination to determine the presence or absence of such objects. Even permanent makeup and tattoos can cause problems because of the metallic salts in some dyes. Patients are asked to remove all metal objects, such as jewelry or hair clips, before the procedure.

Other contraindications include gross obesity, claustrophobia, agitation, inability to cooperate, and inability to lie flat. It may be difficult for the patient to lie in one position for a prolonged period. The patient's need for pain medication should be assessed before the procedure. Use of pillows for positioning may improve comfort. The narrow, tunnel-like structure of the MRI unit causes claustrophobia in some patients. Sedatives can be given or an open MRI unit may be used if one is available. Warn the patient that the procedure involves a noisy "knocking" sound. Encourage the use of deep breathing, guided imagery, and other relaxation techniques.

SAFETY TIP

Educate patients to consider that they may someday need a life-saving MRI before having tattoos or permanent makeup applied! Some pigments do not contain metal and are safer.

Angiogram

An angiogram is an x-ray study of blood vessels that is used when an abnormality of cerebral or spinal blood vessels is suspected or to obtain information about blood supply to a tumor. Following injection of a local anesthetic, a catheter is inserted through the femoral artery and advanced until contrast material can be injected into the appropriate vessels. The dye then shows the vessels on the radiograph and provides information about the structure of specific vessels, as well as overall circulation to the area.

Nursing Care

Before an angiogram, the patient receives a clear liquid diet and has an intravenous (IV) needle placed. Informed consent must be obtained. BUN and creatinine levels are evaluated because the contrast material is excreted through the kidneys. Potential for bleeding is assessed by prothrombin time and partial thromboplastin time tests before the procedure because the procedure involves inserting a large-bore catheter into a large artery. Typically, the patient receives some type of sedation before being transported to the angiography suite. During the injection of the contrast material, the patient may report severe heat sensations and a metallic taste in the mouth. The patient must lie still while the radiographs are being taken, and so should be told about the sensations he or she may experience. Patients who are disoriented or agitated may need sedation to complete the test.

After the procedure, maintain pressure on the catheter insertion site and keep the patient flat in bed for 6 to 8 hours to prevent bleeding from the insertion site. The patient may turn from side to side but must keep the affected leg straight. Assess the patient's vital signs, neurologic status, circulatory status, and insertion site every 15 minutes for 1 hour, then every 2 hours for 4 hours, or as ordered. Report any decrease or loss of the pedal pulse in the affected foot immediately; this may indicate a clot in the femoral artery. Encourage the patient to increase oral intake in addition to the IV fluids that are administered to aid in excretion of the contrast material.

Myelogram

A **myelogram** is an x-ray examination of the spinal canal and its contents. Following a lumbar puncture, cerebrospinal fluid is removed and sent for laboratory analysis. Contrast material is then injected into the subarachnoid space. The patient is moved into various positions and radiographs are taken. Compression of nerve roots, herniation of intravertebral disks, and blockage of cerebrospinal fluid circulation may all be detected by myelogram. Sometimes, CT or MRI is used in place of x-rays for a myelogram.

Nursing Care

After the procedure, keep the patient on bedrest with the head elevated less than 30 degrees. This lessens the possibility of the contrast material getting into the cerebral CSF circulation. The contrast material used for myelograms can lower the seizure threshold in some patients. Any patient with a known seizure disorder should have serum levels of anticonvulsants evaluated and be carefully observed for signs of seizures. Encourage the patient to drink plenty of fluids to help the kidneys excrete the dye.

Because of the invasive nature of these procedures, a separate informed consent form may be required for the lumbar puncture and myelogram. The physician performing the test explains the risks, benefits, and possible complications of the examination. If a patient who needs these diagnostic procedures has cognitive deficits, it may be necessary to obtain consent from the legal next of kin.

Electroencephalogram

Electrical activity of the brain is evaluated by use of an **electroencephalogram** (EEG). Electrodes are attached to the scalp with an adhesive. Electrical activity is transmitted through the electrodes to a computerized tracing. Analysis of the tracing can identify areas of abnormality, such as a seizure focus or areas of slowed activity.

Nursing Care

Before the test, make sure that the patient's hair is clean and dry. The physician may write orders to withhold sedatives to prevent interference with the EEG, and patients may be weaned from their anticonvulsants if the goal of the test is to identify the seizure focus during a seizure. These patients must be very carefully monitored and protected from harm. Typically, they undergo videotaping while the EEG is performed. Following the procedure, the adhesive must be washed from the hair. Assist the hospitalized patient to do this as soon as possible, before it becomes hardened and difficult to remove.

THERAPEUTIC MEASURES FOR THE NEUROLOGIC SYSTEM

Moving and Positioning

Patients who have pain may need help changing positions and ambulating. Use of heat, cold, or analgesics may allow the patient to be more independent in mobility.

• WORD • BUILDING •

myelogram: myelo—referring to the spinal cord + gram—picture

electroencephalogram: electro—electrical activity + encephalo—referring to the brain + gram—picture

If the patient has sensory loss, make sure that no part of the body is inadvertently compressed (e.g., a hand caught under a hip or the scrotum compressed between the legs). Pressure ulcers are of primary concern with the patient who is unable to move independently. Collaborate with the physical therapist to determine positioning techniques that maximize the chance of useful recovery.

Patients with paresis, paralysis, or **paresthesia** (abnormal sensation such as burning or tingling) may be partially or completely dependent in moving and positioning. Take care to maintain the body in functional positions when routine position changes are made. This means keeping the trunk, extremities, hands, and feet in usable positions—for example, hands can be splinted to keep the thumb and fingers opposed, or tennis shoes can be used to keep the feet in an appropriate position for standing or walking.

Contractures and footdrop are complications that are often associated with neurologic disorders. Contractures are permanent muscle contractions with fibrosis of connective tissue that occur from lack of use of a muscle or muscle group. They cause permanent deformities and prevent normal functioning of the affected part. Footdrop occurs when the feet are not supported in a functional position and become contracted in a position of plantar flexion (Fig. 47.10). Use footboards, high-top tennis shoes, and splints to help prevent footdrop. Splints are commonly used to prevent contractures of the upper and lower extremities and to keep the affected parts in a functional position. If splints are used, the patient must be evaluated for discomfort and skin breakdown at the splint site.

Mobilization should be begun as soon as a patient is medically stable. Initially this may involve the use of a cardiac chair if the patient is unable to bear weight. Transfer of the patient to a bedside chair or use of ambulation aids may require a multidisciplinary approach. Be careful to recognize any physical or cognitive deficits that may affect safety and adjust the environment to protect the patient. This includes communicating any safety concerns to unlicensed personnel who interact with the patient.

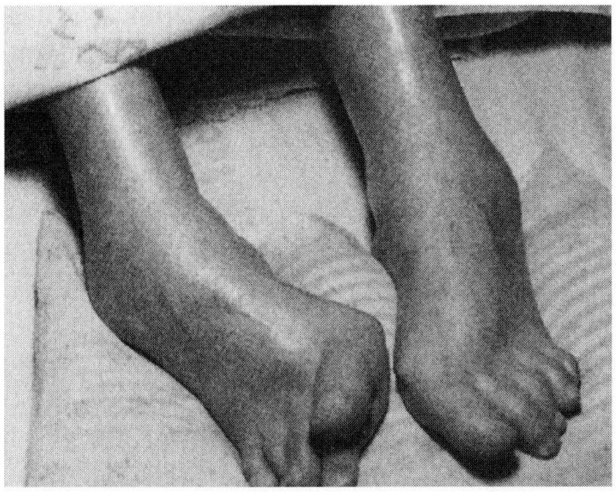

FIGURE 47.10 Contractures, footdrop. (From Hegner, B. [1998]. *Assisting in long term care* [3rd ed.]. Albany, NY: Delmar, with permission.)

Activities of Daily Living

The effects of neurologic disorders on activities of daily living (ADLs) may range from an inconvenience to complete dependence. Patients may have trouble bending over to put on their shoes and socks, lifting a full cooking pot, or caring for an infant. A quadriplegic patient may be completely unable to perform ADLs but can be taught to direct his or her own personal care. Encourage patients to use strategies they learned in occupational or physical therapy.

Assessment of a hospitalized patient should include a discussion of the strategies the patient normally uses at home to accomplish ADLs. Every attempt should be made to continue to use these strategies. This is particularly true if the patient is admitted to a long-term care facility. Patients who have intact cognitive function should be included in care planning and encouraged to work collaboratively with caregivers. If the strategies the patient uses during ADLs must be changed (e.g., if the patient's transfer technique is unsafe), be sure to explain the rationale for the changes to the patient and significant others. If patients have impaired cognitive function, try to maintain a specific routine that is as close to their normal environment as possible. Normalizing routines may help patients adapt to a change in environment and maximize their ability to function.

Communication

The communication problems associated with neurologic disorders have a variety of etiologies. Some neurologic disorders cause difficulty speaking (**dysarthria**). Dysfunction of the lips, tongue, or jaw makes speech difficult or impossible to understand. When dysarthric individuals know what they want to say but cannot be understood, they can become very frustrated. This frustration is compounded if the patients are treated as if they have cognitive deficits merely because they have difficulty communicating.

Patients who have had a stroke can experience different types of aphasia. Expressive aphasia is difficulty or inability to verbally communicate with others. The patient may be able to speak in sentences but inappropriately substitute words, such as "The sky is dish." Word-finding difficulty is another type of expressive aphasia. These patients may tell you "I want a. . . ." and then be unable to complete the sentence. In severe cases of aphasia, the patient may make sounds that resemble words or may only utter sounds. For individuals with no intelligible speech or with word-finding difficulty, a picture board with commonly used items may facilitate communication. (See an example of a picture board in Chapter 49.) Keep in mind that patients with expressive aphasia may answer yes to all

• WORD • BUILDING •

paresthesia: para—beside + asthesia—sensations

dysarthria: dys—dysfunctional + arthria—movement of the joints used in speech questions rather than just those for which yes is correct. The same is true of answering no. This is one reason why a nurse should never ask a patient, "Are you Mrs. Gonzalez?" An aphasic patient may say yes even if that is not her name. Instead, ask the patient to state her name. Always check the identification band.

For patients who substitute words, simply correct the substitution and continue the conversation. Patients with expressive aphasia are often very aware of and frustrated by their difficulty communicating. Give them time to try to express themselves. If you cannot understand them, offer possibilities based on the situation. If the patient is sitting in the chair, ask if he or she wants to go back to bed or wants to use the bathroom. If the patient is restless, ask if he or she is in pain.

Some patients use the same word in response to all questions, and for a few patients that word is a profanity. This is very difficult for significant others to deal with, particularly if swearing is not something the patient normally did. Make it clear to the family that you understand that this behavior is part of the patient's illness.

Receptive aphasia affects the patient's ability to understand spoken language. Again, the severity of the aphasia varies. Some patients may understand simple directions such as "sit down" or "squeeze my fingers." In other cases, the nurse may need to pantomime the action the nurse wants the patient to perform, such as showing the patient pills and then mimicking taking the pills and drinking water.

SAFETY TIP

If the patient has receptive aphasia, assume that he or she cannot understand or follow safety instructions, such as "Do not stand up until I get back." Even going around the corner to get water can give a patient enough time to try to stand up and subsequently fall.

Nutrition

Alterations in the ability to maintain an adequate nutritional intake can have many causes. The level of consciousness may be depressed enough that the patient does not recognize that she or he is hungry or thirsty. Decreased level of consciousness or cranial nerve dysfunction may impair the patient's ability to swallow safely. Severe weakness may limit the patient's ability to take in enough food to meet the body's requirements. These conditions are often compounded by the increased metabolic rate that accompanies neurologic injury or illness.

If there is any question of the patient's ability to swallow, a swallowing evaluation should be performed by a speech therapist. Some institutions use a radiological examination to evaluate the ability to swallow. A small amount of barium is added to food or fluid, and fluoroscopy is used while the patient swallows. This allows visualization of the path of the food or fluid. Patients with swallowing difficulty (dysphagia) may have better success with foods or thick liquids rather than thin fluids. Liquids may be thickened with special thickening agents to allow easier swallowing. All patients should be positioned as upright as possible while eating or drinking, and patients who have difficulty swallowing should be monitored during eating and not left alone.

If weakness or fatigue is the cause of decreased nutritional intake, several modifications are possible. Serving small portions of food more frequently can increase intake. Using high-protein, high-calorie foods and supplements increases the nutritional content of small amounts of foods.

For patients who cannot swallow or who cannot swallow enough food, enteral tube feedings may be needed. If enteral feedings are anticipated to be for a short duration, a nasogastric tube may be used. The disadvantages of nasogastric tubes include impairment of the integrity of nasal skin and the risk of aspiration. The risk of aspiration in neurologically impaired patients who have cognitive impairments is increased because these patients may pull out the nasogastric tube due to their lack of understanding the purpose of the tube. If long-term enteral feedings are anticipated, a gastrostomy tube may be placed directly through the abdominal wall into the stomach. This feeding method has the advantage of reducing the risks of aspiration and eliminating nasal skin breakdown.

Family

When working with patients who have a neurologic deficit, whether acute or chronic, in the hospital, extended care facility, or at home, the family needs to be included in their care and rehabilitation. Depending on the patient's diagnosis and prognosis, the family will need support from staff. It is rewarding to see the patient who has had an accident recover with rehabilitation, but it is also rewarding to promote quality of life for the patient with Alzheimer's disease and his or her family. Communication with the family regarding patient improvements and information about the illness is extremely important. Include the family in the patient's care, such as bathing, feeding, and grooming. Suggest that the family participate in physical therapy sessions. Education is of vital importance, especially if the patient is going to be discharged home. Direct the patient and family to support groups and case managers for information regarding financial assistance and community resources during rehabilitation.

SUGGESTED ANSWERS TO

CRITICAL THINKING

■ *Mrs. Stevens*

Albuterol is an adrenergic agonist (sometimes called a sympathomimetic), which is given to stimulate the sympathetic nervous system, resulting in open airways in patients with respiratory disease. However, it can also stimulate the cardiac system and cause a rapid heart rate and increased blood pressure. Be sure to monitor vital signs in patients receiving medications that affect the autonomic nervous system.

■ *Tim Thompson*

1. He is alert but confused, oriented to person only.
2. The nurse should ask his wife if this has ever happened before; check his medical history for any disorders that may contribute to neurologic dysfunction; do a quick neurologic examination to determine if any additional deficits exist; check vital signs and pulse oximetry if available; and notify the physician immediately if the symptoms are a new finding.
3. Some possible explanations to explore include hypoxemia, stroke, worsening heart problems causing inadequate flow of blood to the brain, hypoglycemia, or even confusion (delirium) related to a sudden transition from home to an unfamiliar environment.

REVIEW QUESTIONS

1. Which neurons carry impulses from the CNS to effectors?
   a. Mixed
   b. Motor
   c. Afferent
   d. Sensory

2. Which structure in the CNS regulates body temperature?
   a. Hypothalamus
   b. Temporal lobe
   c. Pons
   d. Pituitary

3. Which of the following is a symptom of increasing intracranial pressure that should be reported immediately to the primary care provider?
   a. Constricted pupils
   b. Decreasing level of consciousness
   c. Narrowing pulse pressure
   d. Bradypnea

4. What are the normal effects of aging on the CNS? **Select all that apply.**
   a. Increased postural stability
   b. Reduced blood flow to the brain
   c. Impaired short-term memory
   d. Sleep disturbances
   e. Loss of deep tendon reflexes
   f. Decrease in acetylcholine

5. A patient asks what to expect when she has an angiogram. Which response by the nurse is best?
   a. "A small needle will be inserted into your spinal column to withdraw fluid for examination."
   b. "You will be in a large machine that uses magnetic energy to create images; it has a noisy knocking sound."
   c. "Electrodes will be placed on your head to monitor electrical activity in your brain."
   d. "A catheter will be placed in your femoral artery, and dye will be injected that will make your vessels show up on x-ray."

6. Which of the following activities should be encouraged when a patient returns from a CT scan using a contrast medium?
   a. Ambulation
   b. Drinking fluids
   c. Turning side to side
   d. Coughing and deep breathing

7. Which of the following nursing interventions can help prevent footdrop?
   a. Position the patient in the left lateral position.
   b. Provide daily foot massage.
   c. Apply high-top tennis shoes.
   d. Maintain the patient in an upright position as much as possible.

Reference

Waszynski, M. (2007). How to try this: Detecting delirium. *American Journal of Nursing, 107*(12), 50–59.

48

Nursing Care of Patients with Central Nervous System Disorders

DEBORAH L. WEAVER

KEY TERMS

akinesia (AH-kin-EE-zee-uh)
ataxia (ah-TAK-see-ah)
bradykinesia (BRAY-dee-kin-EE-zee-ah)
contracture (kon-TRAK-chur)
contralateral (KON-truh-LAT-er-uhl)
craniectomy (KRAY-nee-EK-tuh-mee)
cranioplasty (KRAY-nee-oh-plas-tee)
craniotomy (KRAY-nee-AHT-oh-mee)
delirium (de-LEER-ee-um)
dementia (dee-MEN-cha)
dysreflexia (DIS-re-FLEK-see-ah)
encephalitis (en-SEFF-uh-LYE-tis)
encephalopathy (en-SEFF-uh-LAHP-ah-thee)
hemiparesis (hem-ee-puh-REE-sis)
hydrocephalus (HEYE-droh-SEF-uh-luhs)
ipsilateral (IP-si-LAT-er-uhl)
laminectomy (LAM-i-NEK-toh-mee)
meningitis (MEN-in-JIGH-tis)
neurodegenerative (new-roh-de-JEN-er-uh-tiv)
nuchal rigidity (NEW-kuhl re-JID-i-tee)
paraparesis (PAR-ah-puh-REE-sis)
paraplegia (PAR-ah-PLEE-jee-ah)
photophobia (FOH-tuh-FOH-bee-ah)
postictal (pohst-IK-tuhl)
prodromal (proh-DROH-muhl)
quadriparesis (KWA-dri-puh-REE-sis)
quadriplegia (KWA-dri-PLEE-jee-ah)
turbid (TERR-bid)

QUESTIONS TO GUIDE YOUR READING

1. What are the causes, risk factors, and pathophysiology of central nervous system infections, including meningitis and encephalitis?
2. What nursing interventions are appropriate for a patient with a central nervous system infection?
3. How do the various types of headaches differ?
4. What education should you provide for the patient experiencing headaches?
5. What are the causes and types of seizures?
6. How would you care for someone during a seizure?
7. How would you recognize a patient who is developing increased intracranial pressure?
8. What nursing interventions can help prevent increased intracranial pressure?
9. What are the causes, risk factors, and pathophysiology of injuries to the brain and spinal cord?
10. What nursing care would you provide for a patient with an injury to the brain or spinal cord?
11. What are the causes, risk factors, and pathophysiology associated with neurodegenerative disorders such as Parkinson's, Huntington's, or Alzheimer's disease?
12. What nursing care would you provide for a patient with a neurodegenerative disorder?
13. What nursing interventions are appropriate for the patient with dementia?

Disorders of the central nervous system (CNS) include problems originating in the brain and spinal cord. Because the CNS is the control center for the entire body, disorders in this system can cause symptoms in any part of the body, ranging from pain to paralysis, confusion, and coma. This chapter presents nursing care of patients with these disorders. Care of patients with cerebrovascular disorders is covered in Chapter 49.

CENTRAL NERVOUS SYSTEM INFECTIONS

Infectious agents can enter the central nervous system via a variety of routes (Table 48.1). Anything that depresses the patient's immune system such as steroid administration, chemotherapy, radiation therapy, or malnutrition can make the patient more vulnerable to infection.

Meningitis

Pathophysiology and Etiology

Meningitis is an inflammation of the brain and spinal cord that may be caused by either bacterial or viral infection. Any microorganism that enters the body can result in meningitis. Bacterial meningitis is a serious infection that is spread by direct contact with discharge from the respiratory tract of an infected person. Viral meningitis, also called aseptic meningitis, is more common and rarely serious. It usually presents with flu-like symptoms, and patients recover in 1 to 2 weeks.

The most common bacteria causing meningitis include *Neisseria meningitidis, Streptococcus pneumoniae,* and *Haemophilus influenzae* type b (Hib). With current immunization standards in the United States, *H. influenzae* type b has decreased in recent years. *N. meningitidis,* the cause of meningococcal meningitis, and *S. pneumoniae,* the cause of pneumococcal meningitis, are the major causes of bacterial meningitis. Bacterial infection generally begins in another area, such as the upper respiratory tract, enters the blood, and invades the CNS, causing the meninges to become inflamed and intracranial pressure (ICP) to increase. Vessel occlusion and necrosis of areas in the brain may occur. Cranial nerve function may be transiently or permanently affected by meningitis. Some of the effects are listed in Table 48.2.

Prevention

Vaccines are available against Hib and *S. pneumoniae.* Hib vaccinations are begun during the newborn period. The vaccine against *S. pneumoniae* is not effective for children younger than age 2; it is recommended for people over age 65 and those who have a chronic medical condition. Chemoprophylaxis is recommended for those who have had significant exposure to anyone currently infected with meningitis. To destroy the organism from the nasopharynx, antimicrobials such as rifampin, the quinolones, and the sulfonamides are used.

Signs and Symptoms

The most common symptom of meningitis is headache, caused by tension on blood vessels and irritation of the pain-sensitive dura mater. A high fever and stiff neck are present and the patient may experience **photophobia** (light sensitivity). The patient with meningococcal meningitis usually presents with petechiae on the skin and mucous membranes.

Nuchal rigidity (pain and stiffness when the neck is moved) is caused by spasm of the extensor muscles of the neck. Positive Kernig's and Brudzinski's signs are often seen in patients suffering from meningitis. Both signs are caused by inflammation of the meninges and spinal nerve roots. To elicit Kernig's sign, the examiner flexes the patient's hip to 90 degrees and tries to extend the patient's knee. The sign is positive if the patient experiences pain and spasm of the hamstring. Brudzinski's sign is positive when flexion of the patient's neck causes the hips and knees to flex (Fig. 48.1). Nausea and vomiting associated with meningitis are caused by direct irritation of brain tissue and by increased ICP.

TABLE 48.1 ROUTES OF ENTRY FOR CENTRAL NERVOUS SYSTEM INFECTIONS

Route of Entry	Examples
Bloodstream	Insect bite Otitis media
Direct extension	Fracture of frontal or facial bones
Cerebrospinal fluid	Dural tear Poor sterile technique during procedure
Nose or mouth	Meningococcus meningitis
In utero	Contamination of amniotic fluid Rubella Vaginal infection

TABLE 48.2 CRANIAL NERVES AFFECTED BY MENINGITIS

Cranial Nerve Affected	Manifestation
III, IV, VI	Ocular palsies Unequal and sluggishly reactive pupils
VII	Facial weakness
VIII	Deafness and vertigo

• WORD • BUILDING •

meningitis: mening—membranous covering of the brain + itis—inflammation

photophobia: photo—light + phobia—fear or intolerance

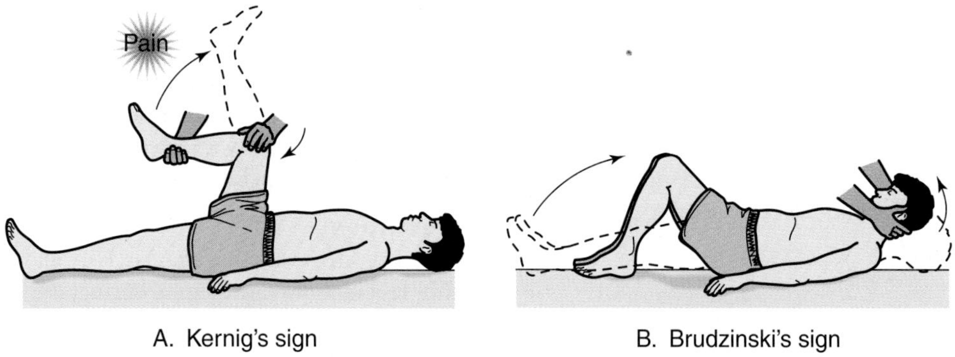
Pain
A. Kernig's sign
B. Brudzinski's sign

FIGURE 48.1 (A) Kernig's sign. (B) Brudzinski's sign.

Encephalopathy refers to the mental status changes seen in patients with meningitis. These are manifested as short attention span, poor memory, disorientation, difficulty following commands, and a tendency to misinterpret environmental stimuli. Late signs of meningitis include lethargy and seizures.

Complications

Resolution of meningitis depends on how quickly and effectively the disease is treated. Some people have no lasting effects, while others have permanent neurologic deficits. Cranial nerve damage may leave the patient blind or deaf. Seizures may continue to occur even after the acute phase of the illness has passed. Cognitive deficits ranging from memory impairment to profound learning disabilities may occur.

Diagnostic Tests

A lumbar puncture is the most informative diagnostic test for a patient with suspected meningitis (see Chapter 47). Viral meningitis is characterized by clear cerebrospinal fluid with normal glucose level and normal or slightly increased protein level. No bacteria are seen, but the white blood cell count is usually increased. In contrast, the cerebrospinal fluid of an individual with bacterial meningitis is **turbid**, or cloudy, because of the elevated number of white blood cells. Bacteria are identified by Gram stain and culture, and a sensitivity test is done to identify the most effective antibiotic. The bacteria utilize the glucose normally found in cerebrospinal fluid (CSF), thereby lowering the glucose level. The amount of protein in the CSF is elevated. A magnetic resonance image (MRI) or computed tomographic (CT) scan may be done to evaluate for complications.

Therapeutic Measures

Meningitis can be fatal if not treated promptly. Antibiotics such as penicillin G and cephalosporins are administered for bacterial meningitis. Symptom management is the same as that for viral or bacterial meningitis. Antipyretics such as acetaminophen are used to control the fever; a cooling blanket also may be used. Care should be taken to avoid cooling the patient too much because shivering increases the metabolic demand for oxygen and glucose. Analgesics are given to lessen head and neck pain. Corticosteroids and anti-inflammatory agents are given to decrease swelling. Nausea and vomiting are controlled with antiemetic medications. The patient with meningococcal meningitis should be placed in isolation for at least the first 24 hours of medication administration to prevent transmission to others.

Patients may become agitated. A quiet, dark environment lessens the stimulation of a patient who has a headache or photophobia and who may be agitated, disoriented, or at risk for seizures. An important aspect of nursing care focuses on keeping patients from harming themselves. It is very upsetting to families to see a loved one acting agitated or disoriented. Therefore, it is important to teach the family about symptoms and treatment goals for the patient. (See Table 48.3.)

Encephalitis

Pathophysiology

Encephalitis is an inflammation of brain tissue. Nerve cell damage, edema, and necrosis cause neurologic findings localized to the specific areas of the brain affected. Hemorrhage in the brain may occur in some types of encephalitis. Increased ICP may lead to herniation of the brain (see later section on increased ICP).

Etiology

Viruses are the most common cause of encephalitis. They may be specifically related to a particular time of year or geographical location. Some viruses, such as West Nile virus, are carried by ticks or mosquitoes. Others are systemic viral infections, such as infectious mononucleosis or mumps, which spread to the brain. Parasites, toxic substances, bacteria, vaccines, and fungi are other potential causes of encephalitis.

Herpes simplex is the most common non–insect-borne virus to cause encephalitis. The majority of individuals harbor herpes simplex virus type 1 in a dormant state. This is the virus responsible for sores on the oral mucous membranes, commonly called cold sores. Infectious diseases,

• WORD • BUILDING •

encephalopathy: encephalo—brain + pathy—illness
encephalitis: encephalo—brain + itis—inflammation

TABLE 48.3 MENINGITIS SUMMARY

Signs and Symptoms	Nuchal rigidity Positive Kernig's and Brudzinski's signs Fever Photophobia Petechial rash on skin and mucous membranes Encephalopathy
Diagnostic Tests	Lumbar puncture with CSF analysis, C&S Complete blood count C&S nose and throat
Therapeutic Measures	Antimicrobials (if bacterial) Seizure precautions Antipyretics Pain management Reduction of environmental stimuli Education
Complications	Seizures Increased ICP Hearing loss Vision impairment Cognitive defects
Possible Nursing Diagnoses	*Hyperthermia* *Acute Pain* related to nuchal rigidity *Risk for Injury* related to positive culture in CSF

CSF = cerebrospinal fluid; C&S = culture and sensitivity; ICP = intracranial pressure.

fever, and emotional stress are possible reasons for the virus becoming active, but the exact mechanism is not known.

Signs and Symptoms

As with many viruses, there is a period of headache, general malaise, nausea and vomiting, and fever. These symptoms usually develop over a period of several days. Additional symptoms include nuchal rigidity, confusion, decreased level of consciousness, seizures, photophobia, **ataxia** (lack of muscle coordination), abnormal sleep patterns, and tremors. The patient may also have **hemiparesis**.

The patient with herpes encephalitis develops edema and necrosis (sometimes associated with hemorrhage), most commonly in the temporal lobes. This significant cerebral edema causes increased ICP and can lead to herniation of the brain. If the patient becomes comatose before treatment is begun, the mortality rate may be as high as 70% to 80%. The first 72 hours is the most likely time for death to occur due to the cerebral edema.

Complications

Patients who have had encephalitis are often left with cognitive disabilities and personality changes. Ongoing seizures, motor deficits, and blindness may also occur. Deterioration in cognition and personality changes are particularly stressful for significant others. The patient's behavioral control is a major factor in determining discharge plans. You can assist significant others to realistically assess the patient's functional level and the family's ability to care for the patient. In-home care, outpatient therapy, and adult day care are options to explore. For some severely impaired individuals, custodial care may be the only feasible and safe discharge option.

• WORD • BUILDING •

hemiparesis: hemi—one side + paresis—partial paralysis

Diagnostic Tests

CT scan, MRI, lumbar puncture to obtain cerebrospinal fluid, and electroencephalogram (EEG) are used to diagnose encephalitis. Cerebrospinal fluid analysis typically reveals increased white blood cell count and protein level and normal glucose levels. Breakdown of blood after cerebral hemorrhage results in yellow-colored CSF. Viral serology may be useful to identify the type of virus and guide treatment options.

Therapeutic Measures

No specific treatment is currently available for insect-borne encephalitis. Careful neurologic assessment and treatment of symptoms may help prevent complications and improve survival. Anticonvulsants, antipyretics, and analgesics are administered to reduce seizures, fever, and headache. Corticosteroids are used to decrease the swelling from the inflammation. Sedatives may be given for irritability. Antiviral medications such as acyclovir (Zovirax) may also be used, especially for herpes simplex.

INCREASED INTRACRANIAL PRESSURE

Pathophysiology and Etiologies

Any patient with a pathological intracranial condition may be at risk for increased ICP. ICP is the pressure exerted inside the cranial cavity by its components (blood, brain, and cerebrospinal fluid). Normal ICP is 0 to 15 mm Hg. This pressure fluctuates with normal physiological changes, such as arterial pulsations, changes in position, and increases in intrathoracic pressure (e.g., coughing or sneezing). Common causes of increased ICP include brain trauma, intracranial hemorrhage, and brain tumors. Prompt detection of changes in neurologic status indicating increased ICP allows intervention aimed at preventing permanent brain damage.

The skull is a rigid compartment containing three components: brain, blood, and cerebrospinal fluid. If an increase in one component is not accompanied by a decrease in one or both of the other components, the result is increased ICP (Fig. 48.2). The consequences of increased ICP depend on the degree of elevation and the speed with which the ICP increases. Patients with slow-growing tumors may have significantly increased ICP before they develop symptoms. Conversely, patients with a subarachnoid hemorrhage may sustain a sudden sharp increase in ICP.

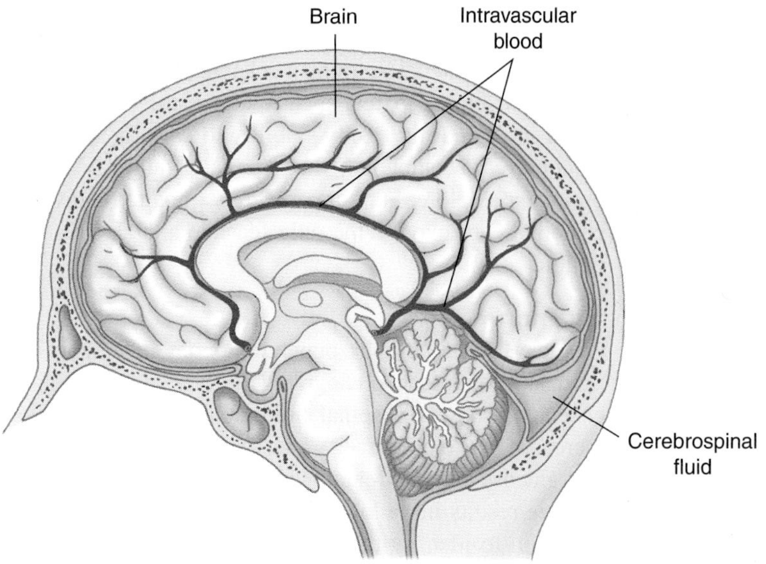
Brain
Intravascular blood
Cerebrospinal fluid

FIGURE 48.2 Any increase in brain tissue, blood, or cerebrospinal tissue can increase intracranial pressure.

The normally functioning body has several methods of compensating for increased ICP. Cerebrospinal fluid can be shunted into the spinal subarachnoid space. Hyperventilation may trigger constriction of cerebral blood vessels, decreasing the amount of blood within the cranial vault. These compensatory mechanisms are temporary and not particularly effective if the increase in ICP is sudden or severe.

Signs and Symptoms

Initial symptoms of increased ICP include restlessness, irritability, and decreased level of consciousness because cerebral cortex function is impaired. If not intubated, the patient may hyperventilate, causing vasoconstriction as the body attempts to compensate. As the pressure increases, the oculomotor nerve may be compressed on the side of the impairment. Compression of the outermost fibers of the oculomotor nerve results in diminished reactivity and dilation of the pupil. As the fibers become increasingly compressed, the pupil stops reacting to light. If the compression continues and the brain tissue exerts pressure on the opposite side of the brain from the injury, both pupils become fixed and dilated.

Vital sign changes are a late indication of increasing ICP. Cushing's triad is a classic late sign of increased ICP and is characterized by bradycardia, irregular respirations, and arterial hypertension (increasing systolic blood pressure while diastolic blood pressure remains the same), resulting in widening pulse pressure. By the time these symptoms appear, the ICP is significantly increased and interventions may not be successful.

Monitoring

ICP monitoring allows for early detection of changes in the pressure on the brain, before changes in symptoms can be seen. The most common method of monitoring ICP in adults is by placing a catheter in the ventricle of the brain, in the cerebral parenchyma, or in the subdural or subarachnoid space. This can be done at the bedside or in surgery. Each of these methods requires anesthetizing the scalp and drilling a hole, called a burr hole, into the skull.

Placement of a catheter into one of the lateral ventricles is referred to as external ventricular drainage (Fig. 48.3). This method allows for pressure monitoring as well as drainage of cerebrospinal fluid to reduce ICP. Disadvantages to this method include difficulty in locating the ventricle for insertion of the catheter and clotting of the catheter by blood in the cerebrospinal fluid.

To allow communication with the subarachnoid space, a subarachnoid bolt can be tightly screwed into the burr hole after the dura has been punctured (Fig. 48.4). The advantage of a subarachnoid bolt is ease of placement. Disadvantages include occlusion of the sensor portion of the bolt with brain tissue and inability to drain CSF. An intraparenchymal monitor is placed directly into brain tissue. Some physicians believe that this most accurately reflects the actual situation within the skull. These monitors cannot be used to drain CSF and may become occluded by brain tissue.

Patients with ICP monitors are cared for in an intensive care unit (ICU) and require aggressive nursing care to prevent complications. These patients are often mechanically ventilated and may be pharmacologically paralyzed and sedated. In addition to meeting the patient's physiological needs and preventing complications, education and emotional support to significant others is important.

Nursing Process for the Patient with an Infectious or Inflammatory Neurologic Disorder

Data Collection

Collaborate with the registered nurse (RN) to obtain a complete history from the patient, if feasible, and from significant others. Pay particular attention to exposure to risk factors. The physical examination must include all body systems because neurologic impairment affects the entire

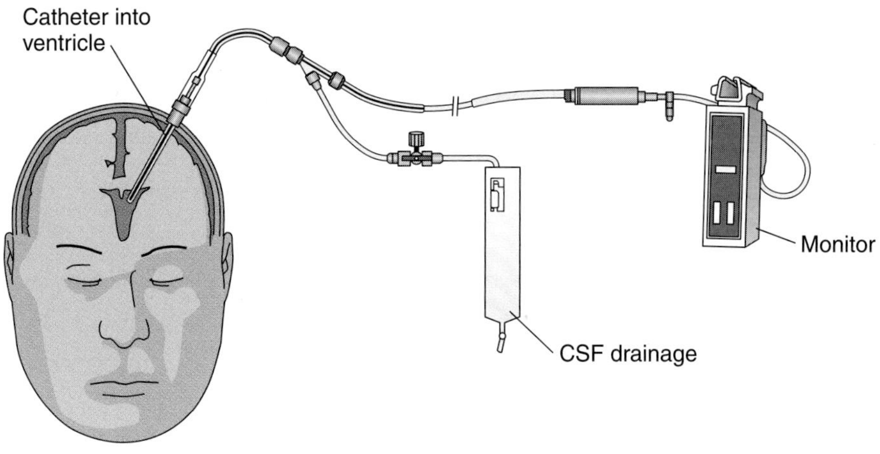
Catheter into ventricle
Monitor
CSF drainage

FIGURE 48.3 Ventricular drain. A catheter into the ventricle allows intracranial pressure monitoring and cerebrospinal fluid drainage.

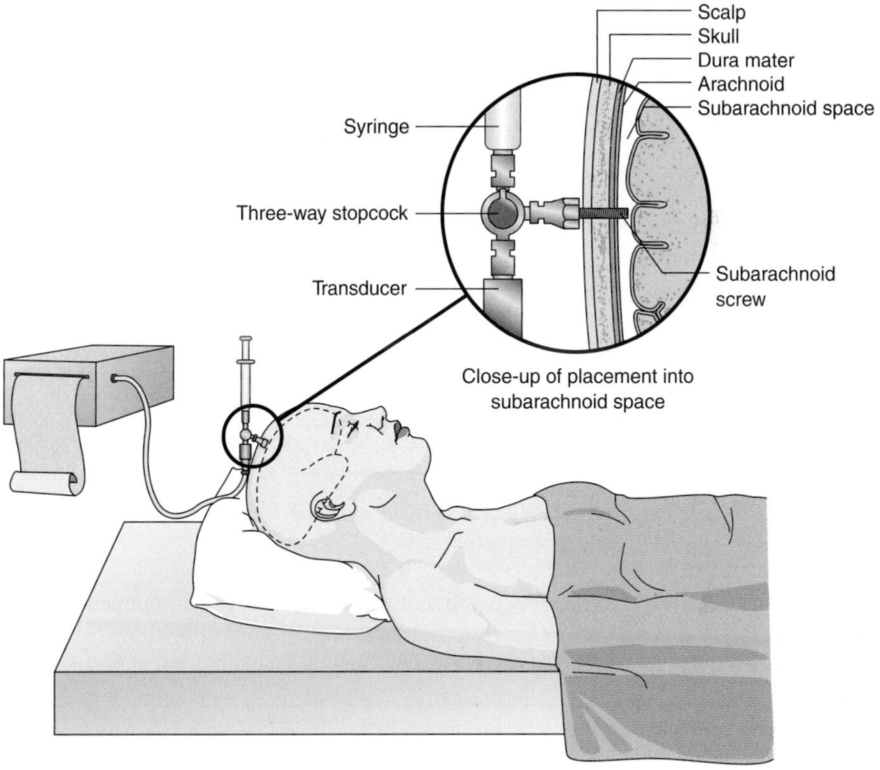
Scalp
Skull
Dura mater
Arachnoid
Subarachnoid space
Syringe
Three-way stopcock
Transducer
Subarachnoid screw
Close-up of placement into subarachnoid space

FIGURE 48.4 Subarachnoid bolt monitor.

person. Following the initial examination, serial neurologic assessments continue to be important to detect and report changes promptly. You can assist with monitoring pupil response, level of consciousness (LOC), and vital signs for signs of increased ICP (Box 48.1). Monitor headache on a pain scale if the patient is able to participate. The Glasgow Coma Scale, presented in Chapter 47, is a valuable tool to monitor level of consciousness.

Nursing Diagnoses, Planning, and Implementation

The patient with increased ICP is usually cared for in an intensive care setting. The LPN/LVN collaborates with the RN in implementing care. For additional interventions for patients with infectious or inflammatory disorders, see the *Nursing Care Plan for the Patient with a Brain Tumor or Injury.*

Box 48.1

Signs and Symptoms of Increased Intracranial Pressure

- Vomiting
- Headache
- Dilated pupil on affected side
- Hemiparesis or hemiplegia
- Decorticate then decerebrate posturing
- Decreasing level of consciousness
- Increasing systolic blood pressure
- Increasing then decreasing pulse rate
- Rising temperature

NURSING CARE PLAN for the Patient with a Brain Tumor or Injury

Nursing Diagnosis: *Risk for Acute Confusion* related to cerebral edema and increased intracranial pressure

Expected Outcomes: The patient will be oriented to person, place, and time; if this is not possible, patient's safety will be maintained.

Evaluation of Outcomes: Is patient oriented to self, place, and time and able to ask for help appropriately to prevent injury?

Interventions	Rationale	Evaluation
Assess level of consciousness (LOC) using Glasgow Coma Scale.	Change in LOC can indicate increased intracranial pressure and should be reported.	Is patient alert and responsive? Is LOC stable?
Monitor orientation and reorient as needed.	Giving correct information to patient will assist in orientation.	Can patient identify who he/she is, location, and month, year, or season?
Observe patient's reaction to simple commands such as "raise your hand."	This helps distinguish between reflexes and purposeful movement.	Is patient able to follow simple commands?
Monitor patient's capabilities as activities increase.	Patient may experience dizziness, imbalance, and confusion; the patient will need assistance with mobilization until stable.	Can patient sit up and ambulate to chair without dizziness?
If patient is not able to be reoriented, assess for safety and implement appropriate safety measures.	Depending on the patient's prognosis, orientation may not be a realistic goal.	Is patient's safety maintained?

Nursing Diagnosis: *Self-Care Deficit,* dressing/feeding/toileting related to mental status changes and inability to perform ADLs independently

Expected Outcomes: The patient will maintain as much independence with ADLs as possible.

Evaluation of Outcomes: Is the patient able to participate in self-care at an appropriate level?

Interventions	Rationale	Evaluation
Assess what the patient was able to do before admission/injury.	The patient's potential for participation will depend on what he or she was able to do prior to injury.	What was the patient able to do? How does that compare with what he or she can do now?
Provide all supplies and equipment needed to carry out ADLs.	Assembling equipment for the patient reserves energy for performing self-care.	Is the patient able to perform the majority of bath and hygiene tasks with appropriate setup?
Encourage the patient to perform activities at own pace.	The patient may need more time to perform activities.	Does the patient gradually increase performance of self-care in a timely fashion?
Teach and encourage family to participate with care.	Including the family in the patient's care promotes support and family interaction.	Is the family involved? Is the patient accepting of their assistance?
Refer to occupational therapy if indicated.	An occupational therapist is trained to assist patients to manage ADLs within health limitations.	Is occupational therapist able to assist patient with strategies to maintain independence?

NURSING CARE PLAN for the Patient with a Brain Tumor or Injury—cont'd

Nursing Diagnosis: *Acute/Chronic Pain* related to cerebral edema and headache as evidenced by patient pain rating or evidence of painful behaviors

Expected Outcomes: Patient's pain is controlled as evidenced by statement that pain level is acceptable, or demonstration of decrease in painful behaviors.

Evaluation of Outcomes: Does patient state pain level is acceptable? Are pain behaviors reduced?

Interventions	Rationale	Evaluation
Assess pain using a scale of 0 to 10, or a faces scale (see Chapter 10). If patient is unable to participate, observe for pain behaviors such as restlessness, agitation, grimacing, or moaning.	The patient's self-report is the best measure of the patient's pain.	Is the patient able to rate pain? Is there evidence that pain is present?
Monitor vital signs.	Pulse and blood pressure may be elevated in acute pain.	Are vital signs elevated?
Administer appropriate pain medication as ordered.	Nonnarcotic medications are preferred because they do not alter the level of consciousness. If these are not effective, codeine preparations, which have a minimal effect on LOC, may be prescribed.	Does patient state pain has decreased? Is sedation minimized?
Keep head of bed elevated at least 30 degrees.	Elevating the head of the bed helps prevent increased intracranial pressure, which can increase pain.	Does keeping head of bed elevated help prevent pain?
Provide alternative comfort measures such as dim lights, a quiet environment, and positioning for comfort.	Decreasing stimuli in the room by dimming lights and decreasing noise can have a calming effect.	Is patient resting quietly, with no reports of pain?

Nursing Diagnosis: *Disturbed Sensory Perception* related to brain injury and cranial nerve involvement as evidenced by alterations in response to stimuli

Expected Outcomes: The patient will be kept safe from injury related to reduced sensation.

Evaluation of Outcomes: Is patient safe? Is skin intact?

Interventions	Rationale	Evaluation
Monitor patient's ability to perceive stimuli.	Changes in patient's perceptions must be incorporated into the plan of care.	What can the patient feel?
Turn patient and assess skin at least every 2 hours while in bed; provide moisturizer as needed. Protect bony prominences.	If the patient cannot determine pressure or dryness, the nurse must evaluate and act to prevent skin breakdown.	Is skin intact, pink, warm, dry, and without redness?
Assist the patient out of bed and into a different environment.	This can help prevent sensory deprivation and social isolation.	How does patient respond to being in a chair or wheelchair and taken to sunroom or common area?

Continued

NURSING CARE PLAN for the Patient with a Brain Tumor or Injury—cont'd

Interventions	Rationale	Evaluation
Teach the patient to monitor own position and skin, and to direct position changes.	This provides a way for the patient to maintain some control over his body and to take part in preventing complications.	Is patient able to direct care activities effectively?

Nursing Diagnosis: *Impaired Physical Mobility* related to motor deficits as evidenced by weakness, inability to change position

Expected Outcomes: The patient will maintain maximum mobility and be free from complications of immobility.

Evaluation of Outcomes: Is patient kept mobile without contractures? Is skin intact?

Interventions	Rationale	Evaluation
Assess degree of mobility limitation.	A good assessment can help determine how much the patient can actively participate in a plan for mobilization.	How much can patient do independently? Is physical/occupational therapy evaluation indicated?
Turn patient every 1 to 2 hours; if postoperative, avoid positioning on the operative site unless specifically permitted by the surgeon.	Turning helps prevent skin and respiratory complications.	Is a turning schedule maintained? Is skin free from redness and breakdown?
Position patient in correct body alignment. High-top tennis shoes, trochanter rolls, and slings can be used to keep the body in alignment.	This keeps the patient in functional position in case function is regained in the future.	Are all joints maintained in correct alignment?
Perform range-of-motion (ROM) exercises; consult physical therapy as ordered.	ROM exercises help prevent contractures.	If patient unable to perform active ROM exercises, are passive ROM exercises provided on a regular schedule?
Consult occupational therapist to assist the patient in learning to perform ADLs.	The patient may be able to participate in self-care with assistive devices.	Do assistive devices help patient mobilize and maintain independence?

Nursing Diagnosis: *Risk for Injury* related to seizures

Expected Outcomes: The patient will remain free of injury if a seizure occurs.

Evaluation of Outcomes: Is safety maintained? Is skin intact, without bruising or discoloration?

Interventions	Rationale	Evaluation
Observe the patient's behavior and time the length of the seizure. When patient is alert following seizure, determine if an aura occurred, and what it was.	Observing the seizure can provide clues for teaching the patient to recognize the warning signs of a future seizure and how to maintain safety.	What did the patient experience? What can be taught to help keep patient safe in the future?

NURSING CARE PLAN for the Patient with a Brain Tumor or Injury—cont'd

Interventions	Rationale	Evaluation
If patient loses consciousness during the seizure, lay patient on his or her side or turn head to the side.	This helps prevent oral secretions from being aspirated.	Did patient maintain a patent airway without respiratory distress?
Remove objects from patient's surroundings to prevent injury during a seizure. If the patient must have side rails, pad them with blankets or foam. See also Table 48.6.	During a tonic-clonic seizure the patient may be harmed by hitting furniture or other objects.	Is patient protected from objects that could cause injury during a seizure?

Pain (Headache and Nuchal Rigidity) Related to Increased ICP

EXPECTED OUTCOME: The patient will not exhibit evidence of pain.

- Monitor pain using a 0 to 10 pain scale if the patient is able to cooperate. *A pain scale is the most accurate way to monitor a patient's pain.*
- If the patient becomes restless, consider pain as a cause. *The patient may not be able to communicate pain sensations.*
- Administer analgesics as ordered. Avoid opioid analgesics. *Opioid analgesics (with the possible exception of codeine) are usually avoided because they mask neurologic symptoms and make detection of changes difficult.*
- Provide a dark, quiet room with few distractions. *Avoidance of extra stimuli may help reduce headache.*
- Implement measures to prevent increased ICP. See Table 48.4 for measures and rationale.

Hyperthermia Related to Infectious Process

EXPECTED OUTCOME: The patient will not exhibit evidence of hyperthermia.

- Assess temperature every 4 hours and prn. *An elevated temperature can increase risk for seizures.*
- Administer acetaminophen or aspirin as ordered *to reduce fever.*
- Provide a cooling mattress or tepid sponge baths as necessary *to reduce fever. Remember these are uncomfortable for the patient. Comfort can be increased and shivering reduced by cooling the patient gradually and wrapping extremities in bath blankets during cooling mattress therapy.*

Evaluation

Successful nursing management of a patient with an infectious or inflammatory neurologic disorder is evidenced by a patient who is comfortable, afebrile, and has no preventable

TABLE 48.4 MEASURES TO PREVENT INCREASED INTRACRANIAL PRESSURE

Preventive Measures	Rationale
Keep head of bed elevated 30 degrees unless contraindicated.	Head elevation reduces ICP in some patients.
Avoid flexing the neck; keep head and neck in midline position.	Neck flexion may obstruct venous outflow.
Administer antiemetics and antitussives as necessary to prevent vomiting and cough.	Coughing and vomiting can increase ICP.
Administer stool softeners.	Straining for bowel movement can increase ICP.
Minimize suctioning. If absolutely necessary, oxygenate first and limit suction passes to one or two.	Suctioning can increase ICP.
Avoid hip flexion.	Hip flexion can increase intra-abdominal and thoracic pressure, which can increase ICP.
Prevent unnecessary noise and startling the patient.	Noxious stimuli can increase ICP in some patients.
Space care activities to provide rest between each disturbance.	Clustering care activities may increase ICP.

ICP = intracranial pressure.

complications such as pressure ulcers or **contractures**. The absence of complications increases the possibility that the patient with a neurologic deficit will benefit from rehabilitation and improve his or her level of functioning following the acute illness.

Patient Education

The nature and focus of teaching depend on the patient's level of consciousness and cognitive status. When appropriate, both the patient and significant others should be included in the education process. If the patient is not able to participate, the significant others become the focus of teaching.

Describing the brain as in control of body functions may help significant others to understand some of the symptoms of neurologic disorders. The spinal cord can be compared to a telephone cord, with hundreds of tiny individual wires (nerves) making up the cord. The specific wires affected by disease determine the symptoms the patient experiences.

> **CRITICAL THINKING**
>
> ***Mr. Chung***
>
> ■ Mr. Chung is an 18-year-old Asian college student. He comes to the emergency department with a headache, stiff neck, and fever. On physical assessment you notice a petechial rash on his legs and torso. The physician diagnoses meningococcal meningitis.
>
> 1. What tests are likely to be performed?
> 2. What patient education should be planned for Mr. Chung?
> 3. What infection control practices should be instituted?
> 4. What comfort measures might you offer to Mr. Chung?
> 5. What concerns do you have about how Mr. Chung contracted his illness?
>
> *Suggested answers at end of chapter.*

HEADACHES

As mentioned throughout this chapter, headache is a common symptom of neurologic disorders. However, most headaches are transient events and do not indicate a serious pathological condition. If headaches are recurrent, persistent, or increasing in severity, the patient should undergo a neurologic evaluation.

Types of Headaches

Because the causes, signs and symptoms, pathophysiology, and treatment of headaches vary based on the type of headache experienced, these subjects are discussed separately for each type of headache.

Tension or Muscle Contraction Headaches

Persistent contraction of the scalp and facial, cervical, and upper thoracic muscles can cause tension headaches. A cycle of muscle tension, muscle tenderness, and further muscle tension is established. This cycle may or may not be associated with vasodilation of cerebral arteries. Headaches of this type may be associated with premenstrual syndrome or psychosocial stressors such as anxiety, emotional distress, or depression. Symptoms typically develop gradually. Radiation of pain to the crown of the head and base of the skull, with variations in location and intensity, is common. *Pressure, aching, steady,* and *tight* are some of the words patients use to describe the pain of tension headaches.

Care must be taken to thoroughly rule out physical causes before attributing the headache to psychosocial origins. Symptom management may include the use of relaxation techniques, massage of the affected muscles, rest, localized heat application, nonopioid analgesics, and appropriate counseling.

Migraine Headaches

A migraine headache is believed to be caused by cerebral vasoconstriction followed by vasodilation. The vasoconstriction may be due to a response triggered by the trigeminal nerve, which stimulates release of substance P, a pain transmitter, into the vessels or by the release of amines such as serotonin, norepinephrine, and epinephrine. A migraine may or may not begin with an aura (visual phenomena, such as a flashing light that precedes an attack). The tendency to develop migraine headaches is often hereditary. Commonly used descriptors of migraine pain include *throbbing, boring, vise-like,* and *pounding*. The pain is usually on one side of the head. Noise and light tend to worsen the headache, leading patients to seek a dark, quiet environment. Triggers for the headache include specific foods, noise, bright light, alcohol, and stress.

There are two types of migraine headaches: a classic migraine and a common migraine. The classic migraine has a preheadache (**prodromal**) phase in which the patient may experience visual disturbances, difficulty with speaking, and/or numbness or tingling. The headache that follows is often accompanied by nausea and sometimes vomiting, and may last for hours to days. A common migraine does not have the preheadache phase, but the patient experiences an immediate onset of a throbbing headache.

Treatment of migraine may be prophylactic or directed at an acute episode. Prophylactic treatment is usually reserved for those patients experiencing one or more migraine headaches per week. Dietary restrictions may be helpful if precipitating foods or beverages can be identified. Nifedipine (a calcium channel blocker) and propranolol (a beta-adrenergic blocker) are prophylactic treatments that are

• WORD • BUILDING •
prodromal: pro—before + dromos—running

usually used to control blood pressure. These medications may help prevent the vascular changes that cause the headache and should be used cautiously because of the potential for lowering blood pressure. Amitriptyline (a tricyclic antidepressant) may also help prevent migraines; however, it may cause drowsiness, dry mouth, and weight gain. None of these medications should be stopped abruptly after long-term use.

Several types of medications are available to treat the acute migraine headache. Nonsteroidal anti-inflammatory drugs (NSAIDs) such as naproxen (Naprosyn, Aleve) may be tried first. Ergot (Cafergot), a vasoconstrictor, is effective only if taken before the vessel walls become edematous, usually within 30 to 60 minutes of headache onset. Triptans such as sumatriptan (Imitrex) and zolmitriptan (Zomig) work at the serotonin receptor sites and have a vasoconstricting action. Treximet combines naproxen and sumatriptan. Opioids are habit forming and are used only as a last resort. The potentially additive nature of multidrug regimens requires careful monitoring.

Cluster Headaches

Vascular disturbance, stress, anxiety, and emotional distress are all proposed causes of cluster headaches. As indicated by the name, these headaches tend to occur in clusters during a time span of several days to weeks. Months or even years may pass between episodes. Alcohol consumption may worsen the episodes.

The patient may state that the headache begins suddenly, typically at the same time of night. *Throbbing* and *excruciating* are often the adjectives used by the patient. The headache tends to be unilateral, affecting the nose, eye, and forehead. A bloodshot, teary appearance of the affected eye is common.

Because of the brief nature of cluster headaches, treatment is difficult. A quiet, dark environment and cold compresses may lessen the intensity of the pain. NSAIDs or tricyclic antidepressants may be prescribed.

Diagnosis of Headaches

Most headaches are diagnosed based on the patient's history and symptoms. MRI, CT, skull x-ray, arteriogram, electroencephalogram, cranial nerve testing, and lumbar puncture to test CSF may be done to rule out other causes for the headaches.

Nursing Process for the Patient with a Headache

Data Collection

The WHAT'S UP? mnemonic is particularly useful in helping the patient provide useful information regarding the headache:

W—Where is the pain? Does it remain in one place or radiate to other areas of the head? Does the headache consistently start in one place?

H—How does the headache feel? Is it throbbing, steady, dull, band-like, or does it have other qualities?

A—Aggravating or alleviating factors should be assessed. Some aggravating factors include red wine, caffeine, chocolate, and foods containing nitrates or monosodium glutamate (MSG). Other factors include particular stages of the menstrual cycle, emotional stress, and tension. Alleviating factors might include lying down in a dark room, cold compresses, or medications.

T—Timing may be a factor for a patient who experiences headaches just before or during her menstrual period. For other patients, there may be no predictive timing. Also ask how long the headache lasted.

S—Ask the patient to rate the severity on a scale of 0 to 10. Is the severity consistent or does it vary from headache to headache?

U—Ask about other useful data. For example, are there associated symptoms, such as nausea, vomiting, or bloodshot eyes?

P—Determine the patient's perception of the headache. Does it interfere with the patient's life? If so, how? Has the patient had a previous evaluation of headaches?

Nursing Diagnoses, Planning, and Implementation

Acute Pain (Headache) Related to Lack of Knowledge of Pain Prevention and Control Techniques as Evidenced by Patient's Pain Rating

EXPECTED OUTCOME: Headache will be prevented or controlled as evidenced by patient statement of no pain or acceptable pain rating.

- Assist the patient to identify and reduce or eliminate aggravating factors. This can be accomplished by keeping a headache diary for a time, recording the time of day the headache occurs, foods eaten or other aggravating factors, description of the pain, identification of associated symptoms such as nausea or visual disturbances, and other factors related to headache symptoms. *Identification of triggers can help the patient lessen the frequency and intensity of attacks.*
- Encourage the patient to use alleviating techniques such as biofeedback or stress reduction. *This helps the patient participate in the treatment of the headache and provides a sense of control over his or her illness.*
- Teach the patient to use relaxation exercises and warm or cool moist compresses. *These interventions may be helpful for tension headaches.*
- Provide a dark room and rest *to reduce stimulation during a migraine headache.*
- Teach the patient about medications, appropriate dosage, expected action, side effects, and consequences of misuse. *The patient will need to understand medication administration for appropriate use at home.*

Evaluation

If interventions have been effective, the patient will understand self-care to prevent and treat headaches, and be able to report a reduction in headache pain and occurrences.

SEIZURE DISORDERS

Seizures/Epilepsy

A seizure may be a symptom of epilepsy or of other neurologic disorders such as a brain tumor or meningitis. Epilepsy is a chronic neurologic disorder characterized by recurrent seizure activity.

Pathophysiology

The normal stability of the neuron cell membrane is impaired in individuals with epilepsy. This instability allows for abnormal electrical discharges to occur. These discharges cause the characteristic symptoms seen during a seizure.

Seizures can be classified as partial or generalized. Partial seizures begin on one side of the cerebral cortex. In some cases, the electrical discharge spreads to the other hemisphere and the seizure becomes generalized. Generalized seizures are characterized by involvement of both cerebral hemispheres.

Etiology

Epilepsy may be acquired or idiopathic (unknown cause). Causes of acquired epilepsy include traumatic brain injury and anoxic events. No cause has been identified for idiopathic epilepsy. The most common time for idiopathic epilepsy to begin is before age 20. New-onset seizures after this age are most commonly caused by an underlying neurologic disorder.

Signs and Symptoms

Symptoms of seizure activity correlate with the area of the brain where the seizure begins. Some patients experience an aura or sensation that warns that a seizure is about to occur. An aura may be a visual distortion, a noxious odor, or an unusual sound. Patients who experience an aura may have enough time to sit or lie down before the seizure starts, thereby minimizing the chance of injury.

PARTIAL SEIZURES. Repetitive, purposeless behaviors, called automatisms, are the classic symptom of partial seizures. The patient appears to be in a dream-like state while picking at his or her clothing, chewing, or smacking his or her lips. Patients may be labeled as mentally ill, particularly if automatisms include unacceptable social behaviors such as spitting or fondling themselves. Patients are not aware of their behavior or that it is inappropriate. If the patient does not lose consciousness, the seizure is labeled as simple partial and usually lasts less than 1 minute. Older terms for simple partial seizures include *jacksonian* and *focal motor.* If consciousness is lost, it is called a complex partial seizure or psychomotor seizure, and may last from 2 to 15 minutes.

Partial seizures arising from the parietal lobe may cause paresthesias on the side of the body opposite the seizure focus. Visual disturbances are seen if the seizure originates in the occipital lobe. Involvement of the motor cortex results in involuntary movements of the opposite side of the body. Typically, movements begin in the arm and hand and may spread to the leg and face.

GENERALIZED SEIZURES. Generalized seizures affect the entire brain. Two types of generalized seizures are absence seizures and tonic-clonic seizures. Absence seizures, sometimes referred to as petit mal seizures, occur most often in children and are manifested by a period of staring that lasts several seconds.

Tonic-clonic seizures are what most people envision when they think of seizures; they are sometimes called grand mal seizures or convulsions. Tonic-clonic seizures follow a typical progression. Aura and loss of consciousness may or may not occur. The tonic phase, lasting 30 to 60 seconds, is characterized by rigidity, causing the patient to fall if not lying down. The pupils are fixed and dilated, the hands and jaws are clenched, and the patient may temporarily stop breathing. The clonic phase is signaled by contraction and relaxation of all muscles in a jerky, rhythmic fashion. The extremities may move forcefully, causing injury if the patient strikes furniture or walls. The patient is often incontinent. Biting the lips or tongue may cause bleeding.

The **postictal** period is the recovery period after a seizure. Following a partial seizure the postictal phase may be no more than a few minutes of disorientation. Patients who experience a generalized seizure may sleep deeply for 30 minutes to several hours. Following this deep sleep, patients may report headache, confusion, and fatigue. Patients may realize that they had a seizure but not remember the event itself.

Diagnostic Tests

An EEG is the most useful test for evaluating seizures. An EEG can determine where in the brain the seizures start, the frequency and duration of seizures, and the presence of subclinical (asymptomatic) seizures. Sleep deprivation and flashing light stimulation may be used to evaluate the seizure threshold. See Chapter 47 for more information on EEGs.

Therapeutic Measures

If an underlying cause for the seizure is identified, treatment focuses on correcting the cause. If no cause is found

• WORD • BUILDING •
postictal: post—after + ictal—seizure

or if the seizures continue despite treatment of concurrent disorders, treatment focuses on stopping or preventing the seizure activity.

Numerous anticonvulsant medications are available, each with specific actions, therapeutic ranges, and potential side effects (Table 48.5). Typically, the patient is started on one drug and the dosage is increased until therapeutic levels are attained or side effects become troublesome. If seizures are not controlled on a single drug, another medication is added. Many anticonvulsants require periodic blood tests to monitor serum levels as well as kidney and liver functions. Most of these medications can cause drowsiness, so teach the patient to avoid driving or operating machinery until the effects of the drug are known. Driving is also contraindicated until seizures are under control. (See *Evidence-Based Practice* box.)

TABLE 48.5 ANTICONVULSANT MEDICATIONS

Medication Class/Action	Examples	Route	Side Effects	Nursing Implications
Anticonvulsants				
Suppress abnormal discharge of neurons, suppress spread of seizure activity from focus to other parts of brain.	carbamazepine (Tegretol)	PO (short-acting and SR forms)	Drowsiness and ataxia, blood disorders	Monitor CBC. Therapeutic level 6–12 mcg/mL. Do not crush SR form.
	gabapentin (Neurontin)	PO	Drowsiness, dizziness	Blood levels not necessary
	levetiracetam (Keppra)	PO, IV	Dizziness, weakness	May need reduced dose for older adults. Assess WBC, RBC, and liver function tests.
	lamotrigine (Lamictal)	PO	Ataxia, dizziness, headache, nausea, vomiting, photosensitivity, rash	Discontinue therapy and notify physician if rash appears. Monitor blood levels.
	topiramate (Topamax)	PO	Dizziness, drowsiness, impaired memory, psychomotor slowing, vision changes, weight loss	Blood levels not necessary.
	phenytoin (Dilantin)	PO, IM, IV	Gingival (gum) hyperplasia, nausea, ataxia, rash, aplastic anemia. Lethargy might indicate high drug level.	Regular dental care essential. Therapeutic level is 10–20 mcg/mL. Binds to tube feedings—hold tube feeding 1 hr before and 2 hr after dose.
	phenobarbital (Luminal)	PO, IM, IV	Drowsiness, respiratory depression	Monitor vital signs. Therapeutic level 15–40 mcg/mL.
	valproic acid (Depakote)	IV, PO (short-acting and SR forms)	GI upset, nausea, vomiting	Therapeutic level 50–100 mcg/mL. Do not crush SR form.
Emergency Agents—Benzodiazepines				
Potentiate GABA, an inhibitory neurotransmitter in the CNS.	lorazepam (Ativan)	IV	Dizziness, drowsiness, respiratory depression	Given to stop a seizure that has not resolved within 5 minutes. Given IM or IV push by emergency personnel. Rectal Diastat may be given at home.
	diazepam (Valium, Diastat)	IV, IM, rectal (Diastat)		

RBC = red blood cell; SR = sustained release; WBC = white blood cell.

EVIDENCE-BASED PRACTICE

Clinical Question

What is the evidence for treatment of the elderly experiencing seizures?

Evidence

The presentation of seizures differs between the elderly and younger adults. Comorbid diseases such as heart and circulatory problems often cloud the presentation of the postictal phase, which may last up to 2 weeks in the elderly versus a few minutes in the younger adult. A diagnosis of transient ischemic attack or mini-stroke is often made rather than that of a seizure. Because of multiple medications and changes in metabolism related to aging, it may be difficult to find an effective anticonvulsant agent. Side effects may be less tolerated by the elderly (Heckenberg, 2008).

Implications for Nursing Practice

Be sure to do a careful assessment of older adults with a seizure diagnosis. Keep in mind that the postictal phase may be prolonged, and assure patient safety. Treatment should be individualized for the elderly, and lower dosages of medications may be required.

REFERENCE

Heckenberg, G. (2008, July 19). *Epilepsy/seizure: Management.* Adelaide, Australia: Joanna Briggs Institute.

If a patient must discontinue an anticonvulsant, it should be tapered slowly according to manufacturer directions. Stopping an anticonvulsant abruptly can result in status epilepticus, discussed below. If seizures continue despite anticonvulsant therapy, surgical intervention may be considered.

Surgical Management

The success of surgical intervention for epilepsy depends on identification of an epileptic focus within nonvital brain tissue. The surgeon attempts to resect the area affected to prevent spread of seizure activity. In some cases, seizures may be cured, but in others, the goal is to reduce the frequency or severity of the seizures. If no focus is identified or if it is in a vital area such as the motor cortex or speech center, surgery is not feasible.

The preoperative assessment for epilepsy surgery is an extensive multistage process. Thorough assessment and teaching are essential. To adequately identify seizure foci, the patient is weaned off anticonvulsant therapy. Increasing the frequency of seizures with weaning is anxiety provoking to patients and significant others.

Emergency Care

Emergency care is required when a seizure occurs. The prime objective is to prevent injury during a seizure. Side rails, if used, should be padded to prevent injury if the patient strikes his or her extremities against them. If the patient falls to the floor, move furniture out of the way. Maintain a patent airway and, if possible, turn the patient on his or her side to prevent aspiration if vomiting occurs. Do not force an airway or anything else into the patient's mouth once the seizure has begun. Do not restrain the individual because this may also increase the risk of injury. Observe and document the patient's behavior during the seizure: which part of the body was first involved, progression of the seizure, and the length of time the seizure lasted (see Box 48.2, *Patient Perspective*). After the seizure, assess the patient for breathing, suction if necessary, and in rare cases, initiate rescue breathing or cardiopulmonary resuscitation (CPR) as indicated.

Status Epilepticus

Status epilepticus is characterized by at least 30 minutes of repetitive seizure activity without a return to consciousness. This is a medical emergency and requires prompt intervention to prevent irreversible neurologic damage. Abrupt cessation of anticonvulsant therapy is the usual cause of status epilepticus.

Seizure activity precipitates a significant increase in the brain's need for glucose and oxygen. This metabolic demand is even greater during status epilepticus. Irreversible neuronal damage may occur if cerebral metabolic needs cannot be fulfilled. Adequate oxygenation must be maintained, if necessary, by intubating and mechanically ventilating the patient. These patients are also at significant risk for aspiration.

Box 48.2 Patient Perspective

Mrs. Rowley

I have had seizures for 35 years and, as a result of falling during seizures, have experienced cuts, bruises, and a broken bone. I usually have an aura that lets me know a seizure is about to occur. This is helpful if I can get myself to a safe place to prevent falling or being injured. When a patient is having a seizure you can best help by using padding such as pillows or blankets for protection, talking calmly, and using gentle touch to prevent injury. You should not sit on or hold down someone during a seizure. I have had the frightening experience of waking up with a nurse sitting on me and holding down my arms. After you have protected the patient, let the person come out of the seizure naturally. When the seizure is over, I usually want to sleep because seizures are exhausting and uncomfortable. I will rest better knowing you are watching over me to keep me safe.

Intravenous diazepam (Valium) or lorazepam (Ativan) is given to stop the seizures. Because both of these drugs can cause respiratory depression, careful airway management is required. After obtaining serum drug levels, anticonvulsant therapy is adjusted to achieve therapeutic levels.

If seizures remain resistant to treatment, a barbiturate coma may be induced with intravenous pentobarbital. The last line of treatment for status epilepticus is general anesthesia or pharmacological paralysis. Both of these therapies require intubation, mechanical ventilation, and management in an intensive care unit (ICU) setting. Continuous EEG monitoring is used to verify that the seizures have actually stopped. A patient treated with neuromuscular blockade drugs may still be seizing but have no visible manifestations.

For more information on seizures, visit the Epilepsy Foundation of America at www.efa.org.

Psychosocial Effects

Finances can be a major concern to patients with seizure disorders. Some patients with epilepsy experience hiring discrimination, or they may not qualify for some jobs in which safety is a concern. Remind patients that falsifying information on job applications may be grounds for dismissal. Refusal of health insurance coverage can create financial hardships for patients on long-term medications. Most patients whose seizures are controlled can work and lead productive lives. You can help patients explore options for financial assistance if needed.

Patients with poorly controlled seizures should not operate motor vehicles. In today's society, a driver's license is a sign of adulthood and independence, and patients who cannot drive may experience lowered self-esteem. Job opportunities may be limited for patients who depend on public transportation. Encourage the patient to obtain a state identification card. This can be used in place of a driver's license for identification.

Patients may limit interpersonal relationships out of fear of having a seizure. The involuntary movements, sounds, and possible incontinence that occur with seizures are embarrassing to patients and can be frightening to laypeople. Role playing may help the patient determine when and how to confide in others.

Nursing Process for the Patient with Seizures

Data Collection

Perform a general neurologic examination of the patient with a history of seizures. Determine the type of seizure manifestations and type of aura if any. Assess the patient's knowledge of the disease and its treatment. It is important to assess whether the patient has the resources to purchase prescribed anticonvulsant medications and whether the medication regimen is adhered to. Drug levels may help determine degree of compliance with therapy.

Nursing Diagnoses, Planning, and Implementation

Risk for Injury Related to Seizure Activity

EXPECTED OUTCOME: The patient will remain free from injury.

- Instruct the patient with generalized seizures to recognize an aura and to get to safety if it occurs. This may mean lying down away from furniture or other objects. *This helps prevent injury during involuntary movements.*
- Institute seizure precautions for the patient admitted to a health care institution. See Table 48.6 for precautions and interventions *to prevent injury.*
- Encourage all patients to wear medical alert jewelry or other identification *to alert others to the presence of seizure disorder.*
- Assist patients to identify conditions that trigger seizures. Hypoglycemia, hypoxia, and hyponatremia are all potential triggers of hypersensitive neurons. Teach the patient the importance of a consistent schedule of eating and sleeping. *The patient may be able to prevent seizures by avoidance of triggers.*

Risk for Ineffective Self Health Management Related to Complex Regimen and Possible Lack of Resources

EXPECTED OUTCOME: The patient will follow medication regimen as evidenced by therapeutic drug levels and controlled seizure activity.

- Assess patient's ability to obtain and pay for medication. *Stopping a medication suddenly can result in status epilepticus.*
- Refer patient to a case manager or social worker, if needed, *to assist with obtaining resources for medications.*
- Teach the patient about medication action, dose, side effects, schedule, and the importance of not

TABLE 48.6 INTERVENTIONS FOR SEIZURES

Seizure Precautions
- Pad side rails of hospital bed with commercial pads or bath blankets folded over and pinned in place.
- Keep call light within reach.
- Assist patient when ambulating.
- Keep suction and oral airway at bedside.

Nursing Care During a Seizure
- Stay with patient.
- Do not restrain patient.
- Protect from injury (move nearby objects).
- Loosen tight clothing.
- Turn to side when able to prevent occlusion of airway or aspiration.
- Suction if needed.
- Monitor vital signs when able.
- Be prepared to assist with breathing if necessary.
- Observe and document progression of symptoms.

stopping treatment suddenly. *Patients with seizures may have several medications to take several times each day. Patients who understand their regimens are more likely to comply.*
- Teach the patient about the importance of regular blood tests if required. *Therapeutic blood levels help prevent seizures (too low) and toxicity (too high).*

Evaluation
Successful care of a patient with epilepsy is manifested by a decrease in seizures to the lowest possible frequency. Patient verbalization of understanding of needed lifestyle changes is another indication of success. Patients should be able to state measures to prevent injury if a seizure should occur and should verbalize understanding of all medications and their administration schedules. Therapeutic drug levels may be measured to evaluate compliance with the medication regimen.

TRAUMATIC BRAIN INJURY

Traumatic brain injury is a major cause of death and disability in adults. Young men make up a large proportion of brain injury victims.

Pathophysiology
Traumatic brain injury is a complex phenomenon with results ranging from no detectable effect to a persistent vegetative state. Trauma can result in hemorrhage, contusion or laceration of the brain, and damage at the cellular level. In addition to the primary insult, the brain injury may be compounded by cerebral edema, hyperemia, or hydrocephalus.

Etiology
Motor vehicle accidents account for the largest percentage of traumatic brain injuries. Falls, sports-related injuries, and violence are also common causes of traumatic brain injury.

The brain is susceptible to various types of injury and can be classified in several ways. The term *closed head injury* or *nonpenetrating injury* is used when there has been rapid back and forth movement of the brain that causes bruising and tearing of brain tissues and vessels, but the skull is intact. An *open head injury* or *penetrating injury* refers to a break in the skull. *Acceleration injury* is the term used to describe a moving object hitting a stationary head. An example of this type of injury is a patient who is hit in the head with a baseball bat. A *deceleration injury* occurs when the head is in motion and strikes a stationary surface. This type of injury is seen in patients who trip and fall, hitting their head on furniture or the floor.

A combination of acceleration-deceleration injury occurs when the stationary head is hit by a mobile object and the head then strikes a stationary surface. A soccer player who sustains a blow to the head and then hits the ground with his or her head may sustain an acceleration-deceleration injury.

Rotational injuries have the potential to cause shearing damage to the brain, as well as lacerations and contusions. Rotational injuries may be caused by a direct blow to the head or may occur during a motor vehicle accident in which the vehicle is struck from the side. Twisting of the brainstem can damage the reticular activating system, causing loss of consciousness. Movement of the brain within the skull may result in bruising or tearing of brain tissue where it comes in contact with the inside of the skull.

Types of Brain Injury and Signs and Symptoms

Concussion
Cerebral concussion is considered a mild brain injury. If there is a loss of consciousness, it is for 5 minutes or less. Concussion is characterized by headache, dizziness, or nausea and vomiting. The patient may describe amnesia of events before or after the trauma. On clinical examination there is no skull or dura injury and no abnormality detected on CT or MRI.

Contusion
Cerebral contusion is characterized by bruising of brain tissue, possibly accompanied by hemorrhage. There may be multiple areas of contusion, depending on the causative mechanism. Severe contusions can result in diffuse axonal injury. The symptoms of a cerebral contusion depend on the area of the brain involved.

Brainstem contusions affect level of consciousness. Decreased level of consciousness may be transient or permanent. Respirations, pupil reaction, eye movement, and motor response to stimuli may also be affected. The autonomic nervous system may be affected by edema or by hypothalamic injury, causing rapid heart rate and respiratory rate, fever, and diaphoresis.

Hematoma
SUBDURAL HEMATOMA. Subdural hematomas are classified as acute or chronic based on the time interval between injury and onset of symptoms. Acute subdural hematoma is characterized by appearance of symptoms within 24 hours following injury. The bleeding is typically venous in nature and accumulates between the dura and arachnoid membranes (Fig. 48.5). About 24% of patients who sustain a severe brain injury develop an acute subdural hematoma. Damage to the brain tissue may cause an altered level of consciousness. Therefore, it can be difficult to recognize a subdural hematoma based only on clinical examination. As the subdural hematoma increases in size, the patient may exhibit one-sided paralysis of extraocular movement, extremity weakness, or dilation of the pupil. Level of consciousness may deteriorate further as ICP increases.

Older adults and people with alcoholism are particularly prone to chronic subdural hematomas. Atrophy of the

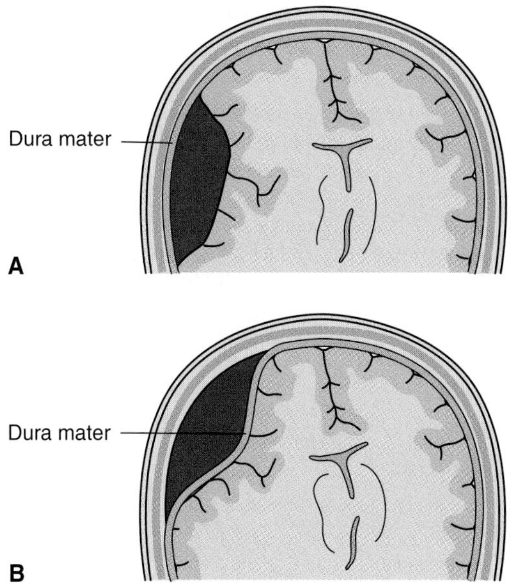
Dura mater
A
Dura mater
B

FIGURE 48.5 (A) A subdural hematoma is usually venous and forms between the dura and the arachnoid membranes. (B) An epidural hematoma is usually from an arterial bleed and forms between the dura mater and the skull.

brain, common in these populations, stretches the veins between the brain and the dura. A seemingly minor fall or blow to the head can cause these stretched veins to rupture and bleed. Often there are no other injuries associated with the trauma. Because a chronic subdural hematoma can develop weeks to months after the injury, the patient may not remember an injury occurring.

The patient with a chronic subdural hematoma may be forgetful, lethargic, or irritable or may report a headache. If the hematoma persists or increases in size, the patient may develop hemiparesis and pupillary changes. The patient or significant other may not associate the symptoms with a previous injury and therefore may delay seeking medical care.

EPIDURAL HEMATOMA. About 10% of patients with severe brain injuries develop epidural hematomas. This collection of blood between the dura mater and skull is usually arterial in nature and is often associated with skull fracture (see Fig. 48.5). Arterial bleeding can cause the hematoma to become large very quickly. Patients with epidural hematoma typically exhibit a progressive course of symptoms. The patient loses consciousness directly after the injury; he or she then regains consciousness and is coherent for a brief period. The patient then develops a dilated pupil and paralyzed extraocular muscles on the side of the hematoma and becomes less responsive. If there is no intervention, the patient becomes unresponsive. Seizures or hemiparesis may occur. Once the patient has symptoms, the deterioration may be rapid. Airway management and control of ICP must be instituted immediately. If ICP is not controlled, the patient will die.

Diagnostic Tests

CT scan is usually the first imaging test performed on a patient with a brain injury. It is faster and more accessible than MRI. This is particularly important for unstable patients or those with multiple injuries. It is easier to identify skull fractures on CT than on MRI. MRI may be used later to identify damage to the brain tissue.

Neuropsychological testing by a trained specialist can be useful in assessing the patient's cognitive function. This information helps direct rehabilitation placement, discharge planning, and return to work or school. Neuropsychological testing identifies problems with memory, judgment, learning, and comprehension. Compensation strategies can be suggested to the patient and significant others based on the results.

Therapeutic Measures

Surgical Management

Surgical treatment of hematomas is discussed under intracranial surgery later in this chapter.

Medical Management

Medical management of traumatic brain injury involves control of ICP and support of body functions. Patients with brain injuries may be partially or completely dependent for maintenance of respiration, nutrition, elimination, movement, and skin integrity.

A variety of techniques are used to control ICP in the patient with moderate or severe brain injury. The first step is to insert an ICP monitor to allow measurement of the ICP. Refer to the section on increased ICP earlier in this chapter for further information.

If ICP remains elevated despite drainage of cerebrospinal fluid, the next step is use of an osmotic diuretic. The most commonly used drug is intravenous mannitol (Osmitrol). Mannitol utilizes osmosis to pull fluid into the intravascular space and eliminate it via the renal system. Serum osmolarity and electrolytes must be carefully monitored when mannitol is being administered. Some patients experience a rebound increase in ICP after the mannitol wears off.

Mechanical hyperventilation may be used if the patient is still experiencing increased ICP. Hyperventilation is effective in lowering ICP because it causes cerebral vasoconstriction. Vasoconstriction allows less blood into the cranium, thereby lowering ICP. Research has demonstrated, however, that aggressive hyperventilation, particularly within the first 24 hours after injury, may induce ischemia in the already compromised brain. Therefore, hyperventilation is now reserved for increased ICP that does not respond to other treatments.

High-dose barbiturate therapy may be used to induce a therapeutic coma, which reduces the metabolic needs of the brain during the acute phase following injury. These patients are completely dependent for all of their needs and care. They will be mechanically ventilated and cared for in an ICU setting. Vasopressors may be required to maintain blood pressure, and the patient's temperature should be kept as normal as possible.

Complications

Brain Herniation

If interventions to control ICP are unsuccessful, the patient may experience uncontrolled edema or herniation of brain tissue (Fig. 48.6). Herniation is displacement of brain tissue out of its normal anatomical location. This displacement prevents function of the herniated tissue and places pressure on other vital structures, most commonly the brainstem. Herniation usually results in brain death.

Patients who experience brain death may be suitable organ donor candidates. For some significant others, the opportunity to donate their loved one's organs provides some sense of purpose in the death. (See Table 48.7.)

Diabetes Insipidus

Edema or direct injury that affects the posterior portion of the pituitary gland or hypothalamus can result in inadequate release of antidiuretic hormone, causing diabetes insipidus. This results in polyuria and, if the patient is awake, polydipsia. Fluid replacement and intravenous vasopressin are used to maintain fluid and electrolyte balance. See Chapter 39 for more information on diabetes insipidus.

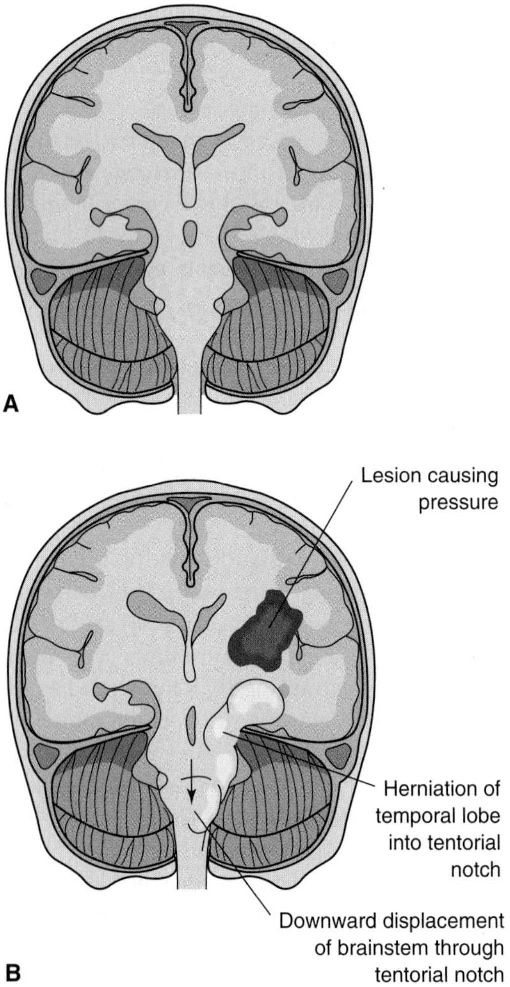
A
Lesion causing pressure
Herniation of temporal lobe into tentorial notch
Downward displacement of brainstem through tentorial notch
B

FIGURE 48.6 Herniation of the brain. (A) Normal brain. (B) Herniation of brain tissue into tentorial notch.

TABLE 48.7 TRAUMATIC BRAIN INJURY SUMMARY

Signs and Symptoms	Loss or decrease in level of consciousness, depending on severity and type of injury Loss of memory before or after the injury Increased ICP Headache, dizziness Nausea and vomiting Unequal pupils Tachycardia, tachypnea Diaphoresis Hemiparesis
Diagnostic Tests	CT scan, MRI Skull x-rays Routine laboratory tests (hemoglobin, electrolytes, coagulation studies, type and crossmatch) Neuropsychological testing
Therapeutic Measures	Control intracranial pressure Surgical management of hematoma Maintain respiratory function Maintain diet/nutrition Maintain skin integrity Prevent complications Education
Complications	Increased intracranial pressure Diabetes insipidus Acute hydrocephalus Post-traumatic syndrome Cognitive and personality changes
Possible Nursing Diagnoses	*Acute Confusion* related to cerebral edema or increased intracranial pressure *Self-Care Deficit* related to increased intracranial pressure *Pain* related to cerebral edema

Acute Hydrocephalus

Cerebral edema can interfere with cerebrospinal fluid circulation, causing **hydrocephalus**. Initial treatment is use of an external ventricular drain, followed by a ventriculoperitoneal shunt if necessary. A shunt drains excess CSF into the peritoneum, where it is reabsorbed into circulation and excreted.

Labile Vital Signs

Direct trauma to or pressure on the brainstem can cause fluctuations in blood pressure, cardiac rhythm, or respiratory pattern. Treatment is aimed at control of ICP.

• WORD • BUILDING •

hydrocephalus: hydro—water + cephalus—head

Post-Traumatic Syndrome

Patients who sustain a concussion may experience ongoing, somewhat vague symptoms. They may report headache, fatigue, difficulty concentrating, depression, or memory impairment. Symptoms may be severe enough to interfere with work, school, and interpersonal relationships. Neuropsychological testing can provide objective evidence of cognitive dysfunction and establish the need for cognitive rehabilitation. Symptoms may take 3 to 12 months to resolve.

Cognitive and Personality Changes

Alterations in personality and cognition may be the most difficult long-term complication for patients and significant others to adjust to. The patient may have significant short-term memory impairment. This limits his or her ability to learn new information and may interfere with ability to function at work or school. Impaired judgment can make the patient a safety risk to self or others. It also affects social functioning.

Emotional lability, loss of social inhibitions, and personality changes may occur. These consequences of traumatic brain injury have a profound effect on the patient and significant others. Spouses may state, "This is not the person I married." If behavior is violent, bizarre, or profane, children may be unwilling to bring their friends home and may become socially isolated. Young children, in particular, have difficulty understanding why a parent is behaving so differently. Disintegration of relationships is not uncommon following traumatic brain injury.

Neuropsychological testing objectively identifies problems. These deficits can then be addressed with cognitive rehabilitation. Individual and family counseling may be of benefit. Support groups for patients and significant others are often helpful.

Motor and speech impairment are additional possible long-term complications of traumatic brain injury. Intensive rehabilitation provides the best opportunity for maximizing recovery. For more information, visit the Brain Injury Association at www.biausa.org.

Nursing Process for the Patient with Traumatic Brain Injury

Acute care is presented below. Also see the *Nursing Care Plan for the Patient with a Brain Tumor or Injury.*

Data Collection

After stabilization in the emergency department, care of the patient with a severe traumatic brain injury is in the intensive care setting, where ICP can be carefully monitored. Frequent data collection is essential, including a Glasgow Coma Scale score, pupil responses, muscle strength, and vital signs. Review Box 48.1, *Signs and Symptoms of Increased Intracranial Pressure*, for additional signs of increased ICP for which to monitor. Once the patient is stabilized, neurologic damage is assessed. Identification of deficits guides nursing care. Assessment of discharge needs should begin as soon as possible. The patient may require extensive rehabilitation, and early referral may speed transfer to an appropriate facility.

Nursing Diagnoses, Planning, and Implementation

Risk for Ineffective Cerebral Tissue Perfusion Related to Increased ICP

EXPECTED OUTCOME: Changes in cerebral tissue perfusion will be prevented or recognized and reported promptly.

- Monitor vital signs for widening pulse pressure or irregular respirations. *These are signs of increased ICP and should be reported promptly.*
- Monitor Glasgow Coma Scale score and report worsening status promptly. *Decreasing level of consciousness (LOC) may indicate increased ICP and may necessitate emergency intervention.*
- Implement measures *to prevent increased ICP*. See Table 48.4 for preventive measures and rationale.

Ineffective Airway Clearance Related to Reduced Cough Reflex and Decreased Level of Consciousness as Evidenced by Adventitious Lung Sounds and Dropping Spo_2.

EXPECTED OUTCOME: The patient will maintain a clear airway as evidenced by clear breath sounds and Spo_2 of 90% or above.

- Monitor airway and breath sounds. *If the patient has excess secretions and is unable to cough effectively, suctioning may be necessary.*
- Limit suction passes to one or two at a time for a maximum of 5 to 10 seconds each time. *Suctioning can increase ICP.*
- Keep head of bed elevated 20 to 30 degrees *to reduce risk of aspirating oral secretions and reduce ICP.*
- Turn the patient frequently *to help mobilize secretions and prevent other complications of immobility.*

Risk for Ineffective Breathing Pattern Related to Pressure on Respiratory Center

EXPECTED OUTCOME: The patient will maintain Spo_2 of 90% or above.

- Monitor respiratory rate and depth, arterial blood gases (ABGs), and Spo_2 and report changes. *If respiratory status is deteriorating, mechanical ventilation may be necessary.*
- Elevate head of bead 20 to 30 degrees *to allow chest expansion and ease work of breathing.*
- Administer oxygen as ordered and needed *to prevent hypoxia. Hypoxia promotes brain death.*

Evaluation

The plan of care has been successful if the patient shows no unexpected worsening of neurologic function and injuries and complications are prevented. The patient's airway should be clear and Spo_2 level should be 90% or above. The patient is kept comfortable, and self-care needs are met.

Rehabilitation

Once the patient is stabilized, evaluation for discharge to a rehabilitation facility is completed. The patient must be able to physically tolerate the rehabilitation program, in which the patient will be taught to function as independently as possible. The family must be prepared for changes in the patient's ability to function and possible changes in personality. It may take months to years before the patient reaches his or her maximum potential. In some cases of severe brain damage or continued comatose state, rehabilitation is not feasible and the patient is discharged to home or a long-term facility for custodial care.

BRAIN TUMORS

Brain tumors are neoplastic growths of the brain or meninges. These tumors may be characterized by vague symptoms such as headache or visual changes or by focal neurologic deficits such as hemiparesis or seizures.

Pathophysiology and Etiology

Brain tumors cause symptoms by either compressing or infiltrating brain tissue. Tumors may arise from central nervous system cells or may metastasize from other locations in the body. Primary brain tumors rarely metastasize; however, if they do, it is to the spine.

There is no established cause for primary brain tumors. It is unclear what causes the cells to begin reproducing in an uncontrolled fashion. Risk factors include age (45 and older), exposure to radiation or industrial chemicals, and family history. Whites are more likely to be diagnosed with a brain tumor than other racial or ethnic groups.

Brain tumors can be classified in several different ways. The traditional distinction of benign and malignant is less helpful when classifying brain tumors than when classifying other cancers. A benign tumor in the brainstem may be fatal, whereas a malignant tumor in the frontal lobe may not be. Location of the tumor can be just as important a factor in outcome as the cell type.

Primary tumors are those arising from cells of the central nervous system. Intra-axial tumors are those that arise from the glial cells within the cerebrum, cerebellum, or brainstem. These tumors infiltrate and invade brain tissue. Extra-axial tumors arise from the skull, meninges, pituitary gland, or cranial nerves; they have a compressive effect on the brain.

Most brain tumors are secondary; that is, they have metastasized from a primary malignancy elsewhere in the body (Fig. 48.7). These tumors commonly spread via the arterial system. If untreated, they cause increased ICP. This may be the cause of the patient's death rather than the primary malignancy.

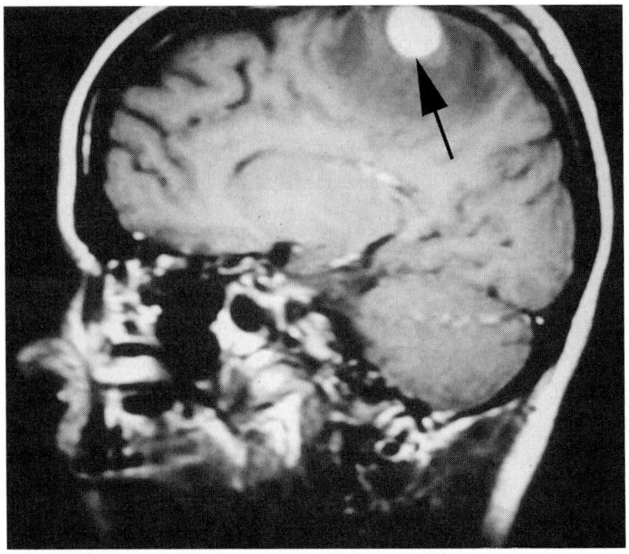

FIGURE 48.7 Metastatic brain tumor. This patient's primary cancer was in the lung.

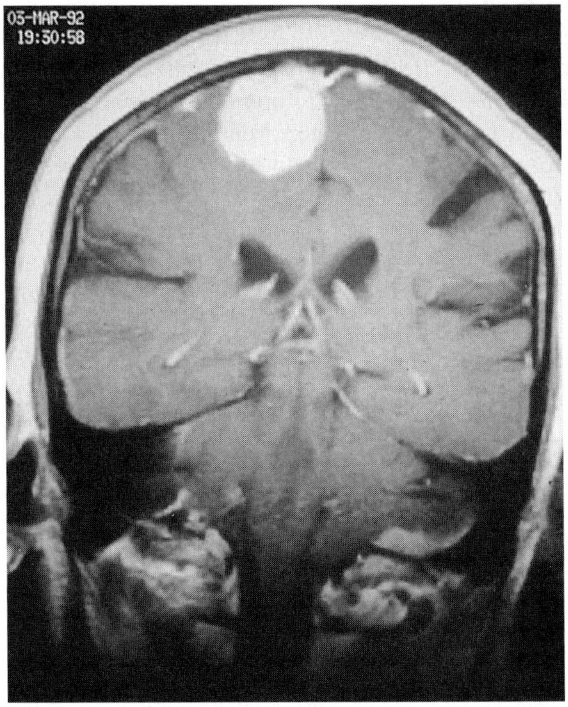
03-MAR-92
19:30:58

FIGURE 48.8 Meningioma.

Signs and Symptoms

The symptoms of a brain tumor are directly related to the location of the tumor in the brain and to the rate of growth. Slow-growing types of tumors such as meningiomas (a tumor arising from the meninges; Fig. 48.8) can get to be quite large before causing symptoms. Conversely, glioblastoma multiforme or metastatic tumors may abruptly cause seizures or hemiparesis. Other types of tumors include oligodendroglioma, astrocytoma, and acoustic neuroma. The suffix *-oma* refers to tumor. The prefix denotes the type of cell from which the tumor arises.

Symptoms of a brain tumor depend on its size and location and can include seizures, motor and sensory deficits, nausea and vomiting, headaches, personality changes, confusion, and speech and vision disturbances. If the pituitary gland is involved, additional symptoms related to changes in hormone secretion occur, such as abnormal growth or fluid volume imbalances.

Diagnostic Tests

MRI gives the clearest images of a brain tumor. If the tumor appears to be highly vascular or in proximity to major blood vessels, an angiogram may be performed. It is now possible to do magnetic resonance angiograms, which involve the intravenous administration of contrast material and is much less invasive than a traditional angiogram. If the tumor is in the region of the pituitary gland, serum hormone levels are evaluated. Biopsy may be done during surgical removal of the tumor, or using needle aspiration. Additional tests may be carried out to find a primary cancer site.

Therapeutic Measures

Surgical treatment involves removal of the tumor or as much of the tumor as possible. Care of the patient undergoing intracranial surgery is discussed later in this chapter.

Medical Treatment

Medical treatment consists of controlling symptoms. Patients who have a seizure are placed on anticonvulsants. If significant cerebral edema is noted on the MRI or if the patient is suffering from headaches or other symptoms, a steroid such as dexamethasone (Decadron) may be prescribed to lessen the edema and reduce symptoms. Typically, patients do not require narcotics for pain relief.

Radiation Therapy

External beam radiation therapy is standard treatment for many patients with a brain tumor. The therapy is typically given 5 days a week for 6 weeks. Some clinicians use a hyperfractionated schedule, in which the patient has therapy twice a day for less time. Brachytherapy is a means of delivering radiation therapy directly to the tumor. Small catheters are implanted in the tumor and then tiny radioactive particles are inserted into the catheters. The treatment typically takes 3 to 5 days. During this time the patient is confined to a private room and interaction with visitors and staff is kept to a minimum because of the radioactivity. This therapy is not appropriate for confused individuals because they may not be able to cooperate with restrictions.

Stereotactic radiosurgery is a technique that utilizes small amounts of radiation directed at the tumor from different angles. A metal frame is affixed to the patient's skull, and the tumor is visualized within the framework on a CT or MRI. A computer plan is generated to direct the radiation. Because multiple small sources are used, the normal brain tissue receives very little radiation while the majority of the radiation accumulates in the tumor.

Chemotherapy

The blood-brain barrier is a protective mechanism that prevents many injurious substances from reaching brain tissue. Unfortunately, it is also effective in preventing most chemotherapy agents from reaching the brain. To penetrate the blood-brain barrier, very large doses of chemotherapy may be required. These doses may not be well tolerated by other body systems. New treatments are currently being investigated. Some clinicians place chemotherapy substances in the cavity left by surgical resection. Others disrupt the blood-brain barrier with mannitol (an osmotic diuretic) and then deliver intra-arterial chemotherapy under general anesthesia. Another newer treatment, called targeted drug therapy, uses bevacizumab (Avastin), a drug that stops formation of new blood vessels that support the tumor. Gene therapy is also being used in an effort to kill malignant cells.

Complementary Therapies

The rate of success for treatment of brain tumors is not as high as treatment of other neoplasms. Patients may be drawn to nontraditional therapies both as cures and for treatment of symptoms. Encourage patients to look at each option in a rational manner. Some questions they should ask themselves include the following:

- Will this interfere with any of my other treatments or medications?
- What is the cost?
- What are the side effects?
- Is there any objective information (research) available?
- What does my physician think of this?

Additional information on evaluation of complementary therapies is found in Chapter 5.

Acute and Long-Term Complications

It is difficult to distinguish between symptoms of a brain tumor and complications of treatment. Seizures, headaches, memory impairment, cognitive changes, and ataxia may be symptoms of the tumor or the result of surgery or radiation therapy. Patients may experience hemiparesis or aphasia following surgery. If the tumor continues to grow despite treatment, the patient will experience further decline in function. Gradually the patient becomes more lethargic and unresponsive. Once the patient becomes comatose, death occurs within a matter of days, particularly if artificial nutrition and hydration are not administered.

Nursing Process for the Patient with a Brain Tumor

Nursing care of the patient with a brain tumor is similar to that for the patient with a brain injury, since both experience neurologic deficits. See the *Nursing Care Plan for the Patient with a Brain Tumor or Injury.*

INTRACRANIAL SURGERY

The primary purpose of intracranial surgery is to remove a mass lesion. These types of lesions include hematomas, tumors, arteriovenous malformations, and, occasionally, contused brain tissue. Other indications for surgery include elevation of a depressed skull fracture, removal of a foreign body, debridement of a wound, or resection of a seizure focus. The term **craniotomy** refers to any surgical opening in the skull. A burr hole is an opening into the cranium made with a drill. **Craniectomy** is the term used to describe removal of part of the cranial bone. **Cranioplasty** refers to repair of bone or use of a prosthesis to replace bone following surgery.

The goal of intracranial tumor surgery is gross total resection of the tumor. This involves removal of all visible tumor, called *debulking*. Even with the use of an operative microscope, viable tumor cells may be left behind that can give rise to recurrence. If the entire tumor cannot be removed, the surgeon debulks as much as possible, thereby giving radiation therapy or chemotherapy less of a burden to combat. In some cases, it is not feasible to attempt more than a biopsy of the tumor. Location of the tumor or the patient's age or medical condition may not allow the patient to tolerate a full craniotomy. The biopsy may be done under local or general anesthesia, depending on the patient's condition. The goal of a biopsy is to obtain tissue that allows pathological diagnosis of the tumor, which then guides any further treatment.

Intracranial surgery is usually performed under general anesthesia. Occasionally, a procedure requires that the patient be awake and cooperative.

Preoperative Care

Preoperative care of the patient undergoing intracranial surgery is similar to that of patients having other surgeries (see Chapter 12). The patient undergoes a laboratory workup and anesthesia evaluation. If the patient has cognitive impairments, it is important that a significant other be available to provide information. A thorough baseline neurologic assessment should be documented.

Patient education is important preoperatively. The extent of education depends on the patient's ability to absorb new information. This is influenced by the disease process, cognitive functioning, anxiety, and educational level. Significant others are involved as needed. Information about the disease process and surgery is provided by the surgeon. The nurse can play an important role in reinforcing and clarifying the information presented.

Anxiety is also a significant concern before surgery. The patient is anticipating serious surgery, as well as an unknown outcome. Allow time for the patient and significant others to express their fears and ask questions. Honest and accurate information should be provided.

Significant others should be prepared for how the patient will look after surgery. A preoperative visit to the intensive care unit may help prevent some anxiety postoperatively. Significant others should be accompanied on this visit by a knowledgeable nurse who can explain what they are seeing.

Surgery may last 2 hours for a biopsy to 12 hours or longer for more involved procedures. Patients and significant others should be prepared for the idea that some or all of the patient's hair will be shaved off. Some people prefer to have all their hair shaved rather than just part. The patient should be prepared to see his or her face swollen after surgery, particularly around the eyes; the periorbital region may be bruised. Many patients wish to wear a scarf or scrub cap after the dressing is removed.

• WORD • BUILDING •

craniotomy: crani—skull + otomy—incision

craniectomy: crani—skull + ectomy—excision, removal

cranioplasty: cranio—skull + plasty—to form

Nursing Process for the Postoperative Care of the Patient Having Intracranial Surgery

Acute care of the postoperative patient is presented below. Also see the *Nursing Care Plan for the Patient with a Brain Tumor or Injury.*

Data Collection

After intracranial surgery, the patient will be cared for in an intensive care unit. Plan to assist the RN with frequent neurologic assessments in addition to routine postoperative monitoring. Patients should have their neurologic status assessed every hour for the first 24 hours or as ordered by the physician. Many patients undergo a CT scan within the first 24 hours following surgery to assess cerebral edema. Also assess the patient's response to changes in body image and the patient's knowledge base related to care that will be required following discharge.

Nursing Diagnoses, Planning, and Implementation

The primary goal following intracranial surgery is prevention of complications. Once the patient is stabilized, goals can change to longer term outcomes such as acceptance of changes in body image and understanding of self-care following discharge. If the patient has severe deficits following surgery, rehabilitation or long-term care may become necessary. A consultation with a social worker can help with planning for this transition. Priority nursing diagnoses are discussed next.

Risk for Ineffective Cerebral Tissue Perfusion Related to Edema of the Operative Site

EXPECTED OUTCOME: The patient will have adequate cerebral tissue perfusion as evidenced by stable or improving neurologic assessments.

- Monitor neurologic status as ordered. Report changes promptly. *Deteriorating status may signify increased ICP.*
- Implement measures *to prevent increased ICP*. See Table 48.4 for preventive measures and rationales.
- Position patient with the head of the bed at 30 degrees or higher, unless ordered otherwise, *to promote venous drainage and minimize increases in ICP.* The exception to this is patients who have had a chronic subdural hematoma removed; these patients must

remain flat. Patients may turn from side to side or lie on their back, but should not lie on the operative side.

- Implement seizure precautions *because the patient is at risk for seizures due to cerebral edema.*
- Use caution to protect the many monitoring systems being used. The patient may have an intracranial monitor in place following surgery *to monitor ICP.* Some patients may also have central venous pressure catheters or pulmonary artery catheters *to monitor fluid status.* Urinary catheters are used during the immediate postoperative period *to accurately monitor fluid balance.*
- Monitor dressings for drainage. *Drainage that is blood tinged in the center with a yellowish ring around it may be CSF leakage. A suspected CSF leak should be reported to the RN or physician immediately.*

Risk for Infection Related to Surgical Procedure

EXPECTED OUTCOME: The patient will remain free from infection as evidenced by temperature and white cell count within normal limits and incision sites clean and dry.

- Monitor patient for rise in temperature, purulence at incision site, and increase in white cell count. *These are signs of infection and should be reported immediately.*
- Use strict aseptic technique for all care of the incision, dressing, and monitoring equipment sites *to reduce risk of infection.*
- Use appropriate hand hygiene *to reduce risk of transmitting infection.*

Disturbed Body Image Related to Changes in Appearance or Function as Evidenced by Patient Statement of Disturbance or Unwillingness to Observe Changes

EXPECTED OUTCOME: The patient will display an accepting attitude toward change in appearance, as evidenced by willingness to look in mirror and/or be seen by others.

- Offer a turban, scarf, or hat if the patient desires *to help conceal a shaved head.*
- Portray an accepting attitude toward the patient. *Patients are likely aware of nurses' nonverbal behavior.*
- Allow the patient to express his or her feelings if desired. *Talking may help the patient work through feelings, but it should not be forced.*

Deficient Knowledge Related to Change in Treatment Regimen Following Surgery as Evidenced by Patient Statement

EXPECTED OUTCOME: The patient and significant others will verbalize correct information for follow-up care at home. They will state they have the resources to manage care effectively.

- Teach the patient and family or significant other home management, including medication regimen, wound care, and ordered activity restrictions, including driving. Have the patient and significant others verbalize the signs of infection or other possible complications to report. *The patient and family will assume responsibility for care after discharge, unless the patient is being transferred to another facility.*
- Teach patient and family seizure precautions and the importance of taking anticonvulsants as ordered. *The patient may be on anticonvulsants to prevent seizures following surgery. If seizure free for 1 year, the physician may discontinue anticonvulsants.*
- Consult social worker or case manager for resources if needed. *The patient may need discharge planning if transfer to another facility is planned. If discharge home is expected, the patient and family will benefit from visiting nurse follow-up. Assistance with obtaining medications can also be provided if necessary.*

Evaluation

Interventions have been effective if the patient's neurologic status is stable, and infection and other complications have been prevented. The patient might be able to look in the mirror and begin to show evidence of acceptance of changes in body image, although this may not happen until after discharge from the hospital. The patient and significant others should be able to describe appropriate follow-up care.

CRITICAL THINKING

Mr. Evans

■ Mr. Evans is a 24-year-old white male who was involved in a motor vehicle crash. His blood alcohol level was 0.24. Mr. Evans has no preexisting medical problems. Emergency medical services personnel report that Mr. Evans was unconscious on their arrival at the scene and then became alert and combative. His CT scan shows a left-sided epidural hematoma. Mr. Evans is admitted to your unit for observation.

1. What symptoms would you expect to see if Mr. Evans' hematoma increases in size?
2. What emergency preparations should you have ready?
3. What psychosocial data should you collect?

Suggested answers at end of chapter.

SPINAL DISORDERS

Herniated Disks

Herniated intravertebral disks are a common health problem. They are characterized by pain and paresthesias that follow a radicular (nerve path) pattern. It is not uncommon for patients to have more than one herniated disk or to have herniated disks in different areas of the spine.

Pathophysiology

When the disk between two vertebrae herniates, it moves out of its normal anatomical position. In most cases, the annulus fibrosus, the tough outer ring of the disk, tears. This allows escape of the nucleus pulposus, the soft inner portion of the disk. Displacement of the disk compresses one or more nerve roots, causing the characteristic symptoms (Fig. 48.9).

Etiology

In some cases, a specific event can be correlated with a herniated disk. The patient may describe a fall, lifting a heavy object, or a motor vehicle accident. In other instances, the patient cannot identify a triggering incident.

Signs and Symptoms

Cervical disk herniation causes pain and muscle spasm in the neck. The patient may have decreased range of motion secondary to pain. Hand and arm pain is unilateral (one sided) and follows the distribution of the spinal nerve root. Patients often report numbness or tingling in the extremity. Asymmetrical weakness and atrophy of specific muscle groups may be detected. If weakness involves the entire extremity, it is unlikely that disk herniation is the etiology. The severity of the pain or paresthesia does not correlate directly with the severity of the nerve compression. However, weakness and atrophy are indicators of significant nerve compression.

Thoracic herniated disks are not common. This portion of the spine is the least mobile; therefore, less stress is exerted on the disks. Patients with herniated thoracic disks may report pain in the back. It is uncommon to detect muscular weakness.

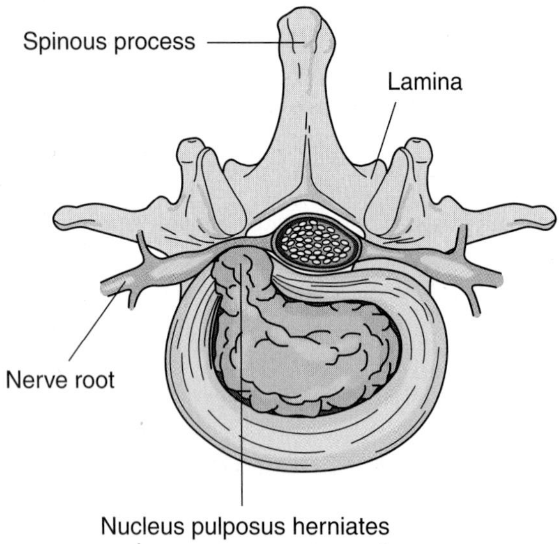
Spinous process
Lamina
Nerve root
Nucleus pulposus herniates
and compresses nerve root

FIGURE 48.9 A herniated disk places pressure on a spinal nerve root.

A herniated lumbar disk is typically characterized by low back pain, pain radiating down one leg, paresthesias, and weakness. The patient may limp on the affected leg or may have difficulty walking on his or her heels or toes. Muscle spasm is often present. Pain and muscle spasm may limit the patient's range of motion. Depending on the disk affected, the knee or ankle deep tendon reflex may be decreased or absent. A severely herniated L5–S1 disk may affect bowel or bladder continence. This is an emergency situation and should be reported immediately.

The WHAT'S UP? mnemonic can be used to assess symptoms of herniated disks at any level:

W—Where is the pain? Does it radiate into an extremity? In what distribution?

H—How does it feel? Sharp, stabbing, burning?

A—Do certain positions or activities alleviate or aggravate the pain? Holding the affected arm above the head may alleviate cervical pain. Sitting places pressure on disks and aggravates lumbar pain. Lying down may relieve it.

T—Is there a correlation between time and pain? Some patients have more pain at the end of the day. Is the pain constant or intermittent?

S—Ask the patient to rate the severity of the pain on a scale of 0 to 10. Which is the most painful, the spine or the extremity?

U—Ask the patient to identify other useful data, such as symptoms of numbness, tingling, or weakness.

P—What is the patient's perception of the pain? Is it interfering with work or other aspects of the patient's life?

Diagnostic Tests

An MRI will detect herniation of a disk and compression or abnormality of the spinal cord. If the patient has previously had surgery in the area of the suspected herniation, the MRI is done with and without contrast to differentiate between scar tissue and a herniated disk.

If the patient cannot tolerate an MRI or if the MRI does not provide enough information, a myelogram may be done. Refer to Chapter 47 for a description of both tests.

Therapeutic Measures

Most clinicians and patients prefer to try conservative medical therapy before performing surgery for a herniated disk.

MEDICAL TREATMENT.

Rest. In the past, bedrest was advised as part of conservative management. The current recommendation is 1 or 2 days of bedrest, followed by a careful, gradual increase in activity.

Physical Therapy. Physical therapy can be very useful for some patients. A gradually progressive course of exercise strengthens the muscles. This is particularly important in the lumbar spine, where the muscles help stabilize the spine. Techniques such as ultrasound, heat, ice, and deep massage can decrease muscle spasm and allow for increased range of motion. Instructions in proper body mechanics and strategies for avoiding reinjury are important components of physical therapy.

Traction. Cervical traction is a noninvasive technique sometimes used by physical therapists for patients with herniated cervical disks. The patient's head is placed in a halter-like device. A series of ropes and pulleys connect the halter to a weight. This gently pulls the head away from the shoulders. The rationale is that this traction slightly separates the vertebral bodies and may allow the disk to return to its proper position. If it is effective in relieving the patient's pain, cervical traction may be done at home on an as-needed basis. Traction is discontinued immediately if it increases the patient's pain. Lumbar traction is not particularly effective because the lumbar paraspinal muscles are very large and strong. The amount of traction needed to overcome the muscular resistance can cause injury.

Medication. Muscle relaxants are often prescribed as a short-term therapy for patients who are experiencing muscle spasms. These medications decrease pain by decreasing the spasm, helping the patient increase range of motion and activity. Muscle spasm is actually a protective mechanism. Muscles tighten and become painful, causing the patient to limit movement. This lessens the chance that the disk will be further injured. However, chronic spasm can cause tearing and scarring of the muscles. It is hard to predict which muscle relaxant will be most effective for a given patient. Patients should be warned that drowsiness is a common side effect of many muscle relaxants. They should be cautioned against driving or operating machinery until they determine how well they tolerate the medication. Diazepam is an effective muscle relaxant; however, it has a strong potential for addiction so it is usually used only if muscle spasm cannot be adequately treated with other medications.

Inflammation of the nerve root is caused by compression and irritation from the herniated disk. Nonsteroidal anti-inflammatory drugs (NSAIDs) can be effective in reducing this inflammation, but there is no way of predicting response to a given drug. It may be necessary for the patient to try several NSAIDs before an effective one is found. Because several of these drugs are now available without prescription, the patient should be cautioned not to use a nonprescription NSAID at the same time as a prescription NSAID. Patients should be instructed to report any stomach upset to the clinician because NSAIDs may cause gastric bleeding. Occasionally, oral steroids are used on a short-term basis for patients with severe inflammation that does not respond to other treatments. A rapidly tapering dose of steroid over 1 week is often prescribed. Steroids may also cause gastric upset, in addition to elevated serum glucose levels. Instruct patients with diabetes to monitor glucose levels closely and consult a physician if the levels are outside their normal parameters.

Epidural injections may be tried for patients who have no relief with more conservative measures. A mixture of medications, typically a steroid, long-acting anesthetic, and long-acting pain reliever, is injected into the epidural space. The anesthetic provides immediate relief, while the steroid reduces swelling for a longer lasting effect. If relief is obtained, the injection can be repeated every 3 to 4 months.

The use of opioid pain medication is a subject of concern in the treatment of patients with herniated disks. Opioids generally are appropriate for short-term treatment of acute pain. However, if treatment is not effective, the pain may become chronic. In that circumstance, the physician and patient must discuss the potential complications of long-term opioid use, such as constipation, tolerance, and dependence. A referral to a pain clinic for alternative strategies may be appropriate.

Some alternatives to long-term use of opioids include topical lidocaine patches or NSAID patches, or use of agents for neuropathic pain such as pregabalin (Lyrica) or amitriptyline (Elavil).

Complementary Therapy. A transcutaneous electrical nerve stimulator (commonly called a TENS unit) is a noninvasive pain-relief technique. Small electrodes are placed on the skin around the area of the pain. The device then transmits a low-voltage electrical current through the skin. The patient feels a tingling or buzzing sensation, which may help block the pain impulses. A physical therapist or pain specialist teaches the patient where to place the electrodes and how to operate the unit. The patient decides when to use it and at what settings. This allows the patient to actively participate in his or her care and have some control over the pain level.

SURGICAL MANAGEMENT. Surgeries are less common today than in the past, because conservative measures have been found to be successful for most patients. If surgery is indicated, several options are available. A **laminectomy** removes one of the laminae, the flat pieces of bone on each side of a vertebra. This may be done to relieve pressure or to gain access for removal of a herniated disk. A diskectomy removes the entire disk. A spinal fusion uses a bone graft to fuse two vertebrae together if the area is unstable. Surgery may be done through a microscope for less scarring and faster recovery. Most patients are discharged within 24 hours of surgery.

A diskectomy is generally done for a herniated cervical disk. This can be accomplished via an anterior or posterior approach. Most surgeons use the anterior approach for cervical herniations because the muscles in the front of the neck are much smaller and more mobile than those in the back of the neck. Therefore, there is less pain and muscle spasm following surgery. It is also safer than the posterior approach, which involves more maneuvering around the spinal cord.

Most surgeons replace the disk with bone or another material. This prevents collapse of the disk space and creates

• WORD • BUILDING •

laminectomy: lamin—posterior portion of the vertebra + ectomy—surgical removal of a spinal fusion. If bone is used, it may be harvested from the patient's iliac crest or donated from a cadaver. Mobility of the spine is lost in the area of a fusion. Spinal fusions may also be done to correct instability of the spine from other causes, such as scoliosis or degenerative disorders.

A posterior approach is used for a herniated lumbar disk. Typically, the vertical incision is 1 to 2 inches long. It is necessary to pull some of the muscle away from the bone, which accounts for some of the postoperative pain that patients experience. A laminectomy is done, and the herniated portion of the disk is resected. The remainder of the disk continues to provide a cushion between the intravertebral bodies. The surgeon removes any free fragments and any disk material that appears unstable.

Percutaneous diskectomy involves insertion of a large needle into the disk under local anesthesia to aspirate herniated disk material. This technique is not used for severely herniated disks. Laser disk surgery may be used to disintegrate the herniated tissue. Laparoscopic techniques may also be used.

In 2004, the FDA approved an artificial disk for use with selected patients. It is made of two plastic disks designed to slide so that mobility is not impaired as with spinal fusion (Fig. 48.10). The artificial disk is attached to the vertebra above and below once the damaged disk is removed. This alternative to spinal fusion has been effective for those with single-disk problems.

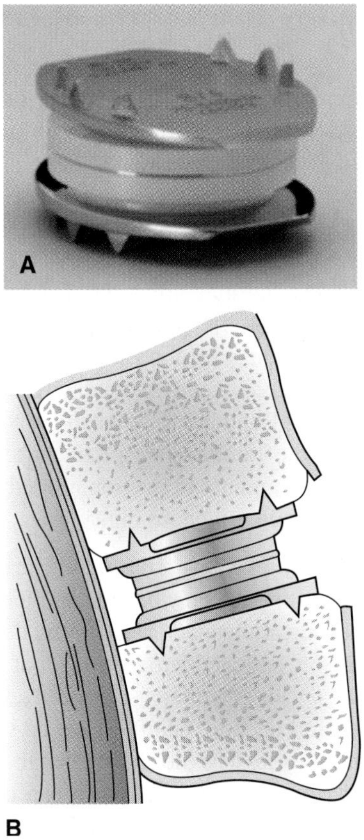
A
B

FIGURE 48.10 (A) The Charité artificial disk can be used to treat pain caused by degenerative disk disease. (B) The disk is approved for use only in the lumbar spine from L4 to S1 for patients who have unrelieved low back pain after at least 6 months of nonsurgical treatment. (Courtesy DePuy Spine, Inc.)

Complications After Surgery

HEMORRHAGE. As with any surgery, intraoperative hemorrhage is possible, although it is not common in disk surgery. If a postoperative hemorrhage occurs in a patient who has had an anterior cervical diskectomy, the airway may become occluded. The patient is monitored for bleeding from the incision and respiratory distress.

NERVE ROOT DAMAGE. If the nerve root is severed during surgery, the patient experiences loss of motor and sensory functions in that nerve's distribution area. This may result in decreased use of the extremity. If the nerve root is damaged or excessive scarring occurs, the patient may experience pain, weakness, or paresthesias. In some cases, physical therapy and NSAIDs may be effective in improving function and reducing pain.

REHERNIATION. Lumbar disks may reherniate. This can occur anywhere from 1 week to several years after the initial surgery. If the reherniation occurs within a few weeks to months after the first surgery, the patient usually undergoes another microdiskectomy. Reherniation of a cervical disk does not occur because the entire disk is removed.

HERNIATION OF ADJACENT DISK. Fusion of the cervical spine results in loss of movement at that motion segment. This can place increased stress on the disks above and below the fusion. This may increase the risk of another herniated disk, especially if the patient already has degeneration of other disks. The patient should be instructed to maintain an exercise program and to frequently move the spine through range-of-motion exercises.

Nursing Process for the Patient Having Spinal Surgery

Preoperative Care

Routine preoperative care is appropriate for the patient undergoing spinal surgery. In addition to routine teaching, instruct the patient in how to logroll following surgery. This procedure involves keeping the body in alignment and rolling as a unit, without twisting the spine, to prevent injury to the operative site.

Postoperative Care

DATA COLLECTION. In addition to routine postoperative data collection, monitor extremities for changes in circulation, movement, and sensation. Monitor color, warmth, and presence of pulses in the extremities. Assess movement by asking the patient to move the extremities. Assess sensation by gently touching the patient's extremity and asking if feeling is present. Report any changes immediately to the physician because this may indicate nerve or circulatory damage.

Monitor pain frequently. The pain that necessitated surgery should be relieved, but the patient may still have muscular and incisional pain. The patient should be reassured that it will gradually subside. Monitor the surgical dressing and drain (if present) for CSF drainage or bleeding. Any sign of CSF drainage or significant bleeding should be reported to the physician immediately. If bone was taken from a separate donor site, this site must also be monitored. Intake and output are measured to ensure that the patient is able to void. Notify the physician if the patient has difficulty voiding.

NURSING DIAGNOSES, PLANNING, AND IMPLEMENTATION. Goals of nursing are to keep the patient safe and free from injury or complications, and free from pain. Gradual return to normal physical activity is expected. Possible postoperative diagnoses are discussed next.

Acute Pain Related to Surgical Procedure as Evidenced by Patient's Pain Rating

EXPECTED OUTCOME: The patient will verbalize an acceptable pain level.

- Monitor pain following surgery using a pain scale. *The patient's self-report is the most reliable method for assessing pain.*
- Administer muscle relaxants, analgesics, and NSAIDs as ordered. If a local anesthetic was injected into the surgical site during surgery, the patient may not have pain immediately postoperatively. *Medications to relieve pain help the patient to mobilize following surgery, which helps prevent complications.*
- Position the patient in bed in correct body alignment. If ordered, keep the patient flat for 6 to 8 hours. *Correct alignment avoids twisting and injury to the operative site.*
- Place a pillow between the legs when lying on the side *to promote alignment and comfort.*

Risk for Impaired Urinary Elimination Related to Effects of Surgery

EXPECTED OUTCOME: The patient will be able to empty bladder without assistance.

- Monitor urine output for retention. *Patients may have difficulty voiding following lumbar surgery because of anesthesia, immobility, or occasionally because of nerve damage related to surgery.*
- If activity orders allow, assist the patient to get up to urinate (or to stand for men). *This may help the patient urinate.*
- If unable to void, try running warm water over the perineum, or taking a warm bath or shower. *This may stimulate voiding.*
- If difficulty urinating occurs, contact the physician for an order for intermittent catheterization until the problem resolves. *Urine retention that is not resolved can lead to bladder rupture. Intermittent catheterization is a safe way to empty the bladder.*

Risk for Impaired Physical Mobility Related to Neuromuscular Impairment

EXPECTED OUTCOME: The patient will be able to ambulate and prevent complications of immobility following surgery.

- Assess mobility of affected extremities following surgery. *A reduction in expected mobility following surgery indicates nerve damage in surgery and should be reported immediately.*
- Assist the patient to logroll to get out of bed and ambulate on the first postoperative day, as ordered. If spinal fusion has been done, the fused area of the spine will be immobile. *Early mobilization after surgery helps prevent complications.*
- Apply a soft cervical collar to the patient with a cervical laminectomy as ordered *for neck support.*

EVALUATION. The patient is expected to be free of complications and pain, be able to urinate, be able to move all extremities, and return gradually to pre-illness activity level.

Spinal Stenosis

Spinal stenosis is a condition in which the spinal canal compresses the spinal cord (Fig. 48.11). Arthritis is a major cause of spinal stenosis. The facet joints of the spine become inflamed and enlarged, narrowing the diameter of the spinal canal and compressing the spinal cord. Patients may report pain and weakness. Compression of the cervical portion of the spinal cord may result in hyperreflexia and weakness of the legs and arms.

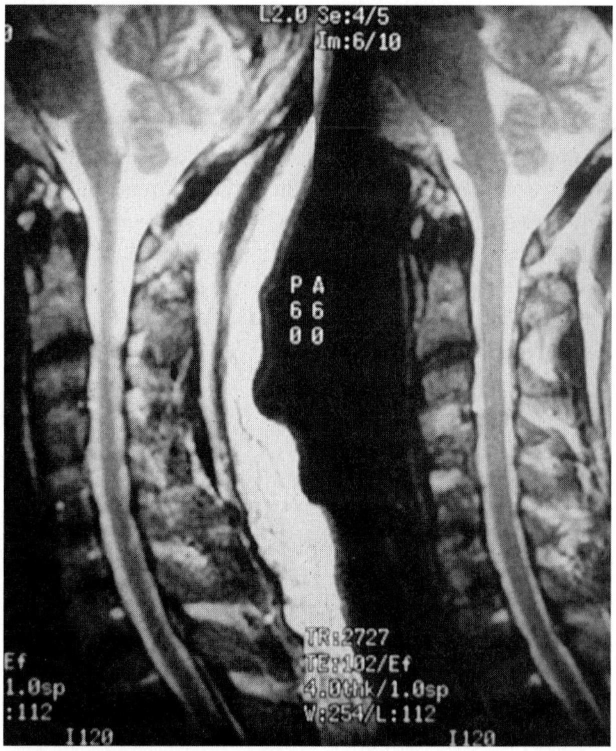
Se:4/5
Im:6/10
P A
6 6
0 0
TR:2727
TE:102/Ef
4.0thk/1.0sp
W:254/L:112
Ef
1.0sp
:112

FIGURE 48.11 Stenosis of the cervical spine (left). Compare with normal spinal column (right).

A laminectomy may be done to relieve pressure on the spinal cord. The size of the incision depends on the number of vertebrae involved. These patients are often older and may have concurrent illnesses. They may require inpatient rehabilitation before returning home.

SPINAL CORD INJURIES

Injuries to the spinal cord affect people of all ages but take their greatest toll on young people. These injuries are characterized by a decrease or loss of sensory and motor functions below the level of the injury.

Pathophysiology

The spinal cord is made up of nerve fibers that allow communication between the brain and the rest of the body. Damage to the spinal cord results in interference with this communication process. Damage may be caused by bruising, tearing, cutting, edema, or bleeding into the cord. The damage may be caused by external forces or by fragments of fractured bone.

Etiology and Types

The causes of spinal cord injury are similar to those of traumatic brain injury. It is not uncommon for a patient to have both a spinal cord injury and traumatic brain injury. Motor vehicle crashes, falls, and sports-related injuries are common causes. Diving into shallow water is a common cause of cervical cord injury. Assaults may cause cord injury if a knife or bullet penetrates the spinal cord.

Spinal cord injuries may be classified by location or by degree of damage to the cord. A complete spinal cord injury means that there is no motor or sensory function below the level of the injury. An incomplete lesion means that some function remains. This does not necessarily mean that the remaining function will be useful to the patient. Some patients find that having areas where sensation is intact may be more painful than useful.

The cervical and lumbar portions of the spine are injured more often than the thoracic or sacral segments. This is because the cervical and lumbar areas are the most mobile portions of the spine.

Signs and Symptoms

Cervical Injuries

Signs and symptoms depend on the level at which the cord is damaged (Fig. 48.12). Cervical cord injuries can affect all four extremities, causing paralysis and paresthesias, impaired respiration, and loss of bowel and bladder control. Paralysis of all four extremities is called **quadriplegia**; weakness of all extremities is called **quadriparesis**. If the injury is at C3 or above, the injury is usually fatal because muscles used for breathing are paralyzed. An injury at the fourth or fifth cervical vertebra affects breathing and may necessitate some type of ventilatory support. These patients typically need long-term assistance with activities of daily living.

Thoracic and Lumbar Injuries

Thoracic and lumbar injuries affect the legs, bowel, and bladder. Paralysis of the legs is called **paraplegia**; weakness of the legs is called **paraparesis**. Sacral injuries affect bowel and bladder continence and may affect foot function. Individuals with thoracic, lumbar, and sacral injuries can usually learn to perform activities of daily living independently.

Spinal Shock

Spinal cord injury has a profound effect on the autonomic nervous system. Immediately following injury, the cord below the injury stops functioning completely. This causes a disruption of sympathetic nervous system function, resulting in vasodilation, hypotension, and bradycardia—called neurogenic shock or spinal shock. Dilation of the blood vessels allows more blood flow just beneath the skin. This blood cools and is circulated throughout the body, causing hypothermia. The patient is unable to maintain control of body temperature. Keep the patient covered as much as possible but avoid overheating. In addition, all reflexes below the level of the injury are lost, and retention of urine and feces occurs. Spinal shock can last from a week to many weeks in some patients.

Complications

Infection

Impaired respiratory effort, decreased cough, mechanical ventilation, and immobility all predispose a patient with a spinal cord injury to pneumonia. Urinary catheterization, whether indwelling or intermittent, places patients at risk for urinary tract infection.

Deep Venous Thrombosis

Lack of movement in the legs inhibits normal blood circulation. Compression stockings, sequential compression devices, and subcutaneous heparin may be used separately or together to reduce the risk of deep venous thrombosis.

Orthostatic Hypotension

Most patients with spinal cord injuries no longer have muscular function in their legs to promote venous return to the heart. They also have impaired vasoconstriction. This leads to pooling of the blood in the legs when the patient moves from a supine to a sitting position. If the movement is sudden, the patient may become dizzy or light-headed. Gradual elevation of the head, use of elastic stockings, and a reclining wheelchair help lessen this response.

• WORD • BUILDING •

quadriplegia: quad—four + plegia—paralysis
quadriparesis: quad—four + paresis—partial paralysis

• WORD • BUILDING •

paraplegia: para—beside + plegia—paralysis
paraparesis: para—beside + paresis—partial paralysis

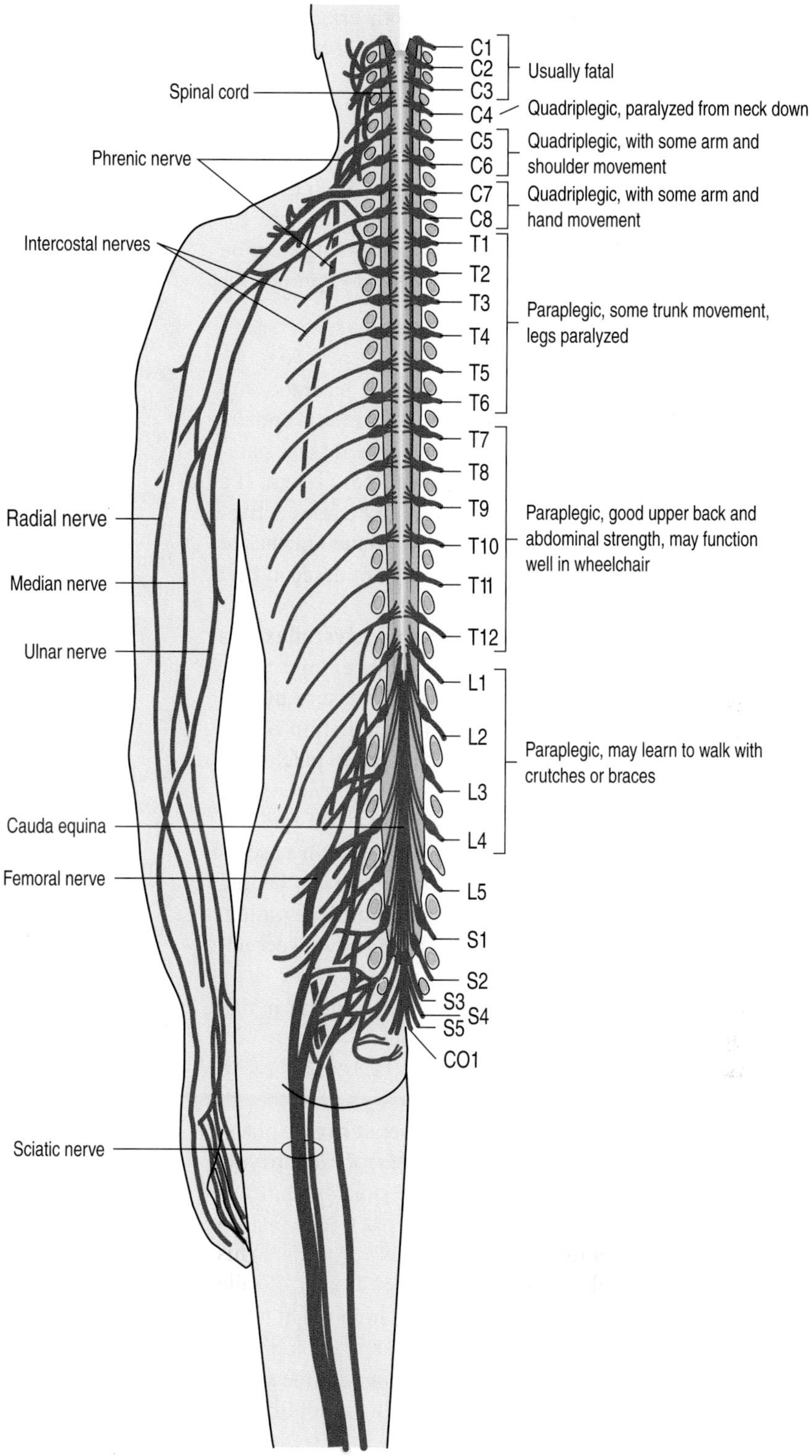
Spinal cord
Phrenic nerve
Intercostal nerves
Radial nerve
Median nerve
Ulnar nerve
Cauda equina
Femoral nerve
Sciatic nerve
C1
C2
C3
C4
C5
C6
C7
C8
T1
T2
T3
T4
T5
T6
T7
T8
T9
T10
T11
T12
L1
L2
L3
L4
L5
S1
S2
S3
S4
S5
CO1
Usually fatal
Quadriplegic, paralyzed from neck down
Quadriplegic, with some arm and shoulder movement
Quadriplegic, with some arm and hand movement
Paraplegic, some trunk movement, legs paralyzed
Paraplegic, good upper back and abdominal strength, may function well in wheelchair
Paraplegic, may learn to walk with crutches or braces

FIGURE 48.12 Spinal cord injury—quadriplegia versus paraplegia. (Modified from Scanlon, V. C., & Sanders, T. [2007]. *Workbook for essentials of anatomy and physiology* [5th ed., p. 163]. Philadelphia: F. A. Davis, with permission.)

Skin Breakdown

Patients or their caregivers must be diligent about relieving pressure on the skin by position changes and cushioning of bony prominences. It is important to realize that the patient may not be able to feel pain and therefore may not ask for position changes. Development of pressure ulcers can lead to infection and loss of skin, muscle, or bone. Treatment of pressure ulcers is time consuming and expensive and may interfere with work or school.

Renal Complications

Urinary tract infections are an ongoing concern for patients with spinal cord injuries. Caregivers as well as the patient need to be taught to observe the color, clarity, and odor of urine and to report changes promptly. Both urinary reflux and untreated urinary tract infections can cause permanent damage to the kidneys.

Depression and Substance Abuse

Patients with spinal cord injury have a higher than average incidence of depression and substance abuse. Both of these factors can interfere with the patient's ability to care for himself or herself. Individual or family counseling may be helpful. Some rehabilitation centers have support groups for patients with spinal cord injuries.

Autonomic Dysreflexia

This life-threatening complication occurs in patients with injuries above the T6 level. The spinal cord injury impairs the normal equilibrium between the sympathetic and parasympathetic divisions of the autonomic nervous system. If a noxious stimulus below the spinal cord injury causes activation of the sympathetic system, it will continue unchecked because the parasympathetic responses cannot descend past the spinal cord injury.

The most common cause of autonomic **dysreflexia** is bladder distention. Other causes include bowel impaction, urinary tract infection, ingrown toenails, pressure ulcers, pain, and labor in a pregnant woman. Stimulation of the sympathetic nervous system results in cool, pale skin, gooseflesh, and vasoconstriction below the level of the injury. Blood pressure may rise as high as 300 mm Hg systolic. The parasympathetic response results in vasodilation, causing flushing and diaphoresis above the lesion, and bradycardia as low as 30 beats per minute. The patient reports a pounding headache and nasal congestion secondary to the dilated blood vessels.

Care of the patient with autonomic dysreflexia is discussed in the care plan later in this section.

Diagnostic Tests

Plain radiographs are done to identify fractures or displacement of vertebrae. A CT scan is also useful for identifying fractures. An MRI may demonstrate lesions within the cord.

Therapeutic Measures

Patients with spinal cord injuries typically are brought to the emergency department. They should be kept immobilized until they are assessed by a physician. If injury to the spinal cord is detected, the patient needs to remain immobilized.

Emergency Management

Emergency management involves careful monitoring of vital signs and airway and keeping the patient immobilized. Intubation and mechanical ventilation may be necessary especially with cervical spine injuries. Intravenous normal saline may be used for fluid replacement and provision of an access site for medication administration. The physician does not rely on fluid administration alone to correct hypotension. It is possible to administer enough fluid to cause pulmonary edema and not correct the hypotension. Vasoactive drugs may be required. The use of various medications to reduce the extent of injury, including intravenous methylprednisolone (a steroid), is routine. Often this treatment is started by emergency medical services (EMS) personnel prior to arrival at the emergency department.

Respiratory Management

Patients with injuries above C4–C5 have some degree of respiratory impairment. The patient may require a tracheostomy and continuous mechanical ventilation or require a ventilator only at night or when fatigued. Some patients are able to breathe by using a phrenic nerve stimulator. This device, similar to a pacemaker, artificially stimulates the phrenic nerve, causing the diaphragm to move. These patients use a mechanical ventilator at night. This lessens the stress on the phrenic nerve and removes the risk of the system failing while the patient is asleep.

Patients may be breathing independently when they first arrive in the emergency department and then experience respiratory compromise as the spinal cord becomes edematous. Edema can compress the spinal cord above the lesion, leading to symptoms at a higher level. This deterioration is usually temporary. Fatigue of the accessory muscles may also cause respiratory compromise. The intercostal muscles are not normally of major importance in respiration. However, if the diaphragm is paralyzed, the intercostal muscles become very important. As these muscles fatigue, the patient's breathing becomes shallow and rapid. Elective intubation and mechanical ventilation protect the patient from expending huge amounts of energy trying to breathe. Feeling their breathing becoming more labored is terrifying to these patients, and they need to be reassured that it is probably a temporary setback. As the edema recedes and the accessory muscles become stronger, the patient is weaned from the ventilator.

Gastrointestinal Management

Absence of bowel sounds is a common finding on examination. Oral or enteral feedings are not started until bowel function resumes. The metabolic needs of the patients are influenced by the work of breathing and the extent of other injuries. If positioning or paralytic ileus precludes oral or enteral feedings, intravenous hyperalimentation is begun.

Genitourinary Management

An indwelling urinary catheter is placed to prevent bladder distention and protect skin integrity until spinal shock resolves. Once it is determined what degree of hand function the patient will have, a bladder management program is devised.

Immobilization

The cervical spine may be immobilized with skeletal traction such as Crutchfield or Gardner-Wells tongs (Fig. 48.13).

• WORD • BUILDING •

dysreflexia: dys—abnormal + reflexia—reflex activity

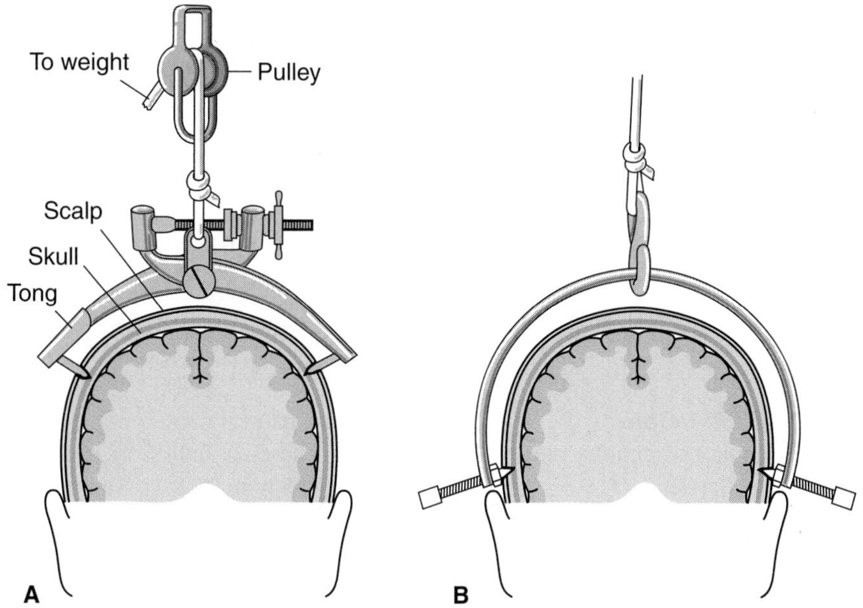
To weight
Pulley
Scalp
Skull
Tong
A
B

FIGURE 48.13 Skeletal traction for cervical injuries. (A) Crutchfield tongs. (B) Gardner-Wells tongs.

Some patients have a halo brace, a device that attaches to the skull with four small pins. The skull ring attaches to a rigid plastic vest by four poles (Fig. 48.14). This device keeps the head and neck immobile while fusion and healing take place. The advantage over traction is that the patient is not confined to bed.

Surgical Management

The goal of surgery following spinal cord injury is to stabilize the bony elements of the spine and relieve pressure on the spinal cord. Surgery may or may not improve functional outcome. Stabilization of the spine allows for earlier mobilization of the patient. This decreases the risk of complications from immobility and speeds the transition to a rehabilitation setting. Patients who have been in cervical traction before surgery may be placed in a halo brace postoperatively.

Unstable thoracic and lumbar fractures may also be treated with surgical implantation of rods to stabilize the spine. It is more difficult to stabilize these areas in the postoperative recovery period. Patients may wear a supportive corset, a rigid brace, or occasionally a body cast to supplement the support provided by the internal fixation devices. For more information, visit the Spinal Cord Injury Information Network at www.spinalcord.uab.edu.

Research is being conducted now with stem cells to help with nerve regeneration. According to the XCell-Center at the Institute for Regenerative Medicine, stem cells are harvested from the bone marrow in the hip. These stem cells are then processed in a laboratory prior to reinjection into the body. Research indicates that of 85 patients who had the stem cell treatment, there was a nearly 60% improvement in mobility and/or sensation. For more information, visit www.xcell-center.com.

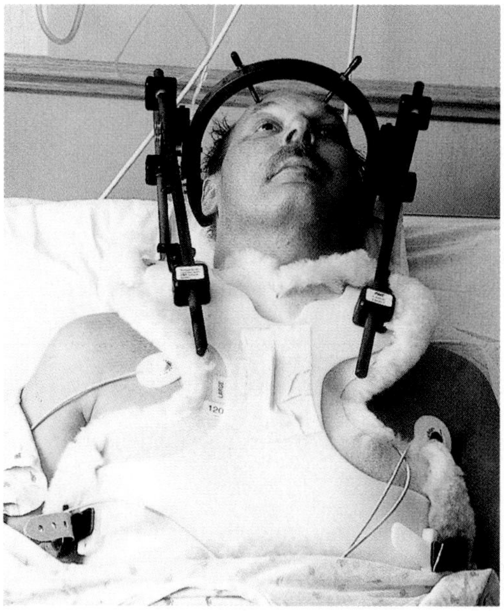

FIGURE 48.14 Halo brace.

Nursing Process for the Patient with a Spinal Cord Injury

Patients with spinal cord injury need ongoing evaluation of all body systems. Frequent neurologic and respiratory assessments are essential. Early assessment of the patient's support systems can help with discharge and rehabilitation planning. Initial goals for the patient include maintenance of safety and prevention of complications. Long-term goals include rehabilitation and maximizing remaining function.

See the *Nursing Care Plan for the Patient with a Spinal Cord Injury,* Box 48.3 (*Gerontological Issues*), and Table 48.9.

NURSING CARE PLAN for the Patient with a Spinal Cord Injury

Nursing Diagnosis: *Impaired Gas Exchange* related to respiratory muscle weakness as evidenced by Spo_2 less than 90%, abnormal ABGs

Expected Outcomes: The patient will maintain oxygenation as evidenced by Spo_2 of 90% or greater, Pao_2 of 75 mm Hg or greater, $Paco_2$ of 45 mm Hg or less.

Evaluation of Outcomes: Are ABGs and Spo_2 within normal limits?

Interventions	Rationale	Evaluation
Monitor respiratory rate, effort, ABGs, and Spo_2.	These are indicators of respiratory function. The patient may have difficulty maintaining normal respiration if diaphragm or accessory muscles are weak related to injury.	Are ABGs and Sao_2 within normal limits? Does patient appear distressed?
Notify physician immediately if Spo_2 or Pao_2 drops, or if $Paco_2$ rises.	If patient is unable to maintain blood gases, mechanical ventilation may be needed.	Are changes recognized and reported promptly?

Nursing Diagnosis: *Ineffective Airway Clearance* related to ineffective cough and decreased muscle control as evidenced by adventitious breath sounds, Spo_2 less than 90%

Expected Outcomes: The patient will maintain a clear airway as evidenced by clear breath sounds and Spo_2 of 90% or greater.

Evaluation of Outcomes: Are breath sounds clear? Is Spo_2 90% or greater?

Interventions	Rationale	Evaluation
Monitor cough and lung sounds.	Patient may not have adequate muscle strength to cough effectively.	Is patient able to cough up secretions? Is there evidence that secretions are retained?
Suction patient prn if unable to cough effectively.	To keep the airway clear.	Is suctioning effective in clearing airway?
Once the patient is stable, try assisting the patient to cough to clear secretions. Gently push upward and inward on the patient's chest while the patient coughs as strongly as possible.	This may help the patient clear secretions without invasive suctioning. This is similar to the Heimlich maneuver but not as forceful.	Does the assisted cough technique help the patient to clear the airway?
Provide humidified air and oral or enteral fluids.	Humidification helps keep secretions thin and mobile.	Are secretions thin and easily expectorated?

Nursing Diagnosis: *Risk for Autonomic Dysreflexia* related to stimuli below the level of injury

Expected Outcomes: The patient will not demonstrate signs of autonomic dysreflexia as evidenced by stable vital signs. If dysreflexia occurs, it is recognized and corrected promptly.

Evaluation of Outcomes: Is patient free of signs or are signs recognized and promptly treated?

NURSING CARE PLAN for the Patient with a Spinal Cord Injury—cont'd

Interventions	Rationale	Evaluation
Monitor for signs of autonomic dysreflexia: sudden high blood pressure, bradycardia, headache, pale skin below the injury, gooseflesh. Remember that patients with spinal cord injury are typically hypotensive, so a finding of even mild hypertension may represent a dramatic increase from their baseline blood pressure.	Autonomic dysreflexia must be recognized quickly in order to remove cause and prevent complications such as seizures, intracerebral hemorrhage, or death.	Are signs of dysreflexia present?
If you suspect autonomic dysreflexia, immediately take the patient's blood pressure and continue to monitor it every 5 minutes.	Blood pressure must be continually monitored until it is under control, to prevent complications.	Is blood pressure higher than normal for patient? Are emergency interventions warranted?
Place the patient in high-Fowler's position. Remove elastic stockings or any other garment that could prevent blood from pooling in the periphery.	High-Fowler's position utilizes the effect of orthostasis to control blood pressure. Allowing blood to pool in periphery can help reduce blood pressure.	Does position change reduce blood pressure?
Evaluate the indwelling catheter for patency. If it is not patent or a catheter is not in place and the bladder is full, obtain an order to insert a catheter immediately. Monitor blood pressure during catheterization.	A full bladder can be the cause of the stimuli causing the dysreflexia.	Is catheter patent? Is bladder full? Does emptying bladder resolve dysreflexia?
Perform a rectal examination to determine if an impaction is present. Apply anesthetic ointment to the rectum before disimpaction. Simultaneously monitor blood pressure and stop disimpaction if the blood pressure increases.	Fecal impaction can be the stimulus causing the dysreflexia. Anesthetic is used because further rectal stimulation may exacerbate symptoms.	Is impaction present? Does removal resolve dysreflexia?
If bowel or bladder distention is not present, examine the patient for other causative mechanisms. If a cause cannot be identified, or removal of the cause does not relieve hypertension, notify the physician immediately.	If the cause cannot be found and removed, an antihypertensive agent may be ordered.	Are other causes identifiable? Is an antihypertensive agent ordered?
If hypertension is treated with medication, continue to carefully monitor blood pressure.	Blood pressure may decrease rapidly once the cause of the autonomic dysreflexia is corrected.	Is blood pressure stabilized?
Once the acute episode is past, work with patient and significant others to devise a plan to prevent reoccurrence. Teach the patient how to direct caregivers in treating autonomic dysreflexia.	Episodes of dysreflexia can recur, and most can be prevented.	Do patient and caregivers verbalize understanding of how to prevent and treat future episodes of dysreflexia?

Continued

NURSING CARE PLAN for the Patient with a Spinal Cord Injury—cont'd

Nursing Diagnosis: *Reflex Urinary Incontinence* related to spinal cord damage and no sensation to void as evidenced by inability to control flow of urine

Expected Outcomes: The patient's skin will be dry and free of urine; urine elimination will be controlled.

Evaluation of Outcomes: Is patient clean and dry at all times?

Interventions	Rationale	Evaluation
Assess patient's ability to control urination.	If patient has some control, a bladder training program may be effective.	Is patient able to sense need to urinate? Is any degree of control present?
Monitor appearance of urine, temperature, and white cell count.	Cloudy urine, and an increase in temperature and white cell count indicate urinary tract infection.	Is urine clear, and temperature and white blood cell count within normal limits?
Implement a bladder training program, utilizing set times for voiding.	Following a voiding schedule can help reduce incontinence.	Is patient able to avoid incontinence with regular voiding?
Use bladder ultrasound to scan bladder for residual urine.	Incomplete voiding can increase risk for urinary tract infection.	Is patient effectively emptying bladder?
Teach the patient or caregiver self-catheterization as ordered, if bladder training is not effective.	Intermittent self-catheterization is associated with fewer complications than an indwelling catheter.	Is patient able to perform self-catheterization correctly?
Consult with physician regarding indwelling Foley catheter if patient is not a candidate for intermittent self-catheterization.	An indwelling catheter can increase risk for infection, but may be necessary as a last resort for some patients.	Is Foley catheter necessary? Are signs of infection avoided?

Nursing Diagnosis: *Constipation* related to immobility and nerve damage as evidenced by passage of hard, dry, or infrequent stools

Expected Outcomes: The patient will return to preinjury bowel pattern.

Evaluation of Outcomes: Does patient pass soft stool at regular intervals?

Interventions	Rationale	Evaluation
Assess previous and current bowel pattern and continence.	Decreased or absent sphincter tone, inability to detect the need to defecate, and immobility put the patient at risk for incontinence and constipation.	What was previous pattern? Is it used to develop goals for patient?
Monitor bowel sounds and abdominal distention.	These are indicators of bowel function.	Are bowel sounds present? Is abdomen soft?
Institute a bowel management program as soon as oral feedings are resumed. Include a suppository on a scheduled daily or every-other-day basis as ordered.	A management program including stool softeners and routine suppository use can help to restore regular defecation.	Does management program keep bowel movements soft and regular and maintain continence?
Provide a high-fiber diet with adequate fluid intake.	Fiber and fluids help keep stool soft.	Is patient receiving adequate fiber and fluids?

NURSING CARE PLAN for the Patient with a Spinal Cord Injury—cont'd

Nursing Diagnosis: *Impaired Physical Mobility* related to hemorrhage, ischemia, and edema of cord as evidenced by paresis or paralysis

Expected Outcomes: The patient will maintain maximum mobility and be free from complications of immobility.

Evaluation of Outcomes: Is patient kept mobile without contractures? Is skin intact? Can patient complete ADLs with assistance?

Interventions	Rationale	Evaluation
Determine patient's ability to move independently.	Assessment should guide interventions.	What can patient do independently?
Assess patient's ability to feel pressure and pain.	If the patient is unable to feel pain or pressure, it will be even more important to monitor skin and prevent prolonged pressure.	Can patient feel pressure and pain?
Reposition every 2 hours, utilizing supportive devices.	Unrelieved pressure on the skin, especially bony prominences, will result in ischemia and necrosis.	Is skin intact without redness?
Change positions slowly; have patient sit at side of bed before standing (if able) or getting up to a chair.	Patients with cervical spine injuries or patients remaining immobile for long periods are prone to orthostatic hypotension.	Does patient become dizzy when getting up?
Perform active or passive range-of-motion (ROM) exercises at least once every 8 hours. If patient has arm mobility, teach patient to participate in doing as much ROM as possible.	ROM exercises maintain mobility and prevent contractures.	Is patient able to perform ROM exercises with minimal difficulty?
Teach patient importance of repositioning self at least every 2 hours.	Patients with some mobility can learn to reposition themselves; this helps prevent total dependence on caregivers.	Does patient demonstrate correct repositioning every 2 hours?
Teach patient to direct own care, if unable to reposition independently.	This allows the patient some control over his or her situation.	Does patient direct own care and prevent complications of immobility?

Nursing Diagnosis: *Self-Care Deficit* related to paralysis

Expected Outcomes: The patient's self-care needs will be met by self or caregivers.

Evaluation of Outcomes: Are patient's needs met? Does patient verbalize satisfaction with care?

Interventions	Rationale	Evaluation
Determine patient's level of function and ability to perform ADLs.	The patient should be encouraged to be as independent as possible.	What is patient able to do? Is it incorporated into plan of care?

Continued

NURSING CARE PLAN for the Patient with a Spinal Cord Injury—cont'd

Interventions	Rationale	Evaluation
Explain the rationale for nursing activities, and encourage the patient and significant others to participate in hands-on care as much as possible.	This will help prepare the patient and significant others to assume responsibility for care at home.	Do patient and significant others verbalize understanding of care? Are they able to demonstrate procedures correctly?
If the patient will not be able to perform self-care, assist him or her to learn to direct care.	This allows the patient some control over his or her care.	Does patient participate by directing care?
Consult with physical and occupational therapists.	Physical and occupational therapists can help the patient learn to adapt to physical limitations; they can provide a wheelchair or other mobility aids.	Is patient adapting to limitations with help?
Discuss discharge to a rehabilitation facility with patient, physician, and discharge planner.	A rehabilitation facility can teach the patient to function independently. Some patients may require long-term care.	Is the patient a candidate for rehabilitation?
Assist patients and caregivers to determine contingency plans. These include what to do in the event of a power failure, fire, or illness of the caregiver.	Planning ahead what to do in an emergency can mean the difference between life and death for an immobile patient.	Do patient and caregivers have a plan to keep the patient safe?
Encourage the patient to establish a relationship with a primary practitioner who is familiar with spinal cord injury.	Patients with spinal cord injuries experience the same basic health care needs as individuals without injuries.	Does patient have a primary care practitioner who understands his or her unique needs?

Nursing Diagnosis: *Risk for Impaired Skin Integrity* related to immobility and possible paresthesias

Expected Outcome: The patient's skin will remain intact without redness or breakdown.

Evaluation of Outcomes: Is patient's skin intact?

Interventions	Rationale	Evaluation
Monitor skin frequently. When permitted by the physician, turn the patient frequently and assess bony prominences for redness.	The patient who does not have sensation is at increased risk of developing pressure ulcers.	Is the patient turned and repositioned at least every 2 hours? Is skin intact?
Start preventive measures in the emergency department by being sure to remove anything between the patient and the backboard.	Patients have developed pressure ulcers from lying on keys or other objects in their pockets.	Are skin surfaces protected from pressure?
Use a pressure-reducing mattress.	Specialty mattresses or beds can reduce pressure, but do not reduce the need to turn the patient.	Is the patient on an appropriate mattress?
If on a self-turning bed, make sure the patient is not sliding as the bed turns. Avoid pulling and friction on skin when repositioning patient in bed.	Sliding can cause friction and shearing damage to the skin.	Is friction damage to skin avoided?

NURSING CARE PLAN for the Patient with a Spinal Cord Injury—cont'd

Interventions	Rationale	Evaluation
Ensure that the patient's extremities do not get caught in side rails or wheelchair spokes.	The patient may not be aware this is happening, and a pressure ulcer can result.	Are all patient's body parts accounted for and safe?
If a patient is in traction or a halo brace, assess pin sites frequently. Keep the sites clean and dry, and report any sign of infection.	Skin sites are at risk for infection and breakdown.	Are pin sites clean and dry?

Nursing Diagnosis: *Risk for Ineffective Role Performance* related to effects of injury

Expected Outcomes: The patient will identify new ways to carry out essential roles.

Evaluation of Outcomes: Is patient able to identify ways to carry out roles?

Interventions	Rationale	Evaluation
Allow the patient to verbalize concerns if he or she wishes.	This may help to clarify potential role problems for the patient, and begin the process of developing a plan.	Is patient able to identify roles he or she has filled in the past that will be difficult to carry out due to injury?
Help patient and family to identify resources.	Interpersonal relationships can be significantly stressed by spinal cord injury. Friends, family, and members of the patient's religious affiliation can provide emotional and physical help.	Does patient have adequate support systems in place to provide help?
Consult a social worker to help the patient gain access to appropriate physical and financial assistance.	Loss of income may be temporary or permanent, and may add to the burden of spinal cord injury. Not all insurance policies cover the extensive inpatient rehabilitation needed by patients with spinal cord injuries. Adaptive equipment is expensive and may not be covered by insurance.	Is patient able to access appropriate financial assistance if needed?
Provide information about area support groups.	Individuals who have been through similar experiences can provide support and information for the patient and family.	Is patient willing to contact support groups?

Nursing Diagnosis: *Risk for Sexual Dysfunction* related to autonomic nervous system dysfunction

Expected Outcomes: The patient will state he or she has an acceptable means for sexual expression.

Evaluation of Outcomes: Does patient state satisfaction with sexual function?

Continued

NURSING CARE PLAN for the Patient with a Spinal Cord Injury—cont'd

Interventions	Rationale	Evaluation
If a male patient has an erection during a bath or catheterization, discontinue the procedure and continue at a later time if possible. Maintain a matter-of-fact attitude.	Male patients with quadriplegia may develop an erection during any penile stimulation.	Is patient's dignity maintained during personal care?
Allow patient to voice concerns about sexual function if desired.	Male patients with paraplegia may have difficulty achieving and maintaining an erection.	Is patient able to voice concerns? Is a consult with a urologist or other specialist needed?
Encourage the patient and partner to explore alternative methods of sexual expression.	Closeness and touching may be a satisfying alternative.	Is patient able to discuss alternative methods with partner?
If a male patient wishes to have children, encourage a consult with a fertility specialist or urologist.	Men with spinal cord injuries may not ejaculate in the normal manner. A specialist may provide some help for conception if desired.	Is patient given information about conception if desired?
Advise women who wish to become pregnant to seek an obstetrician familiar with spinal cord injuries.	A specialist may be needed to meet the unique needs of these patients.	Is the patient interested in pregnancy? Does she have the information needed related to pregnancy with spinal cord injury?
If the patient does not wish to become pregnant, provide information about contraception. See Table 48.8 for contraception for women with spinal cord injuries.	Spinal cord injury does not impair female fertility.	Does the patient have information and resources to prevent pregnancy if desired?
Encourage partners to verbalize feelings about caregiving activities such as catheterizations and make alternative arrangements for care if possible. Some patients with the financial resources to do so may choose to hire an attendant rather than rely on significant others for personal care.	Performing tasks such as catheterization or bowel care may interfere with feelings of intimacy between partners.	Are patient and partner able to discuss feelings about caregiving activities and find alternate arrangements if desired?

Nursing Diagnosis: *Anxiety* related to change in health status as evidenced by behavioral changes such as insomnia, poor eye contact, and irritability

Expected Outcomes: The patient will participate in rehabilitation activities. The patient will be able to verbalize fears, concerns, and expectations.

Evaluation of Outcomes: Is the patient able to participate in rehabilitation? Does patient verbalize that anxiety is controlled?

Interventions	Rationale	Evaluation
Allow patient to voice feelings of fear and anxiety.	Communication is vital to assess the patient's coping abilities.	Is the patient able to verbalize anxiety?

NURSING CARE PLAN for the Patient with a Spinal Cord Injury—cont'd

Interventions	Rationale	Evaluation
Provide information about what is happening to the patient physiologically and about procedures.	Understanding of what is happening can help the patient cope with changes.	Does patient verbalize understanding of what is happening? Does information help keep patient less fearful?
Consult a social worker, pastoral care, and/or support groups.	A social worker or pastor can help provide emotional and spiritual support. Discussing rehabilitation with patients and their families who have had similar experiences can provide insight and encouragement.	Does patient state talking with support persons helps reduce anxiety?
Encourage the patient to participate in physical and occupational therapy.	Seeing progress toward becoming independent may help reduce anxiety and fear about the future.	Does patient participate in therapies? Is anxiety lessening?

TABLE 48.8 BIRTH CONTROL ISSUES FOR PATIENTS WITH SPINAL CORD INJURY

Method	Comments
Oral contraceptives	Contraindicated because of the risk of deep venous thrombosis
Diaphragm	May be difficult to insert for a patient with poor hand function
Intrauterine device	Patient may not feel device move out of position
	Patient may not feel perforation of uterus
Norplant	No contraindications
Condom	No contraindications

Box 48.3
Gerontological Issues

Aging with Spinal Cord Injury

Individuals aging with a spinal cord injury (SCI) have an increased risk for developing complications in the following areas:

- Blood pressure control
- Abnormalities in carbohydrate and lipid metabolism related to immobilization
- Cardiovascular disease
- Respiratory complications
- Osteoporosis
- Bladder infections
- Skin ulcers
- Chronic pain

NEURODEGENERATIVE DISORDERS AND DEMENTIA

Neurodegenerative is a term that can apply to any nervous system disorder that causes degeneration, or wasting, of the neurons in the nervous system. The disorders discussed in this section are some of the most common neurodegenerative disorders that cause chronic illness. By the year 2030, it is estimated that 150 million Americans will have one or more chronic conditions. Management of chronic conditions does not focus on the short-term stay in the hospital due to a exacerbation of the disease process, but rather on the long-term goal of facilitating the patient and family to cope with the disease process and maintain the patient's independence for as long as possible. Nursing care involves providing information on management of the illness, education related to prevention and

• WORD • BUILDING •

neurodegenerative: neuro—nervous system + degenerative—deteriorating

TABLE 48.9 SPINAL CORD INJURY SUMMARY

Signs and Symptoms	Flaccid paralysis and paresthesias (depending on level of the lesion) Loss of reflex activity below the level of the lesion Spinal shock initially Risk for autonomic dysreflexia (injuries above sixth thoracic vertebra)
Diagnostic Tests	Radiograph CT scan MRI
Therapeutic Measures	Immobilization Maintenance of airway and respiratory status Bowel and bladder training Nutrition/diet Activity/rehabilitation Prevention of dysreflexia Prevention of skin breakdown Sexual counseling Education
Complications	Infection Deep venous thrombosis Paralysis Orthostatic hypotension Pressure ulcers Depression
Priority Nursing Diagnoses	*Impaired Gas Exchange* *Ineffective Airway Clearance* *Risk for Autonomic Dysreflexia* *Reflex Urinary Incontinence* *Constipation* *Impaired Physical Mobility*

treatment of complications, and guidance to support groups or case managers. As patients decline, many families will come to a time when they can no longer care for their loved one in their homes and must consider care in a long-term facility.

Dementia

Dementia is not a disease, but rather is a symptom of a number of different disorders. According to the National Institute of Neurological Disorders and Stroke (2009), "People with dementia have significantly impaired intellectual functioning that interferes with normal activities and relationships. They also lose their ability to solve problems and maintain emotional control, and they may experience personality changes and behavioral problems, such as agitation, delusions, and hallucinations. While memory loss is a common symptom of dementia, memory loss by itself does not mean that a person has dementia." Some patients may have mild mental status changes that do not interfere significantly with day-to-day functioning. This is sometimes referred to as mild cognitive impairment, or MCI. However, patients with MCI are more likely to go on to develop Alzheimer's disease than those without MCI.

• WORD • BUILDING •
dementia: de—down or from + mental—the mind

Etiology and Pathophysiology

There are many causes of dementia, including Huntington's, Parkinson's, and Alzheimer's diseases, which are discussed later in this chapter. Multiple "mini-strokes" (multi-infarct dementia or vascular dementia) are another common cause. Chronic alcoholism, neurologic infections, head injuries, and many medications (Box 48.4) also can cause changes in mental status leading to dementia. Although aging is associated with more frequent dementia diagnoses, dementia is not a normal part of aging. Pathophysiologies vary depending on the cause. In general, thinking is affected by changes in the brain that result from reduced blood flow or from structural changes related to disease states.

Much research has been done to determine factors related to dementia; such knowledge helps in its prevention. Some studies indicate that patients who have more education, have higher socioeconomic status, and engage in stimulating intellectual and leisure activities are less likely to develop dementia. Some experts believe these individuals develop a sort of "cognitive reserve" that keeps them functioning at a high level, even when changes in their brains on autopsy indicate dementia. People with less education, fewer leisure activities, and less intellectual stimulation are more likely to develop symptoms of Alzheimer's disease.

Signs and Symptoms

Most people have occasional memory lapses. Students may have memory lapses during examinations, but they

Box 48.4

Some Medications That Can Cause Confusion

- Anticholinergics (atropine, some antihistamines)
- Analgesics (meperidine, morphine)
- Cimetidine (Tagamet)
- Central nervous system depressants (sleeping pills, tranquilizers, alcohol)
- Steroids (cortisone, prednisone)

do not generally have dementia. In patients with dementia, recent memories are usually affected first. Patients may have difficulty recalling whether they ate breakfast, or may accuse a family member of not calling when in reality they called just a few hours earlier. This same patient, however, may easily recall an event or even a phone number from childhood.

As patients become more forgetful, they may ask the same questions repeatedly. They may get lost driving or walking in a familiar neighborhood. They may become disoriented to time, and not be aware of the year. A patient may say that Eisenhower is president, for example, because they remember that as true when they were younger. Later, they may not recognize where they are, and last, they may lose recognition of their own family members.

Later in the course of the dementia, even remote memory may be lost. Patients may forget how to perform simple tasks, such as doing the dishes or making a phone call. They may wander and become lost. Safety is a significant issue with a wandering patient. Patients may develop aphasia and become unable to communicate their needs or follow simple instructions. This can become very frustrating to both the family and nursing caregivers. Behavioral problems may necessitate admission to a long-term care facility. In very late stages, the patient may become totally dependent on caregivers.

Diagnostic Tests

Diagnosis of dementia is twofold: First, dementia must be identified, and then the focus moves to finding the cause of the mental status change. Early diagnosis is essential, because some causes of MCI may be reversible, and early treatment may delay progression. Neuropsychological testing can determine the degree of memory, personality, and behavior changes. The Mini-Mental State Examination is commonly used. The patient should also be tested for depression, because depression can cause mental status changes, but is often easily treated. A review of medications by a knowledgeable nurse, physician, or pharmacist may reveal a medication that can be contributing to the mental changes. MRI, CT scan, positron emission tomographic (PET) scan, and blood tests help diagnose underlying causes.

Therapeutic Measures

Medical interventions depend on the cause of the dementia. See Table 48.10 for medications that may be used to delay progression of Alzheimer's dementia. If medical treatment cannot alter the course of the disease, the focus will shift to delaying progression of symptoms and maintaining patient safety. Excellent nursing care becomes essential for both the patient and family at this point. An important aspect of care in early dementia is determination of the patient's wishes while the patient is still able to make decisions. Some difficult decisions relate to the patient's continued ability to drive and live alone. Other decisions related to resuscitation, guardianship, and powers of attorney for health care and finances are essential to discuss.

Nursing Process for the Patient with Dementia

See the *Nursing Care Plan for the Patient with Dementia.*

Delirium

Whereas dementia is chronic and progressive, **delirium** is a mental disturbance that is temporary, and can have either a rapid or gradual onset. Delirium is considered to be a

TABLE 48.10 MEDICATIONS USED TO TREAT ALZHEIMER'S DEMENTIA

Medication Class/Action	Examples	Route	Side Effects	Nursing Implications
Cholinesterase Inhibitors				
Inhibit cholinesterase, to improve function of acetylcholine in CNS. May improve cognitive function but will not alter course of disease.	donepezil (Aricept) tacrine (Cognex) rivastigmine (Exelon) galantamine (Reminyl)	PO, patch (Exelon)	Headache, diarrhea, nausea	Must be taken regularly; patient may need reminders to take, or family member may need to assist. Monitor for weight loss and report to physician.
NMDA Antagonist				
Reduces binding of glutamate, an excitatory neurotransmitter.	memantine (Namenda)	PO tablets, oral solution	Dizziness	Teach patient and family that improvements may take months.

NURSING CARE PLAN for the Patient with Dementia

Nursing Diagnosis: *Risk for Injury* related to impaired memory, thought processes, and judgment

Expected Outcomes: The patient will remain free from injury.

Evaluation of Outcomes: Is patient safe and free from injury? Is environment safe?

Interventions	Rationale	Evaluation
Monitor patient's ability to maintain safety.	As dementia worsens, the patient's needs change.	Is patient able to make decisions and negotiate the environment safely?
Keep environment simple and familiar; label doors and objects. Keep patient in familiar environment as long as possible.	Change can result in confusion; even a minor change in furniture arrangement can result in falls.	Is patient able to remain in the home with minimum confusion and without injury?
Remove harmful objects (scissors, matches); store medicines in locked cabinet; remove knobs from stoves.	Impaired judgment can make safety a major concern for patients who live at home.	Is the environment safe for the patient?
Make sure patient has eyeglasses and hearing aids if necessary.	Impaired sensory perception can increase confusion and risk of falls.	Is patient able to see and hear effectively?
Use night-lights; remove throw rugs; use safety gates on stairs.	These can reduce the risk for falls.	Is environment set up to reduce risk of falling?
Have identification bracelet on patient and ID tags sewn into clothes, and locks on doors to prevent leaving.	Patients may wander, making them prone to injury.	Is wandering confined to a monitored area? Is environment set up to allow movement within a safe area?
Provide daily walks or exercise.	Exercise can decrease wandering.	Does exercise reduce wandering?

Nursing Diagnosis: *Imbalanced Nutrition: Less Than Body Requirements* related to impaired thought processes and lack of interest or refusal to eat, poor muscle tone, weight loss

Expected Outcomes: The patient will maintain adequate food intake and weight within normal limits for height.

Evaluation of Outcomes: Does patient maintain appropriate weight?

Interventions	Rationale	Evaluation
Monitor intake, weight, and serum albumin.	Loss of weight or a serum albumin level of less than 3.5 indicates poor nutrition.	Are weight and serum albumin level stable and within normal limits?
Develop meal plan to include likes and dislikes, snacks, and protein supplements as necessary.	Using the patient's favorite foods will encourage eating.	Is patient consuming majority of meals?
Offer larger meal when patient has the greatest appetite or serve small meals five to six times a day.	A lot of food at one time may feel overwhelming to the patient.	Is patient eating meals that are served?
Offer one food at a time if patient is not successful with a whole plate full.	Too many choices on a plate may feel overwhelming to the patient.	Does patient eat more if one food at a time is offered?
Offer finger foods.	Utensils may be difficult for the patient to use and may discourage eating.	Does patient eat more when finger foods are offered?
Also see Box 48.5, *Nutrition Notes.*		

NURSING CARE PLAN for the Patient with Dementia—cont'd

Nursing Diagnosis: *Chronic Confusion* related to dementia as evidenced by disorientation and inability to concentrate or follow directions.

Expected Outcomes: The patient will function at optimal cognitive level.

Evaluation of Outcomes: Is patient maintaining optimum cognitive function?

Interventions	Rationale	Evaluation
Monitor changes in thought processes.	As cognitive function declines, care plan will need to be revised.	Is patient able to correctly identify objects, remember tasks, speak clearly, identify person, place, and time?
Provide a box of safe, familiar items, such as empty thread spools, or pretty handkerchiefs for women.	Patients often rummage through drawers, closets, or boxes. These patients may not recognize the difference between their own possessions and those of others. Keeping them occupied with a box of safe items may decrease their need to look for things.	Does a box of items keep patient occupied and content?
Place calendars, clocks, personal items, and seasonal decorations in patient's environment.	These provide orientation to the present.	Can patient identify the season or year?
If patient hallucinates or has delusions, do not attempt to correct. Focus instead on the feelings related to the hallucinations, such as "Do you feel frightened?"	Having feelings validated may help develop trust, while not validating the hallucination.	Does patient respond to refocusing on feelings?
Reduce stressors such as fatigue, overstimulation, or pain.	Stress may increase dysfunctional behaviors.	Are stressors eliminated as much as possible? Is patient's behavior calm?
Maintain patient's usual routines as much as possible.	Familiar routines such as sleeping or eating habits are more comfortable for patients. Change can be stressful.	Are routines organized around the patient rather than the staff?
Communicate clearly. Make eye contact, speak slowly and directly to the patient, use nonverbal gestures.	Unclear communication can increase confusion and stress.	Do all staff communicate clearly and respectfully with the patient?
Involve family in care planning and implementation.	The family knows the patient's preferences and routines best.	Does family presence help patient stay calm and function at optimum level?
Provide video or audiotapes of patient's family members.	Familiar sounds and pictures may reduce agitation when family is not present.	Do video or audiotapes help calm the patient?

Continued

NURSING CARE PLAN for the Patient with Dementia—cont'd

Nursing Diagnosis: *Risk for Caregiver Role Strain* related to demands of caring for patient with declining mental status while balancing other demands

Expected Outcomes: The caregiver will have support needed to safely manage care of patient. The caregiver will be able to identify when the patient is too difficult to care for and requires more structured observation.

Evaluation of Outcomes: Is caregiver managing demands of caring for patient? Is patient safe? Is additional support or a change in environment for patient indicated?

Interventions	Rationale	Evaluation
Allow caregiver to verbalize concerns related to burden of caring for patient.	An assessment of caregiver concerns and challenges can help the nurse plan appropriate support.	Does the caregiver share concerns? What are the caregiver's current support systems?
Observe for signs of depression or stress in the caregiver.	A stressed or depressed caregiver may have difficulty providing safe care for the patient.	Are signs of stress present? Does patient care appear to be suffering?
Encourage caregiver to identify family and friends that can provide support. If they are involved in a local church or religious organization, encourage caregiver to make his or her needs known.	There are often resources in the family or community that can be accessed without cost, and are able to help if they know the need exists.	Can caregiver identify potential resources to contact?
Refer for assistance with caregiving and/or day care utilizing Alzheimer's support groups and resources.	Formal support systems in the community may be available to help relieve some of the caregiver's burden.	Is caregiver able to obtain support and take some time for himself or herself?
Encourage caregiver to use support systems identified to allow him or her time to care for self; encourage to take care of own health needs, and enjoy some respite time doing something enjoyable on a regular basis.	If the caregiver becomes ill due to the stress of caregiving, he or she will no longer be able to assist the patient.	Does caregiver maintain own physical and emotional health?
Allow the caregiver to grieve over the losses he or she is experiencing: losses in the patient as well as loss of control over his or her own life.	As the disease progresses, the patient gradually loses awareness of the neurologic deterioration. Occasional lucid moments can be very difficult for patient and caregiver as they realize what has been lost.	Is the caregiver able to identify feelings of grief, anger, or sorrow?
Discuss progression of the disease process and the possibility of transferring the patient to an extended care facility.	The caregiver may feel guilt over not being able to care for the patient, and may need permission to consider extended care facility placement.	Is caregiver able to identify when home care is too demanding, and choose an alternative arrangement?

Box 48.5

Nutrition Notes

Managing Mealtimes for Patients with Dementia

Dining rooms should be quiet and have adequate lighting. Occupying the same chair for every meal lends familiarity. Serving one course at a time and providing necessary but not extraneous flatware, large handled if needed, limits distractions. Dishes with high sides enable the patient to scoop the food onto a spoon or fork. Finger foods that the patient can manage may increase intake with minimal staff assistance.

Patients with dementia must be reminded of the steps involved in self-feeding:

- Putting the food on the spoon
- Directing it to the mouth
- Swallowing.

Use of verbal cues or guiding the patient's hand to start the necessary movement helps the process. Common courtesies model social expectations and help maintain a person's dignity:

- Introducing the patient to the other persons at the table
- Providing a cup rather than a carton for milk
- Offering foods separately rather than mixing them all together.

Quiet music with a slow tempo may relax the patient and help block out environmental noises that might otherwise be startling. It might help relax staff also!

medical emergency and should be diagnosed and treated promptly. Delirium is characterized by disorganized thinking and difficulty staying focused, and is seen most commonly in older adults when experiencing an illness. Many times response to medications is the cause (see Box 48.4). The disturbance may also be the result of anything that is a stressor to the person's body, such as pain, oxygen deficiency, urinary catheters, fluid and electrolyte imbalances, a change in environment, or nutritional deficiency. Often the most effective nursing intervention is to have a family member present to assist with orientation and reassurance. Additionally, it is beneficial to have continuity in nursing personnel when possible.

It is essential that delirium not be mistaken for dementia. If an older adult is hospitalized and exhibits new-onset confusion, consider that it might be delirium. Correcting electrolyte levels, controlling pain, changing medications, or administering oxygen can be helpful in reversing delirium. See the *Nursing Care Plan for the Patient with Dementia* for nursing interventions.

Parkinson's Disease

Parkinson's disease is a chronic degenerative movement disorder that arises in the basal ganglia in the cerebrum. It usually begins in the fourth or fifth decade of life, with symptoms becoming progressively worse as the patient ages. The disease is characterized by tremors, changes in posture and gait, rigidity, and slowness of movements. Approximately 60,000 new cases of Parkinson's disease are diagnosed each year in the United States (National Parkinson Foundation, 2010).

Pathophysiology

The substantia nigra is a group of cells located within the basal ganglia, which is situated deep within the brain. These cells are responsible for the production of dopamine, an inhibitory neurotransmitter. Dopamine facilitates the transmission of impulses from one neuron to another. Parkinson's disease is caused by destruction of the cells of the substantia nigra, resulting in decreased dopamine production. Loss of dopamine function results in impairment of semiautomatic movements. Parkinson's disease is sometimes referred to as an extrapyramidal disorder because the extrapyramidal tracts in the spinal cord that contain motor neurons are affected.

Acetylcholine, an excitatory neurotransmitter, is secreted normally in individuals with Parkinson's disease. The normal balance of acetylcholine and dopamine is interrupted in these patients, causing a relative excess of acetylcholine, which results in the tremor, muscle rigidity, and **akinesia** (loss of muscle movement) characteristic of Parkinson's disease.

Etiology

The etiology of Parkinson's disease is unknown. It was first described in 1817 by London surgeon James Parkinson. Although scientists now know that the symptoms are caused by death of dopamine-producing cells in the substantia nigra, they do not know what causes the cells to die. There may be a genetic component, especially in younger patients. Certain environmental toxins may also play a role. Parkinson's disease–like symptoms, referred to as parkinsonism, may be associated with use of certain drugs, such as phenothiazines. Parkinsonism was also linked to an outbreak of encephalitis in the 1920s.

Signs and Symptoms

The onset of symptoms in patients with Parkinson's disease is usually gradual and subtle. A substantial percentage of the dopamine-producing cells are nonfunctional before the patient becomes symptomatic. Symptoms may be mistakenly attributed to aging or fatigue. In retrospect, patients and their significant others often identify a long period in which symptoms were present but not identified as symptoms of Parkinson's disease.

• WORD • BUILDING •

akinesia: a—not + kinesia—movement

The primary symptoms of Parkinson's disease are muscular rigidity, **bradykinesia** (slow movement) or akinesia, changes in posture, and tremors. The brain is no longer able to direct the muscles to perform in the usual manner. This lack of communication between the brain and the muscles can have a profound impact on the patient's ability to ambulate safely, perform ADLs and job functions, or enjoy leisure activities. The symptoms may also have a significant negative impact on the patient's self-esteem.

The patient may have difficulty initiating movement; this may be particularly apparent when the patient tries to start walking, rise from a sitting position, or begin dressing. Because considerable effort is required to move the rigid muscles, the patient performs voluntary movements very slowly. At times, the patient may experience "freezing" of gait, and be unable to initiate ambulation or negotiate a turn during ambulation.

The extensor muscles are more affected by Parkinson's disease than the flexor muscles. This impaired function of the extensor muscles results in the stooped posture typical of patients with Parkinson's disease (Fig. 48.15). Flexion of the hips, knees, and neck shifts the center of gravity forward. The gait is characterized by shuffling, short steps that may increase in speed once the patient finally gets walking, and the patient may have difficulty stopping. The patient maintains a broad base when making turns to try to compensate for imbalance. These changes place patients at high risk for falls. Slowness of movement and stiff muscles make it much harder for patients to catch themselves if they start to fall or to relax the muscles to minimize injury.

Tremors typically begin in the hand and then progress to the **ipsilateral** foot. In most patients, the tremor then moves to the **contralateral** side. Many patients identify one side of the body as being more affected by the tremor than the other. Tremor of the hand has been described as a pill-rolling tremor; the thumb typically moves back and forth across the fingers and looks like the patient is rolling a pill. Tremors typically lessen or disappear during movement and are more noticeable when the extremity is at rest or when trying to hold an object still (this is called a resting tremor). The tremors disappear when the patient is asleep. The inability to hold an object still can make simple acts such as drinking a glass of water or reading a book nearly impossible. The signs and symptoms of Parkinson's disease tend to increase in severity when the patient becomes fatigued. Another type of tremor, a benign familial (or essential) tremor, may sometimes be mistaken for Parkinson's disease. Treatment is different for each. See Table 48.11 for differentiation of these tremors.

The secondary symptoms of Parkinson's disease include generalized weakness, muscle fatigue and cramping, and difficulty with fine motor activities. This fine motor dysfunction may make it difficult for the patient to button a shirt or tie shoes. Handwriting typically deteriorates as the disease progresses. A soft, monotone voice

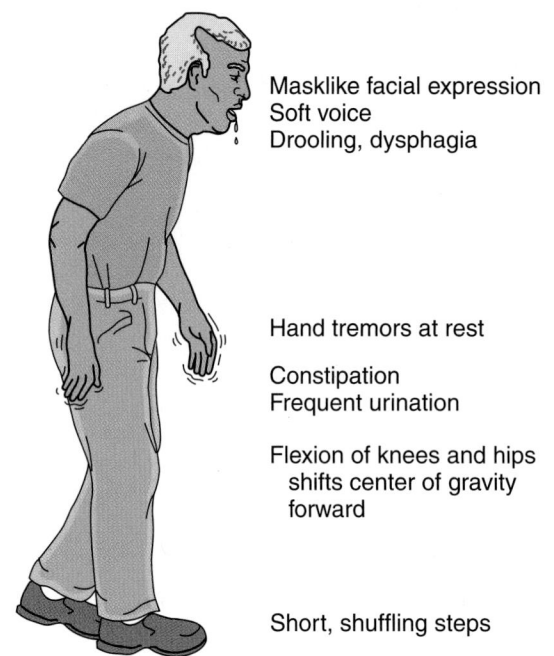

Masklike facial expression
Soft voice
Drooling, dysphagia
Hand tremors at rest
Constipation
Frequent urination
Flexion of knees and hips shifts center of gravity forward
Short, shuffling steps

FIGURE 48.15 Manifestations of Parkinson's disease.

• WORD • BUILDING •

bradykinesia: brady—slow + kinesia—movement
ipsilateral: ipsi—same + lateral—side
contralateral: contra—opposite + lateral—side

TABLE 48.11 SYMPTOMS OF PARKINSON'S DISEASE VERSUS ESSENTIAL TREMOR

Disease	Parkinson's Tremor	Benign Familial
Resting tremor	Yes	No
Intention tremor (with movement)	No	Yes
Pill-rolling tremor	Yes	No
Head/voice tremor	No	Yes
Relieved with beta-blocking medication (propranolol)	No	Yes
Relieved with anti-Parkinson's medications	Yes	No

and mask-like facial expression may make the patient appear to be lacking in emotional responses. It may be necessary to ask patients about their emotional status and help them develop ways of expressing their emotions. The normal blink response is diminished, so the patient and significant others must be educated about eye care to prevent corneal abrasions.

Dysfunction of the autonomic system may cause diaphoresis, constipation, orthostatic hypotension, drooling, dysphagia, seborrhea, and frequent urination. Patients who experience seborrhea and diaphoresis need frequent attention to personal hygiene. Drooling and dysphagia may make the patient reluctant to appear in public. Slowness in initiating walking, balance problems, and frequent urination place the patient at risk for urinary incontinence, which may also increase the patient's reluctance to leave home.

Late in the disease, mental function may become slowed and the patient may develop dementia. This is compounded by the side effects of many anti-Parkinson's drugs. Death is usually from complications of immobility.

Complications

The most typical acute complications of Parkinson's disease are related to the patient's difficulties with mobility and balance. Patients are very prone to falls, which may result in injuries ranging from bruises or fractures to head or spinal cord injuries. Constipation is common because of decreased activity, diminished ability to take in food and fluids, and side effects of anticholinergic medications. Patients are encouraged to increase fiber and fluids in their diet. If constipation is not alleviated by dietary modifications, the patient may need to use stool softeners.

Muscular rigidity and bradykinesia contribute to joint immobility, which decreases patients' ability to ambulate and care for themselves. Position changes may be painful for patients. A turning sheet and adequate personnel are necessary when turning a patient in bed to prevent stress on the joints. Tremors interfere with ADLs, consume immense amounts of energy, and may prevent the patient from working or performing leisure activities. Swallowing may become so impaired that enteral (tube) feeding is required. Depression is a common complication at any stage of Parkinson's disease and may compromise communication, ability to learn, and performance of ADLs. Patients may require counseling or antidepressants.

Diagnostic Tests

No specific tests are used to diagnose Parkinson's disease. The diagnosis is based on the history given by the patient and a thorough physical examination. An MRI may be done to rule out alternative causes of the patient's symptoms.

Therapeutic Measures

There is no cure for Parkinson's disease. Treatment is aimed at controlling symptoms and maximizing the patient's functional level. Drugs used to control symptoms are listed in Table 48.12.

Many patients with Parkinson's disease experience fluctuations in motor function related to their drug therapy. This is referred to as the on-off phenomenon. Patients may experience a decreased response to levodopa, or off period,

TABLE 48.12 MEDICATIONS USED TO TREAT PARKINSON'S DISEASE

Medication Class/Action	Examples	Route	Side Effects	Nursing Implications
Cholinergic Blockers				
Blocks the action of acetylcholine to control tremor and salivation.	trihexyphenidyl (Artane), benztropine (Cogentin)	PO	Urine retention, dry mouth, constipation, blurred vision, dizziness, confusion	Monitor I&O for urinary retention. Teach patient not to discontinue abruptly. Implement measures to prevent constipation.
Dopamine Agonist				
Facilitates release of dopamine.	amantadine (Symmetrel)	PO	Ataxia, hypotension, dizziness, confusion	Use caution with alcohol and other CNS agents.
Dopamine Agonists				
Convert into dopamine in the brain.	levodopa (L-dopa) levodopa/carbidopa combination (Sinemet). Carbidopa prevents peripheral breakdown of levodopa so more is available in the CNS.	PO	Nausea, vomiting, dyskinesias	Teach patient to take food shortly after (not before or with) each dose to prevent gastric irritation. May discolor urine and sweat. Teach patient to take ATC to control symptoms.

Continued

TABLE 48.12 MEDICATIONS USED TO TREAT PARKINSON'S DISEASE—cont'd

Medication Class/Action	Examples	Route	Side Effects	Nursing Implications
Dopamine Agonist				
Stimulates dopamine receptors in the brain.	pramipexole (Mirapex)	PO	Nausea, dizziness, weakness. May cause sudden excessive sleepiness; constipation, dry mouth.	Patients may fall asleep suddenly; caution patient to avoid driving until effects known. Giving with meals may reduce nausea.
	ropinirole (Requip)	PO	Drowsiness, dizziness, syncope, sleep attacks	Caution about drowsiness and sleep attacks (falling asleep during activities that require alertness).
Monoamine Oxidase B Inhibitor				
Blocks metabolism of central dopamine, increasing dopamine in CNS.	selegiline (Eldepryl, Zelapar), rasagiline (Azilect)	PO Zelapar is an orally dissolving tablet.	Nausea, dizziness, confusion, insomnia	May slow progression of Parkinson's disease. Administer daily at noon to prevent insomnia. Can cause dangerous interaction with meperidine (Demerol), alcohol, CNS depressants.
COMT Inhibitor				
Blocks the enzyme COMT to prevent breakdown of levodopa, prolonging levodopa action. For use with Sinemet.	entacapone (Comtan)	PO	Dyskinesias, hallucinations, nausea, diarrhea, yellow-orange urine, rhabdomyolysis, neuroleptic malignant syndrome	Report elevated temperature, muscular rigidity, altered LOC, elevated CPK.

ATC = around the clock; COMT = catechol-*O*-methyltransferase; CPK = creatine phosphokinase; I&O = input and output; LOC = level of consciousness.

Note: With all anti–Parkinson's disease agents, teach patient to check with physician before taking over-the-counter medications, especially cold preparations. Teach to rise slowly to prevent orthostasis.

particularly as the dose is wearing off. As the disease progresses, patients may notice that the off periods become less predictable and occur more rapidly. The patient may have a delayed or absent response to the next dose of levodopa, resulting in the patient being stuck in the off stage and being significantly disabled for that period. Fluctuations in motor function may be accompanied by other symptoms, such as pain, diaphoresis, anxiety attacks, hallucinations, or mood swings. These symptoms significantly increase the disability associated with the episodes.

Patients who are taking maximum doses of medication for Parkinson's disease symptoms may benefit from a "drug holiday." During a drug holiday, patients are taken off all drugs for a time, then restarted on lower doses. Hospitalization may be necessary during this time to maintain patient safety.

Surgical Treatments

Pallidotomy may be an option for patients whose rigidity, tremor, and bradykinesia are uncontrollable by medical management. During this stereotactic procedure, a destructive lesion is placed in the basal ganglia. The surgery is only performed on one side of the brain. The patient remains awake during the surgery to make sure that the lesion is being placed in the appropriate location. These patients need a great deal of education and support before and during the surgery.

Deep-brain stimulation is another surgical treatment, in which a tiny electrode is placed into brain tissue. A generator is then implanted under the skin on the chest, and is connected to the electrode. The generator delivers electrical pulses to the electrode, which may help control symptoms.

Some centers have experimented with implanting stem cells into the brain to develop into dopamine-producing cells; research into gene therapies is also ongoing. These therapies are only experimental at this time. For more information, visit the National Parkinson Foundation at www.parkinson.org.

Nursing Process for the Patient with Parkinson's Disease

DATA COLLECTION. Ask the patient about symptoms of Parkinson's disease and their effect on level of functioning.

Observe ability to move, walk, and perform ADLs safely. Determine risk for injury related to immobility or falls. Assess nutritional status and condition of skin. Identify presence of confusion and side effects of medications. Psychosocial assessment includes the patient's and caregiver's responses to the disease, coping strategies, and support systems.

NURSING DIAGNOSES, PLANNING, AND IMPLEMENTATION. The patient with Parkinson's disease is at risk for many problems. Priority diagnoses are addressed below. If confusion is present, also see the *Nursing Care Plan for the Patient with Dementia.*

Impaired Physical Mobility Related to Muscle Stiffness and Tremor as Evidenced by Unstable Gait, Difficulty with Motor Coordination

EXPECTED OUTCOME: The patient will maintain optimal mobility and ability to ambulate as long as possible.

- Assist patient to plan daily activities based on anticipated response to medications. *Certain times of day may be less troublesome than others.*
- Consult with physical and occupational therapists to provide assistive devices *to help maintain mobility and provide diversional activities.*
- Provide assistance with range-of-motion exercises *to maintain flexibility of muscles.*
- Teach patients who have difficulty initiating walking to pick up one foot as though attempting to step over something to take the first step. It may also help to take several steps in place before starting to walk. *This may help overcome freezing of gait.*

Self-Care Deficit Related to Reduced Mobility as Evidenced by Inability to Carry Out ADLs

EXPECTED OUTCOME: The patient's self-care needs will be met as evidenced by patient statement

- Encourage the patient to participate in ADLs as much as possible. *This helps the patient maintain independence and self-esteem.*
- Consult occupational therapist *to assist with devices and strategies for maintaining independence.*
- Instruct the patient or family to provide clothing without buttons and supply shoes with adherent fasteners, rather than shoelaces, *to help maintain independence.*
- Assist the patient and family to make decisions about long-term care. Consult a social worker as needed for assistance. *As the patient ages, so do the significant others who are providing care. The point may be reached at which the caregiver is no longer able to meet the increasing needs of the patient. The decision to place the patient in a skilled nursing facility is extremely difficult and emotional.*

Risk for Injury Related to Reduced Mobility and Balance

EXPECTED OUTCOME: The patient will remain safe and without injury.

- If the patient is in the hospital or extended care facility, keep the call light within reach at all times. Remind the patient to request assistance with ambulation. *The patient is at risk for injury from falls related to problems with mobility.*
- Maintain bed in the low position, with side rails raised if appropriate (side rails may be prohibited in some institutions). *Maintaining the bed in a low position reduces the risk of injury or fall when getting out of bed. Side rails may increase the risk of injury, and must be used carefully.*
- Use an alarm system that alerts the staff that the patient is getting up *so that staff can assist the patient to get up and ambulate.*
- Avoid use of restraints. *Restraints can increase the risk of injury.*
- Keep environment free from clutter, throw rugs, or other items *that may cause a patient to trip.*
- Provide walkers and other assistive devices *to provide support and prevent falls.*

EVALUATION. The care of the patient with Parkinson's disease has been successful if the patient remains as mobile and independent as possible. Self-care needs should be met by the patient or others, and the patient should remain safe from injury.

CRITICAL THINKING

Ms. Simpson

■ Ms. Simpson is a 47-year-old Caucasian woman. She has had Parkinson's disease for the last 5 years, and the symptoms are becoming progressively worse. She is now admitted for a urinary tract infection.

1. What problems do you foresee when caring for Ms. Simpson?
2. What safety measures should you implement?
3. Ms. Simpson is receiving IV fluids of 5% dextrose in 0.45% saline, 1000 mL over 12 hours. The RN on duty is accountable for her IV, but as you are bathing her you notice that the bag is nearly full and it has been hanging for 4 hours. How many milliliters should still be in her IV bag after 4 hours?

Suggested answers at end of chapter.

Huntington's Disease

Huntington's disease is a progressive, hereditary, degenerative, incurable neurologic disorder. It was first described in 1872 by George Huntington, a general practitioner in

New York. The uncontrolled movements associated with Huntington's disease caused some sufferers in the 17th century to be accused of and executed for witchcraft. Many of the cases around the world can be traced back to specific individuals.

Pathophysiology and Etiology

Huntington's disease (also known as Huntington's chorea) is inherited in an autosomal dominant manner, which means that each offspring of an affected parent has a 50% chance of inheriting the disorder. A mutation in a specific gene has been identified; however, the cause of the mutation is not known. According to a study completed recently at Johns Hopkins in Baltimore, Maryland, a protein called Rhes may be responsible for the activation of a mutant protein that causes destruction of the cells in the corpus striatum (Saey, 2009). Destruction also occurs in the caudate nucleus and other deep nuclei of the brain and portions of the cerebral cortex. This degeneration results in progressive loss of normal movement and intellect. The rate of disease progression varies from person to person.

Signs and Symptoms

Signs and symptoms usually begin in middle age and develop slowly, becoming progressively more apparent. Cognitive signs may be noticed before movement problems. Patients who are not aware of their hereditary risk for Huntington's disease may be incorrectly diagnosed as being mentally ill.

The patient may display personality changes and inappropriate behavior. The patient may be euphoric or irritable and may rapidly alternate between moods. Paranoia is common, and behavior may become violent as dementia worsens. The patient eventually progresses to the point at which he or she is incontinent and totally dependent on others for care. These symptoms are difficult for family and friends as well as professional caregivers to cope with. The disease progression and associated symptoms are particularly devastating for offspring, who may or may not know whether they have inherited the disease.

Physical symptoms also develop slowly. Huntington's disease is characterized by involuntary, irregular, jerky, dance-like (choreiform) movements. Initially these symptoms may take the form of mild fidgeting and facial grimacing. In the early stages of the disease, the patient may try to cover the movements by incorporating them into a voluntary movement such as crossing the arms or scratching. The involuntary movements usually start in the arms, face, and neck and progressively involve the remainder of the body. Patients display hesitant speech, eye blinking, irregular trunk movements, abnormal tilt of the head, and constant motion (Fig. 48.16). The gait is wide, and the patient may appear to be dancing. Emotional upset, stress, or trying to perform a voluntary task can significantly increase the severity and rate of the abnormal movements; the movements typically diminish or disappear during sleep. Dysphagia may significantly impair the patient's nutritional status.

Depression and suicide are common in the earlier stages of the disease, when the patient still has the cognitive ability to carry out a suicidal act. As the disease progresses, the patient becomes more and more dependent. Aspiration resulting in respiratory failure is the primary cause of death. Life span following diagnosis is about 10 to 30 years.

Diagnostic Tests

Huntington's disease has typically been diagnosed based on the clinical examination and a family history of the disease. MRI or CT may be helpful. Genetic testing is available for prenatal use and to determine if an individual has Huntington's disease before he or she becomes symptomatic. This is a significant breakthrough because Huntington's disease does not become symptomatic until patients are in their 30s or 40s, when they may already have children who could be affected (see Box 48.6, *Patient Perspective*).

Therapeutic Measures

Because there is no cure, treatment of Huntington's disease focuses on minimizing symptoms and preventing complications. Antipsychotic, antidepressant, and antichoreic drugs

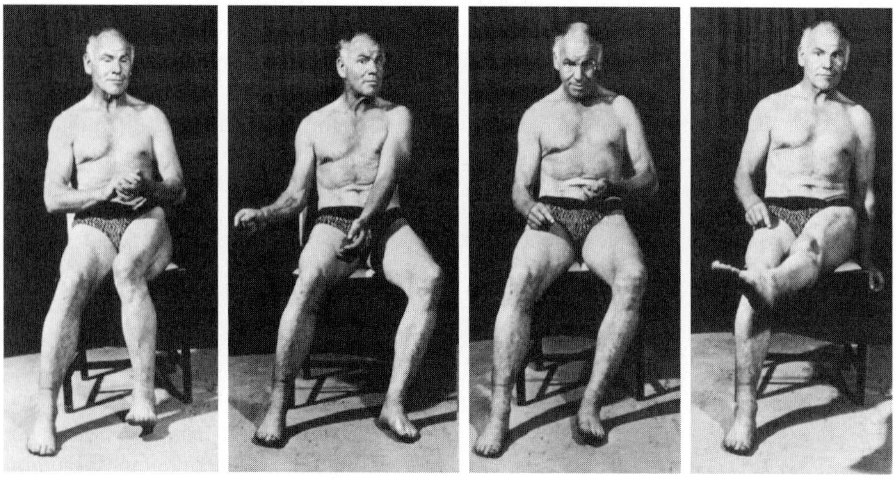

FIGURE 48.16 A 47-year-old patient with Huntington's disease. Note constant fidgety movement. (From Spillane, J. D. [1968]. *An atlas of clinical neurology* [p. 219]. New York: Oxford University Press, with permission.)

Box 48.6

Patient Perspective

Betty

I was born the second of six children. My mom was diagnosed with Huntington's chorea (an old name for Huntington's disease) after she had all of us. My brother was diagnosed with Huntington's disease at the age of 60. He started out with terrible mood swings and a bad temper, but eventually he had a lot of movement problems, including pronounced facial and tongue movements.

By the time we knew the disease had affected our family, many of us had children and grandchildren of our own. My kids wanted me to be tested. It is a hereditary disease and you have a 50/50 chance of having it if a parent has it. If I had Huntington's, then my kids would have a 50/50 chance of having it. If I tested negative, then they and their children would not be at risk.

I was very nervous and afraid of being tested. When I went for the initial visit at the University of Michigan, they observed my movements, how I walked and talked, and my facial movements. They made me go to a psychologist to see if I could handle the results if they did the blood test that would tell for sure. I understand the suicide rate is kind of high for people with Huntington's. After talking for an hour and a half, they decided I could handle the results.

At my next visit they just drew blood, which was sent out for testing. I had to return to the university 6 weeks later for the results. When I went back, I was a nervous wreck. A friend went with me. When the technician came in, she said the doctor would be with me soon. I immediately had bad thoughts. Then when the technician and doctor came back, they were both smiling and had tears in their eyes—I had tested negative. So my friend, the doctor, the technician, and I all hugged and cried.

It is a very hard disease to live with, whether you or another family member has it. My brother has it very bad. Out of my five siblings, four have it for sure, and we think the fifth has it because of mood swings we have observed.

I am the only one of the six who tested clear. I felt very guilty at first that they all had it and I didn't. I'm starting to get over that, but when I see one of them having a bad time with talking, or temper, or movement, the guilt starts to kick in again.

may be used to treat both the involuntary movements and behavioral outbursts. A new medication, tetrabenazine (Xenazine), may help reduce involuntary movements by increasing dopamine in the brain. Physical and occupational therapy can help keep the patient mobile and independent for as long as possible. Research has been done on the benefits of transplanting stem cells into the brains of patients with Huntington's disease, but this is still experimental at this time.

Nursing Care

Patients with Huntington's disease are typically cared for on an outpatient basis. When a patient with Huntington's disease is admitted to an inpatient facility, it is important to obtain as much information as possible about that person's response to medication, daily routine, and emotional and cognitive functioning from the caregivers. For example, knowing that a certain patient is intensely afraid of bathtubs but willingly takes showers can prevent unnecessary struggles and outbursts. Providing some objects from home may make the new environment seem less threatening. The caregivers may relate that the patient has better cognitive functioning at a particular time of day. As the dementia progresses, the patient responds less to attempts at reasoning. Giving directions in a calm but firm tone may help the patient cooperate with activities. The environment should be modified to keep the patient safe. Keep in mind that forceful, involuntary movements of the patient's extremities can happen at any time and should not be misinterpreted as an attempt to harm caregivers.

Difficulty swallowing typically begins toward the middle of the disease course. Patients exhibit trouble swallowing liquids in particular. At this stage, it may still be possible to teach the patient to hold the chin down to the chest while swallowing, which lessens the chance of aspiration. Have patients sit straight upright while eating. Thickening agents may be added to thin liquids to help prevent aspiration. Adaptive devices may prolong the patient's ability to eat independently. Soft foods that are easily manipulated in the mouth are most suitable. These patients may have difficulty taking in adequate calories to maintain a normal body weight, even if a caregiver assists with feeding them. One of the many ethical issues faced by these patients and their significant others is whether artificial feeding should be used and, if so, for how long. Patients and their significant others should be encouraged to discuss end-of-life decisions early in the course of the disease.

See the *Nursing Care Plan for the Patient with Dementia.*

Alzheimer's Disease

Alzheimer's disease (also called dementia of the Alzheimer's type [DAT]) is the most common of several types of dementia. Dementia is a progressive loss of mental functioning that interferes with memory, ability to think clearly and learn, and eventually ability to function (see discussion of dementia earlier in this chapter).

Alois Alzheimer, a German neurologist, first described the disease in 1907. He described pathological changes, now referred to as neurofibrillary tangles and neuritic plaques, that he discovered while performing an autopsy on a patient with dementia. Alzheimer's disease is a progressively degenerative disease that is inevitably fatal. The incidence of Alzheimer's disease is more common in women than men and doubles for every 5 years a person lives beyond age 65.

Etiology and Pathophysiology

Many etiologies have been theorized for Alzheimer's disease, including viral or bacterial infection and autoimmune dysfunction. Markers associated with Alzheimer's disease can be found on several chromosomes. Chromosome 21 in particular has been associated with Alzheimer's disease, and is also the location of the genetic abnormality responsible for Down syndrome. Patients older than age 40 who have Down syndrome usually develop Alzheimer's disease. The exact correlation between the two disorders is still being studied. Lifestyle factors that increase risk of Alzheimer's disease include hypertension, hypercholesterolemia, and poorly controlled diabetes.

Although the exact cause of Alzheimer's disease is unknown, the structural changes associated with it have been well documented. An abnormality exists within the protein of the cell membrane of a neuron. As the axon terminals and dendrite branches disintegrate, they collect in neuritic plaques. Inside the normal brain is a precise arrangement of filaments and tubules that are responsible for cell integrity. Individuals with Alzheimer's disease develop neurofibrillary tangles instead of the normal orderly arrangement. Instead of remaining a small area of abnormality, these neuritic plaques and neurofibrillary tangles spread via axons to other areas of the brain. In addition, patients tend to have a deficiency of acetylcholine in the cerebral cortex. Remember that acetylcholine is a neurotransmitter important for nervous system function.

Advancement of neurofibrillary tangles and neuritic plaques typically affects the hippocampus first, resulting in short-term memory dysfunction. As the tangles and plaques spread to the temporal lobe, the memory impairment becomes more severe. It may be at this point that the patient accesses the health care system. Personality changes and incontinence are inevitable results of Alzheimer's disease. These symptoms can be attributed to the spread of plaques and tangles to the frontal lobes of the brain.

It is believed that the younger the patient is at the time of onset, the faster the neurofibrillary tangles and neuritic plaques spread. Therefore, these patients tend to deteriorate faster, require complete care earlier, and have a shorter life span.

One area of the brain that is left relatively untouched by Alzheimer's is the subcortical area. This structure is responsible for our subconscious urge to survive. The needs for basic requirements such as shelter, food and water, security, and reproduction are controlled by the subcortical area, as are emotional responses to situations. The patient with Alzheimer's disease may experience hunger but no longer know how to meet that basic need. Left to their own devices, these individuals would starve.

Signs and Symptoms

The signs and symptoms of Alzheimer's disease are typically broken down into three stages. The early stage, stage 1, lasts from 2 to 4 years and is characterized by increasing forgetfulness. At this stage, the patient may attempt to cope by using lists and reminders. Interest in day-to-day activities, acquaintances, and surroundings tends to diminish. The patient is reluctant to take on tasks because of uncertainty in how to perform them. If the patient is still working, his or her performance deteriorates and may result in being terminated from the job.

The middle stage, stage 2, is the longest in duration, lasting 2 to 12 years. Progressive cognitive deterioration causes difficulty doing simple calculations or answering questions. Patients may become irritable, particularly when asked to perform a task that they know they should be able to perform but cannot. It may help the patient to break down the task into manageable steps. Depression is common. Aphasia and the resulting inability to make themselves understood may exacerbate patients' irritability. It is during the middle stage, as cognitive function significantly deteriorates, that the patient becomes more physically active. The normal sleep-wake cycle is disrupted, and the patient tends to wander aimlessly, particularly at night. The patient may become lost in familiar surroundings, which compounds the anxiety that typically develops during this stage. Hallucinations and seizures may occur. Management of day-to-day activities such as feeding a pet or paying bills becomes overwhelming. Personal hygiene deteriorates, as does appropriate social behavior. Patients may make up stories to cover for deficits, saying that possessions they misplaced were stolen. Some patients hoard food or money.

The third stage of Alzheimer's disease is characterized by progression to complete dependency. The patient loses the ability to converse or control bowel or bladder function. If the patient is still mobile, constant supervision is required to protect from wandering and avoid injury. Emotional control and the ability to recognize significant others are lost. This lack of recognition is particularly devastating for family members. Eventually the patient is unable to move independently, swallow, or express needs. Death usually occurs from complications of immobility.

The duration of the final stage of Alzheimer's disease, characterized by complete dependence, depends in part on the physical stamina and general health of the individual. The healthier the patient, the longer the body will continue to function. Another factor is the decisions that have been made regarding artificial feeding and respiratory support. Few significant others or health care practitioners advocate intubation and mechanical ventilation for patients with Alzheimer's disease. The issue of enteral (tube) feedings, however, is an emotional one with few easy answers. The use of enteral feedings can prolong the patient's life, despite the absence of cognitive functioning. As with patients suffering from Huntington's disease, every effort should be made to determine the patient's wishes before cognitive impairment makes that impossible. See Table 48.13 for a comparison of the symptoms of Parkinson's, Huntington's, and Alzheimer's diseases.

Diagnostic Tests

The only absolute method of confirming a diagnosis of Alzheimer's disease is by pathological examination at autopsy. In actuality, the disease is diagnosed on the basis of clinical examination, history, and elimination of other possible causes of the symptoms. MRI may reveal the presence of the classic neurofibrillary tangles and neuritic plaques. Positron emission tomography (PET) and single photon emission computed tomography (SPECT) scans show areas of neuronal inactivity. Since researchers in 2007 were able to study patients with Alzheimer's using a variety of diagnostic tests before death and comparing the results to the same tests postmortem, early diagnosis is becoming more promising. Blood tests for specific protein levels and interactions may be the most promising for identifying risk and severity of the disease.

Therapeutic Measures

There is no known cure for Alzheimer's disease. Treatment has traditionally focused on minimizing the effects of the disease and maintaining independence as long as possible. Acetylcholinesterase (AChE) inhibitors such as donepezil (Aricept) or rivastigmine (Exelon) are thought to inhibit the breakdown of the neurotransmitter acetylcholine (see Table 48.10). Increased levels of acetylcholine in the brain allow better functioning of the remaining neurons. They appear to be most effective for those patients who exhibit mild to moderate symptoms of Alzheimer's disease. It may take some time to notice any effects of the drugs. Use of AChE inhibitors diminishes the amount of medical care and social service interventions required and delays admission to skilled nursing facilities. This delay in institutionalization can result in significant positive impact on quality of life, as well as financial savings for the patient and family.

A new class of medications, NMDA (*N*-methyl-D-aspartate) antagonists, may prevent overexcitation of NMDA receptors in the brain and allow more normal function. Memantine (Namenda, Axura) is the only drug currently available in this class. These drugs can be given at any stage of Alzheimer's disease and, like AChE inhibitors, simply slow the patient's decline.

Antidepressants, antipsychotics, and antianxiety drugs may be used as a last resort to control symptoms of depression and behavioral disturbances, but they do not treat the dementia. Patients should be carefully monitored for drug interactions and side effects. For more information, visit the Alzheimer's Association at www.alz.org.

Nursing Process for the Patient with Alzheimer's Disease

See the earlier discussion of dementia and the *Nursing Care Plan for the Patient with Dementia.*

> **CRITICAL THINKING**
>
> ***Mrs. Johnson***
>
> ■ Mrs. Johnson has just become a resident at the Valley Bend extended care facility. She is diagnosed with Alzheimer's disease and is in the second stage with some signs of stage 3 disease. When you check on her during the evening, you find her walking around her room, talking to herself. What other signs and symptoms are typical for stage 2 and stage 3 Alzheimer's disease? How should you address her behavior?
>
> *Suggested answers at end of chapter.*

TABLE 48.13 SYMPTOMS OF PARKINSON'S DISEASE, HUNTINGTON'S DISEASE, AND ALZHEIMER'S DISEASE

Symptom	Parkinson's Disease	Huntington's Disease	Alzheimer's Disease
Tremors	Present	Absent	Absent
Bradykinesia/akinesia	Present	Absent	Absent
Muscle rigidity	Present	Absent	Absent
Memory dysfunction	Late	Late	Early
Cognitive dysfunction	Late	Present	Early
Inability to perform ADLs	Progressive	Progressive	Progressive
Involuntary movements	Absent	Present	Absent
Depression	Present	Present	Present

Home Health Hints

To assess a patient's neurologic status at home:

- Note whether the patient's clothes are matched and properly fastened. Is the patient clean and well groomed?
- Observe the patient during bathing, grooming, or dressing to assess motor function and coordination.
- Assess energy level by noting if the patient makes frequent requests to sit or lie down.
- Observe the patient's gait for steadiness.

To help the patient perform ADLs more easily at home:

- Ask permission to move furniture and small rugs in order to provide a clear path for ambulation.
- Position frequently used items such as a comb, glass of water, eyeglasses, books, tissues, and phone where they are easily accessible.
- Recommend shoes with Velcro closures.
- Use chairs with armrests—the patient can use the armrests to push against to stand.
- Keep the patient cleaner at meals with a clip-on bib such as those used at the dentist's office. Attach clips from suspenders to a piece of elastic and place around the back of the patient's neck. Attach a clean napkin or washcloth for each meal.

To help the patient with Alzheimer's disease who has perceptual deficits:

- Have things used together the same color (e.g., toothbrush and toothpaste).
- Contrast colors in the environment to help patients function independently—slipper color should be different than the floor, a dark-colored placemat can be used under light dishes, and the first and last steps of a stairway can be painted a contrasting color.
- Use a bath or shower seat, handheld shower head, and soothing music to help the patient feel safe and oriented to the task while bathing.
- Cover doorknobs with a piece of cloth to keep the patient from wandering away or have a caregiver purchase inexpensive child safety devices that can fit over doorknobs and/or cabinet latches.
- Family members may require respite care and homemaker services. Discuss with the registered nurse or physician about having social services complete a visit to assist the family with access to community resources.

SUGGESTED ANSWERS TO CRITICAL THINKING

■ *Mr. Chung*

1. Be prepared to assist with a lumbar puncture.
2. You should use short, simple sentences because he may be very anxious or disoriented. Involve his family. Further education can be provided when he is feeling better.
3. Because meningococcal meningitis is contagious, he should be placed in isolation. Gloves, gowns, and masks should be used. Explain the need for these practices to Mr. Chung and his visitors.
4. Comfort measures include tepid baths, a quiet, dark environment, and minimal stimulation. Administer acetaminophen and analgesics as ordered.
5. The health service at his college should be notified of his diagnosis. Close contacts may require prophylactic treatment. If Mr. Chung lives at home rather than at college, his family members should be advised to see their family practitioner and begin prophylactic treatment.

■ *Mr. Evans*

1. You might expect to see impaired speech, right-sided weakness, and a rapid decrease in consciousness if Mr. Evans' hematoma is enlarged.
2. Intubation equipment, mannitol, and intravenous access should be ready. He should be given nothing by mouth (NPO) and the results of laboratory tests should be ready in the event of emergency surgery. The location of Mr. Evans' next of kin must be known.
3. Who are Mr. Evans' support people? Was this drinking episode an isolated incident or a chronic problem that should be addressed if he is discharged safely?

■ *Ms. Simpson*

1. Urinary tract infection is often accompanied by urinary urgency. Ms. Simpson may have difficulty getting to the bathroom quickly and safely.
2. Keep a bedside commode nearby if the bathroom is not close. Assist Ms. Simpson to the bathroom or commode at regular intervals to prevent urgency.

SUGGESTED ANSWERS TO—cont'd

Remind her to ask for help if she needs to get up. Make sure that her call light is within reach.

3. $\frac{1000 \text{ mL}}{12 \text{ hours}} \Big| \frac{4 \text{ hours}}{} = 333 \text{ mL}$

After 4 hours: 1000–333 mL = 667 mL should remain in the bag. Because it is still nearly full, the RN should be notified.

■ *Mrs. Johnson*

Being admitted to a new and unfamiliar facility can increase confusion. Signs of second stage Alzheimer's disease include memory loss, wandering at night, sleeplessness, irritability, loss of way in familiar surroundings, losing possessions and searching for them, and neglect of personal hygiene. During the third stage of the disease, the patient will lose weight, recognize hunger but be unable to eat, be unable to communicate verbally or in writing, lose ability to recognize family, become incontinent of urine and feces, and eventually lose ability to stand and walk. Address Mrs. Johnson by her name and ask her what she needs. Reorient her to where she is and assure her that she is safe and being cared for.

REVIEW QUESTIONS

1. Which of the following problems predisposes someone to develop meningitis?
   a. A sore throat for 3 days
   b. A migraine headache
   c. A muscle injury in the neck
   d. Vision changes

2. A patient with meningitis has photophobia and a severe headache. Which nursing interventions will be most helpful to relieve symptoms?
   a. Administer antibiotics as ordered, and prepare the patient for a lumbar puncture.
   b. Darken the room and administer analgesics.
   c. Administer acetaminophen as ordered and maintain isolation.
   d. Check level of consciousness with the Glasgow Coma Scale and monitor vital signs.

3. Which type of headache is most commonly associated with an aura?
   a. Migraine
   b. Cluster
   c. Tension
   d. Muscle contraction

4. A patient makes an appointment to see a primary care practitioner for recurrent severe headaches. Which instruction by the nurse will help gather the best additional data prior to the appointment?
   a. "Try relaxation and warm moist compresses for your headaches."
   b. "Call and come in the next time you have a headache so you can be examined."
   c. "Keep track of how many headaches you have before you come in."
   d. "Keep a diary of your headaches, recording symptoms, timing, and headache triggers."

5. A patient who has had a generalized tonic-clonic seizure is sound asleep 30 minutes after the seizure. Meals are about to be delivered. Which nursing action is most appropriate?
   a. Wake the patient because nourishment is essential following a seizure.
   b. Wake the patient to do a complete neurologic assessment before the meal.
   c. Let the patient sleep during the postictal state, and keep the meal warm.
   d. Do not attempt to wake the patient because of the risk of a repeat seizure.

6. A patient with a history of seizures reports experiencing an aura and is concerned about an impending seizure. Place the nurse's interventions in the correct order.
   a. Protect the patient from injury during the seizure.
   b. Document the events of the seizure.
   c. Help the patient lie down in a safe place.
   d. Turn the patient on his or her side to sleep.

7. Which patients should be closely monitored by the nurse for symptoms of increased intracranial pressure? **Select all that apply.**
   a. The patient who has a history of epilepsy
   b. The patient admitted with a high fever and severe headache
   c. The patient in the post-anesthesia care unit following craniectomy
   d. The patient with a brain tumor who is admitted for radiation therapy
   e. The patient with a history of migraine headaches, admitted for orthopedic surgery
   f. The patient with Alzheimer's disease admitted with a urinary tract infection

REVIEW QUESTIONS—cont'd

8. Which of the following actions should the nurse take to help prevent increased intracranial pressure in a patient following a traumatic brain injury?
   a. Cluster care so the patient can have long periods of rest.
   b. Keep the head of the bed elevated at 30 degrees.
   c. Suction frequently to keep the airway clear.
   d. Do not give anything by mouth.

9. How much function can be expected in a patient with a spinal cord injury at the L2 level?
   a. Quadriplegic from neck down
   b. Quadriplegic with some arm movement
   c. Paraplegic with some trunk movement
   d. Paraplegic, may learn to walk with a brace

10. A patient is admitted following a T4 spinal injury. When taking morning vital signs, the nurse notes that the patient appears restless and the blood pressure is elevated. Which of the following actions by the nurse is appropriate?
    a. Recheck the patient's blood pressure in 30 minutes.
    b. No action is necessary. This is an expected finding.
    c. Check for a full bladder.
    d. Encourage the patient to express any anxiety.

11. The symptoms of Parkinson's disease are caused by depletion of which neurotransmitter?
    a. Dopamine
    b. Acetylcholine
    c. Serotonin
    d. Norepinephrine

12. Which nursing interventions are appropriate for the patient with a neurodegenerative disorder who has difficulty swallowing?
    a. Show the patient how to tuck his or her chin down to the chest during swallowing.
    b. Provide clear to full liquids; avoid solid foods.
    c. Place the patient in semi-Fowler's position for eating.
    d. Provide adaptive eating utensils.

13. A resident of an extended care facility who has Alzheimer's disease is sitting in a corner, crying loudly that no one is paying attention. Several staff members have tried to find out what's wrong, but the patient won't answer, and just keeps rocking back and forth and crying. Which approach by the nurse might best help the patient?
    a. Say in a quiet voice, "What is wrong? We can't help you if you don't tell us what's wrong."
    b. Sit quietly by the patient and say, "I'm here; you aren't alone."
    c. Say in a firm voice, "Several staff have asked what you need. Now it is time to stop crying."
    d. Ignore the continued crying. Continuing to respond to her will encourage the behavior.

References

National Institute of Neurological Disorders and Stroke. (2009, May 26). Dementia information page. Retrieved June 6, 2009, from http://www.ninds.nih.gov/disorders/dementias/dementia.htm

National Parkinson Foundation. (2010). Parkinson's disease overview. Retrieved May 11, 2010, from http://www.parkinson.org/parkinson-s-disease.aspx

Saey, T. H. (2009, July 4). Huntington's protein may have a crony. Science News, 176(1). Retrieved July 29, 2009, from http://www.sciencenews.org

DavisPlus | For additional resources and information visit http://davisplus.fadavis.com

49 Nursing Care of Patients with Cerebrovascular Disorders

JOHN STURTEVANT AND
WENDY HOCKLEY

KEY TERMS

ataxia (ah-TAK-see-ah)
diplopia (dip-LOH-pee-ah)
embolic (em-BOL-ik)
embolism (EM-buh-lizm)
endarterectomy (end-AR-tur-EK-tuh-mee)
hemiplegia (HEM-ee-PLEE-jee-ah)
hemorrhagic (hem-uh-RAH-jik)
ischemic (i-SKEE-mik)
penumbra (puh-NUM-brah)
thrombolytic (throm-buh-LIT-ik)
thrombosis (throm-BOH-sis)

QUESTIONS TO GUIDE YOUR READING

1. What are the causes, risk factors, and pathophysiology of transient ischemic attack, ischemic stroke, and hemorrhagic stroke?
2. What emergency interventions are used for transient ischemic attack, ischemic stroke, and hemorrhagic stroke?
3. What therapeutic measures are appropriate for transient ischemic attack, ischemic stroke, and hemorrhagic stroke?
4. What outcomes can be expected for a stroke victim?
5. What is the appropriate nursing care for a patient with a cerebrovascular disorder?

Cerebrovascular disorders occur when the supply of blood and oxygen to brain cells is inadequate, allowing brain tissue to die, and causing a cerebrovascular accident (stroke). The most common cerebrovascular disorders include transient ischemic attack, ischemic stroke, and hemorrhagic stroke.

TRANSIENT ISCHEMIC ATTACK

A transient ischemic attack (TIA) is a temporary blockage of blood to the brain that causes a transient (brief) neurologic impairment. The episode typically lasts minutes to hours, and the patient recovers completely. The risk factors, causes and symptoms of a TIA are identical to those of a cerebrovascular accident (CVA), commonly known as a stroke. Indeed, if the blockage that causes a TIA does not reverse, an area of the brain is permanently damaged, and the event is a stroke. About one-third of patients who have a TIA will have a stroke in the future (National Institutes of Health [NIH], n.d.). Urgent evaluation of a TIA is an essential order to decrease the risk of stroke.

Treatment of a TIA is focused on preventing a full stroke. The cause of the TIA may be discovered with diagnostic tests, which can then guide treatment. However, there may be no clear etiology of the TIA. Treatment, therefore, is mostly centered on minimizing the patient's risk factors for a stroke.

CEREBROVASCULAR ACCIDENT

A cerebrovascular accident (stroke) is the disruption of blood flow to the brain, resulting in death of brain cells. In most cases, permanent disability results. A stroke is more likely to happen as one ages; about 795,000 people of all ages are affected each year. Stroke is our nation's number three killer and the leading cause of disability. African Americans, Hispanic Americans, American Indian/Alaska Natives, and multiracial people are at higher risk than non-Hispanic whites (American Heart Association [AHA], 2009).

Pathophysiology

Cerebral function depends on oxygen and glucose delivery to neurons in the brain. The brain cannot store oxygen or glucose, so it relies on a constant supply of these nutrients. If the supply of oxygen and glucose is stopped, brain tissue dies. When a stroke occurs, brain cells begin dying immediately. There is an area of brain tissue surrounding the damage, called the **penumbra**, which contains brain cells that are "stunned" and may be revived if the brain is reperfused quickly. However, they will die if the blood supply is not restored.

• WORD • BUILDING •
penumbra: healthy tissue surrounding infarct

The particular vessel or vessels involved determine the area of the brain affected and the symptoms that result. The duration of ischemia determines whether the symptoms are transient or permanent. A TIA may be a warning of an impending stroke.

Etiology

Strokes are classified as either ischemic or hemorrhagic. Ischemic strokes are more common, accounting for about 87% of all strokes (AHA, 2009). Hemorrhagic strokes account for the remaining 13% of strokes.

Ischemic Stroke

Ischemic stroke occurs when the blood supply to the brain is blocked or significantly slowed. It may be one of two major types: thrombotic or embolic (Fig. 49.1).

THROMBOTIC STROKE. Thrombotic strokes occur when an occlusion builds up in an artery until it significantly decreases or stops blood flow to the brain. Thrombotic strokes most often occur in the internal or common carotid arteries.

EMBOLIC STROKE. An **embolic** stroke is typically caused by a blood clot that is created somewhere in the body, often within the heart, and travels through the arteries until it becomes trapped in a smaller vessel, preventing the passage

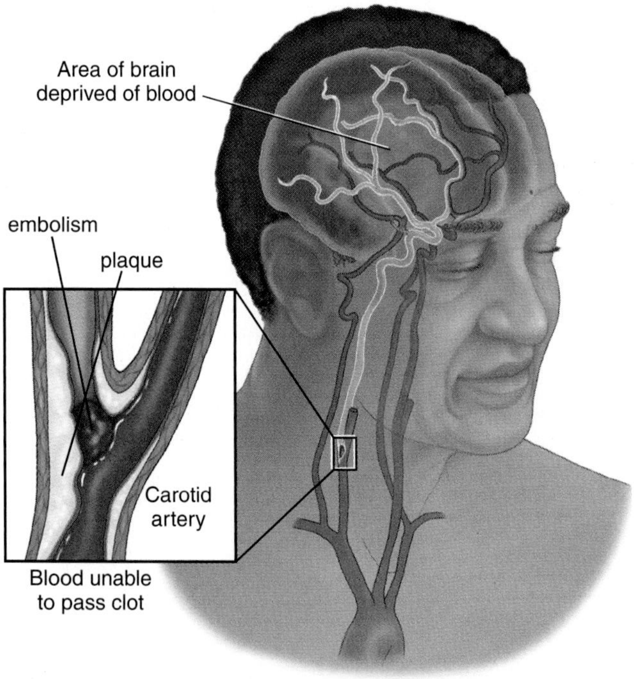
Area of brain
deprived of blood
embolism
plaque
Carotid
artery
Blood unable
to pass clot

FIGURE 49.1 Embolism and thrombosis.

• WORD • BUILDING •
ischemic: isch—to hold back + emia—blood
thrombotic: thrombus—clot + ic—relating to
embolic: embolism—to throw (as in clot or other debris) + ic—relating to

of blood. Typically, the embolism will travel and become lodged in the middle, anterior, or posterior cerebral arteries.

Hemorrhagic Stroke

Hemorrhagic strokes are caused by the rupture of a cerebral blood vessel that allows blood to escape into brain tissue and not travel beyond the point of the rupture. It can be further classified into two major types: subarachnoid hemorrhage and **intracerebral** hemorrhage.

SUBARACHNOID HEMORRHAGE. This type of stroke occurs on the surface of the brain and is most often the result of a ruptured cerebral aneurysm (covered later in this chapter). Strokes caused by subarachnoid hemorrhage usually are very serious and require surgery to correct. They are often fatal.

INTRACEREBRAL HEMORRHAGE. This type of stroke occurs in the deeper tissues of the brain and usually is caused by uncontrolled hypertension. Patients can experience multiple undetected intracerebral hemorrhages, with minimal deficits noted. However, damage will eventually accumulate and the patient will develop major deficits. Maintaining blood pressure below 120/80 mm Hg should be the goal for these patients.

Risk Factors

Risk factors for ischemic stroke are classified as modifiable or nonmodifiable. Nonmodifiable risk factors are those that cannot be altered, such as age or gender. Modifiable risk factors are those that can be changed with treatment, such as high blood pressure. For example, every 15 points of systolic blood pressure above 120 mm Hg doubles the risk of a stroke (Sacco et al., 2006). See Box 49.1 for a list of risk factors. Minimizing or eliminating these risk factors can significantly lower risk of a stroke.

Warning Signs

The five signs or symptoms recognized by the American Heart Association and American Stroke Association are as follows:

- Sudden numbness or weakness of face, arm, or leg, especially on one side of the body
- Sudden confusion or trouble speaking or understanding
- Sudden trouble seeing in one or both eyes
- Sudden trouble walking, dizziness, loss of balance, or coordination
- Sudden severe headache with no known cause (American Stroke Association, n.d.).

Patients and family members should be taught to recognize these signs and symptoms and how to activate emergency medical services (EMS) if these signs occur.

• WORD • BUILDING •

hemorrhagic: blood loss

intracerebral: intra—within + cerebral—cerebrum

Box 49.1

Risk Factors for Stroke

Modifiable Risk Factors

- High blood pressure
- Smoking
- Diabetes mellitus
- Cardiovascular disease
- Atrial fibrillation
- Asymptomatic carotid stenosis
- Transient ischemic attacks
- Sickle cell anemia
- Dyslipidemia
- Obesity
- Excessive alcohol intake
- Poor diet (high sodium, high fat, low potassium)
- Physical inactivity
- Postmenopausal hormone therapy

Nonmodifiable Risk Factors

- Older age
- Gender (more common in men)
- Heredity
- Prior stroke or heart attack

A number of organizations have begun using the acronym FAST (Table 49.1) to teach emergency triage nurses, first responders, nonlicensed personnel, and community members to recognize a stroke and respond quickly. Time is extremely important to preserve brain cells. Utilizing the EMS system is of particular importance. Research has shown that patients arriving by ambulance are admitted and evaluated faster than those who "walk in" on their own. Those arriving by ambulance are also more likely to arrive within 2 hours of symptom onset (Table 49.2).

NURSING CARE TIP

When teaching a stroke victim and family, repetition is very important. Besides the anxiety and stress they may be feeling, the patient's ability to process information may also be altered by the stroke.

Acute Signs and Symptoms

Most patients with stroke symptoms present with sudden or rapidly evolving symptoms. Symptoms are varied and depend on the area of the brain affected (Table 49.3). Common symptoms include visual disturbances, language disturbances, weakness or paralysis on one side of the body, and

TABLE 49.1 RECOGNIZING THE SIGNS OF A STROKE—FAST

Facial droop	Ask the person to smile. Does the face droop or is it uneven on one side?
Arm drift	Ask the person to close his or her eyes and hold both arms out in front. Does one drift downward, or is the person unable to lift one arm?
Speech	Ask the person to say, "It is a bright and sunny day." Are there any difficulties understanding or speaking?
Time	If any signs or symptoms are present, call 911 immediately. These are all indicators of a possible stroke. Brain cells may be dying.

TABLE 49.2 AVERAGE TIME FROM SYMPTOM ONSET TO TREATMENT

Mode of Transportation	Average Time to Treatment
Emergency medical system (911)	1.4 hours
Walk-in to emergency department	3.5 hours
Physician's office	4.5 hours

Source: AANN, 2008.

difficulty swallowing (dysphagia). Signs and symptoms are generally the same for both ischemic and hemorrhagic stroke. Patients may have drowsiness and a severe headache, often described as "the worst headache of my life."

Language Disturbances

Difficulty with language is commonly associated with a TIA and stroke. *Aphasia* refers to the absence of language; *dysphasia* refers to difficulty with speech and is not as severe as aphasia. The patient may experience trouble selecting the correct words, use incomprehensible or non-sense speech, have trouble understanding others' speech, and have trouble writing or reading. Aphasia may be expressive, in which the patient knows what he wants to say but cannot speak or make sense, or receptive, with an inability to understand spoken and/or written words. When both expressive and receptive aphasia are present, it is called global aphasia. Slurred or indistinct speech because of a motor problem (lack of coordination) is referred to as dysarthria.

Motor Disturbances

Motor disturbances include paralysis, weakness, and numbness. Sometimes the first evidence of paralysis or weakness is clumsiness or a feeling of heaviness in a limb. The onset will be sudden and typically involves one side of the body—the side opposite the damaged area of the brain. Deficits may appear on both sides of the body if the patient has had a brainstem stroke or a vertebrobasilar stroke.

TABLE 49.3 POSSIBLE SYMPTOMS OF STROKE ACCORDING TO ARTERY AFFECTED

Artery Affected	Paralysis	Sensory Loss	Mental Status	Visual Changes	Speech
Carotid artery	Contralateral face, arm, leg Dysphagia	Contralateral face, arm, leg	Confusion Amnesia, Personality changes	Same side hemianopsia Temporary blindness	If dominant hemisphere is involved
Anterior cerebral artery	Contralateral face, arm, leg Dysphagia	Contralateral foot and leg			
Middle cerebral artery	Contralateral face, arm Dysphagia	Contralateral face, arm	Unilateral neglect if right hemisphere is affected	Contralateral hemianopsia	Difficulty reading, writing, and calculating if left hemisphere is affected
Posterior cerebral artery	Tremor		Memory deficits Perseveration	Hemianopsia	Dyslexia
Posterior inferior cerebellar artery	Unsteady gait Vertigo Dysphagia	Contralateral pain, temperature, balance		*Same sided:* conjugate gaze paralysis, nystagmus *Bilateral:* visual defects	Dysarthria
Vertebrobasilar/ cerebellar artery	Hemiplegia/ hemiparesis or quadriplegia or quadriparesis Dysphagia	Same side—face	Vertigo Clumsiness Ataxia	Diplopia Hemianopsia Conjugate gaze paralysis	Mutism Dysarthria
Brainstem/ cerebellum arteries	*Motor loss:* all limbs, gait ataxia	All limbs		Bilateral visual defects Nystagmus Dysconjugate gaze	Dysarthria

Source: AANN, 2008.

Most commonly, paralysis or weakness affect the arm and face together. Some patients present with complete hemiparesis, with one entire side of the body flaccid. **Ataxia** may be present, which is poor balance or a stumbling, staggering gait. This can be related to damage to the cerebellum or to poor coordination due to weakness or paralysis. If the swallowing muscles are affected, the patient will have trouble swallowing (dysphagia).

NURSING CARE TIP

Before giving a patient with a suspected stroke anything to eat or drink, including medications, the patient should pass a swallow (dysphagia) screening test to prevent possible aspiration. Evaluate the patient's facial features and, if there is any apparent weakness or asymmetry, stop and do not give the patient anything by mouth. If no weakness is evident, have the patient swallow about 30 mL of water. If the patient coughs, has difficulty swallowing, or has a wet or gurgly voice afterward, keep the patient NPO until evaluated and cleared by a physician or speech and language pathologist.

Visual Disturbances

Visual field disturbances are also a common symptom of a stroke. The vision loss is painless and may involve loss of all or part of the vision in one eye. Patients often describe the change as a curtain dropping, as fog, or as a gray-out or black-out of vision. The involved eye is on the same side as the diseased artery. Potential visual field abnormalities are shown in Figure 49.2. When you are assessing the patient, stop talking and keep moving across the room. If the patient's eyes do not follow you, there is a good chance he or she has a deficit in that visual field.

Diagnostic Tests

On arrival at the emergency department, a computed tomographic (CT) scan will be performed immediately. The purpose of the CT scan is to identify whether symptoms are caused by a hemorrhagic stroke so the physician can determine the appropriate course of treatment. Ischemic stroke changes will not be visible on a CT until several days after the event. Interventions for hemorrhagic strokes are different than for ischemic strokes. Care for hemorrhagic strokes is discussed later in this chapter.

After the CT scan, patients may have an electrocardiogram (ECG) to determine if atrial fibrillation is present. An echocardiogram may be done to determine the presence of other heart disease that may increase the risk of thrombus formation. Other tests that may be performed

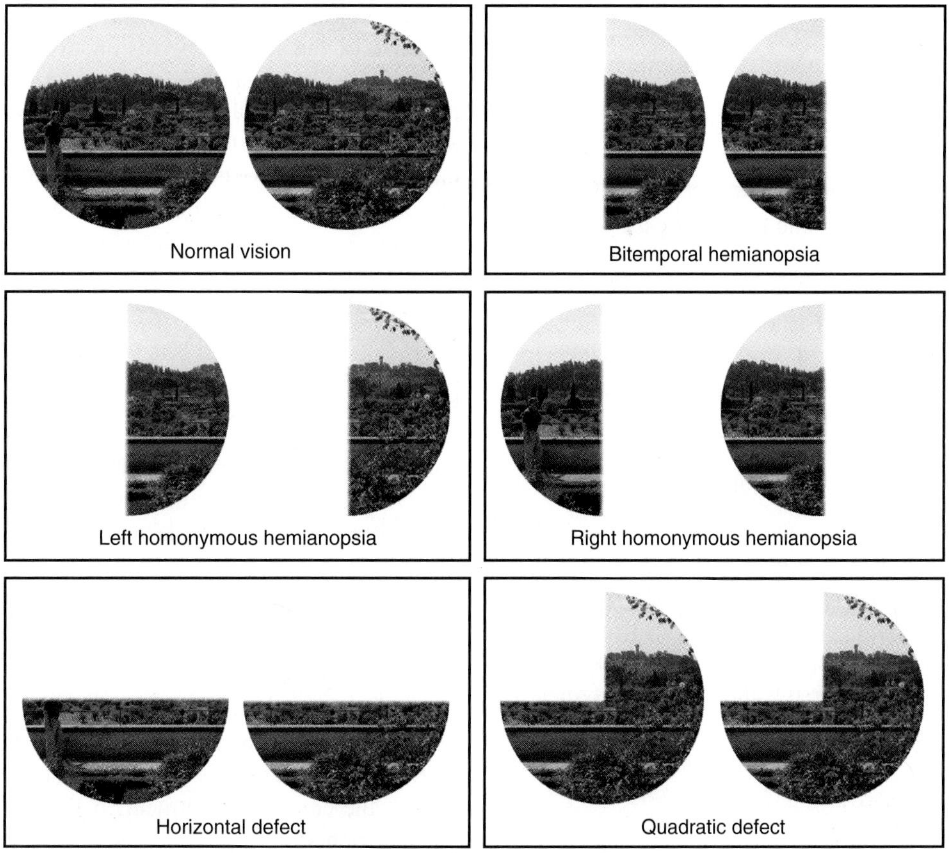

Normal vision
Bitemporal hemianopsia
Left homonymous hemianopsia
Right homonymous hemianopsia
Horizontal defect
Quadratic defect

FIGURE 49.2 Visual deficits in stroke.

in the emergency department (ED) include complete blood count (CBC), blood glucose level, metabolic panel, blood typing, prothrombin time (PT), international normalized ratio (INR), and serum pregnancy if indicated. Stools and emesis may be checked for blood if possible. The patient will be placed on a cardiac monitor and pulse oximeter. The ED nurse will complete a dysphagia screen before the patient consumes anything.

ED staff may complete the National Institutes of Health Stroke Scale (NIHSS) to determine the patient's neurologic deficit level. This 11-point scale determines the severity of a stroke. Nurses can be specially trained and certified to use it. Find out more about the NIHSS at www.nihstrokescale.org.

Once the patient is stabilized, additional tests may be done. Carotid Doppler testing can detect stenosis of the carotid arteries. This noninvasive test involves bouncing sound waves off the carotid arteries to determine the velocity and turbulence of blood flow. Carotid angiography can be done to further determine degree of blockage and help guide treatment.

Therapeutic Measures

Initial emergency care is supportive while test results are pending. ABCs (airway, breathing, and circulation) are monitored. Oxygen is administered if oxygen saturation is less than 92% and the patient's level of consciousness is reduced. Vital signs and heart rhythm are monitored. A temperature greater than 99.6°F is treated because hyperthermia is associated with poorer outcomes. If IV fluids are needed, only solutions without glucose, such as normal saline solution, are used to prevent hyperglycemia. When test results verify whether the stroke is hemorrhagic or ischemic, therapeutic interventions are begun.

Some hospitals have a stroke team that evaluates all patients who arrive at the hospital within 2 hours of symptom onset. The stroke team will assess the patient within the first 15 minutes of arrival and have lab tests, ECG, and CT scans done with results back within 45 minutes after assessment. The physician will make a decision regarding **thrombolytic** therapy within 1 hour of arrival.

Patients suffering from a stroke can often develop increased intracranial pressure (ICP), which further adds to brain damage. Stroke patients are also at risk for repeated strokes. Careful serial neurologic assessments and vital signs are needed to promptly detect and report changes.

Thrombolytic Therapy

Some patients with ischemic stroke may be candidates for thrombolytic therapy. This is a "clotbuster" medication (alteplase [tissue plasminogen activator; tPA]) that can dissolve a clot and potentially completely reverse stroke symptoms. It can only be administered within 3 hours of symptom onset, so it is only an option if the patient arrives at the ED quickly after symptoms begin. Some patients awaken after a night's sleep to discover they have had a stroke; they are considered to have the onset of symptoms at the time they went to bed. Studies are currently being done that suggest it may be safe to treat a patient up to 4.5 hours after symptom onset.

Thrombolytic agents can lyse a thrombus by causing conversion of plasminogen to plasmin. Plasmin is the enzyme that causes thrombi to break down. Patients treated effectively with tPA may be able to leave the hospital within 1 or 2 days with no residual effects from the stroke. Thrombolytics are associated with a significant risk of hemorrhage, so all risk of bleeding must be ruled out before these drugs will be considered. They are used very cautiously.

• WORD • BUILDING •
thrombolytic: thrombo—clot + lytic—causing breakdown

> **LEARNING TIP**
>
> *Remember: Time lost is brain lost.* This means the faster the patient with a stroke receives treatment, the more brain (and brain function) can be saved. Teaching your patients to recognize the signs and symptoms of a stroke and encouraging them to call 911 if needed could mean the difference between leading a normal life and total disability.

Pharmacological Management

Blood pressure control is vital for the stroke patient. Because of the lack of perfusion to certain areas of the brain, the body's response is to increase the systolic blood pressure to force blood into the affected areas. If the patient will receive tPA, the blood pressure must be maintained below 185/110 mm Hg to reduce the risk of bleeding. This is often done through the use of a beta blocker (labetalol) or calcium channel blocker (nicardipine), because of their fast-acting effects and ability to be given IV. See Table 49.4 for medications commonly used for cerebrovascular disorders.

If tPA is not being given, the physician may allow the blood pressure to remain high for a period of time to help salvage brain tissue, depending on the source of the stroke and the location of the clot. This "permissive hypertension" helps blood travel through redundant blood vessels in the brain to reach the affected area. Antihypertensive agents should be given if the systolic pressure exceeds 220 mm Hg or the diastolic pressure exceeds 120 mm Hg (Summers et al., 2009).

Post-Emergent Care

Once emergent treatment is completed, medical management focuses on controlling the cause of the TIA or stroke. The results of the diagnostic tests assist physicians in determining the course of treatment. If the patient has residual physical deficits, the physician will order physical, occupational, and speech therapy consultations to evaluate the

TABLE 49.4 MEDICATIONS USED IN CEREBROVASCULAR DISORDERS

Medication Class/Action	Examples	Route	Side Effects	Nursing Implications
Thrombolytic Agents				
Dissolve existing clots.	tissue plasminogen activator (tPA)	IV	Intracranial, GI, or urinary hemorrhage	Must be administered within 3 hr of symptom onset.
Antiplatelet Agents				
Prevent formation of clots.	aspirin	PO, rectal	Dyspepsia, nausea, vomiting, bleeding	Monitor patient for bruising, change in level of consciousness, prolonged bleeding time.
	clopidogrel (Plavix)	PO	Bleeding, abdominal pain, rash, edema, headache, backache	
	aspirin/dipyridamole (Aggrenox)	PO	Headache, dyspepsia, pain, fatigue	
Anticoagulants				
Prolong time to form clots; prevent new clots.	warfarin (Coumadin)	PO	Hemorrhage, purple toe syndrome, necrosis of skin	Monitor patient for bruising, change in level of consciousness, prolonged bleeding time.
	heparin	Subcutaneously, IV	Hemorrhage, erythema, local irritation, hematoma, ulceration	For warfarin, monitor INR frequently until therapeutic, then monthly.
Statins				
Reduce cholesterol level.	simvastatin (Zocor), pravastatin (Pravachol), atorvastatin (Lipitor), lovastatin (Mevacor)	PO	Irritability, diarrhea, heartburn, hepatitis, dizziness, headache, muscle aches	Patient should notify prescriber if muscle pain or weakness occur.

patient's functional status and make recommendations for further treatment.

The American Stroke Association recommends that patients who have a TIA or stroke receive an antiplatelet drug such as clopidogrel (Plavix), aspirin/dipyridamole (Aggrenox), or aspirin within 24 hours of symptom onset. Decreasing platelet aggregation lessens the likelihood of thrombus formation. The patient in atrial fibrillation may also receive warfarin (Coumadin) to prevent clot development.

Cholesterol-lowering medication, preferably a statin, will be ordered for patients who have a low-density lipoprotein (LDL) cholesterol level greater than 100 mg/dL. This will also help minimize the development of atherosclerotic plaques. Statins also may have a neuroprotective effect and may further decrease risk of a stroke.

Deep vein **thrombosis** (DVT) is of concern when caring for patients who have had a stroke. The decrease in movement, confinement to a hospital bed, and hyper-coagulable state all increase risk of DVT. Not only can DVTs cause severe pain and complications in the affected leg, but the blood clot could dislodge and travel to the lungs and cause a pulmonary **embolism**, or to the brain and cause a repeat stroke. Treatment usually includes medications such as heparin, enoxaparin (Lovenox), or warfarin (Coumadin), or nondrug treatments such as sequential compression devices and elastic stockings.

Patients are at risk for respiratory complications for several reasons. They may be related to an increase in intracranial pressure. Patients with stroke are prone to aspiration because of a decreased level of consciousness and possibly impaired swallowing ability. Patients should be suctioned as needed to keep the airway clear. A patient who vomits should be turned to the side to reduce the risk of aspiration. Oral feedings should be started carefully and progressed slowly and only after the patient is alert and the ability to swallow safely has been determined by an appropriate swallowing evaluation.

Surgery

Patients with warning signs of stroke or patients who have been stabilized following a stroke may be candidates for surgery. In patients with significant carotid artery occlusion, a carotid **endarterectomy** may be performed. This involves a small incision in the neck and surgical removal of the occlusion from the artery.

• WORD • BUILDING •

thrombosis: thromb—clot + osis—condition
embolism: embol—to throw + ism—condition

• WORD • BUILDING •

endarterectomy: endo—inside + arter—artery + ectomy—surgical removal of

Alternatively, a patient who is at high risk for complications with a carotid endarterectomy may have a carotid stent placed. This is placed during a carotid angiogram procedure. A catheter is advanced to the carotid artery, where a balloon is inflated to open the artery by pushing on the plaque. Then, a stent (a tiny metal or polymer-based tube) is expanded inside the artery to keep it open and allow better blood flow to the brain.

CRITICAL THINKING

Mr. Jankowski

■ You are caring for Mr. Jankowski, a 56-year-old man who has been admitted to your orthopedic unit after knee surgery. As you listen to his lungs at the start of the shift, you notice that his lung sounds are diminished. You ask if he is a smoker and find that he has smoked for 40 years. You realize this will place Mr. Jankowski at risk for stroke. What further data should you collect, and what therapeutic measures should you provide?

Suggested answers at end of chapter.

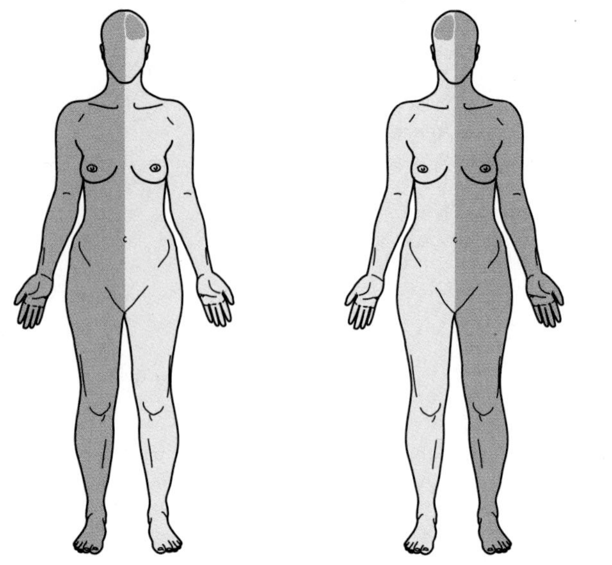
Left-side infarct
Right-side infarct
Right-sided weakness or paralysis
Aphasia (in left–brain-dominant clients)
Depression related to disability common
Left-sided weakness or paralysis
Impaired judgment/safety risk
Unilateral neglect more common
Indifferent to disability

FIGURE 49.3 The side opposite the infarct is affected by a stroke.

Prevention of Stroke

The incidence of stroke can be lessened by reducing risk factors (refer back to Box 49.1). Keeping hypertension, cholesterol level, weight, and diabetes controlled can go a long way toward preventing strokes. Smoking cessation is essential. Emboli may be prevented with warfarin in people at high risk from atrial fibrillation. Aspirin or other antiplatelet agents help prevent abnormal clotting.

It is important to educate all patients about new treatments for stroke and the potential for reversal of symptoms with the use of thrombolytic agents. Patients must be educated about risk factors for a stroke, warning signs, and the importance of immediate EMS transport if symptoms occur.

Long-Term Effects of Stroke

Impaired Motor Function and Sensation

Paresthesias and paralysis are common long-term effects of strokes that were not treated with a thrombolytic agent. The side of the body opposite the side of the cerebral infarct (the contralateral side) is affected because nerve fibers cross over as they pass from the brain to the spinal cord (Fig. 49.3). Paralysis on one side of the body is called **hemiplegia** (Fig. 49.4). The affected limbs may be weak or totally paralyzed (flaccid). The arm or the leg may be weaker, depending on the artery affected. These patients are particularly prone to contractures, which cause permanent immobility of a muscle or joint from fibrosis of connective tissue. Adaptation or assistance with activities of daily living (ADLs) is required.

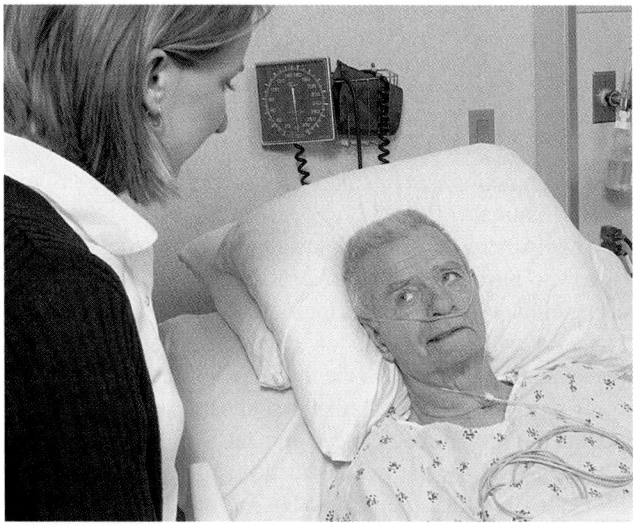

FIGURE 49.4 Note the left-sided weakness in this man's smile as result of a stroke.

• WORD • BUILDING •
hemiplegia: hemi—one side + plegia—paralysis

Motor involvement also often affects swallowing and control of urination and bowel function. Patients should be mobilized within 24 hours if possible to prevent complications of immobility. Physical and occupational therapy are provided to maximize functioning and to progress the patient toward a return to baseline functioning.

Sensation changes may prevent the patient from being aware of pressure, temperature, or injuries on the affected side. Patients must be taught to be aware of these changes and protect the involved limbs.

APHASIA. If a stroke affects the temporal lobe region, especially on the dominant side, the speech center will likely be affected. Aphasia may be expressive, receptive, or global, as described earlier. Patients may be able to say words but be unable to form coherent speech, such as the patient who picks up a fork but calls it a comb. If a patient does not understand what is said, avoid the temptation to speak louder to try to help the patient understand. Remember that it is not the patient's hearing that is affected. You need to be very patient and understanding as the patient tries to communicate with you. Speech therapy can help the patient relearn to communicate. See the *Nursing Process for the Patient with a Cerebrovascular Disorder* section for interventions for the aphasic patient.

Emotional Lability

Emotional lability, or instability, is a common consequence of stroke. Patients may move rapidly from profound sadness to an almost euphoric state and back again. Laughing or crying may have no relationship to the patient's situation at any given moment. Families can be upset by this behavior because they do not understand why a once happy person is now crying all the time or why the patient laughs inappropriately. You can help by explaining that these responses probably do not reflect how the patient is feeling, but rather are caused by the stroke damage.

Impaired Judgment

All patients who have had a stroke, in particular those with right-sided lesions, present a high safety risk. Patients may have poor understanding of their own limitations and believe that they are capable of performing tasks they did before the stroke. Precautions must be taken to protect the patient from injury.

If the frontal lobes are involved, learned social behaviors may be lost. The patient may undress in public, use profanity, or make inappropriate sexual advances. These behaviors are extremely difficult for significant others to cope with. Education and emotional support of significant others are essential. Allowing them to talk about their frustration and anger may facilitate coping. Distracting the patient from inappropriate behavior may help. The patient should never be reprimanded or punished, because he or she no longer has the cognitive ability to control the behaviors.

Unilateral Neglect

The phenomenon of unilateral neglect is seen predominantly in patients who have right hemisphere infarcts. It has been estimated to affect up to 30% of all patients who have had a stroke. These patients do not acknowledge the left side of their environment and may not even be aware of their own body on the affected side. Safety is a primary consideration. Essential items such as the call light and telephone should be placed on the patient's right side. Position the bed so the patient's right side is toward the door. Treatment should focus on providing stimuli to all senses on the patient's affected side, and teaching the patient to focus on the left side. This involves teaching the patient to purposefully check where the left limbs are positioned and to look for safety risks. The patient can learn to turn his or her head and scan the environment. Patients may also need reminders to accomplish simple tasks such as turning their plates during meals to recognize the food on the left side of the plate.

Other Long-Term Effects

The stroke patient may experience other complications after the acute phase of the stroke has passed. These include pneumonia, deep venous thrombosis, pulmonary embolism, pressure ulcers, malnutrition, and depression. For the homeward-bound patient, education for the patient and family regarding prevention and recognition of these complications will assist the patient in a successful recovery. If a patient needs to receive rehabilitation in a skilled nursing facility, prevention of these issues will be a part of the care plan at the facility. For more information, visit the National Stroke Association at www.stroke.org or the American Stroke Association at www.strokeassociation.org.

CEREBRAL ANEURYSM AND SUBARACHNOID HEMORRHAGE

A cerebral aneurysm is a weakness in the wall of a cerebral artery. It may be congenital, traumatic, or the result of disease. If the aneurysm ruptures, the result is often a subarachnoid hemorrhage. It is unknown what causes the formation of congenital aneurysms or what causes them to rupture. Unruptured aneurysms are typically asymptomatic. The exception is a very large aneurysm, which can cause symptoms similar to a brain tumor. Aneurysms often affect young, otherwise healthy adults.

Pathophysiology and Etiology

Aneurysms can occur in any of the cerebral arteries, though most occur in the circle of Willis. The most common site is at the bifurcation of an artery. It is theorized that increased turbulence at the bifurcation can cause an outpouching of a congenitally weak arterial wall.

Subarachnoid hemorrhage is the collection of blood beneath the arachnoid mater following aneurysm rupture. Rupture of an arteriovenous malformation or head trauma may also result in subarachnoid hemorrhage (Fig. 49.5). The presence of blood outside the blood vessels is very irritating to brain tissue. It is believed that irritation from blood breakdown is the major cause of vasospasm, a common complication of subarachnoid hemorrhage.

It is unclear what causes an aneurysm to rupture. Some people develop a subarachnoid hemorrhage while performing Valsalva's maneuver, engaging in sexual activity, or physically exerting themselves. For others, the aneurysm ruptures during a quiet, inactive period. If the aneurysm

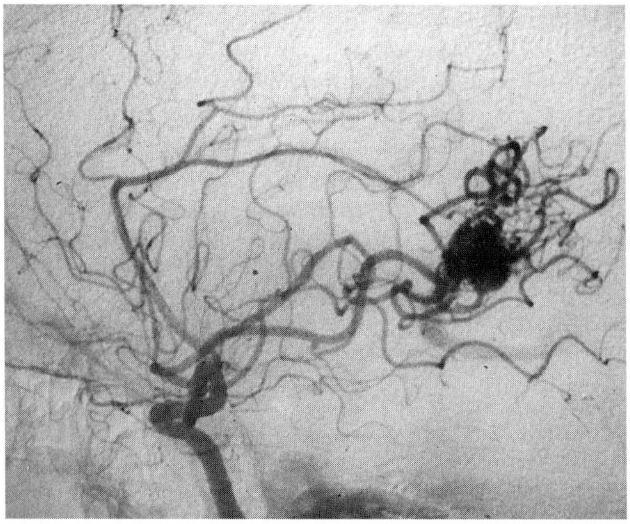

FIGURE 49.5 Arteriovenous malformation. Note tangled vessels.

rupture is associated with a particular activity, the patient may be very frightened of engaging in that activity again. This may have a negative effect on the patient's interpersonal relationships if the associated activity was sexual in nature. The patient's partner may feel guilty or responsible for the hemorrhage. Education, emotional support, and confidentiality are essential to help both the patient and significant other.

Signs and Symptoms

Some patients experience a small hemorrhage before diagnosis of subarachnoid hemorrhage. This leakage of blood may cause a mild headache, vomiting, or disorientation. The symptoms may be attributed to a flu-like syndrome. Patients may dismiss the symptoms and not seek medical care.

The most common presentation of rupture of an aneurysm is sudden onset of a severe headache. Typically, a patient will state, "I have never had a headache this bad in my life." Patients may hold their heads and moan or cry in pain. Sensitivity to light is a common finding. This may make patients reluctant to cooperate with pupil examinations.

Level of consciousness varies based on the severity of the hemorrhage. Patients may be alert and coherent, may lose consciousness immediately, or may gradually become less responsive. The decreased level of consciousness is caused by increased intracranial pressure and impairment of cerebral blood flow. Patients may experience generalized seizures.

Blood in the subarachnoid space causes meningeal irritation. The patient may exhibit nuchal rigidity. The most commonly affected cranial nerves are III and VI. This is manifested as an enlarged pupil or abnormal gaze. Motor dysfunction may involve one or both limbs on the side opposite the hemorrhage.

Diagnostic Tests

Because of the severe nature of the symptoms, patients with subarachnoid hemorrhage almost always come to the emergency department rather than seeking care from a primary health care provider. A CT scan is done to identify and locate a hemorrhage. Precise diagnosis of an aneurysm requires a cerebral angiogram. The contrast material fills the aneurysm if one exists. For a patient with a severe headache and facing a life-threatening illness, this test can be very frightening. If the patient's neurologic status does not allow him or her to cooperate, sedation may be required before and during the examination.

Therapeutic Measures

Patients with subarachnoid hemorrhage are cared for in an intensive care unit setting. They typically have an arterial line and a central venous pressure monitoring catheter. Blood pressure is carefully monitored because high pressures increase the risk of rerupture of the aneurysm and low pressures may be associated with ischemia. Values outside parameters identified by the physician are reported. Typically, the systolic blood pressure is kept between 120 and 160 mm Hg. Vasoactive drugs may be required to maintain blood pressure within the prescribed parameters.

There is no cure for subarachnoid hemorrhage. Treatment consists of correcting the cause of the hemorrhage if possible. Preventing or managing complications and providing supportive care are important aspects of nursing care.

Surgical Management

Definitive treatment of the aneurysm involves performing a craniotomy and exposing the aneurysm. If the aneurysm has a neck (berry aneurysm), it is identified and clamped with a metal clip (Fig. 49.6). An aneurysm without a neck may be wrapped with a sterile plastic or muslin wrap. This provides stability to the aneurysm walls, lessening the chance of rupture. In some situations, it is possible to clamp the artery on either side of the aneurysm, removing that portion of the vessel, and the aneurysm, from the circulation.

Nonsurgical Management

Nonsurgical intervention may be provided for aneurysms that are inoperable because of size, configuration, or the

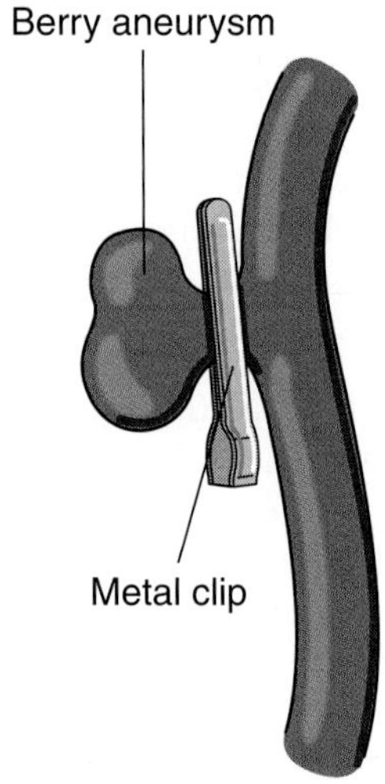
Berry aneurysm
Metal clip

FIGURE 49.6 Surgical management of aneurysms.

patient's medical status. A foreign material such as a metallic or polymer-based coil may be introduced into the aneurysm. A thrombus develops around the foreign body and, if the treatment is successful, occludes the aneurysm. The goal is to fill the aneurysm enough to prevent blood flowing into it, without causing rupture.

Complications

Rebleeding

Recurrent rupture of a cerebral aneurysm carries significant morbidity and mortality rates. Patients are at risk for rebleeding until the aneurysm is surgically repaired. If the aneurysm is wrapped or embolized, there is a risk of rebleeding, but risk is much lower than if the aneurysm is left untreated.

Hydrocephalus

Blood in the ventricular system interferes with the circulation and reabsorption of cerebrospinal fluid (CSF), and hydrocephalus may develop. Early in the course of subarachnoid hemorrhage, an external ventricular drain may be used to treat hydrocephalus.

About 25% of patients with subarachnoid hemorrhage require placement of a ventriculoperitoneal shunt to treat hydrocephalus (Fig. 49.7). This surgical procedure involves placement of a catheter into a ventricle in the brain. The catheter is then connected to a valve, which regulates the rate of CSF drainage. Another catheter connects to the valve and is passed down to the peritoneal cavity. The CSF drains out of the peritoneal catheter and is absorbed into the peritoneal cavity.

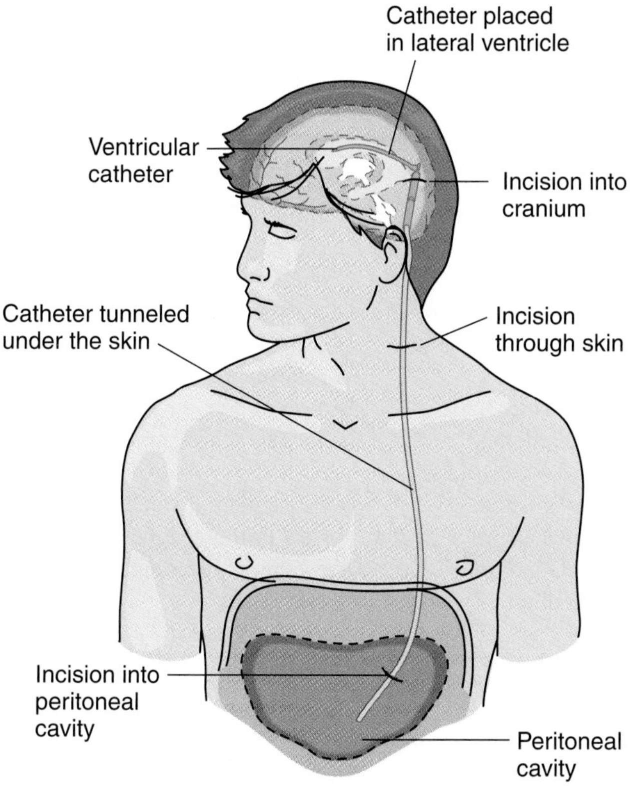
Catheter placed in lateral ventricle
Ventricular catheter
Incision into cranium
Catheter tunneled under the skin
Incision through skin
Incision into peritoneal cavity
Peritoneal cavity

FIGURE 49.7 A ventriculoperitoneal shunt drains cerebrospinal fluid into the peritoneal cavity.

Vasospasm

Vasospasm is responsible for most long-term complications of subarachnoid hemorrhage. Vasospasm causes a blood vessel's diameter to narrow. Although it typically begins in the vessel giving rise to the aneurysm, vasospasm may spread to other vessels. This explains why the ischemia or infarct caused by vasospasm can be so widespread and devastating.

The long-term complications of subarachnoid hemorrhage are similar to those of stroke.

Rehabilitation

If the patient can tolerate intensive therapy, discharge from the hospital may be to a rehabilitation center. Rehabilitation and long-term care are similar, whether the patient has had an aneurysm or an ischemic stroke.

CRITICAL THINKING

Mrs. Washington

■ Mrs. Washington is a 68-year-old African American retired office worker. She was admitted to your unit following a right-sided intracerebral hemorrhage. Her daughter states that Mrs. Washington has taken antihypertensive medication for the past 20 years. However, she states that her mother has been "forgetful" lately and that there are five more pills in the medicine bottle than expected. On admission, Mrs. Washington is oriented only to person and has hemiparesis.

1. What may have precipitated Mrs. Washington's stroke?
2. On which side do you expect Mrs. Washington's extremities to be affected?
3. List two safety concerns and strategies to promote patient safety.
4. List at least two educational needs for Mrs. Washington and her daughter.

Suggested answers at end of chapter.

Nursing Process for the Patient with a Cerebrovascular Disorder

Data Collection

Observe the patient for signs and symptoms of decreased cerebral tissue perfusion: decreased level of consciousness, irritability or restlessness, dizziness, syncope, blurred or dimmed vision, **diplopia**, change in visual fields, unequal pupils or a sluggish or absent pupillary reaction to

• WORD • BUILDING •
diplopia: diplo—double + opia—sight

light, paresthesias, motor weakness, paralysis, or seizures. Reassess frequently and report any decline. Monitor vital signs and oxygen levels. Monitor laboratory tests: CBC, lipid profile, and INR/PT if the patient takes warfarin (Coumadin). Perform a routine respiratory assessment. Monitor lung sounds for adventitious sounds or a change in breath sounds. Assess pain level. Assess swallowing ability before offering oral intake. Promptly report any changes in vital signs, laboratory values, respiratory function, or neurologic status.

Nursing Diagnoses, Planning, and Implementation

See the *Nursing Care Plan for the Patient with Stroke* for nursing diagnoses during acute care. Possible post–acute nursing diagnoses are listed next with outcomes and interventions.

NURSING CARE PLAN for the Patient with Stroke

Nursing Diagnosis: *Ineffective Cerebral Tissue Perfusion* related to interruption of blood supply

Expected Outcomes: The patient will experience improved cerebral tissue perfusion as evidenced by:

- Absence of or reduction in dizziness, syncope, visual disturbances
- Improved level of consciousness
- Pupils equal and reactive to light
- Improved motor and sensory function.

Evaluation of Outcomes: Are the patient's symptoms of ineffective perfusion improving?

Interventions	Rationale	Evaluation
Assess neurologic status at least every 30 minutes initially and then every 4 hours or as ordered. Report changes.	A change in status could indicate decreased perfusion.	Is there a change in neurologic status since the previous documented assessment?
Assess vital signs every 30 minutes initially and then every 4 hours or as ordered.	High or low blood pressure can lead to decreased tissue perfusion and recurrent stroke. Temperature above 99.6°F can worsen ischemic injury to brain tissue.	Are vital signs within normal limits? Are changes reported?
Monitor oxygen saturation and administer oxygen as ordered for Spo_2 less than 92%.	Hypoxemia can increase brain damage.	Is Spo_2 92% or greater?
Monitor blood glucose as ordered and report value greater than 140 mg/dL.	Elevated glucose is associated with worsening of infarct and hemorrhage.	Is glucose level greater than 140 mg/dL? Was physician notified?
Keep head of bed elevated 20 to 30 degrees. Keep neck in neutral position.	This facilitates venous return and reduces risk of cerebral edema.	Is head of bed elevated? Is neck in neutral position?
Monitor medication for therapeutic and nontherapeutic effects. Monitor coagulation studies if appropriate.	Anticoagulant therapy must be closely monitored to make sure it is at a therapeutic level, and not increasing risk for bleeding.	Are coagulation studies within normal or therapeutic ranges? Are signs of bleeding present?

NURSING CARE PLAN for the Patient with Stroke—cont'd

Nursing Diagnosis: *Ineffective Airway Clearance* related to stasis of secretions associated with decreased mobility and poor cough effort; and airway obstruction resulting from tongue falling back in throat

Expected Outcomes: The patient will maintain an open airway as evidenced by respirations quiet and unlabored, 12 to 20 per minute, Spo_2 greater than 92%.

Evaluation of Outcomes: Are respirations quiet, 12 to 20 per minute, with Spo_2 greater than 92%?

Interventions	Rationale	Evaluation
Monitor lung sounds, cough, and respirations.	Assessment provides the basis for intervention.	Are lung sounds clear? Is cough effective? Are respirations quiet and easy?
Position the patient to maintain an open airway.	Side lying may keep tongue from obstructing airway.	Is patient positioned to keep airway clear?
Consult with RN or physician about an oral airway if airway is not clear.	An oral airway will keep tongue from obstructing airway if needed.	Is an airway indicated?
Encourage patient to deep breathe and cough if able.	Coughing and deep breathing will help clear secretions from airway and prevent atelectasis.	Is patient able to deep breathe and cough? Is cough effective?
If cough is ineffective, suction as needed.	Suctioning may be needed if patient is unable to swallow secretions or cough effectively.	Is suctioning indicated? Is airway clear after suctioning?

Nursing Diagnosis: *Risk for Injury* related to seizure, repeat stroke, or hemorrhage secondary to thrombolytic therapy

Expected Outcomes: The patient will remain free from injury.

Evaluation of Outcomes: Is patient free from injury? Are problems recognized and reported quickly?

Interventions	Rationale	Evaluation
Monitor neurologic status frequently and report changes promptly.	Prompt recognition of a repeat stroke is essential.	Are neurologic checks within normal limits? Are changes reported promptly?
Monitor for signs of hemorrhage for 24 to 36 hours following thrombolytic therapy.	Hemorrhage is the most common side effect of thrombolytic therapy.	Are signs of hemorrhage present? Are they reported promptly?
Administer anticonvulsant agent as ordered.	Patient is at increased risk for seizures following a stroke.	Is patient seizure free?
Implement seizure precautions (see Chapter 47).	Precautions help protect patient in event of a seizure.	Are precautions in place and patient protected?
Assist with transfers and ambulation.	Patient is at risk for falls because of motor and sensory deficits and impaired judgment.	Is patient assisted with mobility? Is patient able to call for help when needed?

Impaired Physical Mobility Related to Decreased Motor Function as Evidenced by Weakness or Inability to Move

EXPECTED OUTCOME: The patient will maintain physical mobility as evidenced by maximum physical mobility within limitations of deficits. Patient will not experience complications related to immobility.

- Consult physical and occupational therapists *to assess the patient's abilities and make specific recommendations related to mobility.*
- Discuss use of constraint therapy (see *Evidence-Based Practice* box) with physical and occupational therapists. *Constraint therapy may improve ability to use affected limbs.*

EVIDENCE-BASED PRACTICE

Clinical Question

Should a patient with right-sided weakness be taught how to master his or her environment with only the left side?

Evidence

Recent evidence has shown that following a stroke, a particular limb or muscle group can be "retaught" to function. A technique called *constraint therapy* has been shown to significantly improve a patient's function of an affected limb. Constraint therapy restrains the unaffected side, to force use of the affected side. Wu et al. (2007) showed that constraint-induced movement therapy results in better improvements in daily functional ability, motor function, and quality of life as compared with treatment with standard rehabilitation. Others have shown that the use a constraint mitten on the unaffected hand helps improve function of the hemiplegic arm after a stroke.

Implications for Nursing Practice

While caring for a patient who has experienced a stroke, the nurse should assist the patient in adjusting to his or her disability. Talk to the physical therapist about use of constraint therapy to encourage use of the affected limb.

REFERENCE

Wu, C. Y., Chen, C. L., Tang, S. F., et al. (2007). Kinematic and clinical analyses of upper-extremity movements after constraint-induced movement therapy in patients with stroke: A randomized controlled trial. *Archives of Physical Medicine and Rehabilitation, 88,* 964–970.

- Maintain the patient in correct body alignment *to prevent contractures and promote comfort.*
- Support affected extremities with pillows *to prevent dislocation injuries and promote comfort.*
- Perform range-of-motion exercises as prescribed by the physical therapist *to prevent contractures and atrophy.*
- Follow physical/occupational therapy recommendations for being up in chair or ambulation. *Prolonged bedrest is associated with complications and poor outcomes.*
- If patient is unable to get out of bed, turn and reposition at least every 2 hours *to prevent skin, respiratory, and musculoskeletal complications.*

Imbalanced Nutrition, Less Than Body Requirements, Related to Impaired Swallowing and Motor Deficits, as Evidenced by Weight Loss

EXPECTED OUTCOME: The patient will maintain adequate nutrition without aspiration as evidenced by stable weight at appropriate level for height.

- Keep patient NPO until swallowing can be evaluated *to prevent aspiration.*
- Perform dysphagia screening. *This quick assessment can identify problems before a complete evaluation can be done.*
  - Observe for facial weakness or inability to completely close mouth.
  - Ask patient to stick out tongue and move it side to side.
  - Observe for drooling.
- If swallowing appears to be intact, have patient swallow a sip of water from a cup before offering other foods or fluids. Observe for coughing, choking, or noisy lung sounds. *These are signs of difficulty swallowing.*
- Request speech pathologist evaluation if indicated *to diagnose specific swallowing problems and make recommendations.*
- Implement measures to prevent aspiration. *Aspiration can lead to pneumonia, which will greatly complicate the patient's recovery.*
  - Stay with patient during meals.
  - Ensure that patient is fully alert before feeding.
  - Place the patient in high-Fowler's position or chair for meals.
  - Avoid use of straws.
  - Use a thickening agent if swallowing study recommends.
  - Place food on unaffected side of mouth.
  - Teach the patient to swallow twice after each bite.
  - Check the patient's mouth for pocketing of food.
  - Have suction equipment available.
- Notify primary care provider if patient is unable to take in adequate oral calories. *A feeding tube may be needed if the patient cannot take in enough calories to maintain nutrition. Advance directives should be consulted before a feeding tube is placed.*

- Assist with insertion and care of feeding tube if needed. *If patient cannot swallow effectively, a feeding tube may be needed to maintain nutrition.*
- See Box 49.2, *Nutrition Notes,* for additional interventions.

Box 49.2

Nutrition Notes

Feeding Patients with Swallowing Disorders

Suggestions for persons who have difficulty swallowing include the following:

- Eat slowly.
- Avoid distractions while eating.
- Do not drink with a straw.
- Do not talk while eating.
- Sit up straight while eating.
- Use a teaspoon, taking only half a teaspoonful at a time.
- Swallow completely between bites or sips.

Possible nursing interventions to aid a person with a swallowing disorder include the following:

- Remove loose dentures.
- Position the head correctly. A speech therapist can help determine the optimum head position. A hemiplegic patient often benefits from turning the head toward the weak side.
- When spoon feeding a patient with hemiplegia, place the food on the unaffected side of the tongue.
- Consult a dietitian concerning appropriate textures for liquids and solids. A multidisciplinary assessment may be needed to tailor the diet prescription to the patient's strengths and weaknesses. Foods with mixed textures such as vegetable soup are frequently problematic. Often thicker substances are better managed than liquids. Although infant cereal can be an effective thickener, it may be rejected on a psychological basis in favor of instant potato flakes, unflavored gelatin, or a commercial thickener.
- Be aware that thickening agents may:
  - Cause food to become thicker over time
  - Add significant calories to foods
  - React differently in different foods
  - Affect the palatability of the thickened item.

Disturbed Sensory Perception Related to CNS Damage as Evidenced by Paresthesias or Visual Deficits

EXPECTED OUTCOME: The patient will adapt to sensory-perceptual deficits as evidenced by avoidance of injury to affected areas.

- Assist occupational therapist to assess for visual and/or spatial deficits and decreased sensory perception: heat and cold, position of body parts, pressure. *Identification of specific deficits is the first step in creating a plan of care.*
- Teach patient to scan the environment *to compensate for a visual deficit.*
- Implement plans for skin integrity and mobility *to protect patient from complications related to sensory deficits.*

Risk for Impaired Skin Integrity, Irritation or Breakdown, Related to Immobility and Incontinence

EXPECTED OUTCOME: The patient's skin integrity will be maintained as evidenced by absence of redness or breakdown.

- Examine the skin often for redness or breakdown, especially around bony prominences, dependent areas, and perineum. *Any signs of breakdown must be treated immediately to prevent further damage.*
- Thoroughly cleanse and dry the perineal area after each episode of incontinence. *Urine and feces can be very irritating to the skin.*
- If incontinence is unavoidable, use a barrier cream such as zinc oxide *to protect skin.*
- Turn and position the patient at least every 2 hours, or more often if the patient experiences breakdown. *Pressure impairs circulation and increases risk of breakdown.*
- Use a lift sheet to move patient in bed *to avoid damage from friction.*
- Consider the use of a pressure-reducing mattress if patient cannot be out of bed for long periods. *This helps reduce pressure, but does not eliminate the need to reposition the patient every 2 hours.*
- If breakdown occurs, contact the physician or wound care specialist *to obtain treatment recommendations.*

Incontinence Related to Loss of Voluntary Control of Elimination

EXPECTED OUTCOME: Episodes of incontinence are avoided, or if unavoidable, they will be cleaned up quickly and skin complications avoided.

- Monitor for incontinence of bowel or bladder *so patient can be cleaned promptly and skin protected.*
- Determine usual pattern of urinary and bowel elimination. *Keeping the patient on his or her regular prehospitalization pattern may help prevent incontinence.*
- Provide assistance with toileting according to the patient's usual schedule. *The patient who is unable to get up unaided may wait too long for help or try to get up alone and be injured.*
- Respond quickly to requests for assistance with toileting *to avoid accidental incontinence.*

Self-Care Deficit Related to Decreased Motor Function, Spatial-perceptual Alterations, and Fear of Injury as Evidenced by Inability to Manage Activities of Daily Living (ADLs) Independently

EXPECTED OUTCOME: Self-care will be accomplished as evidenced by patient's ADL needs being met and patient becoming increasingly independent.

- Determine the patient's ability to perform ADLs. *Good baseline data will guide development of a care plan.*
- Work with the patient to create a plan for meeting daily physical needs. *The patient will be more likely to participate in a plan if he or she participated in creating it.*
- Encourage the highest level of independence possible; facilitate patient's ability to do ADLs. *Providing too much assistance can promote dependence and further loss of mobility.*
  - Place objects within reach and within visual field.
  - Place food/fluids within patient's visual field.
  - Encourage use of assistive devices.
- Assist patient with learning to use nondominant side of body. *If dominant side is affected, the patient may have to use the nondominant side.*
- Provide positive feedback *to help reduce discouragement with slow progress.*
- Provide education for family members and significant others regarding patient's deficits and recovery plan. *The family can assist the patient with mobility if they understand what needs to be done.*

Impaired Verbal Communication, Dysarthria, Related to Loss of Motor Function of the Muscles of Speech Articulation, or Aphasia or Dysphasia Related to Ischemia of the Dominant Hemisphere, as Evidenced by Inability to Clearly Speak or Understand Speech

EXPECTED OUTCOME: Communication will be effective as evidenced by the patient communicating needs and desires effectively and by avoidance of frustration.

- Listen for difficulties in verbal communication (difficulty speaking, articulating or incorrect ordering of words, inability to find or name words and objects). *Good baseline data will guide planning of care.*
- Consult a speech pathologist for assistance in determining types of aphasia or dysphasia and need for follow-up treatment. *A speech pathologist is specially trained to diagnose and treat communication problems, and can work with nursing staff to develop a plan of care.*
- Implement measures to facilitate communication. *These measures help assure the patient has his or her immediate needs met while learning to adapt to communication impairment.*
  - Answer call light in person rather than over an intercom.
  - Assess needs frequently.
  - Listen carefully: avoid interrupting patient and allow ample time for communication.
  - When patient is tired, ask questions that require short answers.
  - Provide appropriate aids to communication (picture board, magic slate, pencil and paper). See Figure 49.8.
- Provide education to family members and significant others regarding communication problems and interventions *so they can communicate with patient and participate in care.*
- If the patient is unable to communicate, do not assume that he or she cannot hear and understand. Make every effort to speak to the patient and to keep conversation appropriate when it is within the patient's range of hearing. *The patient may understand exactly what is being said, even if he or she is unable to respond.*
- Contact physician if impairment increases. *This may be a sign of stroke extension.*

Acute or Chronic Confusion Related to Cerebral Ischemia as Evidenced by Inappropriate Responses to Stimuli

EXPECTED OUTCOME: The patient's thought processes will be as clear as possible within limitations of brain damage as evidenced by responses appropriate to situation; the patient's safety will be maintained and patient will feel calm and safe.

- Observe patient for thought process impairment such as shortened attention span, impaired memory, confusion, slowed or quick and impulsive responses, and aggressive and/or inappropriate responses. *Disturbed thinking can be manifested in a variety of ways. See Chapter 48 for interventions for patients with disturbed thought processes.*

Risk for Falls Related to Changes in Mobility, Sensation, or Confusion

EXPECTED OUTCOME: The patient will remain safe and free from falls.

- Perform a fall risk assessment according to agency policy *to identify patients at risk.*
- Instruct the patient and family to call for help before the patient gets up *so staff can assist.*
- Keep call light and other essential items within patient's reach *to prevent falls while trying to access needed items.*
- Provide frequent toileting. *Patients often fall while getting up to use the toilet.*
- Avoid restraints if at all possible. *Restraints are associated with injuries.*

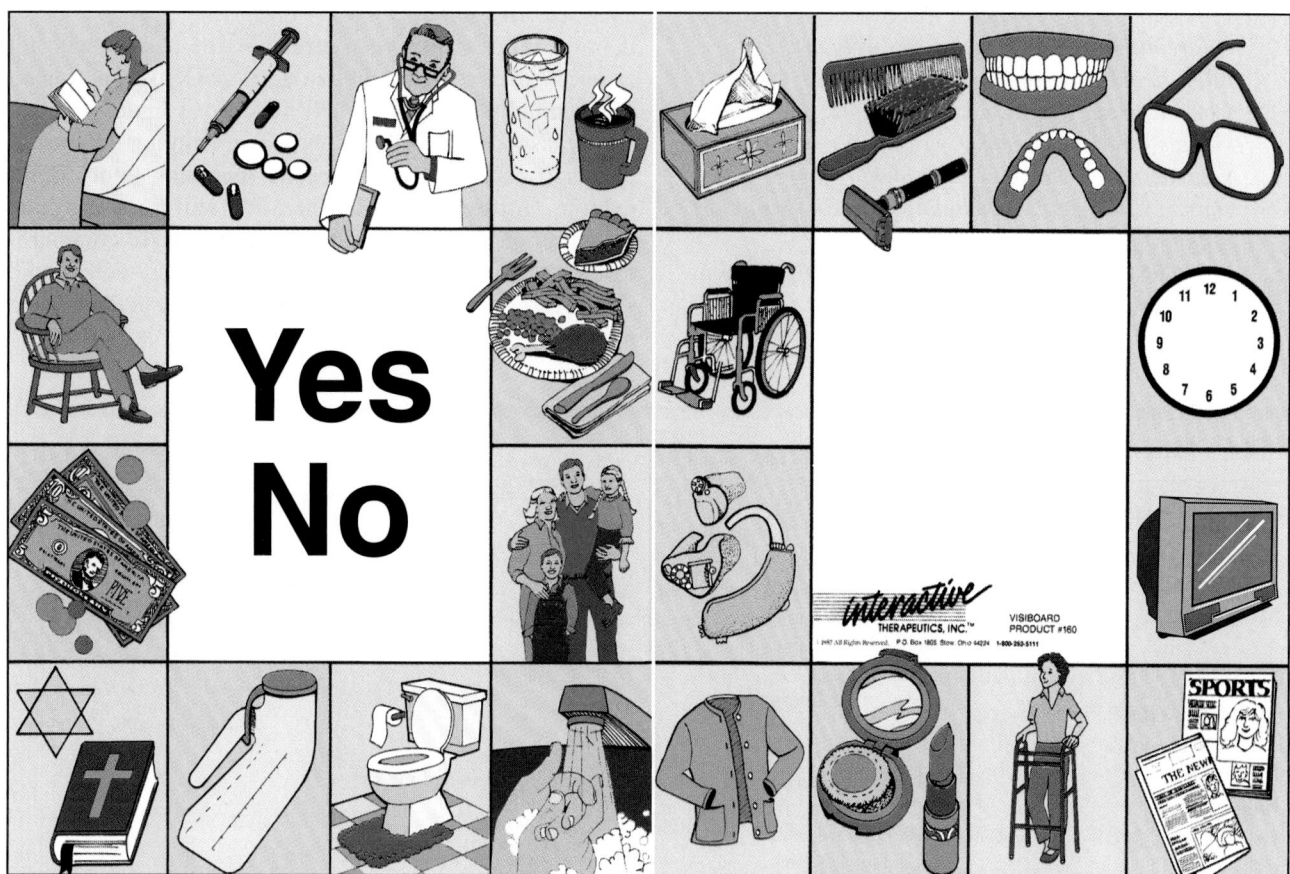
Yes
No
THERAPEUTICS, INC.
VISIBOARD
PRODUCT #160
SPORTS

FIGURE 49.8 Picture board.

Deficient Knowledge Related to Diagnosis and Treatment

EXPECTED OUTCOME: The patient and family will have the necessary knowledge to make decisions and assist with care.

- Explain what has happened to the patient. Explain tests, procedures, and care activities. *The patient and significant others are likely to be very frightened about what is happening. Providing correct information about what a stroke is, tests and procedures, and rationale for care activities helps reduce anxiety.*
- Present information in small amounts and as simply as possible. *The patient may have difficulty managing large amounts of information while acutely ill or if confusion is present.*
- Orient the patient and family to the ICU or other setting and the constant monitoring provided. *This can help reduce anxiety and reassure the patient and significant others that the patient is receiving competent care.*
- If the patient is to be discharged to home, make sure information is provided related to medications, treatments, and follow-up care. *The patient and family need to know how to provide appropriate care at home.*
- Evaluate the need for home nursing, physical therapy, and occupational therapy, and request appropriate referrals. *The patient will likely need continued therapy after discharge to regain as much function as possible.*

Risk for Caregiver Role Strain Related to Changes in Roles, Responsibilities, Finances, and Intimacy

EXPECTED OUTCOME: The caregiver will be comfortable with role as evidenced by statement that she or he understands how to care for the patient and has the needed resources to do so. The caregiver will maintain her or his own health.

- Work with caregiver to identify how the patient's functional level will affect their lives. *Assumption of roles or responsibilities previously fulfilled by the patient may be very stressful to significant others. If the caregiver can anticipate the impact, he or she can plan ahead how to make sure needs are met.*
- Encourage patient and caregiver to identify support systems and make use of community resources.

Provide a list of resources. *If support is in place before discharge, they are more likely to use it after the patient goes home.*

- Consult social worker or case manager. *These individuals have access to many resources, and can help the patient and caregiver identify appropriate sources of assistance, including a caregiver support group.*
- Provide support if transfer to a skilled nursing facility is needed. *This can be a very difficult decision for a patient and caregiver.*

Evaluation

If interventions have been effective, the patient will not experience increased deficits due to decreased perfusion of brain cells. The patient will recover as much physical ability as possible and adjust to remaining deficits to meet self-care needs. Basic needs, including safety, elimination, nutrition, and skin integrity, will be met by the patient or caregiver. The patient will be able to communicate effectively and have needs and desires understood. Caregivers will identify support systems available to help. (See Table 49.5.)

TABLE 49.5 STROKE SUMMARY

Signs and Symptoms	Dizziness Syncope Visual disturbances Irritability, restlessness, confusion Decreased level of consciousness Unequal pupils Paresthesias Motor weakness Paralysis Seizures Difficulty swallowing, understanding language, speaking
Diagnostic Tests	Computed tomography scan Electrocardiogram Carotid Doppler Echocardiogram Cerebral angiogram Laboratory: INR/PT, metabolic panel, glucose, complete blood count, PTT, serum pregnancy (if appropriate), oxygen saturation
Therapeutic Measures	Oxygen for Spo_2 less than 92% Antiplatelet, anticoagulant, or thrombolytic medication Physical, occupational, speech therapy Carotid endarterectomy or stent Knee-high antiembolism stockings
Complications	Stroke evolves, causing more deficits, aspiration pneumonia, skin breakdown, urinary tract infection, malnutrition
Priority Nursing Diagnoses	*Ineffective Cerebral Tissue Perfusion* *Ineffective Airway Clearance* *Risk for Injury*

INR/PT = international normalized ratio/prothrombin time; PTT = partial thromboplastin time; Spo_2 = peripheral oxygen saturation.

Home Health Hints

- Work with a physical therapist, occupational therapist, and speech therapist to assist the patient with rehabilitation.
- Provide assistive devices to aid the patient to function independently.
- Keep home environment clutter free to prevent falls.
- Offer frequent praise for all achievements.
- Keep regularly used items close by. If the patient is using a walker, have him or her tie a small bag to the top to store these items.
- If the patient does not have a portable phone, encourage the purchase of one. Instruct the patient to keep it near at all times in case of an emergency.
- If necessary, assist the patient with obtaining a medical alert device. If the patient falls, he or she can access an emergency medical service by pushing a button.
- Assist with obtaining homemaker or respite care for caregivers if necessary.

Home Health Hints—cont'd

- Patients on a pureed diet can make their own food at home using a food processor. Baby food can also be purchased to meet swallowing guidelines.
- Patients with one-sided paralysis following a stroke should be instructed to wear clothes that are easy to get on and off. Examples include pants with elastic waists, shoes with Velcro closures or slip-on shoes, and pullover shirts without buttons.
- If the patient has difficulty speaking (dysarthria), try using magnetic alphabet letters. Ask questions that require a yes or no answer. The patient can respond with the letter Y or N. You can also help the patient and caregiver develop a communication board of frequently used words and objects.
- Keep bedside commode lids up with patches of Velcro attached to the seat and the frame.

SUGGESTED ANSWERS TO CRITICAL THINKING

■ *Mr. Jankowski*

Ask Mr. Jankowski about other risk factors for stroke, such as his dietary and alcohol habits. Check his chart for history of diabetes, hypertension, or heart disease. Check his weight and cholesterol levels if drawn. Educate him about risk factors for stroke, and how they can be modified. Teach him the FAST acronym (see Table 49.1). Consider a dietitian consultation, and provide written information on stroke prevention and smoking cessation. As a nurse, you will be in a position to recognize risks and help patients modify risk factors for many problems before they occur.

■ *Mrs. Washington*

1. Uncontrolled hypertension, in the presence of a preexisting aneurysm, might have precipitated Mrs. Washington's stroke.
2. Her left extremities will be affected.
3. Mrs. Washington is disoriented. Her room should be as close to the nurse's station as possible. Reorient her to her surroundings and condition frequently. Keep side rails up when Mrs. Washington is alone.

   Mrs. Washington also has hemiparesis. Obtain a commode because Mrs. Washington will probably not be able to walk to the bathroom. Place the call light and telephone on her right side. Assist Mrs. Washington with positioning to prevent injury to her affected limbs.
4. If Mrs. Washington will be going back to her home, you should teach her and her daughter about the relationship of uncontrolled hypertension to intracranial hemorrhage; options for inpatient, outpatient, and in-home therapy; and memory strategies to prevent missed medication doses (e.g., weekly pill box, keeping medications with breakfast food, or an alarm clock or watch).

REVIEW QUESTIONS

1. Which of the following are modifiable risk factors for stroke? **Select all that apply.**
   a. Heredity
   b. Age
   c. Diabetes
   d. Race
   e. High cholesterol
   f. Obesity
2. What is the most important diagnostic test that is completed immediately on the patient with symptoms of stroke in the emergency department?
   a. Head CT scan
   b. Arteriogram
   c. PT/INR
   d. FAST assessment

REVIEW QUESTIONS—cont'd

3. How soon after symptom onset must a person who has had a stroke receive thrombolytic treatment?
   a. 30 minutes
   b. 1 hour
   c. 2 hours
   d. 3 hours

4. A patient is experiencing receptive aphasia. This means that the patient has difficulty with which of the following functions?
   a. Swallowing
   b. Forming words
   c. Hearing
   d. Understanding language

5. A nurse is caring for a patient who is recovering from an ischemic stroke. Upon entering the room to pick up the supper tray, the nurse notes that the patient has only eaten half the meal. What should the nurse do?
   a. Assist the patient by providing finger foods and feeding the patient items that require a utensil.
   b. Remove the tray and do not comment.
   c. Encourage the patient to eat the rest of the meal.
   d. Turn the plate 180 degrees and observe the patient's response.

6. A nurse is doing an afternoon assessment on a patient transferred to a medical unit from intensive care following a subarachnoid hemorrhage. The patient was alert and oriented during the morning assessment, but reported being very tired. Now the patient is difficult to arouse. What action should the nurse take?
   a. Let the patient sleep; transferring from the ICU can be very strenuous.
   b. Reassess the patient in an hour. If the sleepiness continues, notify the RN.
   c. Call the RN immediately.
   d. Call a code.

References

American Association of Neuroscience Nurses. (2008). *AANN clinical practice guidelines series. Guide to the care of the hospitalized patient with ischemic stroke* (2nd ed.). Glenview, IL: Author.

American Heart Association. (2009). Heart disease and stroke statistics 2009 update. A report from the American Heart Association Statistics Committee and Stroke Statistics Subcommittee. *Circulation, 119*(3), e21–e181.

American Stroke Association. (n.d.). *Learn to recognize a stroke.* Retrieved August 1, 2009, from http://www.strokeassociation.org/presenter.jhtml?identifier=1020

National Institutes of Health, National Institute of Neurological Disorders and Stroke. (n.d.). *NINDS transient ischemic attack information page.* Retrieved November 10, 2009, from http://www.ninds.nih.gov/disorders/tia/tia.htm

Sacco, R., Adams, R., Albers, G., et al. (2006). Guideline for prevention of stroke in patients with ischemic stroke or transient ischemic attack. *Stroke, 37,* 577–617.

Summers, D., Leonard, A., Wentworth, D., et al. (2009). Comprehensive overview of nursing and interdisciplinary care of the acute ischemic stroke patient. A scientific statement from the American Heart Association. *Stroke, 40,* 2911–2944. Retrieved August 4, 2009, from http://stroke.ahajournals.org/cgi/content/full/40/8/2911

DavisPlus | For additional resources and information visit **http://davisplus.fadavis.com**

50 Nursing Care of Patients with Peripheral Nervous System Disorders

DEBORAH L. WEAVER

KEY TERMS

amyotrophic (ay-MY-oh-TROH-fik)
anticholinesterase (AN-tee-KOH-lin-ESS-ter-ays)
atrophy (AT-troh-fee)
demyelination (dee-MY-uh-lin-AY-shun)
fasciculation (fah-SIK-yoo-LAY-shun)
neuralgia (new-RAL-jee-ah)
neuropathies (new-RAW-puh-thees)
plasmapheresis (PLAZ-mah-fer-EE-siss)
polyneuropathy (PAH-lee-new-RAH-puh-thee)
ptosis (TOH-sis)
remyelination (ree-MY-uh-lin-AY-shun)
sclerosis (skleh-ROH-sis)

QUESTIONS TO GUIDE YOUR READING

1. What disorders are caused by disruption of the peripheral nervous system?
2. What are the pathophysiology, major signs and symptoms, and complications of selected peripheral nervous system disorders?
3. What therapeutic measures are used for selected peripheral nervous system disorders?
4. What common nursing diagnoses are associated with peripheral nervous system disorders?
5. What are the priority nursing interventions for patients with peripheral nervous system disorders?
6. How will you know if your nursing care has been effective?

The peripheral nervous system (PNS) consists of all nervous system structures outside the central nervous system (CNS). A variety of disorders affect the PNS. Some of these disorders become chronic and cause degeneration of body systems. Some other disorders are more temporary. Two common types of PNS disorders are discussed in this chapter. Neuromuscular disorders compose one group and may include motor or sensory disorders or both. The second group includes cranial nerve disorders. Both types of disorders present a challenge to the nurse caring for the patient and family.

NEUROMUSCULAR DISORDERS

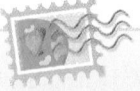

This group of neurologic conditions is chronic and degenerative in nature. Neuromuscular disorders involve a disruption of the transmission of impulses between neurons and the muscles they stimulate. This breakdown in transmission results in muscle weakness. If the muscles of the respiratory system are affected, deadly complications can develop, including pneumonia and respiratory failure. Common neuromuscular disorders include multiple sclerosis, myasthenia gravis, amyotrophic lateral sclerosis, and Guillain-Barré syndrome. An additional neuropathic disorder, Navajo neuropathy, is discussed in Box 50.1, *Cultural Considerations.*

Multiple Sclerosis

Pathophysiology

Multiple **sclerosis** (MS) is a chronic progressive degenerative disease that affects the myelin sheath of the neurons in the CNS. Myelin is responsible for the smooth transmission of nerve impulses. Muscles contract when nerve impulses stimulate the muscle tissue. In MS, the myelin sheath begins to break down (degenerate; Fig. 50.1) as a result of activation of the body's immune system. The nerve becomes inflamed and edematous, causing nerve impulses to the muscles to slow down. As the disease progresses, sclerosis or scar tissue damages the nerve. Nerve impulses become completely blocked causing permanent loss of muscle function in that area of the body.

Etiology

The cause of MS is not really understood. Damage to the myelin sheath is thought to be from an autoimmune process; however, the disease may be related to viral infections, heredity, and other unknown factors. Some research indicates that there is an inherited tendency to develop MS, and the manifestations of the disease only appear in the presence of environmental triggers. This disease affects 400,000 people in the United States and up to 2.5 million people worldwide (National Multiple Sclerosis Society, n.d.). The disease usually starts between ages 20 and 50. Women are affected twice as often as men. The course of the disease is unpredictable, and there are many variations in symptoms, depending on which nerves are affected. Some individuals have mild illness, while others suffer permanent disability or rapid decline and death.

Signs and Symptoms

The patient with MS presents with muscle weakness, tingling sensations, and numbness. Other common symptoms include visual disturbances, usually in one eye at a time. These disturbances may be accompanied by pain with eye movement. Symptoms may begin slowly over weeks to months or start suddenly and dramatically. MS affects many body systems (Box 50.2). Many factors can trigger the onset of symptoms or aggravate the condition, including extreme heat and cold, fatigue, infection, and physical and emotional stress. Hormonal changes after pregnancy may also cause symptom onset or exacerbation.

Periods of exacerbation and remission lead patients with MS to be uncertain about when the disease will flare up and what body system will be affected. Intense fatigue is common; therefore, immobility can become a problem. Accidents and falls are common because of muscle weakness or numbness of the trunk and limbs. Some people with MS experience symptoms such as muscle spasticity, bowel or bladder dysfunction, or paralysis. Difficulty with concentration or forgetfulness can also be problematic. Pneumonia can occur from immobility and from weakness of the diaphragm and intercostal muscles. Death, often resulting from respiratory infection, typically occurs 20 to 35 years after diagnosis.

Box 50.1

Cultural Considerations

Navajo neuropathy is unique to the Navajo Indian population. Characteristics include poor weight gain, short stature, sexual infantilism, serious systemic infections, and liver derangement. Manifestations include weakness, hypotonia, areflexia, loss of sensation in the extremities, corneal ulcerations, acral (extremity) mutilation, and painless fractures (Singleton et al., 1990). Nerve biopsies show a nearly complete absence of myelinated fibers, which is different from other neuropathies that present as a gradual demyelination process. Individuals who survive have many complications and are typically ventilator dependent. None have been known to survive past age 24.

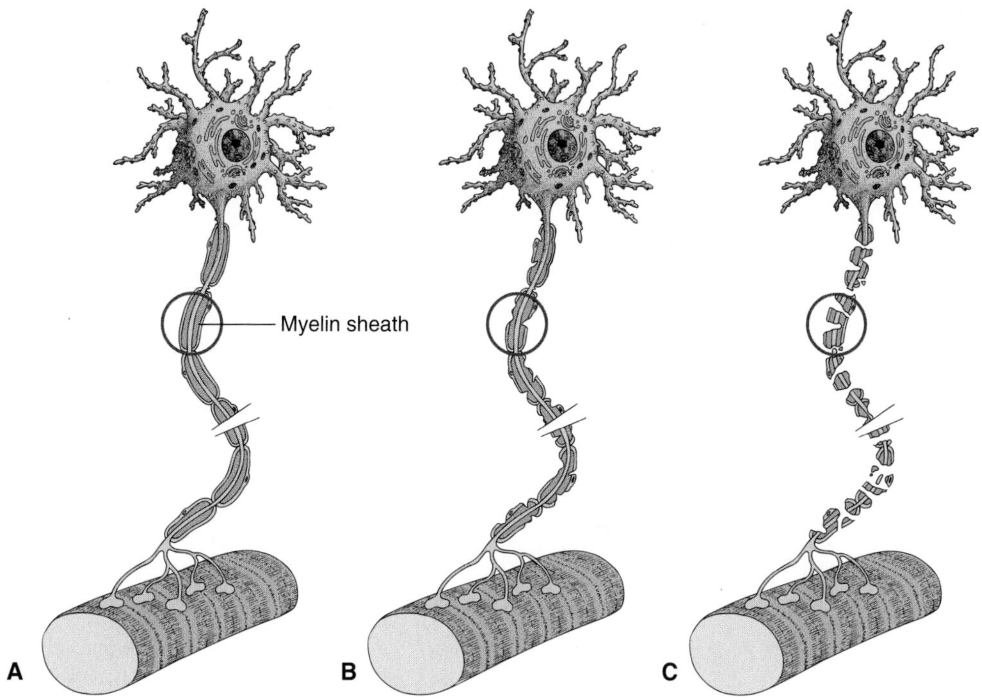
Myelin sheath
A
B
C

FIGURE 50.1 The myelin sheath breaks down in multiple sclerosis, interrupting transmission of nerve impulses. (A) Normal myelin sheath. (B) Myelin beginning to break down. (C) Total myelin disruption. (Modified from Scanlon, V. C., & Sanders, T. [2007]. *Workbook for essentials of anatomy and physiology* [5th ed.]. Philadelphia: F. A. Davis, with permission.)

Box 50.2

Problems Associated with Multiple Sclerosis

- Weakness/paralysis of limbs, trunk, or head
- Diplopia (double vision)
- Slurred speech
- Spasticity of muscles
- Numbness and tingling
- Patchy blindness (scotomas)
- Blurred vision
- Vertigo
- Tinnitus
- Impaired hearing
- Nystagmus
- Ataxia
- Dysarthria
- Dysphagia
- Constipation
- Spastic (uninhibited) bladder
- Flaccid (hypotonic) bladder
- Sexual dysfunction
- Anger, depression, euphoria

Diagnostic Tests

Diagnosis is based on the patient's history and signs and symptoms. Analysis of cerebrospinal fluid (CSF) may show an increase in oligoclonal immunoglobulin G (IgG). Magnetic resonance imaging (MRI) may be helpful in diagnosis because sclerotic plaques can be detected. A new blood test, gMS DX, is now available to help identify people likely to have identifying antibodies associated with MS.

Therapeutic Measures

MS has no cure. Many people with MS do well with no medication at all, though early treatment can delay progression of the disease. Interferon therapy with beta-interferons such as Betaseron or Avonex may reduce exacerbations and delay disability. Steroids such as adrenocorticotropic hormone (ACTH) and prednisone are given to decrease inflammation and edema of the neurons, which may relieve some symptoms. Immunosuppressant drugs such as azathioprine (Imuran) and cyclophosphamide (Cytoxan) may be given to suppress the immune system.

Newer drugs such as glatiramer (Copaxone) and natalizumab (Tysabri) are being used to control progression of the disease. Glatiramer must be injected daily and helps prevent the immune system's attack on myelin. Natalizumab is administered IV once every 4 weeks and is used to prevent immune cells from moving to the brain and spinal cord. Because of serious side effects, it is only prescribed through a special distribution program.

Anticonvulsants such as phenytoin (Dilantin) and carbamazepine (Tegretol) help relieve neuropathic pain. Valium (Diazepam), baclofen (Lioresal), tizanidine (Zanaflex), and physical therapy assist in controlling muscle spasms. Bladder problems are treated with parasympathetic agents such as bethanechol (Urecholine) and oxybutynin (Ditropan). Fatigue may be treated with antidepressants or an antiviral agent such as amantadine (Symmetrel). Table 50.1 reviews additional medications used to treat PNS disorders.

TABLE 50.1 MEDICATIONS USED TO TREAT PERIPHERAL NERVOUS SYSTEM DISORDERS

Medication Class/ Action	Examples	Route	Side Effects	Nursing Implications
Cholinesterase Inhibitors				
Increase acetylcholine at synapses.	neostigmine (Prostigmin) pyridostigmine (Mestinon) edrophonium chloride (Tensilon, used in diagnosis)	PO PO, IM, IV IM, IV	Cholinergic toxicity	Atropine is antidote.
Glucocorticoids				
Reduce inflammation.	prednisone prednisolone prednisolone acetate or sodium phosphate	PO PO IV, IM	Osteoporosis, risk for infection Elevated blood glucose level, sodium and water retention, Cushing's syndrome	Provide calcium supplement. Avoid crowds and others with infections. Monitor fluid balance. May need to treat blood sugar with insulin while on medication.
Immunosuppressants				
Suppress immunity and antibody formation.	azathioprine (Imuran) cyclophosphamide (Cytoxan)	PO, IV PO, IV	Anorexia, hepatotoxicity, nausea, vomiting, anemia, leukopenia, thrombocytopenia, fever, chills	Monitor blood counts. Protect from bleeding and infection. Administer with meals to reduce nausea.
Antispasmodics/Muscle Relaxants				
Relax muscles, reduce pain.	dantrolene (Dantrium) baclofen (Lioresal) diazepam (Valium) tizanidine (Zanaflex)	PO, IV PO PO, IM, IV PO	CNS depression, nausea, constipation, urine retention, sedation, muscle weakness, constipation, diarrhea	Avoid operating machinery or driving until effects are known. Monitor patient for respiratory depression.
Anticonvulsants				
Treat nerve pain.	phenytoin (Dilantin) carbamazepine (Tegretol) gabapentin (Neurontin)	PO PO PO	CNS depression, gingival hyperplasia (phenytoin), ataxia, vertigo	Teach good oral hygiene with soft bristle brush, floss, and gum massage (phenytoin). Monitor for fall risk. Monitor blood counts.
Glutamate Antagonist				
Delays progression of ALS.	riluzole (Rilutek)	PO	Decreased strength, diarrhea, nausea, vomiting, abdominal pain, dizziness, vertigo, sedation, elevated liver enzymes	Rest, monitor for respiratory depression. Give on empty stomach. Avoid large quantities of caffeine. Avoid charcoal-broiled foods. Monitor liver function laboratory values.

For those who suffer sudden severe attacks or who do not respond to high doses of steroids, plasma exchange or **plasmapheresis** may be used to remove from the blood antibodies that may be attacking the myelin (Box 50.3). A new treatment study launched in 2009 includes MS patients willing to have stem cells retrieved, undergo extensive chemotherapy to destroy remaining immune cells, and then have the stem cells re-infused. It is hoped that this process will slow or reverse disease progression (National Multiple Sclerosis Society, 2009).

Rehabilitation after an acute episode includes physical, speech, and occupational therapies. Rehabilitation therapy helps the patient and family adapt the home environment to the patient's special needs. Assistive devices such as braces, canes, wheelchairs, and splints allow the patient increased mobility and independence. Patients who develop speech difficulties benefit from speech therapy. Exercise also may be beneficial (see *Evidence-Based Practice* box).

• WORD • BUILDING •

plasmapheresis: plasma—liquid of blood + pheresis—removal

Box 50.3

Plasmapheresis

Plasmapheresis, also known as plasma exchange therapy, is a procedure that removes the plasma component from whole blood and replaces it with fresh plasma. The goal is to remove antibodies through plasma exchange, suppressing the immune response and inflammation.

Preprocedure Nursing Care

- Teach patient about the procedure and what to expect, including what the machine looks like (similar to but smaller than a dialysis machine), the need for arterial and venous access sites, and the length of the procedure (2 to 5 hours).
- The physician may order medications held until after the procedure.
- Assess baseline vital signs and weight.
- Assess complete blood cell count (CBC), platelet count, and clotting studies.
- Check blood type and crossmatch for replacement blood products.

Postprocedure Nursing Care

- Observe the patient for signs of hypovolemia, such as dizziness and hypotension.
- Apply pressure dressings to the access sites.
- Monitor the patient for infection and bruits at the access site.
- Monitor electrolytes and signs of electrolyte loss. Report imbalances, and administer replacement electrolytes as ordered.
- Compare preprocedure and postprocedure laboratory data, such as CBC, platelet count, and clotting times.

EVIDENCE-BASED PRACTICE

Clinical Question

Can exercise help patients with multiple sclerosis?

Evidence

Several studies have shown that exercise can help preserve muscle strength and exercise tolerance, maintain mobility, and improve mood in patients with multiple sclerosis (Rietberg et al., 2005).

Implications for Nursing Practice

Make sure patients have an exercise plan prescribed by the primary care provider or physical therapist, to be carried out during times when the disease is not exacerbated.

REFERENCE

Rietberg, M. B., Brooks, D., Uitdehaag, B. M. J., & Kwakkel, G. (2005). Exercise therapy for multiple sclerosis. *Cochrane Database of Systematic Reviews 2005, Issue 1* (Art. No. CD003980; DOI 10.1002/14651858.CD003980.pub2).

Nursing Care

See the *Nursing Care Plan for the Patient with a Progressive Neuromuscular Disorder.*

In addition to reviewing routine care, instruct the patient to avoid factors that can exacerbate symptoms. This includes avoiding stressful situations as much as possible. Rest, exercise, and a balanced diet are important self-care steps to control symptoms. In addition, avoiding extreme temperature changes, especially heat, and avoiding infection and illness are important. Any infection, especially respiratory, should be reported immediately to a physician. Two sources of information on MS are the National Multiple Sclerosis Society at www.nationalmssociety.org and the Multiple Sclerosis Foundation at www.msfocus.org.

Myasthenia Gravis

Pathophysiology

Myasthenia gravis (MG) means "grave muscle weakness," or weakness of the voluntary or skeletal muscles of the body. MG is a disease of the neuromuscular junction (Fig. 50.2). Normally, at the neuromuscular junction, the neuron releases

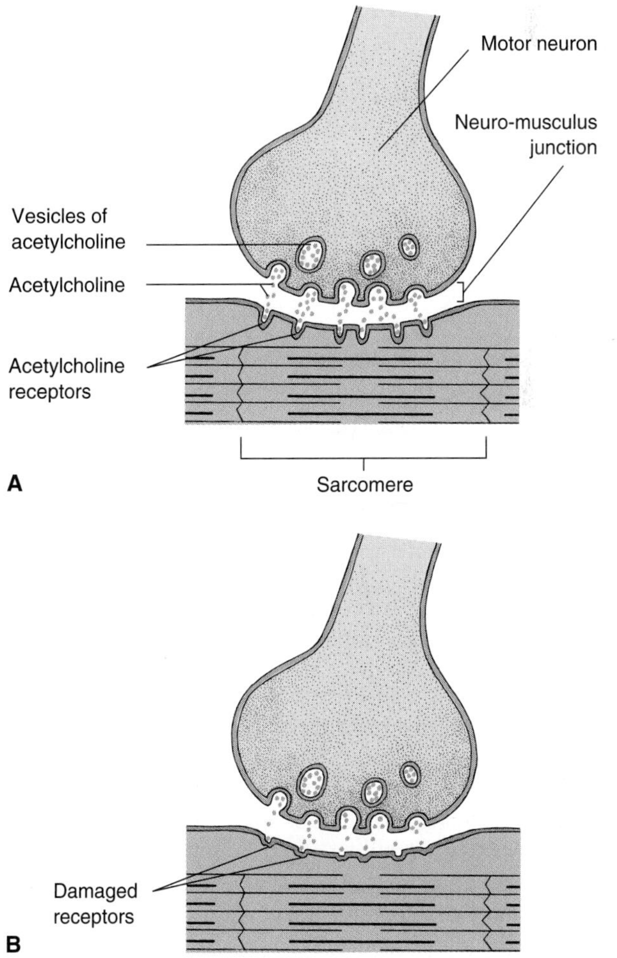
Motor neuron
Neuro-musculus junction
Vesicles of acetylcholine
Acetylcholine
Acetylcholine receptors
A
Sarcomere
Damaged receptors
B

FIGURE 50.2 Myasthenia gravis. (A) Normal neuromuscular junction. (B) Note damaged acetylcholine receptor sites in myasthenia gravis. (Modified from Scanlon, V. C., & Sanders, T. [2007]. *Workbook for essentials of anatomy and physiology* [5th ed.]. Philadelphia: F. A. Davis, with permission.)

NURSING CARE PLAN for the Patient with a Progressive Neuromuscular Disorder

Nursing Diagnosis: *Ineffective Airway Clearance* related to respiratory muscle weakness, impaired cough and gag reflexes as evidenced by crackles, moist cough, inability to clear secretions

Expected Outcomes: The patient will maintain a patent airway as evidenced by clear lung sounds and freedom from signs and symptoms of respiratory distress.

Evaluation of Outcomes: Is patient's airway patent and are lung sounds clear? Is patient free of signs and symptoms of respiratory distress?

Interventions	Rationale	Evaluation
Monitor respiratory rate and depth, breath sounds, oxygen saturation (SpO_2), and arterial blood gases (as ordered). Report deterioration.	Increasing respiratory distress indicates progressing muscle weakness that may require mechanical ventilation or end-of-life decisions.	Is patient's respiratory rate status stable or is intervention indicated?
Encourage patient to cough and deep breathe every 2 hours.	Effective coughing helps keep airway clear.	Does patient have the strength to cough effectively?
Observe patient for breathlessness while speaking.	Inability to speak without breathlessness indicates declining respiratory function.	Is patient able to finish sentences without needing to take a breath?
Elevate head of bed.	Fowler's position improves lung expansion, decreases work of breathing, improves cough efforts, and decreases risk for aspiration.	Does elevation of head of bed help relieve dyspnea and prevent aspiration?
Evaluate cough, swallow, and gag reflexes frequently. Notify physician if absent.	Frequent evaluation of reflexes is needed to prevent aspiration, respiratory infections, and respiratory failure.	Is patient able to cough effectively? Is gag reflex intact?
Suction secretions as needed, noting color and amount of secretions.	Muscle weakness may result in inability to clear airway.	Does patient require suctioning to clear airway? What color are secretions?

Nursing Diagnosis: *Impaired Physical Mobility* related to muscle weakness as evidenced by inability to move independently as desired

Expected Outcomes: The patient will maintain optimum mobility and activity level, identify measures to help maintain mobility, and perform exercises that help maintain current mobility.

Evaluation of Outcomes: Is optimum activity level maintained? Can patient identify measures that will help maintain mobility? Does patient perform exercises that help maintain mobility?

Interventions	Rationale	Evaluation
Determine preillness and current level of mobility.	Provides information to formulate plan of care and goals.	Do assessment findings help determine goals and interventions?
Identify factors that affect ability to be mobile and active.	Some factors that interfere with mobility can be modified.	Are interfering factors modified effectively?
Encourage patient to perform self-care to maximum ability.	Promotes sense of control and independence for patient.	Does patient perform self-care activities? Is assistance required?

NURSING CARE PLAN for the Patient with a Progressive Neuromuscular Disorder—cont'd

Interventions	Rationale	Evaluation
Consult physical therapist (PT) or occupational therapist (OT) to provide assistive devices for walking (canes, braces, walker, wheelchair) and other activities.	Assistive devices decrease fatigue and promote independence, comfort, and safety.	Does patient use assistive devices safely during activities? Do they help keep patient active?
Reposition frequently when patient is immobile.	Prevents skin breakdown and stasis of pulmonary secretions.	Is patient free from complications of immobility?
Provide active/passive range-of-motion (ROM) exercises on a regular basis.	Prevents contractures and disuse atrophy.	Does patient have any contractures or atrophy?
Plan activities with a balance of frequent rest periods.	Rest decreases fatigue.	Is fatigue controlled?
Administer medications as ordered.	Medications may slow progress of disease and reduce symptoms.	Are symptoms controlled?

Nursing Diagnosis: *Risk for Imbalanced Nutrition: Less Than Body Requirements* related to weakness or lack of coordination of muscles for chewing and swallowing

Expected Outcomes: The patient will maintain body weight within normal limits for height and frame.

Evaluation of Outcomes: Is patient's weight stable and within normal limits (WNL)?

Interventions	Rationale	Evaluation
Evaluate cough, swallow, and gag reflexes frequently. Notify physician if absent.	If patient is unable to swallow, a feeding tube may be indicated, depending on patient's wishes.	Does patient eat and drink without aspirating?
Offer soft, easy to chew and swallow foods.	Soft foods require less effort to chew and are less fatiguing.	Is patient able to chew and swallow without excessive fatigue?
Request speech therapist and dietitian consultations as indicated.	Speech therapist can help evaluate swallowing and make recommendations. Dietitian can recommend appropriate foods.	Are consults indicated? Are recommendations implemented?
Institute swallowing precautions as needed.	Swallowing precautions help prevent aspiration and allow patient to maintain oral intake as long as possible.	Do precautions prevent aspiration?

Nursing Diagnosis: *Impaired Verbal Communication* related to impaired respiratory and muscle function as evidenced by inability to articulate needs

Expected Outcomes: The patient will be able to communicate needs.

Evaluation of Outcomes: Does patient indicate that needs are met with a minimum of frustration?

Interventions	Rationale	Evaluation
Assess ability to speak and communicate.	Assessment is essential to planning appropriate communication interventions.	Can patient speak or communicate needs?

Continued

NURSING CARE PLAN for the Patient with a Progressive Neuromuscular Disorder—cont'd

Request referral to speech therapist for assistance if indicated.	Speech therapist can recommend appropriate alternative communication techniques.	Is speech therapy referral indicated? Is referral completed?
Assess for nonverbal signs of pain or distress, such as restlessness, agitation, grimacing.	Patient may not be able to tell you if he or she is in pain or distress.	Are signs of pain or distress present? Are they attended to?
Use picture board or paper and pencil. Ask questions that require a yes or no answer.	These do not require the patient to speak to communicate.	Do alternative methods help patient communicate needs?
Use nonhurried, calm, and caring approach while providing care.	This will help decrease anxiety and provide emotional support to patient and family.	Do patient and family appear anxious? Does calm approach help?
Explain all procedures.	Patient can still hear and needs to know what is happening.	Does patient indicate understanding?

the chemical neurotransmitter acetylcholine (ACh), which crosses the synaptic cleft. Receptors on the muscle tissue take up ACh and contraction of the muscle results. In MG, the body's immune system is activated, producing antibodies that attack and destroy ACh receptors at the neuromuscular junction. Hence, ACh cannot stimulate muscle contraction because the number of ACh receptors has been reduced, resulting in loss of voluntary muscle strength.

Etiology

Myasthenia gravis is a chronic autoimmune process. No specific cause has been found for MG. However, current thought is that a virus may initiate the disease. Disorders of the thymus gland are often associated with MG. Thymomas or tumors on the thymus gland may account for the malfunction of the immune system that initiates the autoimmune process. All ethnic groups and both genders can develop this disease. Peak age of onset in women is ages 20 to 30. Men are affected more often after age 60. MG occurs slightly more often in women than men.

Signs and Symptoms

MG results in progressive extreme muscle weakness. The hallmark of MG is increased muscle weakness during activity and improvement in muscle strength after rest. Muscles are strongest in the morning, when the person is rested. Activity causes the muscles to fatigue easily, but rest allows the muscles to regain strength. Activities affected by MG include eye and eyelid movements, chewing, swallowing, speaking, and breathing, as well as skeletal muscle function. Patients often present with drooping of the eyelids (**ptosis**). Facial expressions become mask-like. After long conversations, the patient's voice may fade. Falls occur because of weakness of the arm and leg muscles. Patients with MG experience periods of exacerbation and remission of symptoms, similar to patients with MS. Exacerbations can be caused by emotional or physical stress, such as pregnancy, menses, illness, trauma, extremes in temperature, electrolyte imbalance, surgery, and drugs that block actions at the neuromuscular junction.

Complications

Major complications associated with MG result from weakness of muscles that assist with swallowing and breathing. Aspiration, respiratory infections, and respiratory failure are the leading causes of death. Sudden onset of muscle weakness in patients with MG resulting from not enough medication is called a myasthenic crisis. Overmedication with **anticholinesterase** (anti-ACh) drugs causes a cholinergic crisis (Table 50.2). Both crises require immediate medical attention.

> **LEARNING TIP**
>
> Symptoms of cholinergic crisis can be remembered with the acronym SLUDGE: salivation, lacrimation, urination, diarrhea, gastrointestinal cramping, and emesis. A severe crisis has been described as "liquid pouring out of every body orifice."

Diagnostic Tests

Diagnosis of myasthenia gravis is based on history of symptoms and physical examination of the patient. A simple test involves the patient looking upward for 2 to 3 minutes. Increased droop of the eyelids (ptosis) occurs if MG is present.

• WORD • BUILDING •
anticholinesterase: anti—against + cholinesterase—chemical that breaks down acetylcholine

TABLE 50.2 COMPARISON OF MYASTHENIC CRISIS AND CHOLINERGIC CRISIS

	Myasthenic Crisis	Cholinergic Crisis
Cause	Too little medication	Too much medication
Signs and Symptoms	Ptosis Difficulty swallowing Difficulty speaking Dyspnea Weakness	Increasing muscle weakness Dyspnea Salivation Lacrimation Urination Abdominal cramping, diarrhea Nausea, emesis Increased bronchial secretions Sweating Miosis (constriction of pupils)

After a brief rest, the eyelids can be opened without difficulty. Another test involves an intravenous injection of edrophonium (Tensilon, an anticholinesterase drug). If muscle strength improves dramatically (e.g., the patient can suddenly open the eyes wide), MG is diagnosed. However, improvement is only temporary. An increased number of anti-ACh receptor antibodies in the blood are present in 90% of patients with MG. Electromyography (EMG) may be done to rule out other conditions. Pulmonary function tests may be done to predict or anticipate potential myasthenic crisis leading to respiratory failure.

Therapeutic Measures

No cure is currently available for MG. Treatment is aimed at controlling symptoms. Removal of the thymus gland (thymectomy) can decrease production of ACh receptor antibodies and decrease symptoms in most patients. Medications used to treat MG include the anticholinesterase drugs neostigmine (Prostigmin) and pyridostigmine (Mestinon). These drugs improve MG symptoms by destroying the acetylcholinesterase that breaks down ACh. Remember that ACh causes muscles to contract. If ACh is allowed more time to attach to muscle tissue receptors, the muscle contracts and strength is increased. Steroids such as prednisone and immunosuppressants are used to suppress the body's immune response. Plasmapheresis can be used to remove antibodies from the patient's blood (see Box 50.3). Use of immune globulin is being researched.

Nursing Process for the Patient with Myasthenia Gravis

DATA COLLECTION. Determine the patient's baseline muscle strength. Ask how much activity is tolerated before fatigue and muscle weakness occur. Identify the patient's support systems and determine whether the patient's needs are being met. Assess the knowledge base of the patient and family. Check respiratory function and swallowing ability.

NURSING DIAGNOSES, PLANNING, AND IMPLEMENTATION

Activity Intolerance Related to Muscle Weakness as Evidenced by Progressive Tiring with Activity

EXPECTED OUTCOME: The patient will improve activity tolerance as evidenced by ability to carry out necessary activities.

- Schedule anticholinesterase drugs so that peak action occurs at times when increased muscle strength is needed *so the patient has strength for activities such as meals and physical therapy.*
- Teach the patient to schedule activities such as grocery shopping or errands at times when medication is at peak action, *so that muscle strength is increased.*
- Be aware of symptoms and treatment of myasthenic and cholinergic crises, *so quick intervention can be carried out to prevent worsening symptoms.*
- Teach the patient and significant others signs and symptoms of crisis conditions *because both crises constitute medical emergencies and require immediate medical attention (see Table 50.2).*
- Teach methods to conserve energy, such as sitting down to do grooming and housekeeping activities whenever possible. *This helps the patient conserve energy to manage ADLs.*
- Teach the patient to rest between activities *to allow time for muscle strength to be restored.*
- Teach the importance of avoiding people with infections and exposure to cold *to minimize risk for respiratory infections, which can exacerbate symptoms and increase risk for ineffective airway clearance.*
- Instruct the patient to eat nutritious, well-balanced meals *to maintain strength and resistance to infections, which can exacerbate symptoms.*
- Teach the patient to only use medications that are prescribed by the physician. If multiple providers are used, all medications should be checked with the provider who is treating the MG. *Many medications can exacerbate muscle weakness* (Box 50.4).
- Provide information about support groups *that can provide encouragement and assistance to patients and their families.*

EVALUATION. If the plan of care has been effective, the patient's activity and self-care needs will be met, either by the patient or by other support individuals.

Also see the *Nursing Care Plan for the Patient with a Progressive Neuromuscular Disorder.* More information can be found at the Myasthenia Gravis Foundation of America website, www.myasthenia.org.

CRITICAL THINKING

Jamie

■ Jamie is referred to a neurologist because of muscle weakness.

1. What history can help differentiate between MS and MG?
2. What physical examination can be done to differentiate between MS and MG?
3. The neurologist prepares to do a Tensilon test and asks you to prepare 2 mg of Tensilon for IV injection. It is supplied as 10 mg per milliliter. How much should you draw up?

Suggested answers at end of chapter.

Box 50.4

Medications That Can Exacerbate Symptoms of Myasthenia Gravis

- Antibiotics (some)
- Alpha interferon
- Anticholinergic agents
- Beta blockers
- Botulinum toxin
- Calcium channel blockers
- Chloroquine
- Lithium
- Magnesium
- Neuromuscular blocking agents (such as those used during surgery)
- Penicillamine
- Prednisone
- Procainamide
- Quinidine

Amyotrophic Lateral Sclerosis

Pathophysiology and Etiology

Amyotrophic lateral sclerosis (ALS, also called Lou Gehrig's disease) is a progressive, degenerative condition that affects motor neurons responsible for the control of voluntary muscles. In the brain and spinal cord, upper and lower motor neurons begin to degenerate and form scar tissue or die, blocking transmission of nerve impulses. Without stimulation, muscles **atrophy,** and muscle strength and coordination decrease. As the disease progresses, more muscle groups, including muscles controlling breathing and swallowing, become involved. The heart and gastrointestinal tract are controlled involuntarily, and so are not affected by ALS. The ability to think and reason also is not affected.

ALS can occur at any age but usually does not appear until adulthood. A specific cause has not been discovered, although ALS may have a genetic predisposition in some cases. About 5000 people in the United States are diagnosed with ALS each year (ALS Association, n.d.). Life expectancy after diagnosis averages about 2 to 5 years; a few patients live as long as 20 years. In a very few patients, the disease slows or stops progressing completely.

Signs and Symptoms

Symptoms are vague early in the course of ALS. Primary symptoms include progressive muscle weakness and decreased coordination. This can begin in the arms, legs, or muscles of speech and swallowing. Atrophy of muscles and **fasciculations** (twitching) also occur. Muscle spasms can cause pain. Difficulty with chewing and swallowing place the patient at a risk for choking and aspiration as the disease progresses. Inappropriate emotional outbursts of laughing and crying may occur. Speech becomes increasingly difficult. Bladder and bowel functions remain intact, yet problems such as constipation, urinary urgency, hesitancy, or frequency may occur.

Late in the disease, communication becomes limited to moving and blinking the eyes in response to questions. Pulmonary function becomes severely compromised to the point of requiring mechanical ventilator assistance if the patient chooses. Other complications may include extreme malnutrition, falls, pulmonary emboli, and congestive heart failure. ALS eventually leads to death from respiratory complications such as atelectasis, respiratory failure, and pneumonia.

Diagnostic Tests

Diagnosis is made based on clinical symptoms. Additional tests such as CSF analysis, electroencephalogram (EEG), nerve biopsy, nerve conduction velocity (NCV), or EMG may be done to rule out other conditions. Blood enzymes may be increased as a result of muscle atrophy.

Therapeutic Measures

Goals of treatment are aimed at improving function as long as possible and emotionally supporting the patient and family through the illness. Baclofen (Lioresal) and diazepam (Valium) may be given to relieve muscle spasticity. Quinine may be used for muscle cramps. Riluzole (Rilutek) slows the progression of the disease and may prolong life. New treatments are constantly being researched.

Nonpharmacological measures such as physical therapy, massage, position changes, and diversional activities may help control pain. Tube feedings via a surgically placed gastrostomy tube help provide adequate nutrition. Prevention of infections, such as pneumonia and urinary tract infection (UTI), is vital. Meticulous skin care minimizes the incidence of pressure ulcers. Rehabilitation therapy, including physical, occupational, and speech therapy, allows the

• WORD • BUILDING •

amyotrophic: a—without + myo—muscle + trophic—nourishment
atrophy: a—without + trophy—nourishment

patient to maximize function and control for as long as possible. Therapy may also decrease the occurrence of complications such as aspiration, falls, and contractures.

Patients with speech problems may benefit from the use of augmentative alternative communication (AAC). A variety of AAC systems are available; most involve laptop computers that patients can use to type in words or symbols to generate speech. Medicare pays at least a portion of the cost for AAC equipment. Support groups and counseling provide emotional support for the patient and family.

Nursing Care

See the *Nursing Care Plan for the Patient with a Progressive Neuromuscular Disorder.*

PATIENT EDUCATION. Reinforce information given by the physician to the patient and family about ALS and its prognosis. Support groups can provide emotional support as the patient and family deal with the likely reality of eventual death. Rehabilitation using assistive devices and exercises helps prevent complications. Teaching family members how to perform physical therapy and other health care activities allows the patient to spend as much time as possible at home. Teach the patient to avoid exposure to persons with infections because an infection can be deadly to a patient with a debilitating disease.

NURSING CARE TIP

When planning care, remember that a person with ALS has an intact mind—it is the body that is deteriorating.

CRITICAL THINKING

Mr. Miller

■ Mr. Miller has been having difficulty swallowing. He is diagnosed with ALS.

1. What are the priority nursing diagnoses for Mr. Miller?
2. How can the patient and his family be supported in coping with this disease?

Suggested answers at end of chapter.

Guillain-Barré Syndrome

Pathophysiology

Guillain-Barré syndrome (GBS) is also called acute inflammatory **polyneuropathy**. This latter term is more descriptive of the actual disease process. GBS is an inflammatory disorder characterized by abrupt onset of symmetrical paresis (weakness) that progresses to paralysis. The myelin sheath of the spinal and cranial nerves is destroyed by a diffuse inflammatory reaction. The peripheral nerves are infiltrated by lymphocytes, which leads to edema and inflammation. Segmental **demyelination** causes axonal atrophy, resulting in slowed or blocked nerve conduction. Typically, the demyelination begins in the most distal nerves and ascends in a symmetrical fashion. **Remyelination**, which is a much slower process, occurs in a descending pattern and is accompanied by a resolution of symptoms.

There are four recognized variants of GBS. The most common form is ascending GBS. It is characterized by progressive weakness and numbness that begins in the legs and ascends up the body. The numbness tends to be mild, but the muscle weakness usually progresses to paralysis. The paralysis may ascend all the way to the cranial nerves or stop anywhere between the legs and head. Deep tendon reflexes are either depressed or absent. In approximately 50% of patients with ascending GBS, respiratory function becomes compromised.

Descending GBS is less common. It affects the cranial nerves that originate in the brainstem first. These patients present with difficulty swallowing and speaking. The weakness progresses downward toward the legs. Respiratory compromise is rapid. Numbness is more problematic in the hands than in the feet, and the reflexes are diminished or absent. Miller Fisher syndrome, a variant of GBS, is rare. Typically, there is no respiratory compromise or sensory loss. The classic symptoms are profound ataxia, absence of reflexes, and paralysis of the extraocular muscles. Some people believe that the fourth form, pure motor GBS, is actually a milder version of ascending GBS. The symptoms are the same except for the lack of numbness or paresthesias.

Etiology

GBS is believed to be caused by an autoimmune response to some type of viral infection or to certain vaccines, although the exact cause is not known. Usually the viral illness affects the respiratory or gastrointestinal system, and occurs within 2 weeks prior to onset of neurologic symptoms. Average age at onset is 30 to 50; men and women are equally affected (National Library of Medicine, n.d.).

Signs and Symptoms

GBS is divided into three stages. The first stage starts with the onset of symptoms and lasts until the progression of symptoms stops. This stage can last from 24 hours to 3 weeks and is characterized by abrupt and rapid onset of muscle weakness and paralysis, with little or no muscle atrophy. Many patients give a history of a recent viral illness or vaccination, supporting the theory that the cause is autoimmune

• WORD • BUILDING •

polyneuropathy: poly—many + neuro—nerves + pathy—disease

• WORD • BUILDING •

demyelination: de—down or from + myelin—sheath surrounding neurons + ation—process

remyelination: re—repeat + myelin—sheath surrounding neurons + ation—process in nature. The degree of respiratory involvement correlates to the type of GBS and the level of paralysis. Patients with ascending GBS may gradually notice a reduced ability to take deep breaths or carry on conversations and may feel short of breath. These patients are terrified that they will not be able to breathe. Patients with either ascending or descending GBS may require intubation and artificial ventilation.

The autonomic nervous system is often affected by GBS. Patients may experience labile blood pressure, cardiac dysrhythmias, urine retention, or paralytic ileus. Patient reports of discomfort range from annoying numbness and cramping to severe pain. The discomfort is exacerbated by the patient's inability to move voluntarily.

The second stage is the plateau stage, when symptoms are most severe but progression has stopped. It may last from 2 to 14 days. Patients may become discouraged if no improvement is evident. Axonal regeneration and remyelination occur during the recovery phase. This stage lasts from 6 to 24 months and symptoms slowly improve. Most patients with GBS recover completely within a few months to a year. A few patients experience chronic disability.

Complications

Complications that can occur include respiratory failure, infection, and depression. Fatigue and paralysis of the respiratory muscles lead to insufficient respiratory effort. Some patients with impending respiratory failure attempt to convince the staff that they are not in distress and do not need to be intubated. It is important to discuss the possible need for intubation early in the patient's illness. The decision to intubate in GBS is different than with the other PNS disorders, because GBS patients are expected to recover. Constant monitoring of respiratory parameters and continuous pulse oximetry provide information indicating the need for immediate intervention.

Patients with GBS are prone to pneumonia and UTIs. Maintaining infection control practices and maximizing the patient's nutritional status help decrease the likelihood of infection. Immobility leads to such problems as skin breakdown, pulmonary embolus, deep venous thrombosis, and muscle atrophy. Patients with GBS have little time to adjust to their illness and deterioration, and often fear they will not recover function. Calm, supportive reassurance is important.

Diagnostic Tests

A lumbar puncture is performed to obtain CSF. The CSF analysis shows a normal cell count with an elevated protein level. Electromyographic and nerve conduction velocity tests are done to evaluate nerve function. Pulmonary function testing helps identify impending respiratory problems.

Therapeutic Measures

During the first stage, patients are partially or completely dependent for all needs. They are often frightened and anxious. Oxygen and mechanical ventilation may be required. Plasmapheresis may be used to remove the patient's plasma and replace it with fresh plasma. This procedure is thought to lessen the body's immune response. To be most effective, plasmapheresis should begin 7 to 14 days from the onset of symptoms. Immunoglobulin therapy may help reduce the severity of the disease. Steroid hormones, although used in the past, are not effective and may be harmful. Supportive interventions include anticoagulants to prevent deep vein thrombosis, and analgesics for pain.

During the plateau phase, patients may become discouraged because they are not getting any better. Emotional support is important during this phase. Axonal regeneration and remyelination occur during the recovery phase. Intensive rehabilitation helps the patient regain function during this phase.

Nursing Process for the Patient with Guillain-Barré Syndrome

See the *Nursing Care Plan for the Patient with a Progressive Neuromuscular Disorder.* In addition, be prepared to teach the patient and family about the disease and treatment (below).

DATA COLLECTION. Assess the patient's vital signs, ABGs, and Spo_2 to monitor respiratory status. Assess gag, corneal, and swallowing reflexes to determine whether safety measures are needed to prevent aspiration or injury to the eyes. Assess the patient's and family's knowledge about the disease and treatment.

NURSING DIAGNOSES, PLANNING, AND IMPLEMENTATION

Knowledge Deficit Related to New Diagnosis and Treatment

EXPECTED OUTCOME: The patient and family will verbalize understanding of what to expect as disease progresses, how treatments will help, and how to participate in care.

- Explain all procedures to the patient and family. *Patients and family members who understand the rationale for assessments or interventions are more likely to cooperate and assist.*
- Educate the patient and family about the need for frequent respiratory assessments and possible need for temporary respiratory support. *Patients may deny respiratory difficulty because of a fear of intubation and mechanical ventilation.*
- Teach and encourage use of diversional activities such as visits from family and friends, listening to music or relaxation tapes, and watching television or videos. *Recovery can be prolonged, and diversional activities can help alleviate boredom, loneliness, and depression.*
- As the patient begins to regain function, assist in teaching patient and family how to participate in patient care and therapies. Encourage family members to attend therapy appointments. *Participation in patient care activities and therapies can provide a sense of control over the situation and helps prepare the patient and family for discharge.*
- Provide information about the disease, treatments, and recovery. *Recovery may take months or years; most of that time will be spent at home.*

EVALUATION. If interventions have been effective, the patient and family will demonstrate understanding of the disease process and participate in care appropriately.

Table 50.3 summarizes and compares MS, MG, ALS, and GB.

Postpolio Syndrome

Pathophysiology and Etiology

Postpolio syndrome is a condition that affects survivors of polio 20 to 40 years after they have recovered from infection caused by the poliomyelitis virus. Up to 80% of patients who previously had polio develop this syndrome. The severity of the syndrome depends on the degree of residual weakness and disability left from the initial illness.

Signs and Symptoms

Postpolio syndrome involves a further weakening of the muscles that were affected with the first involvement with the poliovirus. Symptoms range from fatigue to progressive muscle weakness leading to atrophy. Sleeping problems, joint pain, scoliosis, and respiratory compromise can occur. Some people suffer great debilitation; others have fewer problems.

Diagnostic Tests

Observation and history and excluding other problems are most important in diagnosis of this syndrome.

Therapeutic Measures

No interventions have been found to be effective at this time. Symptoms seem to be best controlled by rest and moderate exercise without pushing the limits of tolerance.

CRANIAL NERVE DISORDERS

Cranial nerves are the peripheral nerves of the brain. There are 12 pairs of cranial nerves. Areas that the cranial nerves innervate include the head, neck, and special sensory structures (see Chapter 48). Cranial nerve problems are classified as peripheral

TABLE 50.3 SUMMARY OF PERIPHERAL NERVOUS SYSTEM DISORDERS

	Multiple Sclerosis	Myasthenia Gravis	Amyotrophic Lateral Sclerosis	Guillain-Barré Syndrome
Signs and Symptoms	Muscle weakness Muscle paralysis Visual disturbances Fatigue	Progressive severe muscle weakness of voluntary muscles Muscles regain strength with rest Mask-like face	Progressive muscle weakness Decreased coordination Muscle twitching Muscle spasms Pain Emotional outbursts Difficulty with speech Intact thought processes	Three stages: 1. Ascending paralysis 2. Plateau 3. Descending resolution Pain, cramping or numbness
Diagnosis	CSF analysis MRI gMS DX	Ptosis test Tensilon test EMG	CSF analysis EEG Nerve biopsy NCV	CSF EMG NCV
Therapeutic Measures	Interferon therapy Steroids Immunosuppressants Plasmapheresis Anticonvulsants Antiviral agents Muscle relaxants Physical therapy Assistive devices for ADLs Speech therapy	Plasmapheresis Thymectomy Anticholinesterase agents Steroids	Antispasmodics/quinine Riluzole (Rilutek) Physical therapy Massage Muscle relaxants Diversional activities Tube feeding Alternative communications devices	Plasmapheresis Ventilation support Physical therapy
Complications	Falls Muscle spasms Bowel and bladder problems, risk for UTI Forgetfulness Extreme fatigue	Aspiration Respiratory infections Respiratory failure Myasthenic crisis or cholinergic crisis	Communication problems Risk for aspiration Pain Respiratory failure	Respiratory infection Respiratory failure Depression Fatigue UTI Complications of immobility
Priority Nursing Diagnoses	*Ineffective Airway Clearance* *Impaired Physical Mobility* *Risk for Imbalanced Nutrition: Less Than Body Requirements* *Impaired Communication*			

CSF = cerebrospinal fluid; EEG = electroencephalography; EMG = electromyography; MRI = magnetic resonance imaging; NCV = nerve conduction velocity; UTI = urinary tract infection.

neuropathies. Disorders can affect the sensory, motor, or both branches of a single nerve. Causes of cranial nerve disorders include tumors, infections, inflammation, trauma, and unknown causes. Two common cranial nerve problems are trigeminal **neuralgia** (tic douloureux) and Bell's palsy.

Trigeminal Neuralgia

Pathophysiology and Etiology

Trigeminal neuralgia (TN), sometimes called tic douloureux, involves the fifth cranial (trigeminal) nerve. This cranial nerve has three branches that include both sensory and motor functions. The branches innervate areas of the face, including the forehead, nose, cheek, gums, and jaw. Trigeminal neuralgia affects only the sensory portion of the nerve. Irritation or chronic compression of the nerve is suspected to initiate symptoms. This condition is seen more often in women and usually begins around age 50 to 60.

Signs and Symptoms

Intense recurring episodes of pain, described as sudden, jabbing, burning, or knife-like, characterize this condition. Episodes of pain begin and end suddenly, lasting a few seconds to minutes. Attacks can occur in clusters up to hundreds of times daily. However, some patients have only a few attacks per year. Pain is felt in the skin on one side of the face. A slight touch, cold breeze, talking, or chewing can trigger attacks of pain. The areas of the face where pain is triggered are referred to as trigger zones. Areas affected include the lips, upper or lower gums, cheeks, forehead, or side of the nose (Fig. 50.3). Sleep provides a period of relief from the pain. Therefore, persons with trigeminal neuralgia may sleep most of the time to avoid painful attacks. They also may refrain from activities such as talking, face washing, teeth brushing, shaving, and eating to prevent pain. Frequent blinking and tearing of the eye on the affected side also occur.

Diagnostic Tests

History of symptoms and direct observation of an attack confirm diagnosis. Radiological studies, including computed tomography (CT) scanning and MRI, may be used to rule out other causes of the pain.

Therapeutic Measures

Initial management includes the use of anticonvulsants such as phenytoin (Dilantin), gabapentin (Neurontin), or carbamazepine (Tegretol) to reduce transmission of painful nerve impulses. Baclofen or clonazepam may also be effective in controlling symptoms. Some patients experience temporary relief from injections of alcohol into painful areas. If medications are not effective, a nerve block using a local anesthetic may be performed. This option offers 8 to 16 months of relief. If medications and nerve blocks do not provide relief, surgical options are available. Surgery is done to identify and remove the cause of irritation and inflammation of the nerve. Radio-frequency ablation is used to destroy some of the nerve branches, resulting in anesthesia of the area. Gamma knife radiosurgery is also an option. The gamma knife creates a lesion on the nerve to block the pain signals.

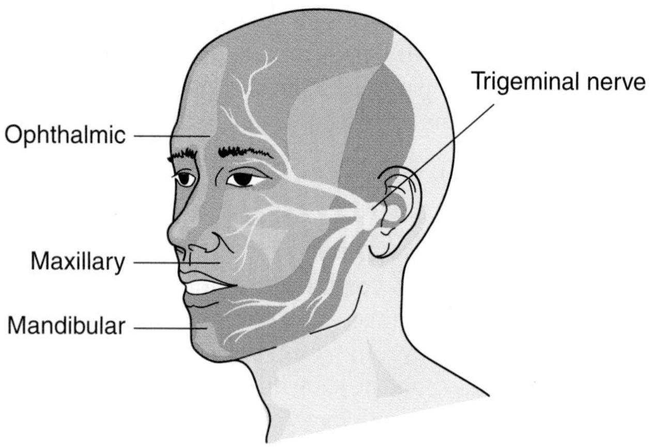
Trigeminal nerve
Ophthalmic
Maxillary
Mandibular

FIGURE 50.3 Areas innervated by the three main branches of the trigeminal nerve (cranial nerve V) are affected in trigeminal neuralgia.

PATIENT EDUCATION POSTPROCEDURE. The patient will need to learn to protect anesthetized areas of the face following nerve block or ablation. If corneal sensation is lost, goggles and sunglasses should be used as needed to protect the affected eye. An eye patch may be needed at night to prevent injury during sleep. Artificial tears may also be needed to prevent corneal damage.

Bell's Palsy

Pathophysiology and Etiology

In Bell's palsy, the facial nerve (cranial nerve VII) becomes inflamed and edematous, causing interruption of nerve impulses. The cause is thought to be nerve trauma from a viral infection such as herpes simplex or herpes zoster. Research is ongoing to determine whether this is an autoimmune disorder. Loss of motor control typically occurs on one side of the face; bilateral facial palsy occurs in less than 1% of cases. Contracture of facial muscles may occur if recovery is slow. Men and women are affected equally. Bell's palsy is more common in women in the third trimester of pregnancy, in people with immune disorders such as HIV infection, and in people with diabetes. It occurs in all ages (including children) and at all times of the year.

Signs and Symptoms

Onset of symptoms may be sudden or may progress over a 2- to 5-day period. The severity of the paralysis usually peaks within several days of onset of symptoms. Pain behind the ear may precede the onset of facial paralysis. Other vague initial symptoms are dry eye or tingling around the lips with progression to the more recognizable symptoms of Bell's palsy. The patient may be unable to close the eyelid, wrinkle the forehead, smile, raise the eyebrow, or close the lips effectively. The mouth is pulled toward the unaffected side (Fig. 50.4). Drooling of saliva occurs, and the affected eye has constant tearing. Sense of taste is lost over the anterior two-thirds of the tongue. Speech difficulties occur. Fifty percent of patients will have

• WORD • BUILDING •

neuropathies: neuro—nerve + pathies—disease
neuralgia: neur—nerve + algia—pain

complete recovery in a short period of time. Thirty-five percent will experience full recovery in less than 1 year (Box 50.5, *Patient Perspective*).

Diagnostic Tests

History of the onset of symptoms is used to diagnose Bell's palsy. Observation of the patient confirms the diagnosis. EMG may be done. The possibility of a stroke must be ruled out.

Therapeutic Measures

Prevention of complications is the goal of treatment. Prednisone may be given over 7 to 10 days to decrease inflammation. Analgesics are given for pain control. Antiviral medication may be prescribed. Moist heat and gentle massage to the face and ear also ease pain. A facial sling may be used to aid in eating and support of facial muscles.

Nursing Process for the Patient with a Cranial Nerve Disorder (Trigeminal Neuralgia and Bell's Palsy)

DATA COLLECTION. Assess attacks using the WHAT'S UP? format, being sure to include factors that trigger pain. Are sensory or motor problems associated with the pain? Assess the effect of the disorder on the patient's life, including

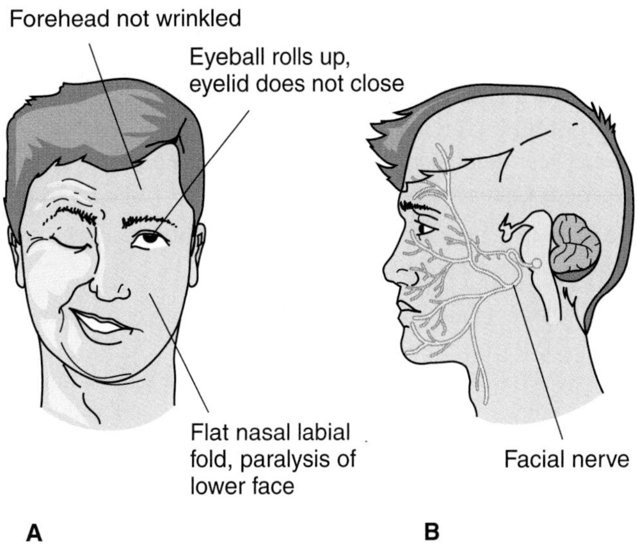
Forehead not wrinkled
Eyeball rolls up, eyelid does not close
Flat nasal labial fold, paralysis of lower face
Facial nerve
A
B

FIGURE 50.4 Bell's palsy. (A) Note weakness of affected side of face. (B) Distribution of facial nerve.

Box 50.5

Patient Perspective

Angela, Bell's Palsy

I woke up that Thursday morning with the same intense pain in my forehead that I had been experiencing for the last week. When I rolled out of bed, I realized that I didn't have morning breath (or so I thought). Knowing that I had not brushed my teeth yet, I proceeded to do so and noticed that I could not taste the toothpaste. The fruit cup I ate for lunch tasted like Clorox. I chomped up and down on each bite, then carefully attempted to swallow. It was like I had been injected with several shots of Novocain. My throat felt like it had closed up, and each swallow took a concentrated effort. Over the course of eating my fruit, I managed to bite my tongue three times.

I was 35 weeks pregnant and on strict bedrest due to pregnancy-induced hypertension and severe edema (which later spiraled into toxemia). We attributed the numbness in my mouth to the edema. I had already swollen up like a balloon and had experienced intense numbness in my extremities since the 12th week of pregnancy. As the afternoon progressed, I grew more and more concerned. I knew something was not quite right. By 5:30 that evening I had lost control of the entire left side of my face. I called my obstetrician and she said to get to the ER because I was either having a stroke or had developed Bell's palsy. The doctor at the ER confirmed that I had Bell's palsy and prescribed Valtrex and prednisone to treat it.

The symptoms of Bell's that I experienced were severe pain in my forehead, not being able to breathe out of the left side of my nose, and difficulty chewing, swallowing, and saying most consonants. I completely lost the ability to smile, blink, close my eye, raise my eyebrow, or use a straw or blow. My eyesight in the left eye blurred, and I could not go out at night due to the intense pain behind my eye triggered by headlights and having to use eyedrops every 5 to 20 minutes.

I delivered my baby (after induction, 2 days of labor, 2 hours of pushing, and emergency C section) 2 weeks after being diagnosed with Bell's palsy. During labor, I continuously asked for my eyedrops and the pain in my head was so fierce that it overshadowed the contractions.

After delivery, I was desperate for my face to be "fixed." I tried everything that anyone suggested: herbal supplements, chiropractic, facial massage, laser treatments, facial exercise, shock treatments, a neurologist consultation, and physical therapy. The only thing that has worked for me is time (and lots of it)!

For the first 15 weeks after being diagnosed, I wanted to hide from the world. However, here it is 7 months later and I have come to terms with it. I am constantly aware of it, though I have regained a tremendous amount of the muscle control. I still have not shared a "real smile" with my daughter and do not blink my left eye. Covering my mouth when I smile or laugh so others do not see has become almost like a reflex now.

nutritional status, general and oral hygiene, behavior, and emotional state. Carefully document all findings.

NURSING DIAGNOSES, PLANNING, AND IMPLEMENTATION

Acute Pain Related to Inflammation or Compression of the Nerve as Evidenced by Pain Rating on a 0- to 10-Point Scale

EXPECTED OUTCOME: The patient will state pain is controlled at an acceptable level.

- Assess pain level and response to interventions prn. *Assessment guides intervention.*
- Administer medications as needed for pain. Anticonvulsant and antidepressant agents used to treat neuropathic pain must be given routinely to prevent pain. *Medications prevent or decrease pain and increase comfort.*
- Discuss and implement alternative and complementary pain relief measures *to complement medications and increase patient's control over pain.*
  - Biofeedback
  - Diversional activities.
- Plan hygiene activities when pain relief is at its peak *to decrease discomfort with activities.*
- Provide alternative communication methods. *The patient may not be able to speak clearly or want to speak due to pain.*
  - Paper and pencil/pen
  - Dry erase board
  - Communication board
  - Pain scales for pointing to level of pain.
- Teach the patient to chew on the opposite side of the face *to avoid triggering pain and injury.*
- Encourage use of an electric razor rather than blades *to prevent injury to numb areas.*
- Provide measures for trigeminal neuralgia *to reduce pain triggers.*
  - Provide soft cloths for facial hygiene using lukewarm water.
  - Avoid touching the patient's face.
  - Provide a soft bristle toothbrush for oral care.
  - Teach patient to protect face from cold or wind.
- Provide measures for Bell's palsy *to reduce pain and prevent muscle atrophy.*
  - Provide warm, moist compresses prn.
  - Massage face.
  - Assist with facial exercises as prescribed by physical therapy.
  - Provide a facial sling.

Imbalanced Nutrition: Less Than Body Requirements, Related to Fear of Triggering Pain as Evidenced by Poor Intake, Weight Loss

EXPECTED OUTCOME: The patient will maintain sufficient nutrition as evidenced by stable weight.

- Weigh patient twice weekly and record *to monitor weight loss or gain.*
- Provide small, frequent meals *to promote nutrition without increasing pain.*
- Provide soft, easy-to-chew foods at lukewarm temperature *to prevent triggering pain.*
- Provide a high-protein and high-calorie diet. *Protein and calories are needed for cellular repair.*
- Avoid hot or cold foods and drinks. *Temperature extremes may trigger pain. If foods are associated with pain, the patient may avoid them.*
- Encourage oral hygiene after each meal and at bedtime *to prevent gum and tooth disease as triggers for pain.*
- Insert a feeding tube as ordered on unaffected side if nutrition is severely impaired *to provide means for nutrient intake while avoiding painful nerve areas.*

Risk for Injury to Eyes Related to Inability to Blink (Bell's Palsy)

EXPECTED OUTCOME: The patient's cornea will remain intact and without injury.

- Administer eyedrops or eye ointment as ordered by the physician *to protect the eye.*
- Teach patient to use a patch over the affected eye *to protect the eye.*
- Advise patient to wear glasses or goggles, especially when outside or in areas with particles in the air, *to protect the eyes.*

EVALUATION. Nursing care has been successful if the patient reports that pain is controlled, nutrition is maintained with no inappropriate weight loss, and the eyes are intact and without injury.

Table 50.4 summarizes and compares trigeminal neuralgia and Bell's palsy.

LEARNING TIP

Trigeminal neuralgia (cranial nerve V) is a sensory disorder; Bell's palsy (cranial nerve VII) is a motor disorder.

Home Health Hints

- If a homebound patient has difficulty speaking (dysarthria), try using magnetic alphabet letters. Ask questions that require a yes or no answer. The patient can respond with the letter Y or N.
- Keep bedside commode lids up with patches of Velcro attached to the seat and the frame.
- Do a thorough nutritional assessment for patients with a history of trigeminal neuralgia to identify if there is a risk for malnutrition.
- Patients with trigeminal neuralgia may benefit from using a small spoon and softer foods for eating during periods of mild to moderate pain.

TABLE 50.4 SUMMARY OF CRANIAL NERVE DISORDERS

	Trigeminal Neuralgia	Bell's Palsy
Cranial Nerve Involved	5th sensory	7th motor
Signs and Symptoms	Intense pain on one side of face: • Sudden onset • Jabbing, burning, knife-like. Sensitive to temperature, air flow, and touch Pain exacerbated by talking or chewing Frequent blinking or tearing of the eye on affected side	Loss of motor control, paralysis on one side of face Variable onset of symptoms Facial droop and inability to close affected eye Drooling Loss of taste over anterior tongue Speech difficulties
Diagnosis	History CT MRI	History EMG
Therapeutic Measures	Anticonvulsants Antispasmodics Nerve block with local anesthetic Surgical radio-frequency ablation	Prednisone Analgesics Moist heat Gentle massage Facial sling
Complications	Corneal damage Poor nutrition Depression	Corneal damage Poor nutrition Depression
Priority Nursing Diagnoses	*Acute Pain* *Imbalanced Nutrition: Less Than Body Requirements* *Risk for Injury* to eye (Bell's palsy)	

CT = computed tomography; EMG = electromyography; MRI = magnetic resonance imaging.

SUGGESTED ANSWERS TO CRITICAL THINKING

■ *Jamie*

1. Muscle weakness caused by myasthenia gravis improves with rest.
2. Have Jamie look up for 2 to 3 minutes. If ptosis occurs, have the patient close her eyes for several minutes. If she can open her eyelids and look up, myasthenia gravis is likely.
3. $$\frac{2\text{ mg}}{} \,\Big|\, \frac{1\text{ mL}}{10\text{ mg}} = 0.2\text{ mL}$$

■ *Mr. Miller*

1. Nursing diagnoses include *Ineffective Airway Clearance* related to muscle weakness and *Risk for Aspiration* related to muscle weakness. If a patient's respiratory system is compromised by a disease, nursing care should be focused on maintaining pulmonary function to preserve life.
2. Providing compassionate care to the patient and providing information about the disease and its prognosis to the patient and family establish an honest and supportive relationship. Support groups provide resources and emotional support.

REVIEW QUESTIONS

1. A patient with trigeminal neuralgia asks the nurse why carbamazepine (Tegretol) has been ordered. Which response is best?
   a. "It will help decrease the inflammation in your nervous system."
   b. "It will depress your immune system, which can slow the progression of the disease."
   c. "It can help relieve nerve pain."
   d. "It is an anticonvulsant to prevent seizures."

2. A patient with amyotrophic lateral sclerosis (ALS) expresses concern about not having enough breath to sing anymore. Which explanation by the nurse is best?
   a. "ALS can damage the nerves to your bronchi and bronchioles, causing constriction and reduced airflow."
   b. "The demyelination of your nerves caused by ALS causes confusion in the impulses to your lungs."
   c. "ALS can affect your vocal cords, making it difficult to form sounds as you speak or sing."
   d. "ALS may be affecting the nerves that go to your respiratory muscles, making them weak."

3. A patient who is newly diagnosed with ALS says to the nurse, "I do not want to be kept alive on machines." Which nursing action is best in response?
   a. Ask the patient if he has advance directives and provide information about preparing them.
   b. Reassure the patient that he will not need to make decisions about machines for a long time.
   c. Inform the patient that individuals with ALS are not candidates for artificial ventilation.
   d. Explain to the patient that a ventilator will be necessary to keep him breathing as his disease progresses.

4. When caring for a patient admitted with Guillain-Barré syndrome, which nursing diagnosis should take priority?
   a. *Anxiety*
   b. *Imbalanced Nutrition*
   c. *Impaired Gas Exchange*
   d. *Impaired Mobility*

5. Which nursing interventions are appropriate for the patient with Bell's palsy? **Select all that apply.**
   a. Administer moisturizing eyedrops.
   b. Apply an eye patch.
   c. Avoid touching the patient's face.
   d. Apply warm compresses.
   e. Provide facial massage.
   f. Teach the patient to protect the face from cool breezes.

6. Which meal would be the best choice for a patient with myasthenia gravis?
   a. Baked chicken sandwich, fresh carrots, apple
   b. Meatloaf, mashed potatoes, canned green beans
   c. Steak, baked potato, green salad
   d. Tacos, fresh vegetables, sliced peaches

7. How will the visiting nurse caring for a patient with myasthenia gravis and severe muscle weakness know if interventions have been effective?
   a. The patient verbalizes satisfaction with the plan of care.
   b. The patient states understanding of the medication regimen.
   c. The patient and family state that no further home visits are needed.
   d. The patient is able to perform ADLs with Sao_2 remaining at 95%.

References

ALS Association. (n.d.). *About ALS.* Calabasas Hills, CA: Author. Retrieved August 8, 2009, from http://www.alsa.org

National Library of Medicine. (n.d.). *Medline plus: Guillain-Barré syndrome.* Retrieved August 11, 2009, from http://www.nlm.nih.gov/medlineplus/ency/article/000684.htm

National Multiple Sclerosis Society. (n.d.). *About MS.* Retrieved June 7, 2009, from http://www.nationalmssociety.org/about-multiple-sclerosis/index.aspx

National Multiple Sclerosis Society. (2009, May 26). *MS trial alert: Sites in Ohio, Texas, and Washington recruiting for a small study of autologous ("self") hematopoietic stem cell transplant underway.* Retrieved June 7, 2009, from http://www.nationalmssociety.org/news/news-detail/index.aspx?nid1510

Singleton, R., Helgerson, S. D., Snyder, R. D., et al. (1990). Neuropathy in Navajo children: Clinical and epidemiologic features. *Neurology, 40,* 363.

unit FOURTEEN

UNDERSTANDING THE SENSORY SYSTEM

51

Sensory System Function, Assessment, and Therapeutic Measures: Vision and Hearing

DEBRA AUCOIN-RATCLIFF, LAZETTE V. NOWICKI, AND JANICE L. BRADFORD

KEY TERMS

accommodation (ah-KOM-uh-DAY-shun)
arcus senilus (AR-kuss seh-NILL-uss)
cochlear implant (KOK-lee-ur IM-plant)
consensual response (kon-SEN-shoo-uhl ree-SPONS)
electroretinography (ee-LEK-troh-RET-in-AW-gruh-fee)
esotropia (ESS-oh-TROH-pee-ah)
exotropia (EKS-oh-TROH-pee-ah)
hearing aid (HEER-ing AYD)
nystagmus (nye-STAG-mus)
ophthalmologist (AWF-thal-MAW-luh-jist)
ophthalmoscope (awf-THAL-muh-skohp)
optician (awp-TISH-uhn)
optometrist (awp-TOM-uh-trist)
otalgia (oh-TAL-jee-ah)
otorrhea (OH-toh-REE-ah)
ototoxic (OH-toh-TOK-sik)
Rinne test (RIH-nee TEST)
Romberg's test (RAHM-bergs TEST)
Snellen's chart (SNEL-enz CHART)
tropia (TROH-pee-ah)
Weber test (VAY-ber TEST)

QUESTIONS TO GUIDE YOUR READING

1. What is the normal anatomy of the sensory system?
2. What is the normal function of the sensory system?
3. What data should you collect when caring for a patient with a disorder of the sensory system?
4. What diagnostic tests are commonly performed to diagnose disorders of the sensory system?
5. What nursing care should you provide for patients undergoing each of the diagnostic tests?
6. What are the common therapeutic measures used for patients with disorders of the sensory system?

Our eyes and ears provide us with a great deal of sensory information. It is difficult to imagine what it would be like not to see or hear the world around us. Nurses have an important role in assessing vision and hearing. Patients depend on health care personnel to assist them in maintaining these primary senses. To learn more about ways to promote vision and hearing health, visit http://web.health.gov/healthypeople.

VISION

Normal Anatomy and Physiology of the Eye

The eye contains the receptors for vision and a refracting system that focuses light rays on these photoreceptors in the retina.

External Structures

The eyelids are the protective covers for the front of the eyeball; on the border of each lid are eyelashes that help keep dust out of the eyes. The eyelids are lined with a thin transparent membrane called the conjunctiva, which is also folded over the white of the eye on its anterior surface.

Associated with each eyeball is a lacrimal gland located within the bony socket at the upper, outer corner of the eyeball. Small ducts take tears to the front of the eyeball, and blinking helps spread the tears over the surface. Tears contain lysozyme, an enzyme that inhibits the growth of most bacteria on the surface of the eye. The lacrimal canals at the medial corner of each eye collect tears, which then drain into the lacrimal sac, to the nasolacrimal duct, to the nasal cavities.

Structure of the Eyeball

Most of the eyeball is within the orbit, the bony socket that provides protection from trauma. The six extrinsic muscles that move the eyeball are attached to the orbit and to the outer surface of the eyeball. There are four rectus muscles that move the eyeball side to side or up and down and two oblique muscles that rotate the eye. The cranial nerves that innervate these muscles are the oculomotor, trochlear, and abducens (third, fourth, and sixth cranial nerves, respectively).

The wall of the eyeball has three layers: the outer fibrous tunic (sclera and cornea), the middle vascular tunic (choroid, ciliary body, and iris), and the inner nervous tunic (retina). The sclera is made of fibrous connective tissue that is visible as the white of the eye. Anteriorly is the transparent cornea (Fig. 51.1), which has no capillaries and is the first part of the eye that refracts light rays.

The choroid layer contains blood vessels and the dark pigment melanin, which prevents glare within the eyeball by absorbing light. The anterior of the choroid is modified into the ciliary body and the iris. The ciliary body has a circular muscle that surrounds the edge of the lens and is connected to the lens by suspensory ligaments. The lens is made of a transparent, elastic protein and, like the cornea, has no capillaries. The shape of the lens is changed by the ciliary muscle, which permits the focusing of light from objects at varying distances.

In front of the lens is the circular iris, which is made of two sets of smooth muscle fibers that change the diameter of the pupil, the central opening. Contraction of the radial fibers is a sympathetic response and dilates the pupil. Contraction

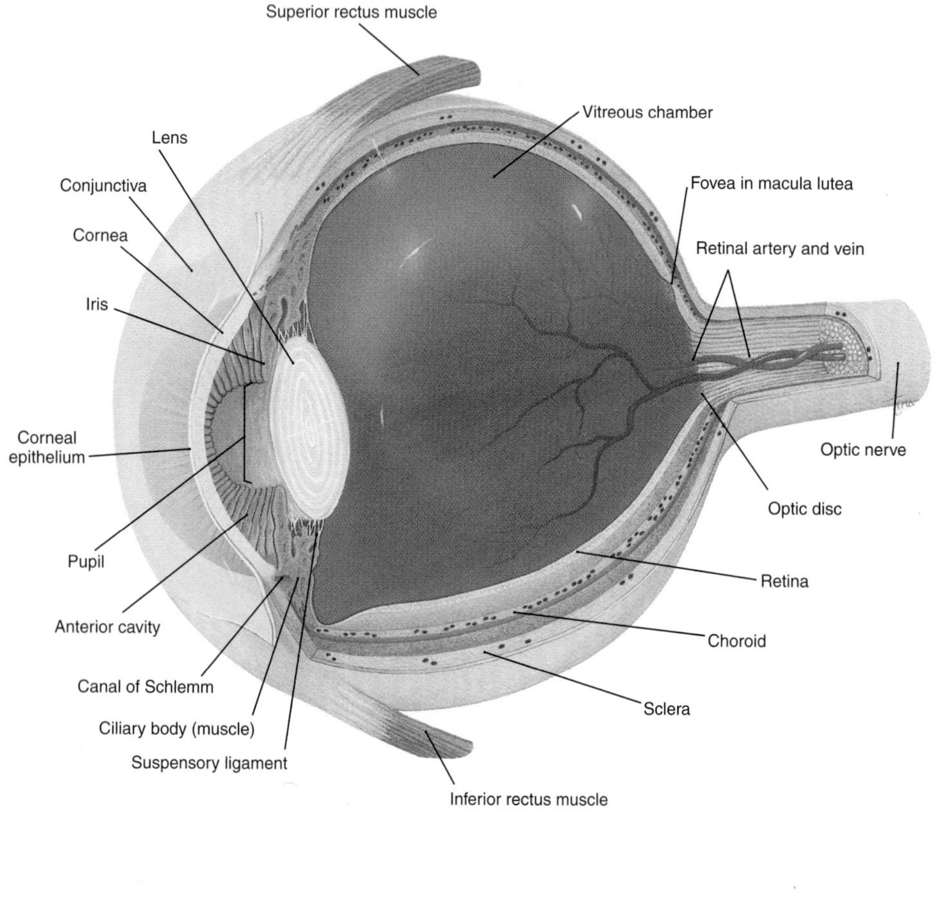
Superior rectus muscle
Vitreous chamber
Lens
Conjunctiva
Fovea in macula lutea
Cornea
Retinal artery and vein
Iris
Corneal epithelium
Optic nerve
Optic disc
Pupil
Retina
Anterior cavity
Choroid
Canal of Schlemm
Sclera
Ciliary body (muscle)
Suspensory ligament
Inferior rectus muscle

FIGURE 51.1 Internal anatomy of the eye. (From Scanlon, V. C., & Sanders, T. [2007]. *Essentials of anatomy and physiology* [5th ed.]. Philadelphia: F. A. Davis, with permission.)

of the circular fibers is a parasympathetic response (mediated by the oculomotor nerves) and constricts the pupil. Pupillary constriction is a reflex that protects the retina from intense light or that permits more acute near vision.

The retina lines the posterior two-thirds of the eyeball and contains the rods and cones, the photoreceptors. Rods detect only the presence of light, whereas cones detect the different wavelengths of light as colors. The fovea centralis is a small depression in the macula lutea of the posterior retina, directly behind the center of the lens, and contains only cones. It is, therefore, the area of most acute color vision. Rods are proportionately more abundant toward the periphery of the retina, and for this reason night vision is best at the sides of the visual field.

Neurons called ganglion cells transmit the impulses generated by the rods and cones. These neurons all converge at the optic disc and pass through the wall of the eyeball as the optic nerve. The optic disc may also be called the blind spot because no rods or cones are present.

Cavities of the Eyeball

There are two cavities divided by the lens within the eye, posterior and anterior. The larger posterior cavity is between the lens and retina and contains vitreous humor. This semisolid substance helps keep the retina in place.

The anterior cavity is between the cornea and the front of the lens and contains aqueous humor, the tissue fluid of the eyeball that nourishes the lens and cornea. Aqueous humor is formed by capillaries in the ciliary body, flows anteriorly through the pupil, and is reabsorbed by the scleral venous sinus (canal of Schlemm) at the junction of the iris and the cornea. The rate of reabsorption normally equals the rate of production.

Physiology of Vision

Vision involves the focusing of light rays on the retina and the transmission of the subsequent nerve impulses to the visual areas of the cerebral cortex.

The refractive structures of the eye are, in order, the cornea, aqueous humor, lens, and vitreous humor. The lens is the only adjustable part of this focusing system. When the eye is focused on a distant object, the ciliary muscle is relaxed and the lens is elongated and thin. When the eye is focused on a near object, the ciliary muscle contracts and forms a smaller circle and the elastic lens recoils and bulges in the middle and has greater refractive power.

When light rays strike the retina, they stimulate chemical reactions in the rods and cones. Receptors contain a light-absorbing molecule called retinal (a derivative of vitamin A) bonded to a protein called an opsin. In the rods, light stimulates the breakdown of rhodopsin into an opsin and retinal; resultant chemical changes generate a nerve impulse for transmission. The cones also contain retinal, and similar reactions take place. The opsins of the cones are specialized to respond to a portion of the visible light spectrum; there are red-absorbing, blue-absorbing, and green-absorbing cones. The chemical reactions within the cones also generate electrical nerve impulses.

The impulses from the rods and cones are transmitted to the ganglion neurons, which converge at the optic disc and become the optic nerve. The optic nerves from both eyes converge at the optic chiasma, just in front of the pituitary gland. Here, the medial fibers of each optic nerve cross to the other side. This crossing permits each visual area to receive impulses from both eyes, which is important for binocular vision.

The visual areas are in the occipital lobes of the cerebral cortex. It is here that the upside-down retinal images are righted and the slightly different pictures from the two eyes are integrated into one image; this is binocular vision, which also provides depth perception.

Aging and the Eye

The most common changes in the aging eye are those in the lens (Fig. 51.2). With age, the lens may become partially or totally opaque. The lens also loses its elasticity with age; most people become farsighted as they get older and by age 40 begin to need corrective lenses. Peripheral vision losses may occur. Depth perception decreases and glare is more difficult to adjust to, which can affect safety. Color vision fades with poorer discrimination of blue, green, and violet colors. Red, yellow, and orange colors are seen best.

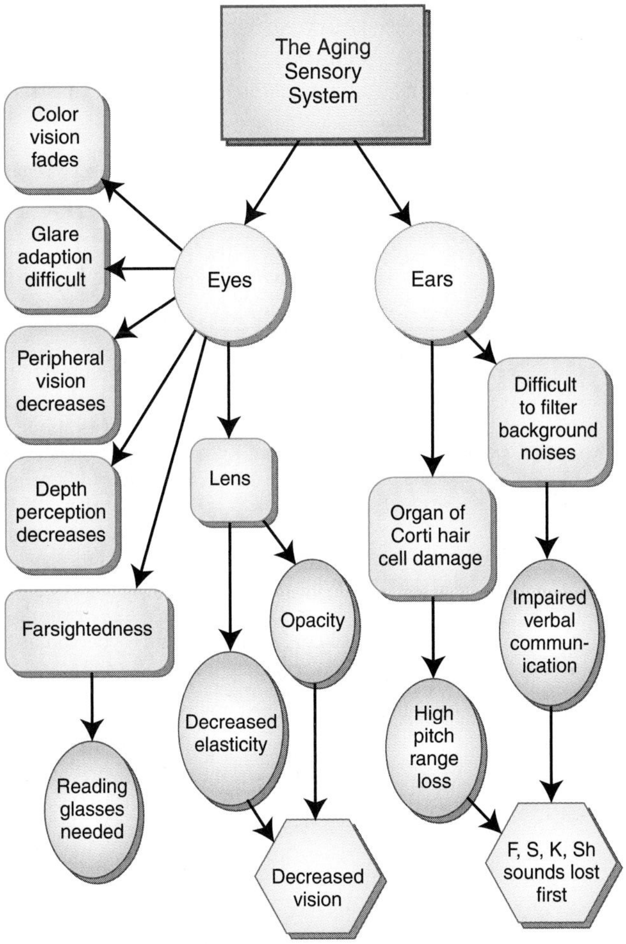
The Aging Sensory System
Color vision fades
Glare adaption difficult
Eyes
Ears
Peripheral vision decreases
Depth perception decreases
Lens
Difficult to filter background noises
Organ of Corti hair cell damage
Farsightedness
Opacity
Impaired verbal commun-ication
Decreased elasticity
High pitch range loss
Reading glasses needed
Decreased vision
F, S, K, Sh sounds lost first

FIGURE 51.2 Aging and the sensory system. This concept map shows the effects the aging process has on the sensory system.

Nursing Assessment of the Eye and Visual Status

As with most examinations, nursing assessment of the eye begins with the collection of subjective data, then moves to observation and testing, and finally a more invasive physical examination is performed. Licensed practical nurses/licensed vocational nurses (LPN/LVNs) usually do not conduct invasive examinations on the eye, but rather assist the advanced practitioner in conducting this portion of data collection.

Health History

The nurse interviews patients and collects data about family history that may affect vision, particularly glaucoma, diabetes, blindness, and cataracts. Because many eye disorders are genetically transmitted, this information alerts the nurse to possible alterations in eye health. Patients should be asked about their general health and the presence of diseases such as diabetes and hypertension. The nurse determines the types of medication the patient is taking to assess for any ocular (eye) effects. Last, the nurse asks the patient about any changes in visual acuity or symptoms of abnormality (Table 51.1).

Physical Examination

VISUAL ACUITY. Objective data collection begins by checking the patient's visual acuity (Table 51.2). Visual acuity is measured in a variety of ways but usually starts with the use of **Snellen's chart**, an E chart, or a handheld visual acuity chart (Rosenbaum's card) to test near and far vision. Snellen's chart is imprinted with alphabetical letters graduating in size from the smallest on the bottom to the largest on the top (Fig. 51.3). The examiner measures 20 feet and marks the distance on the floor. The examiner then asks the patient to cover one eye with a 3 × 5 card or eye cover and then read out loud an indicated line of letters. The lowest line on the chart that the patient is able to read accurately is used to indicate visual acuity for that eye. Normal vision is 20/20, which means the patient can read at 20 feet what the normal eye can read at 20 feet.

Visual impairment occurs at 20/70 and legal blindness at 20/200 or more with correction. An example of findings is the patient who identifies all of the letters correctly on the line marked 30; this patient has a visual acuity of 20/30. This means that the patient can see at 20 feet what the average individual can see at 30 feet. The examination is conducted on both eyes separately, then together, and documented as follows: "oculus dexter (OD) [right eye] 20/30, oculus sinister (OS) [left eye] 20/20, oculus uterque (OU) [both eyes] 20/20."

In addition to identifying the eye tested, the examiner conducts the examination with and without the patient's corrective lenses, if applicable. When corrective lenses are used, documentation reflects this as "OD 20/100 without correction, OD 20/20 with correction." The E chart is used for patients who have literacy problems. The patient is asked to indicate the direction of the E-shaped figure. The handheld visual acuity chart is used to indicate visual acuity by having the patient hold the card approximately 14 inches

TABLE 51.1 SUBJECTIVE DATA COLLECTION FOR THE EYE

Category	Questions to Ask During the Health History	Rationale/Significance
Family History	Do you have any family members with a history of diabetes? Hypertension? Cataracts? Glaucoma? Blindness? Diabetes mellitus? Do any family members wear glasses or contact lenses? Is their vision corrected with the lens?	Many eye disorders are genetically transmitted.
Patient's General Health	How would you describe your general health? What health problems do you currently have? How are they treated? What health problems have you had in the past? Have you ever had trauma to your eyes? What medications do you take? How often do you have eye examinations? When was the last time you had an eye examination?	Some metabolic disorders are precursors to eye disorders, such as diabetes and hypertension. Assess for ocular effects of systemic medications. Assess preventive practices.
Visual Acuity	Do you wear glasses or contact lenses? Have you had any changes in vision such as difficulty seeing distances, difficulty seeing close up, difficulty seeing at night? Do you see things double? Do you have clouded vision? Do you see halos around lights? Does it look like you are looking through a veil or web? Is there sensitivity to light? Is there pain? Itching? Tearing? Burning? Do you have headaches? If so, what are the precipitating events?	Any of these signs and symptoms could indicate visual disorders/disturbances.

TABLE 51.2 OBJECTIVE DATA COLLECTION FOR THE EYE

Category	Physical Examination Findings	Possible Abnormal Findings/Causes
Visual Acuity	Normal vision is 20/20.	Hyperopia, myopia, presbyopia, blurred or cloudy vision Possible causes: refractive error, opacity, or disorder of pathway
Visual Fields	Full peripheral fields	Peripheral field loss
Muscle Balance and Eye Movement	Movement in all six cardinal fields of gaze Corneal light reflex test (Light is at the same place on both pupils.) Cover test–steady gaze	Nystagmus Inability to move in all six fields can indicate cranial nerve impairment Asymmetry could mean muscle weakness Drifting eye indicates muscle weakness
Pupillary Reflexes	Pupillary light reflex Accommodation	Dilated, fixed, or constricted pupils Absence of constriction or convergence
External Structures	Inspection and palpation of eyebrows, orbital area, eyelids, palpebral fissure, medial canthus, irises, corneal clarity, anterior chamber	Ptosis (drooping of eyelid) usually indicates nerve dysfunction. Opaque whitening of outer rim of cornea can indicate arcus senilus. Corneal opaqueness can be from cataract or trauma.

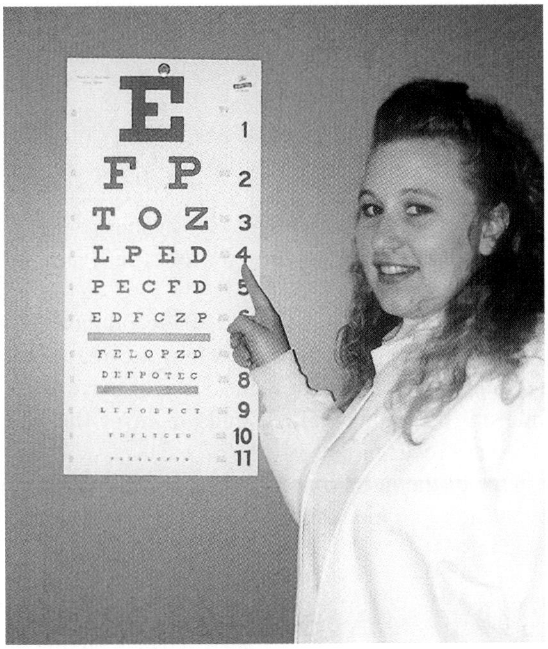
E 1
F P 2
T O Z 3
L P E D 4
P E C F D 5
E D F C Z P
F E L O P Z D
D E F P O T E C 8
9
10
11
FIGURE 51.3 Using Snellen's chart to assess visual acuity.

from the eyes. The test is conducted and documented in the same way as the Snellen's and E chart examinations.

Visual Fields by Confrontation. The examiner also tests peripheral vision, which is the ability of the eye to see objects peripherally while the eye is fixed or kept in one position. This is also known as testing visual fields by confrontation. To do this, the examiner compares his or her own ability to see peripheral objects with that of the patient. This test should be done with an examiner who has normal peripheral vision. The examiner stands 2 feet in front of, and facing, the patient and instructs the patient to cover one eye. The examiner covers his or her own corresponding eye (the eye that is aligned with the patient's eye; e.g., if the patient's right eye is covered, the examiner's left eye is covered). The examiner uses the arm opposite the covered eye, extends it to the space midway between the patient and the examiner, and brings it toward the eye from three directions: superior, inferior, and temporal (middle). The examiner wiggles the finger while moving the arm. The examiner asks the patient to look straight ahead and indicate at what point he or she is able to see the examiner's finger. One eye is tested and then the other. The patient has full visual fields if the point at which the patient sees the finger matches that at which the examiner sees it. The examiner documents the results as "visual fields equal to examiner," "full visual fields," or, if abnormal, "visual fields unequal to examiner in . . ." (identify position, e.g., left superior).

MUSCLE BALANCE AND EYE MOVEMENT. The examiner tests extraocular muscle balance and cranial nerve function by instructing the patient to look straight ahead and follow the examiner's finger movement without moving his or her head. As with the confrontation test, the patient and examiner face each other either standing or sitting. The examiner moves his or her finger in the six cardinal fields of gaze, coming back to the point of origin between each field of gaze (Fig. 51.4). If the patient's eyes are able to follow the examiner's finger in all fields of gaze without nystagmus, the patient is assessed to have adequate extraocular muscle strength and innervation. **Nystagmus** is an involuntary, cyclical, rapid movement of the eyes in response to vertical, horizontal, or rotary movement.

The corneal light reflex test is used to assess muscle balance. This test is conducted by shining a penlight toward the cornea while the patient is staring at an object straight ahead. The light reflection should be at exactly the same place on both pupils. If the eyes lack symmetry, muscle weakness could be present.

The cover test is used in conjunction with an abnormal corneal light reflex test to evaluate muscle balance. The patient

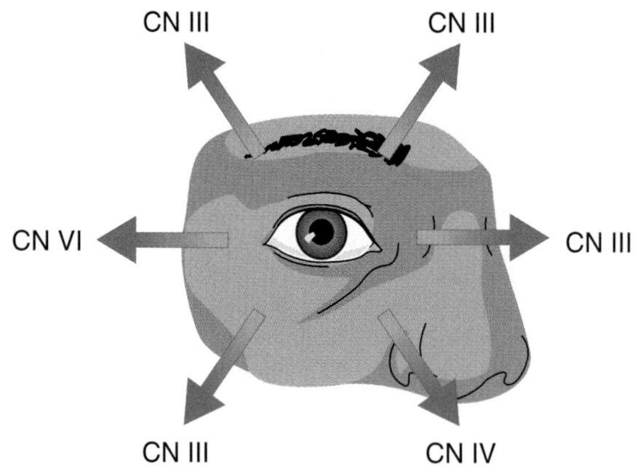
CN III
CN III
CN VI
CN III
CN III
CN IV

FIGURE 51.4 Six cardinal fields of gaze.

is asked to look straight ahead at a far object. The examiner covers one of the patient's eyes with a 3 × 5 card. The uncovered eye should have a steady gaze; if it moves, there may be muscle weakness. Next, the cover is quickly removed and the action of this eye is observed. If this eye moves to fixate on the light instead of staring straight ahead, it indicates a drifting of the eye when it was covered, which is a sign of muscle weakness. This deviation of the eye away from the visual axis is known as **tropia**. Deviation of the eye toward the nose is known as **esotropia**, movement laterally is known as **exotropia**, and downward deviation is hypotropia.

PUPILLARY REFLEXES. The pupils are observed. They should be round, symmetrical, and reactive to light. To test pupillary response to light, both consensual and direct examinations should be completed. A slightly darkened room works best. The patient is asked to look straight ahead, and the size of the pupil is noted. A penlight is shone toward the pupil from a lateral position, and the movement of the pupil is observed. The pupil should quickly constrict. The size of the pupil is noted when it constricts. This is known as direct response.

To conduct a consensual pupil examination, observe the eye just tested for reaction while shining the penlight into the other eye. The observed pupil should constrict. This is known as **consensual response**. Repeat the procedure for the opposite eye.

The examiner now proceeds to test for **accommodation**. Accommodation is the ability of the pupil to respond to near and far distances. The patient is told to focus on an object far away. The size and shape of the pupils are observed. The examiner continues to observe the pupils as the patient focuses on a near object (the examiner's penlight or finger) held approximately 5 inches from the patient's face. Normally, the patient's eyes turn inward and the pupils constrict. These responses, convergence and constriction, are called accommodation (Box 51.1, *Gerontological Issues*). Examiners use the acronym PERRLA to indicate pupils equal, round, reactive to

• WORD • BUILDING •

esotropia: eso—inward + tropia—movement of the eye

exotropia: exo—out + tropia—movement of the eye

Box 51.1

Gerontological Issues

Age-Related Changes in Vision and Hearing

Vision

Older adults commonly have the following changes in their vision:

- Presbyopia, an inability to focus up close because of decreased elasticity in the ocular lens
- Narrowing of the visual field and more difficulty with peripheral vision
- Decreased pupil size and responsiveness to light
- Difficulty with vision in dimly lit areas or at night (requires more light to see adequately)
- Increased opacity of the lens, which causes sensitivity to glare, blurred vision, and interference with night vision
- Yellowing of the lens, which reduces ability to differentiate low-tone colors of blues, greens, and violets (yellow, orange, and red hues are more clearly visible)
- Distorted depth perception and difficulty correctly judging the height of curbs and steps
- Decreased lacrimal secretions

Because visual accommodation decreases with aging, older adults have an increased risk of falling. An older person has difficulty making a visual adjustment when moving from a well-lit room into the evening darkness, for example, or when stepping out of a dark area into the sunlight.

The increased time needed to accommodate to near and far, dark and light, is often the reason that older adults do not drive at night. Usually they say that light from oncoming traffic blinds them or that their eyes do not focus properly.

One of the most simple and effective ways to improve vision for older adults is to ensure that eyeglasses are clean.

Hearing

Presbycusis is an age-related change in which progressive hearing loss is caused by loss of hair cells and decreased blood supplying the ear, resulting in a decreased ability to hear high-frequency sounds. Deafness or decreased hearing acuity is one of the main reasons that older adults withdraw from social activities. The loss of high-pitched hearing causes the older adult to hear distracting background noises more clearly than conversation.

Older adults who are deaf may need adaptive equipment in their home for safety. The use of a hearing aid can increase hearing for those who do not have nerve damage deafness. The use of flashing lights instead of buzzers or alarms increases the safety of an older adult who is not able to hear a smoke detector or fire alarm.

light, accommodation. If accommodation is not tested along with the other tests, the examiner may use the acronym PERRL.

INSPECTION AND PALPATION OF EXTERNAL STRUCTURES. The extraocular structures are inspected beginning with the eyebrows. The presence of eyebrows, symmetry, hair texture, size, and extension of the brow are noted. The examiner inspects and palpates the orbital area for edema, lesions, puffiness, and tenderness. Then the eyelids are inspected for symmetry, presence of eyelashes, eyelash position, tremors, flakiness, redness, and swelling. The patient is asked to open and close the eyelids. When open, the eyelid should cover the iris margin but not the pupil. The distance between the upper and lower eyelid, known as the palpebral fissure, is inspected; it should be equal in both eyes. If the palpebral fissure is nonsymmetrical, observe for ptosis, a drooping of the eyelid, which is commonly seen in stroke patients. Next the medial canthus of the lower lid is gently palpated and observed for exudate. The eyelids are palpated for nodules while the eye is palpated for firmness over the closed eyelid.

The lower eyelid is pulled down, and the patient is asked to look upward. The conjunctiva and sclera are inspected for color, discharge, and pterygium (thickening of the conjunctiva). To inspect the upper eyelid, the upper lid is everted over a cotton-tipped applicator. The patient blinks to return the eyelid to its resting position when the inspection is complete.

The external eyes are inspected for color and symmetry of the irises, clarity of the cornea, and depth and clarity of the anterior chamber. Shining a light obliquely across the cornea assesses the clearness of the cornea. The cornea should be transparent without cloudiness. In individuals older than 40 years of age, there may be bilateral opaque whitening of the outer rim of the cornea known as **arcus senilus**. It is caused from lipid deposits and is considered normal. It does not affect vision. The anterior chamber (the area between the cornea and the iris) of the eye is inspected using oblique light. The anterior chamber should be clear when the light shines on it.

INTERNAL EYE EXAMINATION. Examination of the internal eye is done by the advanced practitioner. The LPN/LVN may be required to explain the procedure to the patient and to assist the practitioner in the examination. To perform the internal eye examination, specialized equipment must be used. It is useful, but not always necessary, to have the pupil dilated for the internal eye examination. Having a dark room allows the pupil to dilate, as does the application of anticholinergic mydriatic eyedrops.

The instrument used to examine the internal eye is called an **ophthalmoscope**. The ophthalmoscope magnifies the structures of the eye, so the examiner can visualize the retina, optic nerve, blood vessels, and macula. The device is handheld and has a light source that is directed into the patient's internal eye. The patient should be instructed to hold the head still with the eyes focused on a distant object. The patient should be notified that the bright light might be uncomfortable. The **ophthalmologist** may examine the eye using a stationary device called a slit-lamp microscope rather than the handheld ophthalmoscope. The patient is seated and rests the chin on a support. This examination allows the examiner to visualize the internal eye by use of a microscope and light source directed into the eye.

Intraocular Pressure. Estimation of intraocular pressure is measured by using one of several types of tonometer. Often, the procedure is performed with anesthetic drops being instilled. One type of tonometer testing uses a puff of air to make an indentation in the cornea to measure intraocular pressure. Readings above the normal range may indicate glaucoma.

Diagnostic Tests for the Eye

Culture

If exudate from any portion of the eye or surrounding structure is present, a culture may be ordered. Results of the culture determine if anti-infective treatment is necessary.

Fluorescein Angiography

Fluorescein angiography is a procedure used to monitor, diagnose, and treat eye diseases. The patient is assessed for dye allergies before the procedure. Then the pupil is dilated and fluorescence dye is injected into the patient's venous system. The dye travels to the retinal arteriovenous circulation, and the eye is examined via a slit-lamp microscope. The blood vessels in the eye are extremely visible with the addition of the dye.

Electroretinography

Electroretinography is useful in diagnosing diseases of the rods and cones of the eye. The procedure evaluates differences in the electrical potential between the cornea and retina in response to light wavelengths and intensity. The test is conducted by placing contact lenses with electrodes directly on the eye.

Ultrasonography

Ultrasound is useful as an examination tool when the internal eye cannot be visualized directly because of obstructions such as corneal opacities or bloody vitreous. The eye is anesthetized with instillation of anesthetic drops, and a transducer probe is placed on the eye to perform the ultrasound. Patients should be instructed to keep the eye and head still during the procedure.

Radiologic Tests

Several radiologic examinations are used to assess eye health. X-ray films are used to view bone structure and tumors. Computed tomography (CT) and magnetic resonance imaging (MRI) are used to visualize ocular structures and abnormalities of the eye and surrounding tissues.

Digital Imaging

Digital imaging is a newer way of viewing the retina without requiring the use of dilating eyedrops. The instrument takes a digital picture of the retina in 2 seconds. The majority of the retina is viewable and assists in early detection of eye disease.

Therapeutic Measures for the Eye and Vision

Nurses have an important role in educating individuals, families, and the community about the care of healthy eyes. Nurses often have the opportunity to screen and educate people about the prevention of disease and impairment. To learn more about ways to promote vision health, visit www.lighthouse.org. For resources to help those persons who are blind, visit the American Foundation for the Blind at www.afb.org or the National Federation of the Blind at www.nfb.org.

Regular Eye Examinations

Regular eye examinations should be encouraged. People who are not known to have visual deficits and do not have diseases associated with visual loss, such as diabetes, should have their eyes examined at regular intervals throughout their life. Screening tests usually are done during an annual physical examination to detect gross visual deficits. Patients who wear corrective lenses or have disease processes that place them at risk for visual loss should have their eyes examined by an eye care provider at least yearly.

Eye care providers include the ophthalmologist and **optometrist**. An ophthalmologist is a physician who specializes in the comprehensive care of the eyes and visual system, including diagnosing and treating eye diseases. An optometrist is a health care provider who specializes in visual examinations, diagnosis, and treatment of visual problems, such as prescribing lenses. The optometrist is not a physician but is identified as a doctor of optometry. An **optician** is a person trained to grind and fit lenses according to prescriptions written by the ophthalmologist or optometrist.

Eye Hygiene

People should be careful to keep debris out of their eyes to prevent scratching of the eye's delicate surfaces. When a foreign object gets into the eye, such as dirt or an eyelash, the person should be taught not to rub the eye but to allow tears to wash out the object. This can be done by pulling the eyelid down over the eye for a brief time. When wiping the eyes, the nurse should wipe from the inner canthus to the outer canthus.

Nutrition for Eye Health

Adequate nutrition is important not only for the whole body but for the eye as well (Box 51.2, *Nutrition Notes*). Eye disorders related to inadequate vitamin intake include corneal damage and night blindness from lack of vitamin A and optic neuritis as a result of vitamin B deficiency.

Eye Safety and Prevention of Injury

Many people in the United States suffer eye injuries each year. Common household activities are responsible for the majority of injuries. Activities such as microwave cooking, lawn care, and shooting rubber bands and BB guns all contribute to eye injury. Many of these injuries could be prevented with education and implementation of safety measures (Table 51.3).

Box 51.2

Nutrition Notes

Interpreting the Role of Antioxidants in Eye Disease

In developing countries, vitamin A deficiency is a leading cause of blindness. In developed countries, antioxidants have been investigated in relation to macular degeneration and cataracts, two conditions that can also lead to severely impaired vision.

Nutrition and Eye Disease

Although observational studies generally have confirmed a protective role for antioxidants in foods (van Leeuwen et al., 2005) or supplements, intervention trials did not limit risk for cataracts or macular degeneration (Chiu & Taylor, 2007). Research in the United States supporting the effectiveness of high-dose antioxidant and zinc supplements in halting the progression of macular degeneration in selected people has not been confirmed in other countries (Evans, 2006). Nutrition-related risk factors for macular degeneration are obesity, high dietary intake of vegetable fat, and low dietary intake of antioxidants and zinc. On the other hand, a high dietary intake of omega-3 fatty acids and fish were shown to decrease the risk of the more severe form of age-related macular degeneration (Jager, Mieler, & Miller, 2008).

Recent research has identified genes involved in lipid metabolism and in innate immunity to the risk of macular degeneration and a particular chromosome to cortical cataract (Delcourt, 2007). Learning more about these factors may help target nutritional interventions to people most likely to benefit from prevention of eye diseases.

Recommendations

Because there are other risk factors for both eye diseases and because whole foods contain many components besides antioxidant vitamins, many researchers conclude by recommending diets rich in fruits and vegetables to prevent disease and also note that health-conscious people who take vitamin supplements often also consume nutrient-dense diets. If a person chooses to take supplements, a multivitamin and multimineral product at Recommended Dietary Allowance levels is advocated rather than separate preparations of individual nutrients.

Eye Irrigation

It is sometimes necessary to irrigate foreign bodies or chemical substances out of the eye. The nurse prepares the patient by explaining the procedure. Usually an isotonic solution is used to irrigate the eye. The solution is delivered using IV tubing or a Morgan lens (Box 51.3 and Fig. 51.5).

TABLE 51.3 EYE SAFETY AND INJURY PREVENTION

To Protect from	Use These Eye Safety Measures
Foreign objects	Wear safety goggles. Avoid mowing over rocks or sticks. Always wear safety goggles when using lawn edging yard devices.
Chemical splashes	Use splash shields when working with chemicals such as cleaning solution or body fluids. Close eyes to avoid getting hair spray in them.
Corneal lens abrasions/infections from contact lenses	Follow manufacturer's or eye care professional's directions for length of use and cleaning procedures. Do not overwear lenses.
Ultraviolet light (UV)	Wear UV-protected sunglasses when outdoors. Instruct patients to wear sunglasses with side shields after administration of mydriatics. Wear a hat to shield sun.
Visual deficits in adult with corrective lenses	Update prescription of glasses yearly. Glasses should fit properly, be clean, and be free of scratches.
Eye strain from computer usage	The position of the bottom of the monitor should be 20 degrees below the line of sight and should be positioned 13 to 18 inches from the eyes. The light in the room should prevent glare. Increase the font size on the screen if letters appear too small. If dry eyes are a problem while using a computer, adjust the monitor to a lower level so the eyes do not have to open as wide, which increases evaporation.
Eye injury from sports	Wear protective eye wear with polycarbonate lenses. Wear face masks or helmets while participating in any high-contact or high-impact sports.

Box 51.3

Eye Irrigation

1. Explain procedure to patient.
2. Wash hands.
3. Gather equipment. For low-volume irrigation, a prefilled squeezable bottle is used. For large-volume irrigation, an intravenous (IV) bag of isotonic solution such as normal saline or lactated Ringer's solution is used. Attach IV tubing to the bag and flush the line.
4. Apply anesthetic drops, if ordered.
5. Place a basin by side of patient's head, and pad area with towels to absorb irrigant.
6. Apply gloves.
7. Eye may be irrigated by holding distal end of IV tubing at inner canthus of the eye, or a Morgan lens may be attached (see Fig. 51.5). Lens is placed directly on the anesthetized eye, and tubing is connected to IV bag tubing. Proceed with irrigation using a slow, steady stream of irrigant. Generally, use of the Morgan lens is more comfortable for patients because eyelids do not need to be held open.
8. Assess patient's tolerance to the procedure.
9. Remove Morgan lens if used.
10. Remove gloves. Wash hands.
11. Document assessment, type and amount of irrigant, and patient's tolerance of procedure.

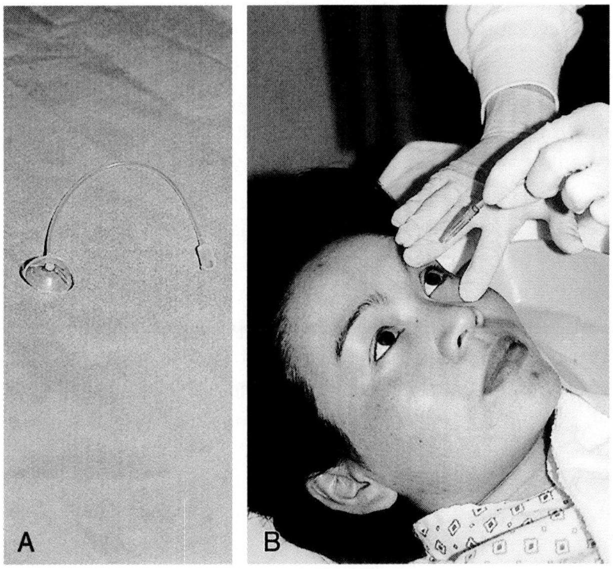
A
B

FIGURE 51.5 (A) Morgan lens is used for eye irrigation. (B) Irrigation of eye.

Medication Administration

A variety of drugs are available for eye application. Most are applied as drops, ointments, or irrigations. The nurse must know the usual dosage and strength, desired action, side effects, and contraindications of the medication being administered to prevent harm to the patient. Systemic adverse reactions can occur and diseases can be exacerbated from the administration of eye medications. The elderly are especially susceptible to this because they have more chronic diseases, as well as long-term use of ophthalmic agents. These agents can interact with other medications the patient is taking. The nurse needs to observe patients for possible reactions.

Chapter 52 discusses specific ophthalmic medications and their uses. To identify the steps in the application of eye medications, see Box 51.4 and Box 51.5. Whenever eye medications, especially eyedrops, are administered, the punctum (tear duct) of the eye should have pressure applied to it by either the nurse wearing gloves or the patient, if able, for at least 1 minute or longer as directed. This reduces systemic absorption of the medication through the punctum. Some eye medications can have serious cardiac or respiratory effects, and patients have had life-threatening reactions to them. The nurse should teach the patient the proper instillation of eye medications to reduce these reactions.

LEARNING TIP

Older patients, when instilling their own eyedrops, may not feel the drops go in. Teaching patients to refrigerate the drops, if not contraindicated, for 15 to 30 minutes before instillation helps them feel if the drops go into the eye or on the face.

EYE PATCHING. After treating an injured or infected eye, the physician may order the eye to be patched. The nurse applies ointment or drops if ordered, asks the patient to keep the eyelid shut, and then places a disposable, cotton gauze eye patch over the depression of the eye socket. If the patient has a deep eye socket, the nurse may need to place two pads over the socket to help the eyelids remain closed. The purpose of eye patching is to protect the eye from further damage by keeping the lids closed. Sometimes an additional metal shield is placed over the soft pads to protect the eye from external injury. The patch is taped in place and the patient instructed to rest the eyes. The nurse should suggest quiet activities, such as listening to music or an audio book, or sleeping. Watching television or reading is not recommended because the patched eye follows the movement of the unpatched eye.

Box 51.4

Administration of Eyedrops

1. Explain procedure to patient. Contact lenses should be removed. They should not be worn if eyes are reddened, and for 10 minutes after drops have been instilled or as directed.
2. Assess allergies, and check medication dosage, strength, side effects, contraindications, and expiration date. Do not use if solution is cloudy.
3. Wash hands, and apply gloves.
4. Avoid touching tip of dropper to anything to avoid contamination that could cause an eye infection. Do not wash or rinse dropper.
5. Instruct patient to tilt head backward and look up toward the ceiling.
6. Gently pull lower lid down and out to form a pocket to catch eyedrop.
7. Approach patient's eye from the side and instill prescribed amount of medication into the pocket. It is helpful (including for patient who is self-administering eyedrops) to use the forehead as a stabilizing area for the hand administering the drop.
8. Release lower eyelid. Have patient close eye.
9. Apply gentle pressure with a tissue to the punctum (over the tear duct) for at least 1 to 5 minutes to keep medication from being systemically absorbed. Nurse or patient can do this.
10. Wipe excess medication off eyelids or cheek.
11. If another eyedrop is to be given, wait 5 to 10 minutes before administering.
12. Remove gloves. Wash hands.
13. Document medication administration and patient's tolerance of procedure.

HEARING

Normal Anatomy and Physiology of the Ear

The ear consists of three areas: the outer ear, the middle ear, and the inner ear (Fig. 51.6). The inner ear contains the receptors for the senses of hearing and equilibrium.

Outer Ear

The outer ear consists of the auricle (or pinna) and the ear canal. The auricle is made of cartilage covered with skin. The ear canal is a tunnel into the temporal bone that curves slightly forward and downward. The canal is lined with skin that contains ceruminous glands. Cerumen, or earwax, is the secretion that keeps the eardrum pliable and traps dust.

Middle Ear

The middle ear is an air-filled cavity in the temporal bone. The eardrum (or tympanic membrane) is stretched across the end of the ear canal and vibrates when sound waves strike it. These vibrations are transmitted through the three auditory bones—the malleus, incus, and stapes. The stapes then transmits vibrations to the fluid-filled inner ear at the oval window.

The eustachian tube (or auditory tube) extends from the middle ear to the nasopharynx and permits air to enter or leave the middle ear cavity. The air pressure in the middle ear must be the same as the external atmospheric pressure for the eardrum to vibrate properly. Swallowing or yawning opens the eustachian tubes and permits equalization of these pressures.

Inner Ear

The inner ear is a cavity in the temporal bone called the bony labyrinth, lined with membrane called the membranous

Box 51.5

Administration of Eye Ointment

1. Explain procedure to patient.
2. Check medication for dosage, strength, side effects, contraindications, and expiration date.
3. Wash hands, and apply gloves.
4. Instruct patient to tilt head backward and look up toward the ceiling.
5. Gently pull lower lid down to form a pocket into which ointment is placed.
6. Express ointment directly into exposed palpebral conjunctiva, moving from inner to outer canthus. Be careful not to touch patient's eye or surrounding structure with tip of ointment tube.
7. Release lower eyelid over the ointment.
8. Instruct patient to gently close eyes.
9. Remove gloves. Wash hands.
10. Explain that vision may be blurred while ointment is in the eye.
11. Document medication administration and patient's tolerance of procedure.

labyrinth. The fluid between bone and membrane is called perilymph, and that within the membrane is called endolymph. These membranous structures are the cochlear ducts, which are concerned with hearing, and the utricle, saccule, and semicircular ducts, which are all concerned with equilibrium.

The cochlea is shaped like a snail shell and is partitioned internally into three fluid-filled canals. The medial canal is the cochlear duct, which contains the receptors for hearing in the organ of Corti (spiral organ). The receptors are called hair cells (their projections are stereocilia), which contain endings of the cochlear branch of the eighth cranial nerve. A membrane called the tectorial membrane hangs over the hair cells.

The process of hearing involves the transmission of vibrations and the generation of nerve impulses. When sound waves enter the ear canal, vibrations are transmitted by the following structures: eardrum, malleus, incus, stapes, oval window of the inner ear, perilymph and endolymph within the cochlea, and hair cells of the organ of Corti. When the hair cells bend, they generate impulses that are carried by the eighth cranial nerve to the brain. The auditory areas, for both hearing and interpretation, are in the temporal lobes of the cerebral cortex.

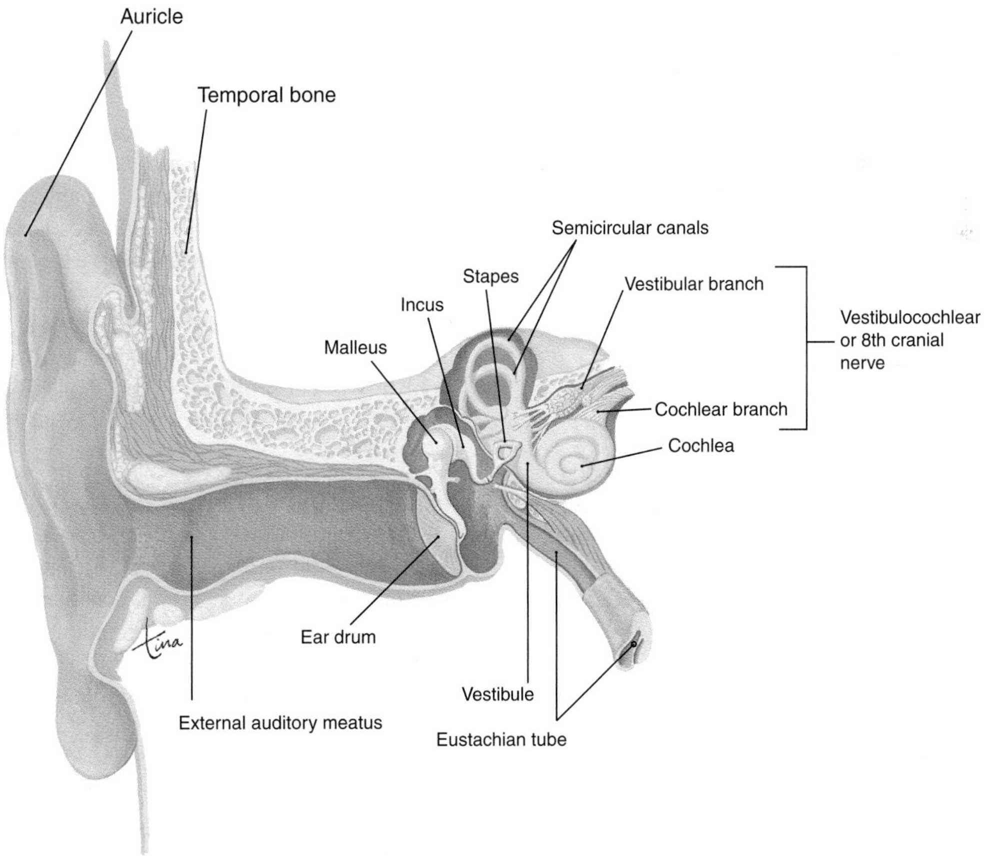
Auricle
Temporal bone
Semicircular canals
Stapes
Vestibular branch
Incus
Vestibulocochlear or 8th cranial nerve
Malleus
Cochlear branch
Cochlea
Ear drum
Vestibule
External auditory meatus
Eustachian tube

FIGURE 51.6 The ear in frontal section through the right temporal bone. (From Scanlon, V. C., & Sanders, T. [2007]. *Essentials of anatomy and physiology* [5th ed.]. Philadelphia: F. A. Davis, with permission.)

The utricle and saccule are membranous sacs within the vestibule, between the cochlea and semicircular canals. Each contains a patch of hair cells embedded in a gelatinous structure that contains otoliths, small crystals of calcium carbonate. The hair cells bend in response to the pull of gravity on the otoliths as the position of the head changes. The impulses generated are carried by the vestibular branch of the eighth cranial nerve to the cerebellum, medulla, and pons. The cerebellum sends this information continuously to the cerebral motor cortex. The cerebellum and brainstem use this information to maintain equilibrium at a subconscious level; the cerebrum provides a conscious awareness of the position of the head.

The three semicircular canals are fluid-filled membranous ovals oriented in three planes. At the base of each is an enlarged portion called the ampulla, which contains hair cells (the cristae) that are affected by movement. As the body moves forward, for example, the hair cells at first bend backward. The bending of the hair cells generates impulses carried by the vestibular branch of the eighth cranial nerve to the cerebellum and brainstem; and then impulses continue on to the cerebral motor cortex. These impulses are interpreted as starting or stopping, turning, or changing speeds, and this information is used to maintain equilibrium while a person is moving.

Aging and the Ear

In the ear, cumulative damage to the hair cells in the organ of Corti usually becomes apparent sometime after the age of 60 (see Fig. 51.2). Hair cells that have been damaged by a lifetime of noise cannot be replaced. Sounds in high-pitched ranges are usually those lost first (presbycusis), whereas hearing may still be adequate for lower pitched ranges. The high-pitched sounds *f, s, k,* and *sh* are usually lost first. It becomes more difficult to filter out background noises, so noisy environments make it difficult to hear conversations.

> **LEARNING TIP**
>
> Presbycusis is the loss of hearing high-pitched sounds (pitch = cycles per second; loudness = decibels [dB]). Because the ability to hear pitch is lost rather than loudness, it is not helpful to talk louder to a patient with this type of hearing loss. In fact, talking louder can make it more difficult to discriminate sounds. It is important to know the type of hearing loss a patient has.

Nursing Data Collection for the Ear and Hearing

Data collection for the ear includes obtaining the patient's health history and performing a physical examination. A quiet environment is helpful for collecting accurate hearing data. Document the patient's behavior because it may provide information related to hearing loss.

Health History

The patient's self-appraisal of his or her hearing or related symptoms is obtained during the health history. Data collection regarding symptoms includes asking the WHAT'S UP? questions: where it is, how it feels, aggravating and alleviating factors, timing, severity, useful data for associated symptoms, and perception of the problem by the patient. Symptoms related to the ear that may be reported include decreased hearing or loss of hearing, **otorrhea** (discharge), **otalgia** (ear pain), itching, fullness, tinnitus (ringing, buzzing, or roaring in the ears), or vertigo (dizziness).

Information about current and past medications is obtained. Many medications are potentially toxic to the ear and can cause hearing loss or decreased hearing. Pay particular attention to any exposure to medications that are potentially **ototoxic**, such as certain antibiotics or diuretics (see Chapter 52).

Ask about **hearing aids** or assistive hearing devices, surgeries, treatments, allergies, sodium and alcohol intake (which can affect the amount of endolymph in the inner ear), and childhood illnesses including mumps, measles, or scarlet fever. Also ask about recent upper respiratory infections, history of infections, injury to the ear, hospitalizations, swimming habits, exposure to pressure changes (flying or diving), medical diseases, and any recent or past exposure to any loud noises.

Family history related to ear disorders includes any hearing problems or hearing loss and family members with Ménière's disease. Significant findings are recorded, including the patient's relationship to the family member with the problem.

Information about the patient's care of the ears is also gathered. It is important to assess what preventive measures the patient practices and what the patient's learning needs are concerning care and protection of the ears. Determine how the patient cleans the ears, any exposure to loud noises during recreational or work activities, any changes in ability to hear, and any exposure to ototoxic medications. Determine if the patient has had a hearing evaluation and if there is a history of ear problems (Table 51.4). Based on findings, instruct the patient in ways to care for the ears and maintain ear health.

Physical Examination

Physical examination of the ear begins by observing the behaviors of the patient (Box 51.6). Note how the patient communicates. Observe how the patient talks, noting any slurred speech or words. Examination of the ear includes inspection, palpation, testing auditory acuity, balance testing, and, for the advanced practitioner, otoscopic examination (Table 51.5).

• WORD • BUILDING •

otorrhea: oto—related to the ear + rrhea—to flow

otalgia: ot—related to the ear + algia—signifying pain

ototoxic: oto—related to the ear + toxic—poison

TABLE 51.4 SUBJECTIVE DATA COLLECTION FOR THE EAR

Category	Questions to Ask During the Health History	Rationale/Significance
Family History	Has any family member had any hearing problems or loss? Has any family member had Ménière's disease?	This may give information about the patient's current ear problem.
Patient Health History	What medications are you currently taking?	Many medications are ototoxic and can cause hearing loss (see Chapter 52).
	Have you had any surgeries or trauma to the ear?	Recent trauma or surgeries can affect hearing.
	Do you have any allergies to food, medications or other substances? Have you had any recent upper respiratory infections? Do you have a history of upper respiratory infections or ear infections?	Can cause nasal congestion leading to middle ear congestion and/or infections.
	Do you have any discharge from the ear (otorrhea), ear pain (otalgia), itching, fullness, tinnitus or vertigo? Do you have a fever, nausea, or vomiting?	May indicate outer, middle, or inner ear infections. May indicate ototoxicity or other ear diseases.
	Are you exposed to pressure changes such as with flying or diving?	Barotrauma may occur due to pressure changes.
	Have you had any recent or past exposure to loud noises?	Can indicate hearing loss and the cause of hearing loss.
	If so, what type and for how long?	Further assessment needed.
Hearing Impairment	Have you noticed any hearing loss? If so, has it been gradual or sudden?	Could indicate hearing loss and further assessment is needed.
	Do you have difficulty understanding certain words or entire conversations? Do you have difficulty hearing when there is a lot of background noise? Do you hear better out of one ear versus the other? Have your friends or family commented on your decreased hearing? Do you wear a hearing aid or other assistive device? If so, what is the device and for which ear is it used?	Patient already may have hearing loss in one or both ears.
	How does your hearing loss affect your daily life? Do you feel embarrassed or frustrated because of your hearing loss? How do your friends and family react to your hearing loss?	Hearing loss can cause social isolation.
	Are you exposed to loud noises, such as with your current or past job, busy traffic, machinery, or loud music?	Can cause damage to the ear leading to hearing loss over time.
Self-Care Behaviors	Have you had your hearing checked? If so, when? How do you clean your ears? How do you protect your ears from loud noises?	Provides information about patient's ear self-care and health.

INSPECTION AND PALPATION OF THE EXTERNAL EAR. Inspection of the external ear begins with examining the auricle. A penlight or otoscope may be used to improve visualization of the external ear. The external ear should be inspected for size, symmetry, configuration, and angle of attachment. Note any obvious deformities or scars. The skin should be smooth and without breaks, particularly behind the ear in the crevice. The color should be uniform, without signs of inflammation. To inspect the external ear canal, tip the adult patient's head to the side and use a penlight or otoscope to inspect the canal. Note any drainage or cerumen (wax), including the color, odor, and clarity of the drainage. The skin should be smooth and without inflammation, edema, or breaks. There should be no lesions, foreign bodies, erythema, or edema in the external ear canal. Inspection of the external ear canal should be completed before obtaining an infrared ear temperature because the presence of cerumen can alter the accuracy of the reading.

Next the auricles are palpated and any tophi, lesions, or masses noted. Tophi are deposits of uric acid crystals that appear as small, hard nodules in the helix (external ear margin); they may also occur in gout. The auricle should be

Box 51.6

Behaviors Indicating Hearing Loss

Adults with hearing loss may show any or all of the following behaviors:

- Turns up volume on the television or radio.
- Frequently asks, "What did you say?"
- Leans forward or turns head to one side during conversations to hear better.
- Cups hand around ear during conversation.
- Mentions that people are talking softly or mumbling.
- Speaks in an unusually quiet or loud voice.
- Answers questions inappropriately or not at all.
- Has difficulty hearing high-frequency consonants.
- Avoids group activities.
- Shows loss of sense of humor.
- Has strained or serious look on face during conversations.
- Appears to ignore people or is aloof; does not participate.
- Is irritable or sensitive in interpersonal relations.
- Reports ringing, buzzing, or roaring noise in the ears.

nontender when it is palpated; tenderness can indicate an external ear infection. A downward protrusion of the helix, called Darwin's tubercle, is a normal finding. The mastoid process should be smooth and hard when palpated. The mastoid process can be of different sizes but should not be tender or swollen.

AUDITORY ACUITY TESTING. Auditory function can be grossly evaluated using three different assessment tests. The whisper voice test is one test to check hearing function in each ear. The patient occludes one ear with a finger, and the nurse stands 1 to 2 feet away on the opposite side. The nurse whispers two-syllable words toward the unoccluded ear. The patient restates the whispered words. The nurse should be by the patient's side to prevent the patient from lip reading. The nurse's voice can be increased from a soft, medium, or loud whisper to a soft, medium, or loud voice. The process is repeated on the other ear. The patient is asked if hearing is better in one ear than in the other ear. The patient should be able to hear a soft whisper equally well in both ears. Findings of one ear hearing better than the other or an inability to hear a soft whisper can be indicative of hearing impairment. Results of the test are documented.

TABLE 51.5 OBJECTIVE DATA COLLECTION FOR THE EAR

Category	Physical Examination Findings	Possible Abnormal Findings/Causes
Inspection and Palpation of the External Ear	Ears should be symmetrical in size, configuration, and angle of attachment.	Asymmetrical size and placement could indicate congenital deformities.
	Skin covering the ear should be intact, smooth, and without edema, erythema, or inflammation.	Discharge, breaks in skin, or inflammation can be caused by trauma, external ear infections, poorly fitting hearing aid or skin disorders.
	Canal should have minimal or no cerumen.	Excessive cerumen may be found. This can alter hearing and cause inaccurate tympanic temperature readings. Excess cerumen may need to be removed.
	No lesions, tophi, or masses should be palpated.	Tophi may be present in the patient with gout.
	No tenderness of auricle when palpated. No odor detected.	Tenderness and odor could indicate an external ear infection.
Auditory Acuity Testing	Patient can hear whispered words at 1–2 feet away. Rinne's and Weber's tests normal (see Table 51.6). Able to understand and converse with examiner.	Patient may have indications of conductive or sensorineural hearing loss.
Balance Testing	Patient can sit and walk without difficulty.	Difficulty sitting and/or walking.
	Patient can complete Romberg's test with minimal swaying.	Increased swaying or falling with Romberg's test due to balance difficulties. May be due to inner ear infection or disorder.
Otoscopic Examination	Ear canal should be smooth and empty, without redness, scaliness, swelling, drainage, excessive cerumen, or foreign objects.	Ear canal may be reddened and swollen; drainage may be present; excessive cerumen or foreign object may be present. Caused by infection, improper care, or excessive cerumen production.
	Internal otoscope examination is completed by experienced practitioner and should reveal a slightly conical, shiny, smooth, pearly gray eardrum.	Eardrum may be dull, bulging or retracted, reddened if caused by middle ear infection or blockage.
Other	Observe the patient's position and posture during the interview and physical exam.	Behaviors may indicate hearing loss and the patient's effort to compensate.
	Does the patient watch the examiner's mouth or lean toward the examiner?	The patient may be unaware of the behaviors.

A second acuity test is the **Rinne test**. This test is performed with a tuning fork and is useful for differentiating between conductive and sensorineural hearing loss. To perform the test, strike the tuning fork and place it on the patient's mastoid process (Fig. 51.7). Verify that the patient is able to hear the tuning fork, and then instruct the patient to say immediately when the sound is no longer heard. When the patient indicates that the sound is not heard, place the vibrating tuning fork 2 inches in front of the ear (see Fig. 51.7). Ask the patient if he or she hears the tuning fork and then to indicate when the sound is no longer heard. Normally, air conduction (AC) is heard twice as long as bone conduction (BC). The patient reports this by hearing the tuning fork when placed in front of the ear (AC) after no longer hearing it when placed on the mastoid process (BC). Normal results are recorded as "AC greater than BC." The test is repeated on the other ear and findings recorded. Abnormal findings can indicate conduction or sensorineural problems (Table 51.6).

The **Weber test** is a third test to assess hearing acuity. The Weber test is also performed using a tuning fork. Place the vibrating tuning fork on the center of the patient's forehead or head (Fig. 51.8). Verify that the patient can hear the tuning fork. If the patient gives a positive answer, ask the patient if he or she hears the sound better in the left ear, better in the right ear, or the same in both ears. It is important to give the patient three choices from which to choose. Normally, the patient hears the sound the same in both ears (see Table 51.6).

BALANCE TESTING. When the patient reports dizziness, nystagmus, or problems with equilibrium, simple tests can be performed to assess vestibular function. The first test is simply to observe the patient's gait by having the patient walk away from the examiner and then walk back. Note the patient's balance, posture, and movement of arms and legs. The patient should be able to walk in an upright position with no difficulties in balance or movement.

Romberg's test, or falling test, is another simple test to assess vestibular function. Instruct the patient to stand with feet together, first with eyes open and then with eyes closed. Normally, the patient has no difficulty maintaining a standing position with only minimal swaying. If the patient has difficulty maintaining balance or loses balance (a positive Romberg's test), the patient may have an inner ear problem. If a fall appears likely, be prepared to support the patient to prevent injury.

OTOSCOPIC EXAMINATION. An otoscope is an instrument consisting of a handle, a light source, a magnifying lens, and an optional speculum for inserting in the ear. Some otoscopes have a pneumatic device for injecting air into the canal to test the eardrum's mobility and integrity. The otoscope is used to visualize the external ear, ear canal, and tympanic membrane. Otoscopic examination is completed to identify specific disorders or infections, remove wax, or remove foreign bodies. Examination of the ear canal should be completed during insertion and removal of the speculum. The ear canal should be smooth and empty. There should be no

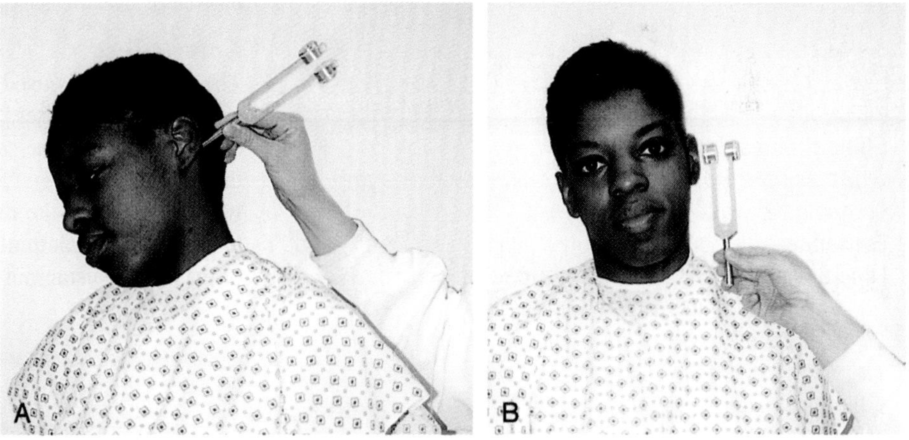
A
B

FIGURE 51.7 Rinne test. (A) Bone conduction. (B) Air conduction.

TABLE 51.6 AUDITORY ACUITY TUNING FORK TESTS

Test	Expected Results	Conductive Hearing Loss	Sensorineural Hearing Loss
Rinne Test	Air conduction heard longer than bone conduction	Bone conduction heard longer than air conduction in affected ear	Air conduction heard longer than bone conduction in affected ear (may be less than 2:1 ratio)
Weber Test	Tone heard in center of the head; no lateralization	Sound heard louder in affected ear	Sound heard louder in better ear

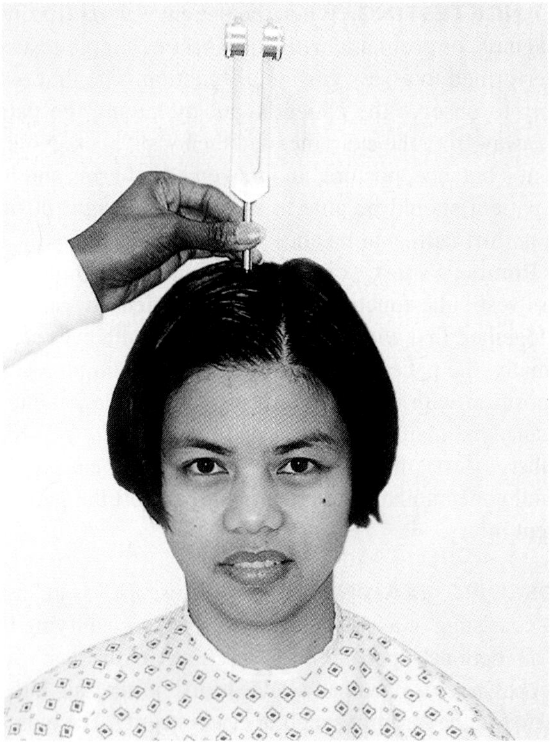

FIGURE 51.8 Weber's test.

redness, scaliness, swelling, drainage, nodules, foreign objects, or excessive wax (see *Evidence-Based Practice* box). The internal otoscopic examination is conducted to examine the eardrum and is done by the experienced practitioner. The eardrum should appear slightly conical, shiny, and smooth and be a pearly gray color.

EVIDENCE-BASED PRACTICE

Clinical Question

What are the best eardrops for removal of symptomatic earwax?

Evidence

Nine clinical trials of various types of eardrops for wax removal were reviewed (Burton & Doree, 2009) and showed that eardrops of any sort can help to remove ear wax, but that water or saline solution drops appear to be as effective as more costly commercial products.

Implications for Nursing Practice

The use of ordered eardrops, including water or saline solution, for symptomatic problems attributed to the accumulation of earwax can be helpful to patients.

REFERENCE

Burton, M. J., & Doree, C. (2009). Ear drops for the removal of ear wax. *Cochrane Database of Systematic Reviews 2009, Issue 1* (Art. No. CD004326; DOI 10.1002/14651858.CD004326.pub2).

Diagnostic Tests for the Ear and Hearing

Audiometric Testing

Audiometric testing is used as a screening tool to determine the type and degree of hearing loss. An audiologist conducts the hearing tests in a soundproof booth. The audiometer produces a stimulus that consists of a musical tone, pure tone, or speech. To test air conduction, the patient is placed in the booth, wears earphones, and signals the audiologist when and if the tone is heard. Each ear is tested separately as the patient is exposed to sounds of varying frequency or pitch (hertz) and intensity (decibels). By varying the levels of the sound, a hearing level is established (Table 51.7). The use of earphones measures air conduction, level of speech hearing, and understanding of speech. During bone conduction testing, a vibrator is placed on the mastoid process and the earphones are removed. Testing proceeds as with air conduction.

A patient with normal hearing should have the same air conduction as bone conduction hearing levels. Alterations in testing air and bone conduction hearing can provide information about the location and type of hearing loss.

Tympanometry

Tympanometry is a test used to measure compliance of the tympanic membrane and differentiate problems in the middle ear. Varying amounts of pressure are applied to the tympanic membrane, and the results create a distinctive response recorded on a graph called a tympanogram. The test is useful in determining the amount of negative pressure within the middle ear. The patient is informed that the tympanometry may cause transient vertigo. The patient should report any nausea or dizziness experienced during the test.

Caloric Test

The caloric test is used to test the function of the eighth cranial nerve and to assess vestibular reflexes of the inner ear that control balance. The test is performed first on one ear and then the other. Warm (112°F [44.5°C]) or cold (86°F [30°C]) water is instilled into the ear canal. This stimulates the endolymph of the semicircular canals, which stimulates movement of the head. Nystagmus is a normal response. The patient also

TABLE 51.7 COMMON NOISE LEVELS

Human hearing threshold	**0–25 dB**
Quiet room	30–40 dB
Conversational speech	60 dB
Heavy traffic	70 dB
Telephone	70 dB
Alarm clock	80 dB
Vacuum cleaner	80 dB
Unsafe noise levels begin	**90 dB**
Circular saw	100 dB
Rock music	120 dB
Jet planes	120–130 dB
Pain threshold	**130 dB**
Firearms	140 dB

may feel dizzy. No nystagmus is seen if the patient has a disease of the labyrinth such as Ménière's disease. The test is contraindicated if the patient has a perforated tympanic membrane. Otoscopic examination should be completed before this test to assess for excessive cerumen or perforated tympanic membrane.

Electronystagmogram

The electronystagmogram is used to diagnose the causes of unilateral hearing loss of unknown origin, vertigo, or ringing in the ears. It is similar to the caloric test. The test is usually completed in a darkened room. Five electrodes are taped to the patient's clean face at certain positions around the eye. The electrodes measure nystagmus in response to vestibular stimulation. Measurements are taken at rest, looking at different objects, with eyes open and closed, in different positions, with water of different temperatures, and with air. Usually tranquilizers, alcohol, stimulants, and antivertigo agents are held for 1 to 5 days before the test. The patient should also avoid tobacco and caffeine on the day of the test. The test is contraindicated in patients who have pacemakers. The patient may experience nausea, vertigo, or weakness following the test.

Computed Tomography

A CT scan produces radiographs similar to those used in conventional radiography. CT is useful for visualizing the temporal and mastoid bones, the middle and inner ears, and the eustachian tube. The patient should remove hairpins and jewelry from the area of visualization.

Magnetic Resonance Imaging

MRI produces cross-sectional images of the human anatomy through exposure to magnetic energy sources without using radiation. The MRI allows the membranous organs, nerve, and blood vessels of the temporal bone to be examined for disease. The test is contraindicated in patients with implanted heart valves, surgical and aneurysm clips, and internal orthopedic screws and rods. The patient should remove dental bridges and appliances, credit cards, keys, hair clips, shoes, belts, jewelry or clothing with metal fasteners, wigs, and hairpieces before entering the magnetic resonance room.

Laboratory Tests

CULTURE. Culture of drainage from the ear canal or surgical incision is important in diagnosis and treatment of acute infections. Identifying the organism responsible for the infection allows the appropriate antibiotic to be used. Often with chronic infections, the culture is less helpful because gram-negative bacilli cover up the original pathogen. Drainage from the external ear is collected using a sterile cotton-tipped or polyester-tipped swab. Samples should be taken to the laboratory immediately.

PATHOLOGY EXAMINATION. Pathology examination of tissue obtained during surgery is completed to rule out a malignancy and identify any unusual problems. A cholesteatoma (cyst of epithelial cells and cholesterol found in the middle ear) is usually documented by a pathology examination.

Therapeutic Measures for the Ear and Hearing

Medications

The medications most often used to treat ear disorders include anti-infectives, anti-inflammatories, antihistamines, decongestants, cerumenolytics, and diuretics. Anti-infectives can be administered systemically or as a topical solution. Ear medications are generally in a liquid form for ease in administration as drops (Box 51.7 and Fig. 51.9). Anti-inflammatories, antihistamines, and decongestants are used with acute infections to reduce nasal and middle ear congestion. Cerumenolytics are used to soften cerumen and remove it from the ear canal. Diuretics are used with some inner ear disorders to reduce pressure caused by fluids.

CRITICAL THINKING

Mr. Frank

■ Mr. Frank's wife expressed concern about his changing behavior during the last 6 months. She reports that Mr. Frank no longer enjoys talking to neighbors or visiting with friends in their church group, is irritable, has lost his sense of humor, and does not always answer her questions appropriately.

1. What do you suspect is happening with Mr. Frank?
2. What examination techniques or tests might you use to gather data related to Mr. Frank's signs and symptoms?
3. What would be the expected findings of these tests?
4. What teaching for these symptoms and their effect on Mr. Frank's lifestyle would be helpful?
5. What safety issues should Mr. Frank be taught to address?

Suggested answers at end of chapter.

Ear Health Maintenance

Routine cleaning and care of the ears should be taught to all patients. Patient education should include prevention of trauma, prevention of hearing loss, and early detection of hearing loss. All patients can benefit from this type of education, as found in Table 51.8.

Assistive Devices

Hearing aids are instruments that amplify sounds (see Chapter 52). Certain hearing aids may be designed to amplify sounds and attenuate certain portions of the sound signal. A microphone receives the sounds and converts them to electrical signals. These signals are amplified, and a receiver then converts the signal to sound. A small battery serves as the energy source. Digital hearing aids contain computers that provide clearer and crisper sound that is

Box 51.7

Administration of Eardrops

1. Explain procedure to patient.
2. Check medication for dosage, strength, side effects, contraindications, and expiration date. Make sure medication is at room temperature.
3. Wash hands and apply gloves.
4. Position patient sitting up with head tilted toward unaffected side or lying down on the unaffected side.
5. For a child, pull auricle down and back. For an adult, pull auricle up and back.
6. Instill prescribed number of drops, being careful not to touch tip of dropper to anything to prevent contamination.
7. Have patient remain in position for 2 to 3 minutes.
8. A small cotton plug may be inserted to prevent medication from running out of ear.
9. Remove gloves. Wash hands.
10. Document eardrop administration and patient's tolerance of procedure.

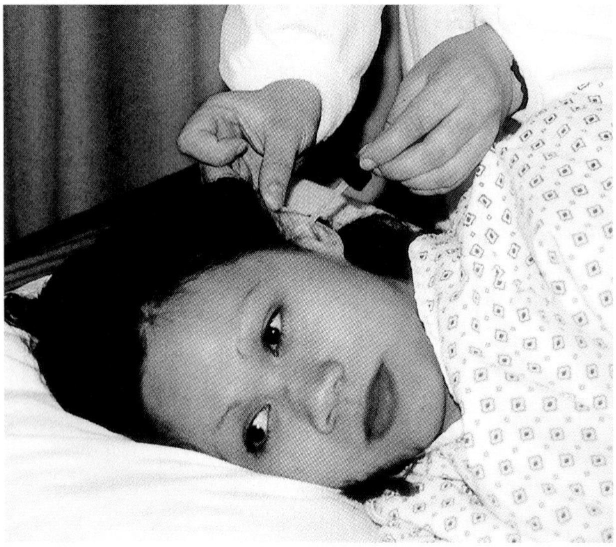

FIGURE 51.9 Eardrop administration.

tailored to the person's hearing loss. Digital hearing aids are more expensive than analog hearing aids. Four types of hearing aids are commonly used:

1. The in-the-ear aid fits into the ear. It is small and unobtrusive to the wearer and others.
2. The behind-the-ear, or postauricular, aid is the most common type. It fits behind the ear and is comfortable to wear.
3. The all-in-one eyeglass aid combines eyeglasses with a hearing aid and is the least commonly used type.
4. The body-worn aid has a fitted earmold inserted into the external ear and is connected to a receiver. The receiver is wired to a transmitter, which is worn around the neck. The wearer is not able to hide the receiver and wires.

To care for a hearing aid, ensure that it is turned off and the battery is removed when it is not in use. This reduces battery expense for the patient, who may be on a fixed income. When turning the hearing aid on, the volume should be turned up just until it squeals and then turned down until the patient indicates it is at the appropriate level for hearing. At least weekly, clean the hearing aid mold portion with either a dry cloth or a damp, soapy cloth and rinse with a damp cloth. A brush may come with the hearing aid for cleaning, or a cotton-tipped swab can be used to clean the small tip that fits into the ear.

Another type of hearing aid is the implantable middle ear hearing device, called the Vibrant Soundbridge (MED-EL, Durham, NC), for those with a sensorineural hearing loss. It provides sound perception by enhancing the normal middle ear hearing function. An audio processor picks up environmental sound and transmits it to the receiver implanted under the skin. The sound is then sent to a tiny floating transducer that directly vibrates the ossicles, which sends the message to the cochlea, as in normal hearing. The hair cells in the cochlea stimulate the auditory nerve, and the brain interprets the message as sound. For more information or to see the Vibrant Soundbridge, visit www.vibrant-medel.com.

A person who is profoundly deaf and has lost all hearing may use a **cochlear implant**. All cochlear implants feature a microelectronic processor for converting the sound into electrical signals, a transmission system to relay signals to the implanted parts, and a long, slender electrode placed in the cochlea to deliver the electrical stimuli directly to the fiber of the auditory nerve. The electrode is surgically placed. Patients commonly have difficulty understanding and learning speech, even with the cochlear implant.

A variety of safety products are available to help people with hearing impairments. These include visual-alarm smoke detectors, which alert by emitting a light. Other models vibrate the bed as a means to alert a person with a hearing impairment of a fire. For resources on helping those with hearing impairments, visit the National Association of the Deaf at www.nad.org.

Diet

The patient with an ear problem usually does not have any diet modifications. However, the patient with Ménière's disease may benefit from a lower sodium diet to prevent retention of fluid. Increased fluid may contribute to Ménière's disease symptoms.

Hearing Ear Dogs

Hearing ear dogs are trained to respond to sounds that the person who is hard of hearing cannot hear. Examples include a crying baby, oven timer, and smoke alarm. These dogs provide a valuable service that enriches the lives of those with hearing problems.

TABLE 51.8 PREVENTION OF EAR PROBLEMS

Activity	Patient Education	Rationale
Care of external ear	Wash external ear with soap and water only. Do not routinely remove wax from the ear canal.	Keeps external ear clean. The ear is generally self-cleaning. Wax is normally removed during showering. Wax serves as a protective mechanism to lubricate and trap foreign material.
Preventing ear trauma	Avoid inserting any objects or solutions into the ear. Avoid swimming in polluted areas. Avoid flying when the ear or upper respiratory system is congested.	Prevents traumatizing the ear and tympanic membrane or exposing the ear to infection. Prevents barotrauma due to pressure changes.
Preventing damage from noise pollution	Avoid exposure to excessive occupational noise levels. Avoid other causes of excessive noise such as use of firearms and high-intensity music.	Normal speech is 60 dB; heavy traffic is 70 dB. Above 80 dB is uncomfortable. If there is ringing in the ear, damage may be occurring. Occupational noise is the primary cause of hearing loss.
	Use protective earplugs or earmuffs if exposure to noise cannot be avoided.	Hearing loss can occur due to exposure to loud noises. Protects ears from hearing loss by decreasing exposure to loud noises.
	Instruct adults to have hearing checked every 2–3 years.	Degenerative changes occur in the ear with aging.
Early detection of hearing loss	Monitor for side effects of ototoxic drugs. Instruct patient to report any dizziness, decreased hearing acuity, or tinnitus when taking ototoxic medications.	Prevents side effects of medications from causing hearing loss.
	Caution older patients who use aspirin that it is ototoxic.	Older patients may have hearing loss and not be able to hear the tinnitus.
	Instruct patient to report to physician any prolonged symptoms of ear pain, swelling, drainage, or plugged feeling.	Many medical problems can be prevented with prompt treatment.
	Instruct patient to blow nose with both nostrils open during upper respiratory infections (colds).	Prevents infected secretions from moving up the eustachian tubes into the middle ear.

SUGGESTED ANSWERS TO

CRITICAL THINKING

■ *Mr. Frank*

1. He is exhibiting behaviors of hearing loss.
2. Ear inspection, a whisper voice test, a Rinne test, and a Weber test might be performed.
3. For inspection of ear, cerumen impaction may be found. For a whisper voice test, the whisper is not heard in affected ear. For a Rinne test, bone conduction is heard longer than air conduction in affected ear. For a Weber test, sound is heard louder in affected ear.
4. Explaining to Mr. and Mrs. Frank symptoms of hearing loss will help them understand Mr. Frank's behaviors. Explore with them the effects of these symptoms in daily life to develop plans for coping with the hearing loss until an intervention is implemented.
5. Mr. Frank may not hear telephones or alarms such as smoke or carbon monoxide detectors, so alternatives such as visual alarms could be considered. If he drives, he may not hear car horns or emergency vehicles of which he should be aware so he can compensate.

REVIEW QUESTIONS

1. In what order does a beam of light pass through the refractive structures in the eye? **Use all items, and place them in the correct order.**
   a. Aqueous humor
   b. Cornea
   c. Lens
   d. Vitreous humor

2. Which of the following methods can be used to assess visual fields?
   a. Inspection with an ophthalmoscope
   b. Fluorescein angiography
   c. Testing vision with Snellen's chart
   d. Comparing the patient's visual fields with the nurse's own

3. Which of the following patient behaviors would the nurse expect to find in the health history of a patient who has a hearing loss?
   a. Turns volume lower on the television.
   b. Is irritable or sensitive in interpersonal relations.
   c. Answers questions appropriately.
   d. Mentions that people talk too loudly

4. The nurse is collecting data during a patient's clinic visit. Which question will best collect data about a patient's preventive ear health?
   a. "What symptoms are you having?"
   b. "Tell me about your ear pain."
   c. "When was your last hearing evaluation?"
   d. "What medications do you take?"

5. Which of the following is the most important nursing intervention during Romberg's test?
   a. Ensure patient safety.
   b. Whisper softly into each ear.
   c. Ensure a quiet environment.
   d. Remove all cerumen from ear canal.

6. Which of the following patient statements indicates that the patient understands ear care teaching?
   a. "I should insert a cotton swab into my ear canal for cleaning."
   b. "I should not get my external ear wet during bathing."
   c. "I should block one nostril when blowing my nose."
   d. "Aspirin can be toxic to the ears."

7. The nurse prepares to provide an eye irrigation to a patient with a methicillin-resistant *S. aureus* (MRSA) infection. Contact precautions are ordered. Which of the following protective items will the nurse need while performing this procedure? **Select all that apply.**
   a. Gloves
   b. Gown
   c. Goggles
   d. Mask
   e. Shoe protectors
   f. Sterile gloves

8. A patient is taking aspirin. Which of the following findings would indicate to the nurse that the patient is experiencing a toxic effect related to the medication?
   a. Halos around lights
   b. Decreased night vision
   c. Tinnitus
   d. Vertigo

References

Chiu, C. J., & Taylor, A. (2007). Nutritional antioxidants and age-related cataract and maculopathy. *Experimental Eye Research, 84,* 229–245.

Delcourt, C. (2007). Application of nutrigenomics in eye health. *Forum of Nutrition, 60,* 168–175.

Evans, J. R. (2006). Antioxidant vitamin and mineral supplements for slowing the progression of age-related macular degeneration. *Cochrane Database of Systematic Reviews 2006, Issue* 2 (Art. No. CD000254).

Jager, R. D., Mieler, W. F., & Miller, J. W. (2008). Age-related macular degeneration. *New England Journal of Medicine, 358,* 2606–2617.

van Leeuwen, R., Boekhoorn, S., Vingerling, J.R., et al. (2005). Dietary intake of antioxidants and risk of age-related macular degeneration. *JAMA, 294,* 3101–3107.

52 Nursing Care of Patients with Sensory Disorders: Vision and Hearing

LAZETTE V. NOWICKI AND
DEBRA AUCOIN-RATCLIFF

KEY TERMS

astigmatism (uh-STIG-mah-TIZM)
blepharitis (BLEF-uh-RIGH-tis)
blindness (BLYND-ness)
carbuncle (KAR-bung-kull)
cataract (KAT-uh-rakt)
chalazion (kah-LAY-zee-on)
conductive hearing loss (kon-DUK-tiv HEER-ing LOSS)
conjunctivitis (kon-JUNK-ti-VIGH-tis)
enucleation (ee-NEW-klee-AY-shun)
external otitis (eks-TER-nuhl oh-TIGH-tis)
furuncle (FYOOR-ung-kull)
glaucoma (glaw-KOH-mah)
hordeolum (hor-DEE-oh-lum)
hyperopia (HIGH-per-OH-pee-ah)
macular (MAK-yoo-lar)
Ménière's disease (ma-NEARS di-ZEEZ)
miotics (my-AH-tiks)
myopia (my-OH-pee-ah)
myringoplasty (mir-IN-goh-PLASS-tee)
myringotomy (MIR-in-GOT-uh-mee)
otosclerosis (OH-toh-skle-ROH-sis)
photophobia (FOH-toh-FOH-bee-ah)
presbycusis (PREZ-by-KYOO-sis)
presbyopia (PREZ-by-OH-pee-ah)
retinopathy (ret-i-NAH-puh-thee)
sensorineural (SEN-suh-ree-NEW-ruhl)
stapedectomy (stuh-puh-DEK-tuh-mee)

QUESTIONS TO GUIDE YOUR READING

1. How would you explain the pathophysiology of each of the disorders of the sensory system?
2. How would you define blindness and the refractive errors of vision?
3. What are the etiologies, signs, and symptoms of sensory disorders?
4. What care would you provide for patients undergoing tests for sensory disorders?
5. What therapeutic measures are appropriate for each sensory disorder?
6. What medications are contraindicated for patients with acute angle-closure glaucoma?
7. What are three ototoxic drugs?
8. What data should you collect when caring for patients with disorders of the sensory system?
9. What nursing care will you provide for patients with disorders of the eye or ear?
10. What nursing care interventions would you use for the patient with a hearing impairment?
11. How will you know if your nursing interventions for sensory disorders have been effective?

VISION DISORDERS

Early detection of visual problems can reduce their impact. Nurses play an important role in assisting the patient with visual problems. (See Table 52.1.)

Infections and Inflammation

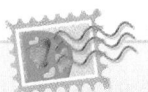

Infections and inflammation of the eye and surrounding structures can be bacterial or viral in origin. The eye may become aggravated by allergens, chemical substances, or mechanical irritation, leading to infection by microorganisms. Mechanical irritation may be caused by sunburn or bacterial infection. Inflammation results from allergies to environmental substances or by irritation of chemical irritants found in perfumes, makeup, sprays, or plants. Viral agents that cause infection include herpes simplex virus, cytomegalovirus, and human adenovirus. Bacterial agents that infect the eye include *Staphylococcus* and *Streptococcus.* The most common type of acute infection is conjunctivitis (Box 52.1, *Cultural Considerations*).

Conjunctivitis

Conjunctivitis is inflammation of the conjunctiva caused by either a virus or bacteria. Viral conjunctivitis occurs more commonly than bacterial conjunctivitis and is highly contagious. The virus is usually transmitted via contaminated eye secretions on the hand that then touches or rubs an eye, which infects the eye. The virus is hardy and may live on dry surfaces for 2 weeks or more. Viral conjunctivitis lasts 2 to 4 weeks. Bacterial conjunctivitis (commonly called pinkeye) usually is due to staphylococcal or streptococcal bacteria and is also highly contagious. Conjunctivitis can also be caused by the organisms *Haemophilus influenzae, Chlamydia trachomatis,* and *Neisseria gonorrhoeae.* Conjunctivitis is commonly transmitted among children and then among family members.

Symptoms of conjunctivitis include conjunctival redness and crusting exudate on the lids and in the corners of the eyes. Patients may report that their eyes itch and are painful. The eyes may tear excessively in response to the irritation.

• WORD • BUILDING •

conjunctivitis: conjunctive—joining membrane + itis—inflammation

TABLE 52.1 EYE DISORDER SUMMARY

Signs and Symptoms	Visual disturbances Pain Redness, secretions, itchiness Sensation of pressure in eyes
Diagnostic Tests and Findings	Visual acuity Ophthalmoscopic examination of internal and external eye Amsler grid (identifies visual field disturbances) Slit-lamp examination (identifies abnormalities on cornea and sclera) Tonometry (identifies intraocular pressure)
Therapeutic Measures	Medications: reduce intraocular pressure, treat infections, anesthetize the eye Surgery
Complications	Worsening vision or loss of vision Acute pain
Priority Nursing Diagnoses	*Disturbed Sensory Perception: Visual* *Anxiety* related to visual-sensory deficit *Risk for Injury* *Deficient Knowledge*

Box 52.1

Cultural Considerations

Vision

Trachoma, a form of conjunctivitis, is a common, chronic disease that affects millions of people worldwide. It is primarily seen among low-income persons in the Mediterranean, Africa, Brazil, and the Far East. Trachoma is caused by a viral strain of *Chlamydia trachomatis* that is highly contagious. Following the acute conjunctivitis phase, the eyelids shrink as a result of scarring. The shrinking tends to pull the eyelashes inward (entropion), which may scratch the cornea. In addition, granulations form on the inner eyelids. This painful condition may eventually lead to corneal ulceration and blindness. Trachoma is medically treated with topical and oral erythromycin or tetracycline.

Viral conjunctivitis is treated by supportive measures, which seek to keep the patient comfortable until the infection resolves on its own. Treatment includes eyewashes or eye irrigations, which cleanse the conjunctivas and relieve the inflammation and pain. Bacterial conjunctivitis is treated with antibiotic eyedrops or ointments (Table 52.2). Eyedrops are generally preferred by adults because they do not impair vision. Ointments are commonly used when the eye is resting (at night) or in children, who may squeeze their eyes shut and cry when ocular medications are applied, thus expelling the medication. With either type of conjunctivitis, hand washing is the best means of preventing the spread of the disease.

TABLE 52.2 OPHTHALMIC MEDICATIONS

Medication Class/Action	Examples	Route	Side Effects	Nursing Implications
Diagnostic Aids				
Fluorescein Sodium				
Staining of eye. Lesions of foreign objects pick up bright yellow-orange stain so abnormality can be detected.	fluorescein (AK-Fluor)	Eyedrop	Transient stinging or burning	Stain needs to be irrigated out of eye when examination is complete. Stain is colorfast, so caution should be used when irrigating.
Topical Anesthetics				
Provide local anesthesia to area, making examination painless. Also used to reduce pain of injury.	tetracaine (Pontocaine)	Eyedrop	Rare	Eye must be protected because blink reflex is temporarily lost. Lid should be kept closed to keep eye moist after examination and treatment.
Antiangiogenetics				
Antivascular Endothelial Growth Factor				
Inhibits growth of new blood vessels and slows progression of wet age-related macular degeneration	pegaptanib (Macugen)	Ophthalmic injection every 6 weeks	Burning, eye pain, redness, light sensitivity, vision loss, cataract, blurred vision, hypertension	Monitor for 1 week after to detect infection early.
Eye Allergy Symptom Relief				
Relieves red, itchy eyes caused by allergies	naphazoline (Naphcon) olopatadine (Patanol)	Eyedrop	Eye redness, blurred vision, burning or stinging, headache	See Box 51.4. Caution patient not to wear soft contact lenses while eyes are red.
Anti-Infectives				
Antibiotics				
Treat bacterial eye infections.	Ciloxan (Cipro)	PO IV	GI upset, dizziness, headache, CNS disturbance, rash, photosensitivity *Rare but serious:* tendon rupture	Give on an empty stomach. Encourage fluids. Urge patient to take with full glass of water.
	polymyxin B and trimethoprim ophthalmic (Polytrim)	Eyedrop	Burning, stinging, eyelid swelling, eye redness, pain, irritation, photosensitivity, drainage	See Boxes 51.4 and 51.5.
	tobramycin (Tobrex) sulfacetamide (Bleph-10, Isopto Cetamide, Sodium Sulamyd)	Eyedrop Ointment Eyedrop Ointment		
Antivirals				
Treat viral eye infections.	trifluridine (Viroptic)	Eyedrop	Burning, stinging, and drug hypersensitivity	See Box 51.4.

Continued

TABLE 52.2 OPHTHALMIC MEDICATIONS—cont'd

Medication Class/Action	Examples	Route	Side Effects	Nursing Implications
Antifungals				
Treat fungal eye infections.	natamycin (Natacyn)	Eyedrop PO	Inflammation, burning, stinging, and drug hypersensitivity	Follow instructions for instillation.
Anti-Inflammatories				
Reduce inflammation of conjunctiva, cornea, or eyelids due to infection, edema, allergic reaction, cataract surgery or burns.				
Steroidal	dexamethasone (Decadron) May be combined with antibiotic, as in TobraDex (tobramycin and dexamethasone)	Eyedrop PO	Transient stinging or burning on application Cataract formation with long-term use	See Box 51.4.
Nonsteroidal	ketorolac (Acular)	Eyedrop PO	Transient stinging or burning on application	See Box 51.4 Use only as prescribed.
	bromfenac (Xibrom)	Eyedrop	Headache, abnormal vision, eye pain, pruritus	Reduces ocular inflammation and pain following cataract surgery usually within 2 days of bid treatment.
Lubricants				
Moisten eyes in healthy and ill persons.	artificial tears (Lacri-Lube, Tears Plus)	Eyedrop Ointment	Rare	Explain that ointment distorts vision.
Miotics				
Lower intraocular pressure by stimulating papillary and ciliary sphincter muscles.	pilocarpine (Pilocar) physostigmine (Isopto Eserine)	Eyedrop	Headache, eye pain, brow pain *Systemic absorption:* nausea, vomiting, diarrhea, asthma attack, respiratory difficulty	See Box 51.4. Expect to see a smaller than normal pupil with little if any reaction to light.
Carbonic Anhydrase Inhibitors				
Reduce intraocular pressure by reducing aqueous humor formation. Used for glaucoma when other miotics have been unsuccessful.	acetazolamide (Diamox)	PO	Dizziness, anorexia, nausea, vomiting, photosensitivity *Severe:* sore throat, fever, bleeding, tingling hands or feet, side pain, rash	Check for sulfa allergy. Instruct patient to avoid excess sun exposure.
Osmotics				
Reduce intraocular pressure in acute open-angle glaucoma.	mannitol (Osmitrol)	IV	Disorientation, especially in elderly, because of change in electrolytes	Monitor for headache, nausea, vomiting, and confusion.
Beta-Adrenergic Blockers				
Reduce intraocular pressure by reducing aqueous humor formation and increasing its outflow.	timolol (Timoptic) betaxolol (Betoptic)	Eyedrop	Transient burning and discomfort Headache, dizziness, cardiac irregularities, bronchospasm	See Box 51.4. Monitor for bradycardia, heart block, and wheezing.

TABLE 52.2 OPHTHALMIC MEDICATIONS—cont'd

Medication Class/Action	Examples	Route	Side Effects	Nursing Implications
Mydriatics				
Dilate pupils for examination or surgical procedures.	atropine	Eyedrop	*Local:* blurred vision, photosensitivity *Systemic:* irregular pulse, confusion, dry mouth, fever	See Box 51.4 Dilated pupils cannot protect eye from bright light, so dark glasses are needed until drug effects have worn off. Monitor for side effects.
Cycloplegics				
Paralyze muscles of accommodation for examination or surgical procedures.	cyclopentolate	Eyedrop	Tachycardia, dry mouth, symptoms of atropine toxicity	Contraindicated in patients with glaucoma because of increase in intraocular pressure.

Blepharitis

Blepharitis, an inflammation of the eyelid margins, is a chronic inflammatory process. The cause may include staphylococcal infection, seborrhea (dandruff), rosacea (a chronic disease of the skin usually affecting middle-aged and older adults), dry eye, or abnormalities of the meibomian glands and their lipid secretions. There are two types of blepharitis: seborrheic blepharitis and ulcerative blepharitis. Seborrheic blepharitis is characterized by reddened eyelids with scales and flaking at the base of the lashes. Ulcerative blepharitis produces crusts at eyelashes, reddened eyes, and inflamed corneas. Eyelids chronically infected with *Staphylococcus* may become thickened and eyelashes may be lost.

Treatment requires a commitment to long-term daily cleansing with cotton-tipped swabs dipped in diluted baby shampoo or sterile eyelid cleanser solutions to prevent infection. If infection occurs, antistaphylococcal antibiotic ointment (bacitracin, erythromycin) is applied to the lid margins one to four times a day after the eyelids have been cleansed. Warm compresses may also be used.

Hordeolum and Chalazion

Another type of eyelid infection is a **hordeolum**. An external hordeolum (sty) is a small staphylococcal abscess in the sebaceous gland at the base of the eyelash (either the glands of Zeis or glands of Moll). Styes are small, raised, reddened areas. Use of cosmetics on the eyes may contribute to hordeolum formation. A second type of abscess, a **chalazion** (internal hordeolum), may form in the connective tissue of the eyelids, specifically in the meibomian glands. A chalazion is larger than an external hordeolum. Styes may be tender; however, a chalazion often puts pressure on the cornea, causing more discomfort.

Hordeolums usually form and heal spontaneously within a few days and require no treatment. Chalazions may require surgical incision and drainage (I&D) if they do not drain spontaneously. If either type of abscess persists, administration of oral antibiotics may be prescribed along with application of warm compresses to aid healing.

Keratitis

PATHOPHYSIOLOGY AND ETIOLOGY. Keratitis is inflammation of the cornea and may be acute or chronic and superficial or deep. The depth of keratitis is determined by the layers of the cornea that may be affected. Keratitis may be associated with bacterial conjunctivitis, a viral infection such as herpes simplex, a corneal ulcer, or diseases such as tuberculosis and syphilis. Herpes simplex keratitis is the most common corneal infection in developed countries, with bacterial and fungal infections being more prevalent throughout the rest of the world. People who have dry eyes, wear contact lenses, practice poor contact lens hygiene, have decreased corneal sensation, or are immunosuppressed are at increased risk of keratitis. Overnight wearing of soft contact lenses increases the risk even more. *Pseudomonas aeruginosa* is the pathogen most commonly associated with infection following the wearing of soft contact lenses overnight. If this infection occurs, the patient may be advised to dispose of the contaminated lenses and be treated with antibiotics.

SIGNS AND SYMPTOMS. The cornea has many pain receptors, so any inflammation of the cornea is painful. This pain increases with movement of the lid over the cornea. Other symptoms of keratitis include decreased vision, **photophobia** (sensitivity to light), tearing, and blepharospasm (spasm of the eyelids). The conjunctiva often appears reddened. In advanced cases, the cornea may appear opaque (cloudy).

DIAGNOSTIC TESTS. Assessment of keratitis or corneal ulcer is made by use of a slit lamp or a handheld light. The cornea is examined by shining the light source obliquely (diagonally) across the cornea to show opacity in the cornea. Fluorescein stain may also be used to outline the area of involvement. When the stained area is viewed with a blue light, the disruption in the corneal surface shows up clear. If the patient is having pain from blepharospasm (contraction

• WORD • BUILDING •
photophobia: photo—light + phobia—fear of

of the orbicularis oculi muscle), the examiner may instill a topical ophthalmic anesthetic such as proparacaine.

THERAPEUTIC MEASURES. Therapeutic interventions may include topical antibiotics, topical corticosteroids, topical interferons, antiviral medications for herpes simplex, cycloplegic agents (to keep the iris and ciliary body at rest), and warm compresses. If the cornea is severely damaged, corneal transplant may be required. The eye may be patched to decrease the amount of eyelid movement over the cornea during healing.

COMPLICATIONS. Corneal infections are usually serious and are often sight threatening. The corneal tissue may become thin and susceptible to perforation. Untreated, keratitis can cause permanent scarring of the cornea, resulting in permanent loss of vision.

Nursing Process for the Patient with Inflammation and Infection of the Eye

DATA COLLECTION. Table 52.3 reviews the subjective data that is collected. Objective data collection includes the condition of the conjunctiva, eyelids, and eyelashes; the presence of exudate, tearing, any visible abscess on the palpebral border, or a palpable abscess in the eyelid; opacity of the cornea; and visual acuity testing comparing unaffected and affected eyes.

NURSING DIAGNOSES, PLANNING, AND IMPLEMENTATION

Acute Pain Related to Inflammation or Infection of the Eye or Surrounding Tissues

EXPECTED OUTCOME: The patient's pain will be decreased or absent as evidenced by lower rating on a pain scale.

- Assess the patient for pain. *Use of dark glasses, rubbing the eye, squinting, and avoiding light may be indicators of pain that should be assessed.*
- Administer eye medications (topical anesthetic drops or ointments, antibiotics, anti-inflammatory agents, or analgesics) as ordered *to relieve eye pain.*
- Apply warm or cool packs as ordered *to assist in soothing the eye.*
- Patching of the affected eye may help reduce pain *by decreasing the movement of the eye across the eyelid.*
- Explore additional methods of pain reduction, *such as guided imagery, relaxation techniques, music, or distraction.*

Disturbed Sensory Perception: Visual, Related to Altered Sensory Reception

EXPECTED OUTCOME: The patient will state that vision has returned to preillness state.

- Reading and television should be discouraged *if the patient is to rest the eye.*
- Encourage quiet activity, such as listening to music, radio, or a recorded book, which can be carried out with the eyes closed *to provide distraction and rest for the eye.*

Risk for Injury Related to Visual Impairment

EXPECTED OUTCOME: The patient will not experience injury as a result of visual impairment.

- Assess and plan for visual impairments that may be present *to promote safety.*
- Advise patient with one eye patched not to drive *to prevent injury because depth perception is altered.*
- Teach caution when ambulating and reaching for things *to prevent injury because inflamed eyes often do not focus well and may have exudate, tearing, or ointment present, which can interfere with vision.*

TABLE 52.3 SUBJECTIVE DATA COLLECTION FOR EYE INFLAMMATION AND INFECTION CONDITIONS

W Where is it?	What part of the eye is affected? Eyelid, conjunctiva, cornea?
H How does it feel?	Pressure? Itchy? Painful? No pain? Irritated? Spasm?
A Aggravating and alleviating factors	Is it worse when rubbing eyes or blinking? Is there photosensitivity?
T Timing	Was there exposure to a pathogen? Previous infection or irritation? How long have symptoms persisted?
S Severity	Is there visual impairment? Does pain affect activities of daily living?
U Useful data for associated symptoms	Is patient infected with lice? Immunosuppression? Do other members of the family or peer group have symptoms? Are eyedrops used? Is there exudate? Are the eyelids stuck together on awakening? Does patient wear contact lenses, soft contact lenses overnight, disposable contact lenses? Does patient have dry eyes? Is patient infected with tuberculosis, syphilis, HIV? What is typical eye hygiene?
P Perception of the problem by the patient	What does patient think is wrong?

HIV = human immunodeficiency virus.

Risk for Infection Related to Poor Eye Hygiene, Use of Contact Lenses

EXPECTED OUTCOME: The patient will not develop an eye infection.

- Administer antibiotics as ordered *to treat infection.*
- Teach not to wear contact lenses when the eye or surrounding structure is inflamed *to prevent irritation.*
- Teach that contact lenses must be sterilized or discarded if not able to sterilize before using after the inflammation resolves *to prevent reinfection of the eye.*

Deficient Knowledge Related to Eye Disease Process, Prevention, and Treatment from Lack of Previous Experience

EXPECTED OUTCOME: The patient will be able to explain the disease process, prevention, and treatment measures. The patient will demonstrate the treatment regimen correctly, such as administration of eyedrops.

- Teach patient prevention, care of the affected eye, medication administration, and safety issues *for understanding and compliance with therapeutic plan.*
- Have patient demonstrate the administration of ointments or drops after teaching has occurred *to evaluate understanding.*
- Teach patient and family how to prevent spreading infection *if it is contagious.*
- Teach patient good eye hygiene *to prevent further complications.*

EVALUATION. The therapeutic measures have been successful if pain is reduced to an acceptable rating, vision improves or returns to preillness level, injury does not occur as a result of visual impairment, infection does not occur as a result of poor eye hygiene or wearing of contact lenses, patient explains disease process, prevention, or treatment regimen accurately, or prescribed treatment is stated or demonstrated correctly (e.g., administering eyedrops or ointments).

Refractive Errors

Pathophysiology and Etiology

Refraction refers to the bending of light rays as they enter the eye. *Emmetropia,* or normal vision, means that light rays are bent to focus images precisely on the macula of the retina. *Ametropia* is a term used to describe any refractive error. When an image is not clearly focused on the retina, refractive error is present. Ametropia occurs when parallel light rays entering the eye are not refracted to focus on the retina. Refractive errors account for the largest number of impairments in vision. There are four common ametropic disorders: **hyperopia**, **myopia**, **astigmatism**, and **presbyopia**.

HYPEROPIA. Hyperopia, also known as farsightedness, is caused by light rays focusing behind the retina (Fig. 52.1).

• WORD • BUILDING •
presbyopia: presby—old age + opia—concerning vision

People who are hyperopic see images that are far away more clearly than images that are close. Physiologically, the globe or eyeball is too short from the front to the back, causing the light rays to focus beyond the retina. Hyperopia is corrected with convex lenses.

MYOPIA. Myopia, commonly referred to as nearsightedness, is caused by light rays focusing in front of the retina. The eyeball is elongated and thus the light rays do not reach the retina. Persons with myopia hold things close to their eyes to see them better. Distance vision is blurred. Myopia is corrected with concave lenses (see Fig. 52.1).

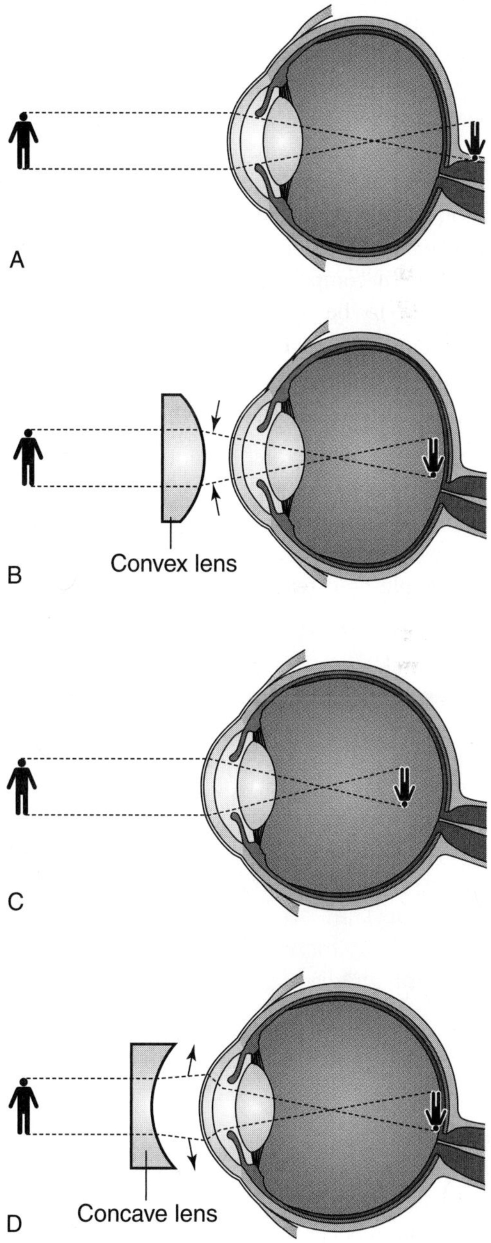
A
B
Convex lens
C
D
Concave lens

FIGURE 52.1 Refractive disorders. (A) Hyperopia (farsighted). The eyeball is too short, causing the image to focus beyond the retina. (B) Corrected hyperopia. (C) Myopia (nearsighted). A long eyeball causes the image to focus in front of the retina. (D) Corrected myopia.

ASTIGMATISM. Astigmatism results from unequal curvatures in the shape of the cornea. When parallel light rays enter the eye, the irregular cornea causes the light rays to be refracted to focus on two different points. This can result in either myopic or hyperopic astigmatism. The person with astigmatism has blurred vision with distortion. The corneal irregularities can be caused by injury, inflammation, corneal surgery, or an inherited autosomal dominant trait.

PRESBYOPIA. Presbyopia is a condition in which the crystalline lenses lose their elasticity, resulting in a decrease in ability to focus on close objects. The loss of elasticity causes light rays to focus beyond the retina, resulting in hyperopia. This condition usually is associated with aging and generally occurs after age 40. If an individual has preexisting hyperopia, the onset of presbyopia may occur earlier than age 40. Likewise, if a person has myopia, presbyopia may correct the myopia by projecting the light rays directly on the retina. Because accommodation for close vision is accomplished by lens contraction, people with presbyopia exhibit the inability to see objects at close range. They often compensate for blurred close vision by holding objects to be viewed farther away. Reports of eyestrain and mild frontal headache are common. These symptoms are relieved with eye rest and corrective lenses.

Signs and Symptoms

People with refractive errors commonly report difficulty reading or seeing objects. Often, the eyestrain that occurs as one attempts to improve visual acuity causes headache. Myopic people may hold reading materials close to the eyes. Hyperopic people hold reading material farther away from their eyes.

LEARNING TIP

To remember the type of vision a person has, use this saying: You are what you say. For example, if you say you are farsighted, this means that you have clear vision of far away images, but difficulty seeing images that are nearer. If you say you are nearsighted, this means that you have clear vision of near images, but difficulty seeing images that are farther away.

Diagnostic Tests

A refractive error can be roughly estimated by use of Snellen's chart. For definitive refractive error measurement, a retinoscopic examination is needed. Before this examination, a cycloplegic drug is often instilled (see Table 52.2). A cycloplegic drug dilates the pupil and temporarily paralyzes the ciliary muscle, thus preventing accommodation. During the examination, an ophthalmologist or optometrist examines the internal and external eye and uses trial lenses via a retinoscope to assess the type of lens best suited to correct the refractive error, which may differ in each eye. If a cycloplegic agent has been used, patients need to be told that blurred vision will be present and sunglasses need to be worn until the agent wears off. In addition, the patient should be instructed that driving and reading are not possible until the effect of the cycloplegic drug is gone.

Therapeutic Measures

Refractive errors are commonly treated with corrective lenses, either eyeglasses or contact lenses. The lenses bend the parallel light rays so that they converge on the macular portion of the retina. Laser-assisted in situ keratomileusis (LASIK) and photorefractive keratectomy (PRK) are surgical procedures also used to correct refractive error. With LASIK and PRK, laser energy is applied to reshape the cornea (Box 52.2). The cornea is made flatter for individuals with myopia and more cone shaped for those with hyperopia.

Complications

Complications of corrective lens use are primarily related to safety. Eyeglasses can be broken. Eyeglass lenses can be made with special polymers that do not break as easily as traditional glass. It is a myth that if corrective lenses are not worn, vision becomes worse. Complications of contact lens use include corneal abrasions, infections, and keratitis. LASIK and PRK both have surgical risks and may not always be successful.

Blindness

Blindness is the complete or almost complete absence of the sense of sight. Some people consider the terms *blind* and *partially sighted* to be negative and prefer the term *visually impaired* to describe their condition. For information or resources, visit the following sites:

- American Foundation for the Blind at http://afb.org
- Canadian National Institute for the Blind at www.cnib.ca
- National Federation of the Blind at www.nfb.org.

Box 52.2

Laser Treatment

Laser is an acronym for "light amplification by stimulated emission of radiation." Lasers are devices that amplify light and produce synchronized light waves. Lasers are based on the principle that atoms, molecules, and ions can be excited by absorption of thermal, electrical, or light energy. After this energy is absorbed, the atoms, molecules, or ions give off a beam of synchronized light waves. By using this extremely intense, highly directional, pure-colored light, lasers can be used for a variety of purposes, such as making incisions, removing tissue, or stopping bleeding.

Pathophysiology and Etiology

Few people are born blind. Blindness is caused by a variety of factors, including trauma, complications from various diseases such as hypertension and diabetes, and conditions such as **cataracts** and **glaucoma**. Blindness is produced when the rays of light on their way to the optic nerve are obstructed, or by disease of the optic nerve or tract of the part of the brain connected with vision. Blindness may be permanent or transient, complete or partial, or may occur only in darkness (night blindness).

Signs and Symptoms

Aside from a general loss of vision, patients may describe their visual image as blurred, distorted, or absent in specific areas of the visual field. Objects may appear dark or absent around the peripheral field in glaucoma or retinitis pigmentosa. Retinitis pigmentosa is a degeneration of the pigmented layer of the retina. The center of the visual field may appear dark for individuals with diabetic **retinopathy** or **macular** degeneration. Half the visual field may be impaired in patients with hemianopia. This results from a defect in the optic pathways in the brain and is often seen with stroke. Patients may report that the visual field appears blurry or hazy in corneal visual problems, cataracts, diabetic retinopathy, or refractive errors (Fig. 52.2).

Diagnostic Tests

Diagnostic tests may include a visual field examination, tonometry, and slit-lamp microscope examination. Retinal angiography is used to follow blood flow through the retinal vessels and to detect vascular changes. Ultrasonography may be used to visualize changes in the posterior eye that cannot be directly examined because of other pathological conditions, such as a cloudy cornea, a bloody vitreous, or an opaque lens.

• WORD • BUILDING •

retinopathy: retino—having to do with the retina + pathy—illness, disease, or suffering

Therapeutic Measures

Therapeutic interventions for blindness center on treating the underlying condition and preventing further impairment. Depending on the cause of the blindness, treatment may include medication prescription, surgical intervention, corrective eyewear prescription, and referral to supportive services.

Nursing Process for the Patient with Visual Impairment

DATA COLLECTION. Table 52.4 reviews the collection of subjective data. Collection of objective data involves observing the patient. Is there squinting? Rubbing of eyes? Is the patient using compensatory measures—magnifying glass, sitting close to television, using large-print reading materials, avoiding reading, using eyeglasses?

Psychosocial data are important because a blind person may be withdrawn or socially isolated, have low self-esteem or poor coping mechanisms, or have poor interpersonal skills as a result of the visual impairment.

NURSING DIAGNOSES, PLANNING, AND IMPLEMENTATION. Nursing care begins by understanding how to interact with a patient who has a visual impairment (Box 52.3). A patient's level of independence must be included in the planning phase. If patients have minimal visual impairment or have attended rehabilitation, they may be able to function independently. If a patient has recently become visually impaired, he or she may be completely dependent until alternative ways of coping with this impairment have been learned.

Planning focuses on meeting self-care needs, keeping the patient safe from injury, supporting the grieving process,

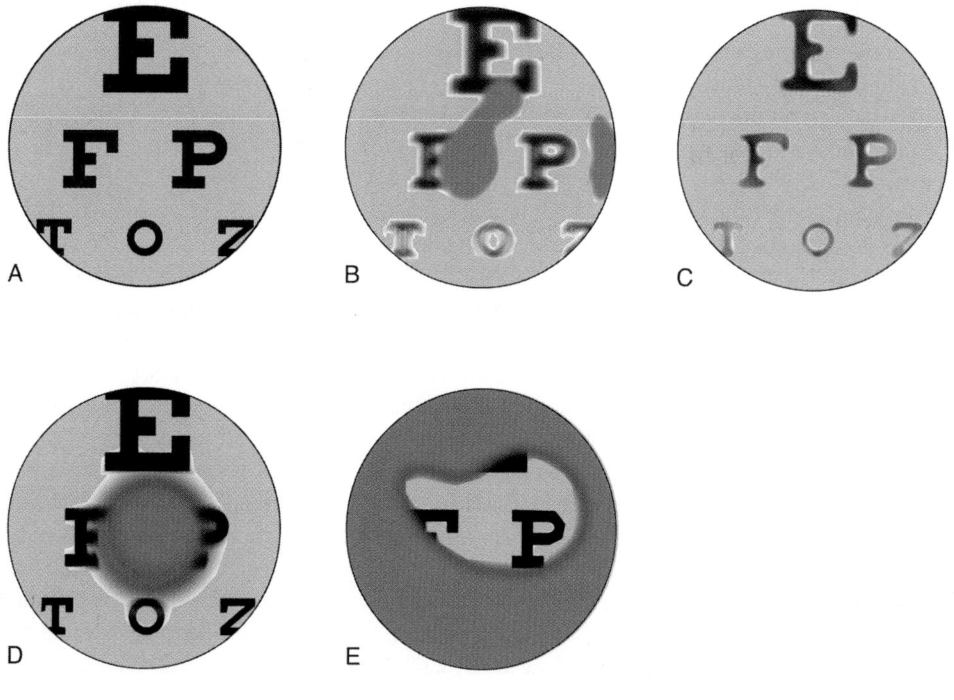
A
B
C
D
E

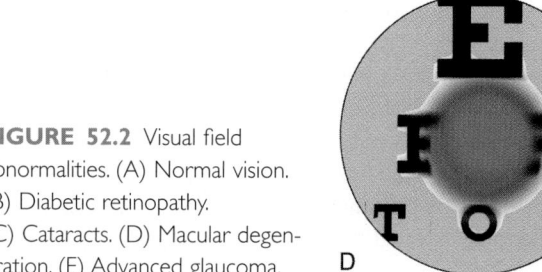

FIGURE 52.2 Visual field abnormalities. (A) Normal vision. (B) Diabetic retinopathy. (C) Cataracts. (D) Macular degeneration. (E) Advanced glaucoma.

TABLE 52.4 SUBJECTIVE DATA COLLECTION FOR VISUAL DISORDERS

W Where is it?	What part of the visual field is affected? If there is vision, what are the characteristics of what can be seen? Blurry? Hazy? Dark? Halos around lights?
H How does it feel?	Is there associated pain with the visual impairment? Headaches? How does it make the patient feel? Fearful? Anxious? Depressed? Helpless? Hopeless? Accepting?
A Aggravating and alleviating factors	Is it worse when reading? Is it worse when watching TV? Does it affect the patient only at night? Is vision better at distances or close up?
T Timing	When did the symptoms start? Do they come and go? Is the impairment progressively getting worse? Was onset sudden?
S Severity	Does the impairment affect the patient's activities of daily living? If so, how severely? Does the patient need assistance to cook, dress, bathe, read mail, pay bills, access health care, obtain transportation, maintain household, shop?
U Useful data for associated symptoms	Does the patient have diabetes, hypertension, a family history of retinitis pigmentosa, a history of eye infection, or eye trauma? Has the patient recently traveled out of the country?
P Perception of the problem by the patient	What does the patient think is wrong? How severe does the patient perceive the impairment to be?

and helping the patient acquire knowledge of agencies, services, and devices that allow maintenance of independence. Families must be included in the planning phase because they need to understand and be supportive of the self-image and role performance changes that may occur (see the *Nursing Care Plan for the Patient with Vision Loss*). Referral to organizations that enhance the independence of people with visual impairments is helpful:

- American Academy of Ophthalmology at www.eyenet.org
- Guide Dogs for the Blind at www.guidedogs.com
- National Association for Visually Handicapped at www.navh.org
- National Eye Institute at www.nei.nih.gov
- National Library Service for the Blind and Visually Handicapped at www.loc.gov/nls/index.html. (This department of the Library of Congress supplies talking books to people who are blind or have other disabilities.)

EVALUATION. The outcomes for a patient with a visual impairment are met if the patient demonstrates the ability to complete activities of daily living with increasing

Box 52.3

Interacting with a Patient Who Has a Visual Impairment

- People entering a room and at each contact with the patient should identify themselves.
- Post a sign on the door or over the bed that identifies the patient's visual status so that others can interact appropriately.
- Remember that the individual is not having hearing problems, so use a normal tone of voice and do not yell.
- Ask patients with visual impairments what their needs are; do not assume they need help with everything.
- Do not hesitate to use the words *blind* and *see*.
- Talk directly to the patient, not through a companion.
- At mealtime, explain the location of items on the tray by comparing their position to the numbers on a clock (e.g., milk is at 2 o'clock, peas are at 7 o'clock).
- Explain any activity going on in the room or within the patient's auditory range.
- Explain procedures before beginning them. Speak to the patient before touching.
- When walking with the patient, allow the patient to grasp an arm and walk a half step behind. Be aware of obstacles on either side when walking.
- When seating a patient, place the patient's hand on the arm of the chair.
- Tell the patient when leaving the room or area so the patient does not continue conversation in an empty room, which may cause embarrassment.
- When orienting the patient to the hospital room, explain the location of items the patient may need, such as the water pitcher, call light, bed controls, urinal, tissues. Attempt to keep these items in the same place at all times.
- If the patient has a seeing eye dog, do not play with the dog, pet it, or feed it without consulting the patient—the dog is working! Make sure the patient's dog is near the bed, on a mat provided especially for the dog, preferably on the side of the bed that is less likely to be used by staff. Instruct staff and visitors about the seeing eye dog.

NURSING CARE PLAN for the Patient with Vision Loss

Nursing Diagnosis: *Disturbed Sensory Perception: Visual*, related to altered sensory reception

Expected Outcomes: The patient will attain optimum level of sensory stimulation. The patient will become aware of visual impairment and ways to compensate. The patient will demonstrate ability to perform activities of daily living, with assistance if necessary.

Evaluation of Outcomes: Patient perceives maximum visual sensory input. Patient is able to compensate for sensory impairment by using other senses and resources. Patient is able to perform activities of daily living as independently as possible.

Interventions	Rationale	Evaluation
Check visual acuity using a standard Snellen's vision chart. If the patient cannot read letters, use directional arrows or pictures.	Determines patient's ability to see.	Does patient have 20/20 vision? Is there an impairment? If so, how severe is it?
Check visual fields using the cover test or confrontation test.	Identifies deficits in visual fields.	Are visual fields of patient equal to examiner's? Is there a deficit? Is it bilateral or unilateral?
Structure environment to compensate for visual loss by adding color and contrast (e.g., chairs and carpeting should be in contrasting colors, bright tape or paint on stairs, medicine bottles color coded with colored dot stickers).	Makes the environment easier to visualize and interpret and assists in depth perception and identifying medications.	Does the environment have clearly delineated walkways, sitting areas, and doorways? Are areas with changes in elevation clearly identified using contrasting tape or paint? Is there a way for patient to safely self-administer medications?
Structure environment to compensate for visual loss by use of large-print directional signs and arrows, well-lit areas, nonglare surfaces, consistent placement of objects, traffic areas free of clutter.	Large directional signs assist the patient in maintaining orientation. Shiny floors or areas with bright window glass can impair vision. Traffic areas free of clutter assist in preventing injury.	Can the patient identify locations such as bathroom, dining room, and office areas? Can the patient ambulate freely without safety hazards?
Provide for optimum care of assistive appliances such as eyeglasses, including maintenance of proper prescription, fit, and cleaning.	Improperly fitting or dirty eyeglasses may impair vision even further. Older adults should have their eyeglass prescription checked yearly.	Do eyeglasses fit properly? Are lenses clean? Is prescription current?
Introduce other assistive devices such as handheld magnifying glasses, tableside magnifiers, television magnifiers, large-print items, and phone dial covers with large numbers, talking watches, alarm clocks, and calculators.	Patients may not be aware of assistive devices that could help them adapt to vision loss and continue previous activities, such as watching TV or reading letters and magazines. Allows people to rely on hearing rather than vision.	Is patient aware of assistive devices that allow participation in previously enjoyed activities such as TV or reading? Is the patient able to pay bills? Read mail? Communicate on the telephone?

Continued

NURSING CARE PLAN for the Patient with Vision Loss—cont'd

Interventions	Rationale	Evaluation
Allow patient to verbalize feelings and grieving about visual loss.	Losing a primary sense such as vision can be devastating. Opportunity to ventilate feelings assists in processing the loss.	Is patient able to verbalize feelings about visual impairment and its loss?
Identify coping strategies that have been successful for patient in the past.	By identifying successful coping strategies, the nurse assists patient in dealing with stress or visual loss. A positive approach focuses on the person's capabilities rather than deficits.	Can patient identify successful coping strategies and use them to deal with the stress of visual impairment?
Refer to specialized clinician such as ophthalmologist or occupational therapist or to specialized resources such as American Federation for the Blind or Prevent Blindness America.	Specialized clinicians can provide detailed examination and treatment for the disorder. Specialized resource groups have networks in place to assist people in coping with loss and assisting with maximizing abilities.	Does patient know who to call for detailed examination and treatment of problems? Does patient know that there are specialized clinicians and resource groups to help with the visual impairment? Does patient know how to access these specialists?

independence, remains free of injury, and demonstrates the ability to assess agencies and services for those with visual impairments.

Diabetic Retinopathy

Pathophysiology and Etiology

Retinopathy is a disorder in which vascular changes occur in the retinal blood vessels. The most common incidence of retinopathy is found in persons with diabetes. The pathological changes that occur with diabetic retinopathy are related to excess glucose, changes in the retinal capillary walls, formation of microaneurysms, and constriction of retinal blood vessels. Three stages of diabetic retinopathy have been identified: background retinopathy, preproliferative retinopathy, and proliferative retinopathy.

Background retinopathy is the earliest stage, in which microaneurysms form on the retinal capillary walls. These microaneurysms may leak blood into the central retina or macula. If the leakage causes edema, the patient may notice a decrease in color discrimination and visual acuity.

The second stage, preproliferative retinopathy, is characterized by swollen and irregularly dilated veins, which results in sluggish or blocked blood flow. Patients generally are not aware of this stage because there are no symptoms.

Proliferative retinopathy, the third stage, is characterized by the formation of new blood vessels growing into the retinal and optic disc area in an attempt to increase the blood supply to the retina. The newly formed blood vessels are fragile and often leak blood into the vitreous and retina. In addition to leaking, the newer vessels may grow into the vitreous, which causes a traction effect, pulling the vitreous away from the retina and subsequently pulling the retina away from the choroid. This condition is called retinal detachment (discussed later).

Signs and Symptoms

Affected people may experience a reduction in central visual acuity or color vision as a result of macular edema (see Fig. 52.2). Many patients with diabetic retinopathy have no symptoms until the proliferative stage, at which point vision is lost. Visual loss at the last stage usually cannot be restored.

Complications

Early treatment for diabetic retinopathy is highly successful in preventing further visual loss; however, visual loss cannot be reversed. For this reason, it is very important for patients with diabetes to have a comprehensive eye examination through dilated pupils at least once each year or as directed by their physician. Careful control of diabetes during the first 5 years following diagnosis reduces the occurrence and delays the onset of diabetic retinopathy.

Diagnostic Tests

Diabetic retinopathy, as well as the other retinopathies, can be diagnosed only on examination of the internal eye. The examination is conducted with an ophthalmoscope following dilation of the pupil using a cycloplegic agent. The examination may be enhanced by use of retinoangiography. In the initial stages, vessels may appear swollen and tortuous (twisted).

Therapeutic Measures

Treatment of diabetic retinopathy focuses on stopping the leakage of blood and fluid into the vitreous and retina. The leaking microaneurysm is sealed by use of laser photocoagulation (see Box 52.2). If blood has already leaked into the vitreous, a vitrectomy is performed. During a vitrectomy, the vitreous humor is drained out of the eye chamber and replaced with saline or silicon oil. The replacement fluid is necessary to support the structures of the eyeball until healing can occur. Further treatment may be needed if the patient has sustained retinal detachment. Use of intravitreal corticosteroids has been shown to be beneficial as well.

Nursing Process for the Patient with Diabetic Retinopathy

DATA COLLECTION. Nursing data collection for diabetic retinopathy focuses on risk factors associated with the incidence of the disease. The patient may not have any symptoms. If patients with diabetes do have changes in perceptions of visual acuity or color discrimination, they should immediately contact their physician.

NURSING DIAGNOSES, PLANNING, AND IMPLEMENTATION. The planning phase of the nursing process focuses on prevention of visual loss by early detection and treatment. If the patient has entered phase three and is already visually impaired, the *Nursing Care Plan for the Patient with Vision Loss* is used. Nursing diagnoses, goals, and interventions for diabetic retinopathy include but are not limited to the following:

Risk for or Actual Ineffective Self Health Management

EXPECTED OUTCOME: The patient will state ability to manage therapeutic regimen.

- Determine if the patient with a visual impairment who is diabetic can monitor blood glucose and draw up and administer the correct amount of insulin. *Specialty devices are available that can be preset to draw up the correct amounts of insulin. Family members may have to assist the patient.*
- Teach patient the importance of yearly comprehensive eye examinations *to detect visual changes for treatment.*

Disturbed Sensory Perception: Visual, Related to Altered Sensory Reception and Transmission

EXPECTED OUTCOME: The patient will adapt to altered visual perception.

- Determine patient's abilities and needs *to develop plan of action and support needed.*
- Assist patient with home and health maintenance as needed *to ensure needs are met.*

EVALUATION. Patient goals are met if the patient is able to manage the therapeutic regimen and visual deficits.

Retinal Detachment

Pathophysiology and Etiology

Retinal detachment is a separation of the retina from the choroid layer beneath it (see Fig. 51.1), allowing fluid to enter the space between the layers. The three causes of retinal detachment are a hole or tear in the retina that allows fluid to flow between the two layers, fibrous tissue in the vitreous humor that contracts and pulls the retina away from its normal position, or fluid or exudate accumulation in the subretinal space that separates the retinal layers.

Signs and Symptoms

Patients experiencing a retinal detachment report a sudden change in vision. Initially, as the retina is pulled, patients report seeing flashing lights and then floaters. The flashing lights are caused by vitreous traction on the retina, and the floaters are caused by hemorrhage of vitreous fluid or blood. When the retina detaches, patients commonly describe it as "looking through a veil" or "cobwebs" and finally "like a curtain being lowered over the field of vision," with darkness resulting. There is no pain because the retina does not contain sensory nerves. On visual examination, the patient typically has a loss of peripheral vision when the visual fields are tested and a loss of acuity in the affected eye.

Diagnostic Tests

Indirect ophthalmoscopy allows the examiner to visualize the retina, which may be pale, opaque, and in folds with retinal detachment to diagnose the type of detachment. If there are lesions in the eye, the slit-lamp examination allows the examiner to magnify the lesions.

Therapeutic Measures

Immediate medical treatment must be sought to prevent loss of vision. One of several procedures may be performed to reattach the retina to prevent blindness:

- Laser reattachment involves focusing a laser beam on the detached area of the retina and causing a controlled burn, which reattaches the layers together by forming an adhesion (see Box 52.2). This procedure is used when only a small area of the retina is involved.
- Cryosurgery involves the placement of a supercooled probe on the sclera. The probe causes injury to the tissue, forming an adhesion—a principle similar to the laser procedure.
- Electrodiathermy, the least used procedure, involves placement of an electrode needle into the sclera to allow fluid that has accumulated to drain. The retina later adheres to the choroid layer.
- Scleral buckling is a surgical procedure that involves placing a silicon implant in conjunction with a belt-like device around the sclera to bring the choroid in contact with the retina. Cryosurgery or laser surgery is used before the buckling procedure to seal the tear

and form a scar that helps adhere the retina and choroid layers together.
- Pneumatic retinopexy is a procedure that can be conducted in the physician's office and is time consuming for the patient. This procedure involves injecting air or gas into the chamber to hold the retina in place. The patient must be extremely compliant with the treatment regimen, reclining for about 16 hours before the procedure to allow the retina to fall back toward the choroid. Because air rises, the patient must maintain a position that keeps the air bubble against the detached area for up to 8 hours a day for 3 weeks.

Complications

With any of the retinal reattachment procedures there is risk of increased intraocular pressure (IOP) and recurrent detachment. The patient is also at risk for future breaks in the retina.

Nursing Process for the Patient with Retinal Detachment

DATA COLLECTION. Subjective data collected include patient observation of the loss of peripheral vision, any change in visual acuity, and the presence of floaters, flashing lights, cobwebs, or veil-like visual impairments. There should be an absence of pain. Objective data collected include the patient's visual acuity, visual fields, ability to perform ADLs, and level of anxiety.

NURSING DIAGNOSES, PLANNING, IMPLEMENTATION, AND EVALUATION. The nursing process for patients with retinal detachment can be found in the *Nursing Process for the Patient Having Eye Surgery* section later in this chapter.

> **CRITICAL THINKING**
>
> ***Mr. Samuel***
>
> ■ Mr. Samuel, age 65, is working in the yard when a branch strikes his right eye. He sees flashes of light and then a short time later a dark shadow out of the right eye.
>
> 1. What should Mr. Samuel do?
> 2. After having a scleral buckling procedure, Mr. Samuel reports nausea. What action should you take?
> 3. Compazine 7.5 mg IM prn every 6 hours is ordered. Available is Compazine 2 mL of 5 mg/mL. How many milliliters should you give?
>
> *Suggested answers at end of chapter.*

Glaucoma

Glaucoma is a group of diseases characterized by abnormal pressure within the eyeball. This pressure causes damage to the cells of the optic nerve, the structure responsible for transmitting visual information from the eye to the brain. The damage is silent, progressive, and irreversible until the end stages, when loss of peripheral vision occurs, followed by reductions in central vision and eventually blindness (see Fig. 52.2). Once glaucoma occurs, the patient will always have it and must follow a treatment regimen to maintain stable intraocular eye pressures.

Pathophysiology

The most common form of glaucoma, called primary, consists of two types: primary open-angle glaucoma (POAG) and acute angle-closure glaucoma (AACG). Secondary glaucoma may be caused by infections, tumors, or injuries. A third form, congenital glaucoma, primarily is due to developmental abnormalities.

AACG occurs in people who have an anatomically narrowed angle at the junction where the iris meets the cornea. When nearby eye structures such as the iris protrude into the anterior chamber, the angle is occluded, which blocks the flow of aqueous fluid. This is considered a medical emergency and results in partial or total blindness if not treated. POAG occurs when the drainage system of the eye, the trabecular meshwork and Schlemm's canal, degenerate and subsequently block the flow of aqueous humor.

Etiology and Prevention

The incidence of AACG is highest among Asians, women older than age 45, and nearsighted people. The incidence of POAG increases in those older than age 40 (older than age 50 for European Americans, older than age 35 for African Americans), in people with diabetes, and in those with a family history of glaucoma, and is four to five times more prevalent in African Americans than European Americans. Those in high-risk groups should have yearly eye examinations for glaucoma detection.

Signs and Symptoms

An ophthalmic emergency, AACG typically has a unilateral, rapid onset. The patient may report severe pain over the affected eye, blurred vision, rainbows around lights, and photophobia and have eye redness, a steamy-appearing cornea, and tearing. The increased IOP can cause nausea and vomiting.

POAG develops bilaterally. The onset is usually gradual and painless, so the patient may have no noticeable symptoms or, after time, may experience mild aching in the eyes, headache, halos around lights, or frequent visual changes that are not corrected with eyeglasses.

Diagnostic Tests

Traditionally, tonometry is used to detect increased IOP (normal IOP: 12 to 20 mm Hg). In AACG, IOP may exceed 50 mm Hg. Tonometry is not adequate to detect glaucoma alone, so three other methods are used. The optic nerve is examined with an ophthalmoscope through dilated pupils, a visual field examination looks for loss of peripheral vision, and the angle where the iris meets the cornea is checked. A newer tool that senses glaucoma much earlier is the GDx Access. This laser device detects nerve damage long before the patient has symptoms of glaucoma.

Therapeutic Measures

The first-line treatment for glaucoma focuses on opening the aqueous flow by administering cholinergic agents (**miotics**) such as carbachol (Isopto) or pilocarpine (Pilocar) to constrict the pupil. When the pupil is constricted, the iris pulls away from the drainage canal so the aqueous fluid can flow freely. A second type of medication may be given to slow the production of aqueous fluid. Types include carbonic anhydrase inhibitors such as acetazolamide (Diamox), adrenergic agonists such as dipivefrin (Propine), and beta blockers such as timolol (Timoptic). Slowing the production of aqueous fluid helps decrease IOP. Additionally, the physician may order steroid eyedrops to reduce inflammation. The patient experiencing an acute attack of AACG is given these types of medications and mannitol, a hyperosmolar agent, to rapidly reduce IOP, as well as analgesics, and is ordered to maintain complete bedrest.

Patients with glaucoma need lifelong use of eyedrop medications twice or more daily. In the absence of symptoms, compliance is often an issue. Other factors that contribute to noncompliance include the patient's age, inability to afford the medication, and lack of understanding of the disease process. Patients need to carry medical alert identification indicating they have glaucoma and what their medications are. This can help prevent administration of contraindicated medications in emergency situations.

Certain medications, regardless of their route, are contraindicated in AACG and can result in blindness if given to a patient with AACG. These medications include any anticholinergics such as atropine and antihistamines such as diphenhydramine (Benadryl) or hydroxyzine (Vistaril) because they are mydriatics. Before a medication is given, the care provider should determine that it is not contraindicated in AACG to prevent blindness from occurring.

> **LEARNING TIP**
>
> - Mydriatic medications are contraindicated in acute angle-closure glaucoma because they can cause an acute episode of increased IOP by dilating the pupil and pushing the iris back, blocking the outflow of aqueous humor.
> - Miotic medications constrict the pupil and so may be given to patients with acute angle-closure glaucoma.
> - To remember what miotic medications and mydriatic medications do, so that the appropriate medication is given and contraindicated ones are never given, remember the following:
>
> **D** = dilate = my**d**riatic = do not.
> No D = constricts = miotic = okay to give.

Surgical Management

When medication is no longer able to control the flow of aqueous humor or reduce the intraocular pressure, surgical intervention may become necessary. Surgery focuses on creating an area where the aqueous humor can flow freely, thus preventing increased IOP (Fig. 52.3). For AACG, laser peripheral iridotomy or surgical iridectomy is performed. Laser iridotomy is a noninvasive procedure utilizing a laser to remove a portion of the iris, thus allowing aqueous fluid to flow through the area. Prophylactic iridotomy may be performed on the other eye to prevent AACG. POAG is treated with laser trabeculoplasty (noninvasive laser beam creates openings in trabecular meshwork), trabeculectomy (part of iris and trabecular meshwork removed), or cyclocryotherapy (cryoprobe destroys part of ciliary body).

Nursing Process for the Patient with Glaucoma

DATA COLLECTION. The patient should be monitored for pain, loss of central and peripheral vision, understanding of disease and compliance with treatment regimen, and ability to conduct activities of daily living.

NURSING DIAGNOSES, PLANNING, AND IMPLEMENTATION. The goal of nursing care for the patient with glaucoma is to prevent further visual loss and to promote comfort if the patient is experiencing pain with acute glaucoma. See the *Nursing Process for the Patient with Visual Impairment* and *Nursing Process for the Patient Having Eye Surgery* sections for additional nursing diagnoses.

Pain Related to Increased Intraocular Pressure

EXPECTED OUTCOME: The patient will report pain is relieved.

- Give analgesics as needed for acute glaucoma *to relieve pain.*

Self-Care Deficit Related to Decreased Vision

EXPECTED OUTCOME: The patient will be able to care for self with assistance if needed.

- Assist with self-care as needed *to ensure activities of daily living are met.*

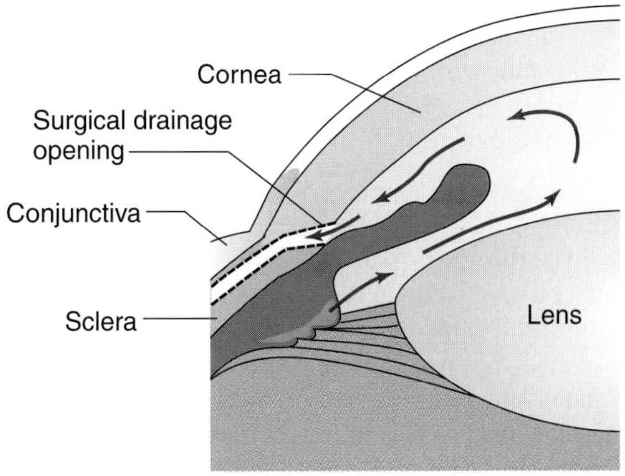
Cornea
Surgical drainage opening
Conjunctiva
Sclera
Lens

FIGURE 52.3 Flow of aqueous humor after trabeculoplasty (arrows).

Anxiety Related to Partial or Total Visual Loss

EXPECTED OUTCOME: The patient will state anxiety is reduced.

- Encourage patient to verbalize concerns about glaucoma *to allow questions to be answered.*

Risk for Injury Related to Decreased Vision

EXPECTED OUTCOME: The patient will not suffer injury as a result of the visual impairment.

- Refer patient to support services that *provide adaptive visual devices.*
- Teach patient and family not to rearrange furniture without patient knowledge *to prevent falls or injury.*

Deficient Knowledge Related to Medical Regimen, Disease Process Due to no Prior Experience

EXPECTED OUTCOME: The patient will demonstrate correct instillation of eye medications and be able to verbalize understanding of condition and treatment.

- Teach need for regular eye examinations through dilated pupils *to monitor disease and detect complications.*
- Teach how to administer medications with a return demonstration *to ensure that eyedrops are administered properly.*
- Teach the patient to rest his or her hand on the forehead *if the patient has trouble keeping the hand steady when administering eyedrops.*
- Consider large-print labels or audiotaped directions *if the patient is unable to see the label on the eyedrop bottle.*
- Consider placing large, multicolored dot stickers on medication bottles and on corresponding instruction cards *for patients with multiple medications.*
- Advise family members that they are at increased risk of developing glaucoma and should have regular eye examinations *because glaucoma can be hereditary.*

EVALUATION. Interventions are successful if the patient maintains an acceptable level of comfort, has no further loss of vision, is able to care for self with assistance, expresses concerns and anxieties, does not suffer injury as a result of the visual impairment, demonstrates correct instillation of eye medications, and is able to verbalize understanding of condition and treatment.

Cataracts

Pathophysiology and Etiology

A cataract is an opacity in the lens of the eye that may cause a loss of visual acuity (see Fig. 52.2). Vision is diminished because the light rays are unable to get to the retina through the clouded lens.

Factors that contribute to cataract development may include age, ultraviolet radiation (sunlight), diabetes, smoking, steroids, nutritional deficiencies, alcohol consumption, intraocular infections, trauma, and congenital defects.

Signs and Symptoms

Cataracts are painless. Symptoms of cataract formation may include halos around lights, difficulty reading fine print or seeing in bright light, increased sensitivity to glare such as when driving at night, double or hazy vision, and decreased color vision.

Diagnostic Tests

Cataracts are diagnosed with an eye examination. Visual acuity is tested for near and far vision. The direct ophthalmoscope and slit-lamp microscope are used to examine the lens and other internal structures.

Surgical Management

When cataracts begin to interfere with daily living and quality of life, treatment is recommended. One eye is treated at a time. The only treatment for cataracts is surgical removal of the cloudy lens. Implantable lenses, which come in various types, are typically inserted after lens removal. Eyeglasses or contact lenses are needed if no lens is reinserted. Eyeglasses may also be needed with some of the lens implants. With the no-stitch cataract operation, there are no postoperative activity restrictions and vision improves in about 1 to 2 days.

Complications

Complications of cataract surgery are rare but include inflammation, increased IOP, macular edema, retinal detachment, vitreous loss, hyphema, endophthalmitis, and expulsive hemorrhage.

Nursing Process for the Patient with Cataracts

DATA COLLECTION. The patient is monitored for visual deficits to assist care planning, as well as knowledge needs about the disease process, surgical intervention, postoperative care, and medical regimen. The majority of patients undergoing cataract surgery have same-day surgery and then go home. So the home situation, the ability of the patient or family member to follow the medical regimen, and transportation to and from the hospital for the patient are evaluated.

NURSING DIAGNOSES, PLANNING, IMPLEMENTATION, AND EVALUATION. Preoperative and postoperative nursing care is the primary nursing responsibility for the patient with cataracts, as discussed next.

Nursing Process for the Patient Having Eye Surgery

DATA COLLECTION. Table 52.5 reviews subjective data to be collected. Objective data may include visual acuity and peripheral field measurements. Visual acuity should be tested with and without any corrective lenses. Eye tearing, redness, or swelling is noted.

Nursing Diagnoses, Planning, and Implementation

Risk for Injury Related to Altered Visual Acuity

EXPECTED OUTCOME: The patient will remain free of injury.

- Explain that depth perception may be affected by eye surgery, which can result in falls, *to help prevent injury.*

TABLE 52.5 SUBJECTIVE DATA COLLECTION FOR PATIENTS HAVING EYE SURGERY

W Where is it?	Where is the visual disturbance? Is it centrally located? Peripherally? Throughout the entire visual field? Unilateral? Bilateral?
H How does it feel?	How does it feel? Painful? Is there an absence of pain?
A Aggravating and alleviating factors	Is it worse in bright light or at night? Better when resting eyes or with head of bed elevated?
T Timing	Was there a sudden onset? Gradual onset?
S Severity	Does it affect activities of daily living? Does it affect close-up work?
U Useful data for associated symptoms	Does the patient suffer from hypertension? Diabetes? Has there been trauma? Vascular disease? What is the level of anxiety? Is the patient older than age 50?
P Perception of the problem by the patient	Will the visual disturbance impair ability to carry out activities of daily living? Ability to comply with medical regimen? Ability to manage home maintenance?

- Ambulate with assistance and use clearly marked stairs *to prevent injury.*
- At home, beverages can be poured and stored in the refrigerator in single-serving glasses *to prevent spills and slippery floors.*

Deficient Knowledge Related to Preoperative and Postoperative Eye Care

EXPECTED OUTCOME: The patient will verbalize preoperative and postoperative care directions.

- Teach disease process, surgical intervention, preoperative and postoperative activity restrictions, use of dark glasses to decrease the discomfort of photophobia, use of correct technique for administering eye medications, need to report for medical follow-up as instructed, and need to protect the eye from further injury *to increase patient knowledge.*
- In some types of cataract surgery, patients may be advised to avoid vomiting, coughing, sneezing, straining, or bending over, if possible, *to prevent IOP.*
- Patients are told to seek medical treatment if they experience sudden, worsening pain, an increase in watery or bloody discharge, or sudden loss of vision *because these are signs of hemorrhage or problems.*

Anxiety Related to Visual Alteration and Surgery

EXPECTED OUTCOME: The patient will report reduced anxiety.

- Give patients the opportunity to discuss their feelings about vision loss and explain any restrictions in activity *to reduce anxiety.*

EVALUATION. The patient goals have been met if the patient is free from injury, verbalizes preoperative and postoperative directions, and reports reduced anxiety.

Macular Degeneration

Pathophysiology and Etiology

Age-related macular degeneration (ARMD) is the leading cause of visual impairment in U.S. residents older than age 50. It involves a deterioration in the macula, the area on the retina where light rays converge for the sharp, central vision needed for reading and seeing small objects. The macula is also responsible for color vision (Fig. 52.4). There are two types of ARMD: dry (atrophic) and wet (exudative). In the dry form, photoreceptors in the macula fail to function and are not replaced because of advancing age. This accounts for 70% to 90% of cases. In the wet form, retinal tissue degenerates, allowing vitreous fluid or blood into the subretinal space. New blood vessels are formed and compromise the macular tissue, causing subretinal edema. Eventually, fibrous scar tissue is formed, severely limiting central vision.

People at risk of developing macular degeneration include those older than age 60, those with a family history of macular degeneration, persons with diabetes, people who smoke, those frequently exposed to ultraviolet light, and Caucasian people.

Signs and Symptoms

Macular degeneration of the dry type is characterized by slow, progressive loss of central and near vision (see Fig. 52.2). Although people usually have the condition in both eyes, each eye may be affected in varying degrees. Macular degeneration of the wet type has the same loss of central and near vision, but the onset is sudden. The loss can occur in one or both eyes. This vision loss is described as blurred vision, distortion of straight lines, and a dark or empty spot in the central area of vision. Some patients may have a decreased ability to distinguish colors.

Diagnostic Tests

Examination of the patient begins with visual acuity for near and far vision and an examination of the internal eye structures with an ophthalmoscope. The examiner uses an Amsler grid (Fig. 52.5) to detect central vision distortion and a color vision test to evaluate color differences. Patients are given an Amsler grid to take home and look at on a regular basis to monitor their vision changes. If any of the grid lines look crooked or disappear, the patient should contact the physician.

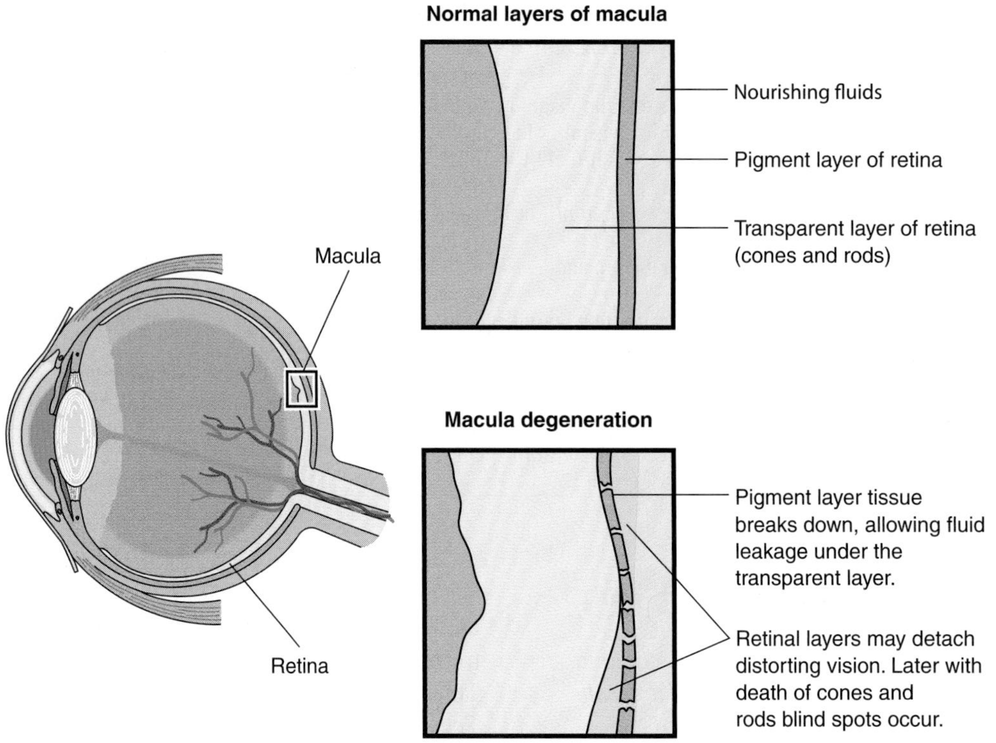
Normal layers of macula
Nourishing fluids
Pigment layer of retina
Transparent layer of retina (cones and rods)
Macula
Macula degeneration
Pigment layer tissue breaks down, allowing fluid leakage under the transparent layer.
Retinal layers may detach distorting vision. Later with death of cones and rods blind spots occur.
Retina

FIGURE 52.4 Macular degeneration. The macula is a small area of the retina responsible for central and color vision.

Intravenous fluorescein (dye) angiography, digital imaging, or optical coherence tomography (similar to a computed tomography scan) may also be utilized to evaluate blood vessel leakage or abnormalities in the eye.

Therapeutic Measures

Unfortunately, there is no treatment for the dry type of ARMD. Most patients with the dry type do not lose peripheral vision or become totally blind, but most are classified as legally blind (less than 20/200 vision with correction). Special low-vision lenses can enhance remaining vision.

If the wet type of ARMD is diagnosed early, laser photocoagulation can seal the leaking blood vessels, slowing the rate of vision loss. If the patient receives laser photocoagulation, there is a small, permanent blind spot at the point of laser contact with the macula. Photodynamic therapy is also available to stop bleeding in blood vessels. Newer evidence-based treatment options for wet type ARMD include antiangiogenesis treatment alone or in conjunction with photodynamic treatment. Drugs that are antiangiogenetic prevent the formation of new blood vessels. Antioxidant vitamins and zinc supplementation have been shown to be beneficial in preventing progression of some macular degeneration. With either type of ARMD, patients have significant visual loss and need to adapt their patterns of daily living.

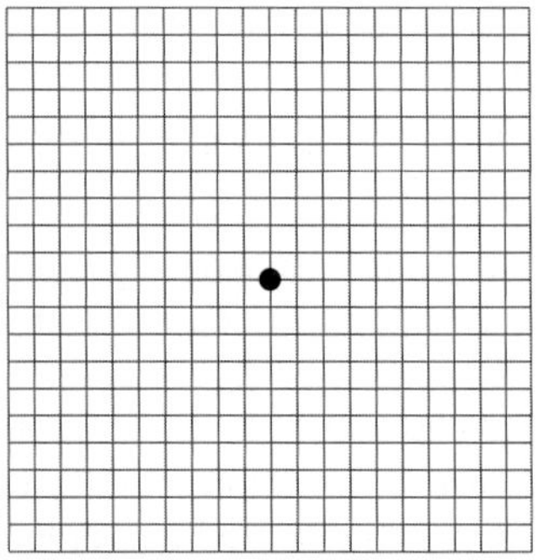

FIGURE 52.5 An Amsler grid is used to identify central vision blind spots or distortions.

Nursing Process for the Patient with Macular Degeneration

See the *Nursing Process for the Patient with Visual Impairment* section.

Trauma

Emergencies and trauma of the eye must be assessed immediately so that proper treatment can be initiated. Injuries to the eye include foreign bodies, burns, abrasions, lacerations, and penetrating wounds. Treatment for chemical burns and sudden, painless loss of vision should be initiated within minutes to preserve vision.

Pathophysiology and Etiology

Foreign bodies are the most common cause of corneal injury. Dust particles or propellants may lodge in the conjunctiva or cornea. Patients automatically rub their eyes to dislodge the object, which further irritates the cornea. Burns may occur from chemical, ultraviolet, or direct heat sources. Depending on the agent causing the burn, it may be superficial or deep. Abrasions and lacerations usually occur as a result of something dragging across the eye, such as a fingernail or clothing. Penetrating wounds are the most serious eye injury. Eye structures may be damaged permanently with complete blindness resulting. A penetrating wound also puts the patient at great risk of infection.

Signs and Symptoms

Foreign bodies produce pain when the eyeball or eyelid moves, causing the foreign body to drag over the opposing surface. Usually the eye tears excessively in an attempt to irrigate the noxious substance out of the eye.

Injuries that irritate or penetrate layers of the cornea range from mild to severe pain. With corneal abrasions, the pain sensation may be delayed for several hours. Other symptoms that may be seen with abrasions, lacerations, and foreign bodies include conjunctival redness, photosensitivity, decreased visual acuity, erythema, and pruritus.

Acute pain and burning are characteristic symptoms of a burn to the eye. Chemical burns must be treated immediately with an eyewash or irrigation to remove the caustic substance from the eye.

Penetrating wounds may result in a variety of symptoms depending on the area of the eye involved and the extent of the damage. If the nerve has been damaged, the patient may have no pain.

Diagnostic Tests

With any eye trauma or injury, visual acuity must be tested. It is important to establish baseline acuity to evaluate effectiveness of treatment, although many patients resist acuity testing because of the discomfort. Testing includes examination by slit-lamp microscope and direct ophthalmoscope. Fluorescein staining is used to evaluate abrasions.

Therapeutic Measures

Foreign bodies are treated with a normal saline flush to irrigate the object out of the eye or to a point where it can be removed with a swab. Topical antibiotic ointment is prescribed to prevent infection.

Most chemical burns are treated with a 15- to 20-minute irrigation of either tap water at the work site or sterile solution in the health care facility. Topical antibiotic ointments are usually prescribed. Burns from heat or ultraviolet (UV) radiation are not irrigated.

Abrasions and lacerations usually are treated with anti-infective ointments or drops after cleansing the eye with a normal saline solution.

An eye specialist treats penetrating wounds. At initial injury, both eyes should be covered to prevent ocular movement. If there is a protruding object, it should be stabilized but not removed until the physician can assess the patient. The nature and extent of the penetrating wound determine treatment.

Complications

If the eye cannot be saved with medical treatment, it may be necessary to surgically remove the eye. This procedure is called **enucleation** (entire eyeball removal).

• WORD • BUILDING •

enucleation: e—removed from + nuclear—center

Nursing Process for the Patient with Eye Trauma

DATA COLLECTION AND EMERGENCY INTERVENTION

Foreign Bodies. The eye is inspected for foreign bodies, which may be visible on the eyeball. The lids should be everted to examine the surface. Then the eye is irrigated.

Burns. Assessment of the type of burn is done because treatment options vary. Immediate irrigation of the eyes is performed once it has been established that a chemical burn has taken place unless contraindicated for the chemical. Medication and eye patching are applied as indicated.

Abrasions and Lacerations. The eye is assessed for visible lacerations and then cleansed, medicated, and patched as indicated.

Penetrating Wounds. The patient is kept calm and relaxed to minimize eye movement and increased IOP. If a protruding object is present, the object is stabilized with tape or other supports.

NURSING DIAGNOSES, PLANNING, AND IMPLEMENTATION

Acute Pain Related to Inflammatory Process and Injury

EXPECTED OUTCOME: The patient's pain level will be within an acceptable range for the patient.

- Administer analgesics as ordered *to reduce pain.*
- Assist patient in remaining calm and relaxed *to reduce pain.*

Risk for Infection Related to Eye Trauma

EXPECTED OUTCOME: The patient will remain free of infection.

- Use sterile technique when irrigating the eye, when applying medications, and during examination *to prevent infection.*

Anxiety Related to Visual-Sensory Deficit

EXPECTED OUTCOME: The patient will verbalize a reduction in anxiety.

- Encourage the patient to verbalize feelings about visual impairment *to reduce anxiety.*
- Reassure patient as appropriate *to reduce anxiety.*

Deficient Knowledge Related to Medical Regimen Due to Lack of Prior Experience

EXPECTED OUTCOME: The patient will be able to verbalize care of the eye.

- Teach patient about interventions and follow-up care *to inform patient.*

EVALUATION. Patient goals have been met if pain level is within an acceptable range for the patient, patient remains free of infection, patient is able to verbalize a reduction in anxiety, and patient is able to verbalize care of the eye.

HEARING DISORDERS

Hearing Loss

Hearing loss is the most common disability in the United States and can be acquired or congenital. Hearing impairment ranges from difficulty understanding words or hearing certain sounds to total deafness. (See Table 52.6.) Hearing impairment can affect communication, social activities, and work activities and can diminish quality of life. Nurses have a responsibility to communicate with patients with hearing impairments and provide needed information regarding health care. For more information on hearing impairment, visit the following websites:

- American Academy of Ear, Nose and Throat at http://entnet.org
- Canadian Hard of Hearing Association at www.cyberus.ca/~chhanational/english.html
- National Information Center on Deafness at www.galludet.edu/~nicd
- National Institute on Deafness and Other Communication Disorders at www.nidcd.nih.gov
- National Organization for the Deaf at www.nad.org.

Conductive Hearing Loss

Conductive hearing loss is any interference with the conduction of sound impulses through the external auditory canal, the eardrum, or the middle ear. The inner ear is not involved in a pure conductive hearing loss. Conductive hearing loss can be caused by anything that interferes with the ability of the sound wave to reach the inner ear. Conductive hearing loss is a mechanical problem. Causes of conductive hearing loss include cerumen, foreign bodies, infection, perforation of the tympanic membrane, trauma, fluid in the middle ear, cysts, tumor, and **otosclerosis**. Many causes of conductive hearing loss, such as infection, foreign bodies, and impacted cerumen, can be corrected. Hearing devices may improve hearing for conditions that cannot be corrected, such as scarred tympanic membrane or otosclerosis. Hearing devices are most effective with conductive hearing loss when no inner ear and nerve damage are present.

Sensorineural Hearing Loss

Sensory hearing loss originates in the cochlea and involves the hair cells and nerve endings. Neural hearing loss originates in the nerve or brainstem. **Sensorineural** hearing loss results from disease or trauma to the sensory or neural components of the inner ear. Some of the causes of nerve deafness are complications of infections (such as measles, mumps, and meningitis), ototoxic drugs (Table 52.7), trauma, noise, neuromas, arteriosclerosis, and the aging process.

Presbycusis is hearing loss caused by the aging process that results from degeneration of the organ of Corti. This degenerative process usually begins in the fifth decade of life. The individual develops an inability to decipher high-frequency sounds (consonants *s, z, t, f,* and *g*). This interferes with the person's ability to understand what has been said, especially in noisy environments. The aging person commonly has more difficulty understanding higher pitched female voices than lower pitched male voices.

Other Types of Hearing Loss

Mixed hearing loss occurs when an individual has both conductive and sensorineural hearing loss. This can be caused by a combination of any of the disorders previously mentioned. Central hearing loss occurs when the central nervous system

• WORD • BUILDING •
otosclerosis: oto—ear + sclerosis—hardening

TABLE 52.6 HEARING LOSS SUMMARY

Signs and Symptoms	Difficulty understanding words or certain sounds Total deafness Changes in social and work activities, turns up volume on TV, asks "What did you say?" Reports people are talking softly, speaks in a quiet or loud voice, answers questions inappropriately. Avoids group activities, loss of sense of humor, appears aloof Reports ringing, buzzing, or roaring noise in ears
Diagnostic Tests and Findings	Abnormal Rinne and Weber tests Audiometric testing indicates hearing loss
Therapeutic Measures	Cerumenolytics Anti-infectives Anti-inflammatories Assistive devices (hearing aids, implantable middle ear hearing devices, cochlear implants)
Complications	Safety issues related to not hearing Withdrawal from social activities and relationships related to hearing loss
Priority Nursing Diagnoses	*Disturbed Sensory Perception: Hearing* related to altered sensory reception and transmission *Impaired Verbal Communication* related to impaired hearing *Impaired Social Interaction* related to impaired hearing and decreased communication skills *Disturbed Body Image* related to impaired hearing and use of assistive hearing devices *Ineffective Coping* related to difficult communication *Deficient Knowledge* related to care of hearing aid due to lack of prior experience

TABLE 52.7 OTOTOXIC DRUGS

Aminoglycoside antibiotics	Amikacin Gentamicin Neomycin Streptomycin Tobramycin
Other antibiotics	Erythromycin Minocycline Vancomycin
Diuretics	Bumetanide Furosemide Hydrochlorothiazide
Other drugs	Cisplatin Indomethacin Methotrexate Quinidine Salicylates

cannot interpret normal auditory signals. This condition occurs with such disorders as cerebrovascular accidents and tumors. Functional hearing loss is a hearing loss for which no organic cause or lesion can be found. It is also called psychogenic hearing loss and is precipitated by emotional stress.

Therapeutic Measures

Medical management consists of improving the patient's hearing. The majority of persons with ear disorders have some degree of hearing loss. With any permanent hearing loss, the use of a hearing aid should always be considered. A hearing aid is designed to amplify sound or attenuate certain portions of the sound signal and amplify other sounds. Various types of hearing aids are available (Fig. 52.6). The in-the-ear aid is a small device that fits in the ear canal. The in-the-ear aid is unobtrusive and may be preferred by the individual. The behind-the-ear aid is worn in a postauricular position. The all-in-one eyeglass aid is attached to glasses and is positioned behind the ear.

Surgical intervention may be available for patients whose hearing is not improved with hearing aids. Implantable middle ear hearing aids can improve sound perception for patients with moderate-to-severe sensorineural hearing loss. Cochlear implants are surgically placed electrical devices that receive sound and transmit the resulting electrical signal to electrodes implanted in the cochlear of the ear. The signal stimulates the cochlea, allowing the patient to hear. The cochlear implants are able to restore up to half of the patient's hearing.

Nursing Process for the Patient with Hearing Impairment

DATA COLLECTION. Nursing care includes identifying those patients at risk for hearing impairment (Table 52.8). Patients with renal or hepatic disease, using two or more ototoxic drugs, or previously having used ototoxic drugs are at risk for developing hearing impairment. If your patient is taking ototoxic medications, assess for tinnitus, sensorineural hearing loss, or vestibular dysfunction, which could indicate ototoxicity. The medications should be discontinued if signs of ototoxicity are present. Monitor for signs of vertigo, horizontal nystagmus, nausea, vomiting, and spinning or rocking sensation while sitting still. To collect data for the patient with hearing impairment, ask family members, as well as the patient, questions related to the patient's hearing status.

Objective data focus on obtaining a gross screening of hearing function. Data collection should start with engaging in normal conversation with the patient. Observe the patient for any difficulty understanding conversation or interview questions. Clarity of the patient's speech is also determined during the interview. Physical examination includes the whisper voice, Rinne, and Weber tests. Test results provide an estimate of conductive or sensorineural hearing loss. The patient should be assessed for the underlying cause of the problem to determine if it is an external, middle, or inner ear problem. Examination of the external ear may reveal an external ear problem. The advanced practitioner may examine the ear canal for impacted cerumen or a tympanic membrane problem. Any assistive hearing devices should be noted and inspected for proper functioning. The results of the examination are documented and communicated to other health team members (see *Evidence-Based Practice* box).

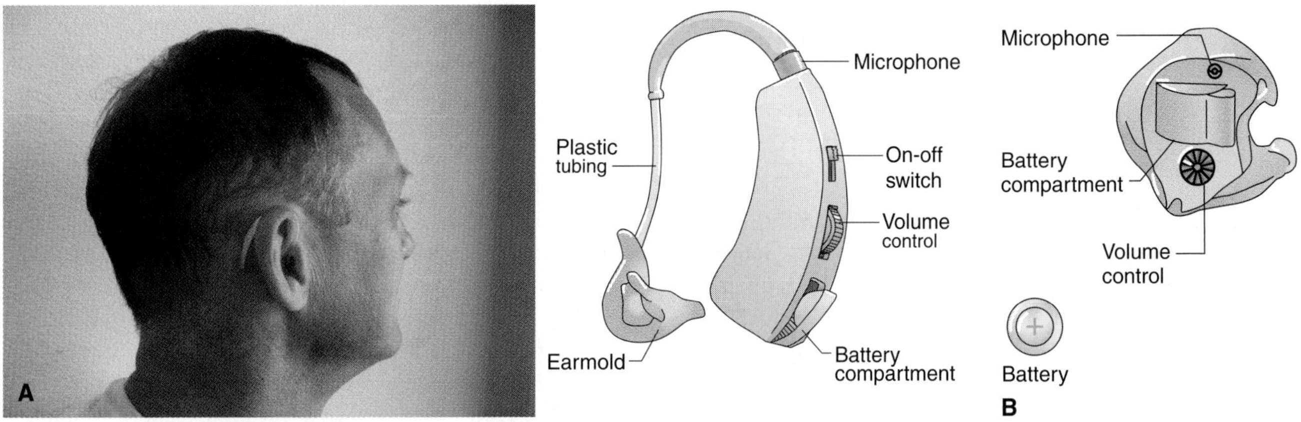
A
Plastic tubing
Microphone
On-off switch
Volume control
Earmold
Battery compartment
Microphone
Battery compartment
Volume control
Battery
B

FIGURE 52.6 Hearing aids. (A) Behind-the-ear hearing aid. (B) In-the-ear hearing aid.

TABLE 52.8 SUBJECTIVE DATA COLLECTION FOR HEARING DISORDERS

W Where is it?	Are both ears affected? Is one side worse than the other?
H How does it feel?	Are certain words unclear, or entire conversations? Are high-frequency sounds (consonants *s*, *t*, *z*, *f*, *g*, and female voices) unclear or difficult to understand? Is any pain associated with the hearing loss? Any tinnitus or vertigo?
A Aggravating and alleviating factors	Is hearing worse in large groups or when there is a lot of background noise? Is hearing improved in a quiet environment or when speaking only to an individual? Is it easier to understand someone when seeing the person's lips move? Does the patient own or use any assistive hearing devices? Are they effective? What type is used?
T Timing	When did the hearing loss start? Was it gradual or sudden? Is the hearing loss associated with any illness or traumatic event? Is it associated with any recent flying? Any history of ototoxic drug use?
S Severity	Does it cause communication impairment? How much? Does it affect activities of daily living? Does it affect or limit usual social activities? Have family or friends commented on decreased hearing? Does patient avoid communication or social activities because of difficulty hearing? Is patient having difficulties hearing telephone voices, radio, television, or movies?
U Useful data for associated symptoms	Is there any fever, nausea, vomiting, or dizziness? Is there any history of occupational or environmental exposure to loud noises? What are the usual ear self-care habits? Any history of impacted cerumen? Has patient ever had cerumen removed from ears?
P Perception of the problem by the patient	What does the patient feel is wrong? Does the patient think that he or she has a hearing problem? How does the patient feel about hearing assistive devices? How does the patient perceive the hearing loss, and how is it influencing the patient's life?

EVIDENCE-BASED PRACTICE

Clinical Question

Can hearing loss predict risk for cardiovascular diseases?

Evidence

A study examined 1,168 patients for underlying cardiovascular disease and low-frequency hearing loss (Friedland, Cederberg, & Tarima, 2009). A significant association was found between low-frequency hearing loss and cardiovascular disease and risk factors.

Implications for Nursing Practice

Patients with low-frequency hearing loss should be referred for cardiovascular disease screening.

REFERENCE

Friedland, D., Cederberg, C., & Tarima, S. (2009). Audiometric pattern as a predictor of cardiovascular status: Development of a model for assessment of risk. *Laryngoscope, 119,* 473–486.

NURSING DIAGNOSES, PLANNING, AND IMPLEMENTATION. Planning focuses on helping the patient optimize hearing, promoting communication, and promoting adjustment to impaired hearing (Boxes 52.4 Box 52.5). Nursing management for the patient with hearing impairment focuses on enhancing communication and quality of life (see the *Nursing Care Plan for the Patient with Hearing Loss*). Families should be included in discussions about therapeutic hearing devices and their care, enhancing communication, and limiting isolation.

EVALUATION. The patient's goals are met if the patient communicates effectively, engages in usual social activities, verbalizes acceptance of an assistive hearing device, copes with emotional reaction to hearing impairment, and demonstrates care of hearing aid.

External Ear

Infections

PATHOPHYSIOLOGY AND ETIOLOGY. Infections are the most common disorder of the external ear, with **external otitis** being the most common infection. Exposure to moisture, contamination, or local trauma provides an ideal environment for pathological growth in the external ear, which results in external otitis. It may be caused by bacterial or fungal pathogens. Staphylococci are the most common causative organisms, but other gram-negative or gram-positive bacteria can cause problems. *Pneumocystis* infections have been seen in patients who have human immunodeficiency virus (HIV). A bacterial or fungal external otitis that occurs when water is left in the ear and washes away protective earwax often after water exposure or trauma is known as swimmer's ear. External otitis occurs more often in the summer months than in the winter months. However, swimmer's ear can be seen year-round in patients who swim indoors.

A localized infection called ear canal **furuncle** or abscess results when a hair follicle becomes infected. A **carbuncle** forms when several hair follicles are involved in forming the abscess. Most furuncles and carbuncles erupt and drain spontaneously. Otomycosis is an infection

Box 52.4

Communicating with a Person Who Has a Hearing Impairment

- Get the person's attention before beginning to speak.
- Face and stand close to the person being spoken to and maintain eye contact.
- Avoid standing in the glare of bright sunlight or other bright lights.
- Speak clearly, at a normal rate and volume. Do not shout or overarticulate.
- Inform the listener of topics to be discussed and when a change of topic occurs. Stick to a topic for a while and avoid quick shifts.
- Use short sentences and assess for understanding. If the listener does not understand after the message is repeated, rephrase the message. If the listener has difficulty with high-pitched sounds, lower the voice pitch.
- Allow extra time for the listener to respond and do not rush the listener.
- Ensure an optimum environment by reducing background noises: turn off television and radio, close the door, or move to a quieter area.
- Encourage nonverbal communication such as touch or gestures as appropriate.
- If the listener uses a hearing device, ensure that it is operational and in place before beginning to communicate. Give the person time to adjust the hearing device before speaking.
- Do not smile, chew gum, or cover the mouth when talking.
- Use active listening with attentive body posture, pleasant facial expressions, and a calm, unhurried manner.
- Do not avoid conversation with a person who has hearing loss.
- Use written communication if unable to communicate verbally.

Box 52.5

Care of Hearing Aids

- Insert hearing aid while over a soft surface such as a pillow to prevent damage if the hearing aid is dropped during insertion.
- Remove hearing aid before showering or bathing. Do not immerse in water.
- Turn the hearing aid off when not in use to conserve battery.
- Do not expose the hearing aid to extreme heat or cold.
- Clean the hearing aid daily with a dry, soft cloth. Clean earmold with small brush or toothpick to keep free of earwax.
- Turn off the hearing aid and turn the volume down before inserting. Turn hearing aid on and increase volume once it is inserted.
- Minimize whistling noise by ensuring that the volume is not too high, the aid fits securely, and the aid is free from earwax.
- Check battery or lower the volume if sound is not clear or is intermittent. Buzzing noise may indicate that the battery door is not completely closed.
- Do not expose the hearing aid to medicinal or hair sprays. Apply sprays before inserting hearing aid.

NURSING CARE PLAN for the Patient with Hearing Loss

Nursing Diagnosis: *Disturbed Sensory Perception: Hearing*, related to altered sensory reception and transmission

Expected Outcomes: The patient will attain optimum level of sensory stimulation. The patient will become aware of auditory impairment and ways to compensate. The patient will demonstrate ability to perform activities of daily living, with assistance if necessary.

Evaluation of Outcomes: Patient perceives maximum auditory sensory input. Patient is able to compensate for sensory impairment by using other senses and resources. Patient is able to perform activities of daily living as independently as possible.

NURSING CARE PLAN for the Patient with Hearing Loss—cont'd

Interventions	Rationale	Evaluation
Begin assessment of hearing by inspecting ear canals for mechanical obstruction. If cerumen is found, use of a softening product is recommended to assist in wax removal.	Hearing loss may result from buildup of cerumen in the auditory canal.	Is ear canal free of mechanical obstruction?
If canal is clear, continue assessment by using a tuning fork, loud ticking clock, or verbal cues to determine auditory ability at various distances.	Determination of hearing ability assists nurse in developing interventions appropriate to patient's hearing level.	Is patient able to hear verbal input? If not, how severe is the impairment?
Enhance hearing by giving auditory cues in quiet surroundings.	The presence of background noise such as television, radio, or large numbers of people makes hearing more difficult.	Are auditory cues being delivered in an environment free of extraneous background noises?
Enhance understanding of auditory cues by getting patient's attention before speaking, speaking slowly with careful enunciation of words, adding hand gestures, speaking face to face with the person with the impairment, and adjusting the voice pitch downward without increasing volume.	Hearing is enhanced when additional cues assist the person in understanding the message. Use of hand gestures to point, lipreading, facial expression, and lower pitch all assist communication.	Are auditory cues being understood by patient? Are instructions given in step-by-step format with written cues?
Structure environment to compensate for hearing loss by adding visual indicators to telephone ringer, doorbell, smoke detectors, and other emergency sounds.	Assists in communication and safety.	Is patient able to receive input in ways other than auditory?
Provide for optimal care of assistive appliances such as hearing aids by making sure that cerumen has been cleaned from the device, that batteries are charged, and that the appliance is placed correctly in ear.	Appliances that are not functioning properly will not assist patient in hearing.	Is patient's hearing aid in place correctly? Is cerumen blocking sound conduction? Do batteries work?
Introduce assistive devices such as hearing amplifiers, telephone amplifiers, telephones with extra-loud bells, written communication, and sign language.	Patients may not be aware of assistive devices that could help them adapt to hearing loss and continue previous activities, such as talking on the telephone or listening to television.	Is patient aware of assistive devices that will allow him or her to continue to verbally communicate with others? Is patient able to use the devices to compensate for auditory impairment?
Allow patient to verbalize feelings and grieving about hearing loss.	Losing a primary sense such as hearing can be devastating. The opportunity to ventilate feelings assists in processing the loss.	Is patient able to verbalize feelings about the auditory impairment and its loss?
Identify coping strategies that have been successful for patient in the past.	By identifying successful coping strategies, the nurse assists the patient in dealing with stress of hearing loss.	Can the patient identify successful coping strategies and use them to deal with the stress of having a hearing impairment?

NURSING CARE PLAN for the Patient with Hearing Loss—cont'd

Interventions	Rationale	Evaluation
	A positive approach focuses on the person's capabilities rather than deficits.	
Refer to specialized clinician such as an audiologist or occupational therapist or to specialized resources such as the National Association of the Deaf or American Speech, Language and Hearing Association.	Specialized clinicians can provide detailed examination and treatment. Specialized resource groups have networks in place to help people cope with loss and maximize abilities.	Does patient know whom to call for detailed examination and treatment? Does patient know that there are specialized clinicians and resource groups to help with hearing impairment? Does patient know how to access these specialists?

caused by fungal growth and is typically seen after topical corticosteroid or antibiotic use. Otomycosis occurs more often in hot weather. An infection of the auricle is called perichondritis, which can result in necrosis of cartilage.

SIGNS AND SYMPTOMS. The most common sign of infection of the external ear is pain. (See Table 52.9.) An early indication of infection is pain with gentle pulling on the pinna. The patient may also experience pain when moving the jaw or when the otoscope is inserted into the ear canal. Pruritus (itching) is also a common symptom and can be an early sign of infection. Signs of inflammation are present on the external ear. The ear canal may become swollen or occluded, and as a result hearing may be diminished. Redness, swelling, and drainage can be observed during otoscopic examination. If drainage is present, it usually starts out clear and becomes purulent as the disease progresses. The patient may also be febrile.

DIAGNOSTIC TESTS. Laboratory tests such as a complete blood cell count (CBC) and cultures of discharge may be completed to diagnose infections. The white blood cell (WBC) count may be elevated. Culture and sensitivity tests isolate the specific infective organism and determine which antibiotics would be most effective to treat the infection. The Rinne and Weber tests can indicate conductive hearing impairment.

TABLE 52.9 EXTERNAL EAR DISORDERS SUMMARY

Signs and Symptoms	Pain Pruritus, swelling, redness Drainage Lacerations, contusion, hematomas, abrasion Erythema, blistering Hearing loss Foreign body
Diagnostic Tests and Findings	CBC with elevated WBC with infections Audiometric, Rinne, Weber, and whisper voice tests (indicate conductive hearing loss with impacted cerumen and trauma) Imaging studies to indicate extent of trauma
Therapeutic Measures	Cerumenolytics to remove earwax Anti-infectives and anti-inflammatory medications (to treat infection) Debridement, surgical repair, or application of protective covering with trauma to external ear
Complications	Spread of infection to other parts of the ear Disfigurement Loss of hearing Scarring
Priority Nursing Diagnoses	*Acute Pain* related to inflammation or trauma *Disturbed Sensory Perception: Auditory*, related to altered sensory reception *Risk for Injury* related to self-cleaning of external ear *Deficient Knowledge* related to care of hearing aid due to lack of prior experience

Impacted Cerumen

PATHOPHYSIOLOGY AND ETIOLOGY. Normally, the ear is self-cleaning. However, cerumen (wax) may become impacted, blocking the ear canal. People with large amounts of hair in the ear canal or who work in dusty or dirty areas are prone to cerumen impaction. Improper cleaning can also result in cerumen impaction. The older adult is at risk to develop impacted cerumen. This occurs because the amount of cerumen secreted is decreased and because of increased amounts of keratin. These two factors cause the cerumen to be drier, harder, and more easily impacted. Patients with hearing aids tend to have problems with impacted cerumen. Patients with bony growths secondary to an osteophyte or osteoma are at risk for cerumen impaction.

SIGNS AND SYMPTOMS. The patient may experience hearing loss, a feeling of fullness, or blocked ear if cerumen has become impacted (see Table 52.6). Otoscopic examination reveals cerumen blocking the ear canal.

DIAGNOSTIC TESTS. Audiometric testing reveals conductive hearing loss in the affected ear. Hearing acuity can be decreased by 45 decibels because of impacted cerumen. Whisper voice, Rinne, and Weber tests also indicate conductive hearing loss (see Chapter 51).

Masses

PATHOPHYSIOLOGY AND ETIOLOGY. Benign masses of the external ear are usually cysts resulting from sebaceous glands. Other benign masses are lipomas, warts, keloids, and infectious polyps. Infectious polyps usually arise from the middle ear and enter the external ear through a hole in the tympanic membrane. Actinic keratosis is a precancerous lesion that can be found on the auricle and may be seen in the elderly. Malignant tumors such as basal cell carcinoma on the pinna and squamous cell in the ear canal may develop and can spread.

SIGNS AND SYMPTOMS. Changes in the appearance of the skin can occur with benign or malignant masses. Usually, impaired conductive or sensorineural hearing loss occurs with masses. Pain is another symptom and is usually described as deep pain radiating inward on the affected side. Ear drainage may be present. As the condition progresses, facial paralysis may occur. Visualization of the mass may be observed during otoscopic examination.

DIAGNOSTIC TESTS. A biopsy may be obtained to determine if the mass is benign or malignant. Imaging studies are also used to diagnose tumors. Audiometric studies reveal any hearing impairment.

Trauma

PATHOPHYSIOLOGY AND ETIOLOGY. Injuries to the external ear are commonly caused by a blow to the head, automobile accidents, burns, foreign bodies lodged in the ear canal, or cold temperatures. Cotton ball pieces and insects are the most common foreign bodies found in adults.

SIGNS AND SYMPTOMS. Lacerations, contusions, hematomas, abrasions, erythema, and blistering are signs seen with thermal or physical trauma. Repeated trauma to the ear can cause swelling, also known as cauliflower ear. This is common among boxers, rugby players, martial artists, and wrestlers. Conductive hearing loss can occur if the ear canal is partially or totally blocked. Patients who have contusions or hematomas commonly report numbness, pain, and paresthesia of the auricle. Symptoms associated with foreign bodies may include decreased hearing, itching, pain, and infection. Care is taken during otoscopic examination not to push the foreign body further into the ear canal.

DIAGNOSTIC TESTS. Imaging studies may be needed to determine the extent of the trauma. Audiometric, whisper voice, Rinne, and Weber tests may demonstrate conductive hearing loss.

Complications of External Ear Disorders

If not treated, infections can spread, causing cellulitis, abscesses, middle ear infection, and septicemia. Metastasis can occur if malignant tumors are not treated. Infection, trauma, and malignant tumors may cause temporary or permanent hearing loss, disfigurement, discoloration, and scarring.

Therapeutic Measures for External Ear Disorders

For external ear infections topical antibiotics are given. Systemic antibiotics are used for severe infections that are localized or have spread to surrounding tissues. Analgesics are used to control pain. Topical or systemic steroids may be used to treat inflammation. The ear is thoroughly cleaned before starting any topical treatment. If the external ear canal has drainage or is swollen shut, a wick may be inserted. The wick serves to aid in removing drainage or to aid in administering medication into the ear canal.

Cerumen may be removed with instillations or irrigation (see *Evidence-Based Practice* box). Instillation or irrigation is not used if the patient has a history of perforated tympanic membrane (eardrum). The irrigation solution, usually water, should be warmed to body temperature. A ceruminolytic is instilled into the ear canal about 15 to 30 minutes before the procedure to soften the cerumen. The patient is draped with a protective plastic drape, and a basin is placed below the ear to catch the irrigating solution. The patient sits with the ear toward the nurse and the head tilted toward the opposite ear. For irrigation, the external ear is pulled upward and backward for an adult, downward and back for a child (Fig. 52.7). A low-pressure stream of water is directed toward the top of the ear canal. Care is taken not to obstruct the canal with the syringe so that the irrigation solutions can flow back out of the canal. Ensure that only the tip of the syringe is in the ear canal and that gentle pressure is used to prevent trauma to the ear canal and eardrum.

EVIDENCE-BASED PRACTICE

Clinical Question

When and how should cerumen be removed from the ear canal?

Evidence

A review of the literature showed strong recommendations for cerumen removal if a patient is symptomatic or if the cerumen prevents examination of the ear canal (Roland et al., 2008). Patients who wear hearing aids were found to be at risk for impaction. A ceruminolytic instilled 15 to 30 minutes before syringe irrigation to ease cerumen removal is recommended. Inappropriate or harmful interventions include cotton-tipped swabs, oral jet irrigators, and ear candling.

Implications for Nursing Practice

Nurses should ensure referral for checkups every 6 to 12 months for patients at risk for cerumen impaction, such as those who wear hearing aids. As ordered, if cerumen impaction exists, use a ceruminolytic 15 to 30 minutes before syringe irrigation. The patient should be taught not to use cotton-tipped swabs, oral jet irrigators, or ear candling in the ear canal.

REFERENCE

Roland, P. S., Smith, T. L., Schwartz, S. R., et al. (2008). Clinical practice guideline on cerumen impaction. *Otolaryngology Head and Neck Surgery, 139*(3 Suppl 2), S1–S21.

Debridement, surgical repair, or application of a protective covering may be done when trauma occurs to the external ear. Surgical management consists of incision and drainage of abscesses. Excision of cysts or cutaneous carcinomas may also be required.

Nursing Process for the Patient with External Ear Disorders

DATA COLLECTION. Subjective data obtained in a patient history include reports of pain, fullness, previous cerumen impaction, itching, or hearing loss, as well as onset, duration, and severity of symptoms. Additional data include patient's occupation, previous ear problems, use of a hearing aid, and typical ear hygiene. Observation for objective data includes redness, swelling, drainage, furuncles, carbuncles, lesions, abrasions, lacerations, growths, cerumen, scaliness, or crusting. The patient may report pain when the ear is palpated. Basic hearing acuity tests are conducted to evaluate hearing loss (see Chapter 51).

NURSING DIAGNOSES, PLANNING, AND IMPLEMENTATION. Possible nursing diagnoses are discussed next.

Acute Pain Related to Inflammation or Trauma

EXPECTED OUTCOME: *The patient's pain will be decreased or absent as evidenced by a lower rating on a pain scale.*

- Assess for nonverbal signs of ear pain *to identify pain.*
- Identify with the patient an optimum analgesic schedule *to promote comfort.*
- Implement nonpharmacological methods, such as relaxation, massage, music, guided imagery, or distraction techniques *to relieve pain.*

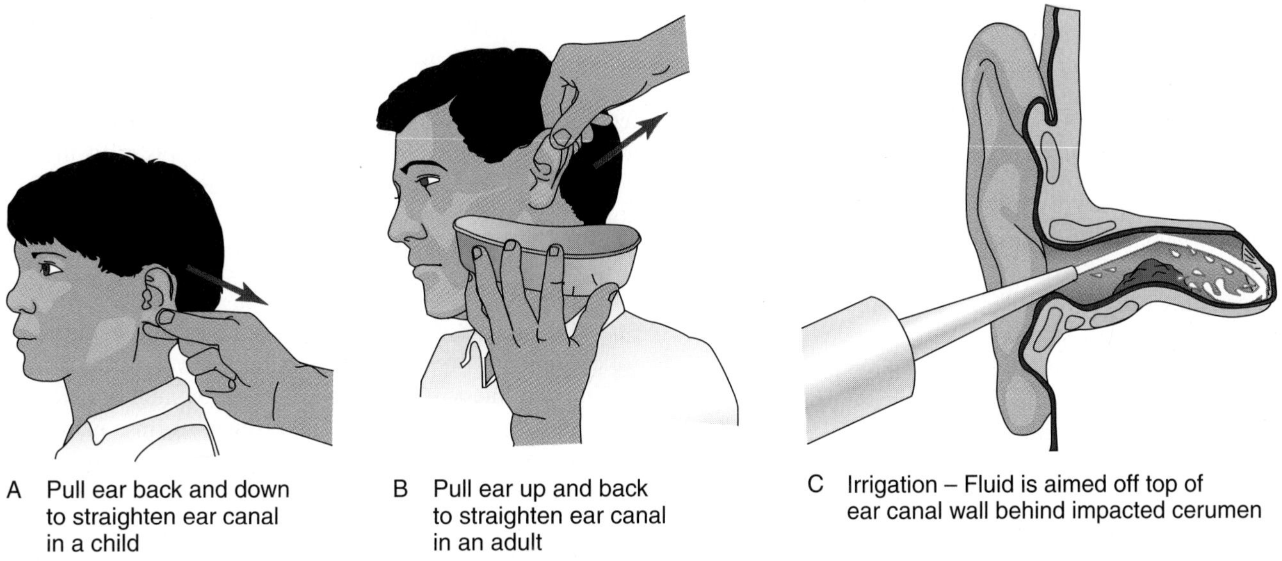
A Pull ear back and down to straighten ear canal in a child
B Pull ear up and back to straighten ear canal in an adult
C Irrigation – Fluid is aimed off top of ear canal wall behind impacted cerumen

FIGURE 52.7 Ear irrigation. (A) Child. (B) Adult. (C) Irrigation.

- Heat may be applied to the area *to promote comfort.*
- Liquid or soft foods may be offered *to relieve pain when chewing.*

Disturbed Sensory Perception: Auditory, Related to Altered Sensory Reception

EXPECTED OUTCOME: The patient's hearing will return to preillness state.

- Teach patient how to administer topical antibiotics and anti-inflammatory medications using aseptic technique *to help restore hearing and relieve blockage of the ear canal.*
- If a wick is inserted into the ear canal, explain to patient that it is used *to monitor for drainage and report excessive drainage to health care provider.*
- Explain procedure before removal of cerumen *to decrease anxiety.*

Risk for Injury Related to Self-Cleaning of External Ear

EXPECTED OUTCOME: The patient will explain or demonstrate prescribed treatment.

- Instruct patient how to care for ear *to prevent injury.*
- Instruct patient how to complete prescribed treatment *to ensure completion of treatment.*

Box 52.6 gives further instructions on ear care.

Deficient Knowledge Related to Lack of Information on Preventive Ear Care

EXPECTED OUTCOME: The patient will explain or demonstrate procedures to maintain wellness of the external ear.

- Instruct patient to keep external ear clean and dry *to prevent problems.*
- Teach patient how to use topical antibiotics, oral antibiotics, and/or anti-inflammatory medications *to promote healing.*
- Teach the patient how to complete the prescribed treatment and maintain ear health (see Box 52.6). Include how to administer eardrops or ointments, keep the ear clean and dry, and use cotton with petroleum jelly or earplugs *to avoid getting water in the ears during an infection.*

EVALUATION. The outcomes for the patient are met if patient indicates pain is decreased or absent as evidenced by a lower rating on a pain scale, hearing improves or returns to preillness level, states or demonstrates prescribed treatment (e.g., administering eardrops or ointments) without injury, and explains or demonstrates measures to maintain wellness of the external ear.

Middle Ear, Tympanic Membrane, and Mastoid Disorders

Infections

PATHOPHYSIOLOGY AND ETIOLOGY. Otitis media is the most common disease of the middle ear. Otitis media is a general term for inflammation of the middle ear, mastoid, and eustachian tube. Inflammation of the nasopharynx causes most cases of otitis media. As inflammation occurs, the nasopharyngeal mucosa becomes edematous and discharge is produced. When fluid, pus, or air builds up in the middle ear, the eustachian tube becomes blocked, and this impairs middle ear ventilation.

There are several types of otitis media in which inflammation can occur alone, with infective drainage, or with noninfective drainage. The first type of otitis media is otitis media without effusion. This is an inflammation of the middle ear mucosa without drainage. The second type of otitis media occurs when there is a bacterial infection of the middle ear mucosa. This is called acute otitis media, suppurative otitis media, or purulent otitis media. The infected fluid becomes trapped in the middle ear. If the infection continues longer than 3 months, chronic otitis media results. The third type of otitis media is otitis media with effusion. Other names include serous otitis media, nonsuppurative otitis media, and glue ear. With this type of otitis media, noninfective fluid accumulates within the middle ear.

SIGNS AND SYMPTOMS. Acute otitis media commonly follows an upper respiratory infection. A fever, earache, and feeling of fullness in the affected ear are common symptoms. (See Table 52.10.) As purulent drainage forms, pain and conductive hearing loss occur. Nausea and vomiting may also be present. Purulent drainage may be evident in the external ear canal if the tympanic membrane ruptures. Mastoid tenderness indicates that the infection may have spread to the mastoid area. Otoscopic examination reveals a reddened, bulging tympanic membrane.

Symptoms of otitis media with effusion may go undetected in adults because there are no signs of infection. The

Box 52.6

Ear Care

1. Cleanse the external ear with a wet washcloth. Gently cleanse the helix.
2. Never insert anything into the ear canal, including hairpins, cotton-tipped applicators, matchsticks, safety pins, toothpicks, paper clips, and fingers.
3. A person with a history of ear infections, perforated tympanic membrane, or swimmer's ear should prevent moisture from entering the ear canal and should avoid swimming in contaminated water. Moisture or water in the ear canal can be prevented by using special earplugs or by using a piece of cotton rolled into a cylinder and covered with petroleum jelly.
4. Avoid home remedies for ear care without consulting a physician.
5. A person with an upper respiratory infection should gently blow the nose with both nares open to prevent microbes from being forced up the eustachian tubes.

TABLE 52.10 MIDDLE EAR DISORDERS SUMMARY

Signs and Symptoms	Fever, earache, and feeling of fullness in affected ear following upper respiratory infection Nausea, vomiting Mastoid tenderness Reddened, bulging tympanic membrane Progressive hearing loss Vertigo Disorientation
Diagnostic Tests	Complete blood count Ear cultures Audiometric, Rinne, Weber, and whisper voice tests
Therapeutic Measures	Antibiotics Analgesics Myringotomy Myringoplasty Stapedectomy
Complications	Perforation of tympanic membrane Cholesteatoma Tympanosclerosis Mastoiditis Permanent hearing loss
Priority Nursing Diagnoses	*Acute Pain* *Deficient Knowledge* *Risk for Infection*

patient may report fullness, bubbling, or crackling in the ear. The patient may have a slight conductive hearing loss or allergies or be a mouth breather. Otoscopic examination can reveal a bulging tympanic membrane with a fluid level, but the eardrum is not reddened.

COMPLICATIONS. A perforation may occur with an acute or chronic infection. Buildup of fluid and pressure in the middle ear can cause a spontaneous perforation of the tympanic membrane. The patient usually experiences pain before the rupture and relief of pain after the rupture. The fluid in the middle ear moves through the perforation into the ear canal, relieving the pressure and pain. A tympanic membrane perforation causes hearing loss. The location and size of the perforation determine the extent of hearing loss. Damage to the ossicles can also occur with perforation.

Repeated infections in the middle ear or mastoid can cause a cholesteatoma, which is an epithelial cystlike sac that fills with debris such as degenerated skin and sebaceous material. The cholesteatoma starts in the external ear canal and spreads to the middle ear through a perforation in the tympanic membrane. Damage occurs in the middle ear structures as a result of pressure necrosis. The cholesteatoma causes conductive hearing loss. As the disease progresses, facial paralysis and vertigo may occur.

Tympanosclerosis is another complication of repeated middle ear infections. Tympanosclerosis consists of deposits of collagen and calcium on the tympanic membrane. The condition can slowly progress over time to the area around the middle ear ossicles. These deposits appear as chalky white plaques on the tympanic membrane and contribute to conductive hearing loss.

Mastoiditis can occur if acute otitis media is not treated. The infection spreads to the mastoid area, causing pain. The use of antibiotics has resulted in acute mastoiditis becoming relatively uncommon. Chronic mastoiditis is still seen with repeated middle ear infections.

DIAGNOSTIC TESTS. An elevated WBC count may be seen and cultures may be done on ear drainage to identify the specific infective organism. Conductive hearing loss is usually present on audiometric studies and Rinne, Weber, and whisper voice tests. Imaging studies may be done to diagnose infection.

THERAPEUTIC MEASURES. Bacterial infections are treated with topical and systemic antibiotics. Topical antibiotics may contain steroids to help with inflammation. Oral analgesics are given to control pain.

A modified Politzer ear device can be used to help equalize pressure in the middle ear and aid fluid drainage. The device, also know as the ear popper, emits a stream of air into the nasal cavity that gently opens the eustachian tubes. This relieves negative pressure and allows pressure to equalize and fluid to drain. For more information, see www.earpopper.com/earpopper/index.htm.

Surgical intervention includes several techniques. Paracentesis may be performed with a needle and syringe. The tympanic membrane is punctured with the needle, and the fluid is drained from the middle ear. A **myringotomy** may also be performed. During this procedure, an incision is made in the tympanic membrane and fluid is allowed to drain out or is suctioned out of the middle ear. Another technique is laser-assisted myringotomy, which vaporizes the tympanic membrane. Various types of transtympanic tubes may be inserted to keep the incision open. The transtympanic tube keeps the incision in the tympanic membrane open, equalizes pressure, and prevents further fluid formation and buildup. The transtympanic tubes are left in place until the infection is cured. Most tubes spontaneously extrude in 3 to 12 months and rarely have to be removed.

Reconstructive repair of a perforated tympanic membrane is called a **myringoplasty**. One technique involves placing Gelfoam over the perforation. A graft from the temporal muscle behind the ear or tissue from the external ear is then placed over the perforation and Gelfoam. The Gelfoam is absorbed, and the graft repairs the perforation.

A mastoidectomy involves incision, drainage, and surgical removal of the mastoid process if the infection has spread to the mastoid area.

• WORD • BUILDING •

myringoplasty: myringo—tympanic membrane + plasty—surgical repair

Otosclerosis

PATHOPHYSIOLOGY AND ETIOLOGY. Otosclerosis, or hardening of the ear, results from the formation of new bone along the stapes. With the new bone growth, the stapes becomes immobile and causes conductive hearing loss. The formation of the new bone growth begins in adolescence or early adulthood and progresses slowly. Hearing loss is most apparent after the fourth decade. Otosclerosis is more common in women than in men. The disease usually affects both ears. Although the exact cause of otosclerosis is not known, most patients have a family history of the disease. It is therefore thought to be a hereditary disease.

SIGNS AND SYMPTOMS. The primary symptom of otosclerosis is progressive hearing loss. The patient usually experiences bilateral conductive hearing loss, particularly with soft, low tones. Usually, medical treatment is sought when the hearing loss interferes with the patient's ability to hear conversations. The patient may also experience tinnitus. Otoscopic examination reveals a pinkish orange tympanic membrane because of vascular and bony changes in the middle ear.

DIAGNOSTIC TESTS. Audiometric testing indicates the type and extent of the hearing loss. Imaging studies indicate the location and the extent of the excessive bone growth. The whisper voice test and normal conversation show decreased hearing. The patient hears best with bone conduction in the Rinne test, whereas lateralization to the most affected ear occurs with the Weber test.

THERAPEUTIC MEASURES. There is no cure for otosclerosis, but hearing aids may be used to improve hearing for the patient. The hearing aid is most effective for conductive hearing loss when there is no sensorineural involvement.

Although total restoration of hearing is not possible, reconstruction of necrotic ossicles is done to restore some of the patient's hearing. Various methods are used to reposition and replace some or all of the ossicles. Unfortunately, the surgeries are not always successful over the long term. Ossiculoplasty is the reconstruction of the ossicles. Prostheses made of plastic, ceramic, or human bone are used to replace the necrotic ossicles. Total or partial ossicular replacement prosthesis may be used.

Stapedectomy is the treatment of choice for otosclerosis. Either part or all of the stapes is removed and replaced with a prosthesis. The prosthesis is placed between the incus and the oval window. Advances in surgical treatment include the use of lasers for improved visualization, less trauma, and greater precision during surgery. The goal is to restore vibration from the tympanic membrane to the oval window and allow sound transmission. Many patients experience improved hearing immediately, others not until swelling subsides. Complications of ossiculoplasty and stapedectomy include extrusion of the prosthesis, infection, hearing loss, dizziness, and facial nerve damage. To view a laser-assisted stapedectomy, see www.mdkiosk.com/Laser%20stapedectomy%20for%20otosclerosis-topicview.php.

• WORD • BUILDING •

stapedectomy: stape(s)—stirrup + ectomy—excision of

NURSING CARE. The operative ear is positioned upward when lying in bed. An earplug may be used to help keep the area aseptic; the proximity of the brain makes this necessary to prevent brain infection. Activity orders may vary. The patient may be dizzy and experience nausea. Antiemetics should be given promptly to prevent vomiting. The patient's safety should be ensured if dizziness occurs. To prevent dislodgment or damage to the prosthesis, patients are instructed not to cough, sneeze, blow their nose, vomit, fly in an airplane, lift heavy objects, or shower. If the patient develops a cold, the physician should be contacted.

CRITICAL THINKING

Mrs. Springhorn

■ Mrs. Springhorn is an 83-year-old woman who is scheduled to be discharged from the hospital following a stapedectomy. She lives alone at home and is able to care for herself.

1. How would you communicate with Mrs. Springhorn to ensure that she understands the discharge instructions?
2. What teaching methods would you use to enhance communication?
3. What ear care instructions would you give her?

Suggested answers at end of chapter.

Trauma

ETIOLOGY AND PHYSIOLOGY. Trauma such as a blasting force, a blunt injury to the side of the head, or sudden changes in atmospheric pressure can cause the tympanic membrane to perforate and middle ear ossicles to fracture. Blast injuries cause injury from the direct pressure on the ear. Blunt injury to the head can cause temporal skull fractures and trauma to both the middle and inner ear. Barotrauma caused by sudden changes in atmospheric pressure in the ears can occur during scuba diving and airplane takeoffs and landings. Pressure changes can occur during normal atmospheric conditions such as nose blowing, heavy lifting, and sneezing. During these rapid changes of pressure, the eustachian tube does not ventilate because of occlusion or dysfunction and a negative pressure develops in the middle ear. The resulting pressure can cause the tympanic membrane to rupture or cause damage to the middle and inner ear.

SIGNS AND SYMPTOMS. Pain and hearing loss are the most common symptoms associated with trauma. Other signs and symptoms of barotrauma include fullness of the ears, vertigo, nausea, disorientation, edema of the affected area, and hemorrhage in the external or middle ear. In severe cases of barotrauma when scuba diving, these symptoms can cause drowning or cerebral air embolism from an overly rapid ascent. Otoscopic examination may reveal a retracted, reddened, and edematous tympanic membrane.

DIAGNOSTIC TESTS. Audiometric studies are completed to determine the hearing loss. Imaging studies may be done to determine the extent of middle and inner ear damage. Conductive or sensorineural hearing loss may be evident, depending on the extent and location of the damage.

Nursing Process for the Patient with Middle Ear, Tympanic Membrane, and Mastoid Disorders

DATA COLLECTION. Table 52.11 reviews the subjective data that should be collected. The external ear should be inspected and palpated to obtain objective data. Pain with palpation is indicative of external ear problems, not middle ear problems. Pain over the mastoid area can indicate a mastoid problem. The middle ear and mastoid cavity cannot be visualized directly. The tympanic membrane is the only middle ear structure that can be directly visualized by the experienced practitioner with an otoscope. Objective assessment also includes vital signs, noting any elevation in temperature. Any drainage from the ear should be noted and described. Hearing acuity should be screened by the experienced practitioner using the whisper voice, Rinne, and Weber tests.

NURSING DIAGNOSES, PLANNING, AND IMPLEMENTATION

Risk for Infection Related to Broken Skin, Pressure Necrosis, Chronic Disease, or Surgical Procedure

EXPECTED OUTCOME: The patient will have no signs of infection (no drainage from ear, no tenderness over mastoid, negative culture, afebrile).

- Explain to patient not to blow nose by pinching off nares *to prevent spread of upper respiratory infections up the eustachian tube.*
- Teach patient to never insert anything into ear canal, and review other ear techniques *to prevent ear damage* (see Box 52.6).
- Teach patient how to correctly remove cerumen from ear *to prevent infection or damage.*

Acute Pain Related to Fluid Accumulation, Inflammation, or Infection

EXPECTED OUTCOME: The patient will indicate pain is decreased or absent as evidenced by a lower rating on a pain scale.

- Monitor pain using a pain scale, and determine optimum analgesic schedule with patient *to maximize pain control.*
- Use nonpharmacological measures such as heat, distraction, and relaxation techniques *for pain reduction.*
- Ensure that the patient knows how to administer eardrops and ear ointment *to help resolve infection and decrease pain.*
- Instruct patient to take all prescribed antibiotics, even after symptoms are relieved, *to ensure that infection is completely resolved.*

Deficient Knowledge Regarding Hearing Loss and Lack of Information or Surgery Related to Lack of Exposure to Information Due to no Prior Experience

EXPECTED OUTCOME: The patient will state an understanding of methods for preventing problems in the middle ear, tympanic membrane, and mastoid process or impending surgery.

- Teach patient to avoid trauma to the ear, loud noise exposure, and environmental or occupational conditions *to prevent damage to the ear.*
- Teach patient to yawn or perform jaw-thrust maneuver (opening mouth wide and moving jaw)

TABLE 52.11 SUBJECTIVE DATA COLLECTION FOR MIDDLE EAR, TYMPANIC MEMBRANE, AND MASTOID DISORDERS

W Where is it?	Are both ears affected? Is it deep within the head?
H How does it feel?	Is there pressure? Fullness? Is it painful; if so, is it sharp, dull, continuous, intermittent, throbbing, localized? No pain?
A Aggravating and alleviating factors	Is it worse with change of position? Worse with movement? Is there relief after drainage? Relief with change of position? Relief with heat or analgesics?
T Timing	When did it start? Has there been any recent upper respiratory infection, airline travel, scuba diving, trauma, or weight lifting? Was it a gradual or sudden onset? How long have symptoms persisted? Has there been a change in symptoms?
S Severity	Does it cause hearing impairment? How much? Does it affect activities of daily living?
U Useful data for associated symptoms	Is there any fever, drainage from the ear canal, nausea, vomiting, dizziness? Is there a family history of otosclerosis? Any previous ear problems or ear surgeries? Any occupational or recreational risk factors, such as scuba diving, weight lifting, or frequent airline travel?
P Perception of the problem by the patient	What does the patient think is wrong? Has problem occurred before? If so, what was the same and what was different?

to equalize ear pressure, which helps maintain ear health.

- Teach patient methods of effective communication *to compensate for hearing loss* (see the *Nursing Care Plan for the Patient with Hearing Loss*).
- Ask about patient's knowledge regarding surgery *to determine learning needs.*
- Include family in teaching sessions *to enhance learning and assist with retention of information.*
- Provide preoperative and postoperative instructions *to promote patient understanding* (Box 52.7).
- Teach patient to avoid getting water in ear postoperatively *to prevent moisture from reaching surgical site.*

EVALUATION. The goals for the patient are met if there is no ear drainage or pain over mastoid and if the patient has negative culture and remains afebrile, states that no pain is present or pain is decreased, verbalizes care of ears and methods to prevent further infection, describes signs requiring medical attention, and verbalizes the rationale and outcome for any upcoming surgery as well as preoperative and postoperative instructions.

Inner Ear

Labyrinthitis

PATHOPHYSIOLOGY AND ETIOLOGY. Labyrinthitis is an inflammation or infection of the inner ear and can be caused by either viral or bacterial pathogens. The bacterium or virus enters the inner ear from the middle ear, meninges, or bloodstream. Serous labyrinthitis is a type of acute labyrinthitis that sometimes follows drug intoxication or overindulgence in alcohol. It can also be caused by an allergy. Diffuse suppurative labyrinthitis occurs when acute or chronic otitis media spreads into the inner ear or after middle ear or mastoid surgery. Destruction of soft tissue structures from the infection can cause permanent hearing loss.

SIGNS AND SYMPTOMS. Vertigo, tinnitus, and sensorineural hearing loss are the most common symptoms. Vertigo, or dizziness, occurs when the vestibular structures

Box 52.7

Preoperative and Postoperative Nursing Interventions for the Patient Having Ear Surgery

Preoperative Care

Nursing care for the patient undergoing ear surgery begins as soon as the decision to have surgery is made. The nurse collects data, determines if the patient understands the events, notes the patient's mental readiness, and obtains baseline physiological data.

- Ask understanding of the surgery and whether local or general anesthesia will be used.
- Help alleviate the patient's fear by encouraging the patient to ask questions. Ensure that all questions are answered before the surgery by appropriate person.
- Explain the type of pain, any packing or dressings that may be in place postoperatively, and any other postoperative restrictions that may be needed.
- Establish baseline vital signs and document findings.
- Ensure that the operative permit is signed.
- Determine current medications the patient is taking and document in the patient's record.
- Determine if the patient understands that surgery does not always correct impaired hearing.
- Leave any hearing devices in place as long as possible before the surgery.

Postoperative Care

Postoperatively the nurse is responsible for assessing the patient's physiological status. The nurse is also responsible for ensuring that the patient and family members understand discharge instructions.

- Some degree of pain may be expected, even with minor procedures. Explain how and when to take pain medication when the patient is discharged.
- Monitor postoperative vital signs and return to presurgical baseline.
- Tell patients that if an occlusive dressing is in place, hearing may be decreased until the dressing is removed.
- Instruct patients with tubes to avoid getting water in the ear. A shower cap or earplugs may be used.
- Instruct the patient to seek medical attention if excessive bleeding or drainage occurs. If a cotton plug is to be left in place, instruct the patient to change it daily.
- Teach the patient, unless contraindicated, to blow the nose very gently one side at a time for the first week after surgery. Instruct the patient to sneeze or cough with the mouth open for 1 week after surgery.
- Avoid airplane flights for 1 week after surgery. For sensations of ear pressure, hold nose, close mouth, and swallow to equalize pressure.
- The patient should avoid strenuous work for several weeks. The patient may return to work in a few days, depending on the type of surgery and the type of work the patient does.
- Tell the patient to take prescribed medication and antibiotics as ordered.
- Have the patient arrange for a follow-up appointment by calling physician's office.

are involved. Tinnitus, or ringing in the ear, occurs when the infection is located in the cochlea. Sensorineural hearing loss can be caused by infections in the cochlea or vestibular structures. Nystagmus on the affected side may occur. Other signs and symptoms include pain, fever, ataxia, nausea, vomiting, and beginning nerve deafness.

DIAGNOSTIC TESTS. A CBC may be done to diagnose infection. A hearing evaluation by an audiologist may reveal mild to complete hearing loss. Rinne and Weber tests indicates conductive or sensorineural hearing loss.

THERAPEUTIC MEASURES. Antibiotics are used to treat bacterial inner ear infections. Viral infections usually run their course in about 1 week. Mild sedation may help the patient relax. Although there is no specific medicine to relieve dizziness, antihistamines can be used if they prove helpful on an individual basis. Patients may be placed on bedrest.

NURSING CARE. Nursing management includes helping the patient manage symptoms and self-care, and educating the patient about safety issues while on bedrest and sedatives to prevent falls and injury. The patient should avoid turning the head quickly to help alleviate the vertigo. The patient is assisted to cope with anxiety that may be present because of the frustration surrounding hearing loss or loss of work.

Neoplastic Disorders

PATHOPHYSIOLOGY AND ETIOLOGY. Inner ear tumors can be benign or malignant. Acoustic neuroma, a tumor of the eighth cranial nerve, is the most common benign tumor. It is slow growing, occurs at any age, and usually occurs unilaterally. As it spreads, it compresses the nerve and adjacent structures. Malignant tumors arising from the inner ear are rare. Squamous and basal carcinomas arise from the epidermal lining of the inner ear.

SIGNS AND SYMPTOMS. Early symptoms of an acoustic neuroma include progressive unilateral sensorineural hearing loss of high-pitched sounds, unilateral tinnitus, and intermittent vertigo. Headache, pain, and balance disorders may also be present. Symptoms progress as the tumor spreads to other structures. Most malignant tumors grow quickly. The symptoms vary depending on the area of the ear that is involved.

DIAGNOSTIC TESTS. Neurologic, audiometric, and vestibular testing are used to diagnose neuroma. Auditory brainstem evoked response (ABR) and electronystagmography (ENG) are completed. Examination of the cerebrospinal fluid shows increased protein. Computed tomography (CT) and magnetic resonance imaging (MRI) are used to determine size and location of the tumor.

THERAPEUTIC MEASURES. The preferred method of treatment involves surgical removal of the tumor. The labyrinth is destroyed, with a resulting permanent hearing loss. Steroids and radiation may be used to decrease the size of the tumor or for inoperable tumors.

NURSING CARE. Nursing management focuses on preparing the patient for surgery and adjusting to the diagnosis and the resulting hearing loss (see Box 52.7).

Ménière's Disease

PATHOPHYSIOLOGY AND ETIOLOGY. Ménière's disease is a balance disorder. Its cause is unknown. With the disease, there is a dilation of the membranous labyrinth resulting from a disturbance in the fluid physiology of the endolymphatic system. The exact etiology is unknown, but is thought to stem from hypersecretion, hypoabsorption, deficit membrane permeability, allergy, viral infection, hormonal imbalance, or mental stress. The disease usually develops between ages 40 and 60. The symptoms range from vague to severe and debilitating.

SIGNS AND SYMPTOMS. A triad of symptoms of vertigo, hearing loss, and tinnitus characterizes Ménière's disease. Recurring episodic bouts of the incapacitating triad of symptoms and nausea and vomiting occur with Ménière's disease. The attacks may occur suddenly, or the patient may experience warning signs such as headache or fullness in the ears. During an acute episode, the patient experiences vertigo that lasts 2 to 4 hours. The vertigo is usually accompanied by nausea and vomiting, followed by dizziness and unsteadiness. The patient is uncoordinated and has gait changes when walking. Hearing loss is often described as a fluctuating fullness in the ears. Tinnitus is present. Irritability, depression, and withdrawal are common. Vital signs usually remain normal. It takes several weeks for symptoms to resolve, and hearing loss in the affected ear remains. The patient then enters a stage of remission until the next attack. The acute episodes occur two to three times yearly. Eventually the patient has complete remission with some degree of permanent hearing loss.

DIAGNOSTIC TESTS. Audiometric studies identify the type and magnitude of the hearing loss. Neurologic testing and radiographic studies are done to rule out other pathological conditions. A caloric stimulation test may demonstrate a difference in eye movement.

THERAPEUTIC MEASURES. Medical treatment consists of symptomatic treatment for acute attacks and prophylactic treatment between attacks. Tranquilizers and vagal blockers may be needed during acute attacks. Salt-restricted diet, diuretics, antihistamines, and vasodilators are used during prophylactic treatment. The patient should avoid alcohol, caffeine, and tobacco use. The patient may be placed on bedrest during acute attacks. The goals of medical treatment are to preserve hearing and reduce symptoms. Some patients who do not respond to treatment may be placed on low doses of methotrexate.

Surgical treatment is used only when medical management has failed. When involvement is unilateral, a labyrinthectomy can be performed. This causes complete loss of hearing in that ear. Another surgical intervention establishes a shunt from the inner ear to the subarachnoid space. This procedure helps drain the fluid and prevent future hearing loss. Another surgical treatment is intratympanic gentamicin injection, which is usually done in the physician's office.

NURSING CARE. Nursing management focuses on managing the patient's symptoms and providing safety during the acute attacks. Because of the unpredictability of Ménière's disease, the nursing care focuses on emotional support for the patient during periods of remission. Provide emotional support and resources to help the patient cope with the unpredictable nature of the disease and the physical impairments associated with the disease.

Nursing Process for the Patient with Inner Ear Disorders

DATA COLLECTION. Table 52.12 reviews subjective data to be collected. Objective data include examination of gross hearing, the whisper voice, Rinne, and Weber tests, a physical examination, and lab data. The patient should be assessed for any nutritional deficiencies, including dehydration, weight loss, or weight gain. An unsteady gait or temperature is also noted.

NURSING DIAGNOSES, PLANNING, AND IMPLEMENTATION. Planning focuses on helping the patient maintain a normal lifestyle, remain free of injuries, cope with the illness or hearing loss, and maintain adequate nutrition and hydration. The major nursing diagnoses and interventions for internal ear disorders include those discussed next.

Anxiety Related to Unpredictability of Sudden and Severe Acute Attacks

EXPECTED OUTCOME: The patient will state that anxiety is decreased.

- Encourage patient to express concerns about hearing loss and the unpredictability of acute attacks *to identify causes of anxiety.*
- Assess for signs of anxiety such as fidgeting, restlessness, apprehension, shakiness, and increased heart rate *to determine if anxiety is present.*
- Explore with patient techniques that have and have not worked in the past *to determine which techniques to use to reduce anxiety.*
- Use a calm reassuring approach *to help instill confidence.*
- Provide quiet environment and diversional activities *to calm patient.*
- Provide factual information regarding diagnosis and treatment *to promote understanding and reduce anxiety.*

CRITICAL THINKING

Mrs. Belmont

■ Mrs. Belmont is a 48-year-old woman diagnosed with Ménière's disease. She is currently in a state of remission. She states that she is fearful that the next attack will occur during her daughter's upcoming wedding.

1. What information would you ask of Mrs. Belmont about her attacks?
2. What instructions can you provide her regarding treatment during her attacks?
3. How will you handle Mrs. Belmont's fears about future attacks?

Suggested answers at end of chapter.

Risk for Injury Related to Impaired Equilibrium

EXPECTED OUTCOME: The patient will not be injured from falling due to alterations in equilibrium.

- Institute fall precautions *to help prevent injury.*
- Ensure that environment is safe and free of obstacles (throw rugs, electrical cords in walkways, and poor lighting) *to prevent falls.*

TABLE 52.12 SUBJECTIVE DATA COLLECTION FOR INNER EAR DISORDERS

W Where is it?	Are both ears affected?
H How does it feel?	Is there pressure? Fullness? Vertigo? Tinnitus? Is it painful; if so, is it sharp, dull continuous, intermittent, throbbing, localized? No pain?
A Aggravating and alleviating factors	Is it worse with change of position? Worse with movement? Is there relief with medications? Is the patient taking current medications? Are there any allergies?
T Timing	When did it start? Was it a gradual or sudden onset? How long have symptoms persisted? Do symptoms progress in a set timing pattern? Do symptoms occur together or separately? Has there been a change in symptoms?
S Severity	Does it cause hearing impairment? How much? Does it affect activities of daily living, nutritional intake, work, or leisure?
U Useful data for associated symptoms	Any fever, nausea, vomiting, or dizziness? Any previous ear problems or ear surgeries? Headache?
P Perception of the problem by the patient	What does the patient think is wrong? Has patient had this problem before? If so, what was the same and what was different?

- Monitor for signs of headache or fullness in the ears *to detect oncoming Ménière's disease attack.*
- Instruct patient to avoid sudden movement of the head during periods of vertigo *to prevent increasing symptoms.*
- Instruct patient on correct dosage and administration of medications *to help ensure resolution of symptoms.*
- Instruct patient to avoid use of alcohol, caffeine, and tobacco *to decrease disruptions of equilibrium.*
- Instruct patient to call for assistance when ambulating *to minimize risk of falling.*
- If indicated, instruct patient to remain on bedrest until symptoms are relieved *to prevent injury.*

Nutrition: Less Than Body Requirements Related to Nausea and Vomiting

EXPECTED OUTCOME: The patient will experience adequate nutrition and hydration with relief of nausea and vomiting.

- Monitor for signs of nausea, vomiting, and inadequate hydration *to determine baseline information.*
- Instruct patient to use deep breathing, voluntary swallowing, and eating slowly *to suppress the vomiting reflex.*
- Medicate as ordered *to relieve symptoms and prevent episodes of nausea and vomiting.*
- Institute salt-restricted diet, if ordered, and instruct patient on low- and high-sodium foods *to reduce fluid retention.*

EVALUATION. The goals for the patient have been met if signs of anxiety are decreased and if the patient remains free from injury and maintains weight within normal range with no signs of dehydration.

SUGGESTED ANSWERS TO CRITICAL THINKING

Mr. Samuel

1. Mr. Samuel should seek assistance, patch both eyes, and have someone take him to receive medical treatment immediately.
2. Ensure that an antiemetic is ordered postoperatively on the patient's return to the unit. When Mr. Samuel reports nausea, the antiemetic should be given promptly.
3. Did you recognize that the concentration is 5 mg/1 mL, and the volume of the vial is 2 mL? The concentration is what is needed to calculate the dose:

$$\frac{7.5\ \text{mg}}{} \left| \frac{1\ \text{mL}}{5\ \text{mg}} \right. = 1.5\ \text{mL}$$

Mrs. Springhorn

1. Gain her attention, face and stand in her visual field, avoid glare, speak clearly, inform her of topics to be discussed, assess for understanding, allow extra time, reduce background noises, use nonverbal communication, and do not cover your mouth when talking.
2. Use active listening. Use written communication to enhance spoken words. Use demonstration and return demonstration. Allow questions. Do not hurry. Provide information in short segments. Reassess understanding at each session.
3. Place the operative ear upward when lying in bed. Use earplug as ordered. Do not cough, sneeze, blow nose, vomit, fly in an airplane, lift heavy objects, or shower. If a cold develops, call the physician. If dizzy, be careful when up.

Mrs. Belmont

1. You would ask Mrs. Belmont about specific signs she may have prior to attacks, such as headache or fullness in the ears. You should also ask her specifically what symptoms she has during attacks. Common symptoms include the triad of vertigo, hearing loss, and tinnitus. She may also have nausea, vomiting, and unsteady gait.
2. Discuss treatment that Mrs. Belmont has used with previous attacks. Ask her which treatments seemed to help. Common treatments you can recommend include taking recommended medication such as tranquilizers and vagal blockers; instruct her to maintain adequate fluid and nutritional intake during attacks; ambulate with assistance; limit salt in diet; avoid alcohol, caffeine, and tobacco use.
3. Discuss with Mrs. Belmont prophylactic treatment such as salt-restricted diet, diuretics, antihistamines, and vasodilators. Discuss the normal progress of the disease. Provide emotional support and discuss methods to help her cope with the disease, such as counseling and relaxation techniques.

REVIEW QUESTIONS

1. A patient is diagnosed with otosclerosis and asks the nurse what this disease is. Which of the following is the most appropriate response by the nurse?
   a. "Infection of the external ear commonly caused by moisture."
   b. "Tumor of the eighth cranial nerve."
   c. "Hardening of the stapes due to new bone growth."
   d. "Inflammation of the inner ear caused by pathogens."

2. A patient is diagnosed with a refractive error and asks the nurse what this means. What would be the appropriate explanation by the nurse?
   a. "You will lose your vision and become blind."
   b. "You will need corrective lenses in order to see clearly."
   c. "The pressure in your eyes is higher than normal."
   d. "Your vision is 20/20."

3. A patient comes to the health clinic for a suspected ear infection. Which of the following data collection findings does the nurse expect with an external ear infection?
   a. Pain
   b. Fullness in ears
   c. Fever
   d. Dizziness

4. A patient has been prepped for an internal eye examination. Anesthetic drops as well as a mydriatic drug have been administered. Which of the following should the patient be taught for eye safety following the examination?
   a. "Wear sunglasses after the exam."
   b. "Rub your eye hourly to increase blood circulation."
   c. "You may reapply contact lenses when the eye exam is completed."
   d. "Flush your eye with water to remove the eyedrops."

5. The nurse understands that which of the following patients needs specific positioning instructions postprocedure to prevent complications?
   a. 19-year-old after removal of congenital cataract
   b. 30-year-old woman after pneumatic retinopexy
   c. 52-year-old man after trabeculectomy
   d. 82-year-old man after corneal transplant

6. Which of the following medications should the nurse question before giving to prevent serious eye complications for a patient who has a history of acute angle-closure glaucoma? **Select all that apply.**
   a. Morphine
   b. Cefazolin (Kefzol)
   c. Atropine
   d. Ranitidine (Zantac)
   e. Hydroxyzine (Vistaril)
   f. Warfarin (Coumadin)

7. Which of the following medications can cause hearing loss?
   a. Furosemide (Lasix)
   b. Acetaminophen (Tylenol)
   c. Warfarin (Coumadin)
   d. Penicillin (Pen-Vee K)

8. Which of the following symptoms would the nurse expect to be in the history of a patient who has macular degeneration?
   a. Loss of peripheral vision
   b. Sudden darkness
   c. Dull ache in the eyes
   d. Loss of central vision

9. Which of the following is the primary goal for a patient with Ménière's disease that the nurse should recommend be included in the plan of care?
   a. Prevent dehydration
   b. Decrease pain
   c. Prevent injury
   d. Preserve hearing

10. The nurse is caring for a patient with presbycusis. Which of the following techniques would be most important for the nurse to use to increase communication with this patient?
    a. Talk in a very loud voice.
    b. Lower voice pitch.
    c. Do not smile or chew gum when talking to the patient.
    d. Allow extra time for patient to respond.

11. A patient with acute angle-closure glaucoma reports use of the following medications. Using which of these medications indicates to the nurse that further instruction is needed?
    a. Acetaminophen
    b. Cefazolin (Kefzol)
    c. Ranitidine (Zantac)
    d. Diphenhydramine (Benadryl)

unit FIFTEEN

UNDERSTANDING THE INTEGUMENTARY SYSTEM

53

Integumentary System Function, Assessment, and Therapeutic Measures

RITA BOLEK TROFINO, MARTY KOHN, AND JANICE L. BRADFORD

KEY TERMS

alopecia (AH-low-PEE-she-ah)
ecchymosis (EK-ih-MOH-siss)
erythema (AIR-ih-THEE-mah)
petechiae (peh-TEE-kee-eye)
turgor (TUR-gur)

QUESTIONS TO GUIDE YOUR READING

1. What is the normal anatomy of the integumentary system?
2. What is the normal function of the integumentary system?
3. What are the effects of aging on the integumentary system?
4. What questions should you ask when you take a history from a patient with a disorder of the integumentary system?
5. What findings do you expect when you inspect and palpate the skin?
6. What laboratory and diagnostic tests are commonly performed to diagnose integumentary disorders?
7. What common therapeutic measures are used for patients with integumentary disorders?

NORMAL INTEGUMENTARY SYSTEM ANATOMY AND PHYSIOLOGY

The skin, its accessory structures, and the subcutaneous tissue make up the integumentary system, the covering of the body that separates the living internal environment from the external environment. The skin itself is considered an organ and consists of two layers: the outer epidermis and the inner dermis (Fig. 53.1).

Epidermis

The epidermis is made of stratified squamous epithelial tissue and is avascular, meaning that it has no capillaries in it. Its nourishment comes from the dermis beneath. The epidermis is thickest on the palms of the hands and soles of the feet. The innermost epidermal layer is called the stratum germinativum, and it is here that mitosis takes place to produce new epidermal cells. The rate of mitosis is fairly constant, but it may be increased by chronic pressure on the skin, as in callus formation. The new cells produce the protein keratin. As they are pushed to the surface of the skin, they die and become the stratum corneum, the outermost of the epidermal layers.

The stratum corneum consists of many layers of dead cells; all that remains is their keratin. An unbroken stratum corneum is an effective barrier against pathogens and most chemicals, although even microscopic breaks are sufficient to permit their entry. Keratin is relatively waterproof, so it prevents the loss of water and therefore dehydration, and it also prevents the entry of excess water through the body surface. As dead cells are worn off the surface of the skin (which contributes to the removal of pathogens), they are continuously replaced by cells from beneath. Loss of large portions of the stratum corneum, as with extensive third-degree burns, greatly increases the risk for infection and dehydration.

Melanocytes are cells in the lower epidermis that produce the protein melanin. The amount of melanin is a genetic characteristic and gives color to skin and hair. When the skin is exposed to ultraviolet (UV) rays from the sun or artificial lighting, production of melanin increases, and it is incorporated into the epidermal cells before they die, making the cells darker. Melanin is a pigment barrier to prevent further exposure of living cells in the stratum germinativum

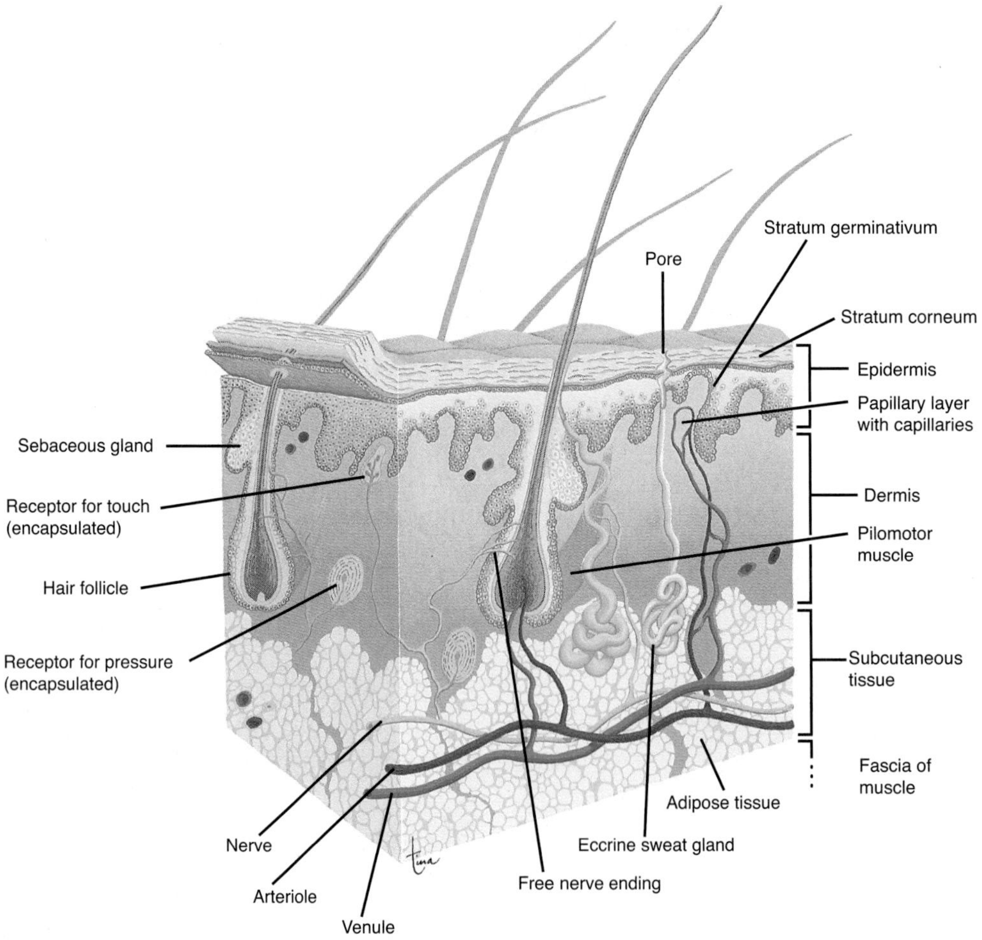
Stratum germinativum
Pore
Stratum corneum
Epidermis
Papillary layer with capillaries
Sebaceous gland
Dermis
Receptor for touch (encapsulated)
Pilomotor muscle
Hair follicle
Receptor for pressure (encapsulated)
Subcutaneous tissue
Fascia of muscle
Adipose tissue
Nerve
Eccrine sweat gland
Free nerve ending
Arteriole
Venule

FIGURE 53.1 Structure of the skin and subcutaneous tissue. (Modified from Scanlon, V. C., & Sanders, T. (2007). *Essentials of anatomy and physiology* [5th ed.]. Philadelphia: F. A. Davis, with permission.)

to UV rays. UV rays are mutagenic; that is, they are capable of damaging the DNA in cells and causing mutations that may result in malignancy.

Also in the epidermis are Langerhans' cells, a type of macrophage that presents foreign antigens to helper T cells. This is the first step in the destruction of pathogens that have penetrated the epidermis.

Dermis

The dermis consists of two layers: The outer papillary region is made of mainly adipose tissue with fine elastin contribution, and the inner reticular region is of dense irregular connective tissue. This reticular region contains cells called fibroblasts, a large contribution of collagen, and some coarse elastic fibers. Fibroblasts produce the protein fibers collagen and elastin. Collagen fibers form the strength of the dermis. Elastin fibers are capable of recoil and make the dermis somewhat elastic. In the dermis are the hair and nail follicles, glands, nerve endings, and blood vessels. The capillaries in the papillary layer of the dermis are important to nourish the stratum germinativum, which has no capillaries of its own.

Hair

Hair develops in epidermal structures called follicles. At the base of the hair root in its follicle is the matrix, a group of cells that undergo mitosis to produce the hair shaft. The cells quickly die after producing keratin and incorporating melanin. Human hair with significant functions includes the eyelashes and eyebrows, which keep dust and sweat out of the eyes, and nostril hair, which filters air entering the nasal cavities. Hair on the head provides thermal insulation.

Nails

Nail roots are found at the ends of the fingers and toes, and growth of nails is similar to growth of hair. Mitosis in the nail root is a continuous process to produce new cells, which contain keratin. As these cells die, they form the visible nail. Nails protect the ends of the digits from mechanical injury and are useful for picking up small objects.

Receptors

The sensory receptors in the dermis are those for the cutaneous senses. Free nerve endings are the receptors for heat, cold, and pain; encapsulated nerve endings are specific for touch and pressure. The sensitivity of an area of skin is determined by the density of receptors present.

Sebaceous Glands

Most of the ducts of sebaceous glands open into hair follicles; a few open directly onto the skin surface. Their secretion is sebum, a lipid substance that inhibits the growth of some bacteria and prevents drying of skin and hair. Skin that is dry tends to crack or fissure more easily, and even these small breaks in the epidermis are potential portals of entry for pathogens.

Sudoriferous Glands

Sudoriferous glands are also known as sweat glands. There are two kinds of sudoriferous glands: apocrine and eccrine. Apocrine glands are really modified scent glands and are most numerous in the axillae and genital area; they are activated by stress and emotions.

Eccrine glands are found throughout the dermis, but are most numerous on the face, palms, and soles. They are activated by high temperatures or by exercise, and they secrete sweat onto the skin surface. The sweat is evaporated by excess body heat, which is a very effective cooling mechanism, although it does have the potential to lead to dehydration if water is not replaced by drinking.

Modified sweat glands called ceruminous glands are found in the dermis of the ear canals. Their secretion is called cerumen or earwax. Cerumen prevents drying of the outer surface of the eardrum. Excess cerumen, however, may become impacted against the eardrum, prevent it from vibrating properly, and reduce hearing acuity.

Blood Vessels

Blood vessels in the dermis serve the usual function of tissue nourishment, but the arterioles are also involved in maintaining body temperature. Blood carries heat produced by active organs and distributes it throughout the body. In a warm environment, dilation of blood vessels in the dermis increases blood flow and loss of heat to air. Constriction of blood vessels in a cold environment decreases blood flow to the skin and conserves body heat.

Stressful situations also cause vasoconstriction in the dermis, which allows blood to circulate to more vital organs, such as the heart, liver, brain, or muscles.

Other functions of the skin are the formation of vitamin D from cholesterol when the skin is exposed to the UV rays of the sun, and the excretion of small amounts of ammonia, urea, and sodium chloride in sweat.

Subcutaneous Tissue

The subcutaneous tissue, between the dermis and the muscles, is made of areolar and adipose connective tissues. Although an unbroken stratum corneum is an excellent barrier to pathogens, even small breaks provide portals of entry. In the subcutaneous tissue are numerous white blood cells that destroy any pathogens that have entered by way of broken skin. Subcutaneous adipose tissue cushions some bones and provides some insulation from cold, but its most important function is energy storage. Excess nutrients are changed to triglycerides and stored as potential energy for times when food intake may decrease.

Aging and the Integumentary System

The effects of age on the integumentary system are often quite visible. Figure 53.2 summarizes the effects of aging.

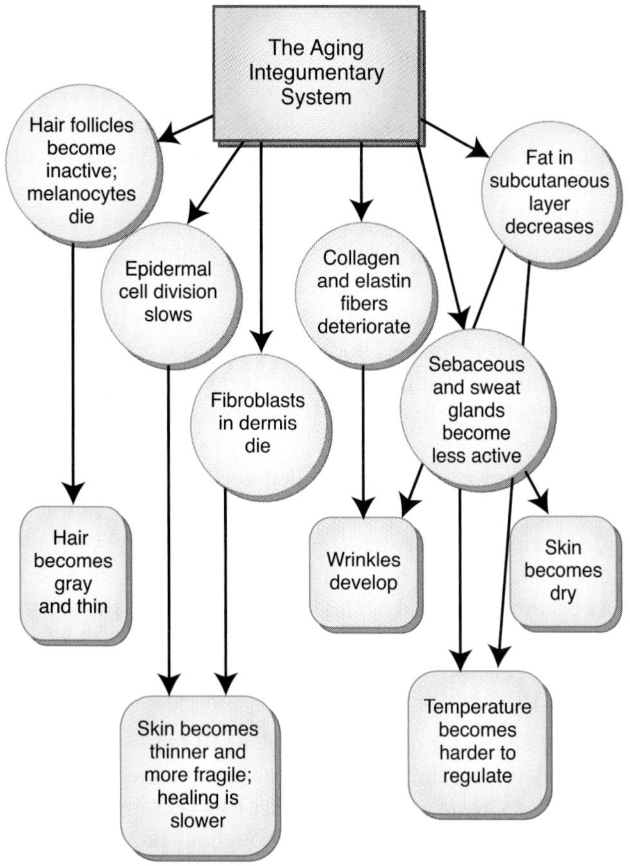
The Aging Integumentary System
Hair follicles become inactive; melanocytes die
Epidermal cell division slows
Collagen and elastin fibers deteriorate
Fat in subcutaneous layer decreases
Fibroblasts in dermis die
Sebaceous and sweat glands become less active
Hair becomes gray and thin
Wrinkles develop
Skin becomes dry
Skin becomes thinner and more fragile; healing is slower
Temperature becomes harder to regulate

FIGURE 53.2 Aging and the integumentary system.

NURSING ASSESSMENT OF THE INTEGUMENTARY SYSTEM

Health History

Skin problems are a fairly common reason for a patient to enter the health system. Many factors can influence the integumentary system. A skin problem may be the only problem the patient has, or it may be a manifestation of an underlying systemic condition or psychological stress. Most important, the skin can visibly communicate the patient's health. Therefore, questions that are posed to the patient are important in determining if the skin problem is a disease entity of its own or a sign of a more systemic disorder. Table 53.1 provides examples of general questions that can be asked of the patient to elicit information.

If further assessment of a particular problem area is needed, the WHAT'S UP? line of questioning can be used. For example, if the patient has a rash, you can respond by pursuing the following information:

- **W**here is it? Is that the only area where you have a rash?
- **H**ow does it feel? Does it itch? Burn? Hurt?
- **A**ggravating and alleviating factors. Does scratching aggravate it? Does anything else aggravate it, such as soaps and detergents? What relieves it? How have you treated it in the past?
- **T**iming. How long have you had this problem? Does it recur?
- **S**everity. How bad is the discomfort on a scale of 0 to 10, with 0 being comfortable and 10 being unable to touch the area?
- **U**seful other data. Do you have other symptoms besides the rash, such as itching, discharge, tingling, or loss of sensation?
- **P**atient's perception. What do you think is causing your rash?

Physical Examination

Examination of the skin involves not only the entire skin area, but also the hair, nails, scalp, and mucous membranes. The main techniques used in physical examination of the skin are inspection and palpation. Make sure the patient is disrobed but adequately draped in a well-lighted and warm environment. Use a handheld magnifying glass or penlight to see small details and further illuminate the area being inspected.

Normally the skin is intact, with no abrasions, and is smooth, dry, well hydrated, and warm. Skin **turgor** (tension) is firm and elastic. The skin surface is flexible and soft. Skin color ranges from light to ruddy pink or olive in white-skinned patients and light brown to deep brown in dark-skinned patients.

You need to be aware of normal developmental changes when performing an examination. The skin of the neonate is

TABLE 53.1 SUBJECTIVE DATA COLLECTION FOR THE INTEGUMENTARY SYSTEM

Category	Questions to Ask During the Health History	Rationale
History	Do you (or does anyone in your family) have a history of dryness, rashes, itching, skin disease, psoriasis, eczema, dermatitis, asthma, hay fever, hives, or allergies?	These conditions may be hereditary.
Risk Factors	Have you noticed any changes in your skin, such as a sore that does not heal, rashes, lumps, or a change in an existing mole?	Sores that do not heal, moles that change color, or lumps may indicate cancer. Slow healing can also be associated with diabetes. Brown staining of the skin in the lower legs is associated with venous stasis.
	Have you had any recent trauma to your skin?	A break in skin integrity can lead to infection.
	Do you have a tendency to sunburn easily? Do you use sunblock? Do you go to tanning salons or use a sun lamp?	Repeat sunburns and tanning are a risk factor for skin cancer.
Hair	Do you wear a wig or hairpiece?	Adequate examination of the scalp requires permission for removal of a wig or hairpiece.
	Have you noticed a change in the growth or loss of your hair?	Hair loss can result from systemic illness or treatment or sometimes from infections or hair care products.
Nails	Have you experienced recent trauma or changes in your nails? Do you wear artificial nails?	Nail changes may be caused by circulatory problems. Artificial nails may mask changes.
Medications	What medications do you take every day (prescription or nonprescription)?	The patient may be taking medication for a skin disorder. Many medications cause skin reactions, from hives and photosensitivity to serious inflammatory conditions.
	What medications did you take most recently? When did you take your last dose?	This might help pinpoint the cause of a new reaction.
Exposures	What is your occupation?	Occupational exposures can lead to skin problems.
	How often do you bathe or shower?	Frequent bathing can cause dry skin.
	What kind of soap do you use?	Some soap may cause allergic reactions.
	What recreational activities do you participate in?	Skin disorders can be caused by gym equipment that was not cleaned properly. Poison ivy may result from jogging in wooded areas.
	Do you or any members of your immediate family or your coworkers have recent skin issues?	Some skin disorders are contagious.
	Have you traveled recently?	This could help to pinpoint causes of suspicious skin changes.
	Is there anything in your current environment, at home or work, that may be causing any skin problems (e.g., animals, plants, chemicals, infections, new carpeting, or new soaps or detergents)?	Various environmental factors cause contact dermatitis; release of some chemicals can cause skin disorders.
	Is there anything that touches your skin that causes a rash?	This may help pinpoint causes of contact dermatitis

very thin and friable (easily broken). During adolescence, the skin becomes thicker, with active sebaceous, eccrine, and apocrine glands. Body hair also changes during adolescence as a result of hormonal influences. In older patients, the skin loses some of its elasticity and moisture. There is decreased activity of sebaceous and sweat glands. The older patient's skin is thinner, more fragile, and more wrinkled.

Inspection

Inspect each area of the skin, including nails, hair, scalp, and mucous membranes, for color, moisture, lesions, edema, intactness, vascular markings, turgor, and cleanliness. This examination should be done in an orderly sequence, such as hair, scalp, nails, buccal mucosa, and then the general skin surface from head to toe.

COLOR. Skin color can be influenced by many factors, including the temperature of the patient, oxygenation, blood flow, exposure to UV rays, and positioning. Because skin color can differ genetically from very light to very dark, skin assessment can be difficult for the novice practitioner.

Commonly noted alterations can include pallor, **erythema** (redness), jaundice, cyanosis, and brown color. Pallor is paleness or decrease in color and can be caused by vasoconstriction, decreased blood flow, or decreased hemoglobin levels from anemia. Pallor is best assessed on the face, conjunctivae, nailbeds, and lips. Erythema, or red discoloration, may indicate circulatory changes and can be caused by vasodilation or increased blood flow to the skin from fever or inflammation. Erythema is best assessed on the face or in an area of trauma.

Jaundice, a yellow-orange discoloration, may result from liver disease. While skin is affected by jaundice, the best place to inspect for jaundice is in the sclera of the eye. Cyanosis, or bluish discoloration, may indicate a cardiac, pulmonary, or perfusion problem. The best places to inspect for cyanosis are the lips, nailbeds, conjunctivae, and palms. People of Mediterranean descent normally have a bluish tone to their lips; this is not cyanosis.

A brown color may be caused by increased melanin production and can indicate chronic exposure to sunlight, or pregnancy. This is best assessed on areas exposed to the sun; changes in pregnancy can be seen on the face, areolae, and nipples. A brownish color also may result from chronic peripheral vascular disease, especially noted on the lower legs.

LESIONS. A lesion is any change or injury to tissue. Assessment of skin lesions helps determine the cause of a skin disorder. Lesions are described as primary or secondary. Primary lesions are the initial reaction to a disease process. Secondary lesions are changes that take place in the primary lesion because of trauma, scratching, infection, or various stages of a disease. Lesions are further described according to type and appearance in Figure 53.3.

When assessing and documenting skin lesions, note the color or colors of the lesion and the size (usually in centimeters), location, distribution, and configuration. Configuration refers to the pattern of the lesions, as shown in Figure 53.4. Also note any exudate, including amount, color, and odor, and any accompanying symptoms. Gently stretching the skin over the rash area makes it stand out more for further assessment.

In general, healthy patients with naturally dark skin have a reddish undertone, with pinkish buccal mucosa, tongue, nails, and lips. If a dark-skinned patient is pale, the mucous membranes have an ash-gray color, lips and nailbeds appear paler than usual, and the skin appears yellow-brown to ash gray. Erythema presents as a purplish gray color. Cyanosis presents as a gray cast to the skin. The nailbeds, palms, and soles may have a bluish cast. Jaundice can be noted in the oral mucosa (particularly the hard palate) and in the sclera closest to the cornea.

MOISTURE/DRYNESS. Assessment of moisture provides clues to the patient's level of hydration. Observe the skin for dryness, moisture, scales, and flakes. Moisture may be found in skinfold areas. The skin should normally be smooth and dry. Flaking and scaling of the skin indicate dry skin, or certain inflammatory disorders.

EDEMA. Edema occurs because of a buildup of fluid in the tissues. Edema can cause the skin to become stretched, dry, and shiny. Examine and document the location, distribution, and color of edematous areas. If edema is unilateral, compare it with the opposite side of the body. Measure edematous extremities to track improvement or worsening of the condition. Dependent edema is edema that occurs in the part of the body that is at the lowest point, typically noted in the feet and ankles or in the sacrum if the patient is lying down.

VASCULAR MARKINGS. Vascular markings can be classified as normal and abnormal. Two common abnormal vascular changes are **petechiae** and **ecchymosis** (see Figures 28.1 and 28.5 in Chapter 28). Petechiae are reddish purple hemorrhagic spots that are smaller than 0.5 mm in diameter. In the darker skinned patient, petechiae are usually not visible on the skin but can be visualized in the conjunctivae and oral mucosa. Ecchymosis is a bruise that changes color from blue-black to greenish brown or yellow over time.

GENERAL INTEGRITY AND CLEANLINESS. Examine the integrity of the skin. Elderly patients have thin, fragile skin that is easily broken or torn. Be sure to check between toes and skinfolds and under a pendulous abdomen or breasts. Check over bony prominences for signs of pressure. Note general cleanliness and odors.

Palpation

Palpation is used with inspection. Use the dorsum (back) of the hand to palpate temperature because this part of the hand is most sensitive to changes in temperature. Use the fingertips to gently palpate over the skin to determine size, contour (flat, raised, depressed), and consistency (soft or indurated) of lesions. If a lesion is moist or draining, wear gloves to protect against the spread of infectious organisms. Note the degree of pain or discomfort associated with light palpation of lesions.

Examine for turgor and observe the texture of the skin. Skin turgor is a measure of the amount of skin elasticity. To assess for turgor, pinch the skin on the back of the forearm or over the sternum between the thumb and forefinger and then release. Normally, the skin lifts easily and then quickly returns to its normal state. Poor skin turgor is indicated by "tenting" of the skin, with more gradual return to its normal state. Poor skin turgor may indicate dehydration. Normal aging of skin produces some loss of skin elasticity; the preferred place to check skin turgor in the elderly is over the sternum.

If edema is suspected, palpate those areas to assess for tenderness, mobility, and consistency. Press the edematous area (against bone, if possible) with your thumb for 5 seconds and then release. When pressure from your fingers leaves an indentation, this is called pitting edema. If the edema is in an extremity, measure and record the circumference in centimeters, and monitor it for increase or decrease in size.

• WORD • BUILDING •

ecchymosis: ec—out + cchymos—juice + is—condition

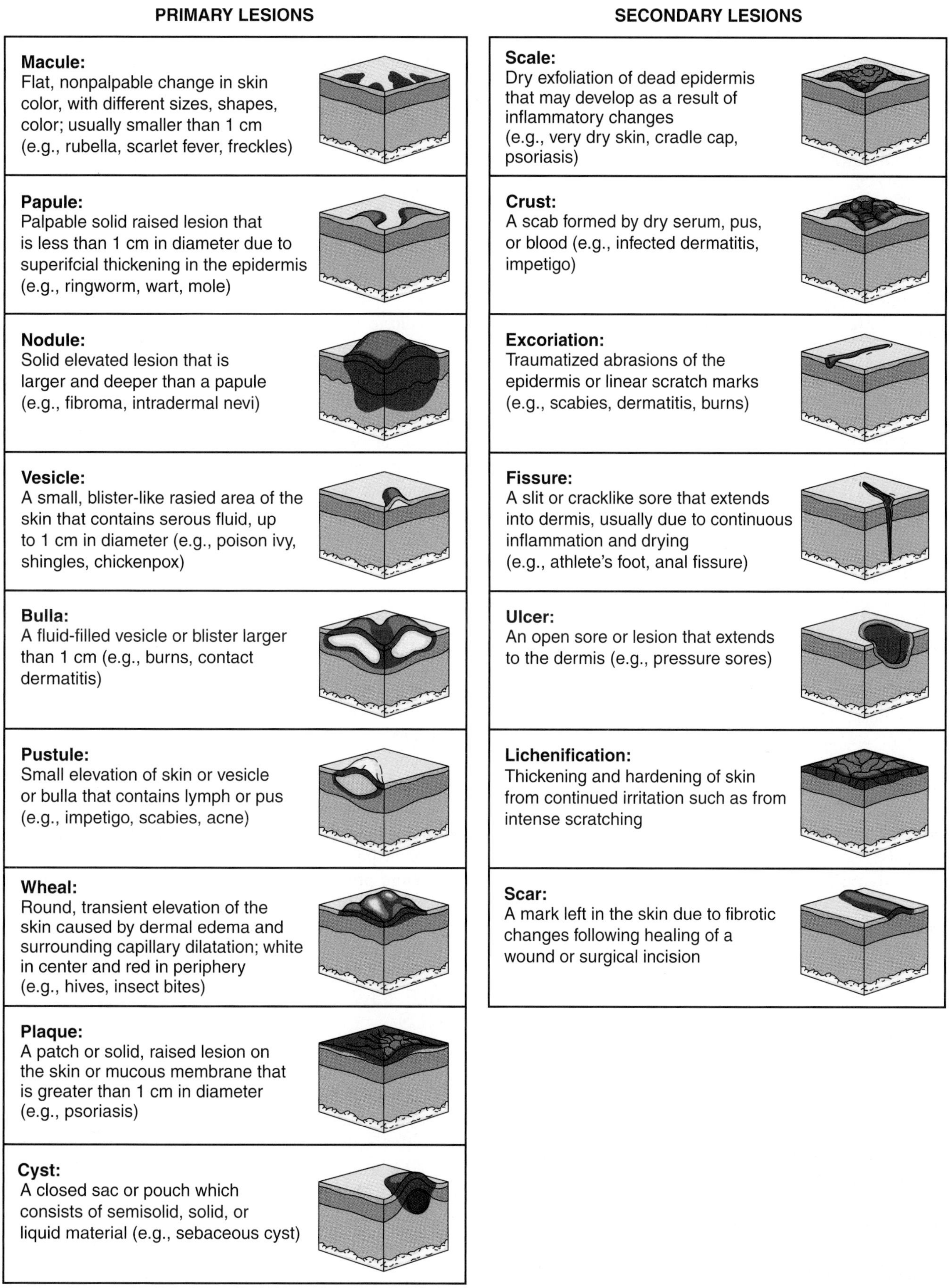
PRIMARY LESIONS
Macule:
Flat, nonpalpable change in skin color, with different sizes, shapes, color; usually smaller than 1 cm (e.g., rubella, scarlet fever, freckles)
Papule:
Palpable solid raised lesion that is less than 1 cm in diameter due to superifcial thickening in the epidermis (e.g., ringworm, wart, mole)
Nodule:
Solid elevated lesion that is larger and deeper than a papule (e.g., fibroma, intradermal nevi)
Vesicle:
A small, blister-like rasied area of the skin that contains serous fluid, up to 1 cm in diameter (e.g., poison ivy, shingles, chickenpox)
Bulla:
A fluid-filled vesicle or blister larger than 1 cm (e.g., burns, contact dermatitis)
Pustule:
Small elevation of skin or vesicle or bulla that contains lymph or pus (e.g., impetigo, scabies, acne)
Wheal:
Round, transient elevation of the skin caused by dermal edema and surrounding capillary dilatation; white in center and red in periphery (e.g., hives, insect bites)
Plaque:
A patch or solid, raised lesion on the skin or mucous membrane that is greater than 1 cm in diameter (e.g., psoriasis)
Cyst:
A closed sac or pouch which consists of semisolid, solid, or liquid material (e.g., sebaceous cyst)
SECONDARY LESIONS
Scale:
Dry exfoliation of dead epidermis that may develop as a result of inflammatory changes (e.g., very dry skin, cradle cap, psoriasis)
Crust:
A scab formed by dry serum, pus, or blood (e.g., infected dermatitis, impetigo)
Excoriation:
Traumatized abrasions of the epidermis or linear scratch marks (e.g., scabies, dermatitis, burns)
Fissure:
A slit or cracklike sore that extends into dermis, usually due to continuous inflammation and drying (e.g., athlete's foot, anal fissure)
Ulcer:
An open sore or lesion that extends to the dermis (e.g., pressure sores)
Lichenification:
Thickening and hardening of skin from continued irritation such as from intense scratching
Scar:
A mark left in the skin due to fibrotic changes following healing of a wound or surgical incision

FIGURE 53.3 Description of skin lesions.

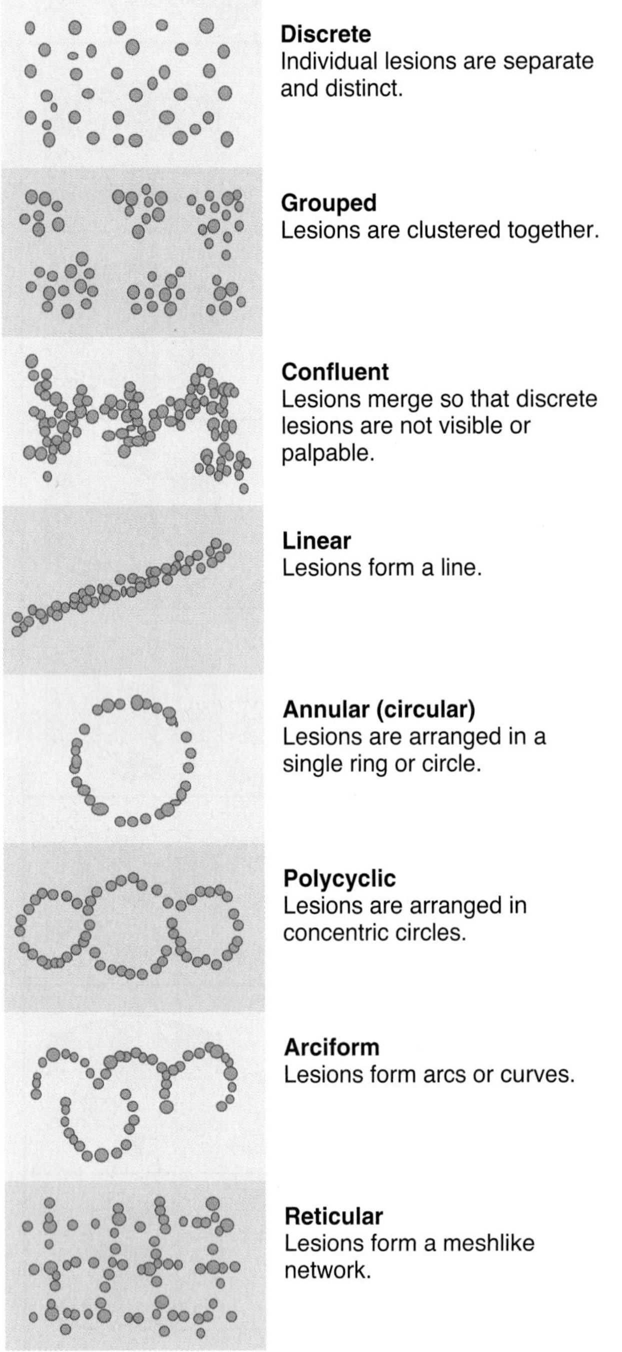
Discrete
Individual lesions are separate and distinct.
Grouped
Lesions are clustered together.
Confluent
Lesions merge so that discrete lesions are not visible or palpable.
Linear
Lesions form a line.
Annular (circular)
Lesions are arranged in a single ring or circle.
Polycyclic
Lesions are arranged in concentric circles.
Arciform
Lesions form arcs or curves.
Reticular
Lesions form a meshlike network.

FIGURE 53.4 To assess configuration, observe the relationship of the lesions to each other. Then characterize the configuration by choosing one of the patterns illustrated in the chart.

Inspect and/or palpate over the entire body for hair color, quantity, thickness, and texture. Note any areas of **alopecia** (hair loss). Determine any recent changes in color and growth pattern. Note cleanliness, redness, scaling, flakes, and tenderness. If lesions or lice are suspected, use disposable gloves to avoid spread of infection.

Terminal hair is the hair on the scalp, eyebrows, axillae, and pubic areas and on the face and chest of men. Vellus hairs are the soft, tiny hairs covering the body. Normally, body hair has a uniform distribution. Note male or female pubic hair distribution. Scalp hair can normally be thick, thin, coarse, smooth, shiny, curly, or straight. Describe scalp hair distribution and cleanliness.

Nails can reflect the patient's general health. Examine fingers and nails for color, shape, texture, thickness, and abnormalities. Normally, the nails appear pink, smooth, hard, and slightly convex (160-degree angle), with a firm base. The nails of elderly patients may have a yellowish gray color, thickening, and ridges. Brown or black pigmentation between the nail and nail base is normal in dark-skinned patients. Abnormal findings include clubbing, which may indicate hypoxia, and spoon nails (concave nails, also called koilonychia), which may be associated with anemia. Thick nails may indicate fungal infection. Palpate for nail consistency, and observe for redness, swelling, or tenderness around the nail area. Table 53.2 describes other nail abnormalities.

Describe any abnormal skin conditions in detail. Include findings such as color of lesion, pain, swelling, redness, location, size, drainage (including amount, color, and odor), and eruption patterns. If equipment is available, an excellent way to supplement documentation is by photographing the area; serial photographs can be mounted in the chart to document healing progression. Box 53.1, *Gerontological Issues,* describes assessment and care specific to the elderly.

DIAGNOSTIC TESTS FOR THE INTEGUMENTARY SYSTEM

Laboratory Tests

Cultures

Skin cultures are done to determine the presence of fungi, bacteria, and viruses. When a fungal infection is suspected, gently scrape scales from the lesion into a Petri dish or other indicated container. The specimen is then treated with a 10 percent potassium hydroxide (KOH) solution to make fungi more prominent. The specimen can remain at room temperature until sent to the laboratory.

TABLE 53.2 ABNORMALITIES OF THE NAILS

Physical Examination Finding	Description	Possible Causes
Beau's lines	Transverse depressions in the nails	Systemic illnesses or nail injury
Splinter hemorrhages	Red or brown streaks in the nailbed	Minor trauma, subacute bacterial endocarditis, or trichinosis
Paronychia	Inflammation of the skin at the base of the nail	Local infection or trauma

Box 53.1
Gerontological Issues

In acute care settings, priorities are determined by medical diagnoses and often center around cardiovascular, respiratory, nutrition, comfort, or other immediate concerns. The feet may be forgotten in the rush to care for the patient and plan a timely discharge.

Feet are also viewed by some as dirty, and washing the feet may be seen as a lowly job. It may be assumed that people take care of their own feet. However, many older people are unable to bend down or bring the feet up high enough to see or care for them.

For these reasons it is especially important for the nurse to assess and care for the feet, both in institutional settings and at home. General guidelines for assessment include the following:

- Inspect feet for redness or pressure ulcers over bony prominences.
- Inspect feet for dryness or cracking.
- Inspect between toes for cracking, wounds, or excess moisture.
- Inspect and palpate for calluses.
- Palpate dorsalis pedis and posterior tibial pulses for circulatory status.
- Assess patient's sensation using a wisp of cotton, monofilament, or light touch.

Hints to promote healthy feet:

- Soak the patient's feet briefly in warm water and wash using a gentle soap. Test the water to be sure it is not too warm, especially for the patient with reduced sensation.
- Thoroughly dry the feet, including between the toes. Water left to evaporate can cause drying and cracking.
- Use a pumice stone to help remove dry dead skin over heels or calluses. Work gently, rubbing the stone in one direction only and removing only a small amount of dead skin at any one time.
- Use a cream or lotion that does not contain alcohol to moisturize the feet. Do not apply between toes. Apply it with gentle massage while moving the patient's feet through range-of-motion exercises. To prevent falls, never apply lotion before the patient steps into the tub or shower.
- Use gauze or a commercially made pad to decrease pressure and friction in areas between toes that cross or other areas where breakdown is likely.
- Encourage the patient to wear cotton or dry weave socks that allow feet to stay dry with perspiration.
- Encourage the wearing of comfortable leather shoes or hard-soled slippers to avoid injury to the feet and prevent falls. Patients with diabetes should be encouraged to wear closed-toe shoes.
- Take extra care to assess and care for feet in patients with diabetes because of their increased risk for injury and slow healing.

NURSING CARE TIP

When scraping scales for culture, position the patient so that the skin lesion is vertical. Place the slide against the skin below the lesion. Be sure to wear gloves when collecting specimens, and wash your hands before and after.

If a viral culture is ordered, the fluid is expressed (gently squeezed) from an intact vesicle, collected with a sterile cotton swab, and placed in a special viral culture tube. If the lesion has crusts, they are removed or punctured before swabbing. The viral culture tube must be kept in ice and sent to the laboratory as soon as possible.

Bacterial cultures may be collected with a sterile swab or wound culture kit. Box 53.2 gives specific instructions.

Skin Biopsy

A skin biopsy is indicated for deeper infections, suspicious lesions, or for evaluation of current treatment. A biopsy is an excision of a small piece of tissue for microscopic examination. Three common types of skin biopsies are punch, shave, and incisional.

A punch biopsy uses a small round cutting instrument, called a punch, to cut a cylinder-shaped plug of tissue for a full-thickness specimen. A shave biopsy removes just the area that has risen above the rest of the skin. An incisional biopsy is performed with a scalpel to make a deep incision and almost always requires sutures for closure. For all biopsies, explain the procedure, assist in preparing a sterile field, calm and comfort the patient during the procedure, and assist in dressing the site following the procedure. The most uncomfortable part of the procedure is usually the injection of the local anesthetic. Explaining the procedure and calming the patient can make the procedure less traumatic.

Other Diagnostic Tests

Wood's Light Examination

Wood's light examination involves the use of ultraviolet rays to detect fluorescent materials in the skin and hair present in certain diseases such as tinea capitis (ringworm). This examination is performed with a handheld black light in a darkened room.

Box 53.2

Steps in Culturing a Wound

1. Use sterile saline to remove excess drainage and debris from the wound. Purulent material may have different bacteria than those actually causing the infection.
2. Using a sterile calcium alginate swab in a rotating motion, swab wound and wound edges 10 times in a diagonal pattern across the entire surface of the wound.
3. Do not swab over eschar.
4. Place swab in culture tube, label, and send to lab.

Skin Testing

Patch and scratch tests are performed when allergic contact dermatitis is suspected. These are usually done by a dermatologist on uninvolved skin, such as the upper back or arms. Any hair in the area must first be shaved.

For the scratch test, the skin is superficially scratched or pricked with an allergen for an immediate reaction. If a reaction such as a wheal occurs, the test is positive for that allergen. Resuscitation equipment should be in the immediate vicinity in the event of a severe allergic (anaphylactic) reaction.

With the patch test, allergens are applied under occlusive tape patches; a delayed hypersensitivity reaction develops in 48 to 96 hours. For this test, the skin should be free of oils to promote patch adhesion, so cleanse the skin first with alcohol. The test site must remain dry and free from moisture. The patch is removed in 2 days. Any reaction is noted, with a final reading in 2 to 5 days.

THERAPEUTIC MEASURES FOR THE INTEGUMENTARY SYSTEM

Open Wet Dressings

Wet compresses may be ordered for acute, weeping, crusted, inflamed, or ulcerated lesions. The purpose of wet dressings is to decrease inflammation, cleanse and dry a wound, and continue drainage of infected areas. They may be ordered either sterile or clean, depending on the risk for infection. The solutions commonly consist of room temperature to cool tap water or normal saline solution, aluminum acetate solution (Burow's solution), or magnesium sulfate. The dressing is saturated with the solution before it is applied. Wet dressings usually are applied every 3 to 4 hours for 15 to 30 minutes.

Wet dressings should not be prescribed for more than 72 hours because the skin may become too dry or macerated. If cool compresses are used, they should be reapplied every 5 to 10 minutes because they become too warm from body heat. If warm compresses are used, monitor the skin closely to prevent burns.

NURSING CARE TIP

To prevent chilling, no more than one-third of the body should be treated at one time. Keep the patient warm during wet dressing treatment.

Balneotherapy

Balneotherapy (therapeutic bath) is useful in applying medications to large areas of the skin, as well as for débridement, or removing old crusts; for removing old medications; and to relieve itching and inflammation. The temperature of the water should be kept at a comfortable level, avoiding hot baths. The bath should last for 15 to 30 minutes, while maintaining its warmth. Fill the tub half full. Keep the room warm to minimize changes in temperature. Advise the patient to wear loose clothing after the bath.

Water and saline solution are utilized for weeping, oozing, and erythematous lesions. Colloidal baths (such as oatmeal or Aveeno) are used for widely distributed skin lesions, for drying, and for relief of itching. Medicated tar baths, such as Almar-Tar or Balnetar, are used for chronic eczema and psoriasis. Any loose skin crusts can be removed after the bath. The room should be well ventilated because tars are volatile.

To increase hydration after the bath, a lubricating agent is applied to damp skin if prescribed. Bath oils, such as Alpha-Keri and Lubath, are used for lubrication and to relieve itching.

NURSING CARE TIP

A bath mat should be used for treatment baths because some of the treatments may make the tub slippery.

Topical Medications

Many types of topical medications are used to treat skin conditions. These include lotions, ointments and creams, powders, gels, pastes, and intralesional therapy. Systemic medications may also be given for more serious conditions.

Lotions tend to cool the skin through water evaporation. They also may have a protective effect and may be antipruritic (anti-itch). Lotions are usually applied with cotton, gauze, gloves, or a soft brush.

Ointments and creams have a varied base (greasy, nongreasy, or penetrating), depending on the drug applied. These medications can protect the skin, provide lubrication, and prevent water loss. They are used for localized or chronic skin conditions. Ointments and creams can cause some reduction in blood flow to the skin. They are applied with a gloved hand or wooden tongue depressor.

Powders usually have a zinc oxide, talc, or cornstarch base and are used to absorb moisture and reduce friction. Powders are usually applied with a shaker top. Powders are avoided for patients with respiratory disease or tracheostomies.

NURSING CARE TIP

Avoid applying too much powder in skinfold areas. Dermatitis can occur with too much powder in these areas. Products with a cornstarch base can provide a good medium for growth of microorganisms.

Gels, or semisolid emulsions, become liquid with topical application. They are usually greaseless and do not stain. Many topical steroids are prescribed in this manner.

Pastes are semisolid substances comprised of ointments and powders. They are used for inflammatory disorders. Mineral oil can facilitate removal of pastes.

Topical corticosteroids are used to reduce or relieve pain and itching by decreasing inflammation. Steroids should be used sparingly and according to package directions. Overuse of topical steroids can cause thinning of the skin. Caution is needed when used on the face to prevent glaucoma, cataracts, and perioral dermatitis.

Intralesional therapy may be used for anti-inflammatory action. This procedure utilizes a tuberculin syringe, most often of a sterile suspension of a corticosteroid, injected just below the lesion. Local atrophy may occur if the injection is made into subcutaneous tissue. Common conditions that are treated with this therapy include psoriasis and keloids.

CRITICAL THINKING

Mr. Evans

■ Mr. Evans comes to the doctor's office with atrophic skin (thin, shiny, pink, with visible vessels) at the area of psoriasis where he is applying his corticosteroid ointment. He says that he has been applying a thick layer of ointment four times a day.

1. What might be the cause of this condition?
2. What should you include when you document his skin condition?

Suggested answers at end of chapter.

Dressings

Dressings may be used to enhance absorption of topical medications, promote retention of moisture, prevent evaporation of medication, and reduce pain and itching. Occlusive dressings (for sealing a wound) are commonly used for skin disorders. For an occlusive dressing, an airtight plastic film is applied directly over the topical agent. Corticosteroids are also available in a special plastic surgical tape that can be cut to size. See the *Nursing Care Plan for the Patient with an Occlusive Dressing.*

Proper application of a plastic wrap dressing includes washing the area, lightly patting it dry, applying the medication to moist skin, covering the medicated area with plastic wrap, and covering with a dressing to seal the edges. Wet dressings and ointments should only be applied to affected areas, not to healthy intact skin, because this can cause maceration of good skin. Plastic wrap dressings should be used for no more than 12 hours a day.

NURSING CARE TIP

Continued use of occlusive dressings can cause skin atrophy, folliculitis, maceration, erythema, and systemic absorption of the medication. To prevent some of these complications, the dressing is removed for at least 12 out of every 24 hours.

Hydrocolloid dressings (e.g., DuoDERM, Tegasorb THIN) can help protect areas exposed to pressure and treat pressure ulcers in early stages. Gels, pastes, and granules can be used to fill in deep wounds to promote granulation and aid healing. See Chapter 54 for dressings used specifically for pressure ulcers. Skin tears should be covered with a nonadherent dressing such as Xeroform and wrapped with gauze. Table 53.3 summarizes various types of wound dressings.

Other items commonly used with topical treatments for skin conditions include gauze or cotton cloth held in place with:

- small, stretchable tubular material (e.g., Surgitube, tube gauze) for fingers, toes, and extremities
- Disposable polyethylene gloves sealed at the wrist for hands
- Cotton socks or plastic bags for the feet
- Disposable diapers or cotton diapers for the groin and perineal areas
- Cotton cloth held in place with dress shields for the axillae
- Cotton or light flannel pajamas for the trunk
- A shower cap for the scalp
- A face mask made from gauze and stretchable dressings with holes cut out for eyes, nose, mouth, and ears.

The patient's primary care provider or a wound care specialist should specify the type of dressing and particular materials needed.

NURSING CARE PLAN for the Patient with an Occlusive Dressing

Nursing Diagnosis: *Impaired Skin Integrity* related to open lesions

Expected Outcome: The patient will experience improved skin integrity as evidenced by reduction in size of lesion.

Evaluation of Outcome: Is there a decrease in wound size?

Interventions	Rationale	Evaluation
Assess areas of lesions for changes in size, color, swelling, and drainage three times a day or as ordered.	Areas of redness, swelling, pain, and drainage may indicate infection.	Are lesions free of redness, swelling, pain, and drainage?
Assess lesions for presence or absence of dead tissue and exudates.	Appearance indicates areas of healing and infection.	Are lesions free of exudates and dead tissue?
Cleanse wound as prescribed (see text for specific bathing instructions). Lightly pat dry.	Cleansing helps provide a healthy granulation area for healing.	Is wound clean and free of debris, crusts, and exudate?
Apply prescribed topical agent (see text for specifics) to moist skin. Apply sparingly or as directed.	Various agents have specific properties (control bacterial growth, prevent itching, have a protective effect, provide lubrication, relieve pain, or decrease inflammation).	Does area exhibit signs of healing (e.g., decrease in size and numbers of lesions, free from infection, less itching)?
Cut plastic film to size and apply. Cover with an appropriate dressing to seal edges.	Film enhances absorption of medication and helps retain moisture.	Is the topical agent adherent to the skin?
Remove dressing for 12 out of 24 hours.	Continued use may cause skin atrophy, folliculitis, erythema, and systemic absorption of medication.	Are there signs of healthy granulation tissue? Is skin pink? Are there less open areas? Is dressing removed for at least 12 hours every 24 hours?

Nursing Diagnosis: *Disturbed Body Image* related to presence of lesion or wound

Expected Outcomes: The patient will verbalize acceptance of condition. The patient will be willing to participate in care of lesion or wound.

Evaluation of Outcomes: Does patient verbalize acceptance of condition? Does patient participate in care of lesions?

Interventions	Rationale	Evaluation
Assess patient's feelings regarding condition.	Assessment provides a baseline for care. If patient denies condition, he or she may not comply with care.	Does patient state willingness to follow care instructions?
Care for patient with an accepting attitude.	Patient will be aware of nuances in nurse's behavior.	Does patient allow nurse to partake in care of lesion or wound?

NURSING CARE PLAN for the Patient with an Occlusive Dressing—cont'd

Interventions	Rationale	Evaluation
Allow opportunities for patient to verbalize concerns about condition.	Verbalization allows patient to begin to accept changes and problem solve.	Does patient verbalize feelings appropriately?
Provide referrals to support groups and counselors as appropriate.	Patient may benefit from talking to others with similar condition or to another professional for objective evaluation.	Is patient receptive to appropriate referrals?
Assist patient in concealing lesion or wound in a safe and appropriate manner.	Long sleeves and long pants may help conceal and protect lesions, and prevent further skin damage.	Is patient accepting of appearance of lesions? Are lesions or wounds visible?

Nursing Diagnosis: *Self-Care Deficit: Bathing/Hygiene* related to presence of lesions or wound and discomfort

Expected Outcomes: The patient will verbalize the importance of good hygiene. The patient will participate in bathing/hygiene.

Evaluation of Outcomes: Does patient verbalize importance of good hygiene? Is patient's skin clean and dry?

Interventions	Rationale	Evaluation
Assess patient's level of hygiene.	Assessment provides a baseline for care.	Is patient's level of hygiene at an acceptable level?
Instruct patient in appropriate bathing/hygiene: • Avoid strong detergents and soaps; utilize gentle emollient soaps or prescribed soaps. • Gently stroke areas of lesions. • Pat dry; avoid friction. • Maintain a little moisture on skin. • Maintain comfortable environmental temperature. • Have temperature of bath at a comfortable level to patient, but not too hot.	Patient needs to be able to properly cleanse lesions to prevent infection. Avoidance of friction and strong soaps prevents further trauma to skin. Patient will not shiver in comfortable temperatures.	Is patient able to verbalize understanding of and also demonstrate good bathing techniques? Are lesions free of infection?

TABLE 53.3 COMMON DRESSINGS

Dressing Type	Description	When Used	Examples
Alginates	Derived from brown seaweed; absorbent and conform and shape to the wound.	When packed into wound, absorb exudate to form a soft gel to maintain a moist environment for wound healing.	Kaltostat SeaSorb Tegagen
Antimicrobial dressings	Topical dressings derived from such agents as silver, iodine, and polyhexamethylene biguanide.	Intended for use in draining, nonhealing wounds that have bacterial contamination, such as burns, surgical wounds, diabetic ulcers, pressure ulcers, and leg ulcers.	Acticoat Aquacel Ag Silversorb gel Tegaderm Ag mesh
Collagen dressings	Collagen is the most abundant protein in the body; its fibers are found in connective tissues, skin, bone, ligaments, and cartilage.	Stimulate new tissue development.	CellerateRX gel BGC Matrix dressing Fibracol plus collagen
Promogran matrix	Oxidized regenerated cellulose and 55% collagen. Binds metalloproteases, which protect growth factors.	Used for diabetic foot ulcers, venous leg ulcers, and surgical wounds.	Prisma
Composite dressings	Combine two or more distinct products into a single dressing.	May absorb and also cover a wound, for example.	Alldress Covaderm
Contact layers	Nonadherent dressing layers often used with other products.	Used to allow exudate to flow through to a secondary dressing; protects wound.	Mepitel Wound veil Profore
Foam dressings	Absorbent; some have a film coating and adhesive border.	Used to provide a moist environment and thermal insulation.	Allevyn Mepilex foam Lyofoam Biatain adhesive dressing PolyMem and PolyMax
Hydrocolloid dressings	Occlusive or semiocclusive dressings made of pectin, gelatin, and carboxymethylcellulose.	Used when a moist environment is needed that allows clean wounds to granulate; provides autolytic debriding.	DuoDERM Tegaderm absorbent Tegasorb THIN Comfeel plus hydrocolloid ulcer dressing Comfeel TRIAD hydrophilic wound dressing Exuderm dressings MPM Excel Restore plus hydrocolloid CarraSmart gel wound dressing
Hydrogels	Water or glycerine-based amorphous gels, impregnated gauzes, or sheet dressings	Used when a moist healing environment is needed to promote granulation and epithelialization and facilitate autolytic debridement.	DuoDERM gel Saf-Gel Amerigel AquaSite CarraDres Curage Silvasorb Vigilon Normlgel 9%

TABLE 53.3 COMMON DRESSINGS—cont'd

Dressing Type	Description	When Used	Examples
Impregnated gauze	Woven or nonwoven material impregnated by the manufacturer with substances such as iodinated agents, petrolatum, zinc, bismuth tribromophenate, chlorhexidine gluconate, crystalline sodium chloride, or aqueous saline.	Used for a variety of conditions, depending on the agent added to the dressing.	Mesalt Xeroform Xeroflo Adaptic Curity nonadherent dressing Dermagran Vaseline petroleum gauze Iodoform packing AMD gauze
Transparent films	Adhesive semipermeable polyurethane membrane dressings that are waterproof and impermeable to bacteria and contaminants yet permit water vapor to cross the barrier.	Used when a moist healing environment is needed, promoting formulation of granulation tissue and autolysis of necrotic tissue.	Bioclusive transparent dressing Tegaderm CarraFilm OpSite Mefilm transparent dressing Polyskin transparent dressing
Wound fillers	Sterile products that absorb exudate and conform to the shape of the wound bed.	Used when wound has exudate and would benefit from debriding.	FlexiGel strands Absorbant wound dressing Iodosorb gel Iodoflex pads

SUGGESTED ANSWERS TO

CRITICAL THINKING

■ *Mr. Evans*

1. He may be sensitive or allergic to the medication. Most likely, he is applying too much too often. This ointment is applied as a thin layer, and usually only twice daily.
2. Note the size (usually in centimeters), location, color, distribution, and configuration of lesions. Describe exactly what you see, avoiding judgments about what you think it is. Document any teaching you provided related to how his medication should be applied.

REVIEW QUESTIONS

1. Which of the following is the protein in epidermal cells that makes the skin relatively waterproof?
   a. Collagen
   b. Keratin
   c. Melanin
   d. Elastin

2. What are functions of subcutaneous tissue? **Select all that apply**.
   a. It nourishes the dermis.
   b. It cushions bony prominences.
   c. It lubricates the epidermis.
   d. It provides insulation.
   e. It stores energy.
   f. It secretes hormones.

3. Older adults have fewer fibroblasts, and epidermal division slows. How do these changes affect nursing care?
   a. The nurse should take care to protect fragile skin.
   b. The nurse should provide blankets to keep the patient warm.
   c. The nurse should apply lubricating lotions to prevent drying.
   d. The nurse should massage the skin to enhance circulation.

4. Which term should be used to document a raised, fluid-filled lesion smaller than 1 cm?
   a. Macule
   b. Papule
   c. Vesicle
   d. Wheal

REVIEW QUESTIONS—cont'd

5. What equipment is most important to have readily available when a patient is undergoing skin testing for allergies?
   a. Resuscitation equipment
   b. Flashlight
   c. Measuring device
   d. Alcohol and cotton swabs

6. Why should wet dressings be applied only to one-third of the body at one time?
   a. So the rest of the body can be observed for reaction to the dressing
   b. To prevent chilling the patient
   c. To prevent absorption of too much water, causing fluid overload
   d. To enable the patient to be more mobile

54

Nursing Care of Patients with Skin Disorders

MARTY KOHN AND
RITA BOLEK TROFINO

KEY TERMS

cellulitis (sell-yoo-LYE-tis)
comedo (KOH-meh-doh)
dermatitis (DER-mah-TYE-tiss)
dermatomycosis (DER-mah-toh-mye-KOH-siss)
eschar (ESS-kar)
lichenified (lye-KEN-i-fyde)
onychomycosis (ON-ih-koh-my-KOH-siss)
pediculosis (peh-DIK-yoo-LOH-siss)
pemphigus (PEM-fih-guss)
pruritus (proo-RYE-tuss)
psoriasis (suh-RYE-ah-siss)
purulent (PURE-you-lent)
pyoderma (PYE-oh-DER-mah)
seborrhea (SEB-uh-REE-ah)

QUESTIONS TO GUIDE YOUR READING

1. How would you explain the pathophysiology of each of the skin disorders listed in this chapter?
2. What are the etiologies, signs, and symptoms of each of the skin disorders?
3. What current therapeutic measures are used for each of the skin disorders?
4. What data should you collect when caring for patients with disorders of the integumentary system?
5. What nursing care will you provide for patients with each of the skin disorders?
6. How will you know if your nursing interventions have been effective?

Skin disorders cover a wide array of diseases and conditions. These disorders can be generalized or localized, acute, chronic, or traumatic. This chapter discusses common skin disorders encountered by nurses. An excellent resource on skin disorders is available at www.nlm.nih.gov/medlineplus/skinconditions.html. The American Academy of Dermatology can be accessed at www.aad.org.

PRESSURE ULCERS

Pathophysiology and Etiology

Pressure ulcers are often referred to by patients with old terms such as *bedsores, decubitus ulcers,* or *pressure sores.* Essentially, a pressure ulcer is a lesion caused by prolonged pressure against the skin. This may result from spending a prolonged period in one position, causing the weight of the body to compress the capillaries against a bed or chair, especially over bony prominences. Pressure ulcers are the result of tissue anoxia and begin to develop within 20 to 40 minutes of unrelieved pressure on the skin. Other causes include pressure from a tight splint or cast, traction, or other device. Those at risk are immobile patients, those with decreased circulation, and those with impaired sensory perception or neurologic function.

Mechanical forces (pressure, friction, and shear) lead to the formation of pressure ulcers. The pressure level that closes capillaries in healthy people is 25 to 32 mm Hg. When pressure applied to the skin is greater than the pressure in the capillary bed, the blood supply to the tissues is decreased, which impairs cellular metabolism. This eventually causes tissue ischemia. This reduction in blood flow causes the skin to *blanch,* or lose color. The longer the pressure lasts, the greater the risk of skin breakdown and the development of a pressure ulcer.

Friction is the rubbing of the skin surface with an external mechanical force. Also referred to as "sheet burns," this can happen when the patient is dragged or pulled across bed linens instead of being lifted.

Shearing occurs when the patient slides down in bed when the head of the bed is raised, or when being pulled or repositioned without being lifted off the sheets. With shearing, the skin and subcutaneous tissue remain stationary and the fat, muscle, and bone shift in the direction of body movement. As a result, damage occurs deep within the tissues.

Any patient experiencing prolonged pressure is at risk for a pressure ulcer. Elderly patients have increased risk because of normal aging changes of the skin. Because thin patients have little padding when pressure is present, they have the greatest pressure applied to their capillaries. Obesity also is a contributing factor because adipose tissue is poorly vascularized and is therefore more likely to develop ischemic changes. Impaired peripheral circulation also makes the skin more susceptible to ischemic damage. See Chapter 24 for more information on problems caused by poor circulation.

Prevention

There are many interventions for the prevention of pressure ulcers (see *Evidence-Based Practice* box). Examine and document the condition of the skin daily, so all are aware of developing problems. Gently cleanse the skin daily with tepid water and mild soap to prevent drying. To reduce friction, pat the skin dry rather than rubbing it dry. After bathing, daily lifelong lubrication of the skin with moisturizers is important to prevent dryness. Thoroughly dry skin-to-skin surfaces, such as under the breasts, skinfolds (especially in the groin and abdominal folds), and between the toes, to prevent prolonged exposure to moisture. If incontinence is a problem, clean the skin promptly with tepid water and mild soap, pat dry, and apply a moisture barrier to prevent breakdown. Avoid massaging bony prominences or reddened skin areas; blood vessels are damaged by massage when ischemia is present or when they lie over a bone.

EVIDENCE-BASED PRACTICE

Clinical Question

What are best practices for preventing pressure ulcers?

Evidence

Researchers at the Joanna Briggs Institute (2008) evaluated 33 research studies to determine which interventions are most effective for preventing pressure ulcers. Their findings showed that the Braden Scale (Table 54.1) had the most supporting research and was better than nursing judgment alone at predicting risk.

Several support surfaces were found to be better than standard hospital mattresses at preventing pressure ulcers, including foam mattresses. Two oral supplements in addition to standard diet were superior to standard hospital diet alone in preventing ulcers in critically ill older adults. Finally, studies evaluating repositioning were limited and did not suggest any changes to the tradition of repositioning every 2 hours.

Implications for Nursing Practice

Position patients every 2 hours and avoid direct pressure on bony prominences. Use a valid risk assessment tool such as the Braden Scale on admission and at least daily. Administer oral nutritional supplements to older adults recovering from acute illness. Apply a foam or other pressure-reducing mattress to the at-risk patient's bed.

REFERENCE

Joanna Briggs Institute (2008). Pressure ulcers: Prevention of pressure related damage. Best Practice, 12(2), 1–4. Retrieved November 20, 2009, from http://www.joannabriggs.edu.au/pdf/BP_Book_Vol12_2.pdf

Teach patients to shift their weight every 15 minutes if possible when lying or sitting. When the patient is immobile, the highest possible level of mobility should be maintained; frequent active or passive range-of-motion exercises should be performed, as well as turning according to a written repositioning schedule. If patients are on bedrest, turn and reposition them at least every 2 hours, but preferably more often because ischemia development begins after 20 to 40 minutes of pressure. Avoid elevating the head of the bed more than 30 degrees, to reduce pressure on the coccyx, and to reduce friction and shear damage from sliding down in the bed. When positioning patients on their side, place them at a 30-degree angle or less and not directly on the trochanter because this area is especially sensitive to pressure and can quickly break down. If patients are placed on the trochanter, they usually become restless and squirm around to get off the trochanter. If the patient is seated in a chair, repositioning every hour is important. A mobility program specific to the patient must be developed.

The patient's heels should not rest on the bed surface. Elevate heels off the bed with pillows placed lengthwise under the calf or with heel elevators. Take care so pressure is not applied on the calf from the pillows. Be sure to also protect the patient's elbows, sacrum, scapulae, ears, and occipital area from pressure.

Avoid the use of donut-shaped cushions. They create a circle of pressure that cuts off the circulation to the surrounding tissue, promoting ischemia rather than preventing it. Pad skin contact surfaces, especially bony prominences, so they do not press against each other. (For example, place a small pillow between the knees when the patient is in a side-lying position.) Provide an appropriate pressure-relieving or pressure-reducing mattress and chair cushion for immobile patients. To avoid friction, use a sheet to lift and move patients; provide an overbed trapeze to assist patients to move themselves. Prevent malnutrition and dehydration by ensuring an adequate intake of protein, calories, and fluid; provide 2500 mL of fluid each day if not contraindicated by other medical problems. Box 54.1, *Gerontological Issues,* summarizes additional preventive measures.

An important aspect of prevention is identification of patients at risk for pressure ulcer development. Most institutions have adopted assessment tools such as the Braden or Norton scales to assess patients for physical condition, mental status, activity, mobility, and incontinence to determine the risk for pressure ulcers. Advanced age, low diastolic blood pressure, elevated body temperature, and inadequate current intake of protein are all risk factors associated with the development of pressure ulcers. See Table 54.1 for the Braden instrument.

NURSING CARE TIP

Implement all preventive measures possible, and be sure to document with photographs all pressure ulcers present on admission to the hospital.

Pressure ulcers are "never events" because they can be prevented. Hospitals will not be paid by Medicare for care of Stage III or IV pressure ulcers acquired during hospitalization.

Box 54.1

Gerontological Issues

Interventions to Prevent Skin Breakdown

- Avoid use of soap and water on dry skin areas. Use a moisture barrier cream or ointment on dry skin areas before bathing to protect the skin from the drying effects of water.
- Regularly wash and dry areas between toes.
- Toilet patient often, and institute a bowel program to prevent incontinence.
- Use perineal cleansing products to cleanse urine and feces residue from the perineum and anal area. These products are specially designed to break down and facilitate the complete removal of urine and feces without irritating the skin.
- Use moisturizing creams that have no alcohol or perfume, which can irritate the skin.
- Avoid areas of skin pressure, especially over bony areas, by assisting the older adult to change positions on a regular schedule.
- Remind the patient to change position or shift weight frequently while sitting in a chair to avoid prolonged pressure.
- Examine skin for areas of redness. If redness occurs, the positioning schedule should be more frequent.
- Keep fingernails short to avoid scratching.
- Use pillows and pads to help maintain alignment with position changes. Use specialized mattresses and chair cushions designed to decrease pressure. Keep the patient's heels off the bed with pillows under the calves for support and to prevent pressure.
- Encourage the older adult to be out of bed and active throughout the day. Remember to assess skin and reposition frequently even when out of bed, because areas of pressure occur whether the patient is in or out of bed.
- Provide a high-protein vitamin-rich diet if not contraindicated.
- Assess for dehydration and encourage fluids if not contraindicated.

Signs and Symptoms

A developing pressure ulcer begins with a reddened area, usually over a bony prominence, that does not blanch with pressure. You have learned to check for capillary refill by

TABLE 54.1 BRADEN SCALE FOR PREDICTING PRESSURE SORE RISK

Patient's Name
Evaluator's Name
Date of Assessment

SENSORY PERCEPTION	**1. Completely Limited**	**2. Very Limited**	**3. Slightly Limited**	**4. No Impairment**
ability to respond meaningfully to pressure-related discomfort	Unresponsive (does not moan, flinch, or grasp) to painful stimuli, due to diminished level of consciousness or sedation OR Limited ability to feel pain over most of body	Responds only to painful stimuli. Cannot communicate discomfort except by moaning or restlessness OR Has a sensory impairment which limits the ability to feel pain or discomfort over 1/2 of body	Responds to verbal commands, but cannot always communicate discomfort or the need to be turned OR Has some sensory impairment which limits ability to feel pain or discomfort in 1 or 2 extremities	Responds to verbal commands. Has no sensory deficit which would limit ability to feel or voice pain or discomfort.
MOISTURE	**1. Constantly Moist**	**2. Very Moist**	**3. Occasionally Moist**	**4. Rarely Moist**
degree to which skin is exposed to moisture	Skin is kept moist almost constantly by perspiration, urine, etc. Dampness is detected every time patient is moved or turned.	Skin is often, but not always moist. Linen must be changed at least once a shift.	Skin is occasionally moist, requiring an extra linen change approximately once a day.	Skin is usually dry, linen only requires changing at routine intervals.
ACTIVITY	**1. Bedfast**	**2. Chairfast**	**3. Walks Occasionally**	**4. Walks Frequently**
degree of physical activity	Confined to bed	Ability to walk severely limited or nonexistent. Cannot bear own weight and/or must be assisted into chair or wheelchair.	Walks occasionally during day, but for very short distances, with or without assistance. Spends majority of each shift in bed or chair.	Walks outside room at least twice a day and inside room at least once every two hours during waking hours
MOBILITY	**1. Completely Immobile**	**2. Very Limited**	**3. Slightly Limited**	**4. No Limitation**
ability to change and control body position	Does not make even slight changes in body or extremity position without assistance	Makes occasional slight changes in body or extremity position but unable to make frequent or significant changes independently	Makes frequent though slight changes in body or extremity position independently	Makes major and frequent changes in position without assistance
NUTRITION	**1. Very Poor**	**2. Probably Inadequate**	**3. Adequate**	**4. Excellent**
usual food intake pattern	Never eats a complete meal. Rarely eats more than 1/3 of any food offered. Eats 2 servings or less of protein (meat or dairy products) per day. Takes fluids poorly. Does not take a liquid dietary supplement OR Is NPO and/or maintained on clear liquids or IVs for more than 5 days	Rarely eats a complete meal and generally eats only about 1/2 of any food offered. Protein intake includes only 3 servings of meat or dairy products per day. Occasionally will take a dietary supplement. OR Receives less than optimum amount of liquid diet or tube feeding	Eats over half of most meals. Eats a total of 4 servings of protein (meat, dairy products) per day. Occasionally will refuse a meal, but will usually take a supplement when offered. OR Is on a tube feeding or TPN regimen which probably meets most of nutritional needs	Eats most of every meal. Never refuses a meal. Usually eats a total of 4 or more servings of meat and dairy products. Occasionally eats between meals. Does not require supplementation.

TABLE 54.1 BRADEN SCALE FOR PREDICTING PRESSURE SORE RISK—cont'd

FRICTION & SHEAR	1. Problem	2. Potential Problem	3. No Apparent Problem
	Requires moderate to maximum assistance in moving. Complete lifting without sliding against sheets is impossible. Frequently slides down in bed or chair, requiring frequent repositioning with maximum assistance. Spasticity, contractures, or agitation leads to almost constant friction.	Moves feebly or requires minimum assistance. During a move skin probably slides to some extent against sheets, chair, restraints, or other devices. Maintains relatively good position in chair or bed most of the time but occasionally slides down.	Moves in bed and in chair independently and has sufficient muscle strength to lift up completely during move. Maintains good position in bed or chair.

Total Score

INTERVENTIONS FOR SPECIFIC RISK LEVEL	SPECIFIC CONDITION MANAGEMENT
AT RISK (15–18)* FREQUENT TURNING MAXIMAL REMOBILIZATION PROTECT HEELS MANAGE MOISTURE, NUTRITION, AND FRICTION AND SHEAR PRESSURE-REDUCTION SUPPORT SURFACE IF BED- OR CHAIRBOUND *If other major risk factors are present (advanced age, fever, poor dietary intake of protein, diastolic pressure below 60 mm Hg, hemodynamic instability) advance to next level of risk.	**MANAGE MOISTURE** USE COMMERCIAL MOISTURE BARRIER USE ABSORBANT PADS OR DIAPERS THAT WICK & HOLD MOISTURE ADDRESS CAUSE IF POSSIBLE OFFER BEDPAN/URINAL AND GLASS OF WATER IN CONJUNCTION WITH TURNING SCHEDULES
MODERATE RISK (13–14)* TURNING SCHEDULE USE FOAM WEDGES FOR 30° LATERAL POSITIONING PRESSURE-REDUCTION SUPPORT SURFACE MAXIMAL REMOBILIZATION PROTECT HEELS MANAGE MOISTURE, NUTRITION, AND FRICTION AND SHEAR *If other major risk factors present, advance to next level of risk.	**MANAGE NUTRITION** INCREASE PROTEIN INTAKE INCREASE CALORIE INTAKE TO SPARE PROTEINS SUPPLEMENT WITH MULTIVITAMIN (SHOULD HAVE VITAMINS A, C, & E) ACT QUICKLY TO ALLEVIATE DEFICITS CONSULT DIETITIAN
HIGH RISK (10–12) INCREASE FREQUENCY OF TURNING SUPPLEMENT WITH SMALL SHIFTS PRESSURE REDUCTION SUPPORT SURFACE USE FOAM WEDGES FOR 30° LATERAL POSITIONING MAXIMAL REMOBILIZATION PROTECT HEELS MANAGE MOISTURE, NUTRITION, AND FRICTION AND SHEAR	**MANAGE FRICTION & SHEAR** ELEVATE HOB NO MORE THAN 30° USE TRAPEZE WHEN INDICATED USE LIFT SHEET TO MOVE PATIENT PROTECT ELBOWS & HEELS IF BEING EXPOSED TO FRICTION

Continued

TABLE 54.1 BRADEN SCALE FOR PREDICTING PRESSURE SORE RISK—cont'd

VERY HIGH RISK (9 or below)*	OTHER GENERAL CARE ISSUES
ALL OF THE ABOVE USE PRESSURE-RELIEVING SURFACE IF PATIENT HAS INTRACTABLE PAIN OR SEVERE PAIN EXACERBATED BY TURNING OR ADDITIONAL RISK FACTORS *Low-air-loss beds do not substitute for turning schedules.	NO MASSAGE OF REDDENED BONY PROMINENCES NO DONUT TYPE DEVICES MAINTAIN GOOD HYDRATION AVOID DRYING THE SKIN

pressing on a fingertip and watching it turn white, then red again. If redness returns within 3 seconds, then capillary refill is considered to be adequate. A pressure ulcer stays red, and does not blanch. If pressure is not relieved and healing does not occur, it can progress to an open, ulcerated area. Stages of ulcers are discussed in the data collection section.

The most common sites for pressure ulcers are the sacrum, heels, elbows, lateral malleoli, greater trochanters, ischial tuberosities, base of the skull, scapulae, and ears. Most patients experience pain at the ulcer site. A report of pain requires continual monitoring, documentation, and treatment.

LEARNING TIP

Pressure ulcers may be described according to a three-color system:

- Black wounds indicate necrosis.
- Yellow wounds have exudate and may be infected.
- Red wounds are pink or red and are in the healing stage.

A wound may contain a mixture of black, yellow, and red colors. Necrotic wounds are the worst because they contain dead tissue. Beefy red wounds are desired because they are healing wounds. It is important to consider treating the worst color present first or healing will be delayed. For example, if a wound is both yellow and black, the dead tissue must be removed first before the infection can be effectively treated. This color system is a helpful system for patients and families to use to describe wounds to the home care nurse because colors are easily recognized and understood by most people.

Complications

Wound infection is a common complication. New ulcers can also appear, and the present ulcer can progress to a deeper wound. Some wounds take a prolonged time to heal or never heal.

Diagnostic Tests

All open pressure ulcers are considered to be colonized with bacteria. This means that bacteria are present, but the wound is not necessarily infected. In most cases, adequate cleansing and debridement can prevent bacterial colonization from advancing to clinical infection. Swab cultures and culture and sensitivity tests may be done to identify the causative organism in suspected infection sites. (See Chapter 53 for instructions for obtaining a culture.) Results need to be interpreted to distinguish between true wound infection and bacterial colonization. If the wound is healing by secondary intention, it becomes colonized by bacterial flora from the skin and from the environment. If, however, the wound is extensive, bacterial growth may exceed the defenses of the local tissue and a true wound infection results.

If the wound does not show signs of healing or if an ischemic ulcer is suspected, noninvasive and invasive arterial blood supply studies are recommended. Wound biopsies may be performed for large, extensive wounds.

Therapeutic Measures

Treatment varies according to the size, depth, and stage of the pressure ulcer; the special needs of the patient; and health care provider preference. All pressure must be removed from the affected area for healing to occur. Cleanliness must be maintained. Basic treatment includes debridement, cleansing, and dressing of the wound to provide a moist and healing environment.

LEARNING TIP

The epidermis "skates" on moisture, so the wound must be kept moist to heal.

Debridement

Debridement is the removal of dead or nonviable tissue from a wound to help clean up the wound and facilitate formation of granulation tissue. It may be done surgically or nonsurgically. Nonsurgical debridement includes mechanical, enzymatic, and autolytic methods. Surgical debridement is used only if the patient has sepsis or **cellulitis**, or to remove extensive **eschar**. Eschar is a black or brown hard scab or dry crust, or thick black leather-like tissue that forms from necrotic tissue. It may hide the true depth of the wound and must be removed for the wound to heal.

MECHANICAL DEBRIDEMENT. Scissors and forceps can be used for mechanical debridement to selectively remove nonviable tissue. Dextranomer beads, another method of mechanical debridement, can be sprinkled over the wound to absorb exudate and all other products of tissue breakdown, as well as surface bacteria. Whirlpool baths and wet-to-dry saline gauze dressings may also be used for mechanical debridement. For wet-to-dry dressings, the wet gauze is placed directly on the wound (avoiding surrounding healthy tissue) and allowed to dry completely. The drying process causes the gauze to adhere to the wound; when it is pulled off, tissue is pulled off with it. This results in nonselective debridement because viable tissue may also be removed in this process. These methods are painful, so the patient should be premedicated for pain and assessed often.

ENZYMATIC DEBRIDEMENT. Enzymatic debridement involves application of a topical enzyme debriding agent. These agents vary as to application methods, so careful reading of instructions is necessary. Most of these debriding agents are proteolytic enzymes that selectively digest necrotic tissue. Be careful to apply them only to the wound and to avoid contact with healthy tissue.

AUTOLYTIC DEBRIDEMENT. Autolytic debridement is the use of a synthetic dressing or moisture-retentive dressing over the ulcer. The eschar is then self-digested via the action of the enzymes that are present in the fluid environment of the wound. This method is not used for infected wounds, because the infection would worsen.

SURGICAL DEBRIDEMENT. Surgical debridement is the removal of devitalized tissue, slough, or thick, adherent eschar with a scalpel, scissors, or other sharp instrument. Slough is loose, yellow to tan stringy necrotic tissue. Slough, like eschar, can be tightly adhered to the wound bed.

Depending on the amount of debridement to be done, this may be performed in the operating room, a treatment room, or the patient's room. Following surgical debridement, grafting may be required to close the wound. This becomes necessary if it is a full-thickness ulcer, if there is loss of joint function, or for cosmetic purposes. For procedures performed without anesthesia, be sure to premedicate the patient for pain. Continually monitor for pain during the procedure, especially if there is a donor site for grafting.

Wound Cleansing

The ulcer should be thoroughly cleansed using a whirlpool, a handheld shower head, or an irrigating system with a pressure between 4 and 15 pounds per square inch (psi). A 30-mL syringe with an 18-gauge needle works well for this purpose. Pressure less than 4 psi does not adequately cleanse the wound, and greater than 15 psi may damage tissue. If an irrigating system is used, 250 mL of normal saline solution (or sometimes tap water for home wound care) should be used to thoroughly cleanse the wound. If the wound is red, gentle irrigation with a needleless 30- to 60-mL syringe should be used to prevent trauma and bleeding. However, if the wound has been diagnosed as being infected, flushing with a 30- to 60-mL syringe and an 18-gauge needle provides the pressure needed to help remove bacteria.

LEARNING TIP

Dilution is the solution to wound pollution!

Once the wound has been cleansed and debrided, apply a dressing. Wounds heal more rapidly in a moist environment, with minimal bacterial colonization and a healing temperature. This takes 12 hours to occur after the wound is covered with an occlusive dressing. If a dressing is frequently removed, the wound may not reach its healing temperature and healing may be impaired. When possible, the dressing should be left in place for extended periods. Infected wounds are not covered with occlusive dressings; draining wounds may require frequent dressing changes.

Wound Dressings

Dressings vary according to size, location, depth, stage of ulcer, and preference of the ordering practitioner. Commonly used dressing materials include hydrogel dressings, polyurethane films, hydrocolloid wafers, biological dressings, alginates, and cotton gauze. See Chapter 53 for more information on dressing types. The use of an appropriate dressing promotes an optimum healing environment. Hypoallergenic tape should be used to secure dressings if tape is necessary. Protective paste may be applied to protect unaffected tissue from topical agents. In all cases, pressure should be kept off the wound. No treatment will be effective if pressure continues to damage the tissue.

Negative Pressure Wound Therapy

Negative pressure wound therapy (NPWT) may be effective for healing large open pressure ulcers (Fig. 54.1). In NPWT, a wound is packed loosely with a sterile sponge and then covered with an occlusive dressing. A vacuum source is placed in the wound and gentle negative pressure is applied. The negative pressure allows excess drainage and infectious material to be removed, which reduces pressure on delicate new tissue. With small vessels decompressed, circulation is increased, and healing is accelerated. NPWT also maintains a moist environment for optimal healing. Research is ongoing to determine best practices for NPWT. A study comparing NPWT with advanced moist wound therapy (AMWT) for patients with diabetes and foot ulcers showed that NPWT was just as

• WORD • BUILDING •

cellulitis: cellu—cell + itis—inflammation

eschar: eschara—scab

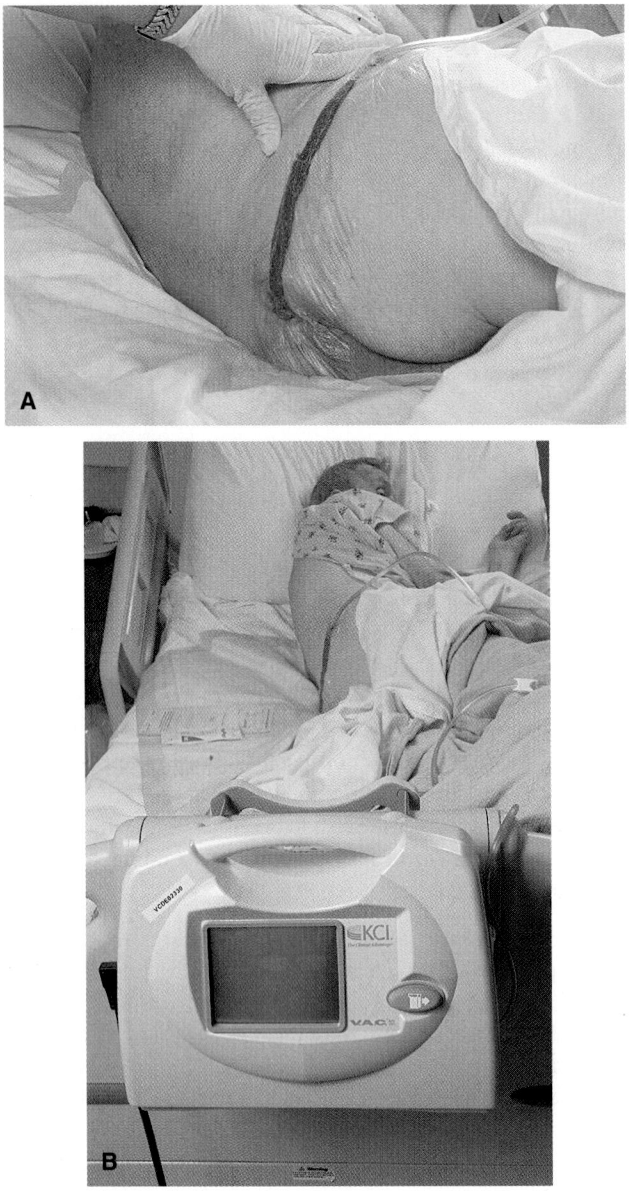
A
B
KCI

FIGURE 54.1 Negative pressure wound therapy. (A) Occlusive dressing is applied to wound with tubing to vacuum source. (B) Vacuum source exerts gentle negative pressure.

safe as, and more effective than, AMWT (Blume et al., 2008).

Nursing Process for the Patient with a Pressure Ulcer

Data Collection

Collaborate with the RN to evaluate the status of the pressure ulcer often, as well as underlying causes and barriers to healing. Monitor for risk factors for impaired healing, such as prolonged immobility, incontinence, and inadequate nutrition and hydration. Also monitor intact skin to prevent development of new pressure ulcers.

Use transparency film or a disposable ruler to measure the diameter of the ulcer in centimeters. Imagine a clock superimposed over the wound with 12 o'clock at the head and 6 o'clock at the feet. Measure in centimeters from 12 to 6 o'clock, and from 9 to 3 o'clock. Depth can be measured with a cotton-tipped applicator. Also, gently probe a cotton-tipped applicator under the skin edges to detect tunneling and measure lateral tissue destruction.

Several staging systems are available for pressure ulcers based on the depth of tissue destroyed. Most staging systems categorize wounds from stage I to stage IV. Additional categories may include deep tissue injury and unstageable (Fig. 54.2).

- *Deep tissue injury:* The National Pressure Ulcer Advisory Panel (NPUAP) defines deep tissue injury as a "purple or maroon localized area of discolored intact skin or blood-filled blister due to damage of underlying soft tissue from pressure and/or shear. The area may be preceded by tissue that is painful, firm, mushy, boggy, warmer, or cooler as compared to adjacent tissue" (NPUAP, 2007). Deep tissue injury is considered unstageable because it is impossible to determine how deep the tissue damage is. This stage can progress quickly to a stage III or IV ulcer, even with appropriate treatment.
- *Stage I:* The skin is still intact, but the area is red and does not blanch when pressed. There may also be warmth, hardness, and discoloration of the skin. A Stage I ulcer may be difficult to detect in a dark-skinned person.
- *Stage II:* There is a break in the skin, with partial-thickness skin loss of epidermis, dermis, or both. The ulcer may appear as an abrasion, a shallow crater, or a blister. Stage II ulcers do not contain slough (yellow fibrous tissue).
- *Stage III:* There is full-thickness skin loss, which extends to the subcutaneous fat, but not fascia. The ulcer looks like a deep crater and may have undermining of adjacent tissue. Bone, tendon, and muscle are not visible.
- *Stage IV:* There is full-thickness skin loss with exposed muscle, bone, or support structures such as tendons. Slough or eschar may be present. There may be undermining and sinus tracts (tunneling).
- *Unstageable:* The base of the ulcer is covered by slough or eschar, so that the depth cannot be evaluated. The wound bed must be debrided before staging and treatment can take place. One exception, according to NPUAP (2007), is stable, dry, intact eschar on the heels. It serves as the body's natural (biological) cover, and should not be removed.

Observe wound exudate. Two common types of wound exudate are serosanguineous and **purulent**. Serosanguineous exudate is fluid consisting of serum and blood. It is blood-tinged, amber-colored fluid. Purulent fluid is a fluid that contains pus. It can vary in color and have different odors,

• WORD • BUILDING •
purulent: purulentus—pus

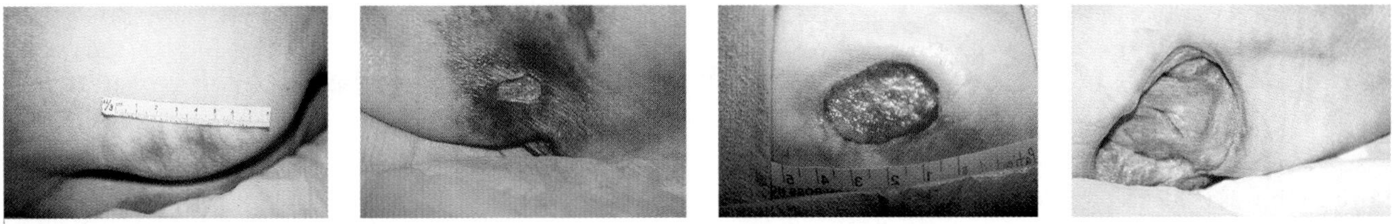

Stage I Stage II Stage III Stage IV

FIGURE 54.2 Stages of pressure ulcers include deep tissue injury, stages I through IV, shown here, and unstageable, as described in the text. (From Dillon, P. M. [2007]. *Nursing health assessment* [2nd ed.]. Philadelphia: F. A. Davis, with permission.)

depending on which bacteria are present. Creamy yellow pus may indicate *Staphylococcus.* Beige pus that has a fishy odor may suggest *Proteus.* Green-blue pus with a fruity odor may indicate *Pseudomonas.* Brown pus with a fecal odor may suggest *Bacteroides.*

Gently palpate the wound with a gloved hand to determine the texture of granulations. Granulation tissue has a budding appearance from the development of tiny new capillaries. If the granulations are healthy, they have a slightly spongy texture.

Document all findings carefully in the medical record, so all health team members can monitor progress of healing. Many institutions have specific forms for drawing pictures of the locations and sizes of wounds, and for photographs to monitor the healing process. Follow policy at the institution where you work.

Nursing Diagnoses, Planning, Implementation, and Evaluation

See the *Nursing Care Plan for the Patient with a Pressure Ulcer.*

> **NURSING CARE TIP**
>
> Many institutions now have nurses who have been specially trained in wound care. Consult one of these nurses for expert wound assessment and treatment recommendations.

> **CRITICAL THINKING**
>
> ***Mr. Russ***
>
> ■ Mr. Russ is an 84-year-old man who was admitted from home to the medical-surgical unit after a fall that fractured his femur. He has a history of type 2 diabetes. He had an open reduction and internal fixation of his femur and is now in a brace. He is 6 ft tall and weighs 160 pounds. His appetite is poor; his wife states he has lost 15 lb in the last 3 months. He is occasionally incontinent of urine. What preventive measures can be taken to prevent skin breakdown in this patient?
>
> *Suggested answers at end of chapter.*

INFLAMMATORY SKIN DISORDERS

Dermatitis

Pathophysiology and Etiology

Dermatitis is inflammation of the skin and is characterized by itching, redness, and skin lesions, with varying borders and distribution patterns. There are three common types of dermatitis: contact dermatitis, atopic dermatitis, and seborrheic dermatitis. Contact dermatitis is caused by exposure to an allergen or irritant such as soap, perfume, or poison ivy. Atopic dermatitis tends to be hereditary and is associated with allergies, asthma, and hay fever. Seborrheic dermatitis occurs most often on the scalp, usually in individuals with oily skin. All types tend to be chronic and respond well to treatment, but are prone to recur. See Table 54.2 for common types of dermatitis.

Prevention

The patient should prevent irritation to the skin by avoiding irritants, allergens, excessive heat and dryness, and by controlling perspiration. Baths should be short, in tepid water. Deodorant soaps should be avoided; mild superfatted soaps are recommended instead. Dry skin can be lubricated with creams, oils, or ointments as appropriate. Itching and scratching should be prevented as much as possible.

Signs and Symptoms

Itching and rashes or lesions are the main clinical manifestations of dermatitis. The lesions vary depending on the type and location of dermatitis. Rashes and lesions may present as dry, flaky scales, yellow crusts, redness, fissures, macules, papules, and vesicles. (These are described in Chapter 53.) Scratching can make any of these lesions worse.

> **NURSING CARE TIP**
>
> Itching and scratching can occur during sleep, causing the rash to worsen. Have the patient wear cotton gloves at night to prevent scratching.

• **WORD • BUILDING** •
dermatitis: derma—skin + itis—inflammation

NURSING CARE PLAN for the Patient with a Pressure Ulcer

Nursing Diagnosis: *Impaired Skin Integrity* related to pressure on skin surface, reduced circulation, or immobility as evidenced by destruction of skin surface or deeper tissues

Expected Outcomes: The patient's skin integrity will be improved as evidenced by decrease in wound size and depth, no development of additional pressure ulcers.

Evaluation of Outcomes: Is there a decrease in wound size? Are there any new pressure ulcers?

Interventions	Rationale	Evaluation
Assess status of pressure ulcer according to stage, color, exudate, texture, size, and depth.	Provides baseline data on which care is based.	What stage is ulcer? Are there any other outstanding characteristics?
Determine and remove cause of pressure (e.g., immobility, friction, shearing).	Allows for correction and also prevents further trauma.	What is the cause of this ulcer?
Cleanse wound gently with warm water; rinse; pat dry gently with gauze. Do not rub the area.	Reduces number of bacteria. Drying prevents maceration of skin. Gentle handling prevents further trauma.	Is wound clean and dry?
Debride wound as prescribed (method depends on patient's condition and goals of care).	Debridement removes drainage and wound debris. Permits granulation of tissue.	Does wound look clean and free of debris?
Apply topical agents and/or dress wound as prescribed. Make sure dressing stays intact with movement and that edges do not roll, causing more pressure.	Protects underlying wound and helps promote healing.	Is dressing applied appropriately?
Position patient off the ulcer.	Prevents further pressure and trauma on ulcer.	Is patient positioned off the ulcer?
If a leg ulcer, provide for frequent rest periods with leg elevated; if immobile, reposition every 2 hours.	Prevents further tissue breakdown.	Is leg elevated? Is patient repositioned every 2 hours?

Nursing Diagnosis: *Risk for Infection* related to open wound

Expected Outcomes: The patient will not experience wound infection or systemic sepsis as evidenced by clean wound bed and by temperature and white blood cell count within normal limits. (Total elimination of bacteria is impossible due to nature of the condition.)

Evaluation of Outcomes: Is patient free from signs and symptoms of local and systemic infection?

Interventions	Rationale	Evaluation
Examine ulcer at every dressing change or at least every 24 hours. Look for areas of tenderness, swelling, redness, and heat; and drainage. Report changes.	Allows for early recognition of infection and response to treatment.	Are signs of infection present?

NURSING CARE PLAN for the Patient with a Pressure Ulcer—cont'd

Interventions	Rationale	Evaluation
Monitor temperature at least every 12 hours.	Elevated body temperature is one sign of infection.	Is patient afebrile?
Provide meticulous wound care (see Impaired Skin Integrity).	Helps decrease the level of contamination and prevent infection.	Is wound showing signs of healing without purulent drainage?
Use thorough hand washing techniques. Use sterile technique for dressing changes.	Prevents cross-contamination.	Does nurse take proper wound precautions?

Nursing Diagnosis: *Pain* related to ulcer and treatments as evidenced by pain rating on 0 to 10 scale

Expected Outcomes: The patient will be as comfortable and as pain free as possible as evidenced by statement of decreased pain and ability to sleep at night.

Evaluation of Outcomes: Does patient express comfort? Does patient express a decrease in pain? Is patient able to sleep?

Interventions	Rationale	Evaluation
Assess level of pain with pain scale and by observing facial expressions and positioning of body.	Monitors level of pain and response to therapy.	At what level is pain? Is it better or worse with treatment?
Offer analgesics as prescribed. Request order for topical analgesics as needed with dressing changes and cleaning of the wound.	Analgesics help relieve pain.	Are analgesics effective?
Decrease anxiety with relaxation techniques (e.g., distraction, music).	Relaxation can lessen pain intensity.	Is patient less anxious? Does patient verbalize less pain?
Maintain a comfortable environment: provide for privacy; position in good alignment and comfortably; and maintain a comfortable room temperature.	Relaxes patient and lessens intensity of discomfort.	Does patient express an increase in comfort?

Complications

The lesion or rash worsens with continued irritation, exposure to offending agents, or scratching. Infections of the skin are common and may be due to the many open areas and breaks in the skin, as well as the patient's reluctance to properly wash the affected area because of pain from the lesions. Some infections can also become systemic.

Diagnostic Tests

Diagnosis is usually based on history, symptoms, and clinical findings. If infection is suspected, cultures of the lesions may be ordered to identify the infecting agent.

Therapeutic Measures

Treatment varies according to symptoms. Basic treatment objectives are to control itching, alleviate discomfort and pain, decrease inflammation, control or prevent crust formation and oozing, prevent infection, prevent further damage to the skin, and heal the lesions as much as possible.

Itching (**pruritus**) and discomfort can be somewhat relieved by antihistamines, analgesics, and antipruritic

• WORD • BUILDING •

pruritus: prur—itch + itis—condition

TABLE 54.2 COMMON TYPES OF DERMATITIS

Type	Description
Contact	Acute or chronic condition; caused by contact with irritant or allergen
Irritant contact	Caused by direct contact with an irritating substance, such as soap, detergent, strong medication, astringent, cosmetic, or industrial chemical
Allergic contact	From contact with an allergen, such as perfume, tanning lotion, medication, hair dye, poison ivy, poison oak; contact results in cell-mediated immune response
Atopic	Chronic inherited condition; may be associated with respiratory allergies or asthma; can vary between bright red maculas, papules, oozing, and **lichenified** or hyperpigmented areas
Seborrheic	Chronic, inflammatory disease usually accompanied by scaling, itching, and inflammation; **seborrhea** is excessive production of sebaceous secretions; found in areas with abundant sebaceous glands (scalp, face, axilla, groin) and where there are folds of skin; can appear as dry, moist, or greasy scales, yellow or pink-yellow crusts, redness, and dry flakiness; can be associated with emotional stress; genetic predisposition may exist

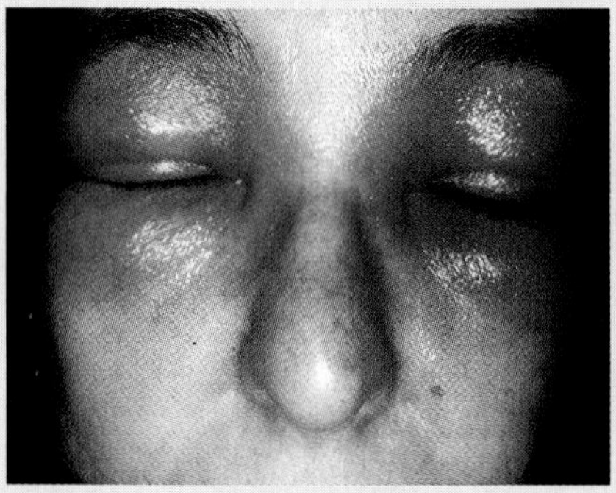
Contact dermatitis caused by nail polish

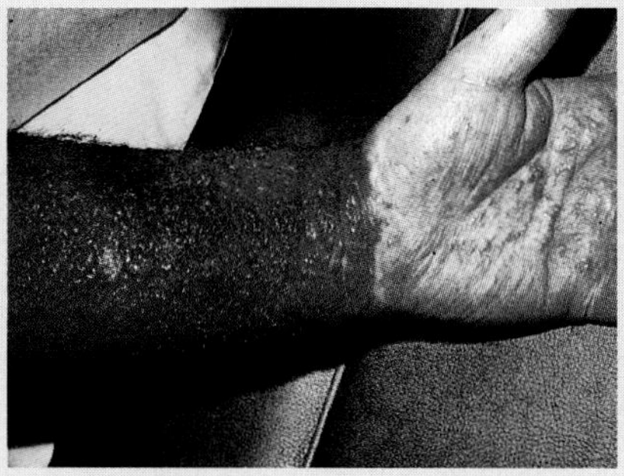
Contact dermatitis caused by topical anesthetic

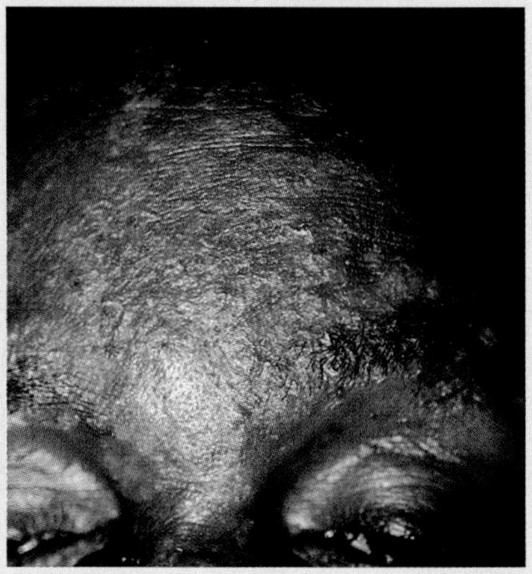
Seborrheic dermatitis

medications as ordered. Colloidal oatmeal preparations added to baths may also help.

Steroids such as hydrocortisone or methylprednisolone may be used to suppress inflammation. They can be administered as a topical, intralesional, or systemic agent. The specific type used depends on the type of lesion, the body area involved, and the extent of the lesion. Topical administration is preferred if possible because systemic steroids can cause serious systemic side effects, including adrenal suppression.

Tub baths and wet dressings help control oozing and prevent further crust formation. These interventions serve to loosen exudates, scales, and other wound debris, providing a clean area for topical application of medication. Skin is protected by lightly patting dry, avoiding friction, avoiding hot water, and using a sunscreen agent when outdoors.

Nursing Process for the Patient with Dermatitis

DATA COLLECTION. You can use the WHAT'S UP? format to assess the rash, as described in Chapter 53. Also refer to Chapter 53, Table 53.1, for specific questions to ask. Observe the rash or lesions for character, distribution, description, skin tenderness, signs of scratching, and other associated problems.

• WORD • BUILDING •
lichenified: leichen—scaly growth + facere—to make
seborrhea: sebum—tallow + rhoia—flow

NURSING DIAGNOSES, PLANNING, AND IMPLEMENTATION

Impaired Skin Integrity Related to Rash, Lesions, and Scratching as Evidenced by Open Lesions

EXPECTED OUTCOME: The patient's skin integrity will improve as evidenced by reduction in lesions; no signs or symptoms of infection.

- Monitor skin condition regularly *to determine if treatment is working.*
- Cleanse the area as ordered by the physician, taking care not to further irritate the skin, *to keep area clean and prevent infection.*
- Provide cool moist compresses, dressings, or tepid tub baths *to help relieve inflammation and itching, debride lesions, and soften crusts and scales.*
- Pat the skin dry rather than rubbing *to prevent further trauma.*
- Apply topical agents as ordered *to help suppress inflammation and itching.*

- Provide skin care at bedtime *to help promote comfortable sleep. Many antihistamines also have a sedative effect.*
- Encourage patient to eat a high-protein diet to promote healing and replace lost protein. *If lesions are generalized, protein can be lost through oozing of serum.* Confirm appropriateness of high-protein diet with primary care provider.
- Encourage use of gloves or mitts, especially at night, *to help prevent scratching.*
- Advise the patient to keep fingernails short *to prevent scratching.*
- Teach the patient that application of slight pressure with a clean cloth *may help relieve itching.*
- Teach relaxation exercises *to help the patient cope with distressing symptoms.*

Disturbed Body Image Related to Visible Rash or Lesions as Evidenced by Verbal or Nonverbal Responses to Lesions, Avoidance of Social Situations

EXPECTED OUTCOME: The patient will have improved body image as evidenced by a statement of acceptance of the condition and ability to socialize with others.

- Allow patients to verbalize concerns if they wish to do so. *Talking about concerns may help patient to begin to work through feelings about body image, but should not be forced.*
- Refer to a support group, if available, *to receive support from others in similar circumstances.*
- Display an accepting attitude while caring for skin lesions. *The patient will be quick to pick up your reaction to the lesions, especially if it is negative.*
- Encourage the patient to participate in skin care *to allow more control over the situation.*
- Encourage the patient to wear long sleeves or other appropriate covering if the patient desires *to make the lesions less noticeable and the patient more comfortable.*

Deficient Knowledge Related to Disease and Treatment as Evidenced by Patient Statement of Need for Information

EXPECTED OUTCOME: The patient will verbalize understanding of the condition and demonstrate ability to perform self-care measures.

- Determine patient's baseline knowledge of condition and treatment. *Teaching should build on baseline understanding.*
- Instruct the patient in application of topical agents and dressings. *Overuse of medications can further traumatize skin; be sure to follow package or prescription directions.*
- Instruct the patient in how to recognize changes, improvement, or flare-ups of the disorder and what symptoms to report to the health care provider. *Because most skin conditions are cared for at home, it is important for the patient to have the skills needed to monitor the condition and carry out treatment appropriately.*
- Advise the patient to avoid overexposure to sun and to use sunscreen agents when outdoors *to prevent skin damage.*
- Encourage use of a humidifier in the home *to help maintain hydration of skin and control itching during dry weather, especially in winter.*
- Teach the patient measures to prevent future flare-ups if possible. *Flare-ups may be avoided if the patient understands what triggers them.*

NURSING CARE TIP

Teach patients that when applying topical medications, more is not better!

EVALUATION. If medical and nursing care have been effective, the lesions will be controlled or in remission, the patient will state that itching and other discomforts are controlled, the patient will be able to socialize without undue difficulty, and the patient will be able to describe and demonstrate self-care measures.

Psoriasis

Pathophysiology and Etiology

Psoriasis is a chronic inflammatory skin disorder in which the epidermal cells proliferate abnormally fast. Usually, epidermal cells take about 27 days to shed. With psoriasis, the cells shed every 4 to 5 days. The abnormal keratin forms loosely adherent scales with dermal inflammation.

The exact cause is not known; however, it is autoimmune in nature, with T cells attacking healthy skin cells, causing an increase in skin cell, T-cell, and white cell production. Often there is a family history. The average age at onset is 27 years, although it can begin at any age. The condition can be severe if the onset is in childhood.

Psoriasis is characterized by exacerbations and remissions. Many factors influence the suppression and outbreak of lesions, but this varies from individual to individual. Sun and humidity may suppress lesions. Aggravating factors include streptococcal pharyngitis, emotional upset, stress, hormonal changes, cold weather, skin trauma, smoking, alcohol, and certain drugs (e.g., antimalarial agents, lithium, beta blockers).

Prevention

Because the exact etiology is not known, measures to prevent exacerbation of symptoms are specific to the patient's circumstances. General preventive measures include avoidance of

• WORD • BUILDING •

psoriasis: psor—itch + iasis—inflammation

upper respiratory infections, especially streptococcal infections; avoidance of or coping with emotional stress; avoidance of skin trauma, including sunburns; and avoidance of medications that may precipitate a flare-up.

Signs and Symptoms

Signs and symptoms vary according to the patient and the particular type of psoriasis. Lesions are red papules that join to form plaques with distinct borders (Fig. 54.3). Silvery scales develop on untreated lesions. Areas most often affected are the elbows and knees, scalp, umbilicus, and genitals. Other signs and symptoms include nail involvement, involvement in the gluteal fold (called intergluteal pinking), itching, and dry or brittle hair.

Complications

Because of the nature of the disease, with its lesions and itching, secondary infections can occur. Psoriatic arthritis may develop after the psoriasis has developed, with nail changes and destructive arthritis of large joints, the spine, and interphalangeal joints. If the psoriasis becomes severe and widespread, fever, chills, increased cardiac output, and benign lymphadenopathy can result.

Diagnostic Tests

Testing depends on the severity of the psoriasis. Normally, this disease is diagnosed by physical assessment alone. Skin biopsy or other diagnostic tests may be performed to rule out concurrent disease or secondary infection.

Therapeutic Measures

Treatment varies according to the type and extent of the disease, as well as patient preference. Psoriasis is a chronic disease with remissions and exacerbations. Basic treatment objectives are to decrease the rapid epidermal proliferation, inflammation, and itching and scaling. Usually, the patient is instructed to bathe daily in a tub, using a soft brush to assist in the removal of scales.

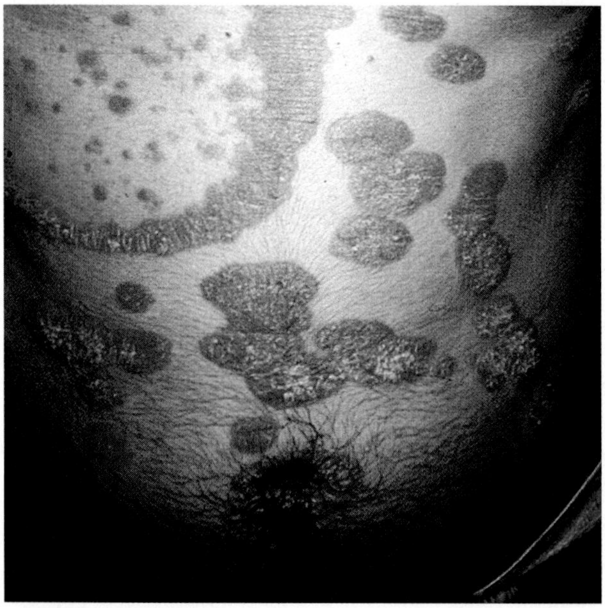

FIGURE 54.3 Psoriasis. Note bright red scaly plaque with silvery scales. (From Goldsmith, L. A., Lazarus, G. S., & Tharp, M. D. [1997]. *Adult and pediatric dermatology* [p. 258]. Philadelphia: F. A. Davis, with permission.)

A variety of topical and systemic agents are used to treat psoriasis. Topical corticosteroids may be used for their anti-inflammatory effect. Occlusive dressings are commonly used to enhance penetration of medications (see Chapter 53). Keratolytic ointments or gels enhance the effects of salicylic acid to loosen or remove scales. Synthetic vitamin D cream slows the proliferation of skin cells. Fish oil supplements may reduce inflammation in some patients.

Tar preparations may be prescribed along with corticosteroids. The tar acts as an antimitotic, slowing the epidermal cell division. Occlusive dressings are not used with tars. Anthralin is a substance extracted from coal tar that suppresses mitotic activity. The anthralin may be mixed with salicylic acid in a stiff paste. The patient must be closely observed because anthralin is a strong irritant and can cause chemical burns. It is usually applied for no longer than 2 hours. Both coal tar and anthralin are commonly used in combination with UV light and are usually administered in inpatient settings or specialized outpatient clinics.

Topical preparations for the scalp are used in shampoo form. Teach the patient to read package instructions; these preparations generally need to be left in the hair for a period of time to work.

Ultraviolet light may be designated as UVB, shorter wavelength, or UVA, longer wavelength. UVA is from an artificial source, such as special mercury vapor lamps. The amount of exposure depends on the patient's condition, pigmentation, and susceptibility to burning. The patient must wear eye guards during treatments. Oral psoralen tablets (a photosensitizing agent) followed by exposure to UVA is called PUVA therapy. PUVA therapy temporarily inhibits DNA synthesis, which is antimitotic. Because psoralen is a photosensitizing agent, the patient must not only wear dark glasses during the treatment period, but also for the entire day after a treatment. The long-term safety of PUVA therapy is still unknown. Possible side effects include increased skin carcinomas, premature skin aging, and actinic keratosis (premalignant lesions of the skin). The patient should be observed closely for redness, tenderness, edema, and eye changes. Initial and follow-up eye examinations, skin biopsies, urinalysis, and blood tests may be ordered.

Retinoids are oral agents such as acitretin (Soriatane) that promote skin cell differentiation and inhibit malignancies from forming in the skin. They may be used in combination with UV therapy.

Antimetabolites, usually used for cancer chemotherapy, are reserved for the most severe cases. Methotrexate is the most common agent given. Because of its hepatotoxicity, it is contraindicated in patients with liver disease, alcoholism, renal disease, and bone marrow suppression. Other systemic agents, such as cyclosporine and etanercept (Enbrel) work by altering the immune system.

CRITICAL THINKING

Mrs. Long

■ Mrs. Long arrives at the health clinic stating that the shampoo prescribed for her scalp psoriasis is not working. She says that she washes her hair thoroughly with the medicated shampoo and then rinses completely. She wants to know why her scalp shows no signs of improvement. What additional information should you collect? What can you tell her?

Suggested answers at end of chapter.

Nursing Care

Nursing care for the patient with psoriasis is the same as nursing care for the patient with dermatitis. Teach the patient how to use prescribed medications and how to identify and avoid triggers. Explain that drinking alcohol can interfere with some treatments. In addition, consult with the physician about recommending small amounts of sunlight to help improve skin lesions.

INFECTIOUS SKIN DISORDERS

A variety of infections can affect the skin. The most common disorders are discussed in this section. See Table 54.3 for a summary of additional skin infections.

Herpes Simplex

Pathophysiology and Etiology

Herpes simplex virus (HSV) infection is a common viral infection that tends to recur repeatedly. There are two types of herpes simplex: that caused by type 1 virus (HSV-1), which occurs above the waist and causes a fever blister or cold sore (Fig. 54.4), and that caused by type 2 virus (HSV-2), which occurs below the waist and causes genital herpes. See Chapter 44 for information on genital herpes.

The primary infection occurs through direct contact, respiratory droplet, or fluid exposure from another infected person. Following the initial infection, the virus lies dormant in nerve ganglia near the spinal column, where the immune system cannot destroy it. The patient is asymptomatic at this time.

Recurrence of symptomatic infection can happen spontaneously or may be triggered by a stressor such as fever, sunburn, illness, menses, fatigue, or injury. The secondary lesion may appear isolated or as groups of small vesicles or pustules on an erythematous base. Crusts eventually form, and the lesions heal in about 1 week. The lesions are contagious for 2 to 4 days before dry crusts form.

Prevention

Avoidance of contact with a known infected lesion during the blistering phase can prevent the primary lesions. Patients should also be taught to avoid sharing contaminated items such as toothbrushes, lipsticks, and drinking glasses. This disease can recur spontaneously. Avoidance of stressors, such as sunburn, injury, and fatigue, may delay a recurrence. The use of sunscreens, especially on the lips, may be helpful.

Signs and Symptoms

Some patients may have a prodromal phase of burning or tingling at the site for a few hours before eruption. The area becomes erythematous and swollen. Vesicles and pustules erupt in 1 to 2 days. There may also be redness with no blistering. Lesions can burn, itch, and be painful. The attacks vary in frequency but diminish with age. The patient is contagious with each outbreak until scabs are formed.

Complications

If herpes simplex is present in the vagina at childbirth, the newborn may be infected (meningoencephalitis or a panvisceral infection may occur). If the person touches the affected area and then rubs the eyes, the eyes can become severely infected. Secondary bacterial infection of lesions can occur. Rarely, herpes encephalitis can occur. This is deadly if not treated promptly.

Diagnostic Tests

Cultures of the lesions provide a definitive diagnosis. Most lesions are diagnosed on the basis of history, signs, and symptoms.

Therapeutic Measures

There is no complete cure for herpes simplex. Recurrences will happen. Topical acyclovir (Zovirax) ointment is the drug of choice for primary lesions, to suppress the multiplication of vesicles. It does not benefit secondary lesions. Oral antivirals (acyclovir, famciclovir, or valacyclovir) may be recommended for severe or frequent attacks (six or more attacks per year) or for patients who are immunosuppressed. Various lotions, creams, and ointments may be prescribed to accelerate drying and healing of lesions (e.g., camphor, phenol, alcohol). Antibiotics may be indicated for secondary infections.

Herpes Zoster (Shingles)

Pathophysiology and Etiology

Herpes zoster, or shingles, is an acute inflammatory and infectious disorder that produces a painful vesicular eruption on bright red edematous plaques along the distribution of

TABLE 54.3 INFECTIOUS SKIN DISORDERS

Type	Description	Complications	Treatment/Nursing Care
Impetigo Contagiosa 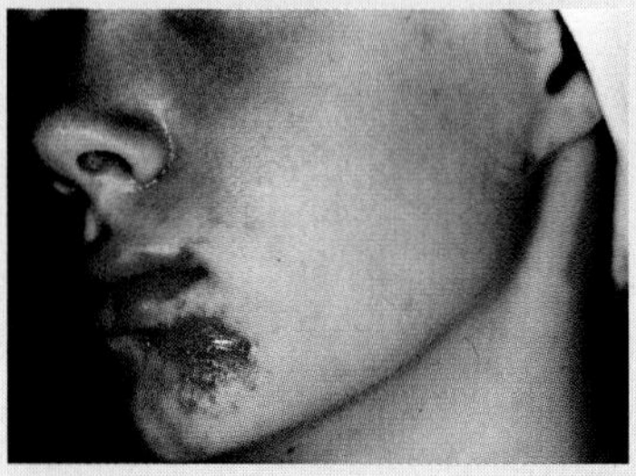 Impetigo on the face	Common contagious, infectious, inflammatory skin disorders usually caused by *Streptococcus* or *Staphylococcus aureus;* sources of infection include swimming pools, pets, dirty fingernails, beauty and barber shops, and contaminated clothing, towels, sheets; may occur secondary to scrapes, cuts, insect bites, burns, dermatitis, poison ivy. Primary skin infection can appear on exposed areas of the body (extremities, hands, face, neck) or skinfold areas (axillae). Rash appears as oozing, thin-roofed vesicle that rapidly grows and develops a honey-colored crust; crusts are easily removed, and new crusts appear; lesions heal in 1 to 2 weeks if allowed to dry.	Glomerulonephritis resulting from a particular strain of streptococcus infection. Lesions may spread from one skin area to another. Lesions may persist if not permitted to dry. Secondary **pyoderma**, or acute inflammatory purulent dermatitis, may occur if lesions are unresponsive to treatment.	Administer systemic antibiotics as prescribed. Topical antibiotics are used after crust removal. Wash gently with a mild soap, or soak with warm, moist compresses, to aid in removal of crusts and debris, and to provide a clean bed for topical therapy. Keep fingernails short and clean. Use gloves or hand mitts as necessary to prevent scratching. Patient must remain home until all lesions are healed. Teach proper disposal or washing of any material that comes in contact with lesions. Teach good hygiene to prevent skin-to-skin or person-to-person spread. Observe client for 6 to 7 weeks for signs/symptoms of glomerulonephritis.
Furuncles and Carbuncles	A furuncle is a small, tender boil that occurs deep in one or more hair follicles and spreads to surrounding dermis; may be single or multiple; usually caused by *Staphylococcus*; usually occurs on body areas prone to excessive perspiration, friction, and irritation (e.g., buttocks, axillae); can recur; the boil eventually comes to a soft yellow, black, or white head; there is localized pain, tenderness, and surrounding cellulitis; lymphadenopathy may be present. A carbuncle is an abscess of skin and subcutaneous tissue; deeper than a furuncle; usually caused by *Staphylococcus*; usually appears where skin is thick, fibrous, and inelastic (e.g., back of neck, upper back, and buttocks); associated symptoms may include fever, pain, leukocytosis, prostration.	Furuncles may progress to more severe carbuncles. Carbuncles may progress to infection of bloodstream. Further spread of infection can occur to self and others.	Assist physician with draining lesion. Administer antibiotics as ordered. Prevent trauma; avoid squeezing or irritation. Cleanse surrounding skin with antibacterial soap, followed by application of antibacterial ointment. Surgical incision and drainage may be performed. Cover draining lesion with dressing. Follow standard precautions. Double bag all soiled dressings and dispose of properly.

• WORD • BUILDING •
pyoderma: pyo—pus + derma—skin

TABLE 54.3 INFECTIOUS SKIN DISORDERS—cont'd

Type	Description	Complications	Treatment/Nursing Care
	Both tend to occur in debilitated clients, and more often with diabetes. Occasionally, scarring may occur. 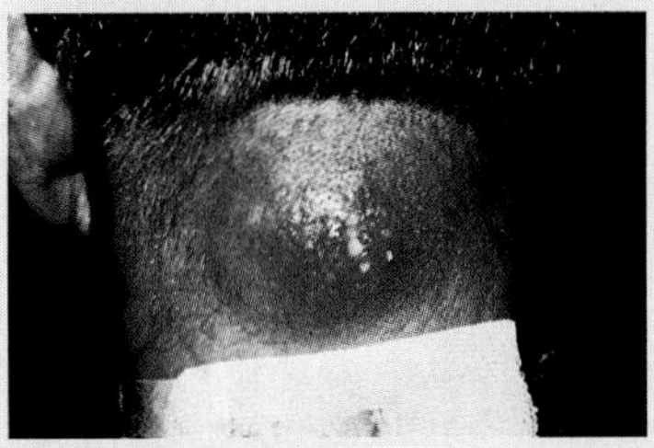 Carbuncle		Systemic antibiotic therapy is instituted for carbuncles or spreading furuncles. Analgesia and antipyretics are ordered as necessary. Bedrest is advised with carbuncles or furuncles on perineal or anal regions. Cover mattress and pillows with plastic and wipe daily with a disinfectant. Wash all linens, towels, and clothing after each use. Properly discard razor blades after each use. Maintain strict hand washing to prevent cross-contamination.

nerves from one or more posterior ganglia. This eruption follows the course of the cutaneous sensory nerve and is almost always unilateral (one sided) (Fig. 54.5).

Herpes zoster is caused by the varicella zoster virus—the same virus that causes chickenpox. After a case of chickenpox, the virus remains dormant in nerve tissue near the brain and spinal cord. Herpes zoster is a reactivation of this latent varicella virus. The incubation period of herpes zoster is 7 to 21 days. Vesicles appear in 3 to 4 days. Eruption usually occurs posteriorly and progresses anteriorly and peripherally along the dermatome. The total duration of the outbreak can vary from 10 days to 5 weeks.

This disease occurs most commonly in the elderly or in those who have a diminished resistance, such as the patient with acquired immunodeficiency syndrome (AIDS), the patient on immunosuppressant agents, or the patient with a malignancy or injury to the spine or a cranial nerve.

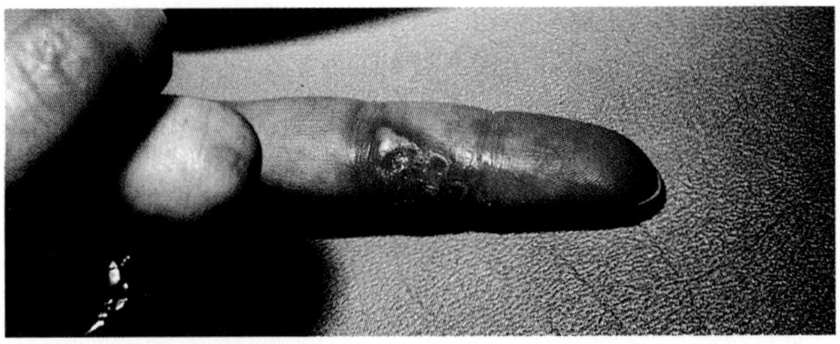

FIGURE 54.4 Herpes simplex. (From Goldsmith, L. A., Lazarus, G. S., & Tharp, M. D. [1997]. *Adult and pediatric dermatology* [p. 306]. Philadelphia: F. A. Davis, with permission.)

Prevention

Avoidance of persons with herpes zoster during the contagious phase (a few days before eruption until vesicles dry or scab) is the best prevention. Varicella vaccine (Varivax) in children and adults who have not had chickenpox can reduce the risk of becoming infected with varicella. Another new vaccine,

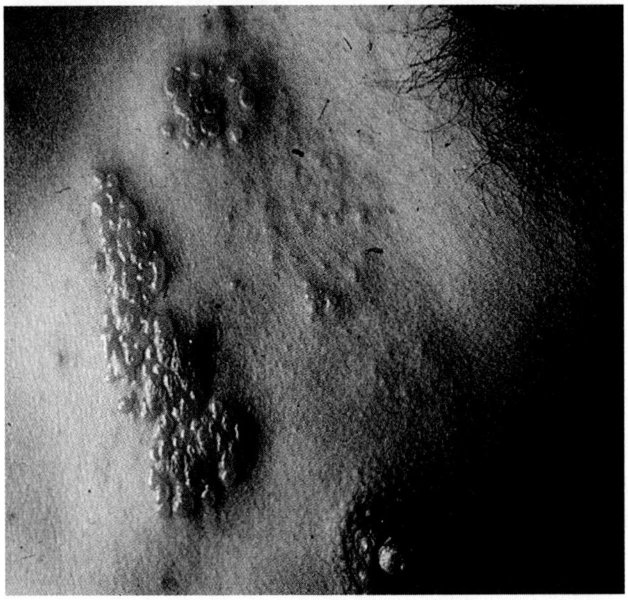

FIGURE 54.5 Herpes zoster (shingles). (From Goldsmith, L. A., Lazarus, G. S., & Tharp, M. D. [1997]. *Adult and pediatric dermatology* [p. 307]. Philadelphia: F. A. Davis, with permission.)

Zostavax, is recommended for all patients over age 60 who have had chickenpox. It reduces the risk of shingles outbreak, and reduces the severity if it does occur.

Signs and Symptoms

In addition to the vesicles and plaques, there may be irritation, itching, fever, malaise, and, depending on the location of lesions, visceral involvement. Lesions may be very painful; the incidence of pain increases with age.

Complications

Post-herpetic neuralgia, persistent dermatomal pain, and hyperesthesia are common in the elderly and can last for weeks to months after the lesions have healed. The incidence and severity of these complications increase with age.

Ophthalmic herpes zoster affects the fifth cranial nerve and can be a serious complication. Consultation with an ophthalmologist is imperative because this complication can affect eyesight. Other complications can occur with facial and acoustic nerve involvement, including hearing loss, tinnitus, facial paralysis, and vertigo. Full-thickness skin necrosis and scarring can occur if lesions do not heal properly; systemic infection can occur from scratching, causing the virus to enter the bloodstream.

Diagnostic Tests

Diagnosis is usually confirmed by history and physical examination of the patient and associated signs and symptoms. Cultures may be ordered if secondary bacterial infections are suspected.

Therapeutic Measures

Treatment is aimed at controlling the outbreak, reducing pain and discomfort, and preventing complications. Mild cases may heal without medication. Antiviral agents such as acyclovir are used for more severe cases, and are most effective if started within 72 hours of the onset of the rash. Analgesics may be prescribed for pain and discomfort. Anticonvulsants (gabapentin/Neurontin) or antidepressants (amitriptyline/Elavil) may also be effective for neuropathic pain.

Use of corticosteroids is controversial, but they may help reduce discomfort and improve quality of life when used with antiviral agents. Topical steroids should not be applied if a secondary infection is present because they suppress the immune system. Antihistamines can be administered to control itching. Antibiotics are prescribed for secondary bacterial infections.

In addition to medications, cool compresses or baths may help with pain and itching. Topical agents containing calamine or lidocaine may also be helpful.

Fungal Infections

Pathophysiology and Etiology

Dermatomycosis, or a fungal infection of the skin, occurs when there is an impairment of the skin integrity in a warm, moist environment. This infection occurs through direct contact with infected humans, animals, or objects. *Tinea* is the term used to describe fungal skin infections; the name used after tinea indicates the body area affected. For example, tinea capitis is a fungal infection of the scalp, and tinea pedis is the term used for athlete's foot. The term *candidiasis* is used when *Candida* is the infecting organism. Common fungal infections and treatments are described in Table 54.4.

• WORD • BUILDING •

dermatomycosis: derma—skin + myco—fungus + osis—condition

Cellulitis

Pathophysiology and Etiology

Cellulitis is inflammation of the skin and subcutaneous tissue resulting from infection, usually with *Staphylococcus* or *Streptococcus* bacteria. Methicillin-resistant *Staphylococcus aureus* (MRSA) is becoming a common cause, and is resistant to many antibiotics. Cellulitis can occur as a result of skin trauma; as a secondary bacterial infection of an open wound, such as a pressure ulcer; or it may be unrelated to skin trauma. It most often occurs in the extremities, especially the lower legs.

Prevention

Good hygiene and prevention of cross-contamination are important. If an open wound is present, preventing infection and promoting healing are critical.

Signs and Symptoms

The initial sign of cellulitis is a localized area of inflammation that may become more generalized if not treated properly. Common clinical manifestations include warmth, redness, localized edema, pain, tenderness, fever, and lymphadenopathy. The infection can worsen rapidly and become systemic if not treated properly.

Diagnostic Tests

Culture and sensitivity testing of any pustules or drainage is necessary to identify the infecting organism. Blood cultures may also be indicated to rule out bacteremia.

Therapeutic Measures

Topical and systemic antibiotics are prescribed according to culture and sensitivity test results. Debridement of nonviable tissue is necessary if an open wound is present. Systemic antibiotics are indicated if fever and lymphadenopathy are present.

Elevation of the extremity may reduce pain and swelling. Monitor vital signs and report hypotension and tachycardia, because such changes can indicate systemic infection. Measure the extremity daily to monitor progress. Outlining the affected area with a marker can also help monitor progress, but may be difficult if the borders are not clear.

Acne Vulgaris

Pathophysiology and Etiology

Acne vulgaris is a common skin disorder of the sebaceous glands and their hair follicles that usually occurs on the face, chest, upper back, and shoulders. The etiology is multifocal. The most common cause is hormonal changes during puberty.

TABLE 54.4 FUNGAL INFECTIONS

Type	Description	Treatment/Nursing Care
Tinea Pedis (Athlete's Foot)	Common fungal infection, most frequently seen in those with warm, moist, sweaty feet; occlusive shoes; or friction/trauma to the feet Four types: interdigital (between the toes), chronic hyperkeratotic (chronic plantar erythema and scaling), inflammatory/vesicular (vesicles on plantar surface), and ulcerative (vesicular lesions and ulcers between toes and on plantar surface).	Administer over-the-counter or prescription topical antifungal agents as ordered; may be oral in more severe or unresponsive cases. Apply topical agents in a thin layer; treat for time specified, even after apparent clearing. Antibiotics may be ordered for secondary bacterial infection. Wet dressings or vinegar soaks may be ordered to dry blisters. Teach patient prevention measures: keep feet dry; dry carefully between toes; apply foot powder to absorb perspiration; wear cotton socks to absorb perspiration; if weather permits, use perforated shoes or sandals; avoid plastic or rubber-soled shoes; wear water shoes in public showers and near swimming pools.
Tinea Capitis (Ringworm of Scalp)	Contagious fungal infection of the scalp; commonly causes hair loss in children. Appears as scattered round, red, scaly patches; small papules or pustules may be evident at edges of patches; hair is brittle at site, breaks off, and temporary areas of baldness result; mild itching, tenderness, and pain may be present. Kerion is a severe inflammation of the scalp with resulting alopecia that sometimes occurs with tinea capitis. 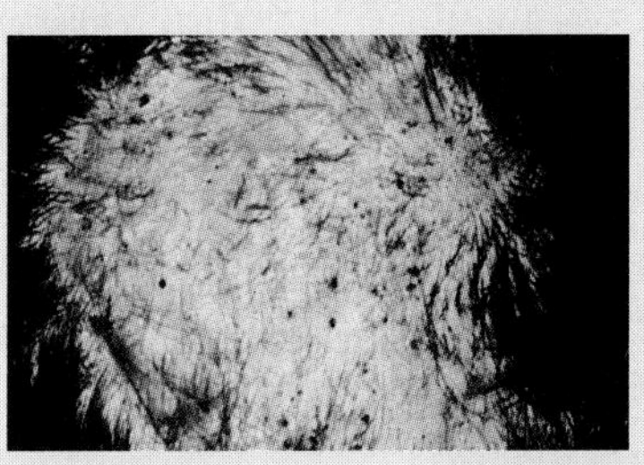 Tinea capitis	Administer systemic antifungals as prescribed; relapse rate is high with topical agents; review side effects with patient. Oral corticosteroids are indicated for kerion inflammation to help prevent alopecia; review side effects with client. Instruct family on contagious aspect of disease; assess other family members and pets for organism. Teach prevention measures: never share combs, brushes, pillowcases, or headgear.
Tinea Corporis (Tinea Circinata, Ringworm of Body)	Fungal infection of the body that appears as an erythematous macule; progresses to rings of vesicles or scale with a clear center that appears alone or in clusters; usually occurs on exposed areas of body; can be moderately to intensely itchy.	Topical antifungals are prescribed for small, localized lesions. Oral antifungals are indicated for severe, widespread, resistant, or follicular cases. Infected pet is common source of infection. Topical corticosteroids are prescribed for itching. Teach patient prevention measures: avoid heat, moisture, and friction; keep skin areas, especially folds, dry; use clean towel and washcloth daily; wear cotton clothing, especially on hot, humid days.

Continued

TABLE 54.4 FUNGAL INFECTIONS—cont'd

Type	Description	Treatment/Nursing Care
Tinea Cruris (Ringworm of Groin, Jock Itch)	Infection of groin, inner thighs, and buttocks area; may occur with tinea pedis; often in obese people who are athletic. Lesion first appears as a small red scaly patch and then progresses to a sharply demarcated plaque with elevated scaly or vesicular borders; itching can range from minimal to severe. 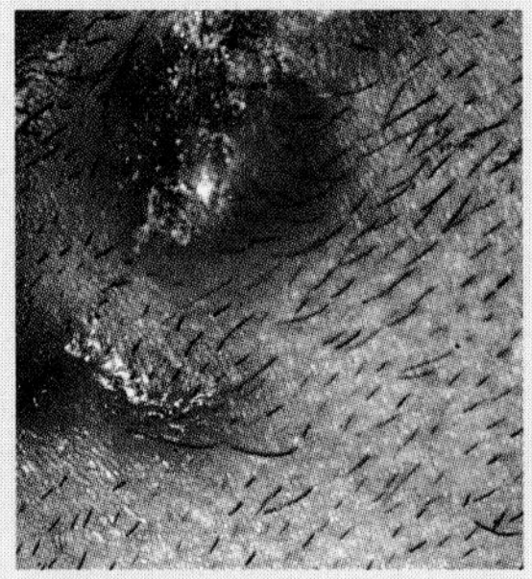 Tinea cruris	Topical antifungals are prescribed; apply in a thin layer to rash and a few centimeters beyond border. Unresponsive cases may require oral antifungal agent. Teach patient prevention measures: bathe daily and change to clean underwear. Avoid tight clothing. Do not share personal items. Treat tinea pedis to prevent spread.
Tinea Unguium (Ringworm of Nails, Onychomycosis)	Chronic fungal infection of nails, usually the toenails; a lifelong disease. There is yellow thickening of nail plate; it is friable and lusterless. Eventually crumbly debris accumulates under free edge of the nail and causes nail plate to become separated; over time, the nail may become thickened, painful, and destroyed. 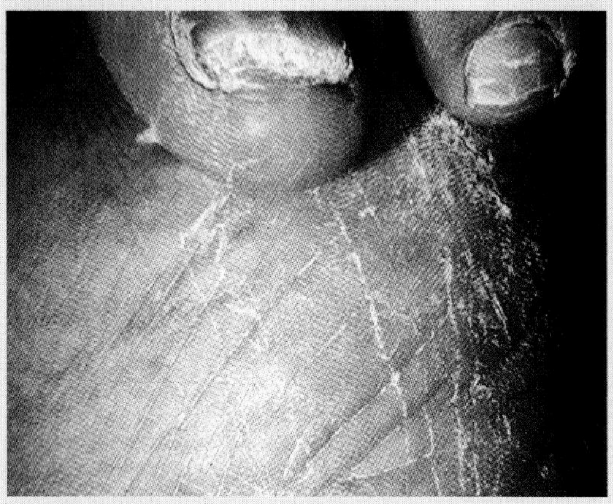 Onychomycosis (tinea unguium)	Systemic antifungals are rarely given for toenail involvement, but may be prescribed for fingernail involvement. Topical antifungals are usually ineffective because they do not penetrate nails. Nail may have to be surgically removed (nail avulsion). Explain high relapse rate to patient. Keep nails neatly trimmed and buffed flat; gently scrape out any nail debris.
Candidiasis/Thrush	Oral candidiasis is called thrush. Infection of skin or mucous membranes with *Candida*. Grows in warm moist areas such as under breasts, in groin, vagina, or oral mucous membranes. Appears as white patches in mouth, white vaginal discharge, or red irritated areas in skinfolds. May occur as a result of antibiotic therapy, because normal flora that usually keep *Candida* in check are destroyed, or with corticosteroid therapy.	Oral or topical antifungal agents are used. Examples include nystatin "swish and swallow" or lozenges for oral thrush, nystatin powder or ointment for skin infection, or vaginal suppositories or creams. Teach patient to keep skin clean and dry, especially in skinfold areas. Treatment is important to prevent systemic infection.

• WORD • BUILDING •

onychomycosis: onycho—fingernail or toenail + myco—fungus + osis—condition

The sebaceous glands are under endocrine control, especially the androgens. Stimulation of androgens (e.g., during adolescence or the menstrual cycle) in turn stimulates the sebaceous glands to increase sebum production. This, along with gradual obstruction of the pilosebaceous ducts with accumulated debris, ruptures the sebaceous glands, which causes an inflammatory reaction that may lead to papules, pustules, nodules, and cysts. Acne occurs when the ducts through which this sebum flows become plugged.

Other factors that influence the occurrence and severity of acne include a hereditary tendency, stress, and external irritants such as strong soaps or cosmetics. Acne is not related to diet, chocolate, sexual activity, or uncleanliness.

Prevention

Acne vulgaris occurs regardless of interventions; however, certain interventions can lessen the severity or prevent complications. Avoidance of "picking" pimples prevents further inflammation and scarring. The patient should avoid excessive washing, irritants, and abrasives.

Signs and Symptoms

The initial lesions are called comedones (singular: **comedo**). Closed comedones, or whiteheads, are small white papules with tiny follicular openings. These may eventually become open comedones, or blackheads. The color is not caused by dirt but by lipids and melanin pigment. Scarring occurs as a result of significant skin inflammation; picking can worsen inflammation and lead to further scarring. The resulting inflammation can lead to papules, pustules, nodules (Fig. 54.6), cysts, or abscesses.

Therapeutic Measures

Medical treatment helps prevent new lesions and helps control current lesions. Effective topical agents include benzoyl peroxide (Desquam-X, Benzagel), which is an antibacterial agent that may help prevent pore plugging; antibiotics (erythromycin, tetracycline) to kill bacteria in follicles; and vitamin A acid (Retin-A, tretinoin) to loosen pore plugs and prevent occurrence of new comedones. Topical agents may be used alone or in combination. It may take 3 to 6 weeks before improvement is seen.

All topical agents should be applied with clean hands to acne-prone areas, not just where the acne occurs. They must be applied to dry skin. Medications should not be applied near eyes, nasolabial folds, or the corners of the mouth because of the potential for irritation. If the patient is ordered a combination of topical agents, unless contraindicated, the tretinoin is used at night and the others in the morning or afternoon. Tretinoin can be neutralized if mixed directly with other agents. The patient must be careful with sun or sunlamp exposure while using tretinoin. Also, remind the patient that it may be necessary to continue treatment even after the skin clears.

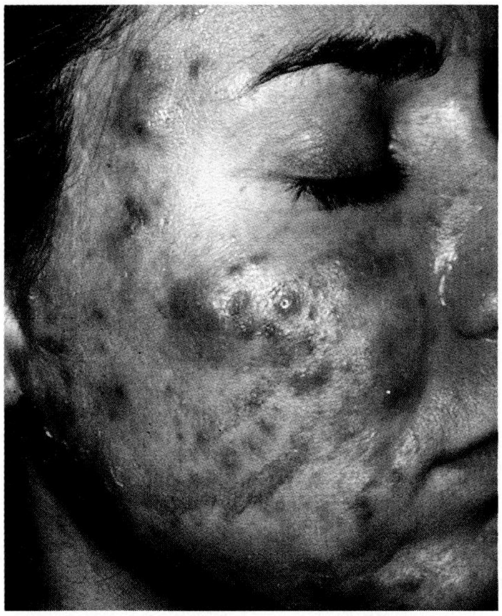

FIGURE 54.6 Acne vulgaris. (From Goldsmith, L. A., Lazarus, G. S., & Tharp, M. D. [1997]. *Adult and pediatric dermatology* [p. 351]. Philadelphia: F. A. Davis, with permission.)

Systemic antibiotics (long term, low dose) and isotretinoin (Accutane) are usually reserved for severe cases of acne; the patient must be closely monitored for side effects. Estrogen therapy (oral contraceptives) may also be prescribed for young women; however, the risks often outweigh the benefits. Women should be aware that some antibiotics reduce the effectiveness of oral contraceptives.

Other medical treatments include comedone extraction, cryosurgery (freezing with liquid nitrogen), mild peeling (UV light, carbon dioxide, liquid nitrogen, mild acid), dermabrasion (deep chemical peel), excision of scars, and injection of fibrin or collagen below the scars. These treatments depend on the severity, age, condition, and physician and patient preference.

> **NURSING CARE TIP**
>
> Topical benzoyl peroxide may bleach colored fabrics. Have the patient wear a white cotton T-shirt under clothing if benzoyl peroxide is used on the back, and use an old or white pillowcase at night.

Nursing Process for the Patient with a Skin Infection

Data Collection

Subjective data collection regarding a skin infection can begin with the WHAT'S UP? acronym. Determine the following:

- **W**here the skin infection is located;
- **H**ow it feels (does it itch, burn, hurt?); what
- **A**ggravates and Alleviates the symptoms; the
- **T**iming, or how long it has been present; how

- **S**evere it is; and
- **U**seful other data, such as whether there is swelling, drainage, or fever. The
- **P**atient's **P**erception is important because he or she may have information about the source or cause of the infection.

Collection of objective data includes observing the affected area and describing the infection in terms of type and configuration of lesions, color, size, and presence of drainage. Also observe for swelling, and check for elevated temperature. If the patient has cellulitis of an extremity, measure and document the circumference of the extremity daily and prn.

Determine the patient's understanding of the cause of the infection, and of infection control measures.

Nursing Diagnoses, Planning, and Implementation

Risk for Infection (Spread to Other Areas)

EXPECTED OUTCOME: The infected area will not spread to other areas on patient or to other individuals.

- Monitor and document size and location of infected area daily and prn. *Careful monitoring can identify improvement or new spread of infection.*
- Monitor temperature every 8 hours and prn. *An increasing temperature can indicate worsening or systemic infection.*
- Monitor for signs and symptoms of systemic spread of infection, such as hypotension, tachycardia, and increasing temperature. *Systemic infection must be reported and treated promptly to prevent complications, including sepsis.*
- Use standard precautions, including careful hand washing, when providing patient care *to prevent transmission to yourself or to others.*
- Implement appropriate isolation precautions for patients with a contagious infection. Contact precautions are usually sufficient, although airborne precautions may be necessary if immunocompromised individuals are present. *Isolation reduces spread of infection.*
- Instruct the patient on wound care, appropriate hand washing, and disposal of soiled dressings. *The patient must follow precautions to protect self and others.*
- Instruct patient on use of prescribed anti-infective agent, including the importance of taking it exactly as directed *to prevent development of a resistant infection.*
- For the patient with acne, advise keeping hands away from the face and avoiding touching or squeezing pimples. Keep hair clean and off the face. *These measures help prevent spread and secondary infection.*

Acute Pain Related to Inflammation as Evidenced by Patient Rating on Appropriate Pain Scale

EXPECTED OUTCOME: The patient will state that pain is controlled at an acceptable level.

- Monitor pain (if present) using a pain scale. *Pain assessment provides a basis for nursing intervention.*
- Administer analgesics as ordered, especially prior to dressing changes or treatments. *Analgesics relieve pain and help prevent pain during dressing changes.*
- For the patient with shingles:
  - Apply cool, moist compresses to painful or itching lesions to help cleanse and dry lesions and reduce itching.
  - Apply firm dressings such as wraps, stockings, or a snug T-shirt to reduce pain from post-herpetic neuralgia.
- For the patient with cellulitis:
  - Elevate affected extremity as ordered to reduce swelling and increase comfort.

Evaluation

If interventions have been effective, the skin lesions will improve, and will not spread to new areas or to others. The patient will state that pain is manageable.

PARASITIC SKIN DISORDERS

Pediculosis

Pathophysiology and Etiology

Pediculosis is an infestation by lice. There are three basic types: pediculosis capitis (head lice), pediculosis corporis (body lice), and pediculosis pubis (pubic, or crab, lice). Generally, the lice bite the skin and feed on human blood, leaving their eggs and excrement, which can cause intense itching. The lice are oval and are approximately 2 mm in length.

In pediculosis capitis, the female louse lays eggs (nits) close to the scalp, where the nits become firmly attached to hair shafts. The most common areas of infestation are the back of the scalp and behind the ears. The nits are about 1 to 3 mm in length and appear silvery white and glistening. Transmission is by direct contact or contact with infested objects, such as combs, brushes, wigs, hats, and bedding. It is most common in children and people with long hair.

Pediculosis corporis is caused by body lice that lay eggs in the seams of clothing and then pierce the skin. Areas of the skin usually involved are the neck, trunk, and thighs.

Pediculosis pubis is caused by crab lice. It is generally localized in the genital region, but it can also be seen on hairs of the chest, axillae, eyelashes, and beard. The lice are about 2 mm in length and have a crablike appearance. It is chiefly transmitted through sexual contact or to a lesser degree by infested bed linen.

Prevention

Prevention involves avoidance of contact with an infected person or object. Brushes, combs, hats, and other personal items should not be shared. Good personal hygiene and routine clothes washing are other preventive measures; however, even someone with meticulous hygiene can develop this infection if there is contact with the organism.

Signs and Symptoms

Pediculosis capitis can result in no itching or intense itching and scratching, especially at the back of the head. Nits may be noticeably attached to hair. A papular rash may be seen.

Pediculosis corporis may appear as tiny hemorrhagic points. Excoriations may be noted on the back, shoulders, abdomen, and extremities. It may also cause intense itching.

Pediculosis pubis results in mild to severe itching, especially at night. Black or reddish brown dots (lice excreta) may be noted at the base of hairs or in underclothing. Gray-blue macules may also be noted on the trunk, thighs, and axillae; this is the result of the insects' saliva mixing with bilirubin.

Complications

Secondary bacterial infections can occur with pediculosis capitis, resulting in impetigo, furuncles, pustules, crusts, and matted hair. Complications of pediculosis corporis include secondary infection and hyperpigmentation. Most important, body lice may be vectors for rickettsial or other systemic disease. Complications with pediculosis pubis include dermatitis and the coexistence of other sexually transmitted diseases.

Diagnostic Tests

Diagnosis is made through history and physical examination. The patient may also be tested for other sexually transmitted diseases if pediculosis pubis is present.

Therapeutic Measures

Medical treatment is aimed at killing the parasites and mechanically removing nits. Over-the-counter (OTC) pediculicides containing pyrethrins or permethrin are the most commonly recommended compounds. These agents should kill the lice and nits, although some lice develop pesticide resistance, making mechanical removal necessary. Permethrin (Nix) remains active for about a week, killing the adult lice immediately and the nits when they hatch days later. Pyrethrins (RID, A-200 Pyrinate) must be reapplied in 1 week to kill newly hatched lice.

If OTC medications are not effective, lindane may be prescribed. Lindane is a controversial, highly toxic topical medication that is only used as a second-line agent.

Complications are treated, as appropriate, with antipruritics, topical corticosteroids, and systemic antibiotics. Physostigmine ophthalmic ointment is applied to affected eyebrows and eyelashes. Other medications should not be applied to eyebrows or eyelashes.

Patient Education

Reassure the patient and family that head lice can happen to anyone, and this is not a sign of uncleanliness. Lice infestations are treated on an outpatient basis, so patient education is important. Package instructions should be followed for correct usage of all medications.

Instruct the patient to bathe with soap and water and to disinfect combs and brushes in hot, medicated soapy water. A fine-toothed comb dipped in vinegar can be used to remove nits from hairy areas. Nits can be removed from eyebrows and eyelashes with a cotton-tipped applicator after treatment. Clothing, linens, and towels should be laundered in hot water and detergent; unwashable clothing should be dry cleaned or sealed in a plastic bag for 10 days. Treatment should be started immediately to prevent rapid spread. Family members and close contacts (sexual contact with pediculosis pubis) should be examined for infestation and should put on clean clothing.

Shampoos and lotions kill nits, but they do not remove them. To loosen nits from the scalp, the hair may be soaked in a solution of equal parts vinegar and water and a shower cap worn for 15 minutes. Then comb the hair with a fine-toothed comb and thoroughly rinse or shampoo to mechanically remove the nits. Children may return to school after adequate medical treatment, even if dead nits are still present.

> **NURSING CARE TIP**
>
> It is not possible to dry clean or wash all infected items, such as mattresses and upholstered furniture. Teach patients to thoroughly vacuum upholstered furniture. The lice die in 3 to 4 days without human contact.

Scabies

Pathophysiology and Etiology

Scabies is a contagious skin disease caused by the mite *Sarcoptes scabiei.* It results from intimate or prolonged skin contact or prolonged contact with infected clothing, bedding, or animals (e.g., dogs, cats, other small animals). The parasite burrows into the superficial layer of the skin (Fig. 54.7). These burrows appear as short, wavy, brownish black lines. The patient is asymptomatic while the organism multiplies, but it is most contagious at this time.

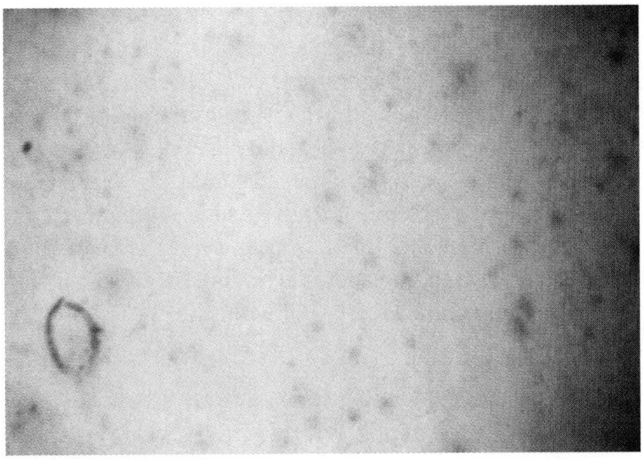

FIGURE 54.7 Scabies. (From Reeves, J. R., & Maibach, H. I. [1997]. *Clinical dermatology illustrated* [p. 236]. Philadelphia: F. A. Davis, with permission.)

Symptoms do not occur until almost 4 weeks after the time of contact.

Prevention

All persons (and animals) in intimate contact with an infected patient should be treated at the same time to eliminate the mites. The mites survive less than 24 hours without human contact. Therefore, bed linens, clothes, and towels should be washed, but furnishings need not be cleaned. Clean clothing and linens should be applied.

Signs and Symptoms

The major complaints are itching and rash. Itching can be intense, especially at night. The itching occurs about 1 month after infestation and may persist for days to weeks after treatment. The rash appears as small, scattered erythematous papules, concentrated in finger webs, axillae, wrist folds, umbilicus, groin, and genitals. Crusts and scales may be present. Male patients may have excoriated papules on the penis and groin area.

Complications

Hypersensitivity reactions to the mite can result in crusted lesions, vesicles, pustules, excoriations, and bacterial superinfections.

Diagnostic Tests

Diagnosis is confirmed by a superficial shaving of a lesion and microscopic evaluation for adult mites, eggs, or feces.

Therapeutic Measures

Topical scabicides (permethrin, crotamiton) are used for chemical disinfection. Usually, the cream or lotion is applied in a thin layer to the entire body from neck to feet (including genitals, umbilicus, and skinfold areas), is left on overnight (8 to 12 hours), and is washed off in the morning; however, package instructions should be referred to for each medication. One or two applications are usually curative, depending on the agent prescribed. Antipruritics may be prescribed for itching.

Patient Education

A warm soapy bath or shower removes scales and skin debris. Advise the patient to apply the topical medication as ordered; not to use scabicides repeatedly, because they can increase itching and cause further skin irritation; to follow medication directions; to treat family members and close contacts simultaneously to eliminate mites; to wear clean clothing; and to use clean linens. Remind the patient that itching may continue for up to 2 weeks after treatment, until the allergic reaction subsides. (Dead mites remain in the epidermis until exfoliated.)

> **NURSING CARE TIP**
>
> Animals infested with scabies should be treated by a veterinarian, so they won't infect humans.

PEMPHIGUS

Pathophysiology and Etiology

Pemphigus is an acute or chronic, serious skin disease characterized by the appearance of bullae (large fluid-filled blisters) of various sizes on otherwise normal skin and mucous membranes. The etiology is unclear, but it is known to be an autoimmune disorder. Sun exposure, genetic predisposition, and certain foods and drugs (e.g., penicillamine, captopril, and enalapril) may trigger the disorder. It usually occurs in patients from middle to older age. One type of pemphigus is associated with malignancy.

The autoimmune response that occurs in pemphigus causes a patient's own antibodies to attack the skin and mucous membranes and destroy the protein "glue" that holds the cells together. The result is skin that separates from itself, causing the characteristic blisters.

Signs and Symptoms

Successive crops of bullae suddenly appear on skin or mucous membranes. The bullae are fragile and flaccid. They enlarge, rupture, and form painful, raw, eroded, partial-thickness wounds that bleed, ooze, and form crusts. Pemphigus usually originates in the oral mucosa and then spreads to the trunk. Large areas of the body become involved.

Besides the appearance of the blisters, the patient experiences pain, burning, and itching. The lesions have a foul smell. Involvement of the oral mucosa can interfere with chewing, swallowing, and talking. The patient is in constant misery.

Complications

The major complication is a secondary bacterial infection. This disease has high associated morbidity and mortality rates.

Diagnostic Tests

A positive Nikolsky's sign is a characteristic finding. This occurs when there is sloughing or blistering of normal skin when minimal pressure is applied. A biopsy of a blister reveals acantholysis, or separation of epidermal cells from one another.

Therapeutic Measures

Treatment is aimed at controlling the disease, healing the skin, and preventing complications. Corticosteroids in large doses and immunosuppressants are prescribed to control the disease and bring about remission. Medicated mouthwashes may be prescribed for mouth lesions. Antibiotic and antifungal agents are prescribed as needed for secondary infections. Analgesics and antipruritics are prescribed according to the patient's specific signs and symptoms. Because of fluid, blood, and protein losses through the partial-thickness skin

• WORD • BUILDING •
pemphigus: pemphix—blister

injuries, a high-protein, high-calorie diet is recommended along with appropriate fluid replacement therapy.

Nursing Care

Monitor fluid balance with regular intake and output, body weight, and blood pressure measurement. Encourage the patient to maintain adequate fluid intake. Offer cool drinks often to lessen discomfort.

Tepid wet dressings or baths help lessen secondary infection, cleanse the area, decrease odor, and increase comfort. Potassium permanganate baths may decrease infection and clean and deodorize the area. Always thoroughly dissolve potassium permanganate crystals in a small container before adding to tub water. Undissolved crystals may further damage and burn the skin. Dry the patient thoroughly after the bath. Do not use tape on the patient because this may cause further blistering. Talcum powder may be used to keep the skin from sticking to linens and bedclothes.

Teach the patient to maintain meticulous oral hygiene. Explain the effects and side effects of medications. Teach the importance of avoiding sun exposure or other triggers. Spicy or acidic foods may exacerbate oral lesions. Even dentures and contact lenses can irritate tissues in some patients. Provide appropriate psychosocial support because of the length of illness, the chronic nature of the condition, and the physical appearance of lesions. Find additional information at www.pemphigus.org.

SKIN LESIONS

Skin lesions can be either benign (noncancerous) or malignant. Benign lesions are described in Table 54.5. Malignant lesions are discussed next. Also see Box 54.2, *Cultural Considerations.*

Malignant Skin Lesions

Pathophysiology and Etiology

The most common skin malignancies include basal cell carcinoma, squamous cell carcinoma, and malignant melanoma. The major cause of skin malignancies is overexposure to ultraviolet rays, most commonly sunlight. Other factors include being fair skinned and blue eyed, genetic tendencies, history of x-ray therapy, exposure to certain chemical agents (e.g., arsenic, paraffin, coal tar), burn scars, chronic osteomyelitis, and immunosuppressive therapy.

TABLE 54.5 BENIGN SKIN LESIONS

Type	Description	Treatment
Cyst	A saclike growth with a defined wall that may contain liquid, semifluid, or solid material. An epidermoid cyst is the most common type of cyst. It results from proliferation of epidermal cells in the dermis. Rarely, it is associated with carcinoma development. 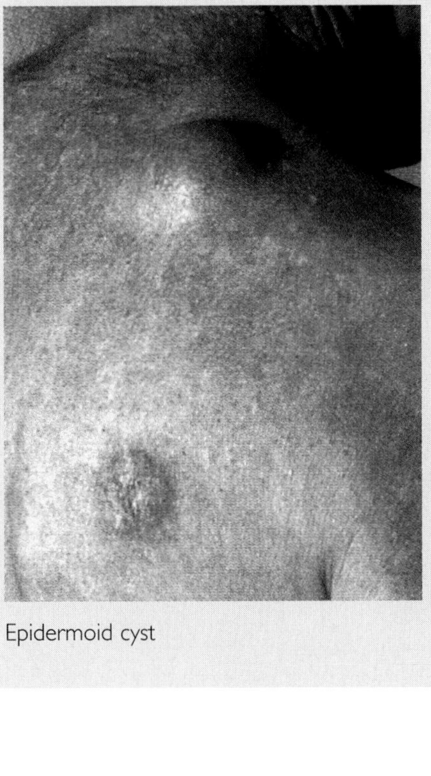 Epidermoid cyst	Not all cysts need to be treated. Treatments include intralesional steroid therapy, and antibiotics if indicated. If bothersome, they may be surgically excised. If excision is done, the entire cyst wall is removed to prevent recurrence.

Continued

TABLE 54.5 BENIGN SKIN LESIONS—cont'd

Type	Description	Treatment
Seborrheic Keratosis	A benign skin lesion with pigmented light tan to dark brown patches. The plaques or papules have a "stuck-on" appearance caused by the proliferation of epidermal cells and keratin piled on the skin surface. Cause is unknown, but it tends to occur in middle-aged to older patients, most commonly on the trunk, scalp, face, and extremities. 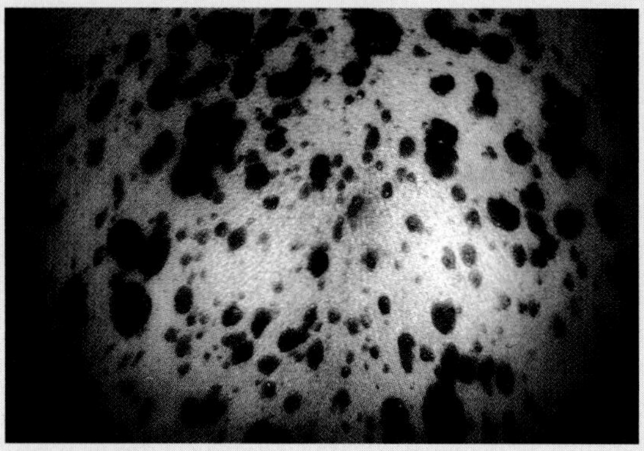 Seborrheic keratosis	Treatment is cosmetic only, or if lesion becomes irritated from friction. Topical agents may be used to reduce lesion size or height. Liquid nitrogen cryotherapy or light curettage may be performed if necessary for removal.
Keloid	A benign growth of fibrous tissue (scar formation) at the site of trauma or surgical incision; occurs in various sizes. Growth of tissue is out of proportion to what is needed for normal healing. The benign wartlike lesion or nodule extends beyond the original injury and occurs mainly in middle-aged and elderly clients and darker skinned patients.	Treatment varies, is not always successful, and is difficult; a larger scar may ensue. Some treatment options include compression therapy, corticosteroid injections into lesions, excision, and laser therapy.
Pigmented Nevus	A benign, flesh-colored to dark brown macule or papule located randomly over the entire skin surface of the body. Can be inherited or acquired and occurs mostly in light-skinned patients. Usually begin to appear between 1 and 4 years of age, increasing in number into adulthood. Some contain a few hairs. There are many variations. Rate of transformation to a malignant melanoma is higher in congenital moles and larger lesions. Clinical signs to observe for in differentiating between a mole and a melanoma include change in color or size; inflammation of surrounding skin; irregular borders; spreading borders; variegated colors, especially a bluish pigmentation; bleeding; and oozing, crusting, and itching. Usually nevi larger than 1 cm should be carefully examined. 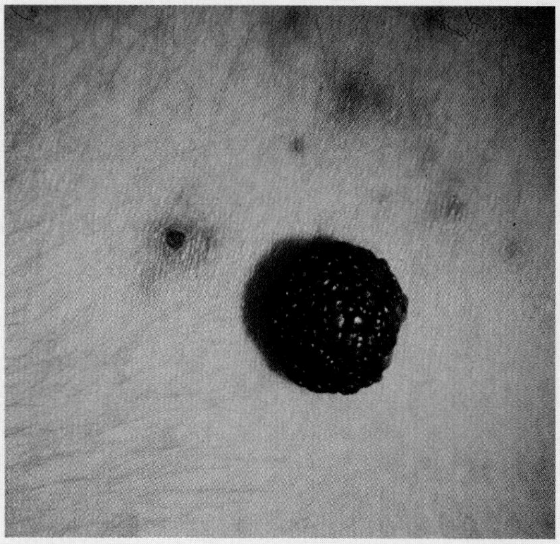 Dermal mole	Treatment is indicated for any of the previously listed indications of melanoma, unsightly nevi (cosmetic), repeated irritation (rubbing from belt, bra), trauma, large moles, and client report of a change in the mole. Surgical removal can include excision (preferred) or surgical shave. All excised moles should be sent for histological examination.

TABLE 54.5 BENIGN SKIN LESIONS—cont'd

Type	Description	Treatment
Wart	Small, common, benign growth of the skin resulting from the hypertrophy of the papillae and epidermis; caused by a virus. Common warts, often seen on hands and fingers, appear as raised, flesh-colored papules that have a rough surface. These warts may crack, fissure, bleed, and be painful to lateral pinching and direct, firm pressure. Plantar warts occur on the sole of the foot. They may appear granular, pitted, or protuberant, with a callous of surrounding normal skin. Incubation period can be several weeks to months. Virus is spread by direct contact into areas of broken skin or to other nails by nail cuticle biting. 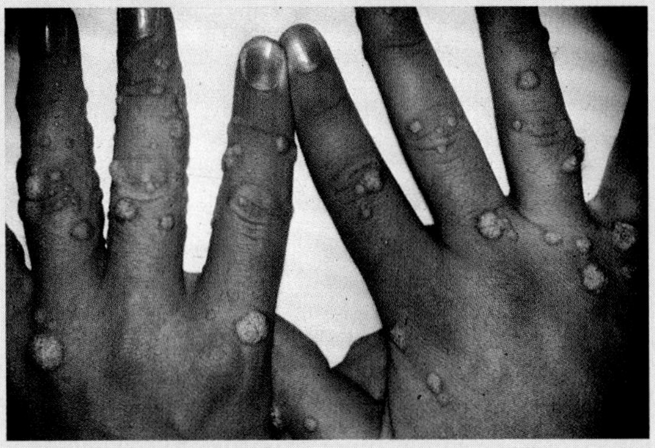 Warts	If no pain or discomfort, no treatment may be indicated. Patient should be cautioned not to spread lesions by picking or biting them. Treatment is indicated for symptomatic warts and for cosmetic purposes. General treatments include kerolytic agents (e.g., salicylic acid plasters) to soften and reduce keratin; cryotherapy (liquid nitrogen); and light electrodesiccation and curettage (requires local anesthesia). Treatment of choice is usually cryotherapy because local anesthesia is not necessary and it leaves little scarring.
Hemangioma (Angioma)	Benign vascular tumor of dilated blood vessels that can have varied clinical manifestations Nevus flammeus involves mature capillaries on the face and neck. It is a congenital neoplasm that appears as a pink-red to bluish purple macular patch. Port-wine stains or port-wine angiomas appear as violet-red macular patches, usually singular lesions, growing proportionately as the child grows. These lesions can persist indefinitely. Cherry hemangiomas are commonly seen in the elderly patient. They appear as small round papules that can vary in color from red to purple.	Nevus flammeus is usually treated for cosmetic reasons. Port-wine stains, if large enough, may require surgical excision with skin grafting. Pulse-dye laser therapy may also be used. Cosmetics to camouflage the affected area are also available. Treatment for cherry hemangiomas is usually not prescribed, except for cosmetic purposes.

Basal cell carcinoma arises from the basal cell layer of the epidermis. It is the most common type of skin cancer. This tumor is mainly seen on sun-exposed areas of the body. The lesion appears as a small pearly or translucent papule with a rolled, waxy edge, depressed center, telangiectasia (lesion formed by dilation of vessels), crusting, and ulceration (Fig. 54.8). Metastasis is rare, although it may be locally invasive.

Squamous cell carcinoma arises from the epidermis. This tumor can occur on sun-exposed areas of the skin and mucous membranes and is mainly seen on the lower lip, neck, tongue, head, and dorsa of the hands. It can occur on normal skin or on a preexisting lesion (actinic keratosis). The lesion appears as a single, crusted, scaled, eroded papule, nodule, or plaque (Fig. 54.9). A neglected lesion appears more rough, scaly, and darker colored. The lesion is fragile and prone to oozing and bleeding. Untreated squamous cell carcinoma can metastasize to distant areas of the body.

Malignant melanoma, as the name implies, is a malignant growth of pigment cells (melanocytes) (Fig. 54.10). It is highly metastatic, with a higher mortality rate than basal or squamous cell carcinomas. This tumor can occur anywhere on the body, and about half arise from preexisting nevi or moles. There are three general types: lentigo maligna, superficial spreading, and nodular.

Lentigo maligna melanoma appears as a slow-growing dark macule on exposed skin surfaces (especially the face) of elderly patients (Fig. 54.11). The lesion has irregular borders and brown, tan, and black coloring. Prognosis is good if treated in the early stage.

Box 54.2

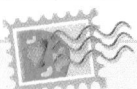

Cultural Considerations

- Some African American men have facial hair that is kinky, curls back on itself, and penetrates the skin, which can result in pustules and small keloids. Many use depilatories or electric razors to prevent nicking the skin, which can also cause keloids.
- Darker skinned people have an increased incidence of birthmarks and Mongolian spots compared with lighter skinned people. Mongolian spots disappear over time. The nurse must be cautious not to mistake these spots for bruising, which can indicate injury or abuse.
- Darker skinned people have a tendency toward an overgrowth of connective tissue components concerned with the protection against infection and repair after injury. Keloid formation is one example of this tendency toward overgrowth of connective tissue. Lymphoma and systemic lupus erythematosus may occur due to this overgrowth of connective tissue.
- For people with light skin, such as those of German, Polish, and Irish descent, prolonged exposure to the sun may increase the incidence of skin cancer. Teach patients to protect themselves from sun exposure to reduce their risk of skin cancer. Nevi (freckles and skin discolorations) occur more often in lighter skinned individuals. They are most common in European Americans, followed by Asians, and then darker skinned African Americans.

Superficial spreading melanoma is the most common melanoma. It can occur anywhere on the body and is usually seen in middle-aged persons. The lesion appears as a slightly elevated plaque with an irregular border. The coloring of the lesion varies in combinations of black, brown, and pink. The fragile surface may bleed or ooze. Eventually the plaque develops into a nodule. The cure rate is excellent when it is in the plaque phase; prognosis is poor with the nodular phase.

Nodular melanoma occurs suddenly as a spherical papule or nodule on the skin or in a mole. Coloration is blue-black, blue-gray, or reddish blue color that may have a rim of inflammation. The lesion is fragile and bleeds easily. Metastasis occurs rapidly. This type of melanoma has the least favorable prognosis. Early diagnosis and treatment is imperative.

Prevention

Risk of most types of skin cancer can be reduced by limiting or avoiding direct exposure to ultraviolet rays (sun, tanning booths). If exposure to the sun is necessary, exposure should be avoided during its highest intensity (10 a.m. to 4 p.m.). The patient should use a protective sunscreen with sun protection factor (SPF) of 15 or more. The patient should also wear sun-protective clothing, such as hats and long sleeves. The patient should seek medical advice if there is a change in color, size, shape, sensation, or character of a lesion or mole.

Diagnostic Tests

A preliminary diagnosis can be based on the appearance of the lesion. A definitive diagnosis is made by biopsy. Other

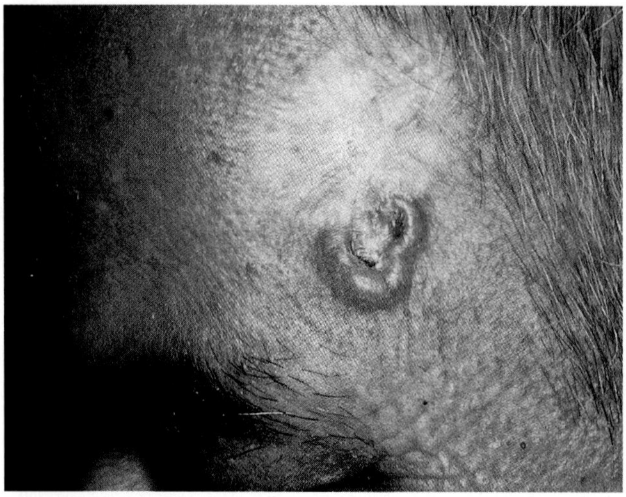

FIGURE 54.8 Basal cell carcinoma. Note pearly, flesh-colored papule with depressed center and rolled edge. (From Goldsmith, L. A., Lazarus, G. S., & Tharp, M. D. [1997]. *Adult and pediatric dermatology* [p. 158]. Philadelphia: F. A. Davis, with permission.)

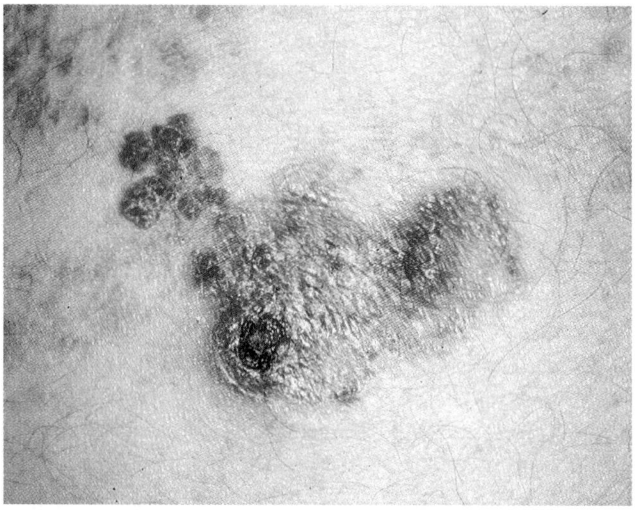

FIGURE 54.9 Squamous cell carcinoma. Surface is fragile and bleeds easily. (From Goldsmith, L. A., Lazarus, G. S., & Tharp, M. D. [1997]. *Adult and pediatric dermatology* [p. 237]. Philadelphia: F. A. Davis, with permission.)

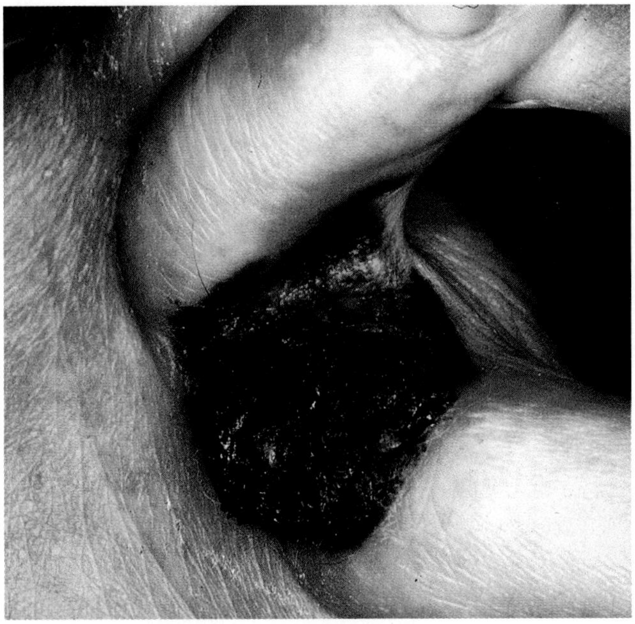

FIGURE 54.10 Malignant melanoma. (From Goldsmith, L. A., Lazarus, G. S., & Tharp, M. D. [1997]. *Adult and pediatric dermatology* [p. 137]. Philadelphia: F. A. Davis, with permission.)

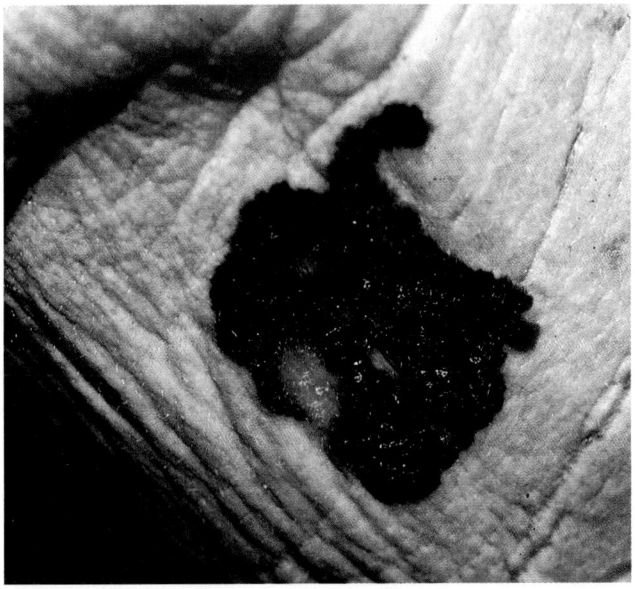

FIGURE 54.11 Lentigo maligna. (From Goldsmith, L. A., Lazarus, G. S., & Tharp, M. D. [1997]. *Adult and pediatric dermatology* [p. 55]. Philadelphia: F. A. Davis, with permission.)

tests are performed based on the results of the pathological examination.

Therapeutic Measures

Medical treatment depends on the type, thickness, and location of the lesion; the stage of the disease; and the age and general health of the patient. Generally, lesions are surgically excised with a 1- to 2-cm margin to make sure no cancer cells remain. Regional node dissection varies; it may be advised if the nodes in the area drain to one group. Grafting may be necessary for closure or repair. Chemotherapy may be used for metastasis. Radiation therapy may be used as adjunct treatment, or may be recommended for patients with a deeply invasive tumor or those who are poor surgical risks. Other therapies that also may be used include cryosurgery and curettage and electrodesiccation.

Nursing Care

Perform a complete skin examination. Palpate lesions to determine texture, size, and firmness. Document size, location, color, surface characteristics, pain, discomfort, itching, and bleeding. Note when the patient first discovered the lesion.

Nursing care of the patient with cancer is documented in Chapter 11. Specific nursing care related to cryosurgery includes preparing the patient for the procedure. Minor discomfort can be expected with little or no local anesthesia. Expect swelling, local tenderness, and hemorrhagic blister formation 1 to 2 days after the procedure. After the procedure, the area is cleansed as ordered and prescribed ointments are applied.

Specific nursing care for curettage and electrodesiccation includes preparing the patient for the procedure. After local anesthesia, a dermal curette is used to scrape away the lesion, followed by electrodesiccation of the remaining wound; the wound heals by secondary intention, usually with minimal scarring. After the procedure the wound is cleansed and dressed as prescribed.

NURSING CARE TIP

To help patients find melanomas as early as possible, encourage them to examine their skin regularly for lesions that fit this profile:

- An asymmetrical shape
- An irregular or poorly defined border
- A variable color
- A diameter larger than that of a pencil eraser
- A changing appearance

Urge patients to contact their physician right away if they find a lesion with these characteristics.

DERMATOLOGICAL SURGERY

Plastic or reconstructive surgery is performed to correct certain defects, scars, and malformations, as well as to restore function or prevent further loss of function. This type of surgery is usually an elective procedure; it may be prescribed by the physician or it may be the wish of the patient in hopes of improving his or her body image. Common types of plastic surgical procedures are listed in Table 54.6. Care of the surgical patient is covered in Chapter 12.

TABLE 54.6 COMMON PLASTIC SURGICAL PROCEDURES

Operation	Description	Purpose	Possible Complications	Postoperative Nursing Care Considerations
Rhinoplasty (Nose)	Removal of excessive nasal cartilage, tissue, or bone; reshaping of nose	Correct congenital or acquired septal defects; improve cosmetic shape of nose	Hemorrhage, hematoma; temporary ecchymosis and edema; infection, septal perforation	Monitor dressing and packing for bright-red bleeding; monitor vital signs and level of consciousness; maintain semi-Fowler's position to minimize edema.
Blepharoplasty (Eyelid)	Incisions on upper and lower lids with excision of fat and skin and primary closure	Removal of bags under eyes and wrinkles and bulges	Corneal injury; hematoma; ectropion; rarely visual loss and wound infection	Eye dressings; antibiotic ointment around eyes and lids; discoloration and swelling usually subside in about 10 days; maintain semi-Fowler's position to minimize edema.
Rhytidoplasty (Face)	Incision anterior to ear with removal of excessive skin and tissue; the subcutaneous tissue and fascia are folded and stretched	Removal of excessive wrinkling or sagging skin	Hemorrhage; hematoma; ecchymosis, and edema (temporary); wound infection, facial nerve damage	Surgical improvement lasts from 5 to 10 years; apply antibiotic ointment to suture line; maintain semi-Fowler's position to minimize edema.
Otoplasty (Ear)	Incision of ear for correction of defect	Correct congenital defects; correct deformities; improve cosmetic shape of ear	Hemorrhage; hematoma; edema; wound infection	Ear dressing for about 1 week; protect ear at times of sleep for about 3 weeks.

Home Health Hints

- A wound-measuring device that will not be misplaced is your hand. Measure your hand, such as the nailbed of a particular finger or the space between joints. Use these as a guide to determine wound measurements.
- Sanitary pads make great cushions for bony prominences. You can also place them in a cotton sock for better molding.
- A handheld shower head is useful for debriding some leg ulcers. Do not use it if it is too painful.
- To relieve pruritus (itchy skin), oatmeal baths are sometimes prescribed. An inexpensive way to do this is to place a half cup of quick-cooking oatmeal in a cotton sock. Put it under the faucet as you fill the tub and ring out the sock.
- Instruct patients to prevent red, dried, cracked skin on hands by wearing gloves outside in the cold or windy weather to prevent chapping, avoiding overheating the house, using a humidifier to keep the air moist, applying hand lotion two or three times a day and after each hand washing, using soaps with added oil and avoiding those with deodorants, using sunscreen with an SPF factor of at least 15, and stopping smoking (smoking reduces blood flow to the skin).
- If necessary, a specialty bed or mattress can be obtained to use in a patient's home.
- Instruct patients who are confined to a wheelchair to rise up briefly, using their armrests, and shift weight every 15 minutes to prevent pressure ulcers.
- Instruct patients with dressings to keep them clean and dry. Unless the patient or caregiver has been instructed on how to perform the dressing change, inform him or her to contact the home care agency if the dressing falls off.
- A patient can wear a cast shoe over a dressing on his or her foot. This will help protect the dressing and provide additional support for the patient while ambulating.
- Surgi-net, or a similar stretchy cover, can be used to cover dressings for patients with tape sensitivities. They are also good for additional support to prevent a dressing from falling off.

SUGGESTED ANSWERS TO

CRITICAL THINKING

■ *Mr. Russ*

- The nurse should assess the patient's mobility and bed surface. A specialty pressure-relieving bed may be appropriate for the patient.
- Change patient's position at least every 2 hours if not more frequently. Keep patient's heels off of the bed at all times by propping them on pillows.
- Request a dietary consult because the body cannot meet the increased healing demands if there is an albumin deficiency. Patients will need increased protein (contraindicated in renal failure). They also need fats, carbohydrates, vitamins, and minerals for wound healing. A dietitian can help determine the amounts of calories and types of foods for the best healing.
- If the patient is able to sit up in a chair, provide a chair cushion to prevent skin breakdown.
- If the patient is wearing a brace or a splint that must be removed, examine the underlying tissue for pressure areas. Braces and splints must be padded to avoid skin breakdown.

■ *Mrs. Long*

You should ask how long she is leaving the shampoo in her hair. For medicated scalp shampoos to work properly, they must remain on the scalp for several minutes. Package instructions should be carefully checked for each product because they vary from product to product.

REVIEW QUESTIONS

1. Psoriasis is an inflammatory skin disorder that is characterized by which underlying pathology?
   a. Epidermal proliferation
   b. Excessive subcutaneous fat
   c. Herpes infection
   d. Excessive melanin production

2. What information is most important for the nurse to teach patients about avoiding malignant skin lesions?
   a. Shower or bathe daily.
   b. Avoid contact with allergens and irritants
   c. Avoid overexposure to ultraviolet rays
   d. Avoid others with malignant lesions

3. Which of the following actions by the nurse is appropriate when caring for the patient with dermatitis?
   a. Bathe in hot oatmeal baths.
   b. Dry vigorously to prevent moisture buildup.
   c. Apply gloves to hands at night.
   d. Apply a thick layer of the prescribed topical agent.

4. A patient develops several wounds on the sacrum and buttocks in spite of being turned and repositioned regularly. Which factors may have contributed to the patient's skin breakdown? **Select all that apply.**
   a. The patient is 20 pounds overweight.
   b. The patient commonly slides down in the chair.
   c. Staff use a lift sheet to move the patient in bed.
   d. The patient sits in a chair most of the day.
   e. The patient is often diaphoretic.
   f. The patient is incontinent of urine and stool.

5. Which instruction should the nurse provide to the patient being treated for scabies?
   a. "Dry-clean all linens, towels, and clothes."
   b. "Wash linens, towels, and clothes."
   c. "Discard infested mattresses."
   d. "Remove infested pets from the home."

6. A patient diagnosed with impetigo contagiosa wants to know when the disease will no longer be contagious. Which response by the nurse is correct?
   a. One week after treatment is started
   b. After spread of lesions has stopped
   c. After all the lesions crust over
   d. When all lesions are healed

References

Blume, P. A., Walters, J., Payne, W., et al. (2008). Comparison of negative pressure wound therapy using vacuum-assisted closure with advanced moist wound therapy in the treatment of diabetic foot ulcers: A multicenter randomized controlled trial. *Diabetes Care 31*(4), 631–636.

National Pressure Ulcer Advisory Panel. (2007). *Pressure ulcer stages revised by NPUAP.* Retrieved May 24, 2010, from http://www.npuap.org/pr2.htm

55

Nursing Care of Patients with Burns

RITA BOLEK TROFINO

KEY TERMS

autograft (AW-toh-graft)
epithelialization (ep-ih-THEE-lee-al-eye-ZAY-shun)
escharotomy (ess-kar-AHT-oh-mee)
hemochromogen (HEEM-oh-KROH-moh-jen)

QUESTIONS TO GUIDE YOUR READING

1. How would you explain the pathophysiology of burns?
2. What current therapeutic measures are used for burns?
3. What data should you collect when caring for patients with burns?
4. What nursing care will you provide for patients with burns?
5. How will you know if your nursing interventions have been effective?

Many people are hospitalized each year for burns. Burns affect not only the skin but every major body system. Smoke inhalation and wound infections complicate care of the patient who has been burned.

PATHOPHYSIOLOGY AND SIGNS AND SYMPTOMS

Burns are wounds caused by an energy transfer from a heat source to the body, heating the tissue enough to cause damage. Locally, the heat denatures cellular protein and interrupts the blood supply. The three zones of tissue damage that occur with burns are described in Figure 55.1.

The amount of skin damage is related to (1) the temperature of the burning agent, (2) the burning agent itself, (3) the duration of exposure, (4) the conductivity of tissue, and (5) the thickness of the involved dermal structures. Alterations in normal skin functioning resulting from a major burn injury include loss of protective functions, impaired ability to regulate temperature, increased risk of infection, changes in sensory function, loss of fluids, impaired skin regeneration, and impaired secretory and excretory functions.

Systemic Responses

Alterations in the functional capacity of the skin in response to a burn affect virtually all major body systems.

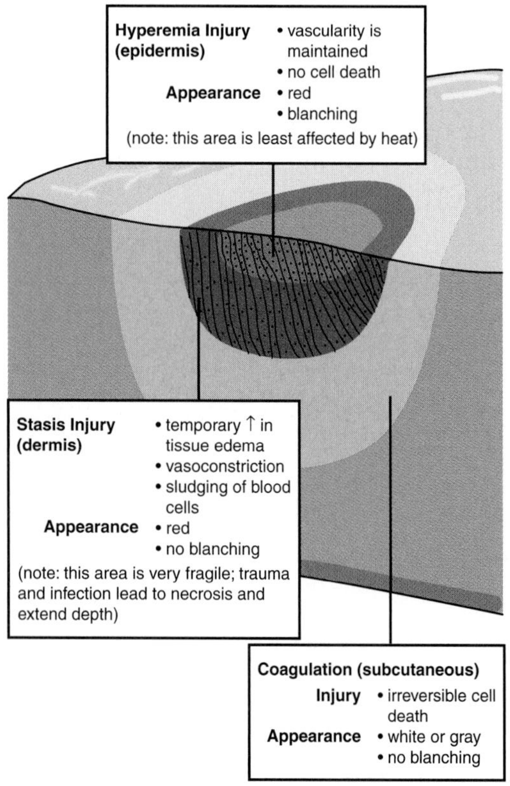
Hyperemia Injury (epidermis)
• vascularity is maintained
• no cell death
Appearance • red
• blanching
(note: this area is least affected by heat)
Stasis Injury (dermis)
• temporary ↑ in tissue edema
• vasoconstriction
• sludging of blood cells
Appearance • red
• no blanching
(note: this area is very fragile; trauma and infection lead to necrosis and extend depth)
Coagulation (subcutaneous)
Injury • irreversible cell death
Appearance • white or gray
• no blanching

FIGURE 55.1 Three zones of tissue damage. (Modified from Ruppert, S. D., Kernick, J. G., & Dolan, J. T. [1996]. *Dolan's critical care nursing* [p. 942]. Philadelphia: F. A. Davis, with permission.)

Fluid Balance

Following a major burn, increased capillary permeability leads to the leakage of plasma and proteins into the tissue, resulting in the formation of edema and loss of intravascular volume. There is also water loss by evaporation through the burned tissue that can be 4 to 15 times normal. Increased metabolism leads to further water loss through the respiratory system.

Cardiac Function

A burn is followed by an initial decrease in cardiac output, which is further compromised by the loss of circulating plasma volume. Severe hematologic changes resulting from tissue damage and vascular changes occur in patients with major burns. Plasma moves into the interstitial space because of increased capillary permeability. In the first 48 hours after a burn, fluid shifts lead to hypovolemia and, if untreated, hypovolemic shock. Loss of intravascular fluid causes a relative increase in hematocrit, and red blood cells are destroyed. The intense heat decreases platelet function and half-life. Leukocyte and platelet aggregation may progress to thrombosis.

Metabolic Changes

Metabolic demands are very high in patients with burns. A high metabolic rate proportional to the severity of the burn is usually maintained until wound closure. This hypermetabolism is further compromised by associated injuries, surgical interventions, and the stress response. Severe catabolism also begins early and is associated with a negative nitrogen balance, weight loss, and decreased wound healing. Elevated catecholamine (epinephrine, norepinephrine) levels are triggered by the stress response. This, along with elevated glucagon levels, can stimulate hyperglycemia.

Gastrointestinal Problems

A few of the gastrointestinal problems that can develop with a major burn include gastric dilation, peptic ulcers, and paralytic ileus. Most of these problems occur in response to fluid shifting, dehydration, opioid analgesics, immobility, depressed gastric motility, and the stress response.

Renal Function

Acute renal insufficiency can occur as a result of hypovolemia and decreased cardiac output. Fluid loss and inadequate fluid replacement can lead to decreased renal blood flow and glomerular filtration rate. With an electrical burn injury, renal damage can occur from direct electrical current or the formation of myoglobin casts (because of the muscle destruction), which can cause acute renal tubular necrosis.

Pulmonary Effects

Pulmonary effects are mostly related to smoke inhalation. However, hyperventilation may occur with any moderate to major burn injury, usually proportional to the severity of the burn. Oxygen consumption increases because of the hypermetabolic state, fear, anxiety, and pain.

Immune Function

With the skin destroyed, the body loses its first line of defense against infection. Major burns also depress immunoglobulins IgA, IgG, and IgM.

Evaluation of Burn Injuries

The severity of a burn injury is determined by the depth of tissue destruction (Table 55.1 and Figs. 55.2, 55.3, and 55.4), percentage of body surface area injured, cause of the burn, age of the patient, additional injuries, medical history (e.g., heart disease, diabetes), and location of the burn wound.

CRITICAL THINKING

Mr. Weinberg

■ Mr. Weinberg is admitted to the hospital with superficial and deep partial-thickness burns. His wife asks how long it will take for the burns to heal. What should you tell her?
Suggested answer at end of chapter.

The size of a burn wound is estimated based on parts of the body affected. A quick and common method is the Rule of Nines. This method divides the body into segments whose areas are either 9% or multiples of 9% of the total body surface, with the perineum being counted as 1% (Fig. 55.5). This formula is easy, but it is not as accurate when assessing children. A more accurate method uses a table with a relative anatomical scale or diagram that estimates total burned area by ages and by smaller anatomical areas of the body.

LEARNING TIP

For a quick estimation of percentage of burn injury, using the Rule of Nines on an adult burn patient, the palm of your hand is about 1%.

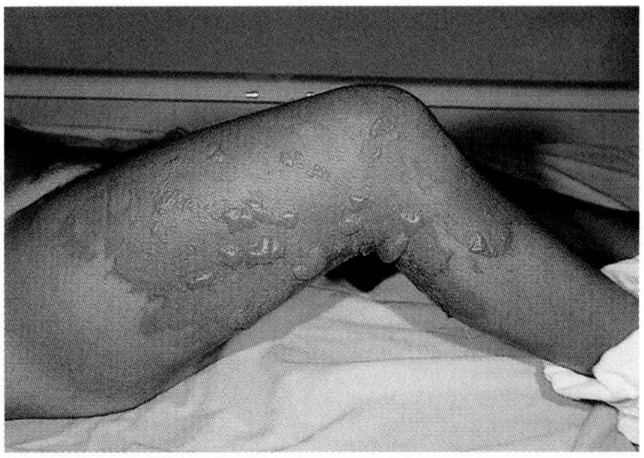

FIGURE 55.2 Partial-thickness burn. (From Trofino, R. B. [1991]. *Nursing care of the burn-injured patient* [plate 1]. Philadelphia: F. A. Davis, with permission.)

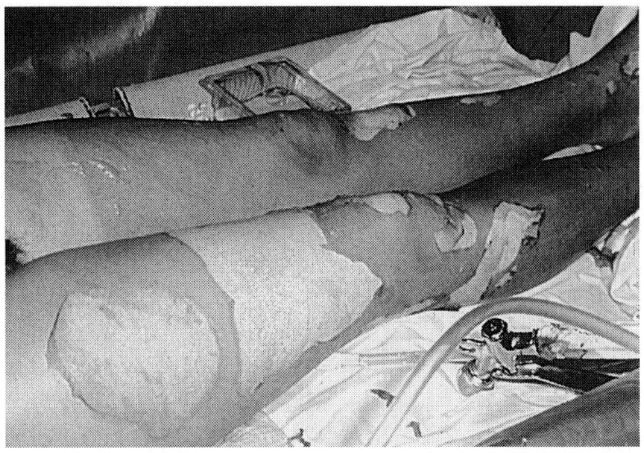

FIGURE 55.3 Partial-thickness burn. (From Trofino, R. B. [1991]. *Nursing care of the burn-injured patient* [plate 2]. Philadelphia: F. A. Davis, with permission.)

TABLE 55.1 CLASSIFICATION OF BURN DEPTH

Classification	Formerly	Areas Involved	Appearance	Sensitivity	Healing Time
Partial thickness (superficial)	1st degree to 2nd degree	Epidermis Papillae of dermis	Bright red to pink. Blanches to touch. Serum-filled blisters. Glistening, moist.	Sensitive to air, temperature, and touch.	7–10 days.
Partial thickness (deep)	2nd degree	Epidermis, 1/2 to 7/8 of dermis	Blisters may be present. Pink to light red to white. Soft and pliable. Blanching present.	Pressure may be painful due to exposed nerve endings.	14–21 days. May need grafting to decrease scarring.
Full thickness	3rd degree to 4th degree	Epidermis Dermis Tissue Muscle Bone	Snowy white, gray, or brown. Texture is firm and leathery. Inelastic.	No pain because nerve endings are destroyed, unless surrounded by areas of partial-thickness burns.	Needs grafting to complete healing.

Source: Trofino, R. B. (1996). Nursing management of the patient with burns. In S. Ruppert, J. Kernick, & J. Dolan (Eds.), *Dolan's critical care nursing* (p. 943). Philadelphia: F. A. Davis.

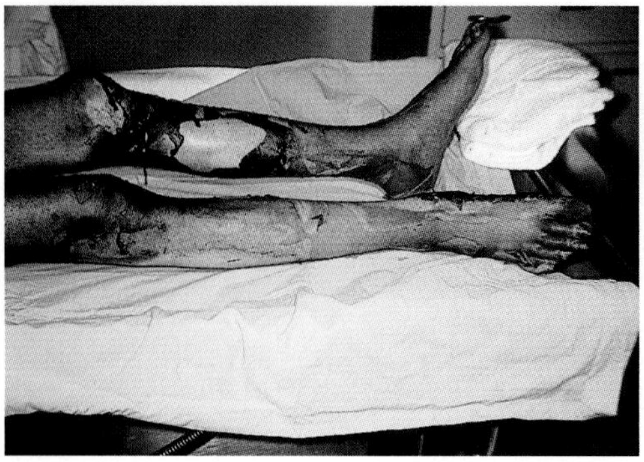

FIGURE 55.4 Full-thickness burn. (From Trofino, R. B. [1991]. *Nursing care of the burn-injured patient* [plate 3]. Philadelphia: F. A. Davis, with permission.)

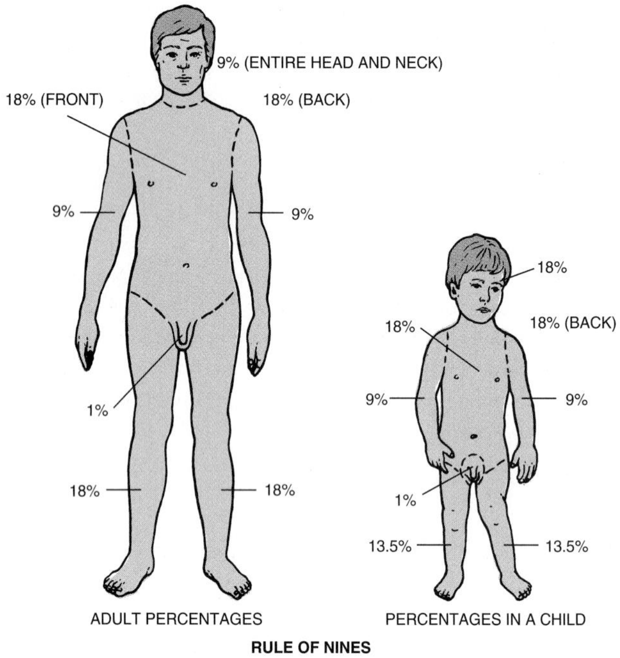
9% (ENTIRE HEAD AND NECK)
18% (FRONT)
18% (BACK)
9%
9%
1%
18%
18%
18%
18% (BACK)
18%
9%
9%
1%
13.5%
13.5%
ADULT PERCENTAGES
PERCENTAGES IN A CHILD
RULE OF NINES

FIGURE 55.5 Estimation of extent of burn injury. (From Venes, D. [Ed.]. [2009]. *Taber's cyclopedic medical dictionary* [21st ed., p. 2057]. Philadelphia: F. A. Davis, with permission. Beth Anne Willert, MS, dictionary illustrator.)

ETIOLOGY

Burn injuries have many causes. The most common causes include flames, contact burns, scalding, and chemical, electrical, and radiation burns. Table 55.2 summarizes common causes; see also Box 55.1, *Gerontological Issues*.

COMPLICATIONS

A major complication that can occur with a flame burn in an enclosed space is inhalation injury. An inhalation injury is a major cause of morbidity and mortality associated with burn injuries. Treatment of an inhalation injury takes precedence over other injuries. Infection is another common complication with a major burn. The incidence of infection increases with the size of the burn wound because the first line of defense against microorganisms is the skin.

Neurovascular compromise can also occur with a major burn. Eschar formation creates pressure and contributes to decreasing blood flow to areas distal to the burned area. Other systemic complications were reviewed in the *Systemic Responses* section earlier in this chapter.

> **CRITICAL THINKING**
>
> ***Mrs. Rivera***
>
> ■ Mrs. Rivera is admitted to the emergency department after sustaining injuries from a house fire. Both arms and hands are burned, she has a right leg fracture and a possible neck fracture, her lips are swollen, her face is sooty, and she is spitting up grayish, blackish sputum.
>
> 1. What is your priority concern with all of these injuries?
> 2. An IV is ordered at 1 L over 4 hours. How many milliliters per hour should be set on the controller?
> 3. Approximately what percent of her body is burned?
>
> *Suggested answers at end of chapter.*

DIAGNOSTIC TESTS

Burns are diagnosed by physical assessment. Various diagnostic tests are performed for systemic reactions, infection, and other complications. Common laboratory tests include complete blood cell count (CBC) and differential, blood urea nitrogen (BUN), serum glucose and electrolytes, serum protein and albumin levels, urinalysis, urine cultures, and clotting studies. If an inhalation injury is suspected, arterial blood gases, bronchoscopy, and carboxyhemoglobin levels are done. X-rays, electrocardiogram, and wound cultures are completed if indicated.

THERAPEUTIC MEASURES

Therapeutic interventions vary according to the severity of the burn and the stage the patient is in. Treatment is managed over three overlapping stages (Table 55.3).

Emergent Stage

At the time of injury, the burning process must be stopped. The clothes are removed, and the wound is cooled with tepid water and covered with clean sheets to decrease shivering and contamination. The burn wound itself is a lower priority than the ABCs (airway, breathing, circulation) of trauma resuscitation. Emergency rescuers at the scene will stabilize

TABLE 55.2 COMMON CAUSES OF BURNS

Flame	House fire is a common cause. Usually associated with an inhalation injury. Flash injury occurs from a sudden ignition or explosion.
Contact	Hot tar, hot metals, or hot grease produce a full-thickness injury on contact.
Scald	A burn from hot liquid. More common in children younger than age 5 and adults older than age 65. With an immersion scald, there are usually no splash marks; usually involves lower regions of body.
Chemical	Usually occurs in an industrial setting. Extent and depth of injury are directly proportional to concentration and quantity of agent, duration of contact, and chemical activity and penetrability of agent.
Electrical	One of the most serious types of burn injury; can be full thickness with possible loss of limbs, as well as cause internal injuries. Entry wound is usually ischemic, charred, and depressed. Exit wound may have an explosive appearance. Extent of injury depends on voltage, resistance of body, type of current, amperage, pathway of current, and duration of contact. Bones offer greatest resistance to the current; can have much damage. Tissue fluid, blood, and nerves offer least resistance; therefore, the current travels this path.
Radiation	Can occur in an industrial setting, as a result of treatment of disease, or from ultraviolet light (sun or tanning salons). Severity depends on type of radiation, duration of exposure, depth of penetration, distance from source, and absorbed dose.

the victim by establishing an airway, ensuring oxygenation, inserting an IV line, and stabilizing fractures, hemorrhage, spine immobilization, and other injuries. Inhalation injury is suspected if the patient sustained a burn from a fire in an enclosed space or was exposed to smoldering materials, if the face and neck were burned, if there are vocal changes, or if the patient is coughing up carbon particles. Intravenous (IV) fluids are given to prevent and treat hypovolemic shock. The patient is treated for pain with appropriate IV opioid analgesics.

Box 55.1 Gerontological Issues

Burn Injury and the Older Adult

According to the Centers for Disease Control and Prevention (2009), unintentional injuries from fires and burns are the fifth most common cause of death in the United States. Older adults are among the six risk groups.

Research by Burton et al. (2009) found that "patients who die from burns tend to be older, present in the hospital during the winter months, and suffer more acute burns to the torso or multiple body regions." Older age was also associated with increased length of hospital stay.

Prevention measures should consider visual and auditory changes as well as mobility impairments the older adult needs to overcome. Individuals must be able to evacuate in case of a fire and seek help if a burn injury occurs. Nurses should target the most common activities that may lead to fire or burn injury: smoking and cooking.

An accurate history of the injury is obtained to determine severity, probable complications, and any associated trauma. The patient's medical history is also obtained. Admission to the facility and burn care treatment are explained to the patient and family.

NURSING CARE TIP

If the patient is unable to communicate effectively, interview all involved family members to determine the cause of the injury, as well as past and current medical history and medications the patient is taking. Getting a full description of the cause of the injury may lead to the detection of other injuries that may not be readily visible.

TABLE 55.3 STAGES OF BURN CARE

Stage	Duration
I (Emergent)	From onset of injury to completion of fluid resuscitation
II (Acute)	From start of diuresis to near completion of wound closure
III (Rehabilitation)	From wound closure to return of optimal level of physical and psychosocial function

Source: Trofino, R. B. (1996). Nursing management of the patient with burns. In S. Ruppert, J. Kernick, & J. Dolan (Eds.), *Dolan's critical care nursing* (p. 948). Philadelphia: F. A. Davis.

Acute Stage

If the patient is in a facility with a special burn unit, multidisciplinary care from a burn team is provided during the acute stage. Management goals include wound closure with no infection, minimum scarring, maximum function, maintenance of comfort as much as possible, adequate nutritional support, and maintenance of fluid, electrolyte, and acid-base balance. The patient continues to be medicated for pain as needed, especially before painful treatments. Patient-controlled analgesia (PCA) is very effective. Nutritional support may be maintained via nasogastric feeding tube (Box 55.2, *Nutrition Notes*).

The wound is cleansed and debrided daily to promote healing, prevent infection, and provide a clean bed for grafting. Wound cleansing is achieved by showering using a shower trolley or shower chair and bedside care.

Debridement, or the removal of nonviable tissue (eschar), can be mechanical, chemical, surgical, or a combination of these methods. Mechanical debridement can involve the use of scissors and forceps to manually excise loose nonviable tissue, or the use of wet-to-moist or wet-to-dry fine-mesh gauze dressings (see Chapter 54). Chemical debridement involves the use of a proteolytic enzymatic debriding agent that digests necrotic tissue. Surgical debridement is the excision of full-thickness and deep partial-thickness burns. This method is followed by application of a skin graft.

If the patient has a circumferential burn (one that surrounds an extremity or area), an increase in tissue pressure secondary to tissue edema occurs. The burn then acts like a tourniquet, impeding arterial and venous flow. Common sites for these burns are the extremities, trunk, and chest. If this occurs on the chest and trunk, respiratory insufficiency can occur as a result of restricted chest expansion. An **escharotomy** may be immediately needed to relieve pressure. An escharotomy is a linear excision through the eschar to the superficial fat that allows for expansion of the skin and return of blood flow or chest expansion (Fig. 55.6).

Box 55.2
Nutrition Notes

Burns

A major burn is the most extreme state of stress a patient can sustain, producing a hypermetabolic state that raises energy needs to as much as 8000 calories per day. Even someone who was well nourished before being burned may rapidly develop protein-calorie malnutrition and remain in a hypermetabolic state for many weeks.

The body's response to severe stress is driven by hormonal changes that affect the storage, breakdown, and utilization of various nutrients. Consequently, multiple means are used to monitor a patient's status, and a team effort is required to frequently revise nutrient prescriptions to avoid both underfeeding and overfeeding (also a cause of complications).

The first concern is replacement of fluid that is lost through the burned area and provision of sufficient fluid to excrete waste products of metabolism. The next concern is meeting the patient's energy needs because, if nutrients are not available from external sources, the body breaks down muscle tissue for energy.

As in other conditions, tube feeding (often into the small intestine rather than the stomach) is preferred to intravenous nutrition if the patient can tolerate it. The patient's condition and ability to use the nutrients dictates the mode of nutrition implemented. A high-protein, high-calorie diet is ordered for most burn patients as soon as oral intake is medically feasible. Complete oral nutritional supplements are commonly used to increase the patient's caloric and protein intake.

NURSING CARE TIP

Remember to provide adequate padding of the bed prior to an escharotomy, because this procedure can be accompanied by copious amounts of drainage. Provide for appropriate disposal of the drainage.

Once the area is cleaned, the burn dressing and topical treatment are prescribed. The type of dressing and topical agent chosen depend on the area involved, the extent and depth of injury, and physician preference. Several common topical agents are listed in Table 55.4.

Dressings may be open, closed, biological, synthetic, or a combination. The open method is the use of a topical agent without any dressing. The closed method involves the

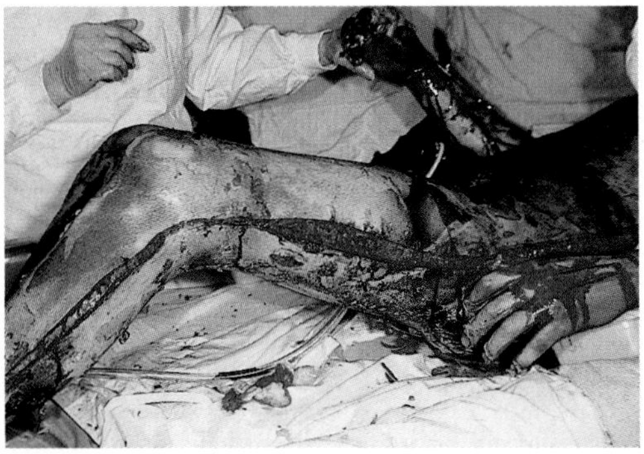

FIGURE 55.6 Escharotomy. (From Trofino, R. B. [1991]. *Nursing care of the burn-injured patient* [plate 16]. Philadelphia: F. A. Davis, with permission.)

• **WORD • BUILDING** •
escharotomy: eschara—scab + otomy—incision

TABLE 55.4 COMMON TOPICAL ANTIBIOTIC AGENTS

Examples	Route	Side Effects	Nursing Implications
Broad-Spectrum Antibiotics			
silver sulfadiazine 1% cream (Silvadene)	Topical	Intermediate penetration of eschar Leukopenia	Buttered on in thick layer. Covered with light dressings once or twice a day.
mafenide acetate (Sulfamylon)	Topical	Pain on application Pulmonary toxicity Metabolic acidosis Inhibited wound healing Hypersensitivity	Buttered on. Open exposure method. Applied three to four times daily.
silver nitrate solution 0.5%	Topical	Poor penetration of eschar Ineffective on established wound infections Can cause an electrolyte imbalance Discoloration of wound and environment makes assessment difficult.	Applied with wet dressings. Change bid. Resoak every 2 hours.
bacitracin	Topical	Poor penetration of eschar Not effective in reducing sepsis in large burns Occasional allergic sensitivity	Buttered on. Reapply every 4–6 hours.
gentamicin	Topical	Pain on application	Apply gently three to four times daily.
mupirocin (Bactroban)	Topical	Burning, itching, pain on application	Apply three times daily.
neomycin/bacitracin/polymyxin (Neosporin)	Topical	Rare allergic reaction	Apply one to three times daily.

use of an occlusive dressing over the wound. General principles for dressings include the following:

1. Limit the bulk of the dressing to facilitate range of motion.
2. Never wrap skin-to-skin surfaces (e.g., wrap fingers or toes separately; place a donut gauze dressing around the ear).
3. Base dressings on the size of wounds, absorption, protection, and type of debridement.
4. Wrap extremities from distal to proximal to promote venous return.
5. Do not wrap dressings too tightly. Check peripheral pulses often.
6. Elevate affected extremities.

The term *biological dressing* refers to a dressing that uses tissue from living or deceased humans (cadaver skin) or deceased animals (e.g., pigskin) or to cellular dressings that may use animal tissue, human tissue, or synthetics. Biological dressings assist with wound healing and stimulate **epithelialization**. These dressings may be used as donor site dressings, to manage a partial-thickness burn, and to cover the clean, excised wound before autografting. Some cellular wound dressings have varied layers that form a matrix onto which the patient's own cells migrate over a few weeks to form a new dermis. A very thin layer of the person's own skin is then grafted onto this new dermis.

Synthetic dressings are used in the management of partial-thickness burns and donor sites. These dressings are more readily available, less costly, and easier to store than biological dressings. They are made from a variety of materials and come in many different sizes and shapes. Most of these dressings contain no antimicrobial agents.

Biological and synthetic dressings are used as temporary wound coverings over clean partial- and full-thickness injuries. They act as skin substitutes to help maintain the wound surface until healing occurs, a donor site becomes available, or the wound is ready for autografting.

Skin Grafts

An **autograft** is a skin graft from the patient's unburned skin that is placed on the clean excised burn. The two common types of autografts are the split-thickness skin graft (STSG), which includes the epidermis and part of the dermis, and the full-thickness skin graft (FTSG), which includes the epidermis and entire dermal layer.

An STSG (0.006 to 0.016 inch, or 0.15 to 0.41 mm) may be applied as a sheet graft or a meshed graft. A sheet graft is used for cosmetic effect, such as for a face, neck, upper chest, breast, or hand burn. It is placed on the area as a full sheet. A meshed graft is passed through a mesher that produces tiny splits in the skin, similar to a fishnet, with openings in the shape of diamonds (Fig. 55.7), to permit the skin to expand one and a half to nine times its original size. The meshing

• WORD • BUILDING •
epithelialization: epi—over + thele—nipple + ization—condition

• WORD • BUILDING •
autograft: auto—self + graft—tissue transplant

allows for coverage of a large burn area with a small piece of skin by stretching it and securing it with sutures or staples. A mesh graft is especially useful when a patient's burns are extensive, resulting in few available donor sites. Graft "take," or vascularization, is complete in about 3 to 5 days.

FTSGs (0.035 to 0.040 inch, or 0.9 to 1.02 mm) can be sheet grafts or pedicle flaps. They are used over areas of muscle mass, soft tissue loss, hands, feet, and eyelids. They are not used for extensive wounds because the donor sites usually require an STSG for closure, or closure from the wound edges. A pedicle graft or flap is a skin flap and subcutaneous tissue that is still attached at one corner by a "pedicle" to a blood supply (artery and vein); it is then attached to an adjacent area in need of grafting. Once the distal part of the graft takes, it remains in place and the flap is divided, with the remainder returning to the original site. Pedicle flaps are not as popular as free skin flaps because they require more than one surgery and take longer for the graft site and donor site to heal. Table 55.5 provides a comparison of split-thickness and full-thickness grafts.

Donor sites are considered partial-thickness wounds. Donor sites usually heal in 10 to 14 days, but this depends on the thickness and method of grafting and the general health of the patient. Treatment for the donor site varies with the individual patient, the area of the body, and physician preference. Considerations for care include promoting comfort and preventing trauma and infection. Use of semiocclusive, transparent dressings, such as Op-Site, Biobrane, or Tegaderm, allows for a moist healing environment and is associated with reduced risk of infection. The donor site is very painful. Appropriate pain medications are provided, along with nonpharmacological measures (e.g., back rubs or distraction).

With any type of graft, the patient must keep the graft site immobilized until the graft takes, to prevent movement or slippage of the grafted skin. Dressings may be bulky to assist in immobilization. These dressings must not be disturbed. The involved area requires frequent circulatory checks, including assessment of color, warmth, sensation, pulses, and capillary refill. Any involved extremities must be elevated to maintain circulation. Table 55.6 describes factors that affect graft viability. A graft has been successful if there is good adherence of the graft to the wound with no evidence of necrosis or infection.

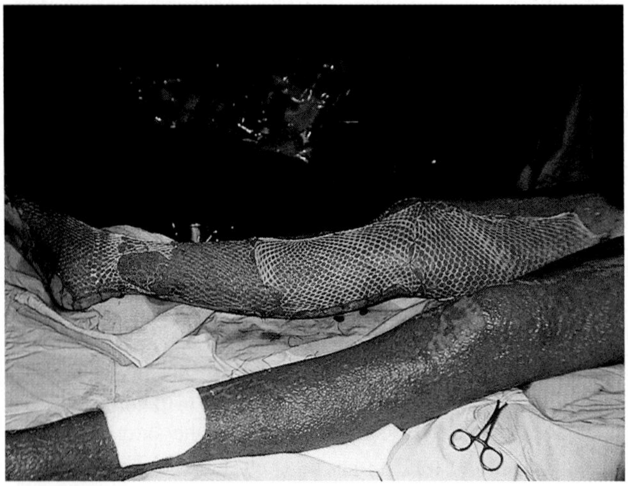

FIGURE 55.7 Meshed graft. (From Trofino, R. B. [1991]. *Nursing care of the burn-injured patient* [plate 17]. Philadelphia: F. A. Davis, with permission.)

TABLE 55.5 COMPARISON OF SPLIT-THICKNESS AND FULL-THICKNESS SKIN GRAFTS

	Split-Thickness Graft	Full-Thickness Graft
Layers	Epidermis Partial layer of dermis	Epidermis. Entire dermal layer.
Advantages	Donor site may be reused. Healing of donor site is more rapid, results in good "take."	Allows more elasticity over joints. Can reconstruct cosmetic defects. Soft, pliable. Gives full appearance. Provides good color-match. Less hyperpigmentation. May allow hair growth.
Disadvantages	Prone to chronic breakdown. Likely to hypertrophy. More likely to contract.	Donor site takes longer to heal. Requires split-thickness graft to heal or closure from wound edges.

Source: Konop, D. (1991). General local treatment. In R. Trofino (Ed.), *Nursing care of the burn-injured patient* (p. 61). Philadelphia: F. A. Davis.

Rehabilitation Phase

The therapy started during the acute phase continues in the rehabilitation phase. There is wound closure, and the goal is to return the patient to an optimum level of physical and

TABLE 55.6 FACTORS AFFECTING GRAFT VIABILITY

Factors That Inhibit Graft Viability	Factors That Promote Graft Viability
Infection	Adequate hemostasis
Necrotic skin (tissue)	Anatomical location of graft
Anatomic location of graft:	Smooth contour
Perineum	Nonjoint areas
Axillae	Graft secured well
Buttocks	Immobilization of graft area
Poor-quality donor skin	Good nutritional status
Poor nutritional status	
Bleeding	
Mechanical trauma	
Shock	

Source: Konop, D. (1991). General local treatment. In R. Trofino (Ed.), *Nursing care of the burn-injured patient* (p. 62). Philadelphia: F. A. Davis.

psychosocial function. This may take months to years to accomplish, depending on the extent of the injury. Reconstructive surgeries may be ongoing for many years.

Two things to keep in mind when caring for the patient with a major burn are that (1) the most comfortable position (flexion) is the position of contracture, and (2) the burn wound will shorten until it meets an opposing force. To avoid contractures (Fig. 55.8), a specific exercise program is begun 24 to 48 hours after injury, along with the use of splinting devices to maintain proper positioning and stretching. Hypertrophic scarring, or a proliferation of scar tissue, can be minimized or prevented through the use of a pressure garment (Fig. 55.9).

As the burn heals, itching may occur and may, at times, be intense. It is important to control itching, because scratching can impair healing and increase risk of infection (see *Evidence-Based Practice* box).

A burn affects the patient's psychosocial status in many ways. The magnitude of these effects are related to the age of the patient, location of the burn (e.g., face, hands), recovery from injury, cause of the injury (especially if related to negligence or a deliberate act), and ability to continue at the pre-burn level of normal daily activities. The patient may experience a disruption of role function and general health and coping ability. Treatment involves the patient and significant others. Referrals to support groups, counselors, and psychiatrists are important during this stage.

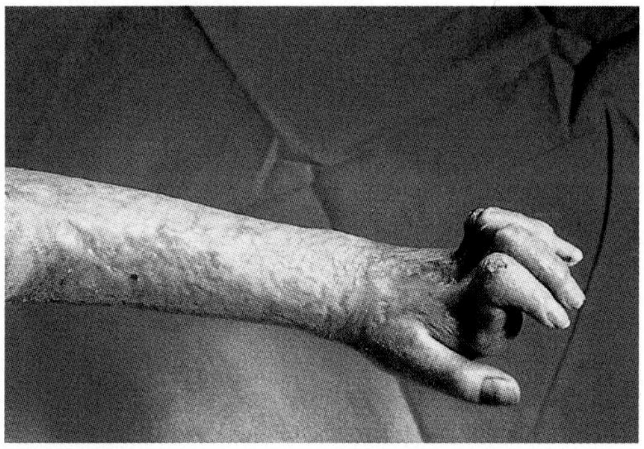

FIGURE 55.8 Burn deformity: contracture. (From Trofino, R. B. [1991]. *Nursing care of the burn-injured patient* [plate 36]. Philadelphia: F. A. Davis, with permission.)

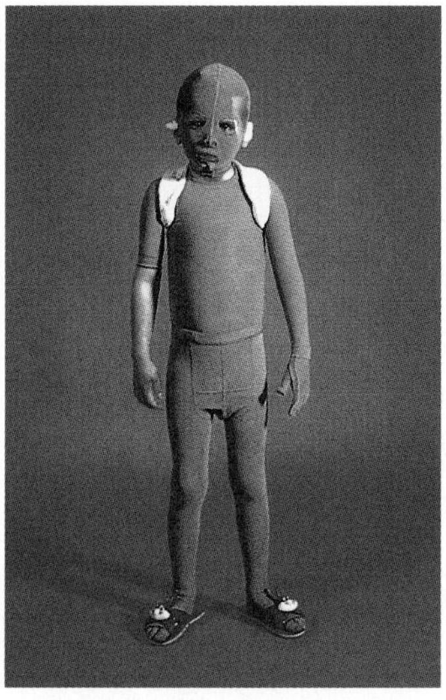

FIGURE 55.9 Full-body pressure garment. (From Trofino, R. B. [1991]. *Nursing care of the burn-injured patient* [plate 39]. Philadelphia: F. A. Davis, with permission.)

EVIDENCE-BASED PRACTICE

Clinical Question

What interventions are helpful for treating itching in a healing burn?

Evidence

More studies are needed to determine best practices for treating itching in burn patients. Some treatments shown to be helpful include cimetidine (an oral antihistamine), colloidal oatmeal baths, and pulsed dye laser therapy (Bell & Gabriel, 2009; UT Southwestern Medical Center, 2009).

Implications for Nursing Practice

Post-burn itching affects about 87% of patients. Nurses can assess the presence and severity of itching on a 0-to-10 scale, and advocate for appropriate orders.

REFERENCES

Bell, P. L., & Gabriel, V. (2009). Evidence based review for the treatment of post-burn pruritus. *Journal of Burn Care & Research 30*(1), 455-461.

UT Southwestern Medical Center. (2009). *Burn rehabilitation experts outline best treatments for post-burn itching.* Retrieved August 30, 2009, from http://www.utsouthwestern.edu/utsw/cda/dept353744/files/518898.html

CRITICAL THINKING

Mrs. Potter

■ Mrs. Potter is recovering from partial-thickness burns and skin grafts. She mentions that she and her family will be going on a much needed vacation to the shore. What concerns do you have?

Suggested answers at end of chapter.

NURSING CARE TIP

Use caution with heating pads, water temperature, and electrical equipment when working with your patients. Burns are "never events" because they can be prevented. Hospitals will not be paid by Medicare for treating burns acquired during hospitalization.

NURSING PROCESS FOR A PATIENT WITH A BURN INJURY

Data Collection

A major burn is painful and frightening to the patient and frightening to the family. Elicit information from the patient, family, and rescuers. If the injury occurred in an enclosed space with flames or smoldering materials, inhalation injury is suspected. If an electrical injury has occurred, ask about voltage, duration of contact, host susceptibility (wet or dry skin), entry and exit sites, and associated falls. With chemical burns, determine type of agent and duration of exposure.

General information to collect for all burns (in addition to normally collected data, such as medical history, allergies, and current medications) includes extent, depth, type, and location of the burn; burn agent; duration of contact with the burning agent; severity and location of pain; and associated injuries. Determine the immediate first aid treatment provided at the scene. Elicit psychosocial information: other people injured, additional losses (home, pets), whether the patient was at fault, and how this injury affects the patient's role function.

Nursing Diagnoses, Planning, Implementation, and Evaluation

See the *Nursing Care Plan for the Patient with a Burn Injury,* and Table 55.7, *Burn Summary.* For more information on burns, go to the American Burn Association Web site at www.ameriburn.org.

NURSING CARE PLAN for the Patient with a Burn Injury

Nursing Diagnosis: *Impaired Gas Exchange* related to upper airway edema, carbon monoxide poisoning, edema of alveolar capillary membranes, as evidenced by abnormal blood gases, elevated CO level

Expected Outcomes: The patient's gas exchange will be improved as evidenced by patent airway, CO level less than 10%, clear lung sounds, PaO_2 80–100 mm Hg, $PaCO_2$ 35–45 mm Hg, responsiveness, and awareness.

Evaluation of Outcomes: Are blood levels improved: CO, PaO_2, $PaCO_2$? Do the lungs sound clear on auscultation? Is patient aware of surroundings? Are there no signs of respiratory distress (e.g., retractions, nasal flaring, use of accessory muscles)?

Interventions	Rationale	Evaluation
Assess respiratory status: auscultate breath sounds every 15 minutes or as needed. Note any adventitious breath sounds. Observe for chest excursion. Monitor ability to cough.	Assessment detects changes in pulmonary function for planning care.	What is patient's respiratory status? Are any adventitious lung sounds noted?
Monitor arterial blood gases and CO level.	Assesses level of oxygenation. Helps guide oxygen therapy.	What are the patient's blood gas levels? Are they abnormal?
Monitor for nasal flaring, retractions, wheezing, and stridor.	Stridor may signal upper airway involvement. Nasal flaring, retractions, and wheezing may indicate lower airway involvement.	Does patient exhibit nasal flaring, retractions, wheezing, and stridor?
Administer humidified 100% oxygen by tight-fitting face mask for the breathing patient.	Provides oxygen for adequate gas exchange.	Is oxygen administered appropriately? Are blood gases improving?
Elevate head of bed (if no cervical spine injuries or no history of multiple trauma).	Decreases swelling of face and neck. Increases ability to expand lungs.	Is head of bed elevated? Is there any change in facial or neck swelling?

NURSING CARE PLAN for the Patient with a Burn Injury—cont'd

Interventions	Rationale	Evaluation
Provide appropriate pulmonary care: turn, cough, deep breathe every 2–4 hours. Provide incentive spirometer every 2–4 hours. Suction frequently as needed.	Mobilizes secretions and promotes lung expansion.	Is patient receiving vigorous pulmonary care? Is it affecting outcomes?
Obtain sputum cultures. Note amount, color, and consistency of pulmonary secretions.	Carbonaceous sputum is diagnostic for smoke inhalation injury. Infection changes color, amount, and consistency of sputum. Culture and sensitivity (C&S) assists in selection of appropriate antibiotic.	Is patient coughing up any sputum? Has character of sputum been reported and documented?
Administer bronchodilators and antibiotics as prescribed.	Bronchodilators decrease bronchospasms and edema. Antibiotics fight infection.	Are medications given appropriately? Are they effective?

Nursing Diagnosis: *Impaired Skin Integrity* related to thermal injury as evidenced by presence of burn lesions

Expected Outcomes: The patient's skin integrity will be improved as evidenced by healing of burned areas with no infection present, stopping of burning process.

Evaluation of Outcomes: Is burned area healed? Is it free from infection? Did burning process stop?

Interventions	Rationale	Evaluation
Obtain history of burning agent.	Provides information related to depth, duration of contact, and resistance of tissues. If fire scenario, consider possible inhalation injury.	What caused this thermal injury? How long was patient in contact with agent?
Assess burning process. If heat is felt on wound, cool with tepid tap water or sterile water.	Depth of injury increases with length of exposure to burning agent.	Is heat felt over wounds? Has burn process been effectively stopped?
Remove clothing and jewelry.	These items can retain heat and thermal agent, therefore increasing depth of injury. Jewelry can be constrictive when edema develops.	Are clothing and jewelry removed and constriction avoided?
Do not apply ice.	Ice causes vasoconstriction, further increasing wound damage. Ice also causes a decrease in core body temperature, which may promote shock.	Has use of ice been avoided?
Cover patient with clean sheet or blanket.	Prevents excessive heat loss. Decreases pain from air exposure. Protects patient from environmental contamination.	Is patient covered?

Continued

NURSING CARE PLAN for the Patient with a Burn Injury—cont'd

Interventions	Rationale	Evaluation
For all chemical burns, initiate immediate copious tepid water lavage for 20 minutes along with simultaneous removal of contaminated clothing. (Do not neutralize chemical because this takes too much time and resulting reaction may generate heat and cause further skin injury.)	Dilution and removal of chemical agent halts burning process. Lavage dissipates heat.	Has lavage been initiated?
Brush off dry chemicals before lavage.	To prevent further burn damage due to reaction of dry chemical with water.	Are dry chemicals removed?
Use heavy rubber gloves or thick gauze for removal of clothing.	To protect health care workers from injury.	Do health care workers remain safe?
Cleanse wound at bedside or via showering.	Promotes healing and helps decrease infection.	Is burn wound clean and free of wound debris?
Assist registered nurse (RN) or physician to assess the burn area for extent (percentage) and depth (partial thickness, full thickness) of injury.	Provides basis for triage of care. Important also for calculating resuscitation fluid therapy.	What is the estimation of percentage of burn injury? What is depth of injury?
Assist RN or physician with debriding wound via surgical, chemical, or mechanical means.	Promotes healing and healthy granulation bed.	Is there any eschar? Is wound free of wound debris?
Apply topical agent as prescribed.	Most agents prevent infection and promote healing.	Is agent applied as directed?
Apply dressing as prescribed.	Dressing types vary and are influenced by area, extent, and depth of injury, as well as by topical agent used. Dressing protects burn area and promotes healing.	Is dressing applied appropriately?
Do not wrap skin surface to skin surface (e.g., wrap fingers and toes separately; donut bandage around ears).	Wrapping separately prevents webbing and contractures.	Are skin surfaces separated? Are webbing and contractures avoided?
Limit bulk of dressings.	Mobility is enhanced with less bulky dressing.	Is patient's mobility maximized?
Wrap extremities distal to proximal.	Circulation is increased when extremities are wrapped distal to proximal.	Is wrapping done correctly? Is edema of distal extremity avoided?

Nursing Diagnosis: *Deficient Fluid Volume* related to evaporative losses from wound, capillary leak, and decreased fluid intake as evidenced by urine output less than 50 mL per hour, hypotension, tachycardia, weight loss

Expected Outcomes: The patient will maintain adequate circulating volume as evidenced by urine output of 50 mL/hr (adult), blood pressure within normal limits, heart rate between 60 and 100 beats per minute (adult), and stabilized body weight.

NURSING CARE PLAN for the Patient with a Burn Injury—cont'd

Evaluation of Outcomes: Is urine output maintained at least at 50 mL/hr? Are the blood pressure and heart rate within normal limits? Is patient's weight stable?

Interventions	Rationale	Evaluation
Obtain admission weight and monitor weight daily.	Helps measure fluid loss or gain.	Is patient's weight documented? Is it stable?
Record intake and output (I&O) hourly.	Serves as guide for fluid loss and replacement.	Is urine output adequate?
Examine for signs and symptoms of hypovolemia (hypotension, tachycardia, tachypnea, extreme thirst, restlessness, disorientation).	Fluid volume loss is multifocal (e.g., through increased capillary permeability, insensible loss).	Does patient exhibit any signs or symptoms of hypovolemia?
Monitor electrolytes, complete blood count (CBC).	Serves as guide for electrolyte replacement and blood product replacement.	What are patient's lab values? Are they within normal limits?
Administer IV fluids as ordered via large-bore IV catheter.	Fluid replacement begins immediately. Large vessels are needed for rapid delivery of fluids.	Is patient's fluid replacement adequate? Is catheter patent?
Insert indwelling urinary catheter.	Fluid replacement is titrated based on accurate urine output.	Is catheter patent?
Monitor urine for amount, specific gravity, and **hemochromogens**.	Specific gravity can predict volume replacement. Hemochromogens can cause renal tubular damage.	What are patient's urine values?
Administer osmotic diuretics as ordered; monitor response to therapy.	Decreased urine output can be caused by decreased renal flow (due to myoglobin in urine).	What is urine output? Has it changed due to therapy?
Assess gastrointestinal function for absence of bowel sounds. Maintain nasogastric tube.	Splanchnic constriction due to hypovolemia can cause a paralytic ileus.	Are patient's bowel sounds normal? Is nasogastric tube patent?

Nursing Diagnosis: *Pain* related to burns or graft donor sites as evidenced by patient's rating on appropriate pain scale, restlessness, sleeplessness

Expected Outcomes: The patient will experience pain control as evidenced by pain rating acceptable to patient and nonverbal cues, such as less restlessness, ability to rest or sleep.

Evaluation of Outcomes: Does patient verbalize pain control? How many hours of rest/sleep does patient have in 24 hours? Does patient state she or he feels rested?

Interventions	Rationale	Evaluation
Assess level of pain: nature, location, intensity, and duration at various times (during procedures, at rest). Rate pain on appropriate pain scale.	Provides baseline to monitor response to therapy.	Is patient's individual response to pain documented?

Continued

• WORD • BUILDING •

hemochromogen: heme—iron + chrom—color + gen—to produce

NURSING CARE PLAN for the Patient with a Burn Injury—cont'd

Interventions	Rationale	Evaluation
Observe for varied responses to acute pain: increase in blood pressure, pulse, respirations; increased restlessness and irritability; increased muscle tension; facial grimaces; guarding.	Responses to pain are variable. These parameters change in response to pain.	What are patient's responses to pain? Do responses change with treatment?
Acknowledge presence of pain. Explain causes of pain.	Encourages trust and understanding.	Is patient more trusting of the nurse and the treatments?
Administer opioids as ordered.	Opioids are needed for severe burn pain.	Is patient being medicated for pain appropriately?
Use patient-controlled analgesia (PCA) as appropriate.	PCA allows patient more control.	
Offer diversional activities (e.g., music, TV, books, games, relaxation techniques).	Helps patient focus on something other than pain.	Does patient use diversional activities? Do they help?
Position patient for comfort in good body alignment.	Increases comfort.	Is patient positioned as comfortably as possible?
Elevate burned extremities.	Elevation decreases edema and pain.	Are extremities elevated? Is pain reduced?
Maintain comfortable environment (e.g., bed cradle; comfortable environmental temperature, 86–91.4°F [30–33°C]; quiet environment).	Pressure from bed linens may cause discomfort; with loss of integument, body cannot self-regulate temperature.	Does patient verbalize comfort of environment?

Nursing Diagnosis: *Ineffective Peripheral Tissue Perfusion* related to circumferential burns, blood loss, decreased cardiac output as evidenced by weak pulses, cool extremities, limited movement and sensation

Expected Outcomes: The patient will maintain adequate tissue perfusion as evidenced by presence of peripheral pulses, minimal edema, intact sensation and motion, and warm extremities.

Evaluation of Outcomes: Are peripheral pulses present? Are extremities warm, with adequate sensation, movement, and circulation? Is edema decreased?

Interventions	Rationale	Evaluation
Assess pulses on burned extremities every 15 minutes.	If pulses diminish, an escharotomy may be indicated.	Are pulses present and documented?
Use Doppler as needed to detect weak pulses. Assess capillary refill, sensation, color, swelling, and movement.	Assesses peripheral perfusion.	Is the extremity warm, with adequate color, sensation, movement, and capillary refill?
Monitor for numbness, tingling, and increased pain in burned extremity.	Can be indicative of increased pressure from edema.	Does patient report numbness, tingling, or pain?
Measure circumference of burned extremities.	Monitors edema formation.	Is there evidence of edema? Is it getting better or worse?
Report changes in assessment promptly.	Emergency intervention may be indicated.	Does patient require an emergency intervention?

NURSING CARE PLAN for the Patient with a Burn Injury—cont'd

Interventions	Rationale	Evaluation
Elevate burned extremity above level of the heart.	Enhances venous return and decreases edema formation.	Are all burned extremities elevated above heart level? Is edema decreasing?
Apply burn dressing loosely.	Prevents constriction and allows for expansion as edema forms.	Is dressing too tight?
Assist with muscle compartment pressure measurement.	Helps determine need for escharotomy (if pressure exceeds 25 mm Hg).	What is patient's pressure?
Assist with escharotomy as needed.	If indicated, removal of eschar allows for edema expansion and permits peripheral perfusion.	Does patient require an escharotomy? Is edema relieved?

Nursing Diagnosis: *Risk for Infection*

Expected Outcomes: The patient will not develop a wound infection or sepsis.

Evaluation of Outcomes: Is there healthy granulation tissue on unhealed areas with no evidence of infection? Are donor sites free of infection? Have skin grafts taken? Is there absence of clinical manifestation of infection (temperature 98.6°F [37°C], normal white blood cell [WBC] count)?

Interventions	Rationale	Evaluation
Use sterile technique with wound care.	The unhealed burn wound is an excellent culture medium for bacterial growth.	Is sterile technique used for all wound care?
Maintain protective isolation with good hand washing technique.	Prevents spread of bacteria from patient to patient or nurse to patient.	Do all persons in contact with patient maintain proper precautions?
Administer immunosupportive medications as prescribed: tetanus and gamma globulin.	Immunoglobulins are depressed at time of severe burn injury.	Does patient require these medications? Have they been administered?
Perform wound care as prescribed, which may include the following: Inspect and debride wounds daily; culture wound three times a week or at sign of infection; shave hair at least 1 inch around burn areas (excluding eyebrows); inspect invasive line sites for inflammation (especially if line is through a burn area).	Provides quick identification of bacterial wound invasion and decreases incidence of infection. Presence of hair increases medium for bacterial growth.	What does wound look like? Is it debrided? What are culture results? Is there any hair near burn or line sites?
Continually assess for and report signs and symptoms of sepsis: temperature elevation, change in sensorium, changes in vital signs and bowel sounds, decreased output, positive blood/wound cultures.	The burn patient is at risk for sepsis until wound is healed.	Does patient exhibit any signs or symptoms of sepsis?
Administer systemic antibiotics and topical agents as prescribed.	Antibiotics prevent or treat infection.	Does patient require systemic antibiotics? Are topical agents applied appropriately? Is wound healing?

TABLE 55.7 BURN SUMMARY

Signs and Symptoms	Pain Superficial partial thickness: pink to red skin, blisters Deep partial thickness: pink to light red or white skin, blisters, blanching Full thickness: white, gray, or brown color, firm and leathery
Diagnostic Tests	Wound cultures Complete blood count, blood urea nitrogen, glucose, electrolytes, urine studies
Therapeutic Measures	IV fluid replacement Antibiotic/antimicrobial agents Analgesics
Complications	Shock Wound infection
Priority Nursing Diagnoses	*Impaired Gas Exchange* *Impaired Skin Integrity* *Deficient Fluid Volume* *Pain* related to burns or graft donor sites *Ineffective Peripheral Tissue Perfusion* *Risk for Infection*

SUGGESTED ANSWERS TO CRITICAL THINKING

■ *Mr. Weinberg*

Superficial partial-thickness burns usually heal in 7 to 10 days. Deep partial-thickness burns may take up to 3 weeks. All of this depends on the location of the injury, the health of the patient, and if he remains infection free.

■ *Mrs. Rivera*

1. Mrs. Rivera has an inhalation injury. This takes precedence over the burn and other injuries.
2. $$\frac{1\text{ L}}{6\text{ hr}} \times \frac{1000\text{ mL}}{1\text{ L}} = 167\text{ mL/hr}$$
3. Approximately 18%.

■ *Mrs. Potter*

The burned and graft areas will be sensitive to sunlight for up to 1 year. These areas should be covered, and she needs to use sunscreen anytime she is out in the sun. Her physician should offer guidance as to whether any exposure is safe, and if so, what type of sunscreen agent is recommended. In addition, if any areas are not completely healed, she will be at risk for infection.

REVIEW QUESTIONS

1. A patient is brought to the emergency department following a house fire. The patient has extensive trunk and lower extremity burns. The areas are blistered and pinkish white, and very painful when pressure is applied. Which type of burn does the patient most likely have?
   a. Superficial partial thickness
   b. Deep partial thickness
   c. Full thickness

2. Which of the following actions is appropriate initial treatment of a chemical burn?
   a. Lavage with water.
   b. Neutralize the chemical.
   c. Apply the prescribed topical agent.
   d. Wrap the patient in sterile sheets.

REVIEW QUESTIONS—cont'd

3. A patient is admitted to the emergency department with flame burns to her entire chest, abdomen, back, and upper extremities. Using the Rule of Nines, what is the approximate percentage of burns?
   a. 36%
   b. 45%
   c. 54%
   d. 64%

4. What nursing interventions are appropriate for a patient with a circumferential burn to an extremity? **Select all that apply**.
   a. Apply compression bandages starting at the distal end of the extremity.
   b. Administer analgesics if numbness or tingling occur.
   c. Check neurovascular status hourly.
   d. Assist with escharotomy if indicated.
   e. Elevate the extremity.

5. How will the nurse know if interventions for impaired gas exchange related to smoke inhalation have been effective?
   a. $PaCO_2$ is greater than 45 mm Hg.
   b. SpO_2 is less than 90%.
   c. pH is 7.34.
   d. PaO_2 is 88 mm Hg.

References

Burton, K. R., Sharma, V. K., Robertson, H., & Lindsay, R. (2009). A population-based study of the epidemiology of acute adult burn injuries in the Calgary Health Region and factors associated with mortality and hospital length of stay from 1995 to 2004. *Burns, 35*(4), 572–579.

Centers for Disease Control and Prevention. (2009). *Fire deaths and injuries: Fact sheet.* Retrieved August 28, 2009, from http://www.cdc.gov/HomeandRecreationalSafety/Fire-Prevention/fires-factsheet.html

unit SIXTEEN

UNDERSTANDING MENTAL HEALTH CARE

56

Mental Health Function, Assessment, and Therapeutic Measures

MARINA MARTINEZ-KRATZ

KEY TERMS

adaptation (ad-dap-TAY-shun)
affect (AF-fekt)
anxiety (ang-ZY-uh-tee)
behavior management (be-HAYV-yer MAN-ij-ment)
cognitive (KOG-nih-tiv)
coping (KOH-ping)
electroconvulsive therapy (ee-LEK-troh kun-VUL-siv THER-uh-pee)
imagery (IM-ij-ree)
insight (IN-syte)
mental health (MEN-tuhl HELTH)
mental illness (MEN-tuhl ILL-ness)
milieu (meel-YOO)
orientation (OR-ee-en-TAY-shun)
psychoanalysis (SY-koh-uh-NAL-ih-siss)
psychopharmacology (SY-koh-FAR-mah-KAWL-luh-jee)
psychotherapy (SY-koh-THER-uh-pee)
stress (STRESS)
stressor (STRESS-ur)

QUESTIONS TO GUIDE YOUR READING

1. What are definitions of mental health and mental illness?
2. What are the components of a mental health status assessment?
3. What is the DSM-IV-TR, and what other methods are used to diagnose mental illness?
4. How can you identify common ego defense mechanisms?
5. What is a therapeutic milieu?
6. How are psychoanalysis, behavior management, cognitive behavioral therapy, person-centered/humanistic therapy, counseling, group therapy, electroconvulsive therapy, and relaxation therapy carried out?
7. What is the LPN/LVN's role in mental health nursing?

REVIEW OF ANATOMY AND PHYSIOLOGY

Although there is much debate about the cause(s) of mental illness, it is important to review and understand the anatomy and physiology of the brain and central nervous system (CNS). The brain is involved in thinking, decision making, speaking, emotion, memory, motor and sensory activity, and the basic functions of temperature regulation and breathing, as well as many other functions. In mental health, it is important to distinguish between a neurologic disorder (such as delirium or Parkinson's disease) and a mental disorder (such as schizophrenia). Sometimes a patient has both a mental disorder and a neurologic or other physical disorder. Refer to Chapter 47 to review the nerves, structure of neurons, synapses, neurotransmitters, and the autonomic nervous system, as well as the structure and function of the brain. Also see Table 56.1 for the possible roles of CNS neurotransmitters in mental illness.

TABLE 56.1 NEUROTRANSMITTERS IN THE CNS

Neurotransmitter	Location/Function	Possible Implications for Mental Illness
Cholinergics		
Acetylcholine	ANS: sympathetic and parasympathetic presynaptic nerve terminals; parasympathetic postsynaptic nerve terminals CNS: cerebral cortex, hippocampus, limbic structures, and basal ganglia Functions: sleep, arousal, pain perception, movement, memory	Decreased levels: Alzheimer's disease, Huntington's disease, Parkinson's disease Increased levels: depression
Monoamines		
Norepinephrine	ANS: sympathetic postsynaptic nerve terminals CNS: thalamus, hypothalamus, limbic system, hippocampus, cerebellum, cerebral cortex Functions: mood, cognition, perception, locomotion, cardiovascular functioning, and sleep and arousal	Decreased levels: depression Increased levels: mania, anxiety states, schizophrenia
Dopamine	Frontal cortex, limbic system, basal ganglia, thalamus, posterior pituitary, and spinal cord Functions: movement and coordination, emotions, voluntary judgment, release of prolactin	Decreased levels: Parkinson's disease, depression Increased levels: mania, schizophrenia
Serotonin	Hypothalamus, thalamus, limbic system, cerebral cortex, cerebellum, spinal cord Functions: sleep and arousal, libido, appetite, mood, aggression, pain perception, coordination, judgment	Decreased levels: depression Increased levels: anxiety states
Histamine	Hypothalamus	Decreased levels: depression
Amino Acids		
Gamma-amino-butyric acid (GABA)	Hypothalamus, hippocampus, cortex, cerebellum, basal ganglia, spinal cord, retina Functions: slowdown of body activity	Decreased levels: Huntington's disease, anxiety disorders, schizophrenia, and various forms of epilepsy
Glycine	Spinal cord and brainstem Functions: recurrent inhibition of motor neurons	Toxic levels: "glycine encephalopathy"; decreased levels are correlated with spastic motor movement
Glutamate and aspartate	Pyramidal cells of the cortex, cerebellum, and the primary sensory afferent systems; hippocampus, thalamus, hypothalamus, spinal cord Functions: relay of sensory information and in the regulation of various motor and spinal reflexes	Increased levels: Huntington's disease, temporal lobe epilepsy, spinal cerebellar degeneration
Neuropeptides		
Endorphins and enkephalins	Hypothalamus, thalamus, limbic structures, midbrain, and brainstem; enkephalins are also found in the gastrointestinal tract Functions: modulation of pain and reduced peristalsis (enkephalins)	Modulation of dopamine activity by opioid peptides may indicate some link to the symptoms of schizophrenia
Substance P	Hypothalamus, limbic structures, midbrain, brainstem, thalamus, basal ganglia, and spinal cord; also found in gastrointestinal tract and salivary glands Function: regulation of pain	Decreased levels: Huntington's disease and Alzheimer's disease Increased levels: depression
Somatostatin	Cerebral cortex, hippocampus, thalamus, basal ganglia, brain stem, and spinal cord Function: inhibits release of norepinephrine; stimulates release of serotonin, dopamine, and acetylcholine	Decreased levels: Alzheimer's disease Increased levels: Huntington's disease

ANS = autonomic nervous system; CNS = central nervous system.

Source: Townsend, M. C. (2004). *Psychiatric mental health nursing: Concepts of care in evidence-based practice* (5th ed., pp. 60–61). Philadelphia: F. A. Davis.

MENTAL HEALTH AND MENTAL ILLNESS

Opinions within the mental health community differ as to what **mental health** and **mental illness** are. Mental health has been defined in many ways. These definitions include the ability to do the following:

- Be flexible.
- Be successful.
- Form close relationships.
- Make appropriate judgments.
- Solve problems.
- Cope with daily **stress.**
- Have a positive sense of self.

Mental illness is defined as experiencing the following:

- Impaired ability to think
- Impaired ability to feel
- Impaired ability to make sound judgments
- Impaired ability to adapt
- Difficulty in coping or inability to cope with reality
- Difficulty in forming or inability to form strong personal relationships.

It is important to remember that mental health and mental illness exist on a continuum. It is natural for emotions to ebb and flow from day to day in response to the degree of stress experienced. People who remain mentally healthy are able to keep their stress in perspective. Others are not able to do so, and over time they may develop physical or emotional illnesses as a result of present and past stresses in their life.

Picture the seesaw that children play on. Mental health and mental illness are like a seesaw. When children of approximately equal weight get on each end of the seesaw, they can balance each other and keep the seesaw even. Mentally healthy people can stay in a state of emotional balance. Sometimes one child weighs just a little more than the other and the seesaw tips just a little to one side. Mentally healthy people can cope with this fluctuation. Sometimes another child gets on or one child greatly outweighs the other, and the seesaw gets out of balance completely; one end goes way up while the other goes way down, and it stays there until someone alters the balance. Ultimately it must be the patient who finds his or her own balance. When a person's moods are way down or way up, he is not in emotional homeostasis.

Etiologies

The discussion surrounding the etiologies of mental illness continues to revolve around the "nature versus nurture" or "organic versus inorganic or functional" arguments. The connections between physical and emotional health are so closely intertwined that it is sometimes hard to decide if emotional causes trigger physical responses or vice versa. It is important to have a basic understanding of both the nature and nurture schools of thought on the causes of alterations in mental health.

Explanations of mental illness in this unit include concepts from the psychoanalytic (or psychological) and the psychobiological (or biological) theories. When pertinent, other theories (e.g., behavioral, environmental) are also presented. Most mental illnesses have no identifiable cause. Some etiological theories have stronger positive correlations to illnesses than others. When appropriate, this unit gives the most current or most widely accepted view of an etiology.

Social and Cultural Environments

Many professionals in the field of psychology believe that social and cultural environments have a great influence on the way people develop and process life experiences. Some psychoanalysts believe that some cultural traditions and beliefs cause disturbances in personal relationships, which can lead to forms of emotional disturbance. It is part of the nurse's role to take time to learn about traits that are common among people and traits that differ. While understanding that each person is a unique individual, it is important to have an understanding of broad customs and beliefs to avoid unrealistic expectations of patients. See Box 56.1, *Cultural Considerations,* for more detailed information about various cultures and mental health issues.

Spirituality and Religion

Spirituality and religion are extremely important to some patients and unimportant to others. A person's success in recuperating from physical or emotional illness may be deeply tied to spirituality. It is necessary to be comfortable talking to the patient about spiritual needs while being careful not to impose personal values on the patient. If you are not comfortable in these situations, you should offer to call the spiritual or religious leader of the patient's choice.

It is important to keep the lines of communication open. People learn by sharing with each other. It is much better to ask a person about something (to clarify or explore what was said) than to make an assumption about it. For more information about mental health and illness, visit the National Institute of Mental Health at www.nimh.nih.gov, the American Psychiatric Association at www.psych.org, the American Psychological Association at www.apa.org, the American Psychiatric Nurses Association at www.apna.org, or the International Society of Psychiatric-Mental Health Nurses at www.ispn-psych.org.

NURSING ASSESSMENT OF MENTAL HEALTH

During the assessment phase of the nursing process, a mental status examination is performed. This is a series of questions, activities, and observations that evaluate eight areas:

- Appearance and behavior
- Level of awareness and reality **orientation**
- Thinking/content of thought
- Memory

Box 56.1

Cultural Considerations

African Americans

African Americans may be at a greater risk for being misdiagnosed with a psychiatric disorder than Caucasians. African Americans with psychiatric disorders are more likely to have hallucinations, delusions, somatization, and hostility, even when controlled for socioeconomic class. Maintaining direct eye contact with some African Americans may be misinterpreted as aggressive behavior. Thus, nurses must take these nonverbal behaviors into consideration when working with the patient with an emotional or mental concern. Additionally, African Americans are more susceptible to the toxic side effects of tricyclic antidepressants.

Smoking, alcoholism, and deaths from suicide or violence are prevalent problems in the American culture. Violent deaths account for high mortality rates among adolescents and young adults of African American, Cuban, Mexican American, and Puerto Rican origin. Programs targeting these populations should be personalized to include adolescents and their families. Given their strong family values, an important approach is to begin early in church groups or family settings.

Haitians

Among many Haitians, some African Americans, and some other groups, conjuring (practicing magic) and root doctors are believed to know more about mental illness than Western-educated physicians. Some depressive and obsessive behaviors are viewed as culture-bound syndromes. These behaviors are expected of some Haitians, and those affected fulfill some expected roles in the society. Some of these illnesses are viewed as having no cure. Thus, the nurse may need to include folk healers when working with African Americans and patients of Haitian descent.

Hispanics

Hispanic patients may need lower doses of antidepressants and experience greater side effects than other Caucasians. Observe carefully for side effects of medications in patients of Mexican heritage.

Asians

Asian patients need lower dosages and have side effects at lower dosages than Caucasians for a variety of psychoactive drugs (e.g., lithium, haloperidol) even when matched with body weight. Asians commonly believe that Western drugs are too strong for them and take less than prescribed. Most Asians are more sensitive to alcohol, resulting in facial flushing, palpitations, and tachycardia.

Navajos

Among the Navajo, mental illness is perceived as resulting from a curse being placed on a person. In these instances, a healer who deals with dreams or a crystal gazer is consulted. People may wear turquoise to ward off evil; however, a person who wears too much turquoise is sometimes thought to be an evil person and someone to avoid. In some tribes, mental illness may mean that the affected person has special powers. Additionally, many Native Americans metabolize alcohol at a faster rate than European Americans, resulting in a higher tolerance for alcohol.

Irish

Newer immigrants from Ireland have a higher incidence of mental illness than the rest of the population. Undocumented Irish immigrants in the United States report more stressors and mental health problems than their legal counterparts. Because many Irish people may have difficulty expressing emotions, health care providers may need to encourage Irish Americans to express their concerns.

Box 56.1

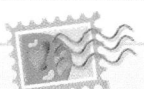

Cultural Considerations—cont'd

Iranians

Mental illness is strongly stigmatized among Iranians and is thought to be genetic. If a family member has mental illness, it is likely to be called a "neurologic disorder" to avoid stigmatizing the family, which may result in daughters having a lesser chance of marrying. Psychotherapy may be avoided because of stigma or because it is perceived as irrelevant. People prefer a medicine that might cure them. There is a tendency to pay more attention to somatic symptoms when under emotional stress; Iranians consider psychopharmacology most effective, and have a high rate of compliance.

Hindus

Because of the stigma attached to seeking professional psychiatric help, many Hindus do not access health care systems for mental health care. Instead, family and friends seem to be the best help, and a general belief is that time is the best healer. Physical and mental illnesses are considered God's will, or karma, and may be associated with a fatalistic attitude.

Greeks

Among Greeks, mental illness is accompanied by social stigma for the afflicted person and the relatives. The shame originates in the notion that mental illness is hereditary, and afflicted people are viewed as having lifelong conditions that pollute the bloodline.

Arabs

Because of social stigma attached to mental illness and retardation, Arabs may keep affected family members from public view. However, when Arab patients suffer from mental distress, they typically seek medical care. They are likely to have reports such as abdominal pain, lassitude, anorexia, or shortness of breath. Arabs have an increased tendency to experience elevated blood levels and adverse affects when customary dosages of antidepressants are prescribed. Patients often expect and insist on somatic treatment, at least vitamins and tonics.

- Speech and ability to communicate
- Mood and **affect**
- Judgment
- Perception

A number of different tools of varying names, lengths, and formats are used to evaluate mental capabilities. See Table 56.2 for a sample mental status examination.

After data have been collected, the licensed practical nurse/licensed vocational nurse (LPN/LVN) collaborates with the registered nurse (RN) to develop nursing diagnoses (Box 56.2).

DIAGNOSTIC TESTS

Physicians use a variety of diagnostic criteria to diagnose mental illness. It is important to rule out physical illness as a cause of symptoms. A primary care provider may choose to refer a patient to a psychiatrist or other mental health professional for further testing and diagnosis.

The diagnostic tool that is used most widely by psychiatrists and other mental health professionals is the *Diagnostic and Statistical Manual of Mental Disorders, Fourth Edition, Text Revision,* or DSM-IV-TR. The DSM-IV-TR groups illnesses into categories of clinical disorders. This is a complex diagnostic tool. Although as an LPN you will not be responsible for completing the assessment or making a diagnosis, you can contribute valuable information.

There are also batteries of psychological tests that can be administered and interpreted by psychiatrists or psychologists. Age, hand tremors, vision, language barriers, educational background, and the interpretation of the psychiatrist, the psychologist, or the advanced practice nurse are some factors that can influence the results of these tests.

Distinguishing Physical Versus Mental Disorders

Many physical disorders can mimic mental disorders, so tests may be performed to either confirm or rule out a diagnosis of a mental illness:

- Laboratory tests can rule out problems such as electrolyte imbalances, hypothyroidism, infections, dehydration, drug toxicity, or pregnancy.

TABLE 56.2 SAMPLE MENTAL STATUS EXAMINATION

Area to Be Examined	Type of Examination	Normal Parameters	Alterations from Normal
Appearance and behavior	Observations about dress, hygiene, posture, and appearance and about the patient's actions and reactions to health care personnel.	Clean, combed hair. Clothing intact and appropriate to weather or situation. Teeth/dentures in good repair. Posture erect. Cooperates with health care personnel.	Displays either unusual apathy or concern about appearance. Displays uncooperative, hostile, or suspicious behaviors toward health care personnel.
Level of awareness and orientation	Subjective and objective assessment of patient's degree of alertness (wakefulness) and degree of patient's knowledge of self.	Awareness is measured on a continuum that ranges from unconscious to manic. "Normal alertness" is the desired behavior. Facilities may provide a standard format for this assessment, but observations can be documented as well if the patient is not able to stay awake for even short intervals or if the patient is overly active and has difficulty staying in one place. Orientation is assessed by asking the patient questions relating to person, place, and time, such as "Who is this sitting next to you?" "Where are you right now?" or "What year is it?"	Outcome is not considered within accepted normal limits if the patient is difficult to arouse and keep awake or if the patient has difficulty feeling calm. Abnormal results of orientation are the patient's inability to correctly answer orientation questions or inability to answer commonly known questions, such as "Who is the president?"
Thinking/content of thought	Subjective assessment of what the patient is thinking and the process the patient uses in his or her thinking.	Formal testing may be done by a psychologist or psychiatrist to determine the patient's general thought content and pattern. Nurses may contribute to the assessment of thought by documenting statements the patient makes regarding daily care and routines.	Abnormal behaviors include flight of ideas, loose associations, phobias, delusions, and obsessions.
Memory	Subjective assessment of the mind's ability to recall recent and remote (long-term) information.	Recent memory: recall of events that are immediately past or within 2 weeks before the assessment, such as a recent news event. One measurement technique is to verbally list five items. After 1 minute, can the patient recall four or five of those items? Continue with the examination, and at 5 minutes the patient should be able to recall three or four of the items. Remote memory: recall of events of the past beyond 2 weeks before assessment. Patients may be asked where they were born, where they went to grade school, etc.	Inability to accurately perform recent or remote (long-term) recall exercises within parameters. May indicate symptom of delirium or dementia.
Speech and ability to communicate	Objective and subjective assessment of how the patient uses verbal and nonverbal communication. Stuttering, repetition of words, and words that the patient makes up (neologisms) are also assessed.	Patient can coherently produce words appropriate to age, education, and life experience. Rate of speech reflects other psychomotor activity (e.g., faster if the patient is agitated). Volume is not too soft or too loud. Speech is fluid and appropriate.	Limited speech production. Rate of speech is inconsistent with other psychomotor activity. Volume is not appropriate to situation (speaks louder or softer than appropriate). Presence of stuttering, word repetition, or neologisms may indicate physical or psychological illness.
Mood and affect	Objective and subjective assessment of the patient's stated feelings and emotions. Affect measures the outward expression of those feelings.	Mood is the stated emotional condition of the patient and should reflect situations as they occur. Facial expression and body language (affect) should match (be congruent with) the stated mood. Affect should change to fluctuate with the changes in mood.	Mood and affect do not match (e.g., facial expression does not appear sad while the patient is expressing sad feelings).

TABLE 56.2 SAMPLE MENTAL STATUS EXAMINATION—cont'd

Area to Be Examined	Type of Examination	Normal Parameters	Alterations from Normal
Judgment	Subjective assessment of a patient's ability to make appropriate decisions about his or her situation or to understand concepts.	When given a proverb or situation to solve, such as "You can't teach an old dog new tricks," the patient should be able to give some sort of acceptable interpretation, such as, "Old habits are hard to break" or "It is hard to learn something new."	Patient cannot interpret the sayings or complete problem-solving questions appropriately. The patient might answer very literally, "Dogs can't learn anything when they get old."
Perception	Assessment of the way a person experiences reality. Observation of the patient's statements about his or her environment and the behaviors expressed in association with those statements. Assessment of the patient's insight into his or her condition.	All five senses are monitored for the patient's perception of reality. Perceptions of environment are accurate. Insight into condition is appropriate.	Presence of hallucinations and illusions may occur with schizophrenia. Patient unable to state understanding of the origin of the illness; associated behaviors inappropriate. Many people with schizophrenia and mania have poor insight.

Box 56.2

Nursing Diagnoses Commonly Used to Address Mental Health Problems

Anxiety (mild to panic)
Compromised Family Coping
Compromised Human Dignity, Risk for
Compromised Resilience
Defensive Coping
Disturbed Body Image
Disturbed Personal Identity
Disturbed Sensory Perception
Disturbed Sleep Pattern
Dysfunctional Family Processes
Fear
Impaired Religiosity
Ineffective Coping
Ineffective Role Performance
Ineffective Self Health Management
Injury, Risk for
Low Self-Esteem (Chronic or Situational)
Post-Trauma Syndrome
Powerlessness
Risk for Violence (Self-Directed or Other-Directed)
Self-Care Deficit (specify)
Self-Mutilation
Sexual Dysfunction
Social Isolation
Stress Overload
Suicide, Risk for

- Computed tomography (CT) scans or magnetic resonance imaging (MRI) can rule out tumors, lesions, or other physical problems.
- Positron emission tomography (PET) scans can identify how the parts of the brain are functioning by showing chemical activity or metabolism.

COPING AND EGO DEFENSE MECHANISMS

"Oh, just learn to cope with it." "Get a grip." "Don't make a mountain out of a molehill." These are pieces of advice that people may have heard or given at some point. But what do they mean? What is **coping**? Coping is the way one adapts psychologically, physically, and behaviorally to a **stressor**. People have different methods of coping or dealing with their stressors. Culture, religion, individual belief systems, experience, and personal choice influence a person's responses to stress. It is not the value of a behavior that we assess as nurses; it is the desired outcome that is important. What is an effective coping skill? Is it healthy? Does it work? How do we as nurses observe and measure it?

Effective Coping Skills

Effective coping skills offer healthy choices for dealing with stressors. Effective coping skills are also conscious mechanisms. Hospitalization is stressful for patients and families. Many things are unknown and unfamiliar. The patient may not understand the illness or the implications of the treatment plan. It is common for patients to use coping mechanisms during hospitalization. The process of effective coping is sometimes called **adaptation**. Allowing the patient to practice new coping techniques will give him or her confidence and will decrease the stress that can accompany change.

Often the dividing line between effective and ineffective coping is the frequency of its use. For instance, mild **anxiety** can be positive. Generally, when there is a little anxiety, people are more alert and ready to respond. The *fight-or-flight mechanism* can actually help one adapt to a new situation. However, too much anxiety begins to cloud the consciousness and interfere with the ability to make appropriate choices and to recall new adaptive tools that have been learned. One of the most helpful roles you can perform is to listen to the patient's thoughts and feelings about the stressor, assist him or her to identify precipitating factors and patterns to the patient's stress, encourage the patient to problem solve, and provide assistance to develop alternative solutions to a problem.

Ineffective Coping Skills

Sometimes coping is ineffective. When conscious techniques are not successful, people may unconsciously fall into habits that give the illusion of coping. These habits are called *ego defense mechanisms* (or coping or mental mechanisms). Ego defense mechanisms act as mental pressure valves. The purpose of ego defense mechanisms is to reduce or eliminate anxiety. They give the impression that they are helping alleviate the stress level. When used in very small doses, ego defense mechanisms can be helpful. When they are overused, or are the only means used to deal with anxiety, they can become ineffective and unhealthy. People are not born with these coping behaviors; they are learned as responses to stress. Many times they develop by age 10. They may appear to be conscious, but they are, for the most part, unconscious mechanisms. Some commonly used ego defense mechanisms are listed in Table 56.3.

CRITICAL THINKING

Mr. Joseph

■ Mr. Joseph is noted wailing loudly and continuously after the death of his wife. It is disturbing the other patients on the hospital wing, and one of the nurses comments, "He is a real nut case. Get him out of here."

What is an appropriate response to this nurse and patient? How would you document his behavior?
Suggested answers at end of chapter.

CRITICAL THINKING

Mrs. Beison

■ Mrs. Beison, a 44-year-old mother of three teenagers, is diagnosed with breast cancer. She is refusing treatment because she does not believe she has cancer. She says if anything is really wrong, her vitamins will take care of it.

What coping mechanism is Mrs. Beison using? Is it effective or ineffective? Why? How can you help?
Suggested answers at end of chapter.

TABLE 56.3 EGO DEFENSE MECHANISMS

Mechanism	Description	Examples
Denial	Usually the first defense learned and used. Unconscious refusal to see reality; not conscious lying.	The alcoholic states, "I can quit any time I want to."
Repression (stuffing)	An unconscious "burying" or "forgetting" mechanism. Excludes or withholds from consciousness events or situations that are unbearable.	A step deeper than "denial." A patient may "forget" about an appointment he or she does not want to keep.
Rationalization	Using a logical-sounding excuse to cover up true thoughts and feelings. The most frequently used defense mechanism.	1. "I made a medication error because the doctor's orders were confusing." 2. "I failed the test because the teacher wasn't clear about what would be on it."
Compensation	Making up for something perceived as an inadequacy by developing some other desirable trait.	1. The small boy who wants to be a basketball center instead becomes an honor roll student. 2. The physically unattractive person who wants to model instead becomes a famous designer.
Reaction formation (overcompensation)	Similar to compensation, except the person usually develops the exact opposite trait.	1. The small boy who wants to be a basketball center becomes a political voice to decrease the emphasis on sports in the elementary grades. 2. The physically unattractive person who wants to be a model speaks out for eliminating beauty pageants.

TABLE 56.3 EGO DEFENSE MECHANISMS—cont'd

Regression	Emotionally returning to an earlier time in life when the patient experienced far less stress. Commonly seen in patients while hospitalized. *NOTE:* People do not go back to the same developmental age. This is highly individualized.	1. Children who are toilet trained begin to wet themselves. 2. Adults start crying and have a "temper tantrum."
Projection (scapegoating)	Blaming others. A mental or verbal "finger-pointing" at another for a patient's own problem.	1. "I didn't get the promotion because you don't like me." 2. "I'm overweight because you make me nervous."
Displacement (transference)	"Kick-the-dog syndrome." Transferring anger and hostility to another person or object that is perceived to be less powerful than oneself.	Parent loses job without notice; goes home and verbally abuses spouse, who unjustly punishes child, who slaps the dog.
Restitution (undoing)	Make amends for a behavior one thinks is unacceptable. Makes an attempt at reducing guilt.	1. A person gives a treat to a child who is being punished for a wrongdoing. 2. The person who sees someone lose a wallet with a large amount of cash does not return the wallet, but puts extra in the collection plate at the next church service.
Conversion reaction	Anxiety is channeled into physical symptoms. Often the symptoms disappear soon after the threat is over.	Nausea develops the night before a major exam, causing the person to miss the exam. Nausea may disappear soon after the scheduled test is finished.
Avoidance	Unconsciously staying away from events or situations that might cause feelings of aggression or anxiety.	"I can't go to the class reunion tonight. I'm just so tired, I have to sleep."

THERAPEUTIC MEASURES

People who experience alterations in their mental health have special treatment needs. When emotional health is threatened, many other daily activities can be altered as well. **Cognitive** ability (the ability to think rationally and to process those thoughts) can be impaired. Emotional responses can be decreased or even absent in some conditions. This can be extremely frightening and can lead to a worsening of the mental disorder or even the development of another disorder. This section will provide an overview of selected therapies to help patients deal with alterations in mental health.

Therapeutic Communication

Many people take communication for granted. In the mental health setting, communication is a tool used to relate therapeutically with patients. It is important to keep in mind what message we want to communicate to patients. Therapeutic communication is accomplished through the deliberate use of verbal and nonverbal techniques. Other areas to consider when communicating are the patient's personal values, attitudes, beliefs, culture, religion, social status, gender, and age or developmental level.

Verbal therapeutic communication techniques can help facilitate an interpersonal interaction. For instance, if you ask a patient to explain something to you in more detail, you are using the therapeutic communication technique of exploring. Verbal communication is also influenced by the tone, pitch, speed, and volume of speech. Some commonly used therapeutic communication techniques are listed in Table 56.4.

Components of *nonverbal communication* include physical appearance, dress, body movement and posture, touch, facial expression, and eye contact. It is believed that most communication takes place nonverbally so it is possible that while you are saying one thing to a patient, your body language could be saying something else.

There are also barriers to effective communication that are commonly called *communication blocks.* A nurse who tells a patient, "Don't worry, everything will be all right," has just given the patient false reassurance. This barrier communicates to the patient that his concerns are not being taken seriously. Some common communication blocks are listed in Table 56.5.

Milieu

One area over which you can have some control is the therapeutic environment. In the mental health setting, this therapeutic environment is called the **milieu** or therapeutic milieu. It is believed that environment has an effect on behavior. Milieu therapy is the systematic management of the social environment as a treatment modality.

A *therapeutic milieu* is an environment that provides containment, support, structure, involvement, and validation during the patient's stay. The goals of milieu therapy are resocialization, ego development, and prevention of regression. Resocialization occurs when patients help govern the running of the unit and attend regular meetings to set rules and assign tasks. Ego development is fostered with

TABLE 56.4 THERAPEUTIC COMMUNICATION TECHNIQUES

Technique	Description	Examples
Encouraging descriptions of perceptions	Asking the patient what he or she is seeing or hearing	"Tell me what the voices are saying to you."
Encouraging comparison	Asking the patient to compare similarities or differences	"How is this medication working for you compared to the last time you used it?"
Exploring	Looking deeper into a subject, idea, or experience	"Tell me more about the last time you were depressed."
Focusing	Concentrating on a single idea or event	"Tell me more about how your divorce made you feel."
Formulating a plan of action	Assisting the patient to come up with a plan to cope with stress	"When this happens in the future how could you handle it more constructively?"
Giving broad openings	Allowing the patient to steer the interaction	"What would you like to work on today?"
Giving recognition	Acknowledging or showing awareness	"I see you went to your therapy group today."
Making observations	Verbalizing what is observed	"I notice you seemed upset after your visit."
Offering self	Extending one's presence	"I am available to talk whenever you would like."
Offering general leads	Giving the patient encouragement to continue	"I see...." "Go on...."
Placing event in time or sequence	Clarification of events in time	"Was this before or after your first hospitalization?"
Presenting reality	Defining reality in simple terms	"The voices may seem real to you, but they are a symptom of your illness."
Restating	Repeating the main idea of what the patient has verbalized	"It sounds as if you are feeling frustrated."
Reflecting	Statements, questions, or feelings are referred back to the patient	"What do you think you should do?"
Seeking clarification	Searching for understanding of what was said	"Tell me if this is what you meant when you said...."
Verbalizing the implied	Putting into words what the patient has implied or said indirectly	"You must be feeling very sad right now."
Using silence	Gives both the nurse and the patient a chance to collect their thoughts and organize what they are going to say	

TABLE 56.5 COMMUNICATION BLOCKS

Mechanism	Description	Examples
Agreeing/disagreeing	Implies that the patient's ideas or feelings are somehow right or wrong	"That is right on target. I agree 100%."
Asking "why" questions	Asking why implies that the patient knows the reason for their behavior and feelings	"Why were you feeling so angry?"
Changing the subject	Changing the subject takes control of the conversation away from the patient	Patient: "I am feeling so hopeless." Nurse: "Did you go to group therapy today?"
Giving advice	Telling the patient what to do implies that the nurse knows what is best	"I think you should...."
Giving approval or disapproval	Passes judgment on the patient's ideas or opinions	"That's right."
Giving false reassurance	Devalues the patient's feelings	"Everything will be all right."
Self-focusing behavior	The nurse focuses on his or her own feelings at the expense of the patient's.	"That happened to me once . . . let me tell you about it."
Double-bind messages	When the nonverbal message doesn't match the verbal message	"I'm listening," as the nurse fidgets in her chair, doesn't make eye contact, and then coughs.

structured activities that are provided to assist the patient to learn coping and social skills. Regression is prevented when patients help with washing dishes or other small jobs that foster independence. Common milieu interventions include role modeling, positive reinforcement, a schedule of events, consistent expectations and rules for behavior, and unit meetings. Milieu therapy is difficult in this era of managed care because of shorter hospital stays.

Psychopharmacology

Psychopharmacology is the use of medications to treat psychological disorders. Since the introduction of the phenothiazine class of drugs in the 1950s (e.g., chlorpromazine), the number of medications available for treating mental health disorders has increased greatly, with newer medications having fewer side effects. The reason for using medications is twofold: First, the medications manage the symptoms, helping the patient feel more comfortable emotionally. Second, the patient is generally more receptive and able to focus on other types of therapy if medications are effective. More information on psychoactive drugs is provided in Chapter 57.

Psychotherapies

Psychotherapy is the term used to describe the form of treatment chosen by the psychologist, psychiatrist, social worker, or advanced practice psychiatric nurse. The goals of psychotherapy include the following:

- Reduce the patient's emotional discomfort.
- Increase the level of the patient's social functioning.
- Increase the ability of the patient to behave or perform in a manner appropriate to the situation.

Several specific types of therapy that are typically used are described next.

Psychoanalysis

Psychoanalysis was developed from Sigmund Freud's psychoanalytic theory. Freud believed that anxiety was the primary motivation for behavior and therefore all behavior had meaning. Psychoanalytic therapy consists of clarifying the meaning of events, feelings, and behavior and thereby gaining **insight** into them. The role of the patient is to provide the psychoanalyst with clues to the unconscious source of problems and to try to develop insights into behavior. The role of the therapist is to uncover these unconscious experiences and interpret their meanings to the patient. Some believe that psychoanalysis will lose popularity as we gain a better understanding of the role of the brain, neurotransmitters, and genetics in mental health.

• WORD • BUILDING •

psychopharmacology: psycho—soul or mind + pharmaco—drug or medicine + ology—study of

psychoanalysis: psycho—soul or mind + analysis—dissolving

Behavior Management

Behavior management (also called behavior modification) is a treatment method that stems from the studies of behavioral theorists such as Skinner and Pavlov. It is a common treatment modality used in long-term care facilities, with children and adolescents, and with individuals who have a low level of cognitive functioning.

According to behavior management theory, all behavior is learned, so it can be unlearned. The belief is that behavior can be changed by either positive or negative reinforcement. *Positive reinforcement* is the act of rewarding the patient with something pleasant when the desired behavior has been performed. For instance, if a patient has the habit of using foul language in an attempt to have a need met, the desired behavior change might be to come to a staff member and ask appropriately for what he or she needs. If this patient loves to be outside but is not allowed out except at supervised times, then a suitable positive reinforcement for her might be to allow 15 more minutes outdoors when the desired behavior is exhibited.

Negative reinforcement is the act of responding to the undesired behavior by taking away a privilege or adding a responsibility. Negative reinforcement can be misinterpreted as punishment. Parents who "ground" their children for unacceptable behavior are using negative reinforcement; requiring the child to perform extra household tasks for a stated period is reinforcing the fact that the behavior has consequences. The child may not repeat the undesired behavior after negative reinforcement has been used. It is necessary to be very careful to avoid violating the Patient's Bill of Rights when performing behavior management with patients. A signed consent from the patient is advised when using this form of therapy.

The patient must understand the consequences of the behavior to be changed and the purpose for the type of consequence that is chosen. If the person is not capable of understanding the situation or is not able to remember the consequences because of some other problem, behavior management could be considered a questionable alternative to other kinds of treatment.

Cognitive Behavioral Therapy

Cognitive behavioral therapists believe that people teach themselves to be ill because of the way they "think" about their situations. Cognitive behavioral therapy stresses ways of rethinking situations. The therapist confronts the patient with certain distortions of thinking and then works out ways of thinking about them differently.

Feeling sad about an unpleasant experience (such as the death of a loved one) is acceptable and normal, but long-term depression about the death is an extreme emotion and therefore considered to be unhealthy. In this situation, the patient might be helped to see the death as a sad loss. Behavioral techniques are also often used with phobias or panic disorders, in which fear may interfere with reasoning.

Cognitive therapies are gaining in popularity because they are usually significantly shorter term than psychoanalysis and therefore less costly to the patient. This type of therapy is commonly performed in groups. The patients are given "homework" that is specific to their needs. Patients practice their assignments between sessions.

Person-Centered/Humanistic Therapy

Abraham Maslow and Carl Rogers are two theorists who are often credited with the concept of person-centered or humanistic therapy. In this form of treatment, caregivers focus on the whole person and work in the "present." It is not important in humanistic treatment to understand the cause of the problem or what happened in the person's past; what is important is the here and now. With this therapy, the patient learns to see himself or herself as a person who has value and who is respected by others.

Nursing is very strongly grounded in person-centered principles. Three qualities are essential for caregivers: empathy, which is the ability to identify with the patient's feelings without actually experiencing them with the patient; unconditional positive regard (respect); and genuineness or honesty. Although you may not be an active participant in the actual therapy sessions with patients, it is important to maintain these three qualities in all therapeutic relationships.

Counseling

Counseling is the provision of help or guidance by a health care professional. The area of counseling is licensed and regulated differently not only state by state but sometimes municipality by municipality. Nurses prepared at an LPN/LVN level or at an RN level can, in some areas and with special advanced education, practice some forms of counseling.

You may be asked or expected to accompany patients to counseling sessions or even to facilitate a group discussion. Remember that these are confidential sessions, even if they are group oriented. Patients are there to work; others are there by invitation for special reasons.

Group Therapy

Groups are formed for many reasons; they can be ongoing or short term, depending on the needs of the patients or the type of disorder. Group therapy is a cost-effective means of providing treatment. For example, Alcoholics Anonymous (AA) and similar 12-step self-help groups are well-established, ongoing groups formed around treatment of a specific problem. Family counseling sessions may occur with individual therapists with a specialty in the problem area for that family. Marriage counseling may be done in a group with other couples. Many times, peer counselors are used.

Therapists and counselors are tools, or facilitators, in the therapeutic process. They do not heal the patient; the patient heals himself or herself. Patients must take the suggestions given by the therapist, try them, and see what works for them. You can help by reinforcing the good work patients do to learn to stay mentally healthy and develop more effective life skills. Also see *Evidence-Based Practice* box.

EVIDENCE-BASED PRACTICE

Clinical Question

Do nurse-led group interventions help patients with schizophrenia?

Evidence

In a study of patients with schizophrenia, participants took part in nurse-led peer support groups to share experiences with each other and to share coping strategies after a psychotic episode (Castelein, Mulder, & Bruggeman, 2008). Study participants and the nurses responded positively to the structure of the nurse-led groups.

Another study of patients with schizophrenia showed that nurse-led cognitive behavioral therapy improved insight, reduced negative symptoms, and decreased hospital readmissions (Turkington et al., 2006).

Implications for Nursing Practice

Nurse-led group interventions are useful for patients diagnosed with schizophrenia. Nurses can use the group setting as a vehicle to implement interventions related to coping, increasing insight, and managing symptoms.

REFERENCES

Castelein, S., Mulder, P. J., & Bruggeman, R. (2008). Guided peer support groups for schizophrenia: A nursing intervention. *Psychiatric Services, 59*(3), 326.

Turkington, D., Kingdon, D., Rathod, S., et al. (2006). Brief cognitive behaviour therapy improved insight and reduced negative symptoms and readmissions in schizophrenia. *British Journal of Psychiatry, 189*, 36–40.

Electroconvulsive Therapy

Electroconvulsive therapy (ECT) is a form of treatment that is used for severely depressed patients who are not responding to psychotropic medications. ECT passes an electric current through the brain to produce a tonic-clonic (grand mal) seizure. Most mental health professionals believe ECT stimulates an increase in circulating levels of the neurotransmitters serotonin, norepinephrine, and dopamine in the brain. In essence, ECT impacts neurotransmitter activity much like the antidepressant medications. ECT may be frightening to patients; it is important for the nurse to provide education and information to the patient and family. Many changes have been made in this form of therapy since the 1940s, and ECT is currently a safe and effective treatment for resistant depression.

Procedure

ECT often takes place in the recovery room of an operating suite, where there is ready access to emergency equipment. Informed consent must be obtained by the physician. About 30 minutes before the procedure, the patient is given a medication to dry secretions and counteract stimulation of the vagus nerve, which can cause bradycardia and syncope. Patients are given a short-acting anesthetic before the treatment and a smooth muscle relaxant to minimize injury. Before giving the muscle relaxant, a blood pressure cuff is placed on one of the patient's lower limbs and inflated. This is to ensure that the seizure activity can be visually monitored in this limb. Blood pressure and pulse are carefully monitored before and after the treatment. The patient is oxygenated with pure oxygen during and after the seizure until spontaneous respirations return. During treatment, an electrical stimulus is delivered to the brain via unilateral or bilateral electrodes. The amount of electrical energy used is individualized to the patient. The seizure must last at least 30 seconds to be effective. The seizure activity is monitored with an electroencephalogram (EEG) and also in the cuffed limb.

Side Effects

Side effects of ECT can be unpleasant, but are usually temporary. The patient may feel confused and forgetful immediately after the treatment. This can be from a combination of the ECT itself and the medication that was used before the treatment. If the seizure was strong, the patient may have some muscle soreness.

ECT is not used indiscriminately. It is used when other therapies have not been helpful, and it is usually reserved for severe or long-term depression and certain types of schizophrenia (Box 56.3, *Patient Perspective*).

Nursing Care

The nurse's responsibilities include careful monitoring of vital signs and accurate documentation of the patient's subjective and objective responses to the treatment. The patient should receive nothing by mouth (NPO) for at least 4 hours before a treatment. Remind the patient to empty his or her bladder and to remove dentures, contact lenses, hair pins, and other items on the body. After the treatment, stay with the patient until he or she is oriented and able to care for himself or herself. Oral medications and food should be withheld until the gag reflex returns. Ensuring that the person is kept safe after therapy is a major concern.

Relaxation Therapy

A variety of relaxation techniques can be taught to help patients manage their responses to stress. Relaxation exercises such as deep, rhythmic breathing can increase oxygenation and provide distraction from stressors. Breathing exercises may be coupled with progressive muscle relaxation exercises. For this technique, patients are taught to start at the head and neck and systematically tense and then relax muscle groups as they progress toward the lower extremities. Soft music may enhance the patient's ability to fully relax.

Imagery is the use of the imagination to promote relaxation. For this technique, the patient is taught to imagine a pleasurable experience from his or her past, such as lying on a beach or soaking in a warm bath. Use of all senses is encouraged—for a beach image, the patient might see a beach, feel the warm sun, smell salt air, and hear waves crashing against the shore. The patient might also be taught to visualize being successful in a problem situation.

Relaxation techniques may be used individually, but they are often used in combination with each other or with other therapies for maximum effect.

Box 56.3

Patient Perspective

A Daughter's Thoughts on ECT

My mom is 83 years old and has had a total of 35 electroconvulsive therapy (ECT) treatments in her lifetime. If you met her, you'd never know; you'd find her delightful. She's a sweet little plump German lady with a big heart. I am a nurse, and when I tell fellow nurses about my mom, they often ask me why I didn't get her on antidepressants. I want to scream, "How dumb do you think I am?!" Of course Mom is on antidepressants. But at intervals they don't work and she sinks into severe depression. My choice then is to help her have ECT or let her stay depressed and miserable and put her in a nursing home. And she would soon die because when she is depressed she refuses to move, doesn't sleep, and is horribly miserable.

The first time my mom was scheduled for ECT, one of the nurses in our local community hospital told her to refuse it, that no one should have to go through that. It was a cruel thing to do. My mom doesn't do well in counseling—she doesn't believe in it. In her mind you don't talk about your "dirty linen." My mom was in an abusive relationship with my father for 47 years, and she hid all the problems away and doesn't talk about them to this day. I'm so grateful to have my mom doing okay and grateful that ECT treatments exist. With ECT my mother is doing well and enjoying life. Without treatment, she would be gone. Please understand that there are times when ECT treatments are the best thing for severely depressed people, when other treatments have been ineffective.

Home Health Hints

Assess the patient and the patient's home for these safety issues:

- Risk of falls (especially if the patient is experiencing orthostatic hypotension from medications)
- Suicide ideation, plan, and means
- Ability to access medications; missed doses; or overdoses
- Need for additional services for activities of daily living (ADLs), such as housekeeping, medication assistance, or safety rails

SUGGESTED ANSWERS TO

CRITICAL THINKING

■ *Mr. Joseph*

Different people cope in different ways. This may be a healthy way to cope in this grieving husband's culture. Gently guide him to a room where he can express his emotions without disturbing others. Ask if he would like you to contact someone to come help support him. Document objectively: "Patient's husband weeping loudly; guided to consultation room for privacy."

■ *Mrs. Beison*

Mrs. Beison is using denial to cope with her cancer diagnosis. Although at times denial can be an effective coping mechanism, if Mrs. Beison continues to deny her disease and refuse treatment, her life will be in danger. You can help Mrs. Beison verbalize her fears about cancer and cancer treatment and can provide accurate information to help her make wise choices. If needed, a psychiatric evaluation can be requested. If she is found to be mentally competent, then her wishes must be respected.

REVIEW QUESTIONS

1. When assessing mental health, which patient behavior would cause the nurse to be concerned or ask further questions?
   a. Patient is always happy and smiling.
   b. Patient can verbalize emotions.
   c. Patient is able to cope with bad news.
   d. Patient maintains some close, personal relationships.

2. Which data are important to collect during a mental health assessment? **Select all that apply.**
   a. Orientation to reality
   b. Mobility
   c. Ability to communicate clearly
   d. Heart sounds
   e. Memory
   f. Appearance

3. A patient being evaluated for depression asks why blood must be drawn. Which response by the nurse is best?
   a. "Your physical illnesses must be under control before your depression can be treated effectively."
   b. "The clinician needs to rule out physical causes for your symptoms."
   c. "Most mental health disorders can be identified with blood tests."
   d. "If your lab work is out of balance, then correcting the imbalance will reverse your depression."

4. A person who always seems to be making excuses is displaying which ego defense mechanism?
   a. Denial
   b. Fantasy
   c. Rationalization
   d. Transference

5. Which of the following best defines a therapeutic milieu?
   a. An environment that is able to provide for all of the patient's physical and emotional needs
   b. An environment that is locked and supervised
   c. An environment that is structured to decrease stress and encourage learning new behavior
   d. An environment designed to be homelike for persons who are institutionalized for life

6. What is the primary reason a patient might be placed on psychopharmacology?
   a. It can provide a cure for mental illness and substance abuse.
   b. It is an easy way to control patients' behavior.
   c. It is used to alter the pain receptors in the brain.
   d. It can decrease symptoms and facilitate other therapies.

7. Which of the following is one of the major skills a chemically dependent person and family can learn during treatment?
   a. Honest communication
   b. Avoidance of difficult topics
   c. Denial
   d. Scapegoating

8. A patient shares some very traumatic life experiences with the LPN. What is the best response by the LPN?
   a. Assure the patient that the staff will not allow such experiences to happen to the patient again.
   b. Ask probing questions about the patient's emotional responses to the experiences.
   c. Encourage the patient to forget the experiences and move on with life.
   d. Listen attentively to the patient and show empathy.

57

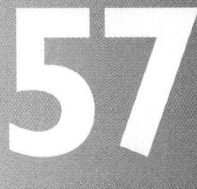

Nursing Care of Patients with Mental Health Disorders

MARINA MARTINEZ-KRATZ

KEY TERMS

abuse (uh-BYOOS)
addiction (ah-DIK-shun)
alogia (ah-LOH-jee-uh)
anhedonia (AN-heh-DOH-nee-uh)
avolition (A-voh-LISH-un)
bipolar (bye-POH-lur)
codependence (KOH-dee-PEN-dense)
compulsion (kum-PUHL-shun)
conversion disorder (kon-VER-zhun diss-OR-der)
delirium tremens (dee-LEER-ee-um TREE-menz)
delusions (dee-LOO-zhuns)
dependence (dee-PEN-dense)
displacement (diss-PLAYSS-ment)
dysfunctional (diss-FUNK-shun-uhl)
eustress (YOO-stress)
hallucinations (hah-LOO-sih-NAY-shuns)
illusions (ih-LOO-zhuns)
mania (MAY-nee-ah)
obsession (ob-SESH-un)
phobia (FOH-bee-ah)
psychosomatic (SY-koh-soh-MAT-tick)
somatoform (soh-MAT-oh-form)
tolerance (TALL-ler-ense)
withdrawal (with-DRAW-ul)

QUESTIONS TO GUIDE YOUR READING

1. What etiological theories have been proposed for mental health disorders?
2. What are the signs and symptoms of common mental health disorders?
3. What therapeutic management can be effective for each of the disorders?
4. What are the classifications, actions, side effects, and nursing considerations for selected classifications of psychoactive medications?
5. What nursing interventions are used to help patients with mental health disorders?
6. What is the role of the LPN/LVN in the care of patients with mental health disorders?

MENTAL HEALTH DISORDERS

Anxiety Disorders

Stress is everywhere in our society. Stress produces anxiety. Most often, stress is associated with negative situations, but the good things that happen to us, such as weddings and job promotions, also produce stress. The stress from positive experiences is called **eustress**. Eustress can produce just as much anxiety as the negative stressors. A stressor is any person or situation that produces an anxiety response. Stress and stressors are different for each person; therefore, it is important to ask patients what their personal stress producers are.

Anxiety is the uncomfortable feeling of dread that occurs in response to extreme or prolonged periods of stress. It is commonly ranked as mild, moderate, severe, or panic. It is believed that a mild amount of anxiety is a normal part of being human and that mild anxiety is necessary to change and develop new ways of coping with stress.

Anxiety may also be influenced by one's culture. It may be acceptable for some people to acknowledge and discuss stress, but others may believe that discussing personal problems with others is inappropriate. This cultural behavior can be a challenge for the nurse when attempting to collect assessment data.

Anxiety is usually referred to as either *free-floating anxiety* or *signal anxiety*. Free-floating anxiety is described as a general feeling of impending doom. The person cannot pinpoint the cause, but might say something like "I just know something bad is going to happen if I go on vacation." Signal anxiety, on the other hand, is an uncomfortable response to a known stressor ("Finals are only a week away and I've got that nausea again.") Both types of anxiety are involved in the various anxiety disorders.

Etiological Theories

Psychoanalytical theorists believe that anxiety is a conflict between the id (the "all for me" part of the personality) and the superego (the conscience), which is repressed in early development but emerges again in adulthood.

Biological theorists view anxiety differently. One biological theory points to the sympathoadrenal (fight-or-flight) responses to stress to explain signs and symptoms of anxiety, and observes that the blood vessels constrict because epinephrine and norepinephrine have been released, causing blood pressure to rise. Another biological theory implicates a lack of the neurotransmitter gamma-aminobutyric acid (GABA) in the etiology of anxiety. GABA is an inhibitory neurotransmitter that prevents postsynaptic excitation.

If the body adapts to the stress, hormone levels adjust and body functions return to a homeostatic state. If the body does not adapt to the stress, the immune system is challenged and risk for physical illness increases.

You may observe psychological responses to physical illness. It is important to recognize the relationship between physical and emotional responses to stress. Some examples of medical conditions that occur because of the body's response to stress are shown in Table 57.1.

Differential Diagnosis

Because there are so many symptoms associated with anxiety disorders, it is important for people to have a complete physical examination before diagnosing an anxiety disorder. Some medical disorders, such as hyperthyroidism, may mimic anxiety. More than one condition may occur at the same time.

Types of Anxiety Disorders

PHOBIA. Phobias are the most common of the anxiety disorders. There are more than 700 documented phobias. *Simple phobias* are defined as irrational fears of specific objects or situations such as snakes or bridges. *Social phobias* are characterized by a persistent fear of behaving or performing in a way that will be humiliating or embarrassing to the individual, such as public speaking, eating in front of others, or using public restrooms. The person is very aware of the fear and even the fact that it is irrational, but is unable to gain control over the stressor and the fear continues.

The psychoanalytic view implies that it really is not the object that is the source of the fear, but rather the fear is a result of a defense mechanism called **displacement**. For example, the person with a phobia of snakes may have seen a frightening movie in which someone died from a snake bite. The stated object of the phobia would be interpreted as a symbol for the underlying cause of the fear, such as fear of dying.

PANIC DISORDER. Panic is a state of extreme fear that cannot be controlled; it is also referred to as panic attack. Panic episodes are recurrent and occur unpredictably. Patients may present themselves at the emergency room because they believe they are having a heart attack or other significant physical illness. Patients must exhibit several episodes within a specified time frame to be given the diagnosis of panic disorder. Some of the symptoms associated with panic disorder include the following:

- Fear (usually of dying, losing control of self, or "going crazy")
- Feelings of impending doom
- Dissociation (feeling that it is happening to someone else or not happening at all)
- Nausea
- Diaphoresis
- Chest pain
- Palpitations
- Shaking.

GENERALIZED ANXIETY DISORDER. In generalized anxiety disorder (GAD), the anxiety itself (also referred to as excessive worry or severe stress) is the expressed symptom. Patients with GAD worry about everything.

• WORD • BUILDING •
eustress: eu—normal or good + stress

TABLE 57.1 RESPONSES TO STRESS

Stress-Related Medical Condition	Pathophysiology	Outcome of Stress on the Body
Lowered immunity	Interferes with effectiveness of antibodies. Possibly related to interactions among the hypothalamus, pituitary gland, adrenal glands, and immune system.	Increased susceptibility to colds and other viruses and illnesses
Burnout	Stress or work-related emotional exhaustion and depression.	Emotional detachment
Migraine, cluster, and tension headaches	Tightening of skeletal muscles. Dilating of cranial arteries.	Nausea, vomiting, tight feeling in or around head and shoulders, tinnitus, inability to tolerate light, weakness of a limb
Stress (peptic) ulcers	Stress contributes to formation of ulcers by stimulating the vagus nerve and ultimately leading to hypersecretion of hydrochloric acid.	Nausea, vomiting, gastrointestinal bleeding, perforation of intestinal walls
Hypertension	Role of stress not positively known. Thought to contribute to hypertension by negatively interacting with kidneys, autonomic nervous system, and endocrine system.	Resistance to blood flow through the cardiovascular system, causing pressure on the arteries. Can lead to stroke, heart attack, and kidney failure
Coronary artery disease	Not fully understood. Stress may be associated with behavioral factors such as overeating, physical inactivity, and obesity.	Hypertension, hypercholesterolemia, atherosclerosis, diabetes
Cancer	Stress lowers the immune response.	Lowered immunity may allow for overcolonization of opportunistic cancer cells.
Asthma	Autonomic nervous system stimulates mucus, increases blood flow, and constricts airways. May be associated with other stress-related conditions such as allergy and viral infection.	Wheezing, coughing, dyspnea, apprehension. May lead to respiratory infections, respiratory failure, or pneumothorax

Symptoms that may be present in GAD include the following:

- Restlessness or feeling "on edge"
- Shaking
- Palpitations
- Dry mouth
- Nausea, vomiting
- Easy frightening
- Hot flashes
- Chills
- Muscle aches
- Hypervigilance (excessive attention to stimuli)
- Polyuria
- Difficulty swallowing.

OBSESSIVE-COMPULSIVE DISORDER. Obsessive-compulsive disorder (OCD) is a different type of anxiety disorder. It consists of two parts: the **obsession** (repetitive thought, urge, or emotion) and the **compulsion** (repetitive act that may appear purposeful). An example of obsessive-compulsive disorder is the need to check that the doors are locked numerous times before one is able to sleep or leave the house. This need to repetitively check the locks may prevent the person from sleeping or leaving the house at all. Some individuals wash their hands compulsively to the point of having raw and bleeding hands. Behaviors become very ritualistic. The person with OCD is unable to stop the thought or the action. Performing the action (such as checking the locks or hand washing) is the mechanism that reduces the anxiety. Although you should not interfere with the repetitive acts, OCD patients can be helped by therapeutic interventions such as cognitive-behavioral therapy or medications (such as fluoxetine).

POST-TRAUMATIC STRESS DISORDER. Post-traumatic stress disorder (PTSD) develops in response to some unexpected emotional or physical trauma when there was the *real threat of death or harm* and the patient was helpless to do anything about it. People who have fought in wars, who have been raped, or who have survived violent storms or violent acts (such as terrorist acts) are examples of those who are susceptible to suffering from this disorder.

A condition that is associated with PTSD is *survivor guilt,* which is the feeling of guilt expressed by those who have survived a tragedy. A survivor of an airline crash may say, "Why me? Why did I make it? I should have died too!" This is especially true if a loved one died in the crash.

Symptoms may appear immediately or may not appear until years later. A key symptom of PTSD is *flashbacks* in which the person may relive the traumatic event as if it were happening at that moment. Sounds and smells associated with the trauma may trigger the flashback.

Signs and symptoms of PTSD include the following:

- Flashbacks
- Social withdrawal
- Feelings of low self-esteem
- Changes in relationships with significant others
- Difficulty forming new relationships
- Hypervigilance
- Irritability and outbursts of anger seemingly for no obvious reason
- Depression
- Chemical dependency.

Therapeutic Measures for Patients with Anxiety Disorders

Treatment for anxiety is individualized and may include one or more of the following: medications (psychopharmacology), individual psychotherapy, group therapy, systematic desensitization, hypnosis, imagery, relaxation exercises, and biofeedback (see *Evidence-Based Practice* box).

EVIDENCE-BASED PRACTICE

Clinical Question

Is the use of guided imagery a useful nursing intervention for anxiety?

Evidence

In multiple studies of patient anxiety, participants who used guided imagery had reduced anxiety and less use of anxiety medications (McCaffrey & Taylor, 2005; Miller, 2003; Toth et al., 2007).

Another study looked at a combination of diaphragmatic breathing and guided imagery in a group of patients undergoing brachytherapy for breast or gynecological cancer. The study used 10 minutes of face-to-face training and a follow-up taped script via audiocassette. Patients in the intervention group had significantly less anxiety at follow-up several weeks later than those in the control group (Leon-Pizarro et al., 2007).

Implications for Nursing Practice

Guided imagery is useful for reducing anxiety in a variety of patient settings. With proper training, guided imagery is an intervention that nurses can deliver at the bedside as an effective anxiety reduction strategy.

REFERENCES

Leon-Pizarro, C., Gich, I., Barthe, E., et al. (2007). A randomized trial of the effect of training in relaxation and guided imagery techniques in improving psychological and quality of life indices for gynecologic and breast brachytherapy patients. *Psychooncology, 16*, 971–979.

McCaffrey, R., & Taylor, N. (2005). Effective anxiety treatment prior to diagnostic cardiac catheterization. *Holistic Nursing Practice, 19*(2), 70–73.

Miller, R. (2003). Nurses at community hospital welcome guided imagery tool. *Dimensions of Critical Care Nursing, 22*(5), 225–226.

Toth, M., Wolsko, P. M., Foreman, J., et al. (2007). A pilot study for a randomized, controlled trial on the effects of guided imagery in hospitalized medical patients. *Journal of Alternative and Complementary Medicine, 13*(2), 194–197.

Psychopharmacology usually involves the benzodiazepines, an antianxiety classification of medications. Alprazolam (Xanax) or lorazepam (Ativan) is commonly used and is effective in most cases. Benzodiazepines are used for short-term treatment because of the strong potential for chemical dependency. Individuals who need longer term therapy for anxiety or who have chemical dependency tendencies can be safely and effectively treated with buspirone (Buspar), clonazepam (Klonopin), the selective serotonin reuptake inhibitors (SSRIs) paroxetine (Paxil) or sertraline (Zoloft), the antihistamine hydroxyzine hydrochloride (Atarax), or the antihypertensive agent clonidine (Catapres). See Table 57.2 for a review of medications.

In *systematic desensitization,* the patient is exposed gradually (rating the fear on a scale from 1 to 10) to the object that causes the anxiety. *Hypnosis* places the patient in a subconscious state, then helps the patient recall events that may be producing anxiety so they can be dealt with. Other therapies were discussed in Chapter 56.

Nursing Process for the Patient with Anxiety

DATA COLLECTION. Observe the patient's anxiety level. Ask about triggers of anxiety and coping mechanisms that have been successful or unsuccessful in the past. Stay alert for physical symptoms, such as changes in vital signs, diaphoresis, or tremor. Assess for the presence of suicidal thoughts and observe for suicidal behavior. It is important to identify anxiety and intervene at the lower levels, before escalation to severe and panic anxiety levels.

NURSING DIAGNOSES, PLANNING, AND IMPLEMENTATION

Anxiety Related to Response to Stressors as Evidenced by Behavioral and Physiological Manifestations (specify) or Statement of Anxious Feelings

EXPECTED OUTCOME: The patient will verbalize that anxiety is controlled. The patient will identify precipitants and

TABLE 57.2 MEDICATIONS USED FOR ALTERATIONS IN MENTAL HEALTH

Medication Class/Action	Examples	Route	Side Effects	Nursing Implications
Typical Antipsychotics				
Block mainly D_2 dopamine receptors (used less often because of serious extrapyramidal side effects).	chlorpromazine (Thorazine) haloperidol (Haldol) fluphenazine (Prolixin) thioridazine (Mellaril) thiothixene (Navane) trifluoperazine (Trilafon) trifluoperazine (Stelazine)	PO, IM PO, IM, long-acting IM PO, IM, long-acting IM PO PO, IM PO, IM PO, IM	Extrapyramidal side effects (EPSEs): pseudoparkinsonism, akathisia, dystonia, tardive dyskinesia, photosensitivity, orthostatic hypotension, gynecomastia, neuroleptic malignant syndrome, anticholinergic effects	For short-term use because of side effects. Monitor for EPSEs. Have patient rise slowly to counter orthostatic hypotension. Offer ice chips, gum or hard candy for dry mouth. Monitor urinary and bowel elimination. Avoid use if patient is in first trimester of pregnancy. Do not use/take with alcohol or other CNS depressants. *Patient teaching:* Use sunscreen when outside.
Atypical Antipsychotics				
Block multiple dopamine and serotonin receptors.	clozapine (Clozaril) risperidone (Risperdal) olanzapine (Zyprexa) quetiapine (Seroquel) ziprasidone (Geodon) aripiprazole (Abilify) paliperidone (Invega)	PO PO, IM, long-acting IM PO, fast-dissolving tablets PO PO, IM	Agranulocytosis (Clozaril); weight gain; type 2 diabetes; dose-related EPSE (especially with Risperdal and in the elderly); lowers seizure threshold; caution with cardiac patients	Monitor CBC (Clozaril). Monitor weight gain. Monitor glucose level for onset of type 2 diabetes.
Antidepressants				
Selective Serotonin Reuptake Inhibitor (SSRIs) Block the reuptake of serotonin at the presynaptic receptor.	fluoxetine (Prozac) sertraline (Zoloft) paroxetine (Paxil) escitalopram (Lexapro) citalopram (Celexa) fluvoxamine (Luvox)	PO, once-weekly dosing PO	Excitation, nausea and vomiting, decreased libido, anorexia and weight loss, increased suicide risk the first few weeks of therapy	Allow time for side effects to subside. Do not administer after 3 p.m. to keep excitation from affecting sleep. *Patient teaching:* It will take 6–8 weeks for therapeutic effects to occur. Do not stop drug abruptly. Do not take with other serotonin-type medications including St. John's wort and SAMe.
Tricyclic Antidepressants Partially block the reuptake of serotonin and norepinephrine at the presynaptic receptor (used infrequently because of side effects).	amitriptyline (Elavil) nortriptyline (Pamelor) imipramine (Tofranil)	PO	Anticholinergic effects, sedation, weight gain, orthostatic hypotension, dysrhythmias, increased suicide risk the first few weeks of therapy	Decreases effects of antihypertensives. Lowers seizure threshold. Will affect oral contraceptives. *Patient teaching:* It will take 6–8 weeks for therapeutic effects to occur. Do not stop drug abruptly. Overdose can cause fatal dysrhythmias.
Selective Serotonin Norepinephrine Reuptake Inhibitors (SNRIs)	venlafaxine (Effexor, Effexor XR) duloxetine (Cymbalta) desvenlafaxine (Pristiq)	PO	Anxiety, abnormal dreams, dizziness, nervousness	Monitor blood pressure for systolic hypertension. *Patient teaching:* Do not take with other serotonin-type medications, including St. John's wort and SAMe. Do not stop drug abruptly.

Continued

TABLE 57.2 MEDICATIONS USED FOR ALTERATIONS IN MENTAL HEALTH—cont'd

Medication Class/Action	Examples	Route	Side Effects	Nursing Implications
Monoamine Oxidase Inhibitors (MAOIs) Block the action of monamine oxidase.	phenelzine (Nardil) tranylcypromine (Parnate) isocarboxazid (Marplan)	PO	Anticholinergic effects, orthostatic hypotension, will interact with foods containing tyramine and cause hypertensive crisis, headache	Rarely used because of side effects and interactions. Interacts with many prescribed and over-the-counter medications. Serious fatal reactions with SSRIs or SNRIs. *Patient teaching:* Follow tyramine-free diet. Do not stop drug abruptly.
Tetracyclic Antidepressants Blocks multiple serotonin and histamine receptors; adrenoreceptor antagonist.	mirtazapine (Remeron) maprotiline (Ludiomil)	PO	Anticholinergic effects, possible increase in blood pressure, sedation, confusion, orthostatic hypotension, increased appetite and weight gain	Administer at bedtime to counteract sedating effects. *Patient teaching:* Do not take with alcohol or other CNS depressants.
Antianxiety Agents				
Benzodiazepines Potentiate effects of GABA, which causes a calming effect.	alprazolam (Xanax) diazepam (Valium) lorazepam (Ativan) clonazepam (Klonopin)	PO PO, IM, IV, rectal PO, IM, IV, SL PO	Sedation, hangover, ataxia, confusion, dizziness, anticholinergic effects	Short-term use only. Addictive. Use cautiously in elderly. Do not use in pregnant patients. *Patient teaching:* Do not operate heavy machinery. Do not stop drug abruptly.
Buspar Action is unknown.	buspirone (BuSpar)	PO	Headaches, dizziness, GI upset, light-headedness	Non–habit forming with little sedating effect. *Patient teaching:* It will take 3–6 weeks for drug to work.
Anticonvulsant Mood Stabilizers				
Antikindling effect, affect GABA receptors.	carbamazepine (Tegretol) lamotrigine (Lamictal) valproic acid (Depakote)	PO	Dizziness, ataxia, drowsiness, blurred vision, nausea, vomiting, headache, weight gain, blood dyscrasias, photosensitivity, rash, Stevens-Johnson syndrome	Loading dose may be ordered for acute mania. Monitor for bleeding. Use cautiously in elderly and in patients with liver or renal disease. Do not use in pregnant or breastfeeding patients. *Patient teaching:* Use sunscreen, and report any signs of rash immediately.
Antimanic Agents				
Lithium Decreases postsynaptic receptor sensitivity.	lithium carbonate (Eskalith)	PO	Thirst, nausea and vomiting, weight gain, tremors, skin rash (acne), hair loss, hypothyroidism	Narrow therapeutic range increases risk of toxicity. Monitor blood levels. Do not use in cardiac or renal disease. Do not use with diuretics. Do not use in pregnant patients. Check interactions with other medications.
Antiparkinsonian Agents				
Restore the natural balance of acetylcholine and dopamine in the CNS to manage extrapyramidal side effects.	benztropine (Cogentin) trihexyphenidyl (Artane) diphenhydramine (Benadryl)	PO, IM	Anticholinergic effects, nausea, GI upset, sedation, dizziness, orthostatic hypotension	Caution in patients with hypersensitivity, glaucoma, history of urine retention.

CNS = central nervous system; GABA = gamma-aminobutyric acid; GI = gastrointestinal; SAMe = S-adenosylmethionine.

patterns for anxiety and demonstrate techniques to control anxiety. Physical signs of anxiety, such as tremors or changes in vital signs, will be absent.

- Assist the patient to identify precipitants and patterns to anxiety. *Recognition of patterns can help guide care and allow the patient to initiate measures to stop anxiety from progressing.*
- Maintain a calm milieu and manner. *A chaotic environment can increase the patient's anxiety. Anxiety is contagious and may be transmitted from staff to patient.*
- Maintain open communication. Encourage the patient to verbalize thoughts and feelings. Observe nonverbal communication. *Honesty in dealing with patients helps them learn to trust others and enhances their self-esteem.*
- Encourage the patient to use positive self-talk, such as "I can do this. Anxiety can't kill me." *This helps the patient replace negative anxious thoughts with positive statements to reduce anxiety.*
- Report and document any changes in behavior, such as positive or negative alterations in the way a patient responds to the nursing staff, to the treatment plan, or to other people and situations. *Any change can be significant to the patient's care.*
- Encourage activities, but avoid placing the patient in a competitive situation. *Activities that are enjoyable and nonstressful provide diversion and give staff an opportunity to provide positive feedback about the progress the patient is making. Competitive situations can produce anxiety.*
- Encourage problem solving and assist to develop alternative solutions. Assist the patient to identify what has worked in the past. *This can help the patient focus on strategies that were effective in the past, and eliminate those that are not effective.*
- Stay with a patient during acute severe or panic levels of anxiety. *Feelings of being abandoned can increase anxiety. The nurse's presence provides a feeling of safety for the patient.*
- Implement suicide precautions if indicated. *The patient may need to be protected from self-harm until treatment is effective.*
- Assess your own level of anxiety. *An anxious nurse may make the patient more anxious.*

EVALUATION. Is the patient able to implement strategies to control anxiety? Does the patient recognize triggers of anxiety? Does the patient state he or she feels less anxious? Are physical signs, such as tremors or changes in vital signs, improved? (See Table 57.3.)

CRITICAL THINKING

Tommy

■ Tommy has come to your clinic with numerous cracks on his hands. They are bleeding and very sore. Tommy tells you that he has to wash his hands all the time. His mother says he washes for 2 to 3 hours at a time and he will not stop when she tells him to. The doctor has diagnosed Tommy with obsessive-compulsive disorder and has explained the illness to Tommy and his mother. When the doctor leaves the room, Tommy's mother begins to cry. "What did he just say? What am I supposed to do? What did I do wrong that Tommy got this illness?" How do you respond?

Suggested answers at end of chapter.

Mood Disorders

Mood disorders (also called affective disorders) are disorders in which the major symptom is extreme changes in mood (emotions) and affect (the outward expression of the mood). Moods involving both highs and lows are bipolar disorders; low moods without any highs are described as depressive disorders. Mood disorders are diagnosed when symptoms begin to interfere with normal day-to-day functioning. People of all age-groups and all ethnic and socioeconomic groups can develop mood disorders.

TABLE 57.3 ANXIETY SUMMARY

Signs and Symptoms	*Phobia:* irrational fear of object or situation *Panic disorder:* extreme fear, feelings of impending doom, palpitations *Generalized anxiety disorder:* worry, restlessness, palpitations *Obsessive-compulsive disorder:* uncontrollable repetitive thoughts, urges, or actions
Diagnosis	History of symptoms; physical causes for symptoms must be ruled out first
Therapeutic Measures	Antianxiety medication Selective serotonin reuptake inhibitors Systematic desensitization Psychotherapy Relaxation exercises
Nursing Diagnosis	*Anxiety*

Etiological Theories

Psychoanalytic theory explains that people who have suffered loss in their lives are at risk for developing depression. Depression is also associated with unresolved anger and has been described as "anger turned inward." In other words, people who cannot or do not deal appropriately with situations that anger them may repress the anger (turn it inside) and become depressed.

Cognitive theorists believe that the way people perceive events and situations may lead to depression. Instead of thinking about failing an examination as being unfortunate and disappointing, some people with tendencies toward depression may exaggerate the emotion and turn the situation into something much deeper, such as thoughts of "I'm stupid" or "I'll never get anywhere."

Biological theories offer genetic links and neurotransmitter dysfunctions as two etiologies. Serotonin, norepinephrine, and dopamine have an effect on mood; if these neurotransmitters are elevated, mood is elevated, and if they are low, mood is low. Biological theorists also believe that there is a connection between these neurotransmitters and female hormones.

Differential Diagnosis

Symptoms of depression may occur in conjunction with other disorders, such as schizophrenia or drug side effects or overuse. Heart failure, nutritional deficiencies, drug toxicity, thyroid disease, fluid and electrolyte imbalances, infections, and diabetes can be associated with depression. Depression related to grief is considered a normal reaction unless it is prolonged (unresolved grief).

Types of Mood Disorders

MAJOR (UNIPOLAR) DEPRESSION. Major depression is an episodic condition, and symptoms interfere with the person's usual social or occupational functioning. Depressed people view the world through "gray-tinted glasses." The *Diagnostic and Statistical Manual of Mental Disorders, Fourth Edition, Text Revision* (DSM-IV-TR) specifies that symptoms of major depression include either a depressed mood or **anhedonia** (the loss of pleasure in things that are usually pleasurable) along with at least five of the following symptoms:

- Significant weight loss or gain
- Increase or decrease in appetite
- Sleep pattern disturbances—insomnia or hypersomnia
- Increased fatigue
- Increased agitation or psychomotor retardation
- Diminished libido
- Anergia
- Social withdrawal
- Decreased ability to think, remember, or concentrate
- Feelings of guilt or hopelessness
- Indecisiveness
- Suicidal ideation.

• WORD • BUILDING •
anhedonia: an—not + hedonia—pleasure

BIPOLAR DISORDER. About 2 million people in the United States have **bipolar** disorder. Formerly called manic depressive illness, bipolar disorder is a mood disorder in which patients experience both **mania** (extreme elation or agitation) and extreme depression. Bipolar disorder is more severe than major depression. Affected people stay depressed longer, relapse more often, display more depressive symptoms, have more delusions and hallucinations, commit suicide more often, require more hospitalizations, and overall experience more incapacitation.

Affected people can cycle slowly (over weeks, months, or even years), or they can be "rapid cyclers" who can change moods several times in an hour. Common signs of depression were covered in the preceding section. Common signs of mania include the following:

- Excessive high (euphoric) moods
- Increased energy, activity, restlessness
- Decreased need for sleep
- Grandiosity (unrealistic belief in one's abilities or powers)
- Extreme irritability and distractibility
- Uncharacteristically poor judgment
- Pressured and rapid speech
- Flight of ideas or subjective experience that one's thoughts are racing
- Increase in goal-directed behavior
- Excessive involvement in pleasurable activities that have a high potential for unpleasant consequences, such as sex, substance abuse, or shopping sprees
- Obnoxious, provocative, or intrusive behavior.

Therapeutic Measures for Patients with Mood Disorders

About 80% of people with major depression respond to treatment. Bipolar disorder is more difficult to treat. Some common medical treatments for *all* mood disorders include the following:

- Antidepressant medications
- Mood stabilizers
- Psychotherapy
- Electroconvulsive therapy.

Lithium was once the drug of choice for treating bipolar disorder. Lithium is an antimanic medication with a very narrow therapeutic range, which means that toxic drug levels can easily develop. Blood must be drawn regularly to assess that serum lithium levels are in the therapeutic range.

Mood stabilizers like the anticonvulsants valproic acid (Depakote) and lamotrigine (Lamictal) are now more commonly used than lithium to treat bipolar disorder. Atypical antipsychotics are also commonly used with a mood stabilizer when the patient is in the acute manic state. Antidepressants should be used carefully because they can induce a manic episode. See Table 57.2 for a summary of medications. Also see Box 57.1, *Nutrition Notes.*

Psychotherapy for the patient and family may be helpful for any type of mood disorder. It can help the patient

Box 57.1 Nutrition Notes

Food-Drug Interactions in Patients with Mental Health Disorders

Monoamine Oxidase Inhibitors

When a patient taking a monoamine oxidase inhibitor (MAOI) consumes foods high in tyramine, the drug prevents the normal breakdown of tyramine, leading to excessive epinephrine levels. Hypertension results, sometimes severe enough to cause intracranial hemorrhage.

All food groups except breads and cereals have some items with sufficient tyramine to cause problems for patients taking MAOIs. The amount of tyramine varies even in different samples of a particular food. Examples of common foods to be avoided are bananas, aged cheese, yogurt, bologna, salami, pepperoni, summer sausage, chocolate, beer, and wine.

Lithium Carbonate

Lithium carbonate, used to treat bipolar disorder, is absorbed, distributed, and excreted alongside sodium. Fluctuations in sodium intake affect lithium metabolism:

- Decreased sodium intake with decreased fluid intake may lead to retention of lithium and overmedication.
- Increased sodium intake from food or medications and increased fluid intake may hasten excretion of lithium, resulting in worsening signs and symptoms of mania.

understand the illness and learn problem solving and other new adaptive coping behaviors. For young children, play therapy is the most common and effective form of therapy. Electroconvulsive therapy is an option for individuals with rapid-cycling bipolar disorder or major depression that is not responsive to conventional treatment.

SAFETY TIP

When collecting data from your patient, be sure to ask about herbal supplements the patient may use in addition to prescription and over-the-counter (OTC) medications. Many people take St. John's wort, an OTC herbal supplement, for depression. Although it may be effective for some people with mild depression, it can interact with many prescribed medications that influence serotonin levels. If combined with prescription antidepressants, it can cause serotonin syndrome, an excess of serotonin resulting in agitation, confusion, diarrhea, muscle spasms, and even death (Boyer & Shannon, 2005).

Nursing Process for the Patient with a Mood Disorder

See the *Nursing Care Plan for the Patient with Depression.* Also see Table 57.4.

CRITICAL THINKING

Mr. Zenz

■ Mr. Zenz is the manager of a busy office. His usual behavior is rather sullen, and he comes across as quiet or sad to various members of the staff. He is in his 40s and married, with three children, ages 4, 5, and 7. He speaks of them proudly but always comments that they "take after their mother." His management style in the office is to let people do their jobs; he rarely interferes, although his door is always open and staff members are told they are welcome any time. Recently, however, staff members have noticed a change in Mr. Zenz. He moves quickly, speaks quickly, and has set unrealistic goals for the staff. He frequently says he has called the president of the company to tell him of his new ideas. He says he has not slept in several days and he feels terrific. He has changed his wardrobe and has begun pointing out specific performance issues to staff. He jokes with staff. Staff members are made aware that he has "bipolar disorder" and has quit taking his medications. His wife has asked for the staff's help. Remember: He is your boss. How do you respond to Mrs. Zenz? How do you approach him?

Suggested answers at end of chapter.

TABLE 57.4 DEPRESSION SUMMARY

Signs and Symptoms	*Unipolar:* depressed mood, weight changes, anhedonia, sleep disturbance, social withdrawal *Bipolar:* signs and symptoms of depression cycling with euphoria; delusions, hallucinations
Diagnosis	History; physiological causes must be ruled out
Therapeutic Measures	Antidepressant medication, mood stabilizers (anticonvulsants), psychotherapy, electroconvulsive therapy
Nursing Diagnoses	*Risk for Suicide* *Ineffective Coping* *Powerlessness*

NURSING CARE PLAN for the Patient with Depression

Nursing Diagnosis: *Risk for Suicide*

Expected Outcome: The patient will not harm himself or herself.

Evaluation of Outcome: Did the patient remain free from self-harm during hospitalization? Does patient have ongoing support following discharge?

Interventions	Rationale	Evaluation
Ask patient directly about suicidal ideations each shift.	Ongoing assessment of suicidal risk is essential to patient safety.	Is the patient verbalizing warning signs of suicide?
Create a safe environment for the patient.	Patient safety is a nursing priority.	Are means of harming self kept from patient?
Initiate suicide precautions according to agency protocol.	The patient must be protected until risk is reduced.	Is increased surveillance of patient implemented and communicated to all staff?
Encourage the patient to seek out nursing staff when experiencing suicidal thoughts.	Active listening and therapeutic communication by staff provide the patient with empathy and alternatives to acting on suicidal thoughts.	Does the patient seek out nursing staff when experiencing suicidal thoughts?

Nursing Diagnosis: *Ineffective Coping*

Expected Outcomes: The patient will cope effectively as evidenced by verbalizing the ability to cope and asking for help when needed and by demonstrating new effective coping strategies.

Evaluation of Outcomes: Does the patient exhibit increased ability to problem solve and cope with stressors?

Interventions	Rationale	Evaluation
Use therapeutic communication techniques to allow the patient to verbalize feelings.	Verbalization of feelings in a supportive environment may assist patient to work through issues.	Does the patient verbalize feelings to nursing staff?
Assist the patient to describe stressors and coping mechanisms used.	Reviewing successful coping strategies can strengthen effective coping and diminish ineffective methods.	Is the patient able to identify stressors and related coping strategies used in the past?
Help the patient set realistic goals and identify his or her existing coping skills and knowledge.	Providing validation of actual stress and available coping resources and strategies aids in positive adaptation to stress.	Does the patient set realistic goals? Does the patient have some effective coping skills on which to draw?
Encourage the patient to make choices and participate in care.	Active involvement in care increases the possibility of positive adjustment.	Is the patient actively involved in care?

NURSING CARE PLAN for the Patient with Depression—cont'd

Nursing Diagnosis: *Powerlessness*

Expected Outcomes: The patient will reduce feelings of powerlessness as evidenced by verbal expression of having control over life, situation, or care, and by participation in care or decision making when opportunities are provided.

Evaluation of Outcomes: Does patient identify feelings of powerlessness? Does patient identify factors that are controllable and actively participate in care?

Interventions	Rationale	Evaluation
Assess for factors contributing to powerlessness.	Correct identification of actual or perceived problems is essential to providing appropriate support.	Is the patient able to identify factors contributing to powerlessness?
Help the patient to identify factors that are or are not under his or her control.	Identifying factors within the patient's control encourages the patient to take some control over the situation.	Is the patient able to identify what is controllable and what is not controllable in his or her life?
Allow ventilation of powerless feelings.	Sharing feelings in groups can lead to the realization that similar feelings are experienced by others and reduce feelings of powerlessness.	Is the patient sharing feelings with nursing staff and in therapeutic groups?
Encourage the patient to actively participate in care with goal-directed activities.	Goal-directed behavior increases self-efficacy and empowerment.	Does the patient set realistic goals daily and achieve them daily?

Somatoform/Psychosomatic Disorders

The **somatoform** (or **psychosomatic**) disorders are conditions in which physical symptoms occur with no known organic cause. It is believed that the physical symptoms are an expression of psychological pain or distress. Because the patient is not able to control the symptoms, they are considered to be caused by some unconscious mechanism.

Etiological Theories

Psychoanalytic theorists believe that the somatoform disorders are rooted in unconscious mechanisms that develop to deny, repress, and displace anxiety. Biological research suggests the possibility of a genetic predisposition to somatic difficulties.

Types of Somatoform Disorders

Several illnesses fall within the category of somatoform disorders, including conversion disorder, hypochondriasis, dysmorphophobia/body dysmorphic disorder, somatization disorder, and somatoform pain disorder. Discussion of all of these disorders is beyond the scope of this book; however, this chapter does give a brief explanation of conversion disorder.

CONVERSION DISORDER. Conversion disorder is an illness that emerges from overuse of the conversion reaction defense mechanism. (See Table 56.3 in Chapter 56.) In conversion disorder there is a loss or change in physical functioning that seems to have a neurologic connection. Paralysis and blindness are the two most common examples of this disorder. Age of onset is usually adolescence and young adulthood, but it can occur later in life as well.

The symptoms, although not caused by organic disease, are very real to the patient. It should not be conveyed to the patient that you think the person is "faking" the illness; this is not true. Patients are truly experiencing the symptoms. It is believed that the symptom is allowing the person to avoid some situation that is unacceptable to him or her. The symptom helps the patient relieve the anxiety. This is called *primary gain. Secondary gain* results from the extra benefits one may acquire as a result of staying ill, such as extra emotional support, sympathy, love, or financial benefits.

• WORD • BUILDING •

psychosomatic: psych(e)—soul or mind + somatic—body

Therapeutic Measures for Patients with Somatoform Disorders

Because of the physical symptoms, hospitalized patients are usually admitted to a medical unit rather than a psychiatric unit. True physiological causes for symptoms must be ruled out before diagnosis of a somatoform disorder can be made. Treatment is individualized for the patient. Hypnosis and relaxation techniques are used with many patients. Methods of stress management are taught. Behavior management may be effective for some patients. Patients may resist accepting the fact that their problem is psychological or emotional in nature and may feel insulted and become resistant to treatment.

Medications are used sparingly. When they are ordered for a patient, the classifications of choice are usually antidepressants, antianxiety agents, or both.

Nursing Management for Patients with Somatoform Disorders

Nursing management for somatoform disorders includes the following:

- *Skillful communication.* Honesty and gaining trust encourage the patient to verbalize thoughts and feelings about the physical and emotional aspects of the disorder. An example of a way to be honest about the situation would be to reinforce what the physician has said to the patient, such as "Ms. Parks, your doctor can find no physical or life-threatening conditions at this time. We will continue to observe and examine you. We will make every attempt to help you improve." Sometimes the practitioner helps the patient find a healthy behavior to substitute for the symptom.
- *Therapy.* Keeping the patient focused on other topics than the symptoms may help in the recovery. Spend time with the patient other than when physical reports are occurring.
- *Support.* When caring for the patient with a somatoform disorder, you must pay attention to the person but must not reinforce the symptoms. Use a matter-of-fact approach, and don't imply that the symptoms are not real. A thorough head-to-toe examination should always be done. Observe and record the frequency of symptom reports. Provide explanations and support during diagnostic tests. The patient will see your concern for his or her health, but you will not be focusing on the area of dysfunction or reinforcing the problem. All findings should be documented objectively.

Schizophrenia

Schizophrenia is becoming more widely viewed as a group of illnesses rather than a single condition. The term *schizophrenia* (which means "split mind") was first used by a Swiss psychiatrist, Eugene Bleuler (1911). Schizophrenia is a serious disorder of thought and association and is characterized by inability to distinguish between what is real and what is not and also by hallucinations, delusions, and limited socialization. People who have schizophrenia may not be able to differentiate between what is "theirs" and what is "everybody else's" in relation to social functioning. Poor self-esteem may be present. It is difficult for them to focus on one topic for any length of time. Schizophrenia is not the same as dissociative identity disorder (once called multiple personality disorder).

Schizophrenia has an insidious onset and often begins during adolescence or young adulthood. It develops over time, and symptoms may go unnoticed for a time before diagnosis. There are four phases of schizophrenia:

1. *Schizoid personality.* Those in this phase are perceived as being indifferent, cold, and aloof. They are often described as loners and don't seem to enjoy close relationships with others. In an adolescent, these behaviors may be dismissed as normal for age. Not all individuals with schizoid personality go on to develop schizophrenia.
2. *Prodromal phase.* Affected people continue to be socially withdrawn and begin to show behavior that is peculiar or eccentric. Role functioning is impaired, personal hygiene is neglected, and disturbances are evident in communication, ideation, and perception.
3. *Schizophrenia.* This is the third and active phase of the disorder. Psychotic symptoms are prominent and include delusions, hallucinations, and impairment in work, social relations, and self-care.
4. *Residual phase.* Symptoms are similar to the prodromal phase, with flat affect and impairment in role functioning.

Positive and Negative Symptoms

Positive symptoms of schizophrenia can be thought of as those symptoms that reflect an "excess" or distortion of normal functioning. Positive symptoms include hallucinations, delusions, disorganized thinking, and disorganized behavior. **Delusions** are fixed, false beliefs that cannot be changed by logic or factual proof. Typically, patients exhibit delusions of grandeur, persecution, or guilt. **Hallucinations** are false sensory perceptions. They can affect any of the five senses; auditory and visual delusions are most common. For example, a person might see a person that no one else sees, or hear voices that no one else hears. In contrast, **illusions** are mistaken perceptions of reality. For example, a person may see a glowing sunset and think the horizon is on fire. Both typical and atypical antipsychotic medications work well to manage the positive symptoms of schizophrenia.

Negative symptoms of schizophrenia can be thought of as a loss of normal functioning. Negative symptoms include affective blunting or flattening, **alogia**, **avolition**, apathy, anhedonia, and social isolation. It is thought that these are the most debilitating symptoms of schizophrenia because

• WORD • BUILDING •

alogia: a—not + logia—(able to) speak

avolition: a—not + volition—energy or initiative to do something they keep the individual from living a normal life. These symptoms respond to atypical antipsychotic medications, but not the typical antipsychotic agents.

Pathophysiology and Etiology

There are psychoanalytical and biological theories of the causes of schizophrenia. The causes of schizophrenia are highly debated on both sides of the nature-versus-nurture theories.

The psychoanalytical, or nurture, theories go back to the anal stage of Freudian theory. The inability to meet the challenge of oral gratification leaves people in the adolescent and young adult years unable to handle their developing sexuality, according to Freud. Lack of nurturing mother-child relationships can also lead to personalities that are cool or indifferent in their relationships. Freud would also attribute the disruption of effective communication to failure to attain oral gratification.

The role of genetics in schizophrenia (psychobiological or nature theory) has been examined in twin studies, family studies, and adoption studies for more than 75 years. Studies of identical twins show that if one twin has schizophrenia, the other has about a 50% chance of developing it. In fraternal twins, the percentage drops to about 10%. It is believed that the more genes twins or family members have in common, the greater the probability of the second twin developing schizophrenia.

Other studies have examined the relationship between neurotransmitters and schizophrenia. Patients with a diagnosis of schizophrenia typically have elevated dopamine levels or a brain that overreacts to the amount of dopamine present. Glutamate is an excitatory neurotransmitter that also appears to be related to schizophrenia. The glutamate theory proposes that there is an underactivity of glutamate of the brain (Patil et al., 2007). Today, schizophrenia is primarily thought of as a series of brain disorders characterized by brain abnormalities and neurotransmitter dysfunction.

Types of Schizophrenia

There are several categories of schizophrenia. This chapter discusses only the most common: paranoid schizophrenia. Paranoid schizophrenia is defined as schizophrenia in which the person exhibits unusual suspicions and fears. The person also may be hostile and aggressive.

Patients with paranoid schizophrenia tend to have delusions of persecution or grandeur. Those with persecutory delusions may state that they feel tormented or followed by people. Patients often integrate people around them into their delusions. They may feel that nursing staff, relatives, or announcers on the radio or television are trying to harm them. In delusions of grandeur, patients may state that they are God or the president of the United States.

Hallucinations often accompany delusions. Hallucinations can affect any of the five senses; the most common are auditory, followed by visual. Patients with paranoid schizophrenia talk about hearing voices. These voices are frightening and derogatory to the patient and are responsible for many of the actions performed by people with paranoid schizophrenia. Patients experience increased fear, anxiety, and suicidal ideation as a result of the voices. You may see or hear patients arguing with what at first appears to be themselves. Actually the patient is arguing with the voices. Describing the voices is difficult, but imagine that you are in a room with six televisions on different stations at the same time. This example comes close to what some patients have described.

Therapeutic Measures for the Patient with Schizophrenia

Medications, social skills training, and individual and family psychotherapy are indicated for patients with schizophrenia. Among the classifications of medications that may be prescribed are the typical and atypical antipsychotics, which block dopamine action in the brain. There are different dopamine tracts in the brain, and typical antipsychotics have a greater effect on the motor function tract, resulting in extrapyramidal symptoms such as parkinsonism (see medications in Table 57.2). Anticholinergic medications such as benztropine (Cogentin) or trihexyphenidyl (Artane) are used to combat the extrapyramidal side effects of the typical antipsychotics by helping return balance between dopamine, acetylcholine, and other neurotransmitters. Newer, atypical antipsychotic medications such as clozapine (Clozaril) and risperidone (Risperdal) have fewer extrapyramidal side effects, but have other side effects. They are effective in treating both the positive and negative symptoms of schizophrenia.

Psychotherapy may include individual, group, and family therapy. Electroconvulsive therapy (ECT) is used in some severe cases or in cases that are difficult to treat; ECT is usually not used until other methods of therapy have been exhausted. Referral of the patient and family to organizations such as the National Alliance on Mental Illness (NAMI) provides helpful education and support (www.nami.org).

Nursing Process for the Patient with Schizophrenia

DATA COLLECTION. Observe the patient with schizophrenia for positive and negative symptoms, including hallucinations, delusions, and illusions. Observe interactions with others. Monitor the patient for response to medications, including side effects. Determine the person's ability to function and manage activities of daily living (ADLs).

NURSING DIAGNOSES, PLANNING, AND IMPLEMENTATION

Disturbed Sensory Perception Related to Abnormalities in Neurotransmitter Function

EXPECTED OUTCOME: The patient will be able to determine what is real and what is not and be able to manage medications, perform ADLs, and function in a community.

- Develop trust. Be honest and consistent in all areas of the patient's treatment plan. *Trust is essential to a therapeutic relationship.*

- Allow the patient to verbalize thoughts and feelings when appropriate to the time and place. *Verbalizing feelings can help the patient clarify concerns and feel supported.*
- Whenever possible, maintain consistent staff assignments *to ensure the best possible continuity of care and to promote the development of a trusting relationship.*
- Never whisper or laugh when the patient cannot hear the whole conversation. Face the patient when having a conversation. *Whispering or turning away may be interpreted as rejection; secretive behaviors can reinforce paranoia and suspiciousness.*
- Avoid placing the patient in situations of competition or embarrassment. *These situations can be threatening to the patient.*
- Never reinforce hallucinations, delusions, or illusions. Orient to reality as needed. *The patient needs to know what is real and what is not.*
- Use distraction to deal with the hallucinations (Table 57.5). Help to connect the delusions and hallucinations to times of increased anxiety. *This models strategies for the patient to use during times of anxiety.*
- Provide a calm and therapeutic milieu *to help reduce anxiety.*
- Provide written instructions and information boards *to help promote reality and self-responsible behavior.*
- Monitor medication use and check the patient's mouth for unswallowed medication as needed. *Patients may have difficulty maintaining a medication schedule or choose to not take medications as prescribed due to paranoia.*
- Keep communication simple. Be brief and clear with all directions. State what is acceptable, giving the rationale and consequences at the same time. State information in positive rather than negative terms: "Eat your food calmly" rather than "Do not throw your food!" *Patients are more likely to process and respond to simple, direct communication.*
- Use touch cautiously. *Perceptions and distortions of reality may cause patients to misconstrue touch.*

EVALUATION. Is the patient oriented to reality? Is he or she able to manage medications, or is there a plan in place to make sure medications are administered? Is the patient able to manage ADLs and live in a community? (See Table 57.6.)

CRITICAL THINKING

Anne

■ While preparing to invite Anne, a young woman receiving chemotherapy on your oncology unit, to a movie in the day room, you observe her standing in the corner of her room trembling. You ask her what's wrong and she responds that she's talking to the woman in the wall. Your first instinct is to giggle, but you ask her, "What woman?" She tells you that you wouldn't understand and says, "You helped put her there and you told me that it is my job to be sure she can't get out." You report this to the charge nurse, who calls the physician. Tests are run, and it is determined that Anne is not experiencing side effects from the chemotherapy. Further work-up delivers the diagnosis of paranoid-type schizophrenia for Anne. What responses are appropriate for the situation above? What special needs might Anne now experience relating to her chemotherapy, if any? How will you get Anne to the movie or to participate in other care activities?

Suggested answers at end of chapter.

TABLE 57.5 SUGGESTED INTERVENTIONS FOR PATIENTS WITH SCHIZOPHRENIA WHO ARE HALLUCINATING

Suggested Action	Rationale
1. "Mr. R., I don't see any snakes. It is time for lunch. I will walk to the dining room with you."	1. Lets the patient know you heard him, but brings him immediately into the reality of time of day and need to go to the dining room.
2. "I see a crack in the wall, Mr. R. It is harmless; you are safe. Susan is here to take you down to occupational therapy now."	2. This is in response to a probable illusion. It lets the patient know that you see something. It validates his fear, but it tells him what you see and then moves him into the here and now.
3. "I know that your thoughts seem very real to you, Ms. C., but they do not seem logical to me. I would like for you to come to your room and get dressed now, please."	3. Again, you are validating the patient's concern without exploring and focusing on the delusion.
4. "Ms. C, it appears to me that you are listening to someone. Are you hearing voices other than mine?"	4. This is a method of validating your impression of what you see. This is as far as you will go into exploring what she may be hearing.
5. "Thank you, Ms. C. I want to help you focus away from the other voices. I am real; they are not. Please come with me to the reading room."	5. Responds to her in the present and reinforces her response to you. Attempts to redirect her thinking.

TABLE 57.6 SCHIZOPHRENIA SUMMARY

Signs and Symptoms	Disorganized speech and behavior Ineffective thinking and decision making Trouble functioning at school and work; self-care deficits Positive symptoms: hallucinations, delusions Negative symptoms: apathy, flat affect, anhedonia
Diagnosis	History Psychiatric evaluation DSM-IV-TR criteria
Therapeutic Measures	Antipsychotic medications Anticholinergic agents to control side effects Psychotherapy Family education Social skills training and therapy
Nursing Diagnoses	*Disturbed Sensory Perception* *Social Isolation* *Impaired Communication*

Substance Abuse Disorders

Alcohol and drug dependency are serious conditions. People start using alcohol and drugs for many reasons, but often it is to feel accepted by a peer group or to feel comfortable and reduce anxiety in a social situation. People mistake the temporary high as a stimulant. In reality, alcohol is a depressant. Any chemical can be potentially dangerous.

It is important to understand the following terms and their definitions:

- **Addiction**—repeated compulsive use of a substance that continues in spite of negative consequences (physical, social, legal).
- **Tolerance**—condition in which increased amounts of a substance are needed over time to achieve the same effect as that previously obtained with smaller doses.
- Physical **withdrawal** syndrome—physiological response to the abrupt stopping or reduction of a substance used (usually) for a long time. Withdrawal symptoms are specific to the substance used.

The general definitions of substance **abuse** and substance **dependence** apply to any substance. *Substance dependence* is a condition in which a person has several (usually three) of the following symptoms for a single 12-month period. The patient:

- needs more of the substance and at more frequent intervals to achieve the same "high," or desired effect of the substance
- spends significant time obtaining the substance
- gives up important social or professional functions to use the substance
- has tried at least once to quit but still obsesses about the substance
- experiences difficulty with job, family, or social activities because of use or withdrawal symptoms
- uses the substance regardless of the problems it causes
- uses the substance to avoid withdrawal symptoms.

Substance abuse is a maladaptive pattern of substance use leading to clinically significant impairment or distress manifested by one or more of the following within a 12-month period:

- Inability to fulfill major role obligations at work, school, or home
- Recurrent legal or interpersonal problems
- Continued use despite social and interpersonal problems
- Participation in physically hazardous situations while impaired, such as driving.

Nurses need to be informed about chemical dependency for several reasons. First, many patients on medical-surgical units are chemically dependent. This affects their healing and the effect of their medications. Second, as part of the human experience, your chance of being in a close personal relationship with a person who is chemically dependent is great. Third, and perhaps most importantly, you are part of a profession whose members are statistically high users and abusers of drugs and alcohol (Box 57.2, *Ethical Considerations*). Studies indicate that 5 to 20 percent of nurses in the United States will be chemically impaired at some point in their lifetime.

Substance abuse is not a one-person illness; it affects personal and professional relationships with people who are associated with the user. The term **dysfunctional** is often used to refer to the relationships in an alcoholic family or work environment. Dishonesty and inability to discuss the situation are strong components of the disease. Many times, people who live or work in the dysfunctional group begin to cover up for the user's behaviors and lack of responsibility. Family members or significant others may take sides, begin to be dishonest with each other, and erode the bond within that group. Eventually this leads to a condition called **codependence**, which can be as serious as the use and abuse of the substance. Codependent members of a family group begin to lose their own sense of identity and purpose and exist solely for the abuser. Their actions take away the opportunity for the user to take responsibility for his or her own actions. This is called *enabling.*

Etiological Theories

Why do some people become addicted or dependent and others do not? Can it be the chemical, or is it the person? Some theorists believe in the existence of an addictive personality, which may begin to explain addictions to food,

• WORD • BUILDING •
dysfunctional: dys—bad or difficult + functional—performance

Box 57.2

Ethical Considerations

Whistle Blowing

Ellen and Julie are LPNs who work on a busy medical unit in a large hospital. They were close friends in nursing school and have been working the night shift together for 3 years. Recently, Ellen began taking care of her mother-in-law who is dying from lung cancer. Julie has noticed that Ellen's personality has changed. Ellen, usually serious and almost compulsive in the completion of her work, has adopted a lackadaisical attitude and often arrives at work looking disheveled. Ellen tells Julie that she is stressed trying to care for her family and her dying mother-in-law. Julie has observed Ellen taking pain medication and fears her friend, in trying to escape the realities of life, has become addicted to the medication.

One evening, Ellen arrives at work with glassy eyes and slurred speech. She asks Julie to watch her patients for her while she "takes a little nap." Julie asks Ellen if she is abusing pain medication. After some initial denial, Ellen admits that she has been taking some of her mother-in-law's old medication to cope with the stress in her life. Ellen pleads with Julie not to tell anyone else about the problem. Because of their friendship, Julie consents to cover for Ellen this night.

The next night, Ellen again comes to work with obvious signs of intoxication. Ellen falls asleep while listening to the taped report for the change of shifts. What should Julie do? How can Julie support her friend through this difficult time while supporting "doing no harm" to the patients in Ellen's care? What ethical principle is most important in this case?

sex, and gambling, as well as alcohol, chemicals, and other dependencies.

Psychoanalytical theorists believe that people who develop addictions to alcohol or other substances are people who failed to successfully pass through the "oral" stage of development.

Biological theories include numerous studies that imply some sort of genetic metabolic disorder. Many of these studies were done on twins born to an alcoholic parent or parents, and who were separated from the parents at birth or shortly after birth. The number of twins who were born of alcoholic parents but raised by nonalcoholic adoptive or foster parents and yet developed alcoholism was consistently elevated.

Cognitive-behavioral theorists suggest the way in which a person perceives being high may influence the act of becoming high. It can be a very innocent beginning: obtaining relief from the medications given by the physician can, according to cognitive theory, leave people perceiving that the drugs offer a miracle cure. It becomes appealing to want that kind of relief again, and very soon a pattern is formed and other substances may be added.

Differential Diagnosis

A patient with a chemical dependency may be admitted to the hospital for problems associated with the addiction (dehydration, liver failure) or for unrelated problems (cancer, diabetes). Nursing assessment, patient need for frequent pain medication, or symptoms of withdrawal may lead you or the physician to pursue the possibility of chemical dependency. Laboratory tests can rule out physiological problems. Drug levels of alcohol or drugs can also be measured. A patient who is uncommonly anxious for early discharge should also be further assessed.

Types of Substance Abuse

ALCOHOL ABUSE AND DEPENDENCE. Use and abuse of alcohol is present in all walks of life, at all economic levels, and in both genders. Sometimes a very fine line exists between a person who is a social drinker and a person who has an abuse condition. One factor used to make that differentiation is the degree of need or compulsion to drink. There is a high incidence of alcohol use and abuse among the elderly, teenagers, and even younger children. Alcoholism either directly or indirectly decreases a person's life expectancy by an average of 10 to 12 years.

Denial is a common ego defense mechanism used by people who are substance abusers. The person who is alcohol dependent often uses statements such as "I can quit anytime I want to" or "I just need a little bump to loosen me up."

Characteristics of dependence were described earlier. In addition, patients with alcohol dependence may experience:

- Binges usually lasting 2 days or more
- Blackouts (unable to recall what happened during a period of drinking)
- Vomiting and dehydration
- Disorientation
- Increased vulnerability to infections, accidents, and other injuries.

Sometimes patients who are actively using drugs or alcohol when admitted to an inpatient setting, or who are cut off from sedatives or alcohol abruptly, experience a condition called **delirium tremens** (DTs). With DTs, hyperexcitability in the sensory activity can cause visual hallucinations, tremors, and possibly tonic-clonic seizures. Elevated blood pressure and pulse and cardiac dysrhythmias also may occur. Symptoms of withdrawal begin within 4 to 12 hours after the patient has stopped drinking and will peak in 24 to 48 hours. Hospitalization is needed to maintain the patient's safety.

Therapeutic Measures. Treatment for and recovery from alcohol dependency and abuse is a slow process. With very few exceptions, a person who has an alcohol dependency and who is recovering cannot ever have another drink, or he or she will risk the chance of returning to previous abusive patterns. Some treatment options are described next. Several forms of treatment may be used together.

Support Groups. A common and effective treatment for alcoholism is involvement in Alcoholics Anonymous (AA). AA is a 12-step program that offers support through others who have stopped drinking. For more information on AA, go to www.alcoholics-anonymous.org. Another program for women only is called Women for Sobriety (www.womenforsobriety.org).

Cognitive-Behavioral Therapy. Cognitive-behavioral therapy (CBT) is used as an adjunct therapy for control of substance abuse. CBT advocates believe that with homework and practice, a person can learn to think differently about the event that led to the drinking. When the person changes the belief system about the activating event and the drinking, the consequences of drinking will be less powerful.

Psychotherapy. Psychotherapy provides one-on-one therapy. Because addiction affects an entire family, family therapy is important in reinstating honesty in communications. A commitment to stop drinking is required, and therapy will only help with some of the issues resulting from years of drinking.

Medications. Medications are used cautiously because of risk for abuse. It is not always wise to substitute another chemical for alcohol. If, however, the anxiety level prohibits participation in therapy, or if a depressive disorder accompanies the abuse, medications may be prescribed. Antidepressant or nonaddictive antianxiety drugs are most often prescribed.

Disulfiram (Antabuse) is a medication that is sometimes prescribed as a deterrent to using alcohol. Disulfiram should never be administered without the patient's full informed consent. If a patient taking disulfiram ingests alcohol, a severe reaction causes chest pain, nausea, vomiting, confusion, and other symptoms. Those taking disulfiram also can be adversely affected if they use products that contain alcohol, such as cologne, mouthwash, aftershave, or cough syrup. The effects of disulfiram last 2 to 3 weeks after the last dose.

Acamprosate (Campral) is a newer drug that is thought to work by helping to restore GABA-glutamate equilibrium. Campral is specifically indicated for maintenance of abstinence from alcohol in patients who have stopped drinking.

Naltrexone (ReVia) may reduce craving, which is the urge or desire to drink. Naltrexone helps patients remain abstinent, and can interfere with the tendency to want to drink more if a recovering patient relapses and ingests alcohol.

Use of benzodiazepines such as diazepam (Valium) and lorazepam (Ativan) can help prevent symptoms of DTs during acute withdrawal, but are not used long term because of risk for dependence.

Hospitalization. Therapy may range from in-house hospitalizations of 2 weeks or more to halfway houses to eventual independence, usually attending AA meetings. It is common for patients to seek treatment multiple times. This should not be interpreted as a weakness in the patient or the treatment program. It is only a sign that the person is learning more about the disorder and the need to help himself or herself. People with all kinds of chronic diseases experience relapse at times.

Nursing Process for the Patient with Alcohol Abuse and Dependence

Data Collection. A common screening tool to determine if a patient has a drinking problem is the CAGE questionnaire (Ewing, 1984):

- Have you ever felt you should ***Cut down*** on your drinking?
- Have people ***Annoyed*** you by criticizing your drinking?
- Have you ever felt bad or ***Guilty*** about your drinking?
- Have you ever had a drink first thing in the morning (as an "***Eye opener***") to steady your nerves or get rid of a hangover?

A "yes" answer to two or more questions suggests a drinking problem.

Alcohol also can have many physiological effects. See Chapter 32 for assessment of patients with liver disorders.

Nursing Diagnoses, Planning, and Implementation

Ineffective Coping Related to Lack of Effective Coping Mechanisms as Evidenced by Abuse of Alcohol

EXPECTED OUTCOME: The patient will accept responsibility for her or his behavior, verbalize acceptance of the relationship between substance abuse and personal problems, and identify effects of alcohol on the body.

- Help patient to identify recent behavior while under the influence of alcohol. *Patients need to see the relationship between their substance abuse and their personal problems.*
- Expect sobriety. *This establishes sobriety as the norm.*
- Teach about the physical impact of drugs and alcohol on the body. *Many patients lack correct information about the effects of substance abuse on the body.*
- Be honest; be aware of your own thoughts and feelings about addictions. *Effective communication is essential for a therapeutic relationship.*
- Provide group support such as a 12-step program. Many chemical dependency units provide group support meetings. *Peer support is an effective treatment that is often more acceptable to patients than other treatments.*
- Confront the patient immediately if projection, rationalization, or denial behaviors are noted. *Projection, rationalization, and denial are ego defense mechanisms that discourage the patient from accepting responsibility for behavior.*
- Use positive reinforcement. Positive reinforcement for successes is important when helping a person with an addiction. *Every step is a big one in this field; every step taken is a new one.*

- Provide a safe environment. *Patients who are chemically addicted may become suicidal or display other bizarre behavior, especially during withdrawal. A patient under the influence of alcohol or another chemical may have poor impulse control or judgment. Maintaining a safe milieu and calm demeanor will help the patient through this difficult time.*
- Remain alert to the possibility that the patient may be using a substance even in the hospital. Express suspicions honestly and nonjudgmentally to the patient. Report and document all findings and behaviors that may be potential safety hazards for the patient. *The fact that a patient is hospitalized does not guarantee that he or she has no access to the chemical or way of using it in your presence. Unfortunately, family members or friends sometimes smuggle drugs or alcohol in to patients.*
- Practice "tough love." "Doing for" patients may be tempting, but it is not in the patient's best interest most of the time. *This encourages patients to be responsible for their own healing.*

Evaluation. Does the patient verbalize acceptance of responsibility for own behavior? Does the patient understand the relationship between personal problems and substance abuse? Does the patient understand the effects of substance abuse on the body?

For additional information, visit the National Institute for Alcohol Abuse and Alcoholism at www.niaaa.nih.gov.

DRUG ABUSE AND DEPENDENCE. Many substances other than alcohol can be addictive. Caffeine and nicotine are two that are very readily available. Coffee, tea, soda, and cigarettes are everywhere in our society and are very addicting. Many experts believe that the single most difficult addiction to overcome is the addiction to nicotine.

Illegal substances such as marijuana, cocaine, crack, PCP, and prescription medications for pain and mental health treatment are also potentially addictive. Methamphetamine (meth) has led to a substantial substance abuse problem affecting families and society. Inhalants such as lighter fluid, paint, paint thinners, and gasoline also can be used to get high; in the United States, these substances are used mainly by teenagers. The term for their use is *huffing*. These are highly neurotoxic substances, potentially lethal, and usually available in the house or garage.

Signs and Symptoms. The signs and symptoms of drug abuse and dependence can be very similar to those of alcohol abuse. Additional signs of drug abuse include the following:

- Red, watery eyes
- Runny nose
- Hostile behavior
- Paranoia
- Needle tracks on arms or legs.

Therapeutic Measures. Therapeutic measures for patients with drug abuse and dependence include the following:

- Narcotics Anonymous
- Group therapy
- Psychotherapy
- Methadone programs.

Methadone acts as a sort of "step down" for people addicted to certain opioid drugs. Methadone can be legally prescribed and dispensed. It, too, is potentially addicting, and its critics believe it is only a substitute for heroin. It is typically given once a day. Psychotherapy is also provided for patients in methadone programs.

Nursing Management. Nursing care for people who are drug dependent is essentially the same as for those who are alcohol dependent. It is important to remember that nurses and physicians cannot "fix" the patient who is chemically dependent. The desire to be chemically free must come from the person who is addicted.

Caring for patients with mental health disorders is challenging and rewarding. You will learn that there are very few absolutes in the area of mental health nursing. There are many guidelines about the illnesses, but caring for the patients who have the illnesses is as individualized as the patients themselves. It is important to remember to care for the whole person. The mind and body work together, so be sure to take care of all aspects of each patient: physical, emotional, cognitive, and behavioral. (See Table 57.7.)

CRITICAL THINKING

Maria

■ You are a school nurse in your local high school. You notice that Maria, a 17-year-old student, is behaving oddly. She has always been rather loud and even has been referred to as "obnoxious" by several of her peers. Lately you have observed her sitting alone, as if waiting for someone, but when you approach her, she barely greets you and then moves away. What are your concerns about Maria? What are some of the possibilities that might be affecting her? How can you approach her more effectively the next time you see her?

Suggested answers at end of chapter.

MENTAL ILLNESS AND THE OLDER ADULT

It is not uncommon for older adults to be admitted to the hospital with a tentative diagnosis of "change in mental status." It is important to distinguish between physical and

TABLE 57.7 SUBSTANCE ABUSE SUMMARY

Signs and Symptoms	Inability to fulfill obligations at work, school, or home Recurrent legal or interpersonal problems Continued use despite social and interpersonal problems Participation in physically hazardous situations while impaired
Diagnosis	History Liver function studies Serum drug or alcohol levels Evaluate for other coexisting disorders (bipolar disorder)
Therapeutic Measures	12-step programs Cognitive behavioral therapy Psychotherapy Disulfiram (Antabuse) Acamprosate (Campral) Naltrexone (ReVia) Benzodiazepines for acute withdrawal
Nursing Diagnoses	*Ineffective Coping* *Ineffective Denial*

mental disorders in these circumstances. Some disorders that affect older adults' mental status are as follows:

- *Dementia* is an impairment of mental functioning that interferes with daily activities and relationships. Causes of dementia include Alzheimer's disease, Lewy body dementia, vascular dementia, Huntington's disease, and others.
- *Delirium* is an acute change in mental status needing immediate evaluation and treatment. This is often due to a physiological condition such as an infection, and can be reversed if recognized and the underlying cause is removed. Read more about dementia and delirium in Chapter 48.
- *Pseudodementia* is a condition in which the patient appears to have dementia but is really depressed. Treating the depression can help reverse the mental status changes.

Depression in the elderly should not be viewed as a normal part of aging; it should be diagnosed and treated. Older adults may be dealing with physical and mental decline, loss of function, isolation, and loss of a marriage partner and friends, and may express their depression through bodily symptoms such as pain. If not evaluated and treated, depression may lead to suicide. (See Box 57.3, *Gerontological Issues.*) Be sure to review Chapter 15, *Nursing Care of Older Adult Patients.*

Box 57.3

Gerontological Issues

Suicide and the Older Adult

Older adults are not immune to suicidal thoughts. White men older than age 75 have an especially high suicide rate. Comments by any older adult referring to hopelessness or desire to die must be explored to assess suicide risk. The following comments could be a reflection of suicide potential in an older adult who is depressed:

- "Living is harder than dying could ever be."
- "I am a used-up old man who is a burden for everyone."
- "I am useless. I can't do anything anymore."
- "I don't know why God won't take me."

To adequately assess suicide potential, ask questions that establish whether the older adult has done the following:

- Thought about ending his or her life
- Attempted to end his or her life in the past
- Developed a plan to end his or her life
- Set the plan into action (i.e., bought a gun, has a full bottle of pills in the bedside table).

Any older adult who has a plan to end his or her life and has the ability or resources to do so must be immediately referred for psychological evaluation. Never leave a person with suicidal thoughts alone.

Crisis Intervention for a Suicidal Older Adult

- Remove any items that the older adult could use to inflict an injury or end his or her life, such as razors, jewelry with pins or sharp points, and mirrors.
- Make arrangements for direct supervision and observation that are reliable, considering personnel and family resources. Often, hospital admission is the most appropriate intervention for a person at a very high risk for suicide.
- Help the older adult talk about the crisis or life event that has devastated his or her desire to live. For example, encourage reminiscence about the patient's spouse, or allow the older person to express the frustration of being unable to physically meet the daily demands of life.
- Develop a "do no harm" or suicide contract with the older adult. Outline a short-term, structured plan to keep the older adult safe. Focus on decreasing social isolation by requiring personal social contacts (e.g., stay at daughter's home for a weekend; go to the senior center for lunch; call a specific person who is willing and wants to listen to feelings and concerns; exercise; take a walk outside; volunteer services at a nursing home, hospital, or school).
- Older adults often need assistance to develop or enhance skills required to cope with life events. Self-care and personal independence in care choices can be encouraged.

Home Health Hints

- Help patients and families identify pharmacies that will deliver medications to the home.
- Set up medications using a system the patient can easily follow.
- Maintain communication with and act as a liaison between the psychiatrist and medical physician.
- Assist the patient and family to identify community resources such as support groups and respite care.
- Assess family members for evidence of caregiver role strain.
- Provide education for family/caregivers related to the patient's illness, medications, and symptom management.

ETHICAL CONSIDERATIONS DISCUSSION

The substance-abusing health professional is one of the most common situations nurses may encounter during their careers. Nurses have easy access to drugs in most work settings. Other factors that contribute to the increased drug abuse among nurses include job stress, short staffing, double shifts, unrealistic expectations, frustration and anxiety, personal problems, and lack of autonomy in practice.

The impaired nurse's colleagues may experience professional and emotional conflicts. Underlying the ethical dilemma is the right of the patient to safe and competent treatment versus the nurse's right to self-determination. However, the nurse does not have a totally unrestricted right to self-determination. This right has limits when it comes to endangering others, especially the patients assigned to this nurse for care and safety. Although the National Association for Practical Nurse Education and Services (NAPNES) Code does not directly address any obligation to protect the public from practitioners who are unsafe, various elements that are related include faithfulness and responsibility to protect patients. In addition, the principle of maleficence can provide guidance so that patients are not exposed to undue harm.

In this particular situation, Julie does have an obligation to do something about Ellen's drug problem. Covering for Ellen will not solve the problem. Julie should document Ellen's behavior and inform her supervisor. If the institution hierarchy does not take any action, Julie should submit the report to the state board of nursing. Some states have programs to assist health professionals to address addiction. They can be helped without fear of losing their jobs or licenses, as long as they comply with treatment.

To allow Ellen to practice while under the influence of drugs puts Julie in a very serious legal position. If Ellen were to do something wrong and harm a patient and Julie knew that Ellen was under the influence of drugs, Julie could be held legally liable.

SUGGESTED ANSWERS TO CRITICAL THINKING

Tommy

You can reassure Tommy's mother that his OCD is not her fault. Tommy can learn to control his illness with medications and therapy. The family must be part of the therapy, for both Tommy's sake and the family's sake. Positive communication between Tommy and his family is encouraged. Tommy's mother can also be encouraged to attend a support group herself.

Mr. Zenz

It is important to be supportive of Mrs. Zenz while maintaining her husband's confidentiality and privacy. Encouraging Mrs. Zenz to talk to Mr. Zenz's physician is appropriate. Showing empathy with statements such as "It must be confusing and difficult to watch your husband change moods so quickly" are good tools to use. It may be a bit more challenging to approach him as your boss. You may certainly ask him if you can speak frankly and share specific observations. You may share your concern, such as "Mr. Zenz, you are a wonderful boss, but I am frightened when you become loud and boisterous." This may help him to reflect. Chances are, however, that if he is in a manic stage, he will not hear your concern. It may require a delicate conversation with the next person up in the corporate chain of command, being careful to objectively report behavior but not share assumptions. This is a tough one. Good luck!

Anne

Appropriate communication skills include being positive, reassuring, and not reinforcing the hallucinations. "I don't see or hear a woman, Anne. It is time for the movie. I'd

SUGGESTED ANSWERS TO—cont'd

like you to come with me for a while at least" is an example of an appropriate verbal interaction. Reinforcing expectations is also appropriate; you might say "Anne, part of your care plan includes attending one unit activity each day. This is the last opportunity for you to meet your care plan objective for today." At all times, nurses need to be aware of drug interactions. Anne will most likely be medicated for her schizophrenia, and those medications may interact unfavorably with her chemotherapy. If she is receiving oral medications, it may be necessary to check her mouth to ensure she is swallowing them. Good nursing data collection skills are essential.

■ *Maria*

A number of options may explain Maria's behavior, including depression, drug use, schizophrenia, or an eating disorder. Next time you see Maria, you might try constructively confronting her behavior by saying something like "Maria, you used to be much more outgoing. We always were friendly and now you leave when I'm near. That change in you concerns me. I'm here if you want to talk." Or, "Maria, I see your behavior is changing. You are loud one moment and very quiet the next. That is unusual for you. What is happening?"

REVIEW QUESTIONS

1. A patient blames a new diagnosis of schizophrenia on a distant maternal-child relationship during youth. Which theory explains this belief?
   a. Psychoanalytic theory
   b. Genetic theory
   c. Biological theory
   d. Cognitive theory

2. A patient suddenly and dramatically experiences a loss of vision. The onset of blindness doesn't seem to bother the patient. This person is most likely experiencing which of the following?
   a. Post-traumatic stress disorder
   b. Schizophrenia
   c. Conversion disorder
   d. Dissociative disorder

3. If an extrapyramidal side effect such as dystonia occurs in the patient on antipsychotic medication, which of the following interventions might help?
   a. Administer anticholinergic agents as ordered.
   b. Discontinue the antipsychotic agent immediately.
   c. Administer prn antianxiety agents as ordered.
   d. Encourage progressive muscle relaxation and imagery.

4. A patient who is a veteran of the Gulf War hears the hospital fire alarm go off during a drill and cries, "There are people hiding behind the pillars! They have guns! Be careful!" What action should the nurse take first?
   a. Tell the patient that his behavior is inappropriate and that he is frightening the other patients.
   b. Administer a prn antipsychotic medication as ordered.
   c. Ask him if he is afraid of the guns.
   d. Stay with the patient while calmly reorienting him.

5. A patient is being treated on the mental health unit for a somatoform disorder. The patient approaches the nurse and reports feeling dizzy and weak, with a sensation of a racing heart. The nursing care plan includes interventions of imagery exercises and prn alprazolam (Xanax) for symptoms of anxiety. What should the nurse do first?
   a. Instruct the patient to sit and breathe deeply.
   b. Give the patient the prescribed prn Xanax.
   c. Measure the patient's vital signs.
   d. Instruct the patient in an imagery exercise.

References

Bleuler, E. (1911). *Dementia praecox or the group of schizophrenias* (p. 26). New York: International Universities Press.

Boyer, E. W., & Shannon, M. (2005). The serotonin syndrome. *New England Journal of Medicine, 352*(11), 1112–1120.

Ewing, J. A. (1984). Detecting alcoholism: The CAGE questionnaire. *Journal of the American Medical Association, 252,* 1905–1907.

Patil, S. T., Zhang, L., Martenyi, F., et al. (2007). Activation of mGlu2/3 receptors as a new approach to treat schizophrenia: A randomized phase 2 clinical trial. *Nature Medicine, 13*(9), 1102–1107.

Appendix A

North American Nursing Diagnosis Association (NANDA) Nursing Diagnoses

Activity Intolerance [specify level]
Activity Intolerance, Risk for
Activity Planning, Ineffective
Airway Clearance, Ineffective
Allergy Response, Latex
Allergy Response, Risk for Latex
Anxiety [specify level]
Anxiety, Death
Aspiration, Risk for
Attachment, Risk for Impaired Parent/Infant/Child
Autonomic Dysreflexia
Autonomic Dysreflexia, Risk for
Bleeding, Risk for
Blood Glucose Level, Risk for Unstable
Body Image, Disturbed
Body Temperature, Risk for Imbalanced
Bowel Incontinence
Breastfeeding, Effective
Breastfeeding, Ineffective
Breastfeeding, Interrupted
Breathing Pattern, Ineffective
Cardiac Output, Decreased
Caregiver Role Strain
Caregiver Role Strain, Risk for
Childbearing Process, Readiness for Enhanced
Comfort, Impaired
Comfort, Readiness for Enhanced
Communication, Impaired Verbal
Communication, Readiness for Enhanced
Conflict, Decisional (specify)
Conflict, Parental Role
Confusion, Acute
Confusion, Chronic
Confusion, Risk for Acute
Constipation
Constipation, Perceived
Constipation, Risk for
Contamination
Contamination, Risk for
Coping, Compromised Family
Coping, Defensive
Coping, Disabled Family
Coping, Ineffective
Coping, Ineffective Community
Coping, Readiness for Enhanced
Coping, Readiness for Enhanced Community
Coping, Readiness for Enhanced Family
Death Syndrome, Risk for Sudden Infant
Decision Making, Readiness for Enhanced
Denial, Ineffective
Dentition, Impaired
Development, Risk for Delayed
Diarrhea
Distress, Moral
Disuse Syndrome, Risk for
Diversional Activity, Deficient
Electrolyte Imbalance, Risk for
Energy Field, Disturbed
Environmental Interpretation Syndrome, Impaired
Failure to Thrive, Adult
Falls, Risk for
Family Processes: Alcoholism, Dysfunctional
Family Processes, Interrupted
Family Processes, Readiness for Enhanced
Fatigue
Fear [specify focus]
Fluid Balance, Readiness for Enhanced
Fluid Volume, Deficient [Hyper/Hypotonic]
Fluid Volume, Deficient [Isotonic]
Fluid Volume, Excess
Fluid Volume, Risk for Deficient
Fluid Volume, Risk for Imbalanced
Gas Exchange, Impaired
Gastrointestinal Motility, Dysfunctional
Gastrointestinal Motility, Risk for Dysfunctional
Grieving, Anticipatory
Grieving, Complicated
Grieving, Risk for Complicated
Grieving, Dysfunctional
Grieving, Risk for Dysfunctional
Growth, Risk for Disproportionate
Growth and Development, Delayed
Health Behavior, Risk-Prone
Health Maintenance, Ineffective
Home Maintenance, Impaired
Hope, Readiness for Enhanced
Hopelessness
Human Dignity, Risk for Compromised
Hyperthermia
Hypothermia
Immunization Status, Readiness for Enhanced
Infant Behavior, Disorganized
Infant Behavior, Readiness for Enhanced Organized
Infant Behavior, Risk for Disorganized
Infant Feeding Pattern, Ineffective
Infection, Risk for
Injury, Risk for
Injury, Risk for Perioperative Positioning
Insomnia
Intracranial Adaptive Capacity, Decreased
Jaundice, Neonatal
Knowledge, Deficient [Learning Need] (specify)
Knowledge (specify), Readiness for Enhanced
Lifestyle, Sedentary
Liver Function, Risk for Impaired
Loneliness, Risk for
Maternal/Fetal Dyad, Risk for Disturbed
Memory, Impaired
Mobility, Impaired Bed
Mobility, Impaired Physical
Mobility, Impaired Wheelchair
Nausea
Neglect, Self
Neglect, unilateral
Noncompliance [Ineffective Adherence] (specify)
Nutrition: Less Than Body Requirements, Imbalanced
Nutrition: More Than Body Requirements, Imbalanced
Nutrition: More Than Body Requirements, Risk for Imbalanced
Nutrition, Readiness for Enhanced
Oral Mucous Membrane, Impaired
Pain, Acute
Pain, Chronic
Parenting, Impaired
Parenting, Readiness for Enhanced
Parenting, Risk for Impaired
Peripheral Neurovascular Dysfunction, Risk for
Personal Identity, Disturbed
Poisoning, Risk for
Post-Trauma Syndrome [specify stage]
Post-Trauma Syndrome, Risk for
Power, Readiness for Enhanced
Powerlessness [specify level]
Powerlessness, Risk for
Protection, Ineffective
Rape-Trauma Syndrome
Relationship, Readiness for Enhanced
Religiosity, Impaired
Religiosity, Readiness for Enhanced
Religiosity, Risk for Impaired
Relocation Stress Syndrome
Relocation Stress Syndrome, Risk for
Resilience, Compromised
Resilience, Impaired Individual
Resilience, Readiness for Enhanced
Role Performance, Ineffective
Self-Care Deficit: Bathing/Hygiene
Self-Care Deficit: Dressing/Grooming
Self-Care Deficit: Feeding
Self-Care Deficit: Toileting
Self-Care, Readiness for Enhanced
Self-Concept, Readiness for Enhanced
Self-Esteem, Chronic Low
Self-Esteem, Situational Low
Self-Esteem, Risk for Situational Low
Self Health Management, Ineffective

Self Health Management, Readiness for Enhanced
Self-Mutilation
Self-Mutilation, Risk for
Sensory Perception, Disturbed (specify: visual, auditory, kinesthetic, gustatory, tactile, olfactory)
Sexual Dysfunction
Sexuality Pattern, Ineffective
Shock, Risk for
Skin Integrity, Impaired
Skin Integrity, Risk for Impaired
Sleep, Readiness for Enhanced
Sleep Deprivation
Sleep Pattern, Disturbed
Social Interaction, Impaired
Social Isolation
Sorrow, Risk for Chronic
Spiritual Distress
Spiritual Distress, Risk for
Spiritual Well-Being, Readiness for Enhanced
Stress Overload
Suffocation, Risk for
Suicide, Risk for
Surgical Recovery, Delayed
Swallowing, Impaired
Therapeutic Regimen Management, Ineffective Family
Thermoregulation, Ineffective
Tissue Integrity, Impaired
Tissue Perfusion, Risk of Decreased Cardiac
Tissue Perfusion, Ineffective (specify type: renal, cerebral, cardiopulmonary, gastrointestinal, peripheral)
Transfer Ability, Impaired
Trauma, Risk for
Trauma, Risk for Vascular
Urinary Elimination, Impaired
Urinary Elimination, Readiness for Enhanced
Urinary Incontinence, Functional
Urinary Incontinence, Overflow
Urinary Incontinence, Reflex
Urinary Incontinence, Risk for Urge
Urinary Incontinence, Stress
Urinary Incontinence, Urge
Urinary Retention [acute/chronic]
Ventilation, Impaired Spontaneous
Ventilatory Weaning Response, Dysfunctional
Violence, [Actual/] Risk for Other-Directed
Violence, [Actual/] Risk for Self-Directed
Walking, Impaired
Wandering [specify sporadic or continuous]

Appendix B

Normal Adult Reference Laboratory Values

BLOOD, PLASMA, OR SERUM VALUES

	Reference Range	
Determination	***Conventional***	***SI***
Aldolase	Less than 7.4 units/L	
Ammonia	12–55 μmol/L	12–55 μmol/L
Amylase	30–110 units/mL	
Atrial natriuretic peptide	20–77 pg/mL	20–77 ng/L

	BNP	Pro-BNP (N-Terminal)
Male	Less than 100 pg/mL	60 pg/mL
Female	<100 pg/mL	12–150 pg/mL

Bilirubin (total)	0.3–1.2 mg/dL	5–21 μmol/L
Calcium	8.2–10.2 mg/dL	2.05–2.55 mmol/L
Carbon dioxide content	23–29 mEq/L	23–29 mmol/L
Chloride	97–107 mEq/L	97–107 mmol/L
Creatine kinase (CK)	*Female:* 26–140 units/L *Male:* 38–174 units/L	
CK isoenzymes		
CK-BB	Absent	
CK-MB	4%–6%	
CK-MM	94%–96%	
CK-MB by immunoassay	10 ng/mL	
Creatinine		
Male	0.6–1.2 mg/dL	53–106 μmol/L
Female	0.5–1.1 mg/dL	44–97 μmol/L
d-Dimer	*Semiquantitative:* No fragments detected. *Quantitative:* Less than 250 ng/mL	
Erythrocyte sedimentation rate (ESR)	(Westergren method)	
Male	*Under age 50:* Less than 15 mm/hr *Over age 50:* Less than 20 mm/hr	
Female	*Under age 50:* Less than 20 mm/hr *Over age 50:* Less than 30 mm/hr	
Glucose	Fasting: 70–100 mg/dL	3.9–5.5 mmol/L
Iron		
Male	65–175 μg/dL	11.6–31.3 μmol/L
Female	50–170 μg/dL	9–30.4 μmol/L
Iron-binding capacity	250–350 μg/dL	45–63 μmol/L
Lactic dehydrogenase	90–176 units/L	
Lipase	0–160 units/L	
Lipids (desirable)		
Cholesterol	Less than 200 mg/dL	Less than 5.18 mmol/L
Low-density lipoprotein	Less than 100 mg/dL	Less than 2.59 mmol/L
High-density lipoprotein	Greater than 60 mg/dL	Greater than 1.56 mmol/L
Triglycerides	Less than 150 mg/dL	Less than 1.70 mmol/L
Magnesium	1.6–2.6 mg/dL	0.62–0.91 mmol/L
Myoglobin	0–85 ng/mL	
Osmolality	275–295 mOsm/kg	275–295 mmol/kg
Oxygen saturation (arterial)	95–100%	
Pco_2	35–45 mm Hg	4.66–5.98 kPa
pH	7.35–7.45	Same
Po_2	80–95 mm Hg	10.6–12.6 kPa
Phosphatase (prostatic acid)	Less than 2.5 ng/mL	

Continued

BLOOD, PLASMA, OR SERUM VALUES—cont'd

	Reference Range	
Determination	***Conventional***	***SI***
Phosphatase (alkaline)		
Male	35–142 units/L	
Female	25–125 units/L	
Phosphorus (blood)	2.5–4.5 mg/dL	0.8–1.4 mmol/L
Potassium	3.5–5.0 mEq/L	3.5–5.0 mmol/L
Protein: Total	6.0–8.0 g/dL	60–80 g/L
Albumin	3.4–4.8 g/dL	34–48 g/L
Sodium	135–145 mEq/L	135–145 mmol/L
Transaminase, alanine aminotransferase (ALT)		
Male	10–40 units/L	
Female	7–35 units/L	
Transaminase, aspartate aminotransferase (AST)		
Male	15–40 units/L	
Female	13–35 units/L	
Troponin I	<0.35 ng/mL	
Troponin T	<0.20 μg/L	
Urea nitrogen (BUN)	8–21 mg/dL	2.9–7.5 mmol/L
Uric acid		
Male	4.4–7.6 mg/dL	0.26–0.45 mmol/L
Female	2.3–6.6 mg/dL	0.14–0.39 mmol/L

URINALYSIS REFERENCE VALUES

Dipstick pH	5.0–9.0
Protein	Less than 20 mg/dL
Glucose	Negative
Ketones	Negative
Hemoglobin	Negative
Bilirubin	Negative
Urobilinogen	Up to 1 mg/dL
Nitrite	Negative
Leukocyte esterase	Negative
Microscopic examination	
Red blood cells	Less than 5/hpf
White blood cells	Less than 5/hpf
Renal cells	None seen
Transitional cells	None seen
Squamous cells	Rare; usually no clinical significance
Casts	Rare hyaline; otherwise, none seen
Crystals in acid urine	Uric acid, calcium oxalate, amorphous urates
Crystals in alkaline urine	Triple phosphate, calcium phosphate, ammonium biurate, calcium carbonate, amorphous phosphates
Bacteria, yeast, parasites	None seen

hpf = high-power field.

HEMATOLOGIC VALUES

Determination	Reference Range *Conventional*	*SI*
Coagulation screening tests		
Bleeding time (template)	2.5–10 min	
Prothrombin time	11–13.5 sec	
International normalized ratio (INR)	Less than 2.0 if no anticoagulation therapy 2.0 to 3.0 with treatment for venous thrombosis, pulmonary embolism, or valvular heart disease 2.5 to 3.5 with mechanical heart valves or treatment for recurrent systemic embolism	
Partial thromboplastin time (activated)	25–38 sec	25–38 sec
Complete blood count (CBC)		
Hematocrit		
Male	43–49	0.43–0.49
Female	38–44	0.38–0.44
Hemoglobin		
Male	13.2–17.3 g/dL	132–173 mmol/L
Female	11.7–15.5 g/dL	117–155 mmol/L
Erythrocyte count		
Male	4.71–5.14 million cells/mm^3	4.71–5.14 × 10^{12} cells/L
Female	4.20–4.87 million cells/mm^3	4.20–4.87 × 10^{12} cells/L

Red Blood Cell Indices	Mean Corpuscular Volume (fl)	Mean Corpuscular Hemoglobin (pg/cell)	Mean Corpuscular Hemoglobin Concentration (g/dL)	RBC Distribution Width Index
Male	85–95	28–32	33–35	11.6–14.8
Female	85–95	28–32	33–35	11.6–14.8

Platelet count	150–450 × 10^3/μL/mm^3	181–521 × 10^9/L

White Blood Cell Count and Differential	SI Units WBC × 10^3/mm^3 or cells/mL	Neutrophils Total (Absolute and %)	Lymphocytes Bands (Absolute and %)	Monocytes Segments (Absolute and %)	Eosinophils (Absolute and %)	Basophils (Absolute and %)
Adult	4.5–11.0	1.8–7.7 59%	0–0.7 3.0%	1.8–7.0 56%	1.0–4.8 34%	0–0.8 4.0%

THERAPEUTIC DRUG LEVELS

Determination	Reference Range *Conventional*	*SI*
Carbamazepine	4.0–12.0 mg/mL	17–51 μmol/L
Digoxin	0.5–2.0 ng/mL	0.6–2.6 nmol/L
Ethanol	0 mg/dL	0 mmol/L
Lithium	0.6–1.4 mEq/L	0.6–1.4 mmol/L
Phenobarbital	15–40 mcg/mL	65–172 μmol/L
Phenytoin (Dilantin)	10–20 mcg/mL	40–79 μmol/L
Salicylate	15–20 mg/dL	1.1–1.4 mmol/L

MISCELLANEOUS VALUES

	Reference Range	
Determination	***Conventional***	***SI***
Carcinoembryonic antigen (CEA)	0–2.5 ng/mL	0–2.5 mcg/L
Gastrin	25–90 pg/mL	25–90 ng/L
Immunological tests:		
Alpha-1-antitrypsin	126–226 mg/dL	1.26–2.26 g/L
Antinuclear antibodies	Negative at a 1:8 dilution of serum	

Reference range values may differ from one institution to another. Most data from Van Leeuwen, A. M., & Poelhuis-Leth, D. J. (2009). *Davis's comprehensive handbook of laboratory and diagnostic tests with nursing implications* (3rd ed.). Philadelphia: F. A. Davis.

Appendix C

Answers to Review Questions

Chapter 1

1. b. Critical thinking is use of cognitive skills or strategies that increase the probability of a desirable outcome.
2. d. Asking a question shows humility. The nurse does not "know it all."
3. a. A respiratory rate of 28 is observable. Selections b, c, and d are patient perceptions.
4. d. Selections a, b, and c all include the nurse's perceptions.
5. c. Shortness of breath is a physiological need and should be addressed first.
6. c, a, d, e, b. These are the steps of the nursing process.
7. a. The LPN implements interventions and assists the RN with the other steps.
8. d. *Acute Pain* is a nursing diagnosis. The others are medical diagnoses.
9. c. The patient who has a specific plan is most likely to be successful.

Chapter 2

1. a, b, f. It is a systematic review of current evidence in many disciplines that looks at the quality of research and considers costs and patient preferences.
2. d. Evidence-based nursing care provides the best and safest patient care.
3. a. Joanna Briggs best practices guideline identifies valid nursing evidence.
4. c. The proposed change will need to go through the policy and procedure committee for evaluation.
5. c. Systematic reviews of randomized controlled trials are the best place to look for evidence.
6. b. A soft toothbrush/fluoride toothpaste is needed to remove plaque from the teeth.

Chapter 3

1. b. The elderly population is growing and will require more complex health care.
2. b, c, d, f. Assessment of conditions present on admission and all care and education to prevent complications, including patient refusal to participate, must be documented during hospitalization.
3. c. All but ambulating a patient are outside the LPN scope of practice.
4. b. Autocratic leaders do not seek input to make decisions.
5. a. LPNs consult with RNs in caring for their patients.
6. d. To understand how to deal with situations that can occur at any stage of life.
7. c. Respectfulness is an attitude of a nurse toward patients that values patients and their feelings as unique individuals.
8. a. Autonomy is the right of self-determination as expressed by the advance directive.
9. b. Clarifying the values of all participants includes checking advance directives.
10. b. Since the nurse believes the wrong choice is being made, it can create moral distress.
11. c. State nurse practice laws explain nursing licensure.
12. a, d, e. See Box 3.3.
13. b. HIPAA requires protection for the privacy of personal health information.

Chapter 4

1. b. Ethnocentrism is thinking one's own ways are the only right and proper ways.
2. d. Allowing parents to stay and pray in the child's room meets the needs of both parents and child.
3. a. American Indians may interpret eye contact as rude; they also tend to be comfortable with silences.
4. c. Islamic Arabs may avoid pork.
5. a. Nonharmful cultural practices should be allowed.

Chapter 5

1. c. "Complement" means "something added."
2. c. Allopathy, or western medicine such as is practiced in the United States, is based on scientific research.
3. d. Ginger, as with all herbs, can interact with other medications.
4. a, c, and e all use some form of relaxation.
5. b. Sharing objective data with patients can help them make informed decisions.

Chapter 6

1. a, e. Sodium is the major cation in the blood and helps maintain serum osmolarity. Sodium is also important for cell function, especially in the central nervous system.
2. b. Dehydration is associated with poor skin turgor because of loss of water in the tissues, and with disorientation because of loss of blood volume in the brain.
3. d. The elderly have reduced kidney function and may not be able to handle excess fluids.
4. c. Daily weights are the best way to monitor fluid imbalances. They are easier to monitor accurately than intake and output.
5. a. Elevating the head of the bed will provide more room for lung expansion and provide the quickest relief for shortness of breath.
6. a. Daily or every-other-day weights are easy to keep track of at home.
7. d. Hypokalemia is associated with muscle weakness.
8. b, c, d.
9. b. Potatoes, tomatoes, and bananas are highest in potassium.
10. a. 7.26 is below 7.35 and is acidotic.

Chapter 7

1. b. Policies may vary slightly by institution. Always use the policies provided by your workplace.
2. a (a man with dehydration requires fluids), b (a woman with an eating disorder will benefit from TPN), c (IV antibiotics may be effective if oral antibiotics have failed), e (prolonged vomiting causes fluid and electrolyte loss and requires replacement), f (IV diuretics will work the fastest on fluid overload).
3. a. Site selection should move from distal to proximal on the arm.

4. b, e, f, a, c, h, i, d, g. See Table 7.1.
5. c. The multiple tourniquet technique will best help visualize veins for cannulation.
6. b. The patient has signs of an air embolism. The cracked tubing must be clamped, and oxygen will support oxygenation until the RN or physician arrives.
7. d. Blood products must be administered with sodium chloride to avoid complications
8. c. The catheter that is palpable under the skin is the tunneled portion of the catheter.
9. 33.

$$\frac{100\text{ mL}}{1\text{ hour}} \Big| \frac{1\text{ hour}}{60\text{ minutes}} \Big| \frac{20\text{ gtt}}{1\text{ mL}} = 33\text{ gtt/minute}$$

10. 83

$$\frac{1000\text{ mL}}{12\text{ hours}} = 83\text{ mL/hour}$$

Chapter 8

1. e, b, c, a, f, d. This is the order in the chain of events leading to an infection (Fig. 8.1).
2. c. Hand hygiene is essential to help prevent infections.
3. b. Applying lotion to skin, the first line of defense, prevents dryness and cracking.
4. c. An elevated low-grade temperature when immunocompromised (neutropenia) can be very significant.
5. a. All patient allergies must be checked to help prevent an allergic reaction.
6. d. Maintaining a closed urinary drainage system is essential to prevent contamination.
7. c. Take all medication as ordered to help prevent relapse and development of bacterial resistance.

Chapter 9

1. c. The sympathetic nervous system (fight or flight) is stimulated to compensate for shock symptoms.
2. a, e, f. Wheezing, urticaria, and bronchospasm are seen specifically in anaphylactic shock.
3. d. Cerebral hypoxia depresses the central nervous system.
4. b. Ineffective tissue perfusion occurs due to shock.
5. b. Restlessness and confusion indicate a need for oxygen, which is started immediately while other treatment is prepared.
6. d. These vital signs indicate moderate shock and require immediate intervention.
7. c. A normal blood pressure would indicate effective treatment for shock.
8. b, c, a. As shock progresses from mild to severe, systolic blood pressure decreases.

Chapter 10

1. b. Pain is whatever the patient says it is, whenever the patient says it is.
2. d. Distraction is an effective method when used with medication for pain control.
3. c. Tolerance is the need for more medication to achieve the same effect.
4. a. Nociceptive pain occurs with tissue injury.
5. b. Chronic pain is least likely to be associated with changes in vital signs, because the patient has adapted to the pain.
6. c. A valid assessment scale is the best way to quantify pain.
7. a, d, e. According to the World Health Organization ladder, adjuvants are always appropriate in addition to analgesics. They are not intended to substitute for analgesics.
8. c. The patient will experience the best pain relief with the combination of an opioid and nonopioid.
9. d. Meperidine should be avoided in elderly patients.
10. b. Gabapentin must be taken continuously to be effective. Chronic neuropathy is not likely to go away, so treatment will be ongoing.
11. d. A placebo should not be administered except in research studies. The supervisor should be involved in educating the physician.
12. 0.7 mL.

$$\frac{10\text{ mg}}{} \Big| \frac{1\text{ grain}}{60\text{ mg}} \Big| \frac{\tfrac{1}{4}\text{ grain}}{1\text{ mL}} = 0.7\text{ mL}$$

Chapter 11

1. b.
2. a, e, f. Malignant tumors are invasive, lack contact inhibition, and have defective communication.
3. a. The blood cell counts, including the white cell count, will be decreased at the nadir.
4. d. Choosing a wig before hair loss will make adaptation easier once it occurs.
5. d. Knowing what has worked in the past will help with planning effective care.
6. c. Patients with bone cancer are at risk for spinal cord compression, which can cause difficulty walking.
7. c. The real goal is intact skin. Selections a, b, and d are interventions.
8. a. Only patients with 6 months or less to live are eligible for hospice care.
9. c. Teach the patient the reason for the isolation. Having a nurse, family member, or another patient in the room would place them at risk for radiation exposure.

Chapter 12

1. a, c, d, e, f. All except b, which can contribute to increasing anxiety and fear, will calm the patient, place the patient in a healthier state, or teach the patient ways to promote recovery.
2. a. Assisting in data collection is an LPN function; selections b and d are the physician's role, and selection c is the RN's role.
3. d, e, f. The LPN may refer questions to the surgeon, read the consent to a patient, and witness the signature of a patient who is informed.
4. b. Large black-on-white printed materials are most easily seen by the older adult.
5. a, e, f. Controlling pain allows the patient to cough and deep breathe more comfortably, which expands the lungs, as does ambulation.
6. c. Clear lung sounds indicate that the lungs are functioning normally.
7. a. Tachycardia is a compensatory sign to maintain cardiac output for fluid volume loss, as in hemorrhage.
8. d. Nausea and vomiting must be controlled before discharge. Pain at a tolerable level is expected in the immediate postoperative period.
9. The home health nurse's role is to assist the patient's recovery.

Chapter 13

1. a, b, c, e. ABCD and vital signs are part of the primary survey, not chronic disability or deformity, which is part of the secondary survey.
2. a. Hemorrhaging is controlled by applying pressure at the site.
3. b. Singed nasal hairs indicate possible inhalation injury from a fire, so the nurse should be alert to possible respiratory complications.

4. c. The immediate need is to remove the patient from the hot environment to allow other interventions to be effective.
5. a, e, f. Inhaled chlorine is irritating to the respiratory tract, which can cause airway obstruction, dyspnea, and pulmonary edema.
6. b. Being respectful will gain trust, while the other choices do not.
7. d. The goal is to treat the most critical yet survivable person first, which is d, because selection c is unlikely to survive and selections a and b are not critical and will survive.
8. c. Airway obstruction can occur in anaphylaxis, which is the most important in ABCs.
9. c. Shock is a condition of progressively decreasing blood pressure.
10. 1.25 mL

$$\frac{500{,}000 \text{ units}}{} \bigg| \frac{1 \text{ mL}}{400{,}000 \text{ units}} = 1.25 \text{ mL}$$

Chapter 14

1. c. Integrity versus despair is the developmental stage for those over age 65. Role changes and coping with these losses are typically experienced in this stage.
2. d. Spiritual distress often occurs with chronic illnesses, along with hopelessness, isolation, and powerlessness.
3. a. The caregiver is exhibiting behaviors indicating *Caregiver Role Strain.* Because behaviors have been exhibited, it is past the risk stage.
4. b. Providing education on the chronic illnesses is most essential for the patient to be able to understand and deal with the illness and achieve a higher level of wellness.
5. b, c, f. Nursing care for a patient who is chronically ill should include encouraging family visits, inclusion of family in teaching, and seeking patient input for plan of care. Education should be increased, patients should set their own goals as able, and socialization with friends should be encouraged.
6. b, c, e, f. The nurse wants to encourage the patient to verbalize feelings of sorrow by having time to listen, actively listening, sharing relevant information to foster coping, and encouraging hope.
7. b. The statement "Maybe tomorrow will be a better day" indicates the patient is hopeful and looking to the future, which is a goal for resolving chronic sorrow.

Chapter 15

1. c. Aging is a maturational process, not a disease, creating the need for individual adaptation because of physical and psychological declines that occur during a lifetime, not a specific age.
2. d. Shortening in height is caused by water loss in the intervertebral disks of the spinal column with aging.
3. b. Offering explanations and active participation with the use of reminders encourages self-care and supports independence for older patients in adhering to a prescribed medication routine.
4. b. Ischemia from unrelieved pressure can begin to develop in 20 to 40 minutes.
5. c. Decreased gag reflex and relaxation of lower esophageal sphincter, increasing the risk of aspiration.
6. a, c, d, e. Adequate fiber and water intake and exercise, including participation in activities of daily living, promote bowel evacuation while some drugs can contribute to constipation.

Chapter 16

1. d. Wald established the Henry Street Settlement in New York City, which laid the groundwork for establishing home care as a nursing specialty.
2. a, b, c, d, f. All are team members except a lawyer.
3. d. The performance of the skills related to the purpose of the visit must be documented for reimbursement.
4. b. Organizing the night before a visit will instill confidence in the nurse and the patient during the visit.
5. a. Infection control is an important function of the home health nurse, and disinfecting the home health bag is important.

Chapter 17

1. c. Difficulty swallowing and weight loss are evidence that the patient is near death.
2. d. A durable power of attorney is a person who can make decisions for a patient when the patient is no longer able to. A living will is the document that outlines a patient's wishes.
3. a. A good death is possible if the patient's wishes are followed and the patient is comfortable.
4. d. There is no one "right" thing to say to a grieving person. Listening is important.
5. b. Scopolamine is an anticholinergic that will dry secretions.
6. a, b, d, f. Positioning, comfort measures, and being present are appropriate.
7. c. Clean the patient and make him presentable for the family. Paperwork can be done later.
8. c. Spending a few minutes with the wife is the most caring.
9. a. A patient can change his mind at any time.

Chapter 18

1. d. Artificially acquired active immunity is provided by a vaccine.
2. a. Older adults should receive an influenza vaccine.
3. a. A splenectomy may reduce immune function.
4. c. Painful enlarged lymph nodes are associated with inflammation and infection.
5. b. For positive ELISA results, which may indicate HIV infection, results must be confirmed by another test, usually the Western blot.
6.

$$\frac{200 \text{ mg}}{} \bigg| \frac{5 \text{ mL}}{125 \text{ mg}} = 8 \text{ mL}$$

Chapter 19

1. c. Viral illnesses and exposure to various chemicals and environmental substances can alter the immune system and its response to previously benign stimuli.
2. a. It is a chronic progressive inflammatory disease of large peripheral joints.
3. a. Glossitis is a sign of pernicious anemia.
4. c. A Schilling test requires 24-hour collection of urine.
5. a, b, c, d, f. All are used for allergic rhinitis except anticholinergics.
6. b. It is important to document the appearance of any skin lesions to note healing over time.
7. d. In an autoimmune disorder, immune cells cannot distinguish "self" from "not self."
8. c, d, e, f. Selection a is not done because the patient may have difficulty swallowing, and for selection b, an IV is needed for medication administration.
9. b. Sun exposure should be avoided and long sleeves, pants, a hat, and sunscreen worn due to photosensitivity.

Chapter 20

1. d. HIV is transmitted from human to human only through infected blood, sexual secretions, and from an infected mother to her unborn baby or to her infant via breast milk.
2. b, c, a. ELISA detects antibodies to the HIV antigen. If positive, the test is repeated. If positive again, the Western blot test detects antibodies to four major HIV antigens and is positive if two antibodies are present.
3. c. HIV is a chronically managed disease with treatment.
4. b, c, e, f. Ways to prevent HIV infection include abstinence, avoiding injection drug use, autologous (self) blood transfusion, and testing for HIV at the time of labor to begin treatment.
5. a, b, e. Preventing infection risk is done with good hygiene (hand washing, toothbrush washing, not reusing dishes, not sharing grooming items), avoiding deli foods that may harbor bacteria, and promptly reporting infection signs.
6. c. HIV causes decreased CD4+ T lymphocytes, so the goal of antiretroviral therapy is to control the virus so CD4+ T lymphocytes will increase.
7. a. A rash and headache are common side effects of delavirdine (Rescriptor).

Chapter 21

1. a. Mitral and tricuspid valves prevent backflow into the atria when the ventricles contract.
2. c. Endocardium prevents abnormal clotting.
3. b. Coronary arteries bring oxygenated blood to the myocardium.
4. d. The medulla is the location of the cardiac centers.
5. b. Angiotensin II causes vasoconstriction and increases aldosterone secretion.
6. c. Increased peripheral vascular resistance increases the workload of the left ventricle and so can contribute to development of left-sided heart failure.
7. d. Tobacco use can be modified through smoking cessation.
8. a. Decreased arterial flow to the extremity is reflected in a slower capillary refill.
9. b. A gait or walking belt should be used for patients who risk falling, which someone with orthostatic hypotension could be.
10. d. On bedrest, edema will be found in dependent areas such as the sacrum.
11. a, d, e, f. *Patient education:* Types of allergies are asked because a dye is used that causes a flushing sensation; firm pressure is applied afterward to prevent bleeding and, therefore, ambulation and flexion are not allowed either for several hours.
12. b. Fiber helps prevent constipation and straining during bowel movements, which reduces cardiac workload.
13. c. Warfarin (Coumadin) affects clotting and is usually stopped before surgery to prevent bleeding issues.

Chapter 22

1. d. There is no known cause for primary hypertension as there is for secondary.
2. a. Reducing weight can help control blood pressure.
3. b. Elevated blood pressure.
4. d, e, f. A healthy diet can control blood pressure and includes eating fresh or frozen fruits and vegetables, reading food labels to make healthy choices, and being aware of safe salt substitutes.
5. c. Prehypertension is 120–139/80–89 mm Hg and should be followed up in 1 year.
6. b. The patient needs immediate treatment for a blood pressure that elevated, so the nurse calls 911.
7. b. Distended jugular veins in semi-Fowler's position are a sign of heart failure.
8. a. To prevent falls from orthostatic blood pressure when on diuretics, the patient rises slowly.
9. c. Blood pressure within normal range indicates effective treatment.

Chapter 23

1. a. Angina indicates cardiac ischemia and requires prompt intervention.
2. b. Symptoms are often not present in MVP.
3. a. In commissurotomy, the valve flaps that have adhered to each other and closed the opening between them, known as the commissure, are separated to enlarge the valve opening.
4. a. Mechanical valves require lifelong anticoagulation to prevent emboli, unlike biological valves, which are less likely to create emboli.
5. a. A streptococcal infection is a bacterial infection treated with the antibacterial agent penicillin.
6. b. Heart failure is a complication of cardiomyopathy.
7. a, d, e, f indicate a blood clot. Selections b and c are seen with heart failure.
8. a. Prothrombin time is monitored during warfarin (Coumadin) therapy.

Chapter 24

1. b. Hypertension is a modifiable risk factor for cardiovascular disease, while the others are nonmodifiable.
2. a. Fatigue is an atypical symptom in the absence of chest pain.
3. b. Coronary artery bypass grafting is done to increase blood flow to the myocardium.
4. c. Intermittent claudication (calf pain with exertion) occurs with peripheral arterial occlusive disease.
5. c. Pentoxifylline (Trental) relieves claudication by decreasing blood viscosity, which increases blood flow in the extremities.
6. c. The patient should keep legs down to promote arterial blood flow to distal extremities.

Chapter 25

1. b, e, a, c, d. The SA node is the primary pacemaker and fires the impulse, which then travels across the atria, to the AV node, bundle of HIS, and Purkinje fibers.
2. a. With a systematic method, it is more difficult to miss abnormalities.
3. c. Defibrillation is used for initial treatment of pulseless ventricular tachycardia to reset the heart's rhythm.
4. c. Teaching for pacemaker care includes having patient take a radial pulse daily and notifying the physician if it is outside expected parameters.
5. b. The patient should be assisted onto a gurney (stretcher) to reduce cardiac workload, promote safety, and quickly begin treatment.
6. d. Bradycardia is the term for a pulse of 59 beats per minute or less.
7. Two tablets should be given per dose.

Chapter 26

1. b. In heart failure, the heart cannot pump enough blood to meet the body's oxygen needs.
2. a. Hypertension contributes to left-sided heart failure because the left ventricle must pump against increased pressure in the aorta from the hypertension.
3. a. A diuretic should be taken in the morning to prevent interference with sleep at night.

4. c. Bumetanide should be given as scheduled because it is working effectively to control the edema.
5. a. Daily weights reflect fluid volume changes as weight gain or loss.
6. 454.5 mg per dose. $160/2.2 = 72.72 \times 12.5 = 909/2 = 454.5$

Chapter 27

1. b. Clotting factors are produced by the liver.
2. c. Erythropoietin is the hormone that stimulates RBC production.
3. b. Blood volume is important for maintenance of circulation and blood pressure.
4. c. Blood cells are suspended in plasma.
5. b. This is a low platelet count; platelets are essential to the clotting process.
6. a. New onset petechiae are associated with bleeding or clotting disorders.
7. a, c, d, f. Name and arm band must be verified against the chart and the unit of blood to ensure correct identification and administration of matching blood. Checking the expiration date is important for patient safety.
8. d. Fever and chills could signify a febrile or a hemolytic reaction. For either, the unit should be stopped immediately and the physician contacted.

Chapter 28

1. b. Anemia means less hemoglobin to carry oxygen to tissues, causing dyspnea.
2. c. Strenuous activity increases oxygen demand, which can cause cells to sickle.
3. d. Disseminated intravascular coagulation uses up clotting factors, which leaves the patient at risk for bleeding.
4. a. A patient with hemophilia should avoid injury; contact sports are too dangerous.
5. d. A patient with leukemia has poor immune function and should not be around someone with a runny nose.
6. a. Multiple myeloma causes bone destruction. A fall increases risk of fracture.
7. a, d, f. IM injections, aspirin, NSAIDs, and walking without shoes or slippers all increase the risk of injury or bleeding in a patient with thrombocytopenia.
8. 1715
9. a. Stage III is diagnosed when lymph nodes on both sides of the diaphragm are affected.
10. d. A high abdominal incision makes deep breathing and coughing difficult, increasing the risk of respiratory complications.

Chapter 29

1. a. The diaphragm contracts and moves downward, creating negative pressure in the chest and pulling air in.
2. c. Cilia move debris up and out of the airway. Damaged cilia are unable to do this.
3. d. 2.5 packs per day $\times$ 10 years = 25 pack-years.
4. b. Wheezes are violin-like sounds made by narrowed airways.
5. d. A normal SpO_2 is 95% to 100%.
6. c, e, b, a, d.
7. b. This delivers the most medication to the lungs.

Chapter 30

1. b. Influenza is caused by a virus. Antibiotics are not effective against viruses.
2. a. Airway is always a priority, especially after surgery that affects the airway.
3. d. Antiviral agents are only effective if they are started within 48 hours of symptom onset.
4. d. Sitting and leaning forward allows the nurse to observe the amount of blood and prevents aspirating or swallowing of blood.
5. a, b, and e all help reduce transmission of influenza.
6. a. The patient with a laryngectomy will suffocate if a finger is placed over the stoma.

Chapter 31

1. c. LTBI is a latent, not active, infection.
2. b. Damaged alveoli and air trapping cause diminished breath sounds.
3. d. Biopsy is always the most definitive test for cancer.
4. c. Pleurodesis is painful; a pain medication should be administered.
5. c. Wheezes and crackles can signify sputum that needs to be coughed up.
6. a. Hypoxia can cause confusion and agitation.
7. b. Diaphragmatic breathing can help make the breathing pattern more effective.
8. a. Spo_2 is the best measure of gas exchange.

Chapter 32

1. b. Pain from a ruptured appendix is located in the right lower quadrant.
2. a. The liver synthesizes plasma proteins.
3. d. Increasing dietary fiber will help regulate normal bowel function.
4. a. Bowel sounds heard at an irregular rate every 5 to 15 seconds are normal.
5. c. Lightly depress the abdomen, not more than 0.5 to 1.0 inch.
6. b. Dehydration must be prevented to avoid a barium impaction.
7. b, c, d. Salem nasogastric tubes are larger bore tubes that are not used for feeding or longer term use.
8. c. A chest x-ray is the only accurate way to verify correct placement of the feeding tube.
9. d. Hyperglycemia may occur due to the high dextrose concentration in TPN.

Chapter 33

1. b. The priority is to provide nourishment and correct electrolyte imbalance, which can be life threatening.
2. c. A body mass index of 31 is defined as obese.
3. d. Topical tetracycline can aid healing canker sores.
4. a. A symptom of gastritis is bloody diarrhea.
5. c. *Helicobacter pylori,* a bacterium, is the most common cause of peptic ulcers.
6. d. H_2 antagonists inhibit secretion of gastric acid.
7. c. To protect the airway, the patient must be placed onto his or her side.
8. b. Fluid and fat intake promote rapid gastric emptying.
9. 25.

Chapter 34

1. a. Report findings because symptoms of dehydration are present along with elevated vital signs.
2. b. Laxatives should be used only occasionally to prevent dependence and complications.
3. a, b, d, f. Control pain and promote lung expansion with activity or coughing and deep breathing.
4. a. Fresh fruit is high in fiber and would promote diarrhea.
5. d. Coughing is contraindicated to prevent damaging the repair, but deep breathing should be done.
6. c. This is the only selection that does not contain a type of grain that must be avoided.

7. a, b, c, d, e. All but edema are a priority to detect pain, dehydration, infection, or shock.
8. a. Black tarry stool is referred to as melena and indicates bleeding above or within the small bowel.
9. a. A high-fat, low-fiber intake increases the risk of colon cancer.
10. a. A dusky color indicates impaired circulation and requires immediate medical treatment to restore blood flow.
11. b. 10 mL

Chapter 35

1. b. Vitamin K is needed for blood clotting, so a low level increases the risk of bleeding.
2. c. Sedatives are potentially toxic to the cirrhosis patient due to impaired hepatic metabolism of these medications.
3. c. Headache, nausea, and flu-like symptoms are symptoms of hepatitis A.
4. d. The serum amylase level is elevated in chronic pancreatitis.
5. d. A low serum albumin level indicates malnutrition.
6. a. Because pancreatitis is very painful, patient satisfaction with pain control is a priority.
7. c. Bile duct obstruction can result in jaundice and dark, amber-colored urine due to bile blockage.
8. a. Roast chicken, rice, and gelatin dessert is a low-fat meal.
9. b, c, e. Pain relief allows comfortable breathing, preventing shallow respirations and guarding. Splinting makes coughing more comfortable, encouraging coughing and deep breathing to keep lungs clear.
10.

$$\frac{12.5\text{ mg}}{} \left| \frac{1\text{ mL}}{50\text{ mg}} \right. = 0.25\text{ mL}$$

Chapter 36

1. a. Urine is formed in the 1 million nephrons of each kidney.
2. a, b, c, d, f. All but selection e are functions of the kidney.
3. c. Provide a night-light in the bathroom to prevent falls.
4. b. Daily weight reflects changes in fluid status.
5. d. To help prevent contamination, women should keep the labia separated while voiding.
6. b, d. Encourage fluids to flush dye from the kidneys, and monitor urine output to detect problems.
7. d. Kegel exercises strengthen the perineal muscles.
8. c. Maintaining a closed catheter system prevents contamination.
9. 912 mL.

Chapter 37

1. a, e. These will help prevent urinary tract infections, while the others do not.
2. b. All urine is strained to detect passage of a stone.
3. a. Tobacco use is a risk factor for bladder cancer.
4. b. Continue changing the pouch because this is normal.
5. a. Fluid intake is increased to flush the kidneys.
6. d. The creatinine level must be reported because it is elevated, and the nephrotoxic gentamicin is held until the physician is notified.
7. b, c, d. Bananas are high in potassium and avoided, while the other options can be given.
8. d. Patency is assessed with palpation for a thrill and auscultation of a bruit over the fistula site.
9. c. Applying pressure to a bleeding site is the first action the nurse takes to control the bleeding.
10. 1600/400 = 4

Chapter 38

1. a, e. Antidiuretic hormone and oxytocin are synthesized in the hypothalamus and secreted by the posterior pituitary.
2. d. T_4 and T_3 regulate metabolic rate and energy production.
3. c. "Calcitonin tones it down" in the blood, and into the bones.
4. a. Excess cortisol (Cushing's syndrome) is associated with moon face and buffalo hump.
5. b. A thyroid scan involves injection of radioactive iodine.

Chapter 39

1. c. Excess cortisol, whether endogenous or exogenous, causes Cushing's syndrome.
2. c. Antidiuretic hormone causes water retention without sodium or potassium retention.
3. b, e, f. Diabetes insipidus is caused by lack of antidiuretic hormone, which results in excess urination, thirst, and dehydration.
4. a. Thyroid hormone is essential to survival. If the thyroid gland has been removed, exogenous hormone replacement is required for life.
5. d. Elevated vital signs can signal the onset of thyrotoxic crisis.
6. a. Routine neurologic assessments are important to detect complications after surgery involving the central nervous system.
7. a. A patient with hypothyroidism typically is fatigued; returning energy is a sign of effective therapy.

Chapter 40

1. a. Diabetes mellitus is characterized by defective insulin secretion or action.
2. b. Obesity is a major risk factor for type 2 diabetes.
3. 126.
4. d. Hyperglycemia causes polyuria, polydipsia, and polyphagia.
5. a. Nephropathy, or damage to the small vessels in the nephrons, causes protein to leak into the urine.
6. c. Tight control of blood glucose levels is the best way to prevent complications. Selections a, b, and d are also helpful, but are not the best way.
7. d. Includes a balance of complex carbohydrates, fats, and protein. Selection a is high fat, low carbohydrate. Selections b and c have minimal fat or protein.
8. c, f, d, e, b, a.
9. a. 48 is below normal and is considered hypoglycemia.
10. a. Sliding scale insulin may be needed during times of stress or illness
11. b. Small, frequent, low-carbohydrate meals will help prevent fluctuations in blood glucose.

Chapter 41

1. c.
2. d.
3. d. An ultrasound can identify fluid-filled cysts.
4. b, c, d, e. A speculum with lubricant for the examination; gloves for the examiner; slides and fixative to send the sample to the lab.
5. b. Young men are at risk for testicular cancer, and so should be taught testicular self-examination.
6. c. Lying flat will reduce discomfort from the carbon dioxide used for insufflation.
7. a. The National Institutes of Health recommends 1200 mg calcium and 400 international units vitamin D for women ages 51 to 70.

Chapter 42

1. c. Mastalgia can be broken down as mast—breast + algia—pain.
2. c. Bleeding again after menopause is always cause for concern.
3. d. Bradycardia and falling blood pressure are signs that the vagus nerve has been stimulated.
4. a. Atropine is an anticholinergic agent that will reverse the cholinergic response initiated by vagal stimulation.
5. b. Relaxation exercises and warm compresses can help relax the patient and reduce the perception of pain, when used with medication.
6. c. Because of compromised circulation in the affected arm, needlesticks and blood pressure measurements should be avoided.
7. b. Because the ovaries are removed in a panhysterectomy, the patient should expect to experience menopause.
8. 240. The patient should eliminate at least 30 mL per hour times 8 hours = 240 mL.
9. a. Douching is ineffective because sperm may already be out of reach. It also may push sperm further upward.

Chapter 43

1. c. Benign prostatic hyperplasia is not cancer, but it must be treated. Telling a patient not to worry is inappropriate.
2. c. Transurethral resection of the prostate (TURP) is most common.
3. a. A B&O suppository will reduce bladder spasms, which often cause pain after TURP.
4. b. Cleaning is important, but be sure to replace the foreskin afterward to prevent paraphimosis.
5. b. A good blood supply is essential for erection.
6. a. Reflecting back and asking the patient if he would like to talk more will identify if there is a concern that should be followed up by a physician or care provider.
7. a, d. Varicocele is like a varicose vein in the scrotum. It can cause pain and infertility.
8. d. Nicotine and alcohol use can interfere with male fertility.

Chapter 44

1. a. *Treponema pallidum* causes syphilis.
2. a, b, c, d, e, f. All symptoms can occur with sexually transmitted diseases and should be assessed.
3. c. Having a sexual relationship with someone is the epidemiological equivalent of engaging in sexual activity with all of that person's previous partners.
4. d. An analgesic is necessary. Wart removal is very painful.
5. c. The man's statement indicates that he would like to talk. Selection c is a therapeutic response that gives the man permission to talk further.
6. a. Alcohol can cloud judgment.

Chapter 45

1. b. Synovial fluid prevents friction in joints as they move.
2. c, e, f. Exercise and diet are important to maintain bone health. Collecting data about them is the first step in planning interventions for the disease.
3. d. Pedal pulses are one of the vascular checks done on the lower extremities.
4. a. Ask if there is any metal or a pacemaker in the patient's body to allow the physician to determine if it is safe to do an MRI.
5. b. Notify the physician because circulation in the extremity may be compromised and require immediate treatment.

Chapter 46

1. b. Turn the patient every 2 hours to expose all sides of the cast to the air for drying.
2. b. Agency protocol specifies pin care.
3. a, e. Washing hands and wearing sterile gloves to apply a new dressing is essential.
4. c. Exercise can help prevent osteoporosis.
5. a. Pain is a classic symptom of Paget's disease. (Remember, P = P).
6. c. Excessive uric acid is formed in gout.
7. a. A classic symptom of systemic lupus erythematosus is a red rash across bridge of nose that resembles a butterfly.
8. b. Maintaining ideal body weight will reduce wear and tear on the knee.
9. b. Maintain legs in abduction to prevent dislocation of the hip.
10. c. Stump dressings should be monitored for bleeding.
11. d. An absent left pedal pulse may be due to circulatory impairment caused by the fracture and requires immediate treatment.
12. d. Notify the physician because the patient may be developing compartment syndrome, an emergency condition.
13. 0.5 mL

Chapter 47

1. b. Motor nerves are efferent nerves. (Remember, efferent—effect.)
2. a. The hypothalamus regulates body temperature.
3. b. Bradycardia, increasing systolic blood pressure with widening pulse pressure, and irregular respirations, commonly referred to as Cushing's triad, are late indications of increasing intracranial pressure.
4. b, c, d, and f are all normal effects of aging.
5. d. An angiogram uses x-ray or other imaging following injection of dye.
6. b. Fluids help the kidneys excrete the dye.
7. c. High-top tennis shoes keep the feet in functional positions.

Chapter 48

1. a. A sore throat is caused by a virus or bacterium, which can spread to cause meningitis.
2. b. Darkening the room will help relieve photophobia, and analgesics reduce pain.
3. a. Some patients experience an aura before a migraine.
4. d. A headache diary provides the best data for diagnosis.
5. c. The patient will be in a deep postictal sleep and can eat when awake.
6. c, a, d, b. The patient should be assisted to lie down before the seizure starts; safety should be maintained; the patient will sleep after the seizure; document last.
7. b, c, d. Fever and headache could indicate encephalitis or meningitis. Craniectomy and brain tumor can be associated with brain swelling.
8. b. Elevating the head of the bed can reduce intracranial pressure.
9. d. An L2 injury is low; the patient may be able to walk with a brace.
10. c. This could be a sign of autonomic dysreflexia.
11. a. Dopamine depletion causes symptoms of Parkinson's disease.
12. a. Tucking the chin may help guide the food into the esophagus.
13. b. This validates her feeling of loneliness in a nonthreatening way.

Chapter 49

1. c, e, f. Diabetes, high cholesterol, and obesity are all treatable to reduce the risk of stroke.
2. a. Computed tomography of the head must be done immediately to determine the course of action.
3. d. Thrombolytic therapy must be given within 3 hours to reverse stroke symptoms and reduce the risk of complications.
4. d. Receptive aphasia is difficulty receiving, or understanding, language.
5. d. The patient may be experiencing unilateral neglect or visual deficits. Turning the plate and observing can help identify the problem.
6. c. Call for help immediately. The patient could be experiencing an extension of the bleed or ischemic area.

Chapter 50

1. c. Anticonvulsants help relieve nerve pain.
2. d. Amyotrophic lateral sclerosis causes weak muscles. If the respiratory muscles are affected, breathing (and singing) may be compromised.
3. a. Advance directives will allow the patient to have his wishes recorded.
4. c. Assessment and maintenance of respiratory function is a nursing priority.
5. a, b, d, and e help with symptoms related to paralysis. Selections c and f are interventions for TN.
6. b. Soft foods are easier to chew and less tiring.
7. d. Ability to perform activities of daily living and effective breathing are signs that muscle strength is adequate.

Chapter 51

1. Cornea, aqueous humor, lens, vitreous humor.
2. d. Comparing the patient's visual fields with your own assesses visual fields.
3. b. Those with a hearing loss are often irritable or sensitive during interpersonal relations because of their inability to hear and interact with others.
4. c. Having regular hearing evaluations helps ensure ear health.
5. a. Ensuring patient safety to prevent injury is essential.
6. d. Aspirin can be toxic to the ears is true, which shows understanding of teaching.
7. a, b, c. Gloves, gown, goggles (if splashing is anticipated) are used in contact isolation for this nonsterile procedure, whereas a mask is used for respiratory isolation.
8. c. Tinnitus occurs with aspirin toxicity.

Chapter 52

1. c. Otosclerosis is hardening of the stapes from new bone growth.
2. b. A refractory error requires corrective lenses to see clearly.
3. a. Pain is experienced with an external ear infection.
4. a. Since the pupils are dilated, the eyes must be protected from bright light.
5. b. After pneumatic retinopexy, the patient is educated on positions to keep the air bubble in place.
6. c, e. Atropine and hydroxyzine are mydriatics, which are contraindicated in acute angle-closure glaucoma to prevent increasing eye pressure.
7. a. Furosemide (Lasix) can cause hearing loss.
8. d. Loss of central vision occurs with macular degeneration.
9. c. Ménière's disease can cause vertigo, which could result in injury.
10. b. With presbycusis, there is an inability to decipher high-frequency sounds, so a lower voice pitch is helpful.
11. d. Mydriatics such as anticholinergics and antihistamines (diphenhydramine) are contraindicated in acute angle-closure glaucoma.

Chapter 53

1. b. Keratin is relatively waterproof, so it prevents the loss of water and therefore dehydration.
2. b, d, e. Subcutaneous tissue is beneath the skin and helps cushion bony prominences, provide insulation, and store energy in the form of fat.
3. a. Slower epidermal division causes thin, fragile skin.
4. c. A vesicle is a fluid-filled lesion.
5. a. A severe allergic reaction may require resuscitation.
6. b. Wet dressings can chill the patient.

Chapter 54

1. a. Psoriasis is a chronic inflammatory skin disorder in which epidermal cells proliferate abnormally quickly.
2. c. Exposure to ultraviolet rays is the major cause of skin malignancies.
3. c. Gloves help prevent scratching, which can worsen lesions.
4. b, d, e, f. Sliding can cause friction and shear damage. Sitting can cause pressure points if weight is not shifted frequently. Diaphoresis and incontinence can cause maceration of the skin and increase risk of breakdown.
5. b. Washing linens should be sufficient, because mites only survive 24 hours without human contact.
6. d. Impetigo is contagious until all lesions are healed.

Chapter 55

1. b. Deep partial-thickness burns are associated with pink to light red or white skin, blisters, and blanching.
2. a. Lavage with water for 20 minutes for all chemical burns, along with simultaneous removal of contaminated clothing. Neutralizing a chemical takes too much time.
3. c. The trunk is 18% front, 18% back, and each arm is 9%.
4. c, d, e. Circulation must be monitored. Escharotomy may be indicated. Elevation promotes venous return.
5. d. PaO_2 88 mm Hg is the only normal value.

Chapter 56

1. a. No one is happy and smiling all the time. It is not an expected behavior.
2. a, c, e, and f can all reflect level of mental health.
3. b. Physical causes of symptoms should always be ruled out before making a mental health diagnosis.
4. c. Rationalization is using logical-sounding excuses to cover up true thoughts.
5. c. A therapeutic milieu is an environment that provides containment, support, structure, involvement, and validation.
6. d. Medications can help manage symptoms so patients can engage in therapies.
7. a. Honest communication is a productive behavior. Selections b, c, and d are defense mechanisms.
8. d. This selection demonstrates therapeutic communication and active listening.

Chapter 57

1. a. Psychoanalytic theory explains disorders based on childhood experiences.
2. c. Conversion disorder describes the patient who experiences a physical symptom to help relieve or avoid psychological stress.
3. a. Anticholinergic agents help restore the balance of neurotransmitters to prevent EPS.
4. d. The patient has post-traumatic stress disorder and needs calm reorientation until the episode is over.
5. c. Checking vital signs verifies that there is not a real physical cause for the symptoms, and reassures the patient.

Appendix D

Medical Abbreviations

ABG	arterial blood gas
ac	before a meal
AD	advance directive
ad lib	freely; as desired
ALT	alanine aminotransferase
AM	morning
A-P	anterior-posterior
AST	aspartate aminotransferase
AV	atrioventricular
bid	twice a day
BM	bowel movement
BP	blood pressure
BUN	blood urea nitrogen
c̄	with
cap	a capsule
CBC	complete blood count
cc	cubic centimeter
cm	centimeter
CNS	central nervous system
CSF	cerebrospinal fluid
CV	cardiovascular
D & C	dilatation and curettage
dc	discontinue
dL	deciliter
DNR	do not resuscitate
DOA	dead on arrival
dr	dram
Dx	diagnosis
ECF	extracellular fluid
ECG	electrocardiogram
ECT	electroconvulsive therapy
ED	emergency department
EEG	electroencephalogram
EMG	electromyogram
EMS	emergency medical service
ENT	ear, nose, and throat
EOM	extraocular muscles
ER	emergency room
ESR	erythrocyte sedimentation rate
F	Fahrenheit
g, gm	gram
GERD	gastroesophageal reflux disease
GI	gastrointestinal
gr	grain
Gtt, gtt	drops
GYN	gynecology
h, hr	hour
Hgb	hemoglobin
hor som, hs	bedtime
IM	intramuscular
IUD	intrauterine device
IV	intravenous
IVP	intravenous pyelogram
J	joule
kg	kilogram
KUB	kidney, ureter, and bladder
L	liter
lb	pound
lmp	last menstrual period
mEq	milliequivalent
mg	milligram
mL	milliliter
mm	millimeter
MRI	magnetic resonance imaging
MS	mitral stenosis; multiple sclerosis
μEq	microequivalent
μg	microgram
npo	nothing by mouth
NSAID	nonsteroidal anti-inflammatory drug
NSR	normal sinus rhythm
OB	obstetrics
O.C.	oral contraceptive
O.D.	right eye
O.S.	left eye
O.U.	both eyes
oz	ounce
p̄	after
pc	after meals
$P\text{CO}_2$	carbon dioxide pressure
PERRLA	pupils equal, regular, react to light and accommodation
pH	hydrogen ion concentration
PM	afternoon/evening
PMI	point of maximal impulse
post	posterior
pr	through the rectum
prn	as needed
qhr	every hour
q2hr	every 2 hours
q3hr	every 3 hours
qid	four times a day
qs	as much as is needed
RBC	red blood cell; red blood count
s̄	without
SA	sinoatrial
SC, sc	subcutaneous(ly)
SOB	shortness of breath
s.o.s	if necessary
sq	subcutaneous(ly)
stat.	immediately
STD	sexually transmitted disease
T	temperature
tab	medicated tablet
temp	temperature
tid	three times a day
top	topically
URI	upper respiratory infection
USP	United States Pharmacopeia
UTI	urinary tract infection
WBC	white blood cell; white blood count
WF/BF	white female/black female
WM/BM	white male/black male
wt.	weight

Adapted from Thomas, C. L. (2005), *Taber's cyclopedic medical dictionary* (20th ed., p. 2463). Philadelphia: F. A. Davis.

Appendix E

Prefixes, Suffixes, and Combining Forms

a-, an-. Without; away from; not.
ab-, abs-. From; away from; absent.
abdomin-, abdomino-. Abdomen.
-ad. Toward; in the direction of.
aden-, adeno-. Gland.
adip-, adipo-. Fat.
-aemia. Blood.
aer-, aero-. Air.
-algesia, -algia. Suffering; pain.
andro-. Man; male; masculine
angi-, angio-. Blood or lymph vessels.
aniso-. Unequal; asymmetrical; dissimilar.
ankyl-, ankylo-. Crooked; bent; fusion or growing together of parts.
ant-, anti-. Against.
ante-. Before.
antero-. Anterior; front; before.
arteri-, arterio-. Artery.
arthr-, arthro-. Joint.
-ase. Enzyme.
-asis, esis, -iasis, -isis, -sis. Condition; pathological state.
aut-, auto-. Self.
axo-. Axis; axon.
bacteri-, bacterio-. Bacteria; bacterium.
bi-, bis-. Two; double; twice.
bili-. Bile.
bio-. Life.
blast-, -blast. Germ; bud; embryonic state of development.
blephar-, blepharo-. Eyelid.
brady-. Slow.
bronch-, bronchi-, broncho-. Airway.
cardi-, cardio-. Heart.
cat-, cata-, cath-, kat-, kata-. Down; downward; destructive; against; according to.
cent-. Hundred.
cephal-, cephalo-. Head.
cervic-, cervice-. Head; the neck of an organ.
chrom-, chromo-. Color.
-cide. Causing death.
contra-. Against; opposite.
crani-, cranio-. Skull; cranium.
cry-, cryo-. Cold.
cyan-, cyano-. Blue.
cyst-, cysto-, -cyst. Cyst; urinary bladder.
cyt-, cyto-, -cyte. Cell.
derm-, derma-, dermato-, dermo-. Skin.
di-. Double; twice; two; apart from.
dors-, dorsi-, dorso-. Back.
-dynia. Pain.
dys-. Difficult; bad; painful.
ec-, ecto-. Out; on the outside.
-ectomy. Excision.
ef-, es-, ex-, exo-. Out.
electr-, electro-. Electricity.
-emesis. Vomiting.
-emia. Blood.
en-. In; into.
end-, endo-. Within.
ent-, ento-. Within; inside.
enter-, entero-. Intestine.
ep-, epi-. Upon; over; at; in addition to; after.
erythr-, erythro-. Red.
eury-. Broad.
ex-. Out; away from; completely.
exo-. Out; outside of; without.
extra-. Outside of; in addition; beyond.
-facient. Causing; making happen.
-ferous. Producing.
ferri-, ferro-. Iron.
fluo-. Flow.
fore-. Before; in front of.
-form. Form.
-fuge. To expel; to drive away; fleeing.
gaster-, gastero-, gastr-, gastro-. Stomach.
gen-. Producing; forming.
-gen, -gene, -genesis, -genetic, -genic. Producing; forming.
glosso-. Tongue.
gluc-, gluco-, glyc-, glyco-. Sugar; glycerol or similar substance.
gyn-, gyne-, gyneco-, gyno-. Woman; female.
hem-, hema-, hemato-, hemo-. Blood.
hemi-. Half.
hepat-, hepato-. Liver.
heter-, hetero-. Other; different.
histo-. Tissue.
homo-. Same; likeness.
hydra-, hydro, hydr-. Water.
hyp-, hyph-, hypo-. Less than; below; under.
hyper-. Above; excessive; beyond.
hyster-, hystero-. Uterus.
-ia. Condition, esp. an abnormal state.
-iasis. SEE *-asis.*
-iatric. Medicine; medical profession; physicians.
in-. In; inside; within; intensive action; negative.
infra-. Below; under; beneath; inferior to; after.
inter-. Between; in the midst.
intra-, intro-. Within; in; into.
ipsi-. Same.
irid-, irido-. Iris.
-ism. Condition; theory.
iso-. Equal.
-itis. Inflammation of.
kera-, kerato-. Horny substance; cornea.
kolp-, kolpo, colp-, colpo-. Vagina.
kypho-. Humped.
leuk-, leuko-. White; colorless; rel. to a leukocyte.
lip-, lipo-. Fat.
-lite, -lith, lith-, litho-. Stone; calculus.
-logia, -logy. Science of; study of.
lumbo-. Loins.
-lysis. 1. Setting free; disintegration. 2. In medicine, reduction of; relief from.
macr-, macro-. Large; long.
mal-. Ill; bad; poor.
med-, medi-, medio-. Middle.
mega-, megal-, megalo-. Large; of great size.
-megalia, -megaly. Enlargement of a body part.
melan-, melano-. Black.
mening-, meningo-. Meninges.
-meter. Measure.
metr-, metra-, metro-. Uterus.
micr-, micro-. Small.
mon-, mono-. Single; one.
muc-, muci-, muco-, myxa-, myxo-. Mucus.
multi-. Many; much.
musculo-, my-, myo-. Muscle.
my-, myo-. SEE *musculo-.*
myel-, myelo-. Spinal cord; bone marrow.
naso-. Nose.
necr-, necro-. Death; necrosis.
neo-. New; recent.
nephr-, nephra-, nephro-. Kidney.
neur-, neuri-, neuro-. Nerve; nervous system.
non-. No.
normo-. Normal; usual.
oculo-. Eye.
-ode, -oid. Form; shape; resemblance.
-odynia, odyno-. Pain.
olig-, oligo-. Few; small.
-ology. Science of; study of.
-oma. Tumor.
onco-. Tumor; swelling; mass.
oo-, ovi-, ovo-. Egg; ovum.
oophor-, oophoro-, oophoron-. Ovary.
ophthalm-, ophthalmo-. Eye.
-opia. Vision.
optico-, opto-. Eye; vision.
orchi-, orchid-, orchido-. Testicle.
orth-, ortho-. Straight; correct; normal; in proper order.
os-. Mouth; bone.
-osis. Condition; status, process; abnormal increase.
oste-, osteo-. Bone.
ostomosis, -ostomy, -stomosis, -stomy. A created mouth or outlet.
ot-, oto-. Ear.
-otomy. Cutting.
-ous. 1. Possessing; full of. 2. Pertaining to.
pan-. All; entire.
para-, -para. 1. Prefix: near; alongside of; departure from normal. 2. Suffix: Bearing offspring.

path-, patho-, -path, -pathic, -pathy. Disease; suffering.
ped-, pedi-, pedo-. Foot.
-penia. Decrease from normal; deficiency.
peri-. Around; about.
perineo-. Perineum.
phaco-. Lens of the eye.
phag-, phago-. Eating; ingestion; devouring.
-phil, -philia, -philic. Love for; tendency toward; craving for.
phlebo-. Vein.
-phobia. Abnormal fear or aversion.
photo-. Light.
phren-, phreno-, -phrenia. Mind; diaphragm.
-phylaxis. Protection.
-plasia. Growth; cellular proliferation.
plasm-, -plasm. 1. Prefix: Living substance or tissue. 2. Suffix: To mold.
-plastic. Molded; indicates restoration of lost or badly formed features.
-plegia. Paralysis; stroke.
pneo-. Breath; breathing.
pneum-, pneuma-, pneumato-. Air; gas; respiration.
-poiesis, -poietic. Production; formation.
poly-. Much; many.
post-. After.
pre-. Before; in front of.
presby-. Old age.
pro-. Before; in behalf of.
proct-, procto-. Anus; rectum.
pseud-, pseudo-. False.
psych-, psycho-. Mind; mental processes.
pulmo-. Lung.
py-, pyo-. Pus.
pyro-. Heat; fire.
ren-, reno-. Kidneys.
retro-. Backward; back; behind.
rheo-, -(r)rhea. Current; stream; to flow; to discharge.
rhino-. Nose.
-(r)rhage, -(r)rhagia. Rupture; profuse fluid discharge.
-(r)rhaphy. A suturing or stitching.
salping-, salpingo-. Auditory tube; fallopian tube.
sclero-. Hard; relating to the sclera.
-scopy. Examination.
semi-. Half.
sero-. Serum.
somat-, somato-. Body.
sperma-, spermat-, spermato-. Sperm; spermatozoa.
steno-. Narrow; short.
-stomosis, -stomy. SEE *-ostomosis*.
sub-. Under; beneath; in small quantity; less than normal.
super-. Above; beyond; superior.
supra-. Above; beyond; on top.
tachy-. Swift; rapid.
tel-, tele-. 1. End. 2. Distant; far.
tendo-, teno-. Tendon.
thorac-, thoraci-, thoraco-. Chest; chest wall.
thrombo-. Blood clot; thrombus.
thyro-. Thyroid gland; oblong; shield.
-tomy. Cutting operation; excision.
top-, topo-. Place; locale.
tox-, toxi-,toxico-, toxo-, -toxic. Toxin; poison; toxic.
tracheo-. Trachea; windpipe.
trans-. Across; over; beyond; through.
-tropin. Stimulation of a target organ by a substance, esp. a hormone.
tympano-. Eardrum; tympanum.
ultra-. Beyond; excess.
-uria. Urine.
uter-, utero-. Uterus.
vaso-. Vessel (e.g., blood vessel).
veno-. Vein.
ventro-, ventr-, ventri-. Abdomen; anterior surface of the body.
vertebro-. Vertebra; vertebrae.
vesico-. Bladder; vesicle.

Adapted from Thomas, C. L. (2001). *Taber's cyclopedic medical dictionary* (19th ed., pp. 2465–2469). Philadelphia: F. A. Davis.

Appendix F

Glossary

ablation: (uh-BLAY-shun) Removal of part, pathway, or function by surgery, chemical electrocautery, or radiofrequency.

abrasion: (ah-BRAY-zhun) A scraping away of skin or mucous membrane as a result of injury or by mechanical means.

abuse: (uh-BYOOS) Misuse; excessive or improper use. May refer to substances or individuals.

accommodation: (uh-KOM-uh-DAY-shun) A reflex action of the eye for focusing.

acidosis: (as-ih-DOH-siss) An actual or relative increase in the acidity of blood caused by an accumulation of acid or a loss of base.

acquired immunodeficiency syndrome (AIDS): (uh-KWHY-erd IM-yoo-noh-de-FISH-en-see SIN-drohm) Suppression or deficiency of the cellular immune response, acquired by exposure to human immunodeficiency virus (HIV).

active immunity: (AK-tiv im-YOO-nih-tee) Acquired immunity attributable to the presence of antibodies or of immune lymphoid cells formed in response to antigenic stimulus.

activities of daily living (ADLs): (ack-TIV-ih-tees of DAY-lee LIH-ving) Those activities and behaviors that are performed in the care and maintenance of self (e.g., bathing, dressing, eating).

acupuncture: (ak-yoo-PUNGK-chur) Technique using needles inserted at specific points to create anesthesia or treat certain conditions.

acute coronary syndromes: (ah-KEWT KOR-un-nah-ree sin-DROMES) Group of conditions, including unstable angina, non-Q-wave myocardial infarction, and ST segment elevation myocardial infarction, caused by a lack of oxygen to the heart muscle.

acute pulmonary hypertension: (ah-KEWT PULL-muh-NAIR-ee HIGH-purr-TEN-shun) An excessive buildup of pressure in the pulmonary arteries caused by sudden obstruction of the pulmonary artery.

adaptation: (ad-dap-TAY-shun) Adjustment to changes in internal or external conditions or circumstances; coping.

addiction: (uh-DIK-shun) Psychological dependence characterized by drug seeking and craving for an opioid or other substance for effects other than the intended purpose of the substance.

adjunct: (ADD-junkt) An addition to the principal procedure or course of therapy.

adjuvant: (ad-JOO-vant) Something that assists something else, such as a second form of treatment added to treat a disease.

administrative laws: (ad-MIN-ih-STRAY-tiv LAWZ) Establish the licensing authority of the state to create, license, and regulate the practice of nursing.

adnexa: (ad-NECK-sah) Appendages or accessory organs.

advance medical directive: (ad-VANS MED-ik-uhl dur-EK-tiv) A set of documents (living will and durable medical power of attorney) that explain a person's end-of-life wishes and direct care when the patient is no longer able to do so.

adventitious: (ad-ven-TI-shus) Abnormal or extra; often refers to extra breath sounds, such as wheezes or crackles.

advocate: (ADD-vuh-kut) Someone who makes sure a person's wishes are adhered to; someone who represents the best interests of the patient.

aerobic: (air-OH-bick) Living only in the presence of oxygen.

affect: (AF-feckt) Emotional tone.

afterload: (AFF-ter-lohd) The forces impeding the blood flow out of the heart (vascular pressure, aortic compliance, blood mass, and viscosity).

agenesis: (ay-JEN-uh-siss) Failure of an organ or part to develop or grow.

agonist: (AG-un-ist) A type of opioid that binds to opioid receptors in the central nervous system to relieve pain.

akinesia: (ah-kih-NEE-zee-ah) Absence or loss of the power of voluntary movement.

alkalosis: (al-ka-LOH-siss) An actual or relative decrease in the acidity of blood caused by loss of acid or accumulation of base.

allopathic: (AL-oh-PATH-ik) Method of treating disease with remedies that produce effects different from those caused by the disease.

alopecia: (AL-oh-PEE-she-ah) The loss of hair from the body and the scalp.

amenorrhea: (ay-MEN-uh-REE-ah) The absence or suppression of menstruation. Amenorrhea is normal before puberty, after menopause, and during pregnancy and lactation.

amputation: (am-pew-TAY-shun) The removal of a limb or other appendage or outgrowth of the body.

anaerobic: (AN-air-ROH-bik) Able to live without oxygen.

analgesic: (AN-uhl-JEE-zik) A drug that relieves pain.

anaphylactic shock: (AN-uh-fuh-LAK-tik SHAWK) Systemic reaction that produces life-threatening changes in the circulation and bronchioles.

anaphylaxis: (AN-uh-fuh-LAK-siss) A sudden severe allergic reaction to an allergen.

anastomose: (uh-NAS-tuh-MOS) To surgically connect two parts.

anemia: (uh-NEE-mee-yah) A condition in which there is reduced delivery of oxygen to the tissues as a result of reduced numbers of red cells or hemoglobin.

anergy: (AN-er-jee) Diminished ability of the immune system to react to an antigen.

anesthesia: (AN-es-THEE-zee-uh) Lack of feeling or sensation; artificially induced loss of ability to feel pain.

anesthesiologist: (an-es-THEE-zee-aw-lah-just) A physician who specializes in anesthesiology.

aneurysm: (AN-yur-izm) A sac formed by the localized dilation of the wall of an artery, a vein, or the heart.

angina pectoris: (an-JY-nah PEK-tuh-riss) Severe pain and pressure in the chest caused by insufficient supply of blood and oxygenation to the heart.

angioedema: (AN-gee-oh-eh-DEE-mah) A localized edematous reaction of the deep dermis or subcutaneous or submucosal tissues appearing as giant wheals.

anion: (AN-eye-on) Electrolyte that carries a negative electrical charge.

anisocoria: (an-ih-soh-KOH-ree-ah) Inequality in size of the pupils of the eyes.

ankylosing spondylitis: (ANG-kih-LOH-sing SPON-da-LEYE-tiss) Inflammatory disease of the spine causing stiffness and pain.

annuloplasty: (AN-yoo-loh-PLAS-tee) Repair of a cardiac valve.

anorexia: (AN-uh-REK-see-ah) Absence or loss of appetite for food. Seen in depression, with illness, and as a side effect of some medications.

anorexia nervosa: (AN-uh-REK-see-ah ner-VOH-sah) Refusal to maintain body weight over a minimal normal weight for age and height.

antagonist: (an-TAG-on-ist) Medication used to counteract the effects of an opioid (e.g., naloxone).

anteflexion: (AN-tee-FLEK-shun) The abnormal bending forward of part of an organ.
anteversion: (AN-tee-VER-zhun) A tipping forward of an organ as a whole, without bending.
anthrax: (AN-thrax) A disease caused by the spore-forming bacterium *Bacillus anthracis* that has three clinical forms in humans: inhalational, cutaneous, and gastrointestinal. It can be used as a biological weapon.
antibodies: (AN-tih-baw-dees) An immunoglobin molecule having a specific amino acid sequence that gives each antibody the ability to adhere to and interact only with the antigen that induced the synthesis.
anticholinesterase: (AN-tih-KOH-lin-ESS-ter-ays) A substance that breaks down acetylcholinesterase.
antidiuretic: (AN-tih-DYE-yoo-RET-ik) Lessening urine excretion.
antigen: (AN-tih-jen) A protein marker on the surface of cells that identifies the type of cell.
antitussive: (an-tee-TUSS-iv) An agent that prevents or relieves cough.
anuria: (an-YOO-ree-ah) Complete suppression of urine formation by the kidney.
anxiety: (ang-ZYE-uh-tee) The uncomfortable feeling of apprehension or dread that occurs in response to a known or unknown threat.
aphasia: (ah-FAY-zee-ah) Defect or loss of the power of expression by speech, writing, or signs, or of comprehension of spoken or written language, caused by disease or injury of the brain centers, such as stroke syndrome.
aphthous stomatitis: (AF-thus STOH-mah-TYE-tis) Small, white, painful ulcers (also known as canker sores) that appear on the inner cheeks, lips, gums, tongue, palate, and pharynx. They tend to recur.
apnea: (APP-nee-ah) Temporary absence of breathing.
appendicitis: (uh-PEN-dih-SYE-tiss) Inflammation of the vermiform appendix.
arcus senilus: (AR-kus seh-NILL-us) A benign white or gray opaque ring in the corneal margin of the eye.
arrhythmia: (uh-RITH-mee-yah) Irregular rhythm, especially heartbeat.
arteriosclerosis: (ar-TEER-ee-oh-skle-ROH-siss) Term applied to a number of pathological conditions in which there is gradual thickening, hardening, and loss of elasticity of the walls of the arteries.
arthritis: (are-THRYE-tiss) Inflammation of a joint.
arthrocentesis: (ar-THROW-sen-tee-sis) Puncture of a joint space with a needle to remove fluid accumulated in the joint.
arthroplasty: (AR-throw-PLAS-te) Repair of a joint. Also called joint replacement.
arthroscopy: (are-THROSS-scop-ee) Examination of the interior of a joint with an arthroscope.
articular: (ar-TIK-yoo-lar) Pertaining to a joint.
artificial feeding: (ART-ih-FISH-uhl FEE-ding) Feeding via a tube into the stomach or intestine when a person is unable to take oral nutrition.
artificial hydration: (ART-ih-FISH-uhl hy-DRAY-shun) Administration of water via intravenous or gastric tube when a person is unable to take oral fluids.
ascites: (a-SYE-teez) Abnormal accumulation of fluid in the peritoneal cavity.
asepsis: (ah-SEP-sis) A condition free from germs, infection, and any form of life.
aseptic: (ah-SEP-tik) Free of pathogenic organisms; asepsis.
asphyxia: (as-FIX-ee-ah) A condition in which there is a deficiency of oxygen in the blood and an increase in carbon dioxide in the blood and tissues.
aspiration: (AS-pih-RAY-shun) Accidental drawing in of foreign substances into the throat or lungs during inspiration.
assessment: (ah-SESS-ment) An appraisal or evaluation of a patient's condition.
asterixis: (AS-tur-ICK-siss) Hand flapping tremor and involuntary movements of tongue and feet; may be present in hepatic encephalopathy.
astigmatism: (uh-STIG-mah-TIZM) An error of refraction in which a ray of light is not sharply focused on the retina but is spread over a more or less diffuse area.
ataxia: (ah-TAK-see-ah) Failure of muscular coordination; irregularity of muscular action.
atelectasis: (AT-eh-LEK-tah-siss) Collapsed or airless condition of the lung or portion of lung, caused by obstruction or hypoventilation.
atheroma: (ATH-er-OH-mah) Fatty deterioration or thickening of the walls of the larger arteries occurring in atherosclerosis.
atherosclerosis: (ATH-er-oh-skle-ROH-siss) A form of arteriosclerosis characterized by accumulation of plaque, blood, and blood products lining the wall of the artery, causing partial or complete blockage of an artery.
atrial depolarization: (AY-tree-uhl DE-poh-lahr-ih-ZAY-shun) Electrical activation of the atria.
atrial systole: (AY-tree-uhl SISS-tuh-lee) The contraction of the atria.
atrioventricular node: (AY-tree-oh-ven-TRIK-yoo-lar NOHD) Located in lower right atrium; receives an impulse from the sinoatrial (SA) node and relays it to the ventricles.
atrophy: (AT-ruh-fee) Without nourishment; wasting.
atypical: (ay-TIP-ih-kuhl) Deviating from normal.
augmentation: (AWG-men-TAY-shun) The act or process of increasing in size, quantity, degree, or severity.
auscultation: (AWS-kul-TAY-shun) Process of listening for sounds within the body, usually sounds of thoracic or abdominal viscera, to detect an abnormality.
autoimmune: (AW-toh-im-YOON) A condition in which the body does not recognize itself and the immune system attacks normal cells.
Ayurvedic: (EYE-ur-VAY-dik) An ancient Hindu system of medicine that improves health by harmonizing mind and body.
azotemia: (AY-zoh-TEE-me-ah) An increase in nitrogenous bodies in the blood, especially urea, as measured by the serum blood urea nitrogen (BUN) level.
bacteria: (back-TEER-ee-ah) One-celled organisms that can reproduce but need a host for food and supportive environment. Bacteria can be harmless, normal flora, or disease-producing pathogens.
balanitis: (BAL-uh-NYE-tis) Inflammation of the skin covering the glans penis.
bariatric: (BEAR-ee-AT-trick) Branch of medicine that deals with the prevention, control, and treatment of obesity.
basal cell secretion test: (BAY-zuhl SELL see-KREE-shun TEST) Part of a gastric analysis; measures the amount of gastric acid produced in 1 hour.
behavior management: (be-HAYV-yer MAN-ij-ment) Treatment method that uses positive and negative reinforcement to alter behavior.
belief: (bee-LEEF) Something accepted as true. Does not have to be proven.
beneficence: (buh-NEF-ih-sens) To provide good care; to do good for patients. One of the oldest requirements for health care providers.
benign: (bee-NINE) Not progressive; for example, a tumor that is not cancerous.
beta-hemolytic streptococci: (BAY-tuh-HEE-moh-LIT-ick STREP-toh-KOCK-sigh) Gram-positive bacteria that, when grown on blood-agar plates, completely hemolyze the blood and produce a clear zone around the bacteria colony. Group A beta-hemolytic streptococci cause disease in humans.
bigeminy: (bye-JEM-ih-nee) Occurring every second beat, as in bigeminal premature ventricular contractions.
bilateral salpingo-oophorectomy: (by-LAT-ur-uhl sal-PINJ-oh-ah-fuh-RECK-tuh-mee) Surgical removal of both fallopian tubes and ovaries.

bimanual: (by-MAN-yoo-uhl) With both hands.
biofeedback: (BYE-oh-FEED-bak) A form of therapy that uses provision of visual or auditory evidence to a person of the status of an autonomic body function such as heart rate, blood pressure, or respiratory rate.
biopsy: (BY-awp-see) A sample of tissue removed for examination.
bioterrorism: (BYE-oh-TEAR-uh-RIZ-um) Biological agent use or threat of use with a pathological organism for terrorist purposes.
bipolar: (bye-POH-lur) Having two poles or pertaining to both poles. Bipolar disorder is characterized by episodes of manic and depressive behavior.
blanch: (BLANCH) To lose color.
bleb: (BLEB) An irregularly shaped elevation of the skin, such as a blister. May also occur in lung tissue.
blepharitis: (BLEF-uh-RYE-tiss) Inflammation of the glands and lash follicles along the margin of the eyelids.
blindness: (BLYND-ness) Lack or loss of ability to see.
bolus: (BOH-lus) A dose of intravenous medication injected all at once.
bone: (BOWN) The hard, rigid form of connective tissue constituting most of the skeleton of vertebrates, composed chiefly of calcium salts.
botulism: (BOTCH-uh-liz-um) A paralytic illness caused by a potent neurotoxin produced by Clostridium botulinum, an anaerobic, spore-forming bacterium. It can be used as a biological weapon.
bowel sounds: (BOW'L SOWNDS) Gurgling and clicking sounds heard over the abdomen caused by air and fluid movement from peristaltic action. Normal bowel sounds occur every 5 to 15 seconds at a rate of 5 to 35 sounds per minute. Absent—no bowel sounds heard after 5 minutes of listening in each quadrant. Hyperactive—bowel sounds that are frequent, high pitched, and loud. Hypoactive—bowel sounds that occur at a rate of one every minute or longer.
bradycardia: (BRAY-dih-KAR-dee-yah) A slow heartbeat characterized by a pulse rate below 60 beats per minute.
bradykinesia: (BRAY-dih-kih-NEE-zee-ah) Abnormal slowness of movement; sluggishness.
breakthrough pain: (BRAYK-throo) Pain that occurs while medicated with long-acting analgesics.
bronchiectasis: (BRONG-key-EK-tah-siss) Chronic dilation of a bronchus or bronchi, usually associated with secondary infection and excessive sputum production.
bronchitis: (brong-KYE-tiss) Inflammation of the mucous membrane of the bronchial airways; may be viral or bacterial.
bronchodilator: (BRONG-koh-DYE-lay-tur) A drug that expands the bronchial tubes by relaxing bronchial smooth muscle.
bronchospasm: (BRONG-koh-spazm) Spasm of the bronchial smooth muscle resulting in narrowing of the airways; associated with asthma and bronchitis.
bruit: (BROO-EE) A humming heard when auscultating a blood vessel that is caused by turbulent blood flow through the vessel.
bulimia nervosa: (buh-LEE-mee-ah ner-VOH-sah) Recurrent episodes of binge eating and self-induced vomiting.
bulla: (BUHL-ah) A large blister or skin lesion filled with fluid. May also occur in lung tissue.
bundle of His: (BUN-duhl of HISS) A bundle of fibers of the impulse-conducting system of the heart. Originates in the atrioventricular (AV) node.
bursae: (BURR-sah) A small fluid-filled sac or saclike cavity situated in tissues such as joints where friction would otherwise occur.
calculi: (KAL-kyoo-lye) An abnormal concentration, usually composed of mineral salts, occurring within the body, chiefly in the hollow organs or their passages. Also called stones, as in kidney stones and gallstones.
cancer: (KAN-sir) A general name for over 100 diseases in which abnormal cells grow out of control; a malignant tumor.
cannula: (KAN-yoo-lah) A flexible tube that can be inserted into the body guided by a stiff, pointed rod. For example, an intravenous cannula is guided by a metal needle.
capillary permeability: (KAP-ih-lar-ee PER-mee-ah-BILL-ih-tee) The ability of substances to diffuse through capillary walls into tissue spaces.
capillary refill: (KAP-ih-lar-ee RE-fill) The amount of time required for color to return to the nailbed after having been compressed; normally 3 seconds or less. Indicator of peripheral circulation.
caput medusae: (KAP-ut mih-DOO-see) Dilated veins around the umbilicus, associated with cirrhosis of the liver.
carbuncle: (KAR-bung-kull) A necrotizing infection of skin and subcutaneous tissue composed of a cluster of boils.
carcinoembryonic antigens (CEA): (KAR-sin-oh-EM-bree-aw-nik AN-tih-jens) A class of antigens normally present in fetal cells; CEA level is elevated in many cancers and is measured to guide cancer treatment.
carcinogen: (kar-SIN-oh-jen) Specific agent known to promote the cancer process.
cardiac output: (KAR-dee-yak OWT-put) A measure of the pumping ability of the heart; amount of blood pumped by the heart per minute.
cardiac tamponade: (KAR-dee-yak TAM-pon-AID) The life-threatening compression of the heart by the fluid accumulating in the pericardial sac surrounding the heart.
cardiogenic shock: (KAR-dee-oh-JEN-ick SHAWK) Occurs when the heart muscle is unhealthy and contractility is impaired.
cardiomegaly: (KAR-dee-oh-MEH-gah-lee) Enlargement of the heart.
cardiomyopathy: (KAR-dee-oh-my-AW-pah-thee) A group of diseases that affect the myocardium's (heart muscle's) structure or function.
cardioplegia: (KAR-dee-oh-PLEE-jee-ah) Arrest of myocardial contraction, as by use of chemical compounds or cold temperatures in cardiac surgery.
cardioversion: (KAR-dee-oh-VER-zhun) An elective procedure in which a synchronized shock is delivered to attempt to restore the heart to a normal sinus rhythm.
cataract: (KAT-uh-rakt) Opacity of the lens of the eye.
cation: (KAT-eye-on) Electrolyte that carries a positive electrical charge.
ceiling effect: (SEE-ling e-FEKT) The dose of medication at which the maximum therapeutic effect is achieved. Increasing the dose beyond the therapeutic dose will not result in increased relief and may result in undesirable side effects.
cell-mediated immunity: (SELL ME-dee-ay-ted im-YOO-nih-tee) Production of lymphocytes by thymus in response to antigen exposure.
cellulitis: (sell-yoo-LYE-tiss) Inflammation of cellular or connective tissue.
cerebrovascular: (sir-EE-broh-VAS-kyoo-lur) Pertaining to the blood vessels of the cerebrum or brain.
chalazion: (kah-LAY-zee-on) A small eyelid mass resulting from chronic inflammation of a meibomian gland.
chancre: (SHANK-er) A hard, syphilitic primary ulcer, the first sign of syphilis, appearing approximately 2 to 3 weeks after infection.
chemotherapy: (KEE-moh-THER-uh-pee) The treatment of disease with medication; often refers to cancer therapy.
chiropractic: (ky-RUH-prak-tik) Treatment modality that uses manual adjustment of the vertebral column and extremities to remove interference with nerve function.
cholecystitis: (KOH-lee-sis-TYE-tis) Inflammation of the gallbladder.

choledocholithiasis: (koh-LED-oh-koh-lih-THYE-ah-siss) Gallstones in the common bile duct.
choledochoscopy: (KOH-LED-oh-KOS-koh-pee) An endoscopic test of the gallbladder and common bile duct.
cholelithiasis: (KOH-lee-lih-THYE-ah-sis) Gallstones in the gallbladder.
chorea: (kor-REE-ah) A nervous condition marked by involuntary muscular twitching of the limbs or facial muscles.
chronic illness: (KRAW-nick ILL-ness) An illness that is long lasting or recurring and usually interferes with a person's ability to perform activities of daily living. Medical care and hospitalization are often required on an ongoing basis.
circumcise: (SIR-kuhm-size) Surgical removal of the foreskin covering the head of the penis.
cirrhosis: (sih-ROH-siss) Chronic disease of the liver, associated with fat infiltration and development of fibrotic tissue.
civil law: (SIV-il LAW) Provides the rules by which individuals seek to protect their personal and property rights.
claudication: (KLAW-di-KAY-shun) Severe pain in the calf muscle from inadequate blood supply.
clubbing: (KLUB-ing) A condition in which the ends of the fingers and toes appear bulbous and shiny, most often the result of lung disease.
cochlear implant: (KOK-lee-er IM-plant) A device consisting of a microphone, signal processor, external transmitter, and implanted receiver to aid hearing.
code of ethics: (KOHD of ETH-icks) A traditional compilation of ideal behaviors of a professional group.
codependence: (KOH-de-PEN-dense) A situation in which the significant others in a family group begin to lose their own sense of identity and purpose and exist solely for the abuser.
cognitive: (KAHG-nih-tiv). The ability to think rationally and to process thoughts.
colectomy: (koh-LEK-tuh-me) Excision of the colon or a portion of it.
colic: (KAH-lick) Spasm of a hollow organ or duct, causing pain.
colitis: (kuh-LYE-tiss) Inflammation of the colon.
collateral circulation: (kuh-LA-tur-ul SIR-kew-LAY-shun) Small branches off of larger blood vessels that will increase in size and capacity next to a main blood vessel that is obstructed.
colonization: (CAW-lin-ih-ZAY-shun) The presence of pathogenic microbes in the body, without development of a symptomatic infection.
colonoscopy: (KOH-lun-AWS-kuh-pee) Examination of the upper portion of the rectum with a colonoscope.
colostomy: (koh-LAH-stuh-me) An artificial opening (stoma) created in the large intestine and brought to the surface of the abdomen for evacuating the bowels.
colporrhaphy: (kohl-POOR-ah-fee) Surgical repair of the vagina.
colposcopy: (kul-POS-koh-pee) Examination of the vulva, vagina, and cervix by means of a magnifying lens and a bright light.
comedone: (KOH-me-doh) Skin lesion that occurs in acne vulgaris (closed form: whitehead; open form: blackhead).
commissurotomy: (KOM-ih-shur-AW-toh-mee) Surgical incision of any commissure as in cardiac valves to increase the size of the orifice.
compliance: (kom-PLYE-ens) The ability to alter size or shape in response to an outside force; the ability of the lungs to distend.
compulsion: (kum-PUHL-shun) A recurrent, unwanted, and distressing urge to perform an act.
conductive hearing loss: (kon-DUK-tiv HEER-ing LOSS) Impaired transmission of sound waves through the external ear canal to the bones of the middle ear.
condylomata acuminata: (KON-dih-LOH-mah-tah ah-KYOOM-in-AH-tah) Warts in the genital region caused by the human papillomavirus (HPV); a contagious sexually transmitted disease.
condylomatous: (KON-dih-LOH-mah-tuss) Pertaining to a condyloma.
confidentiality: (KON-fih-den-she-AL-ih-tee) Maintaining privacy of patient information. Patient and patient's care can be discussed only in the professional setting.
congestive heart failure: (kon-JESS-tive HART FAIL-yur) Results from inability of heart to pump sufficient amounts of blood because of impaired pumping function and sodium and water retention. Congestion refers to the buildup of fluid that ranges from mild to life threatening (pulmonary edema). With left-sided heart failure, the fluid buildup occurs in the lungs and, if severe, immediate treatment is required or death can occur. With right-sided heart failure, the fluid buildup is seen systemically (lower legs/feet, sacral area in bedridden persons, jugular veins, liver, spleen).
conization: (KOH-nih-ZAY-shun) The removal of a cone of tissue, as in partial excision of the cervix uteri.
conjunctivitis: (kon-JUNK-tih-VYE-tiss) Inflammation of the conjunctiva of the eye.
consensual response: (kon-SEN-shoo-uhl ree-SPONS) Reaction of both pupils when one eye is exposed to greater intensity of light than the other.
constipation: (KON-stih-PAY-shun) A condition of sluggish or difficult bowel action/evacuation.
contraceptive: (KON-truh-SEP-tiv) Any process, device, or method that prevents conception.
contracture: (kon-TRACK-chur) Abnormal accumulation of fibrosis connective tissue in skin, muscle, or joint capsule that prevents normal mobility at that site.
contralateral: (KON-truh-LAT-ur-uhl) Originating in or affecting the opposite side of the body.
conversion disorder: (kon-VER-zhun dis-OR-der) An illness that emerges from overuse of the conversion reaction defense mechanism, in which there is impaired physical functioning that appears to be neurologic, but no organic disease can be identified.
coping: (KOH-ping) The process of contending with the stresses of daily life in an effort to overcome or work through them.
cor pulmonale: (KOR PUL-mah-NAH-lee) Hypertrophy or failure of the right ventricle from disorders of the chest wall, lungs, and pulmonary vessels, as with increased pulmonary pressure caused by chronic obstructive pulmonary disease (COPD).
coronary artery disease: (KOR-uh-nah-ree AR-tuh-ree dih-ZEEZ) Narrowing of the coronary arteries sufficient to prevent adequate blood supply to the myocardium.
craniectomy: (KRAY-nee-EK-tuh-mee) Excision of a segment of the skull.
cranioplasty: (KRAY-nee-oh-plas-tee) Any plastic repair operation on the skull.
craniotomy: (KRAY-nee-AWT-oh-mee) Any incision through the cranium.
crepitation: (crep-ih-TAY-shun) A dry, crackling sound or sensation, such as that produced by the grating of the ends of a fractured bone.
crepitus: (KREP-ih-tuss) Crepitation.
criminal law: (KRIM-ih-nuhl LAW) Regulates behaviors for citizens within a country.
critical thinking: (KRIT-ih-kuhl THING-king) Use of knowledge and skills to make the best decisions possible in client care situations.
cryotherapy: (KRY-oh-THER-uh-pee) The therapeutic use of cold.
cryptorchidism: (kript-OR-kih-dizm) A birth condition in which one or both of the testicles have not descended into the scrotum.
culdocentesis: (KUL-doh-sen-TEE-siss) The procedure for obtaining material from the posterior vaginal cul-de-sac by aspiration or surgical incision through the vaginal wall, performed for therapeutic or diagnostic reasons.

culdoscopy: (kul-DOS-koh-pee) Direct visual examination of the female viscera through an endoscope introduced into the pelvic cavity through the posterior vaginal fornix.
culdotomy: (KUL-DOT-uh-mee) Incision or needle puncture of the cul-de-sac of Douglas through the vagina.
cultural awareness: (KUL-chur-uhl a-WARE-ness) Being aware of history and ancestry and having an appreciation of and attention to the crafts, arts, music, foods, and clothing of various cultures.
cultural competence: (KUL-chur-uhl KOM-peh-tens) Having an awareness of one's own culture and not letting it have an undue influence over another person's culture. Having the knowledge and skills about a culture that are required to provide care.
cultural diversity: (KUL-chur-uhl dih-VER-sih-tee) Representing two or more cultures; the differences among cultures. For example, the United States includes people from many different countries.
cultural sensitivity: (KUL-chur-uhl SEN-sih-TIV-ih-tee) Being aware of and sensitive to cultural differences. Avoiding behavior or language that may be offensive to another person's cultural beliefs.
culture: (KUL-chur) The socially transmitted behavior patterns, beliefs, values, customs, arts, and all other characteristics of people that guide their worldview.
curet: (kyoo-RET) A loop, ring, or spoon-shaped instrument, attached to a handle and having sharp or blunt edges; used to scrape tissue from a surface.
custom: (KUS-tum) A custom is the usual way of acting in a given circumstance or something that an individual or group does out of habit. For example, many people in the United States eat turkey on Thanksgiving.
cyanosis: (SYE-uh-NOH-siss) Slightly bluish, grayish, or dark purple discoloration of the skin caused by the presence of abnormal amounts of reduced hemoglobin in the blood.
cystic: (SISS-tik) Pertaining to cysts or the urinary bladder.
cystitis: (siss-TYE-tiss) Inflammation of the urinary bladder.
cystocele: (SISS-toh-seel) A bladder hernia that protrudes into the vagina.
cystoscopy: (siss-TAWS-koh-pee) A diagnostic procedure using an instrument (cystoscope) via the urethra to view the bladder.
cytomegalovirus: (sye-TOW-meg-ul-low-vigh-russ) Species-specific herpesvirus; usually harmless to those with functional immune systems. May cause fatal pneumonia in those who are immunocompromised. Affects retina and may cause blindness in those with acquired immunodeficiency syndrome.
cytotoxic: (SYE-toh-TOCK-sick) Destructive to cells.
data: (DAY-tuh) A group of facts or statistics.
data, objective: See objective data.
data, subjective: See subjective data.
debridement: (day-breed-MAHNT) The removal of foreign material and contaminated and devitalized tissues from or adjacent to a traumatic or infected area until surrounding healthy tissue is exposed.
decerebrate: (dee-SER-eh-brayt) Abnormal extension posture indicating brainstem damage.
decorticate: (dee-KOR-tih-kayt) Abnormal flexion posture indicating cerebral damage.
defibrillation: (dee-FIB-rih-lay-shun) Use of an electrical device that applies countershock to the heart through electrodes placed on the chest wall to stop fibrillation of the heart.
degeneration: (deh-jen-er-AY-shun) Deterioration.
dehiscence: (deh-HISS-ents) A splitting open (i.e., rupture) of an incision.
dehydration: (DEE-high-DRAY-shun) A condition resulting from excessive loss of body fluid that occurs when fluid output exceeds intake.
delirium: (deh-LEER-ee-um) Acute, reversible state of disorientation and confusion without drowsiness, difficulty focusing attention, inability to sleep, and hyperactivity due to an underlying cause. A fairly common acute condition in older hospitalized adults.
delirium tremens: (deh-LEER-ee-uhm TREE-menz) An acute alcohol withdrawal syndrome marked by acute, transient disturbance of consciousness.
delusions: (dih-LOO-zhuns) False beliefs that are firmly maintained in spite of incontrovertible proof to the contrary.
dementia: (deh-MEN-cha) A broad term that refers to cognitive deficit, including memory impairment.
demyelination: (dee-MY-uh-lin-AY-shun) Loss of myelin from neurons.
deontology: (DAY-on-TOL-oh-gee) The study of moral obligations and commitments, including medical ethics.
dependence: (dih-PEN-dens) A state of reliance on something. Psychological craving for a drug that may or may not be accompanied by a physiological need.
depression: (dih-PRESS-shun) A mental disorder marked by altered mood with loss of interest.
dermatitis: (DER-mah-TYE-tiss) Inflammation of the skin.
dermatophytosis: (DER-mah-toh-fye-TOH-siss) A fungal infection of the skin.
dermoid: (DER-moyd) Resembling the skin.
developmental stage: (DEE-vell-up-MEN-tal STAYJ) An age-defined period with specific psychological tasks that need to be accomplished to maintain ego as proposed by Erik Erikson, a psychoanalyst.
diabetes mellitus: (DYE-ah-BEE-tis mel-LYE-tus) A chronic disease characterized by impaired production or use of insulin and high blood glucose levels.
diarrhea: (DYE-uh-REE-ah) Passage of fluid or unformed stools.
diastolic blood pressure: (dye-ah-STAH-lik BLUHD PREH-shure) The amount of pressure exerted on the wall of the arteries when the ventricles are at rest. The bottom number in a blood pressure reading.
diffusion: (dih-FEW-zhun) The tendency of molecules of a substance (gaseous, liquid, or solid) to move from a region of high concentration to one of lower concentration.
dilation and curettage: (die-LAY-shun and kyoor-e-TAHZH) A surgical procedure that expands the cervical canal of the uterus (dilation) so that the surface lining of the uterine wall can be scraped (curettage).
diplopia: (dip-LOH-pee-ah) Double vision.
displacement: (dis-PLAYSS-ment) Transference of emotion from the original idea with which it was associated to a different idea, allowing the client to avoid acknowledging the original source.
disseminated intravascular coagulation: (dih-SEH-mih-nay-ted IN-trah-VAS-kyoo-lar koh-AG-yoo-LAY-shun) A pathological form of coagulation that is diffuse (widespread) rather than localized, as would be the case in normal coagulation. Clotting factors are consumed to such an extent that generalized bleeding may occur.
distributive justice: (dis-TRIB-yoo-tiv JUS-tiss) The right of individuals to be treated equally regardless of race, sex, marital status, sexual preference, medical diagnosis, social standing, economic level, or religious belief.
distributive shock: (dis-TRIB-yoo-tiv SHAWK) Excessive dilation of the venules and arterioles, leading to decreased distribution of blood, resulting in shock.
diverticulitis: (DYE-ver-tik-yoo-LYE-tiss) Inflammation of a diverticulum (a sac or pouch in the walls of a canal or organ, usually the colon), especially inflammation involving diverticula of the colon.

diverticulosis: (DYE-ver-tik-yoo-LOH-siss) The presence of diverticula in the absence of inflammation.
do not resuscitate (DNR): (DOO not re-SUSS-ih-TATE) An order not to do CPR at the end of life.
dormant: (DOOR-mant) Condition of greatly reduced metabolic activity permitting long-term survival and possible reactivation of bacterial endospores, protozoan cysts, larval stages of worm parasites, and viruses.
Dressler's syndrome: (DRESS-lers SIN-drohm) Postmyocardial infarction syndrome; pericarditis.
durable power of attorney: (DUR-uh-buhl POW-ur uv uh-TUR-nee) Person legally designated to speak for a patient when the patient is no longer able to speak for himself or herself.
dysarthria: (diss-AR-three-ah) Imperfect articulation of speech caused by disturbances of muscular control resulting from central or peripheral nervous system damage.
dysfunctional: (dis-FUNCK-shun-uhl) Family or work environment that does not function effectively, sometimes because of other problems of members.
dysmenorrhea: (DIS-men-oh-REE-ah) Pain in association with menstruation.
dyspareunia: (DIS-puh-ROO-nee-ah) Occurrence of pain in the labia, vagina, or pelvis during or after sexual intercourse.
dysphagia: (dis-FAYJ-ee-ah) Inability to swallow or difficulty swallowing.
dysplasia: (dis-PLAY-zee-ah) Abnormal development of tissue.
dyspnea: (DISP-nee-ah) Subjective sense of labored breathing that occurs because of insufficient oxygenation.
dysreflexia: (DIS-re-FLEK-see-ah) State in which an individual with a spinal cord injury at or above T6 experiences an uninhibited sympathetic response to a noxious stimulus.
dysrhythmia: (dis-RITH-mee-yah) Abnormal, disordered, or disturbed cardiac rhythm.
dysuria: (dis-YOO-ree-ah) Difficult or painful urination.
ecchymoses: (ECK-uh-MOH-siss) A bruise of varying size, the color of which may be blue-black, changing to greenish yellow or yellow with time.
ectasia: (ek-TAY-zee-ah) Replacement of normal tissue with fibrous tissue.
ectopic: (eck-TOP-ick) Ectopic hormones are secreted from sites other than the gland where they would normally be found.
edema: (uh-DEE-muh) Collection of excess fluid in body tissues.
ejaculation: (ee-JAK-yoo-LAY-shun) The release of semen from the male urethra.
electrocardiogram: (ee-LEK-troh-KAR-dee-oh-GRAM) A recording of the electrical activity of the heart.
electrocautery: (ee-LEK-troh-CAW-tur-ee) Cauterization using platinum wires heated to red or white heat by an electric current, either direct or alternating.
electrocoagulated: (ee-LEK-troh-coh-AG-yoo-LAY-ted) Coagulation of tissue by means of a high-frequency electric current.
electroconvulsive therapy (ECT): (ee-LEK-troh-kun-VUL-siv THER-uh-pee) A type of somatic therapy in which an electric current is used to produce convulsions to treat such conditions as depression.
electroencephalogram: (ee-LEK-troh-en-SEFF-uh-loh-gram) A record produced by electroencephalography; tracing of the electrical impulses of the brain.
electrolyte: (ee-LEK-troh-lite) A substance that when dissolved in water can conduct electricity.
electroretinography: (ee-LEK-troh-RET-in-AWG-ruh-fee) Measurement of the electrical response of the retina to light stimulation.
emboli: (EM-boh-lie) Solid, liquid, or gaseous masses of undissolved matter traveling with the fluid current in a blood or lymphatic vessel.
embolism: (EM-buh-lizm) Foreign substance or blood clot that travels through the circulatory system until it obstructs a vessel.
empathy: (EM-puh-thee) Objective awareness of and insight into the feelings, emotions, and behavior of another person.
emphysema: (EM-fih-SEE-mah) Distention of interstitial tissue by gas or air; chronic pulmonary disease marked by terminal bronchiole and alveolar destruction and air trapping.
empyema: (EM-pye-EE-mah) Pus in a body cavity, especially the pleural space.
encephalitis: (EN-seff-uh-LYE-tiss) Inflammation of the brain.
encephalopathy: (en-SEFF-uh-LAWP-ah-thee) Dysfunction of the brain.
endarterectomy: (end-AR-tur-EK-tuh-mee) Excision of thickened atheromatous areas of the innermost coat of an artery.
endogenous: (en-DAH-jen-us) Produced or originating from within a cell or organism.
endometritis: (EN-doh-meh-TRY-tiss) Inflammation of the endometrium of the uterus.
endorphins: (en-DOR-fins) Naturally occurring opioids in the body, many times more potent than analgesic medications.
endoscope: (EN-doh-skohp) A device consisting of a tube and optical system for observing the inside of a hollow organ or cavity. Can be flexible or rigid.
enkephalins: (en-KEF-eh-lins) One type of endorphin.
enteritis: (en-ter-EYE-tiss) Inflammation of the intestines, particularly of the mucosa and submucosa of the small intestine.
enucleation: (ee-NEW-klee-AY-shun) Removal of an organ or other mass intact from its supporting tissues, as of the eyeball from the orbit.
epidemiological: (EP-ih-DEE-me-ah-LAHJ-ih-kuhl) The study of the distribution and determinants of health-related states and events in populations and the application of this study to the control of health problems.
epididymitis: (EP-ih-DID-ih-MY-tiss) Inflammation or infection of the epididymis.
epidural: (EP-ih-DUHR-uhl) Situated on or outside the dura mater.
epinephrine: (EP-ih-NEFF-rin) A hormone secreted by the adrenal medulla in response to stimulation of the sympathetic nervous system.
epispadias: (EP-ih-SPAY-dee-ahz) A congenital male defect in which the opening of the urethra is on the dorsum of the penis, instead of the tip.
epistaxis: (EP-iss-TAX-iss) Nosebleed.
epithelialization: (ep-ih-THEE-lee-al-eye-ZAY-shun) The growth of skin over a wound.
equianalgesic: (EE-kwee-AN-uhl-JEE-zik) Drugs having equal pain-killing effect. The same degree of pain relief may require different doses when different medications are given or medications are given by different routes.
erectile dysfunction: (eh-REK-tile dis-FUNCK-shun) Inability to have an erection sufficient for sexual intercourse.
erection: (eh-REK-shun) Enlargement and hardening of the penis caused by engorgement of blood.
erythema: (ER-ih-THEE-mah) Diffuse redness over the skin.
eschar: (ESS-kar) Hard scab or dry crust that results from necrotic tissue.
escharotomy: (ess-kar-AWT-oh-mee) Removal of a slough or scab formed on the skin and underlying tissue of severely burned skin.
esophagogastroduodenoscopy: (eh-SOFF-ah-go-GAS-troh-doo-AW-den-AWS-kuh-pee) An endoscopic procedure that allows the physician to view the esophagus, stomach, and duodenum.
esophagoscopy: (eh-soff-ah-GAWS-kuh-pee) Examination of the esophagus using an endoscope.
esotropia: (ESS-oh-TROH-pee-ah) Strabismus in which there is deviation of the visual axis of one eye toward that of the other eye, resulting in diplopia. Also called cross-eyed.

essential hypertension: (eh-SEN-shul HYE-per-TEN-shun) Chronic elevation of blood pressure resulting from an unknown cause.
ethical: (ETH-ih-kuhl) Describes behavior guided by a system of moral principles or standards.
ethics: (ETH-icks) Branch of philosophy that answers questions about morality such as good, bad or right, wrong.
ethnic: (ETH-nick) Pertaining to a religious, racial, national, or cultural group. For example, individuals may identify with the Jewish, Catholic, or Islamic religions.
ethnocentrism: (ETH-noh-SEN-trizm) The tendency to think that one's own ways of thinking, believing, and acting are the only right ways. People who are different are seen as strange or bizarre. An example is one who believes that his or her religious beliefs are the only right beliefs and other religions are wrong.
eustress: (YOO-stress) Stress from positive experiences.
euthyroid: (yoo-THY-royd) Normal thyroid function.
evaluation: (ee-VAL-yoo-AY-shun) The judgment of anything.
evisceration: (eh-VIS-sir-ay-shun) Extrusion of viscera outside the body, especially through a surgical excision.
exacerbation: (egg-sass-sir-BAY-shun) Aggravation of symptoms.
exophthalmos: (ECKS-off-THAL-muss) Abnormal protrusion of the eyeball.
exotropia: (EKS-oh-TROH-pee-ah) Abnormal turning outward of one or both eyes; divergent strabismus.
expectorant: (ek-SPEK-tuh-rant) Agent that promotes removal of pulmonary secretions.
expectorate: (ek-SPECK-tuh-RAYT) The act or process of coughing up materials from the air passageways leading to the lungs.
external otitis: (eks-TER-nuhl oh-TYE-tis) Inflammation of the external ear.
extracardiac: (EX-trah-KAR-dee-ack) Outside the heart.
extracellular: (EX-trah-SELL-yoo-ler) Outside the cell.
extracorporeal shock wave lithotripsy (ESWL): (EKS-trah-koar-POR-ee-uhl SHAWK WAYV LITH-oh-TRIP-see) Noninvasive treatment using shock waves to break up gallstones or kidney stones.
extravasation: (eks-TRAH-vah-ZAY-shun) The escape of fluids into surrounding tissue.
extrinsic factors: (eks-TRIN-sik FAK-ters) External variables.
exudate: (EKS-yoo-dayt) Accumulated fluid in a cavity; oozing of pus or serum; often the result of inflammation.
fasciculation: (fah-SIK-yoo-LAY-shun) Twitching.
fasciotomy: (fash-ee-OTT-oh-mee) Incision of fascia.
fetor hepaticus: (FEE-tor he-PAT-ih-kus) Foul breath associated with liver disease.
fibrocystic: (FYE-broh-SISS-tik) Consisting of fibrocysts, which are fibrous tumors that have undergone cystic degeneration or accumulated fluid.
filtration: (fill-TRAY-shun) The process of removing particles from a solution by allowing the liquid portion to pass through a membrane or other partial barrier.
fissure: (FISH-er) A narrow slit or cleft, especially one of the deeper or more constant furrows separating the gyri of the brain.
fistula: (FIST-yoo-lah) Any abnormal, tubelike passage within body tissue, usually between two internal organs, or leading from an internal organ to the body surface.
flaccid: (FLAH-sid) Weak, lax, soft muscles.
flail chest: (FLAY-ul CHEST) Condition of the chest wall caused by two or more fractures on each affected rib resulting in a segment of rib that is not attached on either end; the flail portion moves paradoxically in with inspiration and out with expiration.
flora: (FLOOR-a) Microbial life adapted for living in a specific environment such as the intestines, skin, or urinary tract.
fluoroscope: (FLOOR-uh-skohp) A device consisting of a fluorescent screen suitably mounted, either separately or in conjunction with an x-ray tube, by means of which the shadows of objects interposed between the tube and the screen are made visible.
fluoroscopy: (fluh-RAWS-kuh-pee) The use of a fluoroscope for medical diagnosis or for testing various materials by roentgen rays.
full-thickness burn: (FUL-THICK-ness BERN) Burn in which all of the epithelializing elements and those lining the sweat glands, hair follicles, and sebaceous glands are destroyed.
fungi: (FUNG-guy) A general term for a group of eukaryotic organisms (e.g., mushrooms, yeasts, molds).
furuncle: (FYOOR-ung-kull) An acute circumscribed inflammation of the subcutaneous layers of the skin or of a gland or hair follicle.
gastrectomy: (gas-TREK-tuh-mee) Any surgery that involves partial or total removal of the stomach.
gastric acid stimulation test: (GAS-trik AS-id STIM-yoo-LAY-shun TEST) A test that measures the amount of gastric acid for 1 hour after subcutaneous injection of a drug that stimulates gastric acid secretion.
gastric analysis: (GAS-trik ah-NAL-ih-siss) A test performed to measure secretions of hydrochloric acid and pepsin in the stomach.
gastric lavage: (GAS-trik la-VAHJ) Washing out of the stomach; used to empty the stomach when the contents are irritating.
gastritis: (gas-TRY-tiss) Acute—The inflammation of the stomach mucosa; also known as heartburn or indigestion. Chronic—Gastritis that is recurrent; classified as type A (asymptomatic) or type B (symptomatic).
gastroduodenostomy: (GAS-troh-DOO-oh-den-AWS-toh-mee) Excision of the pylorus of the stomach with anastomosis of the upper portion of the stomach to the duodenum.
gastroepiploic: (GAS-troh-EP-ih-PLOH-ick) Pertaining to the stomach and greater omentum.
gastrojejunostomy: (GAS-troh-JAY-joo-NAWS-toh-mee) Subtotal excision of the stomach with closure of the proximal end of the duodenum and side-to-side anastomosis of the jejunum to the remaining portion of the stomach.
gastroparesis: (GAS-troh-puh-REE-sis) Paralysis of the stomach, resulting in poor emptying.
gastroplasty: (GAS-troh-PLAS-tee) Plastic surgery of the stomach. Used to decrease the size of the stomach to treat morbid obesity.
gastroscopy: (gas-TRAHS-kuh-pee) Examination of the stomach and abdominal cavity by use of a gastroscope.
gastrostomy: (gas-TRAWS-toh-mee) Surgical creation of a gastric fistula through the abdominal wall.
gavage: (gah-VAZH) Feeding with a stomach tube or with a tube passed through the nares, pharynx, and esophagus into the stomach. The food is in liquid or semiliquid form at room temperature.
generalization: (JEN-er-al-ih-ZAY-shun) An assumption about a group or an individual item or person that leads to seeking additional information to determine if the generalization fits the individual. Whereas generalizations are true for the group, they may not be true for the individual.
glaucoma: (glaw-KOH-mah) A group of eye diseases characterized by increased intraocular pressure.
glomerulonephritis: (gloh-MER-yoo-loh-ne-FRY-tiss) A form of nephritis in which the lesions involve primarily the glomeruli.
glossitis: (glaw-SYE-tiss) An inflammation of the tongue.
glycosuria: (GLY-kos-YOO-ree-ah) Abnormal amount of glucose in the urine, often associated with diabetes mellitus.

goitrogens: (GOY-troh-jenz) Foods or medications that cause a goiter.

gout: (GOWT) A common group of arthritic disorders marked by deposition of monosodium urate crystals in joints and other tissues.

gravida: (GRAV-id-ah): Number of times a woman has been pregnant.

gummas: (GUM-ahs) A soft granulomatous tumor of the tissues characteristic of the tertiary stage of syphilis.

gynecomastia: (JIN-eh-koh-MASS-tee-ah) Excessive breast tissue on a male.

hallucinations: (huh-LOO-sih-NAY-shuns) False perceptions having no relation to reality and not accounted for by any exterior stimuli.

hand hygiene: (HAND HY-jeen) Cleansing of the hands with hand washing as defined by the Centers for Disease Control and Prevention or an alcohol-based hand sanitizer solution.

health: (HELLTH) A condition in which all functions of the body and mind are normally active.

hearing aid: (HEER-ing AYD) An instrument to amplify sounds for those with hearing loss.

heatstroke: (HEET-strohk) An acute and dangerous reaction to heat exposure, characterized by high body temperature, usually higher than 105°F (40.5°C).

Helicobacter pylori: (HEH-lick-co-back-tur PIE-lori) Bacterium that causes some peptic ulcers.

hemarthrosis: (HEEM-ar-THROH-siss) Bleeding into a joint.

hematochezia: (HEM-uh-toh-KEE-zee-uh) Blood in the feces.

hematoma: (HEE-muh-TOH-mah) A localized collection of extravasated blood, usually clotted, in an organ, space, or tissue.

hematuria: (HEM-uh-TYOOR-ee-ah) Blood in the urine.

hemiparesis: (hem-ee-puh-REE-sis) Weakness affecting one side of the body.

hemipelvectomy: (hem-ee-pell-VEC-toe-me) The surgical removal of half of the pelvis and the leg.

hemiplegia: (hem-ee-PLEE-jee-ah) Paralysis of only one side of the body.

hemodialysis: (HEE-moh-dye-AL-ih-siss) A method for replacing the function of the kidneys by circulating blood through tubes made of semipermeable membranes.

hemolysis: (he-MAHL-eh-siss) The destruction of the membrane of red blood cells with the liberation of hemoglobin, which diffuses into the surrounding fluid.

hemophilia: (HEE-moh-FILL-ee-ah) A hereditary blood disease marked by greatly prolonged coagulation time, with consequent failure of the blood to clot and abnormal bleeding.

hemoptysis: (hee-MOP-tih-siss) Coughing up of blood from the respiratory tract.

hemorrhoids: (HEM-uh-royds) A mass of dilated, tortuous veins in the anorectum involving the venous plexuses of that area.

hemothorax: (HEE-moh-THAW-raks) Blood in the pleural space; may be associated with trauma, tuberculosis, or pneumonia.

hepatitis: (HEP-uh-TYE-tiss) Inflammation of the liver, most often viral.

hepatomegaly: (HEP-uh-toh-MEG-ah-lee) Enlargement of the liver.

hepatorenal syndrome: (hep-PAT-oh-REE-nuhl SIN-drohm) A deadly kidney failure that sometimes accompanies liver disease.

hepatosplenomegaly: (heh-PA-toh-SPLE-noh-MEG-ah-lee) Enlargement of the liver and spleen.

hernia: (HER-nee-uh) The protrusion or projection of an organ or a part of an organ through the wall of the cavity that normally contains it.

herpetic: (her-PET-ick) Pertaining to herpes.

hiatal hernia: (high-AY-tuhl HER-nee-ah) A condition in which part of the stomach protrudes through and above the diaphragm.

high-density lipoprotein (HDL): (HYE DEN-sih-tee LIP-oh-PROH-teen) Plasma lipids bound to albumin consisting of lipoproteins. It has been found that those with high levels of HDL have less chance of having coronary artery disease.

histamine: (HISS-tah-mean) A substance produced in the body that increases gastric secretion, increases capillary permeability, and contracts the bronchial smooth muscle. Plays a role in allergic reaction.

holistic: (hole-ISS-tik) The view that people and other organisms function as complete units that cannot be reduced to the sum of their parts. In health care, holistic care encompasses the person's body, mind, and spirit along with the environment and society in which the person lives.

Homans' sign: (HOH-manz SIGHN) An assessment for venous thrombosis in which calf pain with dorsiflexion occurs if thrombosis is present.

homeopathy: (HO-mee-AW-pa-thee) System of medicine based on the theory that "like cures like," and uses tiny doses of a substance that create the symptoms of disease.

homeostasis: (HOH-mee-oh-STAY-siss) Maintaining a constant balance, especially whenever a change occurs.

hopelessness: (HOHP-less-ness) Subjective state in which a person sees limited or unavailable alternatives; lacking energy.

hordeolum: (hor-DEE-oh-lum) Sty.

hospice: (HOS-piss) A service provided to patients and their families in the last 6 months of life to manage pain and provide emotional support.

host: (HOE-st) The organism from which a parasite obtains its nourishment.

human immunodeficiency virus (HIV): (HYOO-man im-YOO-noh-dee-FISH-en-see VIGH-russ) A retrovirus that causes acquired immunodeficiency syndrome (AIDS).

humoral: (HYOO-mohr-uhl) Pertaining to body fluids or substances contained in them.

hydrocele: (HYE-droh-seel) A collection of fluid in the scrotal sack.

hydrocephalus: (HYE-droh-SEF-uh-luhs) A condition caused by enlargement of the cranium caused by abnormal accumulation of cerebrospinal fluid within the cerebral ventricular system.

hydronephrosis: (HYE-droh-ne-FROH-sis) Abnormal dilation of kidneys caused by obstruction of urine flow.

hydrostatic: (HYE-droh-STAT-ik) Pertaining to the pressure of liquids in equilibrium and to the pressure exerted by liquids.

hypercalcemia: (HYE-per-kal-SEE-mee-ah) An excessive amount of calcium in the blood.

hyperglycemia: (HYE-per-glye-SEE-mee-ah) Excess glucose in the blood.

hyperkalemia: (HYE-per-kuh-LEE-mee-ah) An excessive amount of potassium in the blood.

hyperlipidemia: (HYE-per-LIP-ih-DEE-mee-ah) Excessive quantity of fat in the blood.

hypermagnesemia: (HYE-per-MAG-nuh-ZEE-mee-ah) Excess magnesium in the blood.

hypernatremia: (HYE-per-nuh-TREE-mee-ah) Excess sodium in the blood.

hyperopia: (HYE-per-OH-pee-ah) Farsightedness.

hyperplasia: (HYE-per-PLAY-zee-ah) Excessive increase in the number of normal cells.

hypertension: (HYE-per-TEN-shun) Abnormally elevated blood pressure.

hypertensive emergency: (HYE-per-TEN-siv) Systolic blood pressure above 180 mm Hg and diastolic blood pressure above 120 to 130 mm Hg.

hypertonic: (HYE-per-TAWN-ik) Exerts greater osmotic pressure than blood.

hypertrophy: (hye-PER-truh-fee) An increase in the size of an organ or structure, or of the body, owing to growth rather than tumor formation.

hyperuricemia: (HYE-per-yoor-ah-SEE-me-ah) An excess of uric acid or urates in the blood.

hyperventilation: (HYE-per-VEN-tih-LAY-shun) Increased ventilation that results in a lowered carbon dioxide (CO_2) level (hypocapnia).
hypervolemia: (HIYE-per-voh-LEE-mee-ah) An abnormal increase in the volume of circulating blood.
hypocalcemia: (HYE-poh-kal-SEE-mee-ah) Reduced amount of calcium in the blood.
hypoglycemia: (HYE-poh-glye-SEE-mee-ah) Below-normal amount of glucose in the blood.
hypokalemia: (HYE-poh-kuh-LEE-mee-ah) Reduced amount of potassium in the blood.
hypomagnesemia: (HYE-poh-MAG-nuh-ZEE-mee-ah) Reduced amount of magnesium in the blood.
hyponatremia: (HYE-poh-nuh-TREE-mee-ah) Reduced amount of sodium in the blood.
hypoperfusion: (HYE-poh-pur-FEW-shun) Low blood flow that occurs when the circulatory system cannot deliver adequate oxygenated blood to the organs and tissues, as in shock.
hypophysectomy: (HYE-paw-fih-SECK-tuh-mee) Surgical removal of the pituitary gland.
hypoplasia: (HYE-poh-PLAY-zee-ah) Underdevelopment of a tissue organ or body.
hypospadias: (HYE-poh-SPAY-dee-ahz) A congenital male defect in which the opening of the urethra is on the underside of the penis, instead of the tip.
hypostatic: (HYE-poh-STA-tik) Hypostatic pneumonia occurs from congestion in the lungs associated with lack of activity.
hypotension: (HYE-poh-TEN-shun) Abnormally low blood pressure below 90 mm Hg systolic.
hypothermia: (HYE-poh-THUR-mee-ah) Body temperature below 95°F (35°C).
hypotonic: (HYE-poh-TAWN-ik) Pertaining to defective muscular tone or tension; having a lower concentration of solute than intracellular or extracellular fluid.
hypovolemia: (HYE-poh-voh-LEE-mee-ah) The most common form of dehydration resulting from the loss of fluid from the body; results in decreased blood volume.
hypovolemic: (HYE-poh-voh-LEEM-ick) Low volume of blood in the circulatory system.
hypovolemic shock: (HYE-poh-voh-LEEM-ick SHAWK) Shock that occurs when blood or plasma is lost in such quantities that the remaining blood cannot fill the circulatory system despite constriction of the blood vessels.
hypoxemia: (HYE-pock-SEE-mee-ah) Deficient oxygenation of the blood.
hypoxia: (hye-POCK-see-ah) Diminished availability of oxygen to the body tissues.
hysterectomy: (HISS-tuh-RECK-tuh-mee) Surgical removal of the uterus through the abdominal wall or vagina.
hysterosalpingogram: (HISS-tur-oh-SAL-pinj-oh-gram) Radiograph of the uterus and fallopian tubes.
hysteroscopy: (HISS-tur-AWS-koh-pee) Endoscopic direct visual examination of the canal of the uterine cervix and the cavity of the uterus.
hysterotomy: (HISS-tuh-RAW-tuh-mee) Incision of the uterus.
icterus: (ICK-ter-uss) Yellowing of the skin and the sclera of the eye.
idiopathic thrombocytopenic purpura: (IH-dee-oh-PATH-ik THROM-boh-SYE-toh-PEE-nik PUR-pew-rah) The total number of circulating platelets is greatly diminished, even though platelet production in the bone marrow is normal, resulting in slowed blood clotting.
ileostomy: (ILL-ee-AW-stuh-me) An artificial opening (stoma) created in the small intestine (ileum) and brought to the surface of the abdomen for the purpose of evacuating feces.
illness: (ILL-ness) The state of being sick.
illusions: (ih-LOO-zhuns) Mistaken perceptions of reality.
imagery: (IM-ij-ree) The use of the imagination to promote relaxation.
immunocompromised: (IM-yoo-noh-KAWM-prah-mized) Having an immune system that is not capable of reacting to a pathogen or tissue damage.
impaction: (im-PAK-shun) An immovable accumulation of feces in the bowels.
imperforate: (im-PER-foh-rate) Without an opening.
in situ: (in-SIT-yoo) Localized, not invading surrounding tissue.
in vitro fertilization: (in VEE-troh FER-tih-lih-ZAY-shun) Fertilization in a test tube.
induction: (in-DUCK-shun) The process or act of causing to occur, as in anesthesia induction.
induration: (IN-dyoo-RAY-shun) Area of hardened tissue.
infective endocarditis: (in-FECK-tive EN-doh-kar-DYE-tiss) Inflammation of the heart lining caused by microorganisms.
infiltration: (in-fil-TRAY-shun) The accumulation of an external substance (such as IV fluids) within tissues.
inspection: (in-SPEK-shun) Use of observation skills to systematically gather data that can be seen.
insufficiency: (IN-suh-FISH-en-see) The condition of being inadequate for a given purpose, such as heart valves that do not close properly.
insufflation: (in-suff-LAY-shun) Used to inflate the abdomen during laparoscopic or endoscopic procedures to enhance visualization of structures.
intermittent claudication: (IN-ter-MIT-ent KLAW-di-KAY-shun) A symptom associated with arterial occlusive disease. It refers to pain in the calf of a lower extremity, usually brought on by activity or exercise, and ceases with rest.
international normalized ratio: (IN-ter-NASH-uh-nul NOR-muh-lized RAY-she-oh) The World Health Organization's standard for reporting the prothrombin time assay test when the thromboplastin reagent developed by the first International Reference Preparation is used. The reagent was developed to prevent variability in prothrombin time testing results and provide uniformity in monitoring therapeutic levels for coagulation during oral anticoagulation therapy.
interstitial: (IN-ter-STISH-uhl) Fluid between tissues.
intervention: (in-ter-VEN-shun) One or more actions taken in order to modify an effect.
intracellular: (IN-trah-SELL-yoo-ler) Fluids located within the blood cell.
intracranial: (IN-trah-KRAY-nee-uhl) Within the cranium or skull.
intraoperative: (IN-trah-AWP-er-uh-tiv) Occurring during a surgical procedure.
intravascular: (IN-trah-VAS-kyoo-lar) Fluids located within the blood vessels.
intravenous: (IN-trah-VEE-nus) Within or into a vein.
intrinsic factors: (in-TRIN-sik FAK-ters) Internal variables.
intussusception: (IN-tuh-suh-SEP-shun) The slipping of one part of an intestine into another adjacent to it.
ipsilateral: (IP-sih-LAT-ur-uhl) On the same side; affecting the same side of the body.
ischemia: (iss-KEY-me-ah) Condition of inadequate blood supply.
isoelectric line: (EYE-so-ee-LEK-trick LINE) The period when the electrical tracing is at zero and is neither positive nor negative.
isolated systolic hypertension: (EYE-suh-lay-ted siss-TAW-lik hye-per-TEN-shun) The systolic pressure is 160 mm Hg or more, but the diastolic pressure is lower than 95 mm Hg.
isotonic: (EYE-so-TAWN-ik) A fluid that has the same osmolarity as the blood.
jaundice: (JAWN-diss) Yellowing of the skin and the sclera of the eye.
joint: (JOYNT) An articulation. The point of juncture between two bones.

Kaposi's sarcoma: (ka-POE-sees sar-CO-mah) A vascular malignancy that is often first apparent in the skin or mucous membranes but may involve the viscera.

ketoacidosis: (KEE-toh-as-ih-DOH-siss) A condition in which fat breakdown produces ketones, which cause an acidic state in the body; may be associated with weight loss or diabetes mellitus.

Kussmaul's respirations: (KOOS-mahlz RES-pih-RAY-shuns) Term describing deep respirations of an individual with ketoacidosis.

laceration: (la-sir-A-shun) A wound or irregular tear of the flesh.

lactic acid: (LAK-tik AS-id) By-product of anaerobic metabolism.

laminectomy: (LAM-ih-NEK-toh-mee) The excision of a vertebral posterior arch, usually to remove a lesion or herniated disk.

laparoscopy: (LAP-uh-raw-SKOP-ee) Exploration of the abdomen with an endoscope.

laparotomy: (LAP-uh-RAW-tuh-mee) The surgical opening of the abdomen; an abdominal operation.

laryngeal edema: (lah-RIN-jee-uhl uh-DEE-muh) Sudden swelling of the larynx occurring with severe allergic reactions.

laryngectomy: (lar-in-JEK-tah-mee) Surgical removal of the larynx.

laryngitis: (lare-in-JYE-tiss) Inflammation of the larynx.

laser ablation: (LAY-zer uh-BLAY-shun) Therapeutic destruction of a growth or part of a growth by laser treatment.

lavage: (lah-VAZH) Washing out of a cavity.

law: (LAW) The further formalization of moral considerations.

leadership: (LEE-der-ship) The process of socially influencing others to obtain their assistance and support to accomplish a common task.

leiomyoma: (LYE-oh-my-OH-ma) A myoma consisting principally of smooth muscle tissue.

leukemia: (loo-KEE-mee-ah) A malignancy of the blood-forming cells in the bone marrow.

leukocytosis: (LOO-koh-sye-TOH-siss) An increase in the number of leukocytes in the blood, generally caused by the presence of infection and usually transient.

leukopenia: (LOO-koh-PEE-nee-yah) Abnormal decrease of white blood cells, usually below $5000/mm^3$.

liability: (LYE-uh-BIL-ih-tee) The level of responsibility that society places on individuals for their actions.

libido: (lih-BEE-doh) Sexual drive, conscious or unconscious.

lichenified: (lye-KEN-ih-fyed) Thickened or hardened from continued irritation.

limitation of liability: (lim-ih-TAY-shun OF LYE-uh-BIL-ih-tee) Steps that health care professionals can take to limit their liability.

living will: (LIV-ing WIL) A document instructing health care workers about a patient's preferences when he or she is no longer able to communicate. Implementation of living wills varies by state.

lobectomy: (loh-BEK-tuh-mee) Surgical removal of a lobe of any organ or gland.

low-density lipoprotein (LDL): (LOH DEN-sih-tee LIH-poh-PROH-teen) A lipoprotein that transports cholesterol and triglycerides from the liver to peripheral tissues. LDL allows fats and cholesterol to move within the water-based solution of the blood. Increased LDL cholesterol is associated with cardiovascular disease, so it is often referred to as "bad cholesterol."

lower gastrointestinal (lower GI) series: (LOH-er GAS-troh-in-TESS-tih-nuhl SEER-ees) The use of barium sulfate as an enema to facilitate x-ray and fluoroscopic examination of the colon.

lymphadenopathy: (lim-FAD-eh-NAH-puh-thee) Any disorder of the lymph nodes.

lymphangitis: (lim-FAN-je-EYE-tiss) Inflammation of lymphatic channels or vessels.

lymphedema: (LIMPF-uh-DEE-mah) An abnormal accumulation of tissue fluid (potential lymph) in the interstitial space.

lymphocytes: (LIM-foh-sites) Cells present in the blood and lymphatic tissue that provide the main means of immunity for the body; white blood cells.

lymphoma: (lim-FOH-mah) A usually malignant lymphoid neoplasm.

macrodrop: (MAK-roh-DROP) A large drop (typically 15 to 20 drops per mL). In IV therapy, may refer to an administration device used to deliver large drops of IV solution.

macular degeneration: (MACK-you-lar dee-JEN-uh-RAY-shun) Age-related breakdown of the macular area of the retina of the eye.

maleficence: (ma-LEF-i-cence) Committing harm or evil.

malignant: (muh-LIG-nunt) Growing, resisting treatment; used to describe a tumor of cancerous cells.

malpractice: (mal-PRAK-tiss) A breach of duty arising out of the relationship that exists between the patient and the health care worker.

mammography: (mah-MOG-rah-fee) Use of radiography of the breast to diagnose breast cancer.

mammoplasty: (MAAM-oh-PLAS-tee) Plastic surgery of the breast.

mania: (MAY-nee-ah) Mental disorder characterized by excessive excitement.

marsupialization: (mar-SOO-pee-al-ih-ZAY-shun) Process of raising the borders of an evacuated tumor sac to the edges of the abdominal wound and stitching them there to form a pouch.

mastalgia: (mass-TAL-jee-ah) Pain in the breast.

mastectomy: (mass-TECK-tuh-mee) Excision of the breast.

mastitis: (mass-TYE-tis) Inflammation of the breast.

mastopexy: (MAS-toh-PEKS-ee) Correction of a pendulous breast by surgical fixation and plastic surgery.

mediastinum: (MEE-dee-ah-STYE-num) A septum or cavity between two principal portions of an organ.

megacolon: (MEG-ah-KOH-lun) Extremely dilated colon.

melena: (muh-LEE-nah) Black, tarry feces caused by action of intestinal secretions on free blood.

menarche: (meh-NAR-kee) The initial menstrual period, normally occurring between the 9th and 17th year.

Ménière's disease: (meh-NEARS di-ZEEZ) A recurrent and usually progressive group of symptoms including progressive deafness, ringing in the ears, dizziness, and a sensation of fullness or pressure in the ears.

meningitis: (men-in-JYE-tis) Inflammation of the membranes of the spinal cord and brain.

menopause: (MEN-oh-pawz) The period that marks the permanent cessation of menstrual activity, usually occurring between the ages of 35 and 58.

mental health: (MEN-tuhl HELLTH) State of being adjusted to life; able to be flexible, successful, maintain close relationships, solve problems, make appropriate judgments, and cope with daily stresses.

mental illness: (MEN-tuhl ILL-ness) Any illness that affects the mind or behavior.

metastasis: (muh-TASS-tuh-siss) Movement of bacteria or body cells (especially cancer cells) from one part of the body to another.

microdrop: (MIKE-roh-DROP) A small drop (60 drops per mL). In IV therapy, may refer to an administration device used to deliver small drops of IV solution.

milieu: (me-LYU) Environment.

miotic: (my-AW-tik) An agent that causes the pupil to contract.

morality: (muh-RAL-ih-tee) A social barometer that dictates what is good or bad in a society.

morbidity: (more-BID-ih-tee) State of being diseased.

mortality: (more-TAL-ih-tee) Condition of being mortal; number of deaths in a population.

mucolytic: (MYOO-koh-LIT-ik) Agent that liquefies sputum.
mucopurulent cervicitis: (MYOO-koh-PYOOR-uh-lent SIR-vih-SYE-tiss) Inflammation of the cervix producing mucus and purulent discharge.
mucositis: (MYOO-koh-SYE-tiss) Inflammation of a mucous membrane.
multifocal: (MUHL-tee-FOH-kuhl) Many foci (areas) or sites.
murmur: (MUR-mur) An abnormal sound heard on auscultation of the heart and adjacent large blood vessels.
muscle: (MUSS-uhl) A bundle of long slender cells or fibers that have the power to contract and hence to produce movement.
myalgia: (my-AL-jee-ah) Muscle pain or tenderness.
myectomy: (my-EK-tuh-mee) Surgical removal of a hypertrophied muscle.
myelogram: (MY-eh-loh-gram) The film produced by radiography of the spinal cord after injection of a contrast medium into the subarachnoid space.
myocardial infarction: (MY-oh-KAR-dee-yuhl in-FARK-shun) Death of cells of an area of the heart muscle, myocardium, as a result of oxygen deprivation, which in turn is caused by obstruction of the blood supply. Commonly referred to as a heart attack.
myocarditis: (MY-oh-kar-DYE-tiss) The inflammatory process that causes nodules to form in the myocardial tissue; the nodules become scar tissue over time. Inflammation of the heart muscle.
myocardium: (MY-oh-KAR-dee-um) Heart muscle.
myomectomy: (my-oh-MECK-tuh-mee) Removal of a portion of muscle or muscular tissue.
myopia: (my-OH-pee-ah) The error of refraction in which rays of light entering the eye parallel to the optic axis are brought to a focus in front of the retina; nearsightedness.
myringoplasty: (mir-IN-goh-PLASS-tee) Surgical reconstruction of the tympanic membrane.
myringotomy: (MIR-in-GOT-uh-mee) Incision of the tympanic membrane, usually performed to relieve pressure and allow for drainage of either serous or purulent fluid in the middle ear behind the tympanic membrane.
myxedema: (MICK-suh-DEE-mah) Condition resulting from hypofunction of the thyroid gland.
nasoseptoplasty: (NAY-zoh-SEP-toh-plass-tee) Surgical correction of the nasal septum.
naturopathy: (NAY-chur-AW-pa-thee) System of medicine that uses natural therapies such as nutrition, herbs, hydrotherapy, counseling, physical medicine, and homeopathy to treat disease, promote healing, and prevent illness.
negligence: (NEG-li-jense) An unintentional tort.
neoplasm: (NEE-oh-PLAZ-uhm) New abnormal tissue growth, as in a tumor.
nephrectomy: (neh-FREK-tuh-mee) Surgical removal of a kidney.
nephrogenic: (NEFF-roh-JEN-ick) Caused by the kidneys.
nephrolithotomy: (NEFF-roh-lih-THOT-uh-mee) Incision of a kidney for removal of kidney stones.
nephropathy: (neh-FROP-uh-thee) Any disease of the kidney.
nephrosclerosis: (NEFF-roh-skle-ROH-siss) Hardening of the kidney associated with hypertension and disease of the renal arterioles.
nephrostomy: (neh-FRAWS-toh-mee) Creation of a permanent opening into the renal pelvis.
nephrotoxin: (NEFF-roh-TOCK-sin) A toxin having a specific destructive effect on kidney tissue.
neuralgia: (new-RAL-jee-ah) Nerve pain.
neurogenic: (NEW-roh-JEN-ik) Originating in the nervous system.
neuropathic pain: (NEW-roh-PATH-ik PAYN) Pain resulting from peripheral nerve injury.
neuropathy: (new-RAW-puh-thee) A general term denoting functional disturbances and pathological changes in the peripheral nervous system.
neutrophils: (NEW-troh-fils) Granular leukocytes (white blood cells) having a nucleus with three to five lobes connected by threads of chromatin and cytoplasm containing very fine granules.
nociceptive: (NOH-see-SEP-tiv) Pain sensitive.
nocturia: (nock-TOO-ree-ah) Excessive urination at night.
nodal or junctional rhythm: (NOHD-uhl or JUNGK-shun-uhl RITH-uhm) A cardiac rhythm with its origin at the atrioventricular (AV) node.
nonmaleficence: (NON-muh-LEF-ih-sens) The requirement that health care providers do no harm to their patients, either intentionally or unintentionally.
norepinephrine: (NOR-ep-ih-NEFF-rin) A hormone produced by the adrenal medulla, similar in chemical and pharmacological properties to epinephrine, but chiefly a vasoconstrictor with little effect on cardiac output.
normoglycemia: (NOR-moh-glye-SEE-mee-ah) Normal blood glucose.
normotensive: (nor-moh-TEN-siv) Normal blood pressure.
nosocomial infection: (no-zoh-KOH-mee-uhl in-FECK-shun) Infection acquired in a health care agency.
nuchal rigidity: (NEW-kuhl rih-JID-ih-tee) Rigidity of the nape, or back, of the neck.
nursing diagnosis: (NER-sing DYE-ag-NOH-siss) A standardized label placed on a patient's problem to make it understandable to all nurses.
nursing process: (NER-sing PRAH-sess) An orderly, logical approach to administering nursing care so that the patient's needs for such care are met comprehensively and effectively.
nystagmus: (nih-STAG-muss) Involuntary, cyclical, rapid, movement of the eyes in response to vertical, horizontal, or rotary movement.
obesity: (oh-BEE-sih-tee) Abnormal amount of fat on the body ranging from 20% to 30% over average weight for age, sex, and height.
objective data: (ob-JEK-tiv DAY-tuh) Factual data obtained through physical examination and diagnostic tests; objective data are observable or knowable through the five senses.
obsession: (ub-SESH-un) Repetitive thought, urge, or emotion.
obstipation: (OB-stih-PAY-shun) Intractable constipation.
obstructive shock: (ub-STRUCK-tive SHAWK) Shock caused by indirect pump failure.
occult blood test: (ah-KULT BLUHD TEST) A chemical test or microscopic examination for blood, especially in feces, that is not apparent on visual inspection.
oliguria: (AWH-lih-GYOO-ree-ah) Diminished urination.
oncology: (on-CAW-luh-jee) The study of cancer and cancer treatment.
oncovirus: (ON-koh-VYE-russ) Viruses linked to cancer in humans.
onychomycosis: (ON-ih-koh-my-KOH-siss) Disease of the nails caused by fungus.
ophthalmia neonatorum: (ahf-THAL-mee-ah NEE-oh-nuh-TOR-uhm) Conjunctivitis in the newborn resulting from exposure to infectious or chemical agents.
ophthalmologist: (AHF-thal-MAW-luh-jist) A physician who specializes in the treatment of disorders of the eye.
ophthalmoscope: (ahf-THAL-muh-skohp) An instrument used for examining the interior of the eye, especially the retina.
opioid: (OHP-ee-OYD) A narcotic drug with morphine-like effects. True opioids are derived from opium.
optician: (ahp-TISH-uhn) One who specializes in filling prescriptions for corrective lenses for eyeglasses and contact lenses.
optimum level of functioning: (OP-teh-mum LEV-uhl of FUNK-shun-ing) Highest level of patient activity considering the patient's condition.
optometrist: (ahp-TOM-uh-trist) A doctor of optometry who diagnoses and

treats conditions and diseases of the eye per state laws.

orchiectomy: (or-key-EK-toh-mee) Removal of one or both testicles; a treatment for prostate cancer.

orchitis: (or-KYE-tiss) Inflammation of a testis.

orgasm: (OR-gazm) Pleasurable physical release sensation related to physical, sexual, and psychological stimulation.

orientation: (OR-ee-en-TAY-shun) The ability to comprehend and to adjust oneself in an environment with regard to time, location, and identity of persons.

orthopnea: (or-THOP-knee-a) Labored breathing that occurs when lying flat; relieved when sitting up; associated with left ventricular heart failure.

osmolality: (ahs-moh-LAL-ih-tee) Osmotic concentration; ionic concentration of the dissolved substances per unit of solvent.

osmosis: (ahs-MOH-sis) The passage of solvent through a semipermeable membrane that separates solutions of different concentrations.

osteomyelitis: (AHS-tee-oh-my-LEYE-tiss) Inflammation of bone, especially the marrow, caused by a pathogenic organism.

osteopathy: (AHS-tee-aw-PATH-ee) System of medicine emphasizing the interrelationship of the body's nerves, muscles, bones, and organs; involves treating the whole person, and stresses the importance of diet, exercise, and fitness, with a focus on prevention.

osteoporosis: (AHS-tee-oh-por-OH-siss) A condition in which there is a reduction in the mass of bone per unit volume.

osteosarcoma: (AHS-tee-oh-sar-KOH-mah) A malignant sarcoma of a bone.

otalgia: (oh-TAL-jee-ah) Pain in the ear.

otorrhea: (OH-toh-REE-ah) Inflammation of the ear with purulent discharge.

otosclerosis: (OH-toh-skle-ROH-siss) A condition characterized by chronic, progressive deafness, especially for low tones.

ototoxic: (OH-toh-TOK-sik) Having a detrimental effect on the eighth cranial nerve or the organs of hearing.

pain: (PAYN) An unpleasant sensory and emotional experience associated with actual or potential tissue damage, or described in terms of such damage. Is whatever the patient says it is whenever the patient says it occurs.

palliation: (pal-ee-AY-shun) The relief of symptoms without the intent to cure disease.

palpation: (pal-PAY-shun) Use of the fingers or hands to feel something.

pancreatectomy: (PAN-kree-uh-TECK-tuh-mee) Removal of all or part of the pancreas.

pancreatitis: (PAN-kree-uh-TYE-tiss) Inflammation of the pancreas.

pancytopenia: (PAN-sye-toh-PEE-nee-ah) Abnormal depression of all of the cellular elements of the blood.

panhysterectomy: (PAN-hiss-tuh-REK-tuh-mee) Excision of the entire uterus, including the cervix uteri.

panmyelosis: (PAN-my-eh-LOH-siss) Increased level of all bone marrow components, red blood cells, white blood cells, and platelets.

para: (PAR-ah) Number of deliveries a woman has had from pregnancies after 20 weeks gestation.

paradoxical respirations: (PAR-uh-DOK-si-kuhl RES-pih-RAY-shuns) Chest movement on respiration that is opposite to that expected.

paranoia: (PAR-uh-NOY-uh) Behavior that is marked by delusions of persecution or delusional jealousy.

paraparesis: (PAR-ah-pah-REE-siss) Partial paralysis of the lower extremities.

paraphimosis: (PAR-uh-fye-MOH-siss) Uncircumcised foreskin that has swollen and stuck behind the head of the penis.

paraplegia: (PAR-ah-PLEE-jah) Paralysis of the lower body, including both legs, resulting from a spinal cord lesion.

parenteral: (pah-REN-tur-ul) A medication delivery route that is "beside" rather than in the intestine, such as intramuscular, intravenous, or subcutaneous.

paresis: (puh-REE-siss) Weakness; incomplete paralysis.

paresthesia: (PAR-es-THEE-zee-ah) A heightened sensation, such as burning, prickling, or tingling.

paroxysmal nocturnal dyspnea: (PEAR-ox-IS-mall knock-TURN-al DISP-knee-ah) Sudden attacks of shortness of breath that usually occur during sleep. Person wakes gasping for breath and sits up to relieve symptoms; associated with left ventricular heart failure.

partial-thickness burn: (PAR-shul THICK-ness BERN) Burn in which the epithelializing elements remain intact.

passive immunity: (PASS-iv im-YOO-nih-tee) Reinforcement of the immune system with immune serum for such conditions as tetanus, diphtheria, and venomous snake bite.

paternalism: (puh-TER-nuhl-izm) A unilateral and sometimes unreasonable decision by health care providers that implies they know what is best, regardless of the patient's wishes.

pathogen: (PATH-oh-jen) A microorganism or substance capable of producing a disease.

pathological fracture: (PATH-uh-LAW-jik-uhl FRAHK-chur) Fracture resulting from weakening of the bone structure by pathological processes such as neoplasia or osteomalacia.

patient-controlled analgesia (PCA): (PAY-shent kon-TROHLD an-uhl-JEE-zee-ah) An apparatus that delivers an intravenous analgesic to relieve pain, which is controlled by the patient.

pedicle: (PED-ih-kuhl) The stem that attaches a new growth.

pediculosis: (peh-DIK-yoo-LOH-siss) Infestation with lice.

pemphigus: (PEM-fih-gus) Acute or chronic serious skin disease characterized by the appearance of bullae (blisters) of various sizes on normal skin and mucous membranes.

penumbra: (puh-NUM-bra) An area of brain tissue surrounding damage from a stroke that may be revived if the brain is reperfused quickly.

peptic ulcer disease: (PEP-tick UL-sir di-ZEEZ) A condition in which the lining of the esophagus, stomach, or duodenum is eroded.

perception: (per-SEP-shun) A unique impression of events by an individual. These impressions are strongly influenced by personality, cultural orientation, attitudes, and life experiences.

percussion: (per-KUSH-un) A tapping technique used by physicians and advanced practice nurses to determine the consistency of underlying tissues.

percutaneous: (PER-kyoo-TAY-nee-us) Through the skin; may refer to an injection, a medication application, or a biopsy.

perfusion: (per-FEW-zhun) Supplying an organ or tissue with blood.

pericardial effusion: (PEAR-ih-KAR-dee-uhl ee-FYOO-zhun) A buildup of fluid in the pericardial space.

pericardial friction rub: (PEAR-ih-KAR-dee-uhl FRICK-shun RUB) Friction sound heard over the fourth left intercostal space near the sternum; a classic sign of pericarditis.

pericardial tamponade: (PEAR-ih-KAR-dee-uhl TAM-pon-AID) Compression of the heart by an abnormal filling of the pericardial sac with blood.

pericardiectomy: (PEAR-ih-kar-dee-EK-tuh-mee) Excision of part or all of the pericardium.

pericardiocentesis: (PEAR-ih-KAR-dee-oh-sen-TEE-sis) Surgical perforation of the pericardium.

pericardiotomy: (PEAR-ih-KAR-dee-AH-tah-mee) Incision of the pericardium.

pericarditis: (PEAR-ih-kar-DYE-tis) Inflammation of the pericardium.

perimenopausal: (PEAR-ee-MEN-oh-PAWS-uhl) The phase before the onset of menopause, during which the cycle of a woman with regular menses changes, perhaps abruptly, to a pattern of irregular cycles and increased periods of amenorrhea.

perinatal: (PEAR-ee-NAY-tuhl) Concerning the period beginning after the 28th week of pregnancy and ending 28 days after birth.

perioperative: (PEAR-ee-AW-per-uh-tiv) Occurring in the period immediately before, during, and after surgery.

peripheral arterial disease: (puh-RIFF-uh-ruhl ar-TEER-ee-uhl di-ZEEZ) Disease of the peripheral arteries that interferes with adequate flow of blood.

peripheral parenteral nutrition: (puh-RIFF-uh-ruhl pah-REN-ter-ruhl new-TRISH-un) Nutrition by intravenous injection.

peripheral vascular resistance: (puh-RIFF-uh-ruhl VAS-kyoo-lar ree-ZISS-tense) Opposition to blood flow through the vessels.

peristalsis: (par-is-TALL-siss) Progressive, wave-like movement that occurs involuntarily in hollow tubes of the body such as the alimentary (digestive) canal; causes contents of tube to be moved onward.

peristomal: (PER-ih-STOH-muhl) Area around a stoma.

peritoneal dialysis: (PER-ih-toh-NEE-uhl dye-AL-ih-siss) The employment of the peritoneum surrounding the abdominal cavity as a dialyzing membrane for the purpose of removing waste products or toxins accumulated as a result of renal failure.

peritonitis: (PEAR-ih-tun-NYE-tiss) Inflammation of the peritoneum.

personal protective equipment: (PUR-sun-al proh-TEK-tiv ih-KWIP-mant) Items worn to protect oneself and one's patients from direct transmission of organisms that includes gloves, surgical masks, goggles, gowns, and shoe booties based on the task to be performed and the type of isolation precautions in use.

petechiae: (peh-TEE-kee-ee, puh-TEE-kee-eye) Small, purplish, hemorrhagic spots on the skin that appear in certain illnesses and bleeding disorders.

phagocytosis: (fay-go-sye-TOH-siss) Ingestion and digestion of bacteria and particles by phagocytes, cells that have the ability to ingest and destroy particulate substances such as bacteria, protozoa, and cell debris.

pharyngitis: (fair-in-JIGH-tiss) Inflammation of the mucous membranes and lymph tissues of the pharynx, usually caused by infection.

pheochromocytoma: (FEE-oh-KROH-moh-sigh-TOH-mah) Rare tumor of the adrenal system that secretes catecholamines.

phimosis: (figh-MOH-siss) Uncircumcised foreskin that cannot be moved down from the head of the penis.

phlebitis: (fla-BYE-tiss) Inflammation of a vein; may be due to irritating IV fluids or thrombosis.

phlebotomy: (fleh-BAW-tuh-mee) Entry into a vein for the removal or withdrawal of blood.

phobia: (FOH-bee-ah) A persistent, irrational, intense fear of a specific object, activity, or situation.

photophobia: (FOH-toh-FOH-bee-ah) Abnormal visual intolerance to light.

physical dependence: (FIZ-ik-uhl dee-PEN-dens) A pharmacological phenomenon characterized by signs and symptoms of withdrawal when medication is withdrawn.

phytoestrogens: (FYE-toh-ESS-troh-jens) Naturally occurring plant sterols that have an estrogen-like effect.

pinocytosis: (PIE-noh-sye-TOH-siss) Reabsorption of small proteins from renal filtrate by attachment to the membranes of the tubule cells and then engulfment and digestion.

plague: (PLAYG) A severe febrile illness caused by the gram-negative coccobacillus *Yersinia pestis* that is usually transmitted by the bite of an infectious flea. It can also be used as a biological weapon in which primary pneumonic plague would likely occur.

plaque: (PLAK) A deposit of fatty material on the lining of an artery.

plasmapheresis: (PLAS-mah-fer-EE-siss) Removal of blood to separate cells from plasma.

pleurodesis: (PLOO-roh-DEE-siss) Creation of adhesions between the parietal and visceral pleura to treat recurrent pneumothorax.

***Pneumocystis carinii* pneumonia:** (new-moh-SIS-tiss cah-RIN-ee-eye new-MOAN-yah) An acute pneumonia caused by *Pneumocystis carinii*, a fungus. It occurs in immunodeficient adults and is a defining opportunistic infection of AIDS.

pneumonectomy: (NEW-moh-NEK-tuh-mee) Surgical removal of all or part of a lung.

pneumothorax: (NEW-moh-THORE-raks) Air in the pleural space.

poikilothermy: (POY-kih-loh-THER-mee) The absence of sufficient arterial blood flow, causing the extremity to become the temperature of the environment.

point of maximal impulse: (POYNT of MAKS-ih-muhl IM-puls) The area of the chest where the greatest force can be felt with the palm of the hand when the heart contracts or beats. Usually at the fourth to fifth intercostal space in the midclavicular line.

polycythemia: (PAW-lee-sye-THEE-mee-ah) Excessive red cells in the blood.

polydipsia: (PAW-lee-DIP-see-ah) Excessive thirst.

polymyositis: (PAW-lee-my-oh-SYE-tis) A rare, inflammatory disease of the skeletal muscle tissue characterized by symmetric weakness of proximal muscles of the limbs, neck, and pharynx.

polyneuropathy: (PAW-lee-new-RAW-puh-thee) A disease involving multiple nerves.

polyphagia: (PAW-lee-FAY-jee-ah) Excessive eating.

polyuria: (PAW-lee-YOOR-ee-ah) Excessive urination.

portal hypertension: (POR-tuhl HYE-per-TEN-shun) Persistent blood pressure elevation in the portal circulation of the abdomen.

postcoital: (pohst-KOH-ih-tal) Following sexual intercourse.

postictal: (pohst-IK-tuhl) Occurring after a sudden attack, such as an epileptic seizure.

postmortem care: (pohst-MOR-tum KARE) Care after death.

postoperative: (pohst-AWP-er-uh-tiv) Following a surgical operation.

postprandial: (POHST-PRAN-dee-uhl) After a meal.

powerlessness: (POW-ur-less-ness) Perceived lack of control over a situation.

preload: (PREE-lohd) End-diastolic stretch of cardiac muscle fibers; equals end-diastolic volume.

preoperative: (pre-AWP-er-uh-tiv) Preceding an operation.

preprandial: (PREE-PRAN-dee-uhl) Before a meal.

presbycusis: (PRESS-by-KYOO-siss) Progressive, bilaterally symmetrical perceptive hearing loss occurring with age; usually occurs after age 50 and is caused by structural changes in the organs of hearing.

presbyopia: (PREZ-by-OH-pee-ah) Diminution of accommodation of the lens of the eye occurring normally with aging, and usually resulting in hyperopia, or farsightedness.

pressure ulcer: (PRESS-sure ULL-sir) An open sore or lesion of the skin that develops because of prolonged pressure against an area.

priapism: (PRY-uh-pizm) Erection that lasts too long.

primary hypertension: (PRY-mare-ee HYE-per-TEN-shun) Abnormally elevated blood pressure of unknown cause. Also called essential hypertension.

probiotics: (proh-bye-AWT-iks) Supplements of live bacteria or yeast that assist the body's naturally occurring intestinal flora. Often recommended after antibiotic therapy to reestablish the normal flora.

proctitis: (prock-TYE-tiss) Inflammation of the rectum and anus.

proctosigmoidoscopy: (PROK-toh-SIG-moy-DAWS-kuh-pee) Visual examination of the rectum and sigmoid colon by use of a sigmoidoscope.

prodrome: (PROH-drohm) A symptom indicating the onset of a disease.

prostaglandins: (PRAWS-tah-GLAND-ins) Chemical neurotransmitters usually associated with pain at the site of an injury, periphery.

prostatectomy: (PRAWS-tuh-TEK-tuh-mee) Removal of the prostate gland.

prostatitis: (PRAWS-tuh-TYE-tiss) Inflammation or infection of the prostate gland.

protozoa: (pro-tow-ZOH-ah) Single-celled parasitic organisms that can move and live mainly in the soil.

pruritus: (proo-RYE-tiss) Severe itching.

pseudoaddiction: (soo-doh-ad-DIK-shun) Syndrome in which behaviors similar to addiction appear as a result of inadequate pain control and patients fear not receiving adequate pain medications and pain relief.

psoriasis: (suh-RYE-ah-siss) Chronic inflammatory skin disorder in which epidermal cells proliferate abnormally fast.

psychoanalysis: (SYE-koh-uh-NAL-ih-siss) Form of therapy based on the theories of Sigmund Freud, regarding the dynamics of the unconscious.

psychogenic: (SYE-koh-JEN-ick) Of mental origin.

psychological dependence: (SYE-koh-LAW-jick-al dee-PEN-dens) Obsession of obtaining drugs for use other than medicinal; addiction.

psychopharmacology: (SYE-koh-FAR-meh-KAWL-uh-jee) The study of the action of drugs on psychological functions and mental states.

psychosomatic: (SYE-koh-soh-MAT-ik) Having bodily symptoms of psychological, emotional, or mental origin; illness traceable to an emotional cause.

psychotherapy: (SYE-koh-THER-uh-pee) A method of treating disease (especially mental illness) by mental rather than pharmacological means.

ptosis: (TOH-sis) Drooping of eyelid.

puerperal: (pyoo-ER-per-uhl) Concerning the puerperium, or period of 42 days after childbirth.

pulmonary edema: (PULL-muh-NAIR-ee uh-DEE-muh) Acute heart failure in which there is severe fluid congestion in the alveoli of the lungs; life threatening.

pulse deficit: (PULS DEF-ih-sit) A condition in which the number of pulse beats counted at the radial artery is less than those counted in the same period of time at the apical heart rate.

purpura: (PUR-pur-uh) Hemorrhage into the skin, mucous membranes, internal organs, and other tissues.

purulent: (PURE-u-lent) Fluid that contains pus.

pyelogram: (PIE-eh-loh-GRAM) A diagnostic procedure involving x-ray of the kidneys; may be done after injection of a dye into the bloodstream or directly into the kidneys.

pyelonephritis: (PYE-eh-loh-neh-FRY-tiss) Inflammation of the kidney and renal pelvis.

pyoderma: (PYE-oh-DER-mah) Any acute, inflammatory, purulent bacterial dermatitis.

QSEN project: Quality and Safety Education for Nurses project; focuses on nursing education that promotes the continual improvement of quality and safety in patient care.

quadriparesis: (kwah-drih-par-EE-siss) Weakness involving all four limbs caused by spinal cord injury.

quadriplegia: (KWAH-drih-PLEE-jah) Paralysis of all four limbs caused by spinal cord injury.

radiation therapy: (RAY-dee-AY-shun THER-uh-pee) Cancer treatment with ionizing radiation.

range of motion (ROM): (RANJE of MOH-shun) The range of movement of a body joint.

Raynaud's disease: (rah-NOHZ di-ZEEZ) A primary or idiopathic vasospastic disorder characterized by bilateral and symmetrical pallor and cyanosis of the fingers.

reality orientation: (ree-AL-ih-tee OR-ee-en-TAY-shun) A process to orient a person to facts such as names, dates, and time, through the use of verbal and nonverbal repeating messages.

rectocele: (RECK-toh-seel) Protrusion or herniation of the posterior vaginal wall with the anterior wall of the rectum through the vagina.

regurgitation: (ree-GUR-jih-TAY-shun) A backward flowing, as in the backflow of blood through a defective heart valve.

reminiscence therapy: (rem-uh-NIH-sens THER-uh-pee) Use of life reflection with a therapist to resolve conflicts or bring closure to life events.

remyelination: (ree-MY-uh-lin-AY-shun) Replacement of myelin or neurons.

replantation: (re-plan-TAY-shun) The replacement of an organ or other structure, such as a digit, limb, or tooth, to the site from which it was previously lost or removed.

reservoir: (REZ-er-VWAR) A person, animal, arthropod, plant, soil, or substance in which an infectious agent normally lives and multiplies, on which it depends for survival.

resorption: (ree-SORP-shun) To absorb again, as in removal of bone tissue by absorption.

respiratory excursion: (RES-pih-rah-TOR-ee eks-KUR-zhun) Downward movement of the diaphragm with inspiration.

respite care: (RESS-pit CARE) Short-term, intermittent care for the chronically ill; provides rest for the family members or caregivers from the stress of sustained caregiving.

respondeat superior: (ress-POND-ee-et sue-PEER-ee-or) An institution that employs a worker may be liable for the acts or omissions of its employees.

retinopathy: (RET-ih-NAW-puh-thee) Disease of the retina of the eye.

retroflexion: (RET-roh-FLECK-shun) A bending or flexing backward.

retrograde: (RET-roh-grayd) Moving backward; degenerating from a better to a worse state.

retrograde cholangiopancreatography: (RET-roh-grayd koh-LAN-jee-oh-PAN-kree-ah-TOG-rah-fee) An endoscopic procedure that permits the physician to visualize the liver, gallbladder, and pancreas using an endoscope, dye, and x-ray examinations.

retroversion: (RET-roh-VER-zhun) A turning, or a state of being turned back; the tipping of an entire organ.

rheumatic carditis: (roo-MAT-ick kar-DYE-tiss) Serious complication of rheumatic fever in which all layers of the heart become inflamed.

rheumatic fever: (roo-MAT-ick FEE-vur) A hypersensitivity reaction to antigens of group A beta-hemolytic streptococci.

rhinitis: (rye-NIGH-tiss) Inflammation of the nasal mucosa, usually associated with congestion, itching, sneezing, and nasal discharge.

rhinoplasty: (RYE-noh-plass-tee) Plastic surgery of the nose.

***Rickettsia*:** (rih-KET-see-ah) A genus of bacteria of the tribe Rickettsiae that multiply only in host cells.

Rinne test: (RIN-nee TEST) A test of hearing made with tuning forks.

Romberg's test: (RAHM-bergs TEST) A test to determine if a person has the ability to maintain body balance when the eyes are shut and the feet are close together.

Roux-en-Y: (roo-ehn-WHY) Gastric bypass surgery. A small stomach pouch the size of a thumb is created with staples, then a Y-shaped section of the small intestine is attached to the pouch to allow food to bypass the lower stomach and duodenum.

rule of nines: (ROOL of NYNES) A formula for estimating percentage of

body surface area, particularly helpful in judging the portion of skin that has been burned.
sacral radiculopathy: (SAY-krul rah-DIK-yoo-LAW-puh-thee) Pathology of sacral nerve roots.
salpingitis: (SAL-pin-JIGH-tiss) Inflammation of a fallopian tube.
salpingoscopy: (SAL-ping-AWS-koh-pee) Endoscopic visualization of the fallopian tubes.
scleroderma: (SKLER-ah-DER-ma) A chronic manifestation of progressive systemic sclerosis in which the skin is taut, firm, and edematous, limiting movement.
sclerosis: (skle-ROH-siss) A hardening or induration of an organ or tissue, especially from excessive growth of fibrous tissue.
seborrhea: (SEB-oh-REE-ah) Disease of the sebaceous glands marked by increase in the amount and often alteration of the quality of sebaceous secretions.
secondary hypertension: (SEK-un-DAR-ee HYE-per-TEN-shun) High blood pressure that is a symptom of a specific cause, such as a kidney abnormality.
semipermeable: (SEM-ee-PER-mee-uh-buhl) Partly permeable; said of a membrane that will allow fluids but not the dissolved substance to pass through it.
sensorineural: (SEN-soh-ree-NEW-ruhl) Hearing loss caused by impairment of a sensory nerve.
sensory deprivation: (SEN-suh-ree DEP-rih-VAY-shun) No or minimal stimulation of the senses that creates the potential for maladaptive coping.
sensory overload: (SEN-suh-ree OH-ver-lohd) Excessive stimulation of the senses that creates the potential for maladaptive coping.
sepsis: (SEP-siss) Systematic infection caused by microorganisms in the bloodstream.
serologic: (SEAR-uh-LAW-jick) Study of substances present in blood serum.
serosanguineous: (SEER-oh-SANG-gwin-ee-uss) Fluid consisting of serum and blood.
serotonin: (SARE-ah-TOH-nin) A chemical neurotransmitter important in sleep/wake cycles. Reduced serotonin levels are associated with depression.
shock: (SHAWK) A clinical syndrome in which the peripheral blood flow is inadequate to return sufficient blood to the heart for normal function, particularly transport of oxygen to all organs and tissues.
sinoatrial node: (SYE-noh-AY-tree-al NOHD) Node at the junction of the superior vena cava and right atrium, regarded as the starting point of the heartbeat.
sinusitis: (SINE-u-SYE-tiss) Inflammation of the sinuses; may be due to viral or bacterial infection, or to allergies.
smallpox: (SMALL-pox) A disease characterized by high fever and a rash caused by variola virus, an orthopoxvirus unique to humans that has a 30% fatality rate.
Snellen's chart: (SNEL-ens CHART) A chart imprinted with lines of black letters graduating in size from smallest on the bottom to largest on top; used for testing visual acuity.
somatoform: (soh-MAT-uh-form) Denoting psychogenic symptoms resembling those of physical disease; psychosomatic.
spider angioma: (SPY-dur an-jee-OH-mah) Thin reddish-purple vein lines close to the skin surface.
spirituality: (SPEER-ih-chu-AL-ih-tee) Sense of connectedness with all of life and the universe.
splenectomy: (spleh-NEK-tuh-mee) Excision of the spleen.
splenomegaly: (SPLEE-noh-MEG-ah-lee) Enlargement of the spleen.
standard of best interest: (STAN-derd OF BEST IN-trest) A type of decision made about patients' health care when they are unable to make an informed decision about their own care.
standard precautions: (STAN-derd pre-KAW-shuns) Guidelines recommended by the Centers for Disease Control and Prevention to reduce the risk of the spread of infection.
stapedectomy: (stay-pee-DEK-toh-mee) Excision of the stapes in order to improve hearing, especially in cases of otosclerosis.
Staphylococcus: (STAFF-il-oh-KOCK-uss) A genus of gram-positive bacteria; they are constantly present on the skin and in the upper respiratory tract and are the most common cause of localized suppurating infections.
status asthmaticus: (STAT-us az-MAT-ih-kus) Prolonged period of unrelieved asthma symptoms.
steatorrhea: (STEE-ah-toh-REE-ah) Fat in the stools; may be associated with pancreatic disease.
stenosis: (steh-NOH-siss) The constriction or narrowing of a passage or orifice, such as a cardiac valve.
stent: (STENT) Any mold or device used to hold tissue in place or to provide a support, graft, or anastomosis while healing is taking place.
stereotype: (STER-ee-oh-TIGHP) An opinion or belief about an individual or group that may not be true.
sternotomy: (stir-NAW-tuh-mee) The operation of cutting through the sternum.
stoma: (STOH-mah) A mouth, small opening, or pore.
stomatitis: (STOH-mah-TYE-tiss) Inflammation of the mouth.
stress: (STRESS) The physical (gravity, mechanical, pathogenic, injury) and psychological (fear, anxiety, crisis, joy) forces that are experienced by individuals.
stressor: (STRESS-ur) Any person or situation that produces an anxiety response.
striae: (STRYE-ee) A line or band of elevated or depressed tissue; may differ in color or texture from surrounding tissue.
subarachnoid: (SUB-uh-RAK-noyd) Below or under the arachnoid membrane and the pia mater of the covering of the brain and spinal cord.
subdural: (sub-DUHR-uhl) Beneath the dura mater.
subjective data: (sub-JEK-tiv DAY-tuh) Information that is provided verbally by the patient.
suffering: (SUFF-ur-ing) A state of severe distress associated with events that threaten the intactness of the person. Emotional pain associated with real or potential tissue damage.
summons: (SUM-muns) A notice of suit.
suprapubic: (SOO-pruh-PEW-bik) Bone of the groin (or region) located above the pubic arch.
surgeon: (SURGE-un) A medical practitioner who specializes in surgery.
synovitis: (sin-oh-VYE-tiss) Inflammation of the synovial membrane that may be the result of an aseptic wound, a subcutaneous injury, irritation, or exposure to cold and dampness.
systolic blood pressure: (sis-TALL-ik BLUHD PRESH-ur) Maximal pressure exerted on the arteries during contraction of the left ventricle of the heart. The top number of a blood pressure reading.
tachycardia: (TAK-ih-KAR-dee-yah) An abnormal rapidity of heart action, usually defined as a heart rate greater than 100 beats per minute in adults.
tachydysrhythmia: (TAK-ee-diss-RITH-mee-yah) An abnormal heart rhythm with rate greater than 100 beats per minute in an adult.
tachypnea: (TAK-ip-NEE-ah) Abnormally rapid respiratory rate.
tamponade: (TAM-pon-AYD) Compression of a part.
tension pneumothorax: (TEN-shun NEW-moh-THOR-raks) Abnormal accumulation of air with buildup of pressure in the pleural space.
teratoma: (tare-uh-TOH-muh) A congenital tumor containing one or more of the three primary embryonic germ layers.
terminal illness: (TERM-in-ul ILL-ness) An illness that will probably cause death in 6 months or less.

tetanus: (TET-nus) A highly fatal disease caused by the bacillus *Clostridium tetani* and characterized by muscle spasm and convulsions.
tetany: (TET-uh-nee) Muscle spasms, numbness, and tingling caused by changes in pH and low serum calcium.
thoracentesis: (THOR-uh-sen-TEE-siss) Insertion of a large-bore needle into the pleural space to remove fluid.
thoracotomy: (THOR-rah-KAW-tah-mee) Surgical incision into the chest wall.
thrill: (THRILL) Palpation of a vibration on the surface of the skin. Can be caused by turbulent blood flow through a blood vessel (as with a fistula or graft) or cardiac abnormalities.
thrombi: (THROM-bye) Blood clots.
thrombocytopenia: (THROM-boh-SYE-toh-PEE-nee-uh) Abnormal decrease in the number of blood platelets.
thrombolytic: (throm-boh-LIT-ik) Agent that dissolves or splits up a thrombus, an aggregation of blood factors.
thrombophlebitis: (THROM-boh-fleh-BYE-tiss) The formation of a clot and inflammation within a vein.
thrombosis: (throm-BOH-siss) Formation, development, or presence of a thrombus, an aggregation of blood factors.
tidaling: (TYE-dah-ling) Rise and fall; may refer to water in water-seal chamber of a chest drainage system.
titration: (tye-TRAY-shun) Adjustment of medication up or down to meet patient needs.
tolerance: (TALL-er-ens) The response of the body to medication that requires increased medication administration to achieve the same effect. Often refers to opioids.
torts: (TORTS) Lawsuits involving civil wrongs.
toxemia: (tock-SEE-me-ah) Spread of the poisonous products of bacteria throughout the body.
tracheostomy: (TRAY-key-AWS-tuh-me) A surgical opening in the neck into the trachea to provide an airway when the trachea is obstructed.
tracheotomy: (TRAY-key-AW-tuh-me) An opening in the neck into the trachea.
traditions: (trah-DISH-uns) Practices and customs handed down through the generations, often by word of mouth.
transcellular: (trans-SELL-yoo-lar) Across cell membranes.
transdermal: (trans-DUR-mal) Entering through the dermis, or skin, as in administration of a drug applied to the skin in ointment or patch form.
transillumination: (TRANS-ih-loo-mih-NAY-shun) The passage of strong light through a body structure to permit inspection of an observer on the opposite side.
transjugular intrahepatic portosystemic shunt (TIPS): (TRANZ-jug-yoo-lur in-tra-heh-PAT-ik POR-toh-siss-TEM-ik SHUNT) Shunt that sidetracks venous blood around the liver to the vena cava for treatment of ascites.
transmyocardial: (TRANS-my-oh-KAR-dee-yah) Across all layers of the heart.
trauma: (TRAW-mah) Physical injury caused by an external force.
Trendelenburg's position: (tren-DELL-en-bergz PUH-si-shun) A position in which the patient's head is low and the body and legs are on an elevated and inclined plane.
triage: (TREE-ahj) To sort.
trichinosis: (trick-in-OH-siss) A disease caused by the roundworm *Trichinella spiralis*, which is spread by eating raw or undercooked meat from pigs or wild animals that contains *Trichinella* larvae.
trigeminy: (try-JEM-ih-nee) Occurring every third beat, as in trigeminal premature ventricular contractions.
tropia: (TROH-pee-ah) A manifest deviation of an eye from the normal position when both eyes are open and uncovered.
T-tube: (TEE-toob) A T-shaped tube in the bile duct that allows drainage of bile following gallbladder surgery.
tumor: (TOO-mur) An abnormal growth of cells or tissues; tumors may be benign or malignant.
turbid: (TER-bid) Cloudy.
turgor: (TER-gur) The resistance of the skin to being grasped between the fingers. Dehydration causes poor skin turgor.
unifocal: (YOO-nih-FOH-kuhl) Coming or originating from one site or focus.
upper gastrointestinal (upper GI, UGI) series: (UH-per GAS-troh-in-TES-tih-nuhl SEER-ees) X-ray and fluoroscopic examinations of the stomach and duodenum after the ingestion of a contrast medium.
uremia: (yoo-REE-mee-ah) An excess in the blood of urea, creatinine, and other nitrogenous end products of protein and amino acid metabolism.
urethritis: (YOOR-eh-THRYE-tiss) Inflammation of the urethra.
urethroplasty: (yoo-REE-throh-PLAS-tee) Plastic repair of the urethra.
urinary incontinence: (YOOR-ih-NAR-ee in-KON-tih-nents) Inability to control urine excretion creating accidental urinary leakage.
urodynamic: (YOO-roh-dye-NAM-ik) The study of the holding or storage of urine in the bladder, the facility with which it empties, and the rate of movement of urine out of the bladder during urination.
urosepsis: (YOO-roh-SEP-siss) Septicemia resulting from urinary tract infection.
urticaria: (UR-tih-CARE-ee-ah) Hives signifying an allergic reaction.
utilitarian: (yoo-TILL-ih-TAR-ee-en) Consequences or outcomes of a dilemma are the most important element.
vaginosis: (VAJ-ih-NOH-siss) Inflammation of the vagina caused by *Gardnerella vaginalis*.
values: (VAL-use) Ideals or concepts that give meaning to an individual's life.
valvotomy: (val-VAW-tuh-mee) Cutting through a valve.
valvuloplasty: (VAL-vyoo-loh-PLAS-tee) Plastic or restorative surgery on a valve, especially a cardiac valve.
varices: (VAR-ih-seez) Dilated veins.
varicocele: (VAR-ih-koh-seel) Varicose veins of the scrotum; can lead to infertility.
varicose veins: (VAR-ih-kohs VAINS) Swollen, distended, and knotted veins, usually in the subcutaneous tissue of the leg.
vasculitis: (VAS-kue-LYE-tiss) Inflammation of a vessel.
vasectomy: (vah-SEK-tuh-mee) Surgically cutting and sealing the vas deferens to prevent sperm from getting outside the body. Used as a birth control method for men.
vector: (VEK-tur) Living organism that transmits disease.
venous stasis ulcers: (VEE-nus STAY-siss UL-sers) Poorly healing ulcers that result from inadequate venous drainage.
ventricular diastole: (ven-TRIK-yoo-lar dye-AS-tuh-lee) The period of relaxation of the two ventricles.
ventricular escape rhythm: (ven-TRIK-yoo-lar es-KAYP RITH-uhm) The naturally occurring rhythm of the ventricles when the rest of the cardiac conduction system fails.
ventricular repolarization: (ven-TRIK-yoo-lar REE-pol-lahr-ih-ZAY-shun) Reestablishment of the polarized state of the muscle after contraction.
ventricular systole: (ven-TRIK-yoo-lar SISS-tuh-lee) The contraction of the two ventricles.
ventricular tachycardia: (ven-TRIK-yoo-lar TAK-ih-KAR-dee-yah) A series of at least three beats arising from a ventricular focus at a rate greater than 100 beats per minute.
verrucous: (ve-ROO-kus) Wartlike, with raised portions.
vertebrae: (VER-teh-bray) Any of the 33 bony segments of the spinal column: 7 cervical, 12 thoracic, 5 lumbar, 5 sacral, and 4 coccygeal vertebrae.
vesicant: (VESS-ih-kant) Agent that causes blistering of tissue.
vesicular: (ve-SIK-yoo-lur) Pertaining to vesicles or small blisters.
virulence: (VEER-you-lence) The power of an organism to cause disease.

virus: (VYE-rus) The smallest organism identified by use of electron microscopy; intracellular parasites that may cause disease.
viscosity: (vis-KAW-sih-tee) Thickness, as of the blood.
volvulus: (VOL-view-lus) A twisting of the bowel on itself, causing obstruction.
vulvovaginitis: (VUL-voh-VAJ-I-NYE-tiss) Inflammation of the vulva and vagina.
Weber test: (VAY-ber TEST) A test for unilateral deafness.
welfare rights: (WELL-fare RIGHTS) Also called legal rights; rights that are based on a legal entitlement to some good or benefit.
white blood cells: (WIGHT BLUHD SELLS) Leukocytes; the body's primary defense against infection.
withdrawal: (with-DRAWL) Symptoms caused by cessation of administration of a drug, especially a narcotic or alcohol, to which the individual has become either physiologically or psychologically addicted.
worldview: (WERLD-vyoo) The way individuals look on the world to form values and beliefs about life and the world around them.
xerostomia: (ZEE-roh-STOH-mee-ah) Dry mouth caused by reduction in secretions.

Index

Note: Page numbers followed by f refer to figures; page numbers followed by t refer to tables.

A

B

C

D

F

G

H

J

K

L

N

O

P

Q

R

U

V

W

X

Y

Z

The Wordsworth

Dictionary of Shakespeare

—

Charles Boyce

Editorial Consultant: Professor David White

Foreword by Terry Hands

former Artistic Director, Royal Shakespeare Company

Wordsworth Reference

First published 1990 as *Shakespeare A-Z* by Facts on File, Inc.
460 Park Avenue South, New York, NY 10016

This edition published 1996 by Wordsworth Editions Ltd,
Cumberland House, Crib Street, Ware, Hertfordshire SG12 9ET

ISBN 1-85326-372-9

Printed and bound in Great Britain by Mackays of Chatham PLC

TABLE OF CONTENTS

FOREWORD

Shakespeare is celebrated the world over for the poetry and passion of his plays. He reformed the English language, enriching the vocabulary and increasing the flexibility of verse and prose. Supremely creative himself, he constantly inspired creativity in others. Above all, his profound humanity has enabled succeeding generations to rediscover within the dramatic intensity of his vision their own individual concerns. To many people, in many nations, Shakespeare is still our greatest living author.

All this we take for granted, but Shakespeare's survival was by no means certain. His plays were not published until 1623, some seven years after his death. The Commonwealth ended performance continuity, and with the Restoration in 1660 control of his work passed to the literate only. They decided what the public would or would not receive as Shakespeare. For fifty years, most of his plays were not performed at all, and the remainder heavily adapted. Scenes were cut, characters added or removed, the language rewritten. In this manner the public were treated to John Lacey's *Shrew* not Shakespeare's, Davenant's *Macbeth,* Nahum Tate's *King Lear.* Dryden and Davenant rewrote *The Tempest;* Purcell turned it into a musical.

Sadly the theatre can take little credit for Shakespeare's survival. Occasionally an actor would popularize a play—Betterton's *Pericles* for instance, or Garrick's *Richard III*—but the effects were temporary and the rewriting endemic. Garrick's *Richard III,* for instance, was largely Colley Cibber's, and having promised 'To lose no Drop of that Immortal Man' Garrick proceeded to perform *The Winter's Tale* without three of its five acts.

The seventeenth and eighteenth centuries may have been bad—but they were at least 'lofty' in intention. The nineteenth century made little pretence of presenting Shakespeare for anything other than profit. The plays were 'bowdlerised', rewritten, or if morally irredeemable not performed at all. A famous production of *Henry V* reduced the play to five scenes of which only four appear in the original. Actors pillaged the plays for great roles, great moments, and cut the rest. Managers favoured a few spectacular tableaux. Actor/managers did both. It was not just Kean's acting but Shakespeare himself who was seen only 'by flashes of lightning'.

Paradoxically, throughout this time Shakespeare's reputation continued to grow. The Romantics promoted Shakespeare, but not as a playwright. For them he was a poet to be read rather than seen. Charles Lamb pronounced *King Lear* 'essentially impossible to be represented on a stage'. Considering what the stage was doing to Shakespeare in the nineteenth century, Lamb's assertion was not unreasonable. But where the theatre had failed the publisher was beginning to succeed.

William Poel (1852–1934) first advocated a positive return to Shakespeare's original texts and methods of production. Harley Granville-Barker, in the early twentieth century, took up the theme. But it was not until the post-war years that their principles were generally realised. The key was education. Education and increased literacy created both a new theatre and a new audience. Lilian Baylis's Old Vic and the newly formed RSC re-established the integrity of the plays themselves, while across Europe the principle of state subsidy deferred profit in favour of increased audience accessibility. Today the collaboration of critic, scholar, public and profession in the plays of William Shakespeare is probably higher than it has ever been—thanks to the publisher and the general reader.

The Wordsworth Dictionary of Shakespeare is a remarkable summation of this new Shakespeare awareness. The focus is rigorously upon the plays themselves, with occasional reference to performance, and the tone is at all times individual but rational. It both secures and increases Shakespeare's stature and as such is a brilliant and welcome addition to our knowledge of the man and his works.

Terry Hands,
former Artistic Director and Chief Executive,
Royal Shakespeare Company

PREFACE

This book is not meant as scholarship; my intention has been to assemble conveniently a body of lore for the information and entertainment of the student and general reader. I have not studded the book with references to the scholarship of others that underlies it, for I have presumed that most readers will have little interest in knowing, say, who first suggested that Brian ANNESLEY was a living model for King LEAR's madness. I make no claim to having discovered this possibility, though I do not name the scholar who did. It is enough that someone did, and that the discovery came to my attention, so that I can bring it to yours.

A Note on Cross-References

When a name or term that is entered in this book appears in another entry, it is printed in SMALL CAPITALS, except in the case of Shakespeare himself and the titles of his works (see CANON). Each of these is, indeed, treated in its own entry, but this fact seems self-evident and reference to them is so frequent that to cross-refer each time would produce typographical clutter.

A Note on Citations

Line citations used in this book are taken from the New Arden Shakespeare (Methuen, 1951–1984), except in two instances. For *The Two Noble Kinsmen,* not included in the *New Arden* canon, citations are from the New Penguin edition (Penguin Books, 1977), and for the sonnets, from the exemplary *Shakespeare's Sonnets* of Stephen Booth (Yale, 1977).

A

Aaron Character in *Titus Andronicus,* the chief villain, a vicious criminal who loves evil for its own sake. Aaron, a Moor, is the lover of TAMORA, the Queen of the Goths, and carries out her revenge on TITUS (1) Andronicus, who has permitted her son to be killed. Although Aaron is in the retinue of the captured Queen in Act 1, he is silent. Only in 2.1 does he begin to reveal his character, rejoicing in the advancement of Tamora, who is to marry the Emperor, SATURNINUS, because it will also benefit him. The rich imagery of his first soliloquy (2.1.19–24) suggests that here is a villain who looks forward to catastrophe; it has for him the allure of 'pearl and gold'.

Tamora's two sons lust after LAVINIA, Titus' daughter. Aaron plans their appalling rape and mutilation of the girl that is the centre-piece of the revenge upon her father. Aaron's plots are indeed successful. Not only is Lavinia brutalised, but her new husband, BASSIANUS, is murdered and two of Titus' sons are charged with the crime. Further, Aaron falsely tells Titus that his severed hand is required as ransom for the two sons' lives. Titus submits to the amputation, only to have the sons' heads, and his own hand, delivered to him on a platter. This excessive piece of brutality delights Aaron, and he gloats to himself: 'O, how this villainy / Doth fat me with the very thoughts of it!' (3.1.202–203).

Aaron's blackness was a common symbol of evil in Shakespeare's day (though, as OTHELLO demonstrates, it did not have to have such a connotation). However, even in this early work, Shakespeare doesn't settle for simple conventionality. Later in the play, a NURSE (1) delivers to Aaron Tamora's new-born black infant, his child, calling it 'as loathsome as a toad / Among the fair-faced breeders of our clime' (4.2.67–68). She bears Tamora's orders that Aaron is to kill it to protect her reputation. He refuses and defends the baby at sword's point against Tamora's sons.

The black man's proud defiance of society reflects Shakespeare's awareness that villainy can have ingredients in common with heroism, regardless of race. Although the irony of this extraordinarily evil man cooing over his infant son was probably intended as humorous, it is also a good instance of the playwright's respect for the full humanity of all his characters, even one intended as a demonstration of cruelty.

Aaron's villainy is certainly still active, for he proceeds to kill the NURSE and send the two sons out to buy a white child for Tamora to claim as her own. Aaron attempts to deliver his infant to friends among the GOTHS, but he is captured, and LUCIUS (1) sentences both father and son to hang. Aaron offers to confess all in exchange for the baby's life. Lucius agrees, and Aaron takes the occasion to boast of his evil, declaring, while detailing his crimes, that in his delight with himself, he 'almost broke my heart with extreme laughter' (5.1.113). Lucius, incredulous, asks whether Aaron is not at all sorry for his 'heinous deeds'. Aaron replies: 'Ay, that I had not done a thousand more' (5.1.124). Lucius has Aaron gagged, and the Moor is taken to Rome. After the grisly banquet scene in which Titus' revenge is accomplished, Aaron is brought forth to be sentenced. He is to be buried to the neck and starved to death. This fate only provokes a last outburst: 'If one good deed in all my life I did, / I do repent it from my very soul' (5.3.189–190).

Aaron is the first of Shakespeare's flamboyantly malevolent villains, foreshadowing the likes of RICHARD III, EDMUND, LADY MACBETH, and, most spectacular of all, IAGO. A less developed personality than the later characters, Aaron more clearly represents the conventional figure from which they all descend, the MACHIAVEL. At the time when Shakespeare was writing *Titus, The Jew of Malta,* by Christopher MARLOWE ranked as one of the most successful offerings yet presented in the new world of English theatre, and it featured two very popular Machiavels—Barabas and his assistant Ithamore, racially exotic evil-doers who exult in their criminality. These characters surely influenced the young creator of Aaron. However, some historians of drama see Shakespeare as influenced here by earlier, more purely English theatrical traditions, with Aaron as a descendant of the VICE figure in the medieval MORALITY PLAY. The two propositions are not at all mutually exclusive; the idea of the Machiavel doubtless was influenced by the well-known Vice figure. It is likely that Shakespeare was aware of both and simply used a successful type.

Abbess, The Character in *The Comedy of Errors.* See EMILIA (1).

Abbot of Westminster, William Colchester (c. 1345–1420) Historical figure and character in *Richard II,* a conspirator against BOLINGBROKE (1). After RICHARD II is formally deposed in 4.1, the Abbot conspires with the Bishop of CARLISLE and the Duke of AUMERLE to kill the usurper. The plot is discovered, and the Abbot's death, apparently of a bad conscience, is reported in 5.6.19–21. The historical Abbot was pardoned by Bolingbroke, by then King HENRY IV, after one month in prison, and was permitted to retain his office, which he held until his death. Shakespeare may have confused the Abbot's fate with Carlisle's, as reported (inaccurately) by HOLINSHED. The Bishop is said to have died upon capture, 'more through feare than force of sicknesse'.

Abergavenny, George Neville, Lord (d. 1535) Historical figure and minor character in *Henry VIII,* son-in-law of the Duke of BUCKINGHAM (1). As the play opens, Abergavenny joins Buckingham and the Duke of NORFOLK (3) in their complaints about Cardinal WOLSEY's abuse of power. At the end of 1.1 Abervagenny and Buckingham are arrested for treason, the victims of a plot by Wolsey. Like his father-in-law, Abergavenny calmly accepts his fate, 'The will of Heaven be done, and the king's pleasure / By me obey'd' (1.1.215–216), offering a strong contrast with Wolsey's villainy. Shakespeare took Abergavenny's involvement from HOLINSHED's *Chronicles,* and the lord is merely an echo of Buckingham. At 1.1.211 of the FIRST FOLIO edition of the play, Abergavenny's name is spelled 'Aburgany', indicating its ordinary pronunciation.

Abhorson Character in *Measure for Measure,* an executioner. Abhorson appears in 4.2, where he undertakes to train the pimp POMPEY (1) as his assistant, and in 4.3, where he and Pompey summon the condemned criminal BARNARDINE to be executed, only to be comically frustrated by the victim's refusal to cooperate. Abhorson is part of the comic SUB-PLOT—in 4.2 he drolly claims the status of 'mystery' for his profession—but he serves chiefly to help create the ominous atmosphere of the prison. Abhorson's name, which suggests both the verb 'abhor' and the insulting noun 'whoreson', serves the same two purposes. It conveys clearly the repellent aspects of the man's profession, thereby reinforcing the atmosphere of impending doom that has been established earlier in the play, even as its absurdity helps defuse that tension.

Abram (Abraham) Minor character in *Romeo and Juliet,* a servant of the MONTAGUE (1) family. In 1.1 Abram and BALTHASAR (2) brawl with servants of the CAPULET (1) household. This episode illustrates the extent to which the feud between the two families has upset the civic life of VERONA.

Academic Drama Sixteenth-century literary and theatrical movement, the predecessor of ELIZABETHAN DRAMA. Beginning c. 1540, a body of plays was written and performed, mostly in Latin, by faculty and students of England's two 16th-century universities, Oxford and Cambridge, of its chief graduate school, the INNS OF COURT in LONDON, and of several of England's private secondary schools. The best-known creators of academic drama were Nicholas UDALL and William Gager (c. 1560–1622). Academic plays were secular, but they shared the moralising, allegorical qualities of their medieval religious predecessors (see MORALITY PLAY). They were often intended to improve the Latin and public speech of the students, and compared to the popular theatre of the 1580s they were often quite dull. Nevertheless, they created a generation of theatre-goers and the first important group of English playwrights, the so-called UNIVERSITY WITS.

Achilles Legendary figure and character in *Troilus and Cressida,* a Greek warrior in the TROJAN WAR. Though acknowledged as the greatest Greek warrior, Achilles refuses to fight because he feels he is insufficiently appreciated; he is also motivated by a treasonous desire to please a Trojan lover. Not until Act 5, after his close friend PATROCLUS is killed, does Achilles, enraged with grief, return to the battlefield. Then, he underhandedly has his followers, the MYRMIDONS, kill the chivalrous HECTOR, thereby ensuring the defeat of TROY in the climactic battle. In 5.8 he further discredits himself by declaring that he will mutilate Hector's body by dragging it behind his horse.

Achilles scandalises the Greek camp by ridiculing his superior officers, AGAMEMNON and NESTOR. ULYSSES, in a significant passage, holds Achilles' attitude responsible for the Greek failure to defeat Troy despite seven years of fighting. Societies fail, he says, when hierarchical rankings are not observed. Moreover, Achilles' insubordination has spread, and AJAX is behaving similarly. The prideful warrior thus represents a social defect that is one of the targets of the play's satire—the evil influence of morally deficient leadership. Achilles' selfish, traitorous, and brutally unchivalrous behaviour is the centre-piece of the play's depiction of the ugliness of war and the warrior's life, in principle dedicated to ideals of valour and honour but in fact governed by immorality.

Personally, Achilles is rude and uncivil for the most part, and he falsely claims the honour of having defeated Hector, whom he has merely butchered. His villainy is underlined by the obscene and vicious raillery of his jester, THERSITES, whose remarks include the accurate observation that Achilles has 'too

much blood and too little brain' (5.1.47), and the imputation that he keeps Patroclus as a 'masculine whore' (5.1.16).

The Achilles of classical mythology, recorded first in the *Iliad* of HOMER, is an outsider, the son of a sea-nymph and the leader of a semi-civilized tribe in remote Thessaly—what is now north-eastern Greece. He is disliked as the only Greek leader who still makes human sacrifices, and his treatment of Hector's body is associated with his barbarian ways. He is noted for his uncontrollable anger and his merciless rage in battle. He withdraws from combat during a dispute with Agamemnon over a concubine, Briseis (the original of CRESSIDA), returning, as in the play, upon the death of Patroclus. Apparently under the influence of Homer, cults venerating Achilles as a demi-god were established in several distant regions of the classical world. A later tradition, dating only from Roman times, states that Achilles' mother dipped him in the sacred river Styx, rendering him invulnerable except on the heel by which she had held him. He was later killed by an arrow—fired by PARIS (3)—that struck that heel. This legend gives us our name for the tendon attached to the heel: the Achilles tendon.

Actium Peninsula on the west coast of Greece, and thus the name given to the naval battle fought near it, which is enacted in 3.7–10 of *Antony and Cleopatra*. The battle of Actium marks the downfall of Mark ANTONY, whose fleet, allied with that of Queen CLEOPATRA, is defeated by the forces of Octavius CAESAR (2). In 3.7 CLEOPATRA insists on participating in the battle despite the objections of ENOBARBUS, and Antony supports her by deciding to fight at sea—for the queen has only naval forces—despite the advice of his followers that Caesar is much weaker on land. In 3.8–9 the leaders deploy their men, and in 3.10 Enobarbus, SCARUS, and CANIDIUS witness the climax of the battle as Cleopatra's ships flee and Antony orders his to follow hers. Canidius declares that he will desert Antony and joins Caesar, and though Enobarbus and Scarus remain loyal, they are severely downcast. We are convinced that Antony's fate has been determined by this battle, and this soon proves to be the case.

Shakespeare followed his source, PLUTARCH's *Lives*, fairly closely, though both he and Plutarch—who used an anti-Antony source—laid more emphasis on Antony's misjudgement than do modern scholars. In the summer of 31 B.C. Antony actually had a larger and better-equipped fleet than Caesar, while his land forces were somewhat undermanned. However, his men had not had much recent experience of naval warfare—conducted largely by ramming and boarding the enemy's ships in what amounted to infantry fighting on seaborne platforms—and Caesar's men had just completed a successful compaign against POMPEY (2). Treachery was to be the most important factor, however; in the weeks before the battle Antony's followers, including Enobarbus, began to desert. When the fleets met on September 2nd, it appears that most of Antony's men refused to fight, though scholars are in disagreement over the few details that have survived. In any case, Cleopatra's navy fled to Egypt, and Antony followed with a fraction of his own ships. The actual fighting was therefore confined to minor skirmishes though the outcome was decisive, resulting in Caesar's assumption of complete power over the Roman world.

Adam Character in *As You Like It*, aged servant of ORLANDO. Adam is a figure of unalloyed goodness, loyalty, and faith. In 2.3 the old man volunteers his life's savings to help Orlando flee the evil intentions of his brother OLIVER (1). Orlando equates Adam's virtue with 'the constant service of the antique world, / When service sweat for duty, not for meed' (2.3.57–58). Their flight to ARDEN (1) nearly kills the old man, and Orlando's attempt to steal food for Adam brings him into contact with the exiled court of DUKE (7) Senior. Adam is a sentimental, melodramatic archetype of the loyal servant, but he also has a credible personality. Verbose and nostalgic in the manner of the aged, he boasts a touching combination of moral strength and physical frailty.

A tradition dating from the 18th century asserts that Shakespeare himself performed the role of Adam in the original production by the CHAMBERLAIN'S MEN. This theory is supported by evidence that the playwright played old men on other occasions, but it cannot be proven. Shakespeare derived the character from his source, Thomas LODGE's *Rosalynde*. Lodge in turn followed a medieval English poem, *The Tale of Gamelyn*, which features a faithful servant named Adam Spencer (meaning 'steward' or 'butler'), and the figure seems to be an ancient staple of English folklore.

Adams, Joseph Quincy (1881–1946) American scholar. A longtime professor at Cornell University and director of the FOLGER SHAKESPEARE LIBRARY from 1931 to 1946, Adams wrote a respected biography, *The Life of William Shakespeare* (1923), a volume on Elizabethan theatres, and other works. He was one of the successors to H. H. FURNESS as editor of the *New Variorum* edition of Shakespeare's works (see VARIORUM EDITION).

Addenbrooke, John (active 1608) Debtor to Shakespeare. In December 1608 the STRATFORD court ordered Addenbrooke to pay a debt of £6 that he owed to Shakespeare. This was a sizeable amount of money, perhaps equal to a tenth of the playwright's annual income. In March 1609 the court reported that the debtor had moved from Stratford, and Shakespeare

was forced to sue Addenbrooke's guarantor, the town blacksmith, Thomas Horneby, from whom he received the debt plus damages and court costs. Nothing more is known of Addenbrooke.

Adlington, William (active 1566) English writer, translator of *The Golden Ass* by APULEIUS, a probable inspiration for *A Midsummer Night's Dream* and a possible minor source for *Cymbeline.* Adlington published his translation—from a French translation of Apuleius' 2nd-century A.D. Latin—in 1566, and his book was popular, being reprinted in 1571, 1582, and 1596. Little is known about Adlington's life beyond an apparent association with Oxford University.

Admiral's Men Acting company of the ELIZABETHAN THEATRE, possible employer of the young Shakespeare and later the chief rivals of his CHAMBERLAIN'S MEN. The company was originally organised in 1576 as Lord Howard's Men, under the patronage of Charles HOWARD, later Lord High Admiral of England. After touring the provinces for several years, they are first recorded in LONDON—as the Admiral's Men—in 1585, when the great actor Edward ALLEYN joined the troupe and became its leader. The company quickly established itself as a rival to the QUEEN'S MEN (1) in the London theatre world. They were especially famed for their presentations of the grandiose tragedies of Christopher MARLOWE (1).

By 1590 the Admiral's Men had a new rival, STRANGE'S MEN, but in that year the two companies joined forces at the THEATRE, owned by James BURBAGE (2). In May 1591 a dispute between Alleyn and Burbage disrupted the link, and Alleyn, along with many players of the combined group, moved to the ROSE THEATRE, owned by Philip HENSLOWE. However, when the theatres of London were closed by plague for much of 1593–1594, Alleyn led a combined Admiral's-Strange's company on tour. When the theatres reopened in 1594, the two troupes separated again, with the Admiral's Men settling at the Rose for the next six years. From then on, the Admiral's and the Chamberlain's Men (as Strange's was now known) were the two leading London theatre companies.

The Admiral's Men continued to revive Marlowe, but they also produced many new plays. Among the playwrights employed by the company were George CHAPMAN, Thomas DEKKER, Michael DRAYTON, Thomas HEYWOOD (2), and Anthony MUNDAY. Besides Alleyn, the principal actors included Thomas DOWNTON, Richard JONES (2), Martin SLATER, and Gabriel SPENCER. The company's name was formally changed to the Earl of Nottingham's Men when Howard was awarded the title in 1597, but they are invariably referred to as the Admiral's Men.

In 1598 the Admiral's Men were somewhat weakened when Spenser was killed (by Ben JONSON) and Alleyn retired from acting, though he continued as a partner in the company. He returned in 1600—at the personal request of Queen ELIZABETH (1), according to rumour—and the troupe moved to the new FORTUNE THEATRE, which it and its successors occupied for a quarter of a century. After the accession of King JAMES I in 1603, Howard was succeeded as patron by the new king's son, Prince HENRY (2), after which the Admiral's Men were known as PRINCE HENRY'S MEN. They later became the PALSGRAVE'S MEN, finally closing in 1625.

Scholars believe that Shakespeare was probably a member of the combined troupe of the Admiral's Men and Strange's Men in 1590 and early 1591. This speculation is supported by the texts of *2* and *3 Henry VI,* which were apparently printed from the author's manuscript and included the names of the actors John HOLLAND (3) and John SINCKLO, known to have been part of the combined company. Thus, it is thought that the young playwright wrote these works for production by the Admiral's-Strange's combine at the Theatre in 1590 or 1591. If this was indeed so, then he was doubtless an actor in the company as well.

Adrian (1) See VOLSCE.

Adrian (2) Minor character in *The Tempest,* a follower of King ALONSO of Naples. Adrian hardly speaks; in 2.1 he briefly supports GONZALO in his optimism, which is mocked by ANTONIO (5) and SEBASTIAN (3), and in 3.3 he speaks only half a line, closing the scene. Adrian, with FRANCISCO (2), has been seen by some scholars as evidence for the existence of an earlier version of *The Tempest,* in which his role was more substantial, for there seems no reason to include him in the play as it stands. He may have been intended for scenes that Shakespeare originally planned but then discarded in the course of composition. In any case, minor attendants help establish the high status of royal figures throughout Shakespeare's plays, and Adrian has this function for Alonso; moreover, his reiteration of Gonzalo's position focusses attention on it and helps maintain our sense of good's survival among villains.

Adriana Character in *The Comedy of Errors,* the jealous but loving wife of ANTIPHOLUS OF EPHESUS. Adriana first appears in 2.1, complaining that Antipholus is late for lunch. She argues with her sister, LUCIANA, about the proper obedience owed a husband, in a standard disputation on marital relations that was common in Shakespeare's day. While Luciana adopts the position that a man is rightly the master of his wife, Adriana asserts, 'There's none but asses will be bridled so' (2.1.14). Later in the scene, she bemoans her

husband's attentions to other women, and jealousy is her characteristic trait throughout the play, finally triggering a humorous but acid sermonette by the Abbess, EMILIA, in the final scene (5.1.69–86).

The circumstances of confusion and error that create the atmosphere of the play also stimulate Adriana's jealous streak. In 2.2 she accosts ANTIPHOLUS OF SYRACUSE, thinking him to be her husband, and demands that he come home to eat. Bemused and baffled, he nevertheless goes with her, and there ensues (3.1) the central misidentification of the play; Adriana refuses to admit her real husband to their home, believing him to be an imposter.

In 4.2 Luciana reports to Adriana a declaration of love from the man both believe to be Antipholus of Ephesus; both women thus believe that Adriana's husband is attempting to betray her by courting her own sister. Adriana rails against her husband but concludes: 'Ah, but I think him better than I say, . . . / My heart prays for him, though my tongue do curse' (4.2.25–28).

This note of wifely affection grows stronger as the play hurries to its resolution, for Adriana is truly fond of her husband, irascible and domineering though he may be. She tries to aid him, once she has concluded that he is temporarily insane; the confusions of the plot have led her (and others) to this error. She appears in the final scene just as Antipholus of Syracuse is about to fight a duel, and, thinking him her husband, she implores, 'Hold, hurt him not for God's sake; he is mad' (5.1.33). Antipholus and his servant flee into the PRIORY. Adriana follows her husband there and demands that the Abbess turn Antipholus over to her. The Abbess refuses, however, and Adriana has recourse to the DUKE (8). His investigation triggers the final resolution of the play's confusions, although Adriana plays no great part in that process.

An interesting tradition has it that Adriana was written as a portrait of Anne HATHAWAY, but modern scholarship debunks this idea. Nevertheless, Adriana was clearly an important creation for Shakespeare, for she is a markedly more fully drawn and consequential figure than her predecessor in his source for the play. She is an early example of a Shakespearean character type that recurs often in the plays (e.g., KATHERINA, in *The Taming of the Shrew*, and BEATRICE, in *Much Ado About Nothing*)—an independent woman whose sharp words and sometimes forbidding manner conceal a tender heart. Adriana's dual nature would come to typify Shakespeare's greatest characters. The playwright insisted on presenting multiple points of view about a character or situation, offering his audience varying and often conflicting impressions, and thus re-creating on the stage the inconsistencies of actual life.

Aedile Any of several minor characters in CORIOLANUS, subordinates of the Roman tribunes SICINIUS and BRUTUS (3). The Aediles serve chiefly as messengers for the tribunes. They summon the crowds to rally against CORIOLANUS in 3.1; they announce Coriolanus' approach and are instructed in coaching the crowd in 3.3; and an Aedile brings the tribunes the first report of the VOLSCIANS' advance against ROME in 4.6. They demonstrate the institutional power that the tribunes command.

Aegeon See EGEON.

Aemilia See EMILIA (1).

Aemilius Minor character in *Titus Andronicus.* Aemilius delivers messages between SATURNINUS and LUCIUS (1) and helps acclaim Lucius the new Emperor at the end of the play.

Aeneas Legendary figure and character in *Troilus and Cressida,* a leader of the Trojan forces in the TROJAN WAR. Aeneas serves as an herald, carrying the challenge of HECTOR in 1.3, accompanying the visiting Greek delegation led by DIOMEDES in 4.1–4, carrying a warning of their arrival to TROILUS in 4.2, and announcing Hector's arrival for his duel with AJAX in 4.5. Aeneas represents the Trojan concern for chivalric honour: he is a stiffly correct model of knightly manners. His exchange with Diomedes in 4.1 of courteous declarations of intent to kill is a bleakly humorous picture of mindless warriors who can reduce the horrors of war to an exercise in etiquette.

In the *Iliad* of HOMER, Aeneas is a more important figure; he is a cousin of King PRIAM who is notably favoured by the gods. The sea-god Poseidon predicts that Aeneas shall be a ruler someday. Later tradition developed this forecast into Aeneas' leadership of the Trojan exiles who wandered the Mediterranean world after the fall of their city, and VIRGIL's *Aeneid* makes him the founder of Rome. Shakespeare and his contemporaries saw Aeneas as an ancestor figure because his great-grandson Brut was thought to have settled England and founded London as New Troy. This is reflected in the anti-Greek bias of the play.

Africanus, Leo See LEO AFRICANUS.

Agamemnon Legendary figure and character in *Troilus and Cressida,* the leader of the Greek forces in the TROJAN WAR. Although ULYSSES calls him 'Thou great commander, nerves and bone of Greece' (1.3.55), Agamemnon is in fact an ineffectual leader. He preaches ponderously, but ACHILLES can safely ignore his orders; the Greek forces are accordingly stymied in their siege of TROY. Much of what Ulysses calls the

absence of 'degree' (1.3.83, 101, 109, etc.)—a dissolution of the hierarchy on which Greek society has been based—can be attributed to Agamemnon's recurrent weakness. At the play's close, Agamemnon still lacks authority; in the last line spoken by a Greek, he sends a messenger to request submissively the presence of Achilles, just as he has had to do all along.

The Agamemnon of classical myth and legend probably derives from a historical king who ruled in the Argive, a region of Greece near Corinth, during the Bronze Age. His post as commander of the Greek forces at Troy is recorded in the *Iliad* of HOMER, as are his lack of resolve and his inability to control Achilles. Homer's *Odyssey* and later plays by Greek dramatists continued his tale after the war: upon his return home, he is killed by his wife, Clytemnestra, and her lover. This murder impels Orestes, his son, to kill his mother in revenge. This event and Orestes' subsequent torment by supernatural spirits constitute the *Oresteia*, the subject of works by all the major Greek dramatists and many other writers, into modern times.

Age of Kings, An British Broadcasting Company production (1960) of Shakespeare's two tetralogies (see TETRALOGY) of HISTORY PLAYS. These eight works, which depict a continuous period from 1399 to 1485, were presented in 15 parts. This extraordinary production, which has been called 'the first mini-series', offered a fresh point of view on several stories and characters. For instance, such episodes as the fall of Humphrey, Duke of GLOUCESTER (4), are lent greater coherence by being isolated from their surroundings, and certain characters—notably Queen MARGARET (1), the Duke of YORK (8), and PRINCE (6) HAL, who becomes HENRY V—demonstrate their growth as individuals over the several plays in which they appear.

Agincourt Town in northern FRANCE (1), battle site in the HUNDRED YEARS WAR and location for Act 4 of *Henry V*. The battle of Agincourt provides the climax of *Henry V* and of the second TETRALOGY of Shakespeare's HISTORY PLAYS. The English army, led by King HENRY V, wins an impressive victory over a much larger French force. Henry attributes the triumph to divine intervention in favour of the English. Soundly defeated, FRANCE (1) signs, in 5.2, a treaty granting Henry the inheritance of the French crown, as well as marriage to the FRENCH KING's daughter, KATHARINE (2). England thus achieves a glorious ascendancy over its traditional enemy.

Shakespeare's presentation of the battle focuses on King Henry. Henry may be seen as a chivalric hero, whose courage and high spirits—reflected particularly in his famous 'St Crispin's Day' speech (4.3.18–67)—and democratic identification with his soldiers, shown in 4.1, give his army the morale necessary to defeat the foe. On the other hand, Henry's assertion in the St Crispin's Day oration that he prefers to be outnumbered in order to garner greater honour smacks of the irrational bravado condemned in HOTSPUR in *1 Henry IV*. Similarly, his order to kill the French prisoners (4.6.37) may indicate a praiseworthy decisiveness at a critical moment, but it can also be interpreted as an act of militaristic savagery.

Historians place much more emphasis on the common soldiers than on Henry. A landmark battle in English and military history, Agincourt—fought on October 25, 1415—was indeed an extraordinary event: a crushing defeat was administered by a weary, sick, and badly damaged English force to a French army three times its size. The English victory was chiefly due to the shrewd use of batteries of longbowmen, who cut down the French cavalrymen before they could approach; it was the first victory of massed infantry over the mounted knights who had dominated medieval battlefields. Shakespeare omits this key feature of the battle in order to direct attention towards his protagonist more effectively. Moreover, despite the impressive English victory, Agincourt did not win France for Henry; it merely staved off defeat. He took his army back to England and reinvaded in 1417. Only three years later, after the conquest of Normandy, were the French prepared to negotiate the treaty of TROYES, presented in 5.2 of the play.

Agrippa, M. Vipsanius (63–12 B.C.) Historical figure and character in *Antony and Cleopatra*, a follower of Octavius CAESAR (2). In 2.2 Agrippa displays considerable influence when he suggests the marriage between ANTONY and OCTAVIA, and in 4.6 and 4.7 he is in command of Caesar's army. For much of the remainder of the play he serves as an opposite to Antony's ENOBARBUS, with whom he exchanges remarks on the principal characters; he displays the demeanour of a gruff veteran soldier.

Shakespeare's character does not reflect the importance of the historical Agrippa, who was probably the most important figure—after Caesar himself—in the defeat of Antony and the subsequent establishment of the Roman Empire. Along with MAECENAS, he was one of Caesar's few close friends and advisers. His origins are entirely obscure; even his contemporaries knew nothing of his family or homeland, although he was believed to have been Caesar's schoolmate in Athens before accompanying the future emperor on his return to Italy after the assassination of Julius CAESAR (1) in 44 B.C. (Agrippa does not appear in Shakespeare's *Julius Caesar*.) He was a prominent general throughout the civil wars. He put down revolts in Italy and Gaul and created and commanded the fleets that defeated POMPEY (2) in Sicily and Antony at Actium. After Antony's defeat, Agrippa was Caesar's right-hand man in governing Rome. In 23 B.C. Caesar nearly died of an illness, and he apparently intended that Agrippa

would succeed him as ruler. In 21 B.C. Agrippa married Caesar's daughter. He served as a general and administrator in various parts of the empire until the year of his death.

Ajax Legendary figure and character in *Troilus and Cressida,* a Greek warrior in the TROJAN WAR. For the most part, Ajax is a variant on the ancient MILES GLORIOSUS character type: a braggart soldier, a laughable buffoon who is not to be taken seriously. He presents a comic variation on an important theme: the vanity of the warrior's lust for military glory. At the same time, he has notable redeeming features that offer a counterpoint to the play's generally acerbic tone.

Before he appears, Ajax is humorously described by ALEXANDER (1) as a valiant warrior but a beastlike churl with uncontrollable emotions. (Some scholars believe that this passage [1.2.19–31] is a satirical description of Ben JONSON, though the point is extremely disputable.) When he does appear, Ajax is laughably stupid, incapable of responding to THERSITES' teasing except by hitting him. Selected by ULYSSES as a substitute for ACHILLES, Ajax displays ludicrous pride in his undeserved position, especially since he criticises Achilles for *his* pride, and elicits the amused asides of the other Greeks in 2.3.201–224. One of the play's funniest passages is Thersites' imitation of Ajax' ego in 3.3.279–302. Ajax issues a preposterous parody of a chivalric challenge as he directs his trumpeter to summon HECTOR for their duel, saying, 'Now, crack thy lungs, . . . stretch thy chest, and let thy eyes spout blood' (4.5.7–10).

However, Ajax proves a brave soldier who behaves with valour and chivalrous generosity when he actually faces Hector, getting the better of the fight (according to the cries of the spectators in 4.5.113–115) but accepting the truce his opponent desires. Strikingly, when Thersites describes Ajax as 'a very land-fish, languageless, a monster' (3.3.262–263), we see that this brutish fellow resembles a later Shakespearean figure—also sympathetic in spite of his defects—CALIBAN, the fishy monster of *The Tempest.*

Ajax (Latin for the Greek Aias) is the name of two characters in the *Iliad* of HOMER; Shakespeare combines them. The opponent of Hector corresponds to Aias Telamon, described by Homer as the bulwark of the Greek forces, a courageous warrior who is slow of speech but repeatedly a leader in assault and the last to retreat; he successfully duels Hector, as in the play. Otherwise, Shakespeare's character corresponds to Aias Oileus, often called Aias the Lesser, also a fine warrior but notorious for his pride, rudeness, and blasphemy. In the *Odyssey,* he is drowned by the sea-god Poseidon for cursing the gods while escaping a shipwreck. In a later tradition, he raped CASSANDRA on an altar during the sack of TROY, a misdeed whose punishment accounted for a custom by which his descendants were annually required to provide two virgins who ran a gauntlet of the townspeople and, if they survived, served for life in the temple of Athena. The end of this barbaric practice around 100 A.D. was reported by PLUTARCH, who said it had lasted 1,000 years.

Alarbus Minor character in *Titus Andronicus,* the eldest son of TAMORA. In 1.1, TITUS (1) Andronicus permits the ritual sacrifice of Alarbus, who is killed despite his mother's pleas for mercy. This sparks the cycle of vengeance that comprises the plot of the play.

Albany, Duke of Character in *King Lear,* the virtuous but weak husband of LEAR's villainous daughter, GONERIL. Albany, who does not discover his wife's wickedness until too late, eventually aids the banished Lear and formally restores him to power just before his death. In this way he represents an instance of moral growth in a degraded world. At the play's close he is the ruler of Britain, sharing power with EDGAR and KENT, and intent on repairing the damage to the state that Lear's crisis has produced. In the final lines, Albany offers a possible lesson to be drawn from the tragedy, saying, 'The weight of this sad time we must obey' (5.3.322); he recognises the need to be aware of human susceptibility to catastrophic error, as Lear did not. (Albany's lines here are sometimes given to Edgar, as in the FIRST FOLIO text.)

In his early appearances Albany is ineffectual. He is governed entirely by his wife, who dismisses his question about her rift with Lear by curtly ordering, 'Never afflict yourself to know more of it' (1.4.289). After Act 1 he does not reappear until 4.2, when, having learned of the treacherous blinding of GLOUCESTER (1), he denounces Goneril as an evil-doer. 'You are not worth the dust which the rude wind / Blows in your face', he declares (4.2.30–31). Nevertheless, he goes along with her alliance with EDMUND against CORDELIA's French army, though he privately asserts his intention to revenge Gloucester. Informed by Edgar of Edmund and Goneril's plot against his own life, Albany exposes the villains in 5.3. By this time Albany is clearly intent on rectifying the misdeeds of his wife and her allies, but his earlier weakness has already helped them. His poor judgement in patriotically fighting the French has an unintended and fatal result when Edmund gains control of Lear and Cordelia. Thus, though well-intentioned and finally benevolent, Albany reinforces the play's theme of human fallibility.

Alcibiades (c. 450–404 B.C.) Historical figure and character in *Timon of Athens,* an Athenian general and friend of TIMON. Alcibiades is faithful to Timon in adversity and thereby counteracts the play's theme of false friendship. He is most significant as the central figure in a parallel plot in which he is pitted against the

cold-hearted, legalistic aristocracy of ATHENS. Like Timon he is the subject of ingratitude and a heartless application of the system and its laws. However, Alcibiades takes action and avenges himself. Thus he is placed in sharp contrast with Timon and his passive withdrawal into misanthropy and madness. Then, at the play's close, his humane nature permits a reconciliation, an ending that offers the central lesson of the play: the superiority of mercy over justice in human affairs.

Unlike Timon, Alcibiades realises that good can exist in a world that is evil, and that mercy is a greater corrective for society than revenge. In his final tribute to 'noble Timon' (5.4.80), Alcibiades extends his mercy to the misanthrope himself. Though Timon, as a suicide, cannot participate in the play's ultimate spirit of reconciliation, his extreme hatred is forgiven and finally countered.

For the first half of the play, Alcibiades is clearly an honest friend amidst a group of obviously insincere and hypocritical courtiers that surround Timon, but he is a minor figure. He assumes importance in 3.5, the pivotal scene of the play, when he pleads with the Athenian rulers (see SENATOR [4]) for mercy on behalf of a veteran soldier sentenced to death for murder. Alcibiades argues that 'pity is the virtue of the law' (3.5.8). This reflects a central concern not only of the play but of Shakespearean drama in general. Banished from Athens because he has questioned authority, he promises revenge, and in 5.1 he threatens to sack the city. Thus, he is clearly in opposition to callous ingratitude while at the same time he threatens disaster for the entire city. Such a catastrophe—though here only potential—demonstrates how immoral behaviour among the ruling class leads to trouble for the entire society, a lesson Shakespeare repeatedly offered in the HISTORY PLAYS, the ROMAN PLAYS, and elsewhere. Alcibiades is both opponent and saviour for the 'coward and lascivious' Athens (5.4.1).

Alcibiades is the only character in *Timon of Athens* who is at all fleshed out. He prefers his profession, soldiering, to the banquets of Timon's world, and his controlled anger in his encounter with the Senate is impressive. He knows himself—'I speak like a captain', he says (3.5.42)—and he can plead for a friend. He also understands the self-exiled Timon—as Timon himself cannot—and sees that 'his wits / Are drown'd and lost in his calamities' (4.3.89–90). In these respects Alcibiades seems somewhat at odds with the rest of the play, which relies heavily on the bold symbolism of allegorical characters. Perhaps this unresolvable contrast contributed to Shakespeare's decision to leave *Timon* unfinished.

The fascinating career of the historical Alcibiades is only faintly reflected in Shakespeare's character. Alcibiades was a brilliant though unstable young aristocrat who led an ostentatiously decadent life but nevertheless became an influential general and leading politician. However, despite his political power, he faced banishment for his part in a sacrilegious mutilation of icons. He fled to avoid trial and joined Athens' enemies, the Spartans. They mistrusted him and he moved on and joined their allies, the Persians, whom he tried to win to an alliance with Athens. From exile, he maintained contact with the turbulent Athenian political world and was thus able to assume command of the Athenian fleet, over the objections of the government.

Shakespeare's source, PLUTARCH's *Lives*, states that Alcibiades refused the navy's demand that he attack the city; this is the germ of Shakespeare's account. Actually, though on his return Alcibiades was supported by a revolutionary government that arose in Athens at that time, there was no question of his attacking the city. He fought the Spartans and Persians with such success that the Athenians gave him total command of the armed forces. However, a minor loss permitted his enemies to revive popular resentment against him, and he again left Athens and took refuge with Spartan allies in Phrygia. There, he was murdered by agents of conservative Athenians who had returned to power and made peace with Sparta. Alcibiades was a byword for treachery in the ancient world, though it was also recognised that the Athenians were foolish to follow political loyalties and discard a military genius when they most needed him.

Aldridge, Ira (c. 1807–1867) American actor. The first highly successful black actor, Aldridge was generally acknowledged to be the most accomplished American on the London stage in the 19th century. Particularly noted for his performances as OTHELLO and AARON, Shakespeare's most prominent black characters, Aldridge was also acclaimed as LEAR, HAMLET, RICHARD III, SHYLOCK, MACBETH, and others. He performed in most of the major capitals of Europe and was universally regarded as among the great actors of his generation.

Born to a New York City minister, Aldridge was intended for the ministry himself, but he was attracted to the stage very early, appearing with a black acting company at the age of 14. Befriended by an English actor, Henry Wallack (1790–1870), Aldridge went to England in 1824 when he recognised that racial prejudice would not permit him an acting career in America. He was immediately popular, and his evident talent and sophistication helped promote the growing movement for the abolition of slavery throughout the British Empire. Aldridge underwent a period of apprenticeship in provincial touring companies before he achieved success in London. He remained at the top of his profession for almost 40 years. He died on tour in Poland while preparing for a home-coming to America.

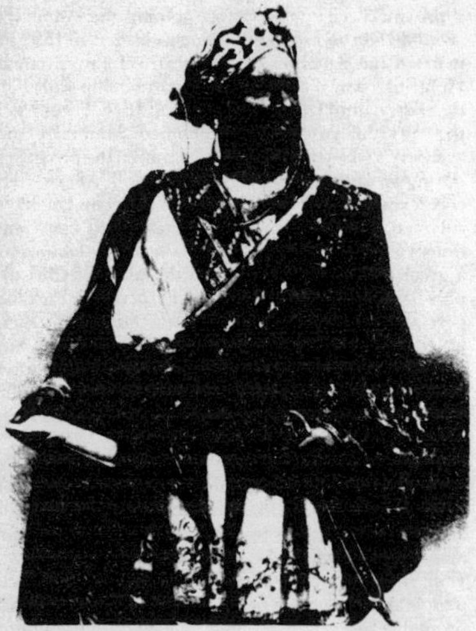

Ira Aldridge as Othello. Denied opportunity in the United States because of his race, the actor found great success on the stages of Europe in the 19th century. (Courtesy of Picture Collection, New York Public Library)

Alençon, John, Duke of (1409–1476) Historical figure and character in *1 Henry VI*, one of the French noblemen who lead the forces of CHARLES VII against the English. Like his fellows, the BASTARD (2) OF ORLÉANS, REIGNIER, and Charles himself, Alençon is depicted as a type, a bragging but inept, treacherous, and cowardly warrior. Alençon's father was the French knight whose glove HENRY V of England is said to have taken during the battle of AGINCOURT (*Henry V*, 4.7.159).

Alexander (1) Minor character in *Troilus and Cressida*, a servant of CRESSIDA. Alexander appears only in 1.2, where he tells his mistress that the Trojan prince HECTOR is furious because he has been humbled in battle by the Greek warrior AJAX. He describes Ajax in humorous terms as a beastlike man. This brief episode introduces the rivalries of the warriors in a fashion that signals the play's satiric intent.

Alexander (2), Peter (1894–1969) British Shakespearean scholar, editor of an edition of Shakespeare's works and author of many works on the playwright and his times. A longtime professor at Glasgow University, Alexander is best known for his *Shakespeare's Life and Art* (1964) and his one-volume edition of the complete works (1951). He also convincingly established Shakespeare's authorship of the *Henry VI* plays in his *Shakespeare's Henry VI and Richard III* (1929).

Alexandria City in Egypt located on the Mediterranean coast at the western edge of the Nile River delta, the setting for many scenes in *Antony and Cleopatra*. Alexandria was the capital of the Ptolemaic Empire inherited by CLEOPATRA, and was the site of her palace, where she conducted her affair with Mark ANTONY. It is to this sanctuary that the lovers retreat after being defeated in the battle of ACTIUM, and it is where they die.

The magnificence of the Ptolemaic capital is implicit in the luxurious decadence of Antony and Cleopatra's life, with its servants and banquets—the reputation of 'fine Egyptian cookery' (2.6.63) is several times admired—and in the pomp of their enthronement 'I' the market place' of Alexandria (3.6.3). The richness of Cleopatra's personal adornment, detailed in ENOBARBUS' famed description in 2.2.190–218 (though she was not in Alexandria at the time), confirms the impression. The city's huge and cosmopolitan population is hinted at in Antony's description of when he and the queen would 'wander through the streets, and note / The qualities of people' (1.1.53–54). Cleopatra's recollections of delightful fishing expeditions, in 2.5.10–18, suggest the pleasures of a great city's riverfront.

Alexandria was the chief city of the eastern Mediterranean from its founding by Alexander the Great in 332 B.C. until its conquest by Arab invaders in the 7th century A.D. Until around the time of the play when its population—probably about one million—was surpassed by that of Rome, Alexandria was the largest city of the entire Western world. It remained the major cultural centre of the Roman Empire and, later, the Byzantine Empire. The library at Alexandria was one of the great treasures of the ancient world, containing at one point around 750,000 volumes. Although the library's final destruction when it was torched by the Arabs c. 640 A.D. is regarded as one of the greatest single acts of vandalism known, the Arab conquest merely completed a process that had begun much earlier; in fact, an early installment occurred when Antony's men, burning their vessels as CAESAR (2) approached after the battle of ACTIUM, accidentally set fire to the library and destroyed an unknown quantity of its contents.

Alexas (Alexas Laodician) (active c. 32 B.C.) Historical figure and minor character in *Antony and Cleopatra*, an attendant to CLEOPATRA. Alexas is a cheerful fellow who jests with CHARMIAN and IRAS in 1.2. He brings Cleopatra a message from ANTONY in 1.5, and attends her—almost without speaking—in 2.5, 3.3, and 4.2.

However, Alexas' desertion to Octavius CAESAR (2), after the battle of ACTIUM, is reported in 4.6, and he appears to be a more important figure than his earlier role would suggest. ENOBARBUS reflects that Alexas had been sent by Antony to 'Jewry' (4.6.12), where he persuaded the ruler, Herod, to join Caesar. He goes on to remark that Caesar, shocked by this treachery, had executed Alexas. The account elaborates on the important Act 4 theme of Antony's fall as many of his one-time followers are seen to have deserted him.

Shakespeare took his account of Alexas Laodician from his source, PLUTARCH's *Lives*, where the Greek servant's promotion to diplomatic status is said to have resulted from the friendship that developed between him and Antony through his job as Cleopatra's message bearer. His surname—found in Plutarch—suggests that he was from the important ancient city of Laodicia, in Asia Minor, but otherwise Alexas is not found in history.

Alice Minor character in *Henry V*, lady-in-waiting to Princess KATHARINE (2) of France. In 3.4 Alice, said to have been in England, gives her mistress a brief lesson in English, telling her the names for such body parts as the hand, the fingers, and so on, in an exchange marked by comical mispronunciation and unintentional sexual references. This oddly charming episode, conducted entirely in French, appears immediately after King HENRY V's dire threats to sack HARFLEUR and thus subtly contributes to the play's sardonic presentation of Henry's career of conquest, parallel to its glorification of him. The scene also foreshadows Henry's aggressive bilingual courtship of Katharine in 5.2, where Alice is also present.

Aliena In *As You Like It*, the name CELIA takes when she and ROSALIND, banished by DUKE (1) Frederick, travel in disguise to the Forest of ARDEN (1). The name suggests her exiled state.

Allde, Edward (c. 1583–1624) London printer, producer of editions of several of Shakespeare's works. In 1597 Allde printed part of the first, pirated, QUARTO edition of *Romeo and Juliet* when the original printer, John DANTER, was suspended by the STATIONERS' COMPANY for another such piracy. Allde himself underwent suspensions later in the same year, and again in 1599, for printing illicit Catholic materials. However, he was generally successful, printing mostly poetry and plays. In 1611 he printed the third quarto of *Titus Andronicus* for publisher Edward WHITE (1), and the second quarto of The Phoenix and Turtle.

Alleyn, Edward (1566–1626) English actor, the leader of the ADMIRAL'S MEN and the foremost actor of Shakespeare's day. The son of a LONDON innkeeper, Alleyn was a teenage actor in WORCESTER'S MEN, then a provincial company, before joining the Admiral's around 1585 and soon becoming its leader. In 1592 he married the daughter of the theatrical entrepreneur Philip HENSLOWE and formed a partnership with him that lasted until Henslowe's death in 1616. From 1590 to 1594 Alleyn led the combined Admiral's and STRANGE'S MEN companies, which toured the provinces during an outbreak of plague in London. Alleyn's letters from this tour to his wife and father-in-law have survived, and they reveal an amiable and conscientious young man. In the 1590s Alleyn was famous as a great tragedian, especially in the plays of Christopher MARLOWE (1); Thomas NASHE declared him the best actor 'since before Christ was borne' and Ben JONSON was later to declare to him, 'others speak, but only thou dost act'. When he retired briefly, around 1598, it was said that Queen ELIZABETH (1) personally asked him to return to the stage. He did so in 1600 but retired for good in 1604.

He retained a financial interest in PRINCE HENRY'S MEN, as the Admiral's was known after the accession of King JAMES I, along with other investments, theatrical and otherwise. By this time Alleyn was quite a wealthy man. With Henslowe, he was a part-owner of the FORTUNE THEATRE, which they had built, and of the licence to operate the London bear-baiting arena. He also had profitable real estate holdings in and around London, and he later inherited Henslowe's interest in the HOPE THEATRE and the Fortune. In 1605 he bought a manor in Dulwich (now a south London suburb, then a rural hamlet), where he moved in 1613. He founded Dulwich College there, a hospital and school for poor families; it is now the site of a small museum, housing a collection of European paintings along with Alleyn and Henslowe's papers, which provide a rich assemblage of 16th-century theatre lore. Alleyn's wife died in 1623; he remarried in the same year, to the daughter of the poet John Donne (1573–1631).

All Is True Alternative title for *Henry VIII*. The play is called *All Is True* in a contemporary account of its performance the day the GLOBE THEATRE burned down. This was probably a subtitle—perhaps to imply a contrast to another play about HENRY VIII, the blatantly fictitious *When You See Me, You Know Me* (1605) by Samuel ROWLEY (1). Some scholars, however, contend that *All Is True* was Shakespeare's original title, which was altered in the FIRST FOLIO (1623) to go with the other HISTORY PLAYS, all named for kings.

All's Well That Ends Well

SYNOPSIS

Act 1, Scene 1

The COUNTESS (2) of ROSSILLION's son BERTRAM is leaving for the court of the KING (17) of FRANCE (1). The

Countess and Lord LAFEW discuss the King's poor health; she regrets that the father of her ward, HELENA (2), has died, because he was a great physician. The Countess bids Bertram farewell and departs, and Bertram, after a cursory farewell to Helena, leaves with Lafew. Helena soliloguises on her seemingly hopeless love for Bertram. Bertram's friend PAROLLES arrives and engages Helena in an exchange of witticisms on virginity. Parolles leaves, and Helena decides that she must act if her love is to be rewarded. She sees an opportunity in the King's illness.

Act 1, Scene 2
The King discusses the war between Florence and Siena, stating that he has decided to permit French noblemen to fight in the conflict if they wish. Bertram arrives and is welcomed warmly by the King. The King remarks on his ill health and regrets the death of the famed doctor who had served in the court at Rossillion.

Act 1, Scene 3
The Countess' jester, the CLOWN (5), requests permission to marry, making obscene jokes and singing songs. The STEWARD (1) wishes to speak about Helena, and the Countess sends the Clown to get her. The Countess remarks on her fondness for Helena, and the Steward confides that he has overheard the young woman musing on her love for Bertram. As the Steward leaves, Helena arrives, and the Countess elicits from her a confession of her love for Bertram and of her intention to go to Paris. Helena asserts that she has secret prescriptions of her father's that she is convinced will cure the King, and the Countess agrees to help her travel to Paris to try them.

Act 2, Scene 1
The King bids farewell to the First and Second Lords (see LORD [6]) and other young noblemen leaving to fight in Italy. Bertram regrets that he is commanded to remain at court. Lafew appears and introduces Helena as a young woman who can cure the King's illness. Helena convinces the King to try her medecine, offering to wager her life that it will work within 24 hours. In return, she asks the King to approve her marriage to the man of her choice.

Act 2, Scene 2
The Clown jests about life at the King's court, and the Countess gives him a message to take to Helena.

Act 2, Scene 3
Lafew, interrupted repeatedly by Parolles, tells of the King's return to health. The King arrives with Helena, who is to choose from among the young gentlemen of the court. She selects Bertram, but he refuses to marry her, saying that her social rank is too low. However, the King orders him to accept, and he acquiesces. Parolles puts on airs, and Lafew disdains him with elaborate insults. Lafew leaves, and Bertram reappears, declaring that he will run away to the wars in Italy before he will consummate his marriage to Helena. He plans to send Helena back to the Countess alone.

Act 2, Scene 4
Parolles conveys Bertram's instructions to Helena.

Act 2, Scene 5
Lafew warns Bertram not to rely on Parolles. Helena tells Bertram she is ready to leave; he pointedly avoids a farewell kiss. She departs, and Bertram and Parolles leave for Italy.

Act 3, Scene 1
The DUKE (4) of FLORENCE receives the First and Second Lords.

Act 3, Scene 2
The Countess reads Bertram's letter declaring that he has run away from his new wife, as Helena appears with the First and Second Lords, who are on leave from Florence. She reads aloud a letter from Bertram: he will not acknowledge her as his wife until she wears his ring and bears his child, which, he insists, will never happen. In a soliloquy, Helena decides that she must leave France and become a wanderer so that her husband may live unhindered by an unwanted wife.

Act 3, Scene 3
The Duke of Florence makes Bertram his general of cavalry. Bertram rejoices to be engaged in war, not love.

Act 3, Scene 4
The Steward reads a letter from Helena stating that she has become a pilgrim. The dismayed Countess orders him to write Bertram, asking him to return, hoping that Helena will eventually come back as well.

Act 3, Scene 5
The WIDOW (2) Capilet, a landlady of Florence, her daughter DIANA (1), and their neighbour MARIANA (1) remark that the new French general, Bertram, has attempted to seduce Diana, sending Parolles as his intermediary. Helena appears, identifying herself as a French pilgrim, and she is told about the general, whom the ladies have heard has rejected his wife. Helena agrees to lodge with the Widow.

Act 3, Scene 6
The two Lords propose to prove to Bertram that Parolles is a coward. They will kidnap him and make him believe he has been captured by the enemy; they are sure that he will betray his comrades out of fear while Bertram overhears his interrogation. Parolles enters and brags that he will retrieve a captured regimental drum, a prized emblem. He leaves, and the First Lord follows to prepare the plan; Bertram invites the Second Lord to visit Diana with him.

Act 3, Scene 7
Helena has told the Widow that she is Bertram's wife, and she proposes a plot: if Diana pretends to accept Bertram as a lover, Helena will substitute for the young woman in bed; Bertram will not recognise her in the dark. The Widow agrees.

Act 4, Scene 1
The First Lord instructs his men to pose as foreign mercenaries, pretending to speak in an exotic language to Parolles. The FIRST SOLDIER volunteers to act as their 'interpreter'. Parolles appears, wondering what excuse he can offer for returning without the drum. He is captured and immediately promises, through the 'interpreter', to reveal military secrets if his life is spared.

Act 4, Scene 2
Bertram attempts to talk Diana into sleeping with him. She demands that he give her his ring, a family heirloom, and also asks him to promise not to speak to her when they meet later that night. He agrees.

Act 4, Scene 3
The First and Second Lords discuss Bertram's disgrace for having left his wife, noting also that he has seduced a young woman by giving her his family ring. They have heard that his wife has died, and they regret that he is probably pleased by this. Bertram arrives, and the blindfolded Parolles is brought in to be 'interrogated'. He reveals military secrets, disparaging both Bertram and the Lords as he does so. The blindfold is removed, and Parolles sees who has exposed him. The Lords, Bertram, and the Soldiers bid him a sardonic farewell and leave for France, the war being over. Alone, Parolles declares that having been proven a fool, he will simply have to become a professional FOOL (1), or jester.

Act 4, Scene 4
Helena intends to take the Widow and Diana to the King's court at MARSEILLES, where she can get an escort to Rossillion and arrive ahead of Bertram.

Act 4, Scene 5
In Rossillion, Lafew, the Countess, and the Clown mourn Helena. Lafew proposes that Bertram marry his daughter, and the Countess agrees. Lafew has learned that the King will visit Rossillion shortly. The Clown reports Bertram's approach.

Act 5, Scene 1
In Marseilles, Helena and her companions encounter a GENTLEMAN (4) who informs them that the King has gone on to Rossillion.

Act 5, Scene 2
In Rossillion, Parolles, now in rags, is teased by the Clown. Lafew appears, and Parolles begs him for assistance. After chastising him for having earned his misfortune through knavery, Lafew promises him a position in his household.

Act 5, Scene 3
The King pardons Bertram for his part in Helena's death and tells him of his prospective marriage to Lafew's daughter. Bertram offers Lafew a ring to give his daughter. The King recognises it as the one he had given Helena, but Bertram claims that it came from an admirer in Florence. The unbelieving King orders him arrested. Diana arrives and asserts that Bertram cannot deny that he took her virginity. She produces his family ring and says that Parolles can testify to her relationship with him. Bertram insists that she seduced him and then demanded his ring; he equates the gift with payment to a prostitute. Parolles appears and states that Bertram's infatuation with Diana extended to promising marriage. Helena appears and claims Bertram as her husband, reminding him that he had said he would accept her when she wore his ring and bore his child. She says these things are done and tells of her impersonation in Diana's bed. The delighted King promises Diana a dowry if she wants to marry. He speaks an EPILOGUE to the audience, asking for applause.

COMMENTARY

All's Well That Ends Well presents the customary material of COMEDY—the triumph of love over obstacles—in a grotesque and ambivalent light, and this has led most scholars to place it with *Measure for Measure* and *Troilus and Cressida* among the so-called PROBLEM PLAYS. Like its fellows, *All's Well* centres on sex and social relations and offers no sure and convincing resolution at its conclusion, leading its audiences to recognise the inadequacy of humanity to live up to the grand ideals and happy endings of literary romance. Nevertheless, *All's Well* is humorous, and it does in the end offer the traditional comedic resolution, albeit in muted form.

Though love is the play's most prominent subject, there is a marked absence of the mutual joy of earlier Shakespearean lovers—as in, say, *Much Ado About Nothing*. Helena is obsessed with a clearly inferior man whose response to her is wholly negative until his grudging and heavily qualified acceptance at the close, and she wins him only through the rather sordid 'bed trick'. The comments of the Lords, the Clown, and other characters deflate the main plot even further. However, although the play supports negative interpretations, it is clear that Shakespeare did not intend such views to predominate. They are effectively countered by the positive attitudes of the Countess, the King, and Lafew. The playwright is careful to build his lovers up and to minimise the vileness of the bed trick, and he provided the traditional reconciliation scene at the close of the play. Moreover, in Helena's persistent

pursuit of Bertram despite his manifest unworthiness, some commentators have seen an allegory of Christian grace, though others disagree. In any case, many critics see an artistic failure in the playwright's attempt to force his naturalistic presentation of Bertram's snobbery and Helena's manipulation into the traditional mould of reconciliation comedy. That *All's Well* is weaker than many other Shakespearean dramas is widely conceded, but it remains of considerable interest precisely because of its conflict between naturalism and romantic fantasy. Though somewhat unsatisfying in its own terms, the play constitutes a step towards the ROMANCES, where a different approach to the same conflict yields more successful results.

All's Well centres on Helena. Though she is sometimes seen by critics as a satirical portrait of a possessive woman, this view seems contrary to Shakespeare's intentions, for he presents her in the most flattering of lights. She is the subject of highly complimentary remarks by the Countess and Lafew at the play's outset, and the King also admires her, both before and after the success of her medicine. In restoring a dying monarch to health, she resembles an heroine of age-old legends, and she takes on an appropriate aura of undoubted goodness. Later, the Widow and Diana welcome her into their lives enthusiastically, and upon her return to those who believe her dead, in 5.3, she is received with the awe due a goddess. Moreover, her immediate resolution of all problems seems to justify this reverence; she is a virtual *deus ex machina*.

The only cause for Bertram's rejection of Helena is her non-aristocratic status. In this respect she becomes an emblem of the play's point: true nobility resides in the spirit of an individual, not in his or her rank in the social hierarchy. This idea is expounded by the King when he chastises Bertram's snobbery, observing that 'From lowest place when virtuous things proceed, / The place is dignified by th' doer's deed' (2.3.125–126). Significantly, Helena's inferior social status was invented by Shakespeare for this purpose. In his source, both lovers were aristocrats of equal rank.

Given Helena's highly positive characteristics, the bed trick places her in less disrepute than it otherwise might. It may be seen as a symbol rather than a realistic manoeuvre, a mere plot device that fulfils our expectation that Helena will get her man. In the source, the bed trick results in the presentation of twin sons to the unwary father, but the playwright purposefully muted this outcome to an almost unnoticeable implication that Helena is pregnant in 5.3.307. Moreover, the extreme artificiality of the device, combined with its familiarity to Shakespeare's audience as an element of traditional folklore, help to distance its squalor from Helena's nobility of spirit. Lastly, its importance is further minimised by the prominence given to the exposure of Parolles while it is taking place. Helena is established as an heroine in the first half of the play, and thereafter—when her actions might not seem heroic—she plays a relatively minor role, becoming a central figure again only in the play's last moments.

Bertram, too, is favourably presented in the first half of the play. The Countess and the King both praise him, the Duke of Florence grants him high command despite his youth, and the First and Second Lords, while deploring his morals, recognise his potential worth and hope that their exposure of Parolles will cause the young count to 'take a measure of his own judgements' (4.3.31–32). Though his faults are plainly evident, Shakespeare's unmistakable position is that Bertram has underlying merit. The possibility that the young man will mature and reform is present throughout the play, helping us to accept his folly.

The nearest character to a villain in *All's Well* is Parolles. He is a braggart and a coward, and the depths of his ignobility are exposed when he proves willing to betray his comrades to save his life. Parolles offers another example of the moral that nobility is a matter of spirit, not rank: although a gentleman, apparently on a par with Bertram, he is presented from the outset as an unworthy man. Much of the blame we might otherwise attach to Bertram is placed on Parolles, who encourages his young friend in his errors and who precedes him in suffering humiliation and downfall. However, Parolles' very villainy makes him an appropriate object of redemption, and his response to his humiliation is telling, for he is resilient; he accepts his own nature and vows to go on as best he can, espousing the highly sympathetic sentiment that 'There's place and means for every man alive' (4.3.328). In this spirit, he falls within range of the play's reconciliation, finding a new career as jester to his old enemy, Lafew.

The basic developments of *All's Well* were provided by the play's source material, but Shakespeare inserted some significant details. Several new characters present distinctive slants on the action. As we have seen, Parolles deflects unfavourable attention from Bertram, while Lafew, the Countess, and the King (who appears in the source material but is much less prominent) are entirely wise and generous, in contrast to the more problematic major characters. They are elderly and are concerned with thoughts of death and fond recollections of their own youth, but, unlike the older characters in standard comedies of the day, they are not the opposition who must be defeated for love to triumph. Instead, they are benign figures who offer understanding and support for the lovers, thus establishing a context that muffles the unpleasant aspects of the story.

We have seen that Shakespeare intended his lovers to be well regarded, and the final reconciliation is in no way rendered impossible by the moral defects of the characters, as it seems to be in *Troilus and Cressida.*

Helena is a paragon of virtue, despite the machinations to which she is driven, and Bertram, who is admittedly sinful, is also forgivable. Nevertheless, the ambiguous nature of the lovers' relations puts a strain on the play's conclusion, and Shakespeare tightens this strain to an almost unbearable pitch as he postpones Helena's reappearance. Bertram disgraces himself ever more fully with lies and evasions, and even Diana is duplicitous in not revealing Helena's presence. The emotional tension that this generates is made evident even as it is relaxed, when Lafew admits that his 'eyes smell onions' (5.3.314) and borrows Parolles' handkerchief. This moment also clinches Lafew's acceptance of Parolles, and thus the two most corrupt characters—Parolles and Bertram—are forgiven. The scene's complex emotional tone reflects the reality of its world: as in life, happiness in *All's Well That Ends Well* is unpredictable and emerges, if at all, only through 'The web of our life [which] is of a mingled yarn, good and ill together' (4.3.68–69). Yet in the play's final line, the King fully expresses the spirit of traditional comedic resolution: 'The bitter past, more welcome is the sweet' (5.3.328).

Nonetheless, though the play's title—a proverb used twice by Helena, in 4.4.35 and 5.1.25—refers plainly to the conventionally happy ending of romantic comedy, Helena's happiness is just as clearly precarious. When she finally asks for Bertram's acceptance, he replies only to the King and only conditionally, in 5.3.309–310. Fittingly, the King's remark in the play's next-to-last line—wittily playing on the title—is ambiguous: 'All yet seems well' (5.3.327) is as far as he can go. Bertram and Helena's marital bliss is doubtful.

The naturalism of the play—its well-drawn characters and credible social milieu—leads us to expect a more plausible dénouement, and we emerge dissatisfied. The romance of an adventurous maiden who can cure kings is unsuccessfully integrated with the more realistic tale of sexual intrigue, and the two components of which the play is made—a psychologically real world versus a conventionally comic one—merge at the end only at a considerable cost in dramatic power.

The conclusion of *All's Well* unquestionably lessens its effectiveness, but if the play is considered in light of Shakespeare's development, its failings seem less significant and its ending less arbitrary. The problem plays are similar to the romances in a number of ways: both depend on unrealistic stories, and both emphasise the power of noble spirituality over circumstances. Particularly in their conclusions, both favour symbolism and ritual over psychological realism. However, in *All's Well* (as in *Measure for Measure*, especially), the latter element still has great power, and the balance between the two is uncomfortable, barring a firm sense that spiritual values have indeed triumphed, despite the play's assertion that they have. *Cymbeline* and *The Winter's Tale*, like *All's Well*, have endings that tax belief and that depend on the evocation of supernatural powers while maintaining the underlying assumption that naturalistic causes have in fact been operating. However, whereas the contradictions of *All's Well* generate an atmosphere of conflict and stress, similar polarities in the later plays yield a pleasurable sense of life's many aspects. In *All's Well That Ends Well*, Shakespeare had not yet developed the capacity to sublimate reality without denying it, but his instincts were leading him in that direction.

SOURCES OF THE PLAY

The main plot of *All's Well That Ends Well*, the story of Bertram and Helena, comes from the *Decameron* (1353) of Giovanni BOCCACCIO, who apparently invented it. Shakespeare used the translation by William PAINTER (2) of Boccaccio's tale in *The Palace of Pleasures* (probably in the 3rd ed., 1575), supplemented by the French translation by Antoine LE MAÇON, which Painter also used. Lord Lafew, the Countess of Rossillion, and the sub-plot concerning Parolles were Shakespeare's inventions, though the last may have been influenced by an episode in *The Unfortunate Traveller* (1594) by Thomas NASHE.

TEXT OF THE PLAY

All's Well was probably written c. 1604. However, no mention of the play prior to its publication in 1623 has survived, and its date of composition has troubled scholars. In the 18th century it was believed to be the mysterious LOVE'S LABOUR'S WON, cited as Shakespearean by Francis MERES in 1598; it was accordingly presumed to have been written before that year. However, *All's Well*'s obvious similarities to *Hamlet, Troilus and Cressida*, and *Measure for Measure* were soon recognised, and Samuel Taylor COLERIDGE introduced another hypothesis: he held that an early version of the play was indeed *Love's Labour's Won* but that Shakespeare rewrote and retitled it between 1604 and 1606. This suggestion was felt to account for perceivable differences in style within the play (as, e.g., the use of a SONNET in 3.4.4–17 and rhymed couplets in several passages). This theory was widely accepted until fairly recently. However, modern scholarship is more inclined to find stylistic variation normal in Shakespeare's plays and to suppose that *All's Well* was a single creation. There is no clear internal evidence to indicate a date for his composition, and estimates have ranged from 1599 to after 1608. However, scholars generally rely on *All's Well*'s close resemblance to the securely datable *Measure for Measure*—in its plot, its heroine, even in its vocabulary—and assign it the same date, 1604.

The play was first published in 1623, in the FIRST FOLIO. The Folio text is believed to have been printed

from Shakespeare's own manuscript, or FOUL PAPERS, for several reasons, most notably its vague and inconsistent speech headings and stage directions and the existence of VIOLENTA, a GHOST CHARACTER. The Folio text, though somewhat flawed, is necessarily the basis of all subsequent editions.

THEATRICAL HISTORY OF THE PLAY

No production of *All's Well* is known before a single performance of 1740, although several references suggest that it had been performed in the early 17th century. The play was popular in the 1740s—Theophilus CIBBER (3) was a popular Parolles, and Peg WOFFINGTON played Helena—but was revived only occasionally during the rest of the century. In the early 19th century a 1794 adaptation by John Philip KEMBLE (3), heavily abridged and censored, was performed from time to time, and this version was also put on by other producers, including Samuel PHELPS. However, the play was not frequently staged in any version.

Only in the second half of the 20th century has *All's Well* become more popular. Among noteworthy productions have been those of Robert ATKINS (1949), Tyrone GUTHRIE (1953 and 1959, in Stratford, Ontario and STRATFORD, England) and John BARTON (1967, Stratford, England). Guthrie's presentation—which in 1959 starred Zoë CALDWELL as Helena and Edith EVANS (1) as the Countess—was highly controversial; it freely abridged Shakespeare's text (the Clown was eliminated entirely) and treated the play as a farce, adding much comic stage business involving such modern props as a radio microphone. The scenes in Paris and Rossillion were set in an Edwardian world, while the Italian wars were startlingly represented by modern desert legionnaires. It was extremely popular at both Stratfords. Another production that evoked the punctilious society of the Edwardian era was Trevor NUNN's (1981–1983), which starred Peggy ASHCROFT as the Countess and moved from Stratford to London to Broadway. *All's Well* has also been produced twice for TELEVISION, in 1968 (Guthrie's version) and 1981.

Alonso, King of Naples Character in *The Tempest*, father of FERDINAND (2). In 2.1, when Alonso and his followers are shipwrecked on the magician PROSPERO's island, Alonso believes his son has drowned and his grief overwhelms him. In 3.3 Prospero's sprite ARIEL, disguised as a HARPY, declares Alonso, ANTONIO (5), and SEBASTIAN (3) to be 'three men of sin' (3.3.53) and reminds the king that he helped Antonio depose Prospero as Duke of Milan (before the play began). Ariel cites the loss of Ferdinand as Alonso's punishment. The three are made insane by Prospero's magic and must be revived at the play's end, in 5.1. Faced with Prospero, Alonso willingly surrenders Milan to him and begs his pardon. When Prospero reveals the surviving Ferdinand, Alonso is overjoyed; his 'I say, Amen' (5.1.204) offers a religious reference that reinforces the play's point that providence can restore human happiness.

Alonso symbolises several of the play's themes. His story demonstrates the Christian pattern of sin, suffering, repentance, and eventual recompense, thus supporting the play's presentation of moral regeneration and contributing to the final aura of reconciliation and forgiveness. His fall into madness and subsequent revival as a purified man is an instance of another important theme, transfiguration. Finally, his innate goodness—exemplified by his grief for Ferdinand and his admission of guilt—contrasts tellingly with the villainy of those around him, especially Antonio.

Ambassador (1) Any of several minor characters in *Henry V*, diplomats representing FRANCE (1) at the court of King HENRY V. In 1.2 one of the Ambassadors conveys the arrogant message of the DAUPHIN (3), including a mocking delivery of tennis balls, implying the king's fitness only for childish games. The insult offers Henry an occasion to declare war.

Ambassador (2) Minor character in *Hamlet*, an emissary from England to DENMARK. The Ambassador arrives at the Danish court, in 5.2, after the deaths of the KING (5), the QUEEN (9), LAERTES, and HAMLET. He reports on the execution of ROSENCRANTZ AND GUILDENSTERN, thereby completing an unfinished element in the play's plot. With FORTINBRAS, the Ambassador offers an outsider's shocked view of the bloody collapse of Denmark's monarchy, reinforcing the play's central theme that evil has a corrupting influence that spreads far beyond its immediate consequences.

Ambassador (3) Minor character in *Antony and Cleopatra*, a representative of ANTONY. In 3.12 the Ambassador carries his master's formal surrender to Octavius CAESAR (2) after the battle of ACTIUM, and in 3.13, after he has reported that Caesar refuses Antony's request for his life but offers leniency to CLEOPATRA if she will abandon Antony, Antony sends him back to Caesar with a challenge of hand-to-hand combat. Antony identifies the Ambassador as the 'schoolmaster' (3.11.71) of his and CLEOPATRA's children. In 3.12 DOLABELLA observes that the use of the schoolmaster as an emissary indicates the totality of Antony's defeat. This schoolmaster is identified by Shakespeare's source, PLUTARCH, as one Euphronius, presumably a Greek scholar but otherwise unknown in history. Plutarch adds that his diplomatic employment was necessary because of the earlier abandonment of Cleopatra by her attendant, ALEXAS.

Amiens Character in *As You Like It*, singer in the court of DUKE (7) Senior. Amiens has no distinct per-

sonality of his own and functions primarily to affirm the duke's sentiments about his exile in ARDEN (1). His songs, which he sings in 2.5.1–8, 2.5.35–42, and 2.7. 174–193, insist on the virtues of life in the woods, compared to life at court: 'Here shall [one] see / No enemy, / But winter and rough weather' (2.5.6–8).

Scholars believe that Amiens may have first been played by Robert ARMIN, a singer/comedian who joined Shakespeare's acting company, the CHAMBERLAIN'S MEN, just before *As You Like It* was written. Armin probably played TOUCHSTONE also, but Amiens' songs may have been created with his abilities in mind.

Amyot, Jacques (1513–1593) French writer and translator of PLUTARCH's *Lives.* Amyot's Plutarch, published in 1559 and now regarded as one of the greatest works of 16th-century French prose, was in turn translated into English by Sir Thomas NORTH and became Shakespeare's primary source for *Antony and Cleopatra, Coriolanus, Julius Caesar,* and *Timon of Athens* and a minor source for other plays. Amyot, born in great poverty, became a leading humanistic churchman and scholar, serving as Bishop of Auxerre and tutor to two French kings-to-be.

Anderson (1), Judith (b. 1898) Australian-born American actress. Anderson came to America in 1918 and began a long and successful career on the New York stage. Perhaps best known for her Medea, she is particularly associated with passionate and ruthless characters. Her Shakespearean roles have included LADY (6) Macbeth—in the 1941 production of Margaret WEBSTER [3] and in a 1960 FILM, both times opposite Maurice EVANS (4)—and Queen GERTRUDE, opposite John GIELGUD's HAMLET, in 1936. Anderson also played Hamlet herself, carrying on a tradition of female Hamlets extending back to the 18th century; she took the part in 1971, at the age of 73.

Anderson (2), Mary (1859–1940) American actress. Anderson, a California native, made her debut as JULIET (1) in Louisville, Kentucky, at 16. She then toured American cities for several years and established herself in New York at 18, in 1877. In 1882 she went to London, where she was successful in a variety of roles, including Juliet and ROSALIND. She returned to New York in 1885 and was regarded as one of the leading lights of the American theatre. In 1887 she was the first actress to play both PERDITA and HERMIONE in *The Winter's Tale.* Two years later she married and retired from the stage. She settled in England, near STRATFORD, where she lived the rest of her life.

Andrew (1) Ship mentioned in *The Merchant of Venice,* a reference that helps scholars to date the play. SALERIO alludes to a shipwreck as an 'Andrew dock'd in sand' (1.1.27); in the original published edition of the play, the name Andrew was printed in italics, evidently denoting a ship. Shakespeare was referring to an event of 1596 in which an English naval force, commanded by the Earl of ESSEX (2) and Charles HOWARD, captured or sank most of the ships in Cadiz, Spain's greatest Atlantic port, and sacked the town. One of the principal prizes of this expedition was the ship *St Andrew,* which was seized after having run aground during the battle; this vessel became an important British warship over the next few years. The news of the battle at Cadiz reached London on July 30, 1596; therefore, Shakespeare could not have completed *The Merchant of Venice* before then. Shakespeare's audiences doubtless recognised the reference, but its sense was lost to later generations until 20th-century scholarship rediscovered its meaning.

Andrew (2) Aguecheek, Sir Character in *Twelfth Night.* See SIR ANDREW.

Andromache Legendary figure and minor character in *Troilus and Cressida,* the wife of HECTOR. In 5.3, disturbed by dire omens, Andromache unsuccessfully tries to persuade Hector not to fight. The episode humanises the warrior by showing that he has a loving spouse, and it also stresses his fatal destiny. According to classical mythology, Andromache became the slave of ACHILLES' son after the fall of TROY, later marrying HELENUS.

Andronicus See MARCUS ANDRONICUS; TITUS (1).

Angelo (1) Minor character in *The Comedy of Errors,* a goldsmith and friend of ANTIPHOLUS OF EPHESUS. Angelo makes the gold necklace that figures in the confusions and misunderstandings at the play's heart. His effort to have Antipholus arrested for debt, having failed to pay for the necklace, results in ANTIPHOLUS OF SYRACUSE retreating into the sanctuary of the PRIORY (5.1.37). This flight triggers the play's final resolution.

Angelo (2) Character in *Measure for Measure,* deputy to the DUKE (9) of VIENNA and lustful pursuer of ISABELLA. Angelo abuses his office by refusing mercy to CLAUDIO (3) when it is obviously due. Then he attempts to extort sex from Isabella with a promise of a pardon for Claudio. Once he has slept with her (or so he thinks), he goes back on the deal and orders Claudio's execution. Angelo is saved, however, from actually committing these unforgivable deeds by the Duke's machinations—MARIANA (2), whom Angelo had deserted years earlier, replaces Isabella in his bed and, instead of Claudio's head, he is shown that of a criminal who has died naturally. Angelo is himself pardoned at the play's close, as part of its emphasis on forgiveness.

Angelo's criminality is a facet of the play's theme of

good government. His downfall results from an excess of zeal. The Duke is too lax, but Angelo errs in the other extreme. At first a righteous public servant—the Duke calls him 'A man of stricture and firm abstinence' (1.3.12)—he proves to be unreasonably stern. A grievous injustice, Claudio's death sentence, is the result. Angelo's rigid personality is seen to be a cause of evil. He ignores pleas for mercy; he is so confident in his own rightness that he never examines his own humanity—a point made by Isabella in 2.2. Blind to human nature, he is not only a bad ruler, he is also incapable of resisting his sudden lust for Isabella. His initial misdeeds lead him further into evil. He sees this himself and cries, 'Alack, when once our grace we have forgot, / Nothing goes right . . .' (4.4.31–32). It is the Duke who saves him from his own intentions and, after he marries Mariana, he is forgiven by the Duke.

Once Isabella's refusal to meet Angelo's demand has left Claudio facing death, in 3.1, the Duke takes over the play, and Angelo is not seen very much until his conviction and reprieve in 5.1. Because Shakespeare wished to employ the happy ending of traditional COMEDY, he was compelled to abandon the psychological portrait of Angelo, though the fallen deputy remains stern at the close, seeking death rather than marriage and forgiveness. Whether the villain's reduced importance is seen as a flaw in the play or simply as a strategy in the service of a non-realistic end depends on one's view of *Measure for Measure,* but in any case Angelo remains a powerful creation.

Angiers City in north-western FRANCE (1), present-day Angers, location for Acts 2 and 3 of *King John* and one scene in *1 Henry VI*. Angiers, capital of ANJOU, the ancient homeland of the PLANTAGENET (1) kings, is presented as a focus of the conflict between FRANCE (1) and England. In 2.1 two armies face each other at the gates of the city, which is acknowledged to be loyal to England. King JOHN (3) of England is opposed by the French ruler, King PHILIP (2), who is backing ARTHUR, whose crown John is said to have usurped. Each side attempts to persuade the town to admit its forces and honour its choice of king. The representative of Angiers—a CITIZEN (4) or HUBERT in various editions—devises a diplomatic solution: John's niece BLANCHE can marry Philip's son LEWIS (1). However, this alliance is quickly dissolved when the papal legate PANDULPH persuades Philip to declare war on John, and Angiers is the scene of a battle in 3.2. England's Queen ELEANOR is almost captured, but John defeats the French and seizes Arthur.

The events of 2.1 are fictitious, devised by Shakespeare to dramatise the disputed succession. He sets the scene in Angiers, the traditional Plantagenet seat, to provide a recognisable symbol of the English holdings in France. Similarly, the events of 3.1 are transferred to Angiers from their historical site at Mirabeau, a castle elsewhere in Anjou. In 5.3 of *1 Henry VI*, JOAN LA PUCELLE, or Joan of Arc, attempts to summon supernatural FIENDS while at Angiers.

Angus, Gilchrist, Thane of (active 1056) Historical figure and minor character in *Macbeth,* a Scottish nobleman. A minor follower of King DUNCAN in Act 1, with ROSSE he brings MACBETH the news that he has been named Thane of CAWDOR, in 1.3.89–116. Angus reappears in 5.2 and 5.4 as one of the Scottish rebels against Macbeth who join the army of Prince MALCOLM. Angus speaks very little, though he does deliver a telling description of the depraved Macbeth, who feels '. . . his title / Hang loose about him, like a giant's robe / Upon a dwarfish thief (5.2.20–22). His mere presence in Malcolm's army is significant, for the rebellion of the nobles demonstrates the extreme disorder in SCOTLAND caused by Macbeth's evil. The historical Thane of Angus, whose surname was Gilchrist, ruled a small territory in eastern Scotland. In 1056, as a reward for his services to Malcolm, he was named Earl of Angus as is anticipated in 5.9.28–30, but little more is known of him; Shakespeare took his name from a list of Malcolm's allies in his source, HOLINSHED's history.

Anjou Region in north-western FRANCE (1), a theatre of operations in the HUNDRED YEARS WAR and the location for several scenes in *1 Henry VI.* Three scenes, 5.2–4, are set in Anjou and concern the capture and trial of JOAN LA PUCELLE, or Joan of Arc. In 5.3 Joan attempts to enlist the aid of FIENDS at ANGIERS, present-day Angers, the capital of Anjou. Angiers is also the location of several scenes in *King John.*

Anne (1) Bullen (Boleyn) (c. 1507–1536) Historical figure and character in *Henry VIII,* the lover and later the wife of King HENRY VIII, and the mother of ELIZABETH (1). At Cardinal WOLSEY's banquet in 1.4, Anne chats pleasantly with Lord SANDS, before meeting Henry. The king is charmed by Anne when he dances with her, though she does not speak. In 2.3 Anne tolerantly accepts the OLD LADY's bawdy jesting about her potential relationship with the king, but her own mind is on the suffering of the rejected Queen KATHERINE. Thus, Shakespeare disassociates Anne's rise from Katherine's fall, which is blamed on Cardinal WOLSEY. Anne appears but does not speak at her own coronation in 4.1, and she is not present at the christening of her daughter Elizabeth in 5.4. She is depicted as a saintly woman, whose Protestantism is said to be a healthy influence on the king and the country. Her role in the play's events, however, is very understated, probably in order to avoid reminding the audience of her well-known fate: only three years later, after failing to produce sons, she was divorced and executed on trumped-up charges of adultery and treason. Any allu-

sion to this would undermine the play's emphasis on King Henry's growth to wisdom and on the general virtues of the TUDOR DYNASTY, of which Elizabeth was so prominent a member

The historical Anne Boleyn was very different from Shakespeare's Anne, and the course of her affair with the king is only sketchily presented in the play. We are not informed that the king had already had an affair with Anne's older sister, Mary, nor that Anne was pregnant with Elizabeth when the king married her. Anne's personality is hard to discern today, after centuries of accusation and defence, but she was certainly not the high-minded virgin of the play. She appears to have had other affairs before Henry—with the poet Thomas WYATT, at least—and her upbringing was notoriously scandalous. Anne's father, Thomas Boleyn (1477–1539), an ambitious merchant who had married a daughter of the Duke of NORFOLK (3), was a determined participant in the power politics of the king's court. His power and influence increased greatly as a result of his daughters' sexual relationships, and it seems likely that both girls were brought up with such possibilities in mind. Boleyn served Henry as ambassador to FRANCE (1), and from the age of about 12, Anne was a lady-in-waiting at the licentious court of King Francis I, where sexual intrigue was a way of life. King Francis later described Mary Boleyn as 'a great prostitute, infamous above all'—and though Anne is not implicated in such accounts, she was certainly close to the participants. Henry knew Anne slightly at this time: he considered having her marry an Irish nobleman as part of a diplomatic settlement, apparently at her father's suggestion.

Anne returned to England around 1522, when her older sister became Henry's mistress. Anne was soon banished from court for a romantic entanglement that interfered with a proposed political marriage, and it was only after her return in 1526 that Henry fell in love with her. She seems to have resisted his desire for sex for several years, probably in the hope of becoming a wife rather than a mistress, but once sure of her eventual legitimacy, she surrendered. In the meantime she and the king scandalised the court and humiliated Queen Katherine with such behaviour as public caresses and mocking remarks. In marked contrast to Shakespeare's portrait, Anne seems to have taken pains to show her disrespect for the older woman. Such behaviour made Anne widely unpopular with both courtiers and commoners, and her ultimate destiny was welcomed by many.

Anne (2), Lady (Anne Neville, 1456–1485) Historical figure and character in *Richard III,* the wife of King RICHARD III. Courted by Richard—the murderer of her late husband, the PRINCE (4) of Wales, and his father, King HENRY VI—Anne is half-hypnotised by his words and accepts a ring from him in 1.2. When she appears again, in 4.1, she is Richard's wife, and she is called to be crowned following his coup d'état. She predicts that he will murder her, and the play implies that he does so.

The historical Anne is alluded to, although in error, in 3.3.242 of *3 Henry VI,* when the Duke of WARWICK (3) agrees that his eldest daughter shall marry the Prince. Actually, Anne was Warwick's younger daughter, and, although she and the Prince were betrothed, they apparently did not actually marry. In any case, she married Richard in 1474. Historically, she did not attend the funeral of Henry VI, and her dialogue with Richard is entirely fictitious; Shakespeare invented it in order to create a scene that contrasts with Richard's later effort to negotiate a marriage with the daughter of Queen ELIZABETH (2). Also, there has never been any evidence that Anne was murdered; she seems to have died a natural death.

Anne (3) Page Character in *The Merry Wives of Windsor,* a marriageable young woman pursued by SLENDER, Dr CAIUS (2), and FENTON. Anne's father, George PAGE (12), favours Slender because he is rich, although completely vacuous. Her mother, MISTRESS (3) Page, prefers Dr Caius, who is an obnoxious but prestigious physician at Windsor Castle. Anne herself is in love with Fenton. A demure daughter, she urges Fenton to do his utmost to win over her father before they consider elopement. However, she has the good sense to see that the other two suitors are totally unacceptable. After Slender has proposed by observing that it isn't his idea to marry her, but that of his uncle and her father, Anne forthrightly pleads, 'Good mother, do not marry me to yond fool' (3.4.81), and when Mistress Page assures her that Dr Caius is more likely, she cries, 'Alas, I had rather be set quick i' th' earth, and bowl'd to death with turnips!' (3.4.85). When her parents each arrange her abduction by their chosen son-in-law, she rebels and urges Fenton to arrange their secret marriage, which her parents accept in the spirit of conciliation that closes the play.

Annesley, Brian (d. 1603) Contemporary of Shakespeare, a possible model for King LEAR. In 1603 Annesley, a one-time gentleman of the court of Queen ELIZABETH (1), had become insane and was the object of a court case; two of his three daughters sought to have him committed and his estates turned over to them. The third daughter, Cordell (a variant form of CORDELIA), opposed them and wrote to King JAMES I's minister, Robert CECIL (1), asserting that her father's service to the late monarch deserved a better reward than the madhouse. Cecil intervened and Annesley lived his final months in the care of a family friend. He bequeathed his estates to Cordell, and the other sisters went to court again but failed to break the will. This family was known to Shakespeare's patron and

friend, the Earl of SOUTHAMPTON (2); in fact, Cordell Annesley married Southampton's stepfather, William HERVEY, not long after her father's death. It is thus quite likely that the playwright—who was writing *King Lear* at the time of or shortly after Brian Annesley's death—knew of this case of madness and filial loyalty and may have incorporated something of it in his play.

Another Lord Character in *Richard II.* See LORD (2).

Antenor Legendary figure and character in *Troilus and Cressida,* a Trojan warrior captured by the Greeks and exchanged for CRESSIDA. This exchange is crucial to the development of the play's love plot, but Antenor's role is otherwise insignificant. He appears in five scenes but never speaks, serving merely to swell the ranks of the Trojan aristocracy.

However, Antenor has a hidden importance, for, in the version of the legend known to Elizabethan England, he later betrayed TROY to the Greeks. Shakespeare does not mention this, presuming that his audience would know it; the knowledge makes evident a striking piece of dramatic irony. When CALCHAS, a Trojan deserter to the Greeks, proposes the prisoner exchange in 3.3, the audience knows, although the characters do not, that he has thus laid the groundwork for two more betrayals beside his own, that of TROILUS by Cressida and, more importantly, that of Antenor against Troy. This irony is signalled by the remarks made about Antenor. He is seen as a very important Trojan—PANDARUS praises him as 'one o'th'soundest judgements in Troy' (1.2.194), and Calchas says that 'Troy holds him very dear . . . their negotiations all must slack, / Wanting his manage' (3.3.19, 24–25).

Anthony Minor character in *Romeo and Juliet,* a SERVING-MAN (2) who helps clear tables in 1.5.

Antigonus Character in *The Winter's Tale,* nobleman at the court of King LEONTES of SICILIA. Antigonus, like his wife, PAULINA, defends Queen HERMIONE against the king's unjust accusation of adultery, and he protests against the cruelty of killing the infant PERDITA, whom the king believes is illegitimate. Leontes threatens him with death for failing to control Paulina's bitter criticism and orders the old man to take the baby and abandon it in the wilderness. Antigonus accepts the king's order and leaves the child on the coast of BOHEMIA, where he is killed and eaten by a BEAR.

Shakespeare has Antigonus die partly so that his knowledge of Perdita's whereabouts will not be available to the repentant Leontes of Act 3. But, more important, the old man's death has a moral point. The bear provides a particularly appalling end for Antigonus, an emblem of the sin of co-operating with evil. Though he is a generally sympathetic figure, humorous when admittedly overwhelmed by Paulina, and courageous in his initial protests to Leontes, he must be compared with his wife, who resists the king's tyranny. Antigonus, though reluctant, is weak; he permits duty to the king to overrule his sense of justice and becomes the agent of Leontes' evil madness. He even comes to believe in Hermione's guilt, as he declares in his soliloquy before abandoning Perdita.

Antigonus' death is part of the workings of providence that underlies the play. At the same time, since he is himself a victim of the king's madness, his death—like that of MAMILLIUS and the MARINER (1)—is an example of the human cost of evil. Antigonus comes to embody the tragic developments of the first half of the play, and his death signals their end, as the drama moves from tragedy to redemption.

Antigonus undergoes a modest redemption himself. The hearty old gentleman who invokes 'the whole dungy earth' (2.1.157) and acknowledges his overwhelming wife with a 'La you now' (2.3.50) is altered by the experiences fate ordains for him. He dares to criticise the king, even if he cannot persist, and he assumes responsibility for Perdita. In his dream of Hermione, he also seems to have a supernatural visitation from the dead. As he leaves Perdita, he recognises his involvement with evil, despairing, 'Weep I cannot, / But my heart bleeds; and most accurs'd am I / To be by oath enjoin'd to this' (3.3.51–53). About to die, he speaks in a poetic diction that elevates him to a nobler level.

Antioch Capital city of the ancient Seleucid Kingdom, located in what is now Turkey, the setting for the first scene of *Pericles.* PERICLES discovers the secret of the incestuous love between King ANTIOCHUS the Great and his DAUGHTER (1), and he must flee the king's anger. Thus, Antioch is the root of the evil that propels Pericles into a wandering exile, the basic premise of the play.

Antiochus, king of Syria (c. 238–187 B.C.) Historical figure and character in *Pericles,* the incestuous father of the DAUGHTER (1) courted by PERICLES. In 1.1 Antiochus proposes a riddle. He who solves it will win the hand of his daughter in marriage, but any who fail will be executed. A row of severed heads attests to many failures. Pericles solves the riddle, but it reveals the king's incest, and, horrified, he withdraws his suit. Antiochus realises that his secret has been uncovered and he decides to kill Pericles, though he attempts to delude his victim by giving him an extra 40 days to answer the riddle. When Pericles flees, Antiochus sends THALIARD in pursuit with orders to murder him. Antiochus appears only in the opening scene and is a conventionally false and vicious villain. In Act 2 the good King SIMONIDES is contrasted with him, and Antiochus' death by 'a fire from heaven' is reported in 2.4.9.

As the play's only historical figure, Antiochus provides us with a date for its action. However, this was unimportant to Shakespeare, who took the name from his sources, which included him because he was one of the most famous rulers of the Greek lands of the eastern Mediterranean. Known as Antiochus the Great, he was a king of the Seleucid dynasty, heirs to a portion of the empire founded by Alexander the Great. Antiochus waged a number of largely unsuccessful wars and is known as 'the Great' because he carried a campaign to 'India' (actually Afghanistan) rather than for any lasting accomplishments. However, he did develop his capital city, and made it one of the great metropolises of its day, after which, as ANTIOCH, it bore his name. No evidence exists that Antiochus was incestuous, though he did have daughters, one of whom, Cleopatra, was married to a ruler of Ptolemaic Egypt and was thus the ancestor of Shakespeare's Egyptian queen. However, the playwright probably did not know of this connection.

Antipholus of Ephesus; Antipholus of Syracuse Characters in *The Comedy of Errors,* long-separated twins who are comically confused with each other and eventually reunited. The twins were parted, each with a different parent, in a shipwreck when they were infants. Twin servants, each called DROMIO, were being brought up with the boys, and they too were separated in the wreck, one going with each master. In 1.1 the twins' father, EGEON, explains their history before they appear, so the audience knows of their relationship, though neither they nor any of the other characters do. In adulthood, the twins have both become merchants, each from a different city, but each bearing the same name.

The two brothers are distinctly different characters. Antipholus of Syracuse arrives in Ephesus, searching the world for his lost brother, for he cannot feel whole until he finds his family. In Ephesus, he is mistaken for his twin, a well-known local merchant, and various strangers startle him by knowing his name and assuming he knows them.

He finds himself dining in his brother's home, and his brother's wife, ADRIANA, believes him to be her husband. Antipholus of Syracuse is so completely mystified by his curious circumstances that he blindly accepts them. Misunderstanding and confusion continue to abound until Antipholus of Syracuse is driven to take refuge in a priory.

Meanwhile, Antipholus of Ephesus has been subjected to similar difficulties, but his responses are characteristically more angry than bemused. For example, when locked out of his house by servants and wife (who believe him an imposter, for the other Antipholus is dining there), he proposes to force his way in with a crow-bar but is dissuaded from this course.

In the end, the brothers are reunited, as the DUKE (3) of Ephesus attempts to resolve the disorders that the confusion has created. The Dromios are brought back together again as well; Antipholus of Ephesus and Adriana are reconciled; Antipholus of Syracuse is free to woo Luciana; and the twins' parents, Egeon and EMILIA (1), rediscover each other, too. The story of the twins presents in an early work a theme that was to be important in Shakespearean COMEDY, the power of providential happenings to defeat potential evil through a general reconciliation. This theme provides the moral ground beneath the farcical atmosphere of *The Comedy of Errors.*

Antium Ancient Italian city on the Mediterranean coast south of ROME, the setting for three scenes of *Coriolanus.* Antium is the home of AUFIDIUS, the leader of the VOLSCIANS. When the Roman general CORIOLANUS is expelled from Rome, he seeks revenge and goes to Antium, in 4.4 and 4.5, and offers his services to his country's enemies. Coriolanus' mother dissuades him from sacking Rome with his victorious Volscian troops, and he makes a treaty instead. After this, in 5.6, he reports to the Volscian leaders in Antium, where Aufidius accuses him of treason and kills him. There is no hint, in dialogue or stage directions, as to the character of the city; Shakespeare merely followed his source, PLUTARCH's *Lives,* when he placed the action there. (There is some confusion as to the location of 5.6, which seems to be Antium in 5.6.50, 73, and 80, and CORIOLES in 5.6.90. However, the latter reference is probably rhetorical, though Shakespeare may have carelessly incorporated two settings. This is the sort of error that recurs throughout the plays, and most editors omit a location in the introductory stage directions or place the scene in Antium.)

The historical Antium—the modern Anzio—was an important Volscian stronghold, but it became a Roman colony in 338 B.C. Several centuries later, as part of the Roman Empire, Antium was an aristocratic resort town. It has provided several artistically significant archaeological sites, including the famed villa of the emperor Nero.

Antonio (1) Minor character in *The Two Gentlemen of Verona,* the father of PROTEUS. Antonio appears only once, in 1.3, to make the decision that he will send his son to join VALENTINE at court, which results in Proteus' encounter with SILVIA and its subsequent complications.

Antonio (2) Title character in *The Merchant of Venice.* Antonio borrows money from SHYLOCK and agrees to let the usurer cut away a pound of his flesh if he defaults on the repayment. Antonio represents the ideal

of selfless generosity that the play advocates. He borrows only in order to help his spendthrift friend BASSANIO, who wishes to appear wealthy as he woos PORTIA (1). Antonio's extravagant willingness to risk his money—and his life—stands in opposition to Shylock's calculating greed. Also, his often expressed fondness for Bassanio represents another literary ideal of Shakespeare's day—that of close friendship between males—which the playwright dealt with more extensively in *The Two Gentlemen of Verona.* Although this motif was a common one, some scholars contend that the intensity of Antonio's affection for Bassanio may demonstrate homosexual tendencies in Shakespeare. Whether or not this is the case, Antonio is a passive, melancholy, somewhat colourless man, stoical in the face of death and lonely amid the lovers' happiness at the play's end.

Antonio (3) Character in *Much Ado About Nothing,* brother of LEONATO. Antonio is a charming old gentleman, especially when he flirts with URSULA at the MASQUE in 2.1, undismayed when his identity is betrayed by his palsy. He is an unimportant member of Leonato's entourage until 5.1, when, sharing his brother's anger at Don PEDRO and CLAUDIO (1) over their humiliation of HERO, he challenges the two younger men to a duel. His extravagant and blustery rage is somewhat comic, particularly since the audience is aware of the imminent resolution of Hero's dilemma, but it is also touching evidence of Antonio's loyalty to his brother and niece.

Antonio (4) Character in *Twelfth Night,* friend of SEBASTIAN (2). After rescuing Sebastian from a shipwreck, Antonio admires the young man so much that he wishes to become his servant. Sebastian rejects this offer, but Antonio follows him to the court of Duke ORSINO of ILLYRIA, although he has many enemies there. In 3.4 he mistakes Sebastian's twin sister, VIOLA, who is disguised as a man, for Sebastian; the episode adds to the play's comic complexities. Antonio's increasing distress—he believes that Sebastian has betrayed him when Viola doesn't acknowledge him, and he is arrested and threatened with death as an old foe of Orsino—contributes to the play's undertone of disquiet and potential violence.

Antonio has had a career at sea, either as a privateer or a naval officer (described in 3.3.26–35 and 5.1.50–61), but otherwise he has little distinctive personality. In addition to participating in minor twists of the plot, he is intended primarily to establish, through his attitude towards Sebastian, the young nobleman's attractive qualities. Indeed, Antonio's references to Sebastian—'I do adore thee so . . .' (2.1.46) and 'how vile an idol proves this god' (3.4.374)—are cited by theorists who believe that Shakespeare intended a religious statement in his portrayal of the young man (see TWELFTH NIGHT, 'Commentary').

Antonio (5) Character in *The Tempest,* villainous brother of PROSPERO. Before the play begins, as we learn in 1.2, Antonio deposed Prospero as Duke of MILAN with the help of King ALONSO of Naples. Fearful of Prospero's popularity, he staged a natural death for the duke, abandoning him and his daughter MIRANDA in a small boat at sea. In the play Antonio, along with Alonso and others, is shipwrecked on the island that Prospero rules in exile. He continues to display his villainy in large and small ways, derogating the optimism of GONZALO and encouraging Alonso's brother SEBASTIAN (3) to assassinate the king and assume the throne of Naples. His manipulation of Sebastian in 2.1.197–285 is a striking demonstration of Macchiavellian villainy, and for this Antonio has been compared to Shakespeare's great villains RICHARD III and IAGO.

Antonio, Alonso, and Sebastian are all captured by Prospero, who casts a spell of witless insanity on them; when he releases them from the spell, he takes back his duchy and forgives them their crimes in an atmosphere of reconciliation. Antonio, however, refuses to accept this reconciliation, remaining silent when even the bestial CALIBAN assents. He thereby represents an important qualification to the play's sense of good's triumph: evil cannot be entirely compensated for in a world of human beings, for there are always Antonios who simply will not accept good.

Antony, Mark (Marcus Antonius) (c. 82–30 B.C.) Historical figure, character in *Julius Caesar* and title character in *Antony and Cleopatra.* In the former play Antony leads the forces opposing the assassins of Julius CAESAR (1), led by Marcus BRUTUS (4). In the latter, his love for CLEOPATRA leads to his downfall and the triumph of Octavius CAESAR (2).

In *Julius Caesar,* Antony is a courageous but crafty schemer whose political skill brings about a civil war. He helps demonstrate the social harm done by the powerful when they pursue their political ends. On the other hand, Antony, a strong personality, is an emotionally honest man and a much more sympathetic character than the virtuous, but cold and domineering, Brutus. Thus, Antony is both a positive and a negative figure who contributes greatly to the moral uncertainty that is at the heart of the play.

Part of Antony's power in *Julius Caesar* comes from Shakespeare's careful presentation of him. In the first two Acts he is an unimportant figure who speaks only 33 words, but other characters refer to him numerous times and acknowledge his potential greatness. Most significantly, Cassius desires that Antony be killed along with Caesar (2.1.155–161). He calls him a

'shrewd contriver' and accurately predicts that if he lives he will be a difficult opponent.

These references prepare us for Antony's sudden dominance of the play in Act 3. Even before he appears, the message he sends to Caesar's assassins (3.1. 126–137) establishes his strong personal style; a confident and powerful tone, both rhetorical and emotional. He soon arrives in person, and his initial response to the sight of Caesar's corpse is direct, uncalculated, heartfelt grief. Even in the presence of the murderers he does not hide his initial outburst. But he quickly turns to the future and takes control when he arranges to speak at Caesar's funeral.

His boldness and fervour are both powerful and charming, but Antony disqualifies himself for our moral sympathy with the long soliloquy (3.1.254–275) in which he proposes to provoke a ghastly civil war—he describes the bloody slaughter of innocent people in detail—in order to avenge Caesar's death. Antony's fine human qualities—his courage and intelligence—bring about tragic consequences.

Our ambivalence about Antony is furthered by his magnificent funeral oration (3.2.75–254), one of Shakespeare's most renowned passages. The speech's virtues—its bold rhetoric, its manipulative presentation of evidence, its appeal to pathos—seem to be clever but cheap effects intended to exploit the passions of the unthinking multitude. Certainly the speech has this effect, as Antony knew it would. But one realises that Antony does not seek to advance himself personally, and that he does not resort to slander against Brutus, or downright dishonesty. Antony is genuinely grieved by Caesar's death, and his expression of it, while extremely inflammatory, is not false. He actually feels the way he brings his audience to feel. And we, too, are moved to share his emotion, even as we are aware of Brutus' virtues in contrast with the mayhem Antony intends.

In 4.1, in an episode invented by Shakespeare to intensify our response to Antony, he bargains away the life of his nephew PUBLIUS (2). In contrast with Brutus' refusal to kill Antony, this action seems particularly detestable. Moreover, Antony also proposes to loot Caesar's bequest to the people, and his attitude to his ally LEPIDUS, whom he regards as no more than a tool, reinforces a sense that he is a cynical politician. As we approach the play's climax at the battle of PHILIPPI, we are inclined to favour Antony's foes, Brutus and Cassius.

However, at the close of the play when Antony delivers his famous eulogy of Brutus (5.5.68–75), he is very generous, and the balance of our sympathy is somewhat restored. Antony not only acknowledges Brutus' noble motive in killing Caesar, he also observes that Brutus was unable to recognise the true nature of his fellow conspirators. Thus, Antony emphasises once more the play's chief theme: that evil can attend good intentions when established rulers are unseated.

In *Antony and Cleopatra*, written about seven years later, Antony again contributes much to the ambivalence that characterises the work. He is both a major political figure and the protagonist of a love story. As a result of his love, his position in the world undergoes great change. Initially, he wields immense power, ruling half the known world—a status that Shakespeare emphasises with a persistent stream of political affairs. However, he wilfully throws this position away for the sake of his passion—a passion whose self-indulgence is stressed by repeated descriptions of the opulent luxury of Cleopatra's court.

As a soldier, Antony has proven himself a model of Roman military virtues—the Romans are dissatisfied with his conduct in Egypt precisely because they value his earlier record as a 'mate in empire, / Friend and companion in the front of war' (5.1.43–44), whose 'goodly eyes . . . Have glow'd like plated Mars' (1.1. 2–4). His earlier successes enacted in *Julius Caesar* are referred to several times, as in 3.2.54–56. Antony values himself for the same reasons and regrets his 'blemishes in the world's report' (2.3.5), but he is trapped in another role by his intense attraction to Cleopatra. Under her influence he has become a voluptuary; he has abandoned his duty for the 'love of Love, and her soft hours' (1.1.44) in Alexandria.

As a lover, Antony offers us a glimpse of the transcendent nature of passion, a theme that Cleopatra will triumphantly present—in Antony's name—after his death. In 1.1 when Cleopatra, as the wily courtesan, demands that he declare how much he loves her, Antony states that love cannot be totalled, for lovers must 'find out new heaven, new earth' (1.1.17). Thus, it is he who introduces the theme of transcendence through love, and this desire is emphasised by hints of the book of Revelation that frame his story in the play. Indeed, 'new heaven, new earth' is very close to the biblical text (cf. Rev. 21:1)—much more familiar to 17th-century audiences than it is to today's—and the imagery that marks his death confirms the association: 'The star is fall'n. / And time is at his period' (4.14. 106–107 [cf. Rev. 8:10; 10:6]).

Although Cleopatra disrupts Antony's loyalty to Rome, he is not totally committed to her either. Though he only tears himself from her with difficulty, in 1.3, he returns to Rome and makes a political marriage to OCTAVIA. Further, his love for Cleopatra is mingled with distrust—with considerable justification, for the Egyptian queen only transcends the behaviour of a courtesan after Antony's death—and he dies presuming she will strike a bargain with his conqueror, Caesar. Moreover, he dies not as a tragically committed lover, but rather more like a clever Roman politician—albeit a loving one—when he offers Cleopatra advice on the politics of Caesar's court. Antony dem-

onstrates that the ideals of love and power are both insufficient, thus manifesting the duality presented by the play as a whole.

Shakespeare followed his source—PLUTARCH's *Lives*—fairly closely in his account of the historical career of Marcus Antonius, with two exceptions. As already noted, the playwright invented Antony's callous sacrifice of a nephew in *Julius Caesar*, and in *Antony and Cleopatra* he placed Antony's involvement with Cleopatra earlier in the sequence of events; in Plutarch the love affair did not actually begin until after Antony's marriage to Octavia. Thus Shakespeare's Antony seems indecisive about his loyalties, if not actually disloyal to Cleopatra as well as to Octavia. However, the change may simply have been motivated by dramatic strategy, for it is obviously better to begin the play with the love affair than to introduce it in the middle, after the political situation has evolved.

However, in *Antony and Cleopatra* Shakespeare departed from the general impression of Antony left by Plutarch. For the ancient historian, Antony was simply a moral failure, a man who threw away his life because he was unable to control his appetites. Antony's catastrophic moral collapse justified Caesar's war against him, and his defeat was entirely for the good. Shakespeare, however, made certain that we would see that Antony's vices contained germs of virtue, that his passion was firmly bound to a noble, if ill-defined, idea of love.

Plutarch depended on pro-Caesar sources (see, e.g., MESSALA) since the victorious Caesar permitted no others to survive, and thus his account is unfairly biased against Antony in the opinion of modern scholars. The debauchery indulged in by Marcus Antonius was rather ordinary among the powerful Roman aristocrats of the time, and we cannot be certain that the political concessions he made to Cleopatra were in fact made at all, nor that they were as foolish as they seem in the sources. In any case, modern scholars generally agree that it was not his affair with Cleopatra that ruined Antonius, but rather his political and military failings—had he been more clever and ruthless, he might have enforced the maintenance of the joint rule that Caesar upset, or he might have triumphed himself, and ruled Rome.

Antony and Cleopatra

SYNOPSIS

Act 1, Scene 1

In ALEXANDRIA the Roman PHILO laments to DEMETRIUS that their leader, ANTONY, is involved with the Egyptian queen, CLEOPATRA, and neglects his military duties. Cleopatra and Antony appear as news from ROME arrives, and she taunts him and accuses him of subservience to his wife and the Roman senate. He therefore refuses to hear the messages.

Act 1, Scene 2

An Egyptian SOOTHSAYER (2) predicts that Cleopatra's waiting-woman CHARMIAN shall outlive her mistress, and adds that she has seen better times in the past than she shall in future. He sees an identical fortune for another waiting-woman, IRAS. The two women laugh over these predictions with their fellow servant ALEXAS. Cleopatra arrives and declares that she will not speak with Antony, who is approaching, and then leaves with her servants. Antony arrives accompanied by a MESSENGER (23) who bears the news that Antony's feuding wife and brother had united to fight against Octavius CAESAR (2), but were defeated. The Messenger also states that a renegade Roman general has led the Parthians in a conquest of Roman territory. Antony is angry with himself, for the conquered lands were lost while he was dallying with Cleopatra. More news arrives: Antony's wife has died. Antony dismisses the messengers and reflects that he had wished his wife dead and now regrets it; he now wishes he could break away from Cleopatra. He summons his lieutenant ENOBARBUS, who makes bawdy jokes about Antony's affair with the queen until Antony sternly orders preparations for a return to Rome where he is needed to aid Caesar against a rebel, POMPEY (2).

Act 1, Scene 3

Charmian advises Cleopatra to accommodate Antony in every way if she wants him to love her, but the queen rejects this idea. Antony appears and announces his departure; Cleopatra taunts him, but he remains determined, and she finally wishes him well. He assures her of his love.

Act 1, Scene 4

In Rome Caesar disgustedly tells LEPIDUS of Antony's debauchery with Cleopatra. News arrives of the rebel Pompey (2), aided by the pirates MENECRATES and MENAS. Caesar hopes that Antony will return to the soldierly ways he was once famous for.

Act 1, Scene 5

In Alexandria Cleopatra grieves over Antony's absence and praises him enthusiastically. Charmian teasingly reminds her that she had once felt the same about Julius CAESAR (1) when he was in Egypt years earlier.

Act 2, Scene 1

In MESSINA Pompey confers with Menas and Menecrates. He states that his chances of defeating Caesar and Lepidus are good since Antony, their ally, dallies in Egypt. News arrives that Antony is about to rejoin his friends; Pompey worries but continues to hope for the best.

Act 2, Scene 2

Lepidus entreats Enobarbus to encourage in Antony a peaceful attitude towards Caesar, but Enobarbus de-

clares that Antony's honour comes first. Antony and Caesar arrive to negotiate. Antony denies any part in the rebellion of his wife and brother. He apologises for not having assisted Caesar against it and admits that he has been too decadent in Egypt. The two leaders agree to put the issue aside and fight together against Pompey, and to further their alliance Antony shall marry Caesar's sister OCTAVIA. The leaders leave together while their followers remain, and Enobarbus tells MAECENAS and AGRIPPA about the gorgeous Cleopatra. He predicts that Antony will never leave her for good.

Act 2, Scene 3
Antony, married to Octavia, promises faithfulness. He consults the Soothsayer who has come to Rome with him. The seer advises him to return to Egypt because Caesar's presence diminishes his prospects for success. Antony decides to follow this advice.

Act 2, Scene 4
Lepidus, Maecenas, and Agrippa prepare to leave Rome; they will meet Antony on campaign against Pompey.

Act 2, Scene 5
In Alexandria Cleopatra receives word that Antony has married Octavia. Raging, she threatens the MESSENGER (25) with death; calming, she sinks into depression.

Act 2, Scene 6
Pompey agrees to a truce with Antony, Caesar, and Lepidus. The leaders leave to attend a celebratory feast aboard Pompey's ship. Enobarbus and Menas stay behind and gossip; they agree that Pompey should have maintained his rebellion while he could. Enobarbus predicts that Antony will abandon Octavia for Cleopatra.

Act 2, Scene 7
At the banquet the drunken Lepidus is teased by the other leaders. Menas takes Pompey aside and suggests that they kill all three Roman leaders, leaving Pompey the sole ruler of the empire, but Pompey declares that while he could approve such an action after it was done, he cannot honourably order it ahead of time. To himself, Menas declares that he will desert this foolishly scrupulous master, for Pompey will obviously lose in the political wars. Caesar declares that their drunkenness is wasteful and leaves. The other leaders follow.

Act 3, Scene 1
Antony's general VENTIDIUS (1), who has defeated a Parthian army, tells his lieutenant SILIUS that he will not pursue the fleeing enemy. He states that he does not want to succeed too thoroughly lest Antony feel overshadowed and in revenge crush his military career. Silius admires Ventidius' political shrewdness. They go to meet Antony in ATHENS.

Act 3, Scene 2
Antony and his followers prepare to depart from Rome. Caesar and Octavia are deeply moved at the separation, while he and Antony exchange tense and suspicious farewells.

Act 3, Scene 3
Cleopatra interrogates the Messenger about Octavia; he tells her that Antony's new wife is an unattractive woman and details her unappealing features. The queen is greatly relieved.

Act 3, Scene 4
In Athens Octavia is upset by the rising enmity between her husband and her brother and begs to be sent as an intermediary between them. Antony agrees, and she prepares to go to Rome.

Act 3, Scene 5
EROS informs Enobarbus that Caesar and Lepidus have defeated Pompey, but that Caesar has arrested Lepidus and sentenced him to death. Enobarbus anticipates war between Antony and Caesar.

Act 3, Scene 6
In Rome Caesar angrily reports that Antony, now in Egypt, has crowned himself and Cleopatra rulers of the eastern empire—a betrayal of both Octavia and Caesar and a virtual act of war against Rome. Octavia appears to negotiate for Antony, whom she believes is still in Athens.

Act 3, Scene 7
At an army camp near ACTIUM Enobarbus tells Cleopatra that her presence is a distraction to Antony, but she insists on remaining. Antony appears and remarks that Caesar has made a very rapid advance. He declares he will accept Caesar's challenge to fight a naval battle, despite the objections of his advisers that they are weakest at sea.

Act 3, Scene 8
Caesar warns his general TAURUS not to fight on land until after the sea battle.

Act 3, Scene 9
Antony orders Enobarbus to establish a post from which to observe the sea battle.

Act 3, Scene 10
Troops from both sides march past; a sea battle is heard. Enobarbus despairs as he sees Antony's flagship retreat. SCARUS reports that just as the battle might have been won by Antony's navy, Cleopatra sailed away from it. Antony followed, and the rest of the fleet followed him. CANIDIUS arrives and confirms the news of defeat. He declares that he will surrender his forces to Caesar.

Act 3, Scene 11
Antony tells his attendants to flee, for he no longer deserves their loyalty. He declares to Cleopatra that though he is filled with despair, his love for her still seems worth all that has been lost.

Act 3, Scene 12
An AMBASSADOR (3) delivers to Caesar Antony's request that he be permitted to live in Egypt or Athens and that Cleopatra continue to rule Egypt. Caesar sends him back with a rejection of Antony's request and an assurance to Cleopatra that she can have whatever she wants if she will kill Antony or drive him from Egypt. Then he sends THIDIAS to her with the same message, telling him to make her any promises he chooses.

Act 3, Scene 13
Thidias arrives and declares to Cleopatra that Caesar believes she had joined Antony out of fear, not love. The queen accepts Caesar's offer of deliverance from Antony. Antony appears as Thidias kisses Cleopatra's hand in acknowledgement of her alliance with Caesar. Antony has his SERVANTS (22) carry Thidias away and whip him, and he accuses Cleopatra bitterly. When the beaten Thidias is returned, Antony sends him back to Caesar with a defiant message. Cleopatra says that despite her surrender to Caesar she still loves Antony. He takes heart and declares that he is prepared to carry on the war against Caesar, who has arrived at Alexandria, with the remnants of his forces. He says that they will have a grand banquet that night, as in the past, and he and Cleopatra leave to prepare for it. Enobarbus reflects on Antony's folly and decides that he will desert him.

Act 4, Scene 1
Caesar describes Antony's contemptuous challenges. Maecenas recommends attacking immediately, for Antony's judgement is clearly clouded by anger, and Caesar agrees.

Act 4, Scene 2
At the banquet Antony declares that he'll fight to the end and either win or recover his honour in death. When he bids the SERVITORS farewell he suggests that this night might be his last. When the servants and Enobarbus weep, he declares that, on the contrary, they will triumph the next day.

Act 4, Scene 3
A group of Antony's sentries hear strange noises that they take to be a bad omen for the forthcoming battle.

Act 4, Scene 4
Antony lets Cleopatra help him into his armour, and he leaves for the battle in high spirits.

Act 4, Scene 5
Antony learns that Enobarbus has deserted to Caesar but he is not angry. He recognises that his own faults have driven his subordinate to despair. He orders Enobarbus' belongings sent to him.

Act 4, Scene 6
At Caesar's headquarters a SOLDIER (10) brings Enobarbus the belongings sent by Antony, and the deserter is stricken by pangs of conscience. He declares that he will die of a broken heart.

Act 4, Scene 7
Agrippa and his troops retreat before Antony and Scarus' forces. Scarus is wounded but insists on continuing the pursuit.

Act 4, Scene 8
Victorious in the day's fighting, Antony returns to Cleopatra. He praises Scarus for his great bravery and prowess.

Act 4, Scene 9
Outside Caesar's camp a SENTRY (2) and his WATCHMEN (4) discover the dying Enobarbus, who regrets his disloyalty and grieves for his lost honour.

Act 4, Scene 10
Antony and Scarus prepare for a combined battle on both land and sea.

Act 4, Scene 11
Caesar decides to concentrate on fighting at sea.

Act 4, Scene 12
Scarus muses on bad omens and on Antony's fretful mood. Antony announces that Cleopatra's navy has deserted to Caesar and that the battle is lost. He sends Scarus to order a general retreat, and he reflects that his desperate condition is the fault of his infatuation with Cleopatra, whom he believes has betrayed him. Cleopatra appears and Antony drives her away with his rage. He declares that he will kill her.

Act 4, Scene 13
Cleopatra flees from Antony and takes refuge in a monument. She sends him word that she has committed suicide, speaking his name as she died.

Act 4, Scene 14
As Antony contemplates suicide, he is brought word that Cleopatra has killed herself, and he decides to do so, too. He orders Eros to kill him, but Eros kills himself instead. Antony then attempts to fall on his sword, but succeeds only in wounding himself. DECRETAS appears and takes Antony's sword to Caesar to ingratiate himself with the conqueror. DIOMEDES (2) brings word from Cleopatra. Realising that Antony might kill himself, she reveals her lie and summons him. Antony orders himself carried to her on a litter.

Act 4, Scene 15
Antony, on his litter, is hoisted up to Cleopatra's hiding place in the monument. He tells Cleopatra that she should trust only PROCULEIUS among Caesar's court.

He proudly states that in killing himself he has prevented Caesar from killing him, and he dies. Cleopatra declares that she too will die in the proud Roman fashion.

Act 5, Scene 1
Caesar sends DOLABELLA to demand that Antony surrender. Decretas arrives with Antony's sword and word of his suicide. Caesar and his friends mourn the death of a great man even though he was their enemy. An EGYPTIAN appears, sent by Cleopatra to receive Caesar's orders. Caesar sends him back with assurances that he offers mercy to the queen; he sends Proculeius and GALLUS to Cleopatra to confirm the message.

Act 5, Scene 2
Cleopatra says that she is content to die. Proculeius arrives and assures her that Caesar will give Egypt to her son. Gallus appears with soldiers to guard Cleopatra. When she sees this, she attempts to stab herself but is disarmed by Proculeius. Dolabella arrives to replace Proculeius; moved by Cleopatra's elegy for Antony, he confides that Caesar intends to parade her ignominiously through the streets of Rome. Caesar arrives and generously offers mercy to Cleopatra, who submits, giving him a list of all her possessions. However, her treasurer SELEUCUS asserts that the list is incomplete. Cleopatra rages at him, but Caesar assures her that it does not matter for she can keep whatever she wants. He leaves, and Cleopatra sends Charmian on a secret errand as Dolabella returns to tell the queen that Caesar intends to transport her to Rome in three days. Charmian returns and a CLOWN (7) arrives with poisonous snakes. After he leaves Cleopatra prepares to die. Iras dies, brokenhearted, as Cleopatra applies two asps to herself and dies when they bite her; Charmian does the same. Dolabella and Caesar return, and Caesar declares that Cleopatra shall be buried with Antony after a grand funeral celebrating the nobility of their love.

COMMENTARY

The opening scenes of *Antony and Cleopatra* establish the basic conflict of the play. Soldierly duty is squarely placed opposite the satisfactions—both physical and emotional—of sexual involvement. The Roman soldiers see Antony as 'a strumpet's fool' (1.1.13), but Antony envisions finding a 'new heaven, new earth' (1.1.17) in the experience of love. Antony refuses to acknowledge the call of duty represented by messages from Rome, and stresses the conflict of the play when he declares, 'Now for the love of Love, and her soft hours, / Let's not confound the time with conference harsh' (1.1.44–45). But when he learns, in 1.2, of a successful revolt against the Roman power he is supposed to be defending, Antony realises that his honour demands that he 'must from this enchanting queen break off' (1.2.125). He returns to Rome but he can only leave Cleopatra with difficulty. He compromises his sense of duty by telling her he is her 'soldier, servant, making peace or war, / As thou affects' (1.3. 70–71), before he wrenches himself away. In 1.4 a purely Roman view of the situation is presented as Caesar and Lepidus regret Antony's neglect of his duty, even as he is returning to Rome.

Thus Shakespeare efficiently establishes the dramatic action of Acts 1–4 of the play: Antony wavers between his Roman heritage of military rigour and his attraction to the 'soft hours' of indolence and lust. Thus, the emotional centre of the work fluctuates between the too-demanding rigours of Roman power and the too-seductive delights of Egyptian luxury, finally escaping to an immortal world created in the imaginations of the lovers—a paradise 'Where souls do couch on flowers' (4.14.51). In Act 5, after Antony's death, Cleopatra, in a striking transformation that constitutes one of Shakespeare's greatest climaxes, raises the lovers' relationship to the level of transcendent love. But the focus returns to Rome's 'great solemnity' (5.2.364), in the play's final words. Even as love triumphs, the final victory of Rome is affirmed in Caesar's closing speech as he translates the tale into a mundane memorial. Shakespeare does not permit the basic conflict, which extends throughout the play, to be overridden by a clearly stated declaration of values.

The fine balance achieved between the values of Rome and Egypt has led to differing interpretations of Shakespeare's play. *Antony and Cleopatra* has been seen on one hand as a romance on the transcendence over the mundane, and on the other as a lesson against neglect of duty; as an exaltation of love and as a rejection of lust. Antony has been seen as a sordid politician who is transfigured by the love of Cleopatra, a courtesan who is similarly transformed. He has also been seen as a fool who sacrifices his nobility to sensual gratification—in more modern terms, a weak individual who indulges in pleasure to escape reality. The play seems to offer no definite conclusion as to the priority of duty or sensuality. This ambiguity has sometimes led to the classification of *Antony and Cleopatra* among the PROBLEM PLAYS, works with disturbingly unresolved attitudes towards issues of love and sex in public contexts.

However, Shakespeare does provide a resolution; it is simply twofold. Social discipline and order—as seen in the order of Caesar's Rome—is presented as a necessary element for society's health and spiritual development. On the other hand, the lovers' fate—paralleled by that of Enobarbus—brings about an awareness of a different level of fulfilment; for the individual, love is more important than political or material success. When love is opposed by the forces of conventional society, as here, its pursuit can result

in an intense realisation of self, which is what happens to Cleopatra in Act 5. Thus, the transfiguration of Cleopatra is not invalidated by Caesar's final triumph because the two climaxes exist in different worlds and point to equally potent but separate resolutions.

After Antony's death in Act 4 the conflict is seen in the opposition of Cleopatra and Caesar—Egypt and Rome, love and duty—and Caesar's victory is stressed in the play's final lines. The virtue of his triumph is made quite plain: Caesar declares as his victory approaches, 'The time of universal peace is near' (4.6.5), a statement that unmistakably refers—though the character is unaware of it—to the imminent coming of Christ. As Shakespeare's original audiences were completely aware, Caesar will found the Roman Empire, which was seen in the 17th century as not only a highlight of history, but as a secular manifestation of the will of God, provided as preparation for the coming of the Messiah.

Although Caesar's victory is thus clearly intended as a genuine resolution and a statement that the tragedy has not been a waste of human potential, his triumph cannot be total. The world of conflicting values that undid the lovers—the world in which Caesar operates—is clearly transcended in Cleopatra's final moments. The lovers, with their jealous quarrels and seeming betrayals, their separations and deceptions, are distinctly of the 'dungy earth' that Antony contrasts to 'the nobleness of life' (1.1.35, 36), but they have the capacity to transcend themselves. Cleopatra's extraordinary vitality leads them beyond death to the 'new heaven, new earth' (1.1.17) that Antony has envisioned. So there are two triumphs: that of Rome, which requires personal sacrifice in the name of the greater good of the world, and that of the lovers, in which individual happiness—particularly as expressed in sexual love—takes precedence over the demands of society.

Cleopatra's ultimate transfiguration cannot be dominated by Caesar's soldiers, and thus the final triumph is that of the individual's aspiration towards transcendence. Cleopatra's vision of reunion with Antony in death is sheer poetry; as such, it can have no effect on the practical, prosaic world of empire building. Her seeming defeat is actually a triumphant assertion of the continuing value of what might have been and what should be. She can, indeed, 'show the cinders of [her] spirits / Through the ashes of [her] chance' (5.2. 172–173). The superiority of the individual imagination over the power of government is stressed, even as the necessities of society maintain their dominance in the real world.

The contrasting elements—power and politics versus pleasure and passion—are mingled and opposed throughout the drama. The political and military developments—first Pompey's rebellion against the Triumvirate and then Caesar's push for sole power—point up the fact that whatever the lovers do has repercussions in the great world, and, conversely, events in the political realm determine their fate. One of the ways in which Shakespeare maintains an even balance between these different worlds is by suppressing the more spectacular aspects of the military situation. The play's two battles occur almost entirely offstage—necessarily so in the case of Actium, a naval battle, but also in Act 4's ground combat—with only glimpses of marching soldiers provided. In fact, the play's only violence is the two suicides. Thus, the love affair is not overwhelmed by the spectacle of clashing powers dividing the known world.

Cleopatra and Antony are not in any sense public figures victimised by the loss of private happiness; their love depends on the political situation that finally destroys them. They value their positions as world figures, and their affection is grounded in this appreciation. Antony promises Cleopatra that he will provide 'Her opulent throne with kingdoms' (1.5.46), and she envisions him as 'an Emperor Antony' (5.2.76). In fact, on his return to Egypt, his gift to her is a political act; as Caesar—who regards the act as a cause of war—observes, Antony 'gave [her] the stablishment of Egypt, made her / Of Lower Syria, Cyprus, Lydia, / Absolute queen' (3.6.9–11). Antony knows that Cleopatra loves power and he delights in giving it to her. But love influences politics as much as politics influences love, and Antony places his power in jeopardy by using it in this way.

The merciless entanglements of power and politics are thus contrasted with the possibility of private withdrawal into sensual pleasure. The aggressive manipulation of society as represented by the armies and ethics of martial Rome has always served an evident social purpose. The nurturing of the individual is an equally pervasive need; it is illustrated extravagantly in the luxuriant court of the Egyptian queen. Antony is absolutely human in his need for both aspects of life; he stands between two principles and he cannot fully reject either. In this lies his grandeur as a tragic hero.

Just as the political world of Rome is both potentially good and a source of tragedy, so love has two aspects, being a manifestation of the life force but also a stimulus towards self-destruction. In the latter mode love demands the renunciation of life, but in the former it glories in life. In this respect, though *Antony and Cleopatra* is unquestionably a TRAGEDY, it displays some of the features of a COMEDY. The structure of the play resembles that of traditional comedy, with Rome and Egypt being similar to the court and the forest of *As You Like It* and *A Midsummer Night's Dream*, or to VENICE and BELMONT in *The Merchant of Venice*. Moreover, comedy traditionally ended in a marriage, typically arranged through the wiles of the leading female character, and *Antony and Cleopatra* closes on a significant reference when Cleopatra, about to die, cries out

'Husband, I come' (5.2.286). Not for nothing are the asps provided by the Clown, a traditional comic rustic.

Further, the comedy of the Clown is only one instance of a feature displayed elsewhere in the play: *Antony and Cleopatra* is often quite funny. In 1.1 Cleopatra's baiting of Antony is humorous, as is her anecdote of dressing her drunken lover in her clothes, in 2.5.19–23. Indeed, in one aspect Antony and Cleopatra embody another ancient comic tradition, that of the infatuated old man enthralled by a scheming young woman. In 1.2 we see an example of the hilarity of Egyptian court pastimes, and in 1.5 the queen jests about the sexlessness of her eunuch, MARDIAN. Cleopatra's mistreatment of the hapless Messenger (2.5. 61–74, 106) may not strike modern audiences as particularly amusing, but such treatment of servants was another traditional comic routine, at least as old as ROMAN DRAMA (compare its use by Shakespeare in *The Comedy of Errors*). The bluff old soldier Enobarbus is at times a quite comical figure, especially when he mocks Lepidus in 2.7 and 3.2. In the former scene Lepidus also assumes a conventional comic role, that of the foolish drunk—a character type in Shakespeare's time that is still seen today. After 3.2 as the political plot comes to fruition and Antony goes down to defeat, the comedy disappears; its re-emergence in 5.2 in the person of the Clown is all the more effective.

The comic aspects of the play point to *Antony and Cleopatra*'s place in the evolution of Shakespeare's work, for the tragic vision of *King Lear, Othello,* and *Macbeth* is here modified by elements from the earlier romantic comedies. The comedies always displayed a potential for tragedy—in the possible success of evil—that was forestalled by the forces of love. In *Antony and Cleopatra* this situation is reversed; tragedy is in the forefront, and the romantic comedy of love amid the Egyptian court remains in a distinctly secondary position. However, the spirit of comedy does recur at the close in support of the final transfiguration of Cleopatra. This treatment foreshadows the magical transcendence that is at the heart of the later ROMANCES.

The mingling of love and politics, lust and strategy, triumph and defeat characterises *Antony and Cleopatra.* In its fusion of the mundane and the exalted—the 'dungy earth' (1.1.35) versus 'fire, and air' (5.2. 288)—*Antony and Cleopatra* is one of the most complex and rewarding of Shakespeare's plays.

SOURCES OF THE PLAY

By far the most important source for *Antony and Cleopatra* was the 'Life of Marcus Antonius' in Sir Thomas NORTH's *Lives of the Noble Greeks and Romans* (1579), which was a translation of Jacques AMYOT's French version (1559–1565) of PLUTARCH's original Greek (c. 125 A.D.). The playwright followed Plutarch's historical account fairly closely, though he gave different emphasis to its incidents. An earlier play on the subject, Samuel DANIEL's *Cleopatra* (1594), apparently influenced Shakespeare in these variations, especially in his treatment of Cleopatra's suicide. Shakespeare's descriptions of Egypt, particularly in 2.7, probably derive from LEO AFRICANUS as translated by John PORY in *A Geographical History of Africa* (1600).

TEXT OF THE PLAY

Antony and Cleopatra was written before the spring of 1608 when it was registered with the STATIONERS' COMPANY by Edward BLOUNT. Samuel Daniel's *Cleopatra* was altered between its editions of 1605 and 1607 in ways that reflect the influence of *Antony and Cleopatra,* which may therefore have been written as early as 1606. Barnabe BARNES' play *The Devil's Charter* contains an apparent echo of *Antony and Cleopatra;* it was performed in February 1607, then revised and published in October, suggesting that Shakespeare's play had been performed in 1607 or 1606. That it was not written earlier than 1606 is clear in light of the unaltered 1605 version of Daniel's work, as well as on stylistic grounds.

Antony and Cleopatra was registered for publication in 1608, but if a printed book was indeed actually produced, no copy of it has survived, and the earliest known text is that published in the FIRST FOLIO (1623). The Folio text was apparently derived from Shakespeare's own manuscript, as is indicated by a number of distinctive mis-spellings and abbreviations, along with elaborate stage directions, often precise yet impractical, unlikely to have been used in a PROMPT-BOOK. As the only authoritative version of the play, the Folio has been the basis for all subsequent editions.

THEATRICAL HISTORY OF THE PLAY

No early performances of *Antony and Cleopatra* are recorded, but a production of c. 1606—presumably the initial staging—is probable in view of the 1607 alterations made to Samuel Daniel's *Cleopatra.* (see 'Text'). Richard BURBAGE (3) is presumed to have originated the role of Antony. No other production is recorded for a century and a half, though John DRYDEN wrote a play about the lovers—*All for Love, or the World Well Lost* (1678)—that was influenced somewhat by Shakespeare's play. Its popularity was so great that it eclipsed *Antony and Cleopatra* until 1759, when David GARRICK staged a version of Shakespeare's text prepared by the noted scholar Edward CAPELL. Though it featured grandiose sets and elaborate costumes and starred Garrick and Mary Ann YATES, two of the most popular players of the day, the production was a failure, closing after a week; the public preferred *All for Love,* which continued to be revived.

In 1813 J. P. KEMBLE (3) presented *Antony and Cleopatra*—using an abridged text that was amply supplemented with Dryden's lines—that starred Helen FAUCIT. Following the taste of the times, this production

featured spectacular effects, including a sea battle and a grand funeral for the title characters, but it was as poorly received as Garrick's. In 1833 William Charles MACREADY starred in his version of the play, likewise spectacular, likewise mixed with Dryden, and likewise unsuccessful. Only in 1849 was Shakespeare's original play produced by Samuel PHELPS, who played Antony opposite Isabel GLYN, though it, too, was a commercial failure.

In the second half of the 19th century *Antony and Cleopatra* increased in popularity, and several productions were ventured, including those of Charles CALVERT (1866), F.B. CHATTERTON (1873), and Ben GREET (1897). Beerbohm TREE's production of 1907 continued the 19th-century tradition of dazzling spectacle requiring many extra players.

In the 20th century *Antony and Cleopatra* has been more widely appreciated, and numerous productions have been staged. The simply staged, textually accurate 1905 presentation of F. R. BENSON (1) was notable for its rejection of the taste for spectacle. This modern tendency was furthered in the 1922 OLD VIC staging by Robert ATKINS, presented on a bare stage. This production starred Edith EVANS (1), who also played Cleopatra in several later productions. In 1936 Theodore KOMISARJEVSKY staged a controversial STRATFORD production starring Donald WOLFIT. Godfrey TEARLE and Katherine CORNELL were acclaimed as the lovers in New York in 1947; Laurence OLIVIER and Vivien LEIGH took the parts in London in 1951; Michael REDGRAVE and Peggy ASHCROFT played them in London and Stratford in a 1953 staging by Glen Byam SHAW (3); and in 1967 Zoë CALDWELL and Christopher PLUMMER triumphed at Stratford, Ontario. In 1972 Trevor NUNN staged all of the ROMAN PLAYS at Stratford, England.

As a FILM, *Antony and Cleopatra* has yielded six movies, three of them silent films. The best-known film version is that directed by and starring Charlton Heston (1972); the fabled flop *Cleopatra* (1962), starring Elizabeth Taylor and Richard Burton, was not derived from Shakespeare's play. An adaptation of *Antony and Cleopatra* was part of SPREAD OF THE EAGLE, a 1963 TELEVISION presentation of the Roman plays, and the play was also produced separately for television in 1981, directed by Jonathan MILLER (2).

Apemantus Character in *Timon of Athens*, an angry, misanthropic philosopher. Apemantus' vulgar insults and remarks offer a strong critique of both the gullible TIMON and the Athenians who sponge off him. In this he resembles a CHORUS (1), and he provides a running commentary on the action of the main plot. Like such similar figures as JAQUES (1) and THERSITES, Apemantus is distinctly unlikeable. This quality ensures his isolation from the other characters and thus assures audiences that his observations are impartial. His cynical attitude, condemned by various characters, proves to be the one adopted by Timon himself in the end. Apemantus disappears after 2.2, and returns in 4.3 to exchange insults with Timon once the former nobleman has retreated to a life of rage and despair in the woods near ATHENS. Though unlikeable, Apemantus still has right on his side, and when he tells Timon, 'the middle of humanity thou never knewest, but the extremity of both ends' (4.3.301–302), he pinpoints the major defect in Timon's personality. Apemantus refuses to alter his opinions or personality to suit the circumstances of his patron, and this gives him great moral stature compared with Timon's false friends. When this is combined with the honesty of his insults, Apemantus counteracts the play's atmosphere of bleak despair. He helps makes it clear that Timon's misanthropic attitude is not that of the play or the playwright.

Apocrypha Works of dubious authenticity, a term usually associated with certain biblical texts but also useful in literary scholarship. Numerous plays have been attributed to Shakespeare at various times, but it is generally thought that they were written by others and are thus outside the CANON; these comprise the Shakespeare apocrypha. While nearly 50 works, in whole or in part, have been assigned to Shakespeare at some time, only 12 have ever been seriously enough proposed to be included in the apocrypha. Six of these were first attributed to the playwright in the Third FOLIO. They are: LOCRINE; THE LONDON PRODIGAL; THE PURITAN; SIR JOHN OLDCASTLE; THOMAS, LORD CROMWELL, and A YORKSHIRE TRAGEDY. The other six are: ARDEN OF FEVERSHAM; THE BIRTH OF MERLIN; EDWARD III; FAIR EM; THE MERRY DEVIL OF EDMONTON, and MUCEDORUS. In addition, the authorship of *Pericles* and *The Two Noble Kinsmen* remains in sufficient dispute that these two plays, though commonly included in the canon (as they are in this book), are sometimes placed among the apocrypha, as is SIR THOMAS MORE, which contains only a few pages by Shakespeare.

Apothecary, the Minor character in *Romeo and Juliet*, the druggist from whom, in 5.1, ROMEO buys a poison with which to kill himself, believing JULIET (1) to be dead. Romeo believes that the poverty-stricken Apothecary can be bribed to break the law and defy common moral sense by selling him this drug. The young hero veers between contempt for the Apothecary and sympathy for another victim in a world of misery.

Apparitions Minor characters in *Macbeth*, supernatural phenomena shown to MACBETH by the WITCHES, in 4.1. These specters are designated as the First, Second, and Third Apparition; each has a distinctive appearance and message. The First Apparition is described in the stage direction at 4.1.69 as 'an armed

head', and it warns Macbeth to beware of MACDUFF. The Second, 'a bloody child' (4.1.76), declares that '. . . none of woman born / Shall harm Macbeth' (4.1. 80–81). The Third Apparition is 'a child crowned, with a tree in his hand' (4.1.86), and it adds that 'Macbeth shall never vanquish'd be, until / Great Birnam wood to high Dunsinane hill / Shall come against him' (4.1.92–94). Macbeth naturally receives these prophecies as 'Sweet bodements!' (4.1.96) and assurances that he will not be killed by his enemies. The tensions of the play tighten with this episode, the first intimation of its climax. Macduff is brought into sharp focus for the first time, yet Macbeth's defeat is made to seem all but impossible. These portents come from the same supernatural agency whose prediction of Macbeth's rise—in the WITCHES' prophecy of 1.3—was gravely accurate.

In Act 5 the prophecies of the Apparitions are borne out, though not as Macbeth anticipates. With hindsight we can see that the Apparitions bear clues as to Macbeth's true fate, for their appearances are symbolically significant The armoured head that is the First Apparition forecasts the severing of Macbeth's own head after 5.8. The Second Apparition, a bloody child, suggests Macduff 'from his mother's womb / Untimely ripp'd' (5.8.15–16). The Third Apparition, the child crowned, foretells the reign of the young Prince MALCOLM with which the play closes, and the tree it bears refers to his decision to have his soldiers bear boughs cut from Birnam wood as they march on DUNSINANE.

Apuleius, Lucius (b. c. 123 A.D.) Roman writer, author of the only surviving Latin novel, a probable inspiration for *A Midsummer Night's Dream* and a possible minor source for *Cymbeline*. Apuleius' *Metamorphoses*, better known as *The Golden Ass*, is a delightful account of a young traveller who dabbles in magic and is accidentally transformed into an ass; in this form he undergoes many adventures before he is restored by the goddess Isis. The transformation of BOTTOM probably comes from this famous tale, still widely read today, and the substitution of a sleeping potion for a poison in *Cymbeline* may reflect Apuleius' use of the same device.

Apuleius specifically identifies his hero—named Lucius—with himself, and his account of an initiation into the sacred mysteries of Isis and Osiris—of great interest to scholars—is presumed to be autobiographical. Apuleius was born in Carthage and in his youth he travelled throughout the Roman Empire. While in Egypt he married and was charged with witchcraft by his bride's disappointed suitor. His defence, which survives as his *Apologia*, offers a tantalising glimpse of provincial life in the ancient world. He returned to his home where he became a noted poet, philosopher, and religious leader. A number of works survive besides *The Golden Ass* and the *Apologia*, mostly miscellaneous philosophical and literary essays, while a great deal more, including his famed poetry, is lost.

Archbishop (1) of Canterbury, Henry Chichele Character in *Henry V*. See CANTERBURY (1).

Archbishop (2) of Canterbury, Thomas Cranmer Character in *Henry VIII*. See CRANMER.

Archbishop (3) of York, Richard Scroop (d. 1405) Historical figure and character in *1* and *2 Henry IV*, a leader of the rebels against King HENRY IV. In *1 Henry IV* the Archbishop appears only briefly, in 4.4, where he confers with his friend Sir MICHAEL (2). He predicts the defeat of HOTSPUR at SHREWSBURY and lays his plans for the rebellions to be enacted in *2 Henry IV*. Shakespeare may have intended the episode as a preparation for the later play, or it may simply have served to remind the audience that the battle of Shrewsbury was not to be the last of Henry's troubles.

In *2 Henry IV* the Archbishop leads the continuing revolt, although his cause is doomed by the treacherous withdrawal of the Earl of NORTHUMBERLAND (1). In 4.1 he states the dilemma of the good man who is provoked into rebellion by poor government but nevertheless believes in the divine right of kings. However, the Earl of WESTMORELAND (1) firmly asserts the point of view of the play: rebellion is a heinous violation of the natural order, and the gravity of the offence is aggravated when the rebel is a clergyman, for a representative of God should not oppose a divinely appointed king. In 4.2 the Archbishop disbands his army, after Prince John of LANCASTER (3) promises that his grievances will be considered, and is then arrested for treason and sentenced to death.

The historical Archbishop had sided with Henry when he deposed RICHARD II, although several members of his family supported Richard, including his brother Stephen SCROOP (3), who appears in *Richard II*. (Later, Stephen's son, Henry SCROOP [1], was executed for treason by HENRY V, as is enacted in *Henry V*.) The Archbishop's cousin William Scroop, Earl of Wiltshire, was one of Richard II's favourites and was executed by Henry in 1399, as is reported in *Richard II* (3.2.142). In 1.3.265 of *1 Henry IV* where Warwick is incorrectly identified as the Archbishop's brother, this execution is said to have sparked the prelate's rebellion against Henry. Although Shakespeare took his information from HOLINSHED, it is not true. The Archbishop supported the new King until 1405, when he and a number of northern barons—among them his brother-in-law Northumberland—joined to oppose the heavy taxes Henry had levied in order to finance his wars against earlier rebels. Once in revolt, the Archbishop was not betrayed by Northumberland; instead, he impetuously began his campaign against the King before his allies were prepared to fight, and

he accordingly found himself outnumbered and then outsmarted—at GAULTREE FOREST.

Archbishop (4) of York, Thomas Rotherham (1423–1500) Historical figure and minor character in *Richard III,* friend of Queen ELIZABETH (2). In 2.4, when news arrives of the imprisonment of the Queen's allies, the Archbishop urges her to seek sanctuary, and he offers her his assistance, even to the illegal extent of giving her the Great Seal of England, with which he has been entrusted. This incident, which Shakespeare took from HALL (2), emphasises the villainy of RICHARD III by presenting opposition to it from a venerable figure.

The historical Rotherham was a powerful clergyman who held a number of secular posts, including that of Chancellor of England, bearer of the Great Seal. He was imprisoned for opposing Richard's accession, but he was soon released. He withdrew from court politics for the remainder of his life, although he remained a prominent churchman.

In some modern editions of the play, the Archbishop of York is eliminated and his lines are given to CARDINAL (2) BOURCHIER, following the 16th-century QUARTO editions. This change was presumably made as an economy for the acting company.

Archidamus Minor character in *The Winter's Tale,* a follower of King POLIXENES of BOHEMIA. In 1.1 Archidamus exchanges diplomatic courtesies with CAMILLO, an adviser of King LEONTES of SICILIA. Their conversation informs the audience of the play's opening situation. Archidamus has no real personality, but his fluent command of courtly language lends the episode a distancing formality, appropriately introducing an extravagant and romantic story. Nevertheless, his last line, 'If the king had no son, they would desire to live on crutches till he had one' (1.1.44–45), closes the scene with a harshness that intimates the misery to come in the play's tragic first half.

Arcite One of the title characters of *The Two Noble Kinsmen,* cousin of PALAMON. In 1.2 Arcite and Palamon are affectionate friends, both nobly concerned with maintaining their honour as chivalrous knights. However, while prisoners of war in ATHENS in 2.1, both fall in love with the beauty of EMILIA (4), sister-in-law of Duke THESEUS (2), and their friendship crumbles as they dispute who may claim her as their loved one. They eventually fight a duel over Emilia, with the stipulation by Theseus that the loser not be killed in the fight, but instead executed. Arcite wins the duel, but he then dies, crushed by a runaway horse, and Palamon gets Emilia.

As the protagonists of a stylised chivalric romance, the two cousins are very similar, and their characterizations tend to blur even more given the unevenness of the play, a collaboration between Shakespeare and John FLETCHER (2). Nevertheless, some distinctions can be drawn. In 1.1 Arcite is the leader of the two, introducing the idea of fleeing the corrupt court of THEBES and attempting to broaden Palamon's military orientation. When they are obliged to fight for Thebes, Arcite draws the deepest conclusion from their situation. Declaring that they will have to trust 'th'event, / That never-erring arbitrator' (1.1.113–114), he presents an important theme of the play, humanity's helplessness to direct destiny. When their quarrel over Emilia arises, he is the more reasonable of the two, attempting to smooth things over in 2.1, when they meet again in 3.1, and as they prepare to duel in 3.3. He is also more sensible about the approach of Theseus, proposing that Palamon hide and they fight later. Nevertheless, he is perfectly willing to fight it out when Palamon insists, and when the combatants offer petitions to the gods in 5.1, Arcite speaks to Mars, the god of war. At his death, Arcite is simply a pawn of the plot, asking forgiveness with his last breath.

Arcite's personality is still further obscured by the fact that in Acts 2 to 4, Shakespeare probably wrote only one scene (3.1), and Fletcher's Arcite is a somewhat different character from Shakespeare's. A sentimentalist, he laments in 2.1 the fact that imprisonment means the cousins will not find 'The sweet embraces of a loving wife' (2.1.84) or produce children, and he thinks achingly that 'fair-eyed maids shall weep our banishments' (2.1.91). When in 2.2 he decides to enter the wrestling and running competition to gain the attention of the duke's court, he is nothing more than a stereotypical hero-in-disguise. Perhaps in light of this, Shakespeare gives him a beautiful meditation on Emilia at the opening of 3.1. However, Arcite's inconsistencies merely reflect the failings of the play as a whole.

Arden (1), Forest of Anglicisation of the Ardennes, a wooded region on the borders of France, Belgium, and Luxembourg, the setting for most of *As You Like It.* Shakespeare's Forest of Arden, like BELMONT in *The Merchant of Venice* and the island in *The Tempest,* is an artificial world, explicitly removed from society. Here, relatively free from pressures and stress, the characters can find themselves and settle conflicts that escape solution in the real world. Arden is equivalent to Arcadia, the land where amorous shepherds and shepherdesses lead an ideal existence in the PASTORAL literary tradition which *As You Like It* both draws on and lovingly parodies.

We first hear of Arden as the place where the exiled DUKE (7) Senior 'and a many merry men with him . . . live like the old Robin Hood of England . . . and fleet the time carelessly as they did in the golden world' (1.1.114–119), referring to the classical myth of

a golden age when an idyllic life was led in the countryside. However, Arden is not a paradise. The duke's praise of his bucolic exile is tempered by his awareness of nature's implacable strength, the 'churlish chiding of the winter's wind' (2.1.7), and his dislike of the need to kill the forest's deer for food. The duke acknowledges that he has 'seen better days' (2.7.120). Moreover, Shakespeare's shepherds are not at all idealised: SILVIUS is a parody of the sentimental Arcadian shepherd, and CORIN is a down-to-earth representative of real rural life. Arden may provide a refuge, but it does not offer a perfect existence. Further, when the duke is restored to power at the close of the play, all of the exiles—except the pessimistic and melancholy JAQUES (1)—are instantly ready to return from Arden to the real world. In the meantime, love has culminated in four marriages, the traditional happy ending in a COMEDY; the artificial world has produced the expected resolutions.

Shakespeare followed his source, Thomas LODGE's *Rosalynde,* in placing his Arcadia in the Ardennes. This forest seemed especially significant in the 16th century because it was a romantic setting in Ludovico ARIOSTO's *Orlando Furioso,* one of the most popular books of its day (from which Shakespeare probably took the name ORLANDO). The name Arden will also have been familiar to the playwright and his audience as that of an ancient wooded area in WARWICKSHIRE—Shakespeare's mother's family took their name from it (see ARDEN [2])—though no forest remained there in Elizabethan times.

Arden (2), Robert (d. 1556) Shakespeare's maternal grandfather. A gentleman-farmer, Arden was a minor member of the gentry. He owned land in both Wilmcote and Snitterfield, villages near STRATFORD, most of which he leased to other farmers. One of these was Richard SHAKESPEARE (12), whose son was to marry Arden's youngest daughter, Mary Arden SHAKESPEARE (11), around 1558.

Arden was one of the most prosperous farmers of the Stratford region. He had eight daughters, six of whom married (and were supplied with dowries), and when he died he left Mary several substantial parcels of land. He is traditionally associated with the Ardens of Park Hall, a lordly WARWICKSHIRE family that was among the very few English families whose ancestry could be traced to before the Norman Conquest. In the Domesday Book (1085 A.D.), an Arden held more land than any other Englishman, and the family took its name from a vast forest that it owned (not to be confused with the Forest of ARDEN [1] in *As You Like It*). However, no records substantiate this connection, and while Robert Arden may have had an ancestor who was a younger son of the Park Hall Ardens, his own circumstances were quite modest by comparison.

Arden of Feversham Anonymous play formerly attributed to Shakespeare, part of the Shakespeare APOCRYPHA. *Arden of Feversham* was published in 1592, 1599, and 1633. It was not until 1770 that a printer and amateur scholar from Faversham—the modern spelling of the play's setting—published a fourth edition of the play in which he attributed it to Shakespeare and sparked a century of debate. Among many notable commentators, only Algernon SWINBURNE favoured the attribution. Modern scholars generally ascribe the play to Thomas KYD, but in any case, it is unlike any of Shakespeare's known works and thus is an unlikely candidate for inclusion in the CANON.

Arden of Feversham is the story of a famous murder that took place in the English town of Faversham in 1551: one Thomas Arden was killed by men hired by his wife, Susan, and her lover, a family servant. The play records Mistress Arden's obsessive intent, through several failures and the withdrawal of several conspirators. She finally succeeds, only to be discovered and sentenced to death with her lover, who romantically declares, 'Faith, I care not, seeing I die with Susan'.

Argument Literary device, a plot summary preceding or concluding a long work. Shakespeare used a prose argument as a preface to his narrative poem *The Rape of Lucrece.* The argument was a conventional attribute of long poems in the 16th century; RENAISSANCE writers adopted it from classical tradition and used it to present the reasons why a work was written and to state the points that the author intended to make. Readers were thus provided with a prior awareness of the contents of the work, freeing them to focus on its purely literary values.

In the argument to *Lucrece,* Shakespeare briefly rendered the story of TARQUIN's lust for LUCRECE and its consequences. This account is somewhat fuller than it is in the poem itself. It describes the despotic and warlike ways of the Roman king and relates how his son, Tarquin, was seized with an uncontrollable desire for Lucrece, the wife of COLLATINE, a Roman general. (It is at this point that the poem begins.) The argument goes on to summarise the poem, and its last sentence makes clear what the poem only implies—that the revenge later taken upon Tarquin resulted in the downfall of the monarchy and the establishment of the Roman Republic. The argument thus offers a larger view of the personal tragedy that the poem details, demonstrating the breadth of political and social concern that also informs many of Shakespeare's plays.

Ariel Character in *The Tempest,* a sprite, or fairy, who serves the magician PROSPERO. Ariel is invisible to all but Prospero, whom he assists in the schemes that

form the plot. He is capable of assuming fantastic disguises and of luring mortals with supernaturally compelling music. He is also something of a theatrical producer, arrangeing the spectacular tableaus that Prospero is fond of, including the magical banquet of 3.3 and the betrothal MASQUE of 4.1. He performs in both, playing a HARPY at the feast and either CERES or IRIS (depending on one's reading of 4.1.167) in the masque. Ariel is eager to please, asking, 'What shall I do? say what; what shall I do?' (1.2.300). To his question 'Do you love me, master?' (4.1.48), Prospero replies, 'Dearly, my delicate Ariel' (4.1.49), and when Prospero returns to MILAN and resumes his role in human society, he regrets departing from the sprite, saying 'my dainty Ariel! I shall miss thee' (5.1.95). A cheerful and intelligent being, Ariel embodies the power of good and is thus an appropriate helper in Prospero's effort to combat the evil represented by ANTONIO (5). In this respect he contrasts strongly with the play's other major non-human figure, CALIBAN, whose innate evil complicates Prospero's task.

Freed by Prospero from a magical imprisonment in a tree trunk, imposed by a witch before the time of the play, Ariel must serve Prospero until the magician releases him. But though he fulfils his tasks cheerfully, he yearns to be free again. Almost as soon as he first appears, he reminds Prospero of his 'worthy service . . . without grudge or grumblings' (1.2.247–249) and requests his liberty. Prospero—more of a grumbler than his supernatural servant—reminds him forcefully of his former torment, and Ariel agrees to continue serving and 'do [his] spriting gently' (1.2.298). He does so, but both he and Prospero frequently mention his coming release. Ariel sings of the future: 'Merrily, merrily shall I live now / Under the blossom that hangs on the bough' (5.1.93–94), and his mingling of nostalgia and fresh spirits is touching. In his last lines before the EPILOGUE, Prospero bids Ariel 'to the elements / Be free, and fare thou well!' (5.1.318). This theme, Ariel's captivity in the human world—along with Caliban's slavery and Antonio's remorselessness—helps maintain a tragic undertone as Prospero's schemes for a final reconciliation are achieved. Shakespeare does not ignore the inexorability of evil, even in a fantasy world, though he can create a charming sprite to combat it.

Ariosto, Ludovico (1474–1533) Italian poet whose work became source material for several of Shakespeare's plays. Ariosto's epic poem *Orlando Furioso* (1516, and a longer version in 1532) was one of the most popular literary works of the 16th and 17th centuries. One of the many stories in it contributed an important element to the plot of *Much Ado About Nothing,* the disguising of MARGARET (2) as HERO in order to deceive CLAUDIO (1). Also, Shakespeare gave the name of Ariosto's title character to the romantic lead in *As You Like It,* knowing that his audience would associate it with the lush enchantment of *Orlando Furioso.* The playwright may have known the work in both an Italian edition (probably that of 1532) and the English translation by Sir John HARINGTON (1591).

Another work by Ariosto contributed to two other Shakespeare plays. His play *I Suppositi* (1509), translated into English as *Supposes* by George GASCOIGNE (performed 1566, published 1575), provided the subplot concerning BIANCA (1) in *The Taming of the Shrew.* Further, *Supposes* provided the device used to fool the PEDANT in the same play, an invented hostility between cities said to endanger the travelling citizen of one of them. A ruse in Ariosto and *The Shrew,* the same situation is real in *A Comedy of Errors,* where EGEON faces the death penalty in consequence.

Italian literature—and the works of Ariosto in particular—was extremely fashionable in Elizabethan England, but behind Ariosto were ancient roots that Shakespeare will also have appreciated. In the original Italian text of *I Suppositi,* a PROLOGUE (1), thought to have been spoken by Ariosto himself at the first performance, expressly refers to *his* sources—the ancient Roman dramatists PLAUTUS and Terence—and also mentions *their* sources in Greek New Comedy. Thus, in deriving his tale of romantic intrigue from Ariosto's work, Shakespeare was adding to a theatrical tradition already almost 2,000 years old.

Aristotle (384–322 B.C.) Ancient Greek philosopher, author of a source for *Troilus and Cressida* and possibly *The Tempest.* Aristotle is one of the few Shakespearean sources to be mentioned in a play using his work. HECTOR cites the philosopher's opinion that young men are 'Unfit to hear moral philosophy' (2.2.168) because in their immaturity they form opinions based on their emotions rather than reason. Shakespeare knew this dictum from the *Nicomachean Ethics,* translated into English by John Wilkinson in 1547. Not only does Shakespeare have Hector employ Aristotle's arguments, scholars surmise that the personalities of Hector and TROILUS, and perhaps other characters, were influenced by the psychological types Aristotle proposed in the *Ethics* to illustrate points of morality.

A related aspect of the *Nicomachean Ethics* may have influenced Shakespeare's creation of CALIBAN in *The Tempest.* Aristotle believed in the necessity of civilisation, seeing humanity as naturally incapable of moral behaviour. He saw 'natural man' as morally defective, unable to distinguish good from bad, and thus 'bestial'. He cited 'canibals', reported among the remote barbarians outside the Greek world, as an instance of such people. The animal-like nature of 'the beast Caliban' (4.1.140), as PROSPERO matter-of-factly calls him, is repeatedly referred to, and he is pointedly incapable

of understanding wrong, as when he casually acknowledges having attempted to rape MIRANDA. His name, moreover, is an anagram of 'canibal', an accepted 17th-century spelling.

Aristotle was the first thinker to analyse the way drama works; his *Poetics* is regarded as the fountainhead of European dramatic criticism. This book on TRAGEDY (a companion work on COMEDY has not survived) assesses the Greek drama of Aristotle's day and concludes that the best tragedies have certain characteristics in common. They focus on characters who are essentially good people but who commit a gross moral error through no fault of their own; these plays also deal with family relationships, thereby intensifying the conflict. A well-written work inspires both pity and fear in the audience, so intensely as to elevate our awareness of these emotions. The release from this highly charged response is called *catharsis*—an idea, in various interpretations, that has influenced most critical thought since Aristotle.

However, although Aristotle and his followers were widely studied in universities throughout the Middle Ages, and his ideas were the common coin of literate society (he is mentioned as an object of study in *The Taming of the Shrew* [1.1.32]), his influence on ELIZABETHAN DRAMA was largely indirect, for the *Poetics* was not translated into English until after Shakespeare's day. The *Nicomachean Ethics* was the only translation of Aristotle available in the playwright's lifetime. Though Sir Philip SIDNEY and others wrote about Aristotle's critical theory, it had a greater effect on poetry than the theatre. Shakespeare and his fellow dramatists knew classical drama chiefly through the works of SENECA, which are very different from those Aristotle analysed. Nevertheless, the similarity between the Aristotelian ideal of tragedy and Shakespearean practice indicates that the ancient thinker's opinions had been effectively transmitted.

Aristotle was, with the slightly earlier Plato (c. 429–347 B.C.), one of the Western world's seminal thinkers. Between the two, they formulated most of the categories and concepts—from theology to aesthetic criticism—that have since governed philosophy. The son of a Macedonian physician, Aristotle began to study in ATHENS under Plato at the age of 17. After Plato's death he headed schools of his own in various locations, and for several years he tutored Alexander the Great (356–323 B.C.). He taught again in Athens after 335, establishing a scholarly community that conducted research on a large scale, on subjects ranging from politics to botany. After Alexander's death, anti-Macedonian sentiment led to Aristotle's flight from Athens, and he died in exile. Much of his writing has been lost, but the remainder constitutes a major component of the Western intellectual heritage, and his work is still studied intensively by students in a variety of disciplines.

Armado, Don Adriano de Character in *Love's Labour's Lost,* a comically pedantic and pompous Spaniard who participates in the humorous sub-plot. Armado's language is ludicrous whether he is ingratiating himself with royalty or wooing his rustic sweetheart, JAQUENETTA. Armado is mocked by his own page, the saucy MOTH (1), and his preposterously rhetorical letters are read aloud as entertainment by the other characters. His pompously inflated language, like that of the similar characters HOLOFERNES and NATHANIEL (1), is a satirical target of the play.

Armado participates in the pageant put on by the comic characters in 5.2. In its course, it is revealed that Jaquenetta is pregnant by the Spaniard, and at the end of the play he announces that he has taken a vow to his beloved similar to the promises made by the aristocratic lovers, thus providing a link between the two plots.

Armado boasts of his acquaintance with the KING (19) of Navarre in a richly comical passage (5.1.87–108) and clearly demonstrates his descent from the comic character type known in ancient Roman drama as the MILES GLORIOSUS, a foolish, bragging soldier. In the Italian COMMEDIA DELL' ARTE, this figure was a Spaniard, an enemy of Italy and also of Shakespeare's England. Armado's very name, attached to so ludicrous a character, is a derisive reference to the Spanish Armada's grand failure to invade England in 1588.

Armin, Robert (d. 1615) Famed English comic actor, probably the original portrayer of TOUCHSTONE, FESTE, and other comic roles in Shakespeare. Listed in the FIRST FOLIO as among the 26 'Principall Actors' of Shakespeare's plays, Armin joined the CHAMBERLAIN'S MEN in 1599, apparently replacing Will KEMPE as the company's chief comic actor. Shakespeare's comic characters changed significantly at that time to exploit Armin's particular talents. Armin was a small man whose skills were verbal and musical, in contrast to the physical humour of Kempe, and he was accordingly better cast as a clever FOOL (1) than a bumbling CLOWN (1). The dialogue Shakespeare provided for him is filled with wordplay and ingenious arguments, and his characters often sing. Among the Shakespearean parts he is believed to have originated, besides Feste and Touchstone, are THERSITES and the FOOL (2) of *King Lear.* Shakespeare may have intended VIOLA's remark upon meeting Feste—'This fellow is wise enough to play the fool' (*Twelfth Night,* 3.1.61)—as a compliment to Armin.

By all reports a highly competent actor, Armin was capable of playing different sorts of comic parts; he is known to have played DOGBERRY, reviving a part originated by Kempe, and he probably played CLOTEN as well. Moreover, outside his Shakespearean roles, Armin specialised in a character type that he devised himself, a doltish simpleton called John of the Hospi-

tal. Armin wrote at least one play, *The Two Maids of Moreclacke* (c. 1598), and two books of comedy routines and jokes, *Foole upon Foole* (1600, reissued as *A Nest of Ninnies* in 1608) and *Quips upon Questions* (1600).

Arne, Thomas Augustine (1710–1787) English composer, creator of music for several Shakespearean SONGS. The leading theatrical composer of the mid-18th century, Arne wrote for operas, MASQUES, and plays. He composed incidental music for seven of Shakespeare's plays and set a number of the songs to music, including 'Under the greenwood tree' and 'Blow, blow, thou winter wind' from *As You Like It* (2.5.1–8, 35–42; 2.7.174–193), 'When daisies pied' from *Love's Labour's Lost* (5.2.886–921), and 'Where the bee sucks' from *The Tempest* (5.1.88–94). However, Arne is probably best known today for having written 'Rule Brittania'.

Arragon (Aragon) Character in *The Merchant of Venice,* Spanish prince and unsuccessful suitor of PORTIA (1). In selecting among the caskets of silver, gold, and lead to win Portia's hand, Arragon reveals the arrogance that his name suggests. He rejects the lead casket as unworthy and the gold because its inscription promises 'what many men desire' (2.9.24), and he feels himself superior to the 'common spirits' (2.9.32). Although Arragon is a somewhat comic figure—he is a caricature Spaniard of a sort familiar to 16th-century English theatre-goers—his failure to select the correct casket illuminates the thematic values of the play. He is presented as a foil to BASSANIO, who chooses the humble lead casket and wins the lottery and whose victory reflects on the Spaniard's vanity. Further, the villainous SHYLOCK resembles Arragon in his pride, refusing to relinquish an iota of what he feels he deserves. An unselfish sense of community with others is necessary for romantic success, in the play's scheme of things, and Arragon demonstrates its opposite.

Artemidorus (active 44 B.C.) Historical figure and minor character in *Julius Caesar,* an ally of CAESAR (1). In 2.3 Artemidorus writes a memorandum detailing the plot against Caesar's life, of which he has learned. However, in 3.1 he is unable to prevail upon the busy general to read it, and moments later Caesar is murdered. According to Shakespeare's source, PLUTARCH's *Lives,* Artemidorus, a professor of rhetoric, knew of the plot through his acquaintance with some of the conspirators, but the playwright ignored this information and simply used the futile warning as an illustration of Caesar's over-confidence.

Artesius Minor character in *The Two Noble Kinsmen,* an officer under THESEUS, Duke of ATHENS. When Theseus' wedding is interrupted by the demands of the Three Queens (see QUEEN [1]) for vengeance against King Creon of THEBES, the Duke instructs Artesius to prepare the army for war in 1.1.159–165. He then disappears from the play. His only function is to lend a military air to the preparations.

Arthur, Prince of England (1187–1203) Historical figure and character in *King John,* nephew and victim of King JOHN (3). John has usurped Arthur's crown as the play opens. A defenseless boy, Arthur is supported by King PHILIP (2) of FRANCE (1) and the Archduke of AUSTRIA, who go to war with England. Arthur is captured and is taken to England in the custody of HUBERT, who is instructed to kill him. However, Hubert grows fond of his prisoner and cannot bring himself to carry out his orders. First, he decides to blind the boy; then, in 4.1, in response to Arthur's heart-rending pleas for mercy, he spares him altogether. To protect himself, Hubert reports that Arthur has died. Arthur, in the meantime, attempts to escape and perishes jumping from a castle wall. His death provokes a rebellion by John's nobles, whose reservations about the royal succession are now reinforced by revulsion at Arthur's murder, as they believe it to be.

Historically, Arthur had little claim to the English crown, although he was the son of John's older brother, for the rule of primogeniture—succession passing to eldest sons of eldest sons—was not yet accepted in England. John was named heir to the throne in Richard I's will, and he succeeded his brother peacefully, as Shakespeare's sources make clear. Philip's sponsorship of Arthur was intended purely to justify a war and had no legitimacy for Englishmen, but the playwright wished to develop the theme of usurpation.

Further ignoring his sources, Shakespeare made Arthur a young boy, said to be about 3 feet tall (4.2.100), so as to stress the pathos of his treatment. The historical Arthur was an adult by medieval standards. He was a soldier, the nominal leader, at 15 years old, of the force that besieged Queen ELEANOR at Mirabeau, Shakespeare's ANGIERS. Captured in battle there, Arthur was at first in the custody of Hubert but was transferred to an English-held castle at Rouen. He was never taken to England, as in the play.

It is unclear how Arthur died. One contemporary account held that John had proposed blinding and castrating his prisoner to make him unfit for kingship; Hubert dissuaded the King from this course and then falsely announced Arthur's death, intending to discourage his followers. Another source reported that Arthur drowned attempting to escape. Shakespeare combined these two anecdotes. According to a third version of the story, John killed Arthur himself in a fit of drunken rage. The detailed truth cannot be known, but guilt for Arthur's death must ultimately lie with John. The murder did not trigger the barons' revolt, as it does in the play—that event occurred many years

later—but it may have contributed to the spate of desertions by various nobles that affected the final year of the war against France, which John lost decisively.

Arviragus Character in *Cymbeline*, one of the two kidnapped sons of King CYMBELINE. Arviragus and his older brother GUIDERIUS have been raised to be woodsmen and hunters in the wilds of WALES (1) by their foster-father BELARIUS, who kidnapped them in infancy when he was unjustly exiled by Cymbeline. When their sister IMOGEN, disguised as a young man, happens onto their cave, the boys immediately love 'him', although they don't know that they are siblings. Like Guiderius, Arviragus is inherently noble and desires to prove himself in the greater world of kingly courts and warfare. When the Romans invade Britain, the brothers have their chance. After they save the British army they are honoured by the king, and then, in the extraordinary sequence of revelations and reconciliations in 5.5, they are reunited with their father.

Both Arviragus and Guiderius are simple fairy-tale figures—lost princes who are eventually discovered and restored to their rightful positions—and they have the princely attributes of courage, sincerity, and high spirits. However, Shakespeare takes care to distinguish them from each other. Arviragus is the more reflective of the two; he also speaks some of the play's best poetry. He responds more strongly to Imogen's beauty, and when Guiderius praises her cooking, the more esthetic Arviragus emphasises her singing. When they believe her dead, Arviragus expresses their grief in a lyrical passage (4.2.218–229) that compares her beauty to the flowers. Arviragus also offers an intellectually grounded, if simple, denunciation of money, in 3.7.26–28. Belarius has given Arviragus the name Cadwal, and this name is occasionally used in dialogue, but he is designated as Arviragus in speech headings and stage directions.

As You Like It

SYNOPSIS

Act 1, Scene 1

ORLANDO reports that his older brother OLIVER (1) has ignored their late father's will, withholding Orlando's inheritance, denying him an education, and treating him like a peasant. Oliver appears and harasses Orlando, finally striking him, at which Orlando seizes his brother and refuses to release him until he vows to reform. Oliver promises and is released, and Orlando leaves. Oliver plots to get rid of Orlando, and the wrestler CHARLES appears with news from the court: DUKE (1) Frederick has usurped his position from DUKE (7) Senior, his older brother; Duke Senior now lives in exile in the Forest of ARDEN (1), although his daughter, ROSALIND, remains at court. Charles goes on to say that he worries about injuring Orlando in the wrestling competition soon to be held at court. Oliver asserts that Orlando, being proud and evil, intends to kill Charles if he can and suggests that Charles should do the same to him.

Act 1, Scene 2

Duke Frederick's daughter, CELIA, attempts to cheer her cousin, Rosalind, who is depressed over her father's banishment, by promising her own friendship and loyalty. TOUCHSTONE, the court jester, or FOOL (1), arrives and jokes on knightly honour. A foppish courtier, LE BEAU, appears and reports that the wrestler Charles has brutally killed several opponents. He says that the matches are to be resumed on the site where they are speaking. The duke's court arrives, accompanied by Charles and Orlando. Rosalind and Celia, taken by Orlando's youth and beauty, attempt to dissuade him from wrestling, but he insists on challenging Charles. They wrestle, and Orlando wins. When Orlando identifies himself, the duke refuses to give him the promised prize because Orlando's father had opposed his usurpation. The duke and his followers leave, but Celia and Rosalind remain and congratulate Orlando. Rosalind is clearly lovestruck, giving Orlando her necklace and attempting to converse further, but the tongue-tied Orlando cannot respond, as he laments once they are gone. Le Beau returns to warn Orlando that the temperamental duke intends evil towards him. Orlando asks him about Rosalind's identity before fleeing.

Act 1, Scene 3

Rosalind tells Celia of her love for Orlando. The Duke announces that Rosalind is banished because her father was his enemy. Celia volunteers to share her cousin's exile, and they decide to join Rosalind's father in the Forest of Arden. Rosalind will disguise herself as a young man, take the name GANYMEDE, and pose as Celia's brother; they will ask Touchstone to join them.

Act 2, Scene 1

Duke Senior and his noblemen discuss the pleasures of their life in the forest. One LORD (4) describes the amusing sight of the melancholy JAQUES (1) lamenting the death of a shot deer.

Act 2, Scene 2

Duke Frederick discovers Celia's absence and mistakenly believes that she and Rosalind are with Orlando. He sends men to arrest Orlando or, if he has fled, Oliver.

Act 2, Scene 3

An old family servant, ADAM, meets Orlando to warn him that Oliver intends to kill him. Adam volunteers to flee with Orlando, offering his savings as a means of support.

Act 2, Scene 4
Weary with travel, the disguised Rosalind, Celia, and Touchstone arrive in Arden, where they overhear CORIN, an old shepherd, in conversation with SILVIUS, a young man who bewails his unrequited love for a girl named PHEBE. Talking with Corin, they learn that they can buy a house, land, and Corin's sheep, hiring him to tend them.

Act 2, Scene 5
AMIENS sings a song of the Spartan virtues of woodland life. Jaques parodies it, mocking the affectation of courtiers who take up rural life.

Act 2, Scene 6
Orlando and Adam arrive in Arden, and Adam, exhausted, collapses. Orlando promises to find him something to eat.

Act 2, Scene 7
Duke Senior and his men are eating dinner as Jaques reports his encounter in the forest with a FOOL (1), whose comical dissertation on Time has inspired him. He wishes to be a fool himself, licensed to satirise without fear of punishment. Orlando appears, demanding food at swordpoint. The duke offers him a place at the table, and Orlando apologises for his thievish conduct, explaining his desperation. He goes to fetch Adam. Jaques moralises on the stages of human life. Orlando returns with Adam, and the dinner is resumed. Amiens sings of the evils of man and the jolly woodland life, and the duke welcomes Orlando to his court-in-exile.

Act 3, Scene 1
Duke Frederick disbelieves Oliver's protestations that he does not know where Orlando is, dispossesses Oliver of his dukedom, and threatens him with death or banishment if he does not find Orlando within a year.

Act 3, Scene 2
Orlando hangs a love poem to Rosalind on a tree and wanders off, intending to decorate the forest with such declarations. Touchstone baits Corin on his lack of sophistication, but the old shepherd is confident of the virtues of his simple life. Rosalind appears in her disguise as Ganymede, reading a poem she has found that celebrates herself; Touchstone parodies it. Celia arrives with another poem to Rosalind and informs her that she has seen Orlando sleeping nearby. Orlando and Jaques appear, and the women eavesdrop. Orlando rejects the melancholy Jaques, who mocks his love for Rosalind. Jaques departs, and Rosalind, as Ganymede, approaches Orlando and interrogates him about his love. She proposes to cure him of his lovesickness by posing as Rosalind and spurning his courtship; he agrees to call on Ganymede each day and pretend to woo him as if he were Rosalind.

Act 3, Scene 3
Jaques observes Touchstone wooing AUDREY, a goatherd; the fool's comical remarks satirise love, women, and marriage. Nevertheless, he and Audrey have decided to marry, and Sir Oliver MARTEXT, a country parson, arrives to conduct the ceremony. Jaques objects to the irregularity of the rite and escorts the couple away.

Act 3, Scene 4
Rosalind is distressed that Orlando is late for his date with Ganymede, and Celia accuses all men of being dishonest breakers of appointments. Corin arrives and offers to show them the courtship of Silvius and Phebe.

Act 3, Scene 5
Rosalind, Celia, and Corin overhear Phebe rejecting Silvius. Rosalind steps forward and castigates the thankless young woman for disdaining a good lover, being ugly and unlikely to find better; Phebe instantly falls in love with Ganymede. Left alone with Silvius, she is kinder to him, understanding and pitying his passion, and she agrees to permit him to share her company if he will carry her letters to her new beloved.

Act 4, Scene 1
Rosalind berates Jaques for his melancholy and dismisses him. Orlando appears, addressing Ganymede as Rosalind, in accordance with their agreement. She pretends to chastise Orlando for being late and to satirise his talk of love. She asks Celia to perform a mock marriage ceremony between them, after which Orlando announces that he must meet the duke but will return at two o'clock. Rosalind confides to Celia that her passion for Orlando grows more intense.

Act 4, Scene 2
Jaques and some of the duke's lords sing a hunting song.

Act 4, Scene 3
Orlando is late, to Rosalind's dismay. Silvius arrives with a letter from Phebe to Ganymede, which Rosalind mocks. She sends Silvius back to Phebe with the message that Ganymede rejects her. Oliver appears, seeking Ganymede and his sister. He carries a bloody bandage. He explains that Orlando, walking through the forest, had seen a sleeping man being stalked by a lion. He had recognised the man as his evil elder brother and had contemplated letting the lion kill him. Instead, however, he had mercy, drove the lion away, and was wounded in the process. Oliver confesses that he is the brother, though he has reformed his evil ways, and he goes on to tell that Orlando, recovering from his wound, has asked him to bear a message to Ganymede offering the bloody cloth as excuse for his lateness. He offers the bandage to Rosalind, and she faints. Reviving, she insists that her faint was counterfeit and that Oliver must tell Orlando so.

Act 5, Scene 1
Touchstone and Audrey encounter WILLIAM (2), who is also a suitor of Audrey; Touchstone poses as a sophisticate and threateningly drives William away.

Act 5, Scene 2
Orlando and Oliver, now reconciled, discuss Oliver's love for Celia, which she has returned; the two are to be married the next day. Oliver asserts that he will surrender all of their father's estate to Orlando and remain with Celia, whom he believes to be a shepherdess. He leaves as Rosalind arrives, still disguised as Ganymede. Orlando declares that his lovesickness for the absent Rosalind is such that he can no longer accept the masquerade of Ganymede as his lover. Ganymede then declares that he knows magic and can summon Rosalind; he promises that Orlando can marry her at Oliver and Celia's wedding the next day. Silvius and Phebe arrive, and Ganymede promises Phebe that, if he will marry any woman, he will marry her, but that if she sees that Ganymede will *not* marry any woman, she must accept Silvius. She agrees.

Act 5, Scene 3
Touchstone and Audrey also plan to marry the next day. Two PAGES (7) appear and sing a love song.

Act 5, Scene 4
Orlando tells the duke that he is unsure of Ganymede's promised magic. Rosalind, as Ganymede, appears with Silvius and Phebe; she elicits the duke's assurance that he will permit his daughter, Rosalind, to marry Orlando if he can produce her, and he has Phebe reaffirm her promise to marry Silvius if she must refuse Ganymede. Then Ganymede leaves. Touchstone and Audrey arrive; Touchstone satirises duelling and courtly honour. HYMEN (1), the Roman god of marriage, leads a festive MASQUE. Rosalind, appearing as herself, enters and identifies herself as the duke's daughter and Orlando's bride. Phebe sees that she must marry Silvius and agrees with good will, as Hymen sings a wedding hymn. JAQUES (2), a brother of Oliver and Orlando, arrives with the news that Duke Frederick, having come to Arden with the intention of killing Duke Senior, has been reformed by a holy man. He has accordingly restored the duchy to his banished brother and intends to retire to a monastery. The melancholy Jaques decides to join him, preferring a solitary life of contemplation to the festive court. He leaves as the wedding celebration begins with a dance. Rosalind then speaks an EPILOGUE, soliciting applause for the play.

COMMENTARY

As You Like It, as its title asserts, has something to offer every taste. On one level it serves as a stock romantic comedy, with disguised princesses, an unjustly deposed ruler, and a handsome leading couple. But the play also offers food for thought on a traditionally entertaining subject, the assets and drawbacks of country life. And the dedicated student of literature can consider the play's relationship to a favourite RENAISSANCE literary mode, the PASTORAL romance, a form of escapist writing with roots in ancient Greece. Further, the play is a sparkling theatrical entertainment, with more SONGS than any other Shakespearean play and several diverting set pieces: an on-stage wrestling match in 1.2, a procession of singing hunters in 4.2 (traditionally carrying a deer's carcass, though a set of antlers has been generally substituted in more modern times), and Hymen's charming masque in 5.4.

These features enliven a work whose plotting is strikingly undramatic. After Act 1 establishes the separate banishments of Duke Senior, Orlando, and Rosalind, Acts 2–4, set in Arden, lack striking change. Adam seems near death in 2.3, but we know that the exiled duke's comfortable establishment is near, and we feel only admiration for Orlando's devotion rather than anxiety for Adam's plight. Orlando invades the Duke's banquet, but we know that he will be graciously received, and we are not chilled by any threat of violence. Oliver's tale of peril and salvation offers no thrilling tension, for we know he survived to tell us about it.

Instead of a plot, the play presents conversations among different combinations of characters. They talk mostly about romantic love, country living, or both. Their remarks weave a shimmering pattern of agreements and contradictions, harmonies and counterpoints, that constitute the substance of Acts 2–4. There emerges from this fabric of ideas an opposition of two points of view: a responsiveness to love and life, represented by Rosalind; and a withdrawal from complexities and commitment, represented by Jaques. The play's climax in Act 5 produces a resolution in favour of the former. Jaques, although no villain, must be defeated if the life-affirming spirit of the lovers is to triumph, for his doctrine of passivity and retreat is ultimately antisocial.

Shakespeare neatly and subtly presents the opposition of Jaques and the lovers by having first Orlando and then Rosalind dismiss the melancholy courtier from the stage with a rebuke, in 3.2.289 and 4.1.36 respectively, before each of the two great wooing scenes. This is a bold instance of the dominant technique in the play; the development of dramatic tension not through plotting, as we have seen, but by juxtaposing encounters among the characters. For the most part, we are not expected to judge the speakers but rather to enjoy their meetings and gradually appreciate their differences.

For instance, the pastoral world of the banished duke in the Forest of Arden is described, even before we see it, as one in which the exiles 'fleet the time carelessly as they did in the golden world' (1.1.118–

119), a reference to the golden age of ancient mythology, analogous to Eden in the Judeo-Christian tradition. However, once the play's action moves to Arden, this proposition is undermined. The duke's praise of his exiled court's woodland life is followed immediately by an account of Jaques' lament for the wounded deer, which critiques human interference with nature. Jaques' comments also present a cynical, distrustful image of human society, as he 'invectively . . . pierceth / The body of country, city, court' (2.1.58–59). In 2.2 Duke Frederick's villainy is once again displayed, supporting Jaques' dark viewpoint but also reaffirming the essential virtue of the exiled Duke Senior's court. Shakespeare establishes Arden as an ideal, pastoral world in which characters criticise the real one, but then other characters criticise *them*, both explicitly and by implication. Further, when Rosalind arrives in Arden with Celia and Touchstone in 2.4, their initial response is humorously unenthusiastic, with Rosalind weary in spirit and Touchstone weary in body; the fool comments that 'at home I was in a better place' (2.4.14). Thus we can ponder several points of view without being diverted from the central situation of the drama.

In 2.5 Amiens sings a song that illustrates the Duke's attitude towards the pastoral life, that those 'who doth ambition shun' (2.5.35) are happy to have no enemies but the weather, but Jaques responds with a comically insulting parody. In 2.7 Jaques' delightfully expressed desire to be a jester like Touchstone, licensed to satirise everyone, provokes a sharp reprimand from the duke for wishing to correct the world's vices when he has sinned himself. Later in the same scene Jaques' position is again rejected. As the melancholy courtier completes his sardonic account of human life with a morbid description of helpless old age, Orlando bears in Adam, whom the duke, who is entirely unaffected by Jaques' speech, treats with reverence. The scene closes with another instance of such subtle contradiction. Amiens sings a song condemning humanity for '. . . ingratitude' and asserting that 'most friendship is feigning, most loving mere folly' (2.7.174–193). Just at that moment, the duke's hospitality is enabling Orlando to express his gratitude for Adam's friendship and loyalty. The bases of the pastoral convention—the idealisation of rustic life and an accompanying cynicism towards sophisticated society—are espoused, but they are just as persistently contradicted and undercut.

Most telling in this respect are the play's comparisons of different lovers. The central figures are Rosalind and Orlando. They are flanked by comic variations: the ridiculously conventional Silvius and Phebe on the one hand, and the equally preposterous yet earthy Touchstone and Audrey (with an assist from William) on the other. The lovesick shepherd and the hard-hearted shepherdess who rejects him were standard figures in pastoral literature, and Silvius and Phebe are absurd manifestations of it. Their exaggeration is emphasised by Rosalind's own overstated realism when she advises Phebe, 'Sell when you can, you are not for all markets' (3.5.60).

Silvius' sentimentality is countered in Touchstone's attitude to Audrey. So far from adoring Audrey, or being in love with love itself, the jester finds only that 'man hath his desires, and as pigeons bill, so wedlock would be nibbling' (3.3.72–73). His detached and resigned submission to human instincts is ironically opposed to the worship of an ideal woman. Touchstone also provides a foil for Rosalind's love for Orlando. When Silvius' plaintive lament reminds the heroine of her seemingly impossible passion (Orlando not yet having arrived in Arden), Touchstone immediately mocks her by saying that his preposterous love for one Jane Smile led him to kiss 'the cow's dugs that her pretty chopt hands had milked' (2.4.46–47).

In another repeated theme, different sorts of rustic characters are contrasted. Silvius and Phebe are essentially stereotypical literary lovers, countrified only vaguely by their occupation as shepherds. Audrey and her hapless swain William are typical rustic buffoons, instances of the Shakespearean CLOWN (1). And Corin is a lifelike peasant, a man who fully understands the realities of extracting a living from the land. In 2.4.73–84 he frankly discusses his poverty and, by implication, the essential falseness and sentimentality of the pastoral convention. At the same time, he does not envy the courtiers their easier but less honest life, and his exchanges with Touchstone in 3.2.11–83 constitute one of the most telling critiques of the pastoral in the play. The country world holds its own against courtly sophistication, yet its hardships and difficulties are clearly stated.

Even the two figures who comment on the activities of the others, Touchstone and Jaques, are pointedly different from each other. They first meet offstage, as we hear in Jaques' enthusiastic report on the 'motley fool' (2.7.13). Touchstone's observations on the human tendency to ripen and then rot appeal greatly to the melancholy courtier. However, the jester ridicules everything and has no philosophy, while Jaques is dedicated to a pessimistic view of life and looks to mockery to 'cleanse the foul body of th'infected world' (2.7.60). His jaded attitude leads him to withdraw from human society at the play's end, whereas Touchstone enters the play's swirl of courtships with enthusiasm, if also with sarcasm. Touchstone eventually joins the 'country copulatives' (5.4.35) and marries, while Jaques departs, declaring himself 'for other than for dancing measures' (5.4.192). The contrast reflects the play's two opposing poles, love and withdrawal.

The play's repeated juxtapositions of ideas and temperaments constitute its overall mood and are perhaps referred to in its title. Each character has an opinion

about love and the good life, but then another personality presents a viewpoint that contradicts or modifies it. Each idea is qualified, and each has some merit. In the end, as the multiple marriages in 5.4 suggest, the dominant theme is the unifying power of love.

Rosalind represents this theme throughout, and perhaps the most telling juxtaposition in the play is that of Rosalind to herself in her disguise as Ganymede. Ganymede insists that Orlando's love is a sickness he can cure. The delightful result is the spectacle of Rosalind, while madly in love with Orlando, telling him that 'love is merely a madness' (3.2.388) and then quite hysterically confiding her love to Celia—'O coz, coz, coz . . . that thou didst know how many fathom deep I am in love!' (4.1.195–196). The climax nears in 5.2, when Ganymede's masquerade can no longer suffice. The love between Celia and Oliver is too much for Orlando to witness without pain; he insists that he cannot go on with the pretence that Ganymede is Rosalind. The disguised heroine realises that her lover has outgrown the conventional attitudes she has been teasing him about, and she prepares to resume her true identity. Her turn to magic—reprised in the appearance of the supernatural Hymen in 5.4—is appropriate to the position she has occupied as the prime manipulator of affairs. Disguised as Ganymede, she has been invisible though entirely in control. She returns accompanied by the solemn magic of Hymen's masque, casting a spell of acceptance and reconciliation; even Jaques, despite his withdrawal, blesses the couples with humour and wisdom.

Hymen's nature is problematic, but whether he is a supernatural being or a costumed human recruited by Rosalind is not as important as his role as a symbol of divine approval for the play's happy ending. This suggestion has been prepared for by various religious references. Some are quite touching evocations of traditional religion, such as Adam's touching prayer, 'He that doth the ravens feed, / Yea providently caters for the sparrow, / Be comfort to my age' (2.3.43–45), and Orlando's equation of 'better days' with times when 'bells have knoll'd to church' (2.7.113–114). Others are more prosaic allusions to biblical episodes. Orlando touches on the parable of the prodigal son in describing his lot under Oliver, in 1.1.37–39; In 2.1.5 Duke Senior likens his exile to the expulsion from the Garden of Eden, and Jaques refers to the plagues of Egypt in 2.5.58. Corin assumes that one may 'find the way to heaven / By doing deeds of hospitality' (2.4.79–80). Duke Frederick is converted by 'an old religious man' (5.4.159), and Rosalind invents an 'old religious uncle' (3.2.336) for Ganymede. The entire episode of Sir Oliver Martext, however ridiculous, raises other issues of churchly doctrine. These references subtly suggest the parallels between Christian ideals of pity and loving-kindness and the play's themes of love and reconciliation.

SOURCES OF THE PLAY

Shakespeare's only important source for *As You Like It* was Thomas LODGE's prose romance, *Rosalynde* (1590, 4th ed. 1598). For the tale of a young heir's mistreatment by his older brother, Lodge drew on a medieval English poem, *The Tale of Gamelyn;* he apparently invented the story of Rosalind and Celia as well as the sub-plot of Corin, Silvius, and Phebe (though Shakespeare changed all of his names except Rosalynde and Phoebe, as Lodge spelled them). Shakespeare added most of the other characters: Jaques, Touchstone, Le Beau, Amiens, Audrey, William, and Martext. Shakespeare also made brothers of the usurped and usurping dukes, providing a parallel to the story of Orlando and Oliver and thus tightening the relationship between the plots. Significantly, the playwright also invented the repentance of Duke Frederick; Lodge's counterpart dies in battle against the denizens of Arden. Shakespeare's atmosphere of reconciliation was to be all-inclusive.

Certain details reflect the playwright's further reading. The name Orlando invokes the hero of ARIOSTO's 16th-century romance *Orlando Furioso.* Another famous romance, Jorge de MONTEMAYOR's *Diana Enamorada,* is actually referred to in 4.1.146, and it may have influenced Shakespeare's creation of a network of lovers here, as it did in *A Midsummer Night's Dream.* Also, *As You Like It* contains echoes of several works by John LYLY, who also influenced Lodge's *Rosalynde.* Finally, the name Corin probably came from an English play of the 1570s, published in 1599, *Syre Clyomon and Clamydes,* as did, perhaps, hints of the characters Audrey and William.

As You Like It is both an example and a parody of PASTORAL literary conventions. The pastoral tradition began with the bucolic idylls of the Greek writer Theocritus (c. 308–c. 240 B.C.), six of which appeared in an anonymous English translation in 1588, and was most famously manifested in the *Eclogues* of VIRGIL, which 16th-century English readers knew well. In the English RENAISSANCE the pastoral achieved its greatest popularity in Sir Philip SIDNEY's *Arcadia,* a work that the playwright drew on in other plays. Although Shakespeare did not draw directly on these pastoral works in composing *As You Like It,* they nevertheless underlie its general nature.

TEXT OF THE PLAY

As You Like It was probably written in 1599, though this date is uncertain. The play was in existence by August 1600, when Shakespeare's CHAMBERLAIN'S MEN registered it with the STATIONERS' COMPANY as a play 'to be stayed'—that is, *not* to be published. This was a tactic that theatre companies used as a defence against piracy, and it is believed to have applied only to new plays, suggesting that *As You Like It* was a recent

work. This theory is supported by circumstantial evidence. The play is not mentioned in Francis MERES' list of Shakespearean plays, published in 1598. More significantly, for Meres could accidentally have omitted it, the role of Touchstone, Shakespeare's first professional FOOL (1), is thought to have been written for the noted comic Robert ARMIN, who did not join the Chamberlain's Men before early 1599. It is also thought that the company may have intended to profit from a vogue for romantic tales of outlaws, stimulated by two plays about Robin Hood—by Anthony MUNDAY and Henry CHETTLE—presented by the rival ADMIRAL'S MEN in 1598. Duke Senior is compared to the celebrated outlaw in 1.1.116, when his exile is introduced. Further, Jaques' satirical bent and his discussion of humour's purpose in 2.7.45–87 may reflect a dispute on the validity of satire that raged in London in early 1599, culminating in a public book-burning in June of that year.

Another theory holds that the play was originally written much earlier, probably in 1593, and reworked later. The strongest evidence in favour of this hypothesis is a pair of references—one certain, one doubtful—to the killing of Christopher MARLOWE (1) on May 30, 1593. Marlowe's death was among the most notorious news items of the year, and some scholars hold that it is alluded to in Touchstone's remark that 'when a man's verses cannot be understood, . . . it strikes a man more dead than a great reckoning in a little room' (3.3.9–12), which may refer to the fatal dispute—a brawl over a tavern bill, or 'reckoning'—and certainly seems to echo a famous phrase in Marlowe's extremely popular play *The Jew of Malta:* 'infinite riches in a little room'. If this passage indeed refers to Marlowe's death, it does suggest an early date, for it can have had news value for only a season or two. The other instance, in which a line of Marlowe's *Hero and Leander* is quoted and ascribed to a 'dead shepherd' (3.5.81–82) is unquestionably an elegiac reference to Marlowe, though it need not have been made in the wake of his murder. Most scholars still find the earlier dating dubious, and in any case Shakespeare may have cannibalised a lost or unfinished earlier work when writing the surviving text of *As You Like It.*

The play was not published in Shakespeare's lifetime; it first appeared in the FIRST FOLIO (1623). Its text is among the clearest and least disordered in the Folio, and it appears to have been taken from a PROMPT-BOOK, with its brief, imperative stage directions and accurate speech headings. The Folio thus provides the only authoritative text of *As You Like It,* and it has remained the basis of all subsequent editions.

THEATRICAL HISTORY OF THE PLAY

As You Like It may have been written expressly for the first season of the GLOBE THEATRE, in the autumn of 1599, but no certain record of an early performance exists. However, an effort was made to discourage pirate publication, which suggests that the play was popular. Robert ARMIN originated the role of Jaques, and tradition holds that Shakespeare himself played Adam.

The earliest definitely known production of *As You Like It* was LOVE IN A FOREST (1723), by Charles JOHNSON (2), a free adaptation eliminating several characters and incorporating elements from several of Shakespeare's other plays. A reasonably faithful version of Shakespeare's text was staged in 1740, with James QUIN as Jaques, Kitty CLIVE as Celia, and Hannah PRITCHARD as Rosalind. This production was a great success, and the play remained popular throughout the 18th century; the part of Rosalind was taken by most of the leading actresses of the period, including Peg WOFFINGTON, Mary Ann YATES (1), Mary 'Perdita' ROBINSON (2), and Sarah SIDDONS. Dorothy JORDAN was especially successful, playing Rosalind many times between 1787 and 1814. Jaques was played by Colley CIBBER (1) and John HENDERSON, among others. Charles MACKLIN and Richard YATES (2) appeared as Touchstone, but the most famous of the 18th-century jesters was Tom KING (26). From 1776 to 1817 *As You Like It* was the most performed Shakespearean play at London's Drury Lane Theatre.

In the 19th century Rosalind remained in the repertoire of most leading actresses, notably including Helen FAUCIT, Mary ANDERSON (2), and Julia NEILSON (2). J. P. KEMBLE (3) and William Charles MACREADY played Jaques, the latter in his own 1842 production, a careful restoration of Shakespeare's text. In Paris, the French novelist George Sand (1804–1876) staged her adaptation of the play (1856), in which Celia marries Jaques instead of Oliver. Late in the century, two important productions were popular in London: Rosalind was played by Neilson in one and by Ada REHAN in the other. *As You Like It* has been often staged in the 20th century, being particularly popular in outdoor performances. Notable productions have included those of Oscar ASCHE (1907), Glen Byam SHAW (3) (1957), and a controversial 1967 version at England's National Theatre, with an all-male cast headed by Ronald Pickup as Rosalind. Among the other notable Rosalinds of the century have been Edith EVANS (1), and Peggy ASHCROFT.

As You Like It was made as a silent FILM three times, but only one modern movie version has appeared, a 1936 film directed by Paul Czinner (1890–1972) and starring Laurence OLIVIER as Orlando. The play has also been produced on TELEVISION several times.

Asche, Oscar (1871–1936) English actor, playwright, and producer. Asche is probably best known as the author and director of *Chu-Chin-Chow* (1916), a musical that ran for five years, setting a record that was

astonishing for its day. However, he was also a notable Shakespearean director and actor, famous for his portrayals of OTHELLO, KING (5) CLAUDIUS, FALSTAFF, and SHYLOCK. In 1906–1907 he staged a season of acclaimed Shakespearean productions: *Measure for Measure, As You Like It, The Taming of the Shrew,* and *Othello.* Another famous presentation was his modern-dress *Merry Wives of Windsor,* notorious for Falstaff's repeated exit line: 'Taxi!'

Asnath Minor figure in *2 Henry VI,* a supernatural spirit or devil summoned in 1.4 by the witch MARGERY JOURDAIN, with help of spells cast by the sorcerers SOUTHWELL and BOLINGBROKE (2). The spirit is questioned by Bolingbroke; the queries are provided by the DUCHESS (1) of Gloucester, who wishes to examine the prospects for a coup. Asnath displays the traditional reluctance of such spirits to answer, but the laws of magic compel him to obey. He is ambiguous about the future of the King; he forecasts a death by water for the Duke of SUFFOLK (3), and he cautions that the Duke of SOMERSET (1) should avoid castles. Bolingbroke then dismisses him. It is thought that Shakespeare intended his name as an anagram of 'Sathan', a common 16th-century spelling of 'Satan'.

Aspinall, Alexander (c. 1546–1624) Resident of STRATFORD and probable friend of Shakespeare. Aspinall was master of the Stratford grammar school for 42 years, beginning in 1582; however, Shakespeare had probably left the school a few years earlier (his period of attendance is unrecorded). Aspinall and Shakespeare both became prominent figures in Stratford—Aspinall was an alderman and a clerk of the town council—and were neighbours when the playwright lived at NEW PLACE. They were certainly among the most literate and cultured citizens of Stratford, and thus they must have been closely acquainted, at least after Shakespeare retired from London in about 1610.

In 1594 Aspinall was married. In courting his wife, he sent her a pair of gloves, accompanied by the following three-line poem that—according to an account written half a century later—Shakespeare composed: 'The gift is small / The will is all / Alexander Aspinall.' The tradition is highly questionable but it has not been disproved, and, if true, it provides a charming glimpse of the newly successful poet and playwright playfully assisting the romance of an older friend.

Aspley, William (d. 1640) Publisher and bookseller in LONDON. In 1600 Aspley, in partnership with Andrew WISE, published QUARTO editions of both *Much Ado About Nothing* and *2 Henry IV.* He was also a member of the syndicates that published the FIRST FOLIO (1623) and the Second FOLIO (1632), apparently by virtue of his rights in these two plays. He also published and sold plays by several other playwrights including George CHAPMAN and Thomas DEKKER.

Ashcroft, Peggy (b. 1907) English actress. Since achieving stardom at 23 playing DESDEMONA opposite Paul ROBESON, Ashcroft, who was created a Dame of the British Empire in 1956, has played most of Shakespeare's major roles for women. In her youth she was acclaimed as virtually all of Shakespeare's romantic heroines. In 1932 alone, she played IMOGEN, JULIET, MIRANDA, PERDITA, PORTIA, and ROSALIND; remarkably, she could still triumph in these roles many years later—for instance, as BEATRICE in 1950 (opposite John GIELGUD) and as Imogen in 1957. She played the great tragic heroines as well: Desdemona, OPHELIA, CORDELIA, CLEOPATRA. Perhaps her most remarkable role—often cited as one of the great performances of all time—was as Queen MARGARET (1) in the BBC's 'The Wars of the Roses' (1964). She portrayed Margaret as she appears in all four plays of the minor TETRALOGY, growing from the naïve young woman of *1 Henry VI,* to a courageous military leader, to the shrieking and cursing, half-insane ex-queen of *Richard III.*

Athens City in Greece, the setting for *A Midsummer Night's Dream, Timon of Athens, The Two Noble Kinsmen,* and two scenes of *Antony and Cleopatra.* Although references in the dialogue and stage directions of the three full plays set in Athens make it clear where the action is occurring, there is nothing distinctively Athenian in any of them. Shakespeare simply followed his sources in placing his stories in the ancient cultural capital of the Mediterranean world, without troubling to depict the city itself. Only in *Timon* is there any hint of the historical Athens, for the controversial career of ALCIBIADES is sketchily presented.

In *Antony and Cleopatra* Mark ANTONY establishes his headquarters in Athens between the re-establishment of his alliance with Octavius CAESAR (2) and its crumbling into the warfare that results in his final defeat in 3.4 and 3.5. Here Shakespeare simply followed history (as presented in PLUTARCH's *Lives*) in establishing Antony in Athens, and again he makes no effort to delineate the city itself.

Atkins, Robert (1886–1972) English actor and producer. Atkins joined the company at the OLD VIC THEATRE in 1915, and between 1919 and 1925 he directed the Old Vic's complete cycle of Shakespeare's plays. His was the first modern production of *Pericles* (1921), and he startled London with an *Antony and Cleopatra* presented on a bare stage (1922). In 1927–1928 he led a Shakespeare company in Egypt. During the Second World War he ran the Shakespeare Memorial Theatre in STRATFORD, and after the war he produced plays in an outdoor theatre in London. Among

his notable later productions was *All's Well That Ends Well* (1949), in which he played LAFEW.

Attendant (1) Any of several minor characters in *Antony and Cleopatra,* servants of Mark ANTONY. In 1.1 an Attendant brings word that news has arrived from ROME, though Antony refuses to hear it. In 3.11 a group of Attendants declare their loyalty following Antony's defeat at ACTIUM, though he grandly insists they should flee, his fortunes being obviously on the decline. The Attendants' function is to demonstrate the grandness of Antony's household and the loyalty that his magnanimous leadership inspires. The Attendant in 1.1 is designated a Messenger in some editions.

Attendant (2) Any of several minor characters in *Cymbeline,* servants of King CYMBELINE. In 3.5 an Attendant is sent to find IMOGEN and returns to report briefly that her chambers are locked and silent. This informs the court of what the audience already knows—that Imogen has fled. The Attendant serves merely as an instrument of communication. Also, a number of Attendants mutely swell the king's retinue when he is informed of the approaching Roman army, in 4.3; their function is purely decorative.

Audrey Character in *As You Like It,* a goatherd loved by TOUCHSTONE. Audrey is a Shakespearean CLOWN (1), a comic caricature of a peasant. She is uneducated to a ridiculous degree—she is unfamiliar with the words 'feature' and 'poetical'—and she says little, being chiefly a butt for Touchstone's humour. She is, however, charming in her simplicity. She acknowledges her homeliness, saying 'and therefore I pray the gods make me honest' (3.3.29–30), and, as her marriage to Touchstone approaches, she rejoices tentatively: 'I do desire it with all my heart; and I hope it is no dishonest desire, to desire to be a woman of the world' (5.3.3–5).

Though she is a minor and somewhat conventional figure, Audrey is a deftly drawn personality who helps fill out the play's satiric presentation of country life and love. Her passivity contrasts tellingly with PHEBE's conventional resistance to SILVIUS; the two couples parody the lovers of the PASTORAL tradition, each in their own ways. Audrey mocks the pretensions of the literary shepherdesses represented by Phebe by being exaggeratedly down to earth.

Aufidius, Tullus Legendary figure and character in *Coriolanus,* the leader of the VOLSCIANS and the murderer of CORIOLANUS. Aufidius is the oft-defeated rival of Coriolanus, and he vows that he will overcome him by dishonourable means, since he cannot win in combat. Therefore, when Coriolanus deserts ROME and joins the Volscians, Aufidius schemes to kill him. After Coriolanus is dissuaded by VOLUMNIA from sacking Rome, Aufidius accuses him of treachery, and the CONSPIRATORS stab the Roman to death in the play's final scene.

Shakespeare found Aufidius in his source, PLUTARCH's *Lives,* but from a single brief mention of their rivalry he constructed the charged relationship of the play. The playwright's villain is a warped mirror image of his protagonist. Aufidius focusses directly on Coriolanus throughout the play, and neither man can forget the other for long. Like Coriolanus—though without his political difficulties—Aufidius is first and foremost a charismatic warrior, motivated by wholly personal, indeed, egotistical drives, and obsessively concerned with his own achievements. When Coriolanus joins the Volscians, the fellowship of warriors leads Aufidius to welcome his rival with the warmth of a lover. 'Let me twine / Mine arms about that body' (4.5.107–108), he says, and compares their encounter with his wedding night. The extraordinary sensuality of this passage offers bizarre evidence of the misplaced emotional thrust engendered by warrior culture.

Frustrated, Aufidius decides to defeat Coriolanus dishonourably, and his grandeur becomes that of a villain rather than a great warrior. He undergoes this change in Act 1, after the siege of CORIOLES, and he admits that his effort 'Hath not that honour in't it had' (1.10.13). In this respect he is a foil to Coriolanus, whose failing is that his pride will not permit him to sacrifice any aspect of his warrior's persona. Also, when compared with the treachery of Aufidius, Coriolanus' betrayal of Rome seems the lesser villainy. However, after he has killed Coriolanus, Aufidius resumes something of his earlier nobility when he acknowledges his enemy's greatness. He grants him a warrior's funeral and declares, 'he shall have a noble memory' (5.6.153), in the play's final statement

Aumerle, Edward York, Duke of (c. 1373–1415) Historical figure and character in *Richard II,* a supporter of RICHARD II. Aumerle is a flattering courtier whose loyalty to King Richard is later undercut by his willingness to betray his fellow conspirators, who attempted to restore the deposed king, in order to save his own life. Aumerle displays his hypocrisy with seeming pride in 1.4, when he boasts of having feigned affection for BOLINGBROKE (1). He offers advice to Richard at several points; in 3.2 he suggests firmness in resisting Bolingbroke but then shifts to less honourable stalling tactics (3.3.131–132). After Bolingbroke has triumphed, BAGOT accuses Aumerle of complicity in Richard's murder of the Duke of GLOUCESTER (6); Bolingbroke postpones the question, but we hear in 5.2 that Aumerle has been stripped of his dukedom (though he continues to be designated Aumerle throughout the play). In this scene Aumerle's father,

the Duke of YORK (4), discovers his son's involvement in the ABBOT's plot against Bolingbroke and angrily declares that he will inform the new king. Aumerle's mother, the DUCHESS (4), sends him to court to beg for mercy before York can expose him. She follows and successfully pleads for his life. This episode contrasts Aumerle's devious character with his father's forthright patriotism, his mother's maternal passion, and Bolingbroke's generosity.

The historical Aumerle was a favourite of King Richard; when the Duke of Gloucester was killed, before the play opens, Aumerle was awarded much of the dead man's property and was created Duke of Albemarle (corrupted to Aumerle in Elizabethan English). Aumerle accompanied Richard to Ireland, and it was apparently his bad advice that led the King to delay his return to England upon Bolingbroke's arrival and then to dismiss his army when he got there. Further, in an episode probably unknown to Shakespeare, Aumerle abandoned Richard for Bolingbroke at that point; therefore, when he joined the Abbot's conspiracy against Bolingbroke, he was being doubly treacherous, and he was shortly to betray his fellow conspirators as well. His father's part in this action is probably not historical, although it is reported in Shakespeare's chief source, HOLINSHED's *Chronicles*. In any case, Aumerle was pardoned by Bolingbroke, by then HENRY IV, but his mother's involvement is entirely Shakespeare's invention; the Duchess had actually been dead for six years. Moreover, to increase the pathos of her plea, Shakespeare presented Aumerle as an only child; the Duke actually had a younger brother, the Earl of CAMBRIDGE, who is a character in *Henry V*. Aumerle himself reappears as the Duke of YORK (5) in that play.

Austria, Limoges (Lymoges), Archduke of Character in *King John*, ally of ARTHUR and King PHILIP (2) of FRANCE (1). Austria undertakes to fight King JOHN (3) and place Arthur on the throne of England. He claims to have killed the former English king, the famed Richard Coeur-de-Lion, and he wears a lion's skin as a trophy of this act. Austria is boastful, but when he is baited by the BASTARD (1), as in 3.1.56–58 (3.1.131–133, for citation, see KING JOHN, 'Synopsis'), he reveals his cowardice. In 3.2 (3.3) the Bastard displays Austria's head.

Shakespeare confused two historical figures in creating the Archduke. In the 16th century Austria was a major European power, and the playwright treats it as such, but in King John's day it was a minor German state. Leopold of Babenberg, a duke of Austria who died in 1194, five years before the earliest events of the play, had feuded with Richard Coeur-de-Lion when they were both Crusaders in Palestine; he then captured and held Richard for two years, until he received a great ransom. Later, in an unrelated battle, Richard died while besieging the castle of Waldemar, Viscount of Limoges (d. 1199), who may have been killed in revenge by Richard's illegitimate son (who did not otherwise resemble the fictitious Bastard of the play). Thus Shakespeare makes the territory of one of Richard's foes the first name of another. The playwright apparently took this error from 16th-century popular romances, which recounted Richard's life with little or no regard for accuracy.

Authorship controversy Dispute surrounding the identity of Shakespeare. Despite a wealth of evidence, a modern cult supports the proposition that someone other than Shakespeare—the identification varies—wrote the plays that are attributed to him. Shakespeare, it is contended, was an ignorant, perhaps illiterate, minor actor who was surely incapable of producing such literature. It is further contended that only an aristocratic, learned person could have done so, and that such a person would not have wished to be associated with the theatre. Therefore, it is concluded, the learned man assumed the actor's name as a disguise. A wide range of people have been nominated as the genuine author. Francis Bacon (1561–1626) was the favourite when the craze first developed, in the mid-19th century, though there have been many others since, including Christopher MARLOWE (1), the Earl of ESSEX (2), the Earl of DERBY (3), the Earl of RUTLAND (2), the Earl of OXFORD (1), and Queen ELIZABETH (1)—to name only some who actually lived during Shakespeare's lifetime. The current trend is towards Oxford, although he was a playwright without benefit of disguise and died midway through Shakespeare's career. Scholars of the period know beyond doubt that Shakespeare wrote Shakespeare, but the authorship controversy remains a minor sideshow of the literary world, and it will doubtless continue to get publicity.

Autolycus Character in *The Winter's Tale*, a vagabond thief who wanders through BOHEMIA. Autolycus appears, singing and bragging about his career as a petty thief, in 4.3. He picks the pocket of the CLOWN (8) and proposes to find further victims at the sheep-shearing festival, making 'the shearers prove sheep' (4.3.117). In 4.4 he attends the festival disguised as a peddler, singing SONGS, selling trinkets, and picking pockets. His songs and patter, his cheerful irresponsibility, and his insouciant delight in life add greatly to our enjoyment of the rustic scene. When King POLIXENES rages against the love of his son FLORIZEL and the shepherdess PERDITA, Autolycus exploits the situation to rob Perdita's foster-father, the SHEPHERD (2), who fears punishment and wants the king to know that Perdita was a foundling. Autolycus terrifies the old man and his son, the Clown, with accounts of the tortures they can expect and then offers, for money, to help them

reach the king. However, he actually turns them over to the fleeing Florizel, in the hope of reward. In this way evidence of Perdita's identity gets to SICILIA—she is the long-lost daughter of the Sicilian King LEONTES—resulting in reunions for the play's major characters and the incidental enrichment of the Shepherd and Clown with vast rewards. In 5.2 Autolycus admits that his life has earned no success, and he turns to flattering his former victims, now newly made gentlemen, in the hope of employment.

Autolycus is for the most part a charming rogue. He contributes greatly to the atmosphere of gaiety that surrounds the shepherds' world and thus to the comic tone of the play's second half. His crimes are petty compared with those of Leontes in the tragic first half of the play, but in any case it is part of the virtue of the pastoral world that it has room for this comical villain. The importance of mercy as a moral virtue is emphasised by the fact that Autolycus' depredations are accepted as a part of life. He even has a place in the play's final forgiveness and reconciliation, though the playwright could easily have left him in Bohemia. Autolycus represents the irrepressible mischievousness of human nature; that he selfishly views the world entirely in terms of his own convenience is deplorable, but he compensates through his contagious pleasure in simple things and the delightful songs in which he expresses this pleasure.

Autolycus resembles traditional comic characters, but he is not quite classifiable. He is too sophisticated for a rustic CLOWN (1), nor is he a FOOL (1), for he is not a professional jester. He does, however, resemble a Fool in his mockery, his songs, and his disinterested position relative to the main developments. He resembles FALSTAFF in his anomalous social position, his predatory nature, and his pretensions to an anti-ethic (he boasts of a piece of 'knavery', 'therein am I constant to my profession' [4.4.682–683]). Both characters, though amoral, are admirably independent, and the conflict of our judgements on the two traits yields subtle humour, as our own pretensions and secret predilections are exposed.

Autolycus' nature (like Falstaff's) gradually changes. At first he charms us, and we are inclined to forgive his crimes. However, as the shepherds' festival closes, he seems less pleasant, crying, 'Ha, ha! what a fool Honesty is!' (4.4.596) and gloating over his victims, who are sympathetic characters. When he plots how to profit from the desperate young lovers' situation, he is still funny, but we can no longer ignore his amorality, for it threatens the hero and heroine. His terrorising of the Shepherd with truly horrible descriptions of torture adds to our unease, and Autolycus acquires a darkly satirical cast as he replicates Polixenes' wrath while himself disguised as a courtier. He has changed sides in Shakespeare's opposition of pastoral innocence and sophisticated machinations. It is the Clown who is the comic character in 5.2, while Autolycus is merely another practitioner of the courtier's bowing and scraping to which he at first seemed antithetical.

Autolycus' only real connection to the plot, his role in preventing the Shepherd from revealing Perdita's origins too early, comes from the play's main source, the novella *Pandosto* by Robert GREENE (2), in which a servant of the prince—and Autolycus was once Florizel's servant—performs this function. However, making this figure a vagabond and thief was Shakespeare's invention. The playwright probably took the idea, as well as the name Autolycus, from OVID's description of the god Mercury's son in *The Metamorphoses.* Shakespeare's Autolycus brags of the connection, 'My father named me Autolycus; who, being as I am, littered under Mercury, was likewise a snapper-up of unconsidered trifles' (4.3.24–26).

Auvergne Region in south-central FRANCE (1), where 2.3 of *1 Henry VI* is set. The COUNTESS (1) of Auvergne attempts to capture the English lord TALBOT there.

Ayscough, Samuel (1745–1804) English scholar, the compiler of the first concordance of Shakespeare's works. Ayscough, a librarian at the British Museum, published his *Index, or Concordance of the Works of Shakespeare* in 1790.

B

Bad Quarto An early edition of a Shakespeare play, usually in QUARTO format, whose text was reconstructed from memory by actors who had performed the play, rather than coming from an authoritative source that accurately reflected what Shakespeare had written, such as his FOUL PAPERS. These texts, which the editors of the FIRST FOLIO described as 'stolen, and surreptitious copies, maimed, and deformed by the frauds and stealthes of iniurious impostors', were presumably made for purposes of piracy. Publishers—or, in some cases, a rival acting company—could profit from a play's popularity even though the script was jealously secreted by the acting company that had produced the play.

The eight undoubted Bad Quarto editions of Shakespeare's plays are: Q1 of *2 Henry VI* (1594); Q1 of *3 Henry VI* (1595); Q1 of *Romeo and Juliet* (1597); Q1 of *Henry V* (1600); Q1 of *The Merry Wives of Windsor* (1602); Q1 of *Hamlet* (1603); Q1 of *King Lear* (1607); and Q of *Pericles* (1609). Q is the only surviving early text of *Pericles;* the other seven Bad Quartos may be compared with the First Folio, and *Romeo and Juliet* and *Hamlet* also appeared as GOOD QUARTOS. In addition, two other plays are often classed as Bad Quartos: THE TAMING OF A SHREW (1594), considered a Bad Quarto of *The Taming of the Shrew,* and THE TROUBLESOME RAIGNE OF KING JOHN (1591), probably a reconstruction of *King John.*

Bad Quartos exhibit certain characteristics that result from errors of memory, including: repetitions and omissions of words; phrases that recollect earlier lines or anticipate later ones; many metrically flawed lines (see METRE); paraphrases and summaries of speeches; stage directions that summarise missing dialogue; and snippets from other plays in which the rememberer had also performed. Also, some passages are less flawed than others. This reflects an actor's firmer recollection of the lines he spoke than of the rest of the play. For instance, the Bad Quarto of *Hamlet* was probably recorded by a man who had played MARCELLUS, since that role is the only one whose dialogue is very accurately rendered.

A Bad Quarto's flaws can be disastrous, as in the notorious misrendering of HAMLET's most famous soliloquy, which in Q1 begins (with modernised spelling): 'To be, or not to be. Aye there's the point, / To die, to sleep, is that all? Aye all: / No, to sleep, to dream, aye marry there it goes . . .' (compare *Hamlet* 3.1.56–65). Although a corrupt text can be replaced by a sound one—except in the case of *Pericles*—a Bad Quarto is nonetheless useful to scholars in establishing a true text, as in another notable instance from *Hamlet* (in 2.2.415). Q1 records 'godly Ballet' (i.e., ballad) for Q2's 'pious chanson' and the First Folio's 'Pons Chanson'; we see that the actors of the day recognised—even if they did not precisely recall—a wry reference to a popular song on a religious subject. The Folio's reading, with its suggestion of the bridges of Paris, is therefore rejected.

Bagot, Sir John (d. c. 1400) Historical figure and character in *Richard II,* a supporter of RICHARD II. Bagot, with his colleagues John BUSHY and Henry GREENE (1), is one of the 'caterpillars' (2.3.165) whose influence on the King is said by BOLINGBROKE (1) to have been disastrous for England. They recognise that their position as favourites of the King is likely to prove dangerous if Bolingbroke defeats him, and in 2.2 they decide to seek safety when Bolingbroke appears. Bushy and Greene are captured and executed, but Bagot joins the King in Ireland and thus lives to appear before the triumphant Bolingbroke at the beginning of 4.1. He brings an accusation against the Duke of AUMERLE, presumably in exchange for clemency, and then disappears from the play.

The historical Bagot was a lesser aristocrat of WARWICKSHIRE and had originally been a supporter of the murdered Duke of GLOUCESTER (6). He was later recruited to Richard's cause and became close to the King; it was at Bagot's residence in COVENTRY that Richard stayed at the time of the trial by combat between Bolingbroke and MOWBRAY (1) that is depicted in 1.3. After the fall of the King, Bagot was imprisoned by Bolingbroke in the TOWER OF LONDON, where he is last known to have been alive.

Balthasar (1) Minor character in *The Comedy of Errors,* a merchant who is a friend of ANTIPHOLUS OF EPHESUS. Balthasar is present when, in 3.1, Antipholus is kept out of his own home by his wife and servants, who

believe he is an imposter. Balthasar dissuades Antipholus from breaking down the door, on the grounds that such an action would damage his reputation in the neighbourhood.

Balthasar (2) Minor character in *Romeo and Juliet,* servant of ROMEO. In 5.1 Balthasar brings Romeo the erroneous news that JULIET (1) is dead, triggering the last phase of the tragedy. In 5.3 Balthasar accompanies Romeo to Juliet's tomb. Romeo sends him away with a letter to MONTAGUE (1), but, concerned about his master, he stays to observe him. At the end of the play he gives the PRINCE (1) the letter, which helps to explain the tragedy to the lovers' parents.

Balthasar is the only servant of the Montagues in the play except for ABRAM and a nameless companion, who participate in the brawl in 1.1. Accordingly, Balthasar is conventionally designated as the companion, who neither speaks nor is named in early texts of the play.

Balthasar (3) Minor character in *The Merchant of Venice,* servant of PORTIA (1). In 3.4 Balthasar is sent with a letter to Portia's cousin, setting in motion her plan to impersonate a lawyer at the hearing of SHYLOCK's suit against ANTONIO (2). Portia later takes Balthasar's name as part of her disguise.

Balthasar (4) Minor character in *Much Ado About Nothing,* a musician and singer employed by Don PEDRO. In 2.3 Don Pedro instructs Balthasar to sing the SONG 'Sigh no more, ladies', though Balthasar insists he is not a good singer. In 5.3 he sings the solemn 'Pardon, goddess of the night', as CLAUDIO (1) mourns the supposed death of HERO. Balthasar makes feeble attempts to be witty, especially when he fishes for compliments in 2.3, but he has no real personality. He is part of the play's atmosphere of aristocratic decorum and hospitality, here expressed through courtly music, a standard feature of the great noble households of both RENAISSANCE Italy and Elizabethan England.

In a stage direction in the FIRST FOLIO edition of the play (1623), Balthasar is identified as 'Iacke Wilson', a reference to the actor who played the part. It cannot be known for certain who this was, but scholars frequently propose both Jack WILSON (1) and John WILSON (2).

Bandello, Matteo (1485–1561) Italian writer, author of tales that served as sources for several of Shakespeare's works. Bandello's collection of tales, *Novelle* (1554), based loosely on the example of BOCCACCIO's *Decameron* (1353), was adapted in French by François BELLEFOREST and in English by Arthur BROOKE (1), Geoffrey FENTON (2), and William PAINTER (2). Various of these versions and, probably, the Italian original were used by Shakespeare. The creation of AARON in *Titus Andronicus* may have been influenced by a Bandello tale in Belleforest; for *Romeo and Juliet,* the playwright adapted a love story taken from Bandello in versions by Brooke and Painter. The tale of HERO and CLAUDIO (1) in *Much Ado About Nothing* was taken from Bandello's Italian original and *his* source, a tale by ARIOSTO. A single passage in *Twelfth Night* may also have been inspired by Bandello.

Bandello led a highly dramatic life. An aristocrat, he joined the Dominican order as a youth and travelled widely with his uncle, a noted theologian who visited monasteries throughout Europe. However, he soon withdrew from the church to pursue a career as a courtier and man of letters—for instance, for eight years he was court poet to the Duchess of Mantua. Here he began to write the tales that were eventually to make him famous. A political intriguer, Bandello was forced in 1525 to flee hastily from Milan, abandoning all he owned including the manuscripts of many tales. He became an adviser to a pro-French Venetian general, but in 1542 the general was exiled to France, and Bandello followed him.

The French king granted Bandello the income from a bishopric, and he was finally free to assemble the novellas he had been writing for almost half a century. The first edition of *Novelle,* containing some 200 tales, was instantly popular throughout Europe. It consists for the most part of romantic legends retold in a racy, briskly journalistic style. Some stories were virtually pornographic by the standards of the day. Today, Bandello's tales are considered to have very little literary merit, but at the time their influence was widespread in Italy, France, Spain, and England. Besides Shakespeare, other English writers who drew upon Bandello include the English dramatists John WEBSTER (2), Francis BEAUMONT (2) and John FLETCHER (2), and Philip MASSINGER.

Bandit (Thief) Any of three minor characters in *Timon of Athens,* thieves who hope to rob TIMON. In 4.3 after Timon has withdrawn from ATHENS to the woods in rage and despair because he has been abandoned by his friends, the Bandits learn that he has found gold and they accost him. They don't know that he intends to give it away in an attempt to corrupt hateful humanity. He ironically praises them for being obvious thieves, and compares them to those who pretend to be good citizens. He gives them gold and encourages them to commit more crimes. 'Cut throats. / All that you meet are thieves. To Athens go . . .' (4.3.448–449), he says. As they leave, the Bandits remark on Timon's misanthropy. Two of the three contemplate giving up thievery since it is advocated by so malicious a man. As the Third Bandit puts it, 'H'as almost charm'd me from my profession, by persuading me to it' (4.3.453–454). Collectively called 'banditti' in the stage direction that introduces them, at 4.3.401, the Bandits are designated as Thieves in many editions.

Bangor Town in WALES (1), possibly the setting for 3.1 of *1 Henry IV.* Some editors of the play, beginning with THEOBALD in the 18th century, have followed Shakespeare's chief source, HOLINSHED, and placed this scene, in which the conspirators against HENRY IV plan to divide the realm among themselves, in the home of the Archdeacon of Bangor. However, Shakespeare made no designation of location, and the host of the meeting appears to be GLENDOWER.

Banquo Character in *Macbeth,* friend and later victim of MACBETH. In 1.3 Banquo and Macbeth encounter the WITCHES, who predict that Macbeth will become Thane of CAWDOR and King of SCOTLAND. They add that Banquo, whom they describe as 'Lesser than Macbeth, and greater' (1.3.65), shall father a line of rulers, though he shall not be one himself. Macbeth, inspired by this encounter to fulfil his ambition, kills King DUNCAN and seizes the throne. He then worries about the possibility that his kingdom will fall to Banquo's heirs, and he orders Banquo and his son FLEANCE murdered. In 3.3 the FIRST MURDERER (3) and his companions kill Banquo, though Fleance escapes. Banquo's GHOST (4) later appears to Macbeth, aggravating his bad conscience. In 4.1 the Ghost confirms the Witches' prediction that his descendants will be KINGS. King JAMES I, England's ruler in Shakespeare's day, was believed to be descended from an historical Lord Banquo.

Banquo is a decent and honourable nobleman who senses that the Witches are evil and thus not to be relied on. He warns Macbeth that 'oftentimes, to win us to our harm, / The instruments of Darkness tell us truths' (1.3.123–124), and his concern contrasts strikingly with Macbeth's susceptibility to the Witches. Banquo's resistance points up Macbeth's failure to resist and stresses his tendency towards evil, the flaw that makes the tragedy possible. When he decides to murder Banquo, Macbeth acknowledges his 'royalty of nature' (3.1.49). He fears that Banquo's righteousness may turn him into an enemy. Thus, we see that Banquo's fate is dictated by his virtue, just as Macbeth's is determined by his villainy.

In Shakespeare's source for *Macbeth,* HOLINSHED's *Chronicles,* Banquo collaborates with Macbeth in the murder of Duncan and is killed because he knows too much. The playwright may have altered Banquo simply to avoid depicting the king's ancestor as a murderer, though Banquo could merely have been omitted to achieve this end. However, Shakespeare probably realised that the play is stronger with only a single villain, and Banquo's supposed ancestry to the king made him an apt choice to stand in opposition to that villain as a pointedly virtuous comrade. That this was Banquo's more important function for Shakespeare is suggested by the playwright's disregard for Fleance's fate or for the question of Banquo's descendants, once Fleance's survival ensures that he could have had some.

Though Holinshed, Shakespeare, and King James himself had no reason to doubt the belief that Banquo was a predecessor of the STUART dynasty, modern scholarship has established that this was not true. Banquo may reflect some ancient chieftain of Scotland, but outside Holinshed's source, the semi-legendary history of Hector BOECE, he has no historical standing.

Baptista Character in *The Taming of the Shrew,* father of KATHERINA and BIANCA (1). Baptista is an ineffectual elderly gentleman, a comic figure in a tradition going back to ancient Roman drama. He is frequently the butt of Katherina's outbursts of temper. He insists on marrying off his elder daughter first, aggravating Katherina's already shrewish nature. In 2.1, once assured that Katherina is betrothed, Baptista literally auctions Bianca to the highest bidder; his calculating behaviour stands in pointed contrast to the infatuation of Bianca's lover, LUCENTIO. These are standard attitudes and actions of a conventional father-of-the-girl figure; otherwise, Baptista has virtually no personality.

Barbary Horse named in *Richard II.* The GROOM (1) who visits RICHARD II in prison in 5.5 tells the deposed King that his successor, BOLINGBROKE (1), has ridden Barbary at his coronation and that the horse carried its new rider 'proudly' (5.5.83). Richard is initially angry with his former steed, but he then berates himself for railing at the animal.

Shakespeare apparently invented this episode, which appears in none of his sources. Barbary is also the name of a highly valued breed of horse exported from North Africa, itself known as Barbary.

Bardolph (1) Character in *1* and *2 Henry IV, The Merry Wives of Windsor,* and *Henry V,* a follower of FALSTAFF. In *1 Henry IV* Bardolph participates in the highway robbery of 2.2, and in *2 Henry IV* he assists the fat knight in his illicit recruiting efforts in 3.2, collecting bribes from men who wish to avoid service. When Falstaff is rejected by PRINCE (6) Hal in 5.5, Bardolph goes to prison with him. In *The Merry Wives* Bardolph is only a minor figure who occasionally delivers messages to Falstaff. In *Henry V* he is a soldier in the army of King HENRY V. In 2.1 he defuses the feud between PISTOL and NYM. In 3.2.28–57 the BOY (3) convincingly describes him as a coward and thief. In 3.6 we learn that Bardolph is to be executed for having stolen a sacramental vessel from a French church, and in 4.4 the Boy reports that Bardolph has indeed been hung.

Despite his swaggering, he has little distinctive personality. His peacemaking role in *Henry V* ironically counters King HENRY V's bellicosity in an anti-war reading of the play, but if one interprets Henry as a epic hero, then Bardolph remains a comic soldier, a

petty villain whose end helps to demonstrate the King's dedication to justice. Bardolph's most prominent characteristic is his diseased facial complexion, florid and fiery, 'all bubukles, and whelks, and knobs, and flames o' fire' (*Henry V,* 3.6.105–106). He is teased mercilessly about his skin disorder by Falstaff and other characters, finding himself compared to lamps, torches, blushing maids, red wine, red petticoats, hell-fire, and even 'Lucifer's privy kitchen' (*2 Henry IV,* 2.4.330).

Bardolph was originally called ROSSILL, but after *2 Henry IV* was written the name was changed, probably to avoid offending a prominent aristocrat, William Russill, Earl of Bedford. The fact that the name Bardolph had already been assigned to another character in *2 Henry IV,* Lord BARDOLPH (2), is only one instance of Shakespeare's tolerance for minor confusions and inconsistencies in his plays.

Bardolph (2), Lord Thomas (1368–1408) Historical figure and character in *2 Henry IV,* a follower of the Earl of NORTHUMBERLAND (1) and a rebel against King HENRY IV. He is invariably referred to as Lord Bardolph to distinguish him from BARDOLPH (1), who appears in the same play. Lord Bardolph brings Northumberland a mistaken report of a rebel victory in 1.1, and he helps to encourage the crestfallen Earl after the real news arrives. In 1.3 he urges caution on his fellow rebels, Lord HASTINGS (2) and the ARCHBISHOP (3) of York, who insist on challenging the King. Although he then disappears from the play, the defeat of Lord Bardolph and Northumberland is reported in 4.4; he thus seems associated with Northumberland's betrayal of the rebel cause.

The historical Lord Bardolph, like Northumberland, did not desert the rebellion. He fought with distinction and died in battle several years after GAULTREE FOREST.

A speech prefix in the QUARTO edition of the play (1600) indicates that Lord Bardolph's part in 1.1 was originally written for Sir John UMFREVILE, another follower of Northumberland's, whose part was assigned to Lord Bardolph in order to reduce the number of actors required.

Barents (Barentz), Willem (c. 1550–1597) Dutch explorer. Between 1594 and 1597 Barents led several naval expeditions to the Arctic in search of a north-east passage to the Orient; the Barents Sea, north of Scandinavia, is named for him. An account of Barents' voyage of 1596–1597 was published in London in 1598 and was very popular, being reprinted for years. FABIAN is believed to allude to Barents when, in *Twelfth Night,* he tells SIR ANDREW, who has earned OLIVIA's disdain, that he has 'sailed into the nor of my lady's opinion, where you will hang like an icicle on a Dutchman's beard' (3.2.25–26).

Barker, Harley Granville See GRANVILLE-BARKER.

Barkloughly Castle Welsh castle seen in 3.2 of *Richard II.* Shakespeare's source, HOLINSHED's history, incorrectly identified Hertlowli, an ancient name for Harlech Castle, as Barclowlie and thus led the playwright into error. Nevertheless, this name indicates that the scene is in WALES (1) and that Richard has returned to Britain from Ireland.

Barkstead, William (active 1606–1629) English poet and dramatist. A very minor figure in English literature, Barkstead is best known for a long poem, *Myrrha, the Mother of Adonis* (1607), in which he modestly (and correctly) referred to Shakespeare as a much greater poet who had dealt with the Adonis story (see VENUS AND ADONIS). He was employed by several minor acting companies, though his only surviving drama is *The Insatiate Countess* (c. 1610), written in collaboration with John MARSTON.

Barnardine Minor character in *Measure for Measure,* a condemned criminal whose undeserved pardon epitomises the play's theme of unqualified mercy. Barnardine is a comical brute who is 'drunk many times a day, if not many days entirely drunk' (4.2.147–148). He declares he will not come forward to be executed on the day appointed—when he is to substitute for CLAUDIO (3)—because he has 'been drinking hard all night, and [needs] more time to prepare . . .' (4.3.52–53). The DUKE (9) postpones the execution, saying that under the circumstances it could only send the victim to instant damnation, a responsibility the Duke will not take. In 5.1 the ruler pardons Barnardine and remands him into the custody of the FRIAR (1) as part of the mercy and forgiveness of the play's dénouement.

Barnardine is funny in his stubborn refusal to be killed and helps provide relief from the oppressiveness of the prison, where much of the middle of the play is set. Yet he is a callous murderer 'unfit to live or die' (4.3.63). Although Barnardine is specifically designated as a proper subject for execution, he is pardoned as part of the play's final conciliation; his evilness then highlights the magnanimity of the Duke's mercy.

Barnardo (Bernardo) Minor character in *Hamlet.* Barnardo and MARCELLUS are the two sentries who have seen the GHOST (3) of HAMLET's father before the play begins. In 1.1 they introduce Hamlet's friend HORATIO to the phenomenon. When the three tell Hamlet about the spirit in 1.2, Barnardo barely speaks, and when Hamlet accompanies Horatio and Marcellus to encounter the Ghost in 1.4, Barnardo has disappeared from the play.

Barnes, Barnabe (c. 1569–1609) English poet and dramatist, author of an influence on *Pericles* and possibly the 'rival poet' of the SONNETS. Barnes' play *The Devil's Charter* (1607) derived from a work by the Italian historian Francesco Guicciardini (1483–1540), and it featured Guicciardini as a CHORUS (1). Shakespeare used this idea in *Pericles,* where the source, the poet John GOWER (3), serves the same function; in fact, some of Gower's speeches echo the words of Barnes' Guicciardini. Because Barnes was a noted SONNET writer who eulogised the Earl of SOUTHAMPTON (2)—Shakespeare's patron—some commentators, following scholar Sidney LEE, consider him a likely nominee for the 'rival poet' of Shakespeare's sonnets.

Barnet Location in *3 Henry VI,* a town near London and a battle site of the WARS OF THE ROSES. King EDWARD IV, having taken London and captured HENRY VI, marches north to meet the army of WARWICK (3). In 5.2–3 their forces meet in a conflict that is depicted as a simple rout of Warwick's troops, in which Warwick dies and the other Lancastrian leaders flee to join the army of Queen MARGARET (1). The historical battle of Barnet, which occurred on Easter Sunday, 1471, was very closely fought; it was won for Edward only when one element of Warwick's army mistakenly attacked another in the heavy fog that shrouded the field. However, Shakespeare chose to emphasise the strength of the Yorkist forces, for the dynamic of his play at this point is directed towards their final victory at the battle of TEWKESBURY, which occurs over the next two scenes.

Barnfield, Richard (1574–1627) Landed gentleman and amateur poet, an early admirer of Shakespeare. Barnfield published his first work, an imitation of *Venus and Adonis* titled *The Affectionate Shepherd,* at the age of 20; he published three more collections of poems over the next four years, but he then retired to his country estate and apparently stopped writing. He wrote the first published verse in praise of Shakespeare, a stanza in a poem called 'A Remembrance of Some English Poets' (1598). Barnfield was a prominent member of the London literary scene in the 1590s, and Shakespeare was probably acquainted with him. Two of Barnfield's poems were published as Shakespeare's in William JAGGARD's spurious anthology THE PASSIONATE PILGRIM (1599), and it is chiefly for this reason that his work is remembered today.

Barrett, Lawrence (1838–1891) American actor. An actor from the age of 14, Barrett established himself in New York in 1857 and became a friend and partner of Edwin BOOTH (2), playing IAGO opposite his OTHELLO, and CASSIUS—the part for which he was best known—opposite Booth's CAESAR (2). He also played RICHARD III, LEAR, and SHYLOCK. Barrett served in the Union army in the Civil War; he then managed a theatre in San Francisco, from 1867 to 1871, before returning to New York to run the Booth's Theatre. In 1884 he took over Henry IRVING's Lyceum Theatre in London, while Irving toured America. Barrett was unusual among actors of his day in taking an intellectual interest in the American theatre; he introduced revivals of several plays and was a theatre historian, the author of *Edwin Forrest* (1881) (see FORREST) and *Edwin Booth and his Contemporaries* (1886).

Barry (1), Ann (1734–1801) English actress. Ann Barry's earliest recorded performances were at the Dublin theatre of Spranger BARRY (3), opposite whose LEAR and OTHELLO she was acclaimed as CORDELIA and DESDEMONA. She went with Barry to London and later married him. Though particularly successful in COMEDY, she played all sorts of parts, both new and classical. She was much admired as JULIET (1), ROSALIND, ISABELLA, IMOGEN, and PERDITA. Highly popular, she was regarded as one of the few rivals of Sarah SIDDONS. She died shortly after retiring and was buried in WESTMINSTER (1) ABBEY.

Barry (2), Elizabeth (1658–1713) English actress. The leading actress of the late 17th century, Barry is sometimes called the first great English actress. Often playing opposite Thomas BETTERTON, she was especially acclaimed as LADY (6) MACBETH, Queen KATHERINE in *Henry VIII,* and CORDELIA in Nahum TATE's version of *King Lear.* She was said to have garnered her first training as an actress while the mistress of the notorious rake, poet, and aesthete, the Earl of Rochester (1640–1680), with whom she bore a child. Throughout her life, she was named in similar scandals, though at least one man, the playwright Thomas OTWAY, is said to have suffered from her rejection.

Barry (3), Spranger (1719–1777) Irish actor. Barry was among the leading Shakespearean actors of the 1750s, especially noted for his portrayal of OTHELLO. His rivalry with David GARRICK was much publicised; the so-called *Romeo and Juliet* war—their simultaneous performances as ROMEO (Barry in the adaptation by Colley CIBBER [1])—was followed by similar matchups as LEAR and RICHARD III. In 1758 Barry attempted to establish a theatre in Dublin but quickly went bankrupt. He did, however, meet and bring back to London a new leading lady, soon his wife, Ann BARRY (1). Upon his return to London, he joined Garrick's company for the remainder of his career.

Barrymore, John (1882–1942) American actor. After establishing himself as a glamorous leading man—a 'matinee idol'—Barrymore stunned the New York theatrical world in 1922 with an electrifying portrayal of HAMLET, repeating the accomplishment in

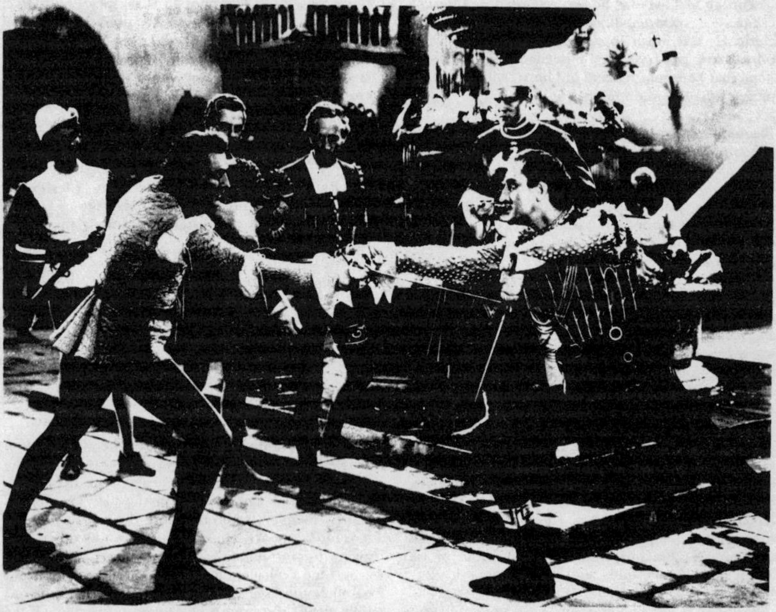

John Barrymore as Mercutio (left) in his swordfight with Tybalt (Romeo and Juliet *3.1). George Cukor's 1936 film also starred Leslie Howard (center) as Romeo and Basil Rathbone (right) as Tybalt.* (Courtesy of Movie Star News)

London in 1925. His Hamlet was regarded as one of the great performances of the day, but Barrymore largely abandoned the stage for film in the remainder of his career. He appeared as MERCUTIO in George Cukor's 1936 film of *Romeo and Juliet.*

John and his siblings, Lionel and Ethel, were regarded as leaders of the American theatre—*The Royal Family,* as the title of a 1927 play about them had it. Both his mother and his father were from long-established theatrical families, and John DREW was his uncle.

Bartholomew Character in *The Taming of the Shrew.* See PAGE (8).

Bartley, George (c. 1782–1858) Nineteenth-century English actor who specialised in playing FALSTAFF. Bartley's success as the fat knight began in 1815 and carried him through to his retirement in 1852. In 1818–1819 he made a triumphal tour of America, although in Hartford, Connecticut, he was arrested by a puritanical official who objected to dramatic readings and enforced a colonial-era 'blue law'.

Barton (1), John (b. 1928) Twentieth-century English theatrical producer. Barton, a long-time director with the Royal Shakespeare Company, has staged many of Shakespeare's plays. Among his most notable productions have been *The Taming of the Shrew* (1960), *Twelfth Night* (1969), *Measure for Measure* (1970), and *Much Ado About Nothing* (1976). With Peter HALL (5), Barton co-directed 'The Wars of the Roses' (1964), the TELEVISION productions that combined the *Henry VI* plays and *Richard III.*

Barton (2), Richard (active 1584–1601) Vicar at STRATFORD. In 1585 Barton baptised Hamnet and Judith SHAKESPEARE (5, 10), the playwright's twin children. Barton, originally from COVENTRY, was vicar in Stratford from 1584–1589. He was apparently a man

of Puritan leanings for he was recorded in a Puritan critique of WARWICKSHIRE ministers as a superior cleric. He was much appreciated by the town, which offered him pay raises and miscellaneous gifts in the hope that he would remain, but he accepted a better-paying post elsewhere after five years.

Bassanio Character in *The Merchant of Venice,* friend of ANTONIO (2) and suitor of PORTIA (1). In requesting money from Antonio in order to court Portia in style, Bassanio is indirectly responsible for the peril in which the merchant finds himself when he borrows from SHYLOCK and risks his flesh. But Bassanio is also an important figure in his own right. He wins Portia by choosing the correct casket in the lottery required by her father, and, in so doing, he demonstrates a 16th-century ideal of romantic love. He distrusts the rich appearance of the gold and silver caskets (3.2.73–107) and instead selects the casket of lead. Such a choice was a conventional indication of selfless love. Only a true lover would value the maid for herself rather than her 'outward shows' (3.2.73), as Bassanio does. He is a leisured gentleman, presumably able to find a wife elsewhere, but he is willing to risk his chances of matrimony in order to win Portia. Like Antonio, he finds value in reaching for the greatest happiness, and is thus placed in opposition to Shylock's stinginess. Similarly, like Antonio and Portia and unlike Shylock, Bassanio gives what he has. He is a good-hearted spendthrift who cannot refuse a request, as when GRATIANO (1) announces that he has a favour to ask and is immediately told, 'You have obtain'd it' (2.2. 169).

Bassanio is sometimes seen in a rather different light. Some critics regard him as an heiress-hunting playboy whose irresponsibility endangers Antonio. However, Bassanio objects to Antonio's acceptance of Shylock's bond (1.3.150–151) and is persuaded only by his friend's assurances that he will certainly be able to repay the loan. And although Bassanio refers to Portia's wealth when he first mentions the idea of marrying her (1.1.161–176), this does not necessarily make him a gold-digger. Such considerations were normal in the 16th century; one would not discuss courtship without bringing up the subject of wealth. For Shakespeare's audience, and for the playwright himself, such behaviour was ordinary, and Bassanio was surely intended as a romantic hero, a personification of good fortune in love.

Bassanio's name—not found in Shakespeare's sources for the play—may have been taken from one of several Bassanios, natives of Venice, who were musicians in the household of Queen ELIZABETH (1) (see LANIER).

Basse, William (c. 1583–c. 1653) English poet. A minor figure in English literature, Basse is best known today for a 20-line EPITAPH on Shakespeare, written c. 1621. This poem was originally published as John DONNE's in 1633; it was credited to 'W. B'. when it appeared in the 1640 edition of Shakespeare's *Poems* (see BENSON [2]). The only other Basse work that is read today is *Angler's Song,* an appreciation of fishing.

Basset Minor character in *1 Henry VI,* a supporter of the Duke of SOMERSET (3). Basset disputes with VERNON (1), a partisan of the Duke of YORK (8), in 3.4 and 4.1. By demonstrating the involvement of lesser figures, these incidents magnify the damage to English morale caused by the dissensions among the noblemen.

Bassianus Character in *Titus Andronicus,* brother of the Emperor, SATURNINUS. In 1.1 Bassianus relinquishes his claim to the throne when TITUS (1) Andronicus declares in favour of his brother, but he will not surrender his fiancée, LAVINIA, to him. The first victim of AARON's plots, Bassianus is killed by CHIRON and DEMETRIUS (1), prior to their rape of Lavinia in 2.3.

Bastard (1), Philip Faulconbridge, The Character in *King John,* illegitimate nephew of King JOHN (3). The Bastard, the most prominent character in the play, is a complicated figure. Early in the play he satirises courtly manners while revealing the self-serving behaviour he mocks. He impulsively insults others and makes humorous asides to himself, yet he is at the same time a calculating social climber. His illegitimacy parallels the king's status as a usurper, and, just as John defies the French challenge to his rule, so the Bastard relies on his strength of character to maintain himself in aristocratic society. Yet while John falls, the Bastard prospers; his rise is concurrent with John's fall, and the contrast lends piquancy to the king's collapse. He begins as a comical figure, but by the end of the play he is clearly the mainstay of the English forces. He has remained true to the king, unlike the other noblemen, and it is he who first acknowledges Prince HENRY (1) as the new king, emphasising the restoration of social order.

The Bastard also functions as a CHORUS (1), commenting on the foibles of society, sometimes contradicting his role in the plot. For instance, he deplores 'commodity', or self-interest, in a famous soliloquy (2.1.561–598), yet he is guilty of commodity himself, as he admits in the last dozen lines of the speech. Shakespeare uses the fictitious Bastard somewhat in the manner of the allegorical figures of a MORALITY PLAY, while at the same time making his spirited courage and loyalty humanly admirable. Most strikingly, while the Bastard bears some resemblance to the ancient dramatic figure of the VICE—in his repeated identification with the devil (e.g., in 2.1.134–

135), and in his presentation of satirical monologues directly to the audience—he is also in some sense the hero of the play, an exemplar of patriotic virtue. He closes the play with a speech (5.7.112–118) that has been a staple of British patriotic literature since it first appeared.

The Bastard is not based on any single historical figure, although elements of his situation are drawn from the lives of several historical bastards. King Richard I did have an illegitimate son named Philip, and, although very little is known of him, he is reputed to have killed the Viscount of Limoges in revenge for his father's death; the Bastard has his first name and kills AUSTRIA, who is identified with Limoges in the play. The name Faulconbridge was borne by another noteworthy bastard, William Neville, Lord FALCONBRIDGE (2), who is mentioned in *3 Henry VI.* An illegitimate Norman nobleman, Faukes de Bréauté (d. c. 1227), led John's armies against the rebellious barons, as the Bastard does in the play, but Shakespeare's character bears no resemblance to this man, a notoriously cruel and oppressive mercenary soldier who finally had to be driven from England by force in 1224. Another famous figure, Jean Dunois, the BASTARD (2) of Orléans, apparently contributed to Shakespeare's character as well. Dunois appears in *1 Henry VI,* but that play does not present this famed general with historical accuracy. However, his proclamation, reported in HOLINSHED's *Chronicles,* that he would rather be the bastard of a great man than the legitimate heir of a humble one, is clearly echoed by the Bastard of *King John* (1.1.164, 259–276).

Bastard (2) of Orléans, Jean Dunois, The (1403–1468) Historical figure and character in *1 Henry VI,* one of the leaders of the French forces. Though the historical Bastard, who was well known by that appellation, was one of the leading soldiers of the 15th century, he is presented in the play as a boastful but cowardly and inept warrior. His personality resembles that of the other French noblemen, whose collective role was simply to demonstrate that France could not have been victorious but for dissensions among the English.

Bastard (3) Character in *Troilus and Cressida.* See MARGARELON.

Bates, John Minor character in *Henry V,* one of the soldiers who encounter the incognito King HENRY V on the eve of the battle of AGINCOURT. Bates is a grumbler who wishes he were elsewhere, even if the King were left alone in FRANCE (1), but he also says, 'yet I determine to fight lustily for him' (4.1.196). He tries to allay the quarrel between WILLIAMS (2) and the stranger (the King), saying, 'Be friends, you English fools, be friends: we have French quarrels enow . . .' (4.1.228–229). Bates is a typical English soldier, part of the scene's varied presentation of the army's morale before the battle.

Bavian Minor character in *The Two Noble Kinsmen,* a performer dressed as a baboon, or bavian. The Bavian is part of an entertainment performed before THESEUS (2), Duke of ATHENS in 3.5. He speaks only two words, 'Yes, sir' (3.5.37), in response to his director, the SCHOOLMASTER (2), who tells him, 'My friend, carry your tail without offence / Or scandal to the ladies; and be sure / You tumble with audacity and manhood, / And when you bark do it with judgement' (3.5.34–37). This directive casts an amusing light on English rustic entertainments of the 17th century. However, most scholars agree that Shakespeare did not write this scene; the Bavian and his instructions are probably the work of John FLETCHER (2).

Bawd Minor character in *Pericles,* the keeper of a brothel in MYTILENE, who, with her husband the PANDAR, buys the kidnapped MARINA. The Bawd is a hard-boiled madam. She coolly assesses her wenches as 'creatures . . . [who] with continual action are even as good as rotten' (4.2.6–9). She rejects her husband's scruples: 'Other sorts offend as well as we' (4.2.34), she says grumpily. She is prepared to be friendly with the newly-bought Marina, and assures her that she 'shall live in pleasure [and] taste gentlemen of all fashions' (4.2.72–76). When Marina grieves at her plight, however, the Bawd turns nasty, and declares, 'you're a young foolish sapling, and must be bow'd as I would have you' (4.2.83–85). The Bawd jokes cynically with her employee BOULT about the venereal diseases of their clients. This was a traditional subject of humour in Shakespeare's day, but placed in contrast with the virginal Marina it seems shocking. When Marina's virtues begin to encourage moral reform among her customers, the Bawd complains comically, 'Fie, fie upon her! She's able to freeze the god Priapus, and undo a whole generation' (4.6.3–4). In her energetic sinfulness, the Bawd resembles such other Shakespearean ladies of the demi-monde as HOSTESS (2) QUICKLY and MISTRESS (2) OVERDONE, though the underworld of Mytilene is not so developed as those of LONDON and VIENNA. The Bawd contributes to the comic—and realistic—relief from the elevated and melodramatic romance of the main plot.

Baylis, Lilian (1874–1937) English theatrical entrepreneur, director of the OLD VIC and SADLER'S WELLS THEATRES. In 1898 Lilian Baylis, the daughter of professional singers, joined her aunt in the management of the Royal Victoria Coffee Music Hall—a temperance organisation dedicated to liquor-free entertainment—in the theatre building already known as the Old Vic. Baylis added opera performances, and the

Old Vic soon became a leading operatic theatre. In 1914, joined by Ben GREET, she added Shakespearean performances to the schedule, and the Old Vic was soon established as a national centre of Shakespearean production. At her instigation and with her support—though she made a point of leaving all artistic decisions to others—the entire CANON of Shakespeare's plays had been staged by 1923. In 1931 Baylis acquired the Sadler's Wells Theatre as a companion theatre in north London for the Old Vic in south London, and put on Shakespeare there as well, although since 1934 it has been chiefly associated with opera. As a leading light of the Shakespearean theatre, Lilian Baylis was regarded as a British national treasure, and she received many honours including one of the first Oxford honorary degrees given to a woman outside academia.

Baynard Castle London fortress, a setting in *Richard III.* In 3.7 RICHARD III receives the MAYOR (3) of London, accompanied by a number of citizens, in Baynard Castle. Manipulated by the Duke of BUCKINGHAM (2), this group offers Richard the crown, insisting that he take it when he cynically feigns reluctance.

Shakespeare took this historical incident and its setting from his sources. Richard's use of Baynard Castle signalled the strength of his drive for the crown, for it was an important bastion of royalty in London, second in strength and importance only to the TOWER OF LONDON. Like the Tower, it was built by England's Norman conquerors to control the city. Looming across the river from SOUTHWARK, Baynard Castle was a familiar landmark in Shakespeare's day; it was later destroyed in the Great Fire of London in 1666.

Beadle (1) Minor character in *2 Henry VI,* a constable of the village of ST. ALBANS who is assigned to whip the imposter SIMPCOX in 2.1.

Beadle (2) Any of several minor characters in *2 Henry IV,* petty London officials assigned to whip the HOSTESS (2) and DOLL TEARSHEET. In 5.4 the Beadles drag the two women across the stage. One of them speaks, remarking that the punishment has been decreed because the women have been involved in a murder. Both women insult the chief Beadle, referring to his skeletal appearance. In the QUARTO edition of the play, a stage direction identified this Beadle as John SINCKLO, a very thin actor, and it is presumed that Shakespeare wrote this scene with him in mind.

Bear Minor figure in *The Winter's Tale,* wild beast that kills ANTIGONUS as he abandons the infant PERDITA on the coast of BOHEMIA. Antigonus is warned by the MARINER (1) that wild animals are present, and as he completes his task, he is attacked. At 3.3.58 one of Shakespeare's most famous stage directions instructs Antigonus, 'Exit, pursued by a bear'. Later in the scene, the CLOWN (8) reports that the bear has 'half dined upon the gentleman' (3.3.105). The startling appearance of a bear makes Antigonus' death a vivid event, forcefully elevating it as a symbol of the consequences of tragedy. At the same time Antigonus' appalling end suggests humanity's helplessness in the face of nature and thus reinforces a major theme of the play, our ultimate dependence on providence.

Carnivores of all sorts figure prominently in Shakespeare's imagery, and bears in particular consistently represent fearsome savagery. Sometimes the image is comical, as in the remark of a stubborn bachelor, 'As from a bear a man would run for life, / So fly I from her that would be my wife' (*Comedy of Errors,* 3.2.153–154); sometimes in earnest, as when PROSPERO describes the tormented ARIEL: 'thy groans / Did make wolves howl, and penetrate the breasts / Of ever-angry bears' (*Tempest* 1.2.287–289). In *The Winter's Tale* Antigonus himself uses such imagery, unconsciously and ironically anticipating his own end, when he hopes that wild animals, including 'wolves and bears' (2.3.186), will be merciful to the abandoned Perdita. This desire is pointedly hopeless, given the nature of wolves and bears. Although the bear does spare the infant, it does so only because it devours Antigonus.

Although Antigonus' death is unquestionably horrific, it also has a slightly comical note. The bear's sudden appearance is as unexpected as a punch line and charged with the awkward unreality of an actor costumed as a bear. The Clown's later description is frankly humorous. The bear's brief appearance thus offers an emotional transition from the tragic first half of the play to the pastoral comedy of Act 4.

Scholars and theatrical directors have speculated on whether Shakespeare intended the use of a live bear on stage. Some scholars have suggested that he did, as live bears attracted crowds to the bear-baiting arena a few doors from the GLOBE THEATRE, where the audience paid to see dogs attack the bears. However, there are many objections to this idea, beginning with the notoriously temperamental nature of bears (tame bears were known in 17th-century England, but they were always leashed—an inappropriate condition for a savage killer). An actor costumed as a bear was most probably what Shakespeare had in mind; a bear is much the easiest wild animal for a human being to imitate, and bear costumes are known to have been used fairly frequently in Shakespeare's day.

Beatrice Character in *Much Ado About Nothing,* sharp-tongued rival in wits—and later the lover—of BENEDICK. Beatrice, who initially disparages love and Benedick, later rejects these attitudes and becomes his betrothed. She in fact loves him all along, as the audience knows; her own awareness comes only with the assurance that he loves her. Their relationship ma-

tures when they act together to defend her defamed cousin HERO at the crisis point of the play.

Beatrice bluntly disdains love, sneering, 'I had rather hear my dog bark at a crow than a man swear he loves me' (1.1.120–122), but her first words (1.1. 28–29) have already betrayed her interest in Benedick, although she covers it with a veneer of witty insults and teasing. She has suffered through an earlier unhappy romance with Benedick, as she suggests in 1.1.59 and 2.1.261–264, and her barbed wit is plainly defensive, disguising her true feelings even from her self. Her brashness is nicely contrasted with Hero's reticence in 2.1: Hero is twice prompted about her response to the expected courtship of Don PEDRO, and on both occasions Beatrice's comments against marriage prevent her reply.

Tricked into believing that Benedick loves her, Beatrice immediately discards her cynicism, saying, 'contempt, farewell, and maiden pride, adieu!' (3.1.109–110), in a lyrical 10-line outburst—almost her only verse lines in the play—that emphasises her elation. Swallowing her pride, she must accept her friends' teasing in 3.4.

When Hero is cruelly rejected on false evidence of promiscuity, Beatrice proves her essential goodness, believing in her cousin's innocence in the face of the evidence and demanding support from Benedick. The two witty lovers become involved in a serious conflict, bolstered by each other's trust. In asking for Benedick's aid, Beatrice confirms her love and acknowledges his.

Nevertheless, once Hero's problem is solved, Beatrice and Benedick briefly retreat from love in 5.4. Their strength is almost not great enough to overcome their old habits, but when their friends produce their love poems, they are forced to reaffirm their true feelings. Beatrice's quick wit cannot resist an attempt at having the last word (5.4.94–96), so Benedick silences her with a kiss.

This rather abrupt close to Beatrice's part suggests an important aspect of the playwright's attitude towards women: Beatrice, like other Shakespearean heroines, such as KATHERINA in *The Taming of the Shrew,* displays a spirited individuality, but in the end she willingly accepts a position subordinate to a man, as was conventionally expected of Elizabethan women. At first, denying that she wants or needs a husband, Beatrice asserts her independence, demonstrating the freedom of will that enlivens Shakespeare's most attractive female characters. However, when she seeks to defend Hero's innocence, she concedes that a male presence is required, saying of the vengeance she desires on her cousin's behalf, 'It is a man's office' (4.1.265). She asks Benedick to fulfil the role that she cannot, reminding us of the ultimately dependent position of women in Shakespeare's world.

Intriguingly, Beatrice shares two further characteristics with Shakespeare's other bold young women, including the 'Dark Lady' of the SONNETS: a sharp wit and a dark complexion. It seems plausible, though altogether unprovable, that these were the traits of a woman (entirely unidentifiable) who was romantically important to Shakespeare.

Beatrice is sometimes seen as shrewish, but this is a misconception; Shakespeare plainly intended to present a delightful young woman—defensive about love but charming and candid. While her repartee can be made to seem malicious or mean-spirited in performance, it is more fittingly delivered with great mirth and gaiety; Don Pedro remarks that she is 'a pleasant-spirited lady' (2.1.320). Shakespeare took Beatrice's name from the Latin name *Beatrix,* meaning 'she who blesses'. She is thus appropriately matched with Benedict (from the Latin *Benedictus,* meaning 'blessed').

Beaumont (1) Minor character in *Henry V,* a French nobleman. Beaumont is a GHOST CHARACTER; i.e., he appears but does not speak. He is named in 3.5.44 and in a stage direction in 4.2.1. His death in the battle of AGINCOURT is reported in 4.8.102. Shakespeare apparently took the name from the list of casualties in HOLINSHED's *Chronicles,* perhaps intending to develop the character further.

Beaumont (2), Francis (c. 1584–1616) English dramatist best known as a collaborator with John FLETCHER (2). As a young man, Beaumont studied at the INNS OF COURT, where he began writing poetry, possibly with the encouragement of Michael DRAYTON, a family friend. He began writing plays under the influence of Ben JONSON, whose friend and protégé he became. His earliest play, a COMEDY OF HUMOURS entitled *The Woman Hater* (1606), was staged by the Children of Paul's (see CHILDREN'S COMPANIES). In 1608 his *The Knight of the Burning Pestle,* a satire on the conventions of drama and literature, flopped dismally, though modern commentators regard it as one of the most endearing Jacobean comedies. In the same year he began his brief but highly successful collaboration with Fletcher. They wrote 15 plays together—one of them, *Philaster* (1610), was among the most important works of the age (see JACOBEAN DRAMA), and in the 1630s, their plays were more popular than Shakespeare's. Their partnership ended in 1613, when Beaumont married a wealthy heiress and retired from the theatre. Beaumont's last dramatic work, written by himself, was *The Masque of the Inner Temple and Gray's Inn* (1613), a courtly MASQUE written to celebrate the marriage of Princess ELIZABETH (3). A scene from it was restaged by Fletcher in *The Two Noble Kinsmen.*

Bedford (1), John Plantagenet, Duke of (1389–1435) Historical figure and character in *1 Henry VI* and *Henry V,* the younger brother of King HENRY V and

uncle of HENRY VI. (The same individual appears as Prince John of LANCASTER [3], in *1* and *2 Henry IV.*) In *1 Henry VI* Bedford is a regent, ruling FRANCE (1) for the infant King Henry. Bedford opens the play memorably, mourning the deceased Henry V in portentous terms: 'Hung be the heavens with black, yield day to night!' (1.1.1). In Act 2 Bedford proves himself a capable warrior when ORLÉANS (1) is captured, but in Act 3 he is an aged invalid, confined to a chair, whom JOAN LA PUCELLE taunts as 'good grey-beard' (3.2.50). He dies happily after witnessing the English victory at ROUEN.

The historical Bedford did die in Rouen, though at the age of 45 or 46, while the city was under English rule; the battle scene in the play is fictitious. He outlived Joan of Arc by several years. In fact, he played a major role in Joan's capture and trial, but Shakespeare transferred this important aspect of his career to YORK (8) in order to lend importance to the character who was to be a leading figure in the civil wars to come.

In *Henry V* a younger Bedford is an inconsequential member of the King's entourage. The historical Bedford, however, played an important role in the English conquest of France. Although he is present at the battle of AGINCOURT in the play, he was actually in England at the time, ruling in Henry's absence. Then he won a crucial naval battle in the second of Henry's campaigns in France. This campaign is ignored by Shakespeare, although it was actually more important than Agincourt in precipitating the final French surrender depicted in 5.2.

Bedford (2), Lucy, Countess of (1581–1627) English literary patron. Lucy Harington was married at the age of 13 to Edward Russell, Earl of Bedford; their marriage is one of several suggested as the occasion of the first performance of *A Midsummer Night's Dream.* Lucy Bedford was the patron of many of the most important English writers of her day, including John Donne (1573–1631), Samuel DANIEL, Michael DRAYTON, John FLORIO, and Ben JONSON. She was also a person of affairs, serving on the council of the Virginia Company and, when her husband was disabled by illness, as a leader of an important political faction in the turbulent 1620s.

Beeston, Christopher (d. 1638) English actor and theatrical entrepreneur. Beeston began his career as an apprentice to Augustine PHILLIPS of the CHAMBERLAIN'S MEN. He may have appeared with STRANGE'S MEN in 1590, though his earliest certain role was with the Chamberlain's Men in 1598. In 1602 he joined the WORCESTER'S MEN, remaining with the company when it became the QUEEN'S MEN (2). He managed the company—ineptly and perhaps dishonestly—from 1612 until it dissolved upon the queen's death in 1619. He then joined PRINCE CHARLES' MEN as its manager and went on to run LADY ELIZABETH'S MEN (1622–1625) and Queen Henrietta's Men (1625–1637). He had already expanded his operations: in 1617 he had built a theatre, the Phoenix, where these and other companies performed. Shortly before his death, he formed his own troupe of boy actors, the King and Queen's Young Company, popularly known as 'Beeston's Boys' (see CHILDREN'S COMPANIES).

His son, William Beeston (d. 1682), also an actor, later provided the antiquarian James Aubrey (1626–1697) with anecdotes about Shakespeare, reporting that his father had found the playwright 'a handsome, well-shaped man; very good company, and of a very ready and pleasant smooth wit . . . [who] wouldn't be debauched'. He also is the source of the report that Shakespeare had briefly been a schoolteacher as a young man.

Beethoven, Ludwig van (1770–1827) German composer, several of whose works were inspired in part by Shakespeare. Like many artists of the Romantic movement of the late 18th and early 19th centuries, Beethoven was deeply moved by Shakespeare and his broad presentation of life that dealt with grand themes and was written in stirring poetry. One movement of a string quartet (opus 18, no. 1; c. 1798) is thought to be based on Beethoven's response to *Romeo and Juliet,* and while his 'Overture to *Coriolanus*' (1807) was composed to accompany a contemporary Viennese imitation of Shakespeare's play, he surely considered the original as well. Beethoven's Piano Sonata no. 17 (1802) is known as *The Tempest* because he once declared that a clue to its meaning could be found by reading Shakespeare's play.

Begger Character in *The Taming of the Shrew.* See SLY (1).

Belarius Character in *Cymbeline,* the foster-father of GUIDERIUS and ARVIRAGUS. Belarius was unjustly exiled from the court of King CYMBELINE many years before the time of the play, and, in revenge, had kidnapped the king's infant sons. He has since raised them in the wilds of WALES (1). When the Roman army invades Britain, Belarius helps his foster-sons save the British army and the three are honoured by the king. However, because Guiderius has killed Prince CLOTEN, he is threatened with the death sentence prescribed for commoners who kill a prince. Belarius, to save the young man's life, reveals the truth. Though he has exposed himself to capital punishment because he had kidnapped the heir to the throne, Belarius is forgiven by the king in the play's final sequence of mercies and reconciliations. Belarius is a good man, unjustly persecuted, who only recovers his position by accident. He thus embodies an important theme of the play, that man is helpless without the aid of providence.

Belarius has taken the name Morgan, but he is designated Belarius in speech headings and stage direc-

tions. His Welsh pseudonym goes well with his comic habit of speaking in moralising clichés, for he fills the 17th-century English stereotype of the dull Welshman.

Belch, Sir Toby Character in *Twelfth Night.* See SIR TOBY.

Belleforest, François de (1530–1583) French author and translator who possibly influenced Shakespeare. An aristocratic courtier, Belleforest wrote poetry and compiled a collection of tales entitled *Histoires Tragiques* (1572), largely translations from the work of the Italian author Matteo BANDELLO. As a young man, Belleforest was a court favourite of Queen Margaret of Navarre (1492–1549), who wrote a famous book of tales, *The Heptameron* (published 1559), that doubtless inspired his own work.

Shakespeare may have taken ideas or details for several of his works—for example, *Hamlet, Titus Andronicus,* and *Twelfth Night*—from the *Histoires Tragiques,* but other sources were available to him in each instance, so we cannot be sure he knew Belleforest's tales. Nevertheless, the fact of several such coincidences suggests that he did, possibly from editions of 1576 or 1582. He may also have known the partial translation by Geoffrey FENTON (2), which was published in English in 1566, before the complete French version had appeared.

Bellini, Vincenzo (1801–1835) Italian composer, creator of an opera based on *Romeo and Juliet.* Bellini was one of the originators of bel canto–style opera in the early 19th century. His *I Capuleti e I Montecchi* was popular for a number of years following its premiere in 1830, but after 1847 it was not performed for almost a century. It now holds a place in modern operatic repertory, though Bellini is much better known for *La Sonnambula, Norma* (both of 1831), and *I Puritani* (1835).

Belmont Location in *The Merchant of Venice,* the estate of PORTIA (1). BASSANIO comes to Belmont to court Portia and succeeds in the lottery of caskets, in 3.2, before being called away by news of SHYLOCK's intended villainy. The estate is also a refuge for LORENZO and JESSICA. At the close of the play, Lorenzo and Jessica rhapsodise romantically about love and the beauties of the night, while ensconsed at Belmont, where the episode of the betrothal rings is played out, and the comedy is concluded, as was proper to a 16th-century comedy, with the union of lovers.

Belmont, a fictitious place, is apparently located on the mainland near VENICE; its name means 'beautiful hill'. Shakespeare simply took the estate and its name from his source, FIORENTINO's *Il Pecorone,* but he made the place his own. Belmont, like the forest of ARDEN (1) in *As You Like It,* is an artificial world, removed from the dreary acquisitiveness and commercialism represented by Shylock, where the conflicts that burden human affairs in the 'real' world can be resolved.

Belott, Stephen (active 1602–1613) Wigmaker of LONDON, plaintiff in a lawsuit in which Shakespeare testified. Belott, the son of French Huguenot immigrants, was apprenticed to Christopher MOUNTJOY, a 'tire-maker'—creator of the elaborate, ornamented headresses worn by aristocratic women. After serving his term and becoming Mountjoy's hired employee, he married his master's daughter. Shakespeare, who was a lodger in Mountjoy's house, participated in the negotiations about the marriage settlement, carrying messages between the father and the prospective bridegroom. After their marriage the Belotts established a rival business, initiating a feud with Mountjoy. After Mountjoy's wife died in 1606, the couple moved back in with him, but arguments over money soon resulted in their departure. Eventually, Belott sued Mountjoy for refusing to relinquish money agreed upon in the marriage settlement. Shakespeare testified in the case (see MOUNTJOY). Belott was eventually awarded a token settlement, though the arbitrators criticised him for debauchery. No more is known of his life.

Benedick Character in *Much Ado About Nothing,* rival of BEATRICE in contests of wit and later her lover. Benedick initially ridicules love, insisting that cuckoldry is the inevitable fate of married men, but he becomes a joyous bridegroom at the play's end. His playful dislike of Beatrice, which predates the beginning of the play, extends to all women, including HERO, whom his friend CLAUDIO (1) loves, but Benedick subtly reveals an underlying readiness to abandon his misogyny when he contrasts his 'custom, as being a professed tyrant to their sex' with his 'simple true judgement' (1.1.154–157). Tricked by Claudio and Don PEDRO into believing that Beatrice loves him, Benedick permits his own suppressed affection to emerge. At the play's climax, when Beatrice asks him to support the maligned Hero, he agrees, though this means turning from the comfortable companionship of Claudio and Don PEDRO. Trusting in his certainty of Beatrice's essential decency, Benedick has grown from shallow misogyny to implicit faith in his lover. His maturation, along with Beatrice's corresponding development, is the chief psychological theme of the play.

Benedick is essentially a comic figure. His friends value him for his sense of humour; Don Pedro says of him, 'from the crown of his head to the sole of his foot he is all mirth' (3.2.9). He is also sometimes a figure of fun. He crosses verbal swords with Beatrice, but she is too quick-witted for him, and he can only respond in her absence, as in the humorous speech that he delivers to Don Pedro in 2.1.223–245. Tricked into

believing that Beatrice loves him, he comically imagines romantic double meanings in her derisive words. Even filled with passion, he can be funny: 'I will live in thy heart, die in thy lap, and be buried in thy eyes; and moreover, I will go with thee to thy uncle's' (5.2. 94–96).

However, Benedick is no buffoon. His essential honour is often displayed. In 2.1, although hurt and humiliated himself, he accosts Don Pedro on Claudio's behalf when it appears that the older man is stealing Hero. When he defends the falsely accused and dishonoured Hero in 5.1, Benedick manfully resigns from Don Pedro's service and challenges Claudio to a duel. At the end of the play, fully committed to marrying Beatrice, he recants his earlier misogyny with no loss of dignity whatever. He admits freely that he had been wrong and is prepared to accept any ridicule that may be attempted against him, saying, ' . . . since I do purpose to marry, I will think nothing to any purpose that the world can say against it' (5.4. 103–105). In acknowledgeing his earlier foolishness, he offers a motto that might well sum up Shakespeare's comedies: 'man is a giddy thing, and this is my conclusion' (5.4.107).

Benedick, a common name in medieval England, comes from the Latin *Benedictus,* meaning 'blessed'; he is thus appropriately matched with Beatrice (from *Beatrix,* or 'she who blesses'). Shakespeare's character has become so firmly entrenched in the imagination of generations of readers and theatre-goers that his name, sometimes spelled 'Benedict', has become a common noun meaning a newly married man who has long been a bachelor.

Benfield, Robert (d. c. 1650) English actor. Benfield was one of the 26 men listed in the FIRST FOLIO as the 'Principall Actors' in Shakespeare's plays. He specialised in dignified figures such as kings and old men. He was with LADY ELIZABETH'S MEN in 1613 and may have joined the KING'S MEN upon the death of William OSTLER in 1614, for he took at least one of Ostler's parts. In any case he was a member of the company by 1619 and remained with the company until its dissolution in 1642, with the opening of the Civil Wars.

Bensley, Robert (1742–1817) English actor. Best known for his portrayal of MALVOLIO, Bensley was a highly mannered actor who frequently played in the productions of David GARRICK. He was a major figure on the London stage of the last decades of the 18th century.

Benson (1), Frank Robert (1858–1939) English actor and producer. F. R. Benson formed a touring company in 1883 that pointedly de-emphasised spectacle in staging Shakespeare, in contrast to the prevailing fashion for lush productions, such as those of Henry IRVING and Herbert Beerbohm TREE. From 1888 to 1919, with few exceptions, Benson directed the annual Shakespeare Festival at STRATFORD. His own performances in leading roles were acclaimed. More important, he presented almost all the plays—only *Titus Andronicus* and *Troilus and Cressida* were omitted—in texts with few cuts or interpolations and on plain stages that focussed attention on Shakespeare's words. In 1900 he staged the complete four- to five-hour-long text of *Hamlet* in London, and at Stratford in 1908 he produced the complete HISTORY PLAYS as a single unit for the first time. In 1916 on the occasion of the tercentenary of Shakespeare's death, Benson was knighted by King George V for his services to the British Shakespearean tradition.

Benson (2), John (d. 1667) London publisher and bookseller, producer of the first collection of Shakespeare's poems. Benson's *Poems* contains most of the SONNETS, *A Lover's Complaint*, *The Phoenix and Turtle*, excerpts from *Measure for Measure* and *As You Like It,* *THE PASSIONATE PILGRIM* (much of which is not Shakespeare's), a few other misattributed works, and a number of poems about Shakespeare by other poets, including MILTON, JONSON, BEAUMONT (2), Leonard DIGGES (2), and William BASSE. Only six of the Sonnets (numbers 18, 19, 43, 56, 75, and 76) are missing, though the remainder are altered to make them appear to be addressed only to a woman. Although the text of Thomas THORPE'S 1609 edition was employed, the Sonnets are arranged in a different order, with titles occasionally assigned to a group of two or three.

Bentley, John (1553–1585) English actor, a member of the QUEEN'S MEN (1). Bentley, one of the original members of the Queen's Men, is best known as the central figure in a brawl of 1583 in which a would-be gate-crasher of a Queen's Men's performance was killed. Though Richard TARLTON attempted to restrain him, Bentley pursued the fleeing miscreant, who hit him with a rock. Bentley and a companion drew their swords, and in the ensuing fight one of them killed the man. There is no record of a criminal prosecution for the killing, which occurred in 1583 during the Queen's Men's first season. As an actor, Bentley was well regarded by his contemporaries, being compared with Tarlton and William ALLEYN, acknowledged leaders of the profession.

Benvolio Character in *Romeo and Juliet,* friend and cousin of ROMEO. Benvolio's good sense and calm temperament are contrasted with the belligerence of Romeo's other friend, MERCUTIO. In 2.1, knowing that Romeo wishes to be alone, Benvolio draws Mercutio away. He attempts to prevent the brawl among the servants in 1.1 and the fight between Mercutio and TYBALT in 3.1; in both cases, he is ineffectual. This courteous and gentle character (whose apt name

means 'good will') appropriately disappears from the play as the tragedy unfolds.

Berkeley (1) Minor character in *Richard III,* one of two named gentlemen among the group that accompanies Lady ANNE (2) and the corpse of HENRY VI in 1.2.

Berkeley (2), Lord Thomas (d. 1417) Historical figure and minor character in *Richard II,* an ally of the Duke of YORK (4). A GLOUCESTERSHIRE nobleman whose castle has assumed strategic importance in the rebellion of BOLINGBROKE (1) against King RICHARD II, Berkeley greets Bolingbroke on York's behalf.

The historical Berkeley apparently allied himself with Bolingbroke when York did, for he served on the commission of noblemen that issued the formal declaration of Richard's deposition, and he opposed the rebellion against the new king, capturing the Duke of SURREY (2) and the Earl of SALISBURY (1). He turned his prisoners over to a mob, who killed them; their deaths are reported in 5.6.8. In later years Berkeley fought for Henry IV, as Bolingbroke became known, against Owen GLENDOWER.

Berlioz, Hector (1803–1869) French composer, creator of several works inspired by Shakespeare's plays. Berlioz, the leading French composer of the Romantic school, wrote the 'King Lear Overture' (1831) and a 'dramatic symphony', as he called it, based on *Romeo and Juliet* (1838). A symphonic fantasy on *The Tempest* (1830) was absorbed into a later work. Two choral works, 'Death March for the Last Scene of *Hamlet*' (with sung but wordless cries of grief) and 'La Mort d'Ophelia' (with a French text after Shakespeare by Ernest Legouvé [1807–1903]), were published in 1848 but may have been written much earlier. Later in his career Berlioz wrote an opera based on *Much Ado About Nothing,* called *Béatrice et Bénédict* (1862), a work that is considered among his finest. Another opera, *Les Troyens* (1859), contains a lyrical episode inspired by the love scene in 5.1 of *The Merchant of Venice.*

Berlioz profoundly influenced 19th-century French culture with dramatic compositions that reflected the romantic spirit of the age. As a young man he abandoned medical studies for music. In 1828 he fell in love with a leading actress, Harriet SMITHSON—famous in France for her OPHELIA—and he may have written his works inspired by *Hamlet* at this time. His *Symphonie Fantastique* (1830)—intended as an expression of his passion for Smithson—established him as a leading composer. He married her in 1833, but then abandoned her for another woman, though he did return to her much later and nursed her through her final illness. His own last days were solitary and unhappy; he proposed for his epitaph MACBETH's despairing cry that life is 'a tale / Told by an idiot, full of sound and fury, / Signifying nothing' (*Macbeth,* 5.5.26–28).

Bernardo Character in *Hamlet.* See BARNARDO.

Berners, John Bourchier, Lord (1467–1533) English translator. Lord Berners' translation (1523–1525) of the 14th-century *Chroniques* of FROISSART may have influenced the composition of *Richard II,* and his English version of a 13th-century French adventure tale, *The Boke of Duke Huon of Bordeaux* (1534), may have inspired something of Shakespeare's OBERON in *A Midsummer Night's Dream.*

Lord Berners was an important political figure; as a young nobleman he supported the Earl of RICHMOND (who appears in *Richard III*) when he seized the throne as King Henry VII in 1485. He was appointed Lord Chancellor by King HENRY VIII in 1516 (though he is not the CHANCELLOR of the play *Henry VIII*), and in his later years served as Deputy of Calais, the English outpost on the coast of FRANCE (1).

Bernhardt, Sarah (1845–1923) French actress. Though not chiefly a Shakespearean actress, Bernhardt scored one of her first great successes as CORDELIA in a French translation of *King Lear.* She also

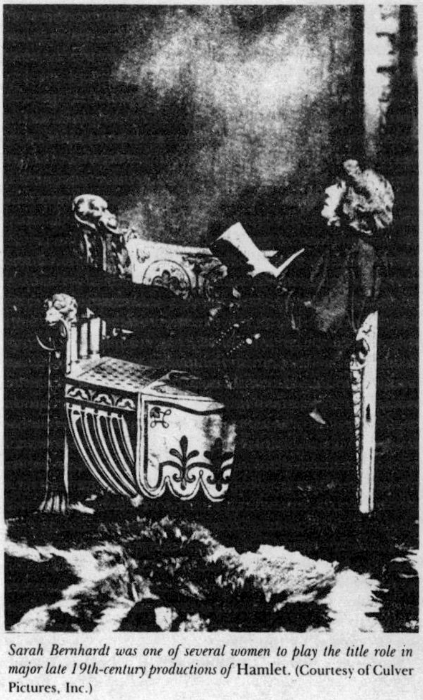

Sarah Bernhardt was one of several women to play the title role in major late 19th-century productions of Hamlet. (Courtesy of Culver Pictures, Inc.)

made an important contribution to the role of LADY (6) MACBETH, as the first to display an overt sensuality that has been heavily stressed by most of her 20th-century successors. In addition, she is strongly associated with HAMLET, a part she played in Paris, London, and New York in 1899 to 1901, as well as in the first FILM of *Hamlet,* a silent movie of 1900.

Berowne (Biron) Character in *Love's Labour's Lost,* one of the gentlemen in the court of the KING (19) of Navarre. Berowne is the witty exponent of the play's two main points: that love is superior to the pursuit of knowledge; and that pretensions, especially verbal ones, cannot be successful. When the King demands that his courtiers follow a three-year ascetic regimen dedicated to scholarship, Berowne argues that this is unhealthy and doomed to failure, because young men will naturally succumb to love. Berowne's common sense is opposed to the affectation of scholarly devotion, and his awareness of real emotion counters the fakery of academic rhetoric.

Unlike the other lovers in *Love's Labour's Lost,* who function simply as vehicles for the conventional proposition that the emotions should take precedence over the intellect, Berowne is a humanly believable character, as well as a funny one. The gentleman mocks himself in a humorous soliloquy at the end of 3.1, confessing that he has fallen under the sway of 'this signor junior, giant-dwarf, dan Cupid' (3.1.175). He is delighted to find that the King and the other courtiers, DUMAINE and LONGAVILLE, are similarly smitten, in the comic high point of the play, a stock eavesdropping scene repeated three times to a height of absurdity (4.3). Berowne proclaims a manifesto in favour of love, using his wit and warmth in a speech that contains perhaps the best verse in the play (4.3.285–361).

The gentlemen attempt to court the ladies with a masquerade and high-flown sentiments, and they are mocked by the women they would woo. Berowne realises that their pretensions have failed them, and he eloquently advances the play's campaign against foolish rhetoric, rejecting: 'Taffeta phrases, silken terms precise, / Three-pil'd hyperboles, spruce affection, / Figures pedantical . . . / Henceforth my wooing mind shall be express'd / In russet yeas and honest kersey noes. . . .' (5.2.406–413).

During the pageant in the same scene, Berowne is merciless in his heckling, perhaps evidencing the essential immaturity of the gentlemen. As a result of his wounding wit, ROSALINE, at the play's dénouement, requires that Berowne must spend a year visiting the sick in hospitals before she will accept him. Berowne, no cardboard character as are his fellows and the King, has human faults that must be corrected, even though he is also the chief exponent of the honest emotional life promoted by the play.

Berowne's name, pronounced 'B'roon', is taken from that of a contemporary French Protestant general, the Duc de Biron, who was a principal adviser to the historical King of Navarre.

Berri, Jean of France, Duke of (1340–1416) Historical figure and minor character in *Henry V,* a follower of the FRENCH KING. Berri does not speak, but he is referred to in 2.4.4 and 3.5.41. The historical Berri was the uncle of Charles VI, the French King of the play, and sometimes served as regent during Charles' bouts of insanity. He was thus an important figure in the French political conflict that resulted from the King's incapacity, although Shakespeare ignored this aspect of HENRY V's conquest. Berri is now famed for his great collection of medieval books of hours, whose beautiful illuminations inspired the costumes and sets for Laurence OLIVIER's well-known FILM of *Henry V.*

Bertram Character in *All's Well That Ends Well,* a young French nobleman, the errant husband of HELENA (2). Bertram is an imperfect man whose decline from callous self-absorption to more serious sin is arrested only by Helena's forceful entrapment. That his peccadilloes make him seem unworthy of Helena's love is one of the play's most bothersome features; as Samuel JOHNSON (7) complained, Bertram is 'dismissed into happiness' that he clearly does not deserve. Moreover, his highly qualified acceptance of Helena in the play's final scene does much to dilute any sense of resolution. This is one of the aspects of *All's Well* that places it among the PROBLEM PLAYS.

Helena persuades the KING (17) to make Bertram marry her as her reward for curing the monarch. Under the influence of the foppish coward PAROLLES, Bertram defies the King and abandons Helena, an act that the other characters uniformly deplore, and he departs from her with casual cruelty in 2.5. Bertram then declines into further immorality as he attempts to seduce the virginal DIANA (1). As his mother, the COUNTESS (2), remarks, he 'cannot thrive' (3.4.26) without Helena's influence.

Our attitude towards this undeniably dubious figure must colour our sense of the play as a whole, and many commentators have felt that he is important evidence that *All's Well* is a bitter satire. However, we can see that Shakespeare took considerable pains to mitigate Bertram's failings: the playwright altered his source, a tale by BOCCACCIO, in Bertram's favour, and he emphasised his youth, by way of excuse for his misdeeds, and his virtues, by way of compensation for them. In Boccaccio, the character corresponding to Bertram goes to the wars expressly to avoid his wife, while Shakespeare's young man displays an earlier desire to leave, a noble urge to distinguish himself in battle. His unwelcome marriage makes flight all the more alluring, and Parolles encourages him in this rebellion. Parolles is himself an addition to the tale, and al-

though Bertram's unthinking acceptance of Parolles' advice reveals his own shallowness, it is also clear that Parolles' chief function is to deflect blame from Bertram. Not only does he encourage Bertram's flight, but he is also the go-between who furthers his seduction of Diana. Other characters, particularly the First LORD (6) and the Countess, explicitly hold Parolles responsible for corrupting Bertram.

Bertram's youth, another plausible excuse for his folly, is repeatedly referred to. He is in his 'minority' (4.5.69), a ward of the King, who feels he is too young be a soldier. Lord LAFEW is asked to advise him for he is 'unseason'd' (1.1.67). When he rejects Helena, the King calls him a 'proud, scornful boy' (2.3.151), and when his mother learns of his flight, she calls him a 'rash and unbridled boy' (3.2.27). Even Parolles describes him as 'a foolish idle boy', 'a dangerous and lascivious boy', 'that lascivious young boy' (4.3.207, 212, 290). In 5.3 the Countess asks the King to forgive Bertram his 'natural rebellion done i' th' blade of youth' (5.3.6), and he himself confesses to having seduced Diana 'i' th' wanton way of youth' (5.3.210).

Not only is Bertram excused for his youth, but he is also aggrandised for his virtues. The DUKE (2) of FLORENCE appoints him a cavalry commander despite his age, and he triumphs, being reported 'high in fame' (5.3.31). (In Boccaccio, his counterpart was merely an officer.) He receives the praise of both the Countess and the King, as well as the intense approval of Helena. Even the First and Second Lords, though they deplore his morals, nonetheless recognise that 'he contrives against his own nobility' (4.3.23–24). Further, Bertram is linked with the virtues of his late father by both the Countess and the King in 1.1 and 1.2. The hope that Bertram will grow into nobility does much to enhance our acceptance of his youthful faults.

In 5.3 Bertram is exposed as a moral coward and a liar, falsely maligning Diana and retreating ignominiously before the King's interrogation. His disgrace is complete. Then suddenly he is rescued by Helena's return. Bertram's wickedness is stressed mercilessly just before he is restored to favour, in order to emphasise the power of his redemption through Helena's love. His central position in the reconciliation that closes the play elevates him to Helena's level of goodness.

However, Bertram's ignominy cannot be completely ignored, and Shakespeare acknowledges the truth of the situation by keeping Bertram in character to the end. His initial response to Helena's arrival is ambiguous: his 'O pardon!' (5.3.302) has been seen as genuine repentance but also as a self-serving effort to lessen his disgrace, for when Helena asks him to acknowledge that he is truly her husband, he does not reply to her but speaks only to the King and only with a qualification: 'If she, my liege, can make me know this clearly / I'll love her dearly, ever, ever dearly' (5.3.309–310). We can hardly fail to doubt the prospects for Bertram and Helena's happiness; even the King, closing the play, can only venture that 'All yet seems well . . .' (5.3.327).

Shakespeare tried to merge the traditional happy ending demanded by comedy with the psychological realism of Bertram's portrayal as a callow, thoughtless youth. The attempt is generally regarded as a failure; that Bertram is all too human is part of the problematic nature of *All's Well That Ends Well.* However, the portrait is an absorbing effort to adapt moral mediocrity to a romantic framework; figures such as POSTHUMUS of *Cymbeline* and LEONTES of *The Winter's Tale* owe something of their development to this less successful predecessor.

Bestrafte Brudermord, Der (Fratricide Punished) Eighteenth-century German version of *Hamlet* thought to derive in part from the UR-HAMLET. This work, fully titled *Tragoedia der Bestrafte Brudermord oder Prinz Hamlet aus Dännemark* but conventionally referred to as *BB*, is known only from the 1789 publication of a manuscript said to have been dated 1710. *BB* is essentially a BAD QUARTO of *Hamlet* with additional scenes, including an allegorical PROLOGUE (1) and several episodes of slapstick comedy. English actors frequently performed in Germany in the 16th and 17th centuries (see, e.g., Robert BROWNE; John GREEN; William KEMPE), and the actors who provided the dialogue translated into German as *BB* knew *Hamlet* in both of its early forms, published as the Q1 (1603) and Q2 (1604) editions; the additional material stems largely from medieval German traditions. However, some details in *BB* do not come from *Hamlet* yet correspond to a source for the play, François BELLEFOREST's version of the story. For instance, the QUEEN (9) blames her remarriage for Hamlet's madness, and Hamlet accuses his mother of hypocritically pretending to cry during their confrontation in her bedroom. These may have been introduced by actors who had performed in the *Ur-Hamlet.*

Betterton, Thomas (1635–1710) English actor, the dominant figure in Restoration theatre. Betterton was apprenticed to a bookseller in 1660, when English theatres reopened with the restoration of the monarchy, after 18 years of Puritan government. His employer opened a theatre, and Betterton was among the actors absorbed into William DAVENANT's troupe when two companies were licensed. Betterton quickly became the leading actor in London. Best known as HAMLET, his versatility was such that his other most appreciated role was as SIR TOBY in *Twelfth Night.* He was also especially acclaimed as MACBETH, MERCUTIO, OTHELLO, and HENRY VIII. After Davenant's death in 1671, Betterton led the company until it merged with the other London company in 1682. In 1695 he estab-

lished a rival company, with which he was successful until he retired shortly before his death.

Betterton wrote a number of dramas; he also adapted Shakespeare's *Henry IV* plays to the tastes of the period. When his version was first staged in 1682, he played HOTSPUR; it was so popular that it was revived repeatedly for 18 years, by which time he played FALSTAFF. Betterton and his wife, Mary SAUNDERSON, were much loved in the London theatre world for their ready assistance to young players, most notably Anne BRACEGIRDLE.

Betterton's talent was viewed as more than extraordinary by his contemporaries. Samuel PEPYS reported that his Hamlet was 'beyond imagination' in 1661; when the actor took the part again in 1668, Pepys described the performance as 'the best . . . that ever man acted'. At the other end of his career, Betterton inspired Colley CIBBER (1) to write that he 'was an actor as Shakespeare was an author, both without competitors, formed for the mutual assistance and illustration of each other's genius'.

Betty, William Henry West (1791–1874) English actor. A famous child prodigy, Master Betty, as he was known, was the greatest sensation of the London theatrical season of 1804–1805, having previously achieved success in Ireland and Scotland. He played several of the great classical roles of English drama that winter, including ROMEO and HAMLET (he was said to have memorised the latter role in a few hours). He also was notable as ARTHUR in *King John.* For a year he was the most popular English actor by far, overshadowing such established figures as John Philip KEMBLE (3). However, his star faded rapidly. In 1808, playing RICHARD III, he was booed off the stage, and he retired long enough to graduate from Cambridge; his subsequent attempt to resume his career was unsuccessful. His father squandered the fortune his earlier success had brought him, and he lived the remainder of his long life in poverty and obscurity.

Bevis, George Minor character in *2 Henry VI,* a follower of Jack CADE. Bevis discusses Cade's rebellion with his friend John HOLLAND (3) in 4.2, and the two men join the revolt. In 4.7 Bevis, here called George, serves as the guard over the captured Lord SAY. Since John Holland is known to have been a minor actor of the early 1590s, George Bevis probably was also, and his name was likely given to this character, by either Shakespeare or the keeper of a PROMPT-BOOK, as a convenience.

Bianca (1) Character in *The Taming of the Shrew,* a young woman courted by three men, LUCENTIO, HORTENSIO, and GRUMIO, in the SUB-PLOT of the play. At first, Bianca seems simply a demure and dutiful foil for her shrewish older sister, the title character, KATHERINA. Katherina's stubbornness prevents Bianca from marrying, since their father, BAPTISTA (1), has ordered that the elder must be wed first. Bianca's sweet submissiveness also seems to make her a perfect object for the stereotypical romantic rapture of Lucentio, who elopes with her at the climax of the subplot.

However, Bianca is more complex than she initially appears. She is catty and self-righteous when she resists Katherina's violence in 2.1, not only declaring her own virtue but also twitting her sister about her age. Furthermore, Bianca draws attention to her supposed moral superiority over Katherina, as when she admonishes her sister to 'content you in my discontent' (1.1.80). Her ambiguous sweetness may help to explain Katherina's generalised belligerence, which has presumably flowered after frequent comparison with her sister's apparent virtue.

When alone with her tutors (not yet revealed to be suitors in disguise), Bianca is decidedly wilful, insisting, 'I'll not be tied to hours nor 'pointed times, / But learn my lessons as I please myself' (3.1.19–20). She is haughtily flirtatious with Lucentio ('presume not . . . despair not' [3.1.43]), and she rejects Hortensio with curt brutality. We are not surprised to find Bianca shrewish herself in the final scene, holding Lucentio up to ridicule for believing in her wifely obedience. This revelation emphasises the ironic contrast between the two sisters' marriages. Katherina has found true love after an explicitly mercenary courtship, whereas Bianca's union with Lucentio, the product of a conventionally idyllic romance, seems likely to be unhappy.

Bianca (2) Character in *Othello,* a courtesan of CYPRUS and the lover of CASSIO. IAGO calls Bianca 'A housewife that by selling her desires / Buys herself bread and clothes' (4.1.94–95), where 'housewife' is intended with the common Elizabethan meaning of 'courtesan'. However, she is not a lowly prostitute; she has her own house (and is thus a literal housewife) and has the pride to be offended by the insults of EMILIA (2) in 5.1. Moreover, her obviously genuine concern for the wounded Cassio in the same scene touchingly demonstrates that she is a fundamentally decent person. This degree of dignity makes it possible for her relationship with Cassio to function as a foil for that of OTHELLO and DESDEMONA. The comparison is emphasised when Iago makes Cassio a part of his campaign to arouse Othello's jealousy of his wife. More pointedly, Bianca is jealous of Cassio—she complains, in 3.4, that he has avoided her and, in 4.1, she rages at him when she suspects that he has another lover. Her emotion echoes Othello's with the pointed difference that it is justified: Bianca's love for Cassio cannot be based on trust for she knows that, in the nature of relations between soldiers and courtesans,

he will eventually leave her. In this context her jealousy seems both entirely rational and entirely vain, thus pointing up Othello's grievous error in two different ways.

Bible The Christian sacred scripture. The Bible was basic reading for Shakespeare and his age, and this is evident throughout the plays. Although the Bible is mentioned by name only once (*Merry Wives*, 2.3.7; it is also referred to as 'Holy Writ' several times) and explicit references to biblical characters or tales are few, Shakespeare, like many other authors, was influenced by biblical idioms and linguistic rhythms.

Several versions of the Bible were available in England in the 16th century. The version Shakespeare knew best was the Geneva Bible, which was translated in the centre of European Calvinism by Protestant exiles during the reign of the Catholic Queen Mary I (1553–1558) and published in England in 1560. He also knew the Bishop's Bible (1568), a revision of an earlier English text that was undertaken in part to counter the influence of radical Calvinism on the Geneva version. However, the Geneva Bible was so powerful a literary text that the Bishop's Bible actually relied on it to some extent, as, later, did the creators of the King James Version (1611), which was prescribed in the Anglican Church until late in the 19th century and is still commonly used and read. Shakespeare doubtless knew it, but only after his career was nearly over. As a reader of Latin, Shakespeare could also refer to the Vulgate of St Jerome, the basic Bible for western Europe from the fifth century to the 16th, when the Reformation stimulated the use of translations.

Bigot (Bigod), Roger (d. 1220) Historical figure and minor character in *King John*, a rebel against King JOHN (3). Bigot is one of the noblemen who oppose the King, responding to the death of ARTHUR, and who treacherously ally themselves with the invading French. Bigot speaks in only one of the four scenes in which he appears.

The historical Bigot was one of the barons who opposed John in 1214 and forced him to sign the Magna Charta. He was a great landowner in eastern England.

Biondello Character in *The Taming of the Shrew*, servant of LUCENTIO. Biondello acts as servant to his fellow employee, TRANIO, who is disguised as their master. His mischievous delight in the situation lends humorous force to his only important passage, the description of PETRUCHIO (2) approaching the wedding (3.2.30–83).

Birmingham Shakespeare Memorial Library Major collection of Shakespeareana in Birmingham, England. Founded in 1864 on the occasion of the playwright's 300th birthday, the library, despite its destruction by fire in 1879, now houses one of the most important collections of early texts, and records of later productions of Shakespeare's plays, with a particular strength in 18th-century materials.

Birnam Wood See DUNSINANE.

Biron See BEROWNE.

Birth of Merlin Play formerly attributed to Shakespeare, part of the Shakespeare APOCRYPHA. The earliest known text of *The Birth of Merlin* is a QUARTO published in 1662 by Francis KIRKMAN, who ascribed the play to Shakespeare and William ROWLEY (2). *Merlin*, a lively entertainment that features dragons, visions, a comet, and a devil, is usually dated to the 1620s based on the evidence of its style and vocabulary. Thus it is too late to be Shakespeare's play. Also, the writing is inferior and it is generally dissimilar to the playwright's known work. However, most scholars believe that Rowley wrote at least part of the play, perhaps in collaboration with Thomas MIDDLETON.

Birthplace, Shakespeare's House in STRATFORD where the playwright was probably born. The birthplace consists of two buildings on Henley Street that were bought on separate occasions by Shakespeare's father, John SHAKESPEARE (9), and joined together. Tradition assigns Shakespeare's birth to the western half, but no actual evidence exists. John Shakespeare lived in an unspecified building on Henley Street in 1552, and in 1556 he bought the eastern half of what was to be the birthplace, but at the same time he bought another house, and it is unclear where he lived. An unrecorded purchase could have been made before the playwright's birth, but John's only other known real estate acquisitions are two houses bought in 1575, one of which may have been the western half. In any case the family was living in the western half by 1597, and the eastern half was used for business.

In 1601 Shakespeare inherited the house upon his father's death. The eastern half was leased to the keepers of an inn called the Maidenhead, and the western half continued to be inhabited by the family; the playwright's sister Joan SHAKESPEARE (8) Hart and her family were living there when Shakespeare died. He left Joan a lifetime lease on it, while leaving the building to his daughter Susanna SHAKESPEARE (14) Hall, who in turn left it to her daughter Elizabeth HALL (3). In the meantime Joan's son and grandsons continued to live there. In 1670 Elizabeth Hall bequeathed it to Joan's grandson George Hart (1636–1702), whose descendants continued to occupy it for another century.

In 1806 the Harts sold the property to one Thomas Court, under whose ownership it became a butcher

shop; his widow auctioned it off in 1846, advertising it as 'the house in which the immortal Poet of Nature was born'. The house was purchased by a nonprofit organisation formed for the purpose and 10 years later was restored, using the public's contributions (among the fund-raisers was Charles DICKENS). In 1891 the Birthplace Trust was incorporated to care for the building and such other properties as NEW PLACE (acquired in 1862), Anne HATHAWAY's cottage (1891), the supposed ARDEN (2) home (1930), and Hall's Croft, the Stratford residence of Dr John HALL (4) (1949).

Bishop (1) Either of two minor characters in *Richard III*, clergymen who accompany RICHARD III as he receives the MAYOR (3) in 3.7. They convey the impression that Richard has been busy with devotional concerns. In fact, this is a contrived deception, and the 'Bishops' are actually unscrupulous lower-ranking clergymen, John SHAA and Friar PENKER, whom Richard has summoned for the purpose.

Bishop (2), Henry Rowley (1786–1855) English composer and conductor. Best known for writing the song 'Home, Sweet Home', Bishop also composed the music for many of Frederick REYNOLDS' operatic adaptations of Shakespeare's plays. In 1842 Bishop became the first musician to be knighted by a British monarch.

Blackfriars Gatehouse House in LONDON owned by Shakespeare. In 1613 Shakespeare bought a residence that had once served as the gatehouse on the estate of the BLACKFRIARS ABBEY. This was his last investment that we know of and his only non-theatrical one in London. He bought the building for £140 from Henry WALKER (1), paying £80 in cash and immediately mortgaging the house to Walker for the remaining £60. He had three trustees who were technically co-owners with him: William JOHNSON (8), John JACKSON (2), and John HEMINGE. They put up no money and had no ownership rights; this arrangement had the effect of eliminating the rights in the property of Shakespeare's wife, Anne HATHAWAY Shakespeare—perhaps because Shakespeare intended to leave the property to his daughter Susanna SHAKESPEARE (14) Hall, which he did in fact do. The trustees surrendered their shares to her in 1618, 'in performance of the confidence and trust in them reposed by William Shakespeare', as the legal document had it.

The gatehouse was very close to the BLACKFRIARS THEATRE, the principal venue for the KING'S MEN, but Shakespeare clearly did not intend to use it. He already lived in STRATFORD full-time, and the purchase was simply an investment. The location, however, suggests how the property could have come to his attention. He leased the gatehouse soon after buying it, to one John ROBINSON (1), who was still living there in 1616. The later history of the building is obscure. It was probably destroyed in the Great Fire of London (1666).

Blackfriars Priory Former Dominican priory building in LONDON, a setting for a scene in *Henry VIII*. In 2.4 the Blackfriars priory houses the proceedings that lead to King HENRY VIII's divorce from Queen KATHERINE, the king having declared it 'The most convenient place [he could] think of / for such receipt of learning' (2.2.137–138). Shakespeare followed his source, HOLINSHED's *Chronicles*, in placing this meeting at the Blackfriars. After England adopted Protestantism, the priory's property was seized by the crown and sold to various private interests. By Shakespeare's time, different buildings of the old priory had become the BLACKFRIARS THEATRE and BLACKFRIARS GATEHOUSE.

Blackfriars Theatre Playhouse in LONDON established by Richard BURBAGE (3), the home from 1600 to 1608 of the Children of the Chapel (see CHILDREN'S COMPANIES), and later of Shakespeare's company, the KING'S MEN. Burbage inherited the Blackfriars from his father, James BURBAGE (2), who died before it was ready for use. The theatre was part of the medieval BLACKFRIARS PRIORY, which had been broken up and sold to private investors at the Reformation. The theatre was rented to Henry EVANS (2) of the Children of the Chapel, but after Evans' failure, Burbage bought back the lease, in partnership with his brother Cuthbert BURBAGE (1), four King's Men—Shakespeare, Henry CONDELL, John HEMINGE, and William SLY (2)—and a relative of Evans. The King's Men used the theatre in the winter from 1609 on. (Before the Burbages' enterprise, between 1576 and 1584 there had been a smaller theatre in part of the same building, which is known as the original, or first Blackfriars Theatre.)

The Blackfriars was called a 'private' theatre, for it had a roof, unlike the King's Men's summer venue, the GLOBE THEATRE, and other public playhouses. Because admission prices were as much as five times greater than in the public theatres, the audiences were higher ranking, socially, and generally better educated. Their tastes were correspondingly different—more influenced by literature and by the courtly MASQUE whose popularity was on the rise in the first decades of the 17th century. All this, combined with the greater intimacy of the theatre itself and its novel and striking candlelit stage, produced important changes in JACOBEAN DRAMA. Shakespeare's ROMANCES and the plays of Francis BEAUMONT (2) and John FLETCHER (2), the King's Men's other main playwrights, were directly influenced by the Blackfriars Theatre.

Blackheath Open land on the south bank of the Thames east of London, a traditional fairground and public meeting place and the location of several

scenes in *2 Henry VI.* Blackheath was famous in Shakespeare's time, as in the period of the play's action, as an assembly point for rebellious bands marching on London, and it figures as such in 4.2–3 of the play. The army of Jack CADE, arriving from KENT, gathers here to be harangued by its leader and to fight its first skirmish before proceeding to the capital. Ironically, when the Duke of YORK (8) returns from Ireland with his army in 5.1—ostensibly to oppose Cade, but also, secretly, to foster insurrection—he also appears at Blackheath.

Blanche (Blanch) of Spain (1188–1252) Historical figure and minor character in *King John,* the niece of King JOHN (3), who marries LEWIS (1), the French Dauphin, after 2.1. Blanche finds herself with mixed loyalties when hostilities break out between her uncle and her new husband. In 3.1 she unsuccessfully attempts to persuade her husband and his father, King PHILIP (2), to refrain from fighting England. She is reduced to a bewildered lament that plaintively expresses the helplessness of the noncombatant.

The historical Blanche of Castile, as she is better known, was raised in Spain. Her mother was John's sister Eleanor, and her father was the King of Castile. A treaty between John and Philip provided for the marriage of Lewis to a princess of Castile, and Queen ELEANOR travelled to Spain and selected Blanche from among several eligible sisters. Thus, at 12, Blanche was taken by her grandmother, whom she had not met before, to another country to marry a man whom she had never met. Although her initial depression in her new home was noted in a contemporary chronicle, she went on to become one of the great women in French history. After the brief reign of Lewis (Louis VIII), Blanche acted as regent for her son, Louis IX, known to history as St Louis. She put down several rebellions and completed the subjection of southern France to royal rule. St Louis spent much of his reign crusading in the Holy Land, and Blanche governed effectively in his absence.

Blank Verse Metrical pattern (see METRE) composed of lines of unrhymed iambic pentameter. The typical pattern in English poetry—though neither exclusively nor originally English—blank verse is the medium of many long poems and nearly all verse dramas, including Shakespeare's, though the plays also contain prose and, more rarely, other forms of verse. Iambic pentameter is especially appropriate for drama and narrative poetry, for it more closely resembles the normal patterns of English speech than does any other sort of poetic pattern (except unmetred free verse). Its stresses imitate the natural flow of clauses and phrases, while the line endings fall at intervals that are easily followed without counting. Unlike rhymed patterns such as, say, the couplet or the limerick, which subtly suggest a point of view by the way they sound, blank verse is neutral in tone and allows the content of the poetry to determine its emotional shading. This is both an advantage and a challenge: blank verse does not easily lend itself to the lively and varied tone that a work of any length requires.

Blank verse was first used in English poetry in the early 16th century in translations of VIRGIL by Henry Howard, Earl of SURREY (1). Surrey was inspired by similar Italian verse and, probably, the example of unrhymed verse in traditional Middle English poetry. The form became popular in England after Christopher MARLOWE (1) established the pattern, in *Tamburlaine* (c. 1587), as the standard for dramatic works. Shakespeare's poetic genius led him to vary the pattern much more freely than his predecessors had, permitting the expression of a wider range of effects, from broad comedy to lyrical ecstasy to raging anger. For the first time, the musical patterns of poetry could approximate the range and specificity of prose.

In Shakespeare's day, blank verse was a very familiar medium; he could expect at least part of his audience to recognise it when spoken, as JAQUES (1) does in *As You Like It,* upon hearing only a single line (4.1.28). Except during the late 17th and early 18th centuries, blank verse remained prominent in English poetry until recent times. It was the favoured medium of such masters of the long poem as John MILTON, William Wordsworth (1770–1850), Robert Browning (1812–1889), and T. S. ELIOT (2). In the 20th century the use of blank verse has declined, due largely to the disappearance of an audience for verse drama and the long poem. To some extent, it has come to be represent conservative poetry, compared to free verse.

Blount, Edward (1564–1632) English bookseller and publisher, a partner in the production of the FIRST FOLIO (1623). In 1601 Blount published LOVE'S MARTYR, including Shakespeare's *The Phoenix and Turtle.* In 1608 he registered two of Shakespeare's plays for publication—*Antony and Cleopatra* and *Pericles*—but did not produce either of them; scholars believe this reflects a 'blocking action' undertaken on behalf of the KING'S MEN to protect their plays from pirated publication. The degree of co-operation with the acting company implied by Blount's action suggests that Shakespeare may have known him personally. Blount and Isaac JAGGARD jointly held the rights to 16 plays in the First Folio—all but two of those that had not been previously published—making them leading members of the syndicate that financed its printing (the others were John SMETHWICK and William ASPLEY). Jaggard and Blount are designated co-publishers of the book on its title page.

Blount became a member of the STATIONERS' COMPANY in 1588, after 10 years of apprenticeship, and he prospered, eventually owning two bookshops and remaining active until at least 1630. He was evidently a

sincere appreciator of literature, publishing prefaces praising his authors and apologising for printer's errors. He published works by Christopher MARLOWE (1) and John LYLY in addition to Shakespeare.

Blunt (1), Sir James (d. 1493) Historical figure and minor character in *Richard III*, a follower of RICHMOND. Richmond uses Blunt as a messenger before the battle of BOSWORTH FIELD. Blunt is the great-grandson of Sir Walter BLUNT (3), who appears in *1 Henry IV*. He may have been selected for his tiny role, from all the possible officers in Richmond's army, as a gesture towards the Blunt family, who were STRATFORD landowners of Shakespeare's day, and were related to the playwright's friends in the COMBE family.

Blunt (2), Sir John (d. 1418) Historical figure and minor character in *2 Henry IV*, an aide to Prince John of LANCASTER (3). Blunt appears only once and says nothing; he is assigned to guard the captive COLEVILE (4.3.73). Blunt was also mentioned in two stage directions in the QUARTO edition of the play (1600), but these references are absent in the FIRST FOLIO (1623) and have generally been omitted since. It is speculated that this alteration may reflect minor cuts made for an early production, perhaps by Shakespeare himself. The historical John Blunt was a minor courtier, the son of Walter BLUNT (3), who appears in *1 Henry IV*.

Blunt (3), Sir Walter (d. 1403) Historical figure and character in *1 Henry IV*, a follower of King HENRY IV. Blunt is a respected adviser and emissary, and his calm personality contrasts with that of the tormented Henry and the temperamental HOTSPUR. In 1.3 Blunt attempts to mediate the quarrel between the King and Hotspur. In 3.2.163–179 he brings the dramatic news that the rebel forces are gathering at SHREWSBURY, a report that propels PRINCE (6) HAL into action. In 4.3 Blunt acts as the King's ambassador, and he is properly short with the bellicose Hotspur. In 5.3 he is dressed as the King, in a standard medieval battlefield tactic, and is killed by DOUGLAS. The sight of his corpse causes FALSTAFF to remark ironically, 'There's honour for you!' (5.3.32).

The historical Blunt was a long-time follower of King Henry's father, John of GAUNT. He was Gaunt's executor, and he naturally became one of Henry's chief advisers. He was indeed killed at Shrewsbury, but he was not among those disguised as the King. He bore the King's standard, a position of honour that suggests a sound reputation as a military man. He was the father of Sir John BLUNT (2), who appears in *2 Henry IV*, and great-grandfather of Sir James BLUNT (1) of *Richard III*.

Boar's Head Tavern Inn in EASTCHEAP, in LONDON, setting for several scenes in *1* and *2 Henry IV* and possibly one in *Henry V*. The Boar's Head, run by the HOSTESS (2) and frequented by FALSTAFF, PRINCE (6) HAL, and their friends, is a haven for petty criminals whose riotous drinking and wenching is depicted with a colourful vigour unmatched until Charles Dickens in the 19th century. In addition to Falstaff's principal followers—BARDOLPH (1), PISTOL, PETO, and DOLL TEARSHEET—numerous minor characters, such as GADSHILL, FRANCIS (1), the VINTNER, the MUSICIANS (4) and the DRAWERS, add verisimilitude to this world.

In *1 Henry IV* the Boar's Head is the scene of several typical episodes in the delinquent career of Prince Hal. In 2.4 he baits Falstaff about his bungled highway robbery, and he joins the fat knight in a mirthful mockery of King HENRY IV. In 3.3 a comical dispute erupts between Falstaff and the Hostess, and the Prince deflects an attempt by a SHERIFF (4) to arrest Falstaff. In 2.1 of *2 Henry IV*, the Hostess attempts to have Falstaff arrested for debt, and a potential brawl is averted only by the timely arrival of the CHIEF JUSTICE. In 2.4 Falstaff hosts an uproarious dinner party at the tavern. Mournful meditations on Falstaff's death are offered by his companions in 2.3 of *Henry V*. This scene is traditionally located in front of the tavern, and, although the original texts provide no site designation, it seems appropriate that the Boar's Head should witness the remembrances for its most famous patron.

The Boar's Head was a famous establishment in Elizabethan London, and, although Shakespeare does not actually name it explicitly (a broad hint is made in *2 Henry IV*, 2.2.138–140), his audiences clearly recognised it, as surviving contemporary references reveal. However, the Boar's Head Tavern is not to be confused with the Boar's Head Theatre, the suburban venue of the QUEEN'S MEN (2), an early 17th-century acting company.

Boas, Frederick S. (1862–1957) British scholar. Boas wrote several important books on Shakespeare, including *Shakespeare and his Predecessors* (1896)—in which he introduced the term PROBLEM PLAY to Shakespeare studies—and *An Introduction to the Reading of Shakespeare* (1927). He also wrote about other figures of the age, including Thomas HEYWOOD (2), Christopher MARLOWE (1), and Sir Philip SIDNEY. He was the longtime editor of *The Year's Work in English Studies*, an annual collection of essays that summarised significant scholarly work.

Boatswain Minor character in *The Tempest*, a crew member of the ship that is wrecked on PROSPERO's island. In 1.1 the Boatswain curses the arrogant SEBASTIAN (5) and ANTONIO (3), who insist on interfering during the great storm that threatens the vessel. Prospero's sprite ARIEL magically preserves the ship and its crew, and in 5.1, as the play closes, the Boatswain is brought to Prospero by Ariel and reports on the ship's miraculous restoration. The Boatswain is a plain-spoken working man whose contrast with Sebastian

nd Antonio helps establish their villainous natures at the outset and whose reappearance at the close suggests the everyday world to which the play's characters will soon return.

Boccaccio, Giovanni (1313–1375) Italian story writer and poet, a frequent source for Shakespeare. The main plots of *All's Well That Ends Well* and *Cymbeline,* as well as details in *The Winter's Tale,* all derive from Boccaccio's *Decameron* (1353), a collection of tales that Shakespeare probably knew in the translations of William PAINTER (2) (into English) and Antoine MAÇON (into French). The *Decameron* may also have provided the main plot of *The Two Gentlemen of Verona,* though this material was heavily modified by other sources. The playwright's other uses of Boccaccio's works were indirect: Geoffrey CHAUCER's *Troilus and Criseyde,* the source for *Troilus and Cressida,* was itself based on Boccaccio's poem the *Filostrato* (1338); Boccaccio's epic poem the *Teseide* (1339–1340) was the source for Chaucer's 'The Knight's Tale', which was in turn the source for both *The Two Noble Kinsmen* and parts of *A Midsummer Night's Dream;* lastly, the stories of Giovanni FIORENTINO, probably sources for *The Merchant of Venice* and *The Merry Wives of Windsor,* were modelled on tales in the *Decameron.*

Boccaccio is considered a founder of Italian RENAISSANCE literature. Among his works are the *Filostrato,* a romance in verse; the *Teseide,* the first epic poem in Italian; the *Fiammetta* (c. 1343), sometimes seen as the earliest European novel; the *Ninfale Fieselano (The Nymph of Fiesole,* c. 1345), a PASTORAL romance in verse that is considered Boccaccio's second greatest work; and the greatest, the *Decameron.* All of these works were written in Italian, but following a religious crisis, Boccaccio decided that writing in the vernacular was sinful and rejected all his works. His later writings in Latin, scholarly works on classical culture, were important to the development of European humanism.

Bodleian Library Major collection of Shakespeareana, at Oxford University, England. The library was founded by the diplomat and scholar Thomas Bodley (1545–1613) in 1597 when an earlier university library, dating to 1445, was reorganised. The Bodleian Library was originally composed largely of theological materials, but in 1821, with the acquisition of the library of Edmond MALONE, it became a great Shakespearean library. It has maintained that status to the present day, with a collection that is especially noted for its early texts of Shakespeare's non-dramatic poetry.

Boece (Boyce), Hector (c. 1465–1536) Scottish historian, author of a source for *Macbeth.* Boece's *Scotorum Historiae,* a history of Scotland in Latin, was the source for Raphael HOLINSHED's Scottish history in his *Chronicles of England, Scotland, and Ireland* (1577), which was Shakespeare's source for the tale of MACBETH, as well as for other materials used in the play.

Boece, a native of Dundee, was a famous professor at the University of Paris when, in 1498, he was invited back to Scotland to participate in the founding of King's College in Aberdeen. His *Scotorum Historiae* was the first work to cover all of Scotland's history (to 1488). It is heavily infused with legendary material—as is much of Macbeth's story—but it was for generations regarded as the best text on its subject. Translated into French, it became well known throughout Europe. In 1536 the King of Scotland commissioned a translation into Scots; this work, by the poet John Bellenden (c. 1500–c. 1548) is the oldest surviving work of Scots prose. In the academic fashion of the times, Boece took a Latin surname and is sometimes still referred to as Hector Boëthius, after the Roman philosopher (c. 480–c. 524).

Bohemia Central European region, part of modern Czechoslovakia, the setting for part of *The Winter's Tale.* In 3.3 ANTIGONUS abandons the infant PERDITA—banished from SICILIA by her father, King LEONTES, who believes her illegitimate—on the Bohemian seacoast. She is found by the SHEPHERD (2) and his son, who raise her as a shepherdess. In Act 4, 16 years later, Prince FLORIZEL, son of the King of Bohemia, falls in love with Perdita, and she with him. The king, however, opposes their marriage, and they flee to Sicilia, where Act 5 takes place.

Bohemia is specified as the setting for the rugged seacoast of 3.3 and the pastoral world of the shepherds in Act 4, but there is nothing nationally distinctive in the text of the play. Shakespeare merely took the name from his source, *Pandosto* by Robert GREENE (2) (though there the princess was exiled from Bohemia and raised in Sicilia). In many ways Shakespeare's Bohemia is a lovingly idealised portrait of English rural life, although the rugged coast and man-eating BEAR of 3.3 add overtones of nature's harshness.

Shakespeare's attribution of a seacoast to Bohemia has inspired much comment, for that land does not in fact have one. It has been argued that the discrepancy points to the playwright's ignorance and provinciality, or to his carelessness in simply accepting the notion from *Pandosto.* The 18th-century scholar Thomas HANMER substituted Bithynia, a region of Asia Minor, for Bohemia, and many later editions of the play followed his lead. Other commentators hold that Shakespeare may legitimately have thought Bohemia bordered the Adriatic Sea, since after 1526 it was part of the Hapsburg Empire, which did so. Also, medieval Bohemia had briefly controlled a stretch of the same coast. However, the actuality of Bohemia's coast is irrelevant; *The Winter's Tale,* as one of the ROMANCES, was expected to dazzle its viewers with exotic locales. Bohemia was very little known in England during Shakespeare's lifetime, for it was small and deep

within continental Europe, in an age of difficult travel and communication. Most of *The Winter's Tale*'s original audience doubtless accepted a Bohemian coastline without thinking about it; it was a satisfying image, providing a dramatic approach to a fabulous land. For those who knew the truth, probably including Shakespeare himself, the anomaly may have been mildly amusing, like modern jokes about the Swiss Navy.

Boito, Arrigo (1842–1918) Italian operatic composer and librettist. Boito, who composed several operas of his own, is best known for two librettos—both adaptations of Shakespeare—that he wrote for Giuseppe VERDI: *Otello* (1887; based on *Othello*) and *Falstaff* (1893; based on *The Merry Wives of Windsor*). These are widely regarded as among the best opera librettos ever written.

Boleyn, Anne See ANNE (1).

Bolingbroke (1) (Bullingbrook), Henry (later King HENRY IV, 1366–1413) Historical figure and character in *Richard II*, the usurper of the throne from King RICHARD II. (The same individual appears as King HENRY IV in *1* and *2 Henry IV*.) Bolingbroke's rise to the throne balances Richard's fall, and Bolingbroke, like Richard, undergoes personal change. In 1.1 he uses elaborate rhetoric to accuse MOWBRAY (1) of murdering the Duke of GLOUCESTER (6) and to challenge him to a trial by combat. We learn in 1.2 that Gloucester's murder was Richard's doing, as Bolingbroke must have known. It is clear that Bolingbroke is hostile to Richard from the very beginning and that the King has no effective response. Bolingbroke's triumph can already be foreseen. (Shakespeare will have assumed that his audience knew that Bolingbroke was to become King in any case.) Although Bolingbroke accepts his banishment, we know that he will shortly reappear as Richard's enemy. Thus Bolingbroke seems an unscrupulous schemer from the beginning.

When he returns from exile to claim his inheritance—the estates of his father, John of GAUNT—his first actions reinforce this impression. In 2.3 he welcomes PERCY (2), ROSS (2), and WILLOUGHBY (3) as his allies with apparently frank gratitude, but, having seen his ambition we doubt his sincerity. Moreover, the playwright will probably have counted on his audience's familiarity with the fate of Percy, who later died in rebellion against Bolingbroke (as is enacted in *1 Henry IV*). Later in this scene, Bolingbroke offers an elaborate rationale for his rebellion against the crown when he is criticised by the Duke of YORK (4); it is clear that he thinks it important to maintain an appearance of justified innocence, masking his ambition with assertions of political rectitude. Further, he proclaims that he has come only to claim his inheritance, but he also proceeds to execute the alleged villains BUSHY and GREENE (1) for 'crimes' that are actually offences against Bolingbroke personally rather than against the state.

Significantly, Bolingbroke's diction changes at this point. As Richard's strikingly poetic manner of speaking becomes prominent in his emotional collapse, Bolingbroke adopts a plainer mode of speech intended to reveal his motives. His practical realism is emblematic of the new era in politics that he represents. Bolingbroke is a Machiavellian leader prepared to take whatever measures are necessary to acquire and preserve power, whereas Richard, relying on long-standing tradition, believes in the ancient theory of divine right. The passing of the romantic medieval world represented by that tradition is a major theme of the play. Bolingbroke's easy reliance on his own strength is a new attribute of kingship, reflected in his speech and manner as soon as he begins to assert his power.

A third Bolingbroke, the generous victor, begins to assume importance in 3.1. Although he undertakes a ruthless act of state in condemning Bushy and Greene, he anticipates his later development in demonstrating his sympathy for Richard's QUEEN (13), instructing that she be treated well. Bolingbroke's magnanimity is further stressed in Act 5, when he pardons CARLISLE and AUMERLE and when he repudiates Richard's murder. The playwright is clearly paving the way for Bolingbroke's appearance as Henry IV.

The historical Bolingbroke was Richard's close contemporary, although the playwright makes the usurper younger than the deposed King (e.g., in 3.3.204–205) to emphasise his greater vitality. Henry Bolingbroke was so called because he was born at Bolingbroke, a castle in Lincolnshire. (The alternative version of his name, Bullingbrook, first used in the Q1 edition of the play, suggests its probable pronunciation in Elizabethan English.) As a young man, Bolingbroke belonged to a political faction, led by Gloucester, that nearly dethroned Richard in 1387. However, he remained aloof from the politics of the court throughout the 1390s, spending much of his time as a Crusader in Lithuania, and he seems to have had nothing to do with the conflict of 1397 that resulted in Gloucester's death. His motivation in challenging Mowbray two years later is unclear, although the play makes it appear to be ambition for the throne. Actually, even after his invasion, Bolingbroke may have intended only to claim his inheritance; it is unclear when he decided to seize power.

Shakespeare invented several aspects of Bolingbroke's assumption of the crown. The deposition scene, in which Bolingbroke formally displaces Richard, is entirely fictitious; the triumphant usurper had no interest in providing his defeated opponent with a public platform. Similarly, his instigation of the murder of Richard by Piers EXTON is unhistorical. The episode, in which Bolingbroke vows to go on crusade to atone for Exton's crime, is intended to introduce

the religious tendencies of Henry IV. Although the playwright took this incident from his chief source and certainly believed it, Bolingbroke's repudiation of Exton after the murder is Shakespeare's fiction. A similar story concerning Thomas à Becket and Henry II was one of several apocryphal anecdotes that the playwright might have used as a model; an account in PLUTARCH was another.

Bolingbroke (2), Roger (d. 1441) Historical figure and minor character in *2 Henry VI*, a sorcerer who, along with John SOUTHWELL and MARGERY JOURDAIN, is hired by HUME to summon and question a spirit for the DUCHESS (1) of Gloucester, who wishes to know the prospects for a coup. Bolingbroke addresses the spirit, ASNATH. He asks it questions, provided by the duchess, about the futures of the king and nobles. They are all arrested by the dukes of YORK (8) and BUCKINGHAM (3). In 2.3 the king sentences Bolingbroke to be strangled.

The historical Bolingbroke was a priest. His execution was of a sort reserved for particularly heinous criminals: he was hanged and then publicly disembowelled and quartered.

Bona, Lady (b. after 1447, d. 1485) Historical figure and character in *3 Henry VI*, the proposed French bride of EDWARD IV, whose rejection of her sparks the defection of the Earl of WARWICK (3). In 3.3 Bona, the sister-in-law of King LEWIS (3), is agreeable to the marriage, having heard good things of Edward, but Edward has instead married an English commoner. Bona adds her voice to a chorus of demands for revenge for this slight, and thus approves of the alliance among Lewis, Warwick, and MARGARET (1), aimed at deposing Edward and reinstating HENRY VI. This episode is one of many in the *Henry VI* plays in which broken oaths result in catastrophe for England—in this case, another phase of the WARS OF THE ROSES. It is analogous to the similar abandonment of a marriage agreement by King Henry in order to marry Margaret at the close of *1 Henry VI*.

The historical Lady Bona of Savoy, Louis XI's sister-in-law, was indeed proposed as a bride for Edward, but the matter never progressed very far. She subsequently married a Duke of Milan, and, after his death, she briefly ruled that duchy as regent for her son.

Bonian, Richard (active 1598–1611) London publisher and bookseller. Bonian began as a printer's apprentice and flourished, becoming a member of the STATIONERS' COMPANY and owning three London bookshops. In 1609 he co-published, with Henry WALLEY, the QUARTO edition of *Troilus and Cressida*. By the time of the publication of the FIRST FOLIO, in 1623, Bonian had died. Little more is known of him.

Booth (1), Barton (1681–1733) English actor. Booth was Thomas BETTERTON's successor as the leading tragic actor on the London stage. He was particularly noted for his portrayal of OTHELLO, but he also played many other Shakespearean roles, including LEAR, HOTSPUR, BRUTUS (4), TIMON, and HAMLET. A reformed alcoholic, he became a co-manager of the Drury Lane Theatre with Colley CIBBER (1) and was one of the most influential figures in the London theatre world of the early 18th century.

Booth (2), Edwin (1833–1893) American actor. Booth, son of Junius Brutus BOOTH (4), was the leading American actor of his day. He first achieved acclaim when he stood in for his ailing father as RICHARD III in 1851. Among Shakespearean roles, he was best known for his portrayal of HAMLET, but he also played most of the other tragic heroes. In 1862 he became manager of a New York theatre, where he staged a number of Shakespeare's plays. In the winter of 1864–1865 he presented a production of *Hamlet* that ran for 100 performances, then a record for the play. Almost immediately thereafter, his brother John Wilkes

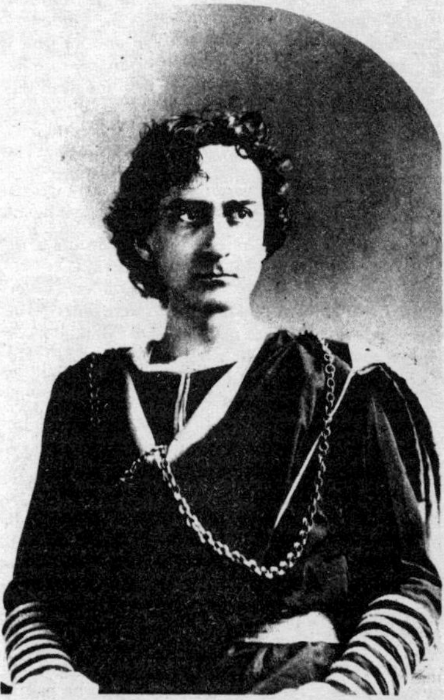

Edwin Booth in the role of Hamlet. Booth's famous 100-night run in this role in 1864 was a record that stood until 1922. In 1865 Booth was forced into temporary retirement by the scandal of Lincoln's assassination at the hand of his brother John Wilkes Booth. (Courtesy of Culver Pictures, Inc.)

BOOTH (3) assassinated Abraham Lincoln, and Booth retired temporarily. He returned to the stage in 1866. The theatre he ran burned down, and he built his own, which opened in 1869, but in four years he was bankrupt. He then toured for several years in America and abroad. In London in 1882, he and Henry IRVING alternated the parts of OTHELLO and IAGO. Returning to America, he became partners with Lawrence BARRETT and performed a variety of roles with him, Helena MODJESKA (in *Macbeth*), and Tommaso SALVINI (who played Othello to Booth's Iago). His last performance was as Hamlet in 1891.

Booth (3), John Wilkes (1839–1865) American actor best known for assassinating Abraham Lincoln. Booth, son of Junius Brutus BOOTH (4) and brother of Edwin BOOTH (2) and Junius Brutus BOOTH (5), Jr., was a well-known actor in 1865—the year of Lincoln's murder. He had played a variety of classical and modern roles, and was particularly noted for his portrayal of RICHARD III. Contemporary opinion varied as to his sanity when he assassinated Lincoln; he himself claimed patriotic motives in support of the Confederacy, which had just lost the Civil War, and for which he may have once been a secret agent. In any case he was at least a competent professional, though in the shadow of his great brother Edwin. He is said to have adopted his father's grandiloquent style in conscious opposition to Edwin's more restrained manner. He was killed while fleeing after the assassination.

Booth (4), Junius Brutus (1796–1852) English actor, father of three notable American stars, Edwin BOOTH (2), John Wilkes BOOTH (3), and Junius Brutus BOOTH (5), Jr. The elder Booth, born to a London lawyer whose republican political sentiments were reflected in his son's name, became a major rival of Edmund KEAN (2) after making his debut as RICHARD III in 1815. He was noted for his portrayals of HAMLET and SHYLOCK. Joining Kean's company in 1820, he played IAGO to Kean's OTHELLO and EDGAR to his LEAR. In 1821 he deserted his wife and son and emigrated to the United States with his lover, a London flower-seller who was to be the mother of the actors and seven other children. Booth helped popularise Shakespeare in America, playing a variety of roles in New York and on extensive tours. He made his last appearance in New Orleans, before dying on a Mississippi River steamboat.

Booth (5), Junius Brutus, Jr. (1821–1883) American actor. Booth, son of Junius Brutus BOOTH (4), was regarded as a lesser actor than either his father or his younger brother Edwin BOOTH (2), though he had a long and successful career in a variety of parts, mostly non-Shakespearean. He played IAGO opposite his father's OTHELLO on several occasions, and once played CASSIUS opposite his two brothers, Edwin and John Wilkes BOOTH (3), who played BRUTUS (4) and ANTONY, respectively. He was respected as a highly competent producer and stage manager.

Borachio Character in *Much Ado About Nothing*, follower of Don JOHN (1). Borachio, Don John's chief lieutenant, receives 1,000 ducats from his master for devising a scheme to prevent the marriage of CLAUDIO (1), whom Don John resents and despises, to the desirable HERO. Borachio masquerades with Hero's waiting-woman, MARGARET (2), as Hero and a clandestine lover. This charade convinces Claudio and Don PEDRO that Hero is promiscuous, and she finds herself publicly humiliated as an unfaithful fiancée. However, when Borachio brags of his success to his friend CONRADE, the WATCHMEN (3) overhear him, and the plot is eventually exposed. In the general reconciliation that closes the play, Borachio repents, confessing his guilt freely and adding that he duped Margaret.

Some modern editors give the lines of BALTHASAR (4) in 2.1.92–102, where he flirts with Margaret, to Borachio. Errors in some of these speech prefixes suggest that the printers of the early editions were confused, and, since Borachio is elsewhere associated with the waiting-woman, he is sometimes given that connection here as well. Borachio's name comes from the Spanish *borracho*, meaning 'drunkard'. This rather undignified appellation reflects the petty villainy of the character, while also implying a relative innocence that makes his acknowledgement of guilt at the end of the play more believable.

Bordeaux City in south-west FRANCE (1), the site of a battle in *1 Henry VI*. In 4.2 TALBOT approaches the walls of Bordeaux and demands its surrender. He is spurned by a French GENERAL, who declares his confidence in the approaching French army. In 4.6 and 4.7, the battle takes place, and Talbot and his son, JOHN (6), are killed.

In reality, Talbot and his forces occupied Bordeaux, which welcomed the English, months before the fatal battle, and the fight took place 50 miles away at Castillon, where Talbot had marched to relieve a siege. The historical battle took place in 1453 and was the last major conflict of the HUNDRED YEARS WAR. Shakespeare placed it earlier in the war in order to suggest that Talbot's death was a direct consequence of the rivalry between YORK (8) and SOMERSET (3). The playwright thereby emphasised the aristocratic discord that led, in the play's sequels, *2* and *3 Henry VI* and *Richard III*, to the WARS OF THE ROSES.

Boswell, James the younger (1778–1822) British scholar, editor of the Third VARIORUM EDITION of Shakespeare's works. Boswell's father (1740–1795), the famed biographer of Samuel JOHNSON (7), was a close friend and colleague of the Shakespearean scholar Edmond MALONE. When Malone died in 1812 while assembling his second edition of Shakespeare's

works, the younger Boswell completed the task. The 21-volume result (1821) added to Malone's many notes and essays much of George STEEVENS' and Isaac REED's 1803 Second Variorum edition. It remained the most comprehensive work of its kind for over a century, until the New Variorum of H. H. FURNESS was completed. The Third Variorum, also known as 'Boswell's Malone', is regarded as one of the most important editions of Shakespeare ever published. Its wide range of scholarship has been basic to virtually all later research on the playwright and his work.

Bosworth Field Battle site in central England, the setting of the final three scenes of *Richard III.* Arguably the most famous battle in English history, Bosworth, fought in August 1485, provides the finale for Shakespeare's first TETRALOGY of HISTORY PLAYS. The army led by the Earl of RICHMOND defeats the forces of King RICHARD III, killing Richard. The WARS OF THE ROSES end, and the TUDOR dynasty is established, as Richmond claims the throne to rule as Henry VII.

Shakespeare's presentation of this event is highly elaborate and symbolic. The prelude to the battle, in 5.3, features councils of war and opposing statements of purpose, climaxed by the appearance of the spirits of Richard's victims (see GHOST [1]). This is far more significant to the narrative than the minor vignettes of combat in 5.4 and the opening action of 5.5, although these scenes encompass the death of Richard. The play is then closed by Richmond's coronation, as he proclaims an end to the wars. Historically, this prediction could not have been certain, of course, and in fact, skirmishes and minor risings were to continue for years. However, the playwright's purpose was not reportorial but dramatic, almost sacramental: the treachery and violence enacted in *Richard III* and the *Henry VI* plays are expiated in a ritual letting of blood followed by a formal reconciliation.

Bottom, Nick Character in *A Midsummer Night's Dream,* a weaver of ATHENS. His comical ignorance and his tendency to mangle language make Bottom a typi-

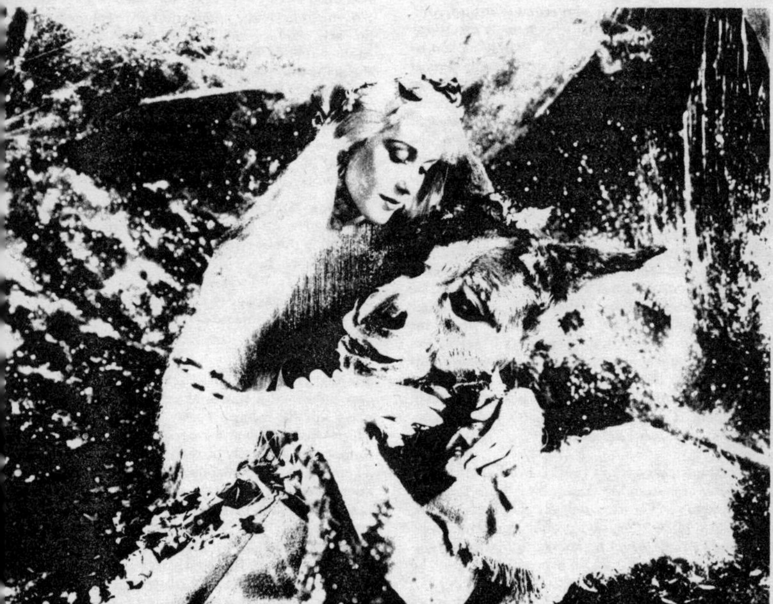

James Cagney as Bottom in Max Reinhardt's 1935 film of A Midsummer Night's Dream. *Given the head of an ass by the mischievous Puck, Bottom temporarily becomes the beloved of the magically charmed Titania.* (Courtesy of Movie Star News)

cal Shakespearean CLOWN (1). He is repeatedly placed in ludicrous situations, but his supremely good opinion of himself is unshakeable. As the leading player in the amateur production of PYRAMUS AND THISBE, Bottom cuts a silly figure as a know-it-all who is unaware of his true ignorance. Given the head of an ass by the fairy PUCK, Bottom temporarily becomes the beloved of the magically charmed TITANIA, and his decorum in this extraordinary situation is ridiculous.

However, Bottom is a sympathetic figure as well. He is not pompous, and he is unfailingly civil to everyone. He is not patronising to his fellow artisans when he lectures them (preposterously) on stagecraft, and he is courteous to his fairy attendants, PEASEBLOSSOM, COBWEB, MOTH (2), and MUSTARDSEED. His self-confidence, though humorous in its fog-like density, is not entirely misplaced: he is a leader among his fellows, as they are quite aware, and we can believe he is surely an excellent craftsman. His comedy lies in the contrast between his circumstances and his lack of awareness, but he is not a victim. His courage makes him admirable as well as amusing.

It is ironic that Bottom, who remains absurdly unperturbed, is the only mortal who actually meets any of the fairies. Yet in the end, he is plainly moved by his experience. Awakening from what he calls 'a most rare vision' (4.1.203), he discovers that he cannot quite recollect it. He expresses his bafflement in comically garbled terms that reflect, among other things, St Paul's description (1 Cor. 2:7–9) of the 'hidden wisdom which God ordained before the world'. We do not need to know the source to sense the power of these words. Bottom aptly observes of his vision, 'It shall be called "Bottom's Dream", because it hath no bottom' (4.1.214–215); he has sensed that something profound has happened to him.

Bottom's name refers to a tool of his trade, the core on which a skein of yarn is wound or, figuratively, the skein itself; its suggestions of the fundamental or basic element of something are equally appropriate to this representative of the common man. To 'get to the bottom' of a subject is to find its essential quality, and Bottom displays the combination of practicality, courage, and blind confidence that underlies much human achievement. The word had no anatomical connotations in Elizabethan English.

Boult Minor character in *Pericles,* brothel employee responsible for training and advertising the kidnapped MARINA. The energetic Boult ('Performance shall follow' [4.2.59], he says proudly) pretends to be cruel and cynical. When he speaks of Marina's modesty, he declares that 'these blushes of hers must be quench'd with some present practice' (4.2.122–124). However, though he threatens to destroy her innocence through rape, in 4.6, she recognises that she can appeal to his inner revulsion at his profession, and tells him his job would shame 'the pained'st fiend / Of hell' (4.6.162–163). He can only plead, 'What would you have me do? go to the wars, would you? Where a man may serve seven years for the loss of a leg, and have not money enough in the end to buy him a wooden one?' (4.6.169–172). This brief, compelling outburst demonstrates the breadth of Shakespeare's humanity: he transforms a minor character's crisis into a striking commentary on a pervasive scandal of his times; the distressing status of military veterans. Boult agrees to help Marina escape the brothel, which we later learn she does. In addition to helping Marina, Boult also contributes to the comic relief from melodrama provided by the brothel scenes.

Bourbon (1), Jean, Duke of (1380–1434) Historical figure and minor character in *Henry V,* a French nobleman. In 4.5, in the confusion of the French defeat at AGINCOURT, Bourbon determines to launch a counterattack. However, in 4.8 he is a prisoner of King HENRY V. Following the QUARTO edition of the play, some editions assign to Bourbon the lines of BRETAGNE in 3.5; this reflects the elimination of Bretagne's part in an early production. The Quarto also gives the lines of the DAUPHIN (3) in 3.7 to Bourbon, suggesting that the actor who played the Duke in the same early production was held in high regard.

The historical Bourbon, after being taken prisoner at Agincourt, spent the rest of his life in captivity in England. The BOURBON (2) who appears in *3 Henry VI* was his illegitimate son.

Bourbon (2), Lewis (Louis), Lord (active 1460s) Historical figure and minor character in *3 Henry VI,* an admiral in the service of King LEWIS (3) of FRANCE (1). In 3.3, when Lewis decides to provide soldiers for MARGARET (1) and WARWICK (3), he orders Bourbon to arrange their passage to England. The historical admiral was the illegitimate son of the Duke of BOURBON (1), who appears in *Henry V.*

Bowdler, Thomas (1754–1825) English editor. Bowdler published a censored version of Shakespeare's plays, his 10-volume *Family Shakespeare* (1818), in which 'those words and expressions are omitted which cannot with propriety be read aloud in a family' or 'by a gentleman to a company of ladies'. A professed admirer of the playwright, he nonetheless felt that without 'profaneness or obscenity . . . the transcendent genius of the poet would undoubtedly shine with more unclouded lustre'. He accordingly changed all expletive uses of 'God' to 'Heaven', and cut extensive passages that he deemed obscene. Some plays involved more drastic action—DOLL TEARSHEET is simply eliminated from *2 Henry IV* and *Henry V,* for instance—and sometimes he had to confess himself defeated,

publishing *Measure for Measure* and *Othello* with warnings.

Bowdler's *Shakespeare* was immensely popular and was reprinted many times. It became so well known—or notorious—that it sparked a new word that is still in use: bowdlerise, meaning to censor a text by omitting vulgarities. Bowdler also produced a bowdlerised version of Gibbons' *The Decline and Fall of the Roman Empire,* published posthumously in 1826.

Boy (1) Minor character in *1 Henry VI,* the son of the MASTER-GUNNER of ORLÉANS (1). In 1.4 the Boy is instructed by his father that their cannon is trained on a tower where the English leaders are known to stand watch, and he subsequently fires the shot that kills the Duke of SALISBURY (3).

Boy (2) (Edward Plantagenet, Earl of Warwick, 1475–1499) Historical figure and minor character in *Richard III,* the son of CLARENCE (1). The Boy appears in 2.2, in which he refuses to believe that his uncle, RICHARD III, has killed his father. He is not seen again, but we hear of his imprisonment by Richard in 4.3.36. Crimes against children are a recurring motif in the *Henry VI* plays and *Richard III,* and this instance is clearly intended to add to the enormity of Richard's crimes. The villain has felt it unnecessary to kill the boy, despite his position as a possible claimant to the throne, only because the boy is 'foolish' (4.2.55), meaning mentally retarded. It is unclear whether or not this was so, but it is known that the historical Boy, Edward of Warwick, was in fact imprisoned not by Richard but by his successor, Henry VII, the RICHMOND of the play. In fact, although the record is obscure, it is thought that Richard may have named Warwick his successor after the death of his own son (who does not appear in the play) in 1484. Later, after a number of people attempted to impersonate the imprisoned Warwick and seize power, Henry finally had him executed.

Boy (3) Character in *Henry V,* servant of BARDOLPH (1), PISTOL, and NYM. Having been employed by FALSTAFF as a page—the same figure appears in *2 Henry IV* as the PAGE (5) and in *The Merry Wives of Windsor* as ROBIN (1)—he accompanies his late master's cronies to France as part of King HENRY V's army. In 3.2.28–57 he elicits our sympathy by regretting his association with such cowardly thieves. At the battle of AGINCOURT he acts as an interpreter between Pistol and the captive FRENCH SOLDIER in 4.4, and after this sorry episode he again bemoans his continued connection with Pistol; he also reveals that Bardolph and Nym have been hung. In this speech (4.4.69–80) he remarks that only he and other boys guard the English baggage train, which would thus make a good target for the French, if only they knew the situation. With this observation the Boy grimly heralds his own death, for in 4.7.5 GOWER (2) reports the French massacre of all these youngsters.

Boy (4) Minor character in *Much Ado About Nothing,* servant of BENEDICK. In 2.3 Benedick sends the Boy on an errand whose sole purpose seems to be to permit the mention that the scene is set in an orchard or garden. The Boy flippantly asserts that his speed will be such that 'I am here already, sir' (2.3.5), an effervescent pleasantry suited to the early action of the play.

Boy (5) Minor character in *Troilus and Cressida,* a servant of TROILUS. In 1.2 the Boy summons PANDARUS to his master's house. The incident leaves CRESSIDA alone to soliloquise on her love for Troilus.

Boy (6) Minor character in *Measure for Measure,* servant of MARIANA (2). At the opening of 4.1 the Boy sings a stanza of the SONG 'Take, O take those lips away' and is dismissed. The Boy provides the relief of a song as the plot tightens and helps, by his presence, to indicate the social status of Mariana.

Boy (7) Minor character in *Antony and Cleopatra,* a singer. Some modern editions include a stage direction specifying that a Boy sings the SONG that accompanies the dance led by ENOBARBUS (2.7.111–116) because Enobarbus stipulates that 'the boy shall sing' (2.7.108), although the authoritative FIRST FOLIO text does not include a specific mention of the Boy.

Boy (8) Minor character in *Coriolanus,* the son of the title character. After CORIOLANUS has been banished, he joins the VOLSCIANS and threatens ROME with destruction. His mother and wife go to beg him to desist, and they bring the Boy with them. Coriolanus addresses his son with a brief homily of the warrior's honour that he himself has lost: 'The god of soldiers . . . inform / Thy thoughts with nobleness, that thou mayst prove / To shame unvulnerable' (5.3.70–73). The Boy speaks only once. With both courage and good sense, he declares that his father 'shall not tread on me. / I'll run away till I am bigger, but then I'll fight' (5.3.127–128). Coriolanus is clearly touched and insists that he must listen no more to his family or he'll give in. Eventually—at the play's climactic turning point—he does indeed surrender to their influence, to which the Boy has added his share.

The Boy is described in 1.3.55–68 as an energetic lad who would rather play at war than go to school and who has a temper like his father's, which leads him to kill a butterfly with his teeth. This image is effectively reprised when MENENIUS describes the fearful approach of the Volscians—led by Coriolanus—who advance confidently, like 'boys pursuing summer butter-

flies' (4.6.95). The image contributes to the anti-war theme that runs through the play.

Boy (9) Minor character in *Henry VIII,* an attendant of Bishop GARDINER (1). Identified in the stage directions opening 5.1 as the bishop's page, the Boy carries a torch for his master and in his three words confirms that it is one o'clock. He thus establishes the time of night, while also indicating by his presence the high rank of Gardiner, once the king's secretary.

Boy (10) Minor character in *The Two Noble Kinsmen,* a singer at the wedding of THESEUS (2) and HIPPOLYTA (2). In 1.1.1–24 the Boy sings the SONG 'Roses, their sharp spines being gone' and strews flowers. He provides a note of decorous festivity before the ceremony is interrupted by the arrival of the three Queens (see QUEEN [1]).

Boydell, John (1719–1804) British engraver and publisher. Boydell founded an art gallery devoted to depictions of scenes from Shakespeare's plays, engravings of which were published for profit. He was supported in this endeavour by Britain's leading artist, Joshua Reynolds (1723–1792), who hoped to promote an indigenous school of English history painting. The gallery was opened in 1789 with a collection of 34 paintings commissioned from a number of notable artists, including Reynolds, Joseph Wright of Derby (1734–1797), and Henry Fuseli (1741–1825). The collection eventually grew to almost 200 pieces, and many engravings were sold. Despite their popularity, however, the venture foundered economically, and Boydell's heirs were forced to sell the collection in 1805.

Boyet Minor character in *Love's Labour's Lost,* a gentleman in the entourage of the PRINCESS (1) of France. Boyet is a smooth courtier, a familiar type in the Elizabethan court. We first see him flattering his mistress and being put in his place. He often serves as a messenger. He happens to overhear the plans of the King and his gentlemen to masquerade as Russians, and he warns the Princess and her ladies. BEROWNE expresses his dislike for Boyet in 5.2.315–327.

Brabantio (Brabanzio) Minor character in *Othello,* DESDEMONA's father. Brabantio, a senator of VENICE, learns from IAGO of Desdemona's secret marriage to the Moorish general OTHELLO and is outraged at the thought of his daughter on 'the sooty bosom / Of such a thing as [Othello]' (1.2.70–71). He accuses Othello of having 'enchanted her . . . with foul charms . . . with drugs or minerals' (1.2.63–74) and seeks his imprisonment as a sorcerer, but he is foiled when Desdemona testifies to her love for the general. Defeated, he departs, but his final speech carries heavy irony as he warns Othello, '. . . have a quick eye to see: / She has deceiv'd her father, [and] may do thee' (1.3.292–293). Brabantio disappears from the play at this point, though we are told in 5.2 that he has died of grief at Desdemona's marriage. He serves chiefly to establish, through his racial prejudice and enmity towards Othello, the extent to which the Moor is isolated in Venetian society.

Bracegirdle, Anne (c. 1673–1748) English actress. Bracegirdle began her career as a child actress and a student of Thomas BETTERTON and Mary SAUNDERSON. She was best known for her roles in the comedies of William Congreve (1670–1729), whose wife or mistress she was (the record is unclear), but she also played many Shakespearean roles, especially CORDELIA, DESDEMONA, OPHELIA, and PORTIA.

Bradley, Andrew Cecil (1851–1935) British critic and scholar. Bradley was a professor of literature at several English universities. He is best known for his book, *Shakespearean Tragedy* (1904), which centres on comprehensive analyses of the characters in *Hamlet, King Lear, Macbeth,* and *Othello.* Though criticised by modern commentators as overly dependent on the idea that the characters—who are, after all, fictions—can have genuinely human psychologies, it was nonetheless a dominant work among students of Shakespeare for almost 30 years.

Bradock (Bradocke), Richard (active 1581–1615) London printer. Bradock, about whom little is known, printed several editions of *Venus and Adonis* for William LEAKE between 1599 and 1603. In 1608 Thomas PAVIER hired him to print the first edition of A YORKSHIRE TRAGEDY, a play that was falsely attributed to Shakespeare.

Brakenbury (Brackenbury), Robert (d. 1485) Historical figure and character in *Richard III,* the commander of the TOWER OF LONDON and thus the chief gaoler of, first, CLARENCE (1) and, later, the young PRINCE (5) Edward and his brother, YORK (7). Some editions of the play follow the first QUARTO and assign Brakenbury the lines of the KEEPER (3) in 1.4.

The historical Brakenbury was a Constable of the Tower, but not at the time of Clarence's death. The inconsistency doubtless resulted from Shakespeare's marked compression of historical time in the early part of the play. Brakenbury was killed at the battle of BOSWORTH FIELD, as is reported in 5.5.14.

Brandon (1) Minor character in *Henry VIII,* an officer who arrests the Duke of BUCKINGHAM (1) and Lord ABERGAVENNY. Brandon appears in 1.1 and instructs a SERGEANT (3) AT ARMS to arrest the two noblemen. Brandon is sorry to have this duty and civilly explains

that they are alleged to be part of a conspiracy against the king. His apologetic attitude helps convey the play's point of view, that Buckingham's enemy Cardinal WOLSEY is in the wrong.

Brandon may be the same person as the Duke of SUFFOLK (1), who appears later in the play and whose name was Charles Brandon. The designation of one character by two names might indicate joint authorship of the play, or it might simply be an instance of Shakespeare's carelessness in such matters, evident throughout his plays.

Brandon (2), Sir William (d. 1485) Historical figure and minor character in *Richard III*, a follower of the Earl of RICHMOND. In 5.3 Brandon is among Richmond's officers and is designated as the Earl's standard-bearer in the forthcoming battle of BOSWORTH FIELD. In 5.5 his death in the battle is reported. Historically, Brandon was the father of the Duke of SUFFOLK (1), who appears in *Henry VIII.*

Bretagne (Britaine, Brittany), Jean, Duke of (1389–1442) Historical figure and minor character in *Henry V*, a follower of the FRENCH KING. In 3.5 Bretagne and other French noblemen marvel at the fighting abilities of the English. Brittany was still an independent state in the 14th century, and the historical Duke of Bretagne (Brittany) was an important ally of FRANCE (1). He was the son-in-law of Charles VI, the French King of the play.

Bretchgirdle, John (d. 1565) Vicar at STRATFORD. Bretchgirdle probably christened Shakespeare, on April 26, 1564. The record does not include the name of the officiating clergyman, but it was probably Bretchgirdle, who was vicar at Stratford from 1561 until his death. A graduate of Oxford, Bretchgirdle had been a vicar and schoolmaster in Cheshire before coming to Stratford. He was a literate man who bequeathed a large library, much of it to the Stratford Grammar School where Shakespeare was educated.

Bright, Timothy (1550–1615) English author of a probable source for *Hamlet.* Bright, a science writer and the inventor of shorthand notation, was a physician and clergyman. His *A Treatise of Melancholy* (1586) analysed depression and mental illness in general; numerous similarities in ideas and wording suggest that this book influenced Shakespeare's portrait of his melancholy prince HAMLET. However, Bright's *Treatise* was one of many contemporary books on mental depression, a subject that fascinated Elizabethan England, and it need not have been the only inspiration for the creation of a melancholy protagonist, as was once commonly asserted.

A successful physician as a young man, Bright became so obsessed with developing his shorthand system—a rather cumbersome one that was soon superseded—that he neglected his medical practice until he was dismissed from his post in a London hospital. He moved to the country to live as a rural clergyman, but he was dismissed from two positions there for similar reasons, and he retired.

Bristol (Bristow) City in western England, a location in *Richard II.* King RICHARD II's cowardly friends BUSHY and GREENE (1) flee to Bristol when BOLINGBROKE (1) appears with an army to challenge the King. Bristol was the principal port for trade with Ireland and thus a logical place for them to meet Richard upon his return. However, Bolingbroke arrives ahead of Richard, and he captures Bushy and Greene. In 3.1 he condemns them to death before the walls of Bristol Castle.

Britten, Benjamin (b. 1913) British composer, creator of an operatic version of *A Midsummer Night's Dream.* Britten began composing orchestral music as a child, and by the 1930s he was an influential modern composer. He has created many operas and choral works including *A Midsummer Night's Dream* (1960).

Brook (1) Name used by the disguised FORD (1) in *The Merry Wives of Windsor.* Ford, unreasonably jealous, believes that his wife, MISTRESS (1) Ford, intends to commit adultery with FALSTAFF. He visits Falstaff posing as Brook, a would-be lover of Mistress Ford, and he encourages Falstaff to seduce his wife, pretending to hope to follow in his footsteps as Brook. He actually wants to catch his wife in her adultery with the fat knight. His assumed name figures in several jokes, as in 2.2.145–146 and 5.5.241–242.

It is thought that this alias was Shakespeare's subtle, jesting reference to an alteration in his work that had recently been forced upon him. A Puritan leader, William Brooke, Lord COBHAM—or perhaps his son Henry Brooke—had been offended by a fat, lecherous, ne'er-do-well character in *1 Henry IV* whose name, OLDCASTLE, was the same as that of one of his revered ancestors. Cobham was a powerful aristocrat, and his complaint was honoured: Oldcastle became Falstaff. However, in the first play in which the new name was used from the outset, *The Merry Wives,* Shakespeare permitted himself a mild revenge, associating the Cobham family name with a character whose foolishness might be said to resemble their own pridefulness. Since the Oldcastle furore was well known in London, the joke, if it was one, would certainly have been widely understood.

However, Shakespeare's jest was itself subject to revision. In the FIRST FOLIO edition of the play (1623), Ford uses the name Broome throughout. Since the 1602 QUARTO uses Brooke, this change must have been made between 1602 and 1623. It may be that

Henry Brooke demanded the change, although its apparent late date seems to distance the alteration from the original controversy. Several other theories have been proposed; the most convincing asserts that the name was changed for a performance at the court of King JAMES I in November 1604, 18 months after his accession. In the previous year both Henry Brooke and his brother George had attempted coups against the new King and had been convicted of treason. George was executed, and Henry was imprisoned for life. Their surname may have been removed from the play to avoid an unnecessary reminder of James' difficulties.

Brook (2), Peter (b. 1925) British theatrical and FILM director. Brook, an innovative director who has consciously attempted to incorporate influences from many times and cultures into his work, is one of the most important figures in contemporary world theatre, as well as in the more restricted context of Shakespearean production. His many stagings of Shakespeare have varied in style from the Watteauesque romanticism of a 1947 *Love's Labour's Lost* to a brutal 1962 *King Lear*—with Paul SCOFIELD in what is acclaimed as one of the greatest Shakespearean performances of modern times—to the dramatically avant-garde 1970 presentation of *A Midsummer Night's Dream,* which incorporated circus routines, played within a set that was a huge white box. Other famous Brook productions include *Measure for Measure* and *The Winter's Tale* in 1951, both with John GIELGUD, and *Titus Andronicus,* starring Laurence OLIVIER, in 1955.

Brook was an adviser on a 1953 TELEVISION version of *King Lear* starring Orson WELLES, and he made his own film of *Lear* in 1969 with Scofield. While filming *Lear* in Denmark, Brook corresponded about the project with Grigori KOZINTSEV, who was also filming the play in Russia. Brook's result is a bleak depiction characterised by the purposefully disconcerting use of such cinematic techniques as montage, hand-held camerawork, and silent-screen titles. It attracted both great praise and disgusted criticism.

In the 1980s Brook was largely concerned with non-Shakespearean projects, the most notable of which was probably his 1987 staging of the ancient Indian epic *The Mahabharata.* Critics sometimes find Brook's experiments pretentious or criticise a disparity between style and content, but all agree that his successes are major ones, and that his energy and daring have contributed greatly to late 20th-century theatre.

Brooke (1), Arthur (d. 1563) English poet, author of the principal source for *Romeo and Juliet.* Brooke's poem *The Tragicall Historye of Romeus and Juliet* (1562)—a loose translation of a French prose tale that was in turn derived from an Italian story by Matteo BANDELLO—served Shakespeare as his chief source for his version of the tale of tragic lovers. The poem also contributed details to *The Two Gentlemen of Verona* and *3 Henry VI.*

Little is known of Brooke's life, except that he drowned while still a young man on a military expedition to aid the Huguenots in the Wars of Religion of FRANCE (1). He may well have entered the military out of religious conviction, for his introductory remarks to *Romeus and Juliet* are moralistic in a Protestant vein.

Brooke (2), C. F. Tucker (1883–1946) American scholar. A longtime professor at Yale University, Brooke wrote several significant books on Shakespeare, including *The Shakespeare Apocrypha* (1908), *The Tudor Drama* (1911), and *Shakespeare's Sonnets* (1936). He was also a general editor of the Yale edition of Shakespeare's works, published in 40 volumes between 1917 and 1927.

Brooke (3), William, Lord Cobham See COBHAM.

Broome See BROOK (1).

Brother (1) Minor character in *2 Henry VI,* brother of Sir Humphrey STAFFORD (2). Accompanying Sir Humphrey on a mission to put down the revolt led by Jack CADE, the Brother supports Stafford in his undiplomatic approach to the rebels in 4.2; they are both killed in the skirmish in 4.3. It is known from historical sources that the brother's name was Sir William Stafford (d. 1450).

Brother (2) Either of two minor characters in *Cymbeline,* the deceased siblings of POSTHUMUS who appear to him as apparitions, in 5.4. The Brothers appear with the spirits of their father, SICILIUS LEONATUS, and their MOTHER. Led by Sicilius, the group pleads with Jupiter for mercy on Posthumus. The Brothers point out Posthumus' qualities in an elaborate poem; the First Brother speaks two stanzas and the Second Brother one. The Second Brother notes that they had both died, with their father, before Posthumus was born. This fact has been previously mentioned in 1.1. 35–36. The episode adds to the romantic strangeness of the play, and the Brothers have the eerie presence of supernatural beings.

Brother (3) Minor character in *The Two Noble Kinsmen,* brother of the GAOLER (4). In 4.1 the Brother accompanies the Gaoler's deranged DAUGHTER (2), who is returning home. He is a mere pawn who speaks only a few lines. He was probably created by Shakespeare's collaborator, John FLETCHER (2), who wrote this scene in the opinion of most scholars.

Browne, Robert (active 1583–1620) English actor and theatrical entrepreneur. Browne was a member of

WORCESTER'S MEN in 1583–1584, Derby's Men (see DERBY [3]) in 1599–1601, and a partner in the Children of the Queen's Revels (see CHILDREN'S COMPANIES) in 1610, but he is best known for his career in Europe, especially in Germany. Between 1590 and 1620 he toured Germany and the Low Countries with a series of his own acting companies. He performed chiefly English plays, at first entirely in English but increasingly in German. His was the most important of a group of English acting companies whose tours were extremely popular and are generally thought to have contributed greatly to the German theatre of the time. Another prominent figure was Browne's follower, John GREEN. Browne's company is known to have performed plays by Christopher MARLOWE (1), and he probably staged Shakespeare's plays as well, for Green is known to have done so. In 1593 while Browne was on tour, his wife and children died in a London epidemic; two years later he remarried, possibly to a sister of William SLY (2), who in 1608 bequeathed his share in the GLOBE THEATRE to a Robert Browne who is thought to be this man.

Brutus (1), Decius Character in *Julius Caesar.* See DECIUS.

Brutus (2), Junius (active 509 B.C.) Quasi-historical founder of the Roman Republic and minor figure in *The Rape of Lucrece*. He avenges TARQUIN's assault on LUCRECE and expels the last king of Rome, Tarquin's father. (The same figure appears in *Coriolanus,* though as a very different character. See BRUTUS [3].) Brutus appears only in the closing stanzas of *Lucrece,* beginning in line 1807. He rallies the grief-stricken husband and father of Lucrece, COLLATINE and LUCRETIUS, to pursue the villain, with the consequence, stated briefly in the last line of the poem, that Tarquin is banished. Shakespeare described this conclusion slightly more elaborately in the final sentence of the ARGUMENT: '. . . the Tarquins were all exiled, and the state government changed from kings to consuls'.

Brutus is said to have been a foolish young man, best known 'for sportive words and utt'ring foolish things' (line 1813), before finding maturity in undertaking this act of revenge and revolution. Shakespeare took this characterisation from his Latin sources, OVID and LIVY. However, these writers lived five centuries after Brutus; very little is actually known of the historical figure, if he actually existed. His name, meaning 'brutish' (like that of HAMLET), was probably an insult, originally, referring to his careless early life. However, Roman tradition revered Brutus as the leader of the revolt that established the republic in 509 B.C., though all that was recorded of him, and only recorded somewhat later, was that he was one of the first two consuls, the officers who replaced the kings and ruled jointly for a year at a time. (The association of the revolution with a rape is entirely legendary.) Marcus BRUTUS (4), the assassin of Julius CAESAR (1), claimed descent from him, as is mentioned several times in *Julius Caesar* (e.g., in 2.1.53–54). Brutus is also mentioned in *Henry V,* 2.4.37, where his legendary mis-spent youth is compared with PRINCE (6) HAL's.

Brutus (3), Junius Quasi-historical figure and character in *Coriolanus,* a tribune of ROME. Brutus shares power with Sicinius Velutus, another legendary tribune, but since they are very similar characters who always appear together (except for a brief final appearance by Sicinius in 5.4), they are both covered here. The tribunes represent the common people's share in political power, and they reject their foe, the aristocratic Roman warrior CORIOLANUS. By orchestrating mob violence—and aided by Coriolanus' foolish actions—they succeed in having him banished from Rome. They enjoy their triumph, but when the exiled Coriolanus attacks Rome, the tribunes deny their responsibility; 'Say not we brought it' (4.6.121), they retort, and insist that the aristocrats resolve the crisis. The tribunes are stereotypes of scurvy politicians and are scarcely distinguishable from each other, but Shakespeare does vary their functions somewhat, with Brutus dominant in the first half of the play.

The shortsightedness of the tribunes' campaign against Coriolanus certainly threatens the city. They are an example of the dangers that result when power is accorded to the common people (see CITIZEN [5]), an important theme of the play. At the same time, however, they are concerned with the health of the city. Their offices were created as a result of the corn riots that open the play. The riots are attributed to the arrogance of Coriolanus and the other aristocrats in the face of the common people's hunger. As Sicinius observes in the wake of Coriolanus' banishment, Rome enjoys 'peace / and quietness' as a result of their victory, while the aristocrats 'blush that the world goes well' (4.6.2–3, 5). When Coriolanus contemptuously asks Brutus, 'What do you prate of service?', the tribune replies with dignity, 'I talk of that, that know it' (3.3.84–85). Indeed, he seems to attempt more service for his people than does the foolish and treacherous warrior for his fellow aristocrats. Nevertheless, the tribunes have a chiefly negative significance in the play's political world, for in a properly run society—as Shakespeare conceived it—the common people would follow the leadership of their social superiors, and have no tribunes. However, Coriolanus' pride has promoted social disruption, of which the tribunes are a result.

The social conflict enacted in *Coriolanus*—taken by Shakespeare from his source, PLUTARCH's *Lives*—is representative of several such episodes that occured in the late 6th century B.C. as the Roman republic came into being. Though the story of Coriolanus is entirely

legendary, Brutus may have been a real person. He appears as Junius BRUTUS (2) in Shakespeare's *The Rape of Lucrece*, though as a very different character. Shakespeare followed Thomas NORTH's translation of Plutarch and erroneously transcribed Sicinius' second name as Velutus, which Plutarch renders as Bellutus. In any case, Plutarch's Sicinius is otherwise unknown in Roman legend, unless he is identifiable with Lucius Sicinius Dentatus, who appears in other sources and is said to have represented the plebeians, though at a somewhat later period.

Brutus (4), Marcus (c. 85–42 B.C.) Historical figure and character in *Julius Caesar*, leader of the assassins of CAESAR (1) and of the forces opposing Mark ANTONY in the subsequent civil war. Brutus, the protagonist of *Caesar*, is representative of the moral ambiguity that is the play's central theme. He seems both good and evil: a patriotic and honourable man who nonetheless brings about Rome's downfall and his own.

When Caesar's apparent ambition to rule alone begins to disturb Roman aristocrats, Brutus is drawn by CASSIUS to lead a plot against him. 'With himself at war' (1.2.45), Brutus debates the murder of his friend and mentor: Shall his patriotism be stronger than his love and respect? He concludes that Caesar must be killed, despite his personal virtues, to save Rome from tyranny. Brutus then approaches the assassination as a moral imperative, but Shakespeare offers much evidence that Brutus is not the wholly selfless figure he believes himself to be. Not only does his decision prove to be politically catastrophic, but it appears to be morally flawed, too, for Brutus is unconsciously in pursuit of power himself.

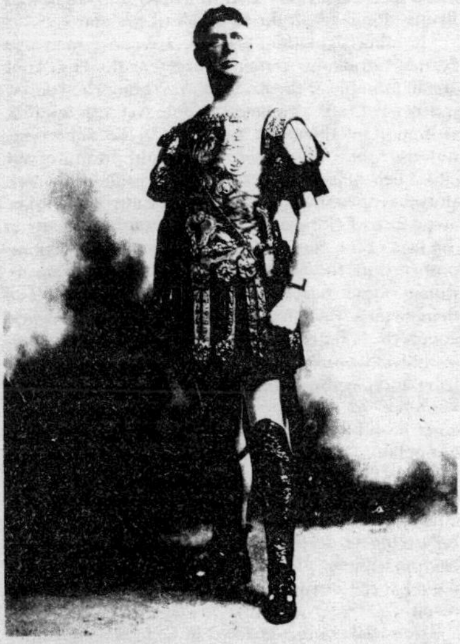

Brutus, the protagonist of Julius Caesar. *While trying to save Rome from Caesar's dictatorship, he becomes, ironically, like a dictator himself.* (Courtesy of Culver Pictures, Inc.)

Brutus' self-appraisal has often been mistaken for Shakespeare's portrait of him, but the playwright, while acknowledgeing his protagonist's patriotism and honourable intentions, presents a host of opposing indications that paint another picture. Brutus is wilful and arrogant, resembling the tyrant he kills and growing more like him as the play unfolds. As leader of the conspiracy, he peremptorily opposes anyone else's initiative, refusing to share leadership with either Cassius or CICERO. His disdainful over-confidence is disastrous when he dismisses Antony as a man of little importance in 2.1.181–183. He overrules Cassius, insisting that Antony be spared and then that Antony be permitted to speak at Caesar's funeral. Both decisions prove fateful. As the battle of PHILIPPI approaches, Brutus once again demands his own way—and leads his cause to defeat. In insisting on his own way at all times, Brutus displays the dictatorial behaviour he had feared in Caesar. But, unlike Caesar, he is not a competent leader. Lacking insight into other men's motives, as he abundantly demonstrates with respect to Cassius and Antony, he is an inadequate politician. He is also an inexperienced and impatient general.

Brutus' self-delusion is startlingly apparent on several occasions. On one level he considers the assassination a high moral duty; yet, subconsciously guilty, he also needs to justify it, saying, 'Let's be sacrificers, but not butchers' (2.1.166). Further, when Caesar has been stabbed to death, Brutus improvises a cleansing ritual—the assassins bathe their hands in their victim's blood—but this act accentuates, not alleviates, the violence of the deed. Brutus does not see the gore through his own vision of rectitude.

Particularly striking is Brutus' unconscious hypocrisy in praising himself for refusing to acquire funds through graft or by accepting bribery, saying, 'I can raise no money by vile means' (4.3.71), while at the same time castigating Cassius for refusing to share with him his own ill-gotten gains. In another instance, in 4.3.180–194, he pretends to accept with great stoicism the news of the death of PORTIA (2'), when he has in fact known of it for some time. (It has been contended that Shakespeare had excised this passage

from the play, it surviving only because of a printer's error; however, the ploy suits Brutus' imperiousness quite well, and the rejection of the passage seems unnecessary.) This deception may be defended as good for the morale of his underlings, but it is nevertheless quite as patronising as Caesar's feigned reluctance to accept a crown, as reported in 1.2.230–263.

A possible source of Brutus' self-deception is his repeated denial of his emotions and thus his inability to recognise his own drives. He rejects his love for Caesar, for Cassius, even for Portia, lest they contaminate the higher faculty of his reason. His errors in trusting Antony and relying on the support of the PLEBEIANS stem from his assumption that they, like he, will act rationally. Not only does he undervalue the significance and power of passion in others, he does not see its operation in himself. Thus blinded, Brutus never sees the error of his attack on Caesar. The unnecessary disaster of the civil war has resulted from his own obsession with controlling the Roman political world, but he honestly sees only his own idealistic point of view. Thus his actions are virtuous in their intent but evil in their consequences. Precisely because of this contradiction, Brutus resembles a tragic hero, attempting great things and failing through his own psychological flaws.

Julius Caesar is not simply the story of a man who injures his society by an illicit rebellion or of a man who murders a friend for bad reasons. Rather, the tragic grandeur of Brutus' moral imperfection lies in his effort to transcend human limitations and create a political world without the potential for evil and exploitation. Like OTHELLO or HAMLET, Brutus possesses an integrity that impels him towards a wrong course. Attempting the impossible, he can produce only chaos, and he brings about the downfall of both his world and himself. Antony's final eulogy not only acknowledges the nobility of Brutus' conscious intentions in killing Caesar but also reminds us of his weakness, observing that he was an honourable man who did not recognise the dishonour of his actions.

The historical Brutus was a rather different person than Shakespeare's patriotic but deluded idealist, and much of his career is neither enacted nor alluded to in *Julius Caesar.* Renowned in his own day as an admirable Roman nobleman—upright in his dealings and grave in demeanour—Brutus was descended from an illustrious patrician family. His mother was Caesar's mistress for many years, giving rise to the rumour that Brutus was Caesar's son (alluded to in *2 Henry VI,* 4.1.136), though the relationship probably began only after Brutus' birth. Brutus had a highly successful political career; he received profitable appointments as an administrator of Roman territories abroad. He was also a prominent player in the factional politics of the period. Prior to the time of the play, Brutus was a follower of Pompey the Great (106–48) in his civil war against Caesar, but after Caesar's decisive victory at the battle of Pharsala (48 B.C.) he switched sides. Caesar rewarded him with appointments to high offices. However, Brutus seems to have regretted his betrayal of Pompey; he published a defence of Cato, a prominent Pompeian, and he married Portia, Cato's daughter, which his contemporaries recognised as a gesture of opposition to Caesar.

Brutus and the conspirators compared themselves to Brutus' ancestor, Junius BRUTUS (2), a legendary Roman patriot, as Shakespeare indicates in 1.2.157 and 2.1.53–54, but in fact their ends were more selfish than patriotic. They stood for the privileges and vested interests of the Roman aristocracy, threatened by Caesar's long-standing dictatorship—normally a temporary office held during a crisis. Caesar seemed to be establishing a new order, in which the nobles would be subordinated to him and to his government.

Brutus' ritual bloodbath, described above, is Shakespeare's invention, intended to emphasise both the violence of the deed and its political nature. PLUTARCH, Shakespeare's source, reports the murder in brutal imagery drawn from hunting, presenting just the sort of picture Brutus attempts, in the play, to avoid. Thus the playwright distorted his source material in order to create a telling effect.

Shakespeare greatly compressed the complicated events following Caesar's death for dramatic reasons, and Brutus' struggles to maintain a political position in Rome are ignored. After the assassination Brutus and the conspirators negotiated with Antony and other Caesarians, and for several weeks the two groups governed Rome jointly, although the citizenry frequently rioted against the assassins. Numerous intrigues, now obscure, dominated Roman politics; Brutus and Cassius attempted to recruit followers among the rural aristocrats with only modest success. In mid-April they left Rome for good. They remained in Italy throughout the summer, during which a possible alliance between Antony and Octavius began to seem threatening. Brutus then left for Macedonia, where he held a government appointment. Negotiations between the assassins and Antony continued throughout the winter, but the civil war began in the spring of 43 B.C., with Antony defeating DECIUS in northern Italy. In November, Antony and Octavius formed the Triumvirate with Lepidus, and the following summer they launched the campaign that led to Philippi.

Except for collapsing two battles into one, Shakespeare's account of Brutus' defeat and death at Philippi is accurately retold from Plutarch, although other sources indicate that Cassius did not oppose the decision to march to Philippi; the conspirators' forces were supported by the local population, while Antony

and Octavius were short of supplies. One other mild distortion of Brutus' nature follows from Shakespeare's compression of events: in the twenty days between battles, Brutus most fully revealed his serious incompetence as a general, for he had only to wait for time and hunger to defeat his enemies and he could not do it.

Bryan, George (active 1586–1613) English actor. Bryan appears in the list of 26 'Principall Actors' who performed in Shakespeare's plays recorded in the FIRST FOLIO (1623), though he is not known to have played any specific rôle. He was among the English actors that visited Denmark in 1586 and was a player in STRANGE'S MEN at least from 1590–1593. He was probably still among them when they became the CHAMBERLAIN'S MEN in 1594, for he is recorded as a co-receiver of a payment to that company in 1596, implying that he was an important member of the group. However, he is not listed among the casts of particular Chamberlain's Men plays; the earliest such list dates from 1598, and scholars speculate that Bryan had retired by then. Apparently successful as a minor courtier, Bryan was recorded as a member of the Queen's household, in an unspecified capacity, in 1603 and in 1611–1613.

Buchanan, George (1506–1582) Scottish poet and historian, Scotland's leading Protestant humanist of the 16th century, and the author of a minor source for *Macbeth.* Buchanan's history of Scotland in Latin, *Rerum Scotiarum Historia* (1582), may have influenced Shakespeare in the development of Macbeth's character, as well as providing several political details.

The history, considered one of the great works of late Latin literature, was the crowning achievement of a long and varied career. As a student at the University of Paris, Buchanan wrote notorious satires aimed at the clerical corruption that was stimulating the Protestant Reformation. Back in Scotland c. 1528, Buchanan was imprisoned for his writings, but escaped and established himself as a professor at a college in Bordeaux, where one of his pupils was MONTAIGNE. He wrote a number of notable Latin plays at this time. In 1548 he was appointed the head of a university in Portugal, but while there he was imprisoned by the Inquisition. In prison he wrote an acclaimed Latin rendition of the Book of Psalms.

Buchanan returned to Scotland in 1560 and converted to Calvinism. Tutor to Mary, Queen of Scots, he later became her enemy, assisting in her prosecution for treason in England. Upon her imprisonment he was made tutor to her son, later King JAMES I of England. During James' childhood as ruler of Scotland, Buchanan was an important figure in the government. In his last years he wrote his major works: a treatise on government that was condemned for its democratic tendencies and the history of Scotland that Shakespeare read.

Buckingham (1), Edward Stafford, Duke of (1478–1521) Historical figure and minor character in *Henry VIII,* a nobleman falsely convicted of treason and sentenced to death, a victim of Cardinal WOLSEY's intrigues. In 1.1 Buckingham's anger at Wolsey's duplicitous misuse of power establishes the cardinal as a villain. His own contrasting goodness is demonstrated as he calmly accepts his arrest for treason, even though it becomes apparent that Wolsey has bribed the duke's former SURVEYOR to commit perjury. In 2.1, on his way to be executed, Buckingham furthers the contrast by forgiving his enemies, wishing King HENRY VIII well, and humbly preparing for death. Buckingham's victimisation marks one end of the play's most important development—the growth of King Henry—for the ease with which the king is deceived by Wolsey and the Surveyor is soon replaced by increasing maturity and wisdom.

In 2.1.106–123 Buckingham compares himself to his father, also falsely executed for treason. That Duke of BUCKINGHAM (2) appears in *Richard III,* and *his* father, this duke's grandfather, is the BUCKINGHAM (3) of *2 Henry VI.*

Buckingham (2), Henry Stafford, Duke of (1455–1483) Historical figure and character in *Richard III,* the most important supporter of RICHARD III before he deserts the King in response to his ingratitude. Buckingham acts as a spokesman for Richard's positions, especially to the MAYOR (3) and the people of London. His style of speaking, bombastic and obscure, is typical of devious politicians, and his wily, conspiratorial nature makes him an important adviser to Richard at several junctures, notably in hatching the plot against HASTINGS (3). He prides himself on his capacity for deceit in the remarkable conversation that opens 3.5.

However, in 4.2, when Richard, now enthroned, proposes to go further and kill the young PRINCE (5) of Wales and his brother, Buckingham is somewhat reluctant, perhaps sensing that a king should be more cautious. Richard, angered, then refuses Buckingham the earldom he had promised him. Buckingham perceives that he is in danger of suffering Hastings' fate, and he decides to abandon the King. He raises an army in rebellion but is quickly captured. In 5.1 Buckingham, about to be executed, formally reflects on his circumstances, recollecting past oaths and prophecies almost in the manner of a Greek CHORUS (1). Thus, in a prelude to the approaching doom of Richard, Buckingham invokes the sense of ordained fate that is central to the play.

Shakespeare's sources offered several possible motives for Buckingham's revolt, but Shakespeare chose one that was definitely untrue, for Richard had given

Buckingham his earldom prior to his defection. The question cannot be answered with the surviving evidence; he may simply have anticipated Richard's overthrow by RICHMOND. It has been suggested that Buckingham was ambitious to rule, for he had a distant claim to the throne himself, being descended from Thomas, Duke of GLOUCESTER (6), the youngest brother of RICHARD II. Buckingham's father was the Duke of BUCKINGHAM (3) of *2 Henry VI,* and his son appears as BUCKINGHAM (1) in *Henry VIII.*

Buckingham (3), Sir Humphrey Stafford, Duke of (d. 1455) Historical figure and character in *2 Henry VI,* an ally of the Duke of SUFFOLK (3) against GLOUCESTER (4) and later of King HENRY VI against the Duke of YORK (8). Buckingham enters Suffolk's conspiracy cheerfully, nominating himself as a possible replacement for Gloucester as Lord Protector (1.1.177–178). When the DUCHESS (1) of Gloucester is driven from the assembled court by Queen MARGARET (1), Buckingham volunteers to follow her, remarking that the woman's anger will make her 'gallop far enough to her destruction' (1.3.151), and in the next scene, indeed, Buckingham is able to arrest the Duchess for witchcraft. When Gloucester himself is arrested, Buckingham impatiently urges on the action (3.1.186–187). In 4.4 Buckingham counsels the King during the rebellion led by Jack CADE, and, with CLIFFORD (2), he later (4.8) defuses that uprising by presenting the rebels with the King's offer of pardon. In 5.1 he acts as the King's representative to the Duke of York. Shakespeare's peremptory, sharp-spoken Buckingham rings one of the notes of individual personality among the group of fractious nobles that mark this play as an improvement over *1 Henry VI.*

The historical Buckingham died in the battle of Northampton, and his death is noted in *3 Henry VI* (1.1), though it is placed at the battle of ST. ALBANS, fought at the close of *2 Henry VI.* His son, Henry, Duke of BUCKINGHAM (2), figures in *Richard III.*

Bullcalf, Peter Minor character in *2 Henry IV,* one of the men whom FALSTAFF recruits for the army in 3.2. Bullcalf claims to be ill, despite the robust appearance his name suggests, but he is recruited anyway. However, his friend Ralph MOULDY secures release for them both by bribing Corporal BARDOLPLH (1). The episode satirises the notoriously corrupt practices of 16th-century recruiters.

Bullen, Anne Character in *Henry VIII.* See ANNE (1).

Bullingbrook Character in *Richard II.* See BOLINGBROKE (1).

Bullough, Geoffrey (1901–1982) British scholar. Bullough, long-time professor of English literature at London University, is best known for his eight-volume *Narrative and Dramatic Sources of Shakespeare* (1957–1975). This definitive work is commonly known as 'Bullough' and is considered a necessary reference for any Shakespearean scholarship. Bullough also edited a collection of the poems and plays of Fulke GREVILLE (2).

Burbage (1), Cuthbert (c. 1566–1636) English theatrical entrepreneur, son of James BURBAGE (2) and brother of Richard BURBAGE (3). Cuthbert, unlike his brother and father, was never an actor, but he was nevertheless an important figure in ELIZABETHAN THEATRE. Cuthbert managed the first LONDON playhouse, the THEATRE, which he inherited when his father died in early 1597, just before the expiration of the lease for the land on which the building was constructed. After fruitless negotiations over its renewal, Cuthbert simply had the building torn down and reassembled as the GLOBE THEATRE, which was owned half by himself and Richard, and half by a group of actors from the KING'S MEN, including Shakespeare. Cuthbert was also a partner in a similar arrangement for the BLACKFRIARS THEATRE.

Burbage (2), James (c. 1530–1597) English theatrical entrepreneur, builder of the first LONDON theatre and father of Cuthbert and Richard BURBAGE (1, 3). A poor carpenter who turned actor, Burbage was a leading member of LEICESTER'S MEN when he decided, in 1575, to construct a building devoted only to the performance of plays, in the hopes of profiting from the admissions fees. His wealthy brother-in-law John Brayne provided the capital for the venture, and Burbage took a 21-year lease on a plot of land just north of the city. On it he built the THEATRE, which was opened sometime in late 1576 or early 1577. Burbage was evidently a fiery and argumentative man, and he and Brayne, and later Brayne's widow, disputed vigorously about the distribution of the profits in court and, on one occasion, in a physical brawl in front of an arriving audience. Burbage prospered at the Theatre, and in 1596 he bought a building that he converted into the BLACKFRIARS THEATRE. At his death he left the Theatre and its ground lease to Cuthbert, and the Blackfriars Theatre to Richard.

Burbage (3), Richard (c. 1568–1619) English actor, son of James BURBAGE (2) and brother of Cuthbert BURBAGE (1), the leading actor of the CHAMBERLAIN'S MEN and the original portrayer of many of Shakespeare's protagonists. With William ALLEYN, Burbage is said to have been the greatest actor of the ELIZABETHAN THEATRE. Contemporary allusions establish that Burbage played HAMLET, LEAR, MALVOLIO, OTHELLO, and RICHARD III, and he probably played many more major Shakespearean roles.

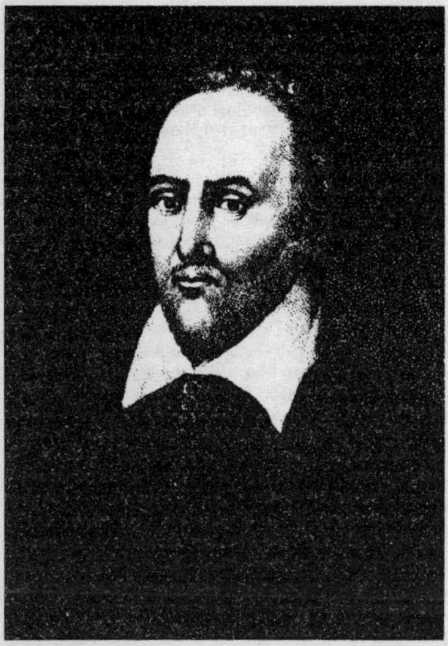

Richard Burbage, the greatest English actor of Shakespeare's time, originated the roles of Richard III, Hamlet, Othello, and Lear. He was the leading tragedian of the Chamberlain's Men. (Courtesy of Billy Rose Theatre Collection; New York Public Library at Lincoln Center; Astor, Lenox and Tilden Foundations)

Burbage's early career is obscure. He probably appeared with the company composed of the ADMIRAL'S MEN and STRANGE'S MEN, who played at his father's playhouse, the THEATRE, in 1590–1591. He first achieved widespread recognition in *Richard III,* the play that also established Shakespeare as a playwright, around 1591. (In connection with this role, Burbage figures in the only surviving contemporary anecdote about Shakespeare; see MANNINGHAM.) He apparently did not tour with this troupe during the plague years, 1593–1594, but he was an early member of the Chamberlain's Men, as Strange's was known after 1594. He may have been with PEMBROKE'S MEN in the interim. He remained with the Chamberlain's Men, later the KING'S MEN, until his death, though the last record of a performance dates from 1610.

When James Burbage died in 1597, he left Cuthbert the theatre (which he tore down and reassembled as the GLOBE THEATRE) and Richard the BLACKFRIARS THEATRE; the brothers shared them through partnerships with each other. Burbage was also a painter. A well-known likeness of him is thought to be a self-portrait and the CHANDOS PORTRAIT, long thought to be of Shakespeare, was traditionally attributed to him. As a painter, he collaborated with Shakespeare on an allegorical shield for the Earl of RUTLAND (2).

Burby, Cuthbert (d. 1607) London publisher and bookseller. In 1594 Burby published THE TAMING OF A SHREW, probably a BAD QUARTO of Shakespeare's *The Taming of the Shrew.* He also published the first edition of *Love's Labour's Lost* (1598) and the second (Q2) of *Romeo and Juliet* (1599). In 1607, just before his death, he sold the rights to all three works to Nicholas LING. Burby was a brother-in-law of the printer Thomas SNODHAM.

Burghley (Burleigh), Lord (William Cecil) (1520–1598) The leading statesman of Elizabethan England, chief minister to Queen ELIZABETH (1); sometimes said to have been a model for POLONIUS in *Hamlet.* An aristocratic courtier, Burghley was the most important member of Elizabeth's government from her accession in 1558 until his death. After the Pope excommunicated the Protestant Elizabeth and encouraged her assassination (and that of her chief minister) in 1570, Burghley set up an early variety of secret police, using espionage and torture in a ruthless and largely successful campaign to cripple the Counter-Reformation in England. Though he privately declared his dislike of these methods, he remains a symbol of unscrupulous state power. He is also remembered for his *Ten Precepts,* a pamphlet of sententious advice on gentlemanly conduct addressed to his son Robert CECIL (1), who succeeded him as the most powerful man in England.

Some scholars nominate Lord Burghley as a possible satirical model for Polonius chiefly because the character was named CORAMBIS—an obviously satirical name—in Shakespeare's source, the lost play called the UR-HAMLET, probably written by Thomas KYD. Polonius resembles Burghley in being a high government official and in delivering 'precepts' (1.3.58) to his son. Also, in 2.1 Polonius sends his servant REYNALDO to spy on his son LAERTES, who is at school in Paris, and a connection has been drawn to Burghley's espionage network and to the fact that his eldest son, Thomas CECIL (2), led a notoriously dissolute life on the continent for several years in his youth. However, if Corambis was intended as a satire on Burghley—or anyone else—it was Kyd's idea, not Shakespeare's; indeed, the name Polonius may have been intended to defuse any such reference.

Even if Kyd's Corambis is linked to Burghley, Shakespeare's Polonius is not. Burghley had been most powerful in the 1570s and 1580s—and had been dead for several years by the time *Hamlet* was written—making a satire on him by Shakespeare almost pointless. Also, Shakespeare was not given to personal

satire—he had been willing to change the names of characters in *1* and *2 Henry IV* to avoid offence (see HARVEY [1]; OLDCASTLE; ROSSILL)—and the likelihood that he would have attempted to mock the father of a powerful member of the court is slim.

Other factors also weigh against the association of Burghley with Polonius. *Ten Precepts* was not published until 1637, and, although the sophisticated literary world may have known of it in 1601, most of the satire's hypothetical audience would not have. In any case, such collections of paternal wisdom were widely popular, and Polonius' version does not particularly resemble Burghley's. A father spying on his high-living son was likewise not unusual in literature, and the episode in *Hamlet* has legitimate dramatic purposes and need not be associated with anything outside the play.

Burgundy (1), Duke of Minor character in *King Lear*, a suitor who rejects CORDELIA when she is disinherited by King LEAR. Burgundy appears only in 1.1; he and the King of FRANCE (2) have been summoned to determine which of them will marry Lear's youngest daughter and thus govern one-third of Britain. Burgundy's concern is with a politically and materially advantageous match, and when Cordelia is disinherited he simply loses interest in her. She dismisses his frank but polite apology cooly, saying, 'Peace be with Burgundy! / Since that respect and fortunes are his love, / I shall not be his wife' (1.1.246–248). Burgundy's conventionally greedy behaviour contrasts tellingly with the response of France, who recognises Cordelia's virtues and marries her.

The Duke's equal footing with the King of France reflects a reality of medieval Europe: the Duchy of Burgundy, though formally a client state of FRANCE (1), was an independent and wealthy country (see BURGUNDY [2]). However, this medieval context is an anachronism, for in the early period in which *King Lear* is set the Duchy of Burgundy did not yet exist.

Burgundy (2), Philip, Duke of (1396–1467) Historical figure and character in *1 Henry VI* and *Henry V*, an ally of the English in the HUNDRED YEARS WAR who defects to the side of FRANCE (1). Early in *1 Henry VI* Burgundy assists the English at ORLÉANS (1) and ROUEN; then in 3.3 JOAN LA PUCELLE persuades him to align himself with France. In *Henry V*, set some years earlier, a younger Burgundy encourages HENRY V and the FRENCH KING to make peace in 5.2.23–67. He speaks at length on the horrors of war, in a passage that contributes much to the play's modern reception as an anti-war work. Burgundy then attends the French King in the final negotiations of the treaty of TROYES, which occur off stage while Henry courts KATHARINE (2). Upon returning, Burgundy jests lewdly with Henry about his forthcoming marriage.

The historical Burgundy was not an ally of France at Troyes, and he was a much more important figure than his role suggests. He was a cousin of Charles VI, the French King of the play, and he ruled the most powerful of the independent French duchies. His father, Duke John (1371–1419), was the Duke of Burgundy mentioned in *Henry V* 3.5.42 and 4.8.99; Duke John fought against Henry at AGINCOURT. He was murdered in the factional disputes over the rule of France during Charles' frequent bouts of insanity, and Philip of Burgundy, upon inheriting the duchy, sought support from outside the circle of French rivalries. He sided with England and thus assured Henry V's victory, a phenomenon that Shakespeare, focussing on the accomplishments of the English King, ignored in *Henry V*. Burgundy's subsequent alliance with England under HENRY VI was marred by many disputes over policy and by his feud with the Duke of GLOUCESTER (4); he eventually restored his family's traditional amity with France, helping to drive the English from the country in the 1450s, as is depicted in *1 Henry VI*. However, both historically and in Shakespeare's sources, Joan of Arc had nothing to do with Burgundy's defection, which took place four years after her death. This alteration serves to amplify the importance of Joan, who is Shakespeare's chief representative of the deceitful and villainous French.

Burleigh, William Cecil, Lord See BURGHLEY.

Burnaby, William (c. 1672–1706) Minor English playwright. Burnaby is remembered primarily because he incorporated adaptations of scenes from *Twelfth Night* into his 1703 comedy *Love Betray'd, or The Agreeable Disappointment*.

Bury St Edmunds Town in the English county of Suffolk, site of a famed medieval abbey and the setting for Act 3 of *2 Henry VI*. Here, in the ancient abbey, the Duke of GLOUCESTER (4) is prosecuted and then murdered by the clique surrounding Queen MARGARET (1) and the Duke of SUFFOLK (3). Consequently, the King exiles Suffolk for life at the insistence of an outraged mob, and CARDINAL (1) BEAUFORT, one of the conspirators, dies with a bad conscience.

Bury St Edmunds was an unusually isolated location for a meeting of Parliament. Although Shakespeare does not mention it, much of his audience will have realised that this town was deep in the home territory of the Duke of Suffolk, far from Gloucester's power base in London. The mob appearing in the play to demand Suffolk's punishment is fictitious; precisely because of its location, Gloucester's arrest went unprotested. Suffolk was not in fact banished until much later, and for different reasons.

As ST EDMUNDSBURY, the town is a location in *King John*.

Busby, John (active 1576–1619) London bookseller and publisher. Busby was associated with apparently pirated publications of three of Shakespeare's plays. In 1600 Busby and John MILLINGTON published the first QUARTO edition of *Henry V.* In 1602 he registered a forthcoming publication of *The Merry Wives of Windsor* with the STATIONERS' COMPANY but immediately sold his 'rights' to his long-time business partner, Arthur JOHNSON (1), whose name appared alone on the title page of the play. In 1607 he registered *King Lear* jointly with Nathaniel BUTTER, though again, when the play was published the next year, Busby's name was dropped. Each of these editions was a BAD QUARTO, that is, it was transcribed from the recollections of actors who had performed in the play. This method was used by publishers who had no access to the proper text of a play—carefully withheld by acting companies in the hope of foiling such pirates as Busby.

Bushy (Bussy), Sir John (d. 1399) Historical figure and character in *Richard II,* a supporter of RICHARD II. Bushy, John BAGOT, and Henry GREENE (1) are the 'caterpillars' (2.3.165) whose influence on the King is alleged by BOLINGBROKE (1) to have been disastrous for England. Bushy attempts to comfort the distraught QUEEN (13) Isabel in 2.2; his elaborate courtier's language seems grotesque even to modern ears, unaware that it parodies 16th-century religious meditations. Later in 2.2 Bushy, Bagot, and Greene recognise that their position as favourites of the King is likely to prove dangerous if their master is defeated by Bolingbroke. The three decide to flee when Bolingbroke approaches; Bushy and Greene seek safety in BRISTOL Castle, but Bolingbroke captures them and sentences them to death.

The historical Bushy was a minor politician; he was frequently Speaker of the House of COMMONS—not an important post in his day—and was also three times Sheriff of London. Originally a supporter of the Duke of GLOUCESTER (6), he was recruited to Richard's party in the 1390s, before the murder of the Duke.

Butcher Minor character in *2 Henry VI.* See DICK THE BUTCHER.

Butter, Nathaniel (d. 1664) London bookseller and publisher who issued the first edition of *King Lear.* In 1607, jointly with John BUSBY, who several times pirated Shakespeare's plays, Butter registered a forthcoming edition of the play with the STATIONERS' COMPANY. However, when the QUARTO edition of the play appeared the next year it was attributed solely to Butter. It was a BAD QUARTO, an inaccurate text assembled from the recollections of actors, a frequent recourse of unauthorised publishers. Butter also published THE LONDON PRODIGAL (1605), a play that was falsely attributed to Shakespeare, and he is known to have pirated a play by Thomas HEYWOOD.

Butter, the son of a printer and bookseller, published his first book in 1604, opened a bookshop (at the sign of the 'Pied Bull') the next year, and sold books at various locations until his death. After 1622 he specialised in publishing news sheets, early predecessors of newspapers, but he did not flourish and is said to have died a pauper.

Butts, Doctor (William Butts, d. 1545) Historical figure and minor character in *Henry VIII,* King HENRY VIII's physician. In 5.2 Doctor Butts leads Henry to an upper room where he can secretly view his council's meeting below, in order to thwart the councillors' attempt to imprison Thomas CRANMER, Archbishop of Canterbury. Butts informs the king that the archbishop has been humiliated by having to wait with the servants outside the meeting room, and this adds to the king's anger. Shakespeare took Butts' role in this incident from his source, FOXE's *Actes and Monumentes.* Butts was King Henry's personal physician for many years, and his death is said to have distressed the king greatly. His personal appearance has been preserved in a fine portrait by Hans Holbein the Younger (c. 1497–1543).

C

Cade, Jack (d. 1450) Historical figure and character in *2 Henry VI,* the leader of a rebellion and pretender to the throne of England. Cade, whose revolt occupies most of Act 4, is presented as a buffoonish but brutal figure. He makes preposterous promises to his followers and proposes to legislate on such matters as the length of Lent. He also whimsically executes people for being literate or for being ignorant of an arbitrary change in his title. He enthusiastically seconds a follower's proposal: 'The first thing we do, let's kill all the lawyers' (4.2.73). In the case of Lord SAY, the victim's actual virtues, such as having been a benefactor of education, are used by Cade as grounds for his death. Cade orders the destruction of London Bridge, the Tower of London, and the INNS OF COURT as well. All this viciousness is explained as having been commissioned by the Duke of YORK (8) in order to give him a reason to bring an army into England and suppress the rebels.

In presenting this episode, Shakespeare took remarkable liberties with history, for not only did the historical York have nothing to do with Cade's rebellion, but the uprising itself is based in part on accounts of a different event, the Peasants' Rebellion of 1381, when there were attempts to destroy London Bridge and the Inns of Court. The proposal to kill the lawyers also dates from the earlier revolt, which was a much more anarchic and bloody affair than the one actually led by Cade.

The historical Cade was probably Irish; he had married into a minor landholding family in KENT (1), and the rebels he led were lesser gentry, artisans, and tradesmen—that is, members of the nascent middle class. Their revolt was intended to achieve well-defined ends that were expressed in a document, the 'Complaint of the Commons of Kent', which demonstrates an informed awareness of real political problems. It refers to the loss of France and subsequent Kentish business losses, and to excessive taxation and the extravagance of the royal household. It complains of the dominance of the Duke of SUFFOLK (3) among the King's councilors, for Suffolk was hated in Kent as an unreasonable and extortionate magnate.

As Cade and his men approached London, in June 1450, they ambushed a party of royal troops and killed the commander, Sir Humphrey STAFFORD (2), and his BROTHER (1), as in the play. At this point, the royal government placed Lord SAY in the Tower of London as a sop to popular sentiment, and fled to the countryside. (Say was a widely detested Kentish landowner and no model aristocrat, as Shakespeare presents him.) On July 4, the people of London welcomed the rebels into the city, and Say was taken from the Tower and executed. After several days, the Kentishmen had seemingly worn out their welcome, for the citizens, aided by the Tower guards under Lord SCALES, who appears in the play, drove them south across the Thames into SOUTHWARK. There, the King's pardon was offered to all who would disperse, and most did. Cade himself did not, and he was pursued and killed by Alexander IDEN, who was the Sheriff of Kent, and not the simple, patriotic landowner of the play.

Shakespeare thus took a real episode from the period of his play and altered its character in order to make certain points. From the prevalent Elizabethan point of view, which Shakespeare shared, Cade and others like him were traitors pure and simple, propagators of vicious and immoral doctrines that could only undermine society. Thus the playwright felt perfectly justified in depicting Cade's undertaking as a more brutal and violent event than it in fact was, for an important point addressed by the history plays is the value of political stability. The distinction between Cade's revolt and the 1381 uprising was unimportant to Shakespeare; each constituted an unacceptable subversion of a properly ordered society.

The episode of Cade, as it is presented, serves three purposes. First, it provides comic relief after the sustained political battle, ending in the murder of GLOUCESTER (4), of Acts 1–3. The buffoonery of Cade and his followers is in an old tradition of comical rusticity that Shakespeare always favoured. However, the humour quickly turns vicious, and the evil of anarchy is abundantly demonstrated, which is the second function of the action. The uncontrolled common people mirror the dissensions of the nobles and demonstrate, conversely Shakespeare's most important political point—that all social good derives from a stable monarchy. Third, the episode is associated with the rise of York and thus serves to introduce the final sequence

of the drama, the ambitious advance to open rebellion by that lord. Thus aristocratic ambition is demonstrated to have directly produced tragic disorder among the common people.

Cadwal In *Cymbeline*, the false name under which King CYMBELINE's son ARVIRAGUS is raised from infancy by his kidnapper and foster-father, BELARIUS.

Caesar (1), Julius (102–44 B.C.) Historical figure and title character of *Julius Caesar*, ancient Roman political leader assassinated by conspirators led by Marcus BRUTUS (4). Caesar's role is not a large one, but the character dominates the play even after his murder early in Act 3. He is an enigmatic figure, representative of the central theme of the play, the moral ambiguity surrounding his murder. The assassination victim is both a valuable leader and an arrogant tyrant; thus the conspiracy against him seems alternately malevolent and noble.

Caesar is undeniably imperious. When he first appears, in 1.2, surrounded by admiring followers, he is clearly accustomed to command. Irritated by the warning of the SOOTHSAYER (1) to beware the ides of March, he coolly dismisses him. Knowing the outcome, as Shakespeare assumed his audience would, we see immediately that Caesar's self-confidence is misplaced. Caesar's smug sense of power is strikingly evident in his language; he frequently refers to himself with the royal 'we', as in 3.1.8, and sometimes even in the third person, as when he declares his intention to defy bad omens and go the Senate, saying, 'Caesar should be a beast without a heart / If he should stay at home to-day for fear. / No, Caesar shall not. Danger knows full well / That Caesar is more dangerous than he' (2.2.42–45). His wife, CALPHURNIA, warns that his 'wisdom is consum'd in confidence' (2.2.49), and we clearly see that he is ripe for a fall. In the last moments of his life Caesar's arrogance extends almost to blasphemy, as he dismisses all argument with the order, 'Hence! Wilt thou lift up Olympus?' (3.1.74). The assassination, which follows immediately, seems entirely justified.

On the other hand, Caesar is also presented as 'the foremost man of all this world' (4.3.22), as Brutus calls him. He is certainly a strong leader; the only weaknesses attributed to him are physical: some deafness and mild epilepsy (1.2.210, 251) and the poor swimming and susceptibility to illness that CASSIUS complains of in 1.2.99–114, matters so patently unimportant that they tell us more about Cassius' petty envy than they do about Caesar. In 2.1.20–21 Brutus observes that Caesar has never let his emotions alter his judgement, and we learn the value of that judgement when we hear his acute portrayal of Cassius in 1.2. 189–207. The funeral orations of Brutus and ANTONY in 3.2 offer evidence of his virtues, and indeed Caesar's greatness is evident in the respect that almost all the other characters show him.

It may seem odd that a figure killed before the halfway point should be the title character of a play, but it is appropriate here, for Caesar's spirit continues to dominate the action after his death. Not only does Antony's revenge for Caesar's murder provide the plot of the play's second half, but the thought of Caesar recurs repeatedly to Brutus and Cassius as well. Notably, each speaks of Caesar at his death. Moreover, Caesar's arrogance is taken up by Brutus in a subtle demonstration of the psychology of power. The survival of Caesar's spirit is made tangible by the appearance of Caesar's GHOST (2) in 4.3 and at the battle of PHILIPPI (reported by Brutus in 5.5.17–20).

Caesar's greatest importance lies in the action he stimulates, his assassination. The murder of the seemingly tyrannical Caesar triggers a civil war and—as Shakespeare and his audiences were aware—would soon lead to much greater despotism under the Empire of OCTAVIUS, later known as CAESAR (2). Thus Caesar symbolises a social good that is flawed by the potential evil of tyranny, as opposed to the social disruption created by Brutus' ideal of a political world in which no such evil exists.

Shakespeare added salient details to the Caesar he found in his source, PLUTARCH's *Lives*, humanising the leader by inventing physical defects that the historical figure did not have: deafness and poor swimming. He also ascribed to Caesar a concern with superstition in his last days, stressing an intellectual corruption produced by power, in preparation for the audience's sympathetic response to the assassins when the murder is committed. On the other hand, he did omit a number of anecdotes from Plutarch that would have portrayed Caesar too negatively, leaving less room for doubt about the killing. For instance, Caesar is said to have looted a famous temple and to have acquiesced in dishonouring an earlier wife in order to divorce her.

More significantly, Shakespeare followed Plutarch in exaggerating Caesar's real threat to the privileges of the Roman aristocracy that spurred the assassins historically. In fact, modern scholars find, Caesar's policies were surely not directed towards creating a monarchy, as the conspirators—and Plutarch—believed. They were to some extent not directed at all, being largely driven by events.

After his well-known conquests in Gaul and Britain, Caesar had, at the time of the play, recently won a civil war against another Roman political and military leader, Pompey the Great (106–48). As the head of a faction intent on admitting new members to Rome's small ruling class, Caesar had fought a group of conservatives and had more nearly represented the republican ideals later associated with Brutus—in part because of Shakespeare's presentation—than Brutus himself did. He was in no sense a revolutionary, how-

ever. In the course of his conflict with Pompey, Caesar had assumed the dictatorship, a legitimate office of the Roman government that carried extensive powers and was temporarily awarded to leading military commanders in times of crisis. Caesar had been dictator briefly in 49 B.C., but this time he had held the dictatorship for several years, using its powers to protect his gains in the civil war. In early 44 B.C. the Senate—which Caesar had greatly enlarged and filled with his followers—declared him dictator for life. This event sealed the conspirators' determination.

It was rumoured that Caesar intended to be crowned and to move the capital to Ilium, a Roman possession in the Near East. However, this was never likely—the ceremony in which he rejected the crown, as reported by CASCA in 1.2, was planned by Caesar expressly to defuse these rumours—and it seems probable that Caesar was more conservative than the nobility feared. He assumed his extraordinary powers because the forces of Pompey's son (the POMPEY [2] of *Antony and Cleopatra*) still threatened him and because he was aware of the threat of assassination. To preserve the government, newly established after years of disorder, Caesar needed dictatorial power to suppress his enemies. He did, however, protect ancient privileges to a considerable degree, resisting pressures from his more radical followers for drastic reforms.

Moreover, Caesar understood the need for a strong ruler to maintain order in a nation that had been disrupted by years of internal strife. He is said (though not by Plutarch) to have anticipated his end, observing that his assassination would produce terrible consequences for Rome; the actual result was the effective elimination of the old Roman aristocracy under the Empire. As Shakespeare felt, although he did not clearly see the underlying historical reality, Caesar's assassination unnecessarily disrupted the Roman state, already weakened by civil wars, and it only led to a much greater tyranny.

Caesar (2), Octavius (63 B.C.–A.D. 14) Character in *Antony and Cleopatra,* the successful rival of Mark ANTONY for control of the government of ROME. (The same figure appears in *Julius Caesar* as OCTAVIUS.) Caesar is to some extent a foil for Antony. He is a coldly ambitious, dispassionate, and manipulative political and military leader whose triumph points up Antony's opposite traits: passion, generosity, and misjudgement. Caesar typically regrets drinking wine at a celebratory banquet, saying 'our graver business / Frowns at this levity' (2.7.118–119). In consequence he is superior to his rivals in action; in war, as CANIDIUS remarks before the battle of ACTIUM, 'this speed of Caesar's / Carries beyond belief' (3.7.74–75). Less attractively, Caesar breaks his treaty with POMPEY (2) and betrays LEPIDUS, while Antony, in contrast, magnanimously forgives ENOBARBUS for deserting. But whatever else Caesar may be, he is successful. At the outset of *Antony and Cleopatra,* Caesar shares power with Antony and LEPIDUS in the Triumvirate, but in the course of the action he defeats each of them in separate civil wars, and before the play's climax he assumes sole power over Rome's vast territories.

However, Caesar's greatest importance comes in Act 5, after Antony's death, when he is powerfully contrasted with CLEOPATRA. His Roman dedication to power stands in opposition to her vivid appeal to passion as the justification for life. Caesar schemes to prevent Cleopatra's suicide. He treacherously assures her of his goodwill, when in fact he intends to exhibit her in a parade of triumph in Rome and subject her to the ultimate humiliation in order to demonstrate Rome's relentless power and his own strength. Though Cleopatra achieves transcendence in death, Caesar commands the stage at the close of the play and Rome's triumph is finally asserted.

However, Caesar is not simply a villain; he clearly cares for his sister OCTAVIA—though he also uses her as a political pawn when he marries her to Antony—and he is capable of appreciating Antony's virtues. In his first lines, opening 1.4, he declares his admiration for his rival, and in his final tribute to the 'pair so famous' (5.2.358) he recognises the 'strong toil of grace' (5.2.346) that Cleopatra has shown in her noble death. Nevertheless, Caesar is a ruler whose actions are not governed by his emotions; he can understand his opponents sympathetically but he makes them his victims all the same.

As the representative of the growing Roman power, Caesar has a significance that is quite independent of his personal qualities. He declares that his victory will usher in a 'time of universal peace' (4.6.5). In a stroke of dramatic irony, Caesar cannot recognise the implications of this remark, but for the playwright and his original audiences its meaning was both profound and obvious. It refers to the imminent coming of Christ, for Caesar went on to found the Roman Empire, whose establishment of political unity in the Mediterranean world—the *pax romana*—was seen in the 17th century as a manifestation of the will of God, the period of peace that ushered in the coming of the Messiah. Thus, Caesar displays a dignity and majesty that seem to reach beyond the world of the play.

Shakespeare's cold and ambitious ruler seems to correspond fairly closely to the historical Octavius Caesar—who took the title Augustus upon becoming emperor—though it is difficult to be certain as Octavius is known in history from only a few biased accounts, one of which is Shakespeare's source, PLUTARCH's *Lives.* However, it is noteworthy that the playwright significantly altered the story he read in Plutarch. Shakespeare's Caesar has failings—particularly moral ones—but is nonetheless a singularly potent figure who personally dominates the political and

military worlds of the play. However, though undeniably a great leader, Octavius Caesar was highly dependent on his subordinates. Only the most notable of these—AGRIPPA, in the military realm, and MAECENAS, as a diplomat—have even minor roles in *Antony and Cleopatra.* The triumphant warrior of the play was in fact a weak and sickly campaigner; this is alluded to by the embittered Antony in 3.11.35–40, but little is made of it. Shakespeare's aggrandisement of an already grand figure reinforces our sense of Caesar's dignity and majesty in support of the religious aspect of his significance.

Caius (1) Minor character in *Titus Andronicus.* Mentioned only in stage directions, Caius does not speak. He is present for the shooting of arrows to the gods in 4.3, and he helps to capture CHIRON and DEMETRIUS (1) in 5.2.

Caius (2), Doctor Character in *The Merry Wives of Windsor,* a French physician and suitor of ANNE (3) Page. Caius is descended from a traditional stock figure, the blustering, arrogant, and ineffective doctor, although his profession is not important in the play; his bad temper and aggressive nature are exemplified by his explosive reiterations of the expletive 'By gar'—e.g., in 5.5.203–207. Caius is also a stereotypical foreigner, mangling the English language and behaving with notable wrong-headedness. He challenges EVANS (3) to a duel for having attempted to assist SLENDER, a rival for Anne's hand. The duel is averted by a group of townsmen, led by the HOST (2). Caius and Evans then conspire against the Host, arrangeing to steal his horses. Although Caius' combativeness is generally amusing, this petty vengeance, combined with his vanity, isolates him from the generally mild temper of the play, and it is probably significant that he and Evans, a Welshman, are WINDSOR's only foreigners. Caius is also the only character to withdraw wilfully from the reconciliations in 5.5.

Caius (3) Ligarius Character in *Julius Caesar.* See LIGARIUS.

Caius (4) In *King Lear,* the name adopted by the Earl of KENT (2) as part of his disguise as a yeoman. This Roman name is inappropriate to the pre-Roman Britain in which the play is ostensibly set, but such anachronisms abound in *King Lear* and the playwright doubtless felt that 'Caius' was appropriately antique for the ancient world in which the work is set. However, Kent only uses his alias at the very close of the play, in 5.3.282, where it attracts little notice. Shakespeare may have thought he had used it earlier; the slip would be typical of the many small errors and inconsistencies to which he was inclined.

Calchas Legendary figure and character in *Troilus and Cressida,* the father of CRESSIDA. Calchas, a Trojan priest, has foreseen the defeat of TROY in the TROJAN WAR and has deserted to the Greeks before the play begins. In 3.3.1–29 he proposes a prisoner exchange: the Greeks can repay him for his treason by trading the newly captured Trojan prince ANTENOR for his daughter. Thus Cressida is removed from her lover, TROILUS, just as their affair has begun, and she is exposed to the temptation that leads her to betray Troilus in favour of the Greek warrior DIOMEDES. Aside from triggering this development, Calchas' role in the play is insignificant.

In the *Iliad* of HOMER, Calchas is a Greek prophet who foretells the length of the war. His transformation into a Trojan occurs in the later, pro-Trojan version of the legend that was the basis for the English accounts on which Shakespeare relied.

Caldwell, Zoë (b. 1933) Australian-born British actress. Caldwell was a prominent actress in Australia in her early twenties, when she went to England and played a variety of roles at STRATFORD. Her first major role was as HELENA (2) in Tyrone GUTHRIE's 1959 production of *All's Well That Ends Well.* She has been acclaimed in many other Shakespearean parts, including CORDELIA—opposite Charles LAUGHTON—OPHELIA, LADY (6) MACBETH, and, perhaps most notably, CLEOPATRA.

Caliban Character in *The Tempest,* the beastlike slave of the magician PROSPERO. Before the time of the play, Prospero and his daughter MIRANDA took Caliban, the illegitimate son of a witch and a devil, into their home and taught him to speak and function as a human, but his response was to attempt to rape the girl. In the course of the play he and STEPHANO (2) attempt to murder Prospero. Though Caliban is powerless to effect his schemes, his villainous nature is an important element in *The Tempest*'s scheme of things. At the play's close a chastened Caliban declares, 'I'll be wise hereafter, / And seek for grace' (5.1.294–295) as part of the general reconciliation engineered by Prospero.

Caliban is only partly human. He is a 'monster' (2.2.66), a 'moon-calf' (2.2.107), a 'born devil' (4.1.188), and a 'thing of darkness' (5.1.275). Because his father was a devil, Caliban is supernatural like ARIEL, but unlike that airy spirit, he has no supernatural powers. He is more like a debased human than like any other supernatural creature in Shakespeare. He has intelligence enough to learn language, but he is seemingly incapable of moral sense; reminded of his attempted rape, he merely asserts his animal drive to procreate. Caliban serves as a foil for the other characters: his foolish credulity in accepting Stephano as a god contrasts with Prospero's wisdom, his viciousness with Miranda's innocence, his amorality with the hon-

ourable love of FERDINAND (2), and, most significantly, his finally regenerate state with the intransigent evil of ANTONIO (5).

Caliban's human qualities illuminate another of the play's themes and, in doing so, shed light on Shakespeare's world, which was just becoming aware of the natives of America (see EPENOW). As Prospero's 'slave' (1.2.310) Caliban is linked with America; his mother's god, Setebos, was known by Shakespeare as a South American deity; in finding Stephano divine and in responding greedily to his liquor, Caliban behaves like the American natives of early explorers' accounts.

The discovery of native American societies in the early 17th century stimulated debate on an ancient question: is 'natural man' a savage whose life is governed only by animal drives, or is he in a blessed state, unspoiled by the manifold corruptions of civilisation? Although the idealism of the latter view is reflected in GONZALO's praise of primitive society in 2.1.143–164 (drawn from remarks on America by the French essayist MONTAIGNE), Caliban's nature contradicts it. He represents 'natural man', but his very name, an anagram of 'canibal' (a legitimate 17th-century spelling of 'cannibal'), lends a negative quality to the connection.

It is precisely his naturalness that condemns Caliban. He is confined to brute slavery because he has refused to accept a civil role in Prospero's household. Prospero says that 'on [his] nature / Nurture can never stick' (4.1.188–189). In a telling comparison, Caliban's resistance to his wood-carrying chores is contrasted with Ferdinand's philosophical delight in similar labours. The young man knows that 'some kinds of baseness / Are nobly undergone; and most poor matters / Point to rich ends' (3.1.2–4). Miranda expressly judges both Ferdinand and Caliban: the first is 'a thing divine' (4.1.421), the second, 'a thing most brutish' (1.2.358).

Yet Caliban has some positive attributes, which qualify Shakespeare's condemnation of 'natural man'. Though he proclaims that his education has merely taught him 'how to curse' (1.2.366), his use of language is in fact quite impressive, and he rises to lyrical poetry—revealing an aesthetic sensibility—in describing his dreams of 'a thousand twangling instruments' (3.2.135). He can imagine a level below himself to which he does not want to descend, for he fears he and his companions will be 'turn'd to barnacles, or to apes / With foreheads villainous low' (4.1.248–249). Though he is foolish enough to follow Stephano and TRINCULO, he is more sensible than they and scorns their frivolous absorption with mere 'luggage' (4.1. 231). His proposed revolt is both repulsive and ineffectual, but Caliban's dislike for his enslavement is one with which we instinctively sympathise. His initial statement of grievance is compelling; he helped Prospero and Miranda survive and is now enslaved. Only then do we learn of his crime, but even afterwards, Caliban is permitted his say on his status: his elaborate complaint of Prospero's harassment in 2.2.1–14 casts his master in a bad light, and his comical enthusiasm for 'Freedom, high-day! high-day, freedom! freedom, high-day, freedom!' (2.2.186–187) is infectious.

For all his villainy, Caliban contributes to the general sense of regeneration with which the play closes. He recognises his folly and expresses his intention to improve himself in a religious metaphor—he will 'seek for grace' (5.1.295). His earlier behaviour certainly makes us wonder if reform is really possible, but Shakespeare pointedly elevates this beastlike character's moral stature before he exits forever. However appalling Caliban's fallen state, he offers the hope for restoration to grace that is part of Shakespeare's sense of human possibility.

Calphurnia (Calpurnia) (active 59–44 B.C.) Historical figure and character in *Julius Caesar,* the wife of CAESAR (1). In 2.2 Calphurnia, alarmed by accounts of dire omens, begs Caesar not to attend the Senate session on the Ides of March. She asserts that his 'wisdom is consum'd in confidence' (2.2.49) and prevails on him to stay home. However, her work is immediately undone by DECIUS, and Caesar goes to his death. The episode demonstrates Calphurnia's devotion to her mighty husband and casts a softer light on him than we would otherwise have. Further, it reminds us that his assassination was a domestic tragedy as well as a political event, thus humanising the play's account of murderous intrigue and civil war.

Caesar married the historical Calpurnia—as her name was spelled in Latin—in 59 B.C. to cement a political alliance with her father. Although Caesar was blatantly unfaithful and came close to divorcing her a few years later in order to make another political marriage, Calpurnia was thought by contemporaries to have been a genuinely devoted wife; the tale of her entreaty, as reported in Shakespeare's source, PLUTARCH's *Lives,* is probably true. After the assassination, Calpurnia assisted Mark ANTONY's campaign against the conspirators by turning over to him Caesar's papers and a large amount of cash. Little else is known of her life.

The spelling Calphurnia, though less familiar than Calpurnia and incorrect in Latin, is increasingly used by modern editors, restoring the style of the FIRST FOLIO (1623), which is also followed by most of Shakespeare's contemporaries in other writings about Caesar. (In Shakespeare's source, NORTH's English translation of Plutarch, both forms are used.) In the 18th century, editors of Shakespeare chose to revert to the Latin form, establishing a different tradition.

Calvert, Charles (1828–1879) British theatrical producer. Calvert was a follower of Samuel PHELPS in restoring Shakespeare's texts and simplifying produc-

tions. After a career as an actor, he became the manager of a theatre in Manchester, England, where he established his reputation as a producer. From 1864 to 1875 he staged many revivals of Shakespeare plays in London, focussing on works that were traditionally less frequently performed, such as *2 Henry IV* and *Henry VIII*, but also presenting popular pieces like *Richard III* and *The Merchant of Venice* (the latter in 1871 with music by Arthur SULLIVAN [1]). However, his theatre was not financially successful, and he returned to touring at the close of his career.

Cambio In *The Taming of the Shrew*, the name LUCENTIO takes when disguised as a scholar of languages in order to be appointed tutor to BIANCA (1).

Cambridge, Richard York, Earl of (1376–1415) Historical figure and character in *Henry V*, a traitor who plans to assassinate King HENRY V but is foiled and condemned to death. In 2.2 Henry, who knows of the intended treason, asks Cambridge and his co-conspirators, Lord SCROOP (1) and Sir Thomas GREY (3), how to deal with a drunken soldier who has spoken against him. They all insist that Henry be firm against any hint of disloyalty. Then Henry reveals his knowledge of their treason and applies their own advice, denying them clemency and sentencing them to death. Cambridge, who has no distinctive personality, welcomes death with conventional remorse, as do the others, in a passage intended to emphasise Henry's godlike majesty.

The historical Cambridge benefited from Henry's benevolence, for the King had restored his older brother to the dukedom of YORK (5), despite his history of rebellion against HENRY IV, and had elevated Cambridge to his earldom. However, the Earl firmly opposed Henry IV's usurpation of the throne from RICHARD II, and he continued to rebel. In *Henry V* French gold alone motivates the traitors, although in 2.2.155–157 Cambridge observes that he wants the cash for a purpose that Shakespeare did not specify because he wished his audience to focus on Henry's enemies in France. The historical traitors, however, planned to replace Henry on the throne with Edmund MORTIMER (1), Cambridge's brother-in-law, whose father was held to have been the rightful heir to Richard II. Mortimer himself was loyal and turned in the conspirators, which Shakespeare does not mention, but his claim to the throne was revived by Cambridge's son, the Duke of YORK (8) of the *Henry VI* plays, and the WARS OF THE ROSES ensued as a result. Thus this minor scene in *Henry V* carries the germ of future English disasters, as many people in Shakespeare's original audiences will have recognised.

Camden, William (1551–1623) English historian, author of a minor source for *Coriolanus*. Camden, a noted educator, scholar, and antiquarian, wrote a massive Latin work on ancient and medieval England, *Britannia* (1586). An English translation by Philemon HOLLAND (4) came out in 1610, but English excerpts had already been published in *Remaines of a greater Worke concerning Britaine* in 1605. From the *Remaines*, Shakespeare took some details for MENENIUS' famous 'belly speech' (*Coriolanus*, 1.1.95–159). The *Remaines* also contains an appreciation of Shakespeare as one of England's greatest writers.

Camden was a longtime secondary school teacher and headmaster, who taught poetry composition to Ben JONSON, among others. He remained a lifelong friend of Jonson and through him may have known Shakespeare personally. He was also a noted authority on heraldry and the chief founder of the Society of Antiquaries, an important intellectual institution of the day. In addition to *Britannia*, Camden wrote a Latin history of the reign of Queen ELIZABETH (1) and an English account of the Gunpowder Plot (see GARNET).

Camillo Character in *The Winter's Tale*, an adviser of King LEONTES of SICILIA. The mad Leontes suspects his best friend, King POLIXENES of BOHEMIA, of committing adultery with his wife, and in 1.2 he orders Camillo to poison Polixenes. Instead, Camillo informs Polixenes and flees with him to Bohemia. Camillo reappears there in the second half of the play, set 16 years later. He has been a faithful adviser to Polixenes, and in 4.4 he helps the king thwart the romance between Prince FLORIZEL and a shepherd girl, PERDITA. However, he then helps the couple flee to Sicilia, where it is discovered that Perdita is the lost daughter of Leontes, and the play ends in an atmosphere of general reconciliation and love.

Camillo represents a familiar character type in the romantic literature on which *The Winter's Tale* is based: the servant who aids his master by disobeying him. As such, he is one of the good people who fight the evil that infects the play's world. Only providence, supported by the power of love, can bring the play's characters through to the happy ending, but human agency, chiefly that of Camillo and PAULINA, is an important auxiliary. Thus, Camillo supports a major theme of the play, that humanity must energetically use its capacity for good. Fittingly, he becomes engaged to Paulina, by royal command, at the play's close.

Campeius, Cardinal Laurence (Lorenzo Campeggio, 1472–1539) Historical figure and minor character in *Henry VIII*, the pope's ambassador to the court of King HENRY VIII. Campeius comes to England to consider the legality of Henry's proposed divorce of Queen KATHERINE; Cardinal WOLSEY has assured the king that Campeius will rule in his favour, but in 2.4 the Roman

cardinal merely postpones a decision. Irritated, Henry complains, 'These cardinals trifle with me: I abhor / This dilatory sloth and tricks of Rome' (2.4.234–235). Here—as throughout—Campeius embodies the untrustworthiness of Catholicism from the play's point of view. The episode also demonstrates Henry's growing mistrust of Wolsey, as he moves from gullibility to wisdom, a principal theme of the play. In 3.2 Campeius is said to have 'stolen away to Rome . . . / [having] left the cause o'th'king unhandled' (3.2.57–58).

The historical Campeggio—Shakespeare uses the Latin form of his name—was responsible for English affairs at the Vatican and had visited England before he arrived to adjudicate Henry's divorce in 1528. In fact, Henry had appointed him absentee Bishop of Salisbury in 1524. Unknown to Wolsey, he was under instructions to delay Henry's divorce as long as possible, for the pope did not want to offend the Holy Roman Emperor, Queen Katherine's nephew. He succeeded in postponing the trial for nine months and then, when it seemed likely that Henry would win his case, he declared an adjournment and left for Rome. Henry eventually declared himself divorced when he assumed papal powers in England as part of the Reformation, and at that time Campeggio lost his English bishopric.

Canidius (Camidius) (Publius Canidius Crassus, d. 30 B.C.) Historical figure and character in *Antony and Cleopatra,* a general in ANTONY's army. Canidius appears only briefly, in 3.7 where he objects to Antony's decision to fight CAESAR (2) at sea, and in 3.10 where he declares that he will surrender his troops to Caesar after Antony has lost the battle of ACTIUM. Antony's power and authority waned due to the influence of CLEOPATRA, and his followers lost their faith in his success. The character Canidius demonstrates this.

The historical Canidius was in fact the only major figure among Antony's followers to stay with him to the bitter end. He fled after Actium and made his way back to ALEXANDRIA, where he was captured and executed upon his leader's final defeat and death. Shakespeare's source, PLUTARCH's *Lives,* was based on an anti-Antony source (see MESSALA), and modern scholars believe that Canidius' impressive record as a hardy and loyal officer makes Plutarch's interpretation of his actions unlikely.

Canon An authoritative list of the works of an author. The canon of Shakespeare's plays varies slightly according to the opinions of various scholars, but it usually includes 38 titles: the 36 plays of the FIRST FOLIO, plus *Pericles* and *The Two Noble Kinsmen.* However, some scholars doubt the Folio's reliability, especially with regard to *Henry VIII*—perhaps written in part by John FLETCHER (2)—while others often relegate *Pericles* or *The Two Noble Kinsmen*—especially the latter—to the APOCRYPHA, a list of dubious titles. Other titles are also occasionally disputed.

This book assumes that the canon consists of the 38 plays specified above; i.e., in alphabetical order: *All's Well That Ends Well, Antony and Cleopatra, As You Like It, The Comedy of Errors, Coriolanus, Cymbeline, Hamlet, 1 & 2 Henry IV, Henry V, 1, 2, & 3 Henry VI, Henry VIII, Julius Caesar, King John, King Lear, Love's Labour's Lost, Macbeth, Measure for Measure, The Merchant of Venice, The Merry Wives of Windsor, A Midsummer Night's Dream, Much Ado About Nothing, Othello, Pericles, Richard II, Richard III, Romeo and Juliet, The Taming of the Shrew, The Tempest, Timon of Athens, Titus Andronicus, Troilus and Cressida, Twelfth Night, The Two Gentlemen of Verona, The Two Noble Kinsmen,* and *The Winter's Tale.*

In Shakespeare studies, the term 'canon' often applies only to the plays. However, a broader usage, equally correct, would also include the 154 SONNETS (though a few of them are disputed), the long poems *Venus and Adonis* and *The Rape of Lucrece,* and various shorter poems, including *The Phoenix and Turtle,* some of the works in THE PASSIONATE PILGRIM, and some EPITAPHS (though other epitaphs are clearly apocryphal). Other poems are sometimes suggested for the canon, e.g., 'SHALL I DIE?'; scholars periodically nominate new discoveries for inclusion, and disputes over the correct list can last for decades without resolution.

Canterbury (1), Henry Chichele, Archbishop of, (1362–1443) Historical figure and character in *Henry V* who gives King HENRY V a rationale for going to war with FRANCE (1). In 1.1 Canterbury, speaking with the Bishop of ELY (2), expresses his hope that a state of war—especially when supported by the large donation he has offered the King—will divert the introduction of legislation requiring a vast state seizure of church property. In 1.2 he presents the King with a long, legalistic argument in support of his hereditary claim to the French crown, and he joins others in encouraging a conquest of France.

Shakespeare's portrayal of Canterbury is flawed, though only because his sources were. The historical Henry Chichele did not become Archbishop until some time after the war began; until then he was Henry's ambassador to France. Shakespeare followed HALL (2) in this error. More significantly, the church was not particularly instrumental in promoting the war, and the Archbishop's motives, although Shakespeare took them from HOLINSHED, are unhistorical. In fact, although the legislation to seize church property had been proposed under King HENRY IV (as Canterbury observes in 1.1.2–3), it was not reintroduced under Henry V. Thus the church had no reason to promote the war, and, although it contributed to the King's war fund, as was customary, its donation was not exceptionally great, as it is in the play.

Canterbury (2), Archbishop of, Thomas Cranmer Character in *Henry VIII.* See CRANMER.

Capell, Edward (1713–1781) Shakespearean scholar. Capell was the first scholar to collate the old editions of Shakespeare's plays to arrive at the most accurately rendered texts possible, and he also introduced the first serious scholarly consideration of Shakespeare's sources. After 24 years of labour, his edition of the collected plays was published in 1768. His *Commentary, Notes and Various Readings to Shakespeare,* begun in 1774, was published posthumously in 1783. Though his judgements are still acclaimed today, he is very little read except by specialists, in part because of his tedious prose. As Samuel JOHNSON (7) put it, 'he doth gabble monstrously'.

Caphis Minor character in *Timon of Athens,* servant of a SENATOR (4). In 2.1 the Senator sends Caphis to collect a debt from TIMON, who he fears will soon be bankrupt. The servant barely speaks and serves simply as a vehicle for the Senator's greed. In 2.2 he joins other servants in asking Timon for payment on their masters' behalf.

Capilet See WIDOW (2).

Captain (1) Minor character in *Titus Andronicus,* the officer who announces the arrival of TITUS (1) Andronicus in 1.1 and praises his virtues as a general.

Captain (2) Minor character in *1 Henry VI,* an English officer. When TALBOT is invited to visit the Countess of AUVERGNE, in 2.2, he rightly suspects a trap and confers with the Captain. Though he is not seen in 2.3, the Captain is presumably responsible for the troop of soldiers who immediately free Talbot when the trap is sprung.

The same character (or perhaps a different Captain) challenges the cowardly FASTOLFE, who is fleeing from the battle in 3.2. And, in 4.4, a Captain precedes Sir William LUCY (2) in seeking reinforcements from the Duke of SOMERSET (3).

Captain (3) Character in *2 Henry VI.* Some editions, following the CONTENTION, or BAD QUARTO, assign this rank to the LIEUTENANT (1), who appears in 4.1. This small difference presumably resulted from an actor or viewer's assumption that the leader of the pirates would be called their captain. The Quarto presents a reconstruction of the play from memory, while the Lieutenant's rank in the FIRST FOLIO edition and its successors is believed to come from the original manuscript.

Captain (4) Minor character in *Richard II,* the Welsh commander of troops who desert the cause of RICHARD II in 2.4, after the King has not appeared for many days. The Captain tells of rumours that Richard has died and cites menacing omens that seem to substantiate them. Shakespeare may have associated the Captain with Owen GLENDOWER, who is mentioned in 3.1.43.

Captain (5) Minor character in *Twelfth Night,* the rescuer of VIOLA. After saving Viola from a shipwreck, the Captain offers her hope that her brother may also have been saved, thereby establishing that SEBASTIAN (2) will eventually appear. The Captain goes on to direct Viola's attention to the court of Duke ORSINO, which she determines to visit, disguised as a man. Unlike ANTONIO (4), who saves Sebastian, the Captain is not a salty mariner; oddly, he is something of a gentleman, speaking familiarly of the duke's affairs and quoting an image from OVID (1.1.15). Otherwise the Captain has no real personality; he simply introduces developments and indicates by his attitude that Viola is an attractive heroine.

Captain (6) Minor character in *Hamlet,* an officer in the Norwegian army of Prince FORTINBRAS. In 4.4 the Captain tells HAMLET of Fortinbras' march with 20,000 soldiers to conquer a small, valueless parcel of land in Poland. Shakespeare may take an ironical stance towards the folly of war in these brief and straightforward lines, but Hamlet seems to accept Fortinbras' goal as reasonable, responding to the Captain's account only by comparing his own scruples and hesitations with the unthinking commitment of the soldiers, who will die fighting for so small a prize. Thus the incident emphasises Hamlet's concern with his failure to avenge his father's death—the central strand of the play's plot—and reminds us of Fortinbras' strength, which will assume greater importance at the end of the play.

Captain (7) Character in *King Lear.* See OFFICER (5).

Captain (8) (Sergeant) Minor character in *Macbeth,* a wounded soldier who describes the brave MACBETH's achievements in battle against the rebels who oppose King DUNCAN. In 1.2 the Captain offers an image of Macbeth as an hero, and the shock of Macbeth's later treason is the greater because this initial image is shattered. The effect is furthered by the Captain's considerable dignity; he speaks in measured rhetorical cadences and his own suffering is bravely suppressed until he closes touchingly with, 'But I am faint, my gashes cry for help' (1.2.43). He is not seen further, however, being important only as a commentator on the opening situation.

Some modern editors note that the Captain is referred to by MALCOLM as 'the Sergeant' in 1.2.3 and designate him with that rank in the stage directions

and speech headings. However, he is called 'Captain' in those places in the first edition of the play, in the FIRST FOLIO (1623), and other editors retain this designation. It is supposed that 'Sergeant' refers to the character's function as a valued but not high-ranking subordinate.

Captain (9) Minor character in *Antony and Cleopatra,* an officer in ANTONY's army. In 4.4 the Captain greets Antony cheerfully on the morning of a battle, listens to his leader's parting remarks to CLEOPATRA, and leaves with him. His function is to add a note of martial bustle to the scene. In the first edition of the play, in the FIRST FOLIO, this character was designated as ALEXAS, but this reflects an error—probably Shakespeare's—for in 4.6.12–16 we learn of Alexas' earlier treason and execution. Nicholas ROWE altered the designation and assigned the Captain his rank in the 1709 edition of the plays, and all subsequent editors have accepted the change.

Captain (10) Minor character in *Cymbeline,* an officer in the Roman army. In 4.2 the Captain reports to LUCIUS (4) that the army has landed in WALES (1). His six terse lines serve to convey information that moves the plot to a new stage.

Captain (11) Either of two minor characters in *Cymbeline,* officers in the British army. In 5.3 after the British victory over the Romans that is described by POSTHUMUS earlier in the scene, the Captains discover Posthumus in his Roman uniform and take him prisoner. They turn him over to King CYMBELINE in a DUMB SHOW that ends the scene. With only a few lines between them, the Captains' function is to further the plot. However, they also inform the audience that in addition to the heroes BELARIUS, GUIDERIUS, and ARVIRAGUS—already described by Posthumus—there was a fourth. This leads us to guess that this man was Posthumus himself, which proves to be the case.

Capuchius (Capucius), Lord (Eustace Chapuys, active 1530s) Historical figure and minor character in *Henry VIII,* ambassador to England from the Holy Roman Empire, a visitor to Queen KATHERINE. In 4.2 Capuchius bears a message from King HENRY VIII wishing good health to the dying Katherine. She observes mildly that the gesture comes too late. She asks Capuchius to take the king a letter, in which she requests that he look after their daughter—and remember her to the child—and treat her followers and servants well. She then retires to die. The episode, which Shakespeare knew from his source, HOLINSHED's *Chronicles,* offers a final demonstration of Katherine's virtue.

Following Holinshed, Shakespeare used the Latin form of the ambassador's name. Chapuys' surviving official correspondence casts light on the intrigues of the period. One letter declares that Cardinal WOLSEY had written to him recommending that the pope excommunicate King Henry and use arms to enforce Catholicism in England. In an unrelated treason trial of 1533, it was alleged that Chapuys had planned an invasion of England in support of Katherine, but that the emperor had vetoed the idea. This may not have been taken seriously, because Chapuys continued in his post and, as we have seen, was permitted to visit Katherine.

Capulet (1) Character in *Romeo and Juliet,* the father of JULIET (1) and the head of the family bearing his name, rivals to the MONTAGUE (1) clan. Though short-tempered, Capulet at first seems benevolent: he resists the marriage proposal by PARIS (2) in 1.2, observing that Juliet is too young, and in 1.5 he orders TYBALT to leave the banquet rather than fight ROMEO. However, in 3.4 he suddenly decides to give Juliet, by now secretly married to Romeo, to Paris and rages furiously at his daughter when she resists; he belongs to the conventional, unfeeling world that opposes the lovers. When he impulsively moves the wedding date up by a day (4.2), Capulet becomes an agent of fate, hastening the play's tragic climax. His humorous involvement in the wedding preparations does not restore him to our affections, nor does his cursory and somewhat stilted mourning when he believes the drugged Juliet to be dead. Only at the end of the play, when his daughter's actual death impels him to seek a reconciliation with Montague, can we again find him humanly sympathetic.

The feud between the Capulets and the Montagues did not in fact occur, although Shakespeare and his sources believed it to have been real. See VERONA.

Capulet (2), Cousin Minor character in *Romeo and Juliet,* an aged relative of CAPULET (1). Cousin Capulet (called 'Old Man' in some editions) speaks only two lines in a brief conversation, at the feast in 1.5, on the rapid flight of the years. This episode, occurring just as ROMEO and JULIET (1) are about to meet, is one instance of the motif of time's passage, which recurs throughout the tragedy.

Capulet (3), Lady Character in *Romeo and Juliet,* mother of JULIET (1) and wife of CAPULET (1). Desiring the marriage of Juliet to PARIS (2), Lady Capulet is curt, imperious, and coldly unsympathetic to her daughter's qualms, even without knowing that they stem from her passion for Romeo; she is a representative of the conventional world that opposes the young lovers. Her grief in 4.5, when she believes the drugged Juliet is dead, elicits our sympathy, but we may remember her enraged demands for revenge on Tybalt's murderer in 3.1. She does not speak in the final scene of reconciliation.

Cardenio Lost play, possibly written by Shakespeare and John FLETCHER (2). In 1613 the KING'S MEN twice performed a play recorded as *Cardenno* or *Cardenna.* In 1653 the manuscript collector and publisher Humphrey MOSELEY claimed the copyright on an old play, *The History of Cardennio,* said to be by Shakespeare and Fletcher, but his copy did not survive. In 1727 Lewis THEOBALD produced a drama titled *Double Falsehood* (published 1728), which he asserted he had adapted from an unpublished play manuscript by Shakespeare. This play derives from a story in Miguel de CERVANTES' *Don Quixote,* whose hero is named Cardenio. Theobald wrote that he owned three manuscript copies of the play, but they subsequently disappeared, and when he published his edition of Shakespeare's plays in 1733, he did not include this one. Moreover, scholars agree that the play, at least in Theobald's version, is very un-Shakespearean. It is speculated that the King's Men's play of 1613 was passed on, in a corrupt form, as far as Theobald, who came to reject its authenticity.

Around 1613 Fletcher and Shakespeare collaborated on *The Two Noble Kinsmen* and possibly *Henry VIII,* so there is nothing unlikely about a third such project. Moreover, a translation of *Don Quixote* was published in 1612. Fletcher used it as a source for later plays, so that his hand in the King's Men's play of 1613 seems likely. However, the play's absence from the FIRST FOLIO (1623) suggests that its editors—King's Men themselves—felt it was not by Shakespeare, either because his part in it was too slight to merit mention or simply because he had nothing to do with it at all.

Cardinal (1) Beaufort, Henry (1374–1447) Historical figure and character in *2 Henry VI,* a leader of the plot against the Duke of GLOUCESTER (4) that dominates the first half of the play. The Cardinal, the illegitimate son of John of GAUNT, is a great-uncle of the King and a powerful secular lord in his own right. (The same historical person appeared in *1 Henry VI* as the Bishop of WINCHESTER (1), where his rivalry with Gloucester is developed; he is sometimes referred to in *2 Henry VI* as Winchester—as in 1.1.56.) In 1.1 the Cardinal smoothly recruits other noblemen to his cause, accusing Gloucester, the heir apparent to the throne, of self-interest, turning against him what should be to his credit—his patriotic anger at the King's foolish cession of lands in his marriage contract. The Cardinal and Gloucester agree to fight a duel in 2.1, but they are interrupted. At the end of that scene, word is brought that Gloucester's wife has been arrested for witchcraft, and the Cardinal gloats that his rival, abruptly humiliated, will not have the heart to fight.

When Gloucester himself is arrested for treason, in 3.1, the Cardinal and his confederates agree that the Duke should be murdered, and the Cardinal volunteers to hire the murderer, although SUFFOLK (3) actually performs that deed. After Gloucester's murder, word is brought to the King that the Cardinal is dying of a sudden illness. When the King and WARWICK (3) visit him in 3.3, he appears to have a bad conscience. The Cardinal's ravings are not quite specific but they nonetheless convict him.

Historically, Cardinal Beaufort, although he was in fact a rival of Gloucester, was not his murderer; in fact, Gloucester was probably not murdered at all. The Cardinal may not even have had anything to do with Gloucester's arrest by Suffolk, which led to the Duke's death, for Beaufort by this time had largely abandoned his political role and retired from public life. Shakespeare's version of the Cardinal's death is pure fiction; he actually died at home in a normal manner at the age of 73, some months after Gloucester's death. However, the playwright held the opinion, along with his sources, that 'good Duke Humphrey' had been victimised by his rivals (see WINCHESTER [1]), and he accordingly made an unscrupulous villain, or MACHIAVEL, of the Cardinal, who was actually a far more prudent and statesmanlike figure than Gloucester.

Cardinal (2), Lord (Thomas Bourchier, c. 1404–1486) Historical figure and minor character in *Richard III,* the Archbishop of Canterbury. In 3.1 the Cardinal is persuaded by BUCKINGHAM (2) to remove the young Duke of YORK (7) from sanctuary in a church. The historical Bourchier was a politically accommodating prelate who crowned EDWARD IV, RICHARD III, and Henry VII, the RICHMOND of the play.

In some modern editions of the play, the ARCHBISHOP (4) of York is eliminated and his lines are given to the Cardinal, following the 16th-century QUARTO editions. This change was presumably made as an economy for the acting company.

Cardinal (3) Campeius Character in *Henry VIII.* See CAMPEIUS.

Cardinal (4), Pandulph Character in *King John.* See PANDULPH.

Cardinal (5) Wolsey Character in *Henry VIII.* See WOLSEY.

Carew, Richard (1555–1620) English scholar and contemporary admirer of Shakespeare. Carew, a country gentleman and self-taught student of languages and early English history, translated poetry from Italian and Spanish and also published his own verse. His major work was a history of Cornwall (1602), but he is remembered today chiefly for a remark in a letter (1603) to William CAMDEN, in which he offered an early assessment of 'Shakespeare', declaring him the

equal of Catullus as a poet. The letter was published in the second edition (1614) of Camden's *Remaines.*

Carey (1), George, Baron Hunsdon See HUNSDON (1).

Carey (2), Henry, Baron Hunsdon See HUNSDON (2).

Carlisle, Thomas Merke, Bishop of (d. 1409) Historical figure and character in *Richard II,* a supporter of King RICHARD II. Carlisle accompanies Richard on his return from Ireland to face BOLINGBROKE (1), and he warns the King against inaction, but his speech is equivocal. His ambivalence is immediately emphasised by the Duke of AUMERLE's much more pointed statement of the same warning. Nonetheless, Carlisle is the only defender of Richard in the deposition scene, 4.1. In a formal speech he appeals to the assembled aristocrats not to violate the sanctity of a King, divinely placed on the throne—'What subject can give sentence on his king?' (4.1.121), he asks rhetorically—and he predicts disaster for England if the deposition is carried out. NORTHUMBERLAND (1) promptly arrests him for treason, and he is placed in the custody of the ABBOT of Westminster. At the close of the scene Carlisle joins the Abbot and Aumerle in a plot against Bolingbroke. At the end of the play he is brought before Bolingbroke, now King HENRY IV, who pardons him, referring to his honourable character.

The historical Carlisle was a Benedictine monk who served Richard ably as an administrator and was rewarded with his bishopric as a result. He did not protest Henry's accession; his speech is drawn from accounts of his opposition to a later proposal to try Richard on criminal charges. These accounts may have been invented, however, for they derive from an unreliable, propagandistic tract, probably written by a member of QUEEN (13) Isabel's French household, that was the source for Shakespeare's source, HOLINSHED's *Chronicles.* However, regardless of its historical reality, Carlisle's speech presents an important aspect of Tudor political dogma: the citizenry may not judge its monarch in any way. This idea is emphasised in Holinshed, and it is present throughout the HISTORY PLAYS.

Carlisle did participate in the Abbot's conspiracy, but he was not willingly pardoned by Henry. Tried and convicted, he was dismissed from his see, and his life was spared only by papal intervention.

Carpenter Minor character in *Julius Caesar,* a COMMONER (1). In 1.1 the Carpenter, who speaks one line (1.1.6), is part of a crowd being dispersed by the tribunes FLAVIUS (1) and MARULLUS. He identifies himself by profession, establishing the social class of the group. In some editions the Carpenter is identified as the First Commoner.

Carrier Either of two minor characters in *1 Henry IV,* freight haulers who prepare to take a cargo to LONDON from ROCHESTER in 2.1. The Carriers comically complain about conditions at the inn. They tellingly distrust the highwayman GADSHILL when he asks to borrow a lantern, but they unwittingly supply him with information, commenting that they expect gentlemen carrying valuables to accompany them on the road. At least one of the Carriers is apparently among the TRAVELLERS who are ambushed in 2.2, for he appears in London with the SHERIFF (4) in 2.4, having recognised FALSTAFF during the robbery.

Casca, Publius Servius (d. 42 B.C.) Historical figure and character in *Julius Caesar,* one of the assassins of CAESAR (1). In 1.2 Casca officiously orders the festival crowds to be silent in Caesar's presence, but later he speaks contemptuously to BRUTUS (4) and CASSIUS about Caesar's rejection of the crown and his fit of epilepsy. In addition, he pokes fun at the pedantry of CICERO and his companions, who had remarked on Caesar in Greek; Casca delivers one of Shakespeare's most-quoted lines, 'It was Greek to me' (1.2.281), implying that he scorned to know a foreign language. Brutus calls him a 'blunt fellow' (1.2.292), but Cassius defends him as a bold man, useful in any difficult enterprise. Casca, who is vain, holds the same opinion, saying, 'I will set this foot of mine as far as who goes furthest' (1.3.119–120). However, earlier in the same scene he has shown himself to be cowardly, trembling at reports of dire omens, in telling contrast to Cicero's coolness. Casca is also a hypocrite; in 2.1, as the conspirators hatch their plot, he swiftly reverses his opinion of Cicero in response to Brutus' ('Let us not leave him out' [2.1.143]; 'Indeed he is not fit' [2.1.153]). In 3.1 Casca is the first of the conspirators to stab the defenseless Caesar, although he disappears from the play thereafter. (It has been speculated that Shakespeare discontinued the role at this point in order to free an actor to take the part of OCTAVIUS, who appears somewhat later.)

Little is known about the historical Casca, aside from his participation in Caesar's murder. Shakespeare's source, PLUTARCH, states that he was the first to stab Caesar and that Caesar called him 'vile' or 'vicious' (in different accounts of the assassination), and these two brief mentions are the basis of Shakespeare's fairly elaborate portrait. The playwright omitted two other episodes concerning Casca—that he almost revealed the conspiracy inadvertently and that he was responsible for the brutal killing of prisoners at PHILIPPI—but these inglorious moments doubtless contributed to the playwright's vision of Casca's unpleasant personality. Plutarch does not record Casca's suicide after the battle of Philippi, an honourable end by Roman standards and an episode that might have altered Shakespeare's characterisation.

Cassandra Legendary figure and character in *Troilus and Cressida*, a princess of TROY, the daughter of King PRIAM and sister to the princes HECTOR, TROILUS, and PARIS (3). Cassandra, a seer, twice foretells the fall of Troy. First, she hysterically interrupts a council of war to warn, 'Troy burns, or else let Helen go' (2.2.113), only to be dismissed as the victim of 'brain-sick raptures' (2.2.123). In 5.3, in calmer tones, she joins ANDROMACHE and Priam in trying to persuade Hector not to enter battle on a day of ill omens. Rebuffed again, she bids her brother a sad farewell. Although the other characters do not believe her, Cassandra's prophecies contribute to the play's atmosphere of fateful destiny, for they are known by the audience to be ironically correct.

In the *Iliad* of HOMER, Cassandra is a minor figure and not a seer. She first appears as a prophet in Greek literature of the 5th century B.C. According to the dramatist Aeschylus, her prophetic power was given to her by Apollo, but when she refused his love, he transformed it into a curse, causing her to be always disbelieved. This myth has been well known since ancient times, and Shakespeare could presume that his audience would recognise Apollo's curse in the Trojans' rejection of Cassandra's warnings.

Cassio Character in *Othello*, a Florentine officer serving under OTHELLO. IAGO is the enemy of both Othello and Cassio because Cassio has been appointed Othello's lieutenant, a post Iago had coveted for himself. Iago gets Cassio drunk and incites RODERIGO to fight him; the lieutenant disgraces himself by brawling drunkenly while on guard duty and is demoted. More important, Iago convinces Othello that his wife, DESDEMONA, is Cassio's lover, going so far as to plant on Cassio a handkerchief that Othello has given Desdemona. The enraged general commissions Iago to kill Cassio, and Iago again employs Roderigo. However, Cassio survives the attack and testifies against Iago in the play's closing moments.

The change in Othello's attitude towards Cassio is paralleled by Cassio's change towards Iago. Before his disgrace, Cassio is distant and refuses to be friendly with Iago, as we see at the beginning of 2.3. However, when Iago befriends him after he is discharged by Othello he accepts him entirely. He calls him 'honest Iago' (2.3.326) and says, 'I never knew / A Florentine more kind and honest' (3.1.40–41). He is grateful for what seems like excellent advice from Iago to ally himself with Desdemona. Though this is to have disastrous consequences, Cassio does not see through Iago until much too late, after the villain is exposed in the wake of Desdemona's murder

Cassio's relationship with BIANCA (2), a courtesan of CYPRUS is another echo of the main plot. Though they are not married we compare them with Othello and Desdemona, partially because Iago employs the unwitting Bianca in deceiving Othello about the handkerchief, in 4.1. More pointedly, though Bianca is jealous on Cassio's account—just as Othello is on Desdemona's—Cassio disdains her, in striking contrast to Desdemona's intense love for Othello. Cassio's tawdry affair casts light on the nature of Othello's blessed but rejected marriage.

Cassio's relationship with Bianca and his account of it to Iago, in 4.1, reflect the worldliness of a professional soldier, accustomed to finding women wherever he is stationed. As a competent soldier, he is respected and valued by Othello before Iago's poison begins its work. We see this in his appointment as lieutenant, and in the general's easy conversational tone as Cassio assumes guard duty, in 2.3. The lieutenant is apparently a gentleman, and he has enough learning to be mocked by Iago for his 'bookish theoric' (1.1.24). In 2.1.61–87 he expresses his reverence for Desdemona in courtly formal rhetoric that reflects his respect for Othello as well, establishing clearly an aura of gentlemanly honour and stately virtue.

On the other hand, while Cassio's soldierly dignity helps stress the vulgarity of Iago, he is often without that dignity, being drunk in 2.3 and awkwardly humiliated most of the time after that. Though his remorse at his irresponsibility is genuine and honourable—he regrets having 'deceive[d] so good a commander, with so light, so drunken, and indiscreet an officer' (2.3.269–271)—he is nevertheless somewhat ridiculous: he foolishly drinks wine he doesn't want and then quickly falls into Iago's next trap. His speech is often ludicrously high-flown; he declares, 'O thou invisible spirit of wine, if thou hast no name to be known by, let us call thee devil!' (2.3.273–275).

Yet Cassio 'has a daily beauty in his life' (5.1.19) that stirs Iago's envy, and his reputation and dignity are restored by the end of the play. He is given the command of Cyprus, and he shows a quiet assurance in insisting to Othello, 'Dear general, I did never give you cause' (5.2.300). At the close it is fitting that Cassio is the only person to recognise the grandeur of the suicidal general, declaring 'This did I fear, . . . For he was great of heart' (5.2.361–362).

Cassius (Caius Cassius Longinus) (d. 42 B.C.) Historical figure and character in *Julius Caesar*, one of the assassins of CAESAR (1) and, with BRUTUS (4), a leader of the forces opposing Mark ANTONY in the subsequent civil war. Cassius presents two quite different aspects in the course of the play. He first appears as a cynical, unscrupulous conspirator whose scheming stresses the evil side of political ambition. However, he later proves to be a courageous fighter, a sensible general, and a friend to Brutus. Cassius can thus be seen as a foil for Brutus and *his* two sides, first as a noble conspirator and then as an increasingly imperious leader; further, Cassius' two faces reinforce the play's insis-

tence that the qualities that make up a political leader result from the continuous interaction of good and evil.

Prior to Caesar's murder, Cassius is bitterly envious of his power, and his diatribes against his leader in 1.2 and 1.3 are hysterically petty. Although it is typical of Brutus that he does not recognise Cassius for what he is, Caesar analyses him with great perceptiveness in his famous remarks on his enemy's 'lean and hungry look. . . . Such men as he be never at heart's ease / Whiles they behold a greater than themselves, / And therefore are they very dangerous' (1.2.191, 205–207).

Cassius knows that Brutus' sense of honour makes him susceptible to manipulation, and his soliloquy at the close of 1.2 reveals his intention to seduce Brutus into leading the conspiracy against Caesar. This speech presents Cassius as a MACHIAVEL, the typical political villain of ELIZABETHAN DRAMA. It also pointedly contrasts Cassius' cynical scheming with Brutus' honourable motives (though these are seriously questioned elsewhere), and it thus establishes two possible points of view towards the assassination of Caesar.

Cassius has an unstable personality. He rages over trifles like Caesar's poor swimming and susceptibility to illness (1.2.99–130). During the assassination, he loses his nerve and Brutus has to reassure him that POPILIUS does not know of their plot. In 5.1.71–89 he wavers in the face of unfavourable omens before PHILIPPI. His weakness has great consequences, for it causes him to give in to Brutus' insistence that Antony should be spared and then permitted to speak at Caesar's funeral. Later, he similarly accedes to Brutus' strategy at Philippi with equally catastrophic results. Cassius' death at Philippi, when he too hastily believes a report of defeat, reflects this character flaw; a stronger man would have resisted longer.

However, in Acts 4 and 5 Cassius is generally a finer figure than he is before the assassination. He is an experienced and sensible general, although he permits himself to be overruled, and he attracts the loyalty and admiration of his officers. He displays a touching affection for Brutus, especially when he learns of his friend's grief over the death of PORTIA (2), and he generously forgives Brutus his fatal errors. When they exchange farewells before the battle, in 5.1.116–122, their mutual affection rings true, reflecting Shakespeare's constant inclination to believe that people are not wholly bad.

The historical Cassius was noted in his own day for his violent temper and sarcastic speech, as is reflected in Shakespeare's source, PLUTARCH's *Lives,* and other ancient documents. Before the time of the play, Cassius had fought against Caesar in an earlier civil war, and Caesar had forgiven him. He apparently originated the plot against Caesar; his motives are unclear, though Shakespeare followed Plutarch's contention that his private dislike for Caesar stimulated his public hatred of tyranny. Shakespeare's account of Cassius' death at Philippi is also accurately retold from Plutarch. However, other sources indicate that Brutus and Cassius did not disagree on the decision to march to Philippi; their forces were supported by the local population, while Antony and OCTAVIUS were short of supplies. The loss of Cassius was decisive. Shakespeare compressed two battles of Philippi, which actually occurred 20 days apart, into one; it is thought that Cassius, a more experienced general than Brutus, would not have fought the second one, in which the forces of Caesar's assassins were finally defeated.

Casson, Lewis (1875–1969) British actor and producer. After a successful career as an actor, Casson turned to production and was especially known for staging ancient Greek drama and Shakespeare, usually in collaboration with his wife, the actress Sybil THORNDIKE. Particularly noteworthy was his 1938 production of *Coriolanus,* starring Thorndike and Laurence OLIVIER, which is widely credited for establishing the play's place in the British theatrical repertory.

Cardinal (4) Pandulph Character in *King John.* See PANDULPH.

Castelnuovo-Tedesco, Mario (1895–1968) Italian composer with a particular interest in Shakespeare. Castelnuovo-Tedesco wrote music in a variety of forms, and was the composer of five operas, two of them based on Shakespeare's plays—*All's Well That Ends Well* (1958) and *The Merchant of Venice* (1961). He also wrote overtures to five more of the plays and settings for all of the SONGS. After 1938 the composer lived in Hollywood, where he wrote music for numerous films.

Castiglione, Baldassare (1478–1529) Italian writer and diplomat, author of *Il Libro del Cortegiano* (*The Book of the Courtier,* 1528), a possible influence on *Much Ado About Nothing.* Castiglione, a nobleman of MANTUA, was a highly successful diplomat, serving the Montefeltro family, dukes of Urbino. When they were dispossessed of their dukedom by the pope in 1516, Castiglione returned to Mantua and served as the city's envoy to Rome. His famous book, on which he worked for 20 years, is one of the most important documents of the Italian RENAISSANCE. In it he describes an ideal courtly society, set in the ducal court of Urbino, renowned in his day as one of the most artistic and intellectually accomplished courts of Europe. Castiglione's vision of excellence included the idea—revolutionary at the time—that women have much to contribute to society. To illustrate this point, he composed a series of sprightly debates between a man and a woman that may well have inspired the battles of wit between BEA-

TRICE and BENEDICK in *Much Ado. Il Libro del Cortegiano* was translated into English by Sir Thomas HOBY (1), appearing in 1561 as *The Courtyer.* Shakespeare may have read Castiglione in Italian, however.

Catesby, Sir William (d. 1485) Historical figure and character in *Richard III,* a follower of King RICHARD III. Catesby is a useful underling who appears in many scenes, mostly as a messenger, and he lacks a distinct personality. The historical Catesby was a lawyer who served as estate manager for Lord HASTINGS (3). He was captured and executed after the battle of BOSWORTH FIELD.

Catherine See KATHARINE.

Cathness (Caithness), Thorfin Sigurdsson, Earl of (active 1014–1065) Historical figure and minor character in *Macbeth,* a Scottish nobleman. In 5.2 Cathness, with MENTETH, ANGUS, and LENOX, marches to join the army led by MALCOLM and MACDUFF against MACBETH. In 5.4 they prepare to march on DUNSINANE, though Cathness does not speak. This Scottish soldier helps to suggest the play's national scope, for the rebellion of which he is a part results in the restoration of good government and social stability in SCOTLAND.

The historical Earl of Caithness was in fact a Viking lord, the powerful independent ruler of the Orkney and Hebrides Islands and parts of mainland Scotland, including Caithness on the northernmost coast. Known as Thorfin the Mighty, he is also a minor figure in *King Harald's Saga,* a classic of medieval Norse literature. His daughter (or possibly his sister) later married Malcolm.

Catling, Simon Character in *Romeo and Juliet.* See MUSICIANS (2).

Cato Minor character in *Julius Caesar,* soldier in the army of BRUTUS (4). In 5.4.4, at the battle of PHILIPPI, Cato's bold battle cry declares that his father was Marcus Cato, a famous opponent of CAESAR (1). He is killed shortly afterwards. Shakespeare took this gallant but fatal exploit—a motif popular with Elizabethan audiences—from PLUTARCH's *Lives.* Cato's sister was Brutus' wife, PORTIA (2).

Cawdor, Thane of In *Macbeth,* a noble title forfeited by a defeated rebel against King DUNCAN of SCOTLAND and granted, with its lands and income, to MACBETH as a reward for valour in 1.2.67. Thereafter, the title refers to Macbeth, though he does not know of this development when the WITCHES predict, in 1.3, that he will become Thane of Cawdor and then king. When he receives Cawdor's title the reinforcement of the prophecy stimulates his ambition to be king. The title thus comes to carry a reference to the aura of evil that attends Macbeth's rise to power. The original Cawdor's repentant acceptance of his execution is reported to Duncan with the famous remark, 'Nothing in his life / Became him like the leaving it' (1.4.7–8). In this the first Cawdor contrasts with his successor, Macbeth, who struggles to preserve his life even after it has become a burden and he is 'aweary of the sun' (5.5.49). On the other hand, there is also irony in the resemblance between the two, as the rebel yields his title to a man who thereupon becomes a usurper himself.

Caxton, William (c. 1422–1491) English translator and printer. In 1475 Caxton produced the first book printed in English, *The Recuyell of the Historyes of Troye,* his own translation (from a French version) of Guido delle COLONNE's Latin history of the TROJAN WAR. This work, probably in its 5th edition (1596), provided Shakespeare with much of the detail for his account of the war in *Troilus and Cressida.* Caxton also translated and published, in 1484, a French tale that may have inspired the husbands' wager on their wives' obedience in 5.2 of *The Taming of the Shrew.*

Caxton, who is known as the father of English printing, began as an apprentice to a cloth merchant. A capable businessman, he became the representative of the Merchants' Guild in the busy European commercial centre at Bruges, eventually being appointed governor of the English commercial and diplomatic colony. In 1469 Caxton became an adviser to the Duchess of Burgundy; as such he had the leisure to devote to literature, and he began his translating career. He also learned printing while in the Duchess' employ, and the *Recuyell* was printed in Bruges. He returned to England in 1476 and continued publishing until his death. His publications (more than 100 titles, including many of CHAUCER's works) were extremely influential on English literature for more than a century.

Cecil (1), Robert, Earl of Salisbury (1563–1612) Elizabethan and Jacobean statesman, one of the most powerful men in Shakespeare's England. The son of Lord BURGHLEY, Cecil was intended for statesmanship from his youth. He was an enemy of the Earl of ESSEX (2) in the 1590s, but after Essex's attempted rebellion, Cecil intervened to save the Earl of SOUTHAMPTON (2), Essex's follower and Shakespeare's patron, from the death penalty. Cecil was acting secretary of state before he turned 30, and he held the office officially from 1596 until just before his death, thus controlling English foreign policy for almost 20 years. He helped prepare for the peaceful accession of King JAMES I in 1603, for which he was rewarded with great wealth and high rank, becoming the first Earl of Salisbury in 1605. After 1608 he effectively ran the government. He was responsible for the downfall of Sir Walter RALEIGH in 1606, but eventually his political rivals brought him

down the same way, by poisoning the king's opinion of him. He fell from favour in 1611, dying not long thereafter.

Cecil spent much of his money on the patronage of art, including the creation of one of the finest Jacobean mansions, Hatfield House. His father is sometimes thought to have been a model for POLONIUS, in part because of the letters of moralistic advice he sent to the young Cecil. If so, Cecil's resemblance to the impulsive fighter LAERTES stops there, for the Earl of Salisbury was deformed and physically weak while being entirely in control of himself emotionally and intellectually.

Cecil (2), Thomas (1542–1623) Soldier, opponent of the Earl of ESSEX (2). The eldest son of Lord BURGHLEY, Cecil led a notoriously dissolute life in Paris and Germany before taking up a military career. He served with distinction in Scotland and the Netherlands and at sea against the Spanish Armada. In 1599 he was appointed military governor of northern England; visiting London while on leave from this post in February 1601, Cecil improvised the military opposition to Essex' abortive uprising, crushing it immediately.

Cecil (3), William See BURGHLEY.

Celia Character in *As You Like It*, ROSALIND's cousin and friend, daughter of DUKE (1) FREDERICK. Celia is a secondary but important figure. In 1.3 she defies her tyrannical father when he banishes Rosalind; her spirited loyalty and sense of morality trigger the central action of the play, the two women's flight to the Forest of ARDEN (1). Thereafter, Celia listens to the disguised Rosalind's professions of love for ORLANDO, which she cannot otherwise express while disguised as a man. Celia responds skeptically in remarks such as, '. . . the oath of a lover is no stronger than the word of a tapster' (3.4.27–28), which maintain the play's ironic stance towards romance until the climactic resolution.

When Celia herself is betrothed to OLIVER (1) in Act 5, the triumph of love is complete. The marriage of the chaste Celia to the once-villainous Oliver has been criticised as unrealistic, unfair to Celia, and unduly generous to Oliver. However, the union is largely symbolic in intent. It serves to confirm the sincerity of Oliver's repentance, and it contributes greatly to the spirit of reconciliation that closes the play.

Censorship Governmental regulation of plays and other works. In Shakespeare's England, plays had to be submitted to the MASTER OF REVELS, who often required revisions both large and small before granting the required licence. After 1606 his powers were extended to the publication of plays as well. As early as 1559, Queen ELIZABETH (1) prohibited the dramatic treatment of religious or political issues. It is believed that the absence of the 'deposition scene' of *Richard II* (4.1) from the first three editions of the play is a result of this law. (As late as 1680, Nahum TATE's adaptation of *Richard II* was suppressed by the government, despite his attempt to disguise the work as *The Sicilian Usurper.*) The 1606 statute—called an 'Act to Restrain Abuses of Players'—outlawed the slightest profanity, and this feature is reflected in many of Shakespeare's plays, where such expletives as 'God', which appear in the earliest published versions, are replaced with 'Jove' or 'heavens' in the FIRST FOLIO (1623).

Sometimes the texts reveal self-censorship practised by the playwright or the acting companies. While not strictly censorship, in not being imposed, the excisions might not have been made but for the possibility of trouble with the authorities. For instance, some scholars believe that a passage deleted from Q2 of *Hamlet*—2.2.335–358, mocking the CHILDREN'S COMPANIES—was removed for fear that it might offend the new king, JAMES I, who had just taken a children's company under royal protection. Another passage, on the drunkenness of Danes (1.4.17–38), does not appear in the FOLIO edition of the play, perhaps to avoid giving offence to King James' queen, Anne of Denmark.

An informal, quasi-governmental censorship sometimes operated alongside the official system, as when pressure from an offended aristocrat apparently brought about the change of a notable character's name from OLDCASTLE to FALSTAFF (see COBHAM). Such efforts were unusual, but their effectiveness was ensured by the threat of official censorship, for the government frequently used a heavy censorial hand. For instance, when a play by Thomas NASHE, *Isle of Dogs* (1597; now lost), was declared seditious, all the LONDON theatres were closed for the summer and three of the actors were given gaol sentences. In 1605 George CHAPMAN and Ben JONSON were gaoled because their play *Eastward Ho!* contained passages that offended King James. (Jonson had been one of the three *Isle of Dogs* actors.) The ultimate form of state censorship came from the STUART DYNASTY's opposition, however, when the revolutionary Puritan government outlawed the theatre at the outset of the Civil Wars in 1642. Drama of any sort (excepting 'opera', see DAVENANT) was illegal until the restoration of the monarchy in 1660.

Ceres Pagan goddess and minor figure in *The Tempest*, a character in the MASQUE presented by the sprite ARIEL, at PROSPERO's orders, to celebrate the engagement of MIRANDA and FERDINAND (2). Ceres, goddess of harvests, is presented by IRIS but declares she will not participate unless she can be assured that Venus and Cupid will not be present. This reminds us of Prospero's insistence on Miranda's virginity before marriage, part of the play's theme of moral discipline.

Once reassured, Ceres joins JUNO in singing a hymn of blessing, wishing 'Earth's increase, foison [abundance] plenty' (4.1.110) for the couple.

In ancient mythology Ceres—from whose name comes our word *cereal*—was a pre-Roman corn-goddess. She became identified with the Greek goddess Demeter, who governed all fruits of the earth, especially grain. According to a central myth of the classical world, Ceres' daughter was stolen by the god of the underworld; the goddess responded by withholding her bounty until a compromise was achieved: her daughter spends half the year in the underworld, during which time Ceres resumes her grief and winter rules. In *The Tempest* Ceres blames Venus and Cupid for her daughter's theft, following the account given in OVID's *Metamorphosis* (the same incident is referred to in *The Winter's Tale* 4.4.116–118).

Cerimon, Lord Character in *Pericles*, a nobleman and physician of EPHESUS who revives the seemingly dead THAISA. Cerimon's benevolence as well as his expertise as a scientist is conveyed in his conversation with two neighbours (see GENTLEMAN [9]), in 3.2. He assists a SERVANT (26) who has suffered the great storm of the night before—the storm during which the unconscious Thaisa was mistakenly buried at sea, in 3.1—and he speaks of his long study of 'physic, [the] secret art [of] the blest infusions / That dwells in vegetives, in metals, stones' (3.2.32–36). Today, we might call him an alchemist. He revives Thaisa by invoking the spirit of Aesculapius, the Greek god of healing, which suggests ancient medical wisdom. Cerimon guides Thaisa to the famous Temple of DIANA (2)—one of the most important ancient pagan temples—when the revived queen, certain she will never see her husband again, desires 'a vestal livery' (3.4.9). In 5.3 when Thaisa, by then a high priestess at the Temple, is reunited with PERICLES, Cerimon is there, and, as the only calm person present, is able to confirm Thaisa's story. This kind and intelligent scholar foreshadows Shakespeare's last great protagonist, the magician PROSPERO of *The Tempest*.

Cervantes Saavedra, Miguel de (1547–1616) Spanish novelist, author of *Don Quixote* (1605–1615), a probable influence on the lost play CARDENIO, possibly by Shakespeare and John FLETCHER (2). The first part of *Don Quixote* was translated into English by Thomas Shelton (active 1612–1620) and published in 1612. A story within it is presumed to be the source for *Cardenio*, and Fletcher used Cervantes' work as inspiration for several of his own plays.

Cervantes had an adventurous military career: he lost a hand at the battle of Lepanto (1571), was later captured, and spent five years as a slave in Algiers before returning to Spain in 1580. He was disappointed not to receive a lucrative appointment as a reward and was reduced to extreme poverty. He struggled through his later life as a petty government employee—he was once gaoled for irregularities in handling funds—but he nevertheless managed to write a number of plays, poems, and novels, including the only one that was successful in his own time, the masterpiece for which he is still famous. He died on the same day as Shakespeare.

Cesario In *Twelfth Night*, name taken by VIOLA in her disguise as a young man.

Chamberlain (1) Minor character in *1 Henry IV*, an inn employee who scouts for the highwayman GADSHILL. In 2.1 the Chamberlain tells Gadshill of two likely victims who are staying at his inn and who will soon be leaving for LONDON. He is promised a share in the highwayman's take. In 2.2 Gadshill, FALSTAFF, and others rob the unfortunate TRAVELLERS. In Shakespeare's day the employees of inns were generally mistrusted, and contemporary writings describe many instances of this particular arrangement among thieves.

Chamberlain (2), Lord Character in *Henry VIII*, an official of King HENRY VIII's household, overseer of the king's travel, entertainment, and wardrobe. In 1.4 he assists Sir Henry GUILFORD with Cardinal WOLSEY's banquet, where he introduces the king to ANNE (1) BULLEN. In 2.2 and 3.2 he appears briefly as a plotter against Wolsey with the Dukes of NORFOLK (3) and SUFFOLK (1), and in 5.2 he is a member of the royal council, though he speaks only a few lines. In 5.3 he helps prepare for the christening of Princess ELIZABETH (1). Throughout he is representative of the elaborate world of courtly entertainment. Historically, the Chamberlain was Sir William SANDS, but Shakespeare mistakenly gave that nobleman another part in the play.

Chamberlain's Men Acting company of the ELIZABETHAN THEATRE, troupe in which Shakespeare was a partner. Though Shakespeare may have been involved with various other acting companies (see ADMIRAL'S MEN, DERBY'S MEN, LEICESTER'S MEN, PEMBROKE'S MEN, QUEEN'S MEN [1], STRANGE'S MEN, and SUSSEX'S MEN), he is most closely associated with the Chamberlain's Men (known as the KING'S MEN after the accession of King JAMES I in 1603). He was a partner in this troupe from at least December of 1594 until his retirement almost 20 years later.

The Chamberlain's Men was created in the spring of 1594 as a reorganisation of Derby's Men—originally Strange's Men—following the death of Lord Ferdinando STRANGE, the patron of the company. A patron was legally necessary for an acting company, so

Henry Carey, Baron HUNSDON (2), agreed to place the actors under his protection. Since Lord Hunsdon was the Lord Chamberlain to Queen ELIZABETH (1), the company was known thereafter as the Chamberlain's Men. In July 1596, when the Lord Chamberlain died, his son, also Lord HUNSDON (1), became patron of the company, which was briefly known as HUNSDON'S MEN. However, Hunsdon became Chamberlain himself, in March 1597, and the troupe resumed its old name.

The earliest surviving mention of the Chamberlain's Men records an appearance at NEWINGTON BUTTS in June 1594, though it soon moved to the THEATRE, whose owner, James BURBAGE (2), had earlier been part of a provincial company patronised by Hunsdon. The original partners in the Chamberlain's Men were probably George BRYAN, Richard COWLEY, John HEMINGE (who functioned as the group's business manager), William KEMPE, Augustin PHILLIPS, Thomas POPE (2), Richard BURBAGE (3), and Shakespeare, though the last two may have joined the others later in 1594. Bryan retired sometime before 1598, and Pope did likewise around 1600. They were replaced by William SLY (2) and Henry CONDELL, both of whom had performed earlier with the company; Kempe left in 1599 (though he may have returned briefly in 1601 or 1602) and was replaced by Robert ARMIN. The makeup of the partnership did not otherwise change until after the creation of the King's Men in 1603.

The Chamberlain's Men originally played at the Theatre in summer and the CROSS KEYS INN in winter, but in 1596 the latter venue was closed by the city, and the company is thought to have moved to the SWAN THEATRE. A year later it played the CURTAIN THEATRE, and a group of the partners built their own house, the GLOBE THEATRE, in 1599; there they remained for the duration of their existence. Each year over the Christmas holidays, the troupe also performed at the court of the queen, whose invitations were a mark of success and prestige. At first their rivals, the Admiral's Men, vied closely with them for this honour, but gradually the Chamberlain's Men dominated the competition; over their nine-year lifetime, the Chamberlain's Men performed at court 32 times and the Admirals' Men only 20. The Chamberlain's Men specialised in plays by their own Shakespeare, though they also performed a number of Ben JONSON's dramas as well as occasional works by others, including Thomas DEKKER and John MARSTON. (For the history of the troupe after 1603, see KING'S MEN.)

Chambers, Edmund Kerchever (1866–1954) English scholar, author of several standard works on Shakespeare and the ELIZABETHAN THEATRE. Chambers was a civil servant who also wrote dramatic criticism. In the 1890s he began writing a small book on Shakespeare that eventually grew to become *The Medieval Stage* (2 vol., 1903), *The Elizabethan Stage* (4 vol., 1923), and *William Shakespeare: A Study of the Facts and Problems* (2 vol., 1930). He also produced critical editions of Francis BEAUMONT (2), John Donne (1572–1631), John FLETCHER (2), John MILTON, and others. He wrote biographies of Matthew Arnold (1822–1888) and Samuel Taylor COLERIDGE, and he edited the *Shakespeare Allusion Book* (1932) (see INGLEBY).

Chancellor Minor character in *Henry VIII*, the highest-ranking official of King HENRY VIII's government and keeper of the Great Seal of England, used to signify royal approval of any document. In 5.2 the Chancellor chairs the meeting of the royal council at which Bishop GARDINER attacks Archbishop CRANMER. He sides with Gardiner, but when the king intervenes for Cranmer, the Chancellor declares that their intention was simply to provide the archbishop with a chance to clear his name. He typifies the malevolence that the king overcomes in the final political episode of the play.

We hear in 3.2.393–394 that Sir Thomas MORE has succeeded Cardinal WOLSEY as Chancellor, but Shakespeare's Chancellor is nameless. In fact, More held the office for only three years, and the Chancellor at the time of 4.1 and 5.2 was Sir Thomas Audley (1488–1544). However, the specific identification is immaterial; the Chancellor is present simply as a representative of the highest levels of government.

Chandos portrait Possible portrait of Shakespeare. The Chandos portrait—named for its long-time owners, the Dukes of Chandos—was traditionally said to have been painted by Richard BURBAGE (3) and given by the artist to Joseph TAYLOR, who in turn bequeathed it to William DAVENANT. However, modern scholars find this tradition improbable. Taylor was 20 years younger than Burbage and not connected with him professionally—he only joined the KING'S MEN after the older man had died. It is therefore unlikely that he was intimate with Burbage. Moreover, he left nothing to Davenant or anyone else, for he died intestate. Nevertheless, the Chandos portrait is a quite competent portrait, almost certainly painted from life—unlike either of the two portraits regarded as authoritative (see DROESHOUT; JANSSEN [2]). However, since it only vaguely resembles the authoritative likenesses, the identity of the sitter is questionable, at best. The Chandos portrait was widely considered to be a picture of Shakespeare until well into the 19th century, and some commentators still argue that it is possibly genuine. In 1856 it became the first possession of the fledgling British National Portrait Gallery. It was the basis for Peter SCHEEMAKER's statue of Shakespeare in WESTMINSTER (1) ABBEY, and a copy of it, painted for John DRYDEN by the renowned portraitist Sir Godfrey

Kneller (1646–1723), now hangs in the FOLGER LIBRARY.

Chapman, George (c. 1559–1634) English poet and playwright, a major figure in both ELIZABETHAN and JACOBEAN DRAMA, a noted translator of HOMER, and the author of minor sources for *The Merry Wives of Windsor* and *Troilus and Cressida.* Chapman may have been the model for the character HOLOFERNES in *Love's Labour's Lost,* and he is sometimes identified with the 'rival poet' of the SONNETS. Scholars who believe that many of Shakespeare's works were written in part by other playwrights (see, e.g., FLEAY and ROBERTSON) have attributed to Chapman passages or whole scenes in a number of the plays, especially *All's Well That Ends Well, Measure for Measure,* and *Troilus and Cressida;* however, modern scholars dispute most such attributions.

Chapman was a melancholy and disputatious man who made many enemies, possibly including Shakespeare, for some scholars believe that the playwright satirised him as the pedantic Holofernes. In any case Chapman's book-length philosophical poem *The Shadow of Night* (1594) is probably alluded to several times in the obscure jests that stud *Love's Labour's Lost,* and the drama may have been conceived as an answer to *The Shadow of Night*'s denigration of pleasure and practicality in favour of a contemplative life. Shakespeare exploited Chapman in other works. NYM's comical use of the word *humour* in *The Merry Wives of Windsor* is borrowed from Chapman's highly successful COMEDY OF HUMOURS, *The Blind Beggar of Alexandria* (1596), and several passages in *Troilus and Cressida* echo Chapman's initial partial translation of Homer's *Iliad* (1598). Some scholars believe that the latter play was also intended to counter Chapman, who rejected the usual English view that favoured the Trojans in the TROJAN WAR.

Chapman's only literary friends appear to have been the equally acerbic Ben JONSON and Thomas MARSTON. His embittered bellicosity emerged in his writing, sometimes with disastrous effects. In 1605 he and Jonson were briefly gaoled when King JAMES I took offence at remarks about SCOTLAND in their play *Eastward Ho!* (1605, written with Marston). He encountered government CENSORSHIP again in 1608, over another play, and he retired from the theatre to concentrate on his translation of Homer, which was only completed in 1615. This was his masterpiece and remained the standard English version for generations, though it is full of inaccuracies and has long been superseded.

Although Chapman was more a poet than a playwright, Francis MERES classed him as a leading writer of both COMEDY and TRAGEDY. *The Blind Beggar of Alexandria* (his first play) was a great success, and his tragedy *Bussy D'Ambois* (1607) is still performed occasionally today. However, despite the appreciative opinions of his contemporaries, Chapman's works are largely ignored by modern readers. He is now probably best known for John KEATS' great sonnet, 'On First Looking into Chapman's Homer'.

Charles Minor character in *As You Like It,* a wrestler. Charles is a professional performer who takes on all comers, under the patronage of the aristocratic OLIVER (1). In 1.1 Oliver's younger brother ORLANDO proposes to challenge Charles at a forthcoming festival, and Oliver falsely informs Charles that Orlando, by nature an evil man, intends to kill him. He promises Charles that he will not be punished if Orlando dies instead, and the wrestler assures Oliver that this will be the outcome. In 1.2, however, Orlando defeats Charles soundly. This scene helps to establish Orlando as an hero. Charles also introduces a major theme in 1.1, informing us—and Oliver—of the fact that DUKE (7) Senior, having been deposed and exiled by his brother, DUKE (1) Frederick, has set up a court in the Forest of ARDEN (1).

Shakespeare derived his wrestler from his source, Thomas LODGE's *Rosalynde,* but toned down the character considerably. The original, an inhumanly strong and cruel villain, takes a bribe to kill Orlando's counterpart, but Charles is led to believe he will be in the right to do so; Lodge's wrestler kills his earlier opponents outright, while Charles' survive. Lodge made much of the contrast between his hero and the gigantic, villainous wrestler; Shakespeare's Charles is a more neutral figure who is simply defeated for the good of the plot.

Charles VI, King of France Character in *Henry V.* See FRENCH KING.

Charles VII, King of France (1403–1461) Historical figure and character in *1 Henry VI.* The historical Charles VII became King of FRANCE (1) upon the death of his father CHARLES VI, as is recorded in 1.1. However, he is throughout the play referred to as the Dauphin (sometimes rendered as Dolphin), a title traditionally applied to the eldest son of a French monarch and not to a king. This reflects the historical English position that the treaties following the conquests of HENRY V gave the French crown to the English king. Charles' enthronement was therefore an act of rebellion, and the French subsequently drove the English from their lands.

In the play, Charles is not readily distinguishable from the other French noblemen, who are all depicted as boastful but inept, treacherous, and cowardly warriors. Charles moons lovingly over JOAN LA PUCELLE at first—for instance, in 1.2.110–117—but he is quick to turn on her at the first misadventure of their campaign (2.1.50–53). In his final scene (5.4), he takes the advice of his nobles and agrees to a peace treaty with the intention of violating it later. (Historically, the treaty

referred to was a mere truce, followed by the fighting—already undergone in the play—that drove the English out of France.)

Charmian Character in *Antony and Cleopatra,* an attendant of CLEOPATRA. In 1.2 Charmian is pleasantly humorous as she banters with her friends ALEXAS and IRAS over the predictions of the SOOTHSAYER (2), and one can understand Cleopatra's obvious fondness for her. The queen addresses Charmian more intimately and much more often than she does her other servants. She confides in her and permits her to offer advice, even if she usually rejects it. Charmian reminisces with her mistress about fishing expeditions she took with ANTONY, in 2.5.15–18; she also boldly attempts to restrain the queen's temper when she says, 'Good madam, keep yourself within yourself' (2.5.75), and she teases her about her past affair with Julius CAESAR (1), in 1.5.67–73. Charmian is a spirited, attractive young woman of a type that Shakespeare often depicted.

In 4.13, however, it is Charmian who makes the ill-fated suggestion that Cleopatra let Antony believe she has committed suicide. This is perhaps a device whereby Shakespeare intended to remove blame from the queen, whose transition from courtesan to transcendent lover is about to take place. Charmian herself undergoes such a change along with her mistress, fulfilling the Soothsayer's prediction that she 'shall be yet far fairer' (1.2.16) than she already is. Her loyalty takes on a grandeur as she accompanies her mistress' grave poetry with cries of grief—'Dissolve, thick cloud, and rain, that I may say, / The gods themselves do weep' (5.2.298–299)—and she cries out to the queen with almost religious intensity, 'O eastern star!' (5.2.307). When Cleopatra dies, Charmian touchingly straightens her mistress' crown before she kills herself in the same way. As she dies, she proudly declares to a Roman soldier that Cleopatra's suicide 'is well done, and fitting for a princess / Descended of so many royal kings' (5.2.325–326). Her coda to Cleopatra's grand declaration of ultimate love adds an echo of ecstasy before Caesar's final triumph.

Shakespeare adapted Charmian from a mere mention in his source, PLUTARCH's *Lives,* and developed the character greatly. Plutarch states that Cleopatra was attended at her death by a serving-woman named Charmian, but this person is otherwise unknown in history.

Chatillon (Chatillion) Minor character in *King John,* the ambassador of King PHILIP (2) of FRANCE (1) to King JOHN (3). A haughty lord, Chatillon opens the play by delivering an ultimatum to John in terms that are obviously meant to be insulting. He reappears only briefly, bearing the news of John's invasion of France in 2.1; while belittling the English, he must speak of their military success. Chatillon's role helps to develop a strong sense of the arrogance of power, heightening the impact of treachery in high places, one of the play's major themes.

Chatterton, Frederick Balsir (1831–1886) English theatrical producer. Between 1863 and 1879, F. B. Chatterton was manager of the Drury Lane Theatre in London, and he was a notable promoter of Shakespeare's plays, especially as presented by Samuel PHELPS. Unfortunately, these productions were not generally profitable, and Chatterton is remembered for a famous witticism, inspired by a production of an ephemeral play by the poet Byron: 'Shakespeare spells ruin and Byron bankruptcy'.

Chaucer, Geoffrey (c. 1340–1400) English poet, Shakespeare's greatest predecessor and the author of sources for several of the plays. Chaucer's *Troilus and Criseyde* was the main source for the Trojan scenes in *Troilus and Cressida.* The same work taught Shakespeare about leitmotifs—recurring images that provide a sense of aesthetic continuity in a work whose tone changes considerably—a technique that he used in *Romeo and Juliet* and elsewhere. Moreover, *Troilus and Criseyde* had influenced the *Romeus* of Arthur BROOKE (1), the chief source for *Romeo and Juliet,* and Chaucer's *Parliament of Fowles* provided material for MERCUTIO's 'Queen MAB' speech in the same play. Chaucer's 'The Knight's Tale' in *The Canterbury Tales* was the main source for *The Two Noble Kinsmen* and for parts of *A Midsummer Night's Dream.* 'The Merchant's Tale' and 'Sir Tophas' from *The Canterbury Tales* contributed further details to the *Dream.* The personality of the HOST (2) in *The Merry Wives of Windsor* was probably influenced by Chaucer's innkeeper in *The Canterbury Tales.* Lastly, various works of Chaucer provided minor details in other plays (e.g., *2 Henry VI* 3.2.115–116).

Chaucer was the son of a vintner with connections to the court of King Edward III (ruled 1327–1377), and he is first recorded as a teenaged page to the Duke of Clarence, the king's son, with whom he went to war in FRANCE (1) at the outset of the HUNDRED YEARS WAR. For the rest of his life he was an employee of the royal courts in one way or another, mostly as an official of the customs service. His greatest patron was John of GAUNT (who appears in *Richard II*), probably because he married a sister of Katherine Swynford, Gaunt's long-time mistress and eventual wife (although the identity of Chaucer's wife remains obscure). Little is known of Chaucer's private life, though passages in his works suggest that he was improvident and a bad administrator, that he had an unhappy marriage but a loving mistress (by whom he probably had a son), and that he possessed a sunny disposition. He had many

friends—among them the poet John GOWER (3)—who attested to his virtues.

Chaucer, who wrote in Middle English (an early dialect), was the first great poet in English and is still considered among the finest English poets of all time. His works cannot be dated precisely as they were not published until after his death (printing did not exist in his lifetime). Nevertheless, his career can be divided into periods. Among his best-known early works is *The Book of the Duchess;* his middle period—following two trips to Italy in the 1370s, when he encountered the works of Dante and BOCCACCIO—produced *The Legend of Good Women, The Parliament of Fowles,* and *Troilus and Criseyde.* Chaucer's final period encompasses the composition of one of the masterworks of the English language, the unfinished *Canterbury Tales.* These lively, often bawdy stories are supposedly told by various pilgrims on their way to the shrine at Canterbury. Though difficult to read without practice, the *Tales* are immensely gratifying, filled with sharp character studies, sly asides on human behaviour, and inimitable descriptions. After his death, Chaucer was the first poet to be buried in what became the famous 'poet's corner' in WESTMINSTER (1) ABBEY.

Chettle, Henry (c. 1560–c. 1607) English printer and dramatist. As a printer, Chettle (briefly a partner of John DANTER) is best known for having published *Groatsworth of Wit* (1592) by Robert GREENE (2), which contains a denunciation of Shakespeare as an arrogant young plagiarist, the first published reference to the playwright. Chettle, who had apparently edited Greene's work, subsequently apologised for it in a pamphlet of his own, and wrote that he knew Shakespeare to be an honest man and a good writer. Chettle had turned to writing plays by 1598, when he was mentioned by Francis MERES as a fine writer of comedies, and he is known to have written or collaborated on at least 48 dramas—one of them being SIR THOMAS MORE—for the ADMIRAL'S MEN and Philip HENSLOWE.

Chester, Robert See LOVE'S MARTYR.

Chichele, Henry, Archbishop of Canterbury Character in *Henry V.* See CANTERBURY (1).

Chief Justice, Lord Character in *2 Henry IV,* the highest-ranking judicial officer of England. The Chief Justice chastises FALSTAFF twice. In 1.2 he observes that only Falstaff's success at the battle of SHREWSBURY has kept him from being prosecuted for the highway robbery at GAD'S HILL in *1 Henry IV,* and he warns the knight against continuing his dissolute life. In 2.1 he orders Falstaff to repay a debt to the HOSTESS (2). In both cases the Chief Justice has enough intelligence and humour to appreciate Falstaff's wit and to recognise that the fat knight cannot be cajoled into an honest life, but his own sense of public morality urges him to make the attempt.

In 1.2.55–56 Falstaff's PAGE (5) calls the Chief Justice 'the nobleman that committed the Prince for striking him about Bardolph', referring to an earlier imprisonment of PRINCE (6) HAL. In 5.2, after HENRY IV's death, the Chief Justice expects to find the new King vengeful, but when he defends his action, noting that he was right to follow the law irrespective of the offender's rank, the former Prince approves entirely and confirms him in his office. The young King asserts that he will be guided by the justice, and when he rejects Falstaff in 5.5, his formal diction seems to reflect the judge's influence. The Chief Justice later implements Hal's decision to banish Falstaff.

The story of Hal's assault on the Chief Justice was part of the popular legend of 'wild Prince Hal': he is said to have been reprimanded by the justice for seeking a favourable ruling on behalf of a delinquent acquaintance, whereupon he struck the judge and was gaoled for it; as in the play, he maintained the justice in office upon becoming Henry V. However, this tale is almost surely fictitious; the earliest written reference to any such event did not appear until 1531, more than a century later, in Thomas ELYOT's *The Boke named the Gouernour.* Moreover, Elyot reports no assault, merely the Justice's reprimand, which the Prince accepted meekly. The assault and incarceration occur only in THE FAMOUS VICTORIES, a 16th-century farce that has no historical validity whatsoever. Shakespeare doubtless knew this, but the tale was too dramatic to waste. The Chief Justice of Hal's day, unnamed in the play or in any of Shakespeare's sources, was Sir William Gascoigne (c. 1350–1419), a distinguished jurist who had long served King Henry IV, having been his attorney when he was in exile as Henry BOLINGBROKE (1) (as enacted in *Richard II*). As King Henry's chief legal officer, Gascoigne had presided over the sentencing and execution of the rebels captured at GAULTREE, although Shakespeare does not associate him with this event in 4.3 of the play.

Children Minor characters in *The Merry Wives of Windsor* who imitate fairies and elves to torment FALSTAFF in 5.5. ANNE (3), WILLIAM (1), and other Children, disguised as diminutive supernatural beings, help to carry out MISTRESS (3) Page's plot for the final humiliation of Falstaff, devised in 4.4.28–64. When the lecherous Falstaff meets Mistress Page and MISTRESS (1) Ford in the forest, seeking double adultery, the Children appear, led by Mistress QUICKLY, PISTOL, and EVANS (3). They dance in a circle (while ceremonial references to the Order of the Garter are made—see *The Merry Wives of Windsor,* 'Text of the Play'), and they hold candles to Falstaff and pinch him, while singing a song condemning 'lust and luxury' (5.5.95).

Children's Companies English acting companies in the 16th and 17th centuries composed of boys. Before the ELIZABETHAN THEATRE became well established in the 1570s, professional companies tended to be troupes of acrobats and mimes, more appropriate to a country fair than to the court of Queen ELIZABETH (1). There, entertainment was often provided by schoolboys from Eton and Westminster, and by the Chapel Royal, a boys' choir that provided schooling for the boys it recruited from church choirs around the country. These groups traditionally staged plays in Latin (the language of their education). The Chapel Royal even had its own dramatic company, known as the Children of the Chapel, as early as the 1520s. In the 1550s two more such groups were created, the Children of Paul's at the school attached to St Paul's Cathedral and the Children of Windsor at the church grammar school in WINDSOR. These groups were very popular at the queen's court: in the first 20 years of Elizabeth's reign, boys performed at court half again as often as did men. Though composed of children, these companies performed plays written for adults and featuring adult characters.

However, by the late 1570s, the adult troupes had become legitimate theatre companies. LEICESTER'S MEN became favourites at court, and one member, James BURBAGE (2), built the first LONDON playhouse, the THEATRE, in 1576. The children's companies appeared to be falling from favour, but their course also changed in 1576. The Children of Windsor and of the Chapel merged, under the direction of Richard FARRANT, who leased rooms at a former priory and created the first BLACKFRIARS THEATRE, where his boys played to the public as well as continuing to perform at court. After Farrant's death, the company was directed by William HUNNIS, but its popularity waned and play production ceased after 1584, when the landlord took back the Blackfriars building. In the final season, another children's company, patronised by the Earl of OXFORD (1), joined the troupe at Blackfriars.

From 1584 to 1600 the children's companies ceased performing plays, as the QUEEN'S MEN (1) and other professional troupes took over, though the choirs were maintained. In 1600, however, Nathaniel GILES and Henry EVANS (2) revived the Children of the Chapel as a theatre company, leasing the second Blackfriars Theatre from Richard BURBAGE (3). They were immediately popular, due in good part to the involvement of Ben JONSON, as both actor and playwright. The Children of Paul's also re-entered the theatrical arena at this time, performing at court and at the school, which had a theatre. They staged plays by George CHAPMAN, Thomas DEKKER, Thomas MIDDLETON, and John WEBSTER (2), and they too competed with the adult companies. The children's companies were fierce rivals, and their competition spilled over into the contents of the plays they staged, in the so-called WAR OF THE THEATRES—a development alluded to in *Hamlet* 2.2.326–258.

In 1602 Giles and Evans were accused of graft and the misuse of the Chapel Royal's recruiting privileges to enroll non-singers; Evans fled the country, and Giles retired from play production. Under King JAMES I, who was crowned in 1603, Evans returned to the theatre, but his connection with the Chapel Royal was severed. Instead, he and Edward KIRKHAM formed the Children of the Queen's Revels, under the patronage of the queen. However, they lost the royal favour by staging controversial plays—especially the allegedly seditious *Eastward Ho!*, by Jonson, Chapman, and Thomas MARSTON (see CENSORSHIP)—and in 1605 they changed their name to Children of the Revels, and then, at the insistence of the crown, to Children of Blackfriars.

In 1606 a new children's company entered the field, the Children of the King's Revels, owned by a group including Michael DRAYTON and managed by Martin SLATER. (This troupe may have been the Children of Paul's, reorganised, for that company disappears from the records at this time.) They performed at a new playhouse founded for the purpose, the WHITEFRIARS THEATRE. The King's Revels company was unsuccessful, however, and died in 1609, amid rancorous litigation among the partners.

In 1608 Evans' old company, now under new direction, moved to the new theatre as the Children of Whitefriars. In 1610—under yet another management group including Robert BROWNE, Richard JONES (2), and others—they were restored to royal favour and once again were known as Children of the Queen's Revels. Their chief actor and playwright was Nathan FIELD (1). This company was absorbed into LADY ELIZABETH'S MEN in 1613. Though troupes of boys were occasionally organised as late as the 1630s, the great era of the children's companies was over.

Chiron Character in *Titus Andronicus,* son of TAMORA. Chiron and his brother DEMETRIUS (1) murder BASSIANUS and then commit the horrible rape and mutilation of LAVINIA, the daughter of TITUS (1) Andronicus; they are encouraged and abetted by AARON. Titus' counter-revenge includes the killing of the two brothers, who are baked in a meat pie and served to their mother in the final scene.

Chorus (1) Dramatic device, originally from ancient Greek drama, employed by Shakespeare in various forms. A chorus is a character or allegorical figure who usually does not participate in the action of the play, but rather provides a commentary on it. He does this either by offering a critique of the actions and attitudes of the other characters or by supplying missing facts or filling in the narrative where it is not actually

enacted. Two such figures in Shakespeare are frankly designated as choruses—the CHORUS (2) of *Romeo and Juliet* and the CHORUS (3) of *Henry V*—while one allegorical figure and one named character are in fact choruses: TIME in *The Winter's Tale* and GOWER (3) in *Pericles*. Also, a number of plays have a figure designated the PROLOGUE (1), whose choric function is limited to the introduction of the action. RUMOUR *(2 Henry IV)* is also a prologue figure. In addition, some regular characters occasionally step aside from the action and speak about it in a choric manner—a good example is the BASTARD (1) of *King John*—and other characters are obviously commentators on the action without stepping back from it, as exemplified by *King Lear*'s FOOL (2), who is often figuratively referred to as a chorus.

The use of a chorus, whether frankly or subtly employed, lets the playwright establish a point of view that the characters themselves, by and large, do not share, thus bringing the audience into the play without making it identify with some characters to the exclusion of others. The chorus also invites the audience to help ensure the success of the drama by willingly engaging its own imagination and sympathies. This is especially important if the play is an allegorical spectacle like *Pericles*, whose story Gower concedes he could not 'convey / Unless your thoughts went on my way' (4.Chorus.49–50). Or, as the Chorus of *Henry V* demands, in an appropriately military tone, we must 'Follow, follow! / Grapple [our] minds to sternage of this navy' (3.Chorus.17–18).

In the Greek theatre, the chorus was a group of actors—originally 50, later as few as 12—who sang lyrical passages of commentary and explanation while dancing; their passages are also referred to as choruses. In RENAISSANCE and later plays, a chorus is usually a single character or small group who speaks similar lyrical explanatory passages. (In a more literally accurate use of the term, a chorus is also the group of singing and dancing background figures in opera or musical theatre.) The ancient Greek use of the chorus probably evolved from singing in religious ceremonies. However, the practice was not transmitted to Roman drama, where choruses appear only in SENECA's works, which were not intended for performance. For Seneca, the chorus was a conscious archaism intended to invoke the spirit of Greece as the fountainhead of Roman culture. However, in Shakespeare's day, ancient drama was known only from Seneca's work; thus, the Renaissance delight in classicism encouraged the use of choruses in English plays, although such a ritualistic device is actually quite inappropriate to the distinctly secular ELIZABETHAN DRAMA. It was never employed in the strict sense of group recitation, let alone singing and dancing; rather, various approximations, like those of Shakespeare, came into use.

Chorus (2) Minor character in *Romeo and Juliet*, the nondramatic figure who comments on the play in each PROLOGUE (1), preceding Acts 1 and 2 respectively. In the manner of an ancient Greek CHORUS (1), this character comments on the drama from outside it, displaying a knowledge that no character could have. In the Prologue to Act 1, the Chorus not only provides a terse account of the tragedy's course but suggests a response to it, pointing out that the feud between families 'makes civil hands unclean' (Prologue.4) and that the 'fearful passage' (Prologue.9) of the love affair will provide the only resolution of the conflict. Prior to Act 2, the Chorus extols the two lovers while outlining the difficulties that the feud will cause them. Each prologue takes the form of a SONNET, traditionally reserved for romantic poetry, preparing the audience (which in Shakespeare's day will have been likely to recognise the form on hearing it) for a love story. This treatment reflects the fact that a tragic love story was a novelty in the 1590s. TRAGEDY ordinarily concerned warriors and kings; lovers were expected to appear in COMEDY, where they would find a happy ending in marriage.

Chorus (3) Allegorical figure in *Henry V*, speaker of the PROLOGUE (1) (where he is identified in a stage direction as the Prologue), an introduction to each act, and the EPILOGUE. The Chorus apologises for the inadequacy of the theatre to present historical events in a sufficiently grand manner, and he therefore offers a supplementary account of the events dramatised. He uses a stylised and artificial diction that is in marked contrast with the realism of the dramatic scenes, and the Chorus' grand rhetoric contributes to the epic quality so important to the play. However, if *Henry V* is considered as an acid satire on politics, then the Chorus' epic voice has an ironic quality, sardonically at odds with the cynical waging of an unnecessary war by an hypocritically religious King. In the Epilogue—a formally correct SONNET—the Chorus again remarks on the inadequacy of historical drama, and he praises the accomplishments of HENRY V anew. Then he goes on to observe that all of Henry's gains in FRANCE (1) were almost immediately lost under HENRY VI, closing with a reference to Shakespeare's well-known *Henry VI* plays, which depict this loss.

The Chorus repeatedly invokes imaginary scenes: in the Prologue he asks the audience to 'piece out our imperfections with your thoughts' (Prologue.23) and thereby to 'carry [characters] here and there, jumping o'er times' (line 29). In 3.Chorus.18 he requests, 'Grapple your minds', and later, 'Work, work your thoughts, and therein see . . .' (line 25), and lastly, 'eke out our performance with your mind' (line 35). Thus the Chorus, by insisting on the audience's part in shaping the narrative, supplying with their imagina-

tions what cannot be provided in a theatre, helps to provide an almost cinematic sweep of time and events.

Christopher (1) Sly Character in *The Taming of the Shrew.* See SLY (1).

Christopher (2) Urswick (1448–1522) Historical figure and minor character in *Richard III,* a follower of RICHMOND. Prior to Richmond's invasion of England, Sir Christopher Urswick makes contact with Lord Thomas STANLEY (3), Richmond's stepfather, who confirms his intention to defect from RICHARD III. The historical Urswick was a priest in the employ of Margaret Beaufort, Richmond's mother and Stanley's wife.

Cibber (1), Colley (1671–1757) English actor, playwright, and producer. Cibber, the son of a Danish sculptor who had moved to England, began his career in 1690 as an actor in Thomas BETTERTON's company, and by 1696 he had his first play staged. He was a successful actor, portraying mostly comical fops, often in his own plays, which were fashionable comedies of sentiment, set in high society. His tragedies were generally unsuccessful, except for his adaptation of *Richard III* (1700)—more than half of which he wrote himself—which was immensely popular and became the standard version of Shakespeare's play for more than a century. As a long-time manager of the Drury Lane Theatre, Cibber staged a number of Shakespeare's plays—or rather adaptations of them—including his own *Romeo and Juliet* and *Papal Tyranny in the Reign of King John.* He played a number of Shakespearean characters, including Cardinal WOLSEY, IAGO, and JAQUES (1) (the last in LOVE IN A FOREST by Charles JOHNSON [2]). His autobiography, *Apology for the Life of Colley Cibber, Comedian* (1740), provides many interesting glimpses of 18th-century theatre life. Cibber was named Poet Laureate in 1730. Theophilus CIBBER (3) was his son.

Cibber (2), Susannah Maria (1714–1766) English actress. Susannah Cibber, a sister of Thomas ARNE, married Theophilus CIBBER (3) in 1734, though they only lived together briefly. Originally an opera singer, she was coached as an actress by her father-in-law, the actor and producer Colley CIBBER (1). Her husband's flight from England, to avoid creditors, exposed the scandalous *ménage à trois* they had maintained with another man, and Susannah retired from the stage for several years. She later returned to a successful career in the productions of David GARRICK. She was especially acclaimed as CONSTANCE in *King John.*

Cibber (3), Theophilus (1703–1758) English actor. The son of Colley CIBBER (1), Theophilus Cibber was best known for comic roles, especially PISTOL and PAROLLES. After the scandalous dissolution of his marriage to Susannah Maria CIBBER (2), Theophilus Cibber's stage career collapsed, and he supported himself as a hack writer. He wrote a brief biography of Shakespeare in his *The Lives of the Poets* (1753)—probably ghost-written—that is the only source for the anecdote that Shakespeare began his career as a 'horse boy', holding horses for members of the audience as they dismounted outside the theatre.

Cicero, M. Tullius (106–43 B.C.) Historical figure and minor character in *Julius Caesar,* a senator of ROME. Cicero appears only to dismiss CASCA's concern about omens in 1.3. Earlier Casca had described in comical terms Cicero's pedantic use of Greek ('It was Greek to me' [1.2.281]), and later BRUTUS (4) rejects the suggestion that Cicero be included in the conspiracy against CAESAR (1) as an elder statesman. Brutus says that Cicero is too independent and will 'never follow any thing that other men begin' (2.1.151–152). Cicero's execution by ANTONY and OCTAVIUS is reported in 4.3. 176–177.

Although he is an interesting background presence, Cicero is of no real importance to the play. Probably his inclusion simply reflects his immense stature as a writer. Cicero was perhaps the most influential of all classical authors. His works were highly respected in his own lifetime and throughout the period of the Roman Empire; during the Middle Ages he was revered as a master of rhetoric. In the RENAISSANCE his works were well known to all educated people, and they influenced humanistic writers on a broad range of subjects. In Shakespeare's time Cicero was certainly one of the best-known ancient Romans, and it was therefore natural for the playwright to present him on stage. Cicero was often known in the 16th century as 'Tully', from his middle name, and he is so referred to in *2 Henry VI,* 4.1.136, and *Titus Andronicus,* 4.1.14.

Cicero was also a highly successful lawyer and politician. He was among the most important men in the Roman world at the time of the play. He was a leader of the opposition to Caesar's party, although he had no part in Brutus' plot, and after the assassination he denounced Antony in a series of speeches. As is reported in the play, he was executed as a result.

Cinna (1), Gaius Helvetius (Helvius) (d. 44 B.C.) Historical figure and minor character in *Julius Caesar,* victim of a mob of PLEBEIANS (1). In 3.3 Cinna, a poet, is mistaken for CINNA (2), one of the assassins of CAESAR (1), and he is killed by the ferocious Roman mob incited by Mark ANTONY's funeral oration for Caesar. The historical Cinna—called Helvetius Cinna for his birth in what is now Switzerland—was a noted poet of his day. His epic poem *Zmyrna* was famous for generations as a difficult 'modernist' masterpiece, but it is

now lost. Not mentioned in Shakespeare's source, PLUTARCH's *Lives*, is Cinna's political role; he was Caesar's ally, and he became a tribune when Caesar deposed FLAVIUS (1) and MARULLUS. His murder by the pro-Caesar mob was therefore all the more ironic, but the playwright did not know this.

Cinna (2), Lucius Cornelius the Younger (active 44 B.C.) Historical figure and minor character in *Julius Caesar*, one of the assassins of CAESAR (1). In 1.3 CASSIUS assigns Cinna to distribute anonymous letters encouraging BRUTUS (4) to join the conspiracy against Caesar. When Caesar is stabbed, Cinna cries, 'Liberty! Freedom! Tyranny is dead!' (3.1.78).

The historical Cinna—whose father (d. 84 B.C.) had been a famous radical leader under whom Caesar had served in the earlier Roman civil wars—had been appointed to high office under Caesar. Shakespeare's source, PLUTARCH, mentioned Cinna as one of the conspirators and reported that, after the assassination, he made a speech against Caesar that infuriated the crowd. It is not historically certain, however, that Cinna was actually one of Caesar's murderers; he may merely have been among those who supported the assassins after the fact. In either case, he was identified with the killing in contemporary minds; as is enacted in 3.3, a pro-Caesar mob encountered Helvetius CINNA (1) and, believing him to be L. Cornelius Cinna, beat him to death.

Cinthio (Giovanni Battista Giraldi) (1504–1573) Italian poet, novelist, and playwright, author of sources for *Measure for Measure* and *Othello*. The story of OTHELLO and DESDEMONA and the main plot of *Measure for Measure* came from two different tales in Cinthio's *Hecatommithi* (1565), a cycle of novellas modelled on BOCCACCIO's *Decamaron*. *Measure for Measure* was also influenced by Cinthio's *Epitia*, a dramatisation of the source novella, published posthumously in 1583. The same tale was translated into English by George WHETSTONE, but Shakespeare does not appear to have used it. The *Othello* source tale was not translated into English until the 18th century, so Shakespeare must have known Cinthio's work elsewhere. He may have read it in the original Italian, or in a French translation of 1584, or there may have been an English translation that is now lost.

Giraldi (known as Cinthio in England from the name Cinzio, which he called himself in his poetry) was a famed professor of philosophy and rhetoric. As a playwright, he was noted for his efforts to reform tragic drama, based in his time on ancient models, so that it reflected tenets of Christian humanism. In his eight published plays, including *Epitia*, a CHORUS (1) commented on the action, which consisted in good part of debates on such subjects as the proper relationship between love and justice. This aspect of his work is reflected particularly in the highly moral character of ISABELLA and the political musings of the DUKE (9) in *Measure for Measure*. On the other hand, Cinthio was also the first RENAISSANCE playwright to present atrocities on stage, which perhaps indirectly influenced Shakespeare to write such noteworthy scenes of violence and gore as those in *Titus Andronicus*, *King Lear*, and *Othello*.

Citizen (1) One of several minor characters in *2 Henry VI*. In 4.5 one of a group of citizens reports to Lord SCALES, the commander of the Tower of LONDON, that the rebels led by Jack CADE are successfully assaulting London Bridge and that the Lord Mayor has requested Scales' assistance.

Citizen (2) Any of several minor characters in *Richard III*, common people of LONDON who respond to the sinister affairs surrounding the crown. In 2.3, three Citizens discuss the death of King EDWARD IV and the ambitions of RICHARD III in tones of anxious foreboding. One of them summarises their viewpoint: 'All may be well; but if God sort it so / 'Tis more than we deserve, or I expect' (2.3.36–37). In 3.7 a number of Citizens accompany the MAYOR (3) to witness Richard's charade of unwillingness to accept the crown, and their silence speaks volumes about the usurper's impropriety.

Citizen (3) Any of several minor characters in *Romeo and Juliet*, townspeople of VERONA who attempt to halt the street fighting between the feuding MONTAGUE (1) and CAPULET (1) families in 1.1 and 3.1. Their presence reflects the importance Shakespeare placed on civil disorder—one of his favourite themes—as an element in his tragedy of young lovers.

Citizen (4) Minor character in *King John*, a citizen of ANGIERS who appears on the walls of the city in 2.1 to explain to the kings PHILIP (2) of France (1) and JOHN (3) of England why the gates are closed. He declares the town's allegiance to the King of England but adds that, until it is established whether John or ARTHUR is properly holder of that office, the citizens have 'ramm'd up our gates against the world' (2.1.272). The Citizen's suspicion of his leaders illuminates the treacherous nature of royal politics, a major theme of the play.

In the FIRST FOLIO, where *King John* was first published, the Citizen departs at 2.1.282 and HUBERT acts as representative of Angiers to the forces outside after entering at line 325. However, in some modern editions, Hubert's lines in 2.1 are given to the Citizen. Conversely, in other editions, the Citizen's part in its entirety is given to Hubert.

Citizen (5) Any of several minor but significant characters in *Coriolanus*, residents of ROME. The Citizens are chiefly important for their fickleness, as their opinions of CORIOLANUS change repeatedly under the influence of various other characters. In this they symbolise a political doctrine that Shakespeare espoused in a number of plays: the common people, however sympathetic as individuals, are politically irresponsible as a class.

The Citizens are most distinguishable as individuals in 1.1. Amid a riot, the First Citizen introduces the play's most important motif: the excessive pride of Coriolanus. He recommends killing him, but the Second Citizen opposes this suggestion, and points out the great services that Coriolanus has performed as the military genius of Rome. He thereby introduces the counter-theme and prepares us for the tragedy that will constitute the main plot, as the noble hero falls victim to his own pride. The riot is halted as the Citizens listen to the aristocrat MENENIUS justify the powers of the aristocracy with a simplistic fable—his famed 'belly speech' (1.1.95–153)—and though the First Citizen offers sensible objections, the crowd as a whole is diverted from its original intentions. The arrival of Coriolanus cows them altogether, and they depart in an initial demonstration of their malleability.

Thereafter, the Citizens serve chiefly to further the same point. They are manipulated by the aristocrats, who influence them to vote for Coriolanus in Act 2, and by their own representatives—the tribunes BRUTUS (3) and SICINIUS—who organise them as a mob in Act 3, and bring about the banishment of Coriolanus. Lastly, in 4.6 some Citizens thank the tribunes for getting rid of their enemy, but when word arrives that the banished Coriolanus is marching on Rome with the army of the VOLSCIANS, they reappear to declare that they had had misgivings about the banishment all along. With the exception of the First Citizen in 1.1, the Citizens are not portrayed as individuals and serve only as pawns, both of the tribunes and the playwright.

Citizen (6) Minor character in *Coriolanus*, a resident of ANTIUM. In three brief lines the Citizen directs CORIOLANUS to the home of AUFIDIUS. He serves merely to advance the plot.

Clarence (1), George York, Duke of (1449–1478) Historical figure and character in *Richard III*, the victimised brother of RICHARD III. Richard reveals in his opening soliloquy (1.1) that he has turned King EDWARD IV, his oldest brother, against Clarence, his next oldest. When Clarence is arrested, in the same scene, Richard sympathises with him and promises him assistance, but in fact, he proceeds to hire two murderers to kill him. Thus Clarence is removed from the succession to the crown, leaving Richard in his place.

In 1.4 we see Clarence in his cell in the TOWER OF LONDON. He has just awakened from a terrible nightmare, in which he was drowned and went to hell. There he encountered the spirits of both the Earl of WARWICK (3), whom he had betrayed, and the one-time PRINCE (4) OF WALES, whom he had helped to murder (Both events are enacted, with Clarence appearing as GEORGE [2], in *3 Henry VI*.) Awake but still afraid, he admits that his conscience is heavy.

The murderers arrive, and Clarence learns that Richard, whom he had thought he might rely on in his distress, has hired them. He piteously bewails his fate. The SECOND MURDERER (2), who had displayed pangs of conscience earlier, is prepared to relent, but the FIRST MURDERER (2) proceeds to stab Clarence and, for good measure, seals him in a cask of wine to ensure that he won't survive.

Clarence's death scene is an emotional highlight of the play. It has tremendous impact, shocking the audience, for Richard's villainy, which has been seductively entertaining up to this point, is now seen to have serious consequences. Clarence's account of his dream reveals a soul in torment; he speaks in passionate verse, the most lyrical in the play. His spiritual suffering—his heavy-hearted loss of hope and fear of death—is intense. The scene anchors much of the action that follows: although Richard's cold-hearted machinations result only in off-stage violence, they nevertheless cannot be witnessed without recalling this chilling evidence of their real weight.

Shakespeare's account of Clarence's death has little relation to history, though the playwright certainly believed it to be true; he took it from his chief source for the HISTORY PLAYS, the account of the WARS OF THE ROSES written by Edward HALL (2). Historically, Richard actually protested against Clarence's imprisonment and execution. However, Clarence's position was irreparable, for he had persisted in involving himself in plots against King Edward. After forgiving his brother several times (one of these occasions is dramatised in *3 Henry VI*), Edward finally ordered Clarence's trial for treason, appearing in person as the prosecutor. Clarence was sentenced to death, and a few days later his death was announced, although there was no public execution, as would have been ordinary. This last detail may account for the persistence of the rumour that Richard had Clarence murdered, which was, by Shakespeare's time, accepted as fact.

Clarence (2), Thomas, Duke of (1388–1421) Historical figure and minor character in *2 Henry IV* and *Henry V*, son of King HENRY IV and younger brother of PRINCE (6) HAL. In *2 Henry IV* Clarence receives advice

from his dying father on dealing with Hal after he succeeds to the throne. In *Henry V*, although he receives a command from the King in 5.2.84, he does not reply, nor is he named in the stage directions or the DRAMATIS PERSONAE in most editions of the play.

The historical Clarence was an important figure in the regimes of his father and brother. A young governor of Ireland in the first years of Henry IV's reign, Clarence replaced Hal on the King's council when the latter was dismissed in 1411, and he led a successful military expedition in GASCONY in 1412. Late in the reign of Henry V, Clarence was killed in battle in FRANCE (1).

Clarke, Mary Cowden (1809–1898) and Charles Cowden (1787–1877) British Shakespearean commentators. The Clarkes, who married in 1828, studied and wrote about Shakespeare throughout their married life. Mary Cowden Clarke prepared a concordance to Shakespeare's work (1844–1845), and wrote a best-selling three-volume collection of short fictions entitled *The Girlhood of Shakespeare's Heroines* (1851–1852). Charles Cowden Clarke published his lectures on *Shakespeare's Characters* (1863). The couple produced jointly an edition of the complete plays (1868), a popular guide to Shakespeare's language entitled *Shakespeare Key* (1879), and editions of the works of George Herbert (1593–1633) and others. Their *Recollections of Writers* (1878) is a memoir of their friendships with such 19th-century luminaries as John KEATS, Charles and Mary LAMB (1), and Charles DICKENS.

Claudio (1) Character in *Much Ado About Nothing*, lover of HERO. Claudio falls in love with Hero on sight, but he rejects her when the deceitful Don JOHN (1) presents him with false evidence of her infidelity. Once aware of his error, and believing that Hero has died of shame, Claudio repents and agrees to marry Hero's supposed cousin, who turns out to be Hero herself, and the couple is at last united. Claudio's apparent lack of awareness and his haste to mistrust his beloved make him seem shallow and insensitive, and modern audiences tend to find him one of the least likeable or interesting of Shakespeare's young noblemen.

However, Claudio may be considered from another point of view that more likely reflects Shakespeare's intentions. Claudio, like Hero, is a model young Elizabethan. Even before he appears, he is extolled by the MESSENGER (14) as a paragon of knightly virtues, 'doing, in the figure of a lamb, the feats of a lion' (1.1.13–14). His youth and inexperience make him a plausible target for Don John's lies; his passive wooing of Hero, dependent on Don PEDRO's assistance, emphasises his vulnerability. He is often faulted for a seemingly mercenary interest in Hero (1.1.274), but his inquiry about her inheritance is merely conventional: any young man of Shakespeare's day would ask such a question of a prospective bride, and the query simply demonstrates his interest in marriage. Gullible, he believes Hero has been unfaithful, but Shakespeare takes care to make his credulousness less ridiculous by having Don Pedro seem duped as well. The viciousness of Claudio's response indicates the extent to which he has been hurt by his seeming rejection. Both Claudio and Don Pedro regret the understandable anger of Leonato and ANTONIO (3) in 5.1, and they refrain from a violent response. Their awkward jesting confirms their embarrassment over the situation. Claudio's repentance and atonement are sometimes regarded as cursory and hypocritical, but Shakespeare treats them seriously. Although the scene at Hero's supposed tomb is brief, it is solemn. In 5.4 Claudio's return to happiness is complete, and he is unquestionably accepted in LEONATO's generous and cheerful court.

This more charitable interpretation of Claudio better suits the play, which is after all a comedy. Don John, the villain, is plainly saddled with all the blame. In any case, the play revolves around BEATRICE and BENEDICK; as Claudio's conventionality suggests, he is a relatively unimportant figure whose personality need not be well developed. Significantly, after the disguised Hero is revealed, the re-united lovers do not speak, as the focus of the play immediately shifts to Beatrice and Benedick. As Claudio's usefulness as a character is spent, he recedes into the background.

Claudio (2) Character in *Julius Caesar*. See CLAUDIUS (1).

Claudio (3) Character in *Measure for Measure*, a condemned prisoner and brother of ISABELLA. Claudio has impregnated JULIET (2) out of wedlock, and has been condemned to death, under an antiquated law, by ANGELO (2), the deputy of the DUKE (9) of VIENNA. This is the basic situation from which the play's central conflict arises—Angelo's demand of sex from Isabella in exchange for Claudio's life. Claudio's intentions are clearly honourable, however; he wants only to marry Juliet. Their sexual relations would have been perfectly legal but for a delay in marriage arrangements, and his condemnation is an evil excess on Angelo's part, as all the other characters agree.

Claudio's situation is a result of the Duke's lax regime in Vienna. Despite his aristocratic upbringing, the young man is familiar with the bordello world of LUCIO, POMPEY (1), and MISTRESS (2) OVERDONE, from whom we first learn of his plight, in 1.2. We recognise the stereotype of an immature young man in bad company, and we are not surprised that his ascetic sister is disappointed in him when his fear of death overcomes his sense of nobility. The moving passage in which he begs her to accommodate Angelo begins, 'to

die, and go we know not where' (3.1.117). His reaction is touchingly human and we do not share Isabella's hysterical condemnation; the episode helps us realise that she is, in her way, as extreme as Angelo. Claudio's moral character is favourably compared with Angelo's in the contrast between his loving relationship with Juliet and Angelo's desertion of MARIANA (1).

Claudius (Claudio) (1) Minor character in *Julius Caesar,* a soldier in the army of BRUTUS (4). Claudius and VARRO, serving as messengers, sleep through the appearance of the GHOST (2) of CAESAR (1) in Brutus' tent and are awakened by Brutus to confirm that they have seen nothing.

In the first edition of *Julius Caesar,* that in the FOLIO (1623), Claudius' name is rendered as Claudio, and some modern editors follow this practice. Others, however, use Claudius, which is correct in Latin and appears in Shakespeare's source, NORTH's translation of PLUTARCH's *Lives.*

Claudius (2), King Character in *Hamlet.* See KING (5).

Cleomenes (Cleomines) and Dion Minor characters in *The Winter's Tale,* followers of King LEONTES of SICILIA. Cleomenes and Dion are virtually indistinguishable, and they share their only significant function, so they are treated together here. Seeking support for his accusation that Queen HERMIONE is guilty of adultery, King Leontes sends them to consult the oracle of Apollo. They describe the oracle in awestruck tones, with Dion ecstatically reminiscing, 'O, the sacrifice! / How ceremonious, solemn and unearthly' (3.1.6–7), and Cleomenes declaring that 'the ear-deaf'ning voice o' th' Oracle, / Kin to Jove's thunder, so surpris'd my sense, / That I was nothing' (3.1.9–11). Their remarks stand in for the actual appearance of a god—a feature of the other ROMANCES—and introduce the climactic moment of the play's first half, the checking of Leontes' madness through the apparent intervention of Apollo. However, when the oracle's pronouncement is delivered in 3.2, Cleomenes and Dion speak only half a line, in unison, swearing that they have not read the message. They reappear briefly in 5.1, but they are merely pawns of the plot.

Cleon Character in *Pericles,* governor of THARSUS and husband of DIONYZA. In 1.4 Cleon bemoans the catastrophic famine that has beset Tharsus, and when PERICLES brings relief, he is very grateful. He curses anyone who may ever harm his benefactor, and includes 'our wives, our children, or ourselves' (1.4.103). This remark proves very ironic when Dionyza attempts to murder Pericles' daughter, MARINA, who has been left in their care. Cleon disapproves of his wife's deed, but he gives in to her harangue against his cowardice, and, as the head of the family, he eventually receives much of the blame for it. The play's spokesman, GOWER (3), tells us in the EPILOGUE that Cleon and his entire family have been massacred by the citizens of Tharsus, who were incensed when they learned of the murder. When his bravery is questioned by Dionyza, Cleon resembles MACBETH (in *Macbeth* 1.7, 2.2, and 3.4) and the Duke of ALBANY (in *King Lear* 4.2), but he is a very minor figure whose function is to depict man's weakness in the face of evil.

Cleopatra, Queen of Egypt (68–30 B.C.) Historical figure and title character of *Antony and Cleopatra,* the Queen of Egypt and the lover of the Roman general, Mark ANTONY. Throughout Acts 1–4 Cleopatra displays the powerful charms of an experienced and thoroughly professional courtesan. She attempts to control her lover with a strategy of alternate taunts and insults and seductive sexuality. Then in Act 5, after Antony is dead, Cleopatra acknowledges the depth of her true feelings for her lover and dedicates her suicide to their joint love. She thereby transcends her earlier nature through the power of passion.

Many commentators, who admire Cleopatra's ultimate nobility do not accept the reality of her earlier role as the exploiter of Antony's sexuality. But Shakespeare's Cleopatra is clearly representative of a familiar dramatic character type: the scheming courtesan. From her first appearance she ridicules Antony, makes outrageous demands for his exclusive affection, declares that his love is insufficient—all classic techniques of emotional domination—and is oblivious to Antony's more romantic interpretation of love. She even uses his devotion against him when she declares that his lack of affection for his wife is evidence that he will eventually desert her as well.

Cleopatra also has great charm and she richly deserves the famous tribute from ENOBARBUS, 'Age cannot wither her, nor custom stale / Her infinite variety' (2.2.235–236). She is witty even in the direst extremity. As the dying Antony is hoisted to her hide-out she can jest, in 4.15.32. In fact, some critics consider her one of the great comic figures in Shakespeare, comparable to FALSTAFF. She has a pleasing delight in mischief; Enobarbus accompanies his description of her magnificence with an account of when she put aside regal dignity and hopped gaily through the streets. Her beauty is enrapturing, and she has in abundance the intoxicating sexuality essential to the successful courtesan; as Enobarbus puts it, 'vilest things / Become themselves in her' (2.2.238–239).

She also has genuine affection for Antony, but even as she reveals her fondness for him—in his absence—she discloses her past history as a courtesan. She speaks in 1.5.18–34 of her earlier affairs with Julius CAESAR (1) and Pompey the Great (father of the play's POMPEY [2]). Her hurt and anger at the news of An-

tony's marriage to OCTAVIA are certainly genuine, but when she learns of Octavia's unattractive physical features her spirits are restored, for, courtesan-like, her confidence in her sexual allure assures her that she will win her lover back. She does, but when her flight from the battle of ACTIUM brings about Antony's disgrace, she once again displays her essentially selfish nature, in 3.13, when she accepts Caesar's offer of an alliance, conveyed by THIDIAS. She coolly waits out Antony's rage—'I must stay his time' (3.13.155)—and resumes the role of docile and playful lover. However, when her sailors again betray Antony and his rage drives her away, she resorts to an extremely cynical ploy, the pretended suicide that sparks Antony's real one. Falsely assumed emotion—the favourite weapon of the courtesan—remains Cleopatra's most characteristic resource.

However, in the end she is transformed through her noble response to the death of her lover. In 4.15.25–26 she first mentions the idea of suicide simply as a way to foil Caesar's potential humiliations, but after Antony's death she refers to it as a noble ideal on the model Antony himself has offered, 'the high Roman fashion' (4.15.87). In refusing to be humiliated, Cleopatra finds herself at one with Antony in the Roman ideal of honourable suicide. SELEUCUS' revelation that she has withheld treasure from Caesar is sometimes taken as evidence that Cleopatra reverts briefly to ideas of survival, though another interpretation is that she chose to deceive Caesar as to her intentions so that he would not prevent them. However, even if we suppose that she does waver, she also returns to the idea of a noble death, and her focus remains on Antony—rather than on Caesar—as she approaches the deed.

Cleopatra accepts death because it is the only end equal to her newly awakened love for Antony. It is in her ecstatic appraisal of him as 'an Emperor Antony . . .' (5.2.76–100) that she first finds the exalted note of commitment to the memory of her lover that carries her through to the end. When she cries, 'Husband, I come' (5.2.286), she completes her transformation into 'fire, and air; my other elements / I give to baser life' (5.2.288–289). When she abandons her actual, earthly relationship with Antony for an eternal union, Cleopatra transcends the mortal world of politics and courtesanship where she and Antony had come to grief.

Cleopatra's personality does not change with her final ecstasy—Shakespeare was too good a writer to exchange one sort of portrayal for another at the close of the play. Cleopatra dies, but she makes her death a luxurious and hedonistic one. She combines the splendour of grand costume—'Give me my robe, put on my crown' (5.2.279)—with an almost sexual surrender to death at the end, when she cries, 'As sweet as balm, as soft as air, as gentle. / O Antony!' (5.2.310–311). Her theatrical nature provides the grandeur that elevates the tragedy provoked by her earlier conduct. Thus we can see Cleopatra's moral defects—her selfishness as a lover and her practice of the courtesan's wiles—in a new light, as inextricable elements of a personality powerful enough to generate the mysterious grace that she brings to her final gesture. Through this grace and power, Cleopatra's vision of reunion with Antony after death is a triumphant affirmation of love and life. Even in seeming defeat she embodies the imagination of the individual and the value of what could have been over what worldly power has insisted on. She knows that compared to her, Caesar is 'but Fortune's knave' (5.2.3), for the conqueror, with his limited vision, can only suppose that 'her life in Rome / Would be eternal in our triumph' (5.1.65–66), but Cleopatra's death is the true triumph celebrated by the play.

The historical Cleopatra bore little resemblance to Shakespeare's character. She was not particularly beautiful—Shakespeare's source, PLUTARCH's *Lives*, attributes her magnetism to her conversation. Nor, in all probability, did she die for the sake of love but rather for the more practical end of avoiding a horrible captivity, and she only killed herself after she attempted to win Caesar with a promise to betray Antony. She was descended from one of the Greek successors of Alexander the Great, and was entirely of Greek ancestry and not African in any degree, despite the modern tendency to classify her among Shakespeare's black characters. Cleopatra inherited the throne of Egypt in 51 B.C., at the age of 17. Deposed by an aristocratic clique in 49 B.C., she was restored with the assistance of Julius Caesar a year later.

She became Caesar's mistress, and she later filled the same function for Pompey the Great and Antony—unlike in the play, however, she did not become Antony's mistress until after his marriage to Octavia. In all three cases her motive is clear; she needed the political support of the forces of Rome present in the eastern Mediterranean, and thus she ingratiated herself with whoever commanded them. Modern scholars think it unlikely that she influenced the policies of any of her protectors, who simply used her as a means of extracting wealth from Egypt. Antony's gifts to her of kingdoms and power that Octavius Caesar complains of in the play were merely ordinary applications of Roman policy by which administrative jurisdictions in conquered lands were consolidated under a client ruler. The arrangement inspired no mistrust at the time. Cleopatra, who was reportedly greedy for even the trappings of power, persistently requested more such titular kingdoms, but Antony refused her.

When Antony found himself at war with Caesar he naturally made use of the Egyptian kingdom that he governed through Cleopatra, but the unreliability of Egyptian forces at Actium and afterwards—as recounted in the play—cannot be attributed to her in-

fluence. It is uncertain whether Antony and Cleopatra were married, but she bore three children by him; the two boys were killed after Caesar's victory, and the girl later became a pawn of Roman politics and was married to a Numidian king.

Clerk Minor character in *2 Henry VI,* a victim executed by the rebels led by Jack CADE. Cade and his men are suspicious of the clerk's literacy, which they construe as a sign of hostility towards the peasantry. They are particularly infuriated by the fact that his given name is Emmanuel, a word often used to head legal documents. Cade orders him hung 'with his pen and ink-horn about his neck' (4.2.103–104). The incident is one of several that Shakespeare uses to depict Cade's rebellion as an anarchic uprising by ignorant peasants concerned only with killing their betters, although historically this was not the case.

Clifford (1), Lord John (c. 1435–1461) Character in *2* and *3 Henry VI,* the obsessed avenger of his father's death, who kills both the Duke of YORK (8) and his young son, RUTLAND (1). As Young Clifford, this character appears briefly in Act 5 of *2 Henry VI* as a supporter of King HENRY VI against the Duke of York and as a participant in the battle of ST. ALBANS. On the battlefield, he sees the dead body of his father, Thomas CLIFFORD (2), whom York has killed, and he delivers a famous speech (5.2.40–65), a rhetorical comparison of this death with the last judgement, closing with a vow of revenge that prefigures some of the most dramatic action in *3 Henry VI.*

In the later play Clifford's bloodthirsty quest for revenge reflects the bestiality that England's aristocracy has descended to as the civil war progresses. 'Patience is for poltroons', he cries (1.1.62), when King Henry tries to placate an angry earl. In 1.3, when he encounters Rutland, a child attempting to flee the battle of WAKEFIELD, he kills the boy, despite his pleas for mercy, citing his own father's death as justification. When York is captured in 1.4, Queen MARGARET (1) can only with difficulty restrain Clifford long enough to enjoy herself tormenting her enemy with an account of Rutland's murder. Finally, unable to wait any longer, Clifford kills York also. In 2.2, before the battle of TOWTON, Clifford chastises King Henry for his 'harmful pity' in a speech filled with the animal imagery that contributes to the impression of savagery that runs so strongly throughout the play. Ironically, it is another bloody deed by Clifford that costs his side the battle: when WARWICK (3) hears that Clifford has killed his brother, that seemingly defeated leader is aroused and inspires the Yorkists to rally and win the day. In 2.6 Clifford appears, wounded in this battle, to deliver a death-bed speech in which he regrets the weakness of the monarch that has brought the country to this bloody pass. He recognises that his enemies are upon him, and he dies daring them to wreak their vengeance on him. When they recognise him, before they realise he is dead, they taunt and mock him.

Shakespeare took his account of Clifford's revenge on Rutland from HALL (2), but it is entirely unhistorical. Rutland was not a child; he was an officer in the Yorkist army. While he did die at Wakefield, it was never known who killed him. Moreover, it is not known who killed Clifford's father at St Albans either; he died in the thick of the battle, as the playwright also reports in *3 Henry VI* (in 1.1.9), in a famous instance of Shakespearean carelessness. Lastly, Clifford did not die at Towton, but in a skirmish several days earlier. He was struck in the neck by an arrow, as in the play, but was reported at the time to have died instantly.

Clifford (2), Lord Thomas (1414–1455) Historical figure and character in *2 Henry VI,* a backer of King HENRY VI against the claims of the Duke of YORK (8). Clifford first appears as a representative of the King, offering a pardon to the rebel followers of Jack CADE in 4.8. Following York's declaration of rebellion in 5.1, Clifford supports the King and exchanges insults and challenges with the Earl of WARWICK (3), but in the ensuing first battle of ST. ALBANS, he is killed by York. His son, Young CLIFFORD (1), on seeing his father's corpse, vows revenge on the followers of York, anticipating events in *3 Henry VI.* In a famous instance of Shakespeare's carelessness, Clifford's death is reported in different ways in *3 Henry VI.* In 1.1.9, it is stated that Clifford was killed by common soldiers, which almost surely is historically accurate. However, in 1.3.5 and 1.3.46, his son declares that he was killed by York. The playwright was following separate accounts in his sources, making good dramatic use of the son's reported remark—probably a rhetorical one—and forgetting to omit the altogether more plausible version.

Clitus (active 42 B.C.) Historical figure and minor character in *Julius Caesar,* a soldier in the army of BRUTUS (4). In 5.5 Clitus—like DARDANIUS and VOLUMNIUS—refuses to help Brutus to commit suicide after the battle of PHILIPPI, saying 'I'll rather kill myself' (5.5.7). The episode shows the fondness with which Brutus' subordinates regard him, fostering an aura of sentiment around his death. Little is known of the historical Clitus, whose role Shakespeare took from PLUTARCH'S *Lives.*

Clive, Kitty (1711–1785) English actress. A great comic actress, Clive spent most of her career playing opposite David GARRICK. She was especially acclaimed as CELIA in *As You Like It,* and she also played OLIVIA. She was perhaps best known for her performances in the title role of Garrick's *Catherine and Petruchio,* an adaptation of *The Taming of the Shrew.* Though she

played PORTIA (to the SHYLOCK of Charles MACKLIN), OPHELIA, and HAMLET (in accordance with the 18th-century vogue for female Hamlets), her strength was in broad COMEDY, and she is said to have fought with Garrick over his reluctance to cast her in TRAGEDY. She was especially popular in the London literary world and was a good friend of Samuel JOHNSON (7) and the writer Horace Walpole (1717–1797).

Cloten Character in *Cymbeline,* the uncouth son of the QUEEN (2) and the rejected suitor of IMOGEN, who then plans to rape her and kill her husband, POSTHUMUS. Cloten is a comic villain for the most part. He is a stupid and vainglorious man who inspires bemused contempt, though he has his threatening moments and reminds us of the potential for tragedy that underlies the fairy-tale ambience of much of the play. He is finally killed when he happens, entirely by chance, on the lost prince GUIDERIUS, who handily beheads him and then remarks, 'This Cloten was a fool, an empty purse' (4.2.113). His function is that of a fairy-tale villain whose fate is to be defeated by the hand of providence.

Cloten's personality and function vary considerably in the course of the play. In Acts 1–2 Cloten is quite simply a boor; a braggart who is mocked by his own companions (see LORD [15]) and by Imogen's LADY (3). Imogen tells him he is not worth the 'mean'st garment' of Posthumus (2.3.132), and complains that she is 'sprited with a fool' (2.3.138). In Act 3 Cloten takes on a different, less inane, air as he blusters patriotically and helps to commit Britain to a foolish war against ROME. Finally, in Act 4 he is the villain who schemes to kill Posthumus in front of Imogen before he rapes her, and who crassly insults Guiderius for his supposed inferiority.

Such changes make it hard to precisely characterise Cloten's function in the play, and this problem offers a hint of Shakespeare's trouble with the ROMANCES, a new genre in which *Cymbeline* was an experiment. The irregularities in Cloten's personality are similar to those of the play as a whole, and they betray the playwright's difficulty in melding the realistic characters to which he was accustomed with the ethereal figures required by the romances. Cloten seems to be a compound of several types of writing, created as Shakespeare struggled with the task of generating a new type of character, a villain who must convincingly represent evil without being so real as to intrude on a world of fantasy. Though a faulty character, Cloten foreshadows a much more successful figure of this kind, CALIBAN of *The Tempest.*

Some scholars have speculated that portions of Cloten's role may have been considerably modified by the actor who played the character, probably Robert ARMIN. Armin wrote plays and was famous for improvisation, so he was capable of creating additional dialogue. Moreover, in addition to his Shakespearean roles, he specialised in playing a character type of his own devising, a mentally limited CLOWN (1) who may be reflected in some of Cloten's doltishness. Cloten's speeches are in both prose and verse, and this theory suggests that the prose passages were written—or at least altered in performance, before publication—by Armin. However, though some such alteration could have contaminated the text—if it was based on a PROMPT-BOOK—this idea cannot be proven. More probably the evidence reflects the difficulties mentioned above.

Clown (1) Character type often used by Shakespeare, a humorously ignorant and unsophisticated figure, usually male and often associated with rustic ways. The clown is to some extent a comic caricature of a peasant; his humour is earthy and simple, often featuring awkwardness and confusion, such as the unintentionally comic misuse of language, but there is an underlying element of shrewdness as well. Shakespeare's clowns include some of his most delightful characters, from such early creations as LAUNCE in *Two Gentlemen of Verona* and COSTARD in *Love's Labour's Lost,* through DOGBERRY in *Much Ado About Nothing* and BOTTOM in *A Midsummer Night's Dream,* to the CLOWN (8) in *The Winter's Tale.* Most common in COMEDY, the clown is usually minor in the HISTORY PLAYS (see, e.g., FEEBLE)—though Mistress QUICKLY has something of the clown and was probably played by an actor who specialised in the type. The clown, however, often appears in TRAGEDY, where he provides comic relief. The CLOWN (2) of *Titus Andronicus* foreshadows such more developed figures as the CLOWN (7) who is the incongruous bearer of CLEOPATRA's deadly asps in *Antony and Cleopatra,* the PORTER (3) in *Macbeth,* and, perhaps most famous of Shakespeare's clowns, the GRAVE-DIGGER in *Hamlet.*

The clown is usually distinguished from another Shakespearean character type, the FOOL (1), although the Elizabethans used the terms synonymously. (For example, FESTE, who is unquestionably a fool, being a professional jester, and who is called a 'fool' by the other characters, is identified as 'Clown' in speech headings and stage directions throughout the play.) Nevertheless, the difference between the two comic roles is unmistakable. Where the clown's comic effects are accidental results of his bumbling nature, the fool is intentionally witty. Clowns, moreover, tend to operate outside the main plots and often—especially in such early figures as Launce and LAUNCELOT (of *The Merchant of Venice*)—address the audience in somewhat elaborate asides, usually narratives. In contrast, the fool is more involved with the main characters and speaks more analytically.

Although, to some extent, these different comic figures may reflect changes in the actors Shakespeare

wrote for (see ARMIN; KEMPE), the distinction is significant in itself. The fool's subtle and intellectual comedy provides a satirical edge, whereas the clown serves a different symbolic function. He is to some extent a parody of the sublimely simple rustic of PASTORAL tradition, but the mockery is not cruel. The clown is ridiculous but worthy; he retains the virtues of nature and is fundamentally sensible, as is demonstrated when Dogberry accidentally discovers the villains, or when Bottom is the only mortal to experience fairyland. To some extent, this is a reflection of his social position—because he has nothing to lose, he can speak the truth as he sees it—but the clown is also closer to nature and thus closer to the unconscious. He manifests our simplest, often 'vulgar' impulses, with the solid strength of one who is relatively uncorrupted by society. With a natural good grace, he accepts his clumsiness, like his inferior social position, as part of his destined lot. Because he is more obviously long-suffering than profound, the clown parallels on a more accessible plane the stoicism of the tragic hero.

Clown (2) Minor character in *Titus Andronicus.* The clown appears in 4.3, carrying two pigeons in a basket. After some conversation, in which the Clown reveals himself to be a comically naïve rustic, a traditional dramatic type (see CLOWN [1]), TITUS (1) offers him a fee to make the pigeons an offering to the Emperor SATURNINUS. Titus includes a taunting message of his own, wrapped around a dagger. When, in 4.4, the hapless Clown delivers his birds, and Titus' message, to Saturninus, the infuriated emperor orders him killed. He is led away, exclaiming, 'Hang'd, by 'r-Lady! then I have brought up a neck to a fair end' (4.4.48–49). This insignificant addition to the play's roster of victims is one of Shakespeare's earliest Clowns, and his realistic, if dim-witted, voice provides a simple, earthy moment of relief from the savagery that dominates the play.

Clown (3) Character in *Twelfth Night.* See FESTE.

Clown (4) Either of two characters in *Hamlet.* See GRAVE-DIGGER; OTHER.

Clown (5) Character in *All's Well That Ends Well,* court jester to the COUNTESS (2) of ROSSILLION. The Clown comments on aspects of the play, both through parody and by direct references. He professes to be a rustic (as his designation as a CLOWN [1] suggests), 'a woodland fellow' (4.5.44) who enjoys ridiculing the royal court, but he is clearly a sophisticated professional FOOL (1). His somewhat cynical worldliness adds an element of realism that counters the improbabilities of the play.

Sometimes the Clown is overtly contemptuous, as in his insults to PAROLLES in 2.4 and his disparagement of Bertram in 3.2, but usually his function is more indirectly carried out; his concerns parallel those of the main plot, drawing our attention to it in odd ways. For instance, he expounds upon his proposed marriage to 'Isbel the woman' (1.3.16) just after we have been introduced to HELENA and BERTRAM. He goes on to equate Helena with HELEN of TROY, a digression that suggests the sexual conflict emerging in the main story line. Later, in 3.2, he rejects Isbel, apparently out of sexual exhaustion, just as the Countess is reading the letter in which Bertram tells of his rejection of Helena. The Clown's parody of courtly manners in 2.2 immediately precedes PAROLLES' assumption of gentlemanly airs in 2.3 and is itself a commentary on the vanity of social rank, a theme of the play. In his final lines, in which he asserts exuberantly that Parolles smells bad, he not only emphasises Parolles' loss of status, but the rankness of his 'similes of comfort' (5.2.24–25) seems to sum up the play's obnoxious developments to this point. At the same time, he offers some sympathy for Parolles, declaring 'I do pity his distress' (5.2.24), thus maintaining our hope of a milder outcome, which is indeed about to develop.

The Clown is an oddly melancholy jester, with his low-key parodies of theology and his claim to be in the service of 'the black prince . . . alias the devil' (4.5.39–40). He is sometimes somewhat nasty, as when he rejects Isbel, and he can be overly wordy, as LAFEW reminds us when he tells him 'Go thy ways; I begin to be aweary of thee' (4.5.53). However, the Countess clearly enjoys him, though she recognises that he is a 'shrewd knave and an unhappy' (4.5.60). He reminds her of her late husband, 'who made himself much sport out of him' (4.5.61–62). The pleasant relationship between the Countess and her jester contributes to our sense of her household as a source of generosity and kindness that helps to offset the unpleasant aspects of the play.

It is presumed that the Clown's part was intended for Robert ARMIN, the actor who specialised in jesters for the KING'S MEN. His name, Lavatch (sometimes rendered Lavache), is not mentioned until 5.2.1. The name is usually regarded as a corruption of the French *la vache* ('the cow'), though some scholars believe it represents the French *lavage* or the Italian *lavaggio* ('washing, cleansing').

Clown (6) Minor character in *Othello,* a jester, or FOOL (1), in the retinue of OTHELLO. The Clown jokes lewdly with the MUSICIANS (6), in 3.1, before dismissing them with Othello's payment. In 3.4 he briefly jests with DESDEMONA before carrying a message for her. As comic relief, the Clown does not do much to interrupt the play's increasing tension; he may well have been merely a conventional figure, expected by Shakespeare's audiences and therefore supplied by the playwright.

Clown (7) Minor character in *Antony and Cleopatra,* the pretended fig seller who provides CLEOPATRA with the poisonous snakes with which she kills herself. The Clown, summoned by CHARMIAN in 5.2, is a CLOWN (1) in the literary meaning of the term in Shakespeare's day. He is a conventional comic figure, the ludicrously naïve country bumpkin who had figured in COMEDY from ancient times. He comically warns Cleopatra that poisonous snakes are dangerous. Solemnly, he states, '. . . his biting is immortal: those that do die of it, do seldom or never recover' (5.2.245–247). Clowns are usually talkative, and he goes on to tell of 'a very honest woman, but something given to lie' (5.2.250–251) who has reported on her own death by snake bite. He further expounds on the tendency of women to be corrupted by the devil—another medieval comic routine—before Cleopatra can get him to leave.

With ANTONY dead and Cleopatra about to kill herself, this episode comes at an agonising point in the play's climax. The scene shatters the fascinated horror of the audience, while at the same time heightening it by the inane and excruciating postponement of the plot's development. Further, the play's sudden comic tone at this crucial moment highlights the triumphant, celebratory aspect of Cleopatra's suicide; the traditional ending of a romantic COMEDY is evoked, and the transcendence of Cleopatra's total commitment to love is emphasised.

Clown (8) Character in *The Winter's Tale,* foster-brother of PERDITA. The Clown is present in 3.3 when the abandoned infant Perdita is discovered by his father, the SHEPHERD (2). In Act 4, 16 years later, the Clown is part of Perdita's pastoral world, though he has no direct contact with her. As his designation implies (see CLOWN [1]), he is an oafish rustic, a likeable and well-meaning fellow who is somewhat stupid and unconsciously comical. In 3.3 he is unwittingly funny when describing the horrible deaths of ANTIGONUS and the MARINER (1), helping to establish the comic tone of the play's second half. A gullible victim, he is robbed by AUTOLYCUS in 4.3, and in 4.4, at the shepherds' festival, his foolish pleasure in buying gifts for his girlfriend, MOPSA, adds to our enjoyment of the scene. He declares to the peddler (Autolycus in disguise), 'If I were not in love with Mopsa, thou shouldst take no money of me; but being enthralled as I am, it will also be the bondage of certain ribbons and gloves' (4.4.233–236).

Later in 4.4, when King POLIXENES, angry at Perdita's love for his son FLORIZEL, threatens the Shepherd with death, the Clown encourages his father to disclaim his adopted daughter. Autolycus offers to take them to the king for a fee, but he tricks them onto the ship carrying Perdita and Florizel to SICILIA, where Perdita's identity as King LEONTES' daughter is discovered. The Shepherd and the Clown are rewarded with a raise in status, and in 5.2 the Clown comically brags of being 'a gentleman born . . . and [having] been so any time these four hours' (5.2.134–136). Despite his foolishness and his single act of cowardice—understandable in a shepherd facing a king's wrath—the Clown is clearly a good person. As such, he contributes to the atmosphere of human virtue that characterises the second half of the play, countering the evil of the first.

Coat of arms, Shakespeare's Heraldic escutcheon signifying the social status of the family as members of the gentry, awarded in 1596 to Shakespeare's father, John SHAKESPEARE (9), by the Garter King of Arms (a government official charged with authorising such honours). This honour was said to reflect the services of an unnamed ancestor to King Henry VII, founder of the TUDOR DYNASTY, but it in fact depended on the growing success of John's son as a playwright. John Shakespeare had applied for a grant of arms 20 years earlier, but his financial reversals derailed the effort. In a class-conscious society such as 16th-century England, such an award was an important symbol of a family's honourable place in society and was commonly acquired by men who had attained social prominence and wealth. As a visual emblem, the coat of arms could be displayed on one's door, on personal items, and the like. Specifically, the Shakespeare coat of arms consists of a gold shield with a diagonal black band bearing the image of a gold spear—a visual pun on the name 'Shakespeare'—with a silver head. Above the shield is a falcon holding another spear. It appears on Shakespeare's tomb in the parish church in STRATFORD.

Cobbler Minor character in *Julius Caesar,* a COMMONER (1). In 1.1, as the tribunes FLAVIUS (1) and MARULLUS disperse a crowd of artisans gathered to cheer CAESAR (1), the Cobbler jests impertinently when they ask about his profession. He calls himself 'a mender of bad soles' (1.1.13) and asserts that he has joined the crowd to encourage the others to wear out their shoes and thus gain extra business. This brief bit of comedy immediately brings the audience into the reality of ancient ROME and prepares them for the contrasting spectacle of the rioting PLEBEIANS (1) in Act 3. In some editions the Cobbler is identified as the Second Commoner.

Cobham, William Brooke, Lord (d. 1597) Contemporary of Shakespeare, powerful aristocrat whose pressure probably resulted in the change of the name OLDCASTLE to FALSTAFF. Cobham was descended from the historical Oldcastle and was offended by the use of the name for a gluttonous lecher and coward in *1* and *2 Henry IV.* His position as Lord Chamberlain, the official responsible for the royal entertainment bud-

get, made him important to the acting companies, and therefore the character's name was altered.

Cobham held his office only from August 1596 until his death in March 1597. His predecessor, Lord HUNSDON (2) had used the position to protect the theatrical profession from the London government, which was dominated by Puritans and thus opposed to public drama. However, under Cobham, the London authorities achieved a long-sought goal and banished the players from the city limits.

The power of his office and his antipathy to the theatre suggest that it was Cobham who instigated the change in Oldcastle's name, but the complainant may have been his son, Henry Brooke. In either case, the family may well have regretted the attempt to protect their ancestor's name, for their protest became a public joke, as various references in surviving letters of the time make clear. Moreover, the substitution of the name Falstaff was in itself another joke, for, in addition to its punning suggestion of sexual impotence, it referred to a notorious coward, Sir John FASTOLFE, or Falstaffe, who appears in *1 Henry VI.* Oldcastle's descendants were now associated not only with the offensive character in the *Henry IV* plays, but also with a second unpleasant character from another very popular work. In addition, in *The Merry Wives of Windsor,* when Frank FORD (1) foolishly worries that he is being cuckolded by Falstaff, he disguises himself and adopts the name BROOK (1), a probable reference to the Cobhams' family name. (Ford's pseudonym was later changed, possibly after further protest by Henry Brooke.) A number of subtle references to Oldcastle are made in *The Merry Wives* (e.g., in 4.5.5), further ensuring that the audience would not forget the increasingly comical conflict. Worst of all, from the Cobhams' point of view, the *Henry IV* plays were frequently performed using the name Oldcastle until well into the 17th century, despite Shakespeare's changes. Further, in other writings of the period the name Oldcastle is linked to the gluttonous, lascivious behaviour we call Falstaffian.

Coburn, Charles Douville (1877–1961) American actor and producer. With his actress wife, Ivah Wills Coburn, Coburn founded the Coburn Shakespearian Players in 1906, and they produced many of Shakespeare's plays, as well as others, with great success. In 1934 they founded one of the first summer theatre festivals at Union College in Schenectady, New York. Coburn retired upon his wife's death in 1937, returning to the stage only once more, in 1946, to play FALSTAFF, the role for which he had been best known.

Cobweb Character in *A Midsummer Night's Dream,* a fairy, an attendant to the Fairy Queen TITANIA. In 3.1 Titania assigns Cobweb to the retinue of the comical rustic BOTTOM because the Queen has been magically induced to love him. Cobweb serves Bottom by hunting for honey in 4.1. His name suggests the spider's short-lived weaving; Bottom also refers to the ancient use of cobwebs to stop small cuts from bleeding (3.1. 176); perhaps the name suggests that Cobweb possesses medicinal lore.

Coleridge, Samuel Taylor (1772–1834) English poet and literary critic. Best known as a poet, Coleridge also lectured and wrote on literature. His lectures on Shakespeare, delivered between 1802 and 1818, were not published until 1849, but they were nevertheless influential in their own time. While regarded as highly uneven in quality, they offer telling insights into the process of creating characters and letting the play evolve through that process. On certain plays—*Richard II,* for instance—Coleridge's opinions are still regarded as among the most stimulating available. He was among the first English critics to acclaim Shakespeare's poetry—as opposed to the theatrical virtues of the plays—since the 17th century, for the intervening generations had tended to ignore this aspect of the playwright's work. Inspired in part by the work of A. W. SCHLEGEL, which he had studied in Germany, Coleridge's lectures were an important stimulus to the literary criticism of the English Romantic movement.

Colevile (Coleville) of the Dale, Sir John (d. 1405) Historical figure and minor character in *2 Henry IV,* a rebel knight captured by FALSTAFF. After the rebels have been tricked into dispersing without a battle, Colevile peaceably surrenders to Falstaff, who makes much of his own valour as he turns his prisoner over to Prince John of LANCASTER (3). Lancaster sends Colevile to be executed. The episode provides a comical glimpse of Falstaff in the long and otherwise entirely political Act 4.

Shakespeare took Colevile's name from HOLINSHED, who lists him among the executed rebels, but it is possible that Colevile was pardoned and lived to be recorded as Sir John Colvyl, who fought in FRANCE (1) with HENRY V.

Collatine (Tarquinius Collatinus) Legendary husband of the Roman matron Lucretia and minor figure in *The Rape of Lucrece,* the husband of LUCRECE. After being sexually assaulted by the king's son, TARQUIN, Lucrece sends for her father and Collatine, or Collatinus, as he is occasionally called (e.g., in line 218). Collatine does not appear until line 1584, and he is mostly tongue-tied by grief for the rest of the poem, for Lucrece informs the men what has happened and kills herself after demanding vengeance. Collatinus is roused to revenge only by another witness of Lucrece's account, Junius BRUTUS (2).

The last words of the poem's introductory ARGU-

MENT observe that the vengeance that Brutus exacted upon Tarquin resulted in the fall of his father's kingdom and the establishment of the Roman Republic. Shakespeare took this conclusion from his sources, OVID and LIVY, but the association of the birth of the republic with a rape has no historical truth. All that is known of the historical Tarquinius Collatinus is that in 509 B.C. he was (with Brutus) one of the first two consuls, the executives who jointly ruled the republican government of Rome. His name suggests that he was Etruscan, like the departing royal family.

Collier (1), Constance (1878–1955) English actress. Constance Collier began her long career playing PEASEBLOSSOM at the age of three. She subsequently became one of the famous Gaiety Girls but left to play in more serious dramas. A member of Beerbohm TREE's company from 1901 to 1908, she played numerous Shakespearean parts. Beginning in 1908 she divided her career between New York and London and was very popular in both cities. She played QUEEN (9) Gertrude to John BARRYMORE's HAMLET in his London production of 1925.

Collier (2), John Payne (1789–1883) English scholar and forger. A one-time journalist and lawyer, Collier established himself as a Shakespeare scholar with a series of books published between 1835 and 1850. He is best known, however, for having forged a number of documents in support of his literary theories: annotations in 17th-century books; contemporary references to Shakespeare; theatrical business records; a source for *The Tempest,* etc. Collier claimed to own an annotated copy of the second FOLIO and published the notations as *Notes and Emendations to the Text of Shakespeare's Plays* (1852). The authenticity of this material was questioned by a number of scholars, and further investigation revealed both its falseness and the existence of other forgeries. Collier's forgeries still have an impact on Shakespearean scholarship, for the extent of his handiwork cannot be precisely established, and any documents to which he is known to have had access must be viewed with scepticism.

Collins, Francis (d. 1617) Lawyer in STRATFORD, the drafter of Shakespeare's will. Collins, who served Shakespeare as a lawyer on a business deal in 1605, was probably also a friend, for he received a sizeable bequest in the playwright's will, though it probably included his fee for drawing it up. He also witnessed the will. Collins held various public offices in Stratford, beginning in 1600, though by 1613 he lived in Warwick. He was a close friend of John COMBE (1) and drew up his will (which contained a bequest to Shakespeare). He moved back to Stratford in 1617, when offered the post of town clerk on the condition that he do so, but he died a few months later.

Colman, George (1732–1794) English playwright and theatrical entrepreneur. Colman was a close associate of David GARRICK, who produced his plays, including *The Jealous Wife* (1761), one of the most popular comedies of its time. After a dispute with Garrick over the casting of a play, however, Colman leased the Covent Garden Theatre, where, from 1767 to 1774, he produced many plays, including those of Oliver Goldsmith (1730–1774). He staged *Cymbeline,* but his most important Shakespearean production was *King Lear,* from which he dropped many of the alterations made by Nahum TATE, though he added some of his own. He later managed another theatre before retiring in 1789. Among the plays Colman produced were the early works of his son, also George Colman (1762–1836), later a notable comic dramatist.

Colonne, Guido delle (active late 13th century) Sicilian writer, author of a source of *Troilus and Cressida.* Colonne translated the *Roman de Troie* by Benoit de SAINTE-MAURE, a 12th-century poem on the TROJAN WAR, into Latin prose. His version, the *Historia destructionis Troiae* (published 1270–1287) became the standard work on the subject until the rediscovery of HOMER during the RENAISSANCE. Colonne's book influenced Shakespeare through two English works. A French translation was re-translated into English by William CAXTON as *The Recuyell of the Historyes of Troye* (1471), and John LYDGATE was inspired by the *Historia* to compose a long poem entitled *Troy Book* (1420, publ. 1512, 1555). These two works provide much of the detail in the account of the war reported in *Troilus and Cressida.*

Combe (1), John (before 1561–1614) Landowner and money-lender in STRATFORD, a friend of Shakespeare. Said to have been the richest citizen of Stratford in his day, Combe was noted for his charities. Though he often sued for repayment of the loans he made, several of these creditors later named him in their wills as their good friend. He died a bachelor, and in his will he left the large sum of £30 to be distributed among the poor of the town. He and his uncle William COMBE (4) sold Shakespeare 127 acres of land near WELCOMBE in 1602. His brother Thomas and his nephews Thomas and William COMBE (2, 3, 5) were also associates of Shakespeare. Combe and the playwright appear to have been close friends. He left Shakespeare £5 in his will—a quite sizeable token. His tomb in Stratford's Holy Trinity Church, like Shakespeare's tomb nearby, was designed by Gheerart JANSSEN (2). Later in the 17th century, two EPITAPHS on Combe were attributed to Shakespeare. One is simply a variant on a traditional rhyme about usurers, and the other seems un-Shakespearean sytlistically, so modern scholars tend to doubt the ascriptions.

Combe (2), Thomas (d. 1609) Landowner in STRATFORD, a business associate of Shakespeare and the brother of his friend John COMBE (1). Thomas Combe was partner with Shakespeare in a lease to collect the tithes—or church taxes—on some agricultural land near WELCOMBE (the rights to such taxes were transferable, like commodities shares). When he died, his share in the lease was passed on to his elder son, William COMBE (5), who proved a difficult business partner. His second son, another Thomas COMBE (3), was a friend of Shakespeare. According to an 18th-century tradition, Shakespeare wrote an insulting poem about this Thomas Combe, by way of a humorous EPITAPH; it was published in 1740. Modern scholars generally reject the attribution.

Combe (3), Thomas (1589–1657) Lawyer in STRATFORD and friend of Shakespeare, son of Thomas COMBE (2). In his will Shakespeare left Thomas Combe his sword, as a mark of esteem and friendship, but nothing more is known of their relationship. Thomas supported his brother William COMBE (5) in the controversy over the enclosure of lands at WELCOMBE, and like William, he seems to have been a violent man; Thomas GREENE (3) recorded an account of Combe 'kicking and beating' a shepherd who demanded his pay.

Combe (4), William (1551–1610) Landowner in WARWICKSHIRE. Combe, the uncle of Shakespeare's friend John COMBE (1), lived in the city of Warwick but owned land in and around STRATFORD and served as a lawyer for that town. In 1602 he and his nephew sold Shakespeare some land near WELCOMBE. Combe was frequently a member of parliament for Warwickshire.

Combe (5), William (1586–1667) Lawyer, moneylender, and landowner in STRATFORD, a business associate of Shakespeare. Combe was a son of Thomas COMBE (2) and brother of Thomas COMBE (3). From his father, he inherited a share with Shakespeare in a tithe lease—the leased right to collect the taxes on a piece of land. In 1611 Shakespeare sued him for tardiness in paying his share of the rent, leaving the lease open to seizure. This was part of a complicated series of legal actions involving a number of others, and it was settled equably between Shakespeare and Combe. Combe supported an attempt to enclose large tracts of cultivated land at WELCOMBE for sheep grazing, an episode in which he played a brutal part. At one point Julian SHAW (4), the bailiff, or mayor, of Stratford, wrote to Combes that it seemed his conscience was 'blinded . . . with a desire to make yourself rich with other men's loss'. In the 1620s he was said to be richer than his uncle John COMBE (1) had been, suggesting a considerable fortune. During the Civil Wars he fought for the Parliamentarian side, and Royalist troops sacked his house in Stratford. His fortunes declined during the decade of the wars, and in 1650 he was reported to be in considerable debt, with all his land up for sale.

Comedy Drama that provokes laughter at human behaviour, usually involves romantic love, and usually has a happy ending. In Shakespeare's day the conventional comedy enacted the struggle of young lovers to surmount some difficulty, usually presented by their elders, and the play ended happily in marriage or the prospect of marriage. Sometimes the struggle was to bring separated lovers or family members together, and their reunion was the happy culmination (this often involved marriage also). Shakespeare generally observed these conventions, though his inventiveness within them yielded many variations.

Eighteen plays are generally included among Shakespeare's comedies. In approximate order of composition, they are *The Comedy of Errors, The Taming of the Shrew, The Two Gentlemen of Verona, Love's Labour's Lost, A Midsummer Night's Dream, The Merchant of Venice, The Merry Wives of Windsor, Much Ado About Nothing, As You Like It, Twelfth Night, Troilus and Cressida, Measure for Measure, All's Well That Ends Well, Pericles, Cymbeline, The Winter's Tale, The Tempest,* and *The Two Noble Kinsmen.* These works are often divided into distinct subclasses reflecting the playwright's development. The first seven, all written before about 1598, are loosely classed as the 'early comedies', though they vary considerably in both quality and character. The last four of these—*Love's Labour's Lost,* the *Dream,* the *Merchant,* and the *Merry Wives*—are sometimes separated as a transitional group, or linked with the next three in a large 'middle comedies' classification. The *Merry Wives* is somewhat anomalous in any case; it represents a type of comedy—the 'city play', a speciality of such writers as Ben JONSON and Thomas DEKKER—that Shakespeare did not otherwise write. The next three plays, *Much Ado, As You Like It,* and *Twelfth Night,* are often thought to constitute Shakespeare's greatest achievement in comedy; all written around 1599–1600, they are called the romantic, or mature, comedies. The next group of three plays, called the PROBLEM PLAYS, were written in the first years of the 17th century, as Shakespeare was simultaneously creating his greatest tragedies. The final cluster, all written between about 1607 and 1613, make up the bulk of the playwright's final period. They are known as the ROMANCES. (The problem plays and romances were intended to merge TRAGEDY and comedy in TRAGICOMEDY, and they are treated separately in this book.) Many minor variations in this classification scheme are possible; indeed, the boundaries of the whole genre are not fixed, for *Timon of Athens* is often included among the comedies, and *Troilus and Cressida* is sometimes considered a tragedy.

Shakespeare's earliest comedies are similar to existing plays, reflecting his inexperience. *The Comedy of Errors*—thought by many scholars to be his first drama, though the dating of Shakespeare's early works is extremely difficult—is built on a play by the ancient Roman dramatist PLAUTUS. Characteristically, Shakespeare enriched his source, but with material from another play by Plautus. The SUB-PLOT of *The Taming of the Shrew* was taken from a popular play of a generation earlier, and the main plot was well known in folklore, though the combination was ingeniously devised. *The Two Gentlemen of Verona* likewise deals with familiar literary material, treating it in the manner of John LYLY, the most successful comedy writer when Shakespeare began his career.

However, the young playwright soon found the confidence to experiment, and in *Love's Labour's Lost*, the *Dream*, and the *Merchant*, he created a group of unusual works that surely startled Elizabethan playgoers, though pleasurably, we may presume. In the first he created his own main plot and used a distinctively English variation on COMMEDIA DELL' ARTE traditions for a sub-plot. He thus produced a splendid array of comic situations. The play's abundant topical humour was certainly appreciated by the original audiences, although today we don't always know what it is about. In any case, the major characters are charming young lovers, the minor ones are droll eccentrics, and the closing *coup de théâtre*, with which a darkening mood brings the work to a close, is a stunning innovation. Already, the eventual turn towards tragicomedy is foreshadowed. *A Midsummer Night's Dream* mingles motifs from many sources, but the story is again the playwright's own; moreover, the play's extraordinary combination of oddity and beauty was entirely unprecedented and has rarely been approximated since. *The Merchant of Venice* mixes a social theme, usury, into a conventional comedy plot to deepen the resonance of the final outcome as well as to vary the formula. Here, the threat that is finally averted is so dire as to generate an almost tragic mood, again anticipating developments later in the playwright's career.

The mastery that Shakespeare had achieved by the late 1590s is reflected in the insouciance of the titles he gave his mature comedies (*Twelfth Night*'s subtitle—'What You Will'—matches the others). That mastery is accompanied by a serious intent that is lacking in the earliest comedies. Shakespeare could not ignore the inherent poignancy in the contrast between life as it is lived and the escape from life represented by comedy. In *Much Ado*, as in *The Merchant of Venice*, a serious threat to life and happiness counters the froth of a romantic farce. Even in *As You Like It*, one of the most purely entertaining of Shakespeare's plays, the melancholy JAQUES (1) interposes his conviction that life is irredeemably corrupt. FESTE's song at the close of *Twelfth Night* gives touching expression to such sentiments, as he sends us from the theatre with the melancholy refrain, 'the rain it raineth every day' (5.1.391). We are not expected to take him too seriously, but we cannot avoid the realisation that even the life of a jester may be a sad one. The mature comedies thus further a blending of comedy and tragedy.

In the end, however, all of Shakespeare's comedies, including the later problem plays and romances, are driven by love. Love in Shakespearean comedy is stronger than the inertia of custom, the power of evil, or the fortunes of chance and time. In all of these plays but one (*Troilus and Cressida*), the obstacles presented to love are triumphantly overcome, as conflicts are resolved and errors forgiven in a general aura of reconciliation and marital bliss at the play's close. Such intransigent characters as SHYLOCK, MALVOLIO, and Don JOHN (1), who choose not to act out of love, cannot be accommodated in this scheme, and they are carefully isolated from the action before the climax.

In their resolutions Shakespeare's comedies resemble the medieval MORALITY PLAY, which centres on a sinful human who receives God's mercy. In these secular works, a human authority figure—Don PEDRO or DUKE (7) SENIOR, for instance—is symbolically divine, the opponents of love are the representatives of sin, and all of the participants in the closing vignette partake of the play's love and forgiveness. Moreover, the context of marriage—at least alluded to at the close of all but *Troilus and Cressida*—is the cap-stone of the comedic solution, for these plays not only delight and entertain, they affirm, guaranteeing the future. Marriage, with its promise of offspring, reinvigorates society and transcends the purely personal element in sexual attraction and romantic love. Tragedy's focus on the individual makes death the central fact of life, but comedy, with its insistence on the ongoing process of love and sex and birth, confirms our awareness that life transcends the individual.

Comedy of Errors, The

SYNOPSIS

Act 1, Scene 1

The DUKE (8) of EPHESUS informs EGEON, a merchant of Syracuse, that he is subject to the death penalty, prescribed for any citizen of Syracuse found in Ephesus, unless he can pay an immense ransom. Egeon tells of the long search that has brought him to Ephesus: 23 years earlier, his wife and one of their infant twin sons had been separated from him in a shipwreck. The other son had set forth, at the age of 18, in search of his lost brother. He took with him his servant, who had also been separated from a twin brother in the same shipwreck. Egeon himself had then begun to

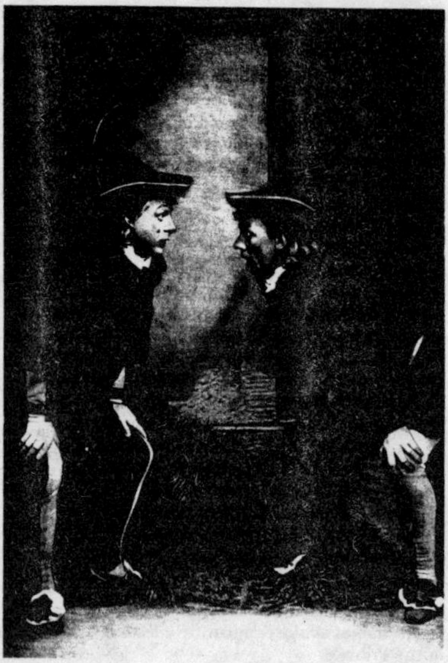

'Methinks you are my glass, and not my brother' (The Comedy of Errors *5.1.417). The two Dromios, brothers separated at birth, are reunited at the end of the play.* (Courtesy of Culver Pictures, Inc.)

roam the world for news of either son. The Duke is sympathetic to this tragic tale; he gives the prisoner the rest of the day to beg or borrow ransom money.

Act 1, Scene 2

A local MERCHANT (1) advises ANTIPHOLUS OF SYRACUSE, newly arrived, not to reveal his origins, telling of the fate of Egeon. Antipholus instructs his servant, DROMIO OF SYRACUSE, to return to their inn and guard their money. In a soliloquy, Antipholus tells of his search for his lost brother, and the audience realises that he is one of Egeon's sons. DROMIO OF EPHESUS enters and mistakes Antipholus for his own master, ANTIPHOLUS OF EPHESUS. Antipholus of Syracuse in turn mistakes this Dromio for his own servant. The presence in the city of the two sets of twins is now known to the audience. Dromio of Ephesus relays his mistress' demand that his master return home. Antipholus of Syracuse asks about the safety of the money, and Dromio denies knowledge of any money. Antipholus beats him, and the mystified servant runs away. Antipholus remarks to himself on the reputation of Ephesus as a centre for witchcraft and thievery, and he hurries back to his inn, fearing theft.

Act 2, Scene 1

ADRIANA, the wife of Antipholus of Ephesus, complains that her husband is late for lunch, thus triggering a disputation on marriage with her sister, LUCIANA; Luciana holds for wifely obedience in all things, while Adriana asserts her independence. Dromio of Ephesus returns to tell of the beating he has received. Adriana sends him out again to fetch Antipholus home. Adriana asserts that her husband prefers the company of other women to her own, though Luciana rebukes her for unjustified jealousy.

Act 2, Scene 2

Antipholus of Syracuse encounters his own servant, whom he berates for the behaviour of the other Dromio and then beats when he declares his innocence. Adriana and Luciana appear, and Adriana, thinking Antipholus of Syracuse to be her husband, chastises him for infidelity. When he responds with natural confusion, he is rebuked by Luciana. The servant also claims ignorance, and the two are jointly condemned by the women. The visitors are mystified and fear that supernatural doings are afoot. However, Antipholus decides to follow the drift of things in the hope of discovering the truth, and he permits himself to be taken to Adriana's home, where Dromio is assigned the gate-guarding duties of his namesake.

Act 3, Scene 1

Antipholus of Ephesus enters with his servant Dromio and two friends, ANGELO (1), a goldsmith, and BALTHASAR (1), a merchant. Antipholus invites his friends to come to his house, but they are turned away at the gate by Dromio of Syracuse, who is obeying his orders to keep out all comers. Another servant, LUCE, and finally Adriana herself, persist in keeping Antipholus out, believing him to be an imposter. The outraged husband announces that he will pay a visit to a COURTESAN he knows and that, moreover, he will give that woman the gold necklace he had commissioned from Angelo as a gift for his wife.

Act 3, Scene 2

Luciana is appalled that Antipholus of Syracuse, whom she believes to be her brother-in-law, Antipholus of Ephesus, has declared his love for her. She concludes that he is mad and flees, announcing her intention to tell Adriana about this turn of events. Dromio of Syracuse enters and tells of the extravagantly ugly kitchen-maid, NELL (1), who has claimed him as a husband. Antipholus sends him to prepare to depart; as he observes in a soliloquy, they must flee the witchery of the place, especially since he has fallen in love with one of the supernatural creatures—

namely Luciana. Angelo appears with the gold chain commissioned by the other Antipholus and turns it over to this one, despite the latter's bewildered protests.

Act 4, Scene 1
A Merchant demands of Angelo the repayment of a debt, and he is accompanied by an OFFICER (1) empowered to arrest debtors. Angelo says that he can satisfy the debt as soon as Antipholus pays him for the gold chain. Just then, Antipholus of Ephesus appears with his servant, whom he sends to buy a rope, with which he proposes to whip his wife for having kept him out of his house. When he sees Angelo, he protests that he has not received the chain. Confusion leads to anger, and Antipholus is arrested. At this point, Dromio of Syracuse appears. He announces that he has arranged passage on a ship and bids Antipholus go aboard. For this seeming asininity, and for not having a rope, Antipholus rebukes Dromio and promises him a future beating. The servant is then sent to Adriana for bail money.

Act 4, Scene 2
Luciana and Adriana discuss the apparent infidelity of Antipholus. Dromio of Syracuse enters and tells of the need for bail. The women, who think he is Dromio of Ephesus, send him back with the required funds.

Act 4, Scene 3
Antipholus of Syracuse is wearing the gold chain provided by Angelo. Dromio of Syracuse arrives with the bail money, but of course his master does not know what he is talking about. Antipholus attributes their confusion to the supernatural qualities of Ephesus. Consequently, when the Courtesan appears, asking if his gold chain is the one he has promised her, he responds by asserting that she must be an agent of the devil. When she demands the return of a ring she had given him, the two Syracusans flee. The Courtesan reflects that Antipholus must surely be mad. She determines to tell Adriana of her husband's state.

Act 4, Scene 4
Antipholus of Ephesus, in the custody of the Officer, sees Dromio of Ephesus and thinks his bail money has arrived. This Dromio, however, has the rope he was sent to purchase. He is struck with it by the furious Antipholus and delivers an elaborate lament on being beaten. Adriana, Luciana, and the Courtesan arrive, with Doctor PINCH, whom Adriana entreats to restore Antipholus to sanity. Antipholus, becoming more and more enraged, attempts to strike Adriana, and he and Dromio are restrained and tied up by a group of passers-by. Pinch takes the two prisoners to Adriana's house for treatment. Antipholus and Dromio of Syracuse appear; the others flee, believing the two have escaped from Pinch and are bent on revenge.

Act 5, Scene 1
Angelo and the Merchant discuss the strange behaviour of Antipholus of Ephesus. Antipholus and Dromio of Syracuse appear; Angelo charges Antipholus with dishonesty, and tempers flare. Antipholus and the Merchant draw their swords. Adriana, Luciana, and the Courtesan reappear, calling for help in capturing Antipholus and Dromio. The two Syracusans flee, taking sanctuary in the PRIORY. The Abbess of the Priory, EMILIA (1), emerges. Adriana demands the return of her husband; the Abbess refuses to permit a violation of the right to sanctuary.

Adriana determines to appeal to the Duke. The Duke appears, with a retinue including the unfortunate Egeon, who is to be beheaded. Antipholus and Dromio of Ephesus arrive, having escaped from Pinch. Antipholus, too, demands justice of the Duke. Charges and counter-charges are exchanged by Antipholus, Angelo, Adriana, and the Courtesan. The extent of the confusion overwhelms the Duke, who sends for the Abbess. Egeon claims Antipholus of Ephesus as his son, but, as it is the wrong Antipholus he addresses, he is repudiated. The Abbess reappears with Antipholus and Dromio of Syracuse. All are stunned by the presence, together for the first time, of the two sets of identical twins. The Abbess recognises Egeon and reveals that she is his long-lost wife, Emilia. The identities of the twins are quickly established, and Emilia invites all the company to a feast of celebration in the Priory.

COMMENTARY

The Comedy of Errors is an early work, lacking most of the features we associate with Shakespeare's masterpieces. It contains no brilliant dialogue or poetry, no very impressive characters, and, most strikingly, its plot line is difficult to take at all seriously. Of all Shakespeare's plays, *The Comedy of Errors* most nearly resembles a FARCE, pure and simple, which the *Oxford English Dictionary* defines as 'a dramatic work (usually short) which has for its sole object to excite laughter'.

This play is both short and funny, but it is also more than that. Shakespeare's genius lies in his concern with what it is to be human and here he elevates a common farce by means of telling depictions of the human condition. He presents and resolves disruptions and anxieties that invite sympathy and stimulate compassion. In watching or reading *The Comedy of Errors,* we experience an awareness of the value to an individual of relationships to other people. Further, the play presents aspects of the situation of women in Elizabethan society, a matter Shakespeare often dealt with. The redeeming power of love, a profound theme in much of the playwright's later work, is also presented here, in an uncomplicated foreshadowing of subtler renderings.

A traditional opinion among scholars and critics,

only lately being revised, is that *The Comedy of Errors* is best regarded as an apprentice work, only marginally related to the greater plays that followed. There is some justification for this point of view. For one thing, the play is very conventional, conforming in staging and general outline to standard Elizabethan ideas, derived from what was known of ancient Roman drama, of what constituted a proper play. In staging his play, Shakespeare was content to abide by most of the ancient conventions of the form. In accordance with accepted neoclassical doctrine, the action of the play takes place in a single place and in a single day. The setting consists of three buildings—the PHOENIX, the PORCUPINE, and the PRIORY, each labelled with a sign or emblem—in imitation of Roman stagecraft as it was understood in Shakespeare's time.

Moreover, Shakespeare's play is undeniably farcical in its assembled absurdities. These are simply conventions of farce, as acceptable to a 16th-century audience as those of the Marx Brothers are acceptable today, and no different in kind. In adding the twin servants to the story he received from PLAUTUS (see 'Sources', below), Shakespeare doubled the chances for misadventure and created a set of complications that has been likened to a Bach fugue, but the principles of farce remain the same.

Another striking addition Shakespeare made, changing the character of the work in a very important way, is the sub-plot featuring Egeon. Egeon's explanation of his family's separation in 1.1 serves as a PROLOGUE (1) to the play, a classical device that Shakespeare used more formally elsewhere. More important, Egeon's pathetic circumstances serve to colour the farcical main plot: we cannot wholly forget this poor, unfortunate father to the Antipholus twins. Because this is a humorous play, we of course presume that all will end well, but we know that before it does this potential tragedy will have to be overcome somehow. Indeed, Egeon experiences a moment of extreme despair, after his seeming rejection by his long-sought son (5.1.298–322). Thus the coming reconciliation scene ends a truly important human crisis, as well as resolving the comic confusions of the central tale. Shakespeare, even as a young man at the beginning of his career, felt that a happy ending should not be divorced from an awareness of mortality and human frailty. In this he utterly transcends the genre of farce.

Some critics have charged that this device damages a play that might have been a fine farce but that, in its present form, is neither tragic nor wholly comic. However, modern opinion has generally held that the Egeon sub-plot is necessary, providing a moral ground for an otherwise unenlightening display of low comedy. In any case, this sub-plot is an early example of an important aspect of Shakespeare's art—the formulation of more than one point of view, generating different and potentially conflicting responses from the audience.

Chief among the characters involved in the central story of *The Comedy of Errors* is Adriana, one of the earliest of Shakespeare's many attractive heroines. Shakespeare developed Adriana from a stereotype of the contentious, jealous shrew, and she conforms to this image. But she is raised from a type to a real human being through the wit her creator gives her. Further, her evident loyalty to and love for her difficult husband render her quite sympathetic and admirable. She resembles such other Shakespearean women as KATHERINA, in *The Taming of the Shrew,* and BEATRICE, in *Much Ado About Nothing,* in being sharp-tongued and independent-minded, but ultimately tender and accepting. The playwright could thus present the reality of Elizabethan women whose personal strengths enabled them to temper, if not overcome, the general subservience of their gender, while at the same time confirming the legitimacy of the system, as his own conservatism inclined him to do. Adriana is contrasted with her sister, Luciana, who is a dimmer figure, demure and passive. The debate between the two women on the proper relation of man and wife (2.1.7–42) is a set-piece disputation of a sort often presented on the Elizabethan stage. Although Adriana is a much more interesting and appealing character, Luciana's attitude to marriage seems to prevail at the play's end, in keeping with the common opinion of the day, which most women and Shakespeare shared.

Many of Shakespeare's plays hinge on a basic political question, the nature of the relationships among the citizen, the ruler, and the state. In this early work, the matter is only touched upon, but in a fashion that reveals an attitude that the playwright was to hold all his life. In a brief but telling passage, the Duke of Ephesus refuses to allow any alteration in the laws (1.1.142–148). He is explicit: his personal honour requires this relationship to the state. This is a kingly ideal that is expressed repeatedly, in much greater elaboration, in later plays. That the young Shakespeare found occasion to present it here, without any compelling reason to do so, suggests its early importance for him.

For Shakespeare and his contemporaries, everyone, not just the king, took his or her identity from a relationship with society as a whole. One was not simply a conscious, individual being, but, more important, one occupied a position in the social framework. Shakespeare was to consider this matter of social identity in a number of ways in later plays; it is touched on in this early work. Antipholus of Syracuse is concerned for his lost selfhood when he regrets the loss of his family in a touching soliloquy (1.2.33–40) on his lack of contentment. Also, it is evident that the distress undergone by the four misidentified twins is caused by the loss of their sense of identity; as the people in their

world fail to recognise them, they experience a painful uncertainty as to who they are themselves.

Antipholus of Syracuse, in his confusion, seeks to be remade, through love, by Luciana. The transforming power of love was always an important theme for Shakespeare; in several later plays, it is a major concern. Here, it is overwhelmed by the farce for the most part, but we see it roughly sketched out with reference to romantic love in the depiction of the marriage of Adriana and Antipholus of Ephesus, and in the wooing of Luciana by Antipholus of Syracuse. Familial love triumphs in the reunion at the close of the play. And Emilia, the Abbess, who provides the resolution when the Duke, for all his power, cannot, represents the strength of Christian grace and mercy, a transcendent form of love.

Shakespeare's interest in the inner and outer worlds of human experience is what makes him great. He writes of the web of relationships, both political and domestic, that make up a society, and his characters have inner lives that we can recognise as realistic. In *The Comedy of Errors,* although it is derivative and rather limited in range, we see his talent already beginning to produce a drama of conflict and resolution in a world of basic human concerns, using themes and materials that would recur in his mature work.

SOURCES OF THE PLAY

Shakespeare's principal source for *The Comedy of Errors* was *The Menaechmi,* a play by the ancient Roman playwright Plautus. The first English translation of *The Menaechmi,* by William WARNER, was not published until 1595, a little later than the date when Shakespeare's play was presumably written, but the playwright may have known the translation in manuscript, as was common at that time, or he might have read it in one of several 16th-century Latin editions. Shakespeare made a number of important changes in the story, as he usually did when using sources. His boldest and best-known alteration was the addition of a second set of misidentified twins, a twist he took from another play by Plautus, *Amphitryon.* A number of other changes result in a general shift in the qualities of the play. For example, a ribald emphasis on a husband's relations with a mistress is elevated to a concern with the virtues of courtship and marriage.

The sub-plot concerning Egeon may derive from any of a number of sources; the motif of separated and reunited families had been familiar since ancient times. Shakespeare surely knew it from the medieval *Gesta Romanorum,* translated by Richard ROBINSON (3)—later a source for *The Merchant of Venice*—and the *Confessio Amantis,* by John GOWER (3)—later a source for *Pericles.* However, the hostility between cities resulting in a traveller's death penalty comes from George GASCOIGNE's *Supposes* (performed 1566, published 1573), where the situation is invented as part of a ruse; it is used in the same way to dupe the PEDANT in *The Taming of the Shrew.*

TEXT OF THE PLAY

The Comedy of Errors is sometimes said to have been the first play that Shakespeare wrote, although this cannot be proven. It was certainly one of his earliest. The play's first recorded performance was held on December 28, 1594, as part of a programme of Christmas revels at Gray's Inn (see INNS OF COURT). This private performance, the play's brevity (with fewer than 1,800 lines, it is Shakespeare's shortest), and its resemblance to ancient Roman comedy have prompted some scholars to suggest that the play was commissioned for this presentation to a particularly learned audience. However, most scholarly opinion holds that it was written at an earlier date; estimates have ranged from the late 1580s to 1594.

The play was initially published in the FIRST FOLIO, in 1623. This version is believed to have been derived from Shakespeare's FOUL PAPERS. The Folio contains the only early publication of *The Comedy of Errors,* and it has been the basis for all subsequent editions of the play.

THEATRICAL HISTORY OF THE PLAY

The Gray's Inn performance of December 1594 and a performance at the court of King James I in the Christmas season of 1604 are the only known early productions, although various references in contemporary plays and books suggest that there were probably other 16th- and 17th-century stagings. In the 18th century and well into the 19th, all presentations of *The Comedy of Errors,* with the possible exception of a brief run in 1741, were adaptations that varied more or less grossly from the original. The brevity of the play, its esoteric relation to classical drama, and a sense that it was more an 'apprentice' piece than a mature work seem to have combined to provide justification for a long series of illegitimate productions, by Thomas HULL and others. Perhaps the strangest of these offspring was the 1819 opera produced by Frederick REYNOLDS (1), whose libretto included songs from *As You Like It, Love's Labour's Lost, King Lear,* and *Othello,* plus two of the SONNETS, and which used additional dialogue and entire scenes from various sources, only some of them Shakespearean.

Shakespeare's play was first restored to the stage in its proper form by Samuel PHELPS in 1855. It has gradually increased in popularity since then and has often been produced in recent years. Variations on the play have also continued to be produced in the 20th century; the 1938 musical comedy *The Boys from Syracuse,* by Richard Rodgers and Lorenz Hart, is an example. In 1976, Trevor NUNN made a FILM of *The Comedy of*

Errors, with Judi DENCH as Adriana, and the play has been made for TELEVISION several times.

Comedy of Humours Genre of ELIZABETHAN DRAMA, plays in which each character possesses some strong, clearly identifiable personality trait or quirk that determines his or her behaviour in any circumstances. For instance, a lecher will find all occasions appropriate for chasing women; a glutton will continually be concerned with food; a jealous husband will always look for evidence of his wife's infidelity. Among Shakespeare's plays, *The Merry Wives of Windsor* and *Twelfth Night* most nearly exemplify the genre, although he tended to combine features of several types of play. The most important practitioner of the comedy of humours was Ben JONSON.

In the late 1580s and early 1590s the term 'humour', referring to striking aspects of personality or patterns of behaviour, became prominent in Elizabethan London. It stemmed from a medieval medical theory—in its last decades of respectability and increasingly recognised as problematical—that held that human health depends on a proper balance among four 'humours', or bodily fluids: black bile, yellow bile, blood, and phlegm. When the balance was upset and one 'humour' dominated, a person was likely to become ill and/or act strangely. The word became associated with all striking behaviour, and it began to take on the association with comedy that it has today.

In the 1590s the attribution of prominent humours to dramatic characters arose as a plausible way to use the elaborate system of character types that occur in ancient Roman drama, especially in the plays of PLAUTUS. Comedies of humours were generally intended to ridicule the 'humorous' behaviour they presented. Elaborate complications involving intrigue and deceit typified their plots. Characters often bore tag names indicating their qualities, as do Shakespeare's SHALLOW and MALVOLIO.

The vogue for comedy of humours—and for using the word 'humour'—was itself a subject for comedy. For example, NYM, who appears in *The Merry Wives of Windsor* and *Henry V,* uses the word 'humour' in almost every speech he makes. He took this trait from a character in a successful play by George CHAPMAN, *The Blind Beggar of Alexandria* (1596). The comedy of humours reached its peak with Jonson's works of the early 17th century, but it remained popular for about another 100 years.

Cominius Legendary figure and character in *Coriolanus,* a Roman general. Cominius is the commander of the Roman troops fighting against the VOLSCIANS at CORIOLES, and his friend MARTIUS (2) (later CORIOLANUS), is a general under him. Cominius is a discreet general who contrasts with the hero. He executes a sensible withdrawal in 1.6, before he is joined by Coriolanus who goads him on to a successful counterattack. In the same scene we see Cominius as the subject of Martius' bizarre enthusiasm. Excited by the fighting, Martius embraces him with the fervour, he says, of his wedding night. The commander accepts this as normal battlefield comradeship, however, and in 1.9 he praises Martius and proposes that he take the honourable name Coriolanus. In 2.2 he nominates Coriolanus to the consulate. However, in Act 3 he cannot prevent Coriolanus' obstinate pride from bringing about his own banishment, and in 5.1 he reports that he has been unable to persuade Coriolanus—now fighting for the Volscians—from his campaign against Rome. Cominius is a representative of the ineffectual aristocracy who cannot control events.

Shakespeare took Cominius from his source, PLUTARCH's *Lives,* but added the intimacy of his relationship with Coriolanus, and thereby established him as a foil to the protagonist. As Coriolanus' friend, Cominius helps us see Coriolanus at his problematical best, early in the play. We recognise his value to his fellows while we acknowledge that he is excessive in his enthusiasm for combat.

Commedia dell' Arte Genre of 16th- and 17th-century Italian COMEDY, probable influence on several of Shakespeare's plays. In commedia dell' arte—which was frequently performed in England by travelling Italian companies, especially in the 1570s and 1580s—dialogue was largely improvised, as the action followed prescribed general lines familiar to both players and spectators; the plays were in any case so obvious that the troupes could find success with non-Italian-speaking audiences. The melodramatic and/or sentimental plots usually featured farcical intrigues involving love and money, though several involved a shipwreck on a magician's island, perhaps suggesting to Shakespeare the basic situation of *The Tempest.* The principal characters wore masks and were thus immediately recognisable; their personalities were understood before they said a word. They represented stock character types, some of which are thought to have influenced Shakespeare's characters.

Among the most important of these types was the pantaloon, an avaricious and lecherous old man, often a miser offering windy and moralistic advice to the young lovers. He may have contributed something to POLONIUS. At any rate, Shakespeare presumed his audiences were at least familiar with this figure, for in *As You Like It* he has JAQUES (1) cite 'the lean and slipper'd pantaloon . . . His youthful hose well sav'd' (2.7.158–160) as a symbol of old age. Another commedia figure was a lawyer, Dr Graziano or the *dottore,* also amorous but distinguished by his preten-

tious pedantry. HOLOFERNES, of *Love's Labour's Lost,* is quite similar to the *dottore,* and his fellow comical rustic in that play, ARMADO, resembles a third commedia figure, the *capitano,* a braggart soldier, the descendant of the ancient Roman MILES GLORIOSUS. Several other Shakespearean characters resemble the *capitano,* including most notably PAROLLES and FALSTAFF.

An important feature of the commedia dell' arte was a group of ostensibly minor comic characters called *zanni*—the root of our word *zany*—who were servants to the major figures but often dominated the action. In fact, another name for the genre is *commedia dei zanni.* They shared the characteristics of greed and shrewdness but evolved into a number of distinctive figures. Chief among them were Arlequino, a clever rascal (who survived the passing of the genre as Harlequin), and Pulcinella (Punch), a violent egotist. The *zanni* were descendants of the stock clever slaves and servants of Roman drama, which Shakespeare knew from PLAUTUS. So, although the DROMIOS of *The Comedy of Errors* and TRANIO of *The Taming of the Shrew* resemble *zanni,* Shakespeare need not have taken them from the commedia. However, the playwright's demonstrable awareness of the Italian players strongly suggests that the commedia dell' arte exercised at least some influence on Shakespeare's characters.

Commoner (1) Any of several minor characters in *Julius Caesar,* working people of ROME. In 1.1 the tribunes FLAVIUS (1) and MARULLUS disperse a crowd of Commoners who have gathered to cheer CAESAR (1). Two of the Commoners speak, the CARPENTER only to identify himself, the COBBLER to bandy crude witticisms with the officers. (In some editions the speakers are identified as the First and Second Commoners.) This pleasingly vital episode comically introduces the urban mob that, as the PLEBEIANS (1), flares into riot in Act 3.

Commoner (2) Any of several minor characters in *Coriolanus,* citizens of ANTIUM who first support and then turn against CORIOLANUS. In 5.6 Coriolanus has spared ROME from destruction at the hands of his Volscian troops, and he reports to the Volscian leaders at Antium accompanied by a throng of enthusiastic Commoners. In ironic contrast to his history in Rome, Coriolanus now has the support of the common people for the first time in the play. However, once AUFIDIUS accuses him of treason, they turn against their hero. 'Tear him to pieces!' (5.6.120), they cry, in an episode that parallels the fury of the populace in 3.3 that led to Coriolanus' banishment from Rome (see CITIZEN [5]). Though mostly mute—their three lines are assigned to the whole group—the Commoners' placement in the play's last moments is crucial. They stress again an important theme of the play, one that has been demonstrated repeatedly by their fellows in Rome: the common people, as a group, are susceptible to inflammatory rhetoric and are therefore unreliable participants in political life.

Commons Group of extras in *2 Henry VI,* members of the parliament assembled at BURY ST EDMUNDS. These representatives of the common people gather in an unruly crowd in 3.2 to protest the murder of the Duke of GLOUCESTER (4) and demand punishment for the Duke of SUFFOLK (3). As is usual in Shakespeare, the common people en masse, as distinguished from individual characters, are presented as a thoughtless rabble, controllable only by aristocrats, here the Earls of WARWICK (3) and SALISBURY (2). Warwick refers to them as 'an angry hive of bees / That want their leader' (3.2.124–125), and Salisbury speaks for them in their address to the King. They prepare the audience for the later appearance of the rebels led by Jack CADE, as the disorder in the state intensifies.

Complaint Poem intended to express unhappiness. A popular genre from the 14th through the 17th centuries, the complaint could take many forms, from meditations on the general sorrows of life to the bewailing of a particular event or situation—especially unrequited love—to humorous laments over trivial subjects, though these last were less common. Shakespeare's *The Rape of Lucrece* is often classed as a complaint—although the form was usually written in the first person—and it was written in RHYME ROYAL, the pattern that theorists prescribed for the genre. After Shakespeare's time the complaint was gradually replaced by the less expressly plaintive lament or elegy.

Compton, Fay (1895–1978) English actress. Fay Compton played numerous Shakespearean parts in her long and distinguished career, most notably appearing as OPHELIA opposite the HAMLETS of both John BARRYMORE and John GIELGUD. She was the sister of the noted novelist Compton Mackenzie (1883–1972), and her own memoirs (*Rosemary,* 1926) were very popular.

Condell, Henry (d. 1627) English actor and co-editor, with John HEMINGE, of the FIRST FOLIO edition of Shakespeare's plays. Listed in the Folio as one of the 26 'Principall Actors' in the plays, Condell became a partner in the CHAMBERLAIN'S MEN in 1598 and had probably acted with the company from its inception in 1594. He remained with its successor, the KING'S MEN, until his death. He acted in both tragedies and comedies, but he is not known for any particular Shakespearean role. His friendship with Shakespeare is evidenced by the playwright's small legacy to him in his will. Condell was one of the original partners in the BLACKFRIARS THEATRE, and he later acquired shares in

the GLOBE THEATRE as well. He apparently invested well, for he died a wealthy man.

Conrade (Conrad) Character in *Much Ado About Nothing,* follower of Don JOHN (1). In 3.3 Conrade listens as his friend BORACHIO tells of the scheme to implicate the innocent HERO as a promiscuous woman. This conversation is overheard by the WATCHMEN (3), which leads ultimately to the exposure of Don John's villainy. Conrade is a simple pawn, needing no personality, but he does display a vehement temper when, irritated by Constable DOGBERRY's interrogation, he blurts out, 'You are an ass, you are an ass' (4.2.70). This triggers one of Dogberry's best comic bits, his indignant repetition of the insult.

Conspirators Minor characters in *Coriolanus,* followers of AUFIDIUS. In 5.6 the Conspirators affirm that they will help Aufidius take revenge on CORIOLANUS. They encourage him in his anger and point out that Coriolanus is overshadowing him. When Aufidius accuses his enemy of treason, they lead the mob in demanding Coriolanus' death, a demand they then fulfil by killing him with their swords. Though the conspirators are designated First, Second, and Third, they are indistinguishable from each other, and their speeches are divisions of a single voice. The Conspirators help to illuminate one of the play's principal themes: the common people (see COMMONER [2]) are susceptible to manipulation, and are thus an unstable and unreliable component of society. On the other hand, because they encourage—even goad—Aufidius to kill Coriolanus in such an ignominious fashion, they also help demonstrate the inadequacies of the warrior class.

Constable of France, Charles d'Albret (Delabreth) (d. 1415) Historical figure and character in *Henry V,* a high-ranking officer in the French army. Although the Constable recognises that King HENRY V is not the dissolute figure the DAUPHIN (3) believes him to be, he nonetheless falls prey to the over-confidence of the French prior to the battle of AGINCOURT. His death in the battle and his name are reported in 4.8.94.

Constance, Duchess of Brittany (d. 1201) Historical figure and character in *King John,* mother of ARTHUR. Before the play begins, Constance has gained the support of King PHILIP (2) of FRANCE (1) in her attempt to place Arthur on the throne of England, from which King JOHN (3), his uncle, has displaced him. In 3.1 she rages furiously at the betrayal of her cause by Philip and the Archduke of AUSTRIA emphasising the theme of treachery that runs throughout the play. However, she then helps persuade Philip to another betrayal, as he turns on his new ally, King John. In 3.3 (3.4; for citation, see *King John,* 'Synopsis'), Constance grieves hysterically over Arthur's capture by King John. She raves about making love to death (3.3.25–36), and Philip fears that she will harm herself. Her death 'in a frenzy' is reported in 4.2.122. Her agonising madness helps to stress the evil of John's usurpation.

The historical Constance was the daughter of a rebellious duke of Brittany whom King John's father, Henry II, defeated. In an effort to assure Brittany's loyalty, Henry insisted that Constance marry his son Geoffrey. After Geoffrey's death Constance ruled Brittany for Arthur, whose name may suggest her ambition to see her son rule England. Her ambition is reflected in Shakespeare's sources, but the playwright altered the details of her life freely. For instance, Constance bemoans her 'husbandless' state in 2.2.14 (3.1.14), but in fact she married twice after Geoffrey's death. Also, in order to continue a deliberate pairing of Constance with ELEANOR, he has the the two women die at the same time, although in fact Constance died three years before.

Contention, The Abbreviated title of the first QUARTO edition of *2 Henry VI.* Published in 1594 by Thomas MILLINGTON, the play was originally titled, in the florid manner of the time, *The First part of the Contention betwixt the two famous Houses of Yorke and Lancaster, with the death of the good Duke Humphrey: And the banishment and death of the Duke of Suffolke, and the Tragicall end of the proud Cardinall of Winchester, with the notable Rebellion of Iacke Cade: And the Duke of Yorkes first claime unto the Crowne. The Contention,* known as the Q1 edition of *2 Henry VI,* is a shorter, inferior version of the F edition in the FIRST FOLIO, published in 1623. The Q2 edition of *2 Henry VI,* varying very little from Q1, was published by Millington in 1600, also as *The Contention.* Q3, a more heavily edited version, appeared in 1619, combined with a BAD QUARTO edition of *3 Henry VI* in one volume now known as THE WHOLE CONTENTION.

The existence of Q1 has generated a number of theories. It has been regarded as an original play, written earlier than *2 Henry VI,* probably by GREENE (2), PEELE, NASHE, MARLOWE (1), or possibly Shakespeare himself (or some combination of these in collaboration). Later, according to this theory, Shakespeare revised the play for a new production, creating the F text.

Another theory holds that *The Contention* is a 'reported' version of *2 Henry VI,* i.e., a bad quarto that was assembled from the recollections of actors or viewers for purposes of unauthorised publication. It has even been speculated that *The Contention* may be a reported version of yet another play, a lost original. *2 Henry VI* would then be a revision of either *The Contention* or of the lost play.

All these theories can be supported in one way or another, and the truth of the matter cannot be ascer-

tained from the existing evidence. However, modern scholarship has generally, though not unanimously, accepted the second of these propositions—that *The Contention* is a reported, or 'memorial', text of *2 Henry VI.* It was perhaps created in 1593, at the time of the bankruptcy and temporary collapse of the PEMBROKE'S MEN, the acting company that originally produced the play.

Cooke (1), Alexander (d. 1614) English actor, one of the 26 men listed in the FIRST FOLIO as the 'Principall Actors' of Shakespeare's plays. Cooke apparently became a member of the KING'S MEN in 1604—having served as a hired actor earlier—and he remained with them at least into 1613. He was probably apprenticed to John HEMINGE, whom he refers to as 'my master' in his will.

Cooke may have appeared with PEMBROKE'S MEN in THE TAMING OF A SHREW, sometime between 1592 and 1594. In that BAD QUARTO of *The Taming of the Shrew* (where the text was assembled from actors' memories), one of the PLAYERS (1) is designated 'San' or 'Sander', and Sander—a common Elizabethan nickname for Alexander—is the name of the equivalent of Shakespeare's GRUMIO. Their speeches are fairly accurately reproduced in *A Shrew,* so if Cooke did play these parts, he was one of the actors who compiled the text.

Cooke (2), George Frederick (1756–1811) English actor. Cooke was a rival of John Philip KEMBLE (3) in the early years of the 19th century. He was especially noted for his OTHELLO, with which he established himself as a respected actor. He played many Shakespearean roles, including RICHARD III, HENRY VIII, and FALSTAFF. He eventually moved to America and died in New York. Remarkably, Cooke played a Shakespearean role nearly 170 years after his death, when his skull—preserved by his physician upon his death and eventually given to a Philadelphia university—was employed as that of YORICK in a 1980 TELEVISION production of *Hamlet.*

Corambis Name given to POLONIUS in the BAD QUARTO (Q1, 1604) of *Hamlet.* Corambis is thought to allude to a well-known Latin proverb on triteness: *Crambe bis posita mors est* ('Cabbage served twice is deadly'); this seems appropriate to the long-winded Polonius but the reason for the variation in names is uncertain. Polonius' servant, REYNALDO (1), is also renamed in Q1 as MONTANO (1), suggesting a satirical point to the names—a cabbage attended by a mountain might caricature a prominent bore and his hulking assistant—but no target is now identifiable, although some scholars nominate Lord BURGHLEY, a leading English statesman.

Q1 is a version of the play compiled from the memories of actors who played in it, and some scholars suppose that Corambis was the name of the equivalent character in an earlier play, now lost, the UR-HAMLET, and that it was inserted in Q1 by an actor who also knew the earlier work. If so, then any satirical point was intended not by Shakespeare but by the author of the *Ur-Hamlet,* probably Thomas KYD; perhaps Shakespeare changed the name in order to dissociate his character from the earlier caricature.

Corambis may be a corruption of Corambus, a form that appears in DER BESTRAFTE BRUDERMORD, a German version of *Hamlet* derived in part from Q1. Shakespeare used this form in passing in *All's Well That Ends Well* (4.3.158), which is sometimes taken as circumstantial evidence that, since he knew the name, he could perhaps have taken it from the *Ur-Hamlet.*

Cordelia Character in *King Lear,* the virtuous daughter whom King LEAR mistakenly rejects. Knowing she will marry, Cordelia refuses to assert that all of her love will forever go to her father, unlike REGAN and GONERIL, her hypocritical sisters. Lear mistakes Cordelia's honesty for a lack of affection and disinherits her, though the King of FRANCE (2) recognises her innate worth and marries her anyway. She leaves Britain with him at the end of 1.1 and does not reappear until Act 4, when she arrives with an army. She intends to restore her father to his throne, for he has been humiliated and banished to the wilderness by Regan and Goneril. Lear and Cordelia are reunited, but are nonetheless defeated in battle, and the villainous EDMUND imprisons them and orders their murder, in 5.3. Although Edmund is defeated by EDGAR it is too late; the assassin has killed Cordelia, though Lear kills him. In the play's final episode Lear grieves over his daughter's corpse and dies of a broken heart.

During her long absence from the play we are not permitted to forget Cordelia, for her goodness and self-sacrifice are central to the tragedy: the FOOL (2) is said to have 'much pined away' for her, in 1.4.72; in 2.2, the loyal KENT (2) reveals that she knows of Lear's situation; Lear himself refers to her in 2.4.211; and her invasion force is mentioned several times, beginning in 3.1.30.

Many commentators believe that Shakespeare specifically intended Cordelia as an example of the Christian virtues of self-sacrifice and acceptance of God's will. Cordelia accepts her undeserved fate while she displays undiminished love for her erring father. In this view she is a Christlike figure in a pagan world who offers a suggestion of Christianity's coming redemption of humanity. Her death thus symbolises Christ's crucifixion, and the tragedy's lesson is the mysterious nature of God's will.

A non-religious interpretation of Cordelia's sacrifice is also proposed by many critics, who see her virtue as its own reward, for as a pagan she lacks the

Christian's promise of recompense in the afterlife. In this humanistic view her goodness inspires our admiration all the more for being unrewarded, and the pure light of her courage offers the most compelling sense that the play's tragedy is not utterly futile. Also, many critics hold that Shakespeare intended Lear to die believing that Cordelia is still alive, in which case his own fate is greatly eased, and we can feel more strongly the redemptive effect of her virtues. A final variation on her importance does not diminish it: some writers hold that *King Lear* reflects a despairing and pessimistic view of life that denies aid for human folly in a tragic universe. In this interpretation Cordelia's virtues, combined with the injustice of both her rejection by her father and her ultimate death, offer striking confirmation of the dire point of view attributed to the playwright.

In almost any view Cordelia's manifest virtue is a dominating element of the play, giving her an importance seemingly unjustified by her relatively few appearances on stage. In her pure honesty and unqualified love she seems almost devoid of ordinary human personality traits, and her saintly qualities are especially stressed by the GENTLEMAN (7) who reports on her in 4.3, preparing the audience for her return to the drama. In a passage rich in imagery and rhetoric he describes her mingled joy and sorrow at news of Lear, saying, for instance, '. . . she shook / The holy water from her heavenly eyes' (4.3.29–30). Later, she is described as one 'Who redeems nature from the general curse' (4.6.203). Evoked in these terms, Cordelia resembles an angel more than she does a worldly character. Her vague personality contributes to our sense of dislocation in *King Lear.* She is remote from the more active figures, even the fighters against evil, Edgar, Kent, and ALBANY, and this draws attention to the failure of human interaction in the play's tragic universe.

Cordelia may also be seen in a more human light. In fact, some writers declare that she exhibits a prideful stubbornness in Act 1, only adopting an attitude of loving generosity when she sees the damage that has been done. In this light her moral progress may be said to parallel that of her father. This is a minority view, however, for most commentators feel that Shakespeare intended her initial insistence on honesty to be an obvious virtue.

Corin Character in *As You Like It,* an honest, elderly shepherd. In 2.4 and in 3.5 Corin is associated with SILVIUS, a conventional shepherd who is filled with literary conceits about love; in most PASTORAL literature the countryside was an idealised setting for amorous tales of shepherds and shepherdesses, such as Silvius and his beloved, PHEBE. Corin, by contrast, is a real shepherd. He describes the economic plight of the shepherd to ROSALIND and CELIA in 2.4.73–84, while at the same time establishing himself as a representative of traditional rural values, offering such modest hospitality as he can.

In 3.2 Corin expresses his down-to-earth relationship to his world, and he can say, 'I am a true labourer: I earn that I eat, get that I wear; owe no man hate, envy no man's happiness . . .' (3.2.71–72). TOUCHSTONE wittily derides this simple life, but he cannot upset Corin. The honest shepherd anchors the rustic life of ARDEN (1) in the real world and thus offsets the high-flown sentiment of pastoral tradition.

Corin's name was commonly applied to shepherds in late medieval and Renaissance romantic literature; it may be a masculine form of Corinna (active c. 500–470 B.C.), an ancient Greek lyric poetess. Shakespeare may have been inspired to use the name by an English play of the 1570s, published in 1599, *Syre Clyomon and Clamydes,* in which a princess disguised as a man serves a shepherd named Corin.

Coriolanus, Martius Legendary figure and title character of *Coriolanus,* a famed Roman warrior whose excessive pride leads him to dishonour and death. His pride is part of his sense of himself as a warrior and aristocrat, a self-image that he has acquired from a rigorous upbringing by his extraordinary mother, VOLUMNIA. When the changing political world of ROME—represented by the tribunes BRUTUS (3) and SICINIUS—demands compromises that his pride will not accept, Coriolanus is driven from Rome and joins the city's enemies, the VOLSCIANS. Finally, when his mother persuades him to spare Rome, he is killed by the Volscian leader, his archrival AUFIDIUS.

Like OTHELLO and MACBETH, Coriolanus is a successful warrior who finds himself in a situation—here, the political world of Rome—to which he is temperamentally unsuited and in which he can be manipulated by others. Politically unsophisticated and emotionally immature, he can neither strike political deals with the tribunes nor resist his mother's insistence that he do so. He is reduced to blind vengeance, but she blocks him in that direction as well. Under these pressures, his great strength can only destroy him. His fate contains the irony found in all Shakespeare's tragedies: with greatness comes great weakness. Coriolanus' pride makes him great, but it also brings about his downfall.

Coriolanus' relationship with his mother makes him one of the most psychologically interesting of Shakespeare's protagonists. He is entirely Volumnia's creation, and thus Coriolanus is psychologically dependent on her good opinion, as is demonstrated in both of their crucial scenes. In 3.2 she bullies him into political compromise as his resistance collapses under her disdain: 'Thy valiantness was mine . . . but owe thy pride thyself' (3.2.129–130). In 5.3 he cannot withstand another personal denial—'This fellow had a

Volscian to his mother' (5.3.178)—and he abandons his life rather than suffer his mother's disapproval. She can manipulate him because when she created him she deprived him of all motives but one, his pride, which depends on her continuing approval. Though he avoids the psychological trauma of her rejection and saves his honour as a Roman warrior, by giving in to her he must accept an ignominious death at the hands of his enemy Aufidius.

Nevertheless, Coriolanus is brave and ready to go beyond his duty as a soldier; he is clearly a noble figure. His name reminds us of this: he is known as MARTIUS (2) through the first eight scenes, and is renamed in honour of his military exploits at CORIOLES. The hero's nobility is made clear throughout the play, in the opinions of both the Romans—friends like MENENIUS all but worship him, and even the tribunes concede that he has 'served well for Rome' (3.3.84)—and of his enemy Aufidius, who calls him 'all-noble Martius' (4.5.107). Moreover, the play's final statement is that Coriolanus 'shall have a noble memory' (5.6.153). However, he lacks a genuine sense of himself, and Volumnia's inflexible creation becomes increasingly dehumanized under the pressure of developments. He is isolated from others—significantly, Shakespeare used the word 'alone' more often in this play than in any other. Strikingly, he characterises himself as a 'lonely dragon' (4.1.30). By the time he has joined the Volscians, he is chillingly described as 'a kind of nothing, titleless, / Till he had forg'd himself a name o'th'fire / Of burning Rome' (5.1.13–15). He wilfully sheds his connection with humanity. 'Wife, mother, child, I know not' (5.2.80), he cries. However, he cannot distance his weakness. As he anticipates his fall, he cries out, 'I melt, and am not / Of stronger earth than others' (5.3.28–29), and he attempts to find strength by imagining himself to be parentless: 'I'll . . . stand / As if a man were author of himself / And knew no other kin' (5.3.35–37).

In the final moments of the play, Shakespeare deftly reminds us of his protagonist's ultimate weakness. Coriolanus protests against being called a 'boy of tears' (5.6.101), and he cites his triumph at Corioles. 'Alone I did it' (5.6.116) he cries, and this 'Alone' only makes clearer the nature of his failure. His perverse dependence on his mother has made him unable to recognise and accept his need for involvement with others—first the people of Rome, and now the Volscians. The result is that his truly noble elements—his bravery and his warrior's achievements—are negated. It is because he has indeed remained a boy, emotionally, that he has been unable to avoid his final calamity.

Shakespeare had long been interested in Coriolanus' tale, as we know from his use of it as a metaphor for revenge in *Titus Andronicus* 4.4.67–68, but in *Coriolanus* the playwright made a subtle but important change in the character he found in his source, PLUTARCH's *Lives.* The ancient historian stated that Coriolanus' pride was the consequence of his father's early death and his resulting lack of guidance. Shakespeare, however, does not present his hero's failings as a function of neglect, but rather as the product of a Roman aristocratic ideal that is applied excessively. The commentary on the potential harm in this situation is strongly made and is one of the play's important themes. Though both Shakespeare and Plutarch believed Coriolanus' story to be historically accurate, modern historians realise that it was based on a pre-Roman fable, probably Volscian, that may have told originally of the local deity who gave his name to Corioles.

Coriolanus

SYNOPSIS

Act 1, Scene 1

Rioting Romans (see CITIZEN [5]) seek the death of MARTIUS (2), a leading aristocrat who is known for his pride. MENENIUS stalls them with a humorous fable that justifies the aristocracy. Martius arrives, and his scathing anger quiets the rioters. He reports that the rioting has resulted in a concession to the commoners: the people have been allowed to elect their own judges, called tribunes, two of whom are Sicinius and BRUTUS (3). News arrives that ROME is threatened by a neighbouring tribe, the VOLSCIANS. A municipal delegation—the generals COMINIUS and LARTIUS, some Senators (see SENATOR [2]), and the new tribunes—seek Martius' support in repelling the invaders. He agrees, and remarks on his desire to fight the noble Volscian general, AUFIDIUS, who is a former foe. The aristocrats all depart to prepare for war and leave the tribunes, who talk of their hatred of Martius.

Act 1, Scene 2

At CORIOLES, the Volscian Senators (see SENATOR [3]) meet with Aufidius to plan their campaign. Aufidius will take the field, and the Senators will defend Corioles.

Act 1, Scene 3

Martius' mother, VOLUMNIA, berates his wife, VIRGILIA, because she is not pleased that he has gone to war. She declares that her son's honourable death would bring her more joy than his birth had. She describes the wounds she hopes her son will receive, which will increase his honour, and she mocks Virgilia's revulsion. Virgilia's friend VALERIA appears, and they discuss the son of Martius and Virgilia, who resembles his father. Valeria brings the news that Martius and Cominius have Corioles under siege.

Act 1, Scene 4

At Corioles, a delegation of Volscian Senators defies the Romans, and combat begins. The Romans retreat.

Martius curses them and charges alone through the city's gates. The Romans believe he has been killed, but he emerges from Corioles, chased by Volscians, and the Romans rally to his defence.

Act 1, Scene 5
Corioles has been taken, and Martius insists, despite his wounds, that he join Cominius who is fighting Aufidius.

Act 1, Scene 6
Martius arrives as Cominius withdraws against superior forces. Full of enthusiasm for battle, Martius insists that he resume the fight and face Aufidius.

Act 1, Scene 7
Lartius places a LIEUTENANT (3) in charge of Corioles and goes to join Cominius and Martius.

Act 1, Scene 8
Martius and Aufidius fight. Several Volscians arrive to assist their general, but Martius drives them all away. Aufidius cries out that he has been shamed by their support.

Act 1, Scene 9
Martius modestly objects to hearing his deeds praised amidst the cheers of the soldiers. Cominius proposes that in honour of his courage at Corioles, he shall hereafter be known as CORIOLANUS.

Act 1, Scene 10
Aufidius rages against Martius, who has now defeated him five times. He swears that next time he will not lose even if he must resort to treachery rather than valour.

Act 2, Scene 1
Menenius berates Sicinius and Brutus for their animosity towards Martius, and he scorns the bad judgement of the common people they represent. Martius, now Coriolanus, returns and is formally welcomed and taken by the aristocrats to the Capitol to receive further honours. The tribunes voice their resentment of Coriolanus, who will now be nominated as consul, the highest office in Rome. However, they reflect that his pride will probably prevent him from displaying his scars to the commoners—as tradition requires—and that as the commoners' representatives, they can then oppose him and keep him from the office.

Act 2, Scene 2
An OFFICER (7) and his two fellows speculate that Coriolanus' pride will lead to his rejection as consul, though they believe him worthy of the office. Coriolanus is nominated for the consulate, but he asks to be excused from exhibiting himself to the common people. The tribunes refuse to accept the idea, and the aristocrats attempt to persuade Coriolanus to go through with it. Though uneasy, he agrees and goes with them to perform the ceremony.

Act 2, Scene 3
A group of citizens decide to support Coriolanus if he will formally ask them to. Coriolanus arrives, dressed in the traditional humble garb, and he asks groups of citizens for their support, though in a surly, begrudging manner. They agree to support him, and Menenius and the tribunes confirm his election. Coriolanus and Menenius leave, and the tribunes upbraid the citizens for supporting the proud Coriolanus. They convince them to rescind their approval before Coriolanus' formal installation as consul.

Act 3, Scene 1
Coriolanus hears that Aufidius has expressed a desire to fight with him, and he wishes for a war. The tribunes report that a mob has risen against Coriolanus. Despite the efforts of the aristocrats to calm him, Coriolanus angrily declares the commoners unworthy of a voice in the selection of a consul. The tribunes declare him a traitor to the laws of Rome and summon the mob. The mob follows Sicinius' lead and demands that Coriolanus be killed. Coriolanus draws his sword, but the aristocrats take him away. Brutus and Sicinius continue to raise the mob's fury, but Menenius convinces them to follow legal procedures and try Coriolanus for treason in the tribunes' court. He promises to get the general to attend it.

Act 3, Scene 2
Volumnia helps the other aristocrats convince Coriolanus to swallow his pride and apologise to the commoners as a matter of practical politics. After lengthy argument, he finally agrees.

Act 3, Scene 4
Brutus and Sicinius instruct a subordinate to prepare the crowd to support whatever line they take in the trial of Coriolanus, who they plan to provoke to anger. Coriolanus and his friends appear, and at first Coriolanus mildly makes the recantation demanded by the tribunes. When Sicinius calls him a traitor, however, he responds wrathfully and rejects the authority of the common people in insulting terms. The tribunes convict him of treasonous hostility to the people's justice and declare him banished from Rome; the mob takes up the cry. Coriolanus replies angrily that he shall be glad to leave a city controlled by such ignorant commoners, and he departs. The tribunes encourage the mob to follow him out the gates of the city.

Act 4, Scene 1
Coriolanus bids farewell to his family and friends and departs for exile.

Act 4, Scene 2
Volumnia rages furiously at the victorious tribunes.

Act 4, Scene 3
A ROMAN (2) gives information to a VOLSCE, telling him of Coriolanus' banishment. He recommends that the

Volscians strike against the city now that it has lost its most illustrious general.

Act 4, Scene 4
Coriolanus, disguised a poor man, arrives in ANTIUM and is directed to Aufidius' house.

Act 4, Scene 5
Coriolanus finds Aufidius and tells him bitterly of his banishment; he offers to fight for the Volscians against Rome. Aufidius is ecstatic at encountering his great enemy and agrees enthusiastically. Aufidius' servants (see SERVING-MAN [7]) marvel that their master has accepted a poor wanderer, but when one of them learns the truth they rejoice at the prospects for a successful war.

Act 4, Scene 6
The tribunes refuse to believe the news that the Volscians are again attacking Roman territory, led by Coriolanus. A crowd arrives, and the citizens declare that they had had misgivings about the banishment all along. The worried tribunes hope that the news will prove untrue.

Act 4, Scene 7
A Volscian LIEUTENANT (4) worries that Aufidius will be overshadowed by Coriolanus' growing popularity among their soldiers. Aufidius confides that he intends eventually to turn against the Roman.

Act 5, Scene 1
Cominius reports that Coriolanus, whose Volscian army threatens the city, has refused to meet with him. The tribunes convince Menenius to attempt to beg mercy for the city. Cominius declares that Menenius will also fail, and that their only hope lies in Coriolanus' mother and wife.

Act 5, Scene 2
Volscian guards declare to Menenius that Coriolanus has specifically refused entry to any Roman. When Menenius insists that he is an old friend and will be accepted, they mock him. Coriolanus appears and pointedly rejects Menenius.

Act 5, Scene 3
Volumnia appears, accompanied by Virgilia, Valeria, and a BOY (8)—Coriolanus' son. Coriolanus becomes increasingly upset as he hears and rejects their petitions for mercy. Finally, a long speech by Volumnia convinces him to make peace with Rome. Aufidius, in an aside, observes that he now has the means to get revenge on Coriolanus.

Act 5, Scene 4
Menenius and Sicinius despair for the city, but news arrives of Volumnia's success and the withdrawal of the Volscian forces.

Act 5, Scene 5
The Senators thankfully welcome Volumnia and the other women back to Rome.

Act 5, Scene 6
Aufidius consults with a group of CONSPIRATORS. They agree to support his charges of treason against Coriolanus and then to help him kill his enemy. Coriolanus appears, followed by an enthusiastic crowd of Volscians (see COMMONER [2]). Coriolanus presents his treaty with Rome as a conquest, but Aufidius accuses him of treachery. He calls him unmanly because he has given up the city in response to a woman's plea. Coriolanus angrily threatens to beat him, but Aufidius turns the crowd against him. When the mob loudly demands that Coriolanus be lynched as an enemy, the Conspirators attack him in a group and kill him. Aufidius defends the killing as motivated by patriotic rage, but he goes on to observe that Coriolanus was a great warrior and stipulates that he should have a noble funeral.

COMMENTARY

Coriolanus is one of the most politically oriented of Shakespeare's plays; it depicts political confrontation between social classes. However, though *Coriolanus* opens with a civil insurrection and features the political manipulations of tribunes and aristocrats, Roman political strife is not the principal subject matter. Rather, it provides a context for the main plot, which is another sort of story. The play is first and foremost a TRAGEDY, the personal story of a great man whose greatness is accompanied by moral and psychological failings that bring about his downfall. As Coriolanus' story unfolds, Roman politics fall away, and the climactic confrontation in 5.3 does not oppose social classes or even political rivals. Rather, it presents an internal conflict within the protagonist, the clash between his pride in himself and his psychological dependence on his mother.

Coriolanus' importance to the plot is immediately established in Act 1, where he is prominently regarded as a brilliant military hero. Moreover, after the tragedy has run its course, the statement that 'he shall have a noble memory' (5.6.153) confirms this status for the protagonist. In between, his excessive pride produces catastrophe. Even before Coriolanus appears, his pride is carefully established as a major theme of the play in the remarks of the First Citizen. Then, it is flagrantly demonstrated with his first entrance. After Menenius has established a truce of sorts with the rioting commoners, Coriolanus appears and destroys it. His first three lines are a burst of anger that immediately creates a gulf between himself and the people that will never be bridged. He has the pride appropriate to a warrior, but he lacks a sense of ordinary social

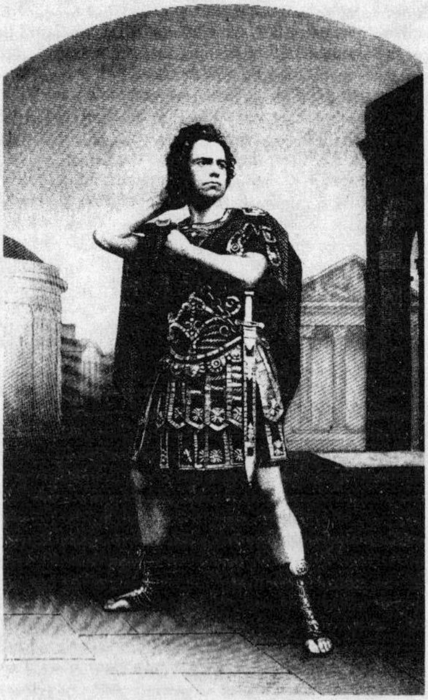

Shakespeare's Coriolanus is a great and noble warrior, but excessive pride leads to his defeat. (Courtesy of Culver Pictures, Inc.)

intercourse, let alone of compromise. He does not consider the justice of the commoners' complaints; he is simply offended that they should question aristocratic authority at all. His response is to suggest a massacre: 'Hang 'em! . . . I'd make a quarry / With thousands of these quarter'd slaves' (1.1.189–198). From this initial outburst to his final anger at Aufidius' taunt that he is a 'boy of tears' (5.6.101), Coriolanus is incapable of flexibility. He has sense enough to see the propriety in other approaches—he understands Volumnia's Machiavellian argument in 3.2, and, too late, he courts the Volscian common people in Act 5—but his pride repeatedly overwhelms his common sense.

The influence of Volumnia is the driving power behind Coriolanus and the play. Well may she boast to her son, 'Thou art my warrior: / I holp to frame thee' (5.3.62–63), for she has bred in her son the pride that makes him believe that he and his class are incontestably superior. Yet Coriolanus is entirely incapable of dealing with the play's developments. At two crucial moments, Volumnia makes demands of her son that are inconsistent with his sense of his own superiority. After her persuasion in 3.2 he attempts to compromise with the political world, but the tribunes trigger his too-ready anger and he is banished from Rome. Thus, he loses his only honourable standing—as a Roman warrior—and he deserts to the Volscians. When his mother comes to plead that he refrain from assaulting the city, in 5.3, he is trapped. If he destroys Rome, he will destroy himself psychologically through his mother's rejection, but by giving in to her he accepts an ignominious death at the hands of Aufidius. His responses are woefully limited, and his inflexibility proves his undoing; he is fragile in his great strength. Yet it was his mother who bred in him the sternly martial pride that brought him to eminence in the first place. This ironic situation demonstrates the basic theme of all Shakespearean tragedy: great strength is inextricably interwoven with correspondingly great weakness.

The changing world of Rome provides the secondary component of the play, its political plot. The heavy political emphasis of much modern commentary on *Coriolanus* is not misplaced, for the conflicts that spark the tragic hero's downfall are representative of the social clashes that constitute much of political history. The play stresses a theme that was important to Shakespeare when he wrote his earlier English HISTORY PLAYS: the impact of immoral behaviour in the ruling class on the peace and prosperity of all of society. As Shakespeare knew from his source, PLUTARCH's *Lives*, the ancient warrior was thought of as a member of peaceful society as well as a leader in war. To maintain his honour, he was obliged to participate in society by submitting to its laws and customs just as did his non-heroic fellow citizens. Coriolanus lacks the moral discipline to honour this social contract; indeed, he would rather abandon the contract altogether and join Rome's enemies than honour it and accept Rome's common people. Not only does he imperil himself, he endangers the city's very existence. Thus, the personality defects of the protagonist have profound political consequences.

The other aristocrats are conscious of the need to compromise with the commoners, and to a certain extent they counteract Coriolanus' ill effects. However, their grudging willingness to accept the need of such an arrangement also corrupts the social contract. Menenius' 'belly speech' (1.1.95–153) is politic and mild, but it is accompanied by an undisguised disdain for the common man, the 'great toe' (1.1.154) of society. In 3.2.41–86 Volumnia recommends that Coriolanus be hypocritical with the people. This Machiavellian speech betrays a cynical disregard for

'th'ignorant' (3.2.76) that flouts the social co-operation that it supposedly furthers. Coriolanus' indignant assumption that Brutus knows nothing of 'service' (3.3.83) is typical of the aristocratic rejection of social co-operation, though the tribune is obviously an industrious representative of his constituency. In fact, one may conclude that Brutus provides more useful service to the commoners than the proud warrior does to his own caste. Coriolanus represents the ideal of one sort of virtue: the warrior's single-minded quest for glory as the military hero of his people. This ideal is no longer desirable in a community that acknowledges the demands of all its people. The emergence of the new political morality causes Coriolanus' fall; put another way, the stresses of that emergence are enacted in his catastrophe and death.

These themes are reinforced by a fascinating and bizarre motif, the confusion of normal love, sexual and maternal, with the warrior's enthusiasm for war. Coriolanus embraces a fellow warrior on the battlefield and declares that his delight equals that of his wedding night (1.6.29–32), and later, Aufidius responds to him in similar fashion, in a passage (4.5. 107–127) of extraordinary sensuality. The general Cominius announces that his patriotic feelings are 'more holy and profound, than mine own life, / My dear wife's estimate, her womb's increase / And treasure of my loins' (3.3.113–115). When we first see Volumnia, in 1.3, she compares the thrill of giving birth to Coriolanus with that of seeing him as a soldier, and goes on to identify the beauty of a mother's breast with the sight of a head wound. She later attributes Coriolanus' fierceness in combat to her nursing of him, in 3.2.129. In her final manipulation of her son, she equates motherhood with the state in a violent image—'. . . assault thy country [and] tread / . . . on thy mother's womb' (5.3.123–124)—that reinforces our sense that she is a horrifyingly abnormal mother. In fact, when Coriolanus attempts to resist Volumnia's influence, he supposes himself outside the procreative process, 'as if a man were author of himself' (5.3.36). This recurring theme of emotional misplacement is a strong reminder that the moral world of Coriolanus and Volumnia is an unhealthy one, and that their story can only come to a tragic end.

The common people are not the cause of the city's near fall. Their objections to the rule of the aristocracy are given a fair presentation, especially in Act 1, where the First Citizen makes a sensible argument against the unfair distribution of corn that is the cause of the commoners' rebellion. Yet the cynicism of the tribunes, combined with the fickleness of the crowd, supports the aristocratic argument that the common people are not worthy of power. The critical element in Rome's catastrophe is Coriolanus' decision to defect, not simply his banishment, and he would not have defected had he not been driven from Rome by the ungrateful people who were manipulated by the tribunes. Moreover, this issue is reprised in the episode of the Volscian commoners in 5.6, where Coriolanus is again abandoned by a fickle mob.

Thus, the faults of both the aristocracy and the plebeians are exposed. The combination has produced a bewildering range of critical assessments, and *Coriolanus* has been declared to be the vehicle of fascist, conservative, moderate/pragmatic, liberal, and communist sentiments. While Shakespeare certainly displayed a conservative bias in favour of the established, hierarchical society, he was aware of, and wished to present, both sides of the political question. As a playwright, he was more interested in dramatic effect than in political science, and in this work he heightened the human foibles that lead to conflicts of the sort that he found in his sources.

The common people as a social and political class are more prominent in *Coriolanus* than in the history plays, which may reflect developments in England just before the play was written. (Also, the Roman plays, set in a remote time and place, offered Shakespeare a chance to explore more fully the fissures in society that government CENSORSHIP might well have disallowed in works dealing with relatively recent English history.) In *Coriolanus,* Shakespeare emphasises a corn shortage as the cause of plebeian discontent, while in Plutarch it was a relatively minor factor. Scholars connect this alteration with the extensive corn riots—called the Midlands Insurrection—that shook much of rural England in 1607. These demonstrations, which extended to brief losses of governmental control of some areas, raised issues of poverty and powerlessness that had not been publicly considered in generations. As a landowner and agricultural investor, Shakespeare may be presumed to have taken a particular interest in the phenomenon. He may even have witnessed a riot—or at least spoken to witnesses—since disturbances erupted near STRATFORD at a time when he may have been there. Thus, the class warfare we see in *Coriolanus* may reflect events in England, which, though Shakespeare could not know it, was only a generation away from a cataclysmic civil war.

Thus, *Coriolanus* displays the political concerns of the history plays within the more grandiose framework of a tragedy. Shakespeare emphasised the stresses that result from these political concerns, rather than attempting to alleviate them, and *Coriolanus* is a very complex and dynamic play. Its rough, spontaneous poetic style is accompanied by structural devices intended to reinforce our sense of crowded conflict. Surprises in tone startle us at several important points: Volumnia's violent manner of speech in a pointedly domestic setting, in 1.3; the banished Coriolanus' unexpected appearance in Antium in 4.4; and the silence at the close of Volumnia's long, final speech. This is one of Shakespeare's most brilliant *coups de théâtre,*

specified in the stage direction, 'Holds her by the hand silent' (5.3.183). All of these serve to keep the audience's attention at a peak, aware that the play's developments do not flow predictably.

The inevitability of events is nevertheless made clear through another structural device, the use of many parallel scenes and images. Menenius' 'belly speech' of 1.1 is repeatedly invoked with images of food and physiology that stud the play. In 1.3 Coriolanus' son is vividly described as like his father when he kills a butterfly with his teeth, and when Coriolanus marches on Rome with the Volscians, their advance is likened to 'boys pursuing summer butterflies' (4.6.95). At the close of Act 3 the plebeians throng to see Coriolanus 'out at gates' (3.3.142); the warrior's banishment reminds us of his triumph in 1.4 when he was similarly repudiated by the commoners—this time, the cowardly soldiers—and alone passed through the gates of a city, Corioles. As we have seen, the Volscian Commoners re-enact the Roman mob's change of heart towards Coriolanus in the play's final episode. Aufidius' welcome to Coriolanus in 4.5 echoes the strange mixture of love and war that Coriolanus displayed to Cominius in 1.6. When he calls him a 'traitor' (5.6.85), Aufidius tempts Coriolanus into the defiance that results in his death with the same technique that Sicinius used to elicit the defiance that resulted in his banishment, in 3.3.66. Most striking, Volumnia's dramatic final plea echoes her earlier effort to move her son to submit to her instructions, in 3.2. These parallel themes are startling as they are recognised on each occasion, and are also cumulatively powerful as Coriolanus' fate inexorably unfolds. The great strength of the play is its complexity, for its similarity to both the history play and the tragedy make possible its difficult presentation of Coriolanus as a tragic hero in a real society.

SOURCES OF THE PLAY

Shakespeare's principal source for *Coriolanus* was PLUTARCH's *Lives*, in Thomas NORTH's translation (2nd ed., 1595). The general course of developments is taken from this account, and several important passages—e.g., Volumnia's appeal in 5.3.94–182—follow North's text very closely. Though Shakespeare invented several minor incidents—including all of Volumnia's other appearances—and developed the psychology of his hero, his fidelity to Plutarch was generally quite close in this play as compared to the other Roman plays.

Only one passage strongly reflects other sources. Menenius' comparison of politics and anatomy in 1.1.95–159—very well-known since ancient times—was derived from several earlier renderings. In addition to North's version, which he followed fairly closely, Shakespeare also took a number of significant details from William CAMDEN's *Remaines* (1605), where the fable is told by a medieval pope, and from another variant of the Coriolanus story found in LIVY's *Ab urbe condita*, translated by Philemon HOLLAND (4) as *The Romane Historie* (1600).

TEXT OF THE PLAY

It is difficult to determine the date *Coriolanus* was written, and estimates range from 1603 to 1612. However, most scholars favour 1605 to 1609, for several reasons. First, the play must be later than Camden's *Remaines*, which was possibly available to Shakespeare in manuscript as early as 1603, though more probably used after its publication in 1605. Second, there is an apparent allusion to *Coriolanus* in Ben JONSON's play *Epicoene*, which was produced in late 1609 or early 1610. This implies that Shakespeare's play was written and staged somewhat earlier.

Further support, especially for the later part of this range of dates, is provided by other evidence. Applications of the VERSE TEST suggest that the play was roughly contemporary with *Antony and Cleopatra* (c. 1606), *Pericles* (c. 1607), *Cymbeline* (c. 1608–1610), and *The Winter's Tale* (c. 1610–1611). Also, some commentators find topical allusions in the text of the play. For example, 'fire on the ice' (1.1.172) may refer to the freezing over of the Thames River in the winter of 1607–1608, and Coriolanus' metaphor for treachery, 'he'll turn your current in a ditch / And make your channel his' (3.1.95–96), may have been inspired by the much-discussed failure of an English canal-building scheme in 1609. Some scholars believe that Shakespeare's treatment of relations between the aristocracy and the plebeians may have been stimulated in part by the Midlands Insurrection of 1607. This featured extensive corn riots suggestive of the similar disturbances that open the play. Further, psychoanalytically minded commentators feel that the prominence of Volumnia may reflect the death of Shakespeare's mother, Mary ARDEN (2), in 1608. Since none of these suggestions can be confirmed or denied, the date of composition of *Coriolanus* remains uncertain, with 1608 as perhaps the best estimate.

The play was initially published in the FIRST FOLIO (1623). The text was probably printed from Shakespeare's own manuscript, or FOUL PAPERS, for it contains elaborate and literary stage directions (e.g., at 1.3.1 and 5.3.183), variable speech headings *(Cor., Corio., Coriol.)*, and idiosyncratic spellings (especially Sc for S in Sicinius, a form closely associated with Shakespeare [see SIR THOMAS MORE]). It also contains other irregularities that would have been omitted or corrected in a copy made by a scribe or in a PROMPTBOOK.

THEATRICAL HISTORY OF THE PLAY

Though no evidence of early productions of *Coriolanus* has survived, an apparent allusion to the play in Jon-

son's *Epicoene* implies that the work was performed c. 1609. Richard BURBAGE (3) was probably the original Coriolanus. The lack of contemporary references suggests that it was staged infrequently, and the play has never been consistently popular. Many productions have been intended primarily as political propaganda, and Shakespeare's text has been persistently altered to serve these ends.

The earliest recorded version of *Coriolanus* is the adaptation by Nahum TATE, *The Ingratitude of a Commonwealth,* which was performed in 1681–1682, an uncertain period in English politics. This version stressed the importance of respectful loyalty, and supported Coriolanus' complaints about the commoners of Rome and de-emphasised the hero's faults. Though it retained some of Shakespeare's text, it was virtually a different play, and included numerous passages of lurid violence. Despite these features, it was a commercial failure. In 1718 John RICH (2) staged a *Coriolanus* that was probably Shakespeare's, but it was immediately followed by another politically motivated adaptation, *The Invader of His Country: or, The Fatal Resentment,* by John DENNIS (2). This work—largely Dennis' text, with insertions of Shakespeare's—was directed against the 1715 invasion of Britain by the exiled STUART DYNASTY. It starred the popular Barton BOOTH (1) but nevertheless lasted only three performances.

Though Dennis' failure apparently triggered presentations of Shakespeare's play—in some form, at least—in each of the next three years, *Coriolanus* was then ignored for a generation. In 1754 Thomas SHERIDAN combined Shakespeare's play with another *Coriolanus*—an entirely independent work by James Thomson (1700–1748)—in an adaptation that was quite popular and was frequently revived for almost 15 years. In 1754 David GARRICK attempted to rival it with an abridged version of Shakespeare's text, but this production lasted only a week.

In the 19th century the play's popularity grew. Between 1789 and 1817 John Philip KEMBLE (3) staged a series of successful versions of Sheridan's adaptation that usually starred himself and his sister, Sarah SIDDONS. In 1819 W. C. MACREADY—and in 1820, Charles KEAN (1)—staged the play with abridged but otherwise genuine Shakespearean texts. Kean's version was a failure, but Macready's was popular, and he revived it frequently for almost 20 years. Samuel PHELPS—who had played Aufidius in one of Macready's productions—put on the play several times in the 1840s and '50s, but after this the play was again ignored in England for years, though Edwin FORREST scored notable successes in New York. In the 1890s Frank BENSON (1) restored the play to the English stage with several successful productions.

The 20th century's apocalyptic history has prompted a continuing interest in this most political of Shakespeare's plays. In fact, *Coriolanus* has played a small part in that history. In the winter of 1933–34 a Paris production—condemned as Fascist and briefly closed by the government—provoked pro- and anti-Fascist street demonstrations. The uproar is said to have contributed to the rallying of public support for the French government at a time when it very nearly fell to Fascist and royalist conspirators. In Nazi Germany *Coriolanus* was taught in schools. The protagonist was identified with Hitler as a model of firm leadership, and the injustice of his banishment was emphasised. After World War II the American occupation forces banned the play until 1953.

On the other hand, a 1935 Moscow production of *Coriolanus* stressed the protagonist's treachery and his aristocratic pride. It was acclaimed by Stalin's propagandists as an excellent lesson in the betrayal of the people by an individualistic leader in the Western mode. Perhaps the most notorious modern adaptation of the play is that of the Marxist German playwright Berthold Brecht (1898–1956), who prepared a text for an East German ensemble that cut all hints of approval of Coriolanus or of disapproval towards the common people. This version is a simplified text that unambiguously celebrates the revolution led by the tribunes. The West German writer Günter Grass (b. 1927) was stimulated by this work to write a play called *The Plebeians Rehearse the Uprising* (1970), in which Brecht is ironically seen rehearsing his *Coriolanus* during the 1953 anti-government riots in East Berlin. However, Brecht's play was not produced until after his death in 1963.

In England, Benson continued to produce the play through 1919, and numerous later productions have confirmed the play's popularity. The most significant of these was probably Lewis CASSON's 1938 production that starred Laurence OLIVIER and Sybil THORNDIKE. This version's success firmly established the play in the repertoire of the modern British theatre. Other notable productions include those of Glen Byam SHAW (3) (1952, with Anthony QUAYLE in the title role), Peter HALL (5) (1959, with Olivier and Edith EVANS [1], and 1984, with Ian MCKELLEN), Joseph PAPP (1965, in New York's Central Park), and Trevor NUNN (1973, with Nicol WILLIAMSON). *Coriolanus* has not been produced as a FILM, though two versions have been made for TELEVISION, and it is included in THE SPREAD OF THE EAGLE, an adaptation of all of the ROMAN PLAYS.

Corioles (Corioli) Ancient Italian city of the VOLSCIANS, located about 25 miles south-east of ROME, setting for four scenes of Act 1 of *Coriolanus.* In 1.2 the Volscians make their plans to defend against the expected siege by the Romans. In 1.4–6 the Roman MARTIUS (2) displays great bravery after an initial success

by the Volscians when he charges single-handed through the city gates and turns the tide of battle. In 1.7 the Roman general LARTIUS leaves a LIEUTENANT (3) in charge of the city. In 1.9 Martius is honoured for his bravery at Corioles with a new name, CORIOLANUS, by which he is known for the rest of the play.

There is nothing to distinguish Corioles from the many other besieged towns in Shakespeare—the gates and walls of a medieval city are called for in the stage directions, and nothing more is shown. Shakespeare presented the town because it was called for in his story. The ancient Volscian city has been lost, but it is believed to have been located near the modern Velletri.

Cornelius (1) Minor character in *Hamlet,* ambassador to the King of Norway from the KING (5) of Denmark. In 1.2 Cornelius and VOLTEMAND are appointed to carry a message to Norway. The two ambassadors return in 2.2, and Voltemand reports Norway's reply. Cornelius barely speaks and serves only to flesh out the play's presentation of courtly diplomacy.

Cornelius (2) Character in *Cymbeline,* a physician to the QUEEN (2) of Britain. In 1.6 Cornelius has provided the Queen with a poison—for experimental purposes, she says—but he informs us in an aside that he distrusts her and has substituted a sleeping potion. IMOGEN later takes this and is mistaken for dead. Later, in the play's final scene, he recounts the dying Queen's confession (5.5.31–61) and explains again about the poison (5.5.243–258). Cornelius' function is to further the plot and highlight the Queen's evilness.

Cornell, Katharine (1898–1974) American actress. Though best known as a leading lady in contemporary romantic dramas, Cornell also played in classic works by Chekhov, G. B. SHAW (2), and Shakespeare. She was closely associated with the role of JULIET (1), which she played several times, perhaps most notably on a 77-city tour of the depression-era U.S. beginning in 1932.

Cornwall, Duke of Character in *King Lear,* the villainous husband of King LEAR's usurping daughter REGAN. Cornwall takes a prominent part in the evil deeds that spark much of the play's action. In 2.1 he declares that EDGAR, who has been falsely accused of a murder plot against his father, GLOUCESTER (1), shall be executed, and he adopts as a follower Edgar's persecutor, EDMUND. He places Lear's loyal follower KENT in the stocks and he supports his wife and sister-in-law GONERIL in their expulsion of Lear. At his most cruel, in 3.7 he puts out Gloucester's eyes when the earl remains loyal to the outcast former king. For this offence he is killed by an appalled SERVANT (19), as is reported in 4.2 by a MESSENGER (20). His death is proof that the triumph of villainy will not be total, but at the same time the enormity of his final deed contributes greatly to the general atmosphere of horror that so distinguishes the play.

Costard Character in *Love's Labour's Lost,* a quick-witted CLOWN (1) who is at the centre of the rustic sub-plot. In 3.1 Costard is employed by Armado to send a love letter to JAQUENETTA and by BEROWNE to send another one to ROSALINE (1). He delivers each to the wrong woman, resulting in two comical outcomes: Armado's pompous rhetoric is read aloud to the amusement of the PRINCESS (1) of France and her retinue; and Berowne's love poem exposes to his fellow courtiers his own susceptibility to romance, just as he is chastising them for the same failing.

To a great degree, Costard is simply a character type derived from the Italian COMMEDIA DELL' ARTE tradition—that of the servant or rustic yokel descended from the comic slave figures of ancient ROMAN DRAMA. He engages in several bits of standard by-play—for instance, when he comes to believe that 'remuneration' means a three-farthing coin and 'guerdon' a shilling. However, he displays realistic touches of humanity that rank among the play's literary gems. A participant in the comical pageant of the Nine WORTHIES, Costard plays Pompey the Great (see POMPEY [2]), but he muffs his lines and shamefacedly apologises, in 5.2.554–555. Some twenty lines later, Costard demonstrates an appreciation for his fellows that exceeds the restricted humanity of a stock figure, when he speaks up for NATHANIEL (1) the Curate, who has been driven away by stage fright.

Costard's name is an old word meaning 'apple' or 'head', which stimulates a cluster of jokes in 3.1.

Cottom (Cottam), John (active 1566–1581) STRATFORD schoolmaster, one of Shakespeare's teachers. Cottom taught at Stratford from 1579–1581 and probably supervised the last years of Shakespeare's formal education (though the records of Shakespeare's attendance have not survived). He was recruited for the job by his predecessor, to whom he paid £6 (about a third of a year's pay) for the opportunity. Cottom's younger brother, a Jesuit priest, was tried for treason in November 1581, for his active opposition to the Protestant state religion. He was executed the next spring. In December 1581 John Cotton resigned his position at Stratford, probably under pressure because of his brother's situation. He eventually inherited a country estate where he lived in retirement and practised Catholicism. His religion may have influenced Shakespeare, who seems to have been at least tolerant of Catholicism in an intolerant age, and who some scholars believe may have been a secret Catholic himself.

Countess (1) of Auvergne Minor character in *1 Henry VI,* a French noblewoman who attempts to capture TALBOT by means of a ruse. She invites him to visit her castle, pretending an innocent desire to meet so valiant an hero in person. He receives the invitation in 2.2, but, suspicious, he plans a counter-ploy. In 2.3 she springs her trap, but following his plan, a troop of soldiers immediately frees him. Talbot gracefully accepts the Countess' apology.

This episode is entirely fictitious, probably derived by the playwright from similar events in the 'Robin Hood' cycle of tales. It serves to emphasise the virtues of Talbot, whose eventual loss to the English is one of the climaxes of the play. In attributing such deceit to the French, implicitly denying their military strength, the episode contributes to the play's chief point—that the successes of the French could not have occurred without dissensions among the English.

Countess (2) of Rossillion Character in *All's Well That Ends Well,* the mother of BERTRAM and guardian of HELENA (2). The Countess comments on the main action of the play, overseeing from her estate at ROSSILLION the relationship between her son and her ward. Loving Helena, she promotes their marriage; loving Bertram, she rues his foolishness in abandoning his bride, and she is present to see them reconciled at the play's close. With Lord LAFEW and the KING (17), the Countess helps to create a world of kindness and generosity that counters the play's unpleasant aspects.

One of her most important functions is to guide the audience's responses to the major characters through her own, exalting Helena and forgiving Bertram. Her love for Helena is as generous as her affection for her son is natural. Her sympathy for Helena's love, based on her 'remembrances of days foregone' (1.3.129), is touching, and her collaboration with Helena serves to start the heroine on her way. She is also aware of Bertram's defects, while at the same time remaining willing to make allowances and forgive. The Countess loves her son, but, when he abandons Helena, she recognises that he is a 'rash and unbridled boy' (3.2.27) and sends letters that she hopes will bring him to his senses. The Countess is an especially sympathetic character in a play full of moral ambiguity. George Bernard SHAW (2) called hers 'the most beautiful old woman's part ever written'.

Countrymen Group of minor characters in *The Two Noble Kinsmen,* peasants. In 2.2 four Countrymen tell ARCITE of wrestling and running competitions at a country fair. The outcast nobleman subsequently distinguishes himself at the fair, coming to the attention of the court of Duke THESEUS (2), and thus meeting his beloved, EMILIA (4). Six Countrymen appear in 3.5, one of them dressed as a BAVIAN, or baboon, as part of the duke's entertainment; five of them, with NELL (2) and her friends, perform a dance under the direction of the SCHOOLMASTER (2). Most scholars agree that neither 2.1 nor 3.5 was written by Shakespeare; thus, the Countrymen are probably the creation of John FLETCHER (2).

Court, Alexander Minor character in *Henry V,* soldier who meets the incognito King HENRY V on the eve of the battle of AGINCOURT. His companions, BATES and WILLIAMS (2), converse with the king, but Court speaks only one line.

Courtesan Minor character in *The Comedy of Errors,* a 'professional entertainer' visited off-stage by ANTIPHOLUS OF EPHESUS after he is mistakenly rejected by his wife, ADRIANA. The Courtesan appears later, in 4.3, to claim a necklace Antipholus promised her in exchange for her ring. She mistakenly approaches ANTIPHOLUS OF SYRACUSE, who rejects her as a sorceress or agent of the devil. She goes to Adriana and accuses her husband of lunacy and of theft of the ring, thus triggering the pursuit that results in Antipholus of Ephesus' treatment for insanity at the hands of PINCH.

Cousin Capulet Character in *Romeo and Juliet.* See CAPULET (2).

Coventry City in WARWICKSHIRE in central England, the setting for a scene each in *3 Henry VI* and *Richard II.* In *3 Henry VI* Coventry is the site of an encounter (5.1) between the Earl of WARWICK (3) and the Yorkist leaders, at which GEORGE (2) is brought to abandon Warwick's cause, prior to a battle in the following scenes. In *Richard II,* Coventry is the scene (1.3) of the scheduled trial by combat between BOLINGBROKE (1) and MOWBRAY (1) that RICHARD II cancels, sending the two disputants into exile instead.

Cowley, Richard (d. 1619) English actor, one of the 26 men listed in the FIRST FOLIO as the 'Principall Actors' in Shakespeare's plays. Cowley is known to have performed with STRANGE'S MEN as early as 1590, and was probably with the CHAMBERLAIN'S MEN from their formation in 1594, though the earliest surviving documentation dates from 1600. He was a member of the KING'S MEN—as the Chamberlain's became—at least through 1605 and probably much later, for several associates of the King's Men witnessed his will in 1618. Speech prefixes in early texts reveal that Cowley played VERGES in *Much Ado About Nothing* and QUINCE in *A Midsummer Night's Dream;* he is thus presumed to have worked well as a straight man to the great comic actor Will KEMPE, who played DOGBERRY and BOTTOM, the respective counterparts to Cowley's roles.

Cox, Robert (d. 1655) English actor, famed for his performances of DROLLS, which were brief playlets at

fairs and in taverns from 1642 to 1660, when English theatres were closed by the revolutionary government, Cox performed his drolls illegally until he was arrested and imprisoned in 1653. A collection of his scripts—some of which he wrote, though most were adaptations of scenes from well-known plays—was published by Henry MARSH and Francis KIRKMAN in 1662.

Crab Dog in *The Two Gentlemen of Verona.* LAUNCE's pet is the subject of his two memorable comic monologues, in 2.3 and 4.4. The name refers to the crab apple, and it suggests an animal small in size and sour in expression.

Craig (1), Gordon (1872–1966) English actor, producer, and theatrical designer. The son of Ellen TERRY (1) and the famed architect and designer Edward Godwin (1833–1886), Craig was a successful child actor and in his late teens and early 20s was a member of Henry IRVING's company. He played many leading Shakespearean roles, but his fame rests on his later career as a producer, designer, and theoretician. He advocated simple productions and aspired to approximate the Elizabethan stage; he was an important influence on Harley GRANVILLE-BARKER. Among Craig's most important books are *The Art of the Theatre* (1905), *Towards a New Theatre* (1911), and *The Theatre Advancing* (1921). He also wrote books on both Terry and Irving.

Craig (2), Hardin (1875–1968) American scholar, author of several important works on Shakespeare. A long-time professor at the University of Missouri, Craig believed that an understanding of the cultural and intellectual world in which Shakespeare lived was crucial to the comprehension of his poetry and plays. Craig's best-known works were *The Enchanted Glass: The Elizabethan Mind in Literature* (1935) and *New Lamps for Old: A Sequel to the Enchanted Glass* (1960).

Crane, Ralph (active 1620s) Professional copyist, or scribe, whose copies of some of Shakespeare's plays were probably published in the FIRST FOLIO. Crane, a legal clerk who chiefly copied documents for lawyers, also did free-lance work copying plays—either from the playwrights' FOUL PAPERS or from a PROMPTBOOK—for private libraries (a common practice of the day). He also worked for the KING'S MEN in the early 1620s. Several signed Crane transcripts survive (though none of a Shakespeare play), so his idiosyncratic style can be identified. On the basis of this style, scholars believe that he provided the copy used in printing five of the plays in the First Folio (1623)—*Measure for Measure, The Merry Wives of Windsor, The Tempest, The Two Gentlemen of Verona,* and *The Winter's Tale.*

Scholars distinguish Crane's work by his peculiar habits of punctuation—especially his use of hyphens to join adjectives and their nouns, as in 'palsied-Eld' (*Measure for Measure* 3.1.36), and his frequent use of parentheses to set off words or phrases, as in 'that same knave (Ford her husband) hath' (*Merry Wives of Windsor* 5.1.18). Scholars also point to Crane's idiosyncratic spellings, like 'sirha' for 'sirrah', and his provision of 'massed entrances', in which all of the characters in a scene are listed in a group at its opening, without regard for when they actually come on stage.

Cranmer, Thomas (1489–1556) Historical figure and character in *Henry VIII,* an adviser to King HENRY VIII and later Archbishop of Canterbury. Cranmer is the central figure in 5.1–2, as Bishop GARDINER (1) and the Lord CHANCELLOR attempt to charge him with heresy at a meeting of the royal council, only to be thwarted by the king's intervention. The episode demonstrates the king's mastery of the situation—Henry's increasing wisdom is an important theme of the play. It also illustrates the triumph of the Protestant leaders—Cranmer and the king—over the pro-Catholic conspirators.

Cranmer is sometimes confused with another Archbishop of Canterbury in the play, whom the king addresses in 2.4.215–217. However, this figure—who remains mute—is Cranmer's predecessor, Archbishop William Warham (d. 1532), for Cranmer is abroad at this point. Henry wishes Cranmer were present in 2.4. 236–237; his return and his appointment as Archbishop are reported in 3.2.64, 74.

At the close of the play, Cranmer's prediction of glory for the infant ELIZABETH (1) even includes praise of her successor, JAMES I, and thus extends *Henry VIII* into Shakespeare's own time. In this, the play differs from all the other HISTORY PLAYS. Cranmer, well known to 17th-century audiences as a martyred religious hero, is a suitable vehicle for such a spiritual evocation of 'the happiness of England' (5.4.56).

The historical Cranmer was a professor at Cambridge University in the 1520s who was influenced by continental Protestant doctrines, especially on papal authority. He proposed that King Henry did not need the pope's permission to divorce Queen KATHERINE if he had the approval of other authoritative clerics. Henry sent Cranmer and others to solicit opinions, some of them approving, from religious thinkers throughout England and Europe. When Cranmer was appointed archbishop in 1533, he declared the king's marriage invalid. Cranmer's greatest historical importance, however, lies in his work as the chief creator of a liturgy for the new Protestant Church of England. He supervised the production of the first two editions (1549, 1552) of a prayer book and promulgated a formal statement of doctrine in 42 articles (1552), later reduced to 39. An oath of adherence to the 39 Articles, as they were known, was required of all Anglican

clergymen and became a bone of contention in English politics for generations. Cranmer also edited and wrote parts of the first book of *Homilies* (1547), intended to be used for sermons in Anglican churches. For these works and his leadership as archbishop, Cranmer is regarded as the principal founder of the Church of England. Under the Catholic Queen Mary (ruled 1553–1558), he was ousted from his archbishopric and charged with heresy. He formally recanted but was condemned anyway and burned at the stake.

Creede, Thomas (active 1578–1617) London printer, producer of editions of several of Shakespeare's plays. Creede printed the first editions of *2 Henry VI* (Q1, 1594, for Thomas MILLINGTON), *Henry V* (Q1, 1600, for Millington and John BUSBY), and *The Merry Wives of Windsor* (Q1, 1602, for Arthur JOHNSON [1]). He also printed second editions of *Henry V* (Q2, 1602, for Thomas PAVIER) and *Romeo and Juliet* (Q2, 1599, for Cuthbert BURBY). Creede also produced four editions of *Richard III* (Q2–Q5, 1598, 1602, 1605, 1612; the first two for Andrew WISE and the others for Matthew LAW). Creede is regarded as among the most skilful printers of the period, and he had a long and successful career. He became a member of the STATIONERS' COMPANY in 1578 and operated his own press from at least 1593. He probably died in 1617 when his partner became sole owner of his company.

Cressida Legendary figure and title character in *Troilus and Cressida,* lover of TROILUS. Because Cressida's betrayal of her lover in favour of the Greek DIOMEDES is the focal event of the love plot, many commentators have seen her role as that of a villain, though in fact Shakespeare did not treat her unsympathetically. Her disloyalty is a necessary element of his story, and she is representative of human or perhaps (for Shakespeare) feminine weakness, but she is certainly not a vicious breaker of hearts, nor, despite ULYSSES' mistaken assumption upon meeting her in 4.5, is she a prostitute, for she shows no hint of mercenary motives. Diomedes courts her in 5.2 with the same wiles she used on Troilus earlier—affecting disinterest and a readiness to ignore her—and she is susceptible, though she resists confusedly. She is a frankly sensual woman, as has been evident from her affair with Troilus, and now, alone in a new world, having just been removed from TROY to the Greek camp, she succumbs to her nature.

Cressida is frequently associated with HELEN (1), the worthless prize of the TROJAN WAR, in order to underscore her similar deficiency as a motive for Troilus. She is a much more alert and interesting personality than Helen, however. She is a knowledgeable flirt, able to consider the tactics of courtship, and she is scornfully aware that PANDARUS is 'a bawd' (1.2.286). Once united with Troilus in 3.2, she frankly confesses her love, but in confusion she regrets abandoning her tactical game. Tellingly, she speaks of her 'unkind self, that itself will leave / To be another's fool' (3.2.146–147). Swept up in the excitement of the moment, she deludes herself that a real romance is in the offing, but her profession of faith is couched in negative terms, allowing the prediction—recognised by the audience to be accurate in a textbook instance of dramatic irony—that the future will call 'false maids in love . . . "as false as Cressid" ' (3.2.188–194). Although she pledges her loyalty to Troilus in the enthusiasm of passion, she recognises her need for Diomedes in Troilus' absence. She admits her guilt, attributing it to her gender: 'Ah, poor our sex! . . . The error of our eye directs our mind' (5.2.108–109). Such simple awareness of guilt is unique in this play filled with hypocrisy and self-delusion.

Cressida's name stems from a character in the *Iliad* of HOMER, Briseis, a slave and concubine of first ACHILLES and then AGAMEMNON and a source of dispute between them; she had nothing to do with Troilus. The name evolved through Briseida, to Griseida, and then Criseyde—in the works of SAINTE-MAURE, BOCCACCIO, and CHAUCER respectively—before Shakespeare used the variant that is now standard.

Créton, Jean (c. 1340–after 1400) French writer whose poem *Histoire du Roy d'Angleterre Richard* may have influenced the writing of *Richard II.* Créton, a French nobleman, was a visitor to RICHARD II's court beginning in 1398. He accompanied Richard to Ireland and was with the King when he was captured by BOLINGBROKE (1). His account is highly favourable to Richard.

Crier Minor character in *Henry VIII,* petty official at the divorce trial of Queen KATHERINE. In 2.4.7 and 10, upon the orders of the SCRIBE, the Crier formally demands the presence of King HENRY VIII and the queen. In this he emphasises the pomp and ceremony with which the king is proceeding against Katherine, thereby increasing our sense of her vulnerability.

Cromer, Sir James (d. 1450) Historical figure mentioned in *2 Henry VI,* the son-in-law of Lord SAY. Cromer himself does not appear in the play, but the rebel Jack CADE orders him executed, along with his father-in-law, in 4.7, and the revolutionaries carry his head on a pole at the end of that scene.

Cromwell, Thomas (c. 1485–1540) Historical figure and character in *Henry VIII,* secretary to Cardinal WOLSEY and later to King HENRY VIII's council. In 3.2, as Wolsey's downfall becomes clear, Cromwell's demonstration of loyalty improves our image of Wolsey. He seems genuinely grieved, crying out, 'O my lord, / Must I then leave you? must I needs forgo / So good,

so noble and so true a master?' (3.2.421–423). The episode also offers an opportunity for the fallen cardinal to display magnanimity—concerning himself with Cromwell's welfare amid the debacle of his own affairs and thereby demonstrating his capacity for moral regeneration in adversity, an important theme of the play. Cromwell's subsequent political rise is mentioned by the Third GENTLEMAN (14), who calls him 'A man in much esteem with th'king' (4.1.109). In 5.2 Cromwell defends Archbishop CRANMER against heresy charges and is himself accused of Protestant leanings by the orthodox Bishop GARDINER (1). The episode points up the political importance of religious rivalries in the play's world. Also, that the one-time aide to Wolsey should become the king's ally demonstrates the progress from evil to good so central to *Henry VIII.*

The historical Cromwell served as Wolsey's secretary, but Shakespeare invented his sympathetic response to the cardinal's plight. Cromwell eventually succeeded Wolsey as the king's chief minister. A vigorous administrator, he devised and oversaw the dissolution of English monasteries to enrich the crown and set up an intensive domestic intelligence service, sometimes called the first prototype of a secret police force. Eventually, however, Cromwell shared Wolsey's fate. He tried to ally England with the Protestant powers of northern Europe, and to that end arranged Henry's fourth marriage, in 1540, to the German princess, Anne of Cleves (1515–1557). The rapid failure of the marriage was the minister's downfall. He was convicted of treason and executed. (His fate is obscurely alluded to in 3.2.449.) His career was the subject of the play THOMAS LORD CROMWELL, at one time attributed to Shakespeare.

Cross Keys Inn Inn in LONDON whose courtyard was used for play performances in the 16th century, and at which Shakespeare performed early in his career. From its foundation in 1594, the CHAMBERLAIN'S MEN, of which Shakespeare was a member, performed in the winter at the Cross Keys and in the summer at the THEATRE—the first true playhouse in England. Plays had been performed at the inn—in summer and winter—since at least as early as 1579. Other entertainments were also conducted there; a performing horse, for example, is recorded sometime before 1588. In 1596 the London government outlawed play performances within the city limits, and the Cross Keys Inn ceased to function as a playhouse.

Crosse, Samuel (active c. 1604) English actor, a member of the CHAMBERLAIN'S MEN or KING'S MEN. Cross is listed in the FIRST FOLIO among the 'Principall Actors' in Shakespeare's plays, but he is unknown elsewhere. He may only have been with the company before it became the King's Men in 1603, for he was not among the nine members listed in the patent granted at that time. On the other hand, he may have joined soon thereafter, since the group numbered 12 in the summer of 1604. However, he was apparently not with the company in May 1605, when Augustine PHILLIPS bequeathed small legacies to twelve named members of the company; some scholars believe he died in the interim.

Crowne, John (c. 1640–1703) English dramatist who adapted *2* and *3 Henry VI.* In 1680 Crowne combined the last two Acts of *2 Henry VI* with *3 Henry VI* in a play entitled *The Misery of Civil War.* This was a topical work, intended as propaganda for the early Whig political party in the disputes of the day, as was its successor, which was based on the earlier parts of *2 Henry VI,* though titled *Henry VI, the First Part* (1681).

Cumberland, Richard (1732–1811) British playwright, creator of an adaptation of *Timon of Athens.* A minor politician, Cumberland also wrote a number of sentimental plays, most of which are now forgotten. His adaptation of *Timon* was unsuccessfully staged in 1771. He was caricatured as Sir Fretful Plagiary in Richard Brinsley Sheridan's play *The Critic* (1779).

Cupid In *Timon of Athens* the name taken by a LADY (2) who leads the MASQUE in 1.2. Her disguise as the Roman god of love demonstrates both the fashionable neoclassicism of such aristocratic entertainments and the slightly lascivious quality that enlivened many of them.

Curan Minor character in *King Lear,* a follower of the Earl of GLOUCESTER (1). In 2.1 Curan tells EDMUND of a rumour that the Dukes of CORNWALL and ALBANY—the husbands of REGAN and GONERIL, to whom King LEAR has foolishly given power—are soon to fall into civil war. This is the first hint that Lear's error, already disastrous for him personally, is also a potential catastrophe for the kingdom as a whole.

Curio Minor character in *Twelfth Night,* a follower of Duke ORSINO of ILLYRIA. Curio has no personality and very few lines, serving to fill out the Duke's retinue. In 1.1.16–18 Curio achieves his greatest prominence when he provides the occasion for a pun by his master.

Curtain Theatre, The Second LONDON playhouse, probably built by Henry LANEMAN in 1577. It was apparently a round or multi-sided three-storey building, located near the first playhouse, the THEATRE, in Shoreditch, a northern suburb of London. Its name refers to its neighbourhood, the Curtain Close, and not to theatre curtains, which were not in use at that time. Between 1590 and 1592 STRANGE'S MEN—perhaps including the young Shakespeare—often played

at the Curtain, and in 1597–1598, the CHAMBERLAIN'S MEN, definitely Shakespeare's company, played there before moving to the new GLOBE THEATRE in the following year. It was during this period that Shakespeare wrote *Henry V*, with its mention of a circular theatre as 'this wooden O' (Prologue, 13). This is often taken as an allusion to the Globe but more probably refers to the Curtain. From 1603 until at least 1609, the QUEEN'S MEN (2) were usually tenants of the Curtain, and PRINCE CHARLES' COMPANY played there after 1621. The theatre is last mentioned in 1627.

Curtis Minor character in *The Taming of the Shrew*, a servant of PETRUCHIO (2). Curtis, who has been in charge of the household in his master's absence, greets the returning GRUMIO and engages him in comical repartee at the beginning of 4.1. Later in the scene, he is one of the servants whom Petruchio abuses as part of his programme to demonstrate to KATHERINA the ugliness of shrewish behaviour. Curtis' name is thought to be that of an actor who played him, possibly Curtis GREVILLE (1).

Cushman, Charlotte (1816–1876) American actress, generally considered the first great American-born actress. Cushman, who began her career as an opera singer, was particularly noted for her fierce portrayals of LADY (6) MACBETH, which she played opposite William MACREADY, Edwin FORREST, Edwin BOOTH (2), and others. She was also highly praised as DESDEMONA and *Henry VIII*'s Queen KATHERINE of Aragon. In addition, she was noted for her successes in male parts, especially ROMEO—opposite the JULIET (1) of her sister, Susan—Cardinal WOLSEY, and HAMLET.

Cymbeline (d. c. A.D. 40) Historical figure and title character of *Cymbeline*, the king of Britain and father of IMOGEN. Though Cymbeline is the title character, he is not an important one. The title of the play suggests the land he rules, rather than him personally. He is a typical king of fairy-tale and romantic literature. He loses his prosperity when he follows evil advisers, and then recovers it in a traditional happy ending through the workings of a benevolent fate. Influenced by his vicious QUEEN (2) and her son CLOTEN, he proceeds unjustly against his innocent daughter and her husband, POSTHUMUS. He loses Imogen as he once lost his sons, by another unjust action, the banishment of BELARIUS twenty years earlier. Moreover, still under the influence of his wife and stepson, he commits Britain to a foolish war against ROME. However, fate intervenes, and Cymbeline is eventually freed from evil. The Romans are miraculously defeated by the king's long-lost sons, and Cymbeline recovers his family and survives to be merciful to his enemies at the play's close.

Cymbeline is a passive figure whose competence as a ruler can only be restored by a happy ending brought about by chance, rather than by himself. On the other hand, his crimes are equally not his own; he is only unintentionally cruel, and though wrongheaded, he is quite willing to admit his folly and accept the mercy of providence. He is a figure from traditional lore who is necessary to the plot but does not contribute to it. His character is not fully developed, and what we see is a feeble store of anger in early scenes, a dumbfounded confusion later on, and a mild exaltation at the end.

The historical Cymbeline, generally called Cunobelinus, was a powerful ruler among the Celtic tribes of south-east England, but Shakespeare's figure bears virtually no resemblance to him. Shakespeare's source, HOLINSHED's *Chronicles*, was rather vague and inaccurate regarding Cunobelinus' reign, but the playwright did not follow his source particularly closely in any case. The most striking difference is that Rome's invasion—a successful one that established Roman rule in Britain—came several years after Cunobelinus' death. Cunobelinus was among the most successful of England's tribal kings in terms of conquering his neighbours, but little else is known of his reign.

Cymbeline

SYNOPSIS

Act 1, Scene 1

One GENTLEMAN (12) tells another that King CYMBELINE's daughter IMOGEN has married a poor but worthy nobleman, POSTHUMUS LEONATUS, whose father had died—before he was born—in the king's service. However, Posthumus has been banished from Britain because the king had wanted Imogen to marry CLOTEN, the boorish son of the QUEEN (2). He adds that Imogen is the king's only child, with the exception of two sons who were kidnapped 20 years earlier and never recovered.

Act 1, Scene 2

The Queen affects friendship for Imogen and the departing Posthumus, but Imogen mistrusts her. The Queen warns them that the king may find them, but in an aside she declares that she will send the king their way. As they bid each other farewell, Imogen gives Posthumus a diamond ring and he gives her a bracelet. The king appears and angrily drives Posthumus away. Posthumus' servant PISANIO reports to Imogen that his master has told him to remain at court and serve her. He adds that Posthumus and Cloten have fought but that Posthumus refrained from hurting his opponent.

Act 1, Scene 3

Cloten boasts to a LORD (15) of his swordplay against Posthumus while a Second Lord mocks him behind his back.

Act 1, Scene 4
Pisanio tells the lovesick Imogen of Posthumus' departure.

Act 1, Scene 5
In ROME the exiled Posthumus meets IACHIMO. They speak of a duel that Posthumus had once fought over his claim that Imogen was superior to all other women, both in beauty and virtue. Iachimo declares that Imogen is not so virtuous. He offers to bet his estate against Posthumus' diamond ring that he can seduce her, and the enraged Posthumus accepts the wager.

Act 1, Scene 6
In Britain; the Queen assures the physician CORNELIUS (2) that the poison he has given her is intended only for experiments on small animals, to further her education in herbal lore. Pisanio arrives, and the Queen muses to herself that she will poison him since he serves Cloten's enemy. In a soliloquy, Cornelius reveals that since he mistrusts the Queen he has substituted a powerful sleeping potion for the poison; a victim will appear dead for a time but will suffer no harm. The Queen tries to recruit Pisanio to convince Imogen to marry Cloten, and as a reward she gives him the poison. She tells him it is a potent restorative.

Act 1, Scene 7
Iachimo arrives at court and meets Imogen. He tells her that Posthumus leads a riotous life in Rome, and that he speaks mockingly of his faithful lover at home. He encourages her to seek revenge by sleeping with him. When she angrily dismisses him, he declares that he did not mean it but had merely been testing her virtue to see if Posthumus' praise had been true. Imogen is mollified and agrees to assist Iachimo. She says she will keep a chest containing valuables that are partly owned by Posthumus safe in the most secure possible location—her own bedchamber.

Act 2, Scene 1
Cloten brags of his ill temper over gambling losses and is mocked behind his back by the Second Lord, who sympathises with Imogen in a soliloquy.

Act 2, Scene 2
In her bedchamber Imogen retires for the night. Iachimo emerges from the chest, which is being kept there as Imogen had agreed. He memorises the nature of the furnishings and decorations, takes a bracelet from the sleeping Imogen's wrist, notices a mole on her breast, and returns to the chest.

Act 2, Scene 3
MUSICIANS (7) hired by Cloten serenade Imogen, but she does not respond. He accosts her. She tries to turn him away politely, but when he persists she lashes out at him and declares that he is not worth the clothes Posthumus wears. She leaves, and Cloten vows revenge.

Act 2, Scene 4
In Rome; Iachimo has returned from Britain and claims the diamond ring Posthumus had wagered. He offers a description of Imogen's bedchamber as proof that he has slept with her. When Posthumus refuses to believe him, he displays the bracelet—which Posthumus had given Imogen—and then clinches his case when he tells of the mole on Imogen's breast. Posthumus believes him and, cursing all women, vows to seek revenge on Imogen.

Act 3, Scene 1
In Britain; LUCIUS (4), the ambassador from the Roman emperor, informs Cymbeline that Britain owes tribute money to the Romans. Cloten boldly insists that the tribute shall not be paid, and the king agrees. Lucius replies with a declaration of war.

Act 3, Scene 2
Pisanio grieves over a letter from Posthumus that orders him to murder Imogen as punishment for her adultery; he is confident that Posthumus has been tricked. Imogen arrives and Pisanio gives her a letter from Posthumus; it tells her to run away and join him at Milford Haven, a port in WALES (1). Delighted, she immediately makes plans to do so.

Act 3, Scene 3
BELARIUS stands outside a cave in Wales and addresses his sons GUIDERIUS and ARVIRAGUS. He praises the wilderness life they lead as infinitely superior to life at a king's court. The two young men respectfully declare that they regret the lack of an opportunity to prove themselves in the great world. Belarius argues that his own unjust banishment justifies his remarks. The sons leave to prepare for the day's hunt, and Belarius soliloguises that their enthusiasm for accomplishment reflects their royal blood. Although they believe him to be their father, they are actually royal princes, the sons of King Cymbeline, kidnapped by Belarius when he was exiled.

Act 3, Scene 4
Near Milford Haven, Pisanio shows Imogen the letter from Posthumus that declares her unfaithfulness and commands her murder. Grief stricken, Imogen raves madly until Pisanio proposes a plan. The deceived Posthumus must be made to believe she is dead until he can learn the truth. Pisanio will claim to Posthumus that he has killed Imogen, and news of her disappearance from court will confirm the account. In the meantime, she should disguise herself as a page boy and take service with Lucius, who is expected in Wales soon. She can then go to Rome and at least maintain contact with Posthumus. She agrees and assumes her disguise. Pisanio gives her the medicine he received

from the queen in case she falls ill while alone, and returns to the court.

Act 3, Scene 5
Lucius regrets the end of his friendship with Cymbeline and leaves the court for Milford Haven where he will sail for Rome. Imogen's absence is reported. Cloten encounters Pisanio and threatens to kill him if he does not tell where Imogen is. He reveals Posthumus' letter to Imogen that tells her to meet him in Wales. Cloten then orders Pisanio to bring him some of Posthumus' clothes. After a soliloquy in which he plans to kill Posthumus in front of Imogen and then rape her, all while wearing the very clothes that she had insultingly compared him with, he sets out for Wales.

Act 3, Scene 6
Imogen, tired and in despair, comes to Belarius' cave. Seeking rest, she calls out; she gets no answer and enters the cave.

Act 3, Scene 7
Belarius, Guiderius, and Arviragus return from the hunt and discover Imogen, disguised as a boy. She identifies herself as 'Fidele' and says that she is travelling to join her master at Milford. Struck by 'his' courtly manners and almost supernatural beauty, the two young men declare their brotherly love for the stranger. They invite Imogen to stay the night before travelling on.

Act 3, Scene 8
In Rome a SENATOR (5) issues plans for the invasion of Britain. Lucius is to command a force raised from the gentry of Rome.

Act 4, Scene 1
In Wales, Cloten wears Posthumus' clothes and compliments himself on his appearance. He believes he will soon find his enemy and have his revenge.

Act 4, Scene 2
Imogen, who is ill, takes the medicine Pisanio has given her and retires to the cave. Cloten appears; Belarius recognises him and believes he has been sent to arrest them. He and Arviragus go to scout for soldiers, and Guiderius addresses the intruder. After Cloten insults him, the two begin to fight and they skirmish their way off stage. Belarius and Arviragus reappear and meet Guiderius, who returns with Cloten's head. Belarius is afraid of the consequences, but the two young men are happily defiant. Their pleasure collapses when they discover that 'Fidele' has apparently died. They sing an elegy for 'him' and leave the body with the headless corpse of Cloten, while they go to prepare a funeral. Imogen awakes and sees a headless body in Posthumus' clothes. She believes that her lover is dead. Grief stricken, she falls insensate on the body. Lucius appears, on his way to join the troops arriving from Rome. He sees Imogen, who identifies herself again as Fidele and says that her master has been killed by brigands. She is taken into Lucius' service, the Roman orders his men to bury the corpse, and he departs with his new page.

Act 4, Scene 3
Cymbeline is distracted because Imogen is missing and the Queen has been stricken with madness since Cloten is also missing. He threatens Pisanio with torture if he does not reveal Imogen's whereabouts. News arrives of the approaching Roman army, and the king goes with his lords to prepare. Pisanio, in a soliloquy, admits bewilderment, having heard nothing from either Posthumus or Imogen. He puts his hope in providence, for he can do nothing.

Act 4, Scene 4
At their cave, Belarius, Guiderius, and Arviragus hear the battle. Belarius wishes to retreat into the mountains, but the young men insist on fighting. They say that it would be dishonourable not to take the opportunity to prove themselves. They convince him, and the three go to join the British forces.

Act 5, Scene 1
Posthumus is serving as a Roman officer. He contemplates the bloody cloth Pisanio has sent him as proof of Imogen's death, and he is stricken with remorse. He wishes he had died rather than she and decides that he will disguise himself as a peasant and fight for the British until he is killed.

Act 5, Scene 2
The Roman army, which includes Lucius and Iachimo, skirmishes with the British army, which includes Posthumus. Iachimo is disarmed by Posthumus but is left alone as the battle shifts off-stage. He laments that he has blackened Imogen's name and supposes that his burden of guilt has made him inept in battle. The battle continues; Cymbeline is briefly captured by the Romans, but Belarius, Guiderius, and Arviragus, aided by Posthumus, rally the British troops and rescue him.

Act 5, Scene 3
Posthumus tells a fleeing Briton that the British, though nearly defeated, have won the battle thanks to an old man and two handsome young ones, who rallied the British troops. Posthumus regrets that he was not killed in battle and decides to resume his Roman garb and be captured by the British. He hopes that they will avenge the day's slaughter by killing their prisoners. A British CAPTAIN (11) appears and talks about the old man and his sons who saved the army, and a Second Captain adds that they were assisted by a British peasant. Posthumus accosts them and is taken prisoner.

Act 5, Scene 4
In gaol Posthumus prays for death. He falls asleep and has a vision. His father, SICILIUS LEONATUS, appears, accompanied by his MOTHER and brothers (see BROTHER [2]). In solemn rhymes they beseech JUPITER to have mercy on Posthumus, who has suffered enough. The god himself appears, riding an eagle, and declares that Posthumus shall recover and marry Imogen. Posthumus awakes, and a GAOLER (2) arrives to escort him to his execution. However, a summons calls Posthumus to the king.

Act 5, Scene 5
Cymbeline knights Belarius, Guiderius, and Arviragus as the heroes of the battle and regrets that he cannot find the peasant who fought beside them. Cornelius arrives with word of the Queen's death and reports her death-bed confession. She had planned to poison the king and place Cloten on his throne. The Roman prisoners include Lucius, Iachimo, the SOOTHSAYER (3), Posthumus, and Imogen, who is still disguised as Fidele. Lucius asks mercy for Fidele; Cymbeline is struck by 'his' appearance and offers the 'boy' a boon. Imogen demands that Iachimo explain where he got the diamond ring he wears. Iachimo tells of his wager for Posthumus' ring, and Posthumus comes forward, declares himself a gullible fool, and confesses that he had Imogen murdered. This leads to a series of explanations that reveal the play's complications to all. Cymbeline, delighted with the return of his sons, forgives Belarius for kidnapping them and then frees the Roman captives. Iachimo begs for death, as punishment for his wager, but Posthumus pardons him. Cymbeline declares that his happiness makes him desire peace, and he agrees to resume paying the Roman tribute. He commands a celebration of the renewed alliance.

COMMENTARY

With *Cymbeline,* Shakespeare continued to develop the ROMANCES, an experiment with a new genre that began with *Pericles* and culminated in his two late masterpieces, *The Winter's Tale* and *The Tempest.* His attempt to blend the features of TRAGEDY and COMEDY with the magical fantasy of romance, a literary mode familiar from 16th-century prose and poetry, was not yet successful. The play is a veritable anthology of motifs and situations from romantic literature: a wicked stepmother, long-lost children, the discovery of bodily identification marks, a decoded riddle, the appearance of a god, and so on. These motifs appear in a profusion intended to generate a seductive fairy-tale world. However, in *Cymbeline* vestiges of earlier modes remain—from the tragedies, in particular—and the effect of the romantic features is seriously undercut. The realism in character and setting that creates our emotional involvement in the tragedies is not appropriate to the idealisation of the new genre, and the domestic pleasantries of comedy are not yet sublimated in the unreal world of romance.

Cymbeline therefore exhibits a jarring set of components that distract from the play's themes. The central message of the play is that order transcends chaos and that ultimately, despite our human ineffectuality, peace and love can triumph in a grand reconciliation of disordered elements. This idea is present throughout the romances. Here, marking an advance on *Pericles,* the emphasis falls on forgiveness of others: it is necessary for humans to act with mercy, rather than justice, in keeping with the behaviour of the gods. However, the potential for catastrophe is too strongly presented in *Cymbeline,* and by the time Jupiter appears to reassure us that all will be well, a state of near chaos has steadily grown and events appear to be entirely out of control. Iachimo's scheme has succeeded; Imogen believes Posthumus has been killed by Pisanio, who is in fact her only ally; Guiderius and Arviragus remain unrecognised as princes; and Britain is locked in a foolish war against Rome. Most dire of all, perhaps, Posthumus is suicidal because he believes Imogen is dead, a situation appallingly suggestive of *Romeo and Juliet.* The generally romantic context suggests that these problems will be resolved, but the tone is almost as anarchic as that of *Macbeth.* The play's final sequence of revelations and reconciliations therefore seems confusing, if not simply arbitrary, and its message is accordingly weakened.

Nevertheless, the play has many real virtues, one of the greatest being its variety of attractive characters. Imogen's considerable charm, which we shall consider later, heads the list, of course, but several of the other characters are also quite entertaining. For instance, Cloten's offensiveness is of an intriguing sort. His vice and violence are accompanied by great foolishness—he inspires the Second Lord's mockery and is several times referred to as a fool—and he is clearly intended to be a humorous grotesque. He is a predecessor of *The Tempest*'s CALIBAN. Along with his mother, the archetypal wicked stepmother of fairy tale, Cloten manifests the other-worldliness of romance. The other comic villain of the piece, Iachimo, is a pleasing creation who also helps maintain the play's tone. He is a stock MACHIAVEL and is often downright comic—for example when he emerges from his trunk like a jack-in-the-box and compares himself vaingloriously to the truly menacing TARQUIN. His humorous aspect takes the edge off his villainy and permits us to recognise that Imogen's disgrace can have no lasting consequences in the world of romance. In 5.5 Iachimo's long confession, as boastful as it is apologetic, constitutes a plea for forgiveness and entitles him to share in the play's final reconciliation. Pisanio is another sort of figure, the loyal and clever servant of tradition who stands firmly for common sense, truth, and resource-

ful continuance. Finally, however, as the chaos of the plot builds, he throws up his hands and commits himself to providence. 'Fortune brings in some boats that are not steer'd' (4.3.46), he declares.

Cymbeline is very exciting to watch on the stage, for the complexities and improbabilities of its plot yield many splendid surprises. The role of the central figure, Imogen, shifts constantly. The plot turns from the theme of separated lovers, to that of a wager on the maiden's chastity (and two different, equally repellent, assaults on it), to the maiden's ambivalent journey—she braves the wilderness to find her lover but is actually being ambushed by him—and finally to a traditional comic ploy, the maiden disguised as a boy. In the meantime, two other plots have been introduced, either of which might be central in a more conventional play. One concerns lost princes raised in the wild, and the other offers high politics and war as Britain refuses tribute to Rome.

Particular episodes offer individual surprises as well. Iachimo's first appearance, in 1.5, is entirely unanticipated, and he later startles us again when he emerges from the trunk in Imogen's bedroom. The first presentation of Belarius' cave suddenly introduces a very different sub-plot, just as the main plot is growing increasingly complicated. We are shocked (though probably delighted) when Cloten's head is borne on-stage by Guiderius, and while we are prepared for Imogen's false death, its conjunction with Cloten's headless corpse is a pleasantly novel complication. Not least, Posthumus' supernatural vision in 5.4 is probably the most spectacular eruption of the unexpected in Shakespeare. Shakespeare's earlier works had occasionally offered surprises—the final episode in *Love's Labour's Lost* is a famous example—but a great emphasis on novelty is distinctive to the romances, and the dramatic excitement produced is strongly felt by audiences.

This emphasis on the playwright's artfulness has inspired many commentators to insist that *Cymbeline* is merely an artistic experiment undertaken for its own sake. However, the play's marked esthetic aspect generates a sense of unreality that is important to the cental theme of the romances—humanity's dependence on providence—and to their major motif—magic and the supernatural. We are notified that the play is *not* about real life, and if we permit it, a state of timeless suspension is the result.

The play's complications and surprises also serve another purpose. Tragedy and comedy each enact events that lead towards a conclusion, be it the triumph of love or of disaster. In *Cymbeline*, however, the pattern is so complicated and the turnings of fate so unpredictable that we can only rely on the final surprise of 5.4 (final to us; 5.5 offers a long series of surprises for the characters), the literal *deus ex machina* of Jupiter's appearance, to resolve the situation. Jupiter's descent is significantly climactic. It follows the battle scene that envelops all the characters, and precedes the all-too-human fumbling that is revealed in the comically complicated final scene. We are reminded of Pisanio's prediction—fortune, not steering, will bring in the boats—and that humanity is dependent on providence.

The play's seeming peculiarities reflect this message. Its variety of characters and tonalities—comic or tragic, realistic or fantastic—all are reconciled in a positive and unifying vision. The comic is never farcical, and the potentially tragic remains merely potential. The realistic does not preclude abstraction, and the elements of romance do not give way to an entirely escapist retreat from reality. *Cymbeline* thus suggests and attempts to demonstrate, in not completely effective fashion, a vision of human weakness transcended. Shakespeare more successfully accomplished this vision in less complicated and more homogeneous plays, *The Winter's Tale* and *The Tempest.* For though its themes are dramatic, *Cymbeline* is nevertheless decidedly flawed. As we have seen, it leans disconcertingly towards tragedy, as if the author's intentions had been uncertain. Similarly, several of the characters seem to reflect too many differing ideas, and are inconsistently presented. Iachimo, for instance, while a conventional comic villain, also offers glimpses of tragedy, as when he envisions infidelity in terms of passion and damnation and invokes 'all the plagues of hell' (1.7.111). Here, as when he fleetingly identifies himself with utter evil—'hell is here' (2.2.50)—he sounds more like OTHELLO or MACBETH than the play can bear. Posthumus, likewise, is presented to us as the traditional romantic hero—the 'most prais'd, most lov'd' of men (1.1.47)—but when he accepts the wager, believes Iachimo, and finally takes revenge through Pisanio, he is immature and ignoble. He resembles Othello, also, in his insecurity; he believes that Imogen would find it easy to betray him. His tirade against women with its vividly bestial image of Imogen and Iachimo strikes a horrifying note that is as unromantic as Iachimo's earlier evocations of evil. Posthumus' ultimate decision to seek death in battle is also unsuitably grim.

Imogen is subject to similar inconsistencies, and the main plot seems to have caused Shakespeare to revert to familiar modes of creation. The heroine is the traditional, idealised princess, 'more goddess-like than wife-like' (3.2.8), and the proper mate to Posthumus' glorious prince. However, in her resourcefulness and wit, Imogen is plainly a typical Shakespearean comic heroine, capable of disguising herself as a man and going in search of her lover. She sharply—and wittily—rejects the unwanted attentions of Cloten; she acknowledges—and overcomes—her feminine fear of swords. She resembles ROSALIND of *As You Like It,* BEATRICE of *Much Ado,* and VIOLA of *Twelfth Night,* rather more than she does the passive object of adoration

and intrigue that is the central figure in traditional romance. Imogen is enchanting, and her transformations onstage are delightful, but while she captures our affections, the fashion in which she does so is contrary to the general direction of the play.

Further, the presence of differing character types seems similarly disjointed. Fairy-tale figures such as the queen and the lost princes coexist with more psychologically developed figures. The more peripheral characters seem more appropriate to the essentially comic optimism of romance, while the central situation has the potential for tragedy. The play is also disjointed in its setting. No fewer than four distinct worlds are evoked: classical Rome, RENAISSANCE Italy, pagan Britain, and the abstracted countryside of pastoral romance (represented by Wales). The intricate reconciliation of these venues in the final scene requires such extraordinary ingenuity that it has inspired equal measures of praise and ridicule, as perhaps no other scene in Shakespeare has. Another device, the use of comic relief, such as in 2.1 (see LORD [15]) and 5.4.152–192 (see GAOLER [2]), reflects the need to dilute a mood of growing tragedy that is counter to the play's general thrust.

In *Cymbeline* the seams of Shakespeare's construction show—they don't in *The Winter's Tale* and *The Tempest.* We should not reject the play altogether, however, for as we have seen, it has magic. Samuel JOHNSON (8) complained of the play that 'to remark the folly of the fiction, the absurdity . . . , the confusion . . . were to waste criticism upon unresisting imbecility, upon faults too evident for detection . . .'. However, these evident faults also provide, along with folly and confusion, the escapist charms of romantic literature in general and of Imogen's world in particular. They need not be apologised for but merely accepted, and *Cymbeline* may be enjoyed for itself as well as for its place as the immediate predecessor of Shakespeare's last two masterpieces.

SOURCES OF THE PLAY

The main plot of *Cymbeline*—a man wagers on his lover's chastity and is fooled, orders her death, which a good servant prevents, and is finally reunited with her—had been popular for centuries in various forms and in several languages. Shakespeare's version drew on two sources: one, an anonymous English translation of a Dutch tale, *Frederyke of Jennen* (Antwerp, 1518; London, 1520, 1560), and, much better known, a tale in the *Decameron* (1353) of Giovanni BOCCACCIO. Although no English translation of Boccaccio's story appeared before 1620, Shakespeare may have read it in Italian (though his capacity to do so is disputed), or in a French translation such as the very popular version of Antoine LE MAÇON (1545). The same tale was to be a minor source for *The Winter's Tale.* Boccaccio's tale and *Frederyke of Jennen* (i.e., of Genoa), apparently stem from the same medieval Italian source, which is now lost. They both tell essentially the same story, but *Cymbeline* reflects details exclusive to each.

Another source was Raphael HOLINSHED's *Chronicles of England, Scotland, and Ireland* (2nd ed., 1587), which provided an account of the historical Cymbeline's reign. However, minor details come from at least two other historical sources, Robert FABYAN's *New Chronicle of England and of France* (1516) and A MIRROR FOR MAGISTRATES (1587), a popular collection of biographies. An obscure, anonymous English play, *The Rare Triumphs of Love and Fortune* (performed in 1582, published in 1589), provided Shakespeare with most of the other important components of *Cymbeline*—Posthumus and Imogen's love, Cloten's jealousy, Posthumus' banishment, Imogen's flight to an unjustly banished courtier who lives in a cave—along with various minor details. Some scholars speculate that a nearly contemporary play, *Philaster,* by Francis BEAUMONT (2) and John FLETCHER (2), may have influenced some of the language in *Cymbeline,* but since the dates of both plays are obscure and since Beaumont and Fletcher were novice playwrights at the time, other scholars believe that the younger men imitated Shakespeare.

TEXT OF THE PLAY

Cymbeline was probably written c. 1608–1610, but firm evidence is lacking. A performance was recorded in the summer of 1611, so the play cannot have been composed later than early in that year. Stylistic evidence makes clear that it was roughly contemporary with the other ROMANCES, especially *The Winter's Tale* (c. 1610–1611), and it seems to represent an advance over *Pericles* (c. 1607) in the development of the genre. Some scholars believe it was written during the plague-imposed closure of the London theatres from the summer of 1608 to December 1609.

The play was not published in Shakespeare's lifetime, and appeared first in the FIRST FOLIO (1623). This text was probably printed from a transcription of Shakespeare's FOUL PAPERS, though some scholars believe it was taken from a PROMPT-BOOK. As the only early version of the play, the Folio text has been the basis for all subsequent editions.

THEATRICAL HISTORY OF THE PLAY

The earliest known performance of *Cymbeline*—probably at the GLOBE THEATRE—was recorded by Simon FORMAN in the summer of 1611; no other early performances are known. Thomas D'URFEY adapted the play as *The Injured Princess or the Fatal Wager* (1682), a popular version with an elaborate sub-plot in which Cloten kidnaps a daughter of Pisanio. It was revived periodically for 80 years.

Colley CIBBER (1) produced a version of Shakespeare's play in 1744, and *Cymbeline* was mildly popu-

lar for the rest of the 18th century, though only with altered texts. David GARRICK, who staged the play several times beginning in 1761, was especially noted for his Posthumus (opposite Sarah SIDDONS, in the 1780s). In 1767 the play was staged in colonial New York. The 19th century saw few productions of *Cymbeline,* but they were very elaborately staged. The most important of these were the productions of John Philip KEMBLE (3) (1806, 1827). Helen FAUCIT played the heroine a number of times up to the age of 48, with great success, and Adelaide NEILSON (1) was also associated with the role. Ellen TERRY (1), in Henry IRVING's production of 1896, was widely acclaimed as the century's greatest Imogen. This production was heavily abridged (as most have been); for example, the vision of Jupiter was cut.

Cymbeline has not been widely produced in the 20th century, either, though George Bernard SHAW (2) staged his own witty version of Act 5, titled *Cymbeline Refinished,* in 1937. Probably the most notable modern productions of the play have been the 1923 modern dress staging by Barry JACKSON (1)—his first such experiment—and the 1957 STRATFORD staging by Peter HALL (5), starring Peggy ASHCROFT as Imogen. Though *Cymbeline* was twice made into a silent FILM—in the United States (1913) and Germany (1925)—it has not been a movie since. The BBC produced a TELEVISION version starring Claire Bloom in 1984.

Cyprus Large island in the eastern Mediterranean, now a country, the setting for much of *Othello.* Although there is nothing especially exotic—let alone specifically Cypriot—about Acts 2–5 of *Othello,* Shakespeare's placement of the action on this remote outpost of the Venetian Empire is significant. After leaving VENICE the characters are removed from the buffering effects of society. In the isolation of Cyprus IAGO's influence over OTHELLO works its poison in the absence of any social or political distractions that might direct the general's attention elsewhere, or suggest different responses. Similarly, DESDEMONA has no peers to turn to for advice or intervention.

To effect this isolation, Shakespeare invented the 'Cyprus wars' (1.1.150) of the play, which do not appear in his source, CINTHIO's tale. Moreover, although conflict between Venice and the Ottoman Turks was constant in the 15th and 16th centuries, the situation described in *Othello*—with the Turks threatening both Cyprus and Rhodes (see 1.3.14)—never arose. The Turks did not attack Cyprus until 1570, long after they controlled Rhodes. However, Shakespeare may have had this attack in mind, mistaking the details while intending to associate his hero with it, for its direct result was the naval battle of Lepanto (1571), in which an alliance led by Venice and Spain defeated the Turkish fleet. This was united Christendom's last great victory over Islam, and in Shakespeare's day and for generations thereafter it was regarded as one of the key events of European history. Its aura of epic victory doubtless influenced early audiences' sense of Othello as a grand figure. Nevertheless, Lepanto was an expensive victory and Venice, retrenching in its aftermath, ceded Cyprus to the Turks in 1573. Thus, for Shakespeare, Cyprus was associated with vulnerability as well as strength, a combination reflected in Othello's personality.

D

Daly, Augustin (1838–1899) American theatrical entrepreneur. Daly operated theatres in both London and New York. With Ada REHAN as the centre-piece of his company, he specialised in classical COMEDY (along with modern drama) and produced most of Shakespeare's comedies, usually with greatly abridged texts and spectacular scenic effects. He was also a playwright with about 100 plays to his credit (though scholars believe his brother may have written most of them, and they are virtually all adapted from earlier plays, mostly French or German). These works were all highly colourful melodramas: his first great success in the theatre was with a famous and often imitated scene of a man tied on railroad tracks in front of an oncoming train.

Dance, James (1722–1774) English actor and playwright, author of an adaptation of *Timon of Athens.* Dance, son of a famous architect, took the name James Love for his acting career. He was best known for his portrayals of FALSTAFF. His version of *Timon* (1768) combined Shakespeare's text with Thomas SHADWELL's earlier adaptation. It was only moderately successful. Dance also wrote a popular long poem on cricket.

Daniel, Samuel (c. 1562–1619) English poet and dramatist, author of sources for several of Shakespeare's plays. Daniel's epic poem *The Civil Wars between the two Houses of York and Lancaster* (1595) influenced Act 5 of *Richard II* and the minor TETRALOGY of HISTORY PLAYS in general. His *The Complaint of Rosamund* (1592), a love story in verse, inspired several passages in *Romeo and Juliet;* moreover, Shakespeare's use of it helps date the play. Daniel's TRAGEDY *Cleopatra* (1594) influenced Shakespeare's treatment of his Egyptian queen, and another Daniel play, *The Queen's Arcadia* (1605), provided minor details for *Macbeth.* Also, Daniel's immensely popular SONNET sequence *Delia* (1592) may have helped inspire Shakespeare to write his SONNETS.

A minor diplomat early in his career, Daniel was later a tutor to William Herbert, Earl of PEMBROKE (3). His connection with Pembroke has inspired speculation that he may be the 'rival poet' of Shakespeare's sonnets. By 1595 Daniel was well established as a major literary figure of the day, and after 1603 he often composed MASQUES for the court of King JAMES I. A play produced by the Children of the Revels (see CHILDREN'S COMPANIES) in 1604 got him in trouble with state CENSORSHIP, for it seemed to express sympathy for the rebellious Earl of ESSEX (2), but Daniel nevertheless continued to write for the court. He also wrote a prose *History of England* (1612) that was very influential during the political turmoil of the 1620s and 1630s, as England approached civil war. In the last years of his life he became reclusive; Shakespeare is said to have been among the few people he would accept as visitors.

Danter, John (d. 1599) London printer, producer of editions of two of Shakespeare's plays. In 1594 Danter printed the first QUARTO edition of *Titus Andronicus* for publishers Thomas MILLINGTON and Edward WHITE (1), and in 1597 he undertook a pirated edition, the first, of *Romeo and Juliet,* only to have his press seized by the STATIONERS' COMPANY for other such piracies before the job was finished. It was completed by Edward ALLDE. Danter was in trouble for piracy throughout his career, but he always re-established himself. However, all of his surviving work is sloppily done. He was also suspended in 1596 for printing illegal Catholic materials. He was a business partner of Henry CHETTLE from 1589 to 1591.

Dardanius (Dardanus) (active 42 B.C.) Historical figure and minor character in *Julius Caesar,* a soldier in the army of BRUTUS (4). At PHILIPPI, Dardanius, along with CLITUS and VOLUMNIUS, refuses to help Brutus to commit suicide, saying, 'Shall I do such a deed?' (5.5.8). The episode demonstrates that Brutus was regarded with affection by his subordinates, adding sentiment to the presentation of his death. Shakespeare mis-spelled the name of the historical figure, Dardanus. Little is known of this individual, whose role Shakespeare took from PLUTARCH's *Lives.*

Dark Lady See SONNETS.

Daughter (1) Minor character in *Pericles,* incestuous lover of her father, King ANTIOCHUS of Syria. PERICLES attempts to win the Daughter in marriage by solving

Antiochus' riddle, but when the solution reveals the incest, he withdraws in horror, repelled by the sin and fearful of Antiochus' wrath. When she appears in 1.1 the Daughter is presented as a personification of fertility, 'apparell'd like the spring' (1.1.13). However, a warning is immediately voiced by her father, who calls her 'this fair Hesperides, / With golden fruit, but dangerous to be touch'd' (1.1.28–29). She speaks only two lines and approves of her suitor, but when Pericles learns the truth, he rejects her and says 'Good sooth, I care not for you' (1.1.87). He later speaks of her and her father as 'both like serpents . . . who though they feed / On sweetest flowers, yet they poison breed' (1.1.133–134). In Act 2 THAISA and her father, SIMONIDES, are implicitly contrasted with the Daughter and Antiochus, whose deaths by divine vengeance are reported in 2.4: 'A fire from heaven came and shrivell'd up / Their bodies . . .' (2.4.9–10). The Daughter has no personality and is a convenient agent of evil in the play's melodramatic plot.

Daughter (2) Character in *The Two Noble Kinsmen,* deranged lover of PALAMON and child of the GAOLER (4). Although she has already agreed to marry the WOOER, in 2.1 the Daughter falls in love with Palamon, a prisoner of war in her father's prison. After remarking to her father on the nobility of Palamon and his fellow prisoner, ARCITE, in 2.1, the Daughter appears alone for her next four scenes, all soliloquies. In 2.3 she declares that she will help Palamon escape, and in 2.5 she reports that she has done so. In 3.2 she is alone in the woods, unable to find Palamon and clearly going mad. She decides that Palamon has been eaten by wild animals and contemplates suicide. Her fourth soliloquy in 3.4 is frankly insane, as she gabbles of shipwrecks and a magic frog and sings scraps of SONG. In 3.5, wandering insanely through the countryside, she is recruited for the rustic entertainment directed by the SCHOOLMASTER. Finally, in Act 4 she returns home, where the DOCTOR (4) prescribes that the Wooer, disguised as Palamon, take her to bed. The treatment apparently works, for her father later reports that she is is 'well restored, / And to be married shortly' (5.4.27–28).

Though she resembles Shakespeare's OPHELIA—both are unlucky in love, both gather flowers by a lakeside (see 4.1.54, 78), and both sing bits of song (in 4.1.108 the Daughter names a song Ophelia sings in *Hamlet* 4.5.184)—the Daughter is a very un-Shakespearean character. Her chief function is clearly as an object of humour, for in Shakespeare's day insanity was regarded as highly amusing (see, e.g., PINCH). Her diatribes are conventional indications of madness, artificial and unconvincing, and her cure is laughable, as it was doubtless intended to be. She was almost certainly not created by Shakespeare but by his collaborator, John FLETCHER (2), who probably wrote all the scenes she appears in (though some scholars attribute 2.1 and the best of her soliloquies, 3.2, to Shakespeare).

Dauphin (1) Charles, the Character in *1 Henry VI.* See Charles VII.

Dauphin (2) Lewis, the Character in *King John.* See Lewis (1).

Dauphin (3) Lewis, the (1396–1415) Historical figure and character in *Henry V,* son of the FRENCH KING. The Dauphin—who bore the traditional title of the eldest son of a king of FRANCE (1)—leads the French nobles in their cocky over-confidence before the battle of AGINCOURT. In 1.2 the French AMBASSADOR (1) delivers a sneering message to Henry from the Dauphin, accompanied by a shipment of tennis balls, said to be appropriate weapons for so foolish a monarch; the insult gives Henry an occasion to declare war on France. When the English invade, the Dauphin and his friends are preposterously boastful and arrogant caricatures, presented only to be put down by events. In 4.5 a hysterically suicidal Dauphin is shown in defeat; his capture is reported in 4.8.78.

Shakespeare's Dauphin, besides being a stock figure, misrepresents the historical Dauphin in several small matters of fact as well. He mocks Henry for his youth, as in 2.4.28, but he was in fact nine years younger than his foe. Nor was he present at Agincourt; too sick to fight, he died two months after the battle.

Davenant (D'Avenant), William (1606–1668) English poet, playwright, and theatrical entrepreneur. Davenant, along with Thomas KILLIGREW, dominated the LONDON theatrical world during the 1660s. When the monarchy was restored in 1660, the theatres of England were reopened after their long closure by the Puritan revolutionary government, and Davenant received one of the two licences to put on plays in London. His Duke of York's Company—named for its patron, the future King James II—staged many plays by Shakespeare and others. Davenant's licence assigned him the rights to 10—later amended to 13—of Shakespeare's plays: *Hamlet,* the *Henry VI* plays (considered as one work), *Henry VIII, King Lear, Macbeth, Measure for Measure, Much Ado About Nothing, Pericles, Romeo and Juliet, The Tempest, Timon of Athens, Troilus and Cressida,* and *Twelfth Night.*

Davenant is notorious for his adaptations of the plays. He combined *Measure for Measure* and *Much Ado About Nothing* in THE LAW AGAINST LOVERS (1662), and he greatly abridged and altered the texts of the others, changing names, rewriting passages, inserting his own words—or sometimes merely inserting Shakespeare's words into his own play—and taking care to 'refine' (his word) Shakespeare's language. This process was particularly egregious in his *Macbeth.* With John DRYDEN, he adapted *The Tempest* as *The Tempest, or The*

Enchanted Island (1667, published 1670), adding many characters and situations from the work of the Spanish playwright Pedro Calderón (1600–1681) and retaining little of Shakespeare's text. This adaptation was hugely popular, especially in Thomas SHADWELL's operatic version (1674; Henry PURCELL provided a new score in 1690). Modern commentators condemn it, but the Davenant/Dryden *Tempest* influenced all other versions of the play for almost 200 years.

As a young man, Davenant was a playwright, composing several tragedies in the style of JACOBEAN DRAMA and a popular comedy of manners, *The Wits* (1633). He collaborated on several MASQUES with Inigo Jones, the royal architect, and when Ben JONSON died in 1637, Davenant was awarded his masque-writing duties and his pension (the equivalent of being named Poet Laureate). He fought for the royalists in the Civil Wars and was knighted for valour by King Charles I. Captured in 1650, he was imprisoned for more than a year before being freed by the poet John MILTON, who was a member of the revolutionary government. (Davenant was to repay the service upon the restoration of the monarchy in 1660, when Milton was sentenced to death.) Upon his release, Davenant wrote plays that he managed to stage despite the ban on theatres, by adding music and calling them operas. His *The Siege of Rhodes* (1656) is considered the first opera performed in England. Thus, when the restored monarchy legalised the theatre again, Davenant was already in business.

Davenant claimed to be Shakespeare's illegitimate son. His parents had run an inn on the road between STRATFORD and London, and Davenant declared that he had been conceived during a stopover. In a variation of this claim—the version reportedly varied with alcohol consumption—he took the status of godson. Neither claim is supported by any evidence.

Davies (1), John, of Hereford (c. 1565–1618) English poet, author of early references to Shakespeare. Davies published several volumes of poetry between 1603 and 1617, including one, *The Scourge of Folly* (c. 1610), containing a poem praising Shakespeare as 'our English TERENCE'. His *Microcosmos* (1603) and *Civil Wars of Death and Fortune* (1605) contain praises of the actors 'W.S'. and 'R.B.', presumed to be Shakespeare and Richard BURBAGE (3). Davies taught writing to the ill-fated Prince of Wales, Henry (1594–1612), son of King JAMES I.

Davies (2), Sir John (1569–1626) English poet and lawyer, author of a minor source for *Julius Caesar.* Davies published several volumes of poetry, including *Epigrams* (1590), *Orchestra, or a Poeme of Dauncing* (1596)—a long poem justifying the pleasures of dancing—and *Hymnes of Astraea* (1599), a collection of acrostics based on the name of Queen ELIZABETH (1). Also published in 1599 was his *Nosce Teipsum* ('Know Thyself'), a long philosophical poem on the nature of the human soul. Several minor echoes of this text in *Julius Caesar* establish that Shakespeare was familiar with the work.

Davies was by profession a lawyer. He was disbarred from 1598 to 1601 after he assaulted a fellow attorney, but he was reinstated under King JAMES I and was highly successful. He was first solicitor general and then attorney general of Ireland from 1603–1619. He supported King Charles I in his early disputes with Parliament and in return was appointed Lord Chief Justice, the highest-ranking judicial post in England, but he died before taking office.

Davy Character in *2 Henry IV,* steward to Justice SHALLOW. In 5.1 Davy makes the necessary arrangements when FALSTAFF visits Shallow and conducts ordinary business—seeing to minor repairs, planting, paying the blacksmith, and so on—at the same time. As a typical resident of GLOUCESTERSHIRE, he is part of the play's delightful presentation of English country life. On behalf of his friend William VISOR, Davy asks his master for a favourable ruling in a lawsuit, offering a humorous look at small-time legal chicanery. At Shallow's drinking party in 5.3, Davy manages to function as host, guest, and servant

Day, John (c. 1574–c. 1640) English playwright, possible collaborator with Shakespeare. Day, a minor figure in the ELIZABETHAN THEATRE, collaborated with many playwrights, including Thomas DEKKER, Samuel ROWLEY (1), George WILKINS, and possibly Christopher MARLOWE (1). He may also have had a hand in *Timon of Athens* and/or *Pericles,* though in both cases the identity—or even existence—of collaborators is uncertain.

Day became a hack writer in LONDON after being expelled from Cambridge University for theft in 1593. Little is known of his life, except that he was chronically in debt, and that in 1599 he stabbed and killed the playwright Henry PORTER (5), apparently in self-defence. Day wrote plays for the ADMIRAL'S MEN from 1599 to 1603, usually in collaboration, though after this period he mostly wrote alone. The later plays, of which six have survived, were generally staged by the Children of the Revels (see CHILDREN'S COMPANIES). One of them, *Isle of Gulls* (1606), a satire on Anglo-Scottish relations, offended the government and resulted in the imprisonment of several of its producers. He also wrote a series of non-dramatic dialogues, *The Parliament of Bees* (1608), that is considered his masterpiece, though it is a minor work.

Decius (Decimus) Brutus (d. 43 B.C.) Historical figure and minor character in *Julius Caesar,* one of the assassins of CAESAR (1). In 2.2 Decius persuades Cae-

sar to proceed with his fateful plans after CALPHURNIA has convinced him to stay at home. Caesar thus goes to the Senate and is assassinated.

The historical figure was named Decimus Brutus, not Decius; the error originated with Jacques AMYOT, who translated PLUTARCH into French. His work was retranslated into English by Sir Thomas NORTH, who transmitted the incorrect name to Shakespeare. Decimus Brutus (a cousin of Marcus BRUTUS [4]) had distinguished himself as a commander under Caesar in Gaul. Although awarded high office under Caesar, he joined the conspiracy against his leader and played the part enacted in the play. He was killed in the ensuing civil war.

Decretas (Decretus, Dercetas, Dercetaeus, Dercetus) (active 30 B.C.) Historical figure and minor character in *Antony and Cleopatra,* a member of ANTONY's personal guard. In 4.14 Antony stabs himself with his sword, and Decretas, seeing that his master's defeat is now complete, takes Antony's sword to CAESAR (2), where he hopes to ingratiate himself with the conqueror by being the first to tell him of his enemy's death. In 5.1.5–26 he makes his presentation to Caesar and praises Antony eloquently, after which he disappears from the play. He demonstrates, by his flight to Caesar, the collapse of loyalty around Antony, and then—somewhat incongruously—he bears witness to the nobility of the hero's end, a major theme of Act 5.

Shakespeare took the name of this minor figure—unknown in history outside this anecdote—from his source, PLUTARCH's *Lives,* and it has been variously rendered. In Plutarch and in Sir Thomas NORTH's English translation his name is Dercetaeus. Shakespeare—or someone else associated with early productions of the play—simplified this spelling, and it appears in the FIRST FOLIO (1623) as 'Decretas' (twice, plus several abbreviations beginning 'Dec') and 'Dercetus' (once). In 1725, Alexander POPE (1) compromised and introduced a new variant, 'Dercetas', and subsequent editors have chosen from among these possibilities.

Deiphobus Legendary figure and minor character in *Troilus and Cressida,* a Trojan warrior. Deiphobus appears in five scenes but speaks only two lines, serving merely to flesh out the Trojan aristocracy. In the *Iliad* of HOMER, Deiphobus, a son of King PRIAM, is a prominent warrior.

Dekker, Thomas (c. 1572–c. 1632) English dramatist. Between 1598 and 1605, Dekker wrote about 44 plays (many of them in collaboration) for the ADMIRAL'S MEN and WORCESTER'S MEN, but only six have survived. He is best known for two comedies, *The Shoemaker's Holiday* (1599) and *The Honest Whore* (1604, with Thomas MIDDLETON). Writing for the Children of Paul's (see CHILDREN'S COMPANIES), he participated in the WAR OF THE THEATRES, an exchange of satirical plays among rival playwrights. His *Satiromastix* (1601, with John MARSTON) was a reply to Ben JONSON's satire of him in an earlier work. Jonson struck again in *The Poetaster* (1601), calling Dekker a 'playdresser and plagiary'.

Dekker went on to write many pamphlets, including a vivid group describing a plague epidemic. In the 1620s he returned to writing plays, mostly for PRINCE CHARLES' MEN and mostly in collaboration with such dramatists as John DAY, John FORD, and Philip MASSINGER. Little is known of Dekker's life, though his works reveal him to have been a pleasant, cheerful man, with an admiration for the strengths of London's poor, of whom he was one. He was perennially in debt; he spent almost eight years in debtors' prison between 1612 and 1619 and may have returned just before his death.

Deloney, Thomas (c. 1550–1600) English writer, possibly the author of a poem sometimes ascribed to Shakespeare. The poem, 'Crabbed age and youth cannot live together', published as number XII in THE PASSIONATE PILGRIM (1599) where it was attributed to Shakespeare, appeared as Deloney's work in a posthumously published anthology, *Garland of Goodwill* (1631). Most modern scholars do not believe the poem was written by Shakespeare, though a minority opinion holds that it might be an early work of the playwright. If Deloney's, it is one of his best poems.

Deloney was a minor poet of the 1580s and 1590s—best known for three long ballads on the Spanish Armada—who turned to prose and wrote several so-called 'craft novels'. These were prose narratives which celebrated various urban occupations. One of them, *The Gentle Craft* (1598), about shoemakers, was the chief source for Thomas DEKKER's well-known play, *The Shoemaker's Holiday* (1599). Deloney's novels are notable for their descriptions of LONDON life, and although they were popular, Elizabethan novelists were ill-rewarded and Deloney died in poverty.

Demetrius (1) Character in *Titus Andronicus,* a son of TAMORA. Demetrius and his brother CHIRON murder BASSIANUS and then commit the appalling rape and mutilation of LAVINIA, the daughter of TITUS (1) Andronicus; they are encouraged and abetted by AARON. Titus' counter revenge includes the killing of the two brothers, who are baked in a meat pie and served to their mother in the final scene.

Demetrius (2) Character in *A Midsummer Night's Dream,* the lover of HERMIA whose affections are magically diverted to HELENA (1). Chosen by EGEUS to be Hermia's husband, Demetrius had wooed Helena earlier, before the opening of the play, but had aban-

doned her. In addition to fickleness, Demetrius shows an unpleasant shortness with Helena, who pursues him, but on the whole he is—like Hermia's beloved, LYSANDER—a colourless young man who exists merely to be manipulated by OBERON's spells.

Demetrius (3) Minor character in *Antony and Cleopatra,* a follower of ANTONY. In 1.1 Demetrius and his friend PHILO discuss Antony's neglect of his military duties while he dallies with the Queen of Egypt, CLEOPATRA. The episode establishes a disapproving Roman view of the love affair.

Dench, Judi (b. 1934) English actress. Dench began her Shakespearean career as OPHELIA in Michael BENTHALL's 1957 *Hamlet* and went on to a much acclaimed JULIET (2) in Franco ZEFFERELLI's 1960 staging of *Romeo and Juliet.* She has played many of Shakespeare's best female roles since, including a remarkable performance as both HERMIONE and PERDITA in *The Winter's Tale* (1969). She played LADY (6) MACBETH both in Trevor NUNN's 1976 production at STRATFORD and in his 1979 TELEVISION version.

Denmark Country in northern Europe, the setting for *Hamlet.* The entire play takes place in and around the royal castle in ELSINORE, a seaport in northern Denmark. Denmark was familiar to English audiences as a rival in the Baltic Sea trade, and Shakespeare offers several glimpses of Danish ways, focussing chiefly on the Danes' reputation for excessive drinking, which HAMLET remarks on disparagingly in 1.4. 13–38. Sixteenth-century accounts confirm bits of information provided in the play, such as the popularity of Rhine wines (1.4.10) and the habit of accompanying a toast with kettledrums (1.4.11) or, more extravagantly, with cannon fire (1.2.126). Further, it is thought that the description of Danish preparations for war in 1.1.74–81 reflects news of contemporary conflicts between Denmark and Sweden.

Scholars have occasionally proposed that Shakespeare's knowledge of Denmark reflects a visit he

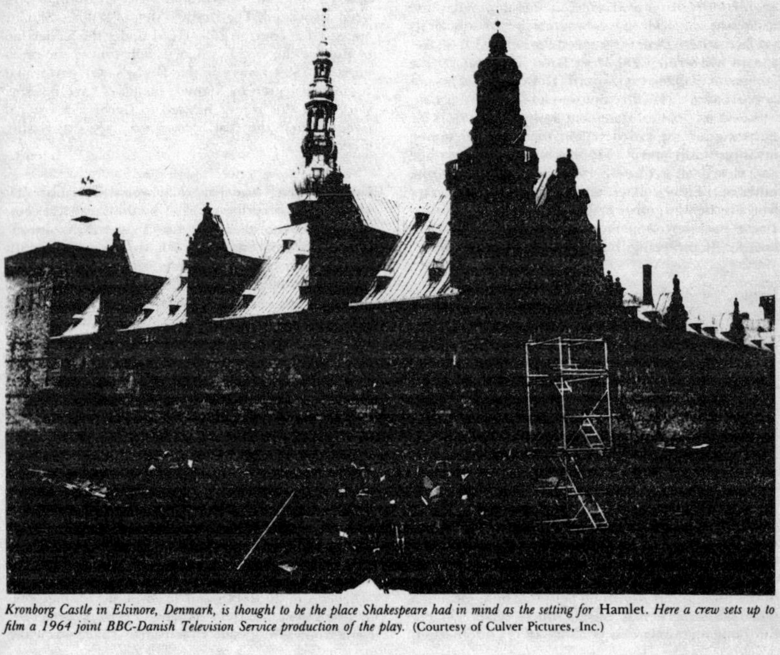

Kronborg Castle in Elsinore, Denmark, is thought to be the place Shakespeare had in mind as the setting for Hamlet. *Here a crew sets up to film a 1964 joint BBC-Danish Television Service production of the play.* (Courtesy of Culver Pictures, Inc.)

made to that country with an English acting company in 1585 or 1586, when such trips are known to have occurred (see e.g. KEMPE), but many contemporary sources provided sufficient information on the country and its customs to account for the play's descriptions. In fact, Shakespeare's extremely faulty knowledge of the geography of Denmark—a flat country with no 'cliff / That beetles o'er his base into the sea' (1.4.70–71) and that is not connected by land to Norway or Poland, as the route of FORTINBRAS' army would imply (see 2.2.75–78; 4.4.10–12)—suggests strongly that he had not been there.

Dennis (1) Minor character in *As You Like It,* servant of OLIVER (1). Dennis appears only to announce the arrival of the wrestler CHARLES in 1.1.88–92.

Dennis (2), John (1657–1734) English playwright. Dennis, a minor poet and dramatist, wrote and produced two unsuccessful adaptations of Shakespeare plays. His *The Comical Gallant* (1702) is a crude version of *The Merry Wives of Windsor.* It was unpopular and disappeared quickly; it is now remembered only for its preface, where Dennis recorded the belief that Shakespeare had written *The Merry Wives* in 14 days at the command of Queen ELIZABETH (1). Dennis' *The Invader of His Country* (1719) employed excerpts from *Coriolanus* in its political statement against FRANCE (1) for having aided the exiled STUART DYNASTY's attempted invasion of England in 1715. It was booed off the stage and closed after three performances. Dennis wrote other anti-French plays, and he amused the literary world by being egotistical enough to ask that a special clause be inserted in the Treaty of Utrecht (1713), specifically protecting him from French reprisals.

Denny, Sir Anthony (1501–1549) Historical figure and minor character in *Henry VIII,* a member of King HENRY VIII's court. In 5.1.80–81 Denny reports that he has brought Archbishop CRANMER to a midnight meeting with the king, as Henry has instructed. After escorting Cranmer to the king, he disappears from the play. Shakespeare took Denny's tiny role from a source, FOXE's *Actes and Monumentes,* and used it to intensify the air of intrigue surrounding the meeting, which begins the major episode of Act 5. The historical Denny was a close friend of the king.

De Quincey, Thomas (1785–1859) English essayist. Best known for his memoir, *Confessions of an English Opium Eater* (1822), De Quincey also wrote many miscellaneous essays in an impressionistic style reflective of the tumultuous Romantic period. These include a remarkable piece that is still widely read, 'On the Knocking on the Gate in *Macbeth*' (1823), interpreting the role of the PORTER (3) in the play. De Quincey also wrote a long article on Shakespeare for the 7th edition of the *Encyclopaedia Brittanica* (1838).

Derby (1), Ferdinando Stanley, Earl of Contemporary of Shakespeare. See STRANGE.

Derby (2), Thomas Stanley, Earl of Character in *Richard III.* See STANLEY (3).

Derby (3), William Stanley, Earl of (1561–1642) English theatrical patron and writer, younger brother and successor of Ferdinando, Lord STRANGE. In 1594 William Stanley succeeded Strange as Earl of Derby, and in January 1595 he married; the wedding may have been the occasion for the first performance of *A Midsummer Night's Dream.* From 1594 to 1618 Derby maintained a troupe of actors known as Derby's Men. This group is not to be confused with his brother's STRANGE'S MEN, who also briefly used that name (see DERBY'S MEN) and with whom Shakespeare may have been associated. The Derby's Men of William Stanley appeared at court in 1599–1601 under the leadership of Robert BROWNE, but they usually toured the provinces. In 1599 it was said that Derby's Men performed comedies written by Stanley; his plays have not survived, but this report has led to Derby's occasional nomination as the 'real' Shakespeare (see AUTHORSHIP CONTROVERSY).

Derby's Men Name used between September 25, 1593, and the spring of 1594 by the theatrical company better known as STRANGE'S MEN or the CHAMBERLAIN'S MEN. Shakespeare may have been a member of the company during this time. The LONDON theatres were closed by a plague epidemic and Strange's Men were on tour when the father of their patron, Lord STRANGE, died; Lord Strange assumed his father's title, Earl of Derby, so the company changed its name accordingly. On the following April 16, the new Earl of Derby also died, and the actors, still on tour as Derby's Men, sought a new patron. When they returned to London, where the theatres had reopened, they found one in Lord HUNSDON (2), the Lord Chamberlain, and they were known thereafter as the Chamberlain's Men. The exact date of the transition is not known, but they performed under the new name on June 5, 1594, at the theatre in NEWINGTON BUTTS. The earliest record of Shakespeare as an actor places him in the Chamberlain's Men in December 1594, but he may have been with the company earlier, when it was still Derby's Men.

Earlier, in the 1560s and 1570s, Lord Strange's father had maintained a company of players, which became known as Derby's Men after 1572, when the

father had become Earl of Derby. This troupe played the provinces exclusively and is not to be confused with the later company, basically a London organisation.

Dering Manuscript Early 17th-century document, the handwritten text of a play combining and abridgeing *1* and *2 Henry IV.* Possibly prepared for a private performance, perhaps at the court of King JAMES I, the Dering manuscript contains various revisions made by Sir Edward Dering (1598–1644), a gentleman from Kent. The manuscript is based on the Q5 edition (1613) of *1 Henry IV* and Q (1600) of *2 Henry IV;* most of the former play is represented, but much of the latter is not. The primary emphasis of Dering's version is the relationship between HENRY IV and PRINCE (6) HAL, especially at the expense of FALSTAFF. For instance, the scenes of *2 Henry IV* set in GLOUCESTERSHIRE are entirely omitted. Dering's alterations seem to incorporate some minor features from the FIRST FOLIO versions of the plays and are thus dated to 1623 or 1624.

Desdemona Character in *Othello,* the wife of OTHELLO. Desdemona is unjustly suspected of adultery and murdered by her jealous husband, who has believed the lies of his villainous aide, IAGO. She is a strong, outspoken woman, unafraid to challenge the racial bias of VENICE or the opinions of her imposing husband, and she is also touching in her sorrow as Othello's love turns to hostility. Desdemona's function, however, is largely symbolic; she represents the spirit of self-sacrifice traditionally associated with the most intense and spiritual love. Indeed, in her martyr-like resignation to an entirely undeserved death, many commentators see her as symbolising Christian love and acceptance of God's will. In Desdemona, Shakespeare created an emblematic figure that was familiar to his original audiences from the medieval MORALITY PLAY, still a well-known theatrical form in the early 17th century. She resembles the angel that opposes the devil in such a play, struggling for control of the central character, who is a symbol of humanity. Like the angel, Desdemona evokes the forgiveness of God, and, as in the medieval play, the good she represents is acknowledged at the close and thus is seen to be the play's central theme.

Desdemona's role is a passive one; her only significant action—marrying Othello—has been taken before the play opens. She is the chief repository of the play's values. Othello knows this when he says, 'I do love thee, and when I love thee not, / Chaos is come again' (3.3.92–93). She alone has recognised his inner worth. She says she 'saw Othello's visage in his mind' (1.3.252), and even when his virtue is obscured she retains her vision. As she puts it, '. . . his unkindness may defeat my life, / But never taint my love' (4.2.162–163), and even as she dies, she declares her love of the inner, obscured Othello, saying, 'Commend me to my kind lord' (5.2.126).

At first, Desdemona's nobility of spirit is matched by that of her new husband. When the couple justify their elopement before the DUKE (5), in 1.3, they display a mature love that is both spiritual, in their mutual appreciation of each other's virtues, and sensual, in their excited anticipation of the physical side of married life. Desdemona's strength of character is evident in her calm resistance to her father, BRABANTIO, who holds that loving a black man is 'Against all rules of nature' (1.3.101). She firmly and courageously stands up to the prejudices of the only society she has ever known. Once committed to Othello she is steadfast; the central fact of the play is her unswerving loyalty. The suspicion that Iago induces in Othello is always seen to be completely unjustified. In 4.3 EMILIA (2) defends adultery, but Desdemona spurns this temptation in an episode that parallels Othello's failure to resist Iago. Desdemona recognises that Othello's jealousy is ignoble, but she continues to give him her love to its fullest extent, saying, '. . . my love doth so approve him, / That even his stubbornness, his checks and frowns, / . . . have grace and favour in them' (4.3.19–21). Her love is literally unconditional, standing in stark contrast to the malevolence of Iago.

Diana (1) Character in *All's Well That Ends Well,* young woman of FLORENCE who assists HELENA (2) to entrap her runaway husband, BERTRAM. The lustful Bertram wishes to seduce Diana, who is respected in FLORENCE for 'a most chaste renown' (4.3.14). She, honourably determined to remain a virgin, resists his advances until in 4.2, as part of Helena's plot, she agrees to sleep with him (though Helena will in fact occupy her bed). She is demure and pliant in making this arrangement, but she expresses herself zestily after Bertram's departure, brusquely critiquing male morals and declaring, '. . . in this disguise, I think't no sin / To cozen him that would unjustly win' (4.2.75–76). In 5.3 she confronts Bertram in the presence of the KING (17) and accuses him of violating his promise to marry her. She is denounced as a whore, and then, when she claims to be a virgin although Bertram has seduced her, she is further subjected to the irritated King's threat of imprisonment before Helena appears and resolves matters. The King thereupon grants her a sumptuous dowry as part of the final reconciliation that closes the play.

Diana has little real personality, being a stereotype of the virginal maiden, but her symbolic importance is considerable. As the object of Bertram's attempts at seduction, she serves by contrast to emphasise his evil nature; as the long-suffering complainant of 5.3, she exemplifies victimisation, making the final outcome more dramatically satisfying.

Diana (2) Pagan goddess and minor character in *Pericles, Prince of Tyre.* After PERICLES has been reunited with his daughter MARINA, Diana appears to him in a vision, in 5.1.238–247. She instructs him to go to her temple at EPHESUS and publicly tell of his continued separation from his wife, THAISA. In 5.3 he does so and is thereby reunited with Thaisa, for she is a priestess at the temple. The play's protagonist thus finds final relief from his suffering through supernatural intervention, and this stresses the play's most important theme: the helplessness of humanity in the face of destiny.

Diana, the ancient goddess of the moon and the hunt, was a familiar theatrical personage in Shakespeare's day. She appears in a number of 16th- and 17th-century dramatic productions, generally clad in a costume decorated in silver with emblems of the moon, and carrying a silver bow (which she mentions here, in 5.1.246). Her appearance in *Pericles,* the first of Shakespeare's ROMANCES, heralds the supernatural atmosphere and dreamlike quality that characterises these late plays.

Dick the Butcher Minor character in *2 Henry VI,* a follower of the revolutionary Jack CADE. After making several small jokes at his leader's expense when the rebels are introduced in 4.2, Dick also delivers the famous line 'The first thing we do, let's kill all the lawyers' (4.2.73). Elsewhere in the depiction of Cade's uprising, Dick further displays the anarchic brutality that Shakespeare attributed to the episode.

Dickens, Charles (1812–1870) English novelist. Dickens lent his prestige as a world-famous novelist to help raise funds to preserve Shakespeare's birthplace in STRATFORD, and he took a prominent part in the project. He also wrote numerous articles on the playwright. Dickens maintained a small theatre in his house where he performed in amateur productions; he was particularly noted for his portrayal of SHALLOW in a production of *The Merry Wives of Windsor* that toured northern England and Scotland to raise money for the birthplace project.

Digges (1), Dudley (1583–1639) English politician, entrepreneur of colonial expeditions, and possible source of inspiration for *The Tempest.* Digges, brother of Leonard DIGGES (2) and stepson of Shakespeare's friend, Thomas RUSSELL, was probably acquainted with Shakespeare. He was closely involved in the exploration of the New World and could have been the playwright's source for the 1610 letter by William STRACHEY (2) describing a shipwreck in Bermuda. Scholars speculate that Digges edited a pamphlet that was another possible source of inspiration for the play, *A True Declaration of the state of the Colonie in Virginia* (1610), which was published by a group of investors defending the colonial enterprise.

Digges was financially and intellectually involved in numerous other foreign expeditions. He was active in the East India and Muscovy companies, as well as the proposed colony in Virginia, and he also promoted geographical exploration with only remote commercial applications. He helped finance Henry Hudson's search for the North-west Passage and wrote tracts asserting the existence of that route to China; he even advocated a purely scientific expedition to the North Pole. In 1618 he travelled to Russia on a combined scientific and diplomatic mission. Politically, he served in parliament intermittently from 1601 to 1628 and in the 1620s was a leader of the opposition to King Charles I that would eventually lead to the Civil Wars. He was twice briefly imprisoned for his opposition, but was reconciled with the king before his death.

Digges (2), Leonard (1588–1635) Poet, translator, and acquaintance of Shakespeare, author of two notable poems commending the playwright. Digges knew Shakespeare through his stepfather, Thomas RUSSELL, and probably wrote the poems about the playwright in 1616 on the occasion of his death. The first was published as part of the preface to the FIRST FOLIO edition of the plays (1623); the other appeared posthumously in the 1640 edition of Shakespeare's *Poems,* published by John BENSON (2). Digges, brother of Dudley DIGGES (1), was a respected poet and a translator of several languages, especially noted for his renderings of Spanish.

Diomedes (1) Legendary figure and character in *Troilus and Cressida,* a Greek warrior and seducer of CRESSIDA. Diomedes plays a very minor role in the TROJAN WAR until he is assigned to oversee the exchange of prisoners whereby Cressida is traded for ANTENOR. When he arrives among the Trojans, he expresses a sharply cynical view of HELEN (1) that makes plain his lack of the romantic idealism that has led TROILUS to deceive himself about love. Thus, when he manipulates Cressida's emotions in 5.2, using an affected disinterest—the tactic with which she herself beguiled Troilus—we recognise him as a cold-blooded seducer. When she agrees to a sexual assignation, he demands from her the love token given her by Troilus, thus climaxing her betrayal. Diomedes is coolly amoral, contributing to our sense of the corruption that infects the play's world.

In the *Iliad* of HOMER, Diomedes is the king of Argos, a Greek state owing allegiance to AGAMEMNON, and he is second only to his overlord in prestige and power. He plays a prominent part in the Trojan War, both as a warrior and strategist, and he is closely associated with Odysseus (the play's ULYSSES). He has no love life in the *Iliad* (his connection to Cressida arose

only with the development of her story in the Middle Ages), though a post-Homeric tradition gave him a wife whose infidelity while he was at Troy causes him to emigrate to Italy after his return; there he founded several cities and chivalrously refused to fight the Trojan refugees who also came there. He was an object of cult worship in Italy, especially on the shores of the Adriatic, where the sea birds were believed to be the souls of his followers.

Diomedes (2) (Diomed) (active 30 B.C.) Historical figure and minor character in *Antony and Cleopatra,* a servant of CLEOPATRA. In 4.14 Diomedes comes to ANTONY with a message which states that his mistress is alive, despite an earlier report that she had committed suicide, but he arrives too late, for Antony has just stabbed himself. Diomedes accompanies the soldiers who carry Antony to Cleopatra and announces their arrival in 4.15. Diomedes appears by name in Shakespeare's source, PLUTARCH's *Lives,* but is otherwise unknown in history.

Dion Character in *The Winter's Tale.* See CLEOMENES AND DION.

Dionyza Character in *Pericles,* would-be murderer of MARINA. In 3.3 PERICLES leaves his daughter Marina in the care of Dionyza and her husband CLEON. However, Dionyza grows jealous of the girl as she overshadows their own daughter, and in 4.1 she forces her servant LEONINE to agree to kill Marina. Though he does not do so, he tells his mistress he has, and in 4.3 Dionyza faces Cleon's horror at her deeds—she has also poisoned Leonine to ensure secrecy. In response to his dread, she says 'I think you'll turn child again' (4.3.4) and compares his qualms to complaining that 'winter kills the flies' (4.3.50). She clearly resembles her forerunner LADY (6) MACBETH but is a much less developed character. In 1.4 we see her as she echoes her husband's distress over a famine, and her transition to evil seems unmotivated. She is merely a stereotype of the wicked stepmother, evil because the plot requires it.

Doctor (1) Character in *King Lear,* a physician who reports to CORDELIA on the condition of her father, King LEAR. In 4.4 he tells Cordelia that Lear's sanity can be restored through rest, saying, 'Our foster-nurse of nature is repose' (4.4.12). He assures her that he can provide drugs to sedate the mad king. Later, he oversees the touching reunion of the rested Lear with his daughter. He ends the meeting for the good of his patient, but again reassures Cordelia that 'the great rage . . . is kill'd in him' (4.7.78–79). His kindly ministrations contrast with the evil that has permeated Lear's world to this point.

Doctor (2) Minor character in *Macbeth,* an English physician serving King Edward the Confessor of England (ruled 1042–1066). In 4.3 the Doctor tells MALCOLM and MACDUFF of King Edward's power to miraculously cure disease by merely touching the victims. This is a reference to a well-known superstition that any English sovereign could cure scrofula, a tuberculosis of the lymph nodes that could leave its victims 'All swoln and ulcerous, pitiful to the eye' (4.3.151), as Malcolm puts it. The positive magic of the saintly king is contrasted with the evil machinations of the WITCHES who support MACBETH. The episode may also have been intended as a compliment to the new King of England, JAMES I; it suggests the sacred status of his office. Some scholars believe that the entire passage, 4.3.139–159—probably written by Shakespeare—may have been interpolated into the original text of the play on the occasion of a performance before the king.

Doctor (3) Minor character in *Macbeth,* a physician who attends LADY (6) MACBETH. The Doctor witnesses Lady Macbeth's hallucinations in the sleep-walking scene (5.1) and understands the allusions to the murders she has on her conscience. He observes, 'Unnatural deeds / Do breed unnatural troubles . . . More needs she the divine than the physician' (5.1.68–71). This emphasises the play's connection of evil with psychological disorders. Further, the Doctor points up the atmosphere of fear and distrust that surrounds the rule of MACBETH when he departs, saying, 'I think, but dare not speak' (5.1.76). In 5.3 at besieged DUNSINANE, the Doctor reports to Macbeth that Lady Macbeth continues to suffer from mental disturbances; he confesses that he cannot cure them and incurs the king's disdain. Again, he has a pertinent exit line: 'Were I from Dunsinane away and clear, / Profit again should hardly draw me here' (5.3.61–62), a salty reminder of Macbeth's evil influence as it was felt by ordinary citizens of SCOTLAND.

Doctor (4) Minor character in *The Two Noble Kinsmen,* a physician who treats the deranged DAUGHTER (2) of the GAOLER (4). The Daughter is obsessed with the nobleman PALAMON, whom she helps escape from gaol but does not see again. In 4.3 the Doctor prescribes that her WOOER humour her by pretending to be Palamon. In 5.2 he adds that the disguised Wooer should sleep with her, to which the young man readily agrees. In 5.4 the Gaoler reports that his Daughter is 'well restored, / And to be married shortly' (5.4.27–28). The comic Doctor was probably created by Shakespeare's collaborator, John FLETCHER (2), to whom scholars usually assign both 4.3 and 5.2.

Doctor (5) of Divinity Character in *Hamlet.* See PRIEST (3).

Dogberry Character in *Much Ado About Nothing*, comical rustic constable in charge of the WATCHMEN (3). Dogberry, his second-in-command VERGES, and the Watchmen are humorously inept, but their apprehension of BORACHIO and CONRADE nonetheless exposes the nefarious plot of Don JOHN (1) against CLAUDIO (1) and HERO. However, Dogberry's officious bumbling postpones this result long enough that Claudio is deceived and Hero humiliated. The tensest moment of the play occurs when Dogberry's tediousness prevents Hero's father, LEONATO, from learning the truth before the wedding, where Hero is to be accused of promiscuity. We are exasperated by the constable's foolishness and infuriated by his preening when he is appointed to interrogate the suspects, but he is nonetheless endearingly amusing.

Although the ridiculous policeman who garbles language was an ancient theatrical character type—Shakespeare had used the figure before in Constable DULL of *Love's Labour's Lost*—Dogberry is one of Shakespeare's most impressive comic creations. A typical Shakespearean CLOWN (1), he affects a more pretentious vocabulary that he can master, misusing the language spectacularly. He is very much a distinctive personality, however. Preposterously long-winded, smugly self-assured, touchingly (though absurdly) incredulous that CONRADE could call him 'an ass' (4.2. 70), Dogberry has a naïve dignity that has charmed audiences and readers for centuries.

In part, this response reflects our gratitude for the relief from melodrama that his comedy produces. Dogberry is an important element in Shakespeare's strategy to lighten Hero's plight and maintain a comic tone throughout the play. His foolish locutions and ideas provide comic relief at several points. In 3.3, just after Don John's scheme has begun to bear fruit, we first encounter Dogberry and the Watchmen; our knowledge that the villain's plot will eventually be exposed makes Hero's humiliation less painful. Dogberry's laughable confusion during the interrogation of Conrade and Borachio takes the edge off the revelation of their evil, and in 5.1 his arrival as a comical *deus ex machina* resolves the plot on a note of hilarity.

In the early texts of the play, a number of Dogberry's speech prefixes in 4.2 refer to 'Kempe' or 'Kemp'; it is accordingly believed that the actor William KEMPE first played the role. Dogberry's odd name refers to the fruit of the wild dogwood, a common English shrub. 'Berry' may also designate fish roe, a common Elizabethan usage. The anomalous reference thus produced—dog roe—seems appropriate to the constable's absurdity.

Dolabella, Cornelius (active 30 B.C.) Historical figure and minor character in *Antony and Cleopatra*, a follower of Octavius CAESAR (2). Dolabella appears as a minor member of Caesar's entourage in 3.12, 4.6, and 5.1; in the third of these scenes we see him sent to ANTONY with a demand for surrender, before it is known that Antony is dead. Attention is brought to this errand later in the scene when Caesar recollects it; thus the focus is drawn to Antony once again. In 5.2, now delegated to guard CLEOPATRA, Dolabella succumbs to her charms and reveals to her that Caesar intends to humiliate her in a triumphal parade in ROME. This furthers her decision to commit suicide.

Little is known of the historical Dolabella beyond the anecdote of his brief encounter with Cleopatra, told in Shakespeare's source, PLUTARCH's *Lives*. Modern scholars believe that Caesar was actually manoeuvring Cleopatra towards suicide. He wanted her out of the way but found the execution of a woman an undignified proceeding for a Roman ruler, so Dolabella may not have been as charitable—or as charmed—as it seems in Plutarch and Shakespeare. Another Roman writer later reported that Dolabella was an intimate of the Emperor Augustus, as Octavius Caesar became known.

Doll Tearsheet Character in *2 Henry IV* and *Henry V*, lover of FALSTAFF. Doll joins Falstaff at his uproarious dinner at the BOAR'S HEAD TAVERN in 2.4. She is clearly a prostitute, but her affection for Falstaff is more than commercial. Although they fight with gusto, Doll's sentimental fondness for the fat knight is evident. She invokes their long-standing friendship in a hard world: 'Come, I'll be friends with thee, Jack, thou art going to the wars, and whether I shall ever see thee again or no there is nobody cares' (2.4.64–66). He feels comfortable enough with her to admit, 'I am old, I am old', and she assures him, 'I love thee better than I love e'er a scurvy young boy of them all' (2.4.268–270). When Falstaff departs to join the troops, Doll is genuinely upset, unable to speak for tears.

In 5.4 Doll and the HOSTESS (2) are arrested for their involvement in a murder, and Doll's capacity for invective and deceit comes to the fore as she berates the BEADLE (2) while claiming a fictitious pregnancy, potentially useful in court. This episode emphasises the criminality of Falstaff's world and indicates a change in the lax moral climate that has existed in LONDON, foreshadowing the crucial scene in which PRINCE (6) HAL rejects Falstaff.

Doll was a name conventionally applied to prostitutes. Moreover, as other allusions in 16th- and 17th-century literature make clear, Doll's last name is also related to her profession, implying vigour in its practice. In *Henry V* PISTOL says that Doll is in hospital with a venereal disease (2.1.74–77), and her death is reported in 5.1.85.

Don (1) John Character in *Much Ado About Nothing*. See JOHN (1).

Don (2) Pedro Character in *Much Ado About Nothing.* See PEDRO.

Donalbain (c. 1033–1099) Historical figure and character in *Macbeth,* the younger son of the murdered King DUNCAN of SCOTLAND. Donalbain plays a very minor part in the play; after he attends his father in three scenes of Act 1, he speaks for the first time in 2.3 after Duncan's murder. He suggests to his brother, MALCOLM, that they flee, lest suspicion fall upon them. He declares that he will go to Ireland while Malcolm goes to England. Malcolm returns to reclaim the kingdom from MACBETH, but Donalbain does not reappear in the play though he is mentioned several times, lastly in 5.2.7–8, where it is observed that he is not with Malcolm's army of invasion. However, in the play's final speech, Malcolm says that he intends 'calling home our exil'd friends abroad' (5.9.32), a remark that may remind us of Donalbain.

The historical Donalbain was a child when Macbeth seized the throne from Duncan in 1039. His name is a corruption of Donald Ban, or Donald the White, which suggests that he was flaxen-haired. For dramatic purposes, Shakespeare altered the story and increased the ages of the brothers, but they did in fact leave Scotland—taken by adults, however—for separate exiles, Donalbain going to the Hebrides Islands off Scotland's north-west coast. He may have spent some time in Ireland, but it is from the Hebrides that he re-entered history years later. Donald became the leader of the conservative Celtic nobility of north-western Scotland who opposed the European orientation that Malcolm, as king, gave the country. When Malcolm died fighting the Norman rulers of England in 1093, Donald invaded Scotland and deposed Malcolm's heir, Duncan II, with the help of one of Duncan's brothers. They ruled jointly for three years. However, another brother reconquered Scotland with the assistance of England—gained by accepting feudal subordination to the English king—and in 1099 Donald was captured, blinded, and imprisoned for the last few months of his life.

Dorcas Character in *The Winter's Tale,* a shepherdess. Dorcas appears only in the shepherds' festival in 4.4. She speaks briefly, chiefly to tease her friend MOPSA about her engagement to the CLOWN (8), and she sings a SONG with Mopsa and AUTOLYCUS. She has no personality to speak of, but she contributes to the festive atmosphere of the occasion. Dorcas' name is from the Bible (see Acts 9:36–39).

Doricles In *The Winter's Tale,* name taken by Prince FLORIZEL of BOHEMIA when he disguises himself to court PERDITA, a seeming shepherdess.

Dorset, Thomas Grey, Marquis of (1451–1501) Historical figure and character in *Richard III,* the son of Queen ELIZABETH (2) by her first marriage. Dorset appears with his mother several times in the early scenes of the play. In 2.2 he offers her the rather cold comfort, on the occasion of the death of King EDWARD IV, that God is simply taking back the gift of royalty that He had given. In 4.1, when the Queen receives word that RICHARD III has seized the crown, Dorset is sent abroad to join RICHMOND. Following the FIRST FOLIO stage directions, many modern editions include Dorset among Richmond's followers at BOSWORTH FIELD in 5.3, although he does not speak. In actuality, the invading Earl had left Dorset in France, as a hostage to ensure the co-operation of his mother's party.

Douglas, Archibald, Earl of (1369–1424) Historical figure and character in *1 Henry IV,* the leader of the Scottish army that joins the rebels against King HENRY IV. Douglas' appearance is preceded by word of his reputation for courage and military prowess. In 3.2 the King speaks of his renown by way of praising HOTSPUR, who has captured him at the battle of HOLMEDON, and FALSTAFF describes him as 'that sprightly Scot of Scots, Douglas, that runs a-horseback up a hill perpendicular . . .' (2.4.339–340). In accordance with WORCESTER's plan, Hotspur frees Douglas and recruits him for the rebellion against Henry. A bold talker ('. . . there is not such a word spoke of in Scotland as this term of fear' [4.1.84–85]) and fighter, Douglas' fiery temperament resembles Hotspur's, and both men urge the rebels into the battle of SHREWSBURY without waiting for reinforcements. During the battle, in 5.3–4, Douglas seeks out Henry, first slaying Sir Walter BLUNT (3). He nearly kills the King, but PRINCE (6) HAL drives him away. He then attacks FALSTAFF, who feigns death. In 5.5 Douglas' capture is reported, but Prince Hal declares that he shall be freed without the payment of ransom, as a tribute to his valour.

Black Douglas, as the historical figure was known, was indeed a famous warrior, although he may have been a bad commander, for he was never on the winning side in a major battle. He was not in fact released at Shrewsbury; he was only freed five years later, after the payment of a very large ransom. Shakespeare followed his source, HOLINSHED, in this error. Douglas later fought against the English for King CHARLES VII of France in the HUNDRED YEARS WAR, and he died in FRANCE (1).

Dover City in south-eastern England, near which much of *King Lear* is set. The invasion of England by an army under CORDELIA and FRANCE (2) draws the play's action to this seaport on the English Channel, famous for the white chalk cliffs overlooking the sea that are vividly described by EDGAR in 4.6.11–24. Some scholars think this description may reflect Shake-

speare's personal response to the natural phenomenon, for he probably visited Dover as an actor; his company—the CHAMBERLAIN'S MEN, later the KING'S MEN—performed there in 1597 and 1605.

Dowden, Edward (1843–1913) Irish literary scholar. Dowden was a long-time professor of English literature at Dublin's Trinity College. He established himself as a significant Shakespearean scholar with his *Shakespeare: A Critical Study of his Mind and Art* (1875), the first book in English (but see GERVINUS) to consider the growth of the playwright through the course of his career. Though regarded by later critics as a sentimental work, too inclined to idealise its subject, Dowden's book influenced all later Shakespearean biography because of its developmental approach. Dowden also published other works on Shakespeare, editions of some of the plays, biographies of other literary figures, and editions of SPENSER and other English poets.

Downton, Thomas (active 1593–1622) English actor, a leading member of the ADMIRAL'S MEN for many years. Downton was probably one of the amalgamated troupe of Admiral's Men and STRANGE'S MEN that toured England in 1593–1594 while the LONDON theatres were closed by the plague. He was a charter member of the reorganised Admiral's Men of 1594, and he was still with the company in 1615 when it was the PALSGRAVE'S MEN, though he had briefly performed for PEMBROKE'S MEN in 1597. He played a variety of roles and was involved in the business affairs of the troupe. In 1618 he married the widow of a wine merchant and took up that profession.

Drawer Any of several minor characters in *2 Henry IV*, servants at the BOAR'S HEAD TAVERN. In 2.4 the Drawers, who 'draw' wine from casks for their customers, prepare for FALSTAFF's dinner party. They enjoy an anecdote in which PRINCE (6) HAL taunts Falstaff about his age, and they plan for entertainment with a musician named SNEAK. Among their number is FRANCIS (1), who also appears in *1 Henry IV*. The Drawers present one of the many glimpses of working-class life in the *Henry IV* plays.

Drayton, Michael (1563–1631) English poet and dramatist. Though best known for his poetry, Drayton also wrote for the stage. In the late 1590s and early 17th century, he wrote about 20 plays for the ADMIRAL'S MEN, all in collaboration with other playwrights, including Anthony MUNDAY and Richard HATHWAY. One of their plays was SIR JOHN OLDCASTLE, later published as Shakespeare's. In 1598 Francis MERES praised Drayton as among England's best writers of tragedies. Drayton helped found the WHITEFRIARS THEATRE in 1608 and joined Martin SLATER in forming a short-lived boy's troupe (see CHILDREN'S COMPANIES) that played there. Drayton was raised as a page in an aristocratic household near STRATFORD and visited there often later in life. He was treated by Shakespeare's son-in-law, Dr John HALL (4), and so may have known the playwright. However, there seems to be no truth in the legend that Shakespeare died after a drinking bout with Drayton and Ben JONSON, for Drayton was well known for his strict sobriety.

Drew, John (1853–1927) American actor. One of the leading actors of his day, John Drew was especially noted for his PETRUCHIO in *The Taming of the Shrew*. For many years he appeared in the productions of Augustin DALY, often opposite Ada REHAN. Through his sister he was the uncle of John BARRYMORE.

Droeshout, Martin (1601–c. 1650) English engraver, creator of the portrait of Shakespeare that illustrates the FIRST FOLIO edition (1623) of the plays. This is one of the two portraits of the playwright considered by scholars to reflect his actual appearance (the other is a sculpture by Gheerart JANSSEN [2]). Droeshout was a poor draftsman, and the portrait is badly flawed—for instance, the head is much too big relative to the torso, and one eye is larger and lower than the other. However, because it was acceptable to Shakespeare's friends, the Folio editors who published it and Ben JONSON who praised it, it is presumed to have provided a reasonable likeness. Scholars believe that Droeshout worked from a drawing or painting and probably never saw the playwright. For all its defects, the Droeshout portrait has been copied many times and is probably the basis for most people's sense of Shakespeare's appearance.

Droeshout was the grandson of a Protestant artist who fled from religious persecution in Brabant (in what is now Belgium) in 1566. His family were members of the same LONDON church as that of Gheerart Janssen, and it is thought that the sculptor may have helped secure the Folio commission for a fellow Netherlander. Droeshout later produced portraits of other notable figures.

Droll Brief playlet, often an adaptation of scenes from full-length plays, performed in 1642–1660, when theatres were closed by the English revolutionary government. Drolls were presented at fairs and in taverns in conjunction with such licensed forms of entertainment as rope dancing. One of the best-known performers of drolls was Robert COX, a collection of whose scripts was published by Henry MARSH and Francis KIRKMAN—after the restoration of the monarchy and the reopening of the theatres—as *The Wits, or Sport upon Sport* (1662). Among the most famous of drolls were 'The Grave-diggers', from *Hamlet*, and

'The Merry conceited Humours of Bottom the Weaver', from *A Midsummer Night's Dream.* The latter was published separately in 1661, when it was described on the title page as having been performed in legitimate, public performances and '. . . lately, privately, presented by several apprentices for their harmless recreation'.

Dromio of Ephesus and Dromio of Syracuse Two characters in *The Comedy of Errors,* twin servants to the twin masters ANTIPHOLUS OF EPHESUS and ANTIPHOLUS OF SYRACUSE. The Dromios were separated from each other in infancy, each with a similarly separated master, in a shipwreck. They share with their masters the confusions and errors that mistaken identities lead to. As comic buffoons, the Dromios receive numerous beatings as their masters' affairs become increasingly disordered, and they respond with quips and quibbles, in a tradition of stock humorous servants and slaves that extends back at least to the Roman drama from which Shakespeare took much of the material for the play. The Dromios also share with their masters the joyful reunion at the end of the play.

Shakespeare may have taken the name Dromio from the play *Mother Bombie* by John LYLY (published 1594), who may, in turn, have based it on the name Dromo, frequently used for slaves in the work of the Roman dramatist Terence.

Dryden, John (1631–1700) English poet, playwright, and literary critic. One of the leading playwrights of the Restoration period (1660–1688), Dryden also wrote extensive assessments of English writers and was an acute appreciator of Shakespeare. However, while admiring 'the divine Shakespeare', he also felt that ELIZABETHAN DRAMA was in general crude, and that Shakespeare shared in its defects. Thus, like many others of his day, he did not hesitate to alter Shakespeare's works. He is notorious for his rewriting of *The Tempest,* in collaboration with William DAVENANT, as *The Tempest, or The Enchanted Island* (1667, published 1670). This adaptation adds whole SUB-PLOTS and retains little of Shakespeare's text. Many of the additions were taken from a Spanish playwright, Pedro Calderón (1600–1681). Although this work was hugely popular, it is deplored by modern commentators. Dryden also adapted *Troilus and Cressida,* which he described in his preface as a 'heap of rubbish', in an equally radical and unfortunate alteration known by its subtitle as *Truth Found Too Late* (1679). His own best play, *All for Love* (1677), was a version of *Antony and Cleopatra;* it has appealed to audiences ever since.

Du Bartas, Guillaume de Sallust (1544–1590) French poet, author of a minor source for *Romeo and Juliet.* A poem by Du Bartas—featured in English translation in the *Ortho-epia Gallica* (1593) of John ELIOT (1)—inspired the debate on bird song between ROMEO and JULIET (1) in 3.5 of *Romeo and Juliet.*

Most of Du Bartas' work was of a more serious nature. Born a nobleman in Gascony, Du Bartas was a friend of the King of Navarre—later Henri IV of France—the leader of the Protestant faction in the civil and religious conflict that tore France apart in the late 16th century. The poet composed monumental poems on religious themes and fought on the battlefield. In 1587 Henri sent Du Bartas on a diplomatic mission to Scotland, where he became a close friend of King James, later JAMES I of England. His works were highly regarded throughout Protestant Europe, were widely translated, and greatly influenced 17th-century religious poetry, including, most notably, John MILTON's *Paradise Lost.*

Duchess (1) of Gloucester, Eleanor Cobham, (d. 1454) Historical figure and character in *2 Henry VI,* the wife of Duke Humphrey of GLOUCESTER (4). The Duchess is ambitious for her husband, the heir apparent to King HENRY VI, but the Duke repudiates her desire that he be king. She therefore proceeds behind his back. In 1.2 she meets with a renegade priest, John HUME, who has hired conjurers for her so that she may see the future in order to plan a coup. Hume, however, is in the pay of Gloucester's enemy, the Duke of SUFFOLK (3), and the Duchess is arrested in 1.4, along with the sorcerers SOUTHWELL and BOLINGBROKE (2) and a witch, MARGERY JOURDAIN. These commoners are sentenced to death in 2.3, but the Duchess' punishment is limited to the humiliation of public exposure in a parade through the streets of London, followed by lifelong banishment to a castle on the Isle of Man, in the Irish Sea. Her unscrupulous attempt to harness the supernatural as an aid to treason marks the first stage in the downfall of 'good Duke Humphrey', the chief business of Acts 1–3.

The historical Eleanor Cobham was a young woman of relatively low standing, compared to the PLANTAGENET (1) lineage of her husband, and her position seemed to some degree scandalous, both to her own contemporaries and to Shakespeare's. The Duke had married her after an earlier marriage, to a Burgundian noblewoman stolen from her husband, had been annulled. The new Duchess dabbled in witchcraft, and she apparently attempted to divine the date of the King's death through the assistance of Hume and the others. However, there seems to be no evidence that she plotted against the King's life. Nor is there evidence that Gloucester's enemies plotted against her; they did not need to, for the Duchess initiated her indiscretions herself. She was tried and convicted of using sorcery, and, as in the play, she was sentenced to public humiliation—a punishment usually reserved

for common prostitutes—and banishment. She died on the Isle of Man some years later, after enforced residence in several other, less remote locations.

Shakespeare's only important departure from the historical record of this incident is chronological. The Duchess' disgrace actually occurred four years prior to the arrival of Queen MARGARET (1) in England, with which the play begins, and while the incident was troublesome for her husband, it did not contribute directly to his own ultimate collapse in fortunes. However, the playwright wished to compress all the Duke's embarrassments into a brief sequence of bad luck, and to associate them with Margaret and Suffolk. In this way, the play emphasises the degree to which selfish ambition undercut the one man whose judgement and honesty, in the light of history as Shakespeare and his contemporaries understood it, might have prevented civil war.

Duchess (2) of Gloucester, Eleanor de Bohun (1367–1399) Historical figure and minor character in *Richard II*, sister-in-law of John of GAUNT and widow of Duke Thomas of GLOUCESTER (6). In 1.2 the Duchess visits Gaunt to discuss her husband's murder. She blames King RICHARD II for his death and passionately entreats Gaunt to avenge it. He insists that vengeance against a king may be taken only by God, and the Duchess wrathfully expresses the hope that BOLINGBROKE (1) will kill MOWBRAY (1), whom she says murdered Gloucester at the king's order. Then she resignedly asserts that she will soon die of grief and departs for her home. Her death is reported in 2.2.97. The episode casts light on the conflicts of 1.1 and 1.3, making clear to the audience that Richard is implicated in Gloucester's murder and that Bolingbroke's accusation of Mowbray is embarrassing to the king.

Although the Duchess appears to be Gaunt's contemporary, she was actually a generation younger, being only 32 when she died, reportedly of grief at the death of her only son. Shakespeare's rendering of her as an older woman helps to heighten the pathos of the vanishing medieval world that colours his story of the king's fall.

Duchess (3) of York, Cicely Neville (1415–1495) Historical figure and character in *Richard III*, the mother of RICHARD III and his brothers, EDWARD IV and CLARENCE (1). The widow of Richard, Duke of YORK (8), a major figure in the *Henry VI* plays, she was also the mother of RUTLAND, who figures briefly in *3 Henry VI*. The Duchess is a symbolic figure, whose role is to lament Richard's evil nature in a stylised manner reminiscent of a Greek CHORUS (1). Shakespeare's sources hardly mention her; it is thought that the playwright was influenced by similar characters in the plays of SENECA. The historical Cicely Neville was a daughter of Ralph, Earl of WESTMORELAND (1), who appears in *1* and *2 Henry IV* and *Henry V*.

Duchess (4) of York, Isabel of Castile (1355–1393) Historical figure and minor character in *Richard II*, mother of the Duke of AUMERLE. When her husband, the Duke of YORK (4), discovers Aumerle's part in a plot against the new king (BOLINGBROKE [1]), he insists on protecting the monarch by revealing the conspiracy, exposing his son to charges of treason. The Duchess' objections go unheeded, and in 5.3, after sending Aumerle ahead, she goes to the king herself and argues against her husband, opposing her motherly anguish to his concern for the state. She receives Bolingbroke's pardon of Aumerle with great gratitude. A powerful dramatic presentation of maternal passion, the episode also serves to stress the magnanimity of Bolingbroke in preparation for his role as King HENRY IV in *1* and *2 Henry IV*.

The incident is entirely fictitious; the real Duchess Isabel had been dead for years before the events depicted in the play took place. The Duke of York had remarried, but the second duchess, besides not being Aumerle's mother, had nothing to do with his being pardoned by King Henry.

Duffett, Thomas (active 1673–1678) English dramatist, author of parodies of two adaptations of Shakespeare. Passages in Duffett's *The Empress of Morocco* (c. 1673) mocked William DAVENANT's extravagant production of *Macbeth*, and his *The Mock-Tempest, or The Enchanted Castle* (1674) was a full-scale comic imitation of Thomas SHADWELL's operatic version of *The Tempest* (1674).

Duffett was a milliner who took up playwrighting with some success. Four of his plays were staged between 1673 and 1676. Three—including the two named above—were burlesques of other works, and the fourth was a MASQUE.

Duke (1) Frederick Character in *As You Like It*, younger brother and deposer of DUKE (7) Senior. Duke Frederick is the villain of the play. A cardboard character with no real personality, he is a conventional bad man, intended simply to anchor one end of the play's scale of values. He not only exiles his brother to the Forest of ARDEN (1), but he also banishes his innocent niece, ROSALIND, thus provoking the flight of his daughter, CELIA. His hostility towards Rosalind is said to be based 'upon no other argument / But that the people praise her for her virtues, / And pity her for her good father's sake' (1.3.268–271). The Duke's reported reformation, after encountering 'an old religious man' (5.4.159) while launching an army against Arden, is entirely unbelievable in human terms. However, it symbolises the play's climactic triumph of harmony and reconciliation.

Duke (2) of Florence Character in *All's Well That Ends Well,* the ruler of FLORENCE. In 3.1 the Duke welcomes the French noblemen who have come to fight for him against Siena, and in 3.3 he appoints BERTRAM to command his cavalry. The Duke is merely an example of a courtly ruler, offering a contrast with the less chivalrous behaviour of Bertram and PAROLLES.

Duke (3) of Milan Minor character in *The Two Gentlemen of Verona,* the father of SILVIA and the ruler of the court where the main action of the play takes place. Informed by PROTEUS that Silvia plans to elope with VALENTINE, the Duke banishes Valentine from the realm. In the final scene, the Duke appears, as ruler and as father of the future bride, to approve the final happy outcome.

Duke (4) of Venice Minor character in *The Merchant of Venice,* the ruler of VENICE. The Duke presides over the trial of SHYLOCK's suit against ANTONIO (2). He is helpless to influence matters, being bound by the laws of the state, a position in which Shakespeare often places his rulers (see, e.g., the DUKE [8] of EPHESUS). In this way the Duke emphasises a principle to which the playwright was strongly committed: the importance of the law in a well-ordered society. Although the Duke is prepared to see Antonio die, as the full rigour of the law dictates, he is merciful to SHYLOCK after the case is resolved in Antonio's favour, thus highlighting another virtue Shakespeare saw in an ideal ruler.

Duke (5) of Venice Character in *Othello,* the ruler of VENICE. In 1.3 the Duke meets with his advisers (see SENATOR [1]) to decide on a response to the Turkish assault on CYPRUS. Summoning OTHELLO, their chief general, they are faced with BRABANTIO's accusation that Othello has used witchcraft to marry his daughter, DESDEMONA. When Desdemona confirms that theirs is a love match, Brabantio is bitter, but the Duke offers wise proverbs on emotional moderation, such as, 'To mourn a mischief that is past and gone, / Is the next way to draw more mischief on' (1.3.204–205). He represents a social wisdom that is markedly lacking in the main plot.

Duke (6) Orsino of Illyria Character in *Twelfth Night.* See ORSINO.

Duke (7) Senior Character in *As You Like It,* ruler deposed by his brother, DUKE (1) Frederick, and exiled to the Forest of ARDEN (1). The father of ROSALIND, Duke Senior is a symbol of authority and wisdom with little distinctive personality. Before we meet him, we are told that he and his followers in exile 'fleet the time carelessly as they did in the golden world' (1.1.118–119), a reference to the rustic life idealised in PASTORAL literature. In his first speech the Duke introduces the audience to Arden and firmly establishes the contrast between the woodland world and the realities of politics and power: 'Hath not old custom made this life more sweet / Than that of painted pomp? Are not these woods / More free from peril than the envious court?' (2.1.2–4). The Duke makes the best of his exile, finding 'tongues in trees, books in the running brooks, / Sermons in stones, and good in everything' (2.1.16–17). Such remarks, like the songs of AMIENS, express the ideal of an escape from the pressures of the real world.

However, the Duke is aware that Arden is no paradise. He acknowledges that he has 'seen better days' (2.7.120), and he shares some attitudes with the alienated and melancholy courtier JAQUES (1). In 2.1.22–25 he regrets having to kill deer for food shortly before an elaboration on the thought is attributed to Jaques. In 2.7.137–139 he suggests to Jaques his famous comparison of human life to the action in a drama ('All the world's a stage, / And all the men and women merely players' [2.7.139–140]). Nevertheless, the Duke also opposes this point of view: in 2.7.64–69, he chastises Jaques for wishing to satirise the world when he is himself hardly free from sin, and, in doing so, he sets a limit on the play's tolerance for Jaques' criticisms. Most important, when Duke Frederick's religious conversion and abdication are reported in 5.4, Duke Senior is immediately ready to resume his dukedom, and, as Jaques remarks, his 'patience and . . . virtue well deserve it' (5.4.186). The Duke's fondness for the pastoral life is less powerful than his sense of social responsibility, mirroring Shakespeare's own view that a ruler's duty to his position is paramount.

Duke (8) Solinus of Ephesus Character in *The Comedy of Errors,* the ruler of the city of Ephesus, where the play takes place. The Duke first appears in 1.1 to condemn EGEON, a wandering merchant from Syracuse who has arrived in Ephesus, unaware of the hostilities between that city and his own, and is sentenced to either death or an immense fine, which he cannot pay. Egeon tells of his separated family and his search for them, and the Duke expresses pity for the old man but says he cannot exempt him from the law.

The sources and use of power are subjects that were important to the playwright, and they are dealt with in a number of the plays. In this early work, the Duke, regrets that he cannot act on his pity, but explains that the law explicitly limits his range of action, while at the same time it is the implicit source of his authority. His crown and his dignity are equated with his oath, a matter of law. However, the Duke will bend as far as he feels he legally can, out of pity for the aged wanderer, and he gives Egeon a day in which to find some

way to raise his ransom money. This day becomes the time in which the play proper takes place.

Neither the Duke nor Egeon reappears until the final scene, when the confusions and mistaken identities that are the chief material of the play have reached a climax. When he re-enters, at 5.1.131, he is still sympathetic to Egeon's plight, although the unfortunate victim is escorted by the EXECUTIONER and seems fated soon to die. The Duke is immediately swept up in the misunderstandings of the central plot, being requested to rule against the Abbess, EMILIA (1), who has granted sanctuary in her PRIORY to ANTIPHOLUS OF SYRACUSE.

When ANTIPHOLUS OF EPHESUS appears, the true complexity of the situation becomes apparent. The Duke, the representative of secular law, is clearly baffled, so he sends for Emilia, who enters with the second Antipholus, bringing the twins together for the first time. Further, Emilia recognises Egeon as her long-lost husband, and the resolution of the play's complexities begins. The intervention of Christian grace and mercy, represented by Emilia and the Priory, has tempered the insensitive cruelties of secular justice. However, the Duke is quite evidently pleased with the outcome, in keeping with his consistently sympathetic attitude. When Emilia proposes a 'gossip feast' or celebratory party, the Duke accepts with enthusiasm and leads the company off-stage to close the play.

Shakespeare may have taken the name Solinus (which appears only in 1.1.1) from that of an ancient geographer, Gaius Julius Solinus, who described (c. 200 A.D.) the seaports of the Mediterranean. His work was published in an English translation in 1587, a few years before *The Comedy of Errors* was probably written.

Duke (9) Vincentio of Vienna Character in *Measure for Measure,* the ruler of VIENNA. The Duke, who appoints the stern ANGELO (2) as his deputy and then spies on his performance, personifies a major theme of the play: the relationship of government to Christian doctrines of forgiveness and mercy. The Duke's government has been lax, as he admits to the FRIAR (1) in 1.3, but in designating Angelo to restore a strict public morality he errs to the opposite extreme. His deputy is incapable of applying the law flexibly, and the result is a harsh injustice, the death sentence for the honourable CLAUDIO (3). However, the Duke is intent on personal improvement—ESCALUS (2) says of him that he 'above all other strifes, contended especially to know himself' (3.2.226–227)—and his effort teaches him to acknowledge the need for mercy to counteract human weakness.

Significantly, the Duke's disguise as he investigates Angelo's governance is that of a friar; in adopting a religious role he manifests the God-given authority that Shakespeare and his original audiences ascribed to all rulers. Angelo's lust for ISABELLA, Claudio's intercessor, produces a seemingly unresolvable conflict. However, the Duke, in his friar's guise, takes over the play and effects two improbable schemes: the substitution of another head for that of the supposedly executed Claudio, and of another woman, MARIANA (2), for Isabella. Having thus negated Angelo's evil intent, the Duke re-emerges, in 5.1, to bring the play to a close in a flurry of pardons and marriages.

Many commentators have found this dénouement lacking in credibility, but Shakespeare's purpose was symbolic, and realism should not be expected. The Duke controls the outcome and thus fulfils the ruler's proper role in the play's scheme of things. He offers the mercy of God to the deserving and undeserving alike. It is he who recognises in BARNARDINE, the vicious murderer, a mere 'creature unprepar'd' (4.3.66), and he forgives LUCIO his slanders, despite the insult to both his personal pride and his authority. Most important, he proves susceptible to the pleas of Mariana and Isabella for mercy towards the villainous Angelo. Finally, though he has earlier claimed immunity from 'the dribbling dart of love' (1.3.2), he proposes marriage to Isabella. In striking contrast to the negative attitudes of both Angelo and Isabella, early in the play, the Duke underscores Shakespeare's belief in the happy marriages that traditionally close a COMEDY.

Duke Humphrey Possible lost play by Shakespeare. In 1660 the publisher Humphrey MOSELEY claimed the copyrights to a number of old plays, including *Duke Humphrey.* The 18th-century antiquarian John WARBURTON reported owning a copy as well, but otherwise the play is unknown, unless the title refers to *2 Henry VI,* which was originally published as 'The First part of the Contention betwixt the two famous Houses of Yorke and Lancaster, with the death of the good Duke Humphrey' (a reference to the Duke of GLOUCESTER [4]; see CONTENTION). However, since both Moseley and Warburton were mistaken in claiming other plays as Shakespeare's, scholars generally do not believe that *Duke Humphrey* was written by him.

Duke of York's Men See PRINCE CHARLES' MEN.

Dull, Anthony Minor character in *Love's Labour's Lost,* the slow-witted rustic constable. Dull is a character type whose name summarises his nature. Dull acts as a foil to the comical pedants ARMADO, HOLOFERNES, and NATHANIEL (1), offsetting their elaborate contortions of language by being himself. At one point, Holofernes observes, '*Via,* goodman Dull! Thou hast spoken no word all this while'. Dull replies, 'Nor understand none neither, sir' (5.1.141).

Dumaine (Dumain) Character in *Love's Labour's Lost,* one of the gentlemen who fall in love and thus dis-

rupt the ascetic academic programme of the KING (19) of Navarre. Although committed to the King's idea at the outset of the play, Dumaine falls in love with KATHARINE (1), a lady-in-waiting of the PRINCESS (1) of France. Along with the King and the other courtiers, he breaks his vows and abandons scholarship for love.

The Duc de Mayenne, well known in Shakespeare's London for his role in the French Wars of Religion, is usually thought to have provided the name Dumaine. Unlike the originals of LONGAVILLE and BEROWNE, he was not an aide to the historical King of Navarre; rather, he was a principal enemy of the insurgent monarch, but this inconsistency would probably not have bothered either the playwright or his audience. An alternative, the less notable General D'Aumont, who was an aide to the King of Navarre at the time, has been proposed.

Dumb Show Scene performed in pantomime, especially as part of an Elizabethan TRAGEDY. Shakespeare employed dumb shows in several scenes of *Pericles,* a single scene in *Cymbeline,* and in *Hamlet.* A dumb show could function as a PROLOGUE (1) or CHORUS (1); it sometimes illustrated an off-stage event, presented plot elements that were not fully acted out, or enacted what was shortly to come in the main action, intimating a symbolic meaning.

In *Pericles* three dumb shows are employed in the choric narrations of GOWER (3). At 2.Chorus.16 a dumb show enacts the reception of a letter by PERICLES, followed by his hasty departure; Gower reveals that the message has warned the hero of danger and he has fled. At 3.Chorus.14 a more elaborate enactment depicts Pericles receiving another letter, read also by his new father-in-law, SIMONIDIES. The attending courtiers kneel to Pericles. He then departs with his new wife, who is pregnant. Gower explains that the letter has summoned Pericles to TYRE, where he is ruler, thus revealing his royalty and sparking another journey. Lastly, in 4.4 a dumb show presents Pericles weeping at the tomb of his supposedly dead daughter, MARINA, though the audience knows that Marina is actually alive. Thus, in *Pericles,* the dumb show is a simple device that compresses the plot by providing brief summaries of what would otherwise require complete scenes.

In *Cymbeline* a brief dumb show occurs at the close of 5.3. In it POSTHUMUS, disguised as a Roman soldier, is brought as a prisoner to CYMBELINE, who turns him over to a GAOLER (2). This may not be a dumb show proper, but rather a survival in the printed play of notes for a scene that was never actually written (see CYMBELINE, 'Text of the Play').

The PLAYERS (2) in *Hamlet* stage a dumb show before their performance of THE MURDER OF GONZAGO, the playlet that HAMLET hopes will inspire an unconscious revelation of guilt in his uncle, the KING (5), who has murdered his father. The dumb show is described in an elaborate stage direction at 3.2.133. After being affectionately embraced by his queen, a king sleeps and a man puts a poison in his ear. The queen returns and mourns the dead king, but she responds to the attentions of the poisoner, who takes her away with him as the king's body is removed. This enactment resembles the real king's crime—as Hamlet has been informed by the GHOST (3)—but the king does not respond until the spoken dialogue of the playlet later in the scene.

This delay presents one of the many small problems that have puzzled commentators on *Hamlet* for generations: have two different renderings of the playlet been accidentally preserved, when only one was intended for performance? Are we supposed to believe that the king was not paying attention or that he did not recognise his crime in the dumb show, only in the more elaborate rendering that followed? Or was he able to stand the sight of his guilty action once but not twice (the so-called 'second tooth' theory)? In Shakespeare's text the king remains inscrutable during the dumb show, perhaps to heighten the buildup of tension, but many productions present him as engaged in conversation with the QUEEN (9) thus not seeing the dumb show, or as silently but visibly aghast, recovering himself only to collapse later.

The 'second tooth' theory has been most widely accepted by scholars, but whatever theory is correct, the King's inscrutability works well on stage and the dumb show serves a definite theatrical purpose: A formal device that is not itself a part of the plot, it outlines the coming playlet, permitting the audience to concern itself with the responses of Hamlet and the King. Moreover, the playlet is never completed after the King's guilty reaction disrupts it, so its closure with the queen's acceptance of the murderer—analogous to the behaviour of Hamlet's mother, the real Queen—is known only through the dumb show.

It is likely that the dumb show originated in RENAISSANCE Italy. Probably always accompanied by music, it was intended as an elaborate and diverting spectacle, and Shakespeare assumed his audience would recognise it as having this function for the Danish court in *Hamlet,* just as it presumably did for the actual viewers of *Pericles.*

Duncan, King of Scotland (c. 1001–1039) Historical figure and character in *Macbeth,* ruler of SCOTLAND who MACBETH murders for his throne. Shakespeare's Duncan is an elderly man, a respected and noble figure; as Macbeth reflects, he 'Hath borne his faculties so meek, hath been / So clear in his great office, that his virtues / Will plead like angels, trumpet-tongu'd' (1.7.17–19). Duncan's generous and trusting nature contrasts strikingly with the evil which surrounds

Macbeth. Though he appears only in Act 1, he is an important symbol of the values that are to be defeated and restored in the course of the play. His generosity and fatherly affection for Macbeth make his murder even more appalling. The unconscious irony is sharp when he greets Macbeth, who is already plotting against him, with a declaration of his *own* ingratitude, in 1.4.14–16. Duncan's faith, misplaced first in the rebellious CAWDOR and then in MACBETH, provides the audience with an introduction to the atmosphere of betrayal that exists throughout the world of the play.

The historical Duncan was a much younger man than Shakespeare's character, only a few years older than Macbeth. The playwright altered Duncan's age to stress the evil of Macbeth's crime, but in fact Macbeth did not murder Duncan; he usurped the crown through a civil war, and Duncan died in battle. The two were first cousins, both grandsons of Duncan's predecessor on the throne of Scotland, King Malcolm II (ruled 1005–1034). Duncan's claim to the throne was somewhat stronger than Macbeth's as it appears that Malcolm II had named Duncan as his heir, although the facts are obscure. However, Macbeth's action was an ordinary political manoeuvre in 11th-century Scotland; King Malcolm II took the throne previously by murdering his cousin, Kenneth III (997–1005). Shakespeare devised his version of Duncan's death from an account of an earlier royal assassination, that of Malcolm II's uncle, King Duff (d. 967), in his source, Raphael HOLINSHED's history.

Dunsinane (Dunsinnan) Castle near Perth in central Scotland, the setting for Act 5 of *Macbeth.* 'Great Dunsinane' (5.2.12), whose 'strength / Will laugh a siege to scorn' (5.5.2–3), is clearly an imposing structure—one appropriate to the grim events of the play's climax. Macbeth resists the army of Prince MALCOLM, Lord MACDUFF, and the English lord, SIWARD, within its walls. A few miles away lies Birnam Wood, the royal forest featured in the WITCHES' prediction Macbeth believes ensures his safety: '. . . until / Great Birnam wood to high Dunsinane hill / Shall come against him' (4.1.92–94). When the camouflage devised by Malcolm seems to bring the wood to the castle, in 5.5, Macbeth's fate becomes apparent. The castle proves to be no hindrance to the invaders, being 'gently render'd' (5.7.24) by all its inhabitants but the doomed king.

Historically, Dunsinane was not the site of Macbeth's final defeat, though Siward did win a battle there in 1054. Malcolm was only finally victorious—and Macbeth slain—at a battle elsewhere in Scotland, three years later. Shakespeare took the error from his source, HOLINSHED's *Chronicles,* and doubtless believed it to be correct.

D'Urfey, Thomas (1653–1723) English dramatist, author of an adaptation of *Cymbeline.* D'Urfey's *The Injured Princess or the Fatal Wager* was staged and published in 1682 (though its EPILOGUE notes that it had been written nine years earlier). Shakespeare's language—including most of the names—was much altered by D'Urfey, but the plot remained fairly close to the original. It differs only in the addition of an elaborate sub-plot in which Cloten kidnaps a daughter of Pisanio, and the fact that Pisanio mistrusts Imogen as much as Posthumus does. *The Injured Princess* was quite popular and was revived periodically for almost 60 years.

Tom D'Urfey wrote plays and song lyrics; the latter were set to music by his composer friends, among them Henry PURCELL. His songs were published in six volumes entitled *Wit and Mirth, or Pills to Purge Melancholy* (1720). He also wrote 29 plays, many of which were very popular.

Dutchman and Spaniard Minor characters in *Cymbeline,* non-speaking witnesses of the wager between POSTHUMUS and IACHIMO. Neither the Dutchman nor his companion the Spaniard does anything at all; they are only mentioned in the stage directions at 1.3.1. Shakespeare found both figures in one of his sources, *Frederyke of Jennen,* but scholars differ on their function in the play. Each may be a GHOST CHARACTER, considered by the playwright but then abandoned and therefore not actually employed in early productions. Alternatively, lines they spoke, probably brief explanatory ones, may have been lost. Finally, Shakespeare may have intended them as comic caricatures of their nationalities—a popular dramatic feature in his day—and perhaps he intended them to be in a drunken stupor, also popular in comedy.

Dutton, Laurence (active 1571–1591) English actor. Dutton was a member of at least five different acting companies, including OXFORD'S MEN and the QUEEN'S MEN (1); his brother John worked with him in three of them. Their reputation for fickleness prompted an anonymous satirist of 1580 to refer to them as the 'chameleon' Duttons.

E

Eastcheap Neighbourhood in LONDON, location of the BOAR'S HEAD TAVERN and setting for several scenes in *1* and *2 Henry IV* and *Henry V.* Eastcheap, an ancient and impoverished commercial district—'cheap' comes from an Anglo-Saxon word for 'bargain'—was noted for its butcher shops and meat markets. It was also known as a dangerous and disreputable area and was thus an appropriate locale for FALSTAFF's world of petty crime and dissipation, which PRINCE (6) HAL samples and rejects. The neighbourhood is specified as the scene of the Prince's delinquencies in Shakespeare's source, the FAMOUS VICTORIES.

Ecclestone, William (active 1610–1623) English actor, a member of the KING'S MEN. Ecclestone is one of the 26 men listed in the FIRST FOLIO as the 'Principall Actors' in Shakespeare's plays. He was with the King's Men from 1610 until at least 1623, except for two years (1611–1613) when he was with the newly formed LADY ELIZABETH'S MEN. He may have played a LORD (6) in *All's Well That Ends Well,* designated as 'E' in the Folio text of the play. He performed in many of the plays of Francis BEAUMONT (2) and John FLETCHER (2), and is thought to have specialised in playing spirited young men given to sword fights.

Eden, Richard (c. 1521–1576) English translator of a probable minor source for *The Tempest.* Eden's *History of Travaille* (1577) provided Shakespeare with several details for his play, including the name of CALIBAN's god, Setebos. The book, which was published posthumously, was composed of two translations; Shakespeare's material came from an account of the first circumnavigation of the globe, led by Ferdinand Magellan (c. 1480–1521).

As a young man, Eden was secretary to the statesman Lord BURGHLEY. He then travelled for several years before taking up a career as a scientific translator from Latin, Italian, and Spanish. He helped advance the capabilities of English seamanship with his *Arte of Navigation* (1561), from the pioneering manual by the Spaniard Martin Cortes (active 1551), and his subsequent translations of various writings on navigation and exploration increased English awareness of the New World. Eden's other books, like the *History of Travaille,* focussed on the exploration of the New World, and he is regarded as the most important predecessor of Richard HAKLUYT.

Edgar Character in *King Lear,* the banished son of the Earl of GLOUCESTER (1). Misled by his illegitimate son EDMUND, Gloucester formally exiles Edgar to the wilderness; this action parallels King LEAR's rejection of his daughter CORDELIA. In 2.3 under threat of execution, Edgar disguises himself as a wandering lunatic. When Lear is banished by his villainous daughters the disguised Edgar accompanies him, in 3.4 and 3.6. When Gloucester is blinded and expelled because he has remained loyal to Lear, Edgar, still disguised, becomes his father's guide, in 4.1, and saves him from suicide and a murder attempt by OSWALD, in 4.6. In Act 5 Edgar finally takes control of the play, exposing Edmund and GONERIL's plot to murder the Duke of ALBANY and defeating Edmund in a trial by combat. At the play's close Edgar is invited by Albany to share in the rule of Britain; with his final lines, he offers a possible lesson to be drawn from the play—that we must be aware of our human susceptibility to folly, as Lear was not—saying, 'The weight of this sad time we must obey' (5.3.322). (In some editions these lines are given to Albany.)

As the insane Tom O'Bedlam, Edgar embodies the play's theme of disease and misery as products and emblems of human folly. Tom blames his insanity on his sexual promiscuity, thus illustrating the morbid attitude towards sex that permeates the world of the play. Similarly, when he is again himself, Edgar attributes Gloucester's tragedy to 'The dark and vicious place' (5.3.171) where Edmund was conceived, that is, to sex outside of marriage.

On the other hand, Edgar's loving loyalty to his father parallels Cordelia's to Lear. Both present a Christlike willingness to sacrifice themselves that is often cited as a lesson in accepting the will of God. Even from a non-religious viewpoint, Edgar is an agent of redemption, preserving order and goodness where chaos and evil have threatened by acting as a guide and saviour first for Lear, then for his father, and finally for Britain as a whole. When he saves his father from suicide, in 4.6, he offers a way to renew

acceptance of life. Deceiving Gloucester into believing he has jumped from a cliff and lived, Edgar declares his father's survival to be 'a miracle' (4.6.55); the blind man concludes that he should not give in to despair, but endure. Thus, Edgar illuminates a basic principle that is at the core of the tragedy: we must struggle to make the best of our lives, accepting death only when its time comes. As he says to his father, 'Men must endure / Their going hence, even as their coming hither: / Ripeness is all' (5.2.9–11).

Edmund Character in *King Lear,* the unscrupulous and ambitious illegitimate son of the Earl of GLOUCESTER (1). Edmund conspires against his legitimate brother EDGAR, who is banished into the wilderness in 2.1; he betrays his father to King LEAR's evil daughter REGAN and her husband, the Duke of CORNWALL, who put out the old man's eyes, in 3.7; and he pursues a love affair with Lear's other daughter GONERIL, with whom, in 4.2, he plots to murder her husband, the Duke of ALBANY. When Cornwall is killed the widowed Regan schemes to take Edmund from Goneril, and this unsavoury love triangle is an important part of the play's atmosphere of moral collapse.

In Act 5 Edmund leads Cornwall's army against the supporters of Lear's faithful daughter CORDELIA; victorious, he thwarts Albany's plans for mercy and imprisons Lear and Cordelia, ordering their execution. Edgar learns of the plot against Albany, charges Edmund with treason and challenges him to a trial by combat, wounding him fatally. The dying Edmund confesses his intention towards Lear, but it is too late to prevent Cordelia's death, and Lear dies of a broken heart soon thereafter.

Edmund's villainy is a central element in *King Lear;* his schemes are crisply executed and do much to provide a dramatic structure in the SUB-PLOT that the more idea-oriented main story lacks. However, Edmund is a stereotypical villain with little human complexity—his deeds are more interesting than he is himself—and his schemes are effective due to the moral weakness of others, not his compelling personality. His declaration of repentance—'some good I mean to do / Despite of mine own nature' (5.3.242–243)—is perfunctory and unconvincing. It serves to spark the final episode—Lear's fatal grief—after which Edmund is carried away to die. Albany's brusque dismissal of the news of his death demonstrates the extent of the villain's defeat; compared to the lessons to be absorbed from Lear's end, Edmund's demise is 'but a trifle here' (5.3.294).

Shakespeare identified Edmund's unscrupulous ambition with a troubling social phenomenon of his own day, the rise of the new commercially active classes—the bourgeoisie of the cities and the lesser landowners, or gentry, of the countryside. The success of these groups depended on their willingness to engage in trade and banking, as opposed to the traditional dependence on the land, and in this they were at odds with the great territorial nobles of the old aristocracy. A worldly emphasis on practical finance characterised the commercial classes, and this was regarded as unscrupulous by hostile eyes. From this point of view, Edmund represents the new man in his lack of chivalric scruples and his concern for his own advancement.

Traditionalists conventionally associated such an attitude with a new, 'modern' strain of thought, and Edmund quite plainly identifies himself with this new mode. In his first soliloquy he declares, 'Thou, Nature, art my goddess' (1.2.1), boldly stating his independence of 'the plague of custom' (1.2.3) and its man-made moral standards. Such sophisticated agnosticism arose in part from the RENAISSANCE rediscovery of classical paganism, and it was reflected in such works as the *Essays* of MONTAIGNE, which Shakespeare had read and which he admired in some respects. However, in placing these sentiments in the mouth of a self-proclaimed villain, Shakespeare declares his alliance with the old world of the aristocracy that is quite clearly represented by Lear, Gloucester, and Edgar, Edmund's enemies.

Edward III An anonymous play perhaps written in part by Shakespeare but generally regarded as part of the Shakespeare APOCRYPHA. Published in 1596 by Cuthbert BURBY, *The Raigne of King Edward the third* was first ascribed to Shakespeare in 1656 by the generally unreliable William LEY. Although the 18th-century scholar Edward CAPELL supported the attribution, modern scholars are sceptical and believe that at most only parts of the play could have been written by Shakespeare. At least two writers seem to have composed the work; the principal evidence suggesting that one of them was Shakespeare is a single line—'Lilies that fester smell far worse than weeds'—that also appears in one of the SONNETS (number 94). However, Shakespeare could have remembered the image from the anonymous play, or the unknown playwright may have known the sonnet in manuscript form.

Edward IV, King of England (1442–1483) Historical figure and character in *2* and *3 Henry VI* and *Richard III.* Known simply as Edward until Act 3 in *3 Henry VI,* King Edward IV receives his crown as a result of the machinations of his ambitious father, the Duke of YORK (1), and his heirs are murdered later by his brother, who succeeds him as RICHARD III.

In *2 Henry VI* Edward appears in 5.1 to support his father in his claim to the throne. Edward has only one line, which Richard immediately tops. In *3 Henry VI,* although Edward comes into his own, he continues to be overshadowed by his brother. He becomes King, but the leadership of the Yorkist cause is clearly provided by WARWICK (3), prior to that lord's defection,

and by Richard. Edward displays the unscrupulous ambition that characterises the aristocrats in all the *Henry VI* plays. He baldly displays his own dishonesty, claiming that '. . . for a kingdom any oath may be broken: / I would break a thousand oaths to reign one year' (1.2.16–17). However, Edward is outclassed in criminality by his brother Richard.

Edward demonstrates a selfish disregard for the responsibilities of kingship, and his behaviour necessitates a renewal of the WARS OF THE ROSES. He ignores the benefits of an alliance with FRANCE (1) and abandons a marriage to Lady BONA in order to satisfy his lust for ELIZABETH (2). In the resulting war, he indulges in pointless bravado and permits himself to be captured in 4.3. After the final Yorkist victory, Edward casually allows Richard to murder the finally displaced King Henry, demonstrating a lack of concern for civil order that typifies England's corrupt public life. In *Richard III* Edward appears only in 2.1, on his deathbed. He learns of the death of CLARENCE (1), and his dismay, it is implied, leads to his own rapid demise. His death is reported in 2.2.

Shakespeare's treatment of the reign of Edward IV is extremely unhistorical, for the playwright wished to emphasise the disruption of English public life that the coming of the TUDOR dynasty repaired. Edward's 22-year tenure is presented as a rapid succession of quarrels and battles. In fact, though, Edward was a very competent ruler. He was judiciously merciful to most of the Lancastrians; he introduced badly needed financial reforms; he withdrew from France—at the cost of considerable personal popularity, but to the immense benefit of the country. His marriage to Elizabeth was not the chief, or even an important, cause of Warwick's rebellion. Although his lusty appetites, given much emphasis in the play, were well known to his contemporaries, they do not seem to have interfered with his public duty, although it has been suggested that over-indulgence in wine and women may have resulted in his early death.

Edwards (Edwardes), Richard (c. 1523–1566) English poet, musician and playwright, author of a minor source for *The Two Gentlemen of Verona* and of a song quoted in *Romeo and Juliet.* Edwards was choral director of the Children of the Chapel (see CHILDREN'S COMPANIES). Under his direction the choirboys performed two of his plays, *Damon and Pythias* (1565) and *Palamon and Arcite* (1566) two of the earliest musical dramas. The former, published in 1571, was a tale of male friendship, an ancient genre, and it provided minor details for Shakespeare's similar effort, *The Two Gentlemen. Palamon and Arcite,* like *The Two Noble Kinsmen,* was based on CHAUCER'S *The Knight's Tale,* but it is not believed to have influenced Shakespeare and his collaborator, John FLETCHER (2). In *Romeo and Juliet,* PETER (2) sings a few lines of a well-known song, 'In Commendation of Musique', written by Edwards and published in his posthumous *The Paradise of Dainty Devises* (1575), an anthology of his and others' works.

Egeon (Aegeon) Character in *The Comedy of Errors,* the condemned man who proves to be the father of the long-separated twins ANTIPHOLUS OF EPHESUS and ANTIPHOLUS OF SYRACUSE. Egeon's tale is presented only in the first and last scenes of the play, framing the principal plot. A wandering merchant from Syracuse, in Sicily, Egeon comes to EPHESUS, on the Aegean coast of Asia Minor, not knowing that hostility has arisen between that city and his home. The penalty of death or a large ransom has been imposed by each city upon any citizen of the other who enters it. Egeon has thus been sentenced to pay a thousand marks of ransom or die.

In 1.1 his situation is revealed in his conversation with Solinus, the DUKE (8) of Ephesus. Egeon elaborates on the tragedy that has enveloped his life, beginning when he was separated from his wife and one of his infant twin sons in a shipwreck 23 years before, never to see them again. The other son, at the age of 18, had insisted on setting out to search for his lost brother. Egeon himself has unsuccessfully spent the last five years looking for news of either twin. The Duke, sympathetic though stern, offers Egeon the freedom of the city for the coming day so that he can beg or borrow the money to pay his ransom. These hours become the time of the action of the play.

Egeon does not reappear until well into the final scene of the play, but the audience cannot forget his desperate plight. Although the comic misadventures and errors that follow are chiefly farcical, they are coloured by our sombre recollection of Egeon's imminent fate.

In the final scene, Egeon is escorted on stage by the Duke, accompanied by the EXECUTIONER and seemingly doomed to die. The Duke reminds us of his plight (5.1.130–132) before being sidetracked into attempting to unravel the confusions of the main plot. Amidst these complexities, Egeon, upon seeing Antipholus of Ephesus, believes him to be the other Antipholus, the son who left Syracuse five years earlier. He identifies himself to this Antipholus, only to be rejected, of course, for Antipholus of Ephesus does not know him. Egeon's stricken response is rendered in a moving passage (5.1.298–322); the Duke concludes that Egeon's 'age and dangers' have driven him mad.

As the confusion and errors are eventually resolved and the play reaches its conclusion, Egeon is a spectator, for the most part; the principals in this dénouement are the two sets of twins and EMILIA (1), Egeon's long-lost wife, whose recognition of her husband begins the resolution. Although he has good lines in both 1.1 and 5.1 and is an important figure, Egeon is not so much a fully developed character as he is a

vehicle for a simple, secondary plot, an evocation of pathos intended to temper our view of the central wrangle of error and delusion.

Egeus Character in *A Midsummer Night's Dream,* the father of HERMIA. Egeus' angry demand for severe punishment of his daughter for refusing to marry DEMETRIUS (2) interrupts the blissful anticipation of marriage with which the play opens. Duke THESEUS hopes to persuade Egeus to abandon his intentions, but we see in 4.1, when Egeus and the Duke discover the sleeping lovers in the enchanted woods, that his attempts have not succeeded. Egeus insists that LYSANDER be executed for having tried to elope with Hermia. His harshness makes him no more sympathetic to the Duke than to the audience, and Theseus takes evident pleasure in announcing, 'Egeus, I will overbear your will' (4.1.178). Shakespeare apparently took the name Egeus from CHAUCER's 'The Knight's Tale' (see *A Midsummer Night's Dream,* 'Sources of the Play'), in which Egeus is Theseus' father.

Eglamour Minor character in *The Two Gentlemen of Verona,* the gentleman who helps SILVIA flee her father's court in search of VALENTINE in 5.1. In selecting Eglamour as her confidant and guide, Silvia acclaims him 'valiant, wise, . . . well-accomplished' (4.3.13) and is certain she can rely on his honour and courage. Yet, when Silvia is captured by the OUTLAWS, he is reported to have fled ignominiously, 'being nimble-footed' (5.3.6). This unlikely inconsistency, along with the fact that one of JULIA's suitors is also named Eglamour (1.2.9), has sparked some debate. This may simply be one of the many instances of Shakespeare's carelessness in matters of detail, or it may reflect the former existence of two versions of the play. Also, it may be that a jocularly presented instance of cowardice is intended to undercut the seriousness of the romantic ideals that the play simultaneously depends on and laughs at.

Egyptian Minor character in *Antony and Cleopatra,* a messenger for CLEOPATRA. The 'poor Egyptian', as he describes himself in 5.1.52, appears before Octavius CAESAR (2), who has just defeated the forces of Cleopatra and Mark ANTONY. He has been sent to learn Caesar's orders to the Egyptian queen; Caesar sends him back with a conciliatory message. This episode demonstrates Cleopatra's changed circumstances; she is no longer mistress of her own fate, a situation that she will find intolerable. The Egyptian's modest mission ushers in the final development of the play.

Elbow Minor character in *Measure for Measure,* a comic constable of VIENNA. Elbow brings POMPEY (1) to court, in 2.1, and attempts to prosecute FROTH for an unspecified insult to his, Elbow's, wife. However, with his comical mispronunciations and unconscious double meanings he is a stereotypical CLOWN (1), and he cannot make a sensible accusation. He is foiled by Pompey's humorous evasions, which result in the dismissal of the case. The episode serves as comic relief from the increasingly tense main plot. It also illustrates vividly the SUB-PLOT's world of petty vice and crime, standing in striking contrast with the more rigid world of the DUKE (9), ANGELO (2), and ISABELLA. In 3.2 Elbow has the satisfaction of bringing Pompey to prison, though his triumph is not so humorous as his defeat. Compared to his better-known predecessor DOGBERRY, Elbow is a less successful version of an ancient character type—the bumbling, foolish constable. His is a familiar figure in traditional English drama: in 2.1.169, ESCALUS (2) compares Elbow and Pompey to Justice and Iniquity, characters in a MORALITY PLAY.

Eld (Elde), George (d. 1624) London printer and publisher, producer of first editions of *Troilus and Cressida* and the SONNETS. In 1609 Eld printed the QUARTO edition of Shakespeare's play for publishers Richard BONIAN and Henry WALLEY, and Thomas THORPE's edition of the Sonnets. Eld himself sometimes published the plays he printed, including THE PURITAN (1607), which was attributed to 'W. S.', perhaps in an effort to falsely associate the work with Shakespeare. Eld, apprenticed to a printer from 1592–1600, acquired his business by marrying a woman twice the widow of earlier owners. He died in a plague epidemic, but little more is known of his life.

Eleanor (Elinor) of Aquitaine, Queen of England (1122–1204) Historical figure and character in *King John,* mother of King JOHN (3). Queen Eleanor is a bold and forthright character, quick to respond to possible insult to her son, whether from CHATILLON (1.1.5) or from King PHILIP (2) of FRANCE (1) (2.1.120). She is fully prepared to fight (1.1.40), but she is also a wise diplomat, equally ready to make peace when it seems profitable (2.1.468–479). It is clear that she is a very important figure in John's life, and his distraction following her death just as the French invade, in 4.2, is completely understandable.

The historical Eleanor of Aquitaine was one of the most remarkable women of the Middle Ages. The daughter of the Duke of Aquitaine, she inherited her father's duchy, a powerful independent territory in what is now the south of France, at the age of 15. Three months later, she married the Dauphin of France; one month after that, her new father-in-law died, and she became Queen of France. However, she bore no heirs to Louis VII. This fact, the great personality differences between herself and the King, and her marital infidelities, referred to in 2.1.125, resulted in their divorce in 1152. Eleanor was publicly humiliated

in the process, but as Duchess of Aquitaine, the greatest heiress in Europe, she was able to avenge herself immediately by marrying Louis' greatest rival, Henry II of England. By Henry she bore four sons, among them both Richard I and John. However, her relations with her second husband were no better than with her first, and she incited her sons to rebel against him. When the revolt failed, she was imprisoned for 15 years, being released only upon Henry's death. She devoted the rest of her life to supporting her sons, and her death in 1204, at 83, must indeed have seemed a monumental loss to John, although it occurred many years before the crisis with which it is associated in the play.

Eliot (1), John (b. 1562) English author and translator, creator of a minor source for *Romeo and Juliet* and several other plays. Eliot's *Ortho-Epia Gallica* (1593) was a collection of lively colloquial essays—written in French and published with Eliot's English translation on facing pages—that dealt with LONDON life, European travel, and contemporary French poetry. It contained a translation of a poem by the French poet Guillaume DU BARTAS that influenced the lovers' debate on bird song in 3.5. Other material in *Ortho-Epia* inspired minor details in other plays as well, most notably elements of PISTOL's roguish speech.

Like Shakespeare, Eliot was from WARWICKSHIRE. After he attended Oxford he became a novice monk, but he withdrew before he took his vows. Instead, he wandered in Europe and supported himself as a schoolmaster, a hack journalist, and, possibly, a spy for one (or more) of the factions in the religious and civil wars of FRANCE (1). He returned to England in 1589—apparently fleeing the aftermath of King Henri III's assassination—and settled in London as a teacher and translator of French. His *Survey or Topographical Description of France* appeared in 1592, followed by the popular *Ortho-Epia*. After this Eliot disappeared from history. Scholars presume he returned to France, possibly when King Henri IV was crowned in 1594. Eliot was probably acquainted with Shakespeare, for they are known to have had mutual friends in the London literary and theatrical worlds.

Eliot (2), Thomas Stearns (1888–1965) American-British poet and critic. T. S. Eliot is best known as one of the leading poets of the 20th century, but he also wrote a great deal of literary criticism. Much of this focussed on the Elizabethan era and included critical essays on a number of Shakespeare's plays. As a Shakespearean critic he is notorious for his assessment of *Hamlet* as 'an artistic failure'. Less controversially, he observed, 'About any one so great as Shakespeare, it is probable that we can never be right; and if we can never be right, it is better that we should from time to time change our way of being wrong'.

References to Shakespearean characters occur in a number of Eliot's poems, and his 'Coriolan' (a suite of two poems: 'Triumphal March' and 'Difficulties of a Statesman') probably helped spark the tremendous increase in critical and theatrical attention given Shakespeare's *Coriolanus* in the 20th century. Eliot's enthusiasm for, and perceptive studies of, Elizabethan literature certainly did much to generate a revival of interest in the subject as a whole. Eliot also wrote several modern plays in verse, the best known of which is *Murder in the Cathedral* (1935).

Elizabeth (1), Queen of England (1533–1603) Ruler of England for much of Shakespeare's life and a very minor character in *Henry VIII*, written 10 years after her death. Elizabeth appears as an infant—that is, as a prop held by an actor—in 5.4 of the play, where she is the subject of a long eulogy by Archbishop CRANMER. Queen Elizabeth was the most important patron of ELIZABETHAN THEATRE: her influence was essential in protecting the theatrical profession from Puritan-inspired prohibitions, and her court provided an

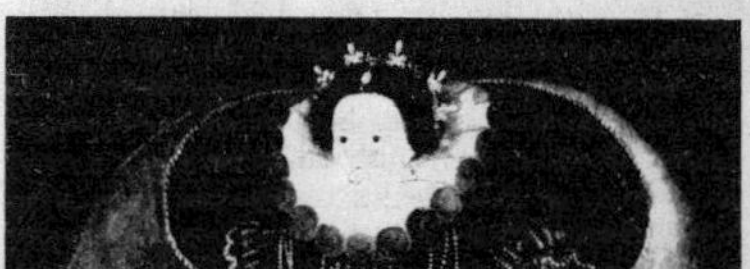

Elizabeth I ruled while England became a world power. The works of Shakespeare are only the most prominent of many great artistic and intellectual achievements that occurred in England during her reign. (Courtesy of Colonial Williamsburg)

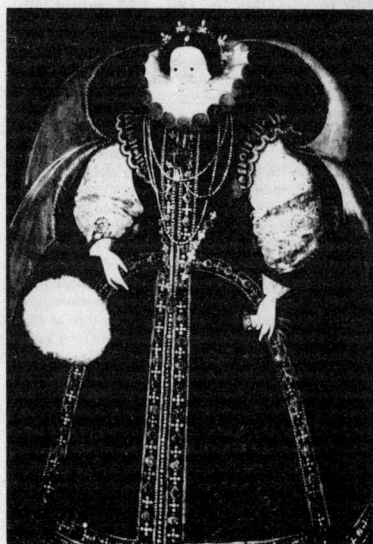

important source of income and prestige for the leading LONDON acting companies. She especially favoured Shakespeare's company, the CHAMBERLAIN'S MEN, and he often performed for her.

The queen is said to have been so pleased with FALSTAFF in the *Henry IV* plays, that she commanded the playwright to produce a play in which the fat knight falls in love; the result was *The Merry Wives of Windsor*—written, according to legend, in two weeks. There may be a germ of truth to the tale, for *The Merry Wives* was probably written for a royal occasion. In any case, Elizabeth's fondness for Shakespeare's plays is testified to in Ben JONSON's accolade, printed in the FIRST FOLIO, in which he refers to the playwright's 'flights . . . That so did take Eliza . . .'.

Shakespeare rendered appropriate tribute. Twice in *A Midsummer Night's Dream,* passages subtly allude to Elizabeth, probably because she was expected to be present at the wedding celebration for which the play is believed to have been written. In 2.1.155–164 she is complimented by a lyrical description that evokes the conventional allegorical representations of the queen in popular prints of the day. In 5.1.89–105 Duke THESEUS (1) praises a monarch's benevolent reception of tongue-tied subjects, behaviour that Elizabeth is known to have prided herself on.

Cranmer's eulogy to Elizabeth in *Henry VIII,* delivered by an important English national hero, doubtless reflects the nostalgia for her reign felt by England a decade after her death. Elizabeth was the only child of King HENRY VIII and Anne Boleyn, the ANNE (1) of *Henry VIII.* After succeeding her stepsister Mary (ruled 1553–1558), she ruled longer than any previous English monarch (only Queen Victoria [1837–1901] has ever outlasted her). Her reign saw Protestantism firmly established in England, and the nation showed its strength against its Catholic enemies with the defeat of the Spanish Armada in 1588. Elizabeth's reign also encompassed magnificent achievements in English literature. Although drama itself was not appreciated as art, the great value of the prose and poetry of Philip SIDNEY, Edmund SPENCER, Thomas NORTH, and others—including the Shakespeare of *Venus and Adonis* and *The Rape of Lucrece*—was recognised and appreciated. In the early 17th century, Elizabeth's reign was already considered—as it has been ever since—England's golden age.

Elizabeth (2) Woodville (Woodvile), Lady Grey (later Queen, 1437–1492) Historical figure and character in *3 Henry VI* and *Richard III,* the wife of King EDWARD IV. Her brother is Lord RIVERS in the same plays, and her father is Richard WOODVILLE in *1 Henry VI.* Known as Lady Grey until Act 4 of *3 Henry VI,* Elizabeth becomes Queen when Edward marries her after she refuses to become his mistress. Edward was already promised to Lady BONA of FRANCE (1), so the marriage becomes a stimulus for warfare. Elizabeth is a pawn in the troubled politics of the time. However, she displays dignity in an awkward position, as in her speech at 4.1.66–73, and her instinct to protect her unborn child in 4.4 is also noteworthy. She quite properly distrusts the treacherous and violent noblemen of the disturbed nation, but she is powerless.

In *Richard III* Elizabeth is cursed in 1.3 by the former Queen, MARGARET (1), and sees her enemy's wishes come true as Edward dies and Richard murders her two sons by Edward. He also has her brother, Rivers, and a son, GREY (2), executed, while another son, DORSET, is forced into exile. However, Richard fails to exploit her family further. Elizabeth resists him in 4.4, when he attempts to win her approval of his plan to marry her daughter. She rejects his efforts to swear an oath, stifling him until he is reduced to wishing ill on himself, fatefully (4.4.397–409). Elizabeth suspends the conversation at 4.4.428–429, leaving the resolution of the matter in doubt. (Her daughter is betrothed by the victorious invader RICHMOND at the play's end.)

Historically, WARWICK's alienation from Edward was provoked by disagreements over policy and not simply by the King's marriage, as Shakespeare would have it, but among the minor causes was the behaviour of the greedy Woodvilles. Elizabeth Woodville was the first commoner to become Queen of England, and her many male relatives exploited her new position by marrying the cream of eligible heiresses. However, Elizabeth attracted supporters when, after the death of King Edward, her son inherited the crown. Edward had appointed Richard the boy's Protector, with ruling power, before he died; Elizabeth's allies attempted to circumvent this arrangement with a coup. They were defeated by Richard, as in the play, though he treated Elizabeth herself with great generosity and provided her with a distinguished place at his court.

Richard repeatedly denied rumours that he planned to marry Elizabeth's daughter. In fact, since he had in part based his claim to the throne on the charge that Edward himself was illegitimate, an attempt to marry his daughter would seem self-defeating. However, Shakespeare's sources reported the rumours, and the playwright expanded them into a powerful scene. Elizabeth herself had other plans; it appears that she secretly allied herself with Richmond (later King Henry VII) before his invasion, with the agreement that, should he succeed, he would marry the daughter, which he did. Elizabeth lived out her life as an honoured dowager at the court of her son-in-law.

Elizabeth (3) Stuart, Queen of Bohemia (1596–1662) Daughter of King JAMES I of England and Scotland, patron of a theatre company, LADY ELIZABETH'S MEN, and somewhat later an international figure by virtue of her ill-starred marriage to a powerful Ger-

man prince, Frederick V, Elector Palatine and briefly King of BOHEMIA. Elizabeth's marriage was celebrated by a season-long series of festivities over the winter of 1612–1613, in which Shakespeare's acting company, the KING'S MEN, had a notable part. They put on 20 different plays, eight of them Shakespeare's, probably including *1* and *2 Henry IV*, *Julius Caesar*, *Much Ado About Nothing*, *The Winter's Tale*, and *The Tempest*. (Some scholars believe that the MASQUE in 4.1 of *The Tempest* was inserted into the play for this occasion.) Her marriage stirred nation-wide enthusiasm and was regarded as the consummation of an idyllic romance.

However, Elizabeth's destiny was tragic. After five years of comfort and pleasure at Frederick's capital in Heidelberg, the couple were swept up in the complex religious politics of the Holy Roman Empire. Frederick unwisely accepted the throne of Bohemia, a Protestant country that had rebelled against the Catholic Hapsburgs, rulers of the empire. After a brief reign—Frederick is known to history as 'the Winter King'—he was deposed by the emperor, in the first phase of the Thirty Years War. Elizabeth spent the rest of her life in exile, mostly in The Hague, attempting to recover her husband's position.

Frederick died in 1632, leaving Elizabeth unhappy and, by royal standards, poor, especially after the STUART DYNASTY was also dethroned by the English revolution. She had 13 children but quarrelled with them all; when her eldest son recovered the Palatine Electorate, he refused to provide her with a home. Finally, with the restoration of the monarchy in England, she returned to London in 1661, only to die within months. Eventually, her grandson ruled England as George I (ruled 1714–1727).

Elizabethan Drama Art of writing for the theatre as practised in England during the reign of Queen ELIZABETH (1) (1558–1603). Shakespeare was undeniably the major figure of Elizabethan drama, but many other playwrights were active, and the period constitutes a Golden Age in English drama, indeed in the drama of the world.

In 1558, when Elizabeth became queen, almost no English drama was being written; Elizabethan drama came of age in the late 1570s, growing out of the competition between the CHILDREN'S COMPANIES, composed of schoolboys, and the adult companies who had come to LONDON under the protection of noble patrons, both seeking the favour of the queen and her courtiers (see ELIZABETHAN THEATRE). The children's companies performed Latin plays (both ancient Roman works and modern imitations) and English works modelled on them. These plays had greater appeal to the educated tastes of the court than did the often bawdy INTERLUDE—derived from native English roots in medieval festivals and the MORALITY PLAY—that was the stock-in-trade of the adult companies, just beginning to perform in public theatres. The adult companies, however, sought playwrights who could appeal to court tastes as well and found them in the literary world growing up in early modern London. A tremendous wellspring of talent was tapped, and thousands of plays were produced over the next several decades.

In the 1580s Elizabethan drama was dominated by a group of playwrights known as the UNIVERSITY WITS, who brought together various influences: classical literature and its contemporary imitation in ACADEMIC DRAMA, morality plays, and contemporary RENAISSANCE literature from Italy and France. In the 1590s a broader range of playwrights emerged, including Shakespeare.

Elizabethan TRAGEDY (which was strongly influenced by the ancient dramas of SENECA) consisted of two general varieties. The REVENGE PLAY was introduced by Thomas KYD in his very popular *Spanish Tragedy* (c. 1588) and was most fully developed in *Hamlet*. John MARSTON was a later practitioner of the revenge play. Another sort of tragedy presented grandiose fantasies about the downfall of powerful rulers; this genre burst forth in the *Tamburlaine* of Christopher MARLOWE (1), in which BLANK VERSE was established as the medium for Elizabethan drama. Shakespeare brought the genre to complex new levels in such works as *Macbeth*, *King Lear*, and the ROMAN PLAYS.

Elizabethan COMEDY took several distinct forms. Romantic comedy, a popular genre centred on young love, reached its pinnacle in Shakespeare's comedies of the 1590s, such as *Much Ado About Nothing* and *As You Like It*. Lesser figures writing this sort of play included Robert GREENE (2) and Thomas DEKKER. Towards the end of the 1590s, a variation arose, the COMEDY OF HUMOURS, in which bold character types were employed to ridicule contemporary behaviour. Ben JONSON was the leading exponent of the comedy of humours. The so-called court comedy was written with an aristocratic audience in mind. These plays often used mythological or classical subjects and were distinguished by their emphasis on refined dialogue and prominent allusions to Renaissance learning. John LYLY was the most important writer of court comedy; his plays influenced Shakespeare's early work, especially *Love's Labour's Lost*. Another category, the chronicle or HISTORY PLAY, while it had roots in didactic, allegorical dramas akin to morality plays, was essentially developed by Shakespeare, in his enactments of the WARS OF THE ROSES.

Elizabethan drama is sometimes considered to include work from the next two reigns, those of Kings JAMES I and Charles I, until the theatres of England were closed by revolution (1603–1642). However, the more restricted sense is used here, for the subsequent period, which includes Shakespeare's late work, saw pronounced changes in taste and in theatrical tech-

niques, making for differences in tone and subject matter (see JACOBEAN DRAMA).

Elizabethan Theatre Professional presentation of dramas as practised in Shakespeare's time, especially during the reign of Queen ELIZABETH (1) (1558–1603). Elizabethan theatre was very different from today's theatre in its organisation, methods, and even in the nature of the buildings used. Before the 1570s English theatre barely existed, but in the course of Shakespeare's lifetime, a thriving centre of dramatic art evolved in LONDON.

At the outset of Elizabeth's reign in 1558, English drama consisted largely of religious enactments such as the MORALITY PLAY presented at medieval festivals, and these were generally performed by members of the trade guilds of different towns. Professional entertainers were mostly wandering acrobats, musicians, and clowns, more like circus performers than actors. They were legally classed with vagabonds and could be jailed merely for pursuing their calling. Some troupes, however, were taken into the households of aristocrats and were therefore exempt from such laws. They provided entertainment for the lord and his guests, often performing an INTERLUDE at a meal, a much more drama-like feature than the 'feats of activitie' commonly recorded. These troupes often travelled, performing for other nobles and gradually taking over the guilds' functions for the dramatic elements of seasonal festivals.

London naturally became a focus for such activities. London companies were still under the patronage of some great nobleman but were no longer closely affiliated with his household, though they might perform at his country home on special occasions. (The law required that actors be members of a noble household, and certain nobles co-operated with the actors, but the patrons generally had nothing else to do with the operations of a company.) Performances in London were usually held in large inns or taverns, most of which were within the walls of the city. However, the London government, largely controlled by Puritans, was particularly hostile to actors, so the companies began to arrange their performances in nearby areas. In 1576 the THEATRE, the first building in England intended solely for the performance of plays, was built by James BURBAGE (2), just north of the city line. Other playhouses soon followed.

In a different social world, Queen Elizabeth catered extensively to performers, and the royal court became a second centre of the nascent theatre world. In 1574 the queen proclaimed one of the acting companies, LEICESTER'S MEN, to be members of her household and thus exempt from even London's laws against performing. Also during this time students at schools, universities, and the INNS OF COURT, affected by the RENAISSANCE revival of classical literature, began to read and perform the plays of ancient ROME and their modern imitations. These sophisticated entertainments were more to the taste of the queen and her courtiers than the interludes of the adult acting companies, so the CHILDREN'S COMPANIES were generally more featured at court. Entrepreneurs such as Burbage and Philip HENSLOWE then began to hire dramatists to produce work that would attract sophisticated patrons and gain them the prestige of association with the court. ELIZABETHAN DRAMA was born.

For almost a decade, Leicester's Men were the most important theatre company in London, but the QUEEN'S MEN, created by Elizabeth in 1583, soon eclipsed them. In the early 1590s, two other companies arose that were to dominate Elizabethan theatre thereafter: the ADMIRAL'S MEN and STRANGE'S MEN, later the CHAMBERLAIN'S MEN, Shakespeare's company. Other companies included OXFORD'S MEN, PEMBROKE'S MEN, and SUSSEX'S MEN. They played at court and at the Theatre and the other public playhouses: the CURTAIN THEATRE (built near the Theatre in 1577), the ROSE THEATRE (the first in SOUTHWARK, which became the most important theatre district), the SWAN THEATRE, the GLOBE THEATRE, and the FORTUNE THEATRE. Plays were also staged at the CROSS KEYS INN, until London outlawed the theatre in 1596, and in an outlying district, NEWINGTON BUTTS.

These theatres were generally roughly cylindrical, three-storied buildings surrounding a central, unroofed space containing the stage, built out from a section of the building that served as a backstage area. (Indoor theatres appeared somewhat later, in Shakespeare's lifetime but during the reign of King JAMES I; they are part of the story of JACOBEAN DRAMA.) The actual appearance of these theatres is obscure, since the only evidence is a single drawing—of unknown reliability—depicting the interior of the Swan Theatre and the contract for the building of the Fortune. Some spectators stood on the ground around the stage, within the 'wooden O' (*Henry V*, Prologue, 13) of the building; the 'groundlings', as they were called, paid a cheap admission price. Each floor of the building was divided into galleries, which offered a better view of the stage and were more expensive. In the most expensive galleries seating was provided, and seats were also available, at the highest price, on the stage itself. A canopy, called the 'heavens' or the 'shadow', extended over the stage from its rear wall. The stage itself probably contained one or more trapdoors, often used to represent graves or the mouth of hell. (Supernatural phenomena were popular on the Elizabethan stage, and Shakespeare often presented them [see, e.g., APPARITION, ASNATH, and GHOST].) Behind the stage, the building contained dressing rooms—the 'tiring [attiring] house'—and upper rooms for musicians and for the machinery used to hoist actors or props in spectacular ascents or descents through the

'heavens'. Atop the whole structure was a hut, or 'penthouse', from which flags were flown and trumpets sounded to announce a performance.

Plays were held outdoors (very few seem to have been cancelled by weather, suggesting a hardy audience). They usually began at two o'clock in the afternoon, and they had to be finished before nightfall, for the only illumination besides the sun were torches to provide partial relief on an overcast day or at the onset of dusk. (This limitation is often incorporated into the texture of the play. For instance, near the end of *Julius Caesar* a character witnesses the suicide of CASSIUS and observes, 'O setting sun, / As in thy red rays thou dost sink to night, / So in his red blood Cassius' day is set / The sun of Rome is set. Our day is gone' [5.3.60–63], and the audience could confirm his remarks with their own eyes.) The average duration of a performance was about two hours—the CHORUS (2) of *Romeo and Juliet* speaks of 'the two hours' traffic of our stage' (Prologue, 12)—though many plays must have taken longer. Often the play was followed by a jig—a brief, often bawdy, miniature comic opera, with wild dancing and simple lyrics set to the melodies of popular SONGS.

A performance in the Elizabethan theatre was very different from one today. The stages were simply raised areas amid the audience, with very little if any scenery. No curtain opened on a prepared scene or closed on a finished one. The actors had to enter at the beginning and immediately command the audience's attention, with the consequence that scenes tended to begin with powerful material. They also had to exit at the end to make room for the next sequence, so scenes generally did not end on a note of crisis, as is common in modern plays.

Acting styles seem to have been very different as well, according to written evidence that values a very formal and artificial style. Rhetorical flourishes and conventional poses created a distance that was felt to enhance the effect of the lines. Realistic portrayals were simply not expected, though some of Shakespeare's characters begin the evolution towards modern dramatic realism. Costumes were contemporary for the most part, regardless of the setting of the play, except for special outfits that conventionally identified figures from the classical world (a toga or a plumed helmet and armour), from the exotic Middle East (billowing trousers, a turban, and a scimitar), or supernatural beings such as gods or ghosts.

The strangest feature of the Elizabethan stage, by comparison with our own, was the absence of women. In the children's companies all the roles were taken by boys, but among the adult companies the effect was even stranger, for the boys played the women (though old, comical women, such as Mistress QUICKLY or the NURSE [3] in *Romeo and Juliet*, could be played by men). Even then boys as the heroines of romance must have seemed somewhat comic, for playwrights often build on this peculiarity by having the heroine disguise herself as a boy. Thus, a boy plays a girl who plays a boy. A further complication was often invoked by having a woman (played by a boy) mistakenly fall in love with the disguised woman (also played by a boy). The situation is not only comical, but also suggestive of hidden depths of human sexuality. The use of boys as women was commonly attacked by Puritan critics as immoral, and many non-Puritans agreed. When the English theatres were reopened in 1660, after being closed by the Puritan revolution, only women were allowed to play women.

In Elizabethan times the boys also played the parts of boys, of course, and some of these roles, though brief, were demanding (see, e.g., BOY [3], SON [1], MOTH). A boy was sometimes apprenticed to an adult actor, who trained, educated, and supported him until he was capable of playing men's roles. The adult recovered his expenses by 'selling' the trained boy to an acting company, perhaps his own. Neither party was bound by strict contracts, as in other trades, for members of noble households—as actors formally were—were not covered by the laws on apprenticeship.

An actor's status as an aristocratic retainer was merely a legal fiction, for acting companies were actually commercial enterprises, with share-holding partners and paid employees. Some companies, including the Admiral's Men, used a performance space owned by an entrepreneur, such as Philip HENSLOWE or Francis LANGLEY, while others, typified by the Chamberlain's Men, controlled their own theatre. Five of the Chamberlain's Men, including Shakespeare, owned half of the Globe, with Cuthbert BURBAGE (1) and Richard BURBAGE (3)—himself an actor in the company—owning the other half. As owners, or 'housekeepers', these men profited from the owner's share of the theatre's receipts and paid the owner's expenses; as partners in the acting company, or 'sharers', they profited from the other side of the arrangement. The housekeepers received half the receipts from the galleries, with which they maintained the building and paid the ground rent for the land on which it stood. The sharers received the company's part of a performance's receipts: all of the income from the cheaper admissions paid by the groundlings and half of that from the more expensive galleries. They shared this as profit after meeting their own expenses. They hired their employees—extra actors, stagehands, musicians, and others—and paid for costumes and props; most important and most expensive, they commissioned dramas.

Playwrights sold plays to acting companies, who then owned the script; unless he was a member of the company, the author received no further income from his efforts. Some playwrights worked under contract,

especially with Henslowe, who employed dozens of writers. Others, most notably Shakespeare, wrote only for a company in which they were sharers. A few, like Ben JONSON, free-lanced, writing for a variety of companies in succession.

Plays were performed in a repertoire that was rotated frequently; a given play was rarely staged more than once a week but might be staged frequently during a season, which might include a dozen or more plays. Popular plays, such as those of Shakespeare or Christopher MARLOWE (1), might be revived periodically over many years or rewritten to appeal to changing fashions.

New plays were in great demand and were produced at an extraordinary rate. It has been estimated that at least several thousand plays were written for London theatre companies during the years of Shakespeare's career; he himself wrote 39 (including CARDENIO), for an average of almost two a year. Thomas HEYWOOD (2) declared that he had written or collaborated on 220 plays. Once a company bought a play, they submitted it, with the necessary fee, to the MASTER OF THE REVELS, who had to approve it for performance. He might refuse or demand changes for political or religious reasons (see CENSORSHIP). The company might sell a script to a publisher, who then profited exclusively from it, but they preferred not to, for as long as they owned it, they could anticipate further profits. Thus, the vast majority of the plays that were written in Shakespeare's time were never published and are lost.

Elsinore Danish seaport (Helsingør in Danish), setting for *Hamlet.* The royal castle of the KING (5) of DENMARK, located in Elsinore, is the setting for every scene in the play except 5.1, which is set in a nearby graveyard; three dramatically striking early scenes (1.1, 1.4–5), are set on its fortified walls. The town is mentioned several times (e.g., in 1.2.174), but it is not described at all.

Elsinore was well known to Elizabethan England, being located on the narrow straits between Denmark and Sweden, an important trade route for English ships. It was the site of a Danish fortress, Kronborg, doubtless the castle envisioned by Shakespeare, from which tolls were collected from all ships entering or leaving the Baltic Sea. The castle is now a maritime museum where Shakespeare's plays are regularly performed. English acting companies travelled to Elsinore in 1585 and 1586—and possibly on other, unrecorded tours—and it has been speculated that Shakespeare may have been among the players who performed there, although there is no clear evidence of this, and his faulty knowledge of the physical place—Elsinore has no 'cliff / That beetles o'er his base into the sea' (1.4.70–71), for example—suggests that he never made the trip.

Ely (1), Bishop of Character in *Henry VIII.* See BISHOP (3).

Ely (2), John Fordham, Bishop of (d. 1435) Historical figure and character in *Henry V* who supports the Archbishop of CANTERBURY (1) in urging war to King HENRY V. In 1.1 Ely and Canterbury express their hope that a state of war—especially when supported by a large donation from the church—will forestall the introduction of legislation requiring a vast state seizure of church property. In 1.2 Ely, Canterbury, and others encourage Henry to invade FRANCE (1).

Ely (3), John Morton, Bishop of (c. 1420–1500) Historical figure and minor character in *Richard III,* a pawn in the scenario arranged by RICHARD III as he strikes at Lord HASTINGS (2) in 3.4. At a council meeting, Richard requests that the genial Ely send for some strawberries from his garden, thereby establishing a mood of cordiality that he shortly shatters with his accusations of treason. Both Hastings and the audience have been lulled into a false sense of security that is rudely smashed, in a manner symbolic of Richard's effect on the entire realm. As ineffectual as Ely seems here, he is later, at 4.3.46, said to have joined the forces of the Earl of RICHMOND, thus contributing to Richard's downfall.

The historical John Morton had been a rising young ecclesiastical lawyer when the WARS OF THE ROSES broke out. He became a firm Lancastrian, to the extent of joining Queen MARGARET (1) in exile. However, after the Yorkist victory, he submitted to the victors and resumed his clerical and legal career with great success. He was appointed Bishop of Ely in 1479, and he was the executor of the will of King EDWARD IV. But under Richard he fared less well. After the incident described above, Ely, as an adherent of the young PRINCE (5), was among those arrested. He was placed in the TOWER OF LONDON, but the Duke of BUCKINGHAM (2) took over his custody after several years and recruited him to his rebellious conspiracy. Ely joined Richmond abroad, and when that Earl was crowned as Henry VII, the Bishop became a prominent member of his government. Morton was also to become the patron of the young Thomas MORE, whose history was Shakespeare's source for the strawberry anecdote. Thus its historical accuracy seems certain.

Ely Palace portrait Possible portrait of Shakespeare. The Ely Palace portrait, discovered in 1845, bears an inscription stating that the anonymous sitter was 39 years old in 1603—as was Shakespeare—when it was painted. It closely resembles the DROESHOUT engraving, one of the two authoritative likenesses of the playwright, and it may be the original from which the engraver worked. However, it may also be a postdated copy of the engraving; scholars remain uncer-

tain. The portrait at one time hung in the official residence of a 19th-century bishop of Ely and is now owned by the Shakespeare's Birthplace Trust and hangs in STRATFORD.

Elyot, Sir Thomas (c. 1490–1546) English author, an influence on several of Shakespeare's plays. Elyot's most famous work is *The Boke Called the Governour* (1531), an extended essay on political morality and the education of statesmen. Echoes of this work appear in a number of Shakespeare's early works, including *The Two Gentlemen of Verona* and *2 Henry IV.* Elyot covers the WARS OF THE ROSES at length, and observes that they represent a deterioration of the English nation's unity that the TUDOR dynasty had fortunately repaired. These ideas were highly important to Shakespeare when he wrote his HISTORY PLAYS. Though such doctrines were also widely available elsewhere, Shakespeare's evident familiarity with the *Governour* makes it clear that he was especially influenced by these ideas through Elyot.

Elyot was an important figure in RENAISSANCE English literature. He translated a number of Latin works, promoted the study of the classics, and compiled the first Latin-English dictionary (1538). He also published a popular health manual. He served King HENRY VIII as a diplomat, and attempted fruitlessly to gain the support of the Holy Roman Emperor for Henry's divorce of KATHERINE of Aragon.

Emery, John (1777–1822) English actor. An actor from childhood, Emery was typically cast as an old man even in his teens, and he became a leading character actor and comedian. He was best known for his portrayal of CALIBAN, and he was also acclaimed as DOGBERRY, the GRAVE-DIGGER in *Hamlet,* and SIR TOBY BELCH. Emery also had a career as a successful painter.

Emilia (1) (Aemilia) Character in *The Comedy of Errors,* the stern and peremptory Abbess of the PRIORY who is revealed to be the long-lost wife of EGEON and mother of the twins ANTIPHOLUS OF EPHESUS and ANTIPHOLUS OF SYRACUSE. She first appears in the final scene (at 5.1.37), after Antipholus and DROMIO of Syracuse take refuge in her Priory, a place of legal sanctuary. She determines that ADRIANA has been jealous of her husband and delivers a short, epigrammatic sermon on the evils of jealous womankind (5.1.69–86). Emilia further declares that the sanctuary of the Priory may not be violated by the return of the two refugees, and she exits briskly.

Later in the scene, having been sent for by the DUKE (8) of Ephesus to help resolve the confusions that have by now come to a head, Emilia returns with Antipholus of Syracuse, placing the twins on stage together for the first time (5.1.329). Ten lines later, she recognises the condemned EGEON as her lost husband. She relates how kidnappers had stolen away the infants who had survived the shipwreck that separated the family years before. The Duke deduces that these infants are now the adults Antipholus and Dromio of Ephesus. After all is revealed, she invites the company to the Priory for a 'gossip's feast' of celebration (5.1.405), to which all depart, ending the play. The term 'gossip's feast' refers to a baptismal or christening party, underlining the importance of Emilia as a symbol of Christian mercy, softening the hard authority of the Duke's laws and embodying the resolution of the play's complexities.

Emilia (2) Character in *Othello,* lady-in-waiting to DESDEMONA and wife of IAGO. Despite Emilia's loyalty to and fondness for Desdemona she is manipulated by Iago, who convinces OTHELLO that Desdemona is having a love affair with CASSIO. Unwittingly, Emilia aids Iago in this deception when she provides him with Desdemona's handkerchief, a love token from Othello that Iago plants on Cassio. In 5.2 after the jealous Othello has been driven to murder, Emilia fearlessly denounces him, and when Iago's involvement becomes apparent she exposes his schemes just as boldly. In reprisal Iago stabs her. Dying, she asks to be placed next to Desdemona and makes a final oath that her mistress was faithful to Othello.

Except in this final scene, Emilia serves principally as a foil to her mistress. A sharp-tongued woman whose worldly cynicism makes plausible her marriage to the ambitious and unscrupulous Iago, her nature contrasts tellingly with Desdemona's loving innocence. Though Emilia does not suspect Iago's motives, their marriage is obviously unhappy. She stoically receives his insults, but when alone with Desdemona she rails against men and marriage, declaring, in 4.3, that she would commit adultery, given the chance. Despite her unhappiness, Desdemona rejects this idea firmly, in contrast with Othello's failure to repudiate Iago's sentiments.

Emilia (3) Minor character in *The Winter's Tale,* a lady-in-waiting to Queen HERMIONE. In 2.2, when PAULINA attempts to visit the unjustly imprisoned Hermione, the GAOLER (3) only lets her see Emilia. She tells Paulina that the queen has given birth and returns to her mistress with Paulina's suggestion that the infant be brought to the king in a bid for mercy. Emilia's role is small, and she is an uncomplicated messenger, a simple tool of the plot without any real personality.

Emilia (4) Character in *The Two Noble Kinsmen,* sister of HIPPOLYTA (2) and the beloved of both PALAMON and ARCITE, the title characters. The subject of the obsession that destroys the friendship of the kinsmen, Emilia is to some extent a pawn of the plot. At first unconscious of the situation, she is inconsequential;

later, as the cousins prepare to duel for the right to marry her, she is emotionally distressed, but the focus remains on the men. However, as a virtuous and noble figure, she is a potent symbol, and she is finally, in her helplessness, an important illustration of the play's central theme, that human beings are unable to control their destiny but must strive to maintain dignity as they confront their fate.

Shakespeare introduces Emilia as an attractive, serious young woman. In 1.1 her pity and magnanimity as she responds to the pleas of the three widows (see QUEEN [1]) establish her as a noble person. In 1.3 she tenderly recalls a close childhood friendship with a girl who has died, and she is quietly confident that she will never love a man as much; later, we realise that her expectation was all too appropriate, for her part in the play's love story is tragically involuntary.

However, as a character, Emilia suffers from the defects of the play, which was written collaboratively by Shakespeare and John FLETCHER (2). Shakespeare's Emilia is a promising figure, but Fletcher, who wrote all of her scenes in Acts 2–4, did not develop her; at first she is simply another young woman of the court, interested in flowers in 2.1, when the two kinsmen fall in love with her beauty, and politely agreeable to the disguised Arcite in 3.5. Then Fletcher alters her radically, but the change is entirely artificial. She agonises over her choice of lovers in a highly rhetorical passage (4.2.1–54) that introduces the arrival of the duellists in a melodramatic manner, but reduces her to a mere illustration of hysteria. Nevertheless, the speech furthers the course of the play, for it demonstrates that she, like the kinsmen, is trapped by destiny. As she puts it, 'my reason is lost in me, / I have no choice' and 'I am sotted, / Utterly lost' (4.2.34–35, 45–46). Emilia embodies humanity's helplessness, both here and in Act 5, where she is again Shakespeare's creation and a more dignified and credible character.

In 5.1, before the duel, Emilia addresses the goddess Diana, seeking assistance in her quandary. She asks the goddess to make sure the winner is the cousin who genuinely loves her the most, adding that she would prefer to remain unmarried. In response, a rose tree with a single rose appears on the altar; supposing that its singleness means she will not have to marry either cousin, Emilia is delighted, but then the rose falls. Chagrined, Emilia remains hopeful, closing touchingly with the plea, 'Unclasp thy mystery.— I hope she's pleased; / Her signs were gracious' (5.1.172–173). In 5.3 she is too distracted to watch the duel, which is reported to her by a SERVANT (30), and we cannot help but sympathise. When she is awarded to Arcite and Palamon is sent to be executed, according to the rules for the duel, Emilia cries out, 'Is this winning? / O all you heavenly powers, where is your mercy?' (5.3.138–139). This despairing cry is the nadir of the play; however, Emilia immediately accepts her fate, rejecting suicide in the next line, because the gods' 'wills have said it must be so' (5.3.140). By the play's end Emilia can accept the final twist of fate—Arcite dies accidentally and Palamon wins her by default—with equanimity. She has learned the lesson that THESEUS (2) declaims in the final line: we must 'bear us as the time' (5.4.137).

Emmanuel Minor character in *2 Henry VI.* See CLERK (1).

Enobarbus (Cnaeus Domitius Ahenobarbus) (d. 31 B.C.) Historical figure and character in *Antony and Cleopatra,* ANTONY's chief lieutenant who later deserts him and joins Octavius CAESAR (2). Antony's closest friend and adviser through Acts 1–3, Enobarbus abandons his leader when he perceives, in 3.13, that Antony's involvement with CLEOPATRA has led to inevitable defeat. However, when he learns of Antony's sympathetic response to the betrayal, Enobarbus feels terrible pangs of guilt and declares that he will 'go seek / Some ditch, wherein to die' (4.6.37–38). In 4.9 a SENTRY (2) and his WATCHMEN (4) listen as Enobarbus praises Antony and prays for death, then they see him collapse and die. Enobarbus realises that he was wrong to permit good sense to overrule loyalty, for by being prudent he has broken his own heart. The episode foreshadows Cleopatra's final transcendence, and demonstrates that the power of love can invalidate questions of military and political success. In fact, Enobarbus' betrayal is loving, for it is clear that he leaves Antony because he cannot bear to witness his leader's slide into weak-willed failure. Enobarbus thus offers another complex angle on the play's themes of love and power.

Enobarbus is a wise and witty figure before his crisis draws him under. He frequently offers frank, sardonic comments on the other characters and fills some of the functions of a CHORUS (1). For instance, his mockery of LEPIDUS, in 3.2, satirises the dishonesty of Roman politics. On the other hand, his persistent criticism of Antony's love affair helps establish the point of view of the rigorously disciplined ROME, as opposed to the pleasure-oriented world of Cleopatra's court. Enobarbus rises to fine poetry, as in his famous description of the first meeting of Antony and Cleopatra—'The barge she sat in, like a burnish'd throne / Burn'd on the water . . .' (2.2.191 ff.), but he is more often a gruff veteran of the civil wars who jests about the conflict's ups and downs and feels comradeship with his one-time and future enemies. His soldier's humour is well developed and provides a significant portion of the play's comic spirit, an important element in Shakespeare's dramatic strategy.

The historical Domitius Ahenobarbus, as he was called, came from an important Roman political and military family. He fought for Pompey the Great (fa-

ther of the character in *Antony and Cleopatra*) against Julius CAESAR (1) and was later convicted of participating in Caesar's murder in 44 B.C. He commanded a naval force for BRUTUS (4) at PHILIPPI in 42 B.C., though he does not appear in *Julius Caesar.* After Philippi, he established himself as a warlord. He controlled the Adriatic Sea with his fleet and issued coins bearing his portrait. In 40 B.C. he allied himself with Antony. He opposed Cleopatra's participation in the war against Caesar, and in 31 B.C. he changed sides, as in the play, but he did it just before the battle of ACTIUM, rather than afterwards. Shakespeare knew this from his source, PLUTARCH, but he preferred that his character be a basically loyal subordinate who only leaves when Antony's failings have made defeat inevitable. Ahenobarbus, on the other hand, deserted when his services must still have seemed valuable to his new master. However, he immediately became too sick to command troops, and he died soon after the battle.

Epenow Historical figure probably alluded to in *Henry VIII,* a Native American who visited LONDON. In *Henry VIII* the PORTER (4) alludes to the enthusiasm of women for a 'strange Indian with the great tool come to court' (5.3.33–34). Scholars believe this lewd reference is to Epenow, a large man of impressive courage and equanimity, whose appearance in London is recorded in several contemporary sources. He was one of a number of American natives brought to England in the first quarter of the 17th century, some under the auspices of Shakespeare's patron, the Earl of SOUTHAMPTON (2). Their celebrity as mysterious visitors from the New World may have influenced Shakespeare's creation of CALIBAN.

Brought to England in 1611, Epenow was lionised for a time, but his hosts soon turned to exhibiting him for a fee in a travelling show. Dissatisfied, Epenow devised an escape from England. He persuaded a group of investors that he knew of a gold mine on an island off New England. A vessel was outfitted, and Epenow sailed with it as a guide, but as soon as the ship reached familiar shores, the guide dove overboard, swam ashore, and disappeared.

Ephesus Ancient city in Greek Asia Minor (now in Turkey), the setting for *The Comedy of Errors* and several scenes of *Pericles.* In Shakespeare's chief source for the play, *The Menaechmi,* by PLAUTUS, the setting is in another city, Epidamnum. The playwright is presumed to have made the change for two reasons. First, Ephesus was certainly better known to his audience through St Paul's Epistle to the Ephesians and other New Testament references. Second, Ephesus was notorious, through these allusions, as a centre of witchcraft and sorcery. This made it an appropriate setting for Shakespeare's tale of strangeness and confusion. In 1.2.97–102 ANTIPHOLUS OF SYRACUSE refers to this characteristic of the city to which he has come.

One reason for this reputation was the importance of Ephesus as an ancient centre of paganism, especially due to the presence of a famous temple to DIANA (2) that figures in *Pericles.* PERICLES' wife, THAISA, is mistakenly buried at sea, near Ephesus. She recovers, but, believing that she will never see her husband again, she decides to enter a convent dedicated to Diana. In Act 5 after the goddess has appeared in a vision to Pericles, he comes to the Temple of Diana where Thaisa has become a priestess and they are reunited. Shakespeare took this episode from his source, and except for the references to the temple, the play does not evoke the actual city. However, the herbal lore with which CERIMON revives the unconscious Thaisa is appropriate to an ancient centre of magical arts.

Epilogue A speech at the end of a play referring to the performance that has just been completed, often asking for applause. The actor who speaks the Epilogue speaks directly to the audience and is often not in character (in which case, he may be designated as 'Epilogue', himself, in stage directions and speech headings). The device provides a sense of closure to the work and acknowledges its artificiality, returning the spectator to the real world. Eleven of Shakespeare's plays conclude with an Epilogue: *All's Well That Ends Well, As You Like It, 2 Henry IV, Henry V, Henry VIII, A Midsummer Night's Dream, Pericles, The Tempest, Troilus and Cressida, Twelfth Night,* and *The Two Noble Kinsmen.*

Epitaph Brief literary work memorialising a deceased person. A number of epitaphs are attributed to Shakespeare, with varying degrees of probability (see COMBE (1); JAMES; JONSON; STRANGE), including one to himself. A number of other poets wrote epitaphs to Shakespeare shortly after the playwright's death (see BASSE; DIGGES (2); HOLLAND (2); JONSON; MILTON).

Although an epitaph is by definition suitable for inscription on a grave marker, it need not be intended for that purpose and may simply be a brief expression of sentiment, ranging from elegiac to humorous, about the deceased. Shakespeare's reputed epitaph on Jonson (said to have been written jointly with Jonson himself) is a 4-line jest; Milton's on Shakespeare, on the other hand, is a 16-line masterpiece on the capacity of art—Shakespeare's plays in particular—to negate mortality.

Eros Character in *Antony and Cleopatra,* servant of ANTONY. Eros first appears in 3.5 where he reports to ENOBARBUS that Octavius CAESAR (2) has defeated POMPEY (2) and imprisoned LEPIDUS, news that foreshadows the conflict with Caesar that will prove fatal to

Antony. Eros appears thereafter several times—in 3.11, 4.4, 4.5, and 4.7—as an obviously devoted servant; in 4.14 the defeated Antony, believing that CLEOPATRA has committed suicide, orders Eros to take his sword and kill him, in accordance with a promise made when Antony had freed the servant from slavery, years earlier. However, Eros cannot bring himself to do it and kills himself instead. Antony, declaring Eros 'Thrice-nobler than myself' (4.14.95), follows his example and stabs himself. This episode, a familiar dramatic exercise (compare, for example, the death of Marcus BRUTUS [4], in 5.5 of *Julius Caesar*), lends pathos to the noble death of Antony.

Erpingham, Sir Thomas (1357–1428) Historical figure and minor character in *Henry V,* officer in the army of King HENRY V. In 4.1, on the eve of the battle of AGINCOURT, Erpingham rejects Henry's suggestion that he is too old to sleep on the hard ground, asserting that he enjoys being able to say, 'Now lie I like a king' (4.1.17). Henry congratulates him on his spirit, thus contributing to the episode's emphasis on the high morale of the English army.

The historical Erpingham supported the King's father, Henry BOLINGBROKE (1), later King HENRY IV, when he deposed King RICHARD II (enacted in *Richard II*) and later served as his chancellor. He was one of the highest-ranking officers at Agincourt.

Escalus (1), Prince of Verona Character in *Romeo and Juliet.* See PRINCE (1).

Escalus (2) Character in *Measure for Measure,* a subordinate to the DUKE (9) of VIENNA. Escalus is a respected elder—the Duke praises the 'art and practice' of 'Old Escalus' (1.1.12, 45). He is appointed ANGELO's (2) second-in-command in the Duke's absence, and serves as his foil in the play. He consistently advocates mercy for CLAUDIO (3), in opposition to Angelo's determination to execute the young man for fornication. Though his pleas are dismissed, he continues to defend the ideal of justice tempered with mercy. On the other hand, in the comical trial scene of 2.1 Escalus represents the opposite failing of government in being too lax when he releases the pander POMPEY (1) with a warning—one for which the pimp has no respect. This produces the anomaly that a hardened promoter of prostitution goes unpunished while the honourable Claudio remains under sentence of death. Escalus contrasts with Angelo in another respect: he is true to his duty while the Duke's deputy is corrupted by his lust for ISABELLA. Though he disagrees with Angelo's severity towards Claudio, he limits his resistance to argument and makes no effort to forestall the decision of his superior officer. The Duke recognises his devotion to duty at the play's close. Escalus' chief function is to serve as a symbol of both dutiful submission and kindness.

Escanes Minor character in *Pericles,* a lord of TYRE. Escanes appears with PERICLES' deputy, HELICANUS, in 1.3 and 2.4—mute in the former scene and speaking two short lines in the latter. In 4.4.13–16 he is said to be governing Tyre while Pericles and Helicanus are abroad. His presence adds dignity to Helicanus, for whom he serves as a retinue.

Eschenburg, Johann Joachim (1743–1820) German scholar. Eschenburg translated all of Shakespeare's plays into German prose. Based in part on the translations of C. M. WIELAND, Eschenburg's edition (1775–1782) was the first complete rendering of the plays in German. It dominated German Shakespeare studies until it was superseded by the verse versions of A. W. von SCHLEGEL in the early 19th century.

Essex (1), Geoffrey FitzPeter (d. 1213) Historical figure and minor character in *King John,* follower of King JOHN (3). Essex appears only in 1.1 and has only one short speech. Textual scholars speculate that Essex' lines were assigned to Lord BIGOT—perhaps in 1601, after the failed rebellion of the later Earl of ESSEX (2)—and that this alteration was overlooked in the one speech in the FIRST FOLIO text. The historical Essex, no relation to Shakespeare's contemporary, had been named an earl by John and remained a loyal follower of the King.

Essex (2), Robert Devereux, Earl of (1566–1601) English aristocrat, a major political figure in Elizabethan England and a close friend of Shakespeare's patron, the Earl of SOUTHAMPTON (2). Essex, long a favourite of Queen ELIZABETH (1), attempted to raise a rebellion against the queen on February 8, 1601. It failed miserably, and Essex was executed in March. The day before the scheduled uprising, Essex's followers hired Shakespeare's acting company, the CHAMBERLAIN'S MEN, to stage a performance of *Richard II,* apparently with the hope that the depiction of a sovereign's deposition might inspire backing among the citizens of LONDON. After Essex's defeat, the company had to send a representative to explain themselves, but they were exonerated and in fact performed for the queen the day before Essex's execution.

Essex succeeded his stepfather, the Earl of LEICESTER, as the queen's closest courtier, and probably was her lover. He fought in the Netherlands in 1589–1590 alongside Philip SIDNEY, whose widow he married on his return. The queen was angry, but she eventually forgave Essex, and he was again in favour. He became involved in the factional politics of the court, emerging as the chief rival of Lord BURGHLEY. Among his

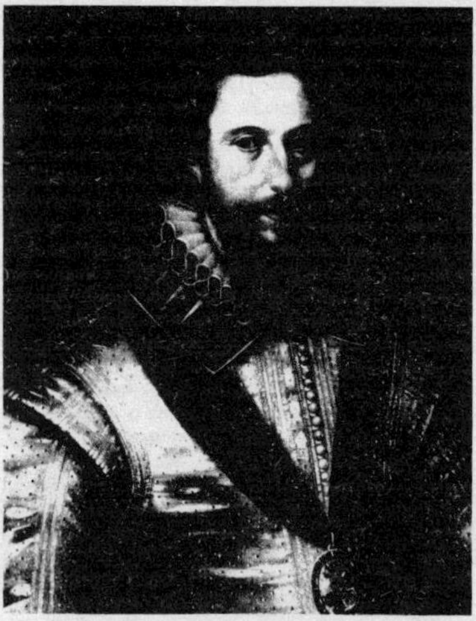

The Earl of Essex was one of the most compelling figures of Shakespeare's time. A daring military victory at Cadiz led to his becoming a national hero and the favourite of Queen Elizabeth. But political intrigues led to his downfall. He was tried and executed for treason in 1601, with Elizabeth herself signing the death warrant. (Courtesy of National Portrait Gallery, London)

enemies was Sir Walter RALEIGH, and it is thought that the many now-incomprehensible inside jokes that stud *Love's Labour's Lost* may have been intended as a satire on Raleigh's circle, on behalf of Essex and Southampton. In 1596 Essex achieved his greatest success, leading, with Charles HOWARD, a successful raid on the Spanish port of Cadiz. Nevertheless, his relations with the queen deteriorated to the point where his rudeness caused her to strike him, and he drew his sword in anger. Another reconciliation took place, and he was given command of a military expedition to put down a revolt in Ireland in 1599.

At this point, probably because Shakespeare's patron was Essex's close friend and political ally, the playwright alluded to Essex flatteringly in a play, one of the few times that contemporary political affairs are noticed at all in the plays. In *Henry V*, written just as Essex left for Ireland, the CHORUS (3) suggests that the audience envision HENRY V's triumphant return to England as though it were that of 'the general of our gracious empress, / . . . from Ireland coming, / Bringing rebellion broached on his sword' (5.Chorus.30–32). However, Essex failed in Ireland; apparently gripped by inertia, he was unable to conquer the rebels and he made a treaty that England regarded as shameful. He returned before he was ordered, in September 1599, and the angry queen arrested him. Eventually, a board of inquiry ordered him deprived of his titles. His rebellion was his last hope, so he attempted to raise the city of London against the government, but found no support, and after one day of minor skirmishing, he surrendered.

Euphronius Character in *Antony and Cleopatra*. See AMBASSADOR (3).

Evans (1), Edith (1888–1976) British actress. One of the most acclaimed actresses of the 20th century, Dame Edith Evans played a great range of parts in plays of all sorts. She made her stage debut in 1912 as CRESSIDA in the first recorded production of the complete text of *Troilus and Cressida*. She eventually portrayed most of Shakespeare's comedic heroines, as well as the NURSE (3) in *Romeo and Juliet*. She was also successful in tragic roles, playing such differing characters as CLEOPATRA, VOLUMNIA, and Queen KATHERINE of Aragon.

Evans (2), Henry (active 1583–1612) Welsh-born LONDON theatrical entrepreneur. In 1583–1584 Evans was a partner with William HUNNIS, master of the Children of the Chapel (see CHILDREN'S COMPANIES), in productions staged at the original BLACKFRIARS THEATRE. Beginning in 1584 Evans was also associated with a boys' company patronised by the Earl of OXFORD (1). In 1600 he joined Nathaniel GILES, the new master of the Children of the Chapel, and they produced plays at the revived Blackfriars, which Evans leased from Richard BURBAGE (3). However, in 1602 Evans and Giles were accused of graft and other improprieties. Evans fled the country. He returned in 1603 after the accession of King JAMES I. He then joined Edward KIRKHAM as director of the successor to the Children of the Chapel, the Children of the Queen's Revels. They again performed at Blackfriars, which Evans continued to lease from Burbage. However, the company lost its royal patronage when it performed allegedly seditious plays, and Evans surrendered the lease of the theatre to Burbage and the KING'S MEN in 1608, though a Thomas Evans, believed to be Henry Evans' representative, retained a one-seventh interest in the proceeds of the theatre. Events of Evans' later life are unknown, though in 1611–1612 he was the subject of several lawsuits filed by his one-time partner Kirkham.

Evans (3), Sir Hugh Character in *The Merry Wives of Windsor*, a Welsh clergyman and schoolmaster. A peaceable busybody, Evans is distinguished by his heavy Welsh accent—FALSTAFF says he 'makes fritters of English' (5.5.144). In 1.1 he volunteers to form a

committee to settle a dispute between Falstaff and SHALLOW, and he repeatedly tries to allay the irrational jealousy of Master FORD (1). When he attempts to promote SLENDER's marriage to ANNE (3), he is challenged to a duel by Dr CAIUS (2). The clergyman is daunted by this prospect, describing himself as 'full of . . . trempling of mind' (3.1.11–12). To calm himself, he sings a popular Elizabethan love SONG (with words by Christopher MARLOWE [1]), comically borrowing a line from the Bible. The HOST (2) defuses the duel by sending the two men to different rendezvous. To preserve his honour, Evans proposes an alliance with Caius against the Host, claiming that they have been made fools of. They later are apparently responsible for the theft of the Host's horses.

Evans also figures in the famous 'Latin scene' (4.1), in which he quizzes young WILLIAM (1) on his Latin lessons. In lines that parody the standard Latin textbook of Shakespeare's day, LILY's *Latin Grammar,* Evans' accent and Mistress QUICKLY's capacity for misunderstanding join to make fritters of Latin. The scene is full of double entendres and bilingual puns, presumably intended especially for the educated audience for whom the play was originally written. The episode may also reflect Shakespeare's own memories of childhood: he learned Latin from Lily's *Grammar* at school in STRATFORD, where he probably had a teacher of Welsh ancestry, Thomas JENKINS.

Evans was popular with London theatre-goers of the late 16th century; when *The Merry Wives* was first published, in 1600, he figured in the subtitle—as 'Syr Hugh the Welch Knight'—for it was thought that his name would attract buyers. Shakespeare was plainly aware of the popular English stereotype of the Welsh as stubbornly foreign and naturally given to music and theft. Also, along with the interest in WALES (1) demonstrated in several other works, especially *1 Henry IV* and *Henry V,* the character of Evans probably indicates that Shakespeare's acting company included one or more Welshmen in the late 1590s.

Evans (4), Maurice (1901–1989) Anglo-American actor, one of the leading Shakespearean performers of the 1930s and 1940s. Though born in England, Evans acted in America for much of his career and became a citizen of the United States in 1941. As a member of the armed forces, he organised entertainment for troops and toured the Pacific in an abridged version of *Hamlet* that he later staged in America as well. Having achieved great acclaim as HAMLET in 1938—in the play's first full-length staging in America, produced by himself and directed by Margaret Webster—Evans was particularly associated with the part. Other notable roles included ROMEO, opposite Katharine CORNELL, RICHARD II in the Margaret Webster production of 1937, and FALSTAFF in her 1939 *1 Henry IV.* In 1962 Evans performed with Helen Hayes in 'Shakespeare Revisited', a programme of excerpts from the plays that was staged in 69 American cities. He also starred in TELEVISION productions of *Hamlet, Richard II,* and *Macbeth.*

Executioner (1) Minor character in *The Comedy of Errors,* the ax man prepared to behead EGEON. The Executioner, who does not speak, appears in 5.1 in the entourage of DUKE (8) Solinus. His presence attests to Egeon's desperate plight.

Executioner (2) Any of two or more minor characters in *King John,* HUBERT's assistants in the preparations to blind ARTHUR. Before Hubert dismisses the Executioners, one of them, the First Executioner, voices the distaste with which these hardened men view the prospect of practising their profession on a boy. His qualms heighten the pathos of the scene.

Executioner (3) Minor character in *The Two Noble Kinsmen,* the ax man prepared to behead PALAMON. The executioner does not speak as he stands ready in 5.4; his presence merely serves to heighten the tension with a visible reminder of Palamon's apparent end, before a pardon arrives.

Exeter (1), Henry Holland, Duke of (1430–1473) Historical figure and minor character in *3 Henry VI,* a supporter of King HENRY VI and Queen MARGARET (1). Exeter acknowledges the claim to rule of the Duke of YORK (8) in 1.1, but he remains loyal to Henry. This may represent a slip by the playwright, or it may be a subtle reminder of the difficulty of the issue for the participants.

Exeter (2), Thomas Beaufort, Duke of (1337–1427) Historical figure and character in *1 Henry VI* and *Henry V,* illegitimate son of John of GAUNT and younger brother of the Bishop of WINCHESTER (1). In *1 Henry VI* Exeter speaks of his position as the 'special governor' (1.1.171) of the infant King HENRY VI, which reflects his historical appointment, under the will of HENRY V, as the new King's tutor. Although the historical Exeter died a few years thereafter, before most of the events of the play, Shakespeare kept him alive to function as a periodic commentator on the action, like a Greek CHORUS (1), predicting disaster for the feuding English. For instance, he closes 3.1 with a grim forecast of the WARS OF THE ROSES, hoping that his own 'days may finish ere that hapless time' (3.1.189–201).

In *Henry V,* set a decade earlier, Exeter is a valued follower of his nephew the King, but he has no distinctive personality. He bears a boldly defiant message from Henry to the FRENCH KING and the DAUPHIN (3) in 2.4, and in 4.6 he recounts the death of the Duke

of YORK (5) at AGINCOURT, in tones reminiscent of courtly epic poetry. Thus Exeter's formulaic speeches help to maintain a distinctive tone in both plays.

The historical Exeter, though born a bastard, was granted princely titles and incomes even before being legitimised by his father at the age of 40. He was an important military commander under both HENRY IV and Henry V, and he was named an executor of the latter's will. As in *Henry V*, 3.3.51–54, Exeter was made Governor of HARFLEUR after its capture by Henry, though it is unclear whether or not he fought at Agincourt. He was not named Duke of Exeter until after most of the events of *Henry V;* Shakespeare took this minor inaccuracy from HOLINSHED's *Chronicles.*

Exton, Sir Piers (Pierce) Character in *Richard II,* the murderer of RICHARD II. Exton, an ambitious nobleman who wishes to curry favour with BOLINGBROKE (1), the new king, decides in 5.4 that he will murder the old one, believing that Bolingbroke has expressed a desire that this deed be done. In 5.5 Exton leads a gang of hired murderers against Richard in his cell at POMFRET CASTLE, and they kill the ex-king, although Exton suffers pangs of conscience. He presents the corpse to Bolingbroke, now HENRY IV, hoping for a reward, but the king rejects him.

Shakespeare took the account of Exton's deed from his chief source, HOLINSHED, but the anonymous French author of Holinshed's source, probably a member of QUEEN (13) Isabel's household, apparently invented the story. No other early source mentions Exton or supposes that Richard died violently; the only other contemporary chronicler asserts that Richard was starved to death, either by his gaolers or by his own will. This source, also French, has its own propagandistic bias, and Richard may well have died of natural causes. His skeleton was exhumed and examined in the 1870s, and no evidence of violence was found.

We cannot say conclusively how the ex-king died, but, in any case, Henry IV's rejection of the murderer appears to be Shakespeare's own addition to the tale, possibly in anticipation of the opening of *1 Henry IV.* A similar story concerning Thomas à Becket and Henry II was only one of several apocryphal anecdotes that might have served the playwright as a model; an account in PLUTARCH was another.

F

Fabian Character in *Twelfth Night,* member of OLIVIA's household and friend of SIR TOBY and MARIA (2). Fabian joins Sir Toby, SIR ANDREW, and Maria (2) in their plot to embarrass MALVOLIO, Olivia's steward. He shares their zest for good times and, like them, represents the spirit of fun that triumphs over Malvolio's stiff ill humour. In his final speech (5.1.354–367) he distinguishes himself as a peacemaker and diplomat, elevating the tone of the comic SUB-PLOT.

As their scheme unfolds and the conspirators observe Malvolio envisioning himself as Olivia's husband, Fabian restrains an outraged Sir Toby from assaulting their victim, saying, 'Nay, patience, or we break the sinews of our plot' (2.5.75–76). He later assists Sir Toby in his practical joke against Sir Andrew, who is manoeuvred into a duel with Cesario (the disguised VIOLA) and shows himself a coward. Fabian's wit and common sense give him an ironic detachment, and in 5.1 he comes into his own, first reading Malvolio's letter (5.1.301–310) and then, more significantly, when quick-wittedly protecting Maria when her forging of Olivia's handwriting becomes evident; he blames himself and Sir Toby, whose marriage to Maria he reveals. He goes on to hope that their plotting 'may rather pluck on laughter than revenge' (5.1.365), forestalling Malvolio's aggrieved cry for vengeance and pointing to the reconciliation that follows.

Fabian's social position is unclear. He seems to be a servant when Olivia addresses him as 'sirrah' (5.1.300), yet he can refer casually to Olivia's kinsman, Sir Toby, as 'Toby' (5.1.358). Shakespeare may have pictured him as a flippant servant or as an impoverished gentleman, dependent on the charity of a wealthy relative or other connection, such as commonly lived in aristocratic households of the 16th and 17th centuries.

Fabyan, Robert (d. 1513) English historian, author of a source for Shakespeare's HISTORY PLAYS. Fabyan, a wealthy merchant, assembled a history book by combining miscellaneous works by earlier writers in his posthumously published *New Chronicle of England and of France* (1516). It has very little historical value, but it includes, at its close, an account of the London of his own times that is of interest to scholars of Tudor England. His chronicle was consulted by Shakespeare, particularly when he wrote *1 Henry VI.*

Fair Copy In textual studies, an amended manuscript of a play prepared for a printer or a theatrical company, usually by a professional scribe. No original Shakespearean manuscript exists (except, probably, three pages of SIR THOMAS MORE), but scholars can determine from what sort of copy the printers of an early edition set their type—whether from a manuscript or an earlier printing, and if from a manuscript, whether fair copy or FOUL PAPERS (the author's uncorrected manuscript). Modern editors can determine from such information how closely a given printed text represents what Shakespeare actually wrote.

If the printers used fair copy as their source, the published text is likely to contain many of the characteristic signs of a copyist's work: uniformity of proper names in speech headings and stage directions, consistent spelling, and edited colloquialisms or contractions. This last feature, editorial intervention, is often identified by a resulting metrical defect. For instance 'Before the game's afoot thou still let'st slip' (*1 Henry IV,* 1.3.272) is a pentameter line (see METRE) as it appears in the early QUARTO editions of the play; someone, however, changed 'game's' to 'game is' in the fair copy from which the FIRST FOLIO edition was printed, and the resulting line does not scan properly. This item alone would mean very little, but numerous such instances indicate that the Quarto edition of *1 Henry IV* presents Shakespeare's foul papers and the Folio the fair copy. Modern editors are therefore inclined to favour the Quarto version over the Folio text when they conflict because it was probably printed from Shakespeare's actual manuscript, rather than a copy.

Fair Em Anonymous play formerly attributed to Shakespeare, part of the Shakespeare APOCRYPHA. *Fair Em* is a romantic comedy set in the time of William the Conqueror. It was published in 1593 by an unknown publisher who declared that the play had been acted by STRANGE'S MEN, by whom the young Shakespeare was probably employed. Though the play was included with MUCEDORUS and THE MERRY DEVIL OF EDMONTON in King Charles II's specially assembled col-

lection of Shakespeare's plays, the 19th-century scholar Richard SIMPSON was the chief supporter of the theory that *Fair Em* was written by Shakespeare. Simpson argued that the comedy was a retort to the 1592 attack upon the playwright by Robert GREENE (2). Modern scholars unanimously reject this idea, for aside from the convoluted quality of Simpson's argument, it fails to address the considerable difference between *Fair Em* and Shakespeare's known works. The anonymous comedy is an extremely feeble play that lacks wit or poetry of any quality and contains only the crudest of characters and two almost totally unrelated plots.

Fairy Any of several minor characters in *A Midsummer Night's Dream,* attendants of TITANIA and Oberon. In 2.1 a nameless Fairy encounters PUCK, and their conversation establishes the nature of the quarrel between Titania and OBERON. In 2.2 Titania is accompanied by several Fairies, who sing her to sleep. Other Fairies in the play are COBWEB, MOTH (2), MUSTARDSEED, PEASEBLOSSOM, and Puck.

Falconbridge (1) (Faulconbridge) Any of several characters in *King John.* See BASTARD (1); LADY (5); ROBERT.

Falconbridge (2) (Fauconberg, Faulconbridge), William Neville, Lord (d. 1463) Historical figure mentioned in *3 Henry VI,* sometimes assigned the lines of the Marquess of MONTAGUE (3) in Act 1. Montague's assertions of kinship with EDWARD (3) would make more sense if spoken by Falconbridge, who was Edward's brother-in-law. His connection with the sea, at 1.1.216, also applies better to Falconbridge, who was at the time a military commander responsible for the English Channel defenses, as is mentioned 30 lines later. It is supposed that Falconbridge was deleted and his lines reassigned, possibly before any performances were given, as an economy measure for the production.

False Folio Collection of 10 pirated or spurious plays published as Shakespeare's in 1619. William and Isaac JAGGARD and Thomas PAVIER produced a group of QUARTO editions of plays attributed to Shakespeare, though only a few were proper texts of Shakespeare's plays. (Though not in FOLIO format, they are named by analogy with the earliest legitimate collection of Shakespearean plays, the FIRST FOLIO.) Two of the False Folio's offerings, A YORKSHIRE TRAGEDY and *Part 1* of SIR JOHN OLDCASTLE, were not by Shakespeare at all, and six more were BAD QUARTOS of Shakespearean plays *(2* and *3 Henry VI* [see WHOLE CONTENTION], *Henry V, The Merry Wives of Windsor, King Lear,* and *Pericles).* The publishers held the rights to only one of the two respectable texts, that of *A Midsummer Night's Dream,* which had been bought by Jaggard as part of his purchase of James ROBERTS' company in 1608. The rights to the other, *The Merchant of Venice,* were held by Laurence HEYES, who protested to the STATIONERS' COMPANY, as did the Lord Chamberlain at the time, Lord PEMBROKE (3), who spoke on behalf of the KING'S MEN. The publishers responded by backdating the unprinted titles (only three had been issued) so that they could pass for the original editions. However, they were printed in a distinctive format, slightly taller than a standard quarto, on paper with the same watermark, and bibliographical scholars have no difficulty identifying these pirated editions. While the publishers seem blatantly dishonest by modern standards, in the world of 17th-century publishing, their behaviour was not particularly unscrupulous and it did not prevent the Jaggards from joining the syndicate that published the First Folio a few years later.

Falstaff, Sir John Character in *1* and *2 Henry IV* and *The Merry Wives of Windsor.* Falstaff—physically huge, stunningly amoral, and outrageously funny—is generally regarded as one of the greatest characters in English literature. Lecherous, gluttonous, obese, cowardly, and a thief, he lies to the world but is honest with himself. His monumental presence, both literal and metaphoric, dominates the plays in which he appears, and he has become one of the most familiar of Shakespeare's creations, having inspired work ranging from pub signs and ceramic mugs to operas and symphonic works.

In the *Henry IV* plays Falstaff, although an entirely credible human being, also functions as a symbol of an extreme lifestyle. In *1 Henry IV* young PRINCE (6) HAL begins to come to grips with his role as the future King of England, and he is presented with strong figures who suggest modes of adulthood. Unlike Hal's father, the calculating and politically shrewd King HENRY IV, and unlike the intensely single-minded warrior HOTSPUR, Falstaff, in the free and dissolute ambience of the BOAR'S HEAD TAVERN, indulges in food, drink, and adventure, whether sexual or criminal, and rejects life's demands for courage or honour. From the beginning the Prince states his intention to reject Falstaff's world, in the famous 'reformation' speech (1.2.190–212). Still, throughout the play he is clearly delighted with his friend's bold effronteries and witty lies; at its close he promises to support Falstaff's claim to have killed Hotspur. In *Part 1* Falstaff is a decided rascal, cowardly and deceitful, but his common sense and tolerance counter the values of Hotspur and King Henry.

In *2 Henry IV* the Prince is closer to his assumption of power, and he is accordingly more remote from Falstaff. Falstaff dominates this play entirely. He is still very funny—as he puts it, 'I am not only witty in myself, but the cause that wit is in other men' (1.2.8–

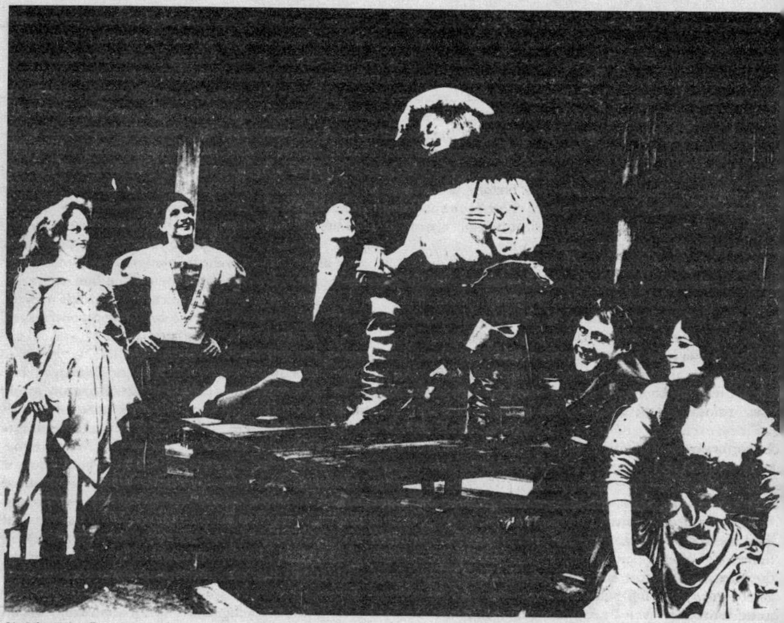

Sir John Falstaff (seated on tabletop) in a scene from a modern production of 1 Henry IV. *Shakespeare's corrupt but outrageously funny knight teaches Prince Hal things he cannot learn from more conventional role models.* (American Shakespeare Festival, Stratford, Connecticut. Photo courtesy of Billy Rose Theater Collection; New York Public Library at Lincoln Center; Astor, Lenox and Tilden Foundations)

9)—but he is presented in a significantly darker light, contributing to the play's atmosphere of disease and death. He is ill; his first words deal with a diagnosis (1.2.1), and he describes himself as sick on several occasions. He refers to his age several times, as when he doubts his attractiveness to DOLL TEARSHEET, saying, 'I am old, I am old' (2.4.268). In *Part 1* he says he is in his 50s (2.4.418–419), while in *Part 2* his acquaintance with SHALLOW is said to date from 'fifty-five year ago' (3.2.205), making him at least 70.

Most important, his misdeeds are distinctly more serious in *2 Henry IV.* In *Part 1* his extortion of bribes from draft evaders is merely reported (4.2.11–48), while we actually see it happen in *Part 2,* 3.2. Moreover, his impressed soldiers, anonymous victims in *Part 1,* take human shape in *Part 2* as such sympathetic, if minor, figures as SHADOW and FEEBLE. The recruiting scene is hilarious, but it remains on the record as evidence of Falstaff's criminality. In fact, the episode was clearly intended as a satirical condemnation of a real practice that plagued the English poor in Shakespeare's time. Perhaps Falstaff's most serious offence is his selfish exploitation of his friends. He promises love but instead bleeds money from his loyal admirer the HOSTESS (2), as she herself describes in 2.1.84–101. The preposterous Shallow is a natural victim, but Falstaff's cynical rationale for fleecing him—'If the young dace be a bait for the old pike, I see no reason in the law of nature but I may snap at him' (3.2.325–326)—is, however wittily put, morally repugnant.

Hal is distant and hostile to Falstaff when they meet in 2.4, and when the knight seeks to profit from Hal's succession to the crown, the new king forbids his presence. Hal is cold and forceful—although he mercifully provides his former friend with a generous pension—and Falstaff's fall seems abrupt, although it has been prepared for throughout both plays. The needs of the greater, political and military world of Prince Hal triumph in the end.

Still, however fully one may endorse Prince Hal's rejection of Falstaff (and many people do not accept it at all), the fat knight remains a generally sympathetic figure. If his misdeeds would be offensive in real life, they are frequently delightful on stage. He deflates pretension with the needle of his satire, and he counters excessive rigour with his entertainingly flexible morals. His combination of grandiose rhetoric, penetrating wit, and common sense shines in such virtuoso passages of comic monologue as his battlefield rejection of courage (*1 Henry IV*, 5.4.110–120)—leading to a particularly outrageous gesture, the stabbing of Hotspur's corpse—and his tribute to wine (*2 Henry IV*, 4.3.85–123), long acclaimed as one of the most delectable discourses in English literature. In the plays' tavern scenes (2.4 in each) he is uproarious and hearty. His ceaseless flow of parody and imitation evokes a wide and enjoyable range of personages from aristocrats to highwaymen.

Falstaff is a figure of immense psychological resonance; through him we can enjoy our own fantasies of life without responsibilities. When it seems he can offer no excuse for some misdeed and must surely be brought down, like the rest of us, he devises some extravagant lie or joke and escapes. His vitality seems limitless; as he puts it himself, 'banish plump Jack, and banish all the world' (*1 Henry IV*, 2.4.473–474). However, Falstaff *is* banished, for he also represents amoral disloyalty, criminal exploitation, and weak social values. Less sternly, he is often compared to springlike weather in autumn (e.g., in *1 Henry IV*, 1.1.154–155, and *2 Henry IV*, 2.2.112), a common metaphor for youthful energy in old age. The fat knight clearly reflects Shakespeare's fond appreciation of tavern life and its pleasurable delinquencies, but one of the values most important to the playwright—as is especially plain in the HISTORY PLAYS—was the maintenance of social order. Thus Falstaff is repudiated in no uncertain terms, both in the *Henry IV* plays and in *The Merry Wives*.

Part of Falstaff's humour lies in his burlesque of the chivalric values of the aristocracy, and part of his vital force in his energetic individuality. These traits lead many modern readers to think of the *Henry IV* plays as ironical satires of war and government and of Falstaff's rejection as proof that human authenticity is tragically at odds with the practice of politics. However, this ascribes to Shakespeare the views of our own age, when the worth of the individual is placed above that of traditional societal values. But in earlier times Falstaff was held to be flatly villainous. The first great Shakespearean editor, Nicholas ROWE, called him 'a Thief, Lying, Cowardly, Vainglorious, and in short every way vicious' in his 1709 edition of the plays. A little later, Samuel JOHNSON (7) wrote that Falstaff 'has nothing in him that can be esteemed'. Although Shakespeare himself was surely less critical of his creation, he certainly would have understood their point of view. In the RENAISSANCE the potential of the individual was beginning to be recognised, as Shakespeare's interest in and respect for human psychology exemplify, but the ancient, biblically sanctioned, hierarchical society of medieval Europe is persistently championed in the plays, as well as in other works of Elizabethan literature. Therefore, necessity—that national order be restored after a civil war—demands the rejection of the thoughtless pleasures and the irresponsibility that Falstaff displays.

Falstaff's popularity on the Elizabethan stage prompted Shakespeare to announce, in the EPILOGUE to *2 Henry IV*, that the fat knight would appear in another play. However, he does not appear in *Henry V*, although he may have been a character in a lost, probably unacted version of that play. A number of textual peculiarities make it clear that *Henry V* was altered after it was first written; most strikingly, PISTOL takes on Falstaffian characteristics in several passages. Following his humiliation in 5.1, he speaks of growing old and of losing Doll Tearsheet, lines that are plainly more appropriate to Falstaff. Also, Pistol's capture of the FRENCH SOLDIER parallels Falstaff's comic achievements in *1* and *2 Henry IV*. Scholars speculate that, in an original draft of the play, Falstaff was the chief comic character, that he was deleted by the playwright—for it appears that the present version of the play derives from Shakespeare's manuscript—and that much of his part was transferred to Pistol. This theory cannot be proven, but it does explain the textual evidence.

Why would Shakespeare have eliminated Falstaff? Two answers present themselves. The first supposes that the controversy surrounding Falstaff's original name, OLDCASTLE, was still current and that pressure from the son of Lord COBHAM necessitated another change, finally ending the enmity of a powerful aristocrat towards the CHAMBERLAIN'S .EN, Shakespeare's company. However, Shakespeare may simply have thought better of resurrecting his mammoth exemplar of immorality in a play that is dedicated to the English triumph at AGINCOURT. Falstaff had already been rejected on well-established grounds, and his powerful presence may have seemed too distracting from the patriotic themes of *Henry V*.

However, the fat knight's death is described in *Henry V*, 2.3, by Pistol, the Hostess, BARDOLPH (1), and NYM, and their affection for him reflects the playwright's. When Bardolph wishes he were with Falstaff 'wheresome'er he is, either in heaven or in Hell!' (2.3.7–8), the Hostess asserts that he is surely in heaven; she goes on to describe his death-bed touchingly: '. . . after I saw him fumble with the sheets and play with flowers and smile upon his fingers' end, I knew there was but one way; for his nose was as sharp as a pen, and a' babbled of green fields . . . a' cried out "God, God,

God!" three or four times . . .' (2.3.14–20). Thus Falstaff's humanly believable end summons our sympathy one last time for the knight who had 'more flesh than another man, and therefore more frailty' (*1 Henry IV*, 3.3.167–168).

The Merry Wives of Windsor was written before *Henry V*, probably during the creation of *2 Henry IV*, and here Falstaff is a less complex figure than the giant of the *Henry IV* plays. His function is more purely comic and stands at the centre of the play rather than in contrast to the realities of history. He is more nearly a traditional character type, the comic villain whose downfall is obvious from the outset. He is also associated with another type, the foolish and boastful would-be lady's man, although in attempting to seduce the wives to get at their husbands' money, Falstaff is not erotically inclined. However, he is thereby linked with the familiar theme of the jealous husband, and the sexual side of his story links him with the sub-plots centred on the courting of ANNE (3) Page.

The complications caused by Falstaff's greedy impulses lead him to receive a humorous retribution and then forgiveness. His personality has not changed—he is still brassy, shrewd, and amorally selfish—but the resourceful prankster and brazen reprobate of the *Henry IV* plays no longer has the initiative. He is easily tricked by the wives, not once but three times. This is sometimes regarded as an unfortunate trivialisation of a great character, but it may also be argued that Falstaff's lesser magnitude in *The Merry Wives* suits his simpler function as a comic butt. In the world of Prince Hal, Falstaff was a shrewd courtier in addition to his other roles, and he never forgot his status—indeed, several of his fantastic excuses for his misbehaviour refer to the exalted position of the Prince. In Windsor he assumes regal attitudes: he tyrannically bullies Pistol and Nym, and he attempts to lord it over the townspeople. His changed behaviour—in addition to demonstrating Shakespeare's acute perception of social relations—makes Falstaff an entirely appropriate target for a comic comeuppance.

This aspect of the character is particularly evident in Falstaff's apologetic confession following his final humiliation (5.5.122–129)—often seen, in its 'un-Falstaffian' quality as evidence of a lost source play. However, in the masquelike finale, where none of the characters present their ordinary characteristics, symbolic expression is given to the play's implicit moral—the triumph of domesticity. Here, then, Falstaff makes the formal surrender that his status as a traditional comic butt requires.

In this respect, Falstaff has been seen as a representation of an ancient fertility spirit in a tradition that in the playwright's time was still alive in remote regions of Britain and was still generally understood. As such, his figurative role was that of the sacrificial victim punished for the sins of society in ancient religious practices. This image need not be taken literally to see that the Falstaff of *The Merry Wives* is identified with common human foibles.

Indeed, Falstaff has the same function in the *Henry IV* plays as well. He moves us, in a way that Hal or Hotspur or Anne Page cannot, because, like him, we all often feel irresponsible, dishonest, selfish inclinations. We know that Falstaff is part of us, like it or not. In the *Henry IV* plays he represents a childish, self-centred universe of pleasure that adults are doomed to leave and that is defeated by a harsh and demanding political ideal, insistent on duty and order. In *The Merry Wives* Falstaff is again opposed by a triumphant principle, in this case the world of domestic security. In both cases, he embodies the need of each of us to rebel against the constraints of society and thus find our individual potential, and his defeat symbolises the need to sublimate that rebellion in light of our innate dependence on each other.

In his first appearance, Hal excuses Falstaff from even an awareness of time, 'unless hours were cups of sack, and minutes capons, and clocks the tongues of bawds, and dials the signs of leaping-houses, and the blessed sun himself a fair hot wench in flame-coloured taffeta' (*1 Henry IV*, 1.2.7–10). The essential nature of Falstaff's personality is revealed in this passage, for the thrust of his wit, and of his life, is to elaborate this fantasy and to defend it against the demands of reality. We delight in the brilliant energy of his efforts, and we mourn the impossibility of their success.

Falstaffe (Falstaff), Sir John Name given to Sir John FASTOLFE in some editions of *1 Henry VI*.

Famous Victories, The Abbreviated title commonly used for *The Famous Victories of Henry the Fifth*, an anonymous late 16th-century play that was an important source for *1* and *2 Henry IV* and a minor one for *Henry V*. *The Famous Victories* is a farce in two parts, the first of which concerns the adventures of PRINCE (6) HAL before he accedes to the throne and the second of which covers his reign as HENRY V.

There are numerous resemblances between the farce and Shakespeare's plays, including appearances by GADSHILL, POINS, the CHIEF JUSTICE, Princess KATHARINE (2) of France, and Sir John OLDCASTLE, which was the original name of FALSTAFF in *1* and *2 Henry IV*. Many of the incidents in *1* and *2 Henry IV* also occur in the *Famous Victories*, though they are presented very crudely by comparison. Such similarities make it clear that Shakespeare used *The Famous Victories* as a source, but he made major alterations, quite aside from his integration of its farcical material with another, more serious plot line. The Prince in the *Famous Victories* is simply a hooligan, wishing his father dead and roaring drunkenly about the stage. Shakespeare's Hal is a reflective young man who states early in *1 Henry IV* his

intention to reform, and his participation in Falstaff's highway robbery is limited to stealing from the thieves. He is generally intent on affairs of state in *2 Henry IV*, his mischief extending only to disguising himself as a DRAWER in 2.4. Oldcastle is an insignificant character who bears little resemblance to his successor. And in *Henry V* King Henry's wooing of Princess Katharine in 5.2 was developed from a similar but less elaborate scene in *The Famous Victories*, which otherwise provided only a few minor details.

The only surviving version of *The Famous Victories* was published in 1598; it is clearly a 'memorial' version of the play, a BAD QUARTO assembled from the recollections of actors. It is a very poor text, commonly judged to be unactable, and it is generally presumed that Shakespeare knew a superior version, perhaps a publication recorded in 1594 that is now lost. However, some scholars hold that *The Famous Victories*, along with Shakespeare's plays, derives from an earlier play on the same subject (perhaps the one published in 1594, perhaps one that Shakespeare himself wrote earlier in his career).

Fang Minor character in *2 Henry IV*, a constable who attempts to arrest FALSTAFF for debt. In 2.1 the HOSTESS (2) employs Fang and his assistant, SNARE, to arrest the fat knight, but when Falstaff and his companion, BARDOLPH (1), draw their swords, the officers are helpless. The CHIEF JUSTICE appears and resolves the situation without their assistance. Fang's name, which in Elizabethan English meant 'snare' or 'trap', is appropriate to his function, if not to his abilities.

Farce A play, usually short, that has no purpose but to generate laughter in the audience. A form of COMEDY, it uses artificial situations, unrealistic plots, and physical humour rather than wit to achieve its end. Common plot components include mistaken identity, overheard information, accidental encounters, reunions of long-separated people, and extraordinary coincidences. Characterisation, meaningful plotting, or any intellectual elements are eschewed. Farce has been widely popular from ancient times to the present. None of Shakespeare's plays is properly called a farce, though *The Comedy of Errors* is very like one but contains additional elements.

Farrant, Richard (d. 1580) English composer and theatrical entrepreneur, founder of the first BLACKFRIARS THEATRE. In 1564 Farrant, a court musician, became director of the Children of Windsor, a boys' choir in the service of Queen ELIZABETH (1). The boys also performed plays (see CHILDREN'S COMPANIES), and in 1576, when Farrant became the deputy of William HUNNIS, director of the similar Children of the Chapel, he was assigned responsibility for the productions of the combined companies. He accordingly leased rooms in the defunct BLACKFRIARS PRIORY and staged plays there, in what became known as the original Blackfriars Theatre. Farrant, who was also the queen's organist, composed church music, some of which is still performed, and may also have composed music for the boys' plays.

Fastolfe, Sir John (c. 1378–1459) Historical figure and character in *1 Henry VI*, an English officer in the HUNDRED YEARS WAR. In the play Fastolfe is depicted as a cowardly soldier whose hasty retreats cause great losses to the English. His retreat at Patay, near ORLÉANS, was recorded in the chronicles that were Shakespeare's sources, but the playwright magnified this single event in order to create a striking contrast to the heroism of the play's most important figure, TALBOT. The defeat at Patay is reported in 1.1 by a MESSENGER (3), who says that Fastolfe has 'play'd the coward' (1.1. 131). In 1.4 Talbot describes his resultant captivity, and he rails against the 'treacherous Fastolfe' (1.4.34). Fastolfe first appears on stage in 3.2; he is fleeing ignominiously during the assault on ROUEN, an entirely fictitious episode. Asked whether he is abandoning Talbot, Fastolfe replies, 'Ay, all the Talbots in the world, to save my life' (3.2.108). Finally, in 4.1, Talbot angrily tears the Order of the Garter from Fastolfe's leg, describing again the action at Patay. The king promptly banishes the coward, who departs in silence.

The historical Fastolfe had a very different career. The incident at Patay, which did not result in Talbot's captivity, is viewed by modern historians as having been chiefly due to bad generalship by Shakespeare's hero, necessitating a sensible withdrawal by Fastolfe, his fellow commander. The Duke of BEDFORD (1) seems to have been most upset by the episode; it is he, not Talbot, who stripped Fastolfe of his Garter (temporarily and probably without authority) while an investigation was conducted at Talbot's request. The investigators exonerated Fastolfe completely, and he went on to complete a distinguished career as a general and diplomat.

The only early text of *1 Henry VI*, that in the FIRST FOLIO of 1623, names this character Falstaffe. Subsequent editors, however, generally have used the historical figure's correct name, thereby avoiding confusion with Shakespeare's great comedic figure FALSTAFF.

Father That Hath Killed His Son, The Minor but significant character in *3 Henry VI*, a participant in the battle of TOWTON in 2.5. The Father, a soldier, prepares to loot the corpse of an enemy he has killed, when he discovers that the body is that of his own son. He mourns for himself and for the times: 'O, pity, God, this miserable age! / What stratagems, how fell, how butcherly, / Erroneous, mutinous, and unnatu-

ral, / This deadly quarrel daily doth beget!' (2.5.88–91).

The Father's discovery and grief are witnessed by King HENRY VI, who has withdrawn from the battle to wish despairingly that he were a rustic shepherd, rather than a combatant. This incident, along with that of the SON THAT HATH KILLED HIS FATHER, is juxtaposed ironically with Henry's pastoral musings to highlight the horrors of civil war.

Faucit, Helen (1817–1898) British actress. Faucit played most of Shakespeare's major female roles, usually opposite W. C. MACREADY, but she was particularly associated with BEATRICE and HERMIONE. She recorded her interpretations in a book, *On Some of Shakespeare's Female Characters* (1885).

Faulconbridge (1) (Falconbridge), Lady Character in *King John.* See LADY (5).

Faulconbridge (2) (Falconbridge), Philip Character in *King John.* See BASTARD (1).

Faulconbridge (3) (Falconbridge), Robert Character in *King John.* See ROBERT.

Faulconbridge (4), William Neville, Lord Character in *3 Henry VI.* See FALCONBRIDGE (2).

Feeble, Francis Minor character in *2 Henry IV,* one of the men whom FALSTAFF recruits for the army in 3.2. Feeble is selected over hardier men who bribe their way out of service, and Falstaff justifies the choice by saying that Feeble will be useful in retreat, being already inclined to run. However, Feeble is willing to fight if he has to, saying, 'I will do my good will, sir, you can have no more' (3.2.155), and '. . . he that dies this year is quit for the next' (3.2.233). Feeble gives his occupation as a 'woman's tailor', which gives rise to ribaldry: 'tailor' was Elizabethan slang for the genitals, male or female.

Fenton (1) Character in *The Merry Wives of Windsor,* suitor of ANNE (3) Page. Fenton, a conventional young romantic lead, has little personality, although we are told that he 'kept company with the wild Prince and Poins' (3.2.66–67). Anne's father, George PAGE (12), objects to Fenton on this ground and on the related one that he is too socially high-ranking to be an appropriate husband for the bourgeois maid. Moreover, Page suspects Fenton is a treasure hunter. Fenton himself admits to Anne in 4.3.12–18 that, although he has fallen in love with her since, Page's money was his original motive for courting her. Nevertheless, he compares favourably with Anne's other suitors, SLENDER and CAIUS (2), and when Anne's parents each plot to have her abducted and married by one of these misfits, her elopement with Fenton comes as a natural course of action. When Fenton announces their marriage in 5.5.216–227, her parents gracefully accept the situation in the spirit of reconciliation that closes the play.

Fenton (2), Geoffrey (c. 1540–1608) English translator, creator of a possible minor source for several of Shakespeare's plays. As a young nobleman living in Paris, Fenton wrote English versions of 13 of Matteo BANDELLO's Italian tales, working from the French translations of Pierre Boaistuau (d. 1566) and François BELLEFOREST. The resulting book, *Certaine Tragicall Discources* (1566), was very popular, and Shakespeare almost certainly knew it. He may have been influenced by it when he wrote *Hamlet, Titus Andronicus,* and *Twelfth Night,* all of which were based on tales that appear in Bandello, though which of several possible versions was used by the playwright is in each case uncertain.

Fenton translated several other French works, mostly religious in nature, including an attack on drama that was popular among English Puritans who opposed ELIZABETHAN THEATRE. He was best known in his day for his *History of the Wars of Italy* (1579), taken from French translations of the writings of the Italian political theorist Francesco Guicciardini (1483–1540). After 1580 Fenton deserted literature for a successful career as a member of the Irish colonial establishment and lived out his life in Dublin.

Fenton (3), Richard (1746–1821) English author. Fenton, a lawyer, wrote and published poetry and essays. In his *A Tour in Quest of Genealogy through several Parts of Wales* (1811), published anonymously, he claimed to have found a copy—in the handwriting of Anne HATHAWAY—of a journal kept by Shakespeare, from which he quotes a number of passages concerning the playwright's career. Though some contemporaries took this material seriously, most scholars, then and now, believe that Fenton's discovery was merely a mild hoax, intended humorously.

Ferdinand (1) Character in *Love's Labour's Lost.* See KING (19).

Ferdinand (2) Character in *The Tempest,* the lover of the magician PROSPERO's daughter, MIRANDA. Prospero arranges the match between Miranda and the son of his old enemy, King ALONSO of Naples, as part of the atmosphere of reconciliation and forgiveness with which he resolves his own exile. Prospero pretends to distrust Ferdinand and puts him to forced labour, but when the young man's love survives this trial, Prospero blesses the future marriage of the couple. Ferdinand's ardour is important to the play's scheme of things, for he and Miranda symbolise the healing value

of love. Ferdinand is accordingly a sterotypical romantic leading man, though his role is relatively small.

Ferdinand is tellingly compared with Prospero's bestial slave, CALIBAN. Miranda explicitly judges the two, in pointedly contrasting terms: Caliban is 'a thing most brutish' (1.2.358) and Ferdinand 'a thing divine' (4.1.421). Caliban has attempted to rape Miranda, but Ferdinand vows to respect her virginity until they are married. Caliban truculently resists his chore of delivering fire wood with whines and curses; Ferdinand is assigned a similar task—carrying logs—but he rejoices in the labour, for it is associated with his love. Ferdinand's mourning for his father, whom he believes drowned, is also part of the play's depiction of goodness and helps (with Alonso's similarly mistaken grief over his son) to ameliorate the king's earlier crime against Prospero.

Feste Character in *Twelfth Night*, jester, or professional FOOL (1), in the household of OLIVIA. Feste represents the play's spirit of festivity, which eventually triumphs over the steward MALVOLIO's chilly ill humour. Outside the coils of the lovers' confusions, Feste can take an ironic view of them and their world. He appears in a number of settings, the better to apply his vision to all. He frequents the courts of both Olivia and Duke ORSINO, encounters both VIOLA and SEBASTIAN (2), challenges the first appearance of Malvolio, and takes part in the revelry of SIR TOBY and SIR ANDREW. He also carries the comic SUB-PLOT to its farthest extreme, disguising himself as a curate, Sir TOPAS, and pretending to exorcise the imprisoned Malvolio. As he himself observes, 'Foolery, sir, doth walk about the orb like the sun, it shines everywhere' (3.1.39–40).

As an officially designated fool, it is Feste's duty to point out with jests and barbs the folly of those who are supposed to be wise. As Viola remarks when she meets Feste, 'This fellow is wise enough to play the fool, / . . . For folly that he wisely shows is fit; / But wise men, folly-fall'n, quite taint their wit' (3.1.61–69), and Olivia tells Malvolio, 'There is no slander in an allowed fool, though he do nothing but rail' (1.5.93–94). Feste wittily demonstrates that Olivia is foolish to mourn her brother's ascent to heaven, and her good humour is immediately restored. Although his jests are less effective against Orsino's foolish self-image as a romantic melancholic, they make the duke's mental disorder plain. Feste compares himself to Sir Andrew, saying, 'Better a witty fool than a foolish wit' (1.5.36), pointing out both Sir Andrew's limitations and his own role. He also cares for the drunken Sir Toby, observing bitingly, 'the fool shall look to the madman' (1.5.138–139).

Finally, Feste's pretended exorcism of Malvolio casts light on the steward's character. Malvolio's humourless ambition and incapacity to love are metaphorically alluded to in Feste's diagnosis: 'I say there is no darkness but ignorance, in which thou are more puzzled than the Egyptians in their fog' (4.2.43–45). The subsequent comic dialogue deals obliquely with Malvolio's underlying deficiency—his lack of concern for anyone but himself. Feste declares that Malvolio will 'remain . . . in darkness [until] thou shalt . . . fear to kill a woodcock lest thou dispossess the soul of thy grandam' (4.2.58–61).

In *Twelfth Night* Shakespeare deliberately undercut the conventions of romantic comedy; one of his techniques was to establish what has long been called 'the problem of Malvolio'; the steward's discomfiture seems out of proportion to his offence, giving rise to an uncertain response in the audience, which responds with both delight at Malvolio's comeuppance and sympathy for his victimisation. Feste's final encounter with Malvolio, upon the steward's release, contributes to this ambiguity. Here, the fool cruelly uses Malvolio's own words against him and then observes that 'the whirligig of time brings in his revenges' (5.1.375-376); while 'whirligig' is funny, 'revenges' is not.

Feste's songs are an important part of his role, illuminating different aspects of the play. In 2.3 he sings a love song for boisterous Sir Toby and Sir Andrew, and the audience shares the delight of the two knights, but the lyrics have a somewhat depressing tinge, for they advocate seizing love while one is young because 'what's to come is still unsure' (2.3.50). This observation is part of the play's disturbing undertone, as is Feste's next song, 'Come away death' (2.4.51–66), which is humorously suited to Orsino's affected sadness but is also strikingly melancholy in itself.

Feste's last song, which closes the play, offers a poignant moment. Left outside the happy ending the lovers enjoy, the fool sings a bitter ditty that sums up the play's anti-romantic secondary theme. He sings of the sorry, loveless life of a drunkard for whom, as the chorus insists, 'the rain it raineth every day' (5.1.391 et al.). These lyrics emphasise Shakespeare's ironic view of the limitations of comedy. However, this message is greatly offset by the music, and the gross exaggeration in the words makes them somewhat comical; also, the song's final stanza presents a standard EPILOGUE, asking for applause and promising that the actors will 'strive to please you every day' (5.1.407). Feste remains a generally sunny character whose darker moments serve to make him, and the play, more complex and humanly interesting.

Ffarington, William (1537–1610) Steward to Ferdinando Stanley, Lord STRANGE, and possibly a model for MALVOLIO in *Twelfth Night* and OSWALD in *King Lear*. Ffarington—whose personality and habits have been recorded in his own elaborate housekeeping accounts and elsewhere—resembled both characters to some

degree. Like Malvolio, he was noted for his severe mode of dress but was also fond of fine fabric and precious stones (see TWELFTH NIGHT, 2.5.48, 61), and he disinherited his son for refusing a financially and socially advantageous marriage, betraying an attitude suggestive of Malvolio's own matrimonial ambition. Ffarington's style of dress also is reminiscent of Oswald, castigated by KENT (2) as a vain and pretentious imitator of gentlemen in *King Lear,* 2.2.13–24. Kent also calls Oswald 'action-taking' and 'super-serviceable' (2.2.16), evoking Ffarington's noted readiness to begin a legal action and undeniable devotion to his master

Ffarington's employer was the patron of an acting company, STRANGE'S MEN, to which the young Shakespeare probably belonged. Strange's Men often visited their patron's home in Lancashire, as did other companies whose members were later Shakespeare's associates. Thus Shakespeare may have known Ffarington personally and almost certainly had at least heard of him. Ffarington was probably a singularly unpleasant figure to the travelling players, for he detested actors and the theatre, as his own accounts make clear (he commented adversely on his employer's enthusiasm). In fact, Ffarington disliked all festivities; in 1580 he attempted to suppress the local May games, a longstanding tradition.

This gentleman certainly seems a plausible target for satire. Moreover, unlike Sir Ambrose WILLOUGHBY (1) and Sir William KNOLLYS—the other chief candidates as models for Malvolio—he was not so high in the social hierarchy as to be too dangerous to satirise (both the others were valued servants of Queen ELIZABETH [1]). However, most scholars regard the true identity of the model for Shakespeare's stewards—and for most other Shakespearean characters—as ultimately unknowable.

Fidele In *Cymbeline,* the name taken by IMOGEN in her disguise as a young man. Fidele is a French name, and this contributes to the multilingual confusion of the play, a characteristic feature of Shakespeare's ROMANCES.

Field (1), Nathan (1587–1620) English actor and dramatist. Field was one of the 26 men listed in the FIRST FOLIO as the 'Principall Actors' in Shakespeare's plays. He joined the KING'S MEN in 1615 or 1616—scholars speculate that he replaced Shakespeare just before or after the playwright's death—after a long association with one of the CHILDREN'S COMPANIES and with the LADY ELIZABETH'S MEN. He was particularly noted in the title role of George CHAPMAN'S *Bussy d'Amboise.* As a playwright he collaborated with Philip MASSINGER, John FLETCHER (2), and perhaps others, and he wrote two comedies himself, along with a defence of the stage.

Field, whose Puritan father had written fiercely against the stage before his death in 1588, was recruited from the choir of a secondary school into the Children of the Chapel (later the Children of the Queen's Revels) in 1600. As a boy actor in this company Field continued his education under the tutorship of Ben JONSON, who was later to name Field and Richard BURBAGE (3) as the finest English actors. After the Children of the Revels were absorbed by the Lady Elizabeth's Men in 1613, Field became the leader of the combined company before he joined the King's Men.

Field (2), Richard (1561–1624) London printer, producer of the first several editions of *Venus and Adonis* and the first editions of *The Rape of Lucrece* and *The Phoenix and Turtle.* A native of STRATFORD whose father knew Shakespeare's father, Field is presumed to have been a friend of the playwright's. Scholars speculate that Shakespeare may have playfully referred to Field when the disguised IMOGEN claims employment with one 'Richard du Champ' (*Cymbeline* 4.2.377), i.e., 'Richard Field' in French. In 1593 Field published the young playwright's first ambitious literary undertaking, *Venus and Adonis,* in a QUARTO edition known today as Q1. He then sold the rights to this work and *Lucrece* to John HARRISON (2), who hired him to print the second, third, and fourth editions (Q2–4, 1594–1596) of *Venus and Adonis* and the first quarto (Q1, 1594) of *Lucrece.* He later printed, for publisher Edward BLOUNT, the first edition of LOVE'S MARTYR (1601), which contained *The Phoenix and Turtle.*

Field's early life in Stratford is unknown, apart from the fact that his father was a tanner. He was apprenticed to a London printer in 1579; on the death of his second master, in 1587, he took over that man's business and married his widow. He doubtless regretted the sale of the rights to *Venus and Adonis* and *Lucrece,* which became very popular, but he prospered nonetheless. Among other works, he produced the first edition of HARINGTON'S translation of *Orlando Furioso,* a 1598 edition of SIDNEY'S *Arcadia,* and several editions of NORTH'S translation of PLUTARCH.

Fiend Any of several minor characters in *1 Henry VI,* the supernatural beings that JOAN LA PUCELLE summons by means of sorcery in 5.3. Joan asks the assistance of these creatures 'cull'd / out of the powerful regions under earth' (5.3.10–11) in fighting England. However, they silently refuse, leading her to realise that all is lost. Her capture follows immediately.

Fife Region in Scotland, the setting for 4.2 of *Macbeth.* When Fife's ruler, Lord MACDUFF, betrays the usurper MACBETH and joins the rebels led by Prince MALCOLM, Macbeth sends murderers (see FIRST MURDERER [3]) to Macduff's castle where they kill his wife,

LADY (7) MACDUFF, and his SON in an episode that marks the depths of Macbeth's evil. Shakespeare took the setting from his source, Raphael HOLINSHED's history, but there is nothing in the scene that particularly denotes Fife.

Film Medium in which most of Shakespeare's plays have been produced. Many of the plays have been filmed more than once, in numerous languages. *Hamlet*, for example, has been filmed more than two dozen times. The earliest movie made from Shakespeare was of a single scene from Beerbohm TREE's stage production of *King John*, but the film has been lost. Oddly, many silent films of Shakespeare plays were made, perhaps because the medium sought respectability in its earliest days. Among the most notable directors and producers of Shakespearean films have been Grigori KOZINTSEV, Akira KUROSAWA, Laurence OLIVIER, Max REINHARDT, Orson WELLES, and Franco ZEFFIRELLI.

Fiorentino, Giovanni (active 14th century) Italian author, writer of a collection of tales that included sources for *The Merchant of Venice* and *The Merry Wives of Windsor*. Little is known of Fiorentino, whose collection of stories, *Il Pecorone (The Simpleton)*, was written in the 1370s but not published until 1558. He was a Florentine clerk, and his tales were closely modelled on the works of BOCCACCIO.

There is no known Elizabethan translation of *Il Pecarone* into English, yet Shakespeare's use of it seems extremely likely, expecially in the case of *The Merchant of Venice*. The playwright may have read the work in Italian, although his ability to do so is not certain. There may have existed an English version that has not survived, or he may have been told the relevant details by someone who had read it. In any case, his knowledge of Latin would have permitted him to struggle through the Italian, once he knew there was material there that he was interested in.

First Clown Character in *Hamlet*. See GRAVE-DIGGER.

First Commoner Character in *Julius Caesar*. See CARPENTER.

First Executioner Character in *King John*. See EXECUTIONER (2).

First Folio Earliest published collection of Shakespeare's plays, appearing in 1623. Produced in the FOLIO format, the First Folio was edited by John HEMINGE and Henry CONDELL, who had been professional associates of Shakespeare in the CHAMBERLAIN'S MEN and its successor, the KING'S MEN. The First Folio contains 36 plays, 18 of which were not otherwise published and would probably have been lost without this edition. These plays are *All's Well That Ends Well, Antony and Cleopatra, As You Like It, The Comedy of Errors, Coriolanus, Cymbeline, 3 Henry VI, Henry VIII, Julius Caesar, King John, Macbeth, Measure for Measure, The Taming of the Shrew, The Tempest, Timon of Athens, Twelfth Night, Two Gentlemen of Verona,* and *The Winter's Tale.*

The editors' intention in publishing Shakespeare's plays was also to counter the imperfect editions that did exist. Since they knew the works intimately, having worked with the playwright for most of his career, their corrections of other editions are significant to scholars, as is their selection of 36 plays. Heminge and Condell would have selected only plays they knew to have been written by Shakespeare—or at least mostly by him, in cases of collaboration. Thus, the First Folio constitutes a basic CANON of the plays. (However, the earliest part of Shakespeare's career may not have been known to them very well, and even in the case of the more mature works, while those included are almost certainly Shakespearean, the editors could have excluded plays for such reasons as defective texts, copyright problems, or CENSORSHIP.)

Besides the plays, the First Folio contains various minor elements: a title page decorated with the DROESHOUT PORTRAIT, facing a poem by Ben JONSON commending the likeness; a brief introduction by the editors, stating their purpose; a dedication to the Earls of PEMBROKE (3) and MONTGOMERY (2); verses on Shakespeare by Jonson, Hugh HOLLAND (2), Leonard DIGGES (2), and 'I.M'. (probably James MABBE); a list of 26 'Principall Actors in all these Playes'; and a table of contents. It was printed in an edition of about 1200, of which about 230 have survived. Oddly, it appears that no two copies are identical (though they have not all been collated), for proof-reading and correction went on simultaneously with printing. The process began in April 1621, but was interrupted and was not completed until December 1623.

The title page contains the information that the book was printed by Isaac JAGGARD and Edward BLOUNT. A colophon on the last page states that it was printed for William JAGGARD (Isaac's father, who died just before the book was issued), Blount, John SMETHWICK, and William ASPLEY. The members of this syndicate held copyrights to the previously published plays. Blount and Isaac Jaggard held most of them, which probably accounts for their joint listing on the title page, for Blount was not in fact a printer. Isaac Jaggard oversaw the publishing process, and Heminge and Condell may have done little more than supply Jaggard with the texts. The actual editing may have been done by Edward KNIGHT (4), the King's Men's book-keeper, who was responsible for maintaining the PROMPT-BOOK of each play.

First Grave-digger Character in *Hamlet*. See GRAVE-DIGGER.

First Lord (1) Character in *As You Like It.* See LORD (4).

First Lord (2) Character in *All's Well That Ends Well.* See LORD (6).

First Murderer (1) One of 'two or three' characters in *2 Henry VI,* the killers of the Duke of GLOUCESTER (4). Several men, two of whom speak, flee the scene of the crime at the beginning of 3.2. The First Murderer calmly accepts payment for the crime from the Duke of SUFFOLK (3), thus distinguishing himself from the SECOND MURDERER (1), who is conscience-stricken.

First Murderer (2) Character in *Richard III,* one of two hired assassins employed by RICHARD III to kill his brother the Duke of CLARENCE (1). The First Murderer coolly accepts his role as a killer, whereas the SECOND MURDERER (2) has an attack of conscience as they approach their victim in 1.4. Later in this scene, when Clarence pleads for mercy and the Second Murderer seems inclined to yield, the First stabs the Duke, carries him off stage, and drowns him in a large barrel of wine.

First Murderer (3) Minor character in *Macbeth,* an assassin recruited by MACBETH. In 3.1 the First Murderer and his accomplice, the Second Murderer, accept Macbeth's assignment to kill BANQUO and FLEANCE. They are virtually indistinguishable from each other. Neither speaks much, although each makes a brief complaint (3.1.107–113) about the desperation of his unfortunate life and his determination to perform any deed that may improve his lot. In 3.3 the Murderers, assisted by the THIRD MURDERER, undertake their commission. They cooly assault their targets and kill Banquo, though Fleance escapes. In 3.4 the First Murderer reports the deed succinctly to Macbeth. He takes pride in their fierceness and describes Banquo's wounds as 'twenty trenched gashes on his head; / The least a death . . .' (3.4.26–27).

In 4.2 an unspecified number of Murderers, probably the First and Second, kill the SON (1) of LADY (7) Macduff and chase her off stage where they kill her, as we learn in 4.3. Their cold-bloodedness is here particularly horrifying as one of them notes his victim's youth, calling the Son an 'egg' (4.2.82) as he kills him.

The Murderers are not distinct from each other as individuals. The First Murderer offers a pleasing description of a sunset in 3.3.5–7, but we do not imagine that he is a man of esthetic sensibility. He is merely a vessel for Shakespeare's poetic lyricism, which here helps to establish the eerie atmosphere of dusk for a scene that, in the playwright's theatre, was performed without modern stage lighting to set the mood.

First Officer Character in *Twelfth Night.* See OFFICER (3).

First Player (1) Character in *The Taming of the Shrew.* See PLAYERS (1).

First Player (2) Character in *Hamlet,* the leading member of the PLAYERS (2), a travelling company of actors who visit ELSINORE and perform before the court of KING (5) Claudius. In 2.2 HAMLET greets the Players with enthusiasm and requests that the First Player recite a speech he remembers hearing him deliver in a play. Hamlet begins the speech, and the First Player takes it up; it is a highly dramatic account of an episode in the TROJAN WAR, the vengeful killing of King PRIAM by PYRRHUS, followed by the grief of Queen HECUBA. The First Player's fine recital is testified to by POLONIUS, who observes approvingly that he has 'turned his colour and has tears in's eyes' (2.2.515–516), effects that were conventionally associated with fine acting in a tradition extending back to Plato. The First Player receives Hamlet's instructions to stage THE MURDER OF GONZAGO before the court in 2.2.531–536, and he presumably appears as the PLAYER KING in the playlet.

First Soldier (1) Character in *All's Well That Ends Well.* See SOLDIER (7).

Fisher, Thomas (active 1600–1602) London publisher and bookseller, publisher of the first edition of *A Midsummer Night's Dream.* Fisher hired an unknown printer (possibly Edward ALLDE or Richard BRADOCK) to produce Q1 of Shakespeare's play, which appeared in 1600. This was Fisher's only noteworthy publication; he was a draper who joined the STATIONERS' COMPANY in 1600 and operated a bookshop for the next two years, but little more is known of him.

Fishermen Three minor characters in *Pericles,* poor men of PENTAPOLIS. In 2.1 the Fishermen assist the shipwrecked PERICLES and inform him that the ruler of Pentapolis is King SIMONIDES, whose daughter, THAISA, is to marry the winner of a jousting tournament. When Pericles' armour is brought up in the Fishermen's net, he decides to use it in the king's tourney, and the Fishermen agree to guide him to Simonides' court.

This episode introduces the next scene in the play, but the Fishermen also have a greater significance, as they reflect the play's major theme. Before they encounter Pericles they speak of the shipwreck and regret their inability to help the victims 'when, well-a-day, we could scarce help ourselves' (2.1.22). They also philosophise on the ways of the world in a humorous way. They observe, for instance, that fish live 'as men do a-land: the great ones eat up the little ones'

(2.1.28–29). Thus, the Fishermen present the idea that people are at the mercy of forces outside themselves, whether natural or social. This helplessness is the central element of the play's world.

The First Fisherman is the leader of the group; he refers to the Second and Third Fishermen by their names—Pilch and Patch-breech—both humorous terms for raggedy clothes. These labels suggest the general appearance of the Fishermen, which is that of a traditional comic character, the rustic CLOWN (1).

Fitton, Mary (1578–1647) Maid of honour to Queen ELIZABETH (1), possibly the model for the 'Dark Lady' of the SONNETS. Mary Fitton joined the queen's court in 1595 through the influence of Sir William KNOLLYS, a friend of her father. Knollys fell in love with her—generating gossip that may have helped inspire Shakespeare's creation of MALVOLIO's courtship of OLIVIA in *Twelfth Night*—but she became the mistress of William Herbert, the Earl of PEMBROKE (3), by whom she became pregnant in 1600. She was banished from the court in disgrace, Pembroke refused to marry her (preferring a prison term instead), and the infant died shortly after it was born. Fitton went on to marry and be widowed twice.

In his 1890 edition of the Sonnets, Thomas TYLER (2) suggested that Mary Fitton was the Dark Lady—on the assumption that the poems were addressed to Pembroke—and the theory was made widely popular by Frank HARRIS (1). However, most scholars now find the hypothesis improbable, chiefly because two surviving portraits of Fitton show that she had a fair complexion, brown hair, and grey eyes.

Fitzwater (Fitzwalter), Lord Walter (c. 1368–1407) Historical figure and minor character in *Richard II*, a supporter of BOLINGBROKE (1). In 4.1 Fitzwater seconds BAGOT's assertion that AUMERLE had boasted of killing the Duke of GLOUCESTER (6), and he challenges Aumerle to a trial by combat. He is in turn challenged by the Duke of SURREY (3), as the scene erupts in charges and counter-charges. The episode reflects England's political chaos, for Bolingbroke has just displaced King RICHARD II. In 5.6 Fitzwater reports the defeat of a rebellion against Bolingbroke, and is promised rewards by the new king.

Flaminius Minor character in *Timon of Athens*, a servant of TIMON. In 2.2 Flaminius is told to ask Lord LUCULLUS for a loan to assist his master, whose extravagant generosity—to Lucullus, among others—has led him to bankruptcy. However, in 3.1 Lucullus refuses, and tries to hide his ingratitude by bribing Flaminius to say he could not be found, but the loyal servant is outraged and flings the offered coins at Lucullus. He follows this gesture with an heated condemnation that helps emphasise one of the play's major themes: the appalling ingratitude of the Athenian aristocracy. Flaminius' major function is to further the unfolding of Timon's abandonment by his friends.

Flavius (1) (L. Caesetius Flavus) (active 44 B.C.) Historical figure and minor character in *Julius Caesar*, a tribune of ROME and an ally of BRUTUS (4). In 1.1 Flavius, with his fellow tribune, MARULLUS, disperses a crowd (see COMMONER [1]) that has assembled to cheer CAESAR (1) upon his triumph over Pompey in a civil war. The tribunes criticise the Commoners for their disloyalty to Pompey, whom they had earlier supported. After the crowd has dispersed, Flavius and Marullus decide to strip the city's statues, which are decorated in Caesar's honour, because they fear the triumphant general will become a tyrant. In 1.2.282–283 CASCA reports that Flavius and Marullus have been 'put to silence' for this deed. The episode establishes a widespread mistrust of Caesar. Flavius also appears briefly in 5.4 as a member of the army of BRUTUS (4) at the battle of PHILIPPI.

Shakespeare followed an error of his source, PLUTARCH's *Lives*—transmitted through the translations of AMYOT and NORTH—in mis-spelling the name of the historical tribune, Flavus. Little is known of Flavus beyond the incident enacted: he and Marullus were dismissed from their positions by Caesar. Flavus' appearance at Philippi is Shakespeare's invention.

Flavius (2) Character in *Timon of Athens*. See STEWARD (2).

Fleance Minor character in *Macbeth*, the son of BANQUO and the intended murder victim of MACBETH. The WITCHES predict to Macbeth that he will be king but that Banquo's descendants will rule, rather than his own, so once Macbeth has seized the throne of SCOTLAND, he decides that he must kill Banquo and Fleance to prevent the prediction coming true. Fleance appears briefly in 2.1, simply to establish his existence, and when Banquo is killed in 3.3 Fleance escapes after an even briefer appearance. Thus, the possibility is preserved that Banquo's line will eventually replace Macbeth's, and this is Fleance's sole function in *Macbeth*. Once his survival is noted, he is not mentioned in the remainder of the play.

Banquo and Fleance are named as forefathers of the STUART dynasty in Shakespeare's source for the play, HOLINSHED's *Chronicles*. A Stuart ruled England at the time *Macbeth* was written in the person of King JAMES I, and the playwright dutifully included the information (the connection to the Stuarts is made by Banquo's GHOST [4]). However, this was simply a legend recorded as fact in Holinshed's source, the semi-legendary history by Hector BOECE. Fleance in fact never existed, although the name may well have been used by some ancient Scottish lord.

Fleay, Frederick Gard (1831–1909) Shakespearean scholar. F. G. Fleay, who turned to the study of ancient Egypt and Assyria after publishing several works on Shakespeare and his world, was among the early advocates of close study of the plays. He helped develop the VERSE TEST as an analytic tool and was one of the first 'disintegrators', a school of critics who believe that many of the plays attributed to Shakespeare were written by more than one person and who attempt to determine by literary analysis who wrote what. Fleay, like J. M. ROBERTSON, approached this question through a subjective comparison of styles, a procedure that is generally frowned on by more scientifically minded scholars.

Fletcher (1), Giles (1546–1611) English diplomat and writer, author of a possible influence on *Love's Labour's Lost.* Fletcher, after a journey to Russia to negotiate trading rights, wrote *On the Russe Common Wealth* (1591). He was highly critical of the Russians, who had treated him badly. English merchants, fearful of insult to their potential customers, attempted to have the book suppressed. However, parts of it were republished by Richard HAKLUYT and others, and the book went on to become quite popular. Scholars believe that Fletcher's book was the stimulus for the pageant of comic Russians performed at the INNS OF COURT in 1594; this performance influenced in turn Shakespeare's comical Russian masquerade in 5.2 of *Love's Labour's Lost.*

Fletcher was born into a clerical family—his brother (the father of the playwright John FLETCHER [2]) became the bishop of London—and he was a prominent lay administrator in the Church of England before becoming a diplomat. He was also noted for a volume of sonnets in the style of SPENSER, published in 1593. In 1600 he served as executor for his brother, the bishop, who had died in debt, and was almost imprisoned for that debt himself. He was saved through the influence of his friend the Earl of ESSEX (2), and when the Earl staged an unsuccessful rebellion against Queen ELIZABETH (1) the next year, Fletcher stood up for his saviour to the extent that he was imprisoned for several years and his diplomatic career was ended.

Fletcher (2), John (1579–1625) English playwright, collaborator with Shakespeare, and a leading figure of JACOBEAN DRAMA. Fletcher wrote parts of *The Two Noble Kinsmen* and possibly parts of both *Henry VIII* and a lost play, CARDENIO. He succeeded Shakespeare as principal dramatist for the KING'S MEN theatre company. Fletcher's earliest works, influenced by Ben JONSON'S COMEDY OF HUMOURS and written for the CHILDREN'S COMPANIES, were not very successful. In 1608 he began to collaborate with Francis BEAUMONT (2), a similarly unsuccessful young writer of COMEDY. The two enjoyed tremendous success and became the closest of friends, sharing the same lodgings—and, reportedly, the same mistress—while writing about 15 plays in eight years. They were the most important English dramatists in the generation that followed Shakespeare's retirement. Beaumont retired in 1613, but Fletcher wrote many more plays, all of them for the King's Men, many in collaboration with other playwrights, especially Philip MASSINGER but also Jonson, George CHAPMAN, and Thomas MIDDLETON.

Beaumont and Fletcher first achieved success with *Philaster* (1610), a TRAGICOMEDY that was hugely popular and influenced English drama for decades. They followed their success with more of the same, as well as with tragedies and romantic comedies. Among their best known works are *Cupid's Revenge* (1608), *The Maid's Tragedy* (1610), *A King and No King* (1611), and *The Scornful Lady* (1613). In the 1630s, and again in the 1660s, the popularity of Beaumont and Fletcher surpassed that of all other English dramatists, including Shakespeare.

Fletcher's own dramas are often difficult to identify, for so much of his work was collaborative. However, scholars believe that he wrote at least 16 works of his own. They included tragicomedies, such as *The Island Princess* (c. 1619–1621), which confirmed the style set by *Philaster,* and comedies of manners, like *The Wild-Goose Chase* (1621), which were to be very influential on Restoration comedy. In all his works, Fletcher's goal is simply entertainment, whether provided in high-flown rhetoric of death and love, farcical romantic entanglements, or graceful songs. His work is part of an escapist and decadent period in English drama, but in its own terms, it is undeniably successful.

Fletcher (3), Laurence (d. 1608) English actor active in SCOTLAND. Fletcher was recorded as an 'English player' employed by the King, later, King JAMES I of England. He was at the head of the list of members of Shakespeare's KING'S MEN when they received their licence in 1603 upon the occasion of the accession of King James to the English throne. However, since there is no other mention of Fletcher in connection with the King's Men, scholars believe that he may have been included on the licence simply because he had headed James' company in Scotland and was never actually an active member of the London company. He was a minor member of King James' household until his death. Some scholars believe that Shakespeare may have performed with Fletcher in Scotland in 1601, but no solid evidence exists to support this notion. Shakespeare may have left London in the wake of the seeming involvement of the CHAMBERLAIN'S MEN in the rebellion of the Earl of ESSEX (2).

Flint Castle Fortified castle in northern WALES (1), location in *Richard II.* In 3.3 BOLINGBROKE (1) takes custody of King RICHARD II at Flint while professing to be his humble subject. Historically Richard was already the prisoner of Bolingbroke's lieutenant,

NORTHUMBERLAND (1), when he was taken to Flint, a notoriously impregnable castle. It was the first of the many castles that the English built in Wales when they occupied the country in the 13th century.

Florence Italian city, a location in *All's Well That Ends Well.* Various French noblemen, including BERTRAM, join the army of the DUKE (2) of Florence in his war with Siena, and HELENA (2), pursuing Bertram, follows them. Much of Acts 3 and 4 take place in Florence and vicinity. However, nothing in the play is distinctively Florentine—or even Italian—and it is clear that Shakespeare merely followed BOCCACCIO, his ultimate source, in setting part of the action there.

Florizel Character in *The Winter's Tale,* son of King POLIXENES of BOHEMIA and suitor of PERDITA. Florizel defies his father's anger at his intention to marry Perdita, a shepherd girl deemed unsuitable for the heir to the kingdom, and the couple flees to SICILIA. There her identity as the daughter of King LEONTES is discovered, leading to the couple's formal engagement and the reconciliation of their fathers. Florizel is present in only three scenes—4.4, 5.1, and 5.3—and he does not speak in 5.3. Moreover, he is something of a cardboard hero, a stereotype of the chivalric young knight of traditional romantic literature—brave, handsome, and passionately loyal to his lover but with little further in the way of personality. Nevertheless, though his emotional range is restricted, Florizel is important to the play, for his cheerful adoration of Perdita is a charming and forceful manifestation of young love, and his courageous persistence in the face of Polixenes' wrath permits the pair to remain together long enough for the solution to emerge. He is thus an emblem of the power of love to withstand tyrannous opposition. His name probably comes from that of a similar hero, Florizel de Niquea, the protagonist of a chivalric romance by the 16th-century Spanish author Feliciano de Silva (c. 1492–1558).

Flower portrait Portrait of Shakespeare, probably a copy of the DROESHOUT engraving. Some commentators hold that the Flower portrait—named for Sir Desmond Flower, who donated it to the Shakespeare Museum in STRATFORD in 1911—was the original from which Martin Droeshout did his engraving, which is considered an authoritative likeness. However, most scholars believe that it is a copy of the engraving, for it more closely resembles a corrected version of Droeshout's work rather than his initial effort. Moreover, the painting's inscription, 'Willm. Shakespeare, 1609', is in a script that did not come into use until somewhat later, and the paint includes a pigment not used until the 18th century. Therefore, the portrait was probably made in the 18th century, as a forgery.

Florio, John (Giovanni) (c. 1553–1625) English translator whose version of the French essays of Michel de MONTAIGNE supplied minor sources for *The Tempest, Hamlet,* and *King Lear.* Florio's *Essayes on Morall, Politike, and Millitarie Discourses* (1603), his most significant work, was an eccentric elaboration of Montaigne's writing rather than a literal translation. Florio indulged in extravagant alliteration and euphuistic imagery (see LYLY), and he frequently included his own pedantic digressions and fantasies. Although a very inaccurate rendering of Montaigne's spare, crisp prose, Florio's book is a minor English masterpiece in its own right. Florio also wrote an Italian-English dictionary, *A Worlde of Wordes* (1598, 1611), and a series of textbooks for the study of Italian.

Florio taught Italian to the Earl of SOUTHAMPTON (2) and was a friend of Ben JONSON; scholars accordingly presume that Shakespeare was at least acquainted with the translator. Less probably, it is sometimes supposed that Shakespeare's comic pedant of *Love's Labour's Lost,* HOLOFERNES, was intended as a caricature of Florio. Holofernes does quote an Italian proverb found in *Second Fruits* (and elsewhere) in 4.2.93–94. Further, an anonymous sonnet in praise of Florio, published with his Italian text *Second Fruits* (1591), is sometimes attributed to Shakespeare.

Florio was born in LONDON to Italian Protestants who had fled from religious persecution. He attended Oxford, where he later taught French and Italian. Florio moved to London sometime before 1600 and became a tutor to the wife and children of King JAMES I. He was a notable member of the London literary world; besides his acquaintance with Jonson and (probably) Shakespeare, he was married to a sister of Samuel DANIEL.

Fluellen Character in *Henry V,* a Welsh officer in the army of King HENRY V. Fluellen, although hot-tempered, rather humourless, and pedantic, is open, honest, and courageous as well. He is further distinguished by a comically extravagant Welsh accent. His prickly insistence on military traditions leads him to speak sharply to Captain MACMORRIS in 3.2, PISTOL in 3.6, WILLIAMS (2) in 4.8, and GOWER (2) at several points. Irked by Pistol's anti-Welsh mockery, Fluellen forces him to eat a leek, the Welsh national emblem, in 5.1. The king remarks that Fluellen is 'touch'd with choler, hot as gunpowder' (4.7.185).

Fluellen's bravery and sense of military honour mark him as a fine soldier, and his enthusiasm for Henry—especially in his humorous comparison of the king and Alexander the Great (4.7.12–55)—supports the play's presentation of the king as an epic hero. On the other hand, his fiery irrationality and suffocating self-confidence are also to be associated with the king and thus colour the alternative view that Henry is a vicious militarist and the play a satirical picture of war and political power. Shakespeare intended both as-

pects of the play to be felt, and Fluellen, in his small way, contributes to this effect.

Fluellen's name is a variant of the more common Welsh name Llewelyn; Shakespeare may have borrowed the surname of one William Fluellen, an associate of his father, John SHAKESPEARE (9). Fluellen's Welshness helps to demonstrate the unity of the peoples of Britain under Henry V, especially in the 'international scene' (3.2), where Wales, England, Ireland, and Scotland are represented by Fluellen, Gower, Macmorris, and JAMY respectively. Also, the emphasis on Fluellen's accent probably reflects the presence of a Welshman in Shakespeare's acting company (see WALES [1]).

Flute Character in *A Midsummer Night's Dream,* a bellows-mender of ATHENS and a performer in the comical amateur production of PYRAMUS AND THISBE staged at the wedding celebration of Duke THESEUS (1) and Queen HIPPOLYTA (1). Flute plays Thisbe in the INTERLUDE, which is directed by Peter QUINCE. In 1.2 Flute resents being cast as a woman, asserting that he has 'a beard coming' (1.2.43–44). His objection makes clear that in fact he is still a beardless youth. Flute's name, like those of his fellow artisans, refers to his trade; the flute is the nozzle through which a bellows expels air. The name also suggests the high-pitched quality of the character's voice, and Shakespeare may well have selected the name, and then the occupation, to suit the player of Thisbe.

Folger Shakespeare Library Major collection of Shakespeareana in Washington, D.C. The Folger Library was founded in 1930 by Henry Clay Folger (1857–1930), an oil executive whose private collection provided the core of the Library's holdings. The Library, which is administered by Amherst College, also offers Shakespearean and modern plays on an Elizabethan-style stage (see ELIZABETHAN THEATRE), and publishes books and pamphlets of general interest on Shakespeare and his world. The Library houses 79 copies of the FIRST FOLIO, over 200 QUARTO editions of the plays, and thousands of other volumes in one of the world's largest and finest collections.

Folio Format for a page or a book. A folio is a sheet of paper that is folded in half to make two leaves—four pages—or a book composed of such pages. (See also QUARTO.) Since printing paper is large to begin with, a folio volume is large in size, usually about 15 inches tall. In Shakespearean studies the term Folio—capitalised—usually refers to the FIRST FOLIO, the earliest collected edition of Shakespeare's plays (1623), which was published in the folio format. Three more folio-size editions appeared in the 17th century, the Second, Third, and Fourth Folios (1632, 1663, 1685). Each was printed from the preceding edition and added its own corrections and errors. Since they have no connection to an original manuscript or other prepublication source, they are of little scholarly interest. However, the Third Folio (copies of which are relatively rare, probably because many were lost in the fire that destroyed much of London in 1666) incorporated *Pericles* for the first time and introduced a number of plays into the Shakespeare APOCRYPHA as well.

Follower Any of several minor characters in *Hamlet,* rebels led by LAERTES. Upset about the killing of his father, POLONIUS, by Prince HAMLET, Laertes has returned to DENMARK from abroad in a fury. When he arrives in 4.5, he and his Followers break down the door to get to the KING (5). However, he immediately dismisses his men, and the King persuades him to seek revenge against Hamlet rather than through revolution. The Followers speak very little and serve primarily to demonstrate the widespread effects of evil, as political rebellion and social disorder arise from the more personal conflict between Hamlet and the King.

Fool (1) Character type often used by Shakespeare, a sharp-tongued comic, usually a professional jester, who wittily insults the other characters and comments on their actions. He often serves as a CHORUS (1), providing a position outside the plot with which we, the audience, can identify. Real jesters were well known in Shakespeare's day—Queen ELIZABETH (1) employed fools, for instance—and the playwright found this recognised social figure, with his well-defined traditional role, a useful embodiment of objectivity to balance the improbabilities of COMEDY.

Shakespeare did not use fools in his early work, though SPEED in *Two Gentlemen of Verona* and the BASTARD (1) in *King John* foreshadow later figures. In *A Midsummer Night's Dream,* PUCK serves as a jester to OBERON, and he demonstrates an important attribute of the fool, a cool detachment from the problems of the plot and a somewhat self-centred focus on his own notions of humour. The FALSTAFF of the *Henry IV* plays also has points in common with the jesters of later plays. Not only does he present some similar attributes—verbal dexterity, a facility for imitation, and an inventive sense of the absurd—but he also shares the fool's deeper significance as an emblem of freedom from convention. It is with the development of Shakespeare's mature comedy that we find his true jesters. FESTE in *Twelfth Night* and TOUCHSTONE in *As You Like It,* are quintessential fools. Delighted by Touchstone, JAQUES (1) describes and defines the fool's profession and purposes at length, in a striking series of speeches (2.7.12–61). The fool's critique is seen as powerful enough to 'cleanse the foul body of th'infected world' (2.7.60).

A fool can also prove useful in TRAGEDY, providing comic relief as well as his customary objectivity. The FOOL (2) who serves King LEAR, for example, develops the character type to a new level of dramatic expres-

sion. He is virtually an alter ego of the king. His jests are a foil to Lear's frenzy, and his riddles, songs, and scraps of rhyme—combined with his ridicule of the king's folly—offer a sense that somewhere outside the terrifying universe of the play, there remains a real world in which sanity still exists.

In Shakespeare's PROBLEM PLAYS, the fools are less attractive figures. In *All's Well That Ends Well,* the jester to the COUNTESS (2) of ROSSILLION—named Lavatch but designated CLOWN (5)—is a melancholy and sometimes slightly obnoxious character; rather strikingly, when PAROLLES, the comic villain of the play, is defeated, he finds recourse in becoming a professional fool, with the hope that his reputation as a hapless knave will seem entertaining. THERSITES in *Troilus and Cressida* is an abusive and rancorous bandier of insults; while funny, he is also somewhat dispiriting. In *Timon of Athens* (sometimes classed with the darker comedies), APEMANTUS, though technically not a fool—in that he is not a jester—is similar to Thersites. *Measure for Measure* has no fool, but the malicious defamation practised by LUCIO gives him something of Thersites' quality also. The fool's objectivity is not desirable in the unreal world of the ROMANCES, Shakespeare's last works, and the only fool to appear in them—TRINCULO of *The Tempest*—is, although a jester, rather more a CLOWN (1) than a fool.

The distinction between clown and fool is significant, although the Elizabethans tended to treat the terms as synonyms (Lavatch and Feste—both professional jesters—are designated 'Clowns'). The clown tends to be outside the plot's main developments, while the fool is involved with the central characters. Whereas the clown's humour is unintentional, the fool's intellectual wit and trenchant observation are deliberate. With his blunt, earthy spontaneity, the clown lacks the fool's satirical edge. Shakespeare's fools may reflect the stage manner of Robert ARMIN, who joined the playwright's troupe just before the creation of Touchstone, but the type also carries meaning: the fool's sardonic attitude towards the defects of human society adds an underlying melancholy to the essentially positive stance of comedy.

Fool (2) Character in *King Lear,* the court jester or FOOL (1) to King LEAR. The Fool sees that Lear should not have rejected CORDELIA and placed himself in the power of REGAN and GONERIL, and he repeatedly reminds his master of this. He employs barbed quips, for instance, having caused Lear to observe that 'nothing can be made out of nothing', the Fool remarks, '. . . so much the rent of his land comes to' (1.4.130–132). He also utters simple truths, such as 'Thou should'st not have been old till thou hadst been wise' (1.5.41–42). He strives to use his wit to ease Lear's mind as the king goes insane, and he accompanies him into the stormy wilderness in Act 3. The Fool is last seen leaving with Lear and KENT after GLOUCESTER (1) has warned them

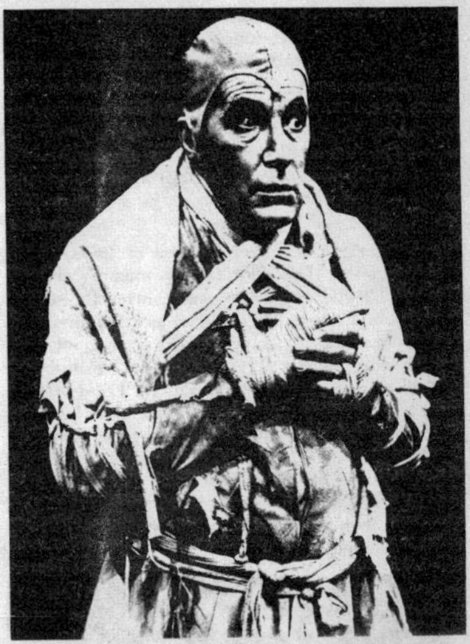

Nicholas Pennell as the Fool in the 1985 Stratford (Ontario) festival production of King Lear. (Photograph by David Cooper)

of a murder plot against the king. His last line, 'And I'll go to bed at noon' (3.6.83), suggests an early death, but his fate is not reported.

The Fool is deeply moved by Lear's plight, but he is capable of detachment from it. Lear's Fool shares with other Shakespearean jesters, such as FESTE and TOUCHSTONE, an irony that permits him to comment on the action of the play, as does a CHORUS (1). With jokes, riddles, and scraps of SONG, he clarifies the central situation by commenting on it more intelligently than the other characters. Especially pertinent is his observation, '. . . the Fool will stay, / And let the wise man fly' (2.4.79–80); with it he makes a declaration of loyalty that helps contrast a moral world with the tragic one that dominates the play. Similarly, his sanity is a foil for Lear's increasing disintegration.

The Fool is closely associated with Cordelia at two significant points. Before his first entrance in 1.4.72, he is said to have 'much pined away' for her, the first mention of Lear's daughter since her departure in 1.1. At the play's close, Lear, grieving over Cordelia's corpse, says, 'And my poor fool is hang'd' (5.3.304). 'Fool' was a common term of endearment in Shakespeare's day, and Lear may simply be referring to his lost daughter, but the playwright nevertheless takes the occasion to compare the two characters. The Fool resembles Cordelia in both his devotion to Lear and

his commitment to a truthful assessment of life. He replaces her as the exponent of these virtues during her long absence from the play; in fact, some scholars suggest that the two roles may have been taken by the same actor in the original productions by the KING'S MEN. Others, however, hold that the part of the Fool was probably played by the famed comedian Robert ARMIN, whose notoriety would have made him an unlikely Cordelia.

Fool (3) Minor character in *Timon of Athens,* a professional jester. This FOOL (1) accompanies APEMANTUS in 2.2 and exchanges witticisms with VARRO'S SERVANT and others. He is apparently employed by a courtesan who is the subject of two jests about venereal disease, but his circumstances and qualities are not developed. His major speech (2.2.112–118) contains a pithy condemnation of ATHENS, which furthers an important theme of the play. However, most commentators believe that he may represent a false start for the playwright, who introduced him with the intention of developing a SUB-PLOT around him and then did not do so before he abandoned this incomplete play.

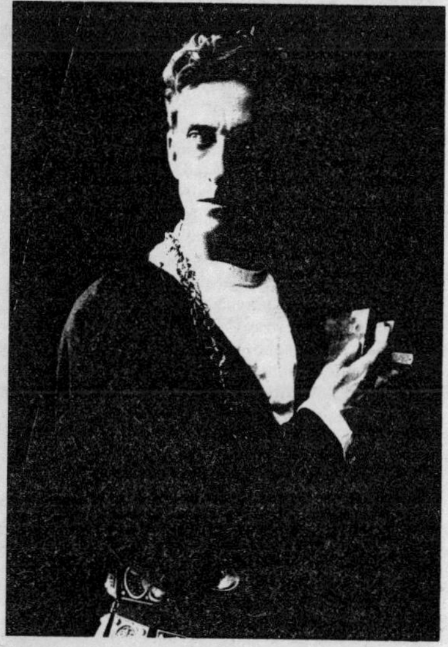

Johnston Forbes-Robertson was renowned for the power of his voice. His portrayal of Hamlet (as seen here) was said to be the greatest of his time. (Courtesy of Culver Pictures, Inc.)

Forbes-Robertson, Johnston (1853–1947) British actor. Forbes-Robertson studied acting under Samuel PHELPS. He was especially noted for his HAMLET, ROMEO, MACBETH, and OTHELLO and often starred in Henry IRVING'S productions. He succeeded Irving as manager of the Lyceum Theatre in 1895 and produced several of Shakespeare's tragedies, including *Hamlet* (1897), to which he restored the closing episode following Hamlet's death, seldom enacted in the 19th century.

Ford (1), Frank Character in *The Merry Wives of Windsor,* jealous husband of MISTRESS (1) Alice Ford. Ford is to some extent a character type, representing a traditional figure in European folklore and literature, the jealous husband, but he is also humanly credible. His emotional excess is not only a source of simple comedy; it also adds to our rich sense of domestic life in Windsor. Ford's jealous tendencies are established before he appears, when his wife remarks on them to her friend MISTRESS (3) Page in 2.1.97–103. Then, in a psychologically masterful manner, Shakespeare demonstrates the growth of an episode of jealousy. At first Ford disbelieves PISTOL'S assertion that FALSTAFF is courting his wife, though only for a rather uncomplimentary reason—'Why, sir, my wife is not young' (2.1.109)—but then he tersely directs himself to look into this possibility, in lines scattered within NYM'S insinuations of a similar adultery to PAGE (12) and he refuses to follow Page in his dismissal of the accusations. When his wife observes that Ford appears preoccupied, he snaps at her. She remarks that he has 'some crotchets in thy head now' (2.1.148), and we are aware that mistrust and anxiety have taken control of him. When Mistress QUICKLY says that his wife 'leads an ill life with him' (2.2.85), we easily believe her.

Ford's strategy—taking the name BROOK (1) and encouraging Falstaff to approach his wife so that he can catch him at it—is a simple-minded device suitable to the jealous husband in a farce, and the wily wives make Ford foolish at the same time that they dupe Falstaff. Although we do not sympathise with Ford, his heartfelt relief when the situation is revealed to him is touching. Moved to impromptu rhetoric, he asserts to his wife, 'I rather will suspect the sun with cold than thee with wantonness' (4.4.7–8), inspiring Page to remark tellingly, 'Be not as extreme in submission as in offence' (4.4.11–12).

Ford (2), John (1586–c. 1639) English dramatist, one of the last playwrights of JACOBEAN DRAMA. Ford began to write plays around 1612, collaborating with Thomas DEKKER, John WEBSTER (2), and others. Of his own works, he is chiefly remembered for several tragedies marked by bitter resignation and despair, the best known of which is *'Tis Pity She's a Whore* (c. 1632), a tale

of incest between brother and sister. His historical drama *Perkin Warbeck* (1633) is also highly regarded. Ford lived much of his life in poverty and is thought to have spent his last years in seclusion.

Ford (3), Mistress Alice Character in *The Merry Wives of Windsor.* See MISTRESS (1).

Forester Minor character in *Love's Labour's Lost,* the guide for a royal hunt. The Forester's naïve honesty provides a foil for the wit of the PRINCESS (1) of France in 4.1.

Forman, Simon (1552–1611) English astrologer and diarist. Forman recorded several early performances of Shakespeare's plays. His records—generally brief synopses—help scholars determine the dates, and in some cases the likelihood of variation from the published texts, of various plays, including three of Shakespeare's works: *Macbeth, Cymbeline,* and *The Winter's Tale.*

Astrology was a more reputable occupation then than now, but Forman may have been less than scrupulous. He was frequently gaoled for practising medicine without a licence, and because of his reputation, it was suspected, when he drowned in the Thames after predicting the date of his death, that he was a suicide.

Forrest, Edwin (1806–1872) American actor. The first great American Shakespearean actor, Forrest helped create popular enthusiasm for Shakespeare in the United States, especially with his performances as OTHELLO and LEAR. He appeared in London in 1836 and 1845, and a rivalry developed between him and W. C. MACREADY. Comparisons of the two took on a nationalistic colour, especially in America, and led to the notorious Astor Place riot in New York in 1849, when a mob of Forrest fans—and opportunistic, anti-England political agitators—stormed a theatre where Macready was playing and the commotion left 22 dead. In the opinion of contemporaries and most subsequent scholars, Forrest personally instigated the affair, and the actor's popularity slowly waned after this incident. He eventually fell from favour entirely, dying an embittered failure.

Fortinbras Character in *Hamlet,* Prince of Norway and enemy of DENMARK. Although he does not appear until 4.4, Fortinbras is described in 1.1.98–107 as a hot-blooded young warrior intent on recapturing lands taken from Norway after the combat in which his father, the late King of Norway, was killed by HAMLET's father, the late King of Denmark. Thus he is immediately established as a parallel figure to Hamlet, one who is also compelled to avenge his father's death. Fortinbras' brief appearance in 4.4 on his way to an invasion of neighbouring Poland energises Hamlet, who sees in this war, directed at no more than 'a little patch of ground . . . a straw . . . an eggshell' (4.4.18, 26, 53), a direct and shaming contrast to his own inaction in taking revenge against his father's murderer, KING (5) Claudius. When Hamlet, nearing death at the play's end, learns that Fortinbras is returning from Poland, he proclaims him heir to the crown of Denmark. When he arrives, Fortinbras takes command and orders a military funeral for Hamlet.

While Fortinbras' example inspires Hamlet to fierce declarations—'My thoughts be bloody or be nothing worth' (4.4.66)—Hamlet's rhetoric is an overreaction to a situation that is not in fact analogous to his own. As the play unfolds, Hamlet comes to realise that an acceptance of fate and its evils is the only way to understand human life; within this context, Fortinbras, who works his will in the world and is doubtless uninterested in such philosophical matters, is clearly a lesser figure. Still, his stalwart resolution and military valour—reminiscent of Shakespeare's HENRY V—are not only admirable but also stand in important contrast to the evil and debased intrigue of Hamlet's world.

When Fortinbras appears after Hamlet's death in 5.2, he reminds us that he comes as a hostile power, declaring that he will claim his revenge as his 'vantage doth invite' (5.2.395), and we realise that Claudius' evil has damaged his kingdom to the extent that an outsider has taken over. Thus Fortinbras symbolises a lesson in political morality that Shakespeare offered in several plays (e.g., *Titus Andronicus, Macbeth, King Lear*): personal evil in powerful members of society will weaken the state as a whole, often resulting in a surrender of sovereignty to another country.

Fortune Theatre Playhouse built in a northern LONDON suburb by Philip HENSLOWE and William ALLEYN in 1600, long the home of the ADMIRAL'S MEN and its successors, PRINCE HENRY'S MEN and the PALSGRAVE'S MEN. The Fortune may have been built in response to the construction of the GLOBE THEATRE near Henslowe and Alleyn's ROSE THEATRE in SOUTHWARK, south of the city. Some scholars theorise that when Cuthbert BURBAGE (1) and the CHAMBERLAIN'S MEN moved to the Globe in 1599, Henslowe and Alleyn saw an opportunity to avoid direct competition while at the same time filling the vacuum created by the Chamberlain's departure from the CURTAIN THEATRE, to the north of London. Moreover, their lease on the ground the Rose was built on was about to expire. In any event, the Fortune was meant to rival the Globe; it was commissioned from the same builder, under a contract requiring that it be 'finished and done according to the manner and fashion of the said house called the Globe'. It took its name from a statue of the Goddess of Fortune over its entrance. When the Fortune

burned down in 1621, it was described as 'the fairest playhouse' in London. It was rebuilt in 1623 and was used for surreptitious play productions after the Puritans' revolutionary government made theatre illegal in 1642, at the beginning of the Civil Wars. The building was pillaged by soldiers in 1649 and finally destroyed around 1656.

Foul Papers In textual studies, a playwright's original, unpolished manuscript from which the printers of an early edition of a play might set the type. This version differs from FAIR COPY, which was used for the same purpose but was provided by a scribe, who might make various corrections to the original manuscript. A published text set from foul papers is therefore distinctively flawed by minor errors and inconsistencies taken from the source.

In the case of Shakespeare, the playwright's careless slips survived into the printed text: his spelling is often irregular, and inconsistent names occur in speech headings and stage directions. Lady CAPULET (3), for instance, is designated in the Q2 edition of *Romeo and Juliet* as *Capu. Wi, Ca. Wi, Wife, Old La., La., Mo.*, and *M.* Sometimes an actor's name will appear as a speech heading—e.g., KEMPE for DOGBERRY in 4.2 of *Much Ado About Nothing*—which is evidence that Shakespeare created the part with a particular player in mind. GHOST CHARACTERS may appear without again being mentioned, like INNOGEN in 1.1 and 2.1 of *Much Ado.* In fair copy most of these problems were corrected. Also, when a text was printed from foul papers new errors resulted from the use of a rapidly composed manuscript that was likely to be difficult to read and was further confused by handwritten amendments and marginal insertions.

Sometimes material was retained by the typesetter that the author intended to cut. For instance, Q2 of *Hamlet* preserves a line Shakespeare had rejected; two lines of similar meaning occur together, and the first one does not rhyme with any other although it is in the midst of a long passage of rhyming couplets. Clearly, the playwright rejected it in favour of the second (3.2. 162) as he was writing, but the substitution was not evident to the printer, who simply reproduced everything he saw. The error was corrected in the FIRST FOLIO edition.

Stage directions in foul papers are sometimes casually imprecise, as in 'Enter . . . others, as many as can be' (*Titus Andronicus,* 1.1.70). They may also reveal the playwright's thoughts on production in more elaborate and specific stage directions than usual, such as: 'Enter VOLUMNIA and VIRGILIA, mother and wife to MARTIUS. They set them down on two low stools and sew' (*Coriolanus,* 1.3.S.D.). These parenthetical remarks were normally abbreviated or eliminated by a copyist.

With the probable exception of three pages of SIR THOMAS MORE, no original Shakespearean manuscript exists, but by observing such features as those mentioned above, scholars can determine what sort of copy was the basis for an early edition—whether a manuscript or an earlier printing, and if a manuscript, whether fair copy or foul papers. Modern editors can determine from such information how closely a given printed text represents what Shakespeare actually wrote.

Foxe (Fox), John (1516–1587) English historian of religion, author of a source for *2 Henry VI, King John,* and especially *Henry VIII.* Foxe's *Actes and Monumentes,* better known as the *Book of Martyrs,* is a history of Protestantism, focussing on the English Protestants who were persecuted during the reign of Queen Mary (ruled 1553–1558), a zealous Catholic. Passages from his account of Thomas CRANMER's life were Shakespeare's principal source for Cranmer's trial in 5.1–2 of *Henry VIII.* Other material provided details for *2 Henry VI* and *King John.*

Foxe's book was written in Latin during his exile from England during Mary's reign. He returned in 1559 and translated and published his work in 1563, enlarging it for a second edition in 1570. It immediately became immensely popular and influential—the 1570 edition was required by law to be available to worshippers in all English cathedrals and for generations it was regarded by English Protestants as a virtual supplement to the Bible. Many houses contained only those two books. The *Book of Martyrs* was republished many times in the 16th and 17th centuries; Shakespeare probably used the fourth edition (1583).

France (1) Country in Europe. France, England's most powerful neighbour and perennial rival, was its enemy in the HUNDRED YEARS WAR and earlier conflicts. It thus provides settings in three of the HISTORY PLAYS and is prominent in several other plays as well.

In *1 Henry V* and *Henry VI,* Shakespeare presented the later phases of the Hundred Years War, the major struggle between England and France in the 14th and 15th centuries. King HENRY V's triumph at the battle of AGINCOURT (1415) is enacted in Act 4 of *Henry V* and followed by the negotiation of the treaty of TROYES in 5.2, completing the English conquest. King Henry V is betrothed on this occasion to Princess KATHARINE (2) of France; their child is to be King HENRY VI.

In *1 Henry VI,* English forces besiege ORLÉANS (1) and ROUEN, and the young Henry is crowned king of France in PARIS (1). However, the English conquest of France is actually being undone under the leadership of JOAN LA PUCELLE and CHARLES VII. The final battle of the war, the English loss at BORDEAUX, occupies most of Act 4, though Shakespeare salvaged a seeming victory by staging Joan's trial at ANGIERS in 5.3.

France is unimportant in the other *Henry VI* plays,

though one scene of *3 Henry VI* (3.3) is set at the court of King LEWIS (3), who offers aid to English rebels. In *King John*, set much earlier in history, King JOHN (3) also fights in France, protecting PLANTAGENET lands against the French King PHILIP (2). This war centres on Angiers, where fighting occurs in 2.1 and 3.2.

Long after the Hundred Years War, rivalry with France remained a prominent feature of English politics. Only in 1564, the year of Shakespeare's birth, did England finally renounce its last claims to French territory, and, during the playwright's lifetime, war between the two countries seemed likely on more than one occasion. Catholic France was seen by Protestant England as a potential religious enemy, for Europe was still plagued by sectarian wars. Thus, along with another rival, Spain, France loomed as large in the fears of Shakespeare's contemporaries as the Soviet Union does to many Westerners today. England and France remained hostile for centuries after Shakespeare's time; only in the 20th century has warfare between them seemed improbable.

Because Shakespeare's audiences shared an interest in France and French affairs, he also used this country and its people outside the history plays. A king of France (FRANCE [2]) finds his way into ancient British myth in *King Lear*. In *Love's Labour's Lost*, the presentation of a KING (19) of Navarre reflects the importance in contemporary French politics of the current King of Navarre, soon to become King Henri IV of France. A comical Frenchman, Dr CAIUS (2), is mocked in *The Merry Wives of Windsor*.

All's Well That Ends Well is set partially in France, in the province of ROSSILLION (the French Roussillon), and Shakespeare elaborates on his sources in providing a realistic political relationship between France and Italy that reflects the French military involvement in Italy throughout the first half of the 16th century.

It has been speculated that Shakespeare travelled in France, although no evidence has survived to confirm this. It is clear, though, that he knew the French language. Not only did he sometimes use French sources that had not been translated into English, but his French dialogue—e.g., in *Henry V*, 3.4, 4.4, 5.2—is only slightly flawed.

France (2), King of Character in *King Lear*, the suitor and later the husband of CORDELIA, King LEAR's rejected daughter. France, as the king is called, appears only in 1.1. He recognises the honesty and virtue in Cordelia and thus emphasises Lear's moral blindness. He agrees to marry her, saying 'She is herself a dowry' (1.1.240), and takes her back to FRANCE (1). Cordelia is thus absent for most of the action as her sisters humiliate and banish their father. The Earl of KENT (1) soon knows that 'from France there comes a power' (3.1.30) to aid Lear, but France himself does not reappear; he has returned home to deal with 'something he left imperfect in the state' (4.3.3), while a French general unsuccessfully attempts to re-establish Lear on the throne. The subject of foreign invasion was a touchy one in Shakespeare's day because Protestant England felt threatened by Catholic enemies, including France, and scholars believe that the playwright found it expedient, in view of government CENSORSHIP, to deemphasise the role of France, both man and country, in *King Lear*.

France (3), Princess of Character in *Love's Labour's Lost*. See PRINCESS (1) OF FRANCE.

France (4), Queen of Character in *Henry V*. See ISABEL (2).

Francesca (Francisca) Character in *Measure for Measure*. See NUN.

Francis (1) Minor character in *1* and *2 Henry IV*, an indentured servant at the BOAR'S HEAD TAVERN. In 2.4 of *1 Henry IV* PRINCE (6) HAL teases Francis, engaging him in conversation while POINS, by pre-arrangement, summons him. The endearingly simple-minded Francis can only reply with the well-known protest of the harried waiter, 'Anon, anon', as Hal has predicted. Hal suggests that Francis might run away from the tavern, and then he extravagantly promises Francis £1,000 for a packet of sugar. He next asks if Francis will rob the innkeeper and goes on to speak of Francis' likely future. 'Why then your brown bastard is your only drink', he says, 'for look you, Francis, your white canvas doublet will sully. In Barbary, sir, it cannot come to so much' (2.4.72–74). Francis is now hopelessly confused, and he exits hurriedly as Poins, Hal, and his boss, the VINTNER, all call him at once.

This puzzling exchange has elicited a number of explanations, the simplest of which is that Hal is merely playing a practical joke on Francis, an example of the idle tavern life that he will later reject. However, while a joke is clearly intended, the Prince is deliberately placing himself on familiar terms with an 'under-skinker' (2.4.24), continuing his exploration of the lives of the common people whom he will later rule. Thus the episode helps to demonstrate that Hal's participation in FALSTAFF's world is part of his preparation for his greater role, and not simply dissipation. He suggests as much when, asked by Poins what the point of the joke was, he replies that he is now 'of all humours' (2.4.90) and compares his good mood with HOTSPUR's mania for war. In Francis' humble life, he has seen a contentment that the warrior can never discover. Further, Hal observes that, if Francis will not be tempted by theft or flight, he must accept the low life of a servant. This may reflect, albeit in a resigned manner, Hal's attitude towards his own destiny to

become a leader, rather than a participant in the easier, irresponsible world of the tavern.

In *2 Henry IV* Francis appears to have been promoted, as he organises the service for Falstaff's dinner in 2.4.

Francis (2), Friar Character in *Much Ado About Nothing.* See FRIAR (2).

Francisco (1) Minor character in *Hamlet,* a sentry on the walls of the castle at ELSINORE. Francisco is relieved from duty by BARNARDO at the opening of 1.1, as the scene's locale is established. He declares himself 'sick at heart' (1.1.9), suggesting immediately that something is amiss in the play's world.

Francisco (2) Minor character in *The Tempest,* a follower of King ALONSO of Naples. In 2.1.109–118 Francisco attempts to reassure the king that Prince FERDINAND (2) has survived their shipwreck. This passage is an extension of GONZALO's efforts to cheer the king, and Francisco speaks only three more words, in 3.3.40, so there seems little reason for his presence in the play. In some editions, in fact, he is deleted and his lines given to Gonzalo. Some scholars have taken him and ADRIAN (2) as evidence of an earlier version of *The Tempest,* in which they played a greater part. He may have been intended for scenes that Shakespeare originally planned but then discarded in the course of composition. In any case, royal figures are conventionally endowed with unimportant attendants throughout Shakespeare's work.

Frederick Character in *As You Like It.* See DUKE (1).

French, George Russell (1803–1881) English architect and amateur scholar, publisher of a genealogy of Shakespeare. French's *Shakespeareana Genealogica* (1869), covered Shakespeare's ancestors, relatives, and descendants, along with genealogical notes on the characters in the HISTORY PLAYS, *Hamlet,* and *Macbeth.* His was the first work in this area, and it is still valuable to scholars. French also wrote genealogies of Admiral Horatio Nelson (1758–1805) and the Duke of Wellington (1769–1852), and he was a well-known campaigner against the drinking of alcohol.

French King (Charles VI of France, 1368–1422) Historical figure and character in *Henry V,* the opponent of King HENRY V. The French King plays an inconsequential role. He presents a brief history of earlier English conquests in FRANCE (1) in 2.4.48–64; he encourages his noblemen before the battle of AGINCOURT in 3.5; and in 5.2 he accepts the terms of the treaty of TROYES, surrendering to Henry the inheritance of his crown, as well as the hand of his daughter, Princess KATHARINE (2). The ineffectual French King complements another model of French inadequacy, the caricature of foolish bravado that is his son the DAUPHIN (3).

This perfunctory portrait omits the most important fact about the historical Charles VI: he was intermittently insane. His illness—later to surface in his grandson King HENRY VI of England—was known to Shakespeare, but the playwright, who had not touched on madness in the *Henry VI* plays either, may have disliked pointing out defects in the ancestral line of his own ruler, Queen ELIZABETH (1). Also, focussing on Henry V's greatness, he probably did not wish to elaborate on France's weakness. For in failing to mention Charles' lunacy, Shakespeare also omitted its most important consequence—a state of virtual civil war in France that made the English conquest much easier.

Two factions vied with each other for the regency of France when the King was sick. When Henry invaded, the party in power at first refused to fight him, fearing that their rivals would seize Paris in their absence. This led to the Dauphin's failure to relieve HARFLEUR, of which its GOVERNOR (1) complains in 3.3. The French pulled themselves together—note the French King's roll-call, including noblemen of both factions, in 3.5.40–45—but the victory at Agincourt saved the English. When Henry again entered France, in 1417, the same situation prevailed; as a result, the English were able to conquer Normandy and claim the French crown. (See HUNDRED YEARS WAR.)

French Soldier Minor character in *Henry V,* a gentleman taken prisoner by PISTOL at AGINCOURT. In a grimly comic scene Pistol, who speaks no French, attempts to extract ransom from the Soldier, who tries to offer it but does not speak English. Finally the BOY (3) interprets, and Pistol agrees not to kill his captive.

Frenchman Minor character in *Cymbeline,* a friend of the Roman gentleman PHILARIO. In 1.5 POSTHUMUS arrives in ROME. He has been exiled from Britain because he married the king's daughter, IMOGEN, and he meets the Frenchman and IACHIMO at Philario's home. The Frenchman has known Posthumus in the past, and he recollects a duel the Briton once fought over the virtues of a woman. This triggers the fateful wager between Posthumus and Iachimo over Imogen's chastity. The Frenchman is a pawn of plot development, and represents the world of gentlemanly duels inhabited by Posthumus and Iachimo.

Friar (1) Character in *Measure for Measure,* helper of the DUKE (9) of VIENNA. In 1.3 the Duke asks the Friar to disguise him as another friar so that he can return to Vienna incognito and observe the administration of his deputy, ANGELO (2). In 4.5 the Duke revisits the

Friar, who assists in his plans to expose the misconduct of Angelo, and in 4.6 the Friar escorts ISABELLA and MARIANA (2) as part of those plans. Finally, in 5.1 he introduces the two women as witnesses to Angelo's evil doings. Though the Duke speaks of him in 1.3 as an intimate friend, the relationship is not developed and the Friar serves merely to further the plot.

The Friar is named Thomas in the stage direction at the beginning of 1.3, but the name is never used elsewhere, and in a later appearance he is named Peter. Shakespeare—who made such minor slips throughout the plays—apparently gave the Friar a name when he first created him, but then forgot about it before writing Act 4 where he gave him another one. The earliest text of the play, that of the FOLIO, was printed from a transcription of Shakespeare's manuscript, and his original note was erroneously included.

Friar (2) Francis Minor character in *Much Ado About Nothing,* clergyman who supports the slandered HERO, restoring her father LEONATO's faith in her. The Friar officiates at the wedding of Hero and CLAUDIO (1), only to see the ceremony disrupted. Claudio (1), misled by Don JOHN (1), rejects his bride, accusing her publicly of promiscuity. Hero faints in response, and Leonato, humiliated, curses her. However, the Friar believes Hero is innocent, and his spiritual authority persuades Leonato. The Friar then proposes a plan intended to rouse Claudio's guilt and sympathy and renew his love for Hero; Hero should be said to be dead. While this plan has no effect on Claudio, it provides an interesting detour in the plot, during which Don John's scheme is exposed by other means. The Friar marries Hero to Claudio and BEATRICE to BENEDICK as the play closes.

Friar (3) John Minor character in *Romeo and Juliet,* an unsuccessful emissary between FRIAR (4) LAURENCE and the exiled ROMEO. In 5.2 Friar John reports that he has been unable to deliver Laurence's letter to Romeo, having been quarantined as a suspected plague carrier. Thus Romeo remains unaware that the death of JULIET (1) is feigned, and the tragic dénouement is launched.

Friar (4) Laurence (Lawrence) Character in *Romeo and Juliet,* the clergyman who assists ROMEO and JULIET (1). Although presented as a respectable, well-meaning old gentleman given to platitudes, the Friar serves as an agent of malevolent fate. In his first speech (2.3.1–26) a sententious bouquet of rhymed observations on plant lore, he demonstrates the conventionality of thought that will lead him to proceed recklessly—to the lovers' destruction—while maintaining an air of caution. Moreover, his remarks on good and bad uses for herbs foreshadow the role of potions and poisons later in the play. He warns Romeo against haste in such passages as 2.6.9–15, but nonetheless agrees to perform the secret marriage of the young lovers. The Friar's flimsy morality is evident when he advises the distraught Juliet in 4.1. Accepting a bigamous marriage as an alternative, though not an ideal one, he proposes a devious capitulation to her parents' wishes, accompanied by the desperate expedient of the sleeping potion. In the final scene, his lack of character is richly demonstrated as he abandons Juliet in the predicament his rash plans have brought about.

Friend Either of two minor characters in *The Two Noble Kinsmen,* acquaintances of the GAOLER (4). In 4.1 the Friends assure the Gaoler that THESEUS (2), Duke of ATHENS, has forgiven him for the fact that PALAMON has escaped from his gaol with the assistance of his DAUGHTER (2), and they sympathise with him when the WOOER brings evidence that the Daughter is deranged. The Friends, mere pawns of the plot, were probably not Shakespeare's creations, for most scholars agree that 4.1 was written by his collaborator, John FLETCHER (2).

Frogmore Village near WINDSOR, the setting for 3.1 of *The Merry Wives of Windsor.* In this scene the curate EVANS (3), challenged to a duel by Dr CAIUS (2), awaits his foe in a field near Frogmore. The duel is averted, and the enemies return to Windsor as allies. Shakespeare used the name Frogmore simply to evoke the neighbourhood of Windsor, which was well known to his original audience, members of the court of Queen ELIZABETH (1).

Froissart, Jean (1338–1410) French chronicler whose work may have influenced the writing of *Richard II,* particularly in presenting a highly favourable account of John of GAUNT. Further, it is speculated that Froissart's romantic presentation of the pomp and pageantry of medieval ceremonies may have helped form Shakespeare's sense of the courtly world of King RICHARD II. The playwright will have known Froissart's work in Lord BERNERS' translation (1523–1525).

In his *Chroniques* Froissart wrote of the contemporary HUNDRED YEARS WAR, interviewing many key participants and observing some events himself. His colourful history ends with the deposition of RICHARD II. Froissart is considered to have been the last great medieval writer; his vivid and exciting description of the traditions and practices of the chivalric aristocracy records a world that was fast vanishing in his own time. His chronicles are still regarded as classics of European literature.

Froth Minor character in *Measure for Measure,* a customer of MISTRESS (2) Overdone's bordello and bar

who is arrested by the comical constable, ELBOW. In an episode of comic relief, Froth is brought to court along with Mistress Overdone's accomplice, POMPEY (1), in 2.1. Froth says very little and serves only as the subject of the humorous dispute between Elbow and Pompey. Dismissed by the judge ESCALUS (2), Froth makes his only substantial remark, a joke that seems to account for his name. He jests that he never enters a tap-room willingly, but is drawn in; a reference to the foam, or froth, 'drawn' by a tapster in the course of serving ale.

Furness, Horace Howard (1833–1912) American scholar, first editor of the *New Variorum* edition of Shakespeare's plays (see VARIORUM EDITION). Furness began work on this annotated collection of the plays in 1871 with *Romeo and Juliet.* In this edition he provided textual notes and excerpts from pertinent critical writings from many eras and several languages. With the assistance of his wife, Helen Kate Furness (1837–1883), and his son, H. H. Furness, Jr. (1865–1930), he had completed 18 volumes before he died. His son succeeded him as general editor of the series, which was not completed until 1953.

Furnivall, Frederick James (1825–1910) English scholar. Furnivall encouraged the study of Shakespeare's works as a whole—still a new pursuit in his day—in his notable introductions written for each play, in his scholarly edition of the *Works* (1876), and with the English translation of G. G. GERVINUS' *Shakespeare Commentaries* (1875). He was particularly associated with the development of the VERSE TEST as a tool for determining the chronological order of the plays. He also edited a 43-volume collection of facsimiles of the QUARTO editions of the plays (1880–1889).

Furnivall was a prolific scholar and educator with many interests besides Shakespearean studies. He founded many scholarly organisations, including the Early English Text, Chaucer, Ballad, New Shakespeare, Wyclif, Browning, and Shelley Societies; he was involved in the creation of the Oxford English Dictionary, and he produced a number of scholarly editions, most notably a collection of six texts of CHAUCER's *The Canterbury Tales* (1868).

G

Gad's Hill (Gadshill, Gads Hill) Geographical feature near the city of ROCHESTER, setting for the highway robbery in 2.2 of *1 Henry IV.* Gad's Hill, on the road from Rochester to London, was a notorious site for highway robberies, both in the 16th century and in the period when the play is set. It is there that GADSHILL, FALSTAFF, and others rob the TRAVELLERS, only to be robbed themselves by PRINCE (6) HAL and POINS.

The name of this infamous setting provided a nickname for a robber who operated there in the playwright's source, the FAMOUS VICTORIES, and Shakespeare simply adopted the name for the Gadshill of *1 Henry IV.* In old editions of the play, the site is spelled as one word, and some modern editors follow this style. Others adopt one of the two-word variants, also used in Elizabethan times, and thus ease the slight confusion that the duplication can produce. Shakespeare's double use of the name is one of many instances of the playwright's toleration for minor confusions and inconsistencies in his texts.

Gadshill Character in *1 Henry IV,* a highway robber and friend of FALSTAFF and PRINCE (6) HAL. In 2.1 of *1 Henry IV* Gadshill uses a well-known highwayman's tactic: an accomplice, the CHAMBERLAIN (1) of an inn, tips him off about the travel plans of rich guests. Then he and Falstaff and others rob these TRAVELLERS in 2.2, only to be robbed in their turn by the Prince and POINS. Gadshill—a professional thief, unlike Falstaff and the Prince—serves to demonstrate the depths of delinquency from which the Prince must emerge.

Gadshill is a nickname taken from Shakespeare's anonymous source, the FAMOUS VICTORIES, where it is applied to a highwayman whose favourite working locale was GAD'S HILL. No proper name is given for Shakespeare's character.

Gallus, Caius Cornelius (c. 69–27 B.C.) Historical figure and minor character in *Antony and Cleopatra,* a follower of Octavius CAESAR (2). In 5.1 Gallus wordlessly follows Caesar's order to accompany PROCULEIUS on his mission to offer mercy to CLEOPATRA, and in 5.2 he arrives at the quarters of the Egyptian queen with a squad of soldiers (see GUARDSMAN [2]). Gallus leaves immediately, but his appearance—and his remark, 'You see how easily she may be surpris'd' (5.2.35)—makes clear that Cleopatra is now entirely in Caesar's control. She responds by attempting to stab herself, but she is prevented by Proculeius. Gallus reappears as part of Caesar's entourage later in the scene, but he does not speak again.

The historical Gallus was an important Roman poet, regarded as the principal inventor of the Roman love elegy, but only a fragment of a single line of his work survives. He abandoned art for war after an unsuccessful love affair and became a leading member of Caesar's military establishment; historians give him much of the credit for Antony's final defeat. After the war he became the first Roman governor of Egypt. He put down several rebellions and traveiled up the Nile into what is now Sudan where he established relations between Rome and Ethiopia. However, he was a notably poor administrator, and a scandal, the details of which are lost, resulted in his dismissal. He was convicted of treason and punished with exile from Rome, to which he responded by killing himself.

Ganymede In *As You Like It,* name taken by ROSALIND when, banished by DUKE (1) Frederick, she travels with CELIA to the Forest of ARDEN (1) disguised as a young man. In Greek mythology Zeus, the king of the gods, became infatuated with Ganymede, a beautiful boy, and took the form of an eagle to kidnap him and carry him to Mount Olympus, where the youth became a cup-bearer to the gods. The name Ganymede thus came to suggest boyish beauty.

Gaoler (1) Minor character in *The Merchant of Venice,* the custodian of ANTONIO (2), who is arrested for debt, in 3.3. The Gaoler, who does not speak, represents the authority of the state, mutely showing that Antonio may not be exempted from the law. Shakespeare believed such rigour to be necessary, however undesirable the personal consequences.

Gaoler (2) Either of two minor characters in *Cymbeline,* keepers of the captured POSTHUMUS, who is believed to be a Roman prisoner of war. In 5.4 the First Gaoler is a CLOWN (1) who interrupts the action with humorous remarks on life and death (the Second

Gaoler speaks only half a line). He provides comic relief as the plot becomes most troubling. He offers a sardonic philosophy of death as a relief from life, a view that encapsulates Posthumus' depressed state.

The placement of this character is significant. The Gaoler (after a mute appearance in 5.3, and a brief one at the opening of 5.4) arrives to summon Posthumus to his execution, at 5.4.152. This is after Posthumus has had his vision of SICILIUS LEONATUS and JUPITER—which we recognise as the climax of the play. Thus, the Gaoler's comic approach to the tragic potential of life comes only after an assurance that the play will have a happy ending.

The Gaoler resembles such predecessors as the PORTER (3) of *Macbeth* and the GRAVE-DIGGER of *Hamlet.* Some scholars believe that the Gaoler's part was written to be performed by the same actor who played CLOTEN—probably Robert ARMIN. This hypothetical idea is based on the clownishness of the two characters and the possibility of one person playing both, since Cloten dies early in Act 4.

Gaoler (3) Minor character in *The Winter's Tale,* the custodian of the imprisoned Queen HERMIONE. When Lady PAULINA visits the unjustly incarcerated queen, the Gaoler is sympathetic—calling her 'a worthy lady / And one who much I honour' (2.2.5–6)—but he sticks to his duty, only allowing her to see Hermione's lady-in-waiting, EMILIA (3), and only in his presence. When Paulina proposes to take Hermione's daughter—born in the prison—to the king, the Gaoler is reluctant, saying, 'I know not what I shall incur to pass it, / Having no warrant' (2.2.57–58), but in the face of Paulina's insistence he accedes. This weak figure provides a foil for Paulina, establishing her as the powerful presence that will dominate several later scenes; at the same time, by reminding us of the authority he represents, he contributes to our growing sense of tragedy.

Gaoler (4) Character in *The Two Noble Kinsmen,* the prison-warden whose DAUGHTER (2) goes mad with unrequited love for PALAMON, a prisoner of war and one of the title characters. The Daughter helps Palamon escape, but when he returns to the aristocratic world, she loses her mind. The Gaoler first appears in 2.1, where he agrees to the WOOER's suit for the Daughter's hand, and where he is a conventional warden to his prisoners. He is unaware of his daughter's state when he reappears in 4.1, worrying that he will be blamed for Palamon's escape. Once informed of the Daughter's madness, he is helpless to ease her plight. In 5.2 he objects mildly to the DOCTOR's (4) prescription—that the Wooer disguise himself as Palamon and sleep with her—but he goes along and reports her cure in 5.4. A simple pawn of the plot, he is believed to have been the creation of Shakespeare's collaborator, John FLETCHER (2).

Gardener Minor character in *Richard II,* a worker in the household of the Duke of YORK (4). In 3.4 the Gardener and his assistants (see MAN [1]) discuss the news of the capture and likely deposition of King RICHARD II by BOLINGBROKE (1). In their conversation the garden is an extended metaphor for the state: just as a garden must be constantly tended if it is to bear flowers and fruits, so must the state be kept in order by its rulers if it is to function healthily. Thus the Gardener summarises one of the play's important moral points.

The episode also has another function. The QUEEN (13) overhears the Gardener's remarks and reacts with hysterical anger. Although she curses him, the Gardener is sympathetic to her grief, and his response neatly emphasises the human side of Richard's story. Up to this point we have been encouraged to judge the King harshly as a self-centred and unreliable ruler; here, the Gardener's pity stirs an awareness that Richard's fall, however deserved it may be, has a personal dimension. Our sympathies begin to shift, preparing us for the tragic and philosophical Richard of the second half of the play.

Gardiner (1), Stephen (d. 1555) Historical figure and character in *Henry VIII,* a follower of Cardinal WOLSEY and later his successor as the play's principal villain. In 2.2 Gardiner appears as King HENRY VIII's new secretary; in an aside he assures Wolsey of his personal loyalty, and the cardinal tells CAMPEIUS that Gardiner will do as he tells him. When we next see Gardiner, in the coronation parade in 4.1, he has become a bishop, and a GENTLEMAN (14) remarks that he is the powerful enemy of the Archbishop of Canterbury, Thomas CRANMER. In 5.1 and 5.2 Gardiner leads an effort to convict Cranmer of heresy, but the king intervenes and he is stymied. In Act 5 Gardiner is the unscrupulous, pro-Catholic schemer that Wolsey was before his fall, but here the king is more than a match for the villain. This indicates Henry's growth from gullibility to wisdom, an important theme of the play.

The historical Gardiner, a bright young priest, was employed by Wolsey to represent him in ROME before becoming the cardinal's secretary. Wolsey promoted his protégé into the king's service, presumably for the reasons given in the play, and Gardiner prospered. He became the king's secretary in 1529 and Bishop of Winchester in 1531. A conservative cleric, his opposition to Cranmer centred on the archbishop's prominent role in the Reformation in England. Henry balanced one against the other, but after the king's death, Cranmer gained power and Gardiner was imprisoned. However, under the Catholic Queen Mary (ruled

1553–1558), Gardiner was restored to power and Cranmer was executed, though Gardiner died before his enemy went to the stake.

Gardiner (2), William (1531–1597) Contemporary of Shakespeare, a wealthy London real-estate investor and Justice of the Peace who figured in a dispute that also involved Shakespeare. Gardiner, who bought his judgeship, seems to have been a notorious swindler; he was also imprisoned several times for abusive and violent actions and even faced charges of murder by witchcraft. In 1596 he feuded for unknown reasons with Francis LANGLEY, the proprietor of the SWAN THEATRE, and Langley sought the protection of the courts against him and his stepson William Wayte. In response, apparently, Wayte sought the same protection against Langley, Shakespeare, and two women who are otherwise unknown. Shakespeare's connection with the quarrel cannot be determined, but some scholars have inferred (though others disagree) that either he lived in BANKSIDE, which was part of Gardiner's judicial jurisdiction or that Shakespeare's acting company at the time, the CHAMBERLAIN'S MEN, played at the Swan, although there is no other evidence of this.

The noted scholar Leslie HOTSON has proposed that Shakespeare intended the comical Justice SHALLOW in *The Merry Wives of Windsor* as a satirical portrait of Gardiner, with his dim-witted relative SLENDER intended as Wayte. Shallow's coat of arms, described in *The Merry Wives,* 1.1.15–25, resembles Gardiner's, and, like Gardiner, Shallow threatens to use the law against an enemy. Moreover, Shallow intends to marry Slender to a rich young woman, a circumstance that might refer to Wayte's marriage to an heiress whom Gardiner subsequently swindled. Since *The Merry Wives* was written a few months after Wayte's complaint against Shakespeare, a literary retaliation, if one were attempted, might reasonably appear there.

However, this evidence is somewhat weak. The Elizabethan era was highly litigious, and the use of the law against one's enemies was quite ordinary. Though the coats of arms of Gardiner and Shallow both include luces, a kind of fish, the heraldic resemblance between them is not especially close (closer to Shallow's arms are those of Sir Thomas LUCY [1]). Moreover, Shallow is losing his memory and based in rural GLOUCESTERSHIRE, whereas Gardiner was a wily London businessman. Further, no slightest resemblance to Gardiner can be found in Shallow's appearance in *2 Henry IV,* written at the same time. Most significantly, although Shallow is a comic figure, his personality seems inappropriate to a scoundrel such as Gardiner appears to have been. Shakespeare's pleasant portrait of a garrulous and gullible but warm-hearted elderly country gentleman seems an unlikely weapon of vengeance.

Gargrave, Thomas (d. 1429) Historical figure and minor character in *1 Henry VI,* an officer who is killed by the same cannon shot that kills the Earl of SALISBURY (3) at the siege of ORLÉANS (1) in 1.4. The historical Gargrave is a minor figure in Shakespeare's sources, a nobleman who is recorded as having been killed at the siege.

Garnet, Henry (1555–1606) English Jesuit priest whose execution for treason is cryptically referred to in *Macbeth.* As the play's horror mounts, the PORTER (3), in a comical interlude, drunkenly pretends to serve as the door-keeper to Hell. He welcomes 'an equivocator, that could swear in both the scales against either scale; who committed treason enough for God's sake, yet could not equivocate to heaven' (2.3.8–11). The word 'equivocate' was highly charged in the English political world at the time that this scene was written (c. 1606), and it had particular pertinence to Garnet's treason trial, a notorious public event. Moreover, the Porter also welcomes to Hell 'a farmer, that hang'd himself' (2.3.4–5), a reference to the name 'Mr Farmer', used by Garnet as an underground alias. Shakespeare's original audiences will certainly have understood these lines as a political joke.

In 1605 England was shaken by the exposure of the Gunpowder Plot, an attempt by radical Catholics to blow up the Houses of Parliament and kill King JAMES I as part of an effort to install a Catholic monarch. Garnet, a Catholic convert, was the director of the clandestine Catholic Church in England. Though not one of the plotters, he was charged with complicity in the scheme for he had known of it ahead of time and had concealed his knowledge, itself a treasonable act under English law. He denied his foreknowledge at first, but when faced with an informer he confessed and justified his perjury with the doctrine of equivocation, a term he used repeatedly at his trial. 'Equivocation' was a Catholic theological term describing morally acceptable perjury, condoned when undertaken in the name of Catholic opposition to Protestantism. This defence was of course rejected, and Garnet was convicted of perjury as well as treason; he was sentenced to death and hanged.

Garrick, David (1717–1779) British actor and producer. For 35 years, beginning in 1740, Garrick dominated the London stage. He led a revolution in acting, rejecting the tradition of formal declamation still employed by James QUIN and others in favour of naturalistic speech and actions. As the longtime manager of the Drury Lane Theatre (1747–1766), he also altered the presentation of plays, introducing realistic scenery and hidden lighting, and eliminating the presence of spectators on the stage. He did much to popularise Shakespeare, producing 24 of his plays. He often re-

stored excised text and eliminated the additions of earlier producers such as Nahum TATE and William DAVENANT. Among the Shakespeare plays he resurrected in this way were *Macbeth, Coriolanus, Cymbeline, Antony and Cleopatra, The Tempest, Romeo and Juliet,* and *King Lear*—though he added his own passages to several of these and altered some of the other plays quite radically. He rewrote two plays as operas—*A Midsummer Night's Dream* (*The Fairies* [1755]) and *The Tempest* (1756)—and his *Catherine and Petruchio* (1754) and *Florizel and Perdita* (1756) were severely altered versions of *The Taming of the Shrew* and *The Winter's Tale,* respectively. His *Hamlet* (1772) was his most notorious adaptation, for he eliminated most of Act 5.

As an actor, Garrick played 17 different Shakespearean roles. He was best known as BENEDICK, RICHARD III (the part that established him as a major actor), HAMLET, MACBETH, and LEAR. In 1769 Garrick organised the Shakespeare Jubilee at STRATFORD, an elaborate celebration of the playwright that did much to make Stratford a mecca for Shakespearean enthusiasts. Garrick also wrote several successful plays, mostly farces, and several volumes of poetry. He was buried at WESTMINSTER (1) ABBEY.

Garter (Garter King-at-Arms) Minor character in *Henry VIII,* an official of the court of HENRY VIII. The Garter, whose duties include making formal proclamations at official ceremonies, is present, though mute, at the coronation of ANNE (1), and he recites a brief prayer after the christening of the future Queen ELIZABETH (1) in 5.4.1–3. His small role adds pomp and circumstance to the picture of the court.

Gascoigne, George (c. 1535–1577) English poet, author, and playwright, creator of a source for several of Shakespeare's plays. Gascoigne's *Supposes* (performed 1566, published 1575), a translation of the Italian drama *I Suppositi* (1509) by Ludovico ARIOSTO, provided the SUB-PLOT concerning BIANCA (1) in *The Taming of the Shrew,* along with many details in *The Comedy of Errors* and *The Two Gentlemen of Verona.*

Gascoigne, who wrote poetry, prose, and plays, was a literary innovator. His *Notes concerning the making of verse* (1575) is one of the earliest examples of literary criticism in English, and his TRAGEDY *Jocasta* (1566) was only the second English play to be written in BLANK VERSE. His adaptation of Ariosto helped introduce a taste for RENAISSANCE Italian literature into England.

Born into a wealthy family, Gascoigne led a dissolute life as a young man. He studied 'such lattyn as I forgat' at Cambridge, and supposedly studied law at the INNS OF COURT. He was chronically in debt and occasionally in trouble for questionable financial dealings. In 1561 he married a wealthy widow—and thus became stepfather to the noted poet Nicholas Breton (c. 1545–c. 1626)—but in 1570 he again had money troubles and was gaoled for debt. In 1572 he joined the English volunteer soldiers aiding the Dutch rebellion against the Spanish. He was intermittently in the Low Countries for the last years of his life, although he returned to England to write and publish several works, among them a final volume—*The Glass of Government* (1575)—that recorded his moral conversion.

Gascony Region in south-western FRANCE (1), an English colony from 1204 to 1453 and the location for Act 4 of *1 Henry VI.* Much of the act focusses on the battle near BORDEAUX, in which the English hero TALBOT is killed; 4.3–4 are set at English camps elsewhere in Gascony. The loss of the region following this battle, fought in 1453, effectively ended the HUNDRED YEARS WAR.

Gaultree Forest Extensive woodland near YORK (2) in northern England, setting for 4.1–3 of *2 Henry IV.* Following his sources, Shakespeare recorded an encounter between the army of King HENRY IV and that of the rebels led by the ARCHBISHOP (3) of York at the ancient royal hunting grounds of Gaultree, or Galtres. Prince John of LANCASTER (3), Henry's son, offers the rebels a fair hearing of their grievances before the King if they will disband their forces. Once they do so, he has them arrested for treason and executed. He justifies this treachery by contending that all he had promised was that the King would hear their complaints, not that they would be safe from prosecution. The episode brings Lancaster to the fore—FALSTAFF delivers an amusing assessment of him in 4.3.84–123—and it offers a closer look at the rebels. The situation is discussed, especially by the Archbishop and WESTMORELAND (1) in 4.1, in terms that offer a human understanding of the rebels' position but that also condemn rebellion as an unjustifiable disruption of society, particularly when linked to religious sentiments.

Shakespeare substituted Lancaster for Westmoreland, who actually conducted the negotiations and perpetrated the betrayal, in order to emphasise the importance of Henry's family in the web of treachery and conflict that followed his usurpation of the throne (enacted in *Richard II*). Otherwise, the historical event is accurately depicted. Lancaster is presented as a cold-blooded Machiavellian, although his ruse is not explicitly disparaged; many such ploys were used in late medieval warfare, and neither the historians whom Shakespeare read nor the playwright himself seem to treat this one as particularly heinous, particularly when compared to the much greater crime of rebellion against an anointed ruler.

Gaunt, John of (Duke of Lancaster, 1340–1399) Historical figure and character in *Richard II,* King

RICHARD II's uncle and father of BOLINGBROKE (1). Gaunt, though he dies in 2.1, is an important figure. He represents a grand tradition of statesmanlike patriotism and honour, encouraging Bolingbroke, in 1.1 and 1.3, towards the ideal of obedience to the King, whom he believes rules by divine right. On the same grounds, he resists the DUCHESS (2) of Gloucester's demands in 1.2 for vengeance against the King for the murder of her husband, Gaunt's brother. Yet he is aware of Richard's failings, and, before dying, he chastises the King severely for ruining the country through overtaxation and self-indulgence. Preparing himself for this final encounter with Richard, he meditates on England in a patriotic passage that has been famous since it was first performed: 'This royal throne of kings, this scept'red isle, . . . This blessed plot, this earth, this realm, this England, . . .' (2.1.40–50).

The historical Gaunt was a very different sort of man from the paragon of virtue presented in the play. Shakespeare altered the much more accurate portrait found in his principal source, HOLINSHED's *Chronicles*, in part because Queen ELIZABETH (1) traced her ancestry to Gaunt, but also in order to hold up an ideal representative of the chivalric age, whose passing is a major theme of the play. Gaunt, named for his birth in English-occupied Ghent, in Flanders, was a greedy and aggressive aristocrat, devoted to his own interests, not to the common welfare. Before the time of the play, he spent several years—and vast amounts of English wealth—fighting in Spain in an unsuccessful attempt to seize the crown of Castile for himself. He was widely detested in England, and during the great revolt of 1381 his palace in London was thoroughly sacked by gleeful crowds.

General Minor character in *1 Henry VI*, a French officer on the walls of BORDEAUX. He rejects TALBOT's demand for the surrender of the city in 4.2.

Gentleman (1) Either of two minor characters in *2 Henry VI*, captives of pirates in 4.1, along with the Duke of SUFFOLK (3). After the gentlemen agree to pay a ransom for their lives, Suffolk is executed by the pirates. One of the gentlemen is released to carry ransom messages to London, and he also receives Suffolk's severed head to deliver to Queen MARGARET (1).

Gentleman (2) Minor character in *Richard III*. The Gentleman vainly attempts to prevent RICHARD III from interrupting the funeral procession of HENRY VI early in 1.2, and then restarts the procession, at Richard's command, later in this scene. He speaks one line on each occasion. His first line is sometimes assigned to a HALBERDIER, for the abuse the character takes from Richard is thought inappropriate for a gentleman. Villainous though he is, it is supposed that Richard would observe the formal distinctions between aristocrats and commoners.

Gentleman (3) Minor character in *Hamlet*. In 4.5 the Gentleman brings QUEEN (9) Gertrude news of OPHELIA's madness, describing her erratic behaviour and confused language, 'That carry but half sense . . . [but] would make one think there might be thought . . .' (4.5.7–12). He thus prepares us to understand the meaning in Ophelia's disconnected songs and talk in the rest of the scene.

Gentleman (4) Minor character in *All's Well That Ends Well*, a nobleman who helps HELENA (2). In 5.1 the Gentleman tells Helena that the KING (17) has left MARSEILLES. He takes her message to the King, appearing in 5.3 with the letter that entraps BERTRAM at the play's climax. The Gentleman is merely a stereotypical courtier and a pawn of plot development.

Gentleman (5) Either of two minor characters in *Measure for Measure*, friends of LUCIO. The Gentlemen appear briefly in 1.2 where they help establish the ambience of the play's SUB-PLOT, the atmosphere of vice and degradation amid good spirits that characterises the underworld of VIENNA. They are soldiers who callously regret the prospects of peace and go on to jest about venereal disease, especially when MISTRESS (2) Overdone appears. The Gentlemen have no distinct personalities and are not distinguishable from each other. After this brief scene they disappear from the play.

Gentleman (6) Any of three minor characters in *Othello*, Venetian noblemen and members of the occupation force on CYPRUS. In 2.1 two Gentlemen talk with MONTANO (2) about the dispersal of the Turkish fleet by storm, then a third appears with news of OTHELLO's arrival to take command of the island. In 2.2 one of the Gentlemen (designated as Othello's Herald in the FOLIO and some other editions) reads the general's formal proclamation declaring a holiday, and in 3.2 another accompanies Othello on an inspection of the fort, uttering a single line. These figures are representative of the Venetian military presence, serving to further the plot.

Gentleman (7) Minor character in *King Lear*, a follower of LEAR. The Gentleman assists the loyal KENT (2) in his efforts to aid the wandering and insane king. Primarily a useful attendant, the Gentleman delivers two important descriptions that help form the audience's responses to the play in significant ways. In 3.1 he reports vividly to Kent on Lear's raging in the storm and prepares the audience for the wild scene to follow. In 4.3 he movingly describes CORDELIA's

haunting response to the news of her wretched father. Rich in religious imagery, this passage provides a strong sense of Cordelia's saintly nature, a central image of the play.

Gentleman (8) Minor character in *King Lear,* a follower of the Duke of ALBANY. In 5.3, the horrified Gentleman announces the deaths of GONERIL and REGAN. Goneril has stabbed herself after confessing that she poisoned Regan. The character adds to the increasing hysteria of the final scene.

Gentleman (9) Either of two minor characters in *Pericles,* neighbours of the physician Lord CERIMON. In 3.2, after a great storm, the Gentlemen encounter Cerimon and he remarks on his medical practise and knowledge of arcane herbal treatments. This establishes the physician's credentials to the audience, in readiness for the next episode—his revival of THAISA—which the Gentlemen observe and comment on briefly. The Gentlemen serve to carry the plot forward.

Gentleman (10) Either of two minor characters in *Pericles,* visitors to a bordello who are converted to virtue through their encounter with MARINA. In 4.5 the two Gentlemen discuss the young woman whose virtuous nature has shamed them. They marvel that 'divinity [has been] preach'd there' (4.5.4), and one of them declares, 'I'll do anything now that's virtuous' (4.5.8). With this very brief (nine-line) scene, Shakespeare establishes Marina's superiority to her circumstances. We have just seen her sold to the bordello by PIRATES who had kidnapped her earlier, and this scene makes it clear that good is in the process of triumphing over evil.

Gentleman (11) Any of several minor characters in *Pericles,* attendants of PERICLES. In 5.1 the Gentlemen are summoned to receive LYSIMACHUS, the governor of MYTILENE, who is visiting Pericles' ship. One Gentleman acknowledges the call in four words, but otherwise these courtiers do not speak. They are extras, intended to increase the atmosphere of ceremonious formality that surrounds Pericles.

Gentleman (12) Either of two minor characters in *Cymbeline,* noblemen at King CYMBELINE's court. In 1.1 the First Gentleman tells the Second Gentleman about the marriage of the king's daughter, IMOGEN, to POSTHUMUS, a poor but noble youth who has been banished from Britain because the king had wanted Imogen to marry the boorish CLOTEN. He adds that Imogen is the king's only child, other than two lost sons, kidnapped 20 years earlier and never recovered. The First Gentleman's excitement is clear in his hurried speech. This stirs interest in the audience, though his companion merely punctuates his monologue with brief questions. The episode, which fills the whole of the play's first scene, establishes the basic situation of the plot.

Gentleman (13) Any of three minor characters in *The Winter's Tale,* courtiers at the court of King LEONTES of SICILIA. They report to AUTOLYCUS on the off-stage encounter of Leontes and his old friend King POLIXENES, whom he had earlier wronged, and of the discovery by Leontes of his long-lost daughter, PERDITA. The First Gentleman knows only that something extraordinary has happened, the Second knows the result, but only the Third Gentleman can describe the events as they happened, which he does at length, in 5.2.31–103. The language of all three Gentlemen is flowery and ornate, typical of the courtly idiom of the 17th century. Although they display little individual personality, they are nevertheless interesting as miniature portraits of Jacobean courtiers. (Some editors presume that the SERVANT [27] of 5.1 is another such courtier and designate him a Gentleman.) Shakespeare's presentation of crucial events through the reporting of minor characters is sometimes criticised, but here he avoids a scene that would repeat much that the audience already knows. He also provides a contrast with the play's true climax, still to come in 5.3.

Gentleman (14) Any of three minor characters in *Henry VIII,* members of the court of King HENRY VIII. In 2.1 two of the Gentlemen discuss the trial and conviction of the Duke of BUCKINGHAM (1). They attribute the duke's fall to Cardinal WOLSEY, who they say is hated by the common people as much as Buckingham is loved. After witnessing Buckingham's moving farewell, they discuss Wolsey's effort to bring down Queen KATHERINE and mention the arrival of Cardinal CAMPEIUS as part of that story. Thus, they convey much important information about the plot, while stirring the audience's responses to the villain and his victims.

In 4.1 the Gentlemen reappear, this time at the coronation of Queen ANNE (1). They speak of the deposed Katherine's exile to KIMBOLTON, and as the royal procession passes by, they identify and remark on its participants. They are then joined by a Third Gentleman, who describes the actual coronation ceremony in exalted terms that foster the play's depiction of Anne as a saintly queen, rejoiced in by the country. They go on to discuss the advancement of Thomas CRANMER and Thomas CROMWELL in the wake of Wolsey's fall, and they mention the rivalry between Cranmer, now Archbishop of Canterbury, and Bishop GARDINER (1). This foreshadows the political developments of Act 5. Once again, the Gentlemen convey information while also suggesting the play's point of view.

Gentleman (15) Minor character in *Henry VIII,* an attendant to Queen KATHERINE. In 3.1 the Gentleman announces the arrival of 'two great cardinals' (3.1.16), WOLSEY and CAMPEIUS, thus introducing the main business of the scene.

Gentleman (16) Minor character in *The Two Noble Kinsmen,* a messenger from Duke THESEUS (2) of ATHENS to EMILIA (4). In 4.2 the Gentleman informs the sorrowing Emilia that ARCITE and PALAMON are prepared to duel for her love. He serves merely to translate the scene from Emilia's soliloquy to the preparations for the duel. Most scholars agree that 4.1 and the Gentleman were the work of Shakespeare's collaborator, John FLETCHER (2).

Gentleman-poet Character in *The Winter's Tale.* See SERVANT (27).

Gentleman Usher Minor character in *Henry VIII,* an attendant to Queen KATHERINE and her official escort at her divorce trial. The Gentleman Usher, accompanied by a lesser servant carrying a silver mace, walks before the Queen with great ceremony, in the stage direction opening 2.4. Later in the scene, he speaks one line, following King HENRY VIII's order that the departing queen be called back. He serves merely to emphasise the pomp of the proceedings. The same figure reappears under his proper name, GRIFFITH, in 4.2.

Gentlewoman (1) Minor character in *Macbeth,* an attendant to LADY (6) MACBETH. The Gentlewoman confers with the DOCTOR (3) on her mistress' somnambulism, and together they witness Lady Macbeth's hallucinatory manifestations of guilt in the famous sleep-walking scene (5.1). Before Lady Macbeth appears, the Gentlewoman refuses to tell the Doctor what she has heard—her mistress' obsession with MACBETH's murders—without a witness to back her up. This demonstrates the distrust that permeates the play's world, one of *Macbeth*'s important themes.

Gentlewoman (2) Minor character in *Coriolanus,* an attendant to VIRGILIA and VOLUMNIA. In 1.3 the Gentlewoman announces the arrival of VALERIA and then escorts her on stage. She speaks only a single line and serves to indicate the prestige and wealth of the ladies she serves.

Geoffrey of Monmouth (c. 1100–1154) English medieval writer, creator of the Arthurian cycle of tales. Geoffrey's *Historia Regum Britanniae* (c. 1140) provided much material for Raphael HOLINSHED's *Chronicles of England, Scotland, and Ireland* (1577, 1587), Shakespeare's principal source for his two plays dealing with pre-medieval Britain, *King Lear* and *Cymbeline.* Geoffrey's book was not actually a history so much as a collection intended to appeal to the fashion for courtly tales—for example, the French stories of Charlemagne—and it immediately became very popular. It claimed to be a Latin translation of a book in Cymric, the language of WALES, that told the history of Britain up to the reign of King Arthur. It was in fact a mixture of various old chronicles, traditional stories and, probably, outright fictions. It established King Arthur as a British cultural hero, and it has been called the most important literary work of the 12th century.

Geoffrey was born into a family of clergymen and was educated at Monmouth's famed Benedictine abbey. He was probably a monk, though he was primarily a writer rather than a man of the cloth. In his old age he was made a bishop due to the influence of his aristocratic patrons—possibly including King Stephen of England—but he had to be ordained a priest for the occasion.

George (1) Character in *2 Henry VI.* See BEVIS.

George (2) York, Duke of Clarence (1449–1478) Historical figure and character in *3 Henry VI,* the untrustworthy younger brother of EDWARD IV. George returns from exile following the death of his father, the Duke of YORK (8). He supports Edward in his pursuit of the crown, becoming Duke of Clarence upon his brother's accession. However, resenting the advancement of his brother's in-laws (see ELIZABETH [2]), he joins WARWICK (3) in his rebellion, leaving Edward's court in 4.1. After helping Warwick reinstate HENRY VI, George is persuaded to defect again by his younger brother Richard (see RICHARD III) in 5.1, and he returns to Edward's cause. After fighting for Edward at BARNET and TEWKESBURY and participating in the murder of the PRINCE (4) of Wales, George is present in the final scene to pledge his rather doubtful loyalty to his elder brother. In *Richard III* the same figure appears as CLARENCE (1), and he is often so called, by himself and other characters, in *3 Henry VI.*

The historical George remained abroad in exile until Edward was crowned, at which time he was still only 12 years old. Shakespeare brings him into the action before that time, and as an adult, in order to establish him as a member of Edward's court well before he deserts it. Also, George's prominence in the play does much to emphasise the disloyalty and lack of honour that prevailed at the time of the WARS OF THE ROSES.

German, Edward (1862–1936) British composer, creator of incidental music for *Henry VIII.* German—whose name is pronounced with a hard 'G'—established himself as a composer for the theatre with three dances created for Henry IRVING's 1892 production of *Henry VIII.* These pieces were immediately popular

and were staples of the music-hall repertoire for years, besides adorning subsequent productions of Shakespeare's play. German went on to a successful career as a composer of light opera—most notably *Merrie England* (1902)—and miscellaneous theatrical music.

Gertrude Character in *Hamlet.* See QUEEN (9).

Gervinus, Georg Gottfried (1805–1871) German scholar. A professor of literature at the University of Heidelberg, Gervinus published a four-volume collection of commentaries on Shakespeare's plays (1849, translated as *Shakespeare Commentaries* in 1863), which was highly influential on Shakespeare scholars in both Germany and England. He was an important advocate of the VERSE TEST, used to determine the chronology of the plays, and he is considered the first writer to study the development of the playwright's work over the course of his career.

Ghost (1) Any of 11 minor but significant characters in *Richard III,* the ghosts of the victims of RICHARD III, who appear to the King and his enemy RICHMOND in 5.3, on the eve of the battle of BOSWORTH FIELD. The ghosts each deliver brief messages, insisting that Richard shall 'despair and die' and assuring Richmond of victory. The ghosts appear in the order in which they died: the ghosts of the PRINCE (4) of Wales and his father, HENRY VI, hark back to murders Richard committed in *3 Henry VI,* the preceding play in Shakespeare's TETRALOGY. Next appears the ghost of Richard's brother CLARENCE (1), followed by those of lords RIVERS, GREY (2), and VAUGHAN. The ghost of Lord William HASTINGS (3) comes forth next, succeeded by those of the two children Richard had ordered killed—another PRINCE (5) of Wales and his brother YORK (7). Richard is then faced by the ghost of his wife ANNE (2), only recently eliminated so that the King could make a politically convenient second marriage. The ghost of Richard's closest ally in his bloody rise to power, the Duke of BUCKINGHAM (2), executed only two scenes earlier, appears last. Shakespeare's source, the history by Edward HALL (2), mentions rumours that Richard had complained of nightmares before the battle, but the content of the dreams appears to be the playwright's invention.

Ghost (2) Character in *Julius Caesar,* the spirit of the assassinated CAESAR (1). In 4.3, as BRUTUS rests in his tent near SARDIS, the Ghost appears to him, identifies itself as Brutus' 'evil spirit', and warns, 'thou shalt see me at Philippi' (4.3.281, 285)—that is, at the subsequent battle of PHILIPPI. In 5.5, defeated and preparing for suicide, Brutus recounts that the Ghost of Caesar has appeared to him a second time and concludes, 'I know my hour is come' (5.5.20). Shakespeare's presentation of the Ghost closely follows the account in PLUTARCH's *Lives.*

Ghost (3) Character in *Hamlet,* the spirit of the murdered King of Denmark, HAMLET's late father. The Ghost, which has been silent in its appearances before the play opens and in 1.1 and 1.4, speaks to Hamlet in 1.5, revealing the secret of his death—'Murder most foul' (1.5.27) at the hands of his brother, Claudius, the present KING (5)—and insisting that Hamlet exact revenge. This demand establishes the stress that disturbs Hamlet throughout the play. The Ghost reappears in 3.4 to remind Hamlet that he has not yet accomplished his revenge, thereby increasing the pressure on the prince.

The Ghost is clearly an awesome presence, as the responses of BARNARDO, MARCELLUS, and HORATIO make clear in 1.1 and 1.4, and we are plainly meant to be impressed by Hamlet's bravery in speaking to it. At first, Hamlet cannot be sure whether it is 'a spirit of health or goblin damn'd' (1.4.40), and his doubts recur when he suspects that its message may be a lie that 'Abuses me to damn me' (2.2.599). Only Claudius' reaction to the playlet re-enacting the murder makes clear that the Ghost is to be trusted.

The Ghost pushes Hamlet to face the trauma of his father's murder and his mother's acceptance of the murderer. It keeps his anguish sharp. However, the Ghost is absent at the end of the drama. It has represented the emotional demands of Hamlet's grief and despair; when Act 5 offers the play's reconciliation of good and evil, the Ghost has no further function.

Belief in ghosts was common in Shakespeare's world—King JAMES I, who was regarded as a competent writer on religious matters, wrote a treatise on their characteristics—though many educated people regarded such beliefs as unfounded superstition. Shakespeare's own opinion cannot be known, for the only evidence is the attitudes he ascribes to his fictional characters; Hamlet certainly accepts the reality of the spirit, doubting only its purposes for a time. In any case, a ghost was a common feature of the REVENGE PLAY, a popular genre in the early 17th century, and Shakespeare took the Ghost in *Hamlet* from one such work, the UR-HAMLET.

Ghost (4) Character in *Macbeth,* the spirit of the murdered BANQUO. The Ghost appears at the banquet hosted by MACBETH and LADY (6) MACBETH in 3.4. It can only be seen by Macbeth, who had ordered Banquo's murder and is the only one present who knows he is dead. It appears again in 4.1 in the company of the ghostly procession of future KINGS shown to Macbeth by the WITCHES. In both cases the Ghost is silent. In 4.1 Macbeth observes that it 'points at them [the Kings] for his' (4.1.124); this confirms the Witches'

prediction that Banquo's descendants will be kings. On both occasions the Ghost appears when Macbeth names Banquo, first, when he hypocritically praises him at the banquet, in 3.4, and then when he demands to know about the prediction, in 4.1. This highlights the connection between the Ghost and Macbeth's internal state. Moreover, in 3.4, the Ghost is seen only by Macbeth, which further points up his disturbed state of mind in the aftermath of his crimes.

That no one else can see the Ghost in 3.4 is sometimes taken as evidence that the spectre does not in fact exist and is merely Macbeth's hallucination. However, it was believed by many in Shakespeare's day that ghosts and other supernatural beings could limit their visibility at will to particular individuals at particular times. (For instance, the GHOST (3) in *Hamlet* is seen by HAMLET and several other characters in Act 1, but is invisible to GERTRUDE when Hamlet sees it again in 3.4.) Banquo's Ghost thus serves as both a supernatural and a natural—that is, psychological—phenomenon, and no conclusions can be drawn as to Shakespeare's belief in ghosts. In any case, whether it is real or not, Banquo's Ghost adds to the eerie supernatural atmosphere that permeates the play and stresses the unnaturalness of Macbeth's evil.

The Ghost is usually played by the actor who has played Banquo, though some productions employ film or slide projections or some other image, like the huge mask in Orson WELLES' controversial 'voodoo' *Macbeth.* In other productions Macbeth is presented as hallucinating, and the Ghost does not actually appear.

Ghost Character Person mentioned in stage directions but not actually appearing in a play, having been excised or possibly simply forgotten about in the course of composition. The existence of such a character is often taken as evidence that the text in which it first appears was printed from the playwright's FOUL PAPERS, for such a superfluous figure would presumably have been deleted from any more evolved text, such as a PROMPT-BOOK. Ghost characters in Shakespeare's plays include VIOLENTA in *All's Well That Ends Well;* LAMPRIUS, RANNIUS, and LUCILLIUS in *Antony and Cleopatra;* BEAUMONT (1) in *Henry V;* INNOGEN in *Much Ado About Nothing;* PETRUCHIO (1) in *Romeo and Juliet;* and the MERCER in *Timon of Athens.*

Gibborne, Thomas (active 1624) English actor. Though known as a member of the PALSGRAVE'S MEN according to a document of 1624, Gibborne is thought by some scholars to have been the actor who played Shakespeare's RAMBURES in *Henry V,* because the character is designated as 'Gebon' in speech headings and stage directions of the BAD QUARTO edition of the play (1600). However, Samuel GILBURNE is generally thought a more likely nominee.

Gide, André (1869–1951) French author and translator of Shakespeare. Gide is best known for his novels (*The Immoralist* [1902], *The Plague* [1947], etc.), but he also translated *Hamlet* and *Antony and Cleopatra* into French and wrote prefaces to translations of several other of the plays. He was awarded the Nobel Prize for Literature in 1947.

Gielgud, John (b. 1904) British actor and director. Gielgud's long and distinguished career began with an appearance as the HERALD (4) in *Henry V* at the OLD VIC THEATRE in 1921. His portrayals of HAMLET and RICHARD II are especially renowned, but he has also played most of Shakespeare's other protagonists. He has produced a number of Shakespeare's plays, including *Hamlet, Macbeth,* and *Romeo and Juliet.* His 1949 production of *Much Ado About Nothing,* with himself as BENEDICK, was revived several times in the 1950s. With Laurence OLIVIER and Ralph RICHARDSON (2), Gielgud is considered one of the greatest Shakespearean actors of the 20th century.

Gilbard, William (d. 1612) Stratford teacher and clerk, possible inspiration for Shakespeare's character NATHANIEL (1) of *Love's Labour's Lost.* Gilbard is recorded as the assistant schoolmaster in 1561–1562 and as the acting schoolmaster on many occasions thereafter, until 1574; thus, he probably taught the young Shakespeare. By 1576 Gilbard was a curate and assisted the parish priest. His literacy enabled him to supplement his income as a clerk—he drew up many wills, for instance, including that of Anne HATHAWAY's father—and from 1603–1611 he was the parish clerk. The records he kept in this capacity contain a much higher proportion of Latin words and phrases than other clerks of the time used, which suggests that he was proud of his education. Gilbard has been suggested as a model for Nathaniel, also a curate, though there is no actual evidence to support the idea.

Gilburne, Samuel (active 1605) English actor. Gilburne is listed in the FIRST FOLIO as one of the 26 'Principall Actors' in Shakespeare's plays, but he is otherwise known only as a beneficiary of Augustine PHILLIPS' will (1605), where he is said to have been Phillips' apprentice, presumably as a boy. Gilburne may have played a LORD (6) in *All's Well That Ends Well*—designated as 'G' in the Folio text of the play—and *Henry V*'s RAMBURES, who is designated as 'Gebon' in the BAD QUARTO edition (1600).

Gildon, Charles (1665–1724) English playwright and critic. Trained as a Roman Catholic priest, Gildon abandoned his calling to become a hack writer. He published popular commentaries on English poetry and drama, including an anthology of biographical

pieces (some written by him, though all unsigned) that included a brief and entirely unreliable life of Shakespeare. In 1699 he produced a play entitled *Measure for Measure, or Beauty the Best Advocate,* based loosely on Shakespeare's play—or rather on William DAVENANT's earlier adaptation, THE LAW AGAINST LOVERS. Gildon dropped much of Davenant's introduced material and replaced it, not with Shakespeare's text, but with a play within a play, an operatic MASQUE on the ancient Roman legend of Dido and AENEAS. In 1710 Gildon published *Poems* by Shakespeare, which was bound as a seventh volume of Nicholas ROWE's six-volume collection of the plays though not published by the same publisher. This piece of near-piracy earned Gildon an insulting passage in the famous literary satire, *The Dunciad* (1728), by Alexander POPE (1).

Giles, Nathaniel (c. 1559–1634) Choirmaster and sometime director of the Children of the Chapel (see CHILDREN'S COMPANIES). Giles, a Protestant minister and musician, was appointed director of the Chapel Royal, the court choir of Queen ELIZABETH (1), which recruited boys from church choirs all over the country and placed them in a school at court, where they were educated while performing for the queen. In 1600 Giles joined Henry EVANS (2) in producing plays performed by the Chapel school's acting company, the Children of the Chapel, at the WHITEFRIARS THEATRE. However, in 1602 Giles and Evans were accused of misusing the Chapel Royal's recruiting power to enroll non-singers for the acting company. Evans fled the country and only returned after the queen's death; Giles continued to run the company, but in 1616 the choir's connection with Evans and the actors was severed by royal command. Giles remained as choirmaster until his death. He also was a noted composer of church music.

Girl (Margaret Plantagenet, 1473–1541) Historical figure and minor character in *Richard III,* the daughter of CLARENCE (1). The Girl mourns her father's murder in 2.2 and is present but silent in 4.1. Richard is fearful that a husband of the Girl might claim the throne, her father having been the heir apparent. He remarks in 4.3.37 that he has therefore married her to a low-ranking husband, who cannot claim the crown. Historically, this manoeuvre was performed by Richard's conqueror and successor, Henry VII, the RICHMOND of the play. At the age of 68, being the last surviving PLANTAGENET, Margaret was beheaded by a paranoid HENRY VIII.

Giulio Romano (Giulio Pippi) (1492–1546) Italian painter and architect, the only RENAISSANCE artist mentioned in Shakespeare. In *The Winter's Tale,* when PAULINA announces that she has a statue representing Queen HERMIONE, believed long dead, the statue is said to be 'performed'—meaning either made or painted—'by that rare Italian master, Julio Romano, who, had he himself eternity and could put breath into his work, would beguile Nature of her custom, so perfectly he is her ape' (5.2.95–99). Since the sculpture turns out not to be a sculpture at all, its ascription to Giulio proves irrelevant; the use of the name merely lends verisimilitude to the gossip surrounding Paulina's cover story.

That Shakespeare should use Giulio's name in such a context suggests that his audience knew the artist's work, but that he should mistakenly make him a sculptor—or a mere finisher of sculptures—suggests that the playwright and presumably his audience did not know his work very well. It is of course an anachronism to name a Renaissance artist in a tale set in ancient times, but Shakespeare was tolerant of such inconsistencies, which appear throughout his plays. In any case, in Shakespeare's ROMANCES, with their welter of languages and exotic settings, a degree of confusion is probably intentional, promoting a sense of timelessness that furthers the playwright's ends.

The historical Giulio Romano (born Peppi but later named for his birthplace, ROME) was the chief pupil and assistant of Raphael (1483–1520), one of the most important Italian painters. Giulio himself became one of the leading painters and architects of his day, an innovator with a boldly pioneering style. He completed a number of Raphael's great decorative programmes at the Vatican on the master's death and then moved to MANTUA, where he was court painter and architect to Duke Federigo Gonzaga (1500–1540). His masterpiece is a ducal palace, the Palazzo del Tè, begun in 1526; both its architecture and its elaborately painted decor broke the conventions of Renaissance art to create bizarre and startling effects—an early example of the Mannerist style that dominated the second half of the 16th century. Giulio's painting, which combined elements from Raphael and Michelangelo (1475–1564), was widely influential.

Glansdale, Sir William (fl. 1429) Historical figure and minor character in *1 Henry VI,* an officer present when the Earl of SALISBURY (3) is killed at the siege of ORLÉANS (1) in 1.4. The historical Glansdale is a minor figure in Shakespeare's sources as well; he was an officer who is recorded as having been present at the siege.

Glendower, Owen (c. 1359–c. 1416) Historical figure and character in *1 Henry IV,* military leader from WALES (1) who joins rebellious English noblemen against King HENRY IV. In 3.1, at a rebel council of war, Glendower boasts of supernatural powers, displaying the superstitiousness traditionally associated with the Welsh, to the disgust of HOTSPUR. The clash of these two personalities almost upsets the alliance, though

Glendower, admiring his hot-headed ally, makes peace several times during the scene. In a lighter vein Glendower interprets for his daughter, LADY (8) Mortimer, who is in love with her husband, Lord MORTIMER (2), but does not speak English. Father and daughter together reveal their lyrical sentimental streak and a love of music, also traits stereotypically associated with the Welsh.

Later, in 4.4.16–18, Glendower is reported to have absented himself from the crucial battle of SHREWSBURY, 'o'er-rul'd by prophecies'. This episode adds Glendower's superstitiousness to the general weakness and incapacity that plague the rebel cause. Also, the account lends Hotspur's defeat an ominous, fated quality that is in keeping with the play's condemnation of rebellion.

Although Shakespeare's sources mention Glendower's training in law and his youthful service at the English court, he is chiefly portrayed as a barbaric and ruthless Welsh outlaw, as is reflected in the report on him by the Earl of WESTMORELAND (1) in 1.1.40–46. However, Shakespeare amplifies and softens this figure, and his Glendower is a composer and scholar whom Mortimer can describe as 'a worthy gentleman, . . . valiant as a lion, and wondrous affable, and as bountiful as mines of India' (3.1.159–163). Traditional English bias against the Welsh may account for the brute of the chronicles; the music-loving sage of the play may reflect Shakespeare's acquaintance with Welsh residents of London. Glendower's superstitiousness may also derive from the playwright's personal knowledge, for the English stereotype of the superstitious Welshman was grounded in the survival of a strong Celtic religious sensibility in Wales. Although Hotspur finds this trait ridiculous (3.1.142–158), Shakespeare himself apparently regarded it more sympathetically, as a humorous failing. Glendower is on the whole a positive figure, if a weak one. Even Hotspur's raillery against him is enjoyable rhetoric.

The historical Glendower led the last and most nearly successful Welsh rebellion against the English. In 1400, shortly after Henry IV's deposition of RICHARD II, Glendower led an uprising that grew from a quarrel with his English neighbour into a full-scale revolt. In 1403 the Welsh rebels joined with those from northern England led by Hotspur, and only Henry's decisive advance on Shrewsbury prevented their forces from combining. That Glendower's superstition led him to abandon the rebels at Shrewsbury is not reported in Shakespeare's sources; HOLINSHED, in fact, mistakenly says that Glendower was at the battle, and DANIEL, like modern historians, attributes his absence only to King Henry's superior generalship. In 1404, with most of Wales under his control, Glendower established a national government at Harlech, where a parliament elected him Prince of Wales, and he entered into an alliance with England's enemy, FRANCE (1). In 1405, with French troops reinforcing his own, he invaded England but was defeated by Henry. This was the high-water mark of his rebellion, and by 1409 Glendower had lost even Harlech and had retreated deep into the mountains. After 1410 he disappears from history, though he is thought to have lived somewhat longer. Although only briefly successful, Glendower united Wales—a land of petty principalities before the English invaded in the 12th century—and led it to an independence it never again attained. He remains a great hero of Welsh culture.

A minor character in *Richard II,* the CAPTAIN (4), is sometimes thought to have been intended as Glendower, and the famous leader is specifically referred to in that play as Glendor (3.1.43). He is also inaccurately said to have imprisoned his son-in-law Mortimer in *2 Henry VI* (2.2.40). His death is reported (several years too early, due to an error in Holinshed) in *2 Henry IV* (3.1.103).

Globe Theatre Theatre in SOUTHWARK built by Cuthbert BURBAGE (1) in 1599, the principal home of Shakespeare's acting company and the site of the first performances of many of his plays. The Globe was built for the CHAMBERLAIN'S MEN when Burbage was unable to renew the ground lease for the land on which their old home, the THEATRE, stood. He therefore had the Theatre, a timber building, taken down

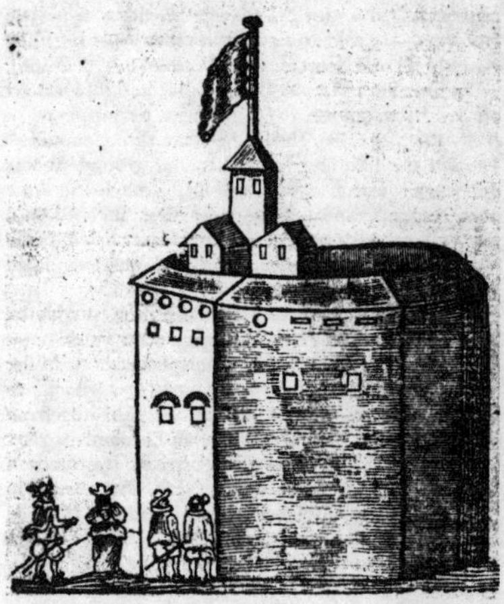

Artists' depictions such as this one, while not fully trustworthy, give us an idea of what the Globe Theatre might have looked like. (Courtesy of Culver Pictures, Inc.)

and reassembled at a new site, in Southwark, on the south side of the Thames River, beyond the jurisdiction of the LONDON government, which was opposed to theatre. The lease for the land was jointly held, half by Burbage and his brother Richard BURBAGE (3), and half by a group of five actors—Shakespeare, John HEMINGE, Augustine PHILLIPS, Thomas POPE (2), and Will KEMPE—who put their shares in trust with William LEVESON and Thomas SAVAGE. The Globe opened in late 1599; *As You Like It* may have been written for the occasion, and when Shakespeare had JAQUES (1) say, 'All the world's a stage . . .' (2.7.139), he may have been slyly alluding to the new theatre.

The Globe was a roughly cylindrical—probably polygonal—three-storey timber building, unroofed over the stage in the centre. Each floor contained open galleries with seats. The galleries extended around much of the circle, and the stage was built out into the centre from the remaining part of the building. In the building behind the stage were dressing rooms—the 'tiring house'—perhaps galleries for musicians, and apparatus for scenery and props. Above the thatched roof rose a tower, or 'penthouse', from which flags were flown and trumpets sounded to announce a production. An 18th-century account asserted that on its facade the Globe sported a painted sign depicting Hercules supporting the planet Earth (one of his legendary tasks was to stand in for Atlas). If this was so—and scholars generally believe it was—this sign may be alluded to in *Hamlet,* where the CHILDREN'S COMPANIES, in a satirical passage on the WAR OF THE THEATRES, are said to have triumphed over both the PLAYERS (2) and 'Hercules and his load too' (2.2.358).

On June 29, 1613, the Globe's thatched roof was set on fire by a cannon fired during a performance of *Henry VIII,* as called for in the stage direction at 1.4.49, and the building burned to the ground. It was open again within a year, rebuilt to much the same plan, but this time the roof was tiled. In 1644, two years after the theatres of England were closed by the revolutionary government, the Globe was torn down and tenements built on the lot.

The appearance of the Globe can only roughly be determined, from several drawings of its exterior (in large-scale city scenes), from the specifications in the builder's contract for the FORTUNE THEATRE (which was modelled on the Globe), and by extrapolating from the only sketch of the interior of an Elizabethan playhouse, the SWAN THEATRE. Nevertheless, two modern replicas of the Globe have been made. One opened in 1988 in Tokyo with a British production of *Henry V,* and the other is scheduled to open in 1991 in London (though at a different location from the original).

Gloucester (1), Earl of Character in *King Lear,* father of EDGAR and EDMUND. Gloucester is the central figure of the play's SUB-PLOT, in which his illegitimate son Edmund's villainy and his own error lead him to disaster and suffering from which he recovers only to die. This progression parallels the story of King LEAR in the main plot. Deceived by Edmund, who wants to inherit the earldom, Gloucester disinherits and banishes his legitimate son Edgar. Because Gloucester is faithful to the outcast and insane Lear, Edmund turns him over to Lear's enemy, the Duke of CORNWALL, who puts out Gloucester's eyes and banishes him into the wilderness. Edgar, disguised as a wandering lunatic, tends to his father. He saves him from suicide, in 4.6, and renews in him the strength to endure. Finally, however, when Gloucester learns Edgar's identity, the old man dies; 'his flaw'd heart, . . . 'Twixt two extremes of passion, joy and grief, / Burst smilingly' (5.3.195–198).

Gloucester's tale offers a significant parallel to that of Lear; like the king's, Gloucester's tragedy is self-induced, for his actual blinding is preceded by figurative blindness when he fails to see either Edgar's virtue or Edmund's villainy. Like Lear, Gloucester recognises his error—'I stumbled when I saw' (4.1.19), he confesses—when it is too late. His helpless wanderings, dependent on the aid of a seeming lunatic, suggest powerfully the similar straits of the mad king. The similarity between the two reaches a horrific climax, in 4.6, when they encounter each other on the beach at DOVER; it is one of the most touching passages in Shakespeare. The mad and the blind old men recognise each other and acknowledge their joint status as victims; their consciousness, though it is flawed by their handicaps, is clearly more acute than it was before.

Their parallel tales, and the close sympathy of Lear and Gloucester when they meet, is highly significant for our interpretation of the play's final moments. Gloucester's death immediately precedes Lear's at the close of the play, and because their parallel development has been stressed, we may read in the king's death the same 'extremes of passion' and presume that his heart, too, 'burst smilingly'. Thus, Gloucester's tragedy helps confirm the nobility of human suffering, a central message of the play.

Gloucester (2), Eleanor Cobham, Duchess of Character in *2 Henry VI.* See DUCHESS (1).

Gloucester (3), Eleanor de Bohun, Duchess of Character in *Richard II.* See DUCHESS (2).

Gloucester (4), Humphrey, Duke of (1390–1447) Historical figure and character in *1* and *2 Henry VI, 2 Henry IV,* and *Henry V,* the youngest son of King HENRY IV and the brother of King HENRY V and the dukes of CLARENCE (2) and LANCASTER (3). He is an important figure in the aristocratic disputes of the *Henry VI* plays, presented as the chief cause of the English loss to FRANCE (1) in the HUNDRED YEARS WAR. In the later

works, where he is a younger man, he is a minor character.

In the *Henry VI* plays Gloucester engages in a running dispute with his uncle the Bishop of WINCHESTER (1). He is depicted as a valorous defender of England's honour, whereas Winchester is an opportunistic politician. Their feud rages through 3.1 of *Part 1,* after which it is replaced in importance by that between YORK (8) and SOMERSET (3). In *Part 2* Gloucester's wife, the DUCHESS (1) of Gloucester, is convicted on charges of witchcraft and banished. Then, in 3.1, Gloucester himself is arrested at BURY ST. EDMUNDS, falsely charged with treason, and killed. Hired murderers flee the scene of the crime at the beginning of 3.2; the SECOND MURDERER (1) regrets the deed because the duke's death had been marked by religious penitence.

After Gloucester's death the country slides into civil war, and we are meant to see him as having been the guardian against such an event. In order to magnify the duke's virtues, two otherwise irrelevant anecdotes are inserted into the story. In 2.1 Gloucester demonstrates his perceptiveness by exposing the imposter SIMPCOX, and in 3.1 he wisely postpones a potentially explosive issue, York's appointment as regent in France, until a marginally related dispute can be resolved (see PETER [1]; HORNER). These incidents demonstrate the qualities of prudence and judgement that are shortly to be denied the country by the duke's murder.

The historical Gloucester was very different from the 'good Duke Humphrey' (*2 Henry VI,* 3.2.322) of these plays. Shakespeare, following his sources and the established opinion of his own time, was opposed to the political position of Gloucester's enemies and he thus depicted Humphrey as a patriot. Winchester headed a 'peace party' that advocated a withdrawal from a war virtually lost. Gloucester and the 'hawks' of the day, however, insisted that the war go on. In the HISTORY PLAYS Shakespeare presents the view that the French were able to drive the English from France only because of English disunity, and Gloucester's insistence on continuing the war was taken to demonstrate a patriotic faith in English arms that the 'peace party' lacked.

Gloucester was in fact selfishly ambitious, quite willing to pursue his own interests at the expense of the country's, once the restraining influence of Henry V was gone. After Henry's death Gloucester's power was restricted by a council of nobles who recognised his headstrong selfishness. He rebelled; the dispute with Winchester at the TOWER OF LONDON (*1 Henry VI,* 1.3) reflects Gloucester's actual coup attempt of 1425. A year later, he eloped with the wife of a close friend of the Duke of BURGUNDY (2), England's most important ally, and then recruited an army to support his new wife's claims. A duel with Burgundy was avoided only by the annulment of the marriage. This affair was among the grievances that Burgundy cited when he eventually defected from the English alliance against France. Later Gloucester scandalously married his mistress, Eleanor Cobham, who, as Duchess of Gloucester, was found guilty of treason and witchcraft.

No evidence has ever been offered to support the belief that Gloucester was murdered. Although he died while in Suffolk's custody, historians generally believe that his death was natural. No question of murder arose at the time, and Suffolk's banishment only occurred some years later, for different reasons.

In *2 Henry IV* and *Henry V,* set years earlier, Gloucester's role is minor. He is present at his father's deathbed in 4.4 and 4.5 of the first play, and in 5.2 he commiserates with the CHIEF JUSTICE on the treatment the jurist expects to receive from the new king, whom he believes is an enemy. In *Henry V* Gloucester is an almost anonymous member of the king's entourage.

Gloucester (5), Richard Plantagenet, Duke of (later RICHARD III, King of England) Title held by RICHARD III after 2.6 of *3 Henry VI* and until he is crowned king in 4.2 of *Richard III.* Some modern editions of these plays follow 16th- and 17th-century practise and designate the character as Gloucester (Gloster) in stage directions and speech headings in Acts 3–5 of *3 Henry VI* and Acts 1–3 of *Richard III.* Other editions name him Richard, throughout.

The prior holder of Richard's dukedom had been the ill-fated Humphrey, Duke of GLOUCESTER (4), whose murder occurs off-stage in 3.2 of *2 Henry VI.* Therefore, as Shakespeare's audience will have recognised, the title bodes evil for its holder. Richard himself points this out in 2.6.107 of *3 Henry VI.* His words ironically prefigure his own fall, in a technique Shakespeare frequently used in the HISTORY PLAYS: references in the dialogue to past or future events serve to heighten dramatic tension, which is threatened by the long period of time over which the action takes place.

Gloucester (6), Thomas of Woodstock, Duke of (1355–1397) Historical figure mentioned prominently in *Richard II,* brother of John of GAUNT, uncle of King RICHARD II, and husband of the DUCHESS (2) of Gloucester. Although he does not appear in the play, the Duke of Gloucester, often called Woodstock, is an important figure in Acts 1–2. His murder, which occurred six months prior to the play's opening, sparks the crises that lead to Richard's deposition.

In 1.1 BOLINGBROKE (1) accuses MOWBRAY (1) of complicity in the death of Gloucester, who died in Mowbray's custody in the prison of the English fortress at Calais. In 1.2 Gaunt and the duchess discuss Woodstock's death: they know that Mowbray did indeed kill the duke, and that he did so under the king's orders. In 4.1, just before Richard's deposition, the murder is again mentioned—Richard's favourite, the

Duke of AUMERLE, is now implicated—to reinforce our sense of Richard's guilt. Gloucester's murder is given importance as a symptom of illness in the body politic, evidence that Richard's fall has been made inevitable by his own misdeeds.

Gloucester is presented as a splendid figure of humanity. Gaunt, in his dying speech to Richard, refers to Gloucester as a 'plain, well-meaning soul' (2.1.128), alluding both to his sturdy, unfashionable dress and his frank and open mode of speech. He is several times referred to as 'noble'. The duchess loved him as a husband, and she calls him 'the model of [his father, the late King Edward III's] life' (1.2.28), thus equating him with England's greatest contemporary hero. Furthermore, the duchess points out that his royal blood should have made him sacrosanct; with his death, an important tradition has been defiled. Gloucester is thus a focus of nostalgia: he symbolises the chivalric ethic of Edward III's day, a glorious age whose passing is one of the major themes of the play.

Shakespeare's Gloucester presents an image of the man that was widely held in the 16th century and that is reflected in a number of the playwright's sources, particularly the anonymous play WOODSTOCK. However, Shakespeare's principal source for *Richard II*, HOLINSHED's *Chronicles*, depicts Gloucester as a wilfully violent man of little judgement. Modern scholarship finds Holinshed much nearer the mark. The historical Gloucester was a scheming, power-hungry aristocrat who clearly attempted to subvert the rule of his nephew.

When Edward III died, in 1377, Gloucester, though young, was markedly abler than his older brothers, and he became the power behind the throne of the pre-adolescent King Richard. As Richard matured, he attempted to assume power himself. The resulting conflict with his uncle escalated into a brief civil war in 1387. Gloucester's faction was victorious, forcing the exile or execution of several of Richard's favourites and effectively ruling the country for a time. In 1389 Richard, now 22 years old, declared that he would rule, and the coalition of nobles accepted his sovereignty. Richard was a successful king, and he cultivated his own group of supporters, including former followers of Gloucester such as Mowbray and Bolingbroke. Another rupture between the king and his uncle came in 1397. This time Richard quickly prevailed, imprisoning his opponents with little difficulty. Gloucester was placed in Mowbray's custody and died in the prison at Calais, as the play states. Whether or not he was murdered under Richard's orders cannot be confirmed, but modern scholarship seconds the contemporary popular opinion that he was.

Gloucestershire County in south-western England, setting for three scenes of *2 Henry IV* and one of *Richard II*.

In 3.2 of *2 Henry IV* FALSTAFF, marching to join the army at GAULTREE FOREST, drafts several recruits from among a number of villagers assembled by the local justice of the peace, SHALLOW. The scene is chiefly a satire of corrupt Elizabethan recruiting practices, but it also presents a collection of humorous provincial portraits, both of the gentry—bluff, silly Shallow and his taciturn cousin SILENCE—and of the villagers MOULDY, SHADOW, WART, FEEBLE, and BULLCALF. A reference to the Lincolnshire market town of Stamford (3.2.38) suggests that this scene may have been intended to be set in that county, which would make much more sense in terms of Falstaff's march from London to Gaultree. However, Shallow's jurisdiction is specified as Gloucestershire in 4.3.80 and 126, as well as in the opening lines of *The Merry Wives of Windsor*. It is thought that Shakespeare changed his mind about the location while writing *2 Henry IV*—possibly while interrupting that task to write *The Merry Wives of Windsor*—and, with his typical inattention to minor contradictions, did not rewrite the earlier scene.

In 5.1 and 5.3 of *2 Henry IV* Shallow's home is the setting for another delightful sampling of rural England, where the daily tasks of a small country estate are attended to and a party honouring Falstaff is arranged and then held. Shallow reminisces windily about his hell-raising student days, while Silence turns mildly boisterous when drunk. Shallow's steward, DAVY, is introduced; he sees to the running of his master's farm and demands a court ruling in favour of a friend, in an amusing vignette of small-time corruption. Place names and family names—e.g., William VISOR of Woncot and Clement PERKES 'a'th'Hill' (5.1.35)—are used with a congenial familiarity. Although this rural ambience is somewhat comical and its inhabitants humorously limited, it is plain that Shakespeare was fond of these people, and the Gloucestershire scenes of the play contribute greatly to *2 Henry IV*'s depiction of English life.

In 2.3 of *Richard II*, Gloucestershire's location, near WALES (1) and the Irish Sea, makes it strategically important. BOLINGBROKE (1) marches there to intercept King RICHARD II as he returns from Ireland. The Earl of NORTHUMBERLAND (1) speaks of Gloucestershire's 'high wild hills and rough uneven ways' (2.3.4), referring to the Cotswold Hills. Although this region seems tame today, it was heavily forested and difficult to cross in Shakespeare's day.

Glover, Julia (1781–1850) English actress. One of the most respected performers of her time, Glover, who claimed descent from Thomas BETTERTON, made her debut as a child, playing the Duke of YORK (7), young nephew of RICHARD III. Although she became quite obese, she successfully portrayed DESDEMONA, LADY (6) MACBETH, HAMLET, and other Shakespearean

characters, and she was one of the few women ever to play FALSTAFF.

Glyn, Isabel (active 1849–1867) English actress. Isabel Glyn was best known for her performances as CLEOPATRA. She played the role in several of the few 19th-century revivals of *Antony and Cleopatra,* most notably that of Samuel PHELPS in 1849, which reintroduced the play to the London stage. She also succeeded as QUEEN (9) Gertrude in *Hamlet.*

Gobbo (1), Launcelot Character in *The Merchant of Venice.* See LAUNCELOT.

Gobbo (2), Old Minor character in *The Merchant of Venice,* father of LAUNCELOT. Gobbo, nearly blind, is teased by Launcelot, who pretends to be a stranger and informs the old man that his son has died. Rewarded by his father's distress, Launcelot tells him the truth and enlists him to help approach BASSANIO about a job. After providing these few moments of incidental mirth, Gobbo disappears from the play.

Goethe, Johann Wolfgang von (1749–1832) German poet, dramatist, novelist, and critic. Goethe was one of the leaders of the Romantic movement that swept Europe in the early 19th century, and he found some of his inspiration in the scale and power of Shakespeare's plays. As the foremost German writer of his day—or any other, in most opinions—his enthusiasm made Shakespeare's position in German literature permanent. His influence in this respect, as in many others, spread beyond Germany to the rest of Europe.

A lawyer, the young Goethe wrote poems and plays, including *Götz von Berlichingen* (1773), a historical drama modelled on Shakespeare's HISTORY PLAYS. His novel *The Sorrows of Young Werther* (1774), the story of an unrequited lover who commits suicide, was a sensation throughout Europe and established Goethe as a leading literary figure. In 1775 he became a government minister in Weimar, one of the many small countries of 18th-century Germany, and remained there for the rest of his life. In addition to serving as the chief aide to the ruling Duke, he also ran a small theatre that was highly influential on subsequent German drama. Oddly, however, he did not find Shakespeare's plays successful on stage, and focussed instead on their literary qualities. The only one he produced was his own radical abridgement of *Romeo and Juliet* (1812), using the translation of August von SCHLEGEL.

Goethe is still regarded as one of the giants of European literature—one of the few writers of Shakespeare's stature—and one of the great men of German history. Among his many works are the play *Iphigenia in Tauris* (1788), the epic poem *Faust* (published at intervals from 1790–1832), and the novel *Wilhelm Meister* (1796). He was also a scientist, and he published respected works on optics, anatomy, and botany.

Goffe (Gough), Matthew (d. 1450) Historical figure mentioned briefly in *2 Henry VI.* In 4.5, during the battle to drive Jack CADE's rebels from London, Lord SCALES asserts that he will assign Goffe to a sector of the fighting, and, in a stage direction at the beginning of 4.7, Goffe is said to be killed in a skirmish. The historical Gough, a renowned warrior in the French wars, had shared command of the Tower of London with Scales, and he was indeed killed while fighting the rebels. His phantom presence in the play may reflect an actual appearance that was deleted in a revision.

Golding, Arthur (c. 1536–c. 1605) English writer and translator. In 1567 Golding published his famous translation of OVID's *Metamorphoses,* which appears to have been one of Shakespeare's favourite books; material derived from it, as well as direct quotations, pepper the plays and poems. The work was widely popular among other Elizabethan readers as well, at least in part because Ovid's poetry is somewhat racy, though Golding was himself a staunch conservative Protestant who allegorised and moralised the ancient poet's mythological tales. He also translated selections from the classical historians and from contemporary Protestant reformers, most notably John Calvin.

Goneril Character in *King Lear,* one of the villainous daughters of King LEAR. Goneril and her sister REGAN declare their great love for Lear, in 1.1, when in fact they merely want the portion of his kingdom that he has foolishly promised to whichever daughter can assure him she loves him most. They share the prize when their honest younger sister CORDELIA enrages the king with a frank admission that her love will be given in part to her future husband. Goneril takes the lead in the two sisters' villainy. She introduces the idea of humiliating Lear, in 1.1, and she orders her steward, OSWALD, to commence the practise, in 1.3. In 1.4 she starts the dispute over Lear's followers that sends the ex-king fleeing into the storm, where he descends into madness. In 4.2 Goneril's wickedness becomes more pronounced as she enters into a love affair with the ambitious EDMUND and hints at the existence of a murder plot against her husband, the virtuous but weak Duke of ALBANY. She and Regan both desire Edmund, and Goneril declares that she would rather lose the battle against the avengeing forces led by Cordelia than lose Edmund to her sister. This rivalry depicts the vicious sexuality that is part of the play's general atmosphere of moral and physical unhealthiness. When Goneril and Edmund's plot against Albany is exposed, she poisons Regan and then commits suicide as the GENTLEMAN (8) reports in 5.3.225–226.

Goneril's extravagantly evil nature is so boldly and unsubtly drawn that only her greater aggression distinguishes her from her sister. Her manipulation of her husband foreshadows Shakespeare's LADY (6) MACBETH, but Goneril, a less sophisticated creation, is simply an imitation of a standard male villain, cruel and ambitious. Unlike Lady Macbeth, she cannot compare herself with conventional femininity, nor does she succumb to illness through a bad conscience, for she is a much less complex character and serves chiefly as an emblem of evil.

Gonzalo Character in *The Tempest*, adviser to King ALONSO of Naples. Gonzalo is a kind and charitable, if ineffectual, figure who is a foil to the cynical villainy of ANTONIO (5), Duke of MILAN, his master's ally. Gonzalo's goodness is an important element in the play. He persistently takes a generous and optimistic point of view, as in his fantasy of an ideal society in 2.1.143–164 (see also MONTAIGNE). At the play's close, when PROSPERO's schemes result in a final reconciliation and the seemingly miraculous restoration of the king's son, FERDINAND (2), it is the ageing adviser—called by Prospero 'Holy Gonzalo, honourable man' (5.1.62)—who cries out, 'O, rejoice / Beyond a common joy!' (5.1.206–207).

In 1.1, as the king's ship sinks, Gonzalo's calm acceptance of fate contrasts with Antonio's arrogant fury and helps establish our sense of the moral polarities with which the play is concerned. In 1.2 we learn that Alonso assisted Antonio in deposing his brother, PROSPERO, and abandoning him and his infant daughter MIRANDA at sea, but that Gonzalo helped the victims by providing them with supplies. The contrast between Antonio and Gonzalo remains throughout the play. In 2.1 Gonzalo is mocked by Antonio and SEBASTIAN (3) for his attempts to cheer the king, and Antonio proposes to kill Gonzalo along with Alonso in his scheme to place Alonso's brother Sebastian on the throne of Naples. At the close Gonzalo's hearty participation in the aura of reconciliation points up Antonio's refusal to accept it.

Good Quarto An early edition of a Shakespeare play, printed in QUARTO format. A Good Quarto was derived from an authoritative source, such as Shakespeare's FOUL PAPERS, and reflects what the author actually wrote, as opposed to a BAD QUARTO, which was reconstructed from memory. Fourteen early editions of Shakespeare's plays are Good Quartos. They are: Q1 of *Titus Andronicus* (1594); Q1 of *Richard II* (1597); Q1 of *Richard III* (1597); Q of *Love's Labour's Lost* (1598); Q0 of *1 Henry IV* (1598); Q2 of *Romeo and Juliet* (1599); Q of *2 Henry IV* (1600); Q1 of *The Merchant of Venice* (1600); Q1 of *A Midsummer Night's Dream* (1600); Q of *Much Ado About Nothing* (1600); Q2 of *Hamlet* (1604); Q of *Troilus and Cressida* (1609); Q1 of *Othello* (1622); and Q of *The Two Noble Kinsmen* (1634). *Romeo and Juliet* and *Hamlet* also appeared as Bad Quartos, and Q1 of *Richard III* is sometimes classed as a Bad Quarto, for its generally sound text contains certain minor flaws that suggest that it was reconstructed from memory.

Goslicius, Laurentius Grimalius (Wawrzyniec Goślicki) (d. 1604) Polish statesman and author, whose chief work was possibly a minor source for *Hamlet* and *Measure for Measure*. Goslicius (sometimes known in English as Grimaldus) is considered the greatest statesman of 16th-century Poland. He wrote in Latin a manual of advice for government officials and diplomats, *De Optimo Senatore* (Venice, 1568), that was among the most admired books of its kind for several generations. An anonymous English translation, *The Counsellor*, appeared in 1598 (2nd ed., 1604), and it is echoed in several passages in *Hamlet*. Goslicius is thought to have inspired the name POLONIUS; the title page of *The Counsellor* declared the work 'consecrated to the Polonian Empire', and it seems likely that Shakespeare whimsically appropriated the author's nationality as a name for his Danish minister. Further, Goslicius' work may have influenced the creation of both the DUKE (9) and ANGELO (2)—for it expounds on both good and bad magistrates—in *Measure for Measure*.

Gosson (1), Henry (active 1601–1640) LONDON publisher and bookseller, producer of the first two editions of *Pericles*. In 1609 Gosson capitalised on the great popularity of Shakespeare's ROMANCE and had William WHITE (2) print a pirated edition of *Pericles*. Known as Q1, it is a BAD QUARTO, whose text was taken from the recollections of actors or viewers. The publication was a great success, and Gosson produced a second edition (Q2) in the same year. This made *Pericles* one of the few Shakespeare plays to appear in two Quartos in the same year.

Gosson, who inherited his business from his father, published mostly short-lived literature such as ballads, news sheets, and joke books. *Pericles* was the only play text he produced. He prospered and owned several shops in London, but little else is known of his life.

Gosson (2), Stephen (1554–1624) English writer, a Puritan opponent of the professional theatre. Gosson, a poet, dramatist, and—probably—actor, changed his life in his early 20s and became a clergyman. He wrote three books (published between 1579 and 1582) that declared poetry and drama unnsavoury influences on society. The theatre—which he called a 'market of bawdry'—came in for particular abuse. He was willing to exclude only a few sober plays, including one of his own, from his general verdict that drama 'was not to be suffered in a Christian common weale'. Thomas LODGE began his literary career with a rejoinder, *De-*

fence of Plays (1581), and Sir Philip SIDNEY may have been inspired by him to write his great *Apology for Poetry* (1583). Several companies revived Gosson's plays, hoping to embarrass him and capitalise on the publicity the controversy had created. Despite his enmity towards his former profession, Gosson remained a lifelong friend of the great actor Edward ALLEYN.

Gosson was among the most prominent of Puritan opponents of the theatre. Although in the 16th century such opinions were merely a nuisance to the profession (see, e.g., COBHAM), they triumphed later during the Civil Wars. Beginning in 1642 the Puritan revolutionary government closed the theatres of England for almost 20 years.

Goths Barbarian European tribe known to the ancient Romans. In *Titus Andronicus* Shakespeare uses the Goths as the enemies of Rome whose forces are necessary to restore order within the empire, which has been disrupted through the villainy of AARON and TAMORA. This device anticipates several later occasions, notably in *Hamlet* and *Macbeth*, when forces from outside the affected society must take charge, thereby heightening the playwright's emphasis on the catastrophic results of social disorder.

Gough (Goughe), Robert (d. 1624) English actor. Gough is one of the 26 men listed in the FIRST FOLIO as the 'Principall Actors' in Shakespeare's plays, but he is not known to have performed in any particular role and was clearly a minor player. He may have played a LORD (6) in *All's Well That Ends Well*, for the character is designated as 'G' in speech headings in the Folio text of the play (but see GILBURNE). Gough was probably a member of STRANGE'S MEN by 1590—'R. Go' appears in a Strange's Men's cast list. He was probably employed by the CHAMBERLAIN'S MEN or its successor, the KING'S MEN, sometime before 1603, when Thomas POPE (2) willed him some of his costumes and stage weapons. He was married to Augustine PHILLIPS' sister in 1603, and he witnessed Phillips' will in 1605. He is recorded as a partner in the King's Men in 1619 and 1621, but no more is known of him. His son, Alexander Gough (1614–after 1655) was also an actor for the King's Men who specialised in female characters. He was with the company until the theatres were closed by the revolutionary government in 1642, after which he participated for some time in clandestine performances at private homes. He eventually became a publisher.

Gounod, Charles François (1818–1893) French composer who wrote an opera based on *Romeo and Juliet*. A popular composer in his own day, Gounod is now considered a minor figure in French music history, best known for *Roméo et Juliette* (1867) and another opera, his masterpiece, *Faust* (1859). Few of his other compositions are still performed.

Governor (1) of Harfleur Minor character in *Henry V*, a French official. The Governor surrenders the town of HARFLEUR to HENRY V, confessing in 3.3.44–50 that, without the support of the DAUPHIN (3), the town is indefensible.

Governor (2) of Paris Minor character in *1 Henry VI*, an official commanding the capital of English-occupied FRANCE (1). The Governor wordlessly takes an oath of allegiance to HENRY VI when the King is crowned monarch of France in 4.1.

Gower (1) Minor character in *2 Henry IV*, a messenger. In 2.1 Gower brings the CHIEF JUSTICE a report that King HENRY IV and PRINCE (6) HAL have returned to London from fighting rebels in WALES (1), and he answers the judge's questions about military news. His knowledge suggests that he is in the army, but there is no other evidence to link him with Captain GOWER (2) in *Henry V* and he is generally regarded as a different character.

Gower (2) Minor character in *Henry V*, an officer in the army of King HENRY V. Gower functions chiefly as a foil to FLUELLEN, a calm and restraining friend of—and audience for—the irascible Welshman. Gower, a stolid military man, reveals his own personality only when he voices his heartfelt disapproval of PISTOL, whom he sees as a petty thief and braggart impersonating a soldier, in 3.6.67–82, his sole substantial speech.

Gower (3), John (c. 1330–1408) English poet, a historical figure and a character in *Pericles*. Gower's major work, the *Confessio Amantis* (1390), was Shakespeare's chief source for *Pericles* and a possible influence on *The Comedy of Errors* and *The Merchant of Venice*. In *Pericles* Gower acts as a CHORUS (1) who summarises off-stage action and moralises on the course of developments. He appears in brief PROLOGUE-like passages before each act, and also in 4.4 and 5.2. At the play's close he delivers a brief EPILOGUE. His manner of speaking is quaintly old-fashioned by the standards of the 17th century, which indicates his historical position as well as clarifying the remote and romantic nature of the story being enacted. Occasionally, Shakespeare's character clearly imitates the real Gower's poetic style, as in 3.Chorus. Also, two passages not spoken by the character—1.1.65–72 and 3.2.70–77—follow the real poet's verse quite closely.

Gower's *Confessio Amantis* contained 141 ancient tales from various sources, rendered in English verse. One of its stories, the Greek 'Apollonius of Tyre', dates to at least the 3rd century A.D., though Gower

took it from the work of a later chronicler, Godfrey of Viterbo (c. 1120–c. 1196). A 1554 edition of Gower's *Confessio* provided Shakespeare with the general outline of events, the locations, and most of the characters of *Pericles*. The same tale may also have inspired the sub-plot concerning EGEON in *The Comedy of Errors* and the episode of the three caskets in *The Merchant of Venice*.

Gower was a minor nobleman who pursued his literary career in London, supported by rents from two small country estates. He wrote major works in Latin, French, and English, though the *Confessio* (which may have been commissioned by King RICHARD II) is by far the most important. Its 33,000 lines of eight-syllable couplets constitutes one of the greatest achievements of 14th-century English poetry. Gower was a contemporary and friend of Geoffrey CHAUCER, who dedicated his *Troilus and Criseyde* to him. However, the two poets may have become estranged, for a tribute to Chaucer in the first manuscript edition of the *Confessio* is omitted from later ones produced in Gower's lifetime.

Grafton, Richard (d. 1572) English chronicler and historian whose works, published between 1562 and 1571, were consulted by Shakespeare when writing his HISTORY PLAYS. They provided the playwright with a number of minor details.

Granada, Luis de (1504–1588) Spanish mystic and writer, author of a minor source for *Hamlet*. De Granada, a Dominican monk and theologian, wrote several works on prayer and mystical contemplation, including *Libro de la Oración y Consideración* (1554), usually translated as *Of Prayer and Meditation*, which probably influenced some of HAMLET's observations on graves and death in 5.1. This book was among the most popular religious treatises of the 16th century, and many English translations were published, beginning with the work of Richard HOPKINS in 1582. De Granada emphasised the presence of God as manifested in nature in lyrical works that are still appreciated; an anthology in English, *The Summa of Christian Life*, was published as recently as 1954.

Grandpré Minor character in *Henry V*, a French nobleman. Grandpré appears only once, to describe, in 4.2.38–55, the listless and dispirited English army just before the battle of AGINCOURT. The speech contributes to the presentation of French overconfidence. Grandpré's death is reported in 4.8.101. Shakespeare apparently took the name from the list of casualties in HOLINSHED's account of the battle.

Granville, George (1667–1735) English dramatist and politician, creator of an adaptation of *The Merchant of Venice*. After graduating from Cambridge University, Granville wrote *The Jew of Venice*, a farce based on Shakespeare's play that was produced in 1701 with Thomas BETTERTON playing BASSANIO and the popular comic Thomas Doggett (c. 1670–1721) as SHYLOCK. Though it has little literary merit, this work was popular for 40 years before it was superseded by Charles MACKLIN's revival of Shakespeare's play.

Granville was elected to Parliament in 1702, which was the beginning of his meteoric political career. He became secretary of war in 1710 and a peer in 1711, but he was imprisoned in 1715 for supporting the Jacobite invasion (see STUART DYNASTY). From 1722–1732 he lived in exile in France.

Granville-Barker, Harley (1877–1946) English actor, director, and Shakespearean commentator. After a successful career in the theatre, Granville-Barker wrote a series of *Prefaces to Shakespeare* (1927–1946) that covered 12 of Shakespeare's plays. He addressed questions of interpretation and staging that arise in actual production in the theatre, rather than taking a scholar's point of view. It is for these well-written and influential texts that he remains best known today.

As a director, Granville-Barker specialised in modern works, chiefly those of Ibsen and George Bernard SHAW (2). He only staged three of Shakespeare's plays—*The Winter's Tale* and *Twelfth Night* in 1912, and *A Midsummer Night's Dream* in 1914—but they were revolutionary and have greatly influenced the modern staging of ELIZABETHAN DRAMA. He used uncut texts and sped up the pace, and he also cut much traditional stage business to focus attention on the plays themselves. He extended the stage into the audience in an effort to simulate the theatre of Elizabethan times. By applying William POEL's notions of simplified staging, though he didn't go so far as to eliminate scenery altogether, Granville-Barker succeeded in making a commercial success of an idealistic approach to Shakespearean production.

As a young man, Granville-Barker acted in the productions of Poel and Ben GREET; he was especially acclaimed as RICHARD II. He also wrote plays, and his *The Voysey Inheritance* (1905), a satirical comedy in the vein of his close friend Shaw, is regarded as one of the best dramas of its period.

Gratiano (1) Character in *The Merchant of Venice*, friend of BASSANIO and lover of NERISSA. Gratiano is a crude and frivolous companion. As Bassanio himself puts it, 'Gratiano speaks an infinite deal of nothing' (1.1.114). He can be tactless, as in 1.1, where he is the only one of Antonio's friends who fails to see the propriety of leaving Antonio and Bassanio to confer privately. Bassanio, fearful that his friend will embarrass him before PORTIA (1), feels constrained to chastise him, 'Thou art too wild, too rude, and bold of

voice . . .' (2.2.172). Gratiano's bluff heartiness turns ugly in the trial scene (4.1), when he baits the desperate SHYLOCK, and his lewd remarks, as in 3.2.216, mark him as a lesser person than the gentlemanly Bassanio. His courtship of Nerissa is simply an echo of Bassanio's wooing of Portia and seems to have no point but symmetry; such doubling was very popular among Elizabethan audiences. Gratiano's name comes from the Italian COMMEDIA DELL'ARTE tradition, where it was used for a stock character, the comical doctor

Gratiano (2) (Graziano) Minor character in *Othello,* a Venetian nobleman, DESDEMONA's uncle. Gratiano is a member of the delegation from VENICE that comes to CYPRUS at the close of the play and witnesses the climax of OTHELLO's madness. He ineffectually responds to the cries of CASSIO and EMILIA (2) for assistance, in 5.1 and 5.2, respectively. In both cases he fails to prevent IAGO's wicked schemes. In this respect he is representative of the society at large, whose racial prejudice has helped make Othello vulnerable to Iago. In his most important remark, Gratiano declares that Desdemona's father, BRABANTIO, has died of grief at her marriage to Othello.

Grave-digger (First Clown, First Grave-digger) Minor character in *Hamlet,* the digger of OPHELIA's grave. At the opening of 5.1, the Grave-digger talks with his friend, called the OTHER, in a comical series of exchanges on suicide, the law, and the profession of grave-digging. HAMLET, meditating with HORATIO in the graveyard, speaks with the Grave-digger, who gives flip and enigmatic answers to his questions. In the course of describing the decomposition of corpses, he presents the prince with the skull of the late court jester, YORICK. This plunges Hamlet into another conversation with Horatio, and the Grave-digger does not speak again.

This scene does not further the plot; indeed, it quite distinctly delays development, providing some needed comic relief in the face of the rapidly approaching climax. The Grave-digger also serves as a subtle commentator on the main action, rather like a CHORUS (1). He frankly suggests the possibility of Ophelia's suicide, and his equally honest and humorous attitude to the world of the aristocrats and 'great folk [who] have countenance in this world to drown or hang themselves more than their even-Christen' (5.1.27–29) reminds us of the extent to which intrigue infects Hamlet's world.

Most important, the Grave-digger's remarks and behaviour reflect the play's attitude towards death: it is the normal human fate to die. The Grave-digger's job makes this an everyday fact rather than a philosophical observation. At a crucial point in the play, his demeanour, both prosaic and comical, helps to make clear to the audience that Hamlet's meditations on death no longer reflect the depression and grief that characterised him in Acts 1–4 but are rather the healthy recognition that death and decay are parts of life that must be accepted.

The Grave-digger is addressed by his companion as 'Goodman Delver' (5.1.14), which may be his surname preceded by the honorific 'Goodman' (roughly equivalent to 'Mister'), or it may simply refer to his occupation as a digger. In his uneducated but knowing humour, he is a good instance of a character type, the rustic CLOWN (1) and some editions, including the earliest ones, designate him accordingly in stage directions and speech headings.

Gravelot, Hubert (1699–1773) French painter and engraver, illustrator of Shakespeare's plays. Gravelot worked on two illustrated editions of Shakespeare, THEOBALD's second edition (1740) and HANMER's deluxe volumes (1744), each of which contained 36 illustrations. For the first of these, Gravelot provided all of the 36 illustrations but engraved only eight of them himself; for the second, he provided only five illustrations but engraved all 36. The other images were provided by Francis HAYMAN.

During his residency in London (1732–1745), Gravelot was for English artists the most important source of the French rococo style in painting and decoration. He was more important as an illustrator than as a painter, and few of his paintings survive, but he was an important influence on painters such as his close friend William Hogarth (1697–1764) and his students Hayman and Thomas Gainsborough (1727–1788).

Green, John (active 1606–1627) English actor active in Germany. Green was a member of one of Robert BROWNE's touring companies as early as 1606, and he had his own company beginning in 1615 until at least 1627. He succeeded Browne as the most important English influence on the roots of German drama, which were influenced by English touring companies between the 1590s and the middle of the 17th century. A listing of Green's repertoire in 1626 has survived; it included plays titled *Romeo and Juliet, Julius Caesar, Lear König von Engelandt,* and *Hamlet einem printzen in Dennemark,* almost certainly Shakespeare's plays or adaptations of them.

Greene (1) (Green), Henry (d. 1399) Historical figure and character in *Richard II,* a supporter of King RICHARD II. Greene, John BAGOT, and John BUSHY are the 'caterpillars' (2.3.165) whose influence on the King is alleged by BOLINGBROKE (1) to have been disastrous for England. In 1.4 Greene, the least prominent of the three, advises the King that he must address the pressing problem of a rebellion in Ireland. The three favourites recognise that their closeness to the King is likely

to prove dangerous if their master is defeated by Bolingbroke. In 2.2 they decide to flee when Bolingbroke appears; Bushy and Greene seek safety in BRISTOL Castle, but Bolingbroke captures them and sentences them to death.

Little is known about the historical Greene, a member of the gentry who was recruited for Richard's faction from among the supporters of the Duke of GLOUCESTER (6) some time before the Duke's murder.

Greene (2), Robert (1558–1592) English writer, author of the earliest literary reference to Shakespeare, as well as of the chief source for *The Winter's Tale* and a minor source for *Troilus and Cressida.* Greene was one of the UNIVERSITY WITS who revolutionised ELIZABETHAN DRAMA in the 1580s. He wrote at least 10 plays, mostly romantic comedies, the best-known of which is *Friar Bacon and Friar Bungay* (1589), still occasionally staged. He also wrote romantic novels—including *Pandosto* (1588), from which Shakespeare took the plot of *The Winter's Tale*—and numerous essays, such as those collected in *Eupheus his Censure to Philautus* (1587), which provided minor ideas and incidents for *Troilus and Cressida.*

Greene's reference to the young Shakespeare was made in *Greene's Groatsworth of Wit* (1592), one of several brief repentant but embittered autobiographies written as he approached death (he had led a dissolute life among criminals and whores after abandoning his wife and child). In this angry tract Greene advised other playwrights not to trust actors, declaring them to be uneducated, dishonest poseurs and citing the example of 'an upstart Crow . . . that with his *Tygers hart wrapt in a Players hyde* [Greene's emphasis], supposes he is as well able to bombast out a blanke verse as the best of you: and . . . is in his owne conceit the onely Shake-scene in a country'.

After Greene's death, his editor, Henry CHETTLE, issued a public apology to Shakespeare, but the power of slander survives retraction: the parody of 'O tiger's heart wrapp'd in a woman's hide' (*3 Henry VI* 1.4.137) has been offered as evidence that Greene wrote the play—or at least part of it, including that line—and that he was complaining of plagiarism, or at least usurped credit. Moreover, Shakespearean commentators who believe that much in Shakespeare's early plays was written by other playwrights (see, e.g., FLEAY and ROBERTSON) have suggested that Greene was also responsible for parts of *Titus Andronicus, 1* and *2 Henry VI, The Comedy of Errors, The Two Gentlemen of Verona,* and sometimes others. Most modern scholars discount these theories, however, and believe that the parody in *Groatsworth of Wit* was simply a mocking of Shakespeare's bold language.

Greene (3), Thomas (c. 1578–1641) Lawyer in STRATFORD, friend and possibly kinsman of Shakespeare. Greene, who was from nearby Warwick, became the town clerk of Stratford in 1602, shortly after becoming a lawyer. He may have known Shakespeare in LONDON when he studied at the INNS OF COURT, for he knew the playwright John MARSTON, but he was in any case close to the Shakespeare family for years in Stratford. His children were named after the playwright and his wife, Anne HATHAWAY Shakespeare, and he and his family lived at Shakespeare's NEW PLACE for a time, perhaps more than a year, while waiting on the renovation of another home. Some of his correspondence has survived, and in it he several times refers to Shakespeare as his 'cousin'. No family connection is known, and the word was used loosely in those days, but Greene may have been a blood relation of the playwright.

Greene was closely involved in the political crisis that gripped Stratford in the years just preceding Shakespeare's death (see WELCOMBE). He and Shakespeare jointly owned a contract to collect the taxes on agricultural lands that were proposed in 1614 for conversion to sheep farming—a politically unpopular process known as enclosure. Shakespeare negotiated an arrangement whereby they were protected against loss if enclosure went through and might profit. However, the town of Stratford opposed enclosure and, as town clerk, Greene worked against it successfully. It has been suggested that disagreements over this political crisis, which gripped Stratford for two years, may have led to the odd fact that Greene is not mentioned in Shakespeare's will. A year after Shakespeare's death, Greene moved to Bristol.

Greet, Philip Barling Ben (1857–1936) British actor and theatrical entrepreneur. As an actor, director, and producer, Ben Greet was dedicated to presenting Shakespeare's plays with fidelity to the playwright's text, after centuries of adaptation and traditional stage business had become attached to virtually all of the plays. He insisted on simple staging, in contrast to the late-19th-century fondness for extravagant spectacle, and he endeavoured to bring Shakespeare's plays to a wide audience. Between 1886 and 1914 he toured Britain and America with a repertory company that he then took to the OLD VIC THEATRE, which he helped establish as Britain's most important centre of Shakespearean production.

Greg, Walter Wilson (1875–1959) British scholar. Widely regarded as among the greatest of Shakespearean scholars, Greg edited the diaries and papers of Philip HENSLOWE (published 1904–1908), and assisted A. W. POLLARD in researching his ground-breaking *Shakespeare Folios and Quartos* (1909). He went on to produce many valuable studies, including *Dramatic Documents of the Elizabethan Playhouses* (1931), *The Editorial Problem in Shakespeare* (1942), *Shakespeare First Folio*

(1955), and the monumental four-volume *A Bibliography of the English Printed Drama to the Restoration* (1939–1959).

Gregory (1) Minor character in *Romeo and Juliet,* a servant of the CAPULET (1) household. Gregory and his fellow servant SAMPSON brawl with servants of the MONTAGUE (1) family in 1.1, after opening the play with a pun-filled comic dialogue in which Gregory taunts his companion for being a coward. The brawl is purely verbal until TYBALT appears and the rival households come to blows. The episode illustrates the lengths to which the feud between the families has gone, with their servants pursuing the quarrel in the streets.

Gremio Character in *The Taming of the Shrew,* an elderly suitor of BIANCA (1). Gremio is referred to as a 'pantaloon' (3.1.36), the humorous figure of a greedy old man in the COMMEDIA DELL'ARTE, and he is indeed simply a character type with little real personality. He is comically cowardly, fearful that the assertiveness of PETRUCHIO (2) will offend BAPTISTA, Bianca's father. His own style is offensively humble; approaching Baptista, he refers to himself as a 'poor petitioner' (2.1.72), in the obsequious language of a minor courtier. He lies about his wealth when Baptista promises his daughter to the wealthiest suitor, but to no avail. Gremio is absurdly ineffective; in fact, in his attempt to win Bianca's hand he actually introduces the successful suitor into her presence, for in 2.1 he hires the disguised LUCENTIO as a tutor for the girl, hoping to impress her father.

Greville (1), Curtis (active 1622–1631) English actor who may have performed in early productions of *The Two Noble Kinsmen* and *The Taming of the Shrew.* In the first edition of *Kinsmen* (Q1, 1634), the stage direction at 4.2.70 designates the MESSENGER (32) as 'Curtis'; in the opening stage direction of 5.3, the Attendants called for—one of whom is presumably the SERVANT (30)—are named, one of them 'Curtis'. Scholars believe that these references are to Greville, indicating that he played the parts in an early production by the KING'S MEN. Greville was with the company from before 1626 until 1631, so this clue (with similar evidence concerning Thomas TUCKFIELD) suggests that Q1 was printed from a PROMPT-BOOK of the 1620s. Some scholars believe that *The Shrew*'s CURTIS similarly takes his name from Greville's portrayal.

Little is known of Greville. In 1622 he moved from LADY ELIZABETH'S MEN to the PALSGRAVE'S MEN, presumably as part of the latter company's effort to reopen the FORTUNE THEATRE, closed by fire. By 1626 Greville was with the King's Men, with whom he is known to have played several minor roles.

Greville (2), Fulke (Lord Brooke) (1554–1628) English poet and author, possibly a patron of Shakespeare. Greville is best known for his biography of Philip SIDNEY, whose close friend he had been since the age of 10. However, he also wrote a considerable body of poetry, two plays, and several treatises on politics, religion, and education. He was a significant figure in RENAISSANCE English literature in other ways, as well. As a member of the 'Areopagus' group of poets—with Sidney, Edmund SPENSER, and others—he helped stimulate the use of classical METRE in English poetry. As a wealthy man he was a patron of writers, and assisted Samuel DANIEL, among others. He also served as a diplomat and economic adviser to both Queen ELIZABETH (1) and King JAMES I. The latter monarch made him a baron on his retirement from government in 1621, and he is sometimes known as Lord Brooke.

The young Shakespeare may have benefited from Greville's largesse. According to a 1665 account, Greville once described himself as worthy only because he had been 'Shakespeare and Ben JONSON's master . . . and Sir Philip Sidney's friend'. Most scholars regard this anecdote as apocryphal, but whether or not he did indeed act as an elder adviser and patron to the young playwright, the remark reflects Greville's famed modesty. His EPITAPH, composed by himself, reads 'Servant to Queen Elizabeth, Counsellor to King James, Friend to Sir Philip Sydney.'

Grey (1), Lady Character in *3 Henry VI.* See ELIZABETH (2).

Grey (2), Sir Richard (d. 1483) Historical figure and character in *Richard III,* a kinsman of Queen ELIZABETH (2) and a victim of RICHARD III. Grey simply functions as a pawn in Richard's game of power politics. He is executed in 3.3 solely because he is the Queen's relative. As he goes to his death, along with RIVERS and VAUGHAN, he recollects the curses of Queen MARGARET (1), who had anticipated this event in 1.3.

Shakespeare was apparently confused about Grey's relationship to Elizabeth, although his habitual carelessness about minor matters suggests that he probably did not concern himself about it. Historically, Grey was Elizabeth's son by her first marriage, but in the play he is implied to be her brother. However, in recalling Margaret's curse, he speaks as though he were DORSET, unquestionably a son of Elizabeth.

Grey (3), Thomas (d. 1415) Historical figure and minor character in *Henry V,* a traitor who plans to assassinate King HENRY V but is captured and sentenced to death. In 2.2 Henry, who knows of their plot, asks Grey and his fellow conspirators, Lord SCROOP (1) and the Earl of CAMBRIDGE, for advice about a drunken soldier who has criticised him. They all recommend

severity, insisting that Henry be firm against any hint of disloyalty. Then Henry reveals his awareness of their treason and applies their own rule against them, sentencing them to death. Grey, like the others, offers a conventionally remorseful speech, thanking God for the defeat of the conspiracy and welcoming death. Grey has no personality; the episode merely serves to emphasise Henry's godlike majesty.

The historical Grey was a landowner in Northumberland and is thought to have been allied to the Percy family, persistent rebels against King HENRY IV. The revolt led by Cambridge may have been a final spasm of the civil conflict enacted in *1* and *2 Henry IV*.

Griffin, Bartholomew (d. 1602) Author of at least one and probably four of the poems attributed to Shakespeare in *THE PASSIONATE PILGRIM* (1599). Little is known of Griffin, who is remembered primarily because one SONNET from his 62-sonnet sequence, *Fidessa* (1596)—a conventional and undistinguished work—was published as no. 11 in William JAGGARD's spurious anthology. Three other poems in the collection (nos. 4, 6, and 9) resemble no. 11 closely enough that they are often attributed to Griffin as well. His preface to *Fidessa* suggests that Griffin may have been a gentleman and a lawyer, and it also asserted that he was writing a long pastoral poem, but, if this was completed and published, it has not survived.

Griffith Minor character in *Henry VIII*, an attendant to Queen KATHERINE. Griffith is the GENTLEMAN USHER to the Queen in 2.4, but in 4.2 he has a more intimate function, as a faithful servant who continues to attend the now-deposed queen in exile at KIMBOLTON. Griffith tells Katherine that Cardinal WOLSEY repented of his evil deeds before dying. As Wolsey's victim, Katherine speaks harshly of him, but Griffith suggests a more charitable view of the cardinal, emphasising his good works. Katherine thanks Griffith for reminding her of the proper Christian attitude towards her enemy, since she is near death herself. Griffith is tender with the dying queen; along with the waiting-woman PATIENCE, he helps surround the queen's death with an atmosphere of virtuous mildness. Griffith is named in Shakespeare's sources, but only in connection with his duties as the queen's gentleman usher; the playwright invented his role in 4.2, as part of his association of Katherine with the themes of forgiveness and patience in adversity.

Groom (1) Minor character in *Richard II*, a supporter of RICHARD II. The Groom visits the imprisoned Richard in 5.5, in a demonstration of allegiance that raises the ex-King's spirits. He tells Richard of the use of the horse BARBARY by BOLINGBROKE (1). This minor incident illustrates that Richard could inspire loyalty in a simple servant and thus heightens the pathos of the deposed ruler's murder, which follows immediately.

Groom (2) Any of two or three minor characters in *2 Henry IV*, servants who strew the London streets with rushes in preparation for the crowds attending PRINCE (6) HAL's coronation as HENRY V. Their presence at the opening of 5.5 sets the scene. They are identified as two Grooms in the FOLIO edition of the play, and as three Strewers in the QUARTO edition; modern editions vary.

Grumio Character in *The Taming of the Shrew*, servant of PETRUCHIO (2). Grumio is a distinctly English comic figure in all respects except his name. At 1.2.28, he even fails to recognise Italian. Grumio represents a long theatrical tradition—the comical servant whose nonsense masks shrewdness. His wily foolishness is a vehicle for humour when, in 1.2, he remarks sharply on the mercenary marriage that his master is pursuing. It can also be a means of manipulating others, as when he feigns incomprehension—first with KATHERINA and later with the TAILOR—in 4.3. His name comes from a character in an ancient Roman play, *The Haunted House*, by PLAUTUS.

Guardsman (1) Any of several minor characters in *Antony and Cleopatra*, soldiers who serve as ANTONY's personal guards. In 4.14 three Guardsmen (designated First, Second and Third Guardsman) discover the wounded Antony who requests that they kill him as he has unsuccessfully attempted suicide. Horrified, they flee from the room. Twenty lines later, when called by DIOMEDES (2), several of them return and carry the wounded Antony to CLEOPATRA. Though dismayed and sorrowful, the Guardsmen have no real personalities; they merely reflect the demoralised state of their leader.

Guardsman (2) Any of several minor characters in *Antony and Cleopatra*, soldiers in the army of Octavius CAESAR (2) assigned to guard CLEOPATRA. In 5.2 they enter with GALLUS at 5.2.34, but none of them speak until 5.2.232, when one of them announces the arrival of the CLOWN (7) who secretly delivers to Cleopatra the poisonous asps with which she will kill herself. After her death the Guardsmen enter as a group to discover the situation and call an officer, DOLABELLA. Two of them speak, and they are designated First and Second Guardsman. Their presence emphasises Cleopatra's captivity and thus helps to justify her suicide.

Guiderius Character in *Cymbeline*, one of the two kidnapped sons of King CYMBELINE. Guiderius and his younger brother ARVIRAGUS have been raised as hunters in the wilderness of WALES (1) by their foster-father

BELARIUS, who kidnapped them in infancy when he was unjustly exiled by Cymbeline. Guiderius shares with his brother the desire to prove himself in war, which is evidence of his inherently regal courage. When their sister IMOGEN, disguised as a boy, appears by chance, both young men immediately love 'him', which stresses to the audience that they are siblings. When the Romans invade Britain, the brothers display their innate capacity for leadership and save the British army. They are honoured by the king and then identified and reunited with him, as part of the revelations and reconciliations at the play's close.

Guiderius, like Arviragus, is a simple fairy-tale figure—a lost prince who is restored to his rightful position—and his personality is mostly seen in courage and high spirits. However, Shakespeare takes care to distinguish the brothers from each other. As the future heir to the throne, Guiderius is more forceful and dynamic than his reflective brother Arviragus. When they discuss Imogen's virtues, Guiderius proves more practical when he mentions her cooking, while Arviragus praises her singing. When they believe her dead, Guiderius cuts short his brother's 'wench-like words' (4.2.23.) and says, 'Let us bury him, / And not protract with admiration what / Is now due debt. To th'grave!' (4.2.230–233). At his most striking, Guiderius kills CLOTEN, earlier in the same scene, with soldierly aplomb. He brandishes his victim's head while he remarks, 'This Cloten was a fool, an empty purse' (4.2.113). Later, he declares he will throw the head into the creek 'to tell the fishes he's the queen's son' (4.2.153). In 5.5 he manfully acknowledges that he has killed Cloten despite the threat of capital punishment for killing a prince (he is not yet known to be a prince himself). His 'I have spoke it, and I did it' (5.5.290) has a kingly simplicity and force. Belarius has given Guiderius the name Polydore, and this name is occasionally used in dialogue, but he is designated as Guiderius in speech headings and stage directions.

Guildenstern Character in *Hamlet.* See ROSENCRANTZ AND GUILDENSTERN.

Guilford (Guildford), Sir Henry (1489–1532) Historical figure and minor character in *Henry VIII,* a steward to Cardinal WOLSEY. In 1.4 Guilford, welcoming the guests to the cardinal's banquet, cheerfully delights in the 'good company, good wine, good welcome' (1.4.6). He speaks briefly as the scene opens and then disappears from the play, having served to establish the mood of this occasion, when King HENRY VIII meets his future bride ANNE (1) BULLEN. The historical Guilford later became a steward to King Henry and functioned as his MASTER OF THE REVELS, before that office was formally created.

Gurney, James Minor character in *King John,* a friend or servant of LADY (5) Faulconbridge. Gurney speaks only half of one line (1.1.231), a friendly response to his dismissal from the scene (and the play) by the BASTARD (1), Lady Faulconbridge's son. This moment illuminates the world of rural informality that the Bastard has come from.

Guthrie, Tyrone (1900–1971) British theatrical producer. Guthrie directed the OLD VIC THEATRE from 1933 to 1945, and he was chiefly responsible for the creation of the Shakespeare Festival in Stratford, Ontario, in 1953 and the Guthrie Theatre in Minneapolis in 1963. His daringly experimental productions sparked controversy in England and America. Particularly noted were his 1937 *Twelfth Night* and his renderings of *All's Well That Ends Well* as a farce (1953 and 1959, in Ontario and STRATFORD, England, respectively). He wrote several books, including *Theatre Prospect* (1932) and *A New Theatre* (1964).

Gwinne (Gwinn), Matthew (c. 1558–1627) English physician and playwright, author of a possible inspiration for *Macbeth.* Gwinne's Latin MASQUE *Tres Sibyllae* was performed on the occasion of King JAMES I's visit to Oxford in 1605. It features prophecies addressed to MACBETH and BANQUO, and alludes to the king's legendary descent from Banquo. Some scholars believe that its success with its royal auditor may have inspired Shakespeare to compose his own version of the Macbeth tale.

Gwinne was closely associated with Oxford, though he also had a medical practise in London. He was the supervisor of theatrical productions at the university in the 1590s, and he was highly respected as an academic dramatist, chiefly on the strength of two Latin plays, *Nero* (1603) and *Vertumnis* (1605). The latter work gained an unfortunate notoriety when it put the king to sleep.

H

Haberdasher, The Minor character in *The Taming of the Shrew,* an artisan whom PETRUCHIO (2) abuses. The Haberdasher, who has been commissioned to make a hat for KATHERINA, speaks only one line before being driven away by his client, who is demonstrating the ugliness of shrewish behaviour to his bride.

Hakluyt, Richard (c. 1552–1616) English geographer. Hakluyt (pronounced 'haklit') was a clergyman, but he devoted his career to the publication of materials concerning the exploration of the New World and the promotion of English efforts in this realm. He learned the major European languages in order to have access to all possible sources of information. In 1582 he published *Divers voyages touching the discoveries of America.* He was also employed as a diplomat and spy by the government, serving as chaplain to the British ambassador in FRANCE (1) from 1583–1589. During this period, he compiled his most important work, *The Principall Navigations, Voyages, and Discoveries of the English Nation* (1589). As revised in 1600, this work contained a well-known map, probably the 'new map with the augmentation of the Indies' referred to in *Twelfth Night* (3.2.76–77). Some of Hakluyt's material was gathered by John PORY, and the collection was further enlarged by Hakluyt's friend Samuel Purchas (c. 1575–1626), who published an account of a shipwreck by William STRACHEY (2) that influenced Shakespeare's *The Tempest.* Hakluyt's *Voyages,* as his book is known, was very influential on the course of English exploration, besides being extremely popular among lay readers. It is still in print. In 1846 the Royal Geographic Society founded the Hakluyt Society, which continues to publish historical accounts of explorations and travels, including new editions of Hakluyt's works.

Hal, Prince Character in *1* and *2 Henry IV.* See PRINCE (6).

Halberdier Minor character in *Richard III,* one of the soldiers guarding the coffin of King HENRY VI in 1.2. The Halberdier vainly attempts to prevent RICHARD III from interrupting the King's funeral procession. (A halberd, the weapon assigned this character in the stage directions, was a combination of lance and battle-ax, mounted on a long pole.)

The Halberdier's single speech is attributed to him by modern editors who feel that older editions err in giving it to the GENTLEMAN (2). A gentleman, it is argued, would neither receive nor accept the abuse that Richard heaps on the unfortunate soldier. Villainous though he is, it is supposed that Richard would observe the formal distinctions between aristocrats and commoners.

Hall (1), Arthur (c. 1540–1604) English writer. Hall completed the first English translation of HOMER; his version of the first 10 books of the *Iliad* was published in 1581. Shakespeare surely knew this work, and it may have influenced his treatment of Homeric materials in *The Rape of Lucrece* and *Troilus and Cressida* (although it is clear that in the latter work he relied chiefly on the translation by George CHAPMAN).

Hall, an orphan, was raised in the household of the leading Elizabethan statesman Lord BURGHLEY. As an adult, he was notorious for riotous living and was imprisoned several times; although he began his translation of the *Iliad* while in his 20s, he did not complete it for many years. Inaccurate and awkward, it was completely overshadowed by Chapman's *Iliad,* which appeared between 1598 and 1611, and has been little read ever since.

Hall (2) (Halle), Edward (c. 1498–1547) English historian, author of an important source for Shakespeare's HISTORY PLAYS. Hall's account of the 15th-century WARS OF THE ROSES, *The Union of the Two Noble and Illustre Families of Lancaster and York* (1548), was particularly influential on the *Henry VI* plays, though echoes of it occur throughout the eight plays (see TETRALOGY) that deal with the wars. Hall's central theme in the *Union* is that the weakness of King HENRY VI and the resulting wars were God's punishment for the sin of Henry's grandfather, HENRY IV, who altered God's intended line of kings when he usurped the throne. This notion is in turn based on the premise that history has a moral purpose, set by God. Both of these

ideas are strongly evident in Shakespeare's plays. However, Hall's work was also employed by Shakespeare's most important source on British history, Raphael HOLINSHED, and it is often difficult to determine which source the playwright was using. Scholars generally feel that Hall was his major source for the history of the wars, while Holinshed was used chiefly for additional details, particularly in the *Henry VI* plays and *Richard III*.

Hall incorporated earlier histories into the *Union*, notably Sir Thomas MORE's *History of Richard III* (published in Richard GRAFTON's chronicles), and Polydore VERGIL's *Historia Anglia* (1534). Hall was in turn incorporated by later writers, including Holinshed and John STOW. Thus, his work is a central element in the 16th century's picture of the 15th. Hall was a lawyer and politician who wrote his history with the specific intention of glorifying the TUDOR dynasty, whose foundation ended the Wars of the Roses. In this, he was part of a well-established tradition of Tudor history writing that was consciously instituted by King Henry VII (see HISTORY PLAYS) as a type of propaganda. Shakespeare, though his own sensibility permeates his work and makes it more interesting and comprehensive, was also a part of this tradition.

Hall (3), Elizabeth (1608–1670) Shakespeare's grand-daughter, child of Susanna SHAKESPEARE (14) and John HALL (4). Elizabeth was eight when Shakespeare died, and the playwright left her most of his silver. After her mother's death she also inherited most of the rest of the Shakespeare estate, including NEW PLACE and the BIRTHPLACE. She married Thomas NASH (2) in 1626 and lived with him at New Place, though probably not until after her father's death in 1635. Nash died in 1647 and she was remarried in 1649 to John Bernard (d. 1674), with whom she moved to Northamptonshire. She had no children by either husband and was Shakespeare's last descendant. She left the Shakespeare birthplace to her cousin George Hart, grandson of Joan SHAKESPEARE (8), and the remainder of her grandfather's estate, including New Place, to Bernard, whose heirs sold it.

Hall (4), John (1575–1635) Shakespeare's son-in-law, the husband of Susanna SHAKESPEARE (14) and father of Elizabeth HALL (3). Hall was a notable doctor who probably treated his father-in-law and was certainly well-regarded by him, for with his wife he was executor of the playwright's will. Hall, the son of a physician from Bedfordshire, studied medicine at Cambridge University and possibly in France, though he never received a formal degree in the subject. He settled in STRATFORD around 1600 and was soon regarded as the region's leading doctor. He was reportedly a very devout Protestant, perhaps with Puritan leanings, and it has been speculated that he did not approve of his famous father-in-law's profession. During the Civil Wars his widow sold one of his Latin medical notebooks—apparently not realising that he had written it—and it was later published as *Select Observations on English Bodies* (1657). It contains accounts of many of his patients—including his wife and Michael DRAYTON—but unfortunately begins only in 1617 and so does not treat Shakespeare.

Hall (5), Peter (b. 1930) British theatrical director. Hall directed the ROYAL SHAKESPEARE COMPANY in STRATFORD from 1960 to 1968 and the National Theatre Company of Britain from 1972 to 1988. Among his most notable Shakespearean productions have been *Henry V* (1960), two stagings of *Coriolanus* (1959 and 1984, starring Laurence OLIVIER and Ian MCKELLEN, respectively), and a rare uncut *Hamlet* (1975).

Hall (6), Susanna Shakespeare Shakespeare's daughter, wife of John HALL (4). See SHAKESPEARE (14).

Hall (7), William (active 1577–1620) English printer, a possible 'Mr W. H'. of the dedication to the first edition (1609) of the SONNETS. Hall was mostly a printer of business papers, and had no known connection with Shakespeare or his works. However, he has been suggested by the scholar Sidney LEE as a possible 'Mr W. H'. on the strength of the coincidence of initials and the fact that the next word in the dedication is 'all'. Lee speculated that Hall acquired for publisher Thomas THORPE the copies of the poems from which the book was published, and was thus called the 'onlie begetter' of the Sonnets. Aside from this supposition there is no evidence to associate Hall with the work.

Halle, Edward See HALL (2).

Halliwell-Phillips, James Orchard (1820–1889) British scholar. A long-time librarian at Jesus College, Cambridge, Halliwell-Phillips was one of the most important 19th-century Shakespeare scholars. He published a *Life of Shakespeare* (1848), an edition of the *Works* (1853–1861), and a collection of documentary materials on the playwright's life, *Outlines of the Life of Shakespeare* (1881). The *Outlines* is a trove of material that has been used by all later biographers. He was a founder of the original Shakespeare Society in 1840 and the first editor of the STRATFORD archives.

Hamlet Title character of *Hamlet*, the crown prince of DENMARK. Prince Hamlet is required by his murdered father's GHOST (3) to take vengeance on the present KING (5), his uncle, who committed the murder and then married the widow of his victim, Hamlet's mother, the QUEEN (9). Hamlet's troubled re-

sponse to this situation, his disturbed relations with those around him, and his eventual acceptance of his destiny constitute the play.

Hamlet is almost universally considered one of the most remarkable characters in all of literature. His language, extraordinary even in Shakespeare's oeuvre, sweeps us up in a seemingly endless stream of brilliant impressions. He does not often use the similes and metaphors of ordinary speech, instead pouring forth fully fleshed images that convey the excitement of his thought. His psychology is stirringly genuine because it is humanly complex; he is filled with passion and contradiction, and his emotional life develops credibly through the course of the play. His personality, his attitudes and ideas, even his subconscious, have intrigued readers and theatre-goers for centuries, and copious commentary on him is still being written. Many writers have supposed that Hamlet's troubled mind reflects a traumatic development in Shakespeare's life, although there is almost no evidence of the playwright's personal life to confirm or refute this theory.

Although Hamlet foreshadows the psychologically realistic characters of modern drama, Shakespeare did not create the prince's emotional life for its own sake but rather as a vehicle for presenting a philosophical attitude. Hamlet's troubled mind demonstrates the development of an acceptance of life despite the existence of human evil, and this is the dominant theme of the play. The critical element in this development is the prince's recognition of evil in himself; in containing both good and evil, he represents the dual nature of humankind. The reconciliation of humanity with its own flawed nature is a central concern of Shakespeare's work, and in Hamlet an evolution of attitudes leading to this conclusion is displayed in a grand and powerful portrait.

Although he can deal in a practical manner with the world of intrigue that surrounds him, Hamlet is more a thinker than a doer, and he directs our attention often to his own concerns, large issues such as suicide, the virtues and defects of humankind, and the possibility of life after death. Above all, his circumstances demand that he consider the nature of evil.

We first encounter the prince as he struggles to deal with his father's death. In 1.2.76–86 he describes his mournful state; dressed in funereal black, conscious that he looks dejected and can be seen to have been weeping, he nevertheless asserts that this appearance cannot convey the depths of his grief. By focussing on the difference between appearance and reality—a difference that here is merely one of degree since his inner state is at least superficially indicated by his dress and demeanour—Hamlet betrays the confused perception that comes with great emotional trauma. In the early stages of grief, the ordinary aspects of existence seem absurdly thin and weak, inappropriate to the mourner's overwhelming sense of pain and loss.

In this state of mind, Hamlet is strongly offended by his mother's hasty and incestuous remarriage, even before he learns from the Ghost of his father's murder. He sees his father as an ideal man and a great king, an assumption supported by other opinions in the play and by the dignity and grandeur of the Ghost. He is thus appalled by his mother's willingness to accept an inferior man, a libertine and—as is soon revealed—a murderer. Hamlet comes to see his mother as evil and is devastated by the idea. Although he is the son of a godlike father, he is also the son of a mother who readily beds with 'a satyr' (1.2.140). Plunged into despondency, he rejects life, saying, 'How weary, stale, flat, and unprofitable / Seem to me all the uses of this world! . . . things rank and gross in nature / Possess it merely' (1.2.133–136). This attitude is further expressed in one of literature's most powerful evocations of mental depression, 'I have of late . . . lost all my mirth [and] this goodly frame the earth seems to me a sterile promontory, this most excellent canopy the air . . . appeareth nothing to me but a foul and pestilent congregation of vapours. What a piece of work is a man, . . . and yet, to me, what is this quintessence of dust? Man delights not me—nor woman neither . . .' (2.2.295–309).

He declares that his life is not worth 'a pin's fee' (1.4.65); indeed, he longs for death, as he declares more than once, wishing, for instance, '. . . that this too too sullied flesh would melt' (1.2.129) and declaring death '. . . a consummation / Devoutly to be wish'd' (3.1.63–64), though in both of these speeches he also rejects suicide, once because of the religious injunction against it and once out of fear of the afterlife.

His disgust with life turns, therefore, to a revulsion against sex, the mechanism of life's continuance. Not only does sex generate life, with its evils, but the attractions of sex have led his mother to adultery and incest. Though some commentators have supposed that Hamlet unconsciously desires his mother sexually, as in the Oedipus complex hypothesised by Freud, such a theory is unnecessary, for the play's world provides the prince with real, not fantasised, parental conflicts: his father is dead, and he is the enemy of his mother's lover. However, the facts of Hamlet's situation, dire as they are, are less important than the interpretation that he puts upon them. Plainly influenced by his disgust with sex, he is obsessed by the image of his mother's 'incestuous sheets' (1.2.157); he virtually ignores the political consequences of his father's murder—the murderer's succession as King—and focusses on the sexual implications, and, most significantly, he transfers his mother's sexual guilt to OPHELIA.

Hamlet denies his love for Ophelia in 3.1.117–119,

though only after affirming it two lines earlier, and Shakespeare plainly intended us to take Hamlet's courtship of Ophelia before the play begins as having been sincere. Ophelia's shy description in 1.3.110–114, along with her regretful one in 3.1.97–99, make this clear. Moreover, Hamlet's intensity and confusion as he parts from Ophelia—in the strange behaviour she recounts in 2.1.77–100 and in his famous insistence that she enter a nunnery in 3.1.121–151—indicate his great emotional involvement. However, although he apparently loved her earlier, Hamlet does not actually respond to Ophelia as a person in the course of the play. Theirs is not a love story but rather a dramatisation of Hamlet's rejection of life, and of love, marriage, and sex. 'Why wouldst thou be a breeder of sinners?' he cries in 3.1.121–122, and he immediately goes on to identify himself with the world's evil-doers. Hamlet cannot avoid his sexual desire for Ophelia, as his obscene jesting in 3.2.108–119 demonstrates, but this episode is also a plain indication of the disgust he now feels for sex. His attitude symbolises his condemnation of life, a viewpoint that he overcomes by the end of the play.

Hamlet's delay in seeking revenge may similarly be seen as a psychological trait emphasised to make a philosophical point. The prince's procrastination is not immediately obvious, for not much time seems to pass and only one plain opportunity for revenge presents itself (in the 'prayer scene', 3.3), but Hamlet insists upon its importance, berating himself as 'a rogue and peasant slave . . . / A dull and muddy-mettled rascal' (2.2.544, 562); his assumption of guilt is clearly excessive. Though committed to the idea that revenge is his duty, Hamlet senses the evil in the obligation, sent from 'heaven and hell' (2.2.580), and he resists.

Once the King's guilt is firmly established by his response to the performance of THE MURDER OF GONZAGO, Hamlet falls victim to a pathological rage. This is first shown in his chilling resolution, ' 'Tis now the very witching time of night, / . . . Now could I drink hot blood . . .' (3.2.379–381). This state of mind persists as he demands eternal damnation for the King, not merely murderous revenge, and therefore avoids killing him at prayer in 3.3. Then in 3.4 he vents his hysterical rage at his mother and kills POLONIUS with a furious gesture in the process. This crime lacks even the justification of revenge. Whatever his faults, Polonius was innocent of Hamlet's father's murder, and, moreover, his death leads to the insanity and subsequent death of Ophelia, whose blamelessness is absolute. Hamlet's avoidance of one evil has thus involved him in another, greater one.

Hamlet's rage and his descent into evil are central to the play, both literally, occurring near its mid-point, and figuratively, for his deeds trigger its climactic development. Polonius' son, LAERTES, seeks revenge and eventually kills Hamlet, and more immediately, Polonius' death results in Hamlet's exile, during which he finds his salvation.

In Act 5 we find that Hamlet has changed. He meditates on death in the graveyard in 5.1, but now death is neither welcoming nor fearful; it is merely the normal human destiny and the prince's remarks are satirical thrusts at the living. His memories of YORICK are pleasurable appreciations of the past, as well as occasions for sardonic humour. Ophelia's funeral triggers a last explosion of emotion as Hamlet assaults Laertes, but although this resembles his fury of Act 3, here Hamlet restrains himself and departs. His outburst has been cathartic, producing two significant declarations. As he challenges Laertes, Hamlet proclaims himself 'Hamlet the Dane' (5.1.251), at last accepting his role as his father's heir—Denmark, once his 'prison' (2.2.243) is now his kingdom—and at the same time implicitly challenging the King. Perhaps given courage or awareness by this pronouncement he goes on to assert the feelings he had suppressed in his anger and depression, stating 'I lov'd Ophelia' (5.1.264). The prince is no longer in the grip of his grief.

In 5.2 Hamlet confides to HORATIO the cause of the change in his sense of himself: by impulsively rewriting his death warrant to save himself, he has realised that his hesitations and ponderings had been beside the point. He sees that 'Our indiscretion sometime serves us well / When our deep plots do pall. . . . There's a divinity that shapes our ends, / Rough-hew them how we will . . .' (5.2.8–11). He acknowledges that he cannot carry out the revenge called for by the Ghost without committing murder, the very crime he must avenge. He accepts that he must be evil in order to counter evil. He senses a basic truth: the capacity for evil exists in him because he is human.

In accepting his destiny, Hamlet also prepares for his own death. He senses his end approaching, as the King's plot takes form, but he remains composed, saying, 'There is special providence in the fall of a sparrow. If it be now, 'tis not to come; if it be not to come, it will be now; if it be not now, yet it will come. The readiness is all. Since no man, of aught he leaves, knows aught, what is't to leave betimes? Let be' (5.2.215–220). This final remark—since we know so little of the world, it is no great matter to leave it early—reflects the prince's awareness of the futility of his earlier philosophical inquiries. It is more important to live and then to die, coming to terms with one's fate.

Hamlet's salvation—his awareness of his human failings—comes only with his death. However, Horatio's prayer for him, '[May] flights of angels sing thee to thy rest' (5.2.365), offers the hope of an eternal release from the stresses the prince has undergone.

The playwright leaves us assured that his tragic hero has finally found peace.

Hamlet

SYNOPSIS

Act 1, Scene 1

On the castle wall in ELSINORE, a sentry, BARNARDO, replaces FRANCISCO (1) on guard and is joined by HORATIO and MARCELLUS. Barnardo and Marcellus tell of a supernatural being they have seen. The GHOST (3) of the late King of DENMARK silently appears and withdraws. The three agree that this visitation seems especially ominous in view of an impending war with Norway. The Ghost re-enters but disappears again when a cock crows. Horatio decides that they should tell Prince HAMLET of the appearance of his father's spirit.

Act 1, Scene 2

Claudius, the KING (5) of Denmark, speaks of the recent death of the late king, his brother, and of his marriage to QUEEN (9) Gertrude, his brother's widow and Hamlet's mother. He also tells of an invasion threat from young Prince FORTINBRAS of Norway, who is acting without the knowledge of his uncle, the Norwegian king. The King therefore sends CORNELIUS (1) and VOLTEMAND with a letter to the King of Norway advocating restraint. LAERTES, the son of the King's adviser POLONIUS, requests permission to return to his studies in France, which the King grants. The King and Queen urge Hamlet to cease mourning his father's death. The King denies Hamlet permission to return to his own studies at Wittenberg; the Queen adds her wish that he stay in Denmark, and Hamlet agrees to do so. The monarchs and their retinue depart. Hamlet remains and muses mournfully on his mother's hasty and incestuous marriage. Horatio, Marcellus, and Barnardo appear and tell Hamlet about the Ghost. With great excitement, he arranges to meet them on the castle wall that night.

Act 1, Scene 3

Laertes, leaving for France, warns his sister, OPHELIA, about Hamlet's affection for her, which he says cannot be permanent in view of the prince's royal status. Polonius arrives and gives Laertes moralising advice on his conduct abroad. Laertes departs with a last word to Ophelia about Hamlet; this triggers a diatribe from Polonius about the suspect morals of young men, and he forbids Ophelia to see the prince.

Act 1, Scene 4

The Ghost appears to Hamlet, Horatio, and Marcellus, and Hamlet speaks to it. It beckons, and Hamlet follows.

Act 1, Scene 5

The Ghost confirms that it is the spirit of Hamlet's father. It declares that the prince must avenge his murder: the King had poured poison in his ear. The Ghost departs, and Hamlet vows to carry out its wishes. Horatio and Marcellus appear, and Hamlet swears them to secrecy—about the Ghost and about his own intention to feign madness—as the Ghost's disembodied voice demands their oaths.

Act 2, Scene 1

Polonius sends his servant REYNALDO (1) to spy on Laertes in Paris. Ophelia reports that Hamlet has come to her and behaved as if he were insane. Polonius concludes that his separation of Ophelia and Hamlet has driven the prince mad, and he decides to inform the King of this.

Act 2, Scene 2

The King and Queen welcome ROSENCRANTZ AND GUILDENSTERN, fellow students of Hamlet, who have been summoned in the hope that the prince will confide in them. They agree to spy on their friend. Voltemand and Cornelius arrive to report that the King of Norway has agreed to redirect Fortinbras' invasion to Poland. Polonius then declares—with comical tediousness—that Hamlet is lovesick, producing a love letter from the prince that he has confiscated from Ophelia. He offers to arrange for the King to eavesdrop on an encounter between Ophelia and Hamlet. Hamlet appears; Polonius advises the King and Queen to leave, and he approaches the prince alone. Hamlet answers him with nonsensical remarks and absurd insults. Polonius interprets these as symptoms of madness and departs, as Rosencrantz and Guildenstern enter. Hamlet greets them with more wild talk, and he badgers them into admitting that they have been sent to observe him. PLAYERS (2) from the city arrive, and Hamlet welcomes them enthusiastically, asking the FIRST PLAYER (2) to recite a dramatic monologue describing an episode of revenge from the TROJAN WAR. Hamlet requests that the Players perform THE MURDER OF GONZAGO before the court that night, inserting lines that he will compose. He dismisses the actors and the courtiers and soliloquises on his delay in avengeing the Ghost. He suspects that the spirit may have lied; he will have the Players enact a killing similar to his father's murder, and if Claudius responds guiltily, he will know that the Ghost has spoken the truth.

Act 3, Scene 1

Polonius instructs Ophelia to meet Hamlet while he and the King eavesdrop. The two men hide themselves as Hamlet approaches, meditating on the value of life, and Ophelia greets him. He passionately rejects her with a wild diatribe against women. He leaves her grieving for his apparent madness. The King tells Polonius that he has decided to send Hamlet on a mission to England, accompanied by Rosencrantz and Guildenstern. Polonius suggests further surveillance in the meantime, proposing that his mother summon

Hamlet after the performance by the Players; he, Polonius, will spy on their conversation.

Act 3, Scene 2
Hamlet lectures the Players on acting, saying that overacting and improvisation are distractions from a play's purposes. The court assembles, and the Players perform an introductory DUMB SHOW, in which a murderer kills a king by pouring poison in his ear as he sleeps. He then takes the king's crown and exits with the king's wife. The PLAYER KING and PLAYER QUEEN then speak; she asserts that she will never remarry if he dies, but he insists that she will. He then rests, falling asleep. Another Player, in the part of LUCIANUS, speaks darkly of the evil powers of poison and pours a potion in the ear of the PLAYER KING. The real King, distressed, rises and leaves in anger. Hamlet exults in the success of his plan. Rosencrantz and Guildenstern, and then Polonius, deliver the Queen's summons to Hamlet, and he agrees to go to her, but not before ridiculing them. He prepares himself to meet his mother, feeling great anger but reminding himself not to use violence against her.

Act 3, Scene 3
Polonius tells the King that Hamlet is on his way to the Queen's chamber, where he, Polonius, will spy on their meeting. He goes, and the King soliloquises about his murder of his brother. He says that he has been unable to pray for forgiveness because he is conscious that he is still enjoying the fruits of his crime—his brother's kingdom and his widow. He tries again to pray; Hamlet enters, sees the King on his knees, and contemplates killing him on the spot. He reflects, however, that, if the King dies while at prayer, he will probably go to heaven and the revenge will be incomplete. He decides instead to wait until he finds the King engaged in some sin, however petty, and then kill him, ensuring that his soul will go to hell.

Act 3, Scene 4
Polonius hides behind a curtain in the Queen's chamber. Hamlet arrives; he attempts to make his mother sit down, and she cries for help. Polonius cries out also, and Hamlet stabs him through the drapery, killing him. After expressing regret that his victim was not the King, Hamlet condemns his mother's behaviour. He compares the virtues of his father to the vices of his uncle; the distraught Queen's cries for mercy only enrage him more. The Ghost appears. The Queen, unaware of its presence, thinks Hamlet is mad as he speaks with the spirit. The Ghost reminds Hamlet of the vengeance he must exact, urges pity on the Queen, and departs. Less violently than before, Hamlet urges his mother to confess her sins and refuse to have sex with the King. He leaves, dragging the body of Polonius with him.

Act 4, Scene 1
The Queen tells the King that Hamlet has killed Polonius. The King sends Rosencrantz and Guildenstern to recover the body.

Act 4, Scene 2
Rosencrantz and Guildenstern confront Hamlet. He mocks them, refusing to tell them where the body is, but he goes with them to the King.

Act 4, Scene 3
The King tells his LORDS (5) that Hamlet is dangerous, yet, because of the prince's popularity, his exile to England must seem routine. Rosencrantz and Guildenstern return with Hamlet under guard. Hamlet expounds humorously on corpses before revealing where he has put Polonius' body. The King tells Hamlet that he is being sent to England immediately for his own safety. The King's entourage escorts Hamlet to the boat, leaving the King alone to muse on his plot: he is sending letters to the English that threaten war unless they kill Hamlet immediately.

Act 4, Scene 4
Hamlet, accompanied by Rosencrantz and Guildenstern, encounters a CAPTAIN (6) from Fortinbras' army, on its way to Poland. The Captain speaks of Fortinbras' war as a fight over a small, insignificant piece of territory. Hamlet compares himself, unable to avenge his father's death, with the 20,000 men who will fight and die for an inconsequential goal. He vows that in the future, he will value only bloody thoughts.

Act 4, Scene 5
A GENTLEMAN (3) tells the Queen that Ophelia is insane, rambling wildly in senseless speeches that yet seem to convey some unhappy truth. Ophelia enters, singing a song about a dead lover. The King arrives, and Ophelia sings of seduction and betrayal. She leaves, speaking distractedly about a burial. A MESSENGER (16) appears with the news that Laertes has raised a rebellion and is approaching the castle. Laertes and several FOLLOWERS break down the door and enter. He demands vengeance for his father's death, and the King promises that he shall have it. Ophelia returns, singing about a funeral, and distributes flowers to the King, the Queen, and Laertes. She sings again, about an old man's death, and departs. The King takes Laertes away to plot revenge on Hamlet.

Act 4, Scene 6
A SAILOR (1) brings Horatio a letter from Hamlet. It tells of his capture by pirates who have agreed to release him; Rosencrantz and Guildenstern continue to sail to England. Horatio goes with the sailor to meet Hamlet.

Act 4, Scene 7
The King tells Laertes that he cannot act directly against Hamlet, out of consideration for the Queen

and because of the prince's popularity. The King proposes a plot: they shall arrange a fencing match between Hamlet and Laertes, in which Hamlet will use a blunted sword intended for sport while Laertes shall secretly have a sharp sword. Laertes agrees and adds that he has a powerful poison that he will apply to his sword point. The King further suggests a poisoned glass of wine to be given Hamlet when the sport has made him thirsty. The Queen appears with the news that Ophelia has drowned, and Laertes collapses in tears.

Act 5, Scene 1
A GRAVE-DIGGER who is a CLOWN (1) speaks with his friend, the OTHER clown, about Ophelia, who has been granted Christian burial although possibly a suicide. He comically misconstrues the law on suicide and jokes about grave-digging. Hamlet and Horatio arrive, and Hamlet meditates on death's levelling of the wealthy and ambitious. He talks with the Grave-digger, who displays a skull that had belonged to YORICK, a court jester whom Hamlet had known. The prince reflects on the inevitability of death. Ophelia's funeral procession arrives, accompanied by Laertes and the King and Queen; the PRIEST (3) declares her death a suicide. When Hamlet realises whose funeral he is witnessing, he rushes forth and tries to fight Laertes, challenging his position as chief mourner. Restrained, he departs in a rage. The King assures Laertes that he will get his revenge.

Act 5, Scene 2
Hamlet tells Horatio how he rewrote the King's letter arrangeing his death, substituting Rosencrantz and Guildenstern's names for his own. He assumes that the two courtiers were killed, but he feels no remorse, since they were schemers. OSRIC, an obsequious and mannered courtier, arrives with the King's request that Hamlet fence with Laertes; the King has wagered that Hamlet can win. Hamlet mocks Osric before sending word that he will fight. He tells Horatio that the proposed match makes him uneasy but says that he is prepared to die. The King and Queen, a group of courtiers, and Laertes arrive for the match. The King pours wine to toast Hamlet's first successful round, and he places a pearl—a congratulatory token, he says—in Hamlet's cup. Hamlet and Laertes fence, but after his first victory Hamlet postpones refreshment and resumes the match. The Queen drinks from his cup, although the King tries to stop her. Laertes wounds Hamlet with the poisoned sword, the two fighters scuffle and accidentally exchange swords, and Hamlet wounds Laertes. The Queen falls, exclaims that she is poisoned, and dies. Laertes, himself poisoned by the exchanged sword, reveals the King's plot. Hamlet wounds the King with the sword and then forces him to drink the poisoned wine. Hamlet and Laertes forgive each other, and Laertes dies. Horatio starts to drink the poisoned wine, but Hamlet demands that he remain alive to tell his side of the story. Osric announces the return of Fortinbras from Poland; Hamlet declares Fortinbras his successor and dies. Fortinbras arrives and takes command, ordering a stately funeral for Hamlet.

COMMENTARY

Hamlet is the most notoriously problematic of Shakespeare's plays, and questions about it still bedevil commentators after almost 400 years. Tremendous amounts of energy have gone into considering its possible interpretations, and the range of opinions on them is immense; as Oscar Wilde wittily put it, perhaps the greatest question raised by *Hamlet* is, 'Are the critics mad or only pretending to be so?'

Hamlet was classed with the PROBLEM PLAYS when that term was first applied to Shakespeare's works of the early 17th century (see BOAS). Like those dark comedies, this TRAGEDY deals with death and sex and with the psychological and social tensions arising from these basic facts of life. And like the problem plays, *Hamlet* treats these issues without providing clear-cut resolutions, thereby leaving us with complicated, highly emotional responses that cause both satisfac-

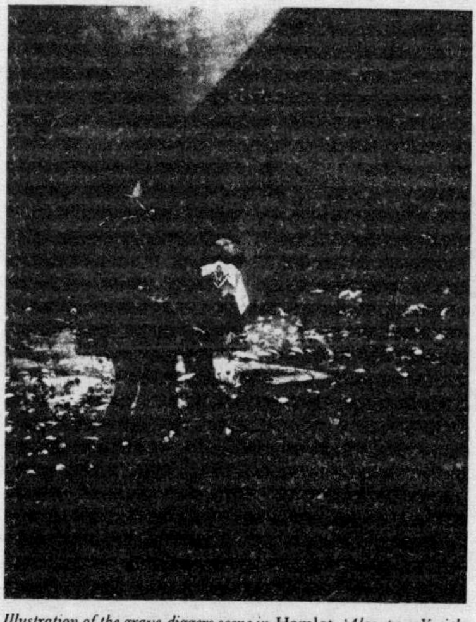

Illustration of the grave-diggers scene in Hamlet. *'Alas, poor Yorick. I knew him, Horatio' (5.1.178). Hamlet confronts the fact of human mortality.* (Courtesy of Culver Pictures, Inc.)

tion—at seeing basic elements of our own lives treated dramatically—and pain—at the nagging persistence of these difficulties, as in real life.

It is precisely through such ambiguity, however, that *Hamlet* offers a robust and vital assertion of human worth, for the play is essentially a moral drama whose theme is the existence of both good and evil in human nature, a central concern in Shakespeare's work as a whole. Although it anticipates modern psychological dramas in some respects, *Hamlet* is not itself such a work; the extraordinary presentation of Prince Hamlet's troubled mind is simply the vehicle—albeit a vivid one—for the development of his acceptance of humanity's flawed nature. Shakespeare's great accomplishment in *Hamlet* was to express the philosophy that underlies this realisation.

Some of the play's many puzzles are interesting but superficial, such as Horatio's status at the Danish court, the identification of Hamlet's inserted lines in *The Murder of Gonzago*, or the determination of the prince's age. These matters chiefly reflect the playwright's lack of concern for minor inconsistencies, a trait seen throughout the plays. Others are deeper matters of plotting and psychology: Is Hamlet's emotional disturbance real or feigned? What is the nature of his relationship to Ophelia? Is King Claudius an unalloyed villain? The 'problem of problems', as it has been called, is Hamlet's unnecessary delay in executing the revenge he plainly accepts as his duty.

The basic story—a young man grieves for his father while faced with the duty to avenge his death—came from Shakespeare's source, the UR-HAMLET, and its genre, the REVENGE PLAY, but Shakespeare's attitude towards vengeance is not the traditionally approving one. Hamlet's regret when he says, 'The time is out of joint. O cursed spite, / That ever I was born to set it right' (1.5.196–197), testifies to this, as does the existence of a parallel revenge plot, that of Laertes' revenge of *his* father's murder by Hamlet. The hero of one plot, Hamlet is in effect the villain of the other, casting an inescapable doubt upon his heroic role. Hamlet recognises the ambivalence of his position when he says of Polonius' death, '. . . heaven hath pleas'd it so, / To punish me with this and this with me' (3.4.175–176).

This paradox suggests the essential duality of human nature, which is both noble and wicked, and numerous comparisons throughout the drama stress this point. Several times Hamlet contrasts his murdered father and his uncle—the former an ideal ruler, just and magnanimous; the latter an unscrupulous killer and lustful adulterer. Similarly, Hamlet juxtaposes his father's virtues with his mother's sin in accepting her husband's murderer and having sex with him. Other polarities abound: the chaste Ophelia versus the incestuous Queen; the faithful Horatio versus the treacherous Rosencrantz and Guildenstern; the devious duellist Laertes versus the manly soldier Fortinbras. Each of these contrasts recalls and reinforces the play's basic opposition between good and evil.

Faced with the awareness of evil, Hamlet longs for death and is disgusted with life, especially as it is manifested in sex, which he not only sees as the drive behind his mother's sin but which he abhors as the force that inexorably produces more life and thus more evil. 'Why wouldst thou be a breeder of sinners?' (3.1.121–122), he cries to Ophelia, and his rejection of her stems from his rejection of sex. Shakespeare did not intend their relationship as a love story; instead, it is an allegory of the condemnation of life, a point of view whose ultimate rejection is central to the play.

Hamlet's notorious procrastination of his revenge has a similar function. Though he accepts the Ghost's orders, he senses the evil in this duty, sent from 'heaven and hell' (2.2.580), and he resists its fulfilment. Though psychologically true to life, Hamlet's delay serves primarily to offer opportunities to stress the duality of human nature: as revenger, Hamlet is both opposed to and involved in evil. His repeated insistence on postponing his highly ambiguous duty emphasises his ambivalence and stimulates our own. Emotionally, Hamlet's procrastination produces in him a growing rage that leads to his killing of Polonius in 3.4, an act that provokes the King and Laertes to set in motion the incidents that lead to the bloody climax and that hastens Hamlet's exile and his escape from the King's execution plot. This event, in turn, jars Hamlet from his absorption in his personal tragedy and prepares him to find the 'divinity that shapes our ends' (5.2.10).

Both Hamlet and the play undergo a sweeping change before the climax, and this change is well prepared for by the establishment of a dominant tone in the play's language that is later varied to quite dramatic effect. Through Acts 1–4, the pervasiveness of evil and its capacity to corrupt human life are conveyed by an extended use of the imagery of illness, evoking a strong sense of stress and unease. In the play's opening moments, Francisco declares himself 'sick at heart' (1.1.9), and Horatio, speaking of evil omens, refers to the moon being 'sick almost to doomsday with eclipse' (1.1.123). Hamlet equates evil with bodily disorder when he speaks of a birthmark, 'nature's livery' (1.4.32), as the 'dram of evil' (1.4.36) that makes a virtuous man seem corrupt and ignoble. He is referring figuratively to the excessive drinking of Danish courtiers, rather than to the more serious evils soon to arise, but he strikes a note of disease, death, and physical corruption that recurs throughout the play.

For instance, Hamlet speaks of the King's prayer as

'physic [that] prolongs thy sickly days' (3.3.96) and of resolution as 'sicklied o'er' (3.1.85); the King refers to those who tell Laertes of his father's death as '. . . buzzers [who] infect his ear / With pestilent speeches . . .' (4.5.90–91). Strikingly, diseases of the skin, where an inner evil is presumed to be present, are often mentioned, as in Hamlet's reference to a 'flattering unction . . . [that] will but skin and film the ulcerous place, / Whiles rank corruption . . . / Infects unseen' (3.4.146–151), or in his image for the outbreak of a pointless war: an abscess 'that inward breaks, and shows no cause without / Why the man dies' (4.4.27–29).

Planning to exile Hamlet, the King observes, 'Diseases desperate grown / By desperate appliance are reliev'd' (4.3.9–10). He refers not only to the danger he faces from an avengeing Hamlet, but he is also thinking of Hamlet's apparent insanity. Hamlet's lunacy seems at times to be real, at least in some respects, such as his hysterical rejection of sex and love, but he himself asserts that it is false on several occasions—e.g., in 3.4.142–146. The question remains one of the play's many enigmas. In any case, Hamlet's insanity, whether feigned or real, is itself a major instance of the imagery of sickness, a constant reminder that 'something is rotten in the state of Denmark' (1.5.90).

A particularly vivid example of disease imagery is the Ghost's clinical description of the action of the poison that first thinned his blood and then produced on his skin 'a vile and loathsome crust' (1.5.72) before killing him. The poisoning is enacted twice in 3.2, first in the Players' dumb show and then by the Player playing Lucianus. Further, a similar fate awaits the four major characters in 5.2.

An extension of the play's imagery of death is the repeated suggestion of suicide, although it is rejected. Hamlet's first soliloquy regrets the religious 'canon 'gainst self-slaughter' (1.2.132). Horatio worries that the Ghost may tempt Hamlet to the 'toys of desperation' (1.4.75) on a cliff overlooking the sea. In 5.1 the Grave-digger discusses the law on suicides, and Ophelia's death is declared 'doubtful' (5.1.220) by the Priest. In his last moment, Hamlet prevents Horatio from killing himself with the poisoned cup. The prince also discusses the possibility of suicide at length in the soliloquy beginning 'To be or not to be . . .' (3.1.56–88) before rejecting the idea. More important, near the crucial mid-point of the play, just before his dramatic rejection of Ophelia and love, Hamlet raises the question of the desirability of life and answers, in effect, that we have no choice but to accept our destiny and live. Thus, while suicide serves as part of the play's imagery of despair, its rejection foreshadows the ultimate acceptance of life and its evils.

Act 5 opens with Hamlet meditating on death in the graveyard, but now death, represented with ghoulish humour by the skulls dug up by the Grave-digger, is not a potential escape, nor is it the fearful introduction to a possibly malign afterlife; it is merely the destined end for all humans. The conversation with the Grave-diggers offers comic relief as the climax draws closer, and Hamlet's recollections of Yorick offer a healthy appreciation of the pleasures of the past as well as a sardonic acceptance of death: 'Now get you to my lady's chamber and tell her, . . . to this favour she must come' (5.1.186–188). The prince is no longer in the grip of his grief. Ophelia's funeral and Hamlet's encounter with Laertes bring a final catharsis, and he is able to assert the love for Ophelia that he once denied and to accept his role in life by taking the royal title 'the Dane' (5.1.251).

In the first episode of 5.2, we hear of the cause of this change as Hamlet tells of the plot he has foiled by sending Rosencrantz and Guildenstern to their deaths in his place; in impulsively acting to save himself, he has learned, 'There's a divinity that shapes our ends, / Rough-hew them how we will . . .' (5.2.10–11). Hamlet finally comes to terms with his duty to exact vengeance, even though he cannot do so without committing the very crime he avenges, murder. In realising that he must be evil in order to counter evil, Hamlet also accepts his own death; although he senses his end approaching as the King's plot takes form, he remains composed, saying, 'There is special providence in the fall of a sparrow. If it be now, 'tis not to come; if it be not to come, it will be now; if it be not now, yet it will come. The readiness is all' (5.2.215–218).

The tragic paradox at the close of *Hamlet* is that the protagonist's psychological liberation comes only with his own death, a death that inspires Horatio's lovely farewell wish to Hamlet that 'flights of angels sing thee to thy rest' (5.2.365). The attitude towards death expressed in this elegiac prayer is unlike anything earlier in the play, and its emphatic placement after the climax clearly marks it as the drama's conclusive statement, a confirmation of the benevolence of fate despite the inevitability of evil and death.

SOURCES OF THE PLAY

Shakespeare's basic source for *Hamlet* was the UR-HAMLET (c. 1588), a play on the same subject that is known to have been popular in London in the 1580s but for which no text survives. This work, believed to have been written by Thomas KYD, was apparently derived from a tale in François BELLEFOREST's collection *Histoires Traqiques* (1580). Although Shakespeare knew Belleforest's work, he adopted a central element of *Hamlet*, the Ghost, from the *Ur-Hamlet*, and this fact, along with the theatrical success of the lost work, suggests that it was Shakespeare's chief source.

Belleforest retold a story from a 12th-century Latin work, the *Historiae Danicae*, by SAXO GRAMMATICUS, first published in 1514. Saxo provides the earliest com-

plete account of a legendary tale—9th-century fragments are known from the Icelandic sagas—of Amleth, a Danish nobleman who took revenge after his uncle killed his father and married his mother. The name Amleth, from Old Norse, means 'dim-witted' or 'brutish', in reference to his stratagem of feigning madness after his father's murder. Many other elements of *Hamlet*—including a dramatic encounter between Amleth and his mother, during which he kills a spy; his love affair with a beautiful woman; his exile to England and his escape by replacing the order for his execution with one condemning his escorts—are present in Saxo's account.

Shakespeare doubtless found much of this in the *Ur-Hamlet,* but this work, to judge by its probable companion piece, Kyd's *The Spanish Tragedy* (1588–1589), lacked *Hamlet*'s dramatic development and thematic unity; Shakespeare may have found hints of a unified point of view in Belleforest's version. In particular, the French writer develops the contrast between the good king who is murdered and his evil, incestuous killer, a comparison that is prominent in Hamlet's thoughts.

Many scholars believe that *The Spanish Tragedy,* also a revenge play, was itself a source for numerous elements in *Hamlet.* For instance, Kyd's play has a procrastinating protagonist who berates himself for talking instead of acting and who dies as he achieves his revenge; it also features a play within a play, a heroine whose love is opposed by her family, and another woman who becomes insane and commits suicide. However, some commentators feel that Kyd took at least some of these elements from the *Ur-Hamlet,* whether he wrote it or not, and that Shakespeare could have done so as well.

Other sources contributed to *Hamlet* in minor ways. A play that provokes a confession of guilt was a well-established literary motif, but Shakespeare's company had recently staged an anonymous drama, *A Warning for Fair Women* (1599), in which it is used, so this work was probably the immediate stimulus for Hamlet's 'Mousetrap' plot. The physician Timothy BRIGHT's *A Treatise of Melancholy* (1586) may have influenced Shakespeare's portrayal of Hamlet's depression. Thomas NASHE's widely popular pamphlet, *Pierce Penniless His Supplication to the Devil* (1592), influenced several passages of the play, especially Hamlet's diatribe on drunkenness in 1.4.16–38. Some of Hamlet's remarks on graves and death in 5.1 echo a popular religious work, *Of Prayer and Meditation,* by the Spanish mystic Luis de GRANADA, which Shakespeare probably read in the translation by Richard HOPKINS. *The Counsellor* (1598), an anonymous translation of a volume on good government by the famed Polish diplomat Laurentius GOSLICIUS is echoed in several passages, most notably Hamlet's speech beginning, 'What a piece of work is man' (2.2.303).

PLUTARCH's *Lives,* always one of Shakespeare's favourite sources, mentions a Greek tyrant, famed for many cold-blooded murders, who wept at a recital of HECUBA's woes, and this may have inspired the recitation by the First Player in 2.2. However, the playwright also knew the tale of Hecuba from VIRGIL's *Aeneid,* where it first appears, and from *The Tragedy of Dido* (1594), a play by Nashe and Christopher MARLOWE (1).

Shakespeare could also have read a retelling of Plutarch's Hecuba anecdote in the *Essays* of Michel de MONTAIGNE, either in French (publ. between 1580 and 1595) or in a manuscript of John FLORIO's translation, (publ. 1603). Echoes of Montaigne occur in several key passages—e.g., both Hamlet and the French essayist liken death to a sleep and to a 'consummation' (3.1.63).

Some scholars believe that an incident of 1577 at the court of Marguerite de Valois, a French princess married to the King of Navarre, influenced Shakespeare's conception of Ophelia's death. A young woman of the court was reported to have died of love for a young nobleman; he was absent from the court at the time and learned of her death only when he accidentally encountered the funeral procession upon his return. This event was widely reported in England at the time, due to the English support of the Protestant forces, led by Navarre, in the French Wars of Religion. The same event is thought to be referred to in *Love's Labour's Lost* (see KATHARINE [1]).

A real event also inspired the murder of Hamlet's father by pouring poison in his ear. In 1538 the Duke of Urbino, one of the leading military and political figures of day, died. His barber-surgeon confessed that he had killed the duke by putting a lotion in his ears, having been hired to do so by one Luigi Gonzaga. Shakespeare gave the name of the plotter to the victim (as *Gonzago* [3.2.233]), but the combination of his name and the unusual method of poisoning point to this actual crime as the stimulus to the playwright's fictional one, although the *Ur-Hamlet* may have used it first.

TEXT OF THE PLAY

Hamlet was probably written in late 1599 or early 1600, though possibly a year later. It followed *Julius Caesar*—performed in September 1599—for it echoes *Caesar* in 1.1.116–118 and alludes to it in 3.2.102–105, and it probably preceded John MARSTON's play *Antonio's Revenge,* staged in late 1600, which recalls *Hamlet* in many places, indicating that Shakespeare's play had been performed by no later than the autumn of 1600.

However, one passage in *Hamlet*—2.2.336–358, describing the competition of the PLAYERS (2) with a troupe of child actors—clearly refers to THE WAR OF THE THEATRES, a rivalry among acting companies that dominated the London theatre in the spring of 1601. If *Hamlet* was written in 1600, then this passage must

have been inserted later. Some scholars, however, hold that *Hamlet* was written in its entirety in early 1601 and that either *Antonio's Revenge* was Shakespeare's source rather than the other way around or both Marston and Shakespeare took their common materials from the *Ur-Hamlet*.

Hamlet was first published in 1603 by Nicholas LING and John TRUNDELL in a QUARTO edition (known as Q1) printed by Valentine SIMMES. Q1 is a BAD QUARTO, a mangled version of the text, assembled from the memories of actors who had performed in the play. It was supplanted by Q2 (1604, with some copies dated 1605), printed by John ROBERTS and published by him and Ling. A sound text, Q2 is believed to have been printed from Shakespeare's own manuscript, or FOUL PAPERS, with occasional reference to Q1 where the manuscript was unclear. However, two substantial passages appear to have been deliberately cut from Q2: Hamlet's reflections on Denmark as a prison (2.2. 239–269), perhaps thought offensive to the Danish wife of England's new king, JAMES I; and the passage on child actors mentioned above, which may have been cut because James patronised a CHILDREN'S COMPANY or perhaps simply because it was out of date by 1604. In 1607 Ling sold his rights to the play to John SMETHWICK, who published three further quartos, Q3 (1611), Q4 (1622), and Q5 (1637), each of which was printed from its predecessor.

Hamlet was published in the FIRST FOLIO edition of Shakespeare's plays (1623). This text, known as F, derives from Q2 but differs from it significantly. It corrects many small errors and improves on Q2's stage directions, but it also contains its own, more numerous, omissions and errors. F 'modernises' words the editors or printers thought old-fashioned, and some bits of dialogue apparently derive from actors' ad libs, such as a cry of 'Oh Vengeance!' in the middle of Hamlet's soliloquy at the end of 2.2. More important, F provides the significant passages cut from Q2. It is thought that the printers of F followed both Q2—probably a copy that had been annotated for production use—and a FAIR COPY, a transcription of Shakespeare's manuscript, with errors and alterations made by a scribe but including the missing material.

Modern editions rely on Q2 because it is plainly closest to Shakespeare's own manuscript, but they turn to F for its restored cuts and for frequent minor improvements. Rarely, Q1 provides a correction of an obvious error in the other two texts or a clarification in stage directions.

THEATRICAL HISTORY OF THE PLAY

From the outset, Hamlet has been recognised as one of the greatest works of the English stage, and it has remained the most widely produced of Shakespeare's plays (though most productions—probably including the original one—have used an abridged text). Most leading actors—and some actresses—of every generation have played the title part. The play has also been frequently performed in other languages.

The first production was that of the CHAMBERLAIN'S MEN in 1600 or 1601, referred to in the registration of the play with the STATIONERS' COMPANY in 1602. Contemporary references, along with many echoes of the play in the work of other playwrights, testify to its early popularity. Richard BURBAGE (3) was the first Hamlet; after his death in 1619 the role was taken, to great acclaim, by Joseph TAYLOR. A tradition first recorded by Nicholas ROWE in 1709 reports that Shakespeare played the Ghost in the original production.

'The Grave-Makers', an adaptation of 5.1 of *Hamlet*, was performed as a DROLL during the period of revolutionary government in England (1642–1660), when the theatres were legally closed. After the restoration of the monarchy, *Hamlet* was revived by William DAVENANT, though with a much abridged text, in a 1661 production starring Thomas BETTERTON, who was celebrated in the role for the rest of the century.

David GARRICK played Hamlet many times between 1734 and his retirement in 1776. Susannah Maria CIBBER (2), who often played opposite him, was regarded as the best Ophelia of the day. Garrick's production of 1772 was one of the most severely altered, and is still notorious for its elimination of much of Act 5. Beginning in 1783, John Philip KEMBLE (3), regarded as one of the greatest Hamlets, played the part often, sometimes opposite his sister, Sarah SIDDONS, as Ophelia.

Siddons herself was the first of many women to play Hamlet, taking the role in 1775. Female Hamlets were most popular in the late 18th and 19th centuries; among the best known were Kitty CLIVE, Charlotte CUSHMAN, Julia GLOVER, and Sarah BERNHARDT. In the 20th century Judith ANDERSON (1) (at the age of 73) and Eva Le Gallienne, among others, have also played the prince.

Most of the major theatrical entrepreneurs of the 19th century produced *Hamlet* at least once. Among the most acclaimed Hamlets of the period were Ira ALDRIDGE, William Charles MACREADY, Edwin BOOTH (1), and Henry Irving (usually opposite Ellen TERRY [1] as Ophelia). Irving had his first great Shakespearean success with the play in 1874, later staging an extravagantly scenic and very popular version (1879). William POEL used the Q1 text in 1881.

F. R. BENSON (1) staged Shakespeare's complete text in 1900, confirming that the resulting four- to five-hour performance was feasible. Other noteworthy 20th-century *Hamlet*s have included the controversial 1925 Barry JACKSON (1) production, which introduced modern dress to the Shakespearean stage; a New York staging by Margaret WEBSTER (3), starring Maurice EVANS (4) (1939); and Joseph PAPP's productions of 1972 and 1987, starring Stacy Keach and Kevin Kline

respectively. Several 20th-century actors are especially well known for their portrayals of Hamlet, including John BARRYMORE, John GIELGUD, Laurence OLIVIER, and Evans.

Hamlet has been acted on FILM at least 25 times—far more than any other Shakespeare play—since 1900, when Sarah Bernhardt played the prince in a silent movie. Among the best-known films are Olivier's heavily abridged version of 1948, with music by William WALTON; the Russian Grigori KOZINTSEV's epic presentation of a prose translation by Boris Pasternak (1964); and the 1969 film by Tony Richardson (b. 1928), with Nicol WILLIAMSON. *Hamlet* has also been presented on TELEVISION five times.

Hamlett, Katherine (d. 1579) Englishwoman whose death may be reflected in that of OPHELIA in *Hamlet.* A resident of Tippington, a village near STRATFORD, Mistress Hamlett was drowned in the Avon River while fetching water, and a coroner's jury hesitated over the possibility of suicide before declaring, two months later, that she had died a natural death. It has been speculated that the coincidental similarity between a family name he once knew and the name of his protagonist might have recalled Katherine Hamlett's death to the playwright—who was 15 when it occurred—as he described Ophelia's death by drowning, declared 'doubtful' (5.1.220) by the PRIEST (3), although the coroner 'finds it Christian burial' (5.1.4–5).

Hands, Terry (b. 1941) British theatrical director. Hands has been associated with the ROYAL SHAKESPEARE COMPANY in STRATFORD since 1966, serving as associate director, joint artistic director from 1978, and artistic director and chief executive since 1986. He has directed many of Shakespeare's plays, at Stratford, in the United States, and on the Continent.

Hanmer, Thomas (1677–1746) Early editor of Shakespeare's plays. Hanmer, a former Speaker of the House of Commons, was the fourth editor of the collected plays. His edition was published in 1744 in an elaborately bound and expensive set of six volumes. It was illustrated by Hubert GRAVELOT and Francis HAYMAN and was intended for a wealthy market. Hanmer was a disrespectful editor who inserted alterations of his own, insisted that passages he did not approve of could not have been by Shakespeare, and failed to annotate adoptions of the readings of earlier editors. In addition, he did not go back to the early texts but simply worked from the collection published by Alexander POPE (1) in 1725.

Harcourt Minor character in *2 Henry IV,* a messenger. In 4.4 Harcourt brings King HENRY IV news that Lord BARDOLPH (2) and the Earl of NORTHUMBERLAND (1) have been defeated, thus ending the rebellion that began in *1 Henry IV.*

Harfleur City on the northern coast of FRANCE (1), location in *Henry V.* Harfleur is besieged by the army of HENRY V. In 3.3 the king describes the bloody terror Harfleur can expect if it continues to resist, and the GOVERNOR (1) surrenders the city. This episode is a good instance of the play's ambiguity. Henry may be seen as merciful and statesmanlike; he spares the town, and he explicitly orders EXETER (2), 'Use mercy to them all' (3.3.54). On the other hand, his brilliant evocation of a sacked city, with vivid descriptions of rape and murder, stresses the horrors of an army gone amok, an emphasis that reinforces a reading of *Henry V* as a mordant anti-war work.

Harington, Sir John (1561–1612) First English translator of ARIOSTO's *Orlando Furioso,* a source for *Much Ado About Nothing.* Harington, a godson of Queen ELIZABETH (1), spent much of his life at court. It is thought that his translation of *Orlando Furioso* (1591) was made at the Queen's command, as an ironic punishment for having independently translated one of its indecent passages.

Harpy Supernatural creature in whose guise ARIEL appears in 3.3 in *The Tempest.* PROSPERO's sprite accuses the 'three men of sin'—ALONSO, ANTONIO (5), and SEBASTIAN (3)—and his disguise makes him more terrifying. The Harpies, three mythological monsters, sisters, were woman-headed birds. They stole things from mortals—especially food (appropriate to the banquet setting of Ariel's appearance)—and defecated vilely as they left. Apparently wind-gods in origin, these semi-divine beings may have derived in part from rumours reaching Greece of an actual creature in India, a large, fruit-eating bat noted for its excrement.

Harris (1), Frank (James Thomas) (1856–1931) British author and editor. Best known today for his sexually explicit autobiography, *My Life and Loves* (1927), Harris also wrote short stories, two plays, a novel, essays, biographies, and other works. Among these were *The Man Shakespeare and His Tragic Life Story* (1909), a biography laced with elaborate interpretations of the SONNETS and various plays as detailed evidence of Shakespeare's life, especially his love life. For example, Harris advocated the theory, first suggested by Thomas TYLER (2), that Mary FITTON was the 'Dark Lady' of the SONNETS, and he furthered this notion in his play *Shakespeare and His Love* (1910) and in another book, *The Women of Shakespeare* (1911). He saw Shakespeare's works as delivering a message to humanity, extolling forgiveness and love, and he equated it with Christ's. Being immensely egotistical, he identified himself with these two personages—and GOETHE—as 'God's spies' (*King Lear,* 5.3.17).

Harris was an adventurer before he became a literary figure; he ran away from his home in Scotland at 14 and worked at various jobs, including cowboy, in America and Europe, before settling in London and establishing himself as a writer of fiction. He became the editor of two of Britain's most important magazines, the *Fortnightly Review* (1886–1894) and the *Saturday Review* (1894–1898), in which he published H. G. Wells, Oscar Wilde, and George Bernard SHAW (2), among others. He later wrote biographies of Wilde and Shaw. He cultivated a scandalous reputation, aided by his persistent campaign against Victorian prudery and his pro-German sentiments during World War I. He made many enemies, and by 1920 he was neglected and impoverished. While his reputation as a writer has improved since his death and his importance in literary history is acknowledged, his scholarship—including his work on Shakespeare—is generally derided; even his autobiography has been found to be grossly inaccurate and self-serving.

Harris (2), Henry (c. 1630–1681) English actor. A leading man in William DAVENANT's theatre company, Harris acted many Shakespearean parts, including Cardinal WOLSEY in *Henry VIII,* for which he was particularly noted. He also played HORATIO opposite the HAMLET of the great Thomas BETTERTON, in the first staging of *Hamlet* (1661) after the reopening of the English theatres following the Puritan revolution. In 1662 he became the first ROMEO to play opposite a female JULIET (1) (Mary SAUNDERSON), as actresses were admitted to English stages. He was felt by some contemporaries, including Samuel PEPYS, to be as fine an actor as Betterton. He joined Betterton in 1671 in the management of London's Dorset Garden Theatre, serving as the artistic director.

Harrison (1), George Bagshawe (b. 1894) English scholar, author of many works on Shakespeare. An authority on the Elizabethan background of Shakespeare's life, Harrison was also the general editor of the Penguin editions of Shakespeare's works, published between 1937 and 1959. His *England in Shakespeare's Day* (1928) and *Shakespeare at Work* (1933) are general studies, and he compiled a wealth of primary material from the period 1590 to 1610 in his *Elizabethan* and *Jacobean Journals* (1928, 1933, 1941), which remain essential references for the Shakespeare scholar.

Harrison (2), John (d. 1617) Highly successful London publisher and bookseller, a founding member of the STATIONERS' COMPANY. In 1594 Harrison purchased the rights to Shakespeare's narrative poems *Venus and Adonis* and *The Rape of Lucrece* from Richard FIELD (2), who had already produced the first edition of the former. Between 1594 and 1596 Harrison published the second, third, and fourth editions (known as Q2–4, though only the first of them was a QUARTO; the others were published in an octavo format), employing Field as the printer. In 1596 he sold the rights to the poem to William LEAKE. Harrison published the first edition of *Lucrece,* printed by Field, in 1594 and the second, printed by Peter SHORT, in 1598. He passed on the rights to this work to his younger half-brother, also named John Harrison, who published Q3 and Q4 (both 1600), printed by Short, and Q5 (1607), printed by Nicholas OKES. The younger Harrison sold the rights to *Lucrece* to Roger JACKSON (3) in 1614.

Harrison (3), William (1534–1593) English historian, collaborator with Raphael HOLINSHED on Holinshed's *Chronicles of England, Scotland, and Ireland* (1577), which in its second edition (1587) was an important source for Shakespeare. Harrison, a clergyman who was personal chaplain to Lord COBHAM, served as Holinshed's assistant editor and contributed greatly to the *Chronicles.* He translated Hector BOECE's Latin history of SCOTLAND and wrote descriptions of the geography of England and Scotland. After his work with Holinshed, Harrison wrote extensively on his theory that Britain had once been inhabited by giants. He left a massive history of the world unfinished at his death.

Harsnett, Samuel (1561–1631) English clergyman and writer, author of a source for *King Lear.* An ambitious clerical politician, Harsnett wrote *A Declaration of Egregious Popish Impostures* (1603), a diatribe against Catholic priests who had claimed to exorcise demons from several lunatics in a famous case of 18 years earlier. Shakespeare took many details of the pretended insanity of EDGAR from this work, who, in his disguise as a wandering lunatic, claims to be pursued by demons. Early in his career Harsnett was denounced as a Catholic, but he recovered and rose to be a leading figure at Cambridge University as well as bishop of several different sees. He was famous for his harsh manner and was forced to resign from his position at Cambridge when his fellow scholars launched a formal campaign against him. However, in 1628 he was named Archbishop of YORK (2), the second-highest position in the Anglican Church.

Hart (1), Charles (d. 1693) Leading actor of the Restoration period, presumed illegitimate son of William HART (3), who was the son of Shakespeare's sister Joan SHAKESPEARE (8) Hart. Shakespeare's grandnephew, Charles Hart was apprenticed to Richard ROBINSON (4) of the KING'S MEN and performed at the BLACKFRIARS THEATRE as a child, playing women's roles. During the Civil Wars, he achieved distinction in combat as an officer in the Royalist forces, and after the war he was

a member of Thomas KILLIGREW's King's Company. He was particularly distinguished as OTHELLO and BRUTUS (4).

Hart (2), Joan Shakespeare Shakespeare's sister. See SHAKESPEARE (8).

Hart (3), William (1600–1639) An actor, Shakespeare's nephew, son of Joan SHAKESPEARE (8) Hart. William Hart was a member of the KING'S MEN in the mid-1630s and played FALSTAFF, among other roles. He apparently died unmarried, though Charles HART (1) is believed to have been his illegitimate son.

Harvey (1) Original name of PETO in *1* and *2 Henry IV.* When the name Peto was substituted for Harvey, shortly after the plays were written, in 1596–1597, one instance of the original designation inadvertently remained in the early texts of *1 Henry IV,* in 1.2.158, revealing that the change had occurred. Since the 18th century this reference has also been altered in most editions. The change of name was made at the same time that OLDCASTLE became FALSTAFF—at the insistence of Lord COBHAM, a descendant of the historical Oldcastle—presumably in the hope of avoiding a similar problem with another prominent aristocrat, Sir William HERVEY (also known as Harvey).

Harvey (2), Gabriel (c. 1545–1630) English writer, a major literary figure of Shakespeare's day and possibly a model for the pedantic HOLOFERNES of *Love's Labour's Lost.* Harvey was a lecturer at Cambridge University and an unpopular gadfly of the academic world. He published his generally critical opinions of the literature of the day and spent much energy futilely advocating the use of Latin prosody in English poetry. Extremely vain and critical of others, he made many enemies, and his disputatious nature hindered his aspirations to higher office in the educational establishment. In the 1590s Harvey quarrelled with both Robert GREENE (2) and Thomas NASHE in a battle of pamphlets that was much talked about in LONDON. This dispute may be the subject of the obscure topical jokes that fill *Love's Labour's Lost,* and some scholars propose that Harvey was satirised as Holofernes, though the point cannot be proven with the existing evidence. Harvey annotated the margins of his books densely, and his *Marginalia* (published 1913) record his opinions of what he read, along with much else, providing scholars with a detailed glimpse of the academic and literary world of the late 16th century. Among other things, Harvey observed that 'the younger sort takes much delight in Shakespeare's *Venus and Adonis,* but his *Lucrece,* and [*Hamlet*] have it in them to please the wiser sort'.

Harvey (3), William See HERVEY.

Hastings (1), Pursuivant Minor character in *Richard III,* a petty official. In 3.2 Lord HASTINGS (3), converses briefly with his like-named acquaintance, conveying the information that his enemies, the allies of Queen ELIZABETH (2), have been imprisoned. The Lord remarks that they had last met when he himself had been under arrest and in danger of execution; the audience is aware that, ironically, he is about to be imperiled again. This curious incident, although it depicts a historical event recorded in Shakespeare's sources, seems to have little point in the drama, unless it is intended to help to emphasise the intricate workings of fate, by virtue of the coincidences of names and circumstances. However, many editions of the play have followed the FIRST FOLIO version in ignoring this character's name, referring to him only by his title, Pursuivant, which signifies a minor subordinate of a herald.

Hastings (2), Lord Ralph (d. 1405) Historical figure and character in *2 Henry IV,* a rebel against King HENRY IV. An ally of the ARCHBISHOP (3) of York, Hastings makes several errors of judgement, first advocating that the rebels proceed against the King despite the desertion of NORTHUMBERLAND (1) and then, when they find themselves outnumbered at GAULTREE FOREST, recommending that they accept the peace offered by Prince John of LANCASTER (3). Lancaster's offer proves treacherous, and Hastings and the other rebels are arrested and sentenced to death. The historical Hastings was a minor nobleman of northern Yorkshire.

Hastings (3), Lord William (c. 1430–1483) Historical figure and character in *3 Henry VI* and *Richard III,* a Yorkist supporter who becomes a victim of political murder. In *3 Henry VI* Hastings is only a minor nobleman attached to EDWARD IV, but in *Richard III* he is more prominent. He exemplifies the pettiness of English public life during the WARS OF THE ROSES. He profits from Richard's rise, as his old enemies are imprisoned and sentenced to death, but he is unwilling to aid his leader's attempt to seize the crown; he is reluctant to oppose the legal heirs. Richard accordingly turns on him, but Hastings, ignoring warnings, has too little imagination to conceive that his situation has changed. In 3.4 Richard fabricates a tale of treason, accuses Hastings, and condemns him to death in one sentence, as his victim sits speechless. In 3.7 Richard justifies Hastings' immediate execution, citing the dangers of the supposed plot.

The historical Hastings played an obscure role in the events surrounding Richard's accession. Shakespeare followed his source in having Richard fabricate Hastings' treason, but it was probably real. In June 1483 he apparently joined in an attempt to unseat Richard from his position as Protector of Edward's

young heir. The plot failed, and Richard arrested Hastings and had him executed without a trial, as in the play.

Hathaway, Anne (Anne Hathaway Shakespeare) (c. 1556–1623) Shakespeare's wife. Anne Hathaway was the daughter of a farmer in Shottery, a village a mile from STRATFORD. (The farmhouse in which she grew up was bought by the Shakespeare BIRTHPLACE Trust, which maintains it as a showplace.) She was eight years older than her husband, with whom she had three children: Susanna SHAKESPEARE (14), born in 1583, and twins, Hamnet and Judith SHAKESPEARE (5, 10), born in 1585. Susanna was born only six months after the wedding, and it is obvious that Anne's pregnancy prompted the marriage, which was arranged in haste (see WHITGIFT; SANDELLS; RICHARDSON [1]). A number of commentators have presumed that the playwright came to regret his marriage to Anne—at 21 he found himself 'saddled' (as some see it) with three children and a wife nearing 30, and the plays contain a number of recommendations against both pre-marital sex and the taking of older wives by young men—but these are conventional remarks by fictional characters, and there exists no actual evidence of such discontent. While Shakespeare conducted his career in LONDON—as he had to—he maintained close contact with Stratford, and he eventually returned there and again lived with Anne. In his will he notoriously left Anne only the 'second best bed', though this probably had no emotional significance, for she was by ancient custom entitled to one-third of the estate, so he knew she was provided for. The special bequest of the bed was most likely made in response to some particular association with it, of which we cannot know.

Hathway (Hathaway), Richard (active 1598–1603) English playwright. In 1598 Hathway was named by Francis MERES as a leading writer of comedies. He wrote plays for the ADMIRAL'S MEN, usually in collabo-

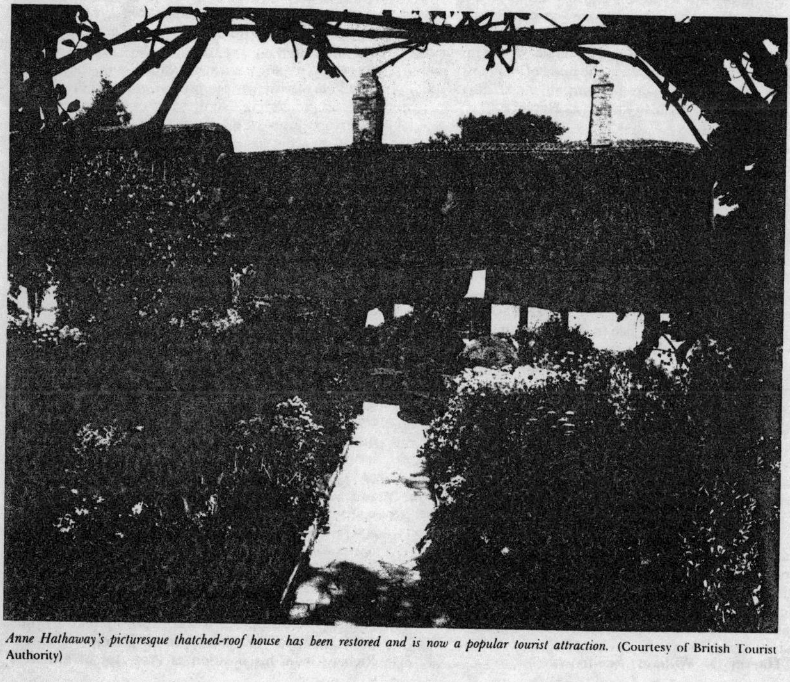

Anne Hathaway's picturesque thatched-roof house has been restored and is now a popular tourist attraction. (Courtesy of British Tourist Authority)

ion with other playwrights such as Michael DRAYTON d Anthony MUNDAY. Payment to Hathway for 18 :h works is recorded, but the only play that has vived is *SIR JOHN OLDCASTLE*, a work that was later ributed to Shakespeare. Hathway, whose name was en spelled 'Hathaway', is sometimes confused with akespeare's brother-in-law, also Richard, but the ywright was no relation to Anne HATHAWAY.

ayman, Francis (1708–1776) English painter, illus- tor of the HANMER edition of Shakespeare's plays. ayman was a one-time scene painter at the Drury ne Theatre. He had become a well-known painter of rtraits and 'conversation pieces'—informal group rtraits—when he was commissioned, along with bert GRAVELOT, to illustrate Shakespeare's plays. ese he executed in a light rococo style. Hayman ovided 31 of the 36 images for the illustrations, but avelot engraved all of them.

Under the influence of his master, Gravelot, Hay- an was one of the artists who translated the French coco style into an English idiom. He was an impor- at influence on the young Thomas Gainsborough 727–1788) and, later, a founding member of the yal Academy.

azlitt, William (1778–1830) English essayist and erary critic. Hazlitt, a journalist who published es- ys on the leading English political figures of the first cade of the 19th century, turned to literary and amatic criticism around 1815. He wrote *Characters of akespeare's Plays* (1817), in which he expressed his light in Shakespeare's poetry, an aspect of the play- ight's accomplishment that was largely ignored in rlier periods. His *Lectures on the English Poets* (1818) d *Lectures on the English Comic Writers* (1819) covered glish literature from the 16th century to his con- mporaries. Like his close friend Charles LAMB (1), azlitt was an early admirer of the Romantic poets. He er turned again to political subjects in *The Spirit of Age* (1825), with its studies of the great public fig- es of his times, and a massive *Life of Napoleon* (1830). e contributed to the Romantic era's idea of Shake- eare as a consummate literary artist as well as simply great dramatist, and he helped begin the systematic udy of the history of English literature.

eadsman Character in *The Comedy of Errors*. See ECUTIONER.

ecate (Hecat, Heccat) Minor character in *Macbeth*, supernatural being allied with the WITCHES. In 3.5 ecate appears to the Witches and chides them be- use they did not include her in their entrapment of ACBETH. She goes on to plan for another encounter ith him and promises to devise extremely powerful ells for the occasion. Then ghostly music begins, and Hecate is called away by invisible singers. In 4.1 she appears briefly to the Witches as they prepare for their second meeting with Macbeth. She praises their witchcraft and leaves to the accompaniment of another spectral song.

Hecate's appearance in *Macbeth* was obviously added to the play after it was originally written (c. 1606) but before it was published (1623). This can be determined because the songs were written by Thomas MIDDLETON for a play, *The Witch*, probably written sometime between 1610 and 1620, and because 3.6 has been moved from its proper chronological position (it should follow 4.1), in order to separate the two Witch scenes, 3.5 and 4.1, which would otherwise be in direct sequence. Because Middleton was associated with the KING'S MEN, the theatrical company that performed *Macbeth* in the early 17th century, and because the Hecate episodes are clearly designed to introduce Middleton's songs, it has been traditionally presumed that he wrote them. However, the Hecate passages of *Macbeth* are quite different in style from Middleton's work, and most modern scholars believe that someone else wrote these lines, possibly—though it is a minority opinion—Shakespeare himself.

Hecate was a familiar figure in classical literature and was frequently invoked, for instance, in SENECA, whose plays were well known to Shakespeare. She was a fearsome goddess of the underworld, associated with witchcraft and other ghostly and uncanny things. The ancients commonly worshipped three-faced statues of her at lonely country crossroads, where she glared down a side lane and both directions of the main trail. She remained well known throughout the Middle Ages, especially in connection with black magic, and Shakespeare was clearly familiar with her. Whether or not he employed her as a character in *Macbeth*, he had his protagonist mention her twice, in 2.1.52 and 3.2.41 (in passages that were definitely written by Shakespeare). Further, she is also invoked in *Hamlet* (3.2.252), *A Midsummer Night's Dream* (5.1. 370), and *King Lear* (1.1.109). Her name is a synonym for witch in *1 Henry VI* (3.2.64), though here the name has three syllables—pronounced *heckity* rather than *heckit*—and, partly for this reason, some scholars think this passage may have been written by someone else.

Hector Legendary figure and character in *Troilus and Cressida*, the crown prince of TROY, son of King PRIAM and brother of TROILUS and PARIS. Hector, the leading Trojan warrior, holds to an ideal chivalric code centred on the notion of personal honour and the possibility of glory. Thus he is a principal element of the play's sardonic presentation of the false glamour of war.

Though he is to some extent a character type—the romantic warrior-hero—Hector is made more humanly interesting through his deviations from the

chivalric norm. He recognises the defects of his position when, at the Trojan council of war, he advocates returning HELEN (1) to the Greeks and ending the fighting, and he points out the evil consequences of permitting 'the hot passion of distemper'd blood [to influence] a free determination / 'Twixt right and wrong' (2.2.170–172). However, he subordinates such wisdom to his enthusiasm for personal honour and glory and agrees with Troilus that they must carry on the conflict. Like his Greek counterpart as a spokesman for sanity, ULYSSES, Hector presents an image of right behaviour that he cannot live up to himself, reinforcing the play's bitter commentary.

Hector's humanly malleable ideals play a part in his death in 5.8, which results from an ironic combination of obsessive adherence to, and temporary abandonment of, his chivalric code. Citing 'the faith of valour' (5.3.69), he ignores dire omens and refuses the pleas of his father, his wife, ANDROMACHE, and his sister, CASSANDRA, that he not fight. On the battlefield he chivalrously permits ACHILLES to recover from exhaustion in 5.6. Then, in an uncharacteristic moment of greed and vanity, Hector kills a Greek soldier in order to loot the corpse of its fine armour. While doing so, he removes his own armour, and in this vulnerable moment he is killed by the MYRMIDONS. Nevertheless, Hector remains one of the most positive figures in the play, self-deluded and weak at a critical moment but essentially honourable.

Hector's name is probably a variation of an ancient Greek word for 'holder' or 'stayer', and this leads scholars to surmise that he is an invention of HOMER or earlier Greek poets, rather than a rendering of a historical person. He has no importance in classical myth and literature outside Homer's *Iliad,* though he was the subject of cult worship in several places, notably at later settlements around Troy. Hector remained famous throughout medieval and RENAISSANCE times. He was one of the panoply of traditional heroes known as the Nine WORTHIES, and as such he is depicted in the comical pageant in *Love's Labour's Lost* (5.2.541–717).

Hecuba Legendary Trojan queen whose famed grief is described dramatically in *Hamlet.* In 2.2 the FIRST PLAYER (2), at HAMLET's insistence, delivers a monologue telling of Hecuba's response to the killing of her husband, King PRIAM, by PYRRHUS; her grief is said to have produced tears in '. . . the burning eyes of heaven / and passion in the gods' (2.2.513–514). Her distress is implicitly compared with the short-lived widowhood of Hamlet's mother, the QUEEN (9), before she married her husband's murderer, KING (5) Claudius. Thus the passage reminds Hamlet and the audience of the central focus of his life and of the play—his need to avenge his murdered father.

Hecuba was well known in Shakespeare's day as one of the great heroines of classical mythology; she appears in HOMER's *Iliad,* where she elaborately mou[rns] the death of her son HECTOR (an episode alluded t[o in] 5.10.15–21 of *Troilus and Cressida*), in several Gr[eek] tragedies, and in VIRGIL's *Aeneid.* PLUTARCH's *Lives*—favourite Shakespearean source—reports that a Gr[eek] tyrant, famed for many cold-blooded murders, o[nce] wept at a recital of Hecuba's woes; this may have [in]spired Hamlet's request for the monologue.

The most famous classical model of the sorrow[ing] woman, Hecuba is often referred to in Shakespear[e's] plays, most frequently in *Troilus and Cressida,* where s[he] is actually said to be present in 1.2.1—though s[he] does not appear on stage—but also in *Titus Androni[cus]* (4.1.20–21), *Coriolanus* (1.3.40–43), and *Cymbeline* (4 313). Also, in a famous passage in *The Rape of Luc[rece]* (lines 1464–1491), the woeful LUCRECE vents her em[o]tions by acting the part of the grieving Hecuba.

Heicroft, Henry (c. 1549–1600) Vicar of STRATFO[RD,] baptiser of Susanna Shakespeare (14). Heicroft w[as] the vicar of Stratford from 1569 to 1584, when he l[eft] for a better paying position. In 1583 he baptis[ed] Shakespeare's first child. Heicroft was a graduate [of] Cambridge University. He married two years after [his] arrival in Stratford, and had five children, three [of] whom died before he moved to his new post. Lit[tle] more is known of his life.

Helen (1) Legendary figure and character in *Tro[ilus] and Cressida,* the mistress of Prince PARIS (3) of TRO[Y.] Years before the play opens, Paris stole Helen fr[om] King MENELAUS of Sparta, thereby sparking the TROJ[AN] WAR. Helen appears only in 3.1, where she is portray[ed] as a simpering lady of fashion whose vapid coque[try] induces PANDARUS to sing a love song while she e[n]tirely misses her guest's transmission of a message [to] Paris. That the object of the conflict should be th[is] inane society hostess illustrates the play's lessons [on] the false glamour of both sex and war, and these le[s]sons are confirmed by the warriors' own opinions [of] Helen. She is repeatedly declared an inadequate cau[se] of war by HECTOR, PRIAM, DIOMEDES (with particula[rly] scathing remarks in 4.1.56–67), and even by TROIL[US] in 1.1.90–94, although elsewhere Troilus, arguing f[or] the continuance of the war, calls Helen 'a pearl Whose price hath launched a thousand ships' (2.2.8[1–] 83). (Shakespeare's alteration of this famous line [by] MARLOWE [1]—even better known then than it [is] now—is significant; Helen's *price,* rather than her *fa[ce],* as in *Dr Faustus,* launches the ships.)

In classical mythology, Helen is one of the offsprin[g] resulting from the rape of Leda by Zeus, who w[as] disguised as a swan. She was accordingly born from a[n] egg, whose shell was reputedly preserved as a relic [in] Sparta into historical times. This cult, and the fact th[at] her name is not Greek, may reflect Helen's status as [a] 'faded' deity, a goddess in an earlier, now lost religio[n]

who survived as a mortal in Greek mythology. Helen's abduction sparks the Trojan War in the *Iliad* of HOMER, as in the play, but in Homer she becomes Paris' wife, rather than his mistress, and she is deeply disturbed by her bigamous status. A later tradition held that Paris, deceived by a friendly goddess, carried off a mere phantom of Helen to Troy. Helen thus preserved her honour, spending the war years in Egypt. After the war, she is reunited with Menelaus in all accounts.

Helen (2) Character in *All's Well that Ends Well.* See HELENA (2).

Helena (1) Character in *A Midsummer Night's Dream,* the lover of DEMETRIUS (2). Helena is obsessed with Demetrius, who has betrayed her, and while she realises she is shaming herself, she cannot stop pursuing him, even to the extent of betraying her friend HERMIA. That she has lost her self-respect is evident in her first words, 'Call you me fair? That fair again unsay!' (1.1. 181). When, through OBERON's magic, both men woo her, she can only construe their praise as ridicule. Her frustration leads her to insult Hermia viciously in the four-way quarrel in 3.2. Her flawed personality has nothing to do with her finally winning Demetrius, as she knows; she treats the outcome as a miracle, saying, 'I have found Demetrius like a jewel, / Mine own, and not mine own' (4.1.190–191).

Helena (2) Character in *All's Well That Ends Well,* the lover of BERTRAM. Helena's pursuit of Bertram constitutes the main plot of *All's Well,* and his lack of interest, combined with her use of the vulgar 'bed trick'—substituting herself for another woman in bed and thus inducing him to father her child—help to give the work the dark and troubling quality that places it among the so-called PROBLEM PLAYS. The central figure in the play, Helena is subject to quite contradictory interpretations, depending largely on one's view of the play as a whole.

Some commentators have found Helena wholly good. Samuel Taylor COLERIDGE called her Shakespeare's 'loveliest character', and her persistent efforts to win Bertram despite his feelings have been seen as an allegorical representation of Christian grace, chiefly on the strength of a remark by the COUNTESS (2), Bertram's mother, that her son 'cannot thrive, / Unless her prayers, whom heaven delights to hear / And loves to grant, reprieve him from the wrath / Of greatest justice' (3.4.26–29). However, other critics have seen in Helena a satirical portrait of an ambitious, possessive woman, intent on marrying a man who does not love her and unscrupulous in using her body to deceive him.

In 1.1 Helena is introduced as a young woman of great energy and determination. She is first seen dressed in mourning, with the elderly Countess and LAFEW. They discuss the late Count's death and then her own father's and the seemingly terminal illness of the KING (17). Helena is especially depressed because her secret love, Bertram, is leaving, and, as she puts it, 'there is no living, none, / If Bertram be away' (1.1.82–83), and she prepares to 'sanctify his relics' (1.1.96). Then PAROLLES, the play's comic villain, appears, and his cynical banter about virginity makes Helena realise that she must fear the influence of such worldly wisdom on Bertram: 'The court's a learning-place', she reflects, 'and he is one—' (1.1.173); she suppresses the observation that Bertram is likely to be an apt pupil. More important, Parolles' vitality stimulates a similar energy in Helena. He leaves, and in the ensuing soliloquy, written in formal couplets intended to suggest her elevated mood, she firmly decides to pursue Bertram.

Thus the main plot opens with the establishment of Helena's initiative. But whether she is an admirably plucky young woman or an ambitious schemer remains a matter of interpretation. This unresolved question is often considered part of the play's larger failure to combine naturalistic elements with the scheme of reconciliation and love that COMEDY traditionally demands. To some extent, the contradictory points of view may be taken to represent different aspects of the same personality, and, as so often in Shakespeare, the resulting paradox offers us a rewarding sense of the complexity of human nature.

However, there are numerous clues that Shakespeare intended Helena as a virtuous and spunky heroine. Most significantly, the play's final resolution is accomplished only by a highly dramatic, carefully planned appearance by Helena late in the closing scene, in which she disentangles the plot's complications in a few lines, like a deus ex machina. A satirical figure used in this manner could only inspire sardonic reflections on the hypocrisy of happy endings, and nothing in the dialogue suggests any such intent on the playwright's part. Further, the fairy-tale motif of the maiden who cures the King is presented in the solemn music of rhymed couplets and mystical language that would be utterly inappropriate to a satirical purpose. Similarly, Helena has several other striking and lyrical speeches, such as her declaration of love in 1.3.186–212 and her dramatic renunciation in 3.2.99–129, whose evident sincerity tends to enforce a view of her as an admirable heroine.

In addition, Shakespeare altered the story that he took from his source, a tale by BOCCACCIO, and some of his changes were plainly designed to elevate the moral character of the heroine. For instance, he added such sympathetic characters as the elderly Countess and her friend Lord Lafew, whose chief purpose is to shape our opinions of the major characters. They convincingly inform us of Helena's virtues, as does the

King. Shakespeare also added another theme to the tale, in which Helena is clearly an heroine: the King, responding to Bertram's rejection of her as a commoner, defends her as an illustration of the value of an individual's spiritual nature regardless of his or her rank in society. In Boccaccio, the pursuer and pursued are aristocrats of equal status, and no social question is raised.

When Boccaccio's protagonist triumphs at the end, she presents her reluctant husband with twin sons. In *All's Well,* only the merest mention is made of Helena's pregnancy, in 5.3.307; Shakespeare plainly wished to de-emphasise the physical aspect of the bed trick because this ruse is clearly the most embarrassing episode of Helena's story. In another significant departure from his source, Shakespeare altered the circumstances of Helena's appearance in FLORENCE. In Boccaccio, she hears of her husband's attempt at seduction, devises the bed trick, and goes to Italy to perform it. In *All's Well,* she wanders to Florence as a pilgrim and must be informed by the WIDOW (2) of Bertram's presence. Thus the bed trick seems a product of fortunate happenstance, rather than a calculated ploy.

Shakespeare also used dramatic structure to mitigate the bed trick's bad impression and maintain Helena's heroic stature. After 3.2 Helena is much less frequently on-stage than before. She appears in only four brief scenes and has no important speeches before returning 30 lines from the end of the play. We remember her in the highly positive light in which she was presented in the first half of the play, and we are influenced by the Countess' observations on the efficacy of Helena's prayers, the similarly complimentary remarks of the two LORDS (6) in 4.3, and the loving regrets of the Countess' household when they believe her dead—even the cynical CLOWN (5) is moved to call her 'the sweet-marjoram of the sallet' (4.5.15). Shakespeare therefore establishes Helena as an heroine early in the play, and later, when her actions seem less heroic, he downplays her, permitting only brief and positive glimpses.

Thus Helena seems intended as a delightful romantic heroine. Lafew says she can 'quicken a rock, and make you dance canary / With sprightly fire and motion' (2.1.73–74)—and her infatuation with Bertram's 'arched brows, his hawking eye, his curls' (1.1.92) is no less endearing for her healthy interest in sex. In this light, she seems to be a lively, virtuous young woman to whom divine favour offers opportunity and then success. And in the second half of the play, the possibly manipulative exploiter of sex is more properly regarded as a contrite, self-sacrificing wife whom fortune has led to a happy resolution of her problems. At the play's conclusion she is received with the awe due a goddess, and her summation of the play's final statement of reconciliation suggests that she deserves this treatment. Indeed, Helena's role is an exalted one: in the course of capturing and keeping a husband, she has saved the King's life, preserved Bertram from a life of idle sin, and brought new life, in the form of their child, into the world. The absorption in death with which the play opened has been dispelled.

Helenus Legendary figure and minor character in *Troilus and Cressida,* a son of King PRIAM. In 2.2.33–36 Helenus challenges TROILUS' insistence on Trojan honour as a justification for retaining the kidnapped HELEN (1) and continuing the TROJAN WAR, but Troilus dismisses him with the remark, 'You are for dreams and slumbers, brother priest' (2.2.37), and an accusation of cowardice, and Helenus is not mentioned again. Shakespeare took this incident—which appears in two of his sources, William CAXTON's *The Recuyell of the Historyes of Troye* and John LYDGATE's *Troy Book*—to help establish Troilus' hot-blooded chivalrousness. Helenus himself is of no consequence and has no personality.

Helicanus Minor character in *Pericles,* adviser to and surrogate ruler for Prince PERICLES of TYRE. In 1.2 Helicanus stands out among a group of flattering courtiers (see LORD [11]) when he makes a speech that stresses the value of honest criticism to a ruler. Impressed, Pericles leaves Helicanus in charge of Tyre when he must flee from the powerful King ANTIOCHUS of Syria. In 2.4 the Tyrian nobles desire a ruler who is in residence, and suggest that Helicanus declare himself Pericles' successor, but the faithful adviser summons Pericles home instead. In Act 5 Helicanus serves Pericles again. He acts as Pericles' spokesman when the grief-stricken prince—he has been separated from his wife and daughter—refuses to speak. He witnesses Pericles' reunions with MARINA, in 5.1, and THAISA, in 5.3. Helicanus demonstrates that loyalty and goodness do continue to exist among humans, despite the misfortunes that plague Pericles. Pericles praises Helicanus' virtues several times, and calls him 'fit counsellor and servant for a prince, / Who by thy wisdom makes a prince thy servant' (1.2.63–64), and 'a grave and noble counsellor' (5.1.182). This wise elder's presence seems appropriate to the play's conclusion in divinely wrought happiness and good fortune.

Heminge (Heminges), John (d. 1630) English actor and a co-editor, with Henry CONDELL, of the FIRST FOLIO edition of Shakespeare's plays. One of the 26 'Principall Actors' listed in the First Folio, Heminge was a member of STRANGE'S MEN, of the CHAMBERLAIN'S MEN (probably from its inception in 1594), and of its successor, the KING'S MEN, until his death. Thus, most of his career was spent alongside Shakespeare. He was apparently the business manager of the com-

pany, probably beginning at least in 1596, and he seems to have stopped acting after 1611.

He served as a trustee in Shakespeare's purchase of the BLACKFRIARS GATEHOUSE, and he was executor or overseer of the wills of several of the King's Men. Shakespeare and most of the other members of the troupe left him small legacies, tokens of their friendship. Heminge was a shrewd businessman and became quite wealthy. At his death, he owned about a quarter of the shares in the GLOBE THEATRE and the BLACKFRIARS THEATRE, including the shares originally owned by his late son-in-law William OSTLER (2), which he had claimed despite a lawsuit by his daughter.

Henderson, John (1747–1785) British actor. Henderson established himself as a fine classical actor in 1777 with a portrayal of SHYLOCK. During his brief career, he was acclaimed as the leading FALSTAFF of his day, and he played a variety of other Shakespearean parts, including MALVOLIO and IAGO.

Henry (1), Prince (later King Henry III of England) (1207–1272) Historical figure and minor character in *King John,* the son of King JOHN (3). Henry appears only in the final scene, 5.7, in which he witnesses the death of his father and accepts the submission of the noblemen to him as the next King. He is thus a symbol of the restoration of social order after the dislocations of John's reign.

Shakespeare's Henry is a young man but definitely an adult, capable of musing on the nature of disease and death. The historical Prince was only nine years old upon his succession. He ruled England well for 56 years. His great-great-great-grandson was RICHARD II (see PLANTAGENET [1]).

Henry (2) Frederick, Prince of Wales (1594–1612) Son of King JAMES I, heir-apparent to the English throne until his death, and patron of PRINCE HENRY'S MEN, formerly the ADMIRAL'S MEN. Though Prince Henry died young, he was already a significant supporter of the arts. He patronised George CHAPMAN and Ben JONSON, and he defended Walter RALEIGH. He was the first major supporter of Inigo Jones (1573–1652), later the royal architect and collaborator with Jonson (see MASQUE). Most significantly for the theatrical world, he became the patron of the Admiral's Men. Unfortunately, the young prince died of typhoid fever, just before the planned wedding of his sister, Princess ELIZABETH (3). Her husband-to-be, a German prince, took over the patronage of Henry's theatre company, which became known as the PALSGRAVE'S MEN.

Henry I* and *Henry II Lost plays attributed, probably wrongly, to Shakespeare and Robert Davenport (c. 1590–1640). In 1653 the publisher Humphrey MOSELEY claimed the copyrights to a number of old plays, including 'Henry ye first, & Hen: ye 2. by Shakespeare and Davenport'. The 18th-century collector John WARBURTON reported owning a copy of *Henry I,* by 'Will. Shakespeare & Rob. Davenport'. However, none of these manuscripts has survived, and their attribution to Shakespeare, even as a collaborator, is extremely doubtful. *Henry I* was licenced for the KING'S MEN to perform in 1624—eight years after Shakespeare's death—but only in Davenport's name. Moreover, Davenport himself is first recorded only in 1620; a much younger and inferior playwright, he would have been an unlikely collaborator for Shakespeare.

Henry IV, King of England (1366–1413) Historical figure and title character in *1* and *2 Henry IV.* (The same figure appears in *Richard II* as BOLINGBROKE [1].) King Henry is not the most prominent character in the plays that take his name, but he is nonetheless an important figure. The major concern of the plays is the growth of his son and successor, PRINCE (6) HAL. The question of what constitutes a good ruler is thus paramount, and as king, Henry personifies the issue. He is viewed from three distinct points of view in *Part 1:* he sees himself as a weary but effective monarch; Hotspur regards him as a dishonourable politician who first deposed a king (as is enacted in *Richard II*) and then betrayed those who helped him do so; and Falstaff considers him a cold, rigid opponent of comfort and licence. By *Part 2* Henry is almost a tragic figure. The cost of power shows itself in his illness and fatigue, while he himself suggests that his decline and death are the deserved fate of a usurper.

Henry is presented as a strong ruler: for instance, his dismissal of Hotspur and NORTHUMBERLAND (1) in 1.3.116–122 of *Part 1* makes it clear that he does not tolerate insubordination, and in 3.1 of *Part 2* he overcomes his illness and melancholy to face the rebellion squarely, saying, 'Are these things then necessities? then let us meet them like necessities' (3.1.92–93). He is also politically astute to the point of cynicism. In *Part 1* (3.2.39–59) he describes the appearance of regal splendour that he assumed during his rebellion against Richard II in order to win the hearts of the populace (Richard also describes this in *Richard II,* 1.4.23–36), and his distinctly Machiavellian deathbed advice to Hal—divert potential rebels by engaging in wars abroad—is chilling.

But, despite his strength, Henry's principal characteristic is weariness. From the first line of *Part 1* Henry presents himself as a sick and tired man who wants to embark on a crusade to the Holy Land to atone for his role in the murder of Richard II. Moreover, his disappointment over Prince Hal's dissolute life embitters him. In 3.1 of *Part 2* he comments that the terrible burden of power prevents him from sleeping; he broods, 'uneasy lies the head that wears a crown' (3.1.31). He goes on to wish, 'Oh God, that one might read

the book of fate . . .' (3.1.45), in tones that foreshadow the darkly brilliant meditations of Shakespeare's tragic heroes.

Hotspur sees Henry as a treacherous usurper who has turned against his allies. Henry himself is very much aware that he has been a rebel. In his deathbed conversation with Hal, he plainly suffers guilt for the 'by-paths and indirect crook'd ways' (*2 Henry IV,* 4.5. 184) by which he gained power, a reference to the deposition and murder of Richard II. He observes that many of his allies against Richard later resented his assumption of power. He anticipates that Hal will have an easier time when he ascends the throne, being legitimately descended from a sitting king. This indeed proves to be so, as the end of *2 Henry IV* and all of *Henry V* demonstrate. However, as Shakespeare and his contemporaries were well aware, the disputes over the royal succession that Henry's actions had triggered were settled only by the disastrous WARS OF THE ROSES, and Henry's sense of guilt is a reflection of the curse that his sinful usurpation has brought upon himself, his family (see LANCASTER [1]), and his country. Nevertheless, Henry is the established power in these plays, and Hotspur and his allies sin in rebelling against him and are repeatedly condemned as a result.

Henry's ultimate significance in the drama is as the holder of the position for which Prince Hal must equip himself. While Henry's cold, Machiavellian world of political manipulation is too rigid and inhumane for the young man to grow up in, he does in the end enter it. In 4.5, in a reprise of the king's lament over the stresses of kingship (*2 Henry IV,* 3.1.4–31), Hal rhetorically addresses Henry's crown and speaks of the burden that kingship demands. He accepts that burden for himself, emphasising his decision by placing the crown on his own head. One consequence of this decision is that he must become like Henry to some degree; he must enact in the real world the disciplinarian's role he had taken in the tavern burlesque of *Part 1.* Hal is often criticised for his icily brutal dismissal of Falstaff in 5.5; readers have thought that, in rejecting Falstaff, Hal also rejects part of his own humanity, but it may equally well be argued that he is simply adopting a different type of humanity, that of his weary, careworn father.

The history of Henry's reign is strenuously compressed in the plays, producing an impression of greater civil disorder than in fact occurred. While the various rebellions of the play did take place, they were widely spaced and relatively easily suppressed. Henry was a strong king, although he was not a competent administrator and his regime had persistent financial troubles. Two significant variations from history in the plays concern Henry personally. First, in *Part 1* Henry is committed from the very beginning (indeed, from *Richard II,* 5.6.49–50) to a crusade to ease his conscience, thus stressing sin and retribution as the ultimate causes of the unrest of Henry's reign. In fact, and in Shakespeare's sources, Henry did not propose a crusade until late in his reign, when it seems to have been intended to expand his influence in European diplomacy. Second, Henry's illness, which he actually developed only a year before his death, plagues him for most of his reign in the plays, dominating all his appearances in *2 Henry IV.* Shakespeare may have been influenced in this direction by Samuel DANIEL, whose *Civil Wars* stresses Henry's deathbed struggles with his bad conscience. The effect produced, a melancholy sense of impending death, makes more fateful and solemn Hal's acceptance of his kingly burden.

Henry IV, PART 1

SYNOPSIS

Act 1, Scene 1

King HENRY IV's plans for a crusade are upset by a report from the Earl of WESTMORELAND (1) that Welsh rebels under Owen GLENDOWER have defeated and captured Edmund MORTIMER (2). There is better news, however: young Henry Percy, nicknamed HOTSPUR, has defeated rebellious Scots under the Earl of DOUGLAS and has taken many prisoners. Henry observes that Hotspur's honourable success in war reflects badly on his own son, PRINCE (6) HAL, who leads a dissolute life in LONDON. However, he goes on to complain of Hotspur's prideful refusal to turn over his prisoners to the king, as is customary. Westmoreland attributes this stubbornness to the influence of Hotspur's uncle, Thomas Percy, Earl of WORCESTER.

Act 1, Scene 2

Prince Hal and FALSTAFF jest about their debauched life of petty crime, drunkenness, and wenching. POINS arrives with a plan for a highway robbery. At first, the Prince does not wish to participate, but, after Falstaff leaves, Poins proposes to Hal that they play a joke on Falstaff: they will go to the scene of the crime but avoid taking part; then, after Falstaff and the others have stolen the money, Poins and the Prince can steal it from them; the cowardice of Falstaff and his friends will make this easy. Later they will have the pleasure of listening to Falstaff lie about the episode, followed by the further delight of exposing the old rogue. Hal agrees, and Poins leaves. In a soliloquy the Prince reveals his intention to eventually abandon his life of idle dissolution and become a sound ruler.

Act 1, Scene 3

Hotspur tells the king that he had not refused to surrender his prisoners, as Henry believes, but had merely responded in hasty anger to the arrogant courtier who had presented the king's claim. Unappeased, the king observes that Hotspur not only still holds the prisoners but also insists that Mortimer be ransomed

om the Welsh before he turns them over. Henry serts that Mortimer, who has married Glendower's ughter, has treasonably defected to the Welsh, and refuses to ransom him. Hotspur defends Mortimer, d the king exits angrily. Hotspur rages against enry's ingratitude to the Percy family, which helped e king depose RICHARD II. With difficulty, Worcester lms Hotspur and proposes that Hotspur should re-ase his Scottish prisoners and enlist them in a rebel-n against the king while his father, the Earl of ORTHUMBERLAND (1), recruits the ARCHBISHOP (3) of ork. Worcester himself will join Glendower when the ne is ripe, and the three forces will rise simulta-eously.

t 2, Scene 1

an inn in ROCHESTER, two CARRIERS prepare to leave r London. GADSHILL, a highwayman, appears and arns from them that they will be accompanied by me gentlemen carrying valuables. The CHAMBER-AIN (1) of the inn tells Gadshill of these potential ctims in more detail. Gadshill boasts of an accom-ice in high places who can get them off if the theft es wrong.

t 2, Scene 2

he robbers assemble at GAD'S HILL. Hal arranges an nbush, placing himself and Poins in a reserve posi-on just down the road. The Prince and Poins leave st before the TRAVELLERS appear. The thieves rob e Travellers and bundle them off-stage; when the ieves return, they are themselves effortlessly robbed the Prince and Poins.

t 2, Scene 3

otspur reads a letter from a nobleman who makes xcuses for not joining the rebellion. LADY (10) Percy opears, and Hotspur announces his imminent depar-re. She speaks worriedly of his absorption in his lans—he even speaks of military matters in his eep—and she demands to be told what they are. otspur playfully refuses to tell her, claiming military ecrecy.

t 2, Scene 4

t the BOAR'S HEAD TAVERN, Prince Hal teases FRANCIS), a waiter, and he laughingly compares his own ood humour with Hotspur's mania for war. Falstaff nters; egged on by Hal and Poins, he tells an elabo-ate tale of his courage in resisting the brigands who obbed him. After leading Falstaff on to ludicrous ex-ggerations, the Prince reveals the truth, and Falstaff omically claims to have recognised Hal at the time nd to have fled so as to avoid harming the heir appar-nt of the realm. A message from King Henry com-ands Hal's presence in the morning; a rebellion, led Hotspur, has begun. Falstaff anticipates the king's nger at Hal and suggests that the Prince rehearse his esponse. Falstaff pretends to be Henry and chastises Hal for the company he keeps, excepting only one commendable man called Falstaff. They change roles, and Hal, as the king, upbraids his 'son' for tolerating so bad a man as Falstaff. Falstaff, playing the Prince, defends Falstaff. He is interrupted by the approach of the SHERIFF (4). Falstaff was recognised at Gad's Hill and has been traced to the tavern. Falstaff hides; the Prince assures the Sheriff that the thief is not present and that he, the Prince, will guarantee that any stolen money will be refunded. The Sheriff leaves, and Hal discovers that Falstaff has fallen asleep in his hiding place. The Prince looks forward to the campaign against the rebels.

Act 3, Scene 1

The rebel leaders convene to make a formal alliance, but friction between Glendower and Hotspur threat-ens to break up the meeting. The discussion turns to the division of the realm after King Henry has been deposed. Hotspur objects that his portion is too small, and his arrogance offends Glendower. They argue again, but the Welshman gives in and a tenuous peace is maintained. Glendower leaves, and Mortimer and Worcester chastise an unapologetic Hotspur for of-fending a valuable ally. Glendower returns with his daughter, LADY (8) Mortimer, and Lady Percy. Morti-mer regrets that he cannot speak Welsh, his wife's only language; Glendower interprets as the couple ex-change loving remarks. Lady Mortimer invites her husband to lie in her lap while she sings to him. Hot-spur humorously mocks this in conversation with his wife, whom he teases affectionately. After Lady Morti-mer's song, the men leave to join their troops.

Act 3, Scene 2

Henry speaks to Prince Hal about his dissipated be-haviour and doubts his son's loyalty in the coming conflict. Hal apologises for his debaucheries and as-sures his father that he intends to conquer Hotspur. News arrives that the rebels have assembled at SHREWSBURY, and the King devises a plan for the cam-paign; Hal is to command one of the armies.

Act 3, Scene 3

At the Boar's Head, Falstaff speaks of repentance for his ways but goes on to praise bawdiness and merri-ment. He teases BARDOLPH (1) about his fiery complex-ion and banters with the HOSTESS (2). The Prince ar-rives, excited about the coming campaign; he tells Falstaff to meet him the next day to receive his orders. He leaves, and Falstaff turns to his meal, wishing he could conduct his part in the war from the tavern.

Act 4, Scene 1

Hotspur, Worcester, and Douglas, encamped at Shrewsbury, receive word that Mortimer is extremely sick and cannot join them with his forces. Sir Richard VERNON (2) reports the approach of the King's armies and reveals that Glendower's troops cannot come for

another two weeks. Although the rebels are seriously outnumbered, Hotspur urges that they fight anyway.

Act 4, Scene 2
Falstaff, marching towards Shrewsbury, soliloquises on the money he has made selling exemptions from the draft. The Prince and Westmoreland meet him and urge him to hurry, for the battle will soon begin. After they leave, Falstaff remarks to himself that he hopes to arrive just as the battle ends.

Act 4, Scene 3
Hotspur and Douglas argue for an immediate attack on the king's forces, but Vernon and Worcester want to wait for reinforcements. Sir Walter BLUNT (3) appears with a message from King Henry offering a negotiated peace. Hotspur condemns Henry's usurpation of the throne and his ingratitude towards those who helped him carry it out. However, he agrees to have Worcester meet with the king the next day.

Act 4, Scene 4
The Archbishop speaks of the likely defeat of the rebels at Shrewsbury, and he begins to prepare for further opposition to the king.

Act 5, Scene 1
Worcester and Vernon arrive to negotiate with King Henry. Worcester justifies rebellion by pointing out the king's ingratitude. Prince Hal offers to fight Hotspur in single combat to settle all issues, but Henry rejects the idea, offering the rebels a last chance for surrender with amnesty: if they reject it, the two armies must fight. Worcester and Vernon depart. Falstaff asks the Prince to protect him in the battle; Hal, leaving, responds that he will have to take his chances. Falstaff muses that he will not follow an honourable course in the battle, for honour is a minor matter compared to life.

Act 5, Scene 2
Worcester insists to Vernon that they not tell Hotspur of the king's offer of an amnesty lest he accept it; he believes that Henry cannot be trusted and that, while Hotspur may be forgiven on grounds of youth and high-spiritedness, he, Worcester, would bear the brunt of the king's wrath. Worcester accordingly reports that the king has elected to fight, and he tells of Hal's challenge. Hotspur responds by preparing for battle.

Act 5, Scene 3
During the battle Blunt, disguised as King Henry, is killed by Douglas. Falstaff meets Prince Hal and lies about his courageous combat, but the Prince discovers a bottle of sack in Falstaff's pistol case.

Act 5, Scene 4
During a lull in the battle the king suggests that his sons Prince Hal and Prince John of LANCASTER (3) retire from the fighting, but they both refuse. Lanc ter rejoins the fray, and Hal lauds his fighting sp before following him. Douglas appears and fights king, nearly killing him; the Prince returns and sl Douglas. The king comments that Hal has prov himself. Henry exits, and Hotspur arrives to exchan challenges and fight with the Prince. Falstaff watch this combat until Douglas enters to fight him; Falst feigns death, and Douglas moves on. The Prince ki Hotspur and eulogises his dead foe. He then sees F staff and, believing him dead, pronounces a more sual benediction before leaving. Falstaff rises, sta Hotspur's corpse with his sword, and declares that will take credit for killing him. The Prince and Lanca ter return and are surprised to see Falstaff alive. F staff claims to have killed Hotspur and supposes th the king will reward him; out of friendship, the Prin agrees to corroborate his lie.

Act 5, Scene 5
King Henry sentences the captured Worcester a Vernon to death, while Douglas is to be set free. T king begins to make plans to fight the remaini rebels.

COMMENTARY

Henry IV, Part 1, was a highly innovative work in 15 for precisely the reasons that make it one of the grea est of Shakespeare's HISTORY PLAYS. It marks an a vance both in Shakespeare's development and in th growth of English drama, for, by repeatedly shifting i focus between affairs of state and bawdy irreverenc the play presents a composite image of a whole soc ety, something that had never been attempted befor In addition to the quarrels and alliances among th aristocracy, the principal interest of the earlier histo ries, here Shakespeare offers the scruffy circle of com mon laborers and petty criminals who frequent th Boar's Head Tavern. Both worlds are more vivid f the contrast, and a dramatic tension is established b tween them. Groundbreaking in its own day, *1 Hen IV* is still impressive in ours, due to the range of pe ple, events, and language, from the most casual r baldry to the boldest rhetoric, realistically presente on stage.

Prince Hal belongs to both worlds; surrounding hi are such boldly drawn figures as the volatile Hotspu and his charming wife, the talkative Hostess, and th many personalities evoked by Falstaff's parodies an imitations: churchmen and highwaymen, knights an knaves. The Prince's significance lies in the choice h must make between worlds, and his dilemma empha sises, as in the other history plays, the question c order in society. Both the Falstaffian delinquents c the Boar's Head Tavern and the rebels led by Hotspu have contributed to the decay of the social fabric, an King Henry believes that both groups have been ser

by heaven in revenge for his own disturbance of society, the deposition of King RICHARD II (as enacted in *Richard II*). Hal's choice is indeed pivotal for the future of the realm. Of course, Shakespeare's original audiences knew that Hal went on to become the highly successful King HENRY V, so there is no suspense about the Prince's choice; the tension lies instead in the presentation of the alternatives.

Although the sub-plot concerning Falstaff is highly diverting, the major concern is Hal's decision to embrace his role as Hotspur's rival, abandoning the life of a barfly for that of a military leader. This central issue is not fully resolved until the end of *2 Henry IV*, when Hal rejects Falstaff, but *Part 1* presents an initial phase of Hal's development, his acceptance of his role as princely hero.

The play's climax is the hand-to-hand combat between Hal and Hotspur at Shrewsbury. Not only does the play build to this climax through a series of episodes depicting the progress of Hotspur's rebellion, but Hal and Hotspur are repeatedly compared, both by the king—as early as 1.1.77–90—and by Hal himself. The king regrets that his own son seems so feckless in comparison to the rebel leader. Hal assures his father that he is not the dissipated playboy he seems and that he will prove superior to Hotspur when the time is ripe. This motif—the potential readiness of the Prince—has already been established in Hal's famous 'reformation' speech (1.2.190–212). Shakespeare makes it abundantly clear that the Prince will indeed prove himself in the traditional terms of chivalry, and in the combat at Shrewsbury, an episode devised by the playwright for this purpose, Hal becomes the hero whom he has promised to be.

Hotspur's defeat attests that chivalry is not an unalloyed virtue, as does his outsised personality, which consists of impatience and an exaggerated sense of honour. Hotspur is a temperamental, driven man who is concerned only about his reputation for bravery in battle. His fixation is as excessive in its way as is Falstaff's licentiousness. This leads to his own destruction, as he cannot bring himself to postpone the battle at Shrewsbury until his side has a better chance.

Hotspur has his redeeming features as well. Hal admits that his military accomplishments are worth aspiring to, and the Prince's eulogy over Hotspur's corpse (5.4.86–100) is genuinely admiring. Moreover, while the rebellious noblemen are certainly self-serving to various degrees, Hotspur's own motive is not personal gain or power; he is driven by an ambition for honourable action that one could admire if it were in better balance in his life. Hotspur's loving marriage to the engaging Lady Percy is presented in 2.3 and 3.1, and we recognise that he is not simply a 'wasp-stung and impatient fool', as his father calls him in 1.3.233, but also a husband who credibly inspires affection. His domestic bliss does not in any way negate the problem of his flawed values, but it makes him a multi-dimensional character.

Falstaff embodies an opposite weakness to Hotspur's, that of an anarchic refusal to accept responsibility. His world of food, women, and wine has no need for 'redeeming time'—as Hal vows to do in the 'reformation' speech (1.2.190–212)—for time is of no consequence when one refuses to acknowledge any obligations. Falstaff staves off all demands and responsibilities—the stuff of history—with humour, continually devising witticisms and preposterous excuses for his behaviour. We are as delighted with his inventive comedy as Hal is in 1.2, but, like the Prince, we can see that a ruler must live a more orderly life. In addition, the fat knight displays a chilling disregard for ordinary values, in an episode that Shakespeare plainly intended as a satire on a military abuse of his own times, when he callously offers the soldiers he has recruited to be 'food for powder, food for powder' (4.2.65–66), meaning that they will be quickly consumed by gunpowder, i.e., combat. He later announces coolly that he has abandoned his troops under fire, where 'there's not three of my hundred and fifty left alive' (5.3.37). Falstaff's anarchy here has an unpleasant, faintly evil edge to it. His crimes and misdemeanours may be forgivable in a comedy—and *1 Henry IV* is somewhat comic—but they are unacceptable in the domain of history, where the hard realities of peace and war are at stake.

Just as Hotspur has an unrealistic view of the world, so does Falstaff. Falstaff lives in an immature universe where one's appetites are gratified immediately and the inevitability of age and death is denied. He has been seen as a re-creation of ancient figures of European folklore who traditionally enlivened holiday celebrations by behaving in perversely loose ways that are normally forbidden. These figures, who returned to ordinary behaviour after the festival, made a great show of eating and drinking to excess, of flouting authority, and, often, of sexual promiscuity. Thus illicit cravings were acknowledged and vicariously satisfied without disrupting the society. Such customs were prominent in pre-modern societies and were still well known, if not widely practised, in Elizabethan England. Falstaff's gluttony, his lechery, and his very fatness are easily associated with such figures.

However, Falstaff is not simply a temptation to be resisted or a negative lesson for Hal. Falstaff's world is also in itself useful for the Prince, offering him an arena in which he can test himself and come to understand the people who will be his subjects when he is king, and learn about himself as well. At the Boar's Head, Hal tries on the roles of robber, of tavern servant, even of king. The other worlds of the play—Hotspur's inflexible, honour-bound world or Henry's tense world of political calculation—do not permit the temporary attitudes and stances necessary to learning.

The world of comedy thus has virtues that the world of history cannot provide.

Just as Hotspur's happy marriage deepens his characterisation, so Falstaff is caught in a revealing moment of uneasiness about his life in 3.3, when he worries that he is wasting away and muses on his long absence from church. When his eventual death is suggested by Bardolph, the fat knight immediately reverts to his more usual comic line, but we have seen that he, too, has a soul and is subject to universal fears.

Both Hotspur and Falstaff are strong figures, and it is not wholly possible to dismiss or accept either of them; with great force of irony, we are made to sympathise with both the impatient firebrand and the irresponsible rogue, even as we recognise the faults of each. When Prince Hal comes fully into his own, it is appropriate that we see him standing between these two extremes; Falstaff lies to one side, rejecting honour by feigning death, and Hotspur lies to the other, dead because he overvalued honour.

Hal's story does not end with this play; *2 Henry IV* is a sequel. Scholars debate whether or not Shakespeare had fully evolved this relationship when he was writing *1 Henry IV,* but the evidence suggests strongly that he had. First, Hal's rejection of Falstaff in *2 Henry IV* hinted at several times in *1 Henry IV*—e.g., in his 'reformation' speech; when he portrays his father in the tavern ('I do, I will' [2.4.475]); when he dismisses Falstaff during the battle (5.3.55)—while the play closes with the fat knight at an acme of both wrongdoing and acceptance, boasting that he has killed Hotspur himself (after stabbing the corpse) and finding the Prince generous enough to let his claim stand. This situation prepares us for a continuation of Falstaff's adventures, when his death, with Hotspur's, could have closed the play effectively. Further, Shakespeare invented an important role for John of Lancaster at Shrewsbury, establishing him as a major figure in apparent anticipation of his function in *2 Henry IV.* Moreover, both the rebels and the king are preparing for further action as the play ends. Each of these points may be explained in some other way, but collectively they strongly suggest that *1 Henry IV* was written with *2 Henry IV* in mind. Nevertheless, *1 Henry IV* is a complete drama, with its own plot line that reaches fruition independently of its sequel.

Shakespeare's great achievement in *1 Henry IV* is the establishment of a sense of community between the audience and the fictional world of the play. Structurally he accomplishes this by a continual oscillation between two poles, the aristocratic and the common or the political and the hedonistic. These elements are sometimes parallel—as in 1.1 and 1.2, where preparations for war are followed by preparations for robbery—and sometimes in opposition, as in the comparison of Hal and Hotspur. Some scenes have analogues in *2 Henry IV*—e.g., Hotspur's farewell to his wife in 2.1 is comparable to Falstaff's departure from DOLL TEARSHEET in 2.4 of the sequel. Such juxtapositions enforce a comprehensive sense of a complex, lifelike fictional world, quite aside from the historical actions of the political plot.

The integration of two genres, comedy and history, permits each to influence the other. The history, presenting issues that impinge on all our lives, is made graver because it affects the lives of the comic figures. The comedy, while providing an ironic slant on social themes, is given sharpness of tone and richness of texture by its proximity to the serious aspects of life. By successfully accommodating two genres, the play—and its implicit tolerance—is made more intense: although one is made aware of human failing, one may also glory in human possibility.

SOURCES OF THE PLAY

Shakespeare's principal source for the historical material in *1 Henry IV* was Raphael HOLINSHED's *Chronicles of England, Scotland, and Ireland* (2nd ed., 1587), but the playwright was also greatly influenced by Samuel DANIEL's epic poem *The Civil Wars Between the Two Houses of York and Lancaster* (1595). In Daniel, the streamlined narrative emphasises the relation of King Henry's troubles to his deposition of Richard II, and it climaxes with the battle of Shrewsbury, compressing the remainder of Henry's reign into a cursory account. Shakespeare's handling of historical events in *1 Henry IV* closely reflects this approach. Daniel also supplied the inspiration for the hand-to-hand encounter between Hal and Hotspur in 5.4 and for the alteration in Hotspur's age. Daniel, while stating no ages, implies that Hotspur was of Hal's generation; Shakespeare makes this explicit. Historically, however, Hotspur was older than Hal's father.

The anonymous play WOODSTOCK (c. 1592–1595) provided various details for the fictitious highway robbery in 2.2, and, more significantly, featured a story of national politics that is integrated with comical doings by a high-ranking criminal, a possible predecessor of Falstaff. Tales of Prince Hal's mis-spent youth had been part of English popular lore since his own time; Shakespeare derived his account chiefly from the anonymous play *The Famous Victories of Henry the Fifth* (see FAMOUS VICTORIES), a farce that was acted at least as early as 1588. Most of the episodes of Hal's dissipated existence in Eastcheap, and of his later rejection of it, were presented in this work, which in turn drew on several earlier accounts, including the historical works of John STOW. Shakespeare probably consulted these independently, finding there the assertion that Hal refunded the victims of his companions' robberies, along with some additional details.

Other sources, including well-known ballads about the Percy-Douglas feuds and a biography of Glendower in the popular collection A MIRROR FOR MAGIS-

TRATES (1559), may have provided incidental material. It has also been suggested that this play and *2 Henry IV* may have been derived from an earlier play by Shakespeare on the same subject, but this speculation is unprovable.

TEXT OF THE PLAY

The date of composition of *1 Henry IV* can only be inferred, but with some precision. It seems to follow closely upon *Richard II;* not only does *1 Henry IV* come next in historical sequence, but *Richard II* contains material that seems to point to a sequel. *Richard II* is generally dated to 1595 or 1596; *1 Henry IV* was therefore composed no earlier than 1596. OLDCASTLE's name was changed to Falstaff as a consequence of protests following performances of the play, and that alteration was apparently made before or during the writing of *The Merry Wives of Windsor,* which was first staged in the spring of 1597. Thus it is likely that *1 Henry IV* was being performed during the winter of 1596–1597 and was probably written in early or mid-1596.

Two QUARTO editions of *1 Henry IV* were printed by Peter SHORT for publisher Andrew WISE in 1598. Only four sheets (1.3.199–2.2) survive from the earlier of these, known as Q0; the other, Q1, was printed from Q0 with minor emendations. Four more quartos were published before the FIRST FOLIO of 1623: Q2 (1599), Q3 (1608), Q4 (1613), Q5 (1622). Although Q2's title page claims that it was 'newly corrected by W. Shakespeare', it was in fact printed—again with minor changes—from Q1, and each subsequent quarto was derived from its predecessor. The Folio version of *1 Henry IV* was printed from Q5; it also contains many minor alterations, some of which may have come from a PROMPT BOOK. Q0 is thought to have been printed from Shakespeare's manuscript, either in the form of a FAIR COPY or his original FOUL PAPERS. Q1 is thus the basis for most modern editions.

In addition to the published texts, there is a handwritten copy of a play that combines *1* and *2 Henry IV,* the DERING MANUSCRIPT. The material it takes from *1 Henry IV* appears to derive from Q5 and the Folio text and is thus dated 1623–1624. Its variations from these texts are not thought to reflect either alterations by the playwright or the practices of early productions, and modern editions do not follow it.

THEATRICAL HISTORY OF THE PLAY

Although no certain records of 16th-century performances of *1 Henry IV* have survived, numerous references in contemporary documents, especially to Hotspur or Falstaff, testify to its popularity. Several actors are said to have played Falstaff during the early 17th century, including John LOWIN, John HEMINGE, and Shakespeare's nephew William HART (3). During the Commonwealth, when the revolutionary Puritan government outlawed the theatre, *The Bouncing Knight,* an abbreviated version of *1 Henry IV,* was performed secretly, as a DROLL. After the restoration of the monarchy in 1660, *1 Henry IV* was among the first plays performed in the reopened theatres, and it remained popular: Samuel PEPYS records productions in 1660, 1661, 1667, and 1668. In 1682 Thomas BETTERTON produced an adaptation of the play in which he played Hotspur; this version was so popular that it was still being revived 18 years later, by which time the 65-year-old producer was playing Falstaff. In the 18th century the play was also frequently staged, and most of the leading actors of the day played Hotspur or Falstaff. David GARRICK, among others, played both; he was acclaimed as Hotspur, but the most successful Falstaffs were James QUIN in the first half of the century and John HENDERSON in the second. In the late 18th century producers twice experimented with a woman, once the famed Julia GLOVER, in Falstaff's part.

In the first half of the 19th century a number of productions of the play were popular. William Charles MACREADY and John Philip KEMBLE (3) were notable Hotspurs, and the latter's two brothers, Charles and Stephen KEMBLE (1,4), played Falstaff. The leading Falstaff of the time, however, was Charles BARTLEY.

Henry IV, Part 1, declined in popularity in the second half of the 19th century, although it was presented by Samuel PHELPS, F. R. BENSON (1), and Beerbohm TREE. However, it has often been staged in the 20th. Among the most successful productions was that of Margaret WEBSTER (3), starring Maurice EVANS (4) as Falstaff, in 1939. Laurence OLIVIER played Hotspur in 1940 and 1945; Ralph RICHARDSON's Falstaff in the latter production is considered one of his greatest successes. Orson WELLES adapted the two *Henry IV* plays in his 1965 FILM *Chimes at Midnight,* in which he starred as Falstaff. Several cycles of the history plays have presented *1 Henry IV,* notably those at STRATFORD in 1906, 1951 (with Michael REDGRAVE as Hotspur), and 1964. A number of TELEVISION productions of the play have been broadcast since the 1950s. The continuing appeal of the *Henry IV* plays was recently demonstrated by a 1987 production in London: the two plays and *Henry V* were staged on different nights of the week, and, most strikingly, theatre-goers responded with enthusiasm to marathon Saturday performances featuring all three works in succession.

Henry IV, PART 2

SYNOPSIS

Induction

A personification of RUMOUR announces that he has put forth a false report, following King HENRY IV's victory at the battle of SHREWSBURY—where PRINCE (6) HAL has killed the rebellious HOTSPUR—that the king

and Prince were killed and the rebels were victorious. This report, Rumour says, is now reaching WARKWORTH CASTLE, home of Hotspur's father, the Earl of NORTHUMBERLAND (1).

Act 1, Scene 1
Lord BARDOLPH (2) brings Northumberland the false news of Hotspur's victory; however, TRAVERS appears with two reports, one corroborating Lord Bardolph's account and the other telling of Hotspur's death and the rebels' defeat. MORTON, an eyewitness, arrives to confirm the truth of the second story. In addition, he says that the victorious king has sent troops, under the Earl of WESTMORELAND (1) and Prince John of LANCASTER (3), to capture Northumberland. The earl rages madly, but his followers counsel calm; the revolt may still be alive. Morton says that the ARCHBISHOP (3) of York has raised a rebel army to avenge the death of King RICHARD II, whom Henry deposed and murdered. Northumberland begins to make plans for the renewal of the war.

Act 1, Scene 2
FALSTAFF jests about the comical disparity between his own huge bulk and that of his diminutive PAGE (5). He encounters the CHIEF JUSTICE, who upbraids him for having refused to answer a summons, observing that, although Falstaff's service at Shrewsbury has allowed earlier offences to be overlooked, he must behave better in the future. Falstaff wittily dismisses this warning. The justice attempts to shame the old man for his foolishness, but to no avail. The knight asks to borrow money from the justice, who leaves. Falstaff then sends the Page with letters to the Prince, Lancaster, Westmoreland, and a woman whom he says he has promised to marry. Complaining of his gout, he declares that a limp will prove useful: he will seem to have been wounded in the war and will get a bigger pension.

Act 1, Scene 3
The rebels, led by the Archbishop, lay their plans. Lord Bardolph advises that they postpone action until they can be sure of Northumberland's support. Lord HASTINGS (2), however, argues that the King's forces are divided, facing threats from the French and the Welsh as well as from themselves, and suggests that the rebels launch their campaign at once. The Archbishop agrees, citing the turn of public opinion against Henry, and they leave to assemble their forces.

Act 2, Scene 1
The HOSTESS (2) of the BOAR'S HEAD TAVERN enlists the officers FANG and SNARE to arrest Falstaff for debt, but when they try to do so, he and his friend BARDOLPH (1) draw their swords and prepare to fight. The furor brings the Chief Justice and his men. He asks the Hostess to explain her claim, and she states that Falstaff has proposed to her, in addition to owing her a great deal of money. Falstaff says that the Hostess is insane, but the Chief Justice insists that he recompense her. Falstaff speaks to the Hostess in private, and he wheedles another loan from her, along with a promise of dinner. The Chief Justice receives word that immediate preparations for battle against the rebels are being made.

Act 2, Scene 2
Prince Hal jests with POINS, but when Poins twits him for not displaying sadness at his father's illness, the Prince observes bitterly that his dissipated life has left him with such a bad reputation that a show of melancholy could only be taken for hypocrisy. Bardolph and Falstaff's Page arrive with a saucy letter from the knight to Hal. The Page reports that Falstaff is dining with the Hostess and a harlot, DOLL TEARSHEET; the Prince and Poins concoct a plot to surprise him at his meal by disguising themselves as DRAWERS.

Act 2, Scene 3
LADY (10) Percy and LADY (9) Northumberland try to dissuade Northumberland from joining the rebel armies. He pleads his duty, but Lady Percy reminds him that he failed to assist his own son, her late husband, Hotspur, whom she eulogises. Humiliated, the Earl agrees to flee to Scotland.

Act 2, Scene 4
At the Boar's Head, the Hostess, Doll Tearsheet, and Falstaff banter drunkenly. PISTOL arrives and makes so much noise that Falstaff drives him away. The Prince and Poins, disguised, overhear Falstaff's assertions that they are inconsequential louts. When Hal confronts Falstaff, the fat knight says that he had disparaged the noblemen only in order to protect them from the ignominy of finding themselves admired by such wicked sorts as Doll and the Hostess. PETO appears with news that the king's army is urgently assembling. The Prince, conscience-stricken that he was indulging himself, hurries away. A further summons arrives for Falstaff, and he departs as well.

Act 3, Scene 1
King Henry sends a PAGE (6) with letters to the earls of SURREY (2) and WARWICK (2). He reflects on his heavy responsibilities, which keep him awake at night while his subjects sleep. Warwick and Surrey arrive and attempt to calm him, but he morosely speaks of the inevitable ravages of time and recalls the prophecy of RICHARD II (in *Richard II*, 5.1) that Northumberland would rebel. Warwick remarks that Northumberland's essentially false nature made such an outcome inevitable, and the observation restores Henry to a sense of the necessity for action. Warwick assures the king that the rebellion seems under control, for the Welsh leader GLENDOWER's death has been reported.

Act 3, Scene 2
The country justices SHALLOW and SILENCE leisurely await the arrival of the king's army recruiter, Falstaff,

for whom they have assembled a group of villagers. Shallow reminisces windily on his student days in London, where he knew Falstaff. Falstaff appears with Bardolph and comically interviews the potential soldiers, selecting several for enlistment before adjourning for a drink with the justices. Bardolph collects bribes from two of the recruits, and upon Falstaff's return tells him which ones are to be released from duty. Falstaff justifies his choice of the least likely recruits in a humorous parody of military standards. After promising another visit, Falstaff leaves. In a soliloquy, he asserts that on his return he shall fleece the gullible Shallow.

Act 4, Scene 1
In GAULTREE FOREST the Archbishop tells his fellow rebels that Northumberland has deserted. Westmoreland appears and demands an explanation for the rebellion. The Archbishop asserts that the illness of the realm requires that they take up the role of surgeons. Westmoreland states that Lancaster, the commander of the king's army, is prepared to hear their grievances during a period of truce. Mowbray is opposed to this offer, but the Archbishop states their complaints against the king, and Westmoreland leaves. Mowbray asserts that the king will always distrust them and that they should continue to pursue victory, for only then can they be safe. The Archbishop and Hastings, however, argue that Henry genuinely desires peace.

Act 4, Scene 2
Lancaster meets the rebels and promises to redress all their grievances if they will disband their forces. The Archbishop and Hastings agree, but Westmoreland arrests them once their forces have dispersed. Lancaster says that he had promised only that their grievances would be redressed, not that they themselves would be pardoned, and he sentences them to death.

Act 4, Scene 3
Falstaff encounters a rebel officer, John COLEVILE, who recognises him and surrenders. Falstaff transfers his prisoner to Lancaster, who sends Colevile to be executed. Lancaster announces that he must go to London, where his father, King Henry, is very sick. Lancaster grants Falstaff permission to return through Gloucestershire, and he leaves. Alone, Falstaff reflects that he cannot make the unconvivial Lancaster laugh because the prince does not drink. In a long, humorous soliloquy he praises strong drink, saying that it both improves the wit and warms the spirit. He asserts that Prince Hal is courageous only because the cold blood he inherited from King Henry has been heated by his drinking.

Act 4, Scene 4
The dying King Henry is attended by his younger sons, the dukes of GLOUCESTER (4) and CLARENCE (2), and by Warwick. Learning that Prince Hal is at his old haunts in London, the king rails against his dissipated son. Warwick defends Hal, asserting that he is merely studying the ways of evil men, the better to judge them as king. News arrives of the final defeat of the rebels, but the king suddenly feels much weaker and is taken into a bedroom.

Act 4, Scene 5
Prince Hal arrives and watches alone at his sleeping father's bedside. He addresses the royal crown, declaring that the cares and stress it represents have killed the king. Believing that his father has died, the Prince meditatively puts on the crown and absently wanders from the room. The king awakes and assumes that Hal has demonstrated an impatience to see him dead. When the Prince is found, weeping in another room, the king predicts dire disorder for England when he succeeds to the throne. The Prince explains why he took the crown and prays for the return of the king's health. The king, convinced, expresses his pleasure with the Prince and offers him advice. Having become king only through usurpation, Henry says he had made enemies. While the Prince, inheriting the crown, will be more widely accepted, he will still have some of the same enemies. The king recommends overseas wars to divert the would-be rebels and to provide an arena in which Hal can prove his valour and undo his sullied reputation. The others return, and the king asks to be taken back to the JERUSALEM CHAMBER, where he wishes to die.

Act 5, Scene 1
Shallow, with the help of his steward, DAVY, prepares to entertain Falstaff with a dinner. Before accompanying his host indoors, Falstaff belittles his intended victim.

Act 5, Scene 2
Warwick and the Chief Justice regret the death of the king and the accession of the delinquent Prince. The Chief Justice expects trouble, for he once gaoled the Prince. The Prince, now called HENRY V, arrives, and he suggests that the Chief Justice may regret that incident. The jurist defends his action, however, asserting the rule of law. Hal agrees and reappoints him to his post, vowing to mend his ways and become a proper king.

Act 5, Scene 3
After dinner Shallow, Silence, and Falstaff drink together in Shallow's orchard. Shallow is drunkenly hospitable, and Silence sings snatches of various songs. Pistol arrives from London with word that the king has died. Falstaff, assuming that Hal, now king, will provide richly for his old friends, makes haste to go to London and claim his fortune. He promises Shallow and Pistol all they desire, and he vows vengeance on the Chief Justice.

Act 5, Scene 4

The Hostess and Doll Tearsheet are under arrest, having apparently been involved in a murderous tavern brawl. They revile the BEADLE who arrested them, but to no avail.

Act 5, Scene 5

Falstaff and his entourage, including Shallow, attend the coronation parade. Falstaff boasts that the new king will welcome him, but when Hal appears, he rejects the old man, promising him a pension but requiring him to live at least 10 miles from court. Falstaff assures Shallow that the king has only put on a public front and will send for him later that night. Shallow is dubious. The Chief Justice, accompanied by Lancaster, arrives and sends the entire group to prison, pending their expulsion from London. Lancaster expresses satisfaction with Hal's kingly behaviour and predicts that the new king will lead a military expedition to France.

Epilogue

A speaker, identifying himself as the author, apologises for a recent unpopular play and hopes that this one has been more satisfactory. He then speaks of himself as a dancer whose performance may make up for the play's defects. He promises that another play featuring Falstaff will continue the story. In closing he observes that Falstaff does not represent the martyr OLDCASTLE.

COMMENTARY

Henry IV, Part 2, is concerned with the demands of kingship, although Falstaff plays a much greater role than he did in *Part 1.* From the Induction and 1.1, with their emphasis on the disruptions of rebellion, to the close, when Prince Hal assumes the heavy mantle of kingship as Henry V, the lessons of *2 Henry IV* are political. Hal rejects Falstaff in 5.5, the final scene, and this incident symbolises the ethic of a ruler: strict justice, though tempered by mercy.

To an even greater degree than in *Part 1,* Shakespeare here presents a picture of all England—the common people who underlie history as well as the aristocrats who make it. Palace chambers and battlefields are set against dissolute EASTCHEAP and bucolic GLOUCESTERSHIRE. In addition to several familiar Eastcheap denizens from *Part 1,* Shakespeare here presents two other extraordinary figures: the Ancient Pistol and Doll Tearsheet. In Gloucestershire, rural England is represented by Justice Shallow and a number of splendid countrymen, including Davy and Silence. In assembling these citizens, *2 Henry IV* continues the unprecedented achievement of *Part 1,* the creation of a comprehensive sense of the diverse life of England in the context of key historical events.

As in *Part 1,* Prince Hal's development is central to the history being presented, though here he becomes a statesman rather than a warrior. However, he is an unimportant character until 4.5, when he meditates on and accepts the burden of kingship. Then, having become king in Act 5, he accepts the Chief Justice, a symbol of honesty and duty, and rejects Falstaff, an emblem of irresponsibility. Hal is committed to becoming a good king, and this is the end to which the rest of the play leads as well, but the focus of the dramatic action is elsewhere, on values opposed to good government, represented by Falstaff on one hand and the rebels on the other.

Falstaff makes quite a different impression than he did in *1 Henry IV.* He is older and in bad health, as he remarks in 1.2.229–233; the prospect of his death looms, as Doll reminds him in 2.4.229–232. He is more distinctly and unpleasantly a swindler, preying on Shallow and the Hostess and sending FEEBLE and his fellows to their probable deaths; in *Part 1* his robbery victims were the anonymous—and supposedly rich and powerful—TRAVELLERS, and his soldiers remained unseen. Further, he justifies his selfishness in *Part 2* with a flagrantly cynical appropriation of 'the law of nature' (3.2.326). He thus seems singularly ripe for a downfall.

The groundwork for Falstaff's rejection by Hal in 5.5 was laid in *Part 1,* and it is anticipated throughout *Part 2.* Falstaff's awkward encounters with the Chief Justice in 1.2 and 2.1 foreshadow this end. In addition, Hal is conspicuously absent from Falstaff's early scenes; their only encounter prior to 5.5 is Hal's somewhat hostile appearance at Falstaff's tavern party in 2.4, which ends with the Prince's cursory farewell to his old friend as he leaves to help suppress the rebellion. Hal shows no interest in Falstaff's world after that point. But after the new king so coldly and firmly dismisses him, Falstaff persists in supposing that Hal is only putting up a public front, although by this time, even the gullible and unsophisticated Shallow sees the truth. Falstaff's rejection comes as no surprise to anyone but himself. His folly in leaping boldly into Hal's coronation scene only seals his fate. His lack of judgement is, of course, the fundamental reason why he is not acceptable company for a king.

It has often been contended that one's response to Hal's rejection of Falstaff reflects one's attitude towards Shakespeare's political sensibility, perhaps towards all political philosophy. According to this theory, the extent to which one sympathises with Falstaff, who represents comic licence and freedom, limits the value that one can simultaneously place on social order. This view, however, not only denies Shakespeare's breadth of vision, which encompassed both freedom and order, but, more important, it also depends on a more sentimental outlook than that of the 16th century. The playwright's plain purpose was to bring Falstaff to a reckoning and to complete the ele-

vation of Prince Hal to his intended destiny as the just King Henry V.

Shakespeare is clearly more sympathetic to the fat scoundrel than the Prince is, for Falstaff is still intended as an essentially delightful character. His inventive humour is still appealing; as he says himself, 'I am not only witty in myself, but the cause that wit is in other men' (1.2.8–9). In his famous praise of wine (4.3.84–123), Falstaff compares himself favourably to the cold and calculating Lancaster, and we are irresistibly inclined to agree with him. At the end of 2.4 the Hostess and Doll Tearsheet touchingly show their affection for him, although they are fully aware of his nature. His ways may bar him from being close to a responsible ruler, but they do not prevent others from appreciating his high spirits. Shakespeare's fondness for Falstaff is further demonstrated by the remarkable leniency with which the new king treats him, however frostily Hal may address him. He is allowed to live as he pleases, with a comfortable pension; clearly, the playwright did not wish to deprive his remarkable creation of sack and capons. Moreover, as the Epilogue indicates, Shakespeare intended to bring him back in another play. Falstaff is very much a part of Shakespeare's England and thus of the historical context within which the play's political questions are set

The rebellion of the nobles is at the political core of *2 Henry IV.* The threat of social disorder runs through all the HISTORY PLAYS, and in *2 Henry IV* it manifests itself both in the petty crimes of Falstaff and in the more grievous offence of the rebels. Rebellion is cast in a highly negative light. Northumberland's apocalyptic rage in 1.1.153–160 demonstrates the anarchic morals of the rebel leaders, who are willing to permit society to collapse. And, to stress his worthlessness, Northumberland is presented as treacherous to his own treacherous cause in the Induction (lines 36–37) and in 2.3. Morton describes, in 1.1.200–209, the Archbishop's sacrilegious use of religion to stimulate armed revolt; Westmoreland elaborates on the Archbishop's particular guilt in 4.1.30–52. However, Shakespeare rarely settled for a single viewpoint on any subject, and the Archbishop makes a plainly sincere response to Westmoreland, in which he states the dilemma of the royalist who nevertheless is provoked into rebellion by misgovernment. Here and in 4.2.30–42, he offers to disband the rebel forces if his complaints are heard by the king, and it is precisely this that is promised when Lancaster deceives and traps the rebel leaders.

Nonetheless, the playwright thoroughly disparages the rebels, and it is striking that he does not similarly deplore Lancaster's treachery against them. Such a scheme, common enough in the histories Shakespeare read, seems acceptable, in the play's terms, because it works against the greater evil of the uprising. It may also serve as an example of the woeful state of public life amid the dynastic struggles that dominate most of the history plays. The rebellion itself is a continuing reminder of King Henry's situation: he is a usurper, under whom the nation cannot be calm. He himself observes this several times (e.g., 3.1.57–79, 4.5.183–186), and in dying he takes comfort that Hal, a legitimate heir, will not encounter the same difficulty.

The play's focus on political turmoil is sharpened by several secondary themes, the most important of which is the unreliability of human knowledge. This motif is repeatedly stressed. At the play's outset, Rumour summons a baffling array of 'surmises, jealousies, conjectures' (Ind. 16) that humanity must face. Among the false impressions that pervade the play are the king's fear that Hal will prove a disastrous heir, Falstaff's contrary assumption that he will prove a delightful one, the rebels' expectation of aid from Northumberland, and their betrayed hopes at Gaultree. The Archbishop seems entirely justified in his plaint 'What trust is in these times?' (1.3.100). Only Prince Hal is aware—from the beginning of *1 Henry IV*—that his own position will be regal. He alone is free of misunderstanding, as befits his ultimate heroic stature as Henry V.

Recurrent references to disease and death add to the atmosphere of urgent uncertainty. Both the king and his rival, Northumberland, are physically ill, and the King's fatal sickness is particularly prominent. Falstaff, as we have seen, encounters his mortality as well; Hal notices his white hairs and says that his 'grave doth gape' (5.5.48–53). Henry says of his kingdom, 'How foul it is, what rank diseases grow' (3.1.39), and the Archbishop constructs an elaborate metaphor on the diseased nation, asserting the need to 'purge th' obstructions which begin to stop our very veins of life' (4.1.65–66).

Animal imagery, a favourite device of Shakespeare's, serves to represent the brutal energy of civil disruption: the Archbishop likens the fickle public to a dog eating its own vomit in 4.1.95–100; Northumberland speaks of the civil conflict as 'a horse [that] madly hath broke loose, and bears down all before him' (1.1.10–11). And, when the king paints a hysterical picture of England under the rule of a profligate Hal, he says, 'the wild dog shall flesh his tooth on every innocent' (4.5.131–132).

Political realities prohibit any festive, comic resolution of *2 Henry IV.* Even Hal's succession to the throne, while an optimistic conclusion to the conflicts that have marred his father's reign, is not a consummation; rather, it points onwards to the wars of Henry V. The several worlds that are juxtaposed in *2 Henry IV*—fictional versus historical, aristocratic versus plebeian, urban versus rural—are each disturbed by political events. Their rich interactions yield a convincing portrait of difficult times, pertinent in the nervous Elizabethan era when fears of rebellion pervaded political

thought, and no less relevant in our own troubled time.

SOURCES OF THE PLAY

Shakespeare's chief source for the historical material in *2 Henry IV* was Raphael HOLINSHED's *Chronicles of England, Scotland, and Ireland* (2nd ed., 1587), modified by the account of Henry's reign in Samuel DANIEL's epic poem *The Civil Wars between the two Houses of York and Lancaster* (1595). In particular the playwright was influenced by Daniel's elaborate treatment of Henry's death-bed and of his guilt as a usurper. In addition, in developing the Chief Justice, who is merely mentioned in his other sources, Shakespeare drew either on John STOW's *Annales of England* (1592), where he found an account of Hal's encounters with the jurist, or on Stow's source, Thomas ELYOT's *The Boke called the Governour* (1531). Additional details seem to have come from the anonymous farce known as the FAMOUS VICTORIES (before 1588) and from the life of Owen Glendower in the popular anthology of biographies A MIRROR FOR MAGISTRATES (1559). It has been suggested that both *Henry IV* plays may have been derived from an earlier play by Shakespeare on the same subject, but this speculation is unprovable.

TEXT OF THE PLAY

The composition of *2 Henry IV* can be dated only approximately. The play was probably begun early in 1597 and completed before the end of 1598. The revised Epilogue refers to *Henry V,* while the version used in the earliest productions does not. We may presume, therefore, that *2 Henry IV* was in performance before *Henry V* was begun, in the spring of 1599. The survival of the name Oldcastle in the QUARTO edition of the play indicates that Shakespeare had at least begun the play before this name was changed to Falstaff. This alteration followed the first production of *1 Henry IV* in the winter season of 1596–1597.

A Quarto edition of *2 Henry IV* was published in 1600 by Andrew WISE and William ASPLEY. Printed by Valentine SIMS, this edition, known as Qa, omitted 3.1. Later, the same individuals published Qb, a reprint of Qa that included the missing scene; although the large number of surviving copies of Qa suggests that it was in circulation for some time before Qb was printed, that interval is unknown. The 1600 Quarto (Q) is considered to consist of Qa plus 3.1 from Qb. Q evidently derives from Shakespeare's FOUL PAPERS; in addition to the usual imperfections of detail associated with foul papers, Q includes the strange spelling Scilens, for the character Silence, an idiosyncracy that helps to identify the 'Hand D' pages of SIR THOMAS MORE as Shakespearean. No other edition of the play was published prior to the FIRST FOLIO of 1623, known as F.

Because it was derived from Shakespeare's manuscript, Q has been the basic text for modern editions, but it is supplemented by material available only from F. Eight Folio passages, ranging in length from 3 to 36 lines, are not found in Q. Some of these apparent cuts in Q may have been intended to shorten the performing time of the play; others may imply CENSORSHIP. The Folio editors took this material from an unknown source, possibly a PROMPT-BOOK, that itself probably derived from Q plus a now-lost manuscript, perhaps the same one that Q was originally printed from. F varies from Q in other ways: many words and phrases are different, its punctuation is greatly reworked, and its stage directions are almost entirely altered and improved.

In addition to the published texts, there exists a 17th-century handwritten copy of a play that combines *1* and *2 Henry IV,* the DERING MANUSCRIPT. With respect to *2 Henry IV,* it derives from Qb. Because it includes minor details from the Folio versions of both plays, it is dated 1623–1624. Its variations from the published texts are not thought to reflect either alterations by Shakespeare or the practices of early productions, and modern editions do not follow it.

THEATRICAL HISTORY OF THE PLAY

The Quarto of *2 Henry IV* (1600) states that it had been 'sundrie times publikely acted' by the CHAMBERLAIN'S MEN, and several references to its characters in various writings of the early 17th century testify that it continued to be staged. The earliest known record of a specific performance is of Thomas BETTERTON's adaptation of 1700 (revived 1720), *The Sequel of Henry the Fourth.* As this title suggests, *2 Henry IV* has generally been less popular than *1 Henry IV,* which has been produced much more frequently. In the 1720 revival Colley CIBBER (1) was a great success as Shallow, a part he took in another adaptation that was staged in 1731 and 1736.

The play was relatively popular throughout the 18th century, and numerous adaptations appeared, frequently in conjunction with *Part 1.* James QUIN played Falstaff several times, and David GARRICK played Henry IV. King George II (incognito) played Henry in a public performance of 1753, to the scandal and delight of London. Theophilus CIBBER (3) played Pistol in his own adaptation, *The Humourists* (1754). The play was produced as part of George III's coronation ceremonies in 1761 (and W. C. MACREADY revived this production for the coronation of William IV in 1821). In 1804 J. P. KEMBLE (3) played the King opposite his brother Charles KEMBLE (1) as Hal; Charles took the same role in Macready's coronation production. In 1853 Samuel PHELPS revived Betterton's version of the play, appearing as both the king and Shallow, a widely acclaimed virtuoso accomplishment. Phelps revived this version again in both 1864 and 1874; in the latter

production the young Johnston FORBES-ROBERTSON played Hal. Another revival of 1874, by Charles CALVERT, was scrupulously Shakespearean.

In the 20th century *2 Henry IV* has been produced as part of the numerous cycles of the history plays that have been popular, notably those at STRATFORD in 1906, 1951, and 1964. Ralph RICHARDSON's performances as Falstaff in a 1945–1946 production of both *Henry IV* plays were particularly admired. Several history cycles on TELEVISION since the 1950s have included *2 Henry IV.* A 1987 London production demonstrated the continuing popularity of the *Henry IV* plays; both parts, along with *Henry V,* were staged on different nights of the week, and, most strikingly, theatre-goers responded with enthusiasm to marathon Saturday performances featuring all three works in succession.

Henry V, King of England (1387–1422) Historical figure and title character in *Henry V,* victorious leader of an English invasion of FRANCE (1) during the HUNDRED YEARS WAR. (The same individual appears as PRINCE [6] HAL in *1* and *2 Henry IV.*) Henry may be seen in two very different ways, in accordance with the play's essential ambivalence. The play may be taken

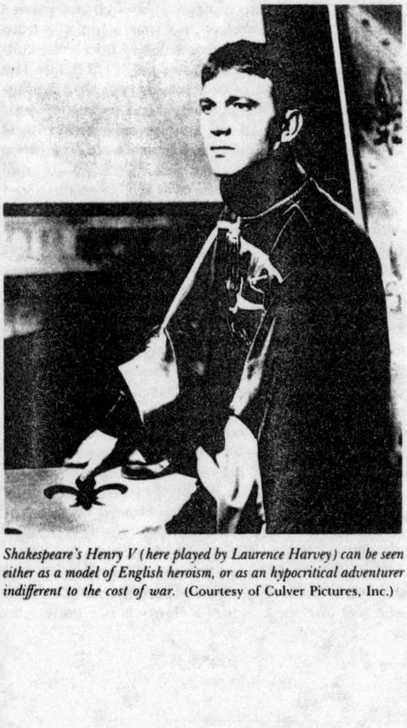

Shakespeare's Henry V (here played by Laurence Harvey) can be seen either as a model of English heroism, or as an hypocritical adventurer indifferent to the cost of war. (Courtesy of Culver Pictures, Inc.)

either as an epic patriotic drama or as a satirical exposure of vicious hypocrisy, depending on one's interpretation of its protagonist; many episodes support both points of view. Henry has two dramatic functions: he is a hero whose exuberant leadership carries England to triumph over a traditional foe, yet he is also a coldly Machiavellian politician who is indifferent to the human costs of war.

Henry's stature as a model of kingship is evident from the outset. In 1.1 the Archbishop of CANTERBURY (1) extols Henry as a thoughtful and devout ruler, praising his understanding of religious, military, and political matters. The king's statesmanship is demonstrated in 2.1, when he solemnly warns of the grave consequences of war. Once agreed that honour requires him to invade France, his inflammatory response to the French AMBASSADOR (1) displays an invincible martial spirit. Henry's rule is secure within his realm, and he easily foils the assassination plot of CAMBRIDGE, SCROOP (1), and GREY (3) in 2.2 and sentences the conspirators to death. The skill with which he manipulates them demonstrates his ability to handle men, while his clemency to the drunken soldier, described in 2.2.39–43, mitigates his severity. On the eve of the invasion of France, we are told, 'all the youth of England are on fire . . . following the mirror of all Christian kings' (2.Chorus.1–6). Henry inspires his forces with one of the most famous patriotic speeches in English literature (3.1.1–34). His chivalric behaviour stands out especially by comparison with his boastful opponents, the vain and foolish French. His anger at the mocking delivery of tennis balls from the DAUPHIN (3) in 1.2 is proportionate to the foolishness of the gift. On the battlefield Henry's dignified refusal to avoid conflict in 3.6 is followed immediately by the prattle of the cocky French nobility.

At AGINCOURT, in Act 4, we see the King at his most heroic. Henry shares the anxieties of the common soldiers in 4.1, and his triumphant courage and high spirits are reflected in his officers, particularly after another famous morale-raiser, the 'St Crispin's Day' speech (4.3.18–67). His weeping response to the deaths of YORK (5) and SUFFOLK (2) in 4.6 belongs to an ancient tradition of vignettes in which great heroes grieve for their slain companions. Displaying the decisiveness of a great general, he reacts harshly in a moment of danger, ordering death for the French prisoners in 4.6.37, but this action is associated in the next two scenes with revenge for a French atrocity. In 4.7 Henry's righteous anger and the approval of GOWER (2) and FLUELLEN reflect the opinion of both Shakespeare's sources and 16th-century military theory that Henry's act was praiseworthy.

Following the battle, Henry is betrothed to Princess KATHARINE (2) of France. This completes the portrait of an epic hero, who, especially if he is a king, must

produce offspring to carry on his line. Henry predicts that their son shall be a great Christian hero, rescuing Constantinople from the Turks. Further, by a dramatic convention of the day, the marriage signifies a happy ending: the war has been resolved, and a bright future is promised.

Most important to Henry's stature as an epic hero, God is on his side. His battle cry asserts, 'God for Harry . . .' (3.1.34), and the traitors acknowledge God's hand in their downfall (2.2.151, 158). Henry utters frequent prayers and assertions that earthly affairs are controlled by God. He is particularly concerned about his relations with heaven in view of his father's sins of usurpation and murder, as he reveals in his prayer for victory on the eve of Agincourt (4.1.295–311). He refuses credit for the subsequent victory, saying, 'Praised be God, and not our strength, for it!' (4.7.89) and orders that psalms of thanksgiving be sung.

Henry seems a proper epic hero, but a contrary view is also suggested from the first. The sincerity of Canterbury's praise in 1.1 is dubious, for the archbishop frankly wants to win the king's support against Parliament. The sentimental 2.1 and 2.3, in which FALSTAFF's followers regret his illness and then mourn his passing, place the king in a moral shadow, for the knight's death is expressly attributed to Henry—'The king hath killed his heart' (2.1.88), the HOSTESS (2) says, referring to Falstaff's rejection in *2 Henry IV*. For many, this act is a coldly ungrateful example of personal betrayal, however appropriate in terms of public policy; a germ of disapproval towards Henry is thus planted before he even appears.

Henry often seems sanctimonious rather than genuinely religious. He chiefly calls on God to justify his own intentions, and he turns ostensibly religious sentiment into a casual anti-French slur in 3.6.166–167. More significantly, Henry's prayer for victory in 4.1.295–311 may be seen as a crass material bargain with God, an invoice, as it were, for the charitable works he has paid for since becoming King. Henry's prayer follows a long passage on the difficulties of kingship, during which it did not occur to him to seek divine assistance. Had Shakespeare intended his hero as a seriously religious person, that would have been a telling and touching moment to have him turn to God. This omission is not in itself very important, but it contributes to a sense that Henry does not truly possess the Christian spirit that he projects.

These suspicions of hypocrisy are supported by the impression that Henry is that most un-Christian figure, the ruthless militarist. The morality of Henry's war is sharply questioned. In 1.1 the play's only formal representatives of Christianity plot to foment a war to protect church property, and we must doubt the propriety of Henry's cause. In Henry's angry speech to the French Ambassadors he justifies himself as an instrument of God's will, but he brandishes ugly threats that are far from Christian in spirit. His God seems to offer an all too convenient excuse to do what he already wants to do—that is, conquer France. At this point we may recall the advice that Henry received from his dying father in *2 Henry IV*—namely, to fight a foreign war to distract potential rivals at home.

The apparent dishonesty of the archbishop's justification for war, noted above, is striking; that it is the archbishop and not Henry who makes the argument is equally telling. Henry has placed the onus on the prelate, having cautioned him, in 1.2.13–28, that the making of war is a mighty responsibility that he refuses to accept himself. This evasion recurs when the soldier WILLIAMS (2) makes a similar point in 4.1. Henry responds with a lecture on the sinfulness of all the soldiers (4.1.150–192), cleverly deflecting moral responsibility away from himself.

Henry's military heroism has a negative side as well, for he repeatedly reveals a nasty viciousness. His spirited reply to the French Ambassadors is also brutally violent, threatening death to 'many a thousand' and grief for those 'yet ungotten and unborn' (1.2.284, 287) as vengeance for a petty insult. His handling of the traitors in 2.2 is effective, but it also suggests a catlike delight in cruelty as Henry toys with his prey. The king's threats to HARFLEUR, though not carried out—the town surrenders and spares him the trouble—are extreme, promising a list of horrors including 'naked infants spitted upon pikes' (3.3.38). The references to his killing of prisoners (4.6.37, 4.7.9–10, 4.7.65), while justifying the act, are all seemingly insistent on the image of the king as executioner. And lastly his cool response to BURGUNDY's plea for peace in 5.2—'. . . you must buy that peace' (5.2.70)—is quite chilling when viewed in light of Henry's demonstrated brutality on the battlefield.

In less political contexts Henry also seems unfeeling. As we have seen, the death of Falstaff raises this point in Act 2, and the fat knight's rejection is referred to again in 4.7.47–53, where it is associated with Alexander the Great's murder of a friend. Moreover, in 3.6.110 Henry lets BARDOLPH (1) die for a petty offence in the name of discipline. The king's cold, Machiavellian nature is thus illustrated several times, contributing to the portrait, alongside that of the epic hero, of a cynical politician.

Henry's aggressive courtship of Princess KATHARINE (2), while possessing a certain bluff charm, may also seem repellent. Not only is the king falsely humble, claiming to be a 'plain soldier', (5.2.153) but he is clearly aware that she is already properly his as a trophy of war. This scene harbours the crowning irony of the play: as Henry crows over the prospective greatness of his and Katharine's future child, we know that this son is to be the hopelessly ineffective HENRY VI, who will lose the conquests Henry is presently cele-

brating. This is bluntly stated in the EPILOGUE, ending the play on a note of resignation and loss that flatly oppose the idea of Henry as an epic hero.

Nonetheless, Henry V was undeniably a monumental figure in the eyes of Elizabethan England, universally accepted as a great king, and Shakespeare took this status as a given. The king is the major figure in the play in either interpretation, and the playwright took pains to emphasise his importance. It appears that Falstaff was removed from the play after it was written, presumably in order to avoid impinging on Henry's significance. Further, Shakespeare altered the historical reality of Henry's reign to the same purpose. The battle of Agincourt, fought in 1415, is the central event of the play and appears to lead directly to the surrender of France. But the decisive campaign in Normandy in 1417–1419, and the importance of naval warfare in its success, is not mentioned; nor is the English alliance with Burgundy, which made Henry's final victory possible five years after Agincourt. In the battle itself the king's role is overstated by the striking omission of a crucial and well-known element, the devastation wrought by the English longbowmen. This aspect of the English victory was already legendary in Shakespeare's time, but it was not suited to the playwright's focus on Henry.

Henry V must dominate the play, for the play's essential ambivalence towards power depends entirely on the extraordinary dual nature of the protagonist, who must function as two quite different figures at the same time. Henry V is in this way unparallelled in Shakespearean drama, though many characters are greater than he in other respects. Thus he brings us to a renewed awareness of the range of his creator's genius.

Henry V

SYNOPSIS

Prologue

The PROLOGUE laments that the players cannot adequately represent such great events as King HENRY V's war against FRANCE (1). But he begs the audience's indulgence and says that he will serve as CHORUS (3).

Act 1, Scene 1

The Archbishop of CANTERBURY (1) and the Bishop of ELY (2) discuss a movement in Parliament to appropriate huge amounts of the church's wealth. Canterbury says that the king, despite his decadent youth (as enacted in *1* and *2 Henry IV*), is likely to support the church; he marvels at length that the king has proved himself a wise statesman. He adds that he has just offered the king an immense sum of church money to support a war in France and assure his support against Parliament, but, before Henry could accept it, the arrival of an AMBASSADOR (1) from France postponed their conversation. Canterbury and Ely leave to witness the king's reception of the Ambassadors.

Act 1, Scene 2

The king summons Canterbury for a conference before receiving the Ambassadors. The archbishop delivers a long and learned justification of Henry's claim to the throne of France. Ely, the Duke of EXETER (2), and the Earl of WESTMORELAND (1) second him in recommending a war to support that claim, and Henry decides to invade. He receives the Ambassadors, who bring an insulting message from the DAUPHIN (3): Henry has gone too far in claiming certain French dukedoms; he should stay home and play games, as suits his dissolute character. A barrel of tennis balls accompanies this insolence. Henry sends the Ambassadors home with a declaration of war.

Act 2, Chorus

The CHORUS tells of English preparations for war in highly rhetorical terms. He also states that three men intend to kill the king in SOUTHAMPTON (1) before he can sail for France. The Chorus assures the audience that the play will transport them to France—without seasickness—after first taking them to Southampton.

Act 2, Scene 1

Lieutenant BARDOLPH (1) encourages Corporal NYM to forgive PISTOL, who has married the HOSTESS (2), to whom Nym had been betrothed. Bardolph wishes them reconciled before they all go to fight in France, but Nym talks of violence against Pistol. Pistol and the Hostess appear, and he and Nym exchange insults and draw swords. Bardolph's threat to kill the first to use his weapon prevents immediate bloodshed. The BOY (3) arrives, summoning the Hostess to help FALSTAFF, who is very ill, and she leaves with him. Pistol and Nym quarrel further, but Bardolph effects a truce. The Hostess returns to report that Falstaff's sickness has worsened, and they all leave to visit him.

Act 2, Scene 2

Exeter, Westmoreland, and the Duke of BEDFORD (1) discuss King Henry's cool pretence that he does not know of the treason intended by the Earl of CAMBRIDGE, Henry SCROOP (1), and Thomas GREY (3). Henry arrives with the three traitors, and he mentions to them his intention to pardon a drunken soldier who has been arrested for speaking disloyally of him. They all recommend severity against any challenge to the king's authority. He then shows them the formal charges against themselves. They plead for mercy, but he cites their own arguments and sentences them to death. They acknowledge his justice before being taken away to be executed.

Act 2, Scene 3

Falstaff's friends mourn him before departing for France. The Hostess touchingly describes his death.

Act 2, Scene 4
The FRENCH KING lays defensive plans against the English. The Dauphin belittles Henry's military potential, but the CONSTABLE and the king remember earlier English triumphs led by Henry's ancestors. Exeter arrives as Henry's ambassador, and he delivers a demand that the French King relinquish his crown or be conquered.

Act 3, Chorus
The Chorus asks the audience to imagine the glorious English fleet sailing to France and, further, to imagine a French ambassador offering Henry a marriage to Princess KATHARINE (2), with a dowry of dukedoms, and being turned away as English cannons begin the fighting.

Act 3, Scene 1
At the siege of HARFLEUR, Henry encourages his troops with a speech extolling the traditional courage of English soldiers, ending with a battle cry.

Act 3, Scene 2
Bardolph enthusiastically shouts a battle cry, but Pistol, Nym, and the Boy seek safety. FLUELLEN appears and harasses the reluctant soldiers up to the front, though the Boy stays behind long enough to soliloquise on the cowardice and dishonesty of his masters, reflecting that he hopes to leave their service soon. GOWER (2), an English officer, talks with Fluellen, MACMORRIS, and JAMY, who are Welsh, Irish, and Scottish, respectively. They discuss the tactics of siege warfare in a conversation made comical by their various dialects and stereotypical temperaments.

Act 3, Scene 3
Henry addresses the citizens of Harfleur, vividly describing the horrors of an army sacking a town. The GOVERNOR (2) of Harfleur appears and surrenders.

Act 3, Scene 4
In French, Princess Katharine receives a comical lesson in English from her waiting-woman, ALICE, enlivened by gross mispronunciations and inadvertent sexual references.

Act 3, Scene 5
The French leaders marvel at the fighting abilities of the English, and the French King orders a massive assault. The Constable remarks that this show of force will surely make the English offer ransom rather than fight, for their forces are sick, hungry, and greatly outnumbered.

Act 3, Scene 6
Gower and Fluellen discuss the English success in taking a bridge. Fluellen praises Pistol's accomplishments there but is disappointed when Pistol appears and seeks his intervention to save Bardolph, who has been sentenced to death for stealing from a church. Fluellen refuses, favouring stern discipline, and Pistol curses him and leaves. Fluellen recollects that Pistol's supposed bravery at the bridge had consisted only of bold words, and Gower elaborately describes the sort of cowardly rogue who avoids fighting and then brags of his heroics in London taverns. Henry arrives, and Fluellen tells him of Bardolph's sentence; the king approves. A French herald, MONTJOY, arrives with a proposed truce if Henry will offer a large ransom. While admitting that he is at a disadvantage, Henry refuses to pay and prepares for battle.

Act 3, Scene 7
The night before the battle, a group of the French leaders converse idly, anticipating an easy victory.

Act 4, Chorus
The Chorus asks the audience to imagine the two opposing camps, busy in the night preparing for battle. The overconfident French play games, gambling prospective English prisoners with each other. The rueful English contemplate defeat and death. However, he says, Henry moves among his troops, raising their spirits. He adds that the actors will depict the ensuing battle of AGINCOURT, although their petty presentation will disgrace the battle's fame.

Act 4, Scene 1
King Henry's cheerful approach to the coming battle is mirrored by an aged knight, Sir Thomas ERPINGHAM. Henry dismisses his attendants, and, incognito, encounters several soldiers in his army. The disguised king is roundly cursed by Pistol when he defends Fluellen. Henry then overhears a conversation between Fluellen and Gower and reflects that Fluellen is a good and careful officer. He next meets three English soldiers, one of whom, Michael WILLIAMS (2), asserts that, while common soldiers will be killed, the king risks only capture, after which he will be ransomed. Henry, speaking as another commoner, insists that this is not so; the king has vowed to die rather than be taken prisoner. Williams doubts that this will happen. After a brief argument, Williams agrees to fight his opponent after the battle, if they both live, and they exchange tokens of identity, so that they can recognise each other in the day time: each will wear the other's glove on his hat. The soldiers depart, and Henry, in a long soliloquy, meditates on the cares of kingship. Erpingham appears and delivers a request that the king confer with his nobles, and Henry sends him to convene a meeting at his tent. Alone again, the king prays that God will not permit his soldiers to fail as punishment for his father's deposition and murder of RICHARD II (enacted in *Richard II*), since he has reburied Richard and made other formal atonements for the crime.

Act 4, Scene 2
The French nobles, about to begin the battle, remark on the feeble opposition.

Act 4, Scene 3
The English nobles, though ready to fight, comment on the degree to which they are outnumbered. Westmoreland wishes they had reinforcements from England, but Henry observes that their triumph will be the greater because they are fewer. He would prefer that the faint-hearted depart so that the honour of the battle need be shared only by those who are worthy. He predicts that the day will be long remembered as a great one for England and that all those present will value the experience for the rest of their lives. Montjoy reappears with another offer of peace for ransom, but Henry sends him back with a proud refusal.

Act 4, Scene 4
Pistol captures a FRENCH SOLDIER and threatens bloody death if he is not paid a ransom, but the soldier doesn't understand English. Pistol comically, but viciously, rants at his helpless prisoner, until the Boy interprets into English the Frenchman's offer of money, and Pistol marches off with him. Alone, the Boy reflects that Pistol has avoided the fate of Bardolph and Nym—both hanged for theft—only through cowardice, having been afraid to steal. He observes that only he and other boys are with the army's baggage train, which makes it a good target for the French.

Act 4, Scene 5
The French nobles hysterically try to organise a counter-attack against the English, who are winning the battle.

Act 4, Scene 6
Exeter gives Henry a touching account of the death of the Duke of YORK (5). When it appears that French reinforcements have entered the battle, Henry orders all prisoners killed.

Act 4, Scene 7
Fluellen and Gower discuss the cowardly French massacre of the unarmed boys tending the baggage train. Praising Henry's response to this outrage—ordering the death of all prisoners—Fluellen presents a long and comical comparison between the king and Alexander the Great. Henry arrives and sends a messenger to tell the remaining French knights that they should prepare to fight or flee, for all French prisoners are to be killed. Montjoy reappears to ask that the fighting stop so that the French can bury their dead, and he concedes that the English have won the battle. Fluellen praises the king, noting his Welsh blood. Williams appears and tells the king of the oath that the glove on his hat represents. Henry sends him with a message to Gower. The king then gives Fluellen a glove to wear on his hat, saying that he had captured it in the battle and that anyone who challenges it is a friend of the French and should be arrested. Fluellen, proud of his assignment, is also sent to Gower. Henry then instructs Warwick and Gloucester to follow Fluellen and prevent a fight between him and Williams.

Act 4, Scene 8
Williams encounters Fluellen and strikes him; Fluellen prepares to fight, as Warwick and Gloucester prevent him. The king arrives, explains the circumstances, and gives Williams a glove full of coins. Fluellen attempts to increase the reward with his own shilling, but Williams rejects it. Henry reads a long list of French noblemen killed in the battle, along with only four English knights, and he orders that religious rites of thanksgiving be observed.

Act 5, Chorus
The Chorus tells of Henry's triumphal return to London, of the peace negotiation between England and France, and of Henry's subsequent return to France.

Act 5, Scene 1
Fluellen tells Gower that Pistol has insulted the leek, symbol of WALES (1), that he wears in his hat. Pistol appears, and Fluellen cudgels him and forces him to eat the leek. The humiliated Pistol decides that he will return to England and take up a life of petty crime. He will pretend the scars from Fluellen's beating were obtained in battle.

Act 5, Scene 2
King Henry, the French King, and their respective entourages, meet to sign a peace treaty. The Duke of BURGUNDY (2) makes an eloquent plea for peace, and Henry replies that peace must be bought, as the treaty provides. The French King requests a final consultation on certain points, and Henry sends his noblemen to negotiate with the French. Henry is left with Princess Katharine and Alice. The king courts the princess, and their language difficulties are humorous. She is uncertain what to think, but she concedes that, if her father agrees to the marriage, she will also consent. The negotiators return, and all parties accept the marriage. Henry orders that wedding preparations begin.

Epilogue
The Chorus states in a SONNET that this ends the presentation of Henry's glory. Conquered France was left to the infant HENRY VI, during whose reign it was lost through English discord and mismanagement, as the actors have often depicted on stage.

COMMENTARY

Henry V completes the second TETRALOGY of Shakespeare's HISTORY PLAYS, and this work restates a prob-

lem first dealt with in *Richard II:* Can sensitivity and warmth—the spiritual values that elevate human life—coexist with the ruthless strength and shrewdness that a ruler needs to govern? In *Henry V* this question can be plausibly answered in two ways that seem to be mutually exclusive. Some readers find the play a patriotic tribute to Henry, who is seen as an ideally heroic leader who takes England to new heights of power and defeats a traditional enemy; he is an hero suited to the threatening times England endured in the late 16th century, when the play was written, and the play has been popular in times of national crisis ever since. Alternatively, though, the play is a mordant commentary on politics and war, in which Henry is a Machiavellian militarist, a cold-blooded, power-hungry hypocrite who uses religion to justify the horrors of an unnecessary war. This anti-heroic view has found its audience primarily in recent decades, but the observations that war is hellish and that it is often conducted for selfish ends are not new, and Shakespeare could easily have found them suitable material for a play.

Both readings are equally valid, and they may reflect Shakespeare's own ambivalence towards the subject of power. In either interpretation, *Henry V* is a powerful dramatic work whose epic quality is plainly intended to invoke the grandeur of the ancient world, whether seriously or sardonically. For instance, the use of the Chorus, itself a direct reference to ancient Roman drama, places the action in a timeless, semi-mythical context. Such lines as the Prologue's desire for 'a Muse of fire' (Prologue.1) and the description of the night as filling 'the wide vessel of the universe' (4.Chorus.3) are unquestionably grand, and they lend a monumental air—ironic or otherwise—to the work. A sense of great moments passing into legend is often called forth in this play, as when Henry declares, 'Then call we this the field of Agincourt, fought on the day of Crispin Crispianus' (4.7.92–93).

However, Shakespeare remains committed to the great portrait of the common people of England that he began so successfully in the *Henry IV* plays. A group of new characters, led by Fluellen, provides a glimpse of Henry's army. Part of their function is to exemplify the stalwart bearing of the common soldier, lending dignity to Henry, but they also offer a frequently humorous cross-section of the British public. In 3.2, known as the 'international' scene, Gower, Macmorris, Jamy, and Fluellen represent England, Ireland, Scotland, and Wales respectively in a tribute to British unity under Henry. Jamy and Macmorris are simple stereotypes, but Fluellen and Gower have more depth. Likewise, Henry's conversation with BATES and Williams in 4.1 is humanly complex and real and stirs our feelings in preparation for his important soliloquy on the difficulties of kingship (4.1.236–290). These vignettes reveal that Henry's strength derives from his subjects, who in turn respond to him and are proud to be British.

However, the world of the BOAR'S HEAD TAVERN, familiar from *1* and *2 Henry IV,* is treated less sympathetically. Falstaff dies off-stage almost immediately, and the Hostess' role is brief, if poignant. Then Bardolph and Nym die ignominiously, and the Boy is killed in an atrocity of war. Finally, Pistol is humiliated by Fluellen in 5.1. These incidents serve both interpretations of the play, for, while they may represent a defeat for anarchy by the new order of the epic hero, at the same time they present Henry as an unforgiving, unfeeling politician who can cite principles of discipline while permitting an old friend to die.

Earlier, the account of Falstaff's death makes this point more explicitly. We hear of his illness and death in two sentimental scenes, 2.1 and 2.3, that give emotional resonance to his EASTCHEAP cronies; Pistol and Nym, in particular, are otherwise little better than mindlessly vicious. Their grief lends them a pathos that helps sustain the epic quality of the play, but, on the other hand, Falstaff's final agony is expressly attributed to Henry's cold and Machiavellian nature—'The king hath killed his heart' (2.1.88), the Hostess says, referring to Falstaff's rejection in *2 Henry IV*—and this contributes to the play's sardonic and cynical viewpoint.

Various sorts of evidence (see FALSTAFF) reflect the likelihood that Falstaff was originally the chief comic character of the play, and Shakespeare's deletion of the fat knight is indicative of his purposes. Henry's central role could only be compromised by the presence of so massive a personality; in either interpretation Falstaff's cheerful immorality would only distract from its primary focus, be it an epic vision of England's greatness or a biting assessment of Henry's calculating militarism.

Henry's invasion of France and the victory at Agincourt were already legendary peaks of English glory in Shakespeare's day, and national pride is patently evident at many points in the play; several passages—especially 3.1.1–34 and 4.3.56–67—have been standard items of patriotic rhetoric since they first appeared. However, the play is not merely rousing pageantry; the morality of Henry's war is questioned throughout. The major justification for the war is presented by the Archbishop of Canterbury in 1.2.33–95, and while this speech may be read with great solemnity, it also has a more ironic side—for example, in Canterbury's assertion that his complicated and legalistic argument makes Henry's claim to the French crown 'as clear as is the summer's sun' (1.2.86). That the archbishop and not Henry makes the argument demonstrates Henry's manipulative nature: he places the onus on the archbishop, cautioning him, in 1.2.13–28, that the justification of war is a mighty responsibil-

ity, but he refuses to accept that responsibility when Williams makes a similar point in 4.1.

More boldly, the play commingles with its sense of heroic chivalry several passages that are explicit condemnations of war, including Henry's 'conjuration' to the archbishop just mentioned. Best known is Burgundy's plea for peace in 5.2.24–67, in which the plight of a war-torn land is movingly evoked. Significantly, Henry's response is the cool insistence that France must 'buy that peace' (5.2.70).

Most important, the savagery of war is repeatedly described in vivid speeches that compellingly counter the heroic idea of warfare that they ostensibly promote, beginning subtly with the archbishop's strangely inappropriate equation of war booty with the peaceful activity of bees gathering honey and quickly escalating to Henry's inflamed response to the Dauphin's mockery in 1.2.261–296. At Harfleur the king describes in grisly detail the fate the town will undergo if his soldiers loot it (3.4.1–41). While Henry is in fact merciful to the citizens—because they do in fact surrender, sparing him the trouble of a battle—his graphic threat is a stark reminder of the horrors of war. Williams' description of a battle also illustrates the terrifying reality of warfare, in terms that are far from conventionally heroic rhetoric: '. . . all those legs and arms and heads, chopped off in a battle' (4.1.137–138).

Moreover, the only actual combat we see involves Pistol, who is systematically deplored throughout the play. He is decried at length for cowardice, vanity, and downright criminality by Gower in 3.6 and the Boy in 3.2 and 4.4. Further, Pistol makes us aware of a frequent consequence of war, the social havoc that can be wreaked by hardened and embittered soldiers returning to a civilian population. Having failed in war, he declares that he will become a professional thief on his return to London (5.1.89–95).

Thus the evils of war are abundantly demonstrated, even as the triumph of English arms is glorified. Both messages are strongly reinforced by the seemingly anticlimactic courtship scene, 5.2. First, Henry's development as an epic hero is brought to its proper climax by his marriage; he woos his bride briskly, with joyous predictions of a happy marriage and fine offspring. He is now a complete hero whose fine traits and accomplishments can be carried forward into the future. Moreover, the supremacy of England over France is again emphasised. However, Henry's aggressive wooing of Katharine may also be seen as an extension of his brutal conquest. In addition, the final bankruptcy of Henry's cause is frankly, if subtly, asserted: Henry predicts great heroism for his son, but we know that this son will become the ineffectual HENRY VI, under whom England's French conquests will be lost; this is expressly mentioned in the Epilogue. These references remind us, as they reminded Shakespeare's original audience—to whom all of these matters were much more familiar—that *Henry V* actually presents a mere interlude in the bloody and tragic tale of England's disruption by the selfish ambitions of feuding aristocrats. This heavy irony chillingly closes the play on a note of failure and resignation that does much to offset the epic nature of the story.

Some critics view the play's ambiguities as unintentional, claiming that Shakespeare intended a portrayal of heroic idealism but failed to present it convincingly, perhaps due to an unconscious revulsion against authority. Others assert that the play's emphasis on Henry's Machiavellian nature conflicts with his status as a national hero, resulting in a confused political statement. Perhaps a compromise position permits the fullest response: Shakespeare may have accepted Henry's status as a hero while also being aware of the sordidness of political life. In the TETRALOGY that closes with *Henry V*, Shakespeare developed his ideal of a King whose human sensitivity matches his capacity for ruthlessness, but in doing so, he perhaps discovered the limitations imposed on this ideal by the nature of power.

Shakespeare's instinctive response to the irreducible complexity of life was to be further reflected in the great plays of the next several years. *Julius Caesar*, another play about power and idealism, followed almost immediately; the great tragedies pose questions about the reliability of human motives, whether political or otherwise—questions that are implicit in the ambiguities of *Henry V*. The need for social order is an important issue throughout Shakespeare's work; however, so is an evident distrust of those who hold authority. We can only conclude that the playwright recognised the paradox that underlies much political thought from the late Middle Ages to the present: the only forms of power that seem fully moral—such as those outlined in Thomas MORE's *Utopia* and its successors—are impossible to achieve. Thus the ambivalence of *Henry V* reflects our most profound political ideals as well as our most disturbing fears of political power.

SOURCES OF THE PLAY

Shakespeare's chief source for the historical material in *Henry V* was Raphael HOLINSHED's *Chronicles of England, Scotland, and Ireland* (2nd ed., 1587), supplemented by *The Union of the Two Noble and Illustre Families of Lancaster and York* (1548) by Edward HALL (2). Other historical details may have come from the chronicles of Robert FABYAN (1516) and John STOW (1592). Shakespeare may also have read several Latin biographies of King Henry, written during the monarch's lifetime or shortly thereafter: the *Henrici Quinti Angliae Regis Gesta*, written by an army chaplain who was pre-

sent at Agincourt; the *Vita et Gesta Henrici Quinti,* whose anonymous author is known as Pseudo-Elmham; and the *Vita Henrici Quinti,* by Tito Livio, which was translated as *The First English Life of King Henry the Fifth* (1513).

Several fictional episodes may have been inspired by other works. The Dauphin's insulting gift of tennis balls in 1.2, Pistol's capture of the French Soldier in 4.4, and Henry's courtship of Katharine in 5.2 probably derive from similar scenes in an earlier play about Henry V, the FAMOUS VICTORIES (before 1588). Also, Katharine's language lesson in 3.4 closely resembles several scenes in 16th-century French farces, suggesting that Shakespeare had read some of these plays, although they were published only in France and never translated into English. Henry's clemency to the drunken soldier, described in 2.2. 39–43, may derive from a similar episode in PLUTARCH's *Lives of the Noble Grecians and Romans,* translated by Thomas NORTH (1579). And the Archbishop's comparison of human society to a hive of bees (1.2.187–204) was probably inspired by a passage in the *Georgics* of VIRGIL.

TEXT OF THE PLAY

We know that *Henry V* was written in the spring or summer of 1599, for it contains a plain allusion to a contemporary event. In 5.Chorus.30–32, the CHORUS (3) refers to the military expedition of the Earl of ESSEX (2) to Ireland, hoping that he would return triumphantly. Essex left London in March 1599 and returned ignominiously in September. The reference was probably made in the spring, for it quickly became known that the expedition was destined for failure.

The play first appeared in print in a QUARTO edition of 1600, printed by Thomas CREEDE for publishers Thomas MILLINGTON and John BUSBY. This edition, known as Q1, is a BAD QUARTO—that is, it was recorded from memory by actors who had appeared in it, and its text is seriously flawed. Moreover, Q1 lacks the Prologue, Epilogue, all of the speeches of the Chorus, three other whole scenes, and long portions of six others. Q2 (1602) and Q3 (1619), both published by Thomas PAVIER, are reprinted from Q1; they differ from it only accidentally and omit the same material. Q3 was part of the notorious FALSE FOLIO and is spuriously dated 1608.

The FIRST FOLIO version of the play (1623) is the first to present the missing material, and it has been the basis of all subsequent editions. Descriptive stage directions, the presence of a GHOST CHARACTER (see BEAUMONT [1]), and idiosyncratic spellings known to have been used by Shakespeare suggest that the Folio text was printed from the playwright's FOUL PAPERS. Minor details derived from Q3 indicate that the printers also used a copy of that edition.

THEATRICAL HISTORY OF THE PLAY

The title page of the 1600 edition of *Henry V* asserts that the play had already been 'sundry times played', but the earliest known performance was held at the court of King JAMES I on January 7, 1605. No other 17th-century production is known, and the play has been popular only intermittently since then. A 1723 adaptation eliminated the comic characters from Eastcheap. David GARRICK produced Shakespeare's text in the 1750s, playing the Chorus. John Philip KEMBLE (3) played the King in his own quite successful version of the play between 1788 and 1811. W. C. MACREADY also played Henry several times, culminating in a memorably spectacular production of 1839. Nineteenth century producers were inclined to extraordinary effects; in 1859 Charles KEAN (1) staged a triumphal march after Agincourt that employed 550 actors. Charles CALVERT presented *Henry V* in both London (1872) and New York (1875).

At about the turn of the 20th century F. R. BENSON (1) played Henry, but the play has not often been staged since. Its patriotic aspect made it successful during both world wars; *Henry V* has been performed frequently as an anti-war play in Britain and America since the 1950s, as the nuclear age and its series of small but vicious conflicts have generated strong pacifist sentiments in Western society. Among the most notable productions was that of Peter HALL (5) at STRATFORD in 1960. The play has also been produced as part of a number of cycles of the HISTORY PLAYS, notably those at Stratford in 1901, 1906, 1951, and 1977 and on British TELEVISION in 1960, one of six television versions of the play. *Henry V* has twice been made a FILM: Laurence OLIVIER's patriotic wartime version (1944; music by William WALTON) contrasts with the bleaker 1989 movie by Kenneth Branagh (b. 1961). A 1987 London stage production demonstrated the continuing public interest in the play: both *Henry IV* plays and *Henry V* were staged on different nights of the week, and, most strikingly, theatre-goers responded with enthusiasm to marathon Saturday performances featuring all three works in succession.

Henry VI, King of England (1421–1471) Historical figure and title character of *1, 2,* and *3 Henry VI.* Despite their titles, King Henry is not the leading figure in any of the *Henry VI* plays. In *Part 1* he is a child, and even the story of the nobles who presume upon his weakness is overshadowed by the account of the military loss of FRANCE (1) and the bravery of TALBOT. In *Part 2* Henry is merely a witness to the political developments that occupy the play: the fall of GLOUCESTER (4) and the rise of YORK (8). In *Part 3* he is more articulate but no less helpless. Pious and plaintive, he is crushed between the contending forces that his

akness has allowed to rise. He is finally killed, and corpse appears early in *Richard III.*

Ienry is a virtuous man; he is gentle, thoughtful, governed by a sense of moral values. However, has placed him on a throne and he lacks the ruth- vigour required of a medieval ruler. In fact, he is aragon of weakness—a vacuum into which disorder hes—and the HISTORY PLAYS are about order and order.

n *1 Henry VI* the king is an infant at the outset and y a young man at the end. He is distressed by the lries he sees around him but is unable to resolve m, being entirely incompetent in worldly matters. his most important scene in the play (4.1.134–173), nry makes a grave error in his haste to defuse the tility between York and SOMERSET (3), dividing the glish military command between the two dispu- s. At the close of the play, he succumbs to the crupulous arguments of the Earl of SUFFOLK (3) agrees to marry MARGARET (1), a decision that the sequent plays demonstrate to have been disastrous England and for Henry himself.

n *2 Henry VI* the king, although an adult, is no more ontrol of his kingdom than he was in his youth. His ef interest is religion, and, in the face of dangerous ensions, his only response is to preach the virtues nity and peace. He is thoroughly manipulated by ers, first by Suffolk and then, after that lord's th, by Queen Margaret. He permits the ruin of ucester, although knows it to be unjust. Even when ed with the bloody rebellion led by Jack CADE, the g cannot take decisive action, but again thinks first is religion. When York rebels, opening the WARS THE ROSES, Henry is again quite helpless. He real- his own unsuitability for command and regrets his ition in life.

n *3 Henry VI* the king attempts to bring about an to the growing civil war, but the leaders of the two ions, York and his son Richard (see RICHARD III) one side and Margaret on the other, will not be eased. Henry protests the barbarities that ensue. is the only important character in the play who s not espouse the principle of revenge, but he not influence the action. His position as king is well mplified during the dispute among the nobles in where he twice demands to speak (at 117 and –120) and has no chance to say another word in scene. In 2.5, a scene central to the play, Henry ndraws from a raging battle to meditate lyrically on virtues of a pastoral existence that is as far oved from his reality as it imaginably could be. In k contrast, he immediately witnesses the grief of SON THAT HATH KILLED HIS FATHER and the FATHER T HATH KILLED HIS SON. He is completely dispirited r these incidents; this gentle man is finally crushed his world. Only as he is killed does Henry again come alive on the stage, prophesying the future crimes of his murderer, in anticipation of the next play in the cycle, *Richard III.*

The character and career of the historical Henry VI are less clearly delineated. While he was certainly not the strong, activist monarch that his father, HENRY V, had been, it is uncertain how much his courtiers manipulated him. He possessed the powers of a medieval king and could not be defied if he were to insist on something. Even in Shakespeare, when he decrees the banishment of Suffolk, the earl leaves. However, it is uncertain when and on what points he stood firm, so we cannot know how much he is to blame for the wartime policies of the 1440s (in *Part 1*), for the unrest of the following decade (in *Part 2*), or for the policies of the civil war period. It is known that, in the early 1450s, Henry was literally incompetent for a time, being beset with a mental illness that rendered him speechless and almost immobile. The playwright chose to ignore this episode (during which York ruled and the country remained stable and at peace)—perhaps because it would have aggrandised York, perhaps becuase he wished to avoid offending the dignity of a ruler.

In any case, Shakespeare was more concerned with drama than with history, and, as Henry's character develops through the plays, we can observe the young playwright learning how to devise a suitable tragic figure whose very virtues are his undoing. The germ of some of Shakespeare's great characters is here: a man who is good finds himself in a situation where his limitations generate an evil that crushes him. In *Richard II,* and later in *Hamlet* and *King Lear,* the drama can rest upon this predicament. However, in the *Henry VI* plays the playwright had not yet honed his skills so finely and Henry VI can merely speak of his woeful ineffectuality while the world sweeps him away.

Henry VI, PART 1

SYNOPSIS

Act 1, Scene 1

The play opens on the funeral of King HENRY V; the Duke of BEDFORD (1) notes astrological portents of disaster. The Duke of GLOUCESTER (4) and the Bishop of WINCHESTER (1) argue, disrupting the ceremony. A MESSENGER (3) arrives with news of disastrous military defeats in FRANCE (1). A second Messenger arrives, bringing news of a general rebellion of France against England, featuring the crowning of the Dauphin as King CHARLES VII, in violation of the treaty enforced by Henry V, and the rallying to his cause of several important noblemen, including the BASTARD (2) OF ORLÉANS, REIGNIER, and the Duke of ALENÇON. Another Messenger arrives to tell of the defeat of England's

leading knight, TALBOT, wounded and captured due to the cowardice of another English commander, Sir John FASTOLFE. Bedford vows to lead reinforcements to France, and the Messenger relates that the army under the Earl of SALISBURY (3) is pinned down outside ORLÉANS (1).

Act 1, Scene 2
At the siege of Orléans, Charles VII, Alençon, and Reignier exult in their recent good fortune and mock the English. An assault occurs, and the French are driven off-stage. The three French leaders re-enter, cursing the English, and decide that they will abandon the town. The Bastard of Orléans arrives. He describes a young woman, JOAN LA PUCELLE, who has been sent by a vision from heaven to aid the French forces. Joan enters and offers to demonstrate her God-given military capacities in single combat with Charles. Charles accepts the challenge and is overwhelmed. He accepts her offer of assistance. Alençon and Reignier ask about plans for Orléans, and the newly inspired Charles declares that they will fight it out.

Act 1, Scene 3
The Duke of Gloucester and the Bishop of Winchester argue about the right to command the Tower of London. They and their men come to blows. The MAYOR (2) OF LONDON enters, with the king's order commanding public peace. The disputants separate with insults and challenges.

Act 1, Scene 4
The MASTER-GUNNER of Orléans instructs a BOY (1) to keep watch on a tower where English soldiers come to observe the besieged city. Several Englishmen, including Salisbury and Talbot, appear on the tower. Talbot explains that he has been exchanged for a captured Frenchman. They begin to plan an attack on the city, but they are struck by a cannonball. Salisbury falls badly wounded, and another man is killed. Talbot cries out against the loss of Salisbury's heroism and leadership. A Messenger arrives with the news that Charles and Joan have arrived with an army to raise the siege.

Act 1, Scene 5
Skirmishing, Joan pursues a group of Englishmen across the stage. Talbot and Joan fight to a draw. Joan says that Talbot's time has not yet come, and she enters the city with the successful French troops, leaving Talbot to bemoan the poor state of English morale. In another skirmish, the English are driven back into their trenches, and Talbot concedes defeat.

Act 1, Scene 6
Joan, Charles, Reignier, and Alençon assemble on the walls of Orléans to celebrate their victory over the English.

Act 2, Scene 1
With a group of soldiers, Talbot, Bedford, and Duke of BURGUNDY (2), an ally of the English, ass Orléans. The French leaders are driven over the w The Frenchmen exchange recriminations, but J encourages them to think of counter-attack. Howe an English SOLDIER (1) enters, shouting Talbot's na as a war cry, and the French party flees in panic.

Act 2, Scene 2
Bedford, Burgundy, and Talbot mourn the dead Sa bury. A Messenger arrives with an invitation for bot from a French noblewoman, the COUNTESS (1 AUVERGNE, who wishes to entertain the valorous queror. Talbot leaves with the Messenger, but he whispers something to a CAPTAIN (2).

Act 2, Scene 3
The Countess of Auvergne gloats over her plan capture Talbot. He arrives, and she mocks his sique. Offended, he begins to leave, and she nounces his capture. But he springs his counter-p blowing his horn to summon a waiting troop of diers, who immediately free him.

Act 2, Scene 4
Richard Plantagenet (see YORK [8]) argues hotly the Duke of SOMERSET (3) in the company of sev other men. Richard plucks a white rose from a gar tree, and calls on those who support him to do l wise. Somerset immediately takes a red rose as his emblem. The Earl of WARWICK (2) joins Plantage Suffolk sides with Somerset. Both Plantagenet Somerset agree that the dispute should be settled a majority vote among the group. However, wh most support Plantagenet, Somerset hints at a d He goes on to cast aspersions on Plantagenet, re ring to the execution of his father, the Earl of C BRIDGE, for treason. Plantagenet counters that the ecution had not been carried out legally. He threat action against Somerset, who replies in kind and parts. Warwick assures Plantagenet that he will reinstated as Duke of York.

Act 2, Scene 5
In the Tower of London, Plantagenet visits a dy relative, MORTIMER (1), who is a prisoner. Plantage wants to know the story of his father's death. Morti tells of the deposition of King RICHARD II by HENRY head of the Lancastrian branch of the royal fam Mortimer, of the YORK (1) branch, had been the leg mate heir to the throne, but an attempt to install h as king has resulted in his imprisonment for life wh still a young man. In the reign of Henry V, Mortime brother-in-law, who had been Richard Plantagen father, had repeated the attempt to crown Mortir and was executed for it. Mortimer names Plantage his successor, and he dies, after cautioning younger man not to act against the house of LANC

TER (1), which is too strong to be removed. Plantagenet vows that he will begin to seek vengeance for his family by becoming reinstalled as Duke of York at the forthcoming Parliament.

Act 3, Scene 1
In the Parliament House, Winchester and Gloucester and their respective supporters argue violently. King HENRY VI, still a child, pleads for peace between the factions. The Mayor enters, reporting that the followers of Gloucester and Winchester are battling in the streets. Two SERVING-MEN burst in, fighting. The king continues to plead for peace; Gloucester says he is willing. Winchester, reluctant, finally agrees, and the servingmen are dismissed. The king agrees to restore Plantagenet as Duke of York. Gloucester announces that all the preparations have been made for Henry to be crowned King of France in Paris. As the others depart, Exeter remains and, in a soliloquy, predicts disaster for the English forces.

Act 3, Scene 2
Outside the gates of ROUEN, Joan and four soldiers gain entrance to the city disguised as tradesmen. She signals to the French troops, who take the city. The French leaders taunt the English, who are now outside the walls. Talbot and Burgundy exchange vows to recapture the town immediately. The dying Bedford, confined to an invalid's chair, refuses to leave the scene of battle. The skirmishing begins, and Fastolfe appears, fleeing in panic. The French are defeated, and Bedford, pronouncing himself satisfied, dies in his chair. Talbot and Burgundy exult in their victory and eulogise Bedford.

Act 3, Scene 3
The French leaders call the Duke of Burgundy to a parley to convince him to desert the English. Joan speaks to him of the misery of his homeland and asserts that the English are not his true friends. While suggesting that he may have been bewitched by Joan, Burgundy does change sides, declaring himself an ally of France.

Act 3, Scene 4
Talbot is knighted by Henry in Paris, where the king has come to be crowned. VERNON (1) and BASSET engage in another round of the York-Somerset rivalry, exchanging insults and threats.

Act 4, Scene 1
Winchester crowns the king, and the GOVERNOR (2) of Paris kneels and accepts the oath administered by Gloucester. Fastolfe arrives with a message from Burgundy. Talbot tears off the Order of the Garter that Fastolfe wears, declaring him a coward, and the king banishes Fastolfe. Gloucester reads Burgundy's letter, in which he declares his changed allegiance. Talbot is ordered to march against Burgundy and departs spiritedly. Vernon and Basset appear, demanding a trial by combat. Their dispute spreads, and York challenges Somerset to a duel. Gloucester intervenes, and the king attempts to restore order. To demonstrate his even-handedness, he foolishly divides the command of the English forces, assigning the infantry to York and the cavalry to Somerset.

Act 4, Scene 2
Talbot appears before the walls of BORDEAUX and demands the surrender of the city. A GENERAL on the walls refuses, confident in the strength of the approaching French army. Talbot recognises danger, and he urges his troops to fight fiercely.

Act 4, Scene 3
York receives a Messenger, who tells of the force that is marching to attack Talbot, and he curses Somerset for not providing cavalry support. Sir William LUCY (2) arrives from Bordeaux with an urgent plea for reinforcements. He is resisted by York, who continues to accuse Somerset.

Act 4, Scene 4
Lucy approaches Somerset with the same plea, and Somerset refuses, criticising York for a bad plan. He refuses to send cavalry without an explicit request from York. Lucy cries out that Talbot will be defeated and killed, and he blames Somerset for feuding.

Act 4, Scene 5
Talbot tells his young son, JOHN (6), that he should flee the certain death to be expected in the upcoming battle. John refuses, citing the honour of the family. They debate the matter, but the boy insists that he will stay.

Act 4, Scene 6
In the midst of the battle, Talbot rescues his son, fighting off surrounding attackers. The father describes the fierce fighting that has occurred, and he renews his insistence that his son should flee, but John again refuses.

Act 4, Scene 7
Talbot, mortally wounded, mourns the death of his son, killed in the battle, and then dies also. The victorious French leaders talk of John Talbot's valour and express thanks for York and Somerset's absence. Lucy appears, under a flag of truce, to retrieve the bodies of the two Talbots.

Act 5, Scene 1
Gloucester tells King Henry that a peace treaty has been arranged, and that a marriage, intended to secure the peace, has been proposed between the king and the daughter of a French nobleman, the Earl of Armagnac. The King agrees to treaty and marriage, and the visiting ambassadors are summoned to receive his formal acceptance.

Act 5, Scene 2
The French leaders rejoice at the news that Paris has risen against the English, but they are then disturbed by further news that the English army, reunited, is approaching.

Act 5, Scene 3
Joan uses witchcraft to summon a group of FIENDS, but these spirits silently refuse to aid her, and she realises that all is indeed lost. After a skirmish, York defeats Burgundy and takes Joan prisoner. He leads her away as Suffolk enters with MARGARET (1) of Anjou as his prisoner. He has already fallen in love with her, and he devises a plot to make her his lover, although he is already married. He offers to marry her to King Henry and make her Queen of England if she will be his lover. She accepts, on the condition that her father, Reignier, agree. Reignier is summoned, and he does agree, provided that he be awarded his home territories, Anjou and Maine. Suffolk promises to arrange this, and he leaves Margaret with her father.

Act 5, Scene 4
Joan, condemned to be burned, encounters her father, a SHEPHERD (1), but she refuses to acknowledge him, claiming descent from royalty. She declares that her death will bring damnation to her executioners. She is nevertheless ordered to the stake. Next, she claims she is pregnant, but she is sent to her death, cursing England. The French leaders arrive to settle the details of the peace. Charles at first refuses to declare himself a subject of the English king, but Reignier and Alençon convince him to sign, for he can always break his word later.

Act 5, Scene 5
Suffolk's description of Margaret's virtues has caused the King to desire her. Gloucester objects, citing the earlier marriage agreement. However, the king orders Suffolk to return to France to arrange a marriage to Margaret. The play closes with a soliloquy by Suffolk, in which he proposes to rule the kingdom himself, through Margaret.

COMMENTARY

1 Henry VI is the first of Shakespeare's HISTORY PLAYS, and it shares with the later works a particular emphasis on the state. The development of individual characters is not very important, for the theme is English history. This play commences the TETRALOGY of dramas dealing with the WARS OF THE ROSES, the great crisis that formed the English nation as it was known to Shakespeare and his contemporaries. Here, the playwright deals with the earliest of the disruptions, beginning during the last phase of the HUNDRED YEARS WAR, a series of conflicts in which the French resisted English attempts to conquer them.

The action starts after the death of King HENRY V, who had led his forces to great victories, establishing English control over large stretches of France (as Shakespeare was later to recount in *Henry V*); in the course of this play, these territories are almost all lost. However, Shakespeare's concern is not with narrative history. Rather, he amplifies the theme that England's misfortunes were the result of selfish ambitions unchecked by a weak monarch's incompetence. King Henry VI is an infant when the play begins and only a young man when it ends. Ambitious noblemen felt they had plenty of opportunity to increase their personal power, and to indulge in feuds that a more assertive monarch would have curtailed.

Shakespeare immediately sets out his themes in 1.1. The outbreak of verbal sparring between the Duke of Gloucester and the Bishop of Winchester introduces the disorder among the nobles. Moreover, the effects of this dissension are already beginning to be felt, as the Messengers arrive to tell of military losses in France, including the catastrophic capture of a great English leader, Talbot.

French successes in the war are juxtaposed with brawling disorders in England. For example, the disagreement between Gloucester and Winchester at the Tower of London in 1.3 follows the arrival of Joan of Arc to boost the morale of the French forces. Similarly, the rock-fight that spreads even into the king's deliberations in 3.1 immediately precedes Joan's successful ruse at Rouen in 3.2. The feuding of Vernon and Basset begins in 3.4, just after the defection of the Duke of Burgundy, and it continues in 4.1, providing a sorry prelude to the death of Talbot.

This disorder in the realm is reflected in the repeated instances of hypocrisy and dishonesty on the part of various characters. Mortimer advises Plantagenet to conceal his opposition to the Lancasters (2.5). The Bishop of Winchester plots to kidnap the infant king, although this strand of the plot goes undeveloped, and he pretends to be reconciled with Gloucester after the fight in Parliament (1.1, 3.1). In the Temple garden dispute (2.4), Somerset refuses to abide by the majority vote he had agreed to honour. Suffolk plots to deceive the king in Act 5, and in the final scene, even the saintly Henry is prevailed upon to go back on his agreement to marry the daughter of Armagnac. Another recurrent motif, representing the English dissension, is the interrupted ceremony. Three times, in 1.1, 3.1, and 4.1, ceremonial occasions are disrupted, each time more than once.

Shakespeare counterbalances these ominous occurrences with the character of Talbot, a model knight who symbolises the lost English supremacy under Henry V. Talbot is the only nobleman who stands out from the array of rhetorical quarrellers. He is knightly courtesy itself at the beginning of the coronation scene, and he personifies righteous indignation when he refuses to tolerate the wearing of the Garter, sym-

bol of valour, by the coward Fastolfe. Talbot's praises are sung repeatedly by English and French alike. But his virtues cannot survive in the prevailing climate of deceit and disorder, and his courageous death in 4.7 is presented as the direct result of the York-Somerset struggle.

Historically, the episode of York and Somerset's divided command took place in Normandy during the 1440s, while Talbot's death occurred in southern France some years later. However, to increase the contrast between the brave and honourable Talbot on the one hand and the selfish, scheming factions on the other, Shakespeare provided a direct connection between the rise of the nobles and the loss of England's hero. Neither the playwright nor his audience was concerned with historical accuracy, but *1 Henry VI* is nevertheless strikingly at odds with the record as Shakespeare knew it. For instance, although the Duke of Burgundy did indeed change sides during the Hundred Years War, he did so some years after Joan's death. Moreover, this defection resulted from two decades of minor disputes and disagreements between the English and the Burgundians. For dramatic reasons, Shakespeare compressed all this into one highly charged, if entirely fictitious, scene; this enabled him to emphasise the duplicity of the French and Joan's associations with sorcery.

Similarly, the play describes, in close succession, Talbot's death, Joan's execution, and Henry's marriage: the fall of the great English hero prepares for that of the French heroine, who in turn is succeeded in the play by another Frenchwoman, the focus of a plot against Henry's power. To achieve these emotionally resonant juxtapositions, Shakespeare wilfully ignored the chronicles, which correctly record a rather different arrangement. Joan was burned in 1431, Henry was married in 1444, and Talbot died in 1453. Smaller distortions of the historical record occur throughout the play.

The playwright also invented a number of scenes for dramatic impact. Talbot's encounter with the Countess of Auvergne (2.3), for instance, points up aspects of the hero's soldierly nature and contrasts his honesty with the Countess' deceit. A more important invention is the confrontation between the future Duke of York and his rival Somerset in the Temple garden (2.4), in which they select as emblems a white and a red rose. This scene objectifies the rivalry that was to develop into civil war in the sequels to this play. Although historically it did not happen, it is so dramatically appropriate that we might wish it had.

Such inventions and obvious errors are much more evident to a reader than to an audience. The Hundred Years War and the English political scene are made real through a highly theatrical counterpoint of formal spectacle and unpredictable violence. The disrupted ceremonies noted above are obvious manifestations of this dramatic tension; the cool equanimity of the dying Bedford amid the hurly-burly of battle in 3.2 is a subtler instance. And Joan's brief dismissal of Sir William Lucy's elegiac recital of Talbot's noble titles brings us with a jolt from the formal dignity of medieval pomp to a renewed awareness of the carnage of battle (4.7. 75–76).

King Henry himself is a humanly interesting character, unlike the caricatures of 'ambitious courtiers' around him, although his personality is more developed in *2* and *3 Henry VI.* The conflict between his nature and the requirements of his situation fuels some of the development in this play and becomes highly significant in its sequels. Henry is gentle and thoughtful. He is distressed by the dissensions around him but is unable to contain them, not only on account of his youth, but also because of his innate dislike of involvement in worldly matters.

In general, however, character development is not a strength of this play, which partly explains its general unpopularity with modern audiences. The play's style is rhetorical and formal, its content is largely expository, and the poetry tends to be somewhat stilted. Another problem arises from the playwright's need to consider the play as one of a series; a certain amount of dramatically undirected material must be used in order to establish concerns that will be dealt with only in the sequels. Most glaring of these incidents is the relationship between the Earl of Suffolk and Margaret of Anjou, which seems unrelated to anything else in the play. It is certainly used to establish a major theme of the next play. However, it also provides a natural climax to this one, completing the devastation of England's position in France with the loss of Anjou and Maine. Also, Margaret becomes the strong adversarial figure that Joan had been. It is typical of Shakespeare's strategies in *1 Henry VI* that Margaret first appears just as Joan is rendered powerless.

Among the conventional stances that the play adopts are a vicious anti-French bias and a contemptuous attitude towards Joan that now seems excessive. In the 18th and 19th centuries they were cited as evidence that the play could not have been written by Shakespeare, such attitudes being thought beneath a great writer. Such virulent Francophobia was in tune with Elizabethan attitudes, however, and the picture of Joan as a whorish sorceress comes from Shakespeare's sources and he doubtless regarded it as historically sound.

On the whole, *1 Henry VI* cannot be regarded as a successful play. It lacks cohesion, being composed of scenes whose connections are more often contrasting than developmental. It is rhetorical to an extent that inhibits an audience's responses, and it does not reflect the insights into human nature that we associate with the mature Shakespeare. On the other hand, the play does present an extensive tract of complicated

history, and it does so in a manner that enables us to apprehend it intellectually and also taste something of the nerve-racking reality of confused warfare. It was probably Shakespeare's first attempt at a new form, the drama of historical narrative, and he was to improve upon it in each of its sequels, before going on to the glories of the major tetralogy.

SOURCES OF THE PLAY

Shakespeare's chief sources for *1 Henry VI,* and its sequels were the best-known English histories of his day, Raphael HOLINSHED's *The Chronicles of England, Ireland, and Scotland* (second edition, 1587) and *The Union of the Two Noble and Illustre Families of Lancastre and York,* by Edward HALL (2) (third edition, 1550). An older text, *The New Chronicle of England and of France,* by Robert FABYAN (1516), provided some supplementary material, such as an account of the stone-throwing skirmish in 3.1.

TEXT OF THE PLAY

In the 18th and 19th centuries a distaste for the treatment of Joan of Arc in *1 Henry VI* led to a tendency to attribute the play to other writers, especially to joint authorship—usually some combination of NASHE, GREENE, (2) and MARLOWE (1)—with only certain elements (especially 2.4, 2.5, and 4.2–7) credited to Shakespeare. Modern scholarship, however, generally finds the play to be largely Shakespearean, although some authorities still assign Act 1 to Nashe.

It is impossible to date the composition of Shakespeare's early HISTORY PLAYS with absolute certainty; the evidence is sparse, complex, and contradictory. However, *1 Henry VI* contains several minor resemblances to Edmund SPENSER's *Faerie Queene,* dated December 1589, and the play was referred to by Thomas Nashe, in the summer of 1592, as already very popular. Since the theatres were closed by plague after June of that year, the play must have been performed that spring. Therefore, we do know that it was written between 1589 and 1592.

Although it is sometimes contended that *Part 1* was written *after* the other *Henry VI* plays, modern opinion tends to support common sense in supposing that the plays of the minor tetralogy, including *Richard III,* were written in the order in which they are read. *Richard III* seems to have been known to Marlowe by early 1592; therefore, it seems likely that the four plays were composed between early 1590 and late 1591, with *1 Henry VI* being written near the beginning of this period.

The only early publication of the play was in the FIRST FOLIO edition of 1623, and this text has necessarily been the basis for all subsequent editions. The Folio version's many errors and inconsistencies have provided grist for much scholarly dispute over minor points, but the text is not seriously flawed. Some characteristics—the casual stage directions and the retention of flagrant contradictions that would probably have been corrected in a performance script—seem to indicate that the Folio was printed from the author's manuscript.

THEATRICAL HISTORY OF THE PLAY

Nashe's reference to the play as an established hit just before the theatres closed in 1592 proves that it had been performed that spring. However, no other early productions are known. After Shakespeare's time, *1 Henry VI* was all but ignored for almost three centuries, being revived only in 1738 and 1899. However, elements from it were occasionally used in abridgements of the complete set of Henry VI plays. In the 20th century it has been somewhat more frequently produced, especially in cycles presenting the history plays in clusters. It has also continued to provide material for abridged combinations, on both stage and TELEVISION. It has never been a FILM, but it was made for television in 1983 and was incorporated in two BBC series: AN AGE OF KINGS (1960) and 'The Wars of the Roses' (1964), which combines the *Henry VI* plays and *Richard III.*

Henry VI, PART 2

SYNOPSIS

Act 1, Scene 1

The court of HENRY VI is assembled to welcome the King's new bride, MARGARET (1) of Anjou, whom the Earl of SUFFOLK (3) has brought to England. The Duke of GLOUCESTER (4) reads aloud the terms of the marriage contract, by which Anjou and Maine, French territories that England had conquered, are ceded to Margaret's father. This so upsets him that he cannot read on. CARDINAL (1) BEAUFORT continues, reading that Margaret shall pay no dowry. The king accepts the terms. He then promotes Suffolk to a dukedom and temporarily suspends the appointment of the Duke of YORK (8) as Regent of FRANCE (1). The royal newlyweds and Suffolk depart. Gloucester, backed by York, the Earl of SALISBURY (2), and the Earl of WARWICK (3), rails against the marriage contract. He leaves, prophesying the loss of France. The Cardinal suggests that Gloucester, the heir apparent to the throne, is quarrelling only because he seeks to replace the king. He observes that Gloucester is popular and thus doubly dangerous. The Duke of BUCKINGHAM (3) agrees and proposes a plot to unseat Gloucester from his position as Lord Protector. The Cardinal leaves to recruit Suffolk for the plot, and in his absence, the Duke of SOMERSET (1) contends that the Cardinal is himself ambitious to fill the Protector's office. Salisbury and Warwick speak of the good of the country and decide to back Gloucester, an honest and competent Protec-

r. They recruit York to their cause, but when they ave, York, in a soliloquy, confides that he thinks of mself as the rightful king and of Henry as a usurper. e determines that he will ally himself with the back- s of Gloucester and await a good time to seize the rone by force.

t 1, Scene 2
he DUCHESS (1) of Gloucester encourages Gloucester aspire to the throne, but he rejects the idea and bukes her for it. A MESSENGER (4) summons the ıke, who leaves. Alone, the Duchess speaks of her tention to pursue the crown for her husband. She mmons HUME and arranges for a séance with a witch d a sorcerer whom he has contacted on her behalf. e pays Hume and leaves, and he reveals in a solilo- y that he is also in the pay of Suffolk and the Cardi- l, arrangeing a scandalous exposure of the Duchess at will bring down Gloucester as well.

t 1, Scene 3
TER (1), an armourer's apprentice, reports that his aster, HORNER, has heard the Duke of York express claim to the throne. Suffolk has Peter taken into stody and Horner sent for. The new queen com- ains to Suffolk that the king seems merely the equal his noblemen. Suffolk assures her that his plots will do the noblemen, but that she must be patient. The ng arrives with the nobles of the court. They discuss e regency of France; Gloucester backs York for the sition. The queen attacks Gloucester, as do Suffolk, e Cardinal, Somerset, and Buckingham. Gloucester orms off, and the queen provokes a quarrel with his fe, striking her, and the Duchess leaves also. Buck- gham follows her. Gloucester returns, his anger oled, and again proposes York for the regency, but ffolk accuses York of treason, and Horner is ought in. Horner denies having said anything about rk and asserts that his apprentice is lying. Glouces- calls for a trial by combat. Peter despairs, saying he nnot fight, but the combat is scheduled.

t 1, Scene 4
ıme assembles the witch MARGERY JOURDAIN and the rcerers BOLINGBROKE (2) and SOUTHWELL to call a irit for the Duchess of Gloucester. The spirit ASNATH pears and is asked about the future of the king. He plies ambiguously. He predicts a death by water for ffolk, and he advises that Somerset should avoid stles. The spirit is dismissed, and York and Bucking- m appear, placing everyone present under arrest.

t 2, Scene 1
ıe members of the court are hunting with falcons. oucester and the Cardinal quarrel to the point of rangeing a duel. The king opposes the dispute but nnot stop it. A Citizen of nearby ST. ALBANS ap- oaches, proclaiming a miracle: a man blind since th can suddenly see. Gloucester interviews the man, one SIMPCOX, suspecting a fraud, and his clever ques- tioning confirms his guess. Buckingham appears with news of the arrest of the Duchess of Gloucester as a user of witchcraft and leader of a conspiracy against the king. When his enemies gloat, Gloucester an- nounces that, if his wife has indeed done these things, he will reject her and leave her to the process of the law.

Act 2, Scene 2
York outlines his claim to the throne to Salisbury and Warwick. Convinced, they swear allegiance to him, but he cautions them that he is not king yet. They should conceal their plot, he says, and wait for Suffolk, the Cardinal, and their allies to bring down Gloucester, who is the most important Lancastrian.

Act 2, Scene 3
King Henry sentences the conspirators who were ar- rested in 1.4. The commoners are sentenced to death. The Duchess of Gloucester will be paraded ignomini- ously through the streets of London and then exiled. The king orders Gloucester to surrender his staff of office. He does so and leaves. Horner and Peter ap- pear for their trial by combat. Horner, expected to win the contest, is too drunk to fight and is killed by Peter. Dying, he confesses having lied and exonerates his apprentice.

Act 2, Scene 4
The Duke of Gloucester witnesses his wife's humilia- tion in the streets. She forecasts that he will soon be threatened with death by Suffolk and his allies. Gloucester asserts that his unblemished loyalty and honesty will be his protection.

Act 3, Scene 1
The queen's clique insists to the king that Gloucester is planning a coup. The king denies it. The Duke of Somerset appears to announce the loss of all the En- glish territories in France. The king accepts this defeat as the work of God, but York is bitter. Gloucester arrives, and Suffolk accuses him of treason. Gloucester leaves under arrest, and the king, saying that he is grief-stricken, relinquishes his authority to the queen's clique and leaves. The conspirators decide that Gloucester is still too dangerous and agree to have him murdered. A Messenger arrives from Ireland with news that a revolt is in progress there. Suffolk assigns York an army and sends him to suppress the rebels. All but York depart, and the duke reveals his plans in a long soliloquy. He exults that he has an army at his disposal, and he plans a rebellion to be staged by his hired agent, Jack CADE. Then he will take advan- tage of the unrest and seize the throne.

Act 3, Scene 2
Several murderers flee from Gloucester's chambers and are met by Suffolk, who promises them their pay

for the deed. The king and his court arrive, and Suffolk is sent to summon Gloucester. He returns to announce Gloucester's death. The king faints, awakening to mourn. Margaret responds with an extravagant plaint, lamenting that she will be slandered with implications of guilt and that Henry now wishes her dead. She is interrupted by Warwick and Salisbury, who arrive with a crowd of commoners. Warwick reports that the people are distressed by rumours that Gloucester has been murdered. Warwick examines the corpse and points out signs that the duke was indeed slain. He accuses Suffolk. The two agree to a duel and depart, but they return immediately, just ahead of a mob. Salisbury reports that the people demand death or banishment for Suffolk. The king formally banishes Suffolk from England and leaves with his loyal noblemen. The queen and Suffolk are left to make their farewells, revealing that they love each other. VAUX (3) enters with news that the Cardinal is dying.

Act 3, Scene 3
The king, Warwick, and Salisbury witness the Cardinal's death. The delirious Cardinal reveals his guilt.

Act 4, Scene 1
On a beach, members of the crew of a pirate ship assemble their three captives, recently seized from another ship. A LIEUTENANT (1) of the pirates awards the prisoners to his men, who will collect ransom from them. Suffolk is awarded to the pirate Walter (pronounced 'water' in Elizabethan English) WHITMORE. Whitmore, having lost an eye in the battle, insists on vengeance and declares that Suffolk must die. Suffolk recalls his predicted death by water. He identifies himself, and the Lieutenant speaks against him, reciting his political crimes. Whitmore takes Suffolk off to be beheaded. The Lieutenant releases one captive, a GENTLEMAN (1), to carry ransom messages to London. Whitmore returns to deposit Suffolk's head and body at the feet of the Gentleman, who vows to carry them to the king and queen.

Act 4, Scene 2
BEVIS and HOLLAND (3) discuss the rebellion of Jack CADE and join the uprising when the rebels arrive. Cade claims to be a PLANTAGENET (1) and the proper heir to the crown. Comically, he promises his followers preposterous rewards. One rebel proposes killing all lawyers, and Cade agrees, ranting against the use of documents. The CLERK of Chatham is brought in as a prisoner, and he is sentenced to death for being literate. A Messenger arrives to warn of the approach of troops led by Sir Humphrey STAFFORD (2). Stafford insultingly demands that the rebels surrender, but they refuse.

Act 4, Scene 3
In a skirmish, Stafford and his BROTHER (1) are slain. Cade proposes to march on London.

Act 4, Scene 4
In the king's palace in London, Margaret, carryi Suffolk's head, mourns her lover's death, while Hen and Buckingham plan how to deal with the rebellio A Messenger reports the approach of the rebels, a Buckingham recommends that the king retreat un the revolt is suppressed. Another Messenger repo that the rebels have reached London and that some the citizens are rising in sympathy with them. The ki and queen depart with Buckingham.

Act 4, Scene 5
A CITIZEN (1) reports to Lord SCALES, the command of the Tower of London, that the rebels are succes fully assaulting London Bridge and that the Lo Mayor has requested Scales' assistance. Scales pro ises to send aid and issues orders.

Act 4, Scene 6
Cade declares himself Lord of London and comman that the water fountain be made to flow wine for year. He further declares that it shall be treason address him as anything but Lord Mortimer. A SO DIER (3) enters, calling out for Cade, unaware of t new regulation. Cade orders him set upon, and he killed. Cade orders that London Bridge and the Tow of London be burned down.

Act 4, Scene 7
Lord SAY is brought to Cade's camp. Cade derisive accuses him of various deeds that are usually consi ered praiseworthy, such as building a grammar scho Say pleads for his life, but, after several exchange Cade sends him off to be beheaded with his son-i law. Some soldiers return with the two heads on pole Cade orders these trophies paraded through t streets.

Act 4, Scene 8
Buckingham and Lord CLIFFORD (2) offer the king pardon to all rebels who will declare allegiance to t throne. A great roar of 'God save the king' goes u Cade counters with a speech that evokes a similar c in his favour. Clifford, however, seduces the fick mob back to the king's side. Cade flees.

Act 4, Scene 9
The king laments his fate. Buckingham and Cliffo enter and announce Cade's flight. They are accomp nied by many former rebels seeking the king's forgiv ness, which he grants. News arrives that York has r turned from Ireland with a strong army, demandi the removal of the Duke of Somerset. The king, d tressed, sends Buckingham to negotiate with York a temporarily orders Somerset to the Tower.

Act 4, Scene 10
Cade hides in the walled garden of an estate and discovered by its owner, Alexander IDEN. After a bri quarrel, the two fight and Cade is killed.

Act 5, Scene 1
York, at the head of an army, announces that he has returned from Ireland to claim the throne, but he observes that he must still pretend loyalty to Henry. Buckingham delivers a message from the king and informs York that Somerset is a prisoner; York accordingly dismisses his soldiers. The king arrives, and York expresses his allegiance. Iden appears with the head of Cade, which he offers to the king. The king knights him. The queen arrives with Somerset. When he sees that Somerset is not in prison, York angrily declares that he shall no longer regard Henry as king and claims the throne for himself. Somerset and Margaret challenge him. York's sons, Edward (see EDWARD IV) and Richard (see RICHARD III), enter to support him, opposing Clifford and his son, John CLIFFORD (1), whom the Queen has summoned. Warwick and Salisbury arrive and side with York. Warwick and Clifford vow to fight each other in the battle that is now necessary, and Young Clifford exchanges insults with York.

Act 5, Scene 2
York kills Clifford on the battlefield. The younger Clifford discovers his father's body and in a lament, compares death to the Last Judgement. He asserts his intention to kill the children of the Yorkists as they have killed his aged father. York and Somerset enter fighting, and Somerset is slain. York notes that the prediction that Somerset should avoid castles has come true; he has been killed beneath a tavern sign depicting a castle. York exists, and the king and queen arrive in retreat. Henry hesitates, but Margaret insists that they must flee in order to fight again.

Act 5, Scene 3
Near the battlefield, Salisbury proposes to York that they should pursue their fleeing enemies. York agrees, as does Warwick, who comments that the battle is likely to become famous.

COMMENTARY

Henry VI, Part 2 is a political play, rather than a drama of human interaction or development. It tells of England's collapse into the anarchy and civil strife of the WARS OF THE ROSES due to selfish ambitions unleashed by the weakness of a young and indecisive ruler. As part of the minor TETRALOGY of HISTORY PLAYS, this work also furthers the underlying themes of inexorable tragedy caused by the usurpation of the crown by the LANCASTER (1) family and of the eventual retribution delivered to that dynasty. In *2 Henry VI* these concerns are developed in two episodes. The first, occupying Acts 1–3, involves the political downfall and eventual murder of Duke Humphrey of Gloucester, who is presented as a just and prudent statesman whose leadership might have preserved the kingdom. The second is an account of the final steps the Duke of York takes towards his own seizure of the crown. This episode begins with a popular rebellion led by York's agent, Jack Cade, a comical affair providing relief after the relentless unfolding of Gloucester's fate. It turns vicious, however, illustrating the evil of anarchy unloosed by the murder of 'good Duke Humphrey'. York capitalises on the uprising to advance his own claim and brings the nation to civil war at the first battle of St Albans, with which the play closes.

Shakespeare was dramatising history in the *Henry VI* plays, but he was not at all averse to altering actual events for dramatic purposes, although *Part 2* uses less such distortion than *Part 1*. The greatest misrepresentation is the depiction of York's ambition, presented as a carefully deliberated plot by a determined usurper. Historically, York, who had nothing to do with the outbreak of Cade's rebellion, made no attempt to seize the crown until very shortly before the war broke out. Prior to that time, he does not seem to have contemplated doing so; he had fiercely competed with the Duke of Somerset for power as a minister under King Henry, but he attempted to rule himself only when it became clear that Margaret's influence on Somerset's behalf was too great to be finally overcome and that Somerset planned to destroy his own power altogether. In order to emphasise the rivalry of the Lancaster and York families, and to stress the evils of aristocratic ambition, Shakespeare humanised the confused political process that had in fact uncoiled in the 1440s and 1450s by making a convincing schemer of York. Much exciting history has simply been eliminated—most notably, York's capable assumption of the regency in 1453–1454, when the king fell helplessly insane and was unable to speak.

The story of Gloucester's fate is tightened and given a melodramatic sense of inevitability by compressing many events, widely separated historically, into a swiftly flowing narrative. The tale of the Duchess of Gloucester's sorcery and exile is historical, but it occurred four years before the arrival of Queen Margaret. The two women are made contemporary, thereby involving Margaret in Gloucester's fall, and the episode is made to contribute directly to that fall, which it did not actually do. Similarly, the exile and death of Suffolk are moved back by several years and are thereby associated directly with Gloucester's death. Thus six years of aristocratic manoeuvrings are collapsed into a matter of months in order to heighten the drama of Gloucester's fall and clearly establish it as the spark for the events that follow.

Though the play's point is made by its sequence of events, Shakespeare created a number of believable, humanly distinct characters to execute them, marking a great improvement on the masses of quarrelling nobles in *1 Henry VI*. King Henry himself—enthralled by religion, well-meaning but ineffectual—is moving towards the pathetic, almost tragic figure he becomes in *3 Henry VI*. Also striking are Queen Margaret and the

Duke of Suffolk, who are convincing as scheming villains and at the same time inspire sympathy as lovers in their farewell scene (3.2). One sees that Shakespeare is developing the capacity to produce such great later characters as the villains IAGO and RICHARD III and the lovers ROMEO and JULIET.

Richard III, in fact, makes his first appearance late in this play. His role is unimportant, and he is present simply as a harbinger of the next two dramas in the tetralogy, but he is a cleanly drawn figure, sardonically epigrammatic. Another minor figure, Buckingham, sounds an aristocratic note of peremptory command, and two men who will figure prominently in the next play, Warwick and Clifford, are strongly delineated minor characters in this one.

Given this range of characters and events, the poetic style in *2 Henry VI* is necessarily varied. The speeches of Cade and his rebels are comically gross, while Margaret and Suffolk's farewells draw on the tradition of courtly love. The vicious repartee of the feuding nobles differs from the high poetry of the pirate Lieutenant. In contrast with *1 Henry VI,* Shakespeare here shows his increasing mastery of the difficult task of writing credible speech in verse.

Shakespeare's wilful manipulation of his historical sources is successful on the whole but does misfire in some instances. Most notable in this respect are two episodes taken from widely separated accounts in the sources and used to illustrate the good judgement of the Duke of Gloucester. The incident involving Horner's reported remarks about York's ambition provides an occasion for the Duke to exercise prudence. He withholds office from York pending resolution of the matter. However, the resolution never comes; the dying Horner admits that he had made the incriminating comment, but no note is made of the obvious implications concerning York's loyalty and the matter is never again referred to; the playwright has left his audience dangling. In the other incident, Gloucester cleverly exposes the impostor Simpcox. Here, the scene is dramatically complete and quite amusing, but it is too trivial to stand up to the more important events with which it is juxtaposed.

Henry VI, Part 2, although it marks a considerable advance on *Part 1,* is still plainly the work of a young, less than masterly, playwright. Moreover, it suffers from its position in a sequence of plays. Much of the early exposition is intended to provide a link to the action of *1 Henry VI,* and several dramatically unnecessary characters, such as Richard and Young Clifford, appear in Act 5, where they foreshadow *3 Henry VI.* Nevertheless, it is an exciting play, composed of varied and interesting scenes that generate two plausible climaxes, and it is full of the promise of greater things to come.

SOURCES OF THE PLAY

As in the other history plays, Shakespeare adapted material from the available chronicles. For *2 Henry VI,* his chief source was *The Union of the Two Noble and Illustre Families of Lancastre and York,* by Edward HALL (2) (third edition, 1550), supplemented by Raphael HOLINSHED's *The Chronicles of England, Ireland, and Scotland* (second edition, 1587). He also used John FOXE's *Book of Martyrs* (fourth edition, 1583), from which he took the story of Simpcox's false miracle, along with other details. Various minor suggestions seem to have come from other chronicles, including those of Robert FABYAN and Richard GRAFTON, along with a popular anthology of biographies, A MIRROR FOR MAGISTRATES.

TEXT OF THE PLAY

It is impossible to date the early history plays with certainty, but since *1* and *2 Henry VI* both contain minor resemblances to Edmund SPENSER's *Faerie Queene,* dated December 1589, these plays cannot have been written earlier than 1590. It is thought by many that the four plays of the tetralogy were written in the order in which they are read, and the last of them, *Richard III,* was apparently known to MARLOWE (1) by early 1592. Therefore, it seems likely that the four plays were composed between early 1590 and late 1591. If the second of them is assigned the second quarter of this span of time, we may date *2 Henry VI* to the latter half of 1590.

The play was first published in the form in which we know it in the FIRST FOLIO, in 1623, and that text has been the basis for all subsequent editions. However, a BAD QUARTO edition, known as THE CONTENTION, was published by Thomas MILLINGTON in 1594 and again in 1600; these editions are known as Q1 and Q2 respectively. Thomas PAVIER published another QUARTO edition (Q3) that included a bad quarto of *3 Henry VI* (see WHOLE CONTENTION), as part of the FALSE FOLIO (1619). While Q3 may have provided some details for the Folio text (notably in the genealogy recited in 2.2, adapted by Pavier from John STOW's chronicles), the quarto editions are chiefly of historical interest.

THEATRICAL HISTORY OF THE PLAY

No specific performances of *2 Henry VI* during Shakespeare's lifetime are recorded, but it is clear that all of the *Henry VI* plays were popular, and they were doubtless performed often. In about 1612 Ben JONSON referred to them as well-known works. The architect and designer Inigo Jones drew a costume for Jack Cade at around the same time or a little later, probably reflecting an unrecorded production. However, the earliest known performances are much later, in 1681 and 1723, and both of these were heavily reworked adaptations.

The first performance of the whole play since at least the early 17th century was given in 1864. The play has been more successful in the 20th century. F. R. BENSON (1) produced it several times, beginning in 1899. It has appeared in a number of history-play cycles, notably in two BBC TELEVISION productions: AN AGE OF KINGS (1960) and 'The Wars of the Roses' (1964), which incorporates the *Henry VI* plays and *Richard III*.

Henry VI, PART 3

SYNOPSIS

Act 1, Scene 1
The Duke of YORK (8), his sons Edward (see EDWARD IV) and Richard (see RICHARD III), and their followers discuss the first battle of ST. ALBANS, with which *2 Henry VI* closed. Richard displays the head of the Duke of SOMERSET (1), whom he killed in the previous play. York seats himself on the throne, which is present for an anticipated meeting of the king's council. The king arrives with a retinue. He restrains his followers from seeking immediate vengeance on the Yorkists, and the two sides parley. York states his claim to rule, based on the proposition that Henry had inherited a usurped crown, taken by his grandfather, HENRY IV, from RICHARD II, whose true heir York claims to be. The king counters weakly that Richard II had voluntarily given the kingdom to Henry IV. Lords CLIFFORD (1) and WARWICK (3) escalate the argument, and Warwick summons his hidden soldiers. The king, hoping to avert further violence, agrees to name York as his heir if he be permitted to retain the throne in his own lifetime. York accepts the offer and vows to refrain from rebellion. York and his men depart, satisfied. The king's supporters leave dissatisfied, expressing their disdain for the king's act. Queen MARGARET (1) and the PRINCE (4) of Wales arrive. Margaret reviles Henry for disinheriting their son the Prince, and declares herself divorced. She and the Prince depart to continue the battle against York.

Act 1, Scene 2
York's sons contend that he may properly seize the crown without violating his oath. Richard makes the case that the oath is invalid because it was not made to a proper monarch but rather to a usurper. York accepts this idea with delight and begins to plan a campaign. News arrives that Margaret's army of 20,000 men is approaching. York decides to engage the queen's army immediately, although he is outnumbered four to one.

Act 1, Scene 3
At the battle of WAKEFIELD, York's young son RUTLAND (1) is taken by Clifford, who declares that he will kill the child in revenge for his own father's death at York's hands. Rutland's pleas for mercy are ignored, and Clifford kills the boy.

Act 1, Scene 4
York appears on the battlefield and describes the courage of his sons in a losing cause. As his pursuers approach, he realises that he is doomed. Margaret and the Prince appear, accompanied by NORTHUMBERLAND (2) and Clifford. The queen mocks York for his failure. She further taunts him by giving him a handkerchief that has been dipped in Rutland's blood. As her mood grows increasingly vicious, she orders him beheaded. York responds with a long condemnation of the queen, and he weeps for the death of Rutland. Northumberland is moved to pity the captive, but the queen and Clifford stab York to death.

Act 2, Scene 1
Richard and Edward, wondering about their father's fate, see three suns in the sky, which they interpret as an omen of success. News arrives of York's capture and death, and Warwick arrives with more bad news: the duke's forces have been defeated by the queen's. However, he assures the brothers that they can still achieve victory and install Edward as king.

Act 2, Scene 2
Outside the walls of YORK (2), Margaret points out the Duke of York's head, which has been placed on the city gate; King Henry is dismayed by the sight. Clifford chastises him for being too soft, encouraging him to fight, if only for the inheritance of his son. Henry is unimpressed, arguing that evil cannot produce success. The Yorkist leaders arrive, headed by Warwick and Edward. Edward claims to be king and demands that Henry kneel to him. Margaret and Clifford respond sharply; Richard and the other lords enter the bitter argument. Henry is ignored by all. Amid a barrage of insults, the parley breaks up.

Act 2, Scene 3
At the battle of TOWTON, Warwick, wounded and exhausted, seeks rest. Edward and his brother GEORGE (2) enter and fear that the battle is lost. Richard arrives to report that Warwick's brother, slain by Clifford, had cried out with his last breath for Warwick to avenge his death. Warwick, reinvigorated, vows to return to the conflict and not rest again before winning or dying. Their morale restored, the brothers go back to the battle with him.

Act 2, Scene 4
Richard and Clifford prepare to fight hand to hand, with declarations of intended vengeance, when Warwick arrives and Clifford flees.

Act 2, Scene 5
King Henry, having withdrawn from the fighting, musingly wishes that he had been born a shepherd whose

time passes uneventfully in the company of his flock. He watches a soldier carry a body from the field in order to loot it, only to discover that his victim had been his own father. Henry, unseen, shares the devastating grief of the SON THAT HATH KILLED HIS FATHER. Another soldier, with another body and the same intent, discovers that he carries the corpse of his own son. Henry is likewise stricken with the horror that fills the FATHER THAT HATH KILLED HIS SON. Margaret and the Prince enter in full retreat from the victorious Yorkists, and they take the king with them.

Act 2, Scene 6
Clifford, wounded in the neck, regrets his own imminent death because he knows it spells disaster for the king's cause. He wishes that the king had been a stronger man, for the war would not have been necessary in that case. He faints just before Edward and his followers arrive, discussing their victory and wondering where Clifford is. They discover his body just as he dies; not realising that he is dead, they revile and taunt him. Once his death is apparent, Warwick orders that his head replace York's on the city gate. Next, Warwick says, Edward shall be crowned. Then he, Warwick, will go to FRANCE (1) and arrange Edward's marriage to the French king's sister-in-law, Lady BONA. Edward agrees, conferring on Warwick the authority to act as though he were king himself.

Act 3, Scene 1
At a game park, two KEEPERS (2) come across King Henry. He is a refugee, having fled after the battle. The Keepers accost him, and, although Henry chastises them mildly for their inconstant loyalty, he goes with them to be taken into captivity.

Act 3, Scene 2
In London, King Edward hears the plea of Lady ELIZABETH (2) Grey that her late husband's sequestered lands be returned to her. He agrees, but only on condition that she become his mistress. She refuses, and he, infatuated, declares that he will marry her. Richard, in a long soliloquy, makes a frank declaration of his intention to become king. He cynically analyses his own capacity for villainy, acknowledgeing that he will have to murder those who precede him in the order of succession.

Act 3, Scene 3
In France, Queen Margaret explains her and her deposed husband's plight to a sympathetic King LEWIS (3). Warwick arrives with Edward's proposal of marriage to Lady Bona, and Lewis, accepting Edward as king, consents. Then Edward's marriage to Elizabeth is announced. Warwick, furious at the dishonourable position this places him in, volunteers to abandon Edward's cause and ally himself with Margaret and the Earl of OXFORD in an effort to restore Henry to the throne. Lewis, seeking to avenge the insult to Bona, agrees to assist them, and an invasion is planned.

Act 4, Scene 1
George and Richard oppose the ill-considered marriage, but Edward insists that his royal prerogative negates all criticism. News of the impending invasion arrives. George's dissatisfaction comes to a boil, and he declares that he will join the rebels; he leaves, along with the Duke of SOMERSET (2). Richard declares his loyalty to Edward, after an aside confirming his true interest—the pursuit of the crown.

Act 4, Scene 2
Warwick and Oxford have landed with the invasion force. They encounter George and Somerset and accept their alliance.

Act 4, Scene 3
Warwick's forces rout the WATCHMEN (1) in Edward's camp and capture the king, although Richard escapes. Warwick plans to march to London and reinstate Henry as king.

Act 4, Scene 4
Queen Elizabeth, as Edward's wife is now known, knows of her husband's capture. Pregnant, she proposes to flee to the legal sanctuary of a church to protect the unborn Yorkist heir to the crown.

Act 4, Scene 5
Richard and others help Edward escape from captivity.

Act 4, Scene 6
Henry, released from the TOWER OF LONDON by Warwick and George, assigns his power of command to them. The young Earl of RICHMOND is present, and Henry acclaims him as a future king. Word arrives of Edward's escape, and plans are made against him. Somerset and Oxford take Richmond into exile abroad to protect him against the possibility of Edward's victory.

Act 4, Scene 7
Edward has arrived at York to find the city gates closed by the MAYOR (5), who cites the town's allegiance to Henry. Edward contends that he claims only his position as Duke of York, and he is admitted. MONTGOMERY (1) arrives with troops to support Edward, but only if he resumes his claim to the throne. Edward agrees and makes a formal assertion of kingship.

Act 4, Scene 8
Warwick deploys various of Henry's supporters to raise troops and meet him in COVENTRY. They all depart, leaving Henry to be captured by Edward and Richard, who suddenly appear on their way to meet Warwick in battle.

Act 5, Scene 1
Warwick, within the walls of Coventry, is besieged by Edward and Richard; he receives reinforcements from several noblemen. George also arrives with troops, but Richard persuades him to abandon Warwick and rejoin Edward.

Act 5, Scene 2
At the battle of BARNET, Warwick lies wounded, meditating on the insignificance of his former power now that he is near death. Oxford and Somerset, retreating, tell him that the battle is lost and that they are going to join Margaret, who has an army in the field. As they speak, Warwick dies.

Act 5, Scene 3
Edward, Richard, and George, triumphant, plan to march to TEWKESBURY and fight the queen's army.

Act 5, Scene 4
At Tewkesbury, Queen Margaret makes a stirring speech, and her courage inspires her followers. The Yorkist leaders arrive, and Edward and Margaret each make brief statements signalling the start of battle.

Act 5, Scene 5
The queen and her followers are prisoners of Edward. The Prince defies his captors, insulting Edward and his brothers, and they stab him. Richard departs for London, stating that he has important business there. Helpless, Margaret rails against the killers of her son.

Act 5, Scene 6
Richard accosts Henry in his cell in the Tower of London. Henry reviles Richard for his villainy, predicting the future tragedy he will cause many people and referring to the evil omens that accompanied his birth. Richard kills him and accepts, in a soliloquy, his own evil nature, proposing to use his capacity for crime to achieve the throne.

Act 5, Scene 7
King Edward rejoices in his resumption of power and delights in his son, the new PRINCE (5) of Wales, and in the support of his brothers. Richard's dark asides demonstrate the king's naïveté.

COMMENTARY

Like Shakespeare's other HISTORY PLAYS, *3 Henry VI* is essentially concerned with civil disorder. As the young playwright's skills matured, his handling of the theme improved, and this third play of the minor TETRALOGY marks a notable advance. Shakespeare's ability to organise a confused mass of material is superior to that in *1* and *2 Henry VI.* Also, and more important in light of his later development, his presentation of chaos includes disorder in the individual as well as in the state; malfunctions of personality underlie those of politics. The painter of tableaux and pageantry is becoming a tragedian.

The dissolution of the state is the major concern of the play, which describes the overthrow of King Henry VI, but this major theme is also reflected in minor keys. Just as the organisational principle of society, the state, is disrupted, so, too, the basic social bond of the family is disturbed. Henry disinherits his own son to purchase relief from York's threats of war, and the action sparks Margaret's unilateral declaration of divorce. The opposing clan, the Yorks, are no better off. George abandons his brother's cause after Edward turns his attentions to the relatives of his new bride. Richard plots the death of both his brothers. The theme of familial collapse is given spectacular exposure in 2.5, the scene involving the Son That Hath Killed His Father and the Father That Hath Killed His Son. Further, an abandonment of individual honesty characterises the world of the play. As Edward quite coolly asserts in 1.2.16–17, '. . . for a kingdom any oath may be broken: I would break a thousand oaths to reign one year'.

These themes, so suggestive of chaos, are developed within a regularly alternating cycle of changes of fortune, beginning and ending with the ascendancy of the house of York. Yorkist success at the outset is countered by the Lancastrian victory at Wakefield and York's ignominious death. However, Warwick rallies the Yorkists, who are victorious at Towton in Act 2. In Act 3 Edward's perfidy triggers the defection of Warwick and the consequent reinstatement of Henry as king. But the last swing of the pendulum produces the defeat and death of Warwick and Richard's murders of Henry and his heir. This easily perceived sequence imposes order on the turbulent events.

Dramatic unity is furthered by the persistence of images that reflect the violence of nature. Throughout the play, the characters refer to their conflicts in terms of the killing of animals by men, as in 1.4.61–62 and 2.4.13, or the taking of prey by animals, as in 2.1.14 and 5.6.7. Even more evocative are references to the power of tempests, such as Henry's striking description of the battle of Wakefield in 2.5.5–9 and Margaret's more elaborate nautical analogy at the beginning of 5.4. Our awareness of the brutality and viciousness of the play's action is constantly reinforced by this recurrent imagery.

Moreover, Shakespeare frequently has his characters refer to the past and predict the future—devices that serve to bring all the parts of the play to the repeated attention of the audience. For instance, in 1.1.130–133 Henry foretells the coming battles and his own death; the dying York, in 1.4.165–166, wishes upon Margaret a fate that comes to pass in 5.5. Clifford, in 2.6, summarises King Henry's hapless reign. Henry, before his murder in 5.6, predicts Richard's

future crimes. Many such allusions, both plain and subtle, reverberate throughout the play.

More important than this clever technique, however, is Shakespeare's increasing ability to make his characters much more convincing. Henry VI in particular has grown greatly as the playwright's skill has advanced. The king's gentleness is touchingly rendered in his revulsion at the sight of York's head in 2.2, in his wish to be a simple shepherd (2.5.1–54), and in his forgiving his prison guard in 4.6. However, Henry's virtue has a negative side, causing him to become more and more dissociated from his surroundings. The consequences are both subtly recorded, as when the king demands to speak but is ignored and remains speechless in 2.2, and obvious, as upon his virtual abdication in 4.6. Henry's position involves a tragic paradox: his goodness ought to be given scope by his power, but it is precisely his power that places him in the way of historical forces that goodness cannot resist. That Henry is believably both weak and good makes this situation humanly tragic as well as politically disturbing.

Queen Margaret also displays greater dimensions than in the earlier plays. The strength that enables her to organise the resistance to York is fuelled by intemperate rage. When she has York at her mercy in 1.4, her viciousness comes to the fore, and we are faced with a fearsome shrew in one of the most powerful scenes Shakespeare had yet written. Though Margaret is undeniably bloody-minded—as in 2.2, where she encourages Henry to gloat over York's severed head—she also possesses a capacity for military leadership and strength that is not without a noble appeal. Her persistence in the face of setbacks and her readiness to resume battle when the tide turns, in 3.3, makes credible her leadership in the face of final defeat at Tewkesbury. Her inspiring speech in 5.4 rings true, for we have seen that she is a real warrior.

Edward, too, is a well-developed figure. His stature as York's heir to the throne proves illusory once he is crowned, for he shows no regard for the responsibilities of kingship. He is wilful in pursuing his lust, and his behaviour brings on further civil war. In the conflict, he indulges in pointless bravado and permits himself to be captured. In 5.5.84, after the final victory, Edward casually permits Richard to murder Henry, evincing a lack of concern for civil order that will eventually result in his own victimisation in *Richard III*.

But Shakespeare's greatest accomplishment in the play is the creation of his first great villain—Richard. Richard's extraordinary personality bursts forth in 1.1, when he abruptly throws down the head of Somerset, saying, 'Speak thou for me, and tell them what I did' (1.1.16). Richard's violence is mixed with sardonic wit throughout the play. He gloats over Clifford's corpse in 2.6, his speech darkening from morbid humour to vicious rhetoric. Later, after killing Henry, Richard raises his bloody sword and sarcastically crows, 'See how my sword weeps for the poor King's death' (5.6.63). Richard is conscious of his own character, and he shares his self-awareness with the audience, enlarging our appreciation of his villainy. In his famous soliloquy at the end of 3.2, he observes that he 'can smile, and murder whiles I smile'; he associates himself with a paragon of atheism and amorality in claiming he will 'set the murderous Machiavel to school'(see MACHIAVEL). His appreciation of his own viciousness seems very modern, as does his psychological motivation: his personality is formed in part by his physical deformity, a hunched back. In 3.2.154–164, he attributes his own malevolence to this defect. Richard, established in *3 Henry VI* as mis-shapen and monstrously evil, will achieve heights of villainy in the following play in the sequence, which bears his name.

Shakespeare ties together his various strands in a spectacularly ironic final scene. The victorious Edward congratulates himself on his success, in pointed contrast to Richard's Judas kiss, which prepares us for the horrors of *Richard III.* In the final line, Edward carelessly rejoices in a future happiness that the audience knows very well to be doomed. The author has combined the consummation of his play's action with a foreshadowing of its sequel.

SOURCES OF THE PLAY

Shakespeare's main source for *3 Henry VI,* as for the other *Henry VI* plays, was *The Union of the Two Noble and Illustre Families of Lancastre and York,* by Edward HALL (2) (3rd ed., 1550). The playwright supplemented Hall's basic information with ideas from other sources, as was his habit. Most notably, the poem *Romeus and Juliet* (1562), by Arthur BROOKE (1), provided the germ of Queen Margaret's rousing speech at the beginning of 5.4, and Edmund SPENSER's *Faerie Queene* influenced the descriptions of the sun in 2.1. Minor elements can also be traced to A MIRROR FOR MAGISTRATES, a popular anthology of biographies, and to *The Spanish Tragedy* (1588–1589) and *Soliman and Perseda* (1590), plays by Thomas KYD.

TEXT OF THE PLAY

It is impossible to date the early history plays with certainty, but since all three *Henry VI* plays contain minor reflections of Edmund Spenser's *Faerie Queene,* published December 1589, they cannot have been written earlier than 1590. It is thought that the four plays of the minor tetralogy were written in the order in which they are read, and the last of them, *Richard III,* was apparently known to MARLOWE (1) by early 1592 (see RICHARD III, 'Text of the Play'); therefore, it seems likely that the four plays were composed between early 1590 and late 1591. If we assume the third of them to have been written in the third quarter of

this span of time, we may date *3 Henry VI* to the first half of 1591.

The play was first published in the form in which we know it in the FIRST FOLIO of 1623, and that text has been the basis for all subsequent editions. However, a BAD QUARTO edition, known as THE TRUE TRAGEDY, was published by Thomas MILLINGTON in 1595 and again in 1600: these editions are known as Q1 and Q2 respectively. In 1619 a third quarto edition, Q3, was published by Thomas PAVIER in the same volume with a bad quarto of *2 Henry VI.* This edition is known as the WHOLE CONTENTION. Its text for *Part 3* is very close to that of Q1. While some minor details of the Folio text of the play may have come from the quartos, these editions are chiefly of historical interest.

Scholars believe that the Folio edition was derived largely from Shakespeare's FAIR COPY, as is indicated by the presence of elaborate stage directions, along with other minor clues. The editors of the Folio probably used a copy made by a scribe, for their text includes various small adjustments of a sort known to have been common in the work of Elizabethan scribes.

THEATRICAL HISTORY OF THE PLAY

Henry VI, Part 3 seems to have been popular in Shakespeare's day, although we have no documentary evidence of any particular performances. However, the title page of *The True Tragedy* informs us that the play had been performed by PEMBROKE'S MEN before they disbanded in 1593. The play's several quarto editions indicate a continuing public interest, as does the remark made by the CHORUS (1) at the end of *Henry V* that 'oft our stage hath shown' (Epilogue, 13) the events of the *Henry VI* plays. Further, Ben JONSON, writing in about 1612, referred to these works as particularly popular.

Subsequently, however, the play has not been notably well received. Favourable critical attention in the second half of the 17th century suggests that it was still read and regarded as a successful work, but the only performances known from the period were greatly altered, containing very little of Shakespeare's text (see, e.g., CROWNE). Two such productions are also known from the 18th century. A German production of *2 Henry VI* to celebrate the tercentenary of Shakespeare's birth in 1864 seems to have provided the only performances of the 19th century. The play has been produced a number of times in the 20th century, generally in cycles with the other plays of the minor tetralogy. It has been made for TELEVISION (1983) and also incorporated in two BBC series that abridge and combine the history plays: AN AGE OF KINGS (1960) and 'The Wars of the Roses' (1964), which presents the *Henry VI* plays and *Richard III.*

Henry VIII, King of England (1491–1547) Historical figure and title character of *Henry VIII.* King Henry is nominally the protagonist of the play, but he does not create the action; rather, he is placed in a series of situations and the change in the nature of his responses—as he grows from an easily influenced tool of evil men to a wise and mature ruler—illuminates the play's themes. The play's dominant moral point concerns the importance of humanity's capacity for good, which is represented in Henry's development. On another level, the play is about the establishment of England as a Protestant country, and as such it is a celebration of the TUDOR DYNASTY. Unlike Shakespeare's other English kings (see HISTORY PLAYS), Henry is not a realistic participant in political or military events, but rather a symbol for the greatness of England.

King Henry is dramatically subordinate to other figures in each of the play's episodes, though he alone appears throughout. In Acts 1 and 2 he is manipulated by Cardinal WOLSEY. First, the cardinal deceives him about the Duke of BUCKINGHAM (1), so that he sends an innocent man to death. However, Shakespeare makes certain that we do not blame Henry. Wolsey's evident villainy and Buckingham's saintly forgiveness indicate that the king's only offence is ignorance. In 1.4 the king meets and falls in love with the virtuous ANNE (1) BULLEN, who will become the mother of ELIZABETH (1) and who, as a Protestant, anticipates the English Reformation. Henry's connection to this righteous woman prepares us to sympathise with his moral qualms about his marriage to Queen KATHERINE of Aragon. He fears his sin in marrying his brother's widow has prevented him from fathering an heir to the throne of England, and this worry makes him susceptible to Wolsey's machinations. The king is again manipulated, but this time only through his own scrupulous morality. Moreover, because Katherine's fall leads to the ascendancy of Protestantism and the birth of Elizabeth, Shakespeare's audience could be expected to find the result satisfactory. When Henry rejects the 'dilatory sloth and tricks of Rome' (2.4.235) in favour of the 'well-beloved servant CRANMER' (2.4.236)—a famous Protestant leader—we see that from the play's point of view, Henry is progressing towards wisdom.

In 3.2 Wolsey is accidentally exposed as a profiteer and an opponent of Henry's marriage to Anne, and Henry responds forcefully, though he mercifully spares the cardinal's life. Wolsey then finds atonement with God, for which he thanks the king. Henry's actions are now unmistakably a force for good, even if it has taken a providential accident to spur him.

Act 4 offers a celebration of Anne—and indirectly of the Tudors generally—along with a restatement of the mercy and forgiveness that characterise the stories of Katherine and Wolsey. These themes further free Henry from blame, in a general atmosphere of blessedness. In Act 5 Henry's actions in support of good are taken on his own initiative, as he preserves

Cranmer from the wiles of Bishop GARDINER (1), Wolsey's successor as villain. Here we see the culmination of Henry's development. He is now a wise and masterful ruler, capable of foiling the evil intentions of Catholic sympathisers and preserving the Reformation's most important leader. It is at this pinnacle of maturity that Henry, in the play's finale, can pass on to the infant Elizabeth a virtuous realm and the prospect of prosperity for England.

The historical Henry VIII was far from the wise, benevolent, and virtuous ruler Shakespeare depicts. Shakespeare de-emphasised Henry's ruthlessness and altered history in order to refocus the play on the themes of forgiveness and mercy. Only a small segment of Henry's reign is dealt with. His expensive, inconclusive wars and his court's wasteful extravagance are not mentioned, and the vicious despotism of his later years is ignored. The future execution of Anne Boleyn (as Anne is known to history) is not so much as hinted at, nor is the existence of Henry's other ill-fated wives.

At the time of his accession in 1509, Henry was an intelligent and well-educated young man who was determined to be a good king. However, his egocentric desire to be a chivalric hero led him to wars and extravagance. He wasted the considerable treasury amassed by his father, the highly competent Henry VII (see RICHMOND), and left his successors with a serious debt problem. Moreover, he was a brutally tyrannical ruler, inclined to suspect treason without cause and to punish without mercy, especially as he got older. In contrast to the play, Henry probably ordered the trumped-up execution of Buckingham, for he feared that the duke, a distant relative, might try to seize the throne. Similarly, he beheaded the last PLANTAGENET (1), 68-year-old Margaret (the GIRL of *Richard III*), simply because she was a theoretical rival.

The divorce of Katherine of Aragon was also Henry's idea, and he was much less kind to his long-time wife than in the play. Katherine, however, was permitted to live out her life in peace; the king was less considerate of his later wives. Anne soon fell victim to Henry's need for a male heir. Henry was already involved with his next wife-to-be when Anne's second pregnancy ended in stillbirth. The king arranged false charges of adultery, incest (with a brother), and treason, and within weeks—less than three years after her coronation—Anne was beheaded. Henry was to marry five other wives, one of whom was also executed. His viciousness extended to others as well: he often chose execution as a punishment for failure or opposition. Thomas CROMWELL and Sir Thomas MORE were among his victims.

The king's behaviour in his later years has often been diagnosed as psychotic. Although this diagnosis is hypothetical, Henry VIII was undeniably a violent and arbitrary ruler. Shakespeare and his contemporaries, however, had a very positive image of Elizabeth's father: he was a national hero who had led England to Protestantism and freed the country from the corrupt influence of the Vatican. This view was widely disseminated by the historians of the Tudor dynasty, including Shakespeare's chief source for the play, HOLINSHED's *Chronicles.* From the playwright's point of view, the title character of *Henry VIII* is a perfectly plausible historical figure.

Henry VIII

SYNOPSIS

Prologue

The PROLOGUE (4) disclaims any attempt at humour. The play, he says, will be serious, full of important issues and unhappiness. Its noble scenes will inspire pity and also present the truth. For those who simply like a splendid show, it will prove satisfying. But it will not be a frivolous play, with foolery and fighting. The audience should prepare to be sad, for they will see great and noble people fall upon misery.

Act 1, Scene 1

The Duke of NORFOLK (3) tells the Duke of BUCKINGHAM (1) about the recent meeting in FRANCE (1) between King HENRY VIII and the French ruler. The two courts competed in displaying their wealth, and elaborate jousts were held. Norfolk notes that Cardinal WOLSEY arranged the meeting. Lord ABERGAVENNY joins the conversation, and the three men criticise Wolsey, especially for having seized too much power over England's affairs. They declare that the peace he negotiated with France is no good, for France is still seizing English trade goods. Norfolk, who has heard that Buckingham is feuding with Wolsey, warns him that his foe is dangerous. Wolsey himself arrives and exchanges glares with Buckingham. He speaks with his SECRETARY about a pending interview with Buckingham's SURVEYOR, or overseer, and declares that its results will cut the duke down to size. When he leaves, Buckingham rages against him, accusing him of treason. He asserts that the cardinal deliberately negotiated a weak treaty with France after being bribed by the Holy Roman Emperor, who feared a genuine peace between France and England. BRANDON (1) appears and arrests Buckingham and Abergavenny for treason; Buckingham says that his Surveyor has doubtless been bribed.

Act 1, Scene 2

At a meeting of his council, the king thanks Wolsey for having suppressed Buckingham's conspiracy. The queen, KATHERINE of Aragon, arrives and speaks on behalf of the people against the unjust taxes introduced by Wolsey. Norfolk adds that uprisings are occurring as a result. The king, who knows nothing of

these taxes, orders Wolsey to invalidate them and pardon the rebels. In an aside the cardinal instructs his Secretary to issue these orders but to make it seem as though the relief came from him. Queen Katherine regrets the arrest of Buckingham, and King Henry suggests she hear the evidence. Buckingham's Surveyor is brought in and testifies that Buckingham had planned to become king if Henry died. Katherine doubts his testimony, but he goes on, reporting that the duke spoke of killing Wolsey and the king. Convinced, Henry rages against Buckingham.

Act 1, Scene 3
The Lord CHAMBERLAIN (2), Lord SANDS, and Sir Thomas LOVELL (2) jest about the recent, deplorable rise of the French influence in manners and clothes. They then leave for a dinner being given by Wolsey, praising the cardinal's bountiful table.

Act 1, Scene 4
The guests gather at Wolsey's banquet and jest bawdily with the young women there. On his arrival Wolsey encourages his guests to drink and enjoy one another. The Lord Chamberlain introduces a group of masquers (see MASQUE) who, dressed as shepherds, dance with the women. One of them is King Henry, who is clearly attracted to his partner. After the dance, the Lord Chamberlain introduces her to him as ANNE (1) BULLEN, one of the queen's ladies-in-waiting.

Act 2, Scene 1
On a street in LONDON, a GENTLEMAN (14) meets a friend, who tells him of Buckingham's trial and conviction. Presuming that Wolsey was behind the duke's fall, the Gentlemen discuss the cardinal's political manoeuvrings. They remark that Wolsey is as hated by the common people as Buckingham is beloved. Buckingham then appears, under guard, and makes a speech, forgiving his enemies and asking for his friends' prayers. He compares himself to his father, who was also betrayed by a servant and unjustly killed as a traitor. After he leaves for his execution, the Gentlemen rue his fate. They go on to talk of a rumour that Wolsey's next victim will be Queen Katherine. The king, they say, has been incited to divorce her by Wolsey, who seeks to embarrass the Holy Roman Emperor—Katherine's nephew—who refused Wolsey an archbishopric he wanted. Another cardinal, CAMPEIUS, has come from ROME, allegedly to oversee the divorce.

Act 2, Scene 2
The Lord Chamberlain discusses the king's possible divorce with Norfolk and the Duke of SUFFOLK (1). They, too, see the influence of Wolsey. They hope the king will come to his senses, remember the virtues of his 20-year marriage, and recognise the cardinal for the schemer he is. After the Lord Chamberlain leaves, the dukes approach the king, who is reading. He is angry at their interruption but welcomes the arrival of Wolsey and Campeius. Norfolk and Suffolk leave, muttering curses at Wolsey. Henry then confers briefly with his secretary, GARDINER (1), and Wolsey informs Campeius that Gardiner will do whatever he, Wolsey, tells him to. Henry sends Gardiner with a message to the queen and announces that a hearing will be convened on the divorce question.

Act 2, Scene 3
Anne Bullen, talking with an OLD LADY, pities the queen and says it would be better to be born poor than to be queen and subject to injustice and rejection. The Old Lady accuses her of hypocrisy and asserts, with bawdy quibbles, that she herself would gladly give up virginity for a crown. Anne declares that she would not. The Lord Chamberlain appears and announces the king's gift to Anne of a rich estate and title; she receives the news with great modesty, and the Chamberlain praises her in an aside. After he leaves, the Old Lady chortles over the gift, predicting that Anne will soon be a duchess. Anne, however, is offended and thinks again of the unfortunate queen.

Act 2, Scene 4
After a grand procession and formal proclamations by a CRIER, the divorce proceedings begin. Addressing Henry, Katherine argues that she has always been a good and faithful wife. When Wolsey and Campeius object to her personal remarks, she replies that she refuses to be judged by an enemy. She demands a hearing from the pope and leaves. Henry, while praising her, also declares Wolsey innocent of any enmity towards her or any influence on himself. He asserts that he fears that his marriage is sinful because Katherine was once married to his elder brother. Though the church approved his marriage to Katherine at the time, he wants another ruling, to clear his conscience. Campeius declares an adjournment until the queen can be made to attend. In an aside Henry deplores these formalities and wishes his adviser CRANMER were present to expedite matters.

Act 3, Scene 1
Wolsey and Campeius visit Katherine and suggest that she abandon her defence and accept the king's decision to avoid the scandal of a divorce trial. Raging at them, she decries her helplessness but finally subsides into acceptance.

Act 3, Scene 2
Norfolk, Suffolk, Lord SURREY (5), and the Lord Chamberlain discuss Wolsey's downfall: Henry has learned that the cardinal secretly opposed the divorce (now completed) and did not wish the king to marry the virtuous Anne Bullen. But Henry has secretly done so and plans to make her queen; moreover, Wolsey's enemy, Cranmer, has been appointed Archbishop of Canterbury. Wolsey appears, seeming troubled, and muses in an aside that he intends to

see the king marry a French duchess and not Anne Bullen. The king arrives and tells the noblemen that Wolsey has mistakenly included personal financial records among state papers sent to the king. Henry is shocked at the cardinal's wealth. He approaches Wolsey and sardonically praises him for putting his duty above personal gain. After giving him a folder of papers, Henry leaves angrily with the noblemen. When Wolsey sees that the papers include his records and his letters opposing the divorce, he realises that all is lost. The noblemen return and recite a long series of formal charges against him, adding that the king has ordered all his possessions confiscated. They leave and the cardinal soliloquises on his loss of greatness, comparing it to humanity's common end in death. He now recognises the futility of his pride and riches. When his follower CROMWELL approaches him, Wolsey declares that his downfall has led him to a fresh, healthier view of life. His conscience is finally free, and he has the fortitude to withstand whatever earthly miseries may be in store. Cromwell grieves for his master's downfall, but Wolsey encourages him to serve as an adviser to the king. For himself, he regrets not having given as much energy to religion as to the state.

Act 4, Scene 1

The two Gentlemen meet again, at the coronation parade of Queen Anne. A grand procession passes by, including Suffolk, Norfolk, and Surrey—all now high officers of the realm—as well as the new queen. A Third Gentleman, who has seen the actual coronation, describes the ceremony in great detail. The discussion turns to political gossip: Gardiner, who is now Bishop of Winchester, is an enemy of Archbishop Cranmer, but the latter has a new and powerful ally in Cromwell, who is a close adviser of the king.

Act 4, Scene 2

At KIMBOLTON, Katherine learns of Wolsey's death from her attendant, GRIFFITH. According to Griffith, the cardinal repented before his death and died at peace with God. When Katherine speaks bitterly of Wolsey, Griffith offers a charitable view of him, describing him as an excellent public servant who, though greedy for wealth, was also generous with his ill-gotten gains—founding two colleges, for instance. Katherine, who is near death, thanks Griffith for pointing to the Christian viewpoint. She falls asleep and sees a vision, which appears on-stage: six dancing figures ceremoniously present her with garlands of bay leaves. When she awakes, her waiting-woman PATIENCE observes that she is near death. She then receives a visitor, Lord CAPUCHIUS, the ambassador to England from her nephew the emperor. She asks him to take King Henry a letter, in which she asks to be remembered to their daughter and requests that he treat her followers and servants well. She then retires to bed, prepared to die.

Act 5, Scene 1

Bishop Gardiner meets Lovell in the middle of the night and learns that Queen Anne is in labour and may die. Gardiner hopes she does and insists, over Lovell's objection, that for them and their allies, it would be best if Anne, Cranmer, and Cromwell were all dead. He adds that he believes he has brought the king's council to move against Archbishop Cranmer's Protestant opinions. The council will interrogate the archbishop in the morning. After Gardiner leaves, the king arrives and meets Cranmer, whom he has sent for. Though Lovell tries to eavesdrop, the king orders him away. Henry tells Cranmer that he will have enemies at the council meeting in the morning. Cranmer declares that he has nothing to fear, but Henry warns him against false witnesses. Observing that the council may try to gaol him, he gives him a ring to signify the king's protection. Cranmer leaves, and Anne's companion the Old Lady arrives to inform the king that he has a daughter. She first comically identifies the infant as a boy and then complains about the size of the tip the king gives her.

Act 5, Scene 2

Cranmer arrives for the council meeting but, insultingly, is kept waiting outside. Doctor BUTTS brings the king to an upper room, where he can watch the proceedings. After Cranmer is admitted, the CHANCELLOR accuses him of spreading heresies; Gardiner adds that severe treatment is called for, lest civil disorders arise from the heresy, like the religious wars then raging in Germany. Although Cranmer asserts his opposition to civil disorder, Gardiner insists that he must be imprisoned. Cromwell says Gardiner is too harsh, and Gardiner accuses him of involvement in heresy himself. The Chancellor then orders Cranmer to prison, but the archbishop produces the king's ring. His enemies are dumbfounded, realising that the king has stymied them. The king then emerges from his vantage point and castigates them mercilessly. He confirms his support for Cranmer by asking him to baptise his daughter.

Act 5, Scene 3

On the day of the christening the PORTER (4) and his MAN (3) are unable to prevent a crowd of celebrating commoners from invading the palace courtyard. They make comical remarks about the riotous celebrants.

Act 5, Scene 4

A grand procession escorts the infant ELIZABETH (1). It is led by the GARTER, who recites a prayer for her. Cranmer addresses the assembled court, predicting a great future for the child and happiness for the coun-

try. The king thanks him and declares the day a holiday for all.

Epilogue
An actor asserts that people may criticise the play for various reasons, but that all must concede that it has glorified good women, and so he supposes it will get applause, for no men will withhold it when their ladies prompt them.

COMMENTARY

Henry VIII, though classed with the HISTORY PLAYS, treats English history in a very different way. The play does not realistically enact a political conflict, as the other history plays do. Rather, it is a symbolic tribute to the TUDOR DYNASTY, presented in the manner of Shakespeare's other late plays, the ROMANCES. Like these plays, it uses an episodic plot line, studded with spectacles and tableaus, and closes with the promise of a new generation. Moreover, *Henry VIII* makes the same moral point as the romances—that humanity depends on divine providence, which requires that we exercise our capacity for good through a steadfast spirit, mercy, and forgiveness. The play celebrates King Henry VIII's attainment of wisdom and the country's simultaneous rejection of the authority of Catholic Rome, but Henry does not guide the play's development so much as he is simply its leading figure. A national myth is embodied in *Henry VIII*—that England is chosen by providence for Protestant freedom—and it is Henry who leads the country there. The final tableau confirms Henry's virtues in those predicted for his daughter Elizabeth, the last and greatest of Tudor monarchs. In the earlier history plays, the qualities of the characters, good and bad, generated events; here, history is driven by destiny.

As in the romantic literature on which Shakespeare's last plays were based, the rise or fall of great personages is displayed in a series of brief, almost actionless scenes that enact a pattern of loss and regeneration. Buckingham (1) is executed and Queen Katherine humiliated because of the Cardinal Wolsey's enmity; then Wolsey is exposed and discredited. Anne Bullen (better known today as Anne Boleyn) is crowned, and Cromwell and Cranmer assume high office. Finally, Cranmer's enemies—led by Wolsey's one-time underling, Bishop Gardiner—are confounded. All these events are given significance in relation to the growth of Henry. The king is easily deceived by Wolsey about Buckingham, and his moral qualms about his first marriage help Wolsey bring about the fall of Katherine. Although the intervention of chance is necessary to expose the cardinal, the king then masterfully subdues him. The king recognises good in the virtuous—and Protestant—Anne, despite Wolsey's attempts to keep her from him, and the king's maturing wisdom contributes to the rise of Cromwell and Cranmer, two fine men, the latter an important Protestant religious hero. Finally, the king saves Cranmer from Gardiner's machinations. When the monarch has thus arrived at a summit of wisdom and maturity, he brings forth a glorious successor in Elizabeth, who is rhapsodically praised by Cranmer in 5.4. Cranmer's eulogy even extends to the monarch ruling at the time the play was written, Elizabeth's successor, King JAMES I.

Henry VIII also resembles the romances in its use of pageantry. The play opens with a description of elaborate ceremonies and closes with the enactment of one. Between the opening and the close there are several spectacular tableaus, often with heavily descriptive stage directions that indicate their importance to the play. These episodes are more than mere entertainment, however. In the first half of the play, they demonstrate the effects of evil on the play's world; in the second, they evidence the exaltation of its recovery from evil.

In 1.1 the meeting of monarchs in France is described in terms that convey greed and corruption. One side's display resembles 'heathen gods' (1.1.19); the other then makes 'a fool and beggar' (1.1.28) of its competitor. The women 'almost sweat to bear' (1.1.24) their jewelry. Most significant, 'these fierce vanities' (1.1.54) are associated with the villainies of Wolsey; moreover, the treaty being celebrated is shown to be worthless. In 1.4 the cardinal's banquet offers an aura of decadence, especially in the risqué conversation before the king's masque, which is important to our sense of Wolsey's evil effect on the court. (On the other hand, the masque, during which Henry falls in love with Anne—a development that counters Wolsey's evil—is a lovely, ordered dance.) In 2.1 Buckingham is solemnly led to execution with 'tipstaves before him, the axe with the edge towards him, halberds on each side' (2.1.53, stage direction); the grandeur of the play's world becomes increasingly ominous. An extremely elaborate stage direction at the opening of 2.4 describes in detail the panoply of Katherine's divorce trial. Particularly gaudy is the ecclesiastical pomp of the two cardinals, clad in their scarlet robes and escorted by 'two Gentlemen bearing two great silver pillars'. However, their rich display cannot help the king, who is attempting to rectify a sin that has deprived the nation of an heir to the throne. As the scene ends, Henry rejects the 'dilatory sloth and tricks of Rome' (2.4.235) in favour of the 'well-beloved' (2.4.236) Cranmer. Here, the play's luxuriant splendour is associated with Catholicism, but the path of recovery is evident.

After Wolsey's downfall and the revelation that Anne is to become queen in Act 3, we again find spectacle in Act 4, but now the association is entirely posi-

tive. In 4.1 a complex, 10-part stage direction presents the coronation procession. The Gentlemen remark on the participants, including Anne: '. . . the sweetest face I ever look'd on . . . an angel' (4.1.43–44). The Third Gentleman then provides a description of another ritual ceremony, the actual coronation, in entirely positive terms. The splendid and spectacular are now associated with the good of England and the triumph of virtue. Although Katherine's vision in 4.2 is in a very different key, it, too, is presented in great detail; it is also entertaining on stage and distinctly linked with virtue, in this case more personal and religious. Lastly, there is another procession preceding Cranmer's speech at Elizabeth's christening. This sumptuous parade provides a fitting culmination to the play's use of ceremony and ritual as expressions of moral tone. Here, the triumph of virtue is confirmed in another formal display of religion, but this time it is a Protestant religion—a distinction immediately evident to Shakespeare's audience, through costume as well as Cranmer's presence.

Divine intervention underlies the play's developments. In the first half this is clear in the way chance brings Anne to the king's attention and exposes Wolsey. It is also evident in the forgiving attitude and acceptance of God's will of Wolsey's victims. In the second half of the play, the religious theme becomes prominent, limiting the importance of personality among the play's chief characters. Henry demonstrates the significance of personal growth—the wisdom and maturity he attains in the course of the play are necessary to its happy conclusion—but he simply displays differing outlooks, without going through a process of internal development.

More striking as personalities are the 'tragic' characters, who embody the importance of patiently accepting fate. However, they are restricted in emotional range, precisely to emphasise their thematic significance. Buckingham, Katherine, and Cardinal Wolsey appear only briefly before meeting their fates; they achieve importance only at their downfalls, when they respond to adversity with dignity and wisdom.

Upon his arrest, Buckingham's anger against Wolsey—his only trait so far—disappears, and he simply says, 'The will of heav'n / Be done . . . I obey' (1.1. 209–210). In this he is supported by his fellow victim, Abergavenny. On his way to be executed in 2.1, Buckingham forgives his enemies and accepts his downfall as a blessing. Though he reveals some bitterness in recollecting his father's similar fate, he controls it and departs with a prayer: 'I have done, and God forgive me' (2.1.136).

Queen Katherine's conduct at her trial—her dignity as she presents her case, her fire as she turns against Wolsey, and her resolute departure—is truly impressive. Even when she recognises defeat, she finds powerful poetry to express it: 'like the lily / That once was mistress of the field and flourish'd, / I'll hang my head and perish' (3.1.152–153). (This episode is introduced with the SONG 'Orpheus with his lute' [3.1.3–14], which in its union of mysticism and music is a typical ploy of Shakespearean romances.) Perhaps most important is Katherine's joint demonstration, with Griffith, of forgiveness towards Wolsey. In her mild way, the deposed and dying queen is bitter towards her enemy, but after Griffith's recital of the cardinal's hidden virtues, she confirms that 'religious truth and modesty' require her declaration, 'peace be with him' (4.2.74, 75). She approaches her death 'meditating / On that celestial harmony I go to' (4.2.79–80). Her vision adds supernatural sanction to our impression of her virtues, as well as reinforcing the importance of divine intervention in the play's world.

Most significant, the play's only important villain, Wolsey, makes a similar demonstration of acceptance. Once his downfall is certain, in 3.2, the cardinal recognises the futility of his struggle for wealth and power, and rejects the 'Vain pomp and glory of this world' (3.2.365). Free from the temptations of intrigue and ambition, he finds 'A peace above all earthly dignities, / A still and quiet conscience' (3.2.379–380), and he thanks the king, who has overthrown him, for his newly found 'fortitude of soul' (3.2.388). He considerately advises Cromwell on both worldly advancement and spiritual health, before departing from the court with the wish that he had 'but serv'd my God with half the zeal / I serv'd my king' (3.2.455–456). In 4.2 Griffith repeats the lesson in describing the cardinal's death: 'His overthrow heap'd happiness upon him, / For then, . . . [he] found the blessedness of being little / And . . . died fearing God' (4.2.63–68). Thus, Wolsey's end, like those of Buckingham and Katherine, points to the ultimate superiority of the divine over the mundane. The eulogies Shakespeare provides for the cardinal are all the more important when we consider what a departure they were from the standard English view of his day. For most English Protestants of the 16th and 17th centuries, Wolsey was a chief villain of pre-Reformation English Catholicism; to present him as a recipient of God's mercy was to make mercy a prominent theme indeed.

Like the romances, *Henry VIII* stresses the triumph of good and the importance of patience in adversity, elevating these propositions by placing them in a schematic plot in which it is clear that God controls all. However, unlike the romances, the plan is set in an historical world, one still very well known to the play's original audience. It is not only a moral tale of suffering borne with dignity, it is a national myth. Here the regenerative pattern of the romances is employed to display the redemption of a particular country at a particular time—England as it acquired the state church—and the anti-Catholic stance—with which its people largely identified in Shakespeare's time. In the

spirit of the romances, this process yields great optimism: old errors are expiated in an atmosphere of reconciliation, and the future offers the promise of a new generation. The providence that lends strength to the allegorical characters of *Pericles, Cymbeline, The Winter's Tale,* and *The Tempest* is here devoted to an entire people. *Henry VIII* is history in a romantic mode.

SOURCES OF THE PLAY

Shakespeare's principal source for most of *Henry VIII* was Raphael HOLINSHED's *Chronicles of England, Scotland, and Ireland* (Second edition, 1587), supplemented by the account of Henry's reign in *The Union of the Two Noble and Illustre Families of Lancaster and York* (1548) by Edward HALL (2). However, for the trial of Cranmer in 5.1–2, the playwright relied on John FOXE's *Book of Martyrs* (1563).

TEXT OF THE PLAY

Since 1850, Shakespeare's authorship of *Henry VIII* has been disputed. Some scholars have thought the play was too badly organised to be the work of a single author and have attributed much of the play to John FLETCHER (2). Some go so far as to hold that Shakespeare did not write any of it, ascribing it to Fletcher and Philip MASSINGER. The question is still argued, but increasingly scholarly opinion tends to find the play wholly Shakespearean for a variety of reasons. For one, the FIRST FOLIO editors accepted *Henry VIII* while rejecting the plays known to be Fletcher-Shakespeare collaborations (*The Two Noble Kinsmen* and CARDENIO). Moreover, the use of sources seems consistent throughout the play, and it is different from Fletcher's practise elsewhere. Finally, the 'disorganisation' of *Henry VIII* seems less significant if one compares the play with Shakespeare's contemporary romances, which are intentionally episodic, rather than with his histories, which are more narrative in structure.

Henry VIII was written between late 1612 and June 1613, when the GLOBE THEATRE burned down during a performance of it. (A report of this event calls the play ALL IS TRUE, apparently a subtitle.) By its style *Henry VIII* can be identified as a very late work, so it was probably written not long before this performance. It may have been composed specifically for the celebration of the marriage of the Princess ELIZABETH (3) in February 1613, as is suggested by its patriotism and its particular attention to the princess' namesake. In any case, its suitability for Elizabeth's marriage also made it an appropriate offering to the public that spring. In sum, most commentators agree that it was first performed in early 1613 and written not long before.

Henry VIII was first published in the First Folio (1623). The text derives from the author's FOUL PAPERS (or possibly from the FAIR COPY made by a professional scribe), for it has elaborate and literary stage directions (some taken directly from source material), which would have been abbreviated in a PROMPT-BOOK. The Folio offers the only early text and has therefore been the basis for all subsequent editions.

THEATRICAL HISTORY OF THE PLAY

As already noted, *Henry VIII* may have been first performed as part of the festivities celebrating the marriage of Princess Elizabeth in the winter of 1612–1613. However, it is not in the list of 14 Shakespeare plays staged by the KING'S MEN during the winter's wedding festivities (though it may have been the play cancelled due to scheduling conflicts on February 16). The earliest recorded performance (but clearly not the first) was on June 29, 1613, when cannon fire—called for in the stage direction at 1.4.49—set fire to the thatched roof of the Globe and burned the theatre to the ground. A tradition first reported in 1708 held that John LOWIN was the original Henry and 'had his instructions' from Shakespeare himself, which suggests that the playwright may have directed the production. One other early staging is known: a private performance in July 1628, commissioned by King Charles I's favourite, George Villiers, Duke of Buckingham. Though no relation to the play's Buckingham, Villiers reportedly left the performance after the duke is led away to be executed in 2.1. (He was himself assassinated a few weeks later.)

After the reopening of the London theatres following 18 years of revolutionary government, *Henry VIII* was staged by William DAVENANT in 1664, with Thomas BETTERTON as King Henry and Henry HARRIS (2) as Wolsey; Samuel PEPYS saw it, but his account of a play about Henry 'with all his wives' suggests that it may have been considerably altered by Davenant. It was recorded as a 'stock play' for Davenant's company over the next few decades, though no specific performance was noted. It then disappeared for a generation.

In 1716 it was revived by Colley CIBBER (1), who produced it frequently during the next decade and added increasingly spectacular scenic effects, especially for the coronation procession in 4.1. Appropriately, Cibber presented the play at the coronation of King George II in 1727. Barton BOOTH (1) played the title role in Cibber's presentations.

The coronation procession from *Henry VIII* was often performed separately in the middle of the 18th century, as part of a programme of pantomimes or even along with other plays. David GARRICK continued the trend to spectacle—his production, revived many times between 1742 and 1768—required 140 actors in 4.1. Other elements were cut to make time for this one, most notably the vision of Queen Katherine in 4.2. Garrick played Henry opposite the Queen Katherine of Hannah PRITCHARD.

After a 20-year hiatus, J. P. KEMBLE (3) revived *Henry VIII* in 1788, with his sister Sarah SIDDONS as Queen Katherine, a role for which she was particularly acclaimed throughout her career. Kemble himself played Cromwell (to whom he assigned Griffith's part, as well). After 1803, as manager of the Covent Garden Theatre, Kemble revived the play numerous times, often playing Wolsey, and after his retirement in 1817, his younger brother Charles KEMBLE (1) continued the tradition. In 1830 Charles' daughter Fanny KEMBLE (2), though only 20 years old, was successful as Queen Katherine.

Henry VIII naturally appealed to the 19th-century taste for spectacle, and the next notable production, that of Charles KEAN (1) in 1855, was probably the most elaborate. His 5.4 opened with (in his words) 'the Lord Mayor and City Council proceeding to the royal ceremonial in their state barges, to give a panoramic view [on a moving backdrop] of London, as it then appeared'. He managed nonetheless to restore material often dropped from earlier productions, such as the role of Griffith and Katherine's vision (in which Ellen TERRY [1], as a small child, played an angel in a revival of 1858). Henry IRVING staged *Henry VIII* in 1892, with Terry as Katherine, Irving himself as Wolsey, and Johnston FORBES-ROBERTSON as Buckingham. Irving's production was no less sumptuous than its predecessors, and it was wildly popular.

In the 20th century, the popularity of *Henry VIII* has waned somewhat, but a number of notable productions have been staged. Beerbohm TREE presented the play in a characteristically extravagant adaptation that cut Act 5 entirely. This spectacular, starring Tree as Wolsey, was a hit in London (1910) and New York (1916). Sir Lewis CASSON produced the play with Sybil THORNDIKE as Katherine in 1925. Margaret WEBSTER (3) presented it in New York in 1946, as the inaugural production of the American Repertory Company, with Eva Le Gallienne (b. 1899) as Katherine. Tyrone GUTHRIE has staged it three times: in 1933 at SADLER'S WELLS THEATRE, with Charles LAUGHTON in the title role; in 1949 at STRATFORD, with Anthony QUAYLE as Henry; and at the OLD VIC THEATRE in 1953, in honour of the coronation of Queen Elizabeth II. Michael BENTHALL's OLD VIC (1958) production starred John GIELGUD as Wolsey and Edith EVANS (1) as Katherine.

Tree's 1910 production of *Henry VIII* was the basis for a brief silent FILM made in 1911, but since only five scenes were filmed, over a period of only two hours including rehearsals, it is fair to say that *Henry VIII* has not yet been produced as a movie. It was made for TELEVISION in 1979, with Claire Bloom (b. 1931) as Queen Katherine.

Henryson, Robert (c. 1430–before 1506) Scottish poet, author of a poem known to Shakespeare as part of Geoffrey CHAUCER's long poem *Troilus and Criseyde*, a chief source for *Troilus and Cressida*. Henryson's *Testament of Cresseid* continued Chaucer's story. Although it is written in a Scots dialect, Henryson's poem, like Chaucer's, is written in RHYME ROYAL, and for centuries it was regarded as Chaucer's work. In every edition of *Troilus and Criseyde* from 1532 to 1710, it was published as part of the poem. In Henryson's sequel to the story, CRESSIDA is stricken with leprosy as a punishment for her faithlessness and TROILUS gives her alms without recognising her. This development is referred to in *Henry V* (2.1.76) and *Twelfth Night* (3.1.56), so we know that Shakespeare had read Henryson, but oddly it is not mentioned in *Troilus and Cressida*, unless Cressida's future status as a beggar is alluded to in Troilus' pained complaint that the 'orts of her love, / The fragments, scraps, the bits, and greasy relics / Of her o'er-eaten faith are given to Diomed' (5.2.157–159).

Henslowe, Philip (d. 1616) English theatrical entrepreneur, owner of the ROSE, FORTUNE, and HOPE THEATRES and the keeper of a record book that has survived as a principal source on ELIZABETHAN and JACOBEAN THEATRE. Henslowe, the son of a gamekeeper, was a servant to the bailiff of a nobleman in the 1570s. He married the bailiff's widow and thereby acquired the money to establish himself in business. He was first a dyer, then a pawnbroker and a dealer in real estate, mostly in SOUTHWARK, just across the Thames River from LONDON. In 1585 he leased a plot of land there, upon which he built the Rose Theatre, which opened in 1588. In 1592 his step-daughter married the great actor William ALLEYN, who became Henslowe's partner. His company, the ADMIRAL'S MEN, played at the Rose for most of the rest of the century, making theatrical history while also making Henslowe and Alleyn rich. Henslowe also had other theatrical properties. By 1594 he either owned or leased the theatre at NEWINGTON BUTTS, and he and Alleyn bought a licence to put on bull- and bear-baiting entertainments, a profitable sideline. In 1600 he and Alleyn built the FORTUNE THEATRE, to which the Admiral's Men moved, while the Rose was abandoned when its ground lease expired. In 1613 Henslowe tore down the old animal-baiting arena and built the HOPE THEATRE, where various companies played, financed by Henslowe. These arrangements resulted in a lawsuit of 1615, in the records of which Henslowe is shown to have had a reputation as a tough businessman. However, his relations with theatrical companies seem otherwise to have been mostly good.

Henslowe's *Diary*, as the collection of his papers is called—though it is actually an account book—covers the years 1592 to 1603, recording the performances at the Rose through 1597 and the revenues each earned, as well as the loans and advances that Henslowe made to acting companies (mostly the Admiral's Men) and

to individual players, for he was essentially a banker to them. Henslowe bought the plays the Admiral's Men performed, as well as their costumes and props, all of which are recorded in the *Diary.* He was repaid—with great interest—from the company's share of the playhouse revenues. His papers were inherited by Alleyn, who left them in the collections at Dulwich College, where they were forgotten until Edmond MALONE discovered them in 1790.

Herald (1) Minor character in *2 Henry VI,* a messenger from the king summoning the Duke of GLOUCESTER (4) to a meeting of Parliament in 2.4.70.

Herald (2) Either of two minor characters in *Richard II,* petty officials at the trial by combat between BOLINGBROKE (1) and MOWBRAY (1) in 1.3. Each Herald cries out a formal statement of purpose for one contestant.

Herald (3) Either of two minor characters in *King John,* the respective representatives of King JOHN (3) of England and King PHILIP (2) of FRANCE (1), to the city of ANGIERS in 2.1. Each Herald formally proclaims the victory of his King in the preceding skirmish and demands that the city declare its loyalty to that ruler and open its gates to his soldiers. The symmetrical opposition of the Heralds emphasises the difficulty in resolving competing claims to power, an important theme of the play.

Herald (4) Minor character in *Henry V,* a messenger who brings King HENRY V a written account of the French fatalities at AGINCOURT. The Herald speaks only one line.

Herald (5) Character in *Othello.* See GENTLEMAN (6).

Herald (6) Minor character in *King Lear,* an official at the duel in which EDGAR kills EDMUND. In 5.3.110–116 the Herald announces to the troops of ALBANY, GONERIL, and REGAN that Edmund will defend himself against any challenger who dares to assert that 'he is a manifould traitor' (5.3.112), as Albany has said someone intends to do. When Edgar, disguised, appears, the Herald formally asks him to identify himself, though once Edgar replies his answer is taken up by Albany and Edmund, and the Herald is not heard from again. His small part helps create a sense of chivalrous order to the final retribution upon Edmund.

Herald (7) Minor character in *Coriolanus.* In 2.1 the Herald accompanies the army's return into ROME, and formally announces that Caius MARTIUS (2) has been awarded a new name. In honour of his extraordinary bravery in taking the city of CORIOLES, he is to be known henceforth as CORIOLANUS. The Herald speaks five grandiose lines and concludes with the cry, 'Welcome to Rome, renowned Coriolanus!' (2.1.165), that is repeated by the assembled crowd. Shakespeare provided the Herald to lend an air of pomp and circumstance to Coriolanus' reception. This heightens the dramatic irony when this same reception turns ugly later in the same act.

Herald (8) Minor character in *The Two Noble Kinsmen,* an attendant to Duke THESEUS (2) of ATHENS. In 1.4, following the defeat of King Creon of THEBES, the Herald informs Theseus of the identity of two of his noble prisoners of war, ARCITE and PALAMON, the title characters of the play. The main plot is thereby begun. The Herald is an extra, whose splendid official uniform provides colour, if not authenticity, to a scene of ancient warfare.

Herbert (1), Henry (1595–1673) Longtime MASTER OF REVELS for King JAMES I and King Charles I. Herbert was a minor nobleman, a cousin of the Earls of PEMBROKE (1, 2, 3) and brother of the famed poet George Herbert (1593–1633). Beginning in 1622 Herbert leased the office of Master of Revels—licenser of theatrical productions and publications—from its appointed holder, Sir John Ashley (d. 1641), a minor courtier. He paid £150 a year and collected for himself the many fees that were paid to the Master. Though Herbert was nominally the Deputy to the Master of Revels, he was formally recognised as the rightful exerciser of the Master's powers and was knighted by King JAMES I in 1623.

Upon Ashley's death Herbert became Master in name as well as fact, but in the summer of 1642, when the civil war erupted and the Puritan government of London closed the theatres, the office ceased to pay. In 1660 when the monarchy was restored, Herbert attempted to reclaim the powers of the Master of Revels, but the new, unfettered licences granted to producers William DAVENANT and Thomas KILLIGREW took precedence. After a series of unsuccessful lawsuits, Herbert retired.

A volume of Herbert's official records, known as his *Office Book,* survived into the 18th century, when it was used and recorded in part by such scholars as George CHALMERS and Edmond MALONE. It was subsequently lost, but extensive quotations from it remain and provide scholars with an important glimpse of the 17th-century English theatre.

Herbert (2), Henry, Philip, or William, Earls of Pembroke See PEMBROKE (1, 2, 3).

Herbert (3), Sir Walter (c. 1462–after 1485) Historical figure and minor character in *Richard III,* an officer under RICHMOND. Herbert, whose father, William of

PEMBROKE (4), has a non-speaking role in *3 Henry VI*, speaks one line in 5.2 and is present but silent in 5.3.

Hermia Character in *A Midsummer Night's Dream*, one of the four lovers whose adventures in the enchanted wood are the centre-piece of the play. In 1.1, when Hermia's father, EGEUS, demands that she be punished for refusing to marry DEMETRIUS (2), her civil but firm response reveals a determined nature. Her first words, a straightforward assertion of her beloved LYSANDER's virtues, indicate that she will not easily be deterred. When Lysander's love is magically diverted to HELENA (1), Hermia is prepared to fight for her man, and she drives her friend away. Several remarks indicate that Hermia is a brunette with a dark complexion, and she has often been associated with the 'Dark Lady' of Shakespeare's SONNETS, which he was writing at about the same time.

Hermione Character in *The Winter's Tale*, wife of King LEONTES of SICILIA and mother of PERDITA. Unjustly accused of adultery by her mad husband, Hermione gives birth in prison to Perdita, whom Leontes condemns to be abandoned in the wilderness; then her son MAMILLIUS dies just as Leontes sentences her to death. The shock of this loss kills her, according to her ally Lady PAULINA. However, Paulina keeps Hermione alive in secret, awaiting the time when Leontes shall have sufficiently repented. In 5.3, after Perdita has miraculously reappeared, Paulina offers to display a statue of Hermione, which is actually the still-living queen herself. As the others watch in awe, Hermione comes to life, and the play closes with reunion and reconciliation.

Hermione is a passive but highly important figure in the play. Her fate in the tragic first half makes her an emblem of a major theme of the play—indeed, of all Shakespeare's ROMANCES—the critical role of providence in securing human happiness in an unreliable world. Even more, she helps illustrate that the efficacy of providence depends on the moral strength of good people in the face of evil. Her dignity in the face of her undeserved fate is highly impressive. Even the steady strength of the poetry she speaks contrasts favourably with the hysterical ranting of Leontes. She puts her faith in providence, saying, 'if powers divine / Behold our human actions (as they do), / I doubt not then but innocence shall make / False accusation blush' (3.2.28–31). Upon her reappearance she restates this attitude when she invokes a blessing on Perdita—'You gods, look down, / And from your sacred vial pour your graces / Upon my daughter's head' (5.3.121–123).

Hermione displays a loving nature that anticipates the role of Perdita in the second half of the play. Her charm is evident in 1.2, when, at Leontes' request, she persuades King POLIXENES of BOHEMIA to extend his visit. This arouses Leontes' jealous suspicions, but it also demonstrates Hermione's fine qualities: a readiness for friendship and an intelligent appreciation of the previous affection between her husband and Polixenes. Her capacity for love is delightfully demonstrated in 2.1, where we see her playing with Mamillius. Her evident goodness makes her apparent death all the more tragic and her apparent resurrection all the more Christlike. Although Hermione's significance diminishes in the second half, in the first—and at the conclusion—she is key to *The Winter's Tale*'s presentation of humanity's capacity for good.

Hero Character in *Much Ado About Nothing*, daughter of LEONATO and beloved of CLAUDIO (1). Hero is a demure and pliant maid, a conventional representative of the Elizabethan ideal of docile womanhood. She accepts an arranged marriage, first to Don PEDRO and then to Claudio. She is pleasant and has enough sparkle to engage in the ploy whereby her cousin BEATRICE is tricked into accepting BENEDICK's love, but she largely lacks personality or spirit. A pawn, first proffered in marriage to Claudio and then rejected by him, she can only faint when unjustly accused of promiscuity. Beatrice, Benedick, and the FRIAR (2) stand up for her, and Constable DOGBERRY's timely exposure of the villainous Don JOHN (1) finally clears her, but she is herself inactive. Significantly, once she and Claudio are finally reunited, they barely speak, as the play's focus immediately shifts to Beatrice and Benedick.

Hero's name—which bears no relation to the common noun *hero*, though it is pronounced the same—comes from an ancient Greek tale of two lovers that was very well known in Shakespeare's day as the subject of the immensely popular poem 'Hero and Leander', by Christopher MARLOWE (1). In naming his tractable heroine after a famous romantic lover, Shakespeare may have intended a mild irony.

Hervey (Harvey), William (c. 1565–1642) English soldier, possible 'Mr W. H'. of the dedication to the SONNETS. Hervey was the stepfather of Shakespeare's patron, the Earl of SOUTHAMPTON (2), and some scholars believe that he provided manuscripts of the Sonnets to the publisher, Thomas THORPE, who therefore dedicated his 1609 edition to him as the 'onlie begetter' of the poems, 'begetter' being taken to mean 'procurer'.

As a young man, Hervey distinguished himself fighting against the Spanish Armada in 1588, and he was knighted for his service under the Earl of ESSEX (2) at Cadiz in 1596. He married the Countess of Southampton in 1599, and after her death in 1607 he married Cordell Annesley, whose concern for her mad father, Brian ANNESLEY, may have helped inspire *King*

Lear. Hervey continued soldiering, mostly in Ireland, and was rewarded with great estates by King JAMES I. He died a wealthy man.

Shakespeare probably had Hervey (also known as Harvey) in mind when he changed the name of his character HARVEY (1), in *1. Henry IV*, to PETO. Several such name changes were made (see OLDCASTLE, ROSSILL) to avoid giving offence to powerful aristocrats.

Heyes, Thomas (d. c. 1604) LONDON bookseller and publisher, producer of the first edition of *The Merchant of Venice.* In 1600 Heyes bought the copyright to *The Merchant* from the printer James ROBERTS. He published a QUARTO edition, known as Q1, and used Roberts as the printer. When he died, Heyes left the rights to the play to his son Laurence (d. 1637), whose protest at Thomas PAVIER's illicit publication in 1619 led to the exposure of Pavier's FALSE FOLIO.

Heywood (1), John (c. 1497–c. 1580) Early English dramatist. Heywood was a musician at the courts of King HENRY VIII, King Edward VI, and Queen Mary I, and wrote dramatic dialogues for the intermissions in musical entertainments (see INTERLUDE). He contributed to the evolution from the medieval MORALITY PLAY towards the secular ELIZABETHAN DRAMA. He was also famous for his ballads. Heywood's four extant interludes—probably written between 1519 and 1528—are comedies in the form of moral debates. They are pious by later standards, but they are significantly different from their predecessors. The allegorical figures of the morality plays are replaced with real characters, drawn from contemporary society. They are inclined to a boisterous and obscene humour that was startling for the day. However, although Heywood's farcelike works stimulated a broader sense of theatrical possibility, Shakespearean COMEDY has different roots.

Heywood was probably the son of a provincial coroner. He was recruited as a boy for the choir of St Paul's School (see CHILDREN'S COMPANIES) and thus began his career. An ardent Catholic and a relative by marriage of Sir Thomas MORE, Heywood feared persecution early in the reign of Queen ELIZABETH (1). Protestantism was forcefully instituted as the state religion, and he fled England for the Spanish Netherlands in 1564. In 1578 when he was in his 80s, he again faced religious persecution when he was among the Catholics expelled from Antwerp by a Protestant mob. This was a minor episode of Protestant revolt against Spanish rule. He lived out his life in nearby Louvain, a more securely Catholic city.

Heywood (2), Thomas (1573–1641) English actor and playwright, possible collaborator with Shakespeare. Heywood acted and wrote for the ADMIRAL'S MEN from 1596 to 1602, and with WORCESTER'S MEN (later the QUEEN'S MEN [2]) until their dissolution in 1619. He then retired from acting but continued to write plays, both by himself and collaboratively. Some scholars believe he may have written parts of *Timon of Athens.* Heywood was astoundingly prolific and claimed to have 'had either an entire hand or at the least a main finger' in 220 plays. However many there may in fact have been, only about 20 have survived, though the names of a dozen more are known. The best-known survivors are *Four Prentices of London* (1600), which was satirised in *The Knight of the Burning Pestle* by Francis BEAUMONT (2), *A Woman Killed with Kindness* (1603), and *If You Know Not Me, You Know Nobody* (1605). Heywood also wrote a prose pamphlet countering Puritan objections to the theatre, *Apology for Actors* (published 1612), which is important for the light it casts on the ELIZABETHAN THEATRE. In a digression in it, he points out that two of his poems had been published in THE PASSIONATE PILGRIM as Shakespeare's, and he objects on Shakespeare's behalf; the publisher, William JAGGARD, withdrew the ascription.

Higgins, John (c. 1545–1602) English poet, author of sources for both *Julius Caesar* and *King Lear.* Higgins was a classical scholar and a writer on early British history. He collaborated with Nicholas UDALL on translations from the Roman dramatist Terence (c. 185–159 B.C.) but he is best known for his contribution to A MIRROR FOR MAGISTRATES, a popular anthology of verse biography that Shakespeare knew well. Higgins edited the third and fourth editions of *A Mirror* (1574, 1578) and contributed to it 16 long poems dealing with 'the first unfortunate Princes of this lande', the quasi-mythical kings and heroes of ancient Britain. His account of 'Leire' provided Shakespeare with a number of significant details for his *King Lear.* For the fifth edition (1587) of *A Mirror,* probably the one Shakespeare used, Higgins provided another 24 poems, all but one on figures from the classical world. Among them was a life of Julius CAESAR (1) that Shakespeare used in composing his play on the Roman leader.

Hilliard, Nicholas (1547–1619) English painter, the foremost English artist of Shakespeare's times and the creator of a portrait formerly believed to be of Shakespeare. The 'Hilliard miniature' was reproduced in James BOSWELL's 1821 edition of Shakespeare's works. It had been brought to the editor's attention by its owner, a descendant of a Mr Somerville, and the painting is also known as the 'Somerville miniature'. Somerville allegedly was a STRATFORD friend of the retired Shakespeare and the commissioner of the portrait. However, the Hilliard miniature does not much resemble the most authoritative portraits (see DROES-

HOUT; JANSSEN [2]), and modern scholars are confident that the portrait is not of Shakespeare.

Hilliard, chiefly a painter of miniature portraits, was inspired by the work of the great German painter Hans Holbein the younger (1497–1593). Holbein had been court portraitist to King HENRY VIII, and Hilliard worked for both Queen ELIZABETH (1) and King JAMES I. His elaborately detailed renderings of jewelry and rich costumes give his portraits an exquisite, gemlike presence that is still admired.

Hippolyta (1) Character in *A Midsummer Night's Dream,* Queen of the Amazons and the bride of Duke THESEUS (1) of ATHENS. Hippolyta's role is small, but she is a sympathetic figure who contributes to the play's theme of domestic love. In 1.1 her distress at the prospect of HERMIA's punishment highlights the young lovers' plight. In 5.1 she disagrees with Theseus about the lovers' accounts of their experiences in the enchanted wood. He has doubted their story, but she observes that 'all the story of the night told over / . . . grows to something of great constancy / . . . strange and admirable' (5.1.23–26). Her mythical origins as leader of the Amazons are hinted at only fleetingly, in her recollected acquaintance with Hercules and Cadmus, in 4.1. Shakespeare took her name and gentle nature from a character in CHAUCER's 'The Knight's Tale'.

Hippolyta (2) Character in *The Two Noble Kinsmen,* Queen of the Amazons, fiancée and later wife of THESEUS (2), Duke of ATHENS. Hippolyta helps establish the tone of magnanimous nobility and pity that dominates Act 1, but she is unimportant thereafter. In 1.1, when her wedding to Theseus is interrupted by the pleas of the royal widows (see QUEEN [1]) who seek the duke's aid, Hippolyta speaks in their support, insisting that her anticipated marital joy must be postponed in their cause. In 1.3 she describes the friendship between Theseus and PIRITHOUS, which offers a parallel to the relationship between the title characters, PALAMON and ARCITE, and which also signifies nobility of spirit. She herself displays a serene spirit in observing without jealousy, in fact approvingly, that Theseus might be unable to choose between Pirithous and herself. In Acts 2–4, where her part is written by John FLETCHER (2), she is an ordinary aristocratic figure, graciously attending the duke at court. She is presumably married to Theseus by this time, although the rescheduled wedding is never mentioned. In Act 5 Hippolyta hardly speaks, but she makes a significant point after the duel fought by Palamon and Arcite for EMILIA (4), when she offers a tender acknowledgement that the play's developments provoke 'Infinite pity' (5.3.144–145).

History Plays Shakespeare's 10 plays dealing with events in English history. In the order in which they were written, the history plays are: (a) the so-called minor TETRALOGY—consisting of *1, 2,* and *3 Henry VI* and *Richard III*—written in 1590–1591; (b) *King John* (1591, possibly 1595); (c) the major tetralogy—*Richard II, 1* and *2 Henry IV,* and *Henry V*—written between 1595 and 1599; and (d) *Henry VIII,* perhaps written in collaboration with John FLETCHER in 1612, one of Shakespeare's last works.

The minor tetralogy deals with the English defeat by FRANCE (1) in the last years of the HUNDRED YEARS WAR (enacted in *1 Henry VI*), followed by the disputes and battles of an English civil conflict, the WARS OF THE ROSES (in the other three plays). The tetralogy begins with the death of King HENRY V in 1422 and ends with the foundation of the TUDOR dynasty in 1485. *King John* presents much earlier events, a series of incidents during the reign of King JOHN (3) (1199–1216). The major tetralogy covers the deposition and murder of King RICHARD II in 1398 *(Richard II),* two unsuccessful rebellions against his usurper, King HENRY IV, and that ruler's death *(1* and *2 Henry IV),* and the invasion and defeat of France by Henry's son and successor, King Henry V, closing with the signing of the treaty of TROYES in 1420 *(Henry V). Henry VIII* consists of a series of tableaux that present various events in the reign of HENRY VIII, ending with the christening of Queen ELIZABETH (1) in 1533. It is very different from the other histories and is generally regarded as greatly inferior to them.

The two tetralogies are Shakespeare's major achievement in the histories. (*King John,* although a fine play, is nevertheless an isolated excursion into an earlier, almost mythic, period.) The tetralogies cover English history from 1398 to 1485. Shakespeare plunged into the disorder of a civil war in the first four plays and then, in the second, delved into the history that preceded this cataclysm, examining its causes and painting a portrait of the nation as it changed, traumatically, from medieval to modern.

The central theme of these plays is political—they deal with the gain and loss of power—but Shakespeare transcended this subject. As he wrote his histories, the playwright increasingly pursued the definition of the perfect king. After presenting two distinctly bad rulers, the ineffectual HENRY VI and the villainous RICHARD III, he turned to a consideration of kingly virtues. He began to explore the psychology of political leaders, and these plays are, at their best, as much psychological as historical.

In *Richard II* a weak king jeopardises the stability of the realm, but, although we recognise his opponent, Henry BOLINGBROKE (1), to be a superior ruler, we nonetheless sympathise with Richard, whose spiritual qualities make him more open and responsive to life.

A conflict is established between human vulnerability and cold political calculation, and the question that dominates the next three plays is whether a successful ruler can combine humane sympathy and ruthless efficiency. Such a monarch would be able to hold the country together, as Richard cannot, while staying in touch with his subjects, a connection Bolingbroke never had and does not acquire as Henry IV.

The *Henry IV* plays focus on the development of the king's son, young PRINCE (6) HAL. In *1 Henry IV* Hal is presented with two alternatives, represented by HOTSPUR and FALSTAFF respectively, and he finds his way between them, seeing both their weaknesses and their virtues. However, in *2 Henry IV* the Prince is psychologically remote, and, as he inherits the crown from his father, he seems to abandon his friends among the commoners in order to focus on his duty as a ruler. Hal's increasing coldness is evident, but the play's great question—is personal loyalty morally superior to public duty?—is left unanswered by the Prince's final rejection of Falstaff, as is shown by the debate that the episode has engendered ever since.

In *Henry V* this basic ambivalence towards Hal—now King Henry V—remains the major theme. On the one hand, he is plainly a successful king, uniting all Britain behind him in a conquest of France and displaying the combination of leadership and camaraderie typical of an epic hero. On the other, he seems a cynical manipulator of war and peace, an hypocrite who uses a religious sensibility to mask his political ends. Both points of view are legitimate in the context of the play; Shakespeare's recognition of political complexities compelled him to explore Henry's defects. His discovery of the psychological limitations of his ideal king was to influence the great tragedies (see TRAGEDY) in the next phase of his career.

Not content to deal with the nature of kingship solely from the point of view of the rulers, Shakespeare also focusses on the lives of the common people of England, especially in the major tetralogy. Sometimes fictitious minor figures, such as the GARDENER in *Richard III* or WILLIAMS (2) in *Henry V*, fulfil an important function simply by offering their own interpretation of political events and historical personalities and thus influencing our own responses. But many common people are developed as characters in their own right. Indeed, in the *Henry IV* plays, often considered the greatest of the histories, Falstaff and a number of fully sketched minor characters offer a sort of national group portrait that is contrasted with political history. The juxtaposition generates a richly stimulating set of relationships.

That secular accounts of the past, neither legendary nor religious, were presented on the stage—and were highly popular—reflects the Elizabethan era's intense interest in history. In the late 16th century, when these plays were written, England was undergoing a great crisis. As a leading Protestant state, it found itself at odds with the great Catholic powers of Counter-Reformation Europe, including its traditional enemy, France, and a new foe, Spain. The latter, at the height of its power, was a very dangerous adversary, and England felt seriously imperiled until the defeat of the Spanish Armada in 1588. This situation sparked a tremendous patriotism among all classes of English society, and with that came an increasing interest in the nation's history, an interest that the theatre was of course delighted to serve.

Written not long after the peak of nationalistic fervour in 1588, the history plays, which were extremely popular, deal with England: the Wars of the Roses were the great crisis that had formed the nation, as Shakespeare and his contemporaries knew it. Its resolution at BOSWORTH FIELD lay in the relatively recent past—closer to the author's own day than the American Civil War or the Crimean War is to ours. Thus Elizabethans were very much aware of the significance of the events depicted in these plays. Moreover, although in hindsight the reign of Queen ELIZABETH (1) seems very different from those of the troubled 15th century, this was not so clear at the time. A number of threats to the government arose—including the failed rebellion of the Earl of ESSEX (2) in 1599, when the rebels used a performance of *Richard II* as propaganda. The English of the late 16th century felt a strong fear of civil war and anarchy; for both moral and practical reasons they valued an orderly society ruled by a strong monarch. The history plays addressed this attitude by presenting a lesson in the evils of national disunity.

This view of English history was held not only by both the playwright and most of his audience, but also by the historians whose works Shakespeare consulted. When the Tudor dynasty came to power, among the policies adopted by King Henry VII (the RICHMOND of *Richard III*) was the use of scholarly propaganda to justify his seizure of the throne. He encouraged and commissioned various works of history and biography to emphasise the faults of earlier rulers and present his own accession as the nation's salvation. Among them was an official history of England by the Italian humanist Polydore VERGIL, which was to have a strong influence on subsequent historians, including Raphael HOLINSHED and Edward HALL (2), whose chronicles were Shakespeare's chief sources. Holinshed's book, the most up-to-date and authoritative work of its kind in the 1590s, provided much of the historical detail, especially in the minor tetralogy. Hall's history of the Wars of the Roses foreshadowed Shakespeare by stressing the theme that England's happiness under its last great medieval king, Edward III, Richard II's predecessor, had been lost through Richard's weak-

ness, which necessitated Henry IV's profoundly sinful act of deposition. This guilty deed brought down God's wrath on England, plunging the country into generations of civil conflict that was ended only by the triumph of Henry VII and the founding of the Tudor dynasty.

Such writings shaped the understanding of the past that was available to Shakespeare when he wrote the history plays. He saw—and passed on—a story of inevitable progress towards the benevolent reign of the Tudors. Shakespeare's account of historical events varies considerably from that developed by later scholarship, in part because the sources available to him were highly unreliable by modern historical standards. In any case, Shakespeare was not writing history; he was concerned with dramatic values more than with historical accuracy.

The history play, a theatrical work dealing realistically with great events of the past, was a novelty in Shakespeare's day. Shakespeare himself is often credited with inventing the genre, although its origins are somewhat obscure, since the texts of most Elizabethan plays are lost. Dramatic works dealing with historical events had been staged somewhat earlier, but these works had treated their materials allegorically, like the MORALITY PLAY from which they derived. Shakespeare was probably the first playwright to depict real events in works expressly intended to illuminate the past, although some lost plays may have anticipated him in some respects.

Other Elizabethan playwrights also wrote histories, whether influenced specifically by Shakespeare or simply by the age. However, most of these works are familiar only to scholars. Shakespeare's work has survived because he was not merely exploiting a current interest; nor was he a mere purveyor of Tudor propaganda. In writing history plays, he pursued his own concerns, exploring political values and social relations. Throughout his career he was preoccupied with the value of order in society; this theme is present in such very early and apparently unlikely works as *The Comedy of Errors,* and it recurs in most of the plays. But nowhere is it as explicitly dealt with as in the histories.

What, then, do the history plays say about this subject? As we have seen, the ideal king of the history plays, Henry V, is a highly ambiguous figure. While Shakespeare's belief in the need for authority is evident in his work, so also is a distrust of those who hold authority. This paradox reflects a fundamental irony: the only rational form of rule—power that is humane yet absolute—is also impossible to achieve. Thus the history plays point up an underlying characteristic of human societies—political power inspires disturbing fears as well as profound ideals.

Hoby (1), Sir Thomas (1530–1566) First English translator of CASTIGLIONE's *Il Cortegiano,* thought to have influenced *Much Ado About Nothing.* As a young man, Hoby travelled widely on the Continent. In 1552–1553, while living in Paris, he translated *Il Cortegiano,* though the resulting work, *The Courtyer,* was not published until 1561. It became immensely popular, being reissued several times before 1588. Hoby died in 1566, while serving as the English ambassador in Paris. Thomas Posthumous HOBY (2) was his son.

Hoby (2), Sir Thomas Posthumous (1566–1640) Contemporary of Shakespeare, Puritan landowner who may have been a model for MALVOLIO in *Twelfth Night.* Born after the death of his father, Sir Thomas HOBY (1), Hoby ran away from home as a young man to pursue a military career; then he settled down as the husband of a wealthy heiress from Yorkshire. He acted as an agent for the Protestant government in his wife's very Catholic district, and his enthusiasm for prosecuting Catholics made him highly unpopular. In 1600 he sued several of his neighbours for coming uninvited to his house, where they drank, played cards, mocked his religious practices, and threatened to rape his wife. The case was notorious (Hoby won), and some scholars believe that it may be reflected in the antagonism between Malvolio and SIR TOBY in the play. (For other possible Malvolios, see FFARINGTON; KNOLLYS; WILLOUGHBY [1].)

Holingshed, Raphael (c. 1528–c. 1580) English historian, compiler and author of a source for several of Shakespeare's plays. Holinshed's *Chronicles of England, Scotland, and Ireland* (probably in its second edition, 1587) was a major source for the HISTORY PLAYS and *Macbeth,* and a minor one for *Cymbeline* and *King Lear.* The *Chronicles*—along with the work of Edward HALL (2)—provided much of Shakespeare's knowledge of the WARS OF THE ROSES, which is the subject of eight of the history plays (see TETRALOGY). With the work of John FOXE, it contributed the history covered in the two others, *King John* and *Henry VIII.* For *Macbeth,* Shakespeare used the *Chronicles'* account of the medieval King MACBETH of Scotland. The ancient British kings CYMBELINE and LEAR were also treated by Holinshed, and details of his treatments are reflected in Shakespeare's plays about them.

Holinshed's *Chronicles* was the most authoritative history of Britain in Shakespeare's day, and other Elizabethan dramatists besides Shakespeare used it as a source. Its three and a half million words were not all written by Holinshed, whose principal contribution was the section dealing with England's history. In writing it, he relied on a number of earlier works, most notably that of Hall. The history of SCOTLAND was a translation by William HARRISON (3) of the Latin chronicle of Hector BOECE, and the history of Ireland was written by Edmund Campion (1540–1581). Prefatory geographical essays were provided by Harrison

for England and Scotland, and Campion and Richard Stanyhurst (1545–1615) for Ireland.

The book was the remnant of a much larger project, led by Reginald Wolfe (d. 1573), a 'cosmography of the whole world [including] the histories of every known nation', for which Holinshed was a translator. Holinshed succeeded Wolfe as editor-in-chief, though only one other volume, an atlas, was published. The *Chronicles* was published in 1578 and again, in a revised and enlarged version, in 1587. Holinshed wrote nothing else—even the second edition of the *Chronicles* was brought out by others (including John STOW)—and he became a steward on a country estate, where he died.

Holland (1), Henry, Duke of Exeter Character in *3 Henry VI.* See EXETER (1).

Holland (2), Hugh (c. 1574–1633) Poet and antiquarian, friend of Shakespeare's. Holland wrote an EPITAPH on Shakespeare, a SONNET that was one of the introductory poems in the FIRST FOLIO (1623). Like Shakespeare, he was a good friend of Ben JONSON and a member of the group that met regularly at the MERMAID TAVERN. Holland wrote in four languages—English, Greek, Italian, and Welsh—and he was a well-known poet in his own time, noted particularly for a long poem on Owen Tudor's courtship of Queen KATHARINE (2).

Holland (3), John Minor character in *2 Henry VI,* a follower of Jack CADE. Holland discusses Cade's rebellion with his friend George BEVIS in 4.2, and they join the rebels when they appear. Holland also makes several joking asides in 4.7. A John Holland is known to have been an actor with STRANGE'S MEN in the early 1590s, and it is believed that he played this part. His name was given to the character as a convenience by either Shakespeare or the keeper of a PROMPT-BOOK.

Holland (4), Philemon (1552–1637) English translator of minor sources for *Othello, Coriolanus,* and possibly *The Rape of Lucrece.* Holland's version of PLINY the Elder's *Natural History* (1601) provided details for *Othello,* mostly in the hero's account of his adventures in 1.3. A passage in Holland's translation of LIVY's history of ROME, *Ab urbe condita,* published as *The Roman Historie* (1600), is echoed in certain details of MENENIUS' famous 'belly speech' in *Coriolanus* (1.1.95–159). The same passage was also influenced by Holland's translation of William CAMDEN's *Remaines* (1605), excerpts from a Latin history of Britain. Holland's Livy may also have inspired parts of *Lucrece,* whose story it tells. However, there are no literary echoes of Holland in Shakespeare's poem, so the playwright may have only used the original.

Holland, the son of a clergyman, practised medicine in COVENTRY. He was famous for his translations from the Latin; in addition to those already mentioned, he produced English versions of three other ancient works of history, published in 1606, 1609, and 1632. After 1608 Holland gave up medicine and became the headmaster of a grammar school.

Holmedon (Homildon) Site of a battle between England and Scotland (1402) that is reported in 1.1.62–74 of *1 Henry IV.* Holmedon, known today as Humbleton, is near the Scottish border. An invasion by the Scots was repelled by English forces under HOTSPUR, who captured many aristocratic prisoners—usually held for ransom under medieval practices of war—including the Scottish commander, Lord DOUGLAS. Hotspur's refusal to turn these prisoners over to King Henry triggers enmity between the two, leading to the rebellion that the play depicts.

Shakespeare alters the chronology surrounding this battle in minor ways. He asserts that the battle occurred simultaneously with another, against the Welsh, in which Lord MORTIMER (2) was captured, but in fact they occurred months apart. His alteration heightens the dramatic impact of their accounts. Both are placed closer to the beginning of Henry's reign than they actually were, thus stressing the connection of the rebellion against Henry to his usurpation of the crown (enacted in *Richard II*).

Holofernes Character in *Love's Labour's Lost,* a comical pedant. Named for Dr Tubal Holofernes, a tutor in Rabelais' *Gargantua,* Shakespeare's scholar is so Latinate in his speech that he can hardly be understood. Holofernes, never without his obsequious follower, NATHANIEL (1) the Curate, is the subject of much mirth on the part of the other characters. MOTH (1) says of Holofernes and his fellow grotesque, ARMADO, that 'they have been at a great feast of languages, and stolen the scraps' (5.1.35–36). Although Holofernes is consistently wrong-headed, conceited, and intolerant of those he considers his intellectual inferiors, we nevertheless feel sorry for him when he attempts to perform in the pageant of the Nine WORTHIES and is mercilessly heckled by the gentlemen. Driven from the stage, he cries, justly, 'This is not generous, not gentle, not humble' (5.2.623).

While Shakespeare's audiences will have made more of Holofernes' ranting than we can, it is nonetheless good comedy, for much of the fun lies in its near-incomprehensibility. Some of his references are clearly to topical jokes that are now hopelessly obscure. It has been speculated that Holofernes was intended as a parody of some contemporary literary figure—John FLORIO and Gabriel HARVEY (2) have been suggested—but this theory cannot be proven.

Homer Ancient Greek poet, a source, through the translation of George CHAPMAN, of *Troilus and Cressida.*

Two great epics—the *Iliad,* an account of the TROJAN WAR, and the *Odyssey,* which tells of the wanderings of Odysseus, known in Latin as ULYSSES—are attributed to Homer, as they have been since remote antiquity. However, Homer may be an apocryphal figure and his works may have been written by more than one unknown author. In the absence of persuasive evidence one way or the other, the works continue to be conventionally regarded as Homer's. In the ancient world, estimates of Homer's dates ranged over many centuries, but by comparing passages in the works with the archaeological evidence, scholars generally believe that the poems were composed in the 8th or 7th century B.C.—i.e., 400–600 years after the era depicted in them. Internal evidence further suggests that the poet(s) lived in Ionia, or Greek Asia Minor.

In the Middle Ages it was believed that other accounts of the Trojan War preceded Homer's, but they were actually written much later. Only in the RENAISSANCE were Homer's works restored to the position of eminence they had held in ancient Greece and Rome. Some of the information Shakespeare used in writing *Troilus and Cressida* came from the medieval tradition, which took a Trojan rather than a Greek point of view. However, Homer entered English literature in Shakespeare's time, and the playwright certainly knew two partial translations of the *Iliad,* that of Arthur HALL (1), taken from a French version (1581), and Chapman's, from the Greek (published in part in 1598 and in full in 1612). Indeed, he could have read nine different translations—five Latin, two French, and two English. However, it is clear that he used Chapman's translation in composing the play (c. 1602), for the incidents from Homer that he used were those covered in Chapman's first edition. Chapman's *Odyssey* was completed in 1615, and numerous translations of both works have been made since, some of them masterful works of English literature in their own right.

Hope Theatre Theatre near LONDON built by Philip HENSLOWE in 1613 on the site of a bear-baiting house—an arena for audiences to watch bears or bulls being attacked by dogs—which was torn down for the purpose. Henslowe held a licence for animal-baiting, a very popular entertainment, and he wished to expand this business while perhaps attracting the audiences of the GLOBE THEATRE, which had just burned down. The Hope thus had accommodations for the animals along with the usual attributes of a theatre. The smell of the animals was apparently offensive, but LADY ELIZABETH'S MEN and other companies played there in 1614–1615. However, disputes between Henslowe and the players resulted in a series of lawsuits, which continued after Henslowe's death, and his heir, William ALLEYN, could not negotiate a settlement. During this period,. few plays were produced at the Hope, and by 1619 it had reverted to animal-baiting exclusively. This pastime was outlawed in 1642, and the Hope was eventually torn down to make way for tenements in 1656.

Hopkins, Richard (c. 1545–c. 1594) English translator of the works of Luis de GRANADA. Hopkins, a Catholic, spent his life abroad in religious exile. A student in Catholic universities in the Netherlands, Spain, and France, he probably lived chiefly in Paris, although details of his life are obscure. His translation of Granada's *Of Prayer and Meditation* was published in London in 1582 and may have influenced Shakespeare's writing of *Hamlet.*

Horatio Character in *Hamlet,* friend and confidant of Prince HAMLET. Horatio is the one person in Hamlet's world whom the prince values and trusts. With Horatio he can speak freely, and in doing so he demonstrates the evolution of his emotions. Further, the presence of Horatio lessens Hamlet's otherwise total alienation and permits relief—for him and for us—from the heightened tension that characterises his existence.

Horatio is a calm and stoical figure whom Hamlet admires as 'A man that Fortune's buffets and rewards / Hast ta'en with equal thanks . . . [a] man / That is not passion's slave' (3.2.67–72). He thus represents a RENAISSANCE ideal—a person with the mental discipline to resist highly emotional responses, which were seen as evidence of humanity's fall from grace. This ideal was considerably influenced by the newly rediscovered Stoic philosophy of the classical world, and Horatio rightly thinks of himself as 'more an antique Roman than a Dane' (5.2.346). His restraint makes Horatio one who 'in suff'ring all, . . . suffers nothing' (3.2.66), and Hamlet, embattled by his own suffering, envies his friend's relative peace of mind. However, it is precisely his vulnerability that gives Hamlet's emotional odyssey the grandeur that makes it worth recording. Horatio is an admirable figure, but he does not spark our imagination or sympathies.

Horatio knew Hamlet at school, as the prince makes plain in welcoming him from Wittenberg as a 'fellow student' (1.2.177), but otherwise his past is unclear. In 1.1 he seems to be an intimate of the Danish court, but at several points—most notably when he must ask if musical accompaniment to drinking toasts is 'a custom' (1.4.12)—he appears to be unfamiliar with local ways. Horatio's status in DENMARK—Danish nobleman or foreign visitor—is an example of the many problematic points in *Hamlet* that scholarship cannot resolve. Shakespeare probably simply formulated the character in different lights as he composed the drama and did not concern himself with the minor contradictions that resulted, as was apparently his habit throughout the plays.

Horner, Thomas Minor character in *2 Henry VI*, an armourer who is reported to have remarked that his client the Duke of YORK (8) was 'rightful heir to the crown' (1.3.26). Horner's apprentice, PETER, informs the Duke of SUFFOLK (3) of Horner's assertion, and Suffolk brings them both before the court in an effort to embarrass York. Horner denies Peter's assertion, and a trial by combat is ordered by the Duke of GLOUCESTER (4), the Lord Protector. Thus a potentially explosive issue is postponed and diverted into what will prove a minor spectacle for the court. Also, at Gloucester's recommendation, the reappointment of York as Regent of FRANCE (1) is withheld until this question should cool off. Thus the episode serves to illustrate Gloucester's qualities of prudence and discretion—ironically not long before his downfall.

Horner, though expected to win the combat against the cowardly Peter, arrives at the contest drunk in 2.3 and is slain by his apprentice. Dying, he confesses that Peter's account had been true, and the apprentice is exonerated. Although the combat is not treated seriously by the court, it prefigures York's rebellion in the WARS OF THE ROSES, which begins later in the play.

Hortensio Character in *The Taming of the Shrew*, a suitor of BIANCA (1). A bland young man who is outsmarted in his campaign to win Bianca, Hortensio is an appropriate character to enter, ludicrously pale 'for fear' (2.1.143), to report KATHERINA's assault on him with a lute, thus providing an image of the 'shrew' of the title at her worst. After losing Bianca, Hortensio turns to a WIDOW (1) who has pursued him. He visits the country house of PETRUCHIO (2) to observe that character's shrew-taming techniques, but it is unclear at the play's end whether Hortensio will be strong enough to use them when he needs them, for the Widow proves, in 5.2, to be a formidable shrew herself.

Hortensius Minor character in *Timon of Athens*, the servant to a creditor of TIMON. In 3.4 Hortensius and other servants unsuccessfully dun Timon and his STEWARD (2) for payment. The servants regret their assignment, for their greedy masters have benefited from Timon's generosity. Hortensius is especially vocal, and he says, 'I know my lord hath spent of Timon's wealth, / And now ingratitude makes it worse than stealth' (3.4.27–28). He thus stresses one of the play's important themes, the callousness of the aristocracy of ATHENS.

Hortensius appears with TITUS (2), PHILOTUS, LUCIUS' SERVANT and two men who are each designated as VARRO'S SERVANT. Since the latter three are addressed as 'Lucius' and 'Varro' (3.4.2, 3), it is presumed that Shakespeare intended the names of the first three to refer to their masters as well, perhaps reflecting a casual linguistic practise of the early 17th century.

Host (1) Minor character in *The Two Gentlemen of Verona*. JULIA, disguised as a boy, converses with the Host in 4.2, having arrived at court to see her lover, PROTEUS. While she observes the infidelity of PROTEUS, the Host falls asleep, subtly isolating the heroine at this crucial moment.

Host (2) Character in *The Merry Wives of Windsor*, the keeper of the Garter Tavern. The bluff and ebullient Host is a peacekeeper whom EVANS (3) nominates to the committee intended to arbitrate between SHALLOW and FALSTAFF and who later leads the effort to prevent the duel between EVANS and Dr CAIUS (2). The would-be combattants, the only two foreigners in Shakespeare's WINDSOR, reward the Host's good intentions by having his horses stolen. The Host's heartiness is evident in his extravagant rhetoric. For instance, when directing a visitor to Falstaff's rooms at the inn, he says, 'There's his chamber, his house, his castle, his standing-bed, and truckle-bed; 'tis painted about with the story of the Prodigal, fresh and new. Go, knock and call; he'll speak like an Anthropophaginian unto thee; knock, I say' (4.5.5–9). His bold language encompasses an extraordinary range of epithets, from 'bully rook' (1.3.2, et al.), 'Cavaliero' (2.1.186; 2.3.70), and 'bully Hercules' (1.3.6), to such fanciful constructs as 'Bohemian-Tartar' (4.5.18) and 'Castalian-king-Urinal' (2.3.31).

Hostess (1) Minor character in *The Taming of the Shrew*, the proprietor of the tavern from which Christopher SLY (1) emerges at the beginning of the INDUCTION. Sly may be referring to her, in Ind.2.21, as Marian Hacket, believed to have been a real person who lived in a hamlet near STRATFORD and whom Shakespeare presumably knew as a boy. In any case, the brief appearance of this angry but businesslike barmaid contributes to the believable rural atmosphere of the Induction.

Hostess (2) Character in *1* and *2 Henry IV* and *Henry V*, the proprietress of the BOAR'S HEAD TAVERN in EASTCHEAP. The Hostess, a good-hearted woman whose affection for FALSTAFF withstands his exploitation of her purse, is comically loquacious. Aspiring to conversational brilliance, she displays a considerable vocabulary, but she unfortunately misplaces one word for another, in an ancient comedy routine, going so far, in a state of great excitement, as to confuse 'honeyseed' and 'honeysuckle' for 'homicide' and 'homicidal' (*2 Henry IV*, 2.1.49–51). She is a denizen of the quasi-criminal underworld of London (she associates with highwaymen and harlots and is arrested when a murder is said to have occurred in her tavern), but no

crimes are explicitly attributed to her. Indeed, her amiable and forgiving nature contains no hint of villainy.

The Hostess' role in *1 Henry IV* is very minor. In 2.4 she is an amused spectator of the mock drama played by PRINCE (6) HAL and Falstaff, and in 3.3 she disputes with Falstaff over his debt to her. He mocks her, and his insults spark her honest indgination.

In *2 Henry IV* the Hostess is a somewhat more substantial character. She escalates her dispute with Falstaff by summoning two officers, FANG and SNARE, to arrest the fat knight for debt. She elaborates on her complaint, remembering at length (2.1.83–101) that he had promised to marry her in order to borrow money. However, Falstaff not only talks her into calling off her legal action but also into lending him more money. She weeps, but she agrees, showing the gullibility and kindness that mark her relationship with him. In 2.4, when Falstaff is called to join the armies assembling to oppose the rebels against HENRY IV, the Hostess displays her sentimental attachment to him, weeping and saying, 'Well, fare thee well. I have known thee these twenty-nine years, come peascod-time, but an honester and true-hearted man—Well, fare thee well' (2.4.379–382). Even the Hostess' credulousness does not extend to a belief in Falstaff's honesty; she is merely expressing her love with conventional sayings that come first to her mind. The Hostess' tolerance and affection for Falstaff are important in Shakespeare's presentation of the fat rogue as an humane, though flawed, person. It comes as a shock when the Hostess and her friend DOLL TEARSHEET are arrested in 5.4, in a demonstration of the rigorous law enforcement of the new regime, anticipating Prince Hal's rejection of Falstaff in 5.5.

In *Henry V* the Hostess (now married to PISTOL) has a small but striking role, as she describes her attendance at Falstaff's death-bed, in a speech (2.3.9–27) that is one of the masterpieces of English comic literature, being simultaneously extremely funny, even bawdy, and touchingly tender. Her efforts to comfort a dying and conscience-stricken sinner reflect Shakespeare's own forgiving humanity.

The Hostess is given the name Mistress Quickly in all three plays (e.g., in *1 Henry IV,* 3.3.90; *2 Henry IV,* 2.1.44; *Henry V,* 2.1.19), but she is plainly a different person from the Mistress QUICKLY of *The Merry Wives of Windsor;* Shakespeare simply reused the name and comical verbal habit of the Hostess with his customary disregard for questions of consistency. Some scholars hold that the correct pronunciation of Quickly should be 'quick-lie', a legitimate Elizabethan variant that carries an obvious implication that she is a prostitute. Falstaff hints that she is (e.g., in *1 Henry IV,* 3.3.128), but, although she consorts with Doll, who is a courtesan, there is no other evidence to support this. It is more probable that her name, pronounced ordinarily (as it commonly was in the 16th century), is simply intended to suggest the hustle and bustle of an innkeeper's life.

Hostilius Minor character in *Timon of Athens,* a visitor to ATHENS. With his companions, the First and Second STRANGERS, Hostilius witnesses the callous rejection of TIMON's request for assistance by the miserly LUCIUS (3), in 3.2. Lucius has just insisted to Hostilius that he would always help his generous former patron. Like his friends, Hostilius represents a detached judgement on the selfish citizens of Athens—the First Stranger explicitly makes the case. This is an episode of a type familiar from the medieval MORALITY PLAY that serves to fix the play's moral point of view. In some editions Hostilius, who is named in 3.2.64, is designated as the Second Stranger.

Hotson, Leslie (b. 1897) Canadian literary scholar. Hotson has specialised in scholarly detective work and distinguished himself with many striking discoveries, including the probable murder of Christopher MARLOWE (1), the likely first performance of *The Merry Wives of Windsor,* and Shakespeare's connections to William GARDINER (2) and Francis LANGLEY. On the other hand, many of his proposals—such as the identification of *Troilus and Cressida* as LOVE'S LABOUR'S WON—have not been generally accepted.

Hotspur (Henry Percy, 1364–1403) Historical figure and character in *1 Henry IV,* a rebel against King HENRY IV. Hotspur, a fiery warrior, is repeatedly contrasted with Henry's son, PRINCE (6) HAL. The Prince's dissipation in the company of FALSTAFF is compared unfavourably with Hotspur's military prowess and chivalric honour. The play's major theme is Prince Hal's decision to abandon the tavern for the field and to compete with Hotspur, whose example inspires the Prince to adopt his proper role as a military hero. At the play's climax, the two young men meet in hand-to-hand combat at SHREWSBURY, where the Prince kills his rival. The play makes clear that Hotspur's volatile temper has led to his defeat and to the failure of his rebellion: he has carried his ideal of chivalric honour to excess. In this sense, he is contrasted with Falstaff, whose self-indulgent cowardice represents an opposite extreme. Hotspur thus resembles a figure from the MORALITY PLAYS, a symbol of a value or attitude.

Even before he appears, Hotspur is associated with military honour and prowess, as well as with excessive pride, in King Henry's account (1.1.66–74, 90–91) of his capture—and arrogant possession—of DOUGLAS. Hotspur begins the play in the service of the king, but the Percy family harbours a simmering resentment over Henry's apparent ingratitude for the help they gave him when he usurped the throne (as enacted in *Richard II*). When a dispute erupts over Hotspur's

failure to relinquish custody of Douglas, and the king refuses to ransom a Percy relative, Lord MORTIMER (2), the Percies decide to rebel. Hotspur's reputation for courage and his proven success in combat, make him the natural leader of the rebellion, but his older relatives—his father, the Earl of NORTHUMBERLAND (1), and his uncle, the Earl of WORCESTER—must struggle to curb the young man's temper. Ultimately, they are unable to do so, and Hotspur's rash insistence on fighting against the odds at Shrewsbury dooms the rebellion to defeat.

Hotspur's virtues are manifest; he is a fine military leader in a world that values this trait highly. King Henry's regret that his own son is not more like Hotspur is genuine, and the Prince himself, after killing his rival, acknowledges his worth in a warm eulogy (5.4.86–100). However, Hotspur represents, like Falstaff, an unbalanced attitude towards life. He lives only for battle and identifies himself entirely with his reputation for military valour. His rhetoric grows windy on the subject, as in 1.3.199–206 and 4.1.112–123. As his wife, LADY (10) Percy, tells us in 2.3.48–63, he even fights battles in his sleep. Utterly single-minded, he rejects even sex, declaring that 'this is no world to play with mammets, and to tilt with lips' (2.3.92–93).

His impetuosity makes him as much a liability as an asset to his allies. He has no control over his emotions, letting his enthusiasm for honour dominate all other considerations; his own father calls him 'a wasp-stung and impatient fool' (1.3.233). At Shrewsbury, messengers present a steady procession of reasons for caution, as the rebel fortunes grow increasingly uncertain, but Hotspur's response is almost ludicrously inappropriate: 'Come, let us take a muster speedily— / Doomsday is near; die all, die merrily' (4.1.133–134). His foolish refusal to wait for reinforcements condemns his cause to defeat; he is so overwrought at the approach of battle that he cannot even read his despatches, saying that life is too short to waste on such petty activity. Hotspur's impulsiveness is evident even in minor details of his speech—e.g., in his habit of interrupting himself, as in 1.3.155–184 and 4.1.13. Characteristically, he dies in mid-sentence. However, he is not merely a stock emblem of fiery and foolish chivalry; he displays intelligence, humour, and high spirits, and he has a loving wife whose affection emphasises his humanity.

The historical Hotspur was as celebrated—and evidently as vain and foolish—as Shakespeare's character, and the play presents his role at Shrewsbury accurately, except in two important respects. First, his death in the battle cannot definitely be attributed to Hal, or to anyone else. Second, and more significant, he was not Hal's contemporary, being in fact older than King Henry. The alteration in his age serves to make him a more satisfying foil to Prince Hal, but at the time of Shrewsbury, when Hal was 16, Hotspur was a veteran soldier of 39, having been a famous warrior on the Scottish border—where he won the nickname Hotspur—for more than 20 years. The alteration in Hotspur's age is established in *Richard II,* in which young PERCY (2), who becomes Hotspur, is introduced as a boy.

A theatrical tradition of playing Hotspur as a stutterer—an effective indication of his excitability—seems to have arisen in 19th-century Germany, where the respected translator SCHLEGEL interpreted Lady Percy's recollection of her husband's 'speaking thick' (*2 Henry IV,* 2.3.24) as 'stammering'. Shakespeare may have been referring to his Northumbrian dialect or, more likely, to his habit of speaking rapidly. In any case, there is no record concerning the historical Hotspur's speech.

Hotspur's son, another Henry Percy, was still a boy when first his father and then his grandfather were killed fighting against King Henry. Prince Hal, upon his accession as King HENRY V, pardoned young Percy and permitted him to resume the family title. As a result, he fought for Hal's son, HENRY VI; he was the Earl of Northumberland whose death in the first battle of ST. ALBANS is reported in 1.1.4–9 of *3 Henry VI.* His son and successor, Hotspur's grandson, appears as the Earl of NORTHUMBERLAND (2) later in that play.

Howard, Charles (1536–1624) English admiral, a leading military figure of the late 16th century and the aristocratic patron of an acting company, the ADMIRAL'S MEN. Howard was a cousin of Queen ELIZABETH (1). He was trained for the admiralty from an early age, and after a successful career as a soldier in the Low Countries and as an English diplomat, he was appointed Lord Admiral of England in 1585. He commanded the country's resistance to the Spanish Armada in 1588, and in 1596 he was a co-commander of the successful English attack on Spain at Cadiz. The latter event is alluded to in *The Merchant of Venice* (see ANDREW [1]). Under King JAMES I, Howard continued to influence naval and foreign policy until his retirement in 1619. He was renowned for his civility and honesty and has always been regarded as one of the finest public figures of the era. Beginning in 1576, Howard was the patron of an important LONDON theatre company known first as Lord Howard's Men and later as the Admiral's Men. His role consisted of permitting them to use his name—necessary under restrictive Puritan laws (see ELIZABETHAN THEATRE)—and he had nothing to do with the company's productions.

Howard's Men or Lord Howard's Men See ADMIRAL'S MEN.

Hubert Character in *King John,* a follower of King JOHN (3) and custodian of ARTHUR. Hubert first ap-

pears as a representative of the city of ANGIERS (see also CITIZEN [4]), proposing a compromise between John and King PHILIP (2) of France. His opening remarks (2.1.325–333) emphasise the balance between opposing forces that recurs throughout the play. By 3.2 (3.3) (for citation, see *King John*, 'Synopsis'), Hubert has joined King John's entourage. When Arthur is captured in battle, Hubert accepts John's implicit order to kill him. In 4.1, one of Shakespeare's most terrifying and moving scenes, Hubert, touched by the boy's innocence, hides Arthur and tells the king that he has died. Arthur's supposed death proves politically catastrophic to the king; yet when Hubert reveals that Arthur is alive, it turns out that the young prince has in the meantime died attempting to escape. Thus Hubert's career mirrors the changes in fortune and the ambiguities of good and evil that are a principal theme of the play.

Shakespeare's character bears almost no resemblance to the historical figure who provided the name. Hubert de Burgh (d. 1243), although he briefly had custody of Arthur, seems not to have been involved in his death; he may have actually tried to prevent it. In any case, he certainly was not the bourgeois opportunist depicted in the play. On the contrary, he was one of the highest-ranking aristocrats in England, being descended directly from Charlemagne, and he was an important administrator both before and during the period of the play and under John's successor, Henry III (see HENRY [1]). Furthermore, he won a great naval victory over a French fleet that was attempting to reinforce the forces of LEWIS (1) in England. Shakespeare translates this battle—the first in Britain's long tradition of naval supremacy—into a storm, reported in 5.3.9–11, rather than give credit to Hubert. The playwright may have felt that depicting Hubert as a commoner made the unscrupulous ambition that leads him to agree to kill a boy more believable, while the character's lack of commitment to the high politics of the realm could make his subsequent mercy credible.

Hughes, Margaret (d. 1719) The first recorded English actress. In 1660, when English theatres were reopened following the Puritan Revolution, actresses were for the first time permitted to take the female parts, previously played by boys (see ELIZABETHAN DRAMA). Margaret Hughes was the first woman to do so, playing DESDEMONA in Thomas KILLIGREW's production of *Othello.* She had a long and successful career, joining William DAVENANT's company in 1676. She was also the mistress of the king's famous cousin, the military hero Prince Rupert (1619–1682), and mother of his illegitimate daughter.

Hull, Thomas (1728–1808) English actor and theatrical entrepreneur, producer of adaptations of two of Shakespeare's plays. Hull produced adaptations of *Timon of Athens* (1786) and *The Comedy of Errors* (1793). The first of these was an economic failure, but his *Comedy* was restaged for many years and only disappeared from the English stage when Shakespeare's original text was restored in the second half of the 19th century. Hull was well known in his own day as a successful actor of secondary parts who spent a nearly 50-year career in one establishment, London's Covent Garden Theatre.

Hume, John (active 1441) Historical figure and character in *2 Henry VI*, a dishonest priest who arranges to hire a witch, MARGERY JOURDAIN, and two sorcerers, John SOUTHWELL and Roger BOLINGBROKE (2), for the DUCHESS (1) of Gloucester. The Duchess wishes to read the future so that she can prepare for a possible coup against King HENRY VI. In 1.2 Hume reveals in a soliloquy that he is also in the pay of the Duke of SUFFOLK (3), who seeks the Duchess' downfall as part of his campaign against her husband, the Duke of GLOUCESTER (4). Consequently, Hume's information leads to the arrest of the Duchess, along with that of Hume and the magicians, at a séance in 1.4. Hume's confederacy with Suffolk does him little good, for the king sentences him to death in 2.3 for his part in the plot.

Historically, Hume, whose first name was actually Thomas, was pardoned, for reasons that the chronicles do not specify; there is, however, no evidence that he was an agent of Gloucester's enemies. Shakespeare's reason for omitting Hume's pardon, seemingly appropriate to his presentation, is not apparent. Perhaps the playwright intended a subtle intimation of treachery on Suffolk's part. Or this may simply be an instance of the petty inconsistencies to which the playwright was persistently susceptible.

Hundred Years War (1337–1453) Fourteenth- and 15th-century conflict between England and FRANCE (1), parts of which are enacted in *1 Henry VI* and *Henry V.* The Hundred Years War, which actually lasted 116 years, consisted of three distinct phases separated by periods of peace. Shakespeare dealt only with the third stage, which began in 1415.

The war was basically a dynastic quarrel between the PLANTAGENET family and France's House of Valois. King Edward III of England claimed the French throne by inheritance through his mother. The French countered that the ancient Salic Law—disparaged by CANTERBURY (1) in *Henry V*, 1.2.33–95—excluded women from the succession. Edward declared war on France in 1337, and the English conquered large tracts of French territory to add to their already vast holdings in GASCONY. In 1360 a peace treaty ended this first phase of the war. Nine years later a revolt broke

out, and the French recovered most of their lost territory. Two decades of sporadic fighting ensued before RICHARD II negotiated a peace treaty in 1396. England conceded its losses, and the second phase of the conflict came to a close.

The third phase of the war began when HENRY V invaded France in 1415, as presented in *Henry V*. In Shakespeare's play the English victory at AGINCOURT leads directly to the French surrender at TROYES, enacted in 5.2, but in fact five more years of fighting were necessary before Henry was granted the inheritance of the French crown. However, when Henry died in 1422, the French rebelled. Their subsequent success is presented in *1 Henry VI;* over the next 30 years, aided by a charismatic leader, Joan of Arc (see JOAN LA PUCELLE), they drove the English from France (except a tiny foothold at Calais, which England held for another century) in campaigns that culminated in the battle of BORDEAUX (1453). The English were soon engaged in the internal WARS OF THE ROSES, and they never attempted another conquest; the Hundred Years War was over.

The Hundred Years War was a watershed in the history of both countries. France, finally free of English colonisation, began to unify the territories that constitute the modern French nation. England, defeated on the Continent, began to develop its naval power. In military history, the war was also decisive. Medieval warfare, which depended on the mounted knight, was now obsolete; the development of tactics involving many archers and foot soldiers—plus the first use of gunpowder in Europe—spelled the beginning of more modern armies, involving masses of common troops. Moreover, the long and bloody war almost wiped out the knights, the traditional feudal nobility of both countries, permitting the monarchs to begin to ally themselves with the rising middle class, a process that was to result in the modern nation-state. This is to some extent reflected in Shakespeare in the fall of the medieval ideal of kingship represented by Richard II, although in the playwright's day this effect was not clearly perceived.

Hunnis, William (d. 1597) English poet and musician, master of the Children of the Chapel (see CHILDREN'S COMPANIES). In 1566 Hunnis succeeded Richard EDWARDS as director of the choirboys. They performed numerous plays at the court of Queen ELIZABETH (1), some of which Hunnis may have written himself. In 1576 he delegated his theatrical responsibilities to his deputy, Richard FARRANT, who organised the first BLACKFRIARS THEATRE where the boys performed. Upon Farrant's death in 1580, Hunnis resumed direction of the troupe which he led until his death, though their play production ceased almost entirely after 1584.

An accomplished composer, Hunnis was a court musician for King Edward VI as early as 1550. Under Queen Mary, his ardent Protestantism led him to join a plot against the queen. For this he was imprisoned, being freed upon Elizabeth's accession in 1558 when he resumed his career. His poetry was largely religious, though he also wrote secular works, including parts of the elaborate festivities held at KENILWORTH in 1575, which may have been witnessed by the 11-year-old Shakespeare.

Hunsdon (1), George Carey, Baron (1547–1603) English diplomat and theatrical patron. George Carey, the second Lord Hunsdon, was the son of Henry Carey (see HUNSDON [2]), Lord Chamberlain to Queen ELIZABETH (1). Upon his father's death in 1596, Hunsdon assumed the patronage of his theatrical company, the CHAMBERLAIN'S MEN, of which Shakespeare was a member. Because Hunsdon did not immediately succeed his father as Chamberlain (see COBHAM), the company was known for nine months as HUNSDON'S MEN. When he was appointed Chamberlain in 1597 the company resumed its old name, which it retained until the patronage was assumed by King JAMES I in 1603, shortly before Hunsdon's death.

George Carey had a successful career as a soldier and diplomat before he succeeded to his father's title. As Lord Chamberlain, he continued his father's policy of protecting the budding ELIZABETHAN THEATRE from the persecution of the puritanical London government. He provided many occasions for performances by the Chamberlain's Men, either at court or in his own home, Hunsdon House.

Hunsdon (2), Henry Carey, Baron (1524–1596) English statesman and theatrical patron. Lord Hunsdon, as he was known, was Lord Chamberlain of England. In 1594 he assumed the patronage of Shakespeare's theatrical company, DERBY'S MEN, after the death of their previous patron. In recognition of Hunsdon's high office, the company was renamed the CHAMBERLAIN'S MEN. As Lord Chamberlain, Hunsdon protected the theatrical profession (see ELIZABETHAN THEATRE) from persecution by the London government, which was controlled by Puritans, an increasingly powerful religious sect that opposed public drama.

In February 1596 Hunsdon's grand-daughter was married, and scholars speculate that her wedding may have been the occasion of the first performance of *A Midsummer Night's Dream,* staged by his company. Upon his death, the company's patronage was assumed by his son George Carey, also Baron HUNSDON (1). The elder Lord Hunsdon was one of the most valued advisers of Queen ELIZABETH (1), and he held a series of high offices in her government. His mistress, Emilia LANIER, is among the women identified by

commentators as the possible Dark Lady of Shakespeare's SONNETS.

Hunsdon's Men Name used by Shakespeare's theatrical company, better known as the CHAMBERLAIN'S MEN, between July 22, 1596, and the following March 17. On the first date, the patron of the Chamberlain's Men, Baron HUNSDON (2), Lord Chamberlain for Queen ELIZABETH (1), died. He left his baronial title and the patronage of the company to his son, also Lord HUNSDON (1), but since the younger Lord Hunsdon did not immediately succeed his father as chamberlain, the company's name was changed to Hunsdon's Men. Nine months later, the new baron was appointed to his father's old office, after the death of the intervening holder, Lord COBHAM, and the company resumed their old name. As Hunsdon's Men, the company continued to be the leading London troupe; during this time, they introduced *Romeo and Juliet*—as is known from the title page of the play's first edition—and they rehearsed *The Merry Wives of Windsor,* which was first staged just after the second Lord Hunsdon became chamberlain.

The elder Lord Hunsdon had maintained another company as early as 1564, also known as Hunsdon's Men. They had been associated with the ADMIRAL'S MEN in the 1580s but had chiefly toured in the provinces and are not to be confused with the brief incarnation of the Chamberlain's Men. The provincial Hunsdon's Men were disbanded around 1590.

Hunt, Simon (active 1571–1575) STRATFORD schoolmaster, Shakespeare's teacher. Hunt was master of the Stratford Grammar School from 1571 to 1575. Sometime during this period, Shakespeare probably advanced in school to the point where he was taught by the master. Younger pupils were taught by an assistant, called an usher, but since no usher's names have survived from the period, Hunt probably is the earliest known teacher of Shakespeare. However, it is uncertain who Hunt was. A Simon Hunt who began a career as a Catholic clergyman in 1578 and died in 1585 is recorded. If he was Shakespeare's teacher, he may conceivably have influenced the religious sensibilities of his pupil and promoted a tolerance for Catholicism. Many scholars see this tolerance in the adult Shakespeare's work, some going so far as to believe that the playwright was a secret Catholic. However, another Simon Hunt is known to have died in Stratford in 1598, and whoever the Simon Hunt of Stratford Grammar School was, he did not teach Shakespeare long before being succeeded by Thomas JENKINS.

Huntington Library Major collection of Shakespeareana in San Marino, California. The Huntington Library was created by Henry E. Huntington (1850–1927), the heir to a railroad fortune. Huntington spent much of his wealth on the art museum and library that bear his name. The library contains the largest American collection of early printed books, including many QUARTO and FOLIO editions of Shakespeare's plays. It also contains other Shakespeareana and a large collection of 16th-century music.

Huntsman (1) Minor character in *3 Henry VI,* a servant assigned to escort the captive EDWARD IV. Surprised by Edward's rescuers in 4.5, the Huntsman elects to travel with the escapee's party, saying, 'Better do so than tarry and be hang'd.' (4.5.26). This one-liner provides a hint of comic relief amid a grim series of political and military manoeuvrings.

Huntsman (2) Either of two minor characters in the INDUCTION to *The Taming of the Shrew,* servants of a local landowner, the LORD (1). In Ind.1 the Huntsmen assist the Lord in his practical joke on Christopher SLY (1), which is the business of the introductory scenes. The Huntsmen's role in the plot could have been filled by servants of any sort, but the Lord's conversation with them on the merits of his hounds contributes to the rural atmosphere of the Induction.

Hyman, Earle (b. 1926) Black American actor. Hyman has played many parts in both classical and modern plays since beginning his career in 1942 at the American Negro Theatre of Harlem. Among his noted Shakespearean portrayals have been OTHELLO and CALIBAN.

Hymen (1) Minor character in *As You Like It,* the Roman god of marriage. In 5.4.107–145 Hymen is the central figure in the MASQUE that accompanies ROSALIND's appearance, undisguised, to resolve the play's complexities. Hymen, after making a formal statement of divine pleasure when earthly confusions are resolved, announces the return of Rosalind. Rosalind in turn declares her true relationship to her father, DUKE (7) Senior, to ORLANDO, and to PHEBE, all hitherto hidden by her disguise as a young man. Hymen then solemnly blesses four couples: Rosalind and Orlando, CELIA and OLIVER (1), Phebe and SILVIUS, and TOUCHSTONE and AUDREY. He then leads a 'wedlock hymn' (5.4.136), which everyone sings. This formal celebration of marriage represents the happy conclusion of the play's various courtships.

It is unclear whether Shakespeare intended Hymen as a human impersonator of a god taking part in a festive tableau arranged by Rosalind or as an actual deity appearing to mortals, as gods do in other Shake-

spearean plays—e.g., in *Cymbeline,* 5.4, and *The Tempest,* 4.1. In either case, Hymen's function is the same: his masque lends a gracefully solemn air to the play's climax. The part of Hymen is often assigned to AMIENS, who is a singer and who is present in this scene, according to the stage direction at 5.4.1, but who has no spoken lines in it.

Hymen (2) Minor character in *The Two Noble Kinsmen,* the Roman god of marriage, as portrayed by a celebrant in the interrupted wedding of THESEUS (2) and HIPPOLYTA (2). Hymen does not speak; he is described in the opening stage direction as entering 'with a torch burning' (1.1.1). He provides a note of formal dignity to the occasion.

I

Iachimo Character in *Cymbeline,* the villain who pretends to have seduced POSTHUMUS' new wife, IMOGEN. He thus provokes the murderous jealousy in Posthumus that stimulates much of the action of the play. Motivated only by an irresponsible pleasure in mischief, Iachimo wagers that he can seduce Imogen. When he fails, he resorts to trickery. He secretes himself in her bedroom, steals her bracelet, and then poses as her lover. He flaunts his knowledge of her intimate surroundings and declares the bracelet a gift. His plan accomplished in 2.4, Iachimo pockets the diamond ring he has won from Posthumus and disappears from the play until very near its close, when he returns to Britain as a member of the Roman army. He proves unsuccessful in combat, and he supposes that his guilt for blackening Imogen's name has weakened him as a warrior. Captured, he confesses to his crime when the disguised Imogen recognises on his hand the ring he has won. In the aura of reconciliation that closes the play, he is forgiven by Posthumus.

Commentators have often compared Iachimo to Shakespeare's most extraordinary villain, IAGO, whose lies are similar in content. His name, the diminutive of Iago, suggests a similarly evil temperament, but Iachimo is a very different sort of villain. He is closer to the likeable AUTOLYCUS, the vagabond thief of *The Winter's Tale.* Iachimo is essentially a stock comic figure, the unscrupulous Italian (see ROME). He has no intention of destroying anyone's life, as Iago does; he barely has any intention at all. He is more like a con man than a rapist, though he compares himself to the genuinely fearful TARQUIN. However, he does so just as he has comically emerged like a jack-in-the-box, from a trunk, in 2.2, and such a ludicrous villain assures us that Imogen will not be permanently damaged. This aspect of Iachimo is important to the play's generally optimistic tone. We are never in doubt that the world of romance is dominant; Iachimo is merely an instrument of fate, which controls the adventures of Posthumus and Imogen. Even in the humiliation of his final exposure, Iachimo remains comic. Our awareness of his harmlessness is reinforced as he shamelessly embroiders the truth, apparently hoping to make himself seem a pleasingly audacious young gentleman. Both boastful and apologetic, he seems an entirely appropriate object of mercy—an immature fool. Unlike the other villains of the piece, the QUEEN (2) and CLOTEN, mercy is granted to him.

Iago Character in *Othello,* OTHELLO's villainous aide. The play centres on Iago's effort to destroy Othello's happiness. He convinces him that his wife, DESDEMONA, has been having a love affair with CASSIO, his lieutenant. One of Shakespeare's most thoroughly villainous characters, Iago has intrigued audiences for generations through his combination of realistic malice and seemingly unjustified lust for revenge, his 'motiveless malignity', in Samuel Taylor COLERIDGE's famous words. However, Shakespeare does provide his villain with stimuli that provoke his evil. In fact, if Iago's motives seem unclear it is because he is motivated in several ways, rather than not at all.

Shakespeare provides us with much evidence of Iago's motives in his soliloquies. He has been passed over for promotion in favour of Cassio, and in his first soliloquy he schemes to reverse this development and considers entangling Desdemona and the lieutenant as a step in this direction. Much later, Iago's wife, EMILIA (2), unknowingly comes close to guessing the cause of Othello's jealousy when she remarks, 'Some busy and insinuating rogue, / . . . to get some office, / [Has] devis'd this slander' (4.2.133–135).

Military ambition is commonplace, and this is an entirely credible motive, but it does not preclude the simultaneous operation of others. A second motive is sexual jealousy, the emotion which Iago transmits to Othello. Iago suspects Emilia's adultery with Othello in 1.3.385–386, and in his second soliloquy jealousy is his only stated motive. His suspicions are sometimes thought to be only a justification in his campaign against the general, but he expresses them in soliloquy, when he need not lie, and he is also jealous of Cassio (2.1.302). Emilia speaks of his suspicions, in 4.2.149, and Iago seems to have some general grounds for his jealousy, as Emilia states explicitly that she would commit adultery, given the opportunity (4.3.70). It is telling that the weapon Iago fashions to destroy Othello is precisely the one that hurts himself. The power of sexuality as a goad is further revealed in Iago's obsessive references to bestial sex (as in 1.1.88–

89), and in his vivid description of Cassio in bed with him (3.3.425–432). It is obvious that Iago's suspicions stem from his morbid imagination, but from Iago's point of view they are no less effective as inducements to action.

Both of these motives reflect an even deeper level of feeling. Iago's professional and sexual jealousies cause him to 'hate the Moor' (1.3.384), but they also stem from a greater, generalised jealous sense, an envy of those who have advantages over him that extend beyond promotions or access to his wife. He senses that the open and virtuous qualities in others may point up his own worthlessness. He cannot 'endure . . . [Othello's] constant, noble, loving nature' (2.1.283–284), and he sees in Cassio 'a daily beauty in his life, / That makes me ugly' (5.1.19–20). Like Satan—and not coincidentally, as we shall see—Iago is envious of those who are spiritually greater than he.

Iago's multiple motives make him a humanly credible character, but these are joined by an inhuman ferocity that adds a dose of terror to our perception of him. His envy and anger are so strong that they compel him to risk his life in his passionate effort to damage Othello. Though he has motives, his response outweighs the stimulus, and thus a less easily understood motive merges with the others: Iago loves evil for its own sake. He clearly delights in what he is doing. He speaks of fooling RODERIGO as 'my sport' (1.3.384); his delighted irony all but bubbles over when he exults, 'And what's he then, that says I play the villain . . .' (2.3.327); and his enjoyment is obvious when he says, 'Pleasure, and action, make the hours seem short' (2.3.369). After his triumph in the temptation scene (3.3), he cannot refrain from returning to manipulate his enemy some more. When accident brings him Desdemona's handkerchief, he comfortably contemplates the damage he may do with it, like an artist savouring a new and exciting idea—'this may do something' (3.3.329), he slyly understates. After reducing Othello to hysteria, he gloats, 'Work on, / My medicine, work' (4.1.44–45), and even in utter defeat his final refusal to talk smacks of self-satisfaction.

With his pleasure in evil Iago resembles the VICE of medieval drama. The Vice was an allegorical figure whose delight in horseplay and mischievous humour made him a popular character. Iago, however, is a realistic, rather than an abstract, embodiment of evil. Although Iago is not a comic character, he is occasionally funny. In 1.1.118, for example, he returns BRABANTIO's 'Thou art a villain' with 'You are a senator', and in his many ironic remarks on his own honesty, as in 2.3.258 and 318, the humour is unrecognised by anyone but himself and the audience. He also adopts a jocular attitude for his own purposes, as in the conventional battle of wits in 2.1.109–166 and the drinking bout of 2.3. Many commentators and theatrical directors agree with the advice of Edwin BOOTH (2), who insisted that actors playing Iago should 'not sneer or glower' and suggested that 'the "light comedian" . . . not the "heavy man" ' should play the part.

Many people have a problem with the plot of *Othello:* the hero is unrealistically gullible, murdering his wife on the strength of a suggestion that has no serious credibility. However, Shakespeare relied on an established dramatic convention: Iago has a double role as villain to the audience but trustworthy friend to the characters in the play. He is seen as good by everyone but the audience, which fosters a high degree of suspense. For this reason, Shakespeare made Iago's villainy evident immediately in his first exchange with Roderigo in Act 1, and his evilness is repeatedly confirmed in his soliloquies. Iago is frank about his double role, saying 'I am not what I am' (1.1.65). Even his name—that of the patron saint of England's great enemy, Spain—indicated his evil nature to a 17th-century audience. Shakespeare's audiences presumed that Iago's victims would be taken in—and most modern audiences believe this as well.

Iago deceives Othello by also manipulating other people to achieve his ends. At Iago's instigation, Cassio urges Desdemona to intervene for him, thus unwittingly inflaming Othello's jealousy, and Roderigo attacks Cassio, who might expose Iago. Iago gets Desdemona's incriminating handkerchief from Emilia, and he exploits the affair of BIANCA (2) and Cassio to mislead Othello further. He describes his schemes aptly as spiderwebs, in 2.1.168. At the close of the play he fails, when his network of villainy begins to unravel. When Cassio fails to kill Roderigo, Iago does it himself—or thinks he does, though actually Roderigo lives to testify against him, as is revealed in 5.2.325–330. Only at this point, significantly, does Iago's cool self-confidence leave him, and he hastily mutters to himself, 'This is the night / That either makes me, or fordoes me quite' (5.1.127–128).

In the end the power of Iago's envy expires, and the forces of trust and love recover, though it is a bleak victory. Othello finally recognises the goodness of Desdemona, and Iago is condemned, but in the meantime Iago has demonstrated the power of evil. His power depends, however, on the weakness in Othello. In his motives, his judgements, and his single-minded savagery, Iago embodies his victim's psychological flaws. Iago can triumph only because Othello rejects his own potential for love and trust in favour of the self-centred desperation of jealousy and envy, the passions that dominate Iago.

Iago is the evil influence on Othello, in opposition to Desdemona's good. This situation closely resembles that of the medieval MORALITY PLAY, still familiar in Shakespeare's day, in which a central character must choose between an angel and a devil. Iago is associated with satanic evil at several points in the play. For example, when Othello, fainting with rage at

the image of Desdemona's infidelity cries out, 'O devil!' (4.1.43), Iago, on cue, exults, 'Work on, / My medicine, work' (4.1.44–45). Iago hints at the hellish nature of his undertaking early on when he openly (to Roderigo) claims as his allies 'all the tribe of hell' (1.3.358), and in his soliloquy declares, 'Hell and night / Must bring this monstrous birth to the world's light' (1.3.401–402). Later, when he says that his 'Dangerous conceits . . . Burn like the mines of sulpher' (3.3.331–334), he reminds us of the conventional metaphor for hellfire.

Finally, at the play's close, Iago overtly identifies himself with the devil. Othello makes the connection first, after Iago's malevolence has been exposed. He looks at the villain's feet to see if they are cloven and says, 'If that thou be'st a devil, I cannot kill thee' (5.2.288), as he attempts to stab him with his sword. Iago, wounded, gloats defiantly, 'I bleed, sir, but not kill'd' (5.2.289), fully accepting the implication. It is the last thing he says before refusing to speak any further. In this final refusal Iago brazenly displays his malice, for all along his power has been in his words, talking his evil ends into existence. In making Iago's nature so strikingly evident at the play's close, Shakespeare helps assuage our horror, for we see that the villain's uncanny malevolence is even more immense than we had thought. It is as vast as hell itself, the abode of infinite evil, and we are therefore doubly glad that his career is finished, not only in relief from the play's agonising developments, but also in satisfaction at the suppression of a truly satanic menace.

Iden, Alexander (active 1450) Historical figure and minor character in *2 Henry VI*, a landowner who kills the rebel Jack CADE, who has hidden in his garden, in 4.10. Iden represents an ideal of the English country gentleman and small landowner. He is the very opposite of the subversive and destructive Cade, and also of the scheming noblemen whose ambitions are the chief business of the play. We see Iden before he knows of Cade's presence, enjoying his garden and rejoicing in his lot. Challenged by the desperate and angry Cade, Iden refuses to send for help. They fight, and Iden kills Cade, cursing the rebel as he does so. In 5.1 he presents King HENRY VI with Cade's head and is knighted.

Shakespeare created this paragon of the minor gentry from a bare mention of Cade's killer in the chronicles. The historical Iden was a sheriff of Kent who presumably killed Cade for the sizeable bounty that was offered for the rebel's head, which he in fact collected.

Illyria Region on the Adriatic coast of present-day Yugoslavia and northern Albania, setting for *Twelfth Night.* As in most of Shakespeare's plays set overseas, there is nothing specifically Illyrian about the surroundings in which the action occurs; Illyria was simply remote and exotic and therefore suitable to a tale of disguise, intrigue, and romance. Like such idealised locales as the Forest of ARDEN (1) in *As You Like It*, Illyria is pervaded with music and song and its inhabitants are concerned chiefly with love and revelry. However, ANTONIO (4) observes that 'these parts . . . often prove rough and unhospitable' (3.3.9–11), reflecting the unnsavoury reputation of the Illyrian coast, which was a notorious den of piracy until the 17th century. There are references to Illyrian pirates elsewhere in Shakespeare (*2 Henry VI*, 4.1.107; *Measure for Measure*, 4.3.70) and in other Elizabethan literature.

Imogen Character in *Cymbeline*, daughter of King CYMBELINE and wife of POSTHUMUS. Imogen, the central character of the play, loses the love of her husband through no fault of her own, is exposed to great danger and wanders in the wilderness, and then is finally restored to happiness. She embodies the play's lesson that while humanity may exhibit courage and an undefeatable spirit of love, our happiness nevertheless depends on providence. Imogen has long been among the favourite heroines in Shakespeare. The Victorian poet SWINBURNE extravagantly called her 'the woman best beloved in all the world of song and all the tide of time'. However, her great charm is also evidence of a failure on the playwright's part as he struggled with a new genre, the ROMANCES.

Imogen is subjected to a harrowing sequence of misfortunes. Her father banishes Posthumus to Italy, and she faces the unwanted courtship of both the boorish CLOTEN and the oily IACHIMO, the latter of whom malevolently convinces Posthumus that she has been unfaithful. Posthumus thereupon arranges for her murder in the wilds of WALES (1). A faithful servant, PISANIO, warns her and provides her with a disguise as a young man, but she finds herself stranded in the wilderness. After several adventurous episodes during which she comes to believe Posthumus is dead and is herself believed to be dead by others, she returns to her father's court in the guise of a Roman prisoner of war. In the final scene's sequence of reconciliations her identity is revealed, and she is reunited with both husband and father.

Though Imogen has always enchanted audiences, her resourcefulness and charm suggest one who battles against destiny rather than the helpless victim of fate. In the literature on which Shakespeare's romances were based, the traditional character type corresponding to Imogen was the fairy-tale princess who is adored for her beauty and passive calm, an object of intrigue but not a participant in it. She represents humanity's helplessness and inspires pity in her plight, rather than admiration for her pluck. Imogen is intermittently presented in terms of this ideal. To Pisanio,

she is 'more goddess-like than wife-like' (3.2.8), and Iachimo compares her to 'th'Arabian bird' (1.7.17), the fabled Phoenix who cannot die. She sometimes seems to be a helpless puppet of the plot, as when she immediately accepts Iachimo's transparently false excuse for having proposed adultery with a humble 'You make amends' (1.7.168). Moreover, she adopts a purely conventional morality when she refuses to sleep with Posthumus even after they are married, presumably because she awaits her father's approval of the match.

However, Imogen has another set of qualities as well. In her spunk, her sharp wit, and her willingness to pursue her lover—as well as in her male disguise—Imogen is typical of Shakespeare's earlier comic heroines. In *Cymbeline* the playwright approached a new sort of character but could not divorce himself from habits of characterisation that he had used earlier. This happened with several of the characters in the play. Imogen is a transitional figure; Shakespeare would soon create female characters whose ethereal serenity would fulfil the romantic ideal. In Imogen he produced an uneasy conjunction of ideal womanhood—seen in HERMIONE of *The Winter's Tale* and MIRANDA of *The Tempest*—and boyish pluck, such as had enlivened ROSALIND of *As You Like It,* and VIOLA of *Twelfth Night,* among others. Imogen, for all her charming virtues, presents an image slightly contrary to the general tone of the play and thus in part contributes to its weakness.

Induction Dramatic device of the 16th and 17th centuries—an introductory scene or set of scenes that frankly announce the presentation of a play—that Shakespeare used at the outset of *The Taming of the Shrew.* In two successive scenes the drunken tinker Christopher SLY (1) is persuaded by the LORD (1) that he is a nobleman, by way of a practical joke, and a group of players performs a play for him; that play is *The Taming of the Shrew.*

Strictly speaking, an induction, though similar in purpose to a PROLOGUE, consists of dialogue instead of a single speech. However, the FOLIO edition of *2 Henry IV* labels the introductory speech by RUMOUR as 'Induction', and it is traditionally separated from 1.1.

An induction was generally found most appropriate in a COMEDY, for it emphasises the artificiality of the presentation to follow and prepares the audience to accept the ridiculous confusions that characterise the genre. It places the audience at a distance from the main action, which effectively becomes a play within a play.

Ingleby, Clement Mansfield (1823–1886) English scholar. In 1859 Ingleby helped expose the forgeries of J. P. COLLIER (2) in his *The Shakespeare Fabrications.* He followed it with *A Complete View of the Shakespeare Controversy* (1861), which is still regarded as a definitive book on Collier. He wrote a number of other books on Shakespeare and assembled *Shakespeare's Centurie of Prayse* (1875), an anthology of references to the playwright in surviving documents from the period 1591–1693. It was the first of its kind, and later editors have expanded and revised Ingleby's collection, which remains at the core of *The Shakespeare Allusion Book* (1932) edited by Sir Edmund CHAMBERS.

Innogen GHOST CHARACTER who is mentioned in stage directions in *Much Ado About Nothing* (at the opening of 1.1 and 2.1) but does not appear, the wife of LEONATO. The existence of a ghost character, apparently reflecting an unrealised intention of the playwright, is evidence that the original published text, the QUARTO of 1600, was printed from Shakespeare's FOUL PAPERS—his unpolished manuscript—and is therefore highly authoritative.

Inns of Court Four law schools in LONDON, in whose buildings at least two of Shakespeare's plays were staged, and which served as a location for a scene in *1 Henry VI.* The Inns of Court—Gray's Inn Lincoln's Inn, the Middle Temple, and the Inner Temple—were so called because part of their function was to prepare young men to be gentlemen of the royal court. In addition to academic and legal studies, students learned dancing and music, and the Inns were famous for their elaborate MASQUES and other entertainments. The masque presented in 5.2 of *Love's Labour's Lost* is believed to be based on a noteworthy pageant presented at the annual Gray's InnChristmas Revels in 1594. Shakespeare presumably saw this event, for *The Comedy of Errors* was performed by his acting company as part of the same festival (the earliest recorded performance of the play). It is thought that the 'houses' (see PHOENIX; PORCUPINE; PRIORY) described in the *Comedy*'s stage directions reflect the classically influenced stage of the Inn. Also, *Twelfth Night* was performed at the Middle Temple in 1602.

In 2.4 of *1 Henry VI,* the antagonists of what will be the WARS OF THE ROSES engage in a dispute in the Temple Garden, a precinct of the Inns of Court. They bait each other by pointedly selecting emblems from two rose bushes, one red and one white. The incident, which is fictitious, is well placed, for the Inns were legally sanctuaries, where violence of any kind was strictly forbidden. Therefore, the dispute could not come to blows but rather had to be fully explicated in words and symbols.

Interlude Sixteenth-century term for a play—especially a short one with few characters—used more specifically to refer to elements in two of Shakespeare's plays. In *The Taming of the Shrew,* the passage 1.1.248–253 is spoken of as an interlude because it is

a return to the story of Christopher SLY (1), begun in the INDUCTION. It is believed that there were originally several other interludes and an EPILOGUE, completing the tale, and that these are presented, although in altered form, in the anonymous play *THE TAMING OF A SHREW* (published 1594), thought to be a BAD QUARTO of Shakespeare's play. These passages are sometimes included in modern editions of the play, although they are missing from the original publication of *The Taming of the Shrew;* they were probably cut from an early production because of a shortage of available actors.

The term 'interlude' is also used in *A Midsummer Night's Dream*—and by writers about the play—to refer to the performance of *PYRAMUS AND THISBE* staged by the artisans of ATHENS. The term was probably old-fashioned in Shakespeare's day and may have carried a connotation of rustic quaintness.

Inverness City in northern SCOTLAND, the site of MACBETH's castle and the location of several scenes in *Macbeth.* Beginning in 1.5 when LADY (6) MACBETH learns of the WITCHES' prediction that Macbeth will be king, through 2.4, when Macbeth's upcoming coronation is abruptly announced, Inverness is associated with the planning, execution, and aftermath of the assassination of King DUNCAN. In 1.6 Duncan and BANQUO describe the castle at Inverness as a lovely building, thronged with birds and characterised by a pleasant atmosphere, but its nature quickly changes as our sense of it is influenced by the evil done there. It is associated with hell in 2.3.1–21, where the PORTER (3) comically portrays a gatekeeper of hell, an ancient dramatic tradition of medieval religious drama. The description of terrible omens in 2.4 leaves us with an impression of Inverness as a castle of horrors. Productions of *Macbeth* have commonly emphasised this idea, with sets that stress darkness and Gothic detail.

Historically, the inclusion of Inverness in the play is an anachronism. Macbeth did not murder Duncan at Inverness—he didn't murder him at all—and there was no castle at Inverness until at least a century later. However, Shakespeare took this error from his source, HOLINSHED's history, and doubtless believed it was correct.

Iras Character in *Antony and Cleopatra,* an attendant of CLEOPATRA. In 1.2 Iras is a pleasantly humorous young woman who jests over the predictions of the SOOTHSAYER (2), but she displays almost no personality thereafter. She is overshadowed by CHARMIAN in the queen's household, as she is on much less intimate terms with her mistress and has a much less developed role. Significantly, the Soothsayer tells Iras only that her fortune will be the same as Charmian's (1.2.52). She appears often with Cleopatra and Charmian but speaks very little. In 5.2 as Cleopatra prepares her suicide, Iras declares her loyalty and says that she will not see the queen as a Roman prisoner, 'for I am sure my nails / Are stronger than mine eyes' (5.2.222–223), but, as elsewhere, she is a faint echo of Charmian. When Cleopatra applies the poisonous asp to herself, Iras falls dead. Perhaps she uses the snake herself, moments earlier, or perhaps she simply dies of grief. In either case, she departs wordlessly. Shakespeare's source, PLUTARCH's *Lives,* states that Cleopatra was attended at her death by a serving-woman named Iras, but she is otherwise unknown in history.

Ireland, William Henry (1777–1835) English forger. In 1794 the 17-year-old Ireland, a lawyer's clerk, forged a number of documents relating to Shakespeare. These included business papers, letters (one to Anne HATHAWAY, with a lock of hair), and the playwright's profession of religious faith. He claimed they had been given by Shakespeare to a friend, a descendant of whom had disclosed them anonymously. Ireland's father, an amateur scholar, exhibited these materials in good faith and published them as *Miscellaneous Papers and Legal Instruments under the Hand and Seal of William Shakespeare* (1796). They caused a sensation, and Ireland responded by creating two Shakespearean plays. One of them, a tragedy entitled *Vortigern and Rowena,* was produced by J. P. KEMBLE (3) in April 1796, although scholars, led by Edmond MALONE, were already suspicious. The play was laughed off the stage, and the second work *(Henry II)* was never performed. Under pressure after the publication of Malone's *Inquiry into the Authenticity of Certain Miscellaneous Papers and Legal Instruments* (1796), Ireland confessed, and wrote *An Authentic Account of the Shakespearian Manuscripts* (1796), in which he described his procedures and cleared his father. He became a hack writer and produced a number of poor novels and a memoir (*Confessions of William Henry Ireland* [1805]), before he died in poverty.

Iris Pagan goddess and minor figure in *The Tempest,* a character in the MASQUE presented by the sprite ARIEL to celebrate the engagement of MIRANDA and FERDINAND (2). Iris—goddess of the rainbow and messenger of the greater deities—functions as the 'presenter' of the masque, which features CERES, goddess of harvests; JUNO, queen of the gods; and a dance of Nymphs and Reapers. Iris' beautiful invocation to Ceres in 4.1.60–75 establishes a tone of serene power appropriate to divinity. Ariel subsequently declares that he 'presented Ceres' (4.1.167), indicating that he played the part of either Ceres or Iris, the presenter; most commentators believe Shakespeare intended the former, with Iris' initial speech providing time for Ariel to costume himself.

In Greek mythology Iris is a hazy figure and was never the object of a cult of worship. Originally simply associated with the rainbow, she was perhaps consid-

ered a messenger of the gods because rainbows seem to connect sky and earth. In classical literature—as distinct from mythology—Iris was particularly associated with Juno, and Shakespeare draws on this tradition when Ariel's masquer speaks of Juno as 'the queen o' th' sky, / Whose wat'ry arch and messenger am I' (4.1.70–71).

Irving, Henry (1838–1905) British actor and producer. Irving was London's leading Shakespearean actor and producer for the last quarter of the 19th century. Though he played few Shakespearean parts during the first 15 years of his acting career, Irving was highly acclaimed as HAMLET in 1874, and over the next few years portrayed MACBETH, OTHELLO, and RICHARD III, establishing himself as one of the best classical actors of the day. From 1878 to 1902 he managed his own company at London's Lyceum Theatre, with himself and Ellen TERRY (1) as the featured performers. They staged many of Shakespeare's plays, including *Hamlet* (1879), *The Merchant of Venice* (1879), *Othello* (1881), *Romeo and Juliet* (1882), *Much Ado About Nothing* (1882), *Twelfth Night* (1884), *Macbeth* (1888), *Henry VIII* (1892), *King Lear* (1892), *Cymbeline* (1896), and *Coriolanus* (1901). He was famous for his extravagant productions, with many extras, elaborate sets and costumes, and special scenic effects. Irving was a tyrannical director by all accounts, 'incapable of caring for anything outside his work', in Terry's words. His business manager at the Lyceum was Bram Stoker, the author of *Dracula,* and it has been thought that Stoker's famous protagonist reflects the actor-producer's domineering personality. Irving's acting and production were not without detractors, but he was generally praised, and in 1895 he became the first actor to be knighted. In 1902 his lease on the Lyceum was not renewed, and he turned to touring. He died a few hours after a performance on the road.

Isabel (1), Queen of England Character in *Richard II.* See QUEEN (13).

Isabel (2), Queen of France (1370–1435) Historical figure and character in *Henry V,* the wife of the FRENCH KING. Queen Isabel appears only in 5.2, where she blesses the marriage of King HENRY V and her daughter, Princess KATHARINE (2).

The historical Queen Isabel was a Princess of Bavaria who married Charles VI, the French King of the play, at the age of 14. She was a notoriously self-indulgent, licentious, and extravagant woman. When it became evident that her husband was insane, Isabel became a leader of the factional strife that was probably most responsible for the victories of Henry V. She went so far as to declare that her second son, the successor to the DAUPHIN (3) as the heir to the throne, was illegitimate, her love life being too rich to permit identification of the father. He nevertheless managed to claim the crown upon the death of the king, and he appears as CHARLES VII in *1 Henry VI.*

Isabella Character in *Measure for Measure,* a would-be nun and the object of the illicit lust of ANGELO (2). Isabella pleads with Angelo to pardon her brother CLAUDIO (3), who has been sentenced to death for sexual immorality; in doing so, she arouses the official's desire, and he demands sex of her in exchange for the pardon. She refuses and asserts that to avoid such a sin is worth a life; she objects hysterically when Claudio begs her to give in. She is, in her strict insistence on morality, as extreme as Angelo was when he sentenced Claudio. She realises her error by the end of the play and requests mercy for Angelo when he is condemned to death by the DUKE (9). Finally, she abandons her earlier intention to become a nun and agrees to marry the Duke, thus bringing about the play's happy ending in marriage, the traditional closing of a COMEDY.

Isabella undergoes a great change of heart in the course of the play, for neither acceptance nor leniency seem part of her nature at first. Like Angelo, before he succumbs to her beauty, she is strictly insistent on virtue. Not only is she about to enter a nunnery, she regrets that its rules are not strict enough. Like Angelo, she wants to see her own ideals applied to others, 'wishing a more strict restraint / Upon the sisters stood' (1.4.4–5) and demanding that Claudio 'Take my defiance, / [and] Die, perish!' (3.1.142–143). When she seeks mercy for Claudio, she holds fast to her morals, pleading that the fault be condemned rather than the doer of it. When this fails to work, she goes on to demand that Angelo behave as God would. Her strict attitudes appeal to Angelo's obsessiveness, sparking his lust as no simple offer of a sexual bribe could. Her extremism matches his.

As with other Shakespearean heroines, Isabella's assertiveness is an attractive feature to audiences, but here it is counterproductive and brings nearer the potential tragedy of Claudio's death. This serves, of course, to further the plot, but it also emphasises an important point: mercy may not be brought about through evil means. If Claudio is to be saved it must be through the action of good, and Isabella, concerned wholly with a rigid sense of morality, cannot provide that action.

Isabella's obsession with her virginity covers her own strong sexuality, which is startingly apparent in her response to Angelo's proposition. She declares that she'd rather die under torture, saying, 'Th'impression of keen whips I'd wear as rubies, / And strip myself to death as to a bed / That longing have been sick for . . .' (2.4.101–103). The strength of her subconscious passion suggests—as does her assertiveness—that she is not a good candidate for the convent,

and at the end of the play when her judgemental attitude has softened, her assent to the Duke's marriage proposal seems appropriate, a step towards fulfilment.

Resolution is only made possible by the substitution of MARIANA (2) in the 'bed trick', permitting the entrapment of the villain without compromising the heroine. Shakespeare's introduction of this device, which is not present in his sources, suggests his attitude towards Isabella. In the original story, the Angelo figure sleeps with the Isabella figure and then is forced to marry her and restore her honour. However, Angelo and Isabella have been shown in the first half of the play to be enemies, and their obsessiveness has been presented with powerful realism. Even within the play's aura of forgiveness, these two characters simply cannot be made to accept each other without losing their dramatic power. Mariana therefore replaces Isabella, and a resolution becomes possible. What is more, Isabella participates in the resolution. She makes the arrangements for the assignation with Angelo, though a message would have sufficed, and then tells Mariana of the plot, a task that could have been performed by the Duke. Shakespeare kept Isabella in the action at this point, thus making her an active force.

Most important, Isabella pleads for Angelo. As the Duke points out, 'Her brother's ghost . . . would . . . take her hence in horror' (5.1.433–434). Isabella's intercession opposes her natural feelings towards Angelo, her intended rapist and the apparent killer of her brother, but she supports Mariana's plea. She argues in rational terms for mercy, in a fashion suited to the case, rather than in the absolute terms in which she had pleaded for Claudio. Isabella is no longer a moral extremist. Perhaps she is under the influence of Mariana's example of love, or perhaps she remembers her claim, in 2.2, that she would be merciful if she had power, or, possibly, she wishes to atone for her willingness to sacrifice Claudio for a principle. Her act flies in the face of common morality with its demand for justice, just as does Christ's command in the Sermon on the Mount to love one's enemies. Isabella has arrived at the giving of a full measure in the spirit of the biblical text that inspired the play's title.

While the play's ending often seems arbitrary to modern readers, its convenient resolution of the impending tragedy was not only perfectly acceptable in Shakespeare's day, it was highly satisfying: the triumph of good, in a clear and traditional manner, gratified the sentimental feelings of audiences. While Isabella is somewhat diminished as a character by her symbolic quality in the play's dénouement, she is nonetheless sufficiently well developed to rank among Shakespeare's most interesting heroines.

Isidore's Servant Minor character in *Timon of Athens*, an employee of Isidore, a creditor of TIMON. In 2.2 Isidore's Servant, with CAPHIS and VARRO'S SERVANT, solicits Timon and his STEWARD (2) for payment, but they are put off. These servants of greedy masters are pawns of plot development; Isidore's Servant speaks even less than the others.

Italy European country, the setting for many of Shakespeare's plays. Though not yet a single nation in Shakespeare's day, Italy was the fountainhead of the RENAISSANCE and the cultural leader of Europe. Many of Shakespeare's sources were Italian, with the consequence that Italian cities were the locations of many of his plays, especially the comedies. Also, Italy had been the centre of the ancient Roman Empire, so Shakespeare's ROMAN PLAYS tended to feature Italian locations, especially ROME. However, there is nothing especially Italian about Shakespeare's settings, and the Italian cities ostensibly shown—such as MANTUA, MESSINA, PADUA, VENICE, and VERONA—tend to resemble Shakespeare's LONDON. The plays in which some or all of the action is set in Italy include *All's Well That Ends Well, Antony and Cleopatra, Coriolanus, Cymbeline, Julius Caesar, The Merchant of Venice, Much Ado About Nothing, Othello, Romeo and Juliet, The Taming of the Shrew, Titus Andronicus, The Two Gentlemen of Verona,* and *The Winter's Tale.*

J

Jackson (1), Barry (1879–1961) British theatrical producer. Jackson was extremely influential on 20th-century Shakespearean production, especially with his modern-dress productions of *Cymbeline* (1923), *Hamlet* (1925), and *Macbeth* (1928), staged at the Birmingham Repertory Theatre, which he founded in 1913. He was director of the Shakespeare Memorial Theatre in STRATFORD from 1945 to 1948.

Jackson (2), John (c. 1574–c. 1625) Friend of Shakespeare in LONDON. Jackson was a partner with Shakespeare and others in the purchase of the BLACKFRIAR'S GATEHOUSE in 1613. He was probably the John Jackson, a shipping magnate from northern England, who was a regular patron of the MERMAID TAVERN and a close friend of Thomas SAVAGE.

Jackson (3), Roger (1601–1625) London publisher and bookseller. Jackson bought the rights to *The Rape of Lucrece* from the younger John HARRISON (2) in 1614, and he published Q6 of the poem, the first edition to bear the full title, in 1616.

Jacobean Drama Art of writing for the theatre as practised in England during the reign of King JAMES I (1603–1625). The drama of this period clearly evolves from ELIZABETHAN DRAMA, and that term is often taken to cover the Jacobean period as well. However, by about 1610, Jacobean drama was quite different. It is usually characterised as decadent, by comparison, in that substantive themes and fine poetry were increasingly subordinated to the titillating effects of the spectacular and bizarre. There are certainly exceptions to this indictment, most notably the late work of Shakespeare, but commentators over the centuries have generally agreed that the period is markedly inferior to its predecessor.

Early in the Jacobean period, Shakespeare manifested the continuing vitality of English TRAGEDY with *Othello, King Lear, Macbeth, Antony and Cleopatra,* and *Coriolanus.* Another major Jacobean tragedy was written early in the period, George CHAPMAN's *Bussy D'Ambois* (1604), but besides Shakespeare, the only great Jacobean writer of tragedies, in most opinions, was John WEBSTER (2), whose *The White Devil* (1612) and *The Duchess of Malfi* (1614) are still frequently performed. He may also have written most of *The Revenger's Tragedy* (1606), though it is frequently attributed to Cyril TOURNEUR, a much lesser talent. Webster's tragedies are all REVENGE PLAYS (as is *Bussy*), a genre that continued to be popular. Thomas MIDDLETON also wrote tragedies, and late in the period another figure arose, John FORD (2).

In line with the decadence of the period, Jacobean tragedies often rely on false starts, sudden changes of motivation, and gratuitous accidents. The artificiality of these devices reflects a different emotional tone: these works largely ignore the implications of human disaster for society or for humanity as a whole, and focus instead on the pathos of the individual. Even that tends to be diminished by a predilection for cheap sensationalism and unnsavoury sexual themes, as the open bawdiness of the Elizabethans yields to a furtive indecency.

Perhaps the best-known Jacobean dramatists are Francis BEAUMONT (2) and John FLETCHER (2), who collaborated on a number of plays that typify the spirit of the era, so much so that in the 1630s they were rated well above Shakespeare by most playgoers. Their *Philaster* (1610) sparked a vogue for a characteristic TRAGICOMEDY that was widely imitated for decades. Its unrealistic protagonist, who changes his motivation repeatedly, rejects his lover on ludicrous suspicions of infidelity. By a series of absurd coincidences, lives and nations are placed at stake while he splits hairs at great length over perverse notions of honour. Only further improbable accidents bring about a final reunion of the lovers. Mysterious in their way, grand in their pretensions, and entirely escapist, *Philaster* and its successors appealed immensely to the decadent court society that made up its audience.

In COMEDY, Shakespeare's ROMANCES, written early in the period, evidence the emerging taste for spectacle, exotic locales, romantic characters, and improbable plots. However, these works are singular for their interest in the virtues of innocence and the role of providence in human affairs. The romance literature at their roots is uproariously satirised in Beaumont's *The Knight of the Burning Pestle* (c. 1608), but Jacobean comedy in general is not so genial as this work. Ben

JONSON's 'city comedies', which evolved from the earlier COMEDY OF HUMOURS, satirised 17th-century LONDON with sharp and biting acerbity. These works—most notably *Volpone* (1606), *Epicoene* (c. 1609), *The Alchemist* (1610), and *Bartholomew Fair* (1614)—are among the greatest English comedies. They represent the positive aspect of Jacobean comedy, which otherwise tended towards coarser works chiefly concerned with the pursuit of money through bald sexual intrigue. Among the other Jacobean dramatists who wrote notable comedies are Middleton, Fletcher, and Philip MASSINGER.

Jacobean drama (the term is taken from *Jacobus,* Latin for James) is often considered to cover Caroline or Carolean drama (1625–1642), that is, during the reign of Charles I until the closure of the theatres by the Civil Wars. The only important playwrights of this period were Ford and James Shirley (1596–1666). The Jacobean tendencies to decadence continued to grow, and Puritan opposition to the theatre grew with it; the result was the 18-year demise of the theatres. The Caroline period is considered the end of the RENAISSANCE in England.

Jaggard, William (c. 1568–1623) and Isaac (1597–1627) London printers and publishers, father and son, producers of the FIRST FOLIO and other editions of Shakespeare's works. In 1599 William Jaggard published THE PASSIONATE PILGRIM, an anthology of poems that he claimed was by Shakespeare, though only about a quarter of them actually were. In 1612 he reissued this work, adding to it two poems by Thomas HEYWOOD (2). When Heywood publicly protested, on his own behalf and Shakespeare's, Jaggard replaced the title page with one that named no author.

Beginning in about 1613, Isaac Jaggard increasingly controlled the firm, due to his father's failing eyesight. In 1619 the Jaggards, with Thomas PAVIER, produced a group of QUARTO editions of 10 plays attributed to Shakespeare, though only a few were proper texts of Shakespeare's plays. These are known collectively as the FALSE FOLIO. Protests prompted the publishers to backdate most of these titles so that they could pass for the original editions.

Such practices were more acceptable then than now, and did not prevent the Jaggards from joining the syndicate that published the FIRST FOLIO edition of Shakespeare's works in 1623. William Jaggard was blind by this time, and Isaac headed the project; William died before it was completed.

Jailor Minor character in *The Comedy of Errors,* a guard. The attendant assigned to the condemned EGEON in 1.1 speaks only one line and functions to emphasise the power of the state and the extremity of Egeon's predicament.

James, Elias (c. 1578–1610) London brewer whose EPITAPH is attributed to Shakespeare. The six-line memorial to James first appeared in a manuscript collection of poems dating from the 1630s, some years after Shakespeare's death. The poem is ascribed to Shakespeare in an unknown hand, but modern scholars are inclined to accept the attribution, for James may well have been a friend or acquaintance of the playwright. James' brewery was located near the BLACKFRIARS THEATRE, and Shakespeare's friend John JACKSON (2) married the widow of James' brother and partner Jacob James.

James I, King of England (1566–1625) Ruler of England during the last years of Shakespeare's life and the patron of his acting company. James and his court were enthusiastic playgoers, and their tastes were highly influential on JACOBEAN DRAMA. James had been interested in the theatre before he came to England; as James VI of SCOTLAND, he had employed English actors led by Laurence FLETCHER (3). As king of England, he took over Shakespeare's CHAMBERLAIN'S MEN, and they performed at his court—as the KING'S

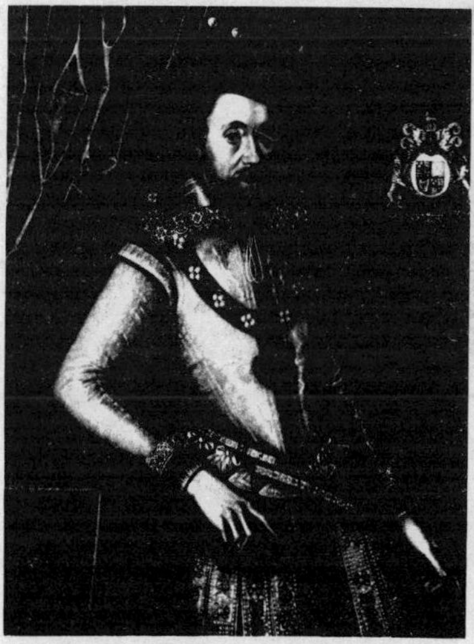

James I was an enthusiastic patron of the theatre, and he particularly enjoyed Shakespeare's works. Ben Jonson, speaking also of James' predecessor Queen Elizabeth, wrote of Shakespeare's 'flights . . . That so did take Eliza, and our James!' (Courtesy of National Maritime Museum, Greenwich)

MEN—more than twice as often as they had for his predecessor, Queen ELIZABETH (1). Moreover, the other two leading LONDON companies came under royal patronage, as the QUEEN'S MEN (2) and PRINCE HENRY'S MEN. The family added two more troupes around 1610, PRINCE CHARLES' MEN and LADY ELIZABETH'S MEN. On the other hand, state CENSORSHIP increased under King James, whose strong religious sentiments combined with his worries as the first ruler of the STUART DYNASTY—especially after the Gunpowder Plot (see GARNET)—to demand strict controls on the public's exposure to ideas.

Twice Shakespeare alluded to James in his plays, both times in the words of characters making auspicious prophecies of Britain's future. In *Macbeth* James' purported ancestor BANQUO is a very positive figure, and eight spectral KINGS appear to MACBETH, who realises they represent Banquo's progeny and notes that some of them carry 'two-fold balls and treble sceptres' (4.1.121). To Shakespeare's original audiences, this was an easily recognised reference to James' royal regalia as the ruler of both England and Scotland. In *Henry VIII* the play reaches its climax with Archbishop CRANMER's eulogy to the infant Elizabeth, and he adds a postscript praising her heir, declaring that he 'Shall star-like rise, as great in fame as she was, / And so stand fix'd' (5.4.46–47). James was presumably flattered by these references; that he enjoyed Shakespeare's works is attested to in Ben JONSON's poem on Shakespeare (published in the FIRST FOLIO [1623]), where he speaks of the playwright's 'flights . . . that did so take . . . our James!'

James was the son of Mary, Queen of Scots (1542–1587), and in 1567, as an infant, he was made King James VI of Scotland, on his mother's forced abdication. He never saw his mother again—after losing a civil war, she fled to England and was eventually executed by her enemy, Queen Elizabeth. He was raised a Protestant by a series of regents. The cornerstone of his policy as king was to secure his succession to the childless Elizabeth, who was his cousin. In 1589 he married Princess Anne of Denmark (1574–1619), and though he was homosexual by preference, they had seven children, three of whom survived infancy, Prince HENRY (2), Prince Charles—later King Charles I (ruled 1625–1649)—and Princess ELIZABETH (3). Though James was at first well liked in England—not least because his accession had been bloodless, despite fears of civil war—soon his popularity waned. His increasingly blatant homosexuality offended many, his sale of monopolies to his favourites angered parliament, and his policy of alliance with Spain enraged the country.

Further, his tendency to preach to his subjects eventually aroused resentment. James was undeniably a pedant; John HARINGTON, meaning no compliment, called him 'schoolmaster of the realm'. He published a number of works on theology, two books asserting the divine right of kings, and a pamphlet denouncing the evils of smoking (*A Counterblaste to Tobacco* [1604]). He also wrote and translated poetry in English, Latin, and Scots, and published a manual of Scots prosody. Though James was an intelligent king who sincerely desired to be a good ruler, he was a failure. Out of touch with the English people and by nature disinclined to compromise, he was a bad politician, and his reign widened the gap between crown and parliament that led to the Civil Wars.

Jamy Character in *Henry V*, a Scottish officer in the army of King HENRY V. Jamy appears only in the 'international' scene, 3.2, with the Welsh FLUELLEN, the English GOWER (2), and the Irish MACMORRIS. The episode emphasises the diversity of British subjects serving together under Henry. Although Fluellen speaks of him as a fine soldier, Jamy merely lends colour, uttering commonplaces in an almost impenetrable brogue.

Janssen (1), Cornelius (Cornelius Johnson or Jonson) (1593–1661) English painter to whom a possible portrait of Shakespeare is attributed. The 'Janssen portrait', or 'Somerset portrait', as it is known (it was owned by a Duke of Somerset in the late 18th century), somewhat resembles the most authoritative portraits of Shakespeare (see DROESHOUT; JANSSEN [2]). However, it is chiefly associated with the playwright for its inscription, which indicates that the anonymous sitter was 46 years old in 1610, the date the portrait was painted, as was Shakespeare. Even so, this could easily be coincidence, and that the painting depicts Shakespeare is regarded as highly questionable by most scholars. The work is apparently a copy of another portrait from the period, also possibly by Janssen—the clothes, elaborately detailed, are exactly identical in the two paintings—with the facial features altered to resemble the known images of Shakespeare. The creation of a portrait of a well-known figure was to be done in this way in both the 17th and 18th centuries, so the altered copy could have been made then.

Janssen, whose name is often Anglicised, was born in England of Dutch parents but probably returned to Holland for his training. He was painting in London at least as early as 1617, and he maintained a thriving practise as a portraitist until he returned to Holland for good in 1643, when he fled from the English Civil Wars. He is regarded as among the leading English painters of his day.

Janssen (2), Gheerart (Gerard Johnson) (active 1600–1623) English sculptor, creator of the memorial bust of Shakespeare in Holy Trinity Church at STRATFORD, one of the two portraits of the playwright considered by scholars to reflect his actual appearance

(the other is an engraving by Martin DROESHOUT). Because the Janssen bust was presumably commissioned and approved by Shakespeare's family, it probably provides a satisfactory likeness, although it is a conventionally stylised image rather than a psychologically revealing portrait. Presumably, it was made from an earlier portrait, probably a drawing or painting that is now lost. Made of painted limestone, the bust depicts a well-dressed gentleman with auburn hair and a quill pen in his right hand. The bust and its elaborate frame were installed sometime between 1616 and 1622; it was whitewashed in the late 18th century, and repainted in its present colours—though they may not be those originally provided by Janssen—in 1861. In 1790 the original pen, made of lead, was replaced with a real goosefeather quill, and a new quill is provided every year on Shakespeare's birthday.

Gheerart Janssen, whose name is sometimes Anglicised, was the son of a Dutch stone carver who arrived in England in the 1560s and established a flourishing business in SOUTHWARK, near the GLOBE THEATRE. This location suggests that Janssen may have known Shakespeare, at least by sight. Janssen inherited the family business in 1611. Another of his clients was Shakespeare's friend, John COMBE (1), whose memorial which he created is also in the Stratford church.

Jaquenetta Minor character in *Love's Labour's Lost,* the young dairymaid wooed by both ARMADO and COSTARD. Jaquenetta receives a love letter that BEROWNE intended for ROSALINE and turns it over to the KING (19), on the advice of HOLOFERNES. This embarrasses Berowne, who must acknowledge his susceptibility to love. In 5.2 Costard reveals that Jaquenetta is pregnant by Armado, and the Spaniard vows fidelity to her at the end of the play.

Jaques (1) Character in *As You Like It,* gloomy follower of DUKE (7) Senior who provides a contrast to the play's comic values. Jaques muses on the viciousness of human hypocrisy, affects to dislike music and dancing, and praises only the satire that can expose the sins of the world. When the duke prepares to return to his dukedom at the play's close, accompanied by most of the other characters, Jaques decides to stay in the Forest of ARDEN (1) and pursue a life of contemplation.

Jaques' pessimism and self-imposed isolation place him at odds with the play's central tenet, that love is the most valued element in human life. However, he never seriously threatens this ideal; his position is consistently undercut, in part because Shakespeare envisioned Jaques to some extent as a parody of a fashionable 16th-century affectation of cynicism and melancholy. People who held this attitude doubtless felt that they appeared intellectually superior and penetrating, but others found them amusingly pretentious.

The ineffectuality of Jaques' ideas is repeatedly pointed up by his repudiation by the other major characters. His elaborately melancholy pose is described even before we meet him, when the duke hears of his lament over a slain deer (2.1.26–66). In 2.5, in his first appearance, Jaques satirises AMIENS' song, which mirrors the duke's sentiments about the virtues of life in Arden. Then, in 2.7, having encountered the jester TOUCHSTONE, he raves about the opportunities for a FOOL (1) to 'cleanse th'infected world' (2.7.60) through satire. However, Jaques is then sternly chastised by the duke for 'chiding sin' (2.7.64) when he has been a sinner himself. Even Jaques' most spectacular speech, his cynical depiction of the seven ages of man, beginning, 'All the world's a stage, / And all the men and women merely players' (2.7.139–140), is undercut. No character bothers to respond to it, and, immediately after Jaques' harrowing description of old age, the ancient ADAM is borne on stage and treated as a respected member of the community.

Jaques is most explicitly contrasted with the lovers ROSALIND and ORLANDO. When he first meets Orlando, Jaques declares he would rather be alone, and he disparages Orlando's poetry, his wit, and his lover's name. Jaques has said that he is seeking a fool, meaning Touchstone, but Orlando invites him to look in the brook, where he will see his own reflection. Insulted, Jaques leaves.

Rosalind is similarly dismissive. In 4.1 Jaques asserts that he is melancholy, saying, 'I do love it better than laughing' (4.1.4). The heroine fiercely insists that those who are excessive in laughter *or* melancholy are 'abominable fellows, and betray themselves to every modern censure, worse than drunkards' (4.1.5–8). Further, when he says that his state of mind has been influenced by his travels, she delivers a standard Elizabethan diatribe on the foolishness of travel. Significantly, these rebukes each occur just before one of the two major courtship scenes between Rosalind and Orlando, 3.2.290–423 and 4.1.40–190. Jaques' negativism must be overcome before the lovers' affirmation can occur.

Touchstone seems to resemble Jaques at first glance; they are both given to satire, wit, and cynicism. However, Touchstone is a professional comic whose statements are usually meant only to be humorous. His comprehension of the world's ways stirs him to amusement rather than despair. Jaques, by contrast, is a philosopher of sorts, and he has a consistently dour viewpoint that opposes sociability; as he remarks, 'I am for other than for dancing measures' (5.4.192).

Jaques wishes for a pristine past, before human societies came to Arden to kill deer, before humans existed at all, perhaps. This is an extreme form of the

PASTORAL literary conventions, a target of the play's parody. Such extravagantly anti-social desires place Jaques beyond the reach of the celebration of love that closes the play. This is a recurring device that Shakespeare uses in his COMEDIES: characters whose actions are not motivated by love and whose presence would mar the harmonious resolution of the play—such as Don JOHN (1) of *Much Ado About Nothing* and MALVOLIO of *Twelfth Night*—are left out of such scenes of reconciliation.

However, Jaques is not a villain, as is Don John. Except in his encounter with Orlando in 3.2, he behaves with civility. In 2.5 he and a group of fellow courtiers listen to music. In 4.2 he sings with others in a ribald interlude celebrating the hunt with jokes about cuckold's horns and deer's antlers (quite forgetful of his distress over the slain deer of 2.1). Even his satire of Amiens' song in 2.5 is good-natured, particularly since the 'gross fools' (2.5.53) he criticises include himself. Also, although he expresses anti-social views, Jaques converses with more different people than any other character. Finally, the blessings that Jaques bestows on the duke and each of the marrying couples in 5.4.185–192 are pleasant and humorous, as well as perceptive.

In fact, Jaques' closing lines reveal that he, too, has been affected by the general awareness of love's power that surrounds him. He knows that he is not destined to be a part of it, but he certainly does not begrudge the lovers their happiness. In fact, his final remarks concern his friends and their prospects; Jaques has become humanised. He remains isolated, but he is no longer a malcontent. He does not disparage the wedding festivities; he simply opts for something else. His reason for remaining in Arden is eminently acceptable: 'There is much matter to be heard and learn'd' (5.4.184).

Jaques' final self-acceptance is in keeping with the play's spirit of conciliation, most vividly represented by the multiple marriage in 5.4. Further, his early cynicism, although inappropriate to the world of Arden and therefore countered by the other characters, sharpens the flavour of a play that might otherwise be overly sentimental. Lastly, Jaques' railing reminds us that outside the magical world of Arden, the ways of the world are all too often wicked indeed.

Jaques (2) de Boys Minor character in *As You Like It*, brother of OLIVER (1) and ORLANDO. Jaques is named in 1.1.5, but he does not appear until 5.4, when he suddenly arrives with the news of DUKE (1) Frederick's armed march on ARDEN (1) and later conversion to a life of religious contemplation. The episode both provides a place for the villain in the play's ultimate reconciliation, and, in its suddenness, intensifies the play's atmosphere of romantic wonder.

The duplication of names with a major character, the pessimistic courtier JAQUES (1), presents a minor difficulty. Jaques de Boys identifies himself only as 'the second son of old Sir Rowland' (5.4.151). In the FIRST FOLIO edition of the play, stage directions identify him as 'Second Brother', and some modern editions follow this practise, avoiding the issue to some extent, but the mention of his name in 1.1 suggests carelessness on Shakespeare's part. Perhaps the playwright originally intended his melancholy courtier to be Orlando and Oliver's brother, established his existence with the reference at 1.1.5, and then developed Jaques as a member of the exiled DUKE (7) Senior's court, neglecting to remove the earlier reference.

Jeffes, Humphrey (d. 1618) English actor. Jeffes may have played a minor role in an early production of *3 Henry VI*, for in the FIRST FOLIO text of the play a KEEPER (2) is designated 'Humfrey' in a stage direction. If this is Jeffes, he was probably a member of PEMBROKE'S MEN in 1592–1593, when they are believed to have staged the play. Jeffes is first recorded, however, as a member of the ADMIRAL'S MEN in 1597, after the Pembroke's Men collapsed in the wake of the ISLE OF DOGS scandal. He remained with his new company for almost 20 years, and finally left its successor, the PALSGRAVE'S MEN, in 1616 to take a company on tour in the provinces, though his company soon had its permit revoked for unknown reasons.

Jenkins, Thomas (active 1566–1579) STRATFORD schoolmaster, Shakespeare's grammar school teacher. Jenkins was master of the Stratford Grammar School from 1575–1579, the period when Shakespeare learned much of the Latin literature that was at the core of the Elizabethan grammar school curriculum. Jenkins was a well-qualified teacher of the material, as he was an Oxford-educated clergyman and an experienced teacher. The Stratford burgesses recruited him from a similar position in Warwick. His Welsh name has suggested to scholars that he may be the inspiration for Shakespeare's creation Sir Hugh EVANS (3), the Welsh schoolteacher of *The Merry Wives of Windsor*. However, Jenkins was born in London, the son of a servant. His education was presumably provided by his father's master, who was a founder of the college at Oxford where he studied. In 1579 he resigned his position at Stratford and recruited his own successor, John COTTOM. Jenkins was married—a daughter died and a son was born during his tenure at Stratford—but little more is known of his life.

Jerusalem Chamber Room in WESTMINSTER (1) ABBEY, the setting for 4.4 of *2 Henry IV*. The dying King HENRY IV talks there with his younger sons and other noblemen about PRINCE (6) HAL, who the king

fears is dissolute and will make a bad heir to the throne. News arrives that the rebels against the king have been defeated, but the excitement causes the king to swoon and he is taken to another room. The encounter between Hal and his father in 4.5 takes place in the second chamber; the king asks the name of the first room. Told that it is the Jerusalem Chamber, he asks to be returned there, thus fulfilling a prophecy that he would die in Jerusalem.

King Henry did in fact die in the Jerusalem Chamber, but the prophecy, which Shakespeare took from HOLINSHED, is not recorded elsewhere. The same story—a prophecy of death in Jerusalem followed by death in a church or room of that name—is told of several medieval figures and is probably apocryphal in most cases, including this one. The name of the room, which was originally part of the Abbot's residence, comes from an inscription surrounding the fireplace.

Jessica Character in *The Merchant of Venice*, daughter of SHYLOCK and lover of LORENZO. Jessica is an apparently demure young woman who nevertheless abandons her father and her religion willingly in eloping with Lorenzo, and she also steals Shylock's money. TUBAL reports her extravagance with these funds in 3.1. In 5.1 the romantic rhapsodies of Lorenzo and Jessica provide the play's finest lyric poetry and establish the triumph of love, a major theme of the work.

Jessica's behaviour to her father has often been criticised, and, if Shylock is viewed as a sympathetic or tragic character, his daughter can only seem immoral. Moreover, her desertion and theft seem to be related to the anti-Semitism that infects this play. Referring to Jessica's enthusiastic readiness to steal from her father, Gratiano avers that she is 'a gentle [i.e., gentile], and no Jew' (2.6.51). That is, she qualifies as a Christian by her actions against a Jew. However, the play is clearly a traditional romantic COMEDY, and Jessica's role in that context is a simple one. She flees to romantic love from the prison of her father's miserly household, which she describes as 'hell' (2.3.2). In doing so, she illustrates a bold example of the opposition between love and greed that lies at the heart of the play. Further, her theft of her father's funds reflects Shylock's traditional function as a comic villain (although Shakespeare enlarged the character considerably) and was probably received by the play's original audiences as a comeuppance to the miser, a traditional subject of comical raillery. Jessica is humorous as she steals, archly asserting that the weight of a purloined casket is 'worth the pains' and saying she will 'gild myself with moe ducats' as she leaves (2.6.33, 49–50). She is essentially a secondary character, graceful but uncomplicated. Only her relationship to Shylock inspires comment.

Jeweller Minor character in *Timon of Athens*, a flatterer of TIMON. As the play opens, the Jeweller proposes to sell a jewel to Timon, confident that the nobleman will pay a good price. Later in 1.1 he flatters his potential client. The Jeweller is simply a representative greedy flatterer.

Joan La Pucelle (Joan of Arc) (c. 1412–1431) Historical figure and character in *1 Henry VI*, a leader of the French forces in the HUNDRED YEARS WAR. The historical Joan of Arc was known as La Pucelle, 'the virgin', in her own lifetime, and Shakespeare takes the name from the chronicles. In Acts 1–4 Shakespeare's Joan is in some respects difficult to distinguish from the other French leaders, CHARLES VII, ALENÇON, and REIGNIER; like them, she is intended to show, by her trickery and lack of military valour, that a French victory would have been impossible without the English dissension that is the play's chief theme. Unlike her fellows, though, Joan can be a charismatic leader. In 1.2 she revives the morale of the French after a lost skirmish, and in 1.5 she leads them in breaking the English siege of ORLÉANS (1), as the historical Joan had done.

This is as much of the real Joan of Arc's life as the play reflects, however. The English capture of Orléans in 2.1 is entirely unhistorical, as is, of course, the French leaders' flight from a single English soldier. Similarly, Joan's devious tactic while taking ROUEN in 3.2, is fictitious; in fact, the actual anecdote that Shakespeare drew upon tells of an *English* strategy in a different battle. In 3.3 Joan convinces the Duke of BURGUNDY (2) to abandon the English cause; in actuality, Burgundy did not withdraw from his alliance with England until well after Joan's death.

In Act 5 the playwright recasts Joan as a villainess in an altogether more absolute manner. Joan's sorcery in 5.3, where she calls up FIENDS, is simply intended to blacken her image. (Similarly, the other characters insult Joan freely throughout the play, casting aspersions on her courage and her virginity and frequently accusing her of witchcraft.) Lastly, in Shakespeare's most glaring misrepresentation of Joan, she makes a cowardly attempt, in 5.4, to avoid execution, first by claiming royal birth and refusing to acknowledge her father, the SHEPHERD (1), and then by disavowing her virginity and claiming to be pregnant. She goes to her death cursing England and the English.

The play's uncharitable attitude towards Joan of Arc has stimulated much hostile criticism. In fact, this feature was once taken as evidence of non-Shakespearean authorship, on the grounds that no great writer would stoop to such propagandistic viciousness. However, such keen anti-French sentiments were common in Elizabethan times, as well as in the play's source material, such as the chronicles of HALL (2) and HOLINSHED,

and modern authorities, whatever their opinions as to the authorship of *1 Henry VI*, do not find it odd that a playwright should have portrayed Englishmen insulting Joan in this manner.

The historical Joan, born Jeanne Darc, began, at the age of 12, to hear voices that she understood to be those of angels and of God, advising her to lead a holy life. Later the voices instructed her to help Charles VII drive the English from FRANCE (1). In 1428 she persuaded a local military commander to take her to Charles' court, where she convinced Charles to permit her to lead a small army to relieve besieged Orléans. Remarkably, her troops were victorious, and she is still known as 'the maid of Orléans'. Her continued participation in the war infused the French with the courage and confidence that turned the tide of the conflict. She was captured by Burgundian forces in 1430. Her captors sold her to the English under WARWICK (2), who arranged for a 'show trial' for heresy before a French ecclesiastical tribunal. She was convicted and burned at the stake on May 30, 1431. Her conduct at the trial was, by all accounts, dignified and honourable, entirely unlike that of the Joan of the play. In 1456 her admirers obtained a retrial, at which her innocence was pronounced. She was declared a saint by the Catholic Church in 1920.

John (1), Don Character in *Much Ado About Nothing*, the villainous brother of the prince, Don PEDRO. With the help of his follower BORACHIO, Don John schemes to mortify CLAUDIO (1) by slandering his betrothed, HERO. After Borachio arranges for an incriminating impersonation of Hero, the would-be bride is humiliatingly rejected by the deluded Claudio, but by a fortuitous accident, the plot is uncovered and Don John flees from MESSINA, only to be captured and brought back. However, his flight and final comeuppance occur off-stage and are only reported (in 4.2.58 and 5.4.123–124); Don John himself is absent at the close of the play, for his vicious nature would be out of place amid the general spirit of reconciliation.

Don John resents Claudio because 'that young start-up hath all the glory of my overthrow. If I can cross him any way, I bless myself . . .' (1.3.62–64). Claudio's advancement in Don Pedro's court has come at Don John's expense, for Claudio has shone in the war that suppressed Don John's rebellion against his brother. However, this motive is relatively unimportant; Don John plots to cause as much trouble to those around him as he can, apparently out of a simply evil nature. He declares that he would 'rather be a canker in a hedge than a rose' and describes himself as 'a plain-dealing villain' (1.3.25, 30). His is a generalised, undirected discontent; he envies other people's happiness and is therefore misanthropic.

Although Borachio compares him to the devil in 3.3.145–151, Don John is a slight figure, a study for a portrait of a villain. He is neither as grandiose as RICHARD III nor as direct as MACBETH. Nor is he as threateningly mysterious as IAGO, whom he anticipates in both his ill-defined motivation and his manipulation of the conventional sexual attitudes of his victims. Most important, he lacks the human complexity of any of these larger, more fully developed characters. Don John is a simple stereotype, intended chiefly to advance the plot of a COMEDY, offering just enough evil to necessitate a triumph for happiness but not enough to evoke terror, as in a TRAGEDY.

John (2), Friar Character in *Romeo and Juliet*. See FRIAR (3).

John (3), King of England (1167–1216) Historical figure and title character in *King John*. John is a complicated protagonist of a complicated play. Not quite hero or villain, he espouses values of English patriotism while his selfish ambition leads the country to catastrophe. John passes from unscrupulous strength to dispirited weakness, and his own moral failings are at the heart of his collapse. He is ultimately an inadequate leader, controlled by events rather than controlling them. As the play opens, John has usurped the English throne from his nephew ARTHUR. Nevertheless, he initially appears to be a strong king: in 1.1 he boldly defies the challenge to his rule from Arthur's supporter King PHILIP (2) of FRANCE (1). However, he soon displays his weakness when, in the treaty concluded in 2.1, he surrenders a great deal of English territory in order to protect his claim to the rest. He exhibits strength again, in a context particularly significant to 16th-century Protestant England, when he refuses to obey the dictates of the pope, conveyed by PANDULPH in 3.1, and renewed war with France results. John's forces capture Arthur, and the king dishonourably orders him killed by HUBERT in 3.2 (3.3) (for citation, see *King John*, 'Synopsis'). He also commands the BASTARD (1) to loot England's religious houses to pay for the war.

Shakespeare's handling of Arthur's death, the central event of the play, illuminates John's ambiguous nature. Before learning that Hubert has not killed the boy, John expresses regret for the crime and dishonestly tries to excuse himself in 4.2.103–105 and 205–248; he rejoices when he discovers that Arthur is alive. Yet Arthur does die when he tries to escape his captors. John is thus blamed for the death anyway and suffers the political consequences.

John's fortunes deteriorate from this point on. His barons desert him; his mother, Queen ELEANOR, dies; a wandering seer, PETER (4), predicts that he will give up his crown. The Dauphin LEWIS (1) of France invades England, and several barons join his forces. In

5.1 John formally acknowledges the supremacy of the pope over England, in return for Pandulph's promise to make the French withdraw. Lewis will not abandon his successful invasion, however, and only the efforts of the BASTARD (1) keep England's defences functioning. Demoralised and sick, John withdraws to SWINSTEAD ABBEY, where a monk, enraged by the king's pillaging of the churches, poisons him. John dies in torment, just as an urgent message of fresh disaster is being delivered. His death returns peace and stability to England, as the French finally withdraw and the Bastard leads the nobles in pledging allegiance to John's successor, HENRY (1).

The sources Shakespeare used in creating his John were not very accurate, according to modern scholarship, and the playwright altered many details in any case. The historical John was not a usurper; he did not lose the support of his barons by killing an innocent boy; he was not murdered. He was indeed an unsuccessful king, though probably due more to the assets of his enemies than to his own defects. Philip Augustus of France was a powerful soldier and statesman, and Innocent III was one of the greatest of medieval popes. John did not, however, lack leadership skills himself. Many of his nobles remained loyal to him, and he never withdrew from the fight against the rebels and their French allies; he died of a sickness contracted on the battlefield. His personality is not well recorded, but he appears to have been highly temperamental, perhaps deranged; according to one account he beat Arthur to death in a drunken rage. However, Shakespeare did not attempt to delineate John's true nature; the character is a fiction designed to illustrate the nature of misused power. The king's moral weakness is central to an intellectual drama of politics, and his personality is not relevant.

John (4) of Gaunt Character in *Richard II.* See GAUNT.

John (5) Plantagenet Character in *1 Henry VI; 1 & 2 Henry IV; Henry V.* See BEDFORD; LANCASTER (3).

John (6) Talbot (also known as Young Talbot, c. 1425–1453) Historical figure and character in *1 Henry VI,* the son of TALBOT, England's heroic general. John appears in 4.5, fighting courageously beside his father. When Talbot realises that the coming battle is a doomed one, he attempts to persuade John to flee and save his life. The young man, citing the family honour, refuses in 4.6.42–57. John does die, and, in 4.7, Talbot, dying himself, addresses his son's corpse, praising John's exploits in the battle.

Shakespeare intended the melodramatic deaths of Talbot and John to contrast with the selfishness of YORK (8) and SOMERSET (3), whose disputes denied the heroes reinforcements. To increase the poignancy of the comparison, Young Talbot is said to be his father's only son, but, in fact, several others carried on the Talbot line. Further, John appears quite young, although the historical figure was in his late twenties and had a number of children.

Johnson (1), Arthur (d. 1631) LONDON bookseller and publisher, producer of the first edition of *The Merry Wives of Windsor.* Johnson published a wide range of literature, including several plays. In 1602 he brought out the BAD QUARTO (Q1) of *The Merry Wives* and in 1608 the first edition of *The Merry Devil of Edmonton,* a play that was later wrongly attributed to Shakespeare. Sometime after 1624 Johnson moved to Dublin, where he became a stationer.

Johnson (2), Charles (1679–1748) English playwright. Johnson wrote 18 plays, several of them quite successful, but he is best known today for two works derived from Shakespeare. *The Cobbler of Preston* (1716), a political play that commented on the Jacobite rebellion of 1715, was embedded in a version of the Christopher SLY (1) episode of *The Taming of the Shrew.* LOVE IN A FOREST (1723) was a loose adaptation of *As You Like It.* A prominent figure in the London literary world of his day, Johnson was among the targets of the satirical *Dunciad* (1728, 1743), by Alexander POPE (1).

Johnson (3), Cornelius See JANSSEN (1).

Johnson (4), Gerard See JANSSEN (2).

Johnson (5), Robert (c. 1585–c. 1634) English musician and composer, probable writer of music for several of Shakespeare's plays. In the *Cheerful Ayres* (c. 1660) of John WILSON (2), Johnson is credited with music for 'Where the bee sucks' and 'Full fadom five' from *The Tempest,* possibly written for the performance of the play given as part of the wedding festivities of Princess ELIZABETH (3) in 1613. Scholars believe that Johnson also composed song music for *Cymbeline* and *The Winter's Tale,* although the surviving sheet music is anonymous. Music he wrote for a MASQUE by Francis BEAUMONT (2), also performed at Princess Elizabeth's wedding, was probably also used in performances of *The Two Noble Kinsmen.* Johnson also composed songs for *The Duchess of Malfi* (1614) by John WEBSTER, *The Witch* (1615) by Thomas MIDDLETON (this music may have been used in early productions of *Macbeth,* as well), and for five plays by Beaumont and John FLETCHER (2).

As a boy, Johnson was a servant in the household of George Carey, Lord HUNSDON (1); his abilities were already recognised, for he was employed as a music teacher. It was doubtless through Hunsdon, who was the patron of the CHAMBERLAIN'S MEN, Shakespeare's

acting company, that Johnson became a theatrical composer. After 1604 he was also the royal lutenist for King JAMES I and King Charles I, composing and performing music for royal masques and other entertainments.

Johnson (6), Robert (d. 1611) Vintner and innkeeper of STRATFORD and Shakespeare's tenant. Johnson owned a tavern, known at different times as the White Lion and the Swan Inn, that abutted the property on which Shakespeare's birthplace stood. He rented a barn on that property from Shakespeare and presumably used it in connection with the inn. This rental is known only because the lease is mentioned in the inventory of possessions accompanying Johnson's will, recorded in October 1611 by Thomas ASPINALL. In 1670 Johnson's son still rented the barn, when it was mentioned in the will of Elizabeth HALL (3), Shakespeare's grand-daughter.

Johnson (7), Samuel (1709–1784) English poet, scholar, literary critic, and lexicographer, the leading figure in English literature in the mid-18th century. Dr Johnson, as he is universally known, wrote poems, biographies, and essays on a wide range of subjects, and he compiled the first great English dictionary (1755). In 1765 he published an edition of Shakespeare's plays. While it is not regarded as significant in terms of scholarship—it was based on an inferior text and added little in the way of notes and commentary—it was nevertheless the basis for the greater edition of George STEEVENS, and it includes a preface that is regarded as one of Johnson's finest works. Johnson's intellectual and social life as a leader of his age are still accessible to us through the *Life of Samuel Johnson* (1791) by James Boswell (1740–1795), a masterpiece of English literature.

Johnson (8), William (active 1591–1616) Landlord of the MERMAID TAVERN in London and a friend of Shakespeare. Johnson, with John HEMINGE and John JACKSON (2), assisted Shakespeare by serving as a trustee in his purchase of the BLACKFRIARS GATEHOUSE in 1613. While no other connection is known, this one presumes a fairly close acquaintance. Shakespeare may have been a member of the Friday Street Club, a literary gathering that met informally at the Mermaid, or he may have stayed there while visiting London after he moved back to STRATFORD.

Johnson had served an apprenticeship with the previous landlord of the Mermaid, taking over the management himself in 1603. Shortly after his involvement in Shakespeare's purchase, Johnson found himself in legal difficulties, charged with serving meat at the tavern during Lent, though the case may not have gone to court.

Jones (1), James Earl (b. 1931) American actor. Jones, one of the leading black actors of the New York stage, made his Broadway debut in 1958 and soon established a reputation as a classic actor. He was especially acclaimed as the title character in a 1973 production of *King Lear* by Joseph PAPP. He was also noteworthy as OTHELLO, opposite Christopher PLUMMER's IAGO, in Nicol WILLIAMSON's 1982 staging.

Jones (2), Richard (active 1583–1624) English actor. Jones was a member of WORCESTER'S MEN in 1583–1584 with the young Edward ALLEYN, and he was probably a member of Alleyn's ADMIRAL'S MEN by 1585. He travelled in Germany with a company headed by Robert BROWNE in 1592–1593, but he rejoined the Admiral's Men again in 1594. Except for a brief period in 1597, he was with them until 1602. He is known to have played PRIAM in *Troilus and Cressida.* In 1610 he was a partner, with Browne and others, in a CHILDREN'S COMPANY that performed at the WHITEFRIARS THEATRE, but by 1615 he was again in Germany, this time with John GREEN. By 1622 he was employed as a musician in a minor German court, but he returned to England the next year. He is last known from a letter of 1624 to his German employer, asking to return, since he had not found work in England.

Jones (3), Robert (active 1590–1615) Composer and theatrical entrepreneur. Jones was a famed lute player and composer of settings for songs. Shakespeare apparently adapted the song 'Farewell, dear heart' (*Twelfth Night,* 2.3.102–112) from a work in Jones' *The First Book of Songes and Ayres* (1600), though the playwright may have known the song elsewhere.

Jones (4), William (d. 1618) LONDON bookseller and publisher, producer of first editions of two plays of the Shakespeare APOCRYPHA. Between 1598 and 1615 Jones published the first six editions of MUCEDORUS, one of the most popular plays of the day; none of these editions attributed the play to Shakespeare. In 1602 Jones published the first edition of THOMAS LORD CROMWELL, which was credited to 'W. S.', though it is unclear whether this attribution was intended to associate the work with Shakespeare. Jones was apprenticed to a printer in 1578, was a member of the STATIONERS' COMPANY by 1587, and when he died in 1618, left a widow who was forced to sell his copyrights. Little more is known of his life.

Jonson, Ben (1572–1637) English poet and playwright, a great satirist and a leading light of JACOBEAN DRAMA. Jonson's greatest achievements were works of satiric COMEDY—especially *Volpone* (1606), *Epicoene* (c. 1609), *The Alchemist* (1610), and *Bartholomew Fair* (1614)—and MASQUES written for the court of King JAMES I. Jonson's satire influenced Shakespeare's own

most nearly satirical works, such as *Troilus and Cressida* and *Timon of Athens,* and the popularity of Jonson's masques helped create the theatrical world in which Shakespeare wrote his ROMANCES. He is regarded as second only to Shakespeare among the playwrights of the period. Jonson also wrote on literary theory, and his stress on clarity over personal style, on classical forms of aesthetic organisation, and on relevance to one's own times influenced English poets and dramatists for a century.

Jonson received a good secondary education at the Westminster School, where he was taught by William CAMDEN, but as the stepson of a bricklayer, he was then apprenticed to that trade. Instead, he enlisted in the army and went to the Low Countries, where he reportedly killed an enemy soldier in a man-to-man combat staged between the opposing armies. By 1592 he was back in LONDON and married, though his life for five years is otherwise unknown. In 1597 he was a member of PEMBROKE'S MEN, gaoled as a player in the 'seditious' play *Isle of Dogs* (see CENSORSHIP), which he may have helped write. A year later he was again imprisoned, this time for killing his fellow actor Gabriel SPENCER in a duel. He escaped the death penalty only through an archaic technicality: clergymen were exempt from punishment, and clergymen were defined as all those capable of reading Latin.

Jonson's first successful play, *Every Man in His Humour,* was staged by the CHAMBERLAIN'S MEN in 1598; Shakespeare may have been responsible for its acceptance by the company, and he was in the cast. One of the finest examples of the COMEDY OF HUMOURS, this work was extremely popular. Unfortunately, its sequel the next year, *Every Man out of His Humour,* was equally unsuccessful. It was one of the first shots in the WAR OF THE THEATRES, an exchange of satirical plays by Jonson on one side and John MARSTON and Thomas DEKKER on the other. Jonson's other efforts in this fray were produced by the Children of the Chapel (see CHILDREN'S COMPANIES). Jonson next worked for Philip HENSLOWE and the ADMIRAL'S MEN, writing additional material for *The Spanish Tragedy* (c. 1588) by Thomas KYD before creating his own major work, *Sejanus* (1603). This TRAGEDY, modelled on SENECA, was staged by the KING'S MEN, again with Shakespeare in the cast (this is the last record of Shakespeare as an actor).

Beginning in 1605, Jonson began his collaboration with Inigo Jones (1573–1652), the royal architect, who designed the settings and machinery for the masques that Jonson composed. Over the next quarter-century, this partnership produced brilliant spectacles that influenced both drama and theatre design for generations. However, near the beginning of this period, Jonson once again courted royal disfavour, this time as co-author with Marston and George CHAPMAN of *Eastward Ho!* (1605), a play containing political remarks that the king declared seditious. Jonson was briefly gaoled again, before the affair blew over. In the next few years Jonson reached his peak of achievement, with *Volpone, Epicoene,* and *The Alchemist.* The first and last of these was produced by the King's Men. *Bartholomew Fair* was staged by LADY ELIZABETH'S MEN in 1614, after Jonson returned from a year's travel in Europe as the tutor to Sir Walter RALEIGH'S son.

In 1616 Jonson issued a collection of his works—poetry, prose, and drama—a deed that was widely ridiculed because plays were not generally considered to have literary value at the time. In the same year the king gave Jonson a pension for life, making him effectively the first Poet Laureate, though the honour was not so named until later. He travelled in SCOTLAND, where William Drummond of Hawthornden noted his conversational remarks on himself and his contemporaries—a record that has served modern historians of the theatre. After his return his career deteriorated. Only one further play was a success, *The Staple of News* (1625), a satire on the newsletter of Nathaniel BUTTER. A bitter fight with Inigo Jones ended his creation of masques. (Characteristically, Jonson recorded the quarrel in *A Tale of a Tub* [1633], a play that flopped in London.) He also suffered from illness and lost his extraordinary library to a disastrous fire. He died with a play half-written and was buried in WESTMINSTER (1) ABBEY.

Shakespeare and Jonson were very different men, with different sensibilities and different attitudes towards life and art, yet they seem to have been friends, beginning with the production of *Every Man in His Humour.* The tradition that Shakespeare died after a drinking bout with Jonson and Michael DRAYTON is almost certainly not true, but it reflects a reality. They probably met often at the MERMAID TAVERN, and they seem to have enjoyed criticising each other. Another story, possibly apocryphal, demonstrates the tone of their friendly rivalry: Jonson and Shakespeare, 'being merry at a tavern', composed an EPITAPH for Jonson. Jonson composed the first two lines, 'Here lies Ben Jonson / that was once one', and Shakespeare devised the final two: 'Who while he lived was a slow thing, / And now, being dead, is nothing'. (Jonson's agonising slowness in writing was often jested about.)

An amateur play about the theatre world, performed at Cambridge University in 1601 (see PARNASSUS PLAYS), refers to Shakespeare's having given Jonson 'a purge' in response to criticism. This may merely express the author's preference for Shakespeare, but it may also echo some otherwise lost piece of gossip. At least once Shakespeare alluded to Jonson in his work. In *Twelfth Night* FESTE remarks that the word *element* is 'overworn' (3.1.60), a casual reference to Dekker's satire of Jonson's alleged overuse of the term. Further, Shakespeare's AJAX, JAQUES (1), and

NYM have all been suggested as possible parodies of Jonson.

For his part, Jonson frequently remarked on Shakespeare, often acknowledgeing his friend's greatness. For instance, after Shakespeare's death, Jonson wrote, 'I lov'd the man, and do honour his memory (this side idolatry) as much as any'. However, this remark followed a criticism of Shakespeare's carelessness as a writer, and most of Jonson's recorded comments on his friend are likewise combinations of praise and censure. Jonson was an arrogant man, by all accounts, including his own, and he was a fierce critic; he once declared that John Donne (1573–1631) 'deserved hanging' for writing poetry in an irregular METRE. While he could not but admire Shakespeare's virtues, he could not refrain from finding things to criticise, particularly when such 'defects' contrasted with his own traits. For instance, Jonson's famous contention (quite untrue) that Shakespeare 'never blotted' a line, implicitly praised his own laborious technique. Similarly, his notorious remark that Shakespeare had 'small Latin and less Greek' was true only by comparison to his own great erudition. Nevertheless, each derogation was coupled with praise—'There was ever more in him to be praised, than to be pardoned', he wrote—and it was Jonson who penned one of the most famous tributes to Shakespeare, in his prefatory verses to the FIRST FOLIO (1623), 'He was not of an age, but for all time!'

Jordan, Dorothy (1761–1816) Irish actress. Mrs Jordan—the adopted name by which Dorothea Bland was known—made her stage debut in Dublin in 1777, playing PHEBE in *As You Like It.* After 1775 she established herself in London, where she mostly played comedic heroines. Her best-known Shakespearean roles were ROSALIND, IMOGEN, and VIOLA. She also played in William Henry IRELAND's forged Shakespearean play, *Vortigern* (1796). She was the long-time mistress of the Duke of Clarence, later King William IV (ruled 1830–1837), by whom she had 10 children.

Joseph Minor character in *The Taming of the Shrew,* a servant of PETRUCHIO (2). Joseph is one of the servants whom Petruchio abuses in 4.1, as part of his demonstration to KATHERINA of the ugliness of shrewish behaviour.

Jourdain (1), Margery Character in *2 Henry VI.* See MARGERY JOURDAIN.

Jourdain (2) (Jourdan), Sylvester (c. 1580–1650) English colonial entrepreneur and writer, author of a probable source for *The Tempest.* Jourdain was a member of an expedition to Virginia that was shipwrecked in Bermuda in 1609. He was marooned for 10 months, and his recounting of his experiences in *The Discovery of the Barmudas* (1610) provided Shakespeare with such details for *The Tempest* as the mysterious 'supernatural' noises that CALIBAN describes in 3.2.133–138. Jourdain's account also confirmed Shakespeare's principal source, a letter by William STRACHEY (2), which stressed the miraculous nature of their survival. Shakespeare follows these accounts in emphasising the role of providence in *The Tempest.* Jourdain was a Puritan merchant from Dorsetshire who settled in LONDON after his adventures.

Julia Character in *The Two Gentlemen of Verona,* the betrayed lover of PROTEUS. Julia disguises herself as a boy and follows Proteus to court, where he has fallen in love with SILVIA. Learning of his infidelity, Julia nonetheless remains true to Proteus, serving, in her disguise, as his messenger to her rival. She is present in the final scene, when VALENTINE offers Silvia to Proteus, and her quick wit tells her to swoon, interrupting the transaction. She reveals herself, her presence restores Proteus to his original loyalty, and he vows his love for her anew.

Julia is an early instance of a type of young woman Shakespeare clearly admired—independent, active, and capable of pursuing a man, even if he is unworthy of her. Other instances include HELENA (2), in *All's Well That Ends Well* and VIOLA, in *Twelfth Night.*

Juliet (1) One of the title characters in *Romeo and Juliet,* the lover of ROMEO. Juliet first appears as a conventional upper-class daughter, affectionately dependent on her NURSE (3) and accepting of the marriage to PARIS (2) that is planned for her. However, when she is gripped by passion for Romeo, she displays a heroic capacity to resist her world, despite the dangers of her love. She accepts death no less readily than Romeo when destiny has destroyed their lives.

When she first meets Romeo, she shows herself to be intelligent and perceptive. She matches wits with him in improvising their joint SONNET (1.5.92–105), and she recognises in him traces of the bookish, artificial lover he has been earlier, remarking that he kisses 'by th'book' (1.5.109). While no less enraptured than her lover during the subsequent 'balcony' scene (2.2), she is nonetheless more aware than he of their danger, as in 2.2.116–120, and it is she who sees that they must commit themselves to marriage if their plight is to be overcome. Although her response to the onset of passion is mature, she does not lose her appeal as a blooming young lover. Her soliloquy at the opening of 3.2, before she learns of Romeo's banishment, is a brilliant and utterly endearing expression of the impatience of the lover looking forward to a tryst.

When faced with Romeo's banishment and the prospect of an enforced marriage to Paris, Juliet agrees to take the sleeping potion offered by FRIAR (4) LAURENCE. In 4.3.15–58, she reviews a roster of possible

terrors she faces in a frightening speech that underlines the courage with which she must and does proceed. She is no less resolute at the tragic climax of the play. Waking to find that mischance has overwhelmed her efforts, she does not hesitate to join her lover in death rather than continue living in a world that lacks their love.

It has often been thought that Juliet's age, 14, represents a typical marriage age for English women of Shakespeare's day, but historians believe that the normal age was the late teens or early twenties. In any case, Shakespeare lowered Juliet's age from that given in his source, 16, and lines such as 1.2.8–13 suggest that she is supposed to be thought of as quite young for marriage, perhaps to emphasise her vulnerability. On the other hand, Lady CAPULET (3) states explicitly that Veronese girls younger than Juliet were mothers (1.3.69–71). The question remains puzzling.

Juliet (2) Minor character in *Measure for Measure,* the pregnant fiancée of CLAUDIO (3). Claudio's death sentence for having illicit sex with Juliet is the central element of the play's plot, but the young woman is nevertheless a shadowy and undeveloped character. She speaks in only one of the three scenes in which she appears (2.3), and though she is touching in her combination of repentance and love, she remains a minor figure.

The role of Juliet is small, and this has suggested to some scholars that the play was at some point extensively revised—by Shakespeare or someone else—and her role was awkwardly cut. However, other commentators feel that her function as a pathetic victim is fully realised by her mere presence, and any enlargement of her role would be distracting.

Julius Caesar

SYNOPSIS

Act 1, Scene 1

Two tribunes, FLAVIUS (1) and MARULLUS, disperse a crowd (see COMMONER [1]) that is celebrating the return of Julius CAESAR (1) to ROME, though not before a COBBLER makes some flippant jokes. The tribunes rebuke the Commoners for disloyalty in welcoming the conqueror of another Roman, Pompey, whom they had also celebrated in the streets. The two officers remove the decorations that have been placed on public statues.

Act 1, Scene 2

At the feast of Lupercalia, Caesar arranges for Mark ANTONY, who is to participate in a fertility rite, to ritually touch CALPHURNIA, Caesar's wife. A SOOTHSAYER (1) warns Caesar to beware the ides (the 15th day) of March; Caesar ignores him and leads his entourage to the festival. CASSIUS and BRUTUS (4) remain behind and speak of Caesar's ambition to rule alone, a violation of the Roman political tradition that all aristocrats share power equally. Cassius says that Rome looks to Brutus for leadership in this crisis, and they hear cheering from the festival, which, they fear, means that Caesar is being acclaimed king by the Commoners. Cassius observes resentfully that he does not wish to be ruled by a man no better than himself, as another cheer erupts. Cassius continues to speak against Caesar's rule and refers to an ancient revolt against a king that Brutus' ancestor had led. Brutus hints that he has contemplated a similar action. Caesar's group returns; Caesar confides to Antony that he distrusts Cassius and then exits. Brutus and Cassius detain CASCA and hear an account of the festival from him. Caesar was offered the crown three times, Casca reports, and he refused it each time, though only with regret. Casca and Brutus leave, and Cassius soliloquises that Brutus, though a very important figure, is easy to manipulate, and he plans to further influence him with letters purporting to be from angry citizens who seek action against Caesar.

Act 1, Scene 3

Amid thunder and lightning, Casca meets CICERO and tells of omens that have accompanied the storm, foretelling extraordinary events. Cicero dismisses this superstitiousness and departs. Cassius appears and recruits Casca for a plot against Caesar, naming a meeting place for later that night. Another conspirator, CINNA (1), arrives, and Cassius directs him to leave messages, which he provides, in places where Brutus will receive them.

Act 2, Scene 1

Brutus, having been awake all night, decides at dawn that Caesar's ambition makes it necessary to kill him. He receives one of Cassius' anonymous letters urging him to protect Rome, and he resolves to lead the conspirators in assassinating Caesar. Cassius and other plotters arrive, and they lay their plans. Brutus insists that Antony not be killed, arguing that they must not seem bloodthirsty and that Antony will be helpless without Caesar. DECIUS volunteers to ensure that Caesar will attend the day's Senate session, where the assassination is to take place. The conspirators depart. Brutus, seeing his sleeping servant, LUCIUS (2), muses on his own sleepless life. His wife, PORTIA (2), appears and asks why he is disturbed. He promises to tell her later, as a last conspirator, LIGARIUS, arrives, and she leaves. Ligarius agrees to follow Brutus in any exploit, and they leave together for the Senate.

Act 2, Scene 2

Calphurnia tells Caesar of the many appalling omens that have been seen and insists that he stay home

rather than go to the Senate. He refuses, insisting that one must face death if it comes, but then he decides to humour Calphurnia and stay at home, pleading illness. However, Decius arrives and claims that the omens are favourable and that the Senate proposes to offer Caesar a crown. Caesar changes his mind again.

Act 2, Scene 3
ARTEMIDORUS reads aloud a message naming the conspirators and warning Caesar against them. He vows to present it to Caesar at the Senate.

Act 2, Scene 4
Portia worries hysterically about Brutus. The Soothsayer appears, saying that he hopes to warn Caesar of impending harm, and he goes on to the Senate. Portia sends Lucius on a pointless errand to Brutus, with orders to return and tell her how he seems.

Act 3, Scene 1
At the Senate, Caesar encounters the Soothsayer, who warns that the ides of March is not yet over. Artemidorus attempts to deliver his message, but Caesar rejects him and proceeds with Senate business. One conspirator draws Antony away from the meeting, while another presents Caesar with a petition that he has already rejected. Caesar's continued refusal is the signal: the conspirators stab him. Caesar, dismayed that his friend Brutus should be among the attackers, dies. The assassins, led by Brutus, ritually bathe their hands in Caesar's blood, declaring their devotion to political liberty. A message arrives from Antony: he is prepared to ally himself with the conspirators if they can provide a rationale for their deed. Though Cassius has reservations, Brutus approves. Antony arrives and volunteers to die with Caesar if the conspirators wish to kill him, but Brutus insists on their alliance, and he grants Antony's request to speak at Caesar's funeral. The conspirators depart, and Antony soliloquises about his intention to avenge Caesar's death by launching a civil war. News comes of OCTAVIUS' approach to Rome.

Act 3, Scene 2
Brutus addresses the PLEBEIANS (1), assuring them that the assassination was necessary in order to preserve the Republic. They applaud him, proposing that he be crowned himself. Antony arrives with Caesar's body, and Brutus tells the crowd to listen to Antony's funeral oration. Brutus leaves, and Antony addresses the Plebeians, praising Caesar while seeming to acknowledge the honour of the assassins. Gradually, Antony generates a mood of hostility towards the conspirators while denying his intention to do so. Introducing Caesar's will, which designates a generous bequest to be distributed among the people, he sparks a riotous response to the assassination. The Plebeians rage into the streets, intending to burn the houses of Brutus and the others. Antony exults. Learning of Octavius' presence in Rome, he goes to join him; as he leaves he hears that Brutus and Cassius have fled the city.

Act 3, Scene 3
A mob of Plebeians encounters the poet CINNA (2) and kills him, mistaking him for the conspirator with the same name.

Act 4, Scene 1
Antony, Octavius, and LEPIDUS decide who must be executed to protect their new power in Rome. Antony sends Lepidus on an errand, and then belittles him as an insignificant man who is not fit to rule but who will be useful for a while. Antony and Octavius begin to plan a campaign against Brutus and Cassius, who have raised an army.

Act 4, Scene 2
At Brutus' camp, LUCILIUS returns from a visit to Cassius' troops and reports that Cassius has not displayed the warmth of earlier meetings. Brutus interprets this as a sign of waning friendship between Cassius and himself. Cassius arrives and immediately asserts that Brutus has wronged him; Brutus suggests that they enter his tent to talk privately.

Act 4, Scene 3
Cassius charges that Brutus has ignored his arguments and punished an officer for taking bribes. He insists that they cannot be overstrict in a time of crisis, and Brutus remarks that Cassius himself is reputed to be corrupt and accuses him of withholding funds. The infuriated Cassius, declaring that he never expected such insults from his comrade, offers his dagger and suggests that Brutus kill him. Brutus gently mocks Cassius' excess but apologises for being overheated himself, and the two shake hands in reconciliation. A POET (1) arrives and chastises the two generals for their disharmony. Cassius is amused, but Brutus dismisses him abruptly. Brutus then tells Cassius that he has been short-tempered in part because he has just learned of Portia's suicide due to her fear of the immense army that Octavius and Antony are sending against her husband. MESSALA arrives with news from Rome: Octavius and Antony have executed many political enemies and are on the march. He also reports Portia's death. Brutus hides his prior knowledge and pretends to receive the news stoically, arousing Messala's admiration. Brutus then proposes marching on PHILIPPI, where their enemies have camped. Cassius argues that they should stay where they are and let Antony and Octavius use up their energy marching, but Brutus insists that his plan is superior and Cassius gives in. Brutus then retires for the night, and the others leave. The GHOST (2) of Caesar appears to

Brutus, announces that they shall meet again at Philippi, and disappears.

Act 5, Scene 1
Octavius and Antony reflect on their good fortune that Brutus and Cassius have taken disadvantageous positions. Octavius insists on commanding the more important right wing, despite Antony's seniority. Brutus, Cassius, and their army appear, and the opposing commanders parley. They quickly begin to exchange insults, and Octavius and Antony leave. Cassius confides to Messala that he is uneasy about the forthcoming battle. Brutus and Cassius tell each other that they will commit suicide rather than be captured.

Act 5, Scene 2
Brutus orders an attack on Octavius' forces, which he can see weakening.

Act 5, Scene 3
TITINIUS and Cassius, hard-pressed by the enemy, see that Brutus has launched his attack too soon and left them at a disadvantage. PINDARUS arrives with news that troops are approaching their headquarters; Cassius sends Titinius to investigate and tells Pindarus to watch from a nearby hill. Pindarus reports that Titinius is captured, and Cassius, believing that his own capture is imminent, impales himself on his sword, assisted by Pindarus. Pindarus flees, as Titinius returns safely with Messala to announce that Brutus has defeated Octavius. They find Cassius' body and realise what has happened. Messala leaves to tell Brutus, who appears and mourns his comrade. He announces that they shall launch another attack before nightfall.

Act 5, Scene 4
Brutus is forced to retreat. Lucilius pretends to be Brutus and is captured. Antony arrives, realises that the captive is not Brutus, and praises Lucilius for courageously diverting attention from his commander.

Act 5, Scene 5
Brutus, defeated, asks several companions to help him to commit suicide, but they refuse. As enemy troops approach, he prevails upon STRATO to help him, and he dies on his sword. Antony and Octavius appear, triumphant, and find Brutus' body. They praise him and order his honourable burial.

COMMENTARY

Julius Caesar is a play about moral ambiguity in a political setting and the personal tragedy that results. It resembles both the HISTORY PLAYS, written somewhat earlier, and the great TRAGEDIES, soon to come. Like the tragedies, it presents a protagonist who aspires to heroism and fails because of his own moral shortcomings. At the same time, *Julius Caesar* also reflects the

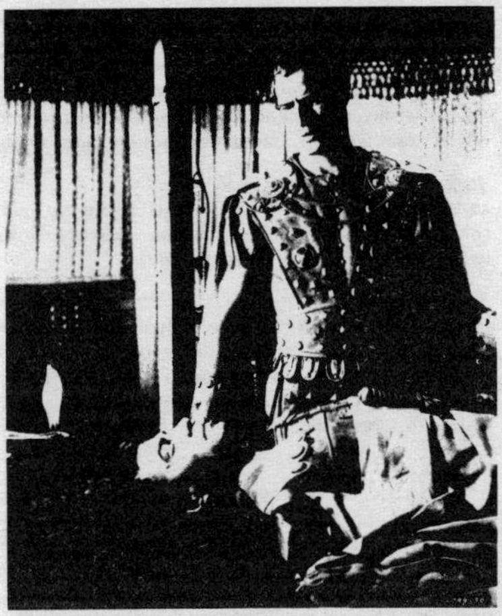

'This was the noblest Roman of them all' (Julius Caesar *5.5.68). Antony (Marlon Brando) eulogises Brutus (James Mason) in the 1953 film version.* (Courtesy of Movie Star News)

political philosophy that had informed the playwright's picture of English civil war in the history plays. Because civil disorder and violence are tragic for the entire society, their avoidance is a higher moral obligation than the pursuit or control of power, even for apparently just or moral purposes. Therefore, for Shakespeare, the preservation of the political status quo is a primary good.

Brutus, the protagonist of *Julius Caesar,* is an ambivalent figure who may be seen as both good and evil—an honourable man dedicated to the good of his country, but also a destroyer of its peace. The play's central action—the murder of Caesar—may seem an act of disinterested idealism or one of inflated self-love. Twentieth-century views of the play reflect these possibilities: with the rise of fascism in the 1920s and 1930s, Brutus was aggrandised as a model of republican virtues and Caesar identified with Mussolini and Hitler. More recently, however, Caesar has been defended as a hero who is destroyed by a neurotically envious Brutus, who pursues glory without regard for the disaster he provokes.

These positions are not as mutually exclusive as they may seem; *Julius Caesar* is sometimes grouped with the PROBLEM PLAYS as a work about the uncertain outcome of human endeavours. In this light, the heart of *Julius Caesar* is the tension between Brutus' idealistic rejection of a dominating leader and the reality that

human society requires the discipline that Caesar imposes. From another angle, the conflict occurs between the protagonist's obsessive demand for a perfect world and the catastrophe that follows in the real, imperfect world. Thus Brutus' actions are both virtuous and disastrous. Precisely because this ambiguity is possible, Brutus is a tragic hero who attempts the humanly impossible and fails.

At first glance, it seems odd that the play's title character is killed less than halfway through the work, but Caesar, though his part is small, dominates the whole drama. First, his assumption of power in Rome stimulates the conspiracy; later, the inescapable memory of him inspires Antony and haunts Brutus.

The telling comparisons between Brutus and Caesar demonstrate the play's most essential ambivalence: the tyrant and his opponent are not easily distinguishable. In this fashion, the morality of the assassination is questioned, and the importance of Caesar's leadership—first resented and then absent—remains evident. Both Brutus and Caesar have great leadership qualities, and, being certain of his virtues, each is susceptible to flattery and manipulation by lesser men. In murdering Caesar, Brutus follows the Caesar-like course of attempting to change society in accordance with his views. Similarly, in the war that follows the assassination, Brutus behaves as imperiously as Caesar did, enacting precisely the failings of autocratic leadership—the isolation from his followers, the presumption of sound decision-making, the potential for tyranny—that he had acted to prevent in killing Caesar. Significantly, Caesar's Ghost identifies itself as Brutus' 'evil spirit' (4.3.281).

Nevertheless, Caesar is superior to Brutus in his analysis of Cassius and in his recognition that a single leader is needed to control Rome. Moreover, Brutus persistently makes bad judgements, and he suffers the consequences, going from error to error. He refuses to share leadership of the conspiracy with Cassius or Cicero. His arrogant overconfidence is plainly demonstrated when he dismisses Antony as an inconsequential underling in 2.1.181–183. Later, he twice rejects the advice of the more experienced Cassius, resulting in the failure of his cause at Philippi. He is persistently blind to reality, following his own superficial rectitude to disaster. The patriotism he invokes is certainly a living ideal for Brutus, but it is also a cover for his vanity and his unacknowledged need to be like Caesar himself.

As Brutus deteriorates morally in the second half of the play, becoming ever more Caesar-like, so Caesar himself seems to grow in worth as Rome collapses in the leadership vacuum created by his death. This important point is made especially clear by the behaviour of the Plebeians after the murder. Ironically, they hail Brutus as an autocrat—'Let him be Caesar' (3.2.52)—just after he has murdered Caesar to prevent him from becoming one. However, the fickle mob is immediately turned against Brutus by Antony's oration, and their brutality in killing the wrong Cinna in 3.3 heralds the disorder that later prevails on a larger scale in the civil war. Brutus has unleashed a whirlwind.

Brutus' attempts to dignify the assassination by invoking the gods through ritual are pointedly undercut. Brutus wishes to make a ceremony of the killing, saying, 'Let's be sacrificers, but not butchers' (2.1.166), but he immediately goes on to reveal an unconscious awareness of public opinion: '. . . so appearing to the common eyes, / We shall be call'd purgers, not murderers' (2.1.179–180). Another attempt to ritualise the murder occurs when Brutus leads the assassins in washing their hands in Caesar's blood, an act that only accentuates the violence of the deed.

In the second half of the play, Antony, heretofore an unimportant figure, suddenly comes into his own. He dominates the conspirators, taking control of Rome by the end of 3.2. In 4.1, where he bargains the lives of his relatives with Octavius and Lepidus, and then disdains the latter as an impotent tool, we see Antony as both a cynical political operative and a strong leader, a complex figure whose ambivalent nature deepens the moral ambiguity of the play's world.

Later developments confirm that Brutus' decision to kill Caesar was wrong both politically and morally. Antony's dire prediction of the bloody course revenge will take, in 3.1.258–275, strongly invokes the conventions of the REVENGE PLAY, a popular genre of ELIZABETHAN and JACOBEAN DRAMA that Shakespeare had exploited earlier in *Titus Andronicus* and would again in *Hamlet* and *Macbeth*. In a revenge play an inexorable rule operates: a murder must be punished with another one, usually under the eye of the victim's ghost; the first murderer is doomed, regardless of politics or personality. Thus such factors as the possible benefit to Rome of Caesar's death are swept aside. Brutus' moralising has been useless; Antony will inevitably triumph. The would-be saviour of Rome has produced only a morally chaotic situation in which final victory goes, not to the high-minded assassin, nor to the hot-blooded avenger, but to the cool opportunist Octavius. This icily commanding figure takes control from Antony in 5.1.20 and disposes of matters at the play's close. Roman history was much more familiar in Shakespeare's time than in ours, and the playwright knew that his audience would immediately recognise the irony that Brutus' attempt to prevent one tyranny merely paved the way for the greater autocracy of Octavius, known to history as the first Roman emperor, Augustus CAESAR (2). (Shakespeare was to dramatise the final consolidation of Octavius' power in *Antony and Cleopatra.*)

As he did in the history plays, Shakespeare altered the historical record considerably in writing *Julius Caesar.* Following PLUTARCH, the playwright accurately

presented the broad outlines of Roman history but altered many details for dramatic purposes. Notably, he compressed the chronology of events from months to a few days or hours in order to achieve a more dramatic sequence of events. For instance, Caesar's triumphant return to Rome occurred in October of 45 B.C., while the feast of Lupercalia fell in the following February. Only some weeks after this event were the tribunes Flavus (the play's Flavius) and Marullus ousted after removing public decorations that honoured Caesar. Shakespeare combined all these events into a single day, enacted in 1.1–2.

Similarly, the aftermath of the assassination covers only several hours in the play. In Plutarch the same events took months. Antony's speech followed Brutus' by several days, rather than immediately, and Brutus, whose flight is reported after the speech, did not in fact leave Rome until mid-April. Similarly, Octavius' arrival coincides with the orations in the play, but he did not actually appear in Rome until six weeks afterwards. And though Antony welcomes Octavius in the play, the two actually quarrelled to the point of warfare, and their alliance was not arranged for almost 20 months, though in the play it follows immediately.

The battle of Philippi is a dramatic example of Shakespeare's compression of events. In the play, the battle directly follows the meeting of Cassius and Brutus in 4.2–3, whereas it actually occurred more than 6 months later. In fact there were two battles at Philippi, as Plutarch reports: the first was a draw, in which Cassius killed himself; in the second, 20 days later, Brutus was defeated and also committed suicide. Shakespeare compresses the two conflicts into a single afternoon.

Other changes involve the historical figures themselves. In 1.2 Cassius refers to an estrangement between himself and Brutus, and Brutus replies that his private worries have made him distant to his friends. In fact, according to Plutarch, the hostility between the two stemmed from their rivalry for a political position. Shakespeare's version draws attention to Brutus' worries about Caesar's aspirations and also makes him seem thoughtful and conscientious, rather than politically ambitious.

Further, Shakespeare substantially elaborated Plutarch's accounts of the speeches of Brutus and Antony in 3.2 and of the riot of the Plebeians in 3.3. Plutarch merely alludes to the two orations, attaching no great importance to their styles, while Shakespeare creates antithetical deliveries—rational versus emotional—that reflect on the characters who speak them and on the very nature of politics. Similarly, while Plutarch mentions the actions of the mob, the playwright gives the crowd life and thus transforms their volatility and fickleness, even their grim sense of humour, into a significant political phenomenon.

Shakespeare had to emphasise politics in *Julius Caesar*, for otherwise Brutus' fate would be meaningless. Brutus himself never sees his mistake in murdering his best friend and the leader of his country. His fate is dramatically satisfactory only in light of the impact of his action on Roman society as a whole, that is, in its political consequences. His error stems from an unconscious desire for a political world in which evil is impossible. Thus his political blindness has a psychological element, reflecting Shakespeare's progress towards the psychological portraiture of the great tragedies.

SOURCES OF THE PLAY

The primary source for *Julius Caesar* was Sir Thomas NORTH's translation of the ancient Roman biographical collection Plutarch's *Lives* in either its first or second edition (1579, 1595). Isolated passages suggest other materials that the playwright knew, including a biography of Caesar by John HIGGINS in A MIRROR FOR MAGISTRATES, the philosophical poem *Nosce Teipsum* ('Know Thyself'), by John DAVIES (2), published in 1599, and several works by CICERO. Nevertheless, three of the lives in Plutarch—those of Caesar, Brutus, and Antony—supply all of the incidents in the play. In addition, English plays about Caesar had been popular since at least the early 1580s, and this tradition must have helped stimulate the writing of *Julius Caesar*. While there is no evidence that any of these plays influenced Shakespeare directly, the famous phrase 'Et tu, Brute' (3.1.77) may have come from such a work, for it does not appear in any Latin source yet was a well-known tag line in Shakespeare's day.

TEXT OF THE PLAY

Julius Caesar was probably written in early 1599. The diary of Thomas PLATTER records a performance of the play on September 21, 1599, and the play is not on the list of Shakespeare's plays published by Francis MERES in September 1598. While Meres' list does not pretend to be complete, *Caesar* was a strikingly popular work, as contemporary references indicate, and is not likely to have been omitted if it had been staged. While it might have been written during the latter part of 1598, it is fairly certain that *Much Ado About Nothing* and *Henry V* were written then, so *Julius Caesar* is thought to have followed them.

Caesar was not printed during Shakespeare's lifetime; the first edition is that of the FIRST FOLIO (1623). This text, known as F1, is relatively error-free—it is generally held to be the least corrupt text in the Folio—indicating that it was probably printed from a copy of Shakespeare's own manuscript, or FOUL PAPERS. This copy had probably been used as or taken from a PROMPT-BOOK, in which the playwright's characteristic mis-spellings and unnecessarily elaborate stage directions had been corrected. The later folios—and a series of late 17th-century QUARTOS—vary

slightly from F1, but all are clearly based on it, as are all modern editions.

THEATRICAL HISTORY OF THE PLAY

The earliest known performance of *Julius Caesar* was held on September 21, 1599, as recorded in Thomas Platter's diary, and many references from 1599 and the early 17th century indicate that the play was very popular with its original audience, as does the existence of a competing play about Caesar produced by Philip HENSLOWE in 1602. Leonard DIGGES wrote about *Caesar*'s enthusiastic audiences as late as the 1620s, and it was performed at the royal court at least twice, in 1613 and 1638. In the 1660s the play was included in the repertoire of Thomas KILLIGREW's company and was one of the few Shakespearean plays to be popular in the late 17th century; Charles HART (1) played Brutus for Killigrew, and later Thomas BETTERTON was successful in the part. The play was published six times between 1684 and 1691.

In the 18th century Spranger BARRY (3) was a notable Antony, while Barton BOOTH (1) and James QUIN played Brutus in several productions. The celebrated Peg WOFFINGTON appeared as Portia in the 1750s, though that small part has not generally attracted leading actresses. In the 19th century most major English actors portrayed one or more of the play's important roles, and the play was also very popular in America, where Lawrence BARRETT, Edwin FORREST, and Edwin BOOTH (2) were particularly associated with it. In 1864 Booth and his brothers Junius Brutus BOOTH (5) and John Wilkes BOOTH (3) played Brutus, Cassius, and Antony respectively, performing on the same stage for the first and only time. In London, a very popular 1895 production, presented by Beerbohm TREE, featured sets and costumes by perhaps the most famous English painter of the day, Sir Lawrence Alma-Tadema (1836–1912).

Perhaps because the rise of totalitarianism in Germany and Russia between the world wars generated a concern with political tyranny, *Julius Caesar* has often been produced in the 20th century. Particularly memorable was Orson WELLES' modern-dress rendering of 1938, in which Caesar was attired as the Italian Fascist leader Benito Mussolini. *Julius Caesar* has also yielded a number of FILMS, notably M.G.M.'s 1953 version starring Marlon Brando as Antony. The play has likewise been produced several times on TELEVISION, beginning as long ago as 1938; in 1963 the British Broadcasting Corporation presented *The Spread of the Eagle,* based on all three ROMAN PLAYS.

Juno Pagan goddess and minor figure in *The Tempest,* a character in the MASQUE presented by ARIEL to celebrate the engagement of MIRANDA and FERDINAND (2). After an introduction by IRIS, Juno joins CERES in singing a hymn of 'marriage-blessing' (4.1.106) to the couple. Though queen of the gods, Juno has the smallest role in the masque. However, in Shakespeare's hierarchy-conscious world, Juno's rank gave her a greater importance than she seems otherwise to have. As a queen, her presence—her 'sovereign grace' (4.1.72)—gives the masque a particularly dignified air appropriate to the betrothal of PROSPERO's daughter. If, as some scholars believe, the masque was added to the play when it was performed as part of the 1613 marriage festivities for Princess ELIZABETH (3), this feature would have had even greater import. Juno's entrance is accordingly a spectacular one. The stage direction at 4.1.72 reads 'Juno descends', indicating theatrical practise in Shakespeare's time, at least in the new BLACKFRIARS THEATRE: the goddess was lowered from the ceiling above the stage, probably seated on a throne decorated with peacocks, as mentioned by Iris in 4.1.74. (Nineteenth-century productions of *The Tempest* often featured live peacocks.)

Jupiter Pagan god and minor character in *Cymbeline.* Jupiter, the Roman king of the gods, appears to the desperate POSTHUMUS in a vision where he assures the spirit of Posthumus' father, SICILIUS LEONATUS, that the young man will be restored to good fortune. He then departs, and leaves a tablet with a cryptic message (5.4.138–145) that is interpreted later by the SOOTHSAYER (3) as an allegory of reunion and renewal. Posthumus does not realise that his chaotic drift towards tragedy has ended with the god's appearance, and he is still intent on death. However, the audience is aware that he shall be 'happier much by his affliction made' (5.4.108), as the god puts it. Thus, Jupiter embodies the play's moral: that humanity depends on providence for happiness.

Jupiter's style is very formal. He speaks in rhyming verse and old-fashioned language unlike anything else in the play. This signifies his supernatural nature. In performance, his lines are sometimes sung. The stage direction at his entrance reads, 'Jupiter descends in thunder and lightning, sitting upon an eagle . . .' (5.4.-92); this makes it clear that either the BLACKFRIARS THEATRE or the GLOBE, or both, were equipped with a mechanical apparatus that permitted characters to enter a scene from above by being lowered from the ceiling. As in the present case, this permitted a literal *deus ex machina,* or 'god from the machine', the phrase for a surprise appearance by a god who resolves the situation of a play. The machine was originally a crane-like device used in ancient Greek theatre to lower actors portraying deities as though they were descending from heaven.

Some scholars believe Jupiter may have been intended as an allegorical representation of King JAMES I, newly crowned as the first joint monarch of England and Scotland. In this light, the cryptic tablet reads as

a tribute to the union of the two countries, a matter that was disputed in the first years of James' reign.

Justice Minor character in *Measure for Measure,* a magistrate of VIENNA. The Justice appears only in 2.1, speaking three lines to his superior, ESCALUS (2). This brief exchange serves to remind the audience of the condemned CLAUDIO (3) after the diversion of the long comic trial of POMPEY (1). The Justice and Escalus depart together at the close of the scene.

Some scholars believe that the Justice's absence elsewhere in the play is evidence that it was considerably revised. Another theory supports only a tiny revision, holding that the Justice's lines had originally been written for the PROVOST, but that in production they had been reassigned. Normal stage practise in Shakespeare's day frowned on an immediate re-entrance after an exit, and since the Provost opens the next scene, he could not close this one by leaving with Escalus. So, possibly, a new character was invented by Shakespeare or someone else. As a matter of economy, the Justice is often cut from modern productions and his lines eliminated or given to the Provost.

K

Katharina Character in *The Taming of the Shrew.* See KATHERINA.

Katharine (1) (Katherine; Catherine) Character in *Love's Labour's Lost,* the beloved of DUMAINE and a lady-in-waiting to the PRINCESS (1) OF FRANCE. Although primarily a stock figure in the play's courtly tableau of lovers, she is given a flash of true human feeling. In 5.2, ROSALINE (1) teases her about a sister who was said to have died of love, and Katharine is overtaken by her memory of the occasion. 'He made her melancholy, sad, and heavy; / And so she died: had she been light, like you, / Of such a merry, nimble, stirring spirit, / She might ha' been a grandam ere she died. . . .' (5.2.14–17). This brief remark gives us not only a glimpse of a young woman's recollected grief, but we receive an impression of Rosaline's character as well.

It is thought that Shakespeare derived the story of Katharine's sister's death from a current account of a similar demise among the attendants of the historical Princess of France of the day, Marguerite of Valois, who was in fact married to the King of Navarre. The same tale may also have influenced the OPHELIA episode in *Hamlet.*

Katharine (2) (Catherine, Katherine), Princess (1401–1438) Historical figure and character in *Henry V,* the daughter of the FRENCH KING, later betrothed to King HENRY V. Princess Katharine is an innocent girl. She is comically instructed in English by her waiting-woman, ALICE, in 3.4, and she is the upright but somewhat baffled subject of King Henry's aggressive courtship in 5.2. Most of her lines are in French or broken English. She has little personality; she is simply the object of King Henry's affections and part of his reward for victory over FRANCE (1).

The historical Katherine of Valois was the youngest child of Charles VI, the French King of the play, and Queen ISABEL (2). She was married to Henry as part of the treaty of TROYES. After Henry's death, she married an obscure Welsh nobleman, Owen Tudor; their grandchild was to become King Henry VII of England, and he appears as the Earl of RICHMOND in *3 Henry VI* and *Richard III.*

Katherina Title character in *The Taming of the Shrew,* the ill-tempered young woman courted, married, and 'tamed' by PETRUCHIO (2). Katherina is sometimes thought of as a representative oppressed woman, dominated by a selfish man and trapped in a loveless marriage. But this point of view is based on modern notions of marital relations (see 'Commentary' on the play), and it obscures the real nature of the character. Katherina undergoes a positive transformation during the play: she is freed from an unhappy emotional state, and she enters a happy marriage.

In Acts 1–3 Katherina is presented as a volatile and distinctly unhappy person. She is a familiar type, a young adult who resents the rejection she receives, yet, in an effort to feel immune to the opinions of others, she simply makes herself less likeable by belligerently taking exception to everything. In addition, she has clearly been compared to her younger sister—the deceptively sweet BIANCA (1)—too often for comfort. The psychological pressure within Katherina bursts forth in violence, both threatened and actual. Not content with curtly dismissing the rudeness of HORTENSIO, for example, she goes on to express a desire to 'comb your noddle with a three-legg'd stool' (1.1.64). Corrected by a music teacher (Hortensio again, in disguise), she assaults him with a lute. Her envy and suspicion of Bianca drive her to physical abuse in 2.1. When she first encounters Petruchio, knowing only that he is a suitor, she repeatedly insults him (2.1.195–259) and she slaps him to 'try' (2.1.217) his gentlemanliness.

In Acts 4–5, however, Katherina changes, under the forceful guidance of Petruchio. His 'taming' consists of demonstrating that she need not continue to be an outcast, disliked and shunned, and that there is indeed a place in the world that she can occupy happily. His persistent references to her calm and sweetness—initially fictitious—make her realise the psychological benefits that such attributes could bring: acceptance and a sense of moral worth. His own behaviour shows her the ugliness of shrewishness. She chooses to reject her bristly defensiveness and assume the role of an ordinary wife. She will admit that the world is not hers to control; in return, she will have the emotional security of a prescribed place in it.

The submissiveness that Katherina accepts, and that troubles modern readers, was simply held to be a conventional attribute of a wife: Shakespeare and his contemporaries of both sexes believed that the Bible, as well as long-hallowed tradition, prescribed hierarchical relationships among humans: husbands ruled wives, as parents ruled children, as monarchs ruled commoners, and as God ruled all. Katherina voices this belief in her banquet speech in 5.2.

Katherina loves Petruchio. She indicates as much in the grace with which she kisses him at the end of 5.1, and her speech in 5.2 is an implicit expression of her love. At the banquet she has already demonstrated her obedience and need not do more; Petruchio has merely asked her for a statement of principle, as much to aggravate the WIDOW (1) and Bianca as anything else. She goes far beyond his intent, specifically referring to her own experience and stating that she is grateful for inclusion in the system she describes. The entirely spontaneous physical act of submission that closes her speech symbolises the wifely duty demanded in this system, but it is also directed to her husband, as an expression of her gratitude. That this gesture is loving is confirmed by his affectionate response to it. Katherina has found not only comfort in an assured position in society, but happiness in a loving marriage. She is thus the vehicle for an elaboration of two of Shakespeare's persistent concerns: the virtue of an ordered, hierarchical social system and the value of marriage as a venue for love. Her psychological transformation also reflects his fascination with the mysteries of the human personality.

Katherina's is a small part, for all its importance, and, while boldly drawn, she lacks the subtlety of later Shakespearean heroines who resemble her, such as BEATRICE in *Much Ado About Nothing.* It is noteworthy that Katherina shares with several of the playwright's most lovingly developed female characters, as well as with the 'Dark Lady' of the SONNETS, a sharp temper and a dark complexion (see 2.1.248–249). It seems possible (though altogether unprovable) that these characters share the traits of a woman (entirely unidentifiable) who was romantically important to Shakespeare. The thought certainly adds resonance to his portrait of a shrew.

Katherine (Katharine) of Aragon, Queen of England (1485–1536) Historical figure and character in *Henry VIII,* the rejected wife of King HENRY VIII. The focus of most of Acts 2 and 3 is on Henry's finally successful effort to divorce Katherine and marry ANNE (1) BULLEN. Katherine appears first in 1.2, where she opposes the unjust taxes introduced by Cardinal WOLSEY. The episode establishes the queen as a good person and Wolsey, already designated a villain, as her enemy—and it is Wolsey's influence that leads the king to divorce her. In 2.4, at her divorce trial, Katherine spiritedly defies Wolsey, refusing to submit to his judgement and demanding an appeal to the pope. In 3.1, when she is visited by Wolsey and Cardinal CAMPEIUS, she concedes her helplessness, but refuses to co-operate in her own downfall. Finally, in 4.2, she is seen dying in exile at KIMBOLTON, after the king has married Anne and crowned her as queen. She hears of Wolsey's death, and though bitter, she accepts GRIFFITH's advice and forgives the cardinal. Throughout she is a spirited woman, insisting on the respect due a queen. Her virtues are stressed in the enactment of her dream, in which supernatural beings crown her with garlands.

Katherine's role in the play is largely symbolic. As a paragon of goodness, she makes a suitable victim for Wolsey, whose villainy dominates the first half of the play. Henry is susceptible to Wolsey's influence, but his evident affection for Katherine makes it clear that he is not himself a villain, despite the divorce. The loss of Katherine is seen as a misfortune that is compensated for by the king's later wisdom and maturity, and by the birth of ELIZABETH (1) at the play's close.

For dramatic purposes, Shakespeare places Katherine's death immediately after Wolsey's death and Anne's coronation, though she in fact lived for six years after the first event and three after the second, almost long enough to see Anne's downfall. Aside from chronology, Shakespeare's presentation of Katherine's story is fairly accurate. The daughter of King Ferdinand and Queen Isabella of Spain (ruled 1479–1516), Katherine was married to Henry's elder brother, Prince Arthur (1486–1502), the heir apparent to King Henry VII, in 1501. Prince Arthur died shortly after marrying Katherine, and she declared, then and later, that the marriage had not been sexually consummated. Henry disputed this later, when he sought an annulment and cited Katherine's marriage to his brother as having disqualified her for marriage to him. (Though traditionally called a divorce, what Henry actually obtained was a declaration that he had never been married in theological terms.) Yet when Henry had acceded to the throne in 1509, he had actually received papal approval to marry Katherine.

In marrying Katherine, Henry had wished to maintain the Spanish alliance that she represented, but he apparently loved her as well. However, when she did not produce a suitable heir to the throne—their only child was a daughter, not considered acceptable at the time—Henry considered a new marriage. Thus, on falling in love with Anne, he proceeded to dispose of his wife of 20 years. Though Katherine was badly humiliated by Henry before and after the divorce, he allowed her to live out her life in some comfort, and it was thought by contemporaries—and most modern

historians agree—that his affection and respect for her never completely disappeared.

Kean (1), Charles (1811–1868) British actor and producer. Charles Kean, the son of Edmund KEAN (2), was acclaimed as HAMLET, but his greatest importance was not as an actor but as the producer of Shakespeare's plays (and others) in a lavish style, incorporating elaborate spectacles that laid claim to historical accuracy. Costumes and sets were designed with scrupulous attention to archaeological detail, and immense casts of extras were used. Among his most notable productions were *Henry VIII* (1855), *The Winter's Tale* (1856), *Richard II* (1857), and *Henry V* (1859). He established a style of production that was to last into the early 20th century in the work of his followers, including Henry IRVING and Beerbohm TREE.

Kean (2), Edmund (1787–1833) British actor. The abandoned son of an actress, Kean was raised in provincial touring companies, by various people—including his guardian, Moses Kean, a comic and ventriloquist who may have been his uncle, though his paternity was never clearly established. He already had many years of acting experience when he achieved a London triumph as SHYLOCK in 1814. His acting style was frenzied and active, in marked contrast to the reigning Shakespearean actor, the dignified J. P. KEMBLE (3). A contemporary, using a political metaphor, declared that Kean was 'one of the people . . . a *radical* performer', and Samuel Taylor COLERIDGE remarked of his 'rapid descents from the hyper-tragic to the infra-colloquial' that 'to see him act, is like reading Shakespeare by flashes of lightning'. His greatest successes were as villains—especially Shylock, RICHARD III, OTHELLO, and Barabas in *The Jew of Malta* by Christopher MARLOWE (1)—while his HAMLET and LEAR were sometimes criticised as unthoughtful. He was a temperamental and undisciplined man who often missed performances, and he figured in a notable sex scandal with the wife of a popular politician. Nevertheless, only Kemble and W. C. MACREADY rivalled him in popular-

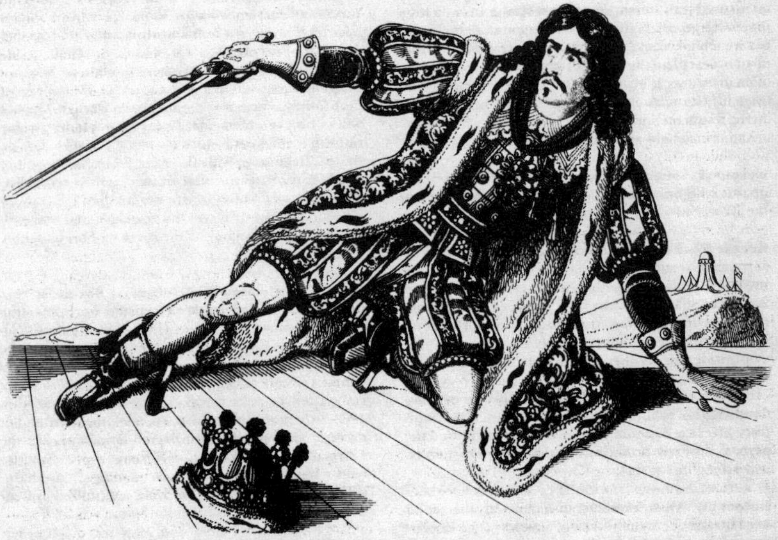

In the early 19th century, Edmund Kean (seen here as Richard III) helped replace the classical ideal of acting that had prevailed through the 18th century with a new, romantic style marked by violent emotion. The poet and critic Samuel Taylor Coleridge remarked that Kean could reveal Shakespeare through 'flashes of lightning'. (Courtesy of Culver Pictures, Inc.)

ity. His success was so great that he has been called the theatre's first star, to whom all other features of a production were subordinated. He collapsed on-stage while playing Othello—opposite the IAGO of his son Charles KEAN (1)—and died a few weeks later.

Keats, John (1795–1821) English poet much influenced by Shakespeare. Generally regarded as among the greatest of all poets, Keats kept a bust of Shakespeare in his study and believed, at least sometimes, that the spirit of Shakespeare presided over his work in a supernatural way, dictating choices as he wrote his poems. In any case Shakespeare's influence on Keats' poetry—in a conventional literary sense—is very evident; his poems are steeped in Shakespearean imagery, and his letters, a literary masterpiece in themselves, abound in allusions to the playwright.

Keats had a set of small volumes of the plays (an 1814 reissue of the 1765 edition of Samuel JOHNSON [7]), which he annotated heavily. His notes have been published by Caroline SPURGEON as *Keats' Shakespeare* (1928). Some of the plays were plainly of greater interest than others: the HISTORY PLAYS, for example, were virtually ignored, while *A Midsummer Night's Dream* and *The Tempest* sparked frequent and enthusiastic commentary. Keats' remarks on Shakespeare in his letters have offered much grist for subsequent writers. In one such comment, still often cited, Keats observed that Shakespeare had the 'quality [that] went to form a Man of Achievement, especially in Literature . . . I mean *Negative Capability,* that is, when a man is capable of being in uncertainties, mysteries, doubts, without any irritable reaching after fact and reason'.

Keeper (1) Minor character in *1 Henry VI,* one of the guards who attends the imprisoned MORTIMER (1) in the Tower of London in 2.5.

Keeper (2) Either of two minor characters in *3 Henry VI,* gameskeepers who capture the refugee King HENRY VI in 3.1. Henry chastises the Keepers for their inconstant allegiance, which they once gave to him but now proclaim to be owed to King EDWARD (4). They respond with rationalisations before arresting him. This incident is another instance of changeable loyalties in the disrupted world depicted in the play.

In the FIRST FOLIO text of the play, the Keepers are designated in a stage direction as 'Sinklo' and 'Humfrey'. These are presumably the actors who played the parts in an early production, probably John SINCKLO and Humphrey JEFFES.

Keeper (3) Minor character in *Richard III,* the gaoler of CLARENCE (1) in the TOWER OF LONDON. The Keeper listens sympathetically to Clarence's report of a nightmare in 1.4. Some editions follow the first QUARTO and assign the Keeper's part to BRAKENBURY. The dropping of the character doubtless reflects an economy measure by a 16th-century acting company.

Keeper (4) Minor character in *Richard II,* the gaoler of the deposed King RICHARD II. The Keeper brings Richard a meal in 5.5, but he refuses to taste it for poison, as had been routine, asserting that Sir Piers EXTON has forbidden him to do so. Richard strikes him in anger, and the Keeper's cries summon Exton and his murderers, who kill the prisoner.

Keeper (5) Minor character in *Henry VIII,* the doorman at a meeting of the king's council. In 5.2 the Keeper, following his orders, prevents CRANMER, the Archbishop of Canterbury, from entering the meeting to which he has been summoned. This is plainly an insult to a person of his rank, as King HENRY VIII realises angrily when he is informed of it by Doctor BUTTS. The incident demonstrates the enmity of Bishop GARDINER and the councillors towards Cranmer, whose support by the king is the theme of 5.1–2.

Kemble (1), Charles (1775–1854) British actor and producer, brother of J. P. KEMBLE (3) and Sarah SIDDONS, and father of Fanny KEMBLE (2). As an actor, Charles Kemble was best known as a player of secondary parts—such as MALCOLM, MACDUFF, MERCUTIO, and LAERTES—opposite his brother, though he was also acclaimed as BENEDICK and ORLANDO. He succeeded his brother as manager of the Covent Garden Theatre, where he presented Shakespeare's works in productions that aimed at historical accuracy in sets and costumes. Beginning with the *King John* staged by him and J. R. PLANCHÉ in 1823, his ideas influenced Shakespearean productions for the rest of the 19th century. Kemble was an unsuccessful manager and was only saved from bankruptcy by the success of his daughter, Fanny.

Kemble (2), Fanny (1809–1893) British actress, daughter of Charles KEMBLE (1). Fanny Kemble's stunning performances as JULIET (1) saved her father's Covent Garden Theatre from bankruptcy in 1829, and she went on to triumphs as BEATRICE and PORTIA (1). Unlike the other members of the family, she was not committed to a theatrical career, and she retired in 1834, when she married a Philadelphian. After her divorce in 1845, she returned to Britain and in the 1850s and 1860s toured both there and in America with a highly popular series of readings from Shakespeare. She finally retired in 1868 and settled in London.

Kemble (3), John Philip (1757–1823) British actor and producer, brother of Charles and Stephen KEM-

BLE (1, 4) and Sarah SIDDONS. J. P. Kemble played most of Shakespeare's protagonists, often opposite his sister, and was especially acclaimed for his portrayals of HAMLET, CORIOLANUS, and HENRY V. He initially established himself as Hamlet in 1783 at the Drury Lane Theatre in London, which he managed from 1788 until 1802. After that he ran the Covent Garden Theatre, finally retiring in 1817. As a producer, he continued the trend towards more realistic costumes and sets, which was begun by David GARRICK and eventually resulted in the elaborately 'historical' productions of Charles Kemble, Charles KEAN (1), and Henry IRVING. A stately and dignified actor, Kemble dominated the English stage until the rise of his only great rival, Edmund KEAN (2). The son of an actor and actress, Kemble was a child performer before training for the priesthood. He abandoned his studies and returned to the theatre in 1776, though the experience is thought to have influenced his deliberate and ascetic acting style.

Kemble (4), Stephen (1758–1822) Nineteenth-century actor, brother of Charles and John Philip KEMBLE (1, 3) and Sarah SIDDONS. A child actor like his siblings, Stephen became a chemist before returning to the stage in his late twenties. Being very heavy, he often played FALSTAFF. His girth and the fact that he was quite overshadowed by John Philip led to the contemporary witticism that they were 'the big Kemble and the great Kemble'.

Kempe (Kemp), William (d. c. 1608) English actor, a member of the CHAMBERLAIN'S MEN and one of the 26 men listed in the FIRST FOLIO as the 'Principall Actors' in Shakespeare's plays. Kempe's name appears in early texts of *Romeo and Juliet* (stage direction at 4.5.99) and *Much Ado About Nothing* (speech headings in 4.2), proving that he was the original portrayer of PETER (2) and DOGBERRY. As a CLOWN (1), he is also believed to have originated such other Shakespearean comic parts as BOTTOM, COSTARD, LAUNCE, LAUNCELOT, and possibly FALSTAFF, before leaving the company in 1599, when he was replaced by Robert ARMIN.

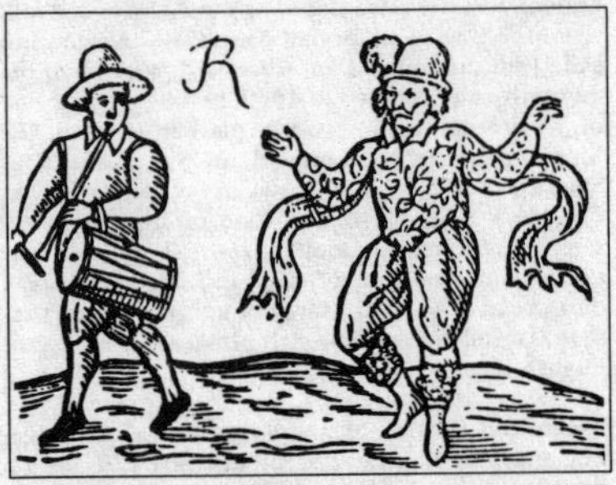

Will Kempe created many of the great Shakespearian comic roles. He also was famous, as shown in this contemporary illustration, for his stunt of dancing a morris along the road from London to Norwich—a distance of almost 100 miles. (Courtesy of Bodleian Library, Oxford)

Based on the differences in such comic parts written before and after 1599, it is clear that Shakespeare wrote the earlier ones with Kempe in mind. From analysis of these characters, combined with other surviving references to Kempe, we know something of his style. He was a big man who specialised in plebeian clowns who spoke in earthy language, with seemingly ingenuous spontaneity, often addressing the audience in frank asides. Kempe's characters have a tendency to confuse and mispronounce their words, and contemporary references to his dancing and his ability to 'make a scurvy face' suggest a physical brand of humour. He was especially famous for an extraordinary publicity stunt, as it would now be called, of 1600, when he performed a morris dance along the road from LONDON to Norwich—a distance of almost 100 miles, which he covered in nine days. He then wrote a book about it, *Kemps nine daies wonder* (1600).

Kempe is first known as the jester, or FOOL (1), to the Earl of LEICESTER, with whom he travelled to the war in the Netherlands in 1585–1586. He may even have been a member of LEICESTER'S MEN at this time. During the summer of 1586 he performed with an English company in DENMARK. He was a member of STRANGE'S MEN by 1593, when he was already a noted comedian, hailed by Thomas NASHE as the successor to Richard TARLTON, another famous Elizabethan comic. Kempe is presumed to have been an original member of the Chamberlain's Men in 1594, for he was a principal partner in it the next year. In 1599 he was one of the original partners in the GLOBE THEATRE, but for reasons unknown, he left the troupe in the same year and sold his share in the theatre to Shakespeare, John HEMINGES, Augustine PHILLIPS, and Thomas POPE (2). He toured in Germany and Italy, before returning to England in 1601. He may have rejoined the Chamberlain's Men briefly, but by 1602 he was with WORCESTER'S MEN. Nothing is known of his life after 1603; he was mentioned as dead in 1608.

Kenilworth Castle in WARWICKSHIRE, a location in *2 Henry VI* and the scene of an extraordinarily lavish entertainment held for Queen ELIZABETH (1) in 1575, when Shakespeare, who lived nearby, was 11 years old. It is thought that he was probably among the

multitudes of commoners from the neighbourhood who were permitted to gather and view parts of the spectacle. This fabulous occasion, which lasted for three weeks, featured many MASQUES and other theatrical entertainments. Contemporary accounts of these have survived, and it is often supposed that one of them may have provided the germ of a passage in *A Midsummer Night's Dream* (2.1.148–154). In 4.9 of *2 Henry VI* King HENRY VI and Queen MARGARET (1) retreat to Kenilworth, in the remote countryside, as CADE's rebellion sweeps London.

Kent (1) County in south-easternmost England, the setting of a number of scenes in *2 Henry VI.* The play reflects the position of the Duke of SUFFOLK (3) as the most powerful aristocrat in Kent. Historically, although Shakespeare does not point out the connection, Suffolk's death on a beach in Kent in 4.1 was a trigger for the rebellion led by Jack CADE, depicted in the following scenes, for Suffolk was a grasping and extortionate landlord and his power was a source of popular discontent. In the play, Cade retreats to Kent when his uprising fails, to be killed by Alexander IDEN in 4.10.

Cade's rebellion was a typically Kentish phenomenon, one of several major revolts to arise in the county between the 14th and 16th centuries. Kent, located on the coast at England's nearest point to FRANCE (1), had since prehistory been a relatively prosperous and cosmopolitan region by virtue of its trade with the Continent. In the late Middle Ages it was thus a centre of political and social discontent, as the growing merchant class combined with artisans and rising small landholders to protest against the inequities and restrictions of feudalism.

Two settings in *1 Henry IV,* ROCHESTER and GAD'S HILL, are also located in Kent.

Kent (2), Earl of Character in *King Lear,* nobleman faithful to King LEAR. Kent attempts to dissuade the king from his catastrophic decision to banish CORDELIA when she honestly admits that her love will go to her husband as well as her father, but Lear banishes him as well for interfering. Kent then disguises himself and attempts to assist Lear when he is rejected by his other daughters, REGAN and GONERIL. He succeeds in keeping Lear safe from possible murder, and he reunites the king and Cordelia at DOVER. His conflict with Goneril's steward OSWALD stresses an important value in the play, the association of virtue with gentlemanly behaviour. Kent's steadfast honesty and loyalty is contrasted with the courtier's self-serving ambition. However, when Cordelia's invasion fails and she and Lear are captured by EDMUND, Kent is helpless. As he witnesses Lear's death at the play's close, he exclaims, 'Break, heart; I prithee, break!' (5.3.311). Whether he refers to his own heart or Lear's, this forsaken cry is emblematic of the sorrowful view of humanity's plight that is an important theme of the play. Yet Kent's final declaration of his own imminent death, 'I have a journey, sir, shortly to go; / My master calls me, I must not say no' (5.3.320–321) also contributes to the play's sense of the nobility of human suffering.

Kent corresponds to a character named Perillus in Shakespeare's chief source for *Lear,* the play KING LEIR (c. 1588). Some scholars think Shakespeare may have played Perillus for the CHAMBERLAIN'S MEN in the 1590s, for a number of passages in the older play are especially closely echoed in *Lear* when Kent is onstage.

Kesselstadt Death Mask Death mask formerly thought to be Shakespeare's. Discovered in 1847 at the estate sale of a Count Kesselstadt, this death mask—a cast made of the face of a dead person—was once widely believed to be Shakespeare's, chiefly because it is inscribed 'WS/1616'. However, it does not resemble either of the most authoritative portraits (see DROESHOUT; JANSSEN [2]), and the date is almost certainly false for no other non-royal death masks are known from that period. Scholars are therefore in agreement that the Kesselstadt death mask is a forgery, but it provides a good demonstration of the appeal of dramatic Shakespeareana.

Killigrew, Thomas (1612–1683) English playwright and theatrical producer. Killigrew, along with William DAVENANT, dominated the London theatre world in the 1660s. Killigrew wrote several moderately successful tragicomedies (see TRAGICOMEDY) before the London theatres were closed by the Puritans in 1642, when the Civil Wars began. A royalist, he went into exile with the future King Charles II, and when the monarchy was restored in 1660, he was granted one of the two licences to produce plays in London. His King's Company was granted the rights to 20 of Shakespeare's plays, but he staged only four of them: *The Merry Wives of Windsor* (one of the first plays staged after the restoration), *1 Henry IV* (at least four times), *Julius Caesar,* and *Othello.* In Killigrew's *Othello,* on December 8, 1660, Margaret HUGHES played DESDEMONA and became the first woman to act on an English stage.

Kimbolton Castle Manor house near Cambridge, England, a setting for a scene in *Henry VIII.* In 4.2 HENRY VIII's divorced and deposed queen, KATHERINE of Aragon, lives in exile at Kimbolton, accompanied by only a few attendants. When she sees a vision of herself receiving garlands from spiritlike creatures, she knows she is near death.

Kimbolton was one of several residences where the historical Katherine lived out her exile. At the time it was a fortified manor built over an ancient castle. Today, a grand neo-classical country house of the early 18th-century overlays the older establishment and is open to the public as a museum.

King (1), Alonso of Naples Character in *The Tempest.* See ALONSO.

King (2) Antiochus of Syria Character in *Pericles.* See ANTIOCHUS.

King (3) Charles VI of France Character in *Henry V.* See FRENCH KING.

King (4) Charles VII of France Character in *1 Henry VI.* See CHARLES VII.

King (5) Claudius of Denmark Character in *Hamlet,* murderer and royal successor of HAMLET's father and husband of his victim's widow, QUEEN (9) Gertrude, Hamlet's mother. The central issue of the play is the conflict between Hamlet's desire for vengeance against the King—to which he has been sworn by his father's GHOST (3)—and his recognition that revenge would involve him in evil himself.

The King's crime, by his own confession, 'is rank, it smells to heaven; It hath the primal eldest curse upon't' (3.3.36–37)—that is, he has followed Cain, the first criminal, in murdering his brother. Cain is referred to several times in the play—e.g., in 1.2.105 and 5.1.76—reminding us of the King's heinous offence.

Hamlet repeatedly compares his father and King Claudius. Although he is surprised when the Ghost tells him of the murder, he is not surprised, a few lines later, to learn the killer's identity, for his 'prophetic soul' (1.5.41) has already apprehended his uncle's character. Earlier, in his first soliloquy, he despises the King as an inferior successor to his father, 'so excellent a king, that was to this / [as] Hyperion [is] to a satyr' (1.2.139–140). He elaborates on this comparison when he upbraids his mother in 3.4.

In 1.1 an ideal of kingship is established in recollections of the heroic achievements of Hamlet's father and in the sense of dread occasioned by his death; the implicit contrast with Claudius persists throughout the play, as we become aware that the King's crime is the source of the evil that permeates the play's world, the 'something . . . rotten in the state of Denmark' (1.4.90). In a telling detail, the King is closely associated with excessive drinking, presented as a characteristically Danish failing. He often proposes toasts, the rowdy behaviour of his court is noted, and Hamlet finds it likely that he would be 'distempered . . . With drink' (3.2.293–294) or 'drunk asleep' (3.3.89). Appropriately, Claudius finally falls victim to his own poisoned wine.

Despite the King's distinctly evil nature, he does have some redeeming features. In fact, some commentators believe that the playwright intended King Claudius as an admirable ruler and man and that Hamlet's contrary opinion is a result of his tragic insanity. Most critics, however, find the King's wicked nature abundantly evident; his good features exemplify Shakespeare's genius for providing fully human portraits. The King is clearly intelligent and quick-witted, particularly in 4.5.112–152, where he defuses the coup by LAERTES with smooth talk and converts the rebel into an accomplice. In 1.2, as he disposes of court business, we see that he is a reasonable man, a competent diplomat, and a generally able monarch. The King even reveals, however fleetingly, his bad conscience about his crimes when he compares his 'deed to [his] painted word' (3.1.49–54) and when he tries to pray in 3.3. However, as he recognises, 'Words without thoughts never to heaven go' (3.3.98), and, unable to repent sincerely, he continues in his evil ways.

Beginning with his recruitment of ROSENCRANTZ AND GUILDENSTERN to spy on Hamlet, the King schemes cruelly against the prince. His two death plots—to have him executed in England and to arrange a rigged fencing match—are particularly vile. The King recruits Laertes after Hamlet escapes from England, but when, at the climax, his follower repents and seeks the prince's forgiveness, the King is left as the sole focus of our sense of evil in the play. When Hamlet kills him, he cries, 'Here, thou incestuous, murd'rous, damned Dane' (5.2.330); his villainy is emphatically described and condemned. HORATIO leaves us with a final summary of the King's role when he refers to his 'carnal, bloody, and unnatural acts' (5.2.386).

Shakespeare may have named Claudius, or the name may have come from his source, the UR-HAMLET, but in either case the King was named for a Roman emperor, Claudius I (10 B.C.–54 A.D.), who was regarded in Shakespeare's day as a prime example of an evil ruler. (His modern reputation is considerably better, in part because of Robert Graves' novel *I, Claudius* [1934].) Upon his accession to the throne in 41 A.D., Claudius married his niece Agrippina, an incestuous relationship that may have influenced the choice of names. Agrippina later poisoned Claudius and was herself murdered by her son, Nero, as Hamlet recollects in 3.2.384–385.

King (6) Cymbeline of Britain Character in *Cymbeline.* See CYMBELINE.

King (7) Duncan of Scotland Character in *Macbeth*. See DUNCAN.

King (8) Edward IV of England Character in *3 Henry VI* and *Richard III*. See EDWARD IV.

King (9) Henry IV of England Title character of *1* and *2 Henry IV*. See HENRY IV.

King (10) Henry V of England Title character of *Henry V*. See HENRY V.

King (11) Henry VI of England Title character of *1, 2,* and *3 Henry VI*. See HENRY VI.

King (12) Henry VIII of England Title character of *Henry VIII*. See HENRY VIII.

King (13) John of England Title character of *King John*. See JOHN (3).

King (14) Lear of Britain Title character of *King Lear*. See LEAR.

King (15) Leontes of Sicilia Character in *The Winter's Tale*. See LEONTES.

King (16) Lewis (Louis XI) of France Character in *3 Henry VI*. See LEWIS (3).

King (17) of France Character in *All's Well That Ends Well*, the ruler of FRANCE (1). The dying King recovers his health through the ministrations of HELENA (2). He rewards her with marriage to the unwilling BERTRAM. Bertram's disdain for a commoner sparks the King's most important speech, a lecture on the value of individual virtues over social rank (2.3.117–141), a trenchant summary of one of the play's important themes. In 5.3 he forgives Bertram's flight from Helena, but he then presides over the exposure of the young man's perfidy towards DIANA (1) and his justice is as stern as his forgiveness had been yielding. When Helena finally unravels the plot and the final reconciliation takes place, the King behaves with great magnanimity, granting a dowry to Diana and offering a final statement that, although qualified, insists on the traditional happy ending of COMEDY: 'All yet seems well, and if it end so meet, / The bitter past, more welcome is the sweet' (5.3.327–328).

With the COUNTESS (2) and Lord LAFEW, the King helps provide an atmosphere of generosity and wisdom that offsets the play's unpleasant aspects. His gracious welcome of Bertram in 1.2 stimulates in the audience a sense that the young man, despite his faults, is basically worthy. Similarly, his immediate appreciation of Helena in 2.1 helps to establish her virtue. The King is himself a wholly sympathetic figure, a stereotypically 'good' ruler: wise and moderate in deciding not to go to war while still permitting his young noblemen to distinguish themselves on campaign in Italy; touching in his nostalgic remembrance of Bertram's father; and generous in friendship and forgiveness to the young people.

King (18) of France Character in *King Lear*. See FRANCE (2).

King (19) Ferdinand of Navarre Character in *Love's Labour's Lost*, the ruler whose decision to make 'a little academe' (1.1.13) of his court leads to the action of the play. Although opposed by the sardonic humour of BEROWNE, the King bans all mirth, banqueting, and even the company of women in order to promote disinterested study. The King's humourless desire to make of his courtiers 'brave conquerors . . . / That war against your own affections / And the huge army of the world's desires' (1.1.8–10) is focussed on an abstract idea, not a love of scholarship, and is therefore vain. This self-centred seriousness is overcome by love as the play develops. The King himself succumbs to the charms of the PRINCESS (1) of France, and when, at the close of the play, she requires that he prove his love with a year of monastic life, he willingly assumes the task, asserting, 'My heart is in thy breast' (5.2.808).

King (20) Philip Augustus of France Character in *King John*. See PHILIP (2).

King (21) Polixenes of Bohemia Character in *The Winter's Tale*. See POLIXENES.

King (22) Priam of Troy Character in *Troilus and Cressida*. See PRIAM.

King (23) Richard II of England Title character of *Richard II*. See RICHARD II.

King (24) Richard III of England Title character in *Richard III*. See RICHARD III.

King (25) Simonides of Pentapolis Character in *Pericles*. See SIMONIDES.

King (26), Tom (1730–1804) English actor, famous as TOUCHSTONE and MALVOLIO. King, one of the most popular members of the acting company run by David GARRICK, played comic roles exclusively, both in Shakespeare and 18th-century works. In the 1770s he managed the SADLER'S WELLS THEATRE. King was very

successful and made a great deal of money in the theatre, but he was addicted to gambling and died in poverty.

King John

SYNOPSIS

Note: Act and scene numbers in *King John* vary significantly from edition to edition. Traditionally editions since THEOBALD's (1726) have altered the FOLIO's scene divisions in Acts 2 and 3; some modern editions revert to the Folio's arrangement, while others do not. In this volume citations to *King John* follow the New Arden edition, which uses the Folio designations. Where there is a difference from the traditional citation, the latter is given in parentheses.

Act 1, Scene 1
King JOHN (3) and his mother, Queen ELEANOR, receive a French ambassador, CHATILLON, who delivers a demand from King PHILIP (2) of FRANCE (1): John must relinquish the crown of England to his young nephew ARTHUR. John replies defiantly that he will invade France, and Chatillon departs. Eleanor supports John's decision, implying that, since his rule is illegal, it must be maintained through force. ROBERT Faulconbridge and his older brother, the BASTARD (1), enter and ask the king to judge a dispute: Robert claims their father's estate, asserting that his brother is illegitimate, having been sired by the late King Richard I. Eleanor and John recognise the strong resemblance of the Bastard to the late king, and they like his bold and saucy manner. They offer him a knighthood if he will leave the Faulconbridge estate to his brother and go to war in France with them. He accepts, and, after the others have left to prepare for the campaign, he soliloquises humorously on the manners of the courtly world he is about to enter. His mother, LADY (5) Faulconbridge, arrives, having followed her sons to court to defend her honour. However, when the Bastard tells her he has renounced his inheritance in favour of greater glories, she admits that King Richard was indeed his father. He revels in his newly discovered patrimony.

Act 2, Scene 1
Outside ANGIERS, an English-occupied city in France, King Philip, his son LEWIS (1), and Arthur greet the Archduke of AUSTRIA, who has agreed to fight in support of Arthur's claim to the English crown. Austria is thanked effusively by Arthur and his mother, CONSTANCE. Chatillon appears with news that an English army, led by John, is approaching. John and his entourage enter, and Philip questions John's legitimacy, noting that Arthur is the son of John's older brother and thus the proper heir. John simply denies Philip's right to judge the matter, and the two parties trade insults. A CITIZEN (4) of Angiers appears on the city walls and states that the city will admit neither ruler until it can be ascertained which one represents the true King of England. The two armies skirmish, but HUBERT, speaking for Angiers, reiterates the city's refusal to open its gates. The Bastard suggests that the two parties ally temporarily and conquer the recalcitrant town. As they prepare to do so, Hubert proposes a peaceful settlement: Lewis can marry John's niece BLANCHE of Spain, uniting the two parties. Lewis and Blanche are agreeable, and a treaty is concluded. John grants many of the English territories in France to Philip, and Philip implicitly recognises John's legitimacy in return. Arthur is to be given high rank and the rule of Angiers. Everyone enters the town to prepare for the wedding except the Bastard, who muses in a soliloquy on the dishonour that the kings have incurred, John for giving away much of his kingdom to secure the rest, Philip for having abandoned an allegedly sacred cause. He rails against 'commodity', or self-interest, but then confesses that he does so only because he has not yet had the opportunity to pursue it himself.

Act 2, Scene 2 (Act 3, Scene 1)
The Earl of SALISBURY (4) brings word to Constance and Arthur of the settlement between France and England. Constance rants wildly against Salisbury for bringing the news, against Philip for abandoning Arthur's cause, and against fortune for favouring King John.

Act 3, Scene 1 (Act 3, Scene 1 continued)
The wedding party appears, and Constance resumes her cursing. A papal legate, Cardinal PANDULPH, arrives with a demand from Rome that King John surrender to the pope's authority in a dispute over the archbishopric of Canterbury. John flatly refuses. Pandulph excommunicates him and insists that Philip abandon his new alliance with England and make war on John—or face excommunication himself. When Philip hesitates, Pandulph delivers an equivocal argument justifying the breaking of an oath. Philip rejects the alliance with John, and the two parties prepare for war.

Act 3, Scene 2
The armies skirmish. Resting from the battle, the Bastard displays the severed head of Austria. John arrives with the captive Arthur, whom the king turns over to Hubert, now allied with the English.

Act 3, Scene 2 continued (Act 3, Scene 3)
After further skirmishing, John and the Bastard enter, accompanied by Arthur, Hubert, and Eleanor. John sends the Bastard back to England with orders to loot the monasteries there. Eleanor takes Arthur aside to comfort him, while John speaks with Hubert. After flattering him and speaking of future rewards, the king

hints that he has a secret desire. Hubert offers to fulfil it, whatever it may be. John observes that Arthur is a potential problem to him, and he speaks the single word 'death'. Hubert responds that Arthur shall die, and John expresses his satisfaction.

Act 3, Scene 3 (Act 3, Scene 4)
Philip and Lewis discuss the English victory with Pandulph. Constance appears, mad with grief at her son's capture. When she leaves, Philip follows her, fearing that she may harm herself. Pandulph tells Lewis not to lose heart and suggests a plan: John will surely kill Arthur and thus alienate his own followers, and Lewis, as Blanche's husband—she being Arthur's cousin—may claim the throne. Moreover, Pandulph urges, the Bastard's ransacking of the monasteries will also antagonise the English so that a French invasion will be welcomed by rebels in England. Pandulph and Lewis go to present this plan to King Philip.

Act 4, Scene 1
Hubert prepares hot irons to put out Arthur's eyes. Hubert summons Arthur, who says that the only comfort he has had in his imprisonment has been the affection of Hubert. The older man, in asides, reveals his torment, but he nevertheless tells Arthur that he must put out his eyes. Arthur pleads for mercy. Hubert relents, but he insists that Arthur's death must be feigned to protect himself, Hubert, from the king's anger.

Act 4, Scene 2
PEMBROKE (5) and Salisbury tell John that many nobles are dismayed that Arthur is kept imprisoned, and they urge him to free his nephew. He agrees, as Hubert arrives to confer with the king. The two noblemen remark that they know Hubert was assigned to kill Arthur. When John announces that Hubert has brought word of Arthur's death, they are not surprised, and they leave angrily. News arrives that the French have invaded and that Queen Eleanor has died. The Bastard appears and reports that the country is inflamed over Arthur's reported murder. John sends him to summon the disaffected nobles; in view of the invasion, he must attempt to win back their allegiance. Hubert returns and tells of superstitious fears among the populace. John blames Hubert for killing Arthur, claiming that he had not ordered him to do so. Hubert confesses that Arthur is not in fact dead, and John, relieved, tells him to carry this news to the rebellious lords.

Act 4, Scene 3
Arthur attempts to escape by leaping off the castle wall, but he dies from the fall. Pembroke, Salisbury, and Lord BIGOT pass by, discussing their plan to join the French invaders, who have offered them an alliance. The Bastard accosts the noblemen with the king's request that they join him. They refuse. Discovering Arthur's body, they rage with increased venom, vowing revenge on John. Hubert enters, claiming that Arthur lives; when shown the body, he is shocked, but the lords do not believe him. They depart, intent on joining Lewis' army.

Act 5, Scene 1
King John yields his crown to Pandulph and receives it back again, thus acknowledgeing the pope as the source of his authority. In return, Pandulph promises to persuade the French to leave England. The Bastard arrives with news of French successes and of Arthur's death. He rebukes the king for inaction. John explains that he has Pandulph's promise to rely on, and the Bastard is mortified, first that a papal alliance has been formed and second that no military response to France has been prepared. John tells him to make such arrangements himself.

Act 5, Scene 2
In the French camp, the dissident nobles seal their alliance with Lewis. Salisbury weeps, lamenting the necessity to fight against his own countrymen. Pandulph appears and reports John's reconciliation with the pope, but Lewis refuses to halt his onslaught. The Bastard arrives under a flag of truce and is informed of Lewis' intransigence; he responds with a challenge to continued war. The two sides prepare for battle.

Act 5, Scene 3
During the battle Hubert reports to King John that his armies are losing. John admits that he is sick, with fever and at heart. A message from the Bastard requests that the king leave the battlefield. John replies that he shall go to SWINSTEAD ABBEY. The MESSENGER (8) adds that French reinforcements have been lost at sea and that their army has retired to defensive positions. John is too ill to respond to this good news, and he departs for Swinstead.

Act 5, Scene 4
A French nobleman, Lord MELUN, mortally wounded and conscience-stricken, tells the rebellious English lords of Lewis' plan to have them executed once John is defeated. Salisbury replies for the group that they will rejoin King John.

Act 5, Scene 5
Lewis receives news of Melun's death, the disaffection of the English lords, and the wreck of his supply ships. He prepares for hard fighting the next day.

Act 5, Scene 6
In the middle of the night Hubert encounters the Bastard and informs him that King John has been poisoned and is dying. The Bastard, whose own forces

have been badly damaged by the storm, hastens to rejoin the king.

Act 5, Scene 7
John, burning with fever and aware that he is near death, is brought to his son Prince HENRY (1). The Bastard arrives with news of the war, but the king dies as he speaks. Salisbury tells the Bastard that Lewis has made offers of peace and has already begun to return his forces to France. The nobles acknowledge Henry as the new king, and the Bastard delivers a patriotic speech, observing that, now that its internal disputes are over, England will once again be invulnerable to invasion.

COMMENTARY

Aside from the very late and uncharacteristic play *Henry VIII*, *King John* is the only one of Shakespeare's HISTORY PLAYS that is not part of a TETRALOGY. Further, its narrative is not linked to the others, which together cover an unbroken 87-year period in English history, but rather deals with a much earlier and more obscure era. Thus *King John* has been somewhat neglected, being viewed as a minor and transitional work between the two tetralogies. However, its subject matter is basically the same—the disruption of English public life by dynastic disputes—and its moral weight is as great as that of most of the other histories. Moreover, it is especially closely linked to the contemporary concerns of the playwright's own time.

One of the issues that Shakespeare's history plays most persistently raised is the nature of good government. In *King John* the playwright impresses us with the need for a sound political ethic by presenting a near-catastrophe that stems from ethical weakness. In *Richard III* a melodramatic villain had generated the problem, and his supernaturally aided defeat at BOSWORTH FIELD had solved it. In this more intellectual work Shakespeare examines political realities and problems that require compromises, not heaven-sent intervention.

The chief political concern in the frequently disrupted monarchy of medieval and early modern England was that of the legitimacy of the ruler, and this is the play's primary focus. Shakespeare felt no compunctions about taking liberties with historical reality, and *King John* is one of his least accurate history plays. Besides using such minor anachronisms as John's threat to use cannon in 1.1.26 (gunpowder did not come into use in Europe until the HUNDRED YEARS WAR, about 150 years later), he simply rewrote the main lines of John's reign. Compressing the events of 17 years into a single brief sequence, the playwright juxtaposes conflicts that were in fact widely separated in time. John's defence of his right to rule against the partisans of Arthur occupied the first few years of his reign and was completed by 1203, when Arthur was killed. Arthur's death is the central event of the play, but it simply closed the earliest epoch of John's actual reign. In the play the death stimulates the rebellious barons to oppose John and join the invading French. But historically the barons' revolt occurred 10 years after Arthur's death and had nothing to do with it; murder was, after all, an ordinary political event in medieval times. Further, the French invasion came only after the barons' revolt had been settled by the signing of the Magna Charta in 1215 and then resumed in the following year.

The most important issue of John's reign, at the time and to Shakespeare's contemporaries, was John's dispute with Pope Innocent III. However, the playwright lessened its importance and interwove it with the other two conflicts, Arthur's claim and the barons' revolt. In fact, John's dispute with Innocent III began several years after Arthur's death, and it ended before the barons rebelled. The king surrendered to the pope—permitting Pandulph to recrown him, as in the play—precisely because he was concerned about the barons, and Pandulph was in fact John's ally against them. As depicted by Shakespeare, Pandulph's opposition to John revives Arthur's claims, which had been rejected by the marriage treaty of 2.1; the papal legate then stirs up a French invasion in anticipation of Arthur's death; and he finally proves incapable of ending the war in return for John's surrender to papal authority. All of this is flagrantly unhistorical; as always, Shakespeare was less concerned with history than with dramatic effect, and he made John's usurpation of the crown from Arthur the dominant issue in the play in support of his all-important theme, political legitimacy.

Shakespeare's John, then, is an illegitimate ruler, and illegitimacy is a recurring motif in the play. Most prominently, the Bastard raises the issue of illegitimate birth, in speech and in person; significantly, he proves nobler in his steadfast loyalty than all of the other characters, whose treachery and dishonour exemplify illegitimacy in a broader sense: illegitimate actions in terms of the courtly code that all of the aristocrats profess. The Bastard is seen as England's saving grace: he maintains the English resistance, and English honour, when John has succumbed to his moral crisis. Most important, the Bastard gives expression to the value of legitimate succession when he leads the nobles in patriotic support of Henry III in 5.7. It is clear that positive results have come from loyalty to John—that is, that this usurper has his own legitimacy.

The issue of legitimacy was not only an historical one: Queen ELIZABETH (1) faced similar political problems to a lesser degree. She was conceived outside marriage, as was well known, and Rome did not recog-

nise her legitimacy, either in birth or as a ruler. Similarly, Innocent III had declared John an illegitimate King against whom revolt was lawful, as Pandulph affirms in 3.1.100–101 (3.1.174–175). Further, on several occasions conspiracies against Elizabeth's life were discovered, and the Earl of ESSEX (2) actually attempted rebellion towards the end of her reign. Advocates of Mary, Queen of Scots, compared her claim against Elizabeth with Arthur's claim against John; their voices were not silenced until Mary was executed. TUDOR monarchs were aware of their own dynastic roots in rebellion (as is enacted in *Richard III*), and they incorporated a new doctrine in their laws, declaring that the holder of the crown is not only in fact the wielder of power, he or she is also the proper ruler in law, despite the legitimacy of any other claim. This is the implicit principle on which the Bastard bases his loyalty to John. John makes the same claim for himself—'Doth not the crown of England prove the king?' (2.1.273)—and the play reinforces it through remarks such as Eleanor's acknowledgement that 'strong possession much more than . . . right' (1.1.40) must secure his throne, and through the analogy that the Bastard's possession of the Faulconbridge estates is sufficient evidence of right, even in the face of a legal bequest (1.1.126–133). Further, Arthur is presented as not only a tool of France, but—inaccurately—as a mere child, clearly unsuited to be king. John's legitimacy, like Elizabeth's, must be continuously reaffirmed.

Parallels between John and Elizabeth abound in the play, and Shakespeare's original audience will have recognised them immediately. Pandulph's excommunication of John (3.1.99) [3.1.173] is plainly a reference to the excommunication of Elizabeth in 1570. His promise, four lines later, of canonisation to an assassin of John was an inflammatory glance at fairly current events: in 1589 Henri III of France had been murdered by a monk who contended that the King was soft on Protestantism; the assassin's canonisation was publicly sought by Catholic groups in France, to the shock and revulsion of Protestants (and some Catholics) throughout Europe. It was widely believed in England that a similar bounty was offered in the case of Elizabeth, and Pandulph's words must have evoked patriotic horror. The conflict between Reformation and Counter-Reformation in the 16th century inspired Protestants to think of John as a predecessor who attempted to rebel against the power of Rome, and they made much of his notorious—but fictitious—poisoning at the hands of a monk. Shakespeare's Pandulph is a stereotype of the malevolent Catholic of fearful Protestant imaginations; John's insulting address to him (3.1.73–86) [3.1.147–160] is an example of 16th-century rhetoric, reflecting the attitudes of Shakespeare's England, not of John's.

Shakespeare is often regarded as sympathetic to Catholicism, and although *King John* would seem to douse that speculation thoroughly at first glance, the religious issue is nevertheless far less prominent in the play than it was in the actual historical period or in the playwright's sources. Although strong public interest would certainly have justified a strong presentation of the struggle between Rome and England, Shakespeare refrained. *King John* is primarily a play about a usurpation that did not in fact occur, rather than about the religious conflict that did. To Shakespeare, the religious question is less important than the issue of political legitimacy.

Readers today are often puzzled to find that *King John* makes no mention of what today seems the most salient feature of John's reign, the signing of the Magna Charta in 1215. However, in Shakespeare's day, when the aristocracy was definitely subordinate to the crown, John's concessions to his fractious noblemen seemed unimportant. Our own conception of the Magna Charta as the wellspring of democratic freedom from royal control was not formulated until shortly after Shakespeare's death. Opponents of King Charles I, seeking legal precedents to cite in their struggle, discovered that King John had made concessions, 400 years earlier, that could be said to establish the principle that a ruler was obliged to consult his subjects. This interpretation helped fuel a dispute that led to civil war in 1642. However, the charter signed by John was rather reactionary, restoring to the barons certain feudal rights that the central government was absorbing and would absorb again, especially under the Tudors. The political establishment of Shakespeare's day, intent on preserving its own relatively unrestricted power, certainly had no use for the Magna Charta, and Shakespeare, a supporter of a strong central government, shared this attitude.

King John is sometimes thought of as a failure, with an episodic, undirected plot and confused characterizations, but these seeming defects are actually purposeful techniques. The play's ambiguities and contradictions illustrate the dangers of an unreliable political world, and this is the principal point of the play. The course of the action continually varies, with the vagaries of fortune constantly before us. The characters change their natures repeatedly: John is variously a patriotic hero, resisting France and Rome; a villain, murdering Arthur; a traitor, surrendering his authority to the pope; and a simple failure, collapsing into pathetic uselessness in the face of a crisis. The Bastard first appears as a satirical baiter of aristocratic society, but he becomes the noblest of the Englishmen at the end. Hubert is first a cagey Angevin diplomat caught between big powers, then a sycophantic courtier prepared to murder a child to gain favour with the king, and finally a sorrowing penitent. Our point of

view changes repeatedly, our sympathies are continually shifting, and we are drawn into the play as if into an intrigue. Such ambiguity is appropriate for a study of political confusion and uncertainty.

SOURCES OF THE PLAY

It has traditionally been assumed that Shakespeare adapted another play, THE TROUBLESOME RAIGNE OF KING JOHN, in writing *King John,* but the proposition that the former play was derived from Shakespeare's work has gained ground in recent years. In any case, the principal source for whichever play came first was Raphael HOLINSHED's *Chronicles of England, Scotland, and Ireland* (2nd ed., 1587). Shakespeare also referred to John FOXE's *Book of Martyrs* (probably in the 4th ed., 1583), and he took various details from other sources as well. For instance, from the *Chronica Majora,* a Latin history by Matthew Paris (d. 1259), Shakespeare reworked the Bastard's account of his losses in a storm (5.6.39–42, 5.7.61–64) and elements of Salisbury's lament in 5.2. Also, Shakespeare probably knew the popular romances concerning Richard Coeur-de-Lion, from which he may have taken the erroneous identification of Austria with Limoges. His attitudes towards John and his reign may have been influenced by further reading, perhaps including the *Annals* of John STOW, in which John is taken to task as a usurper.

TEXT OF THE PLAY

The date of *King John*'s composition is difficult to determine, if *The Troublesome Raigne of King John* was Shakespeare's source for the play. *The Troublesome Raigne* was published in 1591, and *King John* had been performed by 1598, for it appears in the list of Shakespeare's works that Francis MERES compiled then. Every year between those dates has been proposed for the writing of the play. Stylistically, it is generally thought to fall between the two major tetralogies—that is, in the first half of the 1590s.

If *The Troublesome Raigne* was derived from Shakespeare's play, however, then the date of *King John* must be 1590 or 1591: *King John* contains a reference (1.1.244) to a character in a popular play of 1590, *Soliman and Perseda* (probably by Thomas KYD). A dating of 1590 for *King John* is also supported by the play's frequent allusions to the Spanish Armada (1588)—more than in any other work by Shakespeare—suggesting that it was written soon after the attempted invasion.

King John was first published in the FIRST FOLIO edition of the plays (1623), and that text has been the basis of all subsequent editions. It is thought that the Folio was printed either from Shakespeare's FOUL PAPERS, probably slightly emended by the Folio editors, or from a PROMPT-BOOK, perhaps one that Shakespeare himself had revised.

THEATRICAL HISTORY OF THE PLAY

Numerous early 17th-century references to *King John* testify to the play's popularity at that time, but no production of it is known before a revival in 1737. In 1745 Colley CIBBER (1) staged an adaptation emphasising the French invasion, attempting to capitalise on the patriotism stimulated by the defeat of the Jacobite Rebellion in that year. However, Shakespeare's play, starring David GARRICK as John, was produced at the same time, and the Cibber play folded immediately. *King John* was staged several times in colonial America, beginning with a Philadelphia production in 1768. In London in 1803, during the Napoleonic Wars, another adaptation stressing French iniquities appeared. It was wildly popular and played for years throughout Great Britain. Charles KEMBLE's 1823 production of *King John,* designed by J. R. PLANCHE, inaugurated the 19th-century Shakespearean tradition of striving for historical accuracy in costumes and stagings. Kemble's example was followed in William Charles MACREADY's successful production of 1842 and elaborate versions were staged in New York (1846) and London (1852) by Charles KEAN (1).

A great favourite in times of British national crisis, when the Bastard's patriotic speeches have proved inspiring, *King John* has been staged a number of times in the 20th century. In 1945, Peter BROOK (2) directed a striking production featuring Paul SCOFIELD as the Bastard. The play has been produced for television twice, in 1951 (with Donald Wolfit as King John) and in 1984 as part of the BBC's inclusive Shakespearean cycles. Although *King John* has not been made as a movie, excerpts from Beerbohm TREE's 1899 stage production of the play were recorded, when cinema was still experimental, in the earliest appearance of Shakespeare on film.

King Lear

SYNOPSIS

Act 1, Scene 1

The Earl of GLOUCESTER (1) introduces his illegitimate son EDMUND to the Earl of KENT (2) and observes that he has a legitimate son as well. King LEAR arrives with his daughters, GONERIL, REGAN, and CORDELIA, and explains his intention to abdicate and distribute Britain among his sons-in-law, the Dukes of ALBANY and CORNWALL—married to Goneril and Regan, respectively—and either the Duke of BURGUNDY (1) or the King of FRANCE (2), suitors of Cordelia. He will give the largest share of the kingdom to whichever daughter can convince him she loves him the most. Goneril and Regan declare their love effusively, but Cordelia simply states that her love is that of a daughter to a father, and that she will also love her husband when she has one. In-

furiated, Lear disinherits her; Kent attempts to dissuade him, and Lear banishes him. Burgundy rejects the disinherited Cordelia, but France decides to marry her and take her back to France. Regan and Goneril confer on the need to control their obviously senile father lest he turn against them.

Act 1, Scene 2
Edmund bewails his illegitimacy and decides to steal his brother EDGAR's inheritance with the help of the letter he holds. Gloucester enters, and Edmund pretends to hide the letter, but his father insists upon reading it. It is supposedly from Edgar, proposing to Edmund that they murder Gloucester. Edmund pretends to believe the letter is merely a test of his morals, and he offers to arrange for Gloucester to overhear a conversation between the half brothers. Gloucester agrees and leaves; Edmund remarks on his naïveté. Edgar appears, and Edmund tells him that their father is viciously angry with him, warning him to go armed lest he be attacked.

Act 1, Scene 3
Goneril desires to humble her father and instructs her steward OSWALD to treat Lear and his followers disdainfully when they arrive.

Act 1, Scene 4
Kent, disguised, plans to rejoin the king's court at Goneril's castle. Lear arrives with his followers, and Kent is accepted among them. Oswald is surly to the king, and, to Lear's delight, Kent rails against him, knocks him down, and drives him away. Lear's FOOL (2) mocks the king for having surrendered his authority. Goneril appears and scolds Lear for the conduct of his men. She demands that he halve their number, and he declares that he will leave and go to Regan. He departs. Albany protests over Goneril's behaviour, but she silences him and sends Oswald with a letter to Regan that details her tactics with their father.

Act 1, Scene 5
Lear sends Kent with a letter to Regan. The Fool again taunts the king for being at the mercy of his daughters.

Act 2, Scene 1
Edmund encounters Edgar and advises him to flee for his life. As Gloucester approaches, Edmund tricks Edgar by saying that he must pretend to prevent Edgar's flight but that he will actually help him escape. He draws his sword and fakes a fight, hustling Edgar away. He then tells Gloucester that Edgar had assaulted him when he opposed the murder plot. Gloucester declares he will have Edgar captured and executed, and he vows to legitimate Edmund. Cornwall and Regan arrive on a visit to Gloucester; they praise Edmund and take him into their service.

Act 2, Scene 2
Outside Gloucester's castle, Kent insults and pummels Oswald as Edmund, Cornwall, Regan, and Gloucester appear. Asked to explain his behaviour, Kent declares that Oswald is a hypocrite. Cornwall places Kent in the stocks despite his status as messenger of the king. Gloucester protests but is ignored. When the others leave, Kent muses on a letter he has received from Cordelia, who has learned of Lear's humiliation.

Act 2, Scene 3
Edgar has escaped from a search party and overheard a proclamation that he is outlawed. He decides to disguise himself as a wandering lunatic, taking the name Tom O' Bedlam.

Act 2, Scene 4
Lear, seeking Regan, arrives at Gloucester's castle and finds Kent in the stocks. The Fool calls Kent a fool for attaching himself to a powerless master. Gloucester reports that Regan and Cornwall will not receive Lear, who begins to rage but restrains himself. Regan and Cornwall appear and Kent is freed. Regan defends Goneril against Lear's complaints as Goneril arrives. The two unite in demanding that Lear dismiss his retinue. The distressed Lear wavers between tears and anger and rages out into a storm that has arisen, followed by Gloucester and the Fool.

Act 3, Scene 1
Kent meets a GENTLEMAN (7) who reports that Lear is raging madly in the storm, accompanied only by the Fool. Kent asks him to report Lear's situation to Cordelia, who has arrived in DOVER with a French army.

Act 3, Scene 2
Lear raves in the storm, cursing his daughters. Kent appears and urges the king to take shelter in a nearby hovel. The Fool bitterly predicts disruption for England, whatever lies in store.

Act 3, Scene 3
Gloucester tells Edmund that Cornwall, his feudal lord, has forbidden him to take Lear in. He confides, however, that he has received a letter assuring that Lear's revenge is at hand in the form of the French invasion. Edmund decides to inform on his father so he can get his inheritance sooner.

Act 3, Scene 4
Lear, Kent, and the Fool approach the hovel. Lear declares that he prefers the storm to the thoughts he would have if he were sheltered, but he sends the Fool inside. He reflects on the woes of the poor and homeless, whom he had never considered when he ruled. The Fool reappears, terrified of a madman in the hovel. He is followed by Edgar, disguised as Tom O' Bedlam, who raves about being pursued by devils.

Lear sympathises with him, assuming that he too has been betrayed by his daughters. Edgar asserts that his demons are punishment for certain offences: he had been a decadent and immoral servant who slept with his mistress, among other sins. Gloucester appears and offers them shelter. He confides to Kent that Lear's daughters seek the king's death.

Act 3, Scene 5
Edmund has revealed Gloucester's correspondence with the French army, and Cornwall orders him to have his father arrested.

Act 3, Scene 6
Gloucester leaves Kent, Lear, the Fool, and Edgar in a warm room. Lear acts out a criminal trial of Goneril and Regan and finally falls asleep just as Gloucester returns and warns them to flee immediately. Kent and the Fool leave, carrying the sleeping Lear. Edgar, left behind, reflects that his own fate does not seem so bad compared with that of the mad king.

Act 3, Scene 7
Gloucester, under arrest, is brought before Cornwall and Regan. When he says that he will see them punished by fate, Cornwall puts out his eyes. The duke is attacked by a SERVANT (19), who cannot abide such evil. Cornwall kills the Servant, but not before being badly wounded. Regan takes him away, and the remaining Servants agree to take the blinded Gloucester to the wandering madman, who can help him safely escape.

Act 4, Scene 1
An OLD MAN (2) leads the blind Gloucester to Edgar, who grieves to see his father in such condition. However, still an outcast, he resumes his madman's disguise. He agrees to lead Gloucester to the cliffs of Dover.

Act 4, Scene 2
Oswald meets Goneril and Edmund and tells them that Albany has learned of Cordelia's invasion, which pleases him, and that Edmund has informed on Gloucester, which does not. Goneril sends Edmund with a message to Cornwall to hastily muster an army; they exchange loving farewells, accompanied by hints of a murder plot against Albany. Albany appears and berates Goneril for her evil; she replies that he is merely a coward. A MESSENGER (20) arrives with news of Cornwall's death and Gloucester's blinding. In an aside, Goneril worries that Regan has possible designs on Edmund, now that she is a widow. Albany vows privately to revenge Gloucester.

Act 4, Scene 3
In Dover the Gentleman tells Kent of Cordelia's tearful response to news of Lear. Kent replies that Lear is in Dover but refuses to see Cordelia, out of shame.

Act 4, Scene 4
Cordelia hears that Lear has been seen wandering wearing a crown of weeds and flowers, and she orders a search party. The DOCTOR (2) assures her that Lear's madness may be eased by rest, and that sedatives are available. News arrives that the armies of Albany and Cornwall are approaching.

Act 4, Scene 5
Oswald reports to Regan that Goneril has convinced Albany to fight against Cordelia's invasion. He also has a letter from Goneril to Edmund, which sparks Regan's jealousy; she gives Oswald a token from herself to give Edmund with Goneril's letter. She adds that if Oswald finds and kills Gloucester, he will be rewarded.

Act 4, Scene 6
Edgar convinces Gloucester that they have reached the top of the cliffs at Dover and then pretends to leave him. In an aside to himself he says that he must humour his father's despair in order to cure it. Gloucester leaps forward and falls to the ground. Edgar then pretends to be a passer-by at the bottom of the cliff and says that he had seen Gloucester at the top with a hideous demon. Gloucester accepts the idea that the gods have miraculously preserved him from an evil impulse, and he vows to accept his affliction in the future. Lear appears, covered with wildflowers and raving madly. A Gentleman with a search party arrives and takes Lear to Cordelia. Edgar learns from him the location of the British army. Oswald appears and attacks Gloucester, but Edgar kills him. As he dies, Oswald asks his killer to deliver his letters to Edmund. Edgar reads a letter from Goneril proposing that Edmund murder Albany and marry her.

Act 4, Scene 7
Cordelia greets her father, but Lear mistakes her for a spirit and only gradually realises that he is still alive. The Doctor says that he needs more rest, and he is taken indoors, leaving Kent and the Gentleman to discuss the coming battle. Kent declares that his life will end that day.

Act 5, Scene 1
Jealously, Regan interrogates Edmund about Goneril, and Goneril says to herself that she would rather lose the battle than see Regan get Edmund. Edgar appears in disguise, and takes Albany aside. He gives him the letter he got from Oswald. He proposes that after the battle Albany call for a challenger to prove in trial by combat that its contents are true. In a soliloquy Edmund reflects that Albany's leadership will be needed during the battle, but that he hopes Goneril will then see to killing him. He observes that Albany has proposed mercy for Lear and Cordelia, but he, Edmund, will not permit it.

Act 5, Scene 2
Edgar leaves Gloucester and goes to fight. Fleeing soldiers pass by, and Edgar returns, saying that Cordelia's forces have been routed and she and Lear captured. Gloucester fatalistically elects to stay, but he recovers when reminded of his resolution to endure, and the two flee together.

Act 5, Scene 3
Edmund sends the captured Lear and Cordelia to prison. Lear rejoices at being with Cordelia, despite the circumstances. Edmund sends an OFFICER (5) after them, telling him to carry out his written instructions mercilessly. Albany arrives with Regan and Goneril. He arrests Edmund and Goneril for treason, asserting that a challenger will appear to back the charge in trial by combat. Regan departs, suddenly sick. Edgar appears, unrecognisable in full armour, and he and Edmund fight until he wounds Edmund badly. Albany displays the letter, and Goneril departs hastily. The dying Edmund confesses his crimes. Edgar identifies himself and tells of escorting Gloucester, adding that when he finally told his father who he was the emotional shock killed the old man. An hysterical GENTLEMAN (8) reports that Goneril has confessed to poisoning Regan, and then committed suicide. Edmund reveals that he has ordered someone to kill the king and hang Cordelia in her cell, an apparent suicide. Edmund is carried away and a soldier is sent to halt the killer, but Lear appears carrying the dead Cordelia in his arms. He mourns her death, but at intervals believes she may be still alive. He sees Kent but cannot recognise or understand him; the others realise that he is mad again. Edmund's death is reported, and Albany declares that he will return Lear's kingdom to him. Lear suddenly announces that he sees Cordelia breathing, and as he does so, he dies. Albany orders funeral preparations and appoints Kent and Edgar to be his associates in rule, though Kent says that he will

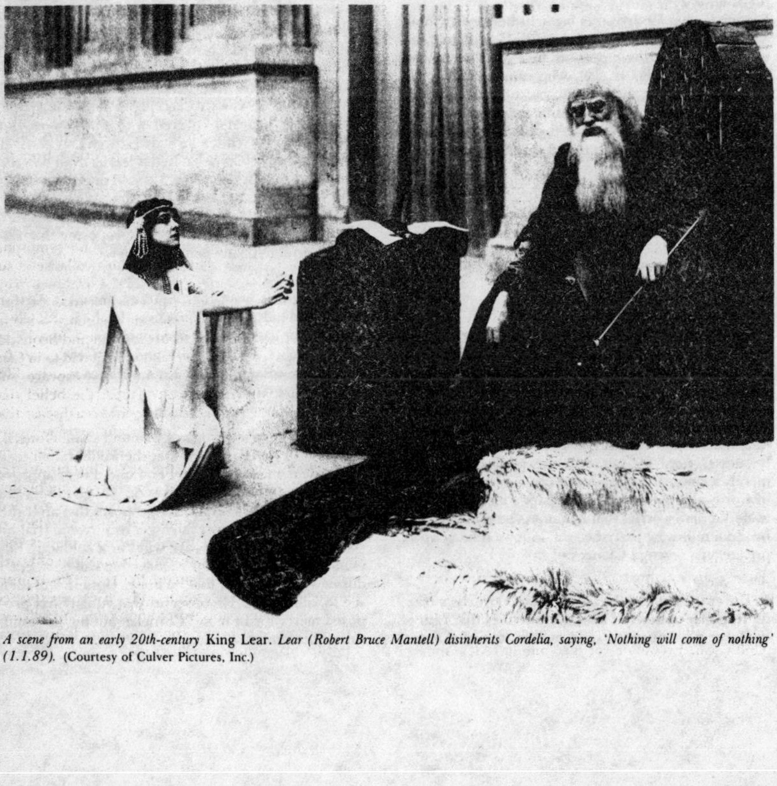

A scene from an early 20th-century King Lear. *Lear (Robert Bruce Mantell) disinherits Cordelia, saying, 'Nothing will come of nothing' (1.1.89).* (Courtesy of Culver Pictures, Inc.)

soon die. Edgar closes the play with the assertion that such woes as Lear's shall not be seen again.

COMMENTARY

As was his habit, Shakespeare altered his sources considerably when he wrote *King Lear,* and his most important alteration changed the nature of the story entirely. In the many versions of the tale that preceded Shakespeare's, Lear does not go mad, but recovers his throne and leaves it to Cordelia. The old story is essentially reassuring: one may make a catastrophic mistake and still survive to live a peaceful and happy life. Shakespeare plainly felt that life makes more strenuous demands than a happy ending can illustrate, and at the core of his story is human failing. Gloucester's blindness is foreshadowed in his lack of judgement about Edgar, and Lear's madness by his egotistical demand for total love. These failings are seen in conjunction with the unscrupulous ambition for power represented by Edmund, Cornwall, Goneril, and Regan, and we are repelled by crimes within families, violations of the most basic human solidarity. Our horror is compounded by the vivid depiction of villainy triumphant, which is only slightly lessened by the villains' deaths, as these are more than matched by those of Gloucester, Lear, and Cordelia. Edmund's remorse at the play's close does little to compensate for his evil, and Regan and Goneril display no final repentance at all. Our pity for Lear and Gloucester is increased by the knowledge that they brought their sufferings on themselves.

The enormity of the tragedy is unmistakable, and the play leaves us with a troubling question: How can we reconcile human dignity with human failure in the face of life's demands? This is finally unresolvable; however, several possible ways of addressing the question emerge through Shakespeare's rich presentation of human tragedy.

Perhaps most striking is the play's obvious religious interpretation, emphasised by numerous allusions to religious matters. These range from the trivial—as in the many mentions of pagan gods—to serious remarks such as Edgar's 'The Gods are just, and of our pleasant vices / Make instruments to plague us' (5.3.169–170). Also, numerous references to the end of the world are made, most strikingly in the cries of Kent, Edgar, and Albany at the horror of Cordelia's death, in 5.3.262–263. Most significantly, Cordelia, who suffers through no fault of her own and accepts her fate with uncomplaining fortitude and undiminished love, is often seen as a personification of the Christian virtues of self-sacrifice and acceptance of God's will. In fact, many commentators have found her to be a Christlike figure whose death symbolises Christ's crucifixion. This offers a positive interpretation of the play's fatal close: the tragedy is a manifestation of God's will, a reminder of the coming redemption of humanity through Christianity. On the other hand, a non-Christian interpretation of Cordelia's sacrifice is also compelling. She lacks the Christian's reward in the afterlife because she is a pagan, thus her virtue is its own reward. Her conduct is therefore all the more stirring, and our admiration of her heroic courage is increased.

The sufferings of Lear and Gloucester, which they have brought upon themselves, may be compared to punishment for sins by God. They recognise that they are at fault and are then reconciled with their children, and this development suggests God's forgiveness for those who are contrite. Their forgiveness is accompanied by death, and this points up the doctrinal importance of the Christian afterlife and its eternal mercy. However, this promise is lacking in Lear's pagan world and, as with Cordelia, a non-religious interpretation could be that Lear's endurance is heroic in itself, and his triumph lies in his recognition and acceptance of his failings before he dies. Most commentators agree, in any case, that the suffering of the characters in *Lear* is finally redemptive, for it is heroic, it leads to heightened consciousness in Lear and Gloucester, and it provides the example of Edgar and Cordelia's undiminished loyalty and love. Also, many commentators hold that Shakespeare intended Lear to die believing that Cordelia is alive, as his last words indicate, which implies a happy resolution in death akin to that of Gloucester, whose heart 'burst smilingly' (5.3.198).

Another positive conclusion can be drawn from the tragedy. Politics are as important in *King Lear* as religion. In fact, in Shakespeare's time, the references to the end of the world carried a political implication, for people commonly believed that the world's end was more or less imminent, and that one of the symptoms of approaching apocalypse would be a collapse of social structures, including political bonds. Much reassurance was found in the peaceful assession of King JAMES I—civil war was feared at the time—with its promise for the unification of England and Scotland. The threat of civil war, several times alluded to in *Lear,* raises a point that was important to Shakespeare, and which dominates the HISTORY PLAYS, the belief that personal immorality in the ruling class is a disease that spreads evil throughout society, in extreme cases causing it to fall apart. Though Lear, Gloucester, and Cordelia do not live to appreciate it, Britain at large is rescued from the evil that has overrun the highest reaches of its society; civil war in Britain is avoided, and the French invasion caused by Lear's lack of judgement is defeated by Albany. The play is thus supportive of civil authority; the catastrophe of Lear's reign might be compared, by the 17th-century playgoer, with the strength and harmony expected from that of James. It is worth noting that in 1606 *Lear* was performed at James' court on a very festive occasion, the day following Christmas.

Another point addressed in *King Lear* is that a sovereign is responsible for his subjects. Raving madly in the storm, Lear realises that he had been unaware of hunger and homelessness when he was king, and he sees that his present experience could have been valuable to him as a ruler. He says to himself: 'Take physic, Pomp; / Expose thyself to feel what wretches feel, / That thou mayst shake the superflux to them, / And show the Heavens more just' (3.4.33–36). Lear recognises that his errors are more important than others' because he is a king.

A more particular social question is also addressed in *King Lear.* In Shakespeare's day, the newly prosperous gentry and the commercially active bourgeoisie were rising in prosperity and power, largely at the expense of the old aristocracy. This conflict is plainly the cause of the extraordinary venom displayed by Kent towards Oswald in 2.2. Oswald is a caricature of a 17th-century social climber, as Kent's accusation, phrased largely in terms of social status, makes clear. Edmund also represents the new classes, with his lack of chivalric scruples and his concern for his own advancement. In his first soliloquy Edmund identifies himself with a typical modern rejection of tradition by declaring, 'Thou, Nature, art my goddess' (1.2.1), a reference to the RENAISSANCE rediscovery of classical paganism and the sophisticated agnosticism that was thought to accompany it. In placing these sentiments in the mouth of a self-declared villain, Shakespeare stresses his alliance with the old world of the aristocracy, just as he does in ridiculing Oswald through Kent.

However, though *King Lear* may lend itself to numerous interpretations, Christian or humanistic, political or moral, our response to the play is largely governed by its conclusion. Act 5 brings no relief for our anguish, despite the expectations raised by the reunion of Lear and Cordelia. The finality of death may suggest that the play reflects a morbidly depressed response to life on Shakespeare's part (without denying that other plays express other responses). Such a viewpoint has led some to compare *Lear* to the Book of Job and see the play as an explication of the power of fate, or God. However, both Edgar and Albany survive to carry on, conscious of the fragility of happiness and on guard against the errors of Lear and Gloucester, for as Edgar (Albany, in some editions) says, 'The weight of this sad time we must obey' (5.3.322).

The extraordinary woe that is at the heart of *King Lear* can make it a harrowing experience for audiences. Shakespeare maintains this atmosphere of wretched despair through a variety of subtle effects. Most striking perhaps is the repeated depiction of pain and disease, capped by Lear's madness and Gloucester's blinding, but also represented by Edmund's self-mutilation in 2.1, Edgar's feigned lunacy, and Lear's convulsion of the throat known as 'Hysteria passio' (2.4.55), among other instances. Further, painful metaphors of torment and sickness are extensively used. For instance, the Fool compares the rejected Lear to a bird that 'had it[s] head bit off' (1.4.214); Edgar speaks vividly of self-mutilation, in 2.3.14–16; and Lear speaks of his daughters' rejection as a 'mouth . . . tear[ing a] hand' (3.4.15). In a famous image, Gloucester compares humanity's relationship to the gods with that of 'flies to wanton boys . . . They kill us for their sport' (4.1.36–37).

Another aspect of the theme of disease is the play's morbid attitude towards sex. In *King Lear* sexual love is seen as evil and is only presented in the monstrous rivalry of Regan and Goneril for Edmund. It is also seen as the source of other evils. The misdeeds of Lear's daughters are firmly connected by Lear to the sexual acts from which they were conceived, and Edgar points out that Edmund was the product of illicit sex. Also, in his disguise as Tom O'Bedlam, Edgar declares that intercourse, 'the act of darkness' (3.4.85), is responsible for his painful madness. Lear goes so far as to condemn human procreation, demanding that the gods 'Crack Nature's moulds, all germens spill at once / That makes ingrateful man!' (3.2.8–9). In the extreme, the raving Lear links female sexual anatomy with evil, saying, 'there's hell, there's darkness, / There is the sulphurous pit—burning, scalding, / Stench, consumption; fie, fie, fie!' (4.6.126–128). This incrimination of a natural drive is an indication of the troubled world in *King Lear* and of the disturbed minds of its inhabitants. Happiness is only offered in the isolated and asexual world of the reunited but imprisoned Lear and Cordelia, where all other human contact is willingly forsworn; the exhausted king declares that 'Upon such sacrifices . . . / The Gods themselves throw incense' (5.3.20–21).

The play's treatment of psychological distortion is well served by its disjointed and varying tone. This is largely provided by its complex SUB-PLOT, whose differing elements include Gloucester's blinding, Edgar's exile as mad Tom, and Regan and Goneril's sexual rivalry. The intercutting of these developments with Lear's story was once much criticised; early 19th-century commentators such as Charles LAMB (1) declared that *Lear* was a bad play in theatrical terms, while acknowledgeing its power as poetry. This was long a traditionally accepted idea, influencing 20th-century critics to elaborately consider the plot's 'failings', despite the play's unquestionable success with modern audiences.

The sub-plot actually anchors the play's dramatic structure. The wanderings of Edgar and Gloucester are presented in sequential incidents, as are the machinations of Edmund and the cruel sisters. Together, they provide a well-defined structure that the main plot—Lear's foolish choice and subsequent isola-

tion—does not offer. Indeed, the principal action can hardly be called a plot at all; it is simply a progression, taking the central character from vanity and folly through deepening madness to a recovered consciousness and ultimate collapse. As we watch this progression, we do not think about the next step in the plot so much as we simply observe Lear's personal qualities and contemplate their evolution. The *events* of Lear's progress are less important and are not presented in a structured way, unlike, for example, in *Julius Caesar*, but are indicated by discrete and almost unconnected subsidiary developments.

The play also offers disconcerting suggestions of comedy that complicate our response and thus increase its emotional power. In *King Lear* Shakespeare employed a number of elements traditionally associated with comedy: a double plot; the use of a jester to comment on the action; the use of disguise; the progression of the action from royal court to country and back to court; and the counterpoint of youth and age. Moreover, Kent's ridicule of Oswald, a number of Edgar's remarks as Tom O'Bedlam, and the Fool's routines are all quite funny. These elements suggest the potential for a different sort of story altogether, not a simple tale of evil triumphant.

King Lear is complex also in its repeated emotional polarities. We are presented with oppositions of weeping and laughing, silence and speech, honesty and guile, madness and intelligence, delusion and clear-sightedness, love and hate. Cordelia's frankness and spirituality is contrasted with the deceit and lasciviousness of her sisters; Kent's moral firmness with Oswald's self-serving oiliness and his strength with Lear's weakness; the merciful Albany with the cruel Cornwall. Individual characters present contrasts, as well, though the playwright is careful to motivate each change so as not to dilute a character's strength as a representative figure. Kent, for instance, announces that he will 'other accents borrow / That can my speech defuse' (1.4.1–2), and he adopts a plain-spoken prose and only reverts to verse when he cannot be heard by Lear or when he expresses his love and concern for his demented master, as in 3.2.42–49, 60–67. Edgar similarly effects prose as Tom O'Bedlam but speaks poetry as himself, and the hypocritical sisters use verse to flatter their father and prose to plot against him. *Lear*'s great range of characters stimulates our strong awareness of the play as a philosophical statement about the human condition.

SOURCES OF THE PLAY

The main plot of *King Lear* was well known in Shakespeare's day—at least 40 versions have been uncovered by scholars—but it is clear that the playwright relied chiefly on an earlier, anonymous play, KING LEIR (c. 1590). This work contains the general story of Lear's relations with his daughters, though at the play's close King Leir is restored to his throne and Cordelia lives. Some scholars think Shakespeare may have acted in *King Leir* in the 1590s, playing a character corresponding to Kent, for a number of passages that are especially closely echoed in *Lear* are spoken when that figure is on-stage.

Shakespeare also knew the story from an account in Raphael HOLINSHED's *Chronicles of England, Scotland, and Ireland* (2nd ed., 1587), which inspired several passages. Holinshed's account of Lear is based on the work of a medieval historian, GEOFFREY of Monmouth. Details of Gloucester's attempted suicide were probably inspired by another story in Holinshed, that of a giant who was thrown to his death from the cliffs of Dover. John HIGGINS' version of the tale in A MIRROR FOR MAGISTRATES (1587) provided Shakespeare with a number of significant details, including France's praise of Cordelia's virtues. Other details can be ascribed to a variety of sources, most notably Edmund SPENSER's *The Faerie Queene* (1589), Ben JONSON's *Sejanus* (1605), Gerard LEGH's *Accedens of Armory* (1562), and, possibly, William CAMDEN's *Remaines* (1605).

Shakespeare found the sub-plot involving Gloucester, Edmund, and Edgar in a tale from Sir Philip SIDNEY's *Arcadia* (1590), about a king who is betrayed by one son and saved by another. It may also have influenced the main plot, for Sidney's tragic hero is not restored to his former glory, like King Leir, but dies of mingled joy and exhaustion, like Shakespeare's Gloucester. Also, Sidney's king is driven out into a storm, like Lear, and lives as a beggar, like Edgar. Another anecdote in *Arcadia* may have influenced Edmund's plot to disgrace Edgar, and a poem in *Arcadia* is a meditation on suicide that is echoed in several passages of the play.

Two other works contributed to the play's themes, though not to the actual plot: Samuel HARSNETT's *A Declaration of Egregious Popish Impostures* (1603), which provided the lore of demons for Edgar's assumed lunacy, and John FLORIO's English translation of the *Essays* of Michel de MONTAIGNE (1603), whose scepticism influenced Edmund's disdain for the conventional attitude towards illegitimacy, as well as his unscrupulous attitude towards morals. It is also possible that a contemporary case of insanity resembling Lear's (see Brian ANNESLEY) may have sparked Shakespeare's imagination, for in no earlier version of the tale is the king mad.

TEXT OF THE PLAY

King Lear was written between the spring of 1603 and early 1606, for one of the play's sources—Samuel Harsnett's book—was published in March 1603, and a play that was influenced by *Lear*—*The Fleir*, by Edward SHARPHAM—was registered for publication in May 1606. A more precise date is difficult to determine; some passages in the play seem to offer clues, but no

agreement can be reached. Similarly, relationships between *Lear* and other works published between 1603 and 1606 are generally problematic, as it is impossible to tell which is in debt to which.

The play was first published in 1608 by Nathaniel BUTTER in a QUARTO edition known as Q1. Twelve copies of Q1 exist, but they encompass 10 slightly different texts, since proof-reading and correction were carried on simultaneously with printing. Q1 is sometimes called the 'Pied Bull Quarto' because its title page refers to Butter's shop 'at the signe of the Pide Bull'. Q1 is a BAD QUARTO, assembled from the recollections of spectators or of actors who had performed in the play, but scholars differ in their conclusions about who these reporters were and whether or not they had access to a manuscript. It is a poor text with many errors, little punctuation, missing or inadequate stage directions, and many passages of verse set as prose and vice versa. A second quarto (Q2), printed from a copy of Q1, was dated 1608 and attributed to Butter, but it was actually produced in 1619 as part of the pirated FALSE FOLIO.

King Lear appears in the FIRST FOLIO (1623), and this version (F) is a far better text than Q1, incorporating many corrections, including amplified stage directions. Most significantly, it is a radically altered script. More than 300 lines of dialogue from Q1 are omitted in F—including a number of significant passages—and about 100 lines are added, including Lear's final lines (5.3.309–310).

It is generally believed that the omissions from Q1 reflect shortening made for performances sometime between 1608 and 1623, and that the additions are Shakespeare's, made before he retired around 1613. Scholars are divided on the form in which the printers of the Folio received the alterations, but the most widely accepted theory is that F was printed from a copy of Q1 that had been heavily annotated with amendments and references from the PROMPT-BOOK used by the KING'S MEN. However, a recently popular theory holds that the Folio text represents a re-writing of the play by Shakespeare, from which it follows that there exist two different *King Lear*s, each distinctive in tone and emphasis. One new edition of Shakespeare's works, that of Oxford University Press (1986), prints them as such, though most editors have combined the two in a single text that omits nothing of consequence while relying on F, the superior text, where the two conflict.

THEATRICAL HISTORY

The earliest known performance of *King Lear* is recorded in the publisher's registration of the play, which asserts that it was performed at the court of King JAMES I on December 26, 1606. Scholars believe that the play was not well received in Shakespeare's day, for there are few surviving references to it in contemporary documents. However, it is known that Richard Burbage (3) was the original Lear.

After the 1660 reopening of the English theatres—they had been closed during the Puritan Revolution—*Lear* was staged only twice, in 1660 (by William DAVENANT) and 1675. It was replaced in 1681 by an adaptation, Nahum TATE's *History of King Lear*. Tate's *Lear* retained much Shakespearean dialogue, but amid vast changes in plot, including a happy ending in which Lear is restored to his throne. Thomas BETTERTON played Lear for Tate. Though modern commentators condemn this version as a travesty, it was one of the most successful plays in the history of the English theatre, continuing to be staged—with Shakespeare's text sometimes restored in varying degrees—until as late as 1843 (and occasionally in modern times as an historical curiosity).

The restoration of Shakespeare's text began with David GARRICK's production of 1742, and the process was furthered by George COLMAN (though he also added his own alterations) in 1768. In the late 18th and early 19th centuries the play was suppressed by the government, which disliked its focus on a mad monarch at a time when King George III was insane. It reappeared in 1809 in a version by John Philip KEMBLE (3) that restored most of Tate's text. Edmund KEAN (2), under the influence of the critics Charles LAMB (1) and William HAZLITT, restored Lear's death in his production of 1823, though the text was still largely Tate's. Not until 1838 were Tate's words completely removed in Charles William MACREADY's production, though Gloucester's travails were still omitted. It remained for Samuel PHELPS to produce a genuinely Shakespearean version in 1845. Edwin BOOTH (2) played Lear with Tate's text early in his career, but by 1876 he was presenting Shakespeare's play. No subsequent production reverted to Tate, but considerable editing of the original text remained common; Henry IRVING, for instance, cut more than half the play in his presentation of 1892 that starred himself and Ellen TERRY (1).

In the 20th century *King Lear* has been extremely popular. Most leading actors have played Lear; among the most notable have been Robert Bruce MANTELL early in the century; John GIELGUD and Donald WOLFIT in the 1940s; Michael REDGRAVE, Orson WELLES, and Charles LAUGHTON in the 1950s; Paul SCOFIELD, especially in a famed 1962 staging by Peter BROOK (2); and James Earl JONES (1) in Joseph PAPP's production of 1973. The role of Cordelia has similarly attracted leading actresses, among them Peggy ASHCROFT and Zoë CALDWELL. *Lear* has been presented on FILM eight times; the two most famous, by Brook and the Russian Grigori KOZINTSEV, were made simultaneously as the two directors, shooting in Denmark and Russia respectively, corresponded, comparing notes on their projects (1969). The play has been made for TELEVI-

SION five times. Also, Akira KUROSAWA's *Ran* (1985) is based on *Lear.* The play has also inspired six operas—though only one, by Aribert Reimann (1978), has entered the general operatic repertoire—and at least one well-known orchestral work, the *King Lear Overture* by Hector BERLIOZ (1831).

King Leir Anonymous play of c. 1588 (publ. 1605) that influenced Shakespeare's version of the same tale, *King Lear.* The earlier play presents the general lines of the king's misjudgement of his daughters and characters who are equivalent to KENT, ALBANY, and OSWALD. Also, many minor details from it are echoed in Shakespeare's play. However, at the play's close Cordelia lives and King Leir is restored to his throne. The authorship of *King Leir* has been attributed to various playwrights, including Thomas LODGE, George PEELE, Robert GREENE (2), and Thomas KYD, but scholars remain divided on the question.

King Leir—fully titled *The True Chronicle History of King Leir and his three daughters*—is now known only in the edition of 1605, but references in the text suggest that it was written around the time an invasion of England was threatened by the Spanish Armada in 1588. It was registered with the STATIONERS' COMPANY in 1594, but if an edition was published at that time no copy has survived. Some scholars believe that Shakespeare knew the play from the stage and simply recalled the elements he employed in *Lear.* He probably knew the play before 1594, in any case, for several minor details in *Richard III* (c. 1591) can be traced to *King Leir.* In fact, Shakespeare may have acted in *King Leir,* playing the character that corresponds to KENT (2), for a number of passages in the old play that are echoed in *Lear* are spoken while that character is on-stage. It is conceivable that Shakespeare consulted the 1605 edition of *King Leir,* though it appeared only very shortly before *Lear* itself, and it is just as likely that it was republished in order to capitalise on the forthcoming appearance of a new play by Shakespeare.

Kings Minor characters in *Macbeth,* eight ghostly figures who appear to MACBETH, representing future rulers. In 4.1 Macbeth seeks to learn from the WITCHES whether their earlier prediction, that BANQUO would father a line of rulers, is still true. In response, the eight spectral Kings appear in a procession led by Banquo's GHOST (4), who indicates, with a smile and a gesture, that they are indeed his descendants. Macbeth observes that some of the Kings carry 'twofold balls and treble sceptres' (4.1.121). This is a topical reference to the coronation regalia of the newly crowned ruler of England and SCOTLAND in Shakespeare's day, King JAMES I. James was of the STUART dynasty and was believed (though inaccurately) to be descended from Banquo. Moreover, the eight Kings correspond to the eight Stuart kings, the first of whom was crowned in 1371. (Shakespeare omits the one queen in the line—Mary, Queen of Scots, James' mother—presumably because she had been the enemy of England's Queen ELIZABETH (1) and had been executed by her in 1587.) These allusions were much more obvious to Shakespeare's original audiences than they are today.

Through this episode Macbeth sees that the Witches' earlier prediction is confirmed. He realises that his ambition must remain incompletely satisfied. Thus, figuratively, Macbeth's downfall has begun. The significant message that MACDUFF has abandoned him—the first step in his actual defeat—follows immediately.

King's Men Acting company in which Shakespeare was a partner, the successor to the CHAMBERLAIN'S MEN. When King JAMES I acceded to the throne of England in 1603, the Chamberlain's Men's patron, Lord HUNSDON (1), surrendered his position to the new king, an enthusiast of the stage. The number of performances at court was much higher for the troupe under James—an average of twelve times a year in Shakespeare's lifetime, versus four during the reign of Queen ELIZABETH (1)—and after 1608, the King's Men had a new winter home, the BLACKFRIARS THEATRE, with a different, more sophisticated audience. Under these influences, a new sort of play evolved and JACOBEAN DRAMA emerged, led by the King's Men.

At the time of the change of patron, the partners in the company were Shakespeare, Robert ARMIN, Richard BURBAGE (3), Henry CONDELL, Richard COWLEY, John HEMINGE, Augustine PHILLIPS, and William SLY (2). Joining them was Laurence FLETCHER (3), a member of the king's household. Fletcher had a theatrical background but seems not to have been an active participant in the King's Men. By 1605 three more members were added, probably Alexander COOKE (1), Samuel CROSSE, and John LOWIN. In 1619 the company's royal patent was renewed, and its members were named in a surviving official document. Only Burbage, Heminge, and Condell remained of the original eight; the other nine partners listed were Lowin, Nathan FIELD (1), John UNDERWOOD, Nicholas TOOLEY, William ECCLESTONE, Robert BENFIELD, Robert GOUGH, Richard ROBINSON (4), and John SHANK. Burbage died in the same month and was replaced by Joseph TAYLOR. The company's business manager was Heminge until his death in 1630, after which it was run by Lowin and Taylor.

The King's Men performed at the GLOBE THEATRE in the summer and, after 1608, at the Blackfriars in the winter. The company was universally regarded as England's best. Their many appearances at court were a measure of their prestige; especially noteworthy is the fact that they performed 20 plays—eight of them

Shakespeare's—during the weeks-long celebration of the marriage of the Princess ELIZABETH (3) in 1613. The King's Men's principal playwrights were Shakespeare and later John FLETCHER (2)—often in collaboration with Francis BEAUMONT (2)—and Philip MASSINGER. The King's Men also staged works by other dramatists, including Ben JONSON and John WEBSTER (2).

King's Revels See CHILDREN'S COMPANIES.

Kirkham, Edward (active 1586–1617) English theatrical entrepreneur. Kirkham was a subordinate to the MASTER OF THE REVELS and was therefore involved in the regulation of ELIZABETHAN THEATRE. He also invested in the profession. Between 1603 and 1608 he was a partner of Henry EVANS (2) in the productions of the Children of the Queen's Revels (see CHILDREN'S COMPANIES) at the BLACKFRIARS THEATRE, which Evans leased from Richard BURBAGE (3), Shakespeare's associate in the KING'S MEN. When the boys' company lost its royal patronage in 1608, Evans relinquished his lease on the Blackfriars to Burbage, who thereupon sold shares in the theatre to a number of people, including Shakespeare and a relative of Evans. Kirkham was effectively abandoned. He sued Evans, Burbage, and others, in unsuccessful attempts to gain from their profits. Modern scholars find in the records of these suits a number of clues as to the nature of the early 17th-century theatre, including the information that the Blackfriars was much more profitable to the King's Men than was the GLOBE THEATRE.

Kirkman, Francis (1632–after 1674) English writer and publisher. In 1662 Kirkman's collection of DROLLS—the brief dramas performed illicitly when the English theatres were closed in 1642–1660—was published by Henry MARSH, his business partner, as *The Wits: or Sport upon Sport*. Kirkman himself published a second edition in 1672 and a supplementary volume in 1673. He also compiled and published a *Catalogue of English Stage Playes,* which listed 690 dramas in its first edition (1661) and added 116 more in the second (1671). Kirkman also published an edition of THE BIRTH OF MERLIN (1662), which he attributed to Shakespeare and William ROWLEY (2). He translated and published romantic tales from French and Spanish and wrote several of his own, as well as at least one play.

Kittredge, George Lyman (1860–1941) American scholar. Kittredge, a longtime professor at Harvard University (1888–1936), was a respected authority on both Shakespeare and CHAUCER. He is best known as a teacher who influenced generations of students to a greater appreciation of English literature in general and Shakespeare's plays in particular. He also edited an edition of Shakespeare's *Complete Works* (1936) and wrote books on Shakespeare, Chaucer, and other subjects ranging from *Sir Thomas Malory* (1925) to *Witchcraft in Old and New England* (1929).

Knell, William (d. 1587) English actor, a member of the QUEEN'S MEN (1). Knell is known to have played Prince Hal in THE FAMOUS VICTORIES, but his significance rests on his place in a theory about Shakespeare's early years. Knell was killed in a fight while the Queen's Men were playing in STRATFORD in June 1587, and some scholars speculate that the young Shakespeare was hired to replace him and accompanied the troupe to LONDON, thus beginning his theatrical career. This intriguing hypothesis is entirely unprovable, but Knell has nonetheless found a niche in literary history. His widow married John HEMINGE.

Knight (1) Minor character in *King Lear,* a follower of King LEAR. In 1.4 the Knight is sent by Lear to summon OSWALD, steward to the king's ungrateful daughter GONERIL. He returns to report that Oswald insolently refuses to come, and he goes on to remark that 'your Highness is not entertain'd with that ceremonious affection as you were wont' (1.4.56–57). This is a summary of the main plot so far: Goneril and her sister REGAN are purposefully humiliating the king. The Knight also mentions CORDELIA, the virtuous daughter whom Lear had rejected in 1.1, and reminds us that the king's plight lies in his own foolishness. Thus the Knight serves to mark the plot's development just before it intensifies with Lear's expulsion into the wilderness in the next scene.

Knight (2) Any of several minor characters in *Pericles,* jousters who compete with PERICLES for the hand of THAISA. In 2.2 five Knights—along with Pericles—are presented to Thaisa and her father, King SIMONIDES, and Thaisa describes their elaborate coats of arms. None of them speak. In 2.3 at the banquet that follows, one of the Knights—designated as the First Knight—offers brief courtly remarks to Pericles and the king. In 2.5 each of three Knights—First, Second, and Third—speaks a single line as they leave Simonides' court, having been told that Thaisa refuses to marry. The Knights are required for the jousting, and they add to the ceremony of Simonides' court, but they do not have individual character attributes.

Knight (3) Any of three minor characters in *The Two Noble Kinsmen,* companions of PALAMON. The Knights have agreed to serve as seconds to Palamon in his duel with ARCITE over the love of EMILIA (4). The rules of the combat, established by Duke THESEUS (2), require that the loser and his escorts be executed, while the winner gets Emilia. In 5.4 Palamon has lost, and his Knights prepare gallantly to die with him, uttering

brave mottos such as, 'Let us bid farewell, / And with our patience anger tottering fortune' (5.4.19–20). They typify the chivalric ethos that the play depicts.

Knight (4), Edward (active 1623–1633) Book-keeper for the KING'S MEN. As the book-keeper for Shakespeare's theatre company, Knight was responsible for maintaining the PROMPT-BOOK of each play the company performed. He must therefore have known their repertoire quite well, and for this reason some scholars believe he may have done much of the actual editorial work on the FIRST FOLIO edition of Shakespeare's plays. Some of the correspondence he carried on with the MASTER OF THE REVELS has survived, and it sheds light on the business side of the theatrical world in Shakespeare's day.

Knight (5), G. Wilson (1897–1985) English literary critic. Knight boldly interpreted Shakespeare's plays as mystical poems that express their ideas through the symbolic use of imagery and themes in meaningful configurations. This view has influenced both commentary and theatrical production beginning in the 1930s. He is regarded as one of the most important 20th-century Shakespearean critics, but his emphasis on religion is not always accepted. For example, he saw *King Lear* as similar to the Book of Job and LEAR himself as symbolic of the crucified Christ. His best-known works are *The Wheel of Fire* (1930, 1949), *The Imperial Theme* (1931), *The Shakespearean Tempest* (1932), *The Crown of Life* (1947), and *The Sovereign Flower* (1958).

Knollys, Sir William (c. 1547–1632) High official in the court of Queen ELIZABETH (1) and possibly a satirical model for MALVOLIO in *Twelfth Night.* After a successful military career, Knollys succeeded his father, Sir Francis Knollys (c. 1514–1596), as comptroller, and later treasurer, of the royal household, a position analogous to that of steward, the office held by Malvolio in the household of OLIVIA. In the late 1590s Knollys was the subject of amused court gossip as he pursued a much younger woman, Mary FITTON, going so far as to dye his beard—a young man's fashion of the day—perhaps suggesting Malvolio's laughable courtship of Olivia. Fitton, however, had another lover, the Earl of PEMBROKE (3), by whom she became pregnant in 1600, bringing the gossip to a peak at about the time *Twelfth Night* was written. The theory linking Knollys and Malvolio was introduced by Professor Leslie HOTSON; detractors think that Shakespeare would have been unlikely to pillory a man who remained powerful at court throughout the playwright's career, particularly if *Twelfth Night* were written for a courtly occasion, as Hotson also proposed. (For other possible Malvolios, see FFARINGTON; HOBY (2); WILLOUGHBY [1].)

Komisarjevsky, Theodore (1882–1954) Russian director. A major figure in the theatre and opera of pre-revolutionary Russia, Komisarjevsky came to Britain in 1919. He is best known in the West for his stagings of Chekhov and for a series of avant-garde Shakespearean productions in STRATFORD in the 1930s. Especially notable were *Macbeth,* played in a severely abstract metallic set (1933), a highly praised *King Lear* (1936), and *The Comedy of Errors,* presented as a COMMEDIA DELL' ARTE play (1939).

Kozintsev, Grigori (1903–1973) Russian stage and FILM director. Kozintsev is best known in the West for his films of *Hamlet* (1964) and *King Lear* (1970). During the shooting of the latter, Kozintsev corresponded with Peter BROOK (2), who was simultaneously making his film of the play. Both movies are characterised by the intimacy of the acting and the epic grandeur of their landscapes, interiors, and costumes. Kozintsev also wrote an influential book, *Shakespeare: Time and Conscience* (1967).

Kurosawa, Akira (b. 1910) Japanese FILM director, maker of famed adaptations of *Macbeth* and *King Lear.* Kurosawa's *Throne of Blood* (1957) is based on *Macbeth,* and his *Ran* (1985) is derived from *King Lear* (*ran* means 'chaos'). These films are set in medieval Japan, and they employ many aspects of Japanese Noh drama and samurai films, unfamiliar genres in the West. Moreover, Shakespeare's tales are altered considerably (for instance, the children of Kurosawa's LEAR equivalent are male, and his LADY [6] MACBETH has a miscarriage), none of the names are the same, and the language is not at all Shakespearean, even in translation. However, these works are nonetheless powerful evocations of Shakespeare's themes, and unlike virtually all other Shakespearean adaptations, they are regarded as great works of art in their own right by nearly unanimous critical consent.

Kyd, Thomas (1558–1594) English playwright, author of an important influence on *Hamlet* and of minor sources for other plays. Some commentators believe that many of Shakespeare's plays were written in part by other playwrights (see, e.g., FLEAY and ROBERTSON) and have attributed passages and scenes in several plays, especially *Hamlet* and *Titus Andronicus,* to Kyd. Modern scholars, however, dispute most such attributions.

With Christopher MARLOWE (1), Kyd was the most important English playwright when Shakespeare began his career, and he was immensely influential on both the younger playwright and on ELIZABETHAN DRAMA in general. With *The Spanish Tragedy* (c. 1588), he virtually invented the REVENGE TRAGEDY, a genre that was to be immensely popular. It and its probable

companion-piece, the now-lost play known as the UR-HAMLET, provided the apparent inspiration—as well as many details—for *Hamlet. The Spanish Tragedy* was also the source of minor elements of *Titus Andronicus, Richard III,* and *3 Henry VI;* the latter play also owes some details to Kyd's *Soliman and Perseda* (1590).

Kyd, the son of a scribe, was not university-educated, but he attended an excellent secondary school, where Edmund SPENSER was a classmate. He was at least conversant with Latin literature, for SENECA's influence on his work is great (though he would have known the Roman playwright in English translations as well). He was a close friend and probable collaborator of Marlowe, and when Marlowe was prosecuted for 'atheism and immorality' in 1593, Kyd was also arrested. Under torture, he recanted and was released, but he received no patronage thereafter and died in deep poverty.

L

Lacy, John (d. 1681) English actor and playwright, author of an adaptation of *The Taming of the Shrew.* Lacy's *Sauny the Scot* (1667) was a farcical revision in which the comical servant GRUMIO—renamed Sauny—was the principal character. The play was written in prose and set in England. Extremely popular, *Sauny* was revived periodically for a century.

Originally a dancing instructor, Lacy turned to the theatre in the 1660s and achieved fame as a comic actor in Thomas KILLIGREW's company. He was particularly noted for his FALSTAFF, and he played the title role in the original production of *Sauny.* He wrote three other comedies.

Lady (1) Either of two minor characters in *Richard II,* attendants of QUEEN (13) Isabel. In 3.4 the Ladies try without success to alleviate the Queen's grief at the fall of King RICHARD II.

Lady (2) Any of several minor characters in *Timon of Athens,* presenters of a MASQUE at TIMON's banquet. In 1.2 the Ladies, led by one who is disguised as CUPID, perform a masque and dance with Timon's guests. They present an elaborate aristocratic entertainment that suggests Timon's extravagant life-style. LUCULLUS' fatuous remark to Timon that the masque demonstrates 'how ample y'are belov'd' (1.2.126) suggests further that the Ladies are among the many spongers off Timon's hospitality.

Lady (3) Any of several minor characters in *Cymbeline,* noblewomen of King CYMBELINE's court. Attendants of IMOGEN or the QUEEN (2), the Ladies serve mostly to signify their mistresses' royal status and to swell the scene at court, though one Lady does offer an amusingly disdainful reception to the boorish Prince CLOTEN in 2.3.76–84, which helps to characterise the play's comic villain.

Lady (4) Any of several minor characters in *The Winter's Tale,* ladies-in-waiting to Queen HERMIONE. Two ladies, designated First Lady and Second Lady, join Hermione and her young son, MAMILLIUS, in the playful exchange that opens 2.1. Mamillius teases the ladies about their cosmetics, and they in turn tease the prince about his prospective younger sibling, pointing out that Hermione is quite pregnant. The episode provides a striking contrast with the mad brutality of King LEONTES, whose arrival interrupts these domestic pleasures. When the king appears, one of the ladies escorts Mamillius away, and the others leave with the queen when she is sent to prison. (EMILIA, who appears by name in the prison scene [2.2], is presumably one of these ladies, but here she is anonymous.) Ladies, again nameless, mutely attend Hermione at the hearing in 3.2. The courtly ladies lend a charming atmosphere to Hermione's household, contrasting with the tragic developments that surround them; at the same time they help maintain the regal atmosphere appropriate to TRAGEDY in Shakespeare's literary world.

Lady (5) Faulconbridge (Falconbridge) Minor character in *King John,* mother of the BASTARD (1) and ROBERT. Lady Faulconbridge follows her two sons to court, where Robert has claimed that his older brother is the illegitimate son of the late King Richard I. She hopes to preserve her reputation, but when the Bastard tells her that he has renounced his status as a Faulconbridge in favour of royal illegitimacy, she confesses that Richard was indeed his father. Her role serves merely to allow her son's spirit to manifest itself.

Lady (6) Macbeth (c. 1005–c. 1054) Historical figure and character in *Macbeth,* the wife of MACBETH. Lady Macbeth shares her husband's lust for power, and her fierce goading in Act 1 leads him to murder King DUNCAN in 2.2 and seize the throne of SCOTLAND. He is reluctant and fears detection. He recognises that the deed is evil, but Lady Macbeth's ferocious will inspires him with the perverse intensity necessary to overcome his scruples. However, the evils unleashed by the murder prove too much for the new queen, and she goes insane. Reduced to sleep-walking and hallucinations in 5.1, she eventually dies, as is reported in 5.5. Her death is declared a suicide in 5.9.

Lady Macbeth's principal importance lies in her ability to influence her husband early in the play when she urges him to murder the king. When she learns of

Lady Macbeth, one of Shakespeare's grandest creations, is played here by Ellen Terry, one of the most acclaimed of all Shakespearean actresses. (Courtesy of Billy Rose Theatre Collection; New York Public Library at Lincoln Center; Astor, Lenox and Tilden Foundations)

Duncan's approach to INVERNESS—which offers the opportunity for murder—she fervently prays, 'Come, you Spirits . . . unsex me here, / And fill me, from the crown to the toe, top-full / Of direst cruelty!' (1.5.40–43), and she asks that the milk of her breasts be changed to gall. This speech introduces an important motif: the distortion of sexuality, which is a symbol of moral disorder. She goes on to summon 'the dunnest smoke of Hell' (1.5.51) to obscure her deeds from Heaven's sight. This invocation of supernatural horrors is chilling, and reminds us of the WITCHES, already established as a source of evil.

With hypocritical charm, Lady Macbeth welcomes King Duncan to Inverness in 1.6, after which she must deal with her husband's qualms. She insinuates that he is not an adequate man if he gives in to his fears. 'When you durst do it, then you were a man' (1.7.49), she taunts. This tactic is another instance of dysfunctional sexuality as a manifestation of evil. She goes on to exploit her own sexuality when she describes the experience of nursing a loving infant. She insists that she would have ruthlessly 'plucked my nipple from his boneless gums, / And dash'd the brains out' (1.7.57–58), if it had been necessary to achieve their goal. Shamed by her vigour, Macbeth agrees to proceed, but in 2.2 it is left to her to break the horror-struck trance into which he falls after he murders Duncan and to bring their plan to completion. Her ruthless intensity has brought the throne within reach, and Macbeth is crowned soon thereafter.

Lady Macbeth's viciousness has horrified generations of readers and audiences. However, her grim fervour not only makes her fascinating—the role has consistently attracted major actresses of all periods—but it also illuminates the most important element of the play: Macbeth's relationship to evil. He clearly would not have carried out the regicide, although he had already considered it, without the impetus from her. She, on the other hand, willingly commits herself to evil. The contrast makes clear the potential goodness in Macbeth that he abandons when he kills his king. Lady Macbeth thus functions as a symbol of evil until she falls victim to it herself.

However, Shakespeare's major characters are never one-dimensional, and Lady Macbeth is not a simple cartoon of villainy. She, too, is repelled by the evil inherent in murder, though only subconsciously. She can only refer to the regicide euphemistically—Duncan must be 'provided for' (1.5.66); the killing is 'this enterprise' (1.7.48) or merely 'it' (5.1.34), and she is unable to bring herself to do the deed because Duncan too closely resembles her father. When Macbeth speaks of evil just after he has killed Duncan, she prophetically declares, 'These deeds must not be thought / After these ways: so, it will make us mad' (2.2.32–33). Finally, her anguish in the sleep-walking scene demonstrates convincingly that she simply cannot tolerate her too-hastily accepted immersion in evil. Lady Macbeth's madness, along with her husband's profound emotional malaise, is essential to one of the play's strongest effects. Because we see their dreadful breakdown so vividly, we must acknowledge that they are victims of evil as well as its instruments. Indeed, Lady Macbeth finally commits suicide, as reported in 5.9.36–37.

There may also be another cause for her madness. She and Macbeth are obviously fond of each other, as

we see when they first meet in 1.5. Macbeth's letter to her—read in her first speech—makes clear that they have long confided in each other, and that their ambitions are closely shared. Yet when they accomplish their long-sought goal it has an unforeseen consequence for her. Once Duncan has been killed, Lady Macbeth becomes increasingly unimportant to her husband as he begins to undergo the emotional collapse that is the play's principal development. She does not become Macbeth's 'dearest partner of greatness' (1.5.11), as both had anticipated, but is instead excluded from his confidence. He does not inform her of his plan to kill BANQUO, and after her ineffectual attempts to control him when he sees Banquo's GHOST (4), in 3.4, she disappears from the plot. The evil she was so willing to accept betrays her—as it betrays Macbeth—and produces only anguish in place of the rewards she had envisioned. Not only does she lose her husband to his increasingly dead emotional life, she also loses the access to power that had motivated her in the first place. Nothing remains to her and she goes insane. When she stimulates action, in Act 1, Lady Macbeth overflows with vitality; in 5.1 she is reduced to fear of the dark. Though she seemed much stronger than her husband, in the end she lacks the animal strength he uses to bear the aftermath of their deed to its fatal conclusion.

The intimacy between Macbeth and Lady Macbeth combined with the use of perverse sexuality as a symbol of moral disorder has led to a theatrical tradition (dating to the interpretation of Sarah BERNHARDT, in the late 19th century) that presents their relationship as highly charged sexually, and she as a bold flaunter of her sexual charms. However, the play could also suggest sublimated passions whose energies have been displaced onto political ambition. In any case, it is clear that their relationship—however construed—withers in the atmosphere of mistrust and emotional disturbance that is unleashed with Duncan's murder.

The historical Lady Macbeth, whose first name was Gruoch, was the grand-daughter of a Scottish king who was murdered in 1003 A.D., 36 years before the time the play begins. Macbeth was Gruoch's second husband. By her first, a nobleman from northern Scotland, she bore a son, Lulach, whom Shakespeare presumably had in mind when Lady Macbeth remembers nursing a child, in 1.7.54–58. When Macbeth seized the throne, his wife's royal descent doubtless supported his pretensions, though it was not necessary to his claim. There is no evidence at all that she attempted to persuade her husband to make such a claim, nor that she needed to. In fact, Gruoch is very little in evidence at any point in the history of Macbeth's reign, though after his fall her influence may be supposed. Lulach ruled briefly after Macbeth's defeat and death in 1057 before being killed by the triumphant MALCOLM. Since Lulach was known as 'the Simple', some historians think that his mother engineered his assumption of power. Perhaps her spirit passed down to Lulach's grandson Angus, Lady Macbeth's last known descendant, who attempted unsuccessfully to seize the throne in 1120.

Lady (7) Macduff Character in *Macbeth*, wife of Lord MACDUFF and a victim of MACBETH's hired Murderers (see FIRST MURDERER [3]). In 4.2 Lady Macduff is afraid that her husband's departure for England to join the rebellion against Macbeth has placed her and her children in danger. Rosse attempts to reassure her, but he can only say 'I dare not speak much further: / But cruel are the times . . .' (4.2.17–18). This exchange makes plain the extent to which evil has triumphed in Macbeth's SCOTLAND. Rosse leaves, and the Lady, in her distress, blurts out to her SON (1) that Macduff is dead. He is an intelligent lad who realises that stress has made her say it, and her loving appreciation of his childish wit shines through her distracted grief. This touching moment is interrupted by the MESSENGER (22) who warns them to flee, and the immediate appearance of the Murderers, who kill the Son and chase Lady Macduff out of the room and off the stage. Her death is reported in 4.3.

Though a minor figure, this pathetic character—created only to be unjustly killed—is a striking example of the well-crafted small role of which Shakespeare was a master. In her brief appearance she is vivid enough to contrast powerfully with LADY (6) MACBETH. As a loving mother, domestic life is more important to her than politics, and she is everything in a woman that Lady Macbeth is not. As she is the only other female character (except the WITCHES), the contrast is firmly impressed on us. She also affects us in another way, for her helpless bewilderment is another of the many instances of the nation's disorder. The terror she experiences in her last moments alive constitutes the depths of the play's horror. Her death is an important turning point, for it motivates Macduff, in 4.3, to undertake the fight against Macbeth with a stronger will than politics alone could prompt.

Lady (8) Catherine Mortimer (active 1403–1409) Historical figure and character in *1 Henry IV*, daughter of GLENDOWER and wife of Lord MORTIMER (2). Lady Mortimer speaks only Welsh (with the consequence that her lines are dropped from many productions of the play) and must converse with her husband through the interpretation of her father. Glendower reports that she is upset that her husband is leaving for battle and that she is likely to cry. Through him, she asks her husband to lie in her lap while she sings to him. She sings in Welsh, to the amusement of the fiery HOTSPUR, in an episode that lends humanity to the rebel cause. It is thought that the scene may have been prompted by the presence

of actors from WALES (1) in the CHAMBERLAIN'S MEN, one of whom played Lady Mortimer.

Practically nothing is known of the historical Lady Mortimer. She is thought to have died in London after being taken prisoner when her father was defeated and her husband killed at Harlech in 1409.

Lady (9) Northumberland (Margaret Neville, d. c. 1400) Historical figure and character in *2 Henry IV*, the wife of the Earl of NORTHUMBERLAND (1). In 2.3 Lady Northumberland and her daughter-in-law LADY (10) Percy plead with the Earl not to join the rebels against King HENRY IV. He bows to their pressure and flees to Scotland. The incident demonstrates the weakness of Northumberland's allegiance. The historical Lady Northumberland died some time before the period of the play, but Shakespeare revived her in order to create a situation in which family loyalties oppose political ones. She was a sister of the ARCHBISHOP (3) of York, a relationship that Shakespeare ignored.

Lady (10) Elizabeth Percy (1371–c. 1444) Historical figure and character in *1* and *2 Henry IV*, wife, and then widow, of HOTSPUR. In 2.3 of *1 Henry IV* Lady Percy is distressed that her husband apparently intends to return to war. She playfully attempts to extract his plans from him, but he teasingly refuses to tell her. In 3.1, just before Hotspur departs for SHREWSBURY, she joins him. He affectionately teases her about her refusal to sing while LADY (8) Mortimer serenades her husband. He finds another target in her mild oath 'in good sooth' (2.3.240), and he fondly scorns her temperance. These episodes reveal that the fiery Hotspur, whose rivalry with PRINCE (6) HAL is the play's major theme, is also a loving husband who has plainly inspired affection in his wife. Hotspur's warm relationship with his wife complements the fierce fixation with battle that otherwise dominates our picture of him. Without these scenes, Hotspur might seem so one-dimensional that we could not accept the favourable opinion of him held by King HENRY IV and Hal. Lady Percy also displays a personality of her own, that of a modest, possibly somewhat stiff, but spirited and pleasant young matron.

In 2.3 of *2 Henry IV* Lady Percy makes a single appearance, joining her mother-in-law, LADY (9) Northumberland, in persuading Lord NORTHUMBERLAND (1) not to rejoin the revolt. Lady Percy bitterly observes that the elderly lord had failed to assist the rebels when Hotspur was still alive, and she goes on to eulogise her late husband glowingly.

Lady Percy's name in Shakespeare's source, HOLINSHED's *Chronicle*, is given inaccurately as Elianor, but Hotspur calls his wife Kate. Shakespeare was decidedly fond of this name—he frequently used it, perhaps most notably for KATHERINA in *The Taming of the Shrew*—and he may have regarded it as an affectionate nickname for a woman, regardless of her real name.

Lady Elizabeth's Men Seventeenth-century LONDON theatrical company. Founded in 1611 and named for their patron, Princess ELIZABETH (3), Lady Elizabeth's Men spent a year touring the provinces before coming to London and playing under contract to Philip HENSLOWE. Among the members were William ECCLESTONE, John RICE, and Joseph TAYLOR. They performed at the ROSE, SWAN, and WHITEFRIARS THEATRES. In 1613 they absorbed the Children of the Queen's Revels (see CHILDREN'S COMPANIES) and, with them, Nathan FIELD (1), who became their leader. After two seasons at the HOPE THEATRE, the company sued Henslowe in 1615; some of the records of the case survive and provide a glimpse of the theatre world's business side. Sometime just before or after Henslowe's death in 1616, the company formed an alliance with PRINCE CHARLES' MEN, but Field had already left and soon the company failed, though it seems to have existed in the provinces for several years. In 1622 a new company called Lady Elizabeth's Men was formed by Christopher BEESTON, and it prospered briefly, but it was stricken by plague in the epidemic of 1625 and was not founded again. Princess Elizabeth had long been gone from England, and Beeston replaced Lady Elizabeth's Men with Queen Henrietta's Men, named for the new queen.

Laertes Character in *Hamlet*, son of POLONIUS, who seeks vengeance against HAMLET for his father's murder. Laertes is placed in direct contrast with Hamlet by the fact that each seeks and finally achieves revenge for his father's murder, although they do so in very different ways. Laertes is distinctly unheroic. He stoops to fraud and poison with no thought for consequences or morality. Yet at the close of the play he regrets his underhandedness, offers forgiveness in place of vengeance, and is himself forgiven.

Laertes is shallow and immature, as shown by the trite moralising that inspires his insistence in 1.3 that OPHELIA distrust Hamlet's love and by his rhetorical and exaggerated responses to his sister's insanity and death in 5.1. As an avenger, he is easily manipulated in 4.5 by the KING (5), who dissuades him from his rebellion with smooth talk about the divine right of kings. He gives no thought to honour as he accepts with grim glee the King's suggestion of a rigged fencing match, adding the idea of poisoning his sword. Moreover, he is thoughtlessly bold, prepared to sacrifice the peace of the country and his own salvation—'Conscience and grace, to the profoundest pit! / I dare damnation' (4.5.132–133), he bellows—to satisfy his rage.

Yet in the end Laertes begs to 'exchange forgiveness' (5.2.334) with Hamlet, and he admits that he is

'justly kill'd with mine own treachery' (5.2.313). 'The King—the King's to blame' (5.2.326), he cries, and, as he renounces his revenge, Laertes shifts the moral balance of the play in its last moments, leaving the King as the sole focus of evil. Laertes and Hamlet each kill his father's killer, while each forgives, and is forgiven by, his own killer. Contrasted earlier in the play—in their differing relationships with Ophelia, in Laertes' return to university while Hamlet is detained, in the contrast of a father's 'double blessing' (1.3.53) for Laertes and Hamlet's father's death and reappearance as the GHOST (3)—they come together at its close to represent the conjunction of good and evil in humanity, a fact whose acceptance is the play's major theme.

Lafew (Lafeu), Lord Character in *All's Well That Ends Well,* friend of the COUNTESS (2) of ROSSILLION. Lafew is an elderly gentleman who comments on the main action. He also introduces Helena to the KING (17), whom she cures, thereby winning BERTRAM as her husband. Lafew counsels Bertram, the Countess' son, to accept marriage to HELENA (2) and to reject the friendship of PAROLLES, but Bertram ignores him. Lafew is most prominent in 2.3.184–260, where he mercilessly insults Parolles, recognising that the foppish, boastful courtier lacks the nerve to fight. Lafew's temper justifies his name, the French for 'fire'. The episode clinches our recognition that Parolles is a coward and blusterer, though Bertram does not see this until later in the play. In 5.3 Lafew accepts the thoroughly defeated Parolles into his household as a FOOL (1), or jester, a generous gesture that exemplifies the play's spirit of reconciliation. Thus Lafew demonstrates the wisdom to be found in the courtly world of honour and patronage, both by exposing Parolles as a scoundrel and by sympathising with him later. Throughout the play, Lafew, with the Countess and the King, represents a world of wisdom and generosity that stands in contrast to the less pleasant major plot.

Lamb (1), Charles (1775–1834) English essayist, best known for his whimsical essays written under the pseudonym Elia. Lamb also wrote commentary on Shakespeare's plays, and with his sister Mary (1764–1847), he compiled prose renditions of the comedies and tragedies in *Tales from Shakespeare* (1807). Lamb's most influential critical work was his *Specimens of English Dramatic Poets who lived about the time of Shakespeare* (1808), which did much to revive interest in ELIZABETHAN DRAMA. He also wrote a notorious essay 'On the Tragedies of Shakespeare' (1811), in which he contended that the plays—especially *King Lear*—were unsuited for performance, though he also insisted that if they were staged, it should be done using Shakespeare's texts rather than adaptations. Lamb wrote essays on contemporary Romantic poetry as well; he was one of the first critics to recognise the genius of John KEATS, and Samuel Taylor COLERIDGE and William Wordsworth (1770–1850) were close friends. He wrote poetry himself, but neither it nor his fiction is widely read today, whereas *Tales from Shakespeare* and the collected *Essays of Elia* (1823, second series 1833) have continued to be popular.

Lamb's life was stricken by personal tragedy. Mental illness ran in his family; Lamb himself was briefly hospitalised for insanity in his youth and suffered from alcoholism all his life. In 1796 his sister Mary Lamb killed their mother in a fit of temporary madness; Lamb refused to have Mary institutionalised and cared for her the rest of his life.

Lamb (2), George (1784–1834) British politician, playwright, and poet, author of an adaptation of *Timon of Athens.* In 1816 Lamb composed an adaptation of Shakespeare's play with the intention of restoring the original text, which was heavily altered in presentations at the time. While Lamb's *Timon* retained some features of its immediate predecessors and failed to restore some omissions, it did employ most of Shakespeare's text. Produced by Edmund KEAN (2), who also took the title role, it was only moderately successful but may have paved the way for the first staging of the complete text, by Samuel PHELPS, a generation later.

Lamb had a varied career. After briefly practising law, he shared in the management of the Drury Lane Theatre in London. He staged two of his own plays—an operetta and a farce—besides *Timon.* He was probably best known for his translation of the poems of Catullus (c. 84–c. 54 B.C.), though both it and his own poetry are generally regarded as mediocre. Introduced into politics by his brother William Lamb, Lord Melbourne (1779–1848), twice prime minister, George Lamb was a member of parliament in 1819–1820 and again from 1826 to his death. He also served briefly as undersecretary of state.

Lambert, John (active 1587–1602) Shakespeare's first cousin and opponent in litigation. In 1588 John SHAKESPEARE (9), acting for himself, his wife, and his son William, sued his nephew John Lambert for the return of a piece of property—a house on 56 acres of land near STRATFORD—which Lambert had inherited from his father Edmund (c. 1525–1587), Mary ARDEN (2) Shakespeare's brother-in-law. This property had been mortgaged to Edmund by John Shakespeare in 1578, in return for a loan of £40 to be repaid in two years. The money was never repaid, and Edmund still owned the land at his death. According to the Shakespeares' complaint, John Lambert had agreed to accept £20 in return for clear title to the land, but Lambert denied this and won his case. John and Mary sued again in 1597 on different grounds but again lost. Lambert sold part of the property in 1602. The nam-

ing of Shakespeare in the legal papers of 1588 is the only surviving mention of the playwright between the baptism of Hamnet and Judith SHAKESPEARE (5, 10) in Stratford in 1585 and the mocking reference by Robert GREENE (2) to the young LONDON playwright in 1592. This mention has sometimes been thought to indicate that Shakespeare was in residence in Stratford or its environs at the time, but scholars generally agree that his technical involvement in the suit has little significance.

Lamprius Minor character in *Antony and Cleopatra*, an attendant of ENOBARBUS. Lamprius appears only once and does not speak; he is mentioned only in the opening stage direction of 1.2. Like RANNIUS and LUCILLIUS who accompany him, he is a GHOST CHARACTER. Some editors assume that Lamprius is the name of the SOOTHSAYER (2)—the stage direction reads '*Enter* Enobarbus, Lamprius, *a Soothsayer,* Rannius . . .'—though the Soothsayer appears to be an Egyptian in 2.3, and Lamprius is a Roman name. Shakespeare may have found the name in his source, PLUTARCH, who states that his own grandfather was named 'Lampryas'.

Lancaster (1) Family Branch of the PLANTAGENET (1) dynasty, major figures in Shakespeare's HISTORY PLAYS. The Lancastrian kings were descended from John of GAUNT, Duke of Lancaster, the third son of King Edward III (d. 1377). In 1399 Gaunt's son, Henry BOLINGBROKE (1), deposed King RICHARD II and ruled as HENRY IV. He bequeathed the throne to his son, HENRY V, in 1413. These events are dealt with in the major TETRALOGY of history plays, comprising *Richard II, 1* and *2 Henry IV,* and *Henry V.* When Henry V died in 1422, his son, HENRY VI, was an infant. In the absence of a strong monarch, opposition to the illegal deposition of Richard II revived, and the YORK (1) branch of the dynasty successfully pressed its claim to the throne, overthrowing Henry VI in 1461 (he was briefly reinstated in 1470–1471). The rivalry between Lancaster and York, culminating in the WARS OF THE ROSES, is the principal subject of the minor tetralogy, consisting of *1, 2,* and *3 Henry VI* and *Richard III.* The Yorkists were finally defeated in 1485 by the last Lancastrian, the Earl of RICHMOND. This distant cousin of Henry VI, who ruled England as Henry VII, founded the TUDOR dynasty.

Lancaster (2), John of Gaunt, Duke of See GAUNT.

Lancaster (3), Prince John of (1389–1435) Historical figure and character in *1* and *2 Henry IV,* son of King HENRY IV and brother of PRINCE (6) HAL. (The same figure appears in *Henry V* and *1 Henry VI* as the Duke of BEDFORD [1].) In *1 Henry IV* Lancaster first appears in Act 5, at the battle of SHREWSBURY, where his energy and valour are praised by the king and Prince Hal. He speaks only five lines, but his presence heralds his greater role in *2 Henry IV.* In that play he negotiates a truce with the rebels led by the ARCHBISHOP (3), only to seize the unsuspecting leaders once they have disbanded their troops. This treachery is followed by Lancaster's self-righteous utterance, 'God, and not we, hath safely fought today' (4.2.121). Then, in 5.5, he sanctimoniously praises Hal's rejection, as King HENRY V, of FALSTAFF.

Lancaster is portrayed as an uncompromisingly cold, calculating, humourless man. Falstaff says of him, '. . . this same young sober-blooded boy doth not love me, nor a man cannot make him laugh; but that's no marvel, he drinks no wine' (*2 Henry IV,* 4.3.85–88). He presents an extreme alternative to Falstaff's irresponsibility. But, although Falstaff is a far more attractive character, Shakespeare clearly felt that Hal's course as king must lie closer to Lancaster. Prince John's ruse at GAULTREE FOREST is not disparaged in the play. Such ploys were common in late medieval warfare, and neither Shakespeare's sources nor the playwright himself treat it as particularly heinous when compared to the much greater crime of rebellion against an anointed ruler.

Shakespeare inaccurately depicts the historical Prince John. His presence in *1 Henry IV* is fictional; he was only 13 years old at the time of Shrewsbury, and he does not appear in Shakespeare's sources until several years later. However, in addition to preparing for *2 Henry IV,* Shakespeare wished to bring the LANCASTER (1) family together at a point of crisis. Also, the 16-year-old Lancaster was not responsible for the negotiations at Gaultree; as Shakespeare knew, they were conducted by the Earl of WESTMORELAND (1). The playwright wished to attach this manoeuvre to King Henry's family, thus focussing on the web of treachery and conflict that followed Henry's usurpation of the throne (enacted in *Richard II*). John was not Duke of Lancaster—Hal bore that title, in fact—but Shakespeare's sources were confused on this point, and the playwright doubtless thought he was correct. The historical Prince John was a successful military leader who achieved distinction against the Scots and who was later, as Bedford, to help govern the kingdom when HENRY VI was a minor.

Lance Character in *The Two Gentlemen of Verona.* See LAUNCE.

Lane (1), John (1590–1640) Resident of STRATFORD who was sued for slander by Shakespeare's daughter, Susanna SHAKESPEARE (14) Hall. In June 1613 Lane allegedly declared that Mrs Hall had committed adultery with a local hatter, Raphael Smith (1577–1621). She promptly sued him, and when he failed to appear for the trial on July 15, she was formally declared innocent of any impropriety and he was excommuni-

cated. Lane was apparently a difficult man; he was tried in 1619 for riot and libel after he attacked—presumably by public verbal abuse—the vicar and aldermen of Stratford, and in the same year he was declared a drunkard by the churchwardens. Stratford was a small town, and the Shakespeare and Lane families were acquainted in other contexts. Lane's uncle, Richard LANE (2), was a business partner of Shakespeare's and his first cousin, Thomas NASH (2), later married Susanna's daughter Elizabeth HALL (3).

Lane (2), Richard (c. 1556–1613) Resident of STRATFORD, a business acquaintance of Shakespeare. Lane was a friend of Shakespeare's father, John SHAKESPEARE (9), who chose him in 1599 to help gather depositions in a lawsuit. In 1611 Lane joined William Shakespeare in a complicated lawsuit over tithe holdings (see COMBE [5]). In his will Lane appointed Shakespeare's son-in-law Dr John HALL (4) as trustee for his children, just a few days before Susanna SHAKESPEARE (14) Hall sued his nephew John LANE (1) for libel.

Laneman (Lanman), Henry (1536–c. 1592) English theatrical entrepreneur, owner and probably the founder of the CURTAIN THEATRE. Laneman was the owner of the Curtain during the period 1585–1592, when he and James BURBAGE (2), owner of the neighbouring playhouse, THE THEATRE, agreed to pool the profits of both theatres. In 1581 he was the lessor of the land on which the Curtain stood, and so he is presumed to have built it in 1577. Nothing else is known of him.

Langbaine, Gerard (1656–1692) English scholar and writer, the author of the first account of Shakespeare's sources. Langbaine's *Momus Triumphans, or the Plagiaries of the English Stage exposed* (1687) is a catalogue of the sources used by various Elizabethan and Jacobean playwrights, including Shakespeare. However, his treatment was brief and pedantic and was greatly superseded by the work of Charlotte LENNOX (2) and more modern scholars.

Langley, Francis (1550–1601) Goldsmith and theatrical entrepreneur in LONDON, owner of the SWAN THEATRE. Langley's name is linked with Shakespeare's in a mysterious lawsuit. Langley bought land on the south bank of the Thames near the ROSE THEATRE in 1595 and built the Swan, despite the opposition of the London government. However, in the summer of 1597, in the theatre's second season, PEMBROKE'S MEN staged Thomas NASHE's allegedly 'seditious' play *Isle of Dogs*, with the result that the royal CENSORSHIP closed all the London theatres for four months. After that Langley kept his theatre open only with difficulty. Upon his death, the theatre was sold to another London investor.

Records show that another company played at the Swan before Pembroke's Men, and the scholar Leslie HOTSON has established a relationship between Langley and Shakespeare, which suggests that the company was probably the CHAMBERLAIN'S MEN. The owner of the Swan and the playwright were named jointly in a legal paper, though their connection is unknown (see GARDINER [2]). The most plausible relationship between the two is that of theatre-owner and representative of an acting company, so it is concluded that Shakespeare's troupe probably performed at the Swan.

Lanier, Emilia (1570–1654) Mistress of theatrical patron Henry Carey, Lord HUNSDON (2), and possibly the Dark Lady of the SONNETS. Emilia Bassano was the illegitimate daughter of an Italian musician at the court of Queen ELIZABETH (1) and became the mistress of Henry Carey, Lord HUNSDON (2), when she was in her teens. In 1593 she became pregnant and was given some money and married to Alphonse Lanier, another court musician. The next year Hunsdon became the patron of Shakespeare's theatrical company, and it is possible that Emilia Lanier might have known Shakespeare through this connection. She might also have known the playwright through her husband's place in the world of court entertainment. The possibility that she was Shakespeare's Dark Lady rests chiefly on these connections, plus a description of her—by the astrologer, Simon FORMAN, with whom she may have had an affair—as a witch-like 'incuba', a characterisation thought to accord well with the poet's 'female evil . . . [who can] corrupt [a] saint to be a devil' (Sonnet 144.5–7).

Lanier's husband Alphonse was a wastrel, and they were soon impoverished. She published a book—a long poem on the women of the Bible—but it was not popular, and when Alphonse died in 1613, she was very poor. She opened a school, but it failed. Her son, Henry, a court musician to King Charles I, may have provided for her, but he died in 1633, and Lanier was left with the responsibility for his two children. She received a pension from the crown but died in near poverty.

La Pucelle See JOAN LA PUCELLE.

Lartius, Titus Legendary figure and minor character in *Coriolanus,* a Roman general. Lartius is a brave and capable officer who, despite earlier wounds, campaigns with MARTIUS (2) (later CORIOLANUS) against the town of CORIOLES, and leads the forces that join the heroic Martius after he has entered the city alone. After the victory, 'busied about decrees' (1.6.34), he commands the occupied town. He delivers a brief elegy when Martius is believed dead, and an even briefer compliment after the hero has triumphed. He

is inconsequential thereafter, a minor member of Coriolanus' entourage who disappears entirely after 3.1. Lartius helps establish our sense of the Roman military establishment; he represents the solid virtues of the Roman aristocracy in a play where the weaknesses of the class are more often seen.

Lartius appears at Corioles in Shakespeare's source, PLUTARCH's *Lives,* but much less prominently. Shakespeare invented his praises of Coriolanus, and, perhaps to make the praiser a more vivid figure, endowed him with the crutches he uses in 1.1.241. His spirited wager with Martius in 1.4.1–7 is also an addition, probably to the same end. Thus, Lartius offers an interesting example of the playwright's manipulation of a minor figure to develop the play's world.

Laughton, Charles (1899–1962) British actor. Laughton, who studied acting under Theodore KOMISARJEVSKY, is probably best known for his performance in the title role of the 1933 film *The Private Lives of Henry VIII* (not based on Shakespeare's play)—for which he won an Academy Award—and other movie roles, such as Captain Bligh in *The Mutiny on the Bounty* (1935) and the *Hunchback of Notre Dame* (1939). However, in the 1930s, Laughton succeeded in a variety of Shakespearean roles at the OLD VIC THEATRE, including PROSPERO, ANGELO, and MACBETH. Also, after years in Hollywood—he became an American citizen in 1941—he returned to England in 1959 and played BOTTOM and LEAR at the Shakespeare Memorial Theatre in STRATFORD.

Launce (Lance) Character in *The Two Gentlemen of Verona,* a CLOWN (1), the servant of PROTEUS. Launce is not involved with the plot of the play. However, the comparison of his jocular common sense with the absurdly rhetorical fancies of the protagonists helps to parody them, thus contributing to the play's tone. Launce's great speeches are his two prose monologues (in 2.3 and 4.4) about his dog, CRAB. In the first he bemoans the dog's lack of sympathy with his misfortune in having to leave his family to travel with Proteus. In the second, he recounts various canine offences that Crab has committed, such as urinating under the Duke's table and on SILVIA's dress. Launce himself has taken punishment for them to spare the dog. He also engages in two humorous dialogues with SPEED, one of which is preceded by Launce's soliloquy on his love life.

Launce prefigures later, more consequential Shakespearean clowns, such as LAUNCELOT Gobbo in *The Merchant of Venice,* DOGBERRY, in *Much Ado About Nothing,* and BOTTOM in *A Midsummer Night's Dream.*

Launcelot (Lancelot) Gobbo Character in *The Merchant of Venice,* comical servant first of SHYLOCK, then of BASSANIO, for whom he is also a professional FOOL (1). Launcelot carries messages and announces impending arrivals, but his role in the action is otherwise unimportant. His humour is clever and resourceful, but often broad and laced with standard devices. In 2.2, when he first appears, he wittily imitates legal precision in describing the overcoming of his conscience; in he same scene he draws on the ancient comic routine of mistaken identity, teasing his blind father, Old GOBBO (2). He frequently misuses words—a regular feature of Shakespearean clowning—as when he mistakes 'reproach' for 'approach' (2.5.20) and 'impertinent' for 'pertinent' (2.2.130). He engages Lorenzo in a battle of puns and deliberate misunderstandings in 3.5, and in 5.1 he raucously imitates the blare of hunting horns. A standard stage CLOWN (1), he has no particular personality aside from his buffoonish wit.

Launcelot is called 'clown' in the stage directions of old editions, but he does not have the rustic qualities sometimes associated with that stock theatrical figure (although the terms 'clown' and 'fool' were somewhat interchangeable), and here the term may merely indicate that the part was played by the clown of the company, who specialised in broadly comic roles.

Launcelot provides evidence of Elizabethan anti-Semitism. In 2.2 he delivers a comic monologue in which he recounts a dispute between his conscience and a fiend as to whether or not he should leave Shylock's service. This passage and Launcelot's subsequent conversation with his father help to establish Shylock's reputation as a miser in virulently anti-Semitic terms. Similarly, in 3.5 he jests with JESSICA on the likelihood of her damnation as a Jew, reflecting centuries of Christian prejudice. Although plainly intended as comical, Launcelot's attitude surely indicates something of the spirit in which Shakespeare's audience received Shylock—as an obvious villain, at least in part because he is Jewish.

Laurence, Friar Character in *Romeo and Juliet.* See FRIAR (4).

Lavatch (Lavache) Character in *All's Well That Ends Well.* See CLOWN (5).

Lavinia Character in *Titus Andronicus,* the daughter of TITUS (1) Andronicus, whose brutal rape and mutilation are the centre-piece of AARON's revenge against her father. After murdering BASSIANUS, her husband, TAMORA's sons CHIRON and DEMETRIUS (1) rape Lavinia and then cut out her tongue and cut off her hands so that she cannot testify against them. Directed by Aaron, they have improved upon OVID's tale of Philomel's rape by Tereus, who removed his victim's tongue but not her hands; she wove a tapestry that told the tale and exposed her attacker. Lavinia's plight is repeatedly compared to Philomel's. In fact, Lavinia

exposes Chiron and Demetrius by inducing Titus to look in a copy of Ovid's tales and find the example. She then spells out the villains' names in the sand with a wooden staff. When Titus kills the two, Lavinia is a witness and she goes with him to cook their bodies into the meat pie that is to be presented to their mother as revenge. Her father himself stabs her to death, emulating an old legend of a man who killed his raped daughter to expunge the family's dishonour

Law, Matthew (active 1599–1629) Publisher and bookseller in LONDON. Law bought the rights to three of Shakespeare's plays from Andrew WISE and then produced the third through sixth editions of *1 Henry IV* (1603, 1608, 1613, 1622), the fourth and fifth editions of *Richard II* (1608, 1615), and the fourth through sixth editions of *Richard III* (1605, 1612, 1622). Errors in the printing of each of these plays in the FIRST FOLIO (1623) point to delays in the setting of type for them; scholars attribute this delay to difficulties involved in securing Law's permission to republish them. Originally a draper, Law joined the STATIONERS' COMPANY in 1599; he had two bookshops for much of his career. He was fined several times for selling books on Sundays and for selling pirated texts.

Law Against Lovers, The Play by William DAVENANT based loosely on *Measure for Measure* and *Much Ado About Nothing*. Produced in 1662, *The Law Against Lovers* had a main plot that was a much altered version of *Measure for Measure:* the SUB-PLOT and MARIANA (2) are eliminated, ANGELO (2) turns out not to be a villain, and he and ISABELLA are married at the end. This was combined with some material from the BEATRICE and BENEDICK plot of *Much Ado:* Benedick is Angelo's brother and Beatrice is his ward. Davenant also introduced many melodramatic plot developments that had nothing to do with Shakespeare's plays and preserved only some of Beatrice and Benedick's banter and part of Isabella's confrontation with the imprisoned CLAUDIO (3). Most of the dialogue is by Davenant. Davenant declared his intention to 'save' Shakespeare by making the plays palatable to a new audience, but this play was unsuccessful, receiving only a few performances and remaining unrevived thereafter. Though Samuel PEPYS liked it, an anonymous satirical poet of the day differed, saying of Davenant that '. . . only he the Art of it had / Of two good Playes to make one Bad'. *The Law Against Lovers* nevertheless inspired an imitation, Charles GILDON's *Measure for Measure, or Beauty the Best Advocate* (1699), in which much of Davenant's text was retained, but the material from *Much Ado* was replaced by an operatic MASQUE.

Lawyer Minor character in *1 Henry VI,* an observer of the quarrel between the Duke of SOMERSET (3) and Richard Plantagenet (see YORK [8]). Called upon by Somerset for an opinion, the Lawyer answers with humorous exactitude, 'Unless my study and my books be false, / The argument you held was wrong in law . . .' (2.4.57–58).

Le Beau Minor character in *As You Like It,* a foppish nobleman in the court of the tyrannous DUKE (1) Frederick. ROSALIND and CELIA mock Le Beau in 1.2.86–114. He is fastidious in his diction but less so in his tastes; his description of brutal wrestling as 'good sport' (1.2.92) provokes TOUCHSTONE's quite sensible reply: 'It is the first time that ever I heard breaking of ribs was sport for ladies.' (1.2.128–129). However, Le Beau's affectations and callousness are offset when he warns ORLANDO of the Duke's evil intentions in 1.2. 251–275.

Leake, William (d. 1633) London publisher of several editions of *Venus and Adonis.* After buying the rights to Shakespeare's poem from John HARRISON (2) in 1596, Leake, a prosperous bookseller and officer of the STATIONERS' COMPANY, published six editions (Q5–Q10) between 1599 and 1617.

Lear Title character of *King Lear,* an ancient king of Britain. Lear rejects CORDELIA, his only honest daughter, when he mistakes her frankness for a lack of affection. He is then rejected by his other two daughters, REGAN and GONERIL, to whom he has granted his kingdom, and finds himself wandering in the wilderness, outcast and insane. His prideful wrath has blinded him to the difference between good and evil, but before the play's end he recovers his sanity in part, although too late to prevent the tragedy of Cordelia's death. However, in the course of his trials he does come to recognise his failings, which constitutes the play's most important lesson.

Lear's descent into madness, the central event of the play, illustrates the extent to which humanity can be degraded by its errors. Lear is both victim and perpetrator, for his own egocentricity has sparked the events that lead to his collapse; his ensuing suffering is a result of his inadequacy as a human being. Thus his story presents to us a powerful demonstration of humanity's frailty, and the consequent potential for tragedy in life.

Our horror at Lear's tale is alleviated somewhat by his partial recognition and acceptance of his failings. Lear's trials have been variously interpreted. They may be seen as comparable to God's punishment for sins; his recognition of his fault is followed by reconciliation with Cordelia, which is suggestive of God's forgiveness following a sinner's repentance. That the relief is accompanied by death suggests the importance of the Christian afterlife and its eternal mercy, but this promise is lacking in Lear's pagan world. In a non-religious interpretation, Lear's endurance is he-

roic in itself, and his triumph lies in his acceptance of his errors before he dies. These two interpretations are not, of course, mutually exclusive: Lear is heroic in both senses. Also, most commentators agree that Lear's suffering is finally redemptive, in that it leads to heightened consciousness on his part. Further, Lear's last words seem to indicate (though the question is disputed) that he dies believing that Cordelia is alive, which implies a happy resolution in death akin to that of GLOUCESTER (1), whose heart 'Burst smilingly' (5.3.198), and whose sufferings conspicuously parallel Lear's.

In the course of his wanderings, both physical and mental, the distracted Lear is able to understand his folly. He first recognises a general lack in his conduct as a ruler. Raving madly in the storm, Lear suddenly realises that he had been previously unaware of hunger and homelessness, and he sees that the knowledge would have been valuable to him as king. He tells himself 'Expose thyself to feel what wretches feel, / That thou mayst shake the superflux to them, / And show the Heavens more just' (3.4.34–36).

Lear comes to a more personal acknowledgement of fault, though his progress is fitful. At first, his guilt takes an unhealthy, morbid form, as he castigates himself for having fathered his daughters, seeing the fault in the sexual process rather than in his egotistical demands. While still on the stormy moor, he declares his torment to be 'Judicious punishment! 'twas this flesh begot / Those pelican daughters' (3.4.73–74). He elaborates on these sentiments when he equates female sexuality with the torments of hell, in 4.6.117–128. Lear's attitude towards sex—also displayed by EDGAR—is evidence of the unhealthy mental and moral state of the play's world.

However, before his lowest point, Lear learns of Cordelia's faithfulness and realises the wrong he has done her. As Kent reports, 'burning shame' (4.3.46) drives him from her camp. While wandering in the fields nearby, he encounters the blinded Gloucester and, stirred by the sight of another sufferer, acknowledges his own weakness—'they told me I was every thing', he says of his former courtly flatterers, adding sardonically, ' 'tis a lie, I am not ague-proof' (4.6.104–105). Later, as part of his remarks on patience, he declares the weakness of all humanity, firmly including himself. He is raving, but the tone of his lament is clear enough; the arrogance that informed his earlier vow of revenge is entirely gone. Finally, in Cordelia's presence, he declares himself 'a very foolish fond old man' (4.7.60) and admits that he has wronged her. He asks her to 'forget and forgive' (4.7.84), and later, as father and daughter are taken to prison, he is pleased at the prospect of perpetual atonement: 'I'll kneel down, / And ask of thee forgiveness: so we'll live . . .' (5.3.10–11).

Still, his insight is at best flawed. That a catastrophe and such a great degree of unhappiness has been necessary to elicit in Lear the acknowledgement of his faults and the existence of human ingratitude has been held against him by many readers. Shakespeare accepted no simple views on the complexities of life, and Lear is distinctly not a perfectly reformed man. Strikingly, no trace of guilt is found in his grief over Cordelia's death, and his enthusiasm for imprisonment with her is disturbingly egocentric in his lack of any sense of her life, as was his original demand for love, in 1.1. This point has been central to much recent feminist criticism of the play. However, Cordelia acquiesces and so do most audiences; the play's emphasis on forgiveness and redemption seems clear, and in this light, Lear's residual defects are perhaps best viewed as evidence of Shakespeare's honesty about human frailty. Finally, *King Lear* is a play that raises more questions than it answers, and the extent to which Lear's tragedy is illuminating to him—as opposed to us, for its potential for illumination is unquestionably clear—remains for us to contemplate.

Shakespeare doubtless believed that there was a historical king of Britain named Lear, as is recorded in his sources, but he is in fact a mythical figure. The name derives from a Celtic god of the sea, Llyr. The legendary king is reported to have founded the town of Leicester, whose name is related to his own (Lear + *castrum,* Latin for 'camp').

Lee, Sidney (1859–1926) British scholar, author of a standard biography of Shakespeare. Lee, an editor and writer of the *Dictionary of National Biography,* elaborated his dictionary article on the playwright into his *Life of William Shakespeare* (1898), which remained the definitive biography for decades. He wrote other books on Shakespeare, including *Shakespeare and the Modern Stage* (1906) and *Shakespeare and the Italian Renaissance* (1915); he also edited a facsimile edition (1902) of the FIRST FOLIO.

Legate Minor character in *1 Henry VI,* the papal ambassador who receives, in 5.1, the money the Bishop of WINCHESTER (1) owes the Pope for his promotion to Cardinal. The episode typifies anti-Catholic sentiment in England in Shakespeare's time.

Legh, Gerard (d. 1563) English antiquarian, author of a minor source for *The Taming of the Shrew* and *King Lear.* Legh's book on heraldry, *Accedens of Armory* (1562), contains a story that probably inspired the episode of the TAILOR in 4.3 of *Shrew;* it also includes one of many versions of LEAR's story, which provided some minor details for Shakespeare's play on the subject. A prosperous draper, Legh was largely self-taught. The *Accedens,* his only work, is a compendium

of miscellaneous heraldic lore in the form of a dialogue between a herald named Gerard and a knight named Legh.

Leicester, Robert Dudley, Earl of (1532–1588) English nobleman and theatrical patron. As patron of the acting company called LEICESTER'S MEN, Leicester was an important figure in the early history of ELIZABETHAN THEATRE, even though he merely gave the troupe the legal standing they needed and did not actively engage in the production of plays. Leicester was a favourite of Queen ELIZABETH (1) and may have been her lover, but the evidence is uncertain. Though already married, he was thought to aspire to a royal wedding; when his wife died suspiciously in 1560, rumour called it murder (historians generally disagree), so it may have been impossible for the queen to marry him even if she had wished to. She continued to demonstrate her favour in any case, giving him KENILWORTH CASTLE and making him Earl of Leicester.

Leicester became leader of an important political faction and intrigued against the queen's chief minister, Lord BURGHLEY. When he remarried in 1578, he acquired a stepson, the Earl of ESSEX (2), who came to share his hostility to Burghley. His marriage offended the queen, and Leicester was out of favour for several years, but resumed his position when given the command of English forces aiding the Dutch rebellion against Spain. The actor William KEMPE was in Leicester's retinue in the Netherlands, and some scholars speculate that the young Shakespeare may have been as well, though no confirming evidence exists. Leicester returned to England to take a high command in the army assembled to resist the Spanish Armada in 1588 and died of an illness soon after the crisis ended.

Leicester's Men Early English theatrical company. From at least 1559, the nobleman Robert Dudley, later Earl of LEICESTER, patronised a company of actors. Known as Dudley's Men until 1564, when their patron received his title, this troupe mostly toured the provinces. It did, however, play at the court of Queen ELIZABETH (1) several times between 1560 and 1562, perhaps because their patron was the queen's favourite, possibly her lover.

In 1572, when actors were declared vagrants unless supported by a nobleman (see ELIZABETHAN THEATRE), Leicester's Men was formally defined and its players named, including James BURBAGE (2) and Robert WILSON (4). In 1574 the queen declared Leicester's Men her own employees as well, licencing them to play anywhere in England, including LONDON. This challenged for the first time the London government's puritanical opposition to public theatre, an important watershed in the history of English drama.

For a decade Leicester's Men were the most important theatrical troupe in England, performing at Elizabeth's court and (after 1577) at Burbage's THEATRE. However, with the creation in 1583 of the QUEEN'S MEN (1), which was permitted to raid some of Leicester's best performers, their prominence diminished. In the summer of 1586, Leicester's Men played in STRATFORD, and this fact has prompted speculation that the young Shakespeare joined them at this time and returned with them to London to begin his career, although no other evidence supports this proposition. Upon Leicester's death in 1588, the company dissolved; some scholars believe that its members joined STRANGE'S MEN.

Leigh, Vivien (1913–1967) English actress. Leigh, the wife of Laurence OLIVIER, is best known as a movie actress, though she also performed a number of major Shakespearean roles on the stage, usually opposite her husband. Her most notable performances were as CLEOPATRA (1951) and LADY (6) MACBETH (1955).

Le Maçon, Antoine (active c. 1550–1580) French writer and translator. Le Maçon's translation of BOCCACCIO's *Decameron* was probably a subsidiary source for *All's Well That Ends Well* and a major source for *Cymbeline.* Shakespeare's chief source for *All's Well* was William PAINTER's translation of a tale from Boccaccio in his *The Palace of Pleasure,* but the playwright probably used Le Maçon's text also. Painter himself used it, alongside the original. The 'wager' plot of *Cymbeline* derives from a *Decameron* tale that was not translated into English before 1620, and Le Maçon's translation is one of several possible versions of the story that Shakespeare may have encountered.

Le Maçon was a courtier at the court of Princess Marguerite of Valois. His translation of Boccaccio was extremely popular throughout Europe as soon as it appeared in 1545; it was reissued 16 times during the 16th century. He also wrote a prose romance, published in 1550. Little else is known of his life.

Lennox (1) Character in *Macbeth.* See LENOX.

Lennox (2), Charlotte (1720–1804) English writer, author of the first substantial analysis of Shakespeare's sources. Lennox, who was also a novelist, wrote *Shakespear* [sic] *Illustrated; or, the Novels and Histories on which the Plays are founded* (1753), which covered more than half of Shakespeare's plays, thus improving greatly on its only predecessor, the work of Gerard LANGBAINE.

Lenox (Lennox), Thane of Character in *Macbeth,* a Scottish nobleman. Lenox functions as an attendant for most of the play. He is a silent companion of King DUNCAN in Act 1, and he speaks only a little when he arrives to join the king in 2.3, at the time of Duncan's

murder. After MACBETH is crowned, Lenox transfers his services to the new king and attends him silently in 3.1, and with a few words in 3.4 and 4.1. Only in 3.6—a misplaced scene (in the FIRST FOLIO text) that should follow 4.1—does Lenox assume any importance. In this scene he speaks against Macbeth and makes clear the extent to which his evil is loathed in SCOTLAND. Like his fellow thanes ROSSE and ANGUS, Lenox' chief significance lies in his rebellion, which demonstrates the extremity of the nation's disorder once evil has been permitted to flourish. In Act 5 Lenox serves the cause of Prince MALCOLM. Shakespeare's use of the name Lenox may have been intended as a compliment to the new English king, JAMES I, who was descended from an Earl of Lenox.

Leo Africanus (Joannes Leo) (active c. 1520) Moorish traveller and writer whose work may have influenced *Othello* and *Antony and Cleopatra.* Leo translated his writings on the regions now known as North, West and East Africa from Arabic into Italian. John PORY translated them into English in 1600 as *A Geographical History of Africa,* but they had been well known in England in Italian (and a French translation) since about 1550. Leo was among the first writers to replace ancient and medieval legends with real facts about the nations south of the Sahara (a word that Pory's translation introduced into English). His writings are still valuable for modern historians, providing a rare source of reliable information on pre-colonial sub-Saharan Africa. Pory's translation was a celebrated work in its day, and surely provided part of Shakespeare's background knowledge of North Africa, especially as reflected in 2.7 of *Antony and Cleopatra.* Moreover, Pory's preface included an account of Leo's life that is thought to have inspired OTHELLO's autobiographical remarks in 1.3.134–145. Leo's works also informed a number of other English writers, including PUTTENHAM, Richard EDEN, and Ben JONSON.

Leo Africanus, or Leo of Africa, was a North African Moor who crossed the Sahara a number of times as a free-lance soldier and scholar. He was captured c. 1520 by Christian naval forces in the Mediterranean and presented to Pope Leo X, who converted him to Christianity from Islam and gave him the baptismal name Joannes Leo.

Leonardo Minor character in *The Merchant of Venice,* servant of BASSANIO. In 2.2 Leonardo speaks one line when he is instructed to arrange Bassanio's trip to BELMONT.

Leonato Character in *Much Ado About Nothing,* father of HERO and uncle of BEATRICE. The governor of MESSINA, Leonato displays the formality that his position demands, but he is clearly a warm person, fond of his daughter and pleasant to all, offering avuncular advice to Beatrice and friendship even to the villainous Don JOHN (1). He enjoys a joke and is quite willing to participate in Don PEDRO's ruse to trick BENEDICK and Beatrice into falling in love. But Leonato displays little real personality until the crisis of the play. The deluded CLAUDIO (1) rejects Hero at the altar, asserting—with the backing of the prince, Leonato's superior, Don PEDRO—that he has seen her with a lover. Leonato is so sensitive about his honour that his immediate reaction is abysmal shame for himself and furious rage at his daughter. In an hysterical passage (4.1.120–154) that foreshadows the laments of King LEAR, Leonato wishes Hero dead. FRIAR (2) Francis quickly restores his belief in her innocence, however, and he sternly proclaims that he shall have vengeance; in 5.1 he challenges Claudio to a duel. However, in 5.4, Leonato presides over the general air of reconciliation that closes the play, forgiving the errant MARGARET (2) and accepting the repentant Claudio with a practical joke, disguising Hero as a mysterious cousin whom the sinner must marry in atonement.

Leonine Minor character in *Pericles,* the murderer hired by DIONYZA to kill MARINA. In 4.1 Dionyza urges Leonine to ignore his conscience, for he is reluctant to murder so fine a young woman; however, he agrees to uphold his sworn oath to do so. A civil murderer, he offers Marina time to say her prayers, and while she is doing so, he is interrupted by the coincidental arrival of marauding PIRATES, who kidnap his intended victim. Relieved to be freed from his obligation, Leonine nevertheless proposes to tell Dionyza he has in fact done the deed. As we learn in 4.3, Dionyza believed him, but she has also poisoned him to ensure secrecy. Leonine's brief appearance is thus filled with surprises, as first his conscience, then his viciousness, and finally his deceit, all prove insufficient. Such ironic changes are found throughout the play, and demonstrate that humanity is helpless before fate, an important theme for *Pericles* and Shakespeare's late plays in general.

In the *Confessio Amantis* of John GOWER (3), Shakespeare's chief source for the play, Leonine, which means lionlike, is the name of the PANDAR. The playwright presumably transferred the name to the murderer to make better use of its reference to a ferocious beast.

Leontes Character in *The Winter's Tale,* the King of SICILIA, husband of HERMIONE and father of PERDITA. Leontes' insane jealousy is the disorder at the centre of the TRAGEDY that comprises the first half of the play. In 1.2, convinced that Hermione has committed adultery with King POLIXENES of BOHEMIA, Leontes orders her tried for treason. In 2.3, believing the newborn Perdita to be Polixenes' child, he condemns her to abandonment in the wilderness. Even when the oracle

of Apollo declares Hermione innocent in 3.2, Leontes refuses to believe it. Finally, the death from grief of his son MAMILLIUS, taken as an act of vengeance by Apollo, convinces him, and he repents. However, Hermione is apparently dead of grief also, and the mournful Leontes 'shuts himself up' (4.1.19), emerging only in Act 5, after 16 years of 'saint-like sorrow' (5.1.2), to learn that both Perdita and Hermione have survived.

Shakespeare gives Leontes some weight as a particular person: he is about 30 in Act 1; he has inspired love in Hermione and Mamillius and demonstrates his own love for his son; he is conscious of public opinion when he sends messengers to the oracle to 'Give rest to th' minds of others' (2.1.191) and holds a trial that he may 'be clear'd / Of being tyrannous' (3.2.5). Nevertheless, his personality is not well developed, for it is not as a person that Leontes has importance. He functions as a symbol of disorder and chaos; he is not intended to be a realistic human being so much as an obstacle to happiness. He is villainous because the story calls for villainy, not from any well-established motive. His madness is as much a surprise to the other characters as it is to the audience or reader. Leontes is thus also a victim, a man rendered suddenly insane, subject to the whims of fate. It is highly significant that it takes an act of divine intervention to effect his cure. One of the lessons of the play—and of the ROMANCES in general—is that humankind depends on providence for happiness in an insecure world.

At the close of 3.2 Leontes subsides into grief, and there is a sense of calm acceptance of evil's consequences that resembles a tragedy's close. However, Leontes' repentance occurs as abruptly as the sin that made it necessary; it fails to produce any spiritual growth or any profound expressions of torment such as those offered by OTHELLO and LEAR. His repentance, like his jealousy, is archetypal. Still, though Leontes' psychology is not explored, his repentance nevertheless serves as a symbol of the gentler world in which the climactic reconciliations can occur.

Lepidus, Marcus Aemilius (d. 13 B.C.) Historical figure and character in *Julius Caesar* and *Antony and Cleopatra.* Lepidus is a member of the Triumvirate, the three-man governing committee that consists of Lepidus, OCTAVIUS (later Octavius CAESAR [2]), and Mark ANTONY. The Triumvirate rules Rome in the aftermath of the assassination of Julius CAESAR (1). Octavius imprisons Lepidus and then fights Antony for sole control of the Empire. In both plays Lepidus is a markedly weaker figure than his colleagues, and their casual dominance of him helps establish an impression of Roman power politics that is important in each work.

A minor character in *Julius Caesar,* Lepidus appears only once, in 4.1, when the Triumvirs decide on a list of political enemies that must be arrested and executed as part of their campaign against BRUTUS (4) and CASSIUS. After a brief exchange, Antony sends Lepidus on an errand and then belittles him to Octavius. He calls him 'a slight unmeritable man' (4.1.12) and a 'barren-spirited fellow' (4.1.36), and says he does not deserve a position as ruler. He compares him to an ass or horse, whose usefulness is limited and who will be turned out to pasture when he has fulfilled his role. Lepidus does not reappear in the play, and Antony's opinion of him seems appropriate. This episode may deepen our impression of Antony as a cynical political manipulator, or, may justify his boldness in seizing leadership in a power vacuum. In either view, Lepidus serves as a foil to sharpen our sense of Antony.

In *Antony and Cleopatra* Lepidus is similarly weak, though he plays a more prominent role in affairs. He is dominated by Caesar as the two confer on Antony's absence, in 1.4. In 2.4 he pointlessly urges reconciliation between Antony and Caesar, who are already intent on it, and he has little to say once negotiations are underway. He is again a minor player in the talks with POMPEY (2) in 2.6, and at the subsequent banquet he is the butt of a humiliating joke as he has been pressured into drinking too much. He makes a fool of himself and finally must be carried away—in pointed contrast to Caesar, who ends the party with a complaint about the ill effects of wine. The episode is comical, but even a SERVANT (21) recognises its significance for Lepidus' position in high politics, saying, 'To be called into a huge sphere, and not to be seen to move in't, are the holes where eyes should be . . .' (2.7.14–15). Lepidus disappears from the play at this point, though his fate is later reported: Caesar has accused him of treason and imprisoned him 'till death enlarge his confine' (3.5.11–12). Once again, Lepidus provides an example of the necessity for sharp wits and hard morals in the world of power politics, though here the contrast reflects more on Caesar than on Antony.

The historical Lepidus was indeed a lesser figure than his colleagues, though Shakespeare exaggerated this to emphasise the brutal competition of Roman politics. Lepidus was from a traditionally powerful Roman family. He supported Julius Caesar in his rise to power, and in the aftermath of Caesar's assassination in 44 B.C. he naturally allied himself with Antony. By chance, he commanded troops in the vicinity of Rome at the time, and he was able to control the city. It was at this point that he probably held as much real power as he ever would. In *Julius Caesar,* events are telescoped; the Triumvirate only came together after an 18-month period, during which Lepidus was courted by Antony and Octavius, and by BRUTUS (4) and CASSIUS. Upon the formation of the Triumvirate Lepidus was given control of Italy and Gaul, but soon Caesar took over these important commands and Lepidus was shifted to Africa, also important but more

remote. From this base, Lepidus assisted—though only slightly—in the defeat of Pompey's forces in Sicily by Caesar's general, AGRIPPA, in 35 B.C., soon after the events of Act 2 of *Antony and Cleopatra.* However, when Lepidus attempted to override Agrippa once the victory was assured, Caesar daringly entered Lepidus' camp, unarmed, and demanded his surrender to arrest. Lepidus' basic weakness was disliked by his own troops, and they seized him. He was forced to publicly plead for mercy, after which he was formally ousted from the Triumvirate. His treatment was better than is implied in Shakespeare, however. He was permitted to retain his post as Pontifex Maximus—the chief clergyman of the state religion—and was mercifully exiled to a comfortable retreat where he lived out his life.

Lessing, Gotthold Ephraim (1729–1781) German playwright and critic, the first important appreciator of Shakespeare in Germany. In 1767–1768 Lessing wrote a series of articles on German theatre that denounced its dependence on French plays and recommended the adoption of the ancient Greek dramatists and Shakespeare as primary models. These articles were extremely influential; they helped popularise the translations of Christoph WIELAND, and the critic J. G. Herder (1744–1803), a follower of Lessing, introduced Shakespeare to GOETHE, whose writings secured the playwright's place in German literary history. Germany's great enthusiasm for Shakespeare is often said to have begun with Lessing.

Lessing studied theology, literature, and philosophy before taking up journalism to make a living while he wrote plays, poems, and essays. He was greatly celebrated in his own time as Germany's leading man of letters. His plays *Miss Sarah Sampson* (1755), *Minna von Barnheim* (1767, considered one of the finest comedies in all literature), *Emilia Galotti* (1772), and *Nathan the Wise* (1769) are still performed in Germany and elsewhere. Lessing was the greatest representative of the German Enlightenment, and the first German writer to establish an international reputation.

Leveridge, Richard (c. 1670–1758) English singer and composer. Leveridge, a noted bass of his day, mostly composed SONGS, including music for several songs from Shakespeare's plays. He also wrote a burlesque of Italian opera, *The Comick Masque of Pyramus and Thisbe* (1716), that took its plot from the PYRAMUS AND THISBE episode in *A Midsummer Night's Dream.* He is one of several composers whom scholars believe may have written the incidental music for *Macbeth* traditionally attributed to Matthew LOCKE.

Leveson, William (active 1580–1612) English merchant, a trustee for Shakespeare's interest in the ground lease for the GLOBE THEATRE. The lease for the land on which the Globe stood was entered into by two parties, the Burbage brothers (see BURBAGE [1, 3]) and five members of the CHAMBERLAIN'S MEN acting jointly—Shakespeare, John HEMINGE, William KEMPE, Augustine PHILLIPS, and Thomas POPE (2). To make their shares independently saleable, the actors assigned their half to two trustees—Leveson and Thomas SAVAGE—who then regranted a fifth to each.

Leveson probably got this job through Heminge, whom he knew as a fellow parishioner of a London church. Leveson was an investor in overseas expeditions, serving at different times a member of the Muscovy Company (which traded to Russia), the Virginia Company, and the North-West Passage Company. Dudley DIGGES (1), son of Shakespeare's friend Thomas RUSSELL, was Leveson's fellow investor in all of these enterprises.

Lewis (1), the Dauphin (later King Louis VIII of France, 1187–1226) Historical figure and character in *King John,* son of King PHILIP (2) of FRANCE (1). Lewis joins his father in supporting ARTHUR, whose rightful inheritance of the English crown has been prevented by King JOHN (3). The French abandon Arthur's cause for a favourable peace, under whose terms Lewis marries John's niece BLANCHE. In 3.1, despite his bride's pleas, Lewis urges his father to support the pope and turn on John, and he later leads an invasion of England. He refuses to cease fighting when John makes his peace with Rome, insisting that France would be dishonoured by retreat. He withdraws only when deserted by the disaffected English lords who had been aiding him. Lewis is a superficially civil but treacherous Frenchman of a type that Shakespeare often depicted; here the stereotype not only heightens the patriotic sentiments of *King John,* but also stresses the motif of faithlessness that runs through the play.

The historical Lewis did invade England and was successful at first. However, the invasion was not prompted by the pope's quarrel with John, which had been settled earlier. In fact, it was undertaken in defiance of a papal prohibition; it was intended to place Lewis on the English throne, at the invitation of rebellious English barons. A reunited England under John's successor, HENRY (1), drove Lewis back to France. Lewis is frequently referred to as the Dauphin, or Dolphin, a title traditionally given to the eldest son of a King of France, as Prince of Wales is given to his English equivalent. However, this practise began only in 1350, so its application to Lewis is inaccurate.

Lewis (2) The Dauphin Character in *Henry V.* See DAUPHIN (3).

Lewis (3), King of France (1423–1483) Historical figure and minor character in *3 Henry VI,* King Louis XI of FRANCE (1). In 3.3 Lewis is insulted when King

EDWARD IV of England voids his agreement to marry the French King's sister-in-law, Lady BONA. Lewis agrees to back an effort by MARGARET (1) and WARWICK (3) to invade England and reinstate the deposed HENRY VI as king, thereby beginning another phase of the WARS OF THE ROSES.

In a gross over-simplification of years of foreign-policy manoeuvrings, Shakespeare presents a cardboard French king who simply wavers from sympathy with Margaret to alliance with Edward and back again. In reality, Louis XI, known as 'the Spider' for ruthless diplomacy, had long enjoyed good relations with Warwick. Upon Edward's accession, Warwick had backed an English alliance with France and had proposed the marriage to Bona, though nothing came of the idea. Edward, on the other hand, had opted for a connection with Louis' enemy, Burgundy. When Warwick initiated his coup in 1469, Louis discreetly provided him funds. Then, when Warwick was forced to flee England, it was Louis who initiated the alliance with Margaret in June 1470, six years after Edward's marriage to Lady Elizabeth. He financed Warwick's invasion and surely regarded the money as well spent, despite Warwick's ultimate failure, because the incident disrupted English politics significantly.

Licio Name employed in *The Taming of the Shrew.* See LITIO.

Lieutenant (1) Minor character in *2 Henry VI,* an officer, sometimes called a CAPTAIN (3), of a pirate ship. In 4.1 the Lieutenant distributes among his crew the prisoners his ship has taken; each crewman is entitled to extract a ransom from his prisoner. When Walter WHITMORE asserts a desire to kill his instead, the Lieutenant counsels mercy. However, upon learning that the prisoner is the Duke of SUFFOLK (3), the Lieutenant patriotically vows to see him slain, knowing that the Duke's ambitious conspiracies have harmed England. He delivers a virulent recital of Suffolk's political offences and sends him off to be executed by Whitmore.

Lieutenant (2) Minor character in *3 Henry VI,* a guard in the TOWER OF LONDON. When HENRY VI is released from the Tower upon his reinstatement as King in 4.6, the Lieutenant asks and receives the monarch's pardon for having been his gaoler. Henry assures him that he appreciates the Lieutenant's civil behaviour as a guard. When Richard (see RICHARD III) comes to murder the re-imprisoned Henry in 5.6, he dismisses the Lieutenant from his guard post.

Lieutenant (3) Minor character in *Coriolanus,* a Roman officer. In 1.7 the Lieutenant receives orders from LARTIUS to maintain control of CORIOLES, which the Romans have captured from the VOLSCIANS. He speaks only half a line in reply, in a episode whose purpose is to tell that the town has been captured.

Lieutenant (4) Minor character in *Coriolanus,* a follower of AUFIDIUS. In 4.7 the Lieutenant tells Aufidius that CORIOLANUS, who has deserted from the Romans, is growing in popularity among the VOLSCIANS. He regrets that Aufidius has permitted Coriolanus to command troops, because Aufidius is becoming overshadowed. The Lieutenant furthers the play's development with these remarks, for they inform us of Coriolanus' successes and spark Aufidius' hostile replies, which foreshadow the play's concluding episode.

Ligarius, Caius (Quintus) (d. 44 B.C.) Historical figure and minor character in *Julius Caesar,* one of the assassins of CAESAR (1). In 2.1 Ligarius (designated Caius in the FIRST FOLIO text and some modern editions), although ill, accepts the invitation of BRUTUS (4) to engage in an honourable exploit, saying, 'By all the Gods that Romans bow before, I here discard my sickness' (2.1.320–321). Though Brutus does not specify the nature of the deed, he refers to the planned assassination of Caesar, and Ligarius is among the conspirators who accompany Caesar to the Senate in 2.2, although he does not appear in the murder scene (3.1). Ligarius represents the stoical Roman virtues in disregarding poor health to follow duty; more important, his immediate, unquestioning acceptance of Brutus' leadership also demonstrates the authority that Brutus holds among the conspirators.

In 2.1.215–216 Ligarius is said to 'bear Caesar hard, who rated him for speaking well of Pompey'. In fact, the historical Ligarius had fought long and hard for Pompey the Great (106–48 B.C.) against Caesar in an earlier civil war and had been pardoned. In Shakespeare's source, PLUTARCH's *Lives,* he is said to have joined the conspirators out of hatred for Caesar's tyranny. He died shortly after the assassination, probably of natural causes. His name was actually Quintus; the error was Plutarch's.

Lillo, George (1693–1739) British dramatist, creator of a crude adaptation of *Pericles.* In his *Marina* (1738), Lillo used only the last two acts of Shakespeare's play, and he altered those almost beyond recognition. The moderate success of Lillo's version of *Pericles* does not attest to any popularity for the original play; on the contrary, it was the only production of *Pericles* (or rather, related to *Pericles*) during the 18th century.

Lillo was among the leading British playwrights of his day. His best-known work, *George Barnwell* (1731), is a melodramatic tale of a young Londoner led by passion to murder, which ends with a morally proper punishment. It is considered a good example of the 18th-century vogue for sentimental dramas set among the urban bourgeoisie.

Lincoln, Bishop of (John Longland, 1473–1547) Historical figure and minor character in *Henry VIII*, confessor to King HENRY VIII. In 2.4.209–214 Lincoln confirms the king's statement that as his confessor, he, Lincoln, advised Henry to pursue a divorce of Queen KATHERINE. His small part helps justify the king's action.

Longland, Bishop of Lincoln and Henry's long-time confessor, was later to record that the king hounded him at length about the divorce, insisting on his consent. Although Longland did consent—and was on one occasion stoned by a disapproving public—he later declared a change of mind. After the establishment of the Church of England, Longland became known for his religious intolerance and his support of the king's supremacy in matters of religious doctrine.

Ling, Nicholas (active 1570–1607) Printer, publisher, and bookseller in LONDON who produced the first two editions of *Hamlet*. In 1603 Ling and John TRUMBELL published the QUARTO edition known as Q1. It is a BAD QUARTO version of the play, recorded from the memories of actors, probably for this pirated edition. James ROBERTS had registered the play earlier, but he probably sold his rights to Ling, who also produced the first legitimate edition of *Hamlet*—employing Roberts as the printer—in 1604. In November 1607, shortly before his death, Ling sold John SMETHWICK the rights to *Hamlet*, along with those to *Love's Labour's Lost, Romeo and Juliet*—which he had bought from Cuthbert BURBY but never used—and THE TAMING OF A SHREW (a Bad Quarto of *The Taming of the Shrew*). Ling had also bought *A Shrew* from Burby, but he produced an edition of it (Q3, 1607) before selling the rights.

Lily (Lilly, Lyly), William (c. 1468–1522) English scholar and co-author of the standard Latin textbook of Shakespeare's day, known as *Lily's Latin Grammar*, which is quoted several times in the plays—e.g., in 4.1 (the 'Latin' scene) of *The Merry Wives of Windsor*, 1.1. 162 of *The Taming of the Shrew*, and 4.2.20–21 of *Titus Andronicus*. Lily's book, written in collaboration with the famous humanist scholar John Colet, was the basic text used at the Grammar School in STRATFORD, where Shakespeare was educated. Lily was a close friend of Sir Thomas MORE and the grandfather of playwright and novelist John LYLY.

Litio (Licio) In *The Taming of the Shrew*, the name HORTENSIO takes when he disguises himself as a music teacher in order to be appointed instructor to BIANCA (1).

Livy (Titus Livius, 59 B.C.–17 A.D.) Ancient Roman author of a Latin history of ROME, a minor source for *Coriolanus* and possibly an inspiration for *The Rape of Lucrece*. Livy's *Ab urbe condita* was translated by Philemon HOLLAND (4) as *The Romane Historie* (1600), and a passage from Holland's book is echoed in MENENIUS' famous 'belly speech' in *Coriolanus*. Livy's history also contains the story of LUCRECE and was probably consulted by Shakespeare in writing his poem on the subject, though whether it initially inspired him is unknown.

Livy was a prominent member of the literary circle surrounding the Emperor Augustus (see CAESAR [2]). His only major work was his immense history, covering Rome from its mythical beginnings until 9 B.C. He began it at the age of 30 and worked on it for 40 years. Of the 142 books that composed the work, only 35 survived into the Middle Ages, though summaries of most of the others were compiled by other Latin authors. The book made Livy famous even before it was completed, and it dominated the Western world's knowledge of Roman history until the RENAISSANCE. Modern scholars, however, give him more credit for his fine literary style than for the accuracy of his account.

Locke, Matthew (c. 1630–1677) English composer of church and theatre music, including incidental music for John DRYDEN and William DAVENANT's 1667 version of *The Tempest*. Locke was long believed to have written the once-famous incidental music to Davenant's *Macbeth* (1663), on the strength of an attribution published in 1708. Modern musicologists disagree, believing on stylistic grounds that the music was probably written by a later composer. (It is in any case based on the much older work of Robert JOHNSON [5] for Thomas MIDDLETON's *The Witch* [c. 1610–1620]; scholars attribute the revision to any of several composers, including Richard LEVERIDGE and Henry PURCELL.) Locke had a highly successful career before his early death. He wrote some of the music for the first English opera, Davenant's *Siege of Rhodes* (1656), and in 1661 he was named composer to the newly restored King Charles II.

Locrine Anonymous play sometimes attributed to Shakespeare, part of the Shakespeare APOCRYPHA. *Locrine*, a melodrama of ancient kings, was published by Thomas CREEDE in 1595 and credited to 'W. S.', possibly in the hope that the public would believe it was by Shakespeare. In 1664 it was published in the Third FOLIO, but modern scholars are confident that Shakespeare did not write the play, for it is very different from Shakespeare's work in style and content. However, a positive attribution has not been agreed upon. On stylistic grounds, Robert GREENE (2), Christopher MARLOWE (1), and various others have been nominated, while W. W. GREG discovered a copy of the 1595 edition with early 17th-century notes that ascribe

it to one Charles Tilney (d. 1586). Tilney is otherwise unknown as a writer.

Lodge, Thomas (c. 1557–1625) English writer, creator of the major source for *As You Like It.* Lodge, one of the UNIVERSITY WITS who dominated ELIZABETHAN DRAMA in the 1580s, wrote only two plays—one in collaboration with Robert GREENE (2). He was best known for his lyric poetry and a prose romance, *Rosalynde* (1590), that provided the central elements of *As You Like It.* Shakespearean scholars who believe many of Shakespeare's early plays were written collaboratively (see, e.g., FLEAY and ROBERTSON) have often cited Lodge as a possible co-author of *1 Henry VI, The Taming of the Shrew,* and others, but this theory is now generally deprecated. Lodge's very popular romantic poetry may have influenced Shakespeare in the writing of *Venus and Adonis,* though specific connections are absent.

Lodge is regarded as a minor writer whose work was chiefly derived from that of others; *Rosalynde,* for instance, is an imitation of John LYLY's novels. Son of the Lord Mayor of London, Lodge attended Oxford University and the INNS OF COURT, before commencing his literary career with a defence of poetry and drama against the attacks of Stephen GOSSON (2). He produced most of his literary work during the 1580s, after which he lived abroad and travelled—he was part of an expedition that explored South America in 1591 to 1593, for example. On his return, he practised medicine and wrote an account of his travels (now lost). A convert to Catholicism, he faced religious persecution and briefly fled the country in 1616. He died in near-poverty.

Lodovico Character in *Othello,* an emissary from VENICE to CYPRUS. Lodovico appears only towards the end of the play, arriving on Cyprus just as OTHELLO's madness approaches its climax. He serves a symbolic function, representing the life of normal society from which the main characters have been isolated since Act 2. On Cyprus, IAGO's influence can work its poison free of social or political affairs that might engage Othello's attention, and DESDEMONA cannot seek advice or intervention from other Venetian aristocrats. Lodovico is unable to prevent the catastrophe of Desdemona's murder, but in the final scene after Iago's duplicity has been exposed and Othello has committed suicide, Lodovico assumes the mantle of leadership and disposes of practical matters in the wake of the tragedy.

Lodowick In *Measure for Measure,* the name taken by the disguised DUKE (9) of Vienna.

London Principal city of England, a location in each of Shakespeare's HISTORY PLAYS and his residence for much of his life. In Shakespeare's time London was not only the great metropolitan centre of England, home to about 300,000 people (almost 10 percent of the nation's population); it was also the third-largest city in Europe (behind Naples and Paris) and was soon to be the largest. Outside the medieval walled city were new suburban expansions; to the south, across the Thames River via London Bridge, was SOUTHWARK, where the GLOBE THEATRE and several other theatres were established during Shakespeare's residency in the city (see ELIZABETHAN THEATRE).

Shakespeare lived in a number of known locales in London. In October 1596 he was assessed for taxes as a resident of Bishopsgate. This neighbourhood was near the north-easternmost city gate, beyond which, in the suburb of Shoreditch, was the THEATRE, where his acting company, the CHAMBERLAIN'S MEN, performed. However, by November he had apparently moved to the southern suburbs, for he was subject to the jurisdiction of the county of Surrey when he was involved in litigation between Francis LANGLEY and William GARDINER (2). The move probably reflects a season spent at the SWAN THEATRE by the Chamberlain's Men in the winter of 1596–1597. Shakespeare's tax bill followed him and was forwarded in 1600 to the diocese of Winchester, which governed the Clink, a neighbourhood in Southwark near the Globe, so Shakespeare probably lived there at the close of the 16th century.

The playwright can next be located in 1604 as the tenant of Christopher MOUNTJOY in Cripplegate, at the north-west corner of the city. He was probably there as early as 1602 and may have remained for some years after 1604, though no later evidence of a London address for him exists. After 1608 his principal theatrical venue was the BLACKFRIARS THEATRE, north of the river near the western wall of the city. Shakespeare probably moved back to Stratford by about 1610. His connections with the city were still strong, however, and he visited London several times after that, possibly staying at the MERMAID TAVERN, whose manager was his friend William JOHNSON (8). In 1613 he invested in London real estate, buying the BLACKFRIARS GATEHOUSE. Both the Blackfriars Theatre and the Blackfriars Gatehouse were on the grounds of the former BLACKFRIARS ABBEY.

London's buzzing life is frequently manifested in Shakespeare's work. In the English history plays, Shakespeare was dealing with events that often occurred in London, so many scenes are set there. Numerous buildings and other landmarks familiar to his London audiences are presented, including the TOWER OF LONDON, the INNS OF COURT, PARLIAMENT HOUSE, BAYNARD CASTLE, ST. JAMES PALACE, and Blackfriars Abbey. Especially common are interiors of WESTMINSTER (4) PALACE, where the political leaders often assembled.

Some scenes in the histories are particularly noteworthy for their vivid glimpses of the London populace. In Act 4 of *2 Henry VI* Jack CADE's rebellion spreads to the city from KENT (1) and we see the citizenry rise up in support of rebellion, as they did historically, not only for Cade but on other occasions as well. Incidents of Cade's rebellion occur at BLACKHEATH and SMITHFIELD, semi-rural areas adjacent to the city. Another aspect of civil disorder that London knew all too well was the helplessness of the common people in the face of aristocratic quarrels and civil war. This is well exemplified in 2.3 of *Richard III,* where several Londoners (see CITIZEN [2]) discuss the political situation in resigned tones. Another view of such politics is given in 5.2.1–40 of *Richard II,* where the Duke of YORK (4) describes a triumphal entrance into London, in which the assembled people hail the conqueror, BOLINGBROKE (1), and ridicule the fallen RICHARD II. Shakespeare's most famous depiction of the life of London is in the *Henry IV* plays, where much of the action is centred on the BOAR'S HEAD TAVERN in the neighbourhood of EASTCHEAP. There a colourful subsection of city life, the world of petty thieves and slumming aristocrats, is presented with infectious gusto.

Sometimes scenes in plays set elsewhere in Europe reflect the realities of life in London in a manner familiar to London audiences. For instance, the VENICE of *The Merchant of Venice* offers a satirical slant on the business world of Shakespeare's London, and the VIENNA of *Measure for Measure* includes a sort of Eastcheap underworld. The outbreak of plague in VERONA, with its 'searchers of the town' (*Romeo and Juliet* 5.2.8), reflects a disaster that was common in London. Further, the politically unruly commoners of London seem to inhabit the ROME of *Julius Caesar* and *Coriolanus* (see CARPENTER, COBBLER, COMMONER [1, 2], PLEBEIANS).

London Prodigal, The Play formerly attributed to Shakespeare, part of the Shakespeare APOCRYPHA. *The London Prodigal,* a domestic comedy of a prodigal husband's reformation by his wife, was published in 1605 by Nathaniel BUTTER, who ascribed it to Shakespeare. This was probably a conscious fraud, for *The London Prodigal* is totally unlike Shakespeare's plays. Its characters are uniformly shallow, its poetry is weak, and it is of a genre unused by Shakespeare—a comedy set in contemporary London. Though the editors of the FIRST FOLIO rejected it, the play was again published as Shakespeare's in the Third and Fourth Folios (see FOLIO) and in the editions of Nicholas ROWE and Alexander POPE (1). The authorship of *The London Prodigal* remains unknown, though some scholars attribute it to Thomas MARSTON.

Longaville (Longueville) Character in *Love's Labour's Lost,* one of the gentlemen who fall in love and thus disrupt the ascetic academic programme of the KING (19) of Navarre. In 1.1 Longaville is enthusiastic about the King's idea, but he falls in love with MARIA (1), one of the ladies-in-waiting to the PRINCESS (1) of France, and, along with the King and the other courtiers, he breaks his vow and abandons scholarship for love.

Longaville's name was taken from that of a French contemporary of Shakespeare, the Duc de Longueville, a well-known figure in the Wars of Religion. Longueville was an aide to Henri de Bourbon, who was the historical King of Navarre and later ruled France as Henri IV.

Longleat Manuscript Single page containing the earliest known illustration from Shakespeare, a scene taken from *Titus Andronicus.* This document, in the library at Longleat, the estate of the Marquess of Bath, bears a semi-legible date, generally held to be 1594 or 1595, and is signed by Henry Peachem (c. 1576–1643), an artist and writer. The illustration, at the top of the page, depicts TAMORA on her knees before TITUS (1) Andronicus, with two bound figures behind her on the right and AARON behind them. At the left, behind Titus, are two soldiers bearing halberds. Below the picture is a text consisting of Tamora's plea for mercy when her son is to be sacrificed (1.1.104–120) and the captive Aaron's defiant proclamation of his own evil (5.1.125–144). These speeches are linked by three lines not from the play, presumably composed by Peachem. It is speculated that the Longleat manuscript may have been created for a private, amateur theatrical production.

Longueville See LONGAVILLE.

Lopez, Roderigo (d. 1594) Contemporary of Shakespeare, a Portuguese doctor living in England whose trial and execution for treason may have helped inspire the composition of *The Merchant of Venice.* Lopez, born Jewish but a Christian convert, fled the Portuguese Inquisition in 1579 and by 1586 was appointed physician to Queen ELIZABETH (1). In 1592 he entered into a dangerous intrigue involving a pretender to the Portuguese throne, and he appears to have antagonised the powerful Earl of ESSEX (2), who accused him of plotting to poison the Queen. Although Lopez was almost certainly innocent, some of his servants testified under torture that the charge was true, and he was hanged on June 7, 1594. His trial stimulated an outbreak of anti-Semitic feeling in London and also spurred a series of revivals of *The Jew of Malta,* by Christopher MARLOWE (1). It has often been thought that when GRATIANO (1) insultingly tells Shylock that his soul is that of 'a wolf . . . hanged for human slaughter' (4.1.134), he was punning on Lopez' name, which means 'wolf'.

Lord (1) Character in *The Taming of the Shrew,* a country gentleman who appears in the INDUCTION. The Lord takes in the besotted and unconscious Christopher SLY (1) and, as a practical joke, installs the rustic tinker in his home as a gentleman. The Lord is not a three-dimensional character, but he offers a plausible picture of a country gentleman amid his pleasures.

Lord (2) Minor character in *Richard II,* an accuser of the Duke of AUMERLE in 4.1. The Lord asserts that Aumerle falsely denied his complicity in an earlier murder plot, and he challenges Aumerle to a trial by combat. His accusation and challenge follow several others and lend a vivid sense of excess and confusion to the scene, thereby suggesting the potential for chaos produced by the victory of BOLINGBROKE (1) over King RICHARD II.

Lord (3) Minor character in *Much Ado About Nothing,* follower of CLAUDIO (1). The Lord walks with Claudio in HERO's supposed funeral procession in 5.3; he speaks only one line.

Lord (4) Any of several minor characters in *As You Like It,* noblemen in the court of the exiled DUKE (7) Senior. In 2.1 two Lords tell the duke of an encounter with JAQUES (1), and in 2.7 they attend the duke's forest banquet. They also seem likely to be the unspecified 'others' of several stage directions—e.g., at the opening of 2.5.

In addition, two other Lords, from the court of the evil DUKE (1) Frederick, tell their master in 2.2 that ROSALIND, CELIA, and TOUCHSTONE have fled his court.

Lord (5) Any of several minor characters in *Hamlet,* members of the court of the KING (5) of DENMARK. In 4.3 the Lords provide an audience for the King's remarks on the danger of Prince HAMLET's madness. In 5.1 they attend the funeral of OPHELIA and help break up the fight between Hamlet and LAERTES. In 5.2 one of the Lords delivers a request from the QUEEN (9) that Hamlet make peace with Laertes before their upcoming fencing match, and the Lords are presumably among the crowd of courtiers—'all the State' in the stage direction at 5.2.220—who witness that contest. As anonymous onlookers, the Lords heighten our sense of Hamlet's isolation, and they also contribute to a sense of the stratified social world in which the prince lives.

Lord (6) Either of two characters in *All's Well That Ends Well,* French noblemen. Though distinguished as the First Lord and the Second Lord, these two characters are very similar and serve the same dramatic purpose. Reappearing throughout the play, they offer a distinct viewpoint on its developments, especially on the progress of BERTRAM and PAROLLES, and they help to mould the audience's opinions. Recognising the dishonourable cowardice of Parolles, they devise a plan to expose him to Bertram. They recognise Bertram's moral weakness, but they believe in his capacity for improvement, thereby offsetting our possible distaste for him. In addition, their fond admiration of the KING (17) in 1.2 and 2.1 stimulates our appreciation of him, which in turn influences our opinions of Bertram and HELENA (2) when the King shows affection for them. The Lords encourage our positive response to Helena when they sympathise with her abandonment by Bertram in 3.2, while at the same time they downplay Bertram's guilt by blaming Parolles for his behaviour.

The Lords are stereotypes of noble courtiers, and they lack individual personalities. Their parts differ slightly only once, when, at the end of 3.6, the First Lord assumes the job of capturing Parolles while the Second Lord leaves with Bertram for an off-stage visit to DIANA (1), thus enabling him to report on Bertram's attempted seduction when the two Lords critique the young count in 4.3.

In the FIRST FOLIO text of the play, the First and Second Lords are respectively designated 'G' and 'E' in speech headings and stage directions. These initials are presumed to refer to actors in the KING'S MEN who played the parts, probably William ECCLESTONE and Samuel GILBURNE or Robert GOUGH.

Lord (7) Any of four minor characters in *All's Well That Ends Well,* young noblemen whom HELENA (2) rejects as possible husbands. In 2.3, having recovered his health through Helena's treatment, the KING (17) offers her the agreed-upon reward: her choice of a husband from among the young men of his court. She speaks to several of the Lords before choosing BERTRAM, as she had intended all along. The rejected Lords merely comprise a tableau of knightly personages; they speak only three lines among them.

Lord (8) Any of several minor characters in *Macbeth,* members of MACBETH's royal court. In 3.4 several Lords are present at a banquet and witness Macbeth's distress at the appearance of the GHOST (4) of BANQUO. They accept LADY (6) MACBETH's explanation—that the king is suffering the effects of an old illness—and depart. In 3.6 a single, unidentified Lord meets with LENOX, and they observe that Prince MALCOLM has arrived in England, and that Macbeth has defected to his cause. In both scenes, the anonymous noblemen bear witness to the unravelling of Macbeth's power.

Some scholars agree with the suggestion of Samuel JOHNSON (7) that the FIRST FOLIO stage direction calling for 'Lenox and another lord' at the opening of 3.6 was an error that resulted from the misinterpretation of a manuscript abbreviation—'An'.—for ANGUS, who was actually intended as Lenox' companion. This idea

cannot be proven, and in any case, as Angus is a minor character like the Lords, the effect would be identical.

Lord (9) Any of several minor characters in *Coriolanus,* noblemen of ANTIUM. In 5.6 AUFIDIUS presents the Lords of the City, as they are designated in the stage directions, with his evidence that CORIOLANUS has betrayed the Volscian army, which he had joined when he was banished from ROME. Aufidius' inflammatory speech rouses the crowd (see COMMONER [2]) into a lynch mob, while various Lords—designated as First, Second, and Third Lord—attempt to keep order without effect. Like MENENIUS in Rome, the Lords are peaceable men whose efforts to control the mob are ineffective when faced with a leader who can manipulate the shifting moods of the common people. Thus, they help demonstrate an important point of the play: that the common people are unreliable participants in political life.

Lord (10) Any of several minor characters in *Timon of Athens,* flatterers of TIMON. In 1.1 two Lords—designated First and Second Lords but indistinguishable from one another—are criticised by APEMANTUS as dishonest flatterers whose intent is to profit from Timon's generosity. As soon as he departs, the Lords laugh over their good fortune in knowing Timon, and it is clear that Apemantus' judgement was correct. In 1.2 a Third Lord joins them and their flattery is again mocked by Apemantus; all are rewarded with expensive gifts. In 3.6 four Lords gather to receive more bounty, even after they have given patently self-serving excuses why they cannot make loans to the newly impoverished Timon. However, Timon curses them and throws them out, and we see no more of them. The Lords have one personality trait between them—they are greedy hypocrites. They talk about their generosity, but are actually misers. Some commentators have identified these characters with Timon's faithless friends, LUCIUS (3), LUCULLUS, SEMPRONIUS, and VENTIDIUS (2).

Lord (11) Any of several minor characters in *Pericles,* gentlemen of PERICLES' court. The Lords appear briefly in 1.2, flattering Pericles. HELICANES denounces them and thereby gains the confidence of Pericles, who puts him in charge when he leaves TYRE. In 2.4 a group of Lords insist that Tyre needs a resident ruler and that if Pericles does not return, Helicanes should take his place. Helicanes puts them off for a year while he sends for Pericles, who returns to Tyre and is thus separated from his wife and child. Thus, the Lords further the inexorable workings of fate.

Lord (12) Minor character in *Pericles,* a gentleman of THARSUS. In 1.4 the Lord brings CLEON word that a convoy of ships approaches. Though Cleon fears invasion, the Lord observes that the ships bear flags of truce. Sent to escort the arrivals to Cleon, the Lord returns with PERICLES. The Lord is not a developed character, though his common sense presents a mild opposition to Cleon's pessimism.

Lord (13) Any of several minor characters in *Pericles,* attendants of King SIMONIDES of PENTAPOLIS. At the king's jousting tournament in 2.2, three of the Lords mock PERICLES who is wearing rusty armour. This elicits Simonides' observation that 'Opinion's but a fool, that makes us scan / The outward habit by the inward man' (2.2.55–57). The Lords speak only eight lines between them and serve to introduce this single point.

Lord (14) Minor character in *Pericles,* an attendant of LYSIMACHUS. In 5.1 Lysimachus confers with HELICANUS about the speechless despair of PERICLES, and a member of his retinue, the First Lord, reminds his master of the extraordinary qualities of MARINA, who may be able to 'win some words of him' (5.1.43). This timely suggestion brings about the climactic reunion of Pericles and Marina. The fact that the suggestion is made by a minor figure maintains the dignity of Lysimachus—who should not seem preoccupied with Marina—and adds to the atmosphere of courtly formality with which the play abounds.

Lord (15) Any of several minor characters in *Cymbeline,* noblemen at the court of King CYMBELINE. In 1.3 and 2.1 two of the noblemen are featured as followers of the uncouth Prince CLOTEN; the First Lord is attentive and flattering, but the Second Lord mocks the obnoxious prince behind his back, which helps to characterise the play's comic villain. In Acts 3–5, the Lords play a smaller part as often-silent figures who swell the scene at Cymbeline's court. A single Lord appears in 5.3 as a soldier who has fled from the battle against the Romans. Though this could possibly be a different person, POSTHUMUS' disdain for him would be appropriate if he were one of Cloten's followers. In any case, this Lord serves to receive information as Posthumus tells him—and the audience—of the battle's outcome.

Lord (16) Any of several minor characters in *The Winter's Tale,* followers of King LEONTES of SICILIA. A Lord, one of several present, objects to Leontes' brutal imprisonment of his Queen HERMIONE for adultery with King POLIXENES of BOHEMIA. When another Lord, ANTIGONUS, supports the first in his certainty that Hermione is innocent, the king goes so far as to admit that he has submitted the question to the oracle of Apollo. The Lords are present in 2.3 when the raging king sentences his infant daughter, PERDITA, to death. Again, they and Antigonus temper the king's course somewhat, although Leontes still orders the baby

abandoned in the wilderness. The Lords are present at Hermione's trial in 3.2 and a Lord announces the return of King Polixenes in 5.1, but their chief function has already been filled. They help maintain a background of outraged virtue against which the madness of Leontes stands out in the first, tragic half of the play.

Lord (17) Bardolph Character in *2 Henry IV*. See BARDOLPH (2).

Lord (18) Chamberlain Character in *Henry VIII*. See CHAMBERLAIN (2).

Lord (19) Chancellor Character in *Henry VIII*. See CHANCELLOR.

Lord (20) Chief Justice Character in *2 Henry IV*. See CHIEF JUSTICE.

Lord (21) Marshal Character in *Richard II*. See MARSHAL (1).

Lorenzo Character in *The Merchant of Venice*, suitor and then husband of JESSICA. A friend of ANTONIO (2) and BASSANIO, Lorenzo is a stock theatrical figure, a stylish young aristocrat with little distinctive personality. However, the rhapsodies of Lorenzo and Jessica on moonlight and music in 5.1 provide the play's finest lyric poetry. Lorenzo's musing on the music of the spheres (5.1.55–65) presents an idea of universal harmony that is appropriate to the play's conclusion, in which the oppositions that have been its principal substance—love versus greed, justice versus mercy—are resolved.

Love in a Forest Play by Charles JOHNSON (2) based loosely on *As You Like It*. Produced in 1723, *Love in a Forest* was the first version of Shakespeare's play to appear for more than a century, but it was a radically changed text. It incorporated elements from several of Shakespeare's other plays—including *A Midsummer Night's Dream, Much Ado About Nothing, Twelfth Night,* and even *Richard II*—and eliminated a number of characters, among them TOUCHSTONE, AUDREY, WILLIAM (2), PHEBE, and CORIN. Colley CIBBER (1) played JAQUES (1). Popular for a time, *Love in a Forest* was superseded in the 1740s by a production of *As You Like It* itself.

Lovell (1) (Lovel), Sir Francis (1454–1487) Historical figure and character in *Richard III*, a supporter of RICHARD III. Lovell is willing to undertake Richard's dirty work; he assists RATCLIFFE in the execution of HASTINGS (3), bringing that lord's severed head to Richard in 3.5.

The historical Lovell was Richard's Lord Chamberlain. He escaped capture after the battle of BOSWORTH FIELD and died two years later, fighting in an uprising against RICHMOND, by then King Henry VII. He was a distant cousin of Sir Thomas LOVELL (2), who appears in *Henry VIII*.

Lovell (2), Sir Thomas (d. 1524) Historical figure and minor character in *Henry VIII*, a follower of Cardinal WOLSEY and later Bishop GARDINER (1). Lovell appears as a member of Cardinal Wolsey's entourage in Acts 1 and 3. In 1.3–4 his bawdy banter helps establish the decadent flavour of King HENRY VIII's court while it is under the influence of Wolsey. In 2.1 he appears briefly to escort BUCKINGHAM (1) to his execution, a fate arranged by Wolsey. Here, however, he expresses sympathy for the Duke, in an incident that provides evidence of Buckingham's virtues, in contrast to Wolsey's vices. In 5.1 Bishop Gardiner has become Wolsey's successor as villain, and Lovell's support signifies as much; a pawn of the plot, he also provides the audience with information on the new political situation. The historical Lovell was a distant cousin of Sir Francis LOVELL (1), who appears in *Richard III*.

A Lover's Complaint Poem accompanying the SONNETS in their first edition (1609). A 329-line poem in RHYME ROYAL, *A Lover's Complaint* has often been declared non-Shakespearean, chiefly due to its inferior poetry, but current scholarly opinion finds it likely to be an early work of Shakespeare's. The poem consists largely of a monologue delivered to an aged shepherd (who never speaks and goes unmentioned after his introduction) by a distraught young woman who has been betrayed by her lover. Her complaint is overheard by an unnamed narrator who also disappears from the poem once he has set the scene.

The woman tells of having encountered a man whom everyone loved, a paragon of male beauty and wit. She realised, however, that he repeatedly broke his vows of love and fathered many illegitimate children, and she vowed not to succumb to him. However, when he approached her, he acknowledged his reputation but insisted that only in knowing her had he experienced true love. He wept because she could not love him, and she gave in and slept with him. Now, in disgrace and apparently abandoned, she regrets having fallen prey to his wiles, while admitting that he was so attractive that she might do the same thing again.

The COMPLAINT, the genre to which the poem belongs, was very popular in the 1590s, and *A Lover's Complaint* may be, like *Venus and Adonis* and *The Rape of Lucrece*, a product of the young playwright's enforced idleness during the period when the London theatres were closed by a plague epidemic (June 1592–May 1594). If Shakespeare wrote it, it is unquestionably an immature and undeveloped work, particularly in its presentation of personality—as a result of which some

have felt it may date from even earlier in Shakespeare's career—but it does contain pleasing passages, and it is in fact a quite respectable example of Elizabethan verse. On the other hand, it is an essentially trivial work—unlike the two narrative poems, most of the sonnets, and *The Phoenix and Turtle,* the acknowledged Shakespearean poems—and it contains a high percentage of words not found elsewhere in Shakespeare's works; these considerations argue against its inclusion in the Shakespearean CANON. The matter cannot be satisfactorily settled unless new evidence appears, which is unlikely, so *A Lover's Complaint* is best appreciated as a piece of good Elizabethan poetry that can suggest something of the poet's relation to the literary world of his day. If it is by Shakespeare, it is certainly among the least of his works.

Love's Labour's Lost

SYNOPSIS

Act 1, Scene 1
The KING (19) of Navarre proposes to dedicate himself and his courtiers to the pursuit of scholarship. He requires his three gentlemen-in-waiting to sign an oath, swearing off revelry, banqueting, and the company of women for three years. LONGAVILLE and DUMAINE sign readily, but BEROWNE argues against such rigour. He points out a problem with forbidding the company of women: the PRINCESS (1) of France is scheduled to arrive shortly. The King agrees that she will have to be an exception. DULL, a constable, appears with COSTARD, a CLOWN (1), and delivers a comically rhetorical letter from ARMADO, a visiting Spaniard whose ludicrous pedantry is well known. The letter accuses Costard of speaking with JAQUENETTA, contrary to the King's proclamation against consorting with women. The King sentences Costard to a week's diet of bran and water, to be overseen by Armado.

Act 1, Scene 2
Armado and his page, MOTH (1), exchange pedantries; the saucy page mocks his master, who is too slow-witted to notice. Armado confesses his love for Jaquenetta, but he feels ashamed of it because she is a common country girl. Costard, Dull, and Jaquenetta appear. Dull announces Costard's scheduled fast. Before Jaquenetta departs with Dull, Armado speaks to her of his love; she is cool. Armado angrily sends Costard away to be imprisoned, in the custody of Moth, and soliloquises ruefully on the power of love.

Act 2, Scene 1
The Princess of France and her entourage arrive. In light of rumours concerning the King's vow to exclude women from his court, the Princess sends her adviser BOYET ahead to announce her approach. She talks with her waiting-women about the King of Navarre's courtiers, whom they have met before. MARIA (1) praises Longaville, KATHARINE (1) admires Dumaine, and ROSALINE (1) is taken with Berowne. Boyet returns and announces that the King, who is arriving with his courtiers, plans to house the visiting women in tents outside the court, in accordance with his vows. The King and his courtiers arrive. The Princess upbraids the King for his poor hospitality, and she delivers a written message from her father. The courtiers converse with the ladies. Berowne and Rosaline exchange witty remarks; she sharply parries his advances. The King apologises for the accommodations he must provide because of his oath, and he and his retinue depart. Dumaine, Longaville, and Berowne each re-enter in turn to inquire of Boyet the name of the gentlewoman he has been conversing with.

Act 3, Scene 1
Armado orders Moth to free Costard, who is to deliver a love letter to Jaquenetta. Moth goes, after teasing his master about his infatuation, and returns with Costard, who is given the letter. Berowne enters and commissions Costard to deliver a letter to Rosaline. Costard departs, and Berowne, in a soliloquy, despairs that he has been captured by love.

Act 4, Scene 1
Costard interrupts the Princess' deer-hunting party to deliver Berowne's letter to Rosaline. The Princess gleefully asks Boyet to open it and read it aloud. However, Costard has delivered the wrong letter; it is Armado's letter to Jaquenetta, and its preposterous style causes great glee.

Act 4, Scene 2
HOLOFERNES, a comically pedantic schoolmaster, and his follower NATHANIEL (1) discuss the deer hunt in absurdly scholastical terms, to the consternation of Dull. Jaquenetta appears with Costard, seeking a literate person to read her the letter she has received. Nathaniel reads it; it is a sonnet by Berowne, intended for Rosaline. Holofernes realises that it has been misdelivered, and he instructs Jaquenetta to take it to the King, for it may be important.

Act 4, Scene 3
Berowne, alone, again bemoans the fact that he is in love. He hides himself as the King approaches. The King reads a poem he has written and reveals that he, too, is in love. The King also hides when Longaville appears, and Longaville does the same thing, hiding in his turn when Dumaine appears and also reads a love poem. As Dumaine finishes, Longaville comes forth to tease him, but the King in turn chastises them both for breaking their ascetic vows. Berowne comes forth to rebuke the King for hypocrisy, and he takes a superior attitude to them all until Jaquenetta arrives with his letter to Rosaline. Admitting his love, Berowne then provides a rationale for romantic behav-

iour. He says that their vows are unnatural for young men, and, further, that love, superior to all else, should be their proper subject of study. The King and the other courtiers rejoice in his solution and lay plans for festive entertainments to help woo their intended lovers.

Act 5, Scene 1

Armado, while bragging grandiloquently of his close relations with the King, announces that he has been asked to arrange a pageant to entertain the Princess. He consults with Holofernes, who proposes a presentation of 'The Nine WORTHIES', a traditional tableau.

Act 5, Scene 2

The Princess and her gentlewomen mock their suitors, comparing the gifts of jewelry and poems they have received. Boyet arrives to report that he has overheard the courtiers planning to approach the ladies disguised as a delegation of Russians. The Princess devises a counter-plot: the ladies shall be masked, and shall each wear the jewelry given to another of them, so each suitor will address the wrong woman. The gentlemen enter, and the ladies teasingly refuse to dance with them. Each suitor then proceeds to take aside the wrong lady and profess his love. The women continue their ridicule, and soon the gentlemen beat a retreat. The ladies exult in their triumph. Shortly, the gentlemen return undisguised. The women tease the men further by jesting about the fools garbed as Russians that had been present earlier. The embarrassed gentlemen realise that the women had known them all along, and Berowne makes a confessional speech disavowing 'perjury'. The King, reaffirming his earlier vows of love, is perplexed when Rosaline claims to have received them, rather than the Princess. Berowne realises what has happened and rails against Boyet as a spy and teller of tales.

Costard arrives, announcing that the pageant of the Nine Worthies is about to begin. The noblemen heckle the commoners; they drive Nathaniel and then Holofernes from the stage. Costard, misunderstanding part of Armado's performance, breaks in and reveals that Jaquenetta is pregnant by the Spaniard. Armado and Costard are egged on towards a duel by the gentlemen, but MARCADE appears with news of the death of the King of France, the Princess' father.

The emotional tone of the play changes instantly. The 'Worthies' are dismissed; the Princess prepares to depart and, in a new mood of sadness, apologises to the king for the ridicule that she and her maids have used. The King, aided by Berowne, persists in courtship; the Princess responds by promising him her love only if he will adopt a severely monastic life for a year. Katharine and Maria also require a year's wait for Dumaine and Longaville. Rosaline, observing that Berowne has an excessively mocking wit, requires that he spend the same year visiting dying patients in hospitals to learn a more proper seriousness. Armado returns and requests that the nobles hear the song intended to close the pageant. The assembled commoners then conclude the play with a song 'in praise of the owl and the cuckoo' (5.2.878–879).

COMMENTARY

Love's Labour's Lost is a difficult play for modern readers, but it can prove to be a rewarding one. Its basic story-line, in which pretensions are deflated and love conquers all, has a universal appeal. It is well plotted and constructed, and it contains a number of attractive lyrical passages and many comical sketches. Its cheerfully unrealistic atmosphere of games and festive play yields, at the last, to a sterner but nevertheless attractive vision of achieved maturity in the real world and the promise of future happiness.

Nevertheless, the play can seem unapproachable. It is full of in-jokes for Shakespeare's contemporaries, and much of its more accessible humour concerns the use of over-elaborate language, which is of course even farther from our own English than most Elizabethan dialogue. Its characters are often types drawn from older traditions and based on social roles that no longer exist. And its four sets of lovers who barely know each other seem implausible, to say the least. However, the playwright's organisational and linguistic genius carries the audience through the development of the play's comic situation to the satisfactions of its resolution.

The reader can dispose of many of the play's difficulties by dealing with them in a fashion that makes its virtues more evident. The witticisms in *Love's Labour's Lost* are frequently baffling to the most committed scholars and may simply be ignored. It is enough to know that they refer to lost controversies that were possibly obscure even to much of the original audience. Similarly, the inflated rhetorical posturings of Armado and Holofernes are amusingly pretentious, although we may not recognise the once-fashionable manners being parodied. Indeed, the greater part of the humour of a scene such a 4.2, which introduces Holofernes and Nathaniel, lies in its incomprehensibility—to the audience no less than to Dull. Shakespeare's point—that pomposity and pretension in language are laughable—is easy to enjoy in itself, and it also is linked to the main plot.

The romance of the gentlemen and ladies provides the main interest. The play begins with the King's unnatural demand for a dry and rigorous asceticism in the name of learning. This strange proposition, counter to common sense and human instinct, is established in order that it may be refuted. Berowne begins, even in 1.1, to oppose it; his sense of reality never completely deserts him, and he is the first to shake off the fakery that the gentlemen have entangled themselves in. We see the extent to which the false

ideal of ascetic scholarship has been manifested in language, and the SUB-PLOT's connection to the main plot emerges. Just as the gentlemen violate their own natures in attempting to emphasise dry learning over real living, so do the lesser characters err in reducing learning itself to foolish verbiage. In a sense, these figures may be said to be parodies of the King's gentlemen as well as of contemporary manners and mores.

The dramatic conflict between the high-flown pretensions of the King and the sensible humour of the Princess of France and her ladies is established early, and the comedy of the main plot lies in two chief manifestations of that tension: the embarrassed attempts by the gentlemen to resist and then deny love; and the practical joke played on them by the disguised ladies. The story alternates with the sub-plot, scene by scene, with very little overlap. A third component, the element of pageantry, integrates the two plots to some degree, although Shakespeare had not yet mastered the complex interwoven plots of his later, richer works.

If the characters in *Love's Labour's Lost* tend to be rather one-dimensional, this is not inappropriate to the somewhat abstract nature of the play. It is a comedy of notions, in which a blatantly false ideal is overcome by common sense and love is permitted to prevail. The humorous characters of the sub-plot derive mostly from the comical archetypes of the Italian COMMEDIA DELL'ARTE; the lords and ladies are simply courtly representatives of the warring ideals. The exception is Berowne, whose humanity provides a foil for the cold, ascetic withdrawal proposed by the King. His humorous self-mocking soliloquy in which he admits to having fallen in love (3.1.168–200) propels the play towards its lively series of climaxes, and his energy drives the comic tour de force in 4.3, when the King and his three courtiers discover that they have all succumbed to love.

Although Berowne is the most fully developed character in the play, several other figures briefly exhibit flashes of Shakespearean life. The Princess, for instance, is also humanly believable; from her first speech (2.1.13–34), she is intelligent and sensible. Rosaline's sharp wit and balanced sensibility also inspire affection. Katharine has one touching moment of reality, when she is reminded of the death of her sister (5.2.14–18). Costard, primarily a character type, a combination of CLOWN (1) and FOOL (1), also engages our sympathy in a more personal way when he shamefacedly apologises for misreading a line in the pageant of the Worthies (5.2.554–555) and when, shortly thereafter, he speaks up for Nathaniel, who is stricken with stage fright (5.2.575–579).

On the whole, however, the play does not exploit or depend on the delineation of character. It is a formal exercise, balancing the fantastic and the actual, and is as near to dance as it is to psychological realism. As such it must be crisply organised. The alternations of verse and prose, of main plot and sub-plot, merge in the pageantry of the final scene. Acts 1–2 constitute the exposition, Acts 3–4 develop both story lines, and Act 5 creates a transcendent world of romance and festivity, enabling the audience to forget the mundane world. The unreal atmosphere of the play is finally shattered by the appearance of Marcade, a messenger from the real world.

This bold and unexpected stroke, a *coup de théâtre*, changes the tone of the play instantly. 'The scene begins to cloud', Berowne observes (5.2.714), and the final few minutes take place in a more sober atmosphere. But although the interval of festive mirth is ended, it is not repudiated. It must be found in a larger universe, the real world that includes grief and business, but it is allowed its place. A maturation that has taken place permits this, for the gentlemen have advanced from a self-absorbed withdrawal in the name of abstract ideas to a more humane involvement with others. The ladies require of the gentlemen a testing period before their loves can be consummated, but, beyond this chastening trial, the prospect of a happy conclusion is unmistakable. The reappearance of the entire company to sing the opposing songs of Winter and Spring expresses the reality of ongoing life.

SOURCES OF THE PLAY

No written source for the plot of *Love's Labour's Lost* has ever been found, although it has been speculated that an earlier play may have been revised, as is true of other Shakespearean dramas. However, there is no actual evidence that such a predecessor existed, and most authorities conclude that the playwright invented his own stories in this play.

Nevertheless, many details may be traced to the general public knowledge of the day concerning the French Wars of Religion, then drawing to a close. English interest in that conflict was very great, largely because English troops participated in it, in 1591–1593, on the side of the Protestant rebel Henri, King of Navarre, later Henri IV of France. Thus Shakespeare and his audience were familiar with the events in France that *Love's Labour's Lost* alludes to. The central figure in the play is also the King of Navarre, and the names of his courtiers correspond to well-known political figures in Henri's world. Also, Henri did receive a delegation from France headed by a princess; although he was married to her at the time, they were on opposite sides in the war and were engaged in renegotiating her dowry, an important component of which was Aquitaine, the focus of the Princess's embassy in the play. Moreover, Henri of Navarre was one of many 16th-century rulers to found an academy based on Italian Renaissance models. All of these facts were common knowledge in England, thanks to the presence there

of many Protestant refugees from the wars and through many printed accounts.

However, a prominent literary work may also have figured in the genesis of the play: it has been theorised that *Love's Labour's Lost* was written as a rejoinder to 'Shadow of Night', a long poem by George CHAPMAN that extols a life of contemplation and study, as opposed to the concerns of mundane existence. According to this theory, the playwright was involved in a literary dispute among politically hostile aristocratic cliques; references to some of the participants in this feud (see, e.g., Thomas NASHE) are certainly hidden in the now-obscure passages of by-play that baffle most modern readers, such as 3.1.81–95. An attack on Chapman, and on esoteric knowledge, was an attack on Sir Walter RALEIGH and his friends, made on behalf of a rival group led by the Earl of ESSEX (2), whose close friend, the Earl of SOUTHAMPTON (2), was Shakespeare's patron.

The Russian masquerade in 5.2 is thought to have been inserted in a revision of the play made no earlier than 1595, for it, too, can be associated with historical evidence. In 1594 the annual Christmas revels at Gray's Inn(see INNS OF COURT) included a comical pageant of Russians (probably stimulated by the publication in 1591 of a popular and influential book on Russia by Giles FLETCHER [1] an early English traveller to Moscow). We may suppose that Shakespeare knew of this event, for *The Comedy of Errors* was performed at the same festival, a production which the playwright probably acted in himself. Moreover, certain details in *Love's Labour's Lost* correspond with accounts of the Gray's Innpageant of Russians.

TEXT OF THE PLAY

Scholars agree, for a number of reasons, that the text of *Love's Labour's Lost* reflects two renderings of the play. Most prominently, there are several passages that are printed in two versions. Also, there is variation in the names provided for several characters in stage directions and dialogue headings, and there is an evident change in the casting of the pageant of the Nine Worthies between its planning in 5.1 and its presentation in 5.2. Further, it has been speculated that the play may originally have ended at 5.2.870, before the anticlimactic songs of Winter and Spring, and that a scene involving Armado and Moth was cut, leaving Costard's puzzling lines at 4.1.145–150. Internal evidence suggests dates for both an original version and a revision. (See 'Sources of the Play'.) The original composition of *Love's Labour's Lost* probably dates from around 1593, at the height of the literary dispute with which it is associated and while England was still involved in the French wars; the play was apparently revised after 1594.

The earliest surviving text of the play is the QUARTO edition of 1598, by William WHITE (2) for publisher Cuthbert BURBY; this is, incidentally, the earliest play text to carry Shakespeare's name on the title page. The phrase 'newly corrected and augmented' also appears on the title page, suggesting that an earlier edition, of which no copy has survived, had been printed. (However, the phrase may simply refer to the revision of the play.) The 1598 edition was very clumsily printed, with many typographical errors, but it has nevertheless served as the basis for all subsequent editions, including that in the FIRST FOLIO of 1623.

THEATRICAL HISTORY OF THE PLAY

The title page of the Quarto edition of 1598 records that *Love's Labour's Lost* was performed at the court of Queen Elizabeth during the Christmas festivities of 1597, and it had probably been staged previously as well. The only other specifically recorded early production was also held at court, in 1604, although the Quarto of 1631 asserts that the play had been performed at the BLACKFRIARS THEATRE, where Shakespeare's works were not produced before 1608. The very existence of the second Quarto edition suggests that the play remained popular through the first decades of the 17th century. It then completely disappeared from the stage for two centuries, although its songs were occasionally adapted in other works.

First revived in 1839, *Love's Labour's Lost* was both staged and published a number of times in the 19th century. In the 20th it has received a great deal of scholarly and critical attention and is now regarded as one of Shakespeare's most important early works. As such, it has been presented in several major productions and has proven to be quite popular with theatre goers. It has not been made a FILM, but it has been presented twice on TELEVISION.

Love's Labour's Won Possible lost play by Shakespeare. In 1598 Francis MERES listed *Love's Labour's Won* among Shakespeare's comedies. This title was for many years identified with *The Taming of the Shrew,* the only pre-1598 Shakespearean COMEDY that Meres omitted. However, the question was raised anew in 1953, with the discovery of a 1603 bookseller's catalogue listing both *Shrew* and *Love's Labour's Won. Won* could still be *Shrew,* published under another title sometime before 1603 in an edition that has not survived. It could also be such an edition of one of the other comedies appearing after 1598—and so not in Meres' list—but before 1603. The most likely nominees are *All's Well That Ends Well* and *Much Ado About Nothing,* though *As You Like It* and *Troilus and Cressida* have also been suggested.

Love's Martyr Allegorical poem by Robert Chester, published in 1601 with a collection of shorter poems by other poets, including Shakespeare's *The Phoenix and Turtle,* in a book of the same name. Nothing is

known of Chester except that he was a member of the household of Sir John SALUSBURY, whose marriage in 1586 this book so commemorates. An allegory, the poem tells of a mystical love between two birds—the turtledove (commonly called 'turtle' in Elizabethan English), a symbol of fidelity, and the mythological phoenix, an ancient emblem of immortality. The allegory is, however, interspersed with discourses on King Arthur, precious stones, natural history, and so on. Eventually, the phoenix and the turtle decide to die together, and they construct a funeral pyre and burn to death.

The love between phoenix and turtledove is also the theme of the poems later added to Chester's, including *The Phoenix and Turtle.* Salusbury was knighted in 1601, and this was probably the occasion for the poem's publication, with the addition of work by much better-known writers, several of them Salusbury's friends; *Love's Martyr* also includes contributions by George CHAPMAN, Ben JONSON, and John MARSTON, among others. Shakespeare's *Phoenix* is now the only well-known piece in the book.

Love's Martyr was first published in 1601 by Edward BLOUNT in a QUARTO edition printed by Richard FIELD (2). Ten years later it was republished with a new title, *The Annals of Great Britain,* but only the title-page varied from the original quarto. The 1601 edition has therefore been the basis of all subsequent editions of both Chester's poem, which was not republished until 1878, and of *The Phoenix and Turtle.*

Lowin (Lowen), John (1576–1653) English actor. One of the 26 men listed in the FIRST FOLIO as the 'Principall Actors' of Shakespeare's plays, Lowin was one of the most noted members of the KING'S MEN in the early 17th century. A very large man, he was famous for his FALSTAFF, and he may have originated the part of HENRY VIII (although this report—that Lowin learned the part from Shakespeare himself—dates from 1708 and is suspect).

Lowin was apprenticed to a goldsmith as a boy, but as soon as he was free he turned to the stage. He was a member of WORCESTER'S MEN in 1602–1603, but in 1603 joined the King's Men, becoming a partner in 1604. After 1630 he was a co-manager of the company, with Joseph TAYLOR, and he remained with them until the closing of the theatres by the revolution in 1642. After retirement he owned a small tavern, but died in poverty.

Luce Minor character in *The Comedy of Errors,* a servant who, with ADRIANA, refuses ANTIPHOLUS OF EPHESUS entrance to his own home in 3.1, believing him to be an imposter. Luce is often identified with NELL (1), who is referred to later in the play.

Lucentio Character in *The Taming of the Shrew,* the successful suitor of BIANCA (1). Lucentio, aided by his servant TRANIO, disguises himself as a tutor of languages and thus gains access to Bianca, against the wishes of her father, BAPTISTA. Eventually, he elopes with his lover. His wealthy father, VINCENTIO (1) assures Baptista that he will provide an adequate financial settlement on the couple, and Lucentio is forgiven, only to find, in the final scene, that Bianca is not the ideally demure young bride he had anticipated.

Although the romance of Bianca and Lucentio is contrasted to the mercenary calculations of her father, Lucentio is a rather bloodless lover. He is simply a stereotype—the handsome young male romantic lead—representing a tradition as old as ancient Roman drama. However, in earlier plays, this character tended to marry for money and extend romantic love to mistresses and courtesans; Shakespeare's alteration reflects his concern with love in marriage, a major theme of *The Taming of the Shrew.*

Lucetta Minor character in *The Two Gentlemen of Verona,* the waiting-woman to JULIA. Like the other servants in the play, SPEED and LAUNCE, Lucetta seems at least as alert and intelligent as her employer. She is aware of her mistress' love for Proteus before Julia is willing to admit it to herself, and she suspects Proteus of disloyalty when Julia is all too trusting.

Lucian (c. 120–180 A.D.) Greek satirist, author of a probable source for *Timon of Athens.* Lucian's *Timon the Misanthrope* is a satirical dialogue that contains numerous elements of Shakespeare's plot, and clearly was known to Shakespeare in some form. Though no English translation of this work existed in Shakespeare's day, he may have known it in Latin, French, or Italian. Alternatively, he may have used another source based on Lucian, perhaps an anonymous English play known as the 'old *Timon*' (c. 1580–1610), or perhaps some work now lost, possibly a source for the 'old *Timon*' that derived from Lucian.

Lucian was originally from a Greek-speaking settlement in what is now Syria. He travelled around the Roman Empire lecturing on philosophy and rhetoric. He settled in Athens around the age of 40, and there wrote the dialogues that made him famous throughout the Mediterranean as a clever satirist of philosophical and religious ideas.

Luciana Character in *The Comedy of Errors,* the sister-in-law of ANTIPHOLUS OF EPHESUS and the beloved of ANTIPHOLUS OF SYRACUSE. Luciana first appears in an argument with her sister, ADRIANA, about marital relations, in a standard disputation of the day. Luciana says that a man is properly the master of his wife and urges: 'O, know he is the bridle of your will' (2.1.13).

Luciana's demure pliancy is apparently attractive to Antipholus of Syracuse, for when he finds himself in his brother's house, not knowing himself to be mistaken for his twin, he meets Luciana, falls in love, and attempts to court the object of his affections. Luciana, believing him to be her brother-in-law, is naturally horrified by his advances and chastises him roundly (3.2.1–70). Moreover, she describes this exchange to Adriana, thereby furthering the confusion and misunderstanding at the heart of the play. Luciana's subsequent importance to the action is slight. Even when Antipholus of Syracuse observes at the play's conclusion that the re-establishment of his identity will permit him to court her in earnest, Luciana remains silent.

Luciana represents a type, rather than a fully drawn human being. She is the modest and subservient female, whose stipulated position in Elizabethan society served to perpetuate an ideal notion of the family (and, by extension, society at large) as a secure and lasting hierarchy, decreed by God and tradition and undisturbed by change or individual assertion. (Such assertion was of course present among Elizabethan womanhood, as represented by Adriana.) The two sisters together constitute an early attempt by the playwright to achieve a complex portrait of contemporary femininity. While Luciana is thus an incomplete character, she foreshadows aspects of later, more successful Shakespearean heroines, such as VIOLA, in *Twelfth Night,* and IMOGEN, in *Cymbeline.*

Lucianus Character in THE MURDER OF GONZAGO, the playlet presented within *Hamlet.* In 3.2 the PLAYERS (2), following HAMLET's instructions, perform before the court of KING (5) Claudius. In their play Lucianus murders the PLAYER KING by pouring poison in his ear, paralleling the murder of Hamlet's father by the real King. The play is interrupted by the King's guilty response—according to Hamlet's plan—and Lucianus does not get to complete his role, which would have involved marrying the PLAYER QUEEN. Significantly, Lucianus is the nephew of the king he kills—not the brother, as a strict analogy with Claudius' crime would require—and thus he presents to the King not only the image of himself as murderer but also that of Hamlet as avenger. Lucianus' only lines—a brief address to his poison 'of midnight weeds collected' (3.2.251)—are in a highly rhetorical style that is designed to highlight the artificiality of the play within a play.

Lucilius (1) (active 42 B.C.) Historical figure and minor character in *Julius Caesar,* an officer in the army of BRUTUS (4). Brutus confides in Lucilius, clearly a trusted subordinate, at SARDIS in 4.2 and 4.3 and at PHILIPPI in Act 5. In 5.4, as Brutus' army is overrun by the soldiers of Mark ANTONY, Lucilius pretends to be Brutus—daring his opponents to kill him and be acclaimed—in an effort to divert attention from his commander. He is taken prisoner, and Antony, who realises his captive is not Brutus, praises Lucilius' bravery and orders that he be treated kindly.

Lucilius' diversionary tactic was admired in ancient and medieval literature (and, presumably, in warfare) and was popular on the Elizabethan stage. Shakespeare had used it in *1 Henry IV,* where Sir Walter BLUNT (3) is killed while impersonating King HENRY IV. The playwright took Lucilius' exploit from PLUTARCH's *Lives,* where the officer is reported to have been a friend of Brutus and to have remained loyal to Antony after Philippi.

Lucilius (2) Minor character in *Timon of Athens,* a servant of TIMON. When an OLD ATHENIAN complains to Timon that the socially inferior Lucilius is courting his daughter, Timon promises Lucilius a fortune and thus makes him acceptable. The episode helps establish Timon's generosity and extravagance. Lucilius speaks very little and serves merely to further the plot.

Lucillius GHOST CHARACTER in *Antony and Cleopatra,* an attendant of ENOBARBUS. Lucillius appears only once and does not speak; he is mentioned only in the opening stage direction of 1.2, along with LAMPRIUS and RANNIUS.

Lucio Character in *Measure for Measure,* a dissolute gentleman who befriends the condemned CLAUDIO (3) and slanders the DUKE (9) of VIENNA. Although, as Claudio's friend, Lucio supports ISABELLA in her encounters with the obsessively strict official, ANGELO (2), he is nonetheless an unnsavoury character. He maliciously defames the Duke and callously admits to having abandoned a pregnant woman; that he is forgiven his crimes in the end is an important part of the play's emphasis on the value of forgiveness.

We first see Lucio in 1.2, jesting lewdly about venereal disease with his friends (see GENTLEMAN [5]). A customer of the bordello run by MISTRESS (2) Overdone and POMPEY (1), Lucio represents the degenerate life that has flourished in Vienna because of the Duke's lax regime. He is not without good qualities, however. In standing by Isabella, in 2.2 and 2.4, he seems a positive figure, but beginning in 3.2 he takes on another aspect. He flippantly refuses to help Pompey avoid imprisonment, and Mistress Overdone declares that he has informed on her; these episodes make us realise that Lucio's Vienna is an ugly one. In 3.2 and 4.3 Lucio amuses himself by making up the libellous stories about the Duke for which he is punished in 5.1. He does not realise that the 'friar' with whom he converses is the disguised ruler himself.

While Lucio's slanderous lies are plainly malicious,

he seems funny, not evil, to modern sensibilities. But abuse of a ruler—believed to be appointed by God to maintain order in society—was a much more serious matter in Shakespeare's day than in our own, and Lucio's offence, although comical, is decidedly criminal. 17th-century audiences would not have been surprised by the severity of the Duke's proposed punishment: 'Let him be whipp'd and hang'd' (5.1.511). Nevertheless, Lucio remains wittily uncompromising at the end. This testifies to Shakespeare's sympathy with the rebellious individual, even in a play which stresses the importance of authority and the values of society at large.

Lucius (1) Character in *Titus Andronicus,* a son of TITUS (1) Andronicus. In 1.1 Lucius demands the ritual sacrifice of TAMORA's son, thus triggering the cycle of vengeance that drives the action. Later, he is banished from Rome and he joins the GOTHS. He returns in Act 5 at the head of the Gothic troops, and, in that capacity, he sentences the captured AARON to death. Continuing to Rome, he is present at the grisly finale, as is his son, YOUNG LUCIUS. Following the deaths of SATURNINUS and his father, he is acclaimed the new Emperor.

Lucius (2) Minor character in *Julius Caesar,* a young servant of BRUTUS. In 2.1 Lucius falls asleep while the conspirators plot the death of CAESAR (1), and Brutus expresses envy of the boy's carefree state. In 2.4 Lucius appears as an innocent foil to the near-hysterical worry of PORTIA (2). In 4.3, at Brutus' camp near SARDIS, Lucius plays a lute at his master's command, and Brutus shows consideration and affection for the boy in a scene that shows the zealous conspirator in an unusually soft light.

The episodes in which Lucius appears have a distinctive emotional tone. His role offers an important touch of domestic tenderness and loyalty in a work that is dominated by the darker themes of murderous politics and civil war.

Lucius (3) Character in *Timon of Athens,* an ungrateful friend to TIMON. In 3.2 Lucius hears that LUCULLUS has refused to assist Timon with a loan after Timon has impoverished himself by showering gifts on his friends. Like Lucullus, Lucius is also the beneficiary of Timon's excessive generosity, and he proudly declares to HOSTILIUS and two visitors (see STRANGER) that he would never turn away a friend. However, when Timon's servant SERVILIUS appears and asks for help, Lucius brazenly declares that he cannot make a loan. The hypocritical Lucius helps demonstrate—with Lucullus and SEMPRONIUS—the callousness of the Athenian aristocrats, one of the play's important themes.

Lucius (4) Character in *Cymbeline,* ambassador from ROME to the Britain of King CYMBELINE, later the commander of the invading Roman army and the employer of the disguised IMOGEN. In 3.1 Lucius informs Cymbeline that Rome demands tribute from Britain. When he receives the king's refusal he transmits his government's declaration of war. However, he adds that he regrets this, for he appreciates the hospitality he has received in Britain. His gentlemanly nature is again evident in 3.5, when he departs from the king's court, and we understand why PISANIO recommends that the disguised Imogen become a page for Lucius. He calls the Roman 'honourable, and . . . most holy' (3.4.178–179). In 4.2 Lucius readily offers employment and protection to Imogen. He believes that she is a young man, FIDELE, and he takes particular care of 'him' when the Romans are defeated in battle in 5.2. Finally, in 5.5 Lucius nobly faces death at the hands of the victorious Cymbeline, before he receives mercy in the play's final aura of reconciliation.

Lucius is a noble person who is unable to influence the course of events in the play. He is contrasted with assorted weak, but not evil, figures like POSTHUMUS and the king, and thus he offers a positive image of humanity's need for the intervention of providence. The ancient tradition that a soldier named Lucius was the first Roman converted to Christianity may be reflected in Shakespeare's choice of name for this positive character. Two of Shakespeare's other characters named Lucius (see LUCIUS [1, 2]) are also right-minded and in the military, so these may well be conscious references to the ancient convert, who was still fairly well known in the 17th century.

Lucius' Servant Minor character in *Timon of Athens,* the employee of LUCIUS (3), a former friend and creditor of TIMON. In 3.4 Lucius' Servant joins a group of colleagues who unsuccessfully dun Timon and his STEWARD (2) for repayment of loans. He and his fellows regret the necessity of serving greedy masters who once benefited from Timon's generosity. However, Lucius' Servant is somewhat more aggressive in demanding payment. He observes that Timon's has been a 'prodigal course' (3.4.12), and rejects an excuse of ill health, offered by Timon's servant, when he says, 'Methinks he should the sooner pay his debts / And make a clear way to the gods' (3.4.74–75). He thus reflects the atrocious behaviour of his master, who in 3.2 hypocritically refuses to assist the impoverished Timon after he has declared that he would help a friend in need.

Lucrece (Lucretia) Legendary Roman matron and central figure in *The Rape of Lucrece,* the victim of a rape by TARQUIN. Lucrece kills herself rather than accept the disgrace of having slept with someone other than her husband. The bulk of the 1,855-line poem—from

her first awareness of Tarquin's menace in line 442 until her death in line 1724—is dedicated to Lucrece's responses, fearful, horrified, ashamed, and determinedly suicidal. Her great wordiness is often considered a weakness of the poem, but her meditations are nonetheless studded with brilliant passages and also reflect an aspect of Shakespeare's attitude towards women.

Sometimes seen as a victim who is further victimised, Lucrece is actually rather like the boldly assertive young women of Shakespeare's work who have charmed COMEDY audiences for generations. She is admittedly less well realised, however, and her situation is less rewarding, both for herself and for modern readers. Lucrece's values, impossibly remote from modern ones, lead her to adopt a course of great bravery against the advice of the men around her (see lines 1709–1710). She realises that only her death can repair the damage done to her self-esteem, and through her suicide she achieves heroic stature. In an aristocratic value system that gives great weight to marital loyalty—especially in women, who bear children and thus transmit the family line—Lucrece has been forcibly removed from the ranks of the pure, a status in which she has plainly taken great pride. She poignantly expresses her sense of her predicament by comparing herself to a damaged tree: '. . . the bark pill'd from the lofty pine, His leaves will wither and his sap decay; So must my soul, her bark being pill'd away' (lines 1167–1169).

In ancient heroic traditions, these situations are no more subject to rationalisation than are natural catastrophes. Lucrece's response preserves her honour, all that remains within her control. Although Lucrece's action is criticised by BRUTUS [2] (lines 1823–1827), she is nevertheless presented as an heroic figure and her actions stimulate an heroic act, the revolution against the Tarquinian kings and the establishment of the Roman Republic. Moreover, Lucrece's tale was so perfectly in accord with notions of honour and heroism that it survived through almost 2,000 years and several upheavals in European civilisation to find continued acceptance among the Elizabethans.

Shakespeare took the story of Lucrece's rape and its political consequences from his Latin sources, LIVY and OVID, but it is not historical, deriving in fact from pre-Latin traditions. Someone involved with the establishment of the republic may have had a wife named Lucretia (the Latin spelling of Lucrece), but nothing at all is known of her.

Lucretius Legendary father of the Roman matron Lucretia and minor figure in *The Rape of Lucrece*, the father of LUCRECE. Lucretius appears only late in the poem. He is implicitly present from line 1583 but is not mentioned until line 1732, after Lucrece has told of TARQUIN's crime against her and killed herself. He delivers a touching, three-stanza outburst of grief (lines 1751–1771), but it is one of the other witnesses, BRUTUS (2), who rallies the mourners to exact vengeance against Tarquin, finally resulting in the fall of the monarchy. Shakespeare took Lucretius from his Latin sources, OVID and LIVY, who lived several centuries after these events supposedly took place; modern historians have found no record of Lucretius from his own time.

Lucullus Character in *Timon of Athens*, an ungrateful friend of TIMON. In 1.2 Lucullus is among the guests at Timon's banquet. In 2.2 when Timon finds that his extravagant hospitality has bankrupted him, Lucullus is among those he presumes he can count on for assistance. However, when Lucullus is approached by Timon's servant FLAMINIUS for a loan, he declares that he had warned his friend. With unconscious irony, he says, 'Many a time and often I ha' din'd with him, and . . . come again to supper to him of purpose to have him spend less' (3.1.23–25). He sums up his position when he observes that 'this is no time to lend money, especially upon bare friendship, without security' (3.1. 41–43). He then tries to hide his ingratitude by bribing Flaminius to say he could not be found. Like LUCIUS (3) and SEMPRONIUS, whose similar responses occur in the next two scenes, Lucullus helps demonstrate the heartlessness of the Athenian aristocrats, one of the play's important themes.

Lucy (1), Sir Thomas (1532–1600) Contemporary of Shakespeare, a WARWICKSHIRE landowner sometimes identified with Justice SHALLOW, a comic character in *2 Henry IV* and *The Merry Wives of Windsor*. According to a local tradition—first published by Nicholas ROWE in 1709—the young Shakespeare was caught poaching deer on Lucy's estate near STRATFORD; he was prosecuted for the crime and took vengeance by writing an insulting ballad about Sir Thomas. The same tradition was also recorded at about the same time by Richard DAVIES (3), testifying to its currency in the 17th century. In the 18th century several versions of the scurrilous ballad were published by various antiquarians.

Sir Thomas Lucy's heraldic emblem of three vertical white fish (luces—i.e., pike) resembles that of Shallow, as described with comic solemnity and confusion in *The Merry Wives*, 1.1.15–25, and Shallow threatens Falstaff with a lawsuit for having killed his deer. It thus appears that, if the tale of young Shakespeare and Lucy is true, the playwright could have been mocking his old enemy. However, there are a number of reasons to doubt that this is the case. No further resemblance to Lucy can be found in *The Merry Wives* or *2 Henry IV*. The heraldic luces may be found in other coats of arms—in fact, they support the argument in favour of a different identification of Shallow (see William GARDINER [2]). Further, *The Merry Wives* was first

presented at the Queen's court, where it would have been foolish of Shakespeare to pillory a powerful nobleman, supposing—improbably—that his audience would have understood the allusions, and pointless if they would not. Lastly, the story itself is subject to considerable doubt. It is impossible to rely on a tale whose earliest known recounting dates from more than a century after the events it describes. Lucy may not have kept deer; he did not have the required licence to do so, although unlicensed deer parks were known in Elizabethan times, and his grandson later took out a licence for the same land. In any case, the poaching tale could well have arisen from the play, rather than vice versa, the seeming allusions to Lucy perhaps being associated with his grandson's recorded prosecution of poachers in 1610. However, perhaps significantly, Lucy himself in 1584 introduced a bill in Parliament that would have made poaching a felony. Incidentally, a separate tradition tells that the grandson, another Thomas Lucy (1585–1640), was a friend of Shakespeare after the playwright's retirement.

Sir Thomas was one of the richest landlords in Warwickshire; in 1572, when Shakespeare was eight years old, Queen ELIZABETH (1) visited his estate. He would have been a powerful enemy. A zealous Protestant, he was a local leader in the persecution of Catholics. Sir William LUCY (2), who appears in *1 Henry VI,* was his great-great-great grandfather.

Lucy (2), Sir William Character in *1 Henry VI,* an officer who seeks reinforcements for TALBOT during that general's fatal battle in Act 4. Lucy approaches both YORK (8) and SOMERSET (3), but these noblemen are feuding; each blames the other for Talbot's position, and each refuses to send assistance. Lucy grieves for the loss of England's conquests in FRANCE (1), emphasising Shakespeare's point that only dissensions among the English made a French victory possible.

Lupton, Thomas (active 1570s and 1580s) English writer, author of a minor source for *Measure for Measure.* Lupton's collection of political anecdotes and utopian tales, *The Second Part and knitting up of the booke entitled Too Good to be True* (1581; *Too Good to be True* appeared in 1580), contains an account of the Italian judicial scandal of 1547 that was the original source of Shakespeare's play, though the playwright also knew of this event from several other sources that were more important. From Lupton came the germ of the encounters between ANGELO (2) and ISABELLA and, perhaps, the sense of urgency conveyed by repeated, precise references to the scheduling of the imminent execution of CLAUDIO (3).

Though Lupton is today remembered chiefly for his contribution to *Measure for Measure,* he also wrote one of the last English MORALITY plays, and a number of anti-Catholic religious tracts. However, he was best known in his own time for a layman's health manual, a collection of recipes and cures entitled *A Thousand Notable Things of Sundry Sorts* (1579), which was immensely popular and was republished at intervals until 1793.

Lychorida Minor character in *Pericles,* the nurse of MARINA, servant of PERICLES and THAISA. Lychorida accompanies the pregnant Thaisa and Pericles as they embark on a sea journey, shown in the DUMB SHOW in 3.Chorus. In 3.1, aboard ship, she presents the newborn Marina to Pericles and reports that Thaisa has died in childbirth. In 3.3 she carries Marina but does not speak when Pericles leaves infant and nurse in THARSUS. Marina's grief at Lychorida's death 14 years later is probably mentioned in 4.1.11, though the text is unclear. In Shakespeare's world the company of a nurse was a regular attribute of a well-born young woman. Through her service to Thaisa and then her daughter, Lychorida embodies dedicated domestic service and contributes to the play's atmosphere of ceremonious and courtly life.

Lydgate, John (c. 1370–c. 1451) English poet, author of a source of *Troilus and Cressida.* Inspired by Guido delle COLONNE's *Historia destructionis Troiae* (1287), Lydgate wrote a long poem on the TROJAN WAR, entitled *Troy Book* (1420, publ. 1512, 1555), which influenced Shakespeare's play, especially in its emphasis on the chivalric aspects of the war.

Though an ordained priest, Lydgate spent much of his life staging pageants for the guilds of London. He was a friend of the great poet Geoffrey CHAUCER, and he enjoyed the patronage of Humphrey, Duke of GLOUCESTER (4), who appears in four Shakespearean plays and through whom Lydgate became the official poet of the court of King HENRY VI. Though his reputation was quite good in his own day, Lydgate is now generally regarded as a bad poet whose medieval religiosity and prosaic language are no longer of interest. However, his translation of BOCCACCIO's *The Fate of Illustrious Men* (1355–1374)—published as *Falls of Princes* (1431–1438, publ. 1494)—was an influence on the compilers of A MIRROR FOR MAGISTRATES, a prominent work in Shakespeare's day that was also a source for the playwright.

Lyly, John (c. 1554–1606) English novelist and playwright, a major influence on Shakespeare's early plays. Lyly's extravagant novels and courtly comedies were quite fashionable in LONDON in the 1580s, and they evidently fascinated the young Shakespeare. In elaborate language Lyly's plays presented tales of conflicting love and friendship often involving journeys to exotic climes frequented by outlaws. Their tone, combining sentimentality and sharp wit, seems to have

contributed much to Shakespeare's early comedies—especially *Love's Labour's Lost*, but also *The Comedy of Errors*, *The Two Gentlemen of Verona*, and *A Midsummer Night's Dream*. Literal borrowings, however, are rare and minor.

Lyly, grandson of the humanist scholar William LILY, was the oldest member of the UNIVERSITY WITS, who revolutionised ELIZABETHAN DRAMA in the 1580s. He first achieved fame as the author of a romantic novel of courtly love and genteel adventure, *Euphues, the Anatomy of Wit* (1578), whose extravagant prose style startled readers with its novelty. *Euphues* was studded with puns, repetitions, alliterations, high-flown rhetorical digressions, and fanciful references to classical mythology and natural history (often invented). So distinctive was the style that it became known (and is still known) as euphuism. It was highly fashionable for years and was much imitated. Shakespeare was as likely to mock euphuism as imitate it, and in *1 Henry IV* 2.4.393–426, FALSTAFF indulges in a delightful parody of it.

After publishing a second volume of his novel—*Euphues and his England* (1580)—Lyly turned to the theatre. He wrote numerous elegant comedies for two CHILDREN'S COMPANIES, primarily between 1584 and 1590, but also occasionally until 1602. He was also associated with Henry EVANS (2) and William HUNNIS in the first BLACKFRIARS THEATRE. He then turned to politics and the court of Queen ELIZABETH (1). He was several times a member of parliament, and for years, he unsuccessfully pursued an appointment as the queen's MASTER OF THE REVELS.

Lysander Character in *A Midsummer Night's Dream*, the lover of HERMIA. When mistakenly anointed with a magical love potion, however, his affections are transferred to HELENA (1). Lysander is the least distinctive of the lovers in the play. His love interest changed from one young woman to another and back again by the magic of OBERON's herbs, Lysander is merely a pawn in Shakespeare's game of rotating lovers.

Lysimachus Character in *Pericles*, the governor of MYTILENE who becomes betrothed to MARINA. In 4.6 Lysimachus visits the brothel to which the kidnapped Marina has been sold. His familiar banter with the BAWD and BOULT suggests that he is a regular customer. Once alone with Marina, he seems baffled by her refusal to acknowledge the situation, and he insists 'Come, bring me to some private place; come, come' (4.6.89–90). She counters, 'If you were born to honour, show it now' (4.6.91) and goes on to express her revulsion for the brothel. Lysimachus is impressed and shamed. He claims to have come 'with no ill intent' (4.6.109), and says that he wished only to observe Marina's already famous virtue. However, his flight is hasty, and without being funny he suggests the comic potential of the exposed hypocrite. In any case, he serves admirably as a foil for Marina's virtue, courage, and wit. The Lysimachus of Shakespeare's sources is much more plainly a lecher, and when the playwright provided him with an excuse, he certainly intended us to take it as an indication of the governor's essential decency.

In 5.1 Lysimachus witnesses the reunion of Marina and her father PERICLES. When he learns that she is a suitable bride for a ruler, he asks Pericles for her hand. In the final reconciliations and reunions of 5.3 his engagement to Marina is formally declared, and the couple is assigned the rule of TYRE, though Lysimachus does not speak. He is merely a conventional high-born figure, a suitable husband for the heroine.

M

Mab Fairy queen referred to in *Romeo and Juliet*. MERCUTIO delivers an elaborate jesting speech (1.4.53–95) describing Queen Mab as a bringer of dreams to humans in a variety of social situations. The passage, a montage of fairy lore, country superstition, and humorous character types, has the chaotic energy that characterises both Mercutio and the violent world that opposes the private universe of the young lovers, ROMEO and JULIET (1). Parts of the speech have literary antecedents—notably in *The Parliament of Fowles*, by CHAUCER—but Queen Mab as 'midwife' (1.4.54) of dreams is known only in this passage and is probably Shakespeare's invention.

The name Mab is associated with fairies; there was a Queen Mabh in Irish fairy lore, and in the dialect of Shakespeare's native WARWICKSHIRE the word 'Mabled' was once current, meaning 'led astray by fairies or elves'. Also, Mab is expressly tiny, and the word 'mab' means 'small child' in Cymric, the language of WALES (1). Shakespeare's interest in Wales and its language at the period when *Romeo and Juliet* was written, and its importance as the origin of many elements of Warwickshire folklore, make it a possible source for the name.

Mabbe, James (1572–1642) English writer, possibly the author of one of the introductory poems to the FOLIO edition (1623) of Shakespeare's plays. Mabbe is best known as the translator of a major work of the Spanish RENAISSANCE, the novel *La Celestina*, by Fernando de Rojas (d. c. 1541). He was a long-time friend of Leonard DIGGES, who knew Shakespeare, and scholars generally believe he is the author of 'To the memorie of M. *W. Shake-speare*', a poem of four rhymed couplets that is signed 'I. M'. in the Folio (but see MAYNE).

Macbeth (c. 1005–1057) Historical figure and title character of *Macbeth*, a Scottish nobleman who kills King DUNCAN of SCOTLAND and rules the country until he is killed in combat by Lord MACDUFF. The evil of Macbeth's deed, and its effects on him and on Scotland, are the central elements of the play. He is conscious of the evil his ambition gives rise to, but he cannot overcome temptation. This is combined with his ambition, the urging of the equally ambitious LADY (6) MACBETH, and the encouragement given him by the WITCHES, whose supernatural powers seem certain to help him though in fact they bring him to his doom. As a man who abandons his own potential for good, Macbeth may be seen as an illustration of the fall of man, the prime Judeo-Christian example of sinful humanity's loss of God's grace. Eventually, Macbeth is destroyed by two virtuous men—Macduff and Duncan's son MALCOLM—who are his opposites in the play's balance of good and evil.

One of the play's manifestations of the power of evil is the collapse of Macbeth's personality. Macbeth commits, or causes to be committed, more than four murders: first, that of the king, which he performs himself in 2.2, and then those of Banquo, in 3.3, and of LADY (7) Macduff and her children, in 4.2. His behaviour during and after each of these events is different, and in this progression is the heart of the drama.

We hear of Macbeth before we see him. In 1.1 the Witches reveal that he is their target, and in 1.2 the king hears of his prowess on the battlefield. He appears to be a brave and loyal follower of the king, but when the Witches suggest, in 1.3, that Macbeth is to become king himself, we see that he has already entertained the possibility of usurping Duncan's crown. However, in 1.7, as he contemplates the prospect of killing King Duncan, he wavers. He still remembers his society's crude discipline, the 'even-handed Justice' (1.7.10) that dictates that if he kills the king, someone else may kill him. He further acknowledges that in simple decency he should not kill the man who is his kinsman and his guest, and who has, moreover, been notably kind to him. On another ethical level, he recognises that it is evil to deprive society of a virtuous man and a fine ruler.

Macbeth still retains the moral sensibility to declare, 'I dare do all that may become a man. / Who dares do more is none' (1.7.46–47), but Lady Macbeth encourages him to overcome his scruples, and in 2.2 he kills the king. He is immediately plagued by his conscience; he tells of how he 'could not say Amen' (2.2.28) and of the voices that foretold sleeplessness. His absorption with his bloody hands foreshadows his wife's descent into madness in 5.1. Nevertheless, he carries his plot through and is crowned between 2.4 and 3.1.

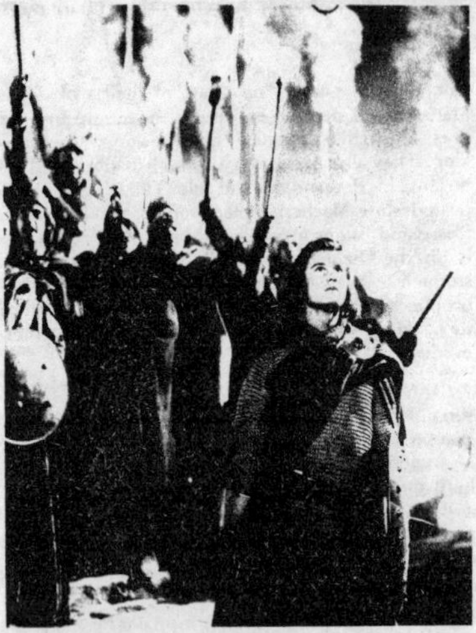

In Orson Welles' 1948 film version of Macbeth, *Malcolm (Roddy McDowell) prepares to lead his army against Macbeth's fortress, Dunsinane, to avenge the murder of his father, Duncan. Malcolm's trick of camouflaging his men with tree branches is instrumental in Macbeth's downfall.* (Courtesy of Culver Pictures, Inc.)

Though the influence of the Witches and of Lady Macbeth is very prominent and reflects different aspects of the ways we can fall into evil, Macbeth is basically not controlled by them. His story is one of a moral choice, and the consequences of that choice. It is clear that Lady Macbeth's influence helps him on his way, but once he has killed Duncan he withdraws from her, and she has no role in his subsequent plots; he plainly *can* get along without her. At the same time, his response to the supernatural is carefully contrasted with Banquo's suspicion of the Witches. Macbeth has every opportunity to avoid his fate: he could have ignored Lady Macbeth, or followed the lead of Banquo. However, he made a different choice, for he is a driven, self-destructive man.

Once installed as king, he considers murdering Banquo. He hopes to dispose of the Witches' prediction that Banquo's descendants will rule. He is troubled and cannot rest; he sees life as a 'fitful fever' (3.2.23), and he cries out, 'O! full of scorpions is my mind' (3.2.36). But he hires murderers (see FIRST MURDERER [3]) to dispose of Banquo and his son FLEANCE. Again, he is tormented by his conscience, especially by the sight of Banquo's GHOST (4). He returns to the Witches a second time and is warned by the APPARITIONS against Macduff. He determines to eliminate this threat also, with the result that the murderers kill Macduff's wife and children, although Macduff has already escaped to England.

By now, however, Macbeth's qualms have disappeared, replaced by a more fundamental disorder. We next see him in 5.3 as he prepares to defend himself against the army of Malcolm and Macduff, and he has become a different person. He veers wildly between rage and despair and has lost any emotional connection to his fellow humans. He declares that he is 'sick at heart' and has 'lived long enough' (5.3.19, 22), and he realises that all that he might once have expected in his old age, 'honour, love, obedience, troops of friends' (5.3.25), is irrevocably lost. Informed of Lady Macbeth's death, he can only reflect on the meaninglessness of life. He has lost his ordinary human repertoire of responses to life and death.

Even his courage, the only virtue he has retained, has an inhuman quality: 'bear-like, I must fight the course' (5.7.2), he growls. Only when he finally understands the deceptive prophecies of the Apparitions does he succumb once again, too late, to a genuine human emotion. He feels sheer terror—'it hath cow'd my better part of man', he cries (5.8.18) when he realises that Macduff is not 'of woman born' (5.8.13). He recovers courage enough to die, and thus in death he is not wholly lost.

His basic strength is also demonstrated in his capacity to face and withstand the ugly truth about himself. He sees the evil to which he has subjected himself and his world. He recognises his own immorality, and he is not satisfied with the position he attains, but he nevertheless defends this position with continued murder. He is aware of this irrational phenomenon; one of his most fascinating features is that he is conscious of the goodness he abandons. When he first contemplates the murder of Duncan, he says its 'horrid image doth unfix my hair' (1.3.135). He recognises the 'deep damnation' to be expected and his hallucination of the dagger confirms the force of this knowledge. After he commits the murder his immediate concern is not with being discovered, but with his conscience. 'To know my deed, 'twere best not know myself' (2.2.72), he says. And at the end of the play he is tormented by the awareness that his life could have been altogether different. It is the contrast with what might have been that makes Macbeth a tragic figure. Though Malcolm understandably refers to 'this dead butcher, and his fiend-like Queen' (5.9.35), the real point of the play resides in the extent to which Macbeth is not simply a monster. He cannot accept his evil callously; he suffers for it.

The historical Macbeth did indeed seize the throne from his cousin Duncan, but Shakespeare's depiction of the man and his reign is otherwise entirely fictional.

Shakespeare took some of his errors from his source, HOLINSHED's *Chronicles,* which itself depended upon the unreliable, quasi-legendary history of Hector BOECE. However, much of the playwright's version varies from Holinshed, anyway, for he was interested in drama, not history.

Though in the play the stigma against Macbeth's action is immense, his usurpation was fairly ordinary in 11th-century Scotland. Duncan's predecessor, King Malcolm II, had taken the throne when he murdered his cousin, Kenneth III. By the standards of the day, Macbeth's claim to the throne was fairly legitimate, as Holinshed makes clear. Macbeth, like Duncan, was a grandson of Malcolm II, and thus a plausible heir. He might also have asserted a claim as the husband of Gruoch (the real Lady Macbeth), who was a granddaughter of Kenneth III. However, there is no evidence that he received—or needed—any prodding from his wife to usurp power. Tradition dictated that any male member of the royal family who could establish that he had regal qualities—usually interpreted as control of an armed force—was qualified to succeed to the crown. In principle, an election within the family settled conflicting claims, though a resort to force was ordinary.

Macbeth, however, did not murder Duncan; he launched a civil war, and Duncan died in battle. Shakespeare took from Holinshed an account of an earlier royal assassination and ascribed it to his protagonist. Further, the play shows Scotland convulsed by the usurper's crime and tormented by his tyranny, but in fact Macbeth was a benign and successful king who ruled in peace for 15 years. Holinshed reported Macbeth's virtues as a king, but Shakespeare ignored them in the interests of drama. As in the play, Macbeth's reign ended when the exiled Prince Malcolm invaded the country with English forces. Malcolm's first attempt at conquest was only partially successful. SIWARD won a victory at DUNSINANE Castle in 1054, but it was not until 1057 that Macbeth was finally defeated in a battle nowhere near Dunsinane.

Macbeth

SYNOPSIS

Act 1, Scene 1
The three WITCHES meet during a storm and declare their intention to encounter MACBETH.

Act 1, Scene 2
The wounded CAPTAIN (8) tells King DUNCAN of SCOTLAND and his son MALCOLM of the bravery of Macbeth and BANQUO in battle against rebels led by the Thane of CAWDOR. ANGUS and ROSSE arrive and report that the battle has been won, and that Cawdor has surrendered. The King orders them to see that Cawdor is executed and to convey the rebel's title and estates to Macbeth.

Act 1, Scene 3
The Witches gather and boast of their evil deeds. Macbeth and Banquo encounter them, and they address Macbeth as Thane of Cawdor and as the future king. They also declare that though Banquo will not be king, his descendants will rule. The Witches disappear despite Macbeth's pleas for more information. Rosse and Angus arrive and inform Macbeth that he is now the Thane of Cawdor. Banquo and Macbeth are stunned by this confirmation of part of the Witches' prophecy. Macbeth muses to himself on his ambition to be king, which has been strengthened by these events.

Act 1, Scene 4
King Duncan praises Macbeth greatly and tells him that he wishes to visit his castle at INVERNESS. Duncan also announces that when he dies, Malcolm shall inherit the throne. Macbeth volunteers to travel ahead and prepare to receive the king; he reflects to himself that his ambition to be king is hindered by Malcolm's new status.

Act 1, Scene 5
LADY (6) MACBETH reads a letter from her husband that tells of the Witches' prophecy and its partial fulfilment. She is delighted, but fears that Macbeth's emotional weakness will prevent him from becoming king. Word arrives of Duncan's approach, and Lady Macbeth exults in this unexpected opportunity to kill Duncan. Macbeth arrives, and he is less enthusiastic, but she declares spiritedly that she will take charge of the murder.

Act 1, Scene 6
Lady Macbeth greets King Duncan courteously on his arrival at Inverness.

Act 1, Scene 7
Macbeth worries about his fate in the afterlife if he becomes a murderer. Lady Macbeth mocks him and fiercely stirs his ambition with the fury of her own. He declares that he will go ahead with the murder.

Act 2, Scene 1
Banquo and Macbeth speak briefly of the Witches. Macbeth discounts their importance as Banquo warns of the temptations that might arise from their prophecies. Left alone, Macbeth sees a hallucination of a bloody dagger. He acknowledges that he is horrified at the prospect of murdering the king, but he forces himself to proceed.

Act 2, Scene 2
Lady Macbeth has drugged the king's guards, and she awaits Macbeth's return. He comes to report that he

has killed Duncan, but he is fearful of divine punishment because when he heard Duncan's sons Malcolm and DONALBAIN praying he could not say 'Amen' to himself. He also says he heard a voice that predicted that he would never again be able to sleep. Lady Macbeth upbraids him because he has brought the bloody daggers with him instead of leaving them in the hands of the guards, as they had planned. She goes to complete the deed, and as she returns they hear a knock at the castle entry. She insists that they must go to bed and pretend they have been asleep.

Act 2, Scene 3
The knocking continues as a drunken PORTER (3) amuses himself with the pretence that he is the doorkeeper of hell. He finally admits MACDUFF and LENOX, and Macbeth arrives to greet them. He pretends to have been awakened by their arrival. Macduff goes to greet the king, while Lenox tells Macbeth of the night's violent and ominous storm. Macduff reappears and cries that the king has been murdered; he raises the alarm as Macbeth runs to the king's chamber. Lady Macbeth, Banquo, Malcolm, and Donalbain arrive in great confusion. Macbeth returns and reports that in his fury at the murder he has killed the guards, who he says are the murderers. As the group departs to dress and meet again, Malcolm and Donalbain confer. They fear that they will be suspected of the murder. They also fear for their lives, and they decide to flee the country.

Act 2, Scene 4
An OLD MAN (3) tells Rosse of the strange omens that had preceded the king's death. Macduff reports that the flight of Malcolm and Donalbain has convinced everyone of their guilt and that Macbeth is to be crowned as Duncan's successor.

Act 3, Scene 1
Banquo, alone, voices his suspicion that Macbeth killed Duncan, and he reflects on the Witches' prophecy that his own heirs will rule. Macbeth, now the king, arrives. He learns that Banquo proposes to go horseback riding with his son FLEANCE, and he insists that they return in time for the evening meal. Banquo leaves and Macbeth plans his murder, lest the Witches' prophecy come true. He sends for the FIRST MURDERER (3) and his companion and arranges for them to kill Banquo and Fleance as the victims return from riding.

Act 3, Scene 2
Macbeth and Lady Macbeth discuss the danger Banquo presents, and Macbeth darkly hints at the plot he has set in motion.

Act 3, Scene 3
The two Murderers, joined by a THIRD MURDERER—sent by Macbeth—attack Banquo and Fleance. Banquo is killed, but Fleance escapes.

Act 3, Scene 4
The First Murderer reports to Macbeth during a banquet. When the king returns to his guests, the GHOST (4) of Banquo appears and sits in his chair. No one sees it but Macbeth, who reacts with horror. Lady Macbeth tells the guests that he is suffering from an old illness, and when the Ghost disappears, Macbeth recovers. But it soon reappears and evokes a strong response from Macbeth; the banquet is disrupted and the nobles leave. Macbeth tells Lady Macbeth that he will consult the Witches, to learn of all possible threats.

Act 3, Scene 5
HECATE chastises the Witches because they have not included her in their dealings with Macbeth. She tells them that they must prepare especially potent spells to delude Macbeth when he consults them.

Act 3, Scene 6
LENOX and another LORD (8) discuss the suspicious deaths of Duncan and Banquo, the exiled Malcolm's support from the King of England, and Macduff's defection to his cause. They hope for aid from England against Macbeth.

Act 4, Scene 1
The Witches and Hecate cast spells, and Hecate departs as Macbeth arrives. The Witches summon three APPARITIONS to answer Macbeth's questions. The first, an armed head, warns Macbeth against Macduff; the second, a bloody child, declares that no man born of a woman can harm him; the third, a crowned child, assures him that he will not be conquered until the forest at BIRNAM marches to DUNSINANE. Macbeth concludes that he is certain of continued success. Macbeth asks if Banquo's descendants shall ever rule Scotland. A parade of eight KINGS appears, escorted by Banquo's Ghost, which smilingly indicates that these are his offspring. The apparitions and Witches disappear. Lenox brings news of Macduff's desertion, and Macbeth decides he will kill all of Macduff's family and followers, as punishment.

Act 4, Scene 2
LADY (7) Macduff bemoans her husband's departure. She tells her SON (1) that his father is dead, but the clever boy realises this isn't true, and engages his mother in a humorous exchange. A MESSENGER (22) appears, quickly delivers a warning of their imminent danger, and flees. The Murderers appear, kill the boy, and chase his mother as she attempts to escape.

Act 4, Scene 3
In England, Malcolm tests Macduff's loyalty to Scotland. He pretends to confess to extreme depravity, and when Macduff mourns for his country, Malcolm knows he is a true patriot. Rosse brings the news that

Macbeth has slaughtered Macduff's family. Macduff vows revenge, and he and Malcolm prepare to launch an army against Macbeth.

Act 5, Scene 1
Observed by a GENTLEWOMAN (1) and a DOCTOR (3), Lady Macbeth walks in her sleep and raves about the blood on her hands. She mentions the murders of Duncan, Lady Macduff, and Banquo.

Act 5, Scene 2
A group of Scottish rebels against Macbeth speak of the approaching English army led by Malcolm, Macduff, and SIWARD. They prepare to rendezvous at Birnam Wood, near the castle at Dunsinane where Macbeth has established his defence.

Act 5, Scene 3
Macbeth boasts that he does not fear the invaders because of the assurances of the Apparitions. The Doctor reports that Lady Macbeth is troubled by hallucinations, which he cannot cure. Macbeth rejects him angrily.

Act 5, Scene 4
Malcolm orders that each of his soldiers, assembled at Birnam Wood, shall carry a branch cut from a tree to provide camouflage and confuse the enemy as to their numbers.

Act 5, Scene 5
SEYTON reports to Macbeth, on the castle walls, that Lady Macbeth is dead. Macbeth laments the nature of life. His Messenger arrives and reports that, unbelievably, Birnam Wood appears to be moving towards the castle. Macbeth recognises the danger predicted in the Apparition's prophecy, but he declares himself ready to die.

Act 5, Scene 6
Malcolm, Siward, and Macduff approach the castle.

Act 5, Scene 7
Macbeth fights YOUNG SIWARD, kills him, and leaves to fight elsewhere. Macduff appears and follows him.

Act 5, Scene 8
Macduff finds Macbeth and they fight. Macbeth boasts that he cannot be killed by any man born of a woman, but his opponent counters with the information that he, Macduff, was taken surgically from his mother's womb before birth, and in this sense was not born of a woman. They fight, and Macduff kills Macbeth.

Act 5, Scene 9
Macduff appears with Macbeth's head and hails Malcolm as King of Scotland. Malcolm declares that when he is crowned his supporters shall be made Earls, in celebration of the defeat of Macbeth.

COMMENTARY

Macbeth is a study of the human potential for evil; it illustrates—though not in a religious context—the Judeo-Christian concept of the Fall, humanity's loss of God's grace. We see the triumph of evil in a man with many good qualities. We are made aware that the potential for evil is frighteningly present in all of us and needs only the wrong circumstances and a relaxation of our desire for good. The good in Macbeth cries out poignantly through his feverish imagination, but his worldly ambition, the influence of Lady Macbeth (though she too has an inarticulate angel struggling against her own evil), and the instigation of a supernatural power all combine to crush his better nature. By the end of the play Macbeth has collapsed beneath the weight of his evil, and the desperate tyrant has so isolated himself from society—and from his own moral sensibility—that for him life seems 'a tale / Told by an idiot, full of sound and fury, / Signifying nothing' (5.5.26–28).

Macbeth's despair strikes a responsive chord in modern audiences and readers partly because it resembles an existentialist response to the uncertainties of modern life. However, Shakespeare was not a philosopher, and in the 17th century existentialism did not exist. Nevertheless, he understood the potential for social and emotional collapse in the absence of morality. Macbeth and his lady chill us with their monstrous perversion of principles so obviously pertinent to people in all periods.

Shakespeare's depiction of evil in *Macbeth* has two aspects, natural and supernatural. The former is the portrait of the man, Macbeth; the latter is the representation of the supernatural world. Evil exists outside the protagonist in the world of black magic, represented most strikingly by the Witches. The appearance of these embodiments of the devil in 1.1 establishes the play's tone of mysterious evil. The Witches cause Macbeth to respond in ways that are 'Against the use of nature' (1.3.137), and his mind 'is smother'd in surmise, / And nothing is, but what is not' (1.3.141–142). When Macbeth finally recognises that their predictions were not what they seemed, he denounces 'th'equivocation of the fiend, / That lies like truth' (5.5.43–44). He thus touches on their most important quality: the Witches deform the lives they interfere with because they disturb a necessary element of human society: its dependence on mutual trust.

Other emblems of the supernatural in *Macbeth* are the omens associated with the murder of Duncan. As he approaches the deed, Macbeth remarks on the ominous night: 'Nature seems dead, . . . Witchcraft celebrates . . .' (2.1.50–51). Moments later, Lady Macbeth hears an owl's hoot and the sound of crickets, both traditional omens of death. Lenox' account of the

night's terrifying storm is full of ancient superstition told in explicit detail, with 'strange screams of death' (2.3.55), earthquakes, and dire prophesies by owls. In 2.4 the Old Man and Rosse intensify the motif when they discuss the day's strange darkness, the killing of a hawk by an owl, and the deadly combat among Duncan's horses. These are gross disruptions of nature that signify the presence of active evil.

The supernatural world is the most extreme example of power that is beyond human control, and it is therefore an apt symbol for the unpredictable forces of human motivation. This larger aspect of evil influences our impression of its more particular manifestation in the man Macbeth. Thus, the pervasive magic in the world of *Macbeth* supports our awareness that the behaviour of the protagonist is, in human terms, unnatural. The portrayal of the evildoer, while convincing, is not psychological in intent; instead, it emphasises the mystery of human behaviour. The play presents possibilities and influences—Macbeth's political ambition, Lady Macbeth's urging, the Witches' bald temptation—but we still wonder why Macbeth does what he does. Macbeth is revolted by himself and his self-awareness makes his descent even more appalling; it also maintains our consciousness of the power of evil. He succumbs to temptation in an almost ritualistic way. He acknowledges each evil and then proceeds, prepared to accept 'deep damnation' (1.7.-20) from the time he first recognises temptation until he is left with no alternative but death.

Macbeth's relation to evil is symbolic. Lady Macbeth, too, though she rejects her husband's scruples, is entirely aware that the proposed murder is evil. She avoids mentioning it too explicitly, and she cannot bring herself to do the deed herself. Finally, her anguished madness—presented in 5.1 and confirmed by her suicide—demonstrates her inability to absorb what she has helped unleash. Thus, she too presents the weakness of humanity in the face of evil. We recognise that they are susceptible to the mental ravages of guilt, and this keeps us from seeing either Macbeth or Lady Macbeth as simply a monstrous sociopath. In fact, much of the play's tension is created because neither of them can simply accept their evil callously. Thus, Macbeth is as much a victim of evil as its instrument, and he is doubly symbolic as a negator of the good in humanity.

Macbeth clearly sees that his evil is a perversion of human values, and the fact that he persists in the face of this awareness demonstrates a profound moral disorder. Indeed, disorder permeates his world. Disrupted sleep—commonly considered a symptom of guilt in Shakespeare's day and in our own—plagues both Macbeth and his wife. He hears a voice predict 'Macbeth shall sleep no more!' (2.2.42) as he commits the murder, and later he speaks of 'these terrible dreams that shake us nightly' (3.2.18–19). Lady Macbeth demonstrates the disorder physically in the sleep-walking scene (5.1). Macbeth even envies the murdered Duncan, for 'After life's fitful fever he sleeps well' (3.2.23).

Emotional disorder is particularly strongly presented in a repeated emphasis on sexual dysfunction. Lady Macbeth makes sex a weapon in her efforts to spur Macbeth's ambition. She casts aspersions on his sexuality when she equates it with his fear. 'Such I account thy love' (1.7.39), she says, and adds 'When you durst do it, then you were a man' (1.7.49). In 3.4 she uses the same technique when she urges him to conquer his fear of Banquo's Ghost. She calls the bloody-handed Macbeth 'My husband!' (2.2.13) when he has just killed the king. This—the only time she calls him 'husband'—suggests that she finds him sexually impressive in his gore. She also distorts her own gender in a startling fashion when she prays, 'Spirits . . . unsex me here' (1.5.40–41), and perversely elevates and then denies her maternal instincts in a vivid description of infanticide in 1.7.54–59. In 2.3.28–35 the Porter delivers a short description of sexual dysfunction from drink just at the moment when Duncan's murder, accomplished but not yet discovered, hangs over the play's world, emphasising the motif. Macbeth's later withdrawal from his wife—he excludes her from his plans for Banquo and she takes no part in his story thereafter—suggests that their marriage has been destroyed, not strengthened, by their immersion in evil.

This motif, combined with the obvious pleasure that Macbeth and Lady Macbeth take in each other upon their first meeting in the play (1.5.54 ff.), has led most modern actors and directors to present their relationship as highly charged sexually, sometimes including sadomasochistic bouts of slapping and grappling. However, the text could also support the suggestion of an icy incapacity to express themselves sexually. In either light, sex is an issue between Macbeth and Lady Macbeth, and the normal marital relationship is pathologically distorted—one way or another—by the force of the evil to which they commit themselves.

The theme of unnatural disorder is reinforced throughout the play. When Macbeth first considers murdering the king, he acknowledges the evil of the deed with a vivid image of the disorder of the elements, 'Stars, hide your fires!' (1.4.50). His doubts are stimulated by his subconscious recognition that there is no possible way to integrate his desires with the proper order of things. Once Macbeth is fully committed to his evil course, this lack of integration is manifested in 3.4. He is horribly isolated at the banquet when only he sees Banquo's Ghost. His response, the decision to return to the Witches, illustrates nicely

the widening difference between himself and other men.

The contrast is stressed in the comparison of Macbeth and Macduff, which becomes an important theme at this point in the play. In 3.6 Lenox and another Lord discuss Macduff's opposition to Macbeth in terms of holiness versus evil. Perhaps most forceful are the parallel impressions of Macduff and Macbeth in grief. Macduff's response to news of the massacre of his family is a powerful demonstration of true humanity—he must 'feel it as a man' (4.3.221). Macbeth's reaction to Lady Macbeth's death—'To-morrow, and to-morrow, and to-morrow, / Creeps in this petty pace . . .' (5.5.19–20)—is the wretched cry of a man so used to evil that he has lost his emotional reflexes. Macbeth's advanced disorder also manifests itself more violently when he alternates between despair and rage in Act 5. He now lacks the capacity for normal emotions.

The force that affects the man also affects the whole society in which he lives. The evil created by the Witches inspires mistrust throughout the world of the play. Significantly, after the Witches' 'overture' in 1.1 the play opens with the suppression of a treasonous rebellion. Duncan's 'absolute trust' (1.4.14) in the Thane of Cawdor was misplaced, and with broad irony, Shakespeare permits the king to award the defeated rebel's title to another man he should not trust. Though trust is still available to the characters, it is already misplaced. Once Duncan has been killed, doubt and confusion grow. This development is signalled by the Porter's allusions to treachery and to the doctrine of 'equivocation', a justification for lying (see GARNET). Duncan's sons feel the world is faithless. They fear that they shall themselves be murdered, and they suspect everyone, particularly one who would be most reliable in a morally sound world, their own relative, Macbeth: '. . . the near in blood / The nearer bloody' (2.3.138–139).

Rosse describes vividly the overwhelming lack of trust that afflicts the land ruled by Macbeth: '. . . cruel are the times, when we are traitors, / And do not know ourselves . . . [and] know not what we fear, / But float upon a wild and violent sea' (4.2.18–21). The subsequent quasi-comical dialogue on treachery between Lady Macduff and her Son offers another slant on the same phenomenon, as does the deliberately false nature assumed by Malcolm to test Macduff, in 4.3. At the play's climax Macbeth discovers that he has been the victim of the 'equivocation of the fiend / That lies like truth' (5.5.43–44), and thus reprises the Porter's motif. Only with Macbeth's defeat and death can honesty return. Siward is proud that his son died having 'paid his score' (5.9.18). When he hails Malcolm as the new king, Macduff wants to express what is in his mind; and Malcolm, in response, declares his wish to be 'even with' his supporters (5.9.28). The malaise generated by Macbeth's evil is dissolved, and 'the grace of Grace' (5.9.38) has returned to the world of the play.

As Malcolm begins to conduct the business of the state, we see that the motif of mistrust has been significant for the play's secondary theme, a political one. Throughout his career, Shakespeare was concerned with the influence on society of the moral quality of its leaders—this issue dominates the HISTORY PLAYS, for instance—and in *Macbeth* he applies his ideas to a tale of ancient Scotland. Like many of the histories, *Macbeth* begins and ends with a battle (one reported, one enacted), and the fate of the country is never ignored. The travails of Scotland while governed by the evil usurper are clearly presented, especially in the conversation among Malcolm, Macduff, and Rosse in 4.3. The fate of Scotland is a parallel development to Macbeth's descent into evil. This strengthens our awareness of his decline, but also stresses the important lesson that the immoral behaviour of a society's leader is a dangerous disease, capable of producing widespread catastrophe.

The political aspect of the play also had a contemporary significance for Shakespeare's original audiences. The alliance of English and Scottish forces against Macbeth predicts the joining of the two countries under King James I in 1603, a recent event still prominent in the public eye, and James' rule is pointed to more directly in the apparition of future rulers presented in 4.1. Moreover, the enormity of regicide, combined with the Porter's allusions to the trial of Henry Garnet, will have brought forcibly to mind the recently exposed Gunpowder Plot, giving the play a thrilling relevance to the biggest political story in many years.

When he devised his drama of personal evil and public affairs, Shakespeare drew on the history of Scotland as presented in his source, HOLINSHED's *Chronicles*, but much of his version varies from Holinshed for he was interested in drama, not history. (See MACBETH, MALCOLM, et al.) These inaccuracies are of no consequence, for the play's bold art generates more power than could a dispassionate presentation of real facts. *Macbeth*, which contains some of Shakespeare's greatest poetry, offers one of literature's most striking accounts of an individual soul's descent into the darkness of evil, and its resulting isolation from society. Macbeth's rejection of morality, and its consequences—the loss of his soul and the disruption of the society that he influences—horrifies us. This is a drama that is as terrifying as the plots and wars of real usurpers and kings.

SOURCES OF THE PLAY

The chief source for *Macbeth* was Raphael HOLINSHED's *Chronicles of England, Scotland, and Ireland* (2nd ed., 1587), whose account of Scotland was

derived from the Latin *Scotorum Historiae* (1527) of Hector BOECE. Shakespeare used Holinshed's report of Macbeth's encounter with witches and subsequent usurpation of the throne, though the playwright altered the story considerably. He also used an account in Holinshed of another Scottish regicide that provided the details of Macbeth's crime and included his wife's involvement. Other details may have come from other Scottish tales in Holinshed. Another history of Scotland, George BUCHANAN's Latin *Rerum Scotiarum Historia* (1582), may also have influenced the playwright in the development of Macbeth's character and in several political details.

Various other sources contributed to *Macbeth* in minor ways. Reginald SCOT's *Discovery of Witchcraft* (1584) contributed to the depiction of the Witches, as did a work by King James I, *Daemonologie* (1599). Another tract by James, his *Counterblast to Tobacco* (1604) provided additional details. The Latin memoirs of Erasmus, *Colloquia* (1500)—which the playwright may have read in school—provided the original version of Macbeth's remarks on dogs and men in 3.1.91–100. Lines from two contemporary plays are echoed in *Macbeth*, Samuel DANIEL's *The Queen's Arcadia* (1605) and John MARSTON's *Sophonisba* (1606). Another play, Matthew GWINNE's Latin work, *Tres Sibyllae* (1605), may have suggested the subject matter in the first place. Some scholars believe, however, that the idea may have come from a lost play on Macbeth thought to have been performed in the 1590s. Also, Shakespeare exploited the plays of SENECA in *Macbeth*, particularly in the depiction of Lady Macbeth. He also used details from three of his own earlier works, *2 Henry VI*, *Richard III*, and, especially, *THE RAPE OF LUCRECE*.

TEXT OF THE PLAY

Macbeth was probably written between 1603 and 1606. It is dated after King James' accession to the throne in the former year and before the publication in 1607 of THE PURITAN, a play whose author—probably Thomas MIDDLETON—had clearly seen *Macbeth*. Some critics feel that the references to James were added later and that the play was written before he came to power, perhaps as early as 1599. However, most scholars believe that the style suggests the later dates. Also, several pieces of evidence—the probable influence of Gwinne and Marston and certain allusions to the treason of Henry GARNET—suggest the summer of 1606 as a more precise date. However, these items could also have been added, and the date of composition remains uncertain.

The scenes involving HECATE in *Macbeth*—3.5 and 4.1.39–43—were obviously added. They include material that came from Thomas MIDDLETON's play *The Witch* (c. 1610–1620), and it is traditionally assumed that Middleton wrote them. However, some scholars point out differences in style and conclude that some other writer, now unknown, was responsible. The scenes were presumably written for a KING'S MEN production sometime after Shakespeare's retirement, but before the publication of the play.

Macbeth was first published in the FIRST FOLIO (1623). At 2,500 lines, it is the shortest of the tragedies, and scholars generally believe that the play was cut considerably before publication and that the surviving text is the acting version of a longer original work. Other alterations are suspected—by Shakespeare or another writer—and the relationship of the published text to the playwright's original manuscript is unknown. The Folio text was probably printed from a PROMPT-BOOK, or a transcript of a prompt-book made for the purpose. As the only old text, the Folio has been the basis for all subsequent editions.

THEATRICAL HISTORY OF THE PLAY

Simon FORMAN recorded the earliest known performance of *Macbeth* in April 1611, but since the play influenced a work published in early 1607, we know it must have been performed at least as early as 1606. Richard BURBAGE (3) is thought to have created the title role. No other early stagings are recorded, but alterations evident in the Folio text (1623) imply that several productions had been mounted by that time.

The English theatres were closed for 18 years while the Puritan government was in power, and when they reopened William DAVENANT produced an adaptation of *Macbeth* (1663) that altered the play greatly. Much of Shakespeare's text was omitted or 'refined' (e.g., 'The devil damn thee black, thou cream-faced loon!' [5.3.11] became 'Now Friend, what means this change of Countenance?'), and musical numbers featuring singers and dancers were added to the Witches' scenes. These scenes were satirised in Thomas DUFFET's *The Empress of Morocco* (c. 1673). Among the actors who were noted for their portrayals of Macbeth in the adaptation were Thomas BETTERTON and James QUIN.

Davenant's version was quite popular, and it was not until David GARRICK's 1744 production that Shakespeare's *Macbeth* was partially restored. Though Garrick consulted Samuel JOHNSON (7) about the text, he still cut some 300 lines, retained many of Davenant's operatic embellishments, and added some lines of his own. Macbeth was one of Garrick's great roles, and he played it for many years. He ceased only upon the death of his longtime Lady Macbeth, Hannah PRITCHARD, in 1768. Another popular 18th-century Macbeth was Charles MACKLIN, who introduced the use of Scottish kilts and plaids in 1773. In the late 18th and early 19th centuries Sarah SIDDONS was a very popular Lady Macbeth, and frequently played opposite her brother, John Philip KEMBLE (3).

Samuel PHELPS' production of 1847 omitted Dave-

nant's operatic elements for the first time. Edwin BOOTH (2) was an especially acclaimed Macbeth in the 19th century, and he often played opposite Helena MODJESKA. Charlotte CUSHMAN played Lady Macbeth opposite both William MACREADY and Edwin FORREST. Cushman and Siddons, in particular, were noted for the ferociousness of their interpretations, but styles changed later in the century when Ellen TERRY (1) played the character as a less assertive partner to Henry IRVING's dominating Macbeth. In the 1890s, Sarah BERNHARDT introduced an explicit sexuality to the role that has been stressed in the 20th century.

Macbeth remains extremely popular with modern audiences, and most leading actors and actresses aspire to the roles of Macbeth and his Lady. There have been many remarkable productions in the 20th century, and one of these was the 1928 modern-dress presentation by Barry JACKSON (1). Another was Orson WELLES' notorious 'voodoo' *Macbeth* of 1936, which was set in 18th-century Haiti and featured a gigantic mask as Banquo's Ghost, a Hecate with a 12-foot bull-whip, and a band of on-stage drummers. The 1941 New York production directed by Margaret WEBSTER (3), which starred Judith ANDERSON (2) and Maurice EVANS (4), and Trevor NUNN's 1976 staging at STRATFORD, with Ian MCKELLEN and Judi DENCH, were both memorable. Other notable Macbeths have included Robert Bruce MANTELL, Laurence OLIVIER, and John GIELGUD. Zoë CALDWELL and Sybil THORNDIKE have been acclaimed as Lady Macbeth. In 1981 a company from the University of Illinois adapted *Macbeth* to kabuki, the traditional, stylised Japanese drama, and performed in several American cities.

Macbeth has been made into a FILM 17 times. The earliest of these was in 1908, when the first of seven silent versions was made. The last of them, by D. W. Griffith, starred Beerbohm TREE. Orson Welles directed and starred in a movie of 1948, and Maurice Evans and Judith Anderson re-created their stage success on the screen in 1960. Probably the best-known (and by virtually unanimous critical acclaim the best) film of *Macbeth* is an adaptation, Akira KUROSAWA's *Throne of Blood* (1957). Five TELEVISION productions of the play have been broadcast, the first in 1949, though one of these simply recorded a performance of Nunn's 1976 stage production.

Macduff, Thane of Fife (active c. 1054?) Quasi-historical figure and character in *Macbeth*, the rival and vanquisher of MACBETH. After Macbeth murders King DUNCAN of SCOTLAND and succeeds him on the throne, Macduff joins Duncan's son MALCOLM in exile in England. There he learns that Macbeth has massacred his family, and when he and Malcolm lead an army against Macbeth, Macduff seeks out the usurper at DUNSINANE to exact personal vengeance. Macbeth relies on the supernatural assurance that no man 'of woman born' (4.1.80, 5.8.13) can harm him, but it turns out that Macduff was 'from his mother's womb / Untimely ripp'd' (5.8.14–15)—that is, delivered by Caesarean section and thus not 'born' in the ordinary construction of the word. In the subsequent fight, Macduff kills Macbeth; he presents the usurper's severed head to Malcolm, in 5.9.

Shakespeare painstakingly builds Macduff up as the play's agent of retribution. We first notice Macduff in 2.4, when he returns to FIFE rather than attend Macbeth's coronation. In 3.4 Macbeth suspects Macduff is hostile, and in 3.6 we hear that he has fled to join Malcolm. Thus, even before he takes a prominent role, Macduff distinguishes himself because he refuses to accept Macbeth's succession to the crown. In 4.1 Macbeth is told by the APPARITIONS to 'Beware Macduff' (4.1.71), and it is evident that the Thane of Fife will be the usurper's rival though Macbeth is calmed by the Apparitions' other predictions. In 4.3 Macduff proves that he is a disinterested patriot. Malcolm fears that Macduff may be Macbeth's agent and tests him. The prince pretends to be a degenerate who would make a terrible king. Macduff despairs for Scotland, and Malcolm accordingly accepts him. Thus, the playwright places Macduff's virtue in clear opposition to the villainy of Macbeth.

As a symbol of triumphant good, Macduff is a somewhat stylised character. He rejects Macbeth, he proves himself dedicated to Scotland, he is able to overcome the magic that Macbeth relies on, and in the end he kills the villain. A multifaceted persona is not required for such a character, and generally we do not see one. However, he has one majestic moment that powerfully evokes our sympathy for him as a man. In one of Shakespeare's most moving episodes, Macduff grieves for the death of his wife, LADY (7) Macduff, and their family, at the hands of Macbeth's hired killers. At first, he can hardly believe it: 'All my pretty ones? / Did you say all?—O Hell-kite!—All?' (4.3.216–217), he cries. When Malcolm encourages him to revenge and says, 'Dispute it like a man' (4.3.220), Macduff replies with great dignity, 'I shall do so; / But I must also feel it as a man: / I cannot but remember such things were / That were most precious to me' (4.3.220–223). We are deeply moved, aware that the grieving thane is profoundly engaged with his love and sorrow. The source of Macduff's virtue is exposed: he is a complete human being who cannot sever the bonds of kinship and love. We see that Macduff's strong acceptance of his grief is the opposite of the cold inhumanity of Macbeth and LADY (6) MACBETH.

It is uncertain whether Macduff existed in history. Shakespeare found him in HOLINSHED's *Chronicles*, which was based on the quasi-legendary history of Hector BOECE, but he cannot be certainly identified with anyone recorded in 11th-century documents. Nevertheless, the name probably represents a histori-

cal ruler of Fife who was an ally of Malcolm against Macbeth. His birth by Caesarean section is even more speculative. The procedure, though known to have existed since ancient times, was certainly extremely rare in medieval Scotland, if practised at all. In pre-modern societies the strangeness of this mode of birth led to its being associated with the extraordinary figures of history and legend—such as Julius CAESAR (1), for whom it is named—and this doubtless accounts for the belief that Macbeth's killer entered the world in this fashion.

Machiavel Villainous but humorous character type of ELIZABETHAN DRAMA, a sly cynic who loves evil for its own sake. A Machiavel is characterised by a delight in evil that makes other motivation unnecessary, the habit of commenting on his own activities in humorous soliloquies, treachery to his own allies, a tendency to lewdness, and a cynical contempt for goodness and religion. By convention, the good characters never recognise the Machiavel's evil intentions until it is too late. OTHELLO's extraordinary gullibility is paradoxically explained, in part, by IAGO's obvious villainy, for its very obviousness to the audience presumes its invisibility to the characters.

Shakespeare's principal Machiavels besides Iago—who is probably the most famous of all such characters—were AARON, EDMUND, and RICHARD III. A number of other Shakespearean characters display the features of the type to a lesser degree—for example, the Bishop of WINCHESTER (1) in *1 Henry VI* and CASSIUS in *Julius Caesar.* The first famous Machiavel—who doubtless influenced Shakespeare—was Barabas, the villain of *The Jew of Malta* by Christopher MARLOWE (1). Also, a character named Machiavel speaks the PROLOGUE (1) to the play. Other dramatists of the period employed the figure as well.

The Machiavel takes his name from the Italian political philosopher Niccolo Machiavelli (1469–1527), who was (and is) popularly misunderstood to have advocated atheism, treachery, and criminality as preferable to other means of statecraft. This model was applied to an already-existing character type, the VICE, a humorous villain from the medieval MORALITY PLAY. Machiavelli added elements of intelligence, craftiness, and political ambition. Shakespeare's Richard, who identifies himself as a superior Machiavel in *3 Henry VI* 3.2.193 (probably referring to Marlowe's prologue-speaker), also describes his methods, 'Plots have I laid, inductions dangerous', and adds for good measure that he is 'subtle, false, and treacherous' (*Richard III* 1.1.33, 37).

Macklin, Charles (c. 1700–1797) Irish actor, a notable SHYLOCK. Macklin is best known as the actor who restored Shakespeare's Shylock after the part had for at least a generation been customarily played for laughs by crude comedians. After Macklin, the dignity and pathos of the figure never again lapsed so far, though even Macklin played him as a melodramatic villain. Macklin played many comic parts in Shakespeare, and in 1754 he delivered a series of lectures on the playwright that are the earliest ever recorded. He was also a playwright who wrote two successful comedies. He retired in 1789, at about age 90, after forgetting his lines while playing Shylock.

Macmorris Character in *Henry V,* an Irish officer in the army of King HENRY V. Macmorris appears only in the 'international' scene, 3.2, with the Welsh FLUELLEN, the Scottish JAMY, and the English GOWER (2). Hot-tempered, Macmorris takes offence at Fluellen's reference to the Irish, presuming he means an insult, and they nearly come to blows, though both respond professionally to the call of duty and postpone their quarrel. The episode exploits ethnic stereotypes to demonstrate the diversity of British subjects working to a common end under King Henry.

Macready, William Charles (1793–1873) British actor and producer. Macready, one of the great tragedians of the 19th century, played all of Shakespeare's great protagonists, as well as numerous other figures, such as HOTSPUR, IAGO, and JAQUES (1). He often played opposite Helen FAUCIT. He helped pioneer the period's return to genuine Shakespearean texts, removing the accretions of earlier centuries, especially in his productions of *King Lear, Coriolanus,* and *The Tempest.* However, Macready's versions were themselves abridgements, in part to make room for the spectacular tableaus for which he was well known, and in part to censor Shakespeare, removing, for instance, the grisly fate of GLOUCESTER (1) from *King Lear.* With Edmund KEAN (2), Macready dominated the English theatre of the 1820s and was alone its major figure in the following decade. His diaries, published in 1875, offer a lively picture of the theatre of his day. Macready played in New York in 1826 and 1848; on the latter occasion, the rivalry of Edwin FORREST led to the notorious Astor Place riots.

Maecenas, Gaius (d. 8 B.C.) Historical figure and minor character in *Antony and Cleopatra,* a follower of Octavius CAESAR (2). Maecenas is a courtier who serves to swell the ranks of Caesar's court. He offers some important advice in 4.1 when he encourages Caesar to advance on ANTONY and finish him off while he is distracted with rage and humiliation after the battle of ACTIUM. This remark helps signal Antony's approaching end.

The historical Maecenas was far more important to Caesar than the play indicates. He was among the future emperor's earliest allies, and he assisted Caesar's arrival in Italy to claim the inheritance of the

assassinated Julius CAESAR (1) in 44 B.C. (Maecenas does not appear in Shakespeare's *Julius Caesar*, however.) Along with AGRIPPA, Maecenas was one of the most trusted friends and advisers of Caesar throughout the civil wars and in the early days of the empire, and he conducted numerous delicate diplomatic missions. He was descended from the ancient kings of Etruria, though his family's fortunes had fallen when his grandfather joined a revolt against Rome. However, Maecenas became one of the highest-ranking and richest men of the early Roman Empire. As such, he was a great patron of Roman literature, the role for which he is now best known. He befriended and supported many poets and writers, including VIRGIL.

Malcolm (Prince Malcolm Canmore, d. 1093) Historical figure and character in *Macbeth*, son of the murdered King DUNCAN of SCOTLAND. In 1.4 Malcolm is named his father's successor to the dismay of MACBETH, who plots to take the crown himself. However, when Duncan is murdered, Malcolm and his brother DONALBAIN fear for their lives and worry that suspicion will fall on them. They flee the country in 2.3 and leave Macbeth to occupy the throne. Malcolm seeks refuge at the court of the English king, where we find him in 4.3. MACDUFF joins him there, and they lead an army to Scotland in Act 5, and defeat and kill Macbeth. At the play's close, Malcolm makes a stately speech that thanks his supporters and announces his forthcoming coronation as King of Scotland.

Like Macduff, the young prince is a figure of goodness placed in opposition to Macbeth's evil, and as such is somewhat two-dimensional. He is clever when he devises a form of camouflage—each soldier carries a branch of a tree as the army marches on DUNSINANE—that proves significant in Macbeth's downfall. However, Malcolm is most distinctive when he tests Macduff's patriotism, in 4.3.1–139. The prospective king describes himself as an intemperate and dishonest degenerate, certain to be bad for the country. When Macduff despairs for Scotland, Malcolm reveals himself as a virtuous prince and accepts Macduff as a leader of his invasion army. This episode has two functions: most important, it stresses the atmosphere of distrust that Macbeth's evil has loosed on Scotland. It also presents Malcolm as a sensible, cautious young man who seems likely to be a successful ruler. This impression, along with our recollection of the clever camouflage, helps establish the sense of healing that comes with his triumph at the play's close. CATHNESS refers to him, appropriately, as 'the med'cine of the sickly weal' (5.2.27).

The historical Malcolm did return from exile to defeat Macbeth, but Shakespeare's treatment of his career is otherwise almost entirely altered. Malcolm was a young child when Macbeth seized the throne in 1039. Duncan was not murdered, so Malcolm did not flee to avoid suspicion. He was in fact sent to his uncle, Earl SIWARD, and he later lived at the court of King Edward the Confessor of England, as in the play. Only 15 years later, once he was a man, did Malcolm attempt an invasion of Scotland in 1054. The attack was repulsed though some territory was taken. Three years later a second attempt succeeded; Macbeth was defeated and killed, and Malcolm took the throne.

Malcolm's reign began a highly important period in Scottish history, the first European orientation for the country. Malcolm's second wife, later known as St. Margaret, was an English princess who had been raised at the cosmopolitan medieval court of the kings of Hungary. Under her influence, Scotland accepted the Roman rather than the Celtic church and the arts and culture of Europe as opposed to those of ancient Britain. Margaret had been a refugee from the Norman Conquest of England in 1066, and Malcolm engaged in periodic warfare against William the Conqueror. He died in battle in 1093, during his fifth invasion of England. His successor was Duncan II, his oldest son by his first wife (the sister or daughter of Cathness). Duncan was overthrown by his uncle, Donalbain, but eventually another of Malcolm's sons (by Margaret) ruled Scotland as King David I (ruled 1124–1153). Through him, Malcolm was an ancestor of JAMES I, the ruler of England in Shakespeare's time.

Malone, Edmond (1741–1812) English scholar. Malone was probably the greatest of 18th-century Shakespearean scholars, and one of the greatest of all time. His *Attempt to ascertain the Order in which the Plays of Shakespeare were written*—the first such effort—was published in George STEEVENS' 1778 edition of the plays, and he edited two volumes added in 1780 to Steevens' collection, containing the poems, the doubtful plays of the third FOLIO, and Malone's history of ELIZABETHAN THEATRE. In 1790 he brought out his own edition of the plays, incorporating a tremendous amount of scholarship, including his massive *Life* of Shakespeare, the basis for all subsequent biographies. In 1796 he led the exposure of the forgeries of William Henry IRELAND, and when he died he was at work on a new edition of the plays. This was eventually completed by James BOSWELL the Younger. Known as the 'Third Variorum' (see VARIORUM EDITION), it has been the foundation of modern Shakespeare studies.

Malvolio Character in *Twelfth Night*, mean-spirited steward to OLIVIA. Malvolio is the focus of the comic SUB-PLOT, in which a group of characters led by MARIA (2) and SIR TOBY conspire to embarrass him, with the result that he is incarcerated as a lunatic. This plot is clearly secondary to the main story of the lovers—VIOLA, ORSINO, SEBASTIAN (2), and Olivia—but Malvolio is such a strongly drawn character that the play sometimes seems to centre on him. In fact, several

documents of the 17th century identify the play as 'Malvolio', and leading actors have always been pleased to take the role. In addition to embodying an ordinary comic villain—an obvious misfit who mistreats others and in the end is humiliated by a crude stratagem—Malvolio is also a humanly interesting victim, and he inspires sympathy as well as derision, thus contributing to Shakespeare's ironic undercutting of the conventional romantic comedy.

Malvolio rejects humour and love in favour of a stern coldness and a consuming personal ambition. His dislike of merriment and his rigorously sober dress and behaviour justify his name, an approximation of the Italian for 'ill will'. (These features also resemble the typical 16th-century—and later—stereotype of the Puritan, but Shakespeare certainly did not consider Malvolio a Puritan, as is clear in 2.3.140–146.) Malvolio opposes the frivolity of Sir Toby, SIR ANDREW, and FESTE in 2.3, inspiring Sir Toby's famous riposte, 'Dost thou think because thou art virtuous, there shall be no more cakes and ale?' (2.3.114–115). Driven away by this assault on his dignity, the angry Malvolio gratuitously threatens Maria, thereby triggering the plot that brings him down.

The steward behaves badly to Viola, who is disguised as a young man, when he brusquely delivers Olivia's ring to her in 2.2, and he is unnecessarily nasty to Feste in 1.5. His churlish behaviour quite plainly foreshadows the comeuppance that he later receives. Even more repellent is the cold ambition of his entirely loveless courtship of Olivia, undertaken in accordance with the comical instructions of Maria's letter but contemplated by him in 2.5, before he finds this missive. His musings on the power and position he hopes to gain strongly illuminate his personality, as he solemnly and pompously contemplates punishing Sir Toby. These boldly unattractive features have inspired scholarly speculations that Shakespeare intended Malvolio as a satire on a particular living person (see William FFARINGTON; Thomas Posthumous HOBY [2]; William KNOLLYS; Ambrose WILLOUGHBY [1]), but these hypotheses have never been convincingly established and they do not alter the character's function in the play.

For all his noxious characteristics, Malvolio is not a serious threat in the manner of, say, SHYLOCK; ultimately he is simply laughed off the stage. Nor does he grow or change in the course of the play; instead he is exposed for what he is by the actions of other characters. There is no question about his destiny; in a comedy such a hypocrite and would-be villain deserves his downfall, and this comes about in an entertaining manner.

Nevertheless, Malvolio's imprisonment and humiliation seem excessive relative to his offence. The 'problem of Malvolio', as this imbalance has long been called, lends the sub-plot a viciousness that contributes to Shakespeare presentation of comedy's limitations. Feste's teasing of the imprisoned Malvolio in 4.2 is undeniably humorous, but even Sir Toby concedes that this continuing torment of their victim may be going too far, remarking 'I would we were well rid of this knavery' (4.2.69–70). Then, provoking the steward's angry final departure in 5.1, Feste mocks the steward even more mercilessly. We sympathise with Malvolio's anger, which seems justifiable, and with his ugly departure and its cry for revenge 'on the whole pack of you!' (5.1.377) Despite the play's happy ending, an aftertaste of bitter feeling remains. A 19th-century critic, Charles LAMB (1), went so far as to find 'tragic interest' in 'the catastrophe of this character'. Although Malvolio lacks the grandeur of a tragic hero, Lamb's comment raises an interesting moral question: How is Malvolio's shabby treatment—or his unrepentant final response—to be reconciled with the happy ending?

While poetic justice requires that Malvolio be brought down, for his rejection of love is insane in the play's scheme of things, Shakespeare softens his actual defeat in several ways. The victim's final cry for vengeance is neutralised by FABIAN's wish that the conspirators' 'sportful malice . . . may rather pluck on laughter than revenge' (5.1.364–365). Moreover, the two leading figures of ILLYRIA offer the promise of reconciliation: Olivia, though amused at the plot against her humiliated steward, is sympathetic towards him, saying, 'Alas, poor fool, how have they baffled thee!' (5.1.368), and Orsino orders that someone follow him and 'entreat him to a peace' (5.1.379).

After Malvolio's exit, the play moves to its happy conclusion; the steward is simply too out of harmony with the joyful spirit of the ending to remain among the celebrants. Though his downfall gives an edge to the romantic comedy—we see that Illyria has its share of the sins of the real world—this point is easily abandoned in the enthusiasm of the lovers. Nevertheless, the 'problem of Malvolio' makes both the character and the play more complex and humanly interesting.

Mamillius Character in *The Winter's Tale,* the son of King LEONTES of SICILIA and Queen HERMIONE, who dies of grief when his father persecutes his mother unjustly. In 1.1 Mamillius is presented as the pride of his parents and the entire kingdom; his future as a man and ruler looks brilliant. These sentiments, however, will soon seem ironic. In 1.2 and 2.1 he appears a likeable boy, especially in 2.1, when he jests with his mother's ladies-in-waiting (see LADY [4]) and tells his mother a story 'of sprites and goblins' because 'a sad tale's best for winter' (2.1.26, 25). The remark confirms our sense of coming tragedy. Mamillius dies of grief, off-stage, during his mother's trial. The shock of his death, reported in 3.2.144–145, stirs his father, too late, to recognise his own injustice. The death of

Mamillius, a completely innocent victim, demonstrates the appalling cost of Leontes' madness; it is the low point of the play's tragic development.

Shakespeare created Mamillius from the mere mention of the analogous figure in his source, the prose romance *Pandosto* by Robert GREENE (2). His name may have been derived from the title of two earlier romances by Greene, *Mamillia* (1583, 1593).

Man (1) Minor character in *Richard II,* the GARDENER's assistant. The Man asks the Gardener why they should bother to tend their plants when the larger 'garden', the country as a whole, is falling into ruin due to neglect. In other words, he maintains that the state must be kept in order by its rulers, just as a garden must by its humbler caretakers.

Man (2) Minor character in *Troilus and Cressida,* a servant of TROILUS. In 3.2 the Man informs PANDARUS that Troilus is waiting for him.

Man (3) Minor character in *Henry VIII,* assistant to the PORTER (4). In 5.3, on the day of the christening of Princess ELIZABETH (1), the Man defends his inability to prevent a crowd of celebrating commoners from entering the courtyard of the royal palace. He comically exaggerates, in military terms, the combats he has undergone.

Manningham, John (c. 1576–1622) English diarist. Manningham, a lawyer and minor official, was an avid theatre-goer who recorded the earliest known performance of *Twelfth Night,* in 1602. In the same year he also preserved the only surviving contemporary anecdote of Shakespeare's life. He had been told, he wrote in his diary, that the playwright, during a performance of *Richard III,* had overheard a message from a female admirer to its star, Richard BURBAGE (2), inviting him to a dalliance later that evening. Shakespeare, according to the story, arrived at the appointment before Burbage and was enjoying the company of the young woman when a servant brought word that 'Richard III' was at the door. Shakespeare then sent back a message that 'William the Conqueror was before Richard III'. While a student at the INNS OF COURT, Manningham knew William COMBE (5), and through him he may have been personally acquainted with Shakespeare.

Mantell, Robert Bruce (1854–1928) Scottish-American actor. Mantell began his career in Ireland and went to America in 1878, joining Helena MODJESKA's company. After a brief return to Britain, Mantell remained in New York for good. A romantic leading man early in his career and a character actor as an older man, he played many Shakespearean parts.

Mantua City in northern Italy, a location in *Romeo and Juliet.* Romeo flees to Mantua when banished from VERONA, and he is seen there in 5.1. Shakespeare took this incident from his source, the poem *Romeus and Iuliet,* by Arthur BROOKE (1). The same source accounts for a reference to the city in *The Two Gentlemen of Verona,* in which SILVIA asserts (mistakenly) that VALENTINE is in exile there (4.3.24). The city is also named in *The Taming of the Shrew* (4.2.77–85); it is referred to as a port, and this has often been cited as an error on Shakespeare's part. But in the 16th century Mantua, situated on the Mincio River, participated in the considerable river-and-canal trade that was prominent in northern Italy until the advent of the railroads in the 19th century.

Marcade (Mercadé) Minor character in *Love's Labour's Lost,* the messenger who brings the PRINCESS (1) of France news of her father's death in 5.2, thus changing the tenor of the play in its closing minutes.

Marcellus Minor character in *Hamlet.* Marcellus, with BARNARDO, has seen the GHOST (3) of HAMLET's father before the opening of the play. In 1.1 they tell HORATIO about the spirit, and in 1.2 Hamlet is informed as well. Marcellus accompanies Hamlet and Horatio when they encounter the Ghost in 1.4; he and Horatio fearfully attempt to dissuade Hamlet from following it, and in 1.5 Hamlet swears them to secrecy. Speculating on the cause of the phenomenon, Marcellus utters the famous observation 'Something is rotten in the state of Denmark' (1.4.90). Scholars believe that the BAD QUARTO of *Hamlet* (Q1, 1603) was recorded by an actor who had played Marcellus, since that role is the only one whose dialogue is very accurately rendered there.

March, Earl of Historically, the hereditary title of the head of the Mortimer family. Several earls of March laid claim to the English throne by virtue of their descent from a daughter of Lionel Plantagenet, Duke of Clarence, the oldest brother of the deposed King RICHARD II. In *1 Henry VI,* this claim is transmitted to the family of the Duke of YORK (8) by Edmund MORTIMER (1), thus helping to lay the groundwork for the WARS OF THE ROSES. Due to confusion in his sources, Shakespeare gave the title, in *1 Henry IV,* to Edmund MORTIMER (2), who was historically a younger brother and thus neither an Earl of March nor in the royal line of descent.

In *3 Henry VI,* Edward of York, soon to be King EDWARD IV, is referred to as the Earl of March, at 2.1.179 and 2.1.192, in connection with his allies among the Welsh, for the Earldom's lands bordered Wales. The word 'march', meaning 'border region', had been added to the title generations earlier.

Marcus Andronicus Character in *Titus Andronicus*, the brother of TITUS (1). Marcus proposes his brother as a candidate for the vacant imperial throne in 1.1, though he accedes to Titus' determination that SATURNINUS should reign. He sides with BASSIANUS and Titus' sons in the dispute over LAVINIA, but a reconciliation is soon effected. In 2.4 Marcus discovers Lavinia in her ravished state, and his seemingly incongruous response—distant and rhetorical despite the extremity of her plight—often puzzles modern readers. It is a good instance of a mode of formal discourse, intended to promote a sense of strangeness and unreality, that was highly prized in Renaissance times but is now quite unfamiliar.

In 3.2, which Shakespeare may not have written, Marcus kills a fly, provoking so manic a response in Titus that he seems unbalanced by grief. Such mania is an important theme in a REVENGE PLAY, which *Titus Andronicus* is. In the rest of the play, Marcus seconds his brother's sentiments of grief and his plans for revenge and mourns Titus at the end.

Mardian Minor character in *Antony and Cleopatra*, a eunuch in the court of CLEOPATRA. Mardian is a minor member of the queen's entourage. In 4.14 he performs his only significant act when, on Cleopatra's orders, he delivers to ANTONY the false message that she has committed suicide. This triggers Antony's suicide attempt. Mardian is the closest thing to a jester, or FOOL (1), in Cleopatra's court. He is referred to as 'saucy' (4.14.25), and he is mildly amusing when he declares that he thinks on 'What Venus did with Mars' (1.5.18) when his mistress jests about his sexlessness. He appears to be the court musician, though he never performs as Cleopatra's willfulness leads her to reject his songs before she hears them. Aside from these semi-official functions, Mardian's function is to swell the ranks of Cleopatra's grand establishment.

Margarelon Legendary figure and minor character in *Troilus and Cressida*, an illegitimate son of King PRIAM. In 5.7 Margarelon challenges THERSITES on the battlefield, identifying himself as 'A bastard son of Priam's' (5.7.15). Thersites declares himself 'a bastard, too . . . bastard begot, bastard instructed, bastard in mind, bastard in valour, in everything illegitimate' (5.7.16–18); he then flees. The episode serves only to display Thersites' coarse wit and cowardice. Margarelon speaks only three lines and has no personality.

In the earliest editions of the play, which reflect Shakespeare's manuscript, this character is identified merely as 'Bastard'. By a tradition dating from the 18th century, he is given the name of a bastard of Priam's that appears in a list of Trojan warriors (5.5.7). Shakespeare took the name from either William CAXTON'S *The Recuyell of the Historyes of Troye* or John LYDGATE'S *Troy Book*, where it is variously spelled Margareton or Margariton. (The change from 't' to 'l' was probably a typesetter's error.) Margareton, one of Priam's many illegitimate sons, had no other importance in classical mythology.

Margaret (1) of Anjou (1430–1482) Historical figure and character in *1, 2,* and *3 Henry VI* and *Richard III*, the French-born Queen, and later widow, of King HENRY VI. Taken as a single role, running through four plays, Margaret is surely the greatest female part in Shakespeare. She develops from an ingenuous young woman thrust into prominence, through a career as a scheming plotter and a courageous and persistent military leader, to a final appearance as a raging, Fury-like crier of curses against her triumphant enemies.

In *1 Henry VI* Margaret plays only a brief role as a French prisoner of war intended as a bride for King Henry by the devious SUFFOLK (3), who loves her himself. Her importance is chiefly to prepare the groundwork for the action of *2 Henry VI*. She replaces JOAN LA PUCELLE (Joan of Arc) as the symbolic Frenchwoman who plagues an England that is divided by the selfish ambitions of the aristocracy. Her appearance marks the completion of one disaster, the loss of FRANCE (1), and begins another, a civil war.

In *2 Henry VI* Margaret's flawed personality is demonstrated early on. She conspires with Suffolk to bring about the fall of Duke Humphrey of GLOUCESTER (4) because she resents Gloucester's influence over the King and her own resulting insignificance. She displays an evil temper when she abuses the PETITIONERS in 1.3; later in this scene she mocks her husband's piety. When Gloucester is forced by his wife's disgrace (see DUCHESS [1]) to leave his position as Lord Protector, Margaret exults, comparing Gloucester's relinquished sceptre of office to an amputated limb (2.3.42). We are not surprised when this bloody-minded woman proposes killing her enemy to ensure against his possible return to power. When the King mourns Gloucester's subsequent murder, Margaret dares to complain that Henry is paying too little attention to her. Henry banishes Suffolk from England for his part in the crime, and, as the Queen and the Duke bid each other farewell, they reveal their passionate love. Shakespeare, aware as always of the complexities of human nature, offsets his portrait of this villainess by evoking a glimmer of sympathy for a woman losing her lover.

In *3 Henry VI* the Queen assumes a major role in the civil war, replacing the ineffectual King at the head of his armies. Her bold and cruel nature reveals itself most fully at the battle of WAKEFIELD, when York has been captured. Margaret insists on postponing his death so that she may torment him with barbs and, most chillingly, with evidence of the murder of his child, RUTLAND (1). Before he dies, York rages at her, calling her a 'she-wolf of France' (1.4.111), an epithet

that has been applied to her by writers ever since, and as a 'tiger's heart wrapp'd in a woman's hide' (1.4. 137), a line that was parodied in the earliest reference to Shakespeare that has survived (see Robert GREENE [2]).

At the crucial battle of TOWTON, Margaret is plainly the leader of the King's forces; in fact, she orders Henry to stay away from the fighting. Although the battle is lost and York's son Edward (see EDWARD IV) is enthroned in Henry's place, Margaret refuses to give up and she goes to France in search of military aid. When she is once again prepared to fight, she sends word to Edward, 'Tell him my mourning weeds are laid aside, / And I am ready to put armour on' (3.3.229–230). Despite her viciousness, this dauntless warrior does command some admiration.

The subsequent battle of TEWKESBURY results in Margaret's final defeat. Forced to witness the killing of her son, the PRINCE (4) of Wales, Margaret is reduced to lamentations and curses ironically similar to those delivered by York just three acts earlier. Richard, later RICHARD III, wishes to kill Margaret, saying, 'Why should she live to fill the world with words?' (5.5.43). He aptly predicts her role in *Richard III.*

Margaret's role in that work is limited to only two scenes, but it is a very powerful element of the play, for she represents Nemesis, the personification of retribution through fate, a theme that underlies the entire minor TETRALOGY, which *Richard III* closes. In 1.3 she heaps elaborate curses upon her victorious foes, reserving for Richard her choicest and subtlest imprecations, hoping that his punishment not come to pass until his 'sins be ripe' (1.3.219). In the formal and theatrical manner of a Greek CHORUS (1), Margaret restates past grievances and suggests future developments. She departs with the prediction that her enemies will come to regard her as 'a prophetess' (1.3. 301). Before her return, in 4.4, many of her curses will have been substantially fulfilled through Richard's murderous malignity, and Richard's own downfall is in progress. Several of Richard's victims reflect on Margaret's curses as they go to their deaths, thereby making more evident her role as Nemesis.

In 4.4 Margaret gloats over the misfortunes of Queen ELIZABETH (2), and leaves for France, content that she has stayed in England long enough to witness the fall of those who brought about her decline. As she departs, the climax of the play is about to unfold, and she has fulfilled her function. As an almost supernatural embodiment of Vengeance, she has represented an amoral world that is now to be overcome by the Christian reconciliation of RICHMOND.

Although Margaret of Anjou was a central figure in the Wars of the Roses, Shakespeare took considerable liberties with her story. He magnified the importance, and the evil, of a Queen who only naturally used her strengths to shore up the fortunes of her incompetent husband. Her foreignness and her gender made her useful as a witchlike figure at the centre of the web of treachery and violence that characterise the plays of the minor tetralogy.

For instance, Margaret's love affair with Suffolk, from its beginnings in *1 Henry VI,* is entirely fictitious. In *Part 2* Shakespeare ascribes to her an important role in English politics almost from the moment she sets foot in England in 1444. In fact, Margaret was a 14-year-old bride with no political experience, placed in an unfamiliar court and country, and she had little or no impact on English affairs for a decade. The fall of the Duchess of Gloucester, which she helps bring about in the play, occurred historically before her arrival. The Duke of Gloucester was probably not murdered, and Margaret had little to do with his political defeat in any case. In 1453 she attempted to assume the Regency of the realm during the period of her husband's insanity (ignored by Shakespeare). However, government by a Frenchwoman was unacceptable to the English aristocracy, and York was appointed Protector. His replacement by the Queen's protégé, SOMERSET (1), eventually led to the opening of the wars, with the first battle of ST. ALBANS.

The Queen was not present at that conflict, as she is in Shakespeare, but in the period immediately following it, she became an important leader of Henry's forces. However, the central incidents in the playwright's version of Margaret's role as a leader are fictitious. The Queen was not present to seize control on the occasion of Henry's concessions to York, enacted in 1.1 of *3 Henry VI;* nor was she a party to the killing of York, depicted with such extravagance in 1.4. Although she was indeed a force behind the later renewal of Lancastrian hopes, WARWICK (3) was far more important. She was in any case neither captured at Tewkesbury nor forced to witness her son's death; he was actually killed in the fighting, and she escaped to be captured a week later. She was imprisoned for several years and then ransomed by the King of France, to whose court she retired for the last six years of her life.

In *Richard III* Margaret's mere presence constitutes a final distortion of history, for she first appears on an occasion that actually took place only after her death in France. Shakespeare ignored this reality in order to use once more, in a highly symbolic manner, the strong but malign character he had developed in the course of the *Henry VI* plays.

Margaret (2) Character in *Much Ado About Nothing,* attendant to HERO. Drawn into Don JOHN (1) and BORACHIO's plan to slander Hero, Margaret dresses in her mistress' clothes and meets Borachio at night, although this occurs off-stage. Hero's betrothed, CLAUDIO (1), is lured to the scene by Don John, and, believing that Hero is seeing a lover, he refuses to marry her.

When the villainy is finally exposed, however, Margaret is judged to have been an unwitting accomplice.

An impersonator of Hero is necessary to the plot, but Shakespeare wished to minimise the villainy in *Much Ado,* stressing comedy over melodrama, and he provided a number of proofs of Margaret's innocence. She is clearly a valued member of the genial circle of friends surrounding Hero; we see her only in scenes of mirthful fun, and she has a playful sense of humour—BENEDICK says her 'wit is as quick as the greyhound's mouth' (5.2.11). Moreover, Borachio's recruitment of Margaret, like the charade itself, is kept off-stage, and when Borachio confesses in 5.1, he insists that Margaret 'knew not what she did . . . but always hath been just and virtuous' (5.1.295–296). Once Hero is finally cleared, Leonato remarks, 'Margaret was in some fault for this, although against her will, as it appears' (5.4.4–5). Her participation resembles, in fact, a well-known masquerading game, recorded in accounts of 16th-century courtly pastimes, in which a woman would dress herself as a bride and thereby demand more elaborate endearments from her sweetheart. In a small but telling touch, Margaret's fondness for clothes is presented in her delighted description of an elaborate gown in 3.4.17–20.

Margery Jourdain (d. 1441) Historical figure and minor character in *2 Henry VI,* a witch hired by HUME to summon a spirit for the DUCHESS (1) of Gloucester. In 1.4, at a séance, Margery summons the spirit ASNATH, and, after it has been questioned by the sorcerer BOLINGBROKE (2), she is arrested, with her fellows and the Duchess, by the dukes of YORK (8) and BUCKINGHAM (3). In 2.3 the King sentences her to be burned at the stake. The historical Jourdain claimed to have magical powers and was convicted of using them in the employ of the Duchess, and she was indeed burned at the stake.

Maria (1) Character in *Love's Labour's Lost,* the beloved of LONGAVILLE and one of the ladies-in-waiting to the PRINCESS OF FRANCE. Maria, like her lover, functions simply as a figure in the courtly pageant of love that constitutes the play's main plot. She has no distinctive personality traits, although she may be said to anticipate more fully developed secondary female characters, such as NERISSA, in *The Merchant of Venice.*

Maria (2) Character in *Twelfth Night,* chambermaid to OLIVIA. With SIR TOBY, SIR ANDREW, and FABIAN, Maria represents the spirit of fun that opposes the humourless severity of Olivia's steward, MALVOLIO, in the play's comic SUB-PLOT. Of the group, Maria is much the smartest. She devises the plot to embarrass the steward, and she composes the remarkably clever forged letter to Malvolio—read aloud by the victim himself in 2.5.92–159—playing on his ambitions and his vanity to impel him to bring about his own downfall. Then in 4.2 she devises a capstone to the joke, disguising the jester FESTE as a curate, Sir TOPAS, to visit and torment Malvolio, who has been locked up as a lunatic.

In witty speeches like those in 3.2.65–80, Maria provides a commentary on Malvolio's actions that establish strongly our favourable, indeed indulgent, attitude towards a 'knavery', as Sir Toby calls it (4.2.70), that might easily turn vicious. When, at the conclusion of the play, we learn that Sir Toby has married Maria out of delight with her wit, we realise that she will be able to control her new husband successfully without repressing his high spirits. Moreover, this marriage provides a parallel to the pairings of the characters in the main plot, ORSINO with VIOLA and SEBASTIAN (2) with Olivia.

Mariana (1) Minor character in *All's Well That Ends Well,* a neighbour of the WIDOW (2) Capilet, a Florentine innkeeper. In 3.5.16–28 Mariana roundly condemns PAROLLES and BERTRAM as unscrupulous womanisers, thus helping to establish the situation when HELENA (2) arrives in FLORENCE. She has no personality beyond that of a stereotypical gossip.

Mariana (2) Character in *Measure for Measure,* the abandoned fiancée and eventual wife of ANGELO (2). By means of the 'bed trick' instituted by the DUKE (9), Mariana replaces ISABELLA—from whom Angelo has attempted to extort sex—in Angelo's bed. When Angelo's evil is exposed, the Duke orders Angelo to marry Mariana—thereby legitimising her action—following which he will be executed. Mariana pleads for mercy, convincing Isabella to join her, and the Duke finally relents in the atmosphere of reconciliation and forgiveness that closes the play. Aside from her rather formal melancholy as she pines for Angelo in seclusion when we first meet her, in 4.1, Mariana is not a developed character, though her plea, in 5.1, is touchingly expressive of the play's charitable point of view. She insists that 'best men are moulded out of faults, / And . . . become much more the better / For being a little bad' (5.1.437–439).

Her plea gives her special significance, for with it she triggers the sequence of pardons and forgiveness that close the play. Perhaps most important, she persuades Isabella to join her. Though Isabella's intercession goes against her natural enmity towards Angelo, she nevertheless proceeds to offer a sensible case for mercy. It is her conversion to this forgiving point of view—one quite removed from her earlier insistence on morality even if it meant the death of her brother—that is the play's climax. Mariana's plea is essentially selfish; she wishes to preserve the husband she has so long sought. But Isabella is totally objective, and it is this that makes her action impressive. Only the exis-

tence of Mariana as a proper mate for Angelo makes this possible.

No hint of Mariana is to be found in Shakespeare's sources for *Measure for Measure,* and the character has particular importance as she is an invention of the playwright that changes the nature of his story in a significant manner. In all of the sources for the play, the Angelo figure successfully extorts sex from the Isabella figure, and then, when exposed, he is forced to marry her. However, in Shakespeare's rendering of the tale, Isabella and Angelo have effectively been presented as intense figures whose opposing psychological strengths make such a union impossible to contemplate. Mariana therefore replaces Isabella. The bed trick, an ancient comedic device that Shakespeare also used in *All's Well,* accomplishes this end. Isabella is preserved as the virtuous counterpart to Angelo's corruption, and Mariana can influence her towards forgiveness as her rigidity relaxes. The device may seem arbitrary to modern readers—like a *deus ex machina,* it disposes of the impending tragedy with ease and convenience—but in Shakespeare's day this conclusion was not only perfectly acceptable, it was highly gratifying to the audience's sentimental feelings.

Marina Character in *Pericles,* daughter of PERICLES and THAISA. Marina appears only in Acts 4–5 (except as a newborn infant—i.e., as a stage prop—in 3.1), but she is nevertheless a major character. Along with her father, she bears the weight of the play's central lesson: the value of patience in the face of fate. Marina, like Pericles, is helpless before her destiny, which subjects her to the loss of her family and great dangers as well. Her name, which implies her birth at sea, suggests her destiny-driven life. Her spirit does not flag, however; she resists despair, as her father does not, and becomes his saviour. Finally, her moral virtues are rewarded by reunion with her parents and a prospective marriage with LYSIMACHUS.

Like Pericles, Marina suffers great misfortune—separation from her parents in infancy, a murder attempt by her foster-mother, a kidnapping and sale to a brothel—through no fault of her own and despite her extraordinary virtue. Also like her father, she is an idealised character, more important as an emblem than as a personality. She represents absolute innocence and purity; she says, 'I never spake bad word . . . never kill'd a mouse, nor hurt a fly . . . But I wept for't' (4.1.75–79). However, though she resembles 'Patience gazing on kings' graves, and smiling / Extremity out of act' (5.1.138–139), she is not without spirit. She demonstrates patience by never giving up on the world, but she is not passive like her father. Her stubborn refusal to surrender her virginity saves her, as she first talks her way out of the brothel and then becomes such a model of grace and kindness that she is called upon to cure the depression of the man who proves to be her father. Marina is typical of Shakespeare's plucky, spirited heroines, even though she does not seek out her adventures but is cast into them by fate.

Marina's ideal virtue and the simplicity and inflexibility of her motives places her in a disturbing contrast with the social reality of the BAWD, the PANDAR, and BOULT. This contrast is often seen as a defect, but the objection ignores the playwright's allegorical purposes, which are emphasised by the contrast. Like Shakespeare's other late heroines, PERDITA and MIRANDA, Marina represents a sort of redemption, a renewal of life. Her spirit revives that of Pericles, who calls her 'Thou that beget'st him that did thee beget' (5.1.195). Through her, he can transcend the buffetings of fate and be reconciled with a life whose disillusionments have been too much to bear. Her healing nature also effects the customers of the brothel (see GENTLEMAN [10]) and even the hard-boiled Boult. Moreover, Marina has been symbolically dead: she was believed dead by Pericles and has undergone a journey through the underworld of the brothel. She thus is representative of resurrection, the play's most important motif. She is an appropriate symbol of the spirit of hope and renewal with which the play ends.

Mariner (1) Minor character in *The Winter's Tale,* seaman who sets ANTIGONUS ashore in BOHEMIA in 3.3 for the purpose of abandoning the infant PERDITA. The Mariner dislikes their task, which has been ordered by the mad King LEONTES, and he fears that the gods will dislike it as well. He warns Antigonus to hurry because bad weather is approaching and because the coast is famous for its wild animals. He is borne out on both points as a storm arises—he perishes in it, as is reported in 3.3.90–94—and Antigonus is eaten by a BEAR. The Mariner offers a point of view outside the story, that of the common man who pities the infant and fears the gods. Like a CHORUS (1), he provides a brief commentary on developments.

The Mariner's death has a dual significance in the play's scheme. A good man, repelled by Perdita's fate, he is himself a victim of Leontes' madness. As such he represents the human cost exacted by evil. On the other hand, as Antigonus' guide, he is Leontes' agent, albeit an unwilling one. His death is part of the necessary workings of providence, for the evil of Leontes' deeds must be thoroughly extirpated as a condition of redemption, and the Mariner, like Antigonus, embodies that evil to some degree.

Mariner (2) Any of several minor characters in *The Tempest,* the crew of the ship that is wrecked on PROSPERO's island. As the play opens, the Mariners receive orders from the BOATSWAIN—'Heigh, my hearts! . . . yare, yare! Take in the topsail' (1.1.5–6). A little later several of them cry out in unison, 'All lost, to prayers,

to prayers! all lost!' (1.1.51), signalling the close of the scene, as the passengers prepare for death. These characters are extras, providing a sense of hysteria aboard the doomed vessel.

Markham, Gervase (Jervis) (c. 1568–1637) English poet and author, writer of possible minor sources for Shakespeare's plays, and perhaps a model for the boastful soldier ARMADO or the 'rival poet' of the SONNETS. Markham was a noted soldier and horseman—he probably introduced the Arabian horse to England—who turned to hack literature after his military career. He wrote copiously on a variety of subjects, especially military tactics, falconry, fishing, housekeeping, and all aspects of owning and breeding horses. His easy, colloquial style made him popular, and he still offers readers a pleasant introduction to the Elizabethan age. Scholars believe that some of his practical information is echoed in Shakespeare's plays, for instance, in PETRUCHIO's elaborate description of falcon training in *The Taming of the Shrew* (4.1.175–198). Markham's easy assurance of infallibility suggests he may have been satirised in Shakespeare's Armado, though the point cannot be proven with existing evidence.

Markham was an extremely prolific author, who sometimes issued almost identical texts under different titles to increase sales. At one point a group of London booksellers, seeing that he was flooding his own market, persuaded him to sign an agreement not to write any more books on blacksmithing, but he soon violated the pact. He occasionally ascended to more serious literature, and because he dedicated one such work to Shakespeare's patron, the Earl of SOUTHAMPTON (2), he has been associated with the 'rival poet', though most scholars find the identification extremely dubious.

Marlowe (1), Christopher (1564–1593) English playwright, Shakespeare's immediate predecessor as leading English dramatist and a considerable influence on his work. Marlowe, with Thomas KYD, virtually invented Elizabethan TRAGEDY, and Marlowe's influence on ELIZABETHAN DRAMA in general was great. In his *Tamburlaine* (1587) he successfully established BLANK VERSE as the standard medium for drama, and the grandeur of his protagonists and themes elevated his successors' aspirations.

Many passages in Shakespeare's early works are clearly modelled on Marlowe; scholars who believe that many of Shakespeare's plays were written in part by other playwrights have even attributed parts of the *Henry VI* plays, *Richard III*, *Titus Andronicus*, and others to Marlowe, though modern scholars mistrust most of these attributions. In *As You Like It*, PHEBE quotes a line from a Marlowe poem, ascribing it to a 'dead shepherd' (3.5.81–82), Shakespeare's only certain reference to a contemporary poet. Further quotations from and allusions to Marlowe's work abound in the plays (e.g., *A Midsummer Night's Dream* 1.1.170, *Merry Wives of Windsor* 3.1.16–35, *Much Ado About Nothing* 5.2.29), attesting not only to Shakespeare's admiration but also to his confidence that his audiences knew and appreciated Marlowe's work. In addition, Marlowe's *The Jew of Malta* (1589) probably helped inspire Shakespeare's SHYLOCK; similarly, Marlowe's *Edward II* (1592) probably informed *Richard II*'s presentation of a flawed ruler, and his poem 'Hero and Leander' offered a model for *Venus and Adonis*. (Marlowe's poem was unfinished at his death and published posthumously—with additions by George CHAPMAN—in 1598, but Shakespeare knew it earlier, in manuscript.)

Marlowe led a violent, dissolute, and dramatic life. A notorious drinker and brawler, he flaunted his homosexuality at a time when homosexuality was a capital crime. He was a soldier in the Netherlands, from which he was deported for counterfeiting gold coins, and he was probably a spy for the government of Queen ELIZABETH (1)—both abroad and in England. In 1589 he was involved in a street fight in which a man was killed. He was one of the earliest Englishmen to publicly admit to atheism, and in 1593 he was charged with blasphemy—along with Kyd—but before he could be tried, he was stabbed to death, reportedly in a dispute over a tavern bill. Some historians believe he was murdered, silenced by a government agent; in any case, his killer, who is known to have been a fellow spy, was immediately pardoned. (Marlowe's death may be alluded to in *As You Like It* 3.3.9–12.)

The son of a shoemaker, Marlowe nevertheless received a good education, graduating from Cambridge University in 1587, in the same year that his first play, *Tamburlaine*, became the talk of LONDON. He followed it with *Tamburlaine, Part 2* (1588), *The Jew of Malta* (1589), *Dr Faustus* (1592), *Edward II* (1592)—the first English historical play—and *The Massacre at Paris* (1593). Most of his plays were probably commissioned by the ADMIRAL'S MEN and his heroic protagonists first played by Edward ALLEYN. At his death Marlowe left another play unfinished—*Dido, Queen of Carthage*, completed by Thomas NASHE and staged in 1594—along with 'Hero and Leander'. His oeuvre was completed by two other short poems (one of them, the delightful 'Passionate Shepherd to his Love', which was falsely attributed to Shakespeare in THE PASSIONATE PILGRIM). While the body of work is small, it encompasses at least three great plays—*Tamburlaine*, *The Jew of Malta*, and *Dr Faustus*—and a magnificent lyric poem, 'Hero and Leander'. Marlowe, who was born the same year as Shakespeare, was only 29 when he was killed.

Marlowe (2), Julia (1865–1950) American actress. Born in Britain, Marlowe came to America at age four, began acting with a touring company at 12, and made her New York debut at 21. She quickly established

herself as a leading actress, especially in Shakespearean comedy, playing VIOLA, ROSALIND, BEATRICE, and PORTIA (1). She also excelled as JULIET (1). In 1904 Marlowe founded a Shakespearean repertory company with E. H. SOTHERN, whom she was to marry. She took on more tragic roles, including LADY (6) MACBETH. Just after her retirement in 1924, she and Sothern staged 10 Shakespearean performances whose proceeds were donated to the Shakespeare Memorial Theatre in STRATFORD.

Marseilles City in southern FRANCE (1), setting for one scene in *All's Well That Ends Well.* HELENA (2) announces her intention to leave FLORENCE and find the KING (17) of France at 'Marcellus' (4.4.9)—indicating the Elizabethan pronunciation of the name—and in 5.1 she is said in the stage directions to be there, only to discover that the King has left for ROSSILLION. No characteristics of Marseilles or southern France are alluded to, but the setting is apt because Marseilles is the major city on either a land or land-and-sea route from Florence to Rossillion.

Marsh, Henry (d. 1665) English publisher. Marsh published the first edition of a famous collection of DROLLS, *The Wits, or Sport upon Sport* (1662), assembled by his partner, Francis KIRKMAN. He may have been a royalist and in exile during the period of the Puritan revolutionary government (1642–1660), for he is absent from the publishing records from 1642 to 1658. When he died he left his business to Kirkman.

Marshal (1) (Lord Marshal) Minor character in *Richard II,* the nobleman who presides over the trial by combat between BOLINGBROKE (1) and MOWBRAY (1) in 1.3. Historically the Marshal on this occasion was the Duke of SURREY (3), a supporter of RICHARD II and thus an enemy of Bolingbroke. Shakespeare apparently forgot this fact, which appears in his chief source, HOLINSHED's history, when he presented the Marshal as a friend of Bolingbroke in 1.3.251–252. This is one of the many minor errors and inconsistencies that appear throughout the plays.

Marshall (2) Minor character in *Pericles,* an official of the court of King SIMONIDES. In 2.3 the Marshall designates a seat for PERICLES at the royal banquet; he speaks only four lines and serves merely to indicate the grandeur of the occasion.

Marston, John (c. 1575–1634) English dramatist. Marston abandoned a legal education to be a writer. In 1598 he established himself in the literary world with two long poems, one erotic *(The Metamorphosis of Pygmalion's Image)* and one satiric *(The Scourge of Villainy).* In 1599 he wrote for Philip HENSLOWE and the ADMIRAL'S MEN, but in the same year he began writing for the CHILDREN'S COMPANIES, where he spent the rest of his short career. He is chiefly remembered for bitter satirical COMEDY, but he also specialised in the REVENGE PLAY. With his best-known work, *The Malcontent* (1604), he managed to combine the two genres. Writing for the Children of Paul's, Marston began the WAR OF THE THEATRES with his *Historio-Mastix* (1599), a comedy containing a satire on Ben JONSON. In reply to Jonson's responses, he added *Jack Drum's Entertainment* (1600) and *What You Will* (1601) to the fray, as well as collaborating with Thomas DEKKER on *Satiromastix* (1601). He was on good terms with Jonson by 1604, when he dedicated *The Malcontent* to his one-time rival. In that year, Marston began writing for the Children of the Queen's Revels, and in 1605 he collaborated with Jonson and George CHAPMAN on *Eastward Ho!* King JAMES I deemed the play seditious, with the result that Marston's collaborators were gaoled, though Marston fled LONDON until the affair blew over, thereby igniting Jonson's enmity anew. In 1608, however, Marston was imprisoned for offending the king again, with a play now lost, and he abandoned the theatre, leaving a final play unfinished. By 1616 he was a Protestant minister.

Martext, Sir Oliver Minor character in *As You Like It,* a country priest. In 3.3 TOUCHSTONE and AUDREY meet with Martext, 'the vicar of the next village' (3.3.37), to be married. Martext speaks only two lines before the ceremony is broken up by JAQUES (1), who belittles the virtues of a marriage performed by a country bumpkin and leads the couple away.

Martext is a parodic figure with particular relevance to Shakespeare's audiences. The English Reformation—instituted about 50 years before the play was written—had produced a shortage of trained clergy, for not only did many Catholic priests refuse to transfer their allegiance to the Church of England, but the new church did not develop training programmes immediately. The quality of the lesser clergy was accordingly poor, even as late as the 17th century, and the illiteracy and ignorance of country priests were subjects of much scandal and humour, of which this scene is an example.

Martext's name not only suggests his incompetence, but it may also be a satirical reference to Martin Marprelate, the central figure in a religious controversy of the late 1580s. Marprelate—a fictitious name with anti-clerical overtones—was the supposed author of a series of anonymous tracts advocating radical Puritanism. Their publisher defied the government's CENSORSHIP for several years, before being captured and hung. Martext's name may therefore suggest that he is a radical as well as an oaf—thus doubly a target for comic insult. However, Shakespeare's humour on religious subjects is never bitter, and the playwright permits Sir Oliver a dignified response to his rejection:

once alone, Martext says, ''Tis no matter. Ne'er a fantastical knave of them all shall flout me out of my calling' (3.3.97–98).

Martius (1) Minor character in *Titus Andronicus,* a son of TITUS (1) Andronicus. Martius, with QUINTUS, is framed by AARON for the murder of BASSIANUS in 2.3. After the two are executed, their heads are delivered to Titus, in 3.1.

Martius (2) (Marcius) In *Coriolanus,* the name by which Caius Martius CORIOLANUS is known before 1.9. 64, when he receives his new name, his 'addition' (1.9.65) of honour for his military exploits in the taking of the city CORIOLES. In the ancient Roman naming system, Martius is a clan name; there is no similar system in modern Western naming. Shakespeare apparently followed tradition (and his source, Thomas NORTH's translation of PLUTARCH's *Lives*) when he used it as a family name in the sense we understand. However, the names Caius and Martius are mistakenly reversed several times in the play—including at 1.9.64—an example of the numerous minor errors to which Shakespeare was prone throughout his career.

Marullus (Murellus), C. Epidius (active 44 B.C.) Historical figure and minor character in *Julius Caesar,* a tribune of ROME and an ally of BRUTUS (4). In 1.1 Marullus and his fellow tribune, FLAVIUS (1), disperse a crowd (see COMMONER [1]) that has assembled to greet the triumphant CAESAR (1). The tribunes criticise their disloyalty to Pompey, whom they had supported earlier and whom Caesar has defeated in civil war. After the crowd has gone, Flavius and Marullus destroy the public decorations that have been put up in Caesar's honour because they fear the triumphant general will become a tyrant. In 1.2.282–283 CASCA reports that Flavius and Marullus have been 'put to silence' for this deed. The episode establishes a widespread mistrust of Caesar from the outset of the play.

Little is known of the historical Marullus, but Shakespeare's source, PLUTARCH's *Lives,* reports that Caesar dismissed the two tribunes from their positions because they had made the gesture dramatised in the play. However, in Plutarch's account this occurred months after Caesar's triumph. Shakespeare compressed these events for dramatic purposes.

In the FIRST FOLIO, where the play was first published, Marullus is identified throughout as 'Murellus', and some modern editions preserve this spelling, though others follow the historically correct rendering of the name.

Masque Courtly entertainment that evolved into a drama-like theatrical genre. Masques appques appear in various forms in a number of Shakespeare's plays. Originally an amateur masquerade in which members of the court put on masks and costumes and fêted the monarch with dancing on holiday occasions, the masque evolved under King JAMES I into a theatrical presentation with extremely elaborate sets and costumes, many professional musicians and dancers in support of the aristocratic amateurs, and highly literary scripts by such writers as Francis BEAUMONT (2), Samuel DANIEL, and most notably Ben JONSON. These productions were staged on significant royal occasions, such as weddings and birthdays. (Non-royal aristocrats also staged masques on such occasions.) The masques were allegorical in nature, with mythological or emblematic characters who represented particular virtues and vices or more or less clearcut ideas, such as marriage or PASTORAL contentment. The great expense of such extravaganzas eventually became a significant political issue, and the courtly masque did not survive the revolution that began in 1642.

The 17th-century masque exerted considerable influence on JACOBEAN DRAMA. Shakespeare's last works—the ROMANCES plus *Henry VIII,* which were written for the aristocratic audiences at the BLACKFRIARS THEATRE—all contain elaborate masquelike elements. Masques also appear in several earlier Shakespeare plays: simple maskings of a social sort are enacted in *Love's Labour's Lost, Romeo and Juliet* (see MASQUERS), and *Much Ado About Nothing,* while more formal stagings, featuring named mythological characters, occur in *As You Like It* and *Timon of Athens.* In addition, there are masquelike elements in other plays, most strikingly in *A Midsummer Night's Dream.*

As in movies that contain scraps of older movies as part of the characters' experience, the appearance of masques in plays amused their audiences with enactments of familiar—or at least notorious—pleasures while also furthering the play's developments. For instance, in *The Winter's Tale,* a masquelike 'dance of twelve Satyrs' (4.4.343) is presented at a sheep-shearing festival. A delightful theatrical spectacle in itself, it demonstrates the vitality of pastoral life and at the same time, by evoking an aristocratic entertainment, expresses the hidden nobility present, for the leading shepherdess is actually the lost princess PERDITA. In *Timon of Athens,* CUPID's brief masque in 1.2 displays the aristocratic elegance of the title character's household while providing an occasion for an irascible complaint against extravagant vanity by the play's philosopher-jester, APEMANTUS. An actual royal masque of 1527 is re-enacted in 1.4 of *Henry VIII,* and the betrothal masque in 4.1 of *The Tempest* resembles contemporary (c. 1611) masques and lends grandeur to the proposed marriage of FERDINAND (2) and MIRANDA, whose status as future royalty has significance in the play's scheme of things. The masque in 3.5 of *The Two Noble Kinsmen* was in fact a scene from a real masque, Beaumont's *Masque of the Inner Temple and Gray's Inn*

(1613) (see INNS OF COURT), though this borrowing was the work of Shakespeare's collaborator, John FLETCHER (2).

The masque was known at least as far back as the 14th century, during the reign of RICHARD II. It was formalised, with prepared scenarios, under Queen ELIZABETH (1), but it only became a literary, quasi-dramatic genre under James. However, even Jacobean masques always contained large elements of dance, the original masque medium, and—at least in life, if not always on the stage—masques were normally preludes to social dancing, in which the participants joined the spectators at a ball. A masque was accordingly an occasion for coquetry and sexual intrigue, as is quite clear in Shakespeare.

Masques were influential on literature, as well as drama. Masquelike elements appear in such works as *The Faerie Queene* by Edmund SPENSER, and some late masques are significant literary works in their own right, most notably John MILTON's *Comus* (performed 1634; published 1637). The courtly masque did not reappear after the Puritan revolution; the last known script was written by William DAVENANT in 1640.

Masquers Group of non-speaking characters in *Romeo and Juliet,* the men who accompany ROMEO to the banquet held by CAPULET (1). In the 16th-century courtly entertainment that evolved into the formal MASQUE, guests often costumed themselves, as Romeo and his friends do in 1.4, and were known as masquers. Arriving in groups and often dressed thematically, the masquers declared themselves to be party-crashers and demanded to dance. Uproarious flirtation was expected to follow. Named characters sometimes appear as masquers elsewhere in Shakespeare's plays (e.g., in *Much Ado About Nothing,* 2.1.78 and *Henry VIII,* 1.4.64–87).

Massinger, Philip (1583–1640) English playwright, a secondary figure of JACOBEAN DRAMA. Massinger's plays are characterised by his imitation of Shakespeare's verse style, to the extent that though no known work of Massinger's can be dated before 1616, he is sometimes thought to have written the parts usually assigned to Shakespeare in his collaborations with John FLETCHER (2), *The Two Noble Kinsmen* and possibly *Henry VIII.* Most scholars, however, deem Massinger's involvement extremely unlikely, though he did collaborate with Fletcher, his close friend, on many plays. He also worked with numerous other playwrights. After Fletcher's death, Massinger became the chief playwright for the KING'S MEN.

Massinger wrote a variety of works. He is best remembered for his satirical comedies, especially *A New Way to Pay Old Debts* (1621), and *The City Madam* (1632). He also wrote tragedies. His *Duke of Milan* (1621), which is based on *Othello,* is regarded as among the better Jacobean tragedies. In the late 17th century, Massinger's *The Roman Actor* (1626) was thought to be by Shakespeare. Massinger often faced governmental CENSORSHIP, for he frequently touched on such sensitive issues as Catholicism (he was himself a Catholic convert), foreign policy, and various public figures.

Master (1) Minor character in *2 Henry VI,* a petty officer on a pirate ship. In 4.1 the LIEUTENANT (1) of the ship awards to the Master the ransom of a GENTLEMAN (1), one of several captured by the pirates.

Master (2) Minor character in *The Tempest,* captain of the ship that is wrecked on PROSPERO's island. The Master speaks only two lines, at the play's opening, instructing the BOATSWAIN to see that the men act swiftly, or they will go aground. In 5.1 he reappears with the Boatswain, who reports on the miraculous restoration of the vessel, but he does not speak himself. He is an extra, helping to provide a realistic depiction of a ship's company.

Master-Gunner Minor character in *1 Henry VI,* a French soldier in the besieged city of ORLÉANS (1). The Master-Gunner instructs his BOY (1) in 1.4 that their cannon is trained on a certain tower where the English leaders are known to stand watch. The Boy subsequently fires the shot that kills the Duke of SALISBURY (3).

Master of Revels English official of the 16th and 17th centuries who regulated the theatre. The Master headed the Revels Office, a department of the royal household that originally dealt with the annual royal entertainments during the Revels season, from All Saint's Day (November 1) to the beginning of Lent in the following spring. The position of Master of Revels was created in 1545 under King HENRY VIII. At first, the Master was simply responsible for hiring and paying entertainers, but gradually the powers of the office were expanded. By Shakespeare's time, the Revels Office consisted of the Master and four full-time subordinates, and it not only hired theatrical companies to perform at court, but provided them with scenery and costumes from its own stores. It also selected the plays they were to perform and oversaw the content of the plays. The Master thus had the authority of a censor (see CENSORSHIP), especially after the passage of the 1606 anti-blasphemy statute, 'Act to Restrain Abuses of Players', which enlarged his authority to cover the publication of plays as well.

The Master collected various fees, as he issued licences for provincial acting companies, for the performance and publication of individual plays, and for dispensations to companies who wished to perform during Lent. In addition, he was frequently bribed.

The office of Master of Revels was accordingly an extremely profitable one. The nominal salary was only £10 a year, but it is known that in 1603 the Master made about £100. Beginning in 1623 Sir Henry HERBERT (1) paid the ostensible Master £150 a year to perform the office and collect the income, which must have been considerably greater. The office of Master of Revels fell into disuse when the theatres were closed at the outset of the civil war in 1642. Herbert tried to revive it upon the restoration of the monarchy in 1660, but his attempt failed, and the office was formally eliminated.

Mate Minor character in *2 Henry VI*, a sailor on a pirate ship. In 4.1 the LIEUTENANT (1) of the ship awards the Mate the ransom of a GENTLEMAN (1), one of several captured by the pirates.

Mayne, Jasper (1604–1672) English writer, possibly the author of one of the introductory poems to the FIRST FOLIO edition (1623) of Shakespeare's plays. Mayne published several poems and two plays (both written c. 1638), one of which contains a scene apparently inspired by the interrogation of PAROLLES in 4.3 of *All's Well That Ends Well.* He also translated the Latin author Lucian. After 1660 he was chaplain to King Charles II. Some scholars attribute to him the poem 'To the memorie of M. *W. Shake-speare*', a poem of four rhymed couplets that is signed 'I. M'. in the Folio. However, because Mayne was quite young in 1623, James MABBE is more commonly believed to be its author.

Mayor (1) of Coventry Minor character in *3 Henry VI*, a supporter of WARWICK (3) in his attempt to reinstate HENRY VI as king. The Mayor, who does not speak, appears on the walls of Coventry with Warwick in 5.1, lending local authority to the effort.

Mayor (2) of London Minor character in *1 Henry VI.* In 1.3 the Mayor breaks up a brawl between the men of the Duke of GLOUCESTER (4) and those of the Bishop of WINCHESTER (1). In 3.1 he tells the king's conference of further disorders. The incidents serve to illustrate the spreading social chaos that aristocratic dissensions have engendered.

Mayor (3) of London Minor character in *Richard III*, a subservient figure who is cowed by RICHARD III. The Mayor appears in several scenes in Act 3. He provides a cover of legality for Richard's actions, approving an execution and acclaiming Richard as king when he moves to seize the throne.

Mayor (4) of St Albans Minor character in *2 Henry VI.* The Mayor accompanies SIMPCOX, a confidence man who is presented to the king's hawking party in 2.1.

Mayor (5) of York Minor character in *3 Henry VI*, the chief officer of the city of YORK (2). In 4.7 the Mayor cites his loyalty to King HENRY VI as the reason for refusing to open the gates of the city to EDWARD IV. Lying, Edward asserts that he will make no claim on the crown but wishes only to be Duke of York. Believing him, the Mayor admits him. The incident illustrates the lack of honour among the feuding royalty during the WARS OF THE ROSES.

McKellen, Ian (b. 1935) English actor. McKellen is noted for a variety of roles, having played most of Shakespeare's protagonists. He played MACBETH in Trevor NUNN's 1976 staging of *Macbeth* in STRATFORD and in the subsequent TELEVISION presentation. He also played the title role in the first known professional performance of SIR THOMAS MORE in 1964.

Measure for Measure

SYNOPSIS

Act 1, Scene 1

As he prepares to leave the city, the DUKE (9) of VIENNA appoints ESCALUS (2) second in command to ANGELO (2), the deputy who will exercise power in the Duke's absence. Angelo receives his orders, and the Duke praises him for his life of devotion to duty.

Act 1, Scene 2

MISTRESS (2) Overdone, a bordello keeper, interrupts the lewd banter of LUCIO and two GENTLEMEN (5) to tell them that CLAUDIO (3) has been sentenced to death for having made JULIET (2) pregnant. POMPEY (1) tells Mistress Overdone of a new law that orders the destruction of bordellos; he assures her that she will survive and that he will continue to work for her. The PROVOST appears and exhibits Claudio in the streets as part of his punishment. Claudio tells Lucio that he slept with Juliet in the belief that they would soon be married, but that her relatives had held up her dowry. Then, after Juliet became pregnant, Angelo began to enforce a long-neglected law making sexual immorality a capital crime. Claudio tells Lucio of his sister who is about to enter a convent, and asks Lucio to ask her to seek mercy from Angelo.

Act 1, Scene 3

The Duke visits the FRIAR (1) and tells him that he has placed Angelo in charge during a revival of disused morality laws. He fears that to revive these laws under his own authority might give them too great a force; this way he can see how they are received and act accordingly. He intends to secretly return to Vienna and oversee the process, disguised as a friar.

Act 1, Scene 4

Lucio visits Claudio's sister, ISABELLA, at the convent. He tells her of Claudio's predicament, and she agrees to plead for mercy from Angelo.

Act 2, Scene 1
Escalus proposes mercy for Claudio, but Angelo refuses. Constable ELBOW brings Pompey and FROTH before the officials; in comically confused speech he charges his prisoners with running a bordello for Mistress Overdone and adds that they attempted to recruit his wife. Pompey's wittily long-winded reply drives Angelo away; he leaves the case to Escalus. After further comical exchanges, Escalus releases Froth and Pompey with a warning that law enforcement is becoming stricter; Pompey leaves sassily.

Act 2, Scene 2
Despite the Provost's pleas, Angelo orders Claudio's execution for the next day. Isabella arrives and pleads at length for mercy. Angelo promises only to reconsider and tell her of his decision the next day. Angelo, alone, reflects distractedly that he has fallen in love with Isabella and is tempted to sin by offering a pardon for Claudio in exchange for her love.

Act 2, Scene 3
The Duke, disguised as a friar, ministers to the inmates of the prison. He encounters Juliet, urges her repentance, and promises that he will visit her condemned lover.

Act 2, Scene 4
Angelo soliloquises that he cannot pray for strength against temptation because his thoughts are filled by Isabella. Isabella arrives and renews her plea. Angelo tells her he will have mercy on Claudio only if she will become his lover. She refuses, and he swears that he will have Claudio tortured. He gives her a day to change her mind and leaves. Alone, she declares her confidence in Claudio. As a man of honour, he will agree that her avoidance of sin is more important than his rescue.

Act 3, Scene 1
The Duke, as a friar, counsels Claudio to prepare for death by considering the ills of life. Isabella arrives, and the 'friar' eavesdrops as she tells Claudio of Angelo's evil ultimatum. Though Claudio at first supports her refusal, he is overcome by fear of death and pleads with her to save him. Furious, she berates him hysterically and leaves. The 'friar' intercepts her and tells her he knows of Angelo's intentions. He proposes to her a plot. Angelo had once abandoned a woman he was supposed to marry named MARIANA (2) and she still loves him. If Isabella arranges to have sex with Angelo on condition that the transaction be silent and in the dark, Mariana could actually keep the appointment. Isabella agrees.

Act 3, Scene 2
Elbow brings Pompey to the prison; Lucio appears, and Pompey asks him for bail but is refused. Lucio speaks with the Duke, thinking he is actually a friar. He claims to be an intimate of the Duke, gossips about him slanderously and leaves. Mistress Overdone is gaoled despite her claim that Lucio has informed on her because she keeps his illegitimate child. Before he leaves to visit Claudio, Escalus observes to the 'friar' that the absent Duke would not have been so merciless as Angelo. Alone, the Duke reflects on the virtues needed in a ruler and rails against Angelo's violation of these standards.

Act 4, Scene 1
The Duke, as the 'friar', visits Mariana. Isabella arrives and reports that she has agreed to meet Angelo that night in his garden. Mariana accepts her part in the plot.

Act 4, Scene 2
The Provost offers Pompey parole if he will serve as assistant to the executioner, ABHORSON, in the beheadings of Claudio and another man, BARNARDINE; he agrees. The disguised Duke arrives and predicts that Claudio will be pardoned. However, a MESSENGER (18) brings the order that Claudio is to be killed immediately and his head sent to Angelo. The 'friar' suggests that Barnardine's head be substituted for Claudio's. The Provost says he cannot do this because of his duty. The 'friar' confides that he knows the Duke's intentions and produces letters from him as proof.

Act 4, Scene 3
Pompey and Abhorson summon Barnardine to be executed, but he refuses because he has a terrible hangover. The Provost appears, and the 'friar' observes that Barnardine is so unrepentant that if he died he would surely go to hell, placing a moral burden on his executioners; the Provost remarks that another prisoner has by chance died that morning, and they agree that his head can be used as the substitute for Claudio's. Isabella arrives, and the disguised Duke decides to postpone telling her of the plot to spare Claudio. He tells her instead that Angelo has demanded and received Claudio's head. He promises her revenge; she is to take a letter to a friar who will bring her to the Duke, and Angelo's guilt will be exposed. As she leaves, Lucio arrives; he brags that he has abandoned a pregnant woman and claims to know the Duke has done the same.

Act 4, Scene 4
Angelo and Escalus discuss the Duke's peculiar instructions: they are to proclaim that any complaints of injustice should be made publicly and then meet him outside the city. Escalus leaves to send out this decree; alone, Angelo bemoans his guilty conscience. Not only did he deflower Isabella, he had Claudio killed for fear he would someday seek revenge. He regrets his decision and cries that one sin leads to more.

Act 4, Scene 5
The Duke visits the Friar again and plans his return to Vienna.

Act 4, Scene 6
Isabella and Mariana ready themselves to encounter Angelo and the Duke; the 'friar' has warned Isabella that she must expect to be mistreated before she triumphs. The real Friar, Friar Peter, arrives to escort them to the Duke's ceremonial return.

Act 5, Scene 1
The Duke returns, and Isabella demands justice. The Duke refuses to believe her tale and has her arrested; she claims that Friar Lodowick can support her. Friar Peter says that he will present the evidence of Friar Lodowick, who is sick. He calls Mariana, who reveals her role as Angelo's sexual partner. Angelo denies having seen her for years and accuses Friar Lodowick of plotting against him. The Duke sends the Provost for Friar Lodowick and orders Angelo and Escalus to handle the investigation while he leaves briefly. The Provost returns with Friar Lodowick—the Duke in his disguise—who loudly declares Angelo's guilt. The Provost and Lucio attempt to arrest the disguised Duke for slander, and in the struggle his identity is revealed. Angelo realises his guilt is known and confesses. The Duke orders him to marry Mariana immediately, and Friar Peter takes the two away to be wed. When Angelo returns with his new wife, the Duke sentences him to death for having killed Claudio. Mariana, joined by Isabella, pleads for his life, but the Duke refuses. The Provost declares that in repentance for having executed Claudio, he has left another prisoner alive. The Duke sends for that man. Barnardine appears, accompanied by Claudio, and the Duke pardons them both. He proposes marriage to Isabella and then pardons Angelo. He declares that Lucio must marry the woman he had abandoned; afterwards, he will be whipped and hung, but in the spirit of forgiveness he withdraws the punishments. He insists on the marriage of Claudio and Juliet, thanks the Provost and Escalus for their good services, and closes the play with an elaboration of his proposal to Isabella.

COMMENTARY

Measure for Measure is a dark play in its focus on evil and its seemingly cynical attitude towards two basic human concerns, sex and the ordering of society. These elements place it among the PROBLEM PLAYS, and like its fellows, *Troilus and Cressida* and *All's Well That Ends Well,* it has generally been among the least popular of Shakespeare's plays during almost four centuries, though they have all increased in popularity during our troubled age. Nevertheless, although its subject matter may have more appeal in the 20th century, the play continues to dissatisfy many readers and viewers. As in the other problem plays, the realistic characters do not readily mesh with the artificial plot or with the happy ending and marriages traditional in COMEDY.

As a TRAGICOMEDY, *Measure for Measure* purposefully combines tragic development with a comic resolution, utilising irony to distance the story line; this technique emphasises the play's symbolic significance. The play addresses its issues—questions of good government and personal morality—through teachings from the Bible, though in a highly secular context. When this is taken into consideration, *Measure for Measure* may seem the least problematic of the problem plays, for its elements then cohere in a convincing manner to justify the traditional happy ending in marriage.

The play's title refers to Christ's Sermon on the Mount, 'measure for measure' being a well-established proverbial abridgement of one of its lessons. In Matt. 7:2 and Luke 6:38 (and in Mark 4:24, in the context of a different sermon) we are taught to use a full, unstinting measure in distributing grain to others, for we shall receive measures in the same way that we distribute them. This lesson was commonly used by preachers and religious books of Shakespeare's day. On a particular Sunday, the version in Luke was by rule the subject of the sermon in all English churches. Thus, we can be sure that Shakespeare was familiar with the text that the proverbial expression referred to, and he could presume that his audience was, too. (He had, in fact, used 'measure for measure' before, in *3 Henry VI,* 2.6.55 and *King John,* 2.1.556–557.)

In Luke and Matthew the 'measure for measure' passages are closely linked to Christ's important pronouncements on the doctrine of Christian forgiveness. The proverb insists on such forgiveness, for only by practising mercy can one expect to receive it. In the play, Angelo's lack of mercy is strikingly compared with Isabella's pleas for it, especially when she seeks mercy for Angelo himself, in 5.1. The biblical passages also contain the familiar instruction not to judge others lest you incur judgement, another lesson in reciprocation. Both ideas were specifically linked with the exercise of power, as well as with personal ethics, by 16th- and 17th-century English Bible commentators. *Measure for Measure* is particularly concerned with the proper exercise of power, at least with respect to the administration of justice; a good ruler, the Duke, uncovers and punishes a bad one, Angelo.

The subject was appropriate in 1604 when Shakespeare wrote *Measure for Measure.* The duties of a Christian ruler were being widely discussed in London, for England had a new king, JAMES I, who was interested in theological matters and had raised the issue himself. In the 17th century it was believed that a ruler's authority came from God, and a good ruler was expected to attempt to be like God in justice and

mercy alike. Because of this relationship, it was almost universally held, a ruler was exempted from the prohibition against vengeance and the exaction of punishment. The ruler was specifically required to use his power to punish wrongdoers, not only to preserve social order but to act as God's weapon in the fight against evil. As such, the ruler could use extraordinary methods that might in others be immoral. Thus, the Duke's disguise and other deceptions, including the bed trick, were entirely acceptable to Shakespeare's audiences. Similarly, the Duke's position justifies his attempts to circumvent the rulings of Angelo, who as a ruler's deputy is also God's appointee. This point is clearly made in the play when the Provost refuses to act against Angelo until the disguised Duke produces a letter indicating that the 'friar' acts for the supposedly absent Duke.

Christian interpretations of the play can be highly literal—some critics have found in it an allegory of divine atonement, in which Angelo is an Everyman figure and the Duke represents Christ, Lucio the Devil, and Isabella the soul. In a more general sense, many commentators have seen Isabella as a particularly Christian figure in her desire to be a nun, her adamant chastity, and her ultimate mercy. However, one need not view the play as purposeful religious doctrine, though it plainly reflects Christian sentiments. Shakespeare's other plays are distinctly *not* allegorical or sermonising, and *Measure for Measure* does not resemble traditional allegory, for most of its characters are believable human beings set in a socially realistic world. The play is easily understood as a traditional secular comedy whose themes have been drawn from a prominent Christian text.

The specifically Christian nature of the play's issues did not have to be raised; the playwright expected his audience to take these ideas for granted and go on to consider their application to the rather grim sex scandal being enacted. As a tale of official misconduct, the play evoked one aspect of the Christian lesson; through its presentation of human psychology a more personal application could be considered. *Measure for Measure* vividly offers both, and in both contexts the final lesson is the same: the power of good (in the form of Christian charity, as stressed by the title) can effect a reconciliation that untangles all plots, rights all wrongs, and leads to marital happiness, just as surely as does secular love in the traditional comedic mode.

As a play on the misuse of authority, *Measure for Measure* opposes two different sorts of bad government, an arrangement appropriate to its title. The Duke's administration of justice prior to the play has been too lax, as he himself admits, saying, '. . . Liberty plucks Justice by the nose, / The baby beats the nurse, and quite athwart / Goes all decorum. / . . . 'twas my fault to give the people scope . . .' (1.3.29–35). It is to rectify this situation that the Duke has transferred his authority to Angelo, but the deputy proves to be the opposite sort of bad governor. He is uncompromisingly strict and cannot apply mercy where it is appropriate, that is, in Claudio's case. The Duke's lax government is also represented in the comic SUB-PLOT by Escalus' release of Pompey. Thus the long comic 'trial' scene featuring Constable Elbow results in freedom for a career pimp, while Claudio, an honourable young man who wishes only to become a husband and father, is still condemned to death. The consequences of the dramatic situation are more extreme than in Shakespeare's other comedies. Angelo's intention towards Isabella is quite simply rape (and he believes he carries it out); then he further blackens himself by going back on his word, and Claudio is very nearly killed.

The remedy begins with the Duke's idea to monitor Angelo, which he actually adopts before the play opens. Significantly, the ruler takes on a religious role. He disguises himself as a friar, thus stressing the divinity of authority. The result, in addition to the preservation of Isabella's honour and Claudio's life, is the emphasis on the Duke's mercy and forgiveness at the play's close. This dénouement might seem exaggerated to modern sensibilities but is utterly fitting to a proper ruler in the world of the play.

In terms of human psychology, the play places Angelo and Isabella in opposition. Angelo's inexcusable refusal of mercy stems from an excess of zeal for the rule of law. This position is related to his notion of himself as a virtuous public servant, one who is beyond examination because he is dutiful. In this Angelo is contrasted with the Duke, who acknowledges his failings and investigates his own government. Because Angelo has not questioned himself, he cannot see the humanity in Claudio, as Isabella points out. His stiff assumption of virtue deprives him of the capacity for honest judgement. Moreover, so confident is he in his own rightness that he is entirely incapable of resisting lust—though he wishes to—when it arises.

The heroine, like the villain, is strictly virtuous. Not only is she prepared to enter a nunnery, she regrets that its rules are not strict enough. Like Angelo, she insists that her own ideas about life be applied to others, 'wishing a more strict restraint / Upon the sisters stood' (1.4.4–5) and demanding that Claudio 'Take my defiance, [and] Die, perish!' (3.1.142–143). Her assertiveness, while attractive in its bold spirit, is uncharitable, also proving Isabella an unlikely nun. Thus, we need not be surprised when she accepts the Duke's proposal of marriage at the close; once her enthusiasm has been allied with a forgiving tolerance she can adopt a more natural destiny than seclusion from the world.

The stiff, unyielding attitudes of the two chief characters establish the play's major conflict. This quality is fittingly expressed in the play's general atmosphere,

for all of Acts 2 and 3 and much of Act 4 take place within a prison or courthouse, and of the nine remaining scenes, three take place in the Friar's cell or the nunnery and one in Mariana's 'moated grange' (3.1.265), a doubly isolated place, both rustic and fortified. Four more scenes (1.1,2; 4.4,6) are in nondescript locales, but they are all distinctly anxious in tone; only the final scene of reconciliation (5.1) takes place in a setting of openness and freedom—'at the gates' (4.4.-4), the site of the Duke's ceremonious re-entry of Vienna.

The play's comic sub-plot both reinforces the claustrophobic atmosphere and relieves it. The shady world of Pompey, Lucio, and Mistress Overdone deals with similar themes as the main plot—sex and criminal justice—but contrasts with it greatly in tone, being bawdy about sex and jocularly dismissive of the courts. The tension of Claudio's fate is thus relaxed, but at the same time the sub-plot offers a dark view of Vienna's civic life that supports a sense of imminent doom. The jesting on venereal disease by Lucio and his friends in 1.2, Mistress Overdone's assertion that Lucio has betrayed her, and the association of Pompey with the executioner Abhorson all contribute to our growing recognition that these humorous figures do not represent an idyllic world of irresponsibility but rather an unpleasant one of commercialised sex and a collapse of values.

In the main story the conflict between Angelo and Isabella becomes unbearably tense. Claudio pleads with Isabella to sin and save him and she denounces him hysterically; by 3.1 it seems painfully clear that either Isabella must break or Claudio must die. The nature of the play changes at this point. No longer an enactment of psychological tension and moral extremism, it becomes a symbolic representation of the power of reconciliation to produce harmony and love where strife had been. The presence of the disguised Duke suggests such an outcome from the beginning. With a balance that is reflected in the title, the second half of the play counters the first. The Duke takes control of the plot, and Angelo, Isabella, and Claudio become much less important. The highly expressive poetry of the first half is replaced by a more mundane mixture of poetry and prose, and the aura of impending tragedy becomes ironic comedy. Through his somewhat absurd plotting, the Duke replaces punishment and death with pardons and marriages. While this development often strikes modern readers as silly, it was for Shakespeare's original audiences a recognisable variant on traditional comedy as well as on medieval MORALITY plays, which generally centred on an undeniable sinner who is forgiven. In Shakespeare's world the fact that Angelo's crime is exceptionally dreadful suggests strongly that he will be forgiven, particularly in light of the play's title.

However, the power of Shakespeare's realistic portrayals of Angelo and Isabella in the first half of the play made a significant change in his source material necessary. In all the variants of the tale the playwright saw, the Angelo figure had his way with the Isabella figure, and then, in the final resolution, was forced to marry her in order that her honour could be restored. However, given the psychological strength with which the two characters have earlier been invested, they simply cannot be made to accept each other without losing their power to move an audience, and much of the play's power also. Mariana therefore replaces Isabella through the use of the bed trick, an ancient comedic device that Shakespeare also used in *All's Well.* Here, the Duke's unquestioned authority makes it seem a less squalid device, though like a *deus ex machina,* this *coup de théâtre* disposes of the impending tragedy with an ease and convenience that is troubling to modern sensibilities. However, in Shakespeare's day this conclusion was perfectly acceptable, the triumph of good had been made explicit in a manner that was satisfying to the sentimental feelings of his audiences.

Mariana also triggers the sequence of pardons in 5.1 by pleading for Angelo's life. More important, she persuades Isabella to join her. Mariana's plea is essentially selfish—she wishes to preserve the husband she has so long sought. Isabella's intercession is, however, more objective; indeed, it goes against her natural enmity towards the man who is her intended rapist and the apparent killer of her brother. The Duke points this out when he says, 'Her brother's ghost . . . would . . . take her hence in horror' (5.1.433–434). But Isabella not only kneels in support of Mariana's plea—which is as much as Mariana asked—but goes on to make a reasoned case for mercy towards her tormentor. Her act flies in the face of common sense, just as does Christ's command in the Sermon on the Mount to love one's enemies. Whether under the influence of Mariana's example of love, or because she remembers her claim to Angelo that she would be merciful if she had his power, or, perhaps, to make up for her willingness to sacrifice Claudio for a principle, Isabella has arrived at the giving of a full measure in the spirit of the text that inspired the play's title.

Thus the play yields a satisfactory outcome on its own terms, those of Christian moral doctrine presented in the form of traditional comedy. The drama is one of ideas, rather than real life. However, Shakespeare's strengths as a dramatist actually diminish this effort, for the psychological and social realism of the play combine to smother the spiritual aura that might otherwise make the play's message more dramatically effective. In the later ROMANCES, Shakespeare more successfully combines the symbolic and the real. Like *All's Well That Ends Well*—which it resembles in many ways—*Measure for Measure* charts the playwright's evolution from a master of personal and societal portrai-

ture towards a more ethereal, intellectual drama. While it is not a successful example of the genre, it marks a significant experiment in its development.

SOURCES OF THE PLAY

Measure for Measure derives from a striking range of sources. The main plot stems originally from a real incident which took place in Italy in 1547: the extortion of sex from the wife of a condemned murderer by a judge who promised mercy and then executed the criminal anyway. The aggrieved widow went to the authorities, and the judge was forced to marry his victim and was then executed. These events were recounted in many works in several languages, and Shakespeare drew on at least one of them, Thomas LUPTON's account in *Too Good To Be True* (1581), which is echoed in the encounters of Angelo and Isabella in Act 2.

More important as a source, however, was a fictional work stimulated by the event, a novella by the Italian author CINTHIO, published in his collection *Hecatommithi* (1565). Here, the criminal's offence is less serious—the seduction of a virgin—and the pleader for mercy is his sister, rather than his wife. At the close she pleads for the life of her violator, now her husband, and a virtuous ruler grants it; a happy ending replaces revenge. Cinthio reworked his novella as a drama, *Epitia* (1583), which also influenced Shakespeare. In *Epitia* the young criminal is spared because a merciful official substitutes a dead man's head for his, as in *Measure for Measure,* and a secondary heroine is featured, a sister of the judge who joins his victim/wife in pleading for his life; she is the original of Mariana.

Miscellaneous details suggest that Shakespeare knew Cinthio's work directly, rather than through the English version of the tale by George WHETSTONE. He could have read Cinthio in the original Italian, in a French translation, or in some now-lost English translation; he certainly did one of these, for another, untranslated Cinthio tale inspired *Othello.* However, Shakespeare was definitely influenced by Whetstone's play on the same subject, *Promos and Cassandra* (1578), which has a comic sub-plot involving harlots and panders who contrast with the virtuous major characters. Also, Whetstone first presents the object of the young criminal's seduction, the model for *Measure for Measure*'s Juliet. Whetstone also elevates the seduction to a respectable act of love that merely precedes formal marriage, as in Shakespeare.

Tales of disguised princes who investigate the workings of their governments were common in 16th-century England, and derived originally from legends concerning the Roman emperor Alexander Severus (reigned 222–235 A.D.). Shakespeare was doubtless influenced by numerous accounts, including one in Whetstone's *A Mirror for Magistrates* (1584). A popular romance dealing with similar material, *The Adventures of Brusanus Prince of Hungary* (1592), by Barnabe RICH (1), was probably the source for Lucio's interactions with the disguised Duke.

The political attitudes of the play, such as those expressed by the Duke in 1.1, may reflect a very popular book on kingship, *Basilicon Doron* (1603), by King James, and the Duke may have been modelled on James himself. At any rate, Shakespeare's remarks on crowd behaviour, in 1.1.67–70 and 2.4.24–30, clearly echo a tract of 1604, *The Time Triumphant,* probably by Shakespeare's fellow actor, Robert ARMIN, describing King James' arrival in London. One further source may have contributed to the political sensibility of the play, the most famous contemporary guide for statesmen, *De Optimo Senatore* (1568), by Laurentius GOSLICIUS (anonymously translated as *The Counsellor* [1598]), which develops criteria to distinguish good and bad public officials that seem reflected in the Duke's opinions on the subject.

TEXT OF THE PLAY

Measure for Measure was written during the spring or summer of 1604. Angelo's remarks on the nuisance of adoring crowds echo a source published in the spring of that year, and Lucio's references to peace talks in 1.2.1–3 are thought to refer to English negotiations with Spain, resulting in a treaty signed in August. Also, Mistress Overdone mentions 'the war, . . . the sweat, . . . the gallows' (1.2.75–76), probably referring to England's continuing war with Spain, an outbreak of plague in London, and the execution of a number of the alleged co-conspirators of Sir Walter RALEIGH, all noteworthy events of early 1604.

The play was first published in the FIRST FOLIO (1623). This text was printed from a copy of the play that had been transcribed by Ralph CRANE, as distinctive punctuation and spelling reveal. Scholars dispute whether Crane's transcription was of Shakespeare's FOUL PAPERS or a later revision of the play—by Shakespeare or someone else—which may have been responsible for irregularities in several scenes, such as the divided soliloquy whose halves appear in 3.2.179–182 and 4.1.60–65. As the only early text, the Folio version has served as the basis for all subsequent editions.

THEATRICAL HISTORY OF THE PLAY

Measure for Measure was performed at court on December 26, 1604, though some topical references in it suggest that it had been performed in public somewhat earlier, perhaps during the previous summer. It was apparently not very popular; the next recorded production was over a century later. It was exploited in two notorious adaptations, one, THE LAW AGAINST LOVERS (1662) by William DAVENENT, which incorporated some material from *Much Ado About Nothing,* and a second, based on the first, Charles GILDON's *Measure*

for Measure, or Beauty the Best Advocate (1699), which featured a full-scale operatic MASQUE (taken from Henry PURCELL) that comprised the sub-plot. Thomas BETTERTON and Anne BRACEGIRDLE starred in the latter work.

Measure for Measure was popular in the 18th century. In 1720 John RICH (2) staged a version that was close to Shakespeare's play, and after more than a decade's popularity it was replaced by a version by Colley CIBBER (1). Like the adaptations, both of these versions and most of their 18th-century successors eliminated all or most of the sub-plot, which was viewed as grossly undignified. Isabella was a particularly esteemed role, and many of the leading 18th-century actresses played it, including Mary Ann YATES (1), Ann BARRY (1), and Sarah SIDDONS.

In the early 19th century John Philip KEMBLE (3) restored the sub-plot in a staging that was much more purely Shakespearean, but the play was not greatly liked nor often produced during the century. Adelaide NEILSON (1) was a noted Isabella in the 1870s. The play has been more popular in the 20th century: among the memorable productions have been those of Oscar ASCHE (1906), Peter BROOK (2) (1950, starring John GIELGUD as Angelo), and John BARTON (1) (1970). *Measure for Measure* has twice been done on FILM, once each in Italian (1942) and German (1963), and has once been broadcast on TELEVISION, in a 1979 BBC production starring Kate Nelligan. The great German composer Richard Wagner's second opera (and his first produced), *Das Liebesverbot* (1836), was based on the play.

Melun (Melune), Giles de, Lord (d. 1216) Historical figure and minor character in *King John.* The fatally wounded Melun, a French lord, relieves his conscience before dying by warning the rebellious English nobles who have aided the French invasion that LEWIS (1), the French leader, intends to kill them after he has defeated King JOHN (3). This information sparks the renewed loyalty of the rebels, led by the Earl of SALISBURY (4).

Shakespeare took this incident from HOLINSHED's history, but it is probably not accurate. In any case, little more is known of Melun. In the play he speaks of his English grandfather, who may have been Robert de Melun, Bishop of Hereford (d. 1164); this cannot be confirmed by known records, however.

Menas (active, c. 40–c. 35 B.C.) Historical figure and character in *Antony and Cleopatra,* a pirate who fights for POMPEY (2). Menas and MENECRATES are called famed buccaneers who make 'hot inroads' (1.4.50) on the coast of Italy in support of Pompey's rebellion. In 2.1 Menas confers with Pompey and predicts accurately the future disputes of ANTONY and Octavius CAESAR (2). In 2.6 he is among his leader's advisers at the signing of the Treaty of MISENUM, though he privately disapproves of it and says, 'Pompey doth this day laugh away his fortune' (2.6.103). In 2.7, during the banquet aboard Pompey's ship, Menas proves himself a true pirate and advises Pompey to cut the throats of the Roman leadership—Caesar, Antony, and LEPIDUS—and seize the state. When Pompey refuses, Menas decides to abandon him as doomed, for 'Who seeks and will not take, when once 'tis offer'd, / Shall never find it more' (2.7.82–83). This shrewdly cynical sailor reveals the mistrust and disloyalty that informs the politics of the play.

The historical Menas is well represented in the play, for he was indeed a notably cynical turncoat. He deserted Pompey at Misenum in 39 B.C. and joined Caesar. Discontented with his rewards, he deserted again and returned to Pompey in time to participate in his defence of Sicily in 36 B.C. Again, however, he disapproved of what he saw as Pompey's lethargy and indecision—an opinion shared by military historians—and he changed sides for a third time and rejoined Caesar. Little more is known of him.

Menecrates (active c. 40 B.C.) Historical figure and character in *Antony and Cleopatra,* a pirate who fights for POMPEY (2). Mentioned with MENAS as one of two 'famous pirates' (1.4.48) who support Pompey's rebellion against Rome with 'hot inroads' (1.4.50) on the coast of Italy, Menecrates turns out to be a mild buccaneer when he appears, in 2.1. He philosophically recommends that Pompey have patience with the slow pace of his success. He then disappears from the play. He is mentioned with the more important Menas as a 'notable pirate' in Shakespeare's source, PLUTARCH's *Lives.*

In the FIRST FOLIO text of the play, all the speeches in 2.1 except Pompey's are designated 'Mene' and seem to belong to Menecrates, though Menas is spelled Menes once elsewhere in the Folio. However, since one of these five speeches—2.1.38–41—clearly belongs to Menas, editors have restored that speech to him and often give him more. In fact, beginning with the 1765 edition of Samuel JOHNSON (7), some editors give all these lines to Menas, leaving Menecrates mute.

Menelaus Legendary figure and minor character in *Troilus and Cressida,* king of Sparta and a leader of the Greeks in the TROJAN WAR. Before the play opens, the theft of Menelaus' wife, HELEN (1), by Prince PARIS (3) of Troy has sparked the war. However, although he is the ostensible beneficiary of the war and the younger brother of the Greek commander AGAMEMNON, he is an inconsequential figure. He speaks more than one line in only one scene, 4.5, where in brief exchanges he is wittily mortified by both PATROCLUS and CRESSIDA. His insignificance makes the cause of the war seem all the more trivial, an important motif of the play. This

theme is further supported by the frequent derisive references to Menelaus' status as a cuckold.

In the *Iliad* of HOMER, Menelaus is intermittently a major figure—defeating Paris in a duel but prevented from killing him by the goddess Aphrodite, for example—but he consciously subordinates himself to Agamemnon. In the *Odyssey* and later works he resumes a comfortable domestic life with Helen after the war.

Menenius Agrippa Legendary figure and character in *Coriolanus,* friend and adviser of the title character. Menenius is an elderly aristocrat who is distinguished by his canny political sense in a time of popular discontent in ROME. In 1.1 he defuses a riot with his clever speech, and he establishes a rapport with the people's tribunes, BRUTUS (3) and SICINIUS. Nonetheless, he cannot prevent CORIOLANUS from destroying himself politically by refusing to compromise his stern aristocratic ideals. In this respect, Menenius' actions are as futile as those of all the aristocrats. Their failure to control Coriolanus is fatal to the hero himself and almost to all of Rome.

Though Menenius' capacity for compromise makes him stand out, and a CITIZEN (5) calls him 'one that hath always loved the people' (1.1.50–51), he nonetheless shares the aristocracy's disdain for the common people. He thereby contributes to the sense of a disturbed society that is one of the play's important themes. He cleverly deflects the mob with his 'belly speech' (1.1.95–153), an elaborate comparison of the body politic to the human anatomy that justifies the hierarchy of Roman society. This was an ancient political fable when it appeared in Shakespeare's source, PLUTARCH's *Lives,* and it was still current in the playwright's time. However, Menenius goes on to dismiss the intelligent remarks of the First Citizen. He calls him the 'great toe' of society (1.1.154), and he insults the tribunes as 'the herdsmen of the beastly plebeians' (2.1.94–95). Like the other aristocrats, Menenius is too proud to contribute to the welfare of the entire city, and instead he contributes to the play's disasters.

After 1.1 Menenius is merely a mildly amusing figure, in his own words a 'humorous patrician, and one that loves a cup of hot wine' (2.1.46–47) ('humorous' here meaning 'temperamental'). He idolises the much younger Coriolanus and greets him with 'A hundred thousand welcomes. I could weep, / And I could laugh, I am light and heavy. Welcome!' (2.1.182–183). He rejoices girlishly over a letter from his hero, and fumes angrily when the tribunes belittle him. However, after Coriolanus has joined the VOLSCIANS and is besieging Rome, he goes to plead with him to spare the city. His rejection yields a moment of genuine pathos and stoic dignity as the elderly gentleman, heartbroken, turns away and says 'He that hath a will to die by himself, fears it not from another' (5.2.102–103).

Menenius Agrippa speaks his 'belly speech' in Plutarch but is otherwise unimportant. Shakespeare made him a paternal friend of his protagonist to lend pathos to the story. Despite Menenius' appearance in Plutarch and other ancient histories, modern scholars recognise him to be entirely legendary.

Menteth (Menteith), Walter Dalyell, Thane of (active 1056) Historical figure and minor character in *Macbeth,* a Scottish nobleman. In 5.2 Menteth, with CATHNESS, ANGUS, and LENOX, joins the army led by MALCOLM and MACDUFF against MACBETH. They are presumably among the 'many worthy fellows' (4.3.183) reported earlier to have risen in arms against Macbeth's tyranny. In 5.4 they prepare to march on DUNSINANE. Though his character is not developed, Menteth's presence helps strengthen the political aspect of the play. The rebellion of the nobles indicates the extent of political and social disruption in SCOTLAND due to Macbeth's evil.

The historical Walter Dalyell ruled Menteith, a territory in central Scotland. Little more is known of him; Shakespeare took his name from a list of Malcolm's allies in his source, HOLINSHED's history.

Mercadé See MARCADE.

Mercer GHOST CHARACTER in *Timon of Athens.* The Mercer is listed in the opening stage direction of 1.1, but he does not appear. Shakespeare apparently listed a number of characters he thought he would make use of in the course of writing the scene, and then when he did not in fact employ a Mercer, he did not bother to delete the reference. Many such minor inconsistencies are found in the plays; *Timon,* as an unfinished play, is naturally subject to them.

Merchant (1) Either of two minor characters in *The Comedy of Errors.* Two Merchants appear in this play (they enter first in 2.2 and 4.1 respectively), and, while Shakespeare apparently made no distinction between them by name, they are plainly different people. The first to appear is familiar with the affairs of Ephesus, offering advice to the foreigner ANTIPHOLUS OF SYRACUSE and warning him not to reveal himself as a Syracusan, lest he be sentenced to death. Having thus reminded the audience of EGEON's desperate plight, this Merchant disappears from the play. He is generally distinguished in modern editions as 'First Merchant'.

The 'Second Merchant', however, seems to be a visitor himself, for he must inquire (5.1.4) about the reputation of ANTIPHOLUS OF EPHESUS, a well-known local figure. Attempting to collect a debt owed ANGELO (1) by one Antipholus, the Merchant mistakenly challenges Antipholus of Syracuse to a duel, precipitating

that twin's flight into the PRIORY, which ultimately leads to the resolution of the play.

Merchant (2) Minor character in *Timon of Athens*, a flatterer of TIMON. In 1.1 the Merchant and his friend the JEWELLER discuss Timon's free-spending nature and intend to profit from it. The Merchant speaks little and serves chiefly as a sounding board for his colleague. Both of them are representative greedy flatterers.

The Merchant of Venice

SYNOPSIS

Act 1, Scene 1
SALERIO and SOLANIO attempt to cheer up their friend ANTONIO (2); they are assisted by BASSANIO, LORENZO, and GRATIANO (1). Antonio denies that he is worried about his investments in far-flung trading voyages, for he is confident of their success. The friends, except Bassanio, depart. Antonio inquires about the love affair Bassanio has promised to speak of. Bassanio replies that his extravagant lifestyle, which he has supported with loans from friends, especially Antonio, may pay off if he can successfully woo and marry PORTIA (1), a rich heiress. However, he wishes to borrow more money in order to present himself as an impressive enough suitor to compete with his wealthy rivals. Antonio assures his friend that he will loan him as much as he needs. Because Antonio's funds are all invested in ships at the moment, he promises to borrow the money to support Bassanio's courtship.

Act 1, Scene 2
Portia discusses her late father's will with her maid, NERISSA. Under its terms, she must marry the man who selects from among three chests or caskets—one each of gold, silver, and lead—the one that contains the consent placed in it by her father. Portia worries about the sort of husband she may win in this lottery. She and Nerissa discuss and humorously dismiss a number of potential suitors, and Nerissa reveals, to the relief of her mistress, that all of them have decided not to choose among the caskets because of a penalty that Portia's father has decreed for those who pick either of the wrong ones. Nerissa reminds Portia of Bassanio, who had visited some time before, and they agree that he would make an acceptable suitor. Word comes that a new suitor, the Prince of MOROCCO, has arrived.

Act 1, Scene 3
Bassanio and Antonio ask the Jewish moneylender SHYLOCK for a loan. Antonio remarks that he is opposed to usury, the lending of money at interest, and Shylock defends the practise. Further, Shylock observes that Antonio has often spat on him and insulted him for being a Jew, and he asks why he should be expected to assist his tormentor. Antonio frankly acknowledges that Shylock must regard the loan as one made to an enemy. Shylock, however, insists that he wishes to be friendly and offers to lend him the money interest-free for three months, requiring only a humorous collateral; if Antonio cannot repay the loan when it comes due, he will permit Shylock to cut from his body one pound of flesh. Although Bassanio is uneasy about this arrangement, Antonio signs a legal contract for the loan, confident that his business ventures will soon bring him nine times the amount required.

Act 2, Scene 1
Morocco declares his love for Portia and agrees to be bound by her father's will: if he selects the right casket, he will marry her, but he must solemnly swear that, if he chooses one of the others, he will never marry anyone.

Act 2, Scene 2
Shylock's clownish servant, LAUNCELOT Gobbo, soliloquises humorously on his desire to run away from his master. His blind father, Old GOBBO (2), appears. Launcelot teases his father, pretending to be a stranger, but finally speaks seriously of his plan to desert Shylock and work for Bassanio, a more liberal and generous master. Bassanio happens by, and Gobbo, with much comical prompting from his son, speaks to him about employing Launcelot. Bassanio, finding the youth amusing, agrees, and Launcelot departs to give notice to Shylock. Gratiano enters and asks to accompany Bassanio when he travels to Portia's estate. Bassanio agrees but insists that Gratiano curb his usual wild humour.

Act 2, Scene 3
Shylock's daughter, JESSICA, bids Launcelot farewell and gives him a letter to deliver to Lorenzo. Alone, she regrets that she is Shylock's daughter but takes heart in the prospect of marrying Lorenzo and converting to Christianity.

Act 2, Scene 4
Lorenzo, with Gratiano, Salerio, and Solanio, are preparing for a masque, when Launcelot arrives with the letter from Jessica. Lorenzo gives him a message for Jessica: he, Lorenzo, shall not fail her. Salerio and Solanio leave, and Lorenzo tells Gratiano that he and Jessica plan to elope that evening.

Act 2, Scene 5
Launcelot delivers an invitation to dinner from Bassanio to Shylock and hints to Jessica that Lorenzo is about to arrive.

Act 2, Scene 6
Lorenzo, accompanied by Gratiano and Salerio, takes Jessica from Shylock's house. Antonio enters and

gives Gratiano the message that Bassanio is preparing to leave for BELMONT, Portia's estate.

Act 2, Scene 7
With Portia, Morocco reads the inscriptions on the caskets. The gold one promises 'what many men desire'; the silver offers as much as the chooser deserves; the lead warns that the chooser 'must give and hazard all he hath'. Morocco rejects the lead as a plainly foolish choice and the silver as inadequate. He selects the gold casket but finds inside it a rhyme informing him that he has lost. He departs, to Portia's relief.

Act 2, Scene 8
Salerio and Solanio gossip about Shylock's hysterical discovery that Jessica has fled and taken much of his money. They reflect that Shylock's anger will affect Antonio if he fails to repay his debt, and they worry that a rich Venetian ship, reported lost, may be one of his.

Act 2, Scene 9
The Prince of ARRAGON ventures to choose one of the caskets and win Portia's hand. He rejects the gold's offer of 'what many men desire' as the choice of the foolish multitudes who value outward appearance. Feeling that he is quite worthy, he elects the silver casket's promise of as much as he deserves. However, a rhyme inside the casket announces his failure, and he leaves. A MESSENGER (10) brings word that a young Venetian intends to enter the lottery of the caskets. Portia and Nerissa hope that he will prove to be Bassanio.

Act 3, Scene 1
Solanio and Salerio discuss the rumoured loss of Antonio's ship. Shylock appears and curses Jessica; he also rails against Antonio, vowing that he will collect his pound of flesh as revenge for Antonio's anti-Semitism. Shylock observes that Jews are like Christians in bodily respects, and he will prove that their desire for revenge is also the same. A message from Antonio causes the gentlemen to depart, and Shylock's friend TUBAL arrives. Tubal reports that he has been unable to find Jessica, but he has heard of her extravagance with her father's money. Shylock is frantic about his lost wealth, but Tubal also tells his friend that Antonio has suffered further losses and is said to be bankrupt. Shylock becomes exultant.

Act 3, Scene 2
Portia asks Bassanio to postpone choosing among the caskets, for he must leave if he fails and she has fallen in love with him. Bassanio, however, cannot tolerate the suspense, and he proceeds to his selection. He rejects the gold and silver as representing false glamour and expensive show, and he opens the lead casket. Inside he finds Portia's picture and a text confirming that he has won her hand. She gives him a ring, which he swears to wear until he dies. Gratiano and Nerissa reveal that they have also fallen in love, and a double wedding is proposed. Salerio arrives from Venice with Lorenzo and Jessica. He tells Bassanio that Antonio has lost all his vessels and that Shylock has said that he will demand the pound of flesh. Portia offers to pay Shylock many times over.

Act 3, Scene 3
Antonio, in the custody of a GAOLER (1), approaches Shylock, but the Jew will not speak to him; he angrily repeats his demand for the pound of flesh and departs. Antonio prepares to die; he hopes only to see Bassanio again.

Act 3, Scene 4
Portia announces her intention to enter a religious retreat while Bassanio tries to help Antonio in Venice. She instructs her servant BALTHASAR (3) to deliver a letter to her cousin in PADUA. He is then to meet her with the documents and clothing the cousin will give him. She tells Nerissa of her plan: they shall go to Venice disguised as men.

Act 3, Scene 5
Launcelot, in his capacity as a professional FOOL (1), impudently jests with Jessica and Lorenzo, who then banter affectionately.

Act 4, Scene 1
The DUKE (4) of Venice convenes a court to try Shylock's claim. Shylock is asked to be merciful, but he refuses. The Duke announces that he has sent to a Paduan scholar for a legal opinion. Portia and Nerissa arrive, disguised as a lawyer and his clerk sent by the scholar. Portia interviews Shylock and Antonio. After Shylock repeatedly demands strict justice, she awards him his pound of flesh but prohibits him from drawing any blood—for blood is not mentioned in the contract—on pain of death. Realising that he is beaten, Shylock says he will accept the money, but Portia rules that he shall have only the exact justice he has demanded: he may attempt to extract his bloodless flesh, or he may withdraw his suit, but he cannot claim the money. Shylock concedes defeat and is about to leave when Portia further rules that, as a non-Venetian who has attempted to take the life of a citizen, he is subject to the death penalty—unless the Duke pardons him—and to the confiscation of all his possessions. The Duke permits him to live, and Antonio suggests that he be allowed to keep half of his earthly goods in exchange for converting to Christianity and deeding the other half to Lorenzo and Jessica. Shylock agrees to these terms. The Paduan lawyer (Portia) refuses a fee but asks Bassanio for his ring as a token of thanks. He refuses, saying that it was a sacred gift from his wife, but he repents after she leaves, accusing himself of ingratitude. He sends Gratiano to give the ring to the lawyer.

Act 4, Scene 2
Gratiano gives the ring to Portia, who asks him to direct her clerk (Nerissa) to Shylock's house to deliver the deed that the money-lender must sign. Nerissa tells Portia that she will contrive to get Gratiano to give her his ring as well.

Act 5, Scene 1
Lorenzo and Jessica enjoy the moonlight and music at Belmont, joyfully comparing themselves to various famous lovers. Word arrives that Portia and Nerissa are returning from the monastery, and Launcelot, comically imitating a hunting horn, heralds the approach of Bassanio. The lovers resume their contemplation, and Lorenzo reflects on the harmony of the spheres. Portia and Nerissa enter, just ahead of Bassanio, Gratiano, and Antonio. The women 'discover' that their husbands no longer have their rings, and they chastise them severely, evoking pained excuses. Finally, Portia reveals the truth, and the party moves indoors to celebrate their reunion.

COMMENTARY

The Merchant of Venice is a richly complicated work in which several themes are presented in the framework of a traditional COMEDY, which calls for the triumph of young lovers over their unromantic elders. Before this end is achieved, three distinct plots are resolved: the winning of Portia by the lottery of the caskets, the settlement of Shylock's claim, and the final complication of the betrothal rings. All of these developments further the traditional romantic purpose of the play.

But before looking at Shakespeare's intentions and devices, let us consider the evidently anti-Semitic nature of the play, which is particularly repellent in light of the Holocaust (1933–1945), in which 6 million European Jews were executed in Nazi concentration camps. Great historical events unavoidably affect the thoughts and sensibilities of later generations, and this terrifying 20th-century manifestation of anti-Semitism must colour our response to *The Merchant of Venice.* Its villain is a stereotypical Jew, and his Jewishness is persistently derided by the Christians in the play. Even though Shylock has his moments of sympathetic humanity, they are rather qualified, and he is finally found deserving of treatment that is unquestionably shabby by modern Western ethical and legal standards. He is deprived of his life's earnings and coerced into renouncing his religion by avowed anti-Semites who preach justice and mercy all the while. Many have asked how Shakespeare could have depicted such behaviour in characters clearly intended to be taken as good people—Portia, Antonio, and their friends—when in the rest of his work his characterisations are so strikingly humane. One must conclude that, to at least some extent, Shakespeare shared in the anti-Semetic biases of his age.

Of course, the anti-Semitism of Shakespeare's England was rather theoretical: practising Jews had been rare there since their expulsion from the country in 1290, and active anti-Jewish bigotry was accordingly unusual. But, while 16th-century Londoners may have found Jews more exotic than malevolent, they also had a generally negative image of Judaism that was the legacy of centuries of bias. Christian tradition, from the New Testament on, stimulated anti-Semitism, and if the 16th-century English version was milder than others, it was nonetheless real. Shakespeare, very much a man of his time and place, probably harboured it to some degree; he was at least willing to accommodate his public, which had responded with great delight to *The Jew of Malta,* by Christopher MARLOWE (1), whose spectacularly villainous title character probably influenced the creation of Shylock. Also, the trial and execution of Roderigo LOPEZ in 1594, not long before Shakespeare wrote this play, generated a spate of more overt expressions of bigotry. (Elizabethan prejudices are similarly addressed in the play's negative presentations of a black man, Morocco, and a Spaniard, Arragon.) In any case, English anti-Semitism was only one expression of a widespread European phenomenon, and there is unquestionably a historical connection across the centuries between the attitudes of Shakespeare's characters and the atrocities of the Holocaust.

Anti-Semitism contributed to the development of Shylock's character simply by providing the only well-known image of a Jew. Sixteenth-century Englishmen tended to attribute to Jews only two important characteristics, both negative: first, that Jews detested Christians and gave much energy to devising evils for gentiles to undergo, and second, that Jews practised usury. The latter assumption was grounded in an old, though disappearing, reluctance on the part of Christians to lend money, due to Biblical injunctions against the practise within one's own religious community. Despite the growth of modern banking in the 16th century, it remained true in much of Europe—including Italy, the source of Shakespeare's story—that lending money at interest was confined by law to non-Christians. In England, however, Christians could and did practise usury, at a legally sanctioned rate of 10 percent. Usury's increasing importance in everyday life was a prominent and widely disliked aspect of economic development in Shakespeare's day, a phenomenon that doubtless led the playwright to adapt a tale that condemned it. That it also condemned a Jew was as much a result of actual Continental practices at the time as of Shakespeare's prejudices. His source featured a Jewish usurer as a villain, and he borrowed this character. He gave the role more life than he found in the source, as he typically did, but he did not alter its anti-Semitic overtones.

Although Shakespeare was influenced by the anti-

Semitism of his day in writing *The Merchant of Venice*, the play was not itself motivated by anti-Semitism, nor was it intended to spread anti-Semitic doctrines. Instead, *The Merchant of Venice* illustrates a theme that occupied Shakespeare in most of his comedies, the triumph of love over false and inhumane attitudes towards life.

The central plot of the play deals with Bassanio's courtship of Portia. Antonio goes to Shylock for a loan only because his friend wishes to woo Portia, and the usurer's undoing comes about through Portia's desire to help the friend of her beloved. The seemingly strange ending of the play is the culmination of Portia and Bassanio's betrothal.

The courtship is based on an ancient folk motif, that of a choice among caskets, the suitor's correct choice being rewarded with marriage to the maiden in question. Bassanio expresses his distrust of rich appearances in 3.2.73–107, as he selects the casket of lead. Such sentiments, attached to similar stories, were common in Elizabethan literature and reflected the ideal of true love. Only a true lover would value the maid for herself and choose the plainest casket, which requires him to 'give and hazard all he hath' (2.7.9). (This ideal is not sullied by Bassanio's frank assessment of Portia's wealth in 1.2.161–176, for such considerations were normal when contemplating marriage in the 16th century; Bassanio could not reasonably bring up the subject with Antonio and fail to mention Portia's wealth, particularly since he was asking to borrow money to accomplish his courtship.)

The tale of the caskets also casts light on another theme of the play, that of the misuse of wealth. The title character of any work may be supposed to represent its essential spirit, and the title character here is Antonio, who risks his wealth—and his life, as it turns out—to aid his friend Bassanio. His enemy, Shylock, is a grotesque miser who loves his ducats more than his daughter. Though his stereotypical Jewishness is essential to his personality, Shylock is more significantly related to another tradition, that of the miser whose mean-spiritedness is contrasted with, and overcome by, the power of love felt by the romantic young. However, the conflict is not simply between money and love, but rather between two different attitudes towards money. Both Antonio and Shylock engage in commerce, but only Antonio is willing to use his wealth in the service of others, resembling Bassanio in his willingness to 'hazard all' for his friends. Shylock has the same blind pride as Arragon, assuming that he deserves as much as he is capable of getting.

In Shakespeare's time, money was a particularly troubling subject. Commercial banking was a relatively new phenomenon in England, where land-based wealth had been the norm for centuries, and it inspired much distrust and resentment. Shakespeare's own position seems somewhat ambiguous: his sympathies with old England and his conservative social and political orientation are evident throughout his work, but he himself was a competent businessman, on good terms with the leading usurer of STRATFORD, John COMBE (1). It has been speculated that his ambivalence may have inspired him to create so three-dimensional a figure as Shylock where a conventional stage villain might have served his traditional comic aims just as well. However, Shylock's humanity gives him great weight; he forcefully represents money's great power to foster hatred and strife, and the open generosity of Antonio and Portia are more convincingly triumphant over Shylock's lust for vengeance when we can clearly see the psychology of his evil need.

As greed is set against love in *The Merchant of Venice*, so is justice placed in opposition to mercy, especially in the trial scene (4.1). The Duke, asking Shylock to excuse Antonio's penalty, asks him, 'How shalt thou hope for mercy rend'ring none?' (4.1.88); he is referring to the usurer's expectations in the afterlife. So is Shylock, when he answers, 'What judgement shall I dread doing no wrong?' (4.1.89). This exchange refers implicitly to a conventional comparison of the Old Testament and the New, in which the former is seen to emphasise strict obedience as humanity's obligation to God while the latter stresses God's mercy. Shylock stands for the strict interpretation of law, for justice in its most rigorous and unbending form. Portia argues for divine clemency, observing, 'The quality of mercy is not strained' (4.1.180), at the opening of her most famous speech.

But Shylock is not wholly evil. His position is defensible, and his demand for vengeance is made humanly understandable. He has earlier traced his own evil to a plausible source in remarking to his tormentors Salerio and Solanio that 'the villainy you teach me I will execute' (3.1.65). Further, Portia, once her battle is won, is not particularly given to mercy, depriving Shylock of any repayment of his loan and then sentencing him to death as well. Shakespeare invented Portia's invocation of a capital punishment statute; it is not in his sources. Thus he emphasised the paradoxical conclusion that Shylock's downfall results from his own insistence on strict justice.

Antonio mercifully rescinds the death penalty, but Shylock is deprived of all his support in life—as Shakespeare permits him to observe in 4.1.370–373. The main thrust of the trial scene is clear: Shylock has been given enough rope to hang himself, and then harsh justice has been tempered by the mercy of the title figure. Antonio, whose affairs have both promoted Bassanio's romantic success and produced his own woes, remains the source of the play's action.

The two primary plots demonstrate and reconcile opposing principles. We see how wealth can aid romance as well as hinder it and that justice can be merciful as well as vengeful. These themes are tied

together in the seemingly gratuitous anecdote of the betrothal rings. Portia's ploy is not simply a practical joke; the rings are carefully presented as tokens first of love, then of gratitude, and finally of forgiveness. Bassanio understands the dilemma he faces when he gives his ring to the lawyer 'Balthasar'; he is not disloyal to Portia, but he recognises that he owes a debt of gratitude to the young lawyer who has saved his friend. Portia knows this, and while she effectively adopts Shylock's position, insisting on the letter of the oath with which the ring was received originally, she clearly intends to forgive Bassanio after teasing him a bit. The story of the rings—a well-known tale in Shakespeare's day—was introduced by the playwright in order to recapitulate in a lightly comic manner the lessons won from the stressful trial. The other elements of 5.1—the rhapsodic musings of Lorenzo and Jessica and the meditations on music—serve a similar purpose. Although often seen as an ill-considered aberration, this scene alleviates the mood of the preceding one. It provides an anticlimax that returns us to the lovers and their world. Without it, *The Merchant of Venice* would resemble the later PROBLEM PLAYS, which tend to deal with unpleasant social phenomena in an ambiguous way. Here, even such a grossly sentimental—and wholly implausible—event as Portia's announcement that Antonio's ships have miraculously survived (5.1.274–279) can be accepted wholeheartedly. The audience is permitted to share in the triumph of love and playfulness—the spirit of comedy—over the selfish and inhumane stinginess that Shylock represents.

Modern readers, aware of the extremes to which anti-Semitism can lead, tend to give Shylock more sympathy than his place in the play's tight structure can bear. Shakespeare and his audiences were comfortable with a formal, allegorical presentation of human truth that often seems obscure to modern sensibilities, which are far more attuned to realism. Shylock's symbolic role, that of an obvious villain opposed to characters representing generosity and love, is more important to the play's themes than is his Jewishness or his personality. Eighteenth- and 19th-century theatrical tradition humanised the character, presenting to our own century a very different figure from the one whom Shakespeare originally conceived.

The Merchant of Venice presents great opportunity for such varying approaches; indeed, it demands them. For example, Shylock can be sympathised with, but he may also be seen as an overdeveloped figure who interferes with a romantic comedy. On the other hand, sometimes 5.1 is seen as a defective scene that draws attention away from Shylock. Portia's strategem of leading Shylock on in his claims to justice can be seen as high-handed and the trial scene regarded as a satire on law and its cruel strictures. Some critics see the focus of the play as the relationship between Antonio and Bassanio; the theme of friendship among men was prominent in medieval literature and was more plainly employed by Shakespeare in *The Two Gentlemen of Verona*. Some go so far as to hold that Shakespeare intended Antonio's affection to be taken as homosexual. These varied interpretations demonstrate the richness of *The Merchant of Venice:* many different views of the play can be plausibly presented. Its diverse complications are not stiffly theatrical, despite their roots in dramatic conventions and old tales. Instead, they derive from the problems and ambiguities of human experience.

SOURCES OF THE PLAY

The primary source for *The Merchant of Venice* was a story in an Italian collection, *Il Pecorone (The Simpleton)*, by Giovanni FIORENTINO, published in Milan (1558). This tale presents all the components of Shakespeare's play in considerable detail, except for the lottery of the caskets and the practise of usury by Shylock (his equivalent loans money at no interest). A possible intervening source has often been proposed: a lost English play, *The Jew*, mentioned in a publication of 1579, may have been reworked by Shakespeare. However, the only reference to *The Jew* is brief and ambiguous, and such complicated plots as that of *The Merchant of Venice* were virtually unknown in the 1570s. This hypothesis is thus increasingly unpopular.

The introduction of the usury theme could have been suggested by several contemporary sources, including Anthony MUNDAY's novel *Zelauto* (1580) and a well-known ballad, 'Gernutus', both of which tell of a similarly forfeited loan, in each case to a usurer. The lottery of three caskets is an ancient motif that the playwright also may have known from a number of sources. The *Confessio Amantis*, by John GOWER (3), which Shakespeare unquestionably knew, contains a variation taken from BOCCACCIO, but the most closely corresponding version is in a translation by Richard ROBINSON (3) of the *Gesta Romanorum*, a famed medieval collection of tales, published in 1577 and 1595. The elopement and conversion of Jessica may have been suggested by similar characters in either *Zelauto* or Marlowe's *The Jew of Malta* (c. 1592). The latter's immense popularity is often thought to have sparked Shakespeare's adaptation of Fiorentino's tale (or *The Jew*) in the first place, and its title character probably influenced the creation of Shylock.

TEXT OF THE PLAY

The Merchant of Venice was written between the summer of 1596 and the summer of 1598. The later date is certain because the play was registered for publication in July of that year, and it is mentioned as a produced play in Francis MERES' book, published in September 1598. The earlier date, though less certain, seems probable in view of Salerio's reference in 1.1.27 to the

ship ANDREW (1)—that is, the *St Andrew*, a Spanish vessel captured by the English in 1596. (Although such a reference could have been added some time after the play was written, earlier dates seem unlikely in view of the play's stylistic similarities to such later works as *1* and *2 Henry IV* and *Much Ado About Nothing.*)

The Merchant of Venice was first published in 1600 in a QUARTO edition known as Q1. It was printed by James ROBERTS for the publisher Thomas HEYES. Its stage directions, which contain many superfluous remarks, suggest that Q1 was printed from Shakespeare's manuscript, though whether from his FOUL PAPERS or from the FAIR COPY, is uncertain. A second edition, Q2, was a reprint of Q1, produced in 1619 by William JAGGARD for Thomas PAVIER as part of the FALSE FOLIO. The publisher, who was reprinting the play without authorisation, asserted on the title page that the edition had been printed by Roberts in 1600—that is, it was in fact Q1. Until the early 20th century, scholars believed it to be the first edition of the play. But, although taken from Q1, Q2 contains several minor alterations of the original text, as well as many new errors. Q3 (1637) and the FIRST FOLIO text of 1623 were based on Q1, and Q1 has also served as the basic text for most subsequent editions. However, the Folio edition contains improved stage directions (probably derived from a text used in early productions), and these have frequently been followed by modern editors.

THEATRICAL HISTORY OF THE PLAY

According to the title page of the first edition of the play in 1600, *The Merchant of Venice* had been performed 'divers times' by that date, but the first performance of which a record has survived was held at the court of King JAMES I in the spring of 1605. It was so well received that the King ordered a second performance several days later, but no other 17th-century performance is known. In 1701 George GRANVILLE produced an adaptation, *The Jew of Venice*, in which Shylock was played for laughs by a popular comic. This version was still quite popular in 1741, when Charles MACKLIN restored Shakespeare's play, portraying Shylock as a melodramatic villain. The play was performed in various versions throughout the rest of the 18th century, with most of the important actors of the day playing the Jew. Shylock was apparently treated as the major figure in the play, and, following Macklin's example, he was depicted as thoroughly malignant.

The first Shylock intended to arouse sympathy was that of Edmund KEAN (2), whose Jew was scornful of his enemies and raged against their pretensions to mercy. William HAZLITT, in a famous review, said of Kean's Shylock, 'He is honest in his vices; they are hypocrites in their virtues'. Other notable 19th-century Shylocks included William Charles MACREADY, Charles KEAN (1), and Edwin BOOTH (2). Beginning in 1879 Henry IRVING was particularly successful playing the villain in a grandly tragic manner. A somewhat later production went so far as to have Shylock commit suicide on stage following his last lines.

In the 20th century the emphasis on Shylock has been modified, and various interpretations have been offered. In a famous 1921 production the German producer Max REINHARDT presented the villain as a buffoon and the play as a farce with a notorious blue and white Cubist-style set, but most attempts have been soberer. In general it has been found that, with Shylock somewhat de-emphasised, productions have been able to assert the essential unity of the play. *The Merchant of Venice* has remained among the most popular of Shakespeare's plays, and many leading players have performed in it, including John GIELGUD and Sybil THORNDIKE. The play had been produced as a silent FILM six times by 1923 but has only once been a movie since, in an Italian version of 1952. It has, however, been presented on TELEVISION five times, including a production by Jonathan MILLER (2) (1970), starring Laurence OLIVIER and Joan PLOWRIGHT.

Mercutio Character in Romeo and Juliet, ROMEO's friend who is killed by TYBALT. Mercutio, a buoyantly ribald and belligerent young gallant, serves as a foil for the maturing Romeo, who is discovering that love offers a more profound world than that of gentlemanly pleasures and enmities. Named for Mercury, the impudent god of thievery, Mercutio embodies an instability inherent in the noble society of Verona. His brilliant comedic monologue on Queen MAB (1.4.53–95) builds to a chaotic crescendo that suggests the violence that is lurking just beneath the surface of Veronese life. He is one of Shakespeare's bawdiest characters; in a mock incantation in 2.1, in which he lists the anatomical parts of Romeo's supposed beloved, ROSALINE (2), he deflates the rhetoric of romance. His unabashedly carnal approach to love contrasts with the pure devotion that Romeo learns, and his hostility is compared with Romeo's intention to make peace with Tybalt after his marriage to JULIET (1).

Mercutio ultimately belongs to the conventional world that opposes the young lovers. He blindly fulfils his role in that world by pointlessly insisting on fighting TYBALT, thereby launching the tragic complications of the play. While we can admire his wit, his loyalty to Romeo, and his courage in death, we also see that Mercutio has little business declaring 'a plague o' both your houses' (3.1.92, 108) when he has himself contributed so dramatically to the final catastrophe.

Meres, Francis (1565–1647) English writer, author of a contemporary assessment of Shakespeare's early career. Meres is considered a pioneer literary critic,

for in his *Palladis Tamia: Wit's Treasury*, an anthology of philosophical and literary maxims, he compares the English writers of his day with classical models. He declares that OVID's soul lives in Shakespeare, citing 'his *Venus and Adonis*, his *Lucrece*, his sugred Sonnets among his private friends'. Thus we know that by 1598, at least some of the SONNETS had been written and circulated in manuscript among Shakespeare's friends. Meres thought Sir Philip SIDNEY was the greatest English poet, but he proclaimed Shakespeare the equal of PLAUTUS in COMEDY and SENECA in TRAGEDY, and 'among the English . . . the most excellent in both kinds for the stage'. Here, he cited six comedies and six tragedies: 'his *Gentlemen of Verona*, his *Errors*, his *Loue labours lost*, his *Loue labours wonne*, his *Midsummers night dreame*, & his *Merchant of Venice* . . . his *Richard the 2, Richard the 3, Henry the 4, King John, Titus Andronicus* and his *Romeo* and *Juliet*'. This list names all of Shakespeare's plays that other evidence indicates had been written by this time, except the *Henry VI* plays and *The Taming of the Shrew* (though the latter may be the mysterious *LOVE'S LABOUR'S WON*). Meres' remarks have helped scholars date the early works and offer evidence of the great respect commanded by Shakespeare among his contemporaries, even early in his career. Meres had only a brief career in LONDON as a writer—he also wrote devotional works—before he became a rural minister and schoolmaster.

Mermaid Tavern Tavern in LONDON, meeting place of a literary club thought to have included Shakespeare. The Friday Street Club, named for the Mermaid's address, was a famous convivial gathering of London writers. Among its members were Francis BEAUMONT (2), John FLETCHER (2), and Ben JONSON. Shakespeare is traditionally counted a member as well, but this is not confirmed in any surviving contemporary accounts, and the club's great days came after the playwright had probably retired to STRATFORD. However, the idea is supported by Shakespeare's close connections with Jonson and Fletcher and his acquaintance at least with the innkeeper at the Mermaid, William JOHNSON (8).

Merry Devil of Edmonton, The Anonymous play formerly attributed to Shakespeare, part of the Shakespeare APOCRYPHA. *The Merry Devil of Edmonton* is a comedy about lovers who elope to escape the bride's parents' plans for a mercenary marriage. It was published in six 17th-century editions, beginning with that of Arthur JOHNSON (1) (1608). It was also popular on the stage, as is shown by many contemporary references to performances. It was first ascribed to Shakespeare by Francis KIRKMAN in 1661, but almost no later scholars have accepted this suggestion. Though *The Merry Devil* is one of the few apocryphal plays that commentators agree is an excellent drama, modern scholars are confident that it is not by Shakespeare. It is not like his work stylistically, and it was never associated with the playwright when it was new, despite the well-established commercial value of his name. Some scholars speculate that it was written by Michael DRAYTON or Thomas HEYWOOD (2), but its authorship remains uncertain.

The Merry Wives of Windsor

SYNOPSIS

Act 1, Scene 1

SHALLOW, in Windsor to sue FALSTAFF, confers with his young relative SLENDER and the local parson, the Welshman EVANS (3). Shallow boasts that his noble ancestry is equal to Falstaff's, and Evans offers to arbitrate the quarrel. Slender mentions his inclination to marry, and Evans suggests ANNE (3) Page, an attractive young woman who has just inherited some money. Shallow suggests that they call on her father, George PAGE (12), whom, Evans says, Falstaff is also visiting. They knock on Page's door and speak with him briefly; Falstaff emerges with BARDOLPH (1), NYM, and PISTOL. Shallow accuses Falstaff of assaulting his men, poaching deer, and breaking into his hunting lodge. Falstaff grandly admits to these deeds and asserts that if Shallow takes the case to the king's council, he will be laughed at. Slender adds that Falstaff's companions have robbed him. They deny it. Evans insists that he, Page, and the HOST (2) of the local tavern shall form a committee to settle these disputes. MISTRESS (3) Page, Anne, and MISTRESS (1) Ford appear with refreshments, and everyone goes indoors except the nervous Slender. Shallow and Evans emerge to say that his marriage to Anne has been proposed. Anne enters to summon the men to dinner, and Shallow and Evans leave her with Slender. Slender is too embarrassed to go in with her, and he makes awkward conversation until Page comes out and insists.

Act 1, Scene 2

Evans sends Slender's servant, SIMPLE, to the house of Dr CAIUS (2) with a letter for his housekeeper, Mistress QUICKLY, asking her to encourage Anne Page to marry Slender.

Act 1, Scene 3

Falstaff persuades the tavern's Host to hire Bardolph as a tapster. He tells Pistol and Nym of his plan to get money: he will seduce both Mistress Ford and Mistress Page. He believes that each woman has found him attractive, and he knows that each controls her family's funds. He has written letters to them, and he asks his followers to deliver them. However, they spurn such a task as unworthy of soldiers, and he dismisses them, giving the letters to his page, ROBIN (1), and then leaving. Pistol and Nym decide to avenge their dismissal by telling FORD (1) and Page of Falstaff's intentions.

Act 1, Scene 4
Mistress Quickly tells Simple that she will assist Slender's courtship. At Dr Caius' approach, Quickly puts Simple in the closet. Caius finds him, and when he tells of his errand, the doctor rages against Evans for sending him, for he—Caius—intends to marry Anne Page himself. Caius writes a letter challenging Evans to a duel and sends Simple back with it. Caius leaves, and FENTON (1) appears. Quickly assures him that his courtship of Anne is going well. Pleased, he gives her money and asks for her continuing assistance.

Act 2, Scene 1
Mistress Page reads Falstaff's love letter. She feels insulted, as does Mistress Ford, who appears with a similar letter. The two women plot revenge: they will tempt Falstaff to spend his money courting them—to no avail—until he is bankrupt. Mistress Ford is particularly irritated with Falstaff because of her husband's quick jealousy. The two women withdraw to discuss their plot, and their husbands appear, accompanied by Pistol and Nym. Pistol and Nym tell the husbands that Falstaff is pursuing their wives, and they leave. The wives reappear as Mistress Quickly arrives, and they decide to employ her as their messenger to Falstaff; the three women leave together. Page and Ford talk; Page doesn't believe the stories of Pistol and Nym, but Ford is worried. The Host and Shallow enter on their way to oversee the duel between Caius and Evans. Shallow tells Page of a plan to interfere with the duel. Ford bribes the Host to introduce him to Falstaff as 'BROOK' (1). He says to himself that he will see what he can find out about Falstaff and his wife.

Act 2, Scene 2
Quickly delivers messages from the wives to Falstaff. Mistress Page writes of her desire for a meeting, but Mistress Ford makes an appointment for that morning. Quickly leaves, and Ford, disguised as 'Brook', arrives. 'Brook' gives Falstaff a gift of money and confesses that he has fallen in love with Ford's wife but that her marital fidelity puts him off. He therefore asks Falstaff to seduce her so that he—'Brook'—may catch her in adultery and thus justify his own advances. Falstaff accepts the bargain; he tells 'Brook' of his appointment with Mistress Ford for that very morning, and he leaves. Ford soliloquises jealously and vows revenge.

Act 2, Scene 3
Dr Caius awaits the arrival of Evans to start the duel. Instead, the Host, Shallow, Slender, and Page appear. All but Slender (who can only moon over Anne Page) talk with the doctor, complimenting him on his valour, while pointing out the good fortune that has kept him from having to kill Evans. The Host tells Shallow and Page to find Evans, who has been sent elsewhere to duel, and they will meet later. He then tells Caius that he will take him to visit Anne Page.

Act 3, Scene 1
Evans awaits the arrival of Dr Caius to start the duel. Page, Shallow, and Slender arrive, and Evans heaps insults on Dr Caius. The Host appears with Caius. The two would-be duellists argue over where they were to meet, and the Host reveals that he has misled them; he proposes that they be friends again. Evans suggests to Caius that they unite in seeking vengeance on the Host, who has made fools of them both. Caius agrees, and they become allies.

Act 3, Scene 2
Ford encounters Mistress Page, accompanied by Robin, who is on loan from Falstaff. He believes that the situation confirms the infidelity of both women. He proposes to himself to unmask Falstaff, disillusion Page, and punish his wife all at once. The group returning from the averted duel appears, and Ford invites them to his house, although Shallow and Slender go to call on Anne Page. Page remarks that he favours Slender as a son-in-law, while his wife prefers Caius. He rejects Fenton as a suitor, observing that the young aristocrat—too high-ranking to marry Anne—is probably a fortune-hunter, being poor despite his rank, and is notably dissolute, having been friends with PRINCE (6) HAL and POINS (of *1* and *2 Henry IV*).

Act 3, Scene 3
The wives lay their plan: they instruct two SERVANTS (10) to be ready to carry away a big basket of laundry and dump it in the river. Falstaff arrives and woos Mistress Ford; Mistress Page appears, and Falstaff hides behind the curtains. Mistress Page announces that an angry Ford is approaching, seeking his wife's lover. Falstaff leaps from his hiding place into the laundry basket, which the two Servants carry out as Ford enters. Ford searches the house, watched by Page, Evans, and Caius, who assert that he is foolish. Left together, the two wives exult over Falstaff's discomfiture and decide to try it again the next morning. Unable to find any lover in the house, Ford admits his error. Page invites the men to go hawking the next morning. Evans and Caius confer about their revenge on the Host.

Act 3, Scene 4
Anne asks Fenton to continue to try to befriend her father before they think of elopement. Quickly arrives with Shallow and Slender. Slender is bashful, but Shallow leaves him to talk with Anne. Anne asks him frankly what his intentions are, and he replies that he himself has none but that others say he should marry her. Anne's parents arrive and announce their approval of Slender's suit and disparage Fenton's presence. Page and Slender leave. Fenton appeals to Mis-

tress Page to support his loving courtship, and Anne states her dislike of both Slender and Caius. Mistress Page relents to the point of promising to consult with Anne, and the two women leave. Quickly takes credit for softening Mistress Page, and Fenton gives her some money. She soliloquises that, having promised to help all three suitors, she will do so, but she favours Fenton.

Act 3, Scene 5
Falstaff laments having been dumped in the river. Quickly brings him an apologetic message from Mistress Ford, who extends another invitation for that morning, while her husband is hawking. Ford arrives, again disguised as 'Brook'. Falstaff tells of his escape in the laundry and of his new opportunity. He leaves, and Ford rages angrily that this time he will catch Falstaff in his house.

Act 4, Scene 1
Evans drills young WILLIAM (1) Page in his Latin grammar, and Quickly listens with comical misunderstanding.

Act 4, Scene 2:
Falstaff calls on Mistress Ford, and once again Mistress Page arrives, sending him into hiding. Again, she tells of Ford's angry approach. The wives disguise Falstaff as the old woman of Brainford, a reputed witch whom Ford particularly despises. Ford arrives with a group of witnesses and ransacks the laundry in search of Falstaff; then in his fury he drives the 'old woman' from the house, beating 'her' mercilessly. He begins to search the house once more, and in his absence the wives decide to tell their husbands of their campaign against Falstaff so that all four may participate in another round of imposture.

Act 4, Scene 3
Bardolph informs the Host that the agents of a German count, soon to arrive at the king's court, wish to hire horses. The Host agrees to let them use his, proposing to overcharge them.

Act 4, Scene 4
The Pages and Fords, with Evans, concoct a plot against Falstaff. They will arrange to have the fat knight meet the women at an ancient sacred oak in the woods at midnight, disguised as a mythological creature, Herne the Hunter, who wears stag's antlers. When he arrives at the rendezvous, he will be accosted by a group of CHILDREN disguised as fairies and elves, led by Anne. They will pinch him and ridicule him until he admits his shabby dealings. Then all the hidden adults will emerge to mock him. As they lay their plans, Ford muses to himself that he may take advantage of the occasion to spirit Anne away with Slender and have them married. Mistress Ford plots similarly with Dr Caius in mind.

Act 4, Scene 5
Simple has followed the old woman of Brainford to Falstaff's rooms to ask her questions of behalf of his master. Falstaff says that he has spoken with the witch, and he gives Simple trick answers when he asks about Slender's chances of winning Anne Page. Bardolph reports to the Host that the Germans have made off with the horses; Evans and then Caius arrive with warnings that the Germans are not to be trusted. Realising that he has been robbed, the Host rages and rushes off. Quickly appears with a message to Falstaff from the two wives, and he takes her to his chamber to hear their proposition in detail.

Act 4, Scene 6
Fenton bribes the Host to help him. Anne has learned of her parents' respective schemes, and the two lovers have hatched a counterplot. The Host agrees to arrange for a minister to marry the couple that night.

Act 5, Scene 1
Falstaff sends Quickly to prepare for his masquerade that night, just as Ford arrives, disguised as 'Brook'. Falstaff assures him that tonight all they had planned will be accomplished.

Act 5, Scene 2
Page, Shallow, and Slender lie in wait, planning for Slender's elopement with Anne.

Act 5, Scene 3
The wives, with Caius, lie in wait, planning for the doctor's elopement with Anne.

Act 5, Scene 4
Evans and the Children lie in wait, planning to accost Falstaff.

Act 5, Scene 5
Falstaff, disguised as Herne, arrives at the rendezvous and compares himself with Jupiter, who took the forms of animals for sexual purposes. The wives appear; Falstaff is jubilant, thinking that his liaison is finally to occur, but the women hear a noise and flee. Evans and the Children, with Pistol and Quickly, all disguised as fairies and elves, come out and conduct a ceremony. They then torment Falstaff, burning him with their candles and pinching him. Slender and Caius arrive, and each steals away with a different fairy; Fenton takes Anne. Page, Ford, and the wives come forward and reveal their hoax to Falstaff, who is mortified. Slender returns to complain that his intended bride has proved to be a boy; Caius appears with the same story. Fenton and Anne return and explain that they have married. The Pages make the best of it and accept Fenton as their son-in-law. In a con-

ciliatory spirit of fellowship, Falstaff is invited to join the others in a festive celebration at the Ford household.

COMMENTARY

The Merry Wives of Windsor was probably written for a ceremonial occasion (see 'Text of the Play'), and it is clearly intended primarily as an entertainment. Unlike such earlier comedies as *The Comedy of Errors* and *The Two Gentlemen of Verona, The Merry Wives* is not coloured by any possibility of serious unhappiness that must be forestalled. In this respect, it is the shallowest COMEDY of Shakespeare's plays, and it is therefore sometimes thought of as an unimportant diversion in Shakespeare's development, an essentially trivial work that does not warrant attention. However, the play's success on the stage—historical and current—has affirmed its value, and modern commentators have increasingly found it to be a particularly interesting work.

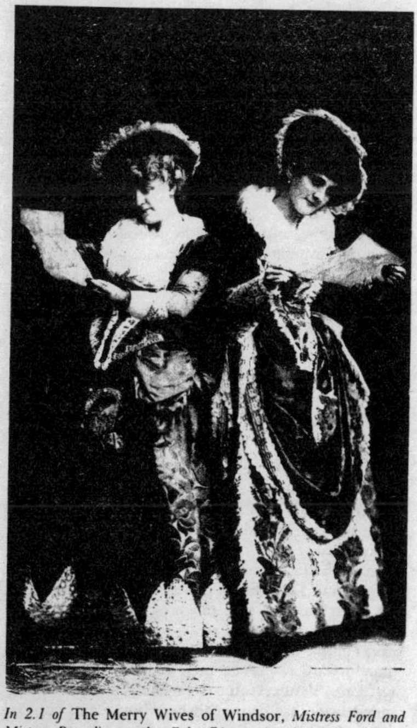

In 2.1 of The Merry Wives of Windsor, *Mistress Ford and Mistress Page discover that Falstaff is courting them both with love letters. They plot their revenge. In this 19th-century production Ada Rehan (left) stars as Mistress Ford.* (Courtesy of Culver Pictures, Inc.)

The Merry Wives is a variation on a medieval moral tale, and thus it draws on the theatrical traditions of Shakespeare's day. But Shakespeare added contemporary elements; it is the only one of his works to focus exclusively on English life in his own time. Moreover, in *The Merry Wives* the playwright gave the initiative in the play's plot to the wives, rather than to male characters, as was normal in earlier comedies, including his own. This points intriguingly to the prominence of heroines in his later comedies.

As a moral tale *The Merry Wives* recounts the triumph of domestic values over the threat of corruption brought in by an outsider, Falstaff, whose amoral selfishness is contrasted with the communal solidarity of the townspeople and whose status as a courtier makes him a social alien. In an ancient tradition, known in Shakespeare's day through both Roman drama and the medieval MORALITY PLAY, satirical comedy exposed human foibles by making fun of them. The happy resolution that defines the genre usually consisted in precisely the sort of humiliation and forgiveness that befall Falstaff in the play. Thus Shakespeare applied a familiar formula, immediately understood by his audience and so self-evident in its intentions that subsequent readers and theatre-goers have responded just as instinctively.

The play also offers another sort of tale, a standard plot in Elizabethan Comedy: the triumph of young lovers—Anne Page and Fenton—over the machinations of the girl's parents and her mercenary suitors. The final comic resolution of this story buttresses that of the Falstaff plot. Moreover, the double dénouement is both forecast and supported by the sub-plot of the enmity and reconciliation of Caius and Evans, whose proposed duel is defused by the collective efforts of various townspeople. Thus the play's theme—the power of good over evil—is developed in several mutually reinforcing ways.

The contemporaneity of *The Merry Wives* is one of its strikingly novel features. In this work, as in the *Henry IV* plays, written at almost exactly the same time, Shakespeare dramatises his own world with unprecedented theatrical realism. He doubtless created the BOAR'S HEAD TAVERN in *1 Henry IV* to strengthen that play's historical themes by associating them with a more mundane aspect of English society. In *The Merry Wives,* which is concerned solely with entertainment, historical markers are almost nonexistent (although a few references are made—e.g., in 3.2.66–67—to the world of Henry IV), and the entire play is a detailed slice of Elizabethan rural life. The characters enjoy such country entertainments as greyhound racing (1.1.81–89) and hunting with small hawks (3.3.214–

215); they are familiar with stiles (3.1.32), goose-pens (3.4.40), bilberries (5.5.46), and the ways of the cuckoo (2.1.121). The specific geographical references—FROGMORE (2.3.81), Eton (4.5.63), Datchet Mead (3.3.12), Herne's oak in Windsor Forest (4.4.53)—lend great realism to the play's setting.

More sophisticated tastes are also provided for in the literary humour of William's Latin lesson (4.1) and in the inside jokes about the Count of MOMPELGARD in 4.3 and 4.5, accessible only to the highest ranks of courtly society. Also, several minor jests involve quotations from the works of SIDNEY and MARLOWE (1), requiring an educated familiarity with contemporary literature, although Shakespeare's audience will have recognised these references much more readily than modern readers can.

Despite its innovativeness, the play was also conspicuously part of the contemporary vogue for the COMEDY OF HUMOURS, in which social types are represented by boldly identifiable characters, each sporting a notable eccentricity of speech or behaviour. Most of the secondary figures in *The Merry Wives* exhibit such traits: Evans and Caius each speak with a comic foreign dialect—Welsh and French respectively. Pistol is an archetypal swaggerer, Slender a foolish bumpkin, the Host a jovial gladhander. Ford, though more humanly complex, belongs to a very ancient tradition, that of the unreasonably jealous husband. Even Falstaff takes on the role of a character type, the unsuccessful lecher, although his motive in approaching the wives is actually mercenary.

The play's many comic characters are ranged around Falstaff, who, although he is a less masterful figure than in the *Henry IV* plays, is nonetheless as brassy, zestful, and humorously rhetorical as ever, brandishing language like a torch to baffle and confuse his intended victims. The difference is that in *The Merry Wives* he does not succeed, even temporarily. He is a comic butt, destined from the outset to be defeated by the forthright and faithful wives. That the resourceful rogue of *1 Henry IV* should be so easily bested, not just once but three times, has been regretted by some, who see in Falstaff's downfall the trivialisation of a great comic figure. However, in *The Merry Wives* Falstaff's function is different. He is not placed in contrast with a historical plot involving politics and war, a circumstance that gives his wit extraordinary resonance in the *Henry IV* plays; here, he has an almost abstract, allegorical role, as the spirit of malevolence that, while comic and releasing, must be roundly crushed. The Falstaff of *The Merry Wives* has been seen as similar to the scapegoat, a sacrificial animal of pre-Christian religious traditions, who is figuratively laden with the misdeeds of the people and then released into the wilderness or killed, taking with it the sins of the community. Certainly 5.5 is suggestive of such rites, which were still remembered and understood in Shakespeare's day, having disappeared only recently—they may, in fact, have still been alive in the remotest parts of Britain. In any case, at the close of the play, Falstaff's humiliation is mitigated by the fact that Page and his wife have also been foiled in their plans for Anne, and the fat villain is included in the final forgiveness and good cheer that embody the spirit of Shakespearean comedy.

The Merry Wives anticipates Shakespeare's later work in its emphasis on women. While the wives, comfortably settled in middle-aged domesticity, are not much like the bold and venturesome heroines that the playwright was soon to create—BEATRICE (*Much Ado About Nothing*), ROSALIND (*As You Like It*), VIOLA (*Twelfth Night*), and HELENA (*All's Well That Ends Well*)—they nonetheless prefigure them. They are clearly the most sensible and competent people in Shakespeare's Windsor. They know who they are, and they firmly assert themselves; we are left in no doubt that they are 'merry, and yet honest too', as Mistress Page says (4.2.96). Falstaff's greed is the first stimulus to the plot, but the wives are his target precisely because they are the important figures in their households, and the initiative in the plot's development lies squarely with them. They repeatedly lead Falstaff on—and thus, indirectly, Ford—although the men think they are imposing their wills on the world. The wives' vigour is evident not only in the execution of their plans but in their language: for instance, Mistress Page passes boldly from technological to classical to sexual imagery in condemning Falstaff's use of identical love letters (2.1.71–78), closing with the ornithological: 'I will find you twenty lascivious turtles [turtledoves] ere one chaste man'. (2.1.78). The merry wives are the defenders of domesticity against promiscuity—of order against misrule, that is—and their symbolic importance clearly indicates, for the first time in the plays, the high value Shakespeare placed on female influence in human affairs, a position that he would reassert, perhaps more strikingly, in later works.

The Merry Wives of Windsor is not one of Shakespeare's greatest plays; it lacks stirring poetry and monumental characters, and its concerns are not so sophisticated as the political philosophy and psychological exploration of some of the more important works. However, it is a bold reminder of the popular morality theatre of medieval England, and it also presents a delightfully picturesque view of 16th-century rural life. An expertly plotted farce that ranges from gentle charm to high hilarity, it deploys a dozen splendid comic characters in a world of solid virtue that is exemplified by its commendable though understated heroines. As such, the play has been appreciated by generations of theatre-goers, and increasing attention from scholars and critics will reinforce its continuing popularity.

SOURCES OF THE PLAY

A number of loose ends in *The Merry Wives of Windsor*—especially Shallow's threatened and then forgotten lawsuit—have suggested to some scholars that the play is based on another one, now lost. This would have been a logical tactic for Shakespeare to use, if it is true that the play was written in two weeks at the Queen's command (see 'Text of the Play'). However, no evidence exists to link *The Merry Wives* to any earlier play, and the inconsistencies within the play may simply be evidence of hasty composition, whether in response to a royal command or not. In any case, nothing in *The Merry Wives* seems beyond the invention of a well-read and creative mind. Its incidents and characters resemble material that had long been current in European literature and folklore. Jealous husbands and lovers who triumph over adversarial parents are staples of Western storytelling, and Shakespeare could simply have thought of stories he had heard or read without referring to particular works. Also, the contemporary vogue for the comedy of humours must have influenced *The Merry Wives*, which, while transcending the genre, certainly incorporates features from it.

Nevertheless, several likely literary sources may be mentioned. A number of details of Falstaff's escapes from the jealous Ford may have been anticipated in a story from Giovanni FIORENTINO's collection *Il Pecorone (The Simpleton)*, published in Milan (1558) and a source for *The Merchant of Venice*. A comical English prose work, Robert Copland's *Gyl of Braintfords Testament* (1560) may have suggested Falstaff's disguise as the old woman of Brainford, and his departure in the laundry basket may derive from a story by Barnabe RICH (1) in his *Farewell to Militarie Profession* (1581). The personality of the Host was probably influenced by Geoffrey CHAUCER's famous innkeeper in *The Canterbury Tales*, and George CHAPMAN's *The Blind Beggar of Alexandria* (1596), a highly successful comedy of humours, contained a character whose comical overuse of the word 'humour' clearly contributed to the creation of Shakespeare's Nym. The famous 'Latin' scene, 4.1, is representative of a set piece in several contemporary French farces, which Shakespeare would have known of and may have read. Lastly, Falstaff's torment at the hands of fairy-impersonators was perhaps based on a scene in John LYLY's play *Endimion* (1588), in which a lecher is punished for his lust by fairies.

TEXT OF THE PLAY

Although absolute proof is lacking, scholars, led by Dr Leslie HOTSON, have convincingly established that *The Merry Wives* was commissioned for a particular occasion, a feast hosted by the Queen on April 23, 1597, in honour of newly elected members of the knightly Order of the Garter. In 5.5.56–75 Quickly, in the guise of the Queen of Fairies, issues instructions to prepare Windsor Castle for the Knights of the Garter. Apparent references to the German Count of MÖMPELGARD also reflect this occasion, as does the setting of the play in Windsor, rather than in Shakespeare's native WARWICKSHIRE or some other rural location. Among the noblemen joining the Order of the Garter on this occasion was George CAREY (1), Lord Hunsdon—patron of Shakespeare's company, HUNSDON'S MEN—who had just become Elizabeth's Lord Chamberlain (the company was called the CHAMBERLAIN'S MEN from then on), and he probably commissioned the play. These circumstances appear to confirm a longstanding tradition that *The Merry Wives* was written in 14 days to fulfil a desire expressed by Queen ELIZABETH (1) to see Falstaff in love. This notion does not appear in print until 1702, but it fits well with the evident purpose of the play's composition: if a play were offered to the Queen, it is quite possible that she would specify a choice of subject. It is known that Hunsdon's Men had performed at court several times in the winter of 1596–1597, and it is likely that they presented their most recent popular success, *1 Henry IV*, in which Elizabeth would have become acquainted with Falstaff.

The play is therefore dated to early 1597. A change in the apparent home of Justice Shallow in *2 Henry IV* (see GLOUCESTERSHIRE) suggests that the composition of that play was interrupted by the writing of *The Merry Wives*, in which Shallow explicitly comes from Gloucestershire (1.1.5). *Henry IV, Part 2*, was probably begun in early 1597, thus pushing the creation of *The Merry Wives* a little closer to the beginning of rehearsals for its April presentation; this allows very little time for the job, perhaps only 14 days, although this cannot be known precisely, of course.

The play was first published in 1602 in a BAD QUARTO edition by Arthur JOHNSON (1), who bought the rights to it from John BUSBY. This edition, known as Q1, was printed by Thomas CREEDE. It was reprinted with minor alterations in 1619 by William JAGGARD, for the FALSE FOLIO of publisher Thomas PAVIER. This edition is known as Q2. The 1623 FIRST FOLIO version of *The Merry Wives* is a greatly superior text. It includes five scenes omitted in the Quartos, and it provides more comprehensible, smoother readings throughout. Scholars believe that the Folio was printed from a transcript of Shakespeare's manuscript, perhaps in a version reflecting a court performance of 1604 (see BROOK [1]); certain idiosyncracies in the text point to the hand of Ralph CRANE, a professional scribe whose work is well known. Q1 represents an already abridged version of the play, one intended for the public theatre rather than for the play's original aristocratic audience at the Queen's banquet. It omits the scenes dealing with the Order of the Garter, along with the 'Latin' scene, presumably thought inap-

propriate for the relatively uneducated public. The Folio was immediately recognised as the superior text, and subsequent editions have been largely based on it, with occasional alterations deriving from Q1.

THEATRICAL HISTORY OF THE PLAY

The Merry Wives was enthusiastically received by its original audience. The subtitle of the 1602 edition of the play asserts that it had been performed 'divers times' both before the Queen and elsewhere, and it specifically mentions Falstaff, Evans, Shallow, Slender, Pistol, and Nym, attesting to the fame of these figures. The earliest specific performance of which a record survives was held at the court of King JAMES I in 1604. An ambiguous record of 1613 may or may not refer to *The Merry Wives,* but the play was certainly played at the court of Charles I in 1638, testifying to its ongoing popularity. After the theatres were reopened following their 20-year closure by the Puritan revolution, *The Merry Wives* was one of the first plays to be staged. Samuel PEPYS saw it in 1660, 1661, and 1667. The programme of an unsuccessful adaptation of 1702, *The Comical Gallant* by John DENNIS (2), implies that *The Merry Wives* had been produced several times in the intervening years, though no late 17th-century performances are recorded. In 1704 Shakespeare's text was staged by Thomas BETTERTON, who played Falstaff, and James QUIN duplicated the project a year later. Since the 1720s the play has been extremely popular both in Britain and America, and many major Shakespearean actors of the 18th and 19th centuries played Falstaff, Ford, or both.

The Merry Wives has remained a favourite in the 20th century; the many productions of the play have included those of Oscar ASCHE and Theodore KOMISARJEVSKY. It was twice a silent FILM (1910, 1917), but has not been a movie since. It has been made for TELEVISION four times, including the 1955 production of Glen Byam SHAW (3), starring Anthony QUAYLE. A number of operas have been based on the play, beginning in 1824, when Fredric REYNOLDS (1) produced an opera with music by Henry BISHOP (2). Among others have been such well-known works as Ralph VAUGHAN WILLIAMS' *Sir John in Love* (1929), and, by general consent the greatest of them, Giuseppe VERDI's *Falstaff* (1893). Another musical work inspired in part by *The Merry Wives* is the English composer Edward Elgar's symphonic study *Falstaff* (1913).

Messala, Marcus Valerius (64 B.C.–8 A.D.) Historical figure and minor character in *Julius Caesar,* a general under BRUTUS (4) and CASSIUS. In 4.3 Messala brings Brutus news of the death of PORTIA (2) and witnesses Brutus' feigned stoicism, to which he responds with admiration, saying 'Even so great men great losses should endure' (4.3.192). Messala appears frequently at the battle of PHILIPPI in Act 5, but his only important moment comes when he discovers the corpse of Cassius in 5.3. In 5.5 he has been captured by OCTAVIUS and ANTONY.

The historical Messala, better known as Messala Corvinus Valerius, was offered the command of Brutus' army as it crumbled at Philippi, but he joined Octavius and Antony instead. Ten years later he fought for Octavius against Antony at ACTIUM (though he does not appear in *Antony and Cleopatra,* where that battle is enacted). Under Augustus CAESAR (2), as Octavius became known, Messala held various offices, was a patron of a group of pastoral poets, and wrote books on history and literature; his work—famous in its day—was a source for Shakespeare's source, PLUTARCH, though none of it has survived.

Messenger (1) Minor character in *The Comedy of Errors.* In 5.1.168–184 he brings ADRIANA a frantic account of the escape of ANTIPHOLUS OF EPHESUS from the custody of PINCH and comically describes Antipholus' revenge on that pseudo-physician. He is identified as a Servant.

Messenger (2) Minor character in *Titus Andronicus.* The Messenger brings TITUS (1) a grisly package—the severed heads of his two sons and the general's own severed hand—that AARON has sent in mockery. The Messenger is sympathetic, remarking on the injustice with a personal note that is rare in this play.

Messenger (3) Any of several minor characters in *1 Henry VI,* mostly soldiers who deliver accounts of battle situations. In the opening scenes, the repeated interruptions of HENRY V's funeral by Messengers bearing tidings of English defeats establish the theme of loss and disruption. In 4.3 a Messenger announces to the Duke of YORK (8) the commencement of the battle that will prove fatal to TALBOT. In 2.2 a French Messenger brings Talbot the deceitful invitation from the Countess of AUVERGNE.

Messenger (4) Any of several minor characters in *2 Henry VI,* whose announcements spark action by greater figures or provide news of events off-stage. In 1.2 a Messenger summons the Duke of GLOUCESTER (4) to a royal hawking party, leaving his wife the DUCHESS (1) alone to pursue the plot that will eventually bring them both down. In 4.4 a Messenger informs the king of the progress of Jack CADE's rebellion, and in 4.7 another man announces to Cade the capture of an important nobleman, Lord SAY. Lastly, in 4.9, a Messenger brings the king the momentous news that the Duke of YORK (8) has returned from his duty in Ireland at the head of an army, an event that heralds the coming civil war.

Messenger (5) Any of several minor characters in *3 Henry VI,* soldiers bringing military reports. The Messengers simply report troop movements, except for the first of two in 2.1, who brings a detailed account of the death of the Duke of YORK (8).

In the FIRST FOLIO text of the play, believed to have been printed from Shakespeare's manuscript, the Messenger is referred to in the stage direction at 1.2.47 as 'Gabriel'. This apparently refers to the actor Gabriel SPENCER, who presumably played the part in the original production.

Messenger (6) Any of several minor characters in *Richard III,* bearers of news. In 2.4 a Messenger brings word to Queen ELIZABETH (2) that her son and brother have been imprisoned, and in 3.2 a Messenger delivers to HASTINGS (3) an account of an ominous dream from STANLEY (3). In a highly dramatic use of messengers, Shakespeare brings four on stage successively in 4.4, within a few lines, to demonstrate Richard's lack of control as news floods in of rebellion against him. In 5.3 one last Messenger brings Richard word of Stanley's desertion at BOSWORTH FIELD.

Messenger (7) Minor character in *The Taming of the Shrew,* the announcer, in the INDUCTION, of the performance by the PLAYERS (1) that begins the play proper. In Ind.2 he informs SLY (1) of the coming presentation and recommends viewing it as a healthy pastime. Various editions of the play have assigned his part to the LORD (1) or a SERVANT (5).

Messenger (8) Minor character in *King John.* In 4.2 the Messenger brings King JOHN (3) news of both the French invasion and the death of John's mother, Queen ELEANOR, and in 5.3 he reappears with a message from the BASTARD (1), urging the king to remove himself from battle. Thus this underling marks the beginning and end of John's collapse.

Messenger (9) Minor character in *King John.* In 5.5 the Messenger brings LEWIS (1) three pieces of bad news: the death of Lord MELUN, the desertion from the French forces of the English barons who had been in revolt against King JOHN (3), and the loss of French ships at sea. These tidings collectively spell doom for the French invasion of England.

Messenger (10) Minor character in *The Merchant of Venice,* servant of PORTIA (1). In 2.9 the Messenger tells Portia that BASSANIO is approaching.

Messenger (11) Any of several minor characters in *1 Henry IV* who bring messages to HOTSPUR. A Messenger informs Hotspur of his father's illness on the eve of the battle of SHREWSBURY in 4.1. Two more Messengers appear in 5.2, just before the battle, in an episode that heightens the excitement of the occasion. One brings letters that Hotspur, in his agitation, refuses to read, and the second brings word that King HENRY IV's army is approaching.

Messenger (12) Minor character in *2 Henry IV,* a soldier. In 4.1 the Messenger brings the rebel leaders a report that the army of Prince John of LANCASTER (3) is approaching.

Messenger (13) Any of several minor characters in *Henry V,* servants in the court of the FRENCH KING. In 2.4 a Messenger announces the arrival of an English ambassador. In 3.7 and 4.2 Messengers, perhaps soldiers, bring word of English troop dispositions prior to the battle of AGINCOURT.

Messenger (14) Minor character in *Much Ado About Nothing,* a servant of Don PEDRO. In 1.1 the Messenger tells Leonato of Don Pedro's successes in war, citing the noble deeds of CLAUDIO (1) and BENEDICK and thus providing expository material on the play's romantic leads. The mention of Benedick subjects the Messenger to BEATRICE's sharp verbal sallies; the passage (1.1.28–83) presents one of the play's major motifs, the witty—though prickly—independence of its heroine. In 3.5.50–51 and 5.4.123–124 the Messenger presents brief reports of off-stage action.

Messenger (15) Minor character in *Julius Caesar,* a soldier in the army of OCTAVIUS and ANTONY. In 5.1 the Messenger announces the approach of the army of BRUTUS (4) and CASSIUS just before the battle of PHILIPPI.

Messenger (16) Minor character in *Hamlet.* The Messenger brings the KING (5) of DENMARK news that LAERTES has raised a rebellion and is approaching. His hysteria emphasises the degree of disruption that the play's developments have produced. In a calmer mood the Messenger brings the King letters from HAMLET in 4.7.

Messenger (17) Minor character in *All's Well That Ends Well,* a servant of BERTRAM. In 4.3 the Messenger tells two gentlemen (see LORD [6]) that his master will soon be returning to FRANCE (1). His single brief speech separates two elements of a long scene: the Lords' critique of Bertram's morality and Bertram's arrival for the interrogation of PAROLLES.

Messenger (18) Minor character in *Measure for Measure,* servant of ANGELO (2). In 4.2 the Messenger delivers to the PROVOST Angelo's command for the execution of CLAUDIO (3), though a pardon has been expected. Angelo's employment of the Messenger

makes his deed seem even more monstrous as he distances himself from it.

Messenger (19) Minor character in *Othello*, bearer of a dispatch from MONTANO (2) to the DUKE (5) of VENICE. In 1.3 the Messenger delivers news of the Turkish attack on CYPRUS that OTHELLO will be sent to oppose. His brief part increases the urgency of the scene.

Messenger (20) Minor character in *King Lear*, a servant of REGAN. In 4.2 the Messenger interrupts a dispute between GONERIL and ALBANY with the news that GLOUCESTER (1) has been blinded and CORNWALL is dead. Goneril immediately withdraws to plan her selfish response to the latter event, in contrast to her husband's shocked dismay over the former. The Messenger then adds that Gloucester had been betrayed by his son EDMUND. The episode stresses the evil that Albany realises he must oppose as the play approaches its climax.

Messenger (21) Minor character in *King Lear*, a follower of CORDELIA. In 4.4 the Messenger brings his mistress the news that the armies of GONERIL and REGAN are approaching. His brief announcement immediately throws the newly arrived Cordelia into the fury of battle, and thereby increases the play's pace as it reaches its climax.

Messenger (22) Minor character in *Macbeth*, a servant of MACBETH. In 1.5 the Messenger brings LADY (6) MACBETH the news that King DUNCAN, whose murder she has just been contemplating, approaches. Her startled response to this sudden opportunity for the crime serves to escalate the plot's tension. In 4.2 the Messenger (or, possibly, another one) betrays his master when he warns LADY (7) Macduff that Macbeth's hired killers approach (see FIRST MURDERER [3]). He is bravely willing to stand up against Macbeth's villainy and his action provides a moment of relief from the growing evil of the plot. In 5.5 the Messenger, still employed by Macbeth (unless, again, he is a different person), brings his master word that the forest appears to be moving. This message signals Macbeth's downfall, and his wrathful response emphasises his desperate position. Though they seem unimportant, all three of the Messenger's appearances mark a change in the play's emotional tone, a striking Shakespearean technique.

Messenger (23) Any of three minor characters in *Antony and Cleopatra*, bearers of news to ANTONY. In 1.2 the First Messenger tells that Antony's wife and brother have been defeated by Octavius CAESAR (2) in the Roman civil wars. He also tells of the conquest of Roman territory in Egypt by a renegade Roman general. A Second Messenger announces the arrival of a Third Messenger, who brings word that Antony's wife has died. The rapid sequence of messages establishes the importance of both the political and personal situation in which Antony lives. Although he seems unnecessary, the Second Messenger, who speaks only five words, contributes to the atmosphere of crisis. One of the Messengers (or, perhaps, a fourth) reappears in 3.7 at the battle of ACTIUM with word of Caesar's troop movements.

Messenger (24) Either of two minor characters in *Antony and Cleopatra*, bearers of news to Octavius CAESAR (2). In 1.4 the Messengers appear, one after the other, with news of the success of POMPEY (2) and of his alliance with the pirates MENECRATES and MENAS. One of the Messengers (or, possibly, a third) appears in 4.6 with word of ANTONY's preparations for battle. The Messengers strengthen our sense of Caesar as an informed and decisive leader.

Messenger (25) Minor character in *Antony and Cleopatra*, a servant who brings CLEOPATRA news of ANTONY's marriage to OCTAVIA. In 2.5 Cleopatra's rage is so great when she hears of Antony's action that she beats the Messenger and threatens to kill him. He naturally flees. He is coaxed to return and repeat his message to the unwilling queen, and he flees again when she is again angry. In 3.3 he assures Cleopatra that he has seen Octavia and knows her to be an extremely unattractive woman whose defects he details. For this tactful report, Cleopatra rewards him with gold and agrees that he is a 'proper man' (3.3.37). The episode demonstrates the mercurial nature of the Egyptian queen. The Messenger represents an ancient theatrical stereotype, the comic servant.

Messenger (26) Character in *Antony and Cleopatra*. See ATTENDANT (1).

Messenger (27) Any of several minor characters in *Coriolanus*, bearers of tidings. In 1.1, 1.4, and 1.6, Messengers who are apparently military men (or perhaps the same man each time), bring reports on the advancing VOLSCIANS to CORIOLANUS or COMINIUS. In 2.1, 4.6, and 5.4, other Messengers who are apparently civilians (or, again, perhaps a single person), bring news of events in ROME to the tribunes, BRUTUS (3) and SICINIUS. The Messengers serve to announce plot developments.

Messenger (28) Any of several minor characters in *Timon of Athens*. In 1.1 two Messengers bring TIMON news, first of the imprisonment for debt of VENTIDIUS (2), and later of the approach of ALCIBIADES. In 5.2 a Messenger reports on Alcibiades' march on Athens. These may well be different men—servants of Ventidius, Timon, and an anonymous SENATOR (4), re-

spectively—but they are indistinguishable and serve to inform the audience of off-stage events.

Messenger (29) Minor character in *Pericles,* a servant of King ANTIOCHUS of Syria. In 1.1 the Messenger informs Antiochus that PERICLES—whom the king intends to kill—has fled the country. The Messenger, who speaks only a single line, helps heighten the melodramatic tension of the scene.

Messenger (30) Minor character in *Cymbeline,* a servant of King CYMBELINE. In 2.3 the Messenger announces the arrival of an ambassador, and in 5.4 he summons POSTHUMUS from his pending execution to an audience with the king. The Messenger's function is to advance the plot.

Messenger (31) Minor character in *Henry VIII,* a servant of Queen KATHERINE. In 4.2 the Messenger, announcing the arrival of Lord CAPUCHIUS, addresses the now-deposed queen as if she were a mere duchess. She instantly rebukes him and orders GRIFFITH to see that he is never sent to her again. The episode, which derives from an historical incident, offers a last demonstration of strength in the victimised and dying Katherine.

Messenger (32) Any of three minor characters in *The Two Noble Kinsmen,* bearers of news. In 4.2 a Messenger reports on the arrival of ARCITE and PALAMON for their duel, describing the combatants and their supporters in elaborately courtly terms. In 5.2 another Messenger (probably played by the same actor, however) tells the GAOLER (4), the DOCTOR (4), and the WOOER about the duel in a few brief lines. Scholars generally agree that Shakespeare's collaborator John FLETCHER (2) wrote both 4.2 and 5.2, but that Shakespeare created the Messenger in 5.4, who dramatically races on-stage to halt the execution of Palamon, crying 'Hold, hold, O hold, hold, hold!' (5.4.40), as PIRITHOUS arrives with a pardon. This bold *coup de théâtre* advances the play to its final episode. In some 17th-century productions, the Messenger was probably played by Curtis GREVILLE (1).

Messina City in Sicily, setting for *Much Ado About Nothing* and one scene of *Antony and Cleopatra.* Although there is nothing particularly Sicilian—let alone Messinian—about the events or locations in *Much Ado,* one of Shakespeare's sources for the play, Matteo BANDELLO's novella, is set in Messina, where an Aragonese army (see PEDRO) is celebrating its conquest of Sicily. Sicily was ruled by the kings of Aragon—and later Spain—from 1282 until 1713. Messina was the site of the first Aragonese victory, in 1282, against the French, who ruled the island until then. This doubtless accounts for Bandello's location, which Shakespeare simply adopted.

In 2.1 of *Antony and Cleopatra* POMPEY (2) confers with MENAS and MENECRATES about their war against Octavius CAESAR (2), LEPIDUS, and Mark ANTONY. Shakespeare did not indicate the locale of this conference, but scholars have identified it. Beginning with Edward CAPELL in 1768, editors have generally provided a stage direction that places this scene in Messina. This follows Shakespeare's source, PLUTARCH's *Lives,* which locates Pompey's headquarters there. Sicily was Pompey's principal base for much of his rebellion against Rome, and his occupation of Messina, which commanded the strait between the island and mainland Italy, was strategically important. His final defeat was only possible through Caesar's blockade of Messina in 36 B.C., in a very difficult campaign that is casually referred to in 3.5.4. of the play.

Metellus Cimber (L. Tillius Cimber) (d. c. 44 B.C.) Historical figure and character in *Julius Caesar,* one of the assassins of CAESAR (1). In 3.1, as part of the assassination plot, Metellus requests that Caesar pardon his brother, who has been banished; since Caesar has refused this plea once, the conspirators are confident that he will do so again, and this refusal is to be the signal—and ostensible stimulus—for their attack. Metellus has no distinctive personality; he simply performs his role and then stabs Caesar along with the others.

The historical figure was actually named Lucius Tillius Cimber; the error comes from Shakespeare's source, PLUTARCH's *Lives,* where Cimber is given two different names, both of them wrong. Cimber had been an associate of Caesar's but abandoned him and joined Brutus' conspiracy. He probably died in combat at PHILIPPI; he fought with Brutus' forces, but no further record of him has survived.

Metre Regular rhythmic pattern in poetry. While some poetry lacks metre—it is called free verse—almost all pre-modern poetry, including Shakespeare's, is metrical; the words are arranged in a definite measurable pattern. The term 'metre' derives from the Greek word for 'measure'. Some metres are *syllabic,* measuring simply the number of syllables in a line; some are *accentual,* measuring only the syllables that are stressed or accented when the poetry is read. *Quantitative* metres measure the duration of the sounds as they are spoken; ancient Greek, Latin, and Sanskrit verse usually follow this pattern. Most English poetry, including Shakespeare's, is composed in accentual-syllabic metres; that is, both the stresses and the syllables are counted.

These patterns of stresses and syllables are generally organised into elements known as *feet.* Six types of feet are most common in English poetry, though very

rarely others—usually taken from quantitative systems—are used. The six feet are the *iamb,* consisting of an unstressed syllable followed by a stressed one, as in the word 'delight'; the *anapest,* consisting of two unstressed syllables followed by one stressed one, as in the word 'intervene'; the *trochee,* one stressed syllable followed by an unstressed one, as in 'hotter'; the *dactyl,* one stressed syllable followed by two unstressed ones, as in 'lovingly'; the *spondee,* two stressed syllables, as in 'amen'; and the *pyrrhic,* two unstressed syllables, as in the syllables '-es of', in the line 'I'll gild the faces of the grooms withal' (*Macbeth,* 2.2.55), where all the other feet are iambs. As this last example demonstrates, a foot does not necessarily correspond to a word or phrase; also, the same word or words may comprise a different sort of foot, depending on the feet surrounding it in the line.

Metres are named according to the number of feet in a line, using the Greek prefixes for numbers—*dimeter* for two feet, *trimeter* for three, *tetrameter* for four, *pentameter* for five, *hexameter* for six, and so on—and according to the kind of foot that dominates in the line—iambic, anapestic, trochaic, dactylic, spondaic, or pyrrhic. Variation is necessary; a poem of any length consisting solely of one sort of foot would sound intolerably mechanical. Thus an iambic pentameter line—typical in Shakespeare's poetry (see BLANK VERSE)—does not always consist only of iambs, and all the lines of an iambic pentameter poem or passage need not have five feet. However, throughout a work that is said to be written in iambic pentameter, iambs will dominate and almost all the lines will have five feet.

Michael (1) Minor character in *2 Henry VI,* a follower of the rebel Jack CADE. In 4.2 Michael brings word that Sir Humphrey STAFFORD (2) is approaching with troops to put down the rebellion.

Michael (2), Sir Minor character in *1 Henry IV,* friend of the ARCHBISHOP (3) of York. In 4.4 the Archbishop and Sir Michael discuss the rebels' likely defeat against King HENRY IV at SHREWSBURY. The episode introduces the Archbishop's subsequent further rebellion against the King, to be enacted in *2 Henry IV.*

No historical Michael is known among the Archbishop's associates. Sir Michael's presence in the play may reflect a lost source that the playwright consulted, or he may be Shakespeare's invention.

Middleham Castle Heavily fortified and moated castle in northern England, a location in *3 Henry VI.* The grounds of Middleham Castle, home to the brother of the Duke of WARWICK (3), are the setting for 4.5, in which the Duke's captive, King EDWARD IV, is rescued by his allies.

Middleton, Thomas (1580–1627) English playwright, a prolific writer of JACOBEAN DRAMA. As a young man, Middleton worked for Philip HENSLOWE, turning out plays in collaboration with Thomas DEKKER, Michael DRAYTON, and Anthony MUNDAY. He wrote comedies for various CHILDREN'S COMPANIES between 1602 and 1608; he then worked with Dekker on *The Roaring Girl* (1610), a highly successful COMEDY of the period. In the 1620s, Middleton collaborated with William ROWLEY (2), who wrote comic SUB-PLOTS, on several plays for PRINCE CHARLES' MEN. These included his greatest play, *The Changeling* (1622), a TRAGEDY of murder, madness, and obsessive love that has frequently been revived in the 20th century. Another of his best works, *Women Beware Women* (c. 1625), is also a tragedy of perverse attractions and grave moral sickness. One of Middleton's last works, *A Game at Chess* (1624), is a boldly anti-Catholic, anti-Spanish allegory that blatantly alluded to King JAMES I's pursuit of a marital alliance with the Spanish Hapsburgs. It was huge success at the GLOBE THEATRE, running for nine days—two days would have been unusual at that time (see ELIZABETHAN THEATRE)—before the government prohibited it and briefly gaoled its author.

Two SONGS from Middleton's tragedy *The Witch* (c. 1610–1620) were printed in the first edition of *Macbeth,* having been interpolated in Shakespeare's play for some early performance. Middleton may have written THE PURITAN and collaborated with William ROWLEY (2) on *THE BIRTH OF MERLIN,* both plays at one time ascribed to Shakespeare, and some scholars give him a role as a collaborator in Shakespeare's unfinished play *Timon of Athens.*

A Midsummer Night's Dream

SYNOPSIS

Act 1, Scene 1

THESEUS (1), Duke of ATHENS, discusses with HIPPOLYTA (1) their forthcoming marriage, only days away. EGEUS arrives with his daughter, HERMIA, and her two suitors, DEMETRIUS (2) and LYSANDER. Since Hermia will not marry Demetrius, whom her father prefers, but insists that she loves Lysander, Egeus wants her subjected to a law that will condemn her to death or a life as a nun for refusing to marry the groom her father has chosen. Theseus reluctantly rules that he must enforce the law, but he gives Hermia until the day of his own wedding to decide what she will do. Lysander, declaring himself the better marital prospect, reveals that Demetrius has earlier courted Hermia's friend HELENA (1) and made her fall in love with him. Theseus leaves, taking with him all but Lysander and Hermia, who decide to elope, agreeing to meet in the woods the next night. Helena appears, pining for Demetrius; Lysander and Hermia encour-

age her by telling of their plan and asserting that, with Hermia gone, Demetrius will be free again. The lovers leave, and the love-sick Helena, in a soliloquy, devises a plot to curry favour with Demetrius: she will tell him of the planned elopement and accompany him to the woods to intercept the pair.

Act 1, Scene 2
QUINCE, with his fellow artisans SNUG, FLUTE, SNOUT, STARVELING, and BOTTOM, gather to rehearse the INTERLUDE they are to perform at Theseus and Hippolyta's wedding. Quince, the director, announces the subject of their playlet—the tale of PYRAMUS AND THISBE—and distributes the parts among the players. Bottom, who is to play Pyramus, is so confident of his acting abilities that he wants most of the other parts as well. Quince declares that, in order to keep their spectacle a surprise, they will rehearse in secret, meeting the next night in the woods.

Act 2, Scene 1
PUCK and a FAIRY discuss the conflict between the King of the Fairies, OBERON, whom Puck serves, and the Fairy Queen, TITANIA, the Fairy's mistress. Titania and Oberon arrive and begin arguing. She refuses to give up a changeling boy whom Oberon covets. She leaves, and Oberon vows vengeance. He instructs Puck to gather for him a certain flower that he will apply to Titania's eyes while she sleeps and that will cause her to fall in love with the first living being she sees when she wakes. While awaiting Puck's return, Oberon overhears Demetrius and Helena, who are now in the woods, and when Demetrius persistently repulses his admirer, the Fairy King decides that he will dose him with the flower also. Puck returns with the magical herb, and Oberon takes some of it to give to Titania. He tells Puck to find the Athenian couple who are roaming in the woods and to apply the rest of the potion to Demetrius.

Act 2, Scene 2
Titania's retinue sings her to sleep. Oberon appears and puts juice from the plant on her eyes. He leaves, and Lysander and Hermia enter, exhausted from wandering. They sleep, though only after Hermia has insisted that they maintain a proper distance from each other. Puck arrives, sees that they are Athenians, and, presuming that their physical separation implies a lack of love, supposes that he has found his target. He administers the juice to Lysander's eyes and leaves. Demetrius appears, pursued by Helena. He shakes her off and goes on alone. Lysander awakes, and, seeing Helena, falls in love with her. She, offended by his seeming fickleness, leaves. He follows her, and Hermia wakes to find herself alone. Titania remains asleep.

Act 3, Scene 1
Quince, Bottom, and their colleagues rehearse in the woods. Puck happens on them and decides to make mischief; he gives Bottom an ass' head, which all but he can see. The other artisans are frightened by this transformation and flee. Bottom, unaware of it, concludes that they are attempting to scare him. To demonstrate his courage, he sings a song, thus waking Titania, who falls in love with him as a result of Oberon's magic. Claiming him, she assigns him an entourage of four fairies, PEASEBLOSSOM, COBWEB, MOTH (2), and MUSTARDSEED.

Act 3, Scene 2
Puck reports on Titania's ludicrous infatuation, to Oberon's delight. Demetrius and Hermia appear, arguing. She leaves angrily, and Demetrius, worn out, falls asleep. Oberon realises that the wrong man has been treated with the magical juice. He commands Puck to lure Helena, while he himself charms Demetrius with the herb. When Helena arrives, Lysander follows, pleading his love. Demetrius wakes; he falls in love with Helena and begins to praise her beauty. She concludes that the two men are mocking her, and she chastises them. Hermia enters in search of Lysander. She expresses bewilderment at her lover's new preference for Helena. Helena takes this as a deliberate insult and concludes that Hermia has joined the men in belittling her. After a series of exchanges, during which first the men and then the women almost come to blows, Lysander and Demetrius stalk off to fight a duel, Helena flees Hermia's wrath, and Hermia leaves baffled. Oberon directs Puck to summon a dense fog and then to impersonate each man to the other and lead them away from any conflict. Then he is to apply an antidote to Lysander's eyes. Puck leads the men on separate chases until each falls exhausted on an opposite side of the stage. Helena and Hermia, both lost in the woods, find spots to sleep. Puck squeezes the juice on Lysander's eyes, singing a song of reconciliation.

Act 4, Scene 1
Watched by Oberon, Titania leads Bottom into the clearing where the lovers sleep. Bottom is pampered by his fairy attendants, and he requests hay to eat. Titania speaks adoringly to Bottom and curls up to sleep with him. Puck appears, and Oberon confides that Titania has surrendered her changeling to him; he decides to release her from his spell. He wakes her and tells Puck to remove the ass' head from Bottom. After casting a spell of deep sleep on the mortals, the fairies leave. Theseus, Hippolyta, and Egeus enter; they are hunting with hounds. They discover the lovers and wake them. Lysander tells of his and Hermia's intended elopement, and Egeus angrily demands his execution for having attempted to prevent Hermia's marriage to Demetrius. However, Demetrius an-

nounces his intention to marry Helena. Theseus is delighted and commands that the two reunited couples shall be married that day, along with himself and Hippolyta. They all return to Athens, leaving Bottom, who awakes amazedly and muses on the strange dream that he can't quite remember.

Act 4, Scene 2
Quince, Flute, Snout, and Starveling wonder at Bottom's absence, and Snug arrives to tell them that the Duke's festivities are about to begin. Their distress is relieved when Bottom arrives, not quite able to recount what he has seen, but prepared to lead them on-stage.

Act 5, Scene 1
Theseus discounts the lovers' experiences in the woods, attributing to them a madness that also affects lunatics and poets. The newlyweds arrive, and Theseus calls for entertainment. Quince's production of *Pyramus and Thisbe* is performed, provoking amusement. Following the performance, everyone departs, and the fairies, led by Puck, arrive to bless the marriages. They leave, and Puck delivers an EPILOGUE suggesting that, if the audience is offended by being asked to believe in fairies, they should simply pretend that they have slept and dreamed.

COMMENTARY

Scholars generally agree that *A Midsummer Night's Dream* was written to be performed at an aristocratic wedding. Everything in the play is related to the theme of marriage. Theseus and Hippolyta's nuptials are the goal towards which all the action is directed—the fairies have come to Athens to bless the occasion; the artisans' performance is intended for it; Hermia's judgement, and thus the climax of the lovers' story, is scheduled to coincide with it, and finally the young lovers are married along with the ducal couple. The very first line emphasises the importance of the forthcoming 'nuptial hour' (1.1.1), and the dénouement is a blessing of the three weddings in terms that suggest a performance within a dwelling, as Oberon orders the

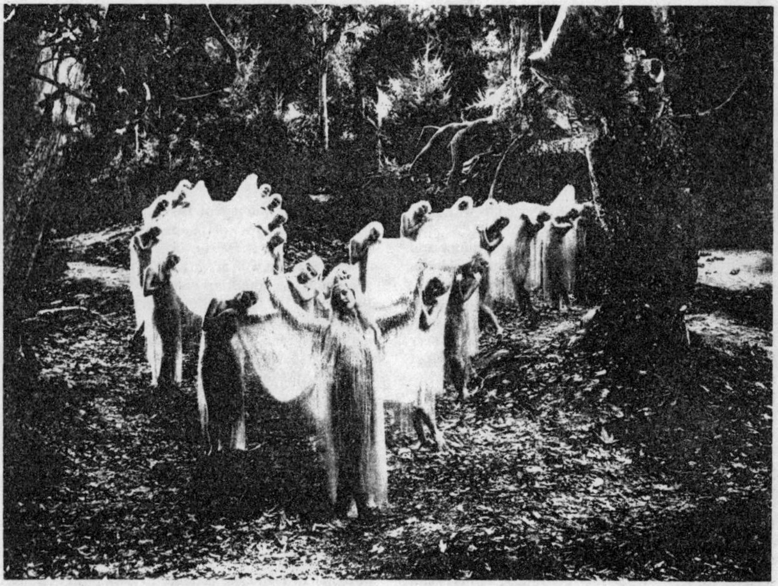

A fairy procession from the 1935 film of A Midsummer Night's Dream *by Max Reinhardt. The Austrian-born director was famous for his lavish sets and costumes.* (Courtesy of Culver Pictures, Inc.)

fairies to distribute blessings 'through this house' (5.1.388). (See 'Theatrical History of the Play'.)

The play suits such an occasion well, for it has the formality of a MASQUE, an entertainment often performed at noble weddings. Like many masques, this comedy presents a world of magic and metamorphosis in brilliant spectacles involving picturesque supernatural beings. It also makes much use of music and dance, and its finale is itself masquelike. It is given over to celebration, with further dancing and a comical performance (*Pyramus and Thisbe*) similar to an anti-masque—the realistic farce that was commonly part of a masque itself. Like a masque again, Acts 1–4 are very symmetrically plotted, moving from the court of Theseus to the woods and back again. In part, this reflects an archetypal plot pattern of withdrawal and return, common in the romance literature preceding Shakespeare and in his own work, but the arrangement here is particularly formal. (Compare, for example, *The Two Gentlemen of Verona* or *Cymbeline*.) There are internal symmetries also. For example, two songs are used—one to put Titania to sleep in 2.2, and the other to wake her in 3.1—and Quince and his cast appear four times, twice on either side of Bottom's adventure.

As is natural in such a formal context, the characters are stylised and unrealistic: they do not interact as people normally do. Theseus and Hipplyta are remote ideals of classical calm; Puck is a typical goblin; and Titania and Oberon are distant in their regal immortality, elemental forces of nature with the power to influence the climate and to bless marriages. Only Bottom and his fellow artisans represent ordinary people, and they are plainly character types with little personality beyond their buffoonery.

The lovers, too, are static; although Lysander and Demetrius are transformed by Oberon's magical herb, they are altered only in their stance towards another character, and in Lysander's case the change is only temporary. Demetrius is left in a position he had held before the opening of the play and thus is ultimately unchanged also. Change occurs only in the pattern of the lovers' relationships, which has often been compared to a dance: first the two men address one of the women while the other woman is alone; then one man's affection is changed, and a circular chase unfolds. Lysander woos Helena, who is still pursuing Demetrius, who continues to court Hermia, who still wants Lysander. Next, when Demetrius is put under Oberon's spell, the two men face the other woman, and the first woman is alone. Finally the only stable arrangement is achieved, with Lysander and Demetrius each returned to his original love interest.

Such intricate masquelike plotting is appropriate not only to a festive occasion but also to the world of dreamy confusion that is central to the story. Much of the action, from 2.1 into 4.1, takes place at night; the lovers assert several times that they are looking at the stars (e.g., 3.2.61, 3.2.188), thus drawing attention to the night-time setting (which was usually enacted in afternoon sunlight in an Elizabethan public theatre). The nocturnal universe of shadowy strangeness is further evoked in the play's imagery. The moon is referred to prominently, beginning in the very first few lines (1.1.3,4,9): Moonlight is mentioned three times more often in *A Midsummer Night's Dream* than in all of Shakespeare's other plays combined. In many different contexts the moon is used in figures of speech: to indicate time of day (1.1.209–210) and of month (1.1.83); with reference to catastrophic flooding (2.1.103) and to the speed of fairies (2.1.7, 4.1.97); cuckoldry (5.1.232) and in connection with chastity (1.1.73, 2.1.162) and opposition to chastity (3.1.191–193). 'Moonshine' is even a character in the artisans' play. The eerie quality of moonlight is reinforced by frequent evocations of the beauty of the woods at night.

Flowers are frequently mentioned as well, as in 1.1.185 and 2.1.110, and of course the magical aphrodisiac is a flower (2.1.166). Even the doggerel of *Pyramus and Thisbe* provides a floral motif (3.1.88–89). Birds, too, are alluded to throughout the play. Afoot (5.1.380) and in flight (3.2.21), as emblems of sight (2.2.113, 3.2.142) and of sound (1.1.184, 1.2.78, 5.1.362), they sing (5.1.384) and soar (3.2.23) in the play's highly lyrical language. Even Bottom, when he sings, brings forth a country ditty about birds (3.1.120–128).

Animals also inhabit the enchanted woods, though they lurk ominously, for the most part. Even a bee poses a threat (4.1.15–16), however slight. The image of preying carnivores is invoked by Helena to describe her desperate pursuit of Demetrius in 2.1.232–233. Dead sheep are part of Titania's vision of disordered nature (2.1.97). Theseus evokes a night-time fear that a bush may be a bear (5.1.22). Potential tragedy is presented in a humorous context only, in the artisans' INTERLUDE, but in that episode tragedy is wrought by a ravening lion. Puck, introducing the fairies' blessings with a reminder of the cruel world that they may also be associated with, remarks that 'the hungry lion roars, / And the wolf behowls the moon' (5.1.357–358).

Indeed, the dream-world of the play involves several hints of nightmare, providing a contrast to its harmonies of love. Hermia awakes from a nightmare at the end of 2.2, and the 'drooping fog, as black as Acheron' (3.2.357) summoned by Puck to deceive Lysander and Demetrius carries a hint of terror, though its purpose is benign. Shakespeare never lets the fairy world seem altogether sweet and light; Puck has a touch of malice to his personality, and he reminds the audience of the fairies' alliance to dark powers in the speech, cited above, that introduces the final ritual, the blessing of the house.

One of the functions of that blessing, indeed, is to

exorcise all potential evil at last. The interlude has just performed a similar task in rendering a lovers' tragedy as farce. In fact, Quince, Bottom, and the boys act as an earthy counterweight to the uncanny airiness of the fairies. This is like an exorcism, because the unreal world of Puck and Oberon, Titania and Peaseblossom is supremely alien and potentially dangerous. The mortals can be manipulated and never know it: the lovers, returning to Athens, believe themselves to have awakened from dreams (4.1.197–198), as does Bottom (4.1.204).

But generations of viewers and readers and critics have felt compelled to ask whether Shakespeare intends us to take the enchanted woods as dream or as reality. The title of the play—related to 'midsummer madness', proverbially a lovers' sickness—suggests that the mortals' experience in the woods is but a figment, perhaps that the whole play is. But we the audience, having witnessed it ourselves, may agree with Hippolyta that 'all the story of the night told over, . . . grows to something of great constancy' (5.1.23–26). Unlike Theseus, who sees only lunacy in the 'forms of things unknown [that] imagination bodies forth' (5.1.14–15), Hippolyta recognises the essential reality, or constancy, that 'things unknown' have, when given by the 'poet's pen . . . a local habitation and a name' (5.1.16–17). We the audience can realise even more: that the play, the poet's embodiment of imaginary things, has made the unreal real.

We must return to our starting point, the occasion for which the play was evidently written. Shakespeare's original audience, guests at a wedding, was removed from the world of reality, just as modern audiences are, and then returned to it by the ritual at its close. The exact definition of reality is not addressed by the play; indeed, the play's ambiguity on the point is deliberate. The experience is all that matters, and the experience, as Bottom knew, is a profound one. When he wakes from his experience in the woods and observes, 'The eye of man hath not heard, the ear of man hath not seen, man's hand is not able to taste, his tongue to conceive, nor his heart to report, what my dream was' (4.1.209–212). Bottom has experienced, though he is unable to express it, the depths of mystery that underlie all things, real and unreal alike. By evoking such awareness, the play fulfils its original and primary function as a celebratory hymn to the beauties of married love.

SOURCES OF THE PLAY

A Midsummer Night's Dream is one of the few Shakespearean plays that seem to have been generated principally from the playwright's own imagination; no known literary work is a source for it. However, it draws on a number of diverse traditions—the courtly spectacle or pageant, the folklore of fairies, and a delight in the antics of the rustic CLOWN (1)—that were common in Shakespeare's day. And the playwright did make use of a number of ideas and images that came from literature, and *A Midsummer Night's Dream*—more, perhaps, than a work that is based firmly on another work, such as *Romeo and Juliet* or *Hamlet*—suggests the range of the author's reading.

At least a dozen works provided general ideas for and/or bits and pieces of this play. Prominent among them is one of the most famous of ancient books, well known to Shakespeare and his audience, *The Golden Ass*, by Apuleius, written in the 2nd century A.D. and translated into English by William ADLINGTON in 1566; this tale tells of a man transformed into an ass. Shakespeare also took ingredients from several works by his greatest English predecessor, Geoffrey CHAUCER, notably 'The Knight's Tale', which provided the characters Theseus and Hippolyta as Duke of Athens and Queen of the Amazons, as well as several situations in the play: the marriage of Chaucer's ducal couple is postponed by the arbitration of a dispute, for example, and Theseus uses his authority to uphold a supernatural resolution of complicated lovers' quarrels. He also interrupts a duel between rivals, as Oberon does in the play. Further, Chaucer's 'The Merchant's Tale' presents a fairy king and queen who are at odds over a human being and who intervene in mortal affairs. Also, his 'Sir Tophas', a satire of knightly romance, features a comical knight-errant who dreams of marrying an 'elf-queene'.

One of Shakespeare's favourite books, OVID's *Metamorphoses* (in the 1567 translation by Arthur GOLDING) was the source of the legend of Pyramus and Thisbe as presented in the interlude in 5.1. That the playwright also knew Ovid in the original Latin is demonstrated by his use of the name Titania, which is not in Golding, but which the Roman poet used several times in contexts relevant to the play's motifs—as another name for Diana, the moon goddess, and for Circe, who transformed men into animals.

The Fairy King, Oberon, was a well-known figure both in folklore and in medieval literature. In *Huon of Bordeaux*, a 13th-century French adventure tale translated by Lord BERNERS (1534), he resembles Shakespeare's character in presiding over a magical forest where mortals become lost and in explicitly distinguishing himself from evil spirits; in both stories he intervenes to bring about a happy ending.

The play incorporates many minor echoes of a work of Shakespeare's own time, *The Discoverie of Witchcraft* (1584) by Reginald SCOT, a tract opposing the prosecution of witches. Shakespeare used Scot's accounts of fairy lore, especially about Robin Goodfellow, or Puck, although Scot derides belief in such things as groundless superstition. Scot also tells of a magical procedure reputed to give a man the head of an ass.

Shakespeare's knowledge of other works is also reflected in the play. These works include Edmund

SPENSER's *Shepheardes Calender* (1579), Bartholomew YONG's translation of *Diana Enamorada,* by the Portuguese author Jorge de MONTEMAYOR (a chief source of *The Two Gentlemen of Verona*), several plays by SENECA and several by John LYLY, plus novels *Euphues* (1578) and *Euphues and His England* (1580). In addition, Thomas NORTH's translation of PLUTARCH's 'Life of Theseus' (1579) provided a number of proper names; this was Shakespeare's first use of a source that would become very important to him.

TEXT OF THE PLAY

Dating the composition of *A Midsummer Night's Dream* precisely is not possible with the existing evidence, but we can assume it was written in 1595 or early 1596. The comical worry about the possible ferocity of a theatrical lion (1.2.70–75, 3.1.26–44, 5.1.214–221) was almost certainly inspired by an account, published in London in late 1594, of a planned appearance by a lion at a christening, cancelled as possibly dangerous and certainly alarming. Further, Titania's description of the cataclysmic weather caused by her dispute with Oberon (2.1.88–114) apparently refers to a series of three extraordinarily cold, wet summers in 1594–1596. This allows us to assume that the play was written between 1595 and 1598, when it was recorded in the list of Shakespeare's works assembled by Francis MERES. However, we know that from 1596 onwards Shakespeare was working on plays—*The Merchant of Venice, 1* and *2 Henry IV,* and *The Merry Wives of Windsor*—very unlike the lyrical *Dream.* The latter work, moreover, is linked stylistically to several plays—*Love's Labour's Lost, Romeo and Juliet,* and *Richard II*—that can be dated to 1593–1595.

The first edition of the *Dream* was published as a QUARTO by Thomas FISHER in 1600. It appears to have been printed from Shakespeare's FOUL PAPERS, with irregular stage directions and other mistakes that would have been corrected in any later manuscript. This edition is known as Q1. The next edition, Q2, was printed by Thomas PAVIER and William JAGGARD in 1619, as part of the notorious FALSE FOLIO; it was dated 1600 in order not to seem a new, unauthorised publication. Q2 was simply an inaccurate reprint of Q1, with many minor errors. It nonetheless served as the basis for the FIRST FOLIO edition of 1623, though its editors also referred to a PROMPT-BOOK of the play, resulting in superior stage directions in their version. Q1, derived from Shakespeare's own manuscript, is regarded as the most authoritative text, and it has been the basis for all modern editions, except with respect to stage directions, for which the Folio text is favoured.

THEATRICAL HISTORY OF THE PLAY

The first performance of *A Midsummer Night's Dream* was almost certainly at an aristocratic wedding of the 1590s, although no record of the event exists. The occasion may have been the marriage in February 1596 of Elizabeth Carey, grand-daughter of Henry CAREY (2) the patron of the CHAMBERLAIN'S MEN, with whom Shakespeare was associated at the time. Another possible wedding was that of the Earl of DERBY (3) a year earlier, for Derby's older brother, Lord STRANGE, had been the same company's patron before his death in 1594.

In 1600 the title page of the first Quarto edition of the play asserted that it had 'been sundry times publickely acted' by the Chamberlain's Men, but the earliest recorded performance, perhaps of an adaptation, was held at the court of King James I in 1604 under the title *A Play of Robin Goodfellow.* No other productions during the playwright's lifetime are known.

A scandal was aroused in 1631 by a Sunday performance of the *Dream* in the house of a bishop, and an excerpt from the play was performed surreptitiously between 1642 and 1660, when the theatres were closed by the revolutionary government. This abridged version was published as a DROLL—*The Merry Conceits of Bottom the Weaver*— in 1661 by Henry MARSH and Francis KIRKMAN. The diarist Samuel PEPYS attended a performance of the *Dream* in 1662 and called it 'the most insipid ridiculous play that ever I saw in my life'.

This was the last recorded performance for more than a century and a half, though many adaptations were popular throughout the period. The first and most successful of these was Henry PURCELL's opera *The Fairy Queen,* produced in 1692 by Thomas BETTERTON. Musical versions continued to be produced in the 18th century, most notably Richard LEVERIDGE's operetta *A Comic Masque of Pyramus and Thisbe* (1716, revived 1745), which satirised the current London enthusiasm for Italian opera. As its title suggests, this work included only the SUB-PLOT of *A Midsummer Night's Dream.* This material was also tapped by Charles JOHNSON (2), who incorporated the comical interlude into LOVE IN A FOREST (1723), his version of *As You Like It.* David GARRICK used the main plot of Shakespeare's play, eliminating Bottom and his friends, in *The Fairies* (1755), an opera incorporating 27 songs by various authors. Frederic REYNOLDS (1) continued the musical tradition in 1816, with an operatic medley based on the *Dream.*

The earliest restoration of Shakespeare's text occurred in 1827, in Ludwig TIECK's Berlin production of SCHLEGEL's German translation featuring the famous overture and incidental music by Felix Mendelssohn (1809–1847), composed in the previous year. Mendelssohn's music also accompanied the first English revival, in 1840. Subsequent 19th-century productions included a grandly scenic staging by Charles KEAN (1) and a more restrained version by Samuel PHELPS. The 19th-century tendency to spectacular

presentations of the *Dream* reached its height in Beerbohm TREE's 1900 production, which featured live rabbits and birds amid dense foliage.

A Midsummer Night's Dream has been among the most frequently performed of Shakespeare's plays in the 20th century. Harley GRANVILLE-BARKER's avant-garde rendering of 1914 (New York, 1915) employed a rigorously Shakespearean text, but it also featured stylised botanical motifs in place of realistic scenery and fairies who were painted gold and used mechanical gestures to emphasise their exotic nature. This highly controversial production was influenced by the *Ballets Russes* of Diaghilev. Max REINHARDT presented highly altered versions of Shakespeare's text on the London stage in the 1920s and in a FILM of 1935, starring James Cagney as Bottom and Mickey Rooney as Puck. More conventional productions have included those of Tyrone GUTHRIE and Peter HALL (5). In 1970 Peter BROOK (2) aroused as much controversy as Granville-Barker had a half-century earlier, with a *Dream* incorporating circus acts and costumes in a bare white set. The musical tradition has continued, with operas by Carl Orff (1895–1982) and Benjamin BRITTEN (1960). Purcell's *The Fairy Queen* was revived in 1946. *Swinging the Dream* (1939) was a jazz version featuring the Benny Goodman Sextet, with Louis Armstrong as Bottom. The play has been made as a FILM seven times (five of them silent movies). It has also been seen on TELEVISION eight times.

Milan City in Italy, possibly the setting of several scenes in *The Two Gentlemen of Verona.* These scenes involve the members of the court of the DUKE (5) of Milan, but the geography of the play is confused, at best, and it is difficult to know where the characters are much of the time. The actual city of Milan is in no way depicted in any case. Elsewhere in Shakespeare's works, Milan is referred to a number of times, though it is nowhere significant. It is most prominent in *The Tempest,* where the magician PROSPERO has been deposed as Duke of Milan and in the course of the play recovers that position. However, the whole play takes place on the magic island where Prospero rules in exile, and Milan is merely mentioned.

Miles Gloriosus Traditional character type, dating from ancient Roman drama, that influenced several Shakespearean character types, most notably ARMADO in *Love's Labour's Lost.* The Miles Gloriosus, a foolish, bragging soldier, was well known in Shakespeare's day through Latin texts and, more important, through the braggart captain of Italian COMMEDIA DELL' ARTE. This *capitano* was usually a Spaniard, a reflection of the Spanish role in the wars that ravaged Italy in the 16th century. His nationality was naturally adopted by Shakespeare, for hostility towards Spain was also a central element of the contemporary English world-view. Besides Armado, the Shakespearean characters who partake of the same ancestry include AJAX and THERSITES in *Troilus and Cressida* and PAROLLES in *All's Well That Ends Well.* Although FALSTAFF is often cited in this connection, he transcends the empty vainglory of the traditional type. Maurice MORGANN—the 18th-century writer on Falstaff—observed that the Miles Gloriosus provides the fat knight with no more than a trace of flavour.

Miller (1), James (1706–1744) Eighteenth-century playwright, author of *The Universal Passion* (1737), a popular adaptation combining Shakespeare's *Much Ado About Nothing* and Molière's *La Princesse d'Élide.* Miller, who became famous for a satire he wrote while he was still a student, later became a clergyman but continued to write plays—generally adaptations of French works. Several of these, including *The Universal Passion,* were successfully produced.

Miller (2), Jonathan (b. 1934) British director, creator of many modern productions of Shakespeare's plays, including a powerful *Merchant of Venice* (1970), with Laurence OLIVIER as SHYLOCK. He is also noted for his numerous Shakespearean TELEVISION productions in the early 1980s, as part of the BBC's complete cycle of the plays.

Millington, Thomas (active 1583–1603) Publisher and bookseller in LONDON, producer of first editions of several Shakespeare plays. In 1594 Millington joined with Edward WHITE (1) to publish the first edition of *Titus Andronicus,* a QUARTO (Q1). The same year, on his own, he published Q1 of *2 Henry VI* (known as THE CONTENTION), and in 1595 he produced Q1 of *3 Henry VI* (THE TRUE TRAGEDY). In 1600 he published a second edition of both these works and, in partnership with John BUSBY, the first edition of *Henry V.* Each of these editions was pirated, for each is a BAD QUARTO, assembled from the memories of actors and published without permission of the acting company that owned the rights.

Milton, John (1608–1674) Major English poet, author of *Paradise Lost, Paradise Regained, Samson Agonistes,* and many shorter works, including a well-known EPITAPH on Shakespeare. The first of Milton's poems to be published was 'An Epitaph on the admirable Dramaticke Poet, W. Shakespeare', which appeared anonymously among the introductory verses in the second FOLIO (1632). It also appeared in the third and fourth Folios (1663, 1685). It is considered one of the poet's best short works (16 lines), an elegiac lyric reflecting on the power of Shakespeare's art to outlast his death. Milton also mentions Shakespeare, in another early work, *L'Allegro,* calling him 'Fancy's child', whose plays 'warble his native wood-notes wild'.

Miranda Character in *The Tempest,* daughter of the magician PROSPERO. Miranda, exiled with her father at the age of two, has lived 12 years with him on the island he rules through sorcery. It is uninhabited except for the supernatural creatures ARIEL and CALIBAN, so when Prospero's magic brings people to the island, Miranda sees her first young man, FERDINAND (2), with whom she falls in love—and he with her—in 1.2. Prospero has planned this—Ferdinand is the son of his old enemy, King ALONSO of Naples—but he pretends to oppose the couple's love to ensure that Ferdinand does not take Miranda lightly. Prospero takes the young man captive, but Miranda contrives to visit him, and they confess their love and plan to marry in 3.1; in 4.1 Prospero declares his approval. As part of Prospero's arrangements for a conclusion of forgiveness and happiness, in 5.1 Miranda and Ferdinand are revealed to King Alonso, who believed his son had drowned. Miranda's marriage plans are confirmed, and Alonso declares that she and Ferdinand will inherit the kingdom of Naples.

Miranda does not speak often or at length, but she is established as a paragon of maidenhood. She displays a touching compassion—fearing for the shipwreck victims, she says, 'O, I have suffered / With those that I saw suffer!' (1.2.5–6). She also shows a capacity for delighted wonder; on first seeing Ferdinand, she cries, 'I might call him / A thing divine; for nothing natural / I ever saw so noble' (1.2.420–422). Her angry disdain for Caliban, who once attempted to rape her, displays the moral sensibility she has learned from her father, but her innocence of society gives her a simplicity that in a less overtly fantastic context would be disconcerting. She ignores the fact that Ferdinand is the son of her father's enemy, and at the play's close she is filled with pleased admiration for all of the king's party, even though some of them are arrant villains, saying, 'How beauteous mankind is! O brave new world, / That has such people in 't!' (5.1. 183–184).

Miranda represents the compassionate, forgiving, and optimistic potential in humanity. She is the only human character in the play who does not undergo some sort of purging transformation, for she does not need to. Innocent of life's difficulties and compromises, she repudiates evil and responds to nobility and beauty. She is most pointedly contrasted with the evil Caliban. Both were raised together by Prospero, but she has become a person of moral sensibility, while he is a would-be rapist who declares that his only use for language is to curse. Their responses to the arrival of strangers on the island are also contrasting: she is filled with demure awe, he with crass fear.

Though innocent, Miranda is nonetheless mindful of sexual propriety, speaking of her 'modesty, the jewel in [her] dower' (3.1.53–54) and declaring that if Ferdinand will not marry her, she will 'die [his] maid' (3.1.84). Her virginity—stressed repeatedly by the men, as in Ferdinand's first declaration of love and in Prospero's emphatic concern about sex before marriage—link her to an ancient archetype, the fertile woman, producer of new generations. The goddesses at her betrothal MASQUE sing of 'Earth's increase' and 'plants with goodly burthen bowing' (4.1.110, 113), making it clear that the occasion concerns reproduction. They also stress Miranda's virginity, for a sure knowledge of paternity has traditionally been very important to the orderly continuation of society. This is especially true among rulers, and Miranda's future as a queen is frequently pointed up. At the play's close, after Prospero's reconciliations have been effected, GONZALO blesses the moment and delights in the prospect that Prospero's 'issue / Should become Kings of Naples' (5.1.205–206). Miranda thus helps fulfil that most ancient of necessities for human societies, continuance into the future. She and Ferdinand embody the regeneration that is the theme of the play's close.

Miranda's name—Latin for 'admirable' (literally, 'to be wondered at')—was coined by Shakespeare. It reflects not only her qualities as an example of innocent womanhood but also her own admiring nature and the extraordinary sense of wonder that the play as a whole conveys. It is punned on by Ferdinand when he calls her 'Admir'd Miranda!' (3.1.37) and, more subtly, when he exclaims 'O you wonder!' (1.2.429).

Mirror for Magistrates, A English anthology of biographies in verse (published in seven versions, from 1559 to 1619) that influenced Shakespeare, especially in the writing of the HISTORY PLAYS. Originally intended as a sequel to John LYDGATE's *Falls of Princes* (1431–1438, publ. 1494)—a translation of BOCCACCIO's *The Fate of Illustrious Men* (1355–1374)—*A Mirror* reflects the RENAISSANCE interest in individual lives, along with a traditional concern for the fates of kings and other monumental figures. Most tales told of the dire fate, usually ending in violent death, of a villainous tyrant or would-be tyrant, for, as its title suggests, the book was intended to exercise a moral influence. The first edition was compiled in 1555, but was suppressed by the government of Queen Mary and not published until 1559 under ELIZABETH (1), and contained 19 such 'tragedies' (see TRAGEDY) by various authors. In 1563 a second edition appeared that featured seven more biographies and included Thomas SACKVILLE's *Induction* and his *Complaint of Buckingham,* the only material in *A Mirror* that has been considered fine literature by later ages.

The material in these first two compilations dealt chiefly with English history from RICHARD II onwards, and it provided Shakespeare with details for most of his history plays. John HIGGINS, whose interests were more antiquarian, issued the third and fourth editions of *A Mirror* (1574, 1578), to which he contributed 16

poems about heroes of ancient Britain. One of these was consulted by Shakespeare in writing *King Lear.* In 1587 a fifth edition (the one Shakespeare knew) appeared. It incorporated with the earlier material new work that included another major contribution from Higgins—an additional 24 lives, all but one from the classical world. His biography of Julius CAESAR (1) provided material for Shakespeare's *Julius Caesar.* Two later editions of *A Mirror*—in 1610 and 1619—included tales of virtue rewarded and added positive lessons to the older accounts of villainy punished.

Misenum Ancient Italian town, location for two scenes in *Antony and Cleopatra.* In 2.6 the co-rulers of Rome—Octavius CAESAR (2), LEPIDUS, and Mark ANTONY—meet with POMPEY (2), whose naval forces have been pillaging Italian coastal towns, and negotiate a peace treaty. Pompey accepts the rule of Sicily and Sardinia in exchange for which he will rid 'all the sea of pirates' (2.6.36), that is, his own followers represented by MENAS and MENECRATES. In 2.7 the negotiators celebrate their agreement with a drunken banquet aboard Pompey's ship, anchored off Misenum. During the banquet, the true colours of several of the participants are revealed.

Located on the northern headland of the Bay of Naples, Misenum was the site of a meeting such as is seen in the play, and it resulted in a pact known as the Treaty of Misenum in 39 B.C. Essentially, Pompey was added to the Roman Triumvirate, but the peace did not last long. Pompey renewed his raids on the Italian coast and provoked Caesar to invade his base at MESSINA and to destroy him for good in 36 B.C., a conquest that is referred to in 3.5.4.

Mistress (1) Alice Ford One of the title characters in *The Merry Wives of Windsor,* wife of Frank FORD (1). When Mistress Ford and her friend MISTRESS (3) Page receive identical love letters from FALSTAFF, they feel their honour has been insulted by a gross lecher, and they plot revenge. In their plan Mistress Ford serves as bait for Falstaff, who comes to her house, where the appearance of her jealous husband causes the lecher's humiliating flight, first in a hamper of dirty laundry and then in disguise as an old woman, pummelled by Ford. Mistress Ford suffers from her husband's neurotic jealousy, but she bears with him, and we sympathise when she quietly observes that Mistress Page's more reasonable man makes her 'the happier woman' (2.1.103). By the same token we share her delight when Ford's jealousy leads him to be made as foolish as Falstaff; 'I know not which pleases me better', she exults, 'that my husband is deceived, or Sir John' (3.3.164–165).

Mistress (2) Overdone Character in *Measure for Measure,* the keeper of a bordello in VIENNA. Mistress Overdone's principal role is as a stereotypical member of Vienna's underworld, which stands in contrast to the world of the major characters. Her servant POMPEY (1) is the most important figure of this comic SUB-PLOT. Mistress Overdone is a familiar figure to LUCIO and his friends; her entrance inspires each GENTLEMAN (5) to jest about venereal disease, establishing the bawdy, depraved tone of the sub-plot. She also introduces a major element of the main plot when she first appears in 1.2 and tells of the prosecution of CLAUDIO (3). She is comically presented as a typical innkeeper, worried about business, though this also includes worrying about the government's attempts to fight prostitution. When she is imprisoned in 3.2 she complains that she has been informed against by Lucio. This reminds us that her world of petty vice is not truly a comic one.

A comic sub-plot featuring a bordello madam and her servant was found by Shakespeare in one of the sources for *Measure for Measure,* George WHETSTONE's *Promos and Cassandra* (1578). However, Shakespeare invented the preposterous names they bear in his play; Mistress Overdone's name reflects her status as a veteran of her profession.

Mistress (3) Margaret Page One of the title characters in *The Merry Wives of Windsor,* wife of George PAGE (12) and mother of ANNE (3) and WILLIAM (1). In 2.1 Mistress Page's response to FALSTAFF's love letter establishes the position of the honest and forthright wives as enemies of Falstaff's amorality. After reviewing the insult to her wifely honour, she concludes, 'How shall I be revenged on him? For revenged I will be, as sure as his guts are made of puddings' (2.1.29–31). When MISTRESS (1) Ford receives an identical letter, the two friends join forces. Mistress Page's role is to break in on Falstaff's visits to Mistress Ford, sparking his humiliating exits, first hidden in a hamper of dirty laundry and then beaten into the streets while dressed in an old woman's clothes. In 4.4 Mistress Page devises Falstaff's final punishment, his torment by children disguised as fairies. If she seems insensitive in seeking to marry Anne to the obnoxious Dr CAIUS (2), she accepts the outcome graciously when Anne elopes with FENTON, saying, 'Master Fenton, Heaven give you many, many merry days!' (5.5.236–237), and she proposes the pleasant resolution of the play, that all the chief characters 'laugh this sport o'er by a country fire, Sir John [Falstaff] and all' (5.5.239–240).

Mistress Page's ebullient strength is well matched with her husband's milder cheerfulness. With him, she contributes a large share of the play's charm, in both her vigorous good humour and her confident assertion of traditional values.

Mistress (4) Quickly Character in *The Merry Wives of Windsor.* See QUICKLY.

Modjeska, Helena (1844–1909) Polish-born American actress. Born Helena Opid in Cracow, she followed her brother into the local theatre, where she got her stage name from a brief first marriage. She became a leading actress in Warsaw and then, in 1876, was forced to flee from Russian-governed Poland with her second husband, who was a Polish nationalist. They went to San Francisco, where Modjeska quickly learned English and played JULIET (1) and OPHELIA, among other parts. Immediately recognised as a superior actress, she made her New York debut the next year and for almost 30 years, despite suffering a stroke in 1897, she was among the most popular of American actresses. Among Shakespearean roles, she was best known for VIOLA, ISABELLA, and LADY (6) MACBETH, playing the latter several times in the 1880s opposite Edwin BOOTH (2).

Mohun, Michael (c. 1625–1684) English actor. Mohun was a boy actor (see CHILDREN'S COMPANIES) in Christopher BEESTON's company in the 1630s. He fought with distinction for the royalists in the Civil Wars, and when the theatres were reopened upon the restoration of the monarchy in 1660, he joined the King's Company under Thomas KILLIGREW. He was among the most admired actors of the period, though he mostly played secondary roles, usually opposite Charles HART (1). He was particularly noted for his portrayals of IAGO and CASSIUS.

Mömpelgard, Frederick, Count of (later Duke of) Württemberg (d. 1608) Historical figure and contemporary of Shakespeare, alluded to in *The Merry Wives of Windsor.* As part of a sequence of anti-German jokes associated with the theft of horses from the HOST (2) in Act 4, several references are made to German travellers in England and particularly to a German Duke who is *not* expected to come to Windsor (4.3.4–5; 4.5.81–84). These obscure allusions have a particular connection both to Mömpelgard and to the occasion for which the play was written.

Frederick of Mömpelgard was heir apparent to the dukedom of Württemberg, then an independent country in what is now south-western Germany. In 1592 he visited Windsor and other English cities (those specified in 4.5.70–74) and developed an enthusiasm for the Order of the Garter. He repeatedly solicited Queen ELIZABETH (1) for membership in the knightly order; finally, after he had inherited the dukedom and achieved some importance in European affairs, she admitted him. However, in what appears to have been a calculated slight, he was not notified of his admission in time for him to attend the investment ceremonies in the spring of 1597. *The Merry Wives* was written for precisely those ceremonies, and thus the references to Mömpelgard's earlier visit, and to a German Duke who is *not* visiting, are quite evidently inside jokes intended for the play's first audience, the knights of the Garter, who will have been well aware of the Queen's action. These references appear only in the FIRST FOLIO edition of the play, which reflects the initial, private performance, and not in the 1602 QUARTO that is derived from early theatrical productions.

Monarcho (d. before 1580) The nickname given to a well-known London lunatic of Shakespeare's day. Monarcho's mad claims to be ruler of the world inspired comment in contemporary documents, including a published epitaph titled 'The Phantasticall Monarke'. ARMADO, the braggart Spaniard in *Love's Labour's Lost,* is thought to have been based on this figure, for he is referred to as 'A phantasime, a Monarcho' (4.1.100). Shakespeare can never have seen Monarcho, who died when the playwright was still a teenager in STRATFORD, but he had clearly heard enough to be impressed.

Monck, Nugent (1877–1958) British theatrical producer. In 1911 Monck founded an important theatrical company for the production of ELIZABETHAN DRAMA in Norwich, England. In 1921, he converted a 16th-century Norwich house into the Maddermarket Theatre, the first modern replica of an Elizabethan playhouse. There he staged many influential productions of Shakespeare's plays, in the crisp, spare manner of William POEL.

Monmouth, Harry (Henry) Another name for PRINCE (6) HAL, later King HENRY V. Both as Prince and King, this character is occasionally called Harry Monmouth, after his birthplace on the Welsh border. (See, e.g., *1 Henry IV,* 5.4.58; *2 Henry IV,* 2.3.45; *Henry V,* 4.7.12–55; *1 Henry VI,* 2.5.23, 3.1.198.)

Montague (1) Character in *Romeo and Juliet,* ROMEO's father and the head of the family bearing his name, rivals to the CAPULET (1) clan. Montague appears only briefly, in the three scenes in which the feud with the Capulets erupts into violence, and on each occasion he accepts in conventional terms the objections of the PRINCE (1) to the fighting. In the final scene of reconciliation (5.3), he offers to commission a golden statue of JULIET (1) as a public memorial to the love that the feud has doomed.

Although Shakespeare believed the Montague-Capulet conflict was a historical event, it in fact never occurred. See VERONA.

Montague (2), Lady Minor character in *Romeo and Juliet,* mother of ROMEO and wife of MONTAGUE (1). Lady Montague appears only twice, beside her husband, and speaks only one line. In 5.3 she is said to have died of grief following Romeo's banishment.

Montague (3), John Neville, Lord (c. 1428–1471) Historical figure and minor character in *3 Henry VI*, a supporter of the Duke of YORK (8) and his sons who deserts their cause to join his brother, the Earl of WARWICK (3), in his revolt. Montague is a Yorkist through 4.1, when he declares his loyalty to King EDWARD IV, although Warwick's rebellion has begun. However, when he next appears, in 4.6, he is with Warwick. His death in the battle of BARNET is reported in 5.2.

The motives of the historical Montague, omitted by Shakespeare, are interesting for the light they cast on the politics of the WARS OF THE ROSES. Upon his accession, Edward had confiscated the estates of the Earl of NORTHUMBERLAND (2) and given them to Montague. After Warwick's defection, seeking allies in the north, Edward gave them back to Northumberland's heir. Edward thought he had appeased Montague with new titles, but he was wrong. When Warwick landed in England with his invasion forces, Montague joined him and a large body of troops was placed under his command. This event is depicted in 5.1.

Montaigne, Michael de (1533–1592) French essayist, author of minor sources for *The Tempest* and perhaps for *Hamlet* and *King Lear*. Shakespeare knew Montainge's essays in the translation by John FLORIO, *Essayes on Morall, Politike, and Millitarie Discourses* (1603). A passage in Montaigne's essay 'Of Cannibals' is echoed in GONZALO's praise of primitive societies in *The Tempest* 2.1.143–164, and another essay, 'Of Crueltie', probably inspired PROSPERO's praise of reconciliation in 5.1.25–30. Montaigne's influence is less direct in the two tragedies. His views seem to inform some aspects of HAMLET's thought, as when he compares death to sleep and calls it a 'consummation' (*Hamlet* 3.1.63), or when he appraises man as 'this quintessence of dust' (2.2.308). In *King Lear* the villainous EDMUND's cynical notions probably reflect Montaigne's scepticism.

For the most part, however, Montaigne's sceptical, 'modern' attitudes are rejected in Shakespeare's work. Gonzalo's theory is decidedly refuted by the play as a whole, Hamlet's musings are obviously the product of despair, and the arguments of so villainous a figure as Edmund can only be disdained by a sympathetic audience. In the playwright's deployment of Montaigne's thought—as in his work in general—we can see that his allegiance lay with the old world of social hierarchy and unquestioned Christianity whose attitudes and customs Montaigne was prepared to question and often rejected. On the other hand, the two writers have in common a tolerant, accepting attitude towards humanity's foibles—reflected more in the use of Montaigne in *The Tempest* than elsewhere. That the playwright should have felt an affinity for the essayist's work is not surprising.

Montaigne was the son of a nobleman and government official of southern France. He became a lawyer in Bordeaux and frequently visited the royal court in Paris on business, once for 18 months. He pursued political ambitions at the court but was unsuccessful, and after his father's death in 1568, he retired to his estate and began writing. Literature occupied much of his time in the 1570s and again between 1586 and his death, but he also travelled, engaged in diplomacy on behalf of Henri of Navarre (later King Henri IV of FRANCE [1]), and was twice elected mayor of Bordeaux. His *Essays* were first published in 1580, with a considerably enlarged collection appearing in 1588; his last work was published posthumously. He also published a travel journal and a translation of a work by the Spanish philosopher Raimundo Sebonde (d. 1436), which sparked his longest and best-known essay, 'Apology for Raimond de Sebonde'.

Montaigne's essays record in an intimate, gossipy style his opinions on a wide range of subjects from minor domestic matters to political issues and philosophical topics. This sort of literary work was previously unknown, and Montaigne indicated the experimental nature of his writings by designating them *essais* (attempts), thus naming the genre as well as inventing it. His scepticism, curiosity, and amiable tolerance yielded essays of a philosophical ambiguity that is reflected in the wide range of critical interpretation they have inspired. Politically, Montaigne has been regarded as reactionary, liberal, and revolutionary, and in religion, as both a devout practitioner and an agnostic (in a famous remark the 19th-century critic Sainte-Beuve declared him a good Catholic but not a Christian). In any case, the *Essays* constitute a self-portrait of a reflective man whose concerns are universal and whose witty and intelligent style has charmed generations of readers. Still regarded as among the greatest works of European literature, Montaigne's essays offer one of the first examples of the individualism that was to dominate Western culture in subsequent centuries.

Montano (1) Name given REYNALDO (1) in the BAD QUARTO (Q1, 1604) of *Hamlet*. The name of Reynaldo's master, POLONIUS, also differs in Q1—it is CORAMBIS. The coincidence makes satire seem likely; the cabbage (Corambis) attended by a mountain (Montano) was perhaps a caricature of some noted figure, now unknown, and his assistant.

Q1 is a version of *Hamlet* compiled from the memories of actors who played in it, and some scholars suppose that Montano was the name of the equivalent character in an earlier play, now lost, the UR-HAMLET, and that it was inserted by an actor who knew that work. The fact that Shakespeare was shortly to use this uncommon name for a character in *Othello* is taken by some scholars as circumstantial evidence: the play-

wright presumably had encountered the name at some point in the early 17th century, perhaps while using the *Ur-Hamlet* as source material for his own play.

Montano (2) Minor character in *Othello,* the governor of CYPRUS who is replaced by OTHELLO. Montano is acknowledged by the DUKE (5) of VENICE to be a competent governor, 'of most allowed sufficiency' (1.3. 224), though Othello, as a tried battle leader, is to replace him. Montano agrees with this judgement and declares his approval of the appointment as soon as he hears of it, in 2.1. He is wounded by the drunken CASSIO in 2.3, and his rank makes Cassio's offence even greater. In 5.2 he witnesses the furor following Othello's murder of DESDEMONA, and he displays soldierly alertness in chasing and capturing IAGO when he flees, but when LODOVICO arrives he takes charge, and it is clear that Montano is an inconsequential figure.

Montemayor, Jorge de (c. 1521–1561) Portuguese-born author of a famous romance that was a source for several of Shakespeare's plays. Montemayor spent most of his life in Spain and wrote in Spanish. Though he was also a poet and composer, his fame rests entirely on his long prose romance, *Diana Enamorada,* which was published in Valencia c. 1559. It soon became popular throughout Europe; Bartholomew YONG translated it into English in 1582. Though this work was not published until 1598, Shakespeare knew the book in manuscript and was able to make use of it in that form. It was among the playwright's chief sources for *The Two Gentlemen of Verona* and *A Midsummer Night's Dream,* and it also probably influenced the writing of *As You Like It* and *Twelfth Night.*

Montgomery (1) John (actually Thomas) (c. 1430–1495) Historical figure and minor character in *3 Henry VI,* a supporter of King EDWARD IV. In 4.7 Montgomery arrives at YORK (10) with troops with which he proposes to aid Edward, but only if Edward will attempt to regain the throne. Edward promptly declares himself king, renouncing his oath that he would not claim the crown, sworn earlier in the scene in order to gain admission to the city. The incident provides one of the many instances of broken promises in these plays.

The historical Montgomery was a loyal Yorkist, having been knighted on the field at TOWTON. He subsequently served Edward as a diplomat on many occasions. He gained great notoriety in 1475 as one of the ministers who negotiated a treaty with FRANCE (1) that aborted an English invasion attempt under terms that were widely viewed as dishonourable to England and that included an annual payment from Louis XI to each of the ministers and to King Edward.

Shakespeare seems to have confused Thomas Montgomery with his father, John (d. 1449), although the BAD QUARTO edition may be the source of the error.

Montgomery (2), Philip Herbert, Earl of (1584–1650) English aristocrat and co-dedicatee of the FIRST FOLIO (1623) of Shakespeare's plays. Montgomery had no connection with Shakespeare and was doubtless included in the dedication—made by John HEMINGE and Henry CONDELL—as a compliment to the other dedicatee, his brother, the Earl of PEMBROKE (3), who as lord chamberlain was responsible for the publication of plays. Also, the publishers may have anticipated Montgomery's becoming lord chamberlain himself, which he did three years later.

Montgomery was a model of the irresponsible aristocrat. He was a courtier from the age of 15, and he became a favourite of King JAMES I, who frequently had to extract him from violent quarrels and extravagant debts. He succeeded his brother as Earl of Pembroke in 1630, but he was offended that James' son, King Charles I (ruled 1625–1649), did not appreciate him sufficiently, and he retired to his country estate, nursing his hostility and eventually joining the Parliamentarian cause in the Civil Wars.

Montjoy Minor character in *Henry V,* a French herald. Montjoy arrogantly delivers the FRENCH KING's challenge in 3.6.122–141 and patronisingly offers mercy on behalf of the CONSTABLE in 4.3.79–88, but he must humbly concede French defeat at AGINCOURT in 4.7.72–85. He is a dramatic pawn without personality, adding to the chivalric tableau of medieval warfare while formally presenting French attitudes to England, a more civil version of the overconfident French nobility represented by the DAUPHIN (3) and the Duke of ORLÉANS (3). Montjoy was actually the title of the chief herald of France, not his name, though 3.6.142–143 suggests that Shakespeare did not know this.

Mopsa Character in *The Winter's Tale,* a shepherdess. Mopsa appears only at the shepherds' festival in 4.4, where she is a charming representative of rustic youth. She is engaged to the CLOWN (8), for which she is teased by her companion, DORCAS. She and Dorcas sing a ballad with AUTOLYCUS, and their enthusiasm is infectious, contributing to the pleasure of the occasion, which contrasts sharply with the pathos and stress of the first part of the play. Mopsa is pleasingly comical as well. When she declares that she wants the Clown to buy her some sheet music, she adds naïvely, 'I love a ballad in print . . . for then we are sure they are true' (4.4.261–262). She then supposes there is truth in a ballad about a usurer's wife who gives birth to bags of money.

The name Mopsa was conventionally rustic, used for peasant women in several 16th-century romantic

works, including the greatest of them, Sir Philip SIDNEY's *Arcadia.* It may have been a feminine version of Mopsus, a name given to several mythological Greek prophets. However, Shakespeare clearly took the name directly from the play's chief source, *Pandosto* by Robert GREENE (2), where Mopsa is the foster-mother of Perdita's equivalent. Oddly, Mopsa is the only name taken from Greene, though Greene's Mopsa is the only character in *Pandosto* that does not reappear, under a different name, in Shakespeare's play.

Morality play Medieval dramatic genre that features allegorical characters who face and overcome personified moral problems or temptations. Morality plays employ one-dimensional characters who represent abstract concepts from which they take their names—Charity, Everyman, Understanding, Perseverance, etc. The plays are constructed with alternating serious and comic scenes that are intended to entertain while they instruct. They use plots that depict the conflict between vice and virtue for the possession of the hero's soul, with virtue triumphant at the close. The moral lesson is uncomplicated and is presented in a direct manner. The best-known surviving Morality plays are *Mankind* (c. 1470) and *Everyman* (c. 1500). The genre arose in the 14th century as a combination of religious sermon and festive entertainment, and Morality plays were still performed in Shakespeare's day, though their popularity was rapidly fading.

In their structure, devices, and themes, Morality plays were influential upon ELIZABETHAN DRAMA. *Dr Faustus,* by Christopher MARLOWE (1), is regarded as the Elizabethan play most similar to a Morality play (though Marlowe pointedly gives the triumph to vice, rather than virtue), but the genre is reflected in a number of Shakespeare's plays, as well. For instance, a number of his villains—perhaps most notably AARON and RICHARD III—display the traits of a stock character from the genre, the VICE. The abstract personages of the genre also appear here and there—for instance, in the disguises of TAMORA and her sons as Revenge, Rape, and Murder (*Titus Andronicus,* 5.2), and in THE SON THAT HATH KILLED HIS FATHER and THE FATHER THAT HATH KILLED HIS SON (*3 Henry VI,* 2.5). More significantly, one of the major themes found in Morality plays, the social evil represented by sin, was to be explored repeatedly by Shakespeare, especially in the HISTORY PLAYS. Other plays where commentators find the particular influence of the genre include *Measure for Measure* and *Timon of Athens.*

More, Sir Thomas (1478–1535) English writer, author of a source for *Richard III.* More is best known for his *Utopia* (1516)—a Latin account of an ideal country, whose name provided our word *utopia.* He also wrote a *History of King Richard the thirde* (written in 1513, it was first published, in part, in Richard GRAFTON's 1543 chronicle and published in full only in 1557). More's account was incorporated by both Edward HALL (2) and Raphael HOLINSHED in their histories, which were Shakespeare's chief sources for his HISTORY PLAYS. Thus, More's account was an important influence on the creation of Shakespeare's villainous RICHARD III. More's chief source for the history of the period was the manuscript of his friend Polydore VERGIL's *Historia Anglia* (1505–1533, published 1534), but he created his own King Richard. It was he who first established the popular image of a cynical and witty villain, a cripple who proves himself through ruthless ambition. More's ironic narrative plainly influenced Shakespeare's similar treatment.

As a youth, More was a page to Cardinal John Morton (1410–1500), who had known King Richard—he appears in *Richard III* as the Bishop of ELY (3). The son of a judge, More became a successful lawyer as a young man, but was also interested in humanism and literature, becoming the intimate friend of such RENAISSANCE luminaries as William LILY, John Colet (1466–1519), and Desiderius Erasmus (c. 1467–1536). He became an adviser to King HENRY VIII and rose quickly in the court hierarchy. In 1529 he succeeded Cardinal WOLSEY as Lord Chancellor (as is mentioned in *Henry VIII* 3.2.393–394), but he resigned the post in 1532 and retired, engaging in literary disputes over the emerging doctrines of Protestantism. Unwilling to support either King Henry's divorce from Queen KATHERINE or his assumption of the pope's authority in religious matters, More was tried for treason, convicted, and executed. He is considered a saint by the Catholic Church, having been canonised in 1935. His life was the subject of the play SIR THOMAS MORE, on which Shakespeare collaborated, and, more recently, of *A Man for All Seasons,* a popular play (1960) and movie (1966).

Morgan (1) In *Cymbeline,* the name taken in exile by the banished courtier BELARIUS.

Morgan (2), McNamara (d. 1762) Irish lawyer and playwright, author of an adaptation of *The Winter's Tale.* Morgan's *The Sheep-Shearing: or, Florizel and Perdita* (1754) focussed on Act 4 of Shakespeare's play, omitting the plot concerning LEONTES' jealousy. In 1761 it was produced as an operetta, with music by Thomas ARNE. Morgan was principally a Dublin barrister who wrote plays as a sideline; both *The Sheep-Shearing* and his tragedy, *Philoclea* (1754, based on part of SIDNEY's *Arcadia*), were produced by his friend Spranger BARRY (3).

Morgann, Maurice (1726–1802) Eighteenth-century English civil servant and writer, author of an influential essay on FALSTAFF. In his *Essay on the Dramatic Character of Sir John Falstaff* (1777), Morgann initiated a

style of impressionistic Shakespearean criticism, centred on a quasi-psychological interpretation of the characters that was popular throughout the 19th century into the 20th. Essentially Morgann ignores the actual evidence of the plays and emphasises one's emotional response to Falstaff. His essay strongly influenced the inclination—powerful ever since in many readers—to defend the fat knight as a bold and courageous character and to fault PRINCE (6) HAL for rejecting his old companion.

Although one of Morgann's purposes in writing was to refute Voltaire, who had called Falstaff a 'drunken savage', his defence of the fat knight displays the humanitarian influence of the French Enlightment, which valued sentiment as evidence of an humane sensibility and opposed the Machiavellian values of statecraft.

Morley, Thomas (1557–1603) English composer, possibly a friend of Shakespeare, who probably wrote music for two of the playwright's songs. Shakespeare's SONG 'It was a lover and his lass' (*As You Like It* 5.3.14–37) was published with Morley's music in the composer's *First Book of Ayres* (1600), but it is uncertain whether he set the playwright's words to music or Shakespeare wrote words to match Morley's tune. Another Morley tune, in his *First Book of Consort Lessons* (1599), bears the title of a Shakespeare song, 'O Mistress mine' (*Twelfth Night* 2.3.40–53); scholars generally believe the song in the play is meant and that this tune was used on stage. However, the composer may have adapted it from an earlier version by his one-time teacher, the notable composer William Byrd (c. 1543–1623).

Morley and Shakespeare were neighbours in 1596 and may have been acquainted. Morley was an organist for St Paul's Cathedral and a musician for the court of Queen ELIZABETH (1). He is best known as a composer of madrigals, contrapuntal songs for several voices that had been introduced into England from ITALY by Byrd. He also composed church music, solo songs with lute accompaniment, and compositions for strings and keyboard. He published five books on music, including *A Plain and Easy Introduction to Practical Music* (1597), the first work of its kind in English.

Morocco (Morochus) Character in *The Merchant of Venice,* an African prince and unsuccessful suitor of PORTIA (1). Faced with the choice among three caskets ordained by Portia's father, Morocco rationalises his choice in a long speech (2.7.13–60) that presents a viewpoint that the play as a whole invalidates. Morocco is attracted by the richness of the gold casket, which promises 'what many men desire' (2.7.5), but he finds within it an image of a death's head and a scroll whose message begins with the now-familiar line 'All that glisters is not gold' (2.7.65). Morocco fails because he equates appearance with inner worth and because he cannot imagine hazarding all in pursuit of happiness, unlike BASSANIO, who wins Portia by selecting the lead casket, and ANTONIO (2), who risks everything for his friend in accepting SHYLOCK's perilous loan.

Portia dislikes the prospect of marrying Morocco because he is black. She makes the conventional Elizabethan association of black skin and evil when she first learns of his approach (1.2.123–125). In 2.1 she politely assures him that she recognises his virtues as a man and a prince, but after his defeat, she is relieved. *The Merchant of Venice* is a play that acknowledges and makes use of Elizabethan prejudices; not only is it distinctly anti-Semitic, but the two unsuccessful suitors—both presented as examples of flawed values—are a black man and a political enemy of England, the Spaniard ARRAGON.

In both the QUARTO and FIRST FOLIO editions of the play, the name Morocco is rendered in Latin, Morochus, and some modern editions follow this practise.

Mortimer (1), Sir Edmund, Earl of March (1391–1425) Historical figure and character in *1 Henry VI,* uncle of Richard Plantagenet (see Duke of YORK [8]), to whom he bequeaths his claim to the throne. In 2.5 Plantagenet visits his aged and dying uncle in the Tower of London, where he is a prisoner. Mortimer tells of the deposition of King RICHARD II by HENRY IV, head of the Lancastrian branch of the royal family. Mortimer, of the York branch, had been the rightful heir to the throne (see LANCASTER [1]). An attempt to install him as king had resulted in his imprisonment for life while still a young man. Mortimer names Plantagenet his successor, and he dies. Mortimer's appearance in the play establishes York's claim to the throne, anticipating developments in *2* and *3 Henry VI.*

Mortimer's claim to royal descent was rather more controversial than the play suggests, for it depended on succession through a woman, a principle of inheritance often not accepted in the medieval world. In any case, the play mistakes this Mortimer for other historical personages, for Shakespeare's sources were likewise confused. By his reference to his mother (2.5.74), this Mortimer seems to be Edmund MORTIMER (2), actually his uncle and neither an earl nor in the royal line of descent. (However, Mortimer [2] appears in *1 Henry IV,* where the confusion continues and he is given this Mortimer's ancestors.) In his lifelong captivity, the character in *1 Henry VI* resembles both a historical cousin of his and a Lord Gray of Ruthven (a brother-in-law of the other Edmund Mortimer), both of whom died in prison late in life. The actual Edmund Mortimer, Earl of March, died a free man at the age of 36. His loyalty to the crown had been demonstrated. In 1415, his brother-in-law (and York's father), the Earl of CAMBRIDGE, plotted to kill King

HENRY V and place Mortimer on the throne. This was the attempt that is inaccurately described in *1 Henry VI.* In fact, Mortimer himself revealed the conspiracy when he learned of it, and Cambridge, with two others, was executed for treason. His sentencing is enacted in *Henry V,* 2.2, though Mortimer is not mentioned.

Mortimer (2), Edmund (1376–1409) Historical figure and character in *1 Henry IV,* a rebel against King HENRY IV. Originally an army commander for the King, Mortimer's capture by GLENDOWER is reported in 1.1. However, the King learns that Mortimer has married Glendower's daughter, and he refuses to ransom him. This becomes a bone of contention between the King and HOTSPUR—whose wife, LADY (10) Percy, is Mortimer's sister—as the revolt begins. Mortimer appears at the rebels' council of war in 3.1, where he proves to be a moderate negotiator among more difficult personalities. He attempts to maintain amity between Hotspur and Glendower. He tries to control Hotspur's temper, and he forthrightly defends his father-in-law against the firebrand's slurs. Mortimer can only speak to his bride, now LADY (8) Mortimer, through the translations of her father, for he speaks no Welsh and she no English. Nevertheless, he sentimentally asserts his love for her in an episode that lends humanity to the rebel cause.

Following errors in his sources, Shakespeare confused Mortimer with his nephew, another Edmund MORTIMER (1), who was Earl of MARCH and thus an heir to the English throne. The rebels speak of his claim several times (e.g., in 1.3.144–157 and 4.3.93–95) in making the case for their fight against Henry. Although an explicit intention to place him on the throne if their rebellion succeeds is not mentioned, Mortimer is to receive England in the division of the kingdom comtemplated at the war council.

The historical Mortimer had supported Henry's usurpation of the crown several years earlier, which Shakespeare depicted in *Richard II,* although Mortimer does not appear in that play. The rebels of 1403, depicted in *1 Henry IV,* intended to place the younger Mortimer on the throne, and this Mortimer acted in support of his nephew, as well as for Glendower. After SHREWSBURY, Mortimer and Glendower were pursued by the King, as Henry stipulates he will do in 5.5.40, and Mortimer died in the unsuccessful defence of Glendower's capital at Harlech in 1409.

Mortimer (3), Sir Hugh (d. 1460) Historical figure and minor character in *3 Henry VI,* an uncle and supporter of the Duke of YORK (8). In 1.2 Sir Hugh arrives with his brother, John MORTIMER (3), to offer aid to York before the battle of WAKEFIELD. Sir Hugh does not speak; the deaths of the brothers in the battle are reported in 1.4.2.

Mortimer (4), Sir John (d. 1460) Historical figure and minor character in *3 Henry VI,* an uncle and supporter of the Duke of YORK (8). In 1.2 Sir John arrives with his brother, Hugh MORTIMER (3), to offer aid to York before the battle of WAKEFIELD. Sir John speaks one line; the deaths of the brothers in the battle is reported in 1.4.2. The historical figures appear only as names in the death list of the battle, where they are mentioned as 'bastard uncles' of York.

Mortimer (5), Lady Character in *1 Henry IV.* See LADY (8).

Mortimer's Cross Location in *3 Henry VI,* an English village near Wales and a battle site of the WARS OF THE ROSES. A plain near Mortimer's Cross is the setting of 2.1, although the battle itself is not referred to. However, an incident from that conflict is depicted; a transient atmospheric effect causes an apparent tripling of the sun in the sky. This omen appears to Edward (see EDWARD IV) and Richard (see RICHARD III), who take it to signify future success. This improbable but historical phenomenon, a type of high-latitude mirage, was indeed seen during the battle, and it inspired Edward to adopt a stylised sun as his emblem.

Shakespeare omitted the battle, which Edward's forces won in February 1461 (historically, Richard was not present, being only nine years old), because he wished to present here a string of Yorkist losses, to be reversed by the battle of TOWTON, which closes the act.

Morton Minor character in *2 Henry IV,* follower of the Earl of NORTHUMBERLAND (1) and rebel against King HENRY IV. In 1.1 Morton arrives at WARKWORTH CASTLE with an eyewitness report—settling a distressing uncertainty—that the rebels have lost the battle of SHREWSBURY and that the Earl's son, HOTSPUR, has been killed by PRINCE (6) HAL. He then joins with Lord BARDOLPH (2) in rousing Northumberland from the despair this news causes him. In doing so, Morton announces (1.1.187–209) the plans of the ARCHBISHOP (3) of York, whose continuation of the rebellion will provide the central action of the rest of the play. Morton's account presents rebellion in terms of subverted religion that help to establish the play's disapproving attitude towards revolt (although Morton himself, as a rebel, finds it acceptable).

Moseley, Humphrey (d. 1661) English bookseller and publisher. In 1653 Moseley claimed the copyrights to a number of old plays whose manuscripts he had collected, including THE MERRY DEVIL OF EDMONTON, CARDENIO, HENRY I AND HENRY 2. In 1660 he added DUKE HUMPHREY, *King Stephen,* and *Iphis and Iantha, or a marriage without a man.* Only *The Merry Devil of Edmonton* has survived, but scholars agree almost unanimously that of these works, only *Cardenio* and

possibly *Duke Humphrey* are connected with Shakespeare.

Moseley was a successful publisher, becoming a high officer in the STATIONERS' COMPANY. He published the first collection of the plays of Francis BEAUMONT (2) and John FLETCHER (2), along with works by John MILTON and others.

Moth (1) (Mote) Character in *Love's Labour's Lost,* a page employed by the Spanish braggart ARMADO. Moth's quick wit is employed to ridicule his master, subtly to his face and blatantly behind his back. Moth appears only in scenes that function as set pieces, humorous sketches intended simply as entertainment. Moth is apparently an energetic teenager or child, small and slight of build. He is described as 'not so long by the head as *honorificabilitudinitatibus*' (5.1.39–40) (the longest word in Latin, and in Shakespeare). His name, pronounced 'mote' in Elizabethan English, suggests both the erratic flight of an insect and the elusiveness of a particle of dust. In the pageant of the Nine WORTHIES (5.2), he plays the infant Hercules. He is the vehicle for a number of the obscure topical jokes that make *Love's Labour's Lost* the most cryptic of Shakespeare's plays. He is believed to have been intended as a parody of the peppery Elizabethan pamphleteer and satirist Thomas NASHE.

Moth (2) Character in *A Midsummer Night's Dream,* a fairy attendant to the Fairy Queen TITANIA. In 3.1 Titania assigns Moth to the retinue of the comical rustic BOTTOM, whom the Fairy Queen has been magically induced to love. As the smallest and least important fairy in the group attending Bottom, Moth is never addressed by his temporary master and is given no particular task. His name means—and in Elizabethan English was pronounced—'mote' and suggests the tiny size of a speck of dust.

Mother Minor character in *Cymbeline,* the deceased parent of POSTHUMUS who appears to him as an apparition, in 5.4. The Mother appears with other ghosts: her husband, SICILIUS LEONATUS, and her two sons (see BROTHER [2]). Led by Sicilius, they plead with JUPITER for mercy on Posthumus. The Mother's part in this ritualistic solicitation is small; she points out that she died when she gave birth to Posthumus and left him an orphan; because of this, he deserves pity. She is a supernatural presence in an episode whose function is to create an air of eerie romance.

Mouldy, Ralph Minor character in *2 Henry IV,* a countryman enlisted by FALSTAFF in his capacity as an army recruiter in 3.2. After joking about his name, Falstaff drafts Mouldy over the man's objections. However, once recruited, Mouldy bribes Corporal BARDOLPH (1) to secure his own release from service, along with that of his friend Peter BULLCALF.

Mountjoy, Christopher (active 1598–1613) Wigmaker in LONDON, Shakespeare's landlord and the defendant in a lawsuit in which Shakespeare testified. In 1612 Mountjoy was sued by his son-in-law and former apprentice, Stephen BELOTT, who claimed that he had not been paid money promised him in his marriage agreement. Belott claimed that in 1604, in the course of the marriage negotiations, Shakespeare, then a lodger in the Mountjoy household, had told him on Mountjoy's behalf that his bride would receive a dowry of £60 plus household goods and that he would inherit £200 on Mountjoy's death. Shakespeare was summoned from STRATFORD in May 1612 to affirm or deny these assertions. He confirmed his residency with the Mountjoys in 1604 (he was probably there a year or two earlier, since he declared that he had first known both Mountjoy and Belott around 1602). He said that he had solicited Belott to marry Mountjoy's daughter at the request of the father, but that he did not remember the amount of the proposed dowry and that he knew nothing of a promised inheritance. The court turned the case over to the arbitration of the men's parish church, which criticised both men but awarded Belott a token payment, though Mountjoy evidently refused to pay it. The records of this episode reveal Shakespeare's London residence around 1602 to 1604 and that he had returned to Stratford by the spring of 1612, as well as offering a glimpse of the private life of the playwright at the period when he was writing *Othello, King Lear,* and the PROBLEM PLAYS.

Mountjoy was a French Huguenot refugee who was a 'tire-maker', or specialist in the elaborate bejewelled ornamental headgear worn by aristocratic women. He was a skilled craftsman in a rich and prestigious trade; he once made a tire for Queen ELIZABETH (1). His wife, Marie, also a Huguenot, was having an affair with a neighbouring cloth dealer during the period that Shakespeare was a lodger, as we know from the diary of the astrologer and physician Simon FORMAN, whom she consulted about a suspected pregnancy. The pregnancy may have been a false alarm or aborted, for she had no child. Shakespeare may have met the couple through his friend Richard FIELD (2), whose wife was also a Huguenot and who lived nearby.

After Marie's death in 1616, Mountjoy evidently took up 'a dissolute and unregulated life', as recorded by the French church. He feuded with his daughter and son-in-law, threatening them with disinheritance, thus sparking the lawsuit that involved Shakespeare.

Mousetrap, The See THE MURDER OF GONZAGO.

Mowbray (1), Thomas, Duke of Norfolk (c. 1365–1400) Historical figure and character in *Richard II,* an

enemy of BOLINGBROKE (1). The play opens with Bolingbroke's accusation to King RICHARD II that Mowbray has committed treason by embezzling military payrolls, engaging in unspecified plots, and, most important, having murdered the king's uncle, Thomas, Duke of GLOUCESTER (6). Mowbray hotly denies these charges, and a trial by combat is scheduled. In their vehement, fiery rhetoric, both contestants evoke the stylised pageantry of a medieval world that was remote even in Shakespeare's day and whose passing is a basic theme of the play. Before the trial by combat begins, in 1.3, two decidedly sympathetic characters, John of GAUNT and the DUCHESS (2) of Gloucester, the widow of the murdered duke, make it clear that Mowbray had in fact killed Gloucester and that he had done so on Richard's orders. The king, presumably hoping to avoid potential embarrassment, cancels the combat and banishes both disputants from England. Mowbray's response is again highly oratorical, but it contains one particularly distinctive passage (1.3.159–173), in which he regrets his departure to non-English-speaking lands, asserting a psychological dependence on the ability to express himself through language. This attitude surely reflects Shakespeare's own. Later CARLISLE declares (4.1.91–102) that Mowbray has died in Venice after fighting bravely against the Saracens in a Crusade.

The historical Mowbray, like Bolingbroke, belonged to a faction, headed by Gloucester, that had rebelled against Richard in the late 1380s, and, with Bolingbroke, he subsequently joined the king's party. When Richard was again opposed by Gloucester, in 1397, the king arrested his uncle and placed him in the custody of Mowbray, who commanded the English fortress at Calais. Gloucester died in prison, and, while it cannot be confirmed, 14th-century rumour and modern scholarship alike agree with Shakespeare that Mowbray most likely had the duke killed at the king's command. When he was expelled from England, Mowbray went on a pilgrimage to the Holy Land, but he did not fight there; the Crusades had ended a full century earlier.

Mowbray's son, Thomas MOWBRAY (2), later rebelled against his father's foe, when Bolingbroke had become HENRY IV. He was captured and executed in 1405, as is enacted in *2 Henry IV.*

Mowbray (2), Thomas, Lord (1386–1405) Historical figure and character in *2 Henry IV*, a rebel against King HENRY IV. An ally of the ARCHBISHOP (3) of York and Lord HASTINGS (2), Mowbray argues against accepting the peace offered by Prince John of LANCASTER (3) at GAULTREE FOREST in 4.1, but he is ignored. When Lancaster's offer proves treacherous, in 4.2, Mowbray is arrested with the others and sentenced to death. The historical Mowbray, not yet 20 years old when he was executed, was the son of Thomas MOWBRAY (1), whose quarrel with Henry BOLINGBROKE (1), later to become Henry IV, was enacted in *Richard II.*

Mucedorus Anonymous play formerly attributed to Shakespeare, part of the Shakespeare APOCRYPHA. *Mucedorus* is a comedy that burlesques pastoral romance and tales of chivalry. It was first published in 1598 by William JONES (4). It was extremely popular and was printed more often than any other work of ELIZABETHAN OR JACOBEAN DRAMA, yielding at least 17 editions by 1668. The play was sometimes ascribed to Shakespeare in the late 17th century, and it was included with *FAIR EM* and *THE MERRY DEVIL OF EDMONTON* in King Charles II's specially prepared collection of Shakespeare's plays. Apparently this ascription is made on the strength of the title pages beginning with the third edition (1610), which stated that the play had been staged by the KING'S MEN. Shakespeare therefore knew the work, and its depiction of a forest-dwelling 'wild man' may have influenced the creation of CALIBAN. However, no modern scholar believes Shakespeare wrote *Mucedorus,* for it is a crude drama that is beneath the standard of even the least of Shakespeare's work. Its authorship remains uncertain, though it is perhaps most frequently given to Thomas LODGE.

Much Ado About Nothing

SYNOPSIS

Act 1, Scene 1

A MESSENGER (14) tells LEONATO, governor of MESSINA, that Don PEDRO, Prince of Aragon, is approaching. He reports the prince's victories in war and tells of the knightly accomplishments of CLAUDIO (1), a young gentleman in Don Pedro's court. Leonato's niece, BEATRICE, asks about another gentleman, BENEDICK; she responds to the Messenger's good report with sharp raillery, which Leonato explains as part of an ongoing rivalry of wits between his niece and the young nobleman. Don Pedro arrives, accompanied by the two young men and his brother, DON JOHN (1). Benedick and Beatrice exchange humorous insults, each of them asserting an extreme aversion to love, particularly for the other. Leonato offers a special welcome to Don John, who has lately been reconciled with his brother. Most of the group departs, leaving Claudio and Benedick alone; Claudio confesses that he has fallen in love with Leonato's daughter, HERO, and wishes to marry her; Benedick derides marriage. Don Pedro returns, and Benedick reveals Claudio's desire. Don Pedro teases Benedick, predicting that he will fall in love one day. Then he helpfully offers to court Hero himself, disguised as Claudio at the MASQUE scheduled for that evening; once assured of Hero's response, he will approach her father on Claudio's behalf.

Act 1, Scene 2
Leonato's brother, ANTONIO (3), reports that a servant has overheard Don Pedro telling Claudio of his intention to marry Hero.

Act 1, Scene 3
Don John complains to his attendant CONRADE of his bitter melancholy. Conrade replies that he should disguise his attitude to preserve his newly restored place in Don Pedro's court. Don John asserts that he can only be himself and that he wishes to be a villain, spreading discontent. Another follower, BORACHIO, brings news of Don Pedro's plan to woo Hero on Claudio's behalf. Don John proposes to make mischief with this information, hurting Claudio, whose advancement he envies.

Act 2, Scene 1
Beatrice acidly compares the ferociously silent Don John to the overly talkative Benedick. Leonato asserts that her attitude towards men will prevent her from getting a husband. He then reminds Hero to respond to the prince's expected wooing, though Beatrice wittily preaches against marriage. Don Pedro and his courtiers arrive for the festivities, and all the participants put on masks. Don Pedro takes Hero aside as other couples flirt. Benedick and Beatrice, in disguise, trade insults, supposedly stating other people's opinions. Don John tells Claudio that he has heard the prince courting Hero. Claudio is shocked, believing that Don Pedro is stealing his prospective bride. He leaves embittered. When Don Pedro appears, Benedick berates him for betraying Claudio, but the prince assures him that he means well by their friend. The talk turns to Beatrice, and Benedick reveals that he is angered and hurt by her sharply expressed disdain for him. Claudio and Beatrice appear, and Benedick leaves. Don Pedro tells Claudio that he has arranged his marriage to Hero, and Claudio rejoices. Beatrice leaves, and the prince reveals a plan to Leonato and Claudio: he will trick Benedick and Beatrice into falling in love with each other.

Act 2, Scene 2
Borachio proposes to Don John a scheme to thwart Claudio's marriage: he, Borachio, will recruit Hero's waiting-woman, MARGARET (2), to disguise herself as Hero and admit him into Hero's window that night. If Don John, pretending concern for Claudio's honour, can get him and Don Pedro to witness this charade, they will believe that Hero has a lover and Claudio will repudiate her.

Act 2, Scene 3
In the garden Benedick reflects on the seductiveness of love. When Don Pedro, Claudio, and Leonato appear, he hides himself in an arbour. They see him, and, following Don Pedro's plan, they speak loudly about Beatrice's passionate love for him. They profess to be reluctant to tell him of her ardour, knowing his hostility towards her. They leave, and Benedick observes that he has misjudged matters and that he will marry Beatrice. Beatrice appears to summon him to dinner. She says that she dislikes her errand and leaves, but Benedick comically imagines that he sees double meanings in her words that prove her love.

Act 3, Scene 1
URSULA, a waiting-woman, is sent to tell Beatrice that Hero and Margaret are talking about her in the garden. As expected, Beatrice eavesdrops on the two, and they speak loudly of Benedick's passion for her, praising him highly as they do so. They profess reluctance to tell her this news, fearing her mockery. They leave, and Beatrice decides that she will return Benedick's love, and she looks forward to happiness with him.

Act 3, Scene 2
Don Pedro and Claudio tease Benedick about his changed appearance, saying that he must be in love. He claims toothache, but he takes Leonato aside to speak privately, presumably about marrying Beatrice. Don John appears and tells Claudio and Don Pedro of Hero's infidelity, offering to prove the truth of his accusation that night.

Act 3, Scene 3
The rustic Constable DOGBERRY, assisted by VERGES, assembles the WATCHMEN (3) for their nightly patrol. In a comically confused passage they assert that all sorts of disorder and dereliction are proper procedures. Then Conrade and Borachio appear. Borachio describes the success of his plan to deceive Claudio and tells of Claudio's determination to disgrace Hero at the wedding. The Watchmen, though perplexed, realise that some villainy has been committed and they arrest the two men.

Act 3, Scene 4
Margaret and Hero tease Beatrice about her seeming love sickness.

Act 3, Scene 5
Leonato, late for Hero's wedding, interrupts Dogberry's comically long-winded account of Conrade and Borachio. He tells Dogberry to interrogate the prisoners and submit a written report.

Act 4, Scene 1
During the marriage ceremony, Claudio rejects Hero, asserting that he has witnessed her rendezvous with a lover. This report is confirmed by Don Pedro, and even Leonato believes it. Hero faints, and Claudio and Don Pedro leave. Leonato rages at her, wishing she were dead, but FRIAR (2) Francis, who had been officiating at the wedding, calms Leonato and states his belief in Hero's innocence. Beatrice and Benedick also support her, and Leonato recovers his faith in his daughter. The Friar suggests that they

pretend that Hero has died, thus silencing gossip and possibly stirring Claudio to grief and reviving his love. Then, if Hero is not exonerated, she can at least be secretly transferred to a nunnery. Leonato and the Friar leave, taking Hero into seclusion. Beatrice and Benedick reveal their feelings for each other, but Beatrice demands that Benedick prove his love by challenging Claudio to a duel in support of Hero. He agrees to do so.

Act 4, Scene 2
Dogberry tries to interrogate Conrade and Borachio, but his comical ineptitude spurs the SEXTON to take over. He questions the Watchmen, who tell of Don John's plot. The Sexton, knowing about the abortive wedding and aware that Don John has fled from Messina, realises that this story is true. He orders the prisoners bound and taken to Leonato, and he goes to report what he has learned. Conrade insults Dogberry, who responds with humorously pompous self-praise.

Act 5, Scene 1
Leonato and Antonio berate Claudio and Don Pedro, exiting just as Benedick arrives. Benedick challenges Claudio to a duel and leaves, declaring that they will fight later. Dogberry arrives with his prisoners, and Borachio confesses all. Leonato returns, having been told the truth by the Sexton, and Claudio begs his forgiveness, promising to perform any penance. Leonato states that he must publicly mourn Hero and then marry Hero's cousin. Claudio assents.

Act 5, Scene 2
Benedick tells Beatrice of his challenge to Claudio, and they tease each other on the subject of love. Ursula tells them that Don John's plot has been exposed.

Act 5, Scene 3
Claudio reads an epitaph for Hero at Leonato's family crypt, believing that she is buried in it. BALTHASAR (4) completes the rite with a mournful song. Don Pedro comes to escort Claudio to his wedding to Hero's cousin.

Act 5, Scene 4
Benedick receives Leonato's permission to marry Beatrice. Claudio prepares to marry the veiled cousin, who reveals herself to be Hero. Benedick and Beatrice cannot bring themselves to admit their love for each other, returning to their barbed wit, but Claudio produces a love poem that Benedick has written about Beatrice and Hero presents a similar lyric by Beatrice about Benedick. Exposed, Beatrice and Benedick agree to be married. As plans are made for a double wedding, word comes that Don John has been apprehended. Benedick promises to devise some suitable punishment, but he turns to celebration in the meantime. The assembled people dance.

COMMENTARY

Much Ado About Nothing shares a theme common to Shakespearean COMEDY: a romance is disrupted, but love triumphs. However, unlike such earlier works as *The Two Gentlemen of Verona* and *A Midsummer Night's Dream*, this play is a comedy of character, rather than of situation; its major development—the defeat of the threat to romantic happiness—comes about through a psychological change on the part of the major characters, rather than through changes in their circumstances. While elaborate and melodramatic coincidences bring the play to its climax, that climax—Beatrice and Benedick's commitment to each other—is one of personal crisis and response.

The conflict between Beatrice and Benedick is the central element of the play, although it is sometimes seen as a SUB-PLOT, being humorous and lacking the villainous interference that adds suspense to the story of Hero and Claudio. The two scorners of love are unquestionably the brightest and most vital characters in the play, and their lively battle of wits engages much of our attention. It is introduced before Claudio and Hero even meet, and Claudio's feebly motivated love at first sight has none of its appeal. The comic trap that brings the former foes together holds our interest in the second half of the play; the tale of the foolish Claudio and his passively victimised lover seems most important as the stimulus for the growing trust between Beatrice and Benedick, who are much more fully developed characters.

The gulf that at first separates Beatrice and Benedick is not created by any outside interference; rather, the lovers themselves have established it. We are immediately aware that they love each other, despite their protestations to the contrary: in 1.1 Beatrice cannot refrain from asking after Benedick's fate in battle, though she affects scorn in doing so, and Benedick thinks first of Beatrice as a model with which to compare Hero (unfavourably) when he mocks Claudio's intention to marry. Beatrice and Benedick have apparently quarrelled in the past; she speaks of 'our last conflict' (1.1.59) and implies an earlier unhappy romance in 2.1.261–264. He is overly sensitive to her criticism, declaring himself unable to abide her company in 2.1.257–258. These hints lead us to believe that both parties are trying to protect themselves against a repetition of their previous unhappiness.

Thus their relationship develops in a way that makes it stirringly real. When Don Pedro's plot makes them fall in love with each other, it seems entirely appropriate and their responses are convincing. Each, once convinced of the other's love, accepts affection and reciprocates it. Their reactions are both comical and humanly touching, as they half-heartedly attempt to disguise their new feelings with transparent complaints of toothache (3.2.20) and head cold (3.4.40).

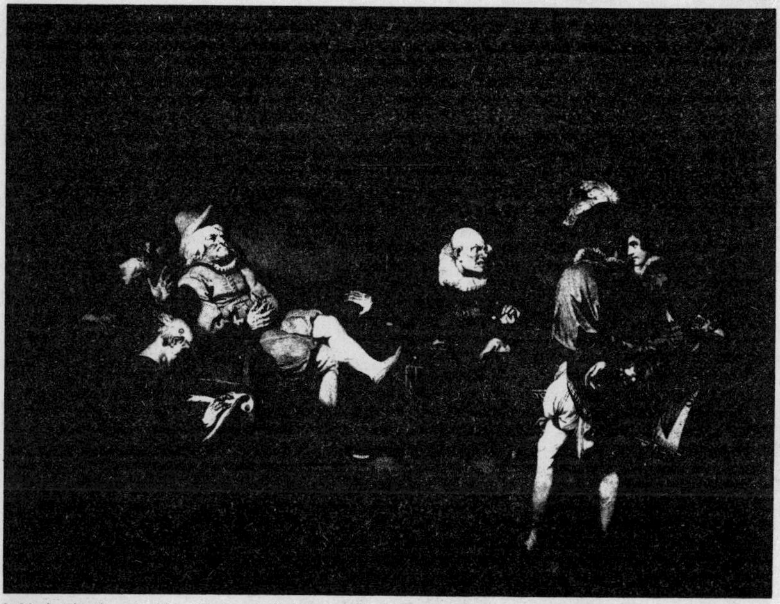

In Much Ado About Nothing *4.2, the comically inept constable Dogberry attempts an interrogation of Borachio and Conrade.* (Courtesy of Culver Pictures, Inc.)

When their friends tease them, we feel a pleasurable sense of escape, seeing on stage, at a safe distance, a kind of foolishness to which we ourselves might be susceptible.

The reaction of these vital and good-humoured figures to the denunciation of Hero lies at the moral heart of the play. The scene of Hero's rejection in church (4.1), which alludes to such religious concepts as 'grace' and 'damnation' (4.1.171, 172), presents a crisis of spiritual values. Beatrice acts on her faith in her cousin, and Benedick acts on his faith in Beatrice. This involvement in a serious issue brings them together utterly, completing the work of their friends' earlier ploys. This process permits them to return to the world of normal relations, where earlier they had isolated themselves from it.

Although Beatrice and Benedick dominate the play—significantly, it was long known by the title 'Beatrice and Benedick'—Claudio and Hero reinforce their lesson of love and faith. While these lovers are undeniably shallower than Benedick and Beatrice, this very fact makes them effective in their own way. Hero and Claudio are conformists who believe in the romantic norms that their more spirited friends reject. Their conventionality supports the comic tone of the play by preventing our emotional or sentimental involvement in their situation.

Hero is a typically pliant and acquiescent young Elizabethan woman. She shows no interest in Claudio until Don Pedro tells her that she is betrothed to him. She is mildly charming, and she is spirited enough to help trick Beatrice into loving Benedick, but she is mostly a docile participant in an arranged marriage. Claudio plays a more prominent role; if Benedick and Beatrice must learn that their opposition to love is a false sentiment, Claudio must also be freed from the naïve pseudo-love that he at first declares for Hero, an emotion not grounded in experience. Claudio has often been condemned as a cad, a mere cardboard figure, or both. However, he should be taken at his word when he professes love for Hero; even as he rejects her, he does so in sorrow, regretting that his love has been disappointed. His vicious attempt to humiliate Hero reflects the extent of his hurt. More-

over, as a conventional young man, Claudio is concerned about the offence to his honour—and to that of his prince, Don Pedro—caused by what he believes to be a plot to foist a promiscuous bride on him. While this consideration is almost meaningless today, it will have been appreciated by Elizabethan audiences, and thus we should recognise that, while Claudio is plainly foolish and gullible, he may reasonably plead in his own defence that he has sinned 'but in mistaking' (5.1. 269).

His repentance at Hero's supposed tomb is often criticised as cynical, too slight and superficial to be taken seriously, but the text of the scene (5.3) offers no justification for this view; it presents a solemn, if brief, ritual of grief and atonement, followed by a formal quatrain, spoken by Don Pedro (5.3.24–27), that invokes hope for the future. However, even though Claudio is properly repentant, he remains uninteresting and it is fitting that he and Hero are simply ignored at the end of the play, when attention turns to Benedick and Beatrice.

Don John is also a conventional figure, a 'plain-dealing villain' (1.3.30), for whom 'any bar, any cross, any impediment will be medicinable to me' (2.2.4–5). His true nature is hidden even from his brother, Don Pedro, even though he has recently rebelled against him. (In 16th-century melodrama, the evil of a villain often remains unknown to his victims until he is overtly exposed.) He is a plot device more than a truly complex character—a sort of anti-comic symbol who opposes the happy ending. Such a mechanical villain is necessary, because a true villain, like RICHARD III or IAGO, would destroy the comic assurance that all will be well for the crossed lovers. Significantly, Don John is not present at the final reconciliation, for his nature is utterly at odds with it.

Much Ado's central plot device is the readiness of the characters to accept error and misinformation: Don John's false presentation of Hero is merely the most important incident in a series of erroneous reports and misunderstandings. While Don John maliciously misleads his intended victims, Don Pedro benevolently tricks Benedick and Beatrice. Dogberry is fully capable of confusing himself and everyone else.

Disguise, another source of error, is also a prominent motif. At the MASQUE in 2.1, Beatrice and Benedick converse in masks, and their dialogue, more vitriolic than usual, marks the extreme extent of their hostility. In the same scene Claudio is pretending to be Benedick when Don John tells him that Don Pedro loves Hero. More important, the play turns on Margaret's use of a disguise, Hero's clothes, as part of Don John's plot to slander Hero. This episode is lent further mystery by being only reported (twice—by Borachio in 3.3 and, slightly differently, by Claudio in 4.1) and not actually shown on stage.

The theme of error and confusion is also enhanced by various other dramatic devices. Prominent is the repeated importance of overhearing, an act that lends itself to misinterpretation and error. Don Pedro's plan to help Claudio woo Hero is overheard and misunderstood by Antonio's servant, as is retold by Antonio in 1.2, and it is also overheard—correctly but with malice—by Borachio, leading to Don John's first piece of villainy. Don John's scheme involves the invention of another overheard conversation, with which he deceives Claudio. Don Pedro uses overhearing benevolently to convince Beatrice and Benedick that each is loved by the other, and the Watchmen overhear Borachio's account of Don John's second villainy, leading to the eventual exposure of his plot. The frequent recurrence of this motif lends strength to the role of luck and timing in the comedy's gratifying resolution.

The very title of the play may contain a pun on this subject, for 'nothing' was probably pronounced like 'noting', which in Elizabethan English could mean 'overhearing' or 'eavesdropping'. This possibility seems to be supported by the wordplay in 1.1.150–152 and 2.3.157. The casual title serves a thematic purpose in any case, affirming the play's comic nature by implying that the lovers' trials will prove in the end to have been of no consequence.

The various plots of *Much Ado* are intricately interwoven in a fabric that both suggests and reinforces the complex confusions that are central to the play. From the beginning our attention is repeatedly transferred from one set of lovers to the other. One plot is conventionally melodramatic, while the other is a series of clever rejections of conventional romance; each of these qualities contradicts the other, preventing a single tone from dominating. The Claudio-Hero plot is written entirely in verse, whereas Beatrice and Benedick spar in particularly loose and lively prose. (An exception, Beatrice's lyrical outburst when she hears that Benedick loves her [3.1.107–116], is sometimes seen as evidence that Shakespeare adapted *Much Ado* from a lost play in verse, [see 'Sources of the Play'] though it is just as likely to have been intended as a sign of her sudden receptivity to romance.)

While the two stories are thus antithetical in some ways, they are similar in others. Both plots feature heroes who err in renouncing their lovers out of pride in both cases—Benedick's pride of overvalued independence, Claudio's pride required by a conventional sense of honour. Both men, however, are plainly going to end up married. Similarly, Beatrice and Hero are alike in destiny and opposed in personality. The two stories combine when they both come to their dissimilar climaxes in 4.1. In fact, Claudio's rejection of Hero sparks the co-operation and trust between Beatrice and Benedick.

Other features of plotting emphasise the play's confusions. Strikingly, Don John's villainy is first spent on a scheme that goes nowhere, the attempt to make

Claudio believe that Don Pedro is taking Hero for himself. This ruse makes us aware of important aspects of both the villain and his victim. Similarly, the third plot element, that of Dogberry and his Watchmen, is also full of confusion. But it is handled with a precision that makes *Much Ado* respected as among the most deftly plotted of Shakespeare's works. Dogberry's Watchmen appear exactly at the crucial moment when Don John's second, more potent villainy has been unfolded to us, though not to its victims. When the Watchmen overhear Borachio and Conrade, we are assured that Hero will be exonerated. Yet Dogberry's comical ineptitude ensures that she won't be cleared immediately, and the lovers' stories are allowed to continue to their resolutions.

Thus hints of tragedy alternate with comical reassurances. We learn the truth while the characters operate in ignorance of it; thus we laugh, preserving the comic nature of the play. Our emotions are insulated from the distress that the deluded characters would evoke in a tragedy or in real life. Nevertheless, the melodrama of Hero's unjust disgrace, shockingly brutal because it is set at her wedding, forbids escapism. Like the later PROBLEM PLAYS, *Much Ado* has the capacity to disturb, and we are morally engaged. The happiness that is finally attained is made more valuable by the difficulty with which it is achieved. At the end, though, as in *The Merchant of Venice,* these hardships are forgotten, and love and happiness prevail. The final reconciliation stems from the essential goodness of the world of Leonato's court: its denizens are cheerfully at home with each other, too witty to be sentimental and too kind to be unfeeling. While Claudio and Don Pedro prove vulnerable to Don John's manipulations, their error is rectified. Evil is undone through the redeeming power of love and faith and through the timely grace of chance. We can agree with Benedick when he says, 'man is a giddy thing, and this is my conclusion' (5.4.107), but perhaps it is Dogberry who most truly, if unwittingly, states the play's nature when he chastises Borachio, asserting, 'Thou wilt be condemned into everlasting redemption' (4.2.53–54).

SOURCES OF THE PLAY

The main plot of *Much Ado About Nothing* is an example of an old European tradition—dating at least to late classical times—of stories in which a lover is deceived into believing that his beloved is unfaithful. Shakespeare drew on a version that first appeared in Ludovico ARIOSTO's massive poem *Orlando Furioso,* which he may have known in both an Italian edition (probably that of 1532) and the English translation by Sir John HARINGTON (1591). He also used another Italian rendering, itself an adaptation of Ariosto, a story by Matteo BANDELLO that was published in a 1554 collection. Between the two Italian texts, most of the details of Claudio's courtship of Hero, its villainous thwarting, and the final happy reunion of the protagonists are foreshadowed. An English version of Ariosto's story, in George WHETSTONE's collection of tales *The Rocke of Regard* (1576), may have suggested Claudio's rejection of Hero at her own wedding.

Some scholars have argued that Shakespeare modified an earlier play to create *Much Ado,* but this viewpoint is highly speculative and largely unpopular, particularly since no existing text is offered as the missing source, although the mysterious LOVE'S LABOUR'S WON is sometimes suggested.

Ariosto and derivative texts account only for the Hero-Claudio plot, while it is the other plots in *Much Ado*—the romance of Benedick and Beatrice and the crucial intervention of the comical constabulary—which make the play a comedy; the older works are straight melodramas. Dogberry is certainly a Shakespearean original, in that no particular literary source provides a forerunner. However, humorous constables—characterised by confused speech and ludicrous logic—were a very old theatrical staple. Indeed, Shakespeare had already used the type in a more minor character, Constable DULL, of *Love's Labour's Lost.* Just as important as any model for Dogberry, in all probability, was Shakespeare's awareness of the on-stage personality of Will KEMPE, the actor for whom the role was written.

As witty scorners of romance, Beatrice and Benedick are also part of a tradition that was well established in the 16th century, but an important stimulus probably came from the Italian Baldassare CASTIGLIONE's *The Book of the Courtier* (1528), one of the most important and widely read works of the time. Shakespeare almost certainly read it, either in Italian or in the popular English translation by Thomas HOBY (1) (1561, three eds. by 1588). Castiglione presents an ideal of courtly life that included the revolutionary idea that women had much to contribute to it. To illustrate this point, he composed a series of sprightly debates between a man and a woman that may well have inspired the verbal sparring between Beatrice and Benedick.

TEXT OF THE PLAY

Much Ado About Nothing is thought to have been written in mid- or late 1598, although this date cannot be proven. Francis MERES omits *Much Ado* from his list of Shakespearean comedies, published in the summer of 1598 (though it is sometimes maintained that the title LOVE'S LABOUR'S WON refers to *Much Ado*). Meres' omission suggests that the play did not exist when he wrote, although he may simply have omitted it. However, a late date is supported by the fact that the play was registered with the STATIONERS' COMPANY in 1600 as 'to be stayed'—that is, *not* to be published. This ploy was generally associated with new work, being an attempt to protect a currently

popular play from piracy by unlicensed publishers. Still, even if *Much Ado* was a recent success in 1600, it was certainly written somewhat earlier, for Will KEMPE, for whom the role of Dogberry was written, left Shakespeare's company, the CHAMBERLAIN'S MEN, in January or February 1599.

The company apparently sold the rights to Andrew WISE and William ASPLEY, for they published a QUARTO edition of the play (known as Q) late in 1600. This text was probably printed (by Valentine SIMMES) from Shakespeare's own manuscript, or FOUL PAPERS, as is evidenced by casual stage directions, some of which name the actors who played Dogberry and Verges, and some of which name INNOGEN, a GHOST CHARACTER.

The next publication of the play was in the FIRST FOLIO of 1623, where it was printed from a copy of Q that had been partially amended, particularly with respect to stage directions. The Folio also made two brief cuts in the play, probably to avoid offending the court or violating the 1606 statute against profanity (see CENSORSHIP). The two texts remain very similar, and modern editions are based on both.

THEATRICAL HISTORY OF THE PLAY

The 1600 edition of *Much Ado About Nothing* asserts that the play had been 'sundrie times publikely acted'. Although it was not reprinted between 1600 and 1623, it is evident that *Much Ado About Nothing* was immediately popular, for many references to it have survived from the early 17th century. When Leonard DIGGES (2) compared the popularity of the plays of Shakespeare and JONSON in 1640, he observed, 'let but Beatrice and Benedick be seen, lo, in a trice the Cockpit, Galleries, Boxes, all are full'. Several performances at the court of King JAMES I are recorded, among them a presentation at the wedding festivities of Princess ELIZABETH (3) in 1613. Later, King Charles I was sufficiently familiar with the play to amend the table of contents of his copy of the Second Folio (1632) by changing its name to 'Benedik and Betrice' (sic).

In the Restoration period William DAVENANT owned the rights to produce the play, but he merged it with *Measure for Measure* in *THE LAW AGAINST LOVERS* (1662). Another production of *Much Ado* itself is not recorded until 1721, when John RICH (2) revived it, restaging it several times over the next quarter-century. The play was again cannibalised in two popular adaptations of this period: *LOVE IN A FOREST* (1723) by Charles JOHNSON (2), a rendering of *As You Like It*, contained bits of *Much Ado;* and James MILLER (1) combined Shakespeare's play with one by Molière in 1737.

Much Ado was very popular throughout the rest of the 18th century and has remained so ever since. David GARRICK played Benedick many times between 1748 and 1776, and it was often said to be his best role. Among the notable Benedicks of the 19th century were Charles KEMBLE (1) and Henry IRVING; Beatrice was principally associated with two actresses, first Helen FAUCIT and then Ellen TERRY (2). Hector BERLIOZ wrote an opera—*Béatrice et Bénédict* (1862)—based on *Much Ado;* it omitted the Claudio-Hero plot.

Among the most notable of many 20th-century productions of *Much Ado* have been John GIELGUD's highly successful London presentation of 1949, revived in 1950, 1952, and 1955; Franco ZEFFIRELLI's production of 1965; Joseph PAPP's 1972 New York version, set in the turn-of-the-century United States, and a more conventional presentation of 1988; and the 1976 STRATFORD staging by John BARTON (1), set in British India. The play has been a film four times—once in the United States before the advent of sound (1926), once in East Germany (1963), and twice (1956, 1973) in the Soviet Union. Several recent productions have been adapted for TELEVISION, including Zeffirelli's (1967) and Papp's (1973).

Munday, Anthony (c. 1560–1633) English playwright, author of a possible influence on Shakespeare and a co-author of SIR THOMAS MORE. Munday, originally a printer apprenticed to John ALLDE, turned to acting but was unsuccessful—he appeared with OXFORD'S MEN in the late 1570s and early 1580s. He began a notorious career as a hack writer with a series of anti-Catholic tracts (c. 1578–1580). His first book was *Zelauto* (1580), a novel written in imitation of John LYLY's famed *Euphues.* Its treatment of usury and Jews may have influenced *The Merchant of Venice.* Between 1594 and 1602 he wrote plays for the ADMIRAL'S MEN. Three of these works have survived: *John à Kent and John à Cumber* (1594) may have suggested elements of the comic sub-plot of *A Midsummer Night's Dream,* and a pair of plays on Robin Hood (both 1598) may have influenced *As You Like It.* Francis MERES referred to Munday as one of England's leading comic dramatists. Munday also wrote numerous plays, including SIR JOHN OLDCASTLE, in collaboration with others. He was probably the principal author of *Sir Thomas More,* which contains a scene by Shakespeare.

Murder of Gonzago, The Playlet presented within *Hamlet.* In 3.2 Prince HAMLET arranges for the PLAYERS (2) to perform *The Murder of Gonzago* for his uncle, the KING (5). The plot of the playlet resembles the actual murder of Hamlet's father by the King, and Hamlet expects the King's response to reveal his guilt. For this reason, he refers to the brief play as *The Mousetrap* (3.2.232).

First, in a DUMB SHOW, a man pours poison in the ear of a sleeping king and then consoles his grieving queen, exiting with her. Then, in dialogue, the PLAYER KING denies the PLAYER QUEEN's assertion that she would not remarry if he died. In the next scene, LUCIANUS, said by Hamlet to be 'nephew to the King' (3.2.

239), poisons the sleeping Player King in his ear, just as the real King had poisoned Hamlet's father. The play has its intended effect at this point, as the King flees the room; the performance is never completed.

Hamlet speaks of a source for *The Murder of Gonzago*—which he calls 'the image of a murder done in Vienna' (3.2.233)—as 'extant, and written in very choice Italian' (3.2.256–257), but if such a document existed, scholars have not discovered it. However, the murder of Hamlet's father—and thus the playlet—is clearly based on a real murder, committed in Italy in 1538 (see *Hamlet*, 'Sources of the Play').

Murderer See FIRST MURDERER; SECOND MURDERER; THIRD MURDERER.

Murellus Character in *Julius Caesar*. See MARULLUS.

Musicians (1) Minor characters in *The Two Gentlemen of Verona*, players hired by THURIO to assist him in wooing SILVIA by performing a SONG in her honour.

Musicians (2) Minor characters in *Romeo and Juliet*, three players hired by PARIS (2) to provide music at his wedding to JULIET (1). However, Juliet is found apparently dead, and they are not needed. They are then accosted by the servant PETER (2), who demands free music and engages them in a comic exchange (4.5. 100–141). Their names, Simon Catling, Hugh Rebeck, and James Soundpost, indicate the instruments they play. A catling is a small, lutelike string instrument; a rebec, an early violin; a soundpost, for the singer in the group, is an internal component of a string instrument.

Musicians (3) Minor characters in *The Merchant of Venice*, servants of PORTIA (1). The Musicians appear in two important episodes. In 3.2 their song 'Tell me where is Fancy bred' provides an interlude that heightens the suspense as BASSANIO contemplates his fateful choice among the three caskets, and it also makes a point about the nature of beauty. Further, it may offer Bassanio a clue as to which casket to select. In 5.1 the Musicians add to the romantic charm of BELMONT, dissipating the disturbing and anxious atmosphere of the preceding courtroom scene. Musicians were a normal feature of a wealthy household in Shakespeare's day.

Musicians (4) Minor characters in *2 Henry IV*. In 2.4 the Musicians, led by SNEAK, perform for FALSTAFF at his drunken dinner with the HOSTESS (2) and DOLL TEARSHEET at the BOAR'S HEAD TAVERN.

Musicians (5) Minor characters in *Much Ado About Nothing*, entertainers hired by LEONATO. In 5.3 the Musicians accompany BALTHASAR (4) when he sings the mournful SONG 'Pardon, Goddess of the night' as CLAUDIO (1) grieves at HERO's tomb, believing her dead. They may also accompany 'Sigh no more, ladies' in 2.3, though the stage direction is ambiguous. Musicians were a normal feature of a grand household in Elizabethan times, and their presence here helps to maintain the splendidly festive atmosphere of Leonato's court.

Musicians (6) Minor characters in *Othello* (6), strolling players hired by CASSIO to serenade OTHELLO, with whom he is out of favour. Cassio's gesture is rejected, however, when Othello's CLOWN (6) pays them to leave, saying 'If you have any music that may not be heard, to 't again, but . . . to hear music, the general does not greatly care' (3.1.15–17). The Clown jests lewdly on the sexual symbolism of their instruments and associates them with venereal disease, suggesting a criticism of the courtly flattery their performance represents.

Musicians (7) Minor characters in *Cymbeline*, players who serenade IMOGEN for CLOTEN. One of the Musicians sings the song, 'Hark, hark, the lark' (2.3.19–25), but otherwise they do not speak and leave as soon as they have completed their performance. The episode offers a musical diversion that is appropriate to a comedy. It also relieves the sense of menace from the previous scene—IACHIMO's trespass in Imogen's bedchamber—and from the approach of Cloten. Additionally, it provides time for Imogen to change her costume from nightclothes to daytime garb.

Mustardseed Character in *A Midsummer Night's Dream*, a fairy attendant to the Fairy Queen, TITANIA. Titania assigns Mustardseed to the retinue of the comical rustic BOTTOM, whom the Queen has been magically induced to love. Bottom has been endowed by PUCK with the head of an ass, but he does not know of his new adornment, and Mustardseed serves him by helping to scratch his strangely itching face. The fairy's name suggests the several references to the tiny mustard seed in the Gospels (e.g., Luke 17:6).

Mutius Minor character in *Titus Andronicus*, a son of TITUS (1) Andronicus. In 1.1 Mutius is killed by his father during the dispute with BASSIANUS over LAVINIA. His murder is symptomatic of a flaw in Titus, whose sense of honour can lead him to such a crime.

Myrmidon Any of several minor characters in *Troilus and Cressida*, followers of the Greek warrior ACHILLES. In 5.7 Achilles orders the Myrmidons to avoid combat in order to save themselves for a confrontation with HECTOR, and when the Trojan leader is encountered without his armour on, in 5.8, the Myrmidons kill him. The episode, presenting an ex-

treme of unchivalrous behaviour, caps the play's picture of the dishonour of war in general and of the TROJAN WAR in particular.

In the *Iliad* of HOMER, the Myrmidons were an ethnically distinct group of soldiers from Thessaly, in what is now north-eastern Greece; they were named for a legendary ancestor, Myrmidon. Like Achilles, the Myrmidons came from beyond the world of ancient Hellenic civilisation and were seen as somewhat barbaric and cruel by the more cosmopolitan Greeks. This attitude survives in Shakespeare's presentation.

Mytilene City on the Greek island of Lesbos, a location for several scenes of *Pericles.* MARINA, the lost daughter of PERICLES, is sold to a brothel in Mytilene in 4.2, and she remains there in 4.5 and 4.6. In 5.1, when she has escaped the brothel but remains in Mytilene, her father arrives there and they are reunited. Marina later marries the Governor of Mytilene, LYSIMACHUS. Shakespeare followed his sources in placing these episodes in Mytilene, and no specific attributes of the city are referred to in the text. The historical Mytilene was a minor port city of the Aegean Sea, famous chiefly as the home of the poet Sappho (active c. 590 B.C.).

Mytilenian Sailor Character in *Pericles.* See TYRIAN SAILOR.

N

Nash (1), Anthony (d. 1622) Farmer in STRATFORD and friend of Shakespeare. Nash was a wealthy farmer who witnessed several business deals made by Shakespeare and managed some of his farm lands. He and his innkeeper brother John (d. 1623) were among the seven close friends to whom the playwright willed money to buy a commemorative ring. His eldest son was Thomas NASH (2), later the husband of Shakespeare's grand-daughter.

Nash (2), Thomas (1593–1647) First husband of Shakespeare's grand-daughter Elizabeth HALL (3). The son of Shakespeare's friend Anthony NASH (1), Thomas Nash may have been acquainted with the playwright as a child. He married Elizabeth Hall in 1626. They probably lived at first in his home, next door to the Shakespeare-Hall home at NEW PLACE. (Known as Nash's House, it is today maintained as a museum by the Shakespeare BIRTHPLACE Trust.) The couple were living in New Place, however, at the time of Nash's death. Nash was a lawyer, but he did not practise after inheriting his father's fortune. He also owned an inn in STRATFORD, inherited from an uncle. He was a committed Royalist in the Civil Wars. At their outset in 1642, he was noted as by far the greatest Stratford contributor of money to the king's cause, and in 1643 he hosted the harried Queen Henrietta Marie at New Place. At his death he willed Nash's House to his wife; he bequeathed New Place to another relative, but Elizabeth and her mother, Susanna SHAKESPEARE (14) Hall, fought the will in court and won.

Nashe (Nash), Thomas (1567–c. 1601) English writer, author of the earliest specific reference to a Shakespeare play and of minor sources for *Hamlet* and *All's Well That Ends Well.* In addition, he may be a model for the character MOTH (1) in *Love's Labour's Lost.* Nashe's popular satirical pamphlet *Pierce Penniless His Supplication to the Devil* (1592) influenced several passages in *Hamlet,* especially HAMLET's remarks on drunkenness in 1.4.16–38. *Pierce Penniless* also contains a reference to the popularity of TALBOT in *1 Henry VI,* the earliest surviving literary remark on a particular Shakespearean work (though Nashe does not mention either title or playwright). An episode in Nashe's novel *The Unfortunate Traveller* (1594) may have influenced the exposure of PAROLLES in 4.3 of *All's Well That Ends Well.*

As the first English picaresque novel, *The Unfortunate Traveller* is an important literary monument, but Nashe is probably best known for his biting satirical pamphlets. Nashe was also the anonymous author of several government counterblasts to the rebellious religious tracts of the pseudonymous Puritan Martin Marprelate (see MARTEXT). In the course of the Marprelate controversy, Nashe's avid anti-Puritanism earned him the enmity of Gabriel HARVEY (2), and the two pamphleteers conducted a long feud in print, which may be the subject of a number of obscure topical jokes in *Love's Labour's Lost.* Moreover, many scholars believe that the diminutive Nashe was satirised as the sharp-tongued and tiny youth Moth.

Nashe was one of the UNIVERSITY WITS, the playwrights who dominated ELIZABETHAN DRAMA in the 1580s, but he wrote only two plays of his own—a satirical MASQUE entitled *Summer's Last Will and Testament* (1592) and *The Isle of Dogs* (1597)—though he also collaborated with Robert GREENE (2) and Christopher MARLOWE (1). The *Isle of Dogs,* whose text is now lost, was among the most controversial of Elizabethan plays, a notable subject of government CENSORSHIP. The government found it 'seditious' and not only suppressed it, but closed all the LONDON theatres for several months; three of the actors in the play—Ben JONSON, Robert SHAW (5), and Gabriel SPENCER—were gaoled briefly, though Nashe fled London and escaped punishment. He only returned in 1599, to face a blanket condemnation of his works by the government. His last years are obscure, and we know of his death only through an elegy published some time later, in 1601.

Nathaniel (1) Character in *Love's Labour's Lost,* the obsequious companion of the comical pedant HOLOFERNES. Nathaniel emulates his friend, seconding his opinions with less Latinity but no less pretension. Although Nathaniel is no more than an object of derision

for the most part, COSTARD presents him in a more human light, standing up for him in 5.2, when he has fled the pageant, stricken with stage fright.

Nathaniel (2) Minor character in *The Taming of the Shrew,* a member of the household staff of PETRUCHIO (2). Nathaniel is one of the servants whom Petruchio abuses in 4.1 as part of his demonstration to KATHERINA of the ugliness of shrewish behaviour.

Neighbour Any of three minor characters in *2 Henry VI,* supporters of Thomas HORNER when he appears, in 2.3, to defend himself in a trial by combat with his apprentice, PETER (1). Unfortunately for Horner, his friends ply him with liquor, by way of cheerful support, and, drunk, he is slain.

Neilson (1), Adelaide (1846–1840) British actress. Neilson was best known for her dramatic adaptations of stories from the works of Sir Walter Scott (1771–1832), but she also played many Shakespearean roles, including JULIET (1), VIOLA, ISABELLA, and IMOGEN. She was noted for her great beauty.

Neilson (2), Julia (1868–1957) British actress, the wife of Fred TERRY (2). A comic actress who played ROSALIND and other Shakespearean parts, Neilson is best known as the co-star and co-manager, with her husband, of a theatre company that presented a variety of plays between 1900 and 1930.

Nell (1) Minor character in *The Comedy of Errors,* a servant in ADRIANA's household. DROMIO OF SYRACUSE refers to Nell in his account to his master of the 'kitchen wench' who claims him as her husband. This parallels Adriana's mistaken identification of the master, ANTIPHOLUS OF SYRACUSE. In a long, broadly comic passage (3.2.71–154), Dromio describes Nell as so grotesquely fat that her other, equally unattractive features are best equated with the continents of the globe.

Nell is described here (and in 5.1.414–416) as the kitchen-maid. LUCE, who appears in 3.1.48–64, is also identified as the kitchen-maid (at 4.4.72–73). This has produced confusion; the two are often thought to be the same character. Some editors of the play have gone so far as to rename Luce as Nell in both stage directions and text.

The different names may be the result of an error on Shakespeare's part; such inconsistencies are common throughout the plays. On the other hand, Dromio may be sarcastically using a pointedly common woman's name to refer to Luce, who is, to his mind, a very common woman. Most simply, the playwright may have expected us to conclude that Adriana had more than one kitchen-maid. If this is the case, and Luce and Nell are not identical, then Nell never actually appears in the play.

Nell (2) Minor character in *The Two Noble Kinsmen,* a country lass who performs in a dance before Duke THESEUS (2). In 3.5 the five young women assemble for the dance; Nell is the only one who speaks, assuring her director, the SCHOOLMASTER (2), that they will do well. Her half-line—a scoffing 'Let us alone, sir' (3.5.31)—contributes to the scene's sense of rustic festivity. However, most scholars agree that Shakespeare did not write 3.5, so Nell is probably the creation of John FLETCHER (2).

Nerissa Character in *The Merchant of Venice,* lady-in-waiting to PORTIA (1). Nerissa is a pert and lively companion to her mistress. In the early scenes involving the lottery of the three caskets, she assures the uneasy heiress that all will be well, and she seconds Portia in the practical joke of the betrothal rings in 5.1. Her courtship by GRATIANO (1) echoes that of Portia by BASSANIO; such symmetrical couples were quite popular in the Elizabethan theatre.

Nestor Legendary figure and character in *Troilus and Cressida,* the oldest of the Greek leaders in the TROJAN WAR. Though respected for his great age, Shakespeare's Nestor is a faintly ludicrous old man who boasts about his longevity and is full of platitudes and long-winded speeches. For instance, agreeing with ULYSSES that another character's purpose is plain, Nestor says, 'True; the purpose is perspicuous as substance / Whose grossness little characters sum up' (1.3.324–325). He is chiefly a supporter of Ulysses' schemes to coax ACHILLES into battle and does very little otherwise.

Nestor was first presented in the *Iliad* of HOMER, where he is the same self-righteous and ineffectual old man we see in Shakespeare. In Homer he is somewhat more than 60, a very respectable age in the ancient world; in the Roman poet OVID's *Metamorphoses,* which Shakespeare read, he is an improbable 200 years old.

New Place Shakespeare's home in STRATFORD from 1597 until his death, and that of his descendants until 1649. The purchase of New Place had considerable personal significance for Shakespeare, advertising to Stratford that his success as a LONDON playwright had restored the family fortune after the financial collapse suffered by his father, John SHAKESPEARE (9), some years earlier. It was the second-largest residential building in the town, built around 1490 by one of Stratford's most famous citizens, Hugh Clopton (d. 1496), a one-time lord mayor of London. Shakespeare bought it from William UNDERHILL in 1597, and despite difficulties created when Underhill was mur-

dered by his son, took possession and began making repairs. Documents relating to the sale reveal that the house was 60 by 70 feet in area and that it had 10 fireplaces (and surely more rooms than fireplaces, as the latter were taxed as luxuries). On its property were two barns, two gardens, and two orchards. An 18th-century drawing shows a three-storied, five-gabled mansion.

Shakespeare did not live at New Place full-time until he retired from the theatre, around 1611, but his wife, Anna HATHAWAY Shakespeare, and his daughters doubtless moved in as soon as the repairs were completed, probably in 1598. Mary Arden SHAKESPEARE (11), the playwright's mother, may have lived at New Place after her husband's death in 1601. Shakespeare retired to New Place and died there in 1616.

Shakespeare left New Place to his daughter Susanna SHAKESPEARE (14) Hall, who lived there until her death in 1649. She in turn left it to her daughter, Elizabeth HALL (3), who had lived there with her first husband, Thomas NASH (2), and did so briefly with her second, John Bernard, whom she married just before her mother died. However, she soon moved to Northamptonshire with Bernard, and the house may have been vacant for some years. Elizabeth left New Place to her husband when she died in 1670, and on his death in 1674 the house was sold to one Edward Walker, whose daughter married a Clopton in 1699, so that the house returned to the family of its builder.

The Cloptons altered the house, virtually rebuilding it to a different ground-plan. In 1756 the property was sold to the Reverend Francis Gastrell, who demolished the house in 1759, reportedly because he felt its taxes were too high. Today, the site of New Place, encompassing the foundations of the house and a series of gardens, is owned by the Shakespeare BIRTHPLACE Trust and is open to the public.

Newington Butts Suburb of LONDON, site of an early theatre. Little is known of the theatre, which was located near an archery practise field—archery targets were called butts—in the village of Newington (then a distant suburb, now well within London). The theatre was in existence by 1580, when it was ordered closed during a plague epidemic. At some point it was apparently bought or leased by Philip HENSLOWE, who hired troupes to play there in June 1594, including the earliest known performance by the CHAMBERLAIN'S MEN, Shakespeare's company. However, the only later record of this theatre is a 1631 reference to its former existence.

Nicanor See ROMAN (2).

Nicholas Minor character in *The Taming of the Shrew,* a member of the household staff of PETRUCHIO (2). Nicholas is one of the servants whom Petruchio abuses in 4.1 as part of his demonstration to KATHERINA of the ugliness of shrewish behaviour.

Nobleman Minor character in *3 Henry VI,* a messenger. In 3.2 the nameless Nobleman brings word to King EDWARD IV of the capture of HENRY VI.

Norfolk (1), John Howard, Duke of (c. 1430–1485) Historical figure and minor character in *Richard III,* commander of the forces of RICHARD III at the battle of BOSWORTH FIELD. A quiet follower of orders, Norfolk brings Richard a note warning of treachery in the forthcoming battle, in 5.3. His death in the fighting is noted at 5.5.13. His son, his second-in-command, is the Earl of SURREY (4). Norfolk was a grandson of Thomas MOWBRAY (1), who appears in *Richard II.*

In 1483 the historical Norfolk received his dukedom for his services in securing for Richard the office of Protector. This may account for his silent presence in the stage directions to 3.4.

Norfolk (2), John Mowbray, Duke of (1415–1461) Historical figure and minor character in *3 Henry VI,* a supporter of the Yorkist cause in the WAR OF THE ROSES. Norfolk's paternal grandfather was the Thomas MOWBRAY (1) of *Richard II.* His uncle was the Lord MOWBRAY (2) of *2 Henry IV.*

Norfolk (3), Thomas Howard, Duke of (1443–1524) Historical figure and character in *Henry VIII,* a nobleman at the court of King HENRY VIII. Through the first three acts, Norfolk is an enemy of Cardinal WOLSEY. In 1.1 he warns the Duke of BUCKINGHAM (1) against Wolsey's power, and in 1.2 he supports Queen KATHERINE's complaint against Wolsey's illicit taxes. In 2.2 he leads a group of noblemen in railing against the cardinal, and in 3.2 he delightedly levels formal treason charges against Wolsey, whose downfall has finally come to pass. Finally, in 5.2, he takes a small part in resisting the attack on Archbishop CRANMER by Bishop GARDINER (1). Though he is no longer prominent, he remains on the side of right in the play's scheme of the things.

The historical Norfolk—one of the great English military heroes of his day—died in 1524, before most of the events in the play took place. He was succeeded as Duke of Norfolk by his son, the play's Earl of SURREY (5). Shakespeare ignores Norfolk's death, perhaps through error or perhaps to keep this dignified hero as a fitting opponent of Wolsey and Gardiner.

Norfolk gained heroic stature by leading the English army to a decisive victory over SCOTLAND at the battle of Flodden Field in 1513. Earlier, however, he was an enemy of the TUDOR DYNASTY, for he fought for RICHARD III in 1485 at BOSWORTH FIELD, where Henry VII (see RICHMOND) established the Tudors as English monarchs. Norfolk appears in *Richard III* as the Earl

of SURREY (4); his father, *Richard III*'s NORFOLK (1), was killed at Bosworth Field. Henry VII deprived the family of its ducal rank, but at the age of 70, this Norfolk won it back at Flodden.

Norfolk (4), Thomas Mowbray, Duke of Character in *Richard II.* See MOWBRAY (1).

North, Sir Thomas (c. 1535–c. 1601). English translator of PLUTARCH's *Lives.* North's *Lives of the Noble Grecians and Romans* (1579)—a retranslation of Jacques AMYOT's French rendering of Plutarch's original Greek—became Shakespeare's primary source for *Antony and Cleopatra, Coriolanus, Julius Caesar,* and *Timon of Athens* and a source for minor elements in other plays. North, a nobleman educated at Cambridge and the INNS OF COURT, translated various works from Spanish, French, and Italian, but he is chiefly known for his Plutarch, which, besides having inspired Shakespeare, also influenced several generations of English prose writers; it is regarded as one of the major works of 16th-century English literature.

Northumberland (1), Henry Percy, Earl of (1342–1408) Historical figure and character in *Richard II* and *1* and *2 Henry IV,* a supporter of BOLINGBROKE against RICHARD II in the first play, and a rebel against him—after he has begun to rule as HENRY IV—in the two later works. In *Richard II* Northumberland is Bolingbroke's chief lieutenant; in 2.1 he leads others into rebellion against Richard by providing a rationale for revolt: 'The king is not himself, but basely led by flatterers . . .' (2.1.241–242). In 2.3 Northumberland himself resorts to flattering his leader unctuously, and in 3.3 he hypocritically conveys Bolingbroke's false declaration of loyalty to Richard. In 4.1 Northumberland takes on the most boldly disrespectful functions in the process of removing the king from his position, and in 5.1 he is the hard-hearted deputy who separates Richard and the grieving QUEEN (12). On that occasion he tersely states a cruel principle that aptly represents the new world of Machiavellian politics that Bolingbroke has inaugurated: replying to a request for mercy, he observes, 'That were some love, but little policy.' (5.1.84)

In the *Henry IV* plays he is a less prominent but no more likeable figure. Northumberland and his son, the fiery HOTSPUR, join in rebellion against King Henry, whom they perceive as ungrateful to the Percy family. However, the earl fails to appear with his forces at the crucial battle of SHREWSBURY, sending word that he is ill; the rebel forces are defeated there and Hotspur killed. At the outset of *2 Henry IV* the personification of RUMOUR claims that Northumberland was 'crafty-sick' (Ind. 37), and in 2.3 LADY (10) Percy, Hotspur's widow, chastises her father-in-law for having dishonorably abandoned his son; no other evidence is presented that Northumberland's illness was feigned, however. The earl then deserts the rebels again, fleeing to Scotland rather than supporting the renewed efforts of the ARCHBISHOP (3) of York. His final defeat is reported in 4.4.97–101.

The historical Northumberland did first rebel with Bolingbroke and then against him, but Shakespeare exaggerates his treachery and alters the facts of his life considerably. A man of King Henry's age in the play, Northumberland was actually a generation older; this change is part of Shakespeare's development of the rivalry between Hal and Hotspur by making them contemporaries. Northumberland, a major landowner in northern England and a distinguished warrior in the Scottish border conflicts, was a close friend and supporter of King Henry's father, John of GAUNT. Like Gaunt, he had supported Richard II against Thomas of GLOUCESTER (6), but he was alienated by Richard's seizure of Gaunt's estate, and when Bolingbroke returned from exile, the earl became one of his chief allies, as in *Richard II.* His despicable personality as Bolingbroke's lieutenant may derive from the playwright's knowledge of a famous incident that, surprisingly, he did not use. Sent by Bolingbroke to negotiate with Richard, Northumberland swore a sacred oath that Bolingbroke intended to allow Richard to remain in power if he were restored to Gaunt's title and estates. Richard was thus induced to forgo escape by sea and leave the castle in which he had taken shelter. He was promptly ambushed by Northumberland and taken to London, where he was deposed. It is not known whether or not Northumberland used this ploy under orders, but it was reported in Shakespeare's source, HOLINSHED's *Chronicles,* as a heinous betrayal.

Once Henry was in power, disputes arose between him and the Percies, eventually leading to their revolt. However, Northumberland's role in it in the *Henry IV* plays is almost wholly fictitious. According to Shakespeare, his unforeseen illness shocks the rebels, disturbs their plans, and contributes to their defeat at Shrewsbury, but in reality he had been sick for some time and his absence had been anticipated. The playwright's version is dramatically more interesting, and it allows the rashness of Hotspur and DOUGLAS to be emphasised. The earl's pretending to be ill is also unsupported by Shakespeare's sources; it is simply an appropriately nasty rumour to associate with his Machiavellian character. Further, his betrayal of the Archbishop is untrue; Northumberland was the elected leader of the renewed rebellion, and the Archbishop commenced the uprising prematurely, before Northumberland could join him. Only after the disaster at GAULTREE FOREST, when Henry marched on his headquarters at WARKWORTH CASTLE, did Northumberland flee to Scotland. Several years later, after recruiting arms and money in Flanders and FRANCE (1), he again revived the rebellion and invaded England,

dying in unsuccessful but valorous combat, according to Holinshed. This account of tenacious courage did not at all suit Shakespeare's model of a contemptible rebel, and he simply ignored it.

Northumberland (2), Henry Percy, Earl of (1421–1461) Historical figure and minor character in *3 Henry VI*, a supporter of King HENRY VI. Northumberland is among the nobles who depart from Henry in anger, when the king agrees to bequeath the throne to YORK (8) in 1.1. He appears with Queen MARGARET (1) and Lord CLIFFORD (1) in 1.4, when the captive York is murdered; his sympathy for York, who is tormented with evidence of his young son's murder before his own, is chastised by the queen. He later dies at the battle of TOWTON.

This Northumberland was the grandson of Henry PERCY (2), known as HOTSPUR, who figures in *Richard II* and *1 Henry IV*. His father, Hotspur's son, died at the first battle of ST. ALBANS, as is described in the opening lines of *3 Henry VI*.

Northumberland (3), Henry Percy, Earl of (1446–1489) Historical figure mentioned in *Richard III*, an apparent follower of RICHARD III. On the eve of the battle of BOSWORTH FIELD, Richard refers to 'the melancholy Lord Northumberland' (5.3.69) as one of his officers. This is the son of the NORTHUMBERLAND (2) of *3 Henry VI*, who had died in the battle against the Yorkist King EDWARD IV (and against Richard) at TOWTON and whose lands and title had been seized by the victors. After the defection of WARWICK (3), King Edward sought new allies and he returned the Northumberland fiefdom to this Northumberland, who was accordingly with Richard at Bosworth. However, Shakespeare did not mention the dénouement of the relationship: Northumberland refused to bring his many troops into the fighting, and after the battle he immediately found favour with RICHMOND.

Northumberland (4), Lady Character in *2 Henry IV*. See LADY (9).

Northumberland (5), Siward, Earl of Character in *Macbeth*. See SIWARD.

Nun Minor character in *Measure for Measure*, a member of the convent that ISABELLA intends to join. The Nun appears only briefly, in 1.4, when she listens to Isabella's complaint that the restrictions imposed on the nuns seem insufficient. When she hears LUCIO's voice she asks Isabella to receive him, for she may not speak to a man except in the presence of the prioress and then only while hiding her face; if showing her face, she must be quiet. Having established these regulations for the audience, the Nun disappears from the play; except for a momentary disturbance at the approach of Lucio, she displays only the quiet of the stereotypical nun. The episode illustrates Isabella's extremism, as we see that she is determined to adopt a sterner rule of withdrawal than that required of the Nun.

The Nun is named Francisca (or Francesca) in the stage direction at the beginning of 1.4, but the name is not used thereafter. Scholars believe that Shakespeare named his character when he created her but then never used the name. Its survival in the earliest published text, the FIRST FOLIO (1623), is viewed as evidence that the printed text came from Shakespeare's manuscript.

Nunn, Trevor (b. 1940) British theatrical director and producer. As the artistic director of the Royal Shakespeare Company since 1968 (and its chief executive since 1978), Nunn has been responsible for numerous notable Shakespearean productions, including a cycle of the ROMAN PLAYS in 1972, a 1973 *Coriolanus* starring Nicol WILLIAMSON, a 1976 *Macbeth* with Ian MCKELLEN and Judi DENCH, and a 1981 *All's Well That Ends Well* that was successful in STRATFORD, London, and New York. In the 1980s Nunn's career centred on contemporary theatre, as he produced such trans-Atlantic hits as *Nicholas Nickleby, Cats,* and *Les Misérables*.

Nurse (1) Minor character in *Titus Andronicus*. In 4.2 the Nurse delivers to AARON his infant son by TAMORA. Aaron kills the Nurse to ensure her silence about the birth.

Nurse (2) Minor character in *3 Henry VI*. A non-speaking character, the Nurse tends to the infant PRINCE (5) of Wales in the final scene.

Nurse (3) Character in *Romeo and Juliet*, a servant in the CAPULET (1) household, the nanny and former wet-nurse of JULIET (1). The longwinded Nurse, a broadly comical figure who repeatedly resorts to the low humour of sexual innuendo, functions as a foil for Juliet's delicacy and openness; in 1.3 the anecdote she relates from Juliet's childhood illuminates the heroine's background. But as the tragedy deepens, the Nurse loses her humorous qualities and becomes a symbol of the conventional world that opposes the private realm of the lovers. Further, her crass recommendation that Juliet simply ignore her union to the banished ROMEO (3.5.212–225) serves to isolate the heroine at a crucial moment. In her last appearance the Nurse cackles mindlessly about sex as she attempts to wake the drugged Juliet, and she echoes the uncomprehending grief of the family when it appears that the girl is dead.

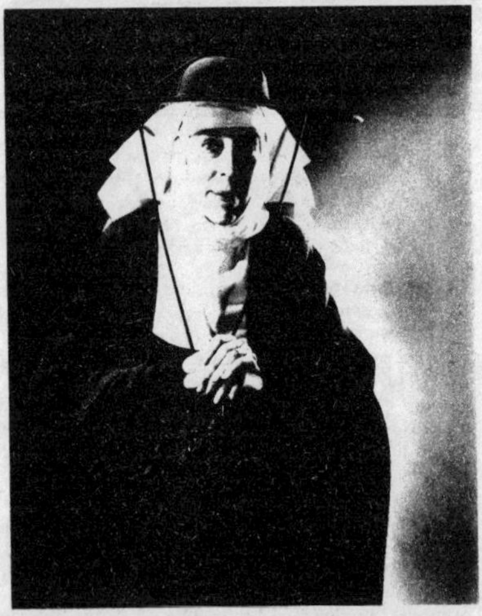

Juliet's Nurse (played by Edna May Oliver in the 1936 film of Romeo and Juliet*) is one of the most famous comedy roles in all of Shakespeare. A perfect foil for Juliet's idealism, the Nurse represents the crassness of the conventional world.* (Courtesy of Culver Pictures, Inc.)

Nym Character in *The Merry Wives of Windsor* and *Henry V*, a follower of FALSTAFF. In *The Merry Wives* Nym is a minor figure, being dismissed by his master early in the play for refusing to deliver love letters. But in three brief scenes he is memorably established as an eccentric character, using the word 'humour' in almost every speech, applying it in every imaginable way, to the point where it ceases to have meaning. This word was a fashionable and widely parodied term in late 16th-century London (see COMEDY OF HUMOURS); in fact, a character in a play of 1596, George CHAPMAN's *The Blinding Beggar of Alexandria,* had the same verbal habit and clearly seems to have influenced Shakespeare's creation of Nym.

In *Henry V* Nym feuds with PISTOL, who has married the HOSTESS (2), to whom Nym was engaged. BARDOLPH (1) reconciles the two. Nym is one of the companions of Falstaff who mourn his death in 2.3, but he says little. In 3.2, as part of King HENRY V's army in France, Nym is cowardly and is upbraided by FLUELLEN. The BOY (3) comments on the villainous characters of Nym, Pistol, and Bardolph in 3.2.28–56, describing them as braggarts, petty thieves, and cowards. In 4.4.72 the Boy reports that Nym has been hung, apparently for theft.

In *The Merry Wives,* Nym's function is comical, although he remains an undeveloped character. In *Henry V,* his more unnsavoury aspects are stressed; he is part of the underworld that is put down by King Henry. His very name suggests petty villainy; it meant 'steal' or 'filch' in Elizabethan English.

O

Oatcake, Hugh Minor character in *Much Ado About Nothing,* one of the WATCHMEN (3). Oatcake, with SEACOAL, is nominated in 3.3.11 for the post of constable, for both are literate, but DOGBERRY appoints Seacoal. Oatcake is presumably one of the Watchmen who reappear in 4.2 and 5.1, but he is not again mentioned specifically. His comical name—which helps heighten the Watchmen's comical foolishness—is typical of a Shakespearean CLOWN (1).

Oberon Character in *A Midsummer Night's Dream,* the Fairy King who works the magic that ensures the triumph of love that is the focus of the play. Oberon gives an unpleasant first impression in 2.1, quarrelling with his queen, TITANIA, and resolving to 'torment' her (2.1.147) because she will not surrender to him a changeling he desires to raise. However, it is clear that he intends his revenge, a dose of a magic aphrodisiac, to be only temporary. Once he knows he will have his way, he is a gentle king, overseeing the confusions of the lovers' plot with good-natured amusement. When Titania, magically enchanted with the ass-headed BOTTOM, has surrendered the changeling, he feels sorry for her and lifts his spell, as he had said he would. For the remainder of the play, he is a benign figure, blessing the marriages and the palace of Duke THESEUS (1). Oberon was the traditional King of Fairies, and Shakespeare must have known of him from several sources, though the one most prominent in the play is a 13th-century French adventure tale, *Huon of Bordeaux.*

Octavia (d. 11 B.C.) Historical figure and character in *Antony and Cleopatra,* the sister of Octavius CAESAR (2) and wife of Mark ANTONY. In 2.2 Octavia's marriage is arranged as part of a treaty; she appears briefly in 2.3 and 3.2 as a dutiful wife. She accompanies Antony to ATHENS, where, in 3.4, she learns of renewed enmity between her husband and brother and volunteers to help negotiate a new truce. However, when she arrives in Rome in 3.6, she is greeted with the news that Antony has returned to CLEOPATRA. Once Antony's desertion is established Octavia disappears from the play. Her docile, peaceable nature makes her a suitable victim, while she also serves as a foil both to Caesar, the cynical politician, and to Cleopatra, the irresistible sensualist.

The historical Octavia had a more prominent and complex role in Roman affairs than she does in the play. The most striking difference in Shakespeare's account concerns the timing of her marriage to Antony, which occurred in 40 B.C. This was before he had begun his affair with Cleopatra—he actually had another mistress at the time, in Athens. Also, Shakespeare telescopes events in his play and gives short shrift to Octavia's success as a diplomat. She in fact brought about a treaty between her husband and brother in 37 B.C., and it lasted for several years. After Antony deserted her, Octavia remained loyal to him. Even after he divorced her in 32 B.C., she continued to care for his children by two prior marriages. Her nobility and humanity won her widespread fame as a sympathetic and estimable figure, a reputation that is reflected in Shakespeare's source, PLUTARCH's *Lives* and survives in the 'beauty, wisdom, [and] modesty' (2.2.241) of the peaceable if ineffectual woman of the play.

Octavius (Gaius Octavius Caesar; Octavian) (63 B.C.–14 A.D.) Historical figure and character in *Julius Caesar,* ANTONY's ally against BRUTUS (4) and CASSIUS. (The same figure appears as CAESAR [2] in *Antony and Cleopatra.*) Octavius is a cool, self-possessed, and efficient leader, whether hearing out Antony's criticisms of LEPIDUS in 4.1, claiming command of the right wing—properly Antony's—before the battle of PHILIPPI in 5.1, or ordering the honourable burial of Brutus in 5.5. Though his part is small, it is boldly drawn and clearly anticipates the briskly calculating victor of the later play.

Shakespeare captures something of the personality of the historical Octavius but ignores the events of his life for the most part. In his will, Julius Caesar formally adopted Caius Octavius—the grandson of his sister—and made him the heir to his name and three-quarters of his immense fortune. (In legally accepting this inheritance after Caesar's murder, Octavius changed his name to Caius Julius Caesar Octavianus, and to English-speaking historians he is generally known as Oc-

tavian from this time until his assumption of the title Augustus in 27 B.C. However, Shakespeare was probably unaware of this distinction, and the character is called Octavius throughout *Julius Caesar.*) Octavius, who had been a physically frail child, was a 19-year-old student in Athens when Caesar died. When he returned to Italy to claim his inheritance, he immediately asserted himself politically but was not taken seriously at first. However, the name of Caesar was a powerful one, and he was soon at the head of an army of the pro-Caesar forces assembling to combat the assassins.

Unlike in *Julius Caesar,* Octavius was a rival of Antony's from the outset, and their alliance—joining with Lepidus in the Triumvirate—was sealed only after 18 months of antagonism that approached full-scale war. While his political acumen was considerable, Octavius was still inclined to illness and was not a competent military man; at Philippi he was notably unsuccessful, and the defeat of Brutus and Cassius was largely the work of Antony. However, Octavius was soon to assume the leadership of much of the Roman world—the situation with which *Antony and Cleopatra* opens—and his cool efficiency in the closing lines of *Julius Caesar* effectively foreshadows this achievement.

Officer (1) Minor character in *The Comedy of Errors,* an agent empowered to arrest debtors. In 4.1 a MERCHANT (1) engages the Officer to arrest ANGELO (1), who owes him money. ANTIPHOLUS OF EPHESUS owes Angelo enough to cover his debt to the Merchant, so Angelo in turn pays the Officer to arrest Antipholus. In 4.4 the Officer turns Antipholus over to PINCH.

Officer (2) Minor character in *The Taming of the Shrew,* a constable. The Officer is summoned in 5.1 to arrest VINCENTIO (1), who is thought to be an imposter. The matter is settled shortly after his entrance, and he does not speak.

Officer (3) Either of two minor characters in *Twelfth Night* who arrest and later act as custodians of ANTONIO (4). In 3.4 the Officers seize Antonio, who was an enemy of Duke ORSINO of ILLYRIA in a recent war. In 5.1.58–63 one of them describes Antonio's achievements as a naval warrior.

Officer (4) Either of two minor characters in *Othello,* soldiers of VENICE. In 1.2 an Officer tells BRABANTIO of the council meeting called by the DUKE (5), and in 1.3 another Officer announces the arrival of news from the Venetian fleet. They serve merely to increase the frantic activity surrounding the prospect of war.

Officer (5) Minor character in *King Lear,* the murderer of King LEAR's daughter CORDELIA. In 5.3 EDMUND orders the Officer, a captain (designated as 'Captain' in some editions), to kill the captured king and his daughter, hanging Cordelia to make her death seem a suicide. The officer is a petty representative of the evil that permeates the play. He responds to Edmund's promise of reward in a cynically mercenary spirit, saying 'I cannot draw a cart nor eat dried oats; / If it be man's work I'll do 't' (5.3.39–40). He succeeds in disposing of Cordelia, but he is killed by her father as he does so as we learn from Lear himself in 5.3.273.

Officer (6) Any of several minor characters in *King Lear,* followers of the Duke of ALBANY. In 5.3.109 an Officer relays Albany's order for a trumpet blast. A little later, an Officer (perhaps the same one) is sent after the fleeing GONERIL, but he does not speak. When it is learned that an assassin has been ordered to kill CORDELIA and LEAR, a different Officer (the pursuer of Goneril does not return) is sent to prevent him. He returns and confirms, in half a line (5.3.274), Lear's account of how he killed Cordelia's murderer. The Officers, whether two or three in number, function merely to swell the ranks of the victorious Albany's entourage in the busy climactic moments of the play.

Officer (7) Either of two minor characters in *Coriolanus,* petty officials who prepare for a meeting at which CORIOLANUS is to be honoured. They speak of Coriolanus' nomination to the post of consul, and remark on the possibility that the general may be rejected by the commoners of ROME (see CITIZEN [5]) because of his aristocratic disdain for them. As the First Officer puts it, 'he's vengeance proud, and loves not the common people' (2.2.5–6). They remark on the fickleness of the crowd and on the obstinacy of Coriolanus, but they agree that the warrior hero's long record of extraordinary service makes him more worthy of the post than the politicians who achieve the office by currying favour with the electorate.

Like a CHORUS (1), the Officers are anonymous and outside the action of the play. They interrupt the progress of the plot to provide a commentary on the merits and faults of Coriolanus and on the Roman political situation. Their interruption breaks the intensity of the political developments and thereby promotes a more objective attitude in the audience, permitting us to see both sides of the issue.

Officer (8) Any of several minor characters in *The Winter's Tale,* officials of the law court assembled by King LEONTES to try Queen HERMIONE for adultery. In 3.2.12–21 an Officer reads the formal indictment of Hermione, and in 3.2.124–129 he (or another) swears in CLEOMENES AND DION, who bring a message from the oracle of Apollo. He then reads the oracle's proclama-

tion that Hermione is innocent. As extras, merely providing an official presence to a trial scene, the Officers have no personality.

Okes, Nicholas (active 1596–1639) Printer in LONDON, producer of two editions of works by Shakespeare. Okes printed the fifth edition of *The Rape of Lucrece* (Q5, 1607) for the publisher John HARRISON (2) and the first edition of *Othello* (Q1, 1622) for Thomas WALKLEY. In the 1620s Okes was prosecuted several times for publishing forbidden political satires.

Old Athenian Minor character in *Timon of Athens,* a citizen of ATHENS. In 1.1 the Old Athenian asks the wealthy nobleman TIMON to protect his daughter from the courtship of Timon's servant LUCILIUS (2), who is socially inferior to his intended bride. The magnanimous Timon solves the problem by providing Lucilius with enough money to be considered eligible. The episode helps establish Timon's extravagant generosity. The Old Athenian is a crude caricature of a social type; the snobbish minor gentleman willing to marry his daughter off for money.

Old Clifford Character in *2 Henry VI.* See CLIFFORD (2), THOMAS.

Old Gobbo Character in *The Merchant of Venice.* See GOBBO (2).

Old Lady Minor character in *Henry VIII,* a waiting-woman to ANNE (1) BULLEN. In 2.3 the Old Lady jests bawdily with Anne, who insists that she would not trade her virginity for a throne. The Old Lady contradicts her, declaring that for 'England / You'ld venture an emballing: I myself / Would for Carnarvonshire' (2.3.46–48). The episode exploits the spicy aspects of a courtly romance while not sullying the play's presentation of Anne as a saintly woman. Anne's tolerance of the Old Lady's sharp tongue also keeps her saintliness from seeming stiff-necked and inhumane.

In 5.1, where Anne is the wife of King HENRY VIII, the Old Lady informs the king of the birth of his and Anne's daughter. Confronted with the king's demand for news of a son, she fudges her announcement: '. . . a lovely boy: the God of heaven / Both now and ever bless her: 'tis a girl / Promises boys hereafter' (5.1.164–166). As she had anticipated, the traditional tip for the bearer of news is a small one, and she complains vigorously, 'I will have more, or scold it out of him' (5.1.173). The Old Lady gives a light and comic touch to the introduction of the play's final motif, the auspicious birth of the future Queen ELIZABETH (1).

Old Man (1) Character in *Romeo and Juliet.* See CAPULET (2).

Old Man (2) Minor character in *King Lear,* a vassal of the Earl of GLOUCESTER (1). In 4.1 the Old Man escorts the blind Gloucester who has had his eyes put out by the evil Duke of CORNWALL. The demoralised and fatalistic Gloucester orders him away, but the Old Man observes that he has been tenant to the Earl and his father for 'fourscore years' (4.1.14) and does not obey until he has turned his master over to an escort, the wandering lunatic Tom O'Bedlam (who is actually Gloucester's son, EDGAR, in disguise). The frailty of the Old Man emphasises Gloucester's weakness, while at the same time his devotion offers evidence that some good remains in the increasingly violent and evil world of the play.

Old Man (3) Minor character in *Macbeth.* The Old Man converses with ROSSE in 2.4 and comments on the evil omens that have accompanied the murder of King DUNCAN. This conversation, like a Greek CHORUS (1), offers a commentary on the action so far. The description of the omens—especially that of Duncan's horses eating each other—stresses an important theme of the play: Duncan's murder and its perpetrator are horribly unnatural. The Old Man states the theme explicitly when he describes the eerie darkness of the day. ' 'Tis unnatural, / Even like the deed that's done' (2.4.10–11), he says.

The Old Man presents himself as venerable but unsophisticated—'Threescore and ten I can remember well' (2.4.1), he says when he introduces himself. This, along with his distinctively rustic image of the 'mousing owl' (2.4.13) that killed the falcon, helps establish that the play's catastrophe is universal. SCOTLAND's collapse due to MACBETH's evil is a major motif of the play, and the country as a whole is represented by this ageing peasant.

The episode is a good instance of a technique that Shakespeare was fond of: the plot is interrupted by the introduction of an anonymous figure who comments on it and then disappears from the play. In *Macbeth* the PORTER (3) serves a similar function in a more elaborate manner; the GRAVE-DIGGER of *Hamlet* is another particularly well-known example.

Old Vic Theatre London theatre, famous for its tradition of Shakespearean productions. The Old Vic was built in south London as the Coburg Theatre in 1818. For years it was noted for extravagant melodrama and staged little or no Shakespeare. In 1833 it was renamed the Victoria Theatre after Princess Victoria (later Queen, ruled 1837–1901) attended a performance. In 1871 the Victoria, by now familiarly known as the Old Vic, became a music hall. In 1880 Emma Cone, a prominent opponent of alcohol, bought it and re-opened it as a temperance hall. Her niece, Lilian BAYLIS, joined her in 1898 and introduced to the rep-

ertoire first opera and, beginning in 1914, Shakespeare. By 1923, under the leadership of Baylis, Ben GREET, and Robert ATKINS, the entire CANON of Shakespeare's plays had been performed at the Old Vic, for the first time in any theatre. Under the direction of Atkins (1919–1925), Harcourt WILLIAMS (1) (1929–1933), and Tyrone GUTHRIE (1933–1945), most of the leading actors and actresses of pre-war Britain performed in Shakespeare's plays at the Old Vic. In 1940 a bomb destroyed the theatre. It was reopened in 1950, and between 1953 and 1958, the entire canon was again staged. In 1963 the Old Vic Drama Company was reorganised as the National Theatre, and in 1976 this company moved to the new National Theatre building. The Old Vic Theatre remains in use as a successful repertory theatre.

Oldcastle Original name of FALSTAFF in *1* and *2 Henry IV*. Shakespeare called one of PRINCE (6) HAL's companions Sir John Oldcastle, following his source, *The Famous Victories of Henry the Fifth*. In the FAMOUS VICTORIES Oldcastle speaks very little and does not resemble his successor in any important way. Shakespeare simply took over the name and applied it to his own creation, the extraordinary figure we know as Falstaff. Soon after writing the plays (1596–1597), the playwright changed the name of the character, evidently in response to protests from William Brooke, Lord COBHAM, a descendant of the historical John Oldcastle. The name was changed before *1 Henry IV* was registered for publication, in early 1598, for Falstaff is referred to in its subtitle at that time. (The names HARVEY [1] and ROSSILL were also changed in this text for similar reasons.)

Several traces of the name Oldcastle survive in the plays. For example, the alteration from three syllables to two produces anomalies in the METRE at several points (e.g., in *1 Henry IV*, 2.2.103). There are more overt clues as well: in *1 Henry IV*, 1.2.41, Falstaff is called 'old lad of the castle'; in the QUARTO edition of *2 Henry IV* (1600), a single speech prefix (1.2.119), inadvertently uncorrected, retains the name Oldcastle; in *2 Henry IV*, 3.2.25, Falstaff is said to have been a page to Thomas MOWBRAY (1), which is thought to have been true of the historical Oldcastle. Moreover, the EPILOGUE to *2 Henry IV* specifically dissociates Falstaff from the historical Oldcastle. Also, another play, SIR JOHN OLDCASTLE was produced by the ADMIRAL'S MEN in 1599, clearly in response to the popularity of Falstaff. It presented the life of Oldcastle in a glowing light, and it opened with a prologue drawing an express distinction between its hero and Shakespeare's character. (Oddly, this play was published as Shakespeare's work by William JAGGARD in the FALSE FOLIO of 1619, and it later appeared in the third and fourth FOLIO editions of Shakespeare's work.)

The historical Oldcastle (c. 1375–1417) had been a friend of Prince Hal. His surname referred to a family estate on which there was a ruin, probably of a Roman fort. The extent to which Oldcastle was involved in the Prince's youthful excesses is unknown. He converted to Lollardy, a proto-Protestant religious movement, was convicted of heresy in 1413, and imprisoned. He escaped and led an unsuccessful religious rebellion against Hal, now King HENRY V, and was captured and executed in 1417. After the Reformation, Oldcastle came to be regarded as a Protestant martyr and was held in great respect by the strict English Protestants becoming known, in Shakespeare's time, as Puritans. That Shakespeare applied the name of a Lollard hero to a criminally debauched character seems to reflect his satirical disapproval of the growing Puritanism in English life.

Despite the name change, the association of Oldcastle with Shakespeare's celebrated reprobate lingered. The name Oldcastle was sometimes used in 17th-century performances of *1* and *2 Henry IV* despite Shakespeare's alteration, and in several other writings of the period the name appears as a humorous reference to the vices we associate with Falstaff.

Oliver (1) Character in *As You Like It*, older brother of ORLANDO. Oliver is plainly a villain from the outset. In 1.1 he is seen to have deprived Orlando of his birthright, then he plots to have Orlando killed by the wrestler CHARLES. His malice derives from envy, as he admits when he observes that Orlando's virtues are so great that he, Oliver, is 'altogether misprised' (1.1.168–169). In 3.1 Oliver becomes a victim himself, as the tyrannous DUKE (1) Frederick seizes his estate and threatens him with banishment if he does not capture Orlando. Oliver protests, asserting that he 'never lov'd my brother in my life' (3.1.14) (to which the Duke replies concisely, 'More villain thou' [3.1.15]).

Yet in 4.3 Oliver is a reformed person, a gentleman of sufficient virtue to attract the love of CELIA, whom he marries in 5.4. This turnabout has no humanly credible motivation, nor is it meant to; Oliver is a cardboard character, intended to play a purely symbolic role. His villainy serves to heighten the malevolence from which the Forest of ARDEN (1) offers escape, and the change in him testifies to the power of love, as found in this idyllic wood, to defeat evil. However, Oliver's conversion is not simply magical; it is the result of Orlando's humane decision to forswear revenge and save his sleeping brother from the serpent and lioness, as Oliver describes in 4.3.102–131. This unselfish act, undertaken at the risk of Orlando's life, provokes Oliver's utter total repentance. Oliver decides to give his estates to Orlando, and his loving relationship with Celia, incredible though it is in realistic terms, is the ultimate symbolic confirmation of—and reward for—his sincerity.

Oliver (2), Sir Character in *As You Like It.* See MARTEXT.

Olivia Character in *Twelfth Night,* wealthy mistress of an estate in ILLYRIA, the lover of Cesario—who, although she does not know it, is VIOLA in disguise—and later the bride of SEBASTIAN (2). Olivia is the object of Duke ORSINO's unrequited romantic fantasies. Like Orsino, she impedes the drama's triumph of love; she, too, has a false view of herself that she must overcome. Olivia moves from one illusion to another, beginning with a wilful withdrawal into seclusion and denial of life and then falling headlong into a passion that is based on a mistake. Only the course of events, beginning with the appearance of Sebastian, can correct matters, for Olivia is never aware of her errors.

Mourning her late brother, Olivia adopts an exaggerated, irrational stance that is acutely described by VALENTINE (3): '. . . like a cloistress she will veiled walk, / And water once a day her chamber round / With eye-offending brine' (1.1.28–30). Ironically, her withdrawal gives her something in common with her steward, MALVOLIO, who scorns pleasure and love.

However, grief is counter to Olivia's true nature. In 1.5 the glee with which she responds to the jester FESTE's comical teasing reveals that she is unsuited to the ascetic pose she has adopted, and she has the common sense to see Malvolio for what he is, saying, 'O, you are sick of self-love, Malvolio, and taste with a distempered appetite.' (1.5.89–90). She forgets her brother once she has been smitten with the charms of Cesario, and her pent-up instinct for love plunges her into a 'most extracting frenzy' (5.1.279). However, her passion is misplaced, not only because a disguised woman is its object but also because she is excessively self-involved, using what she knows to be 'shameful cunning' (3.1.118) to win her beloved. She admits, 'There's something in me that reproves my fault: / But such a headstrong potent fault it is, / That it but mocks reproof.' (3.4.205–207). Olivia has gone from scorning love in the name of propriety to being possessed by love beyond the reach of conscience.

Once Sebastian has replaced Cesario, Olivia remains impetuous, though she still recognises the irrationality of her course. 'Blame not this haste of mine' (4.3.22), she pleads as she leads Sebastian to the altar. At the play's near-hysterical climax in 5.1, Olivia struggles to keep Cesario, though he denies their marriage, until Sebastian reappears to claim her and identify Viola. Olivia is almost silent as this occurs, for her role in the tale of tangled romances is over. She comes to herself only when she realises that she has lost track of Malvolio, now incarcerated as a lunatic. She sees to his release and elicits the truth of the comic SUB-PLOT that has been going on beyond her distracted attention. When the steward flees in rage, she is sympathetic but amused; she has become the humane lady of her establishment that the frenzy of misplaced love had prevented her from being.

Olivier, Laurence (1907–1989) British actor and director. Olivier—whose career covered a wide range of roles, both classical and modern, on stage and in FILM and TELEVISION—is often regarded as the greatest actor of the 20th century. Only John GIELGUD and Ralph RICHARDSON (2) are ranked with him among the great Shakespearean actors of the age. Among Olivier's best-known Shakespearean roles are HAMLET, RICHARD III, HENRY V, SIR TOBY BELCH, and TITUS (1) ANDRONICUS, and he played many other Shakespearean characters.

At the age of nine, playing BRUTUS (4) in a schoolboy production of *Julius Caesar,* Olivier was by chance observed by Sybil THORNDIKE and Lewis CASSON, who recorded their opinion that he was clearly a great actor. Similarly, he attracted rave reviews playing KATHERINA in *The Taming of the Shrew* at 14. In 1926 he joined the Birmingham Repertory Company, under Barry JACKSON (1), where he mostly played non-Shakespearean parts. His fame as a Shakespearean actor began in 1935, when he and Gielgud alternated roles as ROMEO and MERCUTIO in a famous production of *Romeo and Juliet.* In 1936 he played ORLANDO in a movie version of *As You Like It* and then, in a remarkable 1937–1938 season at the OLD VIC THEATRE, he played Hamlet, Sir Toby, Henry V, MACBETH, and IAGO. He also played Hamlet at ELSINORE in 1937. In the late 1930s Olivier made a number of popular and critically acclaimed movies, such as *Wuthering Heights* (1939) and *Pride and Prejudice* (1940). His romance with Vivien LEIGH began in 1936—a subject of extensive gossip, since both were married to others—and they married in 1940.

In 1944 Olivier returned to the Old Vic, where he played RICHARD III to great acclaim and began directing plays. In the same year he produced, directed, and starred in a film of *Henry V.* He made two more films, *Hamlet* (1948) and *Richard III* (1955), starring in each. *Hamlet* won two Academy Awards, for best film and best actor. (Olivier's *Hamlet* was a radically abridged version of Shakespeare's play, however, eliminating almost half the text, including all of ROSENCRANTZ AND GUILDENSTERN's part.) In 1947, Olivier was knighted, and in 1948 he was awarded another Oscar for his achievement throughout his career.

Olivier starred in the *Titus Andronicus* of Peter BROOK (2) (1955), a production that is credited with creating a renewed interest in the play. In 1961, divorced from Vivien Leigh, he married Joan PLOWRIGHT. From 1963 to 1972 he was the founding director of the British National Theatre Company, producing notable stagings of *Othello* and *The Merchant of Venice*—with himself as OTHELLO and SHYLOCK—and many other plays, both Shakespearean and otherwise. Suffering from a de-

generative muscle disease, Olivier gave his last stage performance in 1974, but he continued working in films and television. He won an Emmy for his performance in the 1983 television production of *King Lear*. His last role was a cameo appearance in a 1988 television show, *War Requiem,* based on a work by Benjamin BRITTEN. Olivier published an autobiography, *Confessions of an Actor* (1982), and another book, *On Acting* (1986).

One (1) Minor character in *2 Henry VI,* a citizen who approaches the royal hawking party in 2.1, proclaiming that a miracle has occurred: a blind man, who proves to be the imposter SIMPCOX, has recovered his sight.

One (2) Minor character in *Troilus and Cressida,* an anonymous Greek warrior killed by HECTOR. In 5.6 Hector spies the Greek fighter wearing a sumptuous suit of armour, and he declares he will take it from him. The Greek flees, but in 5.8 we see that Hector has killed him, and as the triumphant warrior takes off his own armour to put on his prize, he is treacherously killed by ACHILLES and the MYRMIDONS.

While stripping the dead Greek, Hector addresses the corpse as, 'Most putrefied core, so fair without' (5.8.1), contrasting the dead body with the pomp and splendour of his armour (in words reminiscent of Christ's condemnation of the Pharisees as 'whited sepulchres' [Matthew 23:27]). The symbolic significance of the One is thus clear: he sums up the hypocrisy of the warriors' pretensions throughout the play. At the same time, the episode also reveals Hector's death to be the result of his abandonment of his code of honourable combat to pursue a rich prize.

One (3) Within Minor character in *Henry VIII,* LONDON commoner. The One Within is part of a crowd of enthusiastic celebrants of the christening of Princess ELIZABETH (1), who invade the royal courtyard, despite the efforts of the PORTER (4). He speaks from off stage, claiming to be a worker in the court of King HENRY VIII in 5.3.4 and baiting the Porter in 5.3.27. His voice contributes to the riotousness of the occasion. The speech prefixes in the FIRST FOLIO edition of the play designate this character as 'Within'; however, most subsequent editors have prefaced this with 'One'.

Ophelia Character in *Hamlet,* lover of Prince HAMLET. In 1.3 Ophelia's brother, LAERTES, cautions Ophelia against believing Hamlet's professions of love, and her father, POLONIUS, forbids her to see him. A demure and obedient daughter, Ophelia returns Hamlet's letters, and, under the pressures of the main plot, Hamlet turns on her with a seemingly insane revulsion against women in general and her in particular. She reports his behaviour in 2.1 and encounters it

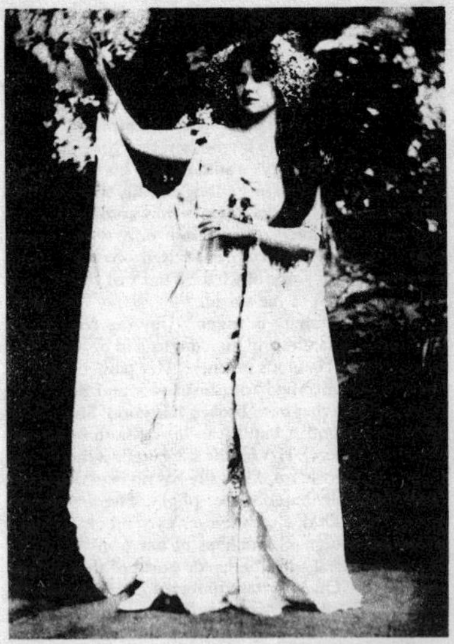

Unable to reconcile her love for her father, Polonius, with her love for her father's murderer, Hamlet, the innocent Ophelia is driven to madness in Hamlet. *The actress in this early photo wears wildflowers in her hair, a standard device to suggest the disorder of Ophelia's mind.* (Courtesy of Culver Pictures, Inc.)

in even more virulent form in 3.1. After her former lover kills her father, Ophelia becomes insane, babbling about funerals and singing scraps of songs in 4.5. Her death by drowning is reported by the QUEEN (9) in 4.7, and her funeral in 5.1—abbreviated by the PRIEST (3) because the death seems a suicide—triggers an encounter between Hamlet and Laertes that foreshadows the play's climax.

Ophelia's nature is abundantly affectionate; her wounded but faithful love—both for her father and for Hamlet—makes her one of the most touching of Shakespeare's characters. As Laertes observes about Ophelia's lunacy: 'where [love] is fine / It sends some precious instance of itself / After the thing it loves' (4.5.161–163). He refers to her love for the dead Polonius, which has caused her to send herself figuratively (and later literally) after him to a world beyond life, but the remark is equally appropriate to her love for Hamlet.

However, the relationship between Hamlet and Ophelia is not a love story, for Hamlet has rejected love. He loved Ophelia before the play opens, as is

attested first by her touching recollection of his gifts and the 'words of so sweet breath compos'd / As made the things more rich' (3.1.98–99) and then by his admission at her funeral in 5.1.264–266. He remains sexually attracted to her—as is shown by his obscene jesting in 3.2.108–117—but he has displaced on her much of his anger with his mother, the Queen. She has become for him simply a stimulus for his disgust with women and sex, and he no longer really sees her as an actual person. Ophelia's fate is thus an outgrowth of Hamlet's emotional collapse; not only is her life diminished—and ultimately destroyed—by his actions, but she is a measure of what he has lost through his mistaken vision of the world.

Ophelia's insanity is triggered by the crushing of her love for Hamlet and then intensified by the loss of her father to Hamlet's madness. Her pathetic ravings in 4.5 are concerned with lost loves and death, the grim realities that have broken her mind. She cannot absorb the conflict implicit in loving both her father and his murderer. Her bawdy songs reflect the lusts of the outside world, of which she has no experience but that have contributed to her plight. The flowers she obsessively alludes to, themselves symbols of innocence, are poignant emblems of her own youth and inability to deal with the harsh world of the play.

While the Queen's description of Ophelia's drowning in 4.7.165–182 permits us to view it as accidental—a tree branch broke as she fell—she also reports that the victim made no effort to save herself. In 5.1 the GRAVE-DIGGER and the Priest view her as a suicide, and her death is certainly a result of her madness. But her insanity is the consequence of the actions of others, and Ophelia is unquestionably a victim of the tragic events that beset DENMARK throughout the play.

Some scholars believe that Ophelia's name—which means 'succor' in Greek, a seemingly inappropriate designation for so victimised a character—may have been used in error instead of Aphelia, meaning 'simplicity' or 'innocence'. Both names were rare in Shakespeare's time.

Orlando Character in *As You Like It,* the lover of ROSALIND. Orlando is first seen as a victim of his older brother, OLIVER (1), who has seized Orlando's rightful inheritance and plots to have him killed by the wrestler CHARLES. After defeating Charles (and meeting Rosalind) in 1.2, Orlando is warned by his faithful servant, ADAM, that Oliver still intends to harm him, and the two flee in 2.3. As they arrive in the Forest of ARDEN (1), Orlando's noble spirit is stressed as he stoops to robbery in order to find food for the feeble Adam. Fortunately, his efforts lead him to the court-in-exile of DUKE (7) Senior, where, in 2.7, he is welcomed as a gentleman. He recalls Rosalind in a juvenile and conventionally romantic way, as he hangs love poems to her from the trees, but he encounters her only in her disguise as GANYMEDE, who scoffs at his professed love and suggests that he might be cured of it if he pretends to woo 'him' and is rebuffed. Orlando is consistent in his avowals, however, though only later does he come to a mature sense of what love means.

The growing power of love in him is demonstrated when he resists the temptation to let a lioness kill his evil brother and instead risks his own life to save him, as Oliver reports in 4.3.98–132. Orlando has become aware of his own need for love and reconciliation in all aspects of his life. His full maturation is triggered by the love that arises between CELIA and the reformed Oliver. Faced with the real thing, Orlando tells Ganymede, 'I can live no longer by thinking' (5.2.50), and Rosalind realises that she can now discard her disguise, for Orlando is unquestionably committed to her and not simply to the idea of romantic love. Though Rosalind is the spokesperson for most of the play's position on the nature of love, Orlando's development is a powerful secondary demonstration of love's link to self-knowledge.

Orlando is something of a cardboard character. As a handsome leading man without a very well-developed personality, he contributes to the play's parody of PASTORAL literary conventions. Shakespeare's original audiences will have recognised Orlando as a romantic hero immediately, for reasons that are less evident to modern readers and viewers. His name is a version of Roland, one of the greatest heroes of medieval legend and literature, and an Orlando was also the hero of the most popular and well-known of 16th-century pastoral romances, Ludovico ARIOSTO's *Orlando Furioso* (1516, translated into English by Sir John HARINGTON in 1591). Further, Shakespeare's Orlando is identified with two great heroes of classical legend, Aeneas and Hercules. In 2.7 Orlando carries the weak and starving Adam to the Duke's banquet, a tableau that, to a classically educated reader or theatre-goer, must have brought to mind the well-known image, from VIRGIL's *Aeneid,* of Aeneas carrying his father to safety during the sack of Troy. And, to an Elizabethan audience, Orlando's conquests of Charles and the lioness will have immediately suggested the myths of Hercules wrestling Antaeus—depictions of which were extremely popular throughout RENAISSANCE Europe—and his killing the Nemean lion barehanded. In addition, Shakespeare dropped a broader hint when Rosalind, says to Orlando, 'Now Hercules be thy speed, young man!' (1.2.198).

Orléans (1) Location in *1 Henry VI,* a city in FRANCE (1). The English siege of Orléans, part of the HUNDRED YEARS WAR, is the subject of 1.2 and 1.4–2.2. Although JOAN LA PUCELLE (Joan of Arc) arrives among the

French and inspires them, and the English commander, the Earl of SALISBURY (3), is killed, the English, led by TALBOT, take the city in a night-time attack.

Shakespeare's treatment of the siege of Orléans was intended to expand Talbot's role and exalt his heroism, and the playwright took extraordinary liberties with the historical record. Most strikingly, the English never actually took Orléans; besieged for six months, the city withstood the English troops. The English were led by Salisbury for only the first few weeks of the siege, and Talbot was not with the army at the time. After Salisbury's death, command was assumed by the Earl of SUFFOLK (3), a much less competent general; 10 days after Joan arrived, the revived French drove his forces away. Neither CHARLES VII nor REIGNIER was present. Talbot's night-time attack was derived from accounts of another battle—the capture of Le Mans.

Orléans (2), Bastard of See BASTARD (2) of Orléans.

Orléans (3), Charles, Duke of (1391–1465) Historical figure and character in *Henry V*, one of the fatuously over-confident French nobles before the battle of AGINCOURT. Like his fellows, Orléans has no distinctive personality; he joins them in feeble humour and idle insults to the English. They are simply caricatures, braggarts set up to take a fall.

The historical Orléans, nephew of Charles VI, the FRENCH KING of the play, was an important figure in the complicated French politics of the time. He was married to the former English QUEEN (13) Isabel, the widow of RICHARD II. He was seriously wounded and captured at Agincourt (as is reported in 4.6.78), and he was imprisoned in England for 26 years. During his captivity, he began to write poetry, continuing to do so after his release, and he is regarded as one of the greatest French medieval poets.

Orsino Character in *Twelfth Night*, the Duke of ILLYRIA, lover first of OLIVIA and then of VIOLA. Orsino, like Olivia, presents a false view of love that must be corrected in the course of the play. Orsino is infatuated with Olivia, who has repeatedly rejected him, while Viola, who is disguised as Cesario, Orsino's page, loves the duke but cannot tell him so. Utterly involved in his self-image as a brooding, rejected lover, Orsino cannot accept the fact that his passion for Olivia is misplaced. Though he is a humorous figure, a parody of the melancholy lovers of conventional 16th-century romances, he also displays aspects of psychological disorder—as FESTE observes, he is irrationally changeable, his 'mind is a very opal' (2.4.75)—and his wrong-headedness contributes to a sense that all is not well in Illyria.

When we first see the duke, he demonstrates his amusingly distorted slant on reality. In his absurdly romantic pose, he demands music to satiate his lovesick soul, insists that a particular phrase be repeated, then immediately orders that the music be stopped, saying, ' 'Tis not so sweet now as it was before' (1.1.8). He tellingly reverses the image of Olivia as the object of a hunt, making himself the hunted. By the end of the scene, Olivia has almost no importance herself; Orsino is totally absorbed in his own fantasies. But Orsino is not in love with himself; he is in love with love. In 1.4 Viola, as Cesario, vainly tries to induce a sensible attitude in the duke. He boasts of his 'unstaid and skittish' (2.4.18) behaviour, which he associates with love. Feste amusingly sings him a dirge of a love song, 'Come away death' (2.4.51–66), but Orsino does not recognise the implicit critique of his exaggerated melancholy.

The duke resembles such earlier Shakespearean lovers as SILVIUS in *As You Like It* and VALENTINE (1) in *The Two Gentlemen of Verona*. As those figures are mocked by ROSALIND and SPEED respectively, so Orsino is taken to task, comically by Feste and ironically by Viola, but like his predecessors, Orsino is hardheaded and resistant. Only the course of events can make things right for him, for he does not even recognise that they are amiss.

At the play's climax, the disquieting side of Orsino's misplaced emotions erupts in threatened violence, as Olivia's continuing rejection precipitates a menacing demonstration of frustrated masculine dominance as he decides to kill Cesario in a romantic gesture combining love and death. Proposing to 'sacrifice the lamb that I do love, / To spite a raven's heart within a dove' (5.1.128–129), he inadvertently acknowledges his affection for Cesario. His blindness has kept him from recognising this, but his instincts have nonetheless directed him truly, and once Viola's identity is revealed, Orsino is immediately ready to love her.

At the close of the play, when he orders that someone 'pursue [MALVOLIO], and entreat him to a peace' (5.1.379), Orsino achieves something of the quality of THESEUS (1) in *A Midsummer Night's Dream*, or PROSPERO in *The Tempest* (though in a lesser key), wise rulers who understand the uses of power and mercy. He becomes the man his position requires once he is brought to a state of loving grace.

Osric Minor character in Hamlet, a foppish nobleman in the court of KING (5) Claudius of DENMARK. In 5.2 Osric carries the King's request that HAMLET meet LAERTES in a fencing match adding that the King has made a wager on Hamlet. Osric's highly mannered language and behaviour inspire Hamlet's amused derision, and the prince mocks the messenger, demonstrating the ease with which the courtier can be made to agree to contradictory assertions and making

fun of his high-flown language. Osric later umpires the fencing match, though no further attention is paid to him.

Osric functions as comic relief in the face of the King's rapidly unfolding plot against Hamlet, which hinges on the fencing match. Further, the distraction offered by Osric subtly suggests Hamlet's own detachment from the danger that threatens him. The prince's bemused handling of the silly fop is reminiscent of his healthy appreciation of YORICK in 5.1. He is no longer in the grip of grief, and, newly aware of the importance of providence in human affairs, Hamlet can *enjoy* Osric. Osric is an ancient Anglo-Saxon name that was still used occasionally in Shakespeare's day.

Ostler (1) Minor character in *1 Henry IV,* groom at an inn. The Ostler shouts his one brief line from off stage, lending an impression of hectic activity to the inn yard depicted in 2.1.

Ostler (2), William (c. 1588–1614) English actor, a member of the KING'S MEN. One of the 26 men listed in the FIRST FOLIO as the 'Principall Actors' in Shakespeare's plays, Ostler began his career as a boy actor (see CHILDREN'S COMPANIES). He and John UNDERWOOD probably became members of the King's Men at the same time, replacing William SLY (2) and Laurence FLETCHER (3) upon their deaths in 1608. John DAVIES (1) called Ostler 'sole King of Actors' in a poem (1611) that also implied that he had been involved in a brawl. In 1611 Ostler married Thomasine, daughter of John HEMINGES, and at the same time became a partner in the BLACKFRIARS THEATRE; a year later he acquired a share in the GLOBE THEATRE as well. After Ostler's early death, Heminges claimed Ostler's shares in the theatres, despite a lawsuit by Thomasine.

Oswald Character in *King Lear,* the steward of King LEAR's villainous daughter GONERIL. In 1.3 Oswald coolly accepts Goneril's instructions to treat her father insolently, for she wishes to humiliate him thoroughly. In 1.4 Oswald acts upon these orders. Thus, the steward is identified with his mistress as a villain, and when Lord KENT (2) beats him and drives him away, we approve. In 2.2 Kent encounters Oswald again and berates him in a long, comical series of insults that focus on the steward's pretensions to gentlemanly status. Kent's speech is a scathing critique of the vain, self-serving 'glass-gazing, super-serviceable' (2.2.16–17) courtier that Oswald seems to be. Less prominent after these encounters, Oswald principally serves Goneril as a messenger, until, in 4.5, he delivers a letter to REGAN and accepts her implied commission to kill the outcast and blinded Earl of GLOUCESTER (1). When he encounters Gloucester in the next scene he attempts to do so, only to be killed himself by the blind man's son, EDGAR. With his dying breath he begs his killer to make amends by delivering his letters. He thus demonstrates loyalty to his mistress—he is indeed 'super-serviceable'—while at the same time he reveals her secrets and provides for her ultimate downfall in the final scene.

Oswald represents a familiar character type found in the satirical comedy of JACOBEAN DRAMA, a caricature of an ambitious commoner attempting to climb into aristocratic social circles. The rise of the gentry and the birth of the bourgeoisie during the reigns of Queen ELIZABETH (1) and King JAMES I resulted in a crisis of confidence among the aristocracy, who attempted to distinguish themselves from the newly rich by insisting on proper manners and values. This social conflict is the subject of humour in many plays of the period (see, e.g., MALVOLIO, of *Twelfth Night*). In the clash between Kent and Oswald the advantage is given clearly to the old nobility at the expense of the rising class, reflecting Shakespeare's conservative social instincts. Some scholars have speculated that Oswald is further intended as a satire on an actual person, perhaps William FFARINGTON, the obnoxious steward of the Elizabethan theatre patron Lord STRANGE, but this cannot be proven.

Othello Title character in *Othello,* the husband of DESDEMONA, whom he murders because he has been misled by the villainous IAGO. A Moorish general in the service of VENICE, Othello has just married the much younger Desdemona as the play opens. The central dynamic of the drama is his alteration from a noble lover to a raving killer under the malevolent influence of his aide, Iago, who convinces him that his wife is having a love affair with another officer, CASSIO. Unable to trust Desdemona—he lacks this basic element of love—Othello disintegrates morally. His destructiveness extends to his own suicide when his error is exposed. He suffers emotional agonies throughout this process, and we suffer with him, grieving for the destruction of his inherent nobility and the beauty that his marriage exemplifies at its outset.

Through 3.2 Othello is a grandly positive character—a leading figure in the Venetian establishment, a respected military man, and a loving husband. He carries himself with impressive dignity while frankly delighting in his young wife, whose love he values above 'the sea's worth' (1.2.28). When the couple defend their elopement, in 1.3, we see that their love is both spiritually satisfying and imbued with a healthy sexuality. However, in the second half of the play he abandons this transcendent love for a blind jealousy too strong to see reason. He loses faith not only in Desdemona but also in himself. When he rejects her love and trust, Othello also rejects his own capacity for love, in favour of a demanding but unsatisfiable self-centredness.

When he collapses in 4.1, Othello can only babble

as he falls at Iago's feet in a trance. He recovers his wits, but from this point he has only one goal: the deaths of Desdemona and Cassio. In his single-minded malice, Othello now shares Iago's malevolent spirit. Indeed, as the play progresses he even comes to resemble the villain in his speech, using staccato repetitions, broken sentences, and Iago's violent, sexual animal imagery. By 4.1 he cruelly insults his wife publicly, and in 4.2, the so-called 'brothel' scene, he indulges in a savage exaggeration of his jealousy when he says he believes Desdemona a harlot and EMILIA (2) her bawd. In the end, though he can still contemplate his love for his wife when he sees her asleep, he kills her with a coolness that stresses the power of his fixation. His reaction once Desdemona's innocence has been established is just as potent. He recognises that he is no longer noble—he calls himself 'he that was Othello' (5.2.285)—and equating himself with the heathen enemies he used to conquer, he kills himself.

Iago can effect this extraordinary response only because Othello is lacking in trust. This lack is implicit in the Moor's situation from the outset, for he cannot partake of the social solidarity that encourages and reinforces trust between humans. He is an outsider in Venice because of his profession—a mercenary soldier, unacquainted with civilian society 'even from [his] boyish days' (1.3.132)—and his race. Though Othello's military skills are valued and he is not denied the protection of a hearing on BRABANTIO's charge of witchcraft, he is nonetheless an alien in a prejudiced society. He is isolated from the world he has married into. Iago can convince him that Desdemona might have come to detest him because he is black; he lacks the support of a solid position in Desdemona's world that might temper the fear of rejection that his jealousy feeds on.

Though the evidence in the play is clear, some commentators have declared that Othello is not actually black—usually on the racist grounds that so noble a figure could not be a 'veritable negro', as Samuel Taylor COLERIDGE put it. Most frequently, a Moor is held to be of an Arab-related racial type, rather than a Negro. However, Shakespeare (like his contemporaries) drew no such distinction, and Othello is clearly a black African; decisively, RODERIGO calls Othello 'the thicklips' (1.1.66). (Significantly, Shakespeare's other notable Moor, AARON of *Titus Andronicus,* calls his child 'thick-lipp'd' and himself 'coal-black', and he refers to his 'fleece of woolly hair' [*Titus* 4.2.176, 99; 2.3.34].)

Shakespeare plainly intended Othello's race to have a great impact on his original audiences, many of whom, he knew, were as prejudiced as Brabantio. Othello is the earliest black character in English literature with a credible personality, let alone a sympathetic one. Shakespeare deliberately emphasised this, for in CINTHIO's tale, his source, Othello's race has little importance, while in the play it is frequently mentioned, especially in Act 1 where the nature of Venetian society is stressed. The obvious racist caricature offered before Othello appears is entirely in line with the standard English stereotypes of the day, but his actual bearing is strikingly noble. This is emphasised numerous times—Othello even claims royal birth in 1.2.21–22, a point that had much greater importance in Shakespeare's day than in ours—and the playwright must have been aware of the impact of this bold departure. For one thing, Desdemona's strength is greatly magnified by her willingness to courageously defy society's biases. Further, Shakespeare's sympathetic portrait of an alien figure, combined with the compassionate presentation of his repentance and suicide at the play's close, emphasises that the potential for tragic failure is universal.

Othello's race helps determine his status as an alienated outsider in Venice, and this makes him susceptible to Iago's persuasions, for he is grievously naïve about Desdemona's world. Iago assures him, 'I know our country disposition well' (3.3.205), and Othello, reminded of his own ignorance, accepts at face value the preposterous claim that adultery is the moral norm among Venetian women. Iago is absolutely correct when he says to Emilia, 'I told him . . . no more / Than what he found himself was apt and true' (5.2.177–178). Most significantly, once distracted, Othello is not capable of appreciating Desdemona; he knows enough of Venice to see its prejudice, but he does not recognise her steadfast courage in opposing it. Like CORIOLANUS and MACBETH, Othello has succeeded as a soldier and is accordingly endowed with dignity and pride but can only misunderstand the world outside the military camp.

With his suicide Othello acknowledges his fault, but his final recognition of Desdemona's goodness offers us—if not him—the consoling sense that in dying he recovers something of his former nobility. He honestly admits that he 'lov'd not wisely, but too well' and was 'perplex'd in the extreme' (5.2.345, 347). We see a vestige of pride when he refers to his former service to the state, and when he identifies his errant self with the 'malignant . . . Turk' (5.2.354) he once slew, we see that in dying he is as triumphant, in a way, as he was 'in Aleppo once' (5.2.353).

Othello has returned to sanity too late, but that he returns at all provides us with some sense of reconciliation. Othello's fate shows us that a noble person may fall to the depths of savagery, but that an essential humanity remains within the troubled soul. The tradition of the medieval MORALITY PLAY was still familiar in Shakespeare's day and certainly influenced him. Othello's striking placement between Iago and Desdemona resembles the situation of the central character in a morality play: symbolic of the human soul, he was placed between an angel and a devil who each demanded his loyalty. Though the devil succeeded for

a time, and the character sinned (entertainingly), the mercy of God nevertheless prevailed, and the character was reclaimed by the angel and forgiven in the end. Similarly, *Othello* offers redemption at its close. Othello is emblematic of one aspect of human life; he incarnates the inexorable guilt and ultimate death that we recognise as the tragic element in humanity's fate, but his eventual awareness offers a redeeming catharsis.

Othello

SYNOPSIS

Act 1, Scene 1

RODERIGO, who has been courting DESDEMONA, is distressed at IAGO's news that she has eloped with OTHELLO, a Moorish general in the service of VENICE. Iago, who is Othello's aide, assures Roderigo that he also hates the Moor because Othello has denied him a promotion that went instead to CASSIO. He says that he only continues to serve the general in the hope of revenge. Iago and Roderigo awaken Desdemona's father, BRABANTIO, to inform him of the elopement.

Act 1, Scene 2

Iago tells Othello of Brabantio's anger, as Cassio arrives with word that the general has been summoned by the DUKE (5) to a council of war. Brabantio and Roderigo arrive. The angry father, informed of the Duke's council, plans to accuse Othello there.

Act 1, Scene 3

The Duke and several SENATORS (1) receive news of an immanent Turkish attack on the Venetian island of CYPRUS. Othello and Brabantio arrive and Brabantio makes his accusation. Othello replies that Desdomona loves him and has married him of her own free will. When she is summoned she supports his account. Brabantio concedes, and the meeting turns to business: Othello is ordered to leave for Cyprus. Desdemona is to live there with him, and Iago is to escort her in a later ship. Privately, Iago assures Roderigo that Desdemona will soon repent marriage to a Moor, and that if Roderigo will come to Cyprus he will continue to help him with his suit by delivering presents to Desdemona. Roderigo agrees and leaves; Iago reflects on how easy it is to get money from this fool. Saying that Othello is rumoured to have cuckolded him, he goes on to plot revenge upon both Othello and Cassio; he will make the general believe that Cassio is the lover of his new wife.

Act 2, Scene 1

In Cyprus the Venetian governor, MONTANO (2), and two friends discuss the great storm that may have destroyed the Turkish fleet. A third GENTLEMAN (6) brings news that Cassio has arrived with word that this has indeed happened, but that the ship carrying the new governor, Othello, has also disappeared. Iago arrives with Desdemona, his wife, EMILIA (2), and Roderigo. Iago engages the two women in a courtly exchange of witticisms while they await word about Othello. The general arrives safely and greets Desdemona with affection. The group moves indoors, except for Iago and Roderigo. Iago proposes a plot: he says that Desdemona is in love with Cassio and proposes that Roderigo pick a fight with the lieutenant while he commands the guard that night, in the hopes that fighting on duty will disgrace Cassio and remove him as potential competition for Desdemona. Roderigo agrees. Alone, Iago meditates on the course of his plans: he will abuse Cassio to Othello and get credit from the general, while at the same time making him sick with jealousy.

Act 2, Scene 2

A gentleman reads Othello's proclamation of a public holiday. All the soldiers are at liberty until eleven at night, when they must return to duty.

Act 2, Scene 3

Despite Cassio's insistence that a little wine will make him very drunk, Iago convinces him to drink for the sake of the holiday. They join some others, including Montano, and when Cassio goes to take his guard post he is drunk. Iago sends Roderigo after Cassio; he shortly reappears, pursued by the drunken lieutenant, who gets into a fight with Montano. Iago sends Roderigo to sound the alarm, and Othello appears and angrily dismisses Cassio from his post. Left alone with a dismayed Cassio, Iago convinces him that his only hope of recovering his position is to get Desdemona to present his case to Othello. Cassio agrees and leaves, and Iago exults in the success of his scheme: now Othello will witness—and jealously misconstrue—Desdemona's interest in Cassio.

Act 3, Scene 1

Cassio has hired MUSICIANS (6) to play before the general's quarters in the hope of influencing his mood. Iago sends Emilia to Cassio; she assures him that Desdemona favours his cause and agrees to take him where he may meet with the general's wife.

Act 3, Scene 2

Othello prepares to conduct an inspection of the fortifications.

Act 3, Scene 3

Desdemona assures Cassio she will plead his case to Othello. Cassio withdraws as Othello and Iago approach; Iago pretends to regard this suspiciously. Desdemona asks Othello to take Cassio back, and he agrees, saying that he loves her and can deny her nothing. She leaves, and Iago begins to ask seemingly innocent questions about Cassio. He pretends to be reluctant to express his suspicion, but goes on to in-

flame Othello with the idea of a sexual affair between Cassio and Desdemona. He suggests that if Othello delays Cassio's reappointment he can see if Desdemona supports the lieutenant to an excessive degree. Othello fears that Desdemona has been unfaithful because he is black or because he is old, but he tries to resist the thought. Desdemona and Emilia arrive to accompany him to a state banquet, and Othello disguises his distress. As they leave, Desdemona drops a handkerchief that was Othello's first gift to her. Emilia picks it up, and Iago takes it from her as she leaves. He states his intention to plant it on Cassio. Othello returns and angrily demands proof of Desdemona's infidelity. Iago asserts that Cassio has Desdemona's handkerchief. Enraged, Othello goes on his knees to formally swear vengeance, and Iago affirms his loyalty and joins him in the oath, promising to kill Cassio himself and to help Othello kill Desdemona.

Act 3, Scene 4
Desdemona speaks of Cassio, but Othello demands his handkerchief. He says it was charmed by an Egyptian sorceress so that the woman who lost it would be damned in the eyes of her lover. Desdemona denies that it is lost. She tries to change the subject back to Cassio, and Othello leaves in a rage. Iago and Cassio appear; Desdemona remarks on Othello's strange anger, and Iago volunteers to go see the general. Emilia observes that Othello may be jealous of his wife, even though he has no reason, and Desdemona decides she must approach him again. The women leave Cassio as BIANCA (2) appears. She humorously chastises Cassio for not seeing her more often. He asks her to make him a copy of the embroidered handkerchief he has found.

Act 4, Scene 1
Iago says that Cassio has admitted to sleeping with Desdemona. Beside himself with rage, Othello babbles incoherently and then faints. Cassio appears, and Iago tells him he has important news that he will give him once Othello has recovered and they can speak alone. Cassio leaves, and when Othello awakens Iago tells him that if he eavesdrops on the meeting he has arranged with Cassio, the general will hear Cassio speak of his affair with Desdemona. Cassio returns, and Iago speaks to him of Bianca, his lover. With amused disrespect, Cassio laughs about how she presumes to think she'll marry him, and Othello, crying out in asides, believes he is speaking of Desdemona. Bianca arrives, angry about the handkerchief, which she believes was given to Cassio by another woman. Othello now thinks that Cassio has given Desdemona's love token to a harlot. Bianca and Cassio leave, and Othello says he will kill Desdemona; Iago promises to kill Cassio that night. Desdemona appears with LODOVICO, who brings a message from Venice calling Othello back and placing Cassio in command of Cyprus. When Desdemona is pleased, Othello hits her; enraged, he can barely speak. He orders her away and then leaves. Lodovico is surprised at this behaviour, but Iago confides that it is sometimes much worse.

Act 4, Scene 2
Othello quizzes Emilia who says there is no reason to suspect Desdemona and Cassio. He does not believe her and sends her to summon his wife. When Desdemona appears he accuses her and ignores her denials. He leaves in a rage as Emilia reappears. When Desdemona tells Emilia of Othello's state, she fetches Iago, and the two try to reassure her. Desdemona and Emilia leave as Roderigo arrives. He complains that Iago has taken his money and jewels and done nothing for him. Iago tells him that because Cassio is to replace Othello as governor, the general is leaving and will take Desdemona with him. Iago promises to help Roderigo kill Cassio so that Othello will have to stay, and Desdemona will remain within reach.

Act 4, Scene 3
On his way out, Othello tells Desdemona that she is to prepare for bed and dismiss Emilia. Desdemona says that she loves Othello despite his unreasonable anger, though she also has a presentiment of tragedy; she sings a song that was sung by an abandoned woman while she died. Though Desdemona is revolted by the idea of sexual infidelity, Emilia declares that men deserve it.

Act 5, Scene 1
Iago sets Roderigo up to ambush Cassio; he hopes that Roderigo and Cassio will kill each other, for Roderigo may claim repayment from him and Cassio may disprove his story. Cassio appears and Roderigo attacks him, but is wounded by Cassio. Iago then wounds Cassio from behind and flees. Othello sees the wounded Cassio crying for help and exults in the sight. He leaves as Lodovico and GRATIANO (2) arrive. Iago returns, pretends to be enraged at the assault on Cassio, and kills Roderigo. Bianca arrives. Iago declares that she is probably involved in the attempted murder and places her under arrest.

Act 5, Scene 2
Othello, at the bed of the sleeping Desdemona, is overcome with love for her and declares that he will not harm her beauty, but will kill her bloodlessly. She wakes, and he tells her to prepare for death. He says the handkerchief is proof of her adultery. She says that Cassio will clear her, but Othello triumphantly reports his death. She pleads for mercy, but Othello smothers her. Emilia appears, and Desdemona recovers enough to declare that she is dying in innocence. She dies, and Othello proclaims that he has murdered her because she was unfaithful. Emilia denies it, and Othello declares that Iago has proved it. She calls for help, and

Montano, Gratiano, and Iago appear. Othello speaks of Desdemona's handkerchief, and Emilia reveals the truth. Iago kills her and flees. Montano chases him, leaving Othello to his mounting grief. When Lodovico brings Iago back, Othello attacks him and wounds him before he is disarmed. Othello declares himself a fool but not a dishonourable one, stabs himself with a hidden weapon and dies.

COMMENTARY

The most striking difference between *Othello* and Shakespeare's other tragedies is its more intimate scale. The terror of the supernatural is not invoked, as it is in *Hamlet* and *Macbeth;* extremes of psychological derangement, as in *King Lear,* are not present. Kingdoms are not at stake, and the political consequences of the action are not emphasised as they are in varying degrees in all of the other tragedies. Here, Shakespeare focusses on personal rather than public life; Othello's plunge into obsession occurs mostly in private—only he and Iago know it is happening—and he murders Desdemona in the seclusion of their bedroom. The play has been described as a domestic comedy gone wrong. Its tragedy lies in the destruction of the happy personal lives of the general and his bride by the perverse malice of a single unsatisfied man. Yet *Othello* is profoundly social, for the human quality that Iago lacks and that he destroys in Othello is trust, the cement that holds people together. Jealousy, the play's central motif, is simply a particularly virulent form of interpersonal distrust. The tragedy of *Othello* is that a noble man loses faith and is reduced to a bestial frenzy. As a result, a love and a life are destroyed, and this loss inspires horror in the audience, which, combined with our pity for Desdemona, gives the play tremendous power. Significantly, *Othello* stands out as one of Shakespeare's plays that has been altered very little over the centuries by its producers, for its capacity to overwhelm audiences has always been recognised.

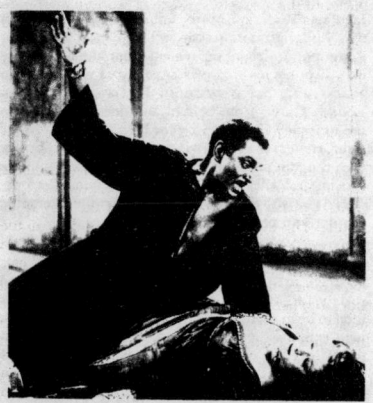

A scene from the 1965 film of Othello *with Laurence Olivier as the Moor and Maggie Smith as Desdemona. The same great passion with which Othello loves his wife leads him to murder her when his faith turns into jealousy.* (Courtesy of Culver Pictures, Inc.)

The central dynamic in *Othello* is the hero's change in attitude towards Desdemona. At first the couple are happily matched; when they defend their elopement, in 1.3, they establish themselves as mature lovers whose passion is both spiritual and sexual, mutually satisfying and based on self-knowledge. But Othello's weakness destroys his happiness as his trust in his wife turns to jealousy and then murderous hatred under the influence of Iago. On the other hand, his trust in his aide never flags until he is finally exposed. Othello comes to see love through Iago's eyes rather than Desdemona's. In a sense, Iago and Desdemona represent internalised features of the hero: he rejects his loving and generous self—that aspect of humanity that makes society possible—in favour of the dark passions of his self-centred ego. In the end, the forces of trust and love regain their strength as Othello finally recognises the goodness of Desdemona, and Iago is formally condemned, but in the meantime the action of the play has demonstrated the power of evil.

The motif of trust destroyed dominates the interactions of Iago and Othello on one hand and Othello and Desdemona on the other. Othello is placed between Iago—who cannot trust or love—and Desdemona—who offers an ideal, unconditional love. This situation closely resembles the traditional MORALITY PLAY, whose central character, usually symbolic of the human soul, is placed between an angel and a devil who each demand his loyalty. This dramatic form was still familiar to Shakespeare and his audience, and *Othello* reflects it in its distinctly allegorical quality. Iago is associated with the devil several times, and Desdemona—in her martyrlike acceptance of her entirely undeserved end—may be seen as a symbol of Christian love and resignation to the will of God.

In its structure *Othello* continually focusses our attention on its main theme, jealous mistrust. The relationships of Othello to Iago and Desdemona are paralleled in those between several minor characters in the play. For instance, Othello's credulousness is foreshadowed in that of Roderigo, whose victimisation by Iago is established in the opening scene, and makes clear the nature and extent of his villainy from the outset. Similarly, later in the play, Cassio's disastrous reversion from distrust to trust of the villain echoes the development of the main plot. Also, Cassio's ad-

miring recognition of Desdemona's virtues offers the opposite image to Othello's loss of perception, while her appreciation of Cassio reflects ironically on Othello's mistaken opinion of Iago.

Perhaps most striking are the two 'marriages' paralleling that of Othello and Desdemona. Cassio is linked with Bianca, and while they are not formally married, a comparison is irresistible because Iago substitutes Bianca for Desdemona when he deceives Othello about the handkerchief, in 4.1. More pointedly, Bianca's jealousy of Cassio—expressed in her complaint that he has avoided her, in 3.4, and her anger when she thinks that he has been given Desdemona's handkerchief by another woman—echoes Othello's emotion but in a context where jealousy seems justified. Iago and Emilia's marriage, while plainly lacking affection, let alone love, is not immune from sexual jealousy. Iago remarks several times that he is suspicious of his wife's adultery with either Othello in 1.3. 385–386) or Cassio (2.1.302). His assumption that his wife's lover was Othello sounds intended only to justify his campaign against the general, but he seems to have some cause for suspicion: Emilia clearly states that she would indeed commit adultery, in 4.3.70–76, 84–103, as she believes that unfaithfulness is a woman's only weapon against a bad husband. The mutual distrust in which these two live offers another instance of the play's major motif, jealousy. All three marriages, with their stress on this emotion, demonstrate abundantly the fragility of trust between humans.

Iago's jealousy is particularly significant, as it suggests that when he misleads Othello he is simply transferring his own psychic ailment. In fact, Iago's jealousy extends beyond a purely sexual context; he is motivated in large part by envy, the jealous sense that others have advantages over him. He fears that the free and virtuous natures of the other characters, especially Desdemona, may demonstrate his own worthlessness. It is precisely Othello's 'constant, noble, loving nature' (2.1.284) that he cannot endure, and he recognises that Cassio 'has a daily beauty in his life, / That makes me ugly' (5.1.19–20). He accordingly proposes to 'out of [Desdemona's] goodness make the net / That shall enmesh 'em all!' (2.3.352–353).

The parallels that reinforce the theme of jealousy illustrate the craftsmanship of the playwright, and indeed, *Othello* is a particularly well-constructed play. Most strikingly, Shakespeare introduces—and then contrives to disguise—what seems to be a serious defect of the plot, namely that Desdemona's infidelity should be utterly implausible to Othello for the simple reason that she has had absolutely no opportunity for it. Iago presents this fictional 'love affair' as though it had been going on for some time, while in fact Othello and Desdemona have only been married a few hours when they depart for Cyprus—on different ships, with Cassio on a third—and once there, Othello passes the first night with Desdemona and kills her on the second. The haste with which the plot unfolds contributes tremendously to its almost unbearable tension, and for this reason Shakespeare chose an unrealistic time span rather than a weeks-long scenario in which an adulterous affair could evolve realistically. He carries it off by means of a clever device that critics refer to as 'double time'. While the two days' development is nonsensical, it is effectively disguised by a number of strategic references suggestive of a different time frame. For instance, Iago speaks of '. . . how oft, how long ago, and when' (4.1.85) Cassio and Desdemona have made love, and Othello later justifies her murder with the claim that this love-making had occurred 'a thousand times' (5.2.213); Emilia says that Iago has asked her 'a hundred times' (3.3.296) to steal Desdemona's handkerchief, and she suggests that Desdemona has had 'a year or two' (3.4.100) to become acquainted with Othello; Cassio is said to have been absent from Bianca for a week, with the implication of an established relationship before that; orders recalling Othello to Venice arrive, reflecting time enough for news of the situation on Cyprus to have reached Venice and the orders returned. These hints, among numerous others, serve to keep before us a convincing sense that more has transpired than could actually be the case.

However, 'double time' is unworkable for exposition, and Act 1 differs from the rest of the play in being performed in real time. Here, in Venice, we are introduced to the characters and their world under more realistic circumstances. Events are not compressed into a short time for before the main action is underway the playwright does not need to deceive us about the pace of events, and he can properly establish the nature of his characters, especially Iago. In the long interchanges between him and Roderigo in 1.1 and 1.3, in his lie that opens 1.2, and especially in his soliloquy that closes the Act, Iago's villainous nature and his enmity towards Othello are made clear, and we are primed for the developments to follow.

Act 1 also differs from the rest of the play in its setting. This is very telling, for Othello's place in the society of Venice plays an important, if subtle, role in his downfall. As Brabantio's response to Desdemona's marriage makes abundantly clear, Venice is a closed society, racist in its distrust of Othello. Also, Venice is seen to be influenced by inhumane commercial values. Iago exploits the degraded values of Roderigo, who thinks love is a commodity, and many commentators have seen a satire on mercantile society—Venetian and English, both—in Iago's repeated advice to Roderigo to 'put money in thy purse' (beginning at 1.3.342). This is a world that cannot appreciate Othello's virtues. The general is thus isolated from the world he has married into; Iago can convince him that

Desdemona might 'repent' the 'foul disproportion' (3.3.242, 237) of a mixed marriage, and Othello lacks the assurance of a respectable social position that might temper the fear of rejection that his jealousy feeds on.

The racial bias of Shakespeare's Venice is important and quite prominent, especially in Act 1. Brabantio's belief that Desdemona could not love 'the sooty bosom / Of such a thing' (1.2.70–71) is based on the racist assumption that such love would be 'against all rules of nature' (1.3.101). Iago and Roderigo have stimulated Brabantio's rage with labels, such as 'old black ram' (1.1.88), 'Barbary horse' (1.1.111), and 'lascivious Moor' (1.1.126), associating race with animals, sex, and the devil, characteristically racist ploys, even today. No one disputes Brabantio's statement that Desdemona has subjected herself to 'general mock' (1.2.69) by marrying a black man; prejudice is plainly widespread in Venice.

Othello is the earliest sympathetic black character in English literature, and the play's emphasis on prejudice must have had particular impact in Shakespeare's LONDON, which was a distinctly biased society. Though Africans were present in London in some numbers beginning around 1550—especially once the English slave trade got underway in the 1560s—little distinction was drawn between North African and sub-Saharan blacks. Africa and Africans had figured in English drama from an even earlier date; dozens of 16th-century plays made use of African settings or characters, though virtually all of them were wildly inaccurate and blatently racist, depicting Africans in simple stereotypes as idle, lustful, and likely to be treacherous. Not surprisingly, the biases of English society as a whole was equally blatant. In 1599 and 1601 the government made an effort to deport all of the 'Negars and Blackamores which [have] crept into this realm'.

The Venice of *Othello,* like London in its greed and racism, has another aspect, however. As represented by the Duke and the Senators, the society offers a model of trust and co-operation. In 1.3 we see these figures arriving through consensus at a collective response to the Turkish threat, and in the same workmanlike spirit they insist that Othello be permitted a defence against Brabantio's charges. They recognise his innocence and accept him as their general, and Brabantio agrees entirely, accepting his society's collective judgement. On the whole, Venice is not a promising milieu for Iago's purposes; significantly, Shakespeare removes the action from Venice when the main plot is to get under way. On Cyprus the action is isolated; no social or political distractions remove Othello from Iago's influence, and Desdemona can have no recourse to advice or intervention. It is only when Venetian envoys come to Cyprus that the truth can be unfolded, though too late.

In another manipulation of time, Shakespeare tightens the tension rapidly as we approach the play's climax by subtly increasing the pace with which things seem to occur. As Iago puts it, 'Dull not device by coldness and delay' (2.3.378). For instance, when Iago first makes Othello desire revenge against Desdemona and Cassio, the general demands Cassio's death 'within these three days' (3.3.479) and Desdemona's death is not scheduled. But when the matter is next discussed, Othello insists on killing Desdemona 'this night . . . this night' (4.1.200–202) and Iago promises to kill Cassio 'by midnight' (4.1.207). This sudden acceleration creates an effect of heightened tension that reflects Othello's mental state. It also diverts attention from the illogicality of time's so-swift passage while increasing the pace.

Only once, and in a very telling manoeuvre, does Shakespeare slacken the pace of events—in the famed 'willow' scene (4.3), in which Desdemona prepares for bed and, unknowingly, for death. This lull prepares us for the final storm of Act 5's violence. Desdemona's melancholy at Othello's changed and angry manner yields a morbid fantasy that is, in effect, a slow, grand elegy of her innocence and virtue. She imagines herself dead, shrouded in her wedding sheets, and she remembers her mother's maid, who died of love, singing 'a song of "willow", / An old thing [that] express'd her fortune' (4.3.28–29). Ominously, Desdemona sings it herself, and its plaintive sadness soothes her even as it chills us with its portent of her death. Her calm and beautiful acceptance of fate is contrasted at the scene's close with Emilia's cynical speech on adultery. Our appreciation of Desdemona in this scene makes the approaching climax all the more horrible. Despite its languid tone, this brilliantly conceived interlude actually succeeds in heightening our anxiety.

Through a simple plot with minimal comic relief, Shakespeare avoids distractions that would permit the audience to recuperate temporarily from the increasing tension into which they are drawn. The few diversions from the main plot are mostly anxiety-producing disturbances. The midnight brawl of 2.3 that results from Cassio's drunkeness; Othello's cruel rudeness as he pretends to take his wife's bedroom for a bordello, in 4.2; another fight scene, in which Roderigo wounds Cassio and Iago kills Roderigo—all of these events offer the reverse of comic relief, tightening our emotional screws for the next stage of Iago's plot against Othello. Even at the play's close, the tension is similarly maintained as the eerie privacy in which the murder of Desdemona takes place is followed by the raucous tumult in which Iago kills Emilia and Othello wounds Iago and kills himself. Only in the very last lines of the play is there relief when Lodovico disposes of practical matters in the wake of the death of the Venetian commander on Cyprus.

Not only is the rule of society re-established at the close, but Iago's triumph over Othello is undercut by

the hero's recognition of his error. The trust that had been violated is at least acknowledged in the end. In the world of tragedy, death and defeat are inescapable, thus mirroring the tragic aspects of human existence. Othello is not a hero through triumph, but because he is an incarnation of basic human energies, both good and bad. When he joins Desdemona in death he offers recompense for his grievous self-centredness earlier, and while this compensation is obviously useless to her, it offers *us* a cathartic sense of reconciliation with tragedy. The lives—and deaths—of Othello and Desdemona are in the end transcended by their involvement with each other. She sacrifices herself to her love and he himself to his grief that he was inadequate to it. Without the support of his love for Desdemona, Othello could only say, 'Chaos is come again' (3.3.93); with his recognition of his error, order is implicitly restored as the ethical meaning of the story is revealed.

SOURCES OF THE PLAY

The source for *Othello* was a novella by the Italian author, CINTHIO, published in his collection *Hecatommithi* (1565). No surviving English translation of the tale was made until much later, and scholars dispute whether the playwright read Cinthio in Italian, in a French or Spanish translation, or in some now lost English translation. In any case, Shakespeare made a number of significant changes in Cinthio's tale. He accelerated the course of events to produce a tauter drama, and he altered the personalities of the major characters, making Othello and Desdemona nobler and Iago more coldly malevolent. He also added such minor characters as Roderigo, Brabantio, and the Venetian officials.

An actual murder may also have been a source for the play. In 1565 an Italian serving the French government was diverted from a diplomatic mission by false reports of his wife's infidelity, circulated by his enemies. Returning home, he accepted her denials, but, after earnestly seeking her forgiveness, strangled her anyway in the name of honour. Scholars speculate that knowledge of this historical event may have influenced Shakespeare in his choice of Cinthio's tale, though no known English source can be cited.

Other minor literary sources include LEO AFRICANUS' *A Geographical History of Africa* (translated by John PORY; publ. 1600) and the *Natural History* of PLINY the Elder (translated by Philemon HOLLAND [4]). Also, Shakespeare's odd mention of two otherwise unknown characters—'Signior Angelo' and 'Marcus Luccicos' (1.3.16, 44)—suggests the existence of some minor source material that is now lost.

TEXT OF THE PLAY

Othello was probably written in 1603 or 1604, just before its earliest recorded performance. Some scholars believe that the BAD QUARTO of *Hamlet* (Q1, 1603) is contaminated by recollections of lines from *Othello*, favouring an earlier date (possibly 1602) for *Othello*, though others find the evidence uncertain. On grounds of style and content, *Othello* cannot be dated earlier than 1602.

The play was first published in 1622 by Thomas WALKLEY, in a QUARTO edition, known as Q1, printed by Nicholas OKES. It was printed from a manuscript whose nature has been the subject of considerable scholarly debate. It may have been a FAIR COPY of Shakespeare's manuscript, or it may have been a transcript of either his FOUL PAPERS or of the PROMPT-BOOK kept by the KING'S MEN. The transcription may originally have been made for Walkley's publication, or for use by the King's Men, or, possibly, for an individual, a theatre enthusiast. Given the surviving evidence, none of these theories can be positively proven or disproven.

In 1623 *Othello* appeared in the FOLIO edition of plays, and this text (known as F) was probably printed from Q1, but amended according to another manuscript whose nature is also perplexing. It may have been Shakespeare's fair copy; it may have been a prompt-book; it may have reflected alterations resulting from years of productions; it may have included errors made by someone relying on their memory of performances; it may have incorporated Shakespeare's own alterations. Again, no hypothesis can be established firmly.

Whatever this manuscript was, it differed significantly from Q1. There are over a thousand variants, most of them minor, but F contains about 160 lines not present in Q1, including a few substantial passages. The longest fragment (4.3.31–52, 54–56) contains much of the 'willow' song, for instance. On the other hand, Q1 contains ten brief passages (the longest being four lines) not in F. Whether these variations represent additions to one text or cuts from the other is debated by scholars; in practise, modern editors have generally found F to be the superior text and have used it as the basis for their versions, while also using variants from Q1 in many particular instances. However, some editors reverse the priority.

THEATRICAL HISTORY OF THE PLAY

The earliest known performance of *Othello* took place at the court of King JAMES I on November 1, 1604. Numerous other performances in various theatres and at court are recorded prior to the closure of the theatres by the civil war in 1642; and it appears to have been among the most popular of Shakespeare's plays in his own lifetime, as it has been ever since. Richard BURBAGE (3) was the first Othello, and though the original Iago was not recorded, it is known that after 1619 Joseph TAYLOR was famous in the role.

After the Restoration, *Othello* was among the first

plays to be staged in the re-opened theatres. On Dec. 8, 1660, Thomas KILLIGREW's version, in which Margaret HUGHES played Desdemona, featured the first woman to perform on an English stage. William DAVENANT's company performed the play as well, attesting to its continuing popularity. A number of anecdotes from this period tell of enthralled spectators leaping onto the stage to prevent the murder of Desdemona. Charles HART (1) played Othello, but Thomas BETTERTON was acknowledged the greatest Moor of the day. Michael MOHUN was a notable Iago.

In the 18th century *Othello* continued to be among the most often performed of Shakespeare's plays. Most leading actors undertook the title roles, with Barton BOOTH (1), James QUIN, and Spranger BARRY (3) prominent among them, while John HENDERSON and Charles MACKLIN were successful Iagos. In the early 19th century Edmund KEAN (2) was acclaimed as the greatest Othello of all time, a status that some critics believe may still apply, though his legend has doubtless been enhanced by the fact that he collapsed on-stage while playing the part (into the arms of Iago, played by his son Charles KEAN [1]) and never recovered, dying a few weeks later. Othello was a natural vehicle for Ira ALDRIDGE, the first great black Shakespearean actor. William MACREADY played both Othello and Iago at various times, as did Edwin FORREST and Edwin BOOTH (2). Forrest's performances as Othello in New York in 1826 are said to have inaugurated the popularity of Shakespearean tragedy in America. Charlotte CUSHMAN was acclaimed as Desdemona, opposite Forrest, in London in 1846. Booth alternated playing Othello and Iago with Henry IRVING in a famous London run of 1881, with Ellen TERRY (1) as Desdemona, and the soon-to-be-famous playwright Arthur Wing Pinero as Iago. Tommaso SALVINI played Othello in Italian, often with an English-speaking company, in productions that were immensely popular in both England and America throughout the 1870s and 1880s.

Among many noteworthy 20th-century stagings of *Othello,* perhaps the most renowned have been two American productions featuring extraordinary performances: that of Paul ROBESON as Othello—directed by Margaret WEBSTER (3) (1943)—and Christopher PLUMMER as Iago opposite the Othello of James Earl JONES (1) in Nicol WILLIAMSON's presentation (1982). Other 20th-century Othellos have included Oscar ASCHE, Earle HYMAN, Ralph RICHARDSON (2), and Donald WOLFIT. In 1981 an American company under a Japanese director adapted *Othello* to Kabuki, the traditional, stylised Japanese drama, and performed in several American cities. Eleven films have been made of *Othello*—seven of them silent movies. An Italian film shot in Venice in 1909 was the first attempt to film Shakespeare on location. The best-known films are those starring Orson WELLES (who also directed; 1952) and Laurence OLIVIER (1965). *Othello* has also been made for TELEVISION three times, all in Great Britain (1946, 1955, 1981). In addition, *Othello* has inspired several operas, the most notable being Guiseppe VERDI's *Otello* (1887), with libretto by Arrigo BOITO, which is considered among the greatest of all operas.

Other (Other Clown, Second Clown, Second Grave-digger) Minor character in *Hamlet,* the GRAVE-DIGGER's friend. The Other is a straight man whose simple remarks and questions give rise to the ripostes of his companion in 5.1.1–60. Although theatrical tradition dating to the 17th century makes the Other—his designation in early editions of the play—a second grave-digger, some modern editors point out that he seems to belong to another, unspecified profession when he addresses the Grave-digger in 5.1.14. Like the Grave-digger, the Other is a CLOWN (1), and some editions identify him accordingly in stage directions and speech headings.

Otway, Thomas (1652–1685) English playwright, author of an adaptation of *Romeo and Juliet.* Otway's *History and Fall of Caius Marius* (1670) combined elements of Shakespeare's play with a drama based on a biography in PLUTARCH's *Lives.* Set in ancient ROME, *Caius Marius* tells of two lovers on opposite sides of a political conflict between patricians and plebeians. His ROMEO was Caius Marius (157–86 B.C.), an historical Roman commoner who rose to high political rank, marrying the daughter of a consul, one Julia (Otway's JULIET [1]), the aunt of Julius CAESAR (1). He later led one side in the first Roman civil war. Otway's *Marius* was so popular that *Romeo and Juliet* was not revived until well into the 1740s.

Otway was best known for two works that dominated the age of Restoration TRAGEDY: *The Orphan* (1680) and *Venice Preserved* (1682). Both are still revived occasionally. Though he was prolific, and his plays were produced by Thomas BETTERTON, Otway ended in poverty, dying quite suddenly at 33, after a short but dramatic life consumed by an unrequited love for Elizabeth BARRY (2). According to one report, he died in a pub; according to another, in a debtor's prison.

Outlaws Minor characters in *The Two Gentlemen of Verona.* The three Outlaws capture VALENTINE (2) and SPEED in 4.1. They are recognisable romantic types, gentlemen whose youthful hot-bloodedness has resulted in their exile. They are also comic figures to some extent, as is shown by their prompt election of Valentine as their chieftain because he is a handsome gentleman who is versed in foreign languages.

Ovid (Publius Ovidius Naso) (43 B.C.–17 A.D.) Roman poet, author of sources for many of Shakespeare's

works. The story of Philomel, in Ovid's *Metamorphoses*, a collection of poems telling tales from Greek and Roman mythology, provided the germ of LAVINIA's fate in *Titus Andronicus*, and in fact Ovid's work is explicitly cited in 4.1.42. *The Metamorphoses* was also the source for *Venus and Adonis*, which has a couplet from Ovid's *Amores* (love poems) as an epigraph. Another work by Ovid—the *Fasti*, an almanac in verse with legends and historical anecdotes for each month—was the principal source for *The Rape of Lucrece*. In addition, many references to and quotations from Ovid are scattered throughout the plays, particularly the early ones. Shakespeare undoubtedly read Ovid in school, as his work figured largely in the Latin curriculum of the times, but he also made use of Arthur GOLDING's translation of *The Metamorphoses*. A Latin copy of *The Metamorphoses* in the BODLEIAN LIBRARY bears a note declaring that it was once owned by Shakespeare, but the accompanying Shakespearean signature is rejected as inauthentic by scholars and handwriting experts.

Ovid, a minor aristocrat who abandoned the practise of law for poetry, lived comforably in Rome. He was respected for his poetry and patronised by the emperor Augustus CAESAR (2), until he was suddenly exiled in 8 A.D., partly for having written some erotic poems (his *Ars Amatoria*, or *Arts of Love*) that allegedly led the emperor's daughter to promiscuity and partly for some other, now obscure scandal. He spent the remainder of his life in a remote colonial outpost on the Black Sea. His boast at the close of *The Metamorphoses* that 'immortality is mine to wear' has proven justified, for that work has inspired poets and artists ever since.

Oxford (1), Edward de Vere, Earl of (1550–1604) English aristocrat, poet, and playwright. Oxford was a patron of poets and players (see OXFORD'S MEN) and wrote verse and plays himself. John LYLY was his secretary and wrote plays for his boys' company (see CHILDREN'S COMPANIES). Oxford's own plays are lost, but he was ranked with Shakespeare by Francis MERES as a good COMEDY writer.

Oxford was renowned as a violent and irresponsible nobleman. Orphaned at 12, he was raised in the household of Lord BURGHLEY, the chief minister of Queen ELIZABETH (1), and he married Burghley's daughter, though against her father's will. He may have killed a servant when he was 17, though the affair was hushed up, and his brawling was notorious. However, he was also an accomplished musician and dancer, and he was a favourite courtier of the queen, until he converted to Roman Catholicism. He then made one of the queen's ladies-in-waiting pregnant, for which he was imprisoned in 1581. After his release, he brawled and duelled with the woman's family, finally leaving the country to fight for the Dutch Republic and incurring Elizabeth's wrath for doing so without seeking her permission. By 1590 he had spent his fortune, but when his wife died and he remarried—to another of the queen's ladies—the queen granted him a pension.

Oxford (2), John de Vere, Earl of (1443–1513) Historical figure and minor character in *3 Henry VI* and *Richard III*, a follower of Queen MARGARET (1) and King HENRY VI in the former play, and of RICHMOND in the latter. In *3 Henry VI* Oxford supports Margaret against WARWICK (3) at the French court in 3.3. When Warwick changes sides and joins Margaret, Oxford participates in the campaign to reinstate Henry. He is captured at the battle of TEWKESBURY and sentenced to imprisonment. The historical Oxford was not present at Tewkesbury, having fled the country after the earlier battle of BARNET. Several years later, he attempted another invasion but was defeated and captured, beginning the imprisonment mentioned in the play. After 10 years, he escaped and joined the Earl of RICHMOND in Paris. In *Richard III* Oxford, though historically an important general in Richmond's campaign, speaks only two lines.

Oxford's Men Acting company of the ELIZABETHAN THEATRE. In 1580 a troupe of players previously patronised by the Earl of Warwick—the Earl of LEICESTER's brother—transferred their allegiance to Edward de Vere, the Earl of OXFORD (1), though it is unclear whether they joined an extant company or constituted the founding members of Oxford's Men. Their best-known member was Laurence DUTTON. They do not seem to have been successful—mostly touring in the provinces and playing at the court of Queen ELIZABETH (1) only occasionally. Their history, however, is not clear, for Oxford also patronised a CHILDREN'S COMPANY managed by Henry EVANS (2) and a troupe of tumblers and acrobats. In some cases the surviving records are unclear about which of Oxford's groups they refer to. In 1602 Oxford's Men—the troupe of adult actors—received a licence to join WORCESTER'S MEN and were absorbed by that company, probably in the same year.

P

Padua City in northern Italy, setting for *The Taming of the Shrew.* Shakespeare transferred the scene of his story from Ferrara, where it is set in his source, GASCOIGNE's play *Supposes,* for Padua was better known to his audience, enjoying a reputation as a major seat of learning. In fact, many English students of Shakespeare's day attended the university at Padua, which had been founded in the 13th century. The town's academic ambience is not important to the play—although in 1.1.1–24 LUCENTIO speaks of the desire for learning that has brought him to Padua—but a university town seems an apt setting for a tale of young love.

In *The Merchant of Venice* Padua is the home of PORTIA's cousin, a scholar known for his legal wisdom, and it thus figures (in 3.4.59 et al.) in the heroine's presentation of herself as a lawyer. It is also the hometown of BENEDICK in *Much Ado About Nothing.*

Shakespeare's apparent assumptions that Padua was a port (*Shrew,* 1.1.42, 4.2.83) and in Lombardy (1.1.3) have often been cited as serious errors, since Padua is neither on the coast nor in Lombardy. However, while the playwright's European geography is sometimes mistaken, here he may be excused: in his day the term Lombardy was often taken to refer to all of northern Italy, and Padua, while it is some 20 miles from the Adriatic, was a 16th-century canal port of some significance. An intricate canal network covered much of northern Italy in the Middle Ages and Renaissance; it operated until it was superseded by railroads in the 19th century. In fact, Padua can still be reached by water in small craft.

Page (1) Minor character in *Richard III,* an attendant to RICHARD III. In 4.2 Richard asks the Page to recommend an ambitious nobleman to do a desperate deed. The youth names James TYRELL, whom Richard commissions to murder his nephews.

Page (2) Minor character in *Romeo and Juliet,* a young servant of MERCUTIO. Mortally wounded in 3.1, Mercutio sends the Page, who does not speak, to summon a surgeon.

Page (3) Minor character in *Romeo and Juliet,* a servant of PARIS (2). The Page accompanies his master on his nocturnal visit to the grave of JULIET (1) in 5.3; when ROMEO arrives and fights with Paris, the Page summons the WATCHMAN and later testifies to the PRINCE (1).

Page (4) Minor character in *The Taming of the Shrew,* servant of the local LORD (1), who directs him to masquerade as the wife of the deluded Christopher SLY (1) in the INDUCTION. He humorously discourages Sly's sexual advances, and his performance as a wife foreshadows the ideal of womanly obedience that the main play advocates. His instructions are to request, as a real wife would, 'What is't your honour will command, / Wherein your lady and your humble wife / May show her duty and make known her love?' (Ind.1.112–115), and he presents himself to Sly as 'your wife in all obedience' (Ind.2.108). These attitudes are precisely those prescribed for wives by the converted KATHERINA in 5.2.

Page (5) Character in *2 Henry IV,* FALSTAFF's attendant. For the most part, the Page simply performs routine tasks and says little. However, in 2.2, where he bests BARDOLPH (1) in a battle of wits and is rewarded with money by PRINCE (6) HAL and POINS, the Page saucily comes into his own, in the manner of the pert young pages in the plays of John LYLY, whose works were well known to Shakespeare.

The Page's diminutive stature is frequently referred to in humorous terms by the other characters; e.g., in 1.2.1, he is a 'giant'; in 2.2.82, an 'upright rabbit'; in 5.1.55–56, 'my tall fellow'. It is thought that these references, with others in other plays, reflect the presence of a particularly small boy actor (see ELIZABETHAN THEATRE) in the CHAMBERLAIN'S MEN, for whom Shakespeare wrote the play. The same character appears in *The Merry Wives of Windsor* as ROBIN (1) and in *Henry V* as the BOY (3).

Page (6) Minor character in *2 Henry IV,* a servant of King HENRY IV. The Page, who does not speak, carries messages for the King in 3.1.

Page (7) Either of two minor characters in *As You Like It,* singers in the court of DUKE (7) Senior. In 5.3 the

Pages sing a parody of a love song for TOUCHSTONE and AUDREY that provides a brief interlude of pure entertainment before the play reaches its climax.

Page (8) Minor character in *All's Well That Ends Well,* a servant of the COUNTESS (2) of ROSSILLION. In 1.1.183 the Page summons PAROLLES for BERTRAM, then exits. He evokes the world of an aristocratic household but is otherwise of no consequence.

Page (9) Minor character in *Timon of Athens,* an illiterate messenger who asks APEMANTUS to read the addresses on letters he is to deliver. The Page is an employee of the same courtesan as the FOOL (3), and has no place in the play's plot. His brief appearance is sometimes taken as evidence of a non-Shakespearean hand in the composition of the play. However, the episode closely resembles that of the illiterate SERVANT (4) in *Romeo and Juliet,* and most scholars now conclude that the Page is Shakespeare's invention. He was probably part of a SUB-PLOT that remained undeveloped when the playwright abandoned this incomplete play.

Page (10) Character in *Henry VIII.* See BOY (9).

Page (11), Anne Character in *The Merry Wives of Windsor.* See ANNE (3).

Page (12), George Character in *The Merry Wives of Windsor,* the husband of MISTRESS (3) Margaret Page. Unlike his jealous friend FORD (1), Page believes in his wife's fidelity. He is consistently mild and cheerful, pleasant evidence of the solid virtues of the bourgeois life of Windsor. He is part of the group, led by the HOST (2), who mediate the quarrel between EVANS (3) and CAIUS (2), and he repeatedly tries to cajole Ford out of his irrational jealousy. If Page seems unpleasantly mercenary in attempting to marry his daughter ANNE (3) to the ridiculous SLENDER, we should remember that such motives were ordinary, indeed expected, in Elizabethan fathers, and we note that Page accepts Anne's elopement with FENTON with good grace. Page's solid common sense is exemplified in his dry reply to Ford's exaggerated protestations of trust in his wife once he has been proven wrong. Page suggests, ' 'Tis well, 'tis well; no more. Be not as extreme in submission as in offence' (4.4.10–12). Once FALSTAFF is properly humiliated for his deeds, in 5.5, it is Page who ends the punishment, saying, 'Yet be cheerful, knight: thou shalt eat a posset to-night at my house . . .' (5.5.171–172).

In 1.1.42 Evans gives Page the name Thomas, though he is called George by his wife in three places (2.1.143, 2.1.151, 5.5.199). While this may represent an error by Evans, it is more probably just a typical instance of Shakespeare's tolerance for minor inconsistencies.

Page (13), Mistress Margaret Character in *The Merry Wives of Windsor.* See MISTRESS (3).

Page (14), William Character in *The Merry Wives of Windsor.* See WILLIAM (1).

Painter (1) Minor character in *Timon of Athens,* a flatterer of TIMON. In 1.1 the Painter and his friend the POET (2) anticipate that they will profit from Timon's generosity when they present him with examples of their art. The Painter speaks much less than his friend, but shares his pride and false modesty. He agrees with the Poet that though Timon is now prosperous, this can change, and the 'quick blows of Fortune' (1.1.93) may reduce their host to poverty and friendlessness. Though the Painter is not among the disloyal friends depicted in Timon's downfall, he is not unlike them. In 5.1 he joins the Poet in an attempt to resume their approach to their one-time benefactor in the belief that his fortunes have again improved. 'Therefore', says the Painter, ' 'tis not amiss we tender our loves to him' (5.1.12–13). He is unconcerned that he has never painted anything for Timon. He imagines that a promise of future work is as 'Good as the best. Promising is the very air o' th' time . . . To promise is most courtly and fashionable' (5.1.22–27). However, Timon understands what they are up to, and drives them away. The Painter, like his friend the Poet, is a satirical emblem of the greed and hypocrisy of courtiers.

Painter (2), William (c.1525–1590) English translator, creator of source material for several of Shakespeare's works. Painter produced an anthology of more than 100 tales from Italian and Latin authors, including LIVY, PLUTARCH, BOCCACCIO, and CINTHIO, in his *Palace of Pleasure* (1566–1567). A Boccaccio story from Painter was the principal source for *All's Well That Ends Well,* and other tales provided material for *Romeo and Juliet, Timon of Athens,* and *The Rape of Lucrece.* Many other Elizabethan and Jacobean playwrights turned to Painter as well, and he may deserve credit for the abundance of Italian settings and stories in their plays. Painter was a government official in charge of military supplies at the TOWER OF LONDON.

Palamon One of the title characters of *The Two Noble Kinsmen,* cousin of ARCITE. As introduced in 1.2, Palamon and Arcite are young noblemen whose chief concern is with their knightly honour and whose lives revolve around their friendship with each other. However, while prisoners of war in ATHENS, they both fall in love with EMILIA (4), the beautiful sister-in-law of Duke THESEUS (2), and they argue over who saw her first. Eventually they fight a duel for Emilia, in which, following Theseus' rules, the loser is not to be killed but rather executed afterwards. Palamon loses, but just before he is to be beheaded, Arcite is killed by a

runaway horse, and Palamon prepares to marry Emilia at the play's close. As stylised knightly protagonists, Palamon and Arcite resemble each other fairly closely, but Palamon can be distinguished as the generally more belligerent of the two. On the other hand, he also seems somewhat disillusioned at the close of their story, making him the more interesting character finally.

In 1.2 Palamon is a shallow fellow whom Arcite criticises for his narrow military outlook. In 2.1 he insists that their enthusiasm for the same, seemingly unapproachable woman is grounds for unsparing enmity, despite Arcite's efforts to find some other approach. Palamon escapes from prison with the help of the warden's DAUGHTER (2)—whom he immediately abandons—and in Act 3 he persistently pushes Arcite to duel, until Theseus intervenes and establishes the rules under which they finally fight.

Palamon's long prayer to Venus in 5.1 marks a turning point, for instead of the enraptured plea for Emilia's heart that we might expect, he vents a satirical recital of the ridiculous behaviour love inspires. He mocks the tyrant who weeps to a girl and the old man who is confident his young wife is faithful, and he recites all the ugly betrayals and offences a lover might commit, though he disclaims them. The pleasant aspects of love are not mentioned. He closes his prayer by apostrophising the goddess as one 'whose chase is this world / And we in herds thy game' (5.1.131–132). Such cynicism reflects the weight that the conflict has had—he wears Venus' 'yoke, . . . [that is] heavier / Than lead itself [and] stings more than nettles' (5.1. 95–97), for in the end he loses his friend. At the close, engaged to Emilia, he addresses his dead cousin with a plaint that typifies the confusion and helplessness of humanity in the hands of unpredictable fate, the play's most important theme: 'O cousin, / That we should things desire which do cost us / the loss of our desire! that naught could buy / Dear love but loss of dear love!' (5.4.109–112).

Palsgrave's Men Theatrical company in LONDON, previously known as PRINCE HENRY'S MEN and the ADMIRAL'S MEN. When Prince HENRY (2) died in November 1612, the patronage of his theatre company was taken over by Frederick V, Elector Palatine, the German fiancé of Princess ELIZABETH (3). The couple married early in 1613, and the actors took one of Frederick's titles. A palsgrave, literally 'palace count', was a noble of the Holy Roman Empire who ruled with imperial powers within his own territories. The new royal patent for the Palsgrave's Men listed the members of the company, including Samuel ROWLEY (1)—who also wrote plays for the company—Thomas DOWNTON, Humphrey JEFFES, and John SHANK. They continued to play at the FORTUNE THEATRE and at the royal court, but in 1621 the Fortune burned to the ground, and the company lost all its costumes and props, and even many play scripts. The company struggled along for several years, but never completely recovered. After a bad season in 1625—complicated by the combination of a plague epidemic and the death of King JAMES I—the company disbanded.

Pandar Minor character in *Pericles,* the keeper of a brothel who, with his wife, the BAWD, buys the kidnapped MARINA. The Pandar is somewhat less hard than his wife. He contemplates retirement from a trade whose practise puts them on 'sore terms . . . with the gods' (4.2.33). However, he does have a business to run, and when Marina's glorious innocence begins to produce moral reform among the clientele he despairs. He moans 'I had rather than twice the worth of her she had ne'er come here' (4.6.1–2). He then curses her with a contradictory pair of sexual problems: 'the pox upon her green-sickness' (4.6.13). Thus, the Pandar offers comic relief from the melodramatic romance of the main story.

Pandarus Legendary figure and character in *Troilus and Cressida,* uncle of CRESSIDA who encourages her love affair with TROILUS. Pandarus, though a comic character, is also a conventional representation of a procurer of prostitutes. As such, he is a symbol of the moral corruption that permeates the world of the play. (Although Pandarus promotes only a single, non-mercenary affair, in both Shakespeare's play and its sources, he was already well established in Shakespeare's day as a symbol of the profession.)

Pandarus uses a variety of humorously exaggerated dictions: the rather affected language of the court (as when he uses the word 'fair' is several ways in one sentence, composing an elaborate compliment to HELEN [1] in 3.1.42–45); babytalk ('Come, come, what need you blush? Shame's a baby' [3.2.39]); and the bold language of braggadocio—e.g., in his deprecation of the SOLDIERS (6) as 'Asses, fools, dolts, chaff and bran, chaff and bran; porridge after meat . . . crows and daws, crows and daws' (1.2.245–248). In these passages Pandarus resembles such other Shakespearean comic characters as FALSTAFF, FESTE, and the NURSE (3) of *Romeo and Juliet.* AENEAS parodies him in 4.2.56–59, emphasising both his comic aspect and his inferior social status.

Pandarus insinuates himself into other people's lives and is capable of outrageous interruptions, as in his interception of Cressida's despairing cry to Troilus, 'Have the god's envy?' with the thoughtless 'Ay, ay, ay, ay, 'tis too plain a case' (4.4.27–28), and even of physical intrusiveness ('Let me embrace, too' [4.4. 13]). As we know from the eventual result of the liaison he arranges, Pandarus is ultimately malevolent. This is strikingly conveyed by his association with venereal disease in 5.4 and 5.10.

In the EPILOGUE, Pandarus steps somewhat out of character, speaking verse for the first time, as the formality of the device demands. However, he is still comically reprehensible. His recital on the humble-bee, whose 'Sweet honey and sweet notes together fail' (5.10.42–45) is a completely appropriate ending for this play of mistakes, misunderstandings, and failures. His flippant insults serve to distance the audience from the play as it closes. Because the audience is actually not composed of 'traitors and bawds . . . traders in the flesh . . . Brethren and sisters of the hold-door trade' (5.10.37, 46, 52), it need not identify with the play's discouraging ending and can feel itself superior to its corrupt world. The satirical nature of the play is confirmed, implicitly allowing for the existence of human virtues in contrast to the vices depicted on stage. Thus Pandarus provides some sense of the high-spirited resolution typical in COMEDY.

Pandarus appears in the *Iliad* of HOMER, but although he is an unpleasant character in that epic, he has nothing to do with Troilus or any other lovers (Cressida does not appear in Homer). It was in the Middle Ages that Pandarus first acquired his role as the lovers' go-between. By Shakespeare's day his name had become a common noun (and later a verb), although the spelling had changed slightly to *pander*, in which form it is still in common use.

Pandulph (d. 1226) Historical figure and character in *King John,* papal legate and enemy of King JOHN (3). Pandulph appears in 3.1 to demand John's submission to the pope in the appointment of an archbishop. When John refuses, Pandulph threatens King PHILIP (2) of France with excommunication if he does not break his new alliance with England and declare war on John. Pandulph offers an elaborate and specious argument (3.1.189–223) justifying the breaking of an oath. In 3.3 he offers the Dauphin LEWIS (1) a plan whereby he may conquer England and claim the throne. Having thus launched an invasion of England, Pandulph promises John that he will call it off in exchange for his oath of submission to the pope. John agrees, and he relinquishes his crown to Pandulph, who recrowns him, thus symbolically asserting papal supremacy over the government of England. However, in 5.2 Lewis refuses to withdraw and is defeated only when his traitorous English allies return to King John's side. Pandulph's unscrupulous warmongering and his inability to fulfil a promise fit the stereotype he represents: that of the steely, hypocritical Jesuit, capable of arguing any side of a question to suit the ends of the Catholic Church.

The historical Pandulph, a native of Rome, was sent to England in 1211—long after the marriage of Lewis and BLANCHE in 1200, with which his arrival is associated in the play—to insist that the papal candidate be installed as Archbishop of Canterbury, as in the play. But Shakespeare's condensation of history has skewed Pandulph's subsequent role, for by the time of the barons' revolt he was John's ally. After receiving John's submission to the pope in 1213, Pandulph supported him against his rebellious nobles, excommunicating those of them who extracted the Magna Charta from the king. John rewarded him with the bishopric of Norwich. Pandulph attempted unsuccessfully to prevent Lewis' invasion in 1216. He remained an influential bishop in England after John's death, serving as one of the regents for the young King HENRY (1) until 1221, when Henry exiled him, apparently on personal grounds. Pandulph died in Rome, but he was buried in Norwich, at his own request.

Pandulph was never a cardinal, the rank he holds in the play. Shakespeare may have taken this error from an early 16th-century play on King John, but there is no other evidence that he knew the work. It is more likely that Pandulph was elevated in rank for a simple and sensible theatrical reason: to dress him in the boldly dramatic scarlet robes of a cardinal, an ordinary item in the wardrobes of acting companies.

Panthino Minor character in *The Two Gentlemen of Verona,* the servant of ANTONIO (1). Panthino helps his master arrive at his fateful decision to send his son PROTEUS to court. Later, at the close of two successive scenes (2.2, 2.3), he furthers the action, appearing in order to hasten the departures of Proteus and LAUNCE respectively.

Papp, Joseph (b. 1921) American theatrical producer. Papp's New York Shakespeare Festival—originally (1953) the Shakespeare Workshop—has produced almost all of Shakespeare's plays. Since 1962 the Festival has offered summer performances free of charge in the Delacorte Theatre in New York's Central Park. In 1986 Papp began a six-year cycle of productions encompassing the 36 plays in the FIRST FOLIO.

Paris (1) Capital of FRANCE (1) and a location in several of Shakespeare's plays. In 3.4 and 4.1 of *1 Henry VI,* English forces occupy Paris, and King HENRY VI of England is crowned King of France there as part of the English diplomatic effort in the HUNDRED YEARS WAR. A number of scenes in *All's Well That Ends Well* (1.2, 2.1, 2.3, 2.4, 2.5) are located in the Paris palace of the KING (17) of France. One scene of *3 Henry VI* (3.3) is set at the court of King LEWIS (3), which is perhaps most plausibly assumed to be in Paris.

Paris (2) Character in *Romeo and Juliet,* a nobleman who wishes to marry JULIET (1). Paris, who is forced on Juliet by her parents, confidently assumes that he will wed her. He is closely juxtaposed with ROMEO throughout the play. Though no villain, Paris is nonetheless an agent of the world that opposes the private

universe of the lovers, and this is indicated by his staid and predictable behaviour and speech. His sentiments are those of the conventionally poetic lover, the type of lover Romeo was before he met Juliet. Lady CAPULET (3) even compares him to a book in 1.3.81–88. His smug exchange with Juliet in 4.1 can only stiffly approximate the brilliant poetry of her dialogue with Romeo. In his final appearance—at Juliet's tomb in 5.3—this well-meaning but vapid gentleman declares his grief in a formal sestet that is reminiscent of Romeo's word play in Act 1; the contrast is completed when the mature Romeo arrives, desperate and resolute. Paris honourably opposes the man whom he believes is desecrating Juliet's tomb, but he dies without comprehending, or even seeing, his rival's passion.

Paris (3) Legendary figure and character in *Troilus and Cressida,* a prince of TROY, son of King PRIAM, and brother of TROILUS and HECTOR. Before the play opens, Paris' theft of HELEN (1), wife of the Greek leader MENELAUS, has caused the TROJAN WAR. Thus his story is one of the examples of human folly that comprise a leading theme of the play. Paris is a decadent figure; his father calls him 'besotted on your sweet delights' (2.2.144), referring to Helen, and Paris confirms this judgement when he avoids the battlefield, claiming, 'I would fain have armed today, but my Nell would not have it so' (3.1.132–133). In his other appearances, he is merely one among the Trojan warriors, remarking on the events of the war; he also aids Troilus' courtship of CRESSIDA, covering for his absence from a state dinner and sending a warning to the lovers that a diplomatic delegation is approaching in 4.1. In Act 5 Paris fights with Menelaus, provoking sardonic remarks from THERSITES on 'the cuckold and the cuckold-maker' (5.7.9).

In classical mythology, Paris was bribed by Aphrodite to select her as the most beautiful of three quarrelling goddesses. She rewarded him by helping him to kidnap Helen. Though this well-known legend was pre-Homeric, HOMER does not mention it, saying only that Paris abducted Helen because of her beauty. In the *Iliad,* Paris is an effective warrior, specialising in archery, though he flees Menelaus in a moment of cowardice. Recovering, he challenges Menelaus to a duel but is defeated and must be rescued by Aphrodite. According to a later legend, Paris was the eventual killer of ACHILLES, placing an arrow precisely in his only vulnerable spot, his heel.

Parliament House Building housing the English Parliament in London, a location in one scene each of *1* and *3 Henry VI.* A part of WESTMINSTER (4) PALACE, this structure was a predecessor to the present Houses of Parliament, which were built in the 19th century. In 3.1 of *1 Henry VI,* an episode in the feud between GLOUCESTER (4) and WINCHESTER (1) occurs in the Parliament House, and in 1.1 of *3 Henry VI* YORK (8) claims the crown of HENRY VI there, pre-empting a meeting of Parliament called by Queen MARGARET (1).

In Shakespeare's day, as in the times he depicted in the HISTORY PLAYS, Parliament did not play the important policy-making and legislative role that we associate with the institution. Although Parliament's power to levy taxes made it a necessary nuisance to the monarch, the aristocracy largely controlled elections to the COMMONS (1), and, in any case, the actual administration of government was entirely in the hands of the royal ruler and his or her advisers. The first great advances towards modern representative government were to come in the quarter-century following the playwright's death.

Parnassus Plays Group of three amateur plays containing several references to Shakespeare and the LONDON theatrical world. These anonymous works are titled *The Pilgrimage to Parnassus, The Return from Parnassus* (Part 1), and *The Return from Parnassus* (Part 2), and they are referred to as *1, 2,* and *3 Parnassus.* They were performed at Cambridge University, probably on Christmas 1598, 1599, and 1601. *1 Parnassus* is an allegory of travel to Mt Parnassus, sacred to the Muses; *2* and *3 Parnassus* are set in London. In *2 Parnassus* a lover quotes from *Venus and Adonis* and declares, 'I'le worshipp sweet Mr Shakspeare, and to honoure him will lay his Venus and Adonis under my pillowe'. In *3 Parnassus* Richard BURBAGE (3) and Will KEMPE appear as characters. Burbage auditions someone who recites the opening lines of *Richard III,* and another character praises both *Venus and Adonis* and *The Rape of Lucrece.* Most strikingly, Kempe declares of inferior playwrights that 'our fellow Shakespeare puts them all downe . . . and Ben Ionson too', adding that Ben JONSON 'is a pestilent fellow . . . but our fellow Shakespeare hath given him a purge'. The play's date, 1601, suggests a reference to the WAR OF THE THEATRES, in which Jonson figured, but except for an obscure allusion in *Twelfth Night* 3.1.60, Shakespeare took no part in this exchange of satires. No 'purge' he might have given Jonson has been identified. The remark may merely express the author's preference for Shakespeare, or it may reflect some lost piece of theatre gossip.

Parolles (Paroles) Character in *All's Well That Ends Well,* a cowardly follower of BERTRAM. As his name, the French for 'words', suggests, Parolles is a blusterer who pretends to be a warrior and nobleman but whose deeds cannot match his boasts. Shallow and thoughtless, he influences Bertram to follow his worst instincts. Parolles aggravates Bertram's tendencies to self-indulgence, and he encourages him to disobey the KING (17) and run away to the wars in ITALY. After Parolles' humiliation in 2.4 by Lord LAFEW, who has

seen through his pretensions to gentlemanly status, he is ready to leave the court; he sees his chance in Bertram's wish to abandon HELENA (2), whom the King has made him marry. 'A young man married is a man that's marr'd. / Therefore away' (2.3.294–295), he urges. Once in Italy, Parolles again supports Bertram's inclinations to vice, serving as a go-between in the young man's attempt to seduce the virginal DIANA (1). Bertram's friends, led by the First LORD (6), then 'capture' Parolles and expose his cowardice and treachery in 4.3.

Parolles' defects have been recognised all along by everyone around Bertram. Upon his first appearance, Helena calls him 'a notorious liar . . . a great way fool, solely a coward' (1.1.108–109), and the Lords agree with Bertram's mother, the COUNTESS (2), that her son has been corrupted by Parolles, who is a 'very tainted fellow, and full of wickedness' (3.2.87). Parolles thus serves an important dramatic function, deflecting the negative image that might otherwise be attached to Bertram, whose stature must not sink too low, lest the central element of the plot—the determination of Helena to marry him—become ludicrous.

In his evil influence on Bertram, Parolles is most nearly the play's villain.

However, after his exposure as a charlatan, Parolles shows a striking resilience. Though his self-promoted career as a noble warrior is over, he will make the most of his new situation. 'Simply the thing I am / Shall make me live' (4.3.322–323), he observes, realising that he can, 'being fool'd, by fool'ry thrive' (4.3.327). He resolves to become a jester, or FOOL (1), among the French lords, a role well suited to his nature. In a line that is richly suggestive of Shakespeare's generous vision of humanity, he declares that 'There's place and means for every man alive' (4.3.328). In becoming a fool and acknowledgeing his defects, Parolles shows himself wiser than Bertram, preceding him in self-knowledge, just as he has preceded him in delinquency. His acceptance of life on any terms demonstrates a tremendous vitality, and he is certainly the most dynamic character in the play, with the possible exception of Helena.

Significantly, Parolles sparks Helena's energy in 1.1. In this scene Helena is understandably depressed; the household is in mourning for both Bertram's father and her own, and Bertram, her secret love, is leaving. Then Parolles appears, and his broadly humorous exercise in fashionable cynicism about virginity has a two-fold effect on the heroine. First, she sees that the courtly life that Parolles represents will offer sexual opportunities for Bertram, which she fears he will accept. Second, Parolles' vitality inspires Helena to declare, 'Our remedies oft in ourselves do lie' (1.1.212), and to decide to pursue Bertram. Thus Parolles' energy pervades *All's Well,* infusing the spirits of both major characters for good and evil alike. Finally, in becoming the jester for his old enemy Lafew at the close of the play, Parolles accepts—unconditionally, in contrast to Bertram—the reconciliation that is at the heart of Shakespearean COMEDY.

Although he has a distinct and credible personality, Parolles is descended from an ancient comic character type, the MILES GLORIOSUS of ancient Roman drama and the braggart soldier of Italian COMMEDIA DELL'ARTE; he shares his ancestry with several other Shakespearean characters, most notably FALSTAFF.

The Passionate Pilgrim Collection of poems published as Shakespeare's in 1599, though only a quarter of the works in the anthology are known to have been written by him. William JAGGARD assembled this miscellany, apparently without Shakespeare's participation or knowledge, presumably to capitalise on the popularity of *Venus and Adonis* and *The Rape of Lucrece.* All of the poems deal with love; the title refers to a commonplace image of the seeker of love as a worshipper at a sacred shrine.

The first two poems in *The Passionate Pilgrim* are SONNETS by Shakespeare (Nos. 138 and 144), and Nos. 3, 5, and 16 (in the modern numbering of the *Pilgrim*'s poems) are versions of passages from *Love's Labour's Lost* (4.3.57–70; 4.2.101–114; 4.3.98–118). Most scholars believe that Shakespeare wrote none of the remaining poems (there are 21 poems in the early editions, in which one poem is broken into two, and 20 in modern editions, in which the reassembled poem is No. 14).

Several of the remaining poems are attributable, with varying degrees of certainty, to other poets. No. 19 combines four stanzas from a poem by Christopher MARLOWE (1), 'The Passionate Shepherd to his Love', with one from Walter RALEIGH's 'The Nymph's Reply to the Shepherd'; these were not published until 1600, but they circulated in manuscript, a common practise at the time. No. 11 had already been published (1598) as the work of Bartholomew GRIFFIN, and Nos. 4, 6, and 9, similar in content and style, are usually attributed to him as well. Nos. 8 and 20 had already been published as the work of Richard BARNFIELD.

Seven of the remaining eight poems are generally considered by critics and scholars to be grossly inferior, unlikely to have been written by Shakespeare, even in his earliest years; only one, No. 12, seems possibly authentic, and, although it has charm, it differs considerably from known Shakespearean poems in its simple assertiveness and unsophisticated poetic technique. In 1631, it appeared as one stanza of a Thomas DELONEY poem.

Two editions of *The Passionate Pilgrim* were published by Jaggard in 1599; they are known conventionally as Q1 and Q2, although they appeared in OCTAVO, not QUARTO, format. Q1 is known only through the existence of isolated pages, bound with pages from Q2

in a single surviving copy, and its date is uncertain. Q2 appears to have been printed from Q1, and it is dated. Modern editions follow the combined texts.

Jaggard published a third edition, Q3 (also an octavo), in 1612 with additional material—also ascribed to Shakespeare—that he had culled from a book by Thomas HEYWOOD (2), which he had published three years earlier. Heywood protested publicly, asserting that not only he, but also Shakespeare was 'much offended' by Jaggard's high-handedness. Jaggard then issued Q3 with a new title page omitting Shakespeare's name.

Pastoral Popular RENAISSANCE literary genre that influenced a number of Shakespeare's works, especially *As You Like It* and *The Winter's Tale.* The term may be used as either an adjective or a noun. In general, pastoral literature encompasses all works that depict an idealised vision of rural life, usually within the context of a love story. Such works are frankly escapist, though they are occasionally vehicles for more elevated literary aims.

The pastoral originated in a genre of ancient Greek poetry that dealt with the lives of shepherds. It was continued in ancient Roman poetry that contrasted the urban and the rural in order to satirise the sophisticated life of urban courtiers, and it was rediscovered and imitated by Italian poets in the Renaissance. The pastoral romance, a long tale in verse or prose, begins with works by BOCCACCIO and was widely popular throughout Europe. In English, Sir Philip SIDNEY's *Arcadia* is among the greatest of pastorals, and Thomas LODGE's *Rosalynde,* the source of *As You Like It,* is a lesser example.

In the English pastoral dramas of Shakespeare's age, the delights of rustic life are conventionally idealised, and the amorous shepherds and shepherdesses are often portrayed as natural philosophers. Many dramatists essayed the genre in one form or another, notably Ben JONSON, John FLETCHER (2), and Samuel DANIEL. *As You Like It* gently parodies the conventions of the pastoral, but in Act 4 of *The Winter's Tale* they are treated more seriously, as a demonstration of human potentiality.

Patch-breech Character in *Pericles.* See FISHERMEN.

Pater, Walter (1839–1894) English essayist and novelist, author of several significant essays on Shakespeare. An apologist for the 'aesthetic' point of view represented by the phrase 'art for art's sake', which he helped introduce into the language, Pater was among the most noted writers of his day and an acknowledged master of English prose. He was best known for his *Studies in the History of the Renaissance* (1873)—the book that made him famous—and a novel, *Marius the Epicurean* (1885). Three notable essays on Shakespeare—on *Measure for Measure* (1874), *Love's Labour's Lost* (1878), and the HISTORY PLAYS (1889)—were highly influential, contributing to a revaluation of the playwright's work during the period.

Patience Minor character in *Henry VIII,* an attendant to Queen KATHERINE. In 4.2 Patience faithfully attends the deposed and dying queen in her exile at KIMBOLTON. Patience speaks very little, remarking on Katherine's ghastly appearance as she approaches death and saying, 'Heaven comfort her' (4.2.99); her mere presence—with that of GRIFFITH—tells us of the loyalty the good Katherine inspires. Her name is so striking that it is often thought Shakespeare created her for its sake. Griffith addresses her, 'Softly, gentle Patience' (4.2.82), as they watch their mistress sleep, and Katherine, approaching death, says, 'Patience, / You must not leave me yet' (4.2.165–166). The quality her name evokes is Katherine's signal trait and an important theme in the play: the virtue of patience in adversity. In gentle Patience, Shakespeare created an embodiment of the virtue itself, an allegorical figure like thsoe of the medieval MORALITY PLAY. This technique is characteristic of *Henry VIII,* which is filled with tableaus, MASQUE, and other emblematic episodes.

Patricians See SENATOR (2).

Patroclus Legendary figure and character in *Troilus and Cressida,* a Greek warrior in the TROJAN WAR and friend and follower of ACHILLES. While he himself is not an important figure, Patroclus' death is a key event in the plot, for it sparks Achilles to abandon his withdrawal from the combat and resume fighting, with the result that TROY loses the climactic battle. Patroclus represents Achilles in his dispute with the Greek leader, relaying his friend's statements of non-cooperation and carrying messages back to him. And, in an incidental episode that heightens the aura of decadence that surrounds the warriors, Achilles' jester, THERSITES, taunts Patroclus with a piece of malicious gossip, saying, 'Thou art said to be Achilles' male varlet . . . his masculine whore' (5.1.14, 16), though the imputation is carried no further and has no dramatic significance.

In the *Iliad* of HOMER, which contains the original version of Patroclus' story, Patroclus was somewhat older than Achilles. He was an attendant of the warrior because, as a boy, he had been taken under the protection of Achilles' father after accidentally killing someone. In Homer, Achilles' devoted friendship for Patroclus is one of the warrior's fine attributes, and there is no hint of a homosexual relationship. However, the tradition that the two were lovers was established by the 6th century B.C.

Paulina Character in *The Winter's Tale,* defender of Queen HERMIONE against the injustice of her husband, King LEONTES, and later the instrument of their reconciliation. Paulina boldly criticises the king for accusing Hermione of adultery, and her courage and common sense contrast tellingly with the king's jealous madness. After failing to prevent the king from exiling PERDITA, the infant daughter he believes illegitimate, Paulina enters into an amazing scheme: she stages Hermione's death and isolates her for 16 years, against the time when Leontes will have thoroughly repented. Perdita's return signals the ripeness of this plan, and Paulina reveals Hermione's existence in 5.3—in a stage-managed presentation of the long-lost queen as a statue. This revelation brings about the play's final reunion. Thus, Paulina, despite her bluff worldliness and overpowering manner, is an agent of redemption.

Paulina thinks clearly and acts decisively; she courageously takes it on herself to defend the queen as soon as she hears of her plight, and she handles the GAOLER (3) with the powerful courtesy of the *grande dame* that she is. Her criticism of the king is excoriating; he is reduced to insult—calling her a 'witch' (2.3.67), a 'callat [prostitute]' (2.3.90), and a 'gross hag' (2.3.107). When he threatens to burn her as a witch, she boldly replies, 'I care not' (2.3.113). Her boldness, however, does not always produce the envisioned results; her tactic of presenting the infant Perdita to the king merely aggravates his anger and results in the child's abandonment. Paulina alone cannot remedy the defect in the play's world—providence must see to that—but her efforts are important evidence that good has not died and may be restored.

Paulina has often been compared to King LEAR's faithful KENT (2). Like him, she offers a cure for the king's madness, declaring, 'I / Do come with words as medicinal as true' (2.3.35–36). Her therapy is a raw and intrusive one. In Act 5 she continues her powerful ministrations. She reinforces Leontes' repentance by continually reminding him of the supposedly dead Hermione and demands that he vow never to take a wife without her approval. She reveals Hermione's survival with a fine theatrical sense, raising dramatic expectations of sorcery by disclaiming 'wicked powers' (5.3.91), and she prevents Hermione from disclosing too much with a hasty 'There's time enough for that' (5.3.128). At the close, within the atmosphere of love and reconciliation, Paulina finally permits herself to lament the loss of her own husband, ANTIGONUS, which stirs the king to ordain her remarriage to CAMILLO. Her value in the world of the play is acknowledged when the king calls her one 'whose worth and honesty / Is richly noted' (5.3.144–145). The central theme of *The Winter's Tale* is that human moral energy must support divine providence, and Paulina's valiant efforts are a prime source of this ingredient.

Pavier, Thomas (d. 1625) English bookseller and publisher associated with the publication of several of Shakespeare's plays. Pavier is notorious for his involvement in the FALSE FOLIO of Shakespeare's works (1619), to which he contributed pirated texts of *2* and *3 Henry VI* (jointly, as the WHOLE CONTENTION), *Henry V*, *Pericles,* and two plays not actually by Shakespeare, SIR JOHN OLDCASTLE and A YORKSHIRE TRAGEDY. Pavier had earlier published the first editions of *Sir John Oldcastle* (1600) and *A Yorkshire Tragedy* (1608), and attributed the latter to Shakespeare at that time. In 1600 Pavier had purchased the 'rights' to a pirated edition of *Henry V* from Thomas MILLINGTON and John BUSBY, and he reissued their BAD QUARTO as Q2 of the play in 1602. Though Pavier's practices seem dubious from a modern point of view, the evolving world of 17th-century publishing was not so strict, and Pavier was an honoured member of the STATIONERS' COMPANY.

Peaseblossom Character in *A Midsummer Night's Dream,* a fairy attendant to the fairy Queen TITANIA. In 3.1 Titania assigns Peaseblossom to the retinue of the

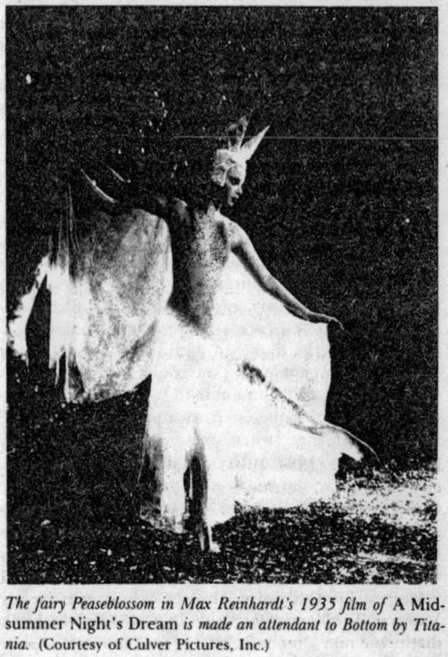

The fairy Peaseblossom in Max Reinhardt's 1935 film of A Midsummer Night's Dream *is made an attendant to Bottom by Titania.* (Courtesy of Culver Pictures, Inc.)

comical rustic BOTTOM, whom the Queen has been magically induced to love. Bottom has been endowed by PUCK with the head of an ass, but he does not know of his new adornment, and Peaseblossom serves him in 4.1 by scratching his strangely itchy face.

Pedant, The Minor character in *The Taming of the Shrew* who impersonates VINCENTIO (1). The Pedant has no personality; he serves merely to fill out the plot of deception and disguise. He flees when his imposture is revealed and is not mentioned again.

Pedro, Don Character in *Much Ado About Nothing,* the Prince of Aragon, who attempts to promote romances on behalf of two of his followers, CLAUDIO (1) and BENEDICK. Visiting the court of LEONATO, governor of MESSINA, Don Pedro volunteers to help Claudio marry Leonato's daughter, HERO, whom he courts on the younger man's behalf. He also decides on the scheme that tricks Benedick and BEATRICE into falling in love. However, his success as a cupid is qualified at best.

The prince has just defeated an uprising led by his brother, Don JOHN (1), whom he has forgiven and who accompanies him. However, Don John remains a villain, and his plot to trick Claudio into believing that Hero is promiscuous fools Don Pedro as well. The prince is offended, as is Claudio, at the dishonour involved in having courted such a woman; he encourages Claudio's humiliating rejection of his bride and coolly accepts her apparent death from shame.

Benedick, like Beatrice, remains loyal to Hero and severs his relations with Don Pedro. The prince and Claudio seem decidedly at fault, for the audience knows that Hero is innocent. When Don John's trickery is exposed, Don Pedro is genuinely remorseful, and he leads Claudio to his penitential marriage to Hero's cousin, who proves to be Hero herself. The two couples are reunited and the play ends in a spirit of reconciliation, in which Don Pedro joins.

The original of Don Pedro in the playwright's source, Matteo BANDELLO's novella, is completely insignificant; Shakespeare elaborated the character to create an elderly, dignified figure who presides over the action, thus enhancing the courtly air that suffuses the play. Although vulnerable to Don John's machinations, being too concerned with personal honour to respond humanely when presented with apparently convincing evidence of Hero's guilt, Don Pedro is otherwise a gentle and likeable figure. His initial forgiveness of Don John after subduing his revolt testifies to his good will, and he participates prominently in the celebration of renewed harmony that closes the play. Like Claudio, he may be defended as having sinned 'not but in mistaking' (5.1.268–269). With the two young couples united, Don Pedro, somewhat poignantly, is left single himself. His awareness of this misfortune is evident a few lines from the end of the play, when the exultant Benedick teasingly enjoins, 'Prince, thou art sad; get thee a wife, get thee a wife!' (5.4.121).

Shakespeare took Don Pedro's name from Bandello's tale, in which the King of Aragon, who has just conquered Sicily, is named Piero. The playwright used the Spanish form of the name, but there is no reason to believe that he was aware of the historical figure whose name he was borrowing. Aragon, one of several medieval kingdoms located in what is now Spain, ruled Sicily beginning in 1282, when a great rebellion arose there against the French. King Pedro III (1236–1285)—generally known in English as Peter the Great of Aragon—was invited by the rebels to assume the crown. He invaded and quickly drove out the French, beginning a period of Aragonese—and later Spanish—rule that was to last until 1713.

Peele, George (c. 1557–1596) English playwright, a possible collaborator with Shakespeare. Peele was one of the UNIVERSITY WITS, the group of dramatists that dominated the LONDON theatre in the 1580s. After attending Oxford, Peele pursued an impecunious and dissipated life in London, writing plays and other works. His most successful work was *The Old Wives' Tale,* a romantic play based on folk stories. Scholars such as FLEAY and ROBERTSON, who believe that many of Shakespeare's early plays were written by more than one person, have often attributed scenes and passages to Peele, especially in *1 Henry VI* and *Titus Andronicus.* However, most modern scholars dispute such propositions, and Peele is chiefly remembered as one of Shakespeare's immediate predecessors.

Pembroke (1), Henry Herbert, Earl of (c. 1534–1601) English aristocrat and theatrical patron. Pembroke was the patron of PEMBROKE'S MEN, with whom Shakespeare may have acted early in his career. Though willing to lend his name to the players, who performed sometimes at his estate, Pembroke took no active part in their operations. His interests were chiefly political and military. An important figure in the court of Queen ELIZABETH (1), he was president of the council of WALES (1) and spent much time in that land. He also took part in several important treason trials under Elizabeth, including that of Mary, Queen of Scots (see JAMES I). He was married to Mary Sidney, sister of Sir Philip SIDNEY, but he did not share the literary interests of that great patron of the arts. If Shakespeare was a member of the Pembroke's Men, it is possible that Pembroke was acquainted with the young playwright, though there is no specific evidence for any personal relationship. Some scholars believe that a continuing connection between Shakespeare and Pembroke may account for the pointed interest in Wales that appears in some of the plays. Also, there is a posthumous connection between the family and

Shakespeare, for Pembroke's sons, William and Philip (see PEMBROKE [3] and MONTGOMERY [2]), were co-dedicatees of the FIRST FOLIO.

Pembroke (2), Philip Herbert, Lord See MONTGOMERY (2).

Pembroke (3), William Herbert, Earl of (1580–1630) English aristocrat, a dedicatee of the FIRST FOLIO of Shakespeare's plays and a possible model for the young man to whom the SONNETS are addressed. Pembroke's father, also the Earl of PEMBROKE (1), may have been acquainted with Shakespeare in the 1590s; this, along with Pembroke's known rejection of possible brides in 1595 and 1597, and the match between his initials and the 'Mr W. H'. of Thomas THORPE's dedication to the Sonnets, has suggested to some commentators that he may have been the young man whose marriage is advocated in Sonnets 1–17. However, no certain connection between Shakespeare and Pembroke is known—the dedication of the Folio was made long after Shakespeare's death, by John HEMINGE and Henry CONDELL, doubtless because Pembroke was the lord chamberlain and therefore responsible for the publication of plays. In the absence of new evidence, Pembroke's association with the Sonnets must remain purely speculative.

Pembroke had other literary connections from an early age, however. His mother was the sister of Sir Philip SIDNEY and the patron of Edmund SPENSER and others. Samuel DANIEL was among his tutors, and as a young man, Pembroke wrote poetry himself. In the 1590s he was a courtier to Queen ELIZABETH (1), but he lost her favour in 1600 when he refused to marry his pregnant mistress, Mary FITTON. He was gaoled for this offence, but Elizabeth's successor returned him to favour, and he became a prominent member of the new court. Pembroke was a patron of Ben JONSON and the poet George Herbert (1593–1633), a distant cousin; he was also an active investor in colonial development. He was a long-time chancellor of Oxford University—Pembroke College there is named in his honour—and he contributed many volumes to the BODLEIAN LIBRARY (there is still a statue of him outside it).

Pembroke (4), William Herbert, Earl of (d. 1469) Historical figure and minor character in *3 Henry VI,* a supporter of EDWARD IV. Pembroke, who does not speak, is present when the Yorkist leaders learn that WARWICK (3) has deserted their cause in 4.1. He is ordered, with Lord STAFFORD (1), to raise an army.

In 1469, the historical Pembroke, who received his title from Edward for his services in the civil war, was commissioned, with Stafford, to put down a local rebellion that Warwick had sponsored; because of a personal dispute, Stafford withheld his forces from a battle, and the rebels captured and beheaded Pembroke. The historical Pembroke was the father of Sir Walter HERBERT (3), who appears in *Richard III.* Through an illegitimate son, he was also the great-grandfather of Henry Herbert, Earl of PEMBROKE (1), the sponsor of PEMBROKE'S MEN, the actor's company with which Shakespeare was probably associated when he wrote this play.

Pembroke (5), William Marshall, Earl of (c. 1146–1219) Historical figure and minor character in *King John,* a rebel against King JOHN (3). Pembroke, like Lord BIGOT, is merely a representative rebellious baron with no distinctive personality.

The historical William Marshall was a famous soldier who in fact remained loyal to John throughout his reign. Shakespeare confused him with his son, who did join the French invasion forces.

Pembroke's Men Acting company of the ELIZABETHAN THEATRE, possible employer of the young Shakespeare. In late 1592 a troupe of actors sponsored by Henry Herbert, Earl of PEMBROKE (1), performed at the court of Queen ELIZABETH (1), and the following year, with the LONDON theatres closed by the plague, the company toured England. The tour was a financial failure, however, and in September 1593 their rival Philip HENSLOWE recorded that they were forced to sell costumes to pay their debts. A number of plays known to have been in their repertoire (see below) were published by other people in 1594, suggesting that they were forced to sell their rights in them as well.

A revived Pembroke's Men played in the provinces from 1595 to 1597, and in the latter year they began a year's engagement in London, at Francis LANGLEY's new SWAN THEATRE. However, their July production of Thomas NASHE's allegedly seditious play, *Isle of Dogs,* resulted in the brief imprisonment of three members of the company—Gabriel SPENCER, Ben JONSON, and Robert SHAW (5)—and the enforced closure of all the theatres for the summer. When they reopened in October, several actors had left Pembroke's for the ADMIRAL'S MEN. Soon the remnant of Pembroke's returned to the provinces, no longer able to compete in London. In 1600 two performances at Henslowe's ROSE THEATRE were flops, spelling the end of the company.

The repertoire of Pembroke's Men can be deduced in part. We know from the title-page of the BAD QUARTO of *3 Henry VI* (published as THE TRUE TRAGEDY in 1595) that this play—and, by implication, its companion, *2 Henry VI*—were staged by the company. As in any Bad Quarto, the actors' faulty memories have been supplemented by their recollections of performances in other plays. Thus, the other works echoed in these texts were probably part of the company's repertoire, including *1 Henry VI* as well as works by Christopher MARLOWE (1), Thomas KYD, and others. The title-

pages of *Titus Andronicus* and THE TAMING OF A SHREW (1594)—a Bad Quarto of *The Taming of the Shrew*—declare that Pembroke's Men also performed these works. The association of Pembroke's Men with five of Shakespeare's early works has led scholars to presume that the young playwright was himself part of the company at some point during the mysterious beginnings of his career, leaving them before their collapse in 1593. The extremely poor quality of *The Taming of a Shrew* suggests that he was no longer with Pembroke's Men when it was prepared in the summer of 1592.

Penker (Pynkie), Friar (active 1483) Historical figure and minor character in *Richard III,* one of two clergymen who, disguised as BISHOPS (1), accompany RICHARD III as he receives the MAYOR (3) in 3.7. This imposture is intended to lend an air of religiosity to the would-be usurper. Penker and Doctor SHAA were summoned by Richard in 3.5.

In Thomas MORE's history, one of Shakespeare's sources for this anecdote, Penker's name is Pynkie, and he is described as a Provincial of the Augustine friars, a fairly high-ranking administrator.

Pentapolis Ancient Mediterranean land, the setting for most of Act 2 of *Pericles.* Pentapolis is the domain of King SIMONIDES, whose daughter THAISA marries PERICLES. At the end of the play, Pericles learns of Simonides' death and announces that he and Thaisa shall rule in Pentapolis. Pericles' encounter with three FISHERMEN in 2.1 establishes that Pentapolis has a seacoast, but the country is otherwise undistinctive and serves purely as an exotic locale.

In classical times, Pentapolis—Greek for 'five cities'—referred to any of five different locales, all of them political entities centred on five towns. None of them were independent kingdoms at the time of the play's only historical figure, ANTIOCHUS the Great, and it is impossible to be certain which of them Shakespeare had in mind. He may not have considered the matter, for he simply took the name from a source, the *Confessio Amantis* of John GOWER (3).

In an early Latin version of the tale—unknown to the playwright—the term clearly refers to the region also known as Cyrenaica, a Greek colony on the shores of North Africa in what is now eastern Libya. Since this was much the best known ancient Pentapolis, scholars generally associate it with the 'country of Greece' (2.1.64) of *Pericles.* (However, it could also be the Pentapolis of Greek Asia Minor, on the Aegean coast of what is now Turkey, rather closer to the other territories represented in the play.)

Pepys, Samuel (1633–1703) Seventeenth-century diarist and long-time administrator of the Royal Navy. Pepys kept his famous diary between 1660 and 1669. An inveterate theatre-goer, he recorded his impressions of many Restoration period adaptations of Shakespeare's plays.

Percy (1), Henry Character in *Richard II.* See NORTHUMBERLAND (1).

Percy (2), Henry (1364–1403) Historical figure and character in *Richard II,* a supporter of BOLINGBROKE (1), son of the Earl of NORTHUMBERLAND (1). The same historical figure appears as HOTSPUR in *1 Henry IV.* In *Richard II* Percy is a minor figure who primarily delivers information. He is plainly introduced solely in anticipation of his far greater importance in *1 Henry IV.* Presented as younger by a generation than he really was, Percy is thus made the contemporary of Bolingbroke's son, PRINCE (6) HAL, who is to be his great rival. Significantly, it is Percy who tells Bolingbroke the disreputable news of his son in 5.3.13–19. Percy's role is clear evidence that Shakespeare had already formulated the general outline of *1 Henry IV* while writing *Richard II.*

Percy (3), Henry Character in *3 Henry VI.* See NORTHUMBERLAND (2).

Percy (4), Lady Character in *1* and *2 Henry IV.* See LADY (10).

Percy (5), Thomas Character in *1 Henry IV.* See WORCESTER.

Perdita Character in *The Winter's Tale,* long-lost daughter of King LEONTES and Queen HERMIONE of SICILIA. The love of Perdita and Prince FLORIZEL of BOHEMIA is the central element in the romantic COMEDY that constitutes the second half of the play, balancing the TRAGEDY of Leontes' mad jealousy in the first. Though she is prominent only in 4.4, her virtue, beauty, and charming personality make Perdita a powerful symbolic force in the remainder of the play.

At the turning point of the play, in 3.3, the infant Perdita is abandoned in the wilderness because Leontes believes she is the offspring of Hermione's alleged adultery with King POLIXENES of Bohemia. A SHEPHERD (2) adopts Perdita, and by Act 4, 16 years later, she has become a charming young woman, the 'Mistress o' th' Feast' (4.4.68) at the shepherds' festival. Florizel's father, King Polixenes, disapproves of the love between his royal son and a peasant girl. When he attends the feast in disguise, he is charmed by Perdita, finding her 'Too noble for this place' (4.4. 159), but he will not accept her as a daughter-in-law. He threatens her with death, and the couple flees to Sicilia, where Perdita's identity is discovered. This leads to their formal engagement, the reconciliation of Leontes and Polixenes, and the restoration of Queen Hermione, who has been kept in hiding. The proph-

ecy of the oracle of Apollo—that only Perdita can restore the happiness Leontes has destroyed—is thus fulfilled. Perdita's love is essential to the workings of providence in the play's outcome, thereby supporting the play's major theme, that the moral virtue of good people is necessary for providence to function as a saviour in human affairs.

Raised as a shepherdess, Perdita is an honest, open young woman with no trace of pretension or sentimentality. She is embarrassed to be 'most goddess-like prank'd up' (4.4.10) in a fancy costume for the festival, and she is frankly worried about Polixenes' opposition to her, though more for Florizel's sake than her own. A clever lass, she briskly counters CAMILLO's flattery in 4.4.110–112 and more than holds her own in the debate with Polixenes in 4.4.79–103, in which she defends the simple ways of nature against the sophistication of art. She values a maidenly decorum in sexual matters, while acknowledgeing the physical side of love. She mentions, for example, a 'false way' of love (4.4.151) and speaks against 'scurrilous words' (4.4. 215) in ballads, yet when Florizel jests that strewn with flowers he would be like a corpse, she replies, 'No, like a bank, for love to lie and play on: / Not like a corpse; or if—not to be buried, / But quick, and in mine arms' (4.4.130–132).

This lovely passage is suggestive of primordial rituals of death and rebirth. Along with her remarks on the Proserpina myth and mythological flower lore in 4.4.116–126, it links her with the ancient veneration of natural fertility, of which the shepherds' festival is a survival. As Florizel puts it, 'This your sheep-shearing / Is as a meeting of the petty gods, / And you the queen on 't' (4.4.3–5). All this reinforces Perdita's association with providence. It was the protection of providence that brought the tragic first half of the play to an end, and it is the love Perdita represents that proves instrumental in effecting the final reconciliations of the second.

Pericles Title character of *Pericles*, the ruler of TYRE. Through no fault of his own, Pericles undergoes tremendous misfortunes. He is driven into exile and becomes separated from both his wife and daughter, only to be finally reunited with them at the play's close. He accepts his fate passively, and thus he embodies a major theme of the play: that we cannot control our destiny, and the acceptance of suffering is humanity's only choice.

Pericles encounters love three times, but each time he loses it. In 1.1 he loves the DAUGHTER (1) of ANTIOCHUS, but when he learns of her incestuous relationship with her father, he withdraws his suit in horror. He is sullied by her sin although he is innocent, for the 'gods . . . inflame'd desire in [his] breast / To taste the fruit' (1.1.20–22). Disillusioned, he loses his youthful assurance and flees into exile, a tribulation that ends when he is shipwrecked on the coast of PENTAPOLIS, in 2.1. He finds love again when he meets and marries THAISA, but suffers a great loss when he wrongly believes that she has died in childbirth during a storm at sea. This is eased by the compensation of MARINA's birth, but he leaves Marina with CLEON and DIONYZA because he fears for her survival at sea. When he returns for her in 4.4, he learns—again wrongly—of her death. Significantly, he endures another storm at this point, but it happens off-stage and is merely mentioned, in 5.Chorus.14, for his fortunes have now begun to turn. Distraught and without hope, he succumbs to despair. He only recovers when he accidently encounters Marina. The goddess DIANA (2) then guides him to a reunion with Thaisa. Thus, in the course of his life Pericles manifests youthful illusions, the misery of incomprehensible suffering, and the ultimate happiness that follows from his patient acceptance of the will of the gods.

His passiveness makes Pericles a strange hero to modern tastes. However, this trait should not be seen as an aspect of his personality, but rather as an emblematic feature that offers an allegory of a possible human relationship to the universe. Like most of the play's characters, Pericles is more emblematic than real and does not have a complex, fully developed personality. He is wholly good and without flaws. Unlike Antiochus, he *is* 'a man on whom perfections wait' (1.1.80). He does not cause his misfortunes, nor does he resist them. He expresses his resignation clearly after the shipwreck. He addresses the tempest and says, 'earthly man / Is but a substance that must yield to you; / And I, as fits my nature, do obey you' (2.1. 2–4). His marriage is not his own doing, either. Thaisa courts him more than he does her, and though he loves her, he declares that he has 'never aim'd so high to love' her (2.5.47). He is not without spunk—he responds with fiery indignation when SIMONIDES pretends to believe him a 'traitor' (2.5.54)—but in the world of the play he must suffer or prosper as fate decrees. Finally, his passiveness leads to his complete withdrawal when he believes Marina is dead. He retreats into speechlessness, a deathlike trance of despair from which only Marina can revive him. The play's theme of regeneration is embodied in part by this, Pericles' resurrection.

The play's strongest treatment of evil is its presentation of incest. Here, Pericles is pointedly contrasted with Antiochus and proves himself a vessel of goodness. The episode is confined to 1.1, but it is mentioned at several points throughout the play, and it makes the point that humanity is capable of gross unnaturalness. It is countered by the example of Simonides and Thaisa, but more dramatically, we see the father-daughter relationship reformulated in the reunion of Pericles and Marina. Pericles recognises her impact on his despair and calls Marina 'Thou that

beget'st him that did thee beget' (5.1.195); thus, incest's horror is reversed. At the play's close, Pericles, unlike Antiochus, willingly surrenders Marina to a husband. He demonstrates the healthy paternal love that promotes the natural cycles of regeneration that are an important theme of the play.

In his summary of *Pericles,* Gower (3) speaks of the hero and his family in words that could refer to Pericles alone. He calls them 'Led on by heaven, and crown'd with joy at last' (Epilogue.6). Pericles is an extremely simple character, and Shakespeare, like many readers, may have found him a little too simple, for the subsequent ROMANCES were to contain a pattern of sin and remorse from which Pericles' story is exempt. Nevertheless, in this first of the late comedies the title character is a fine example of an allegorical protagonist, and is a dramatic success when viewed in the terms set by the play.

The play stems from the ancient Greek tale 'Apollonius of Tyre', and the protagonist's name remained Apollonius in Shakespeare's main sources for the play. The new name was probably suggested by Pyrocles, a hero of Sir Philip SYDNEY's *Arcadia,* one of the play's minor sources. Shakespeare's hero bears no resemblance at all to the Athenian statesman named Pericles (c. 495–429 B.C.), though the playwright undoubtedly read the Athenian's biography in PLUTARCH's *Lives.* The great stature of the historical Pericles may have made his name seem appropriately grand for a fictional ruler of Tyre.

Pericles, Prince of Tyre

SYNOPSIS

Act 1, Chorus

The ghost of John GOWER (3) identifies himself and introduces the play as the enactment of an ancient tale. It opens in ANTIOCH, where King ANTIOCHUS practises incest with his beautiful DAUGHTER (1). He has stipulated that she may only marry the suitor who can solve a certain riddle, and that any suitor who attempts to do so and fails will be executed.

Act 1, Scene 1

PERICLES, Prince of TYRE, hears the riddle, and realises that its solution reveals Antiochus' incest. He declines to give his answer, but he makes it clear that he knows the secret. The king decides to humour him and grants him a 40-day respite before he must answer. Pericles realises that Antiochus will attempt to silence him, and he decides to flee. Antiochus orders THALIARD to kill Pericles, but word comes that Pericles has left Antioch. Thaliard is sent in pursuit.

Act 1, Scene 2

In Tyre, Pericles fears that Antiochus, who is a much more powerful ruler, will attack and devastate his country. A group of fawning courtiers appears, but among them is HELICANUS, who strongly disapproves of flattering a monarch. Pericles admires his spirit and confides his fears to him. Helicanus advises him that he should travel for a time, until Antiochus' rage has cooled. Pericles agrees and decides to go to THARSUS. He appoints Helicanus to rule in his absence.

Act 1, Scene 3

Thaliard has come to Tyre. He learns of Pericles' departure and leaves to inform Antiochus.

Act 1, Scene 4

CLEON, the Governor of Tharsus, and DIONYZA, his wife, are worried because a famine has overtaken their once-rich country. Pericles has heard of their plight, and arrives with shipments of food.

Act 2, Chorus

Gower tells the audience that Pericles is adored in Tharsus. In a DUMB SHOW, Pericles receives a message, which Gower tells us is from Helicanus, who warns the prince of Thaliard's evil intent and suggests further flight. Gower tells us that Pericles fled by sea and was shipwrecked.

Act 2, Scene 1

Shipwrecked, Pericles encounters three FISHERMEN, who inform him he is in PENTAPOLIS. They tell him that their king, SIMONIDES, is holding a tournament the next day at which knights will joust for the hand in marriage of his daughter. Pericles' armour is brought up in the Fishermen's net, and he decides to use it in the king's tournament.

Act 2, Scene 2

At the tournament, the king's daughter, THAISA, receives greetings from each KNIGHT (2) who will compete for her hand. Pericles' rusty armour is ridiculed by some courtiers, but cheers celebrate his victory off-stage.

Act 2, Scene 3

At a celebratory banquet, Pericles is welcomed by Thaisa as the victor and therefore her fiancé.

Act 2, Scene 4

In Tyre, Helicanus tells ESCANES that the gods have punished Antiochus and his daughter by killing them with a heavenly fire. A group of noblemen declare that they cannot be without a king any longer and ask Helicanus to declare himself king. He refuses, but agrees to do so if Pericles has not returned after another year.

Act 2, Scene 5

To test Pericles, Simonides pretends to be angry that the young man has falsely gained the affection of Thaisa, and he calls him a traitor. Pericles rejects the insult manfully, to Simonides' secret delight. Thaisa appears and says it would please her if Pericles loved

her. Simonides reveals his pleasure and declares that she and Pericles shall marry.

Act 3, Chorus
Gower reveals that Thaisa, now married to Pericles, is pregnant. In a dumb show, Pericles receives another letter, which he shows to Thaisa and Simonides. Gower tells us that the letter is from Helicanus, summoning Pericles to Tyre. He goes on to report that Pericles and Thaisa leave by ship, only to be caught in a great storm.

Act 3, Scene 1
Aboard ship, during the tempest, the nurse LYCHORIDA tells Pericles that Thaisa has died in childbirth. She shows him the infant, a daughter. A SAILOR (3) insists that Thaisa must be buried at sea or the ship is cursed, and the distracted Pericles agrees. Pericles orders the ship to stop at Tharsus where he will leave the infant. He is afraid she may not survive a longer voyage.

Act 3, Scene 2
At EPHESUS a chest washed up by the great storm is brought to the nobleman and physician CERIMON. He opens it and finds the apparently dead Thaisa, but he recognises that she is merely unconscious and revives her with medicines.

Act 3, Scene 3
At Tharsus Pericles leaves his daughter MARINA in the care of Cleon and Dionyza.

Act 3, Scene 4
In Ephesus, Thaisa decides to enter a convent devoted to the goddess DIANA (2) since she will never find her husband again.

Act 4, Chorus
Gower tells us that Marina has grown into a gracious and beautiful young woman. So fine a person is she, he says, that she overshadows Cleon and Dionyza's daughter. Dionyza has become so jealous that she decides to have Marina killed.

Act 4, Scene 1
Dionyza reminds LEONINE of his oath to murder Marina, for he is reluctant. Marina appears and is persuaded to take a walk on the beach with Leonine. As he prepares to kill her, a boat-load of PIRATES come ashore and kidnap her. Leonine escapes and is relieved not to have to kill Marina. He plans to tell Dionyza that he has done so anyway.

Act 4, Scene 2
In a brothel in MYTILENE the PANDAR, the BAWD, and their servant BOULT discuss the sorry state of business. They regret that they don't have more attractive young women to offer. A Pirate appears and offers to sell them Marina, and they accept. Despite Marina's pleas and objections, they make plans to offer her to their customers.

Act 4, Scene 3
In Tharsus Cleon is distressed to learn that Dionyza has had Marina murdered. She has also poisoned Leonine to keep him quiet. She is cynically pleased with the success of her plan, and tells Cleon that they will inform Pericles that Marina died naturally.

Act 4, Scene 4
Gower appears by Marina's gravestone in Tharsus with the information that Pericles has come to get his daughter. A dumb show presents his grief when he is shown the tomb by Cleon. Gower reads the flowery epitaph on the monument, and contrasts its flattery with Marina's unhappiness in Mytilene.

Act 4, Scene 5
Two gentlemen of Mytilene discuss the wondrous virtue of a harlot they have encountered, and they vow to reform their lives.

Act 4, Scene 6
The Bawd, the Pandar, and Boult despair at the damage Marina is doing to their business. LYSIMACHUS, the Governor of Mytilene, appears and is offered Marina. She implores him as an honourable man not to use her as a harlot, and he declares that his intention has merely been to test her virtue, of which he has heard. He leaves, but he refuses to give money to Boult. Boult angrily threatens to deflower Marina himself so that her virtue will not further upset the brothel's business. However, she shames him into agreeing instead to help her establish herself as a teacher of music, dance, and handicrafts to young women.

Act 5, Chorus
Gower tells of Marina's success in Mytilenian society. He adds that the grief-stricken Pericles, who has been wandering at sea, has arrived in Mytilene.

Act 5, Scene 1
Lysimachus boards Pericles' ship to greet the visitor, but he is informed by Helicanus that the prince has been made speechless by his grief. A Mytilenian courtier suggests that the charms of Marina could cure Pericles, and she is sent for. When she arrives she is left alone with Pericles, and he speaks because he is startled by her resemblance to Thaisa. In the course of their conversation their relationship becomes apparent and they are happily reunited. Exhausted by the excitement, Pericles is left alone to sleep and the goddess Diana appears to him in a vision. She directs him to go to her temple in Ephesus and proclaim the history of Marina's birth and their separation and reunion.

Act 5, Scene 2
At the Temple of Diana in Ephesus, Thaisa, the High Priestess, stands by the altar. Gower appears and tells us that Lysimachus and Marina are engaged but will

not marry until Pericles fulfils Diana's instructions, so the couple have accompanied Pericles to Ephesus.

Act 5, Scene 3
At the Temple altar, Pericles identifies himself and tells of Marina's birth and adventures. Thaisa recognises him and faints. Cerimon is present, and he reveals her identity to Pericles. When Thaisa recovers, she and Pericles are reunited, and Thaisa and Marina meet for the first time since Marina's birth. When he learns of Simonides' death, Pericles declares that he and Thaisa shall reign in Pentapolis and Lysimachus and Marina will rule in Tyre.

Epilogue
Gower compares the heavenly destruction of Antiochus and his daughter with the ultimate happiness of Pericles, Thaisa, and Marina. He goes on to praise Helicanus and Cerimon, and adds that the people of Tharsus were enraged when they heard of Marina's murder, and massacred Cleon and Dionyza. He then announces that the play is now over.

COMMENTARY

Pericles, Prince of Tyre is the first of Shakespeare's ROMANCES. Even though the opening acts are probably not his work (see 'Text of the Play'), Shakespeare took this opportunity to develop several ideas and techniques. These techniques—such as the melding of COMEDY and TRAGEDY, and the use of strange, elaborate plots and boldly symbolic characters—are the ones that he began to use in the PROBLEM PLAYS and continued to experiment with in works such as *Timon of Athens.* Most important is the growth of a theme that runs through all of the late plays; that humankind cannot alter its destiny in an inexplicable but finally benevolent universe. *Pericles* is flawed, in part due to collaboration, or a very faulty text, or both, but also due to the nature of its imperfectly combined elements. However, it constitutes a significant step towards the magnificent achievements of *The Winter's Tale* and *The Tempest.*

Though *Pericles* was extremely popular in the early 17th century, it has since been considered one of the least satisfying of Shakespeare's plays. Despite the flawed surviving text, it contains much good poetry, especially in the reunion of Pericles and Marina in 5.1, but the play's virtues are largely outweighed by its defects. Its major figures seem lifeless; it is episodic; its events are often described rather than enacted; and all this is presented in a nearly shapeless plot that is full of extreme improbabilities and absurd situations. For instance, why would Antiochus describe his sin in the riddle he invites the world to solve? Why does Thaisa enter a convent instead of going on to Tyre to rejoin her husband? Why does Pericles leave Marina in Tharsus for 14 years? Each question can be answered by reference to the conventions of folklore and narrative romance, but taken together, the whole story lacks plausibility and dramatic interest.

Nevertheless, *Pericles* has increased in popularity in the 20th century. The bold extremes of characterisation and theme found in folklore and narrative romance may be more acceptable to a century familiar with abstraction. The play is more rewarding on the stage than in print, in any case, for it depends in good part on MASQUElike spectacle. It also entertains us with a wide range of human behaviour—however baldly represented—and of good and bad fortune. Its very conventionality is reassuring: we can suspend our sense that life cannot be both randomly threatening and neatly resolved and simply enjoy its bizarre episodes and its happy ending.

Pericles centres on the title character—and, late in the play, on Marina—but it features a number of boldly drawn minor figures. These are not, for the most part, endowed with real human personalities, but they demonstrate the nature of humanity. Antiochus is a regal villain, full of power and sin, while Dionyza represents the archetypal evil stepmother. On the other hand, Helicanus is a paragon of loyalty and strength, while Cerimon is a benevolent nobleman and a master of the far reaches of human knowledge. These figures are not realistic, but this is part of their point. They are symbols of the human potential for good and evil that is so much more complex and obscure in reality, or even in realistic drama. The Fishermen of 2.1 and the staff of the Mytilenian brothel in Act 4 not only provide comic relief, they also remind us of our own parallel universe, mirrored allegorically in the play.

The play is unified by a repeated pattern of loss and recovery. On the largest scale, Pericles loses his confident idealism and is tainted by sexual evil; he suffers as a result, and he recovers goodness and love at the end of his life. This pattern is repeated within the overall development, as Pericles encounters love and loses happiness three times, only to recover each time. The cycle is strikingly punctuated with storms. When he flees the horror represented by Antiochus' daughter, Pericles becomes a shipwrecked exile, but he finds love anew in Thaisa. Beset by another tempest, Pericles loses Thaisa, but takes comfort in the birth of Marina. Finally, though he is driven to despair by the apparent loss of Marina as well, fate changes its course and he recovers both daughter and wife. Significantly, the storm that Pericles endures at this point is merely mentioned briefly, in 5.Chorus.14, and is not given the emphasis of the first two. Like ancient festival rituals, *Pericles* offers an analogy to the eternal cycles of winter and spring, death and rebirth. This pattern is the play's plot.

Our sense of this 'plot' is reinforced by the play's most prominent motif, resurrection. First Thaisa and then Marina seem to die, only to be revived, literally

in Thaisa's case and figuratively with Marina's release from the brothel (after which 'she sings like one immortal' [5.Chorus.3]). When Pericles discovers that his daughter is dead, he withdraws into himself and may be said to have suffered a mock death, from which he is revived by Marina. Once restored, he cries that Marina 'beget'st' him (5.1.195), which suggests his reborn state, and demands 'fresh garments' (5.1.213). The symbolic value of this gesture is difficult to ignore. He has been returned from death as surely as Marina and Thaisa seem to have been. Finally, at the play's close, the ritual cycle of death and birth is brought full circle, and Pericles' mourning for his daughter is forgotten in plans for her marriage. The recurring theme is touched on one last time when Simonides' death is reported. This allows Marina and Lysimachus to take their destined place—once that of the play's protagonist—as rulers of Tyre.

Another major motif of the play, incest, appears only once, but the issue is raised again at sensitive moments. In the play incest suggests the deepest evil to which humanity is susceptible. Pericles, drawn to Antiochus' daughter, is tainted by her sin although he is innocent, for the 'gods . . . inflame'd desire in [his] breast / To taste the fruit' (1.1.20–22). The episode's place at the opening of the play gives it great weight, and its point is further made by contrast when the hero encounters Thaisa and Simonides. Their healthy love is apparent when Simonides delightedly surrenders his daughter to Pericles in marriage. The theme is subtly and dramatically reworked in Pericles' cry to Marina: 'Thou . . . beget'st him that did thee beget' (5.1.195). The horrifying potential of incest—inbred offspring—is inverted. Finally Pericles, like Simonides and unlike Antiochus, can willingly separate himself from Marina as she joins her husband in a new life.

At the play's close, then, the influence of evil has been destroyed and the misfortunes of the hero have been ended, but neither he nor Marina have been responsible for the happy ending. Dramatic coincidence, good luck, and the intervention of the gods have propelled events. Marina, in resisting the brothel world, influences her fate to some degree, but only sheer accident reunites her with her father. The other characters, especially Pericles—who is extraordinarily passive throughout—simply suffer or succeed as fate decrees. The play emphasises that the characters cannot control their destiny, and that the patience to accept the misfortunes of life is the best way to survive them. The most important of the external forces that drive the action is the sea. Its impersonal violence is both the occasion and the symbol of Pericles' recurring losses. Further, help comes to famine-beset Tharsus by sea in 1.4; in 2.1 the shipwrecked Pericles' only remaining emblem of princely dignity, his inherited armour, is brought up in the Fishermen's net; and in 4.2 Marina's unlikely rescuers appear from the sea. Not for nothing does the reunion of Pericles and Marina take place on a feast day dedicated to Neptune. This fact is emphasised by pointed repetition (5.Chorus.17; 5.1.17), and by reiteration of the word 'sea' and references to the sea throughout the scene. The spectacular appearance of Diana makes the divine influence on the play's events completely clear. It is only sensible that Gower should summarise the tale of Pericles' family by saying that they have been 'Led on by heaven' (Epilogue.6).

Another aspect of the characters' dependence on fate is the element of surprise that recurs throughout the play. In 1.1 Pericles is shockingly disillusioned about Antiochus' daughter; in 1.3 Thaliard finds his prey escaped; in 1.4, Cleon is astonished by the arrival of succor from famine, and so on. In almost every scene but Gower's narrations, which serve to anchor us amid seas of uncertainty, are instances of such startled amazement. Indeed, Marina feels that 'This world to me is as a lasting storm, / Whirring me from my friends' (4.1.19–20). The sublimely spiritual quality of the last act owes much to the appearance of a cause for the play's random surprises. As mistrust yields to confidence that the promised joy is real, we, like the characters, can believe that the irrational brutality of the world is a survivable danger; such a solace is to be valued as much as any human achievement.

SOURCES OF THE PLAY

The original source for *Pericles, Prince of Tyre* was an ancient tale known as 'Apollonius of Tyre'. Though the earliest surviving version is a Latin text of the 5th–6th centuries, scholars recognise from its style that it is a translation of a Greek work of 300 years earlier. This tale was extremely popular throughout the Middle Ages and the RENAISSANCE, and Shakespeare (and his collaborators, if any) surely knew it in several different versions that were current in 17th-century England. However, only two of these possible sources are specifically represented in the play: the 14th-century *Confessio Amantis* of John GOWER (3) in a 1554 edition, and Laurence TWINE'S *The Patterne of Painefull Adventures* (c. 1576).

Gower's version of the tale, which was derived from a history of the world in Latin verse by the medieval chronicler Godfrey of Viterbo (c. 1120–c. 1196), was most important to the play. It provided the general outline of events, the locations, and most of the characters. Moreover, a number of passages—including Antiochus' riddle (1.1.65–72), Pericles' note in Thaisa's coffin (3.2.70–77), and Gower's lines in 3.Chorus—follow Gower fairly closely.

Twine's rendering of Apollonius' adventures, which he translated from a French version of the famous *Gesta Romanorum*, a medieval collection of Latin tales, was less important. It was only used extensively in Marina's story, especially in 4.3, where Dionyza cyni-

cally defends the supposed murder of Marina (though similar arguments made by LADY (6) MACBETH and GONERIL also foreshadow this episode). Minor echoes of Twine's words occur elsewhere in the play as well.

Though Shakespeare's Gower resembles and must have been influenced by the allegorical CHORUS (3) of the playwright's own *Henry V*, the idea of using the author of a well-known source as a ghostly CHORUS (1) was probably stimulated by a contemporary play, *The Devil's Charter* (1607), by Barnabe BARNES. This play was derived from a work by the Italian historian Francesco Guicciardini (1483–1540) and featured Guicciardini as a choric narrator. Several of Gower's speeches contain echoes of the words of Barnes' Guicciardini.

Lastly, the hero's name—and thus that of the play—was probably inspired by Pyrocles, a major character in Sir Philip SIDNEY's pastoral romance, *Arcadia* (1590). Two passages in the play—Pericles' appearance in rusty armour in 2.2 and Marina's description of a storm in 4.1—reflect episodes in *Arcadia*.

TEXT OF THE PLAY

Most scholars believe that *Pericles* is the work of more than one author; one or more who wrote Acts 1–2 and, perhaps, 5.2, and another—Shakespeare—who wrote the remainder and completed or revised the earlier version. However, some scholars believe that the faults of the first edition account for all discrepancies, and that the text is wholly Shakespeare's. In any case, if Shakespeare had a collaborator or collaborators, their identities are unknown, though they have been the subject of scholarly dispute since the 18th century. John DAY and Thomas HEYWOOD (2) are considered the likeliest nominees, but no identification has proven entirely satisfactory.

Pericles was probably written in 1607. The likely influence of Barnes' *The Devil's Charter* on the play suggests that *Pericles* was probably not completed before Barnes' play was staged early in 1607. It apparently had been completed, and probably performed, by May 1608, when the text was registered with the STATIONERS' COMPANY as 'A booke called *The booke of Pericles prynce of Tyre*'. This wording almost certainly refers to a theatrical PROMPT-BOOK. Also, there are no surviving references to this extremely popular play that date from before 1608, which implies that it appeared in or just before that year.

Edward BLOUNT registered the play, but he did not publish it, a manoeuvre that scholars believe was a 'stopping action', intended to prevent publishing piracy. The effort was unsuccessful, however, for *Pericles* was published the next year by Henry GOSSON (1) in a QUARTO edition printed by William WHITE (2) known as Q1 (1609). Q1 is a BAD QUARTO, an inaccurate text put together from the recollections of actors or viewers. Some scholars believe that two different recollections were used, which produced the difference between Acts 1–2 and Acts 3–5. Based on this hypothesis, the text may be wholly Shakespeare's. Q1 was so popular that Gosson produced another edition (Q2) in the same year. (*Richard II* was the only other Shakespeare play to appear in two quartos in one year.) An unknown publisher brought out Q3 (1611), and Q4 (1619) was part of Thomas PAVIER'S FALSE FOLIO. Q5 and Q6 appeared in 1630 and 1635. *Pericles* was not published in the FIRST FOLIO (1623) for reasons that are unknown. Perhaps the editors knew that much of the play was not written by Shakespeare, or they may have found the bad quarto too poor a text to reproduce. *Pericles* does appear, along with several other non-Shakespearean works (see APOCRYPHA), in the Third FOLIO (F3; 1664). F3 was printed from Q6, and Q2–Q6 are all derived from Q1. The original quarto, therefore, despite its faults, has been the basis of all subsequent editions.

THEATRICAL HISTORY OF THE PLAY

Undated diplomatic papers record that a performance of *Pericles* was attended by the Venetian and French ambassadors to England sometime between May 1606 (when the French delegate arrived in London) and the closure of London's theatres by a plague epidemic in July 1608. Scholars generally date the play to 1607, so the initial production probably opened during that year or early in 1608. The KING'S MEN made an unsuccessful effort to prevent the pirated publication of *Pericles* in 1608 because the play was already extremely popular. George WILKINS' 1609 novel based on the play capitalised on this popularity, which is further stressed by contemporary references. These include a 1609 remark that great crowds attended the play, and the 1619 record of an elaborate production and intermission banquet with which the government entertained visiting dignitaries. As late as 1631, Ben JONSON complained in print that *Pericles* was outdrawing his own works.

However, though *Pericles* was the first Shakespearean play revived when the theatres were reopened following the English civil war—Thomas BETTERTON was acclaimed in the title role in 1660 and 1661—the play was not popular thereafter. In fact, it was not produced again—except in a very un-Shakespearean adaptation by George LILLO (1738)—until Samuel PHELPS revived it in 1854. Phelps' version was greatly abridged; Gower was eliminated entirely, for instance. It was also sanitised; Victorian tastes could not tolerate the brothel scenes, in particular, so Phelps condensed Act 4 and 'disinfected it of its impurities', as a contemporary reviewer put it.

Only three other productions—two of them German—are known from before World War I, but since then the play has grown somewhat in popularity. Among the most notable 20th-century productions

have been the first modern staging of the unaltered play by Robert ATKINS at the OLD VIC THEATRE (1921), and two productions starring Paul SCOFIELD (1947, 1950). *Pericles* has never been made into a FILM, though it has been produced once for TELEVISION, in 1983.

Perkes, Clement GLOUCESTERSHIRE countryman named in *2 Henry IV,* a legal adversary of DAVY's friend William VISOR of Woncot. Davy, the steward of Justice SHALLOW, asks his master to rule in Visor's favour in his lawsuit against 'Clement Perkes a'th'Hill' (5.1.35), in a glimpse of rural corruption that is part of the play's depiction of English manners and mores. Perkes is thought to represent someone Shakespeare knew, a member of a family named Purchase or Perkis that lived near Woodmancote, the play's 'Woncot', in an area traditionally called 'the Hill'.

Peter (1) Minor character in *2 Henry VI,* an apprentice to an armourer, Thomas HORNER. In 1.3 Peter reports that his master has said that the Duke of YORK (8) is 'rightful heir to the crown' (1.3.26). This bit of hearsay is seized upon by the Duke of SUFFOLK (3), who accuses York of treason and has Peter repeat his account later in the scene. Horner denies having said such a thing, and the question is referred to a trial by combat. This procedure, a judicious postponement of a potentially explosive issue, is ordered by the Lord Protector, the Duke of GLOUCESTER (4). In the meantime, at Gloucester's suggestion, York's reappointment as Regent of FRANCE (1) is postponed until the matter is resolved. Thus, as his downfall approaches, 'good Duke Humphrey' is given an opportunity to display the qualities of prudence and judgement that are shortly to be denied the country through the selfish ambitions of Suffolk and others.

Although Peter is desperately afraid to fight, Horner arrives for the contest drunk in 2.3, and Peter slays him. The dying armourer confesses the truth of Peter's report, and the apprentice is exonerated. Although the nobles do not take this clownish incident seriously, the episode prefigures York's actual treason, which sparks the WARS OF THE ROSES, later in the play.

Peter (2) Minor character in *Romeo and Juliet,* a servant in the CAPULET (1) household, the assistant of the NURSE (3). Peter appears with the Nurse in 2.4 and makes a brief speech that both furthers a sexual innuendo and displays comical cowardice. His principal appearance, however, is in 4.5. When the MUSICIANS (2) hired for the wedding of JULIET (1) are dismissed because she is believed to have died, Peter accosts them. He demands free music and then engages them in a comic exchange, insulting them and playing on their names. A stage direction in the Q2 edition of the play (see *Romeo and Juliet,* 'Text of the Play') indicates that Peter was portrayed by Will KEMPE, a famous comic of the day.

Peter (3) Minor character in *The Taming of the Shrew,* a servant of PETRUCHIO (2). Peter is one of several servants whom Petruchio abuses in 4.1. The servants realise that their master's oppressive behaviour is part of his strategy for taming his shrewish bride, KATHERINA, and Peter delivers a succinct analysis of it in the longer of his two lines: 'He kills her in her own humour' (4.1.167).

Peter is not named in any of the several lists of Petruchio's servants that are recited in the scene. This fact, combined with the mute appearance in 4.4 of a servant of LUCENTIO identified as Peter in a stage direction, suggests that his name may be that of an actor who took both small parts, the second of which appears to have been cut. However, no scholar has been able to identify the actor, and there is nothing inherently improbable in the existence of two Peters.

Peter (4) of Pomfret (d. 1213) Historical figure and minor character in *King John,* a wandering 'prophet' whose public forecasts of the fall of King JOHN (3) are recounted by the BASTARD (1) in 4.2. Peter himself, who has been brought to the King, speaks only one line, affirming his belief that John will have surrendered his crown by the following Ascension Day. John orders him imprisoned, to be hung on Ascension Day, and he does not reappear. On Ascension Day, when John does indeed give up his crown—only to receive it again from the papal legate PANDULPH—he recalls the prophecy and observes that it has been fulfilled, in an unanticipated way. We are not informed of Peter's fate, however. The incident illustrates popular dissatisfaction with John's reign and also suggests that his fall was inevitable.

Shakespeare read of this prophecy in HOLINSHED's *Chronicles,* where Peter, a hermit 'in great reputation with the common people' for his powers of prophecy, offered himself to be executed if he proved wrong. On Ascension Day, John still being in power, he was hung, along with his son. Holinshed thought that the prophet was a fraud, but he records that Peter's death was popularly held to be an injustice in light of John's temporary surrender of his crown to Pandulph, which had occurred the day before and seemed to fulfil the prediction.

Peter (5), Friar Character in *Measure for Measure.* See FRIAR (1).

Petitioners Any of several minor characters in *2 Henry VI* who arrive at court in 1.3 with pleas for justice. The Petitioners, two of whom have spoken lines, join with PETER (1) in planning to address their

grievances to the Duke of GLOUCESTER (4). Queen MARGARET (1) and the Duke of SUFFOLK (3) appear instead and demand to see their petitions; one is personal and the other requests protection from Suffolk himself, who has incorporated common lands into his estates. Peter's business proves useful to Suffolk, but Margaret scornfully rejects the other Petitioners, tearing up their written pleas and abusively ordering them to leave.

Peto Minor character in *1* and *2 Henry IV,* a follower of FALSTAFF. Peto participates in the highway robbery in 2.2 of *1 Henry IV,* and he later tells PRINCE (6) HAL how Falstaff attempted to disguise his cowardice. In 2.4 of *2 Henry IV* Peto brings the Prince news of the King's preparations against the rebellion, stirring Hal to action.

Peto was originally given the name HARVEY (1), but the name was changed after early performances, probably to avoid offending a prominent aristocrat, William HARVEY (3). (See also OLDCASTLE and ROSSILL.)

Petruchio (1) GHOST CHARACTER in *Romeo and Juliet,* a follower of TYBALT. Petruchio appears only in a stage direction at 3.1.34, though he is also mentioned as a guest at the CAPULET (1) banquet (1.5.130). Shakespeare presumably intended to develop Petruchio as he wrote 3.1, but did not in fact do so. Then, with his typical inattention to details, the playwright let the stage direction stand. Such a Ghost character is taken as evidence that the published text in which he first appears—in this case Q2 (1599) of *Romeo and Juliet*—was printed from Shakespeare's own manuscript, or FOUL PAPERS, and is thus especially authoritative.

Petruchio (2) Character in *The Taming of the Shrew,* the suitor, bridegroom, and tamer of KATHERINA, the shrew of the title. Petruchio is sometimes seen as a tyrannical male, selfishly dominating a woman who cannot escape him. However, this view reflects certain modern attitudes towards marriage and ignores both the world in which the character was created and the actual text of the play. Petruchio does not physically abuse her or humiliate Katherina, and in 'submitting' to him, she merely assumes the conventional role of a wife. At the end of the play she is quite evidently grateful for the change that he has wrought in her life. Theirs is a love story, though this is a subtle element set among the play's several comic plots.

Bluff and hearty, Petruchio is a humorous figure—seen in ludicrous clothes while indulging in spectacular tantrums, he provides laughs in an age-old fashion—but his primary role in the play is more serious. Although his attitude towards marriage is distinctly mercenary—'I come to wive it wealthily in Padua', he says (1.2.74)—he is also attracted to Katherina. He is unafraid of her shrewishness, and he sees that the high spirits that underlie her terrible temper may be a positive character trait. His ironic response to the account of her assault on HORTENSIO (2.1.160–162) reflects a willingness to deal with such a person—he is attuned to Katherina even before he has met her. After the 'taming', when they enjoy their first loving kiss (5.1. 137–138), his sentimental reaction reflects his real affection for her. His response to her whole-hearted commitment to a wifely role, in her banquet speech in 5.2, is simple delight, better expressed in a kiss than in words.

However, Petruchio's importance is not as Katherina's lover but as her 'tamer'. He is the instrument of the personality change that is the central event of the play. He overrides her outbursts with his insistence that she is actually gentle and mild, and he behaves with all the virulence any shrew could ever summon. He perceptively senses in Katherina both her desire for appreciation and her instinctive distaste for shrewish conduct, and he induces her to assume the role of a normal Elizabethan wife. He does not simply bludgeon her into submission—as is common in the literature of shrewish wives, before and after Shakespeare's time—but rather functions as a teacher and guide. For much of his time on stage, Petruchio is explicitly playing a part—like many of Shakespeare's protagonists—and only pretends to be a comical tyrant. It is significant that his most important actions in this role occur off-stage and are described by other characters; in 3.2 BIONDELLO describes his outrageous appearance on his wedding day, and then GREMIO describes his outlandish behaviour at the ceremony; in 4.1 GRUMIO tells of his intemperate behaviour on the journey from Padua, and CURTIS recounts his ranting delivery of an immoderate lecture on moderation. This forces the audience to think about Petruchio's ploys rather than simply watch them and emphasises that Petruchio's shrew-taming is a kind of education: he teaches Katherina that her evil-tempered ways are not desirable and that another behaviour pattern is superior. He is training Katherina as he would a hawk, as he describes in 4.1.175–198, and the conceit, although comically grotesque, becomes a metaphor for the socialising process.

Petruchio carries out his functions somewhat mechanically—he states his purposes and accomplishes them, and as a lover he is simply sentimental—but he nevertheless possesses a distinct personality. A genially self-confident aristocrat, he delights in the good life. He understands the appeal of excellent food and fine clothes, and in the final banquet scene he is clearly at home amid the pleasures of merry company. Petruchio doubtless incorporates traits of Elizabethan gentlemen who had hosted the young Shakespeare.

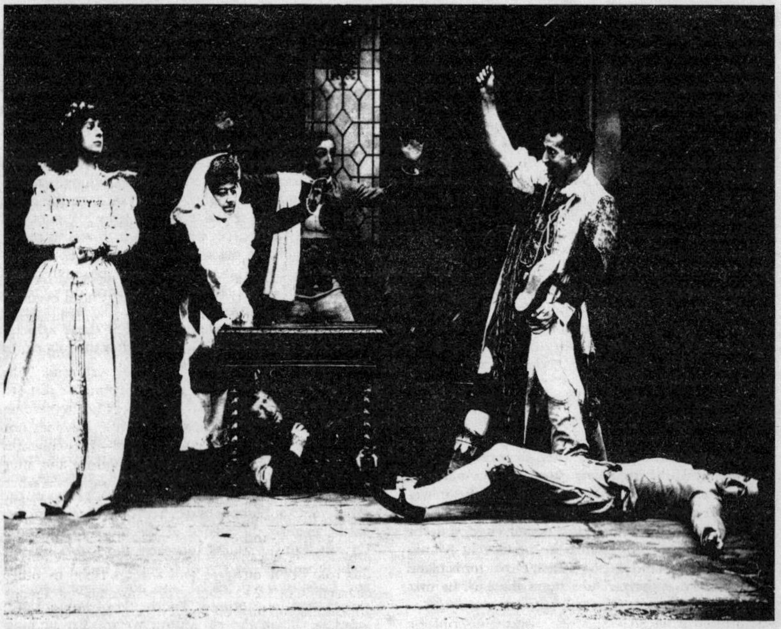

In this early 20th-century production of The Taming of the Shrew, *Petruchio (Frank Benson) terrorises the servants before an unimpressed Katherina.* (Courtesy of Culver Pictures, Inc.)

Phebe (Phoebe) Character in *As You Like It,* shepherdess loved by SILVIUS. Phebe is a caricature of the cruel shepherdess of the PASTORAL tradition, who rejects the love of the shepherd. In spurning Silvius, Phebe scorns romantic passion and denies that her coldness can wound her wooer. In presenting such a perfect parody of literary lovers, Shakespeare permits his hero and heroine, ROSALIND and ORLANDO, to seem relatively normal and to conduct their own courtship free from the extravagant posturing of traditional romances.

Rosalind, disguised as a young man, GANYMEDE, chastises Phebe for her attitude, pointing out that, being homely, she would do better to take Silvius than mock him. She advises Phebe, 'Sell when you can, you are not for all markets' (3.5.60). This extreme candour parodies the exaggerations of conventional sentiment. Then Phebe falls in love with Ganymede and thus assumes the same role as Silvius—that of the love-struck suitor. When Rosalind eventually discloses her true identity and holds Phebe to her promise to take Silvius if she could not have Ganymede, she points up the lesson of the parody: love is falsified by an excessive insistence on doting or rejection.

Phelps, Samuel (1804–1878) British actor and producer. Phelps was among the most influential of 19th-century producers of Shakespeare's plays, restoring much of the original text to plays encumbered by two centuries of adaptations. In an age of lavishly spectacular sets and scenic effects, which often required Shakespeare's texts to be cut to allow time for them, Phelps introduced relative simplicity. His followers William POEL and Harley GRANVILLE-BARKER transmitted these ideas to the 20th century.

Originally a journalist, Phelps moved from amateur theatricals to the professional theatre. He was well established in the British provinces as a tragic actor

before triumphing in London as SHYLOCK in 1837. After several years under Benjamin WEBSTER (1) and W. C. MACREADY, Phelps became manager of the SADLER'S WELLS THEATRE, where in 18 years (1844–1862) he staged most of Shakespeare's plays. In 1845 he presented the first staging of Shakespeare's text of *King Lear* in almost 200 years, finally superseding the radical adaptation of Nahum TATE, and his 1847 presentation of *Macbeth* did away with William DAVENANT's operatic additions. Similarly, he revived *Antony and Cleopatra* in 1849, and his 1851 *Timon of Athens* is believed to have been the initial staging of the play, which was apparently not produced in Shakespeare's time. Phelps was the leading player of his company, and he continued to act under various directors after he left Sadler's Wells. He portrayed most of the great tragic protagonists—OTHELLO and LEAR were thought to be his best parts—while also playing many other characters as well, such as MALVOLIO, PERICLES, and SHALLOW. He was particularly acclaimed as BOTTOM.

Philario Minor character in *Cymbeline*, POSTHUMUS' host in ROME. In 1.5 the gentlemanly Philario attempts to defuse the argument that leads to Posthumus' fatal wager with IACHIMO. In 2.4 when Iachimo claims to have won the bet by seducing IMOGEN, Philario tries to convince the enraged Posthumus not to believe him. He has no success in either endeavour. He thus represents human virtue, a force that promises good in the world but that proves useless in the face of evil. As such, he reinforces the play's theme that humankind is dependent on providence more than on its own efforts.

Philemon Minor character in *Pericles*, a servant of Lord CERIMON. Philemon, summoned by Cerimon, leaves immediately to carry out his master's orders to 'Get fire and meat' (3.2.3) for the victims of a storm. He speaks only four words and helps illustrate Cerimon's concerned care for others.

Philip (1) Minor character in *The Taming of the Shrew*, a member of the household staff of PETRUCHIO (2). Philip is one of the servants whom Petruchio abuses in 4.1 as part of his demonstration to KATHERINA of the ugliness of shrewish behaviour.

Philip (2) Augustus, King of France (1165–1223) Historical figure and character in *King John*, enemy of King JOHN (3) and supporter of ARTHUR. Philip is presented as an opportunist intent on political and military advantage over England by any means available, while mouthing graceful sentiments about honour. In 2.1 he backs Arthur's claim to the English throne, which John has usurped, but he willingly enters into a treaty by which his son LEWIS (1) marries John's niece BLANCHE, receiving in her dowry a large grant of English-held territory. Philip then breaks this alliance—under PANDULPH's threat of excommunication—and launches a war that results in Lewis' invasion of England in Acts 4–5. Philip himself disappears from the play in 3.3 (3.4), (for citation, see *King John*, 'Synopsis'), after Arthur's mother, CONSTANCE, delivers a fierce tirade against his treacherous abandonment of the boy.

The historical Philip is regarded as one of the great kings of FRANCE (1). He was a successful general who regained much of English-held France, to the north and west of Paris, seized territories from Flanders, and began the Albigensian Crusade, which was to result, under Blanche, in the accession of what is now southern France. Philip also successfully opposed the independence of the great barons of France, doing much to establish the powerful monarchy that was to bring France into early modern times. For these achievements he was known as Augustus, after the founder of the Roman Empire (see CAESAR [2]).

Philip (3) Character in *King John*. See BASTARD (1).

Philippi Ancient city in what is now northern Greece, a battle site in the Roman civil wars and a location in *Julius Caesar*. The armies of BRUTUS (4) and CASSIUS on one hand, and ANTONY and OCTAVIUS on the other, meet at Philippi in Act 5. Brutus risks all on this battle, against the advice of the more experienced Cassius, but he attacks too early and leaves Cassius without support, as TITINIUS remarks in 5.3.5. Brutus and Cassius are defeated, and both commit suicide rather than be captured. The battle of Philippi provides the climax wherein Antony avenges Brutus' murder of CAESAR (1).

Shakespeare altered the account of the battle that he found in his source, PLUTARCH's *Lives*. In 5.1 he invented the pre-battle meeting of the opposing generals, at which they trade insults and challenges. This exchange followed a well-known convention of medieval and Renaissance battle accounts, in which the credentials, as it were, of the warriors were established. More important, the playwright also compressed the events of several weeks into a single day to provide a dramatically more cohesive chain of events, as he had done in the HISTORY PLAYS.

There were in fact two battles at Philippi. In the first, fought on October 23, 42 B.C., the forces of Brutus and Cassius won a slight advantage. Antony's forces routed some of Cassius' troops and raided his headquarters, as is reported in 5.3.10; however, as Shakespeare also recounts, Brutus' premature attack was successful, and Octavius' men were defeated. Nevertheless, Cassius, believing mistakenly that all was lost, killed himself; an early account attributed the error to his defective eyesight. The loss was crucial, for Brutus was a bad general. Although Antony and

Octavius' forces were short of supplies in enemy country, Brutus could not control his impatience, and, after 20 days, he fought the second battle of Philippi, which, in the play, takes place on the same afternoon as the first, as per Brutus' order in 5.3.109–110. This second encounter, a bloody day-long battle, resulted in Brutus' defeat and suicide.

The combined battles were decisive; the civil war that followed the assassination of Julius Caesar had been won by the supporters of his style of dictatorial government. Moreover, the remnants of the old Roman aristocracy were largely wiped out in this campaign, which was particularly bloody by the standards of the day. Although more strife was to follow between the victors of Philippi (as is enacted in *Antony and Cleopatra*), the stage was set for the establishment of the Roman Empire under Octavius CAESAR (2).

Phillips, Augustine (d. 1605) One of the 26 men listed in the FIRST FOLIO as 'Principall Actors' in Shakespeare's plays, though not identified with any particular Shakespearean role. Phillips was in STRANGE'S MEN from about 1590 to 1593 and was probably an original member of the CHAMBERLAIN'S MEN. He was one of the original partners in the GLOBE THEATRE in 1599, and he was still with the Chamberlain's Men when it became the KING'S MEN in 1603. Thus, most of his professional life was spent with this troupe. This is reflected in his will, which has survived. The executors were John HEMINGE, Richard BURBAGE (3), and William SLY (2), all King's Men, and he left small bequests to many of his fellow actors, including Shakespeare. Also, Phillips' sister married another member, Robert GOUGH, who witnessed the will just days before Phillips died. Among the items Phillips bequeathed were several musical instruments, suggesting that he had been a musician as well as actor.

Philo Minor character in *Antony and Cleopatra,* a follower of ANTONY. In 1.1 Philo and his friend DEMETRIUS (3) discuss Antony's neglect of his military duty due to his infatuation with the queen of Egypt, CLEOPATRA. Philo's angry complaint opens the play with an emotional flourish. The episode establishes a disapproving Roman view of the love affair.

Philostrate Minor character in *A Midsummer Night's Dream,* the MASTER OF REVELS under Duke THESEUS (1). Philostrate arranges the entertainment for the wedding of Theseus and HIPPOLYTA (1) and presents the Duke with a list of prospective acts. A pompous courtier, Philostrate argues against Theseus' selection of the artisans' production of PYRAMUS AND THISBE on the grounds that it is blatantly undignified. Shakespeare apparently took the name Philostrate from CHAUCER'S 'The Knight's Tale', in which one character uses it as an alias.

Philotus Minor character in *Timon of Athens,* the employee of a usurer who duns TIMON for payment of a loan. In 3.4 Philotus joins other servants when they approach Timon and his STEWARD (2) for repayment, but they are put off. They regret that they must solicit for their greedy masters, who have benefited from Timon's generosity but are now merciless when he is in need.

Philotus appears with HORTENSIUS, TITUS (2), LUCIUS' SERVANT and two men designated as VARRO'S SERVANT. Since the latter three are addressed as 'Lucius' and 'Varro' (3.4.2, 3), it is presumed that Shakespeare intended the names of the first three to refer to their masters, as well. This perhaps reflects a casual linguistic practise of the early 17th century.

Phoenix Name of a house, one of three on stage, in *The Comedy of Errors.* The Phoenix, which may be distinguished in a stage set by a sign above its door, is the home of ANTIPHOLUS OF EPHESUS and ADRIANA. The other houses that comprise the setting are the PORCUPINE and the PRIORY. This arrangement of three structures, each with an entrance onto the stage, was standard in ancient Roman stage design, as it was understood in Shakespeare's time, and it is quite appropriate to this play, which, of all Shakespeare's works, most closely resembles Roman drama.

The Phoenix and Turtle Shakespeare's allegorical poem on the mystical nature of love. *The Phoenix and Turtle* consists of 13 quatrains (four-line stanzas) rhyming *abba,* followed by five triplets (stanzas of three rhyming lines) all in iambic tetrameter (see METRE). The poem tells of the funeral of two lovers: the phoenix, a mythological bird associated with immortality, and the turtledove (usually called 'turtle' in Elizabethan English), a symbol of fidelity. The two birds have burned themselves to death in order to be forever joined in love. The allegory celebrates an ideal of love in which an absolute spiritual union of the lovers, defying rationality and common sense, is chastely achieved through death, the ultimate rejection of the world.

The first five quatrains summon various birds to the funeral. The owl and other birds of prey—considered omens of evil—are refused admittance, while the crow and the swan, whose colour and song, respectively, are traditionally associated with death, are welcomed. The next eight stanzas comprise a funerary 'anthem' (line 21). The lovers are praised for having successfully achieved a total union, defying reason in the process. This defeat of worldly wisdom is celebrated in lyrical paradoxes, such as 'Two distincts, division none; Number there in love was slain' (lines 27–28) and 'Either was the other's mine' (line 36). Reason itself is constrained to cry out, 'Love hath reason, reason none' (line 47). Reason composes a funeral song, the

'threnos', which is presented in the last five stanzas, the solemn triple rhymes. The phoenix and the turtle are said to have embodied truth and beauty and, through their deaths, to have conveyed these qualities to all who 'are either true or fair' (line 66).

This allegory reflects a notion that was widespread in the RENAISSANCE: ideal love was felt to transcend reason and thus to represent a truer state of being than that of the material world. This idea, whose roots lay in the writings of Plato, is also related to the Christian concept of the state of grace that God offers to believers, and *The Phoenix and Turtle* has been interpreted as a specifically Christian allegory. More generally, it may be seen as illustrating the possibility of transcendence through love, an ideal that informs much of Shakespeare's work, particularly the COMEDIES.

The Phoenix and Turtle does not have a literary source, although the idea of an assembly of birds was a common one; for example, it appears in CHAUCER's *The Parliament of Fowls* and a famous mock funeral in OVID's *Amores,* to name only two great authors whom Shakespeare is known to have read and admired. The more specific motif of love between phoenix and turtledove was determined by its use in Robert Chester's LOVE'S MARTYR, a long allegorical poem celebrating the marriage of Sir John SALUSBURY and his wife; Shakespeare's poem was apparently written to be published with that work in 1601. The idea of love between these two symbolic birds was novel, originating with either Chester or his patron.

Salusbury and his wife are the likeliest subjects of any specific symbolism the phoenix and the turtledove may carry, in addition to their joint role as an emblem of ideal love. In addition, scholars have long speculated on possible hidden meanings in *Love's Martyr* and/or *The Phoenix and Turtle,* and various obscure references have been proposed. The two birds have been seen as Queen ELIZABETH (1) and the Earl of ESSEX (2) and as Essex and the Earl of SOUTHAMPTON (2), among other pairings. However, such hypotheses are not provable, and in any case the poem transcends whatever particular purposes it may have had, surviving as a mystical and powerful invocation of love.

Phrynia and Timandra Minor characters in *Timon of Athens,* concubines of ALCIBIADES. In 4.3 Phrynia and her colleague Timandra are travelling with Alcibiades and encounter TIMON in the woods. They generally speak in unison, and are entirely indistinguishable from each other. In his misanthropic fury, Timon has decided to corrupt humanity by distributing the gold he has found. He gives some to the courtesans and accompanies the gift with vicious insults. They laughingly encourage his abuse so long as it is accompanied by gold. This mildly humorous passage satirises greed, and also provides a slight respite from Timon's grim misanthropy. Both women represent a stock comic figure, the greedy whore.

Picardy Region in northern FRANCE (1), location of the battle of AGINCOURT and the setting of several scenes in *Henry V.* In 3.6 and 3.7 the English and French armies, respectively, are shown in camp prior to the crucial battle, which itself occupies all of Act 4. Picardy is the historical term for an area north and east of the River Seine along the English Channel.

'Pied Bull' Quarto See *KING LEAR*, 'Text of the Play'.

Pilch Character in *Pericles.* See FISHERMEN.

Pinch, Dr Character in *The Comedy of Errors,* a quack physician. Dr Pinch is consulted when ANTIPHOLUS OF EPHESUS, as a result of the confusion and mistaken identities that are the chief business of the play, is presumed to be insane. Antipholus later describes him as: '. . . one Pinch, a hungry lean-fac'd villain; / A mere anatomy, a mountebank, / A thread-bare juggler, and a fortune-teller, / A needy-hollow-ey'd-sharp-looking-wretch; / A living dead man. . . .' (5.1.238–242).

Pinch is not a physician in any modern sense; he is merely a man of some learning. He is identified as a 'schoolmaster' (in a stage direction in 4.4.38) and as a 'conjuror', or exorcist (4.4.45 and 5.1.243). Both references are to the fact that he can speak Latin, which was commonly believed in Shakespeare's day to be the language of spirits and ghosts.

Whatever his appearance or qualifications, Dr Pinch's prescription for a case of lunacy ('They must be bound and laid in some dark room' [4.4.92]) was widespread in the 16th and 17th centuries. Although it now seems inhumane, both insanity and this particular treatment of it were common subjects of humour on the Elizabethan stage. The same regime is meted out to MALVOLIO, in *Twelfth Night,* for instance. If Pinch seems a brutal doctor to us, no less so seems his fiery, filthy comeuppance (5.1.171–178), though we may be sure the original audience delighted in it, for such abuse was a comic staple. Shakespeare at least keeps it off-stage.

Pindarus (active 42 B.C.) Historical figure and minor character in *Julius Caesar,* a captured Parthian slave belonging to CASSIUS. In 5.3, at PHILIPPI, Pindarus helps Cassius to commit suicide. Pindarus mistakenly reports the capture of TINTINIUS, and Cassius, in despair, decides that, rather than be captured himself, he will die. He gives Pindarus his freedom in exchange for holding the sword upon which he falls. Pindarus, now free, 'yet would not so have been' (5.3.47), elects to run far away and disappears from the play. Shakespeare took the episode, which fittingly ends the ca-

reer of the emotional Cassius, from PLUTARCH's *Lives*, where Pindarus is reported to have beheaded Cassius before disappearing and to have been suspected by some of having murdered his master.

Pirates Three minor characters in *Pericles*, buccaneers who kidnap MARINA. In 4.1 the Pirates interrupt LEONINE, who is about to murder Marina, and take her from her would-be killer. In 4.2 they sell her to a brothel in MYTILENE and disappear from the play. When they effect this melodramatic change in the heroine's fortunes, the Pirates bring about one of the play's many surprises, which helps demonstrate the human dependence upon fate, an important theme. The Pirates, who speak four short lines between them, display an abrupt vigour ('A prize! A prize!' cries the Second Pirate [4.1.93], in his only speech) but their function is mainly to further the plot.

Pirithous Minor character in *The Two Noble Kinsmen*, friend of THESEUS (2), Duke of ATHENS. Pirithous attends Theseus in every scene in which the duke appears; he also provides commentary on ARCITE in 2.4 and, as a messenger, dramatically halts the execution of PALAMON in 5.4. However, he is significant only as the subject of a conversation in his absence. In 1.3 HIPPOLYTA reflects on the long friendship of Theseus and Pirithous, saying 'Their knot of love, / Tied, weaved, entangled ... May be outworn, never undone' (1.3.41–44). This striking parallel to the tie between Palamon and Arcite helps establish the theme of male friendship that is woven through the play. Hippolyta's remarks also spark a variant on the theme, the account by EMILIA (4) of her similar childhood friendship with a girl.

Pisanio Character in *Cymbeline*, the faithful servant of POSTHUMUS. When his master is exiled for having married IMOGEN, King CYMBELINE's daughter, Pisanio remains at court to serve her. He embodies a well-known figure of folklore and literature: the faithful servant who serves his master best by disobeying him. When Posthumus is deceived by IACHIMO and believes that Imogen has betrayed him, he orders Pisanio to murder her. Instead, the servant helps Imogen escape and provides her with a disguise as a page, in which she has further adventures. However, for all his steadfastness and common sense, Pisanio cannot provide further assistance. He loses contact with both Posthumus and Imogen and finds himself under suspicion at court. Fearful and confused, he resigns himself to whatever fate may bring. 'The heavens still must work' and 'Fortune brings in some boats that are not steer'd' (4.3.41, 46), he says. He thus states neatly the play's central lesson: that humanity is dependent on providence.

Pistol Character in *2 Henry IV*, *The Merry Wives of Windsor*, and *Henry V*, a braggart soldier and follower of FALSTAFF. The comical Pistol serves as Falstaff's aide in King HENRY IV's campaign against the rebels in *2 Henry IV*. He first appears at Falstaff's dinner party at the BOAR'S HEAD TAVERN in 2.4, and he offends everyone present with grandiose insults while asserting his chivalric honour with distorted snatches of rhetoric from Elizabethan drama and literature. This vigorous mode of address is Pistol's principal attribute in all of his appearances. To some extent, Pistol satirises military pretensions, but his rhetoric is more pointedly a literary parody; Shakespeare exaggerates the florid language of MARLOWE (1) and his followers. Pistol is called an ancient; ancient, or ensign (standard-bearer), is a military rank, the equivalent of lieutenant, which BARDOLPH (1) calls Pistol in *Henry V*, 2.1.38. Pistol may actually be an ancient, or he may have simply appropriated the title, for part of his absurdity is his singular unsuitability for command.

Like the 16th-century sidearm for which he is named, Pistol is violently loud but incapable of serious damage. Also, the pistol was commonly associated, in Elizabethan humour, with the penis; much is made of this in *2 Henry IV*, 2.4.109–135. When the Quarto edition of *2 Henry IV* was published in 1600, its subtitle made particular reference to Pistol, whose appeal was already recognised, and he has been among Shakespeare's most popular characters ever since. His extravagant rhetoric makes him hilarious even to audiences for whom the original parodies are meaningless.

In *The Merry Wives* Pistol is again in Falstaff's entourage (apparently as a civilian), but he refuses to deliver his master's love letters, rejecting the task as unsoldierly, and Falstaff fires him. He and NYM seek revenge, and they inform FORD (1) and PAGE (12) that Falstaff has designs on their wives, thereby triggering the principal sub-plot of Ford's jealousy. Pistol is insignificant thereafter, although he does appear in the final MASQUElike scene, disguised as a fairy. This may simply reflect the employment of the actor who played Pistol in another role, but Pistol's appearance in character might have been taken by 16th-century audiences as a clue to the ceremonial nature of the scene, in which personality is wiped out.

In *Henry V*, Pistol mourns the passing of Falstaff with his new wife, the HOSTESS (2), whom he has presumably dazzled with his extravagant braggadoccio. Once on campaign in France, he proves himself a coward in 3.2; following this episode, the BOY (3) remarks on the villainy of Pistol, Nym, and Bardolph. In 3.6 Pistol pleads unsuccessfully for FLUELLEN's intercession on behalf of Bardolph, who has been sentenced to death for looting; in 4.1 he is one of the soldiers whom the incognito King HENRY V encounters the night before the battle of AGINCOURT, though

he has little to say, merely making a nasty remark about Fluellen.

In 4.4 Pistol captures a FRENCH SOLDIER and demands ransom of him, threatening to kill him otherwise. Since he speaks no French and the soldier no English, the scene is comical, but Pistol is unquestionably an unpleasant character, vicious and overbearing. The Boy acts as interpreter, saving the soldier's life, and he remarks afterwards of Pistol, 'I did never know so full a voice issue from so empty a heart' (4.4.69–70). Pistol is last seen in 5.1, where Fluellen forces him to eat a leek. The last survivor of Falstaff's followers, Pistol in *Henry V* serves to show that the anarchic element represented by Falstaff is finally rendered both harmless and completely disreputable. On the other hand, Pistol may also be seen as a symbolic parallel to King Henry's militarism: he satirises notions of military honour, while most of the combat actually presented involves Pistol at his most degenerate. Most strikingly, his threat to kill his prisoner in 4.4 foreshadows Henry's own order that 'every soldier kill his prisoner' (4.6.37).

It is thought that Falstaff appeared in an early, unacted version of *Henry V* and was then excised by Shakespeare, with remnants of his part going to Pistol, who displays Falstaffian characteristics in several scenes, particularly 5.1. This theory cannot be proven, but it is supported by textual evidence (see FALSTAFF).

Planché, James Robinson (1796–1880) British playwright and theatrical designer. Planché wrote many successful burlesques and pantomimes, as well as a few legitimate dramas, over a period of 50 years, beginning in 1818. He was also a serious antiquarian—a founder of the British Archaeological Association—specialising in the history of costume. His *History of British Costume* (1834) was a standard work in the field for many years. In this capacity, he helped create the 19th-century enthusiasm for historically accurate productions of Shakespeare's plays. He designed the costumes for the first such staging, the *King John* staged by Charles KEMBLE (1) in 1823. He also was credited with much of the success of the 1840 *Midsummer Night's Dream* of Charles Mathews and Elizabeth VESTRIS; he designed the Athenian costumes and a famous finale featuring dozens of twinkling lights. Lastly, he designed the 1844 production by Benjamin WEBSTER (1) of *The Taming of the Shrew*, which is said to have legitimised the presentation of Shakespeare's plays in their original form.

Planché, the son of a watchmaker of Huguenot descent, had many other talents. He was a good professional musician and a respected authority on heraldry; he wrote opera librettos; and, following the unauthorised production of one of his plays, he became largely responsible for the first law granting modern copyright protection to dramatists.

Plantagenet (1) family English ruling dynasty in 1154–1484, parts of whose history form the subject matter of most of Shakespeare's HISTORY PLAYS. *King John* deals with an early Plantagenet monarch, and the feuding between the YORK (1) and LANCASTER (1) branches of the family, culminating in the WARS OF THE ROSES, is the subject of two sequences of four plays each (see TETRALOGY) that cover the reigns of the last Plantagenet rulers.

The earliest Plantagenet was a French nobleman, Geoffrey, Count of Anjou, and the family was originally known as the Angevin dynasty. Geoffrey's badge was a representation of a white flower, *planta argent,* from which the later family name derives. (The use of this name began only in the 1460s, when Richard, Duke of YORK (8), assumed it as part of his campaign to claim the throne for his branch of the family.)

In 1127 Geoffrey of Anjou married the daughter of Henry I of England, a younger son of William the Conqueror; Geoffrey's son, Henry II, became the first Plantagenet king. As in most medieval dynasties, the ancient rule of primogeniture provided that the crown was to be inherited by an eldest son or his descendants, or by a next-eldest son if the eldest had no sons or had died before the king. This eventually caused great difficulties for England, but for two centuries the Plantagenets transmitted their power peaceably.

Richard I, the Lionhearted, succeeded his father, Henry II. Dying childless, Richard was succeeded by his younger brother, JOHN (3), in 1199. Beginning with John's son Henry (see PRINCE [3]), son succeeded father through five generations, in a sequence ending with RICHARD II. The dynasty subsequently broke down.

The York and Lancaster branches of the Plantagenet family descended from two of the seven sons of Edward III, who died in 1377. The eldest of these sons died before his father did, and the crown passed to his son, Richard II. King Edward's second son, the Duke of Clarence, did not have a son; his daughter married into the Mortimer family. The third son was John of GAUNT, Duke of Lancaster, whose son, Henry BOLINGBROKE (1) deposed his cousin Richard in 1399 and ruled as HENRY IV, the first Lancastrian King. The fourth son of King Edward, Edmund Langley, Duke of YORK (4), could entertain no claim to rule under a normal succession. However, after Richard's deposition, the Mortimers attempted to claim the throne by virtue of their relation to King Edward's second son, who would have succeeded Richard under any circumstances but usurpation, and York's son, the Earl of CAMBRIDGE in *Henry V,* married a Mortimer and inherited their claim. Thus by the mid-15th century the Yorkist faction was the chief rival to the Lancastrians. The remaining sons of Edward III had no importance in the Plantagenet succession, though the murder of one of them, Thomas, Duke of GLOUCESTER (6),

helped spark the fall of Richard II, which, along with the reigns of the first two Lancastrian monarchs, is dealt with in *Richard II, 1* and *2 Henry IV*, and *Henry V*.

When Henry V died in 1422, his son, HENRY VI, was an infant, and the illegality of Richard II's deposition was still a living issue that only a strong monarch could silence. The Yorkist claim was pressed, and the resulting wars are the principal subject of Shakespeare's earliest history plays, *1, 2,* and *3 Henry VI* and *Richard III.* Beginning in 1461, three members of the York family ruled England: EDWARD IV, Edward V (see PRINCE [5]), and RICHARD III. In 1485 Richard III was overthrown by a distant cousin of Henry VI, the Earl of RICHMOND, who ruled as King Henry VII, the founder of the TUDOR dynasty.

Two Plantagenets survived the Wars of the Roses, a BOY (2) and a GIRL, great-great-grandchildren of the original Duke of York. The boy, Edward, Earl of Warwick, was imprisoned for most of his brief life to prevent him from claiming the crown; Henry VII executed him in 1499, after rebels had made several attempts to impersonate him and seize the throne. His sister, Margaret, the last Plantagenet, lived until 1541, when she was beheaded, at the age of 68, by HENRY VIII, who also feared a rebellion in favour of the former dynasty.

Plantagenet (2), Richard In *1 Henry VI,* the name by which the future Duke of YORK (8) is known until, at 3.1.159, he is restored to the dukedom, lost by the treason of his father, the Earl of CAMBRIDGE.

Plantagenet (3), Richard In *King John* the name granted to the BASTARD (1) in acknowledgement that he is the illegitimate son of the late King Richard I. The Bastard is fictitious; King Richard did have an illegitimate son, but his name was Philip.

Platter, Thomas (1574–1628) Swiss doctor from Basel who travelled widely in 1595–1600 and published an account of his journeys (in German) in 1604. He was in England in September–October 1599 and recorded a performance of *Julius Caesar* at the GLOBE THEATRE and an unnamed play at the CURTAIN THEATRE. His remarks are among the few sources of detail about the ELIZABETHAN THEATRE.

Plautus, Titus Maccius (c. 254–184 B.C.) Ancient Roman dramatist, author of sources for *The Comedy of Errors* and *The Taming of the Shrew.* Plautus' *Menaechmi* was the principal source for *The Comedy of Errors,* providing the central plot of long-lost twins who are farcically mistaken for each other, and another of his works, *Amphitryon,* provided the second set of twins. Numerous details in *The Shrew,* including the names of GRUMIO and TRANIO, came from Plautus' *Mostellaria (The Haunted House).* Minor elements in other plays also reflect Shakespeare's knowledge of Plautus.

Moreover, many other writers and dramatists had relied on Plautus' plays as sources, so elements from Plautus could have reached Shakespeare indirectly. For instance, one of the main sources for *The Shrew,* ARIOSTO's *I Suppositi* (1509), was itself based on Plautus' *The Captives.* The first English comedy, *Ralph Roister Doister* (c. 1553) by Nicholas UDALL, is based on Plautus' *Miles Gloriosus* (after whose hero the character type MILES GLORIOSUS is named). Plautus was still very well known in Shakespeare's day, and the playwright clearly assumed that his audience was familiar with his work, as when he had POLONIUS tritely observe that 'Plautus [cannot be] too light' (*Hamlet,* 2.2.396–397). Plautus continues to provide stimulation to writers of comedy; for instance, elements from several of his comedies were incorporated in the American musical *A Funny Thing Happened on the Way to the Forum* (1962).

Plautus wrote many plays, of which 21 survive, all of them comedies and all free translations of older Greek works, especially those of Menander (c. 342–292), some of whose plays are known only through their Plautine versions. Plautus' works are generally characterised by a casually cynical tone, complicated plots, and stereotyped characters (his character types helped stimulate the 17th-century COMEDY OF HUMOURS). Some works are merely farcical (see FARCE), while others have sentimental or social themes. He was highly popular in the Roman world, and his plays continued to be produced for centuries after his death. Many later plays were falsely ascribed to him—more than 100 have been reattributed by modern scholars. Plautus was ignored during the Middle Ages, and his rediscovery was an important stimulus to RENAISSANCE literature and drama throughout Europe.

Player King Character in THE MURDER OF GONZAGO, the playlet presented within *Hamlet.* In 3.2 the PLAYERS (2) stage a play in which the Player King anticipates that his wife, the PLAYER QUEEN, will remarry if he dies, despite her protests to the contrary. Then he is murdered by LUCIANUS, who pours poison in his ear while he sleeps. This scenario resembles the actual murder of HAMLET's father by KING (5) Claudius—as the GHOST (3) has recounted it the prince—and the King reacts to it with great distress, fleeing from the room. Thus, as he had planned, Hamlet is presented with proof that the Ghost had told the truth.

The Player King speaks in a highly rhetorical style that distances the play within a play from the action of the play itself, emphasising its artificiality. The part of the Player King is presumably taken by the FIRST PLAYER (2), who demonstrates his dramatic gifts when the Players first arrive at ELSINORE in 2.2.

Player Queen Character in THE MURDER OF GONZAGO, the playlet presented within *Hamlet.* In 3.2 the PLAYERS (2) perform before the court of KING (5) Claudius. Following HAMLET's instructions, they stage a play in which the Player Queen assures her husband, the PLAYER KING, that she will never remarry if he dies before her. He insists that she will; in the next scene he is murdered. The play parallels the murder of Hamlet's father by the King and the remarriage of his mother, the QUEEN (9), so it is obvious that the Player Queen's part would include her marriage to the killer. However, the performance is interrupted by the King's guilty reaction, and she never reappears.

The Player Queen is merely a symbolic character. Her highly rhetorical diction helps to emphasise the extreme artificiality of the play within a play.

Players (1) Group of minor characters in *The Taming of the Shrew,* a travelling company of actors. In the INDUCTION the Players are hired by the local LORD (1), who is amusing himself by providing gentlemanly amenities to a drunken tinker, Christopher SLY (1). The Players perform 'a pleasant comedy' (Ind.2.130) for Sly; this play is *The Taming of the Shrew.*

One of the Players, identified in various editions as 'A Player', 'First Player', and 'Second Player', is designated by the name of a real Elizabethan actor in a speech heading in the FIRST FOLIO edition of the play; the part was played by John SINCKLO in an early production. In Ind.1.86 he speaks of a role he had played, naming a character in a play by John FLETCHER (2) that was written in about 1620. This is probably a late insertion into Shakespeare's text, not long before its publication in 1623, but it may be original and refer to an otherwise unknown play of the 1580s or early 1590s that served Fletcher as a source.

Players (2) Characters in *Hamlet,* touring actors who are hired by Prince HAMLET to perform a play that he hopes will shock the KING (5) into an unconscious revelation of guilt. After commissioning the Players to perform THE MURDER OF GONZAGO, a brief drama that enacts a crime similar to the King's killing of Hamlet's father, the prince makes his famous remark 'The play's the thing / Wherein I'll catch the conscience of the King' (2.2.600–601). The playlet—featuring the PLAYER KING, the PLAYER QUEEN, and LUCIANUS—achieves the expected result in 3.2.

There are at least three Players, enough to play the three parts in the playlet, with one of them doubling as the speaker of the PROLOGUE (1) and all three participating in the DUMB SHOW that precedes the spoken play. The elaborate stage direction at 3.2.133 calls for extra players in the dumb show, but this requirement may be ignored in production.

The troupe is led by the FIRST PLAYER (2), who demonstrates his art when he recites a monologue on PYRRHUS and HECUBA in 2.2. He presumably plays the Player King in 3.2, where he also receives Hamlet's opinions on acting—thought to reflect Shakespeare's own—in 3.2.1–45.

In 3.2.330–358 ROSENCRANTZ AND GUILDENSTERN report that the Players' popularity has suffered due to the success of a boys' acting company. This incident reflects the WAR OF THE THEATRES, the competition between the professional players and the CHILDREN'S COMPANIES that raged in London in 1601.

Plebeians (1) Minor but significant characters in *Julius Caesar,* the citizens of ROME who react to the assassination of CAESAR (1). In 3.2 the Plebeians are addressed at Caesar's funeral, first by BRUTUS (4) and then by ANTONY, and they respond enthusiastically to the orations of each. First, when Brutus explains the rationale behind the assassination (3.2.13–48), the crowd excitedly approves his assertions. Ironically, however, the Plebeians shout, 'Let him be Caesar' (3.2.52), and speak of crowning Brutus, who has just killed Caesar in order to prevent a crowning and preserve the Republic. Conversely, they can now say of Caesar, whom earlier they had hailed, 'This Caesar was a tyrant' (3.2.71). Moreover, their change in attitude merely foreshadows another one.

Antony's famous oration (3.2.75–254) plays on the emotions of the Plebeians, whereas Brutus had appealed to their reason, and Antony's impact is much greater. Before he is halfway through, the Plebeians are calling Brutus and the conspirators '. . . traitors . . . villains, murderers!' (3.2.155–158), and they go on to raise a confused cry of 'Revenge! . . . Burn!—Fire!—Kill!—Slay!' (3.2.206–207). Finally, the Plebeians run amok, hurrying to burn the houses of the conspirators, and Antony exults, 'Mischief, thou art afoot' (3.2.262). Almost immediately he receives news that Brutus and Cassius have had to flee the city.

In 3.3 the mob encounters CINNA (1), and simply because he has the same name as one of the assassins—CINNA (2)—they beat him to death. In this brief and grimly humorous scene, the Plebeians are almost incoherent, asking questions of their victim without listening to his answers and finally, realising that he is not their proper prey, declaring, 'It is no matter, his name's Cinna; pluck but his name out of his heart' (3.3.33–34). Having demonstrated their irrational power, they disappear from the play. The civil war that Antony had hoped to foment (in 3.1.254–275) has begun with their riot.

The term 'plebeian' was an ancient designation for the ordinary citizens of the Roman Republic, as distinguished from the patricians, or aristocrats. Its use suggests the intense political context of the play at this point, in contrast to the use of COMMONER (1) in 1.1. Shakespeare valued individual humans regardless of social standing—as is evidenced by many of his char-

acters, including, in this play, the COBBLER—but he distrusted the common people as a class. Two of the most important political points he made in *Julius Caesar* are that the masses are unreliable and that their ascendancy is a key symptom of social disorder. The Plebeians of the play, in their fickleness, brutality, and manipulability, demonstrate the dangers of a political world that includes them. In this respect they resemble the rebels led by Jack CADE in *2 Henry VI* and the rabble (see CITIZEN [5]) of *Coriolanus.*

Plebeians (2) Characters in *Coriolanus.* See CITIZEN (5).

Pliny the Elder (c. 23–79 A.D.) Roman author of an encyclopaedia of natural history that served as a minor source for *Othello.* Pliny's *Naturalis Historia,* translated by Philemon HOLLAND (4) as *Natural History* (1601) provided several details for OTHELLO's description of his adventures in 1.3.

Pliny's vast work assembles a tremendous body of lore, and though much of it is inaccurate, it remained an important reference into the RENAISSANCE. A career military officer and a close friend of the emperor Vespasian (ruled 69–79 A.D.), he wrote many books, mostly on military subjects, but only the *Natural History* survives. His scientific curiosity was so great that during the eruption of Vesuvius in 79 A.D., he travelled to Pompeii and was killed. His death is described by his nephew Pliny the Younger (61–c. 114) in a famous passage from his *Letters.*

Plowright, Joan (b. 1929) English actress, widow of Laurence OLIVIER. Plowright often played opposite her husband, perhaps most notably as PORTIA (1) to his SHYLOCK in his 1970 London production of *The Merchant of Venice* and again in the 1974 TELEVISION version. Her most striking Shakespearean part was also on television, the double role of SEBASTIAN (2) and VIOLA in a 1969 production of *Twelfth Night.*

Plummer, Christopher (b. 1929) Canadian actor. Plummer has played many Shakespearean roles in Stratford, Ontario, and elsewhere. At Stratford in 1972, he starred opposite Zoë CALDWELL in a memorable *Antony and Cleopatra.* He also won particular acclaim for his IAGO, opposite James Earl JONES (1), in Nicol WILLIAMSON's 1982 New York production of *Othello.*

Plutarch (c. 46–c. 130 A.D.) Greek philosopher and biographer whose *Lives*—as translated by Sir Thomas NORTH—was Shakespeare's primary source for *Antony and Cleopatra, Coriolanus, Julius Caesar, Timon of Athens* and a source of minor elements in other plays. Plutarch, after studying in Athens, became a teacher of philosophy in Rome, where he received the patronage of the emperors Hadrian and Trajan and wrote (in Greek) many works on ethical, religious, and political questions. Following Trajan's death, Plutarch returned to Greece, where he wrote his famous biographies of Greek and Roman heroes of history and legend. These works, intended as moral lessons in greatness and failure, have inspired many generations of readers. Among Plutarch's most important admirers, besides Shakespeare, have been Michel de MONTAIGNE, Ralph Waldo Emerson, and Napoleon Bonaparte.

Poel, William (1852–1934) English theatrical producer. Beginning in 1894, with the founding of the Elizabethan Stage Society, Poel revolutionised the theatrical presentation of Shakespeare's plays with productions that attempted to replicate the experience of 16th- and 17th-century playgoers. Using a projecting stage, very little scenery, and original texts, his group staged numerous works by Shakespeare, Christopher MARLOWE (1), Francis BEAUMONT (2) and John FLETCHER (2), Ben JONSON, Thomas MIDDLETON, and others. Financial losses closed the society in 1905, but Poel continued to produce such works elsewhere, including DER BESTRAFTE BRUDERMORD in 1924 (its first English production) and ARDEN OF FEVERSHAM in 1925. His work influenced others, notably Nugent MONCK and Harley GRANVILLE-BARKER, and furthered a long-lasting trend towards scrupulously preserved texts produced in rigorously simple stagings that countered extravagant spectacles of the late 19th century. His work also influenced critical attitudes towards Shakespeare's work; for instance, he was the first director to stage all three PROBLEM PLAYS, thereby helping to stimulate their acceptance in a world that had previously spurned them (Poel had been instructed in college never to read *Measure for Measure* or *Troilus and Cressida* because of their gross impropriety). Poel also wrote several plays himself and a number of books on the theatre.

Poet (1) Minor character in *Julius Caesar,* a wandering bard who accosts BRUTUS (4) and CASSIUS and advises them against discord. He is plainly a fool, and in any event he arrives (in 4.3.122) after the two generals have reconciled. While Cassius tolerates the Poet, Brutus arrogantly dismisses him, demonstrating in a small way the deterioration in his character that is a major theme of the play. Also, the brief episode provides a moment of needed comic relief between the dispute between the two leaders' and the revelation of the death of PORTIA (2).

Shakespeare took this episode from PLUTARCH's *Lives,* where the figure was not a poet but a self-declared philosopher, a seemingly lunatic imitator of the wandering ascetics known as Cynics. (Cynicism, founded by Hellenistic philosophers in the 4th cen-

tury B.C., held that independence and self-control constituted the only human good, and they preached a 'natural' life-style, ostentatiously rejecting wealth, prestige, and even the comforts of ordinary life.) Cassius calls the Poet a 'cynic' in 4.3.132. In Plutarch, the would-be Cynic quotes a line from the Iliad of HOMER, which, after being transmuted through AMYOT and NORTH, appears comically in 4.3.130–131, where Shakespeare—perhaps mistakenly—attributes it to the speaker himself, who is therefore called a poet.

Poet (2) Minor character in *Timon of Athens,* a flatterer of TIMON. In 1.1 the Poet and his friend the PAINTER (1) discuss Timon's generosity, which each hopes to exploit when he presents the nobleman with an example of his art. Pompously self-satisfied, the Poet congratulates himself on being a poet from whom art 'oozes' (1.1.21). He anticipates the play's truths when he tells that the poem he is writing, in which Timon is shown as a favourite of the goddess Fortune, contains the warning that when Fortune changes, her ex-favourites are abandoned by their seemingly loyal followers. Though the Poet is not mentioned in Timon's downfall, he is presumably among the deserters, for in 5.1 he and the Painter attempt to reingratiate themselves with him because they have heard that their one-time benefactor has found gold. Timon overhears him planning 'what I shall say I have provided for him' (5.1.32), though in fact he has written no poems for him. When he and the Painter fawningly assure Timon of their friendship, he mocks them and drives them away. The Poet is an emblematic character, satirically representative of the greed and hypocrisy of courtiers.

Poetomachia See WAR OF THE THEATRES.

Poins, Ned Character in *1* and *2 Henry IV,* friend of PRINCE (6) HAL. Poins suggests the two jokes that he and Hal play on FALSTAFF. In *1 Henry IV,* 1.2.156–185, he devises the plan to rob Falstaff of his takings in the highway robbery of 2.2, and in *2 Henry IV,* 2.2.164–165, he proposes that he and the Prince disguise themselves as DRAWERS and spy on Falstaff. He also participates in the Prince's joke on FRANCIS (1) in 2.4 of *1 Henry IV.* In 2.4 of *2 Henry IV* Falstaff, unaware of Poins' presence, describes him, insultingly but with considerable accuracy, in a hilarious presentation of a rowdy, empty-headed party boy (2.4.241–250). In 2.2.42 Poins demonstrates his blindness to Prince Hal's true character, expecting him to be pleased at the imminent death of his father, King HENRY IV. But in 2.2.61–65 he is conscious of his position as part of the world of delinquency that the Prince must reject, and he accepts his own limitations.

Poins is Shakespeare's version of a character named Ned in the FAMOUS VICTORIES, his chief source for the material on Hal's riotous early life. His last name may refer to the lace ribbons, known as points, that were a prominent feature of a 16th-century courtier's elaborate garb.

Polixenes Character in *The Winter's Tale,* the King of BOHEMIA. In 1.2 Polixenes, visiting his old friend King LEONTES of SICILIA, is persuaded by Leontes' wife, Queen HERMIONE, to extend his stay. However, Leontes goes mad and imagines adultery between Polixenes and Hermione. Warned by CAMILLO that Leontes intends to poison him, Polixenes flees to Bohemia and is not seen again until late in the play. Leontes believes his infant daughter, PERDITA, is the illegitimate child of Polixenes, and orders her abandoned in the wilderness. In Act 4, 16 years later, Polixenes' son, Prince FLORIZEL, falls in love with Perdita, who has been raised by shepherds in Bohemia. Polixenes opposes the match of a prince and a shepherdess, and the couple, pursued by the king, flees to Sicilia. There Perdita's identity is revealed, the couple becomes engaged, and Polixenes is reconciled with his old friend in 5.3, the play's final scene.

Polixenes is a rather colourless victim in 1.2—though his perspicacity in reading the situation contrasts sharply with Leontes' obtuseness—and he is mostly an observer in 5.3. In Act 4 he is more prominent, even though his role is a stereotype of the status-conscious adult who opposes young love. He is charmed by Perdita at the shepherds' festival, but after he removes his disguise, he threatens her with 'a death as cruel for thee / As thou art tender to 't' (4.4.441–442). Thus, in the romantic COMEDY of the play's second half, Polixenes takes the role of villain that Leontes had in the TRAGEDY of the first half.

Pollard, Alfred William (1859–1944) British scholar, a founder of modern textual criticism. Pollard's major contributions to Shakespearean scholarship were his *Shakespeare's Folio's and Quartos 1594–1685* (1909), a groundbreaking consideration of the various texts of the plays, and *Shakespeare's Fight with the Pirates* (1917), a study of the illicit publication of play texts in Shakespeare's time. He helped establish that Shakespeare was a collaborator on SIR THOMAS MORE. He was also a major authority on Geoffrey CHAUCER.

Polonius Character in *Hamlet,* a minister of the KING (5) of DENMARK. Polonius, the father of OPHELIA and LAERTES, loves intrigue and resorts to espionage whenever possible. He volunteers to spy for the King on HAMLET's conversation with his mother, the QUEEN (9), in 3.4, and when Hamlet discovers the intruder, he kills him. The prince stabs through a curtain, so he does not know who his victim is until he is dead, but he feels no remorse for the deed, remarking coolly that his victim has learned that 'to be too busy is some

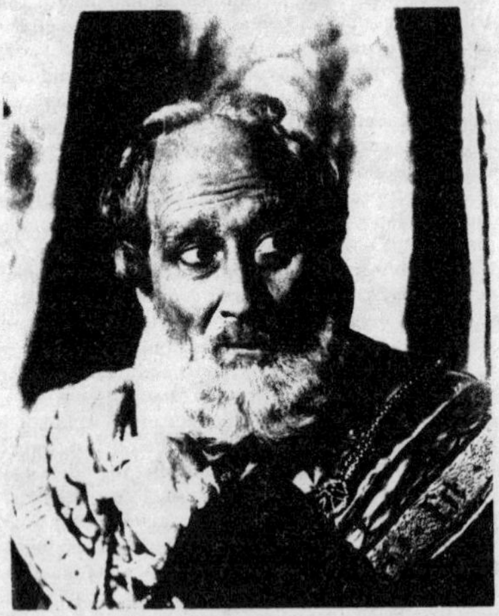

In Hamlet, *Polonius is a pedantic bore and an hypocrite. These traits may derive from the comical Pantaloon of the Italian commedia dell'arte.* (Courtesy of Culver Pictures, Inc.)

danger' (3.4.33). This killing is the central event of the play, hastening Hamlet's exile to England and triggering Laertes' vengeance on the prince.

Polonius' deviousness and dishonesty exemplify the state of moral decay in Denmark. After he offers Laertes his famous advice, 'to thine own self be true . . . Thou canst not then be false to any man' (1.3.78–80), his hypocrisy reveals itself, for in 2.1 he sets a spy on Laertes, offering detailed instructions in espionage and duplicity to REYNALDO (1). He bars Ophelia from any contact with Hamlet, presuming that the prince's professions of love cannot be truthful, perhaps arguing from self-knowledge, and when it appears that he was wrong and that the prince has gone mad from frustrated love, he spies on the lovers himself.

However, Polonius' murder is not to be taken as justifiable; much of its point depends on our recognition of it as an evil act, leading us to the further awareness that Hamlet is capable of evil. Also, Polonius is not completely without good points, making his killing more reprehensible than it would appear if he were an absolute villain. For example, while his means are deplorable, Polonius clearly cares about his son, and his involvement in his welfare serves to cause Laertes to remain memorable through his long absence from the play (between 1.3 and 4.5); similarly, Polonius is a fool in his handling of Ophelia, but there is no doubt of his paternal concern, even if it can be overlaid with ulterior interests at the same time. Ophelia's evident heartbreak at his death in her 'mad scene' (4.5) testifies to his adequacy as a parent.

Polonius is also a comic character at times. Speaking to the King and Queen of Hamlet's alleged madness, he begins by stating an ideal that he proceeds to demolish, asserting '. . . since brevity is the soul of wit, / And tediousness the limbs and outward flourishes, / I will be brief', and then goes on to use such verbiage as 'Mad call I it, for to define true madness, / What is't but to be nothing else but mad?' (2.2.93–94). When this amusing long-windedness is challenged by the Queen's request for 'More matter with less art', Polonius replies with unwitting candour, 'Madam, I swear I use no art at all' (2.2.95–96). The passage, in which Polonius repeatedly interrupts himself and loses his train of thought, parodies a popular tendency of the day to overelaborate rhetoric, and it softens the portrait of Hamlet's victim. In creating Polonius, Shakespeare may have been influenced by the Pantaloon, a comically windy moraliser from the Italian COMMEDIA DELL'ARTE.

Polonius appears as CORAMBIS in the Q1 edition of the play, and scholars believe that this reflects the name of the analogous character in Shakespeare's chief source, the UR-HAMLET. Shakespeare often changed the names in his sources for no particular reason, but here he may have wished to avoid using the caricature probably intended in the *Ur-Hamlet.* However, the name Polonius itself makes a clear reference to Poland, also known as Polonia in Elizabethan England. Scholars believe that the playwright probably intended an allusion to one of the play's minor sources, a well-known book on good government, *The Counsellor* (1598), an English translation from the Latin work of a Polish statesman, Laurentius GOSLICIUS.

Polydore In *Cymbeline,* the false name under which King CYMBELINE's son GUIDERIUS is raised from infancy by his kidnapper and foster-father BELARIUS.

Pomfret (Pontefract) Castle Strong fortress in northern England, the site of a number of political murders and executions in the 14th and 15th centuries, two of which are presented in Shakespeare's HISTORY PLAYS. RICHARD II is murdered in his cell by EXTON in 5.5 of *Richard II,* and lords RIVERS, GREY (2), and VAUGHAN are led to execution in 3.3 of *Richard III.* The historical Earl of SALISBURY (2) was also executed at Pomfret. Lord Rivers refers to the castle's bloody history when he exclaims, just before his death in *Richard III,* 'O Pomfret, Pomfret! O thou bloody prison, / Fatal and ominous to noble peers!' (3.3.9–10).

Pompey (1) Bum Character in *Measure for Measure,* a pimp and servant of MISTRESS (2) Overdone. Pompey

is a humorous petty criminal, a representative of the underworld of VIENNA, and the major figure in the comic SUB-PLOT, which contrasts with the main story and offers relief from its tensions. Tried as a procurer by ESCALUS (2), in 2.1, he outwits Constable ELBOW, who testifies for the prosecution, with long-winded evasions and subtle double entendres. He sassily asks the judge if he intends, through laws against prostitution, 'to geld and splay all the youth of the city' (2.1. 227–228). His bawdy wit makes a mockery of the court, helping to establish that the authority of the DUKE (9) has degenerated due to his lax regime. Pompey is eventually gaoled in the same prison as CLAUDIO (3), whose condemnation for illicit sex is at the centre of the main plot's conflict. As assistant to ABHORSON, the executioner—a position taken in return for a promise of parole—Pompey continues to jest, and his comedy lightens the oppressive atmosphere as Claudio's execution approaches.

As Escalus observes in 2.1.169, Pompey resembles Iniquity, a character from the medieval MORALITY PLAY. He represents a type that was well known, the clownish criminal (he is designated as a CLOWN [1] throughout the FOLIO text of the play). A comic subplot featuring a madam and her servant was found by Shakespeare in a principal source for *Measure for Measure*, George WHETSTONE's *Promos and Cassandra* (1578), and its appeal was surely immediate for the creator of FALSTAFF. Pompey's preposterous name was Shakespeare's invention: an ancient Roman hero, Pompey the Great (see POMPEY [2]), is provided with a surname that is slang for buttocks.

Pompey (2), (Sextus Pompeius) (d. 35 B.C.) Historical figure and character in *Antony and Cleopatra*, a rebel against the co-leaders of ROME, Octavius CAESAR (2), LEPIDUS, and Mark ANTONY. Pompey's threat spurs Antony to action when he is luxuriating with CLEOPATRA in Act 1, but the rebel displays his weakness in Act 2. In 2.6 he negotiates a truce with the Roman leaders, but the remarks of his follower MENAS make clear that he is foolish not to continue his rebellion while he is in a strong position. In 2.7 he refuses Menas' suggestion that he murder his opponents during the feast that celebrates the truce. Pompey is unwilling to seem dishonourable and lets the opportunity go by. Menas observes that 'Who seeks and will not take, when once 'tis offer'd, / Shall never find it more' (2.7.82–83), and decides to abandon his alliance with this weak leader. Pompey is not seen again in the play, but we hear of his fate. After being defeated by the forces of Lepidus and Caesar he retreats to Antony's territory where he is murdered, as is reported in 3.5. Pompey's career offers a case study in the cold realities of Roman politics and war. He cannot win because he is not unscrupulous enough and he lacks good sense. No vestiges of the ancient Roman concept of honour survive, and only a cool and unsentimental manipulator can triumph. It is in this context that we must weigh the conduct of Antony and the triumph of Caesar.

Antony surveys the rebel's strength in 1.2 and outlines Pompey's background. He is continuing a rebellion originated by his father—a famous and popular leader of an earlier generation—and he therefore commands a dedicated following. This is an accurate assessment of the historical Pompeius Sextus, whose father, Pompey the Great (106–48 B.C.), was one of the major figures of early Roman history. He was the defeated opponent of Julius CAESAR (1), as is mentioned several times in Shakespeare's *Julius Caesar.* The renown of Pompey the Great was such that Shakespeare could mention him in three non-Roman plays *(Henry V, 2 Henry VI, Love's Labour's Lost)* and name a comic character after him in *Measure for Measure* (see POMPEY (1) Bum), which presumes that audiences would still know of him after 1,700 years. Pompeius Sextus fought with his father's forces, and after their defeat—and Pompey the Great's murder—in 48 B.C., he reorganised the rebellion around a naval force, which he centred first in Spain and later in Sicily. After Julius Caesar's assassination in 44 B.C., Pompey continued to fight against Caesar's successors, though as part of his policy he briefly supported Antony against Octavius Caesar not long before the period of the play. The peace of Misenum, enacted in 2.6, was negotiated in 39 B.C. but did not last long. Caesar attacked Pompey the next year and totally defeated him in 36 B.C. The loser retreated to Asia Minor and attempted to reestablish himself but was captured and killed by Antony's lieutenant, probably on Antony's orders, though Shakespeare protects his hero's honour by having EROS report his distress at the execution, in 3.5.18–19.

Pope (1), Alexander (1688–1744) British poet and editor of Shakespeare. Best known as a poet, Pope also produced the second scholarly edition of Shakespeare's plays in 1725. He is regarded by modern scholars as a bad editor, however. He claimed to have corrected, by following QUARTO texts, many instances in which the playwright's words had been corrupted by the FOLIO editors; in fact, he mostly followed the 1709 edition of Nicholas ROWE (based on the Fourth Folio), though he did make numerous 'improvements' in his own words. Lewis THEOBALD, the first great Shakespearean scholar, pointed out many of Pope's errors in a 1726 essay, for which he was pilloried in Pope's famous literary satire, *The Dunciad* (1728). Pope, however, did incorporate many readings from Theobald's critique when he reissued his own collection in 1728. Moreover, Pope is credited with some scholarly accomplishments: he first established firmly the locations of many scenes, and he corrected the rhythm of many lines that had been improperly

printed. He was also the first commentator to recognise that *The Troublesome Raigne of King John* was derived from Shakespeare's *King John* rather than the other way around.

A childhood disease left Pope a hunchback, and he was embittered by it, once describing his life as one long disease. His sharp wit and penchant for invective made him a close friend of the satirist Jonathan Swift (1667–1745), but his social relations tended to end in mutual hostility. His talent for recrimination against former friends earned him the epithet 'The Wicked Wasp of Twickenham' (where he lived). He was England's leading poet in the first half of the 18th century, with such works as *An Essay on Criticism* (1711), *The Rape of the Lock* (1712), translations of *The Iliad* and *The Odyssey* (1720, 1725), *Moral Essays* (1731–1735), and *An Essay on Man* (1732–1734).

Pope (2), Thomas (d. c. 1603) English actor, member of the CHAMBERLAIN'S MEN. Though he is one of the 26 men listed in the FIRST FOLIO as the 'Principal Actors' in Shakespeare's plays, it is not known what roles he played. They must have been comic parts, for he was a clown and acrobat. He toured DENMARK and Germany with William KEMPE and others in 1586–1587, and he was a member of STRANGE'S MEN beginning in about 1591. He was probably an original member of the Chamberlain's Men, with whom he remained until at least 1599, when he became an original partner in the GLOBE THEATRE. He was not part of the troupe when it became the KING'S MEN in 1603, having probably retired. He died in late 1603 or early 1604. As late as 1612 he was still described as a memorable actor.

Popilius Lena (active 44 B.C.) Historical figure and minor character in *Julius Caesar*, a senator of ROME. Popilius Lena, present as the assassins prepare to kill CAESAR (1) at the Senate, alarms CASSIUS by conversationally hoping his 'enterprise to-day may thrive' (3.1.13) and then speaking to Caesar; Cassius fears the plot is known. However, it proves a false alarm. The episode, which Shakespeare took from PLUTARCH's *Lives*, heightens the tensions of the moment. Little is known of the historical Lena.

Porcupine (Porpentine) Name of a house, one of three on stage, in *The Comedy of Errors*. The Porcupine, which may be distinguished in a stage set by a sign above its door, is the home of the COURTESAN. The other houses that comprise the setting are the PHOENIX and the PRIORY. This arrangement of three structures, each with an entrance onto the stage, was a standard device of ancient Roman stage design as it was understood in Shakespeare's time, and it is quite appropriate to this play, which, of all Shakespeare's works, most closely resembles Roman drama. It has been speculated that Shakespeare called the Courtesan's house 'Porcupine' ('Porpentine' in Elizabethen English) after a well-known London brothel in an inn of that name.

Porpentine See PORCUPINE.

Porter (1) Minor character in *1 Henry VI*, a servant of the COUNTESS (1) of AUVERGNE who assists in her attempt to capture TALBOT in 2.3.

Porter (2) Minor character in *2 Henry IV*, gatekeeper at WARKWORTH CASTLE, home of the Earl of NORTHUMBERLAND (1). The Porter admits Lord BARDOLPH (2) in 1.1. At the outset of the play, he embodies ordinary lives amid the doings of the aristocracy, an important aspect of the play.

Porter (3) Minor character in *Macbeth*, a doorkeeper at the castle of MACBETH. In 2.3, immediately following Macbeth's murder of King DUNCAN, the Porter appears in response to a knocking at the gate. His humorous drunkenness contrasts strikingly with the grim murder scene, and thus he reinforces the suspenseful horror that we have just been exposed to. Also, in his drunkenness the Porter pretends to be the gatekeeper of hell, and this motif emphasises the fact that Macbeth has just lost his soul.

Shakespeare's original audiences will have recognised immediately that the Porter was imitating a familiar figure of the medieval MORALITY PLAY; the gatekeeper of hell who admits Christ to Limbo in the ancient legend of the 'Harrowing of Hell'. This gatekeeper guarded the literal mouth of hell—a familiar image from the painted backdrops of a gigantic, flaming lion's mouth (derived from Rev. xiii:2) used in the morality plays. The Porter makes it clear that we are to see Macbeth's castle as hell, and leaves no doubt whatever that the enormity of Macbeth's evil is of the greatest importance in the play. When the Porter finally opens the door and admits MACDUFF, a subtle analogy between Macduff and Christ is suggested. This foreshadows Macduff's role as the final conqueror of the evil Macbeth.

The Porter also provides comic relief. His humour is both topical, with references to a contemporary treason trial (see GARNET)—a resonant theme in a play of regicide—and simply vulgar, as in his remarks on the effects of drink, in 2.3.27–35. This vulgarity inspired high-minded commentators such as Alexander POPE [1] and Samuel Taylor COLERIDGE to declare the Porter a non-Shakespearean addition, on the grounds that a genius of literature would not stoop to such low comedy. However, modern critics recognise that the Porter is a typically humorous Shakespearean representation of unsophisticated humanity. With his comedy and his simple mind that nevertheless offers im-

portant commentary on the situation, the Porter is the nearest thing to a FOOL (1) in *Macbeth*. Also, like the OLD MAN (3) of 2.4, he serves the function of a CHORUS (1), and offers a point of view entirely outside that of all the other characters.

Porter (4) Minor character in *Henry VIII*, a doorman at a royal palace in LONDON. In 5.3, on the day when Princess ELIZABETH (1) is to be christened, the Porter and his MAN (3) are unable to prevent a crowd of celebrating commoners from invading the palace courtyard. They make comical remarks about the riotous celebrants, until the Lord CHAMBERLAIN (2) announces the arrival of the royal party, and they return to their efforts to control the crowd. The incident demonstrates the enthusiasm of the common people for Elizabeth and the TUDOR DYNASTY, an important theme of the play, and it offers comic relief that separates the intrigue of 5.1–2 from the grand ceremony of 5.4, with which the play closes.

Porter (5), Henry (d. 1599) English dramatist. Porter wrote at least six plays for Philip HENSLOWE and the ADMIRAL'S MEN, some of them in collaboration with Henry CHETTLE and Ben JONSON. He was praised by Francis MERES as among the best English writers of COMEDY. Only one play written solely by Porter has survived: *The Two Angry Women of Abingdon* (c. 1596), a comedy that resembles *The Merry Wives of Windsor*. Though greatly inferior, it was very popular in its day, and it may have stimulated Shakespeare's interest in writing a busy comedy of town life. Porter was perennially poor, and he died deep in debt. He was stabbed to death in a fight by fellow playwright John DAY.

Portia (1) Character in *The Merchant of Venice*, lover of BASSANIO and defender of his friend ANTONIO (2). Portia, disguised as a lawyer, saves Antonio from the revenge of SHYLOCK. Initially a passive young woman at the mercy of her father's odd matchmaking device, the lottery of caskets, she emerges as a touching lover with Bassanio in 3.2 and achieves a grand maturity when she defends Antonio in 4.1. Her address to Shylock on the virtues of mercy (4.1.180–198) is renowned as one of the finest passages Shakespeare wrote; it is certainly his most effective presentation of Christian ideals. Her tactics in the trial—leading Shylock to believe he can win his case and thus eliciting from him his demands for the strictest interpretation of the law—have been deplored as high-handed, and they are certainly unethical by modern standards. But Shakespeare was composing an allegory, not a legal precedent, and Portia's strategy emphasises the instructive paradox that Shylock's rigid insistence on the letter of the law proves to be his own undoing. Portia, defending Antonio because he is the friend of her beloved, evidences the power of love itself, conquering Shylock, whose calculating usury is opposed to the generosity of the young lovers and Antonio.

Portia's final act—accepting, in the person of the young lawyer 'Balthasar', her own ring from Bassanio and then twitting him with disloyalty—has been seen as arbitrary and graceless, but the episode fittingly closes the play. It recapitulates the play's lesson that love and forgiveness are superior to self-centred greed. By invoking Shylock's attitude, insisting on the letter of Bassanio's oath, Portia reasserts a negative value that she immediately repudiates when she forgives her new husband, and the play closes on a note of loving reconciliation.

Before she appears, Portia is described by Bassanio in extravagantly poetic terms (1.1.161–172), and we envision her as an almost supernatural ideal of womanhood. However, with her opening line, '. . . my little body is aweary of this great world' (1.2.1–2), she instantly becomes human. Her simultaneously grand and companionable nature charms us throughout the play. She is an open young woman who can describe herself as 'an unlessoned girl, unschooled, unpractised' (3.2.159) and who can giggle with NERISSA over the disguises they will wear (3.4) and over the trick they will play on their husbands-to-be (4.2). At the same time, she inspires Bassanio's rhapsody and, most important, she is a resourceful and commanding figure who takes Antonio's fate in hand and delivers him. Shakespeare thus enshrines in virginal youth a gallant, courageous, and worldly woman.

However, Portia has an unattractive feature, to modern sensibilities: she clearly partakes of the 16th-century English racial prejudice and anti-Semitism that are reflected in this play. Addressing Shylock in court, in 4.1, she repeatedly calls him 'Jew', and she is frank about her distaste for MOROCCO's black complexion in 1.2.123–125 and 2.7.79. On the other hand, she is willing to marry the African prince if he wins the lottery of caskets, as she declares in 2.1.13–22, and her attitude towards Shylock's Jewishness—manifested only in the trial scene—is extremely mild, compared to that of other characters. *The Merchant of Venice* accommodates the prejudices of its original audiences, but Portia is not a significant bearer of this theme, and we are in no doubt that Shakespeare intended her as a delightful heroine.

Portia is a fine example of the frank and fearless young women who appear in many of the plays; like ROSALINE (1), BEATRICE, ROSALIND, and HELENA (2), she seems to embody an ideal of femininity that the playwright held and put forth often. Spirited and capable, she is willing to enter a man's world—in this case, that of the law—in pursuit of her aims, yet she ultimately accepts the conventional Elizabethan woman's status, that of a wife, at least theoretically subservient to her husband.

Portia (2) Historical figure and character in *Julius Caesar,* the wife of BRUTUS (4). In 2.1, observing her husband's great emotional distress, Portia insists on sharing his trouble. He has in fact been agonising over the assassination of CAESAR (1), and he is reluctant to reveal this grave plan. She insists that her stature as the wife of a great Roman and the daughter of another warrants her inclusion in matters of importance. She shows Brutus a wound in her thigh that she has given herself to demonstrate that she has the Roman virtue of self-control. He is impressed, saying, 'O ye gods, render me worthy of this noble wife!' (2.1.302–303), and he agrees to take her into his confidence, but then they are interrupted.

Although we do not see him tell her of the conspiracy against Caesar, he evidently has done so by the time she reappears in 2.4, where she is almost hysterical with concern. In both scenes Portia's concern for her husband's welfare is strong, giving the audience another positive viewpoint of Brutus, and her distress also raises the emotional pitch of the play as the first great climax, Caesar's murder, approaches.

In 4.3 we learn that Portia, in Rome as her husband campaigns against Caesar's successors, ANTONY and OCTAVIUS, has committed suicide, convinced that he cannot survive against the tremendous power that she knows has been sent against him. Portia is intended to exemplify the Roman virtues of courage and self-sacrifice. Her virtues were legendary by Shakespeare's time; he also used the name for the splendid heroine of *The Merchant of Venice,* PORTIA (1). There, her suitor alludes to her namesake, asserting that his love is 'nothing undervalu'd to Cato's daughter, Brutus' Portia'. (*Merchant,* 1.1.165–166).

The historical Portia was the daughter of Marcus Porcius Cato (95–46 B.C.), a tribune famous for his honesty and dedication; the CATO of the play is Portia's brother. Their father had opposed Caesar in an earlier civil war, committing suicide rather than be captured, only two years before the time of the play. Her own suicide was regarded as similarly honourable. In the play she is said to have 'swallow'd fire' (4.3.155). This reference follows Shakespeare's source, PLUTARCH's life of Brutus, where Portia is said to have put hot coals in her mouth and kept her mouth closed until she choked to death. This seems improbable, and scholars have speculated that this report may reflect her actual death by carbon monoxide poisoning, produced by a smoky charcoal fire in a closed room.

Portraits of Shakespeare Only two depictions of Shakespeare—both posthumous—are believed to have been based on genuine portraits: the DROESHOUT engraving, which illustrates the title-page of the FIRST FOLIO, and the sculptural bust by Gheerart JANSSEN (2) that is part of the poet's memorial in Holy Trinity Church, in STRATFORD. However, numerous other images have been thought of as portraits of Shakespeare, though modern scholars generally reject them. The most significant of these is probably the CHANDOS PORTRAIT, which was accepted as genuine for many years; it was the basis for the sculpture by Peter SCHEEMAKERS in WESTMINSTER (1) ABBEY. Other portraits of note include the ELY PALACE PORTRAIT, the FLOWER PORTRAIT, the KESSELSTADT DEATH MASK, and works by Nicholas HILLIARD and Cornelis JANSSEN (1).

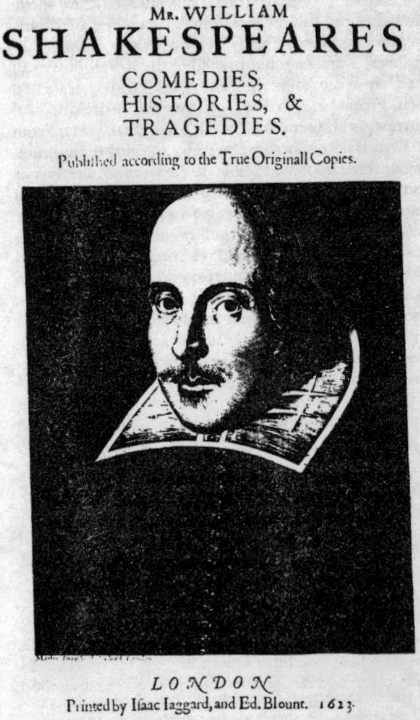
MR. WILLIAM
SHAKESPEARES
COMEDIES,
HISTORIES, &
TRAGEDIES.
Published according to the True Originall Copies.

LONDON
Printed by Isaac Iaggard, and Ed. Blount. 1623.

The title page of the First Folio has on it what is probably a reliable likeness of Shakespeare, an engraving by Martin Droeshout.

Pory, John (1572–1636) English writer, the translator of the work of LEO AFRICANUS, a possible influence on *Othello.* Pory was an associate of Richard HAKLUYT, who suggested he translate Leo's Italian account of his African travels. The translation was published as *A Geographical History of Africa* (1600), and Pory's prefatory biography of Leo probably influenced OTHELLO's autobiographical remarks in 1.3.

Pory also produced a version of a famous early atlas,

The Epitome of Ortelius (1602), but until 1612 he made his living publishing newsletters, accounts of Parliamentary and court events that he sent to private subscribers, a practise that preceded the development of modern newspapers. He was a very widely travelled man. From 1612 to 1617 he travelled in Ireland and Europe as a agent for Sir George CAREW (1); from 1617 to 1619 he was employed by an English diplomat in Constantinople; and in 1619 he went to Virginia as secretary to the governor. Pory was on the governing council of the colony and served as the speaker of the initial session of the Burgesses, the first legislative assembly in the New World. He returned to England in 1623—after being shipwrecked and imprisoned in the Azores—and resumed his newsletter business, retiring a few years before his death.

Post (1) Minor character in *2 Henry VI,* a messenger who brings word of an Irish rebellion in 3.1.

Post (2) Either of two minor characters in *3 Henry VI,* express messengers. One Post carries messages between King EDWARD IV and the French court in 3.3, and returns with answers in 4.1. The replies are quite venomous, and the Post asks assurance that he will not be punished for the contents of his report. In 4.6 another Post carries word to Warwick of Edward's escape from captivity.

Posthumus Character in *Cymbeline,* the husband of IMOGEN. Banished from Britain for secretly marrying the daughter of King CYMBELINE, Posthumus goes to ROME. There, he boasts of Imogen's virtues and wagers the diamond ring she has given him that the courtier IACHIMO cannot seduce her. Iachimo is unsuccessful, but he deceives Posthumus, who foolishly believes him and vows revenge on Imogen. By letter, he instructs his servant, PISANIO, to murder her. Once he has established the situation that faces Imogen in Acts 3–4, Posthumus disappears from the play until, near the end, he reappears, stricken with guilt over the murder he believes has been committed. He seeks death in battle and fights for Britain against ROME, but he is not killed. He then seeks death as a Roman prisoner of war, but while in captivity he dreams of his family (see SICILIUS LEONATUS) and the god JUPITER, who promises that his story shall end happily. Unaware of this when he awakes, Posthumus appears before the king as a Roman captive, but he reveals himself when Iachimo confesses his deception. Posthumus, in his turn, confesses to Imogen's murder before he discovers that she is alive and he is reunited with her. In the aura of reconciliation that closes the play, the king accepts Posthumus as a son-in-law.

In the course of the play, Posthumus' qualities vary enormously from the ideal to the seriously flawed. In this respect he offers clues to the difficulties Shakespeare faced when he wrote the ROMANCES, a new genre of plays in which *Cymbeline* was an experiment. The playwright faced the problem of integrating realistic settings and characters, which he was accustomed to creating, with the ethereal, almost abstract characters of fairy tale and traditional romantic literature on which the romances were based. Posthumus, like other characters in *Cymbeline,* demonstrates that he was not always successful.

As the play opens, Posthumus is praised by a GENTLEMAN (12) who declares, 'I do not think / so fair an outward, and such stuff within / Endows a man, but he' (1.1.22–24); here, he is simply a traditional romantic prince and a proper mate for Imogen. However, once on his own in Rome he is ludicrously immature, intent on an inflated idea of masculine honour. In 1.5, he, Iachimo, and the FRENCHMAN almost seem to offer a satire on duelling. His wholly unnecessary defence of Imogen's chastity is no less ridiculous than his readiness to disbelieve in it later, and his response is ignoble when he instructs his servant to murder Imogen in revenge. Nevertheless, he is once again the traditional princely hero when he helps the king's long-lost sons, GUIDERIUS and ARVIRAGUS, defeat the Romans, and it is certainly to his credit that he comes to regret his earlier actions and feel guilt. However, the basic problem with his character is most evident here. His elaborate attempts at suicide detract from our appreciation of his real personal distress. On one hand, it is difficult to accept Posthumus as a real figure like the victimised OTHELLO, while on the other, he does not provide a bold allegorical representation of human error, like, say, LEONTES, of *The Winter's Tale.* Shakespeare had not yet learned to permit the symbolic to dominate, and Posthumus' human reality interferes with his value as an archetype of jealousy. This makes him a somewhat ridiculous and unsympathetic figure.

The name Posthumus indicates that its owner was born after his father's death. It is so rare today that it seems intended to convey some extra meaning, perhaps comical. However, though unusual (like the phenomenon it commemorates), the name was regularly given in Shakespeare's day (see, e.g., Thomas Posthumous HOBY [2]).

Potpan Character in *Romeo and Juliet.* See SERVINGMAN (2).

Prentice Either of two minor characters in *2 Henry VI,* apprentices and friends of the armourer's apprentice PETER (1), who must fight his master, Thomas HORNER, in a trial by combat. The Prentices encourage Peter before the event, in 2.3.

Preston, Thomas (1537–1598) Sixteenth-century playwright parodied by Shakespeare. Preston's play *Cambyses* (1569), whose full title described it as 'A la-

mentable Tragedie, mixed full of pleasant mirth . . .', is mocked in the comical presentation of PYRAMUS AND THISBE in *A Midsummer Night's Dream* (1.2.11–12, 5.1) and by FALSTAFF in *1 Henry IV* (2.4.382–389). *Cambyses*, though highly bombastic and melodramatic, represents a significant development from the MORALITY PLAY towards TRAGEDY. Preston was primarily an educator; he served as vice-chancellor of Cambridge University.

Priam, King of Troy Legendary figure and character in *Troilus and Cressida*, the ruler of the city besieged by the Greeks in the TROJAN WAR. Despite his regal position, Priam plays an insignificant role, calling to order the war council in 2.2—but participating very little—and unsuccessfully attempting, along with ANDROMACHE and CASSANDRA, to persuade HECTOR not to fight on a day of disastrous omens in 5.3.

Priam was a well-known figure in classical mythology and is referred to in a number of Shakespeare's plays and in *The Rape of Lucrece*. His name was proverbial for someone who has experienced extremes of good and bad fortune. In the *Iliad* of HOMER, Priam is an old man, the father of 50 sons by various wives and concubines. His harem, along with his non-Greek name, suggests to scholars that he represents a folk-memory of some real Asiatic monarch of the second millennium B.C. His death at the hands of Neoptolemus (see PYRRHUS) is the most important incident of his life, both in Homer and in later literature. It is described in the dramatic monologue recited by the FIRST PLAYER (2) in 2.2.464–493 of *Hamlet*.

Priest (1) Minor character in *Richard III*, a friend of Lord HASTINGS (3). Hastings engages in small talk with the Priest in 3.2, demonstrating his naïve lack of concern about the danger from Richard that he has been warned about.

Priest (2) Minor character in *Twelfth Night*, a clergyman. The Priest speaks only once, in 5.1.154–161, to confirm that he has married OLIVIA and SEBASTIAN (2)—whom he and the bride have both mistaken for Cesario, the disguised VIOLA—thereby adding further confusion. At the same time, he provides comic relief from the intensifying crisis, for he is preposterously high-flown, using the most elaborate possible language to say a very simple thing; for instance, he observes, 'Since [the marriage], my watch hath told me, towards my grave / I have travell'd but two hours' (5.1.160–161).

Priest (3) Minor character in *Hamlet*, the officiating clergyman at OPHELIA's funeral. In 5.1 the Priest denies Ophelia the full ceremony because her death appears to have been a suicide. He asserts that even an abbreviated service is too much—only 'great command' (5.1.221), presumably KING (5) Claudius', has made it possible—and suggests that, instead of prayers, 'shards, flints, and pebbles should be thrown on her' (5.1.224). He insists that the rites for the dead would be profaned if Ophelia received them. This ugly episode heralds the mood of gloom and anger that dominates the conclusion of the play.

In some editions of the play the Priest is called the Doctor of Divinity, based on the speech heading 'Doct.', used for both of his speeches in the Q2 edition (1604). Some scholars conjecture that this makes him a Protestant.

Prince (1) Escalus of Verona Character in *Romeo and Juliet*, the ruler of VERONA, where the play is set. The Prince is a representative of civil order, an important ideal for Shakespeare. The Prince appears three times in the play. First, in 1.1, he describes the feud between MONTAGUE (1) and CAPULET (1). In 3.1 he banishes Romeo and precipitates the climax of the tragedy; rather too late, he states a principle of statecraft that has been too little observed in Verona: 'Mercy but murders, pardoning those that kill' (3.1.199). At the close he summarises the fateful resolution of the feud, accepting blame 'for winking at . . . discords' (5.3.293). This acknowledgement of the state's responsibility for order was not present in Shakespeare's sources; it reflects the playwright's interest in the civic as well as the purely personal ramifications of tragedy. This theme recurs throughout Shakespeare's work in dramas ranging from *Richard II* to *King Lear* to *The Tempest*.

In the stage direction that introduces him at 1.1.79, and nowhere else, the Prince is given a name, Escalus. This is a Latinisation of Della Scala, the name of the princely family that ruled Verona in the late Middle Ages.

Prince (2) HAL (also Henry, later King Henry V) Character in *1* and *2 Henry IV*. See PRINCE (6) OF WALES, HENRY.

Prince (3) Henry Character in *King John*. See HENRY (1).

Prince (4) of Wales, Edward (1453–1471) Historical figure and character in *3 Henry VI*, the heir apparent to King HENRY VI. The young Prince Edward, son of Henry and Queen MARGARET (1), has inherited his mother's bold and courageous spirit, and, unlike his father, strongly opposes the efforts of YORK (8) and his sons to seize the throne. He reproaches his father for his weakness on several occasions, and he presents a consistently fiery front to the usurpers; in consequence, he is stabbed to death by Edward and the other York sons after being taken prisoner in the battle of TEWKESBURY in 5.5. The young Prince is a model of chivalry and thus rather dull, but he is intended as

a symbolic figure, rather than a developed personality. He serves as a foil for his father's more complex and human weakness, and, further, as a suggestion of what might have been—an instance of the rigour and pride kingship demands. Shakespeare saw its absence in Henry VI as having been tragic for England. The GHOST (1) of the young Prince appears in *Richard III.*

The murder of the captive Prince was part of the Tudor version of the WARS OF THE ROSES, but it is apparently fictitious. Shakespeare took it from his chief source, Edward HALL (2) but according to earlier accounts, he was killed in the battle, a much more likely end.

Prince (5) of Wales, Edward (Edward V, King of England) (1470–c. 1483) Historical figure and character in *Richard III,* the son and heir of King EDWARD IV whom RICHARD III murders. The Prince appears only once, when he arrives in London after his father's death. Although technically king, he is never crowned and is known as the Prince throughout the play. Being taken to the TOWER OF LONDON and his eventual death, the Prince, 12 years old, impresses us with his serious concern for history. He also provides an ironic commentary on the way the story of his own death has been transmitted, officially unrecorded but nonetheless known. 'But say, my lord, it were not register'd / Methinks the truth should live from age to age . . .' (3.1.75–76). The murder—at Richard's instigation—of the Prince and his younger brother, the Duke of YORK (7), is reported in 4.3 and mourned thereafter. It is clearly intended to be taken as the most heinous of Richard's crimes.

Shakespeare had no doubt as to Richard's guilt, and posterity, greatly influenced by Shakespeare, has agreed. Modern scholarship, however, has thrown doubt on the whole question of the fate of the princes. It is known that they entered the Tower in June 1483 and never emerged, but how they died and who was responsible are not clear (see TYRELL) and may never be, except in the unlikely event that new evidence is uncovered.

In *3 Henry VI* the Prince appears in the final scene as an infant, virtually a stage property, to be displayed by his father. The baby is kissed by his uncles, as a token of loyalty to King Edward. This incident is noteworthy for the behaviour of Richard, who characterises himself in an aside as comparable to Judas, in kissing one to whom he intends harm.

Prince (6) of Wales, Henry (Hal, later King HENRY V) (1387–1422) Historical figure and character in *1* and *2 Henry IV,* the oldest son of King HENRY IV. The central concern of the *Henry IV* plays is Prince Hal's preparation for assuming the throne. (He appears as the king in Act 5 of *2 Henry IV* and in *Henry V.*) The Prince must find his way between two undesirable extremes—anarchy and obsessiveness—represented respectively by the irresponsible debauchery of FALSTAFF and the exaggerated sense of honour of the war-loving HOTSPUR. In neither play is the Prince the most prominent character, but Hotspur in *Part 1* and Falstaff in both plays derive their importance from their relationship to the Prince. In *Part 1* the Prince becomes a chivalric hero by conquering Hotspur, though he remains friendly with Falstaff. In *Part 2* he integrates himself more fully into the world of statecraft, assumes the crown upon his father's death, and makes the final, irrevocable break with Falstaff in his famous 'rejection' speech in 5.5.

The comparison of Hal and Hotspur is foreshadowed in *Richard II,* when Hotspur, then known as PERCY (2), tells of Hal's disreputable life among harlots in London (5.3.13–19). In *1 Henry IV* the dissolute Prince is contrasted with the valorous Hotspur. However, Hal assures Henry that 'the time will come' (3.2.144) when he will conquer Hotspur. Significantly, the Prince does not have to change his character to arrive at this resolution, for he is conscious of his destiny from the outset. As he makes clear in his famous 'reformation' speech (1.2.190–212), he intends to fulfil his inherited duties. He simply chooses to remain in EASTCHEAP until 'being wanted he may be more wonder'd at' (1.2.196). Once Hal has asserted his readiness to assume his proper position as Prince when the time comes—and of course, Shakespeare and his original audiences were very much aware of Hal's future success as Henry V—the ground is laid for the climactic hand-to-hand combat in which the Prince kills Hotspur.

Shakespeare took care to have Hal spurn some of the temptations offered by Falstaff, as when he rejects the old man's lascivious suggestions about a barmaid in 1.2.46. The playwright thus establishes that the Prince is not the reckless and vicious playboy of the well-known farce *The Famous Victories of Henry the Fifth* (see FAMOUS VICTORIES), but rather a good king in the making.

The essential question of the *Henry IV* plays is: can a ruler successfully combine cold-blooded political skills with the spiritual values that derive from social contacts and appreciation of one's fellows. Hal's development take place in the irresponsible world of Eastcheap because the Machiavellian world of King Henry cannot nurture humane values. At the BOAR'S HEAD TAVERN, however, Prince Hal learns about the lives of ordinary people, and he knows that this education has a purpose. 'When I am King of England, I shall command all the good lads in Eastcheap', he says in 2.4.13–14). At the same time, the Prince is learning about himself as well. He places himself in different contexts: highway robbery, in 2.2 of *Part 1,* and menial service in 2.4 of both plays. In the mock drama he enacts with Falstaff in 2.4 of *Part I,* he even samples

the role of king. In Eastcheap the Prince is free to make mistakes, to take positions he will later reject—in short, to learn.

In *Part 1*, although Hal plans to forsake Eastcheap life at some point, he still participates fully in it. He rejects duty in favour of pleasure, sending Falstaff to dispose of the king's messenger, and when the rebellion against his father is introduced, he boldly suggests, in the callous manner of a soldier, that a campaign brings the opportunity to 'buy maidenheads . . . by the hundreds' (2.4.358–359). His merriment in the same scene includes a disrespectful charade of his father. While he does go to SHREWSBURY and defeats Hotspur, the battle seems to be only an interval in his life with Falstaff. At the end of the fighting, he is ready to corroborate Falstaff's lie about his courage 'with the happiest terms I have' (5.4.156).

However, as his kingship draws closer, the Prince avoids Falstaff. In *Part 2* Hal returns to Eastcheap only once. The Prince arrives in London from the battlefield in 2.2, and the uproarious tavern scene (2.4) closes with his being called back to action. Falstaff's world is now an interlude for the Prince, rather than a primary focus. Moreover, his exchange with Falstaff is more hostile than friendly; he does not accept Falstaff's bantering excuses, as he has in the past, and Hal departs with only a cool 'Good night, Falstaff.' Therefore, when, as Henry V, Hal coldly spurns Falstaff in 5.5, we have no reason to be surprised.

Prince Hal's rejection of Falstaff is often considered callous and unfair, but in its historical context it may be seen as both necessary and relatively mild. Falstaff's behaviour is downright criminal in both plays—in fact, the scenes dealing with his corrupt recruitment of troops (*1 Henry IV*, 4.2; *2 Henry IV*, 3.2) were designed as incriminating satires of contemporary practises—yet Hal merely dismisses him with a pension. (The imprisonment imposed by the CHIEF JUSTICE—to an institution reserved for aristocrats—was understood by the playwright and his audience to be lenient and temporary.) While Hal can be thought to be rejecting part of his humanity in order to make himself fit for power, he is in fact simply adopting a different humanity, that of his weary father. In *Henry V* the new king will apply the capacity for fellowship he has learned in Eastcheap; first, in *2 Henry IV*, he becomes a king.

The crucial moment of Hal's development, and the climax of *2 Henry IV*, is Hal's encounter with his dying father in 4.5. Addressing the crown as it lies beside the king, Hal recognises the burden that kingship demands and he accepts that burden, emphasising his decision by placing the crown on his own head. Henry, thinking that Hal has selfishly desired his death in order to wear the crown, delivers an impassioned speech on the dangers England will face once his son is king, crying, 'The wild dog shall flesh his tooth on every innocent' (4.5.131–132) and regretting the collapse of the order he has striven to preserve. This speech asserts powerfully, if negatively, the value of social discipline. After Hal has sworn loyalty to his father—and, implicitly, to the values just expressed—the king advises that Hal keep would-be opponents busy with overseas wars. This militarist solution—honourable in Shakespeare's world, though reprehensible in our own—is related to Henry's view of a ruler's basic duty, the maintenance of order and the avoidance of civil war. The Prince accepts this lesson and receives his father's wishes for a peaceful reign and a final blessing (4.5.219).

Shakespeare altered Hal's biography to suit his dramatic ends. Hal is introduced as an adult at a time when he was only 12 years old, as part of the playwright's strategy of presenting him and Hotspur as contemporaries, though Hotspur was in fact a generation older. Also, Hal did not fight Hotspur at Shrewsbury; the rebel died at the hands of an anonymous warrior. Shakespeare may have believed that the two heroes had met—his sources are ambiguous—but he would surely have had them do so in his play, even if they had not historically done so, to enhance the play's impact.

Prince Hal's wild life was evidently real, for contemporaries recorded his conversion to good behaviour upon being crowned. It was reported that the Prince was given to drunken brawling—and even gang warfare—in Eastcheap. Shakespeare and his contemporaries believed in the truth of a tradition that Hal had hit the Chief Justice and been imprisoned for it, but since this story cannot be traced earlier than 1531 (to an account that omits physical assault), its authenticity is dubious. A more reliable early account stated that Hal had robbed his own agents on the highway; a later version changed the victims to bearers of the king's money. Shakespeare omitted a striking anecdote, well known to the Elizabethans, that is probably true: Hal, perhaps in a spirit of atonement, approached his father wearing a dog collar and a strange garment with many needles sewn to it. This mystifying story has never been explained, and Shakespeare may have simply found it too distracting to use. Hal's unwise wearing of his dying father's crown came from Shakespeare's sources, but it is quite plainly apocryphal.

In any event, reports of 'wild Prince Hal' probably reflect only isolated incidents, and not a committed way of life, in the youth of a privileged and high-spirited soldier. Certainly, much of the Prince's energy was devoted to serious military training, for he fought in Wales beginning in 1400, and he was considered competent at the age of 16 to command a wing of Henry's army at Shrewsbury. He governed part of Northumberland shortly thereafter, and he served in increasingly important offices over the next eight years. In 1411 Hal was dismissed from the king's council, an event that is alluded to in *1 Henry IV*, 3.2.

32, where it is associated with the supposed assault on the Chief Justice. In fact, it appears that King Henry suspected his son of treasonous disloyalty; a reconciliation was effected a year later, not long before Henry's death, and this appears to be the germ of the reconciliation scenes in the plays.

Prince Charles' Men Seventeenth-century LONDON theatrical company. Prince Charles' Men were organised in 1608 as a provincial company called the Duke of York's Men in honour of their patron, King JAMES I's younger son, later King Charles I (ruled 1625–1649). The company began staging plays at the royal court in London in 1610. Among their members were the dramatist William ROWLEY (2), who wrote most of their plays and directed the company, and Joseph TAYLOR, their leading actor. In 1612, when Charles' older brother HENRY (2) died, he became the heir-apparent and was known as the Prince of Wales; the company he patronised changed its name accordingly. Around 1614–1616 the company was briefly allied with LADY ELIZABETH'S MEN. They played at a variety of London playhouses as well as at the court. In 1619 Christopher BEESTON joined the company as its manager, and for several years they played regularly at his theatre, the Phoenix and then, after 1621, at the CURTAIN THEATRE. Taylor left for the KING'S MEN in 1619, and in 1623 Rowley followed him. The company dispersed when Prince Charles became king in 1625 and transferred his patronage to the King's Men.

Prince Henry's Men Seventeenth-century LONDON theatrical company, formerly the ADMIRAL'S MEN. In 1603, after King JAMES I succeeded to the crown of England, his son Prince HENRY (2) assumed patronage of the company, which changed its name accordingly. Their new royal patent lists the members of the company, including Edward ALLEYN—their long-time leader—Thomas DOWNTON, Humphrey JEFFES, and Samuel ROWLEY (1), who also wrote plays for the company. By 1606 Alleyn had retired, though he kept a financial interest in the company and was part owner of the FORTUNE THEATRE, where they appeared, so he probably retained some influence on the company's affairs. In November 1612 Prince Henry died, and his patronage was taken up by the German fiancé of Princess ELIZABETH (3), Frederick V the Elector Palatine. When the royal couple married in early 1613, the company formally took on one of Frederick's titles and was known as the PALSGRAVE'S MEN.

Princess (1) of France Character in *Love's Labour's Lost,* the head of an embassy from France to the court of the KING (19) of Navarre, who falls in love with her. When we first encounter the Princess, in 2.1, she reprimands her courtier, BOYET, for his flattery in sharp but sensible terms that immediately establish her as a straightforward woman. But, although we do have a sense of the Princess as a real person, her chief role in the play is as a participant in the courtly tableau of lovers that draws the King and his gentlemen to an awareness that their narrow world of asceticism is insufficient compared to the power of love.

In 5.2, when she learns of her father's death, the Princess prepares to leave Navarre immediately. She responds to the King's suit by requiring him to live as a hermit for a year to test the strength of his love. She recognises that the process of maturation that the gentlemen have undergone in the course of the play is not complete—a recognition that makes her the character who perhaps most clearly represents the play's point of view.

Princess (2) Katharine of France Character in *Henry V.* See KATHARINE (2).

Priory Name of a house, one of three on stage, in *The Comedy of Errors.* The Priory, which may be distinguished in a stage set by a cross or other sign above its door, is the religious house headed by EMILIA (1), its Abbess. ANTIPHOLUS and DROMIO OF SYRACUSE take refuge there early in 5.1. (Until well into the 17th century in England, a criminal or a defendant in a civil suit could take sanctuary from the law in a church or other sacred building.)

The other houses that comprise the setting are the PHOENIX and the PORCUPINE. This arrangement of three structures, each with an entrance onto the stage, was standard in ancient Roman stage design, as it was understood in Shakespeare's time, and it is quite appropriate to this play, which, of all Shakespeare's works, most closely resembles Roman drama.

Pritchard, Hannah (1711–1768) British actress. Pritchard began her career as a fairground singer and was recruited for the stage by Theophilus CIBBER (3). She went on to achieve fame playing with David GARRICK. She played many Shakespearean roles and was acclaimed for her comedic heroines—especially ROSALIND—which she continued to play well into middle age. She also played tragic roles, and her greatest fame came as LADY (6) MACBETH, which she played opposite Garrick for many years. After her death, he never played MACBETH again.

Problem Plays Three of Shakespeare's comedies—*All's Well That Ends Well, Measure for Measure,* and *Troilus and Cressida*—that are potent satires characterised by disturbingly ambiguous points of view and seemingly cynical attitudes towards sexual and social relations. The problem plays—all written around 1602–1604—are concerned with basic elements of life, sex, and death, and the psychological and social complications

they give rise to. These issues are problematic, and the plays further stress this by pointedly offering no clear-cut resolutions, leaving audiences with a painful awareness of life's difficulties.

Many people find the plays difficult to enjoy because of various other disturbing qualities. All three feature a number of unpleasant characters, villainous or misanthropic or both, such as THERSITES and PANDARUS of *Troilus and Cressida,* PAROLLES and BERTRAM of *All's Well That Ends Well,* and ANGELO (2) of *Measure for Measure.* They all end unsatisfactorily to most tastes, with a bleak and inconclusive dénouement for *Troilus and Cressida,* and with arbitrary and unconvincing 'solutions' imposed on the other two. Perhaps most dismaying to modern tastes, psychologically astute characterisations clash with extremely artificial plotting in a disjunction that seems to weaken both the realism and fantasy in all three plays.

The unpleasant aspects of the problem plays have led some commentators to suggest that they reflect some corresponding unpleasantness in Shakespeare's life, and that they were written by an embittered man who had recently undergone some psychological trauma the nature of which can only be guessed at. Lack of evidence has not inhibited speculation, and a romantic crisis such as that described in the SONNETS, the execution of the Earl of ESSEX (2), and the death of Shakespeare's father in 1601 have all been suggested as causes of the playwright's presumed unhappiness. However, most scholars believe that no such personal explanation is necessary. The problem plays are not so much sad as they are scathing; each is placed in a distinctive and highly stylised social milieu, and their plots do not present realistic personal situations. In all these respects it seems more likely that their peculiar nature was generated by dramatic considerations rather than personal ones. The period saw a strong fashion for social satire, led by the biting comedies of Ben JONSON, and the problem plays are clearly part of this trend in JACOBEAN DRAMA. Moreover, the accession of JAMES I in 1603 stimulated a lot of theorising about society that is reflected in the problem plays, especially *Measure for Measure.*

The origin of the term 'problem play' lends support to the view that the plays were conceived as public discourse rather than private lament. The phrase was first applied to these plays—plus the slightly earlier TRAGEDY, *Hamlet*—by the Shakespearean scholar Frederick S. BOAS in his book *Shakespeare and his Predecessors* (1896). He took the term from the contemporary theatre of his day. In the 1890s 'problem play' was a new expression coined to deal with a new sort of drama—for example, the work of Ibsen, George Bernard SHAW (2), and others—that dealt frankly and purposefully with social problems. Thus, the term as applied to Shakespeare's plays has implications about the playwright's intentions: these works are, indeed, profoundly concerned with society and its discontents.

At the close of both *All's Well* and *Measure for Measure,* villainy is exposed, its effects are corrected, and faults are forgiven in an air of general reconciliation. The effect is one of moral instruction, and, in fact, all three plays are distinguished by a pronounced emphasis on ethical questions. In *All's Well* the native worth of an individual is valued above aristocratic social standing, and the value of forgiveness is stressed in its conclusion. *Measure for Measure* addresses the nature of good and bad governance, the evils of extreme and inflexible moral positions, and, again, the value of forgiveness. *Troilus and Cressida* offers a scathing critique of the soldierly pretensions to honour and of the dishonesties of fashionable courtship in a context that exposes the futility of war.

Less baldly satirical than Jonson's work, the problem plays were perhaps found too serious and troubling by their original audiences, for all three plays were badly received when they were new, and they continued to be decidedly unpopular for three centuries thereafter. They have only been widely accepted in recent times, perhaps because the modern era is inclined both to the analysis of human problems and to a fear that they may not be easily solved. Commentators such as Shaw and Walter PATER instituted a reappraisal of the problem plays in the 1870s and '80s, and William POEL's productions of all three, between 1895 and 1905, began a process of theatrical rediscovery that has not stopped. Since the 1930s the plays have been staged regularly, and they will doubtless continue to attract producers and audiences. Their problematic aspects seem fitted to our problematic times; Shaw, writing in 1907, said that in these works Shakespeare was 'ready and willing to start at the twentieth century if the seventeenth would only let him'.

With greater acceptance, the positive aspects of the problem plays have become more evident. Certain seeming defects have more virtue than is immediately apparent. For instance, the employment of the 'bed trick' by HELENA (2) in *All's Well* and ISABELLA in *Measure for Measure,* along with CRESSIDA's hasty abandonment of TROILUS, are often seen as ill-motivated perversions of the characters' personalities. However, these events have significant symbolic functions, though they may not make sense psychologically. In the problem plays the point is not simply personality but also situation, not merely reality but also ideas. These intellectual aspects need not inhibit theatrical pleasure, for all three plays contain inspiring parts for actors. These include some unattractive figures, such as Thersites and Parolles, and also such splendid non-villains as Isabella, Helena, and ULYSSES. Even some of the lesser parts, such as the COUNTESS (2) of *All's Well,* are notable for fine speeches and a sympathetic pres-

ence. Moreover, all three plays offer genuinely funny passages, and several roles—such as LUCIO, AJAX, Thersites, Pandarus, and Parolles—which are fine vehicles for good comic actors. Especially in performance, the plays have a comedic focus that makes them less dark than the ideas they deal with.

This bright aspect lends its emotional tone to another important factor, one that was more popular in the 17th century than it is today. Except in the case of *Troilus and Cressida,* the plays display marked religious overtones, specifically suggestive of Christian redemption. Both Helena and Isabella have been seen as intentionally symbolic of God's grace, and the title of *Measure for Measure* alludes to the Sermon on the Mount. The appallingly deficient moral character of Bertram and Angelo, the male protagonists of these two plays, is also a powerful symbol in such a context, for these undeserving cads have but one purpose: to sin and be forgiven. These characters are similar to the central figures in medieval MORALITY PLAYS, which were still a living tradition for Shakespeare and his original audiences.

Once we understand that moral issues are the plays' *raison d'être,* we can adjust to the symbolic aspects of character and the allegorical nature of some of the plotting. The extent to which moral questions are stressed makes clear their importance to Shakespeare, and his refusal to provide easy answers to them makes them particularly potent. Shakespeare recognises, as always, the complexity of life and the difficulty in making moral judgements. The capacity of these plays to disturb causes us to be more engaged in these questions; we become aware of the need to strive after ideals, to pursue and believe in virtue even though we, like the figures in the plays, may not fully achieve it.

Proculeius, Caius (active c. 40–c. 20 B.C.) Historical figure and character in *Antony and Cleopatra,* a follower of Octavius CAESAR (2). When he advises CLEOPATRA to surrender to Caesar, ANTONY tells her, 'None about Caesar trust but Proculeius' (4.15.48). In 5.1 Caesar sends Proculeius to the Egyptian queen with instructions to promise her anything. Caesar wishes to prevent her from committing suicide so that he can triumphantly display her in ROME. In 5.2 Proculeius prevents Cleopatra from stabbing herself. He counsels her to be temperate, and tells her she will receive good treatment from Caesar. Because he has been recommended for his trustworthiness, his lies stress the isolation of Cleopatra in defeat, which helps motivate her suicide.

The historical Proculeius, a military commander, had a reputation as a forthright and honest man. This doubtless accounts for Antony's mistaken assumption (Shakespeare took the entire incident from PLUTARCH's *Lives*), but his loyalty was entirely with Caesar. He was a close personal friend of his leader, and he remained so for many years, though he never attained—or, apparently, aspired to—high office in the empire that Caesar was to found.

Prologue (1) Dramatic device in ELIZABETHAN DRAMA, a speech introducing a play. Sixteenth-century plays often opened with a prologue spoken by an allegorical figure—also called the Prologue (e.g., PROLOGUE [2])—commonly dressed in a distinctive black velvet cloak. He remarked briefly on the action to come, preparing the audience to respond appropriately. Elizabethan playwrights borrowed the prologue from Roman drama, which in turn had taken it from ancient Greek drama. Five of Shakespeare's plays begin with a Prologue: *Romeo and Juliet* (see CHORUS [2]), *Henry V, Troilus and Cressida, Pericles* (see GOWER [3]), and *The Two Noble Kinsmen;* in addition, three plays within a play present brief Prologues, those in *A Midsummer Night's Dream* (5.1.108–117), *Hamlet* (3.2.143–146), and *The Two Noble Kinsmen* (3.5.101–135).

Prologue (2) Allegorical figure in *Henry V,* the speaker of the PROLOGUE (1) that opens the play. Although he is designated in the opening stage direction as the Prologue, he identifies himself as the CHORUS (3) in line 32, and his rhetorical invocation of the Muses is taken up again, in remarks delivered under that designation, before each subsequent act (2–5) and in the EPILOGUE.

Prologue (3) Allegorical figure in *Troilus and Cressida* who speaks the PROLOGUE (1) that opens the play. The Prologue tells how the TROJAN WAR stemmed from the abduction of MENELAUS' wife, HELEN (1), by PARIS (3). He commences in the heroic style of traditional chroniclers of war, only to sum up, 'Ravished Helen, Menelaus' queen / With wanton Paris sleeps—and that's the quarrel' (Pro. 9–10). This stylistic jolt, both rhythmic and rhetorical, serves notice that this account of the ancient epic will not be conventional. He goes on to caution the audience that it may not like what the play depicts, for its contents vary with 'the chance of war' (Pro.31). In belittling his warlike costume, the Prologue further hints at the satire of soldiery that is to come. Some scholars believe that the provision for an 'arm'd' Prologue was inspired by, and perhaps was intended as an allusion to, the armoured Prologue in Ben JONSON's play *Poetaster* (1601).

Prologue (4) Allegorical figure in *Henry VIII,* the speaker of the PROLOGUE (1) that opens the play. The Prologue tells the audience that the play will be serious and sad, containing 'Such noble scenes as draw the eye to flow' (Prologue 4), and that it purports to tell the historical truth. It will include pleasing spectacles, but it will not be 'a merry bawdy play' (Prologue 14). (Scholars believe this last remark refers to an

earlier, decidedly non-serious play about King HENRY VIII by Samuel ROWLEY [1].) The Prologue prepares the audience for the solemnity of the play to come, which was a different sort of history play than Shakespeare's audiences were accustomed to. Scholars who believe that *Henry VIII* was written by more than one author usually ascribe the play's prologue to Shakespeare's collaborator.

Prologue (5) Allegorical figure in *The Two Noble Kinsmen,* the speaker of the PROLOGUE (1) that opens the play. The Prologue tells that the play derives from a famous poet, CHAUCER, and that it cannot compare with the original. He hopes, in the name of the acting company, that their production will be good enough to avoid disgrace. Scholars generally believe that the Prologue was written by Shakespeare's collaborator, probably John FLETCHER (2).

Prompt-book Copy of a play used during performances by the prompter, called the book-holder in ELIZABETHAN THEATRE. A prompt-book contained notes for entrances and exits, music cues, cuts in the text made by the company during rehearsals, and so on. Because the author's manuscript, or FOUL PAPERS, was often difficult to use in this way, a prompt-book was usually a transcript made for the purpose and then annotated. Sometimes, however, if a play was already published when a prompt-book was required, a printed copy would be annotated. The prompt-book was usually the text presented to the MASTER OF REVELS for approval, before a play could be staged. Since the prompt-book was the acting company's official copy of a play—and probably the only one—its loss was too dangerous to risk by lending it to a publisher to be printed from. Thus only a few of Shakespeare's plays were first printed from a prompt-book, presumably when another version was not available. Texts printed from prompt-books are characterised by the appearance of actors' names for those of characters, the placing of stage directions a few lines before they are needed, instructions for sound effects, and warnings of upcoming requirements for stage properties.

Prospero Character in *The Tempest,* the magician-ruler of a remote island. Prospero, once the Duke of MILAN, lives in exile with his daughter MIRANDA and two supernatural inhabitants of the island, ARIEL and CALIBAN. Through magic, Prospero controls this world completely, and he is the central figure of the play, simultaneously the sparker and spectator of its various SUB-PLOTS. He has freed Ariel from a magic spell, in exchange for his service as an assistant; he also befriended Caliban at first but enslaved him after he attempted to rape Miranda. Though embittered by his exile, Prospero has gained wisdom through his sorcery, and when chance places his one-time enemies in his power, he uses his magic to create an atmosphere of reconciliation and forgiveness, providing for the future in the union of Miranda with FERDINAND (2), the son of his enemy.

Having accomplished these things, Prospero sacrifices both his dominion over the island and his love of magic, choosing to return to Milan. In doing so, he restores a measure of justice to human society, for he had been unjustly deposed from authority before the play began. He also restores himself to a sound moral footing, for he had earlier placed a private concern—his study of magic—above his duty as a leader of society, with disastrous results. However, Prospero's success is not complete; he remains a melancholy figure at play's end, haunted by Caliban's enmity and his evil brother ANTONIO (5), who refuses regeneration. Thus Prospero brings out an important subtheme of *The Tempest* and of the ROMANCES in general: that life is an admixture of good and evil and that good cannot completely eradicate bad.

Prospero is a philosopher as well as a ruler. His magic is referred to as his 'Art' (1.2.1), consistently spelled with a capital A; this is a conventional allusion to Neoplatonic doctrines of the occult, familiar ideas in the 17th century. The Neoplatonic philosopher/magician attempted to elevate his soul through arcane knowledge of the divine, whether through alchemy, the reading of supernatural signs, or communication with spirits. If these efforts led to a magical manipulation of the real world, it was only as a byproduct of the search for spiritual knowledge. Prospero's original goal was to transcend nature, not control it. Nevertheless, it is clear that the pursuit of this goal was culpably selfish, for it resulted in his exile and the disruption of sound government in Milan, as he recounts in 1.2. He had insisted on studying magic rather than governing and as a result had been deposed by Antonio. Conscious of his failing, regretful at leaving Ariel and the beauties of 'rough magic [and] heavenly music' (5.1. 50–52), distressed by his evident failure to educate Caliban, and, most important, frustrated by the intransigence of Antonio, Prospero returns to Milan at play's end without the satisfaction the conclusion brings to most of the other characters. Though restored to power, and though he has provided a hopeful future for others, he is a partial failure, and he knows it.

Prospero is not a pleasant character. He is a distant and uncommunicative father and a tyrannical master. His unjustified complaints that Miranda is not listening to him in 1.2 and his anguished disruption of the MASQUE in 4.1 are evidence of his temperamental nature. Only in his affection for Ariel is he a pleasant figure, but he is also capable of rounding vituperatively on the sprite —'Thou liest, malignant thing!' (1.2.257)—and threatening him—'I will . . . peg thee [to a tree] till / Thou hast howl'd away twelve winters'

(1.2.294–296). His programme of petty harassments of Caliban, recounted in 2.2.1–14, is equally repellent.

Prospero's exploitation of the island's inhabitants is a clearly established element of the play. Ariel, a free spirit by nature, is restive in his service, and Caliban even attempts a revolt. Some modern commentators go so far as to make this exploitation a central concern, and *The Tempest* has been presented as an allegory of colonialism and oppression. However, it is clear that Prospero's control has been employed for good, for he has undone the dominance of evil that he found on his arrival, when the villainous Caliban prevailed, and Ariel, a good spirit, was imprisoned by Caliban's mother. The inhumane treatment of Caliban and Ariel's dissatisfaction provide evidence of the inexorability of evil; good ends must often be compromised by morally unsatisfactory means.

A central theme of the play is transfiguration, as the characters undergo transformations that suggest the varying human capacity for improvement. Prospero's magic effects these alterations in the others, but he himself also undergoes a highly significant change. His transformation occurs largely before the time of the play, but evidence of it remains. His decision that 'the rarer action is / In virtue than in vengeance' (5.1. 27–28) implies a temptation from which he refrains. We recognise that he has grown: first a scholar of magic, he became a seeker of revenge through supernatural means, but finally he has transcended magic altogether. Once he could say 'my library / Was dukedom large enough' (1.2.109–110), but at play's end he returns to Milan to resume his proper position as a leader of society. In so doing, he renounces his magical powers and discards his semi-devine status as the island's omnipotent ruler. Prospero accepts his humanity and comes to terms with the prospect of his own death, to which he will devote 'every third thought' (5.1.311). He leaves the future in the hands of Ferdinand and Miranda.

Prospero's 'Art' fittingly takes the form of drama, the art practised by Prospero's creator. Assisted by Ariel, Prospero produces three distinctly theatrical illusions—the HARPY's banquet of 3.3, the betrothal masque of 4.1, and the presentation of Ferdinand and Miranda at chess in 5.1. As producer of these spectacles, Prospero comments on their nature at the close of the masque, in his famous speech beginning 'Our revels now are ended' (4.1.148). He points out the illusion involved and goes on to equate such an 'insubstantial pageant' (4.1.155) with life itself, which disappears once it is performed. 'We are such stuff / As dreams are made on', he concludes, 'and our little life / Is rounded with a sleep' (4.1.156–158). Many commentators have regarded Prospero's remarks as Shakespeare's personal valedictory to a career in the theatre. While this notion is imprecise, in that Shakespeare continued to write for the theatre after *The Tempest*, the passage does seem to reflect the experience of an artist whose long career has led to the belief that art's inherently illusory nature is analogous to, and probably related to, the impossibility of understanding life. Here we have a clue to the philosophy underlying a prominent feature of Shakespeare's work, his persistent attention to ambiguity.

Shakespeare may have taken Prospero's name from Prospero Adorno (active 1460–1488), a deposed duke of Genoa, of whom he could have read in William Thomas' *History of Italy* (1549). However, this is uncertain, for another source was nearer to hand: Ben JONSON's *Every Man in His Humour* (1600). This play, in which Shakespeare acted, contains a character—though not a deposed duke—originally named Prospero (the name was later changed to Wellbred, as it appears in modern editions).

Proteus One of the title characters in *The Two Gentlemen of Verona,* the villain who simultaneously betrays his lover, JULIA, and his friend, VALENTINE (2), by pursuing Valentine's lover, SILVIA. Proteus initially presents himself as wholly in love with Julia. His father, ANTONIO (1), forces him to attend the court, for such a sojourn is proper for a young gentleman, and he bids farewell to his beloved, pledging to be faithful. Once at court, however, he falls in love with Silvia, who is already secretly betrothed to Valentine. Proteus knows his love is disloyal, but he is prepared to forsake both Valentine and Julia. Proteus plots against Valentine and even attempts to rape Silvia, but Valentine thwarts and forgives him. Reunited with Julia, who has followed him, Proteus vows renewed fidelity, and the play ends with the planning of a double wedding.

Shakespeare took this character's name from HOMER's *Odyssey,* in which Proteus is a sea god who can change his shape at will. The Proteus of *The Two Gentlemen of Verona,* whose attitudes towards others change with his appetites, is thus fittingly named.

Provost Character in *Measure for Measure,* the warden of the prison in which CLAUDIO (3) is gaoled. From his first appearance—when he exposes Claudio to public humiliation at the orders of ANGELO (2) but declares, 'I do it not in evil disposition' (1.2.110)—we see the Provost to be a kind and honourable man. He pleads with Angelo to be merciful towards Claudio and clearly presents a sensible view of the young man's offence, thereby emphasising Angelo's extremism. Nevertheless, the Provost is prepared to do the duty of his office and oversee the young man's execution. In this way, he offers a contrast to the moral laxity that created the problem in the first place.

In a telling episode the Provost demonstrates Shakespeare's position that social order has a high value. This clearly sympathetic character who obviously favours mercy for Claudio nevertheless resists

the attempts of the disguised DUKE (9) to find a way to save the young man until the Duke produces letters that reveal his authority. Then, supported by the knowledge that he will not be opposing the ruler—Shakespeare and his original audiences believed that rulers were appointed by God—he can enthusiastically help.

Prynne, William (1600–1669) Puritan pamphleteer and opponent of the theatre. In his *Histriomastix, The Players Scourge* (1633), Prynne declared that 'popular stage-plays . . . are sinfull, heathenish, lewde, ungodly Spectacles' and called people who wrote, acted in, or attended plays 'unlawful, infamous and misbeseeming Christians'. Prynne's attack was only one example of Puritan hostility towards drama, and Puritan culture increasingly dominated English life from the 1580s on. After 1642 as the civil wars began and a revolutionary government controlled first London and later the country, the theatres of England were closed for 18 years (but see DROLLS).

Prynne's career also offers an impressive demonstration of the barbarous rigour of the law in 17th-century England. *Historiomastix* contained references to the just downfalls of monarchs, and insulted the queen for appearing in MASQUES. Because of this, Prynne was imprisoned for life, fined a huge amount of money, and had his ears cut off. He managed to publish from prison a pamphlet that attacked English bishops, and was therefore branded on both cheeks with the letters 'S. L'. (for 'seditious libeller'). With the approach of the revolution, he was freed in 1640. He was elected to Parliament, but he continued to attack various aspects of the revolution itself, and in 1650 he was again imprisoned for three years. Prynne finally mellowed somewhat and avoided further prosecution, though he did not cease his public commentaries. In the course of his career he published over 200 books and pamphlets. He supported the restoration of the monarchy in 1660, served again in Parliament, and was appointed to a clerical position at the TOWER OF LONDON, where he had once been imprisoned.

Publius (1) Minor character in *Titus Andronicus,* the son of MARCUS ANDRONICUS. Publius participates in the seemingly mad TITUS (1) Andronicus' plan to shoot message-laden arrows to the gods in 4.3, and he helps capture CHIRON and DEMETRIUS (1) in 5.2.

Publius (2) Minor character in *Julius Caesar,* a witness to the assassination of CAESAR (1). In 3.1 Publius accompanies Caesar to the Senate, and when the killing takes place, he watches horrified; he is the only figure on stage not in violent action. BRUTUS (4) reassures him that no harm is intended to him or any other citizen, and he is sent to pass along this message to others. He remains silent throughout the episode.

Publius is usually designated as a senator in the list of characters, but the text offers no indication of his status; the first such list only dates from ROWE's 1709 edition of the plays. The same Publius may be referred to when Antony consents to the condemnation of his nephew, Publius, in 4.1.4–6. Although no such relationship has been mentioned before, the name recalls the earlier figure and intensifies the picture of Antony as a ruthless politician. Not only does he condemn his own relative to solidify his political position, but he also undoes Brutus' explicit mercy of 3.1.

Publius, unlike the other named characters in *Julius Caesar,* does not appear in Shakespeare's source, PLUTARCH's *Lives.* Antony had no nephew named Publius, and no one of that name appears in Plutarch's account of the assassination. Having decided to present an innocent bystander in 3.1, Shakespeare simply invented an extra character and gave him a handy Latin name (one that he also used in 3.1.53 to identify the brother of METELLUS, who is also unnamed in Plutarch). His various uses of the name may simply be an instance of the minor carelessness that recurs throughout his plays.

Pucelle, La See JOAN LA PUCELLE.

Puck (Robin Goodfellow) Character in *A Midsummer Night's Dream,* a fairy and aide to OBERON, the Fairy

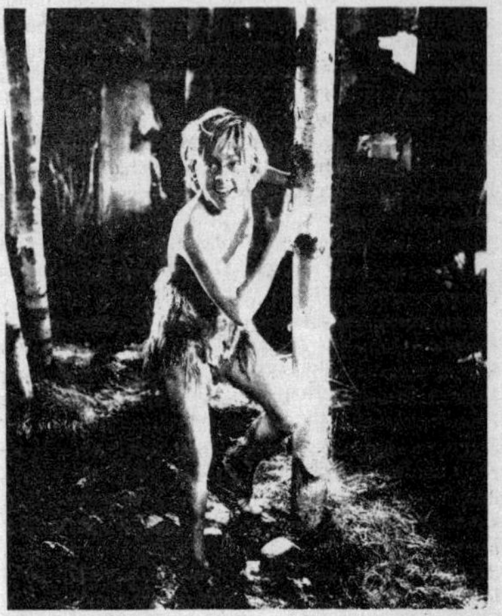

In A Midsummer Night's Dream, *Puck (played here by Mickey Rooney in the 1935 film) is a mischievous trickster who creates trouble by anointing Lysander with a love potion.* (Courtesy of Culver Pictures, Inc.)

King. Puck is a powerful supernatural creature, capable of circling the earth in 40 minutes (2.1.176) and of manipulating the elements—for example, he summons a fog in 3.2—but he is more mischievous than awe-inspiring. He reminds us of a small boy when he boasts of his talents as a trickster in 2.1.42–57 and when he calls out, 'I go, I go, look how I go!' (3.2.100). Like BOTTOM, he is a humorous character, but where Bottom is a CLOWN (1), intended to be laughed at, Puck more closely resembles a FOOL (1), like Shakespeare's jesters TOUCHSTONE and FESTE. He is removed from the practical world and expresses himself through an idiosyncratic sense of humour. He prefers 'things that befall prepost'rously' (3.2.121).

There is some malice in Puck's taste for pranks, and Puck reminds us that the fairy world is not all sweetness and light; this contributes to an undertone of potential evil that makes the comedy, while still benign, a more richly textured tale. He speaks in horrifying terms of the cruel and awesome world that is also the domain of the fairies (5.1.357–373), only to assure us that 'we fairies . . . / Now are frolic'. However, when his error in anointing LYSANDER causes trouble, Puck is immune to Oberon's regret that this has happened, replying only, 'Then fate o'er-rules' (3.2.92). He is coolly indifferent to human suffering.

While Puck explicitly calls himself a fairy in 5.1.369, quoted above, and elsewhere, there is some ambiguity in his relationship to the FAIRY in 2.1, and in 3.2.399 he is identified as a 'goblin'. Shakespeare did not care about such minor inconsistencies, and they do not interfere with Puck's effectiveness in the drama. They do, however, reflect the fairy lore known to Shakespeare, who combined in Puck two supernatural creatures that had earlier been thought of as separate beings: Robin Goodfellow, a name interchangeable with Puck in the 16th century, was a household spirit also associated with travellers; a 'puck' was not a fairy, but a small elf or goblin fond of playing practical jokes on mortals, especially at night. The puck was originally a Norse demon, identified in England with the devil.

Purcell, Henry (c. 1659–1695) English composer, creator of music for several adaptations of Shakespeare's plays. Perhaps the greatest English composer, Purcell led the creation of an English baroque style in music. He is best known today for two operas: *The Fairy Queen* (1692), with a libretto taken by Thomas BETTERTON from *A Midsummer Night's Dream,* and *Dido and Aeneas* (1689), parts of which were incorporated in Charles GILDON's 1699 adaptation of *Measure for Measure.* He also composed music for a 1690 revival of Thomas SHADWELL's *The Enchanted Island,* an operatic version of *The Tempest* (as adapted by John DRYDEN and William DAVENANT), and Shadwell's 1694 adaptation of *Timon of Athens.* However, in all these works, the only words of Shakespeare set to music by Purcell are two SONGS in *The Tempest,* 'Come unto these yellow sands' (1.2.377–389) and 'Full fadom five' (1.2.399–407).

Puritan, The Anonymous play formerly attributed to Shakespeare, part of the Shakespeare APOCRYPHA. *The Puritan,* sometimes called *The Puritan Widow* (its full title was *The Puritan or The Widdow of Watling-Streete*), is a farce with a pointed anti-Puritan bias. It was published by George ELD in 1607 as 'written by W. S.', possibly with the intention of associating the play with Shakespeare. It was also included among Shakespeare's plays in the Third and Fourth FOLIOS and in the editions of Nicholas ROWE and Alexander POPE (1). Scholars are confident, however, that *The Puritan* was not written by Shakespeare. Although it is a better drama than most of the apocryphal plays, it bears no resemblance to Shakespeare's known works as it is a topical satire set in contemporary London and written mostly in prose. Stylistically, it is tentatively ascribed by many scholars to John MARSTON or Thomas MIDDLETON.

Pursuivant Character in *Richard III.* See HASTINGS (2).

Puttenham, George (c. 1529–1590) or Richard (c. 1520–1601) English writer, author of a book of literary theory that is parodied in *King Lear. The Arte of English Poesie* (1589) appeared anonymously; William CAMDEN referred to it as the work of 'Maister Puttenham', but it is not known which brother wrote the book, so it is traditionally ascribed to 'Puttenham'. Puttenham's manual of style critiques the best-known English poets and is considered the first important work of English poetry criticism. It also analyses rhetorical and poetic devices, and advises on language usage. Puttenham inveighs against the use of archaic or foreign terms, and suggests adopting the accents of LONDON and the royal court. Several passages in Shakespeare's plays (e.g., *All's Well* 2.3.293–294) echo Puttenham's wording, and the prophecy of the FOOL (2) in *King Lear* (3.2.79–96) is a parody of some lines attributed to CHAUCER in the book. *The Arte of English Poesie* was published by Shakespeare's friend, Richard FIELD (2), and it is possible the playwright knew its author.

Pyramus and Thisbe Title of the play within *A Midsummer Night's Dream,* an INTERLUDE performed at the wedding of Duke THESEUS (1) and Queen HIPPOLYTA (1). The play is enacted in 5.1 by a group of artisans of ATHENS—led by Peter QUINCE—whom Shakespeare portrays as humorous English rustics. Nick BOTTOM, an excellent Shakespearean CLOWN (1), plays the romantic lead in a comic manner. Theseus generously

gives a dignified reception to the preposterous production, although his bride is less tolerant, declaring the play to be ridiculous, which of course it is meant to be.

The story of Pyramus and Thisbe was familiar to Shakespeare through OVID's *Metamorphoses*, but even illiterate members of his audience will have known it, for Pyramus and Thisbe figured in several Elizabethan popular songs. The ancient Greek myth tells of the love of a boy and girl, Pyramus and Thisbe, who live in neighbouring buildings but whose parents have forbidden them to meet. Able to communicate only through a hole in the wall between their homes, the lovers agree to elope. Thisbe arrives at their rendezvous early. Frightened by a lion, she hides in a cave but loses her cloak as she flees. The lion has just eaten and has a bloody mouth; nuzzling her garment, he bloodies it. When Pyramus arrives, he sees the bloodstained cloak and lion's tracks and concludes that Thisbe has been killed by the animal. Heartsick, he kills himself with his sword. When Thisbe reappears and sees what has happened, she seizes his sword and kills herself.

This tale, although burlesqued by the artisans' production, provides an illuminating counterpart to the elopement of LYSANDER and HERMIA earlier in *A Midsummer Night's Dream.* It demonstrates, in a harmless context, the potential for tragedy that the lovers' predicament harboured. The contrast heightens our pleasure in the benevolent outcome that has actually occurred.

Shakespeare's parody is not directed at Ovid's classic version, but rather at the bombast and theatrical heroics in 16th-century drama, especially that of Thomas PRESTON. In addition, two minor modifications of Ovid's tale stand out. Quince's original casting of the interlude (1.2.56–59) includes the lovers' parents, who are merely mentioned in Ovid, and Bottom's assertion that the wall had 'parted their fathers' (5.1.338) introduces an inter-family feud that does not exist in Ovid. Both additions suggest aspects of *Romeo and Juliet,* and it is thought that Shakespeare's use of the legend in this fashion reflects his recent composition of that play.

Pyrrhus Legendary Greek warrior whose bloody killing of King PRIAM of TROY is recalled as an example of regicide in *Hamlet.* The FIRST PLAYER (2), at HAMLET's request, recites a dramatic monologue in which this episode from the TROJAN WAR is vividly recounted. Pyrrhus at first hesitates, as 'his sword . . . seem'd i'th' air to stick' (2.2.473–475) and he 'like a neutral to his will and matter, / Did nothing' (2.2.477–478). This inaction parallels that of Hamlet, who has so far failed to avenge his father's murder by KING (5) Claudius. But then Pyrrhus' 'aroused vengeance' (2.2.484) impels him to complete his deed, and the recital implicitly stimulates Hamlet to action.

Pyrrhus appears as Neoptolemus in HOMER and other early accounts of Priam's death, but he is Pyrrhus in VIRGIL's *Aeneid,* which was probably more familiar to Shakespeare. He was the son of ACHILLES, and he is mentioned as such in *Troilus and Cressida* (3.3.208). In one version of his myth, he founded a dynasty of kings, one of whom, also called Pyrrhus, is now much better known than he, as the general who achieved a costly, or Pyrrhic, victory.

Q

Quarto Format for a book or page. A quarto is a sheet of paper that is folded in half twice, yielding four leaves or eight pages. It is also a book composed of such pages (see also FOLIO). Most of the early editions of Shakespeare's plays were produced in this format, and the term is often used to refer to these editions. Some of these came from authoritative sources that accurately reflected what Shakespeare wrote, such as his FOUL PAPERS; these are known as GOOD QUARTOS. Others, whose text was reconstructed by actors from memory, are seriously flawed in various ways and are known as BAD QUARTOS. Of the 38 plays in the CANON, 22 were initially published as Quartos. However, there are 10 Bad Quartos and 14 Good Quartos, for *Romeo and Juliet* and *Hamlet* appeared in both Good Quarto and Bad Quarto editions.

Quayle, Anthony (1913–1989) British actor and director. On both stage and screen Quayle played a variety of Shakespearean parts—including BOTTOM, PANDARUS, OTHELLO, and FALSTAFF—as well as other roles in both classic and modern drama. He was director of the Shakespeare Memorial Theatre at STRATFORD from 1948 to 1956. He wrote two novels—*Eight Hours from England* (1945) and *On Such a Night* (1947)—based on his wartime service as a leader of guerrilla bands behind Nazi lines in Europe. Quayle is probably most widely remembered for several non-Shakespearean movie roles, in *The Guns of Navarone* (1961), *Lawrence of Arabia* (1963), and *Anne of a Thousand Days* (1970). In the latter he played Cardinal Thomas WOLSEY.

Queen (1) Any of three minor characters in *The Two Noble Kinsmen,* deposed monarchs who seek the aid of THESEUS (2), Duke of ATHENS. The Queens interrupt Theseus' wedding to tell him that their husbands have been defeated and killed by King Creon of THEBES, who has refused to bury the kings' bodies, thereby exposing their souls to torment. They ask Theseus to avenge this deed by conquering Creon. The First Queen, as she is designated, implores Theseus; the Second Queen addresses his intended bride, the Amazon HIPPOLYTA (2), and the Third speaks to Hippolyta's sister, EMILIA (4). All three respond favourably, but the Queens are not satisfied with anything but instant action, and their petitions are restated. Finally, the wedding is postponed and Theseus sets out. In 1.4, the conquest completed, the Queens thank Theseus, and in 1.5 they proceed with their husbands' funerals.

The Queens are part of the ritualistic aspect of the play that links it to other Shakespeare ROMANCES. They are highly significant figures in 1.1, Shakespeare's spectacular opening scene. Their sudden appearance, all in black at a festive ceremony, is a *coup de théâtre,* with a grand effect on stage. Their repeated approaches, first to one character and then another, form a dancelike, stylised sequence, a kind of liturgy that reinforces the high seriousness of their purpose. In 1.5 they again offer an impressive tableau, as Act 1 closes in tragic triumph.

Queen (2) of Britain Character in *Cymbeline,* the wife of King CYMBELINE and stepmother of his daughter IMOGEN. The Queen, one of several villains in the play, is the most purely vicious of them. She had planned that Imogen marry her son, the oafish CLOTEN, but Imogen eloped with POSTHUMUS instead. Posthumus is banished, and the Queen directs her malice towards Imogen and PISANIO, Posthumus' servant who has stayed with Imogen. She is the archetypal wicked stepmother, and her villainy is clear from her initial appearance, in 1.2, when she pretends to protect Imogen but reveals her malice in an aside. Imogen is undeceived and notes the Queen's 'dissembling courtesy' (1.2.15); thus, the Queen's wickedness is immediately established. In 1.6 the Queen collects poison from the physician CORNELIUS (2) and offers it to Pisanio as a health-giving potion in the hope that he will take it and die. However, Cornelius 'will not trust one of her malice' (1.6.35), and has substituted a sleeping potion for the poison. The Queen is ultimately ineffective, but her evil intent is a prominent element of the first half of the play.

Once her nature is well established, the Queen plays a lesser role. At the play's close we learn of her death from an illness caused by her despair at Cloten's sudden disappearance. Her final confession of sins—including an intent to poison the king himself—prepares

for the final sequence of reconciliations in 5.5. The Queen has only been forestalled by the whim of fortune: Cloten has been killed by a chance encounter that is the result of a long series of events that began with the exile of Posthumus. She has therein fulfilled the villain's role in this play, which is to be defeated by the intervention of providence.

Queen (3) Anne of England Character in *Henry VIII*. See ANNE (1).

Queen (4) Anne of England Character in *Richard III*. See ANNE (2).

Queen (5) Cleopatra of Egypt Title character of *Antony and Cleopatra*. See CLEOPATRA.

Queen (6) Eleanor (Elinor) of England Character in *King John*. See ELEANOR.

Queen (7) Elizabeth of England Contemporary of Shakespeare. See ELIZABETH (1).

Queen (8) Elizabeth of England Character in *3 Henry VI* and *Richard III*. See ELIZABETH (2).

Queen (9) Gertrude of Denmark Character in *Hamlet*, HAMLET's mother, who has married the brother, successor, and murderer of her late husband, the King of DENMARK. Hamlet is horrified by the Queen's acceptance, soon after her husband's death, of 'incestuous sheets' (1.2.157), and he is moved to conclude, 'Frailty, thy name is woman' (1.2.146). His disgust at her behaviour is heightened when he learns from the GHOST (3), in 1.5.42–52, that she had been the lover of Claudius, the new KING (5), before he had killed Hamlet's father. Hamlet's detestation of his mother's part in these evils is transformed into a revulsion against women in general and against the love—and sex—that they offer, which lead only to the creation of more humanity and thus more wickedness. His own beloved, OPHELIA, tragically comes to bear the brunt of the prince's misogyny.

Although the Queen provides an example of the evil that infects Denmark, she herself is a somewhat faceless character. She is basically evil through weakness rather than inclination. The Ghost attributes her wickedness to Claudius and tells Hamlet to exclude her from his revenge—'Leave her to heaven' (1.5.86). In her main scene, in which Hamlet repudiates her for her adultery and her acceptance of the King as a husband, she acknowledges her guilt, crying out that her soul is contaminated by '. . . such black and grained spots / As will not leave their tinct' (3.4.90–91). After Hamlet leaves and the King returns in 4.1, the Queen resumes her role as his accomplice. But in 5.2, when the Queen turns on her husband and cries out a warning to Hamlet as she dies, we may suppose that her son has had some effect on her.

Queen (10) Hermione Character in *The Winter's Tale*. See HERMIONE.

Queen (11) Hippolyta of the Amazons Character in *A Midsummer Night's Dream*. See HIPPOLYTA (1).

Queen (12) Hippolyta Character in *The Two Noble Kinsmen*. See HIPPOLYTA (2).

Queen (13) Isabel of England (1389–1409) Historical figure and character in *Richard II*, the wife of RICHARD II. The Queen is so completely different from her historical counterpart that she is virtually fictitious. Shakespeare introduces her to help provide a human context for the political events of the play. In 2.3 she glumly regrets the temporary absence of her husband—'so sweet a guest as . . . sweet Richard' (2.2.8–9)—casting the vain and headstrong King in a very different light than he has yet been seen. Later, after she overhears the GARDENER's remarks on Richard's capture and likely deposition by BOLINGBROKE (1), she responds with hysterical grief. She last appears in the famous farewell scene with Richard (5.1), which restates, on a personal level, the breach in the political fabric that Bolingbroke's usurpation has effected. (Richard refers to this in his speech beginning with the expostulation 'Doubly divorc'd!' [5.1.71].) The Queen's pleas that she be permitted to accompany her husband are rejected by the stony Earl of NORTHUMBERLAND (1), and the sorrowing couple are forcibly separated, just as Richard has been parted from his crown. The historical is presented on a human level, with a degree of poignancy far greater than any dismay we may feel for Richard's fall from worldly greatness or for the collapse of England's feudal traditions.

The historical Isabel was no happier than Shakespeare's Queen, but she was a child of 10 when these events occurred. The daughter of Charles VI, the FRENCH KING of *Henry V*, she was married to Richard when she was 7. While this couple seem to have been genuinely fond of one another, they had no opportunity to develop the mature relationship that Shakespeare depicts. Although she is banished to France in the play, she was actually detained in England for two years following Richard's deposition, virtually a prisoner, because the new government was reluctant to return her dowry. When she finally returned home, Isabel was still an eminently eligible princess, and she was married in 1404 to Prince Charles of ORLÉANS (3) (who appears in *Henry V*). She died in childbirth five years later, at the age of 20.

Queen (14) Isabel of France Character in *Henry V*. See ISABEL (2).

Queen (15) Katherine of England (and of Aragon) Character in *Henry VIII.* See KATHERINE OF ARAGON.

Queen (16) Margaret of England Character in *1, 2,* and *3 Henry VI* and *Richard III.* See MARGARET (1).

Queen (17), Player Character in *Hamlet.* See PLAYER QUEEN.

Queen's Men (1) (Queen Elizabeth's Men) Acting company of the ELIZABETHAN THEATRE, possibly Shakespeare's first theatrical home. The Queen's Men were created by order of Queen ELIZABETH (1) in 1583; at the queen's command, her MASTER OF REVELS raided other acting companies for some of their finest players. The Queen's Men consequently became the most popular and important LONDON acting company for almost a decade. Its original members included John BENTLEY (who killed a man at an early Queen's Men performance), the great comic actor Richard TARLTON, John SINGER (another comic actor), and Robert WILSON (4). The Queen's Men performed in London in the winter, at the THEATRE and at the court, and toured the provinces in the summer. In the summer of 1587, they played in STRATFORD, a fact that has encouraged speculation that Shakespeare may have gone with them to London to begin his career (see KNELL).

After Tarlton's death in 1588, the fortunes of the Queen's Men declined, and two newer companies, the ADMIRAL'S MEN and STRANGE'S MEN, began to dominate the theatrical scene. Between 1591 and 1594 the Queen's Men performed only twice at court, a measure of their declining prestige. In the latter year, they allied themselves with SUSSEX'S MEN, but to no avail; unable to compete in London, they converted themselves into a full-time provincial touring company, surviving until the queen's death in 1603.

Queen's Men (2) Seventeenth-century LONDON theatrical company, successor to WORCESTER'S MEN. Upon the accession of King JAMES I in 1603, his family assumed the patronage of the three London theatre companies. His queen, Anne of Denmark (1574–1619), gave her name to Worcester's Men, the least important of the three, whose chief members were the actor Christopher BEESTON and the playwright Thomas HEYWOOD (2). When the company's royal patent was issued the next year, they were said to perform regularly at an inn, where they had existed as Worcester's, and at the CURTAIN THEATRE, a new venue for them. In 1609, when the patent was renewed, the locations named are the Curtain and the Red Bull Theatre, a new playhouse. After 1617 they performed at the Phoenix Theatre, owned by Beeston. Beeston managed the company from 1612—ineptly and perhaps dishonestly, as the records of several lawsuits reveal—until the company dissolved on the death of Queen Anne in 1619.

Queen's Revels See CHILDREN'S COMPANIES.

Quickly, Mistress Character in *The Merry Wives of Windsor,* housekeeper of Dr CAIUS (2). Mistress Quickly is a shrewd yet comically foolish servant who meddles in other people's affairs. She serves as a messenger between the merry wives and FALSTAFF, and she impartially supports three different suitors in their pursuit of ANNE (3) Page. Quickly is a traditional, humorously loquacious comic character, given to the misuse of fancy words and the misinterpretation of other people's speeches. For instance, in the famous 'Latin scene', 4.1, Quickly finds bawdy puns in Latin grammatical exercises.

In 5.5 Quickly takes the part of the fairy queen in the ceremonial taunting of Falstaff that is his final humiliation at the hands of the wives. Quickly is entirely out of character in this scene, and her presence in the texts of the play may merely reflect the playhouse practise of having the actor who played Quickly also play the anonymous fairy imitator. Alternatively, her distinctively uncharacteristic presence may have been intended by Shakespeare to suggest the MASQUElike unreality of the scene, emphasising its ritualistic quality.

Mistress Quickly bears the same name as the HOSTESS (2) of *1* and *2 Henry IV* and *Henry V,* and she shares the Hostess' comical way with words, but she is nonetheless best considered as a different person, living in a different world. She is unacquainted with Falstaff when she encounters him in *The Merry Wives,* and she has certainly never had anything to do with the BOAR'S HEAD TAVERN in London. It seems likely that, in the haste with which *The Merry Wives* was written, Shakespeare simply made use of an earlier creation in a new way. Neither he nor his audience was distressed by the inconsistencies this involves.

Quin, James (1693–1766) British actor. The chief rival to David GARRICK in the 1730s and 1740s, Quin was renowned for his portrayal of FALSTAFF, though he also played BRUTUS, OTHELLO, MACBETH, the GHOST (3) in *Hamlet,* and other parts. He is considered the last great representative of the formal and declamatory school of acting that had been popular in the second half of the 17th century but was supplanted by the more naturalistic and active mode of Garrick. Quin appears in Tobias Smollett's great novel *Humphrey Clinker* (1771).

Quince, Peter Character in *A Midsummer Night's Dream,* a carpenter and the director of the comical production of PYRAMUS AND THISBE, performed by several artisans of ATHENS. Quince organises an INTERLUDE to be performed at the wedding of Duke THESEUS

(1) and Queen HIPPOLYTA (1). Though overshadowed by his leading man, BOTTOM, he directs the performances of SNUG, FLUTE, SNOUT, and STARVELING, and he reads the PROLOGUE himself. Despite the supposedly Athenian setting of *A Midsummer Night's Dream,* Quince and his fellows are typical English artisans, excellent representatives of the humorous workers Shakespeare was fond of creating.

Quince comically performs several of the tasks of a real Elizabethan acting company. Not only the director, he has also written the script and is responsible for the properties and staging. He is something of a pedant, given to such high-flown locutions as 'I am to entreat you, request you, and desire you . . .' (1.2.92–93), but he is a tactful director, flattering Bottom into accepting his role in 1.2.79–82, and a resourceful reviser, prepared to create additional dialogue in 3.1. Less talented as an actor, he misreads his initial speech (5.1.108–117). (Quince's comical mispunctuation of the passage was a standard Elizabethan routine dating from the first English COMEDY, Nicholas UDALL's *Ralph Roister Doister* [c. 1553].)

The name Quince refers to certain tools of the carpentry trade, wooden wedges called 'quoins' or 'quines'. Quince is thought to have been originally played by Richard COWLEY.

Quiney (1), Judith Shakespeare (1585–1662) Shakespeare's daughter, wife of Thomas QUINEY (3). See SHAKESPEARE (10).

Quiney (2), Richard (before 1557–1602) Businessman in STRATFORD, an acquaintance of Shakespeare. Quiney was a dealer in fine cloth, a partner with his father, Adrian (d. 1607; a friend of Shakespeare's father John SHAKESPEARE [9]). He was evidently a respected businessman, for he represented the town of Stratford at the court of Queen ELIZABETH (1), on several occasions, and sought government relief for the town after the great fires of 1594 and 1595.

Quiney's surviving correspondence contains several references to Shakespeare as well as the only extant letter addressed to the playwright (though it was apparently never delivered). While in LONDON in January 1598, Quiney received a letter from another Stratford businessman suggesting that he try to interest Shakespeare in a real estate deal they were contemplating, and in October, again in London, he wrote a letter to the playwright asking for a loan to cover extra expenses resulting from an unforeseen delay. He apparently did not deliver this missive, which remained among his papers still sealed, probably because he was able to make his request in person; another letter of the same date, to a friend in Stratford, reports that Shakespeare promised assistance. Later during the same visit, Quiney received a letter from his father that mentions Shakespeare in connection with an otherwise obscure business deal. In addition to establishing Shakespeare's presence in London at these times, these letters also make clear the playwright's continuing involvement with the affairs of his home town.

Quiney opposed the attempt of a neighbouring nobleman, Sir Edward Greville, to enclose the town commons for sheep grazing. A drunken group of Greville's followers roughed him up one night in May 1602, and he died from his injuries. His widow was left with nine children under the age of 20, one of whom, Thomas QUINEY (3), became Shakespeare's son-in-law.

Quiney (3), Thomas (1589–c. 1652) Vintner in STRATFORD and Shakespeare's son-in-law. Quiney, the son of Richard QUINEY (2), ran a tavern and apparently had a reputation as a rake when he married Judith SHAKESPEARE (10) in February 1616. They were wed during Lent without obtaining the necessary special licence, for which he was briefly excommunicated. Within a month he was in worse trouble, for when one Margaret Wheeler died in childbirth in March, Quiney was named as the father of the child (who also died). He was ordered to appear as a penitent, wearing a white sheet, in the parish church on three successive Sundays, though he avoided this public disgrace by paying a fine. It has been speculated that this scandal may have hastened Shakespeare's death, for he died a few weeks later, after changing his will to protect Judith's inheritance from Quiney. Quiney established a wine and tobacco shop, but he was an unsuccessful businessman, and the shop was eventually run by trustees who assigned him a yearly allowance. The Quineys' three sons all died young. Quiney is thought to have died while visiting a brother in London sometime after 1652, though no record of his death has survived.

Quintus Minor character in *Titus Andronicus,* a son of TITUS (1) Andronicus. Quintus, with MARTIUS (1), is framed by AARON for the murder of BASSIANUS in 2.3. The two are executed, and their heads are delivered to Titus in 3.1.

R

Raleigh (Ralegh), Walter (c. 1552–1618) English soldier, seaman, explorer, and writer. Raleigh, son of an obscure country gentleman, became a favourite of Queen ELIZABETH (1) through a combination of personal charm and a successful military career, including naval raids against Spanish overseas territories. During the 1580s Raleigh organised and financed several colonising expeditions to the New World—including the famous lost colony on Roanoke Island, Virginia—but no successful settlements resulted. He also explored the Orinoco River in South America, in search of El Dorado, the legendary city of gold.

In addition Raleigh was a poet, accepted as a literary equal by his friends Edmund SPENSER and Christopher MARLOWE (1). He wrote many poems that were circulated in manuscript, and those that have survived place him among the better poets of his day. (At least one of Raleigh's poems, 'The Nymph's Reply to the Shepherd', was attributed to Shakespeare in the *Poems* published by John BENSON [2] in 1640; also, one stanza of it—linked with the Marlowe poem to which it replies—was attributed to Shakespeare in THE PASSIONATE PILGRIM.)

A man of great intellectual curiosity, Raleigh dabbled in the magical doctrines and esoteric knowledge that were part of the budding science of the RENAISSANCE. These activities raised widespread suspicion that he was an atheist; combined with his arrogant disdain for other people's opinions, this made him generally unpopular. In 1597 he quarrelled with the Earl of ESSEX (2) over the conduct of the naval war against Spain, and they remained enemies thereafter. This feud aggravated Raleigh's unpopularity. Shakespeare may have subtly sided against Raleigh in the obscure jests of *Love's Labour's Lost,* where he seemingly parodies the circle of George CHAPMAN—which included Raleigh—for its interest in magic. The playwright may have taken such a position on behalf of his patron, the Earl of SOUTHAMPTON (2), a follower of Essex, but he may also have felt a personal aversion to the reputedly irreligious and arrogant Raleigh.

King JAMES I certainly felt such an aversion, and he accepted the accusations of conspiracy brought by Raleigh's enemies, especially Robert CECIL (1), and imprisoned him. Raleigh was held in the TOWER OF LONDON from 1603 to 1616, during which time he began his *History of the World,* which is now considered, though incomplete, to be one of the best prose works of the day. He was released in order to conduct another search for El Dorado, on the king's behalf, but with the condition that he not attack the Spanish, whom James was pursuing as allies. However, while in South America, he raided a Spanish settlement, and on his return he was executed for treason.

Rambures, Lord Minor character in *Henry V,* a French nobleman. Rambures, who speaks only a few lines, shares in the French over-confidence prior to the battle of AGINCOURT in 3.7 and 4.2. His death is reported in 4.8.96, where he is said to have been the 'master of the cross-bows'. Shakespeare took this information—and the character's name—from the account of the battle in the *Chronicles* of HOLINSHED. In speech headings and stage directions of the BAD QUARTO edition of the play (1600), Rambures is designated 'Gebon', presumably indicating the actor who played the part. Scholars suppose he was either Thomas GIBBORNE or Samuel GILBURNE.

Rannius GHOST CHARACTER in *Antony and Cleopatra,* an attendant of ENOBARBUS. Rannius appears only once and does not speak. He is mentioned in the opening stage directions of 1.2, along with LAMPRIUS and LUCILLIUS.

The Rape of Lucrece Narrative poem by Shakespeare that retells the ancient Latin story of the sexual assault on Lucretia—Anglicised as LUCRECE—a high-ranking Roman woman, by Sextus Tarquinius, or TARQUIN, the son of the Roman king. Tarquin, tormented by an awareness of his own evil, proceeds to rape his victim nonetheless. Lucrece's distress is described at length, and her subsequent suicide is presented as a high-minded response to the dishonour of having slept with a man other than her husband. Before dying, Lucrece tells her husband and others of Tarquin's crime and elicits an oath of vengeance from them. The last stanza reports that they subsequently drove Tarquin and his

father from Rome. An introductory ARGUMENT makes clear that, in expelling the royal family, the avengers, led by Junius BRUTUS (2), replaced the kingdom with the Roman Republic.

Lucrece complements the slightly earlier *Venus and Adonis,* and it is clearly the 'graver labour' promised in *Venus'* dedication to the Earl of SOUTHAMPTON (2). Both works deal with sexual desire, but the reluctant male of *Venus* is a comic subject, while the ravished female of *Lucrece* is tragic. In contrast to the essential frivolity of the earlier poem, *Lucrece* is an expressly moral work, offering the lesson that disaster will result from a serious moral offence. Scholars speculate that the notoriety achieved by the somewhat salacious *Venus*—a notoriety that is evident in many surviving references—encouraged Shakespeare to appease those possibly offended—including patrons of literature or the theatre—with a second effort of greater propriety. If this was indeed his intent, he succeeded: the critic Gabriel HARVEY (2) noted, 'The younger sort takes much delight in Shakespeare's *Venus and Adonis,* but his *Lucrece* and his tragedy of *Hamlet* . . . have it in them to please the wiser sort.'

The association with *Hamlet* is no accident, for *Lucrece* is an example of a genre that 16th-century theorists classed with tragedy, the COMPLAINT, a poem intended to reflect on the hardships of life or of a particular event. Samuel DANIEL's *The Complaint of Rosalind* (1592), an extremely popular poem, is thought to have influenced Shakespeare's choice of genre. RHYME ROYAL, the verse pattern in which both *Lucrece* and Daniel's work were composed, was regarded as the most appropriate vehicle for such elevated expressions of dismay.

The bold rhyme scheme, with each stanza ending in two couplets, is also appropriate to formal rhetoric, and *Lucrece* is extremely rhetorical, filled with antitheses, virtuoso digressions, and elaborate comparisons. Often a reader can feel overwhelmed by these forced effects and tire of Lucrece's seemingly endless laments. Such baroque passages as the 26-line description of Lucrece's complexion (lines 52–77) seem excessive to modern taste, for example. In general, however, the poet's techniques enhance his points, often in ingenious ways.

But the poem is clearly more than simply a clever technical exercise. Shakespeare was fascinated by the story, and references to it recur in his plays. The character of Junius Brutus is compared to that of the king in *Henry V* (2.4.37); MACBETH, contemplating his intended murder, thinks of Tarquin approaching his victim in terms quite similar to those used in lines 162–168. In a more casual way, Lucrece is cited as a model of chastity in *The Taming of the Shrew* (2.1.289).

Although *Lucrece* is tragic, it is not like the great plays that followed it. Instead, it resembles the early tragedy *Titus Andronicus*—a drama whose central event is a rape and which contains several references to the story of Lucrece. Both works are crude and unsubtle, contrasting absolute good and absolute evil in a context of horrible violence. Nevertheless, in *Lucrece* several of the most important themes and motifs of Shakespeare's later work appeal. In writing *Macbeth* Shakespeare expanded on an interest in the psychology of evil that is presented forcefully in Tarquin's tortured self-awareness. Tarquin's inability to resist an impulse he detests also foreshadows OTHELLO's similar plight. Moreover, the same episode of the poem, in which Tarquin's emotions and motives and indecisions are intensely explored, seems likely to have established a precedent that the playwright followed in creating HAMLET. (Perhaps significantly, both Hamlet and Lucrece refer to the same symbol of despair, Hecuba—he in 2.2.552–553, she in lines 1447–1456.) As late as the writing of *Cymbeline* (1609), Shakespeare was still intrigued with Tarquin. As the subtle villain IACHIMO enters the heroine's bedchamber, he compares himself to Tarquin (2.2.12). Clearly, Shakespeare was fascinated with individuals who are willing to cut themselves off from basic morality, and his portrayal of Tarquin merits attention as an instance of that interest.

Lucrece also illustrates a type of which Shakespeare was fond, for although at first glance she may seem simply a passive victim, she is actually an interesting variation on the bold young women who star in the COMEDIES, such charmingly independent characters as BEATRICE in *Much Ado About Nothing* and PORTIA (1) in *The Merchant of Venice.* Lucrece, though she is indeed victimised, dictates the ultimate outcome of the catastrophe with a resolute will that demonstrates the same strength of character as Shakespeare's other Roman suicides, such as BRUTUS (4), 'the noblest Roman of them all' (*Julius Caesar,* 5.5.68). Her decision may disgust or perplex modern readers, but in terms of ancient Roman psychology and ethics, at least as understood by Shakespeare, she is a true heroine; her sense of honour guides her to the only response she could find correct. Realising that her despair is vain, she determines to take action (lines 1016–1029) and she lays a plan as efficiently as Portia devised hers against SHYLOCK; ignoring the opinions of the men around her (lines 1708–1710), she displays the confidence in her own sensibility that Beatrice shows when she defends her slandered cousin HERO. Like many of Shakespeare's plays, *The Rape of Lucrece* has a female lead.

Numerous touches in *Lucrece* reveal the poet's experience as a playwright. The poem begins at a point well along in the narrative provided by the Argument, reflecting a theatrical instinct to grab the reader with immediate excitement. The long digression to describe the painting of the siege of Troy (lines 1366–1561) allows time for Lucrece's messen-

ger to perform his errand, a feature that will naturally have occurred to a playwright. Tarquin and Lucrece both question themselves in sharp exchanges that resemble the stichomythia that Shakespeare and other Elizabethan dramatists took from the plays of SENECA. And Shakespeare builds sympathy for one of his characters at the expense of the other. Lucrece's extensive pleading with Tarquin serves to further deepen his villainy when he remains untouched. The more reasonably she pleads, the more monstrous is his refusal to heed her. In a like fashion, Jack CADE is blackened by refusing mercy to Lord SAY in *2 Henry VI* (4.7); CLIFFORD (1) behaves similarly to RUTLAND in *3 Henry VI* (1.3).

Also, *Lucrece* contains many passages of considerable power. The detailing of the Trojan painting, mentioned above, is extraordinary; Tarquin's torch-lit approach to Lucrece's chamber (lines 302–371) is a vivid vignette of evil on the prowl, and Lucrece is touchingly vulnerable in the four stanzas of lines 386–413. Another four-stanza passage, in which Lucrece rhetorically addresses the mythological Philomel—another rape victim—is a fine Elizabethan poem in its own right. Thus, although the poem's antique rhetoric and great length can be frustrating, *The Rape of Lucrece* deserves closer examination than it usually gets, for in it the young Shakespeare demonstrated that much greater work was to come.

Lucrece was written between April 1593, when *Venus and Adonis* was registered for publication with the STATIONERS' COMPANY, and May 1594, when it was registered itself. During the period from June 1592 to May 1594, when the London theatres were closed because of a plague epidemic and the young Shakespeare's playwriting career was interrupted, the young dramatist turned to a more prestigious mode of literature. Poetry was then regarded as the only serious form of literature—the stage was still somewhat disreputable (see ELIZABETHAN DRAMA)—and poetry was potentially much more profitable under the patronage system that prevailed at the time. As was customary, Shakespeare offered his poems to a patron by formally dedicating them to him. Shakespeare chose to address both *Venus* and *Lucrece* to the Earl of Southampton, and the earl apparently accepted them, as the dedication to *Lucrece* implies, for its air of intimacy between writer and patron is unlike any other such passage in the literature of the time. Shakespeare's friendship with Southampton is accordingly regarded as a certain feature of the playwright's life, at least in the 1590s; this is one of the few biographical facts not supported by documentary evidence that almost all scholars accept without reservation.

The tale of Lucrece and Tarquin was well known to readers in Shakespeare's day, and the poet drew on a number of familiar sources. He used two Latin texts: OVID's *Fasti* and LIVY's *Ab urbe condita,* the two earliest surviving versions of the story. Shakespeare also used an English translation of Livy from *Palace of Pleasure* (1566), by William PAINTER (2), and he was also indebted to CHAUCER's *The Legend of Good Women* (c. 1386), which was itself based on both Ovid and Livy. At least one detail in the description of the siege of Troy was taken from the *Aeneid* of VIRGIL.

The Rape of Lucrece was first published in 1594 by John HARRISON (2) in a QUARTO edition (known today as Q1) printed by Richard FIELD (2). All subsequent early editions of *Lucrece* were published in octavo format, though they are conventionally known as Q2 and so on. Q6 (1616) was the last edition to appear in Shakespeare's lifetime. Each of these editions was simply a reprint of one of its predecessors, incorporating such minor changes as the printers saw fit to make, and, while they all contain variant readings, none is thought to reflect any changes that Shakespeare made. Q1 is therefore regarded as the only authoritative text, and it is the basis for modern editions.

Ratcliffe, Sir Richard (d. 1485) Historical figure and character in *Richard III,* a follower of RICHARD III. Ratcliffe is a minor underling, distinctive chiefly for his efficient executions of RIVERS, GREY (2), and VAUGHAN in 3.3 and HASTINGS (3) in 3.4. The historical Radcliffe was a long-time and trusted adviser of Richard who had fought with him at TEWKESBURY. He died at the battle of BOSWORTH FIELD.

Ratsey, Gamaliel (d. 1605) English highwayman and theatre-goer. Ratsey was hung for his crimes in March 1605, and later in the year an anonymous biography of him, *Ratseis Ghost,* appeared, of which a single copy survives. In one episode of it, Ratsey displays a fondness for theatre and an awareness of current LONDON enthusiasms. The highwayman reportedly hired a travelling company of actors to perform for him at an inn. He delivered a detailed critique of their profession in which he complained of actors who 'are grown so wealthy that they have expected to be knighted'—a possible reference to Shakespeare's acquisition of a COAT OF ARMS. Nevertheless, he paid his players 40 shillings, twice what they expected. However, the next day he robbed them on the highway, getting back his 40 shillings and more. Before he left them he amused himself by advising the leading actor to go to London to pursue his career. He remarked on the fame of 'one man'—meaning Richard BURBAGE (3)—as HAMLET and elaborated on the possibility of earning enough money to 'buy thee some place or lordship in the country'. He was perhaps referring to the success of Shakespeare—who had bought NEW PLACE in STRATFORD eight years earlier—or, more probably, that of

William ALLEYN, who had bought a country manor in 1603.

Rebeck, Hugh Character in *Romeo and Juliet.* See MUSICIANS (2).

Redgrave, Michael (1908–1985) British actor. Redgrave, the son of actors, was briefly a teacher before turning to the theatre in 1934. After World War II he divided his time between stage and FILM. His Shakespearean parts included HAMLET—on several stages, including that at ELSINORE—LEAR, MACBETH, SHYLOCK, and ANTONY. He also wrote two plays and a book on acting. He was knighted in 1959. His daughters Vanessa (b. 1937) and Lynn (b. 1943) are well-known actresses of stage and film.

Reed, Isaac (1742–1807) British scholar, editor of the First VARIORUM EDITION of Shakespeare's works. Reed, the son of a London baker, became a lawyer but eventually focussed largely on literature. He published editions of old plays and wrote *Biographia Dramatica* (1782), a collection of critical biographies of English playwrights. Reed was a close friend of the Shakespearean scholar George STEEVENS, and he helped edit Steevens' 1785 edition of Shakespeare's works. As his friend's literary executor, he posthumously expanded his 1778 edition of Shakespeare into the First Variorum, and revised and augmented Steevens' already copious annotations.

Regan Character in *King Lear,* one of the villainous daughters of King LEAR. In 1.1 Regan and her sister GONERIL hypocritically claim to love their father in order to share the portion of the kingdom lost by the honest CORDELIA, their younger sister, who frankly admits that her husband as well as her father will receive a share of her love. Regan follows Goneril's lead, and they humiliate Lear once he has surrendered power to them and their husbands. She is led on also by her husband, the Duke of CORNWALL, and supports him when he performs the play's most appalling act of cruelty and puts out the eyes of the Earl of GLOUCESTER (1), in 3.7. Cornwall is killed while performing this deed, and Regan sets her sights on Goneril's lover, the ambitious EDMUND, but her stronger sister poisons her. Regan is last seen as she withdraws, overcome by sickness. Only later is word of her death, and of Goneril's confession as to its cause, brought to the other characters. Regan is the least distinguished of the play's villains, being chiefly a follower of her sister and her husband, though her somewhat cool and aloof quality presents a contrast with the more energetic Goneril.

Rehan, Ada (1860–1916) American actress. Born Ada Crehan (a printer's error in a playbill gave her a stage name), Rehan was for many years the leading actress in Augustin DALY's New York company. She specialised in classical comedy and played several of Shakespeare's heroines, including ROSALIND, VIOLA, and the part for which she was best known, KATHERINA in *The Taming of the Shrew.*

Reignier, Duke of Anjou and King of Naples (1409–1480) Historical figure and character in *1 Henry VI,* one of the French leaders and father of MARGARET (1). Like the other French leaders, Reignier is depicted as a boastful but ineffectual warrior who demonstrates that the French could not have defeated England but for dissensions among the English. He is not himself of any importance in the play, but his presence paves the way for the appearance of his daughter in Act 5. She will marry HENRY VI and become a principal character in *2* and *3 Henry VI.*

The historical figure on whom Reignier is based is better known as René the Good, a proverbially popular ruler of Anjou and parts of Provence, who governed his territories wisely and displayed a penchant for literature and the arts. He wrote the text and may have painted the illustrations of one of the most beautiful of late medieval manuscripts, known as *King René's Book of Love.* René inherited the kingdom of Naples, including most of southern Italy, from a distant relative, but he ruled there for only four years; he was driven out in 1442 by Alfonso of Aragon, who ruled in Sicily. However, while René retained no kingly income or power (from Naples or from more remote claims to the kingdom of Hungary and the former Crusader kingdom of Jerusalem), his royal status made him an important figure in European international relations. His daughter was thus a fitting bride for a king of England.

Reinhardt, Max (1873–1943) German theatrical producer. In the early 20th century, after 10 years as a notable character actor (specialising in old men), Reinhardt began his career as a leading avant-garde director of the classics, especially Shakespeare and the ancient Greek drama. To involve the spectators more closely than before, he extended the stage into the auditorium, where it was surrounded on three sides by seats, and he used rhythmic movements of crowds of players to sweep the audience into the world of the play (he is still considered the greatest master of crowd scenes). His use of a revolving stage quickened the pace and variety of scenes; he also added dramatic lighting and scenic effects.

Reinhardt worked mostly in Berlin until 1920 and in Vienna until 1933, but periodically produced plays in London and New York as well. In 1933 he fled the Nazi regime and lived in America for the rest of his life. Reinhardt's revolutionary techniques were both acclaimed and condemned. Particularly notable

among his Shakespearean productions were his 1912 staging of *A Midsummer Night's Dream* (which he later made as a FILM starring James Cagney and Mickey Rooney [1935]) and his 1921 presentation of *The Merchant of Venice* in a notorious blue and white cubist set.

Renaissance Period of rich development in European culture that marked the end of the Middle Ages and the beginning of the modern era. The Renaissance arose in ITALY in the 14th century and spread throughout Europe over the next 300 years, continuing its development in peripheral regions such as England through the first half of the 17th century. Characterised by humanism, which proposed a focus on human nature and individual expression in art and literature, the Renaissance was sparked by an enthusiasm for the newly rediscovered cultural worlds of classical Greece and Rome. The period saw extraordinary developments in more mundane areas as well, as secular governments emerged from the dominance of the medieval church, the modern commercial world of banks and debt-financed expansion arose, and Europe's expansion into the New World and Asia began. Printing magnified all these effects by permitting an unprecedented diffusion of ideas. The Reformation translated the age's spirit into new religious movements in many parts of northern Europe, including England, and a revitalised Counter-Reformation Catholic Church elsewhere.

In England, the Renaissance began in the early 16th century, though its greatest development was during the reign of Queen ELIZABETH (1) (1558–1603). The grandest accomplishments of the English Renaissance were in literature, especially in poetry and ELIZABETHAN DRAMA. Its leading figures in poetry were Edmund SPENSER, Philip SIDNEY, and Shakespeare and in drama, Shakespeare, Christopher MARLOWE (1), and Ben JONSON. The leading writers of prose included Thomas MORE and Francis Bacon (1561–1626). A flood of translations from Latin, Greek, and contemporary European languages enlivened England's intellectual life. John FLORIO's translation of MONTAIGNE, Arthur GOLDING's version of OVID's *Metamorphoses*, and Thomas NORTH's rendering of PLUTARCH stand out. In philosophy, *The Laws of Ecclesiastical Polity* (1593–1597) by Richard Hooker (c. 1554–1600) established a Protestant doctrine of religious government in elegant prose.

Revenge Play Genre of ELIZABETHAN and JACOBEAN DRAMA, represented in Shakespeare's work by *Titus Andronicus* and *Hamlet*. A revenge play is a drama of retribution in which an evil is avenged—and often the vengeance itself repaid—in a series of bloody and horrible deeds. Often called the horror movies of their time, revenge plays were intended to be spectacular theatrical events, and they were extremely popular. On stage they typically featured murders and physical mutilations, insanity (or feigned insanity), and supernatural visitations, all enacted in a bravura style coloured by extravagant imagery and bold rhetoric. Thomas KYD, with his *The Spanish Tragedy* (c. 1587), led English playwrights in the development of the genre, which was based largely on the works of the Roman dramatist SENECA. Other notable revenge plays include *The White Devil* (1612) and *The Duchess of Malfi* (1613–1614) by John WEBSTER (2), George CHAPMAN's *Bussy D'Ambois* (c. 1604), and the mysterious UR-HAMLET.

Of Shakespeare's two full-scale revenge plays, *Titus* is a perfect example of the genre, but *Hamlet* is somewhat restrained by a more complex attitude towards retribution. Shakespeare also included elements from the genre in other works, especially *Richard III*, *Julius Caesar*, and *Macbeth*.

Reynaldo (1) Minor character in *Hamlet*, servant of POLONIUS. In 2.1 Reynaldo is assigned to spy on his master's son, LAERTES, who is studying in PARIS (1), to make sure he is not engaging in 'such wanton, wild, and usual slips / As are companions . . . / To youth and liberty' (3.2.22–24). Reynaldo hears out his employer's long-winded instructions and departs, disappearing from the play.

This brief episode humorously illustrates the corrupt moral tone of HAMLET's DENMARK, paralleling the later, more sinister use of spies—ROSENCRANTZ AND GUILDENSTERN—by the KING (5). It also displays the intrusiveness and love of spying that eventually bring Polonius to his death. Reynaldo is clearly more sensible than his master, hesitating at times over his orders, but he has little real personality.

In the BAD QUARTO of *Hamlet*, Reynaldo is named MONTANO and Polonius, CORAMBIS. Scholars speculate that these names may reflect a satirical intention in the creation of Polonius and Reynaldo—either in Shakespeare's original conception or in his source, the UR-HAMLET—that the playwright decided not to pursue.

Reynaldo (2) Character in *All's Well That Ends Well*. See STEWARD (1).

Reynolds (1), Frederick (1764–1841) English playwright and theatrical entrepreneur, producer of operatic versions of several of Shakespeare's plays. Reynolds altered Shakespeare's texts freely, cutting large sections and often combining elements from several plays. Most of the scores for these light operas were written by Henry Rowley BISHOP (2), though he sometimes employed music written for other purposes by such composers as Mozart and Thomas ARNE. Reynolds' Shakespearean productions were *A Midsummer*

Night's Dream (1816), *The Comedy of Errors* (1819), *Twelfth Night* (1820), *Two Gentlemen of Verona* (1821), *The Tempest* (1821), *The Merry Wives of Windsor* (1824), and *The Taming of the Shrew* (1828). As a young man, Reynolds was educated as a lawyer but turned to the theatre instead. He wrote more than 200 plays, the first of which was produced in 1785. They were mostly light comedies and melodramas; his most popular work, *The Caravan* (1803), featured a live dog that performed an on-stage rescue of a child from a tank of water.

Reynolds (2), William (1575–1633) Resident of STRATFORD and friend of Shakespeare. In his will, Shakespeare left Reynolds money to buy a memorial ring, a common gesture of friendship, but no more is known of their relationship. Reynolds was a Catholic whose family sheltered a Jesuit priest in the dangerous days of the early 17th century, when anti-Catholic feeling ran high in England. He prospered, however, and died one of the principal landowners of Stratford.

Rhyme Royal Verse pattern in which a stanza has seven lines, each in iambic pentameter (see METRE), rhyming *ababbcc.* Rhyme royal is used in *The Rape of Lucrece* and *The Lover's Complaint;* each of these works is a COMPLAINT, a genre for which the pattern was recommended by 16th-century treatises on poetry. This practise was doubtless inspired by CHAUCER's great use of rhyme royal, which is still sometimes called the Chaucerian stanza. Rhyme royal dominated English poetry in the 15th and 16th centuries. It went out of style entirely in the early 17th century, although it has reappeared occasionally in recent times—e.g., in long poems by John Masefield and W. H. Auden. Rhyme royal is a form of great flexibility and power, capable of carrying a sustained narrative without becoming monotonous, and its subtle rhyming is well suited to a wide range of effects, from simple description to ironic witticism.

Rice, John (active 1607–1630) English actor, a member of the KING'S MEN and one of the 26 men listed in the FIRST FOLIO as the 'Principall Actors' in Shakespeare's plays. As a boy actor, Rice was the apprentice of John HEMINGE in 1607. He is thought to have been considered the best boy actor in the company, for twice, in 1607 and 1610, the King's Men paired him with their leading actor, Richard BURBAGE (3), when they provided players for ceremonial occasions. In 1611 Rice was a member of the LADY ELIZABETH'S MEN, but he rejoined the King's Men in 1619. No record of Rice as an actor has survived after 1625, but he is probably the 'John Rice, clerk of St Saviour's' mentioned by Heminge in his will (1630), so it appears that he retired from the stage and became a church official.

Rich (1), Barnabe (Barnaby Riche) (c. 1540–1617) Contemporary of Shakespeare, author of the principal source of *Twelfth Night.* Rich was a soldier who retired from a career of active campaigning in Europe and Ireland and turned to literature. He wrote several tracts on military and political matters, but he is best known for a collection of romantic tales, derived mostly from Italian originals. One, entitled 'Apolonius and Silla'—taken from a tale by François BELLEFOREST, who had it from an anonymous Italian play, *Gl'Ingannati*—provided Shakespeare with the main plot of *Twelfth Night.* Another of Rich's tales may have inspired FALSTAFF's departure in a laundry basket in 3.3 of *The Merry Wives of Windsor.*

Rich (2), John (1692–1761) British theatrical producer. Rich was a comic actor who popularised the COMMEDIA DELL'ARTE character Harlequin in England, but he is much better known as a theatrical entrepreneur. Rich staged a number of Shakespeare's plays with a company whose leading player was James QUIN. Rich's productions of *Measure for Measure* (1720) and *Much Ado About Nothing* (1721) were especially important, in that they restored much of Shakespeare's text after William DAVENANT's radical alterations. Rich was the founder of London's Covent Garden Theatre in 1733. In the 1750s he produced *Romeo and Juliet* with Spranger BARRY (3) as ROMEO, in rivalry with David GARRICK's presentation, in the '*Romeo and Juliet* war'.

Richard II, King of England (1367–1400) Title character of *Richard II,* king deposed by Henry BOLINGBROKE (1). Richard is a self-centred man and an inept ruler; his fall seems both deserved and inevitable. Nevertheless, Shakespeare elicits strong sympathy for the fallen king as he suffers painful psychological trauma before coming to accept his fate.

It is quickly established that Richard is an incompetent king. In 1.2 we learn that Richard, before the play begins, had arranged the murder of his uncle the Duke of GLOUCESTER (6), an admired member of the royal family. Furthermore, his ordinary conduct as king is persistently disastrous. When his 'coffers, with too great a court / And liberal largess, are grown somewhat light' (1.4.43–44), he turns to extortionate abuses of the public. And he seizes the estate of John of GAUNT, rightly the inheritance of the exiled Bolingbroke. This not only stimulates Bolingbroke's rebellion, but it alarms many other nobles, who fear that their own holdings may similarly be in jeopardy. Richard's wrong-headedness is exemplified by his obstinate refusal to heed the good advice of his uncles Gaunt and the Duke of YORK (4). He delights in ceremony and the trappings of power, and his rhetoric is windy. Narcissistic and arrogant, he does not rule; he enjoys himself in the role of ruler.

Despite all his boasting, Richard cannot use the power of his position, and Bolingbroke's triumph, when it comes, is almost effortless.

However, in political decline Richard becomes a more sympathetic character. His speech is no less extravagant, but now his mannered style is plainly a manifestation of inner distress. He is a more complex person than he had seemed earlier; in his isolation, he is intensely introspective and racked with anxiety, alternating between unjustified hope and exaggerated despair. Finally, imprisoned and due to be killed, he acknowledges that his own failings have played some part in his fall: 'I wasted time, and now doth time waste me' (5.5.49). Richard, with his penchant for strong imagery and elaborate metaphor, is the first of Shakespeare's protagonists to demonstrate an extraordinary imagination and artistic sense. A complex and ambiguous personality, Richard foreshadows the great heroes of Shakespeare's later TRAGEDIES.

Richard's poetic language and love of ceremony place him in striking opposition to the prosaic and practical Bolingbroke. This powerful contrast reflects a basic human conflict between the doer and the dreamer. It also enhances Richard's strong symbolic role as the last representative of the medieval England of Edward III, in which the ethos of chivalry was still dominant. The passing of this nostalgically romantic period is a major theme of the play.

The historical Richard is for the most part ignored by Shakespeare, who focusses entirely on the last year of a 22-year reign. When Edward III died, Richard, his grandson and heir (see PLANTAGENET [1]), was only 10 years old. The young king seems to have been fond of pomp and splendour, and he had a reputation as a dilettante, but he was also courageous. At 14 he faced a murderous crowd during the great peasants' rebellion of 1381 and convinced them to disperse. However, England was governed during Richard's minority by his uncles, especially the Duke of Gloucester. When Richard attempted to assert himself 10 years later, an armed conflict ensued and Richard was nearly forced from the throne. A coalition of nobles ruled for two years, but Richard gathered supporters and successfully began to rule at the age of 22. He seems to have governed well. His reign was noted for his emphasis on peace; he concluded truces in Ireland in 1394 and, more important, in the HUNDRED YEARS WAR against FRANCE (1) in 1396. (By the latter treaty, he agreed to marry the young Princess Isabel, who was a child, not the adult QUEEN [13] of the play.) In 1397 another rupture between the king and Gloucester resulted in the duke's imprisonment and death. Modern scholarship tends to confirm the contemporary opinion that Richard was responsible for his uncle's murder, but the truth cannot be ascertained.

The political events of the play are roughly accurate—Shakespeare followed his sources, for the most part—but the emphasis on Richard's incompetence is distinctly overdrawn. His departure for Ireland, shortly after seizing Gaunt's estate and alienating the nobility, was a grave error, but even worse was his delay in returning once Bolingbroke's invasion had begun. This procrastination, as well as the dismissal of much of his force upon arrival in England, appears to have been advised by Richard's second-in-command, AUMERLE, who promptly deserted his master, an event that Shakespeare omits. Richard was given sworn oaths by NORTHUMBERLAND (1), who was speaking for Bolingbroke, that the latter did not intend usurpation and would disarm if Gaunt's titles and estates were restored to him. Richard accepted these terms and unknowingly allowed himself to be taken prisoner. Thus his final fall was due as much to treachery as to wrongdoing on his part. The deposition scene (4.1) is entirely fictitious; Bolingbroke certainly could not afford to give his enemy a platform, and he did not. Sir Piers EXTON's murder of Richard is also a fiction, although Shakespeare took it from his source and doubtless believed it. A contemporary report states that Richard died of starvation, either deprived of food by his gaolers or refusing to eat. The actual circumstances of Richard's death are not known, although his bones were exhumed in 1871 and no signs of violence were found.

Richard II

SYNOPSIS

Act 1, Scene 1

Henry BOLINGBROKE (1) appears before his cousin King RICHARD II and accuses Thomas MOWBRAY (1) of treason for having embezzled funds, hatched unspecified plots, and murdered Thomas, Duke of GLOUCESTER (6), Bolingbroke and the king's uncle. Mowbray claims innocence and demands a trial by combat. Despite Richard's appeals seconded by Bolingbroke's father, John of GAUNT, the two noblemen insist on fighting; Richard gives in and designates a time and place for the encounter.

Act 1, Scene 2

The DUCHESS (2) of Gloucester, widow of Thomas, demands that Gaunt avenge her husband's murder, but he replies that, since the murder was ordered by the king, God's deputy, vengeance can be exacted only by God. The Duchess then prays that Mowbray shall be killed in the trial by combat.

Act 1, Scene 3

Mowbray and Bolingbroke prepare for the trial by combat, but at the last moment the king rules that the two disputants shall be banished from England—

Bolingbroke for 10 years, Mowbray for life. Before departing, Mowbray asserts that Bolingbroke's disloyalty will eventually surface, to Richard's regret. Richard, seeing Gaunt's despair at his son's banishment, reduces the sentence to six years, but Gaunt replies that he shall die before that time is up. The king, unmoved, departs. Gaunt attempts to cheer up his disheartened son, but to no avail.

Act 1, Scene 4
The Duke of AUMERLE, who has pretended friendship with Bolingbroke, reports to the king that that nobleman has left England. Richard reveals his enmity towards Bolingbroke, on account of the latter's widespread popularity. Sir Henry GREENE (1) remarks that a rebellion in Ireland requires the king's attention, and Richard says that he will lead an army there. This expedition will be financed by selling to entrepreneurs the right to collect taxes and by forcing loans from wealthy noblemen. Sir John BUSHY brings news that John of Gaunt is very sick and has asked to see the king. Richard hopes for his immediate death so that he may confiscate his wealth for the Irish campaign.

Act 2, Scene 1
The dying Gaunt confides to his brother the Duke of YORK (4) his desire to give good counsel to Richard before he dies, and he goes on to rage against the king's shady financial practises. The king arrives with a group of nobles. Gaunt reprimands him, and the angry Richard reminds his uncle of his power to have him killed; Gaunt dares him to do so, accusing him of the murder of Gloucester and asserting that the shame the king has brought on the family will kill him in any case. Gaunt retires to bed, asserting that he will soon die. The Earl of NORTHUMBERLAND (1) brings word that Gaunt has in fact died, and Richard immediately declares that he will confiscate his late uncle's wealth. York, horrified, chastises the king for this illegal seizure, comparing it ominously with the usurpation of a crown. He then exits. The king, ignoring this outburst, plans his departure for Ireland and appoints York to be governor of England in his absence. He leaves with his entourage. The remaining nobles—Northumberland, Lord ROSS (2), and Lord WILLOUGHBY (3)—discuss the king's abuses. They fear that the seizure of Gaunt's estate will set a precedent that threatens all aristocrats. Northumberland reveals that Bolingbroke is returning to England with an army, and the noblemen decide to join him.

Act 2, Scene 2
The QUEEN (13) speaks to Bushy and BAGOT of her strange grief and depression, stimulated by Richard's departure for Ireland. Greene arrives with news that Bolingbroke has invaded England and been joined by several noblemen. York arrives, bewailing the difficulty of defending the realm when Richard has taken all available armed forces with him. A SERVANT (7) brings word of the death of the Duchess of Gloucester, from whom York had hoped to borrow money. York, undone by this news, wishes Richard had cut off his head so that he would not have to deal with his present dilemma: both king and invader are his kinsmen, and he feels he owes loyalty to each of them. Uncertain what to do, York leaves with the Queen. Bushy, Bagot, and Greene decide to flee, realising that trouble lies ahead for the king's favourites.

Act 2, Scene 3
Bolingbroke and Northumberland, on the march, meet Northumberland's son Harry PERCY (2), who brings news that York and a small force are stationed nearby at Berkeley Castle. Ross and Willoughby also join the invading army. Lord BERKELEY enters. He bears York's demand that Bolingbroke explain his presence in England. York himself follows, and he castigates his nephew for disloyalty to the king. Bolingbroke insists that he has returned only to claim what is rightfully his—the estate of his father, Gaunt. Bolingbroke's supporters back him up. York continues to insist on the treasonous nature of their opposition to the king, but he declares that he will remain neutral, lacking power enough to oppose them, and he offers them the hospitality of the castle. Bolingbroke says that he must first go to BRISTOL to capture Bushy and Bagot.

Act 2, Scene 4
A Welsh CAPTAIN (4) tells the Earl of SALISBURY (1) that his troops cannot be prevented from deserting Richard's cause, after 10 days with no word from the king. He tells of rumours that Richard is dead and cites dire omens that seem to support them. Salisbury foresees Richard's fall.

Act 3, Scene 1
Bushy and Greene are prisoners of Bolingbroke, who condemns them to death, asserting that they have misled the king and caused bad relations between the king and his queen. Further, Bolingbroke alleges that they caused the king to banish him and that they then took his property in his absence.

Act 3, Scene 2
Richard, having returned from Ireland, responds to news of Bolingbroke's successes with wild emotional swings, veering between confidence in divine support and dark despair. Finally, informed that York has joined Bolingbroke, he subsides into resignation and concedes defeat.

Act 3, Scene 3
Bolingbroke, outside FLINT CASTLE, learns that the king has sequestered himself within, and he sends

Northumberland to negotiate with him, offering to submit completely to Richard provided that Gaunt's estates are restored to him and that his banishment is repealed. Richard appears with kingly pomp and arrogance, but he immediately agrees to Bolingbroke's terms. Awaiting Bolingbroke himself, Richard falls into despair, ranting about his own deposition and death. When Bolingbroke appears, Richard accepts the successful rebel's pretended submission but remarks that he has merely yielded to strength.

Act 3, Scene 4
The disconsolate Queen hides herself in a garden, hoping to overhear political news in the conversation of the GARDENER and his assistants. The Gardener tells of the executions of Bushy and Greene and speculates that the king, having been seized by Bolingbroke, will soon be deposed. The Queen erupts in anger, demanding to know why the Gardener thinks this; he asserts that Richard's situation is common knowledge in London. The Queen, enraged and in despair, leaves for the city.

Act 4, Scene 1
In WESTMINSTER (3) HALL Bolingbroke holds court. Bagot, who has turned informer, accuses Aumerle of having plotted to murder the Duke of Gloucester. After much argument, the debate is postponed, to be settled at a future trial by combat. York brings word of Richard's willingness to abdicate. The Bishop of CARLISLE speaks against the deposition of God's appointed ruler, predicting civil war as a consequence. He is arrested by Northumberland and placed in the custody of the ABBOT of Westminster. Richard is summoned, and he reluctantly surrenders his crown and sceptre to Bolingbroke. Looking in a mirror, he reflects on the fragility of kingly glory, and he smashes the glass to prove his point. Richard is taken away, and Bolingbroke, departing with his entourage, sets the date for his own coronation. Aumerle, the Abbot, and Carlisle are left behind, and they agree to plot against Bolingbroke's usurpation.

Act 5, Scene 1
The Queen intercepts Richard as he is escorted to the TOWER OF LONDON and tries to raise his spirits. He recommends patient resignation. Northumberland appears with a change of plans: Richard is to be taken to POMFRET CASTLE, and the Queen is to be banished to FRANCE (1). Northumberland resists their pleas that they be permitted to remain together, and the royal couple bid each other an emotional farewell.

Act 5, Scene 2
The Duke of York, after describing Bolingbroke's triumphant entry into London to the DUCHESS (4), asserts his adherence, however dismayed, to the new king. He discovers that his son, Aumerle, is part of a plot against Bolingbroke, and he sets off to warn the king and, to alleviate the stain on his honour, turn in his son. The Duchess fails to persuade him against this course; she then tells Aumerle to ride at top speed and reach the King before his father can and plead for mercy.

Act 5, Scene 3
Bolingbroke laments that his delinquent son, the PRINCE (6), spends his time with criminals and harlots, but he hopes for better behaviour in the future. Aumerle enters and extracts a promise of a pardon for an offence that he wishes to confess. York arrives and warns the king of the plot against him, recommending severity. The Duchess enters and pleads for mercy for Aumerle, and Bolingbroke grants it.

Act 5, Scene 4
Sir Piers EXTON, reflecting on remarks made by Bolingbroke, believes that the new king wants Richard killed, and he resolves to do the deed himself.

Act 5, Scene 5
Richard, in his prison cell, meditates on his lonely, defeated state. A former GROOM of Richard's appears, offering sympathy and raising the prisoner's spirits. However, he is ousted by the KEEPER (4), who brings Richard's meal. The Keeper refuses to taste the food for poison, as is his usual practise, citing orders from Exton. Aggravated, Richard strikes him, and the Keeper's cries summon a group of murderers, led by Exton, who assault Richard. He fights back but is killed. Exton, conscience-stricken, regrets the deed.

Act 5, Scene 6
Bolingbroke receives word of the final defeat of resistance to his rule, including that of the Bishop of Carlisle, who is brought in as a prisoner. Bolingbroke forgives him magnanimously. Exton arrives with a coffin bearing Richard. He expects thanks, but Bolingbroke repudiates him, deploring the deed and regretting that his words had sparked it. He declares that he will lead a crusade to the Holy Land to atone for his part in Richard's death.

COMMENTARY

Shakespeare wrote *Richard II* entirely in verse. The measured cadences of iambic pentameter lend a musical grandeur to the play's most didactic and explanatory passages, and the medium of verse is natural to its highly charged language. In this play emotions are expressed by means of heightened rhetoric. For instance, the parting of Richard and the Queen in 5.1 sparks an exchange of mechanical couplets that may seem emotionally sterile. But taken over the entire work, such language impels respect, for it is

boldly apparent that the characters are in the grip of something higher and more important than their own personalities. The total dominance of poetry lends the play a pointedly aesthetic tone, in striking contrast to its ostensible subject matter, a military coup. The play depicts no battles; in fact, there is little action of any kind. A trial by combat is scheduled but does not take place; an army is assembled but does not fight. York vows to resist Bolingbroke but lacks the strength to do so, and Richard crumbles immediately. Action is systematically thwarted until Richard's murder in Act 5. Language, in the form of poetry, is paramount. The disparity between political history and poetic tone points to the existence of a second level of meaning: this play is about more than the deeds of historical figures. *Richard II* basically deals with the disturbing nature of historical change rather than the events themselves.

In addition, *Richard II* is a moving human document. Richard's personality is the most prominent feature of the play, and, in one of his most brilliant portraits, Shakespeare shows us a gallant but failing human effort to come to terms with change. Richard marks a significant stage in the development of the playwright's art, for he is the first of Shakespeare's tragic heroes whose personal flaws help to bring about his own downfall. His own inadequacies as king lead inexorably to his deposition. However, Richard's greater significance lies in his response to his fate. He does not resist his destiny but accepts it. In 5.5, stirred by the beauty of music and by the love of the Groom who visits him, the imprisoned Richard comes to terms with his humanity and the suffering that goes with it. With this acceptance, Richard—and we who respond to him—transcend the universal fate and thus triumph over death.

Furthermore, Richard is persistently contrasted with the world around him. At the most superficial level, the play depicts the fall of one king and the rise of another, and this automatically invites comparison between the two rulers. Richard's poetic diction and his assertion of transcendent values stand in marked contrast with the prosaic speech and practical concerns of Bolingbroke and York, and even of the Queen, who exhorts him to fight. The play presents a bold juxtaposition of utilitarian and artistic temperaments.

Yet the play also involves a comparison of worlds. Richard's sensibility, his poetic utterances, and his self-conscious awareness of his royal status are grounded in a world of ceremonious spectacle. The gorgeous tournament of 1.1 and Richard's brilliant rhetoric on the divine right of kings, as in 3.2.36–62, have a heavy grandeur that is reinforced by such formal speeches as the conventionally high-flown grief of the Queen in 3.4 and the elaborate metaphor constructed by the Gardener in the same scene. Richard is a medieval king, fully conscious of his divine appointment to rule; his personal weaknesses emphasise the pathos of being the last such ruler in history. Bolingbroke represents a new world, that of the Renaissance. He is a Machiavellian, ready to assume any posture required by the needs of the moment. This brings him political success, but it also makes him an unknowable personality, a symbol of faceless ambition. By contrast, Richard's emotional self-exposure is much more humanly sympathetic. The rising and falling monarchs are most strikingly opposed in 4.1, in which the mere presence of the nearly silent Bolingbroke has as powerful an effect as Richard's polemics. Each regal figure attempts to impose his own reality on the scene: Richard plays the tragically overthrown representative of God, while Bolingbroke maintains the importance of legal rights and social order.

It is profoundly ironic that the anointed ruler has subverted public order, while the blasphemous rebel upholds legality. Richard, though legitimate, has failed to lead his nation and moreover has exploited the kingdom shamelessly, while the usurper Bolingbroke acts in the name of legal redress and proves to be a strong leader who brings England into a new era. Underlying this paradox is a question that was posed by Shakespeare's portrayal of King HENRY VI and that was to be answered by that of HENRY V: can the spiritual qualities that seem to offer the greatest human rewards coexist with the practical, manipulative skills needed to govern a society? In *Richard II* a potentially successful government has been created, but only at the cost of eroding the spiritual underpinnings of society. The civil disorders to come are the direct result, as Carlisle's predictions in 4.1.136–147 and 322–323 remind us.

Both principal figures of *Richard II* achieve their potential yet remain ungratified: Richard's spiritual depths open upon an abyss, while Bolingbroke's political success is dampened by the need for suppression, beginning with Richard's murder This situation reflects a contradiction at the heart of the Elizabethan conception of power: a monarch was still considered to be ordained by God, as had been true in medieval times, but a newer notion dictated that he or she was expressly sent to serve the people. This concept, which was part of early modern Europe's emergence from feudalism, was related to political developments—in England, it was part of the TUDOR dynasty's justification of Henry VII's conquest (enacted in *Richard III*): the deposed king had failed to serve the people, and the new king had been sent by God to do so. Thus a ruler should not be deposed, but, if he were, the usurper should not be replaced either. In this conundrum rested the legiti-

macy of the reign of Queen ELIZABETH (1) and the established politics of Shakespeare's own day. In *Richard II* it is demonstrated in the ultimate inadequacy of both the usurped king and the successful rebel.

Possible solutions to this puzzling irony are offered by Shakespeare, but only as hints concerning the play's sequels. *Richard II* was consciously written as the first in a series of plays, and it is not intended to come to a conclusion. Bolingbroke, soon to be King HENRY IV, becomes more magnanimous as the play closes, pardoning Carlisle and Aumerle and spurning Exton. He turns to religion as well. Thus an improvement in the character of the usurper is at least tentatively proposed. However, Bolingbroke's essential cynicism in this play makes such a solution difficult to believe. More promising is the introduction of a character who does not actually appear, Bolingbroke's son, PRINCE (6) HAL. His bold ridicule of his father's success, as reported by Percy in 5.3.16–19, may seem immature and unproductive, but it is undeniably fresh and youthful; Hal, at least, is entirely outside the coils of politics. His time will come (as the audience knows)—as Henry V, he will be a successful king. Thus history generates its own solution to history's dilemma: whatever may befall a king or a world, youth is always preparing new history.

Finally, too, the invocation of the future suggests the larger framework of *Richard II* and of all the HISTORY PLAYS. *Richard II* introduces the grand theme of the entire cycle: the passage of England from prosperity lost through lack of respect for a divinely ordained order, to civil disruption and war, to a resumption of prosperity under the Tudors.

As was his custom, Shakespeare took some liberties with the history his play chronicles, tightening the pace where it is dramatically desirable—particularly in 2.1 and 4.1, where in each case the happenings of months are compressed into a single day—but the treatment of historical events is much more straightforward than is the case in the earlier histories. Bolingbroke is probably a more deliberate rebel than the playwright's sources demand, and Richard is certainly a more ineffective king, but these distortions serve an aesthetic purpose, illuminating greater issues. Shakespeare always subordinates historical details to a playwright's values, and *Richard II* is, above all, a dramatic presentation of human responses to inexorable change.

SOURCES OF THE PLAY

Shakespeare's primary source for the historical material in *Richard II* was Raphael HOLINSHED's *Chronicles of England, Scotland, and Ireland* (2nd. ed., 1587). In addition, Act 5 was particularly influenced by an epic poem, *The Civil Wars between the two Houses of York and Lancaster*, by Samuel DANIEL, which was published in early 1595, just as Shakespeare was working on this play. Another important source was a popular anthology of biographies in verse, A MIRROR FOR MAGISTRATES (1559), which contains lives of Richard, Northumberland, Mowbray, and the Duke of Gloucester. Shakespeare's John of Gaunt, very different from Holinshed's, was probably derived from the characterisation of the Duke of Gloucester in the anonymous play WOODSTOCK (c. 1592–1595), which provided many other small hints to Shakespeare. Another influence may have been the Gaunt presented in Jean FROISSART's *Chroniques*, a French history that Shakespeare could have known in the English translation (1523–1525) by Lord BERNERS. Two French works written in defence of Richard in his own time, an anonymous chronicle known as the TRAÏSON and a poem by Jean CRÉTON, *Histoire du Roy d'Angleterre Richard*, may have been available to Shakespeare and have been suggested by scholars as possible sources for minor elements. *Edward II* (c. 1592) by Christopher MARLOWE (1) may have influenced Shakespeare's general conception of a flawed king whose downfall is triggered by immoral behaviour.

TEXT OF THE PLAY

Shakespeare completed the text of *Richard II* sometime before its publication in mid-1597 and after the publication of Daniel's *Civil War* in early 1595. The similarity of its lyrical tone to that of *Love's Labour's Lost*, *Romeo and Juliet*, and *A Midsummer Night's Dream*, all written in 1594 and 1595, suggest that *Richard II* was probably written in 1595.

The play was published by Andrew WISE in a QUARTO edition, known as Q1, in 1597. The play must have been popular, because Wise brought out two more quartos (Q2, Q3) in 1598. (*Pericles* is the only other Shakespeare play to have appeared in two quartos in the same year.) These editions were reprinted from Q1 and are inferior to it, having many more errors, although some corrections were also made. Wise sold his right to print the play to Mathew LAW in 1603, and Law produced Q4 (1608) and Q5 (1615), each drawn from its immediate predecessor. Q4 contains the first printing of the deposition scene (4.1.154–318), which had earlier been withheld, presumably due to government CENSORSHIP. It seems to have been printed from a 'memorial' version, dictated or written from memory by an actor. In 1623 the FIRST FOLIO contained a version of the play (F1) that appears to have been printed from Q3, except for its last few columns, taken from Q5. (This peculiarity is thought to reflect a damaged copy of Q3, repaired with two pages from Q5.) However, F1 contains a version of the deposition scene that is greatly superior to that in Q4 and Q5, where it is clearly corrupt. This is presumed to have come from a

PROMPT-BOOK that was also used to correct the Quarto copy.

Q1 is thought to have been printed from a transcript of Shakespeare's own manuscript, for it contains irregular stage directions and other signs of the author's informal version, along with errors that seem likely to have been made by someone who already knew the play, probably a member of the cast in an early production. Thus Q1 is the basis for most modern editions, supplemented by F1, from which is taken, in particular, 4.1.154–318.

THEATRICAL HISTORY OF THE PLAY

Its repeated publication in the 1590s and early 17th century suggests that *Richard II* was quite popular with early audiences. The earliest surviving record of a particular performance is a startling one. On February 7, 1601, the CHAMBERLAIN'S MEN were commissioned by backers of the Earl of ESSEX (2) to perform the play at the GLOBE Theatre. The Earl's abortive rebellion against Queen ELIZABETH (1) took place on the following day, and it was apparently thought that the enactment of Richard's deposition would encourage the population of London to support a latter-day usurpation. It had no such effect, and, although inquiries were made by the government, no action was taken against the acting company or Shakespeare.

The second known performance of the play is also surprising: in 1607 it was performed aboard an English ship off the coast of Africa. No other particular performances during Shakespeare's lifetime are known, although the play was staged at the Globe again in 1631.

In 1681 Nahum TATE produced an adaptation of *Richard II, The Sicilian Usurper,* that was suppressed by a nervous government, despite its changed setting. Other adaptations were produced over the next century, often with material borrowed from other plays, including *King Lear* and *Titus Andronicus.* Shakespeare's play was produced several times in the late 1730s, but the play was not generally popular again until the 19th century. In a highly successful production of 1857, Charles KEAN (1) used more than 500 extras in a spectacular rendition of Bolingbroke's triumph. Beerbohm TREE and William POEL also directed versions of the play. *Richard II* has been extremely popular in the 20th century. John GIELGUD and Maurice EVANS (4) have been particularly successful Richards. The play has been produced many times in recent years, both by itself and in cycles with other history plays, on stage and on TELEVISION.

Richard III, King of England (1452–1485) Character in *2* and *3 Henry VI* and title character of *Richard III.* Known simply as Richard or Gloucester (see GLOUCESTER [5]) until he is crowned in 4.2 of *Richard III,* his ambition never ceases to drive him towards that moment. Richard is more than simply a villain; his dazzlingly evil nature, combining viciousness and wit, makes him as important and valuable to the drama, especially in *Richard III,* as any hero. He was Shakespeare's first great creation, marking a tremendous advance over earlier, more ordinary characters.

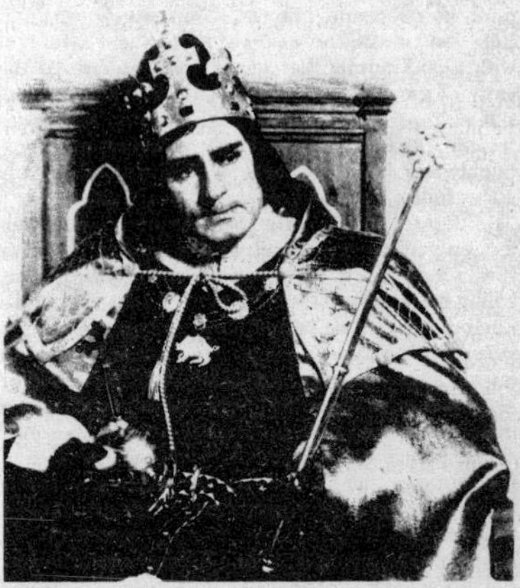

Richard III (played here by Laurence Olivier) was Shakespeare's first great creation. A dazzlingly evil villain, he is as dramatically rich as many of the heroes of later plays. (Courtesy of Culver Pictures, Inc.)

Richard makes his first appearance late in *2 Henry VI,* when he is called to support his father, the Duke of YORK (8). His role is minor; he is present chiefly as a foreshadowing of the sequels to the play. He is nevertheless a cleanly drawn figure, sardonically epigrammatic. For instance, he encourages himself in battle with the cry, 'Priests pray for enemies, but princes kill' (5.2.71). His bold and wilfully, even pridefully, cruel nature is already evident, after only a few lines.

In 1.1 of *3 Henry VI* Richard's extraordinary personality bursts forth. As the nobles recount their exploits at the battle of ST. ALBANS, Richard abruptly throws down the head of SOMERSET (1), saying, 'Speak thou for me, and tell them what I did (1.1. 16).' Richard's blood-thirstiness, not unmixed with dry humour, is evident throughout the play, pointing towards the horrors he is to commit in *Richard III.* In his famous soliloquy at the end of 3.2, he describes himself as able to '. . . smile, and murder whiles I smile'; he will 'set the murderous Machiavel to

school' (3.2.182, 193). Killing the imprisoned King HENRY VI, Richard raises his bloody sword and sarcastically crows, 'See how my sword weeps for the poor king's death' (5.6.63). This bloody villain is fully conscious of his own viciousness and savours it with a cocky irony that seems very modern. At the close of the play, he even delightedly identifies himself with the arch-traitor of Christian tradition, Judas Iscariot. Richard's monstrously evil nature is thoroughly established in *3 Henry VI,* in order that it may attain fullest fruition in *Richard III.*

In *Richard III* the title character has the second-longest part in all of Shakespeare's work (only HAMLET speaks more lines). He murders his way to the throne, killing his brother, his young nephews, his wife, and a number of political opponents. He is still a spectacular villain, with a fondness for commenting humorously on his atrocities before committing them. Once he becomes king, however, his wit and resourcefulness desert him; he clumsily alienates his allies, and quite simply panics when he first learns of the approach of RICHMOND. In Act 5 he dies in battle, defeated at BOSWORTH FIELD. Richmond's triumph releases England from the violence and treachery of the WARS OF THE ROSES.

The personality of Shakespeare's Richard is formed in part by his physical deformity—a hunched back—referred to many times in the plays, often by Richard himself. At the end of *3 Henry VI,* for instance, he says, '. . . since the heavens have shap'd my body so, / Let hell make crook'd my mind to answer it' (5.6.78–79). He rationalises his rejection of human loyalties by theorising that his physical nature has placed him beyond ordinary relationships. Thus he can claim, 'I am myself alone' (5.6.83). Others agree with him: a number of characters associate Richard's deformity with his evil nature. Queen MARGARET (1), for example, asserts, 'Sin, death, and hell have set their marks on him . . .' (*Richard III,* 1.3.293), and various of his enemies identify him with a range of carnivorous animals and with such repulsive creatures as spiders, toads, and reptiles.

However, our fascination with Richard derives largely from the disturbing reality that he has undeniably attractive qualities as well. He has charisma and self-confidence, and he is plainly quite intelligent. He has great energy combined with immense self-control, and, probably most tellingly, he is extremely witty. He cracks a joke even as he plots the murder of his brother in 1.1.118–120 of *Richard III.*

Richard wins admiration even as he repels because he plays to the audience directly. Through his monologues and asides, he brings us into an almost conspiratorial intimacy with him. He sometimes tells us what is shortly going to occur, and then comments on it afterwards. In practising deceit, he also takes on different roles, much as an actor does: he plays a loyal follower of his brother King EDWARD IV, a lover opposite Lady ANNE (2), a friend to his brother CLARENCE (1), and a pious devotee of religion before the MAYOR (3) and his entourage.

With the collapse of his fortunes, Richard's personality changes. He loses his resilience and subtlety; he panics and is disorganised in the face of crisis. We learn that his sleep is troubled; such insomnia was a traditional consequence for royal usurpers, and Shakespeare's sources impute it to Richard conventionally, but the playwright makes more of it, letting both Anne and Richard himself remark on it, before presenting us with an actual nightmare vision in 5.3 of *Richard III.* At this low ebb, Richard seems almost deranged. He recognises his terrible isolation from humanity and despairs, crying out in anguish that his death will neither receive nor deserve pity from anyone. However, Richard recovers his spirit later in the scene and leads his men into battle with renewed flippancy.

Richard represents a well-known type who was a popular figure on the Elizabethan stage, the grandiose villain, first embodied in *Tamburlaine,* by Christopher MARLOWE (1), still popular when *Richard III* premiered. However, the character has a longer pedigree than that. The medieval MORALITY PLAY featured a villain figure, the VICE, whose resemblance to characters in Shakespeare and Marlowe is not coincidental; both writers must have been familiar with the Vice since childhood. But Richard also incorporates a more modern archetype, the MACHIAVEL, a calculating politician whose misdeeds are directed towards particular ends. The Vice's lewd jests and common horseplay give way to a grave assessment of political interest, although verbal wit is part of the Machiavel's character. The Machiavel is a naturalistic figure—a human being, if a depraved one—while the Vice is more allegorical in nature. Thus Richard's personality has a humanly believable quality that is lacking in the criminal-king of traditional history.

It is plain that Shakespeare's character bears very little resemblance to the actual King Richard III, who ruled only briefly. Surviving accounts of his times were written largely by his enemies, and modern scholarship has discovered that the reality of his reign bore little resemblance to the version Shakespeare received and popularised.

Richard has long been envisioned as the physically repellent hunchback of legend. Thomas MORE first wrote of Richard's physical deformity, and Shakespeare followed suit. However, at his coronation Richard was stripped to the waist for anointing, in accordance with tradition, and this exposure seems to have provoked no comment. In fact, a hunched back is nowhere evident in contemporary portraits or accounts of the man. It appears to have been a malicious fiction, although Shakespeare surely believed it to be true.

More interesting are the playwright's purposeful alterations of the historical record as he had it. As was his usual practise, Shakespeare took many liberties with his already unreliable sources. For instance, at the end of *2 Henry VI,* Richard is made to participate in a battle that occurred when he was only three years old. Richard actually lived in exile until after Edward was crowned. His part in history did not begin until the battle of BARNET, enacted in Act 5 of *3 Henry VI.* Shakespeare wrote him into the action earlier, in order to begin to approach the grand denouncement in *Richard III,* which he must have foreseen as he wrote the *Henry VI* plays. Richard also provides an interesting foil for Edward's tenderer character.

This premature introduction is magnified by giving Richard the desire to rule long before the question arises in the sources. Shakespeare's Richard begins to think, 'How sweet a thing it is to wear a crown' (*3 Henry VI,* 1.2.29), fully 23 years before he comes to put one on. Not only does this generate a long, slow rise in tension, but it also emphasises Richard's nefarious ambition early. Thus, when he is finally brought down, the resolution of England's predicament is a clear one: Richard's career has been so strikingly criminal that his death stimulates no further fighting in revenge.

The historical Richard was a very different man, innocent of most, if not all, of the crimes imputed to him. Shakespeare's sources attributed the murder of HENRY VI to Richard, and the playwright added urgency to his villain's action by inventing an impetuous journey to London for the purpose. Modern scholars hold that Edward gave the order for the ex-king's death; Richard, as Constable of England, would have been responsible for seeing the order carried out. Henry's son, the PRINCE (4) of Wales, murdered by Richard and his brothers in 5.5 of *3 Henry VI,* actually died in battle. Richard appears to have opposed the execution of Clarence, which was definitely Edward's doing, historically. Richard's wife, Lady Anne, died naturally.

That Richard did seize the throne is indisputable; that he had long plotted to that end seems unlikely. He could not have anticipated Edward's death at 40, and he seems to have been committed to a career as a ranking prince. He was clearly a trusted and reliable subordinate to his brother, governing the difficult northern provinces with marked success for 12 years. Edward had named Richard, the obvious choice, to serve as Protector after his death, ruling for his son, the PRINCE (5) of Wales. But when Edward died, Queen ELIZABETH (2) and her relatives attempted a coup, keeping the news of the king's death from his brother, assembling military forces, and arrangeing for the Prince's hasty coronation. However, Richard overcame these manoeuvres and assumed his role as Protector. He apparently had plans for Parliamentary confirmation of this arrangement, along with the boy's later coronation, when another coup was attempted. Richard crushed this plot, but he now decided to forestall a third coup by taking the crown himself. It is impossible, with the evidence that is known today, to reconstruct the events of June 1483 precisely, but, as far as history indicates, this marks the beginning of the process that Shakespeare presents as starting two decades earlier. Also, *Richard III* compresses Richard's two-year reign into a few frantic weeks. He seems to have been a quite competent king, though the shortness of his troubled reign makes judgement difficult. Shakespeare was unconcerned with the strengths or weaknesses of Richard as ruler; he simply wanted to introduce Richard's splendid crash immediately after his seeming success.

Richard may or may not have murdered Edward's two sons. Once presumed guilty—at least in good part on the strength of Shakespeare's evidence—Richard has attracted defenders in recent years. It has been observed that, once securely in power, he did not need to have them killed; that the Duke of BUCKINGHAM (2), thought to have coveted the crown himself, had a better motive; that Richmond, as Henry VII, might well have killed them, as he did a number of other possible pretenders to the crown. However, the two youths were never seen again after entering the Tower in 1483, and responsibility must lie with Richard.

This does not make him the fierce killer of the plays, of course; if he did have the princes murdered, he was simply following a fairly ordinary political convention of the day. However, what Shakespeare's rendering of Richard's career lacks in historical validity, it more than makes up for in theatrical success. Richard as a magnificent evildoer has entered our cultural consciousness, and there he remains; we can hardly wish it otherwise.

Richard III

SYNOPSIS

Act 1, Scene 1

RICHARD III observes in a soliloquy that the victory of the YORK (1) faction has ended England's civil strife. He says that he himself is unsuited for times of peace, being deformed and thus not able to engage in the games of love that occupy the court. Therefore, he proposes to be a villain, and he reveals that he has convinced his eldest brother, King EDWARD (IV), that his other brother, the Duke of CLARENCE (1), intends treason. Clarence appears, under arrest; Richard hypocritically sympathises with him and promises to secure his release. As Clarence is taken away, Richard

reveals in another soliloquy that he intends to have him killed. He discusses with Lord HASTINGS (3) the news that the king is near death from illness. In a third soliloquy, Richard details his plans to kill Clarence and to marry Lady ANNE (2), whose late husband Richard helped to murder in *3 Henry VI.*

Act 1, Scene 2
Lady Anne, attending the funeral procession of her father-in-law, the late King HENRY VI, who was also murdered by Richard in *3 Henry VI,* curses the murderer. Richard appears and accepts her scorn, asserting that his proper place in the world is in her bed and claiming that it was the thought of her beauty that caused him to kill her husband. She spits in his face as he asserts his love. He offers her his sword with which to kill him, but she cannot do it. He continues to talk, gradually hypnotising her with words, and she finally accepts a ring from him and agrees to meet him again. She leaves, and in a soliloquy Richard hoots at her susceptibility.

Act 1, Scene 3
Queen ELIZABETH (2) tells her brother RIVERS and her sons DORSET and GREY (2) of her fear that, when the king dies, Richard will rule in the name of her son the PRINCE (5) of Wales. Other noblemen appear, including Richard, who argues with Elizabeth. Queen MARGARET (1), the widow of Henry VI, enters and heaps curses on her old enemies. She desires an early death for the king and the Prince of Wales, as well as for Dorset, Rivers, and HASTINGS (3). She wishes on Elizabeth her own fate—to continue living after seeing her husband and sons killed and herself deposed. She curses Richard most elaborately, and, before departing, goes on to warn BUCKINGHAM (2) against him. The others are called away, and Richard instructs two murderers whom he has hired to kill Clarence.

Act 1, Scene 4
Clarence, in the TOWER OF LONDON, tells of a nightmare in which he was drowned and went to hell, where he encountered the spirits of men whom he had betrayed and murdered. The murderers arrive. The SECOND MURDERER (2) feels pangs of conscience; in a comic exchange, the FIRST MURDERER (2) reminds him of the money that Richard has promised them, and he recovers. Clarence pleads for mercy, and the Second Murderer begins to relent. But the First stabs Clarence and carries him off-stage to drown him in a large barrel of wine.

Act 2, Scene 1
The ailing King Edward orders reconciliation among the peers, and vows of friendship are exchanged. Richard arrives and announces the death of Clarence, to the consternation of the king, who had cancelled the death warrant. Edward is stricken by remorse.

Act 2, Scene 2
The son of Clarence, a BOY (2), reveals that Richard has told him that the king is responsible for his father's death. The DUCHESS (3) of York curses Richard, her son, but the Boy refuses to believe that his uncle has lied. The queen arrives with news of the king's death, and mourning becomes general. Richard arrives with other nobles, and plans are made to bring the young Prince of Wales to London to be crowned. When the others depart, Richard and Buckingham conspire to join the Prince's escort and keep him from his protecting relatives.

Act 2, Scene 3
Three CITIZENS (2) discuss the rivalry between Richard and the queen's relatives. They conclude that there is trouble ahead for England.

Act 2, Scene 4
The queen, the Duchess of York, and the Prince's younger brother, the Duke of YORK (7), await the arrival of the Prince. They are told that Richard has imprisoned several of the queen's allies. The queen decides that she and her son York must enter a church and claim sanctuary.

Act 3, Scene 1
The Prince is formally welcomed. CARDINAL (2) Bourchier goes to remove his brother from his sanctuary. Richard informs the Prince that he and York will be housed in the TOWER OF LONDON, a prospect that disturbs the boy. The younger prince arrives, and the two are escorted to the Tower. Richard makes plans with Buckingham and CATESBY: if Hastings resists Richard's proposed seizure of the throne, he is to be executed. Richard promises that when he is king, he will reward Buckingham with an earldom.

Act 3, Scene 2
Hastings receives a message from STANLEY (3) telling of an ominous dream of danger from Richard, but he dismisses it. Catesby enters and suggests Richard's enthronement; Hastings disapproves. Stanley arrives, still full of misgivings. The naïve Hastings engages in small talk, before leaving for a scheduled council meeting.

Act 3, Scene 3
Richard RATCLIFFE leads Rivers, Grey, and VAUGHAN to execution. The victims recollect Margaret's seemingly clairvoyant curses.

Act 3, Scene 4
The council is in session. Richard withdraws to confer with Buckingham about Hastings. He re-enters, raging about plots against himself, and, when Hastings speaks reassuringly, Richard accuses him of protecting the supposed plotters and sentences him to death.

Act 3, Scene 5
Richard explains to the MAYOR (3) that the danger presented by Hastings' plot had made it necessary to execute him immediately, without a trial. The Mayor assures Richard of his approval and leaves. Richard instructs Buckingham to spread the rumour that the imprisoned princes are illegitimate sons of the late king's illicit liaisons.

Act 3, Scene 6
A SCRIVENER shows a document approving the execution of Hastings. He knows that this justification was prepared long beforehand. He grieves that such deceitfulness should prevail.

Act 3, Scene 7
Buckingham reports that the Mayor has been induced to discuss the possibility of Richard's becoming king. He recommends that Richard feign reluctance to rule. When the Mayor arrives, he is told that Richard is engaged in religious devotions and cannot be disturbed. Buckingham leads the Mayor to insist, and finally Richard appears, accompanied by clergymen. Buckingham, purporting to speak for the Mayor and people, asks Richard to take the throne. Richard refuses, and Buckingham leads the delegation away, but Richard has them called back and accepts their acclaim as king.

Act 4, Scene 1
Queen Elizabeth and the Duchess of York, with Dorset, meet Lady Anne, now Richard's wife. They are not permitted to enter the Tower to visit the princes, by Richard's order. Stanley arrives to say that Richard has been declared king. He helps the women make plans: Dorset is sent abroad to join the Earl of RICHMOND; Anne goes to be crowned, having no choice; Elizabeth will return to sanctuary.

Act 4, Scene 2
Buckingham shows reluctance as Richard, now king, insinuates that the princes should be murdered. Richard, angry, summons TYRELL. Richard orders a rumour started that Anne is deathly ill; he reveals his intention to marry the daughter of Queen Elizabeth. Tyrell agrees to murder the princes. Buckingham returns and wishes to claim the earldom promised him in 3.1; Richard refuses him and departs. Left alone, Buckingham plans his desertion of Richard.

Act 4, Scene 3
Tyrell reports that he has killed the princes; Richard reflects that he has imprisoned Clarence's son and married his daughter to a commoner who cannot claim the crown, and that the princes and Anne are all dead. Knowing that Richmond thinks of marrying Queen Elizabeth's daughter, he proposes again to do so himself. News arrives that the Bishop of Ely has fled to join Richmond, and that Buckingham has raised an army against Richard.

Act 4, Scene 4
Margaret joins Elizabeth and the Duchess of York, who are bewailing Richard's murder of the princes. Margaret thanks God for this development but goes on to call for vengeance on Richard. She gloats over Elizabeth's misfortunes and departs, just before Richard arrives, with a military entourage. Elizabeth and the Duchess confront him with his misdeeds; he orders his drummers and trumpeters to drown them out with noise. The Duchess delivers a tirade against her son before departing. Richard now proposes to Elizabeth that he marry her daughter. After an extended argument, she pretends to agree and leaves. News arrives of Richmond's invasion fleet, and Richard panics, blurting out confused orders and curses. Fearing treachery from Stanley, Richard orders him to leave his son as a hostage. More news arrives of Buckingham's growing rebellion, but then comes a message that his forces and Richmond's fleet have been dispersed by a great storm, followed by word that Buckingham has been captured. His spirits restored, Richard takes command and orders his troops to march.

Act 4, Scene 5
Stanley meets with Sir CHRISTOPHER (2), a representative of Richmond, and says that he will have to postpone his intended defection to the invading Earl because Richard has seized his son.

Act 5, Scene 1
Buckingham is escorted to his execution. He remembers Margaret's warning to him in 1.3.

Act 5, Scene 2
Richmond, in England, speaks cheerfully of the coming battle with Richard's forces.

Act 5, Scene 3
Richard arrives at BOSWORTH FIELD and has his tent pitched at one side of the stage. Richmond arrives and has his tent pitched at the other side. He sends a messenger to Stanley. Richard sends his own message to Stanley, a threat that his son will be killed if he deserts. Richard retires to his tent. Stanley comes to Richmond, promising at least to delay his troops. Richmond prays and goes to bed. Between the tents, a succession of spirits appears, each the GHOST (1) of a character murdered by Richard. Each delivers a similar set of messages: they remind Richard of his misdeeds and bid him 'despair and die'; turning to Richmond, they assure him of supernatural aid. Richard wakes and despairingly acknowledges his guilt. Richmond awakens, refreshed by the visions, and addresses his troops, asserting that Richard's soldiers

will willingly lose, to escape being governed by such a villain. Richard curses his pangs of conscience and speaks to his army, heaping insults on his foes. A messenger reports that Stanley refuses to march; Richard orders the hostage killed but postpones the action, for the combat has begun.

Act 5, Scene 4
During the battle, Richard enters, crying out for a horse, rhetorically offering his kingdom in exchange for one.

Act 5, Scene 5
Richmond kills Richard in hand-to-hand combat and declares victory. Stanley offers him Richard's crown. Richmond proclaims an end to England's civil wars. He announces his intention to marry Elizabeth's daughter, thus uniting the feuding factions, and prays for continued peace.

COMMENTARY

Richard III seems at first glance to be a fairly simple work in its general outlines: a drama with a striking central character whose rise and fall provide a straightforward entertainment, set within a context that lends moral weight to the tale. This description is adequate up to a point, and it suggests the playwright's interest in individual human capacities for good and evil, a characteristic concern of the RENAISSANCE. But because our experience of the play is dominated by its protagonist, we may lose an appreciation of its primary theme, which is a social one: the redemption of English public life through the coming of the TUDOR DYNASTY. Only secondarily, in the magnificence of its dazzling villain-hero, does it concern individuality.

Richard's immense capacity for crime is a final, climactic instance of the disruptive aristocratic ambitions that have spurred the action in all the plays of the minor TETRALOGY. Thus Richard exemplifies something larger than his own fascinating personality. Further, even more important than his negative relationship to peace and public order is the role of fate, which inexorably brings Richard's dominance to an end. Divine providence punishes the fractious Plantagenets, through the crimes of their own last representative, and grants England a restoration of grace with the advent of the Tudors. The workings of fate are revealed in the developments of the plot, of course, but they are also reflected in the organisation of the drama. The play is powered by subtle tensions, generated by contrasting its bold protagonist with its equally bold structural symmetry.

In *Richard III* Shakespeare twice used the potent device—a favourite of his—of two matching scenes, one early in the play and the other late. The second scene echoes the first but differs in revealing ways. In one instance, Richard's attempt in 4.4 to gain Queen Elizabeth's approval of his plan to marry her daughter recalls his courtship of Lady Anne in 1.2. This time, however, Richard is in decline; not only have we seen his downfall begin in earlier scenes, but here he is not the same wooer. He apologises for his deeds, in 4.4.291–298, whereas with Anne he had boldly attributed them to his love (1.2.125ff.). Elizabeth baffles him with rejections of his oaths, stifling his assertions until he is reduced to wishing ill on himself (4.4.397–409). Elizabeth suspends the conversation in 4.4.428–429, leaving its resolution in doubt, where Anne was told where to await Richard's later visit (1.2.214–220). We feel the difference and know that Richard will not have his way this time; in fact, as soon as Elizabeth departs, his downfall resumes with quickened speed. The repetition of motifs increases the strength with which we respond to the differences in situation; we feel that there lurks something fateful in the coincidences linking success and failure.

Similarly, the appearance of the Ghosts to the sleeping Richard in 5.3 reminds us of Clarence's dream in 1.4. Again, a situation where Richard's downfall is imminent is compared with an earlier one in which his villainy is triumphant. In using this device, Shakespeare took each later incident from his sources and invented the earlier ones, which makes his intention very clear. These links unite the different stages of the narrative.

This quality in the play is heightened by the repeated presentation of fulfilled predictions. For instance, the dreams of Clarence and Richard both deal with the dreamer's later death. Moreover, much is made of specific forecasts. Queen Margaret in particular is used by Shakespeare as 'a prophetess', as she calls herself in 1.3.301. In 1.3 she predicts a rash of deaths. As Richard's victims fall, they allude to Margaret's prophecy, and, when she reappears in 4.4, we recollect the the truth of her predictions (which she refers to, in case we don't) with some degree of awe. When she asserts that Richard nears 'his piteous and unpitied end' (4.4.74), we believe her. Similarly, characters predict the future even when they are unaware of it, as when Richard names his own fate to Elizabeth, even as he thinks he is warding it off, in 4.4.397–409.

Omens are equally evocative of a world governed by fate, and *Richard III* is rife with them. Hastings' tendency to ignore them is almost comical. A Citizen of London couches his uneasiness about the political future in terms of augury (2.3.32–35); the young Duke of York's request for Richard's dagger has a foreboding quality, as Richard's reply (3.1.111) makes clear. The strawberries so pointedly introduced in 3.4 had an emblematic association with serpents and the devil that was quite familiar to Shake-

speare's audiences. Most ominous of all are the omens that had attended Richard's birth, which are mentioned several times.

All of these devices create an air of myth that is supported by the uniform tone that persists throughout the play. There is no sub-plot, nor faintest evidence of romantic interest. Aside from Richard's sardonic enthusiasm for his own villainy, there is very little humour. Even the violence takes place off-stage, for the most part. The plot and themes unfold largely through talk—however absorbing and varied—rather than action. The only exceptions are the stabbing of Clarence (though not his drowning) and Richard's death in single combat, each of which constitutes a climactic moment in the play's development. Each is fairly stylised. Such a restrained rendering, despite the many opportunities for bloody tableaux—which were as popular in Shakespeare's day as they are now—produces a pronounced solemnity. Combined with the flavour of sorcery discussed above, the play's pervasive calm contributes to a sense of ritual, of magical demonstration. This surreal aura supports the mythic dénouement: Richard and Richmond—opposing paragons of Evil and Good—face each other in a grand trial by combat.

These ideas might in lesser hands have yielded a set of sermons illustrating the inevitability of divine providence. However, *Richard III* is animated by the presence of Shakespeare's first great protagonist, Richard himself. Not only does this astonishing villain speak nearly one-third of the play's lines, but he delivers all of the major soliloquies as well. Significantly, many of his prominent speeches appear early in the play so that we become accustomed to his point of view. Thus he seems to be in control of the action, until fate intervenes. His wit, his acute political acumen, and his energy enthrall us at the same time that we are appalled by his diabolical sadism. The final defeat of this extraordinary figure makes the power of fate seem all the more awesome.

Richard was a product of a newly established 16th-century tradition of magnificent villain-heroes that stemmed from MARLOWE's Tamburlaine. Marlowe's works were wildly popular when *Richard III* was written, and Shakespeare was not the only playwright to exploit the example they set. Shakespeare's superior talent produced a greater character, a figure whose language is not only more credibly idiomatic but also has greater lyrical power. However, Richard's dominance of the play reminds us of the somewhat derivative character of the young playwright's work. He was later to develop the capacity to create believable characters of greatly varying types in a single play, thereby surpassing Marlowe utterly.

In fact, a number of the lesser characters in *Richard III* testify to that developing talent. Buckingham's woolly rhetoric marks him as a politician who prefers evasiveness to clarity; if he were not malevolent, he would be funny. Clarence is a moving psychological portrait of a tormented sinner whose fear of hellfire makes him writhe in agony. The unfortunate but fatuous Hastings inspires both disdain and pity. None of these figures is fully developed, but each animates effective episodes.

Richard III is a very unreliable guide to the history of the period it purports to describe. As he did in all of the HISTORY PLAYS, Shakespeare took liberties with his sources, and these were themselves biassed and unreliable. The last 12 years of Edward's reign are compressed into 1.1–2.1 as a cluster of related incidents. Richard's career has been notably distorted, first by Tudor historians, especially Thomas MORE, whose account was the basis for much of the tale as Shakespeare received it, and then by the playwright himself, who was concerned not with historical accuracy but rather with the aggrandisement of his villain. At the end of the play, Richard's two-year reign is collapsed into a few frantic weeks, as the success of the usurper is immediately superseded by his fall. Thus the sequence of plays that began with *1 Henry VI* comes to its close. Where King HENRY V had just been lost to England at the beginning of the cycle, Richmond arrives to play the part of a new hero at its end. The death of TALBOT, accompanying the loss of English hopes in the first play, is balanced by Richard's death and their renewal in the last one. Patriotic history is combined in *Richard III* with grand entertainment, creating a drama that has always been popular.

SOURCES OF THE PLAY

Shakespeare's chief source for *Richard III* was *The Union of the Two Noble and Illustre Families of Lancaster and York* by Edward HALL (2) (1548), supplemented by Raphael HOLINSHED's *Chronicles of England, Scotland, and Ireland* (1587 edition). Hall's account is itself an adaptation of Thomas MORE's *History of King Richard the thirde* (1543). More's chief source, in turn, was Polydore VERGIL's Latin *Historia Anglia*. Shakespeare also adapted various details from a number of other works, including several of the plays of SENECA, OVID's *Metamorphoses*, Thomas KYD's *The Spanish Tragedy* (1588–1589), Edmund SPENSER's *Faerie Queene* (1590), and a popular anthology of biographies, A MIRROR FOR MAGISTRATES. In addition, the influence of the plays of Christopher MARLOWE (1) was plainly felt by the young Shakespeare. An anonymous play of the 1590s, *The True Tragedie of Richard the Third*, has sometimes been thought to be a source for *Richard III*. However, most current scholarly opinion holds that the slight similarity between the two plays, if it reflects any relationship, shows an influence of Shakespeare on the other playwright.

TEXT OF THE PLAY

It is impossible to date the early history plays exactly, but several echoes of *Richard III* in Marlowe's *Edward II* indicate that Shakespeare's play was the earlier of the two. The title-page of *Edward II* reports that it was performed by PEMBROKE'S MEN, presumably before the closing of the theatres by plague in June 1592. It cannot have been written, therefore, after early 1592, nor can *Richard III* have been written after late 1591. All three *Henry VI* plays contain minor reflections of Spenser's *Faerie Queene,* published in December 1589. Thus the composition of Shakespeare's cycle seems to span the years 1590–1591, and it is thought that the four plays were written in the order in which their events occur. *Richard III,* the last of them, would therefore have been written in late 1591.

The play was not published until 1597, when Andrew WISE published the first QUARTO edition (known as Q1). It was followed by seven subsequent quarto editions (known as Q2–Q8) over the next four decades. Each of these later editions was derived from its predecessor, adding progressively greater numbers of errors; they all derive ultimately from Q1. Q1 differs considerably from the version of the play that appeared in the FIRST FOLIO in 1623. The Folio text (F1) is much superior. Not only does it contain some 200 lines missing from Q1, but its lines are more metrical, its grammar better, and its poetry more impressive. Thus, F1 is the basis for most modern editions. But Q1 remains important, for it contains some material, both dialogue and stage directions, that F1 omits.

Close study of the texts has revealed that Q1 is a 'memorial' version of the play—that is, it consists of the lines as recollected by actors who had performed them—and thus it is sometimes classed as a BAD QUARTO. However, unlike most such editions, this is a solid, actable version of the play. It even includes elaborate and accurate stage directions that are generally superior to those of F1. It has been concluded that this version was prepared by an entire acting company, rather than by only a few players, as in the more corrupt quartos. This was probably done because the company lost its copy of the play. (Only a single copy of a play was ordinarily kept, to discourage pirate publishers.) The company that performed *Richard III* in the years just prior to 1597 was Shakespeare's own group, the CHAMBERLAIN'S MEN, and the playwright may have had a hand in reconstructing the play.

Textual study further suggests that the printers of F1 worked from a manuscript, probably Shakespeare's FOUL PAPERS, that was collated with one or more quarto copies of the play, certainly a copy of Q3 (of 1602) and possibly a copy of the then-newest edition, Q6 (1622).

THEATRICAL HISTORY OF THE PLAY

Richard III has always been among the most popular of Shakespeare's plays. The very large number of editions published in the late 16th and early 17th centuries suggests immediate enthusiasm for the work, and this is confirmed by many allusions to it in surviving documents of the period. Richard BURBAGE (3) is known to have played the title role in the 1590's (see MANNINGHAM), but a 1633 performance at the court of King Charles I is the earliest performance to be mentioned explicitly. The play is presumed to have been staged until the closing of the theatres by the Puritan Revolution in 1642, and several productions are mentioned in records of the Restoration period, later in the 17th century.

In 1700 Colley CIBBER (1) introduced a radically altered version of the play, which was the basis for subsequent productions for more than 150 years. It was much shorter than Shakespeare's, and more than half its lines were written by Cibber himself. This version of Richard III, presented in New York in 1751, was the first Shakespeare play staged in America, in any form. In the 19th century, elaborate productions using scores of extras were in vogue. Shakespeare's text resumed the stage in the 1870s, though it has often been considerably cut. It has been made a FILM five times, four of them silent films, including Max REINHARDT's 1919 version. Laurence OLIVIER's notable movie of 1956 has introduced many people to the play, but it is a significantly altered version—most strikingly in its elimination of Queen Margaret's furious raging. *Richard III* has been made for TELEVISION once by itself, in 1983, and twice as part of BBC series incorporating groups of the history plays: AN AGE OF KINGS (1960) and 'The Wars of the Roses' (1964), which combines the *Henry VI* plays and *Richard III.*

Richardson (1), John (d. 1594) Farmer near STRATFORD, a friend of Anne HATHAWAY's family. In 1581 Richardson witnessed the will of Anne's father, Richard Hathaway, and in November 1582 he and Fulk SANDELLS posted a bond necessary for Anne's marriage to Shakespeare, who was a minor; they agreed to pay £40 to the church if the wedding proved unlawful. Nothing more is known of Richardson, except that he was a prosperous husbandman who owned £87 and 130 sheep when he died.

Richardson (2), Ralph (1902–1983) British actor. Richardson began his career in 1921, playing LORENZO in *The Merchant of Venice.* By 1926 he was acting under Barry JACKSON (1) in the Birmingham Repertory Theatre. In 1930 he joined the OLD VIC THEATRE, with which he was chiefly associated until 1949. Among his best-known Shakespearean roles

were FALSTAFF, BOTTOM, and SIR TOBY BELCH, though he also played a wide range of other parts. He appeared as BUCKINGHAM (2) in Laurence OLIVIER's FILM of *Richard III.* With Olivier and John GIELGUD, Richardson is considered one of the greatest Shakespearean actors of the 20th century.

Richmond, Earl of (Henry Tudor, later King HENRY VII, 1457–1509) Historical figure and character in *3 Henry VI* and *Richard III,* the victor over King RICHARD III at the battle of BOSWORTH FIELD and his successor on the throne, as Henry VII. In *3 Henry VI* Richmond plays a very minor but significant role. In 4.6 he appears as a child before the newly reinstated King HENRY VI, who predicts that the boy will become a ruler and the salvation of England. This entirely fictitious episode, which Shakespeare took from his sources, reveals the extreme pro-TUDOR bias of Elizabethan historiography and therefore of the HISTORY PLAYS.

In *Richard III* Richmond's appearance in Act 5 is prepared for by Richard's panic in Act 4 at messages announcing his approach. Richmond himself arrives in 5.2; in 5.3 he is addressed by the spirits (see GHOST [1]) that appear to Richard on the night before the battle. In 5.5 he kills Richard in hand-to-hand combat, and in the final episode, he pronounces an end to the WARS OF THE ROSES, which had beleaguered England for a generation. He is a somewhat bloodless, if energetic, leader, pious and filled with an awareness of his own high mission. In addressing his troops, he can claim as allies, 'The prayers of holy saints and wronged souls' (5.3.242). He closes the play with a speech declaring a new era of peace and prosperity for England, ending with the sentiment, '. . . peace lives again. / That she may long live here, God say Amen.'

Richmond is plainly an instrument of heavenly providence rather than a three-dimensional human being, as indicated by his rather stiff bearing and stuffy diction. He must be taken at his symbolic, ritualistic value: he is the antithesis of the ambitious nobility, exemplified by Richard, that has plagued England throughout the reign of Henry VI. He brings redemption for the crimes and sins that have been committed in the names of YORK (1) and LANCASTER (1). In a confrontation reminiscent of a medieval MORALITY PLAY, whose traditions still lived in Shakespeare's time, Richmond represents Good, winning a classic showdown against Evil.

The historical Richmond was descended, through his maternal grandfather, from John of GAUNT, the original head of the Lancaster family, and he attracted the support of such former followers of Henry VI as the Duke of OXFORD (2). He was the last surviving Lancastrian male and therefore fled England in 1471, after the battle of TEWKESBURY, and lived in Brittany and FRANCE (1). His mother, Margaret Beaufort, Countess of Richmond, remained in England, married Lord STANLEY (3), and conspired against the Yorkist kings. She is mentioned in 1.3.20–29 of *Richard III.* She negotiated her son's marriage, announced by him in the final speech of the play, to the daughter of ELIZABETH (2), thus uniting the York and Lancaster branches of the PLANTAGENET family.

Richmond's other grandfather was Owen Tudor, a minor Welsh nobleman who had married the widow of HENRY V, the Princess KATHARINE (2) of France who appears in Shakespeare's *Henry V.* Richmond inherited from his father his title and descent from the kings of France.

After the time of *Richard III,* Richmond was to rule as Henry VII, the first monarch of the Tudor dynasty. He was a highly capable ruler, sometimes called England's greatest. He restored order following the wars and administered soundly, eventually leaving a large financial surplus to his heir, HENRY VIII. Unhinted at in Shakespeare is the historical reality that Henry VII was every bit as ruthless as the Richard of the plays. While he adopted reconciliation as a general policy, he killed troublesome people when he saw fit. In fact, Shakespeare's Richard is saddled with several reprehensible deeds that Henry actually committed. For example, Richard says that he has imprisoned Edward of Warwick, the BOY (2) of *Richard III,* at 4.3.36. But Henry incarcerated him because he was a potential claimant to the throne. After a number of people attempted to impersonate Warwick and seize power, Henry finally executed him in 1499. Shakespeare has Richard manipulate the life of Warwick's sister as well, marrying the GIRL to a low-ranking man who cannot claim the crown. This was actually Henry's doing, too.

Henry also sought to ensure the popularity of his usurpation by blackening the reputation of his predecessor, Richard. He encouraged the writing of vicious biographies that contributed to the legend embodied in Shakespeare's character. He also commissioned an official history of England from the Italian humanist Polydore VERGIL; this work, published in 1534, helped create the understanding of the English past that was available to Shakespeare when he wrote his history plays.

Rinaldo Character in *All's Well That Ends Well.* See STEWARD (1).

Rivers, Anthony Woodville, Earl of (c. 1442–1483) Historical figure and character in *3 Henry VI* and *Richard III,* the brother of Queen ELIZABETH (2) and one of the victims of RICHARD III. He is the son of Richard WOODVILLE, who appears in *1 Henry VI.* Rivers plays a very minor role in *3 Henry VI;* in *Richard III* he is a pawn in a political game, being executed for no other

offence than being the queen's brother and so a presumptive defender of her son, the PRINCE (5) of Wales, who stands in the way of RICHARD III's climb to power. As he is led to his death with GREY (2) and VAUGHAN in 3.3, Rivers functions as a sort of CHORUS (1), referring to POMFRET CASTLE, scene of many such events, and recollecting the curses of Queen MARGARET (1), who had foretold his end in 1.3.

The historical Rivers served King EDWARD IV as a viceroy, governing rebellious WALES (1) with great success. After the king's death, Richard assumed the office of Protector, ruling for the new heir, as Edward had stipulated. Rivers participated in an attempt to unseat the Protector; he was imprisoned and later, after a second coup failed, was executed.

Robert Faulconbridge (Falconbridge) Minor character in *King John*, younger brother of the BASTARD (1). Robert comes to King JOHN (3) in 1.1, seeking to claim his father's estate. He asserts that his brother is illegitimate, having been fathered by the late King Richard I. When the Bastard accepts this lineage and joins the royal court, Robert is awarded the estate and disappears from the play. Content with comfortable nonentity, he is depicted as inferior to the Bastard, who seeks glory.

Much is made of Robert's extraordinarily thin face, as in 1.1.138–147. This is thought to indicate that the actor who originally played Robert was John SINCKLO, whose appearance is similarly noted in several other roles.

Roberts, James (active 1564–1608) Printer and publisher in LONDON, producer of several editions of Shakespeare's plays. Roberts' play publications are complicated by unusual circumstances and have been the subject of much scholarly controversy. As a publisher, he specialised in almanacs and playbills, but otherwise mostly printed for other publishers. In his long career he only registered five (possibly nine) plays with the STATIONERS' COMPANY—all within five years and all belonging to Shakespeare's CHAMBERLAIN'S MEN. Four of them were registered as 'to be stayed' (i.e., explicitly not to be published without further authorisation); in any event he did not publish any of them. Scholars speculate that Roberts was attempting either to protect the plays from piracy on behalf of the Chamberlain's Men or to pirate them himself, though both theories are difficult to sustain. One of the five plays (two if he registered nine) was in fact pirated, so the first theory seems weak. Yet since Roberts himself didn't publish any and printed only two—both from reliable and thus presumably unpirated texts—the second idea seem misplaced. The problem is probably insoluble without further evidence.

In 1598 Roberts registered *The Merchant of Venice* to be stayed; in 1600 he transferred his rights in the play to Thomas HEYES, who then hired him to print an apparently legitimate edition of the play (Q1, 1600). Also in 1600 the printer registered two more Chamberlain's Men plays to be stayed, neither of them by Shakespeare and neither eventually printed by Roberts. (An adjoining entry names four other Chamberlain's Men plays—including *As You Like It*, *Henry V*, and *Much Ado About Nothing*—that may or may not have been registered by Roberts. One was immediately pirated, one legitimately published in the same year, and one remained unpublished until the FIRST FOLIO [1623].) In 1602 Roberts registered *Hamlet*, and though no staying order is recorded, he did not publish the play. A BAD QUARTO was put out by Nicholas LING in 1603, and then Roberts printed a good quarto for Ling (Q2, 1604). In 1603 Roberts registered one more Shakespeare play, *Troilus and Cressida;* it, too, was to be stayed, and it too was neither published nor printed by him.

In 1600, in a straightforward, uncontroversial arrangement that is unrelated to the others, Roberts printed the second edition of *Titus Andronicus* (Q2) for Edward WHITE (1). In 1619 Thomas PAVIER'S FALSE FOLIO erroneously ascribed a backdated edition of *A Midsummer Night's Dream* to Roberts, though he is not otherwise associated with that play. Roberts sold his business to William JAGGARD in 1608 and is not recorded thereafter.

Robertson, John Mackinnon (1856–1933) English literary critic. Robertson was a leading member of the school of so-called 'disintegrators' among Shakespearean scholars. He thought that passages he considered to be of inferior quality must have been written by other, lesser authors, most frequently MARLOWE (1) or CHAPMAN. Robertson thought that only one play, *A Midsummer Night's Dream*, was entirely by Shakespeare. He expressed his views in his five-volume *The Shakespeare Canon*, published over 10 years beginning in 1922, and a smaller work, *The Genuine in Shakespeare* (1930). While Robertson's work has been valuable to later scholars, his overall thesis is generally thought to be exaggerated. Robertson was first a journalist and later a leading Member of Parliament. His enthusiasm for Shakespeare led him to scholarship.

Robeson, Paul (1898–1976) Black American actor. Robeson played only one Shakespearean part, OTHELLO, but his American appearances as the Moor were significant to the history of 20th-century theatre. Robeson was already well known—both as an actor and singer and as a committed socialist and opponent of racism—when he triumphed in a 1930 London production of *Othello*, opposite Peggy ASHCROFT as DESDEMONA. However, American racism blocked a tour of the United States. Eventually, in 1942, Margaret WEB-

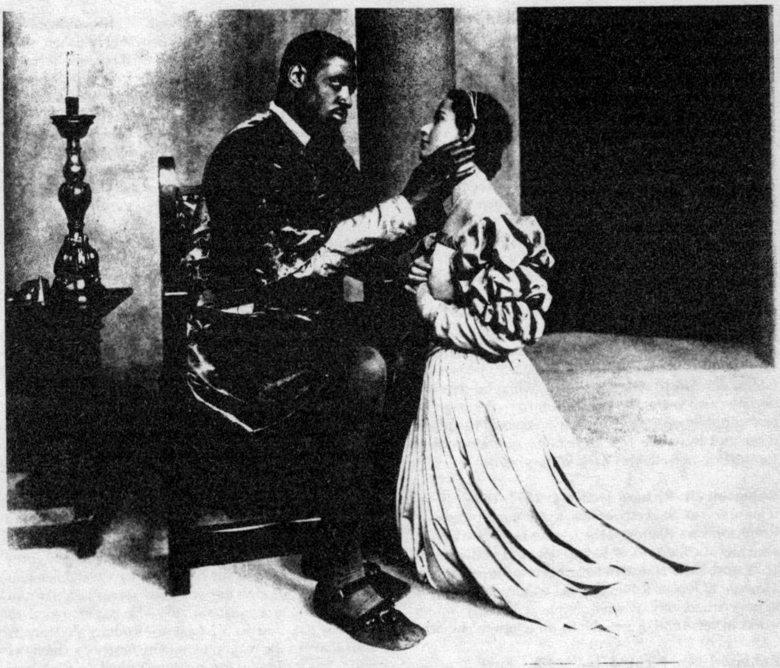

Paul Robeson in the title role of the 1930 London production of Othello. *Peggy Ashcroft is Desdemona.* (Courtesy of Billy Rose Theatre Collection; New York Public Library at Lincoln Center; Astor, Lenox and Tilden Foundations)

STER (3) directed a Robeson *Othello* in America. It played in several cities before it ran for almost 300 performances on Broadway in 1943, then an American record for a Shakespeare play. The production, which was widely publicised in *Life* magazine, sparked controversy as bigots objected to interracial casting, and it considerably advanced the cause of civil rights in the American theatre. Robeson again played the part in 1950 at STRATFORD.

Robin (1) Character in *The Merry Wives of Windsor,* FALSTAFF's page. Robin is briefly loaned by Falstaff to MISTRESS (3) Page and is let in on their plot against his master, which he enters with apparent enthusiasm. His role is minor, limited to announcing entrances, with the exception of a remark in which he both displays his own spirit and casts a mocking aspersion on Falstaff's size and, possibly, arrogance. Speaking to Mistress Page, he says, 'I had rather, forsooth, go before you like a man than follow him like a dwarf' (3.2.5–6).

The same character appears in *2 Henry IV* as the PAGE (5), and in *Henry V* as the BOY (3). Robin's small size is alluded to several times in *The Merry Wives*—e.g., in 3.3.19—where he is called an 'eyas-musket', or baby sparrow hawk. Along with similar references in the other plays, these are thought to reflect the presence of a particularly small boy actor in the CHAMBERLAIN'S MEN.

Robin (2) Goodfellow Character in *A Midsummer Night's Dream.* See PUCK.

Robinson (1), John (active 1616) Witness to Shakespeare's will. A number of John Robinsons appear in STRATFORD records, but no information—save that one was a 'labourer'—is provided about any of them.

Like another of the will's witnesses, Robert WHATCOTT, he may have been a servant in the household of either Shakespeare or his daughter Susanna SHAKESPEARE (14) Hall. In LONDON a John Robinson leased Shakespeare's BLACKFRIARS GATEHOUSE in 1616; possibly he was visiting his landlord when the will was signed. In any case, nothing more is known of him.

Robinson (2), Mary ('Perdita') (1758–1800) English actress. After a short but successful career on the stage, Mary Robinson became the mistress of the Prince Regent, later King George IV (ruled 1820–1830), in 1779. He became infatuated with her when she played PERDITA in David GARRICK's version of *The Winter's Tale,* and their love affair—he referred to himself as her FLORIZEL—was followed with delight by the public, who gave her the name by which she is still best known. After Garrick, struck by her great beauty, trained her for a 1776 debut as JULIET (1), she played several other parts, including ROSALIND, before her fateful encounter with the prince. When he deserted her after two years, she did not return to the stage for fear of public ridicule. She soon contracted rheumatic fever and lived the rest of her life in various spas, supporting herself with hack literary work.

Robinson (3), Richard (active c. 1577–1600) Contemporary of Shakespeare, a writer and translator. Robinson's translation of the famous *Gesta Romanorum,* a medieval collection of Latin tales, was published in 1577 and 1595 and may have been a source for *The Merchant of Venice.* Robinson was an unsuccessful and impoverished writer who composed many minor works in verse and prose, chiefly on religious subjects.

Robinson (4), Richard (d. 1648) English actor, member of the KING'S MEN. Robinson is one of the 26 men listed in the FIRST FOLIO as the 'Principall Actors' in Shakespeare's plays, though it is not known which Shakespearean roles he played. He was in part a comedian—though he played straight dramatic roles as well. Robinson first appeared with the King's Men in 1611 as a boy playing women's roles. He was still known as a 'lad' in 1616, when Ben JONSON praised his impersonation of a woman in what was apparently a practical joke. By 1619, however, he was old enough to be a witness to the will of Richard BURBAGE (3), and in the same year he succeeded Richard COWLEY as a partner in the King's Men. He was noted for his collection of 'pictures and other rarities'. Sometime before 1635, he married Burbage's widow.

Roche, Walter (c. 1540–after 1604) Schoolmaster, lawyer, and clergyman in STRATFORD. Roche was master of the Stratford grammar school between 1569 and 1571, before resigning to practise law; he was replaced by Simon HUNT. Roche almost certainly did not teach Shakespeare, who was still one of the younger students and thus taught by an assistant, or usher, when Roche resigned. Nevertheless, Shakespeare certainly knew him in later years, for he remained in Stratford and lived near the Shakespeare household, even during his rectorship of a church in a nearby town (1574–1578). He mostly practised law (on one occasion representing a cousin of the Shakespeares). Later, when Shakespeare was a successful LONDON playwright whose Stratford home was NEW PLACE, Roche lived only three doors away.

Rochester City in south-eastern England, setting of 2.1 of *1 Henry IV.* In an inn in Rochester, the highwayman GADSHILL learns from two CARRIERS that rich TRAVELLERS are soon leaving for London, and he gets further details on these potential victims from an accomplice, the CHAMBERLAIN (1) of the inn. In 2.2 Gadshill, FALSTAFF, and others rob the Travellers at nearby GAD'S HILL and are then robbed themselves by PRINCE (6) HAL and POINS. Rochester was the half-way point on the pilgrims' route between London and Canterbury and was thus fruitful territory for highwaymen.

Roderigo Character in *Othello,* a Venetian gentleman who is duped by IAGO. Roderigo believes Iago is serving him as a go-between in his attempted seduction of OTHELLO's wife, DESDEMONA, though Iago has simply pocketed the expensive presents intended for the young woman. Iago's exploitation of Roderigo figures prominently early in the play, helping to establish him as a villain. Though he eventually serves as a pawn in Iago's scheme against Othello—he is persuaded to attempt the murder of CASSIO—Roderigo's story is subsidiary to the main plot, and he functions chiefly as a foil. His gullibility foreshadows Othello's credulous acceptance of Iago, and his crass attempt to buy Desdemona's affections contrasts with both the mature love of Othello before he is corrupted and the gentlemanly adoration of Cassio.

Rogers (1), John (active 1605–1619) Vicar in STRATFORD during Shakespeare's later years. Rogers came to Stratford in 1605, after serving in a church in nearby Warwick. After 1611 he lived near Shakespeare's home at NEW PLACE. He was probably the 'Jo. Rogers' who witnessed Shakespeare's contract with Arthur Mainwaring during the WELCOMBE enclosures crisis in October 1614. In 1615 the town asked Rogers to intercede with one of the enclosers, William COMBE (5), but he was unsuccessful. He probably presided at Shakespeare's funeral, though no record has survived. In 1618 the town awarded Rogers a gift of a fur-lined robe but at the same time hoped that he would 'amend his former faultes and faylinges'. This may be a reference to a scandal alluded to in Francis COLLINS' will, written in 1617, in which he declares that he and Ro-

gers had been co-trustees of a legacy left for the poor, but that the vicar and another lawyer had looted it. On the other hand, when Rogers was removed from office in 1619, public outrage led to riots and accusations of Puritan influence.

Rogers (2), Phillip (active 1603–1604) Apothecary in STRATFORD, a debtor to Shakespeare. Rogers, a neighbour of the Shakespeares, bought twenty pounds of malt from the household supply of NEW PLACE between March and May of 1604, agreeing to pay later. He also borrowed a small amount of money. The total debt came to a little over £2. He repaid only sixpence, and Shakespeare, at an unknown date, sued him to collect. At his apothecary shop, Rogers sold drugs, tobacco, and—after getting a licence in 1603—ale, for which he presumably used the playwright's malt.

Roman (1) Any of three minor characters in *Coriolanus,* soldiers in the Roman army. At the opening of 1.5 each soldier—designated as the First, Second, and Third Roman—speaks one brief line about the loot they are carrying away from the battle of CORIOLES. CORIOLANUS appears and remarks sarcastically, 'See here these movers, that do prize their hours / At a crack'd drachma!' (1.5.4–5). These Romans, like the civilians of the city (see CITIZEN [5]) and some of their fellow warriors (see SOLDIER [11]), serve to demonstrate the unreliability of the common people, a primary theme of the play.

Roman (2) Character in *Coriolanus,* a traitor who gives information on the affairs of ROME to a VOLSCE, whose tribe, the VOLSCIANS, is at war with the city. In 4.3 the Roman, named Nicanor, meets the Volsce, named Adrian, to whom he has transferred intelligence before. He tells of the banishment of CORIOLANUS, and he advises that the Volscians attack Rome at this moment of weakness. His cool treachery is an appropriate preparation for the next scenes, in which Coriolanus joins the Volscians against Rome.

Roman Plays Shakespeare's three plays set in ancient ROME. In the order in which they were written, they are: *Julius Caesar, Antony and Cleopatra,* and *Coriolanus.* The much earlier *Titus Andronicus,* though Roman in setting, is generally excluded from this classification because it is a timeless tale that neither needs nor involves any real, historical world. Each of the Roman plays is a TRAGEDY, but they are unlike the other tragedies, which are placed in virtually imaginary historical situations. These works are complicated by the history of ancient Rome, which is reasonably accurately presented, and they are thus similar to the HISTORY PLAYS. The first two plays depict episodes of the civil wars that sundered the Roman Republic in the first century B.C., while the third involves legendary events of the republic's first days, about 450 years earlier.

Julius Caesar deals with the assassination of the title character, CAESAR (1), by Marcus BRUTUS (4), and with Brutus' defeat at the battle of PHILIPPI (42 B.C.) by Caesar's followers, led by his nephew OCTAVIUS and Mark ANTONY. At the play's close the victors rule Rome and its territories. However, the play is less concerned with this development than with the moral ambivalence of Brutus, a highly righteous man whose action—the killing of his ruler and personal benefactor—is intended to produce good for Rome but yields instead the evil of civil war.

Antony and Cleopatra, set about a decade later, tells of Antony's love affair with CLEOPATRA, queen of Egypt; of the enmity this arouses in Antony's co-ruler, now known as Octavius CAESAR (2); of Antony's defeat at the battle of ACTIUM (31 B.C.); and of the subsequent suicides of the title characters. More clearly a tragedy, *Antony and Cleopatra* centres on the moral conflict in Antony as he is torn between the stern call of Roman duty and the irresistible compulsion of love for Cleopatra and her opulent life. At the play's climax Cleopatra's suicide transfigures both lovers as she seems to transcend the play's world by approaching death as intensely as she had lived.

Coriolanus enacts the rejection of a great warrior, CORIOLANUS, by the people of Rome who are provoked by his prideful arrogance. It goes on to tell of his desertion to the enemy VOLSCIANS with whom he attacks the city, and of his submission to his mother's entreaties that he spare the city, after which he is killed by the Volscians. On one hand, *Coriolanus* is the most distinctly personal tragedy of the Roman plays—from beginning to end, the psyche of the doomed warrior is the central concern. On the other, it offers a broader political canvas as background for its story, and features a sharply drawn struggle between aristocrats and plebeians, where *Julius Caesar* and *Antony and Cleopatra* deal only with the high politics of the ruling class.

When he wrote plays about ancient Rome, Shakespeare dealt with material that was highly meaningful to his age, and this fact is reflected in the works. Due to the RENAISSANCE rediscovery of classical literature and art, the Roman era in the Mediterranean world was seen as the high-water mark of western culture, and the general outlines of its history were familiar to all educated people. Thus, the politics of that world, and the lives of its illustrious personages, were viewed with great interest. The moral questions found in the careers of Coriolanus, Brutus, and Antony had particular importance as they were examples taken from the most important epoch in the development of western politics.

Rome's history also had importance to Christians because it was thought of as the period of Christian-

ity's birth. In particular, the establishment of the empire was often perceived as evidence of God's intervention in human affairs. It provided a period during which the birth of Christ and the early growth of the religion named for him could take place in relative peace and stability. This belief is acknowledged in *Antony and Cleopatra,* 4.6.5–7. Thus, the events depicted held additional meaning for the original audiences.

In fact, it is important to the Roman plays that the Roman Republic was pre-Christian. Shakespeare's repeated allusions to suicide as an honourable alternative to defeat marks a striking difference in pre-Christian morality. The allusions were unavoidable in light of Roman history, but the playwright's emphasis on it suggests that these deaths had particular significance. They point to the most important distinction of the Roman tragedies: they lack Christianity's belief in divine providence as a final arbiter of human affairs. This was a very important aspect of ancient history as it was understood in Shakespeare's day. Without God's promised redemption, the moral questions of the classical world had to be resolved within an earthbound universe of references. The protagonists of the Roman plays look to their relations with Rome and its history and cannot consider the more 'cosmic' viewpoint to which we are accustomed—and that we see in such other tragic figures as HAMLET, LEAR, and OTHELLO. Thus, Brutus' course of action can only be ambiguous; he cannot recognise an error and gain divine forgiveness, nor can he be confident that he is right in the face of worldly defeat. Similarly, the final transfiguration of Cleopatra does not involve the presumption of divine judgement that attends, say, Othello's conviction that he faces eternal punishment, or Hamlet's dying confidence that Horatio can justify his life. Cleopatra's achievement is especially admirable for its dependence on pure human spirit

The consequence is that Rome's conflicts are never clearly organised on lines of good and evil; each side contains elements of both. We cannot identify individual figures of pure evil, like IAGO, or of complete good, like DESDEMONA, because, from the Christian point of view shared by Shakespeare and his audiences, these categories simply could not exist prior to God's illumination of the world through Christ. VOLUMNIA, for instance, is not evil but is merely blind to the effects of her actions, and Brutus is a wholly moral man who even so cannot be seen as good, either by himself or by others. The deaths in defeat of Brutus, Antony, and Coriolanus all leave us aware of the limited spiritual possibilities they have had available to them, and Cleopatra's death offers only a partial exception. The Roman tragedies elicit sympathy for their protagonists because they cannot achieve fulfilment, as that idea is understood in the world of Shakespeare's plays as a group.

Surprisingly, the moral ambiguity found in the Roman plays makes them excellent for ethical discussion. In the absence of absolute values, comparisons must be made, and the three plays present a considerable range of political conduct. *Julius Caesar* simply and boldly presents a conflict of opinions about the government and the morality of resistance to despotism. It also offers a demonstration of the differing political techniques of Brutus and Antony. *Antony and Cleopatra* opposes the concerns of the state with the individualism of its protagonists, who insist on the value of private aspirations and satisfactions. In *Coriolanus* an individualist revolts against the demands of the state to the extent of treason, but in this pessimistic work neither the state nor the individual is strong, and a failure to achieve wholeness constitutes both the private tragedy and the public disaster.

Like the histories, the Roman plays reflect a widespread enthusiasm in Shakespeare's England for the study of the past. However, because they were set in remote times and places, they offered the playwright an opportunity to speculate broadly on political possibilities that English settings actually inhibited. *Coriolanus* is particularly noteworthy in this respect, for its picture of class conflict is more realistic and sober than are the glimpses of it that occur in the histories (see, e.g., Jack CADE). The government CENSORSHIP that loomed over Shakespeare's theatre would probably have found English class relations too sensitive a subject to discuss seriously in public. Ancient Rome, however, presented a more intellectual, and therefore discreet, context in which to contemplate an event such as the corn riots, similar to those found in *Coriolanus,* that raged in England not long before the play was written. Similarly, *Julius Caesar*'s central—and unresolved—moral debate on assassination is not found in the histories, nor is Cleopatra and Antony's sexual immorality observed among Shakespeare's English rulers—PRINCE (6) HAL's rejection of FALSTAFF's world at the end of *2 Henry IV* confirms this.

Commentators have often remarked that the Roman plays have points in common with two other Shakespearean genres; the tragedies and the history plays. In the tragedies a distinctively great person, because of some aspect of that greatness, suffers a crushing downfall. This causes us to reflect on the vulnerability of human existence. In the histories the uses and abuses of government are demonstrated in various ways. This causes us to consider the exercise of power and the value of political loyalty. The Roman plays' greatest strength lies in their combination of these themes. They raise important issues about the individual and society while they stimulate our awareness of both disturbing political questions and profound social ideals.

Romances Shakespeare's late comedies—*Pericles, Cymbeline, The Winter's Tale,* and *The Tempest*—consid-

ered as a group. *The Two Noble Kinsmen* is also often considered a Shakespearean romance, although it is largely the work of John FLETCHER (2) and deviates strongly from the group's general pattern. Written between about 1607 and 1613 (1611, if *The Kinsmen* is disregarded), the romances, with *Henry VIII,* are the works of the playwright's final period. Each is a TRAGICOMEDY, in the broadest sense of the term: elements of TRAGEDY find their resolution in the traditional happy ending of COMEDY.

All of the romances share a number of themes, to greater or lesser degree. The theme of separation and reunion of family members is highly important. Daughters are parted from parents in *Pericles, Cymbeline, The Winter's Tale,* and *The Two Noble Kinsmen,* and wives from husbands in the first three; sons are also lost, to a father in *The Winter's Tale* (permanently) and *The Tempest,* and to parents of each sex in *Cymbeline.* The related idea of exile also features in the romances, with the banished characters—usually rulers or rulers-to-be—restored to their rightful homes at play's end. Another theme, jealousy, is prominent in *The Winter's Tale, Cymbeline,* and *The Two Noble Kinsmen,* and it has minor importance in *Pericles* and *The Tempest.* Most significant, the romances all speak to the need for patience in adversity and the importance of providence in human affairs. This visionary conception outweighs any given individual's fate or even the development of individual personalities.

Compared with earlier plays, realistic characterisation in the romances is weak; instead, the characters' symbolic meaning is more pronounced. The plots of these plays are episodic and offer improbable events in exotic locales. Their characters are frequently subjected to long journeys, often involving shipwrecks. Seemingly magical developments arise—with real sorcery in *The Tempest*—and supernatural beings appear. These developments are elaborately represented, and all of the romances rely heavily on spectacular scenic effects.

In all these respects, the romances are based on a tradition of romantic literature going back at least to Hellenistic Greece, in which love serves as the trigger for extraordinary adventures. In this tradition love is subjected to abnormal strains—often involving jealous intrigues and conflicts between male friendship and romantic love—and there are fantastic journeys to exotic lands, encounters with chivalric knights, and allegorical appearances of monsters, supernatural beings, and pagan deities. Absurdly improbable coincidences and mistaken identities complicate the plot, though everything is resolved in a conventional happy ending. The protagonists are also conventional, their chief distinction being their noble or royal blood. They lack believable motives and are merely vehicles for the elaborate plot, whose point is frankly escapist. Such tales were extremely popular in Shakespeare's day, especially in the increasingly decadent world of the court of King JAMES I, who succeeded Queen ELIZABETH (1) in 1603.

The genre had long influenced the stage, but its impact was particularly strong in the early 17th-century MASQUE, a form of drama that was popular at James' court. In the masque, lush and exotic settings framed strange, often magical tableaus and episodes. With the advent of JACOBEAN DRAMA, the taste for such allegorical presentations expanded beyond the court to the so-called private theatres. These differed from the 'public' playhouses, such as the GLOBE THEATRE, in being enclosed against the weather. They were smaller and more intimate, lit by candles and equipped with the mechanical apparatus necessary for elaborate scenic effects. To support all this, they charged a much higher admission price, and they attracted wealthier, better-educated, and more sophisticated audiences.

Shakespeare had made use of romance material throughout his career—*The Two Gentlemen of Verona* is based on a famous romance, for instance, and small-scale masques are performed in a number of plays, while others contain masquelike elements. He had not, however, applied it so fully and systematically before. Any personal motives the playwright may have had for turning to romance late in his career cannot be known, but adequate reasons were available in the theatrical world. Around 1608, his acting company, the KING'S MEN, took over the BLACKFRIARS THEATRE, a private playhouse, and began to produce plays in this new, more remunerative but more demanding venue. Shakespeare was a thoroughgoing theatrical professional—he made his living from the success of every aspect of the company's business, not simply from writing plays for pay—and he responded to the new situation by creating a drama to match it. The exotic locales, supernatural phenomena, and elaborate masques of the romances are clearly intended to satisfy the tastes of the time, and they succeeded. However, though the playwright considered popular demand, he also followed his own artistic sensibility. Unlike many similar works of the period, Shakespeare's plays build a meaningful symbolic world on the escapist premises of romance literature.

In the romances, Shakespeare returned to an idea that had been prominent in his earlier comedies: young lovers are united after various tribulations. Now, however, the focus is not only on the young lovers, but also encompasses the older generation, once the opponents of love. At the end of these plays, the emphasis is not on reward and punishment—with the young lovers wed and the obstructive elders corrected—but rather, on the reunion of parents and children and the hopeful prospect of new generations to come. The romances concern themselves with the lovers not for their own sake but for their effect on the

whole continuum of life. The focus is on family groupings rather than on individuals or couples, and the action is spread over many years (except in *The Two Noble Kinsmen*), making this aspect especially clear. (*The Tempest* and *Cymbeline* take place over shorter periods—*The Tempest* within a single day—but narrations of pre-play events produce the same effect.) This broader canvas is enlarged even further with its many images of the supernatural—gods and goddesses, rituals and oracles, apparent resurrections—which add a sense of infinite mystery.

The prominence of resurrection as a motif in the romances points to their similarity to the ancient festivals celebrating the rebirth of spring each year. The mock death and staged resurrection so common in such rites are re-enacted in each of the romances. In *The Two Noble Kinsmen* the reference is oblique, but PALAMON, sentenced to death, is reprieved, and the Gaoler's DAUGHTER is restored to normal life from her descent into insanity, an emblematic death. In *Pericles* the prince undergoes a similar restoration from catatonia, and two reported deaths, MARINA's and THAISA's, prove false. Similarly, in *The Tempest*, Ferdinand and ALONSO each mistakenly believe the other is dead, as do IMOGEN and POSTHUMUS in *Cymbeline* (Posthumus' very name suggests resurrection). Also, PERDITA and HERMIONE are believed dead in *The Winter's Tale*, where an elaborate resurrection scene is staged by PAULINA.

Winter is represented as well as spring. Compared to the earlier comedies, increased importance is given to separation and bereavement, to error and conflict, in short to the anxieties associated with tragedy. A tone of resignation and grief prevails until a sudden reversal brings an ending of joy and renewal that had seemed impossible. PERICLES, LEONTES, CYMBELINE, and PROSPERO all suffer grievously. Each experiences a painful separation from all he holds dear (while Prospero, unlike the others, retains his daughter, he is isolated from everything else in his once-secure world). Each then undergoes a penance before the final reconciliation (except Pericles, an omission that Shakespeare may have consciously corrected in the subsequent plays). Here, too, the play encompasses the entire community, for each sufferer is also a ruler, so his welfare has great symbolic resonance. His winter of struggle gives way to the spring of resurrection—and regeneration, through the marriage of the young people who have been resurrected. As in ancient ritual, temporary death turns to hope for the future.

The pagan religious component of these plays is quite overt, with the appearances of DIANA (2) in *Pericles* and JUPITER in *Cymbeline*, the vivid evocation of Apollo's oracle in 3.1 of *The Winter's Tale*, the goddesses enacted in the betrothal masque in *The Tempest* (4.1), and the stunning scenes of worship at the altars of Mars, Venus, and Diana in 5.1 of *The Two Noble Kinsmen*. In such an ambience, the merits of the characters are generally of less importance than the good will of the gods—or of Prospero, their surrogate (and even Prospero is dependent on 'bountiful Fortune' [1.2.178] to bring his enemies within range of his magic).

The plays insist that a patient acceptance of the accidents of fate is necessary to survive. The several shipwrecks in these plays and their imagery of the ocean's power make this point clear, for the impersonal violence of the sea is beyond humanity's influence. The characters are often passive and in any case are helpless to improve their situations. Their strength in adversity is supported by faith—not that the gods will save them but that the gods are great—and therein lies their eventual salvation. As Paulina puts it, 'It is requir'd / You do awake your faith' (*Winter's Tale*, 5.3.94–95). Only providence can bring about the destined resolution through strange turns of fate, whose very improbability stresses the irrelevance of human desires. In the unreal world of the romances, the characters—and we as spectators—must, like Pericles, make our 'senses credit . . . points that seem impossible' (*Pericles* 5.1.123–124).

However, more is also required. It is necessary for humankind to act with mercy, in emulation of the gods. Imogen accepts Posthumus despite his viciousness towards her; Hermione also forgives Leontes; and Prospero's forgiveness motivates the entire action of *The Tempest*. Even where repentance is not offered, most flagrantly in the case of ANTONIO in *The Tempest*, vengeance—even justice—is foresworn. All of the romances—like many of Shakespeare's comedies—have points in common with the medieval MORALITY PLAY, in which a sinful human receives God's mercy through no merit of his own. Although the romances are secular works (their pagan gods were presumed by Shakespeare and his audiences to be fictional), their Christian content is nonetheless clear. Our receptivity to such abstract philosophical concerns is eased by the fantasy inherent in the romance genre, for it offers a different level of imagination from which to view the complexities of life.

The romances conclude in a spirit of hope, as the main characters are reunited in an aura of reconciliation—a favourite motif throughout Shakespeare's career. Wrongs are righted and errors amended, exiles return to their homes, and even death is frustrated. The natural good in humanity is put under pressure but preserved through the action of providence. An emphasis on the cycle of regeneration—both in the traditional comedic emphasis on marriage and in the theme of reunited families—offers a guarantee that the preservation will be lasting.

Romano, Giulio See GIULIO ROMANO.

Rome Capital city of the ancient Roman Empire and the setting for much of *Julius Caesar, Antony and Cleopatra,* and *Coriolanus*—collectively called the ROMAN PLAYS—as well as all of *Titus Andronicus* and three scenes of *Cymbeline.* Especially in the Roman plays, Shakespeare places great importance on the idea that ancient Rome relied on a highly developed ethic of public duty. Conflicts between the demands of Roman government and the personal motives of individuals are central to the Roman plays. Though less dominant, the empire is significant in *Titus Andronicus* and *Cymbeline,* as well.

The early *Titus Andronicus* is not classed among the Roman plays for it does not deal with a factual Rome. However, even in this melodrama, Shakespeare deals with the clash between individual drives and public issues that Rome's significance evoked. TITUS (1) insists on pursuing what he sees as the correct moral action for a Roman, and the result is tragic chaos. Titus' unquestionable ethic has failed, and for him, Rome itself has failed. He declares that 'Rome is but a wilderness of tigers' (3.1.54), a line that has often been quoted as a condemnation of vicious power-seeking. The hero's inability to reconcile the Roman ideal with political reality drives him insane. Because the ideal is specifically Roman, an element of grandeur is added to his plight. The significance of Rome was much greater to RENAISSANCE audiences than it is today.

In *Julius Caesar,* the civil order of Rome is disturbed by BRUTUS (4), whose personal morals lead him to kill CAESAR (1). Civil war ensues; thus, society suffers because an individual is unwilling to compromise. On the other hand, it is evident that Brutus also represents a traditional model of Roman political morality. The individual is thus seen to relate to the state in an ambiguous manner. Here, too, the play's themes are given resonance by the fact that the state is Rome, an age-old symbol of authority. The city is the location for all of the scenes prior to 4.2, and actual sites in ancient Rome are evoked—the Forum, the Capitol, the Senate, etc.—though the people of Rome (see COMMONER [1]) seem comparable to the populace of Shakespeare's LONDON.

In *Antony and Cleopatra,* Rome is contrasted with another political venue, the luxurious court of CLEOPATRA. The demanding ethic of Rome is set against the sensual indolence of Egypt. ANTONY finds himself wavering between a Roman ideal—rigorous response to 'the strong necessity of time' (1.3.42)—and an alien one, 'the love of Love, and her soft hours' (1.1.44). This conflict is seen immediately, in 1.1, as Antony rejects the call of duty—represented by messages from Rome—in favour of the irresponsible pastimes of Cleopatra. The city is less in evidence than in *Caesar,* for fewer scenes are set there—1.4, 2.2–2.4, 3.2, and 3.6—and they are located on anonymous streets or in interiors. However, the symbolic weight of Roman power and the energy and rigour of the men who wield it is omnipresent.

Another aspect of classical Rome as it was understood by 17th-century English audiences is important in *Antony and Cleopatra.* The Roman Empire was regarded as not only a great achievement in political history but as a significant phenomenon theologically as well. Christian doctrine held that God permitted Rome to rule the Mediterranean world in order that its power might provide peace for a long period, during which Christ was to be sent to humankind and the Christian church established. CAESAR (2) makes a reference to this doctrine that would have been unmistakably clear in Shakespeare's day. He observes of his imminent victory over Antony, 'The time of universal peace is near' (4.6.5). Thus, the power of Rome was considered a manifestation of God's will. This theme recurs in *Cymbeline.*

Coriolanus takes place in the legendary early days of the Roman Republic as the city is convulsed by the rise of the common people to political power. The conflict between aristocrats and plebeians permits a more detailed depiction of the city's people than in the other plays. In about half of the play's scenes the setting is stated to be Rome, but the physical city is left to the imagination of the reader or theatrical producer. The domestic life of the city is alluded to, as in 4.6.8–9, and the commoners (see CITIZEN [5]) are vividly present in the form of several well-drawn minor figures, but they are essentially no different from the common folk of the English HISTORY PLAYS.

The glory of Rome is much less evident in *Coriolanus.* The idea of a great power is evoked when MENENIUS says, '. . . you may as well / Strike at the heaven with your staves, as lift them / Against the Roman state . . .' (1.1.66–68), but in fact Rome does not fare well here. Its messy politics encompasses the cynicism of tribunes and aristocrats, and the thoughtless unreliability of the common people. The result is the expulsion of the city's greatest warrior, CORIOLANUS, who joins Rome's enemies, the VOLSCIANS. He brings defeat to the city and—because he refuses to destroy Rome utterly—death for himself. The tragedy of *Coriolanus* offers a sense of Rome's greatness in Coriolanus' power and pride, and its later corruption and fall in his foolish politics and ultimate fate. As he is driven from Rome, Coriolanus hurls a curse upon the city that predicts its history—which was entirely familiar to Shakespeare's audiences. He says, '. . . remain here with your uncertainty! / . . . [until you become] captives to some nation / that won you without blows!' (3.3.124–133). The fall of Rome is invoked, which increases the grandeur of the hero's tragic collapse.

Rome has less importance in *Cymbeline,* but the city nevertheless has two different and interesting histori-

cal aspects. Though we see only a domestic interior, 1.5 and 2.4 are set in Rome. We meet there the villainous IACHIMO, whose delight in deceit along with his decadent world of duels and drink were probably intended to suggest an idea commonly held by 17th-century English playgoers. The home of Machiavelli and of Reformation England's enemy, the Catholic Church, contemporary Rome was seen as a sink of duplicity and corruption. In this light, *Cymbeline*'s Rome is closer to SHYLOCK's VENICE than to the ancient imperial capital. On the other hand, we see the familiar toga-clad officials of ancient Rome in 3.8, and we also know from developments at the court of King CYMBELINE that the play's Rome is the capital of Augustus Caesar, whose name is pointedly repeated. Caesar's representative in Britain is the courtly LUCIUS (4), who is clearly a sympathetic character. Here, as in *Antony and Cleopatra*, Shakespeare invokes the Rome that was admired by Christian humanism, the powerful provider of good government and peace appropriate to the birth of Christianity. In this light, the brief war between Britain and Rome that takes place in *Cymbeline* has great symbolic significance. British patriotism is valued only by villains, the QUEEN (2) and CLOTEN, and though (unhistorically) the Britons successfully resist Rome, they finally yield anyway. Part of the play's joyful conclusion in 5.5 is the king's decision to 'submit to Caesar, / And to the Roman empire' (5.5.461–462), for Rome's peace must be accepted by Britain. Thus, here as in the other plays, Shakespeare gilds his drama with the glory of ancient Rome as understood by the Renaissance humanism of his own time.

Romeo One of the title characters in *Romeo and Juliet*, the lover of JULIET (1). Romeo progresses from posing as the melancholy lover of ROSALINE (2) to a more mature stance as Juliet's devoted husband, committed to her despite the world's displeasure. Romeo's early speeches declaiming his affection for Rosaline are parodies of conventional courtship; preposterously bookish and artificial, they emphasise by contrast the depth of his later love for Juliet. And Romeo undergoes another maturation as well: from helpless hysteria in 3.3, after his banishment, he comes in 5.3 to a resolute acceptance of what he sees as his only choice, death with Juliet.

Romeo's growth is clearly brought about by his love. When he and Juliet first meet, he has not yet found a stronger mode of expression than the conventional SONNET, as she recognises when she observes, 'You kiss by th'book' (1.5.109). In their mutual ecstasy in the 'balcony' scene (2.2), it is Juliet who, though no less enraptured, is the more aware of the likely consequences of their love. Further, we recognise the impulsive boy in Romeo as he urges FRIAR (4) LAURENCE to haste in 2.3. Once married, however, Romeo begins his transformation: in his attempt to make peace with TYBALT, he wishes all the world to love as he does, although to no avail. As he departs from Juliet into banishment, after their abbreviated wedding night, he offers hope to his despairing bride and displays a true maturity in sharing the mutual consolation necessary in their seemingly hopeless situation. At the end of the play, he has achieved the capacity to stand alone in the face of tragedy, as is demonstrated in the contrast between himself and PARIS (2). Paris contents himself with formal rhymed verses reminiscent of Romeo's speeches in Act 1, whereas Romeo himself burns brightly with desperate determination.

Romeo and Juliet

SYNOPSIS

Act 1, Prologue

The CHORUS (2) tells, in a SONNET, that the play will concern a pair of lovers whose deaths shall end the conflict between their feuding families.

Act 1, Scene 1

SAMPSON and GREGORY (1), servants of the CAPULET (1) family, encounter ABRAM and BALTHASAR (2), of the MONTAGUE (1) household, in a street in VERONA. They fight; BENVOLIO appears and tries to stop them, but TYBALT enters and insists on duelling with him. Some CITIZENS (3) attempt to break up the brawl, as Capulet and Montague join in, to the dismay of their wives, Lady CAPULET (3) and Lady MONTAGUE (2). The PRINCE (1) arrives and chastises both families. He declares that any further fighting will be punished with death. The Prince and the Capulets depart, and the Montagues discuss with their nephew Benvolio the mysterious melancholy that afflicts their son ROMEO. As Romeo approaches, his parents leave Benvolio to interrogate him. Benvolio learns that Romeo is in love with a woman who is sworn to chastity and ignores him. Benvolio recommends that his cousin consider other women, but Romeo declares that his love's beauty will eclipse all others.

Act 1, Scene 2

PARIS (2) seeks Capulet's permission to marry his daughter JULIET (1). Capulet argues that Juliet is too young, but he says that, if Paris can win Juliet's affections at the banquet planned for the coming night, he will give his consent. He gives a SERVANT (4) a list of guests with instructions to deliver invitations, and he and Paris depart. Romeo and Benvolio pass by, and the Servant seeks their assistance, for he is illiterate. Romeo reads the list of guests, which includes the name of his beloved, ROSALINE (2). He and Benvolio decide to attend the banquet in disguise, Romeo wishing to see Rosaline and Benvolio hoping that the sight of many beautiful women will cure his friend's love-sickness.

Act 1, Scene 3
The NURSE (3) reminisces at length about Juliet's childhood. Lady Capulet tells Juliet about her father's plans for her marriage, and Juliet coolly agrees to consider Paris out of filial duty.

Act 1, Scene 4
Romeo, Benvolio, and MERCUTIO arrive at the banquet. Romeo asserts that he will not dance, due to his melancholy, and he is teased by Mercutio, who humorously enlarges on his probable enchantment by Queen MAB. The group proceeds to the party, although Romeo expresses darkly ominous feelings.

Act 1, Scene 5
Four servants (see SERVING-MAN [2]) joke among themselves as they clear away the dinner. While the guests dance, Romeo first notices Juliet and is enthralled by her beauty. Tybalt recognises him and rages against his presence. Capulet orders him to be peaceful, and he leaves in disgust. Romeo addresses Juliet, and their love immediately blossoms as they kiss. Juliet is called to her mother, and Romeo learns who she is from the Nurse. He is dismayed to learn that her family is his family's rival, and she, when learning his identity from the Nurse, is similarly distressed.

Act 2, Prologue
The Chorus recounts, in another sonnet, that Romeo and Juliet cannot easily meet, their families being enemies, but their passion enables them to find a way.

Act 2, Scene 1
Romeo separates himself from his friends as they leave the party. Presuming he has gone in search of Rosaline, they depart.

Act 2, Scene 2
Juliet appears at a high window and Romeo, in the garden below, admires her beauty. Believing herself to be alone, she soliloquises about her love for Romeo, regretting that he is a Montague. He reveals himself, and they speak of their love and exchange vows. Juliet is called away by the Nurse, but she returns to say that she will send a messenger to Romeo the next day, to whom he can convey a plan for them to marry. She leaves but returns once more, and they exchange loving farewells.

Act 2, Scene 3
FRIAR (4) LAURENCE, picking herbs, muses on their capacity to kill or cure. Romeo arrives and tells him of his new love and asks his help in marrying her. The Friar agrees, hoping that their alliance will end their families' feuding.

Act 2, Scene 4
Benvolio and Mercutio discuss Tybalt, who has challenged Romeo to a duel. Tybalt is well known for his skill with the sword, and Romeo's friends wonder whether the lovesick youth is up to the challenge. Meeting their friend, they banter with him about his love. The Nurse appears; Romeo's friends depart. Romeo gives the Nurse a message for Juliet: she is to go to Friar Laurence that afternoon, and they shall be married. He arranges for the Nurse to receive a rope-ladder for Juliet to lower for him that night.

Act 2, Scene 5
The Nurse returns to an impatient Juliet. She teases her charge by withholding the message briefly; when she delivers it, Juliet departs at once.

Act 2, Scene 6
Juliet comes to Romeo in Friar Laurence's cell, and they greet each other joyfully. The Friar prepares to marry them.

Act 3, Scene 1
Benvolio and Mercutio encounter Tybalt, and Mercutio begins to pick a fight. Romeo appears and is immediately insulted by Tybalt, who wishes to challenge him to a duel. Romeo excuses himself, citing mysterious reasons why he and Tybalt should be friends, but Mercutio cannot tolerate such conciliatory behaviour and draws his sword on Tybalt. Romeo attempts to separate the combatants, and Mercutio is mortally wounded by Tybalt, who flees. Mercutio, after bravely jesting about his wound and cursing both Montagues and Capulets for their feuding, is carried away by Benvolio, who returns to report his death. Tybalt returns, and Romeo fights and kills him. At Benvolio's urging, Romeo flees. The Prince appears and interrogates Benvolio. Judging Tybalt to be guiltier than Romeo, he spares the latter the death sentence but banishes him from Verona.

Act 3, Scene 2
Juliet longs for night, when Romeo is to come. The Nurse brings her word of Tybalt's death and Romeo's banishment. Doubly grieved, Juliet speaks of suicide, and the Nurse volunteers to bring Romeo to her.

Act 3, Scene 3
Romeo, in hiding with Friar Laurence, learns of the Prince's edict and raves that death would be more merciful than life without Juliet. The Nurse arrives with word of Juliet's distress, and Romeo's grief reaches new heights; he too speaks of suicide. The Friar chastises him for his weakness and proposes that, after a night with Juliet, Romeo should flee to MANTUA, where he can live until his marriage becomes known, the families reconciled, and he pardoned. Romeo recovers his spirits and leaves to go to Juliet.

Act 3, Scene 4
Capulet ordains that Juliet, whose grief he finds excessive, shall be married to Paris in three days.

Act 3, Scene 5
Romeo and Juliet reluctantly bid farewell, regretting that dawn is near. The Nurse warns that Lady Capulet is coming, and Romeo departs for Mantua. Her mother tells Juliet of the proposed marriage, and Juliet refuses, objecting to the hastiness of the plan. Her father enters and flies into a rage on hearing of her refusal. Her parents leave angrily, and the Nurse advises that Juliet ignore her marriage to Romeo, which no one else knows about, and marry Paris. Juliet resolves to seek aid from Friar Laurence.

Act 4, Scene 1
Paris confers with a reluctant Friar Laurence about his coming wedding. Juliet arrives and coolly deflects Paris' courtesies. Once alone with the Friar, she desperately craves assistance. Her talk of suicide suggests a plan to him: he will provide her with a potion that will make her seem to be dead. She will be placed in the family crypt, where Romeo will meet her so that they can flee together.

Act 4, Scene 2
As the Capulet household is busy with her wedding arrangements, Juliet appears and apoligises to her father, promising to obey him and marry Paris. Capulet moves the wedding up a day to the next morning.

Act 4, Scene 3
Juliet, alone in her bedroom, is afraid that the Friar's potion may actually kill her. She is also filled with revulsion at the prospect of awakening in the vault, perhaps to encounter the spirits of the dead and with the certain company of Tybalt's fresh corpse. But she steels herself and drinks the potion.

Act 4, Scene 4
The next morning, the wedding day, the Capulet household is astir with last-minute preparations. Capulet sends the Nurse to awaken Juliet.

Act 4, Scene 5
The Nurse, unable to rouse Juliet, raises the alarm that she is dead. Her parents and Paris—who arrives with Friar Laurence and the MUSICIANS (2) intended for the wedding festivities—grieve for her. Friar Laurence counsels acceptance of God's will and ordains her solemn interment in the family vault. PETER (2) then engages the Musicians in a bit of humorous byplay.

Act 5, Scene 1
Balthasar arrives at Romeo's refuge in Mantua with the news that Juliet has died. Romeo immediately plans to return to Verona and join his beloved in death; he buys a fast-acting poison from an APOTHECARY.

Act 5, Scene 2
FRIAR (3) JOHN reports to Friar Laurence that he has been unable to deliver Laurence's letter to Romeo. Laurence sends John to fetch a crow bar, planning to open the vault and take Juliet into hiding in his own cell until Romeo can be summoned.

Act 5, Scene 3
Paris visits Juliet's tomb at night. His PAGE (3), posted as a lookout, whistles a warning that someone is coming, and Paris hides. Romeo appears with Balthasar, whom he sends away with a letter to Montague. Balthasar leaves but hides nearby to observe. Romeo breaks into the tomb, and Paris steps forth to challenge him. They fight, as the Page leaves to call the WATCHMEN (2), and Romeo kills Paris. He addresses Juliet, whom he believes to be dead, saying that he will remain with her forever. He drinks the poison and dies. Friar Laurence arrives and views the carnage just as Juliet awakens. He tells Juliet what has happened and begs her to flee, for he can hear the Watchmen coming. She refuses and stays. She kisses her dead lover and stabs herself with his dagger, as the Watchmen appear. They arrest Balthasar and the Friar as the Prince arrives, followed by Juliet's parents and Romeo's father, all of them drawn by the news of the tragedy. The Friar gives an account of Juliet's feigned death and Romeo's misinformation. His tale is confirmed by Balthasar and by Romeo's letter to his father. The Prince points out that the feud between the two families has led to this moment, and Montague and Capulet forswear their hostility and vow to erect golden statues of the two lovers.

COMMENTARY

Romeo and Juliet is justly famed for the quality of its lyric poetry, but it is no less extraordinary for its sophisticated organisational devices, which enhance its vivid evocation of a world of love and death. Shakespeare compressed the elapsed time of the story from more than nine months in his source (see 'Sources of the Play') to less than five days: Romeo and Juliet meet on a Sunday, marry the next day, and die in the predawn hours on the following Friday. The progression of the days is clearly marked by a succession of dramatic daybreaks: before he appears, Romeo is described as wandering at dawn (1.1.116–121); the next sunrise finds him below Juliet's window in the famous 'balcony' scene (2.2), and the following morning he leaves by that window after the couple's surreptitious wedding night. The Nurse finds Juliet's drugged body at sunrise on Thursday, and at the play's end, a gloomy daybreak accompanies the discovery of the tragedy by the Prince and the couple's parents. The playwright uses a virtuoso display of techniques to heighten the explosive speed of the plot development.

The many symmetries of the play strengthen the spectator's sense of exorably passing time. The Prince appears on three carefully spaced occasions: in 1.1 he describes the Montague-Capulet feud; in 3.1, the piv-

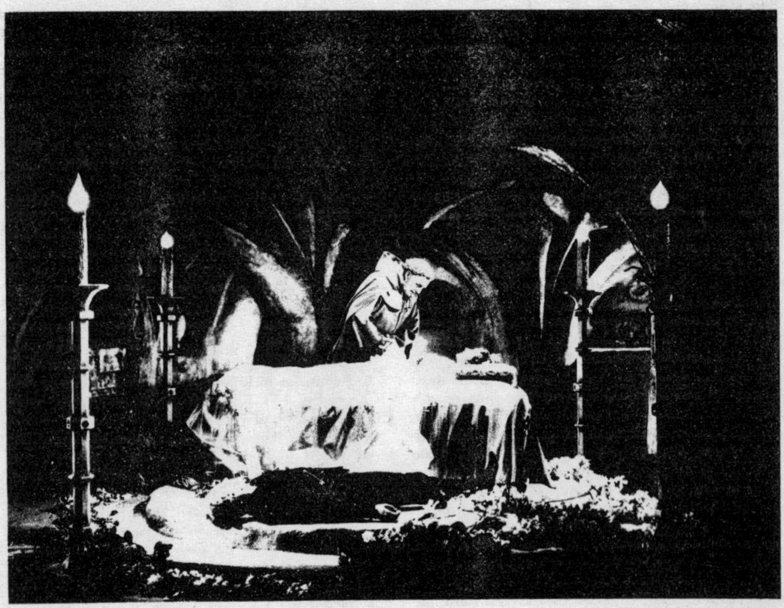

George Cukor's 1935 film version of Romeo and Juliet. *In 5.3 Friar Laurence arrives in the vault to find Juliet (Norma Shearer) awakening to the sight of her dead lover, Romeo (Leslie Howard).* (Courtesy of Culver Pictures, Inc.)

otal scene in which Tybalt is killed, he banishes Romeo and triggers the tragic conclusion; and in 5.3 he summarises the play's course. Other matching scenes link the events of the tragedy, as when the Nurse delivers a message to Juliet, delaying its contents each time, in 2.5 and in 3.1. The first message is a happy one: Romeo has summoned Juliet to their marriage; the second instead reveals Romeo's disastrous duel with Tybalt.

Telling juxtapositions also catch our attention, perhaps most strikingly when the fury and desolation of the duel scene is immediately followed by the lyrical brilliance of Juliet's soliloquy that opens 3.2. Moreover, the duel itself follows Romeo and Juliet's marriage; Romeo falls into the depths of the feud just as he ascends to seeming bliss. His very effort to effect a reconciliation with Juliet's kinsman leads to the death of Mercutio, which in turn requires vengeance. These connections do not occur in his source; Shakespeare added them to heighten the dramatic tension. In another such alteration, the playwright has Romeo first encounter Juliet before his presence at the Capulet feast is discovered, rather than afterwards, as in the source. In this way, Romeo's ecstatic expression of love (1.5.43–52) itself provokes Tybalt's wrath, sparking the violent chain of events that follows.

An effective contrast in 4.4 emphasises a basic opposition between the lovers and the world, while also conveying the sense of hastening hours. In this scene the Capulet household hums with pre-nuptial excitement, completely unaware that Juliet lies in fateful slumber under the same roof. In another striking juxtaposition of scenes, Romeo, having learned of his bride's apparent death, exits with his newly purchased poison at the end of 5.1; at the beginning of 5.2 Friar John immediately enters to explain why he could not inform Romeo of the truth.

The repeated use of certain motifs also unites the events of the play. One such motif is the passage of time. Initially, time passes slowly. Romeo, lost in his infatuation with Rosaline, moans that 'sad hours seem long' (1.1.159). But the tempo quickens: Mercutio

complains of wasted time as he and Romeo approach the Capulets' feast, and just before Romeo first sees Juliet, Capulet complains to an aged relative, Cousin CAPULET (2), that the years fly by too rapidly. As Romeo leaves the party, now in love, Capulet remarks with surprise that it has grown late. As Romeo spies Juliet at her window, he compares her with the sun and with 'a winged messenger of heaven' (2.2.28). However, the accelerating passage of events begins to take on an ominous tone. Juliet, after she and Romeo have first acknowledged their love, says fearfully: '. . . Although I joy in thee, / I have no joy of this contract tonight: / It is too rash, too unadvis'd, too sudden, / Too like the lightning, which doth cease to be / Ere one can say "It lightens".' (2.2.116–120) Hearing of Romeo's love for Juliet, the Friar warns, 'Too swift arrives as tardy as too slow' (2.6.15). From this point, the pressures of time only intensify: Romeo and Juliet must end their wedding night suddenly; Capulet impulsively moves the wedding date forward a day; Friar John's delay deprives Romeo of the truth about Juliet's apparent death; Friar Laurence arrives only seconds too late to prevent the fatal dénouement.

Several times feverish haste is described as resembling the flash of lightning or gunpowder, combining the image of fleeting seconds with that of light, the second major motif in the play. When Romeo first encounters Juliet, he compares her to the brilliant light of torches, and in the balcony scene he associates her with sunlight (2.2.3), starlight (2.2.15–17), daylight (2.2.20–22) and the brightness of an angel (2.2. 26). Juliet proposes that Romeo, if she 'cut him out in little stars' (3.2.22), could fill the sky and cause the night to outshine the day. But light, with time, comes to work against the lovers. As dawn arrives to end their wedding night and signal the beginning of Romeo's exile, he moans, 'More light and light; more dark and dark our woes' (3.5.36).

Images of contrasting light and darkness colour the play's tragic climax. The Friar describes the action of the potion he gives the desperate Juliet as 'Like death when he shuts up the day of life' (4.1.101), but when Romeo opens the tomb he calls it a 'lantern' lit by Juliet's beauty, making 'This vault a feasting presence, full of light' (5.3.86). Finally, the Prince's closing speech in 5.3 begins with the observation that 'A glooming peace this morning with it brings; / The sun for sorrow will not show his head' (5.3.304–305).

As the prominence of darkness and light suggests, *Romeo and Juliet* is a play about extremes and oppositions: the union of the lovers versus the feud between their families; age against youth; the weight of the past versus the promise of the future. Most important, the lovers themselves stand in opposition to the rest of the world—Juliet's irritable father, her match-making mother, the bawdy Nurse, the volatile Mercutio, and the self-righteous Friar, all of whom are content to enact the roles required by their places in society. The lovers, however, experience another, private world, in which they feel a finer degree of responsibility to each other and to their love. Their isolation gives their dying a sacrificial quality, atoning for the sins of their families and of Verona at large.

The lovers are especially distinguished from their fellow citizens by their speech. Their expressions of love are filled with the intense language of lyric poetry: striking images, exaggerated comparisons, and the use of rhetorical figures traditionally associated with love. Among these is the use of the sonnet, whose formal organisation and lyrical fervour suggest the nature of the play itself: rigorously paced and emotionally high-pitched. Acts 1 and 2 are each introduced by a sonnet, spoken by the Chorus, suggesting to the audience (which in Shakespeare's day, more than now, will have been likely to recognise the form on hearing it) that they will witness a structured presentation of emotion. Following a number of sonnet fragments (as in Romeo and Benvolio's exchange at the end of 1.2), Romeo and Juliet's first encounter takes the form of a sonnet (1.5.92–105) that they deliver jointly. Their subsequent dialogue is in blank verse, less stylised and more dramatically powerful, but the use of the sonnet form in the opening scenes suggests the poet's private recollection of emotion. This permits an exhibition of the lovers' intimate experience, inexpressible in ordinary speech. Shakespeare was writing his early SONNETS while he was composing *Romeo and Juliet;* the idea of integrating love lyrics within his romantic love story must have seemed delightful.

As a tragedy of love, ultimately derived from the prose fiction of RENAISSANCE Italy, *Romeo and Juliet* was a novelty in its day; Elizabethan audiences expected to find lovers in COMEDY, whose complicated plots led to happy endings in marriage. Although the tale of *Romeo and Juliet* was well known in prose versions (see 'Sources of the Play'), tragic destinies in the theatre were customarily reserved for ancient rulers and quasi-mythical figures, in dramas (such as Shakespeare's own *Titus Andronicus*) that imitated those of the Roman playwright SENECA. However, despite its unusual protagonists, *Romeo and Juliet* also reflects the traditional values of medieval melodramas of the Wheel of Fortune and, like them, carries catharsis with its load of woe. Fortune, to the medieval mind, brought down the mighty and thus demonstrated that humanity was subject to forces beyond its control, but this was not necessarily a pessimistic notion, for it expressed the certainty of a world of fate beyond human suffering. This ancient tradition was strongly reinforced by the Christian concept of heaven, which was still a vital force in Shakespeare's day. *Romeo and Juliet* concerned the destiny of two young people—not that of, say, an emperor—but it demonstrated the

turnings of the Wheel of Fortune equally well. Thus the play was both conventional and novel.

Romeo and Juliet seems somewhat out of place in the line of Shakespeare's development as a writer of tragedy. Shakespeare's extraordinary later tragedies, such as *Hamlet, Othello,* and *King Lear,* are centred on magnificent but flawed individuals whose personalities lead them to attempt to control their destiny and thereby succumb to an inevitable downfall. Romeo and Juliet bear no resemblance to these mighty protagonists; although they have faults, it is not their weaknesses that bring them to their unhappy end but their 'inauspicious stars' (5.3.111). The young lovers are victims of fate. Thus the play does not belong in the continuum of works, from *Titus Andronicus* to *Macbeth,* that concern themselves with the relationship of evil and personal character. Rather, in its emphasis on fulfilment, its final reconciliation, and its celebration of the power of love, *Romeo and Juliet* anticipates the ROMANCES, Shakespeare's strange and great last plays.

SOURCES OF THE PLAY

The tale of *Romeo and Juliet* had been popular in the literatures of England and the Continent before Shakespeare adapted it. His chief source was *The Tragicall Historye of Romeus and Iuliet,* a poem by Arthur BROOKE (1) (1562). He also knew the story from *Palace of Pleasure,* by William PAINTER (2), which appeared in several editions prior to 1580. In addition, George GASCOIGNE had made the tale the subject of a MASQUE in 1575, and Brooke mentions in his preface a play of the 1550s.

Brooke's poem is a free translation of a French prose work by Pierre Boaistuau (d. 1566), published in Paris in 1559. This in turn was derived from a story (1554) by the Italian writer Mateo BANDELLO, who had adapted the work of another Italian, Luigi Da Porto, whose version was published in 1530. Several variations of the tale existed before that (elements of the plot appear in Latin literature as early as the 3rd century A.D.), but Da Porto was the first author to name the lovers Romeo and Giulietta and to set the action in Verona in the midst of a feud between the Montagues and Capulets. He was also the first to assert that the tale was historical, a belief that persisted into modern times. Bandello, Boaistuau, and Brooke all added elements of plot and character, whereas Shakespeare simply rearranged the material, changed the pace considerably (see 'Commentary', and expanded the roles of several characters, notably Mercutio and the Nurse.

Brooke's chief contribution to the tale was to emphasise the role of fate. In this he was influenced by CHAUCER's *Troilus and Creseyde,* which was then the most famous of English love stories. Shakespeare, perhaps influenced by Brooke, was also affected by this work; he took from it the use of recurrent motifs that is so strong an element in *Romeo and Juliet.* Also, Chaucer's *Parliament of Fowles* was the source for part of Mercutio's 'Queen Mab' speech (1.4.53–95).

Various other sources include Samuel DANIEL's *Complaint of Rosamund* (1592), from which Shakespeare derived Romeo's description of Juliet's body in the tomb (5.3.92–96), as well as several minor ideas and images. The well-known French poet Guillaume DU BARTAS, in a 1593 translation by John ELIOT (1), influenced the lovers' debate on bird-song in 3.5. It is also likely that the playwright was inspired by Sir Philip SIDNEY's great sonnet sequence *Astrophel and Stella* (1591) in seeing the lovers as maturing in isolation through awareness of the power of their love. And the setting of the 'balcony' scene (2.2) may derive from a similar situation in Sidney's work.

TEXT OF THE PLAY

We can deduce that Shakespeare wrote *Romeo and Juliet* after 1593, when the latest of its sources was published, and before 1596, for the first edition of the play appeared in early 1597, bearing on its title-page the boast that the play was already popular on stage (see 'Theatrical History of the Play'). *A Midsummer Night's Dream* contains numerous phrases and ideas that resemble material in *Romeo and Juliet;* since these passages are scattered throughout *Romeo and Juliet* but mostly appear early in the *Dream,* it is presumed that Shakespeare began his comedy with the newly completed tragedy in mind. *A Midsummer Night's Dream* is dated to 1595 or early 1596; *Romeo and Juliet* is therefore thought to have been written in 1594 or early 1595.

The first edition of the play, the QUARTO of 1597, known as Q1, was a pirated edition produced by John DANTER and Edward ALLDE. It is a BAD QUARTO; that is, it was transcribed from the recollections of actors who had performed in it. It is thought that this text was originally prepared for an acting company's provincial tour, for which the play was shortened. Q1 was superseded in 1599 by a second edition (Q2), published by Cuthbert BURBY and printed by Thomas CREEDE. It is nearly 50 percent longer and includes numerous corrected passages. Q3 (1609) was a reprint of Q2, and Q4 (1622) reprinted Q3, although Q1 was also used in places. The FIRST FOLIO edition of 1623 was based on Q3 and Q4. A fifth Quarto edition, Q5, a reprint of Q4, appeared in 1637.

Q2 was probably printed from Shakespeare's FOUL PAPERS, as is indicated by its many inconsistent stage directions and other peculiarities. Therefore, it is generally regarded as the most authoritative text and is the basis for most modern editions, although Q1, which clearly reflects early performances, is often consulted, especially with reference to its more elaborate stage directions.

THEATRICAL HISTORY OF THE PLAY

Romeo and Juliet has always been among the most popular of Shakespeare's plays. The title-page of the first Quarto edition asserted (in 1597) that the play had 'been often (with great applause) plaid publiquely' by HUNSDON'S MEN, and its frequent publication testifies to its continued popularity well into the 17th century. However, the earliest surviving record of a particular performance is from 1662, when William DAVENANT revived the play in an adaptation now lost. Later 17th-century productions altered Shakespeare's play greatly; for instance, in the 1670's an adaptation that preserved the lives of the lovers played in a London theatre on every other night, alternating with another version in which they died. Thomas OTWAY's *Caius Marius* (1680), a version that was staged regularly for 70 years, was set in ancient Rome. In the mid-18th century rival adaptations by Colley CIBBER (1) and David GARRICK, both somewhat truer to the original, were extremely popular. They played London at the same time in 1750—starring Spranger BARRY (3) and Garrick, respectively—in the notorious '*Romeo and Juliet* War'. Shakespeare's text was re-established on the stage in the 1840s, and it has continued to be performed frequently. In 1845, Charlotte CUSHMAN played Romeo opposite the Juliet of her sister, Susan. Henry IRVING's production of the 1880s, John GIELGUD's of 1935, and Franco ZEFFIRELLI's of 1960 were particularly notable. *Romeo and Juliet* has been very popular with movie-makers. At least 17 FILM versions have been made (only *Hamlet* has been more filmed), in 6 languages, including Arabic and Hindi, by directors such as Francis X. Bushman (1916), George Cukor (1936), Paul Czinner (1965), and Zeffirelli (1968). It has also been produced for TELEVISION 6 times, beginning as long ago as 1947.

Vincenzo BELLINI's *I Capuleti e I Montecchi* (1830) and Charles GOUNOD's *Roméo et Juliette* (1867), two of the several 19th-century operas derived from Shakespeare's play, remain in the opera repertory today. In addition, *West Side Story*, the popular American musical drama of stage (1958) and screen (1961), is an adaptation of *Romeo and Juliet*, set among street gangs in modern New York City. Shakespeare's play has also inspired classical composers, including Hector BERLIOZ, who created a 'dramatic symphony' with voices (1838), and P.I. TCHAIKOVSKY, who composed a symphonic fantasy (1864), both entitled *Romeo and Juliet*. The ballet (1936) by Serge Prokofiev (1891–1953) is a staple of modern classical dance.

Rosalind Character in *As You Like It*, lover of ORLANDO and daughter of the exiled DUKE (7) Senior. Rosalind is the play's most important character. She symbolises the love and commitment that finally prevail when her manipulations result in the multiple marriages of 5.4. Both a counsellor and a learner about love, she presents many of the play's themes.

Although her banishment by DUKE (1) Frederick in 1.3 necessitates her masquerade as GANYMEDE, Rosalind retains the disguise in the Forest of ARDEN (1). As a young man she escapes the restrictions that were traditionally placed on women and can control her relationship with Orlando and influence that of SILVIUS and PHEBE, conventional shepherds of PASTORAL literature. Playing the parts of both a man and a woman, both an expert on love and its victim, she simultaneously mocks love and feels it, and she can test Orlando's feelings and her own. The result is both moving and comical, as she finds herself arguing against the conventions of love, saying, 'love is merely a madness' (3.3.388), even as she herself feels 'many fathoms deep . . . in love!' (4.1.196).

Rosalind is a natural and unpretentious figure who opposes affectation both in Phebe and her own Orlando. She punctures the unworthy Phebe's lofty scorn for Silvius, rebuking her in down-to-earth terms that satirise the conventions of the hard-to-get lover, telling her to '. . . sell when you can, you are not for all markets' (3.5.60). And when Orlando says he will die if Rosalind refuses him, she, speaking as Ganymede, denies it: '. . . men have died from time to time, and worms have eaten them, but not for love' (4.1.101–103). Similarly, his conventional assertion that he will love Rosalind 'for ever, and a day' (4.1.137) brings her reply, 'Say a day, without the ever . . . men are April when they woo, December when they wed. Maids are May when they are maids, but the sky changes when they are wives.' (4.1.138–141). This recognition that emotions evolve through time does not deny the virtue of affection or imply a lessening of the intensity of her own love for Orlando. She is herself at a peak of loving good humour as she speaks; she simply wishes to counter the egotistic intensity of love-cults, knowing that a more human approach will yield a truer affection. Our final sense of the love between Rosalind and Orlando is enhanced by this evidence of its freedom from illusion.

Rosalind, in seeking Orlando's love, commits herself to an involvement in life that is directly opposed to the isolation of the melancholy JAQUES (1), the play's other major figure. She criticises Jaques' excessive pessimism when she lumps him with all other extremists, who are, she says, '. . . abominable fellows, . . . worse than drunkards' (4.1.5–8). Her repudiation of his negativism is emphasised by its juxtaposition to a passage of elated love talk with Orlando, which follows immediately. Similarly, Jaques' earlier rejection by Orlando is followed by Rosalind's initial encounter with her lover in Arden. Rosalind's love replaces Jaques' antisocial reserve repeatedly. Rosalind's opposition to Jaques thus comes across indirectly as well as in explicit dialogue.

When we first meet Rosalind, in 1.2, she is sad because of her father's banishment, but her spirits rise throughout the play, as first she meets Orlando at the wrestling match in the same scene and as she later tests and accepts his love. Her attitude towards love grows more mature as well. In 1.2 she treats love as a lark, saying, 'I will . . . devise sports. Let me see, what think you of falling in love?' (1.2.23–24). She is clearly ripe for love, but her attitude is naïve.

In Arden, Rosalind acquires a fuller understanding of love. She absorbs the jester TOUCHSTONE's bawdy parodies of love in his account of Jane Smile (2.4.43–53) and in his comic love poem 'If a hart do lack a hind' (3.2.99–110). As Ganymede, Rosalind acquires a growing sense of what love can be, as her responses to both Orlando and Phebe indicate. Then, when Orlando's own growth makes him impatient with his 'courtship' of Ganymede, in 5.2, Rosalind is ready to reintroduce herself undisguised and claim his love.

Rosalind's association with magic in Act 5—in claiming, as Ganymede, the ability to 'do strange things' (5.2.59) and in invoking the blessing of HYMEN in the MASQUE in which she appears in 5.4—suits the role she has played among the lovers. Disguised as Ganymede, she has been invisible in a sense and has been able to control the situation entirely, guiding the development of Orlando's love through the playful fantasy of portraying herself, bringing together Silvius and Phebe with her 'magical' change of sex, and overseeing the union of OLIVER (1) and CELIA as the latter's supposed brother. She embodies comic pleasure, and her humorous tricks and deceits result in the play's happy ending centred on marriage.

In the EPILOGUE, Rosalind speaks as a man, saying, 'If I were a woman . . .' (5.4.213), referring to the fact that the part was originally played by a boy. This offers a piquant twist to her final manipulations, for we are reminded of the equally magical theatrical illusion that has given us one of Shakespeare's most charming heroines.

Rosaline (1) Character in *Love's Labour's Lost,* the beloved of BEROWNE and one of the ladies-in-waiting to the PRINCESS (1) of France. Rosaline is largely a stock figure—a witty, charming lady who takes part in the courtly pageant of love that is the main business of the play. However, at times we are made to sense her humanity. For instance, we hear a real person, a mischievous young woman, as she contemplates tormenting the lovestruck Berowne: 'How I would make him fawn, and beg, and seek, / And wait the season, and observe the times, / And spend his prodigal wits in bootless rimes, / And shape his service wholly to my hests / And make him proud to make me proud that jests! / So Pair-Taunt like would I o'ersway his state / That he should be my fool, and I his fate. . . .' (5.2.62–68).

Described as having a strikingly dark complexion, and demonstrating a provoking wit, Rosaline is presumed to have been linked, in Shakespeare's mind, to the DARK LADY of the SONNETS, although this cannot be proved. She does seem to anticipate later Shakespearean heroines who are plainly among his favourite types—attractive and assertive young women such as BEATRICE, PORTIA (1), and her near-namesake ROSALIND.

Rosaline (2) Character who is mentioned but does not appear in *Romeo and Juliet,* the object of ROMEO's infatuation before he meets JULIET (1). Early in the play, Romeo asserts his love for the apparently indifferent Rosaline in immature, self-consciously poetic terms. The episode emphasises by contrast the depth of his passion for Juliet when it develops.

Rose Theatre Playhouse built by Philip HENSLOWE in 1587, the first theatre south of the River Thames, in what later became the most important theatre district of LONDON. Henslowe leased a property that had formerly been a rose garden, in partnership with a grocer named Cholmley, who put up capital in exchange for the food concession at the theatre. The theatre was built by early 1588, but the earliest surviving records of the Rose date only to its repair in 1592, from which we known that it was built of timber and plaster on a brick foundation. (In February 1989 these foundations were uncovered during construction of a modern office building and have been partially preserved.)

Henslowe's *Diary* records the companies that played for him, presumably at the Rose, after 1592. STRANGE'S MEN—possibly including the young Shakespeare—were there that spring and during the next winter season; *1 Henry VI* and *Titus Andronicus* probably premiered during this period. SUSSEX'S MEN played there briefly during 1593, when the theatres were mostly closed by a plague epidemic, and shared the stage with the QUEEN'S MEN (1) in the spring of 1594. In that season the ADMIRAL'S MEN, led by Henslowe's son-in-law and partner William ALLEYN, moved to the Rose for a seven-year stay. PEMBROKE'S MEN gave their final two performances at the Rose, just after the Admiral's Men departed in 1600, and WORCESTER'S MEN played there in 1602–1603. The *Diary* goes no further, but it is known that Henslowe did not renew his ground lease in 1605. Authorities differ on the Rose's later history, but it was probably torn down around 1606.

Rosencrantz and Guildenstern Two characters in *Hamlet,* courtiers who assist the KING (5) of DENMARK in his plots against HAMLET. Only once, and only in some editions, does one appear without the other. (In 4.3.11–15 some editors follow the FIRST FOLIO text and have Guildenstern enter four lines after Rosencrantz.)

So familiar as a couple, and so similar to each other are this pair, that they are best dealt with as a unit.

We first encounter Rosencrantz and Guildenstern as the King recruits them to spy on Hamlet in 2.2, where he refers to them as the prince's childhood friends. They respond in the smooth and unctuous language of courtiers, assenting readily and thus establishing themselves immediately as toadies. When they first encounter Hamlet, he sees them as his 'excellent good friends' (2.2.224), but they will not 'deal justly' (2.2.276) with him about their mission from the King, which he has guessed, and he realises that he in fact lacks allies, except HORATIO. This disappointment triggers his impressive monologue on depression (2.2. 295–310). As foils to Horatio, the courtiers point up Hamlet's alienation. As agents of the rottenness that infects the Danish court, they help establish a polarity between the prince and the King.

Hamlet quickly ends friendly relations with the two courtiers, to their eventual doom. When they summon him to a meeting with his mother, he dismisses them by coldly using the royal 'we' for the only time in the play (3.2.324–325). He speaks of them to his mother as 'my two schoolfellows, / Whom I will trust as I will adders fang'd' (3.4.205). His distrust of them leads to his discovery of the documents ordering his execution in England and his plot to send the courtiers to this fate in his stead. Their deaths are bluntly reported in 5.2.376: 'Rosencrantz and Guildenstern are dead'.

This line was to provide the title for Tom Stoppard's 1967 comedy of existential dread. In *Rosencrantz and Guildenstern Are Dead* the two courtiers are innocent, facing death in a play they know nothing about, and the question of their innocence in *Hamlet* is often raised. Rosencrantz and Guildenstern almost certainly did not know of the King's deadly plot and may thus be seen as innocent victims of Hamlet's counterstroke. However, the two have unquestionably been the willing allies of the King; Hamlet has long recognised them as such and can say 'They are not near my conscience, their defeat / Does by their own insinuation grow' (5.2.58–59). The playwright plainly expects us to see the poetic justice in their end; the fate of Rosencrantz and Guildenstern reflects their involvement in the evil environment of the Danish court.

Guildenstern and Rosencrantz were notable Danish family names of the 16th century; it is recorded that at the Danish royal coronation of 1596, fully one-tenth of the aristocratic participants bore one name or the other. Moreover, several students of each name were enrolled in the university at Wittenberg—the *alma mater* of both Hamlet and the two courtiers—in the 1590s. Shakespeare was surely as delighted as we are by the faintly comical tone conveyed by the combination of these grand names (see, e.g., 2.2.33–34), but they also help to convey the foreignness of the play's locale.

Roses, Wars of the See WARS OF THE ROSES.

Ross (1) Character in *Macbeth.* See ROSSE.

Ross (2) (Ros), William de (d. 1414) Historical figure and minor character in *Richard II,* a supporter of BOLINGBROKE (1). In 2.1 Ross, Lord WILLOUGHBY (3), and the Earl of NORTHUMBERLAND (1) agree to join Bolingbroke's rebellion against King RICHARD II. They fear that their own estates are endangered by such acts as Richard's illegal seizure of Bolingbroke's inheritance. In 2.3 they accompany Bolingbroke as he marches against the King. The historical Ross, a prominent landowner in northern England, went on to serve for a time as Lord Treasurer of England during Bolingbroke's reign as King HENRY IV.

Rosse (Ross) Thane of Character in *Macbeth,* a Scottish nobleman. Rosse is a pawn of the plot; he often is the bearer of news. In 1.2 Rosse tells King DUNCAN of MACBETH's success in battle, and in 1.3 he conveys to Macbeth the king's thanks. In 2.4 he discusses evil omens with the OLD MAN (3) and speaks with MACDUFF of Macbeth's coronation. In 4.2 he attempts to encourage the bereft LADY (7) Macduff. In this scene he delivers a speech that stresses the play's motif of fear and mistrust. 'Cruel are the times, when we are traitors, / And do not know ourselves' (4.2.18–19), he says. In 4.3 he reports her murder to her husband and joins him in revolt against Macbeth. In 5.9 he tells SIWARD of the death of his son, YOUNG SIWARD. Rosse's greatest significance is seen in his gradual revolt against Macbeth. He represents SCOTLAND as a whole, which suffers from Macbeth's evil and then rejects him.

Historically, the Thane of Ross (the correct spelling, which has been adopted by many editors instead of the FIRST FOLIO's 'Rosse') was Macbeth himself, who had received the title years before the time of the play. Shakespeare took his error from his source, HOLINSHED's history, where the name appears in a list of Scottish noblemen who revolted against Macbeth.

Rossill (Russell), Sir John Original name of BARDOLPH (1) in *1* and *2 Henry IV.* When the name Bardolph was substituted for Rossill, shortly after the plays were written in 1596–1597, several occurrences of the original name inadvertently remained in the early texts of the plays, revealing that the change had taken place. Since the 18th century these references have also been altered in most editions. The change of name was made at the same time that OLDCASTLE became FALSTAFF—at the insistence of Lord COBHAM, a descendant of the historical Oldcastle—presumably in the hope of avoiding a similar problem with another prominent aristocrat, William Russell, Earl of Bedford (c. 1558–1613). (See also PETO.)

Rossillion (Rousillon) Region in south-western FRANCE (1), a location in *All's Well That Ends Well.* The castle of the COUNTESS (2) of Rossillion is the setting for many scenes in the play, but no specific characteristics of the region are mentioned; Shakespeare simply took the location from his sources, translations from BOCCACCIO. The Countess' son, BERTRAM, is the Count of Rossillion, and he is occasionally called this, as in 4.3.39.

Rossillion is an Anglicisation of the French Rousillon, a medieval state whose capital was Perpignan, the present-day capital of the province of Pyrénées-Orientales. Independent until 1172, Rousillon was then governed at various times by France and Aragon (later Spain), before finally becoming French in 1659. In Shakespeare's day it had been Aragonese since 1493. His placement of it under French rule derives from Boccaccio, but it may also have been designed to emphasise that the action takes place in a remote time and thus, perhaps, to make the play's improbable elements more plausible. Another Count of Rossillion was a familiar legendary figure, a follower of Charlemagne who appeared in the play *Orlando Furioso* (1594), by Robert GREENE (2).

Rouen French city occupied by the English during the HUNDRED YEARS WAR, the site of a battle in *1 Henry VI* and a location for two interior scenes in *Henry V.* In *1 Henry VI,* the French take the city through a ruse by JOAN LA PUCELLE (Joan of Arc), and then the English, led by TALBOT, take it back by assault the same day (3.2). Historically, Rouen remained under English rule from 1419, when HENRY V conquered it, until 1449, 18 years after Joan had been burned there. The French retook it only when the English were driven from Normandy for good; Talbot was actually captured at the fall of Rouen in 1449 and was not ransomed until a year later. Although the incident in the play is wholly fictional, it includes details of other battles, which Shakespeare based on the chronicles of HALL (2) and FABYAN. The episode was created to heighten the contrast between the heroic Talbot and the cowardly FASTOLFE, and to emphasise Joan's trickery.

In 3.4 of *Henry V,* Princess KATHARINE (2) is comically instructed in the English language by ALICE (1), and in the next scene, the French leaders demonstrate over-confidence about facing the English in battle. Both of these interior scenes take place in Rouen, not long before its conquest by the English.

Rowe, Nicholas (1674–1718) First critical editor of Shakespeare's works. Rowe, a successful though minor playwright, issued an edition of Shakespeare's plays in 1709; a second edition in 1714 included the poems. Working from the highly corrupt text of the Fourth FOLIO, Rowe made many emendations, and he also created lists of the *dramatis personae* and act and scene divisions, the first time these features were provided for most of the plays. While many of Rowe's textual emendations continue to be accepted, he was at times rather arbitrary and intrusive in a manner not tolerated by modern scholarship. For instance, where Shakespeare has HECTOR cite ARISTOTLE in *Troilus and Cressida* (2.2.167), Rowe—offended by the anachronism (for Aristotle lived centuries after the TROJAN WAR)—substituted the phrase 'graver sages' for the philosopher's name. Rowe introduced his collection with a brief biography, which he acknowledged was based largely on the lore collected by Thomas BETTERTON. Though filled with anecdotal information that modern scholars reject, Rowe's biography remained the standard life of the playwright until Edmond MALONE's work.

Rowley (1), Samuel (d. c. 1630) English playwright, author of a possible precursor of *Henry VIII.* Rowley wrote plays for the ADMIRAL'S MEN (later PRINCE HENRY'S MEN and the PALSGRAVE'S MEN), for whom he was also an actor. He mostly worked collaboratively, with a variety of playwrights, including John DAY and Thomas DEKKER. The only play known to have been written wholly by him was *When you see me, You know me* (1605), a comic history play dealing with the reign of King HENRY VIII. Scholars believe Shakespeare may have been alluding to Rowley's play in *Henry VIII* when the PROLOGUE (4) promises the audience that they will see a serious work and not 'a merry bawdy play' (Prologue 14). The possible subtitle to *Henry VIII*—ALL IS TRUE—may have been intended to make the same comparison. Rowley may have written some of the comic prose that was added in 1602 to *Dr Faustus* by Christopher MARLOWE (1), and he may have written similar scenes in THE TAMING OF A SHREW and THE FAMOUS VICTORIES OF HENRY V.

Rowley (2), William (c. 1585–1626) English actor and playwright, sometimes held to have been a collaborator with Shakespeare. Between 1607 and 1625, Rowley appeared with or wrote for the QUEEN'S MEN (2), PRINCE CHARLES' MEN, and the KING'S MEN. Rowley was best known in his own time as an actor, and playwriting seems to have been a sideline. He generally provided low comedy scenes in prose. He collaborated several times with Thomas MIDDLETON, most successfully on *The Changeling* (1622). He has been nominated as a co-author of *Pericles* and of THE TROUBLESOME RAIGNE OF KING JOHN, though most scholars dismiss both attributions. In 1662 Francis KIRKMAN published THE BIRTH OF MERLIN as the work of Shakespeare and Rowley, but the ascription to Shakespeare was false; scholars believe that the play is by Rowley alone or by Rowley and Middleton.

Royal Shakespeare Company Modern British theatrical company famous for productions of Shakespeare's plays. In existence since the 1879 founding of the Shakespeare Memorial Theatre in STRATFORD, the Company assumed its present name in 1961. Led by such major Shakespearean directors as Frank BENSON (1), Barry JACKSON (1), Anthony QUAYLE, and Glen Byam SHAW (3), the Company achieved international fame, and since 1961, during the directorships of Peter HALL (5), Trevor NUNN, and Terry HANDS, it has continued to play a leading role in world theatre, with remarkable production of both Shakespeare and a wide range of classical and contemporary playwrights. It employs several theatres in both Stratford and London.

Rugby, John Minor character in *The Merry Wives of Windsor,* servant of Dr CAIUS (2). Rugby, who says little, merely attends his bullying master, a court physician.

Rumour Allegorical figure in *2 Henry IV,* the speaker of the INDUCTION (Ind.). Rumour serves as a CHORUS (1) and introduces the play. Rumour wears a costume 'painted full of tongues' (Ind. 1, stage direction), in a medieval tradition ultimately derived from a description in VIRGIL's *Aeneid,* written in the 1st century B.C. An unpleasant figure full of scorn for human credulity, he describes his own potential to cause disruption and states that he is now going to give the Earl of NORTHUMBERLAND (1) the false news that the rebels against King HENRY IV, led by the Earl's son, HOTSPUR, have won the battle of SHREWSBURY. Act 1 then commences with Northumberland's receipt of this news.

Rumour serves three functions. First, he recounts that Henry has won the battle and that there remain other rebels, under Northumberland, who are still active. Then, in asserting that Northumberland has missed the battle by being 'crafty-sick' (Ind. 37), he introduces the idea that treachery infects the rebel cause, part of the play's unfavourable presentation of revolt. Most significantly, Rumour, introduces the idea that uncertainty cannot be avoided, saying, 'which of you will stop the vent of hearing when loud Rumour speaks?' (Ind. 2). This pessimistic proposition reflects the play's dark mood and is an underlying element of the play's message that order must be maintained in society.

Russell, Thomas (1570–1634) Landowner in WARWICKSHIRE and a friend of Shakespeare. In his will Shakespeare left Russell the sizeable token of £5 and appointed him an overseer of the will. Russell's first wife was a cousin of Henry WILLOUGHBY (2), who may thereby have known Shakespeare and thus possibly written about him in his mysterious poem 'Willobie his Avisa'. Russell may well have known Shakespeare in LONDON, where he lived in 1599. At this time, a widower, he was courting his second wife, who lived near the playwright. She was the widowed mother of Dudley and Leonard DIGGES (1, 2), whom Shakespeare almost certainly did know: the former may have provided information used in writing *The Tempest,* and the latter contributed dedicatory verses to the FIRST FOLIO edition of the plays. After marrying Mrs Digges in 1603, Russell lived with her at her estate near STRATFORD. The couple had already lived together for three years, marrying only when their lawyers could devise a way to break certain provisions in her late husband's will, intended to discourage remarriage. Dudley Digges later came to resent this and harried Russell for years with a long, acrimonious lawsuit.

Rutland (1), Edmund York, Earl of (1443–1460) Historical figure and character in *3 Henry VI,* the murdered son of the Duke of YORK (8). Rutland, though only a child, is killed by the vengeful Lord CLIFFORD (1) as he attempts to flee from the battle of WAKEFIELD in 1.3, accompanied by his TUTOR. His blood, preserved on a handkerchief, is used in 1.4 to torment his father, whom Clifford kills as well. These highly dramatic encounters exemplify the barbarity of the WARS OF THE ROSES. Shakespeare took the incident from his source, Edward HALL (2), but it is entirely fictitious. Rutland was not a child, but, at 17 years old, was an adult by the standards of the time. He fought in the battle of Wakefield and was slain there, but, as is normal for 15th-century warfare, no particular combatant can be positively identified as his killer.

Rutland (2), Francis Manners, Earl of (1578–1632) English aristocrat, a minor patron of Shakespeare. Rutland's records reveal payments to Shakespeare and Richard BURBAGE (3) for the preparation of a ceremonial shield that the Earl used at a tournament held on the 10th anniversary of King JAMES I's accession in 1613. This type of coat of arms bore a painted allegorical composition called an *impresa,* or emblem. It was not used in fighting, but was carried by a knight's page who recited a poetic interpretation of the emblem when the nobleman presented himself for the joust. Each KNIGHT (2) in 2.2 of *Pericles* bears such a shield, and the emblems are interpreted by THAISA. Presumably, Shakespeare wrote the poetic interpretation for Rutland's emblem, and Burbage painted the image, for which each man received 44 shillings in gold. This was a substantial sum of money in the 17th century, at least several month's wages for most workmen.

Rynaldo Character in *All's Well That Ends Well.* See STEWARD (1).

S

Sackville, Thomas (1536–1608) English author and statesman, co-author of the first English TRAGEDY and the author of a source for Shakespeare's HISTORY PLAYS. Sackville's literary activity came early in his career. With Thomas Norton (1532–1584), the first English translator of Calvin and later a Puritan opponent of the theatre, Sackville wrote *Gorbuduc* (1562), the first tragedy written in English. He also wrote poetry and contributed two essays, the 'Induction' and 'Complaint of Buckingham', to the second edition (1563) of A MIRROR FOR MAGISTRATES, a collection of biographies from which Shakespeare derived material for several of the histories. Sackville's work was especially important for *2 Henry VI.*

Sackville was an extravagant young nobleman, and around 1563 he had to flee England to avoid imprisonment for debt. In ROME he was briefly gaoled on suspicion of espionage. He returned after inheriting a fortune. A cousin and favoured courtier of Queen ELIZABETH (1), he was granted an estate at Knole in KENT (1), which he renovated into one of the grandest of surviving English homes. As a diplomat, he represented the queen in several important matters, including her relations with Mary, Queen of Scots. He eventually became her lord treasurer, and he was kept in this position by her successor, King JAMES I. However, in 1608 he was accused of taking excessive bribes, and he died suddenly at his trial on these charges.

Sadler, Hamnet (d. 1624) and Judith (d. 1614) Couple in STRATFORD, probable godparents of Hamnet and Judith SHAKESPEARE (5, 10). Hamnet Sadler was a baker and a lifelong friend of Shakespeare. The Sadler's son, born in 1598, was named William. In Shakespeare's will, which Sadler witnessed, the baker was one of seven friends to whom the playwright left money to buy a commemorative ring (though his name appears to have been inserted as an afterthought, replacing that of Richard TYLER [1]). Sadler's family had been in Stratford for more than two centuries. Hamnet and Judith Staunton were married between 1578—when Hamnet inherited his bakery—and 1580. They had 14 children, of whom seven survived to adulthood. Sadler suffered severe losses in the Stratford fire of 1595, from which he never entirely recovered; several subsequent lawsuits by creditors are recorded. Sadler appears in the records as both Hamnet and Hamlet—he is named Hamlet in Shakespeare's will but he witnessed it as Hamnet—suggesting that the two names were actually variants of one. (In any case Shakespeare took the name for his great tragic hero from his sources, not from his friend or his son.)

Sadler's Wells Theatre London theatre, once a centre of Shakespearean productions. In 1684 an ancient medicinal spring was discovered on a plot of land in open country north of London. Its owner, one Mr Sadler, created on the site a 'pleasure garden', or private park where refreshments and light entertainment were sold. A few years later he built a theatre, where a variety of entertainment was offered. In 1765 a stone theatre was built—it was managed in the 1770s by Tom KING (26)—but it was not particularly distinguished until Samuel PHELPS leased it in 1844 and used it for 20 years to stage his famous and influential series of Shakespearean productions. After subsequent service as a part-time skating rink and boxing arena, as well as, from time to time, a legitimate stage, the theatre became a virtual ruin early in the 20th century. In 1931 Lilian BAYLIS bought and refurbished it, and Shakespearean productions were again resumed, though since 1934 it has chiefly been associated with opera and ballet.

Sailor (1) Any of several minor characters in *Hamlet,* bearers of a letter to HORATIO. In 4.6 a group of Sailors bring Horatio a message from Prince HAMLET. The First Sailor speaks for them all; he seems to lack sophistication because he delivers the missive and afterwards ascertains Horatio's identity. Horatio reads the message aloud, in an aside, and we realise that the Sailors are probably part of the pirate crew mentioned in it. Horatio leaves with them to find the prince. The episode announces Hamlet's return to Denmark and the approach of the play's climax.

Sailor (2) Minor character in *Othello,* a messenger. In 1.3 the Sailor brings news of the Turkish attack on CYPRUS and disappears from the play; he has no per-

sonality and serves only to increase the frantic activity of the scene.

Sailor (3) Either of two minor characters in *Pericles,* seamen aboard whose ship MARINA is born and THAISA apparently dies. In 3.1, during a raging storm, the Sailors believe that PERICLES' wife Thaisa has died, though in fact she is merely unconscious. They demand that she be buried at sea, for they believe that a corpse aboard ship will bring disaster. The distracted Pericles agrees, and Thaisa is cast overboard in a watertight coffin. Thus begins the long separation of husband and wife, a central development in the play's sequence of exiles and disconnections. The Sailors are hearty seamen, conspicuously unafraid of the storm. The First Sailor addresses it contemptuously, 'Blow, and split thyself' (3.1.44), to which the Second Sailor responds, 'But sea-room, and the brine and cloudy billow kiss the moon, I care not' (3.1.45–46). Shakespeare makes it clear that they are not evil; they are merely unknowing implements of fate.

Sailor (4) Character in *Pericles.* See TYRIAN SAILOR.

St Albans Village near London, near which several scenes of *2 Henry VI* occur. Now a city of more than 50,000 people, St Albans was in Shakespeare's day a small village whose chief attraction was a shrine to St Alban, the first British martyr. In 2.1 the imposter SIMPCOX, having staged a 'miraculous' cure at the shrine, is encountered nearby by the king's hawking party. In 5.2 and 5.3 the fields near the town are the scene of the first battle of St Albans, which began the WARS OF THE ROSES in 1455. The Duke of YORK (8), attempting to enforce his claim to the crown of King HENRY VI, defeats the forces of the king and forces him to retreat to London, closing the play. The battle is then alluded to in *3 Henry VI* (1.1). The second battle of St Albans occurred in 1461, and it is described in *3 Henry VI* (2.1).

St Edmundsbury (Bury St Edmunds) English town in Suffolk, the setting for 5.2 of *King John.* The French camp here is the site of the treasonous alliance between the Dauphin LEWIS (1) and several English noblemen, led by the Earl of SALISBURY (4), who are rebelling against King JOHN (3).

St Edmundsbury was the location of an assembly of John's rebellious nobles in 1214, as Shakespeare knew from HOLINSHED's history. The lords swore an oath to oppose the king—a prelude to the signing of the Magna Charta the next year; it was entirely unrelated to the French invasion of 1216. However, Shakespeare associated the two, both to compress the sequence of events in the interest of fast-moving drama, and in order to identify treason with the threat of foreign conquest.

As BURY ST EDMUNDS, the town is a location in *2 Henry VI.*

Sainte-Maure, Benoît de (active c. 1150–1175) French poet, author of a source of *Troilus and Cressida.* In about 1160 Sainte-Maure (also known as Sainte-More or Benoît) wrote his *Roman de Troie,* a very long poem (30,000 verses) on the history of Troy. This work, which derived from a 6th-century account by the pseudonymous Dares Phrygius (Dares the Trojan), was translated into Latin prose by Guido delle COLONNE, and, as his *Historia destructionis Troiae* (pub. 1270–1287), it became the standard work on the TROJAN WAR throughout the Middle Ages, until the rediscovery of HOMER in the RENAISSANCE restored the oldest account of the war to its current prominence. Colonne's *Historia* influenced Shakespeare's Greek and Trojan warriors through two English works—William CAXTON's *The Recuyell of the Historyes of Troye* (1471) and John LYDGATE's long poem *Troy Book* (1420, publ. 1512, 1555). Further, Sainte-Maure's poem inspired BOCCACCIO's *Filostrato* (1338), which, through CHAUCER's *Troilus and Criseyde* (c. 1482), gave the playwright the story of his ill-fated title characters. Sainte-Maure's work was the first to introduce this tale, which is not in Dares Phrygius or Homer.

Sainte-Maure is thought to have been a wandering troubadour, serving as court poet in one aristocratic household after another. He spent many years in England at the court of King Henry II (1133–1189). He probably wrote the *Roman de Troie* there, for it is dedicated to Henry's queen, ELEANOR of Aquitaine.

Salarino Character in *The Merchant of Venice.* See SALERIO.

Salerio (Salarino) Character in *The Merchant of Venice,* a friend of ANTONIO (2). Salerio, whose conversation in elegant verse reflects his position as a cultured gentleman of VENICE, is difficult to distinguish from his companion SOLANIO. They present certain facts to the audience, as when, consoling the melancholy Antonio in 1.1, they refer to his status as a wealthy and successful merchant. In 2.8 the same figures discuss SHYLOCK's despair and rage at JESSICA's elopement (which Salerio has assisted) and speculate that the Jew will vent his anger on Antonio if he can. In 3.1 they tease Shylock, eliciting from him his famous speech claiming equality with Christians. Salerio is simply a conventional figure whose role is to further the development of more significant characters.

In some editions Salerio's part, except in 3.2, is assigned to Salarino, who is thought of as a separate character. However, most modern scholarship holds that the latter name is simply a 16th-century typographical error.

Salisbury (1), John Montague (Montacute), Earl of (c. 1350–1400) Historical figure and minor character in *Richard II,* a supporter of King RICHARD II. In 2.4 Salisbury receives notice from the Welsh CAPTAIN (4) that his troops will no longer remain in Richard's army, and he mourns the likely downfall of the king. He himself stays loyal and is eventually killed fighting against Bolingbroke; his death is reported by the Earl of NORTHUMBERLAND (1) in 5.6.8.

The historical Salisbury was a trusted adviser to Richard for many years; in 1396 he negotiated the king's marriage to QUEEN (13) Isabel. A year after Richard's deposition, Salisbury was captured in battle, along with the Duke of SURREY (2), by Lord BERKELEY, who turned his prisoners over to a mob, which beheaded them. Salisbury's son was the Earl of SALISBURY (3) in *Henry V* and *1 Henry VI.*

Salisbury (2), Richard Neville, Earl of (1400–1460) Historical figure and character in *2 Henry VI,* a patriotic nobleman, distinguished from the selfishly ambitious aristocrats around him. In 1.1 Salisbury and his son, the Earl of WARWICK (3), determine to support the Duke of GLOUCESTER (4), an honest and capable minister, against his enemies. In general, Salisbury is overshadowed by Warwick, who is to be a major figure in *3 Henry VI.* For example, in 3.2 Salisbury, speaking for the enraged COMMONS, demands that SUFFOLK (3) be punished for Gloucester's murder. However, it was Warwick, a hundred lines earlier, who had established Suffolk's guilt.

Salisbury's finest moment comes in 5.1, when he announces his support of York's claim to the throne. Reminded by King HENRY VI of his oath of allegiance, Salisbury replies, 'It is great sin to swear unto a sin, / But greater sin to keep a sinful oath . . .' (5.1.182–183).

The historical Salisbury was the son of the Earl of WESTMORELAND (1), who appears in *1* and *2 Henry IV.* He was also the son-in-law, and thus successor to the title, of the SALISBURY (3) who dies at the siege of ORLÉANS in *1 Henry VI.* Shakespeare distorted Salisbury's political career considerably. Although he was not an enemy of Gloucester, he was not a notable ally of that lord either. As a great magnate of northern England, Salisbury was rather more limited in his concerns than the patriot depicted in *2 Henry VI.* His chief rivals were the Percy family, of neighbouring Northumberland, and he did not become close to York until, well after most of the events in the play, York's rival, SOMERSET (1), fell into a dispute over land with Warwick. As Somerset's enemy, York became the Nevilles' friend, and the family allied itself with York in time for the beginning of the WARS OF THE ROSES. Salisbury was later captured at the battle of WAKEFIELD and executed at POMFRET CASTLE, although this is not mentioned when the battle occurs in *3 Henry VI.*

The early backing of York's cause by Warwick and Salisbury in *2 Henry VI* seems intended to show how even the apparently upright patriots among the aristocracy became caught in the web of hypocrisy and falsehood that pervades all of these plays. It also serves to foreshadow Warwick's importance as the chief Yorkist in *3 Henry VI.* It is sometimes argued on textual grounds that Salisbury originally had a small role in 1.2 of *3 Henry VI,* but that the character was eliminated, perhaps before any performance was given, as a measure of economy for the acting company, and Salisbury's lines were given to MONTAGUE (3).

Salisbury (3), Thomas Montague (Montacute), Earl of (1388–1428) Historical figure and minor character in *1 Henry VI* and *Henry V,* an English general. In *1 Henry VI* Salisbury appears only in 1.4, to be killed by a cannon-ball fired from the walls of ORLÉANS (1), dying in the arms of TALBOT. The incident emphasises the increasing revival of French fortunes in the HUNDRED YEARS WAR. In his even briefer appearance in *Henry V,* set 13 years earlier, Salisbury adds a note of epic valour to the victory of the badly outnumbered English at AGINCOURT, saying, just before the battle, 'If we no more meet till we meet in heaven, then, joyfully, . . . adieu!' (3.3.7–10).

The historical Salisbury chiefly served King HENRY V as a diplomat and administrator, and under HENRY VI he was one of England's most successful generals. Salisbury was indeed killed by a cannon-ball at Orléans, but he did not die immediately, lingering in pain for a week. Talbot was not present, and Salisbury's funeral in 2.2 is also fictitious, for his body was in fact brought back to England for burial.

Salisbury (4), William Longsword, Earl of (d. 1226) Historical figure and character in *King John,* the leader of the English noblemen who rebel against JOHN (3). Salisbury is the spokesman for the other rebels, the Earl of PEMBROKE (5) and Lord BIGOT. They desert John and join a French invasion force, believing that the king has foully murdered young Prince ARTHUR. They return to John's side when they learn from MELUN that the French leader, LEWIS (1), plans treachery against them. The rebellious barons represent an evil consequence of John's evil behaviour, and Salisbury effectively expresses their motives, both in disrupting the realm and in returning to loyalty.

The historical Salisbury was King John's half-brother, an illegitimate son of King Henry II. He was not a leader of the rebellious barons, but remained loyal to the king through the settlement that produced the Magna Charta in 1215. However, upon the resumption of civil war, Salisbury joined the alliance of the barons and the invading French, leaving it only after John's death. He was no relation to the other earls of Salisbury who appear in Shakespeare's plays.

Salusbury (Salisbury), John (c. 1566–1612) Contemporary of Shakespeare, minor nobleman whose marriage was the subject of an allegorical poem, LOVE'S MARTYR (1601), that was published with Shakespeare's *The Phoenix and Turtle.* Originally from Denbighshire, in WALES (1), Salusbury studied law in London and remained there in the court of Queen ELIZABETH (1). He became friends with a number of writers and dramatists, including Ben JONSON, John MARSTON, and probably Shakespeare. Salusbury was knighted by the Queen in 1601, possibly for his loyalty during the attempted rebellion by the Earl of ESSEX (2). This honour is thought to have been the occasion for the publication of *Love's Martyr,* written 15 years earlier by a member of Salusbury's household, with additional works by his more illustrious literary friends.

Salvini, Tommaso (1829–1915) Italian actor. Salvini was Italy's leading Shakespearean actor of the 19th century, playing most of the tragic heroes but specialising in OTHELLO. In the 1870s and 1880s Salvini, a massive man with a booming voice, achieved great success touring Britain and America as Othello (with Edwin BOOTH [2] as IAGO in 1886). Until 1880 these productions were wholly in Italian, and later he continued to perform in Italian while the rest of the company spoke English, but this did not interfere with his great popularity with English-speaking audiences, who admired his stage presence and great vocal power.

Sampson Minor character in *Romeo and Juliet,* a servant of the CAPULET (1) household. Sampson and GREGORY (1) brawl with servants of the MONTAGUE (1) family in 1.1, after opening the play with a pun-filled dialogue in which Sampson boasts of his bold fighting spirit, while Gregory taunts him for being a coward. They both content themselves with verbal battle until TYBALT inspires them to bring matters to blows. Shakespeare presumably gave Sampson an heroic name to add another touch of humour to his role, but the thought went undeveloped; the name is not spoken in the dialogue.

Sandal Castle Castle in Yorkshire, location in *3 Henry VI.* Now a total ruin, in the 15th century Sandal Castle was a fortification belonging to the Duke of YORK (8). In 1.2 York's sons persuade him to renew his claim to the crown, just as an army led by Queen MARGARET (1) approaches, intending to besiege them in the castle. A battle is fought over the next several scenes at nearby WAKEFIELD.

Sandells, Fulk (1551–1624) Farmer near STRATFORD, a friend of Anne HATHAWAY's family. In 1581 Sandells was made of supervisor of the will of Anne's father, Richard Hathaway, in which he was described as Hathaway's 'Trustee friend and neighbour'. He was responsible for paying Anne her inheritance 'at the day of her marriage'. In November 1582 he and John RICHARDSON (1) posted a bond guaranteeing the legality of Anne's intended marriage to Shakespeare, who was a minor; they agreed to pay £40 to the church if the wedding were not properly conducted.

Sands, Lord (William Sands [Sandys], d. 1540) Historical figure and minor character in *Henry VIII,* a nobleman at the court of King HENRY VIII. Sands jests with the Lord CHAMBERLAIN (2) in 1.3 and attends Cardinal WOLSEY's banquet in 1.4, where he flirts with ANNE (1) BULLEN. He helps establish the cheerfully decadent tone that characterises the king's court while still under the influence of Wolsey in the early part of the play.

Shakespeare was confused about the status of the historical Sands. At the time of the play's events, Sands was the Lord Chamberlain, though Shakespeare adds an anonymous holder of that office. Though he is designated as 'Sir Walter Sands' in the stage direction at 2.1.53, this nobleman's name was William, as Shakespeare knew from his source, HOLINSHED's *Chronicles;* the error probably resulted from a printer's misreading of an abbreviation for the name.

Sardis Ancient city in Greek Asia Minor, in what is now western Turkey, a location in *Julius Caesar.* A few days before the fatal battle of PHILIPPI, the rebel generals BRUTUS (4) and CASSIUS meet at Sardis, where they argue over dominance and where Brutus is visited by the GHOST (2) of Julius CAESAR (1). Historically the meeting at Sardis took place many months before Philippi, but Shakespeare compressed events for dramatic purposes.

Sardis was an important city at least as early as the 6th century B.C.; it was ruled by ROME and then the Byzantine Empire from 133 B.C. until the Turks conquered it in the late 11th century A.D. In 1402 the Mongols, under Tamurlane, destroyed the city, which has been a ruin ever since.

Saturninus Character in *Titus Andronicus,* the villainous Emperor. Saturninus becomes Emperor through the support of TITUS (1) Andronicus, but turns against him, fearing his popularity. He becomes a willing accessory to the plots against Titus spun by the Empress, TAMORA, and her lover, AARON. He sentences MARTIUS (1) and QUINTUS to death without a trial in 2.3, and, in a fit of temper, he has the CLOWN (2) killed in 4.4. In the final scene he kills Titus and is himself killed by LUCIUS (1). Saturninus is an early depiction by Shakespeare of an evil ruler who violates the ethics of kingship, an important issue for the playwright.

Saunderson, Mary (d. 1712) English actress. Wife of the leading actor of the time, Thomas BETTERTON, Mrs Saunderson, as she was known, was generally considered the leading actress. She was the first woman to play many Shakespearean parts, after the legalisation of women on stage in 1660, and was particularly notable as OPHELIA, JULIET (1), and LADY (6) MACBETH.

Savage, Thomas (c. 1552–1611) English businessman, a co-trustee with William LEVESON of Shakespeare's interest in the ground lease for the GLOBE THEATRE. Half of the lease for the land on which the Globe stood was entered into jointly by five actors in the CHAMBERLAIN'S MEN, Shakespeare, John HEMINGE, William KEMPE, Augustine PHILLIPS, and Thomas POPE (2). To make their shares independently saleable, the actors assigned their half to two trustees—Leveson and Savage—who then regranted a fifth of it to each of them.

Savage, a goldsmith whose principal occupation was as a minor official governing the coal trade, was Heminge's neighbour and landlord, which is probably why he was one of the trustees. He was also a close friend of Shakespeare's friend John JACKSON (1).

Saxo Grammaticus (c. 1150–c. 1206) Danish poet and historian, author of a remote source of *Hamlet*. Saxo Lange—known posthumously as Grammaticus for his scholarship—wrote in Latin a quasi-mythical history of the Danes, called the *Historiae Danicae*, which contains the earliest complete version of the legendary tale of Amleth, the predecessor of HAMLET, though earlier fragments appear in the Icelandic sagas. Saxo was a monk, the secretary of an archbishop who was chief minister for the king of DENMARK; little more is known of him. His history, though well known in medieval times through manuscript copies, was not published until 1514, in Paris; the Amleth material was then used by a French writer, François BELLEFOREST, in a story that subsequently influenced the author of the UR-HAMLET, Shakespeare's immediate source.

Say, James Finnes, Lord (d. 1450) Historical figure and character in *2 Henry VI*, Treasurer of England who is captured and killed by Jack CADE's rebels. Lord Say is presented as a noble and courageous man who volunteers to stay in London when the rebels approach in 4.4, although he knows that they particularly hate him, for unspecified reasons. He refuses to retreat with the king, lest his presence endanger the monarch. Seized by the rebels and taken before their leader in 4.7, Say is roundly insulted by Cade and accused of deeds ordinarily considered good, such as founding a school. He pleads his own virtues, but is beheaded by the rebels.

Shakespeare incorporated this merciless execution of a patently good man into his version of Cade's rebellion in order to paint it as thoroughly evil. Just as the reality of the revolt was different (see CADE), so was Say a different sort of nobleman than the one depicted here. He was a widely despised landowner in Kent, greedy and oppressive, and a close associate of the equally detested Duke of SUFFOLK (3). Moreover, as Treasurer, he was generally held responsible for the high taxes necessitated by the same misrule that had sparked the rebellion. When the rebels neared London, the King's government did not hesitate to imprison Say in the Tower as a sop to public sentiment before fleeing itself. When the rebels were welcomed into the city, one of their first acts was to execute Say, who made no defence that was recorded.

Scales, Lord Thomas de (d. 1460) Historical figure and minor character in *2 Henry VI*, the commander of the Tower of London during the rebellion led by Jack CADE in 4.5. Scales, whose historical role is accurately presented, helps drive the rebels from London. Scales is also mentioned in passing in *1 Henry VI* as having been captured by the French (1.1.146), as indeed he had been historically.

Scarus Character in *Antony and Cleopatra*, a follower of ANTONY. Scarus first appears at the battle of ACTIUM, in 3.10; he reports on the catastrophic rout of Antony's forces by the navy of Octavius CAESAR (2). Despite the defeat and the desertion of CANIDIUS, Scarus remains faithful to Antony. He fights bravely in his master's brief victory of 4.7 and makes light of his wounds—'I had a wound here that was like a T, / But now 'tis made an H' (4.7.7–8)—and Antony praises him to Cleopatra after the battle. He accompanies Antony to final defeat in 4.12, before he disappears from the play. This scarred veteran—his 'honour'd gashes' (4.8.11) are cited by Antony—illustrates the courageous conduct in Antony's followers to the last, even after the desertion of Canidius and ENOBARBUS. Antony's ability to hold such an honourable soldier allows us to see him and his fate as noble.

Scarus' name, which does not appear in Shakespeare's source, PLUTARCH's *Lives*, apparently is a pun referring to his scars, unless it was a mis-spelling of M. Aemilianus Scaurus (active c. 40–30 B.C.). He was a stepbrother of POMPEY (2) who joined Antony after his kinsman's final defeat in 36 B.C.—referred to in 3.5.4—and remained with him to the end. Scaurus was pardoned by the triumphant Caesar, and though he never held high office in the empire that Caesar established, his son did under the second emperor, Tiberius (ruled 14–37 A.D.).

Scheemakers, Peter (1691–1770) Flemish sculptor, creator of the statue of Shakespeare in WESTMINSTER (1) ABBEY. In 1740 Scheemakers was commissioned to sculpt Shakespeare in the Abbey's 'Poet's Corner' as

part of a memorial designed by the architect William Kent (1684–1748) and financed by a public subscription. He based his depiction of the playwright on the CHANDOS PORTRAIT.

Scheemakers spent most of his career in London, where he was among the most popular sculptors of the mid-18th century. Fourteen of the other Westminster Abbey memorial sculptures are his work. His brother Henry (d. 1748) and nephew Thomas (1740–1808) were also well-known London sculptors.

Schiller, Johann Christoph Friedrich (1759–1805) German poet, dramatist, and philosopher, creator of an adaptation of *Macbeth.* In 1800 at GOETHE's Weimar theatre, Schiller staged his own translation of *Macbeth.* He altered the play radically, making Shakespeare's grand villain into a noble victim of the malignant WITCHES. For the sake of 'purity', the humorous monologue of the PORTER (3) was replaced by a pious hymn. For all his own dramatic genius, Schiller could not accept the complex, full-blooded world of Shakespeare. This reflected the limitations of the developing German theatre of the day.

Schiller is generally regarded as second only to Goethe among German writers. His first play, *The Robbers* (1781), is about a brave man who unsuccessfully defies tyranny. It established Schiller as a defender of liberty in a revolutionary age, and its dramatic virtues—it remains popular today—marked him as a leading literary figure. He also wrote poetry: his 'Ode to Joy' (1785) was used by BEETHOVEN in the chorale movement of his Ninth Symphony. In 1787 he settled in Weimar where he taught history and developed an aesthetic philosophy. Influenced by his friendship with Goethe and his study of the philosopher Kant, he stressed the sublime nature of creativity and was a formative influence on the Romantic movement. He continued to write plays and many of them were staged at Goethe's theatre. The most notable of these were *Mary Stuart* (1800), *Wilhelm Tell* (1804), and his greatest masterpiece, a trilogy of historical plays about a famous general, *Wallenstein* (1798–1799).

Schlegel, August Wilhelm von (1767–1845) German scholar and poet, the most important translator of Shakespeare into German. With his wife, Karoline Michaelis Schlegel (best known as Karoline Schelling; 1763–1809), also a notable writer, Schlegel translated 16 of Shakespeare's plays (published 1797–1801; a 17th was issued in 1810). Following the Schlegels' divorce in 1803 the remaining plays were translated by a group led by Ludwig TIECK. The complete set was published between 1823 and 1829. It immediately became the standard German Shakespeare, replacing the prose versions of J. J. ESCHENBURG. The Schlegel-Tieck Shakespeare is considered to be one of the masterpieces of German literature, and it confirmed the stature that Shakespeare has since held among Germans as history's premier poet and dramatist.

Though best known for his Shakespeare translations, Schlegel also wrote poetry—some of it set to music by Franz SCHUBERT—and translated from Italian and Spanish. He produced the definitive German text of the plays of the great Spanish dramatist Pedro Calderón (1600–1681), as well as works by Dante Alighieri (1265–1321), Ludovico ARIOSTO, and Miguel de CERVANTES. He and his brother the philosopher Friedrich von Schlegel (1772–1829) are regarded as among the most important founders of German Romanticism, a literary and artistic movement that swept Europe in the early 19th century.

Schoolmaster (1) Character in *Antony and Cleopatra.* See AMBASSADOR (3).

Schoolmaster (2) Minor character in *The Two Noble Kinsmen,* the director of a country dance performance. In 3.5 the Schoolmaster directs a group of COUNTRYMEN and women, including NELL (2), in an entertainment presented to the court of Duke THESEUS (2). He is comically pedantic, both in instructing his charges and in his PROLOGUE (1) to the performance. Since most scholars believe that Shakespeare did not write 3.5, the Schoolmaster is probably the creation of John FLETCHER (2).

Schröder, Friedrich Ludwig (1744–1816) German actor and producer. In a series of productions beginning in 1776, Schröder introduced Shakespeare to the German theatre; except for an occasional flawed adaptation, such as *Der* BESTRAFTE BRUDERMORD, the playwright's works had not been performed in Germany since the early 17th century, when English touring companies may have presented some of them. However, beginning with Schröder's *Hamlet* (in which the producer played the GHOST [3]), Shakespeare became a staple of the German stage. Schröder was one of the leading lights of the German theatre, both as an actor and a producer. Born into a family of travelling players, he began his career at the age of three and eventually became a major figure in German cultural affairs of the late 18th and early 19th century.

Schubert, Franz (1797–1828) German composer of the Romantic movement whose many famous works include settings for three of the best-known songs from Shakespeare's plays (see SONG). In the summer of 1827 Schubert composed music for a *Standchen,* or 'Serenade', a translation of 'Hark, Hark, the Lark' (*Cymbeline,* 2.3.19–25), a *Trinklied,* or 'Drinking Song' (*Antony and Cleopatra,* 2.7.111–116), and, the most famous of the three, *An Sylvia,* or 'Who Is Silvia?' (*The Two Gentlemen of Verona,* 4.2.38–52). The first of these was translated by August Wilhelm von SCHLEGEL; the

others by a friend of the composer, Edouard von Bauernfeld. According to a famous—though probably untrue—story, Schubert wrote *An Sylvia* on the back of a menu during a meal.

Schubert, a very prolific and highly influential composer, also set to music a great deal of poetry by J. W. von GOETHE, Friedrich SCHILLER, and Schlegel, as well as German translations of the work of such varied authors as Aeschylus, Petrarch, Alexander POPE (1), and Sir Walter Scott. Best known for his songs and chamber music, he also wrote important symphonic works.

Schücking, Levin Ludwig (1878–1964) German scholar. Schücking was a leading member of the so-called 'realist' school of Shakespearean criticism, which attempted to relate the plays to the traditions and practises of ELIZABETHAN DRAMA and ELIZABETHAN THEATRE, rather than simply analysing the characters and their actions. Schücking's most influential work, translated as *Character Problems in Shakespeare's Plays* (1922), deals with the techniques the playwright inherited from earlier drama, such as having characters comment on the play's developments in the manner of a CHORUS (1).

Scofield, Paul (b. 1922) British actor. Scofield is especially noted for his portrayals of LEAR, directed by Peter BROOK (2), both in the 1962 stage production and the 1970 FILM. As a young man, Scofield joined the Birmingham Repertory Theatre under Barry JACKSON (1), and he went with Jackson to the Shakespeare Memorial Theatre in STRATFORD in 1945. There, he established himself as a classical actor, playing ARMADO, FESTE, MERCUTIO, and HAMLET, among others. He has since played many classical and modern parts. He has only taken movie roles occasionally, but he is probably most widely known as Sir Thomas MORE in the film *A Man for All Seasons,* a part he had previously played on the stage and for which he won an Academy Award in 1966.

Scot (Scott), Reginald (c. 1538–1599) English writer, author of a source for *A Midsummer Night's Dream, Macbeth,* and *The Tempest.* Scot's *The Discovery of Witchcraft* (1584) provided Shakespeare with items of folklore about witches and fairies that he used in his plays, especially in his depictions of PUCK in the *Dream,* the WITCHES in *Macbeth,* and ARIEL in *The Tempest.* Scot himself, however, derided the information as silly superstitions.

Scot, a country gentleman and justice of the peace for KENT (1), was appalled by the persecution of 'witches'—mostly poor or retarded people—that was raging in his time, and he wrote his book against the practise, attempting to disprove the existence of witchcraft. He was a century ahead of his time, for witches continued to be persecuted in England until the early 18th century. Scot's work was attacked by 'authorities' on witchcraft, including King JAMES I. Scot also wrote a pioneering technical manual on the growing of hops, a major Kentish industry.

Scotland Country to the north of England, setting for most of *Macbeth.* The importance of the Scottish nation is stressed at the beginning of the play. Act 1 details the suppression of a revolution supported by foreigners from Norway and Ireland. MACBETH's murder of King DUNCAN is repeatedly associated with a catastrophic decline in Scotland's fortunes and the rebellion against him is specifically intended to restore 'a swift blessing [to the] suffering country' (3.6.47–48). The trials of the nation, especially as described in the conversations of the exiled lords in 4.3 demonstrate the growth of evil that Macbeth's deed triggers. As ROSSE puts it, Scotland under Macbeth seems no longer 'our mother, but our grave' (4.3.166). Shakespeare had a specific lesson in mind here: that immorality in the leaders of a country leads to its social and political disruption. This is a lesson that is very prominent in the HISTORY PLAYS, also.

Scotland loomed large in English political considerations in Shakespeare's day. It was traditionally allied with England's enemy, FRANCE (1), especially since Scotland's ruling family was Catholic, and Scottish plots were feared throughout the reign of Queen ELIZABETH (1). Mary, Queen of Scots, was imprisoned in England for many years and eventually executed. However, her son King James VI of Scotland was a Protestant, and he succeeded Elizabeth as JAMES I in 1603 and united the two lands under a single ruler for the first time (though a full merger was still a century away).

James' accession was probably the reason that Shakespeare wrote a play set in Scotland, and allusions to James' reign are scattered throughout *Macbeth.* Some scholars believe that the playwright may also have been inspired by a trip to Scotland as an actor. He and other members of the CHAMBERLAIN'S MEN may have fled to Scotland in the wake of their seeming involvement in the rebellion of the Earl of ESSEX (2) in February 1601. They may have performed with Laurence FLETCHER (3) in Aberdeen. John Dover WILSON (3) went so far as to propose that *Macbeth* was written in Scotland and first performed in Edinburgh. However, these theories cannot be convincingly supported with any known evidence.

Scout Minor character in *1 Henry VI,* the French soldier who brings news of the English army's approach in 5.2.

Scribe Minor character in *Henry VIII,* petty official at the divorce trial of Queen KATHERINE. In 2.4.6 and

8–9, the Scribe orders the CRIER to formally demand the presence of King HENRY VIII and the queen, thus opening the proceedings. His tiny role stresses the pomp and ceremony of the occasion, thereby pointing up Katherine's vulnerability to the king's power.

Scrivener, The Minor character in *Richard III,* a clerk who learns of a crime committed by RICHARD III. In 3.6 the Scrivener, whose job is to make formal written copies of documents, knows that a certain indictment he has copied is false. Supposedly the record of a proceeding justifying the hasty execution of Lord HASTINGS (3), it was actually written before Hastings had even been accused of any misdeed. The Scrivener realises that Richard has arranged for the death of an innocent man through legal means, and he grieves that the state of public affairs permits such a ploy to succeed.

This incident, like one in 2.3 (see CITIZEN [2]), serves to emphasise that corruption can never be secret. The common people become aware of such cynical machinations, and society comes closer to political chaos as its leaders seem increasingly untrustworthy. This pattern grows more evident as Richard's ambitions come to dominate public life.

Scroop (1) (Le Scroop, Scroope, Scrope), Henry (c. 1376–1415) Historical figure and minor character in *Henry V,* a traitor who plans to assassinate King HENRY V but fails and is sentenced to death. Scroop and his fellow conspirators, the Earl of CAMBRIDGE and Sir Thomas GREY (3), are asked by Henry to advise him on punishing a drunken soldier who has defamed him. They all recommend severity. Then the king reveals his knowledge of their plot and applies their own rule to them, refusing them mercy. They each thank God for preventing their success, in conventional speeches intended to emphasise Henry's own majesty.

Henry judges Cambridge and Grey in a few words, but he chastises Scroop at great length (2.2.93–142). Scroop's treason is deemed particularly heinous, for he has been Henry's close friend and confidant for many years. Henry goes so far as to call Scroop's offence 'another fall of man' (2.2.142). The combination of Henry's grief at his friend's betrayal and his unswerving sternness demonstrates both the humanity and the maturity of the king.

The historical Scroop was indeed close to Henry, but he was also associated with a history of rebellion against the LANCASTER (1) dynasty. Although Shakespeare does not mention it in *Henry V,* Scroop's father, Stephen SCROOP (3), had been a supporter of RICHARD II, who was deposed by Henry's father, Lord BOLINGBROKE (1), later King HENRY IV, as is enacted in *Richard II.* Further, Scroop's uncle, the ARCHBISHOP (3) of the *Henry IV* plays, led two revolts against Henry IV. Scroop and his father disassociated themselves from the Archbishop, and Scroop was given high office under Henry V. Accordingly, his involvement in Cambridge's plot was punished with particular rigour: Grey and Cambridge were each beheaded, while Scroop was drawn and quartered.

Scroop (2), (Scroope, Scrope) Richard Character in *1, 2 Henry IV.* See ARCHBISHOP (3).

Scroop (3), (Le Scroop, Scroope, Scrope) Stephen (c. 1350–1406) Historical figure and minor character in *Richard II,* a supporter of RICHARD II. In 3.2 Scroop tells Richard of the popular acceptance of BOLINGBROKE (1), the execution of BUSHY and GREENE (1), and the defection of the Duke of YORK (4). These tidings undo the king, plunging him into near-hysterical despair, and Scroop remarks pointedly on the king's state; 'Sweet love, I see, changing his property, / Turns to the sourest and most deadly hate' (3.2.135–136).

The historical Scroop family did not accept Bolingbroke's rule. Stephen's brother, the ARCHBISHOP (3) of York, appears as a rebel in *1* and *2 Henry IV.* Stephen dissociated himself from that rebellion, but his son, Henry SCROOP (1), betrayed Bolingbroke's son, HENRY V, and is executed for treason in *Henry V.*

Seacoal, George Minor character in *Much Ado About Nothing,* one of the WATCHMEN (3) of MESSINA. In 3.3.11 Seacoal is recommended to DOGBERRY, the chief constable, as a likely leader of the watch because he is literate, and he is appointed to the position. He has no particular personality and cannot readily be distinguished from the other Watchmen. However, Seacoal may be presumed to be the speaker of commands—such as 'We charge you in the Prince's name, stand!' (3.3.159)—by virtue of his office.

A Francis Seacoal is mentioned by Dogberry at 3.5. 54; he is apparently the SEXTON, who appears in 4.2. The unnecessary and unlikely coincidence of surnames is best explained as one of the many minor errors in the plays. Here, the playwright hastily gave an inconsequential character a name that happened to be handy, forgetting that he had just used it for another such figure.

Sebastian (1) In *The Two Gentlemen of Verona,* the name JULIA takes while disguised as a boy.

Sebastian (2) Character in *Twelfth Night,* lover of OLIVIA and twin brother of VIOLA. Sebastian and Viola's virtually perfect resemblance to each other—a convention of romantic comedy—permits the traditional comic confusion of mistaken identities, but it also provides for two different presentations of love's restorative power. Sebastian resolves issues that his sister has raised, and his entrance stimulates the play's

climax and helps both Olivia and ORSINO to fulfil their potential.

Much of Sebastian's tale is similar to his sister's: both are shipwrecked and saved by helpful seamen—ANTONIO (4), in Sebastian's case—who direct them to the court of ILLYRIA; both are pursued by Olivia; both are threatened with combat by SIR ANDREW; and both are betrothed in the play's happy ending. These parallels heighten the effect of the comic confusions that ensue when Sebastian is mistaken for Cesario, the disguised Viola, and it also emphasises the function Sebastian serves when the mistakes are cleared up in 5.1. While Viola's pose as Cesario has inspired love—hers for Orsino and Olivia's for Cesario—Sebastian's arrival is necessary for these passions to be properly directed.

The correct relationship among the play's lovers—skewed at first by Viola's disguise and Orsino's misplaced passion for Olivia—begins to take shape when Sebastian meets Olivia, who believes him to be Cesario, in 4.1. He is naturally mystified by this ardent woman, but he recognises the value of her love, even knowing that it is based on some mistake, and he boldly plays along. In the same spirit, Sebastian immediately accepts Olivia's proposal of marriage in 4.3.

Sebastian's situation in Illyria differs from Viola's in one highly significant way: while Viola is disguised as a man, Sebastian's gender is unconfused and permits him a forthrightness not available to his sister. When Sir Andrew and SIR TOBY oppose him, his response is squarely in the tradition of masculine assertiveness: he fights and drives them away, in both 4.1 and 5.1. His clear-cut sexual identity allows Sebastian to provide the missing elements in the lives of the other characters. He is the manly youth of Viola's disguise, and he is the lover whom Olivia thought she had found in the disguised Viola. He is the dominant male that Orsino should be but has lost sight of through his romantic affectations. He is also to become the aristocratic husband that MALVOLIO has inappropriately aspired to be.

Sebastian thus helps to redeem other characters, and this fact, combined with Viola's capacity for devotion and sacrifice, has suggested to some scholars a religious interpretation of the play. In any case, his role in the resolution of the play's entanglements makes him the central figure of Acts 4–5, although he says relatively little and lacks a vibrant personality. He is not one of Shakespeare's more endearing heroes, but he is certainly a powerful one.

Sebastian (3) Character in *The Tempest,* brother of King ALONSO of Naples. Sebastian is led by ANTONIO (5), the villainous deposer of PROSPERO, into greater crimes than he would otherwise have contemplated. In 1.1 Antonio and Sebastian arrogantly curse the seamen of their storm-wracked vessel, and after they are shipwrecked on Prospero's magical island they are equally offensive in ridiculing GONZALO's attempts to cheer Alonso, who believes his son is dead. However, Sebastian demonstrates no more than crude offensiveness until Antonio suggests that they kill the sleeping Alonso, so that he, Sebastian, may inherit the crown of Naples. Sebastian accepts the idea greedily, but Antonio's primacy in evil is demonstrated in their plan: Antonio will stab Alonso, while Sebastian takes on Gonzalo. This is Sebastian's moment of greatest involvement. Prospero's sprite ARIEL prevents the assassinations and reduces Sebastian and the others to madness. In 5.1, free from the spell, Sebastian has one more significant line. When Prospero restores Alonso's son, Sebastian cries, 'A most high miracle.' (5.1.177). In acknowledgeing the spiritual power of the moment, Sebastian contrasts with Antonio, who remains unmoved. Thus, Sebastian, like Alonso, finally comes to exemplify humanity's capacity for redemption.

Second Clown Character in *Hamlet.* See OTHER.

Second Commoner Character in *Julius Caesar.* See COBBLER.

Second Grave-digger Character in *Hamlet.* See OTHER.

Second Murderer (1) One of 'two or three' characters in *2 Henry VI,* the killers of the Duke of GLOUCESTER (4). Several men, two of whom speak, flee the scene of the crime at the beginning of 3.2. The Second Murderer regrets the deed because their victim had died religiously. (See also FIRST MURDERER [1].)

Second Murderer (2) Character in *Richard III,* one of the two assassins hired by RICHARD III to kill his brother the Duke of CLARENCE (1). The Second Murderer has an attack of conscience as the two approach their victim in 1.4, but the FIRST MURDERER (2) reminds him of the money they are to receive, and he recovers. Their short exchange provides the only real comic relief in the play. Later in this scene, in an entirely serious vein, the Second Murderer shows an inclination to grant Clarence the mercy he pleads for. The First Murderer thereupon finishes off the duke, and the Second declares that he is too remorseful to accept payment and leaves the reward to his colleague.

Second Murderer (3) Character in *Macbeth.* See FIRST MURDERER (3).

Secretary Minor character in *Henry VIII,* an aide to Cardinal WOLSEY. In 1.1 the Secretary speaks two half-lines, to inform the cardinal that the SURVEYOR who is to testify against the Duke of BUCKINGHAM (1) is ready to be interrogated. As part of Wolsey's businesslike

retinue, the Secretary contributes to our sense of the cardinal's energy and power.

Segar, William (d. 1633) Contemporary of Shakespeare, a scholar of chivalric lore and heraldry. Segar's treatise *The Booke of Honour and Armes* (1590) probably influenced Shakespeare's humorous parodies of duelling in *Love's Labour's Lost* (1.2.167–170), *Romeo and Juliet* (2.4.19–26), and *As You Like It* (5.4.67–102), as well as his more serious treatment of trial by combat in *Richard II* (1.3.1–122). Segar held several important positions as a herald, including that of Garter King of Arms, the chief herald of England. As a result, he played an important part in arrangeing entertainments at the courts of Queen ELIZABETH (1) and King JAMES I and may thus have been personally acquainted with Shakespeare.

Seleucus (active 30 B.C.) Historical figure and minor character in *Antony and Cleopatra,* CLEOPATRA's treasurer. In 5.2 Cleopatra calls upon Seleucus to confirm the inventory of her household that she has submitted to the conqueror of Egypt, Octavius CAESAR (2). Instead, he tells Caesar that she has withheld more than she has listed. Caesar, who is amused by Cleopatra's ploy, tells Seleucus to leave as Cleopatra subjects him to a tirade of insults.

This episode has been variously interpreted. It can be seen as evidence of Cleopatra's shallow character. It continues the play's earlier portrayal of a grasping courtesan who here attempts to salvage what she can from the wreck of her and ANTONY's fortunes. On the other hand, it may actually demonstrate her cool—and, in the play's scheme of things, noble—intention to die rather than live on in humiliating defeat without Antony. Once Caesar has the idea that Cleopatra wishes only to retain a comfortable existence, he leaves her alone, free to arrange her suicide, whereas if her real intention were known, he would prevent her. Shakespeare may have intended Seleucus as the the queen's pawn in a successful effort to deceive the conqueror. The playwright's source, PLUTARCH's *Lives,* states that this was her plan, and though Shakespeare changes many of the details in Plutarch's account of the episode, he may well have included it for the same purpose.

Sempronius (1) Minor character in *Titus Andronicus.* Sempronius is present at the shooting of arrows to the gods (4.3), but he does not speak, though his name is mentioned by TITUS (1) in 4.3.10.

Sempronius (2) Minor character in *Timon of Athens,* an ungrateful friend of TIMON. Sempronius is among the friends to whom Timon sends for assistance when he faces bankruptcy after he has showered his friends—including Sempronius—with expensive gifts. However, when Sempronius is approached by Timon's SERVANT (23), he pretends to be offended that Timon has gone to other friends first and he refuses to lend him money. 'Who bates mine honour shall not know my coin' (3.3.28), he declares. Sempronius—with LUCIUS (3) and LUCULLUS who have similarly rejected Timon's request in previous scenes—helps demonstrate the hypocrisy and cold-heartedness of the Athenian aristocracy, one of the play's important themes.

Senator (1) Any of several minor characters in *Othello,* lawmakers of VENICE. The Senators meet with the DUKE (5), in 1.3, to discuss the threat presented by a Turkish attack on CYPRUS. When they summon their chief general, OTHELLO, they hear BRABANTIO's complaint that Othello has stolen his daughter DESDEMONA. With the Duke, they find Othello innocent of any crime, appoint him commander of Venetian forces in Cyprus, and order him abroad. The Senators are spoken for by the First Senator (except for one brief passage by a Second Senator), who asks appropriate questions. The Senators and the Duke illustrate the pomp and power of the Venetian state; they also demonstrate a collective capacity for social co-operation and judgement by consensus, aspects of society that are notably absent when the main plot unfolds on Cyprus.

Senator (2) Any of several characters in *Coriolanus,* lawmakers of ROME. The Senators appear in 1.1 to summon CORIOLANUS to fight for the city against the VOLSCIANS, and in 2.2 they honour him by nominating him to be a consul. In all three scenes of Act 3 they fruitlessly attempt to calm Coriolanus in his encounter with the tribunes, SICINIUS and BRUTUS (3). After Coriolanus is banished, takes arms against Rome, and is dissuaded from destroying the city by the arguments of his wife and mother, two of the Senators welcome the women back from their successful intercession, in 5.5. These lawmakers are ineffectual aristocrats, and their presence in the play serves to illustrate the weakness of authority in a disordered society.

In the FIRST FOLIO edition of the play, the stage entrance at 2.2.36 designates the Senators as 'the Patricians', and speech headings for a Senator at 3.1.252 and 259 specify 'Patri'. 'Noble' also appears in 3.2. Shakespeare knew the terms were not interchangeable—they are used separately in 4.3.14 and 5.4.54—so this minor carelessness simply indicates his awareness that the Roman Senators were aristocrats.

Senator (3) Any of several minor characters in *Coriolanus,* lawmakers of the VOLSCIANS, enemies of ROME. In 1.2 the Senators confer with the general AUFIDIUS; two of them, designated First and Second Senator, do most of the talking. They agree that Aufidius should

command the field army, while they govern the besieged CORIOLES, their capital. In 1.4 the Senators ineffectually defy the Romans. The presence of the Senators makes clear that the Volscians have a viable state, rather like that of Rome, and their role as Aufidius' nominal superiors helps establish the general's position as CORIOLANUS' opposite.

Senator (4) Any of several minor characters in *Timon of Athens,* the aristocratic legislators of ATHENS. The Senators benefit from Timon's hospitality, but in 2.1 a Senator begins the process of the protagonist's downfall. He recognises that Timon is losing his wealth in reckless generosity, and he decides to dun his one-time benefactor for a debt before 'Lord Timon will be left a naked gull' (2.1.31). The Senators' cold ingratitude is made vivid by Timon's STEWARD (2), who tells that they refused aid for his master 'in a joint and corporate voice [and] . . . After distasteful looks . . . and cold-moving nods, / They froze me into silence' (2.2.208–217). In 3.5 this hard-heartedness is displayed in a different way when the Senators refuse to accept ALCIBIADES' argument for mercy towards an honourable veteran. Instead, they banish the pleader, who in response vows to conquer the city. In Act 5 the Senators unsuccessfully attempt to win back Timon as an ally against Alcibiades, and in 5.4 they are reduced to begging for mercy. The avengeing general Alcibiades grants them mercy in the play's closing atmosphere of reconciliation. Thus, the Senators' callousness has informed both of the play's plot lines, and helps to demonstrate a favourite lesson of Shakespeare's: that the immorality of the ruling class can produce disorder and potential ruin for the society as a whole.

Senator (5) Either of two minor characters in *Cymbeline,* Roman legislators. In 3.8 the Senators inform two TRIBUNES (3) that the emperor has ordered them to raise an army from the gentry of ROME to be sent against King CYMBELINE. The First Senator does all the speaking—apart from the Second Senator's single word in 3.8.11—and he serves to convey information to the tribunes and to the audience.

Seneca, Lucius Annaeus (c. 4 B.C.–65 A.D.) Roman philosopher and playwright, an important influence on Shakespeare and ELIZABETHAN DRAMA in general. Seneca wrote nine tragedies that were widely adapted in 16th-century England. He followed ancient Greek TRAGEDY in his subject matter and his effort to produce a catharsis through pity and terror (see ARISTOTLE), but his focus on bloody incidents and his attention to ghosts and magic rather than divinity gave his works a very different tone. He did not intend his plays for performance, but rather as moral lessons to be read and studied, but his English followers did not know this. In 16th-century England, ancient Greek plays were almost unknown, and Seneca was taken as a model of the classical drama.

The REVENGE PLAY constitutes the purest Elizabethan use of Seneca, for his works generally centre on vengeance taken for the murder of a parent or child and depict bloody killings and physical mutilations. A number of other Senecan devices were popular with Elizabethan playwrights, including Shakespeare: soliloquies, exaggerated rhetoric, insanity and feigned insanity, and the use of ghosts. After the 1560s Seneca's plays were staged infrequently, but Shakespeare presumed his audiences were at least familiar with their reputation and general character, for he has POLONIUS, tritely evaluating theatrical styles, remark that 'Seneca cannot be too heavy' (*Hamlet* 2.2.396).

Highly organised and formal, Seneca's plays observe the classical unities—that is, the events take place within a few hours and occur in a single location. There are five acts, which progress from exposition to anti-climax in a prescribed sequence. The plays are filled with moralising and instructive passages and employ formal devices such as the PROLOGUE (1) and the CHORUS (1). Seneca concentrated on the failings of the evil and powerful; as Sir Philip SIDNEY remarked of his works, 'high and excellent Tragedie . . . maketh kings fear to be tyrants'. *Titus Andronicus* is very Senecan in subject matter and tone, and Shakespeare employed Senecan elements in many other works, especially *Richard III, Hamlet,* and *Macbeth.* Later in his career, however, Seneca's influence diminished.

Seneca, the aristocratic son of a famous rhetorician and historian, also became a famous orator and writer. In 41 A.D. he was exiled by the emperor Claudius, for reasons that are not known; called back in 49, he became tutor to the future emperor Nero. He was probably mentally ill to some extent, as the content of his plays suggests. He nevertheless wrote a number of works on law and philosophy—the plays themselves were meant as works of moral philosophy—but many have been lost. He advocated a stoic detachment and contempt for death that was later praised by Christian thinkers. As a minister under Nero, Seneca was reluctantly involved in the emperor's crimes. For instance, he composed a defence for Nero's murder of his own mother. Implicated in a conspiracy against Nero—probably unjustly—Seneca was sentenced to death. He was permitted to commit suicide, which he did with a serenity that became legendary.

Senior Character in *As You Like It.* See DUKE (7).

Sentry (1) Any of several minor characters in *1 Henry VI,* French soldiers. Posted on the walls of ORLÉANS (1) at the beginning of 2.1, the Sentries fail to warn their superiors of the English assault, which retakes the town. This episode, along with others, serves to ridi-

cule the French, thus furthering the central point that only dissensions among the English could have resulted in the loss of France.

Sentry (2) Minor character in *Antony and Cleopatra,* a soldier in the army of Octavius CAESAR (2). The Sentry and his two underlings, the WATCHMEN (4), are guards at Caesar's camp outside ALEXANDRIA. They discover the dying ENOBARBUS and bring him into the camp. The Sentry demonstrates the intelligence expected of a good non-commissioned officer when he holds the Watchmen back, at first, to discover what Enobarbus will say, in case he should reveal useful information. He helps demonstrate the high morale in Caesar's forces as they approach their final victory. In some editions of the play, the Sentry and the Watchmen are designated as the First, Second, and Third Soldiers.

Sergeant (1) Minor character in *1 Henry VI,* a French soldier. In 2.1, just before the English retake the town of ORLÉANS (1), the Sergeant posts SENTRIES who then fail to warn the others of the English attack. This, with numerous other incidents, points up the military inadequacies of the French, thus helping to emphasise the importance of dissensions among the English in promoting France's victories.

Sergeant (2) Character in *Macbeth.* See CAPTAIN (8).

Sergeant (3) Minor character in *Henry VIII,* a soldier who formally arrests the Duke of BUCKINGHAM (1). In 1.1.198–202 the Sergeant follows the orders of BRANDON (1) and reads a formal charge of treason against Buckingham. He then disappears from the play. His small role adds a note of pomp and ceremony that stresses the great power underlying Buckingham's downfall.

Servant (1) Character in *The Comedy of Errors.* See MESSENGER (1).

Servant (2) Minor character in *1 Henry VI.* In 4.7 the Servant aids the mortally wounded TALBOT on the battlefield and mournfully announces the arrival of the corpse of the hero's son, JOHN (6), killed in the fighting.

Servant (3) Minor character in *2 Henry VI* who accompanies the Duke of GLOUCESTER (4) in 2.4 when he watches his wife, the DUCHESS (1) paraded ignominiously through the streets of London as part of her punishment for conspiring against the king. The Servant suggests that he and his fellows could rescue the Duchess, but the duke rejects the idea.

Servant (4) Minor character in *Romeo and Juliet,* a worker in the CAPULET (1) household. In 1.2 the Servant is given a list of guests to Capulet's banquet and instructed to deliver invitations. However, he is illiterate and seeks the help of ROMEO, who happens to be passing by. Thus Romeo learns of the banquet, which he will attend in search of ROSALINE (2) but where he will meet JULIET (1). At the banquet the Servant (or perhaps another one) is unable to identify Juliet in 1.5.42.

Servant (5) Any of several minor characters in *The Taming of the Shrew,* workers in the home of the LORD (1) who takes in Christopher SLY (1) in the INDUCTION. On the Lord's instructions, the Servants offer Sly the pleasures of gentlemanly life, encouraging him to believe that he has been insane in believing himself a poor drunkard.

Servant (6) Minor character in *The Taming of the Shrew,* a worker in the household of BAPTISTA. The Servant escorts the disguised suitors of BIANCA (1) in 2.1 and, in 3.1, brings Bianca a message about the imminent wedding of her sister, KATHERINA.

In the FIRST FOLIO text of the play, the name 'Nicke' designates the Servant in the speech heading at 3.1.80. Scholars recognise a reference to the actor who played the part, perhaps Nicholas TOOLEY.

Servant (7) Minor character in *Richard II,* a messenger serving the Duke of YORK (4). In 2.2 the Servant brings news of the death of the DUCHESS (2) of Gloucester. This poignant moment emphasises the duke's helplessness in the face of onrushing events.

Servant (8) Minor character in *Richard II,* the attendant of Sir Piers EXTON. The Servant supports Exton in his assumption that BOLINGBROKE (1) wants to have the deposed RICHARD II murdered.

Servant (9) Minor character in *1 Henry IV,* a member of HOTSPUR's household. In 2.3 Hotspur summons the Servant to question him about the availability of a new horse. This brief episode helps quicken the pace of a scene—otherwise involving only the nobleman and his wife—that points to the forthcoming military crisis of Hotspur's rebellion.

Servant (10) Either of two minor characters in *The Merry Wives of Windsor,* workers in the FORD (1) household. In 3.3 MISTRESS (1) Ford has the Servants, whom she addresses as John and Robert, carry FALSTAFF out of the house in a laundry basket and dump him in the river. In 4.2 they again carry out the basket, and they remark humorously on the great weight it contained before. The Servants contribute to the sense of bourgeois prosperity that pervades Shakespeare's WINDSOR.

Servant (11) Minor character in *Julius Caesar,* messenger for CAESAR (1). In 2.2.5–6 Caesar sends the Servant to request an augury—a forecast of the future through the ritual examination of an animal's entrails—from the priests. He returns to report a disastrous outcome in 2.2.37–40: an animal was sacrificed and discovered to have had no heart. The episode reinforces the sense of mounting tension as Caesar's death approaches. However, Shakespeare's source, PLUTARCH's *Lives,* states that Caesar performed the augury himself; rather than attempt a spectacle—probably impractical to stage—that would distract the audience by providing a false climax before the assassination scene, the playwright moved the event offstage and added this character to convey its essence.

Servant (12) Minor character in *Julius Caesar,* a messenger employed by Mark ANTONY. The Servant delivers a speech in his master's name to Caesar's assassins, offering them an alliance. In an eloquent passage (3.1. 125–134) that anticipates Antony's funeral oration, the Servant establishes a sense of Antony's cunning and strong personal style before he makes an important appearance himself.

Servant (13) Minor character in *Julius Caesar,* a messenger for OCTAVIUS. In 3.1 the Servant tells Mark ANTONY of Octavius' approach to ROME. Arriving just after the assassination of CAESAR (1), his shock reminds us of the enormity of the deed. The Servant reappears in 3.2, after Antony's oration at Caesar's funeral, to report that Octavius has arrived. His brief appearances indicate the onset of Rome's future, in the person of the emperor-to-be, and remind us of the inexorability of the events that unfold in the wake of Caesar's murder.

Servant (14) Minor character in *Twelfth Night,* an employee of OLIVIA. In 3.4, just as MALVOLIO appears to have turned lunatic, the Servant announces VIOLA's arrival, contributing to a sense of the busyness of Olivia's household at a moment of comic crisis.

Servant (15) Minor character in *Hamlet.* The Servant tells HORATIO that some 'seafaring men' (4.6.2) (see FIRST SAILOR [1]) have letters for him. Beginning with the earliest productions of the play this part has often been cut.

Servant (16) Minor character in *Troilus and Cressida,* an employee of Prince PARIS (3). In 3.1 PANDARUS asks the Servant about Paris; the Servant replies with saucy witticisms that go over Pandarus' head. The episode exposes Pandarus' foolish and supercilious manner.

Servant (17) Minor character in *Troilus and Cressida,* follower of DIOMEDES. In 5.5 the Servant is instructed to take TROILUS' captured horse to CRESSIDA as Diomedes' testament to his superiority to her ex-lover.

Servant (18) Minor character in *Measure for Measure,* an attendant to ANGELO (2). The Servant receives the PROVOST in 2.2 and announces ISABELLA's arrival in 2.4. His presence reminds us of Angelo's importance and power.

Servant (19) Any of several minor characters in *King Lear,* members of the household of the Duke of CORNWALL. In 3.7, one of the Servants, designated the First Servant, attacks Cornwall in an effort to prevent him from barbarously putting out the eyes of the Earl of GLOUCESTER (1). The First Servant is killed, but he wounds the duke, who dies later. The Second and Third Servants assist the wounded Gloucester and they comment on the evil natures of the duke and his wife REGAN. The episode stresses the horror that has been loosed by King LEAR's folly in granting power to Regan and her sister GONERIL. At the same time, the Servants demonstrate that good still resides in some people, and thereby offer some relief from the increasing violence and terror of the plot.

Servant (20) Any of several minor characters in *Macbeth,* workers in MACBETH's household. In 3.1 a Servant is sent to bring the Murderers (see FIRST MURDERER [3]) to Macbeth; in 3.2 LADY (6) MACBETH sends a Servant (possibly the same one) to summon her husband; and in 5.3, a Servant (again, perhaps the same one) reports to Macbeth that the woods appear to be advancing on DUNSINANE. In all three instances, the Servant's function is to effect a transition or provide information, though in the final scene, Macbeth's fury at the innocent Servant demonstrates his desperate and baleful state of mind.

Servant (21) Any of several minor characters in *Antony and Cleopatra,* workers in the household of POMPEY (2). The servants are waiters at a banquet that celebrates the truce between Pompey and the Roman leaders—ANTONY, LEPIDUS, and Octavius CAESAR (2). At the opening of 2.7 two of the Servants—designated the First and Second Servants—gossip about Lepidus' drunkenness at the feast. They observe that Lepidus has weakened himself in relation to the others. Their conversation prepares us for the comic scene of Lepidus' intoxication that follows and points up the treachery that lurks in the world of high policy and warfare, also illustrated in the remainder of the scene.

Servant (22) Any of several minor characters in *Antony and Cleopatra,* workers in the household of the title characters. In 3.13 a Servant announces the arrival of THIDIAS, an ambassador from Octavius CAESAR (2) to CLEOPATRA; when ANTONY discovers the ambassador

kissing her hand, he summons Servants to whip him. Later, one of them brings Thidias back and declares that he has been punished. The actions of the Servants demonstrate that there is still a remnant of pomp and power available to Antony as he approaches his end.

Servant (23) Any of several minor characters in *Timon of Athens*, workers in TIMON's household. In 4.2 the Servants, under the STEWARD (2), remain faithful to Timon when his false friends desert him. Though they must leave the bankrupt household to find other work, they remain 'fellows still, / Serving alike in sorrow' (4.2.18–19), as one of them puts it. In their loyalty they contrast tellingly with Timon's unfaithful aristocratic friends, and they emphasise one of the play's main themes: the callous heartlessness of ATHENS' ruling class. The Servants are mostly anonymous, though two of them, FLAMINIUS and SERVILIUS, are named in 2.2 and Act 3 and may be present in 4.2. Also, a Third Servant—as he is designated in the stage direction at 3.3.1—distinguishes himself with a scathing monologue criticising the miserly hypocrite, SEMPRONIUS, in 3.3.29–43.

Servant (24) Minor character in *Timon of Athens*, worker in the household of LUCULLUS. In 3.1 the Servant greets FLAMINIUS, who has come from TIMON to borrow money from Lucullus. Lucullus ignobly refuses to make the loan. The Servant, who brings wine and speaks one line when he reappears, serves to indicate the affluent life of his miserly master.

Servant (25) Minor character in *Pericles*, the victim of a storm who is aided by the physician CERIMON. In 3.2 Cerimon informs the Servant that his master will soon die, apparently making the diagnosis based on information the Servant has given him before the scene opened. The Servant then leaves, having spoken only briefly. He serves to help illustrate Cerimon's talents as a physician.

Servant (26) Any of several minor characters in *Pericles*, employees of Lord CERIMON. The Servants deliver a large chest that has been washed ashore by a storm. It proves to be a coffin that contains the body of the supposedly dead THAISA. A Servant is sent to fetch the medical supplies with which Cerimon revives her. One Servant speaks briefly, but they serve mainly to bring stage properties into the scene.

Servant (27) Any of several minor characters in *The Winter's Tale*, workers in the household of King LEONTES of SICILIA. In 2.3 a Servant informs the king of the progress of his son, MAMILLIUS, who is ill, thereby preparing the ground for the announcement by another Servant (or perhaps the same one) of the boy's death in 3.2. In 5.1 a Servant announces the approach of FLORIZEL and PERDITA, describing Perdita's charms rapturously. This last Servant seems to be a GENTLEMAN (13) of the court, the king speaks with him of his poems about Queen HERMIONE. He is probably one of the Gentlemen who appear in 5.2, and many editions designate him as such. He is often referred to by commentators as the Gentleman-poet.

Servant (28) Minor character in *The Winter's Tale*, the employee of the SHEPHERD (2). The Servant appears twice in 4.4, to announce the arrival of AUTOLYCUS and the presentation of a MASQUE at the shepherds' festival. His comical enthusiasm heightens our pleasure in the festivities. He comments, for instance, on Autolycus' singing 'O master! if you did but hear the pedlar at the door, you would never dance again after a tabor and pipe; no, the bagpipe could not move you' (4.4.183–185). He is a rustic CLOWN (1) whose naïveté contributes to the fun; for example, he foolishly construes Autolycus' songs as 'without bawdry', but adds that they contain 'delicate burdens [choruses] of dildoes and fadings, jump her and thump her' (4.4.195–196).

Servant (29) Minor character in *Henry VIII*, a worker in the household of Cardinal WOLSEY. At the cardinal's banquet, the Servant announces the arrival of 'A noble troop of strangers' (1.4.53), who prove to be the masquers (see MASQUE) led by King HENRY VIII. The Servant lends an air of opulence to the occasion.

Servant (30) Minor character in *The Two Noble Kinsmen*, a member of the household of EMILIA (4). In 5.3 the Servant reports to his mistress on the progress of the duel between ARCITE and PALAMON, who are fighting over her. In this way the audience is able to experience the duel while the actual combat is kept off-stage.

Servilius Minor character in *Timon of Athens*, a servant of TIMON. In 2.2 Servilius is sent to ask Lord LUCIUS (3) to assist Timon with a loan, but in 3.2 Lucius refuses, though he has benefited from the extravagant generosity that has created Timon's money troubles. The episode serves to demonstrate the miserly ingratitude of the Athenian aristocracy, an important theme of the play. Servilius, though he appears briefly elsewhere, simply serves to further the plot.

Serving-man (1) Any of several minor characters in *1 Henry VI*, feuding servants of the Bishop of WINCHESTER (1) and the Duke of GLOUCESTER (4). In 3.1 the king and his noblemen, assembled in the Parliament House to settle the feud between the bishop and the duke, learn that the large household staffs of these two are fighting in the streets. These Serving-men have been forbidden to carry arms because of earlier con-

flicts, but they are now pelting each other with rocks. Several Serving-men burst into the meeting, still fighting, and refuse to stop. One asserts, '. . . if we be forbidden stones, we'll fall to it with our teeth' (3.1. 89–90). The episode serves to point up the increasing disorder that has arisen in England because of rivalries among the aristocracy.

Serving-man (2) Any of several minor characters in *Romeo and Juliet,* members of the staff of the CAPULET (1) household. A Serving-man summons Lady CAPULET (3) to dinner in 1.3. In 1.5 four Serving-men, one of whom is comically named Potpan, jestingly clear away the banquet while preparing for a backstairs party of their own. In 4.2 and 4.4 Serving-men joke with Capulet as they assist in his preparations for the wedding of JULIET (1). These mellow and humorous domestics serve to suggest an atmosphere of bourgeois solidity to the Capulet household.

Serving-man (3) Minor character in *The Taming of the Shrew,* a servant of the country LORD (1) who informs his master of the arrival of the PLAYERS (1) in the INDUCTION.

Serving-man (4) Any of several minor characters in *The Taming of the Shrew,* servants at the banquet in 5.2. The Serving-men do not speak.

Serving-man (5) Minor character in *The Merchant of Venice,* servant of PORTIA (1). The Serving-man brings his mistress word that four unwanted suitors are leaving and that another suitor, the Prince of MOROCCO, is arriving.

Serving-man (6) Minor character in *The Merchant of Venice,* servant of ANTONIO (2). In 3.1 the Serving-man tells SALERIO and SOLANIO that his master wishes to see them.

Serving-man (7) Any of several minor characters in *Coriolanus,* servants of AUFIDIUS. In 4.5 when CORIOLANUS arrives at Aufidius' home disguised as a poor man, the Serving-men—designated as First, Second, and Third—attempt to throw him out. He beats one of them, who runs out of the room before Aufidius arrives and the other two Serving-men withdraw. At the close of the scene, two of them reappear to discuss the stranger. They pretend to have recognised Coriolanus' worth from the beginning, and, comically, they hesitate to speak before sounding each other's opinion. The Third Serving-man reappears with news of Coriolanus' identity and of his defection to the VOLSCIANS, for whom he will fight against ROME. The Serving-men are pleased with the prospect of an easy triumph and welcome the coming war. They make humorously greedy predictions of excitement and loot.

In the opening of 4.5 the Serving-men fill an ancient role of foolish servants who emphasise the nobility of their social betters when they mishandle a situation. The episode may have seemed more humorous to its original audiences than it does today, for the beating of servants was a traditional comic routine, dating back to ROMAN DRAMA. At the close of the scene the Serving-men's comical nature is more evident. Their pleasure at the prospect of war is a sharp piece of social satire that keeps our attention on the political themes of the play.

Servitor Any of several minor characters in *Antony and Cleopatra,* servants of ANTONY. In 4.2 Antony bids farewell to these attendants while they serve a banquet before his final battle against Octavius CAESAR (2). He announces that their allegiance to him may be at an end, and says 'Perchance to-morrow / You'll serve another master' (4.2.27–28). They respond with tears, and ENOBARBUS, also weeping, chastises Antony for causing 'discomfort' (4.2.34). Antony laughs and declares that he intends to be victorious in the next day's battle. He rousingly calls for the banquet to begin as the scene ends. The episode demonstrates the disturbed state of Antony's mind as the play's climax approaches. The Servitors, who speak only three words in unison, are merely extras who witness this demonstration.

Sexton Minor character in *Much Ado About Nothing,* a scribe who records Constable DOGBERRY's comically inept interrogation of CONRADE and BORACHIO in 4.2. Exasperated, the Sexton assumes control of the investigation and deduces that the WATCHMEN (3) have uncovered the plot by which the villainous Don JOHN (1) has slandered HERO. His common sense thus allows the exposure of wrongdoing that Dogberry's antics cannot.

The Sexton seems to be referred to in 3.5.54, where Dogberry calls him Francis Seacoal, giving him the same distinctive surname as George SEACOAL, one of the Watchmen. The minor confusion brought about by this unlikely coincidence is hardly noticeable on stage; it is probably simply one of the many minor slips that Shakespeare made throughout his career.

Seyton Minor character in *Macbeth,* an attendant to MACBETH. Seyton appears briefly in 5.3, where he endures Macbeth's impatient abuse, and even more briefly in 5.5, where he informs Macbeth of the death of LADY (6) MACBETH. This triggers Macbeth's famous soliloquy on 'to-morrow, and to-morrow, and to-morrow' (5.5.19). He is a patient servant who functions as a sounding board for Macbeth's increasing dementia.

The men of a Scottish family named Seyton (Seton,

Seaton) were hereditary armourers to the kings of Scotland, and Shakespeare may have intended Seyton as one of them. However, the Seytons' position did not exist until the rule of King Edgar (ruled 1097–1107), who was a son of Macbeth's foe and successor MALCOLM. Some scholars think Shakespeare may also have intended the name to be a pun on 'Satan', a reference to Macbeth's last loyal servant that stresses the king's depravity as he approaches his end.

Shaa (Shaw), Ralph (or John) (d. 1484) Historical figure and minor character in *Richard III*, one of two clergymen who, disguised as BISHOPS (1), accompany RICHARD III as he receives the MAYOR (3) in 3.7. This imposture is intended to create an air of religiosity about the would-be usurper. Shaa and Friar PENKER were summoned by Richard in 3.5. The historical Shaa, sometimes thought to have been named John, was a minor clergyman. He is known to have been a brother of the Mayor.

Shadow, Simon Minor character in *2 Henry IV*, one of the men whom FALSTAFF recruits for the army in 3.2. Shadow is extremely thin, and much is made of the appropriateness of his name. While hardier men bribe their way out of service, Falstaff justifies his choice of Shadow by observing that he will be as hard for a marksman to hit as 'the edge of a penknife' (3.2.262). It is thought that Shadow was originally played by John SINCKLO, an exceptionally thin actor who was among the CHAMBERLAIN'S MEN, the company for whom Shakespeare wrote the play.

Shadwell, Thomas (1642–1692) English playwright and theatrical entrepreneur, producer of adaptations of *Timon of Athens* and *The Tempest*. Shadwell was a successful writer of comedies, usually modelling his work on that of Ben JONSON. He undertook to make an opera of William DAVENANT and John DRYDEN's adaptation of *The Tempest*. The result, *The Enchanted Island* (1674), employed music by several composers, including Matthew LOCKE, though in 1690 Henry PURCELL composed a new score. In this form the work remained popular for well over a century, influencing subsequent adaptations of Shakespeare's play. Shadwell also wrote a dramatic adaptation of *Timon of Athens*. His *Timon of Athens, the Man-Hater* (1678) altered the tone of Shakespeare's play considerably, chiefly by adding two lovers—one faithful, one not—for the title character. It was popular for more than 50 years.

Shakespeare (1), Anne (1571–1579) Shakespeare's sister. Anne Shakespeare was born when the future playwright was seven and died when he was 14. There is evidence that her loss may have been particularly grievous to the family, for the record reveals that her funeral was unusually elaborate and costly, although the financial difficulties of John SHAKESPEARE (9) were great at the time. Nothing else is known of her.

Shakespeare (2), Anne Hathaway Shakespeare's wife. See HATHAWAY.

Shakespeare (3), Edmund (1580–1607) Shakespeare's brother, probably an actor in LONDON. The playwright's brother is only recorded as such at his christening, but he is thought to have been the 'Edmund Shakespeare, a player' who was buried in St Saviour's Church, SOUTHWARK, on December 31, 1607. In addition to the coincidence of name, his very expensive funeral, presumably unaffordable by the estate of an unknown actor, suggests a prosperous relative such as the playwright. Four months earlier, the burial of an illegitimate child, 'Edward, sonne of Edward Shackspeere' was recorded at a different London church; this may be Edmund, mistakenly given the boy's name (similar errors are known in this parish register). Edmund was probably named for his uncle Edmund Lambert (father of John LAMBERT).

Shakespeare (4), Gilbert (1566–1612) Shakespeare's brother. Gilbert Shakespeare was recorded as a haberdasher in LONDON in 1597, but he also lived in STRATFORD, or at least had returned there by 1602, when he stood in for William by receiving a deed to land the playwright had bought from John and William COMBE (1, 4). In 1609 he was summoned to appear in a Stratford court concerning a lawsuit, though neither its subject nor Gilbert's connection to it is known, and in 1610 he witnessed a document in Stratford. He was buried there and recorded as a bachelor.

Shakespeare (5), Hamnet (1585–1596) Shakespeare's son. The birth of Hamnet and his twin sister Judith SHAKESPEARE (10) around the end of January (they were christened on February 2) 1585, offers a datable association of the future playwright with STRATFORD before he left to pursue his career in LONDON, for they must have been conceived around April 1584. Their father is next known as an established actor and playwright in London in 1592. Hamnet's death at age 11 must have been shattering to his father, but there is no certain trace of it in the playwright's work (except possibly in the touching response of HUBERT to the death of Prince ARTHUR in 4.3.105–106 of *King John:* under a generally discredited but still possible hypothesis, this play could have been written as late as 1596). Hamnet was probably named for Shakespeare's friend (and the boy's likely godfather) Hamnet SADLER.

Shakespeare (6), Henry (d. 1596) Shakespeare's uncle. Henry, the brother of the playwright's father, John SHAKESPEARE (9), was a tenant farmer on a manor

near STRATFORD. He was sued several times over money matters—in 1587 John, as his guarantor, was sued as well, at a time when his own finances were in trouble. Henry was in trouble with the law on several occasions. He was fined for fighting in 1574 and in 1583 for improper garb in church, and he was gaoled in 1591 for trespass and in 1596 for debt—three months before his death. At this time his creditor went to his farm and confiscated a team of oxen. This may have paid the debt and secured his release, but he was fined a month later for not properly maintaining his land and the neighbouring highway, as he was required to do. However, despite such problems, he was reported to have been a prosperous man at his death, with money and a barn full of fodder.

Shakespeare (7), Joan (b. 1558) Shakespeare's sister. Nothing is known of this Joan Shakespeare except her christening date, but she certainly died before the birth of the second Joan SHAKESPEARE (8) in 1569. She was probably named for her mother's sister Joan Arden Lambert (mother of John LAMBERT).

Shakespeare (8), Joan (Joan Shakespeare Hart) (1569–1646) Shakespeare's sister. Joan Shakespeare was the only one of the playwright's siblings to survive him, and she was apparently the only one who married. She married a hatter, William Hart (d. 1616, a week before Shakespeare), about whom no more is known. In his will Shakespeare left his sister £20, all of his clothes, and a lifetime lease on the house in which she lived (the playwright's BIRTHPLACE, which he left to his daughter Susanna SHAKESPEARE [14] Hall). She lived there for the rest of her life, and her surviving son, Thomas Hart (1605–before 1670), lived there after her. Her descendants lived there until 1806. Joan had four children in all, the eldest of whom was the actor William HART (3). The other two died in childhood.

Shakespeare (9), John (before 1530–1601) Shakespeare's father. John Shakespeare left the farm of his father, Richard SHAKESPEARE (12), and became an apprentice glover and tanner of fine leathers in STRATFORD. He prospered; he is recorded as a householder in 1552 and had bought more property by 1556 (possibly including the house that was to be the playwright's BIRTHPLACE). Between 1556 and 1558 he married Mary Arden (see SHAKESPEARE [11]), the youngest daughter of his father's landlord. He inherited his father's leasehold on the land, but he sold it to a brother-in-law of Mary, preferring his shop in Stratford. He eventually became a broker of wool and other commodities, in addition to his leather business. He was respected among his fellow citizens and was appointed and elected to a variety of increasingly important civic positions, including that of chamberlain, supervising the town's finances. In 1565 the year after William's birth, he was elected an alderman—entitling his children to a free education at the Stratford Grammar School—and in 1568 he became bailiff of Stratford, the equivalent of mayor. He always signed his name with a mark, but this did not necessarily signify illiteracy (literate men of the time are known to have signed in this fashion). Given John Shakespeare's success as a town official, he was almost certainly literate, though he may have been able to read only. Around 1570 he began the process of applying for a COAT OF ARMS and establishing a position in the gentry.

In 1575 he bought two more houses in Stratford, but thereafter his fortunes declined. After 1577 he stopped attending the aldermen's meetings, at which he had regularly been present. In 1578 he was delinquent in taxes, and in the same year he mortgaged an estate Mary Shakespeare had inherited and sold other property that she owned. In 1580 he was fined the considerable amount of £40—more than his father had possessed at his death—for failure to appear in court and guarantee that he would keep the peace. The cause of this proceeding is unknown, but the size of the fine suggests the court's opinion that he was still a man of wealth. In 1586 he was finally removed from the board of aldermen because of inattendance. By 1590 his real estate holdings had been reduced to the Henley Street house, and in 1592 he was fined for not attending church, with the notation that he was thought to be staying home in fear of arrest for debt. On the other hand, he was still a valued neighbour, and he was several times called on to evaluate people's estates, a position of trust.

It has been speculated that John Shakespeare succumbed to alcoholism in this period, but this cannot be confirmed. In any case the family's situation improved only after 20 years, presumably in consequence of Shakespeare's success in the theatre. In 1596 John was finally awarded his coat of arms. In 1597 John and William attempted unsuccessfully to recover Mary's mortgaged estate (see LAMBERT), but William bought NEW PLACE in the same year. Just before his death, John Shakespeare reappeared on the town council.

Shakespeare (10), Judith (Judith Shakespeare Quiney) (1585–1662) Shakespeare's daughter. The birth of Judith and her twin brother Hamnet SHAKESPEARE (5) in late January, 1585, offers evidence that Shakespeare was in STRATFORD around the previous April, when they were conceived. He must soon thereafter have left to pursue a career in LONDON, but no record of him between then and 1592 has survived.

Judith married at 31, rather late by the standards of the day. She and Thomas QUINEY (3), who was four years younger, were wed in February 1616. Her father evidently disapproved of the match, for he changed

his will to protect her portion from her husband (though the marriage is not mentioned in the will). Dying two months later, he left Judith £100 as a dowry, but a further £150 was held in reserve, and she received only the interest on it as long as Quiney lived. If she died, the sum would revert to Susanna SHAKESPEARE (14) and her heirs and not to Quiney, unless he had by then legally endowed his and Judith's children with land.

Judith and Thomas Quiney were married during Lent without obtaining the special licence required, and he, at least, was briefly excommunicated (the record is unclear about her). In November their first child, Shakespeare Quiney, was born, but he lived only five months. Their two subsequent children also died young, at 11 and 19, both in 1639.

Shakespeare (11), Mary Arden (c. 1540–1608) Shakespeare's mother. Mary Arden was the youngest of the eight daughters of Robert ARDEN (2), a gentleman farmer who owned land in several villages near STRATFORD. In 1556 she was the executor of her father's will though she was 16 and probably illiterate, suggesting her recognised capabilities. Her father left her some money, an estate that included a farmhouse and about 60 acres of land, and a share in another property, part of which was leased for farming by Richard SHAKESPEARE (12). He had also already given her other properties before he died. When she married John SHAKESPEARE (9) sometime between 1556 and 1558 (no record has survived), she moved from the Arden farm to the town of Stratford, where she lived for the remainder of her life. She had two children who died in infancy before William was born in 1564. Of five later children, four lived to adulthood (see Anne, Edmund, Gilbert, Joan, and Richard SHAKESPEARE [1, 3, 4, 8, 13]). All of her inherited property was lost in the course of her husband's financial difficulties. After John's death in 1601, she either lived with her married daughter Joan in the playwright's BIRTHPLACE, her home for more than 40 years, or at NEW PLACE with William's family. Little more is known of her life.

Shakespeare (12), Richard (d. 1561) Shakespeare's paternal grandfather. Richard Shakespeare was a farmer in Snitterfield, a village a few miles from STRATFORD. Nothing is known of him before 1529 (though a Richard 'Shakyspere' was resident in another village, eight miles away, in 1524). He was a tenant farmer working land on several different manors (as was common), one of which was owned by Shakespeare's maternal grandfather, Robert ARDEN (2). The records mentioning Richard Shakespeare reveal the ordinary life of an English yeoman: he was frequently fined for failure to attend a manor court held twice a year—rather than travel six miles there and back, he, like many farmers, preferred to pay the nominal fine—and for grazing too many cattle on the commons (though the vicar of Snitterfield was also fined for forcibly removing them).

He was a solid citizen who was several times called on to value the estates of his deceased neighbours, a position of trust. When he died, his property was valued at more than £38, making him a prosperous though not wealthy husbandman. Richard's wife is unknown, but with her he had at least two sons (records on two other Shakespeares of the neighbourhood are unclear), John SHAKESPEARE (9), the playwright's father, and Henry SHAKESPEARE (6), his uncle.

Shakespeare (13), Richard (1574–1613) Shakespeare's brother. Nothing is recorded of this younger brother of the playwright between his christening and his burial. He was presumably named for his paternal grandfather, Richard SHAKESPEARE (12). He probably lived in STRATFORD all his life and apparently did not marry.

Shakespeare (14), Susanna (Susanna Shakespeare Hall) (1583–1649) Shakespeare's daughter. Susanna Shakespeare was born only six months after her parents' marriage (see HATHAWAY). Her name, taken from the biblical Apocrypha, had only recently appeared in STRATFORD and was associated with strong religious sentiment, especially Puritan leanings. Twenty-four years later, she married a man of strong Puritan sentiments, Dr John HALL (4). (However, a year earlier, she was cited as absent from church on Easter, a criminal offence that was associated with Catholic dissent. The case was dropped, either because she was deemed innocent or because she had formally repented.) Susanna's only child, Elizabeth HALL (3), was born in February 1608, eight and a half months after her wedding. The Halls are only known to have lived at NEW PLACE, which Shakespeare bequeathed to Susanna, but another STRATFORD house, Hall's Croft (now owned by the Shakespeare BIRTHPLACE Trust) is traditionally regarded as the couple's first home. In 1613 Susanna successfully sued John LANE (1) for libel when he declared in public that she had committed adultery, but otherwise she appears only in business records associated with her inheritance. Shakespeare left her most of his estate: New Place (where she lived for the rest of her life), the family home on Henley Street (the 'Birthplace'), the BLACKFRIARS GATEHOUSE, and several leases on other properties. She and Hall were also residuary legatees. She survived her husband by 14 years and was buried with a gravestone declaring that she was 'witty above her sex' and attributing that quality to her father.

Shakespeare (15), William (1564–1616) The few available facts about Shakespeare's life are mostly

mundane details, reflecting the ordinary existence of an Englishman of his day and social position. He exemplified the enterprising yeoman advancing to gentleman status, a common phenomenon in his day. Like many ambitious early modern Englishmen, he was attracted to LONDON without surrendering his roots in the countryside. In terms of day-to-day life, the only unusual feature was that he was a part of the theatrical world. In his day, actors, playwrights, and theatrical entrepreneurs were only just emerging from an era in which they were stigmatised by both law and custom (see ELIZABETHAN THEATRE). Though in the course of Shakespeare's lifetime, the courts of Queen ELIZABETH (1) and King JAMES I gave prestige to acting, and a few theatre people—including Shakespeare—got rich, protest against drama and acting was still very strong in England. The fascination with theatrical lives that resulted in memoirs and biographies in later periods did not yet exist. Nevertheless, the broad outlines of Shakespeare's life can be discerned.

Shakespeare's life falls into three main periods. His first 20 years were spent in STRATFORD, where his father was a member of the local establishment. His career as an actor and playwright in London lasted about 25 years. Finally, he retired to Stratford where for about five years before his death he was a moderately wealthy member of the local gentry. The first two periods are linked by several years about which we know absolutely nothing—the so-called dark years—and the transition between the last two was gradual and cannot be precisely dated.

Shakespeare was baptised on April 25, 1564, and since the normal lag between birth and baptism was several days, his birthday is conventionally regarded as April 23—also the date of his death 52 years later. His father, John SHAKESPEARE (9), was the son of a farmer who lived near Stratford. A member of the yeoman class, John became a tradesman and moved to the town. He prospered and became one of the leading figures of Stratford's establishment, only to encounter serious financial difficulties, for unknown reasons. These began during Shakespeare's adolescence and were only resolved 20 years later, with the money Shakespeare earned in the theatre. However, the family was evidently never impoverished, for the family home (see BIRTHPLACE) was never sold, and John's status in the community was probably not seriously diminished. Shakespeare's mother, Mary Arden SHAKESPEARE (11), was a member of the gentry, the next higher social class. Her father, Robert ARDEN (2), was an owner of inherited property that he both farmed himself and leased to other farmers. The boundary between the gentry and yeoman classes was notably permeable in the 16th century, and John Shakespeare's rise in status through marriage was quite typical.

No record of Shakespeare's education has survived, but he doubtless attended the excellent Stratford Grammar School, which was appropriate to his family's status and free of charge, since his father was an official of the town. Under the guidance of a series of schoolmasters—Simon HUNT, Thomas JENKINS (the most important in terms of time spent with Shakespeare), John COTTOM, and possibly Walter ROCHE and Alexander ASPINALL—Shakespeare studied mostly Latin literature, in Latin. Fragments of the standard textbook of the day, William LILY's *Latin Grammar*, appear in the plays, most amusingly in the famous 'Latin scene' (4.1) of *The Merry Wives of Windsor.* Also, the Latin authors he studied, such as OVID, LIVY, and VIRGIL, are echoed, quoted, and occasionally mentioned in the plays.

Shakespeare probably left school at the normal age, about 15, in 1579. It seems likely, particularly in view of his father's financial problems, that young William took a job of some sort at this point. A number of possibilities have been envisioned—based on various traditions and on references in the plays that imply familiarity with certain occupations—including assistant schoolmaster, law clerk, gardener, and, perhaps the most natural supposition, assistant to his father, who was a glover and dealer in commodities. In any case, John Shakespeare's business activities left the playwright with specialised knowledge that he was later to put to good use—for instance, when the CLOWN (8) in *The Winter's Tale* puzzles over the market price of wool in 4.3.32–34, or when a beard is described as 'round . . . like a glover's paring-knife' (*Merry Wives,* 1.4.18–19). Recollections of life in the countryside around Stratford are also frequently found in the plays (see, e.g., DAVY, HAMLETT, PERKES, VISOR), especially in the INDUCTION to the early *Taming of the Shrew* (see also SLY [1]). The town life he knew in Stratford itself is not often appropriate to his dramas, but it too is convincingly portrayed in *The Merry Wives of Windsor.*

Within a few years after leaving school, Shakespeare had an affair with Anne HATHAWAY, which led to her pregnancy and a hasty marriage, late in 1582. Anne, eight years older than her 18-year-old husband, was the daughter of a farmer in a nearby village. In May 1583 their first child, Susanna SHAKESPEARE (14), was born; twins, Hamnet and Judith SHAKESPEARE (5, 10), soon followed. The christening of the twins in February 1585 provides assurance that Shakespeare was in Stratford nine months earlier, but no record of his activities between then and 1592 has survived. That period, utterly opaque to modern investigation, constitutes the 'dark years'.

Scholarly speculation has not been wanting, of course. Most notoriously, there was a local tradition—first published in the 18th century—that Shakespeare had been caught poaching by a local nobleman, Sir Thomas LUCY (1), and had thus departed for London

as a fugitive. Modern scholarship finds both story and conclusion highly dubious, and attention has instead focussed on Shakespeare's likely occupation during the dark years. In addition to the various possibilities already outlined, suggestions have included a term as a soldier—in the Netherlands under the Earl of LEICESTER or as part of the defence forces assembled against the Spanish Armada in 1588—or a job in the London publishing industry, perhaps with his fellow Stratfordian, the printer Richard FIELD (2).

A 17th-century writer established a tradition that Shakespeare had been a butcher during this period, reporting that young Will had been known to 'kill a calf' in uproarious spirits. His conclusion was based on a misunderstanding: to 'kill a calf' was Elizabethan theatrical slang for a particular comic routine, the details of which are lost. Nevertheless, the anecdote points to the only certain fact about the dark years: at some point Shakespeare became involved with a theatrical company. Many travelling companies played at Stratford, an important provincial town, during Shakespeare's youth, and LEICESTER'S MEN were there in 1586, followed by the QUEEN'S MEN (1) (who possibly had a vacancy [see KNELL]) in 1587. However, there is no evidence that such troupes ever recruited on the road, and Shakespeare probably had to go to London to begin his career.

He was probably in London no later than 1589, for he was established as an actor and playwright by 1592, when the scurrilous criticism of Robert GREENE (2) makes it clear that he was well known. The response by Henry CHETTLE makes it just as clear that he was respected and admired. Several of the plays were already popular—*3 Henry VI* is quoted from by Greene—and while the earliest plays are notoriously difficult to date, it seems likely that they included *The Comedy of Errors, Titus Andronicus,* the three *Henry VI* plays, and probably *Richard III* and *The Taming of the Shrew.* Several of these plays were performed by an acting company called PEMBROKE'S MEN, and it seems likely that early in his career Shakespeare wrote and acted for them. Similar considerations also suggest links with the ADMIRAL'S MEN, SUSSEX'S MEN, and STRANGE'S MEN. The latter seems especially likely, because the earliest sure evidence of his employment is a document of 1594, in which he is listed as a principal member of Strange's Men's successor, the CHAMBERLAIN'S MEN.

In the meantime his career was affected by a plague outbreak that closed the theatres in London for about two years beginning in 1592. Shakespeare may have toured the provinces with a company under William ALLEYN, but he may have left the theatre for a period. He turned his attention to a purely literary endeavour, the writing of book-length poems. His virtues as a writer had by now been established, and the theatre was not regarded as the best career for a serious literary artist in the 16th century. The likeliest avenue to fame and fortune was to write major works of poetry or prose. Writers offered their works as tokens of esteem to wealthy nobles, who, if they were pleased, might respond with a gift of money or even some extended financial support. It was the aristocracy that supported the literary world, for the most part, with publishing playing only a small role. A writer might live quite comfortably with a generous patron, and it is evident that Shakespeare attempted to tap this market during the long layoff due to the plague. He wrote his two long poems, *Venus and Adonis* (1593) and *The Rape of Lucrece* (1594), during this period and dedicated them to the Earl of SOUTHAMPTON (2). Some scholars believe he lived at Southampton's estate for some part of the time. The first of his dedications, in 1593, is an ordinary approach to a potential patron, conventionally flattering and self-deprecating, while the second suggests a warm friendship and makes it clear that the earl had responded positively to the young poet's work. In fact, that the two men were friends is one of the few undocumented aspects of Shakespeare's life that virtually all scholars accept.

However—whether out of concern for his independence or from love of the theatre or in view of some unknown factor—Shakespeare returned to the stage in 1594. Strange's Men were reorganised as the Chamberlain's Men in June of that year, and the playwright is presumed to have joined them then or shortly thereafter, since he was a prominent member of the company in December, when he was a representative of the troupe at court. He was to remain with this company for the rest of his career. During his first few years with them, he wrote a long string of successful plays, probably including (though dates continue to be uncertain) *Love's Labour's Lost, Romeo and Juliet, Richard II,* and *King John.* An earlier play, *Richard III,* was extremely popular as performed by the Chamberlain's Men; later tradition had it that it established both Shakespeare and its leading man, Richard BURBAGE (3), as important figures in the London theatre world. They became subjects of gossip, at least, for the only surviving personal anecdote of Shakespeare that can be certainly dated to his lifetime concerns Burbage and a female admirer, during a production of *Richard III* (see MANNINGHAM).

Tax assessments (see LONDON) and the records of an obscure lawsuit (see GARDINER [2]) reveal some of Shakespeare's residences during this period. He apparently moved across the city when the Chamberlain's Men moved from the THEATRE, in a northern suburb, to the SWAN THEATRE, in southern SOUTHWARK. Some scholars believe that his tax bill in the first of these homes was too large for a single man's dwelling, suggesting that his wife and children spent time with him in London. There is no further evidence to confirm this, however.

Shakespeare continued to turn out plays at a great rate, probably completing the following between 1596 and the death of Queen Elizabeth in 1603: *The Merchant of Venice,* the two *Henry IV* plays, *The Merry Wives of Windsor, Henry V, Much Ado About Nothing, Julius Caesar, As You Like It, Hamlet, Twelfth Night,* and *Troilus and Cressida.* In 1598 an edition of *Love's Labour's Lost* was the first publication to have Shakespeare's name on it, as booksellers realised the value of his growing fame. In the same year Francis MERES cited him as among England's best playwrights for both COMEDY and TRAGEDY and compared his poetry to the greatest of the ancients.

Throughout the 1590s, and perhaps somewhat later, Shakespeare wrote his SONNETS, a complex sequence of love poems that is one of the masterpieces of English poetry. These poems are often taken to reflect a real love for a man and a woman, but they probably represent merely Shakespeare's pursuit of a fashionable genre. In any case, if they are autobiographical they are deliberately obscure and can contribute little to our knowledge of his life; they recount no events or incidents, and they offer little concrete information about the persons depicted. Shakespeare also composed an allegorical poem, *The Phoenix and Turtle,* written for LOVE'S MARTYR, an anthology of poems (1601) celebrating an aristocratic marriage. In addition, a number of brief EPITAPHS are sometimes ascribed to Shakespeare by various scholars.

In 1596, after the first years of Shakespeare's theatrical success, John Shakespeare was awarded a COAT OF ARMS. Such tokens of gentlemanly status were nominally awarded for a family's services to the nation, but they were in fact bought, and it is presumed that the playwright paid the fees for the Shakespeare escutcheon. Such a public assertion of his family's recovery from their earlier troubles must have been satisfying to Shakespeare, especially when it was confirmed by the purchase of a grand Stratford mansion, NEW PLACE, in 1597. However, Shakespeare's triumphs were not unalloyed, for in 1596 his son Hamnet died at the age of 11. Shakespeare presumably returned to Stratford for Hamnet's burial, though his appearance went unrecorded; the earliest surviving documents indicating his presence in the town after 1584 are those recording the sale of New Place. The absence of any certain association of Shakespeare and Stratford for 13 years has sparked suggestions that the playwright had turned his back on his home, perhaps because of an unhappy marriage. However, the grant of arms, the purchase of New Place, and Shakespeare's continuing close involvement with Stratford thereafter constitute so firm a commitment to the town as to imply a strong earlier involvement as well. Later tradition recorded that he had all along returned frequently, and there is no reason to doubt it. That only the later visits can be substantiated merely points up the impact of wealth, for it is Shakespeare's money matters that are mostly recorded. He was soon a force in Stratford, being recorded in 1598 as a leading owner of grain and figuring several times in the correspondence of Richard QUINEY (2) as a man of business. His father died in 1601, and Shakespeare inherited the birthplace, in half of which his family continued to live, while the other half—formerly his father's shop—was leased as an inn. New investments were made in Stratford in 1602 (see COMBE [1]) and land was added to the property surrounding New Place.

In London in 1599, Shakespeare became one of the partners in the new GLOBE THEATRE, a successful enterprise that furthered his prosperity. Most Elizabethan playwrights only wrote, and of the few who also acted—such as Thomas HEYWOOD (2) and Nathan FIELD (1)—Shakespeare alone was a partner in an acting company, deriving his income from the long-term success of the enterprise, rather than merely from the production of single plays. After the accession of King James in 1603, the company was part of the royal household—the number of courtly performances per year more than doubled—and in the first five years of the new regime, Shakespeare produced an astonishing sequence of major plays: *Othello, Measure for Measure, All's Well That Ends Well, King Lear, Macbeth, Coriolanus, Antony and Cleopatra,* and possibly *Pericles,* plus the unfinished *Timon of Athens.* Similarly, when in 1608, the company acquired the BLACKFRIARS THEATRE, with its unusual new scenic capabilities and its sophisticated clientele, Shakespeare responded with plays in a new genre, the ROMANCES. These, with *Henry VIII* and the lost play CARDENIO, comprise his final period.

Late in his career, Shakespeare was acquainted with the young Christopher BEESTON, whose son, retelling his father's reminiscences years later, left us one of the few glimpses we have of the living playwright. Beeston described Shakespeare as 'a handsome well shap't man—very good company, and of a very readie and pleasant smooth Witt'. Beeston also said that the playwright 'understood Latine pretty well, for he had been in his younger yeares a Schoolmaster in the Countrey' (the earliest such statement), and added that he was 'the more to be admired that he was not a company keeper [and] wouldn't be debauched'.

In late 1603 Shakespeare appeared in a play by Ben JONSON; this may have been his last appearance on stage, for he does not appear on later cast lists. His career as an actor is obscure. He certainly began as one—Robert Greene complained in 1592 that it was presumptious of him, as an actor, to write plays—and he appears in the cast lists of several plays put on by the Chamberlain's Men. We do not, however, know of any role he played or even that he ever appeared in one of his own works (though as a member of the company he probably did). He may have played the title character in George PEELE's *Edward I* (c. 1593),

for another character, referring to the king, says, 'Shake thy spears in honour of his name'. Several ambiguous contemporary references seem to associate him with kingship, and scholars have supposed that he played DUNCAN, HENRY IV, or HENRY VI (the great kingly protagonists such as RICHARD III and LEAR were played by Burbage, however). Later traditions ascribed to Shakespeare the roles of ADAM in *As You Like It* and the GHOST (3) in *Hamlet.* From all this it seems likely that he specialised in roles of older, dignified men, but that his contribution as an actor was not a great one.

Late in his career, Shakespeare wrote collaboratively (as he may also have done in the obscure early years) with at least one other playwright, John FLETCHER (2), who wrote parts of *Cardenio, The Two Noble Kinsmen,* and possibly *Henry VIII.* This almost surely reflects Shakespeare's retirement to Stratford; he was certainly in residence there by 1612 (when he visited London to testify in a lawsuit [see MOUNTJOY]), and some scholars believe he may have made the move as early as 1610, writing *The Tempest* in the country. He presumably visited the city to confer with Fletcher on the other late plays.

In 1607 his older daughter, Susanna, married a prominent Stratford physician, Dr John HALL (4), who seems to have become Shakespeare's friend if he was not already, and in 1608, the couple had a child, Elizabeth HALL (3). As the master of New Place, Shakespeare was one of the social leaders of the town; when visiting preachers came for high holy days, they stayed at Shakespeare's home. He continued to invest in Stratford real estate. In 1605 he bought a share of the tax revenues of some agricultural land (a purchasable commodity in those days), was involved in a lawsuit about it in 1611, and astutely managed the investment during the enclosure controversy of 1614 (see WELCOMBE). Also, in 1613 he bought an investment property in London, the BLACKFRIARS GATEHOUSE.

In January 1616 Shakespeare's lawyer, Francis COLLINS, prepared a draft of the playwright's last will and testament. In February his younger daughter Judith married the scandalous Thomas QUINEY (3), and Shakespeare rewrote his will to protect her portion from her husband, signing it on the 25th of March. On April 23 he died. We do not know the cause; a later tradition that he caught a chill drinking with his fellow playwrights Ben Jonson and Michael DRAYTON is almost certainly apocryphal. On April 25 he was buried—52 years to the day after his baptism—in the chancel of Holy Trinity Church. Sometime before 1622, the chancel wall received a memorial relief featuring a portrait bust by Gheerart JANSSEN (2), presumably commissioned by his family.

This bald recitation of facts is as much as we can know about Shakespeare's life, unless further evidence is uncovered. Over the centuries speculative scholars and fantasising enthusiasts have added a great variety of suppositions, extrapolating from the plays to make a more fully motivated, psychologically credible human being—or perhaps simply a more interesting person—than the simple documents allow. This is most easily done by assuming that the opinions expressed by the major characters in the plays—and by the persona of the poet in the Sonnets—are those of the author. However, efforts to interpret the works as fragments of autobiography are generally mistaken; the characters are imaginary, and because they must occupy all the niches of various fictional worlds, they naturally hold a wide range of attitudes and opinions. Even very broad interpretations are highly problematic. For instance, some critics have seen *The Winter's Tale,* in which unjust jealousy is followed by reconciliation, as an autobiographical rendering of the playwright's relationship with his wife. Though the story is in the play's source material, it is argued that Shakespeare must have been driven to choose that source by some similar experience of his own. However, in the absence of evidence, such a hypothesis remains untestable, and it certainly seems unnecessary. A writer who could produce almost two plays a year for 20 years and make real such diverse characters as, say, FALSTAFF, HAMLET, VOLUMNIA, and the NURSE (3) in *Romeo and Juliet,* can have had no serious problem finding material outside his own life. To argue that specific experiences are necessary for Shakespeare's art suggests that, on the evidence of *Hamlet,* he must have suffered from writer's block.

Nevertheless, if considered with care, Shakespeare's works can help us to a fuller comprehension of the man. Repeated motifs and concepts in the plays permit us to draw a few conclusions, however tentatively, about Shakespeare's sensibility and his general ideas on certain subjects. The HISTORY PLAYS and ROMAN PLAYS reflect a political conservatism—in the sense of resistance to changes in the existing system of social organisation—that we might expect of a man of his time and social position. The late 16th and early 17th centuries were an anxious period in England, for the newly Protestant country was at odds with the Catholic powers of continental Europe—to the point of repelling an attempted invasion—and internal strife bubbled up in such episodes as the rebellion led by the Earl of ESSEX (2). Indeed, civil war was regarded as a serious prospect during the last years of Elizabeth's reign (and after a brief respite it became reality, not long after Shakespeare's death). On a more personal level, the playwright's social position was newly achieved and, as his father's experience had demonstrated, precarious.

In these circumstances Shakespeare's politics were naturally conservative. For instance, the plays clearly demonstrate that he places a high value on the preservation of social order and distrusts the disorder that he sees in popular political assertiveness. From Jack

CADE, through the PLEBEIANS (1) who kill the wrong man in *Julius Caesar* and the shifty Junius BRUTUS (3) of *Coriolanus*, to *The Tempest*'s rebellious CALIBAN, the common man in his political aspect is generally a villain, though the playwright's fondness for the common people of England is evident in his many sympathetic characterisations, from the very early DROMIOS to the very late BOATSWAIN. Still, the violent and fickle common man is only a secondary villain. In both the history and Roman dramas popular disorder is seen as a *symptom* of moral sickness rather than a cause. The rulers of the state are the major focus, as aristocratic shortsightedness, greed, and ambition lead to usurpations and civil war. Shakespeare clearly found the greatest threat to society in disruption of the system at the top. Perhaps for this reason, he is sometimes interpreted as representing a proto-revolutionary strain of thought; however, his notions actually reflect the political orthodoxy of the TUDOR DYNASTY, which naturally feared the threat of an opposing aristocratic faction, having come to power as one itself. Shakespeare's work and life considered together do not show us a member of the rising bourgeoisie who is nervous about the crown's overweening power—the proto-revolutionary image—but rather the unmistakable lineaments of a country gentleman and a social conservative.

An interpretation of Shakespeare's life from his work that sparks great controversy is the suggestion that the Sonnets indicate Shakespeare was a homosexual. However, the love for a man expressed in the Sonnets is not sexual (as is specified in Sonnet 20), though sexuality is important in the world of the poems. Sonnet sequences were a fashionable vehicle for comments on love, and they conventionally took unrequited passion as their topic. The love triangle implicit in the Sonnets is probably such a convention—albeit more complex and involving than most (as we might expect of Shakespeare) and so more convincing. In any case it does not involve a homosexual relationship. Here, seeming biographical data have been forged from nothing, by applying modern values to pre-modern materials.

Moreover, the plays repeatedly focus on heterosexual love and its culmination in marriage. Shakespeare's heroines are frankly interested in sex. JULIET (1) longs for her wedding night and its 'amorous rites' (*Romeo and Juliet* 3.2.8); ROSALIND envisions ORLANDO, whom she has just met, as 'my child's father' (*As You Like It* 1.3.10); and PERDITA describes FLORIZEL's body as 'like a bank, for love to lie and play on' (4.4.130). Throughout the plays, Shakespeare celebrates sexuality in marriage, and he plainly sees marriage as a vehicle for the fulfilment of humanity's place in the natural order of things. Nothing that can be seen of his own marriage suggests that he regarded it in any different light, and there seem no grounds for the idea that he was not a conventional husband with a conventional sex life.

Propositions based on the work are necessarily speculative, but a few elements from the plays do seem related to what we know of Shakespeare's life. For instance, we have seen that Stratford is reflected in the early plays, and the playwright's love of country life is evident throughout his work. English rustics reappear in such unlikely settings as ATHENS (in both *A Midsummer Night's Dream* and *The Two Noble Kinsmen*), DENMARK (*Hamlet*), and BOHEMIA (*The Winter's Tale*). More personal concerns may also emerge. Looking at Shakespeare's remarkably similar doomed boys, the SON (1) of MACDUFF in *Macbeth* and MAMILLIUS in *The Winter's Tale*, both charming and intelligent lads seen in touching conversation with their mothers, it is easy to suppose that the playwright was remembering Hamnet. Also, we can surmise that Shakespeare's consciousness of his own increasing age is reflected in his remarkable sequence of tragic lovers. ROMEO and JULIET (created c. 1595, when Shakespeare was around 30) are virtually children, powerless in the face of adult society; TROILUS and CRESSIDA (1602) are young adults and have roles in their societies, but those roles are themselves oppressive and help undo their love; OTHELLO and DESDEMONA (c. 1604) are fully adult, married, and entirely in control of their positions in the world, though not of themselves; ANTONY and CLEOPATRA (c. 1608, Shakespeare was 44) are quite mature and have had adult lives full of incident and accomplishment. Shakespeare seems to have identified himself with different age groups as he grew older; this is of course natural, and in observing it, we are not learning about Shakespeare's life through the plays but rather confirming our awareness that he made his plays out of life.

'Shall I die?' Ninety-line poem recently and controversially attributed to Shakespeare. 'Shall I die?' was stated to be an early Shakespearean work by Professor Gary Taylor in November 1985. Professor Taylor is co-editor of the 1986 Oxford University Press edition of the complete works of Shakespeare, where 'Shall I die?' is included under the title 'A Song', in its first publication anywhere. The poem was first designated as Shakespeare's in a manuscript anthology of poems—such as were commissioned by many wealthy patrons of the 16th and 17th centuries—dated 1630. (It is only known to appear in one other such manuscript, also of the 1630s, where it is unattributed.) Earlier scholars were aware of this attribution but felt that the source was unreliable: such manuscripts commonly contain misattributed poems and were compiled by unknown anthologists whose knowledge was often limited.

Taylor's attribution has generated much controversy: some scholars assert that not only does the

poem fail to resemble any known works by Shakespeare, but it is bad poetry, filled with trite observations and feeble rhymes, too weak as verse to have been written by the author of *Romeo and Juliet,* say, with which Taylor says it is roughly contemporary. On the other hand, defenders point out that 'Shall I die?' contains a number of words that Shakespeare was fond of using, and, while contrived and artificial, it may nonetheless be seen as a virtuoso exercise in technique, employing a complicated rhyme scheme over nine stanzas, no easy feat.

However, while scholars now tend to believe that 'Shall I Die?' is not Shakespearean, a definitive verdict will probably not be reached for years. If ultimately accepted, the poem will become the first addition to the Shakespearean CANON since the 17th century.

Shallow, Robert Character in *2 Henry IV* and *The Merry Wives of Windsor,* a GLOUCESTERSHIRE Justice of the Peace. A garrulous old man who thinks himself sophisticated but is in fact very gullible, the Shallow of *2 Henry IV* is a perfect victim for FALSTAFF's exploitation. Given to lying about his youthful adventures with Falstaff and pluming himself on his status as a justice, he is somewhat ridiculous. As Falstaff remarks in a soliloquy at 3.2.296–322, he remembers the youthful Shallow as a laughing-stock, and he is certainly a comical figure in old age. However, he is never simply laughable, despite Falstaff's elaborate and comically uncomplimentary description. Upon their initial appearance, Shallow and his cousin SILENCE seem amusingly empty-headed as their conversation shifts from the deaths of old acquaintances to the price of livestock in 3.2.33–52, but while the exchange is a tour de force of subtle comedy, the characters are also movingly human: two old men whose minds wander as they confront mortality. Shallow's age and something more of his earlier life are mentioned in 3.2.205, where Silence remarks that it was 'fifty-five year ago' that Shallow entered Clement's Inn, a law school. Supposing him to be about 20 years old at that time, we see that he is about 75 at the time of the play. Clement's Inn, as Shakespeare's audience will have known, was an institution similar to the INNS OF COURT but less socially and intellectually elite. As his capacities in old age suggest, he was not accepted by the top law schools in youth. Such a circumstantial biography helps make Shallow a real person and not simply a comic butt.

Throughout the play, Shallow is a sympathetic character. He presents the pleasant world of the small landowner in *2 Henry IV*'s remarkable panoply of English scenes, hosting Falstaff and his men with a bountiful dinner of home-grown food. His incautious friendship is repaid when he is gaoled along with Falstaff in 5.5, when Falstaff is banished by PRINCE (6) HAL.

In *The Merry Wives,* although Shallow is more prominent and appears in far more scenes than in *2 Henry IV,* he is less strikingly drawn. He is the avuncular promoter of a marriage between his dim-witted young relative SLENDER and the desirable ANNE (3) Page. Also, seconding the HOST (2) in 2.1, 2.3, and 3.1, he helps avert the duel between EVANS and CAIUS, in a sub-plot that contributes to the play's conciliatory quality.

As *The Merry Wives* opens, Shallow—making pompous claims of aristocratic ancestry—threatens a lawsuit against Falstaff; this suit is immediately forgotten in the play, and it is sometimes thought that its purpose was solely to link the laughable country justice with some real person whom Shakespeare had disputed with and was now making fun of (see William GARDINER [2]; Thomas LUCY [1]). However, this is highly questionable, and the episode's peculiarly truncated quality probably reflects the haste with which the play was apparently written, or perhaps it survives from a lost play sometimes hypothesised as a source for *The Merry Wives.*

Shank, John (c. 1565–1636) English actor, a member of the KING'S MEN, one of the 26 men listed in the FIRST FOLIO as the 'Principall Actors' in Shakespeare's plays. Shank was a veteran comedian, especially noted for his antic dancing, when he joined the King's Men. Earlier, he had performed with PEMBROKE'S MEN, the QUEEN'S MEN, and PRINCE HENRY'S MEN (later the PALSGRAVE'S MEN). Though he does not appear in documents as a King's Man before 1619, he may have joined the company in 1615 upon the death of Robert ARMIN, whose roles he presumably played. He seems to have acted very little after 1629, and in 1631 he disappears from the cast lists. In 1635 he was successfully sued by several members of the company for having illegally acquired shares in the GLOBE and BLACKFRIARS THEATRES; in a countersuit, he claimed that the company was punishing him by keeping him off the stage. However, it is likely that he had simply been retired because of his age.

Sharpham, Edward (1576–1608) English playwright. Edward Sharpham wrote several plays, two of which have survived: *The Fleir* (1606) and *Cupid's Whirligig* (1607). The former includes a passage that echoes dialogue from *King Lear,* and this fact helps date Shakespeare's play, which had to have been written before Sharpham's work was registered with the STATIONERS' COMPANY in May, 1606.

Shaw (1) Character in *Richard III.* See SHAA.

Shaw (2), George Bernard (1856–1950) British playwright and essayist. As part of his persona as a crusty opponent of hidebound orthodoxy, Shaw adopted a

disparaging tone towards the conventionally admired Shakespeare. He coined the term *bardolatry* to mock the attitude of such hero-worshippers as the poet Algernon SWINBURNE, and he delighted in such observations as, 'With the single exception of Homer, there is no eminent writer, not even Sir Walter Scott, whom I despise so entirely as I despise Shakespeare.' Moreover, he rewrote the final scene of *Cymbeline* (as *Cymbeline Refinished* [1937]), declaring that Shakespeare's version was simply too poor to be tolerated any longer.

However, Shaw could not help admiring Shakespeare; for instance, he wrote that *As You Like It,* though a 'cheap and pleasant falsehood', was 'one of the most effective samples of romantic nonsense in existence'. He purported to admire Shakespeare's poetry while deprecating his intellect. He wrote that 'Shakespeare's power lies in his enormous command of word-music, which gives fascination to his most blackguardly repartees, and sublimity to his hollowest platitudes.' Essentially, his attitude is egotistical, for in making Shakespeare seem both magnificent and ludicrous, he could claim him as an artistic equal while appearing to be his intellectual superior. This attitude is perhaps best represented in his one-act play *The Dark Lady of the Sonnets* (1910) and his puppet play *Shakes versus Shav* (1949).

While Shaw has been considered Shakespeare's equal by no one but himself, he was nevertheless a very good dramatist and a highly important writer. His criticism, mostly of drama and music, was a strong influence in late-19th- and early-20th-century Britain, helping to introduce modernism to a wide audience. A grand eccentric, he made himself as prominent as possible while advocating vegetarianism, antivivisection, a mystical religion based on evolutionary theory, and spelling reform. He was also an active socialist who promoted his political ideals in all his works, including a body of explicitly political essays. However, his most important role was as a dramatist. Shaw wrote more than 50 plays, among the best known of which are *Mrs Warren's Profession* (1898), *Caesar and Cleopatra* (1901), *Man and Superman* (1903), *Major Barbara* (1905), *Androcles and the Lion* (1912), *Pygmalion* (1913), *Heartbreak House* (1919), and *Saint Joan* (1923). Following the great Norwegian playwright Henrik Ibsen (1828–1906), Shaw dealt with such modern issues as the status of women and the problems of the poor, employing barbed wit and an elegant prose style. He was awarded the Nobel Prize for Literature in 1925.

Shaw (3), Glen Byam (b. 1904) British actor and producer. Director of the Shakespeare Memorial Theatre in STRATFORD from 1952 to 1959 (with Anthony QUAYLE until 1956), Shaw mounted a number of noteworthy productions of Shakespeare's plays, including a particularly acclaimed *Antony and Cleopatra* of 1953, starring Michael REDGRAVE and Peggy ASHCROFT.

Shaw (4), Julian (July) (1571–1629) Wool trader in STRATFORD, a friend of Shakespeare's and a witness to his will. Shaw's first name was recorded as July at his christening, his marriage, and his burial, though he signed himself 'July', 'Julynes', 'Julyns', and 'Julyne' (the *n*'s approximate the Latin rendering 'Julianus' or 'Julinus'). He leased a house near NEW PLACE and was thus Shakespeare's neighbour. He prospered trading wool and malt, becoming an important Stratford landowner, and he served in many public offices in the town, being bailiff, or mayor, at the time he witnessed Shakespeare's will. He was a stepson of Alexander ASPINALL.

Shaw (5) (Shaa), Robert (d. 1603) English actor. Shaw was one of the three members of PEMBROKE'S MEN imprisoned for staging the allegedly seditious *Isle of Dogs* in July 1597. Upon his release he joined the ADMIRAL'S MEN, with whom he remained until 1602. He played a major role in the company's business affairs while he performed in minor parts. In 1602 he joined WORCESTER'S MEN, though in the same year he sold a play—*The Four Sons of Aymon*—to the Admiral's Men, who performed it in 1603; however, this work may have been an old text rather than Shaw's creation.

Shepherd (1) Minor character in *1 Henry VI,* the father of JOAN LA PUCELLE, or Joan of Arc. This humble figure encounters his daughter after she has been captured and condemned to death, but she refuses to acknowledge him, claiming to be descended from a long line of kings. He responds by cursing her. This incident, entirely fictitious, is simply part of the play's strong anti-French bias.

Shepherd (2) Character in *The Winter's Tale,* the foster-father of PERDITA. The mad King LEONTES of SICILIA, believing his infant daughter, Perdita, to be illegitimate, orders her abandoned in the wilderness. In 3.3 the Shepherd discovers her, wrapped in rich fabrics and supplied with identifying documents. He raises her as his daughter. In 4.4, 16 years later, the Shepherd hosts a country festival, at which King POLIXENES threatens him with death, for Prince FLORIZEL has fallen in love with Perdita, offending the royal dignity. The Shepherd and his son, the CLOWN (8), try to show Perdita's documents to the king, to prove that they are not related to her and should not be punished, but they are tricked by AUTOLYCUS into joining the fleeing couple and sailing to Sicilia. There, Perdita's identity is discovered and the Shepherd is amply rewarded; in 5.2 he and the Clown display their new finery, having been created gentlemen by King Leontes.

The Shepherd is one of Shakespeare's most charming minor creations, a true English rustic. He speaks in an upcountry dialect, remarking, 'Mercy on 's, a barne!' on discovering Perdita (3.3.69). In his touching reminiscence of his late wife (4.4.55–62), he conveys a strong and pleasant sense of rural domesticity. He is carefully distinguished from his buffoonish son by his gravity and sense of responsibility. Barring his understandable cowardice when threatened by a king, the Shepherd is a fine, upstanding man. As such, he helps maintain the play's insistence on the essential goodness of humanity in the face of evil.

Sheridan, Thomas (1719–1788) Irish actor. Sheridan played numerous Shakespearean parts in London, beginning in 1744. He especially distinguished himself as HAMLET, and was generally regarded as second only to David GARRICK among the actors of the day. In 1754 Sheridan adapted Shakespeare's *Coriolanus* by combining it with another play of the same title—an entirely independent work by James Thomson (1700–1748)—and played the title role himself, to great acclaim. His production was quite popular and was frequently revived for almost 15 years and was later adapted by J. P. KEMBLE (3). In the 1770s Sheridan was a notable worker for educational reform.

Sheriff (1) Minor character in *2 Henry VI,* an officer who is assigned the task of parading the DUCHESS (1) of Gloucester through the streets of London in 2.4 as part of her sentence for dabbling in witchcraft and conspiring against King HENRY VI.

Sheriff (2) Minor character in *Richard III,* the officer who escorts the Duke of BUCKINGHAM (2) to his execution in 5.1. In the QUARTO editions, this part is assigned to RATCLIFFE, apparently reflecting an economy measure in some early productions.

Sheriff (3) Minor character in *King John,* a petty official who escorts ROBERT Faulconbridge and the BASTARD (1) into the King's presence in 1.1.44. The Sheriff, who does not speak, represents the world of country gentry from which the brothers come.

Sheriff (4) Minor character in *1 Henry IV,* a policeman who investigates the highway robbery committed by FALSTAFF. The Sheriff, who has a witness who knows Falstaff, accepts PRINCE (6) HAL's word that Falstaff is not present at the inn and that the Prince will guarantee the return of any stolen money; he then leaves.

Shirley, Anthony (1565–c. 1635) English traveller and adventurer alluded to in *Twelfth Night.* Shirley, originally a soldier and a follower of the Earl of ESSEX (2), was famous for his unofficial embassy in 1598 to the court of the shah (or sophy) of Persia, Abbas the Great (1571–1629). Shirley made the treacherous overland voyage from the Mediterranean to Isfahan and negotiated rights for Christian merchants in Persia in exchange for assistance in building a modern army for the Sophy's government. (Shirley's brother Robert [c. 1581–1628] served the shah as a military adviser for 20 years.) Shirley conducted several unsuccessful diplomatic missions on behalf of the shah between 1599 and 1601, before moving on to other adventures, chiefly as a mercenary soldier fighting for Spain against the Turks. In the meantime, two books on his adventures in Persia were published in London in 1600 and 1601. These were extremely popular, and Shakespeare included two references to the sophy in *Twelfth Night* (2.5.181, 3.4.284).

Short, Peter (d. 1603) English printer, producer of several editions of Shakespeare's plays and poems. In 1594 Short printed THE TAMING OF A SHREW—a BAD QUARTO of Shakespeare's *The Taming of the Shrew*—for Cuthbert BURBY, and in 1595 he printed the TRUE TRAGEDY—a bad quarto of *3 Henry VI*—for Thomas MILLINGTON, but in both cases the piracy was the publisher's doing, not Short's. Short also printed the first edition of *1 Henry IV* (1598) for Andrew WISE, the second through fourth editions of *The Rape of Lucrece* (1599, 1600) for John HARRISON (2) and his brother, and the third and fourth editions of *Venus and Adonis* (both 1599) for William LEAKE. He also printed the *Palladis Tamia* of Francis MERES. Little is known of his life.

Shrewsbury Town in western England, site of a battle that occupies much of Acts 4–5 of *1 Henry IV.* The battle of Shrewsbury was fought between King HENRY IV and rebellious noblemen led by HOTSPUR, allied with Scotsmen under DOUGLAS. In 4.1 Hotspur receives news that his armies will not be reinforced by the troops of his father, NORTHUMBERLAND (1), nor by those of his Welsh ally GLENDOWER. However, the fiery warrior insists on fighting anyway. In 4.3 the rebels accept an offer to negotiate, and in 5.1 Hotspur's uncle, WORCESTER, meets with the King, who offers clemency. Worcester, fearful of treachery after a truce, does not convey this message to Hotspur, however, and the battle begins. In 5.3 and 5.4 several hand-to-hand combats take place, climaxing with a fight between Hotspur and King Henry's son, PRINCE (6) HAL. Hotspur's death at Hal's hands demoralises the rebels, and they flee, as is reported in 5.5.17–20.

Shakespeare followed his sources in relating the general course of the battle, and his account largely agrees with those of modern scholars, but he invented the close combat between Hal and Hotspur, along with other, less important details. Although Hotspur would not withdraw his outnumbered army, he did not start the battle; King Henry began the fight by break-

ing off the negotiations that preceded it. Hotspur's death did precipitate the rout; the two sides are thought to have sustained about the same number of casualties, and had their leader survived, the rebels might have won.

Shylock Character in *The Merchant of Venice,* Jewish money-lender who seeks to kill the title figure, ANTONIO (2), by claiming a pound of his flesh, as provided for in their loan agreement. Shylock is a stereotypical Jew, shaped by anti-Semitic notions that were prevalent in Shakespeare's England. He accordingly possesses the two standard features ascribed to Jews at the time, a vicious hatred of Christians and the practise of usury, the latter entailing an obsessive miserliness. However, Shakespeare's portrayal of Shylock does not demonstrate his intent to promote or display anti-Semitism; he simply took the figure from his anti-Semitic source and used it for traditional comic purposes. But his genius also transformed the character into something far grander. Shylock has so fascinated generations of readers and theatre-goers that, although his name has become a byword for the warped personality of the unscupulous miser, few can avoid feeling sympathy for him.

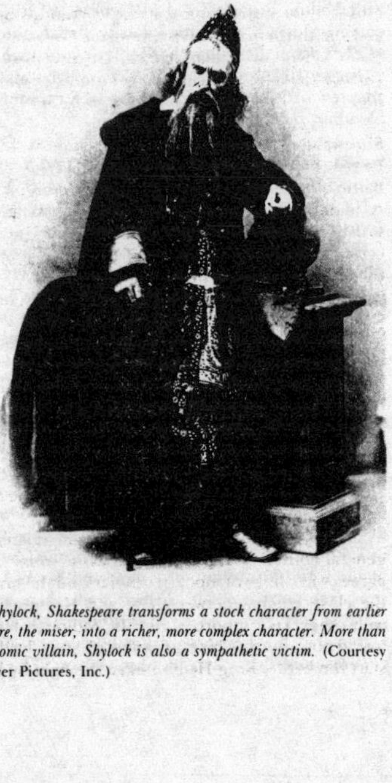

With Shylock, Shakespeare transforms a stock character from earlier literature, the miser, into a richer, more complex character. More than just a comic villain, Shylock is also a sympathetic victim. (Courtesy of Culver Pictures, Inc.)

The miser was a frequent comic villain in the drama and literature of the Middle Ages and early RENAISSANCE, and Shylock belongs to this lineage. He represents the killjoy against whom pleasure-loving characters unite. He is a schemer whose icy shrewdness daunts BASSANIO in 1.3. When Antonio enters in the same scene, Shylock reveals in an aside (1.3.36–47) his deep-seated hostility towards the merchant, 'for he is a Christian'. Yet his first words to Antonio are fawning compliments, and we immediately recognise the cruel usurer as a hypocrite as well. Throughout the play he is repeatedly associated with the devil (e.g., in 3.1.19–20). The famous speech in which he seemingly asserts his basic humanity—'Hath not a Jew eyes? . . .' (3.1.47–66)—is actually a baleful and chilling assertion of his intention to murder Antonio. Shylock grows more and more malevolent until, in the trial scene (4.1), he melodramatically hones on his shoe the knife with which he hopes to kill the merchant while obstinately refusing to grant mercy, even for huge sums of money.

As is true of all comic villains there is never any doubt that Shylock will be defeated in the end, and he is therefore never truly threatening. Further, Shylock is broadly comical at times; in this respect he somewhat resembles the VICE of the medieval MORALITY PLAY. His stinginess has a humorous quality of caricature to it, and he is depicted as a subject for ridicule in all but one of his scenes, even in the trial scene. In his first meeting with Antonio he justifies his usury by citing instances from the Bible, but he comically selects stories of crafty dealing (1.3.66–83) that actually cast him in a bad light. In 2.5, his dream is mocked by LAUNCELOT, and his obsessive insistence on locking his house is humorosly crotchety. In 3.1, following the renowned speech in which he asserts his thirst for revenge, a change of tone—preparing the audience for a return to BELMONT in 3.2—presents him as a farcical villain who becomes ludicrous as he oscillates hysterically between rage and delight when TUBAL tells him of JESSICA's extravagance and Antonio's misfortune. Even at the trial, Shylock repeatedly makes himself clownish, chortling over the absence of a surgeon, naïvely exulting in the pretence of PORTIA (1) that he will win his case, and hastily trying to recover his money when he finds he has lost. Only in 3.3 is Shylock purely evil, making more imperative the development of Portia's counterplot in 3.4.

As villain, Shylock embodies the negative element in several sets of opposing values whose conflicts provide the major themes of the play. First, he is the crabbed old man who opposes the expansive young lovers. His daughter flees him, saying that his 'house is hell' (2.3.2), and his contrast to Bassanio is carried forward to Portia's victory over him in the courtroom.

The final scene (5.1) rings with Shylock's absence, as young love triumphs. Further, he represents justice, as opposed to mercy, insisting on the letter of the law and refusing to accept any reduction of the terms of his contract with Antonio. Most significantly, he personifies greed, in contrast to the generosity of Antonio and Portia. In comically crying, 'My daughter! O my ducats! O my daughter!' (2.8.15), Shylock reveals that he loves money as much as, if not more than, Jessica. Among the reasons he gives for hating Antonio is a commercial one: the Merchant, in making interest-free loans, has depressed the going rate. Thus Shylock's love of money generates acrimony and strife.

It is evidence of Shakespeare's creative empathy that even an evil stereotype is developed to the extent that Shylock is. Not content with a conventional stage villain, the playwright gives Shylock's personality an extraordinary duality. Many of his speeches, even the most humorous and/or malicious, can be construed as cries of anguish: the villain is also a victim, we sense. It is easy to deride the two-faced miser who comically equates his daughter and his ducats, but it is also easy to perceive an old man, enraged by betrayal, who has begun to lose his mind. The usurer is given an opportunity to justify his practise in 1.3, and his solemn citations from the Bible have dignity and are not to be taken as only self-incriminating. He is finally subjected to a total and humiliating defeat: his oaths on his religion are nullified, and he is forced to convert. Yet our response to him remains complex. When the crushed moneylender last exits at the close of 4.1, he may be seen as an unrepentant malingerer ('I am not well . . .' [4.1.392]), as a hopeful Christian convert ('I am content' [4.1.389]), or simply as a properly beaten cur and an appropriate target for the cruel jests of GRATIANO (1). The scene may also be effectively played so as to give Shylock his pride, broken but not vanquished; this image diminishes the righteous triumph of Antonio's defenders. Most strikingly, perhaps, Shylock so vividly evokes Venetian anti-Semitism in 3.1.47–66 that this speech is generally taken as a plea for fair and humane treatment, when it is in fact a justification for an extremely inhumane demand. Repeatedly, the playwright offers the possibility of contradictory responses (as he did, at about the same time, in creating FALSTAFF). However, it is basic to the nature of the character that, although Shylock has come to his extreme behaviour through suffering, his behaviour is nonetheless unacceptable: he is fundamentally a ruthless villain who plans to kill Antonio. Shakespeare does not ignore the process whereby Shylock has become what he is, but he is nonetheless appallingly vicious. Shylock himself says, '. . . since I am a dog, beware my fangs' (3.3.7).

This complex and powerful character dominates the play, despite his relatively small part: he appears in only five scenes and speaks fewer than 400 lines. His multi-faceted nature complicates the work substantially, and it has sometimes inspired criticism on the grounds that it upsets the graceful development proper to a romantic comedy. Shakespeare may have been aware of this problem when he disposed of his villain in Act 4; the final act affirms the triumph of the lovers without his disturbing presence.

Like many of Shakespeare's characters, Shylock lends himself to many interpretations, and he remains as compelling as ever; he anticipates the power and pathos of such later protagonists as OTHELLO and LEAR. But although we may recognise the deformed grandeur and nobility of Shylock, we must not lose our awareness of the ideal of loving community that is at the heart of the play, an ideal to which Shylock at bottom runs counter. Nevertheless, the playwright's complex and humane sensibility brought forth a villain whose downfall cannot be wholeheartedly enjoyed. We are forced to recognise the moral cost involved in his defeat, and to acknowledge that hatred is not easily overcome.

Shylock's name has puzzled scholars. Shakespeare may have derived it from *shallach,* the Hebrew word meaning 'cormorant', a term often used abusively to describe usurers, who were equated with that greedy fish-eating bird. The name has also been associated with Shiloh, a name used in Genesis 49:10 for the coming Messiah, and with Salah or Shelah, the father of Eber, from the whom the Hebrews took their name (Genesis 10:24, e.g.). Also, Shakespeare may have adapted a 16th-century English word for a contemptible idler, *shullock* or *shallock.*

Sicilia Latin for Sicily, the Italian island that is the setting for much of *The Winter's Tale.* Acts 1-2 and 3.1-2 are all set in Sicilia, where King LEONTES unjustly accuses his wife of adultery, leading to a tragic aftermath. Eventually, the action returns to Sicilia in Act 5, when a resolution is achieved. Sicilia is merely specified as Leontes' kingdom, and nothing Sicilian, or even Italian, about the realm is suggested in the text or stage directions. Shakespeare simply took the name from his source, *Pandosto* by Robert GREENE (2), though there Sicilia was the place of exile (not BOHEMIA, as in Shakespeare). Sicilia was suitable for use in a romantic drama (see ROMANCES) because it was on the fringe of familiar European geography and was thus appropriately exotic.

Sicilius Leonatus Minor character in *Cymbeline,* the deceased father of POSTHUMUS, who appears as a ghost in 5.4. The spirit of Sicilius is accompanied by those of his wife, Posthumus' MOTHER, and his two elder sons (see BROTHER [2]). Sicilius leads them as they plead to JUPITER on behalf of Posthumus. Sicilius observes that he died before Posthumus was born, a circumstance that earns pity for his son. The family

demands that Jupiter show mercy and restore Posthumus to happiness, or else, Sicilius declares, they will appeal to 'th' shining synod of the rest' of the gods (5.4.89). Jupiter appears and promises mercy, Sicilius responds with awe and wonder, and all the apparitions disappear.

Sicilius' appearance is foreshadowed at the beginning of the play. In 1.1 a GENTLEMAN (12) tells of Posthumus' parentage. We learn that Sicilius Leonatus gained his surname, which means 'lionlike', for his bravery in battle, and that he died fighting for Britain against the Romans. Posthumus inherited the name and the bravery—as he demonstrates in battle in 5.2—so when Sicilius appears, we see him as an emblem of his son's virtues combined with the awesome presence of a supernatural creature. The episode contributes to the bizarre and romantic atmosphere of the play. Sicilius and the other ghosts employ a rhyming, singsong mode of speech that has encouraged some scholars to speculate that the passage may not have been written by Shakespeare, who was certainly capable of much more elegant poetry. However, the ghosts' language is ritualistic, and establishes an eerie air of the occult prior to the appearance of Jupiter.

Sicinius Character in *Coriolanus.* See BRUTUS (3).

Siddons, Sarah (1755–1831) British actress, sister of Charles and John Philip KEMBLE (1, 3), the leading tragic actress of the late 18th and early 19th century. Daughter of the manager of a travelling acting company, Mrs Siddons, as she was known throughout her career, was a child actress who at 18 married a member of the troupe. An early attempt at success in London failed, but in 1782, she triumphed in a non-Shakespearean play and was quickly regarded as the finest tragic actress of the day, a position she never relinquished. Her most famous Shakespearean parts were CONSTANCE, Queen KATHERINE of Aragon, DESDEMONA, OPHELIA, VOLUMNIA, and, most of all, LADY (6) MACBETH. In 1775, while still touring the provinces, Mrs Siddons became the first of many actresses to play HAMLET, initiating a vogue that has lasted 200 years. She continued to play the Prince of Denmark periodically until she was almost 50, though her evident age and increasing girth provoked some ridicule. She retired in 1812, after a farewell performance as Lady Macbeth, though she briefly returned to the stage several times—to terrible reviews—the last in 1819.

Sidney, Philip (1554–1586) English poet, author, and soldier, whose works influenced several of Shakespeare's plays. Sidney's massive PASTORAL, *Arcadia* (c. 1580, published 1590), introduced romantic literature, a genre of the Italian RENAISSANCE, to England. It was widely influential and helped inspire a number of Shakespeare's works, notably *Two Gentlemen of Verona, As You Like It,* and the ROMANCES. It provided the SUB-PLOT concerning EDMUND and EDGAR, along with various details, to *King Lear,* and one of its heroes, Pyrocles, is thought to have inspired the name of Shakespeare's PERICLES. Sidney also wrote one of the most famous SONNET sequences, *Astrophel and Stella* (c. 1580–1584; published 1591), a work that inspired the great vogue for the genre in the 1590s, when Shakespeare wrote his SONNETS. *Astrophel and Stella* probably influenced *Romeo and Juliet* as well.

Sidney was widely regarded in his own day as an ideal Renaissance gentleman. Born into the aristocracy, he was one of the most admired gentlemen at the court of Queen ELIZABETH (1). Sidney went to war in the Low Countries, on the staff of his uncle the Earl of LEICESTER, and he was killed there. His death sparked general mourning in England; one result was a great poem, 'Astrophel', by his friend Edmund SPENSER.

Silence Character in *2 Henry IV,* a rural justice of the peace, cousin of Justice SHALLOW. Silence, as his name suggests, says very little. In 3.2 he clearly admires his cousin's youthful career as 'lusty Shallow' (3.2.15), and he politely responds to Shallow's remarks. In 5.3, at Shallow's delightful garden party, Silence comes to life under the influence of wine: six times, he breaks into song—two of these excerpts are from known 16th-century ballads, and the others are presumed to derive from lost works—and he has to be carried to bed at the end of the evening. Although we hear of his daughter Ellen and his son William (3.2.6,8), Silence's own first name is never mentioned.

In the QUARTO edition of *2 Henry IV,* Silence's name is spelled Scilens on 18 occasions. This edition derives from Shakespeare's manuscript, and therefore the spelling is presumed to have been used by the playwright. Its only other known occurrence is in the 'Hand D' pages of the manuscript of SIR THOMAS MORE (where it is a common noun); this piece of evidence, along with others, leads scholars to conclude that Shakespeare wrote these pages.

Silius Minor character in *Antony and Cleopatra,* a lieutenant of VENTIDIUS. Ventidius has just defeated a Parthian army in the name of Mark ANTONY, and in 3.1 he explains to Silius why he will not pursue the fleeing enemy. He does not want to succeed too thoroughly, lest Antony feel overshadowed and in revenge crush his military career. Silius admires Ventidius' political acumen. He has no personality and serves merely as a sounding board for his superior officer.

Silvia Character in *The Two Gentlemen of Verona,* VALENTINE's lover, also loved by PROTEUS. Proteus betrays both Valentine and his own lover, JULIA, for Silvia's sake. She has the good sense to recognise the rogue

in Proteus and reject him, and Julia, disguised as a page, is pleased with the sympathy Silvia expresses for Proteus' abandoned lover. After Valentine's banishment, Silvia bravely resolves to follow him. Captured by the OUTLAWS whom Valentine now leads, she is rescued first by Proteus, who attempts to rape her, and then by Valentine. However, her lover, in a rapturous gesture of forgiveness to his friend, presents her to Proteus as a gift. Julia's intervention forestalls this development, and at the play's end, Silvia is betrothed to Valentine. Silvia is chiefly a conventional figure, intended only as the focus of the actions of the two men. Nevertheless, she anticipates later, more humanly interesting Shakespearean women in her forthrightness and pluck.

Silvius Character in *As You Like It,* a young shepherd, lover of PHEBE. Silvius is a caricature of the ardent lover in the PASTORAL tradition that the play satirises. Silvius' courtship of Phebe is presented as 'a pageant truly played' (3.4.48), and as such it follows well-established traditions. Using a familiar gambit of the Elizabethan sonneteer, Silvius insists that, in rejecting his love, Phebe is harder on him than an executioner. ROSALIND calls him 'a tame snake' (4.3.70); his weakness, an exaggeration of the stock posture of the unrequited lover, is part of the play's mockery of literary conventions.

Simmes, Valentine (active 1576–1622) Printer of a number of early editions of Shakespeare's plays. Simmes, the best of the early LONDON printers of Shakespeare, printed nine of his plays in seven years. He printed the first edition of *Richard III* (Q1, 1597) and the first three editions of *Richard II* (Q1, 1597; Q2 and Q3, 1598), all for Andrew WISE. In 1600, working for the partnership of Wise and William ASPLEY, Simmes printed the first editions of *2 Henry IV* and *Much Ado About Nothing* (both Q, 1600). In the same year he printed Q2 of *2 Henry VI* (see THE CONTENTION) for Thomas MILLINGTON. In 1603 he printed the first edition of *Hamlet* (Q1) for Nicholas LING and John TRUNDELL. This was a BAD QUARTO or pirated edition, though the printer was not responsible for that. In 1604 Simmes printed the third edition (Q3) of *1 Henry IV* for Matthew LAW, and in 1607, another bad quarto for Ling, Q3 of THE TAMING OF A SHREW.

Simmes was often in trouble with the law. In 1589, only four years after completing his apprenticeship, he was arrested for assisting in the printing of the seditious 'Martin Marprelate' tracts (see MARTEXT), and in 1595 for pirating books. His press was seized and his type melted down, but he somehow got back in business, for in 1599 he was one of a group of printers expressly forbidden to print satires. In 1622 he was finally forbidden to work at all, though he received a pension from the STATIONERS' COMPANY.

Simonides Character in *Pericles,* king of PENTAPOLIS and father of THAISA. In 2.2 Simonides hosts a tournament, the winner of which is to have his daughter's hand in marriage. He welcomes the anonymous PERICLES to the contest despite his poor appearance in rusty armour. 'Opinion's but a fool, that makes us scan / The outward habit by the inward man' (2.2.55–56), he says. Pericles wins the tournament and Simonides is delighted. Pericles admires Simonides and compares him to his own royal father. In 2.5 Simonides tests the couple's readiness for marriage and pretends to distrust Pericles' motives. This elicits a manly denial from Pericles and a declaration of affection from Thaisa, following which Simonides announces his approval.

Simonides appears only in Act 2, but his symbolic importance is great. We are reminded of this when his death is reported in 5.3 after the perils and separation of Thaisa and Pericles are finally ended. His virtues are made clear before he appears, in the remarks of the FISHERMEN in 2.1. Most important, Simonides' healthy love permits him to be pleased with his daughter's marriage. This presents a powerful contrast to the relationship of ANTIOCHUS and his DAUGHTER (1), the incestuous love with which the play opens and which causes Pericles' exile. The hero's encounter with Simonides and Thaisa signals the beginning of the recovery of his fortunes, and this connection is confirmed at the play's end when Pericles cries, 'Heaven make a star of him!' (5.3.79).

In Shakespeare's sources for the play, the character corresponding to Simonides has another name. Why Shakespeare adopted the name Simonides is not known, but he presumably knew that the name belonged to two ancient poets, Simonides of Amorgos (active c. 660 B.C.) and Simonides of Ceos (c. 556–468 B.C.).

Simpcox, Saunder Minor character in *2 Henry VI,* an imposter who claims to have been blind and had his sight miraculously restored. The gullible villagers of ST. ALBANS present him to the king's hawking party and the equally credulous HENRY VI begins to congratulate him, but the Duke of GLOUCESTER (4) exposes the fraud through clever interrogation. Simpcox, who has also said he is lame, is whipped on Gloucester's orders, and he naturally runs away from the whipper, further revealing his imposture. Gloucester orders Simpcox and his WIFE to be whipped through every town until they arrive at the remote village they have claimed to come from. The incident, besides providing a bit of low comedy, was intended by Shakespeare to demonstrate the sound judgement of Gloucester.

Simple, Peter Minor character in *The Merry Wives of Windsor,* the servant of SLENDER. Simple reveals himself to be no smarter than his name suggests, as he

carries messages and announces arrivals. In his most developed scene, 4.5.24–53, he is fooled by FALSTAFF's elementary verbal tricks.

Simpson, Richard (1820–1876) British scholar. Simpson was a Protestant clergyman who converted to Catholicism and became a literary scholar. He wrote *An Introduction to the Philosophy of Shakespeare's Sonnets* (1868), and he pioneered the study of the playwright's politics in *The Politics of Shakespeare's Historical Plays* (1874). He also edited a series of plays not usually attributed to Shakespeare (see APOCRYPHA) that he nonetheless felt the playwright had written, at least in part. Simpson was the first to suggest that part of SIR THOMAS MORE was Shakespeare's, an idea that is now generally accepted. On the other hand, his elaborate analysis of FAIR EM as Shakespeare's allegorical attack on Robert GREENE (2) has been universally rejected.

Sincklo (Sinklo, Sincler), John (active 1590–1604) English actor who originated several Shakespearean roles. The inclusion of Sincklo's name in stage directions or speech headings of various texts reveals that he played a KEEPER (2) in *3 Henry VI,* one of the PLAYERS (1) in *The Taming of the Shrew,* and a BEADLE (2) in *2 Henry IV.* The Beadle's extraordinary thinness is a source of humour in 5.4.8–30, and it has thus been concluded that Sincklo was notable for this feature and may therefore have been cast as particularly thin men. Indeed, it is possible that Shakespeare wrote extremely thin men into his plays because he knew that Sincklo would be impressive in the parts. A number of characters that he may have played include Dr PINCH in *A Comedy of Errors* ('a hungry, lean-fac'd villain . . . A needy-hollow-ey'd-sharp-looking-wretch' [5.1. 238–241]); FEEBLE, a tailor, and SHADOW, both in *2 Henry IV* (Shadow is compared to 'the edge of a penknife' [3.2.262], and tailors were proverbially skinny, but Sincklo could only have played one of them for they appear together); the TAILOR in *Shrew;* the APOTHECARY in *Romeo and Juliet;* STARVELING in *A Midsummer Night's Dream;* and ROBERT FAULCONBRIDGE in *King John.*

Singer, John (d. c. 1605) English actor, a noted CLOWN (1). A member of the QUEEN'S MEN (1) from their founding in 1583 and after 1594 a member of the ADMIRAL'S MEN, Singer was regarded by his contemporaries as the equal of such better-known theatrical clowns as Richard TARLTON and William KEMPE. He also wrote at least one play, for which the Admiral's Men paid him in 1603, but no other record of it survives.

Sir Andrew Aguecheek Character in *Twelfth Night,* friend of SIR TOBY. Sir Andrew carouses with his friend while they visit the home of OLIVIA, Sir Toby's rich young niece, whom Sir Andrew is courting. Sir Toby takes merciless advantage of Sir Andrew, but it is impossible to pity such a ridiculous figure. He fancies himself a wit, though he is a dolt; a ladies' man, though he is gaunt and repulsive, as his name suggests; and a fighter, though he proves a coward.

Sir Andrew's inanity is well demonstrated when he tries to imitate VIOLA's rhetoric, though he clearly has no idea of its meaning. He proudly recites, ' "Odours", "pregnant", and "vouchsafed": I'll get 'em all three all ready' (3.1.93). He is foolishly ignorant of ordinary references, as when he calls Jezebel a man in 2.5.41, and he mistakes FESTE's drinking song—'a song of good life' (2.3.36–37)—for a hymn to virtue and rejects it, saying, 'I care not for good life' (2.3.39). When Sir Toby offers to marry MARIA (2) out of delight with her plan against MALVOLIO, Sir Andrew duplicates the offer, forgetting his alleged love for Olivia, and then he seconds the next several remarks made (2.5.183–208) in a delicious example of comic slavishness.

Sir Andrew's combination of quarrelsomeness and cowardice—referred to by Maria in 1.3.30–33—typified the braggart, a character type dating to ancient ROMAN DRAMA. Traditional, too, is the comeuppance Sir Andrew receives when he assaults SEBASTIAN (2) and is pummelled in 4.1 and 5.1. When Sir Toby receives the same treatment, he lashes out at Sir Andrew, calling him, accurately if not charitably, 'an ass-head and a coxcomb and a knave, a thin-faced knave, a gull!' (5.1.204–205).

However, Sir Andrew is sufficiently developed to have a few poignant and sympathetic moments. Rejected by Maria, he despondently (though comically) despairs, 'Methinks sometimes I have no more wit than a Christian . . . I am a great eater of beef, and I believe that does harm to my wit' (1.3.82–85). When he wistfully remarks, 'I was adored once' (2.3.181), we suddenly see that he has a past, a remembered youth. We may not need to know more, but we recognise his humanity.

Like many Shakespearean buffoons, Sir Andrew is a foil for other characters. Sir Toby's underlying selfishness manifests itself in his exploitation of Sir Andrew. As a ridiculous suitor, Sir Andrew magnifies by contrast the somewhat slender virtues of ORSINO, who also pursues Olivia. And his self-image as a grand fellow is subtly similar to Malvolio's fantasies of aristocratic stature.

Sir John Oldcastle Play formerly attributed to Shakespeare, part of the Shakespeare APOCRYPHA. Thomas PAVIER first published *The First Part of Sir John Oldcastle* as an anonymous play in a QUARTO edition known as Q1 (1600). Later in the same year, however, he released a second edition (Q2) in which the play was credited to Shakespeare, as it also was in Pavier's noto-

rious FALSE FOLIO (1619). Pavier's false attribution also led to the play's inclusion in the Third and Fourth FOLIOS. The records of Philip HENSLOWE, who produced the play, reveal that its authors were Michael DRAYTON, Richard HATHWAY, Anthony MUNDAY, and Robert WILSON (4). *The Second Part of Sir John Oldcastle,* which is now lost, was written by Drayton alone.

Sir John Oldcastle concerns an historical figure, a proto-Protestant religious martyr. It was conceived in response to a controversy surrounding Shakespeare's great character, FALSTAFF. In *1* and *2 Henry IV,* Falstaff had originally been named OLDCASTLE. The historical Oldcastle's descendants were horrified, and their influence was such that the name was changed. Henslowe presumably saw a way to capitalise on the popularity—and notoriety—of Falstaff, and at the same time ingratiate himself with the historical Oldcastle's chief defender, Lord COBHAM. The prologue of *Sir John Oldcastle* expressly contrasts its hero with Shakespeare's 'pampered glutton', and Falstaff himself is twice mentioned in the play in disapproving terms.

Sir Thomas More Play attributed in part to Shakespeare. *Sir Thomas More* presents episodes from the life of Thomas MORE, a Catholic martyr who was executed by King HENRY VIII for his refusal to accept the English Reformation. It was probably written around 1593 or 1600 (scholarly opinions differ) for the ADMIRAL'S MEN. The manuscript of *Sir Thomas More,* which was assembled around 1595 (or 1603), is mostly in the handwriting of Anthony MUNDAY, but with additions in five different hands, one of which—known as 'Hand D'—is generally accepted as Shakespeare's. If so, this is the only surviving sample of the playwright's handwriting, aside from six signatures on legal documents. For *Sir Thomas More,* he wrote three pages of script comprising one scene of 147 lines, in which More subdues a riot with a moving oration.

That this is Shakespeare's composition is demonstrated through several lines of evidence. First, the handwriting is very like that of the playwright's six known signatures. Further, peculiar spellings—such as *'scilens'* for *'silence'*—occur both in Hand D's pages and in editions of Shakespeare's plays that are known to derive from the author's FOUL PAPERS. Perhaps most tellingly, the imagery used in Hand D's text resembles Shakespeare's, especially in lines that are very similar to passages in both *Coriolanus* and *Troilus and Cressida.* Lastly, the political ideas expressed in Hand D's scene agree with what we know of Shakespeare's thinking, for they demonstrate a respect for social hierarchy combined with sympathy for the common people and stress the malleability of the commoners through oratory.

The odd manuscript of *Sir Thomas More* was the result of government CENSORSHIP; apparently, the play was originally submitted to Edmund Tilney, the MASTER OF THE REVELS, who refused to permit its performance without major revisions. Accordingly, several pages were torn from the original manuscript and replaced with others. Scholars believe that the six hands that recorded the text were those of the three collaborators on the original play plus two revisers and a professional scribe. It is generally held that the original text was written by Munday, Henry CHETTLE, and possibly Thomas HEYWOOD (2), while the revisions were written by Chettle, Thomas DEKKER, and Shakespeare. The revisions did not have their intended effect; Tilney was not moved, and *Sir Thomas More* was not performed until 1964, when it was staged in Nottingham, England.

Sir Toby Belch Character in *Twelfth Night,* uncle of OLIVIA. The self-indulgent Sir Toby drinks and roars through life, and, with MARIA (2), SIR ANDREW, and FABIAN, he represents a jocular, festive spirit that triumphs over the cold and humourless rigidity of Olivia's steward, MALVOLIO, in the play's comic SUBPLOT. His position is boldly presented in his first speech, when he complains of Olivia's mourning for her deceased brother, saying, 'What a plague means my niece to take the death of her brother thus? I am sure care's an enemy to life' (1.3.1–3). Sir Toby laughs and carouses mightily and counters Malvolio's insistence on order with the famous rebuke, 'Dost thou think because thou art virtuous, there shall be no more cakes and ale?' (2.3.114–115). Like another, greater drunken knight, Sir John FALSTAFF, Sir Toby enacts a variety of comic roles: he is Sir Andrew's mentor in debauchery and joins the jester, FESTE, in mockery and jokes. He is a singer of songs and a fierce master of the duelling code. He makes repeated references to dances in 1.3.113–131, 2.3.58, and 5.1.198.

However, Sir Toby has a darker side as well. His selfishness is very apparent. He exploits both his friend and his niece. He spends the foolish Sir Andrew's money while pretending to promote his mercenary marriage to Olivia, boasting that he has taken his dupe for 'some two thousand strong, or so' (3.2.52–53). His drunkenness turns belligerent and incoherent in 1.5.121–122, 129–130. His practical joking has a vicious edge: he forces two unwilling combatants to a duel in 3.4, and he also pushes Maria's plot against Malvolio to a new extreme, gloating, 'we'll have him in a dark room and bound . . . we may carry it thus for our pleasure' (3.4.136–138). This course is criticised in his own fear of reprimand in 4.2.70–74 and by the efforts of Olivia and ORSINO to mitigate Malvolio's humiliation in 5.1. Moreover, Sir Toby's final departure is ugly: he curses Sir Andrew as 'an ass-head and a coxcomb and a knave, a thin-faced knave, a gull!' (5.1.204–205) after his own scheme to humiliate his friend has resulted in both of them being beaten by SEBASTIAN (2).

Sir Toby's somewhat unpleasant traits offer a parallel in the sub-plot to the problematic elements of the main plot. As a result, some critics who view *Twelfth Night* as an ironic social satire regard Sir Toby as a vulgar parasite, a hanger-on in the household of his niece, concerned only with his debauched existence. Sir Toby's attitudes towards Sir Andrew and Olivia corroborate this theory somewhat, but it is surely too extreme. The knight is made to submit to his niece's anger at his ways—'Ungracious wretch . . . Out of my sight! Rudesby, be gone!' she shouts in 4.1.50—but on the other hand, the playwright permits him satisfaction at the defeat of Malvolio. While he is not present at the final scene of recognition and reconciliation, he marries the delightful Maria, as is reported in 5.1.363, again paralleling developments in the main plot. Sir Toby, though he has his faults, is basically a symbol of the values of humour and joyous living and is therefore a representative of the triumphant spirit of comedy.

Siward (Sigurd the Dane), Earl of Northumberland (d. 1055) Historical figure and minor character in *Macbeth,* English ally of MALCOLM and MACDUFF against MACBETH. Siward, a famous soldier who commands an army of 10,000 men, is provided by England's king to the exiled Prince Malcolm of SCOTLAND. As a noble and knightly figure, Siward stands for the virtues lost to the world of the play through Macbeth's evil, and as a foreigner who must be brought in to restore the country's health, he points up the extremity of Scotland's need. He appears briefly several times in Act 5 and is a direct and simple soldier. His most notable moment comes when he is informed that his son, YOUNG SIWARD, has died in combat. With noble fortitude he observes, 'Why then, God's soldier be he! / Had I as many sons as I have hairs, / I would not wish them to a fairer death.' (5.9. 13–15).

The historical Siward, or Sigurd, was of Danish royal descent. His family had seized Northumberland during the Danish conquest of England a few generations earlier; in Northumberland it was traditionally said that his grandfather was a bear. Siward was a famous warrior who had fought for the English kings Hardicanute (ruled 1040–1042) and Edward the Confessor (1042–1066), and he was thus a fitting choice to command Malcolm's army of invasion, quite aside from his kinship to the prince. He was either Malcolm's brother-in-law or uncle—11th-century references differ. Shakespeare's source, HOLINSHED's history, mistakenly called him Malcolm's grandfather, for he was considerably older than Malcolm's father, King DUNCAN. The playwright made him Malcolm's uncle—perhaps thereby unknowingly correcting an error—to place him in the same generation as Duncan.

Much more than the legendary BANQUO, Siward deserved to be called 'the root and father / Of many kings' (3.1.5–6). His oldest son, Osberne, died fighting against Macbeth, as in the play. His younger son, Waltheof (d. 1075), led the last British resistance to William the Conqueror and was later canonised for it as Saint Waldeve. He had a daughter, Matilda, who married Malcolm's son, later King David I of Scotland (ruled 1124–1153). Two of their sons were kings of the Dunkeld dynasty, as were a grandson and great-grandson. A third son of Matilda and David was an ancestor of King Robert II (1371–1390) who was the founder of the Stewart (later STUART) dynasty. Thus Siward is an ancestor of Shakespeare's sovereign, King JAMES I, whose supposed descent from Banquo is celebrated in the play. All this was certainly unknown to Shakespeare, who simply followed Holinshed, and presumably to King James as well, for he seems to have enjoyed his supposed connection to Banquo.

Slater (Slaughter), Martin (active 1594–1625) English actor. A leading member of the ADMIRAL'S MEN from 1594–1597, Slater was then associated with Laurence FLETCHER (3) in England and Scotland, and with other provincial companies. In 1608 he was co-manager with Michael DRAYTON of a CHILDREN'S COMPANY that performed at the WHITEFRIARS THEATRE. In the records of a lawsuit that resulted from this enterprise, Slater is described as an ironmonger with eight children, which suggests that he had need of a sideline. He had returned to touring companies by 1610, and in 1616 he was cited for staging plays without a licence. He continued to perform with provincial troupes until at least 1625.

Slender, Abraham Character in *The Merry Wives of Windsor,* dull-witted suitor of ANNE (3) Page. For financial reasons, a marriage between Anne and Slender is supported by Anne's parents and by Slender's elderly relative Justice SHALLOW, but Slender himself, although attracted to the idea, can only sigh vacantly at the prospect—'. . . sweet Anne Page!' (3.1.38, 66, 105)—and make awkwardly embarrassed conversation. When he finally proposes, he can only blurt that it isn't his idea, 'Truly, for mine own part, I would little or nothing with you. Your father and my uncle hath made motions. . . . You may ask your father . . .' (3.4.61–64). Anne beseeches, 'Good mother, do not marry me to yond fool' (3.4.81), and the audience can only sympathise. However, MISTRESS (3) Page arranges for Slender to elope with Anne during the mock fairy ceremonies in 5.5. Fortunately, Anne and her true love, FENTON, foil the plan, and Slender has a boy foisted off on him, as he only discovers during the marriage ceremony.

Slender's name suggests both his appearance and his lack of self-reliance. Such feeble characters were

stock figures in Elizabethan comedy. It has been speculated that Slender was also intended by Shakespeare as a satirical portrait of the stepson of his enemy William GARDINER (2), but this cannot be proven.

Sly (1), Christopher Character in *The Taming of the Shrew,* a drunken tinker and the principal figure of the INDUCTION. In these two scenes, Sly is found asleep outside a tavern by a local landowner, the LORD (1), who decides to play a practical joke and has him installed as a gentleman in his home. Sly awakes to find himself treated like an aristocrat and told he has been insane to imagine himself a poor drunkard. As part of the joke, a troupe of PLAYERS (1) performs 'a pleasant comedy' (Ind.2.130) for Sly; this drama is *The Taming of the Shrew.* Sly is last seen dozing in an INTERLUDE (1.1.248–253).

Sly is a boldly drawn minor figure, full of drunken pretensions and country sayings, comically ready to assume his new life of ease, though insisting on his poor man's taste for ale over the gentry's wine. His succinct autobiography—'by birth a pedlar, by education a cardmaker, by transmutation a bear-herd, and now . . . a tinker' (Ind.2.18–21)—gives representation to a multitude of obscure lives among the 16th-century poor. Sly makes numerous explicit references to people and places in the STRATFORD area, and this portrait of a rustic sot clearly derives from the young Shakespeare's recollections of his old home.

Although Sly's story ends abruptly after 1.1 in the oldest edition of *The Taming of the Shrew,* in the FIRST FOLIO of 1623, it is complete in THE TAMING OF A SHREW, believed to be a BAD QUARTO of Shakespeare's play and to contain Shakespeare's original rendition of Sly's adventure: in three further interludes, Sly remarks on the play, eating and drinking all the while. In a fifth episode, he has fallen asleep and the Lord orders him returned to the spot where he had been found. In a 23-line EPILOGUE to *A Shrew,* Sly is discovered by the Tapster of the tavern, who remarks that Sly's wife will be angry with him for staying out all night. Sly replies that he need not fear his wife, for he has had a dream that has taught him how to deal with her. Sly was probably played by William SLY (2).

Sly (2), William (d. 1608) English actor, member of the CHAMBERLAIN'S MEN and the KING'S MEN. Sly is one of the 26 men listed in the FIRST FOLIO as 'Principall Actors' in Shakespeare's plays. He was with either STRANGE'S MEN or the ADMIRAL'S MEN around 1590, for he appears in the combined company of that year. Between 1592 and 1594, he was probably associated with PEMBROKE'S MEN, for he apparently helped compile their text for THE TAMING OF A SHREW, a BAD QUARTO (text assembled from memory) of *The Taming of the Shrew.* Sly played—and was presumably the namesake of—Christopher SLY (1) in *The Shrew,* and that part is fairly accurately reproduced in *A Shrew.* His next documented appearance was with the Chamberlain's Men in 1598, though he may have been a member of the company at its inception in 1594. He remained a member after it became the King's Men, until his death. He may have played OSRIC in *Hamlet,* though except for Christopher Sly, no Shakespearean role can be assigned with certainty to him. He was not an original partner in the GLOBE THEATRE, but he had acquired a share by 1605. In 1608 he was an original shareholder in the BLACKFRIARS THEATRE, but he died a week after the agreement was signed and his share was redistributed among the other partners. He left his share in the Globe to Robert BROWNE, who was probably his brother-in-law.

Smethwick (Smithweeke), John (d. 1641) English bookseller and publisher, producer of several editions of Shakespeare's plays and a partner in the FIRST FOLIO. In 1607 Nicholas LING sold Smethwick the rights to *Hamlet, Romeo and Juliet, Love's Labour's Lost,* and THE TAMING OF A SHREW. Smethwick is only known to have produced editions of two of these, however: Q3 of *Romeo and Juliet* (1609) and Q3–5 of *Hamlet* (1611, 1622, 1637). He had a share in both the First and Second Folios of Shakespeare's collected plays (1623, 1632).

Smethwick finished nine years of apprenticeship and became a member of the STATIONERS' COMPANY in 1597. Early in his career, he was fined several times for pirating copyrighted books, but he presumably changed his ways, for he eventually became a high officer in the Stationers' Company.

Smith (1) (Smith the Weaver) Minor character in *2 Henry VI,* a follower of the revolutionary Jack CADE. As the rebels are introduced in 4.2, Smith indulges in several joking asides at the expense of his leader, exhibiting the buffoonery that was one aspect of Shakespeare's characterisation of Cade's uprising. As 'Weaver', he gets one more such line in 4.7.

Smith (2), Morgan (c. 1833–1882) African-American actor in Britain. Like Ira ALDRIDGE before him, Smith made a living in the English theatre at a time when black American actors could not surmount racial prejudice at home. Though not the major figure Aldridge was, he had a successful career as a touring performer, often reading a miscellany of speeches in lieu of a play production. A native of Philadelphia, Smith trained with a Welsh actor in Boston, but, when he was refused employment there, he emigrated. Four days after his arrival in England in 1866, never having appeared in public before, Smith performed successfully as OTHELLO. He also played RICHARD III, MACBETH, HAMLET, SHYLOCK, IAGO, and ROMEO, as well as a range

of non-Shakespearean roles, until ill health compelled him to retire in about 1879.

Smithfield An open field to the north of London, the location, in 4.7 of *2 Henry VI,* of a skirmish won by Jack CADE's rebels, after which they execute Lord SAY. This choice of location, not necessitated by Shakespeare's sources, was appropriate: Smithfield, which was London's great livestock market, was frequently the site of public executions.

Smithson, Harriet (1800–1853) Irish actress, successful in France. Smithson was a relatively unknown London actress when she played OPHELIA in a production mounted in Paris by William Charles MACREADY in 1827. She was a great success, both in this role and others, notably DESDEMONA, and she toured Europe to continued acclaim. A leading Parisian critic of the day declared that she had introduced Shakespeare to France. She soon abandoned her career, however, to marry the composer Hector BERLIOZ in 1833. It was an unhappy marriage, and he eventually left her for another woman, though when she became an invalid in her last years, he returned and stayed with her until her death.

Snare Minor character in *2 Henry IV,* subordinate to the constable FANG. In 2.1 Fang and Snare are hired by the HOSTESS (2) to arrest FALSTAFF for debt. Snare is nervous about the likelihood of armed resistance, and, indeed, when Falstaff and his companion, BARDOLPH (1), draw their swords, Fang and Snare are helpless. Snare's name, like Fang's, indicates his function, if not his capabilities.

Sneak Musician referred to in *2 Henry IV,* the leader of the MUSICIANS (4) who play at FALSTAFF's dinner at the BOAR'S HEAD TAVERN. In 2.4.11 'Sneak's noise' is stipulated as the desired music, and in line 21 a DRAWER goes in search of him. Another reference to Sneak, in a play of 1613, suggests that there was an historical Sneak who enjoyed some renown in London, but nothing more is known of him.

Snodham, Thomas (d. 1625) London printer. Snodham, who established his printing business in 1603, printed an edition of THOMAS LORD CROMWELL—a play spuriously attributed to Shakespeare—in 1613, and in 1616 he printed Q6 of *The Rape of Lucrece* for publisher Roger JACKSON (3). Snodham was a brother-in-law of publisher Cuthbert BURBY.

Snout, Tom Character in *A Midsummer Night's Dream,* a tinker of ATHENS and a performer in the comical amateur production of PYRAMUS AND THISBE staged at the wedding of Duke THESEUS (1) and Queen HIPPOLYTA (1). Snout plays the Wall in the INTERLUDE, which is directed by his fellow artisan Peter QUINCE. Snout's name, like that of his fellow artisans, refers to his trade; a tinker's most common task was repairing the spouts, often called snouts, of kettles and teapots.

Snug Character in *A Midsummer Night's Dream,* a joiner of ATHENS and a performer in the comical amateur production of PYRAMUS AND THISBE staged at the wedding of Duke THESEUS (1) and Queen HIPPOLYTA (1). Snug plays the Lion in the INTERLUDE, which is directed by his fellow artisan Peter QUINCE. Snug presents himself as 'slow of study' (1.2.63), and he is mute during the rehearsal scene (3.1), but he carries off his role commendably at the performance in 5.1. In the woodworking trades, Snug's name means 'tightly fitting', an appropriate name for a joiner.

Solanio Character in *The Merchant of Venice,* friend of ANTONIO (2). Solanio is a cultured gentleman of VENICE whose conversation in elegant verse reflects the advanced civilisation of his city. He is difficult to distinguish from his companion SALERIO. In commenting on the action, these two gentlemen present facts and ideas. For instance, consoling the melancholy Antonio in 1.1, they speak of his status as a wealthy and successful merchant, and in 2.8 they offer a picture of Shylock's despair and rage at JESSICA's elopement and speculate that the Jew will vent his anger on Antonio if he can. In 3.1 they tease Shylock, eliciting from him his famous speech claiming equality with Christians. Solanio is simply a conventional figure whose main purpose is to further the development of more significant characters.

Soldier (1) Minor character in *1 Henry VI,* an English infantryman. In 2.1, during the retaking of the town of ORLÉANS (1) by the English, the Soldier, crying the name of the great English warrior TALBOT, drives the French leaders, including CHARLES VII and JOAN LA PUCELLE, from the stage. He gleefully claims the clothing they have left behind in their panic. This episode, entirely fictitious, emphasises the importance to the English cause of the noble Talbot. It also serves to ridicule the French, thus furthering the play's point that only dissensions among the English could have resulted in French victories.

Soldier (2) Any of several minor characters in *1 Henry VI.* Four French Soldiers, disguised as peasants, accompany JOAN LA PUCELLE and gain entrance to the English-held city of ROUEN in 3.2. They spy out the weakest gate and signal the other French troops, who enter and capture the city. This episode emphasises the treacherous nature of the French by contrasting Joan's deceitful ruse with the unalloyed valour of the English hero, TALBOT.

Soldier (3) Minor character in *2 Henry VI*, a messenger who enters the camp of the rebel leader Jack CADE in 4.6, unaware that Cade has just declared it an act of treason to address him as anything but 'Lord Mortimer'. The Soldier, knowing no better, calls out for 'Cade'; the leader orders him set upon, and he is killed. This incident serves to present a vicious side of the uprising, which has earlier been treated as a focus of broad humour. Now Cade, in addition to being a buffoon, is shown to be a blood-thirsty tyrant in the making.

Soldier (4) Minor character in *3 Henry VI*. When EDWARD IV decides to declare his renewed claim to the crown, in 4.7, he calls on the Soldier to read his proclamation.

Soldier (5) Any of several minor characters in *Julius Caesar*, members of the armies of ANTONY and OCTAVIUS on one hand, and BRUTUS (4) and CASSIUS on the other, in the civil war that follows the assassination of CAESAR (1).

Soldier (6) Any of several minor characters in *Troilus and Cressida*, Trojan troops. In 1.2 the Soldiers, who do not speak, march in front of PANDARUS and CRESSIDA, provoking Pandarus to sneer, 'Asses, fools, dolts, chaff and bran, chaff and bran; porridge after meat . . . crows and daws, crows and daws' (1.2.245–248). This is one of the comically inhumane remarks that pepper the play.

Soldier (7) Any of several characters in *All's Well That Ends Well*, troops in the army of FLORENCE. The First Soldier is the pretended interpreter during the interrogation of PAROLLES. In 4.1 and 4.3 Parolles is captured by the First LORD (6), who proposes to demonstrate the foppish courtier's cowardice and treachery to his deluded friend, BERTRAM. The captors pretend to speak a foreign language so that their victim will not realise that they are French, and the First Soldier pretends to interpret between the Lord and the prisoner. Parolles treasonably discloses secrets, and the First Soldier induces him to insult the Lords and Bertram, which maintains a humorous tone to the scene. The Second Soldier is a messenger who is sent in 4.1 to tell Bertram of Parolles' capture. His submission to orders helps suggest the strength and efficiency of the military, which is contrasted with the cowardice and treason of Parolles.

Soldier (8) Minor character in *Antony and Cleopatra*, a member of ANTONY's army. In 3.8 the Soldier pleads with Antony not to fight the forthcoming battle against Octavius CAESAR (2) at sea, where the opponent has the advantage. However, Antony's pride demands that he accept Caesar's challenge to naval warfare, and he engages in the fatal battle of ACTIUM. The Soldier reappears in 4.5, and Antony acknowledges that he was right. The Soldier then reports that ENOBARBUS has deserted, an event that signals the utter collapse of Antony's fortunes just before what is to be his final battle. The Soldier thus serves as a measure of Antony's declining destiny.

Soldier (9) Any of several minor characters in *Antony and Cleopatra*, members of ANTONY's army. In 4.3 a group of Soldiers gather to perform sentry duty. They hear strange, wailing, musiclike noises—seemingly under the street—and they interpret this phenomenon as a bad omen that portends the loss of the next day's battle. Four of them speak and are designated as the First, Second, Third, and Fourth Soldiers. In 4.4 the Soldiers (or, perhaps, other soldiers) appear the next morning and march to the battle without complaint, but the earlier episode tells us that Antony's end is fast approaching.

Soldier (10) Minor character in *Antony and Cleopatra*, a member of the army of Octavius CAESAR (2). In 4.6 the Soldier brings a message to ENOBARBUS, who has deserted Mark ANTONY and joined Caesar; his former master has sent his belongings after him. The Soldier, though busy with his battle preparations, pauses to remark, 'Your emperor / Continues still a Jove' (4.6.28–29). This disinterested praise from an enemy confirms the play's image of Antony as a great man while it also furthers the plot for it plunges Enobarbus into the guilt that will break his heart and kill him in 4.9.

Soldier (11) Any of several minor characters in *Coriolanus*, members of the Roman army. The Soldiers retreat before the VOLSCIANS at the gates of CORIOLES, and they refuse to follow MARTIUS (2)—later given the name CORIOLANUS—when he enters the city. 'Foolhardiness! Not I' (1.4.46) is the reply in the words of the First Soldier, who speaks for the group apart from one line given to a Second Soldier. However, when they observe Martius' return they are inspired to join him and fight their way into the city. Another group of Soldiers accompanies COMINIUS in 1.6, and they too are inspired by the arrival of the battle-torn Martius. The Soldiers say very little except in unison, and their chief function, much like that of the CITIZENS (5), is to demonstrate the changeable nature of the common man, an important theme of the play.

Soldier (12) Any of several minor characters in *Coriolanus*, members of the Volscian army. In 1.10 one of the Soldiers—designated the First Soldier—interjects four single lines into AUFIDIUS' long speech on CORIOLANUS' recent victory over the VOLSCIANS at CORIOLES. The First Soldier is merely a sounding board who provides the occasion for the audience to see his

leader's vengefulness and rancour towards Coriolanus.

Soldier (13) Minor character in *Timon of Athens,* a messenger for ALCIBIADES. In 5.3 the Soldier, sent with a message to TIMON, discovers Timon's grave. Unable to read the inscription on it, he decides to copy it and bring it to Alcibiades. He does this in 5.4, and thus inspires the play's final passage, in which Alcibiades translates Timon's last statement and remarks on it.

Soliloquy Speech made by a character, usually when alone on the stage, revealing his or her inner thoughts. Originally a device of ancient Greek and Roman drama, the soliloquy was popular in the RENAISSANCE and was widely used in ELIZABETHAN DRAMA. Shakespeare frequently used this device to present the audience with material that could not be realistically delivered in dialogue. Sometimes the soliloquy simply provides information on the plot—as when villains such as AARON, IAGO, and RICHARD III comment on their own schemes—but more often it functions to reveal character through the expression of private emotional drives. This technique is particularly striking in *Hamlet* and *Macbeth,* whose soliloquies are among Shakespeare's greatest poetic achievements. The two uses can of course apply simultaneously, as when Iago both directs our knowledge of the central plot and displays his own tortuous nature. While Shakespeare's most famous soliloquies are given to his great tragic characters, the effect of a soliloquy can also be comic, as in those of MALVOLIO and BENEDICK.

Though artificial, the soliloquy nevertheless supports our sense of the play's truth to reality, for we recognise that a character has no motive for lying in a soliloquy and accordingly accept the passage as a legitimate revelation. In Shakespeare, a character's use of soliloquy often in itself demonstrates an introspective personality; Hamlet and Macbeth are actively molding their psychological and spiritual natures, whereas others, such as CORIOLANUS and ANTONY, do not concern themselves with these matters and seldom reveal themselves to the audience.

Solinus Character in *The Comedy of Errors.* See DUKE (8).

Somerset (1), Edmund Beaufort, Duke of (1406–1455) Historical figure and character in *2 Henry VI,* a Lancastrian rival of the Duke of YORK (8). (See Lancaster [1]; York [1].) Edmund, the younger brother of John Beaufort, the Duke of SOMERSET (3) in *1 Henry VI,* inherited both the rivalry and the title after John's death in 1444. The Somerset-York feud is a central feature in *1 Henry VI;* however, *2 Henry VI* focusses first on the fall of the Duke of GLOUCESTER (4) and later on the sudden rebelliousness of York, and this Somerset is a relatively minor figure.

He is sufficiently consequential, however, that the DUCHESS (1) of Gloucester, seeking political advice from the supernatural world, questions a SPIRIT (1) about his future in 1.4. It is prophesied that Somerset should fear castles, a warning that at the time seems incomprehensible. In 1.3 Somerset is appointed the King's Regent in FRANCE (1), and he reappears in 3.1 to announce the loss of France, evidencing the harm that infighting among ambitious noblemen has done to England. When York returns from Ireland with an army, he demands Somerset's imprisonment. Somerset volunteers to go to the Tower if the king wishes, and York is placated. However, York encounters Somerset, still free, in 5.1 and takes the fact as cause for an armed rebellion. In the ensuing battle, the first of the WARS OF THE ROSES, Somerset is killed by York's son (later RICHARD III) beneath a tavern sign depicting a castle, thus fulfilling the prophecy. (In 1.1 of *3 Henry VI,* Richard displays Somerset's head as a demonstration of his prowess in battle.)

One theme of *2 Henry VI* is the death of 'good Duke Humphrey' at the hands of scheming nobles, who thereby deprived England of its only chance of avoiding the civil war that erupted during Henry's weak reign. Shakespeare desired to compress the events that led to that war, and he eclipsed Somerset's political importance in the process. Somerset was the favourite of Queen MARGARET (1) after the fall of SUFFOLK (3) in 1450. However, Somerset had been the commander under whom Normandy was lost in the late 1440s, and he was Henry's chief minister in 1453, when England was irrevocably defeated in southern France. He was therefore in extreme disfavour at the time. So, even though Margaret would have preferred Somerset to act as Regent in the summer of 1453, when King Henry succumbed to a disabling form of insanity, his unpopularity with both the aristocracy and the public inhibited her, and York was given the post. He governed well and faithfully until late in 1454, when the King recovered. At this point, Somerset was restored to office, and it was this action, probably taken at Margaret's insistence, that led York to gather an army and eventually declare himself king. Shakespeare thus omits several years of intricate political manoeuvring in order to clarify York's drive for the throne.

Somerset (2), Duke of Character in *3 Henry VI*—a combination of two historical figures—who betrays King EDWARD IV to support WARWICK (3) in his rebellion. Shakespeare confused two dukes of Somerset who participated in the WARS OF THE ROSES, Henry (1436–1464) and his younger brother Edmund (c. 1438–1471), both of them sons of the Duke of SOMERSET (1) of *2 Henry VI.* In 4.1 of *3 Henry VI* Somerset

leaves Edward's court with GEORGE (2) to join Warwick and fight for the reinstatement of the deposed King HENRY VI. This Somerset must be Henry, who deserted the Lancastrians and then rejoined them, at which point he is depicted here. Henry was finally captured and beheaded by the Yorkists. All of the subsequent appearances of Somerset in the play occur well after the date of Henry's execution and thus must portray Edmund, who succeeded to his brother's title. Edmund was always a firm Lancastrian, and it is he who is shown aiding the young RICHMOND in 4.6, supporting Warwick and MARGARET (1) in Act 5, and being sentenced to death after the battle of TEWKESBURY, in 5.5, as Edmund in fact was.

Somerset (3), John Beaufort, Duke of (1403–1444) Historical figure and character in *1 Henry VI,* the rival of the Duke of YORK (8). Somerset selects a red rose as his emblem in response to Plantagenet's adopting a white one in the Temple garden scene (2.4). Thus, fictitiously, do the WARS OF THE ROSES begin. Somerset is depicted as dishonourable. He is unwilling to fulfil his agreement to accept the opinion of a majority in his dispute with Plantagenet, declaring that his argument was 'here in my scabbard' (2.4.60), and he goes on to taunt his rival about his father's execution some years earlier. When their quarrel erupts again at HENRY VI's coronation in Paris (4.1), the king unwisely attempts to settle it by dividing the command of the French troops between them. Then the death of TALBOT is attributed to York's and Somerset's refusal to provide him with reinforcements.

The historical Somerset quarrelled with York over the divided command in Normandy in the early 1440s, and Shakespeare uses this material in the sequence culminating in Talbot's death, which actually took place nine years after Somerset's own. Moreover, Somerset was a prisoner in FRANCE (1) in 1421–1438 and thus could not have had taken part in the quarrel with York at the king's coronation or in the Temple garden scene. Thus John Beaufort's younger brother Edmund, his successor as Duke of SOMERSET (1) and a character in *2 Henry VI,* is sometimes considered to have been a co-model for the Somerset of *1 Henry VI.* However, Edmund did not succeed to the title until 1448—later than all the events in *1 Henry VI* except the death of Talbot, which Shakespeare linked to an episode that unquestionably involved John, the divided command. Therefore, it seems best to regard John Beaufort as the Somerset of this play.

Somerville, Sir John (d. 1492) Historical figure and minor character in *3 Henry VI,* a supporter of WARWICK (3) in his rebellion against King EDWARD IV. Somerville reports to Warwick on troop movements in 5.1.

Son (1) Minor character in *Macbeth,* LADY (7) Macduff's child who is killed by MACBETH's hired Murderers (see FIRST MURDERER [3]), in 4.2. The Son sees that his mother is distressed by MACDUFF's departure to England to join the rebellion against Macbeth, and he attempts to understand the situation with pertly humorous questions and remarks. His wit and intelligence make his slaughter all the more vicious and contribute greatly to the power of the episode, which stresses the depths of evil to which Macbeth has descended. The boy's courage in death—he calls one of the Murderers a 'shag-hair'd villain' (4.2.82), and with his last breath he futilely attempts to warn his mother—contrasts tellingly with the villainy of his killers.

Son (2) That Hath Killed His Father, The Minor but significant character in *3 Henry VI,* a participant in the battle of TOWTON in 2.5. The Son, a soldier, begins to loot the corpse of an enemy he has killed, only to discover that the fallen foe is his own father. He bewails his fate and prays, with an allusion to the Crucifixion, 'Pardon me, God, I knew not what I did: / And pardon, Father, for I knew not thee' (2.5.69–70). He is witnessed by King HENRY VI, who has withdrawn from the battle to wish despairingly that he were a rustic shepherd, rather than a combatant. This incident, along with that of THE FATHER THAT HATH KILLED HIS SON, is juxtaposed ironically with King Henry's pastoral musings to highlight the horror of civil war.

Song Short poem accompanied by music, often used in Shakespeare's plays, though not always written by the playwright. Many of these songs are versions or fragments of popular songs known from other sources, a few were probably written by collaborators, and some may have been inserted into a play by someone other than the playwright, in the course of a theatrical run. However, scholars generally believe that the following songs (in approximate order of composition) were written by Shakespeare: 'Who Is Silvia?' *(Two Gentlemen of Verona);* 'When daisies pied' *(Love's Labour's Lost);* 'You spotted snakes' *(A Midsummer Night's Dream);* 'Tell me, where is fancy bred' *(The Merchant of Venice);* 'Sigh no more, ladies' and 'Pardon, goddess of the night' *(Much Ado About Nothing);* 'Under the greenwood tree', 'Blow, blow, thou winter wind', 'What shall he have that killed the deer?' and 'It was a lover and his lass' *(As You Like It);* 'O mistress mine', 'Come away, death', and 'When that I was and a little tiny boy' *(Twelfth Night);* 'Take, O take those lips away' *(Measure for Measure);* 'Hark, hark, the lark' and 'Fear no more the heat o' the sun' *(Cymbeline);* 'When daffodils begin to peer', 'Get you hence, for I must go', and 'Lawn as white as driven snow' *(The Winter's Tale);* 'Come unto these yellow sands', 'Full fadom five thy

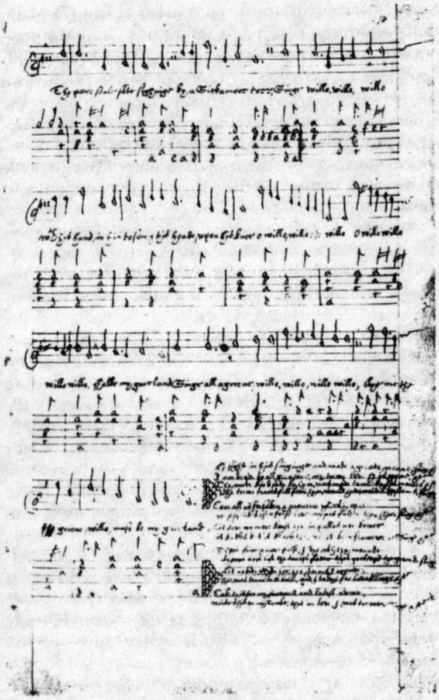

A 17th-century setting of Desdemona's song in Othello. *Songs were elements in many of Shakespeare's plays, whether they were composed by the playwright himself, or, like this one, popular ballads of the day.* (Courtesy of the Trustees of the British Museum)

father lies', and 'Where the bee sucks' *(The Tempest);* 'Orpheus with his lute' *(Henry VIII);* and 'Roses, their sharp spines being gone' *(The Two Noble Kinsmen).*

Shakespeare's early songs mostly served to adorn a COMEDY and generally had little if any importance to the plot or characterisations. However, beginning with the songs of AMIENS and TOUCHSTONE in *As You Like It* (1599), the songs begin to relate to character and to the play's theme. This change probably reflects the talents of Robert ARMIN; before he joined the CHAMBERLAIN'S MEN, the availability of a good singer for a play was uncertain, so the playwright may have been reluctant to give a song much significance. Shakespearean TRAGEDY uses song dramatically—as in the songs of the FOOL (2) in *King Lear,* OPHELIA in *Hamlet,* and DESDEMONA in *Othello*—but these were popular ballads of the day, recognisable by the original audiences and thus even more potent dramatically.

In the last plays, the ROMANCES and *Henry VIII,* the influence of the MASQUE demanded songs, most of which Shakespeare wrote.

Little of the original music for Shakespeare's plays has survived. The tunes of currently popular songs were doubtless used for at least some of the songs, even among those Shakespeare wrote, but other melodies were composed by Robert JOHNSON (5), Thomas MORLEY, John WILSON (2), and possibly others. Shakespeare was plainly conscious of the composer's task, for he was careful to write lyrics with short, rhymed lines of varying lengths, and he emphasised vowel sounds rather than consonants, especially at the ends of lines. Many notable composers have subsequently set Shakespeare's songs to music (see, e.g., ARNE; SHUBERT; SULLIVAN [1]).

Sonnet Verse form, a 14-line poem, usually in iambic pentameter (see METRE) and with any of several traditional rhyme schemes. The sonnet has been widely popular ever since its evolution from medieval Italian verse and is still used by poets in most European languages. Shakespeare's SONNETS are among the best known, and he also employed sonnets in several of his plays, most notably in *Romeo and Juliet* and *Love's Labour's Lost.*

A sonnet usually consists of two parts, an eight-line section (the octet) followed by a six-line section (the sestet). Three rhyme schemes are most commonly employed in English sonnets: the Shakespearean sonnet (abab cdcd efef gg), which is named for Shakespeare's use of it to the exclusion of other schemes; the Spenserian sonnet (abab bcbc cdcd ee), which was developed by Edmund SPENSER; and the Italian sonnet (abba abba cdecde; the sestet may have a different arrangement as long as it does not end with two rhyming lines, a couplet). The Italian sonnet, the oldest variety, is also called the Petrarchan sonnet, after its most famous exponent, Petrarch (1304–1374).

In the Petrarchan sonnet, the pattern of rhymes changes completely in the sestet. This arrangement encourages a two-part division of content; an important component of the Petrarchan sonnet is the *volta* (an Italian musical term), or 'turn of thought', the change of direction that often occurs in line 9. This change may be a feature of non-Petrarchan sonnets as well, as in Shakespeare's 'But thy eternal summer shall not fade' (Sonnet 18.9). However, the Spenserian and Shakespearean schemes—which are more appropriate to English, a language with fewer rhymes than Italian—offer another pattern of development: a progression through three quatrains to a concluding or summarising couplet. These two developments are not, of course, mutually exclusive. Sonnet 18, in fact, exemplifies both: its quatrains lead like stepping stones to a strong concluding couplet.

The sonnet, which developed in medieval Italy, first became known to English poets in the love poems of Dante (1265–1321) and Petrarch. Thomas WYATT introduced the form to England, but it was the Earl of SURREY (1) who popularised the English quatrains-and-couplet arrangement. Spenser's rhyme scheme compromises between the stricter Italian and the looser English. In Elizabethan England, sonnets were a fashionable pastime and sonneteers flourished (they are amiably satirised in *Love's Labour's Lost*). In Elizabethan poetry the sonnet was conventionally associated with love poetry; John Donne, in the early 17th century, expanded its range to encompass religious themes, and John MILTON continued this development, composing sonnets on various personal and public matters. In the 18th century, the form fell into disuse. Revived with the rise of romanticism, the sonnet has adapted well to the less formal modern world. Today it is often used with less rigorously prescribed rhyme and metre, for every imaginable subject.

Sonnets Body of 154 poems, each a SONNET, written by Shakespeare over an unknown period of time, probably around 1592 to 1598. The Sonnets are love poems. They describe aspects of two different loves experienced by the poet, one for a young man and the other for a woman. Some of the Sonnets are great poems (Sonnets 18, 29, 55, 116, and 138 are among the most praised), while a few are poor, but it is as a sonnet sequence—a new genre at the time—that they are particularly fascinating, offering an extraordinary range of love poems. They encompass several distinct points of view on love, unified by a series of delightful observations on the power of poetry to record them.

The Sonnets comprise two groups of poems: the larger group (Sonnets 1–126) is addressed to the young man, the other (127–154) to the woman. (Although the sex of the addressee is unspecified in most of the Sonnets, all those that do address a man precede Sonnet 126, which as the only 12-line variation on sonnet form seems to close the initial group. Similarly, all of the Sonnets that explicitly address a woman fall in the second group.)

In the first group, the poet manifests his love for the young man in a variety of ways. In Sonnets 1–17 he speaks of his friend's beauty and insists that he should marry and have children in order to perpetuate that beauty beyond his eventual death. In the next group of poems (and in many of the others) the poet describes his love in brilliant variations on traditional love poetry, often referring to the poetry love stimulates. However, as the sequence progresses, the poet speaks of his disappointment that his friend has left him, or at least does not love him in return. In 40–42 it appears that the friend has even stolen the poet's (female) lover. In 78–86 the poet fears that his place in his friend's affections (and perhaps in his literary patronage) has been taken by another, superior poet. In 110–111 the poet worries that his friend resents his public displays (probably a reference to Shakespeare's career as an actor). Gradually, however, over the course of the last several dozen poems of this group, the spirit of love returns, apparently reflecting a reconciliation between the friends. Sonnet 126 closes the series with a return to the subject of the young man's beauty and mortality.

Sonnets 127–154 address a woman of dark complexion and metaphorically dark morals (often referred to as Shakespeare's 'dark lady'), who has betrayed the poet's love by loving other men. She may be married, in which case the love she *has* given the poet also constituted betrayal. In 133–134 the poet complains that not only has she been unfaithful to him, she has done so with his friend, thereby leaving him abandoned by both of his loves. Apparently the situation in Sonnets 40–42 is seen here from another angle. The 'dark lady' Sonnets bemoan the poet's plight as an unrequited lover, and they often rail against the woman and against love in general. These poems are sometimes called the 'vituperative sonnets'.

In these two sets of poems, a love triangle is compellingly, if only implicitly, portrayed. There is no actual evidence that the situation was not simply a literary creation, but many of the poems are so convincingly delighted or aggrieved with love that most readers find themselves assuming that the Sonnets are autobiographical, or at least based on personal experience, and that the young man, the 'dark lady', and the 'rival poet' are representations of real people. Despite the lack of evidence, a wide range of suppositions about Shakespeare's life have been engendered by the Sonnets.

The most contentious conclusion that has been drawn from the Sonnets is that Shakespeare was homosexual. However, the poems offer no unambiguous evidence on the subject. The poet refers to and addresses his friend as his 'lover', but in Shakespeare's day the word had many non-sexual connotations, and its meaning varied greatly with context. It could mean sexual partner, but it could also be used in the formal close of a letter—'Thy lover' was as common and as sexually neutral as 'Sincerely yours' (it is so used in *Julius Caesar* 2.3.7). Moreover, in the context of friendship, the word *lover* was synonymous with the word *friend.* Shakespeare often used it as such in the plays (e.g., in *The Merchant of Venice* 3.4.7; *2 Henry IV* 4.3.13; *Coriolanus* 3.3.213). Sexual puns and innuendos of all sorts, indiscriminate in their references to male and female genitals, are common throughout the Sonnets—as they are throughout Elizabethan secular literature in general—but they serve chiefly to promote an

atmosphere of licentiousness rather than to suggest particular acts or attitudes. Sonnet 20 is frequently cited as evidence of Shakespeare's homosexuality, because in it the poet ascribes many feminine attributes to his friend, plays with clever references to his penis, and calls him 'the master mistress of my passion' (20.2). However, in this poem the poet actually disclaims a sexual relation with his friend—whose penis is 'to my purpose nothing' (20.12)—and willingly surrenders sex with him to women. While scholarly opinion remains varied, it is safe to say that the Sonnets do not clearly demonstrate homosexuality in its lovers, quite apart from the likelihood that Shakespeare, like other sonneteers of the day, wrote of an invented relationship.

In any case, the identity of the young man intrigues those who read the Sonnets as autobiographical. The assumption is generally drawn that he is identical with the mysterious 'Mr W. H'. described as the 'onlie begetter' of the Sonnets in the dedication to the first edition (see below). The two models most frequently suggested have been Henry Wriothesley (W. H. reversed), Earl of SOUTHAMPTON (2), and William Herbert, Earl of PEMBROKE (3). Each was a literary patron connected with Shakespeare: *Venus and Adonis* and *The Rape of Lucrece* are dedicated to Southampton and the FIRST FOLIO to Pembroke, who was also a son of the patron of PEMBROKE'S MEN, a theatrical company with which Shakespeare may have acted. Thus, they suit the implied references to patronage in several of the Sonnets. Also, each declined to marry a proposed bride—Southampton in 1590, Pembroke in 1595—making him suitable for the pleas of Sonnets 1–17. However, various commentators point to disqualifying attributes of each. In any case, the point cannot be proved, and so there have been many more nominees. Almost any near-contemporary of Shakespeare with the initials W. H. or H. W. has been proposed. A William Hughes—supposedly the object of a pun in Sonnet 20 but otherwise unrecorded—has been hypothesised (that he should be named William is suggested by the 'Will Sonnets' [135–136], where the word *will* appears 19 times, possibly echoing the names of the poet and his rival for the dark lady's love—the young man). Other possibilities emerge if the young man of the Sonnets is not considered identical with Mr W. H.; among the nominees have been the poet's son Hamnet SHAKESPEARE (5), the Earl of ESSEX (2), and Queen ELIZABETH (1) (heavily disguised).

Many proposals have been also made for the identity of the 'dark lady'. However, none has even the superficial credibility of Southampton and Pembroke, and scholars often simply ignore the question. The most frequently named dark ladies are Mary FITTON and Emilia LANIER. Others include Lucy Morgan (active 1579–1600), a one-time lady-in-waiting to Queen Elizabeth who became a brothel keeper; Penelope Rich (1563–1607), the sister of the Earl of Essex; and William DAVENANT's mother (chiefly because Davenant claimed to be Shakespeare's illegitimate son).

Speculation has similarly surrounded the 'rival poet' of Sonnets 78–86. Most poets of the period have been named, George CHAPMAN and Christopher MARLOWE (1) most often, with honourable mention to Barnabe BARNES and Gervase MARKHAM. However, none of these questions can be profitably pursued: not only is evidence entirely lacking, it is not even clear that Shakespeare had any real people in mind. All three figures function well as literary constructs—characters placed in a quasi-narrative, such as appear in many other sonnet sequences of the day.

The dates of the Sonnets are undetermined and are the subject of continuing scholarly debate. Though the only certainty is their existence before 1609, when they were published, a generally accepted view holds that they were probably all written between 1592 and 1598. These years saw a vogue for sonnet sequences—at least 20 were published—stimulated by Sir Philip SIDNEY's *Astrophel and Stella* (1591), and Shakespeare's poems were apparently part of this trend. In 1598 Francis MERES mentioned the Sonnets, and versions of two of them (138 and 144) were published in 1599 as part of THE PASSIONATE PILGRIM. Of course, it is not known that all of them had been written by then. Nevertheless, parallels to the Sonnets in Shakespeare's other works are most frequent in *Venus and Adonis* (1592–1593), *The Rape of Lucrece* (1593–1594), *Love's Labour's Lost* (c. 1593), *Romeo and Juliet* (1594–1595), and *Richard II* (1595), so the years of the sonnet craze seem the likeliest period of composition for the entire group of poems.

Commentators occasionally doubt the authorship of a few of the Sonnets, especially 145, which is a poor poem and the only Sonnet written in tetrameter (see METRE), as well as 153 and 154, which seemingly have little to do with the others and are the only ones that derive from a specific source (see below). However, each of these poems bears some relationship to its neighbours, and most scholars accept them as genuine.

The collected Sonnets were first published in 1609 by Thomas THORPE, in a QUARTO edition (printed by George ELD) known as Q. They were printed in the order described above, which has subsequently been considered standard (though various editors have altered it), and followed by *A Lover's Complaint.* An introductory page reads: 'TO THE ONLIE BEGETTER OF THESE INSVING SONNETS MR. W.H. ALL HAPPINESSE AND THAT ETERNITIE PROMISED BY OUR EVER-LIVING POET WISHETH THE WELL-WISHING ADVENTVRER IN SETTING FORTH.' This enigmatic message, signed 'T.T.', is unpunctuated (in that there is a period after every word),

ungrammatical, and generally difficult to interpret. The term 'onlie begetter' may signify the inspirer of the Sonnets (presumably the young man of 1–126, as discussed above), or it may simply refer to the procurer of the manuscripts from which they were printed; some commentators find other, more arcane possibilities. In any case, the dedication has been subjected to great scholarly scrutiny, but in the absence of further evidence, it must remain intractably obscure.

As noted above, only Sonnets 153 and 154 have a clear source: they are variations on a well-known classical epigram dating to at least the 1st century A.D. (this epigram was variously rendered in several languages and Shakespeare's immediate source is not known). OVID's *Metamorphoses,* a favourite Shakespearean source, is echoed in wordings and conceits here and there throughout the Sonnets, but the overall scheme of the group as a whole—the accounts of the poet's two loves—has no literary source. However, that Shakespeare wrote a sequence of sonnets can be attributed to the influence of Sidney's *Astrophel and Stella.* Also, an earlier convention required that sonnets be devoted to love, and Shakespeare followed this tradition, though he approaches the subject in an unconventional manner. The love relationships of the Sonnets are reconfigurations of the courtly love usually depicted in love sonnets: the object of the poet's love is addressed in the formal terms of the tradition and is beautiful and virtuous, as expected, but he is, unconventionally, a man; the expected woman is present, but she is neither beautiful nor virtuous. Each Sonnet is concerned with love, as is the collection as a whole, but the points of view taken and the aspects of love dealt with vary greatly, sometimes even within an individual poem. Shakespeare's characteristic recognition that life is complicated and that contradictory ideas and impulses often coexist is very well demonstrated in these works. The Sonnets, like the best of Shakespeare's dramas, offer an experience that transcends both scholarly disputes and the differences between the poet's world and our own.

Soothsayer (1) Minor but notable character in *Julius Caesar.* The Soothsayer bids Julius CAESAR (1), 'Beware the ides of March' (1.2.18, 23). Later, when the overconfident Caesar remarks that the ides of March have arrived without bringing harm, the Soothsayer replies ominously, 'Ay, Caesar, but not gone' (3.1.2). Seventy-five lines later Caesar is killed.

In Shakespeare's source, PLUTARCH's *Lives,* the Soothsayer is reported to have delivered his warning long before; the playwright compressed this account in order to achieve greater dramatic impact. The Soothsayer was probably not a real person; predictions such as his were commonly devised after the fact in ancient accounts of great events.

Soothsayer (2) Minor character in *Antony and Cleopatra,* a seer patronised by Mark ANTONY. In 1.2 the Soothsayer predicts that Cleopatra's waiting-woman CHARMIAN shall outlive her mistress but will see a worse time in the future than in the past. He adds that he sees an identical fate for another waiting-woman, IRAS. He accompanies Antony to ROME, and in 2.3 he recommends that they return to Egypt to get away from Octavius CAESAR (2). He declares that Antony's spirit is bested by Caesar's when the two are together. Antony dismisses the Soothsayer curtly, but muses to himself on the truth of his observation. In both episodes the Soothsayer's remarks prove pertinent, and in hindsight the audience can recollect his words.

In 2.3 the Soothsayer appears to be an Egyptian whom Antony has brought to Rome. Some scholars, however, believe that he may be the otherwise unknown Roman LAMPRIUS, for the stage direction opening 1.2 reads, in part: *'Enter* Enobarbus, Lamprius, *a Soothsayer,* . . . '. Thus, the Soothsayer can be construed syntactically as being named Lamprius.

Soothsayer (3) Minor character in *Cymbeline,* a priestly fortune-teller who serves the Roman army. In 4.2 the Soothsayer tells of his dream of 'Jove's bird, the Roman eagle' (4.2.348), which he interprets as an omen of victory for the forthcoming battle against King CYMBELINE's British forces. Though he is mistaken—the Britons win—this reference may be recalled by the audience when JUPITER (or Jove) appears to POSTHUMUS, in 5.4. In 5.5 the Soothsayer, who is now a prisoner of war, interprets the text that Jupiter left behind. He offers an interpretation that formulates the play's symbolic values of reunion and renewal. The Soothsayer's name, Philarmonus (5.5. 434), suggests the joyful conclusion that he foretells.

Sothern, Edward Hugh (1859–1933) British-born American actor. At 20 Sothern began his career by joining his father, a comedian who was performing in America. Himself a comedian and romantic leading man, he was best known as MALVOLIO and also played HAMLET. From 1904 to 1926 he and Julia MARLOWE (2) headed a Shakespearean company; they married in 1911.

Soundpost, James Character in *Romeo and Juliet.* See MUSICIANS (2).

Southampton (1) Seaport in southern England, a location in *Henry V.* In 2.2, just before invading FRANCE (1), King HENRY V entraps three treacherous noblemen—the Earl of CAMBRIDGE, Lord SCROOP (1), and Sir Thomas GREY (3)—who have conspired with the enemy and plan to assassinate him. Shakespeare himself did not indicate the setting, but the historical event took place in Southampton, and modern editors

have generally followed POPE (1) in placing the scene there.

Southampton (2), Henry Wriothesley, Earl of (1573–1624) Contemporary of Shakespeare, a patron of the arts to whom Shakespeare dedicated *Venus and Adonis* (1593) and *The Rape of Lucrece* (1594). These two dedications are the only certain connection between Shakespeare and Southampton; they were written in the hope of patronage—financial support—from the young nobleman. The first dedication is an ordinary approach by a poet seeking backing from someone he does not know well, but the second reflects considerable friendship between patron and poet. Unlike any other dedication of the period, it is confident of the support it seeks and it radiates an air of intimacy. The poet may have spent some time during the plague years of 1592 to 1594—the period during which he wrote the poems—at Southampton's estate. An 18th-century account attributed to William DAVENANT the information that Southampton had given Shakespeare £1000, and though the amount is much too large to be believed—perhaps 10 to 20 times Shakespeare's annual income at the time—there may be a germ of truth to the story. Some scholars believe that Southampton may be the young man to whom most of the SONNETS are addressed, or the mysterious 'Mr W. H'. to whom they are dedicated by the publisher. This cannot be proven, but that the two men were friends is accepted by most scholars.

A favourite courtier of Queen ELIZABETH (1), Southampton was a patron of John FLORIO and other writers. He became a follower of the Earl of ESSEX (2) and accompanied him on his successful expeditions to Cadiz and the Azores in 1595 and 1596. Essex's cousin was his mistress, and he married her in 1598, when she became pregnant. The queen was angered at the match and briefly imprisoned him; he never recovered the favour of the monarch. In 1599 he joined Essex on his ill-fated mission to Ireland and shared in his subsequent disgrace. He helped plan Essex's rebellion and with him was condemned to death on its failure, but his sentence was commuted to life imprisonment on the intervention of Robert CECIL (1). Southampton spent the rest of Elizabeth's reign in the TOWER OF LONDON. King JAMES I released him and made him a favoured courtier. He became a promoter of colonising enterprises and was an important member of the Virginia Company. In 1624, commanding English troops against the Spanish in the Netherlands, he died of plague. His family name is pronounced 'Risley'.

Southwark Southern suburb of LONDON, the location of a scene in *2 Henry VI,* and Shakespeare's residence between 1597 and sometime before 1602. In Shakespeare's day, Southwark was a raw, newly developed area, with crude roads and a nearby swamp. Beginning in 1587 several theatres—including the SWAN THEATRE, the ROSE THEATRE, and Shakespeare's GLOBE THEATRE—were built in Southwark because it was outside the jurisdiction of London, whose Puritan government was opposed to professional drama. Shakespeare probably moved there when his company, the CHAMBERLAIN'S MEN, left the THEATRE, to the north of London, and began to perform at the Swan. His exact residence in the district is unknown.

Southwark is also the setting for 4.8 of *2 Henry VI,* the depiction of an historical event that took place there in 1450. In 4.8 the rebellion led by Jack CADE has been driven from London across the Thames into Southwark, and the rebels are offered amnesty if they will disband, which most of them do, ending the uprising.

Southwell, John (d. 1441) Historical figure and minor character in *2 Henry VI,* a sorcerer whom HUME employs, along with BOLINGBROKE (2) and MARGERY JOURDAIN, to summon a spirit for the DUCHESS (1) of Gloucester, who wishes to see the future to prepare for a possible coup. In a séance in 1.4 Southwell helps Bolingbroke to cast a magic spell that summons the spirit ASNATH, who answers questions about the king and certain noblemen. Southwell is arrested, along with his fellows and their client, by the dukes of YORK (8) and BUCKINGHAM (3). In 2.3 the king sentences him to be strangled. The historical Southwell was a priest. He died in prison the night before his scheduled execution.

Spalding, William (1809–1859) Scottish scholar. Spalding was a professor of logic at the University of Edinburgh, but early in his career he published an essay that assigned authorship of different parts of *The Two Noble Kinsmen* to Shakespeare and John FLETCHER (2) by studying the verse techniques employed in the play. This ground-breaking study of 1833 contributed greatly to the use of the VERSE TEST in the study of Shakespeare plays.

Spaniard Character in *Cymbeline.* See DUTCHMAN AND SPANIARD.

Speed Character in *The Two Gentlemen of Verona.* Speed, the page of VALENTINE (2), is saucy and impertinent, teasing his master about his infatuation with SILVIA and engaging in witty exchanges with LAUNCE. He is an example of a character type frequently used by early Elizabethan dramatists, especially by John LYLY, whose comedies influenced the young Shakespeare.

Spencer, Gabriel (d. 1598) English actor, a colleague of Shakespeare. Spencer was one of three members of PEMBROKE'S MEN—another was Ben JON-

SON—imprisoned briefly for staging the allegedly seditious play *Isle of Dogs* in July 1597. Upon his release he joined the ADMIRAL'S MEN as a principal actor. In September 1598 Jonson killed Spencer in a rapier duel. Little more is known of Spencer's life except that he himself had killed a man in a fight two years earlier.

Spencer is probably referred to in the FIRST FOLIO text of *3 Henry VI,* where a stage direction at 1.2.47 refers to the MESSENGER (5) as 'Gabriel', apparently meaning Spencer, who must have played the part. The title-page of the 1595 edition of the play states that it had been performed by Pembroke's Men, so we may conclude that Spencer was with them before that date. However, it is possible that the stage direction was written for a later production by the CHAMBERLAIN'S MEN, in which case Spencer may have been a member of that troupe between 1594 and 1597.

Spenser, Edmund (c. 1552–1599) English poet, a major figure in English literature, the first great writer to succeed CHAUCER, and the author of works that influenced Shakespeare. Spenser's monumental epic poem *The Faerie Queene* (published 1590, 1598) provided the playwright with the inspiration for many passages, especially in the earlier plays and poems. The PASTORAL poems in Spenser's *Shepheardes Calendar* (1579), and possibly his great wedding poem *Epithalamion* (1595), did the same for *A Midsummer Night's Dream.* Another of Spenser's poems, 'The Teares of the Muses' (1591), may be alluded to in the *Dream* (5.1.52–53).

The son of a LONDON merchant, Spenser attended Cambridge University, where he met Gabriel HARVEY (2), through whom he was introduced to the literary circle centred on Sir Philip SIDNEY, whose close friend he became. His *Faerie Queene* has been recognised since its first appearance as one of the greatest accomplishments of English poetry. A vast tapestry of chivalry and adventure, it is simultaneously a nationalistic epic, a mythic romance, and an allegory on the human soul. Spenser was also an important influence on the development of the English SONNET.

Spirit Character in *2 Henry VI. See* Asnath.

The Spread of the Eagle TELEVISION production based on Shakespeare's ROMAN PLAYS. The British Broadcasting Corporation presented *The Spread of the Eagle* in 1963, combining *Coriolanus, Julius Caesar,* and *Antony and Cleopatra* in a nine-segment depiction of Roman history from the 5th century B.C. to the defeat of Mark ANTONY by Octavius CAESAR (2) in 31 B.C.

Spurgeon, Caroline (1869–1941) British scholar. A long-time professor of English literature at the University of London, Spurgeon is best known for her book *Shakespeare's Imagery and What it Tells Us* (1935). This groundbreaking study examines the patterns of images in certain plays and attempts to determine aspects of Shakespeare's personality by analysing the imagery he was most inclined to use. Spurgeon also edited *Keats' Shakespeare* (1928), a seven-volume edition of Shakespeare's works as annotated by the poet John KEATS.

Stafford (1), Lord Humphrey (1439–1469) Historical figure and minor character in *3 Henry VI,* a supporter of King EDWARD IV. Stafford, who does not speak, is present when the Yorkist leaders learn that WARWICK (3) has deserted their cause, and he is ordered, with Lord PEMBROKE (4), to raise an army. The historical Stafford, who was knighted by Edward during the battle of TOWTON, was sent with Pembroke in 1469 to subdue a local uprising that Warwick had incited. Because of a personal dispute between the two commanders, Stafford withheld his forces from a battle, with the result that Pembroke was captured and beheaded by the rebels. Stafford was declared a traitor and was hunted down and executed by the local authorities.

Stafford (2), Sir Humphrey (d. 1450) Historical figure and minor character in *2 Henry VI,* a nobleman sent, in 4.2, to deal with the rebellion led by Jack CADE. An arrogant aristocrat, Stafford takes the position *least* likely to defuse an uprising, addressing the mob as 'Rebellious hinds, the filth and scum of Kent . . .' (4.2.116). He and his BROTHER (1) are killed in the skirmish that follows in 4.3. Stafford was not related to the Duke of BUCKINGHAM (3), another figure in the play, although he bore the same name.

Stafford (3), Simon (active 1596–1626) LONDON printer who produced editions of several of Shakespeare's plays. Stafford, who mostly printed ballads and sermons, also printed the second QUARTO (Q2) of *1 Henry IV* (1599) for Andrew WISE, and Q3 of *Pericles* (1611) for an unknown publisher. He also printed the 1605 edition of KING LEIR, a possible source for *King Lear.*

Stafford (4), Sir William (d. 1450) Character in *2 Henry VI.* See BROTHER (1).

Stanley (1), Ferdinando, Lord Strange Contemporary of Shakespeare. See STRANGE.

Stanley (2), Sir John (actually Thomas) (c. 1406–1459) Historical figure and minor character in *2 Henry VI,* a nobleman to whose castle on the Isle of Man the DUCHESS (1) of Gloucester is banished in 2.3.-13. In 2.4 Sir John escorts the Duchess from London after she has been humiliated by being paraded through the streets. He is sympathetic to her for her

husband's sake, and promises to treat her 'Like to a duchess, and Duke Humphrey's lady' (2.4.98). The Isle of Man, in the middle of the Irish Sea, is remote and isolated even now; in the 15th century it was an ideal place of exile. Sir Thomas Stanley inherited the island from his father, Sir John, with whom Shakespeare confused him. John had received it in 1406 from HENRY IV, as a reward for supporting the deposition of RICHARD II.

Stanley (3), Sir Thomas (c. 1435–1504) Historical figure and character in *Richard III,* a nobleman who betrays RICHARD III. Richard, suspecting a defection to the Earl of RICHMOND, requires Stanley's son as a hostage. Stanley allies himself with Richmond; at the battle of BOSWORTH FIELD, he refuses to march with his forces, to Richmond's advantage, but Richard's order to kill the hostage son is not carried out. After Richmond kills Richard in combat, Stanley places Richard's crown on the victor's head.

Shakespeare's Stanley is a judicious, if not a very bold, politician. The career of the historical Stanley was rather less honourable, if similarly successful. He held a powerful position in the north of England, but he was difficult to trust. During the WARS OF THE ROSES, he fought, and on occasion refused to fight, for both sides, as he strove to ally himself with the winning faction at any point. He accordingly ended up with high office under King EDWARD IV, and then under Richard. His wife, Richmond's mother, was implicated in the revolt of BUCKINGHAM (2), but Stanley maintained his position by turning against her, receiving custody of her estates. However, it is clear that he knew of Richmond's invasion before it happened. As a result, Richard took George Stanley hostage. George, who was an adult, not the boy spoken of in the play, was captured while attempting to escape; he saved his life by incriminating his uncle, William STANLEY (4). Thomas Stanley did indeed withhold his troops at Bosworth, as Shakespeare reports, and Richard did order George killed but was ignored. Stanley was amply rewarded with high offices under Henry VII.

In some editions, Stanley is designated Derby, for Shakespeare used that title in introducing him in 1.3. However, he is Stanley in all dialogue thereafter. The use of the title in the play is an anachronism, for Stanley only received it after the accession of Henry VII. Most editors have made the correction in the dialogue headings and stage directions.

Stanley (4), Sir William (c. 1436–1495) Historical figure and minor character in *3 Henry VI,* a supporter of King EDWARD IV. In 4.5 Stanley helps Edward to escape from captivity. He is mentioned in *Richard III,* in 4.5.13, as one of the supporters of the Earl of RICHMOND.

The historical Stanley was the son of Sir Thomas Stanley, misnamed by Shakespeare as John STANLEY (2) in *2 Henry VI,* and he was the younger brother of Sir Thomas STANLEY (3), a prominent figure in *Richard III.* William Stanley had been a consistent Yorkist prior to Richmond's invasion, when he joined his brother in supporting the usurper. His nephew George, Richard's hostage, betrayed him, and Richard declared him a traitor prior to the battle of BOSWORTH FIELD. Nevertheless, following a family tradition of ambivalent loyalty, he held his troops back during that fight until he saw that he could join the winning side. Then his appearance with 3,000 troops turned the tide for Richmond, who amply rewarded him after acceding to the throne as Henry VII. Ten years later, however, Stanley became associated with another attempted coup and was beheaded.

Starveling, Robin Character in *A Midsummer Night's Dream,* a tailor of ATHENS and a performer in the comical amateur production of PYRAMUS AND THISBE staged at the wedding of Duke THESEUS (1) and Queen HIPPOLYTA (1). Starveling plays the Moonshine in the INTERLUDE, which is directed by his fellow artisan Peter QUINCE. The least competent of the actors, Starveling can utter only two of his lines before reverting to prose to inform the audience what the rest of his verses would have said.

Starveling's name refers to the proverbially skinny nature of tailors, and Shakespeare's choice of name and occupation probably reflects the presence in the acting company of John SINCKLO, a strikingly thin actor who is presumed to have played the part.

Stationers' Company English guild of booksellers, publishers, and printers, an organisation licenced by the government to protect the interests of its members by policing the publishing industry (with the exception of the university presses of Oxford and Cambridge). For such offences as printing outlawed works or publishing works properly claimed by another member, the company could fine a printer or publisher, seize his press and type, suspend his right to conduct business, or even, in extreme cases, revoke it altogether (see DANTER; SIMMES). A member of the company could secure the rights to a work once it was licenced by the government—by the MASTER OF REVELS, in the case of plays—by registering it for a fee with the company. Where the publisher got his text was immaterial to the company, for the point was not to prevent piracy but to create copyright for the members. Also, it was not necessary to register a work with the company to publish it; however, an unregistered work could be freely reprinted by anyone. The Stationers' Company made no effort to protect the rights of an author, and even so far as it went it was inefficient—many violaters of the system went unpun-

ished—but it marks the crude beginning of English copyright law.

Steevens, George (1736–1800) English scholar. Steevens published the texts of 20 QUARTO editions of the plays in 1766, and his edition of the collected plays came out in 1773. This edition was based on the text published by Samuel JOHNSON (7), with the addition of his own corrections and notes. It was reprinted with revisions in 1778 and 1785, with the assistance of Isaac REED. In response to Edmond MALONE's 1790 edition, Steevens undertook a final edition of his own in 1793. His 1778 edition was the basis for the first two VARIORUM EDITIONS. To his assiduous scholarship, Steevens added a sardonic wit—inventing scholarly sources to which he attributed indecent interpretations, for instance. For this, he is known as 'the Puck of Commentators'.

Stephano (1) Minor character in *The Merchant of Venice,* a servant of PORTIA (1). In 5.1 Stephano tells LORENZO and JESSICA that his mistress will be returning to BELMONT shortly.

Stephano (2) (Stefano) Character in *The Tempest,* the drunken butler of King ALONSO of Naples, and the ally of CALIBAN in his plot to kill PROSPERO. Stephano is a loutish fellow who is drunk throughout his time on stage, bullies Caliban and TRINCULO, and is ludicrously ineffective in carrying out the plot. In 3.2, when Stephano accepts Caliban's suggestion that after killing Prospero he take MIRANDA for himself, we see that a supposedly civilised man is capable of villainy as deep as that of a bestial savage (for Caliban had already attempted to rape the young woman). Stephano's bluff—and drunken—courage distinguishes him from his companions, but when he is comically distracted from the assassination by the trivial vanity of fancy clothes in 4.1, he seems inferior to even the subhuman Caliban, at least in discipline. He offers an interesting sidelight on one of the play's themes, the relative merits of civilised and natural humanity; in his drunken foolishness, Stephano demonstrates the potential for evil inherent in civilisation's pleasures.

Nevertheless, Stephano is basically a comic villain, contrasting with the more seriously evil ANTONIO (5) in the play's network of comparisons. When he is finally punished, Stephano is reduced to punning on his name, Neapolitan slang for 'belly', by saying 'I am not Stephano, but a cramp.' (5.1.286). This jest has seemed to some scholars to confirm speculation that Shakespeare found inspiration for *The Tempest* in Italian COMMEDIA DELL'ARTE scenarios, while others point to the appropriate definition of 'stefano' in John FLORIO's Italian-English dictionary, *A Worlde of Wordes* (1598).

Steward (1) Minor character in *All's Well That Ends Well,* the chief officer of the household of the COUNTESS (2) of ROSSILLION. The Steward twice offers information about HELENA (2). In 1.3 he reports having overheard her musing on her love for BERTRAM, stimulating the Countess to assist Helena's plan to pursue Bertram. In 3.4 he reads aloud Helena's letter to the Countess telling of her departure from Rossillion so that Bertram, now her unwilling husband, may live there in peace. This letter touchingly reveals the wretchedness of Helena's position.

The Steward's name—rendered by different editors as Rynaldo, Rinaldo, and Reynaldo—is mentioned only (in 3.4.19, 29) after his role is almost complete. Many commentators think that this offers a glimpse of Shakespeare's creative processes, for he appears to have been continually developing even this minor character as he wrote.

Steward (2) Character in *Timon of Athens,* the manager of TIMON's household. The Steward cannot make Timon refrain from the extravagant generosity that finally bankrupts him, but he nevertheless remains loyal to his master when he loses all. In 4.2 the Steward leads Timon's employees (see SERVANT [23]) as they regret their master's fate, and in 4.3 and 5.1 he visits his exiled master, who has withdrawn to the woods outside ATHENS. Timon is misanthropic in his mad despair, but he must make an exception for this faithful servant. He declares, 'I do proclaim / One honest man', and adds, 'How fain would I have hated all mankind' (4.3.500–501, 503). The Steward's virtue counters Timon's absolute hatred of humankind. The Steward is thus very important to the play, for it is through this character that Shakespeare most clearly demonstrates that Timon's bleak view of humanity is not the vision of the play. Like most of *Timon*'s characters, the Steward is not a complex human being, but is rather an emblematic figure who embodies the virtues of pity and loyalty.

Stoll, Elmer Edgar (1874–1959) American scholar. E. E. Stoll, as he is generally known, was a leading Shakespearean critic of the so-called 'realist' school, which focussed on the relationship of Shakespeare's plays to the playwright's times, especially to the practises of the ELIZABETHAN THEATRE. Stoll was a longtime professor at the University of Minnesota; his best-known work is *Art and Artifice in Shakespeare* (1933).

Stow, John (c. 1525–1605) English historian whose works provided Shakespeare with minor details for the HISTORY PLAYS, perhaps especially influencing *King John.* Stow, a self-educated tailor, became an 'antiquarian under the influence of his friend William CAMDEN. He published a collection of the works of

CHAUCER and a summary of early English chronicles, but his major work was his *Annales* (1580), a history of Britain from its mythological foundations to the year of publication. This popular work was reissued five times by 1631, with new additions by other authors. Stow also helped prepare the 1587 edition of Raphael HOLINSHED's *Chronicles*, Shakespeare's most important historical source. He also wrote a book on the LONDON of his day, *Survey of London* (1598), that offers scholars many telling glimpses of Shakespeare's world.

Strachey (1), Lytton (1880–1932) English biographer and critic. Strachey wrote an important work, *Shakespeare's Final Period* (1906), that helped revolutionise Shakespearean criticism in the early 20th century. He influenced subsequent commentators—such as E. E. STOLL and Levin SCHÜCKING—to consider the plays in light of the circumstances under which they were produced, rather than by focussing exclusively on the worlds of the characters. A major figure of the Bloomsbury group—along with novelist Virginia Woolf (1882–1941) and economist John Maynard Keynes (1883–1946)—Strachey is best known for his biographies, such as *Eminent Victorians* (1918), *Queen Victoria* (1921), and *Elizabeth and Essex* (1928).

Strachey (2), William (c. 1567–c. 1634) English colonial entrepreneur and author, writer of sources for *The Tempest* and possibly *King Lear*. In June 1609 Strachey sailed for Virginia as part of a group of investors and adventurers involved in the newly established colony in Jamestown. One of the three ships in the expedition was wrecked in Bermuda, and Strachey, with Sylvester JOURDAIN (2), was marooned for 10 months before going on to Virginia. From Jamestown he wrote to England of his experiences. His letter was circulated among interested investors, and Shakespeare saw it, probably through Dudley DIGGES (1). It provided the playwright with details of the shipwreck in *The Tempest* 1.1 and ARIEL's description of St Elmo's fire in 1.2. 196–206. Perhaps more important, it emphasised the providential survival of the voyagers and stressed the fact that an island previously notorious for evil spirits turned out to be a pleasant and productive place (partly in consequence Bermuda was soon settled by the English and is now the oldest British colony). Both the role of providence and the sequence of deviltry succeeded by blessedness are paralleled in Shakespeare's depiction of PROSPERO's realm. Strachey's letter was eventually published in *Purchas his Pilgrimes* (1625), a famous anthology of exploration literature (see HAKLUYT).

Strachey was acquainted with Ben JONSON and wrote a laudatory poem for the preface to Jonson's *Sejanus* (1605). This poem may have influenced some of the wording in *King Lear*. Strachey's connection with *Sejanus*, a work Shakespeare acted in, suggests that he may well have known the playwright personally.

Strachey returned to England in 1611 and helped write the first code of laws for Virginia. By 1613 he had completed a *Historie of Travell into Virginia Britania*, but this work, valued by modern historians, was not published until 1849.

Strange, Ferdinando Stanley, Lord (c. 1559–1594) English theatrical patron, the sponsor of a theatrical company, STRANGE'S MEN, with whom Shakespeare may have been associated. Lord Strange (the name rhymes with 'sang') was a courtier and minor poet. He patronised a provincial company of acrobats and tumblers that eventually evolved into an important theatrical company, though his involvement was not an influence on its development. As his 'servants', the performers were protected from antitheatrical legislation (see ELIZABETHAN THEATRE), and he could call on the company for private performances, but the personnel and repertoire of the company were determined by its members. Strange's Men visited their patron's Lancashire home often, and Lord Strange may thus have known the young Shakespeare personally, though doubtless distantly. Some scholars believe that the visits (or accounts of them from other players) later influenced Shakespeare to create his comic stewards MALVOLIO (of *Twelfth Night*) and OSWALD (of *King Lear*), who may have been modelled on Strange's steward, William FFARINGTON.

Strange succeeded his father as Earl of Derby (and the company therefore took the name DERBY'S MEN) in 1593. Now that he was a leading nobleman, a conspirator against Queen ELIZABETH (1) approached him to suggest that he seize the crown on the strength of his mother's descent from Henry VII. Derby, as Strange was now known, denounced the traitor, who was executed. When the earl died a few months later it was rumoured that he had been killed in revenge, though modern scholars believe he died naturally. He was succeeded as earl by his younger brother, William Stanley (see DERBY [3]).

At Tong, in Shropshire, is the tomb of some of Lord Strange's relatives; on it are two epitaphs said to have been written by Shakespeare. This tradition, however, was first recorded years after Shakespeare's death and seems highly doubtful. Only one of the two epitaphs is of a literary quality that can plausibly be associated with Shakespeare, and in any case, the occupants of the tomb died either long before or long after the playwright's connection with the family, which existed only through Strange's Men. The traditional attribution of these texts is probably a product of local pride.

Strange's family had long been prominent in the English aristocracy, and Shakespeare depicted several of his ancestors in the HISTORY PLAYS. Ferdinando Stanley, Lord Strange, was the great-great-grandson

of Sir Thomas STANLEY (3), who appears in *Richard III*, and thus Thomas and William STANLEY (2, 4) were also his relatives.

Stranger Either of two minor characters in *Timon of Athens*, visitors to ATHENS. In 3.2 the Strangers accompany HOSTILIUS, who is also a visitor, and they witness the callousness of LUCIUS (3), who refuses to assist his former patron, TIMON. The First Stranger's appalled remarks capture the play's condemnation of the heartless greed of Timon's faithless friends. 'I never tasted Timon in my life', he says, 'Yet I protest' (3.2.79, 81). Because he is detached, he assumes the position of a judge. He protests against 'the monstrousness of man' (3.2.74), and declares 'Men must learn now with pity to dispense, / For policy sits above conscience' (3.2. 88–89). The Second Stranger speaks only half a line, but its quiet condemnation—'Religion groans at it' (3.2.78)—powerfully reinforces his companion's critique. The episode resembles scenes found in medieval MORALITY PLAYS. It stresses the play's moral point of view and also helps the audience recognise that *Timon*'s characters are at least as much didactic models as they are psychological types.

The Strangers are sometimes considered to be three in number. In the FIRST FOLIO text of the play and some other editions HOSTILIUS is designated as the Second Stranger, in which case the religious remark in 3.2.78 is given to a Third Stranger.

Strange's Men Acting company of the ELIZABETHAN THEATRE, possible employer of the young Shakespeare and predecessor of the CHAMBERLAIN'S MEN (later the KING'S MEN), undeniably the playwright's long-time professional home. Named for its patron, Ferdinando Stanley, Lord STRANGE (the name rhymes with 'sang'), Strange's Men was apparently a troupe of acrobats and tumblers when it first appeared in LONDON in the early 1580s, but in 1588, when its leader joined the QUEEN'S MEN (1), the company was reorganised; henceforth, it emphasised acting over acrobatics.

By 1590 Strange's Men was allied with the other major London troupe, the ADMIRAL'S MEN, performing at the THEATRE, owned by James BURBAGE (2), whose son, Richard BURBAGE (3), was to become the company's leading tragedian. Strange's and the Admiral's Men were associated off and on for several years; the former often played at the CURTAIN THEATRE, whose owner, Henry LANEMAN, was James Burbage's partner at the time. A cast list of 1591 shows that among the members of Strange's—or at least acting with them—were Richard Burbage, George BRYAN, Richard COWLEY, Thomas GOODALE, John HOLLAND (3), Augustine PHILLIPS, Thomas POPE (2), John SINCKLO, and William SLY (2). Bryan, Phillips, Pope, and Cowley are also recorded as members in 1593, and these four plus Burbage were charter members of the Chamberlain's Men, when Strange's was reorganised under a new patron following Lord Strange's death in the spring of 1594. Less than a year earlier, Strange had become the Earl of Derby, so the company was also known briefly as DERBY'S MEN.

Scholars believe that Shakespeare was involved with Strange's Men, probably as both author and playwright. (He may, however, have been associated with other companies as well. See ADMIRAL'S MEN, LEICESTER'S MEN, PEMBROKE'S MEN, QUEEN'S MEN (1), and SUSSEX'S MEN.) The troupe produced *Titus Andronicus* and *Harey vj* (almost certainly *1 Henry VI*); the combined Strange's-Admiral's company probably staged both *2* and *3 Henry VI*. Further, though the earliest surviving documentary evidence linking Shakespeare with the company dates only from December 1594, after Strange's Men's demise, the playwright was already a leading figure in the Chamberlain's Men when first mentioned, receiving the company's fee for a performance at court, suggesting that he had already been involved with them for some time.

Stratford Town in WARWICKSHIRE, England, Shakespeare's home town and his residence upon retirement from LONDON. Stratford-on-Avon, to give it its full name, was a simple market town of 1,500 to 2,000 people in Shakespeare's day. It was the centre of a rich farming area and the locus of its trade. Its population consisted largely of farmers, the artisans and craftsmen who served them, and the businessmen who ran stores and inns, retailed manufactured goods, and marketed the farmer's crops. John SHAKESPEARE (9), the playwright's father, advanced economically through all of these groups. The son of a farmer, he became a tanner of fine leathers, a maker and seller of gloves, and a trader in various commodities such as grain and wool. Stratford's principal industry in Shakespeare's day (and until this century) was the brewing of beer and ale (among the commodities John Shakespeare traded was barley, the brewer's basic raw material). At the top of the social scale were wealthy landowners, the class to which Shakespeare advanced when he returned to Stratford a rich man after his career in the theatre.

Stratford was a very ancient rural centre. Taking its name from its location where an ancient road—a *straet* in Anglo-Saxon—crossed the Avon River at a *ford*, it was first settled by bronze-age Celts. It was recognised as an independent market town in medieval times. A religious organisation, the Guild of the Holy Cross, provided its government and a variety of civil services, including its schools. The guild was abolished in 1547, after the coming of Protestantism under King HENRY VIII, and a secular government with elected officials was established in its place. During the 1560s and 1570s Shakespeare's father was among those officials. The guild's headquarters, the Guild Hall, built in

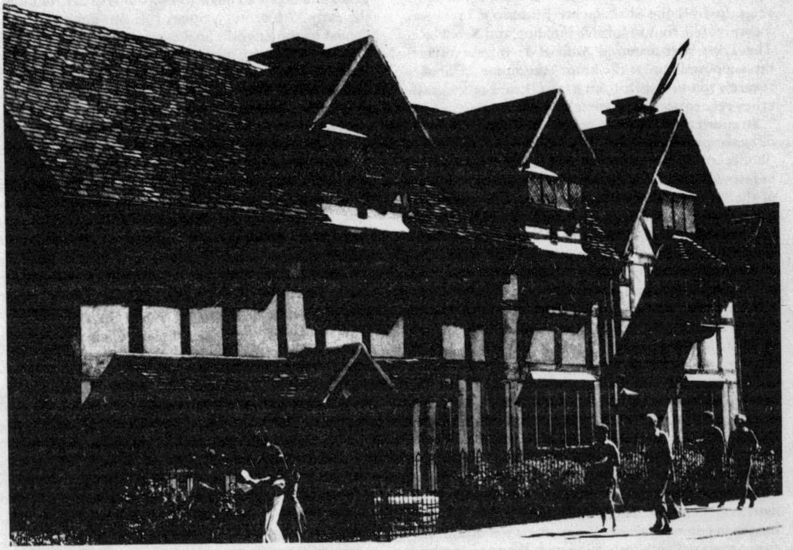

Shakespeare's birthplace, Stratford-on-Avon. (Courtesy of British Tourist Authority)

1417, still survives. A two-storey half-timbered structure, it was the central building of the town in Shakespeare's day, with the meeting rooms of the town government on the street floor and the Stratford grammar school above, in a single large classroom. Shakespeare must have attended the grammar school between approximately 1570 and 1580, though the records for these years have not survived.

The Shakespeares lived in a neighbourhood of prosperous tradesmen on the northern side of the town, in a house that was composed of two modest buildings joined to make a more substantial dwelling. Because the playwright was probably born in this house, it is known as the BIRTHPLACE and it has been renovated as a museum. Shakespeare's other home in Stratford, the mansion called NEW PLACE, no longer survives. It was the second-largest house in the town (the largest had once been a dormitory for the medieval guild).

At the south end of the town was Stratford's most important institution, the Church of the Holy Trinity. The most prominent building in Stratford, then and now, Holy Trinity is regarded as among the loveliest of England's small medieval churches. Its construction began around 1200 A.D., with different parts being added on over the centuries. Indeed, the prominent spire that tops its square tower was built long after Shakespeare's day. At the time of Shakespeare's birth, the rector of Holy Trinity was John BRETCHGIRDLE, who bequeathed to the grammar school much of its library. The first rector that Shakespeare could have known was Henry HEICROFT, who arrived when the future playwright was five and was still there to christen Susanna SHAKESPEARE (14) in 1583. The rector for most of the period after Shakespeare's return from London until after his death was John ROGERS (1). Another important man at Holy Trinity was its longtime curate, or assistant to the rector, William GILBARD, a possible model for NATHANIEL (1) in *Love's Labour's Lost.*

Soon after Shakespeare's death, Stratford's fame as the playwright's home became central to its existence. As early as 1630 a visitor described it as 'most remarkable for the birth of famous William Shakespeare'. In

the centuries since, it has become a mecca for greater and greater numbers of Shakespeare enthusiasts. In 1847 a non-profit organisation was formed to buy and maintain the birthplace, which was then a butcher's shop. In 1891 the Shakespeare Birthplace Trust was incorporated, to care for this building and New Place. The Trust later acquired Anne HATHAWAY's cottage, the supposed ARDEN (2) home, the home of Shakespeare's son-in-law Dr John HALL (2), and other properties related to the playwright.

Stratford also became a centre for the performance of Shakespeare's plays. In 1769 David GARRICK held a 'Jubilee' of performances there, and in 1827 a series of festivals was instituted, though the financial failure of the first one killed the idea. However, as an outgrowth of the elaborate 1864 celebration of Shakespeare's 300th birthday, the Shakespeare Memorial Theatre was created, opening its own building in 1879 with a performance of *Much Ado About Nothing* starring Barry SULLIVAN (2) and Helen FAUCIT. A permanent company evolved under the leadership of Frank BENSON (1) from 1886 to 1919, and Stratford today enjoys an annual theatre season running from April to November. Reorganised in 1961 as the Royal Shakespeare Company, the troupe performs in London in the winter and sends road companies on tour as well, producing Shakespeare's works and other plays, both classical and modern.

Strato (active 42 B.C.) Historical figure and minor character in *Julius Caesar,* a soldier in the army of BRUTUS (4). At the battle of PHILIPPI, Strato helps Brutus to commit suicide. When OCTAVIUS' troops arrive, Strato defiantly proclaims that they are too late to capture his master. The victorious Octavius, admiring his spirit and Brutus', takes Strato into hi service. Strato represents an ideal of Roman martial virtue, confirming the sense of grim rectitude that surrounds the defeat and death of the conspirators who killed CAESAR (1). Little is known of the historical Strato, whose role Shakespeare took from PLUTARCH's *Lives.*

Strewers Characters in *2 Henry IV.* See GROOM (2).

Stuart Dynasty Ruling dynasty in England from 1603 to 1714 (except from 1649 to 1660). King JAMES I (ruled 1603–1625), the first Stuart monarch to govern England, ruled during the last 13 years of Shakespeare's life. James, already King James VI of SCOTLAND, succeeded to the English throne when his cousin Queen ELIZABETH (1), the last monarch of the TUDOR DYNASTY, died childless. Although the Scottish dynasty, which dated to the 14th century (see SIWARD), spelled their name Stewart, James VI's mother, Mary Queen of Scots (1542–1587), married a cousin whose branch of the Stewart family resided in FRANCE (1) and had adopted the French spelling Stuart.

James' ascension provided a Protestant ruler for England and offered the prospect of unity for the two kingdoms he ruled (though the formal union of England and Scotland did not come until 1707). Thus, in the early 17th century, Stuart rule was generally welcomed by the English. Shakespeare reflected this attitude in *Henry VIII,* where a prediction is made that James shall rule with 'Peace, plenty, love, truth, terror' (5.4.47, where 'terror' simply means 'awe-inspiring power').

However, after Shakespeare's time, the Stuart dynasty had a difficult history, in good part because of religious disputes. Though James was strongly Protestant, the next three kings were more sympathetic to Catholicism and all three married Catholic princesses from European countries. English Protestants, a vast and often militant majority, distrusted them. James' son Charles I (ruled 1625–1649) proved unable to prevent the Civil Wars of 1642–1651, in the course of which he was executed and a revolutionary government established in Britain. When the new government eventually collapsed, however, Charles' exiled son was called back and ruled as Charles II from 1660 to 1685. His reign was marked by strong anti-Catholic sentiment in English politics, and while generally popular, he was suspected of pro-Catholic leanings. He was thought to have secretly converted on his deathbed, and his successor, his brother James II (ruled 1685–1689), was suspected of practising Catholicism even before he acceded. James' first wife was a Protestant and their children, Mary and Anne (later to rule), were raised as Protestants, but his second wife was an Italian Catholic. Popular opinion suspected Vatican-inspired plots to impose Catholicism on the country. For this and other reasons, James was deposed and exiled in the Glorious Revolution of 1689, so-called for its bloodlessness.

The thoroughly Protestant Mary Stuart and her Dutch husband, William of Orange, were installed as Mary II and William III, known jointly as William and Mary (ruled 1589–1702). They were succeeded by Mary's sister Anne, during whose reign England and Scotland were formally united as the Kingdom of Great Britain. Anne died childless in 1714, the last Stuart monarch in Britain. However, the Catholic branch of the Stuarts had not yet disappeared. On three occasions—in 1689–1691, 1715, and 1745–1746—rebellions were launched in favour of James, his son, and his grandson, respectively. All were suppressed. Finally, with the defeat of James II's grandson 'Bonnie Prince Charlie' at the battle of Culloden (1746), all hope of restoring the dynasty was abandoned, even by its most fanatical adherents.

Sub-plot Sequence of developments secondary in importance to the main line of action in a drama. The sub-plot is a common feature of ELIZABETHAN and

JACOBEAN DRAMA—indeed, of virtually all pre-modern English drama—and few of Shakespeare's plays lack one. Sometimes his sub-plots offer a pointed contrast with the central material, as in *Love's Labour's Lost*, where the buffoonery of COSTARD and the other rustic characters emphasises the elegance of BEROWNE and the other courtiers. On the other hand, a sub-plot can parallel a main plot, offering different angles on the same theme, as in the sub-plot involving GLOUCESTER (1) in *King Lear*.

Suffolk (1), Charles Brandon, Duke of (c. 1485–1545) Historical figure and character in *Henry VIII*, a nobleman at the court of King HENRY VIII. Suffolk is among the enemies of Cardinal WOLSEY. In 2.2 he joins the Duke of NORFOLK (3) and the Lord CHAMBERLAIN (2) in hoping for the cardinal's downfall, and in 3.2 he takes part in the formal recitation of Wolsey's crimes and punishments. Suffolk is also present but unimportant in Act 5.

The historical Suffolk was the son of Henry VII's devoted follower, Sir William BRANDON (2), who dies at BOSWORTH FIELD in *Richard III*. From childhood on, Suffolk was a close friend of Henry VIII, as their friendly card game in 5.2 suggests. He married Henry's younger sister Mary, widow of the King of France, in 1515; their grand-daughter was the unfortunate Lady Jane Grey, executed in 1554 after the failure of a conspiracy to place her on the throne.

Suffolk (2), Michael de la Pole, Earl of (1394–1415) Historical figure mentioned in *Henry V*. This Earl of Suffolk was one of the few English noblemen killed at the battle of AGINCOURT; his death is described grandly in 4.6.7–32. He is not to be confused with his younger brother, SUFFOLK (3), who succeeded to the title and appears in *1* and *2 Henry VI*.

Suffolk (3), William de la Pole, Earl, later Duke, of (1396–1450) Historical figure and character in *1* and *2 Henry VI*, an ambitious nobleman. Suffolk attempts to control King HENRY VI through his influence on Queen MARGARET (1), whose marriage to Henry he engineers in *1 Henry VI*. With CARDINAL (1) BEAUFORT, Suffolk leads the plot against Duke Humphrey of GLOUCESTER (4) and personally engineers his murder. The downfall and death of 'good Duke Humphrey', presented as a man whose judgement and honesty might have saved the country from the WARS OF THE ROSES, dominates the first half of *2 Henry VI*. Suffolk is thus largely responsible for a national catastrophe, and he is accordingly treated as an arch-villain, calculatingly treacherous and unscrupulous, who will stop at nothing.

In *1 Henry VI* Suffolk emerges as a figure of importance for the first time in 5.3. He has captured MARGARET (1) of Anjou in battle and has fallen in love with her on sight. Plotting to make her his paramour, although he is already married, he decides to marry her to King Henry. He offers her a bargain; he will make her Queen of England if she will be his lover. She defers to her father, REIGNIER, who demands the cession of two territories, Anjou and Maine, before he will give his consent. Suffolk agrees to arrange it. In 5.5 Suffolk overcomes the scruples of the Duke of GLOUCESTER (4) and convinces the king to break a previous marriage agreement and wed Margaret. Suffolk closes the play with a soliloquy in which he proposes to rule the kingdom through Margaret when she is queen. Thus Suffolk's ambition lays the groundwork for the disasters of the civil strife to come.

At the outset of *2 Henry VI*, Suffolk presents Margaret to Henry, who is delighted with his bride, although the terms of the marriage contract include the cession of Anjou and Maine, to the anger and disgust of the assembled nobility. Suffolk's capacity for intrigue is immediately made evident in 1.2, when the renegade priest HUME, having agreed to recruit sorcerers for the DUCHESS (1) of Gloucester, reveals that he is being paid by Suffolk to set the Duchess up for arrest and prosecution. (The Duchess' séance produces a prediction that Suffolk will die by water.) In 1.3 Suffolk takes advantage of the minor episode of the armourer HORNER to embarrass the Duke of YORK (8), a potential rival. When Margaret complains to Suffolk of the arrogance of various nobles, he replies that his plots will conquer all her enemies. One of them, the Duchess, is banished in the next scene. In 3.1, after Gloucester has been arrested for treason, Suffolk urges that he be murdered by any means necessary, lest he be acquitted of the charge.

Suffolk hires the Murderers, and we see him arrangeing to pay them in 3.2. However, he has gone too far; King Henry, stimulated by a furious reaction from the COMMONS and his own grief at Gloucester's death, banishes Suffolk from England for life. Suffolk proceeds to vent his anger with a bloodcurdling series of imprecations on his foes (3.2.308–327).

The farewells of Suffolk and Margaret at the end of 3.2 reveal their passionate love. Shakespeare often, as here, made a point to emphasise the complexities of human character by evoking some sympathy for a villain. We can, astonishingly, forget Suffolk's viciousness for a moment as he laments the prospect of dying without Margaret.

Suffolk comes to an appropriate end. We see him for the last time, on a beach in KENT (1), as the prisoner of pirates who have captured the ship carrying him into exile. The LIEUTENANT (1) of the pirates assigns each captive to a different crewman, who can collect a ransom for each life. However, the pirate who receives Suffolk has lost an eye in the battle for the ship; he wants vengeance and proposes to kill his prisoner. He identifies himself as Walter WHITMORE, and, as Walter

was pronounced 'water' by the Elizabethans, Suffolk sees that his death could fulfil the prophecy made to the Duchess of Gloucester in 1.4. The Lieutenant proves to be an English patriot who detests Suffolk for the damage his ambitions have done the English cause in France, and he recites Suffolk's political offences in virulent terms before turning him over to Whitmore for execution. Suffolk dies with an arrogant courage that can be admired.

The historical Suffolk was a grasping, ambitious, and extortionate aristocrat, but he probably did not earn the place he occupies in Shakespeare and in the chronicles that were the playwright's sources. He was an inept general and unsuccessful minister who bore some of the responsibility for the loss of France at the end of the HUNDRED YEARS WAR, and he did receive a dukedom, which he abused monstrously, for his role in arrangeing the marriage of Henry and Margaret. But his love affair with the queen is entirely fictitious, based on a passing remark in the chronicle of Edward HALL (2). The cession of Anjou and Maine occurred some time after the marriage, on the king's initiative; while Henry was doubtless influenced by Margaret, who was possibly supported by Suffolk, the duke did not arrange the matter himself. Suffolk was Gloucester's enemy, and he instituted his arrest at BURY ST. EDMUNDS, having called Parliament to that remote location, within his own territories, in order to do so. But Gloucester was probably not murdered, although rumour immediately and ever after laid his death to Suffolk. In any case, Suffolk was neither charged nor punished; in fact, his position grew stronger than ever after the deaths of Gloucester and Cardinal Beaufort. Not until three years later, when Normandy was finally and irrevocably lost, did Suffolk's enemies find their opportunity to undo him, and even then he was banished for only five years, not life. However, as in the play, his ship was captured by another one, whose crew took it upon themselves to execute the man they believed had slain 'good Duke Humphrey'. This murder proved to be the opening event in the revolt of Kentishmen led by Jack CADE.

Sugarsop Name mentioned in *The Taming of the Shrew.* Sugarsop is cited by GRUMIO as one of the servants of PETRUCHIO (2) in 4.1.80, but he never appears or is referred to again. This may reflect an abbreviated text, from which roles were cut because of a shortage of actors, but it is more probable that Grumio was being humorous; a sugarsop was a piece of bread soaked in a sweet or spiced sauce.

Sullivan (1), Arthur Seymour (1842–1900) English composer. Best known as the collaborator of W. S. Gilbert in their famous operettas, Sullivan first achieved renown with his incidental music for *The Tempest* (1862). For the tercentenary celebrations of Shakespeare's birth in 1864, he wrote the *Kenilworth Cantata,* which incorporates LORENZO's lovely speech on the beauties of the night (*Merchant of Venice* 5.1.53 ff). He also wrote accompaniments for several of Shakespeare's songs and composed incidental music for *Henry VIII* (1877) and *Macbeth* (1888).

Sullivan (2), Barry (1821–1891) Irish actor. Sullivan played in more than 300 Shakespearean productions. He was best known as HAMLET and RICHARD III. In 1879 he played BENEDICK opposite the BEATRICE of Helen FAUCIT in the premiere performance at the Shakespeare Memorial Theatre in STRATFORD.

Surrey (1), Henry Howard, Earl of (c. 1517–1547) English poet, important developer of the English SONNET and the introducer of BLANK VERSE into English poetry. Surrey studied the poets of the Italian RENAISSANCE, especially Petrarch (1301–1374), and shortly after his close friend Thomas WYATT introduced the sonnet into English, Surrey developed a variant more appropriate to the relatively rhyme-poor English language. This was the rhyme scheme that Shakespeare was to use in his SONNETS, the so-called English, or Shakespearean sonnet. In his partial translation of VIRGIL's *Aeneid* (published 1557), Surrey first used blank verse in English.

Surrey was a cousin of King HENRY VIII and a close friend of his illegitimate son. As a young man, he naturally became involved in the political intrigue of the court. In 1540 he helped his father—the SURREY (5) of *Henry VIII*—bring about the downfall of Thomas CROMWELL. Surrey fell victim to the increasing paranoia of King Henry, who was dying and feared that a promising young man of royal blood might want to hasten the process. Surrey was tried for treason on trumped-up charges and executed, only a few days before the king's death.

Surrey (2), Thomas Fitz-Alan, Earl of (1381–1415) Historical figure and minor character in *2 Henry IV,* a follower of King HENRY IV. In 3.1 Henry sends for Surrey and WARWICK (2) and tells them of his troubles. Surrey does not speak.

The historical Surrey was much more important than this slight role suggests. His father had been executed in 1397, along with Thomas of GLOUCESTER (6), by King RICHARD II in the conflict that was to trigger the events enacted in *Richard II.* Surrey, who fled to Flanders after his father's arrest, joined Henry IV, when, as BOLINGBROKE (1), he deposed Richard, and he remained a strong supporter of the king against the rebellions enacted in *1* and *2 Henry IV.* He was a friend of PRINCE (6) HAL who later, as King HENRY V, entrusted him with the command of major military expeditions.

Surrey (3), Thomas Holland, Duke of (1374–1400) Historical figure and minor character in *Richard II,* a supporter of King RICHARD II. In 4.1 Surrey disputes Lord FITZWATER's account of the Duke of AUMERLE's role in the murder of the Duke of GLOUCESTER (6). Fitzwater challenges him to a trial by combat, one of many similar conflicts that erupt in this scene. The episode serves to demonstrate the widespread disorder that the illicit assumption of power by BOLINGBROKE (1) has engendered.

Although he is not seen again in the play, Surrey subsequently joins the revolt against Bolingbroke, for his execution is announced by NORTHUMBERLAND (1) in 5.6.8, where he is called Kent. Thomas Holland had been named Duke of Surrey by Richard in 1397, but Bolingbroke revoked that status at the time of the rebellion, so Northumberland refers to him by his lesser title, the Earl of Kent. Kent and the Earl of SALISBURY (1) were captured in battle by Lord BERKELEY (2), who turned them over to a mob, who beheaded them.

Surrey (4), Thomas Howard, Earl of (1443–1524) Historical figure and minor character in *Richard III,* a general under RICHARD III at the battle of BOSWORTH FIELD. Surrey, second in command to his father, the Duke of NORFOLK (1), appears briefly in 5.3. He seems despondent just before the fighting, but, when questioned by Richard, assures the King that his heart is lighter than his looks.

The historical Surrey was restored to his father's titles by King Henry VII, the RICHMOND of the play, following a period of disgrace. He appears in *Henry VIII* as the Duke of NORFOLK (3). He was the father of another Earl of SURREY (5), who also appears in that play, and he was the grandfather of the poet Henry Howard, Earl of SURREY (1).

Surrey (5), Thomas Howard, Earl of (1473–1554) Historical figure and character in *Henry VIII,* a nobleman at the court of King HENRY VIII. In 3.2 Surrey joins his father, the Duke of NORFOLK (3), in bringing down Cardinal WOLSEY; he thus avenges the death of his father-in-law, the Duke of BUCKINGHAM (1), who was earlier framed and sent to execution by Wolsey. In 2.1 the First GENTLEMAN (14) asserts that Wolsey has had Surrey assigned to a post in Ireland 'lest he should help his father[-in-law]' (2.1.44); this circumstance makes him a doubly appropriate addition to the play's roster of Wolsey's enemies. Surrey is present but inconspicuous in 5.2.

The historical Surrey was indeed sent to Ireland by Wolsey, almost certainly because the cardinal wanted an enemy out of England, but this occurred some time before Buckingham's treason trial and may not have been directly related to it. Shakespeare took Wolsey's motive from HOLINSHED's *Chronicles* and certainly believed it was true. However, the playwright gave Surrey a wrong name and rank, for by the time he appears in the play his father had died and he had become the Duke of Norfolk. However, since Norfolk remains alive in the play, Surrey must remain an earl. Surrey was an uncle of Anne Boleyn (see ANNE [1]), whose mother was his sister. He was the father of the famed poet Henry Howard, Earl of SURREY (1).

Surrey (6) Horse belonging to King RICHARD III in *Richard III,* his mount at the battle of BOSWORTH FIELD. In 5.3.65, Richard calls for 'white Surrey', who is reported killed in battle in 5.4, before Richard's famous cry, 'My kingdom for a horse' (5.4.13). Surrey's presence is based on several references in the chronicles to a great white charger ridden by Richard, but the name appears to be an invention of Shakespeare's.

Surveyor Minor character in *Henry VIII,* a treacherous steward to the Duke of BUCKINGHAM (1). The Surveyor, bribed by Cardinal WOLSEY, gives false testimony that convicts Buckingham of treason and leads to his execution. After performing his task in 1.2, the Surveyor disappears from the play. The episode emphasises the atmosphere of duplicity that surrounds Wolsey in the first half of the play. Historically, the Surveyor was one William Knyvet or Knevet, otherwise unknown, who had been fired by Buckingham in response to his tenants' complaints that he mistreated them.

Sussex's Men Acting company of the ELIZABETHAN THEATRE, possibly employers of Shakespeare early in his career. An acting company employed by Robert Radcliffe, Earl of Sussex (1573–1629), they performed at the court of Queen ELIZABETH (1) in 1592. In the winter of 1593–1594, Sussex's Men performed for Philip HENSLOWE, probably at the ROSE THEATRE, for a short interval when plays were permitted during the plague year. *Titus Andronicus* was in their repertoire at that time; some scholars think the young Shakespeare may have been a member of the company and may have written it expressly for them. In the spring of 1594, Sussex's Men performed jointly with the QUEEN'S MEN (1), and the two may have coalesced at this time, for Sussex's Men disappear from the record until 1602, when they reappear as a provincial touring company.

An earlier Sussex's Men had been employed by Robert's father, Thomas Radcliffe (c. 1530–1583), and they had appeared regularly at court, as well as on tour in the provinces, between 1572 and 1583. Because Thomas was Elizabeth's chamberlain after 1572, the company was sometimes called the Chamberlain's Men, but they are not to be confused with the later CHAMBERLAIN'S MEN, Shakespeare's company for many years.

Swan Theatre Playhouse in LONDON built by Francis LANGLEY around 1595 and depicted in the only surviving drawing of a 16th-century English theatre interior. Johannes de Witt, a Dutch traveller who visited London around 1596, made a drawing of the Swan, of which a copy has survived. Its accuracy has been questioned, but its major features are probably correct. They include a circular building with three stories of seats, each containing three rows, overlooking an unroofed central area into which a stage thrusts. The stage is half-covered by a canopy extending from its rear wall and supported by massive columns on stage; there are two doors in the back wall of the stage, with a set of box seats above these doors, behind the stage. At the top of this rear structure is a roofed hut, from which a flag flies and a man blows a trumpet, both signs that a play is scheduled. On the stage are three performers.

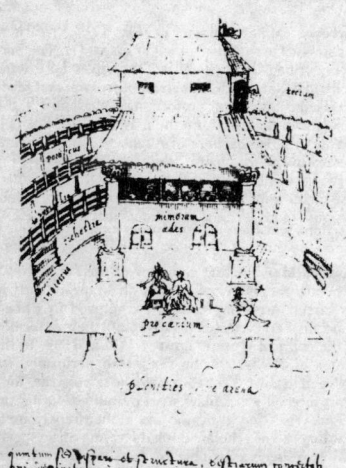

This drawing of the Swan Theatre is the only known contemporary image of the interior of an Elizabethan theatre.

If de Witt was in fact in London in 1596—the record is obscure—then the performers may be members of Shakespeare's company, the CHAMBERLAIN'S MEN, who probably played at the Swan for a season that year. In 1597 the PEMBROKE'S MEN came to London and engaged the theatre for a year, but their production of an allegedly seditious play, *Isle of Dogs* by Thomas NASHE, resulted in the government's closure of all the London theatres for four months. When the theatres reopened, Langley was unable to recruit another company, and the Swan was not used regularly for theatre thereafter. After Langley's death in 1601, the theatre was sold to another London investor, who had no greater success. Only one play besides *Isle of Dogs* is known to have been staged there. Miscellaneous entertainments—a fencing match, a poetry improvisation contest—are also recorded, but in 1632, a writer declared the Swan was 'now fallen to decay'.

Swinburne, Algernon Charles (1837–1909) English poet. Best known as a major late-Victorian poet, Swinburne also wrote literary criticism and enthusiastically encouraged a renewed interest in ELIZABETHAN DRAMA. Swinburne's Shakespearean commentary is regarded as more of a curiosity than a resource, however, for his adulation was extreme. For instance, he called *Cymbeline*'s IMOGEN 'the woman best beloved in all the world of song and all the tide of time'. Such sentimentality spurred a response led by George Bernard SHAW (2), who coined the word 'bardolatry' to mock it.

Swinstead (Swineshead) Abbey Religious establishment in Lincolnshire, setting for 5.6–7 of *King John*, the site of the death of King JOHN (3). Sick and dispirited, John withdraws from the fighting against the French and is poisoned by a monk. He dies the next day, and the BASTARD (1) leads the other noblemen in swearing allegiance to his successor, HENRY (1).

Swinstead Abbey, which Shakespeare misnamed following John FOXE, was not the historical site of John's death, nor was the King poisoned, although Shakespeare took the tale from HOLINSHED and Foxe. John, stricken with dysentery while battling the French-supported rebels, spent a few days at Swineshead Abbey in October 1216, but he died several days later in nearby Newark.

T

Taborer Minor character in *The Two Noble Kinsmen*, a drummer. The Taborer accompanies the COUNTRYMEN and the lasses led by NELL (2) in their dance performed before Duke THESEUS (2) in 3.5. The Taborer speaks only one line, a boisterous greeting in 3.5.24. Since most scholars agree that Shakespeare did not write 3.5, the Taborer is probably the creation of John FLETCHER (2).

Tailor, the Minor character in *The Taming of the Shrew*, an artisan whom PETRUCHIO (2) abuses. Commissioned by Petruchio to provide a gown for KATHERINA, the Tailor is driven away by his client. Petruchio's mistreatment of this innocent man is simply part of his demonstration to his bride of the ugliness of shrewish behaviour. Although the Tailor defends himself before being routed, he otherwise has no distinctive personality.

Talbot, Lord John (before 1388–1453) Historical figure and character in *1 Henry VI*, the principal English military hero in the HUNDRED YEARS WAR. In 1.1 Talbot's reported capture seems to magnify English woes. The MESSENGER (3) who brings this news describes how Talbot's actions in battle had raised English morale. Talbot's account of his captivity, related in 1.4, after he has been ransomed, further demonstrates his capacity to daunt the French enemy. The king acknowledges Talbot's virtues when he repeats his father, HENRY V's, remark, 'A stouter champion never handled sword' (3.4.19).

Talbot's fate is closely linked with that of JOAN LA PUCELLE in an alternating sequence of victories and defeats that closes with Joan's ignoble capture and death in Act 5, presented in contrast to Talbot's own glorious fall in the immediately preceding battle. The war reaches its theatrical climax in these scenes (4.2–7), in which the brave Talbot fights and dies, along with his young son, JOHN (6). He is doomed by the dispute between the dukes of YORK (8) and SOMERSET (3), which prevents reinforcements from reaching him. Sir William LUCY (2), who comes to collect his corpse, delivers a formal, elegiac recital of Talbot's feudal titles, reminding us how little removed Shakespeare was from the Middle Ages.

Throughout the play, Talbot carries the burden of destiny for the English in their struggle with the French. He is also contrasted with the selfish noblemen whose ambitions cause dissensions within the English leadership that lead to the losses to FRANCE (1). While the noblemen engage in squabbles and arguments, Talbot is consistently virtuous. Heightening the contrast, Shakespeare rearranged history so that the jealous rivalry of York and Somerset becomes a direct cause of Talbot's death.

In his *Pierce Penniless*, a book of social commentary published in 1592, Thomas NASHE remarked on the contemporary theatre's capacity to thrill its public with works depicting patriotic stories 'long buried in rusty brass and worm-eaten books'. He chose a single example as sufficient to prove his point: 'How would it have joyed brave Talbot, the terror of the French, to think that after he had lien two hundred years in his tomb he should triumph again on the stage, and have his bones new-embalmed with the tears of ten thousand spectators at least, at several times, who in the tragedian that represents his person imagine they behold him fresh bleeding.' This passage, the earliest known literary reference to *1 Henry VI*, suggests to us how successful the young Shakespeare had been when he created Talbot, a clean-cut hero for his times similar to those played by John Wayne in ours.

The Taming of a Shrew Anonymous play first published in 1594, probably a BAD QUARTO of *The Taming of the Shrew* but once thought to have been the principal source of that play. *A Shrew*, as the play is conveniently known, differs most strikingly from *The Shrew* in having a simpler SUB-PLOT. *The Shrew* features a contest among three suitors for the hand of the younger of two sisters; *A Shrew* adds a third sister and matches each sister with a suitor, eliminating the rivalry. This sub-plot is equally filled with romantic intrigue, as the suitors of the younger sisters conspire to outwit the father of the girls, but it lacks the comical confusions of Shakespeare's work. The main plot is the same, and the dialogue corresponds closely throughout much of the play.

A Shrew is, however, a generally inferior drama, and this, combined with the difference in sub-plots, used

to be taken to indicate that Shakespeare had used *A Shrew* as his chief source for *The Shrew,* unless both were derived from an earlier, subsequently lost play, designated the UR-SHREW. However, close examination of the two texts offers convincing evidence that *A Shrew* was compiled from the recollections of actors who had performed in *The Shrew*—that is, that the former is a Bad Quarto of the latter. This theory renders the Ur-Shrew hypothesis unnecessary.

Although similarities in wording occur throughout the two plays, including their sub-plots, *A Shrew*'s versions of particular passages are consistently garbled or misinterpreted renderings of the corresponding lines in *The Shrew.* Even the introductory moments of the sub-plot of *A Shrew* bear signs of its derivative nature; it appears that its complexities were not well remembered, so the compilers fell back on a more conventional love plot. Further, *A Shrew* contains echoes of other plays, especially *Tamburlaine* and *Doctor Faustus,* by Christopher MARLOWE (1). This is characteristic of reconstructed texts, reflecting faulty memories on the part of the actors. And some scenes in a Bad Quarto are invariably closer to the original text than others, indicating that the principal compilers played the characters whose roles are most accurately recollected and appeared on stage during the best-rendered scenes. It thus seems likely that much of the text of *A Shrew* was the work of the actors who had played Christopher SLY (1) and GRUMIO in *The Shrew,* probably William SLY (2) and Alexander COOKE (1), respectively. The title-page of *A Shrew* asserts that it had been performed by PEMBROKE'S MEN. This acting company toured the provinces for most of the period 1592–1594 and probably produced the text for that tour.

One of the most striking differences between the two texts is the presence in *A Shrew* of four INTERLUDES and an EPILOGUE dealing with Christopher SLY (1), whereas *The Shrew* abandons the tale after one interlude. It is presumed that the editors of the FIRST FOLIO (1623), in which *The Shrew* was first published, used a manuscript that reflected a production that cut these episodes due to a shortage of actors. Thus *A Shrew* apparently presents a version of Shakespeare's original interludes and epilogue, and this material is sometimes included in editions of *The Shrew.*

Marlowe's *Doctor Faustus* was probably written in the spring of 1592, and a compiler of *A Shrew* had acted in it, or at least seen it, so that the the text of *A Shrew* must have been assembled between the summer of 1592 and the spring of 1594, when it was registered for publication. It was published by Cuthbert BURBY, who also published QUARTO editions of several of Shakespeare's other plays. It was reissued in 1597, and Nicholas LING published a third edition in 1607.

The Taming of the Shrew

SYNOPSIS

Induction, Scene 1

Christopher SLY (1) drunkenly falls asleep on the ground. As a practical joke, the local LORD (1) decides to take the unconscious man into his home and have him awaken in the lap of luxury. He orders his servants to inform Sly that he is a gentleman who has been insane for many years, believing himself a poor drunkard. A travelling company of PLAYERS (1) arrives, and the Lord directs them to perform for Sly. He further arranges for his PAGE (4) to pose as Sly's wife.

Induction, Scene 2

Sly awakens in a bedroom of the Lord's house, and the servants offer him delicacies. His 'illness' is explained to him by the Lord, but Sly denies it and briefly describes his true place in the world. The Lord and his servants offer the gentlemanly pleasures they insist are properly his, including a beautiful wife, and Sly accepts their version of his life. The Page appears, dressed as a woman. Sly's lusty instincts are laid to rest by the assertion that sex will produce further delusions of poverty. The Players' performance is announced, and Sly prepares to enjoy it.

Act 1, Scene 1

LUCENTIO, accompanied by his servant TRANIO, has just arrived in PADUA. They observe BAPTISTA telling HORTENSIO and GREMIO that their courtship of his daughter BIANCA (1) is inappropriate, for he will not permit her to be wed until her older sister, KATHERINA, is married. The suitors state that this is an unlikely prospect, as Katherina is a notorious shrew, unacceptable to any man. Katherina's aggressive response seems to justify their remarks, while Bianca demurely accepts her father's order. Baptista asks the suitors to help him find tutors in music and poetry to keep Bianca happy, and he and his daughters depart. Hortensio and Gremio agree to try to find a husband for Katherina so that they can resume their rivalry for Bianca, and they, too, leave. Lucentio tells Tranio of his immediate and intense love for Bianca. The two devise a plan to permit him to court the girl: Lucentio shall disguise himself as a scholar and become Bianca's tutor, and Tranio shall pretend to be Lucentio. Lucentio's other servant, BIONDELLO, arrives and is told of the plan. In addition, Lucentio decides that the disguised Tranio shall declare himself a suitor to Bianca and convince Baptista to accept him. Christopher Sly, who has been dozing, is awakened by the Page and another servant, and he readies himself to watch more of the play.

Act 1, Scene 2

PETRUCHIO (2) arrives in Padua and calls on his old friend Hortensio. He announces that he has come in search of a wife, and Hortensio suggests Katherina,

while warning that she is intolerable. Petruchio is undaunted, for he says he knows how to deal with shrews; he insists on meeting Baptista immediately. Hortensio decides to masquerade as a music teacher, to be recommended by Petruchio as Bianca's tutor. On their way to Baptista's, they encounter Gremio and Lucentio, who is dressed as a scholar. Gremio declares that he will ingratiate himself with Baptista by presenting Lucentio as a language teacher for Bianca. Tranio, disguised as Lucentio, appears and reveals, in his master's name, his intention to court Bianca.

Act 2, Scene 1
Katherina torments Bianca until Baptista stops her, and the sisters go their separate ways. Gremio, Petruchio, and Hortensio arrive. Petruchio introduces himself as a suitor for Katherina's hand and proposes Hortensio as a music teacher to entertain his prospective bride; similarly, Gremio presents Lucentio as a language teacher, intended for Bianca. Tranio arrives, calling himself Lucentio, and declares himself a suitor of Bianca; he bears a gift of a lute and several books. Baptista distributes these to the appropriate tutors and sends the teachers to their pupils. Petruchio, saying that he is in a hurry, arranges a marriage agreement with Baptista, contingent on Katherina's acceptance. Hortensio reports that Katherina has broken the lute on his head in a fit of anger. Petruchio praises Katherina's spirit and wants to meet her. The others leave, and Petruchio reveals his plan in a soliloquy: he will assert Katherina's sweetness, no matter how shrewish her behaviour, and treat their wedding as agreed upon, whatever her protests. She appears, and he immediately takes a familiar tone, addressing her as Kate and complimenting her effusively. They engage in a bantering battle of wits, but he ignores her insults; even when she hits him he responds with moderation. She calls him a fool, but he insists that she shall marry him and he shall tame her. Baptista, Gremio, and Tranio return, and, despite Katherina's protests, Petruchio insists that she has agreed to their marriage and has been very affectionate to him. She calms down as Petruchio confirms with her father his plan to marry her on the next Sunday, and Petruchio takes her with him to get a ring. Baptista asserts that the wealthiest of Bianca's suitors shall marry his younger daughter, and they attempt to outbid each other. Tranio, speaking as Lucentio, offers far more than Gremio, citing the vast fortune of his father, VINCENTIO (1). Baptista agrees that he shall have Bianca once his parent comes to Padua and substantiates his claim. The older men leave, and Tranio plans to recruit a stand-in for Lucentio's father.

Act 3, Scene 1
Lucentio and Hortensio refuse to leave each other alone with Bianca. Lucentio pretends to construe a passage in Latin and reveals his identity and purpose to Bianca. She is demurely wary, but she doesn't dismiss him, telling him not to despair. Hortensio gives her a love note couched as a lesson in the musical scale, but she rejects him altogether.

Act 3, Scene 2
Petruchio, dressed in ridiculous clothes, arrives very late for his wedding to Katherina and goes in search of her. The wedding guests follow, and Tranio has a chance to tell Lucentio of his plan to find a substitute Vincentio. Gremio tells of Petruchio's obnoxious behaviour at the wedding. The rest of the wedding party appears, and Petruchio announces that he is leaving immediately with Kate, rather than staying for the banquet. Furious, Katherina resists, but he carries her off.

Act 4, Scene 1
Petruchio's servant GRUMIO arrives at his master's house in bitter cold, having been sent ahead to arrange for the newlyweds' reception. He tells CURTIS, another servant, of the unchivalrous behaviour of Petruchio, who has allowed Katherina to lie in the mud after falling from her horse and has beaten Grumio needlessly, to his bride's horror. The couple appear. Petruchio orders dinner for Katherina, but he rails at the servants for not presenting it properly, throwing the food at them; his wife gets none. He ignores her pleas for patience and takes her off to bed. A servant reports that Petruchio continues to rant and rave, disconcerting Katherina completely. Petruchio returns, and the servants flee; in a soliloquy he describes his plan: he will continue to insist ferociously that nothing is good enough for his wife so that she will get no food, no drink, and no rest. He likens his strategy to the taming of a wild falcon.

Act 4, Scene 2
In Padua, Hortensio brings Tranio, whom he thinks is Lucentio, to overhear Bianca's loving conversation with the real Lucentio. Tranio pretends to be affronted and joins Hortensio in criticising Bianca as frivolous and unworthy. Hortensio vows to marry a WIDOW (1) who has pursued him, and he leaves. Tranio encounters the PEDANT, a newcomer to Padua, and, after learning that he is from MANTUA, tells him that an outbreak of hostilities has resulted in a new law condemning to death any Mantuan found in Padua. He offers to protect the stranger if he will agree to pose as Vincentio. The Pedant gratefully accepts.

Act 4, Scene 3
Petruchio brings food for Katherina, but she won't speak to him. He refuses to give it to her until she thanks him. She thanks him, but, before she can eat much, he brings in a TAILOR and a HABERDASHER to provide her with fine clothes. Petruchio rejects these garments, although Katherina likes them. He asserts

that she shall have a gentlewoman's clothes only when she is gentle, and, raging, he drives the Tailor and Haberdasher away. Planning their journey to a feast at her father's house, he asserts that it is seven o'clock; when Katherina responds that it is only two, he insists that she must stop contradicting him.

Act 4, Scene 4
Tranio and the Pedant, as Lucentio and his father, call on Baptista. The Pedant asserts his willingness to provide a dowry, and Baptista agrees to the betrothal of Bianca and Lucentio; they leave to sign a marriage contract at Lucentio's house. The real Lucentio, who is present in his role as the tutor, is sent to fetch Bianca. Biondello informs him of Tranio's plan: a priest is ready at a certain church, and Lucentio may now elope with his beloved.

Act 4, Scene 5
On the road to Padua, Petruchio remarks that the moonlight is very bright. When Katherina observes that it is daylight, he threatens to cancel the trip if she does not stop disagreeing with him. She gives in to him, calling the sun the moon, and he says it is the sun. She concurs and states that she will agree to whatever he says. Petruchio asserts that things are now as they should be. When an elderly man approaches, Petruchio calls him a lovely maid, and Katherina, true to her promise, addresses the old gentleman as though he were a girl. Petruchio then changes his mind, and Katherina begs the man's pardon for her mistake. As they travel together, the older man identifies himself as Vincentio.

Act 5, Scene 1
Bianca and Lucentio enter a church to be married. Petruchio, Katherina, and Vincentio arrive at Lucentio's house, where the Pedant poses as Vincentio. Petruchio and Katherina withdraw to witness this development. The clamour brings Baptista and Tranio. Tranio continues to brazen it out, and Vincentio is about to be arrested as an imposter, when Lucentio and Bianca arrive, married. Lucentio identifies himself and explains what has happened. Baptista's anger is cooled by Vincentio's assurance that he will approve Lucentio's marriage. The discussion becomes more cordial and moves indoors. Petruchio wishes to kiss Katherina before following the others inside but she is embarrassed to kiss in the street. He speaks of returning home, and she kisses him. Affectionately, they go to join the others.

Act 5, Scene 2
A banquet celebrates the marriages of Lucentio to Bianca, Hortensio to the Widow, and, belatedly, Petruchio to Katherina. The Widow shrewishly argues with Katherina. The ladies withdraw, and the men gamble on whose wife is the most obedient. Bianca is sent for, but she sends word that she is busy and cannot come. Similarly, the Widow sends the message that, suspecting some joke, she will not come. Petruchio sends Grumio to 'command' that Katherina come, and she does. Petruchio sends her back to fetch the other women. When the women return, the Widow says she is glad not to be so compliant as Katherina, and Bianca calls Lucentio a fool for having bet on her obedience. At Petruchio's order, Katherina lectures the other women on the virtues of submissiveness. She says that the natural order of things places men in authority and that a woman's virtue and beauty are marred by revolt against nature. A husband takes risks in the world to maintain a home, whereas a woman lives in relative comfort, owing no more for her situation than obedience. She compares a woman's proper devotion to a husband with the allegiance that a subject owes a prince, and she observes that she has rebelled herself and has learned that nothing is to be gained from it. She makes a formal gesture of submission, placing her hand beneath Petruchio's foot. Petruchio, exulting in his fine wife, takes her off to bed; the others marvel at the taming of the shrew.

COMMENTARY

The Taming of the Shrew is sometimes seen as an account of the tyranny of man over woman, but this is a misinterpretation stemming from our distance from the assumptions of Shakespeare's day. In Elizabethan England it was almost universally agreed that it was a God-given right, confirmed in the Bible, for a husband to dominate his wife in all things, just as a king could dictate to a citizen or a human being could control an animal. Katherina's famous speech in 5.2.137–180 expresses this belief quite plainly. However, it is a mistake to think that the story of Katherina and Petruchio is intended to make this point; rather, it takes the point for granted. Instead, the play's main plot concerns the development of character and of love in a particular sort of personality.

Shakespeare's version of the 'battle of the sexes' is a striking advance on its predecessors. In treatments of this classic theme both before and since Shakespeare, a woman is commonly beaten into submission or is tormented in some more sophisticated manner. The violence in *The Shrew*—except for conventional beatings of servants, a staple of theatrical humour dating back to Roman drama—is limited to Katherina's own assaults on Bianca and Petruchio, which demonstrate her shrewishness. Petruchio 'tames' Katherina by means of a clever strategy that startlingly resembles modern behaviour-modification therapy.

In fact, the psychology of *The Taming of the Shrew* is highly evolved, evidence that, even early in his career, Shakespeare had the capacity to delineate personalities. Acts 1–3 contain a convincingly familiar portrait of a highly defensive young woman who shields her-

self from criticism by attacking others first, and she is strong enough to make her father and sister regret any effort to reform her. The portrayal of the deceptively demure Bianca, who slyly taunts her sister in 2.1 and who displays her own wilfulness when she is alone with her suitors in 3.1, suggests that Katherina has been compared to her younger sister too often for her temper to tolerate. Petruchio understands this and, although he is motivated to marry for mercenary reasons, he values Katherina's high spirits. Thus he can manoeuvre her into abandoning her shrewishness, and his technique, although comically overdrawn, is psychologically sophisticated.

Petruchio persistently assures Katherina that she is a rational and loving person. On the other hand, he himself behaves terribly, throwing tantrums and flying in the face of good sense—in fact, he exaggerates the behaviour by which she has distinguished herself. She finally succumbs to him and adopts conventional wifely behaviour, represented by the humorous tests she passes in 4.5. Her transformation comes about not because Petruchio has forced her to feign acceptance of a repugnant role, but because she has seen in his antics the ugliness of her own shrewish behaviour and has also come to recognise the emotional rewards for herself in being a dutiful wife. He has understood her, and now she understands both herself and him.

That Katherina and Petruchio are in love before the play ends is sometimes disputed on the grounds that she becomes too servile to allow any relationship between them other than master and slave. However, her servility exists only in the minds of observers from another age, our own; for Shakespeare's audience, and for Katherina herself, her new position is simply a conventional one. It does not at all preclude love. Petruchio and Katherina demonstrate their growing affection, rather than declare it outright, but it is no less real. At the end of 5.1 they express affection for each other for the first time: she kisses him, and she calls him 'love'; he responds by calling her his 'sweet Kate', an epithet he has earlier used only sarcastically.

The 'submission' speech is not delivered in slavish resignation to a demand, but as a duty, carrying with it the rewards of a solid place in the world, a place described with approval in the speech itself. Petruchio has not tried to humiliate Katherina, and she is not humiliated. Instead, he has asserted her superiority to other wives and offered her a podium from which to lecture the Widow. He has not asked her to speak of her own relationship to him; it is entirely her idea to assert that her own experience of rebellion has been barren and pointless. To close the speech, she freely offers a symbolic enactment of her acceptance of the traditional wifely role. Flabbergasted, almost at a loss for words, Petruchio can only sputter, 'Why, there's a wench' (5.2.181), and kiss his bride. Shakespeare consistently gives his heroines the last word in his comedies, and in *The Shrew,* as always, that word confirms the triumph of love, specifically conventional married love.

It is ironic that Petruchio's frankly mercenary interest in marriage yields a love match, whereas Lucentio's rapture for Bianca lands him with a shrew. This twist reinforces the contrasts between the main plot and the SUB-PLOT. Petruchio's tactics and their happy outcome are juxtaposed with the more conventional romancing of Bianca. The sub-plot consists of an assemblage of traditional dramatic situations; youth is pitted against age; the romanticism of intrigue and disguise is compared to courtship conducted in business terms. These comparisons are familiar ones, deriving from Italian and ancient Roman models, and the participating characters are mere stereotypes, with the single exception of Bianca, who is humanly complex. Lucentio and Hortensio are stock young men of Italian romances; Tranio is part of a tradition of cunning servants that dates back to ancient Greek comedy; Baptista is a standard father-of-the-girl; and Gremio is referred to several times as a 'pantaloon', the comic old man of the COMMEDIA DELL'ARTE. These predictable characters make the eccentric individuality of Petruchio and Katherina particularly attractive.

The conventionality of the majority of the characters is just one of several features of the play that intentionally stress its artificiality. The Induction asserts that the tale is a fiction, intended for light entertainment. The final scene serves a similar function. By 5.2 the strands of the plot have all been woven together, and all that remains is a formal summation of the play's themes. The ritualistic setting of a wedding feast and the presence of most of the play's cast strengthen the element of magic in the thrice-repeated summons of the wives and their triple responses, and in the crowning gesture of Katherina's statement of proper martial relations. While it not does not do so as explicitly as the Sly plot, the ceremonial nature of this scene also emphasises the artificiality of the fantasy it closes.

The Taming of the Shrew relies heavily on accepted dramatic conventions, and it approaches traditional farce in many respects. It lacks the depth of Shakespeare's later comedies, but it also foreshadows them; Katherina in particular anticipates BEATRICE in *Much Ado About Nothing.* In its presentation of several psychologically resonant portraits, as well as in its strong organisation and thoughtfully developed themes, it is a remarkable early work.

SOURCES OF THE PLAY

No specific source is known for the main plot of *The Taming of the Shrew.* Folk tales and songs about a husband disciplining a troublesome wife have been common in most cultures, and many were well known in Elizabethan England. A doggerel ballad, *A Merry Jest of*

a Shrewde and Curste Wyfe, printed in 1550, is often cited as a possible source, and it resembles the play in that its shrew is the elder of two sisters: in most such works, she is the youngest of three. However, it differs from *The Shrew* in other respects. The playwright will have known many such tales and ballads, and it is unlikely that any one of them was his specific source. His own version is significantly less brutal than all of its antecedents, and it seems most likely that he simply devised a story line from his recollections of a common popular theme.

Similarly, the Induction's tale of a poor man placed in a rich man's world had widespread currency. Like the shrew theme, this was also the subject of a number of 16th-century English ballads, and a version was published in a London jest-book in 1570. The details of Christopher Sly's existence are plainly taken from the young playwright's own WARWICKSHIRE background, and it seems clear that, again, Shakespeare created his own version of a widely recognised story.

For the Bianca sub-plot, the playwright turned to the play *Supposes* (performed 1566, published 1573, 1587), by George GASCOIGNE, a translation of an Italian drama, *I Suppositi* (1509), by Ludovico ARIOSTO. Knowledgeable members of Shakespeare's audience doubtless enjoyed the coy reference to 'supposes' in 5.1.107.

Various other works have been suggested as sources of certain features. The names Grumio and Tranio appear in *The Haunted House,* by PLAUTUS. Gervase MARKHAM's writings on falconry may have contributed to Petruchio's elaborate description in 4.1.175–198. Gerard LEGH's book on heraldry, *Accedens of Armory* (1562), to which Shakespeare would refer in writing *King Lear,* contains a story similar to that of the Tailor in 4.3. In 1484 William CAXTON translated and published a French tale that might have inspired the husbands' wager in 5.2. However, such bets often appear in the folklore of marital relations. In fact, although literary sources may have provided various details, Shakespeare might just as easily have derived any of the play's minor episodes from some popular tale or ballad now lost.

TEXT OF THE PLAY

It is difficult to determine when *The Taming of the Shrew* was written, as it is for all of Shakespeare's early plays. Estimates have ranged from the late 1580s to 1600, although the later dates reflect an assumption that Shakespeare used *The Taming of a Shrew* as a model. Most scholars now regard *A Shrew* as a BAD QUARTO of *The Shrew* and accordingly conclude that the original play must have been written before the summer of 1592, when *A Shrew* was compiled. The numerous references in the Induction to the playwright's native Warwickshire suggest that the work may have been written not long after his arrival in London, probably in 1588 or 1589. *The Taming of the Shrew* is sometimes cited as Shakespeare's earliest work, but this proposition is unprovable.

The Shrew was not published until it was included in the FIRST FOLIO (1623). The first QUARTO edition was published in 1631. The Folio text appears to be derived from Shakespeare's FOUL PAPERS, as transcribed by a scribe hired to make a copy for the use of an acting company. It has served as the basis for all subsequent editions, although, beginning with POPE (1) in 1723, some editors have included the interludes and the epilogue from *A Shrew* to complete the tale of Christopher Sly.

THEATRICAL HISTORY OF THE PLAY

Little evidence of early productions of *The Taming of the Shrew* has survived. However, Shakespeare's play was certainly popular at least into the 1630s. In about 1611 *The Woman's Prize, or the Tamer Tamed* by John FLETCHER (2), offered a sequel to Shakespeare's work. This play depicts Petruchio's second marriage, following Kate's death, to a woman who applies to him the treatment he had meted out to his first wife. This could have had point only if Shakespeare's play were in vogue at the time. Moreover, the appearance of a Quarto edition of the play in 1631 implies a continuing public interest, and its title-page tells of the play's performance by the KING'S MEN at both the BLACKFRIARS and GLOBE theatres. The play was also acted at the court of King Charles I in 1633.

After a revival in 1663, no performance of Shakespeare's play was recorded for almost 180 years. *The Taming of the Shrew* was replaced by a series of adaptations, none resembling the original very closely. The first of these, John LACY's *Sauny the Scot,* appeared in 1667. A crude farce, it was extremely popular for a century. It stimulated its own spin-off—a musical entitled *A Cure for a Scold* (c. 1735)—which was itself performed until the 1760s. The episode of Christopher Sly, deleted from *Sauny,* was used in *The Cobbler of Preston* (1716), by Charles JOHNSON (2), a political play about the Jacobite Rebellion of 1715. Its popularity stimulated another, non-political, play with the same title in the same year, also based loosely on the Induction.

Sauny was finally replaced on the English stage by David GARRICK's *Catherine and Petruchio* (1754), an abbreviated version of Shakespeare's play, eliminating both the Induction and the Bianca sub-plot. This popular play was regularly staged for more than a century and Frederick REYNOLDS (1) made an opera of it in 1828. An even shorter version, by John Philip KEMBLE (3), competed with Garrick's production in the late 18th century and introduced a piece of stage business—Petruchio cracking a horsewhip—that became

standard in subsequent productions and was probably the public's strongest image of the play into recent times.

It was not until 1844 that Shakespeare's text was revived, in a historic production by Benjamin WEBSTER (1) and J. R. PLANCHE that established the use of legitimate Shakespearean texts as a norm. By the end of the 19th century Shakespeare's version of *The Shrew* was well established on both sides of the Atlantic. Ada REHAN was particularly acclaimed as Katherina. The play has continued to be popular in the 20th century, and notable productions have included a modern-dress staging by Barry JACKSON (1) in 1928 and Joseph PAPP's 1978 presentation starring Raul Julia and Meryl Streep. *The Taming of the Shrew* has been made as a FILM eleven times, six as a silent movie. Two of the talkies are in English. The first, which featured Mary Pickford and Douglas Fairbanks, is remembered chiefly for a credit line that has become a favourite show-business joke: 'Written by William Shakespeare with additional dialogue by Sam Taylor'. Franco ZEFFIRELLI's 1966 film starring Richard Burton and Elizabeth Taylor was a box-office success. Also, the play has been produced for TELEVISION twice, most recently by Jonathan MILLER (2) in 1980.

Tamora Character in *Titus Andronicus,* the villainous queen of the Goths. Tamora, her three sons, and her lover, AARON the Moor, have been captured by the Roman general TITUS (1) Andronicus before the play begins. When in 1.1, her captor permits her eldest son to be ritually sacrificed despite her eloquent plea for mercy, Tamora vows revenge and the play's bloody cycle begins. Tamora find her chance for vengeance, when the new Roman emperor, SATURNINUS, falls in love with her and marries her. Saturninus fears Titus, who is very popular, and wishes to break with him, but Tamora advises her new husband to make peace with the general until his own hold on the throne is more secure. She will see to Titus' downfall herself, she adds.

After this flamboyant introduction, Tamora recedes from the forefront of the play for a while. Her revenge is implemented largely by Aaron, though she helps him frame two of Titus' sons for a murder, and she is particularly villainous in refusing LAVINIA's pleas for mercy in 2.3. Later, in 4.4, when she and Saturninus learn of an approaching army under Titus' son, her husband is stricken with fear, but she reproves him, in a well-known speech emphasising the power held by rulers (4.4.81–87). She goes on to boast that she will 'enchant the old Andronicus', that is, Titus, and prevail upon him to cancel his son's invasion.

With her sons, Tamora goes to Titus in disguise, pretending to be Revenge, a spirit from within the earth come to help the mad old man achieve his vengeance. In her impersonation, she anticipates later Shakespearean witches and ghosts. She believes that Titus is mad, but he is sane enough to see through her plot and pretend to be taken in. Thinking she has won, she leaves her sons with Titus, but he kills them and serves them to her at the banquet in the last scene, before killing her as well.

Tamworth Village in central England, about 10 miles from BOSWORTH FIELD, setting for 5.2 of *Richard III.* As the Earl of RICHMOND approaches the forces of RICHARD III, he mentions the hamlet (in 5.2.13).

Tarlton, Richard (d. 1588) English comic actor, a leading figure in ELIZABETHAN THEATRE when Shakespeare's career began. Tarlton was a member of the QUEEN'S MEN (1) from its foundation in 1583 until his death. He was a particular favourite of Queen ELIZABETH (1) and served also as her personal jester or FOOL (1), though she began to dislike him when he went too far in jokes about her favourites. He also wrote plays, and his *The Seven Deadly Sins* (1585) may have been revived in the 1590s by Shakespeare's STRANGE'S MEN. His greatest accomplishment, however, was the establishment of a popular style for the stage CLOWN (1)—earthy, awkward, comically confused in speech—that became standard. He was a great influence on William KEMPE, for whom Shakespeare wrote a number of parts. Tarlton was especially noted for his ability to improvise, and HAMLET's complaint about 'clowns [who] speak . . . more than is set down for them' (*Hamlet* 3.2.39) was a joke at the expense of Tarlton and his successors. The great clown became something of a cult figure after his death; taverns were named for him, and ballads and joke books about him—or allegedly by him—appeared for at least 40 years. An unproven tradition holds that Shakespeare was thinking of Tarlton when he had Hamlet reminisce fondly of the jester YORICK.

Tarquin (Sextus Tarquinius) Semi-legendary Roman prince and figure in *The Rape of Lucrece,* the rapist who assaults LUCRECE. In the first quarter of the poem, Tarquin, though aware that his act will dishonour him forever, is gripped by sexual desire and continues, 'pawning his honour to obtain his lust' (line 156). He condemns himself at some length (lines 190–245, 260–280), but he finally commits himself to satisfying his lust. He is held between 'frozen conscience and hot burning will' (line 247), in the grip of an evil impulse 'strong past reason's weak removing' (line 243). In this respect Tarquin's story anticipates a major theme of *Macbeth,* and he is specifically referred to in that play (2.1.55).

Once Tarquin assaults Lucrece in her bedroom, the poet's attention turns to the victim (line 442), and,

after committing his crime, Tarquin flees (line 740). He does not reappear, though in the last line of the poem it is reported that Lucrece's avengers, led by Junius BRUTUS (2), expel him from Rome. Earlier, in the last sentence of the ARGUMENT to the poem, Shakespeare also mentions this development, saying, '. . . the Tarquins were all exiled, and the state government changed from kings to consuls'. Thus Tarquin's crime is said to have led to the establishment of the Roman Republic.

In Shakespeare's sources, OVID and LIVY, Sextus Tarquinius is the son of the last king of the Romans, Tarquinius Superbas, and the king, deposed in favour of the Republic in 509 B.C., may have had a son who bore this name. However, the tale of Lucrece's rape has its roots in pre-Roman traditions, and Tarquin may well be totally legendary. In any case the name Tarquinius suggests that these rulers of Rome were Etruscans, whose principal city was Tarquinia.

Tate, Nahum (1652–1715) English poet and playwright, best known for his adaptations of Shakespeare's plays. Tate wrote a number of plays, most of them based on the works of various Elizabethan dramatists, but he is chiefly remembered for his version of *King Lear.* His *History of King Lear* (1681) retained some of Shakespeare's dialogue, but only in a drastically revised play. Tate eliminated the blinding of GLOUCESTER (1) and his suicide attempt, and he added a love affair between EDGAR and CORDELIA. He deleted the king's FOOL (2), and, most notoriously, he provided a happy ending in which LEAR is restored to his throne, abdicating in favour of Edgar and Cordelia. Though modern commentators condemn Tate's adaptation as a travesty, it was one of the most successful plays in the history of the English theatre, performed for over 150 years in successive revivals. (Shakespeare's text was restored in bits and pieces by various producers, but his ending was not again enacted until 1823, by Charles KEAN (1); and the original play as a whole was staged only in 1838, by W. C. MACREADY.)

Tate's play was not simply a tasteless avoidance of the tragic; composed in the wake of a revolution and civil war, it carried a strong moralising endorsement of civil order, which doubtless accounted in part for its original popularity. His Lear, in being both martyred and restored, recalled the recent history of the STUART DYNASTY, and assured its partisans—the establishment of the day—that disaster could be overcome. Later, its generally optimistic stance, combined with the power of Shakespeare's poetry, endeared it to generations; it continued to be staged as late as 1843.

In 1680 Tate also adapted *Richard II,* but the state CENSORSHIP was even more nervous about this story of a king's deposition than it had been in Shakespeare's day—for in the interval the reality had occurred in England. Though Tate changed the scene and characters, calling it *The Sicilian Usurper,* it was suppressed by the government. In 1681, just after his *Lear* was staged, Tate took on *Coriolanus,* again making great alterations. His *The Ingratitude of a Commonwealth* retained some of Shakespeare's text, but it was essentially a different play, most conspicuously in its passages of sensationalistic violence. It too addressed the conservative political sensibility of the day, stressing the value of respectful loyalty, supporting CORIOLANUS' complaints about rebellious commoners, and de-emphasising the hero's faults. However, unlike *The History of King Lear,* it was a commercial failure.

Taurus, Titus Statilius (active 36–16 B.C.) Historical figure and minor character in *Antony and Cleopatra,* a general under Octavius CAESAR (2). Taurus appears briefly at the battle of ACTIUM, and receives, in 3.8, Caesar's order to maintain his army ashore, without fighting, while the naval battle is fought. He marches wordlessly through 3.10 and avoids contact with ANTONY's forces under CANIDIUS, which stresses the inconclusive nature of the land fighting. He is a pawn of Caesar's stategy and speaks only two words.

The historical Taurus was a highly successful general, second only to AGRIPPA among Caesar's military men. His background is unknown, though his name suggests descent from the pre-Roman Lucanians of southern Italy. He is first recorded as an admiral who commanded a unit in the defeat of Sextus Pompeius—the POMPEY (2) of the play. He went on to lead numerous other campaigns and governed conquered territories in North Africa and Spain.

Taylor, Joseph (d. 1652) English actor, a member of the KING'S MEN. Though Taylor only joined the King's Men in 1619, he is listed among the 'Principall Actors' of Shakespeare's plays in the FIRST FOLIO of 1623. He was hired away from PRINCE CHARLES' MEN to replace Richard BURBAGE (3) within a few weeks of that star's death. He took over Burbage's most famous role, HAMLET, and was acclaimed in it. He was also noted as IAGO. In 1630 he became a partner in both the BLACKFRIARS and GLOBE THEATRES. In the same year, he became a co-manager of the company, with John LOWIN, and remained in that position until the theatres were closed down by the Puritan revolution in 1642.

Tchaikovsky, Peter Ilyich (1840–1893) Russian composer. One of the most popular and influential composers of the 19th century, Tchaikovsky was inspired by Shakespeare on several occasions. He wrote brief symphonic pieces for both *Hamlet* and *The Tempest,* and his symphonic fantasy *Romeo and Juliet* (1864) is one of his best-known works.

Tearle, Godfrey (1884–1953) British actor. The son of theatrical entrepreneurs who had staged Shakespeare at STRATFORD in the late 19th century, Tearle had a long and illustrious career on stage and screen. He was especially noted for his portrayals of HAMLET, OTHELLO, and the ANTONY of *Antony and Cleopatra.*

Television Medium for which all of Shakespeare's plays have been produced (except *The Two Noble Kinsmen,* which many people do not admit to the CANON of the playwright's works). Many of the plays have been produced several times. Since the earliest days of the medium, television executives have been frank about using Shakespeare to provide a veneer of high seriousness to their operations, but it is also clear that there is a widespread audience for the plays. The British Broadcasting Corporation, at the forefront of Shakespeare production for television, has broadcast the standard canon of plays more than once, including special series such as THE SPREAD OF THE EAGLE and AN AGE OF KINGS.

The Tempest

SYNOPSIS

Act 1, Scene 1
On a storm-wracked ship, the BOATSWAIN exchanges curses with two arrogant passengers, ANTONIO (5) and SEBASTIAN (3), who are travelling with King ALONSO of Naples. The king's counsellor GONZALO remains calm, however, as the ship goes down.

Act 1, Scene 2
On a nearby island MIRANDA is upset by the shipwreck, but her father PROSPERO, a magician, assures her that the seamen will be safe. He reveals to her that he was once the Duke of MILAN. He studied magic in preference to governing and was deposed by his brother, Antonio, who was aided by King Alonso. The conspirators put Prospero and Miranda, then two years old, in a small boat and abandoned them at sea, but the kindly Gonzalo had given them supplies, including Prospero's books of magic. They then found the island and have lived there since. Through magic, Prospero has raised the storm to bring his old enemies to the island. He magically puts Miranda to sleep and summons his servant, a sprite named ARIEL. Ariel reports that he has entranced the vessel's passengers and dispersed the people around the island, taking particular care, as instructed, with FERDINAND (2), the son of King Alonso. When he complains about his tasks, the magician sternly reminds him that he must work in exchange for his rescue from magical imprisonment in a tree trunk, imposed by the now-dead witch who formerly occupied the island. Prospero promises that if his present scheme is successful, he will release the sprite. He then instructs Ariel to wear a cloak of invisibility, so that he can be seen only by Prospero, and report for further duty. After Ariel leaves, Miranda awakes and Prospero summons CALIBAN, his half-human slave, son of the late witch. Ariel returns, invisible to Miranda, and is sent away again with whispered orders. The surly Caliban reluctantly appears and complains of his slavery, but Prospero declares that he has earned it, for after being taken in and educated by the magician, he attempted to rape Miranda. Caliban is sent to gather wood. Ariel returns, leading Ferdinand by singing fairy songs. Miranda is amazed and delighted by this the first young man she has ever seen. Ferdinand is equally charmed to encounter her. Prospero observes in an aside that they are already in love, as he has planned. However, to ensure that Ferdinand will not take Miranda lightly, he adopts a stern attitude and pretends to distrust the young man. Despite Miranda's pleas, he imprisons him.

Act 2, Scene 1
Gonzalo attempts to cheer King Alonso with assurances that Ferdinand has survived, but he is mocked by Antonio and Sebastian. Ariel appears, invisible to the men, and puts Gonzalo and the king to sleep. Antonio suggests to Sebastian, who is the king's brother, that they should kill the sleeping men and make Sebastian king. Sebastian agrees, but as they draw their swords, Ariel reappears and awakens Gonzalo and the king. The four men go off in search of Ferdinand.

Act 2, Scene 2
Caliban tries to hide from TRINCULO, a FOOL (1) who has survived the shipwreck, but Trinculo sees him. Frightened by thunder, Trinculo takes refuge under Caliban's cloak. Another survivor, STEPHANO (2), appears, drunk on salvaged wine. Seeing Trinculo and Caliban, he decides they are a single, two-headed, four-legged monster. He feeds Caliban wine, hoping to tame the monster. Trinculo identifies himself, and the two friends rejoice at their reunion. Caliban is delighted with his first taste of wine and tipsily volunteers to serve the two men as though they were gods, if they will give him more. They agree and leave with him. Caliban sings drunkenly of his pleasure at leaving Prospero.

Act 3, Scene 1
Ferdinand, forced by Prospero to move a large pile of logs, reflects that though his princely nature rebels against such labour, the work seems joyous because he knows his master's daughter sympathises with him. Miranda appears, and they confess their love for each other, agreeing that they will marry. Prospero, overhearing them, is pleased.

Act 3, Scene 2
Caliban, Stephano, and Trinculo are drunk and squabble comically. Caliban proposes that Stephano

kill Prospero, stealing his magic books and taking possession of Miranda. Stephano decides to do so, envisioning himself as king of the island, with Caliban and Trinculo as viceroys. Ariel leads them away with fairy music.

Act 3, Scene 3
Prospero causes a magical banquet to appear. Alonso, Sebastian, and Antonio step greedily forward, but the banquet disappears. Ariel, disguised as a HARPY, declares that they are evil men and that destiny has therefore stranded them on this island and taken Alonso's son. They shall be tormented until they atone and adopt a sin-free life. Alonso leaves, declaring that he will find his dead son and die beside him. Sebastian and Antonio go with him, angrily intent on fighting the spirits of the island. Gonzalo, believing that their guilt has made them crazy, follows them, to keep them from harming themselves.

Act 4, Scene 1
Prospero consents to the engagement of Miranda and Ferdinand. He calls on Ariel to provide entertainment to celebrate the bethrothal, and several sprites impersonate the goddesses IRIS, CERES, and JUNO in a MASQUE. Prospero, recalling Caliban and Stephano's plot, sends Ariel to gather some fine clothes he has prepared, which are hung in full view. Caliban, Stephano, and Trinculo arrive, still drunk. Trinculo and Stephano, seeing the fine clothes, cannot resist trying them on, despite Caliban's warnings that Prospero will catch them. Spirits disguised as hunting dogs chase the comical villains away. Prospero reflects that his enemies are now all at his mercy. Soon his task will be complete, and Ariel can be freed.

Act 5, Scene 1
Ariel reports that the captive Alonso, Sebastian, and Antonio are insane, while Gonzalo is grief-stricken. Ariel says he feels sorry for them, and Prospero declares that he will be merciful to them, despite the losses he has suffered at their hands. After sending Ariel to fetch them, he asserts in a soliloquy that he will renounce magic once he has cured his victims. He exchanges his magician's robes for the garments he wore as Duke of Milan, and as the victims recover their senses they recognise him. He forgives their offences, and they concede him his duchy. Alonso still mourns the loss of his son, and Prospero reveals Ferdinand and Miranda. Miranda is delighted to see so many humans, Ferdinand is reunited with his father, and the future succession of the engaged couple to the throne of Naples is proclaimed. Ariel appears with the Boatswain and MASTER (2) of the king's ship; they report that the vessel has been miraculously restored to shipshape condition. Ariel fetches Caliban, Stephano, and Trinculo—still drunk—and Prospero sends them to restore the stolen clothes to his closet. He then invites the king and his followers indoors, to hear the story of his time on the island. He gives Ariel a last order—to prepare auspicious winds and weather for the return to Milan—and sets him free.

COMMENTARY

With *The Tempest* Shakespeare reached new heights in a recently developed genre, the ROMANCES; indeed, some commentators find it the greatest accomplishment of his career. After progressively more successful attempts—in *Pericles, Cymbeline,* and *The Winter's Tale*—at mingling elements of TRAGEDY and COMEDY within a framework of magic and exoticism taken from literary romances, the playwright created in *The Tempest* a stunning theatrical entertainment that is also a moral allegory of great beauty and emotional power. Unlike the traditional medieval MORALITY PLAY, Shakespeare's work does not merely present symbols of already understood Christian doctrines; rather, it offers a vision as complex and ambiguous as human nature itself. Such is the inclusiveness of Shakespeare's sensibility and the power of the play's characters as emblems of humanity that *The Tempest* cannot be pinned down by any particular interpretation, but must instead be taken as the embodiment of a variety of propositions. The themes of *The Tempest* are multifarious and mingled, but nevertheless the various ele-

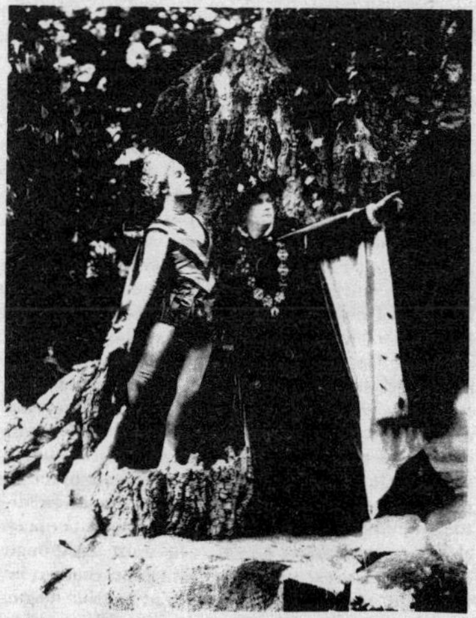

A scene from The Tempest. *A stunning mix of tragedy, comedy, and magic,* The Tempest *is considered by some to be Shakespeare's greatest accomplishment.* (Courtesy of Culver Pictures, Inc.)

ments come together in a traditional comedic happy ending of reconciliation and regeneration.

The Tempest has very little actual plot: the love of Ferdinand and Miranda meets only token—and feigned—opposition, and the proposed assassinations of Alonso and Prospero are never plausible, due to Prospero's overwhelming mastery of the situation. However, Shakespeare makes up for the lack of suspense with bold theatre. Bizarre characters and extravagant effects abound in a spectacular presentation that plainly reflects the influence of the courtly masque, an increasingly popular form in the early 17th century. Striking tableaus figure in almost every act: the shipwreck in 1.1, the supernatural banquet in 3.3, the formal betrothal masque and the spectral hounds in 4.1, and the sudden appearance of Ferdinand and Miranda in 5.1. These elements are almost independent of the dialogue, but their visual imagery adds meaning to the story.

Magic is a vital ingredient of *The Tempest.* The supernatural qualities of Caliban and Ariel are particularly impressive on stage—Caliban is usually costumed to resemble a sea monster and Ariel sometimes flies on cables. The text describes a number of remarkable feats of magic that add to our sense of wonder, as do Ariel's appearances with goddesses and as a harpy. Music is another strong component of the play, which incorporates many songs and several dance numbers. Indeed, music is part of Prospero's magical repertoire, as all of the visitors to the island are manipulated at some point by Ariel's tabor and pipe. The island itself seems haunted by 'sounds and sweet airs [of] a thousand twangling instruments' (3.2.134–135).

Another unifying feature of *The Tempest* is the way the conspiracies that compose the action reflect each other. Before the time of the play, Antonio stole Prospero's dukedom; on the island, that original crime is re-enacted as Antonio offers Sebastian the prospect of a kingdom if he murders Alonso and as Caliban recruits Stephano against Prospero. Each of these conspiracies is finally defused by Prospero, as order is systematically restored. Just as important, they all lead to the reconciliation with which the plays closes.

Yet another important theme is the contrast between Art and nature. Prospero rules through his magical 'Art' (1.2.1), consistently spelled with a capital A in the conventional 17th-century usage associated with the RENAISSANCE image of the magician as philosopher. Such a *mage,* as they were called, attempted to elevate his soul through arcane knowledge of the divine, whether through alchemy, the lore of supernatural signs, or communication with spirits. Although Prospero's goal was originally to transcend nature, he gains control of nature as a byproduct of his magic. This, then, provides for his control of the island.

The contrast of 'Art' and nature is furthered by the comparison of Prospero, whose learned sorcery is Art, and the 'natural' Caliban, with his lust and his beast-like resistance to education. Caliban's naturalness leads him to attempt rape—he would have 'peopled . . . this isle with Calibans' (1.2.352–353)—whereas Prospero and Ferdinand, with civilised sensibilities believe in celibacy before marriage. They understand marital happiness to depend on discipline; the satisfactions of sex are to be preceded by a formal declaration of intention, in the 'full and holy rite' (4.1.17) sanctified by tradition. Put another way, we must intelligently assert what we are doing and not simply plunge. Ferdinand, Miranda, and Prospero all exercise the self-discipline that Caliban lacks, and their success and happiness are compared with his misery. Nature is insufficient and must be built upon by civilisation.

When Prospero arrived on the island, he found it in a state of barbarity; Ariel was imprisoned and the amoral beast Caliban ran free. At the close Ariel is liberated as Caliban returns to the bondage he briefly evaded. The contrast between these two characters spans the play. Both are supernatural, and they are similar in their dislike for being under an obligation to mortals, but otherwise they are antithetical creatures—one airy and beautiful, pleasant, and allied with good; the other dank and ugly, sullen, and inclined to evil. Ariel is a spiritual being, composed of air, uninhibited by normal physical restraints, while Caliban is utterly material, confined to the earth, without the power to resist even the 'urchin-shows' (2.2.5) of Ariel's minor underlings. Explicitly non-human, Ariel and Caliban are essentially allegorical, representing human possibilities. Ariel embodies our potential spirituality, Caliban our propensity to waste that potential in materialism or sensual pleasure.

Ariel is Prospero's analogue and like him is rather isolated; except as a seeming hallucination, he has no contact with anyone but his master. Caliban, however, is pointedly compared to many other characters. He is the baseline from which all else is measured. As we have seen, his conspiracy parallels Antonio's. His inability to learn more than curses contrasts with Miranda's high moral sensibility, even though they were educated together. His response to Miranda's beauty contrasts with Ferdinand's. Caliban resists carrying wood in 1.2, while Ferdinand rejoices in his similar labour in 3.1. When Miranda judges her admirers, she finds Caliban 'a thing most brutish' (1.2.358) and Ferdinand 'a thing divine' (4.1.421).

As already suggested, the ultimate comparison is between Caliban and Prospero. The black magic of Caliban's mother Sycorax contrasts with Prospero's employment of sorcery for a good end, after which it is abjured. Caliban wishes only for 'a new master' (2.2. 185) and even encourages murder to get one; Prospero pits his 'nobler reason 'gainst [his] fury', seeking 'the rarer action [that] is / In virtue' (5.1.26, 27–28).

The ineducable monster can only approach the least of humanity's capacities, while the learned magician aspires to high moral accomplishment.

Caliban represents the 'natural man' that enthralled Europeans as the New World was opened up and its natives became known. He is pointedly associated with the New World through allusions to the Patagonian god Setebos, the island of Bermuda, and such familiar anecdotes of exploration as the reception of explorers as gods and their offering liquor to the natives. With these associations, Shakespeare raised an issue that concerned thinking people throughout Europe: the relative merits of nature and civilisation. Many of Shakespeare's contemporaries viewed 'natural man' as a healthy counter to the ills of civilisation—an attitude that has survived to the present day—but the playwright disagreed. One of the chief spokesmen for the admiring view of natural man was Michel de MONTAIGNE, and Shakespeare gave his position a place in *The Tempest*—a passage from Montaigne's essay 'Of Cannibals' is echoed in Gonzalo's remarks on an ideal commonwealth in 2.1.143–164, but only as a foil to the play's point of view. The ineffectual Gonzalo envisions 'all men idle [and] women . . . innocent and pure' (2.1.150–151), but Caliban, whose name is a pointed anagram of 'cannibal', has in his idleness attempted to rape Miranda and thus represents a standing refutation of Montaigne's thesis. Caliban cannot, like Ferdinand, make the commitment of a 'patient log-man' (3.1.67), and his undisciplined lust is naturally rejected by Miranda. Similarly, Prospero's learning, the key to his power, is rejected by Caliban, and the monster is accordingly powerless. His slavery is a function of his defects as well as of Prospero's magic.

That Caliban and Ariel are non-human is part of the play's masquelike spectacle, but their supernatural quality also serves another function. The role of providence in human affairs, an important idea throughout Shakespeare's romances, is particularly emphasised by the prevalence of magic in *The Tempest.* Moreover, the references to the New World, along with the unspecific location of Prospero's island, add a sense of exotic climes in which the supernatural is to be expected. The eeriness of the play's world—'as strange a maze as e'er men trod' (5.1.242)—virtually requires divine intervention. Action by a specific divinity (provided in the other romances) is lacking here, but it is alluded to in the betrothal masque with its goddesses. They are merely portrayed—although by supernatural creatures—but their capacity to bless is evoked in striking fashion. When all has been resolved, it is natural for 'Holy Gonzalo' (5.1.62) to attribute the outcome to the gods in 5.1.201–204, and for Alonso to cry, 'I say, Amen' (5.1.204).

Prospero's magic leaves both characters and audience unclear about what is real and what is not, and the boundaries of reality constitute another important theme of the play. Mistaken beliefs abound: Ferdinand and Miranda each mistake the other for a supernatural being, and Caliban takes Trinculo and Stephano for gods. Alonso and Ferdinand each believe the other dead. Stephano thinks Caliban and Trinculo a two-headed, four-legged creature. (These three buffoons befuddle their senses with liquor and are then led astray by Ariel, so their capacity to recognise reality is doubly damaged. In a remarkable passage that encompasses both sorts of unreality, Ariel relates his supernatural effects on the trio in a delightfully naturalistic description of drunkenness.) Most strikingly, the audience shares the difficulties of Prospero's subjects. We see Ariel when the characters do not, but other illusions are designed to take us in, too. At the outset we are fooled by the supernatural storm and shipwreck. The sudden appearance of the banquet in 3.3 is obviously supernatural, but like Alonso and his party, we believe it is for eating until Ariel's Harpy makes it disappear. The king and his party, surprised to have survived the shipwreck, remain baffled throughout, until Prospero finally permits them to shed the 'subtilties o' the isle, that will not let you / Believe things certain' (5.1.124–125).

Prospero's 'subtilties' are manifested in several miniature plays, each itself a pretence of reality, reflecting Shakespeare's interest in this aspect of theatre. Prospero stages the banquet of 3.3, the masque of goddesses in 4.1, and the tableau of Ferdinand and Miranda in 5.1. After the masque he points out to his audiences—both on stage and in the theatre—that a masque is an illusion. He then adds, in one of Shakespeare's most famous passages, that reality is too; we ourselves, we are told, 'are such stuff / As dreams are made on' (4.1.156–157). The number of levels of reality exposed here is startling to contemplate: the goddesses we have just been delighting in are supernatural, but they are merely portrayed by actors presenting a masque. However, those actors are themselves supernatural, Ariel's cohorts. Yet in reminding Ferdinand of this, Prospero reminds us that these sprites are themselves actors, in *The Tempest.* Then Prospero goes on to dissolve that reality as well, along with 'the great globe itself' (4.1.153). Although we are not permitted to dwell on this proposition—Prospero immediately dismisses it as merely a 'vex'd . . . weakness' (4.1.158–159)—the point has been made, and the many veils of illusion that have been evoked remain to tantalise us.

The shifting realities of *The Tempest* are appropriate, perhaps even necessary, to its presentation of a multiplicity of themes. Comparisons of art and nature, imagination and reality, discipline and laxity, civilisation and savagery combine to yield a powerful image of the moral nature of humankind. At the same time the play's extraordinary complexity permits quite differing interpretations of what that nature is. For exam-

ple, Prospero's total control over the events of the play, combined with Ariel's and Caliban's desire for freedom from his rule, has suggested political readings to many commentators, especially in the 20th century, with its concern for oppression and imperialism. Another modern interpretation, influenced by the advent of psychology, sees the characters as representing various aspects of Prospero's unconscious enacting an internal conflict. A related, less scientific idea is that the play is an allegory of Shakespeare's own life, or at least of his artistic career. A large body of interpretation has been devoted to religious readings: the play has been seen as a work of Christian mysticism or as an explication of ancient pagan mystery cults or of the cabala. Specific interpretations have ranged widely; among other things, *The Tempest* has been said to be about Neoplatonism, 16th-century French politics, Renaissance science, the creative impulse, and the discovery of America.

Obviously, not all of these interpretations can be correct—possibly none of them are—but whether psychological or political, religious or secular, all reflect an underlying quality of the play. *The Tempest* is about the inner nature of human beings revealed in circumstances of crisis and change. The characters are subject to startling personal transformations: Miranda, Alonso, and Gonzalo are magically put to sleep and awakened; for much of the play, Alonso is stricken by a grief that is based on an illusion; Ferdinand, faced with Miranda, finds that his 'spirits, as in a dream, are all bound up' (1.2.489), and he forgets his own false mourning. All of the island's visitors are subjected to a purging experience of some sort: Ferdinand is put to log-carrying, Stephano and Trinculo find themselves in a 'pickle' (5.1.282), the king and his followers are rendered 'distracted' (5.1.12). Prospero's 'insubstantial pageant' (4.1.155) is a fitting metaphor for the play's fluid, transitory world. Not for nothing does Gonzalo rejoice at the end that 'all of us [found] ourselves / When no man was his own' (5.1.212–213).

Even Prospero, the agent of transformation in others, is not immune to change, although his occurs largely before the time of the play. His decision that 'the rarer action is / In virtue than in vengeance' (5.1. 27–28) implies a temptation to avenge himself from which he has refrained. We recognise that he has undergone a series of changes: from a student of magic, he became a seeker of revenge through it, and finally he has found his way to a transcendence of it. At the end he abandons his godlike status on the island and, embracing his own humanity, returns to Milan and his proper position as duke. Like the others, he is subject to alteration in the depths of his being. These processes of transfiguration enact human possibilities; while *The Tempest* points out the clay of which we're made, it also insists on our divine potential.

Strikingly, however, one character, Antonio, is not transfigured. Shakespeare never accepted a single, simple point of view on life's complexities, and *The Tempest* does not provide a clear and unambiguous conclusion. Prospero does not entirely succeed in effecting his reconciliation, for Antonio remains silent (except for one snide witticism). The defeat of evil is not complete; perhaps Prospero's dry response to Miranda's 'O brave new world' (5.1.183)—' 'Tis new to thee' (5.1.184)—reflects his awareness of this. And while Prospero brings happiness to others, he himself remains melancholy. As in the other late plays, Shakespeare in *The Tempest* acknowledges that an evil once committed can never be entirely compensated for; there are Antonios who will refuse virtue, and Prosperos who cannot forget injustice.

Nevertheless, *The Tempest* has the traditional happy ending of comedy. Prospero is reconciled with his old enemies—he forgives Antonio despite his intransigence—and reassurance is thus offered that redemption is possible in a sinful world. The marriage of Ferdinand and Miranda is especially significant in light of this reconciliation: the daughter of the victim of an injustice marries the son of its perpetrator. The auspiciousness of the marriage is strengthened by the declaration that the couple will inherit the crown of Naples. The focus on the future suggests the rebirth of the world.

SOURCES OF THE PLAY

The general situation in *The Tempest* may derive from the plays of the Italian COMMEDIA DELL'ARTE, several of which depict seamen shipwrecked on islands inhabited by magicians. However, Shakespeare's play is much deeper than these farcical entertainments, and the features that make it so—Ariel and Caliban, Prospero's relationship to and forgiveness of his enemies, and the importance of philosophical themes—are the playwright's inventions. Although various themes in *The Tempest* were treated in earlier works, no specific literary or theatrical sources can be associated with the central material of the play.

Nevertheless, there are various minor sources for particular elements within it. The exploration of the New World inspired Shakespeare and his contemporaries in many ways, and one event in particular probably stimulated the playwright's adoption of a remote island for his drama's setting. A shipload of Virginia-bound colonists was wrecked at Bermuda in 1609; a survivor, William STRACHEY (2), described his experience in a letter—circulated in manuscript—that Shakespeare read and exploited for *The Tempest.* The shipwreck in 1.1, Ariel's description of St Elmo's fire in 1.2.196–206, and some other details derive from this document. It was supplemented by two public accounts of the same disaster, *The Discovery of the Barmudas* (1610) by Sylvester JOURDAIN (2) and *A True Declaration of the state of the Colonie in Virginia* (1610),

possibly by Dudley DIGGES (1). Besides offering historical details, these accounts all emphasise the providential survival of everyone aboard the vessel and the fact that Bermuda, previously notorious as an abode of devils and other evil spirits, turned out to be a pleasant and productive island. Both themes are paralleled in Shakespeare's depiction of Prospero's realm.

Another essay on the New World was exploited by Shakespeare, though in a different way. As already mentioned, Montaigne wrote about the native societies being discovered abroad in his essay 'Of the Cannibals', describing them as utopian societies free of the defects of civilisation. Shakespeare apparently respected Montaigne's clarity of thought, and it finds expression in Gonzalo's remarks on ideal government (2.1.143–164)—although Montaigne's ideas are rejected in general by the play. A passage in another Montaigne essay, 'Of Crueltie', probably inspired Prospero's praise of reconciliation in 5.1.25–30. In both cases Shakespeare used John FLORIO's translation of Montaigne, *Essayes on Morall, Politike, and Millitarie Discourses* (1603).

Other minor sources supplied additional material. OVID's *Metamorphoses,* either in the original Latin or as translated by Arthur GOLDING, provided much of Prospero's catalogue of supernatural beings in 5.1.33–50. Robert EDEN's *History of Travaille* (1577) also provided several details, including the name of Caliban's god, Setebos. Ferdinand's delight in the pain of worthwhile labour, in 3.1.1-14, may owe something to a similar passage in the *Confessions* of St Augustine (354–430 A.D.). MUCEDORUS (c. 1590), a comedy revived by the KING'S MEN in 1610 (and later wrongly attributed to Shakespeare), features a 'wild man' (a traditional medieval figure) whose savage nature may have influenced the creation of Caliban. Caliban may also reflect Shakespeare's reading of ARISTOTLE's *Nicomachean Ethics.* Contemporary demonology and spirit lore, from common opinion as well as literary sources, are evident throughout; in particular, Reginald SCOT's *Discovery of Witchcraft* (1584) may have provided hints for Ariel's nature.

TEXT OF THE PLAY

The Tempest was written in late 1610 or 1611, for several of its sources were not available until at least the late summer of 1610; a performance—not necessarily the first—occurred on November 1, 1611. Some scholars believe that *The Tempest* may be a revision of an earlier work by Shakespeare—perhaps from as early as the 1590s—but the evidence for this theory is highly tenuous, and most modern commentators assume that the play was written in a single effort.

The play was first published in the FIRST FOLIO (1623). The copy used in printing it was a transcript of either a PROMPT-BOOK or Shakespeare's FOUL PAPERS. The transcript—probably made by Ralph CRANE, whose idiosyncratic spelling and punctuation are present in the printed text—was probably made expressly for the Folio printing. As the only early version of the play, the Folio text has served as the basis for all subsequent editions.

One peculiarity of the Folio text may be suggestive of the circumstances in which the play was written: commentators have speculated that the play's elaborate stage directions may indicate that Shakespeare wrote the play in STRATFORD. Distant from the workaday world of the theatre, where the desired behaviour on stage could be established at rehearsals, Shakespeare may have felt compelled to be more specific than in earlier plays. On the other hand, these directions are like those of the courtly masque, and Shakespeare may have merely intended to stress the resemblance between masques and his play. It is also possible that the stage directions were not written by Shakespeare but were added later.

THEATRICAL HISTORY OF THE PLAY

The earliest recorded performance of *The Tempest* was at the court of King JAMES I on November 1, 1611, and it was also staged as part of the festivities surrounding the marriage of Princess ELIZABETH (3) in February 1613. (Some scholars believe that the masque of goddesses in 4.1 may have been added to the play for this performance.) No early performances in public theatres are recorded, although John DRYDEN remarked—in the preface to his adaptation of the play—that it had been performed at the BLACKFRIARS THEATRE early in the century. It is believed that Richard BURBAGE (3) originated the role of Prospero.

Dryden's adaptation, in which William DAVENANT collaborated, was called *The Tempest, or The Enchanted Island* (1667, publ. 1670). Dryden added many characters—including siblings of the opposite sex for Miranda and Ferdinand, a female monster for Caliban, and a female spirit for Ariel—and little of Shakespeare's language was retained. Also, the additions were in good part plagiarised from the Spanish playwright, Pedro Calderón (1600–1681). Though modern commentators unanimously condemn it, *The Enchanted Island* was very popular. In 1674 Thomas SHADWELL turned it into an opera, with music by several composers, including Matthew LOCKE; this work inspired a burlesque, Thomas DUFFET's *The Mock-Tempest, or The Enchanted Castle* (1674). In 1690 Henry PURCELL composed a new score for *The Enchanted Island.* This opera remained popular for a century and continued to influence later adaptations of *The Tempest* until well into the 19th century. It was revived in London in 1959, on the tercentenary of Purcell's birth.

In 1745 a brief revival of Shakespeare's play failed, and the Dryden-Davenport version reappeared the following season. David GARRICK produced another operatic version, *The Tempest* (1756), with words by

himself and Shakespeare (though very little of the original text was used) and music by John Christopher Smith (1712–1795). Immense dance numbers—one involving 60 children—were a prominent feature of this production. However, perhaps repenting, Garrick also staged Shakespeare's text in 1757, with Hannah PRITCHARD as Miranda. John Philip KEMBLE (3) revived the Dryden-Davenant version in 1789, but he included some additional Shakespearean passages and in 1806 restored much more of the original text.

In 1821 Frederic REYNOLDS (1) produced a new version of *The Enchanted Island*, with William Charles MACREADY as Prospero and with music from miscellaneous works by seven composers including Purcell, Mozart, and Rossini. The vogue for such musical pastiches of Shakespeare was past, however, and this production was not a success. Macready also played Prospero in another revival of the Dryden-Davenant *Tempest* in 1833, and then in 1838 he staged his own revival of Shakespeare's play. He cut the dialogue from 1.1 to emphasise a spectacular scenic rendering of storm and shipwreck but was otherwise reasonably faithful to the text, establishing a tradition that has not lapsed. He again played Prospero, opposite Helen FAUCIT as Miranda. Charles KEAN (1) staged a less complete but still wholly Shakespearean text in 1857, playing Prospero in a very elaborate production involving complex 'scenic appliances', as he called them, necessitating more than 140 stagehands. In the same fashion, Samuel PHELPS presented the play in 1871, with himself as Prospero, in a production featuring a proliferation of peacocks and dancers, with music by Arne and Purcell. In 1900 F. R. BENSON's *Tempest* helped introduce a more modern restraint in staging, although Beerbohm TREE continued with 19th-century extravagance in his 1904 staging, in which he played Caliban.

Among 20th-century actors, John GIELGUD has been particularly associated with *The Tempest*, playing Prospero in four noteworthy productions: two at the OLD VIC THEATRE (1930, 1940); a STRATFORD staging by Peter BROOK (2) in 1957, and a London production of 1974. James Earl JONES (1) was acclaimed as Caliban in Joseph PAPP's New York Shakespeare Festival presentation (1962). Peter HALL (5) made his directorial debut at London's National Theatre with a *Tempest* production in 1973 and ended his tenure there with another, in 1988.

In an early experiment with FILM, the opening scene of Tree's production was filmed in 1904, and the silent screen saw two full-length presentations of the play (1911, 1912). However, *The Tempest* has only once been made into a movie with sound—a purposefully bizarre version by Derek Jarman, set in an abandoned church (1970)—although a famous science-fiction film, *The Forbidden Planet* (1954), was based on it. In contrast the play has been done for TELEVISION six times, including a 1960 offering with Maurice EVANS (4) as Prospero and Richard Burton as Caliban.

Besides the operas mentioned above, *The Tempest* has inspired a number of other musical creations, including symphonic fantasies by Hector BERLIOZ (1830) and Peter Ilyich TCHAIKOVSKY (1873), and a setting by Ralph VAUGHAN WILLIAMS (1951) of Prospero's 'revels' speech and Ariel's song, 'Where the bee sucks' (4.1. 148–158; 5.1.88–94).

Terry (1), Ellen (1848–1828) British actress. Terry, the daughter of actors, was the leading Shakespearean actress of the last quarter of the 19th century and the first years of the 20th. She began her career at the age of eight, as MAMILLIUS in the *Winter's Tale* of Charles KEAN (1), and she retired after playing the NURSE (3) in a 1919 production of *Romeo and Juliet.* Between, she was chiefly associated with the company led by Henry IRVING, opposite whom she played many of Shakespeare's most important female roles, as well as many other parts, between 1878 and 1902. She was particularly noted as BEATRICE, IMOGEN, PORTIA (1), and LADY (6) MACBETH, but in all her roles she was acclaimed as one of the great actresses of all time. After a brief early marriage, she lived for a number of years with the famed architect and designer Edward Godwin (1833–1886), with whom she had two children, Gordon CRAIG (1) and the actress Edith Craig (1869–1947). She also had two later, childless marriages. Terry was a member of a sprawling theatrical family. Both her parents and her eight siblings—including Fred TERRY (2)—were in the theatre, and when she celebrated her fiftieth year on the stage, 24 relatives appeared with her in a special performance. John GIELGUD is her great-nephew.

Terry (2), Fred (1863–1933) British actor, brother of Ellen TERRY (1) and husband of Julia NEILSON (2). Terry established himself as an actor playing SEBASTIAN (2) opposite his sister's VIOLA, but he is best known as the co-star and co-manager, with his wife, of a popular theatrical company that performed in London and the British provinces between 1900 and 1930.

Tetralogy Either of two groupings of four HISTORY PLAYS that together deal with English dynastic history from just before the fall of King RICHARD II in 1399 until the battle of BOSWORTH FIELD on August 22, 1485, when the rule of the PLANTAGENET (1) family ended and that of the TUDOR family began. The two tetralogies are usually distinguished as the 'major' and the 'minor', one being regarded as much superior to the other, both as literature and as drama. The minor tetralogy, which was written in 1590 and 1591, consists of *1, 2,* and *3 Henry VI* and *Richard III,* and covers the later part of the historical period, from 1422 on. The major tetralogy is composed of *Richard II, 1* and

2 Henry IV, and *Henry V,* and it is concerned with the earlier history. It was written between 1595 and 1599.

Tewkesbury (Tewksbury) Location in *3 Henry VI,* a town near Gloucester and a battle site in the WARS OF THE ROSES. The army of Queen MARGARET (1) is defeated at Tewkesbury by that of King EDWARD IV. The battle takes place between 5.4 and 5.5; the fighting itself is not staged. In the former scene, the Queen delivers a stirring speech to her followers, and in the latter they are all captives of Edward, who, with his brothers, kills Margaret's son, the PRINCE (4) of Wales. This incident is taken from the chronicle by Edward HALL (2), but earlier accounts report the Prince was killed in combat. The battle, which was fought in May 1471, three weeks after the battle of BARNET, marked the end of Lancastrian hopes and firmly secured Edward on the throne of England.

Thaisa Character in *Pericles,* wife of PERICLES and mother of MARINA. The daughter of King SIMONIDES of PENTAPOLIS, Thaisa is the prize of a knightly tournament won by Pericles in 2.2. She marries him and sails with him to TYRE. En route, Marina is born, and Thaisa is mistakenly declared dead in childbirth and is buried at sea, in 3.1. She is revived by CERIMON in 3.2, but in 3.4, convinced she will never find Pericles again, she enters a convent dedicated to the goddess DIANA (2). She does not appear again until 5.3, when Diana sends Pericles to the temple where Thaisa serves and the two are reunited.

Thaisa's resurrection in 3.2 is one of the play's semi–supernatural marvels. What seems to be an ill-motivated retreat into a nunnery is merely a convention of romantic literature, as is her final reunion with her husband. However, she is not simply a cardboard figure. In Act 2 we see that she is a delightful, strong-minded young woman, like many of Shakespeare's other, more developed, heroines. She is delighted by Pericles' victory in the tournament, for though the exiled prince hides his identity, he seems to her 'like diamond to glass' (2.3.36). He is reluctant to press his right to marry her, so she pursues the matter and insists to her father that she'll marry Pericles 'or never more to view nor day nor light' (2.5.17). When Simonides pretends to be angry that Pericles has allegedly proposed to her, she declares, 'who takes offence / At that would make me glad?' (2.5.70–71). In the final scene, this strength of personality lends resonance to her speech as she recognises Pericles: 'Did you not name a tempest / A birth and death?' (5.3.33–34)

In the *Confessio Amantis* of John GOWER (3), Shakespeare's chief source for the play, Thaise is the name of Pericles' daughter, and his wife is nameless. Having selected the name Marina for his heroine, the playwright adapted the daughter's name for the mother The name is traditionally associated with the legendary beauty of Thais, the mistress of Alexander the Great.

Thaliard Minor character in *Pericles,* assassin sent by King ANTIOCHUS of Syria to kill PERICLES. In 1.1 Thaliard accepts his assignment with cool professionalism, but in 1.3, once he has followed Pericles to TYRE, he expresses reluctance. He declares that he only contemplates committing the deed out of fear of punishment if he refuses and a sense of obligation to his oath of loyalty to Antiochus. He is relieved to learn that his quarry has fled. Thaliard, as a potential assassin, represents an unjust fate, but he is also a victim, trapped by his place in the world. He thus is a part of a major theme of the play: that humanity is helpless in the face of destiny.

Tharsus Ancient river port, the present-day Turkish city Tarsus, the setting for a number of scenes in *Pericles.* Governed by CLEON, Tharsus is saved from imminent starvation when PERICLES arrives with supplies, in 1.4. In 3.3 Pericles leaves his infant daughter, MARINA, in the care of Cleon and his wife, DIONYZA, and in Act 4 Dionyza attempts to murder the child, who is now 14 years old. The location was provided by Shakespeare's sources, and the actual city is not in evidence.

The historical Tarsus was a wealthy city, the centre of a prosperous linen industry. First important as part of the Persian Empire and later a wealthy Hellenistic and Roman centre, it was a commercial centre of the Seleucid Empire at the time of the play. It straddled the Cydnus River and was the site of the first meeting of Mark ANTONY and CLEOPATRA (described in *Antony and Cleopatra,* 2.2.186 ff.), and the hometown of St Paul. It was notorious in classical literature for the luxurious life-style of its upper class, as is reflected in 1.4.21–31 of *Pericles.*

Theatre, The First LONDON playhouse, built by James BURBAGE (2) in 1576. The Theatre was built on leased land in Shoreditch, a northern suburb just beyond the jurisdiction of the London city government, which was controlled by Puritans who were opposed to theatrical entertainment on moral grounds. Before the Theatre was built, plays were performed in inn yards or other buildings not intended for the purpose. No reliable image of Burbage's theatre exists, but it was apparently a polygonal, roughly cylindrical, three-story structure built around an open, unroofed central space. There were rows of galleries overlooking the centre at each level. The stage projected from one sector of the building into the centre, with the building above it reserved for backstage areas (see ELIZABETHAN THEATRE). A number of acting companies played at the Theatre during its lifetime: LEICESTER'S MEN from 1576 to 1578, one of the groups known as OXFORD'S MEN on occasions between 1579 and 1582, the

QUEEN'S MEN (1) between 1583 and 1589, both the ADMIRAL'S MEN and STRANGE'S MEN in 1590–1591, and the CHAMBERLAIN'S MEN after 1594. The Theatre was also used for fencing competitions and other activities. When the theatres were closed by the royal government in July 1597 after the *Isle of Dogs* scandal (see NASHE, PEMBROKE'S MEN, CENSORSHIP), the Theatre did not reopen. Burbage's ground lease had expired the previous April, just after he had died and left the Theatre and its lease to his son Cuthbert BURBAGE (1). After long negotiations, Cuthbert could not come to terms with the landowner, and in December 1598 he and a group of associates disassembled the building and used the lumber to build the GLOBE THEATRE.

Thebes Ancient Greek city, setting for several scenes of *The Two Noble Kinsmen.* In 1.2 the noblemen PALAMON and ARCITE contemplate the evils of life at the court of King Creon of Thebes and decide to leave the city. However, before they can do so, THESEUS (2), Duke of ATHENS, attacks Thebes, and the two young men are honour-bound to fight. Thus, they become prisoners of war in Athens, where most of the play takes place. In 1.4–5 Theseus permits Creon's victims to bury their dead, presumably outside the walls of the city.

There is nothing specifically Theban, or even Greek, about any of these scenes. Shakespeare took the location, along with the idea of Theban corruption, from his source, Geoffrey CHAUCER's 'The Knight's Tale'; Chaucer in turn was responding to an ancient tradition of conflict between the heroic Theseus and the villainous Creon over the latter's refusal to allow the burial of his slain foes.

Theobald, Lewis (1688–1744) English scholar, the third editor of Shakespeare's collected works. A hack writer, translator, and minor producer of theatrical pantomimes, Theobald published a critique of the edition of the plays published by Alexander POPE (1)—for which he was made the protagonist of Pope's scathing satire *The Dunciad* (1728). He went on to produce his own edition in 1733. He was the first scholar to point to the importance of PLUTARCH and Raphael HOLINSHED as sources for the plays. Though Theobald's work was superseded later in the century by such great scholars as Edward CAPELL and Edmond MALONE, his work was extremely valuable, and many of his emendations have remained standard.

Thersites Legendary figure and character in *Troilus and Cressida,* the jester, or FOOL (1), to AJAX and ACHILLES. Thersites rails against everyone he encounters, and his diatribes are vicious and hateful. He is also a coward who avoids combat by unashamedly declaring himself too roguish a person to be fought by a chivalrous knight. The unhealthy aura of disgust that distinguishes this play and contributes greatly to its satire owes much to Thersites' outbursts. Thersites is not likeable, but his language is inventive and funny, and he is capable of amusing imitations of his targets, especially when he enacts the prideful Ajax in 3.3.279–302. Further, his perception of the follies of the warriors of the TROJAN WAR is refreshingly acute, and we respect his capacity to see through the combatants' pretensions to reason and honour when they persist in fighting a sordid, irrational war.

Thersites is a composite of two ancient character types: the boastful MILES GLORIOSUS, a braggart soldier; and the scathing critic, a sort of CHORUS (1), whose usually comic commentary provides telling asides on the main action. As a court jester, he is licenced to insult his superiors, and he thus resembles, in a perverse way, other Shakespearean fools such as FESTE and the FOOL (2) in *King Lear.* However, unlike them, Thersites is 'lost in the labyrinth of [his] fury' (2.3.1–2), and his obscene jests often tell us more about his own disturbed nature than about the warriors he mocks. He displays a morbid excitement when other characters are suffering most, as when he cries out, 'Now the pledge: now, now, now!' (5.2.65), when TROILUS witnesses CRESSIDA surrendering to DIOMEDES (1) the token he had given her. Moreover, he often directs his venom at himself, declaring, for example, 'I am a rascal . . . a very filthy rogue' (5.4.28–29), and 'I am a bastard . . . I am bastard begot, bastard instructed, bastard in mind, bastard in valour, in everything illegitimate' (5.7.16–18). Thersites' pathology has dramatic value, heightening the sense of disease that the play's world conveys.

Thersites plays a similar, though much less prominent, role in the *Iliad* of HOMER, the ultimate source of the drama. In one episode, he rails at AGAMEMNON until Odysseus (Shakespeare's ULYSSES) beats him into silence. In a later tradition, Achilles kills him for insulting him while he is in mourning for an Amazon queen he has slain in combat.

Theseus (1) Character in *A Midsummer Night's Dream,* the Duke of ATHENS. Theseus' wedding to Queen HIPPOLYTA (1) is the climax towards which the play moves. He is a sympathetic lover, though, as a middle-aged man, he is not given to the passions of youth. He is responsive to Hippolyta's moods, noting, for example, her distress at the plight of HERMIA in 1.1.122. Hermia's situation disturbs Theseus, too; it raises an issue that was important to Shakespeare—the relationship between authority and the law. Theseus is a model ruler who respects the laws of his domain, but he regrets the harsh consequences that they may entail for Hermia. He will attempt to help her by persuading EGEUS and DEMETRIUS (2) with 'private schooling' (1.1.116); but if that effort fails, he is committed to carrying out the law.

Theseus is a constitutional monarch, as the TUDOR rulers of England declared themselves to be. Thus he is associated with Queen ELIZABETH (1). A closer identification of the two is implied in 5.1.89–105, in which Theseus proclaims that he responds favourably to his citizens' speeches of welcome, even when, hopelessly tongue-tied, they fail to speak at all. Elizabeth was known to take great pride in doing the same thing, and this passage is thought to embody a compliment to the sovereign and thus to suggest that she was present to receive it at the first performance of the play.

Theseus (2) Character in *The Two Noble Kinsmen,* Duke of ATHENS. Theseus presides over the events of the main plot. He sets an example of noble action when he aids the royal widows (see QUEEN [1]) who petition him in 1.1; in doing so, he undertakes a war against Creon of THEBES, in the course of which he captures the title characters, ARCITE and PALAMON, creating the basic situation of the plot. In 3.6 he intervenes in the quarrel between them, overseeing their duel for EMILIA (4); and at the play's close, he sounds the note of dignified acceptance of fate that is the play's central lesson. Recognising that the fortunes of humanity are incomprehensible, and that we have no choice but to live with them, he rhetorically addresses the gods: 'O you heavenly charmers, / What things you make of us! . . . Let us be thankful / For that which is, and with you leave dispute[s] / That are above our question' (5.4.131–136). He adds, in the play's final words, 'Let's go off, / And bear us like the time' (5.4. 136–137)—that is, accept our circumstances.

Theseus is particularly dominant in Acts 1 and 5, written by Shakespeare, while in Acts 2 to 4, written by John FLETCHER (2), he is a less significant figure and his speeches are far less powerful as poetry. Theseus' importance as a model of nobility is particularly notable in Act 1, where he establishes a tone of magnanimity that would perhaps have dominated the play, had Shakespeare written it in its entirety. Throughout Shakespeare's portions of the play, Theseus' actions are quintessentially chivalrous: he aids the widowed Queens at their request; having triumphed in their cause, he offers to cover the expenses of their husbands' funerals; he demands the finest treatment for his noble prisoners of war; he orders the most opulent temple preparations for the 'noble work in hand' (5.1.6), the duel; he 'adopts' (5.4.124) Palamon's seconds at the play's close; and his concluding remarks offer an example of serene courage. On the other hand, the somewhat ignoble provision that the loser be executed was devised by Fletcher's Theseus.

With respect to aristocratic birth—a necessary component of nobility in chivalric romance—Theseus is literally of supernatural stature and can casually refer to 'Hercules our kinsman' (1.1.66). He is pointedly contrasted with the vicious Creon, to his considerable advantage, and the Second Queen says that he was 'Born to uphold creation in that honour / First Nature styled it in' (1.1.82–83). As the highest-ranking figure in the play's world, and especially since he is presented as a strikingly noble leader, Theseus carries great moral weight; his closing remarks are thereby clearly signalled as the play's essential position.

Thidias Character in *Antony and Cleopatra,* a diplomat who represents Octavius CAESAR (2). In 3.12 Caesar sends Thidias to CLEOPATRA—in the wake of her and ANTONY's defeat at the battle of ACTIUM—to promise her whatever she wishes if she will abandon Antony. In 3.13 Thidias receives from Cleopatra a lavish declaration of allegiance to Caesar, but as he kisses her hand as a formal token of this new diplomatic relationship, Antony appears. 'I am Antony yet' (3.13.93), he says furiously, and he has Thidias taken away to be whipped. A SERVANT (22) returns to report that Thidias begged for mercy during this punishment. Antony sends him back to Caesar with an angry message of defiance, and tells him that if he wants revenge he should whip one Hipparchus, a freed slave of Antony's now in Caesar's service. The episode demonstrates Antony's continuing vitality, but also the disturbed state of his mind.

In Shakespeare's source, Thomas NORTH's translation of PLUTARCH's *Lives,* Caesar's representative is named Thyreus, and many editions of the play, beginning with that of Lewis THEOBALD (1733), use this name. Presumably, Shakespeare simply misremembered the name of this minor character. (In fact, North himself was mistaken, for the ambassador in Plutarch is named Thyrsus, a figure otherwise unknown in history.)

Thief Character in *Timon of Athens.* See BANDIT.

Third Murderer Minor character in *Macbeth,* one of the assassins hired by MACBETH to kill BANQUO and FLEANCE. The Third Murderer joins his colleagues as they approach their targets. He was not with them when they were recruited in 3.1, and they initially distrust him, but his exact instructions convince them that he has been sent by Macbeth. His presence suggests that with the distrust typical of despots, Macbeth has felt the need to plant an agent among his hired assassins. The Third Murderer is indistinguishable from his fellows and speaks only a few brief lines.

Thomas, Friar Character in *Measure for Measure.* See FRIAR (1).

Thomas Lord Cromwell Anonymous play formerly attributed to Shakespeare, part of the Shakespeare APOCRYPHA. *Thomas Lord Cromwell* is a historical drama set in the time of King HENRY VIII. It was published by

William JONES (4) in 1602 as 'written by W. S.', possibly with the intention of associating the play with Shakespeare. It was also included among Shakespeare's plays in the Third and Fourth FOLIOS and in the editions of Nicholas ROWE and Alexander POPE (1). Scholars are certain, however, that Shakespeare did not write it, for it is a badly structured, poorly written drama that is clearly not as good as even the least of Shakespeare's genuine work. Its authorship remains uncertain, though Michael DRAYTON and Thomas HEYWOOD (2) are often nominated.

Thorndike, Sybil (1882–1976) British actress. Thorndike was noted for a number of Shakespearean roles, especially LADY (6) MACBETH, Queen KATHERINE, CONSTANCE, and VOLUMNIA. Much of her career was spent on tour, from her travels to America with Ben GREET's company in the early days of the century to her performances in occupied Europe in 1945. She also played often with the OLD VIC THEATRE company.

Thorpe, Thomas (active 1584–1625) Bookseller and publisher in LONDON, producer of the first edition of Shakespeare's SONNETS. Thorpe's 1609 QUARTO edition of the *Sonnets*, known as Q, bears the obscure dedication to 'Mr W. H'. that has baffled commentators ever since. Signed 'T. T.', this gnomic utterance seems to justify Thorpe's nickname, 'Odd'. Thorpe published a variety of other works, including John MARSTON's *The Malcontent* (1604).

Thurio Minor character in *The Two Gentlemen of Verona*, a suitor of SILVIA. Thurio is inveigled by PROTEUS into hiring a group of musicians to serenade Silvia, but Proteus takes credit with the lady. At the close of the play, Thurio claims Silvia's hand, but beats a cowardly retreat when challenged by VALENTINE (2).

Thyreus Character in *Antony and Cleopatra*. See THIDIAS.

Tieck, Ludwig (1773–1853) German poet, novelist, and literary critic, editor of the German translation of Shakespeare's plays begun by A. W. SCHELEGEL. The Schlegel-Tieck translation, as it is known in Germany, was not actually translated by Tieck. The 19 plays left undone by Schlegel were translated by his daughter, Dorothea Tieck, and another translator, Wolf Baudisson. They produced German texts which Tieck edited. The plays were published between 1823 and 1829. The completed collection is still regarded as a major masterpiece of German literature. Tieck was considered the leading German scholar of Shakespeare and ELIZABETHAN DRAMA, and his *Anglisches Theatre* (1811) was for many years a basic text. He was called upon to participate in productions of English plays, and in 1827 he staged *A Midsummer Night's Dream* in Schlegel's translation. This was the first presentation of the complete play since Shakespeare's time.

As a creative writer, Tieck was an important figure in the German Romantic movement and was especially noted for stories dealing with horror and the supernatural, as well as with the glorification of art as the only thing in life worth pursuing. He was at one time considered the equal of GOETHE, though his reputation declined before his death, and little of his work has appeal for modern readers.

Tillyard, E. M. W. (1889–1962) English scholar. Tillyard is best known for *The Elizabethan World Picture* (1943), an analysis of the political thought underlying the HISTORY PLAYS and Shakespeare's work in general. He argued that the plays endorse the pervasive ideas of Shakespeare's period, offering a conservative view of society and placing a high value on an orderly hierarchical system guaranteed by divine authority. More recent scholars tend to find this view too rigid in light of the rapidity of change in 16th-century England. Tillyard also wrote other influential works on both Shakespeare and John MILTON.

Timandra Character in *Timon of Athens*. See PHRYNIA AND TIMANDRA.

Time Allegorical figure who appears as a CHORUS (1) in *The Winter's Tale*. Time appears only in 4.1, where, alone on the stage, he informs us that 16 years will have passed before the play resumes in BOHEMIA. He briefly sums up the intervening years for King LEONTES and PERDITA and tells us we shall meet FLORIZEL, the son of King POLIXENES. After wishing the audience a good time, he withdraws. This isolated speech, which is virtually a PROLOGUE (1), makes it clear that we are about to witness a new drama altogether. From Time's pleasant, mildly humorous manner, we sense that the TRAGEDY of the first half of the play will be replaced by a COMEDY.

Time's stilted language, which sounded somewhat old-fashioned even in Shakespeare's day, is arranged in rhyming couplets, unlike the speech of any other character. This is appropriate to his singular role, for as a chorus, Time is outside the world of the play and should not sound like anyone in it. Time says, 'remember well / I mentioned a son o' th' king's' (4.1. 21–22), referring to earlier passages (1.2.34, 165–170) where Florizel was spoken of but not named; the use of the first person singular here has suggested to some commentators that Time represents the author of the play—Shakespeare himself. However, this is unlikely, for as a virtually abstract figure, Time is distinctly not human. He is expressly immune from the change he brings to others—'The same I am, ere ancient'st order was, / Or what is now receiv'd' (4.1.10–11)—and as he is winged, he is visually non-human as well. The refer-

ence to his having 'mentioned' simply means—with the mild humour that characterises this figure—that the mentioning occurred in the past, which is a function of time.

Timon Title character of *Timon of Athens*, a benevolent nobleman of ATHENS who is abandoned by his false friends when he is bankrupted by his extravagant hospitality and gift giving. He then sinks into rage and despair. He withdraws to the wilderness where he rages against humanity and dies in abject misery, an apparent suicide. He is the victim of his own excesses of both goodness and hatred.

Timon's excessive generosity is based in misplaced pride, for he attempts to embody an unrealistic ideal of friendship. When he refuses to be repaid for a debt, he says irrationally that 'there's none / Can truly say he gives, if he receives' (1.2.10–11). This absoluteness is unhealthy, for it leaves no room for a sensitive and intelligent approach to life. Timon is blind and gullible, and he ignores the sound, if unpleasantly put, advice of APEMANTUS. When he is rejected by his so-called friends he assumes an extreme degree of misanthropy, a response that is excessive even given his great provocation. Timon presumes that all of humankind is greedy and dishonest, but this is clearly contradicted by the virtues of his own household (see SERVANT [23]), especially his STEWARD (2). He refuses to accept this evidence, however, and drives himself to a death as unnecessary as his financial losses were. At the play's close, the reconciliation effected by ALCIBIADES cements our awareness that Timon has tragically wasted his life.

Nevertheless, Timon is a noble figure, for he tries to live up to an ideal conception of humanity. Before his collapse he desires the finest in human relationships, and while this has the effect of insulating him from reality, it also exalts him. It is both symbolically and psychologically appropriate that when he becomes disillusioned Timon succumbs to another excessive vision of humanity. Obsessive by nature, he can only go from one extreme to another. In both cases, the position he takes is grandiose, capable of inspiring awe along with dismay.

Like most of the characters in the play, Timon is not a fully fleshed-out human being. He is more like an allegorical figure, similar to those of the medieval MORALITY PLAY, a probable influence on Shakespeare's creation of this work. In fact, Timon assumes two such roles in the course of the play, first representing ideal friendship and then extreme despair. As a misanthrope, Timon had been a famous figure for many centuries before Shakespeare's time, but the playwright attempted to demonstrate the defects of the character both before and after his catastrophe, and thus to make a profound moral statement of the sort presented in the morality plays. Although *Timon* is an unfinished play, we can still recognise in its title character the representation of a human truth: that we are susceptible to vain and prideful extremes of behaviour.

Timon of Athens

SYNOPSIS

Act 1, Scene 1

In ATHENS a POET (2), a PAINTER (1), a JEWELLER, and a MERCHANT (2) expect payment from the generous nobleman, TIMON, for their efforts to please him. Timon arrives and promises a MESSENGER (28) that he will pay the debts of VENTIDIUS (2), which will free him from prison. He promises a fortune to his servant LUCILIUS (2) so that he may marry the daughter of an aristocratic OLD ATHENIAN. The philosopher APEMANTUS appears, and the company prepares to be insulted by his heavy wit. Indulged by Timon, Apemantus denounces each of them as a dishonest flatterer. ALCIBIADES arrives, and Timon invites them all to dinner.

Act 1, Scene 2

At Timon's great banquet, Ventidius, whose father has left him a fortune, offers to repay Timon the money he had lent him, but Timon refuses to accept it. Apemantus criticises Timon's greedy followers who consume his banquet, but Timon praises them for the help he knows they would give if it were needed. A MASQUE is performed, and Apemantus rages against the vanity of such things. Timon offers expensive gifts to his guests. His STEWARD (2) worries that such generosity has put Timon deep in debt. Apemantus refuses to seek gifts from Timon because it would be sinful to encourage the nobleman's fondness for flattery.

Act 2, Scene 1

A SENATOR (4) who knows of Timon's excessive generosity decides to send his servant, CAPHIS, to collect the debt Timon owes him before it is too late.

Act 2, Scene 2

Caphis, VARRO'S SERVANT, and ISIDORE'S SERVANT accost Timon when they arrive to collect debts from him. He is astonished, and his Steward has to point out that he has refused to oversee his accounts despite all urging, and that now the debts caused by his generosity cannot be paid because even his lands are already mortgaged. Timon hopes to borrow money from his friends, and sends FLAMINIUS, SERVILIUS, another SERVANT (23), and the Steward to LUCIUS (3), LUCULLUS, SEMPRONIUS, and Ventidius, respectively.

Act 3, Scene 1

Lucullus refuses to lend money to Timon and offers to bribe Flaminius if he will say he could not find him to request the loan. Flaminius curses him.

Act 3, Scene 2
Lucius hears of Lucullus' behaviour and swears that he would have loaned Timon the money, but when Servilius arrives to ask him for a loan, he refuses and claims to have no funds available.

Act 3, Scene 3
Timon's Servant tells Sempronius that his master's other friends have refused to lend money, whereupon Sempronius claims to be offended that he was not asked first and therefore refuses to help.

Act 3, Scene 4
LUCIUS' SERVANT meets the Servants of Varro, TITUS (2), HORTENSIUS, and PHILOTUS, all of whom hope to collect money from Timon. They regret the thanklessness of their masters, who have benefited by Timon's generosity and now will not forgive him his debts. Timon appears in a rage and insists that they will have to cut up his body as payment; the servants realise they will get no money, and they leave. Timon tells the Steward to send out messages to all of his friends inviting them to an immense banquet.

Act 3, Scene 5
Alcibiades seeks mercy from the Senators for a friend who has killed someone in a fight. They refuse, but he continues to argue, and claims that his friend should be spared because he has served as a soldier. Offended that he will not accept their decision, the Senators banish Alcibiades from Athens. He vows to take revenge on the city with his army.

Act 3, Scene 6
Timon's friends assemble at the banquet and make excuses for not having assisted him. They hope to receive expensive gifts, as before. Timon formally curses the guests and drives them away.

Act 4, Scene 1
As he leaves Athens, Timon maliciously wishes evil on all elements of society.

Act 4, Scene 2
Timon's Steward and several of his former Servants part sorrowfully. The Steward soliloquises on the pointlessness of wealth and the foolishness of man. He vows to find Timon and to continue serving him.

Act 4, Scene 3
Timon, alone in the wilderness, denounces humanity. As he digs for roots, he finds gold. He curses it as a great evil and decides to distribute it and thereby destroy society. Alcibiades appears; Timon rejects his offer of friendship but is pleased to hear of his plan to conquer Athens, and he urges him to be brutal. Alcibiades departs, and Apemantus arrives. He offers food, but Timon refuses it with curses, and Apemantus observes that Timon is as extreme in his disgust as he once was in his generosity. The two misanthropes remark on the faults of humanity and then fall into an exchange of insults. As Apemantus leaves, a group of thieves arrives. Timon sarcastically praises them for taking what they want and compares them with thieves who purport to be good citizens. He gives each BANDIT gold. They leave, as the Steward arrives. His compassion moves Timon to relent and concede that one honest man lives, but he refuses to be served by him and drives him away.

Act 5, Scene 1
The Poet and the Painter have heard that Timon has gold, and they seek him in the woods. They intend to promise him great works so that he will give them gifts. Timon overhears their plans and pretends to trust them. He gives them gold as he denounces them and drives them away. Two Senators arrive and ask for Timon's help against Alcibiades. They offer to restore his wealth if he will return to Athens. He refuses and grimly delights in the atrocities he anticipates Alcibiades will visit on the city. He advises Athenians to hang themselves, and declares that he will leave a gravestone with further advice.

Act 5, Scene 2
Some Senators hear of Alcibiades' approach with a large army and then of Timon's refusal of support.

Act 5, Scene 3
As he seeks Timon with a message from Alcibiades, a SOLDIER (13) finds a bitter note that announces Timon's death. He also sees a gravestone inscribed in a language he cannot read. He makes a copy of it to take to Alcibiades.

Act 5, Scene 4
A delegation of Senators seeks mercy from Alcibiades, and he promises that he will only take revenge on the few people who had offended him. The Soldier arrives with the gravestone text, which restates Timon's hatred of humanity. Alcibiades mourns for his friend's state of mind at death as he enters the city and vows to make a lasting peace in Athens.

COMMENTARY

Timon of Athens is an experimental and ambiguous play. So much so, in fact, that this bleak picture of misanthropy is sometimes classed as a COMEDY by editors and commentators. Though its presentation of a grand figure whose downfall results from his own shortcomings is chiefly tragic, *Timon* is also like a comedy in its final statement of reconciliation and in its considerable dose of social satire. In his attempt to combine such different themes, Shakespeare was continuing a line of experiments that included the PROBLEM PLAYS and was to culminate in the ROMANCES. *Timon* is an important step in this development, though its own contradictions remain unresolved.

The play reflects a 17th-century enthusiasm for social satire. Its crass Athenian money-grubbers, who coolly resort to preposterous excuses when they refuse to return Timon's generosity, resemble the Londoners of Ben JONSON's more overtly satirical comedies. Shakespeare's Athenians are very bitterly drawn—Alcibiades illustrates the play's tone when he solemnly calls the city a 'coward and lascivious town' (5.4.1). The critique of Timon's false friends is often straightforward and uncompromising, as in the First Stranger's remarks in 3.2, but sharp comedy is nonetheless present.

In particular, Apemantus' speeches are full of crude jokes, as when he counters the insult, 'Y'are a dog' with 'Thy mother's of my generation' (1.1.200–201). Though the level of his humour is low, he is a typical ill-tempered buffoon of the 17th-century stage and is clearly intended as a comic figure. In fact, Apemantus' viciousness is often so exaggerated that it is comical in itself, which is characteristic of *Timon,* for the play's humour resides more in its situations than in its dialogue. Apemantus closely resembles Shakespeare's THERSITES, of *Troilus and Cressida.* In Act 3 the sequence of hypocritical excuses offered by Timon's supposed friends as they refuse him assistance is amusing; we appreciate these men as comic misers. Timon's story was well known in Shakespeare's time, and he knew his audience would gleefully anticipate the absurd refusals of these familiar character types. Timon's mock banquet in 3.6 is likewise comic in its use of surprises anticipated by the audience but not by the guests. The hypocrisy of his miserly friends as they make excuses to each other for being unable to help their host—though they can find time to dine with him—is broadly humorous. Even in the midst of Timon's grimly inhuman transformation in Act 4, we see humour when Phrynia and Timandra encourage gross insults about themselves, so long as those insults are accompanied by gold. This behaviour was traditionally associated with a comic stage figure, the greedy whore.

Timon's humorous aspects serve a serious purpose, and Shakespeare emphasised this by fashioning the drama to resemble the medieval MORALITY PLAY, which was intended to educate by combining moral lessons with vibrant, often comical entertainment. Because of this resemblance, *Timon* would have reminded 17th-century audiences that such a lesson was being offered. Following the morality tradition closely, *Timon* presents an hero who is totally involved in the material world and only realises its deficiencies when he encounters catastrophe and is rejected by his materialistic friends. Also like a morality, the play features many allegorical characters who symbolise particular vices and virtues. Timon symbolises two: ideal friendship at first and misanthropy later. It is even thought that the most famous morality play, *Everyman,* may have particularly influenced the creation of *Timon.* However, in contrast with morality plays—a contrast much more obvious in the 17th century than it is today—*Timon* does not end with the hero's triumphant return to a proper appreciation of spiritual values, but rather with his decline into despair and a miserable death.

Timon can also be classed as a comedy because it culminates in a spirit of reconciliation. The traditional comedy ended in a spirit of wholesale reconciliation usually represented by a marriage, for like the morality play, it was intended to impart a sense of moral worth. Though *Timon* contains no hint of romantic love, it does nevertheless end in reconciliation and is therefore comedic in this most basic sense. With Alcibiades' ultimate rejection of vengeance when he declares he will 'use the olive with my sword, / Make war breed peace, make peace stint war' (5.4.82–83), the play offers a final contrast with Timon's story. Alcibiades' response to the cold ingratitude of Athens is to take action in the real world rather than to dwell in helpless rancour. All along, this response inspires our sympathy more than Timon's monstrous misanthropy, and Alcibiades' story culminates on a fittingly positive note. Timon's decline has ended tragically, but the playwright gives us a final statement that demonstrates the play's ultimate theme: the greater importance of mercy as opposed to justice.

Nevertheless, *Timon* is also distinctly tragic. The protagonist is elevated above his fellow Athenians by his conspicuous kindness and generosity, and comes to his downfall through the same traits. We are made aware of the fateful vulnerability of human existence, as we are in such greater tragedies as *King Lear* and *Othello.* However, unlike in *King Lear,* with which *Timon* is commonly compared, compassion is seemingly defeated, as Timon rejects the efforts of the loyal Steward to offer comfort and turns instead to brooding exile. Alcibiades' reconciliation at the play's close comes too late for Timon. Like CORIOLANUS, Timon insists on a world of moral absolutes—he prides himself first on his ideal generosity and then on his extreme bitterness—and he is unable to accept that moral absolutes are not reliable guides to social behaviour. He is isolated from the realities of the world, and his retreat into misanthropy is a psychologically plausible response to his disillusion—from one extreme, he can only leap to another. His moral sensibility is arguably noble in that it is superior to ordinary life, but this is also his tragic failing, for he cannot understand the practicality and compromise on which social behaviour rests.

Significantly, it is a Senator, one of the governors of Athens, who first decides to call in Timon's debts, in 2.1, for the role of the state in *Timon* is crucial. In 3.5 the Senators banish Alcibiades when he seeks mercy for a deserving veteran. Here they demonstrate a basic failing, a legalistic and uncharitable demand for abso-

lute obedience. In this absoluteness they parallel Timon; also, their ingratitude to the veteran is like the ingratitude that they (and others) show to Timon. Later, their hypocrisy when they attempt to recruit Timon to help defend the city against Alcibiades reminds us of the Lords who flock to Timon's banquet in 3.6 after they have refused to help him. Thus, the evils of the play's world are summed up in the behaviour of its leaders. This is highly important, for the callousness of the Senators and the other aristocrats produces a potential civic disaster—Alcibiades' threatened sack of the city—and thus demonstrates one of Shakespeare's favourite lessons; the immorality of a ruling class leads to catastrophe for the society as a whole. This theme is central both to the comedic tale of Alcibiades' exile and return, and to the tragic story of Timon's psychological collapse.

Like the problem plays, *Timon* addresses public issues with a disconcerting combination of humour and villainy. With its tragicomic mingling of themes, combined with its seemingly old-fashioned allegorical quality and the startling bitterness of its main plot, *Timon* was definitely an experimental play. For centuries, commentators have generally felt that the experiment was a failure, despite the play's many fine moments. (However, 20th-century readers tend to find its ambiguities—often the focus of earlier criticism—more intriguing than faulty.) Because it is centred on a character whose shallowness is evident both before and after his catastrophe, the play does not achieve the grandeur of the great Shakespearean tragedies. Timon's madness is not resolved through any final self-awareness, as in the cases of the other tragic heroes. A lesser figure, Alcibiades, provides the reconciliation at the end, and though his mercy extends to the 'fault forgiven' of 'noble Timon' (5.4.79, 80), Timon himself is excluded from it. Finally, the excesses that define Timon—his belief first that humanity is worthy of ideal friendship and then that it is only capable of evil—prevent him from having any meaningful interaction with his fellow human beings, to the detriment of the play. The hero is initially aloof, and when brought low, his response is essentially withdrawal rather than opposition; such a moral and psychological progression is perhaps better illuminated in an essay or novel than on the stage.

Shakespeare presumably shared such misgivings, for it seems probable that he abandoned the play before it was complete. However, the experiment was not wasted, for *Timon* marks a stage in the evolution of the playwright's work. The romances, soon to come, treat the same themes—exile and return, the deficiency of moral absoluteness, the transcendent value of mercy—and they do so in a fashion that may reflect lessons learned from *Timon.* The inhuman response of an aggrieved protagonist is no longer the dominant element in the plot; instead, attention centres on the innocent victims of such inhumanity, who typically are driven to the exile that Timon chooses for himself. Even so, the exile is not the crucial phenomenon that it is in *Timon.* In the romances, Shakespeare expands his concerns and explores communal attitudes with a focus on many characters. The somewhat esoteric, allegorical figures of *Timon* evolve into the symbolic yet lifelike caricatures of injured innocence and vague, impersonal villainy that animate the later plays. Moreover, the effect of change on behaviour, an imperfectly developed aspect of *Timon,* becomes increasingly important, for the world of the last plays is powerfully charged with changeability.

The Tempest is a partial exception to some of these ideas, but it is there, in Shakespeare's final triumph, that a theme from *Timon of Athens* is displayed most spectacularly. The humane and conciliatory attitude of Alcibiades becomes the essential theme throughout, while in *Timon* its development is late and insubstantial. Thus, this flawed work retains its interest—aside from its many fine passages and strong theatrical presence—as an excellent demonstration of Shakespeare's continued growth as a playwright late in his career.

SOURCES OF THE PLAY

Shakespeare employed several sources in writing *Timon of Athens.* Numerous elements of the plot come from a Greek comic dialogue of the 2nd century A.D., *Timon the Misanthrope,* by LUCIAN. While Shakespeare may have known this work in Latin, French, or Italian translation, no English version existed in his day. He may merely have been told of its features, for actual echoes of Lucian in the play are obscure, if present at all.

Alternatively, he may have used another source based on Lucian, the so-called 'old *Timon*', an anonymous English play of uncertain date (c. 1580–1610). This work, which has survived in manuscript, contains material that is found only in itself and Shakespeare's *Timon*—such as the mock banquet of 3.6—and thus appears to be a source. However, it may be *later* than Shakespeare's *Timon* and is in any case very different, being a farce. Scholars think that if it is earlier than Shakespeare's play, both works are based on a yet earlier work, now lost, derived from Lucian.

Shakespeare certainly knew Timon's story from the 'Life of Marcus Antonius' in Thomas NORTH's translation of PLUTARCH's *Lives* (1579), the chief source for *Antony and Cleopatra.* Mark ANTONY after losing the battle of ACTIUM is compared to the famous Athenian misanthrope, whose story is briefly recounted. Some details appear in *Timon.* Plutarch's 'Life of Alcibiades', though it contains nothing specifically reflected in Shakespeare, may have provided some ideas for that character as well. Also, many of the incongruously Latin names of *Timon*'s Athenians come from else-

where in Plutarch. Lastly, Shakespeare may have taken minor elements from another version of Timon's story, that in *Palace of Pleasure* (1566) by William PAINTER (2).

Another possible source for some details and perhaps an overall concept is the MORALITY PLAY *Everyman* (c. 1500). This work contains passages that correspond to the introductory observations on prodigality by the Poet, in 1.1.53–90, and to the triple rejection of Timon by his friends in 3.1–3. Also, *Timon* reflects the morality play's overall theme of a representative sinner who is urged to reform by various figures that correspond to Apemantus, the Steward, and Alcibiades, with the important difference that in *Everyman* the hero does reform, while Timon dies in despair. This was perhaps intended as a purposeful contrast, for the morality play model was extremely familiar to Shakespeare's audience.

TEXT OF THE PLAY

The many flaws of *Timon*—irregularities of verse, confusion as to the names of many minor characters, the presence of a GHOST CHARACTER, and so on—inspired the traditional hypothesis that the play was written collaboratively: either Shakespeare completed someone else's work or someone else completed his. Many possible co-authors have been suggested—including George CHAPMAN, John DAY, Thomas MIDDLETON, and George WILKINS—but scholars have generally come to the conclusion that the play is simply incomplete. Its difficulties make it clear that no one fixed up anyone else's text, for the play is not fixed. In fact, among the play's fascinations are a number of passages in which we can see Shakespeare's drafts for BLANK VERSE, with many lines still metrically irregular but carrying their information (e.g., 1.2.190–202). Shakespeare had not yet polished this work to his usual standards when he stopped working on it.

Just when he did so cannot be determined at all precisely, but scholar's assign *Timon* to c. 1606–1608. It contains no datable references to the real world, and there are no surviving references to it prior to its publication, which came after Shakespeare's death. However, its stylistic and thematic similarities with the later tragedies favour the idea that it was written around the same time as those works. The common source with *Antony and Cleopatra* (1606–1608) seems to narrow the date still further.

Timon was first published in the FIRST FOLIO (1623). The varied speech headings and obviously literary stage directions make it clear that the text was taken from Shakespeare's FOUL PAPERS, perhaps as transcribed for the purpose. As the only early text, the First Folio's *Timon* has been the basis for all subsequent editions.

THEATRICAL HISTORY OF THE PLAY

No record of any early performance of *Timon* has survived, and since the play seems unfinished, it was probably never staged in Shakespeare's day. It has indeed been very infrequently performed in any period and has always been one of the least popular of Shakespeare's plays. Thomas SHADWELL presented an adaptation, *Timon of Athens the Man-Hater* (1678), that incorporated a love interest and made other great changes. This production, in which Thomas BETTERTON played Timon, was reasonably popular and was restaged several times until 1745. At different times, Barton BOOTH (1) played both Alcibiades and Timon in this version, and James QUIN was a notable Apemantus. It is believed that Shakespeare's text was staged in Dublin in 1761, though little is known of this production. Unsuccessful adaptations that combined Shadwell and Shakespeare and new material in various proportions were produced by James DANCE, Richard CUMBERLAND, and Thomas HULL, in 1768, 1771, and 1786, respectively.

Another version, close to Shakespeare's play but incorporating some of Cumberland's text, was devised by George LAMB (2) and produced in 1816 by Edmund KEAN (2), who was acclaimed in the title role. The original Shakespearean text was not finally staged until 1851—its earliest known production in England—by Samuel PHELPS, who likewise triumphed as Timon. This extremely popular presentation was revived in 1856. In 1892 F. R. BENSON (1) offered a three-act version at the SADLER'S WELLS THEATRE.

The play has continued to be unpopular, and it has been performed only rarely in the 20th century. Perhaps the best-known production starred Ralph RICHARDSON (2) as Timon at the OLD VIC THEATRE in 1956. *Timon* has never been a movie and has only been produced for TELEVISION once, by Jonathan MILLER (2) in 1981, as part of the British Broadcasting Corporation's complete cycle of Shakespeare plays.

Titania Character in *A Midsummer Night's Dream,* the Fairy Queen, wife of OBERON and, temporarily, the magically charmed lover of BOTTOM. Titania's infatuation with Bottom is Oberon's revenge on her for having persisted in keeping a changeling whom he wants. She asserts that she will keep the boy in memory of his mother, who died in childbirth. She is icily haughty and insists on having her way, although, since she and Oberon are elemental forces of nature, their dispute is causing bad weather, as she vividly describes in 2.1. 88–117. During her enchantment she is a vapid lover, and afterwards she merely serves a decorative role. Her chief qualities are regal pride and grand diction. She is a highly stylised character, generally magnifi-

cently costumed, who symbolises the supernatural at its most glamorous.

Titinius (d. 42 B.C.) Historical figure and minor character in *Julius Caesar,* friend of CASSIUS. In 5.3, during the battle of PHILIPPI, Cassius sends Titinius to determine the status of a group of approaching horsemen, and PINDARUS' mistaken report of Titinius' capture shocks Cassius. Grieving that he has sent his 'best friend' (5.3.35) to be captured, and believing that he himself is liable to be taken, Cassius kills himself. Titinius returns to find his friend and commander dead, and he kills himself also. Shakespeare took this illustration of stoic Roman military virtue from PLUTARCH's *Lives,* where Titinius is said to be one of Cassius' closest friends.

Titus (1) Andronicus Title character of *Titus Andronicus,* a Roman general and the central figure in the cycle of vengeance that comprises the play. Titus is initially presented as an admirable patriot whose life has been spent largely in the service of his country, but his inflexible pride and overly developed sense of honour cause him to kill one of his own sons in a dispute over loyalty to the Emperor. In 1.1 Titus permits the ritual sacrifice of the son of TAMORA, who consequently seeks revenge against him and his family. Tamora's vengeance (implemented primarily by her lover, AARON) results in the false conviction of two of Titus' sons for the murder of his son-in-law BASSIANUS and the horrible rape and mutilation of his daughter, the newly widowed LAVINIA. Further, Titus is tricked by Aaron into having one hand chopped off, and then, when his two sons have been executed, their heads are brought to him, along with his own severed hand, on a platter. His grief turns to madness, though when Tamora attempts to take advantage of his apparent lunacy, by posing as the spirit of Revenge, he shows that he has retained enough sanity to turn the tables on her. However, Titus' own revenge is anything but sane. He kills Tamora's two surviving sons, Lavinia's attackers, and bakes them into a meat pie that he serves to their mother at a banquet. First, however, he kills Lavinia herself, citing a legend in which a father kills his raped and dishonoured daughter Titus then slays Tamora and is killed himself. His only surviving son, LUCIUS (1), becomes the new Emperor.

It is thought that the name Andronicus may suggest a remote origin for the tale, although Shakespeare will not have known of it. The 12th-century Byzantine Emperor Andronicus Comnenus, famous for his cruelty, was killed by a mob after having had his right hand cut off. Perhaps the playwright's unknown source derived ultimately from medieval accounts of this ruler.

Titus (2) Minor character in *Timon of Athens,* the employee of a creditor of TIMON. In 3.4 Titus and other servants dun Timon and his STEWARD (2) for repayment of various loans, but they are put off. Titus introduces the theme of the episode when he observes that their masters, who solicit Timon for money, wear jewels that Timon had given them before he went bankrupt. The other servants join him, and together they regret that they must serve such greedy men, who were once the beneficiaries of Timon's generosity but are now his merciless creditors.

Titus appears with HORTENSIUS, PHILOTUS, LUCIUS' SERVANT and two men designated as VARRO'S SERVANT. Since the latter three are addressed as 'Lucius' and 'Varro' (3.4.2, 3), it is presumed that Shakespeare intended the names of the first three to refer to their masters as well. This perhaps reflects a casual linguistic practise of the early 17th century.

Titus Andronicus

SYNOPSIS

Act 1, Scene 1

SATURNINUS and his brother BASSIANUS both claim to succeed their father as Roman Emperor. TITUS (1) Andronicus, a vastly popular general and patriot, is expected to return shortly from a successful war against the Goths. Titus appears, mourning the loss of several sons in the campaign. A surviving son, LUCIUS (1), declares that their religion demands a human sacrifice, and he nominates ALARBUS, a son of TAMORA, the captive Queen of the Goths. Tamora's plea for mercy is ignored, and Alarbus is killed. Titus is asked to choose the new Emperor. He declares in favour of the technically legitimate successor, Saturninus, the elder of the two brothers. In gratitude, Saturninus declares that he will marry Titus' only daughter, LAVINIA. Titus then turns his prisoners over to Saturninus, who comments lyrically on Tamora's beauty. Bassianus claims Lavinia as his own betrothed, as had earlier been arranged, and Titus' sons back him. Titus accuses them of treason for opposing the will of the new Emperor. The sons and Bassianus take Lavinia away by force, and Titus kills one of his own sons in the skirmish. Saturninus, however, seizes on the chance to reject Titus, whose popularity he fears, claiming him to be associated with his family's treason. The Emperor then declares his intention to marry Tamora. Tamora purports to defend Titus, but, in an aside to Saturninus, she recommends that he take revenge later, when his throne is more secure. She assures him that she will see to it herself to avenge her son's death. Saturninus therefore pretends to forgive Titus and his family. A double wedding is proposed, and a festive hunt is planned for the next day.

Act 2, Scene 1
AARON, a Moor in Tamora's court, exults in his mistress' newly exalted position, from which he will profit, for he knows she loves him completely. Tamora's sons DEMETRIUS (1) and CHIRON enter, arguing over Lavinia, whom each desires. Aaron suggest that they may both have her; he proposes that they rape her during the next day's hunt.

Act 2, Scene 2
Titus and his sons and Saturninus and his court go festively to the hunt. The two couples, Saturninus and Tamora, and Bassianus and Lavinia, are married.

Act 2, Scene 3
Aaron arranges an encounter in which Demetrius and Chiron kill Bassianus and carry Lavinia off to rape her. Then, with the help of a forged letter, he frames MARTIUS (1) and QUINTUS, sons of Titus, for the murder Titus pleads for mercy, but Saturninus decrees that the sons shall be executed.

Act 2, Scene 4
Chiron and Demetrius taunt Lavinia, whose tongue and hands they have cut off, and abandon her. She is discovered by MARCUS ANDRONICUS, Titus' brother, who responds with elaborately rhetorical grief.

Act 3, Scene 1
Martius and Quintus are marched across the stage on their way to be executed. Titus describes his grief to Lucius in extravagant terms. Marcus appears with the ravished Lavinia, and more expressions of woe ensue. Aaron arrives to announce that the Emperor has declared that Titus' severed hand will be accepted as ransom for the lives of the two sons, and Titus lets Aaron cut it off and take it away. Titus' paroxysms of rhetoric are interrupted by the delivery of the two sons' heads, accompanied by his own hand, and he realises that Aaron has viciously tricked him. Titus' grief turns to a thirst for revenge; he sends Lucius to the Goths to raise an army with which to wreak vengeance.

Act 3, Scene 2
At dinner, Titus rants of the injuries his family has suffered. Marcus kills a fly with his knife, prompting an effusive speech against murder by Titus, but, when Marcus observes that the fly resembled Aaron, Titus seizes the knife and rhapsodises about slaying the Moor. Marcus remarks sadly that grief has unbalanced Titus.

Act 4, Scene 1
Mute Lavinia conveys to Titus and Marcus that she wants them to consult a book. It is Ovid's *Metamorphoses,* and she directs them to the tale of the rape of Philomel. They deduce that her case is the same, and they get her to write the names of her attackers in the sand with a wooden staff. She does so, and new vows of vengeance are sworn.

Act 4, Scene 2
A NURSE (1), sent by Tamora, seeks Aaron. She holds the black infant just born to Tamora, and she tells Aaron that the Empress wants him to kill it so that no one knows of her adultery with the Moor. Aaron refuses. He kills the Nurse to ensure her silence, and sends Chiron and Demetrius to buy a white baby and take it to Tamora to be passed off as the child of Saturninus. They depart, and Aaron plans to take his own child to friends among the Goths.

Act 4, Scene 3
Titus, seemingly mad, insists that his family shoot arrows into the sky, each bearing a message to the gods seeking justice for his wrongs. Marcus suggests that the arrows be aimed so as to land in the Emperor's courtyard. A CLOWN (2) appears, carrying two pigeons. Titus persuades the Clown, for a fee, to deliver the pigeons as an offering to the Emperor, and Titus includes with the birds a message wrapped around a dagger.

Act 4, Scene 4
Saturninus, who has received several of the message-arrows, asserts that Titus' madness is feigned and threatens to punish him. The Clown arrives, bearing the pigeons and Titus' message. Saturninus orders the Clown hanged and vows to execute Titus personally. AEMILIUS appears, reporting that a Gothic army under Lucius is approaching. Tamora proposes to trick Titus into halting his son's onslaught. Aemilius is sent to arrange a parley with Lucius at Titus' house.

Act 5, Scene 1
Aaron, who has been captured with his child, is brought before Lucius, who decrees that both be hanged. Aaron says that he will confess the truth about all his misdeeds if Lucius will spare the child. Lucius agrees, and Aaron insolently brags of his evil actions, regretting only that death will keep him from doing more. Aemilius arrives with the offer of a parley, and Lucius accepts.

Act 5, Scene 2
Tamora and her sons, in disguise, approach Titus' house, where she plans to delude the old man that she is Revenge, a spirit sent to aid him. Titus recognises them, but he pretends to be taken in. Tamora proposes to bring the Emperor to a banquet, where Titus can wreak his vengeance. She goes, leaving Chiron and Demetrius, whom Titus promptly has bound and gagged. He reveals his plan to cook them and serve them to Tamora at the proposed banquet. He then cuts their throats.

Act 5, Scene 3
Lucius, arriving at Titus' house for the parley, turns Aaron over to Marcus. Saturninus and Tamora arrive with their noble retinue, and all are seated at the banquet table. Titus welcomes them, dressed as a cook. Referring to a famous legend of a father who killed his raped daughter to remove his family's shame, he kills Lavinia before the horrified guests. He declares that she had been raped by Chiron and Demetrius. He reveals their heads baked in a meat pie that Tamora has already sampled, and then he stabs Tamora to death. Saturninus promptly kills him and is himself immediately dispatched by Lucius. The assembled nobles declare Lucius to be the new Emperor, and Titus is formally mourned. Aaron is brought forward and sentenced by Lucius to be buried to his neck and starved. He responds with a last boastful refusal to repent.

COMMENTARY

Although *Titus Andronicus* is certainly the least satisfying Shakespearean tragedy, it was also his first attempt at the genre, and it has features that suggest the grander achievements to come. Although it is inferior to later work, it is a fine play by the standards of 1590; the young Shakespeare was already a successful professional playwright.

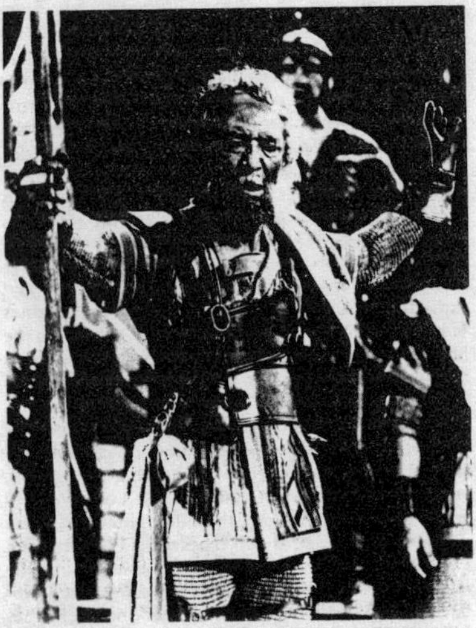

Filled with barbaric crimes and horrible slaughter, Titus Andronicus *was the first tragedy Shakespeare wrote. Titus is an admirable patriot, but his overdeveloped sense of honour causes him to kill one of his own sons.* (Courtesy of Billy Rose Theatre Collection; New York Public Library at Lincoln Center; Astor, Lenox and Tilden Foundations)

The play is based on ancient Roman drama; its format and general character were taken from SENECA. The violence and degradation to which the characters are exposed stand in marked contrast to the highly decorous language in which these excesses are depicted. Also, references to classical literature, especially to OVID, abound. All this was very much in the manner of academic drama that dominated the pre-Shakespearean stage, a tradition that the playwright was soon to outgrow. At the time, still learning his trade, Shakespeare applied the tenets of Senecan drama in a polished and professional manner, using grand rhetoric and precise plotting. He was content to attempt a standard melodrama, plainly geared to box-office success, and he had two recent, immensely popular predecessors to model his work on. One was *The Jew of Malta,* by Christopher MARLOWE (1), which had created a vogue for exotic villains that the character of Aaron clearly exploits. The other was Thomas KYD's *The Spanish Tragedy,* the first great Elizabethan REVENGE PLAY, a favourite genre of the day; *Hamlet* was to be the greatest of them. In fact, *Titus* and *The Spanish Tragedy* remained the two most popular English plays for the rest of the 16th century and into the early 17th.

Glimpses of later, greater plays may be found in *Titus.* For instance, the combination of shrewdly feigned lunacy with some degree of real insanity, applied rather baldly and unconvincingly in the depiction of Titus, is a profoundly compelling trait in HAMLET. Titus also anticipates OTHELLO in being a simple man out of his depth, a successful but easily manipulated military leader. Titus also foreshadows King LEAR in that he commits crimes in the name of honour, but Titus never becomes aware of his errors, as does Lear. The villainous Aaron plainly prefigures such paragons of malevolence as IAGO and RICHARD III. Most important, *Titus* reveals Shakespeare's concern for political ethics. It opens with a question of hereditary succession to a throne, the crux of most of his later HISTORY PLAYS, and concludes with the restoration of orderly rule after disruptions caused by human frailties. Though dealt with very crudely here, these themes suggest the mature presentation to come.

However, *Titus Andronicus* in no way generates the powerful responses we associate with Shakespeare's great works. For one thing, there is no development towards a climax, but rather an assemblage of episodes, all rather similar in tone. Also, the extremely rhetorical dialogue inhibits the development of the characters, who do not reveal their feelings so much

as describe them. In any case, the extremely melodramatic plot makes character development all but impossible; for one thing, more than half of the play's characters are killed, often on stage (including a prodigious three in four lines in the final scene).

This combination of academic formalism and blatant gore has appealed to few theatre-goers since the 17th century. Scholarly opinion used to deny Shakespeare's authorship of the play on the grounds that it was clearly beneath the sensibility of a great writer. However, modern scholarship has rejected this assertion and reminds us that the young Shakespeare's taste was naturally that of his time. *Titus Andronicus* may be seen as roughly equivalent to today's horror movies. As such, it was a major success; it appealed to its audience, and it established the playwright as superior to most, if not all, of his contemporaries.

SOURCES OF THE PLAY

No source for the story of *Titus Andronicus* is known, although it has been suggested that an older play, now lost, was rewritten by Shakespeare. The tale itself, although presented as historical (in accordance with a standard convention of Elizabethan TRAGEDY), is fictional, and Shakespeare may have invented it. However, scholars have noted an 18th-century chapbook, of which only one copy exists, that contains a version of the same story that seems not to be based on Shakespeare's play. It may reflect pre-Shakespearean material that the playwright knew. If so, Shakespeare made notable alterations, emphasising the political issues, especially in adding the role of Lucius and asserting the restoration of Roman authority at the conclusion.

OVID's tale of the rape and mutilation of Philomel is obviously a forerunner of Lavinia's fate in the play; this story is expressly referred to several times. *Thyestes,* by Seneca, probably influenced the general atmosphere of horror pervading *Titus Andronicus* and may have provided certain details as well. While the chapbook has a character analagous to Aaron, another source, a story by the 16th-century Italian author Matteo BANDELLO, features a Moor whose crimes are similar and whose delight in his own evil is much more like the Shakespearean character. Shakespeare may have known the Bandello tale in François BELLEFOREST's French translation or in the English of Geoffrey FENTON (2); also, the tale is known to have been rendered in a popular English ballad. Shakespeare's conception of Aaron surely owes something to Marlowe's *The Jew of Malta* (1589). Lastly, the feigned madness of Titus may derive from that of Hieronymo in Thomas Kyd's *The Spanish Tragedy* (1588–1589).

TEXT OF THE PLAY

Titus Andronicus has been said to be Shakespeare's first play; although this cannot be proved, it is certainly among his earliest. The precise date of composition is unknown; estimates have varied from 1588 to the year of its initial publication, 1594. The play appeared in three QUARTO editions (Q1, Q2, and Q3) before being included in the FIRST FOLIO (F1) in 1623. Q1 was printed in 1594 by John DANTER for publishers Thomas MILLINGTON and Edward WHITE (1); only one copy is known to exist. Although sloppily produced, it contains a seemingly accurate text, and it is the ultimate source for the other early texts and thus for all modern editions. Q2, printed in 1600 by James ROBERTS for White alone, was apparently taken from Q1, but from a damaged copy, for it is missing lines in a number of places. Two copies of Q2 are known. Q3, from 1611, was taken from Q2 and provides a small number of corrections to it, but with a much larger number of errors. Unfortunately, this corrupt text, printed for White by Edward ALLDE, was the basis for F1, which became the best-known Shakespeare edition for centuries. F1 contains several lines and one whole scene (3.2) that are in no other edition. These were presumably written, perhaps not by Shakespeare, after the play had been in production for some time.

Since none of the Quarto editions name a playwright, and since the crudely gory tale has often seemed to post-Elizabethan sensibilities to be beneath a great writer, some controversy has arisen over its authorship. Attributions have been made to many other Elizabethan playwrights, especially George PEELE. However, both the Folio editors, who knew Shakespeare and were members of the same theatrical company, and Francis MERES, the contemporary writer on theatre whose list of Shakespeare's works appeared in 1598, include *Titus Andronicus* among the playwright's works. Twentieth-century scholarship has generally accepted their judgement, with the proviso that the play may be Shakespeare's elaboration and expansion of a Peele work that survives chiefly in Act 1. In any case, *Titus Andronicus* securely belongs in the Shakespearean CANON.

THEATRICAL HISTORY OF THE PLAY

Titus Andronicus was immediately popular; the title-page of its first edition boasted that it had been performed by three different companies: DERBY'S MEN, PEMBROKE'S MEN, and SUSSEX'S MEN. For about 30 years, it remained among the most popular English dramas and was performed repeatedly. For three and a half centuries thereafter, however, it was among the most neglected of Shakespeare's plays. It was not produced at all between 1721 and 1852, nor again between 1857 and 1923; the brief revival was due to the popularity in Britain of a black American actor, Ira ALDRIDGE, who played Aaron. Several 20th-century productions—including a notable 1955 staging by Peter BROOK (2), featuring Laurence OLIVIER as Titus—have helped revive interest in the play, but it remains an oddity. It has never been made as a FILM

and has only once been produced for TELEVISION, in 1985.

Toby Belch, Sir Character in *Twelfth Night.* See SIR TOBY.

Tooley, Nicholas (c. 1575–1623) English actor, member of the KING'S MEN. Tooley was one of the 26 'Principall Actors' of Shakespeare's plays listed in the FIRST FOLIO, though no important role is associated with him. He may have played the SERVANT (6) in *The Taming of the Shrew,* who is designated as 'Nicke' in a speech heading in the first edition of the play. He is known to have played a madman in a non-Shakespearean play. He was a member of the King's Men from 1605 until his death, but he had probably appeared with the company earlier, for he was apprenticed to Richard BURBAGE (3). When he died, he was lodging in the home of Cuthbert BURBAGE (1), who was executor of his will, along with Henry CONDELL.

Topas In *Twelfth Night,* name taken by FESTE in 4.2, when he disguises himself as a Puritan clergyman and visits MALVOLIO, who has been imprisoned as a madman. The name refers to the topaz, a semi-precious gem believed in Shakespeare's day to be capable of curing lunacy.

Torchbearers Group of non-speaking characters in *Romeo and Juliet,* men who accompany ROMEO and the MASQUERS to the banquet given by CAPULET (1). Romeo, mooning over ROSALINE (2), says he wishes to join the Torchbearers (1.4.11–12) because they were expected to watch from the sidelines and not participate in the dancing.

Touchstone Character in *As You Like It,* a professional FOOL (1) and follower of ROSALIND. Touchstone is initially in the service of DUKE (1) Frederick, but he joins Rosalind and CELIA when they flee to the Forest of ARDEN (1) after Act 1. He uses his unbridled humour to satirise all targets. In particular, Touchstone parodies the romances of the other characters, in his own courtship of the goatherd AUDREY.

A touchstone is a mineral used to test gold and silver alloys; when the alloy is rubbed with a touchstone, a discoloration, whose precise shade indicates the metal's purity, is produced. Similarly, something of the quality of the other characters is revealed through Touchstone's mockery of them. Jesting and mimicking, he tests their approaches to the worlds of PASTORAL love and country life, the themes of the play.

Unlike JAQUES (1), who also mocks the other characters, Touchstone presents no alternatives and has no clear-cut vision of the world. Also unlike Jaques, he is consistently funny; his cynicism is amused, not despairing, and his enthusiastic approach to love and rusticity stands in marked opposition to Jaques' isolation. Significantly, while Jaques withdraws from the world at the play's close, Touchstone marries and is part of the climactic festival of love and reconciliation.

The jester is a courtier, both by inclination and profession, a point he explains satirically when he says, 'I have trod a measure, I have flattered a lady, I have been politic with my friend, smooth with mine enemy, I have undone three tailors, I have had four quarrels, and like to have fought one.' (5.4.43-47). In 1.2.58–74 his first jest of the play is at the expense of knightly 'honour', and he mocks LE BEAU's callous enthusiasm for brutal sports in 1.2.127–129. In his encounter with the shepherd CORIN in 3.2.11–83 he cannot keep his arguments for the superiority of courtly wit from backfiring upon himself, so extravagant are they. His extraordinary send-up of duelling (5.4.67–102) has lost much of its point for modern readers, but it is a virtuoso satire of the handbooks of gentlemanly combat that flourished in Shakespeare's day.

Touchstone also turns his humour on the supposedly idyllic country life; when he first arrives in Arden, he exclaims, 'Ay, now am I in Arden, the more fool I; when I was at home I was in a better place . . .' (2.4.13–14). His feet hurt, and he will not let his discomfort go unnoticed. He mocks the dimness of Audrey's rustic swain, WILLIAM (2), in 5.1, and his pursuit of Audrey satirises peasant life by caricaturing an unconsidered, merely biological mating.

However, Touchstone's courtship of Audrey is most strikingly a comical contrast to the relationship of SILVIUS and PHEBE, who present the literary ideal of pastoral love. Touchstone's forthrightness and Audrey's passivity enable these lovers to achieve a very direct and uncomplicated match, whereas only Rosalind's elaborate machinations can unite the shepherd and shepherdess. Earlier, Touchstone mocks both Silvius and Rosalind, after they remark on the pathos of love, by offering the preposterous example of his own romance with 'Jane Smile' (2.4.43–53).

Touchstone's romance is also contrasted with the genuinely moving love between Rosalind and ORLANDO. In 3.2.99–110 his bawdy parody of Orlando's love poetry is intended to embarrass his mistress. She responds with an apt comparison of the jester and a soft fruit, insinuating that Touchstone will be rotten with age before his mind is ripe. The fool has the last word, however, when he says, 'You have said; but whether wisely or no, let the forest judge' (3.2.119–120). Like the forest, Touchstone's indiscriminate comedy is a force of nature, and all manner of things are 'judged' by exposure to it.

Significantly, Touchstone's initial encounter with Audrey follows immediately after Orlando's meeting with the disguised Rosalind. Orlando's promise 'by the faith of my love' (3.2.416) to demonstrate his passion for the supposedly absent Rosalind is thus juxta-

posed with Touchstone's insistence on animal desire as the motive for his own romance. The jester is detached about and resigned to his role as a husband: 'As the ox hath his bow . . . so man hath his desires, and as pigeons bill, so wedlock would be nibbling' (3.3.71–73). His assumption that any wife will assuage his physical desire is the opposite extreme to Orlando's proposition that only Rosalind can possibly serve. The idealism of the latter point of view lacks the acknowledgement of instinct that Touchstone offers. As Rosalind and Orlando's relationship evolves, the play moves beyond Touchstone's simplistic position, but first it must also offer this stance as a specimen of pastoral love.

Touchstone is a professional jester, a performer who was expected to make fun of the members of an aristocratic court for their entertainment and as living proof that they did not fear criticism. His profession required a jester to seem incapable of common sense, and he was accordingly excused from ordinary social life. He developed a purposeful detachment from the real lives of the people around him in favour of a concern with the artificialities of wit. Touchstone is seen only in the light of his calling; though delightful, he is not a fully developed person. His amalgam of fast talk and brash earthiness is dazzling, but he is merely doing his job. As such, he can parody the rest of the characters, but the play is not at all dependent on him, as it is on Rosalind or Jaques. If he were absent, we would be poorer for not knowing him, but *As You Like It* would still make its key points.

Jesters were familiar figures in the drama and literature of the 16th century, obvious vehicles for parody and satire. It is thought that the part of Touchstone was written for Robert ARMIN, an actor who specialised in these parts and who joined the CHAMBERLAIN'S MEN at about the time when *As You Like It* was written. Touchstone was the first of Shakespeare's jesters, and in Jaques' speeches describing an off-stage performance by the 'motley fool' (2.7.12–61), one can almost hear the playwright exulting in the potential of this new sort of role.

Tower of London Fortification and prison, a famous London landmark and a setting in several of the HISTORY PLAYS. Originally a military base built by the Norman conquerors of England, the Tower, actually a complex of several buildings, was a combination of prison, warehouse, and royal residence by the 15th century, when the plays are set. The sinister reputation of the Tower is reflected in (and to some extent inflated by) its role in Shakespeare's plays as the site of RICHARD III's notorious political murders. Richard kills HENRY VI in his Tower cell in 5.6 of *3 Henry VI.* He arranges for the imprisonment of his own brother the Duke of CLARENCE (1), and then hires murderers who kill the prisoner in 1.4 of *Richard III.* Later in the same play, though not on stage, a similar fate befalls Richard's young nephews the PRINCE (5) of Wales and the Duke of YORK (7). In 2.5 of *1 Henry VI,* another political prisoner, Edmund MORTIMER (1), dies in the Tower, though of old age. Also, in *Richard II,* a later play, the deposed King RICHARD II is condemned to the Tower, although his subsequent murder occurs elsewhere.

Aside from its use as a prison, the Tower was a military storehouse and, as such, an important centre of royal power. In Shakespeare's earliest depiction of it, in 1.3 of *1 Henry VI,* two feuding aristocrats dispute its control, and, during Jack CADE's rebellion, depicted in Act 4 of *2 Henry VI,* the commander of the Tower, Lord SCALES, plays a leading role in driving the rebels from London in 4.5.

Towton Location in *3 Henry VI,* a town near YORK (10), a battle site of the WARS OF THE ROSES. The battle of Towton constitutes the action of 2.3–2.6. Although Shakespeare includes several fictitious incidents, such as the death of CLIFFORD (1) and the response of WARWICK (3) to his dying brother's call for revenge, he nonetheless accurately depicts the battle as by far the bloodiest battle of the civil war. In 2.5, a major scene, King HENRY VI withdraws from the fray and comments on its fury, its confusion, and the uncertainty of its outcome. The actual battle was fought in a raging snowstorm on the afternoon of Palm Sunday, in 1461, and, by the time it ended, hours later, about 40,000 men had been slaughtered. Its violence remained a byword in Shakespeare's time, and it was commonly asserted that soldiers had killed their own fathers or sons in the fight, a tradition that the playwright used in King Henry's moving encounters with the SON THAT HATH KILLED HIS FATHER and the FATHER THAT HATH KILLED HIS SON, also in 2.5.

Tragedy Drama dealing with a noble protagonist placed in a highly stressful situation that leads to a disastrous, usually fatal conclusion. The 10 plays generally included among Shakespeare's tragedies are, in approximate order of composition, *Titus Andronicus, Romeo and Juliet, Julius Caesar, Hamlet, Othello, Macbeth, King Lear, Antony and Cleopatra, Coriolanus,* and *Timon of Athens.* A central group of four plays—*Hamlet, Othello, Macbeth,* and *King Lear*—offer Shakespeare's fullest development of tragedy, and they are sometimes collectively labelled the great or major tragedies. These plays focus on a powerful central character whose most outstanding personal quality—his tragic flaw, as it is often called—is the source of his catastrophe. He is the victim of his own strength, which will not allow accommodation with his situation, and we are appalled at this paradox and at the inexorability of his fate. These works—sometimes with the addition of *Antony and Cleopatra*—are often

thought to constitute Shakespeare's greatest achievement as a playwright.

Naturally, Shakespeare wrote his tragedies concurrently with other plays, and the group is not isolated within his oeuvre. In fact, its boundaries are not clear cut. *Timon of Athens* is sometimes classed as a COMEDY, and the FIRST FOLIO edition of the plays (1623) listed *Cymbeline* and *Troilus and Cressida,* usually thought of as comedies, among the tragedies. Moreover, two of the HISTORY PLAYS, *Richard III* and *Richard II,* offer protagonists who have tragic aspects, though the plays themselves, with their pronounced political and social aspects, are not tragedies. Also, three of the tragedies, *Julius Caesar, Antony and Cleopatra,* and *Coriolanus,* are similarly historical in orientation and may be separately grouped as the ROMAN PLAYS.

Shakespeare's tragedies developed out of earlier 16th-century tragedies, which had antecedents in the 'tragedies' of medieval poetry—verse accounts of disaster, suffering, and death, usually of mighty rulers. The poems emphasised the fate of kings and emperors partly because of their importance in a hierarchical society, but also because, from a purely literary point of view, the contrast between their good and bad fortune was highly dramatic. These tragedies, however, did not lend themselves to the stage because they simply made a single point—that suffering and death come even to the great, without regard for merit or station—in the same fashion every time. The emotional tone remained in accord with the doctrine voiced by Aelius Donatus, a 4th-century Roman critic who was influential throughout the Middle Ages: 'The moral of tragedy is that life should be rejected.'

However, at least as early as BOCCACCIO's *The Fate of Illustrious Men* (1355–1374), RENAISSANCE authors, imbued with a sense of the value of human experience, began to alter the pattern. A wider range of subjects was assembled, and, more important, moral lessons were adduced from their lives. A good instance, and an important inspiration for Shakespeare, is the English biographical compilation A MIRROR FOR MAGISTRATES, in which the settings range from the classical and biblical worlds to quite recent history. The typical subject is a villainous tyrant whose fall is obviously and amply deserved. Retribution becomes the theme rather than simple inevitability. This material lent itself to dramatic development, as the tables were turned on the villain. It also lent itself to theatrical effect, as the villainy and the retribution alike were generally bloody. The ancient plays of SENECA were similar in subject and tone; already a part of the Renaissance fascination with the classical world, these works were exploited by 16th-century playwrights. The immediate result was the REVENGE PLAY, which offered the spectacle of the avenger being bloodily dispatched along with the original villain. Christopher MARLOWE (1) and Thomas KYD pioneered this development.

However, the emphasis on evil figures was gradually eroded by an awareness of the dramatic value of virtue, providing the moral contrasts so important to Shakespearean tragedy. The medieval heritage of the MORALITY PLAY was an important influence on this development. Sometimes the good were simply victims, as in *Titus Andronicus;* sometimes virtuous deeds resulted in death or disaster, as in the story of LUCRECE, which Shakespeare treated poetically in *The Rape of Lucrece* and which others dramatised; and sometimes the two motifs combined, in virtuous victims whose deaths are redemptive, spiritually cleansing the world of the play. *Romeo and Juliet* offers a fine example.

Shakespeare's first tragedy, *Titus Andronicus,* is a simple melodrama, frankly imitative of Seneca. With *Romeo and Juliet,* the young playwright advances considerably, developing humanly credible protagonists, virtuous young lovers who are ennobled as love triumphs over death. An essential tragic theme is established in *Romeo and Juliet:* the superiority of the human spirit to its mortal destiny. At about the same time Shakespeare takes another important step. In RICHARD III he first creates a mighty protagonist who can dominate a play by force of personality, though Richard's features are somewhat stereotyped and his tragic defect is simply a given of the plot rather than a plausibly developed personal trait. However, RICHARD II constitutes a new phenomenon, a hero who is not merely 'star-cross'd' (*Romeo,* Prologue 6) but, rather, psychologically flawed. His inner conflicts are exposed in his introspective soliloquies and self-revealing actions, and we see a complex consciousness tragically unable to deal with external circumstances. Nevertheless, Richard's fall depends chiefly on those circumstances. It is in *Julius Caesar* that Shakespeare first achieves the distinctive element of the major tragedies, a protagonist, BRUTUS (4), who is undone precisely by his own virtues, as he pursues a flawed political ideal. A paradoxical sense of the interconnectedness of good and evil permeates the play, as the hero's idealism leads to disaster for both him and his world.

Only with *Hamlet* does the hero's personal sense of that paradox become the play's central concern. In *Hamlet* and its three great successors, Shakespeare composes four variations on the overarching theme that humanity's weaknesses must be recognised as our inevitable human lot, for only by accepting our destiny can we transcend our mortality. HAMLET, unable to alter the evil around him because of his fixation on the uncertainties of moral judgement, falls into evil himself in killing POLONIUS and rejecting OPHELIA but finally recovers his humanity by recognising his ties to others. He accepts his own fate, knowing that 'readiness is all' (*Hamlet* 5.2.218). LEAR, his world in ruins of his own making, can find salvation only through mad-

ness, but in his reconciliation with CORDELIA, he too finds that destiny can be identified with, 'As if we were God's spies' (*Lear* 5.3.17). As EDGAR puts it, sounding very like Hamlet, 'Ripeness is all' (5.2.11). OTHELLO, drawn into evil by an incapacity for trust, recognises his failing and, acknowledgeing that he 'threw a pearl away' (*Othello* 5.2.348), kills himself, 'to die upon a kiss' (5.2.360). The power of love—the importance of our bonds to others—is again upheld. In *Macbeth* the same point is made negatively, as the protagonist's rejection of love and loyalty leads to an extreme human isolation, where 'Life's but a walking shadow' (5.5.24). In each of the four major tragedies, a single protagonist grows in self-awareness and knowledge of human nature, though he cannot halt his disaster. Hamlet's thoughtfulness, Lear's emotional intensity, Othello's obsessive love, MACBETH's ambition—each could be a positive feature, but each is counter to the forces of the hero's world. We find human dignity in a tragic protagonist's acceptance of a defeat made necessary by his own greatest strengths.

In the later Roman tragedies, *Antony and Cleopatra* and *Coriolanus*, we see the same pattern. Both CLEOPATRA and CORIOLANUS face their ends with equanimity. For the Egyptian queen, death is 'as sweet as balm, as soft as air, as gentle' (*Antony* 5.2.310); Coriolanus, in his more stoical way, says only, 'But let it come' (*Coriolanus* 5.3.189). However, these plays differ from their predecessors in that the central figures are placed in a complex social and political context, and the plays are strongly concerned with the relationship between the individual and society, with correspondingly less focus on the emotional development of the tragic hero. *Timon of Athens*, considered the last tragedy (though perhaps written at the same time as *Coriolanus*) is a flawed effort that Shakespeare left incomplete. Also quite socially oriented, it has a strong satirical quality that allies it as much with the comedies known as PROBLEM PLAYS as with the great tragedies. Nevertheless, as in the other tragedies, TIMON is a central figure whose decline stems from a mistaken sense of virtue. Shakespeare's attempt to integrate elements of tragedy and comedy was to be more successful in the later ROMANCES.

Shakespeare's tragedies are disturbing plays. We feel horror at the stories—a horror that is aggravated by such scenes as the blinding of GLOUCESTER (1) in *King Lear*—and we feel pity for the victims. That this pity extends to doers of evil as well—Macbeth, Othello, Lear, Coriolanus—attests to Shakespeare's power. We recognise the nobility of the human spirit, which may err catastrophically but which does so through an excess of strength, challenging its own limits. Hamlet loses his humanity before he learns to accept destiny; Lear in his madness assumes the burden of his evils and thus achieves remission. Othello, recognising the evil he has fallen to, uses his strength to compensate in the only way remaining to him. Even Macbeth, the most explicitly villainous of the tragic protagonists, resumes his humanity at the play's close and seizes his sole virtue, courage, to face his end with vigour. The essence of these plays is that blame is not the appropriate response to evil that derives from human weakness. In a tragic universe, we are all flawed precisely because we are human, and Shakespeare's tragic heroes embody this inexorable feature of life.

Tragicomedy Genre of drama combining elements of TRAGEDY and COMEDY, especially when a tragic plot results in a happy ending. The genre was popular in JACOBEAN DRAMA, for its odd composition lent an ironic distance from its themes—usually a combination of sexual love and violent death in a socially significant setting—that appealed to the age's audiences. John FLETCHER (2), an accomplished practitioner of the genre, provided a neat formulation of it: 'A tragicomedy is not so called [because it combines] mirth and killing, but [because] it wants [i.e., lacks] deaths, which is enough to make it no tragedy, yet brings some [characters] near it, which is enough to make it no comedy'. Though most Jacobean tragicomedies are obsessed with grotesque rhetoric and bizarre acts of violence, in a fashion far removed from Shakespeare's work, a number of his plays may nevertheless be classed as tragicomedies in a structural sense, especially *Measure for Measure*, *Cymbeline*, and *The Winter's Tale*.

Traïson Abbreviated title of an early 15th-century French prose work that may have influenced the writing of *Richard II*. The anonymous *Chronicque de la Traïson et Mort de Richart Deux* may have been written by a member of the household of QUEEN (13) Isabel. It records the last three years of the reign of RICHARD II, closing with his murder and burial. It includes the only early account of Sir Piers EXTON, who is otherwise unknown. (Shakespeare probably took the tale from HOLINSHED, who had it from *Traïson*.) If Shakespeare did know this work, which existed only in manuscript in his day (though at least a partially complete copy is known to have circulated among his contemporaries), he took from it directly only a few minor elements; however, its positive attitude towards Richard may have helped to shape the playwright's portrait of the King.

Tranio Character in *The Taming of the Shrew*, a servant who impersonates his master, LUCENTIO. In 1.1 Tranio proposes that Lucentio disguise himself as a humble tutor in order to approach BIANCA (1), and when he is assigned to take Lucentio's place and maintain his household in PADUA, Tranio is entirely at ease in the role. He plays a smooth young nobleman with educa-

tion and wit enough to cite classical authors while ingratiating himself with BAPTISTA. His initiative propels the SUB-PLOT: he launches Lucentio's courtship; in 2.1 he outbids GREMIO for Bianca's hand in his master's name; he conceives (2.1) and carries out (4.2, 4.4) the impersonation by the PEDANT of Lucentio's father, VINCENTIO (1); and he arranges for Lucentio and Bianca's elopement (4.4). And he is sufficiently bold to carry on with his plot even when the real Vincentio appears (5.1). However, for all his cleverness, he has little personality; he is a stock character, a comically deceitful servant deriving ultimately from ancient Roman drama. In fact, Shakespeare took the name Tranio from *The Haunted House*, by PLAUTUS, where it is given to a witty and resourceful slave who tells inventive lies in his master's behalf.

Traveller Either of two minor characters in *1 Henry IV*, victims of highway robbery at the hands of FALSTAFF and others. The Travellers are presumably the Kentish franklin and the auditor described to GADSHILL by the CHAMBERLAIN (1) of the inn in ROCHESTER in 2.1.52–59.

Travers Minor character in *2 Henry IV*, follower of the Earl of NORTHUMBERLAND (1) and a rebel against King HENRY IV. In 1.1 Travers brings Northumberland the mistaken news that the rebel forces have won the battle of SHREWSBURY, an account shortly belied by the eyewitness account of MORTON. The episode helps to develop a secondary theme of the play, the uncertainty of knowledge.

Trebonius, Gaius (d. 43 B.C.) Historical figure and minor character in *Julius Caesar*, one of the plotters against CAESAR (1). In 3.1 Trebonius plays an important, if silent, role in the assassination, drawing Mark ANTONY away from the scene at the critical moment.

The historical Trebonius was a Roman aristocrat who had been an ally of Caesar in his earlier conflicts and had served as a general in Caesar's conquest of Gaul. Turning against him, he performed the part in the assassination that is enacted in the play. He died in the ensuing civil war.

Tree, Beerbohm (1853–1917) British actor and producer. Born Herbert Beerbohm, Tree was a successful actor when he became manager of London's Haymarket Theatre in 1887. There, he staged several of Shakespeare's plays, including *The Merry Wives of Windsor*, in which he played FALSTAFF, and *Hamlet*, with himself in the title role. He built a new playhouse, Her (later His) Majesty's Theatre, and in 1897 he began to put on extravagant productions in the tradition of Charles KEAN (1) and Henry IRVING, with lavish sets and costumes and spectacular processions and tableaus. For *Julius Caesar* he employed elaborate scenic

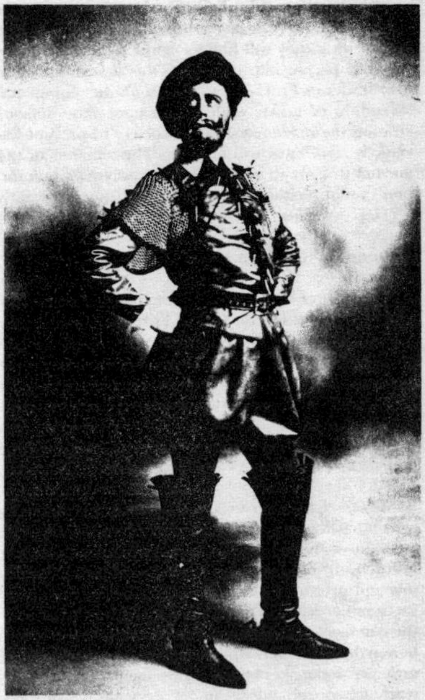

Beerbohm Tree—seen here in his role as Benedick, the confirmed bachelor who comes to marry Beatrice in Much Ado About Nothing*—was a prominent actor and manager of the late 19th century.* (Courtesy of Culver Pictures, Inc.)

designs by the most prominent (and expensive) British artist of the day, Sir Lawrence Alma-Tadema (1836–1912). His *Midsummer Night's Dream* (1900) featured live rabbits and birds on stage, and the coronation parade in 4.1 of his *Henry VIII* (1910, 1916 in New York) was so time-consuming that he had to cut Act 5 entirely. He is the last major exponent of this characteristically 19th-century style, and it was in part rebellion against his work that inspired such modern pioneers as William POEL and Harley GRANVILLE-BARKER.

Tressel Minor character in *Richard III*, one of two named gentlemen among the group accompanying Lady ANNE (2) and the corpse of HENRY VI in 1.2.

Tribune (1) Either of two minor characters in *Titus Andronicus*, officials of the Roman Empire. The Tribunes are present throughout much of 1.1, largely as

mute witnesses to the foolish pride of TITUS (1). In 1.1.220–222 they speak in unison, their only lines, and declare that they will honour Titus' achievements in war and permit him to choose the successor to the deceased emperor. They represent the pomp and splendour of ROME, while at the same time demonstrating the inadequacy of the society to prevent the tragedy that Titus will unleash. The tribunes of the ancient Roman government were always two in number, though neither the text nor the stage directions of *Titus Andronicus* indicate this.

Tribune (2) Characters in *Coriolanus*. See BRUTUS (3).

Tribune (3) Either of two minor characters in *Cymbeline*, Roman officials. In 3.8 the Tribunes are informed by a SENATOR (5) of the emperor's orders: They are to recruit an armed force from among the gentry of ROME that will be sent against King CYMBELINE. Only the First Tribune speaks; he asks two brief questions and tersely accepts the orders. These two figures serve as recipients of information intended principally for the audience.

Trinculo Character in *The Tempest*, a jester to King ALONSO of Naples and a follower of STEPHANO (2) and CALIBAN in their plot to kill PROSPERO. Trinculo is a buffoon, drunk most of the time, and alternately servile and presumptious. He is ridiculously terrified of the weather when he first appears in 2.2 and is a butt for humour when Stephano sides with Caliban against him in 3.2, especially when the invisible ARIEL imitates his voice and makes him seem argumentative when he is in fact entirely docile. In 4.1 Trinculo is comically obsequious towards Stephano, in a parody of the relationship between courtier and king. When the trio of would-be assassins is finally punished, Trinculo can only observe ruefully, 'I have been in such a pickle . . . that, I fear me, will never out of my bones' (5.1. 282–283).

Trinculo is less vicious than Stephano; he is a follower in a conspiracy he could not have conceived himself. Stephano and Trinculo are thus respectively like ANTONIO (5) and SEBASTIAN (3), within the play's various parallels and oppositions. As a professional jester, Trinculo is technically a FOOL (1), but in his buffoonery, his cowardice, and his lack of conscious irony, he more nearly resembles the rustic CLOWN (1).

Troilus One of the title characters of *Troilus and Cressida*, a prince of TROY, a Trojan leader in the TROJAN WAR, and the lover of CRESSIDA. As the only character to have a major part in both of the play's plot lines—a fighter for the honour of Troy in the warriors' plot and the victim of Cressida's betrayal in the ill-fated love story—Troilus contributes greatly to the play's central theme: the inadequacy of good intentions in a corrupt world. Self-deluded both as a lover and a warrior, Troilus is a principal component of, and a sufferer from, the play's atmosphere of error and misdirection.

He is a typical romantic hero, but his complex and credible responses make him interesting as well. Most important, he is mistaken in his attitude towards Cressida. Although PANDARUS' lewd jests and salacious attitude make perfectly plain what sort of game is afoot, Troilus persists in pretending to himself that Cressida is 'stubborn-chaste' (1.1.97). In fact, their relationship is never more than a sexual affair that cannot be expected to last long. Subconsciously, he is aware of the truth; from the outset he is suspicious that Cressida will prove unfaithful. His language is also revealing. With romantic rhetoric, he describes Cressida as a 'pearl' (1.1.100), Pandarus as a ship, and himself as a merchant; unconsciously, he devalues his lover to the status of an object and the consummation of their love to that of a commercial transaction. When he approaches his long-sought rendezvous with Cressida, his thrill is distinctly sensual rather than emotional (as compared to, say, ROMEO). He hopes to 'wallow in the lily beds' (3.2.11) when his 'wat'ry [i.e., salivating] palate tastes . . . Love's . . . nectar' (3.2.18–19). But he does not acknowledge this, preferring to see himself as a romantic figure, 'a strange soul upon the Stygian banks' (3.2.8).

His capacity for self-deception is also important in the warriors' plot. Just as he deludes himself about Cressida, he also deludes himself about the pointless war for HELEN (1). He feels that *she* is a 'pearl' (2.2.82) and the Trojans doers of 'valiant and magnanimous deeds' (2.2.201) in defence of her. In both cases he confuses the real world with a grander, more ideal situation—like that of traditional literature and legend.

As a self-deluded warrior arguing for the continuation of the war, Troilus unconsciously presents an important theme: the unreliable nature of value judgements that are likely to change with time. In the Trojan council of 2.2 he argues that circumstances determine worth: Helen is valuable enough to fight over simply because she has been fought over already. 'What's aught but as 'tis valued?' (2.2.53), he says, but he is unaware that this argument applies to himself. Cressida will eventually value him differently, compared to the more available man, DIOMEDES (1).

When Troilus witnesses Cressida's betrayal while eavesdropping on her conversation with Diomedes in 5.2, his self-delusion becomes strikingly evident. He will not acknowledge Cressida's flighty nature, or that he was wrong about their romance. Instead, he hysterically insists that to do so would indict all womanhood, and further, that all 'beauty', all 'sanctimony . . . the gods' delight', and 'unity itself' (5.2.136, 139, 140) would be flawed. His grief and confusion are real,

but his expressions of it are shallow and rhetorical. His focus is on literary images of betrayal, rather than on the particular betrayal that has just taken place. He avoids admitting that his romance was merely a sexual affair by translating it into high-flown abstractions.

His final response is just as displaced; he translates his love for Cressida into hatred for Diomedes. Significantly, when the berserk Troilus encounters Diomedes on the battlefield, he has completely forgotten why he was so enraged and demands that his foe 'pay the life thou ow'st me for my horse' (5.6.7), a line that is both funny and ironically revealing.

At the close of the play, Troilus has forgotten Cressida and is instead caught up in the death of HECTOR and Troy's loss of the climactic battle. Convinced that all is lost, he proposes to fight to the death. His despair is even more pitiful because, ironically, Troy will actually survive this immediate crisis. Just as when he refuses to fight, in 1.1, because his love seems so much more valuable than the war, Troilus attributes unwarranted grandeur to events concerning himself. In this way he demonstrates in his own person the central theme of the play.

In the *Iliad* of HOMER, Troilus was merely one of the many sons of PRIAM; he dies well before Hector does, and his role in the tale is insignificant. His connection with Cressida arose only in legends from the Middle Ages.

Troilus and Cressida

SYNOPSIS

Prologue

A PROLOGUE (3), dressed in armour, states that the scene of the play is TROY. The Greeks have invaded by sea and pitched camp outside the city. The play omits the first battles, he adds, and begins in the middle of the TROJAN WAR.

Act 1, Scene 1

TROILUS, a Trojan prince, is sick with love for CRESSIDA and declares he cannot join the fighting against the Greeks. He rebukes Cressida's relative, PANDARUS, who speaks of her beauty and thus aggravates his pain. Pandarus replies that he will no longer carry messages for Troilus if he is to be reprimanded, but he continues to remark on Cressida's virtues. He observes that Cressida's father has deserted to the Greeks. Troilus regrets that he must depend on Pandarus to approach Cressida. A Trojan general, AENEAS, reports that Troilus' brother PARIS (3) has been wounded by the Greek MENELAUS. This shames Troilus into returning to the battlefield.

Act 1, Scene 2

Cressida's servant, ALEXANDER (1), tells her that the Trojan crown prince, HECTOR, wounded by AJAX the previous day, is raging for a fight on the battlefield. Alexander comically describes Ajax as a brute though a valiant warrior. Pandarus arrives; he and Cressida watch the Trojan warriors returning from the field while Pandarus praises Troilus. Cressida denounces Pandarus as a procurer after he leaves, but confesses that she is attracted to Troilus. She decides not to reveal her feelings, however, declaring that a man will cease desiring a woman once he knows she loves him.

Act 1, Scene 3

AGAMEMNON, the Greek commander-in-chief, counsels the other Greek leaders not to be discouraged by Troy's survival after seven years of warfare. The Greeks' failure to conquer, he insists, is a test imposed by Jove, who supports them. ULYSSES asserts that Troy stands only because the Greeks are weakened by disorder and faction. He sees this as a consequence of a lack of respect for rank. This is what preserves a society, he says, just as the cosmos would be weakened by insubordination of one of the planets. As an example, he points out the disrespectful behaviour of the warriors ACHILLES and PATROCLUS, who amuse themselves with insulting imitations of their superiors. NESTOR adds that Ajax and THERSITES, his jester, or FOOL (1), do the same. Aeneas arrives from Troy bearing a challenge from Hector daring any Greek to fight him in hand-to-hand combat the next day. Ulysses proposes a plot: although Hector's challenge is clearly directed at Achilles, the most renowned Greek warrior, the leaders should instead select another combatant, Ajax, through a fixed lottery. This might teach Achilles a lesson.

Act 2, Scene 1

Thersites subjects Ajax to witty but crude insults. He mocks him for envying Achilles' reputation. Too slow-witted to retort, Ajax beats the jester, who taunts him for it. Achilles and Patroclus appear and intervene, and Thersites insults them too, to their amusement. Achilles tells Ajax that Hector's challenge is to be met by a warrior selected by lottery.

Act 2, Scene 2

Hector recommends to the Trojan leaders that HELEN (1)—whose abduction by Paris from her husband Menelaus was the cause of the war—be released and the war ended. He says she is not worth further loss of life. Troilus counters that this would sully the Trojan honour. The princess CASSANDRA appears, hysterically predicts disaster for Troy unless Helen is released, and leaves. Troilus states that Cassandra should not influence them because she is insane. Paris argues for keeping Helen in the name of his honour. Hector criticises Troilus and Paris for their immaturity. He then goes on to observe that while absolute right demands that they return Menelaus' wife, he will concede that their honour is a proper issue, and con-

cludes that they must continue fighting. He tells of the challenge he has issued to the Greeks.

Act 2, Scene 3
Thersites, alone, rails against Ajax and Achilles and then insults Achilles and Patroclus when they arrive. When the Greek leaders and Ajax appear, Achilles enters his tent and refuses to see them. After rejecting several messages, he sends word that he refuses to fight the next day. Ajax criticises Achilles for his pride, while, in humorous asides, the other Greeks remark on Ajax' own. They then flatter him extravagantly to his face.

Act 3, Scene 1
Pandarus calls on Paris and Helen and gives Paris a message from Troilus requesting that he make an excuse for him to King PRIAM for missing dinner that night. Paris assumes that Troilus intends to visit Cressida, but Pandarus denies it. This conversation is held in asides so that Helen does not hear it. Helen prevails on Pandarus to sing, and he delivers a song about love.

Act 3, Scene 2
Pandarus brings Cressida to Troilus and they kiss passionately. Troilus swears undying love, and Pandarus promises the same on his niece's behalf. Cressida confesses that she has loved Troilus for a long time. He observes that although he distrusts the fidelity of women, he is himself by nature faithful; she insists that she will be also. Pandarus declares himself the formal witness to their vows and takes them to a bedroom.

Act 3, Scene 3
Cressida's father, CALCHAS, asks the Greek leaders to reward him for having deserted to their side by exchanging Trojan prisoners for his daughter. Agamemnon agrees, and DIOMEDES (1) is told to conduct the exchange. Ulysses suggests that the Greek leaders pointedly ignore the arrogant Achilles to create an occasion for Ulysses to deliver a lecture he has prepared. They agree, and Achilles receives a lengthy talk on honour and reputation from Ulysses. A person's value can only be defined in terms of other people's applause, Ulysses says, adding that Achilles is becoming less valuable since the applause is going to Ajax. Although still relatively unknown, Ajax will now become famous through fighting Hector. Patroclus seconds the lesson, observing that Achilles' refusal to fight has diminished his reputation. Thersites arrives and comically describes Ajax' strutting pride. Achilles wishes to meet Hector and tells Patroclus to ask Ajax to arrange a meeting. Patroclus rehearses this message with Thersites playing a ludicrously inarticulate Ajax. Achilles decides to write Ajax a letter instead.

Act 4, Scene 1
Paris escorts Diomedes and ANTENOR, the captured Trojan who is to be exchanged for Cressida, and they encounter Aeneas. Aeneas and Diomedes exchange chivalrous challenges. In asides, Paris tells Aeneas to go ahead of them and get Troilus away from Cressida's house. Talking with Paris, Diomedes denounces Helen as the cause of a pointless war.

Act 4, Scene 2
Troilus bids farewell to Cressida at dawn; she unhappily begs him to stay. Pandarus appears and teases his niece about having lost her virginity. Aeneas arrives and tells Troilus that Cressida is to be exchanged for a prisoner and will depart immediately. Shocked and aggrieved, Troilus goes with Aeneas to meet the deputation as if by chance. The horrified Pandarus breaks the news to Cressida, who vows never to leave.

Act 4, Scene 3
Paris sends the heartsick Troilus ahead of the deputation to bring Cressida out to be delivered to Diomedes.

Act 4, Scene 4
Troilus assures Cressida that he will try to visit her secretly in the Greek camp. They exchange tokens of love: he gives her a sleeve, and she gives him a glove. He asks her to be faithful, and she assures him she will be, but he cautions her that the Greeks are seductive men. Diomedes arrives to accompany Cressida to the Greek camp. Troilus and Diomedes exchange rather sharp courtesies as the group leaves for the city gates. Paris and Aeneas hurry to accompany Hector to the battlefield.

Act 4, Scene 5
Diomedes arrives with Cressida as the Greeks assemble to view the combat of Ajax and Hector. They greet her merrily, kissing her and engaging in witty repartee and sexual innuendo. After Diomedes takes her to her father, Nestor praises her wit, but Ulysses calls her sexually provocative. The Trojans arrive. Hector says he does not wish to fight to the death because Ajax, part Trojan and part Greek, is his cousin. After a brief fight he chivalrously declines to continue. Ajax introduces Hector to the Greek leaders. Achilles insults him, and the two exchange challenges and agree to a hand-to-hand combat the next day. Troilus asks Ulysses to guide him to the tent of Cressida's father.

Act 5, Scene 1
Achilles tells Patroclus that he intends to get Hector drunk so he can defeat him more easily the next day. Thersites arrives with a letter for Achilles and engages Patroclus in an exchange of insults. Achilles announces that the letter, from his lover in Troy, has reminded him of an oath he made to her that he will not fight. He and Patroclus leave to prepare for the banquet. A number of the Greeks arrive for the banquet with Hector and Troilus. Diomedes excuses him-

self, and Troilus follows him accompanied by Ulysses with Thersites following them.

Act 5, Scene 2
Diomedes meets Cressida, spied upon by Troilus and Ulysses from one direction and Thersites from another. Diomedes reminds Cressida of a promise she has made, but she tries to revoke it and beseeches him not to tempt her further. He insists on taking from her the sleeve she had been given by Troilus. She refuses to tell him who it was from, but she finally gives it to him and agrees to a later rendezvous. Thersites comments keenly on these developments; Ulysses quiets Troilus' growing anger. Diomedes leaves, and Cressida, thinking herself alone, laments her unfaithfulness to Troilus and her susceptibility to romance. After she leaves Troilus mourns the collapse of his world and swears he will kill Diomedes in the next day's fighting.

Act 5, Scene 3
Hector's wife, ANDROMACHE, King Priam, and Cassandra attempt to persuade him not to fight on a day of terrible omens, but he insists he will. Troilus vows he will kill mercilessly. Pandarus brings Troilus a letter from Cressida, but he tears it up.

Act 5, Scene 4
Thersites watches the fighting and describes it in disrespectful terms. Diomedes and Troilus appear, fighting, and continue off-stage. Hector challenges Thersites, but he claims he is a coward and is left alone.

Act 5, Scene 5
Diomedes tells his SERVANT (17) to take Troilus' captured horse to Cressida. Agamemnon arrives with news of Trojan triumphs on the battlefield. Nestor appears with the corpse of Patroclus, which he sends to Achilles. Ulysses reports that Achilles, inflamed by the death of Patroclus, is arming for battle. Ajax, Diomedes, and Achilles arrive and immediately go to join the fighting.

Act 5, Scene 6
Troilus fights Ajax and Diomedes simultaneously, as they disappear off-stage. Achilles and Hector fight; Achilles is winded, and Hector chivalrously offers him a respite, but Achilles insults him and leaves, vowing to return. Hector fights an anonymous Greek in splendid armour. He swears to capture his fine equipment.

Act 5, Scene 7
Achilles instructs the MYRMIDONS to accompany him but to fight as little as possible. They are to save their strength for an encounter with Hector where they are to surround him and kill him. Thersites watches a running skirmish between Menelaus and Paris, cheering them on with vulgar remarks. The Trojan MARGARELON identifies himself as a bastard son of Priam and challenges Thersites to fight, but the jester flees, saying that he, too, is a bastard and a coward to boot.

Act 5, Scene 8
Hector, having killed the Greek warrior, starts to exchange sets of armour and is thus unprotected when the Myrmidons appear. They kill Hector as Achilles looks on. As night falls, the armies separate, and Achilles announces that he will drag Hector's body behind his horse as he returns to camp.

Act 5, Scene 9
The Greek leaders reflect that if Achilles has truly defeated Hector, then they have finally won the war.

Act 5, Scene 10
Troilus announces Hector's death to Aeneas and other Trojans, but he insists they continue to fight the next morning. Pandarus arrives, but Troilus spurns him and leaves with the other soldiers. Pandarus delivers an EPILOGUE in which he bemoans that the fate of the procurer is to be despised. He declares that the audience are pimps too and asks their sympathy for his venereal diseases. He says that in two months he intends to draw up his will and bequeath them his ailments.

COMMENTARY

Although *Troilus and Cressida* contains humorous material and is conventionally classed as a COMEDY, its bleak ending and its bitter picture of love and power place it among the PROBLEM PLAYS. These works are troubling and ambiguous in their treatment of society and sexuality, and they lack the clear triumph of love that is usually associated with comedy. *Troilus and Cressida* offers an extravagantly corrupt and artificial world. A venomous parody of a classic legend, it satirises the glamorous attitudes people often have towards sex and/or war. Pretensions to romantic love and to military glory are thoroughly deflated.

The basic satirical technique employed in *Troilus and Cressida* is the use of character types. The dim-witted and prideful oaf, the deluded lover, the cruel and ambitious noble, the voyeur, the coward, the abusive critic—all are presented boldly in Shakespeare's play as (respectively) Ajax, Troilus, Achilles, Pandarus, and, combining the last two, Thersites. Shakespeare makes these character types interesting, but the depiction of personality was of secondary importance as the playwright's purpose in this play was not psychological but philosophical.

Another device that helps establish the satire is the skewed presentation of familiar material. As presented by Shakespeare, the heroes of the TROJAN WAR and the figures in the famous tale of Cressida's betrayal are seen inhabiting a corrupt world. They are either agents of corruption or deluded and ineffectual victims of it. The contrast between the familiar heroic legends and Shakespeare's satire is so great that the comic intent of the work is obvious. Thirdly, the role

of Thersites resembles that of the traditional CHORUS (1) and boldly emphasises the satire's critique.

The two plot lines interact very little, but they echo each other and are thematically related, for both illustrate foolish self-deception and emotional dishonesty. The human tendency to succumb to illusions about life is isolated and exaggerated by the play. The two lovers proclaim great emotional involvement, but Cressida's infidelity is hinted at from the outset, and Troilus' self-deception does not hide the true nature of their purely sexual affair. It offers no hint of the fulfilling mutual enjoyment of real love. It seems more tawdry because it is dependent on Pandarus as procurer. Though she undeniably betrays her lover, Cressida is not portrayed harshly. Rather than being a vicious breaker of hearts, she is seen as a representative of human, or perhaps feminine, weakness—'Ah, poor our sex!' (5.2.108), she cries. Troilus is the principal object of satire. His self-deception is extensively developed in both the love story and the warriors' plot, in which he is also a major figure. Just as he deludes himself about romantic love, calling Cressida a 'pearl' (1.1.100), he also deludes himself about the pointless war for Helen on the ground that *she* is a 'pearl' (2.2.82) and the Trojans doers of 'valiant and magnanimous deeds' (2.2.201) in defence of her.

The warriors talk of honour and glory, but they too are self-deluded. However, the Trojans and the Greeks are gripped by different illusions. Troilus and Hector believe the war is a chivalric game and the stakes are the personal reputations of the warriors—though in the end both succumb to other motives. Ulysses, on the other hand, believes that an orderly social hierarchy can be maintained through clever reasoning, such as he attempts to employ with Achilles. He, too, abandons his own truth and eventually argues to Achilles that the only merit is in the fleeting glory of reputation. He thus takes a position rather like Hector's, and this ironically reinforces the play's emphasis on human error. The Greek failure to observe Ulysses' ideal of social organisation leads to internal squabbling and a collective inertia that is only broken by Patroclus' death; the Trojans have a false idea of honour that leads to their utter defeat at the play's close. By the end of the play, neither honour nor reason controls the warriors; only greed, injured pride, and revenge motivate the action.

Both Troilus' violent despair and Hector's death are results of their illusions. These two idealistic, if foolish, characters represent the traditional codes of romantic love and military honour that are being deflated by the play's satire, and in the end they find themselves completely at the mercy of ugly reality. Troilus, unable to accept the reality that his romance was only a sexual encounter, takes refuge in violence, to the point of comically forgetting what he is fighting about when he demands of Diomedes 'the life thou ow'st me for my horse' (5.6.7). Hector, who insists on the worth of chivalric honour, dies because Achilles does not observe the code. His own behaviour, however, is just as important, for he is only vulnerable to Achilles because he has abandoned his ideals long enough to pursue a rich piece of booty, the Grecian armour that he is about to don when he is attacked.

Considered alone, the warrior plot amounts to a scathing indictment of warmongers—Hector and Ulysses serving to point up the wickedness of the others—and the play is often taken as an anti-war manifesto. However, the depiction of war serves a more general purpose. War in the play has an equivalent function to that of sex—in the 17th century it was a commonly glamorised human activity—and as such is a telling venue for satire.

The delusions and misjudgements that plague the characters stem from a simple yet inexorable factor: the passage of time. The characters are aware of this, though usually unconscious of its particular effect on themselves. In 4.5, just before the warrior plot begins to build to its bloody climax, Agamemnon stresses the value of the temporary peace in terms of its impermanence: 'What's past and what's to come is strew'd with husks / And formless ruin of oblivion . . . [by contrast with] this extant moment' (4.5.165–167). This emphasis on the value of things as they are at the present moment, without respect to what they were or will be later, echoes Ulysses' claim that 'Love, friendship, charity, are subjects all / To envious and calumniating Time' (3.3.173–174).

The audience's familiarity with the legendary tales on which the play is based strengthens the irony. For instance, we are startled by a stark truth when Helen, intending only an idle pleasantry, observes that 'love will undo us all' (3.1.105). And when Pandarus unwittingly predicts the lovers' fate to become symbols of the betrayed and the betrayer (with himself the panderer), we can only hold our breath as each affirms, 'Amen' (3.2.203–205). These ironies are not only powerful theatrical moments, they also contribute to our awareness that the characters are undone by a process—time—over which they have no control.

Time also changes the value placed on things or people. Cressida observes that 'Things won are done; joy's soul lies in the doing' (1.2.292), suggesting that the value of a goal diminishes as it is achieved. Further, Ulysses proposes to Achilles that time brings the destruction of glory through forgetfulness: 'good deeds past . . . are devour'd / As fast as they are made, forgot as soon / As done' (3.3.148–150). Troilus argues that circumstances over time determine worth: once a woman becomes a man's wife, his evaluation of her must rest on that relationship, which once did not exist but is undeniable once it does (in the age before divorce). Therefore, he declares, Helen is valuable enough to fight over simply because, as 'a theme of

honour and renown' (2.2.200), she has been fought over already. 'What's aught but as 'tis valued?' (2.2. 53), he says, but he doesn't apply this argument to himself: Cressida will, at another time, value him differently, placing him below the more available man.

The idea that values can change is extremely troubling because it contradicts the stabilising belief in a constant reality. The development of this difficult theme over the course of the play prepares us for the emotional tone of its chaotic culmination in Act 5. In 5.1 Achilles is reminded of his lover in Troy and decides his reputation is less important than she and refuses to fight. In 5.2 Troilus learns of Cressida's revaluation of him and is driven to berserk combat. Forecasts of disaster in 5.3 remind us of the effect time will eventually have on Troy, and the remaining scenes present brutal fighting where all is devalued. Reversing his decision of 5.1, Achilles goes to battle, the raging Troilus attaches Cressida's value to his horse, and Thersites rejects all honour. Most distressingly, perhaps, Hector is betrayed by his own chivalric values, which lead him to courteously refuse his advantage over Achilles, in 5.6, who then kills him in 5.8. Worse, Hector betrays his vision himself in chasing after loot, which leaves him vulnerable to Achilles.

The play's relativism strikes a responsive chord in modern sensibilities, and this may contribute more to its popularity in the 20th century than does its reputation as an anti-war piece. It may also account for its origins, for when it was written, England was undergoing unprecedented change as it entered the 17th century; massive revolution and civil war were only forty years away. A changing economic world generated great uneasiness (as is especially reflected in *The Merchant of Venice*). The reformation was only a few generations old, and religious tensions still pervaded society; moreover, religious beliefs placed England at odds with the two most powerful nations in Europe, FRANCE (1) and Spain. Though the Spanish Armada had been defeated in 1588, the threat of war still loomed, particularly in light of the imminent death of Queen ELIZABETH (1). Though old and in poor health, the queen refused to name a successor; the possibility of civil war or invasion by opportunistic foreign monarchs was widely discussed. This atmosphere of crisis—combined with the appearance of CHAPMAN's translation of the *Iliad*—generated a vogue for tales of Troy, and several plays on the subject were written before Shakespeare's. The English identified with the Trojans (see TROY), and the legend was regarded as a clear example of disaster. The disturbing quality of *Troilus and Cressida* is thus part of England's catharsis; the nation's uneasiness found an outlet in the re-enactment of an ancient battle.

Some critics find the play to be an assertion that life is essentially meaningless and that chaos is the inevitable outcome of humanity's futile endeavours. However, this point of view ignores what Shakespeare does in the play to undercut this. For instance, the idea that Cressida is representative of all women is introduced by Troilus, who insists that the fact of her betrayal must be denied 'for [the sake of] womanhood' (5.2. 128). However, his raving is effectively countered by its senselessness in denying what is obviously true, and by the deprecating remarks of Ulysses and Thersites. And elsewhere the tendency towards outright misanthropy is checked—the Greeks and Trojans fraternising in the peaceful 'extant moment' (4.5.167) of their truce; Ulysses evoking a world without the 'envious fever / Of pale and bloodless emulation' (1.3.133–134); Hector's commitment, however flawed, to an ideal of chivalry—such images, woven into the play's general critique of human society, collectively offer an idea of what man might be in a better world than that of the play. Ulysses and Hector, spokesmen for sanity, map out principles for such a world in their famous speeches in the war councils of the Greeks and Trojans. Ulysses advocates a social order like that of the 'heavens themselves' (1.3.85), and Hector cites the 'law in each well-order'd nation' (2.2.181). Each leader fails to institute such principles or even to be true to them himself, but they stand as ideals against which their conduct is measured by the audience. It is an essential characteristic of satire that its critique of human failings implies the possibility of improvement. Though honour and love are corruptible, they can still exist.

While it is a harshly critical work, *Troilus and Cressida* contains much humour and sympathy. For instance, the vicious anger of Thersites and the sly lewdness of Pandarus may not be likeable, but they are inventive and undeniably funny characters. Helen presents a humorous caricature of a thoughtless society hostess, and Ajax is a comical buffoon, especially as impersonated by Thersites in 3.3.279–302. Also, a number of the characters are, at times, humanly sympathetic: the lovers in their aspirations to happiness; Hector in his chivalric idealism; and Ulysses as a commonsense, reasonable man. Even the abrasive Thersites can be respected for his capacity to see through the pretensions of the Greek warriors.

The Epilogue highlights the play's essentially positive intentions. Pandarus' flippant insults make an obvious distinction between the real world of the audience—which of course is not composed of 'traitors and bawds' (5.10.37)—and the fictional world of the play. Shakespeare's comical pairing of the audience with the pander serves as a release from the bleak last moments of the play. The satire is thereby stressed a last time, contrasting the existence of human virtues—our own, at least—to the vices that have been depicted on the stage.

Thus, despite its bleak and bloody dénouement, the play shares the essential optimism of all comedy. The

characters are defeated by the imperfections of themselves and their world, but most playgoers and readers care less about their fate than they do about the more general picture of human folly that the satire has so convincingly presented. *Troilus and Cressida,* like all satire, is to some extent educational, and we find ourselves more thoughtful and aware, perhaps in some sense morally elevated, through our experience of the play.

SOURCES OF THE PLAY

Three chief sources—George CHAPMAN's translation of HOMER's *Iliad* (where the Trojan War was first recorded), and two English renderings, by William CAXTON and John LYDGATE, of a different versions—inspired Shakespeare's presentation of the war in *Troilus and Cressida.* The tale of Cressida's betrayal came from Geoffrey CHAUCER's great poem *Troilus and Criseyde.*

The incidents from Homer in *Troilus and Cressida* tend to be those covered in Chapman's translation (1598), and several verbal echoes confirm that Shakespeare used this work, though nine translations were available to him—five Latin, two French, and two English. Some scholars believe that the play may have been intended in part as a satire against Chapman, whose great admiration for the Greeks, rooted in Homer, was counter to the ordinary English reader's identification with the Trojans.

Homer was not the immediate source for English knowledge of the Trojan War. Traditionally, another work was regarded as more authoritative than the *Iliad* because it was supposedly written by a Trojan eyewitness to the war, Dares Phrygius (Dares the Trojan), himself a minor character in the *Iliad.* This Latin prose account was actually written in the 5th or 6th century A.D. It inspired a 12th-century French poem by Benoît de SAINTE-MAURE, which in turn was rendered into Latin prose by Guido delle COLONNE, a Sicilian. His *Historia destructionis Troiae* (1270–1287) was the standard work on the subject for centuries.

A French version of Colonne's *Historia* was translated by Caxton as *The Recuyell of the Historyes of Troye* (1475, 5th ed. 1596). Lydgate's long poem entitled *Troy Book* (1420, publ. 1512, 1555) was inspired directly by Colonne. Caxton provided much of the detail in Shakespeare's account of the war, while Lydgate drew attention to the chivalric aspects of the warriors' encounters.

The story of Cressida and Troilus first appeared in Saint-Maure's poem, where Diomedes and Troilus are rivals for the love of Briseis, the original of Cressida; all of them are only minor figures in Homer. BOCCACCIO's poem *Filostrato* (1338) was inspired by Saint-Maure; here Pandarus was first given prominence. *Filostrato* in turn inspired Chaucer's *Troilus and Criseyde* (c. 1482), which provided Shakespeare with his version of the story, though the playwright eliminates many incidents to achieve a fast-paced plot.

One of Shakespeare's favourite works, OVID's *Metamorphoses,* in the translation by Arthur GOLDING, probably inspired a number of passages, especially parts of Ulysses' speeches. Also, several ideas and incidents—especially in the debate among the Trojans in 2.2—may owe something to *Euphues his Censure to Philautus* (1587) by Robert GREENE (2), a work consisting of philosophical dialogues ascribed to Greek and Trojan warriors meeting during a truce.

TEXT OF THE PLAY

Troilus and Cressida was registered with the STATIONERS' COMPANY by James ROBERTS in February 1603 but was not published then. Such a blocking action was commonly used to prevent piracy of a new play, so *Troilus and Cressida* was probably new in early 1603 and written in the previous year. However, the play contains considerable evidence of rewriting before publication.

It was finally published in 1609 by Richard BONIAN and Henry WALLEY, in a QUARTO edition (known as Q) printed by George ELD. Q appeared in two versions, the second of which has a different title-page and an attached 'Epistle' preceding the text of the play. These alterations were apparently made in the course of printing the edition, though sometimes the two versions are referred to as separate editions. Q is thought to have been printed from a scribal copy of Shakespeare's FOUL PAPERS, or possibly from the manuscript itself; the evidence is obscure and disputed.

In 1623 *Troilus and Cressida* was included in the FIRST FOLIO, and this text (known as F) was based on Q, but it incorporates numerous minor corrections and adds the Prologue as well as about forty other smaller passages. The manuscript used for F had probably been prepared for the KING'S MEN, the acting company that produced the play, for the Folio has many more and markedly superior stage directions.

What the manuscripts were that were used for Q and F, and how they differed, remains uncertain; subsequent editors of the play have been forced to regard both as authoritative, adopting specific readings on a case-by-case basis.

THEATRICAL HISTORY OF THE PLAY

The early history of *Troilus and Cressida* is quite mysterious. The registration of the play in 1603 states that it had been staged by the CHAMBERLAIN'S MEN (soon to become the King's Men), indicating at least one performance in 1602 or 1603. However, while the first title-page of Q (1609) observes that the play had been acted by the King's Men, the second omits this claim and the Epistle expressly denies it. These contradictions combined with the play's philosophical themes, its high-flown rhetoric, bawdy humour, and legalistic

jokes, have sparked a theory that the play was commissioned for a private performance at one of the INNS OF COURT, or that an early version was altered for this purpose and Q was occasioned by this performance. In any case, the play seems to have been unpopular with 17th-century audiences, for the claim that it had not been publicly staged could not have been made if it had been widely performed. In fact, no records of any early performances of *Troilus and Cressida* have survived.

Indeed, no English production is recorded until 1907 (though it was staged in German at Munich in 1898). However, in 1679 John DRYDEN produced an abridged *Troilus and Cressida*, generally known by its subtitle, *Truth Found Too Late*, which featured a faithful Cressida and a conventionally tragic ending in which Cressida, Troilus, and Diomedes all die. This version, in which Thomas BETTERTON played Troilus, was popular for a few years, and several editions of the text were published before it disappeared from the stage.

Troilus and Cressida has proven popular in the 20th century; its criticisms of war and its relativistic values seem natural to modern audiences, and a number of distinctive productions have resulted. William POEL first produced an uncut text, with Edith EVANS (1) as Cressida (1912–1913). In 1938 Barry JACKSON (1) emphasised the play's anti-war message by costuming the Greeks as Nazis; similarly, Tyrone GUTHRIE's 1956 staging was set early in this century in an imaginary Central European country, and his Greeks wore the spiked helmets of 19th-century Prussian soldiers. In 1960 Peter HALL (5) produced the play on an abstract set, while John BARTON (1) used many startling properties and costumes—along with some near-nudity—in a notorious production of 1976. *Troilus and Cressida* has never been a FILM but has been produced for TELEVISION three times.

Trojan War Legendary conflict between the ancient Greeks and the Trojans, often mentioned in Shakespeare's works, most notably in *Troilus and Cressida*, which enacts part of it. In classical myth and legend, beginning with the *Iliad* of HOMER, the Trojan War was fought by the city of TROY against invaders from Greece, who were attempting to avenge the abduction of a Greek queen, HELEN (1), by a Trojan prince, PARIS (3). The story was quite familiar to Shakespeare's audiences.

As the PROLOGUE (3) declares, *Troilus and Cressida* begins well into the conflict, with the Greeks continuing a seven-year-long siege of Troy, and it ends with the Trojan forces in disarray, facing apparent defeat. However, as the playwright and his audience both knew, that defeat was to be deferred until, in a later episode, Greek troops were smuggled into the city inside the famed Trojan Horse, ostensibly a gift signifying the Greeks' abandonment of their siege. The subsequent sack of Troy is described in a long passage in *The Rape of Lucrece* (lines 1366–1533). Another striking use of the war occurs in *Hamlet*, where the FIRST PLAYER (2) delivers a dramatic account of the killing of King PRIAM of Troy and the grief of Queen HECUBA (2.2.448–514).

According to Greek mythology, Zeus arranged the Trojan War as a cure for overpopulation. With the assistance of Eris, goddess of discord, he sparked a dispute among three goddesses as to which was the most beautiful. Paris was appointed to decide; bribed with the promise of the world's most beautiful woman as a bride, he chose Aphrodite. She rewarded him by helping him to kidnap Helen. Though this well-known legend arose before Homer's time, he ascribes Paris' abduction of Helen to his love for her beauty, with no mention of divine aid.

The Troublesome Raigne of King John Anonymous Elizabethan play published in 1591, probably derived from Shakespeare's *King John* but traditionally regarded as its source. It was long argued that *The Troublesome Raigne*, as the play is known, was adapted by Shakespeare in writing *King John*, but modern scholars—and others, beginning with Alexander POPE (1)—have challenged this assumption, noting the many respects in which the anonymous play resembles a BAD QUARTO: it contains echoes of other plays, including *3 Henry VI*, *Richard III*, and works by MARLOWE (1) and PEELE; its published text is riddled with errors, including ambiguous or missing stage directions; and it contains passages in which stage directions summarise and describe missing dialogue. Moreover, the 1591 title-page associates *The Troublesome Raigne* with an acting company, the QUEEN'S MEN (1), that is known to have put on a number of such derivative plays, including THE TAMING OF A SHREW.

Troy Ancient city of Asia Minor, the site of the TROJAN WAR of Greek legend and the setting for *Troilus and Cressida*. In the play Troy and its people are decadent and immoral. Although they know that HELEN (1) is a worthless prize, the aristocratic warriors carry on a costly conflict simply because they wish to achieve military renown. Love in Troy is represented by the sexual encounter of CRESSIDA and Prince TROILUS as arranged by the voyeuristic PANDARUS. Once the Trojans' great hero HECTOR is killed the city is helpless, and at the play's bleak close, the Greeks are on the verge of victory.

While the Troy of the play is seen as corrupt, the leaders of Troy are distinctly less evil than the Greeks, and it is clear that the playwright felt a bias in favour of the Trojans. This may seem surprising to modern readers familiar with the pro-Greek sentiments of

Troy's first chronicler, HOMER. However, like most western Europeans at the end of the Middle Ages, the English identified with Troy, believing themselves the descendants of Trojan refugees scattered by the defeat of the city. This legend sprang from the ancient Roman belief found in the *Aeneid* of VIRGIL that Rome had been founded by AENEAS. In English tradition the British Isles were first colonised by a great-grandson of AENEAS named Brut, who was said to have founded London, naming it New Troy, and for whom Britain was believed to be named. Accordingly, the English derived the history of Troy from pro-Trojan accounts.

All histories of Troy are legendary—Homer composed his work centuries after its fall—and the historical city is known only through archaeology, principally the famous excavations by Heinrich Schliemann (1822–1890). In the north-west corner of what is now Turkey, Troy occupied a strategically important location overlooking the Dardanelles, a strait that provided access to the Black Sea and was a major route for trade. Troy's location is thought to have been the likeliest stimulus for a Greek invasion. A long succession of ancient cities stood on the same site from as early as 5,000 years ago. Each of these was a rich and heavily fortified town, presumably the capital of the surrounding territory. The seventh of these settlements is believed to have been the one besieged by the Greeks because it was destroyed by a great fire and because it existed at the right time, c. 1200 B.C. Other cities continued to occupy the site until early Christian times.

Troyes City in eastern FRANCE (1), location for 5.2 of *Henry V.* In 1420 the treaty that confirmed King HENRY V's conquest of France was signed at Troyes, located in the domains of the Duke of BURGUNDY (2), England's ally. This event is presented in the play, though the principal action in the scene is Henry's courtship of Princess KATHARINE (2). The only clause of the treaty alluded to, besides the marriage of Henry and Katharine, is the declaration of Henry as the heir to the French crown, pronounced in French and Latin, in 5.2.356–360.

Historically the treaty of Troyes did not result from the English victory at AGINCOURT, as the play suggests. Simplifying his drama, and emphasising the glory of Agincourt, Shakespeare omitted the events that actually produced the treaty, several years of campaigning in Normandy and, crucially, Burgundy's alliance with England. In the play the Duke of Burgundy appears to speak for the FRENCH KING at Troyes.

The True Tragedy Abbreviated title of the BAD QUARTO version of *3 Henry VI,* originally titled *The true Tragedy of Richard Duke of Yorke, and the death of good King Henrie the Sixt, with the whole contention betweene the two Houses Lancaster and Yorke, as it was sundrie times acted by the Right Honourable the Earle of Pembrooke his servants.* It was published twice by Thomas MILLINGTON, in 1595 and 1600; these are known as the Q1 and Q2 editions, respectively, of *3 Henry VI.* (Although the 1595 edition, of which only one copy has survived, was actually published in octavo format, the term *quarto* is retained for convenience.)

It was once believed that *The True Tragedy* was the text of an earlier play, by Shakespeare or someone else, that Shakespeare revised. However, it is now generally agreed that it is a 'reported' copy of *3 Henry VI,* probably recorded mostly by the actors who played WARWICK (3), CLIFFORD (1), and YORK (8). *The True Tragedy* is a good deal shorter than *3 Henry VI,* probably to reduce the playing time; the omitted sections are chiefly passages of rhetoric and poetic description that do not affect the progress of the plot. It is also possible that some passages, dealing with treason or usurpation of the crown, may have been subject to CENSORSHIP.

Q3 of *3 Henry VI,* a slightly edited version of *The True Tragedy,* was published in 1619 by Thomas PAVIER, in a volume with a 'bad quarto' version of *2 Henry VI.* This edition is known by its abbreviated title as THE WHOLE CONTENTION.

Trundell, John (active 1603–1626) London publisher and bookseller. Trundell co-published the first edition (Q1) of *Hamlet* with Nicholas LING in 1603. Little else is known of him.

Tubal Minor character in *The Merchant of Venice,* friend of SHYLOCK. In 3.1 Tubal tells Shylock that he has been unable to find his friend's daughter, JESSICA, who has eloped, but that he has heard reports of her extravagance with the money she has stolen from her father. Tubal also discloses that ANTONIO (2) has suffered grave commercial losses, thus putting him at the mercy of Shylock, who has loaned him money. Shylock's responses, alternating from delirious anger to exultant delight, are grimly humorous. Tubal's name occurs among the list of descendants of Noah in Genesis 10:2; Biblical scholars of Shakespeare's day thought it meant 'confusion' or 'slander', though modern scholars believe it refers to an ancient tribe.

Tuckfeild, Thomas (active 1624) English actor who may have performed in early productions of *The Two Noble Kinsmen.* In the first edition of the play (Q1, 1634), the stage direction opening 5.3 names the Attendants called for; one of them is named 'T. Tucke'. Scholars believe that this refers to Tuckfeild, indicating that he played the part in an early production by the KING'S MEN. Tuckfeild was with the company in 1624, so this clue (with similar evidence concerning Curtis GREVILLE [1]) suggests that Q1 was printed from a PROMPT-BOOK of the 1620s. Tuckfeild is known

from a single document, listing him among the King's Men's 'musicians and other necessary attendants'.

Tudor Dynasty Ruling family in England from 1485 to 1603. The first Tudor monarch was King Henry VII, who seized the throne after winning the final phase of the WARS OF THE ROSES by defeating RICHARD III at the battle of BOSWORTH FIELD. This event is the climax of the long period of conflict dealt with in Shakespeare's HISTORY PLAYS. Henry VII appears in *Richard III* as the Earl of RICHMOND. His son, King HENRY VIII, who ruled from 1509 to 1547, is depicted in *Henry VIII* as a symbol of good kingship, in a play that emphasises his part in introducing Protestantism to England. Henry's son ruled as King Edward VI from 1547 to 1553 but died at 15. His sister Mary was queen from 1553 to 1558; a Catholic, she persecuted Protestants, and it was only under her younger sister ELIZABETH (1) that English Protestantism was finally and firmly established. Queen Elizabeth, who reigned during most of Shakespeare's lifetime, was the last Tudor monarch; upon her death in 1603 the STUART DYNASTY came to the throne. The 16th century saw the country emerge from medieval economic and political practises into the early modern period. Thus, the Tudors presided over a crucial transition in the country's history.

Tutor Minor character in *3 Henry VI,* adult companion of the child RUTLAND (1), the son of the Duke of YORK (8). The Tutor unsuccessfully attempts to spirit the boy away from the battle of WAKEFIELD, but Lord CLIFFORD (1) captures them and, in his pursuit of vengeance against York, declares he will murder Rutland. The Tutor tries to dissuade the killer, but he is unceremoniously taken away by Clifford's soldiers and the avenger does indeed slay the child.

Twelfth Night

SYNOPSIS

Act 1, Scene 1
ORSINO, duke of ILLYRIA, speaks of his consuming passion for OLIVIA. His messenger, VALENTINE (3), reports that Olivia has turned him away, saying that she proposes to enter seclusion for seven years in memory of her late brother. Orsino marvels at her dedication, hoping it will someday be directed towards himself.

Act 1, Scene 2
VIOLA, shipwrecked but safe, is assured by the CAPTAIN (5) that her brother may have been saved also. The Captain informs her that they have landed in his home, Illyria, where the duke, Orsino, is courting a lady who has entered seclusion. Viola decides to become a follower of Orsino and pays the Captain to help disguise her as a man and introduce her to the duke.

Act 1, Scene 3
SIR TOBY Belch complains of the asceticism of Olivia, his niece, with whom he is living. Olivia's chambermaid, MARIA (2), suggests that he and his visiting friend SIR ANDREW Aguecheek, who hopes to woo Olivia, lead less riotous lives, for her mistress dislikes their drunken behaviour. Sir Andrew appears and announces that he will depart, given Orsino's rivalry for Olivia's hand, but Sir Toby assures him that Olivia disdains the duke, and he decides to stay.

Act 1, Scene 4
Valentine assures Viola, who is disguised as a boy, Cesario, that Orsino likes 'him'. The Duke appears and sends Cesario to try to persuade Olivia to marry him. Once alone, Viola muses on her distress: she has fallen in love with the man in whose behalf she must woo.

Act 1, Scene 5
Maria chastises Olivia's jester, FESTE, for his absence from court. Olivia appears with her steward, MALVOLIO. She is angry with the truant Feste, but his witticisms cajole her into a friendly mood. Malvolio berates Feste, but Olivia accuses the steward of an egotistical dislike of anything contrary to his own grumpiness. Maria announces that a messenger from Orsino has arrived; she and Malvolio are sent to keep him away. Sir Toby has encountered the messenger, but he is too drunk to report on him. Malvolio returns and says that the emissary has refused to depart, describing him as more a boy than a man. Olivia decides to greet this youth, who is the disguised Viola. Cesario speaks for Orsino in poetic terms that charm Olivia. She sends him back to the duke with another refusal, but after he leaves, Olivia confesses to herself that she has fallen in love with him. She sends Malvolio after Cesario with a ring, which she asserts the duke's messenger had forced on her.

Act 2, Scene 1
SEBASTIAN (2) tells ANTONIO (4), who has saved him from a shipwreck, that his sister died in the same disaster. Now fully recovered, he proposes to visit Duke Orsino. He insists that Antonio not accompany him; he already owes his saviour too much, he says, and his own bad luck might prove contagious. Sebastian then leaves alone, but Antonio decides that, although he has enemies at Orsino's court, he will follow his new friend.

Act 2, Scene 2
Malvolio gives Olivia's ring to the disguised Viola and departs. Viola realises that Olivia has fallen in love with Cesario. She reflects on the complexity of the situation—she loves Orsino, Orsino loves Olivia, and

Olivia loves her—and she observes that time will have to undo the tangle because she certainly cannot.

Act 2, Scene 3
Sir Toby, Sir Andrew, and Feste carouse drunkenly in Olivia's courtyard, when first Maria and then Malvolio appear to chastise them. Sir Toby mocks the steward, who departs, including Maria in his threats of reprisal as he goes. Maria proposes revenge upon Malvolio: she will write him love letters in Olivia's handwriting, and he will make a fool of himself when he responds to the supposed love of his mistress.

Act 2, Scene 4
Orsino talks of love with the disguised Viola; Cesario speaks of his affection for someone who resembles the duke. At Orsino's request, Feste sings a sad love song. Orsino sends Cesario on another mission to Olivia.

Act 2, Scene 5
Maria leaves a spurious love letter to be found by Malvolio. She, Sir Toby, Sir Andrew, and FABIAN, a fellow conspirator, spy on the steward, who preens himself on Olivia's love. He pictures himself married to Olivia, and he envisions a future when, as her husband, he will chastise Sir Toby; Sir Toby is furious, and his friends must restrain him. Malvolio finds the planted letter and responds as predicted; he will follow the letter's instructions, behaving oddly and wearing peculiar clothes, to signify that he has received the message. Malvolio leaves, and the conspirators rejoice in the success of their scheme.

Act 3, Scene 1
Viola, as Cesario, bandies wit with Feste; Sir Toby and Sir Andrew take her to Olivia, whom she is visiting on behalf of Orsino. Olivia confesses her love to Cesario, who rejects her suit, and she accepts rejection as her melancholy lot.

Act 3, Scene 2
Sir Andrew, seeing that Olivia favours Cesario, prepares to abandon his suit, but Sir Toby and Fabian reassure him, asserting that Olivia's behaviour towards the young man is intended to make Sir Andrew jealous. Sir Toby suggests that Sir Andrew challenge Cesario to a duel; Sir Andrew leaves to write a challenge to the youth. Fabian and Sir Toby chortle over the prospect of watching two cowards—Sir Andrew and Cesario—try to get out of the duel. Maria appears with word that Malvolio is ridiculously dressed, in response to the spurious love letter, and about to meet Olivia. They all run to watch.

Act 3, Scene 3
Sebastian thanks Antonio for rejoining him; Antonio observes that, because he had once been an enemy of Duke Orsino's, he cannot afford to be seen in Illyria. He decides to seclude himself at an inn and meet Sebastian there later.

Act 3, Scene 4
Malvolio, garishly costumed, leers and flirts with Olivia, who is mystified. When word arrives that Cesario has arrived, Olivia leaves but insists that Malvolio, obviously demented, be treated with care. Malvolio interprets her concern as evidence of her love. Sir Toby and Fabian enter, suggesting that Malvolio may be possessed by the devil; he sneers at them and leaves. The exultant plotters plan to have their victim locked up as a lunatic. Sir Andrew appears with a comical letter challenging Cesario to a duel. Sir Toby sends him to find the youth, then declares that the letter is too foolish to scare anyone, so he will deliver his own version of it directly to Cesario. The plotters withdraw as Olivia and Viola enter. Olivia repeatedly offers her love, and Cesario insists that she should grant it to Orsino. Olivia leaves, and Sir Toby ferociously challenges Cesario, allegedly on behalf of a famous swordsman; Viola, alarmed, attempts to find an excuse to leave. Sir Toby fetches Sir Andrew and tells him that Cesario has responded fiercely; he and Fabian encourage the reluctant duellists to fight. Antonio appears and draws his sword in defence of Viola, believing her to be Sebastian, but two OFFICERS (3) appear and arrest him. He asks Viola to repay an earlier loan, which he now will need, but Viola naturally denies that she knows him. As he is taken away, Antonio accuses Viola of ingratitude and calls her Sebastian. Viola realises that her brother must be alive, and she departs, ecstatic with hope. Sir Toby and Fabian point out that Cesario is a coward; Sir Andrew takes heart and sets out to resume the duel.

Act 4, Scene 1
Feste mistakes Sebastian for Cesario and is astonished to be treated as a stranger. Sir Andrew enters, and, making the same mistake, he strikes Sebastian, who responds by beating him. Sir Toby intervenes, and he and Sebastian draw their swords, as Olivia appears. Ordering everyone else to leave, she speaks with Sebastian, whom she also believes to be Cesario. She apologises for the assault and invites him inside; mystified but delighted, he goes with her.

Act 4, Scene 2
Feste disguises himself as Sir TOPAS, a Puritan clergyman, and visits Malvolio in prison. He insists that Malvolio is indeed mad and denies the steward's complaint that his cell is dark. Sir Toby congratulates the jester on his performance but says that it is time to end the joke, for he is in enough trouble with Olivia already. Feste again visits Malvolio, this time undisguised. Malvolio asks him for pen and paper so that he can write to Olivia about his predicament. Feste teases him before agreeing to help.

Act 4, Scene 3
Sebastian muses happily on the bewildering fact that he is apparently loved by a beautiful noblewoman.

Olivia appears with a PRIEST (2) and suggests that she and Sebastian marry. He agrees.

Act 5, Scene 1

Orsino calls on Olivia with Viola and other followers. Antonio appears in the custody of the Officers and is identified as the duke's enemy. He tells of Sebastian's disloyalty, referring to Viola's behaviour in 3.3. Orsino does not believe him because he knows that Cesario has been with him during the time Antonio claims to have spent with Sebastian. Olivia arrives and again rejects Orsino, who responds hysterically that he will kill Cesario, not only because he knows of Olivia's fondness for him but also because he loves the youth himself, and he seeks the pain of sacrifice. Viola declares herself willing to die for the duke, and Olivia cries out to her husband, as she believes Cesario to be. Viola denies this, and Olivia summons the Priest, who testifies to their marriage two hours earlier. As the duke berates Cesario, Sir Andrew and Sir Toby appear, wounded, claiming to have been assaulted by him. They are followed by Sebastian, whose appearance confounds everyone. Sebastian and Viola identify each other and rejoice in their reunion. The duke declares that he will marry Viola. Malvolio is summoned and shows Olivia the letter that he believes she sent him. Olivia realises that Maria has written it; Fabian defends Maria, saying that the plot was Sir Toby's idea and that Toby has married Maria. Feste teases Malvolio, who storms out vowing revenge. The duke declares that a double wedding shall soon occur, and all go indoors to celebrate, except Feste, who is left alone to sing a song of worldly resignation.

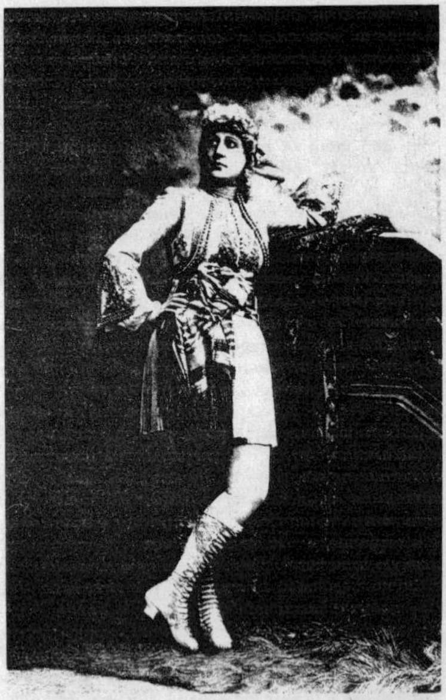

Viola, a character in Twelfth Night, *in a 19th-century illustration. Viola is put at the centre of the play's conflict when she poses as a young man, 'Cesario'.* (Courtesy of Culver Pictures, Inc.)

COMMENTARY

Twelfth Night was the last of Shakespeare's three 'mature' COMEDIES, as it, *Much Ado About Nothing*, and *As You Like It* are called, and it was followed shortly by the first of the major TRAGEDIES, *Hamlet.* This crucial position in Shakespeare's *oeuvre* is reflected in the play's subtle complexity. It sustains the celebration of triumphant love that characterises its predecessors, yet it is distinguished by a troubling undertone that suggests the playwright's need to deal with deeper realms of the human psyche.

Twelfth Night may be read or seen with pleasure on the level of traditional romantic comedy alone. Shakespeare assembles some stock features—separated twins, disguises, impediments to love—and freshly arranges them in a sequence that resembles a stately dance, all accompanied by a lusty SUB-PLOT with a comic villain, Malvolio. The characters are exaggerated examples of human nature, placed in comically preposterous situations whose improbability we willingly accept as necessary for the retelling of a familiar tale. The world of the play is an undemanding one; there is always time for leisurely courtship, for songs, and for practical jokes; Malvolio deserves his lot, because he arrogantly and egotistically refuses to enter the fun.

However, Malvolio is merely a nuisance and not a threat; the triumph of love depends on opposition—such as that offered by the villainous Don JOHN (1) in *Much Ado*—and at first glance that opposition is not present in *Twelfth Night.* It turns out to be Orsino and Olivia, two of the lovers themselves, who inhibit the fulfilment of love, assuming wholly literary self-images as romantic lover and mourning lady respectively. Their self-defeating posture suggests that something is amiss in the idyllic world of romantic comedy. The other important characters inspire a certain disquiet as well. Viola, the most clear-sighted and honest figure, is nevertheless tangled in the lie of her disguise, which prevents her from expressing her love. Sir Toby, for all his humour, is a parasite and, worse, a victimiser of the hapless Sir Andrew, as well as of Malvolio. Even the apparently frivolous Feste betrays a weary cynicism at times, as in his final song. Most

significantly, Malvolio's humiliation and imprisonment seem so out of proportion to his offence that they lend the comic sub-plot a vicious air that adds to our uneasy sense that the play's comedy is darker than it seems at first.

This disturbing quality is subtly reinforced by the repeated motif of madness. Olivia asserts that Sir Toby 'speaks nothing but madman' (1.5.107), and Feste, pretending to excuse Toby's drunkenness, allows that 'he is but mad yet . . . and the fool shall look to the madman' (1.5.138–139). When Sebastian arrives in Illyria, only to be pointlessly assaulted, he cries out, 'Are all the people mad?' (4.1.26), and when Olivia mysteriously treats him as her lover, he exclaims, '[Either] I am mad, or else this is a dream' (4.1.60). Malvolio is especially associated with lunacy. His ludicrous behaviour towards Olivia—induced by Maria's letter—is received as 'midsummer madness' (3.4.55) by his mistress, and he is later imprisoned as a lunatic (the commonest treatment for mental disorder in Shakespeare's day).

These elements have led some critics to regard the play as a social commentary resembling in spirit *Troilus and Cressida* or the satirical comedies of Ben JONSON. Olivia and Orsino may be taken as comic portraits of egotists, Olivia in her extravagant withdrawal from life, and the duke in his absurd pose as a romantic lover. Most of the other Illyrians can be seen as socially ambitious and thus fit subjects for satire: In this view, Feste curries favour with Orsino because he may marry Olivia; Toby is a vulgar glutton who seeks a continued life of ease in Olivia's household; Malvolio, Sir Andrew, and Maria each seek a profitable marriage. Viola alone offers honest love in a society where affectation dominates.

Such propositions seem excessive, however, for the play lacks the acid taste of satire—although they accurately set off Viola, the drama's central figure, from the other characters. Viola is not invulnerable to love's irrationality, but, unlike the others, she recognises and acknowledges her blindness. She admits that the situation is beyond her control as soon as the three loves—hers for Orsino, Orsino's for Olivia, Olivia's for her—have become evident, saying, 'O time, thou must entangle this, not I, / It is too hard a knot for me t'untie' (2.2.39–40). She knows what she wants, however—Orsino's love—and she maintains her disguise as the duke's page and waits for a miracle. In doing so, she is a splendid example of the Shakespearean comic heroine, resourceful and aggressive in pursuit of her man.

Her effect on her fellow lovers is positive also. As the spirited Cesario, her youthful good looks and imaginative compliments to Olivia bring out the would-be recluse's capacity to love. Similarly, the irrepressible femininity beneath her disguise offers Orsino the devotion and loyalty that he subconsciously desires and to which he unwittingly responds. Thus she rescues the two leading figures of Illyria from their own illusions and paves the way for the dénouement. Moreover, Viola is the only character—aside from Feste, who is essentially an observer of the plot's intrigues—whose point of view includes a perspective on the whole action. She enters into the dramatic possibilities of her disguised state with enthusiasm, missing no opportunity for telling remarks on Orsino and Olivia or for double entendres about her ambiguous gender.

The sexual confusion implicit in Olivia's response to Cesario was of course magnified on the Elizabethan stage, where Viola and Olivia were played by boys. The humour in seeing a woman (played by a boy) respond sexually to another woman (also played by a boy) depends chiefly on the absurdity of the confusion, but it also has overtones of both male and female homosexuality. Homosexuality was rarely referred to in ELIZABETHAN DRAMA, but here it is certainly suggested implicitly. The modern use of actresses dampens our perception of this situation, but even so more complicated patterns of desire lurk beneath the surface of the conventional love comedy.

Thus, both socially and sexually, tremors of unease accompany the development of a classical comic complication that reaches its breaking point only in the final scene. Then, equally disquietingly, it generates potential violence on several fronts. Antonio is threatened with death, and Orsino hysterically threatens to 'sacrifice the lamb that I do love' (5.1.128) by killing Cesario. The crisis is heightened by the appearance of Sir Andrew and Sir Toby, both of whom have been wounded in actual violence.

The giver of these wounds follows, and he brings the play's resolution with him. Sebastian's entrance provides not only Viola's missing brother, the return of Olivia's new husband, and the correct identification of Cesario; it also makes possible the final alignment of the lovers; his first encounter with Olivia in 4.1 had begun the process, and he unhesitatingly married Olivia when she suggested it in 4.3. His sudden reappearance in 5.1, confirms his power to dissolve the network of ambiguity that has entrapped the other lovers.

Shakespeare emphasises Sebastian's sound sexual identity, a feature whose absence has heavily influenced the action thus far. In both 4.1 and 5.1 Sebastian displays the ancient warrior mystique of the wholly masculine man, overwhelming weaker males who affront his honour. More subtly, and more significantly, Sebastian represents fulfilment in the incomplete lives of the other characters. He is the figure Viola has masqueraded as and the lover Olivia subconsciously desired before Cesario awakened her. He is the dominant male whom Malvolio sought to impersonate and whom Orsino, in his romantic role-playing,

has forgotten he can be. Thus Sebastian—a rather wooden traditional leading man himself—embodies the positive capacity for love that has been needed to crystallise the swirling vapours of romance that have disturbed Illyria.

Yet our earlier uneasiness is not totally dispelled. Aside from the uncanny ease with which Olivia settles for a look-alike and Orsino translates his affection for a boy into love for a wife—these are part of the improbabilities to be expected in romantic comedy, even if they have here a slight taste of the perverse—there remains the difficult resolution of the sub-plot. The 'problem of Malvolio', as it has long been termed, has attracted attention for centuries; in the 17th century the play was sometimes known as 'Malvolio', and in the 19th century Charles LAMB (1) found 'tragic interest' in 'the catastrophe of this character'. This is an overstatement, for Malvolio lacks the grandeur of a tragic hero, but it reflects the potency of the part and of the moral question the steward's unjust imprisonment raises: how is his undeniably shabby treatment—or his unrepentant final response—to be reconciled with the happy ending?

It is true that Malvolio is a comic character, the villain of a rollicking sub-plot powered by the wit of Maria and the lusty excesses of Sir Toby. He has deserved his comeuppance, and it has been delivered in a comical fashion. Nevertheless, his anger at his humiliation makes him humanly sympathetic, and his raging departure seems justified, if ugly, leaving us with an ongoing sense of disturbance. Shakespeare's purpose here is subtle but effective: our appreciation of the loving aura that closes the play is strengthened by our simultaneous sense of sadness that happiness is never pure.

Feste provides a final statement of the play's anti-romantic undertone in his bitter song (5.1.388–407), which outlines the sorry life of a drunkard. For him, the loving resolution of the main plot seems to count for nothing: 'the rain it raineth every day'. Feste's song expresses the jester's loneliness, for he remains outside the lovers' world, but it also reminds us of the limitations of comedy, which has been part of Shakespeare's message in other ways, as we have seen. Tellingly, another stanza of the same song is sung by the tragic FOOL (2) of *King Lear* (3.2.74–77).

However, the form of Feste's summation—a song—eases the burden of its message; the song is never as painful in performance as its unpleasant lyrics suggest it might be. Music's charms leave us with an echo of the happy ending's harmony. The final stanza of Feste's song also has another function: to end the play formally and send the audience on its way. Like an EPILOGUE, it makes a bid for applause and promises that the actors will 'strive to please you every day' (5.1.407).

This dénouement suggests that, although the play has unsettling aspects, the triumph of love is *Twelfth Night*'s major theme. Its subtitle, 'What You Will', obviously points to the possibility of different interpretations of the work, but its promise of that which 'you will' also hints at the dominance of a positive view. The main title itself remains mysterious. To playgoers of Shakespeare's day, the term 'Twelfth Night' designated January 6, or Epiphany, the last day in the traditional Christmas season, celebrated as the anniversary of the Magi's visit to the birthplace of Christ. In 16th-century writings, the polarity of earthly setting and heavenly signal—the manger in Bethlehem and the magical star that led the Magi—was seen as a powerful symbol of Christ's dual nature, part human and part divine. The twins Sebastian and Viola may be symbolic of this duality as well. Viola, through her patient offering of love to Orsino—expressed most vividly in her declaration 'I . . . to do you rest a thousand deaths would die' (5.1.130–131), a remark that has distinctly Christian overtones—may illustrate Christ's suffering human aspect, while Sebastian, who brings redemption within the play's scheme of things, can be taken to represent Christ's divine dimension. This interpretation may seem somewhat strained, however, given the lack of explicit religious references in the play and the fact that there is little, if any, unambiguously religious content elsewhere in the plays. *Twelfth Night*'s title, as has often been observed, may simply advertise the festive, comic quality of the work by naming a great holiday, as another title, *A Midsummer Night's Dream,* did. Also, the play was probably first performed in the autumn or early winter, as the Christmas holidays were approaching.

We have seen that the romantic comedy in *Twelfth Night* is the play's most powerful component, but the work's disturbing reverberations cannot be overlooked. In this respect the comedy points to the PROBLEM PLAYS, soon to be written. In the meantime, the play tells us that while comedy cannot dispel the pains of life, this knowledge only makes the genre a more necessary solace.

SOURCES OF THE PLAY

Shakespeare's chief source for *Twelfth Night* was a romantic tale, 'Apolonius and Silla', in *Farewell to Militarie Profession* (1581), by Barnabe RICH (1). Shakespeare simplified this rambling narrative considerably, but it provided the essence of the relationships among Orsino, Olivia, Viola, and Sebastian (though the playwright took none of these names from his source). Rich himself took his tale from a French romance, a story in François BELLEFOREST's *Histoires Tragiques* (1570); Belleforest in turn took it from an Italian version in Matteo BANDELLO's collection of romances, *Novelle* (1554), and Bandello drew on the original source, an anonymous Italian play of the 1530s, *Gl'Ingannati* ('The Deceived Ones'). Shakespeare probably did not

know the original play, and, although he did know both Bandello's and Belleforest's collections—he used them in writing other plays (notably *Hamlet* [Belleforest] and *Much Ado About Nothing* [Bandello])—they were not important for *Twelfth Night.* Only one passage—Viola's ironic evocation of a frustrated lover of Orsino (2.4.90–119)—may have been influenced by Bandello.

Gl'Ingannati spawned other works, including two plays by an Italian playwright, Nicolo Secchi (active c. 1550), *Gl'Inganni* and *L'Interesse,* which both contain passages resembling Viola's description of a woman whom she claims to love in her male persona (2.4.25–28). Shakespeare may have consulted these works, though some scholars believe the similarity derives simply from their exploitation of the same source.

TEXT OF THE PLAY

Twelfth Night was written between 1599—the publication date of the 'new map with the augmentation of the Indies' referred to in 3.2.76–77—and late 1601, in time for the earliest recorded performance in February 1602. The play may have been written for a performance on January 6, 1601, when Queen ELIZABETH (1) paid the CHAMBERLAIN'S MEN to entertain a visiting Italian nobleman named Orsino. If so, then the play must have been written in late 1600, but most scholars believe that this theory is inaccurate, although the much-talked-about visitor may have inspired Shakespeare's choice of a name for his duke, suggesting 1601 as the date of composition.

Two pieces of evidence point to the latter half of that year. First, the play's subtitle, 'What You Will', may have been Shakespeare's original title, altered when another *What You Will,* by John MARSTON, appeared in the spring of 1601. Second, Feste's remark that the word 'element' is 'overworn' (3.1.60) refers to a controversy of 1601. As part of the so-called WAR OF THE THEATRES, Thomas DEKKER's play *Satiromastix* made much fun of Ben JONSON's alleged overuse of the term. *Satiromastix* was performed by the Chamberlain's Men in the summer or fall of 1601 in answer to a Jonson play of the spring season; this suggests that Shakespeare was writing *Twelfth Night* no earlier than mid-1601.

Twelfth Night was first published in the FIRST FOLIO edition of 1623. The text was printed from a transcription of Shakespeare's FOUL PAPERS, made by a scribe employed by either the acting company that performed it (the Chamberlain's Men until May 1603, the KING'S MEN thereafter) or the publishers of the Folio. As the only early text of the play, it has been the basis of all subsequent editions.

THEATRICAL HISTORY OF THE PLAY

Twelfth Night was performed at one of the INNS OF COURT on February 2, 1602, according to the diary of John MANNINGHAM. This is the only record of a performance in Shakespeare's lifetime, though the King's Men presented the play at the court of King JAMES I in 1618 and 1623, suggesting its popularity. Robert ARMIN is believed to have created the role of Feste and Richard BURBAGE (3) that of Malvolio. During the Restoration, William DAVENANT staged the play in 1661, 1663 and 1669, though he may have altered Shakespeare's text considerably, as was his practise; Thomas BETTERTON played Sir Toby.

In 1703 William BURNABY's *Love Betray'd* incorporated several scenes from *Twelfth Night,* but the play itself was not again performed until 1741, when Charles MACKLIN staged it and played Malvolio. Somewhat later in the 18th century Richard YATES (2) was a popular Feste as a youth and played Malvolio later in his career. John HENDERSON also appeared as the steward with notable success. Dorothy JORDAN played Viola in 1790, opposite her brother as Sebastian, providing a natural similarity of looks.

In the 1810 production by J. P. KEMBLE (3), 1.1 and 1.2 were reversed, a practise that has continued intermittently to the present. Charlotte CUSHMAN was a popular Viola in 1846, Samuel PHELPS played Malvolio in his own productions of 1848 and 1857, and Henry IRVING's production of 1884 starred himself as Malvolio and Ellen TERRY (1) as Viola. Ada REHAN played Viola in Augustin DALY's production (New York, 1893; London, 1894). Nineteenth-century stagings of *Twelfth Night* tended to have elaborate sets and costumes, often based on images of aristocratic English country life, a practise that reached an extreme with Beerbohm TREE's 1901 set, featuring a terraced garden with real grass and fountains.

In 1820 Frederick REYNOLDS (1) produced a musical version incorporating, in the words of the producer, 'Songs, Glees, and Choruses . . . from the Plays, Poems, and Sonnets of Shakespeare'. Other 19th-century productions also introduced extra songs to the text; notable among these was Daly's usurpation of 'Who Is Silvia?' from *The Two Gentlemen of Verona* (4.2.38–52), which had earlier (1827) been set to music by Franz SCHUBERT.

Among the most famous 20th-century productions of *Twelfth Night* was Harley GRANVILLE-BARKER's revolutionary rendering of 1912, which attempted to evoke the Elizabethan stage. Tyrone GUTHRIE's 1937 production featured Laurence OLIVIER as Sir Toby, and, in an experiment that was generally decried, Jessica Tandy (b. 1909) played both Sebastian and Viola, a non-speaking actor taking the former part in the reunion scene (5.1). Peggy ASHCROFT was acclaimed as Viola in 1950. Other notable productions have included John GIELGUD's (1955), starring Olivier as Malvolio and Vivien Leigh as Viola, and that of John BARTON (1) (1969), with Judi DENCH as Viola.

A silent FILM of *Twelfth Night* was made in 1910, and

Russian and German films were made in 1955 and 1963 respectively. The play has been broadcast six times on TELEVISION, beginning in 1939 with a BBC production featuring Michael REDGRAVE and Peggy Ashcroft. Another British production of 1969—with Ralph RICHARDSON (2) as Sir Toby and Joan PLOWRIGHT as both Viola and Sebastian (a feat more plausible on television than on the stage)—was also notable.

Twine, Laurence (active 1564–1576) English translator, creator of a source for *Pericles.* In his prose romance, *The Patterne of Painefull Adventures . . . That Befell unto Prince Apollonius,* Twine translated the tale of Apollonius of Tyre from a French version of an ancient story found in the *Gesta Romanorum,* a medieval Latin collection. Shakespeare drew from Twine's book in composing his play. *The Patterne of Painefull Adventures* was written c. 1576, but if it was published then, no copy has survived; Shakespeare probably knew it in either an undated edition of c. 1594 or a reprint of 1607.

The Two Gentlemen of Verona

SYNOPSIS

Act 1, Scene 1

A young gentleman, VALENTINE (2), preparing to travel to the court of the DUKE (3) of Milan, teases his lovesick friend PROTEUS about the infatuation that keeps him home. Valentine departs, and Proteus, in a brief soliloquy, expresses his love for JULIA. Valentine's young page, SPEED, enters. Speed has carried a letter from Proteus to Julia, and he reports that she made no response to it.

Act 1, Scene 2

Julia asks her waiting-woman, LUCETTA, her opinion of the suitors who are wooing her. Lucetta favours Proteus, but Julia affects to disdain him. Lucetta gives her a letter from Proteus, delivered by Speed, but Julia pretends to take offence, eventually tearing the letter to pieces and sending Lucetta away. Alone, Julia berates herself and confesses that she loves Proteus.

Act 1, Scene 3

Proteus' father, ANTONIO (1), decides that Proteus shall join Valentine at court, as befits a gentleman's son. Proteus enters, mooning over a love letter from Julia. Antonio reveals his plan to Proteus, leaving the young man to bemoan his misfortune.

Act 2, Scene 1

Speed gives Valentine a glove that has been dropped by the Duke's daughter SILVIA, with whom Valentine appears to be in love. The witty Speed tauntingly diagnoses his master's condition. Valentine reports that Silvia has asked him to write a love letter to an unknown person for her. Silvia arrives, and Valentine gives his composition to her. She promptly returns it to him; Valentine is disturbed, but Speed, in an aside, immediately sees that she loves Valentine himself. When Silvia leaves, Speed attempts to explain this, but Valentine cannot understand.

Act 2, Scene 2

Proteus and Julia say farewell and exchange rings. Proteus vows to be faithful while he is away.

Act 2, Scene 3

LAUNCE, a CLOWN (1) who is Proteus' servant, appears with his dog, CRAB, whose hard-heartedness he complains about in a comic monologue. Launce is upset because he must leave his family and go to court with his master, but Crab shows no distress.

Act 2, Scene 4

The Duke reports that Proteus has arrived at his court, and Valentine praises his friend warmly. Valentine tells Silvia of the love between Proteus and Julia. Proteus enters and meets Silvia, who is then called away. Valentine reveals that he and Silvia are planning to elope. Proteus confesses in a soliloquy that he has fallen madly in love with Silvia, so much so that he is willing to betray both Valentine and Julia.

Act 2, Scene 5

Speed welcomes Launce to court. With clownish wit, the two servants gossip about their masters' love affairs.

Act 2, Scene 6

In a soliloquy, Proteus plots to steal Silvia from Valentine, finding justifications for his disloyalty to his friend and Julia. He proposes to reveal the intended elopement of Valentine and Silvia, scheduled for that night, to the Duke.

Act 2, Scene 7

Julia plans to journey to court to see Proteus. She will travel disguised as a page. Lucetta warns that Proteus' love may have diminished, but Julia is confident he will remain faithful.

Act 3, Scene 1

Proteus tells the Duke of the intended elopement, exiting as Valentine approaches. The Duke 'discovers' the rope ladder hidden under Valentine's cloak, and angrily banishes Valentine from his domain. Proteus arrives with Launce and offers to help Valentine flee. The two friends depart, leaving Launce, who speaks of his own love for a milkmaid. He has a written list of her good qualities. Speed appears, and the two comic figures review this document.

Act 3, Scene 2

The Duke speaks with THURIO, whom he has chosen to marry his daughter. Thurio complains that Silvia loves him even less than she did before Valentine's banishment. Proteus recommends maligning Valentine to

her, and he volunteers for the job, observing that such slander will only be credible coming from someone believed to be Valentine's friend.

Act 4, Scene 1
Valentine and Speed are captured by OUTLAWS. Learning that Valentine is an educated gentleman, as they claim to be themselves, these desperadoes elect him their captain.

Act 4, Scene 2
Proteus soliloquises that his ongoing career of betrayal, now directed at Thurio, has only brought him Silvia's scorn. Thurio arrives with MUSICIANS (1). Also present, unknown to the others, is Julia, disguised as a page. The SONG 'Who Is Silvia?' is performed, and Julia sees that Proteus loves its subject. Thurio and the Musicians depart, and Proteus converses with Silvia, who has appeared on her balcony. He takes credit for the serenade and speaks of his love, but Silvia rebukes him, referring to his former love, Julia. He claims that Julia has died, not knowing that she is listening, and adds that he has heard that Valentine is dead as well. He asks Silvia for a picture, and she agrees to give him one in the morning.

Act 4, Scene 3
Sir EGLAMOUR agrees to accompany Silvia on a journey to find Valentine.

Act 4, Scene 4
In a monologue, Launce complains of Crab's doggy behaviour, for he has urinated at the Duke's dinner. Proteus agrees to employ the disguised Julia as a page, ordering 'Sebastian' to deliver a ring to Silvia, in exchange for the promised picture. Julia makes the exchange and learns that Silvia knows of and feels pity for Proteus' abandoned lover.

Act 5, Scene 1
Eglamour and Silvia flee.

Act 5, Scene 2
The Duke reports Silvia's flight. Thurio, Proteus, and Julia all join him in pursuit.

Act 5, Scene 3
The Outlaws have captured Silvia and are taking her to their captain.

Act 5, Scene 4
Valentine, alone, muses that his lonely exile is appropriate to his grief over his lost Silvia. Hearing a commotion, he hides himself, and Silvia, Proteus, and Julia enter. Proteus demands Silvia's love as a reward for having rescued her from the Outlaws; when she refuses, he attempts to rape her. Valentine comes forth and prevents him, cursing his supposed friend's disloyalty. Proteus, stricken with remorse, begs forgiveness. Valentine is so moved that he offers to yield Silvia to him; hearing this, Julia faints. Revived, she reveals her identity, and Proteus falls in love with her again. The Outlaws arrive with the Duke and Thurio as captives, whom Valentine releases. Thurio claims Silvia, but when Valentine offers to fight him, he fearfully declines. The Duke pardons Valentine and awards him Silvia's hand.

COMMENTARY

The Two Gentlemen of Verona is certainly among the most poorly received of Shakespeare's comedies. Some parts, especially the comic monologues of Launce, are accomplished, but the play as a whole is unconvincing. It is perhaps best viewed as the work of a young and inexperienced playwright who was only beginning to experiment with comedy, a genre he was to master at a later date.

In the past, some scholars have claimed that the play was simply too bad to have been written by Shakespeare, that at most he may have touched up someone else's feeble effort. Modern criticism holds that the play, while an unsuccessful early effort, is nonetheless genuinely Shakespearean. Supporters of this opinion have focussed on the young playwright's intelligent application of the literary conventions current in his day as he developed his own approach to comedy, or they have seen the play as at least in part a deliberate parody of these conventions. These two propositions are not mutually exclusive; a parodist may make use of a style for its entertainment value at the same time that he or she subverts it.

The play draws on two literary traditions: the 'friendship literature' of the Middle Ages; and romantic narrative. 'Friendship literature' told tales of manly companionship, sometimes disrupted by romance but generally restored. The account of the relationship between Valentine and Proteus is an instance of this long-popular plot line. For instance, Valentine's renunciation of Silvia (5.4.82–83), though comically abrupt in context, represents a conventional demonstration of magnanimity that was standard in this tradition.

Romantic narrative derived ultimately from classical roots and was popular throughout the Middle Ages in the form of poetry and prose dealing with courtly love and adventure. Such narratives continued to be written and widely read during the Renaissance; Sir Philip SIDNEY's *Arcadia* was the best-known English example. This tradition was already familiar in the early Elizabethan theatre. A number of plays written in the 1570s and 1580s share several of its characteristic devices: accounts of travels in several different settings; girls or women, abandoned by lovers, who assume disguises; a cynical villain; a mocking servant who comments on the romantic action; eventual reunion at the close. The audience finds in these exotic settings and stylised characters a life that seems both bolder and finer than its own, governed by values that are impossible

in the real world. It is this body of conventions that Shakespeare uses in this play.

In *The Two Gentlemen of Verona,* lovers are separated through a flagrantly evil act of betrayal. After trials and rigours have been undergone, a happy ending reunites them and villainy is overcome. The promised escape has been provided. However, Shakespeare holds up the stereotype of romantic narrative to good-humoured ridicule, especially in the treatment of his hero, Valentine, who is presented throughout as a gullible and foolish young man, a comic and ridiculous hero. When we first see him, he is ridiculing love, and we know, if only from his suggestive name, that his comeuppance surely lies ahead. Valentine's ineptness as a lover is demonstrated, for instance, when he fails to comprehend Silvia's flirtatious letter-writing ploy; when Speed attempts to explain it, he proves too slow-witted to appreciate it.

Valentine's high-flown rhetoric of love, as he recounts his infatuation to Proteus in 2.4, is the voice of exuberant enthusiasm, and he presents a pleasant picture of a young man in the first blush of romance. However, his bubbling account of his planned elopement seems indiscreet at best. Later in the scene, when Proteus reveals his plan to betray his friend, we pity Valentine for the blunder he has unknowingly committed in confiding in this villain, but at the same time, we may chuckle that his effervescent 'braggardism' (2.4.159) was so untimely.

We are not surprised when Valentine steps so neatly into the Duke's trap in 3.1, for his combination of naïveté and feigned sophistication seems entirely in character. So does his helplessness once the Duke rages off; he can only bemoan his fate until Proteus bundles him out of town.

We next see Valentine in the wholly comic scene (4.1) of his capture by the Outlaws, who immediately make him the leader of their gang, in what is clearly a broad parody of romantic adventure stories. He rescues Silvia from attempted rape by Proteus, but he is so silly a hero that it does not occur to him to claim his heroine at this obvious climax. In fact, he does not even speak to her for the remainder of the play. Instead, he responds only to his former friend, who is begging forgiveness, and he goes so far as to turn Silvia over to the would-be rapist. This absurd conclusion is prevented only by the quick-witted Julia, who wants Proteus for herself, and Valentine is united with his beloved only by default.

Only two of the characters in *The Two Gentlemen of Verona* anticipate the magical figures of later works. Launce, an early clown, voices the best writing in the play in his monologues concerning his dog, Crab. The general artificiality of the play is countered to a considerable degree by the presence of this commonsensical man. However, Launce has literally nothing whatsoever to do with the plot; he simply provides intermissions, as it were, in the main action. Later, Shakespeare was to integrate his comic characters more fully. Julia, whose best material is in prose, is also something of a foil to Valentine and Proteus. Her pragmatic assumption of control over events begins with her intention to overcome her enforced separation from Proteus by following him to court, and it triumphs when she abandons her disguise and reconquers his love. She clearly foreshadows such later enterprising heroines as ROSALIND, in *As You Like It,* and VIOLA, in *Twelfth Night.*

SOURCES OF THE PLAY

The two strands that make up the plot of *The Two Gentlemen of Verona* came to the playwright from specific sources, although one derivation is not altogether clear, for Shakespeare made the material his own to a great extent. The relationships among Proteus, Valentine, and Silvia seem to be based on the story of Titus and Gisippus, a 'friendship' tale, originally found in Boccaccio's *Decameron* and very famous in Shakespeare's day. Gisippus bestows his fiancée on his friend Titus, who has fallen in love with her. This tale lacks the betrayal theme, but, as his love develops, Titus contemplates such a course, in terms remarkably similar to those Proteus uses in his soliloquy in 2.6. Also, there are English variants of this tale, and several passages that resemble lines in the play appear in one of them, published in Sir Thomas ELYOT's *The Boke named the Governour* (1531). One such passage seems to have inspired Valentine's notorious couplet of renunciation. Just how Shakespeare knew the tale, and just what he took from which source, cannot be determined.

However, the story of the betrayed love of Proteus and Julia clearly came from *Diana Enamorada,* a prose romance written in Spanish by the Portuguese author Jorge de MONTEMAYOR and first printed in 1542. Although the first English translation, by Bartholomew YONG, was not published until 1598, Shakespeare probably knew the manuscript, which had been completed 16 years earlier, for there are many echoes of it in the play.

A third source was a long poem by Arthur BROOKE (1), *The Tragical History of Romeus and Juliet,* which was also the chief source for *Romeo and Juliet.* Here, Shakespeare's only important adoption was Valentine's rope-ladder, but there are suggestions of the later play in Silvia's conspiratorial visit to a friar's cell (4.3.43–44) and in the mention of a Friar Laurence (5.2.36).

Launce was apparently a Shakespearean invention, although his character type, the rustic clown, was already well established. The early plays of John LYLY offered models for Speed; also, some details of Speed's role derive from *Damon and Pithias* a play of 1571 by Richard EDWARDS. The comical 'catalogue' scene (3.1) seems to have been suggested by a scene

in Lyly's *Midas* (1588–1589). Lyly's immensely popular novel *Euphues* (1578) offered a famous instance of male friendship disturbed by sexual jealousy and, as the sensation of the age, doubtless helped form the young Shakespeare's sense of romantic atmosphere.

TEXT OF THE PLAY

The Two Gentlemen of Verona is known to have been written by 1598, when it was mentioned by MERES, but features of its style suggest that it was written earlier. It has been nominated as possibly the first play Shakespeare wrote, but this cannot be proved. Proposed dates for its composition have ranged from 1590 to 1595, not counting a sometimes hypothesised rewrite of 1598. The only early publication of the play was in the FIRST FOLIO of 1623, and this text has therefore been the basis for all subsequent editions.

THEATRICAL HISTORY OF THE PLAY

No performance of *The Two Gentlemen of Verona* is recorded before 1762, although it is presumed to have been acted in the 16th century—at least on the strength of its inclusion in the list of plays complied by Meres in 1598. The production of 1762, by David GARRICK, was of an altered text, as have been most of the scattered subsequent attempts. The play's many discrepancies have been amended to a greater or lesser extent, and additional material has often been added for Launce and Speed. The only version to achieve even a modest success with 19th-century audiences was a highly altered operatic version produced by Frederick REYNOLDS (1) in the 1820s. There have been successful 20th-century stagings—such as Joseph PAPP's musical adaptation of 1971, and a New York production of 1988 that featured a troupe of jugglers—but it remains one of the least performed of Shakespeare's plays. *Two Gentlemen of Verona* was made as a FILM in Germany (1963) and has been made for TELEVISION once, in 1983, as part of the BBC's complete cycle of Shakespeare's plays.

The Two Noble Kinsmen

SYNOPSIS

A PROLOGUE (5) declares that the play has a noble predecessor, in a work by CHAUCER, that it cannot hope to live up to.

Act 1, Scene 1
As THESEUS (2), Duke of ATHENS, prepares to marry Queen HIPPOLYTA (2) of the Amazons, the ceremony is interrupted by a QUEEN (1) who falls on her knees before Theseus, followed by two more who address Hippolyta and her sister, EMILIA (4). The Queens tell of their husbands' deaths fighting King Creon of THEBES, who has refused to bury the kings' bodies, thereby exposing their souls to torment. They ask Theseus to conquer Creon, insisting that any delay is dishonourable. The wedding is then postponed as Theseus prepares for war.

Act 1, Scene 2
Two noblemen of Thebes, the cousins ARCITE and PALAMON, decide to leave the court of the villainous King Creon. VALERIUS brings word that Duke Theseus has declared war. The cousins realise that their honour requires them to stay and fight for Thebes.

Act 1, Scene 3
Hippolyta and Emilia bid farewell to PIRITHOUS, who is about to join Theseus in Thebes. Hippolyta remarks on the long-standing friendship of Pirithous and Theseus. Emilia recalls her own, similar affection for a childhood girlfriend and declares that she will never love a man so well.

Act 1, Scene 4
The Queens thank Theseus for his victory over Creon, and he sends them to bury their husbands. A HERALD (8) informs Theseus that Palamon and Arcite, both badly wounded, are among his prisoners of war.

Act 1, Scene 5
The Queens lead funeral processions for their husbands.

Act 2, Scene 1
The GAOLER (4) negotiates a marriage settlement with the WOOER of his DAUGHTER (2). The Daughter appears on her way to see the new prisoners, Palamon and Arcite, whom she admires for the spirit with which they bear their imprisonment. The three commoners leave as the two prisoners appear, reflecting on the comfort they can take in each other's company; they believe that their honourable friendship will sustain them throughout their lives. Below their windows, in a courtyard, they see Emilia conversing with a WOMAN (2). First Palamon and then Arcite fall in love with Emilia on sight. After she leaves, they quarrel over who has the right to claim her as his beloved. Each feels that his honour is offended by the other, and they vow to fight a duel if they ever have the opportunity. The Gaoler appears and takes Arcite to the duke. Palamon muses on his love for Emilia until the Gaoler returns to report that Arcite has been freed but banished from Theseus' realm, on pain of death.

Act 2, Scene 2
Arcite, free, decides to stay in Theseus' realm and attempt to meet and woo Emilia. He encounters a group of COUNTRYMEN, who tell him of the wrestling and running competitions to be witnessed by Theseus and his court at a nearby country fair. Arcite decides to enter the competitions in order to come to the attention of the court and thus meet Emilia.

Act 2, Scene 3
The Gaoler's Daughter reflects on her hopeless love for Palamon. She realises that he will never love a commoner, but she decides to help him escape from prison.

Act 2, Scene 4
The disguised Arcite, having won the competitions, is interviewed by Theseus, who accepts him as a courtier. He is assigned to serve as an attendant to Emilia.

Act 2, Scene 5
The Daughter reveals in a soliloquy that she has freed Palamon, who waits in a nearby wood until she can bring him food and a file to remove his shackles. She hopes he will come to love her.

Act 3, Scene 1
Alone in the wood, Arcite reflects on his good fortune in having become Emilia's attendant. Overhearing this, the fugitive Palamon emerges from the trees, and they resume their argument. Though their affection for each other still stands, they agree that they must duel to uphold their respective honours. Arcite declares he will bring Palamon food and a file to remove his shackles, and then they will fight.

Act 3, Scene 2
The Daughter cannot find Palamon and concludes that he has been eaten by wild animals. Hysterical, she reflects that her father will be hanged for her treachery in letting Palamon escape, and she will be reduced to beggary if she does not commit suicide. She wishes she were already dead.

Act 3, Scene 3
Arcite returns to Palamon with food and a file. They agree not to mention Emilia but cannot refrain and fall to quarrelling again. Arcite leaves, saying he will return when Palamon has removed his shackles, and they will fight.

Act 3, Scene 4
Raving wildly about Palamon, her father, and other things, the Daughter sings scraps of SONG.

Act 3, Scene 5
A SCHOOLMASTER (2) instructs a group of peasants, one of them costumed as a BAVIAN, or baboon, on the dance they are to perform before the duke. One of the women of their group is missing, however, so they despair about being able to perform. The Daughter appears, and although they see that she is mad, the dancers recruit her for their performance. Theseus and his court appear and, after a lengthy PROLOGUE (1) from the Schoolmaster, the dance is presented.

Act 3, Scene 6
Palamon and Arcite meet to duel. As they put on their armour, they reminisce fondly, but they continually renew their quarrel. They begin to fight, but Theseus and his court arrive. The cousins identify themselves, and Theseus condemns them to death: Arcite for having violated his banishment and Palamon as an escaped prisoner of war. They plead to be permitted to finish their duel, with the survivor then being executed, and Theseus agrees. However, when Hippolyta and Emilia beg for mercy for them, Theseus compromises. He decrees that the cousins shall return to Thebes and recruit seconds, come back within a month, and then duel for Emilia's hand. The duel shall not be to the death, but rather consist of a contest to force the opponent to touch a pillar erected for the purpose. The winner will marry Emilia; only the loser and his seconds will be executed. The cousins agree and depart.

Act 4, Scene 1
The Gaoler hears of the duel from a FRIEND and worries that he will be blamed for Palamon's escape. A Second Friend arrives and assures him that the duke, encouraged by Palamon, has pardoned the Gaoler and his Daughter. The Wooer then arrives with the news that the Daughter is mad. She appears, ranting about marrying Palamon and taking a sea voyage to meet him.

Act 4, Scene 2
Regretting the upcoming duel, Emilia reviews the virtues of each cousin in turn and admits that she loves them both. She is joined by Theseus and the court. Pirithous and a MESSENGER (32) have witnessed the arrival of the cousins and their seconds, and they describe the gallantly arrayed KNIGHTS (3) in detail.

Act 4, Scene 3
The DOCTOR (4) witnesses the Daughter's ravings and prescribes that the Wooer should dress as Palamon and court her, in the hope that the apparent fulfilment of her fantasy will shock her out of it.

Act 5, Scene 1
In a temple Arcite and Palamon prepare to duel. They bid each other an affectionate farewell. When Arcite and his seconds make a sacrifice to Mars, the altar resounds with thunder. Palamon and his followers make one to Venus, and the altar gives forth doves. After the knights leave for the duel, Emilia appears and makes a sacrifice to Diana. A rose tree bearing a single rose emerges, but the rose falls from it. Emilia is confused by this omen.

Act 5, Scene 2
The Wooer, in the guise of Palamon, reports that he has kissed the Daughter. The Doctor directs that he go on to sleep with her, and he readily agrees. The Daughter emerges from the Gaoler's house and talks of a dancing horse Palamon has given her and how

another horse loves it in vain. Still pretending to be Palamon, the Wooer proposes to her, and she accepts, adding that they should go to the end of the world for the wedding. She returns indoors, and the men go to witness the duel.

Act 5, Scene 3

Emilia, resisting all arguments, refuses to witness the duel, so a SERVANT (30) is left with her to report. Going to and fro, he periodically recounts the action: first one cousin seems to be winning, then the other. Finally, he reports Arcite the victor. The court returns, and Arcite and Emilia are formally declared engaged. Emilia declares that only her duty to comfort Arcite, who has lost his noble kinsman, keeps her from killing herself with grief.

Act 5, Scene 4

Palamon and his seconds prepare to be executed. Palamon asks the Gaoler about his Daughter; he reports that she has recovered and is to be married. As Palamon is about to be beheaded by the EXECUTIONER (3), Pirithous arrives with a pardon, reporting that Arcite is dying after being crushed by a runaway horse. Theseus, Hippolyta, and Emilia appear, with Arcite in a litter. Arcite accepts Palamon's grieving farewell, bequeaths Emilia to him, receives a final kiss from her, and dies. Theseus declares a period of mourning, to be followed by the marriage of Emilia and Palamon.

Epilogue

An anonymous actor, pretending to have stage fright, jests about the audience's hisses and laughter. He asks for their pardon, promises a better play some other night, and bids farewell.

COMMENTARY

The Two Noble Kinsmen is probably the least known of Shakespeare's plays, in good part because (in the opinion of all but a few scholars) much of it was written by someone else, probably John FLETCHER (2). It has rarely been performed or even published over the centuries, though modern commentators' growing interest in Shakespeare's ROMANCES encompasses this work.

Considered separately, the parts of *The Two Noble Kinsmen* written by Shakespeare present the germ of a better and more interesting work than the play as a whole turned out to be. Shakespeare wrote Acts 1 and 5—with some exceptions—plus 3.1 and perhaps some other minor passages. With the beginning and the end of the play, he could introduce characters and themes and bring them to the climax of the action. Scenes 1.1 and 5.1 are especially strong, containing much good poetry and several spectacular theatrical effects. Shakespeare's only substantial contribution to the development between these phases is the encounter between Arcite and Palamon, when they prepare to duel even as they recognise their profound affection for each other. A number of fine passages of verse in 3.1—especially Arcite's lyrical praise of Emilia—sharpen the audience's appreciation that the developing story is more than an assemblage of clichés about knighthood and courtly love enlivened by a comic subplot.

In Shakespeare's portions of the play, *The Two Noble Kinsmen* displays many of the characteristics of his other late works, and it is properly grouped with the romances. The playwright was clearly employing the techniques of spectacle, exotic characters and settings, and bizarre plotting with much the same intention as in other romances—to demonstrate humanity's dependence on providence in the face of inscrutable destiny and to evoke the nobility of the human spirit in the face of this knowledge.

The spectacular is less dramatic and effective in *The Two Noble Kinsmen* than in, say, *The Tempest,* but it is nonetheless present. Theseus and Hippolyta's elaborate wedding opens the play on a ceremonious note, only to be interrupted by the extraordinary sight of the three Queens, all in black and thus contrasting strikingly with the wedding party's festive finery. The Queens' manner is sternly formal, as they first address Theseus and receive his response, then do the same in turn with Hippolyta and Emilia. This ritualistic exchange makes the gravity of their plea unmistakable. The effect is augmented as the plea is repeated with variations: when they receive a promise of support, they demand instant action; when ARTESIUS is assigned to the task, they demand Theseus. The importance of this presentation becomes clear when we consider how Shakespeare has altered his source. In CHAUCER's tale (see 'Sources' below), Theseus is already married, only a single Queen pleads—and only with him—and he consents immediately. In contrast, Shakespeare delayed the process, for action is less important in *The Two Noble Kinsmen* than emotion, here manifested in an almost religious atmosphere of courtliness and mystery. It is appropriate that the first character on stage should be HYMEN (2), a god.

This religious atmosphere recurs in the funeral procession of 1.5. Throughout the play, references to rituals of various sorts, along with manifold allusions to the pagan gods, both singly and collectively, maintain our awareness of the need for harmony with the divine, a consideration that underlies the action. In 5.1 the play's evocation of religion and mystery is at its most intense. The three petitions to pagan gods and the divine responses are in themselves meaningful, as we shall see, but they are also important for the atmosphere they create. Highly elaborate, with startling sound and physical effects—doubtless devised with an eye to the increased technical capacities of the BLACKFRIARS THEATRE—they evoke awe and wonder appropriate to the extraordinary twists of fate in the coming

climax. The supplicants' prayers comprise the best poetry of the play, and the divine responses are gratifyingly spectacular. They are mysterious yet, as the baffled Emilia observes, 'gracious' (5.1.173). The exotic beauty of this scene is generally considered the high point of *The Two Noble Kinsmen.*

Such spectacle is effective simply for its own sake—Shakespeare was certainly inspired in part by the increasing popularity of the MASQUE—but it also helps further the themes of the play. As in the other late plays, the central proposition of *The Two Noble Kinsmen* is that humanity is dependent on providence. In the face of a destiny we cannot understand, we can only accept our fate and hope the gods will refrain from destroying us. This point of view is less pessimistic than it sounds when reduced to its essentials, for the nobility of humanity's continuing survival in the face of such knowledge is impressive. At least, we see the potential for such nobility in each individual.

We are repeatedly reminded of fate's importance. Even the celebratory, flower-filled opening hymn finishes with a sinister hint of fatality in its allusions to birds of ill omen. Theseus recalls the wedding day of the grieving Queen and rhetorically addresses destiny, 'O grief and time, / Fearful consumers, you will all devour!' (1.1.69–70). In 1.2 Palamon declares that Creon is corrupting Thebes by making 'heaven unfeared' (1.2.64); nevertheless, the young men seem powerless to avoid entanglement in Creon's corruption. Admitting that helplessness, Arcite entrusts their future to 'th'event, / that never-erring arbitrator' (1.2. 113–114). Hippolyta hopes that Theseus, in combat, will be able 'To dure ill-dealing fortune' (1.3.5), and a defeated knight, facing execution, declares that the winners have 'Fortune, whose title is . . . momentary' (5.4.17). Even after victory Theseus speaks of 'Th'impartial gods, who from the mounted heavens / View us their mortal herd' (1.4.5). Using a different metaphor for human helplessness before fate, Pirithous describes Arcite's flagging life as 'a vessel . . . that floats but for / The surge that next approaches' (5.4. 82–84). At the end, reviewing the final twist of fate, Theseus declares, 'Never fortune / Did play a subtler game' (5.4.112–113). Fortune is omnipresent in the play's world, yet it is entirely beyond human control or understanding.

Tellingly, the gods answer the eloquent prayers of 5.1, but not in a way that could have been anticipated; fortune is certain but unpredictable. Arcite prays that he may 'Be styled the lord o'th'day' (5.1.60), and he is indeed declared the winner of the duel, but he loses Emilia and his life, as the horse she gives him proves deadly. Palamon asks Venus for victory as 'true love's merit' (5.4.128), but he only gains Emilia through Arcite's accidental death. Emilia prays that the cousin who loves her best should win. This would appear to be Palamon, for he is associated with Venus rather than Mars; moreover, since he saw her first and is more rightly her lover—as Arcite finally admits—he is more truly fighting in the cause of love, with Arcite more intent on defending his personal honour. Yet it is Arcite who wins, even though Emilia does in the end have her wish granted. As expectations are upset and then fulfilled, but fulfilled only tragically, our sense of the incomprehensibility of providence is compounded.

The play, however, counters any implicit fatalism by repeatedly stressing the importance of human nobility. The emphasis begins in the Prologue with the assertion that the story being told has in itself a 'nobleness' (Prologue, 15) that the creators of the drama are striving to uphold, and that Chaucer was its 'noble breeder' (10). The nobility of Palamon and Arcite—explicit in the play's title—is repeatedly confirmed by the other characters. Their friendship is bound up in their appreciation of each other's noble qualities, and it is itself conventionally noble in a literary tradition that was still very much alive in Shakespeare's day. From medieval times into the 17th century, intense friendship between noble young warriors, especially when disrupted by heterosexual love, was the subject of many novels, poems, and plays—including *Two Gentlemen of Verona* and some of the SONNETS. The theme of these works was the essential nobility—the spiritual superiority—of such a relationship. Arcite and Palamon had been celebrated in this light before—even before Chaucer—and Shakespeare obviously intended to do so again. The theme is paralleled in Hippolyta's description of the friendship of Theseus and Pirithous in 1.3.26–47, and in Emilia's touching account of her own childhood relationship with the deceased Lavinia in 1.3.49–82.

Emilia herself is another instance of nobility. In Act 1 she and Hippolyta demonstrate their inherent magnanimity in their response to the Queens, and in Act 5 Emilia displays a noble combination of heightened emotion and disinterested concern for honourable propriety, which is pointedly isolated by the playwright in 5.3, when the duel is held off-stage and reflected in her responses.

It is Theseus, however, who is the central figure at the play's opening and again at its end (although he is a less significant figure in Fletcher's portions of the play). His nobility is strongly emphasised. At least in Acts 1 and 5, his actions are strikingly courtly and generous at every turn: towards the Queens, towards his wounded prisoners of war, in his arrangements for the religious petitions of the duellists, and in his responses to them after the duel and its tragic aftermath. Most important, at the play's close, he adopts a pointedly serene and courageous attitude towards the buffetings of fate to which the play's world has been subjected. This stance has great moral weight, not simply because Theseus closes the play—as its highest-rank-

ing figure, he would do that anyway in the theatrical protocol of Shakespeare's day—but because he has been established as a highly noble man.

The play's emphasis on nobility, while part of an old tradition of chivalric heroes in romance literature, also has a more immediate point: in the face of destiny, human beings are helpless, and it is necessary to accept this. In *The Two Noble Kinsmen* the nobility of the title characters lies in their unhesitating acceptance of their situation. Forced by circumstances to fight for Creon, they 'follow / the becking of our chance' (1.2. 115–116). Seized by an obsession, Arcite strives only to 'maintain [his] proceedings' and 'clear [his] own way with the mind and sword / Of a true gentleman' (3.1.53, 56–57). Palamon also accepts his fateful love, with its corollary of enmity to Arcite, 'As 'twere a wreath of roses, [though it] is heavier / Than lead itself, stings more than nettles' (5.1.96–97). The kinsmen's seemingly senseless system of honour provides them with a recourse: in the face of an inexorable destiny, nobility consists in accepting our losses and maintaining our dignity. Although Emilia can cry, 'Is this winning? / O all you heavenly powers, where is your mercy?' (5.3.138–139), she immediately concedes that if the gods' 'wills have said it must be so' (5.3.140), then she must accept it. In the play's last lines, Theseus addresses the divinities, 'O you heavenly charmers, / What things you make of us! . . . Let us be thankful / For that which is, and with you leave dispute[s] / That are above our question' (5.4.131–136). The characters in the play accept their circumstances, and therein lies their significance.

Had Shakespeare written the middle of the play as well as its introduction and close, *The Two Noble Kinsmen* might convey more of the mystery and beauty of human existence, with the power of *The Winter's Tale* or *The Tempest.* As it is, the play is greatly weakened by Fletcher's contribution. Shakespeare's resonant themes are diminished by a series of SUB-PLOTS, and his emphasis on ceremony and ritual is abandoned in favour of melodrama, comedy, and pathos. The story of the Gaoler's Daughter is weakened by the omission of any contact between her and Palamon, and her madness is an unconvincing pastiche of conventional symptoms. The Doctor's lewd prescription is at best vulgar humour; it has no function but comic relief and bears no relation to lunacy, even to the unrealistic madness depicted. The second sub-plot, the presentation of the Schoolmaster's rustic entertainment, barely deserves to be called a sub-plot, for it is merely an excuse to present a popular dance number. Pleasant but irrelevant, it lacks the vigour of the real personalities that fill Shakespeare's equivalent scenes, most notably in *The Winter's Tale.*

More important, Palamon and Arcite are much less impressive figures. In 2.1, when they fall in love with Emilia and begin to quarrel, furthering the plot and observing the chivalric conventions, they are different men from the pair met in 1.2. Their revulsion at Thebes' corruption—their most prominent characteristic in 1.2—has been replaced by a nostalgia for 'our noble country' (2.1.61). The reliance on personal honour that permitted them to entrust themselves to the 'never-erring arbitrator' (1.2.114) is superseded by thoughts that 'fair-eyed maids shall weep our banishments' (2.1.91). Sentiment takes precedence over character. Shakespeare's maintainance of the cousins' nobility in 3.1 is utterly wasted in 3.3, a scene filled with stale jests about 'the wenches / We have known in our days!' (3.3.28–29). Only in 3.6, where they assist each other before beginning the duel and then face Theseus, do the kinsmen approach their earlier nobility. However, this scene is somewhat redundant thematically—combining the fondness and enmity already presented in 3.1—and Fletcher's poetry is distinctly more pedestrian than Shakespeare's.

The Two Noble Kinsmen has its virtues. It contains scattered passages of good poetry in Shakespeare's complex late style, especially in 1.1 and 5.1. The spectacles in 1.1 and 5.1, as well as the funeral procession of 1.5 and dance of 3.5, are theatrically impressive in a good production. Most important, enough of Shakespeare's premise comes through in Acts 1 and 5 that a fine performance permits an audience to experience some sense of awe at the inexorability of the human condition. However, one has only to compare this work with Shakespeare's undiluted efforts to realise how inadequate it is. It may be best seen as a business venture: Shakespeare, about to retire—possibly already living in STRATFORD—was called upon by his company, the KING'S MEN, to collaborate with its rising creative star, Fletcher, and the two produced a workmanlike job, which seems to have had at least a modicum of success. As such, it is an interesting demonstration of early 17th-century tastes, and since it incorporates what is quite possibly Shakespeare's last dramatic writing, it merits more attention than it would otherwise get.

SOURCES OF THE PLAY

The source for the main plot of *The Two Noble Kinsmen*—the conflict between Arcite and Palamon—was taken by Shakespeare and Fletcher from Geoffrey Chaucer's 'The Knight's Tale', one of the most popular of *The Canterbury Tales* (c. 1482). Chaucer had taken the story from an epic poem by Giovanni BOCCACCIO, *Teseide* (c. 1340). The playwrights altered their source considerably, adding the interrupted wedding in 1.1 (perhaps deriving it from the similar disruption in *A Midsummer Night's Dream,* which was also altered from 'The Knight's Tale'). More significantly, they added the stipulation that the loser of the duel over Emilia must be executed. Another *Dream* source, the 'Life of

Theseus' in PLUTARCH's *Lives* (1579; translated by Thomas NORTH), provided hints for Theseus' depiction, especially in 1.1.

The tragicomic sub-plot of the Gaoler's Daughter was apparently invented for the play, probably by Fletcher, who (according to most scholarly opinion) wrote most of the scenes in which it figures. The lesser sub-plot, the Schoolmaster's presentation of a rustic entertainment, is a restaging of a scene from a popular contemporary masque by Francis BEAUMONT (2), the *Masque of the Inner Temple and Gray's Inn (1613).*

TEXT OF THE PLAY

Modern scholars usually believe that *The Two Noble Kinsmen* was written jointly by Shakespeare and John Fletcher, though a few hold that Shakespeare wrote none of it and a few that he wrote it all. While precise agreement is lacking on the authors' distribution of labours, it is generally thought that Shakespeare was responsible for Act 1, 3.1, and all of Act 5 except 5.2. Many variations of this arrangement are proposed, most commonly the addition of 2.1 or the Daughter's soliloquy at the beginning of 3.2, or the deletion of 1.4 and 1.5. Also, some ascribe the remaining portions not to Fletcher but to Francis Beaumont or Philip MASSINGER, or to some combination of the three.

The Two Noble Kinsmen was almost certainly written in 1613. The rustic entertainment in 3.5 was taken from a masque by Beaumont that was staged on February 20, 1613; the same troupe of dancers probably performed in both productions. A theatrical character named Palamon—presumably the hero of *The Two Noble Kinsmen*—is mentioned in Ben JONSON's 1614 play, *Bartholomew Fair,* suggesting that Fletcher and Shakespeare's play had already been staged by that date.

The Two Noble Kinsmen was the latest to be published of all Shakespeare's plays. It was omitted from the FIRST FOLIO (1623), probably because the editors knew that more than half of it was written by another playwright. The play was first published in a QUARTO edition of 1634 (known as Q1) by John WATERSON. Q1 was ascribed to Shakespeare and Fletcher on its title-page and in its registration with the STATIONERS' COMPANY. Beginning in 1679, however, *The Two Noble Kinsmen* was often published as the work of Beaumont and Fletcher, and it did not appear in a collection of Shakespeare's plays until 1841. It is frequently omitted from modern collections.

Q1 is an excellent edition, with little garbling of text and relatively few misprints. It was based on a PROMPT-BOOK, as is evident from some of the stage directions, which include instructions for the preparation of props. Two actors—'Curtis' and 'T. Tucke'—are named in place of their characters; they are probably Curtis GREVILLE (1) and Thomas TUCKFEILD, which suggests that the prompt-book was prepared for a production of the 1620s. It may derive from the co-authors' FOUL PAPERS. Q1, as the only early text, has been the basis for all subsequent editions.

THEATRICAL HISTORY OF THE PLAY

Jonson's 1614 reference (see 'Text of the Play') implies a performance of *The Two Noble Kinsmen* before that date, and the play was considered for performance at the royal court in 1619 (the choice made is unknown). Further, it was still in the King's Men's repertoire in the 1620s, when Q1 was printed from a prompt-book (see 'Text'). The Q1 title-page asserts that the play had been staged at the BLACKFRIARS THEATRE, but no specific record of an early performance is known.

In 1664 William DAVENANT produced his own version of the play, entitled *The Rivals.* He altered it immensely, changing all the names and locations and supplying a new beginning and a new conclusion. He replaced much of the text—including most of what is attributed to Shakespeare—with his own (which was influenced in part by passages from *Macbeth*). The only known performance is that reported by Samuel PEPYS in 1664, but since *The Rivals* was published four years later, it was probably at least somewhat popular.

The Two Noble Kinsmen was not seen again until 1928, when it was produced at the OLD VIC THEATRE. It has only been staged occasionally since then, and it remains among the least performed of Shakespeare's works.

Tybalt Character in *Romeo and Juliet,* a cousin of JULIET (1). The belligerent Tybalt insists on fighting for the CAPULET (1) family against the MONTAGUE (1) clan on any occasion. His arrival turns the humorous verbal confrontation between servants in 1.1 into a violent brawl. When he recognises ROMEO at the feast in 1.5, he wants to duel with him on the spot. The next day he fights and kills MERCUTIO, thus inciting Romeo to slay Tybalt in revenge, the act for which he is banished. In Shakespeare's source, Tybalt is merely a name, appearing only to be killed by Romeo in a street fight. The playwright elaborates the character to generate dramatic tension in the first half of the play; Tybalt serves to emphasise the potential for violence that accompanies the developing love between hero and heroine.

Tyler (1), Richard (1566–1636) Resident of STRATFORD and friend of Shakespeare. Tyler, two years younger than Shakespeare, probably knew Shakespeare at the Stratford grammar school, for his father, as an alderman, was entitled to send his children there without charge. However, his most significant connection with Shakespeare lies in his removal from the

playwright's will. Though he was originally one of seven close friends given bequests of money to buy a commemorative ring, Tyler's name was scratched out and replaced with that of Hamnet SADLER. This may have been Shakespeare's response to Tyler's involvement in a scandal: as a collector of relief funds after the great Stratford fire of 1614, Tyler was charged with enriching himself. However, he apparently continued to be a friend of the family, participating in the transfer of the BLACKFRIARS GATEHOUSE to Susanna SHAKESPEARE (14) Hall in 1618.

Tyler (2), Thomas (1826–1902) British scholar. Tyler was best known as a biblical scholar, but he also wrote several works on Shakespearean topics, most notably *The Philosophy of Hamlet* (1874). In his edition of the SONNETS (1890), Tyler identified Mary FITTON as Shakespeare's 'Dark Lady'. This theory was popularised by Frank HARRIS (1), but scholars now generally reject it.

Tyre City of the ancient Seleucid Empire on the coast of what is now Lebanon, the setting for three scenes of *Pericles, Prince of Tyre.* The title character is the ruler of Tyre, and 1.2–3 and 2.4 are set within interiors located in the city. Shakespeare simply followed his source in placing his hero in Tyre, and the actual Mediterranean seaport is in no way present in the text of the play.

Of cities surviving today, Tyre is among the most ancient, as it has existed since prehistoric times. A famous producer of dyes—'Tyrian purple' cloth was proverbially rich and fashionable—and a significant port, Tyre was a wealthy city-state that maintained its independence while paying tribute to the succession of empires that ruled the region after its conquest by Alexander the Great in 332 B.C. At the time of Antiochus—the play's only historical figure—Tyre was actually a republic, but Shakespeare was not concerned with Middle Eastern history, and his Tyre is merely an exotic locale, appropriate to a tale of romantic adventures.

Tyrell (Tirell), Sir James (c. 1450–1502) Historical figure and character in *Richard III,* an unscrupulous and ambitious nobleman who agrees to arrange the murder of the PRINCE (5) of Wales and his brother the Duke of YORK (7). RICHARD III, directed to Tyrell by a PAGE (1), commissions the killings in 4.2. At the beginning of 4.3, Tyrell returns to report that the deed has been accomplished by his hired ruffians.

The historical Tyrell was not the unknown minor aristocrat depicted by Shakespeare. He had served the Yorkist cause and been knighted at the battle of TEWKESBURY, and, at the time the princes were imprisoned, he was Richard's Master of Horse. After the accession of Henry VII, Tyrell continued to hold military posts until he was executed, on unrelated charges, in 1502. He was reported to have admitted at that time to arrangeing the murders, and Shakespeare follows Thomas MORE's account of his alleged confession. Modern scholars generally find the story unconvincing, however, and the mystery of the princes' disappearance (and probable death) remains unsolved.

Tyrian Sailor Minor character in *Pericles,* a seaman on PERICLES' ship. As 5.1 opens the Tyrian Sailor tells Pericles' aide, HELICANUS, of the visit of LYSIMACHUS, the governor of MYTILENE. He then relays Helicanus' request for courtiers to greet the governor, and he finally introduces the visitor to Helicanus. This busy episode points up the formality with which Pericles is surrounded, and adds to the ceremonious atmosphere of the play.

The designation of this character as Tyrian is the consequence, first, of the QUARTO edition of the play, which provided two sailors. Later, scholars presumed that one of them was in Lysimachus' service and was thus Mytilenian; the other, Pericles' sailor, was therefore distinguished in like fashion. Editors have varied in their distribution of the episode's lines: sometimes 5.1.11–13 are given to the Mytilenian Sailor, but he is often dropped, and the Tyrian (or First) Sailor speaks all the lines. Sometimes a First and Second Sailor are provided who are both assumed to be Tyrian.

U

Udall, Nicholas (1504–1556) English author and playwright, author of the earliest English COMEDY. Udall translated the Latin plays of Terence (c. 185–159 B.C.) (with John HIGGINS) and essays of the great humanist Erasmus (c. 1456–1536). He also wrote theological works, along with a number of plays, all but one of them lost. His *Ralph Roister Doister* (c. 1553, published 1566) is generally considered the earliest English comedy; only a single copy of it survived in 1825, when its importance was recognised by John Payne COLLIER (2). In boisterous rhymed dialogue, Udall borrowed elements from Terence, PLAUTUS, and crude English farces to create a distinctively original work. Among other comic touches, Udall invented a device—the mischievously mispunctuated reading of a document—that Shakespeare used in *A Midsummer Night's Dream* (5.1.108–116). Udall was discharged from his position as headmaster of Eton for homosexuality, but recovered his social standing sufficiently to find favour with Queen Mary (ruled 1553–1558), who collaborated with him in a translation, licenced him to write plays, and provided him with another headmastership, shortly before his death.

Ulysses Legendary figure and character in *Troilus and Cressida,* a Greek leader in the TROJAN WAR. Ulysses is a voice of sanity among the Greeks, who are fighting a dishonourable war for a pointless cause. Yet such is the corruption of the world of the play that Ulysses fails to influence his fellows and, indeed, gives up his own ideals. In both his idealism and his failure he corresponds to HECTOR among the Trojans.

However, the common sense and political wisdom of Ulysses provide a background against which to view the corrupt world of the play. He diagnoses the Greek failure in the war as due to their departure from strict adherence to a system of social hierarchy, like that of the 'heavens themselves' (1.3.85). However, in his effort to convince ACHILLES that he should return to the battle he abandons this idea and instead encourages the reluctant warrior to consider the loss of status he risks by permitting AJAX to receive the laurels he could receive himself. In giving up his ideals to promote this rivalry, Ulysses reveals himself to be a pragmatist, but the event contributes to our sense of disorder in the play's world. Moreover, his compromise fails in its purpose, for Achilles again withdraws from the battle, and only Patroclus' death finally brings his sword into play. Ulysses, though wise, is no less subject to the chances of war than anyone else.

Ulysses' judgements of the other characters, though firmly stated, are distinctly, if slightly, mistaken, adding to the play's network of self-deception and error. In 4.5, on the strength of his first impression, he declares CRESSIDA to be a prostitute; while he has perceived her sexuality, he has misread it, for she is merely a frankly sensual woman whom circumstance has placed in temptation's way. Ulysses praises DIOMEDES for a spirit that 'In aspiration lifts him from the earth' (4.5.16); he recognises an intensity of purpose, but he fails to see that Diomedes' energies are to be expended on an extremely earthly aspiration: the seduction of Cressida. Similarly, Ulysses says of Troilus that he 'gives not till judgement guide his bounty' (4.5.102), yet we know that Troilus has committed himself to Cressida without judgement. However, Troilus is an idealist in love, and Ulysses' opinion is not wrong, merely uninformed. We are made aware that wisdom and objectivity are no guarantee of knowledge in the world of the play.

Ulysses (better known by his Greek name, Odysseus) is a principal character in the *Iliad* of HOMER. He is noted for his wisdom and good sense as a strategist, and he is also a valiant warrior. He is the central figure in the *Iliad*'s successor, the *Odyssey,* which recounts his long series of adventures after the war. In Homer, Odysseus was famous for craftiness—reflected in the play in Thersites' reference to him as 'that . . . dog-fox Ulysses' (5.4.11). Although he lies fluently when he needs to he is essentially honourable. In later tradition, however, especially in the ancient Greek dramatists, he appears as a cowardly rascal. He was worshipped as a demi-god in the cults of later antiquity.

Umfrevile, Sir John (active 1403) Historical figure mentioned in *2 Henry IV* as an ally of the rebel Earl of NORTHUMBERLAND (1), perhaps the original speaker of some lines assigned to Lord BARDOLPH (2). In 1.1, as TRAVERS approaches WARKWORTH CASTLE with news of the battle of SHREWSBURY, Lord Bardolph tells of hav-

ing encountered Travers and given him such news as he had. When he arrives, Travers reports that he met Umfrevile en route and that Umfrevile had gone ahead of him with his news, which he accordingly omits, proceeding to tell of a later encounter. The QUARTO edition of the play (1600) gives a speech prefix to Umfrevile at 1.1.161—later editors give the line to either Lord Bardolph or Travers—and in 1.3.81 Lord Bardolph reveals his ignorance of information provided in this scene. Scholars conclude that Lord Bardolph's part in 1.1 may originally have been written as Umfrevile's, and that Umfrevile's lines were later assigned to someone else in order to eliminate one character as an economy measure for an acting company.

Underhill, William (1556–1597) Landowner in and around STRATFORD, the seller of NEW PLACE to Shakespeare. Underhill was a member of the gentry who held a remunerative position in the county court at Warwick and had inherited New Place and much other land at the age of 14. He sold New Place to Shakespeare in May 1597, but in July he was poisoned by his eldest son, Fulke (b. 1579), who was executed for the murder in 1599. The Underhill properties were sequestered by the state, and when the second son, Hercules (b. 1581), came of age in 1602, he had to reconfirm the sale of New Place to Shakespeare.

Underwood, John (d. 1624) English actor, member of the KING'S MEN. Underwood was one of the 26 men listed in the FIRST FOLIO as 'Principall Actors' in Shakespeare's plays, though no specific Shakespearean role is associated with him. He and William OSTLER (2) probably became members of the King's Men at the same time, replacing William SLY (2) and Laurence FLETCHER (3), who died in 1608. When Underwood died, he held shares in the GLOBE, CURTAIN, and BLACKFRIARS THEATRES. He left them to his five children, all minors, for whom his fellow actor Henry CONDELL acted as trustee.

University Wits Group of English playwrights credited with the development of ELIZABETHAN DRAMA in the 1580s. Called the University Wits by modern scholars, these men were distinguished by their superior educations in a profession that had always been somewhat disreputable at best (see ELIZABETHAN THEATRE). The most notable of them were Oxford graduates Thomas LODGE, John LYLY, and George PEELE, and Cambridge alumni Robert GREENE (2), Thomas NASHE, and Christopher MARLOWE (1). These men purposefully went beyond the didactic chronicles and shapeless, knockabout farces of the existing English stage. They combined the influences of ancient Roman drama, the medieval MORALITY PLAY, ACADEMIC DRAMA, and contemporary Italian and French drama, to create plays with intelligible structure, vigorous plotting, and vital poetry. The plays of the University Wits were very popular and helped establish the flourishing theatrical world that Shakespeare entered as a young man.

Ur-Hamlet Name given to a lost Elizabethan play resembling *Hamlet* and believed to have been used by Shakespeare as a source. Several references prove that there was an earlier play involving HAMLET. In 1589 Thomas NASHE, mocking plays derived from SENECA and especially those of Thomas KYD, referred to '. . . whole Hamlets, I should say handfuls of tragical speeches'. The context of this remark leads most scholars to conclude that Kyd wrote the *Ur-Hamlet.* A performance of a play called *Hamlet* by Shakespeare's acting company, the CHAMBERLAIN'S MEN, is recorded in 1594, and a famous reference by Thomas LODGE printed two years later implies that the work was still current and provides an image from it: '. . . ghost which cried so miserably . . . *Hamlet, revenge'.*

Little more is known of the play's contents, for no text survives. However, it presumably followed the tale by François BELLEFOREST that was probably its major source. It seems it included most, if not all, of the following elements: Hamlet seeking revenge against his uncle for the murder of his father and the seduction of his mother; his feigned madness and his romantic involvement with a woman; his dramatic encounter with his mother during which he kills a spy; his exile to England and the trick whereby he arranges for the execution of his escorts instead of himself; and his killing of his uncle in a long-deferred vengeance.

Thus the *Ur-Hamlet* was plainly a REVENGE PLAY like Kyd's *The Spanish Tragedy* (1588–1589), to which it may have been a companion piece. Scholars comparing *Hamlet* and *The Spanish Tragedy* find further clues concerning the *Ur-Hamlet:* some elements of *The Spanish Tragedy,* a play that also centres on a postponed revenge, suggest themes found in Shakespeare's *Hamlet* in more developed forms, and it is thought these elements may also have been used by Kyd in the *Ur-Hamlet.* Thus, the *Ur-Hamlet* may have included a procrastinating Hamlet who dies at the play's close, an heroine whose love for Hamlet is opposed by her family and who eventually becomes insane and commits suicide, and a play within a play, all of which resemble components of *The Spanish Tragedy* yet are not present in Belleforest. Further, the sub-plot in which Hamlet kills the father of the man who kills him and of the woman who loves him is not in Belleforest and thus may have been in the *Ur-Hamlet.* However, Shakespeare may very well have devised this himself, and *The Spanish Tragedy* may simply have been an influence on *Hamlet* rather than containing the same ideas as the *Ur-Hamlet.*

One further minor source of information may exist. DER BESTRAFTE BRUDERMORD, a German version of

Hamlet gleaned from the recollections of English actors who toured Germany in the 17th century, offers certain minor details which do not come from *Hamlet* yet correspond to Belleforest, and it is thought these may have been remembered by actors who had also performed in the *Ur-Hamlet.*

Ur-Shrew Hypothetical play sometimes assumed to be the source for both *The Taming of the Shrew* and THE TAMING OF A SHREW. The *Ur-Shrew* is usually attributed to Shakespeare, but it is presumed to have been revised by the playwright in order to incorporate the SUB-PLOT involving BIANCA (1) and her suitors. The revised play, according to this theory, is *The Taming of the Shrew,* whereas *The Taming of a Shrew* is a BAD QUARTO of the *Ur-Shrew,* whose original text has been lost. The *Ur-Shrew* hypothesis exists to account for inconsistencies between *A Shrew* and *The Shrew,* especially the differences between their sub-plots. However, most recent scholarship finds that these questions can be resolved without assuming the existence of a play for which no evidence exists, and the *Ur-Shrew* theory has generally been rejected in favour of the idea that *The Shrew* is Shakespeare's original play and *A Shrew* a Bad Quarto of it.

Ursula Minor character in *Much Ado About Nothing,* attendant to HERO. A cheerful member of LEONATO's court, Ursula has no important function and little personality. She flirts with the aged ANTONIO (3) at the MASQUE in 2.1, and she helps her mistress fool BEATRICE into believing that BENEDICK loves her in 3.1.

Urswick, Sir Christopher Character in *Richard III.* See CHRISTOPHER (2).

Usher Minor character in *Coriolanus,* a servant of VALERIA. The Usher accompanies the lady he serves when she visits VIRGILIA and VOLUMNIA, in 1.3. He does not speak and serves merely to indicate the prestige and wealth of his mistress. He is often dropped from productions of the play. In medieval and RENAISSANCE times an usher was a servant whose function was to precede his employer and open doors, prepare seats, etc.

V

Valentine (1) Minor character in *Titus Andronicus.* Mentioned only in a stage direction, Valentine helps to capture CHIRON and DEMETRIUS (1) in 5.2.

Valentine (2) One of the title characters in *The Two Gentlemen of Verona,* the lover of SILVIA, whom his disloyal friend PROTEUS attempts to steal. Valentine is both a romantic leading man and an object of fun. At first resistant to love, he then becomes an inept suitor. Once Silvia has given him her affection, he naïvely brags of it to Proteus, whose plotting quickly sends Valentine into exile. Later, after he rescues Silvia from an attempted rape by Proteus, only JULIA's intervention prevents him from inanely giving away his beloved to the man from whom he has just saved her.

Valentine (3) Minor character in *Twelfth Night,* a follower of Duke ORSINO of ILLYRIA. Valentine serves as Orsino's emissary to OLIVIA before VIOLA, disguised as Cesario, takes over the job. His name is appropriate to this task, and his flowery language in 1.1.24–32 matches his master's. In this speech he introduces the audience to the play's first development, Orsino's unrequited love for Olivia, and at the opening of 1.4 he informs Cesario that Orsino is fond of him, thus introducing a major complication of the plot.

Valeria Minor character in *Coriolanus,* a friend of CORIOLANUS' wife, VIRGILIA. Valeria is a cheerful, but somewhat insensitive young noblewoman who visits Virgilia in 1.3. Her bland acceptance of the Roman aristocratic ideal, combined with her charming vivacity, contrasts forcefully with the melancholy of her friend, who is distressed by the martial fervour of her mother-in-law, VOLUMNIA. Valeria describes the BOY (8), son of Coriolanus and Virgilia, in 1.3.57–65, and she is not aware that she presents a disturbing picture of the Boy killing a butterfly with his teeth. She does not speak in the three remaining scenes in which she appears, having served her function as a foil for Virgilia.

Valeria accompanies Volumnia and Virgilia on their crucial mission to dissuade Coriolanus from invading Rome, and though she does not speak, she is described in 5.3.64–67 as a particularly noble Roman woman. This allusion reflects the greater role that Valeria plays in Shakespeare's source, PLUTARCH's *Lives,* where she stirs Volumnia to action. However, the playwright preferred to have Volumnia stand alone, and Valeria's role remains minor.

Valerius Minor character in *The Two Noble Kinsmen,* a gentleman of THEBES and friend of ARCITE and PALAMON. In 1.2 Valerius informs his friends of the challenge to King Creon of Thebes issued by Duke THESEUS (2) of ATHENS, who intends to conquer Thebes and avenge the king's evil behaviour in refusing burial to his defeated foes. Valerius thereby provides the link between the two title characters and Athens, where, as prisoners of war, they will enact the main plot of the drama. Having fulfilled this function, Valerius disappears from the play.

Variorum edition Annotated edition of an author's work. The name comes from the Latin *cum notis variorum,* meaning 'with the notes of various [people]'. Several editions of Shakespeare's works are so designated, but in the 20th century the term usually refers to the New Variorum, edited by H. H. FURNESS and his successors, and published beginning in 1871.

The First Variorum was based on the 1778 edition of George STEEVENS' Shakespeare, which was posthumously expanded and published by Isaac REED in 1803. The collected essays and notes included in this 21-volume work offer a copious representation of 18th-century Shakespearean scholarship, though the edition omits the playwright's poems. The Second Variorum (1813) was simply a reprint of the First, but the Third Variorum incorporated the work of Edmond MALONE. James BOSWELL the younger completed Malone's second edition of Shakespeare's works after the older scholar's death in 1812 and grafted it onto Reed's work. The Third Variorum, also known as 'Boswell's Malone', was published in 1821, also in 21 volumes. It encompasses annotated texts of all the plays and the poems, Malone's life of the playwright (a basic reference for all subsequent biographers of Shakespeare), his history of the English stage, and other materials.

The New Variorum consists of one or more volumes

per play, two for the SONNETS, and one for the other poetry. Furness had produced 18 volumes before he died in 1912. The work was completed in 1953 by a series of successors, including his son H. H. Furness Jr, and J. Q. ADAMS.

Varrius (1) Minor character in *Measure for Measure,* a follower of the DUKE (9) of Vienna. Varrius is addressed by the Duke in 4.5 and is mentioned in the stage direction opening 5.1, the Duke's formal entry to Vienna, but he does not speak, nor does he appear in the list of characters in the first published text of the play, in the FIRST FOLIO. Some scholars believe that this is evidence that the play had been cut before it was published. On the other hand, Varrius may be seen as a representative of the Duke's entourage whose tiny part in 4.5 prepares the audience to perceive the Duke's return in 5.1 as a ceremonious occasion.

Varrius (2) Minor character in *Antony and Cleopatra,* a follower of POMPEY (2). In 2.1 Varrius brings the disquieting news to Pompey, MENAS, and MENECRATES that ANTONY has left Egypt to rejoin the coalition against Pompey. Varrius' function is to introduce a development of the plot.

Varro (Varrus) Minor character in *Julius Caesar,* a soldier in the army of BRUTUS (4). In 4.3 Varro and CLAUDIUS (1) are ordered to sleep in the same tent with Brutus to be available as messengers They sleep through the visitation of the GHOST (2) of CAESAR (1), and Brutus wakes them to confirm that they have seen nothing.

In the first edition of *Julius Caesar,* that in the FIRST FOLIO, Varro's name is rendered as Varrus, and some modern editors follow the Folio in this respect. Others, however, use Varro, which is correct in Latin and appears in Shakespeare's source, NORTH's translation of PLUTARCH's *Lives.*

Varro's Servant Either of two minor characters in *Timon of Athens,* employees of Varro, a creditor of TIMON. In 2.2 Varro's Servant joins two colleagues, ISIDORE'S SERVANT and CAPHIS. Together they approach Timon and his STEWARD (2), hoping for repayment of the debts Timon owes their masters, but they are put off. In 3.4 two of Varro's servants—distinguished in speech headings as First Varro's Servant and Second Varro's Servant—join LUCIUS' SERVANT, HORTENSIUS, PHILOTUS, and TITUS (2) on the same errand, again without success. In the latter scene the Servants express their reluctance to solicit for their greedy masters who have benefited in the past from Timon's generosity, but are now merciless.

Varrus Character in *Julius Caesar.* See VARRO.

Vaughan, Sir Thomas (d. 1483) Historical figure and minor character in *Richard III,* an ally of Queen ELIZABETH (2). Vaughan appears only to be executed by Richard (see RICHARD III) in 3.3. In going to his death, he speaks one line.

The historical Thomas Vaughan was a member of the official household of the PRINCE (5) of Wales, son of Elizabeth and King EDWARD IV. The dying king had stipulated that Richard should rule for the boy when he inherited the crown, but Vaughan participated in an attempt to unseat Richard as Protector. He was executed as a result, although the play makes his condemnation seem arbitrary.

Vaughan Williams, Ralph (1872–1958) English composer. Best known for his symphonies and choral works, Vaughan Williams also wrote several operas, among them *Sir John in Love* (1929), based on *The Merry Wives of Windsor.* He often set poetry to music, including many passages from Shakespeare. Among his best known Shakespearean works is a 1951 setting for PROSPERO's famous 'revels' speech (*Tempest* 4.1. 148–148), and he declared that the last movement of his famous Sixth Symphony was based on this passage. He composed music for many of Shakespeare's songs, beginning as early as 1891 and returning to them often. In 1913, he composed incidental music for *2 Henry IV, Henry V, The Merry Wives of Windsor, Richard II,* and *Richard III,* and in 1944 wrote the score for a radio play of *Richard II.*

Vaux (1), Sir Nicholas (d. 1523) Historical figure and minor character in *Henry VIII,* member of the court of King HENRY VIII. In 2.1 Vaux, with Sir Thomas LOVELL (2), escorts the Duke of BUCKINGHAM (1) to the TOWER OF LONDON. He speaks only three lines, suggesting that the prisoner should be treated in accordance with his rank, but Buckingham contradicts him, humbly accepting the loss of his duchy as his fate. Vaux's tiny part helps point up the virtues of Buckingham, which contrast with the evil of his enemy, Cardinal WOLSEY.

Vaux's father, Sir William VAUX (3), who appears in *2 Henry VI,* had lost his estates for having supported King HENRY VI in the WARS OF THE ROSES, but they had been returned to Sir Nicholas by Henry VII. Nicholas Vaux's son was the courtier-poet Thomas VAUX (2).

Vaux (2), Sir Thomas (1509–1556) English poet. Vaux was a cultivated aristocrat who was a member of the courts of several English monarchs, beginning with HENRY VIII. Although his poetry was superior to that of most of his fellow courtiers, he is noteworthy today only for having written 'The aged lover renounces love', which appears, in a very garbled form, as the GRAVE-DIGGER's song in *Hamlet* (5.1.61–64, 70–73, 92–95). Vaux' poem, said to have been written on

his deathbed, was still well known in Shakespeare's day as a popular song.

Vaux' father, Sir Nicholas VAUX (1), likewise a courtier, appears in *Henry VIII,* and his grandfather, Sir William VAUX (3), has a role in *2 Henry VI.*

Vaux (3), Sir William (d. 1471) Minor character in *2 Henry VI,* a messenger who announces the terminal illness of CARDINAL (1) Beaufort in 3.2. Vaux gives a vivid account of the Cardinal's guilty raving about the murder of the Duke of GLOUCESTER (4). The historical Sir William Vaux was a minor member of the entourage of the Cardinal. He later died fighting for HENRY VI at the battle of TEWKESBURY. His son was the Sir Nicholas VAUX (1) who appears in *Henry VIII,* and his grandson was the poet Sir Thomas VAUX (2).

Venice City in northern Italy, setting for *The Merchant of Venice* and the opening scenes of *Othello.* In Shakespeare's day Venice was already famous for the sumptuous beauty that still astonishes the world today. A great commercial centre, it stood for luxuriant culture and the power of money, and Shakespeare pictures it vividly—without describing it—by presenting his audience with its wealthy and self-confident citizens and exotic foreign figures. Significantly, in both *The Merchant* and *Othello* the prosperous society of Venice relies on an outsider—one a Jew and the other a Moor—who is not fully admitted to the society's fellowship and whose alien status is important to the drama's central conflict.

Venice was present in Shakespeare's sources, but he may also have been influenced by the image Elizabethans had of the fabled city in developing his themes of generosity and greed in *The Merchant,* and of human dignity versus envy and malice in *Othello.* Venice is frequently presented in Elizabethan literature as a symbol for a hypercommercial society in which the acquisitive instinct rules to the detriment of finer impulses. Shakespeare was not concerned with presenting an accurate Venetian setting, and he plainly invoked this stereotype, especially in *The Merchant of Venice,* where all of his Venetians express themselves in financial and commercial terms. For example, the clown LAUNCELOT employs legalistic language in 2.2; BASSANIO claims PORTIA in mercantile terms in 3.2. 139–148; and Portia can remark of her lover, 'Since you are dear bought, I will love you dear' (3.2.312). The point is less prominent in *Othello,* but the envious IAGO 'know[s his] price' (1.1.11), and RODERIGO's mode of courtship consists of conspicuous expense. Even the despairing OTHELLO compares his dead DESDEMONA to 'a pearl . . . Richer than [a] tribe' (5.2.348–349), and the saintly Desdemona says of the crucial loss of Othello's love token, 'I had rather lose my purse / Full of crusadoes' (Portuguese gold coins) (3.4.21–22).

Of course, such characteristics are not difficult to find in any cosmopolitan society. Venice was certainly a colourful and exotic locale with its commercial connections to the remote and glamorous East. It was a likely place to encounter such strange sights as a Rialto money-lender in his 'Jewish gaberdine' (*Merchant,* 1.3.107) or a Moorish general, but it surely seemed familiar in its vices to the Londoners of Shakespeare's day. In fact, Venice's success as a commercially based empire was about to be imitated on a larger scale by England. The wealthy and cultivated classes in 16th-century London regarded Venice as something of a prototype of their own developing society, and the satirical thrust of *The Merchant*'s Venice was surely not lost on its original audiences.

Ventidius (1), Publius (c. 90–38 B.C.) Historical figure and minor character in *Antony and Cleopatra,* a Roman general. In 2.3 Ventidius is sent by Mark ANTONY to put down a rebellion in Parthia; in 3.1, he has accomplished his task. He appears with SILIUS, who encourages him to pursue the fleeing Parthians and conquer all of Mesopotamia. Ventidius replies with a lesson in military politics: he will not attempt to do as well against the Parthians as he might, for if he does too well, he may seem to show up his superior, Antony, who may seek vengeance and destroy his career. These remarks stress the cynicism demanded by the Roman world of politics, a cool and unemotional calculation that Antony rejects in his infatuation with CLEOPATRA.

The historical Ventidius was famous in his own day for his extraordinary rise in society amid the chronic turbulence of the time. As an infant he had been enslaved, for his family—from a pre-Roman tribe—had been involved in the last attempted revolt against Roman dominance in Italy. After serving as a Roman soldier, he became a contractor of military supplies. Like many defeated Italians, Ventidius became a backer of Julius CAESAR (1) in the Roman civil wars, and he was granted a senate seat as a reward; after Caesar's assassination he allied himself with Antony. However, despite his caution in victory—which Shakespeare took from PLUTARCH's *Lives*—his success against the Parthians ended his career. He returned to Rome where his triumph was extravagantly celebrated, but Antony discharged him amid rumours of bribes taken from a Mesopotamian ruler, and he died shortly thereafter.

Ventidius (2) Minor character in *Timon of Athens,* an ungrateful recipient of TIMON's generosity. In 1.1 Timon sends the money needed to free Ventidius from debtor's prison, and in 1.2 Ventidius thanks him and offers to return the money, but Timon refuses repayment. Ventidius observes: 'A noble spirit!' (1.2. 14), and he does not speak again. However, when

Timon has bankrupted himself through extravagant generosity, he sends to several friends for help, and Ventidius—who has in the meantime inherited a fortune—is among them. Act 3 begins with Timon being repudiated by a series of his miserly friends, in the course of which it is mentioned that Ventidius has also denied assistance. Ventidius does not reappear after 1.2, and he is simply an emblem of the callous greed that permeates the aristocracy of ATHENS.

Commentators have often remarked on the oddity of Shakespeare's having so dramatically established Ventidius' indebtedness, only to omit, on-stage, his refusal to help his benefactor. In fact, this peculiarity has been offered as evidence that the authorship of the play is divided: Shakespeare may have introduced Ventidius' story and another playwright disposed of it too casually, or vice versa. However, if this is an error—and a case can be made that the anticlimax is effective because it reinforces Act 3's message—then it may simply reflect the fact that *Timon* is an incomplete work, as most scholars believe.

Venus and Adonis Narrative poem by Shakespeare that tells of the goddess Venus' infatuation for a mortal human, the young hunter Adonis. In erotic and humorous passages, Venus courts the youth, attempting to persuade him to make love. Adonis resists her advances, being unmoved by what he sees as simple lust; he prefers to go hunting. The next day, at dawn, Venus discovers the body of the dead Adonis, who has been killed by a wild boar. The poem closes with her lament.

Venus and Adonis has less relevance for most modern readers than do Shakespeare's dramas. Conventions that largely lack meaning today contribute to the overall tone and texture of the poem, and the work is now often perceived as frigidly artificial and remote from real human experience. But although its characterisation and plotting are feeble by comparison with the plays, *Venus* boasts many charming passages. Moreover, and much more important, the poem does in fact deal with a humanly significant theme, sexual love.

Shakespeare dedicated *Venus and Adonis* to the Earl of SOUTHAMPTON (2)—a classically educated and highly sophisticated patron of the arts—thus indicating his intention that the poem be received as a fashionable exercise in delicate eroticism, deftly constructed in an artificial and elaborately rhetorical classical manner. From the literature available to Elizabethan readers, the poet turned to the best source for such a poem, the works of the Latin master of erotic poetry, OVID, which he probably knew both in Latin and in the English translation by Arthur GOLDING (1567). In Ovid's *Metamorphoses,* Adonis reciprocates Venus' love, but Shakespeare followed a variant of the tale that was also well known in England, incorporating elements from other Ovidian stories and portraying the mortal's rejection of the goddess. The epigraph to the dedication—promising a work meant for a select audience—comes from another work by Ovid, *Amores.* Classical literature was entirely familiar to 16th-century readers, and, in associating his work with Ovid's, Shakespeare was plainly declaring his intention to be similarly witty, charming, and delicately sensual. Some details, especially the episode of the stallion and the mare, were probably inspired by passages in the *Georgics* of VIRGIL, the greatest of Latin poets.

Shakespeare was probably also influenced by *Hero and Leander,* by Christopher MARLOWE (1). The date of composition of this poem is unknown—it was unfinished when the poet died in early 1593—and it was not published until 1598, but Shakespeare had probably read it in manuscript; certainly *Hero and Leander*'s unprecedented combination of wit and luxuriant sensuousness was unique before Shakespeare wrote his poem. Like *Hero and Leander, Venus and Adonis* was scandalously popular, to judge by the many references to it, both delighted and disapproving. It has often been speculated that the ferocity of the controversy impelled Shakespeare to follow *Venus* with a much primmer narrative poem, *The Rape of Lucrece.*

Venus and Adonis may be seen as simply a trivial entertainment, intended to attract the patronage of a cultured aristocrat. Or the poem may be given more weight and viewed as a scintillating example of RENAISSANCE art, an evocation of ancient ideals equivalent to, say, the paintings of Botticelli. Still, the thematic richness of the plays, which even at their weakest are intent on exploring ideas and human relations, suggest that a work by Shakespeare must have more point than simple entertainment or beauty. However, the moral to be found in *Venus and Adonis* has proven elusive, and the poem has been assessed in many different ways. Some critics feel that *Venus* is a failure, an immature effort that is confused and uncertain because the author was himself unclear about the nature of love and lust and therefore resorted to humour to patch up his undeveloped work. Others see the poem as a delightfully erotic comedy, a celebration of sexual passion. Although Adonis dies, his story is couched in humour, and his death is not a tragic one—his corpse vanishes into air and his blood becomes the goddess' nosegay. Still other readers find one of two tragic lessons in *Venus.* Accepting the erotic passages as indicative of the poet's attitude, one may see Adonis' death as the pathetic outcome of his cold and foolish aversion to love and sex. On the other hand, the horror of his death and Venus' condemnation of love at the end of the poem may be thought to condemn lust as a primal force of destruction.

All of these viewpoints offer salient truths about the poem; as is so often the case when considering Shakespeare, the most productive response combines various theories. Like *Romeo and Juliet* and *Antony and Cleo-*

patra in particular, *Venus* deals with perhaps the most difficult emotion to understand, love, and all three works present an essential paradox: love, an obvious manifestation of an elemental life force, is often tied to a self-destructive inclination towards death. Thus two irreconcilable attitudes about love are established, and the poem, like the plays, attempts to resolve the opposition between them.

One must start with a pervasive and obviously positive aspect of *Venus and Adonis:* the poem is unquestionably funny. Venus' overbearing seizure of Adonis, beginning in line 25, is a virtual parody of male aggressiveness; the description of the stolid Adonis as a tiny, terrified waterbird (lines 86–87) provides a droll juxtaposition; Venus' erotic characterisation of her own body as landscape (lines 229–240) is sufficiently amusing to extract a smile even from Adonis. Even at a moment of revulsion, as Venus first sees Adonis' corpse, the famous simile of the shrinking snail (lines 1033–1036) offers an irresistibly whimsical image that softens the blow; the situation is not permitted to inspire horror.

In a similar spirit, the poem boasts frequent vivid and sensual representations of country life—from such minor images as the comparison of the captive Adonis to a trapped bird (lines 67–68) or that of Venus to a 'milch doe, whose swelling dugs do ache' (line 875), to the more elaborate descriptions of the boar (lines 619–630), the boar hounds (lines 913–924), and the hunted hare (lines 679–708). Particularly impressive is the fully developed anecdote of Adonis' stallion in pursuit of a mare (lines 258–324), the last couplet of which is itself a handsome miniature landscape. Venus' repeated enthusiasm for physical love (e.g., in lines 19–24) is part of the same charming presentation of the sensual life. The poem offers an idyllic world populated by delightful plants and animals, needing only the consummated love of man and goddess—or so Venus asserts—to complete the picture.

However, a distinctly darker strain complicates matters. Venus' attraction to Adonis is not simply a delightful infatuation, but rather a fever of the soul; she tears at her beloved like a bird of prey (lines 55–58) and, when she refuses to stop kissing him, he is compared to a forcibly tamed hawk and a deer pursued to exhaustion (lines 560–561). Conversely, Adonis rejects not only Venus herself but also her idea of love, which he equates with lust, in a passage (lines 787–798) strikingly reminiscent of Sonnet 129, which decries lust as 'Th' expense of spirit in a waste of shame' (see SONNETS). For Venus, love is entirely involved with physical life, but it is only in death that Adonis can find love, as he conceives it; he says, 'I know not love . . . unless it be a boar, and then I chase it' (lines 409–410). Thus Venus and Adonis represent opposing points of view: the goddess finds fulfilment in the delights of sensuality, while the mortal man conceives of an ideal spiritual state.

We can see that the poem often supports Adonis' position by subtly undercutting that of Venus, and vice versa. The comical sight of Venus plucking Adonis from his horse (line 30) reflects the more serious point that her powers of seduction are so inadequate that she is reduced to this undignified action. When Venus argues—as Shakespeare himself does in several of the sonnets—that love is the most appropriate human activity because it leads to reproduction (lines 163–174), she seems to represent the life force, but in the very next line all such high purpose is lost, as 'the love-sick queen began to sweat'. Even one of Venus' most delightful tactics—her somewhat lewd yet humorous description of herself in terms of landscape (lines 229–240)—results only in her further humiliation; Adonis smiles in disdain, she is reduced to helplessness by his dimples, and the poet remarks, 'being mad before, how doth she now for wits?' (line 249). However, Adonis' ideal is similarly weakened. Although he rejects the animal nature of love that Venus extols, he is himself associated with animals throughout the poem, from the early parallels between him and birds, mentioned above, through the symbolism of his runaway horse as a male lover, to his almost sexual union with the boar in mutual death. The attitude of each protagonist is therefore compromised by the manner in which it is presented.

Thus the apparently hopeless dichotomy between Venus and Adonis is resolved even as it is presented, for Shakespeare's ultimate purpose here is to present opposing views as intertwined principles. The poem opens with a paradoxical introduction of the two protagonists: in the first stanza 'rose-cheek'd Adonis' is contrasted with 'sick-thoughted Venus' (lines 3, 5). A standard romantic convention—lovesick male pursues uninterested woman—is here reversed, and this switch is at the heart of Shakespeare's strategy. Venus is a parody of a typical male suitor, while Adonis is presented in a traditionally feminine role, a sex object, especially in lines 541–564, where he is virtually raped. He is also associated with imagery suggestive of women's physical charms, as in lines 9, 50, 247–248, and, most strikingly, 1114–1116, where the boar's death blow is described in sexual terms. (Adonis' femininity is sometimes taken as evidence of a homosexual inclination in Shakespeare, but the image seems to function quite well in the poem without such a conclusion. However, it does certainly suppose the acceptability of homoerotic ideas to both the poet and his audience.) The confusion of gender anticipates the conjunction of the two points of view that is reached in the closing stanzas.

The poem simultaneously views love in contradictory ways. Though love is the noblest of imaginable

states of mind, as Adonis insists, it also utterly prosaic, even ridiculous, grounded as it is in the physical desires embodied by Venus' lust. Although Adonis' death is brought about by his rejection of Venus' idea of love, it does not discredit her essentially comic approach; instead, it adds to it a tragic element, that of humanity's unachievable aspiration. Love's complicated blend of opposing qualities is asserted in the description of love in Venus' closing lament: 'Sorrow on love hereafter shall attend, [and it] shall be raging mad, and silly mild, make the young old, the old become a child. . . . It shall be merciful and too severe, and most deceiving when it seems most just' (lines 1136–1156). While Venus is 'weary of the world' (line 1189) at the tale's end, yet she also has been able to realise that, for all its pain, love may 'enrich the poor with treasures' (line 1150). This is the theme that the poem offers its readers, in as fine and showy a setting as the young Shakespeare could devise.

Venus and Adonis is a flawed, youthful work. The two protagonists display little credible personality; differences in tone within the poem seem to reflect indecisiveness on Shakespeare's part; in particular, Venus' final position, in which she seems to reject love in light of Adonis' death, is uncomfortably at odds with her earlier, much lighter attitude. Therefore, many readers simply accept the pleasures of the poem's numerous delightful passages and disregard an otherwise seemingly unrewarding text. However, the poem is much richer than this. Like Shakespeare's greater works, it is concerned with the human predicament, and it illuminates the young playwright's attitude towards one of his most important concerns, sexual love.

In the poem's dedication Shakespeare calls his work 'the first heir of my invention', and this is sometimes taken as evidence that *Venus and Adonis* was written before any of the plays. However, most scholars agree that it is much more likely to have been written between June 1592, when the London theatres were closed because of a plague epidemic, and April 1593, when the poem was registered with the STATIONERS' COMPANY. During this enforced break in his promising career, the young playwright turned to a mode of literature that was far more prestigious at the time. Thus the reference in the dedication is taken to allude to the poet's first effort at 'serious' writing. Not only was poetry regarded as the only important branch of literature, while the stage was still somewhat disreputable (see ELIZABETHAN DRAMA), but, under the patronage system that prevailed until long after Shakespeare's death, it was potentially much more profitable than a career in the theatre.

Venus and Adonis was first published in 1593 by the printer Richard FIELD (2) in a QUARTO edition (known today as Q1), of which only one copy—in Oxford's Bodleian Library—has survived. Field, who also printed *The Rape of Lucrece,* was probably a friend of Shakespeare's, and this fact, plus the great care with which both texts were printed, suggests that the narrative poems were the only works whose publication was supervised by Shakespeare himself. *Venus* was very popular, and eight more editions were published during Shakespeare's lifetime. These are known as Q2–Q9 (plus one that is unnumbered, since only a title-page has survived), though all but Q2 were actually published in an octavo format. A tenth edition, Q10, appeared shortly after Shakespeare's death. Each of these editions was simply a reprint of one of its predecessors, incorporating such minor alterations as the printers saw fit to make, and, while they all contain variant readings, none is thought to reflect any changes that Shakespeare made. Q1 is therefore regarded as the only authoritative text, and it is the basis for all modern editions.

Verdi, Giuseppe (1813–1901) Italian composer of several operas inspired by Shakespeare's plays. After creating his first Shakespearean opera, *Macbeth* (1847), Verdi declared his intention of composing for all of the playwright's major works. He planned a *King Lear,* but never actually wrote it, for lack of an adequate libretto. Although his ambition was unfulfilled, his two remaining Shakespearean operas, *Otello* (1887) and *Falstaff* (1893)—the latter based on *The Merry Wives of Windsor,* with additions from the *Henry IV* plays—are great accomplishments in themselves. With libretti by Arrigo BOITO, they are the twin masterpieces of Verdi's old age and in the opinion of most commentators, two of the best operas ever written.

Verges Character in *Much Ado About Nothing,* Constable DOGBERRY's second-in-command. Verges is chiefly a straight man for Dogberry to play against; his eager assistance is rejected by his superior, who prefers to do things himself. Though praised as 'an old man, . . . honest as the skin between his brows' (3.5.10–12), Verges has little personality, being rather like the other WATCHMEN (3)—and Dogberry—in his confusion and comical misuse of language.

Speech prefixes in 4.2 give Verges' lines to 'Cowley'. It is therefore assumed that the actor Richard COWLEY first played the part. Verges' name is traditionally said to be a rustic pronunciation of the word *verjuice,* meaning 'the acid juice of green or unripe fruit', but the character is not notably acid. Verges' name is more probably associated with his office, a *verge* being a rod or staff symbolising authority, usually carried by an underling or assistant to the holder of power.

Vergil, Polydore (1470–1555) Italian-born English author, writer of an history of England that informed Shakespeare's sources for the HISTORY PLAYS. Vergil's *Historia Anglia,* a Latin history commissioned by King Henry VII (see RICHMOND), focussed on the WARS OF THE ROSES and emphasised the influence of divine providence in punishing HENRY IV's sin in usurping the crown from RICHARD II with the civil conflicts. Thus, he aggrandised the TUDOR DYNASTY by presenting its founder, Henry VII, as an instrument of God. This point of view was adopted by Edward HALL (2) and Raphael HOLINSHED, Shakespeare's chief sources, and so became the dominant theme of the history plays.

Vergil, born in Urbino, came to England in 1501 as a representative of the pope. Henry commissioned the *Historia Anglia* in 1505, and the Italian became an English citizen in 1510, though he returned to Urbino in 1551. He was a friend of Sir Thomas MORE, who read Vergil's history in manuscript and was influenced by it in writing his biography of RICHARD III, which was also influential on Shakespeare through Hall and Holinshed.

Vernon (1) Minor character in *1 Henry VI,* a follower of Richard Plantagenet, later Duke of YORK (8). Vernon backs Plantagenet against the Duke of SOMERSET (3), in the scene (2.4) that establishes the rivalry that will eventually lead to civil war. Later, in 3.4 and 4.1, he disputes with BASSET, a backer of Somerset. By demonstrating the involvement of lesser figures, these incidents illustrate the damage to English morale caused by the dissensions among the noblemen.

Vernon (2), Richard (d. 1403) Historical figure and character in *1 Henry IV,* a supporter of HOTSPUR. Vernon arrives at the rebel camp before the battle of SHREWSBURY with news that the the King's armies are approaching. He describes PRINCE (6) HAL's forces in a speech (4.1.97–110) famous for its vivid imagery. In 4.3 he advises vigorously against Hotspur's insistence on entering battle before his reinforcements arrive, and in 5.1 he participates, with WORCESTER, in the negotiations that precede the battle. Captured in the battle, he is sentenced to death by King HENRY IV in 5.5.

The historical Vernon, a powerful magnate of Cheshire, in western England, was in fact captured and beheaded at Shrewsbury, although he was not a participant in the negotiations between the two sides.

Verona City in Italy, the setting for *Romeo and Juliet*. The PRINCE (1) of Verona is named Escalus, a Latinisation of Della Scala, the name of the princely family that ruled the city in the late Middle Ages, but there is nothing specifically Veronese in the play, and Shakespeare simply took the location from his source.

The feud between the MONTAGUE (1) and CAPULET (1) families was long thought to have been historical, but in fact it never occurred. The root of the error, which first appears in a story published in 1530 (see *Romeo and Juliet,* 'Sources of the Play') may be a line in Dante's *Inferno,* in which two families, the Capelleti and the Montecchi, are cited for fomenting civil disorders. However, while the Montecchi lived in Verona, the Capelletti came from Cremona, and there was no connection between them.

While the title of *The Two Gentlemen of Verona* suggests that the title characters come from that city, and several scenes (1.1–2.3 and 2.7) are presumed to take place there for the same reason, there is no textual reference to confirm these suppositions. On the other hand, at 3.1.81 and 5.4.127, it is suggested that the court of the DUKE (3) of Milan is in Verona, clearly an error. The geography of this play is confused at best, and its settings have no specificity.

Verona is mentioned in passing elsewhere in the plays. It is the home of PETRUCHIO (2) in *The Taming of the Shrew,* and several scenes take place in his nearby country house. It may also be the home of Michael CASSIO, though the reference, if it is one, is made in an apparently corrupt line (*Othello,* 2.1.26).

Verse test Scholarly method used to determine the authenticity and the chronological order of Shakespeare's plays. The verse test is a statistical analysis of the playwright's use of poetic devices. At its simplest, a verse test of a work determines the relative quantities of prose and poetry, and of rhymed and unrhymed lines within the poetry, and compares the result to other plays. Additional elements that are generally noted are the number of lines with feminine endings (i.e., that do not end on a stress; see METRE), the number of speeches that end in the middle of a line; and the quantitative ratio of BLANK VERSE to rhymed verse.

Verse tests were first applied by Edmond MALONE and others in the late 18th century, but they were most important in the Shakespearean studies of the 19th century, when a body of comparisons was developed by such scholars as Frederick FURNIVALL, G. G. GERVINUS, F. G. FLEAY, and William SPALDING. In the 20th century verse tests are much less important to scholars, who apply other concepts to the same questions and find the results of verse tests to be inconclusive.

Vestris, Elizabeth (1797–1856) British actress. Madame Vestris, as she was known, was born Lucia Elizabeth Bartolozzi. She kept the name of her first husband, a ballet dancer who deserted her, and became a successful comic actress, specialising in farces and burlesques. She married the actor Charles James Mathews (1803–1878). Beginning in 1839, they managed a theatrical company at the Covent Garden Theatre. They began by presenting the first performances of *Love's Labour's Lost* since the early 17th cen-

tury—Madame Vestris played ROSALINE (1)—followed by *The Merry Wives of Windsor,* in which she played MISTRESS (3) PAGE and used her fine voice to sing a number of interpolated songs. In 1840 Vestris and Mathews presented *A Midsummer Night's Dream,* and though their version was abridged, it was entirely Shakespearean, again for the first time in 200 years. It was also the first English production to use the famous incidental music by Felix Mendelssohn (1809–1847). Unfortunately, these productions were not financially successful, and the couple went bankrupt. Though they never again produced Shakespeare, they continued to perform—indeed, they had to, for Madame Vestris died before their finances were restored. Mathews eventually recovered and followed a less demanding career as a minor comic actor.

Vice, the Conventional figure from the medieval MORALITY PLAY, an influence upon the development of both Shakespeare's villains and his comic figures. The Vice attempts to seduce the soul of the protagonist, who represents mankind, into evil ways. An hypocrite, deceit and guile are his weapons—he is able to weep at will—and he employs them with great pleasure. At the same time, the Vice is a comic figure, designed to entertain while he instructs. He typically makes lewd jokes, puns outrageously, engages in physical horseplay, and brandishes his wooden sword with comic ineffectuality (both FALSTAFF [in *1 Henry IV,* 2.4.133] and PISTOL [in *Henry V,* 4.4.73–74] are associated with this feature). Especially in the more sophisticated 16th-century morality plays, he resembles the FOOL (1). The Vice also evolved into another, more distinctly Elizabethan character type, the MACHIAVEL.

At his most striking, the Vice advertises his villainy to the audience. He revels in viciousness in extravagant, humorous asides filled with demonic laughter. It is a convention of the morality plays that his victims are the only ones who cannot see through his obvious dishonesty; thus, the Vice demonstrates the habitual blindness of the sinner. A number of Shakespeare's early villains are distinctly Vice-like. The most notable of these, perhaps, is RICHARD III, who in fact describes himself as '. . . like the formal Vice, Iniquity' (*Richard III,* 3.1.82). The character's influence is still detectable in the later Shakespearean figure IAGO.

Vienna City in Austria, the setting for *Measure for Measure.* Dramatic convention called for a foreign locale for Shakespeare's sensational tale, and he probably chose Vienna because it was much better known to an English audience than its neighbour, Innsbruck, where the story takes place in his chief source, CINTHIO's novella. Much of the play occurs indoors—mostly in a prison, where local colour is distinctly lacking—and no Viennese ambience is achieved or even attempted.

In fact, Shakespeare's Vienna—presented chiefly in the comic SUB-PLOT—resembles Shakespeare's London, by no coincidence, for the play's satirical edge is intended to expose the immorality and cynicism of 'modern' life of the early 17th century. The humorous catalogue of petty criminals recited by POMPEY (1), in 4.3.1–20, offers a sampling of current London stereotypes. The idle, war-loving noblemen (see GENTLEMAN [5]) who condemn peace and laugh at venereal disease are our introduction to Vienna's streets, in 1.2, and probably reflect the negotiations for peace with Spain that were held in London from May to August of 1604. During this time the citizenry were troubled with the presence of disorderly soldiers, and professional officers bemoaned the prospective interruption of their careers. Similarly, MISTRESS (2) Overdone's complaint about 'the war . . . the sweat . . . the gallows' (1.2.75–76) reflects the same situation, as well as a plague that raged in London over the winter of 1603–04, and a series of treason trials and executions that enlivened the news. Further, the proclamation for the destruction of brothels, reported by POMPEY (1) in 1.2, corresponds to a London law of 1603 ordering the razing of whole districts inhabited by 'dissolute and idle persons'—ostensibly an antiplague effort, but one that was especially directed at whorehouses and gambling dens.

Vincentio (1) Minor character in *The Taming of the Shrew,* the father of LUCENTIO. Vincentio, described as 'a sober ancient gentleman' (5.1.65), arrives in PADUA to find himself impersonated by the PEDANT and Lucentio by his servant TRANIO. He is understandably angry, but otherwise he has no distinctive personality traits.

Vincentio (2) Character in *Measure for Measure.* See DUKE (9).

Vintner Minor character in *1 Henry IV,* an employee of the BOAR'S HEAD TAVERN. The Vintner appears only briefly, to chasten FRANCIS (1) and announce the arrival of FALSTAFF. He contributes to the atmosphere of a busy tavern.

Viola Character in *Twelfth Night,* lover of Duke ORSINO of ILLYRIA and twin sister of SEBASTIAN (2). Viola is at the centre of the play's confusions. Separated from Sebastian in a shipwreck, Viola finds herself in Illyria. Disguised as a young man, Cesario, she meets and falls in love with Orsino, but her adopted persona prevents her from expressing her love for him except through service as his page. Orsino wishes her to court OLIVIA for him, placing her in a strange and difficult position that becomes worse when Olivia falls in love with Cesario. Viola, alone among the characters, knows the truth of this situation. While she is like the

other Illyrians in her susceptibility to passion, she alone can honestly assess it, saying simply, 'O time, thou must untangle this, not I, / It is too hard a knot for me t'untie' (2.2.39–40).

Viola's capacity for love is extreme: when Orsino, hysterical over Olivia's continued rejection, proposes to kill Cesario in a grand gesture, she calmly acquiesces, saying to him, 'I . . . to do you rest, a thousand deaths would die' (5.1.130–131). Such self-sacrificing devotion strikes some readers as Christlike, and, along with the powers of restoration displayed by Sebastian at the play's climax, it has influenced a religious interpretation of the play by some scholars, although an entirely secular reading is probably more appropriate to the comedy and Viola's personality.

Though extravagant, Viola's attitude towards love is much more wholesome than the posturings of Orsino and Olivia, and her effect on these characters is positive. Her spirit and candour arouse love in Olivia, who has been withdrawing into grief-filled seclusion. Similarly, although Orsino is wrapped up in his self-image as a melancholy rejected lover, he responds unconsciously to Viola's devotion, conceiving a fondness for Cesario that he eventually transforms into husbandly affection for the sort of loving wife he truly needs. Viola is the heroine of the play, performing the monumental task of liberating Olivia and Orsino from their misconceived selves and thus making the play's climax possible.

In the meantime, her frank good humour keeps the audience aware of the potential realignment of the lovers. She is not afraid to make telling remarks to Olivia on her unmarried state, arguing that '. . . you do usurp yourself: for what is yours to bestow is not yours to reserve' (1.5.188–190), and she is unafraid to counter Orsino's dramatic and boastful insistence that male love is grander than female, observing (while speaking as a man herself), 'We men may say more, swear more, but indeed / Our shows are more than will: for still we prove / Much in our vows, but little in our love' (2.4.117–119). She entertains herself and the audience with ironic remarks on her own disguised state, asserting to Olivia that 'what I am, and what I would, are as secret as maidenhead' (1.5.219) and, flatly, that 'I am not what I am' (3.1.143). Speaking as Cesario, she ironically tells Orsino that she loves someone 'of your complexion' and 'about your years, my lord' (2.4.26, 28), hiding the fact, which the audience knows, that the object of her love is Orsino himself.

However, there is also an aspect of Viola's position that contributes to *Twelfth Night*'s disturbing undertone. She cannot openly express her love, for her disguise inhibits her, and she thus embodies a disorder in the world of romantic comedy, just as Orsino and Olivia do in their self-delusion, though less blatantly. She herself laments, 'Disguise, I see thou art a wickedness' (2.2.26). Also, her disguise raises questions of sexual ambiguity that can be psychologically unnerving. In Shakespeare's time, Viola would of course have been played by a boy (see ELIZABETHAN THEATRE), making her situation both funnier and more troubling. The spectacle of one woman, played by a boy, mistakenly responding sexually to another one, also played by a boy, makes implicit reference to both male and female homosexuality, as well as to heterosexual love, in a way that is comical but also suggestive of hidden depths of human sexuality. While the modern use of actresses tends to obscure this point, the complexity of the situation retains some of its powerful and upsetting strength.

Nevertheless, these dark aspects do not interfere with Viola's essentially positive role. Until Sebastian arrives and resolves the play's intrigues, she alone has found an appropriate passion, and her strength and determination assure us that love will surely triumph. Whether recovering from disaster at sea, plunging into love and intrigue as Cesario, or turning to her betrothal at the play's close, Viola is one of Shakespeare's most attractive heroines—plucky, adventurous, and committed to the pursuit of love.

Violenta Character named but not present in *All's Well That Ends Well.* Violenta appears in the FIRST FOLIO in the stage direction that opens 3.5. It reads, 'Enter old Widow of Florence, her daughter, Violenta, and Mariana. . .'. Violenta could be the daughter's name, set off by commas, but DIANA (1) is certainly the Widow's daughter. Shakespeare may have originally named Diana differently, or he could have intended a fourth character whom he did not in fact use, in which case Violenta is a GHOST CHARACTER. In either case, the name survived in the text through an error on the part of the printer.

Virgil (Vergil) (70–19 B.C.) Ancient Roman poet, an important influence on Shakespeare's art in general—indeed, on all of English literature—whose works were also a source for details in a number of Shakespeare's plays and poems. For instance, Virgil's *Aeneid,* an epic poem on the founding of ROME, provided imagery and occasional episodes, most prominently in *The Rape of Lucrece, Hamlet,* and *The Tempest.* When the Archbishop of CANTERBURY (1) compares society to a beehive in *Henry V* (1.2.187–204), he is echoing a famous passage in Virgil's *Georgics,* a collection of hymns to the traditional rural life of Italy. Virgil's PASTORAL *Eclogues* were among the finest examples of a genre that particularly influenced *As You Like It* and *The Winter's Tale.*

However, the general impact of Virgil on the playwright's age is more important than any specific contributions. In the RENAISSANCE the works of Virgil, especially the *Aeneid,* were regarded as literature's highest achievement, and every 16th-century writer

felt their impact. The stately, measured pace of Virgil's verse was an important influence on the tone of Shakespeare's poetry and that of all his contemporaries. In fact, BLANK VERSE was introduced to England in the translations of Virgil by the Earl of SURREY (1). Virgil's themes, the patriotism of the *Aeneid* and the rustic beauties of the *Eclogues* and the *Georgics*, informed Elizabethan notions of genre.

Moreover, Virgil was a great literary nationalist—not only in the *Aeneid*'s grand history, but in the local pride of place displayed in the *Eclogues* and *Georgics*. As England emerged from the Middle Ages to find itself a distinctive nation, Virgil's nationalistic vision seemed remarkably appropriate. As if to demonstrate this, more than 50 English writers translated some part of Virgil's works during the 16th and 17th centuries. Shakespeare may have read the renderings of Surrey, Thomas Phaer (c. 1510–1560), or Richard Stanyhurst (1545–1615), but he surely knew the works best in the original Latin, for he studied Virgil in school.

Virgil was born near MANTUA, the son of a prosperous peasant—a potter and beekeeper, according to some traditions. He studied rhetoric and philosophy in Milan and Rome from 55 to around 42 B.C. At this time he began writing, and he also made friends with the poet GALLUS, who introduced him to a patron, MAECENAS, the friend and adviser of Augustus CAESAR (2). Maecenas probably encouraged the publication of the *Eclogues*, which appeared around 39 B.C., and he definitely urged the poet to compose the *Georgics*, which are written in his honour, though they contain many passages eulogising Augustus. The poet read the *Georgics* to Augustus upon his return from the campaign of ACTIUM in 29 B.C. and sparked the future emperor's enthusiasm and support. Both the *Eclogues* and the *Georgics* reflect their troubled times in a nostalgia for a simpler world combined with a hopeful anticipation of better times in the peace that has been wrought by Rome's new ruler. Their patriotic tone anticipates the *Aeneid*, on which Virgil worked for the last 10 years of his life. He died with the epic still incomplete and left instructions in his will that it be burned, but the emperor overruled this stipulation and had the poem published in its unfinished state.

Virgilia Legendary figure and character in *Coriolanus*, the wife of CORIOLANUS. When we first see her in 1.3, Virgilia makes her strongest impression, as she worries over her husband's return to war. She can only respond feebly to the martial enthusiasm of her powerful mother-in-law, VOLUMNIA, who calls her weak because she fears for her husband's safety. Virgilia has the inner strength, however, to refuse to continue her social life. She speaks very little in the remainder of the play—Coriolanus calls her his 'gracious silence' (2.1.174)—but though her role is small, her modesty offers a distinct and significant emotional note that contrasts with and emphasises the more strident tone of her husband and her mother-in-law.

Virgilia acts as a foil to Volumnia and makes clear that her mother-in-law's war-loving, masculine nature is not the only one possible for a Roman matron—rather, we see that Volumnia is not normal. Virgilia is also a foil to Coriolanus: in contrast with her, he seems crude. This is especially obvious when he returns from combat in 2.1 and he jokes with her about coffins and death. He is clearly not aware of her sensibilities, which we have been exposed to just a few scenes earlier.

Her presence also sheds light on her husband in a subtler fashion. He doesn't understand her or perhaps even perceive her clearly, but his recollection of their farewell kiss, 'Long as my exile, sweet as my revenge' (5.3.44–45), is touching, if also twisted. That his demure wife inspires such affection suggests to us a softer, undeveloped aspect of Coriolanus' nature. Virgilia stands for a world that might have been, and the latent presence of that world makes the dramatic reality of the tragedy more wrenching.

Visor, William GLOUCESTERSHIRE countryman named in *2 Henry IV*, a friend of DAVY. Davy, steward of Justice SHALLOW, wishes his master to rule in favour of his friend 'William Visor of Woncot' (5.1.34) in a lawsuit against one 'Clement PERKES a'th'Hill' (5.1.35). Shallow observes that 'Visor is an arrant knave' (5.1.37), but Davy disingenuously asserts the greater right of a knave to favour, since, being a knave, he is likely to be denied it. He goes on to claim the privilege of a loyal servant to 'once or twice a quarter bear out a knave against an honest man' (5.1.44), and Shallow promises that Visor 'shall have no wrong' (5.1.49). We are given a humorous glimpse of small-time country corruption, one of the many vignettes of common life that the play features.

Visor is thought to represent a real person, a member of a family named Visor or Vizard, known to have lived for centuries in the village of Woodmancote, the 'Woncot' of the play. Why Shakespeare chose to present William Visor as 'an arrant knave' is not known.

Volsce Character in *Coriolanus*, a spy who receives information for his tribe, the VOLSCIANS, from a ROMAN (2). In 4.3 the Volsce, named Adrian, meets the Roman, named Nicanor, from whom he has gathered intelligence before. He learns of the banishment of CORIOLANUS. The episode emphasises the atmosphere of intrigue that pervades Coriolanus' world, and prepares us for his defection in the next scenes.

Volscians In *Coriolanus*, an Italic tribe that makes war against ROME. CORIOLANUS receives his name for his bravery when he besieges and takes the Volscian town

of CORIOLES. When the Romans banish him, he joins the Volscians and leads them in a successful campaign. Under him, the Volscians almost take Rome, but the ex-Roman gives in to the pleas of his mother and spares the city. Though the resulting treaty requires large retributions from Rome, the Volscian leader AUFIDIUS has Coriolanus killed. This brings to a close the tragedy of a leader whose uncontrolled pride, combined with civil disorder, leads to catastrophe for himself and for Rome. Shakespeare employs the Volscians in this tale as he does the GOTHS in *Titus Andronicus,* FORTINBRAS in *Hamlet,* and the English in *Macbeth*—they are all foreigners who dominate a society once it succumbs to weaknesses that result from the shortcomings and misdeeds of its rulers. Thus, the Volscians are a sort of nemesis, a punishing fate that confirms the evil of selfish ambition or pride among the privileged. This was an important political point for Shakespeare throughout his career.

The historical Volscians were enemies of Rome throughout its early history. The record is obscure but many hints—including the legends surrounding Coriolanus—imply Volscian successes. They were finally defeated by the Romans during the 4th century B.C., and after 304 B.C.—about 200 years after the time of the play—they were politically incorporated into the Roman state. The Volscians were so thoroughly assimilated that almost all traces of their ancient culture had disappeared before the earliest surviving Roman accounts of them were written.

Voltemand (Voltimand, Valtemand) Minor character in *Hamlet,* ambassador to the King of Norway from the KING (5) of DENMARK. In 1.2 Voltemand and CORNELIUS (1) are appointed to deliver the King's message demanding that the Norwegian king's nephew, FORTINBRAS, who is preparing an invasion of Denmark, be restrained. The two ambassadors return in 2.2, and Voltemand delivers a document of agreement that he summarises in courtly language. The episode introduces the audience to Fortinbras while demonstrating the state of national crisis in which the play takes place.

This character's name was spelled both Voltemand and Valtemand in the most authoritative early edition of the play (Q2, 1604); Voltumand and Voltemar appear in other early editions. The second FOLIO edition (1632) used Voltimand, and this became the established practise until recently, when a compromise version became popular. In any form it is a corruption of Valdemar, the name of several Danish kings.

Volumnia Legendary figure and character in *Coriolanus,* the mother of the title character. Volumnia, an aristocratic Roman matron, has raised her son to be a proud warrior above all else. She dominates her son, for she has so thoroughly bred her own values in him that he is psychologically dependent on her approval and cannot oppose her. As she claims, 'There's no man in the world / More bound to's mother' (5.3.158–159). Desiring that Coriolanus receive the consulate, ROME's highest honour, Volumnia bullies him until he agrees to sacrifice his pride and solicit the approval of the common people. This is one of Shakespeare's most Machiavellian passages—3.2.41–86. However, because Coriolanus is what Volumnia has made him, he cannot restrain his proud contempt, with the result that he is banished from Rome. When he joins the VOLSCIANS, Rome's enemy, and threatens to sack the city, Volumnia again uses her influence over him with an elaborate appeal in 5.3, a virtuoso passage that is the high point of the play, dramatically. She convinces him to withdraw his forces, though he knows this means he will be killed by the Volscians.

Volumnia controls her son by withdrawing her approval: in both 3.2 and 5.3 she disdainfully disowns him—'Thy valiantness was mine . . . but owe thy pride thyself' (3.2.129–130), and 'This fellow had a Volscian to his mother' (5.3.178). While her advice to him is sound, it is only necessary because her influence has made him incapable of functioning sensibly. Because he has only the rigorous pride she has developed in him, he goes to his destruction. He is a tragic hero precisely because his greatness is mingled with his weakness. He is incapable of being anything except what his mother has made him. The influence of Volumnia is thus central to the play.

Volumnia is correct when she boasts to Coriolanus, 'Thou art my warrior: / I holp to frame thee' (5.3.62–63). Her upbringing of him has made him both the charismatic warrior who becomes a great Roman hero and the inflexible aristocrat who sparks the hatred of the Roman people. Her rigorous martial code is revealed on her first appearance, in 1.3, where she delights in Coriolanus' return to combat. She sternly rejects the concern for his safety displayed by his wife, VIRGILIA, and rejoices in the prospect of her son's wounds, or even his death, for the sufferings of war are badges of honour to her mind.

Volumnia's moral code—and thus that of Coriolanus—is seriously flawed, and this is made clear in Shakespeare's depiction of her warped sense of maternal love. In 1.3 her thirst for glory leads her to equate her joy at Coriolanus' birth with her pleasure in his fighting, and she compares the beauty of a mother's breast to that of a head wound. This obviously pathological attitude helps demonstrate the unhealthiness of the rigorous aristocratic ideal that Volumnia upholds, and it is part of the play's critique of the aristocracy. We are not surprised when the results of Coriolanus' upbringing prove catastrophic.

Shakespeare invented all of Volumnia's appearances save that in 5.3—her dramatic appeal to save

Rome—which occurs in the play's source, PLUTARCH's *Lives.* When he devised a powerful mother-son relationship to account for Coriolanus' submission, Shakespeare not only added psychological weight to his protagonist's sudden reversal, he found a basic component of his tragedy.

Volumnius (active 42 B.C.) Historical figure and minor character in *Julius Caesar,* a soldier in the army of BRUTUS (4). In 5.5 Volumnius—like CLITUS and DARDANIUS—shrinks from helping the defeated Brutus to commit suicide, saying 'That's not an office for a friend, my lord' (5.5.29). The episode illustrates the fondness with which Brutus is regarded by his subordinates, thereby contributing to the aura of sentiment surrounding his death. Little is known of the historical Volumnius, though Shakespeare's source, PLUTARCH, asserts that he had been a schoolmate of Brutus.

W

Wakefield Location in *3 Henry VI,* a town in Yorkshire and a battle site during the WARS OF THE ROSES. The battle, fought in December 1460 between the army of the Duke of YORK (8) and a considerably larger force led by Queen MARGARET (1), takes place in 1.2–4. It results in the capture and death of York and a catastrophic loss for his troops. In depicting the conflict, Shakespeare took considerable liberties with the recorded accounts. York's son RUTLAND (1), who died in combat, is incorrectly depicted as a child and a brutally murdered non-combatant. York's oldest son, Edward (see EDWARD IV), whose exploits the playwright describes, was not present at the battle; he was with another armed force, one that might have relieved York had he been patient and waited for it. However, the Duke undertook to fight despite the odds, probably underestimating the leadership of Queen Margaret, and suffered the loss, which is accurately portrayed. Another son, Richard (see RICHARD III), is made to encourage the hasty decision to fight; in reality, Richard was only eight years old at the time and lived in exile in Burgundy. The playwright made these alterations for various reasons: Rutland's murder emphasises the theme of revenge; the presence of Edward and Richard tightens the succession of incidents that the play must depict; and Richard's role further reflects his importance as a major character.

Wales (1) Ancient kingdom to England's west, a location used in *Cymbeline* and *Richard II,* and an important subject in *1* and *2 Henry IV* and *Henry V.* A Welsh character appears in *The Merry Wives of Windsor,* and Wales is referred to occasionally in other plays as well.

In the history plays Wales is strategically important in the civil conflicts fought by King HENRY IV. In *Richard II,* when BOLINGBROKE (the future king) arrives in England with an army, intent on challenging King RICHARD II, Richard is in Ireland. Bolingbroke therefore marches to Wales to intercept him upon his return. Scenes 2.4, 3.2, and 3.3 take place in this important location, although no fighting takes place. In 2.4 Shakespeare first presents, in the person of the CAPTAIN (4), the archetypal Welshman who appears in these plays, a cautious and superstitious figure. The Captain deserts Richard's cause, and he may represent Owen GLENDOWER, a famous Welsh warrior who appears in 3.1 of *1 Henry IV,* where his superstition is a significant factor in the unfolding of the plot.

Wales became a part of Britain by conquest over the course of the 11th to 13th centuries, but periodic revolts lasted until the time of the history plays when Glendower led a rebellion that produced the last few years of Welsh independence, c. 1405–1409. In both of the *Henry IV* plays the political importance of Wales is apparent: as well as being a hotbed of rebellion, it was a fertile source of soldiers. The courage and military prowess of the Welsh were well known, as was their inclination towards feuding and personal disputes. Other characteristics of the archetypal Welshman of Shakespeare's day are embodied in Glendower and his daughter, LADY (8) MORTIMER: a sentimental streak and a love of music. Also, various peculiarities of spelling and syntax in Glendower's speeches, as they were originally published, probably reflect a Welsh accent.

Shakespeare was clearly aware of the popular English stereotype of the Welsh as distinctly foreign, but in *Henry V* Wales is specifically included in a united Britain. Shakespeare depicted HENRY V as a king of all the British peoples, especially in the so-called 'international scene' (3.2). Here the Welsh representative is Captain FLUELLEN, who is notable for his comically powerful Welsh accent. Fluellen is a hot-tempered but honest and courageous soldier; in 5.1, when PISTOL mocks him by saying he smells of leeks—the Welsh national symbol—Fluellen forces him to eat one.

Another Welsh character appears in *The Merry Wives of Windsor,* the village clergyman and schoolmaster, Sir Hugh EVANS (3). He also has a pronounced accent and a tendency towards clichés, another allegedly Welsh characteristic. Also, he is partly responsible for a theft of horses, an episode that reflects another, less attractive English stereotype of the Welsh as inveterate thieves. In the famous 'Latin scene' of *The Merry Wives* (4.1), Evans comically drills a student in the ancient language. This perhaps reflects the playwright's own experience at STRATFORD, where he may have had a schoolmaster of Welsh ancestry, Thomas JENKINS. In any case, the creation of Evans, Glendower, Lady Mortimer, and Fluellen indicates that in the late 1590s

Shakespeare's acting company, the CHAMBERLAIN'S MEN, included one or more Welshmen.

In *Cymbeline*, a much later play, Wales is the location for most of Acts 3 and 4 of the play. It is the land of exile for BELARIUS, who has been unjustly exiled from the court of King CYMBELINE, and it is also the site of a battle between the British and an invading Roman army. In addition to being a wilderness, Wales is again a military venue, as the Romans use Milford Haven, a Welsh port, as their point of invasion. However, these features are not developed in the play, and the only specifically Welsh element in *Cymbeline* is a minor one: the pseudonym, Morgan, taken by Belarius. Since Belarius/Morgan, like Evans, is given to clichés, he may also have been intended to suggest a comic Welsh stereotype.

Welsh material crops up elsewhere in the plays as well. For instance, the fairy lore of *A Midsummer Night's Dream* probably came from Wales, perhaps through the traditions of WARWICKSHIRE, Shakespeare's home, but perhaps also through the Welsh players in the Chamberlain's Men. The *Dream* was written around the same time as *Richard II*, where matters Welsh are first found in Shakespeare. In an intriguing sidelight, it is often thought that 'Ducdame, Ducdame, Ducdame' (*As You Like It*, 2.5.51), the mysterious 'nonsense' refrain in the parody song by JAQUES (1), is a version of a phrase in Cymric, the Welsh language, that means 'Come to me', and which was used in a well-known children's game. The date of *As You Like It* is uncertain, but it is thought to have been written in the same period as *The Merry Wives of Windsor*, *1 Henry IV*, and *Henry V*.

Wales (2), Prince of See PRINCE (4); PRINCE (5); PRINCE (6).

Walkley, Thomas (active 1618–1649) London bookseller and publisher. Walkley published the first QUARTO edition of *Othello*, hiring printer Nicholas OKES. He owned two London bookstores, but little more is known of him except that he published Royalist propaganda during the civil wars.

Walley, Henry (active 1608–1655) London publisher and bookseller, co-publisher of the first edition of *Troilus and Cressida*. With Richard BONIAN, Walley published the QUARTO edition of the play in 1609. When the FIRST FOLIO edition of Shakespeare's works was produced in 1623, Bonian had died and Walley alone held the rights to *Troilus and Cressida*. Textual evidence reveals that printing of the play was delayed once begun, and scholars conclude that Walley drove a difficult bargain with the Folio publishers, led by Isaac JAGGARD. Walley enjoyed a long career; he entered the STATIONERS' COMPANY in 1608 and was elected its master, or chief officer, in 1655.

Walker (1), Henry (d. 1616) Musician in LONDON, seller of the BLACKFRIARS GATEHOUSE to Shakespeare. Walker bought the gatehouse for £100 in 1604 and sold it to Shakespeare for £140 in 1613, issuing a short-term mortgage for £80 of it. Like Shakespeare, he had owned the house as an investment and had not lived in it. He was a musician by trade—a 'Minstrel' in the language of the deed—though he also had a shop and apprentices and was a wealthy man.

Walker (2), William (1608–1680) Shakespeare's godson. Walker, the son of a prosperous cloth dealer who had served three times as bailiff, or mayor, of STRATFORD, received a cash bequest in his namesake's will. Little more is known of him, except that he too was elected bailiff, in 1649.

Walton, William (b. 1902) British composer, creator of music for the FILMS of Laurence OLIVIER. Walton composed the striking scores for *Henry V* (1944), *Hamlet* (1947), and *Richard III* (1954). Walton is best known for his orchestral works; he also composed several well-known operas, including a *Troilus and Cressida*, though it is based on CHAUCER's version of the tale, rather than Shakespeare's.

War of the Theatres Rivalry between playwrights—Ben JONSON versus John MARSTON and Thomas DEKKER—marked by satirical plays written and produced between 1599 and 1602. Also called the Poetomachia—Dekker's comical Greek term for 'combat of the poets'—the War of the Theatres involved seven plays produced by three acting companies. It is difficult to tell whether the rivalry was based on real animosity or was a publicity stunt. Jonson later remembered his hatred for Marston, but he was peacefully collaborating with him just a few years after this conflict, and by all accounts no one felt hostile towards the genial Dekker, either then or ever. And the contest certainly did generate publicity for the CHILDREN'S COMPANIES as they recovered their position in the public theatres in the early years of the 17th century.

The War of the Theatres began with Marston's *Histrio-mastix* (1599), staged by the Children of Paul's, which contained a humorous character modelled on Jonson. Though Marston may have meant no offence, Jonson replied by satirising his bombastic style in *Every Man out of His Humour* (1599), produced by Shakespeare's CHAMBERLAIN'S MEN (who were otherwise uninvolved in the fray). Marston countered by portraying Jonson as a cuckold in *Jack Drum's Entertainment* (1600), a Paul's play. Jonson's reply encompassed Dekker, Marston's fellow writer for Paul's, in *Cynthia's Revels* (1601) (he depicted himself in it as 'a creature of a most perfect and divine temper'); this work was staged by the Children of the Chapel. Marston immediately replied with an uncomplimentary

Jonson-figure in *What You Will* (1601), and Dekker and Marston together began to write another satire. Jonson learned of this, however, and rushed out *The Poetaster* (1601), in which Dekker is presented as a 'play-dresser [i.e., reviser of other people's dramas] and plagiary' and Marston as a 'poetaster and plagiary'. This time Jonson depicted himself as the Roman poet Horace (65–8 B.C.), and in Dekker and Marston's *Satiromastix* (1601), Horace is ridiculed. The battle of plays ended at this point, as the participants moved on to other work. By 1604 Marston even dedicated a play to Jonson.

Shakespeare alluded to the War of the Theatres twice in the plays he was writing at the time. In *Hamlet* the children's companies of DENMARK are said to 'berattle the common stages', with 'much to do on both sides', and 'much throwing about of brains' (2.2. 340, 350, 356). In *Twelfth Night* FESTE's remark that the word *element* is 'overworn' (3.1.60) alludes to Dekker's satire in *Satiromastix* on Jonson's use of the word.

Warburton, John (1682–1759) English antiquarian and manuscript collector. Warburton recorded his ownership of many play manuscripts, including copies of DUKE HUMPHREY (by 'Will. Shakespear') and *Henry I* (by 'Will. Shakespear and Rob. Davenport'; see HENRY I AND HENRY II). Neither manuscript survives—most of Warburton's collection was destroyed by a servant who mistook it for waste paper—but scholars doubt that either was by Shakespeare.

Warders Minor characters in *1 Henry VI*, soldiers manning the Tower of London who refuse admittance to the Duke of GLOUCESTER (4) in 1.3, citing orders from the Bishop of WINCHESTER (1). The term *warder* referred to a soldier whose duty was to act as a guard, especially at the entrance to a building or fortification.

Warkworth Castle Fortified dwelling in northern England, a setting in *1* and *2 Henry IV*. The principal home of the Percy family, this castle served as a headquarters for the rebellion against King HENRY IV led by HOTSPUR and his uncle WORCESTER. In 2.3 of *1 Henry IV* Hotspur here prepares for the forthcoming campaign and bids an affectionate farewell to his wife, LADY (10) Percy. In *2 Henry IV* the INDUCTION, in which RUMOUR tells of the contrary reports that the Earl of NORTHUMBERLAND (1) will soon receive, and 1.1, in which they arrive, are both set at Warkworth, as is 2.3, in which Northumberland is persuaded by LADY (9) Northumberland and Lady Percy to abandon the rebels' hopeless cause.

Warkworth Castle was built in the 12th century and remodelled in the 14th by the Earl of Northumberland of the play. A strategically important fort on England's northern border, Warkworth saw much warfare and was often besieged. In 1405 Henry IV, mopping up the Percy rebels, damaged the castle considerably with his artillery. Today, still owned by the Percy family, it is a picturesque ruin (though still habitable in part) that is open to the public.

Warner, William (c. 1558–1609) English author whose translation of *The Menaechmi* by PLAUTUS, the principal source for *The Comedy of Errors*, may have been known by Shakespeare. Although Warner's translation was not published until 1595, somewhat later than the presumed date of composition of Shakespeare's play, the playwright may have read it in manuscript, a common practise at that time. This speculation is strengthened by the fact that Warner's book was dedicated to Henry CAREY (2), Lord Hunsdon, the patron of the CHAMBERLAIN'S MEN, Shakespeare's theatrical company.

Wars of the Roses English dynastic wars of 1455–1485, in which are set the first four of Shakespeare's HISTORY PLAYS: *1, 2,* and *3 Henry VI* and *Richard III.* The wars were a struggle between two branches of the PLANTAGENET (1) family, the houses of YORK (1) and LANCASTER (1). Traditionally (though inaccurately), the Yorkists were thought to have used white roses as their emblem and the Lancastrians to have worn red ones.

In the mid-15th century a Lancastrian, HENRY VI, ruled England. A weak king, crowned while only an infant and heavily influenced by aristocratic cliques, Henry lost most of England's conquests in FRANCE (1) in the last phase of the HUNDRED YEARS WAR—the principal subject of *1 Henry VI.* These losses, along with evident corruption and extravagance at the royal court, resulted in recurring popular unrest. An opposition party of aristocrats arose, led by the Duke of YORK (8). In the political manoeuvring depicted in *2 Henry VI,* York gained ascendancy over the faction led by Queen MARGARET (1), and he ruled the country while the king was temporarily insane in 1453–1454 (Shakespeare does not mention this episode). York was excluded from power when Henry recovered, and he resorted to war, winning the battle of ST. ALBANS, with which *2 Henry VI* closes, in 1455.

York reclaimed power, but the rivalry continued, and the two sides resumed warfare in 1459. After a Yorkist victory in July 1460, the duke claimed the throne. However, this action produced resistance among the aristocracy, and York had to accept a compromise, as is enacted in 1.1 of *3 Henry VI:* Henry was permitted to continue ruling, though York would succeed him. Queen Margaret retaliated by raising an army; she won the battle of WAKEFIELD in December 1460, in which York was killed. However, her triumph was short-lived: she alarmed the aristocracy by claiming the right to dispossess her enemies of their estates, and she alienated the common people by permitting

her army to loot and pillage after the battle. York's son EDWARD IV assumed his father's claim to the throne, and after a bloody victory at TOWTON in March 1461 he was crowned, ending the first phase of the Wars of the Roses.

Edward ruled England with considerable success for 22 years, though his reign was interrupted in 1470 by a Lancastrian invasion, led by Margaret and the Earl of WARWICK (3), a one-time Yorkist. They placed Henry VI back on the throne for six months, but Edward recaptured the crown in 1471 after winning the battles of BARNET and TEWKESBURY, completing the second cycle of the wars. These events occupy Acts 3–5 of *3 Henry VI.*

Richard III deals with the last stage of the Wars of the Roses. Edward died in April 1483. In his will he appointed his brother Richard (see RICHARD III) as Protector, ruling for the 12-year-old PRINCE (5). However, Edward's widow, Queen ELIZABETH (2), led an attempt to displace Richard, and he responded by seizing the throne in July 1483. He probably had the Prince and his younger brother murdered, although the evidence is inconclusive. In any event, his coup spurred the last, brief campaign of the Wars of the Roses: the only surviving Lancastrian claimant to the crown, the Earl of RICHMOND, invaded England and defeated Richard at the battle of BOSWORTH FIELD. Richmond took the throne as Henry VII and established the TUDOR dynasty.

The Wars of the Roses constituted an important historical watershed, bringing feudalism to an end in England. The feudal aristocracy, exhausted by the conflict, was unable to resist the establishment of a strong, centralised monarchy by the Tudors, who, under Richmond's grand-daughter Queen ELIZABETH (1), still ruled England in Shakespeare's day. One consequence of the Tudor's consolidation of power was the development of a bias in the subsequent writing of English history. Shakespeare's principal sources, the histories by HALL (2) and HOLINSHED and Thomas MORE's biography of Richard III, are fairly reliable with respect to the chronology of the wars, but they are markedly prejudiced in favour of the winning side, depicting Richmond's predecessors, especially Richard, as particularly vicious and villainous.

Shakespeare followed his sources in this respect, but he took important liberties with their account of the wars. In general he altered history in two chief ways: he compressed the time scale during which events occurred, and he exaggerated the ambitions of the Yorkists. The compression, eliminating the long stretches when the conflict was on hold, serves to maintain a high level of dramatic excitement, but it also virtually eliminates the successful reign of King Edward and thereby overstates the extent of England's disruption and over-emphasises the importance of the Tudor 'rescue' of the country. In the plays the conflict seems both horrifying and relentless, though in fact it consisted of only four campaigns, widely scattered over 30 years, and included only one episode of civil plundering, that of Margaret's army after Wakefield, and only one strikingly bloody battle, Towton.

Furthermore, Shakespeare stresses the evil of the Duke of York's attempt to rebel against an anointed king. York is shown conspiring for many years to seize the throne, when in fact his attempted usurpation was almost impulsive. Similarly, Richard III is depicted as scheming to wear the crown at a time when he was actually an infant, and his villainy, although derived from the sources, is magnified to spectacular effect. Thus sinful human greed is presented as the cause of grievous social disruption, when the actual situation, even as reported in the biased sources, was much more complex.

Wart, Thomas Minor character in *2 Henry IV,* one of the men whom FALSTAFF recruits for the army in 3.2. Wart, who is dressed in rags, is initially rejected as being too poor a specimen of soldier. However, after two draftees offer bribes to Falstaff's assistant, BARDOLPH (1), they are released from service and Wart is taken. He is put through an incongruous marching exercise in 3.2.267–272. The episode satirises the notorious greed of 16th-century recruiters.

Warwick (1), Edward Plantagenet, Earl of Character in *Richard III.* See BOY (2).

Warwick (2), Richard Beauchamp, Earl of (1382–1439) Historical figure and character in *1 Henry VI, 2 Henry IV,* and *Henry V.* In *1 Henry VI* Warwick declares for Plantagenet (see YORK [8]) in 2.4, and in 3.1 he presents King HENRY VI with a petition in favour of Plantagenet's restoration as Duke of York. He is present but unimportant in later scenes. In *2 Henry IV* and *Henry V* we see Warwick as a younger man. In *2 Henry IV* he is an adviser to King HENRY IV. He soothes the king's melancholy and rouses him to action in 3.1, and he defends PRINCE (6) HAL in 4.5, asserting that his debauchery is instructing the young man in the ways of evil, from which he will reform himself. This passage is intended to confirm the essential nobility of the future King HENRY V. In *Henry V* Warwick speaks only one line as a member of the King's court.

The historical Warwick was much more important in the affairs of his time than the character is in the plays. As a young man, under Henry IV, he distinguished himself in the army, serving against GLENDOWER's Welsh rebellion and at the battle of SHREWSBURY. He was a highly successful general under Henry V and governed the occupied towns of Calais and ROUEN at various times. Upon the king's death, the infant Henry VI was placed in Warwick's care. In *1*

Henry VI Warwick is overshadowed by York, whom Shakespeare wished to emphasise, although the earl was actually a more successful and prominent figure. When he died, Warwick was governing occupied FRANCE (1) as regent for Henry VI.

Shakespeare confused Richard Beauchamp with Richard Neville, a later holder of the same title (see WARWICK [3]): in *2 Henry IV,* 3.1.66, Beauchamp is misnamed Neville, and in *2 Henry VI,* 1.1.117–120, episodes from his military career are claimed by Neville. It is sometimes thought that Neville was expressly intended as the Warwick of *1 Henry VI,* but, although the chronology of that play is hopelessly skewed, certain key features point to Beauchamp. Although Shakespeare was seemingly unaware of the distinction, it seems likely that Richard Beauchamp is the Warwick depicted.

Warwick (3), Richard Neville, Earl of (1428–1471) Historical figure and character in *2* and *3 Henry VI,* the chief backer of the Duke of YORK (8) and then the leader of an effort to dethrone York's son EDWARD IV after he has become King. The Earl of WARWICK (2) in *1 Henry VI* was his father-in-law, Richard Beauchamp, and Shakespeare confused the two. Early in *2 Henry VI,* Shakespeare has Neville laying claim to certain of Beauchamp's military accomplishments (1.1.118–120).

The young nobleman of *2 Henry VI* is a bold, hot-tempered soldier, unswerving in his devotion to serving the cause of right. A proud and spirited youth, Warwick is unafraid to contradict such high-ranking lords as CARDINAL (1) BEAUFORT. Like his father, the Earl of SALISBURY (2), he seeks the good of England rather than personal advancement, in contrast to the other aristocrats. York confides in the Nevilles his intention to seize the throne, claiming descent from RICHARD II, whose crown had been usurped by HENRY VI's grandfather (see YORK [1]; LANCASTER [1]). Warwick and his father agree to support York, accepting the validity of his right to rule. In Act 5 Warwick distinguishes himself as a warrior, fighting with York's forces at the opening battle of the WARS OF THE ROSES. He closes the play exulting in their success and hoping for more to come, thus anticipating the action of *3 Henry VI.*

It is in the later play that Warwick becomes a major figure in the wars. After York is murdered by Queen MARGARET (1), Warwick becomes the leading lieutenant for the Duke's sons. He boosts their spirits, encouraging Edward to claim the throne himself, and he leads them to war against Margaret. When the battle of TOWTON is all but lost, Warwick's rousing vow to revenge the death of his brother restores Yorkist morale and the day is saved.

In consequence, Edward is crowned and Warwick seems to have accomplished his goal. He goes to FRANCE (1) and negotiates a political marriage for Edward, thus securing the Yorkist position by acquiring a strong ally. However, his arrangements are peremptorily cancelled when word arrives that Edward has married an English commoner, who becomes Queen ELIZABETH (2). Warwick, furious that his plans have been dismissed and that his promises to the French king have been dishonoured, immediately allies himself with Margaret and the displaced HENRY VI. He succeeds in capturing Edward and restoring Henry to the throne, but Edward escapes and himself captures Henry. In 5.2 Warwick is mortally wounded at the battle of BARNET. He dies musing on the insignificance of his former power and influence.

The historical Warwick, known as the 'kingmaker', was indeed the chief architect of Yorkist success, and Shakespeare's account of his drive and ambition ring true. However, in his need to compress the sequence of historical events, the playwright distorted the developments behind Warwick's defection to Margaret, which in the play seems so sudden as to be almost frivolous. Shakespeare preserved the essential features of the story, but Warwick's motives were rather more complicated and humanly interested than those of the fickle figure in the play.

Relations between the kingmaker and his former protégé became strained once Edward was in power. Although Warwick disapproved of Edward's marriage, it did not occur while he was in Paris arrangeing another one; nor was it the principal cause of their split, which did not occur until years later. The two fought over foreign policy, and Warwick's opinions were increasingly ignored. Moreover, when Warwick tried to arrange a marriage between his daughter and Edward's brother GEORGE (2), the king angrily rejected the idea. In 1469, eight years after Edward's coronation, George and Warwick staged a coup. Warwick ruled for nine months in Edward's name, but the king gathered loyalist supporters and drove the usurpers from the kingdom. It was at this point that Warwick, desperate, accepted the proposition of King LEWIS (3), Louis XI of France, that he ally himself with Margaret and restore Henry to the throne. Accordingly, his other daughter, ANNE (2), was betrothed to the one-time PRINCE (4) of Wales, Margaret and Henry's son. As in the play, this alliance briefly placed Henry back on the throne before losing the battle of Barnet, where Warwick did indeed die.

Warwickshire County in England, location of STRATFORD, Shakespeare's home, and a setting in *3 Henry VI.* In 4.2 the Duke of WARWICK (3) comes to Warwickshire, his home territory, with a French army, judging his own locality to be the safest place to commence a conquest of England on behalf of the deposed King HENRY VI. One of the chief towns of Warwickshire, COVENTRY, also figures as a location in several of the

HISTORY PLAYS. In addition, in the INDUCTION to *The Taming of the Shrew,* there are numerous references and allusions to the Stratford neighbourhood. This suggests that the play may have been written shortly after Shakespeare's arrival in LONDON.

Watchmen (1) Three minor characters in *3 Henry VI,* soldiers who guard the tent of King EDWARD IV. On guard in 4.3, the Watchmen remark on Edward's insistence on courting danger when he could be housed in greater safety, but they claim pridefully that they will protect their king. WARWICK (3) and his soldiers appear and capture Edward, routing the guard instantly. The episode offers an instance of Edward's immaturity, as his bravado makes difficulties for his cause. It also provides a touch of rustic humour when the Watchmen comically fly just as they proclaim their own virtues as guards.

Watchmen (2) Minor characters in *Romeo and Juliet,* guards who patrol the streets of VERONA at night. In 5.3 the Watchmen are summoned to the tomb of JULIET (1) by the PAGE (3), who has seen his master, PARIS (2), fighting with ROMEO. They find the bodies of Paris and the two lovers and arrest the witnesses, the FRIAR (4) and BALTHASAR (2). The Watchmen represent the general population of VERONA in opposing the bloody feuding of the MONTAGUE (1) and CAPULET (1) families.

Watchmen (3) Minor characters in *Much Ado About Nothing,* the police patrol of MESSINA. In 3.3 the Watchmen prepare for their night's patrol in a comical sequence in which all of the obvious duties of watchmen are denied. For instance, when their commander, DOGBERRY, orders, 'You shall also make no noise in the streets', a Watchman replies, 'We will rather sleep than talk' (3.3.34–36), and Dogberry responds to a query about 'laying hands' on a thief with the observation, '. . . by your office you may, but I think they that touch pitch will be defiled' (3.3.55–56). It has been suggested that this passage parodies a London statute of 1595 that attempted to control nighttime activity in the city.

However, for all their foolishness, these absurd lawmen play a significant role in the drama: they overhear BORACHIO speaking of the deception he has staged as part of the plot of Don JOHN (1) against HERO and CLAUDIO (1). Although still confused, they recognise villainy, and they arrest Borachio and his companion, CONRADE, and testify against them in 4.2 and 5.1, acts that lead to the exposure of the scheme and the happy resolution of the play.

Most of the Watchmen's speeches were not specifically assigned by Shakespeare to one or another of them, and they are largely indistinguishable, though Hugh OATCAKE and George SEACOAL are said to be literate and the latter is appointed the leader of the night's patrol. Scholars speculate that Shakespeare may have been inspired to create the Watchmen by a similar group in John LYLY's play *Endimion* (c. 1588, published 1591).

Watchmen (4) Two minor characters in *Antony and Cleopatra,* soldiers in the army of Octavius CAESAR (2). Commanded by a SENTRY (2), the Watchmen guard the perimeter of Caesar's camp outside ALEXANDRIA, in 4.9. They discover the dying ENOBARBUS and bring him into the camp. These guards, designated First and Second Watchman, are alert and active soldiers, examples of the higher morale among Caesar's forces after Antony's defeat at ACTIUM, an important development in the play. Some editions follow 18th-century editorial practise and designate the Sentry and the Watchmen as First, Second, and Third Soldiers.

Watchmen (5) Several minor characters in *Coriolanus,* soldiers in the Volscian army. In 5.2 the Watchmen guard the Volscian camp when it is approached by MENENIUS. He seeks to persuade CORIOLANUS, who has deserted ROME and is fighting for the VOLSCIANS, not to attack the city. Two of the Watchmen—designated First and Second Watchman—declare that Coriolanus has banned all Roman emissaries, and they mock Menenius when he claims to be an old friend who will be welcomed by the general. When Coriolanus emerges and rejects Menenius, the Watchmen redouble their taunts as the ambassador departs. This episode provides a mildly comic way to portray the depth of Coriolanus' vengeful hatred for Rome, while reserving the protagonist for the climactic scenes that follow.

Waterson, John (active 1634) Publisher in LONDON, producer of the first edition of *The Two Noble Kinsmen.* In 1634 Waterson published *The Two Noble Kinsmen* as a work by Shakespeare and John FLETCHER (2), in a QUARTO edition (known as Q1). Waterson is known to have been a reputable publisher who handled other plays in the repertoire of the KING'S MEN; these factors support the attribution of the play to Shakespeare and Fletcher, a point that is disputed by some scholars.

Weaver Minor character in *2 Henry VI.* See SMITH (1).

Webster (1), Benjamin (1797–1882) British actor, playwright, and producer. Webster was a successful playwright and character actor, but he is most remembered for a single production from his equally successful career as a theatre-manager In 1844, in collaboration with J. R. PLANCHÉ, he staged *The Taming of the Shrew* and made history by presenting the uncut text of Shakespeare's play. The experiment was well received by the public and the use of legitimate Shake-

spearean texts eventually became the norm. Webster's great-granddaughter was Margaret WEBSTER (3).

Webster (2), John (d. 1634) English dramatist, a leading figure of JACOBEAN DRAMA. Webster is chiefly known for two plays that are generally considered the greatest Jacobean tragedies after Shakespeare's: *The White Devil* (1612) and *The Duchess of Malfi* (1614). These striking REVENGE PLAYS, which feature obsessed and passionate heroines, are still frequently performed. Webster's poetry, filled with leitmotifs and entrancing imagery, is more finely crafted than that of any dramatist of the period except Shakespeare. Only two other plays by Webster—lesser works—can be surely identified, but he may also have written *The Revenger's Tragedy* (1606), a gruesome and bizarre revenge play that ranks with *The White Devil* and *The Duchess of Malfi.* Published anonymously, it is sometimes attributed to Thomas MIDDLETON or, following a late-17th-century ascription, to Cyril Tourneur (d. 1626), a much lesser talent.

Webster (3), Margaret (1905–1972) British actress and producer, active in the United States. The daughter of two well-known actors—and the great-granddaughter of Benjamin WEBSTER (1)—Webster made her professional debut as an actress with Sybil THORNDIKE and Lewis CASSON. She subsequently toured with Ben GREET and performed at the OLD VIC THEATRE in the early 1930s. In 1936 she moved to New York and became a leading director, especially of Shakespeare. Often employing Maurice EVANS (4) as leading man, Webster mounted many noteworthy productions, including *1 Henry IV* and *Hamlet* in 1939, *Macbeth* in 1941—with Judith ANDERSON (2) as LADY (6) MACBETH—and a controversial *Othello* starring Paul ROBESON. She also lectured widely in America and supervised the Shakespearean productions at the New York World's Fair in 1939. While she popularised Shakespeare to a great extent, she was also criticised for tampering with his texts, perhaps most notoriously when she replaced the EPILOGUE of *The Tempest* with PROSPERO's famous 'revels' speech, relocated from 4.1.148–158, in her otherwise well-received production of 1945. She wrote on her experiences as a director in *Shakespeare Without Tears* (1942).

Weelkes, Thomas (c. 1575–1623) Composer of madrigals, the text to one of which was ascribed to Shakespeare in William JAGGARD's spurious anthology *The Passionate Pilgrim* (1599). 'My flocks feed not', published in Weelkes' *Madrigals to 3, 4, 5 & 6 Voices* (1597), appears as poem no. 17 in Jaggard's collection. However, since madrigalists did not usually write the lyrics to their songs, the creator of this poem remains unknown; scholars agree that it—like many of the poems in the *Pilgrim*—is definitely not Shakespearean.

Weelkes was one of the leading composers of his day, but little is known about him. He was also a noted organist, playing at Chichester Cathedral for the last two decades of his life. He published four collections of songs before 1608 but later devoted himself chiefly to church music.

Welcombe Village near STRATFORD, the site of a real estate investment of Shakespeare's and the centre of a political crisis that gripped Stratford from 1614 to 1616. Shakespeare owned property near Welcome, and he also subleased tithes to lands in the village, in partnership with Thomas GREENE (3). That is, he paid a fee for the right to collect the taxes—a percentage of the profits—on specified fields, to a man who had purchased a long-term lease on these rights from the town of Stratford.

In August 1614 a proposal was made by Arthur Mainwaring, a nobleman from Shropshire who owned a large tract of land in Welcombe, to enclose the farmlands in the area and use them to raise sheep. This idea, known as enclosure, was one of the major sources of conflict in 16th- and 17th-century England. Under the traditional medieval system, agricultural lands were owned in units no larger than a few acres and generally much smaller, organised in clusters within which a given owner's or renter's holdings were scattered randomly. This system was extremely uneconomic, for such techniques as crop rotation were impractical and no one would introduce capital improvements such as irrigation when his neighbours would benefit as much or more than he. Under enclosure, these units were grouped together in larger lots that were 'enclosed' by ditches and hedges and used for grazing sheep, whose wool was sold to the burgeoning cloth industry. Though grazing was less productive per acre, it required much less labour, and when enough acres were involved, it was extremely profitable. Its eventual widespread adoption boosted England's economy into the modern world. However, the conversion of lands from agriculture to pasturage was invariably fiercely resisted, for its immediate, local effects were negative. It raised the price of grain by reducing its supply, and it produced unemployment, for herding sheep required only a few shepherds for hundreds of acres.

In 1614 in Stratford, Mainwaring was joined by a local landowner, William COMBE (5), in promoting enclosure, against the opposition of the town of Stratford, protecting the majority of its citizens. Shakespeare's opinion was doubtless ambivalent, for as a tithe holder, he stood to gain if the overall productivity of the area rose, yet he might take immediate losses as arable land was converted to pasture. In any case he had the foresight to strike a deal with Mainwaring's agent, who guaranteed him and Greene against any such losses, thus forestalling their potential opposi-

tion. Greene, however, was the town clerk of Stratford and as such was opposed anyway. His correspondence on the matter has survived, and his continuing attempts to recruit Shakespeare to his side reflect the playwright's cool distance from the subject. In November 1614 he records a conversation in which Shakespeare assured him that Mainwaring's proposal would probably be dropped and need not be worried about.

However, Mainwaring and Combe proceeded, evicting tenant farmers from their lands and preparing ditches and hedges for sheep fields. They countered opposition with violence, Combe being particularly arrogant in his encounters with opponents. In March 1615 the WARWICKSHIRE court issued an injunction against the enclosure, and Mainwaring withdrew, but Combe, incensed, appealed the case and continued to persecute the tenant farmers, destroying their crops, seizing their livestock, beating them, and even briefly imprisoning some of them. He bought up lands and houses in an express attempt to depopulate Welcombe. The crisis dragged on for another year, before the chief justice of England ruled firmly against Combe, only refraining from punishing him because he was the sitting sheriff of Warwickshire at the time. Combe finally dropped his efforts, though he was to reinstitute the proposal several times.

Welles, Orson (1915–1985) American actor, director, and producer of stage and FILM. Welles is probably best remembered for his movies—especially his first, *Citizen Kane* (1940)—and his panic-inducing radio play *The War of the Worlds* (1938), but he was also a significant Shakespearean actor and director. He established himself as an actor playing MERCUTIO in Katherine CORNELL's *Romeo and Juliet* (1933). Working for the Depression-era Negro Theatre Project, Welles directed a controversial *Macbeth* (1936), with an all-black cast, that was set in 18th-century Haiti and featured a gigantic mask as BANQUO'S GHOST (4), a HECATE with a 12-foot bullwhip, and a band of on-stage drummers. In 1937 he and John Houseman (1902–1988)

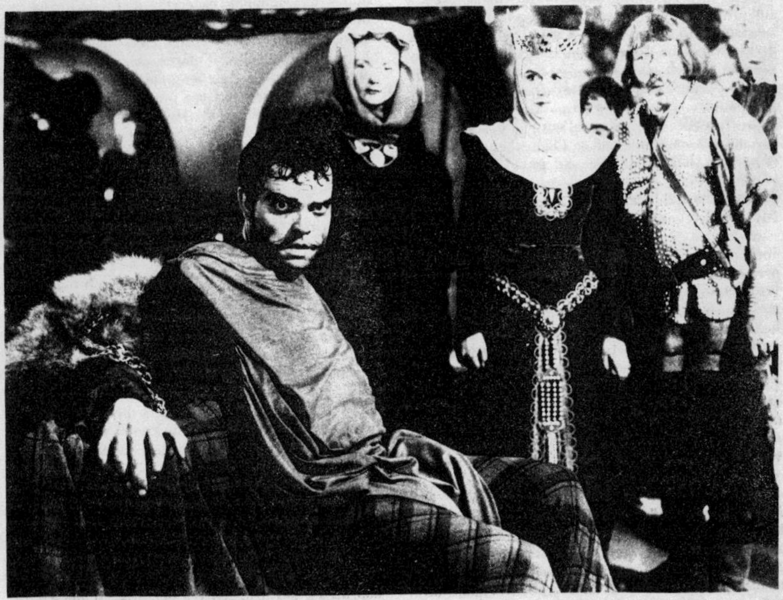

Orson Welles directed and starred in a film version of Macbeth *and another movie,* Chimes at Midnight, *that followed the career of Falstaff through three plays. Welles brought a new, expressionistic language to Shakespeare films.* (Courtesy of Culver Pictures, Inc.)

founded the Mercury Theatre—having lost their federal financing for political reasons—and their first production was a famous, politically oriented, modern-dress *Julius Caesar* (1938), directed by Welles, who also played BRUTUS (4). The Mercury Theatre successfully presented many modern and classic plays and is regarded as a milestone in Broadway history, but Welles turned his attention to films. He went to Hollywood, where he directed several masterpieces of American cinema, including *Citizen Kane, The Magnificent Ambersons* (1941), and *Lady from Shangai* (1948). In 1948 he also filmed *Macbeth,* with himself in the title role. However, these movies were not successful at the box office, and Welles went abroad to make low-budget films, including *Othello* (1952), shot in Morocco. In 1956 he returned to the Shakespearean stage a final time, to direct and star in *King Lear.* Perhaps his finest Shakespearean film was his last one, *Chimes at Midnight* (1965; known as *Falstaff* in Europe) a combination of FALSTAFF's episodes from the *Henry IV* plays, *The Merry Wives of Windsor,* and *Henry V.*

Westminster (1) Abbey London church, the location for 1.1 of *1 Henry VI* and the site of a well-known monument to Shakespeare. A masterpiece of Gothic architecture, the Abbey contains memorials to many famous English men and women, including, in the 'Poet's Corner', a monument incorporating a statue of Shakespeare by Peter SCHEEMAKERS. Westminster Abbey has been the traditional setting for British royal ceremonies since long before 1425, when the funeral of HENRY V took place there, as depicted in *1 Henry VI.*

Westminster (2), Abbot of Character in *Richard II.* See ABBOT OF WESTMINSTER.

Westminster (3) Hall Room in WESTMINSTER (4) PALACE, London, location in *Richard II.* King RICHARD II is forced to abdicate in Westminster Hall in 4.1. This massive chamber (70 by 240 feet) was already famous in Shakespeare's day as the site of many famous trials, including the historical deposition of Richard, although the king was not present on the actual occasion. Shortly after the play was written, the Earl of ESSEX (2) was sentenced to death in the same room. Its famous timber roof, still one of the grandest sights in London, was commissioned in 1394 by Richard himself, following flood damage. Ironically, the work was still in progress when Richard was deposed.

Westminster (4) Palace Complex of buildings constituting the seat of England's royal government and the setting for many scenes in Shakespeare's HISTORY PLAYS. Often, the events depicted in Westminster Palace are of a governmental nature, whether confidential, as when the Earl of SUFFOLK (3) persuades King HENRY VI to marry the future Queen MARGARET (1) in 5.5 of *1 Henry VI,* or public, as when RICHARD III is crowned in 4.2 of *Richard III.* However, since the palace was also a royal residence in the era depicted—as it was in Shakespeare's day—some of the events set within it are private. For instance, in 2.4 of *Richard III,* Queen ELIZABETH (2) prepares to flee with her young sons into the sanctuary of a church, and in 4.5 of *2 Henry IV,* PRINCE (6) HAL encounters his father, King HENRY IV, on his death-bed.

The following scenes—some of them only specified by such stage directions as 'a room in the Queen's apartments' (*Henry VIII* 3.1.1) but some more specifically—take place in Westminster Palace: *1 Henry VI* 3.1 (in PARLIAMENT HOUSE, a separate building within the palace), 5.1, 5.5; *2 Henry VI* 1.1; *3 Henry VI* 1.1 (in Parliament House), 3.2, 4.1, 4.4, 5.7; *Richard II* 4.1 (in WESTMINSTER [3] HALL); *Richard III* 1.3, 2.1, 2.4, 4.2–4; *1 Henry IV* 1.1–2, 3.2; *2 Henry IV* 3.1, 4.5, 5.2; *Henry V* 1.1–2; and *Henry VIII* 1.1–3, 2.2–3, 3.1–2, 5.1–4.

The palace at Westminster, built by William the Conqueror (ruled 1066–1087), was added to and embellished over the centuries, gradually disappearing under the rebuilding, especially after a disastrous fire in 1298. At the time of the history plays, England's monarchs knew Westminster Palace as a warren of buildings that included offices, churches, residences, and meeting halls. Another great fire in 1834 resulted in the construction of the present-day Westminster Palace, encompassing the Houses of Parliament, one of the masterpieces of 19th-century architecture designed by Charles Barry (1795–1860) and A. W. N. Pugin (1812–1852).

Westmoreland (1), Ralph Neville, Earl of (1364–1425) Historical figure and character in *1* and *2 Henry IV* and *Henry V.* In *1* and *2 Henry IV* Westmoreland is a loyal adviser to King HENRY IV, though he is rather faceless. In 1.1 of *1 Henry IV* he brings grave news of military setbacks, introducing the unrest that besets Henry's reign. He later appears briefly at the battle of SHREWSBURY. In *2 Henry IV* Westmoreland is again a solid supporter of the king, defending Henry against the rebellious noblemen's claims of mistreatment. In 4.2 he seconds Prince John of LANCASTER (3) in his fraudulent offer of a truce to the rebels at GAULTREE FOREST, and he arrests the leaders after they have unsuspectingly sent their troops home. In 4.4 he brings news of the final defeat of the rebels, closing the history of revolts against Henry.

In *Henry V* Westmoreland has a minor role and is notable only for expressing a wish for reinforcements just before the battle of AGINCOURT, provoking King HENRY V's famed 'St. Crispin's Day' speech (4.3.18–67). The historical Westmoreland was not present at Agincourt, having been placed in command of the Scottish border. His more prominent role in the *Henry IV* plays reflects his historical position more accu-

rately, though here, too, Shakespeare altered reality. Westmoreland backed BOLINGBROKE (1), later Henry IV, in his deposition of RICHARD II, although Richard had granted him his earldom. He served the new king loyally, as the plays show. It was he who actually tricked the rebel leaders at Gaultree, not Prince John, who was a youth at the time. Shakespeare de-emphasised Westmoreland in order to keep the focus on Henry's family.

Westmoreland married twice and fathered 16 children, and several of his descendants appear in Shakespeare's plays. By his first wife he was the grandfather of the WESTMORELAND (2) who appears in *3 Henry VI;* by the second he was the father of the Earl of SALISBURY (2) of *2 Henry VI* and grandfather of the Earl of WARWICK (3), known as the 'kingmaker', of *2* and *3 Henry VI.*

Westmoreland (2), Ralph Neville, Earl of (c. 1404–1484) Historical figure and minor character in *3 Henry VI,* a Lancastrian nobleman (see LANCASTER [1]). Westmoreland is one of the supporters of King HENRY VI who angrily leave the monarch's presence when he agrees to bequeath the throne to YORK (8) in 1.1. Following his sources, Shakespeare erred in assigning this Westmoreland a role in the WARS OF THE ROSES. He took no part in the conflict and is thought to have been an invalid. He was the grandson of the Earl of WESTMORELAND (1) who appears in *1* and *2 Henry IV* and *Henry V.*

Whatcott, Robert (active 1613–1616) Witness to Shakespeare's will. In 1613 Whatcott appeared as a witness for Susanna SHAKESPEARE (14) Hall in her libel suit against John LANE (1). He may have been a servant in the Hall household.

Whetstone, George (c. 1544–c. 1587) English author and playwright whose works were sources for Shakespeare. Whetstone's play *Promos and Cassandra* (1578), based on a novella by the Italian writer, CINTHIO, was a principal source for *Measure for Measure.* A story in his *The Rocke of Regard* (1576) may have inspired an aspect of *Much Ado About Nothing,* the fact that HERO is rejected at her own wedding.

Whetstone, the son of a London haberdasher, was best known for *Promos and Cassandra* and for *An Heptameron of Civil Discourse,* which describes his travels in Italy in 1580 and includes a version of the Cinthio tale the play was based on. His later works, including *A Mirror for Magistrates* (1584), which also may have had some influence on *Measure for Measure,* were more didactic and sermonising as he came under the influence of Puritanism. An adventurous man, he sailed on an abortive expedition to America in 1578, and he entered the military in 1587, serving under LEICESTER in the Low Countries, where he was killed in a duel with another English officer.

White (1), Edward (active 1577–1612) London publisher of early editions of *Titus Andronicus.* Chiefly a publisher of ballads, White joined Thomas MILLINGTON in publishing the first edition (Q1) of *Titus* in 1594, and he published Q2 (1600) and Q3 (1611) himself. The son of a Suffolk retailer, White was a successful publisher, becoming an officer of the STATIONERS' COMPANY.

White (2), William (active 1583–1615) LONDON printer. White printed plays by Shakespeare and others, as well as numerous ballads. He printed first editions of *Love's Labour's Lost* (1598, for publisher Cuthbert BURBY) and *Pericles* (1609, for Henry GOSSON [1]), and later editions of *3 Henry VI* (Q2, 1600, for Thomas MILLINGTON), *Richard II* (Q4, 1608, for Matthew LAW), *Pericles* (Q2, 1609, for Gosson), and *1 Henry IV* (Q5, 1613, for Law).

Whitefriars Theatre Seventeenth-century LONDON playhouse. The Whitefriars Theatre, named for its site on the grounds of a former priory of the Carmelite, or White Friars, was established by Michael DRAYTON and others in 1608, as a venue for the short-lived King's Revels Company (see CHILDREN'S COMPANIES). The Queen's Revels, another boys' troupe, played there from 1609 to 1613, and an adult company, LADY ELIZABETH'S MEN, in 1613–1614, after which Drayton's lease expired. PRINCE CHARLES' MEN may have played there occasionally until at least 1621, but the later history of the theatre is obscure. It was replaced in 1629 by another theatre on the same site.

Whitgift, John (c. 1530–1604) English clergyman, issuer of Shakespeare's marriage licence and later a powerful leader of the Church of England. As Bishop of Worcester, the diocese that included STRATFORD, Whitgift signed the licence authorising the marriage of Shakespeare and Anne Whateley—a clerical error for Anne HATHAWAY—without the usual three banns or formal announcements of intention to marry. This dispensation was required because Advent season was beginning, during which time banns could not be declared, and a quick marriage was desired, for Anne was pregnant. Whitgift was a famously stern churchman, and that he approved the avoidance of banns indicates that it was not a shady procedure, as some have thought.

Whitgift was shortly to occupy the most powerful position in the English church. A graduate and longtime professor and administrator of Cambridge University, Whitgift forcefully opposed a strong strain of Puritanism among the faculty and students. Queen ELIZABETH (1) was pleased with his opinion on this

subject, which was becoming increasingly divisive in the nation, and she appointed Whitgift Bishop of Worcester in 1577, and then Archbishop of Canterbury in 1583. As archbishop, he was most noted for his repressive campaign against Puritanism, but he was also a highly competent administrator and instituted valuable reforms. He became a close adviser to the Queen, and later officiated at the coronation of her successor, King JAMES I.

Whitmore, Walter Minor character in *2 Henry VI*, a sailor on a pirate ship and the executioner of the Duke of SUFFOLK (3) in 4.1. The LIEUTENANT (1) of the vessel gives Whitmore the authority to collect a ransom from Suffolk, whom the pirates have captured from another ship. Whitmore, having lost an eye in the battle for the ship, wants revenge, not ransom, and he insists, over the Lieutenant's protests, that he will kill Suffolk. When he identifies himself by name, it is as 'Water' Whitmore, the Elizabethan pronunciation of his name, and Suffolk is reminded of the prediction made by a SPIRIT in 1.4 that he would die by water. When the Lieutenant learns who Suffolk is, he denounces the Duke's political crimes and sends him with Whitmore to be beheaded. Whitmore returns with Suffolk's head and body and gives them to a released prisoner, a GENTLEMAN (1), who is to take them to London.

The Whole Contention Abbreviated title of a publication of 1619 containing BAD QUARTO texts of *2* and *3 Henry VI*. The full title of the volume is *The Whole Contention between the two Famous Houses, Lancaster and Yorke. With the Tragicall ends of the good Duke Humfrey, Richard Duke of Yorke, and King Henrie the sixt. The Whole Contention* was printed by William JAGGARD and published by Thomas PAVIER as part of the FALSE FOLIO. It consists of slightly edited earlier versions of the plays; THE CONTENTION (Q1 of *2 Henry VI*) is combined in one volume with THE TRUE TRAGEDY (Q1 of *Part 3*). *The True Tragedy* was altered only slightly by Pavier, but *The Contention* underwent many minor changes, along with the substantial addition of elaborated genealogical material, taken from the 1615 edition of John STOW's *Chronicle*.

Each of the texts in *The Whole Contention* is known as the Q3 edition of its play. For both plays, the FIRST FOLIO text is basic to all modern editions. The *Whole Contention* texts evidently had only minor influence on the composition of the Folio, except for the introduction of the new genealogical material into 2.2 of *3 Henry VI*.

Widow (1) Minor character in *The Taming of the Shrew*, the bride of HORTENSIO. The Widow first appears at the banquet in 5.2. She is unwilling to obey her new husband, although he believes he is able to control her, having watched PETRUCHIO (2) handle the shrewish KATHERINA. When the men bet on the obedience of their wives, the Widow flatly refuses Hortensio's mild request, and Katherina gives her a lengthy lecture on a wife's proper duties. The Widow has no developed personality; she serves simply as a foil for the newly obedient Katherina.

Widow (2) Capilet Character in *All's Well That Ends Well*, a landlady of FLORENCE who befriends HELENA (2) and is the mother of DIANA (1). The Widow permits Diana to make a sexual assignation with BERTRAM, Helena's runaway husband, though Helena will occupy Diana's bed. When she first appears, in 3.5, the Widow has charm as a stereotypical gossip, and she shrewdly recognises Bertram for the cad he is, but thereafter she serves merely as a pawn of the plot.

Wieland, Christoph Martin (1733–1813) German poet and translator. Wieland produced the first German translations of Shakespeare, and rendered 22 of the plays into prose between 1762 and 1766. His work inspired and was superseded by that of J. J. ESCHENBURG.

As a young man, Wieland was known for poetry that supported Pietism, a popular religious and esthetic cult of the day. He later achieved a European reputation as the creator of sophisticated, elegant, and mildly erotic verses and novels that celebrated an ideal of the Enlightenment movement, the combination of intellect and sensuality. He was regarded for a time—until the advent of GOETHE—as Germany's greatest writer. However, with the rise of Romanticism in the early 19th century, Wieland's reputation declined catastrophically, and it is only in recent years that critics have once again taken him seriously.

Wife Minor character in *2 Henry VI*, the wife of the imposter SIMPCOX. In 2.1 the pair appear before the king's hawking party near ST ALBANS. She supports her husband's false story of miraculously repaired blindness, and, when the Duke of GLOUCESTER (4) unmasks their fraud, she is condemned with her husband to be whipped through every town between St Albans and the distant village they had claimed as their home.

Wilkins, George (active 1603–1608) English author and dramatist. Wilkins was a hack writer who penned pamphlets, plays, and a novel; virtually nothing more is known of his life. As a playwright, he collaborated with John DAY, Thomas DEKKER, Samuel ROWLEY (1), and others, and some scholars attribute parts of *Timon of Athens* or *Pericles* to him, though these suggestions are very uncertain and much disputed. Wilkins also wrote a play on his own, *The Miseries of Enforced Marriage* (1607), which dealt with the same notorious murder that was the subject of A YORKSHIRE TRAGEDY. Wilkins' novel, *The Painful Adventures of Pericles Prince of Tyre*

(1608), was written to capitalise on the popularity of Shakespeare's *Pericles*. It is the principal reason for speculation that he wrote parts of the play, but the novel does not much resemble the parts of *Pericles* that can be attributed to a collaborator, so most scholars believe that Wilkins is unlikely to have had a hand in the play.

William (1) Page Character in *The Merry Wives of Windsor*, son of George PAGE (12) and MISTRESS (3) Page. William appears only in the famous 'Latin' scene (4.1), where he is quizzed by his schoolmaster, EVANS (3). Evans' Welsh accent and the confusion of an observer, Mistress QUICKLY, combine to produce a parody of the standard Latin textbook of Shakespeare's day, LILY's *Latin Grammar*. William stumbles through the interview, none too well prepared, until he is finally forced to admit, 'Forsooth, I have forgot' (4.1.-67). He is then excused from the impromptu lesson. The scene, with its bevy of double entendres and bilingual puns, was presumably intended especially for the educated audience for whom the play was written, but the episode may also reflect Shakespeare's childhood memories. He had himself learned Latin from Lily's *Grammar* at school in STRATFORD; perhaps William's name was not without sentimental significance for the playwright.

William (2) Minor character in *As You Like It*, a rustic swain whom TOUCHSTONE intimidates into abandoning his courtship of AUDREY. Like Audrey, William is a CLOWN (1), a comic caricature of a peasant as imagined by the London audience for whom he was created. He fancies he has 'a pretty wit' (5.1.28), but he is preposterously ill-spoken; the longest word he speaks is his own name, and his longest speech has only seven words. He has no substantial personality; he simply offers a humorous contrast to the courtly ways of the major characters. William's unsophisticated weakness parodies the conventions of love in his own way, as the attitudes of Touchstone and SILVIUS satirise them in others.

Williams (1), Harcourt (1880–1957) English actor and director. Williams, a successful actor who appeared mostly in modern plays—although he was the FIRST PLAYER (2) in John BARRYMORE's London presentation of *Hamlet* (1925)—was the director of the OLD VIC THEATRE from 1929 to 1934. A follower of Harley GRANVILLE-BARKER, he insisted on staging the full texts of Shakespeare's plays, with little or no scenery. He encouraged rapid speaking of Elizabethan English, both to make clear its colloquial nature in the characters' mouths and to keep the performances from flagging. In 1935 he published a memoir of his directorate, *Four Years at the Old Vic*. He resumed his acting career and returned to the Old Vic as an actor in 1946.

Williams (2), Michael Character in *Henry V*, a soldier who unknowingly disputes with King HENRY V, who is disguised as a common soldier, in 4.1. Henry finds that Williams doubts the virtue of the English invasion of France and asserts that, if Henry's cause is not righteous, the king must accept responsibility before God for the sin of unjustifiable killing committed by his men. Henry argues irrelevantly that the king cannot be held accountable for the soldiers' sins committed before the battle, and Williams concedes the point but doubts the king's reputed promise to fight to the death rather than be ransomed. The two men exchange gloves, to be worn on their hats as identification, and each agrees to challenge the other to a fight if he sees him after the forthcoming battle of AGINCOURT. However, when Henry, undisguised, sees Williams in 4.7, he does not acknowledge their prior meeting but sends the soldier on an errand. He then gives the glove that he holds to Fluellen and sends him to the same place as Williams, ensuring an encounter. When the two meet in 4.8, they prepare to fight; Henry appears and explains matters but demands a defence from Williams for having dared to abuse the monarch. Williams makes the obvious explanation—that he could not have known the king—and Henry returns him his glove, filled with money. Williams sharply rejects Fluellen's offer of a further gratuity.

This episode may be viewed in either of two lights, depending on one's interpretation of the play, which Shakespeare deliberately made ambiguous. If King Henry is seen as an epic hero, his encounter with Williams may be seen as evidence of the king's commendable ability to relate to the common soldiers of his army. The dispute in 4.1, from this point of view, offers the king a lesson in humility by displaying the virtues of forthright courage that may be found in all men, and it leads to the king's great soliloquy (4.1.236–290) in which he regrets his royalty. When the king generously rewards Williams in 4.8, he recalls the magnanimity of his youth as PRINCE (6) HAL, enacted in *1* and *2 Henry IV*. On the other hand, if the play is taken as a satire on war and politics, and Henry as a hypocritical militarist, then emphasis shifts to Williams' scepticism about the morality of Henry's war. The soldier's honest doubt is shuffled off by a sophistic evasion. The business of the gloves displays Williams as a courageous commoner who is patronised by a superior who first makes a riskless challenge and then diverts it to Fluellen, seemingly for mere entertainment. Shakespeare set up a number of such ambivalent situations in this play, and Williams, a convincing British soldier—his name suggests that he may be Welsh—contributes much to the realism of this one.

Williamson, Nicol (b. 1938) British actor and director. Williamson has been acclaimed in a number of major Shakespearean performances, most notably

perhaps as CORIOLANUS in Trevor NUNN's 1973 Royal Shakespeare Company production, as MACBETH on stage in 1974 and 1982 and on TELEVISION in 1983, and as HAMLET in London, New York, and on an American tour in 1968–1969 and in FILM in 1970. In 1982 he directed a highly successful *Othello,* with James Earl JONES (1) in the title role.

Willoughby (1), Sir Ambrose (active 1598) High official in the court of Queen ELIZABETH (1) and possibly a satirical model for MALVOLIO in *Twelfth Night.* Willoughby was the queen's chief sewer, the official in charge of the service of meals at court. In 1598 Willoughby had a dispute with Shakespeare's patron, the Earl of SOUTHAMPTON (2), that has been proposed as the source of Malvolio's famous encounter with SIR TOBY, SIR ANDREW, and FESTE in 2.3. After having chastised the earl and Sir Walter RALEIGH for their noisy midnight carousing in the queen's courtyard, Willoughby was physically accosted by Southampton but successfully drove the earl from the palace. The queen later publicly thanked Willoughby for the deed.

This incident's resemblance to the one in the play is the basis for the link between Willoughby and Malvolio that some scholars make. Others, however, point out that Elizabeth supported Willoughby very strongly and that the playwright was therefore unlikely to pillory him. (For other possible Malvolios, see FFARINGTON; HOBY (2); KNOLLYS.)

Willoughby (2) (Willobie) Henry (b. c. 1575) English poet and possibly the Mr W. H. of the SONNETS. Willoughby is believed to have been the author of the poem 'Willobie his Avisa' (1594), a long account of the attempts of various suitors, including the poet, to seduce the chaste Avisa. In an anonymous commendatory poem published with 'Willobie', Shakespeare is named as the author of *The Rape of Lucrece,* in the earliest surviving reference to him as a poet. In 'Willobie' itself, the poet, 'H. W.', tells of his conversations with his friend, the 'old player', 'W. S.', who has similarly fallen a victim to passion. Some commentators believe that Shakespeare was W. S., that the frustrating love affair of W. S. is that described in the Sonnets, and that H. W. is the Mr W. H. of Thomas THORPE's dedication to the Sonnets. Further, Avisa is sometimes held to be the 'dark lady' of the Sonnets (although it is unclear in 'Willobie' whether W. S. has loved Avisa or another woman). However, both W. S. and Avisa remain unidentified—even Willoughby is hardly known—and these speculations remain entirely unprovable. Willoughby may conceivably have known Shakespeare, however, for he was a cousin by marriage of the playwright's friend Thomas RUSSELL.

Willoughby (3), William de (d. 1409) Historical figure and minor character in *Richard II,* a supporter of BOLINGBROKE (1). In 2.1 Willoughby and Lord ROSS (2) join the Earl of NORTHUMBERLAND (1) in rebellion against King RICHARD II, agreeing that their status as aristocrats is imperiled by Richard's seizure of Bolingbroke's inheritance. In 2.3 they accompany Bolingbroke as he marches against the King.

The historical Willoughby, a prominent landowner in Lincolnshire, was descended from a knight in the army of William the Conqueror and thus had great prestige among the aristocracy. He later married the widow of the Duke of YORK (4), Joan of Kent—the successor to the DUCHESS (4) of the play—who went on to marry a third Shakespearean character, Henry le SCROOP (1).

Wilson (1), Jack (c. 1585–c. 1641) Singer and actor who may have played BALTHASAR (4) in *Much Ado About Nothing.* A stage direction in the FOLIO edition of the play (1623) refers to 'Iacke Wilson', plainly an actor who played the part—though perhaps not in the original production. Although an otherwise unknown Wilson may have been the man, Jack Wilson is known to have been an actor and singer and is thus generally favoured (but see WILSON [2]). He was the son of a travelling minstrel but was probably a lifelong resident of London himself. Little more is known of him, though he is recorded as a singer whom the city of London hired on ceremonial occasions.

Wilson (2), John (1595–1674) Noted composer, musician, and singer. Early in his career Wilson composed music for the stage, including settings for two Shakespearean songs, 'Take, o take those lips away' (*Measure for Measure,* 4.1.1–6) and 'Lawn as white as driven snow' (*The Winter's Tale,* 4.4.220–232). He may have been the 'Iacke Wilson' who played BALTHASAR (4), according to a stage direction in the FIRST FOLIO edition of *Much Ado About Nothing* (1623). Though he was too young to have originated the part, he could have taken the role in a later production (but see WILSON [1]). In 1635 he became a royal musician under King Charles I; in 1642, at the beginning of the Civil Wars, he fled with the king to Oxford, where he received a doctorate in music, becoming a professor of music in 1656. He published a collection of English songs, *Cheerful Ayres or Ballads* (c. 1660), which contains the pieces mentioned above, along with works by Robert JOHNSON (5) and others. Upon his death Wilson was buried in WESTMINSTER (1) ABBEY, a measure of his eminence.

Wilson (3), John Dover (1881–1969) English scholar. Editor of many of the plays in the New Cambridge edition of Shakespeare's plays, Dover Wilson also wrote a number of books on the playwright and his works, including *The Essential Shakespeare* (1932),

What Happens in Hamlet (1935), and *The Fortunes of Falstaff* (1943).

Wilson (4), Robert (c. 1550–c. 1600) English actor and dramatist. Wilson, associated with LEICESTER'S MEN and the QUEEN'S MEN (1), was highly respected as an actor—he was classed with the great Richard TARLTON in his ability to extemporise witty verse—and he was also noted as a playwright. He apparently retired from the stage before 1594 to concentrate exclusively on writing. He probably wrote *The Three Ladies of London* (1584), *The Three Lords and Three Ladies of London* (1590), and *The Cobbler's Prophecy* (1594), and he collaborated with others on SIR JOHN OLDCASTLE. He is also known to have written or collaborated on a number of other plays that are now lost, many of them created for the ADMIRAL'S MEN.

Winchester (1), Henry Beaufort, Bishop of (1374–1447) Historical figure and character in *1 Henry VI*, illegitimate son of John of GAUNT, older brother of the Duke of EXETER (2), and uncle of the dukes of SOMERSET (1, 3). The same historical figure appears in *2 Henry VI*, where he is known as CARDINAL (1) BEAUFORT. In *1 Henry VI*, 1.1, Winchester's feud with the Duke of GLOUCESTER (4) interrupts the funeral of HENRY V, introducing dissension as a major theme of the play. Winchester reveals depths of criminality by plotting to kidnap the infant king, HENRY VI, although this plan is not followed up; it seems to be presented solely as an indication of the bishop's character, although it may constitute a remnant inadvertently left in place after a revision. The bishop and Gloucester wrangle further, until their followers are battling in the streets. The king pleads for peace and, while Gloucester is willing, Winchester only reluctantly and hypocritically agrees to a truce.

The quarrel between YORK (8) and Somerset takes precedence in the rest of the play, and the bishop's role diminishes. In 5.1 he turns over to the papal LEGATE a bribe owed to the pope for his promotion to cardinal. This does not affect the course of the play, but it confirms Winchester's image as an unscrupulous villain.

Shakespeare depicts Winchester as a MACHIAVEL, unscrupulously ambitious and persistently at odds with 'good Duke Humphrey' of Gloucester. The historical Winchester led a 'peace party' that opposed Gloucester in the 1440s. To some extent, Winchester's stance was dictated by his rivalry with Gloucester; each aspired to power in the vacuum created by the king's extreme youth. On the other hand, Gloucester, as brother of HENRY V and a veteran of the battle of AGINCOURT, was committed to total victory in France and adamantly opposed any compromise. Winchester favoured an accommodation with the enemy to end the long and costly conflict. Shakespeare's position, which his sources and most of his contemporaries shared, was that England lost France as a result of internal dissension that counteracted English valour, which would otherwise have won out. Thus both the sources and the playwright favoured the 'hawk' Gloucester—in reality something of a monomaniac whose actions significantly hurt the English cause—over the 'dove' Winchester, probably the sounder statesman.

Winchester (2), Stephen Gardiner, Bishop of Character in *Henry VIII*. See GARDINER.

Windsor Town west of London, setting for *The Merry Wives of Windsor*, several scenes in *Richard II*, and one scene in *1 Henry IV*. In *The Merry Wives* the town is a typical English rural community in which the intrusion of a comical but cynical and exploitative outsider, FALSTAFF, is defeated by the homespun wiles of the title characters. *The Merry Wives* was written for a ceremonial occasion at the court of Queen ELIZABETH (1), a banquet in honour of new members of the the Order of the Garter. The banquet was held in London, but the formal induction ceremonies were scheduled for a later date at Windsor Castle—an occasion referred to in 5.5.56–74—and this doubtless accounts for the use of Windsor as the setting.

Modern scholars have determined that the events enacted in certain scenes of the HISTORY PLAYS actually took place in Windsor Castle, a principal headquarters for British sovereigns since the days of William the Conqueror, who began its construction; thus in many modern editions the castle is designated as the setting for scenes that are not explicitly located in the original texts. These scenes are 1.1, 2.2, 5.3, 5.4, and 5.6 of *Richard II* and 1.3 of *1 Henry IV*.

The Winter's Tale

SYNOPSIS

Act 1, Scene 1

The courtiers CAMILLO and ARCHIDAMUS speak of their respective kings, LEONTES of SICILIA and POLIXENES of BOHEMIA, who have been friends since childhood. Polixenes has been visiting Sicilia and is about to leave. The courtiers also speak of the good qualities of Leontes' young son, MAMILLIUS, who will certainly make a fine ruler.

Act 1, Scene 2

Leontes tries to persuade Polixenes to extend his visit, but he insists he must return to Bohemia. Leontes then asks Queen HERMIONE to convince him. When she does, Leontes suspects that they are lovers. He sends them away and talks with Camillo, who forcefully rejects his suspicions. Insisting that he is correct, Leontes orders Camillo to poison Polixenes. Camillo

reluctantly agrees, but instead informs Polixenes, and they leave together for Bohemia.

Act 2, Scene 1
When a LORD (16) tells Leontes of the flight of Polixenes and Camillo, the king rages about treachery. He formally accuses Hermione of adultery and treason, declaring that she is currently pregnant with Polixenes' child. She defends herself, but he sends her to prison. Although ANTIGONUS and the other lords try to dissuade the king, he insists that she is an adulteress and adds that he has sent messengers to the oracle of Apollo for confirmation of this.

Act 2, Scene 2
Antigonus' wife, PAULINA, tries to visit Hermione in prison but is only permitted to see her attendant, EMILIA (3), who reports that the queen has given birth to a daughter. Paulina resolves to take the infant to Leontes and convince him that the child is his.

Act 2, Scene 3
When Paulina brings the baby to Leontes, he is enraged. He sends her away and orders the baby killed. Antigonus pleads for the infant's life, and Leontes tells him to take the child—but only to abandon it in some wilderness, where it may or may not survive. Antigonus then leaves with the baby.

Act 3, Scene 1
CLEOMENES AND DION return from the oracle and describe its awe-inspiring appearance. They bear a proclamation answering the king's inquiry.

Act 3, Scene 2
Hermione, accompanied by Paulina, is brought to trial for adultery; she again defends herself and appeals to the oracle. Cleomenes and Dion read the oracle's judgement, which proclaims the innocence of Hermione, Polixenes, and Camillo, but Leontes refuses to believe it. Word then arrives of Mamillius' sudden death from fright at his mother's fate. Leontes interprets this event as a supernatural confirmation of the oracle and repents, but Hermione faints and must be taken away by Paulina. Just as Leontes resolves to welcome Camillo back and apologise to Polixenes, Paulina returns and reports Hermione's death. She excoriates Leontes, and he accepts her criticisms as entirely just.

Act 3, Scene 3
In stormy weather, on a remote part of the Bohemian coast, Antigonus reports a vision in which the ghost of Hermione instructed him to take the baby there and to name her PERDITA. He is attacked and driven away by a BEAR, but a SHEPHERD (2) finds the infant. He is joined by his son, the CLOWN (8), who has seen Antigonus being eaten by the bear and his ship sinking in the storm. They discover that Perdita is wrapped in rich fabrics, which contain a supply of gold.

Act 4, Scene 1
TIME appears and announces that 16 years have passed, that Leontes has shut himself off from the world in grief, and that the story continues in Bohemia. There, he tells us, we shall see Polixenes' son, FLORIZEL, and the 16-year-old Perdita, who lives as the Shepherd's daughter.

Act 4, Scene 2
Camillo wishes to return to Sicilia, but Polixenes declares that he is now too important to the government to be permitted to leave. Moreover, he wants Camillo's help in preventing Prince Florizel from embarrassing the monarchy by marrying a shepherd girl.

Act 4, Scene 3
A vagabond, AUTOLYCUS, sings merrily and brags that he is now a petty thief, although he was once a servant to Florizel. The Clown appears on his way to market to buy supplies for the upcoming shepherds' feast, and Autolycus scents prey. He lies on the ground and pretends to have been robbed; then, as the Clown helps him rise, he picks his pocket. The Clown leaves, and Autolycus decides to attend the festival, which is likely to produce further loot.

Act 4, Scene 4
Perdita reveals her uneasiness at being courted by Florizel, for she knows that his father, the king, will oppose the match. Florizel insists he will marry her even if he has to abandon his royal status. The Shepherd and the Clown arrive for the festival, along with a group including the shepherd girls MOPSA and DORCAS, and the disguised King Polixenes and Camillo. Perdita, as hostess, distributes flowers among the guests. Mopsa and Dorcas lead a country dance, and Autolycus appears as a wandering peddler. Mopsa and Dorcas flirt with the Clown, who buys them presents, while Autolycus entertains them with SONGS; they all leave together, to continue singing and trading. At this point Polixenes reveals himself and demands that Florizel renounce Perdita. Threatening her and the Shepherd with death if she sees the prince again, he departs in a rage. The frightened Shepherd flees, and Perdita is in despair, but Florizel declares that he will not leave her. Camillo proposes that the couple should go to Sicilia, where they will be welcomed as emissaries of King Polixenes. Once there, they may eventually gain Polixenes' forgiveness. Autolycus returns, gloating over the purses he has stolen while selling his goods. Camillo makes him change clothes with Florizel, providing the prince with a disguise, and Perdita dresses as a young man. In an aside Camillo reveals that he intends to inform the king of the couple's flight and, in pursuit of them, get to Sicilia himself. When they leave, Autolycus, who has realised what is going on, plots how to profit from it. He then overhears the Shepherd and Clown planning to ex-

plain to the king that Perdita is not actually their relative, but a foundling. They have proof in the rich fabrics Perdita was found in, years before. Autolycus emerges and promises to take them to the king, for money. Privately, he plans to take them to Florizel and accept the prince's reward for keeping them from the king.

Act 5, Scene 1
In Sicilia, Paulina insists that King Leontes should never remarry until he encounters Hermione's equal, and he agrees not to marry without Paulina's approval. Florizel and Perdita arrive, asserting that they are married. Leontes is delighted to renew relations with the son of his one-time victim, but then word arrives that Polixenes himself has come to Sicilia, to arrest his son for eloping with a shepherd's daughter. Florizel confesses that he and Perdita are not married, but he pleads with Leontes to defend their love to Polixenes, and Leontes agrees, being greatly attracted by Perdita.

Act 5, Scene 2
Autolycus hears from a GENTLEMAN (13) and his friends that the king's missing daughter has been found, as the papers among the Shepherd's bundle of fabrics attest. The Third Gentleman describes the joy and reconciliation among the kings and their children, who are now considered engaged. He adds that the royal party has gone to Paulina's home to view a statue of Hermione. They go off to see it also, leaving Autolycus to bemoan his bad luck: he had brought the Shepherd and Clown to Florizel's ship, whereby they had come to Sicilia with their extraordinary evidence, and yet he cannot profit from it. When the Shepherd and Clown appear, dressed in new clothes and full of comical pretensions to gentlemanly status, Autolycus flatters them abjectly.

Act 5, Scene 3
Leontes, Polixenes, Florizel, Perdita, and Camillo all accompany Paulina to see her sculpture. They marvel at its lifelike qualities, and Leontes regrets again his injustice to Hermione herself. Paulina asserts that she can make them marvel further; she tells the statue to move, and it walks down off its pedestal and takes Leontes by the hand. She then explains that the statue is Hermione herself, alive all these years but awaiting the proper moment for her return. Hermione confirms this account, identifying herself to Perdita. The king, ecstatic at being reunited with his wife, and conscious that Florizel and Perdita are soon to marry, insists that Paulina and Camillo should also wed. The three couples withdraw to savour their happiness.

COMMENTARY

With *The Winter's Tale,* Shakespeare achieved his first great success in a new genre, the ROMANCES. After flawed endeavours in *Pericles* and *Cymbeline,* the playwright found a way to integrate the various elements of romance literature—the exotic and magical mingled with stereotypical characters and situations—with his own strengths as a realistic playwright. *The Winter's Tale* combines the grim psychopathology of Shakespearean TRAGEDY with the visionary optimism of his earlier COMEDY. It is a play with its own distinctive moral tone, balancing the divine and the human.

The most obvious way in which this conjunction is effected is structural; the play falls neatly into two halves, with the hinge at 3.3, the first scene set in Bohemia. The first half is a tragedy centred on the madness of King Leontes, whose jealousy resembles OTHELLO's and appears to have the same result, the death of his wife. The second half, however, is a traditional romantic comedy of young love triumphant and old love restored, complete with a PROLOGUE (1)—the address by Time in 4.1—and a conventional happy ending in multiple marriages. The two halves of the play present a striking opposition between the sins of the powerful and elderly and the natural goodness of youth, but the two halves also offer another, more significant contrast. The tragic first half depends for its resolution on a supernatural phenomenon, the message from the oracle, while the second relies chiefly on the fine qualities of its young lovers to carry things through to the happy conclusion. While humanity is ultimately dependent on providence—a theme that pervades the romances—here divine intervention serves chiefly to enable human virtue to exercise itself and triumph over vice.

Although Leontes' madness is cured only by Apollo, Camillo, Paulina, Hermione, and Antigonus all oppose it, and the forthright dignity of Hermione is never sullied by the abuse she undergoes. Moreover, the human opposition is much more prominent than the brief intercession of the god. Similarly, the healing process that follows remains in the characters' hands; it is accomplished through Paulina's delaying tactics, the Shepherd's kindness, Camillo's craftiness, and Florizel and Perdita's exemplary courage and devotion. In Act 4 love, charm, and humour—abetted by luck and the plotting of the wily Camillo—triumph over the injustice of Polixenes (who here re-creates in a milder key the tyranny of Leontes). The human component in the triumph of good—almost entirely absent in *Pericles* and but fitfully brought to bear in *Cymbeline*—is here given an importance that permits us to identify much more fully with the process.

Providence, however, is by no means ignored. The play is studded with overt references to the gods. Hermione's embattled confidence that 'powers divine / Behold our human actions' (3.2.28–29) is particularly striking, but it is supported by many other instances. Leontes vows daily chapel visits in 3.2.238–243, Florizel cites the love stories of the gods in 4.4.25–31, and Perdita refers to the Proserpina myth and

mythological flower lore in 4.4.116–127. Paulina's mystifications as she reveals the survival of Hermione create an atmosphere of spirituality and magic in an entirely secular scene. Although theophany, or the actual appearance of a god, is avoided—in contrast to the two earlier romances (see DIANA [2], JUPITER)—the descriptions of the 'ceremonious, solemn and unearthly' rituals of Apollo (3.1.7) and 'the ear-deaf'ning voice o' th' Oracle, / Kin to Jove's thunder' (3.1.9–10) have a similar effect. The dramatic intensity of religious experience is evoked, and we are forcefully reminded of humanity's impotence before the divine.

Moreover, although the play's world is pre-Christian, some distinctly Christian ideas are alluded to, notably grace and redemption through suffering. Perdita and Hermione are associated with the words 'grace' and 'gracious' (e.g., in 1.2.233, 2.3.29, 4.1.24, and 4.4.8), as is the oracle itself (in 3.1.22). As the play ends, Hermione invokes a consummate blessing: 'You gods, look down, / And from your sacred vials pour your graces' (5.3.121–122). Leontes' story is a virtual parable of sin redeemed. He blasphemes his saintly wife and the divine oracle, and he is punished by the death of his son and (he believes) his wife. After Leontes spends years in 'saint-like sorrow' (5.1.2), Paulina (whose name is suggestive of Christianity's great preacher) effects the seemingly miraculous return of Hermione, which takes place in a 'chapel' (5.3.86). Not for nothing does Paulina assert, 'It is requir'd / You do awake your faith' (5.3.94–95). Of course, Hermione's apparent resurrection has obvious Christian overtones, and it becomes the central focus of the play's final scene, taking precedence over the more traditional conclusion of a comedy in marriage rites (though these are referred to).

Accompanying these expressly religious motifs is an implicitly sacred theme, a subtle emphasis on the cycles of nature. At the broadest level, the play is about the basic pattern of life and growth. Polixenes remembers when he and Leontes 'as twinn'd lambs did frisk i' th' sun / And bleat the one at th' other' (1.2.67–68). Later, when their dire adult drama of hatred and death is replaced by the pastoral comedy of the shepherds' festival, a cycle has been completed. The festival itself, celebrating the annual wool harvest, is an ancient marking of the passage of the seasons. (Such rustic festivals were still common in pre-industrial England, and Shakespeare could be sure that his audience would be familiar with them and at least aware of the pre-Christian religious sentiment behind them.) Perdita's enumeration of the different seasonal flowers is another potent evocation of nature's cycles. Most compelling of all is her re-enactment of the passage from winter to spring—the original resurrection—when she wishes she had spring flowers for Florizel, 'to strew him o'er and o'er!' He exclaims, 'What, like a corpse?' and she replies, 'No, like a bank, for love to lie and play on: / Not like a corpse; or if—not to be buried, / But quick, and in mine arms' (4.4.129–132). Such references point to our primitive awareness of nature as the source of religious awe.

However, the cycle of the seasons is a natural, not a supernatural phenomenon, and its celebration is a human one. In line with this the play's religious allusions and motifs are never permitted to overshadow the central theme, the power of human virtue. The role of the oracle is critical, but it is the main characters who complete the task and achieve happiness through their virtue. It is not Paulina's magic but her foresight that leads to the 'revival' of Hermione; human intervention, not divine, produces the outcome. That Paulina's scheme seems singularly harebrained to the rational observer is irrelevant; romances are supposed to be illogical. It is only important that a happy ending of reconciliation and love has been reached, without the need for a *deus ex machina*. Given a single assist from Apollo's oracle, the essential good in humanity defeats life's potential for disorder and unhappiness. Leontes hopes Paulina's magic will prove as 'lawful as eating' (5.3.111) and—because it is not magic after all, let alone black magic—it does. The moral drive of ordinary people is what powers *The Winter's Tale*.

Though Leontes certainly lacks such drive, he is nonetheless the central figure in the play's scheme. His sin sparks the action, and his consciousness of sin is necessary to its conclusion. That the king comes to recognise his susceptibility to error reflects Shakespeare's abiding concern for the responsibilities of rulers. Like such differing characters as RICHARD II, HENRY IV, CYMBELINE, and PROSPERO, Leontes learns about himself through the exercise of power. Especially in the romances, the lesson is that the most valuable human capacity is the capacity for mercy, for, more than justice, mercy acknowledges human equality before the divine. Like the medieval MORALITY PLAY, centred on God's mercy to humankind, Shakespeare's late works insist that the relationship between a secular ruler and subject must follow the same pattern.

Leontes moves from sin to remorse and finally finds forgiveness in the pastoral world of love represented by Perdita and Florizel. The most important moral lesson of the play is the power of love. Love is elaborately glorified and briefly threatened in 4.4—the longest scene in Shakespeare—where the pleasures of country life, a traditional romantic motif, are associated with the deep affection shared by Florizel and Perdita. As we have seen, connections are drawn to the divine, and Perdita is strongly linked to ancient emblems of fertility. The lovers acknowledge their sexuality, but recognise the spiritual side as more important. Perdita notes that love can take a 'false way' (4.4.151), and Florizel insists that his desire does not

'Burn hotter than my faith' (4.4.35). In the crisis of Polixenes' wrath against Perdita, Florizel declares that if his faithful love fails, 'let nature crush the sides o' th' earth together, / And mar the seeds within!' (4.4.480–481). The tragedy of the first half of the play results from jealousy, a gross distortion of sexual affection; the love of the second half contrasts in its purity.

The world of the lovers is a blessed one, as the play's transition from Sicilia to Bohemia makes clear, even before the powerful charm of 4.4 is exercised. In a passage that several commentators have pointed to as the pivotal moment of the play, the Shepherd, having just found Perdita and heard from the Clown of the death of Antigonus, says to his son, 'Now bless thyself: thou met'st with things dying, I with things new-born' (3.3.112–113). The old world of Leontes' despotic madness is passing away, and a new dispensation has begun. The Shepherd appreciatively declares, ' 'Tis a lucky day, boy, and we'll do good deeds on 't' (3.3.135–136). The contrast with Leontes' despairing plea, 'Come, and lead me / To these sorrows' (3.2. 242–243)—spoken just moments before—could hardly be greater. A new world has been introduced, and the shepherds' festival is to be at its centre.

Autolycus, his victim the Clown, and the shepherdesses Mopsa and Dorcas, all contribute to a delightful slice of English rustic life, viewed idealistically but not entirely unrealistically. Like the Forest of ARDEN (1) and the GLOUCESTERSHIRE of *2Henry IV*, Shakespeare's Bohemia evokes nostalgia for the solid virtues of country life, and the sense of community of that world is part of the moral regeneration of the second half.

It is interesting to note the care Shakespeare took to emphasise the importance of the human element in his play by altering the story that he found in his source, *Pandosto.* In the fashion typical of 16th-century romances, *Pandosto* is full of events and schemes that are not just improbable but absolutely impossible; credibility is not an issue, any more than in a fairy tale. Shakespeare, however, changed such features enough to create a plausible tale (if only just barely to our modern sceptical minds), a tale shot through with the fabric of real life. For example, we are prepared for Mamillius' death with reports of his illness, whereas in *Pandosto* the son of the unjustly accused queen simply drops dead of dismay. In the book the infant is abandoned in an open boat at sea; her survival—let alone her arrival in the homeland of the Polixenes figure—is entirely a whim of fate. Similarly, when the aggrieved lovers—the equivalents of Perdita and Florizel—flee the king, they simply wander about, ending up in the woman's homeland purely by chance. In Shakespeare, chance is eliminated in favour of human plans; it is Antigonus who brings the infant to Bohemia and Camillo who directs the couple to Sicilia. Another telling difference is in the fate of the Leontes figure. In *Pandosto* an angry Apollo strikes him dead, but, as we have seen, Shakespeare keeps the god at a distance and permits Leontes to survive to regret his deed.

The triumph of good in *The Winter's Tale* is accomplished only with grave difficulty, and the world of the play is shrouded with losses. The 'things dying' encountered by the Clown in 3.3 are human beings, the Mariner and Antigonus, both faultless except for their association with Leontes' sin. Their deaths seem gratuitous, but as agents of the king's wrath they embody the evils of the play's first half, and those evils must be done away with. Even more shocking is the death of the utterly innocent Mamillius—surely the greatest cost of Leontes' madness. Shakespeare here insists on the seriousness of sin. Other serious consequences include Paulina's widowhood and Camillo's exile (both presumably eased by their marriage at the conclusion) and the irretrievable loss of 16 potentially happy years for Leontes and Hermione. For all its joy, the final scene does not restore the unsullied world of the play's opening. The observation of wrinkles on the Hermione statue acknowledges that. The possibility of happiness is limited by evil and its consequences.

Shakespeare's picture of a moral world in *The Winter's Tale* is not, of course, a dry dissertation on faith and good works but rather an entertainment. The very title insists on the play's intention to entertain. Although the article *the* suggests a tale as harsh as the season, in Shakespeare's day the title also conjured up the festive Christmas season, for the connection of tale-telling to celebration was much stronger then than now. Both connotations are supported when the title is alluded to in the play: Mamillius announces 'A sad tale's best for winter' (2.1.25), but he does so in play with his loving mother, and the telling of his tale is plainly fun. The play as a whole also fulfils both interpretations of its title: the cold and dark of winter dominate the the tragedy of the first half, and the warmth and light of holiday festivities suffuse the comedy that follows.

Referring to the play's title in the dialogue is one of several ways in which Shakespeare insists on the artificiality of his romance. Allusions to the artfulness of the story are scattered throughout the play: Hermione, for example, compares her plight to a drama, 'devis'd / And play'd to take spectators' (3.2.36–37); dressed for the festival, Perdita muses, 'Methinks I play as I have seen them do / In Whitsun pastorals' (4.4.133–134); and the Third Gentleman speaks of news that 'is so like an old tale that the verity of it is in strong suspicion' (5.2.27–29). The naïveté of Mopsa, who declares, 'I love a ballad in print . . . for then we are sure they are true' (4.4.261–262), is a playful jab at the willing self-deception of romantic literature's audience. Moreover, there are several highly theatrical episodes set within the play: Hermione's trial, Time's prologue, the shepherds' festival,

and Paulina's dramatic unveiling of the supposed statue, at which Leontes declares, rightly, 'We are mock'd with art' (5.3.68). The very structure of the play reinforces the point, as tragedy changes abruptly to comedy. In stressing the obvious, that *The Winter's Tale* is an artifact and not real life, Shakespeare adds another layer to the basic theme of the play. The very play that points out the need for goodness in human endeavours is itself a human endeavour. Art joins with virtue in challenging the threat to happiness presented by social and psychological disarray. Art, and *The Winter's Tale* in particular, orders human affairs so that we can see how they resist destruction, even the natural decay that comes with time.

SOURCES OF THE PLAY

Shakespeare's main source for *The Winter's Tale* was a prose romance, *Pandosto* (1588) by Robert GREENE (2). The play follows *Pandosto*'s plot fairly closely and Greene's language is reproduced almost verbatim in some passages, but there is much that Shakespeare invented. Autolycus, for instance, was derived from a colourless character, and the shepherds' festival in 4.4 was sparked by a mere hint in *Pandosto.* Most significantly, Shakespeare deviated from Greene's plot in two important respects. In *Pandosto* Hermione's counterpart dies and Pandosto (Leontes) commits suicide. Shakespeare's spirit of reconciliation at the end is not paralleled in Greene's work.

Two passages probably owe their genesis to specific models. Polixenes' argument justifying art in 4.4.79–103 resembles a similar passage in PUTTENHAM's *Arte of English Poesie* (1589). Autolycus' descriptions of torture in 4.4.773–793 were adapted from a tale in Giovanni BOCCACIO's *Decameron* (1353), which Shakespeare may have read in the original Italian or in a French translation, perhaps that of Antoine LE MAÇON (1545). The same tale was the source for *Cymbeline,* written shortly before.

Other minor sources, reflected in various references and word choices, include OVID's *The Metamorphoses* (an old favourite of the playwright), other stories by Greene, passages from *The Knight of the Burning Pestle* by Francis BEAUMONT (2), and possibly two stories, themselves based on *Pandosto,* by a very minor writer, Francis Sabie (active 1595). Most of the names in the play were taken from PLUTARCH's *Lives,* another favourite source.

TEXT OF THE PLAY

The Winter's Tale was probably written in 1610 or early 1611. It must have been written by May 1611, when a performance is recorded, but how much earlier it was composed cannot be precisely determined. Stylistically, it is unquestionably among the late plays, and its greater mastery of the romance genre suggests that it followed *Cymbeline* (1608–1610). Some scholars believe that Shakespeare's mention of a royal performance by the play's dancing satyrs in 4.4.337–338 is a sly reference to the presentation of Ben JONSON's *Masque of Oberon*—which has a similar scene—at the court of King JAMES I on January 1, 1611. If so, then the play may have been begun in late 1610 and completed early in 1611, in time to be staged in May. Alternatively, the play could have been completed in 1610, with the reference to *Oberon* added in the course of early performances.

The play was not published in Shakespeare's lifetime but appeared in the FIRST FOLIO (1623). It was apparently printed from a transcript of Shakespeare's FOUL PAPERS (or possibly of a PROMPT-BOOK) by Ralph CRANE, a professional copyist whose peculiar punctuation and other idiosyncracies can be recognised in the printed text.

THEATRICAL HISTORY OF THE PLAY

The earliest known performance of *The Winter's Tale* was at the GLOBE THEATRE on May 15, 1611, as recorded by Simon FORMAN. The play apparently was popular, for it was performed at the courts of Kings James I and Charles I at least seven times; in 1613 it was one of the plays put on by the KING'S MEN for the wedding festivities of Princess ELIZABETH (3). However, there is no record of a 17th-century performance after 1640 (though the play inspired a popular ballad, published in 1664). The next recorded production, in 1741, was advertised as the first in a century.

The 18th century saw a number of adaptations of the play that excluded or diminished Leontes and Hermione and focussed on the love story of Act 4. Among the best known was *The Sheep-Shearing: or, Florizel and Perdita* (1754) by McNamara MORGAN (2). In 1761, this was produced as an operetta with music by Thomas ARNE. Also well known was David GARRICK's *The Winter's Tale* (1756), with Garrick as Leontes and Hannah PRITCHARD as Hermione (though these parts were reduced to a few lines each). Susannah CIBBER (2) played Perdita, the central role, and Richard YATES (2) played Autolycus, whose part was greatly expanded in this and other adaptations. Garrick's version remained popular throughout the century, though Shakespeare's original text (except for some minor alterations by Thomas HULL) was staged in 1771.

In the 19th century *The Winter's Tale* was staged with spectacular sets and lavish costumes. John Philip KEMBLE (3) produced the play in 1811. His sister Sarah SIDDONS, who had played Hermione in a staging of Garrick's version, finally took on Shakespeare's much greater part in her final season. William Charles MACREADY produced the play in 1837, and Samuel PHELPS followed in 1845, using a text very close to the original. Perhaps the most memorable *Winter's Tale* of the century was that of Charles KEAN (1) in 1856. His elaborate sets and costumes, intended to reproduce an-

cient Sicily and Bithynia (see BOHEMIA) with archaeological exactitude, were accompanied by a lengthy set of programme notes. This production was both immensely popular and widely ridiculed, and a satirical burlesque, *Florizel and Perdita* by William Brough (1826–1870), enjoyed a successful run in a rival theatre. In Kean's play, Ellen TERRY (1), aged eight, spoke her first lines from a stage, as Mamillius. In another noteworthy production, in 1887, Mary ANDERSON (2) played both Hermione and Perdita, with Johnston FORBES-ROBERTSON as Leontes.

The Winter's Tale has been less popular in the 20th century, though there have been a number of notable stagings, beginning with Beerbohm TREE's 1906 effort. Still in the 19th-century vein, it starred Ellen Terry as Hermione, 50 years after her Mamillius. Harley GRANVILLE-BARKER's 1912 production featured a formally stylised, almost bare stage that scandalised traditionalists. Robert ATKINS has produced the play twice, in 1937 and 1950. The most important 20th-century production to date is probably that of Peter BROOK (2) in 1951, starring John GIELGUD as Leontes. The play was produced as a FILM three times (all silent) before 1915, but only once since, a 1960 version starring Laurence Harvey (1928–1973). It has been made for TELEVISION twice, in Great Britain (1962) and the United States (1980).

Wise, Andrew (active 1580–1603) London publisher and bookseller. Wise published five of Shakespeare's plays. He produced the first three editions of *Richard III* (1597, 1598, 1602) and *Richard II* (1597, 1597, 1598), and the first two of *1 Henry IV* (1598, 1599). He sold the rights to these plays to Matthew LAW in 1603. In partnership with William ASPLEY he also published the first editions of *2 Henry IV* and *Much Ado About Nothing* (both 1600). Aspley alone held these rights when the FIRST FOLIO was published in 1623, and Wise may have been dead by that date. After nine years of apprenticeship, Wise became a member of the STATIONERS' COMPANY in 1589, but little more is known of him.

Witches Group of characters in *Macbeth,* supernatural beings who encourage MACBETH in his evil inclinations. In 1.1 three Witches appear in the thunder and lightning of a storm; they say that they will meet again to encounter Macbeth. In 1.3 they boast of their evil deeds before they accost Macbeth and BANQUO. They greet the former with titles he does not possess: Thane of CAWDOR and 'King hereafter' (1.3.50)—though we already know that Macbeth has been named Thane of Cawdor—and they assure Banquo that he shall not be a king but that his descendants shall. After they make these puzzling remarks, they disappear. When Macbeth and LADY (6) MACBETH learn that he is in fact Thane of Cawdor and the Witches' prophecy is corroborated, their ambition is sparked to murder King DUNCAN so that Macbeth can rule SCOTLAND. Then, once he is king, Macbeth worries over the Witches' pronouncement that Banquo's heirs would replace his own, and he murders him, as well. Thus, the Witches inspire the central action of the play.

In 3.5 we see the three Witches with a more powerful spirit, HECATE, who is accompanied by several more witches. (However, most scholars believe that this scene was not written by Shakespeare, and that *Macbeth*'s Witches were originally only three in number.) In 4.1 the Witches concoct a magical brew in a cauldron. They are preparing for another visit from Macbeth, who wishes to learn what he must do to assure his safety now that he is king. They summon the APPARITIONS, whose predictions seem to promise safety but actually foretell his destruction. Finally, in a passage that may be a non-Shakespearean interpolation, the Witches perform a ritual dance, after which they vanish.

Though their appearances are brief, the Witches have an important function in *Macbeth.* The play opens with their grim and stormy meeting, and this contributes greatly to its pervasive tone of mysterious evil. Moreover, they offer another important theme of the play, the psychology of evil. The Witches are an enactment of the irrational. The supernatural world is terrifying because it is beyond human control, and in the play it is therefore symbolic of the unpredictable force of human motivation. At their first appearance, the Witches state an ambiguity that rules the play until its close: 'Fair is foul, and foul is fair:' (1.1.11). Their deceptive pictures of the future—both in their initial predictions of Macbeth's rise, and in the prophecies of the Apparitions—encourage in Macbeth and Lady Macbeth a false sense of what is desirable or even possible. The magic of the Witches is thus an image of human moral disruption. Through their own uncertain nature, they demonstrate—and promote—the disruption in the world of the play. When Macbeth meets them a second time, he describes their capacity for disorder: they 'untie the winds, and let them fight / Against the Churches . . . palaces and pyramids, do slope / Their heads to their foundations . . . Even till destruction sicken' (4.1.52–60). They declare that their activity comprises 'A deed without a name' (4.1.49). Their world is without definition; similarly, Macbeth's disordered sense of the world comes to encompass the assumption that 'Life's . . . a tale / Told by an idiot, full of sound and fury, / Signifying nothing' (5.5.24–28).

Many people in Shakespeare's day believed in the reality of the supernatural world, but at the same time, a recognition that many folk beliefs were merely superstitions had arisen as well. Shakespeare's opinion on the subject cannot be determined, for his handling of the Witches is ambiguous. Banquo asks them,

'Are ye fantastical, or that indeed which outwardly ye show?' (1.3.53–54). After they leave, he wonders if he and Macbeth have 'eaten on the insane root' (1.3.84) and have simply imagined them. Their nature is never clearly stated. Moreover, the extent to which they have powers other than those of persuasion is also uncertain, which perhaps reflects—or exploits—the generally uncertain sense of such things in the playwright's original audiences. Shakespeare may have shared his audiences' ambivalence as to the supernatural, or he may simply have played on it to devise a dramatic grouping of characters. Despite a modern disbelief in the supernatural, we can respond to its dramatic use in *Macbeth,* and find in it a symbol of obscure regions of the human psyche. In this light, the Witches can be thought of as manifestations of Macbeth's ambition and guilt. That Banquo also sees them and Lady Macbeth accepts their reality does not argue against such an interpretation of Shakespeare's intentions; it merely points up the ambivalence of 17th-century attitudes towards the supernatural (see also GHOST [4]).

It is interesting to note that Shakespeare altered the nature of the Witches considerably when he took them from his source, HOLINSHED's *Chronicles.* There, the beings who appear to Macbeth are described as 'nymphs or fairies' who could read the future through magic. A number of references connect them with the three Fates, ancient goddesses who are figures of dignity and grandeur, quite unlike the hags of British folklore. Nymphs and female fairies were traditionally beautiful, but the Witches of *Macbeth* are 'So wither'd and so wild in their attire, / That [they] look not like th'inhabitants o'th'earth' (1.3.40–41). Scholars have surmised that Shakespeare replaced Holinshed's classical spirits with his own, earthier creatures in light of King JAMES I's well-known interest in contemporary witchcraft. However, the traditionally horrifying creatures of folklore are entirely appropriate to the association in *Macbeth* of these beings with the potential evil in humankind.

Within Character in *Henry VIII.* See ONE (3) WITHIN.

Woffington, Peg (Margaret) (1714–1760) English actress. Born in Ireland, Woffington was a child actress who went on to become the leading comedienne of her day. She was famous for a male part, the hero of a popular contemporary comedy that she repeatedly revived to great enthusiasm, but she also played most of Shakespeare's comic heroines, including PORTIA (1), ROSALIND, VIOLA, and HELENA (2). In addition, she took some non-comic parts, such as CONSTANCE in *King John* and PORTIA (2) in *Julius Caesar.* She was David GARRICK's mistress for a number of years and had many other lovers, in a notorious life that still enthralled the public a century later, when it was the subject of a popular novel of 1853 (*Peg Woffington* by Charles Reade [1814–1884]). She became ill in 1757, during her last performance (as Rosalind), and never recovered.

Wolfit, Donald (1902–1968) British actor and director. Wolfit's long career was spent chiefly as a performer and director of Shakespeare's plays. He made his debut in 1920 as BIONDELLO and in 1929 joined the OLD VIC THEATRE company, with whom he played many major parts, including HAMLET, KING (5) CLAUDIUS, and OTHELLO. He played ANTONY in Theodore KOMISARJEVSKY's 1936 production of *Antony and Cleopatra.* In 1937 he formed a touring company and travelled in Canada and the British provinces, performing mostly Shakespeare and other 16th- and 17th-century English dramas. In 1960 he toured around the world, giving recitals of famous Shakespearean passages.

Wolsey, Thomas Cardinal (c. 1475–1530) Historical figure and character in *Henry VIII,* the overpowerful chief adviser to King HENRY VIII. Wolsey is the villain of the first half of the play. He sends his enemy BUCKINGHAM (1) to execution by buying the perjured testimony of the SURVEYOR, and then, to further his foreign policy aims, he encourages the king to divorce Queen KATHERINE. Moreover, he opposes the king's marriage to the saintly ANNE (1) BULLEN. His arrogance and pride are vividly presented in such vignettes as his vicious rebuff of Buckingham in 1.1 and his later disdain for a good man he is said to have driven mad: 'He was a fool, / For he would needs be virtuous' (2.2.131–132). However, when his evils are uncovered and he is brought low, Wolsey comes to realise that his life has been wasted in the pursuit of wealth and power. He reflects that now, removed from politics and its temptations, he can rejoice in a 'still and quiet conscience' (3.2.380). Further, we learn from GRIFFITH's touching description that on his death-bed, the cardinal has 'found the blessedness of being little' (4.2.66) and made his peace with God. Good has arisen from evil, with right balancing wrong in a spiritual sense—an important theme of the play.

Wolsey's evils contribute strongly to several of the play's other themes. His victims are good people and offer important images of forgiveness and forbearance. In the play's opposition of justice and injustice, Wolsey exemplifies the latter. He also represents Catholicism, as understood by the Protestant England of Shakespeare's day. Greedy, proud, and corrupt, he is allied with ROME, in the person of Cardinal CAMPEIUS, against the virtuous—and Protestant—Anne Bullen. Perhaps most significant, early in the play the role of King Henry is defined in terms of his response to Wolsey. About Buckingham, the king is completely duped; with respect to Katherine, he finds his own approach—a blameless one, from the play's point of view—and when he finally realises Wolsey's faults, es-

pecially his opposition to Anne, he angrily drives him from office. Thus, the king's growth from immaturity to wisdom begins with his increasing awareness of the cardinal's evil influence.

Wolsey was one of the great villains for the historians inspired by the TUDOR DYNASTY, including Shakespeare's chief source for the play, Raphael HOLINSHED's *Chronicles,* and the playwright's treatment of the cardinal is particularly noteworthy in this light. The dignity the cardinal is permitted in his fall and the virtue the audience is clearly expected to find in his repentance had a great impact in the 17th century because of the contrast with the expected picture of a wholly evil figure. As in his other late plays, the ROMANCES, Shakespeare's emphasis was on the restoration of good, rather than on the evil that had prevailed earlier. His humanly forgivable Wolsey helps him present this theme in *Henry VIII.*

The historical Wolsey was the son of a prosperous, middle-class livestock dealer and wool merchant. (Wolsey's enemies habitually labelled his father a butcher—Buckingham calls the cardinal a 'butcher's cur' [1.1.120]—and this became an historical commonplace, but it was not true.) As a bright young priest, he was a tutor to the sons of the Marquess of DORSET (who appears in *Richard III*). His intelligence and drive impressed the aristocrats he met, and he was repeatedly advanced until he became Henry VII's chaplain. When Henry VIII became king in 1509, Wolsey was one of his most important advisers. He promoted Henry's invasion of FRANCE (1) in 1512, supplied the army, and negotiated the highly advantageous peace of 1514. He was rewarded with the archbishopric of York; then in 1515 the pope made him a cardinal and he became lord chancellor of England. At this point he virtually governed England for the king. He became very wealthy by accepting bribes and keeping for himself the feudal incomes from various church properties. This was perfectly normal in the 16th century, but as a non-aristocrat, Wolsey aroused great enmity by displaying his power and wealth with extravagant houses, clothes, and entertainment. He was thought, perhaps rightly, to aspire to the papal throne and to have cultivated foreign alliances to that end.

Among Wolsey's principal enemies was Buckingham, who was a leader of the aristocratic clique that had been displaced as the king's main source of advice. However, Buckingham's fate was probably ordered by Henry, who feared him as a relative of the Plantagenets and a potential claimant to the throne. Wolsey doubtless manipulated the surveyor, and he may have been pleased with the outcome, but the motivating force was the king's. Shakespeare, however, followed Holinshed in attributing the deed entirely to Wolsey.

It was the power of the emperor, which Wolsey vainly sought to harness, that finally brought about his fall. Henry ordered Wolsey to see to his divorce from Katherine—Wolsey almost certainly did not instigate this scheme; the play's intimations to that effect come from Holinshed. However, the opposition of Katherine's nephew, the Holy Roman Emperor Charles V (ruled 1519–1555), proved insuperable. Charles controlled the papacy—his troops sacked Rome in 1527, just as Henry's divorce effort began—so approval from that quarter was never possible. Wolsey probably realised this, but Henry persisted, and the cardinal's failure to achieve the impossible meant his ruin. Henry—who knew of and accepted the cardinal's other activities—could not accept frustration, and once the failure was evident, he disposed of his minister quickly in 1529. The cardinal's accidentally revealed inventory in 3.2 is an anecdote from Holinshed, but it happened to a different person, 20 years earlier; it is an excellent demonstration of Shakespeare's inventive use of his sources. In actuality, Henry simply invoked the laws defining papal interference in English affairs as treason. He dismissed Wolsey from office and confiscated most of his possessions but spared his life. The cardinal continued to communicate with Rome and the emperor, in the hope of retrieving his situation; within a year this was discovered and he was again charged with treason. He died while travelling to London for his trial.

Wolsey's contribution to history was great, though it is generally overshadowed by his role in the story of Henry's divorce. He reformed the English judiciary to establish more control for the central government, thereby contributing to England's growth into a modern nation-state, free from the dominance of feudal lords. In foreign policy he was less successful in the short term, but we see in his strategies the first experiment in balance-of-power politics in Europe, with England providing a potential counterweight to any expansion of either French or Hapsburg power. This arrangement was to characterise European international relations for centuries.

Woman (1) Any of several minor characters in *Henry VIII,* attendants to Queen KATHERINE. In 3.1.3–14 one of the women sings a SONG, 'Orpheus with his lute', in an effort to cheer the despairing Katherine. The incident helps establish a melancholy atmosphere around the defeated queen.

Woman (2) Minor character in *The Two Noble Kinsmen,* an attendant of EMILIA (4). In 2.1 the Woman converses with her mistress, who speaks of the maidenly virtues. They are overheard by PALAMON and ARCITE, who fall in love with Emilia. The Woman's decorous conversation simply offers openings for Emilia in an incident that furthers the plot. Since most scholars believe that 2.1 was not written by Shake-

speare, the Woman is probably a creation of John FLETCHER (2).

Woodstock (Thomas of Woodstock) Anonymous play, written circa 1592–1595, that was a source for *Richard II* and *1 Henry IV*. *Woodstock* deals with earlier events than does *Richard II*, focussing on the murder of Thomas of Woodstock, Duke of GLOUCESTER (6). It is sometimes referred to as *1 Richard II;* Shakespeare did not write it, but it has been speculated that he may have known a sequel to *Woodstock*—now lost, if it ever existed—on which he based his own play. The influence of *Woodstock* on *Richard II* is most evident in 2.1, which echoes the earlier work's emphasis on Richard's extravagance and extortionate financial measures. It is also thought that Shakespeare's John of GAUNT is derived from *Woodstock*'s Duke of Gloucester; both are depicted as wise elders and exemplary patriots.

Woodstock has a comic sub-plot involving a corrupt Chief Justice who is also a cowardly highwayman, a possible prototype of FALSTAFF. In its relationship of sub-plot to main plot, the play may also have influenced the structure of *1 Henry IV*. In any case, a number of wordings found in *Woodstock* are apparently echoed in Shakespeare's highway robbery scene, *1 Henry IV*, 2.2.

Woodville (Woodvile), Lieutenant Richard (d. c. 1440) Historical figure and minor character in *1 Henry VI*, the commander of the WARDERS at the Tower of London who refuse to admit the men of the Duke of GLOUCESTER (4); Woodville cites orders from the Bishop of WINCHESTER (1). The historical Woodville became the father of ELIZABETH (2) Woodville, Lady Grey, later Queen of England, and of Lord RIVERS, both of whom appear in *3 Henry VI* and *Richard III*.

Wooer Minor character in *The Two Noble Kinsmen*, the suitor of the DAUGHTER (2) of the GAOLER (4). In 2.1 the Wooer agrees with the Gaoler on a marriage contract, saying that he has the Daughter's consent to marry him. He is not seen again until Act 4, after the Daughter has gone mad with unrequited love for the nobleman PALAMON. Though unafflicted with jealousy and sympathetic to her plight, the Wooer is helpless to ease it, until in 4.3 the DOCTOR (4) prescribes that he disguise himself as Palamon and woo her, adding in 5.2 the instruction that he sleep with her, to which he readily assents. He proposes to her and is accepted, but she suggests bed before he can. The Doctor's ploy works, for the Daughter is later reported to be 'well restored, / And to be married shortly' (5.4.27–28). Slightly buffoonish, the Wooer is a gentle but undistinguished fellow, merely a necessary part of the subplot. He is probably the creation of Shakespeare's collaborator John FLETCHER (2), to whom the scenes he appears in are ascribed.

Worcester, Thomas Percy, Earl of (1343–1403) Historical figure and character in *1 Henry IV*, HOTSPUR's uncle and a leader of the rebels against King HENRY IV. Worcester is presented as a malevolent figure who introduces the idea of rebellion against Henry, beginning in 1.3.185, and formulates its strategy later in the same scene. In 5.2, in an illustration of the evil that attends rebellion, Worcester destroys the rebels' last chance for peace on the eve of the battle of SHREWSBURY by concealing Henry's offer of amnesty, fearing that in a state of peace, the king would single him out for punishment. Although his efforts to control Hotspur's impetuosity in 4.1 and 4.3 show that Worcester well understands the likelihood of catastrophe in the coming battle, he calculatingly permits his cause to court defeat because his personal interest may be at stake. After the battle, in which he is captured, Henry sentences him to death, and he justifies himself, saying, 'What I have done my safety urg'd me to' (5.5.11).

Shakespeare followed his primary historical source, HOLINSHED, in presenting a perfidious Worcester. Modern scholarship finds the truth unclear, but, while Worcester was certainly a leader of the revolt, he was probably not its instigator. He was in fact executed after Shrewsbury, but the tale of the negotiations is probably untrue. On the day of the battle it was apparently Henry who broke off the talks and began fighting. Before the time of the play, Worcester had served ably in the government of King RICHARD II, who had made him an earl in 1397. Two years later he allied himself with BOLINGBROKE (1) when he usurped the crown and became Henry IV (as is enacted in *Richard II;* although Worcester does not appear in that play, his actions are described in 2.2.58–61 and 2.3.26–28).

Worcester's Men Seventeenth-century LONDON theatrical company. Worcester's Men was originally a provincial company, sponsored by the Earl of Worcester, that toured intermittently between 1555 and 1585. They played in STRATFORD several times during Shakespeare's youth. In 1584 William ALLEYN was a teenage member of the troupe, though he soon left for London. In 1589, under a new earl, the company renewed its existence, and in 1602, they staged a play at the court of Queen ELIZABETH (1). William KEMPE and Thomas HEYWOOD (2), who wrote the play, were its leading members In the same year, Worcester's Men absorbed OXFORD'S MEN, and the enlarged troupe received a licence to play before the public at an inn. Thus they became the third theatre company of London, after the ADMIRAL'S MEN and Shakespeare's CHAMBERLAIN'S MEN. Christopher BEESTON, the future manager of the company, joined them at this point. In February 1603 they performed a Heywood play at Philip HENSLOWE'S ROSE THEATRE. Upon Queen Elizabeth's death in March 1603, Worcester's Men came under the patronage of Anne of Denmark (1574–

1619), the wife of England's new ruler, King JAMES I, and were known thereafter as the QUEEN'S MEN (2).

Worthies, The Nine Traditional array of medieval heroes, often presented in dramas or tableaux at fairs and festivals. The comical characters in *Love's Labour's Lost* enact such a tableau (5.2.541–717). Traditionally, the Nine Worthies were divided into three groups of three, representing Old Testament leaders, pre-Christian warriors and medieval notables. They were, respectively: Joshua, David, and Judas Maccabeus; HECTOR of Troy, Alexander the Great, and Julius CAESAR (1); and King Arthur, Charlemagne, and Godfrey of Bouillon (in England, Godfrey was sometimes replaced by Guy of Warwick). The line-up of Worthies in *Love's Labour's Lost* is quite different, which Shakespeare probably intended as a humorously ignorant error on the part of his unsophisticated characters.

Wyatt, Thomas (c. 1503–1542) English poet, the introducer of the SONNET into English and possibly the author of a minor source for *Twelfth Night.* Wyatt, while serving as a diplomat in Italy, translated some of the sonnets of Petrarch (1304–1374), producing the first English sonnets, around 1530. Wyatt and his friend the Earl of SURREY (1) subsequently became the first English poets to compose their own poems in this form. Wyatt also wrote in other forms and may have written the SONG sung by FESTE in *Twelfth Night* 4.2.75–80, though some scholars dispute the attribution.

Wyatt was a successful courtier who achieved high office under King HENRY VIII despite two periods of imprisonment in the TOWER OF LONDON. He was probably an early lover of the king's wife Anne Boleyn (see ANNE [1]), and his incarceration in 1536, as part of Queen Anne's trial for adultery, may have been connected with this.

Y

Yates (1), Mary Ann (1728–1787) English actress, wife of Richard YATES (2). Mrs Yates, as she was known, succeeded Susannah CIBBER (2) as London's favourite tragic actress, though she also played comedic heroines, including VIOLA, ROSALIND, and ISABELLA. She was a famous LADY (6) MACBETH, and she played CLEOPATRA opposite David GARRICK in the first recorded performance of *Antony and Cleopatra* since Shakespeare's day; she was thus the first woman to play the part.

Yates (2), Richard (c. 1706–1796) English actor, husband of Mary Ann YATES (1). Yates, who was considered the finest comedian of his day, specialised in his version of the COMMEDIA DELL'ARTE figure Harlequin. He also played many of Shakespeare's comic characters, including TOUCHSTONE, AUTOLYCUS, FESTE, and MALVOLIO.

Yong (Yonge, Young), Bartholomew (c. 1555–c. 1612) English translator, creator of a work that was a source for *Two Gentlemen of Verona* and *A Midsummer Night's Dream* and may have influenced *As You Like It* and *Twelfth Night.* Yong's version of the Spanish prose romance *Diana Enamorada* by Jorge de MONTEMAYOR was not published until 1598, but it was completed in 1582 and circulated widely in manuscript. Shakespeare knew it well, as its importance to *Two Gentlemen* indicates. Yong, an alumnus of one of the INNS OF COURT, spent two years in Spain, 1577 and 1578, and became familiar with the language, though he apparently encountered Montemayor's *Diana* only after his return. His patron was Penelope Rich (1563–1607), the sister of the Earl of ESSEX (2). Yong also translated BOCCACCIO's *Fiammetta* from Italian, as *Amorous Fiammetta* (1587).

Yorick Figure mentioned in *Hamlet,* the deceased court jester (see FOOL [1]) whose bones are dug up by the GRAVE-DIGGER in 5.1. Yorick's skull sparks a monologue by Prince HAMLET on the inevitability of death. The prince also responds with pleasure to his recollection of Yorick in life, 'a fellow of infinite jest, of most excellent fancy' (5.1.178–179). With the Grave-digger's earlier remarks, the passage on Yorick presents the familiar religious theme of earthly vanity: given the inevitability of death, the things of this life are inconsequential. In fact, Hamlet meditating on the skull of Yorick immediately became a popular symbol of this theme, and it has remained so.

That Hamlet can turn to this doctrine, and at the same time indulge in the healthy nostalgia of reminiscing about Yorick, a friendly figure of his youth, reflects his recovery from the racking grief that has tortured him in Acts 1–4. Thus Yorick is an emblem of the spirit of acceptance that prevails at the close of the play.

Scholars differ on the etymology of Yorick's unique name. It may be a corruption of Eric, a name appropriate to the play's setting in DENMARK; of Jörg, the Danish equivalent of George; or of Rorik, the name of Hamlet's maternal grandfather in older forms of the tale (Rorique in BELLEFOREST; Roricus in SAXO).

York (1) Family Branch of the PLANTAGENET (1) dynasty, major figures in Shakespeare's HISTORY PLAYS. The Yorkist kings were descended from Edmund, Duke of YORK (4), the fourth son of King Edward III (d. 1377). In the WARS OF THE ROSES the house of York fought for control of the throne with another line of the Plantagenets, the house of LANCASTER (1).

Three members of the York family ruled England: EDWARD IV, from 1461 to 1483; Edward V (see PRINCE [5]), briefly and only nominally in 1483; and RICHARD III, from 1483 to 1485. When the Earl of RICHMOND overthrew Richard III, he married Richard's niece, the daughter of Edward IV and Queen ELIZABETH (2), incorporating the York lineage into the new TUDOR dynasty.

The rivalry between York and Lancaster is the subject of Shakespeare's earliest history plays, the minor TETRALOGY, consisting of *1, 2,* and *3 Henry VI* and *Richard III.* The roots of the conflict lie farther back in history, and Shakespeare used this material in the major tetralogy—*Richard II, 1* and *2 Henry IV,* and *Henry V.* Although the Yorks are less important in this historical period, several members of the family figure in these plays as well.

York (2) City in northern England, a location in *3 Henry VI* and *1* and *2 Henry IV*. Second in economic and political power only to London during the Middle Ages, York figured heavily in the history of the time and thus naturally appears in the HISTORY PLAYS.

In 2.2 of *3 Henry VI* Queen MARGARET (1) and King HENRY VI march their army to the walls of York, and the queen points out the severed head of the Duke of YORK (8), which has been placed above the city gate. In 4.7 the duke's son EDWARD (3) comes to York after the reinstatement of Henry, whom he had earlier deposed. The MAYOR (5) declares the city's loyalty to Henry, and Edward is admitted only after he swears he is not pursuing the crown. Once within the walls, he reneges on his pledge and declares himself king. The incident illustrates the treachery and dishonesty of the period's political life, an important theme of the *Henry VI* plays.

In the *Henry IV* plays York is important as the headquarters of the ARCHBISHOP (3) of York, a leading rebel against King HENRY IV. In 4.4 of *1 Henry IV* the Archbishop, at his home in York, plans to continue the failing rebellion, thus anticipating the events of *Part 2*. In 1.3 of *2 Henry IV* the rebels hold a council of war and formulate their strategy in the same location.

York (3), Cicely Neville, Duchess of Character in *Richard III*. See DUCHESS (3).

York (4), Edmund of Langley, Duke of (1341–1402) Historical figure and character in *Richard II*, uncle of King RICHARD II. Like his brother John of GAUNT, York deplores the misguided rule of their nephew but believes strongly in the divine appointment of kings and is doggedly loyal to Richard. Richard, even as he is censured by York, appoints him Governor of England to rule in the king's absence, observing that 'he is just' (2.1.221). However, he is helpless to prevent the usurpation of the crown by BOLINGBROKE (1), and, once this is accomplished, he transfers his loyalty to the new king, despite his own grief at Richard's fall. He even denounces his son, the Duke of AUMERLE, as a traitor.

York is a representative of a vanishing medieval world of inviolable political and social hierarchies. In 2.3.96–105 he consciously identifies himself with that system, nostalgically recalling his comradeship with the Black Prince in the days of King Edward III. Ironically he speaks just as Bolingbroke is preparing the triumph of a more modern world of opportunistic, Machiavellian politics. York's sympathetic character is intended to heighten the pathos that colours the passing of that older world, one of the principal themes of the play.

The historical York apparently resembled Shakespeare's character. He was noted for his gentle, peace-loving nature, combined with a marked incapacity in political and military matters. He was the founder and namesake of the YORK (1) branch of the PLANTAGENET (1) family; through a younger son than Aumerle, the Earl of CAMBRIDGE, who appears in *Henry V*, York's great-grandson would eventually claim the crown and rule as King EDWARD IV.

York (5), Edward, Duke of (c. 1373–1415) Historical figure and minor character in *Henry V*. (The same figure appears as the Duke of AUMERLE in *Richard II*.) In 4.3 York asks King HENRY V for permission to lead the vanguard at the battle of AGINCOURT, offering an instance of English valour. His brave death in combat is touchingly reported by the Duke of EXETER (2) in 4.6. 7–32, a passage that helps to maintain the epic tone of the play's presentation of the battle.

The historical York inherited the title from his father, the YORK (4) of *Richard II*, several years after the time of that play. He was pardoned by Henry V for his rebellions against HENRY IV (one of which is enacted in *Richard II*). As he demonstrated at Agincourt, he remained loyal to the new king, but his younger brother, the Earl of CAMBRIDGE, was executed for treason, as is enacted in *Henry V*, 2.2. When York died childless, the title passed to Cambridge's son, the Duke of YORK (8) of the *Henry VI* plays. The York of *Henry V* died at Agincourt, but not in the courageous manner described in the play. Quite fat, York suffered a heart attack or some other sort of fatal seizure after falling from his horse. His heroic death is Shakespeare's invention; he may have had in mind the great popularity of his earlier description of JOHN (6) Talbot's death in battle in *1 Henry VI*, 4.7.

York (6), Isabel of Castile, Duchess of Character in *Richard II*. See DUCHESS (4).

York (7), Richard, Duke of (1473–c. 1483) Historical figure and character in *Richard III*, the murdered nephew of RICHARD III. The younger brother of the PRINCE (5) of Wales and his successor to the throne, York is a flippant youngster, given to ill-considered jokes about Richard's deformity. He appears with his mother, Queen ELIZABETH (2), and grandmother, the DUCHESS (3) of York, in 2.4 and with his brother and others in 3.1. In the latter scene, he jests about Richard's dagger, in an ominous foreshadowing of his fate. At the end of the scene, the two young brothers are escorted to the TOWER OF LONDON, from which they will never emerge. Although their murder is commonly attributed to Richard, modern scholarship finds the fate of the princes to be impenetrably obscure, barring the unlikely emergence of new evidence (see TYRELL).

York (8), Richard Plantagenet, Duke of (1411–1460) Historical figure and character in the three *Henry VI* plays, claimant to the throne of England against the Lancastrian branch of the PLANTAGENETS (1) (see YORK [1]; LANCASTER [1]). York attempts to seize the throne at the end of *2 Henry VI*, launching the WARS OF THE ROSES. He fails, dying early in *3 Henry VI*, but his son becomes King EDWARD IV. The Yorkist cause thus succeeds, only to be brought to ruin (in *Richard III*) by the greedy machinations of York's younger son, RICHARD III, who inherits his father's ruthless ambition.

In *1 Henry VI* York's claim to the throne is established. His father, the Earl of CAMBRIDGE, has been executed for treason (as is depicted in Shakespeare's *Henry V*) for supporting the royal claims of Edmund MORTIMER (1). The dying Mortimer bequeaths his claim to York, his nephew, in 2.5 of *1 Henry VI*, thus laying the groundwork for the conflict to come. York feuds with the Duke of SOMERSET (3), even at the expense of military disaster in the HUNDRED YEARS WAR.

In *2 Henry VI* York's story is at first overshadowed by that of Humphrey, Duke of GLOUCESTER (4), whose murder is seen as making the civil war inevitable. Early in the play, York reveals his ambition to seize the throne, but this crafty planner keeps a low profile, even when his appointment as Regent in FRANCE (1) is given to another SOMERSET (1), the brother and successor to his old rival. York participates in the plot against Gloucester, but the chief conspirators are the Duke of SUFFOLK (3) and CARDINAL (1) Beaufort.

York is placed in command of an army and sent to crush a revolution in Ireland. He sees that these troops will permit him an opportunity to seize the crown. Despite the grand boldness of his scheme and his demands on himself for extraordinary courage, York's morality is sorely limited; he is prepared to expend any number of lives in the pursuit of his own ambition. He arranges for Jack CADE to foment a revolt in England, providing an excuse for him to bring in his army.

After Cade's rebellion, staged in Act 4, York returns with his army, demanding the imprisonment of Somerset. When this is not done, he announces his claim to the throne and proceeds to battle the King's troops at ST ALBANS. York's forces are victorious, but the King escapes to London. Thus the civil war has begun as the play ends.

In *3 Henry VI* York compromises: King Henry will be permitted to rule in his own lifetime but will pass the crown to York or his heirs. Richard persuades his father to seize the throne anyway, just as Queen MARGARET (1), who has herself rejected Henry's deal, arrives with an army. In the ensuing battle, York is captured; after a dramatic scene (1.4) in which Margaret mocks him viciously, the Queen and Lord CLIFFORD (1) stab him to death. In his last moments, York heaps insults on Margaret and weeps over the death of his young son RUTLAND, with whose fate the Queen had taunted him.

York generally functions more as a foil for other characters or incidents than as a well-developed figure himself. In *1 Henry VI* his ambitious rivalry with Somerset functions as a dark backdrop to the upright and patriotic career of Lord TALBOT; in *Part 2* his machinations are similarly contrasted with the fate of 'good Duke Humphrey' of Gloucester. In the latter half of *Part 2* and in *Part 3*, York simply exemplifies aristocratic ambition in a mechanical manner dependent largely on mere assertion, backed by the tableaux of the battlefield. Even his death scene serves chiefly to present Margaret in the vicious, warlike personality she assumes in that play. Only in his darkly malevolent speeches of *Part 2* is he a stimulating villain, and even then he is overshadowed by Suffolk. In any case, as an agent of evil York pales before the grand MACHIAVEL that his son Richard is to embody.

York's function as an archetype of selfish ambition is achieved at the expense of historical accuracy. The historical York actually had little role in the action of *1 Henry VI;* his presence is magnified in order to prepare for his role in *Parts 2* and *3*. The character's rise begins with the return of his dukedom to him in 3.1 of *Part 1*, but in fact, York had never been kept from that title and so could not be restored to it. York and the Duke of Somerset launch their quarrel in *Part 1*, though in reality the contest between York and Lancaster was not consequential until many years later. Further, the quarrel is made the cause of Talbot's defeat and death, but the divided command depicted by Shakespeare had occurred elsewhere and 10 years earlier. Also, York is assigned elements of the career of the Duke of BEDFORD (1). All of these fictions serve to foreshadow the conflict to come, establishing as a longstanding feud a rivalry that actually only developed some years later.

The greatest difference between the historical York and Shakespeare's character is a basic one: York's ambition is presented as a long-meditated plot to usurp the king's power. In fact, although he was undeniably a powerful figure who attempted to dominate the political world of England in the 1450s, York has nonetheless been considerably misrepresented by Shakespeare. He showed no intention to seize power until very shortly before he actually attempted to do so in 1455, the action that sparked the fighting at St Albans. He had competed fiercely with Somerset for power, but only for power as a minister under King Henry. He seems to have acted to usurp royal authority only when it became evident that his career and very possibly his life would be in great danger from Somerset and Margaret if he did not. Shakespeare has simply eliminated a great deal of intricate and fascinating politics, most notably any reference to York's capable

rule in 1453–1454, when King Henry was insane and unable to speak.

It was not the playwright's concern in composing the *Henry VI* plays to render history accurately. He depicted unscrupulous aristocratic rivalry leading to civil war, thus demonstrating the importance of political stability. One of the ways in which he achieved his end was to make of the Duke of York a simple paragon of selfish ambition, and his success is demonstrated in the effectiveness of this fairly one-dimensional character in providing the impetus for a great deal of complicated action in the three *Henry VI* plays.

York (9), Richard Scroop, Archbishop of Character in *1* and *2 Henry IV.* See ARCHBISHOP (3).

York (10), Thomas Rotherham, Archbishop of Character in *Richard III.* See ARCHBISHOP (4).

A Yorkshire Tragedy Play formerly attributed to Shakespeare, part of the Shakespeare APOCRYPHA. *A Yorkshire Tragedy* was published by Thomas PAVIER in 1608 and again in 1619 (in the FALSE FOLIO) as a play by Shakespeare that had been performed by the KING'S MEN. It was also published in the Third and Fourth FOLIOS of Shakespeare's plays, and in the editions of Nicholas ROWE and Alexander POPE (1). However, although it is a respectable play—unlike most of the apocryphal works—scholars agree that it is not in fact by Shakespeare. This very brief play is quite dissimilar from the playwright's known works in its setting and its subject. It is set in contemporary England and concerns a sensational murder case of 1605 in which a man killed two of his children and attempted to kill his wife and a third child. Moreover, the play's poetry is distinctly inferior to Shakespeare's—especially his late work—and its only important characters, the murderer and his wife, are two-dimensional caricatures who are not even given names, and are thus entirely beneath the level of Shakespeare's characterisations. Its actual authorship remains unknown.

Young Cato Character in *Julius Caesar.* See CATO.

Young Clifford Character in *2 Henry VI.* See Lord John CLIFFORD (1).

Young Lucius Minor character in *Titus Andronicus,* son of LUCIUS (1) and grandson of TITUS (1). Young Lucius attends Titus in his grief and as he plans his revenge. In 4.2 he delivers to CHIRON and DEMETRIUS (1) a gift of weapons containing a cryptic message, the first of Titus' taunts to Tamora's family. He also participates in mourning Titus at the end of the play.

Young Siward (Osberne of Northumberland, d. 1054) Historical figure and minor character in *Macbeth,* an English soldier killed by MACBETH. Son of SIWARD, the English ally of MALCOLM and MACDUFF, Young Siward appears with the leaders in 5.4 but does not speak. In the ensuing battle he bravely challenges Macbeth to personal combat in 5.7, and dies in the encounter. The youth has no personality and serves only as a foil to Macbeth, whose evil is emphasised by the contrast with Young Siward's noble bravery, and whose malign nature is demonstrated in the otherwise unnecessary death of so fine a young man. The actual son of Siward was named Osberne. He did indeed die in combat at an early age during Malcolm's invasion of Scotland, but nothing more is known of him.

Young Talbot Character in *1 Henry VI.* See JOHN (6).

Z

Zeffirelli, Franco (b. 1923) Modern stage and FILM director, creator of a number of noteworthy productions of Shakespeare's plays. Although he has produced many plays and operas, Zeffirelli is most widely known for his films. He produced *Romeo and Juliet* on the stage in 1960 and the screen in 1968, and his film of *The Taming of the Shrew* (1966) was extremely popular. His production of *Much Ado About Nothing* (1965) appeared on TELEVISION two years later. He is often criticised for the lavish spectacle of his productions, which are said to distract from the underlying play, but he has undeniably brought Shakespeare to a very wide audience.

SUGGESTED READING

A comprehensive bibliography on Shakespeare would be many times the size of this book. The following is simply a selection of books that seem particularly interesting and appealing.

Adams, John Cranford. *The Globe Playhouse.* New York: Barnes & Noble, 1966.

Adams, Joseph Quincy. *Shakespearean Playhouses: A History of English Theatres from the Beginning to the Restoration.* Magnolia, MA: Peter Smith, 1959.

Alexander, Peter. *Shakespeare's Life and Art.* Westport, CT: Greenwood Press, 1979.

Baldwin, Thomas Whitfield. *The Organisation and Personnel of the Shakespearean Company.* Princeton: Princeton University Press, 1927.

Barber, Cesar Lombardi. *Shakespeare's Festive Comedy.* Princeton: Princeton University Press, 1972.

Bentley, Gerald Eades. *The Profession of Player in Shakespeare's Time, 1590–1642.* Princeton: Princeton University Press, 1984.

———. *Shakespeare: A Biographical Handbook.* New Haven: Yale University Press, 1974.

Boas, Frederic Samuel. *Shakespeare and His Predecessors.* Brooklyn, NY: Haskell, 1969.

Bradbrook, Muriel C. *The Artist and Society in Shakespeare's Time.* Totowa, NJ: Barnes & Noble, 1982.

———. *Elizabethan Stage Conditions.* Hamden, CT: Archon, 1962.

———. *The Rise of the Common Player.* Cambridge, Eng.: Cambridge University Press, 1979.

———. *Shakespeare and Elizabethan Poetry.* London: Chatto & Windus, 1951.

Bradley, Andrew Cecil. *Shakespearean Tragedy.* Cleveland: World, 1964.

Brown, Ivor. *How Shakespeare Spent the Day.* London: Bodley Head, 1963.

———. *Shakespeare.* Garden City, NY: Doubleday, 1949.

Brown, John Russell, and Bernard Harris, eds. *Early Shakespeare.* New York: Schocken, 1966.

Bullough, Geoffrey. *Narrative and Dramatic Sources of Shakespeare,* 8 vols. New York: Columbia University Press, 1957–1975.

Chambers, Sir Edmund Kerchever. *The Elizabethan Stage,* 4 vols. Oxford: Clarendon Press, 1961.

———. *William Shakespeare: A Study of Facts and Problems,* 2 vols. Oxford: Oxford University Press, 1989.

Chute, Marcel. *Shakespeare of London.* New York: Dutton, 1957.

Clemen, Wolfgang H. *The Development of Shakespeare's Imagery.* Cambridge, MA: Harvard University Press, 1951.

Coleridge, Samuel Taylor. *Coleridge's Criticism of Shakespeare,* ed. R. A. Foakes. Detroit: Wayne State University Press, 1989.

Colie, Rosalie. *Shakespeare's Living Art.* Princeton: Princeton University Press, 1974.

Cooper, Duff. *Sergeant Shakespeare.* New York: Haskell, 1972.

Craig, Hardin. *The Enchanted Glass: The Elizabethan Mind in Literature.* Westport, CT: Greenwood Press, 1975.

Dean, Leonard Fellows, ed. *Shakespeare: Modern Essays in Criticism.* New York: Oxford University Press, 1967.

Drakakis, John, ed. *Alternative Shakespeares.* New York: Routledge, Chapman & Hall, 1985.

Eccles, Mark. *Shakespeare in Warwickshire.* Madison: University of Wisconsin Press, 1963.

Edwards, Philip. *Shakespeare: A Writer's Progress.* Oxford: Oxford University Press, 1987.

———, ed. *Shakespeare's Styles: Essays in Honour of Kenneth Muir.* Cambridge, Eng.: Cambridge University Press, 1980.

Empson, William. *Essays on Shakespeare.* Cambridge, Eng.: Cambridge University Press, 1986.

Foakes, R. A. *Illustrations of the English Stage 1580–1642.* Stanford, CA: Stanford University Press, 1985.

Ford, Boris, ed. *The Age of Shakespeare.* New York: Penguin, 1982.

Fripp, Edgar I. *Shakespeare, Man and Artist,* 2 vols. London: Oxford University Press, 1938.

———. *Shakespeare's Stratford.* Salem, NH: Ayer, n.d., reprint of 1928 ed.

Frye, Northrop. *Fools of Time: Studies in Shakespearean Tragedy.* Toronto: University of Toronto Press, 1967.

———. *The Myth of Deliverance: Reflections on Shakespeare's Problem Comedies.* Toronto: University of Toronto Press, 1983.

Greg, Walter Wilson. *The Editorial Problem in Shakespeare.* Oxford: Clarendon Press, 1954.

———. *The Shakespeare First Folio.* Oxford: Clarendon Press, 1955.

Gurr, Andrew. *Playgoing in Shakespeare's London.* New York: Cambridge University Press, 1987.

———. *The Shakespearean Stage 1574–1642.* Cambridge, Eng.: Cambridge University Press, 1981.

Granville-Barker, Harley. *Prefaces to Shakespeare,* 2 vols. Princeton: Princeton University Press, 1978.

Greenblatt, Stephen. *Renaissance Self-Fashioning.* Chicago: University of Chicago Press, 1980.

Halliday, F. E. *Shakespeare and His Critics.* London: Duckworth, 1958.

———. *A Shakespeare Companion: 1564–1964.* Baltimore: Penguin, 1964.

———. *Shakespeare in His Age.* London: Duckworth, 1956.

Harbage, Alfred. *As They Liked It: A Study of Shakespeare's Moral Artistry.* Philadelphia: University of Pennsylvania Press, 1972.

———. *Conceptions of Shakespeare.* Cambridge, MA: Harvard University Press, 1966.

———. *Shakespeare and the Rival Traditions.* New York: Macmillan, 1952.

———. *Shakespeare's Audience.* New York: Columbia University Press, 1961.

Harrison, George Bagshawe. *Elizabethan Plays and Players.* Ann Arbour: University of Michigan Press, 1956.

———. *Shakespeare at Work.* London: Routledge, 1933.

Hartnoll, Phyllis, ed. *The Oxford Companion to the Theatre.* London: Oxford University Press, 1983.

Hill, Errol. *Shakespeare in Sable: A History of Black Shakespearean Actors.* Amherst: University of Massachusetts Press, 1986.

Hillebrand, Harold Newcomb. *The Child Actors.* Urbana: University of Illinois Press, 1926.

Hodges, Cyril W. *The Globe Restored.* New York: Somerset, 1973.

Honigmann, E. A. J. *The Stability of Shakespeare's Text.* London: Arnold, 1965.

Hotson, Leslie. *Shakespeare's Motley.* Brooklyn, NY: Haskell, 1970.

———. *Shakespeare's Sonnets Dated and Other Essays.* New York: Oxford University Press, 1949.

———. *Shakespeare's Wooden O.* London: Hart-Davis, 1959.

Hunter, George K., *Dramatic Identities and Cultural Tradition: Studies in Shakespeare and His Contemporaries.* Liverpool: Liverpool University Press, 1978.

Jones, Emrys. *The Origins of Shakespeare.* Oxford: Oxford University Press, 1977.

Jones, Ernest. *Hamlet and Oedipus.* New York: Norton, 1976.

Kirschbaum, Leo. *Shakespeare and the Stationers.* Columbus: Ohio State University Press, 1955.

Knight, George Wilson. *The Crown of Life: Essays in Interpretation of Shakespeare's Final Plays.* London: Methuen, 1947.

———. *The Wheel of Fire: Essays in Interpretation of Shakespeare's Sombre Tragedies.* New York: Routledge, Chapman & Hall, 1949.

Knights, Lionel Charles. *How Many Children Had Lady Macbeth?* New York: Haskell, 1973.

———. *Shakespeare's Politics.* London: Oxford University Press, 1957.

Lee, Sidney. *A Life of William Shakespeare.* New York: Macmillan, 1931.

———. *Shakespeare and the Modern Stage.* New York: AMS, 1974.

Leech, Clifford. *Twelfth Night and Shakespearean Comedy.* Toronto: Dalhousie University Press/University of Toronto Press, 1965.

Levin, Harry. *Shakespeare and the Revolution of the Times.* New York: Oxford University Press, 1976.

Merchant, William Moelwyn. *Shakespeare and the Artist.* London: Oxford University Press, 1959.

Miriam Joseph, Sister. *Shakespeare's Use of the Arts of Language.* New York: Columbia University Press, 1947.

Morozov, Mikhail Mikhailovich. *Shakespeare on the Soviet Stage.* London: Soviet News, 1947.

Muir, Kenneth. *Last Periods of Shakespeare, Racine, and Ibsen.* Liverpool: Liverpool University Press, 1961.

———. *Shakespeare's Sonnets.* London/Boston: Allen & Unwin, 1979.

———. *The Sources of Shakespeare's Plays.* London: Methuen, 1977.

Nagler, Alois M. *Shakespeare's Stage.* New Haven: Yale University Press, 1981.

Naylor, Edward Woodall. *Shakespeare and Music.* London: Dent, 1931.

Nevo, Ruth. *Comic Transformations in Shakespeare.* New York: Routledge, Chapman & Hall, 1981.

———. *Tragic Form in Shakespeare.* Princeton: Princeton University Press, 1972.

Noble, Richmond Samuel Howe. *Shakespeare's Biblical Knowledge.* New York: Gordon, n.d., reprint of 1935 ed.

Odell, George C. D. *Shakespeare from Betterton to Irving,* 2 vols. New York: Dover, 1966.

Onions, Charles Talbut. *A Shakespeare Glossary.* Oxford: Clarendon Press, 1986.

Orell, John. *The Quest for Shakespeare's Globe.* Cambridge, Eng.: Cambridge University Press, 1983.

Palmer, Alan, and Veronica Palmer. *Who's Who in Shakespeare's England.* New York: St Martin's, 1981.

Parker, Patricia, and Geoffrey Hartman, eds. *Shakespeare and the Question of Theory.* New York/London: Methuen, 1985.

Partridge, Eric. *Shakespeare's Bawdy.* London: Routledge & Kegan Paul, 1968.

Quennell, Peter. *Shakespeare: The Poet and His Background.* London: Weidenfeld & Nicolson, 1963.

Rabkin, Norman. *Shakespeare and the Common Understanding.* Chicago: University of Chicago Press, 1984.

———. *Shakespeare and the Problem of Meaning.* Chicago: University of Chicago Press, 1982.

Reese, Max Meredith. *Shakespeare: His World and his Work.* New York: St Martin's, 1980.

Ribner, Irving. *The English History Play in the Age of Shakespeare.* New York: Barnes & Noble, 1965.

Righter, Anne. *Shakespeare and the Idea of the Play.* Westport, CT: Greenwood Press, 1977.

Saccio, Peter. *Shakespeare's English Kings.* Oxford: Oxford University Press, 1977.

Schoenbaum, Samuel. *Shakespeare's Lives.* New York: Oxford University Press, 1970.

———. *William Shakespeare: A Compact Documentary Life.* New York: Oxford University Press, 1987.

———. *William Shakespeare: A Documentary Life.* New York: Oxford University Press, 1975.

Siegel, Paul N. *Shakespearean Tragedy and the Elizabethan Compromise: A Marxist Study.* Lanham, MD: University Press of America, 1983.

Simmons, Joseph Larry. *Shakespeare's Pagan World: The Roman Tragedies.* Charlottesville: University Press of Virginia, 1973.

Sisson, Charles Jasper. *Lost Plays of Shakespeare's Age.* Cambridge, Eng.: Cambridge University Press, 1936.

———. *The Mythical Sorrows of Shakespeare.* London: Milford, 1934.

———. *New Readings in Shakespeare.* Cambridge, Eng.: Cambridge University Press, 1956.

Smith, Hallett. *Shakespeare's Romances.* San Marino, CA: Huntington Library, 1972.

Smith, Irwin. *Shakespeare's Blackfriars Playhouse.* New York: New York University Press, 1964.

———. *Shakespeare's Globe Playhouse.* New York: Scribner's, 1956.

Smith, Logan Piersall. *On Reading Shakespeare.* New York: Somerset, n.d., reprint of 1933 ed.

Snyder, Susan. *The Comic Matrix of Shakespeare's Tragedies.* Princeton: Princeton University Press, 1979.

Speaight, Robert. *Shakespeare on the Stage: An Illustrated History of Shakespearean Performance.* Boston: Little, Brown, 1973.

Spencer, Theodore. *Shakespeare and the Nature of Man.* New York: Macmillan, 1942.

Spivack, Bernard. *Shakespeare and the Allegory of Evil.* New York: Columbia University Press, 1958.

Sprague, Arthur Colby. *Shakespeare and the Actors.* New York: Russell & Russell, 1963.

Spurgeon, Caroline. *Shakespeare's Imagery.* Cambridge, Eng.: Cambridge University Press, 1975.

Thompson, Peter W. *Shakespeare's Theatre.* London/ Boston: Routledge & Kegan Paul, 1983.

Tilley, Morris Palmer. *A Dictionary of the Proverbs in England in the Sixteenth and Seventeenth Centuries.* New York: AMS, 1982.

Tillyard, E. M. W. *The Elizabethan World Picture.* New York: Random House, 1959.

Traversi, Derek. *Shakespeare, The Last Phase.* Stanford, CA: Stanford University Press, 1955.

Trewin, John Courtenay. *Shakespeare on the English Stage 1900–1964.* London: Barrie & Rockliff, 1964.

Vickers, Brian. *The Artistry of Shakespeare's Prose.* London: Methuen, 1968.

———. *Classical Rhetoric in English Poetry.* Carbondale: Southern Illinois University Press, 1989.

Walker, Alice. *Textual Problems of the First Folio.* Cambridge, Eng.: Cambridge University Press, 1953.

Wells, Stanley, ed. *The Cambridge Companion to Shakespeare Studies.* Cambridge, Eng.: Cambridge University Press, 1986.

Welsford, Enid. *The Court Masque.* Cambridge, Eng.: Cambridge University Press, 1927.

———. *The Fool: His Social and Literary History.* Garden City, NY: Anchor, 1961.

Whitaker, Virgil Keeble. *Shakespeare's Use of Learning: An Inquiry into the Growth of His Mind and Art.* San Marino, CA: Huntington Library, 1953.

Wickham, Glynne. *Early English Stages,* 2 vols. New York: Columbia University Press, 1980.

Wilson, J. Dover *The Essential Shakespeare.* New York: Haskell, 1977.

Wright, Louis B. *Middle Class Culture in Elizabethan England.* New York: Hippocrene, 1980.

Yates, Frances. *Majesty and Magic in Shakespeare's Last Plays.* Boulder, CO: Shambhala, 1978.

APPENDIX

Actors and Other Theatre Professionals, Composers, and Musicians

Admiral's Men
Aldridge, Ira
Alleyn, Edward
Anderson (1), Judith
Anderson (2), Mary
Armin, Robert
Arne, Thomas Augustine
Asche, Oscar
Ashcroft, Peggy
Atkins, Robert
Barker, Harley Granville (*see* Granville-Barker)
Barrett, Lawrence
Barry (1), Ann
Barry (2), Elizabeth
Barry (3), Spranger
Barrymore, John
Bartley, George
Barton (1), John
Baylis, Lilian
Beeston, Christopher
Beethoven Ludwig van
Bellini, Vincenzo
Benfield, Robert
Bensley, Robert
Benson (1), Frank Robert
Bentley, John
Berlioz, Hector
Bernhardt, Sarah
Betterton, Thomas
Betty, William Henry West
Bishop (2), Henry Rowley
Boito, Arrigo
Booth (1), Barton
Booth (2), Edwin
Booth (3), John Wilkes
Booth (4), Junius Brutus
Booth (5), Junius Brutus, Jr.
Bracegirdle, Anne
Britten, Benjamin
Brook (2), Peter
Browne, Robert
Bryan, George
Burbage (1), Cuthbert
Burbage (2), James
Burbage (3), Richard
Caldwell, Zoe
Calvert, Charles
Casson, Lewis
Castelnuovo-Tedesco, Mario
Chamberlain's Men
Chatterton, Frederick Balsir
Children's Companies
Cibber (1), Colley
Cibber (2), Susannah Maria
Cibber (3), Theophilus
Clive, Kitty
Coburn, Charles Douville
Collier (1), Constance
Colman, George
Compton, Fay
Condell, Henry
Cooke (1), Alexander
Cooke (2), George Frederick
Cornell, Katherine
Cornwall, Duke of
Costard
Cowley, Richard
Cox, Robert
Craig (1), Gordon
Crosse, Samuel
Cushman, Charlotte
Daly, Augustin
Dance, James
Davenant (D'Avenant), William
Dench, Judi
Derby's Men
Downton, Thomas
Drew, John
Duke of York's Men (*see* Prince Charles' Men)
Dutton, Laurence
Ecclestone, William
Emery, John
Evans (1), Edith
Evans (2), Henry
Evans (4), Maurice
Farrant, Richard
Faucit, Helen
Field (1), Nathan
Fletcher (3), Laurence
Forbes-Robertson, Johnston
Forrest, Edwin
Garrick, David
German, Edward
Gibborne, Thomas
Gielgud, John
Gilburne, Samuel
Glover, Julia
Glyn, Isabel
Gough (Goughe), Robert
Gounod, Charles François
Granville-Barker, Harley
Green, John
Greet, Philip Barling Ben
Greville (1), Curtis
Guthrie, Tyrone
Hall (5), Peter
Hands, Terry
Harris (2), Henry
Hart (1), Charles
Hart (3), William
Heminge (Heminges), John
Henderson, John
Henslowe, Philip
Heywood (2), Thomas
Howard's Men or Lord Howard's Men (*see* Admiral's Men)
Hughes, Margaret
Hull, Thomas
Hunnis, William
Hunsdon's Men
Hyman, Earle
Irving, Henry
Jackson (1), Barry
Jeffes, Humphrey
Johnson (5), Robert
Jones (1), James Earl
Jones (2), Richard
Jones (3), Robert
Jordan, Dorothy
Kean (1), Charles
Kean (2), Edmund
Kemble (1), Charles
Kemble (2), Fanny
Kemble (3), John Philip
Kemble (4), Stephen
Kempe (Kemp), William
King (26), Tom
King's Men
King's Revels (*see* Children's Companies)
Kirkham, Edward
Knell, William
Knight (4), Edward
Komisarjevsky, Theodore
Kozintsev, Grigori
Kurosawa, Akira
Lacy, John
Lady Elizabeth's Men
Laneman (Lanman), Henry
Langley, Francis
Laughton, Charles
Leicester's Men
Leigh, Vivien
Leveridge, Richard
Locke, Matthew
Lowin (Lowen), John
Macklin, Charles
Macready, William Charles
Mantell, Robert Bruce
Marlowe (2), Julia
McKellan, Ian
Miller (2), Jonathan
Modjeska, Helena
Mohun, Michael
Monck, Nugent
Morley, Thomas
Neilson (1), Adelaide
Neilson (2), Julia
Nunn, Trevor
Olivier, Laurence
Oxford's Men
Palsgrave's Men
Papp, Joseph
Pembroke's Men
Phelps, Samuel
Phillips, Augustine

Actors and Other Theatre Professionals, Composers, and Musicians

Plowright, Joan
Plummer, Christopher
Poel, William
Pope (2), Thomas
Prince Charles' Men
Prince Henry's Men
Pritchard, Hannah
Purcell, Henry
Quayle, Anthony
Queen's Men (1) (Queen Elizabeth's Men)
Queen's Men (2)
Queen's Revels (*see* Children's Companies)
Quin, James
Redgrave, Michael
Rehan, Ada
Reynolds (1), Frederick
Reinhardt, Max
Rice, John
Rich (2), John
Richardson (2), Ralph
Robeson, Paul
Robinson (2), Mary ('Perdita')
Robinson (4), Richard
Rowley (2), William
Royal Shakespeare Company
Salvini, Tommaso
Saunderson, Mary
Schroder, Friedrich Ludwig
Schubert, Franz
Scofield, Paul
Shank, John
Shaw (3), Glen Byam
Shaw (5) (Shaa), Robert
Sheridan, Thomas
Siddons, Sarah
Sincklo (Sinklo, Sincler), John
Singer, John
Slater (Slaughter), Martin
Sly (2), William
Smith (2), Morgan
Smithson, Harriet
Sothern, Edward Hugh
Spencer, Gabriel
Strange's Men
Sullivan (1), Arthur Seymour
Sullivan (2), Barry
Sussex's Men
Tarlton, Richard
Taylor, Joseph
Tchaikovsky, Peter Ilyich
Tearle, Godfrey
Terry (1), Ellen
Terry (2), Fred
Thorndike, Sybil
Tooley, Nicholas
Tree, Beerbohm
Tuckfeild, Thomas
Underwood, John
Vaughan Williams, Ralph
Vaux (1), Sir Nicholas
Verdi, Giuseppe
Vestris, Elizabeth
Walton, William
Webster (1), Benjamin
Webster (3), Margaret
Weelkes, Thomas
Welles, Orson
Williams (1), Harcourt
Williamson, Nicol
Wilson (1), Jack
Wilson (2), John
Wilson (4), Robert
Woffington, Peg (Margaret)
Wolfit, Donald
Worcester's Men
Yates (1), Mary Ann
Yates (2), Richard
Zeffirelli, Franco

Characters

Aaron
Abbess
Abbot of Westminister, William Colchester
Abergavenny, George Neville, Lord
Abhorson
Abram (Abraham)
Achilles
Adam
Adrian (1) (*see* Volsce)
Adrian (2)
Adriana
Aedile
Aegeon (*see* Egeon)
Aemilia (*see* Emilia)
Aemilius
Aeneas
Agammemnon
Agrippa, M. Vipsanius
Ajax
Alarbus
Albany, Duke of
Alcibiades
Alencon, John, Duke of
Alexander (1)
Alexas (Alexas Laodician)
Alice
Aliena (Celia)
Alonso, King of Naples
Ambassador (1)
Ambassador (2)
Ambassador (3)
Amiens
Andrew (2) Aguecheek, Sir (*see* Sir Andrew)
Andromache
Andronicus (*see* Marcus Andronichus, Titus [1])
Angelo (1)
Angelo (2)
Angus, Gilchrist, Thane of
Anne (1) Bullen (Boleyn)
Anne (2), Lady (Anne Neville)
Anne (3) Page
Another Lord (*see* Lord [2])
Antenor
Anthony
Antigonus
Antiochus, King of Syria
Antipholus of Ephesus; Antipholus of Syracuse
Antonio (1)
Antonio (2)
Antonio (3)
Antonio (4)
Antonio (5)
Antony, Mark (Marcus Antonius)
Apemantus
Apothecary, the
Apparitions
Archbishop (1) of Canterbury, Henry Chichele (*see* Canterbury [1])
Archbishop (2) of Canterbury, (*see* Cranmer)
Archbishop (3) of York, Richard Scroop
Archbishop (4) of York, Thomas Rotherham
Archidamus
Arcite
Ariel
Armado, Don Adriano de
Arragon (Aragon)
Artemidorus
Artesius
Arthur, Prince of England
Arviragus
Asnath
Attendant (1)
Attendant (2)
Audrey
Aufidius, Tullus
Aumerle, Edward York, Duke of
Austria Limoges (Lymoges), Archduke of
Autolycus
Bagot, Sir John
Balthasar (1)
Balthasar (2)
Balthasar (3)
Balthasar (4)
Bandit (Thief)
Banquo
Baptista
Bardolph (1)
Bardolph (2), Lord Thomas
Barnardine
Barnardo (Bernardo)
Bartholomew (*see* Page [8])
Bassanio
Basset
Bassianus
Bastard (1), Philip Faulconbridge, The
Bastard (2) of Orleans, Jean Dunois, The
Bastard (3) (*see* Margarelon)
Bates, John
Bavian
Bawd
Beadle (1)
Beadle (2)
Bear
Beatrice
Beaumont (1)
Bedford (1), John Platagenet, Duke of
Begger (*see* Sly [1])
Belarius
Belch, Sir Toby (*see* Sir Toby)
Benedick
Benvolio
Berkeley (1)
Berkeley (2), Lord Thomas
Bernardo (*see* Barnardo)
Berowne (Biron)
Berri, Jean of France, Duke of
Bertram
Bevis, George
Bianca (1)
Bianca (2)
Bigot (Bigod), Roger
Biondello
Biron (*see* Berowne)
Bishop (1)
Blanche (Blanch) of Spain
Blunt (1), Sir James
Blunt (2), Sir John
Blunt (3), Sir Walter
Boatswain
Boleyn, Anne (*see* Anne [1])
Bolingbroke (1) (Bullingbrook), Henry
Bolingbroke (2), Roger

Characters

Characters

Characters

Gratiano (1)
Gratiano (2) (Graziano)
Grave-digger (First Clown, First Grave-digger)
Greene (1) (Green), Henry
Gregory (1)
Gremio
Grey (1), Lady (*see* Elizabeth [2])
Grey (2), Sir Richard
Grey (3), Thomas
Griffith
Groom (1)
Groom (2)
Grumio
Guardsman (1)
Guardsman (2)
Guiderius
Guildenstern (*see* Rosencrantz and Guildenstern)
Guilford (Guildford), Sir Henry
Gurney, James
Haberdasher, The
Hal, Prince (*see* Prince [6])
Halberdier
Hamlet
Harcourt
Harpy
Harvey (1)
Hastings (1), Pursuivant
Hastings (2), Lord Ralph
Hastings (3), Lord William
Headsman (*see* Executioner)
Hecate (Hecat, Heccat)
Hector
Hecuba
Helen (1)
Helen (2) (*see* Helena [2])
Helena (1)
Helena (2)
Helenus
Helicanus
Henry (1), Prince (later King Henry III)
Henry IV, King of England
Henry V, King of England
Henry VI, King of England
Henry VIII, King of England
Herald (1)
Herald (2)
Herald (3)
Herald (4)
Herald (5) (*see* Gentleman [6])
Herald (6)
Herald (7)
Herald (8)
Herbert (3), Sir Walter
Hermia
Hermione
Hero
Hippolyta (1)
Hippolyta (2)
Holland (1), Henry, Duke of Exeter (*see* Exeter [1])
Holland (3), John
Holofernes
Horatio
Horner, Thomas
Hortensio
Hortensius
Host (1)
Host (2)
Hostess (1)
Hostess (2)
Hostilius
Hotspur (Henry Percy)
Hubert
Hume, John
Huntsman (1)
Huntsman (2)
Hymen (1)
Hymen (2)
Iachimo
Iago
Iden, Alexander
Imogen
Innogen
Iras
Iris
Isabel (1), Queen of England (*see* Queen [3])
Isabel (2), Queen of France
Isabella
Isidore's Servant
Jailer
Jailor
Jamy
Jaquenetta
Jaques (1)
Jaques (2) de Boys
Jessica
Jeweller
Joan La Pucelle (Joan of Arc)
John (1) Don
John (2), Friar (*see* Friar [3])
John (3), King of England
John (4) of Gaunt (*see* Gaunt)
John (5) Plantagenet (*see* Bedford; Lancaster [3])
John (6) Talbot (Young Talbot)
Joseph
Jourdain (1), Margery (*see* Margery Jourdain)
Julia
Juliet (1)
Juliet (2)
Juno
Jupiter
Justice
Katharina (*see* Katherina)
Katharine (1), (Katherine, Catherine)
Katharine (2) (Catherine, Katherine)
Katherina
Katherine (Katharine) of Aragon, Queen of England
Keeper (1)
Keeper (2)
Keeper (3)
Keeper (4)
Keeper (5)
Kent (2), Earl of
King (1), Alonso of Naples (*see* Alonso)
King (2) Antiochus of Syria (*see* Antiochus)
King (3) Charles VI of France (*see* French King)
King (4) Charles VII of France (*see* Charles VII)
King (5) Claudius of Denmark
King (6) Cymbeline of Britain (*see* Cymbeline)
King (7) Duncan of Scotland (*see* Duncan)
King (8) Edward IV of England (*see* Edward IV)
King (9) Henry IV of England (*see* Henry IV)
King (10) Henry V of England (*see* Henry V)
King (11) Henry VI of England (*see* Henry VI)
King (12) Henry VIII of England (*see* Henry VIII)
King (13) John of England (*see* John [3])
King (14) Lear of Britain (*see* Lear)
King (15) Leontes of Sicilia (*see* Leontes)
King (16) Lewis (Louis XI) of France (*see* Lewis [3])
King (17) of France
King (18) of France (*see* France [2])
King (19) Ferdinand of Navarre
King (20) Philip Augustus of France (*see* Philip [2])
King (21) Polixenes of Bohemia (*see* Polixenes)
King (22) Priam of Troy (*see* Priam)
King (23) Richard II of England (*see* Richard II)
King (24) Richard III of England (*see* Richard III)
King (25) Simonides of Pentapolis (*see* Simonides)
Kings
Knight (1)
Knight (2)
Knight (3)
Lady (1)
Lady (2)
Lady (3)
Lady (4)
Lady (5) Faulconbridge (Falconbridge)
Lady (6) Macbeth
Lady (7) Macduff
Lady (8) Catherine Mortimer
Lady (9) Northumberland (Margaret Neville)
Lady (10) Elizabeth Percy
Laertes
Lafew (Lafeu), Lord
Lamprius
Lancaster (2), John of Gaunt, Duke of (*see* Gaunt)
Lancaster (3), Prince John of
Lance (*see* Launce)
La Pucelle (*see* Joan La Pucelle)
Lartius, Titus
Launce (Lance)
Launcelot (Lancelot) Gobbo
Laurence Friar (*see* Friar [4])
Lavatche (Lavache) (*see* Clown [3])
Lavinia
Lawyer
Le Beau
Lear
Legate
Lennox (1) (*see* Lenox)
Lenox (Lennox), Thane of
Leonardo
Leonato
Leonine
Leontes
Lepidus, Marcus Aemilius
Lewis (1), the Dauphin (later King Louis VIII)
Lewis (2), the Dauphin (*see* Dauphin [3])
Lewis (3), King of France
Licio (*see* Litio)
Lieutenant (1)
Lieutenant (2)
Lieutenant (3)
Lieutenant (4)
Ligarius, Caius (Quintus)
Lincoln, Bishop of (John Longland)
Litio (Licio)
Lodovico
Lodowick
Longaville (Longueville)
Longueville (*see* Longaville)
Lord (1)
Lord (2)
Lord (3)
Lord (4)
Lord (5)
Lord (6)
Lord (7)

Characters

Lord (8)
Lord (9)
Lord (10)
Lord (11)
Lord (12)
Lord (13)
Lord (14)
Lord (15)
Lord (16)
Lord (17) Bardolph (*see* Bardolph)
Lord (18) Chamberlain (*see* Chamberlain [2])
Lord (19) Chancellor (*see* Chancellor)
Lord (20) Chief Justice (*see* Chief Justice)
Lord (21) Marshal (*see* Marshal [1])
Lorenzo
Lovell (1) (Lovel), Sir Francis
Lovell (2), Sir Thomas
Luce
Lucentio
Lucetta
Luciana
Lucianus
Lucilius (1)
Lucilius (2)
Lucillius
Lucio
Lucius (1)
Lucius (2)
Lucius (3)
Lucius (4)
Lucius' Servant
Lucrece (Lucretia)
Lucretius
Lucullus
Lucy (2), Sir William
Lychorida
Lysander
Lysimachus
Mab
Macbeth
Macduff, Thane of Fife
Macmorris
Maecenas, Gaius
Malcolm (Prince Malcolm Canmore)
Malvolio
Mamillius
Man (1)
Man (2)
Man (3)
Marcade (Mercade)
Marcellus
March, Earl of
Marcus Andronicus
Mardian
Margarelon
Margaret (1) of Anjou
Margaret (2)
Margery Jourdain
Maria (1)
Maria (2)
Mariana (1)
Mariana (2)
Marina
Mariner (1)
Mariner (2)
Marshall (1) (Lord Marshal)
Marshall (2)
Martext, Sir Oliver
Martius (1)
Martius (2) (Marcius)
Marullus (Murellus) C. Epidius
Masquers
Master (1)
Master (2)
Master-Gunner
Mate
Mayor (1) of Coventry
Mayor (2) of London
Mayor (3) of London
Mayor (4) of St. Albans
Mayor (5) of York
Melun (Melune), Giles de, Lord
Menas
Menecrates
Menelaus
Menenius Agrippa
Menteth (Menteith), Walter Dalyell, Thane of
Mercade (*see* Marcade)
Mercer
Merchant (1)
Merchant (2)
Mercutio
Messala, Marcus Valerius
Messenger (1)
Messenger (2)
Messenger (3)
Messenger (4)
Messenger (5)
Messenger (6)
Messenger (7)
Messenger (8)
Messenger (9)
Messenger (10)
Messenger (11)
Messenger (12)
Messenger (13)
Messenger (14)
Messenger (15)
Messenger (16)
Messenger (17)
Messenger (18)
Messenger (19)
Messenger (20)
Messenger (21)
Messenger (22)
Messenger (23)
Messenger (24)
Messenger (25)
Messenger (26) (*see* Attendant [1])
Messenger (27)
Messenger (28)
Messenger (29)
Messenger (30)
Messenger (31)
Messenger (32)
Metellus Cimber (L. Tillius Cimber)
Michael (1)
Michael (2), Sir
Miranda
Mistress (1) Alice Ford
Mistress (2) Overdone
Mistress (3) Margaret Page
Mistress (4) Quickly (*see* Quickly)
Montague (1)
Montague (2), Lady
Montague (3), John Neville, Lord
Montano (1)
Montano (2)
Montgomery (1) John
Morocco (Morochus)
Mortimer (1), Sir Edmund, Earl of March
Mortimer (2), Edmund
Mortimer (3), Sir Hugh
Mortimer (4), Sir John
Mortimer (5), Lady (*see* Lady [8])
Morton
Moth (1) (Mote)
Moth (2)
Mother
Mouldy, Ralph
Mowbray (1), Thomas, Duke of Norfalk
Mowbray (2), Thomas, Lord
Murderer (*see* First Murderer, Second Murderer, Third Murderer)
Murellus (*see* Marullus)
Musicians (1)
Musicians (2)
Musicians (3)
Musicians (4)
Musicians (5)
Musicians (6)
Musicians (7)
Mustardseed
Mutius
Myrmidon
Mytilenian Sailor (*see* Tyrian Sailor)
Nathaniel (1)
Nathaniel (2)
Neighbour
Nell (1)
Nell (2)
Nerissa
Nestor
Nicanor (*see* Roman [2])
Nicholas
Nobleman
Norfolk (1), John Howard, Duke of
Norfolk (2), John Mowbray, Duke of
Norfalk (3), Thomas Howard, Duke of
Norfolk (4), Thomas Mowbray, Duke of (*see* Mowbray [1])
Northumberland (1), Henry Percy, Earl of
Northumberland (2), Henry Percy, Earl of
Northumberland (3), Henry Percy, Earl of
Northumberland (4), Lady (*see* Lady [9])
Northumberland (5), Siward, Earl of
Nun
Nurse (1)
Nurse (2)
Nurse (3)
Nym
Oatcake, Hugh
Oberon
Octavia
Octavius (Gaius Octavius Caesar; Octavian)
Officer (1)
Officer (2)
Officer (3)
Officer (4)
Officer (5)
Officer (6)
Officer (7)
Officer (8)
Old Athenian
Old Clifford (*see* Clifford [2], Thomas)
Old Gobbo (*see* Gobbo [2])
Old Lady
Old Man (1) (*see* Capulet [2])
Old Man (2)
Old Man (3)
Oldcastle
Oliver (1)
Oliver (2) (*see* Martext)
Olivia
One (1)
One (2)
One (3) Within
Ophelia
Orlando
Orleans (2), Bastard of (*see* Bastard [2] of Orleans)
Orleans (3), Charles, Duke of
Orsino
Osric

CHARACTERS

Ostler (1)
Oswald
Othello
Other (Other Clown, Second Clown, Second Gravedigger)
Outlaws
Oxford (2), John de Vere, Earl of
Page (1)
Page (2)
Page (3)
Page (4)
Page (5)
Page (6)
Page (7)
Page (8)
Page (9)
Page (10) (*see* Boy [9])
Page (11), Anne (*see* Anne [3])
Page (12), George
Page (13), Mistress Margaret (*see* Mistress [3])
Page (14), William (*see* William [1])
Painter (1)
Palamon
Pandar
Pandarus
Pandulph
Panthino
Paris (2)
Paris (3)
Parolles (Paroles)
Patch-breech (*see* Fishermen)
Patience
Patricians (*see* Senator [2])
Patroclus
Paulina
Peaseblossom
Pedant, The
Pedro, Don
Pembroke (4), William Herbert
Pembroke (5), William Marshall, Earl of
Penker (Pynkie), Friar
Percy (1), Henry (*see* Northumberland [1])
Percy (2), Henry
Percy (3), Henry (*see* Northumberland [2])
Percy (4), Lady (*see* Lady [10])
Perdita
Pericles
Perkes, Clement
Peter (1)
Peter (2)
Peter (3)
Peter (4) of Pomfret
Peter (5), Friar (*see* Friar [1])
Petitioners
Peto
Patruchio (1)
Petruchio (2)
Phebe (Phoebe)
Philario
Philemon
Philip (1)
Philip (2), Augustus, King of France
Philip (3) (*see* Bastard [1])
Philo
Philostrate
Philotus
Phrynia and Timandra
Pilch (*see* Fisherman)
Pinch, Dr.
Pindarus
Pirates
Pirithous
Pisanio
Pistol
Plantagenet (2), Richard
Plantagenet (3), Richard
Player King
Player Queen
Players (1)
Players (2)
Plebeians (1)
Plebeians (2)
Poet (1)
Poet (2)
Poins, Ned
Polixenes
Polonius
Polydore (Guiderius)
Pompey (1) Bum
Pompey (2) (Sextus Pompeius)
Popilius Lena
Porter (1)
Porter (2)
Porter (3)
Porter (4)
Portia (1)
Portia (2)
Post (1)
Post (2)
Posthumus
Potpan (*see* Servingman [2])
Prentice
Priam, King of Troy
Priest (1)
Priest (2)
Priest (3)
Prince (1) Escalus of Verona
Prince (2) Hal (also Henry, later King Henry V) (*see* Prince [6] of Wales)
Prince (3) Henry (*see* Henry [1])
Prince (4) of Wales, Edward
Prince (5) of Wales, Edward (Edward V, King of England)
Prince (6) of Wales, Henry (Hal, later King Henry V)
Princess (1) of France
Princess (2) Katharine of France (*see* Katharine [2])
Proculeius, Caius
Prologue (2)
Prologue (3)
Prologue (4)
Prologue (5)
Prospero
Proteus
Provost
Publius (1)
Publius (2)
Puck
Pursuivant (*see* Hastings [2])
Pyrrhus
Queen (1)
Queen (2) of Britain
Queen (3) Anne of England (*see* Anne [1])
Queen (4) Anne of England (*see* Anne [2])
Queen (5) Cleopatra of Egypt (*see* Cleopatra)
Queen (6) Eleanor (Elinor) of England (*see* Eleanor)
Queen (8) Elizabeth of England (*see* Elizabeth [2])
Queen (9) Gertrude of Denmark
Queen (10) Hermione (*see* Hermione)
Queen (11) Hippolyta of the Amazons (*see* Hippolyta [1])
Queen (12) Hippolyta (*see* Hippolyta [2])
Queen (13) Isabel of England
Queen (14) Isabel of France (*see* Isabel [2])
Queen (15) Katherine of England (and of Aragon) (*see* Katherine of Aragon)
Queen (16) Margaret of England (*see* Margaret [1])
Queen (17), Player (*see* Player Queen)
Quickly, Mistress
Quince, Peter
Quintus
Rambures, Lord
Rannius
Ratcliffe, Sir Richard
Rebeck, Hugh (*see* Musicians [2])
Regan
Reignier, Duke of Anjou and King of Naples
Reynaldo (1)
Reynaldo (2) (*see* Steward [1])
Richard II, King of England
Richard III, King of England
Richmond, Earl of (Henry Tudor, later King Henry VII)
Rinaldo (*see* Steward 1)
Rivers, Anthony Woddville, Earl of
Robert Faulconbridge (Falconbridge)
Robin (1)
Robin (2) Goodfellow (*see* Puck)
Roderigo
Roman (1)
Roman (2)
Romeo
Rosalind
Rosaline (1)
Rosaline (2)
Rosencrantz and Guildenstern
Ross (1) (*see* Rosse)
Ross (2) (Ros), William de
Rosse (Ross) Thane of
Rossill (Russell), Sir John
Rugby, John
Rumour
Rutland (1), Edmund York, Earl of
Rynaldo (*see* Steward [1])
Sailor (1)
Sailor (2)
Sailor (3)
Sailor (4) (*see* Tyrian Sailor)
Salarino (*see* Salerio)
Salerio (Salarino)
Salisbury (1), John Montague (Montacute), Earl of
Salisbury (2), Richard Neville, Earl of
Salisbury (3), Thomas Montague (Montacute), Earl of
Salisbury (4), William Longsword, Earl of
Sampson
Sands, Lord (William Sands [Sandys])
Saturninus
Say, James Finnes, Lord
Scales, Lord Thomas de
Scarus
Schoolmaster (1)
Schoolmaster (2)
Scout
Scribe
Scrivener
Scroop (1) (Le Scroop, Scroope, Scrope), Henry
Scroop (2) (Scroope, Scrope), Richard (*see* Archbishop [3])
Scroop (3) (Le Scroop, Scroope, Scrope), Stephen
Seacoal, George
Sebastian (1)

Characters

Characters

Warwick (2), Richard Beauchamp, Earl of
Warwick (3), Richard Neville, Earl of
Watchmen (1)
Watchmen (2)
Watchmen (3)
Watchmen (4)
Watchmen (5)
Weaver (*see* Smith [1])
Westminister (2), Abbot of (*see* Abbot of Westminister)
Westmoreland (1), Ralph Neville, Earl of
Westmoreland (2), Ralph Neville, Earl of
Whitmore, Walter
Widow (1)
Widow (2) Capilet
Wife
William (1), Page
William (2)
Williams (2), Michael
Willoughby (3), William de
Winchester (1), Henry Beaufort, Bishop of
Winchester (2), Stephen Gardiner, Bishop of
Witches
Within
Wolsey, Thomas Cardinal
Woman (1)
Woman (2)
Woodville (Woodvile), Lieutenant Richard
Wooer
Yorick
York (3), Cicely Neville, Duchess of (*see* Duchess [3])
York (4), Edmund of Langley, Duke of
York (5), Edward, Duke of
York (6), Isabel of Castile, Duchess of (*see* Duchess [4])
York (7), Richard, Duke of
York (8), Richard Plantagenet, Duke of
York (9), Richard Scroop, Archbishop of
York (10), Thomas Rotherham, Archbishop of (*see* Archbishop [4])
Young Cato
Young Clifford (*see* Lord John Clifford [1])
Young Lucius
Young Siward (Osberne of Northumberland)
Young Talbot (*see* John [6])

Contemporaries and Near-Contemporaries of Shakespeare

Addenbrooke, John
Africanus, Leo (*see* Leo Africanus)
Allde, Edward
Alleyn, Edward
Amyot, Jacques
Annesley, Brian
Armin, Robert
Aspinall, Alexander
Aspley, William
Bandello, Matteo
Barents (Barentz), Willem
Barkstead, William
Barnes, Barnabe
Barnfield, Richard
Barton (2), Richard
Basse, William
Beaumont (2), Francis
Bedford (2), Lucy, Countess of
Beeston, Christopher
Belleforest, Francois de
Belott, Stephen
Benfield, Robert
Benson (2), John
Bentley, John
Berners, John Bouchier, Lord
Bevis, George
Blount, Edward
Bonian, Richard
Bradock (Bradocke), Richard
Bretchgirdle, John
Bright, Timothy
Brooke (1), Arthur
Brooke (3), William, Lord Cobham (*see* Cobham)
Browne, Robert
Bryan, George
Buchanan, George
Burbage (1), Cuthbert
Burbage, (2), James
Burbage (3), Richard
Burby, Cuthbert
Burghley (Burleigh), Lord (William Cecil)
Burleigh, William Cecil, Lord (*see* Burghley)
Busby, John
Butter, Nathaniel
Camden, William
Carew, Richard
Carey (1), George, Baron Hunsdon (*see* Hunsdon 1)
Carey (2), Henry, Baron Hunsdon (*see* Hunsdon 2)
Cecil (1), Robert, Earl of Salisbury
Cecil (2), Thomas
Cecil (3), William (*see* Burghley)
Cervantes Saavedra, Miguel de
Chapman, George
Chettle, Henry
Chester, Robert (*see* Love's Martyr)
Cinthio (Giovanni Battista Giraldi)
Cobham, William Brooke, Lord
Collins, Francis
Combe (1), John
Combe (2), Thomas
Combe (3), Thomas
Combe (4), William
Combe (5), William
Condell, Henry
Cooke (1), Alexander
Cottom (Cottam), John
Cowley, Richard
Cox, Robert
Crane, Ralph
Creede, Thomas
Crosse, Samuel
Daniel, Samuel
Davenant (D'Avenant), William
Davies (1), John of Hereford
Davies (2), Sir John
Day, John
Dekker, Thomas
Deloney, Thomas
Dennis (2), John
Derby (1), Fernando Stanley, Earl of (*see* Strange)
Derby (3), William Stanley, Earl of
Digges (1), Dudley
Digges (2), Leonard
Downton, Thomas
Drayton, Michael
Droeshout, Martin
Dryden, John
Du Bartas, Guillaume de Sallust
Dutton, Laurence
Ecclestone, William
Eden, Richard
Edwards (Edwardes), Richard
Eld (Elde), George
Eliot (1), John
Elizabeth (1), Queen of England
Elizabeth (3) Stuart, Queen of Bohemia
Essex (2), Robert Devereaux, Earl of
Evans (2), Henry
Farrant, Richard
Fenton (2) Geoffrey
Ffarington, William
Field (1), Nathan
Field (2), Richard
Fisher, Thomas
Fitton, Mary
Fletcher (1), Giles
Fletcher (2), John
Fletcher (3), Laurence
Florio, John (Giovanni)
Ford (2), John
Forman, Simon
Foxe (Fox), John
Gardiner (2), William
Garnet, Henry
Gascoigne, George
Gibborne, Thomas
Gilbard, William
Gilburne, Samuel
Giles, Nathaniel
Giulio Romano (Giulio Pippi)
Golding, Arthur
Goslicius, Laurentius Grimalius
Gosson (1), Henry
Gosson (2), Stephen
Gough (Goughe), Robert
Grafton, Richard
Granada, Luis de
Green, John
Greene (2), Robert
Greene (3), Thomas
Greville (1), Curtis
Greville (2), Fulke (Lord Brooke)
Griffin, Bartholomew
Gwinne (Gwinn), Matthew
Hakluyt, Richard
Hall, Arthur
Hall (7), William
Hamlett, Katherine
Harington, Sir John
Harris (2), Henry
Harrison (2), John
Harrison (3), William
Harsnett, Samuel
Hart (3), William
Harvey (2), Gabriel
Harvey (4), William
Hathway (Hathaway), Richard
Heicroft, Henry
Heminge (Heminges), John
Henry (2) Frederick, Prince of Wales
Henslowe, Philip
Herbert (1), Henry
Herbert (2), Henry, Philip, or William, Earls of Pembroke (*see* Pembroke [1, 2, 3])

Contemporaries and Near-Contemporaries of Shakespeare

Hervey (Harvey), William
Heyes, Thomas
Heywood (1), John
Heywood (2), Thomas
Higgins, John
Hilliard, Nicholas
Hoby (1), Sir Thomas
Hoby (2), Sir Thomas Posthumous
Holinshed, Raphael
Holland (2), Hugh
Holland (4), Philemon
Hopkins, Richard
Howard, Charles
Hunnis, William
Hunsdon (1), George Carey, Baron
Hunsdon (2), Henry Carey, Baron
Hunt, Simon
Jackson (2), John
Jackson (3), Roger
Jaggard, William and Isaac
James, Elias
James I, King of England
Jamy
Janssen (1), Cornelis (Cornelius Johnson)
Janssen (2), Gheerart (Gerard Johnson)
Jeffes, Humphrey
Jenkins, Thomas
Johnson (1), Arthur
Johnson (3), Cornelius (*see* Janssen [1])
Johnson (4), Gerard (*see* Janssen [2])
Johnson (5), Robert
Johnson (6), Robert
Johnson (8), William
Jones (2), Richard
Jones (3), Robert
Jones (4), William
Jonson, Ben
Jourdain (2) (Jourdan), Sylvester
Kempe (Kemp), William
Kirkham, Edward
Kirkman, Edward
Knell, William
Knight (4), Edward
Knollys, Sir William
Kyd, Thomas
Lane (1), John
Lane (2), Richard
Laneman (Lanman), Henry
Langley, Francis
Lanier, Emilia
Law, Matthew
Leake, William
Legh, Gerard
Leicester, Robert Dudley, Earl of
Le Macon, Antoine
Leo Africanus (Joannes Leo)
Leveson, William
Ling, Nicholas
Locke, Matthew
Lodge, Thomas
Lopez, Roderigo
Lowin (Lowen), John
Lucy (1), Sir Thomas
Lupton, Thomas
Lyly, John
Mabbe, James
Manningham, John
Marlowe (1), Christopher
Marsh, Henry
Marston, John
Massinger, Philip
Mayne, Jasper
Meres, Francis
Middleton, Thomas
Millington, Thomas
Milton, John
Mömpelgard, Frederick, Count of (later Duke of) Wurttemberg
Monarcho
Montaigne, Michael de
Montgomery (2), Philip Herbert, Earl of
Montjoy
Mopsa
Morgan (1) (Belarius)
Morley, Thomas
Mountjoy, Christopher
Munday, Anthony
Nash (1), Anthony
Nash (2), Thomas
Nashe (Nash), Thomas
North, Sir Thomas
Okes, Nicholas
Ostler (2), William
Oxford (1), Edward de Vere, Earl of
Painter (2), William
Pavier, Thomas
Peele, George
Pembroke (1), Henry Herbert, Earl of
Pembroke (2), Philip Herbert, Lord (*see* Montgomery [2])
Pembroke (3), William Herbert, Earl of
Phillips, Augustine
Platter, Thomas
Pope (2), Thomas
Porter (5), Henry
Pory, John
Preston, Thomas
Prynne, William
Puck (Robin Goodfellow)
Puttenham, George
Queen (7) Elizabeth of England
Quiney (1), Judith (*see* Shakespeare [10])
Quiney, (2), Richard
Quiney (3), Thomas
Raleigh, (Ralegh), Sir Walter
Ratsey, Gamaliel
Reynolds (2), William
Rice, John
Rich (1), Barnabe (Barnaby Riche)
Richardson (1), John
Roberts, James
Robinson (1), John
Robinson (3), Richard
Robinson (4), Richard
Roche, Walter
Rogers (1), John
Rogers (2), Phillip
Rowley (1), Samuel
Rowley (2), William
Russell, Thomas
Rutland (2), Francis Manners, Earl of
Sackville, Thomas
Sadler, Hamnet and Judith
Salusbury (Salisbury), John
Sandells, Fulk
Savage, Thomas
Scot (Scott), Reginald
Segar, William
Shank, John
Sharpham, Edward
Shaw (4), Julian
Shaw (5) (Shaa), Robert
Shirley, Anthony
Short, Peter
Sidney, Philip
Simmes, Valentine
Sincklo (Sinklo, Sincler), John
Singer, John
Slater (Slaughter), Martin
Sly (2), William
Smethwick (Smithweeke), John
Snodham, Thomas
Southampton (2), Henry Wriothesley, Earl of
Spencer, Gabriel
Spenser, Edmund
Stafford (3), Simon
Stanley (1), Ferdinando, Lord Strange (*see* Strange)
Stow, John
Strachey (2), William
Strange, Ferdinando Stanley, Lord
Tarlton, Richard
Taylor, Joseph
Thorpe, Thomas
Tooley, Nicholas
Trundell, John
Twine, Laurence
Tuckfield (Tuckfeild), Thomas
Tyler (1), Richard
Underhill, William
Underwood, John
Walker (1), Henry
Walker (2), William
Walkley, Thomas
Walley, Henry
Warner, William
Waterson, John
Webster (2), John
Weelkes, Thomas
Whatcott, Robert
Whetstone, George
White (1), Edward
White (2), William
Whitgift, John
Wilkins, George
Willoughby (1), Sir Ambrose
Willoughby (2) (Willobie) Henry
Wilson (1), Jack
Wilson (2), John
Wilson (4), Robert
Wise, Andrew
Wyatt, Thomas
Yong (Yonge, Young), Bartholomew

Documents and Artifacts

Chandos portrait
Coat of arms, Shakespeare's
Contention, The
Dering Manuscript
Ely Palace portrait
False Folio
First Folio
Flower portrait
Kesselstadt Death Mask
Longleat Manuscript
'Pied Bull' Quarto (*see King Lear*, 'Text of the Play')
Portraits of Shakespeare

Historical References

Andrew (1)
Hundred Years War
Lancaster (1) Family
Plantagenet (1) Family
Renaissance
Roses, Wars of the (*see* Wars of the Roses)
Stuart Dynasty
Trojan War
Tudor Dynasty
Wars of the Roses
Welcombe
York (1) Family

Places

Actium
Agincourt
Alexandria
Angiers
Anjou
Antioch
Antium
Arden (1), Forest of
Athens
Auvergne
Bangor
Barkloughly Castle
Barnet
Baynard Castle
Belmont
Birmingham Shakespeare Memorial Library
Birnam Wood (*see* Dunsinane)
Birthplace, Shakespeare's
Blackfriars Gatehouse
Blackfriars Priory
Blackfriars Theatre
Blackheath
Boar's Head Tavern
Bodleian Library
Bohemia
Bordeaux
Bosworth Field
Bristol (Bristow)
Bury St Edmunds
Corioles (Corioli)
Coventry
Cross Keys Inn
Curtain Theatre, The
Cyprus
Denmark
Dover
Dunsinane (Dunsinnan)
Eastcheap
Elsinore
Ephesus
Fife
Florence
Flint Castle
Folger Shakespeare Library
Fortune Theatre
France (1)
Frogmore
Gad's Hill (Gadshill, Gads Hill)
Gascony
Gaultree Forest
Globe Theatre
Gloucestershire
Harfleur
Holmedon (Homildon)
Hope Theatre
Huntington Library
Inns of Court
Inverness
Italy
Jerusalem Chamber
Kenilworth
Kent (1)
Kimbolton Castle
London
Mantua
Marseilles
Mermaid Tavern
Messina
Middleham Castle
Milan
Misenum
Mortimer's Cross
Mytilene
New Place
Newington Butts
Old Vic Theatre
Orléans (1)
Padua
Paris (1)
Parliament House
Pentapolis
Philippi
Phoenix
Picardy
Pomfret (Pontefract) Castle
Porcupine (Porpentine)
Porpentine (*see* Porcupine)
Priory
Rochester
Rome
Rose Theatre
Rossillion (Rousillon)
Rouen
Sadler's Wells Theatre
St Albans
St Edmundsbury (Bury St Edmunds)
Sandal Castle
Sardis
Scotland
Shrewsbury
Sicilia
Smithfield
Southampton (1)
Southwark
Stratford
Swan Theatre
Swinstead (Swineshead) Abbey
Tamworth
Tewkesbury (Tewksbury)
Tharsus (Tarsus)
Theatre, The
Thebes
Tower of London
Towton
Troy
Troyes
Tyre
Venice
Verona
Vienna
Wakefield
Wales (1)
Warkworth Castle
Warwickshire
Welcombe
Westminister (1) Abbey
Westminister (3) Hall
Westminister (4) Palace
Whitefriars Theatre
Windsor
York (2)

The Plays

All Is True (Henry VIII)
All's Well That Ends Well
Antony and Cleopatra
As You Like It
Cardenio
Comedy of Errors, The
Coriolanus
Cymbeline
Hamlet
Henry IV, Part 1
Henry IV, Part 2
Henry V
Henry VI, Part 1
Henry VI, Part 2
Henry VI, Part 3
Henry VIII
Julius Caesar
King John
King Lear
Love's Labour's Lost
Love's Labour's Won
Macbeth
Measure for Measure
Merchant of Venice, The
Merry Wives of Windsor, The
Midsummer Night's Dream, A
Much Ado About Nothing
Othello
Pericles, Prince of Tyre
Richard II
Richard III
Romeo and Juliet
Taming of the Shrew, The
Tempest, The
Timon of Athens
Titus Andronichus
Troilus and Cressida
Twelfth Night
Two Gentlemen of Verona, The
Two Noble Kinsmen, The
Winter's Tale, The

The Poems

Lover's Complaint, A
Phoenix and Turtle, The
Rape of Lucrece, The
Sonnets, The
Venus and Adonis

Related Works

Age of Kings, An
Arden of Feversham
Bestrafte Brudermord, Der (*Fratricide Punished*)
Bible
Birth of Merlin, The
Contention, The
Duke Hnmphrey
Edward III
Fair Em
Famous Victories, The
Henry I and *Henry II*
King Leir
Law Against Lovers, The
Locrine
London Prodigal, The
Love in a Forest
Love's Martyr
Merry Devil of Edmonton, The
Mirror for Magistrates, A
Mucedorus
Passionate Pilgrim, The
Puritan, The
"Shall I Die?"
Sir John Oldcastle
Sir Thomas More
Spread of the Eagle, The
Taming of a Shrew, The
Thomas Lord Cromwell
Traïson
Troublesome Raigne of King John, The
True Tragedy, The
Ur-Hamlet
Ur-Shrew
Whole Contention, The
Woodstock (*Thomas of Woodstock*)
Yorkshire Tragedy, A

Relatives of Shakespeare

Arden (2), Robert
Hall (3), Elizabeth
Hall (4), John
Hall (6), Susanna (*see* Shakespeare[14])
Hart (2), Joan (*see* Shakespeare[8])
Hart (3), William
Hathaway, Anne (Anne Hathaway Shakespeare)
Lambert, John
Nash (2), Thomas
Quiney (1), Judith (*see* Shakespeare [10])
Quiney (3), Thomas
Shakespeare (1), Anne
Shakespeare (2), Anne Hathaway (*see* Hathaway)
Shakespeare (3), Edmund
Shakespeare (4), Gilbert
Shakespeare (5), Hamnet
Shakespeare (6), Henry
Shakespeare (7), Joan
Shakespeare (8), Joan (Joan Shakespeare Hart)
Shakespeare (9), John
Shakespeare (10), Judith (Judith Shakespeare Quinley)
Shakespeare (11), Mary Arden
Shakespeare (12), Richard
Shakespeare (13), Richard
Shakespeare (14), Susanna (Susanna Shakespeare Hall)
Shakespeare (15), William

Scholars, Authors, Translators, Artists, Printers, and Publishers

Adams, Joseph Quincy
Adlington, William
Africanus, Leo (*see* Leo Africanus)
Alexander (2), Peter
Allde, Edward
Amyot, Jacques
Apuleius, Lucius
Ariosto, Ludovico
Aristotle
Aspley, William
Ayscough, Samuel
Bandello, Matteo
Barkstead, William
Barnes, Barnabe
Barnfield, Richard
Basse, William
Beaumont (2) Francis
Belleforest, Francois de
Benson (2), John
Berners, John Bourchier, Lord
Blount, Edward
Boas, Frederick S.
Boccaccio, Giovanni
Boece (Boyce), Hector
Bonian, Richard
Boswell, James the younger
Bowdler, Thomas
Boydell, John
Bradley, Andrew Cecil
Bradock (Bradocke), Richard
Bright, Timothy
Brooke (1), Arthur
Brooke (2), C. F. Tucker
Buchanan, George
Bullough, Geoffrey
Burby, Cuthbert
Burnaby, William
Busby, John
Butter, Nathaniel
Camden, William
Capell, Edward
Carew, Richard
Castiglione, Baldassare
Caxton, William
Cervantes Saavedra, Miguel de
Chambers, Edmund Kerchever
Chapman, George
Chaucer, Geoffrey
Chester, Robert
Chettle, Henry
Cibber (1), Colley
Cicero, M. Tullius
Cinthio (Giovanni Baptista Giraldi)
Clark, Mary Cowden and Charles Cowden
Coleridge, Samuel Taylor
Collier (2), John Payne
Colonne, Guido delle
Craig (2), Hardin
Crane, Ralph
Creede, Thomas
Créton, Jean
Crowne, John
Cumberland, Richard
Daniel, Samuel
Davies (1), John of Hereford
Davies (2), Sir John
Day, John
Dekker, Thomas
Deloney, Thomas
Dennis (2), John
De Quincey, Thomas
Derby (3), William Stanley, Earl of
Dickens, Charles
Digges (2), Leonard
Dowden, Edward
Drayton, Michael
Droeshout, Martin
Dryden, John
Du Bartas, Guillaume de Sallust
Duffett, Thomas
D'Urfey, Thomas
Eden, Richard
Edwards (Edwardes), Richard
Eld (Elde), George
Eliot (1), John
Eliot (2), Thomas Stearns
Elyot, Sir Thomas
Eschenburg, Johann Joachim
Fabyan, Robert
Fenton (2), Geoffrey
Fenton (3), Richard
Field (2), Richard
Fiorentino, Giovanni
Fisher, Thomas
Fleay, Frederick Gard
Fletcher (1), Giles
Fletcher (2), John
Florio, John (Giovanni)
Ford (2), John
Foxe (Fox), John
French, George Russell
Froissart, Jean
Furness, Horace Howard
Furnivall, Frederick James
Gascoigne, George
Geoffrey of Monmouth
Gervinus, Georg Gottfried
Gide, Andre
Gildon, Charles
Giulio Romano
Goethe, Johann Wolfgang von
Golding, Arthur
Goslicius, Laurentius Grimalius

Scholars, Authors, Translators, Artists, Printers, and Publishers

Gosson (1), Henry
Gosson (2), Stephen
Grafton, Richard
Granada, Luis de
Granville, George
Greene (2), Robert
Greg, Walter Wilson
Greville (2), Fulke (Lord Brooke)
Griffin, Bartholomew
Gwinne (Gwinn), Matthew
Hakluyt, Richard
Hall (1), Arthur
Hall (2) (Halle), Edward
Hall (7), William
Halle, Edward (*see* Hall [2])
Halliwell-Phillips, James Orchard
Hanmer, Thomas
Harington, Sir John
Harris (1), Frank (James Thomas)
Harrison (1), George Bagshawe
Harrison (2), John
Harrison (3), William
Harsnett, Samuel
Harvey (2), Gabriel
Hathway (Hathaway), Richard
Hayman, Francis
Hazlitt, William
Henryson, Robert
Heyes, Thomas
Heywood (1), John
Heywood (2), Thomas
Higgins, John
Hilliard, Nicholas
Hoby (1), Sir Thomas
Holinshed, Raphael
Holland (2), Hugh
Holland (4), Philemon
Homer
Hopkins, Richard
Hotson, Leslie
Hunnis, William
Hunnis, William
Ingleby, Clement Mansfield
Ireland, William Henry
Jackson (3), Roger
Jaggard, William and Isaac
Janssen (1), Cornelis (Cornelius Johnson)
Janssen (2), Gheerart (Gerard Johnson)
Johnson (1), Arthur
Johnson (2), Charles
Johnson (3), Cornelius (*see* Janssen [1])
Johnson (4) Gerard (*see* Janssen [2])
Johnson (7), Samuel
Jonson, Ben
Keats, John
Killigrew, Thomas
Kirkman, Francis
Kittredge, George Lyman
Knight (5), G. Wilson
Kyd, Thomas
Lacy, John
Lamb (1), Charles
Lamb (2), George
Langbaine, Gerard
Law, Matthew
Leake, William
Lee, Sidney
Legh, Gerard
Le Maçon, Antoine
Lennox (2), Charlotte
Leo Africanus (Joannes Leo)
Lessing, Gotthold Ephraim
Lillo, George
Ling, Nicholas
Lily (Lilly, Lyly), William
Livy (Titus Livius)
Lodge, Thomas
Lucian
Lupton, Thomas
Lydgate, John
Lyly, John
Mabbe, James
Malone, Edmond
Markham, Gervase
Marlowe (1), Christopher
Marsh, Henry
Marston, John
Massinger, Philip
Mayne, Jasper
Meres, Francis
Middleton, Thomas
Miller (1), James
Millington, Thomas
Milton, John
Montaigne, Michael de
Montemayer, Jorge de
More, Sir Thomas
Morgan (2) McNamara
Morgann, Maurice
Moseley, Humphrey
Munday, Anthony
Nashe (Nash), Thomas
North, Sir Thomas
Okes, Nicholas
Otway, Thomas
Ovid (Publius Ovidius Naso)
Oxford (1), Edward de Vere, Earl of
Painter (2), William
Pater, Walter
Pavier, Thomas
Peele, George
Pepys, Samuel
Planché, James Robinson
Plautus, Titus Maccius
Pliny the Elder
Plutarch
Pollard, Alfred William
Pope (1), Alexander
Porter (5), Henry
Pory, John
Preston, Thomas
Puttenham, George
Raleigh (Ralegh), Sir Walter
Reed, Isaac
Reynolds (1), Frederick
Rich (1), Barnaby (Barnabe Riche)
Roberts, James
Robertson, John Mackinnon
Robinson (3), Richard
Romano, Giulio (*see* Giulio Romano)
Rowe, Nicholas
Rowley (1), Samuel
Rowley (2), William
Sackville, Thomas
Sainte-Maure, Benoit de
Saxo Grammaticus
Scheemakers, Peter
Schiller, Johann Christoph Friedrich
Schlegel, August Wilhelm von
Schücking, Levin Ludwig
Scot (Scott), Reginald
Segar, William
Seneca, Lucius Annaeus
Shadwell, Thomas
Sharpham, Edward
Shaw (2), George Bernard
Short, Peter
Sidney, Philip
Simmes, Valentine
Simpson, Richard
Smethwick (Smithweeke), John
Snodham, Thomas
Spalding, William
Spenser, Edmund
Spurgeon, Caroline
Stafford (3), Simon
Stationers' Company
Steevens, George
Stoll, Elmer Edgar
Stow, John
Strachey (1), Lytton
Strachey (2), William
Surrey (1), Henry Howard, Earl of
Swinburne, Algernon Charles
Tate, Nahum
Theobold, Lewis
Thorpe, Thomas
Tieck, Ludwig
Tillyard, E. M. W.
Trundell, John
Twine, Laurence
Tyler (2), Thomas
Udall, Nicholas
University Wits
Vaux (2), Sir Thomas
Vergil, Polydore
Virgil (Vergil)
Walkley, Thomas
Walley, Henry
Warburton, John
Warner, William
Waterson, John
Webster (2), John
Whetstone, George
White (1), Edward
White (2), William
Wieland, Christoph Martin
Wilkins, George
Willoughby (2) (Willobie), Henry
Wilson (3), John Dover
Wilson (4), Robert
Wise, Andrew
Wyatt, Thomas
Yong, Bartholomew

Theatrical and Literary Terms

Academic Drama
Apocrypha
Argument
Authorship controversy
Bad Quarto
Blank Verse
Canon
Censorship
Chorus (1)
Comedy
Comedy of Humors
Comedia dell' Arte
Complaint
Droll
Dumb Show
Elizabethan Drama
Elizabethan Theatre
Epilogue
Epitaph
Fair copy
Farce
Film
Folio
Foul Papers

Theatrical and Literary Terms

Ghost Character
Good Quarto
History Plays
Induction
Interlude
Jacobean Drama
Machiavel
Masque
Master of Revels
Metre
Miles Gloriosus
Morality play
Parnassus plays
Pastoral
Poetomachia (*see* War of the Theatres)
Problem plays
Prologue (1)
Prompt-book
Quarto
Revenge Play
Rhyme Royal
Roman Plays
Romances
Soliloquy
Song
Sonnet
Sub-plot
Television
Tetralogy
Tragedy
Tragicomedy
University Wits
Variorum edition
Verse test
Vice, the
War of the Theatres
Worthies, The Nine